Contents in Brief

D0086500

Your guide to
BASIC NURSING
Concepts, Skills, & Reasoning

Think.

Key Concepts guide your reading and highlight the information you'll need to know.

Critical-thinking exercises

enhance your clinical decision-making skills and prepare you for your new nursing career.

- ☐ **Clinical Reasoning** lets you safely apply the information you've just learned.
- ☐ **Think Like a Nurse** helps you connect theory to practice.
- ☐ **Toward Evidence-Based Practice** gives you an in-depth look at research that supports nursing practices.

Enrichment icons direct you to the **Fundamentals of Nursing Skills Videos** and your chapter learning resources on the **Electronic Study Guide** online at **DavisPlus**

 Go to Chapter 25, **Tables, Boxes, Figures: Box 25-1,** on DavisPlus.

Concept Maps visually summarize the key aspects you learned in each chapter and show you how they relate to one another.

Knowledge Check divides the material into small sections—perfect for review and exam prep.

Knowledge Check 25-16
- List three errors in technique that can occur when giving parenteral injections. State their possible consequences.
- Describe at least four ways to minimize the discomfort of an injection.
- Name two reasons for giving an intradermal injection.

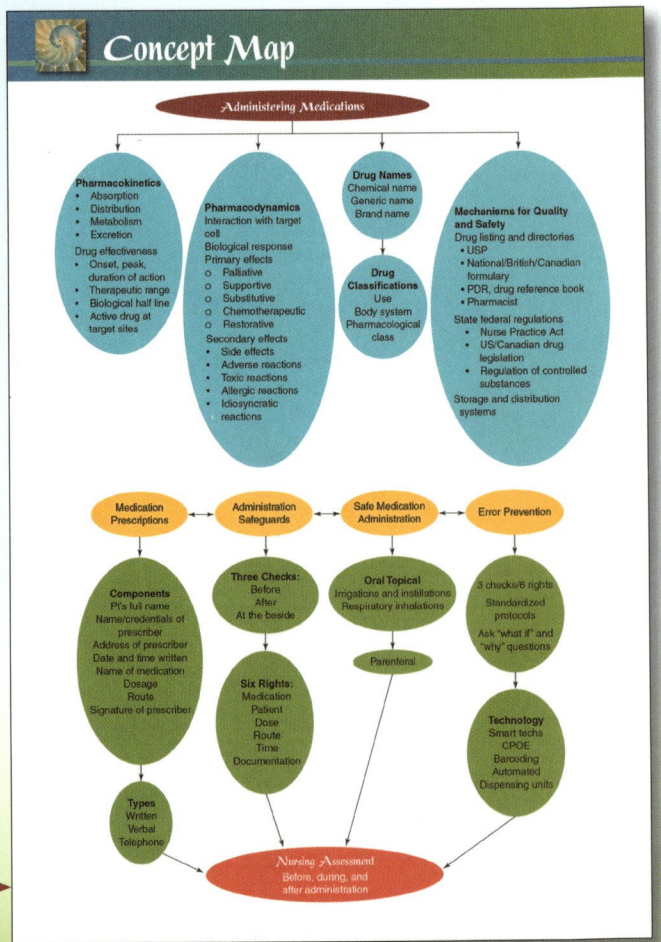

Do.

Procedures teach you nursing skills step by step.

- ☐ **What If...** shows you what to do in special situations.

- ☐ **Thinking About the Procedure** relates each procedure to the corresponding demonstration in the **Fundamentals of Nursing Skills Videos** and the chapter learning resources on the **Electronic Study Guide** online at 🌐 Davis*Plus*.

- ☐ **Documentation** shows you how to provide written or electronic explanations of your care.

Care Plans show you the nursing process in action, incorporating NANDA-I diagnoses and NIC & NOC labels and definitions.

Procedure 25-7 ■ Applyin[g] [ed)

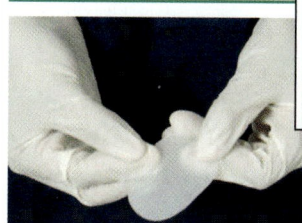

? What if . . .

- ■ **The medication is packaged as an ointment form with calibrated paper?**

  Wear gloves; apply the ointment in a continuous motion along those marks to measure the required dose. Fold the paper in half to distribute the ointment evenly on the patch.

[W]h[at if . . .]

[me]dication is packaged as an [ointme]nt form with calibrated

Wear gloves; apply the ointment in a continuous motion along those marks to measure the required dose. Fold the paper in half to distribute the ointment evenly on the patch.

6. **Apply the patch** to a clean, dry, hairless (or little hair), intact skin area, pressing it down for about 10 seconds with your palm. Be sure the area is free of scars, lesions, and irritation.
   A smooth surface maximizes the contact between medication and the skin. Areas of the skin that are disrupted can become irritated by topical medication. Other lesions involving thickened layers of skin should be avoided to avoid compromised absorption.

7. **Rotate application sites.** Common sites are the trunk, lower abdomen, lower back, and buttocks.
   Rotating sites prevents irritation to local areas of the skin

8. **Teach the patient to** *not* **use a heating pad** over the area.
   Heat can cause some ointments to irritate or even burn the skin.

9. **Write the date, the time, and your initials on the new patch.**
   Complete documentation helps reduce medication errors.

10. **Remove gloves and wash your hands again.**

11. **Observe for local side effects,** such as skin irritation, itching, and allergic contact dermatitis.
    If an adverse response occurs at the local site, remove the patch, wipe the skin clean, and notify the prescriber.

- ■ **My patient is a child who does not want the medication to be applied?**

  Hold the child securely while medication is applied. Then cover the site with a dressing to keep the child from disrupting the application of medication.

- ■ **My patient is an older adult and has fragile skin?**

  Avoid areas where penetration of the cream or ointment is likely to be reduced or cause irritation. Be gentle with application of anything to the skin and diligent with your assessment of the skin response to medication.

Evaluation

- ■ Assess for rash, excoriation, hives, redness, swelling, or signs of allergy or skin sensitivity to topical medication.
- ■ Ask the patient if he feels burning, itching, pain, tenderness, or other sensation to skin where medication was applied.
- ■ Assess for improvement in the patient's condition.

- ■ Record the condition of skin if abnormalities are present and any complaints of discomfort during or after administration.
- ■ Document responses to medication (e.g., symptom relief, side effects).

Patient Teaching

- ■ Explain that topical medication may take up to 30 minutes to be absorbed, depending on the medication.
- ■ Tell the patient to never ingest or inhale topical medication.
- ■ Advise the patient to avoid touching his eyes after handling topical medication.
- ■ Inform the patient to not use more medicine than prescribed or directed.

Thinking About the Procedure

 Go to the *Fundamentals of Nursing Skills Videos,* **Medication Administration: Transdermal Medications.**

1. Where does the nurse apply the transdermal patch?
2. Why does the nurse apply the medication in this location?

For suggested responses, go to Chapter 25, **Thinking About the Procedure Suggested Responses,** on Davis*Plus.*

Documentation

- ■ Refer to Medication Guidelines: Steps to Follow for All Medication (Regardless of Type or Route).

Safety icons alert you to important aspects of safe care.

➕ You can usually recognize an incompatibility when the mixed solution takes on a changed appearance. However, you should always consult medication resources and compatibility charts *before* mixing medications. Then, after mixing, double-check the medication for changes in appearance.

Care Maps visually connect the phases of the nursing process to help you plan patient care.

Care.

Case Studies
show you how theory applies to practice.

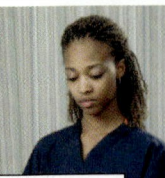

Meet Your Patients

You are scheduled to administer medications to five patients on the medical–surgical unit today. You will be administering medications unsupervised for the first time. Your clinical instructor will be available as a resource. Your

- Rebecca Jones, an 84-year-old woman with compression fractures of two lumbar vertebrae

Caring for the Nguyens

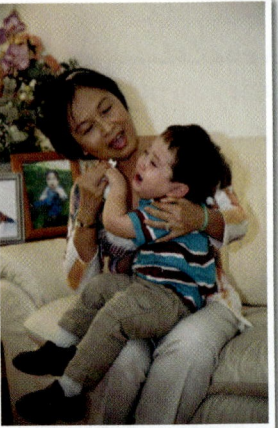

This feature allows you to practice the kind of thinking you will use as a full-spectrum nurse. There is usually more than one correct answer to a critical-thinking question, so we do not provide answers for these features. It is more important to develop your nursing judgment than to "cover content." Discuss the questions with your peers. If you are still unsure, consult your instructor.

Kim Phan, the 3-year-old grandson of Nam and Yen Nguyen, has been tired and observed to be sitting down a great deal at preschool. Last week, he developed coughing, wheezing, shortness of breath, nasal congestion, and extreme fatigue. The pediatrician at the Family Medicine Center diagnosed asthma. He prescribed a 5-day tapering course of prednisone, a leukotriene inhibitor (Singulair) 4 mg orally daily at bedtime, and periodic treatments with albuterol through a home nebulizer system.

Nam's mother, Mai Nguyen, became very upset when she saw the bottle of prednisone elixir. She was even more upset when she learned that Kim received an injection of the medicine in the office. She advised Yen not to give Kim the medicine because, she said, it causes weak bones and stunts growth. Yen has called the clinic asking for advice on how to handle this problem.

Home Care, Self-Care, and Complementary and Alternative Medicine teaching boxes provide important
information that ties classroom instruction to real-world clinical practice.

Self-Care

Teaching Your Patient About Self-Medication

- Do not take medications prescribed to others, and do not share your medications with others.
- Keep a list of your medications, including doses and times taken. Take this list with you when you visit any primary care provider or an emergency department.
- If you take a variety of medications, post a list of them in a prominent place that is easy to get to in the event of an emergency.
- Wear a medical alert bracelet or necklace if you are a diabetic, take anticoagulants, or have allergies to any medication.
- When you are prescribed a new medication, ask why you are taking it, how long you should take it, what side effects you should expect, whether you should take it with food, and whether there are any special precautions.
- Take the medication for the prescribed length of time to make certain you receive the full benefit of the drug. For

QSEN

Understanding the Limitations of Technologies for Medication Safety

Competencies: Safety (Knowledge); Informatics (Knowledge, Skills, Attitudes)*

It is important for you to understand the limitations of safety-enhancing technologies so that you can apply the technologies correctly (Informatics) and reduce the risk of patient harm (Safety).

Computerized physician order entry (CPOE). CPOE was hailed as the answer to prescribing errors and it has had many positive effects. However, several studies have reported mixed results, one documented 22 new types of errors, and one reported an *increase* in mortality after CPOE implementation. Factors contributing CPOE errors include the following:
- "Alert fatigue": the tendency for users to ignore frequent interruptions from warning messages
- Rigid programs that take users through multiple unnecessary screens or force unnecessary decisions. These encourage users to bypass decision points.
- False sense of security generated by the belief that automated systems prevent errors

Quality and Safety Education for Nurses (QSEN) competencies will
help you build the knowledge and skills you need to succeed in professional practice.

Your Learning Resources
Online at  DavisPlus

Premium Resources

Redeem the *Plus* Code on the inside front cover to unlock these Davis*Plus* Premium learning resources...

- **Electronic Study Guide: Chapter Resources**—it's like having a **500-page workbook** at your fingertips! Enhance your learning experience with...
  - IQ Student Test Bank with NCLEX-style review questions
  - Learning Outcomes
  - Knowledge Maps
  - Concept Maps
  - Mastery Exercises
  - Care Plans
  - Care Maps
  - Important tables, boxes, and figures
  - Suggested responses to case studies
  - Responses and answers to all questions and exercises in the textbook
- **Davis Digital Version**—your complete text online! Quickly search for the content you need and add notes, highlights, and bookmarks.
- Interactive Clinical Scenarios
- Animations and Body Sounds Library
- Audio Glossary
- Procedure Checklists
- NANDA-I Nursing Diagnoses
- NIC Interventions Labels and Definitions
- NOC Outcome Labels and Definitions
- **And more!**

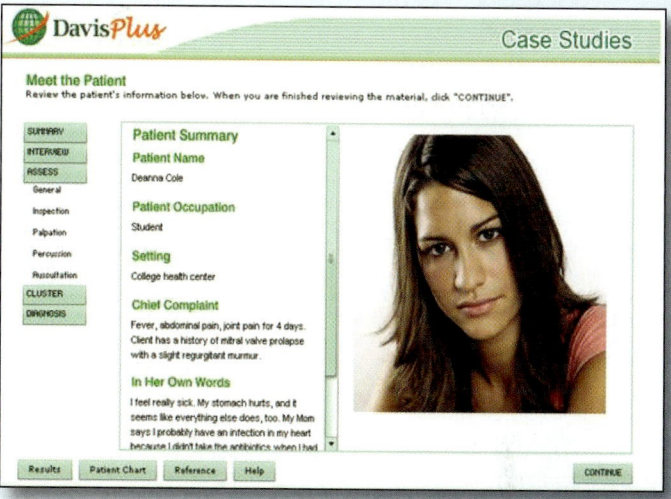

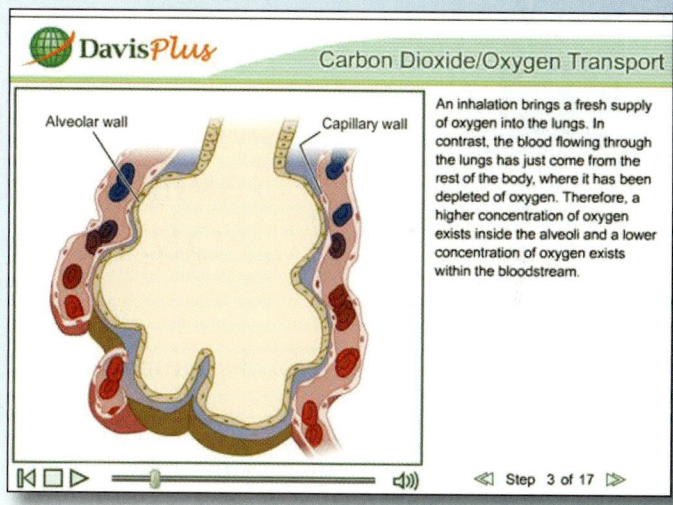

Additional Resources

- Podcast to help you get the most from your learning resources
- Dosage Calculator
- Concept Care Map Creator
- Preventing Medication Errors Tutorial
- Wound Care Tutorial
- Paragraph Matching exercises
- **And more!**

Visit **DavisPlus.FADavis.com** today!

NOTE: Each *Plus* Code may only be redeemed one time. If your code has already been used, visit DavisPlus.FADavis.com to purchase access.

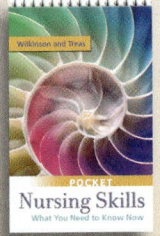
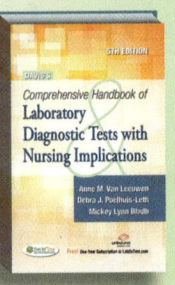
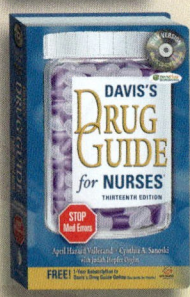
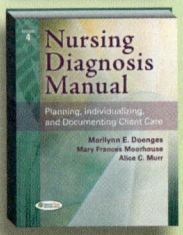
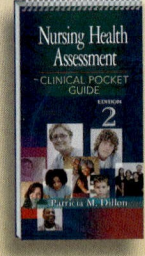
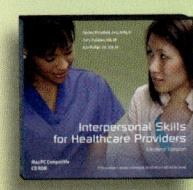
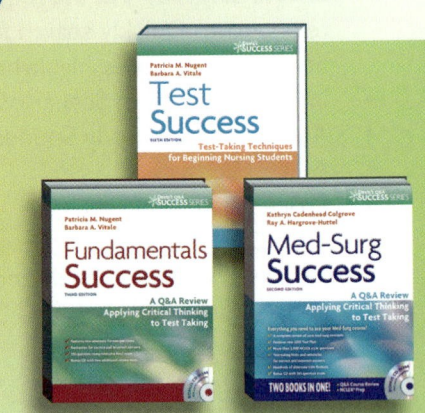
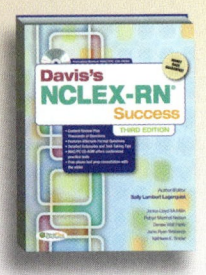
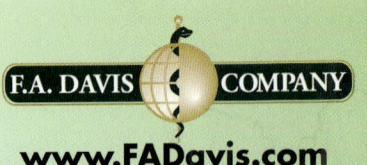

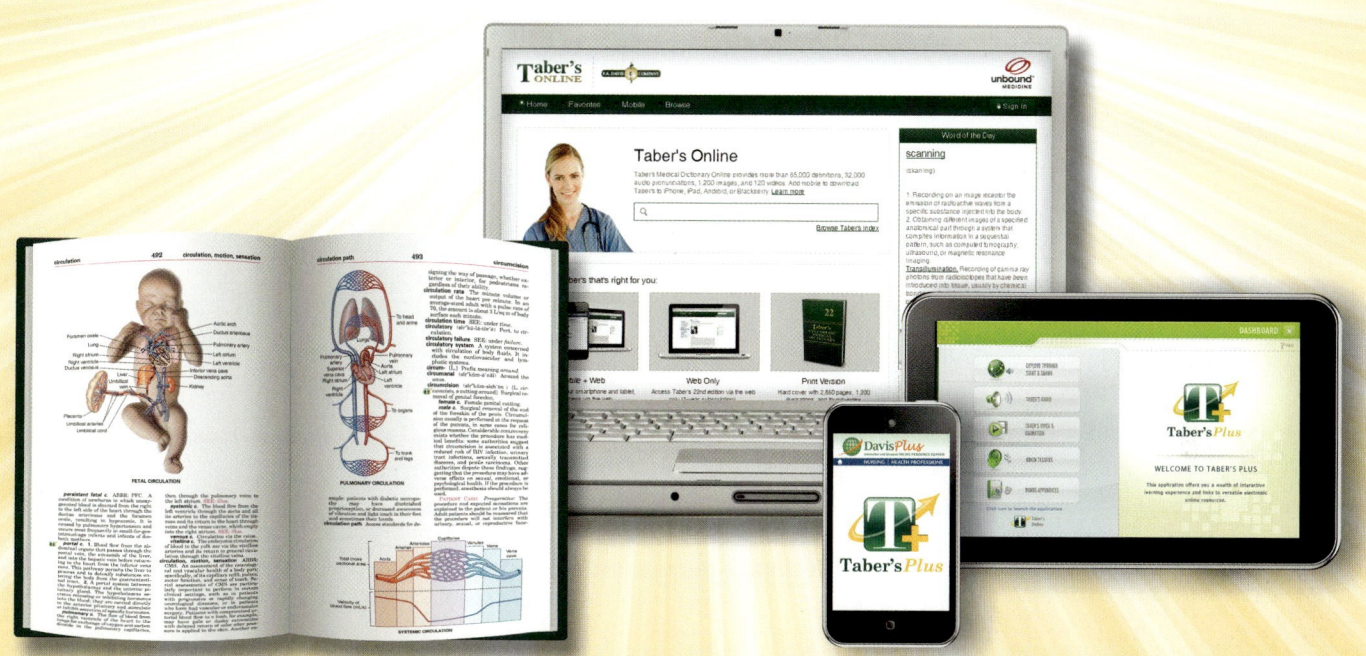
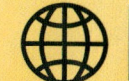
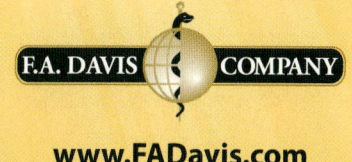

BASIC NURSING

Concepts, Skills, & Reasoning

Leslie S. Treas, PhD, RN, CPNP-PC, NNP-BC
Judith M. Wilkinson, PhD, ARNP

F.A. Davis Company • Philadelphia

F. A. Davis Company
1915 Arch Street
Philadelphia, PA 19103
www.fadavis.com

Copyright © 2014 by F. A. Davis Company

Printed in the United States of America

Last digit indicates print number: 10 9 8 7 6 5 4 3 2

Publisher, Nursing: Lisa B. Houck
Director of Content Development: Darlene D. Pedersen
Project Editor: Jamie M. Elfrank, M.A.
Electronic Project Editor: Katherine E. Crowley
Design and Illustrations Manager: Carolyn O'Brien

As new scientific information becomes available through basic and clinical research, recommended treatments and drug therapies undergo changes. The author(s) and publisher have done everything possible to make this book accurate, up to date, and in accord with accepted standards at the time of publication. The author(s), editors, and publisher are not responsible for errors or omissions or for consequences from application of the book, and make no warranty, expressed or implied, in regard to the contents of the book. Any practice described in this book should be applied by the reader in accordance with professional standards of care used in regard to the unique circumstances that may apply in each situation. The reader is advised always to check product information (package inserts) for changes and new information regarding dose and contraindications before administering any drug. Caution is especially urged when using new or infrequently ordered drugs.

Library of Congress Cataloging-in-Publication Data

Treas, Leslie S.
  Basic nursing : concepts, skills, & reasoning / Leslie S. Treas, Judith M. Wilkinson.
      p. ; cm.
  Includes bibliographical references and index.
  ISBN 978-0-8036-2778-9
  I. Wilkinson, Judith M., 1939- II. Title.
  [DNLM: 1. Nursing Care. 2. Nurse's Role. 3. Nursing Assessment. WY 100.1]
  RT49
  610.73—dc23

                        2013007349

Leslie S. Treas, PhD, RN, CPNP-PC, NNP-BC

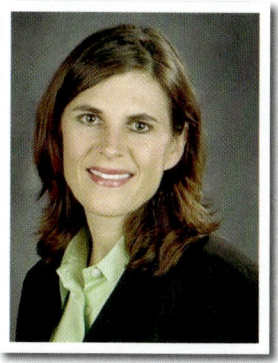

Dr. Leslie Treas, one of the founders and former vice-president of Research and Development of Assessment Technologies Institute™, LLC (ATI), demonstrated leadership and expertise forecasting and directing the design and development of ATI product testing and educational product line since the formation of the company. In this role, Dr. Treas planned and implemented norming, test validation, and standard-setting studies to support data-driven product development, creating tests with sound psychometric properties. Under her management, ATI produced a series of NCLEX®-review books and nursing skills DVD set. She has conducted clinical and educational research, publishing in peer-reviewed journals of health and education.

Dr. Treas was involved in the start-up of a continuing education company for nurses, physicians, and allied health professionals, serving as Director of Education and Accreditation, AcaMedic Institute™, LLC.

Dr. Treas earned a BSN from Pennsylvania State University and an MSN degree with emphasis in maternal–child health at the University of Kansas. She obtained a PhD from the University of Kansas in the Educational Psychology and Research Department with dual areas of study of testing and measurement and nursing education. Her primary area of clinical expertise is the care of sick newborns in the NICU and labor and delivery settings in the clinical role of a neonatal nurse practitioner for 13 years. Dr. Treas obtained dual pediatric and neonatal nurse practitioner certifications at the Cleveland Metropolitan General Hospital, an affiliate of Case Western University.

Her journal and textbook publications have featured various clinical topics ranging from care of neonatal patients to education-based areas related to nursing licensure preparation and prediction, critical thinking, and others. Leslie has also written articles geared to new graduate readers, addressing contemporary issues involving role change, employment, and communication. She is also the co-author of the F. A. Davis text, *Fundamentals of Nursing* (2nd ed.).

Dr. Treas has presented papers at annual conferences for Sigma Theta Tau, National Association of Associate Degree Nurses, National Association of Neonatal Nurses, American Association of Colleges of Nursing, National Conference on Professional Nursing Education and Development, and the Association for the Advancement of Educational Research, to name a few.

She has test-writing expertise; she is a former test-item writer for the National Certification Examination for Pediatric Nurse Practitioners and Nurses as well as the National Certification Corporation for Neonatal Nurse Practitioner Exam.

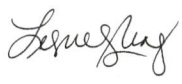

Judith M. Wilkinson, PhD, ARNP

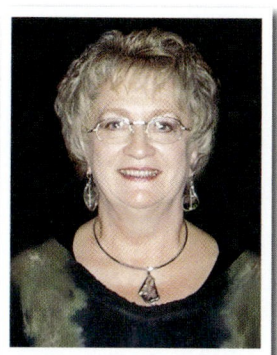

Judith Wilkinson taught fundamentals of nursing for 22 years and, more recently, has taught graduate-level courses in theory, research, and health policy. She also developed, and taught for many years, an LPN-to-RN transition course. She has given numerous presentations and provided consultation and faculty development workshops for nursing and other schools—primarily in the areas of critical thinking and nursing ethics, but also in standardized nursing languages, teaching strategies, testing, evaluation, and curriculum.

She obtained her PhD in Nursing from the University of Kansas School of Nursing, and master's degrees in Education and Nursing from the University of Missouri–Kansas City School of Nursing. Her basic nursing degree is an ADN from Johnson County Community College, followed by a BSN from Graceland College. She was granted a National Endowment for the Humanities fellowship to study nursing ethics, and a Nurses' Educational Fund (Isabel Hampton Robb) scholarship for her nursing doctoral study. Her master's thesis was a seminal work in moral distress; her doctoral dissertation also focused on nursing ethics.

Dr. Wilkinson's broad clinical background includes emergency, critical care, med-surg (float), and obstetric nursing. While engaged in full-time teaching, she also maintained certification in inpatient obstetric nursing; her advanced practice license is in nursing care of women.

Her other publications include F. A. Davis's *Fundamentals of Nursing*; a nursing process text and a nursing diagnosis handbook (each having been published in multiple editions); a maternal–newborn care planning book (as a coauthor); and journal articles on the topics of curriculum, critical thinking, and nursing ethics. Over the years, she has contributed chapters to several textbooks and authored many ancillary materials, including test banks, learning modules, and review modules.

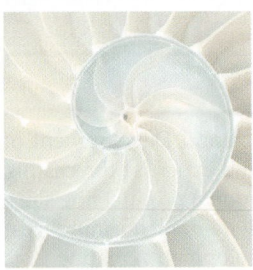

We dedicate this book to:

■ The creative, dedicated nurse educators, who give so much of themselves to help prepare their students for providing care across the full spectrum of nursing.

■ Nursing students, as they strive to acquire the knowledge, skills, and attitudes that they must transfer to their imminent practice.

■ Practicing nurses, who struggle with daily realities to provide comfort and care.

The health of the nation depends on all of us.

—Leslie S. Treas
—Judith M. Wilkinson

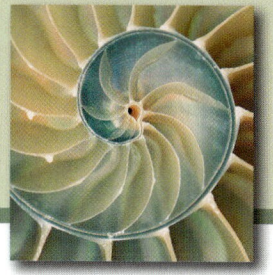

Preface

We chose our book title carefully. We used the words *concepts*, *skills*, and *reasoning* because we believe that excellent nurses use an equal mix of knowledge, thought, and clinical reasoning to translate their caring into action. It is knowledge and its application—not just the tasks nurses do—that delineate the various levels of nursing. Even so, skillful performance of tasks is essential to full attainment of the nursing role.

We used *basic nursing* in the title because this text, and its concomitant course, is truly that: the basis for all that follows. In that sense, and because this basic, fundamental content will be used throughout the nurse's career, we believe it is—or should be—the most important course students take. We want them to say, "Everything I need to know, I learned in fundamentals—all I needed to know about how to think, what to do, and how to care" (at a basic level). You will see those themes integrated throughout each chapter.

We have kept the same open, user-friendly, easy-to-read style that students have been telling us they love in our other fundamentals products.

ORGANIZATION

Enrichment (Supplemental Material)—This book provides comprehensive content that will meet the needs of most students and instructors. However, to minimize weight and bulk, and to keep the content manageable for students, we have put some enrichment material on the Electronic Study Guide located on the DavisPlus Web site for students who need it or who wish to pursue a subject in more depth. Our chapters are self-contained and rich in cross-references so that teachers and students can use them in any order that fits their needs.

Optional Chapters—We anticipate this text will be used as a reference throughout the student's career—and we intended it to be comprehensive but not overwhelming. To that end, we have included two complete chapters on the Electronic Study Guide located on the DavisPlus Web site: Chapter 45, Leadership & Management, and Chapter 46, Holistic Nursing. We recognize that curricula differ—that, for example, many schools have a separate leadership course and do not need that chapter in a basic nursing text. However, for those who do need it, the complete chapter is on DavisPlus.

Within-Chapter Organization—Content within each chapter is generally organized into two major sections: Theoretical Knowledge: Knowing Why, and Practical Knowledge: Knowing How. There is some overlap in these concepts because the two types of knowledge are interdependent. We have made the general distinction because many nursing programs begin with content learned in supporting prerequisite classes and then layer on additional Theoretical Knowledge to explain the rationale for nursing actions and activities (Practical Knowledge). This distinction also affords more flexibility in teaching fundamentals. For example, it is useful to teachers who believe students are more motivated when they present first the concrete (Practical Knowledge), and then the abstract (Theoretical Knowledge); it is equally useful for those who teach from the theoretical to the practical.

Procedures (Nursing Skills)—These are placed at the end of the chapter for two reasons: (1) So they do not interrupt the logical flow of content when the student is studying didactic material, and (2) So they will be easier to locate when the student is looking for a particular procedure.

FEATURES

The chapters have numerous pedagogical features to facilitate student learning. These features include:

- *Learning Outcomes* – These focus the student's study and provide repetition to facilitate retention of material. In addition, a the learning outcomes are reinforced by (1) a Chapter Overview podcast on the DavisPlus Web site and (2) the feature What Are the Main Points? on the Electronic Study Guide located on the DavisPlus Web site.

- *Interactive Approach* – The text is written in an engaging style that speaks directly to the student. Critical-thinking and recall questions are integrated throughout the content to break chapters up into small, manageable segments and maintain interest. They also occur in the clinical reasoning exercises in each chapter and in other activities on the Electronic Study Guide located on DavisPlus.

- *Caring for the Nguyens* – This chapter-opening feature is an ongoing case study that appears in every chapter. It allows students to become familiar with a single family and to experience vicariously the continuity of care they may encounter in outpatient settings. As with all exercises, response sheets are provided on the Electronic Study Guide located on DavisPlus.

- *Key Concepts List and Concept Map* – The key concepts are the umbrella concepts for the chapter—right after the opening features. We listed them to help students begin to use concepts to organize content in their memory. In the section About the Key Concepts we explain how those concepts relate to or can be used to organize chapter content. At the very end of each chapter is a Concept Map, which shows the relationships among the key concepts and many subordinate, related chapter concepts.

- *Meet Your Patient* – This feature, following Caring for the Nguyens, introduces one or more patients, as you might see in "real life" nursing. It is used throughout the chapter to illustrate theoretical points and to make the content come alive. These patients are often followed in the set of clinical reasoning questions near the end of the chapter, as well as in the Think Like a Nurse questions found throughout the chapter.

- *Knowledge Checks* – These questions allow students to test their recall of the material presented in the text. Answer sheets and answers are provided on the Electronic Study Guide located on DavisPlus.

- *Critical-Thinking Exercises* – Thought-provoking questions (Think Like a Nurse) allow the student to synthesize content and explore personal beliefs. Response sheets are provided on the Electronic Study Guide located on Davis*Plus*; suggested responses are found in the Instructors' Guide.

- *Safety Features* – Safety is an important concern in nursing care. To emphasize and help students remember important aspects of safe care, we have specially marked the most important points about safety to make them visible and memorable. They are color-shaded, with an icon to draw attention to them. We do, of course, have an entire chapter on promoting safety.

- *QSEN Competencies* – We have introduced the Quality & Safety Education for Nurses (QSEN) competencies for nurses in the early chapters, and reinforced them where relevant throughout the text. To remind students that these competencies have practical implications, many of the chapters have a QSEN box, providing an example of how a particular competency is expressed in practice.

- *What if . . .* – Where applicable, procedures include a section to aid students in knowing what to do in special situations that require decisions during a procedure. For example, what if you perform a fingerstick to monitor blood glucose, and the monitor shows a very unusual result or an error message? What should you do? We provide the answer.

- *Thinking About the Procedure* – Procedures include exercises that require students to watch the associated Wilkinson & Treas's *Fundamentals of Nursing* skills videos to answer the questions. Answers are provided on Davis*Plus*.

- *Toward Evidenced-Based Practice Boxes* – In every chapter, we describe research related to the chapter topic and pose critical-thinking exercises for students to examine these findings. The concept of evidence-based practice is introduced in Chapter 6 (Planning Interventions), further explained in Chapter 8 (Theory, Research, & Evidence-Based Practice), and mentioned frequently in other chapters as well.

- *Care Plans* – Seventeen care plans integrating NANDA-International, NIC, and NOC are found in the book and on Davis*Plus*. They are based on case studies that allow students to see the nursing process in action. Evidence-based rationales are provided for interventions.

- *Care Maps* – Care Maps associated with each care plan allow visual learners to grasp the connection between the phases of the nursing process. They also provide an alternative method of care planning.

- *Care Planning and Care Mapping Exercises* – Cross-references in the book link students to the Davis*Plus* Web site for practice in constructing care plans both in columnar format and as concept maps, using the Concept Map Generator on the Web site. Sample responses are provided.

- *Practice Documentation* – Cross-references in the book link students to Practice Documentation exercises on Davis*Plus*.

- *Teaching: Self-Care Boxes* – Self-care boxes are similar to the traditional "teaching boxes," but focus on equipping patients to perform self-care.

- *Home Care Boxes* – These provide guidelines for safely modifying care for delivery in the home. Many of the procedures also have a Home Care section for adapting the procedure in the patient's home.

- *Complementary & Alternative Modalities (CAM) Boxes* – Included in several chapters, these describe a complementary therapy related to the chapter topic or present research concerning a complementary therapy (e.g., intercessory prayer in the spirituality chapter).

- *Clinical Reasoning: Applying the Full-Spectrum Nursing Model* – These clinically based exercises guide students to safely practice their clinical reasoning skills, and at the same time reinforce the full-spectrum model concepts of thinking, doing, and caring introduced in Chapter 2 and integrated throughout the book.

- *Diagnostic Testing Boxes* – These are found in applicable chapters. We believe it is more meaningful to place the diagnostic test information near the related content rather than in an isolated chapter. If students need a more comprehensive reference, we recommend a diagnostic testing book.

- *Knowledge Maps* – These are a type of concept map. On the Electronic Study Guide located on Davis*Plus*, in the Student Resources for each chapter, are maps of chapter content. Rather than demonstrating relationship among chapter concepts, the maps show the relationships among the various topics covered in the chapter.

- *Critical Thinking* – An additional set of clinically based exercises (found in each chapter of the Electronic Study Guide located on Davis*Plus*) helps students safely practice their critical-thinking skills in preparation for doing so in the clinical area. Frequently, these clinical exercises further analyze material related to the Meet Your Patient scenario in the textbook.

THEMES

The following are themes are integrated and stressed throughout this text, some of them in every chapter:

- *Critical Thinking, Clinical Reasoning, and the Full-Spectrum Model of Nursing.* In addition to the critical-thinking questions and exercises, we promote critical thinking by often presenting content in an inductive manner, or by posing a question to the student (e.g., "What would happen if . . .?"). The full spectrum model of nursing is a comprehensive approach to care that uses critical thinking in all aspects of care. It is not rigidly overlaid on each chapter. Because students cannot focus on everything at once, different parts are stressed at different times. Sometimes the discussion asks, "What theoretical knowledge do you need to . . .?" In other instances they might be asked, "What biases do you have that might interfere with . . ." The full-spectrum model is reinforced in every chapter, as well as in the feature Clinical Reasoning: Applying the Full-Spectrum Nursing Model, which requires students to use the model concepts of thinking, doing, and caring.

- *Nursing Process.* Chapter 2 explains the relationship between nursing process, critical thinking, and clinical reasoning; Chapters 3 through 7 make up a comprehensive presentation of the nursing process, which is presented as reflexive rather than linear. The Practical Knowledge sections are organized according to the nursing process phases; and the procedures all have assessment and evaluation components. In addition, many of the questions and exercises provide opportunity for using the nursing process.

- *Caring.* Caring is thoroughly integrated within many chapters. Chapter 1 provides historical examples of nursing as a caring profession. Chapter 8 describes the important caring theories. The case study introduces Watson's theory, and that theory is used throughout Chapter 8 to illustrate how theory is applied in nursing. As well, the

Clinical Reasoning: Applying the Full-Spectrum Nursing Model features all have questions involving caring.

- **QSEN (Quality and Safety Education for Nurses).** To remind students of the knowledge, skills, and attitudes needed to achieve the QSEN competencies (patient-centered care, teamwork and collaboration, evidence-based practice, quality improvement, and informatics), we have included QSEN boxes, which provide examples of how a particular competency is expressed.
- **Culture.** Cultural diversity is highlighted throughout the text in clinical scenarios, illustrations, and theoretical discussion. Chapter 15 focuses on culturally sensitive nursing care. The Caring for the Nguyens opening scenario features a Vietnamese family; and ethnic variations are described, as applicable, in procedures.
- **Gerontology.** To allow for an in-depth discussion of aging and gerontology, provided by an expert on this topic, Chapter 10 is entirely devoted to the older adult developmental stage. Common health problems include dementia, depression, elder abuse, and ageism. Assessments and interventions specifically for the young-old, middle-old, oldest-old, and frail elderly are provided. We have also included interventions specific to older adults in clinical chapters where they apply (e.g., assessing for pain, in Chapter 32; variations for older adults in the physical assessment procedures in Chapter 21). You will also find that many features and exercises use an older adult as the patient.
- **Developmental Stage.** Chapter 9 is devoted entirely to growth and development from conception through middle age. The Theoretical Knowledge section in most chapters devotes a portion to the discussion of the effects of the life span on the chapter topic. In addition, the procedures include variations for children and older adults.
- **Documentation.** All chapters include reference to documentation, where relevant. The procedures all have guidelines for documenting the procedure. In addition, we have included some Practice Documentation exercises on the Electronic Study Guide located on DavisPlus.
- **Informatics.** Chapter 44 is an excellent introduction to nursing informatics. Standardized languages and computerized care planning and documentation are interspersed throughout the book (e.g., in the nursing process and medications chapters), and especially in standardized language tables on the Electronic Study Guide located on DavisPlus for the clinical chapters. We also emphasize electronic documentation in Chapter 18. We further encourage use of technology by providing students with links to material on DavisPlus and many other Web sites related to the chapter topic.
- **Contemporary Issues.** We have included information about bioterrorism (Chapter 22, Infection Prevention & Control; and Chapter 41, Community & Home Nursing). Chapter 22 also includes updated and expanded material on drug-resistant pathogens, emerging infectious diseases, and healthcare-acquired infections. The chapter on safety includes ways to assess for and cope with violence in the healthcare setting.
- **NANDA-I, NIC, and NOC Standardized Languages.** Thorough discussion of these taxonomies occurs in the nursing process and other chapters. NOC outcomes and NIC interventions are included in every chapter, and many more are presented in tables on DavisPlus. The Omaha System and the Clinical Care Classification are also used in the community and home health chapters.

- **Wellness.** Many examples used in this text refer to people who are not ill. Chapter 11 emphasizes health, and Chapter 27 talks about the nurse's role in health promotion.
- **Spirituality.** Chapter 16 is probably the most extensive presentation of spiritual care available in a fundamentals text. Spirituality is integrated within various chapters in scenarios, examples, and exercises.
- **Delegation.** Delegation is introduced early, in the nursing process chapters, and is a thread woven through most chapters. All procedures have guidelines for delegating. Chapter 45, Leadership & Management, on the Electronic Study Guide located on the DavisPlus Web site, also discusses delegation.
- **ANA Standards.** Nursing and other healthcare standards (e.g., The Joint Commission, Medicare) are frequently referenced. Links to pertinent Web sites are given so students can keep up with changes to standards.
- **Ethics.** In addition to the comprehensive treatment in Chapter 42, ethical knowledge is an aspect of our full-spectrum model. As such, many of the critical-thinking exercises ask students to grapple with ethical issues. Good examples are found in Chapter 6 and in the feature Clinical Reasoning: Applying the Full-Spectrum Nursing Model in every chapter.
- **Legal Issues.** Chapter 43 is devoted to legal issues that nurses face in their practice. Legal issues are integrated in many other chapters as well (e.g., licensing in Chapter 1, end-of-life legal considerations in Chapter 17).
- **Community and Home Nursing.** Chapter 41 is devoted exclusively to these topics. In other chapters, clinical scenarios and examples involve nurses in these settings; we include special feature boxes regarding these topics; and the procedures have sections for adapting skills to home care, where applicable.
- **Complementary Therapies.** Nursing is presented as holistic throughout. Chapter 46 (found on the Electronic Study Guide located on DavisPlus) is devoted exclusively to complementary and alternative therapies; and several chapters in the book (e.g., Chapter 15, Culture & Ethnicity) contain material and/or boxes related to this topic.

THE TEXT AS A RESPONSE TO CHANGE

This book was developed to address the needs of today's nursing students and in response to the following changes in nursing education and practice.

Changes in Students

- **Nontraditional Students.** Students range from traditional, younger students to older, second-career students. Many are older and have work or family responsibilities that compete with the time needed for classes and studying. To address this change we have followed two principles of adult learning: Learning must be relevant and it must be efficient. For example, we have made good use of the Electronic Study Guide located on the DavisPlus Web site to deliver enhancements to the printed text, knowing that highly motivated and computer-literate students will welcome the chance to use these technologies to maximize their learning.
- **Variety in Learning Styles.** Students learn in different ways. To address this, we have used over 1,400 photos and as many diagrams to assist visual learners. Podcasts, animations, and sound files of heart sounds and many other clinical assessment findings are included on DavisPlus for auditory learners. To teach psychomotor skills, we have, in addition to

step-by-step procedures, skills videos and checklists that students can print out for practicing procedures or teachers to use in evaluations.

Because learning improves when content is meaningful to the learner, each chapter opens with a patient scenario or story of a practicing nurse. This story is woven throughout the chapter to provide context for factual information and to show how concepts are applied and how nurses think. We stress practical application throughout the text because adults want to apply knowledge in real-life circumstances. The Nguyen family case, which is introduced in Chapter 1 and continues throughout all chapters, is a prime example.

- **Reading Comprehension.** Whether because of changes in admission requirements, students having English as a second language, or other reasons, some schools are finding students' reading abilities to be on a lower level than in the past. We address this change by writing in an informal style, addressing the student directly ("you will . . ."). We have not made the content more superficial, but have made reading about it more inviting and user friendly. We define new terms (in bold type) at their first use in each chapter, and include a glossary on Davis*Plus* for additional terms the student may not know.

To aid in retention we have interspersed Knowledge Checks and critical-thinking (Think Like a Nurse) questions frequently in the text to allow students to check their recall and understanding of the material as they progress through a chapter. Recognizing that repetition aids retention, we provide Learning Outcomes at the beginning of each chapter. In addition, each chapter on Electronic Study Guide includes a list called What Are the Main Points In This Chapter? and a full-page Knowledge Map of the chapter content. To accompany each chapter, there is also a podcast on the Davis*Plus* Web site that provides an overview of the chapter content. Finally, an Audio Glossary is available on the Davis*Plus* Web site.

- **The Technology Generation.** The newer generation of students is accustomed to using technology and multitasking. To hold their attention, in addition to our easy-to-read style, we have presented information in an interactive manner, and in relatively short segments interspersed with review questions and critical-thinking questions. For this same reason, the text frequently directs students to find related information on the Davis*Plus* Web site, and on the Internet, often in the form of podcasts or sound files.

The e-Edition of *Basic Nursing* lets student access their textbook anytime, anywhere. Also available from the same authors is a set of skills videos that can be purchased as DVDs or as an application from iTunes.

Changes in Curriculum

- **Concepts-Based Learning.** Even if a curriculum is not entirely concepts based, there is a trend to teaching and learning in a more concepts-based manner. We believe that all fundamentals books are, by nature, concepts based. That is, each chapter consists of the explication of one or two basic concepts (e.g., nutrition, evidence-based practice). To assist teachers and students in adopting a more concepts-based approach, in each chapter we have listed the key concepts, included an explanation of their use (About the Key Concepts), made use of Example Problem sections (e.g., urinary retention in Chapter 30), and included a Concept Map at the end of each chapter to illustrate the relationships among the key concepts and subconcepts in the chapter.

- **Teachers say they do not have enough time to "cover the content."** A concepts-based approach is one way to limit the amount of content that must be presented. See the preceding discussion. Another way to address this problem is to not re-teach material students have had in other classes. We provide, for example, just enough anatomy and physiology in each chapter to aid students who need to review A&P, or who are taking A&P concurrently with nursing courses. You should not need to "cover" it in class. Many students do take a separate course in leadership; so we have included of that material on the Electronic Study Guide located on Davis*Plus* (Chapters 45 and 46).

- **Some curricula have de-emphasized mental health; mental health may be taught in other (e.g., medical–surgical) clinical areas, with no separate mental health course.** Chapter 13 includes tools for psychosocial assessment. In addition to the usual concepts of self-concept and self-esteem we have included basic assessments and interventions for anxiety and depression, which students will encounter regularly in all areas, not just on mental health units. We include content specific to older adults (e.g., differentiating between depression and dementia). In Chapter 20, Communication & Therapeutic Relationships, you will find excellent content on the nurse–patient relationship and communication techniques that mental health teachers find so essential. Chapter 12, Stress & Adaptation, includes information about defense mechanisms.

- **The curriculum does not include separate pharmacology, nutrition, ethics, or nursing process or leadership courses.** Because all nurses need grounding in these topics, we have provided extensive coverage of them. Chapter 25, Medicating Patients, provides in-depth pharmacology information. Chapter 28, Nutrition, provides a basic foundation for understanding patients' nutritional needs. Chapter 42 is a comprehensive look at nursing ethics. Chapter 45 (on the Electronic Study Guide located on Davis*Plus*) is a thorough presentation of leadership. We have, arguably, the most useful and thorough presentation of the nursing process available in a fundamentals text. These chapters, as well as most others, will be a valuable reference for students when they take other clinical nursing courses.

Changes in Nursing and Healthcare

- *The nursing role is increasingly complex, requiring management, decision-making, delegation, and supervision skills early in the career.*

To address this change, the critical-thinking and clinical decision-making exercises, as well as the Nguyens feature, help students to develop clinical decision-making skills. Delegation is presented early, in the nursing process chapters, and stressed in the rest of the chapters as applicable. The procedures each contain a Delegation section. We have included a comprehensive discussion of leadership and management in Chapter 45, on Electronic Study Guide located on Davis*Plus*.

- *Healthcare has moved increasingly from the hospital to the home and community.*

To address this change we have included a provocative discussion about the evolving healthcare system in the supplementary material for Chapter 1 on Davis*Plus*. In addition, Chapter 41 discusses community and home nursing. Home and community care are integrated throughout the book (e.g., *Healthy People 2020* goals are cited). The procedures include home care adaptations, as well as patient teaching

points that will enable patients and caregivers to assume more responsibility for care.

- *Nurses need to be critical thinkers and life-long learners.* To address this change we have organized the text around a model of full-spectrum nursing, a comprehensive approach to care that uses critical thinking in all aspects of care. The model is reinforced in each chapter in the feature Clinical Reasoning: Applying the Full-Spectrum Nursing Model. Critical thinking is integrated throughout both volumes of the text, both in discussion and in Think Like a Nurse exercises. Discussion of this model follows.

THE FULL-SPECTRUM MODEL OF NURSING

We believe that nursing knowledge is a fusion of theoretical knowledge, practical knowledge, self-knowledge, and ethical knowledge. To function at the highest level, nurses use critical thinking and the nursing process to blend thinking and doing to put caring into action. We refer to this blend as **full-spectrum nursing.** We have organized our learning package to reflect this philosophy. This model includes the major concepts of thinking, doing, and caring, patient situation, and patient outcomes. It is presented in Chapter 2 and referred to and used throughout the text.

THE LEARNING PACKAGE

This well-integrated and cross-referenced package contains both a text and the student and instructor resources on the Davis*Plus* Web site. Available from the same authors, for purchase to expand the learning package, are a comprehensive set of skills videos (which can be purchased as DVDs or as an application in iTunes), and a small *Pocket Nursing Skills* book (a handy review of skills to be used in the clinical setting).

The Textbook

The textbook contains all the theoretical and conceptual material typically present in a fundamentals text, presented in a clinically focused, user-friendly manner, and incorporating many examples. The nursing process is used as the model to organize the Practical Knowledge sections in most chapters.

Unit 1—focuses on how nurses think. It begins by showing the evolution of nursing: how our history relates to our present. Chapter 2 focuses on critical thinking, and Chapters 3 through 7 provide an extensive treatment of the nursing process. This unit prepares students to follow the organization of subsequent chapters and provides the thinking tools and processes they need to apply the content of the other chapters. Chapter 8 contains an overview of the processes of theory building, nursing research, and evidence-based practice as they relate to the nurse in practice.

Unit 2—integrates the internal and external factors that affect an individual's health (e.g., life stage, health and illness status, stress, psychosocial health, family, culture, and spirituality). Internal factors are personal beliefs or attributes that influence how the client views health, healthcare, and nursing. A groundbreaking feature is Chapter 11, which describes the health–illness–wellness continuum in an experiential way, encouraging self-knowledge, personal growth, and affective learning of that content.

Unit 3—examines essential nursing interventions. We consider these skills essential because nurses use some or all of these skills in *all* areas of nursing, regardless of setting or patient diagnosis. The unit begins with documentation and includes communication, teaching, taking vital signs, physical assessment, asepsis, safety, hygiene, and medication administration.

Unit 4—concentrates on nursing care that supports physiological function. We examine broad categories of physiological function (e.g., nutrition, elimination, oxygenation) and discuss related nursing care. Most of these chapters make use of Example Problems to help focus on concepts-based learning and the importance of *nursing* problems and interventions.

Unit 5—looks at the context for nurses' work. This includes chapters on perioperative nursing, and home and community and care, as well as the ethical and legal contexts for nursing work. Chapter 44 is a more thorough introduction to informatics than is usually found in a fundamentals text. In addition, we include, on Davis*Plus*, excellent chapters on leadership and management (Chapter 45) and on holistic healing (Chapter 46).

Electronic Study Guide

The Electronic Study Guide is included on the Davis*Plus* Web site at http://davisplus.fadavis.com, keyword Treas. It contains expanded discussions of content in some of the chapters, mastery questions, answers to the Knowledge Check features and other such study questions, a panel of NCLEX®-style test questions for practice, a glossary, additional care plans and care maps, and procedure checklists. Also included are forms that students can print out to write their answers to Knowledge Check questions, Critical-thinking questions, and mastery questions as well as clinical reasoning exercises. It also provides other types of forms that students can print and use in clinical (e.g., assessment tools). The questions themselves have expandable space so that answers can be typed in on the electronic form and then printed out. The large glossary provides definitions of all bolded terms used in the text as well as supplementary terms that may be helpful to students.

Procedure checklists can be used to study for clinical or skills lab experiences, or as a means to assess skill mastery. Checklists are provided in two formats: as a detailed list of steps for each procedure and as a generic, principles-based list that instructors can use to evaluate all procedures.

INSTRUCTOR'S GUIDE

The Instructor's Guide contains everything on the Davis*Plus* Web site plus additional features to assist faculty. These include an image bank of illustrations from the book, lesson plans, and PowerPoint lecture outlines with illustrations. The PowerPoint lecture outlines also include "clicker" questions and a critical-thinking question. The Instructor's Guide also includes teaching strategies to accompany each chapter, suggested responses for critical-thinking exercises (e.g., Caring for the Nguyens), instructions for using concept mapping, and a test bank of over 1,100 NCLEX®-style questions, including the newer NCLEX® formats.

Web Site

The text Web site, for both students and teachers, is available at http://davisplus.fadavis.com/keyword Treas. The site also contains additional content mastery activities, clinical animations, and sound files.

- *Podcasts* – For auditory learners, podcasts for each chapter summarize the main ideas for convenient prep for class or

review for quizzes or exams. There are 12 "stress buster" podcasts: one for each month. You will also find 24 clever and revealing test-taking tips to give you the "one-up" on getting a better test result.

- *NCLEX®-style practice questions for students* – We have added more questions to help students right from the beginning of their nursing studies to become comfortable answering NCLEX®-style questions.
- *E-book* – Tired of lugging around heavy books? Now you can access this textbook electronically.

HOW TO USE THIS LEARNING PACKAGE (FOR TEACHERS)

You are fortunate to be working with students at perhaps the most formative point in their nursing education: the fundamentals course. We are certain that each of you will bring your own special style to the teaching of this most-important-of-all nursing course, and that you will find new and creative ways to use the many teaching and learning features we have provided. We hope your enjoyment of this new and improved learning package is equal to our pride in it.

For suggestions about how to use this integrated learning package,

 Go to **How to Use This Learning Package** on the Instructors Resource located on Davis*Plus*.

We have also prepared for you a PowerPoint slide presentation and a podcast explaining how to use the learning package. You can use either or both to orient new teachers and students so they can easily navigate the entire learning package.

GETTING THE MOST OUT OF THIS LEARNING PACKAGE (FOR STUDENTS)

For ideas about how to use your textbooks and the Electronic Study Guide (ESG) located on the Davis*Plus* Web site to get the best results from your studying,

 Go to **Getting the Most Out of This Learning Package** on the Electronic Study Guide located on Davis*Plus*.

For those times you'd rather listen than read, we offer podcasts that describe ways for you to use the different components of your learning package—that is, your book, nursing skills DVD set, your student Electronic Study Guide, NCLEX®-style practice questions, animations, documentation exercises, Care Mapping Exercises, Concept Map generator, and many more worthwhile learning tools.

 Go to **Getting the Most Out of This Learning Package podcast** on the Davis*Plus* Web site.

We also know that being a student in a nursing program is hard work and can be overwhelming. Log on to the Davis*Plus* Web site for 12 useful strategies to reduce your stress while you are on your journey to becoming a nurse.

 Go to **Stress Busters podcast** on the Davis*Plus* Web site.

Your goal is to do well in your courses. Knowing that testing is an important part of your experience while in school, we now offer clever test-taking tips to help you to take tests with excellence and show what you know!

 Go to **Test-Taking Tips podcast** on the Davis*Plus* Web site.

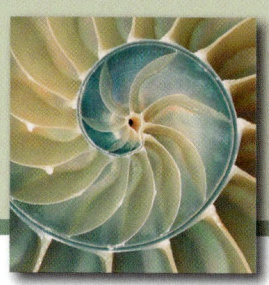

Contributors

The following contributors provided their knowledge and expertise in creating this learning package. We are grateful for their assistance.

Dr. Karen Barnett, DNP, RN
Assistant Professor, Nursing
Southern Connecticut State University
New Haven, Connecticut
Concept Maps

Diane Breckenridge, RN, PhD, MSN
Associate Research Director, Department of Nursing,
    Abington Memorial Hospital
Associate Professor of Nursing, La Salle University
Philadelphia, Pennsylvania
Chapters 3 and 4

Tracey B. Hopkins, BSN, RN
Freelance Author
QSEN boxes

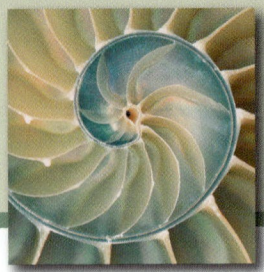

Contributors to Previous Wilkinson and Treas Textbooks

The following people previously contributed material that was used in creating this learning package. We are grateful for their assistance.

Julia Aucoin, RN, DNS, BC, CNE
Clinical consultant and literature reviews

Linda Blazovich, RN, MSN
Procedure checklists

Diane Bligh, RN, MS, CNS
Knowledge Maps, Instructors Guide, Lecture Outlines, Care Planning Exercises

Leanne Cowin, RN, PhD
Literature searches

Lisa Culliton, MSN, CPN
Literature searches

Debbie Ellison, RN, MSN
Nursing care plans; oxygenation procedures

Garrett Fardon
Clerical assistance

Mary Gant, APN, ACNS-BC, RRT
Oxygenation procedures

Kathie Hayes, DNSc
Test bank items

Lisa Lyons, RN, BSN
Procedures for sensory-perception, pain management, activity and exercise, and skin integrity chapters

Lisa LaMothe Melo, RN, BSN
Procedures for sensory-perception, pain management, activity and exercise, and skin integrity chapters

Mary N. Meyer, MSN, ARNP-BC
Procedures for safety and bowel elimination chapters

Lori Ormsby, MSN, GCNS-BC, APRN, CWOCN
Skin integrity content

Pamela Owen, BSN
Healthcare in Canada

Jessica Pedersen, ARNP, FNP-C
Procedures for nutrition chapter

Cynthia Pivec, BS
Procedure checklists

Linda Puetz, RN, BA, BSN, MEd
Documentation chapter content

Veronica Rempusheski, RN, FAAN, PhD
Older adults, Expanded Discussion (ESG)

Elizabeth Richmond, BSN, MEd
Hygiene procedures

Sarah Kennedy Roland, RN, MSN
Documentation exercises, sample nurses notes, test bank items

Susan Simmons, ARNP-BC, PhD
Clinical consultant, literature reviews

Mable H. Smith, RN, JD, PhD
Legal issues chapter

Lynne Sullivan, RN, MS
Procedures for sensory-perception, pain management, activity and exercise, and skin integrity chapters

Mary Pat Szutenbach, RN, CNS, PhD
Nutrition chapter content

Janet Terra, RN, MSN
Chapter 22 procedures

Cynthia Thompson, RN, BSN
Hygiene procedures

Diana Tilton, RN, MSN
Asepsis procedures

Lisa Watkins, RN, MS
Urinary elimination procedures

Janis Watts, RN, MSN
Nursing informatics content

Michelle Williams, RN, MSN
Nursing Care Plans

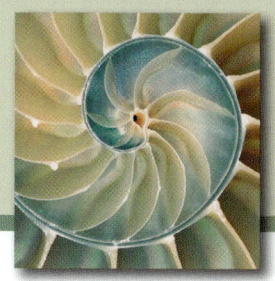

Reviewers

Special thanks to the following content reviewers:

Jocelyn Amberg, MSN, RN
Albuquerque, New Mexico

Elizabeth M. Andal, PhD, PMHCNS-BC, FAAN
Bakersfield, California

Deborah A. Andris, MSN, APNP
Milwaukee, Wisconsin

Patrice Balkcom, RN, MSN
Milledgeville, Georgia

Barbara Bonenberger, RN, MNEd, CNE
Pittsburgh, Pennsylvania

Wanda Bonnel, PhD, RN
Kansas City, Kansas

Colette Dieujuste, RNC, MS
Boston, Massachusetts

Joyce Arlene Ennis, RN, MSN, ANP-BC
Waukesha, Wisconsin

Sally Flesch, BSN, MS, EdS, PhD
Moline, Illinois

Deborah L. Galante, RN, MSN, CNOR
Newark, Delaware

Deborah B. Hadley, RN, MSN, CNOR
Natchez, Mississippi

Linda K. Heitman, PhD, RN, ACNS-BC
Cape Girardeau, Missouri

Gladys L. Husted, RN, PhD, CNE
Pittsburgh, Pennsylvania

Kathleen C. Jones, MSN, RN, CNS
Greeneville, Tennessee

Jeanie Krause-Bachand, EdD, MSN, RN
York, Pennsylvania

Janice Garrison Lanham, RN, MS, CCNS, FNP
Seneca, South Carolina

Dawn LaPorte, BSN, RN, CRRN
Salem, New Hampshire

Maureen Mc Donald, RN, MS
Brockton, Massachusetts

Laura Smith McKenna, DNSc, RN
Concord, California

Mary N. Meyer, RN, MSN
Kansas City, Kansas

Pamela S. Miller, MS, RN
Columbus, Ohio

Christine Ouellette, MS, NP
Quincy, Massachusetts

Linda Pasto, MS, RN, CNE
Dryden, New York

Carla E. Randall, RN, PhD
Lewiston, Maine

Debra L. Renna, MSN, CCRN
North Miami, Florida

Patsy M. Spratling, MSN, RN
Ridgeland, Mississippi

Lynn M. Stover, RN, BC, DSN, SANE
Morrow, Georgia

Mary Pat Szutenbach, PhD, RN, CNS
Denver, Colorado

Marcy Tanner, RN, MSN
Weatherford, Oklahoma

Pamela K. Weinberg, RN, MSN
Sumter, South Carolina

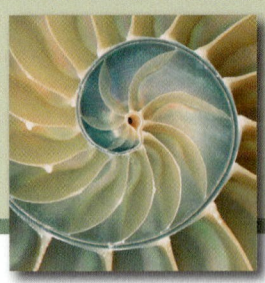

Acknowledgments

We wish to extend sincere thanks to the exceptional team who helped us create this learning package, and especially to the following people:

- **Lisa Deitch,** Acquisitions Editor and friend, for her vision in helping to create this one-volume book, which is different from, but still preserves the integrity of, the two-volume version.
- **Meghan Ziegler,** Senior Project Editor, for her amazing ability to organize and retrieve information and files, all the while churning out a mountain of work. She kept chaos at bay, made our lives easier, and never let us down.
- **Jamie Elfrank,** Project Editor, for her smooth transition into our team during a hectic phase of the production process.
- **Beth LoGiudice,** Developmental Editor, for keen eye for detail and amazing attitude, making this project an enjoyable endeavor.
- **Shirley Kuhn,** Special Projects Editor, for pouring oil on troubled waters (mostly ours) and facilitating communication between the authors and all elements of the production team, including the seamless photo shoot of illustrations for our new Meet the Nguyens feature. We so appreciate her integrity, work ethic, and sense of humor.
- **Darlene Pedersen,** Director of Content Development, for her continued support of the fundamentals projects.

Contents

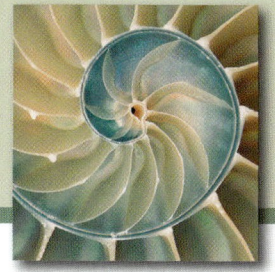

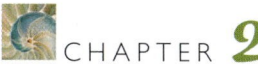
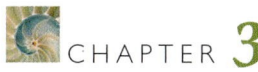

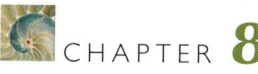
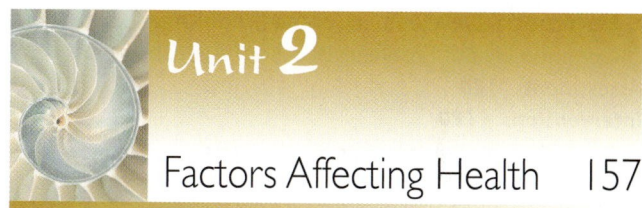
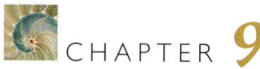

CHAPTER **13**

Psychosocial Health & Illness   272

CHAPTER **14**

Family   299

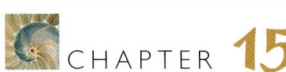
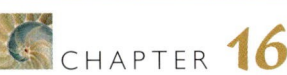
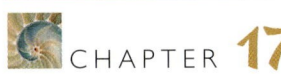

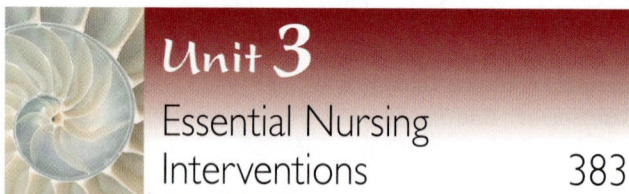

Unit **3**
Essential Nursing
Interventions　　383

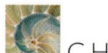
CHAPTER **18**

Documenting & Reporting 384

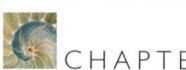
CHAPTER **19**

Vital Signs 412

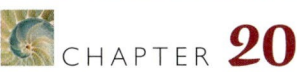

CHAPTER **20**

Communicating & Therapeutic Relationships   462

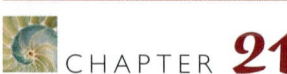

CHAPTER **21**

Physical Assessment   485

CHAPTER **22**

Infection Prevention & Control   604

CHAPTER **23**

Safety 651

CHAPTER **25**

Medicating Patients   744

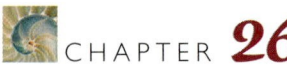

CHAPTER **26**

Teaching & Learning   853

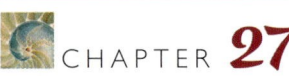

CHAPTER **27**

Health Promotion   877

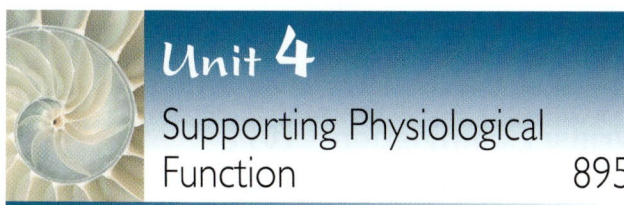

Unit **4**

Supporting Physiological
Function 895

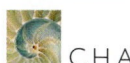 CHAPTER **28**

Nutrition 896

 CHAPTER **29**

Bowel Elimination 964

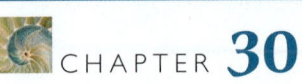

CHAPTER **30**

Urinary Elimination   1011

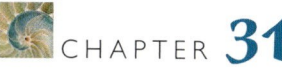

CHAPTER **31**

Sensory Perception   1066

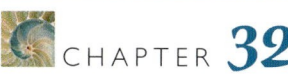

CHAPTER **32**

Pain   1089

CHAPTER **33**

Activity & Exercise   1118

CHAPTER **34**

Sexual Health   1170

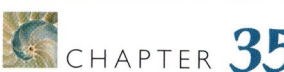

CHAPTER **35**

Sleep & Rest   1200

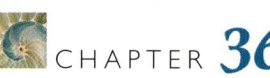

CHAPTER **36**

Skin Integrity & Wound Healing   1221

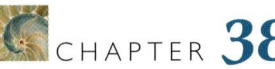

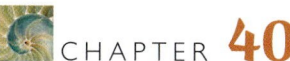

CHAPTER 39

Fluids, Electrolytes, & Acid–Base Balance 1381

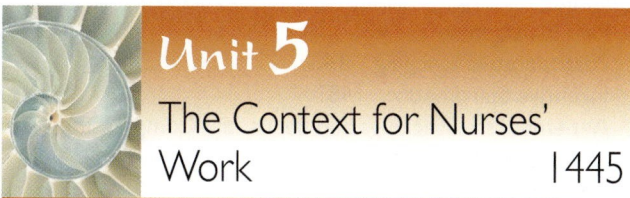

Unit 5
The Context for Nurses' Work   1445

CHAPTER 40

Perioperative Nursing 1446

CHAPTER **41**

Community & Home Nursing   1497

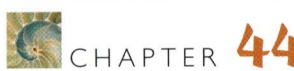
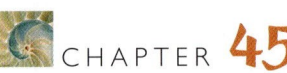
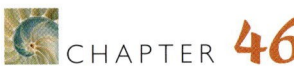

Meet the Nguyens

throughout this text, you will be applying what you have learned as you care for the Nguyen family. In Chapter 1, you will meet Nam Nguyen, a construction work supervisor, who arrives at the Family Medicine Center for his first physical exam in 10 years. It is Mr. Nguyen's knee pain that causes him to seek help because it affects his work. But as you will see, Mr. Nguyen will discover he has other serious health problems that require him to be more vigilant about his health. As you read and work through the exercises in Caring for the Nguyens, you will also get to know Nam's wife, Yen Nguyen, his grandchild Kim Phan, other members of his extended family, and his friends, as they deal with health issues and life changes.

Your experience in caring for the Nguyens will show you that patients come to you with symptoms, but each person brings unique values, lifestyle, and relationships to the encounter. From the Nguyens, you will learn what it means to care for the whole person and how to be a full-spectrum nurse.

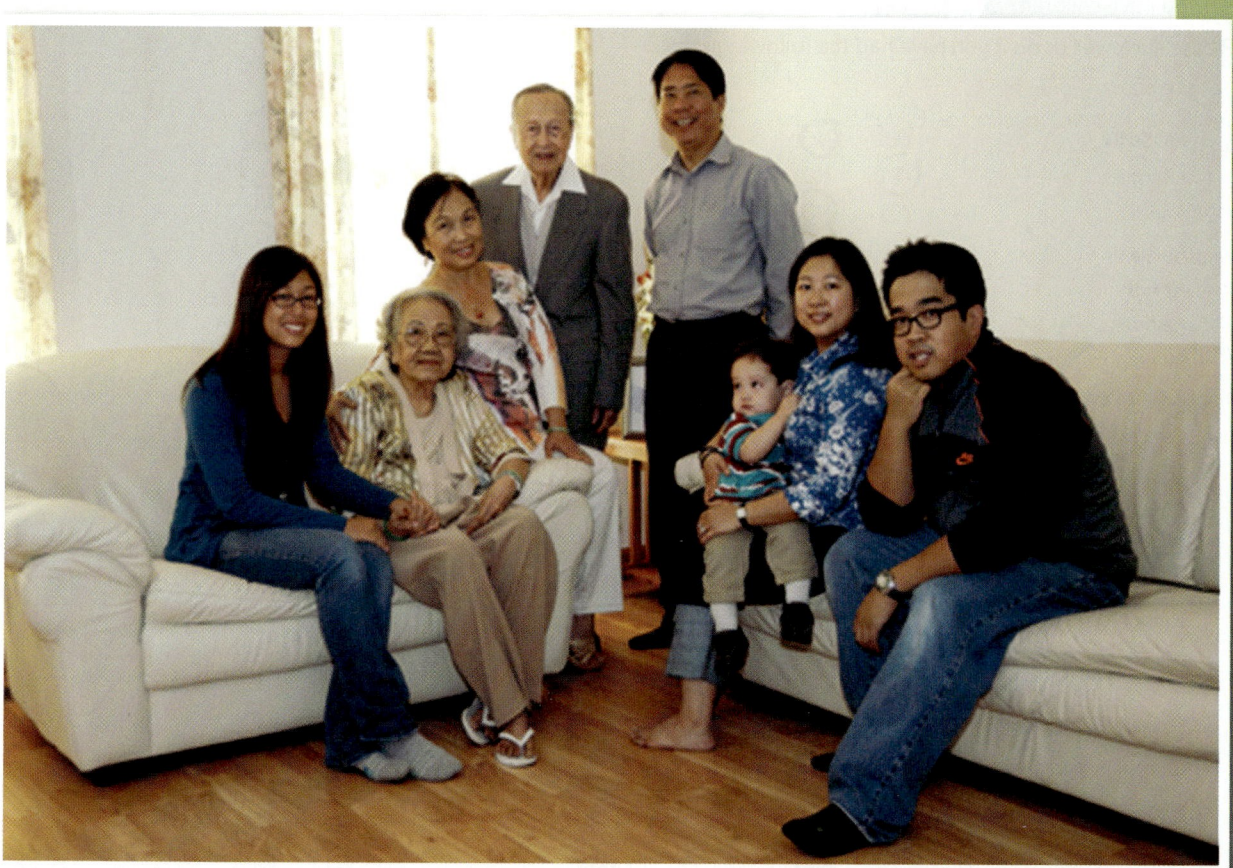

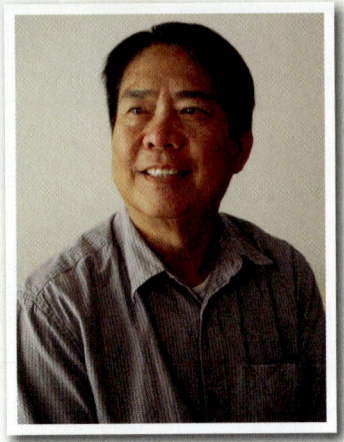

Mr. Nam Nguyen is a new patient at the Family Medicine Center. He arrives at the center for a scheduled physical exam and completes the following admission questionnaire.

Name: *Nam Nguyen*   DOB: *7 / 12 / 50*

Marital Status   S   (M)   W   D   Partnered

If applicable, spouse/partner name: *Yen*

Occupation: *Construction supervisor*   Spouse/partner occupation: *Daycare teacher*

Does your spouse or partner have any health care problems? If so, please list:

High blood pressure

Do you have children? *Yes*   Ages? *30, 27, 22*

Please circle yes or no if you have had the following:

AIDS/HIV +	YES	**(NO)**	Headaches	YES	**(NO)**
Allergies	**(YES)**	NO	Heart Disease	YES	(NO)
Anemia	YES	(NO)	Hernia	(YES)	NO
Anorexia	YES	(NO)	Herpes	YES	(NO)
Anxiety	YES	(NO)	High Cholesterol	YES	(NO)
Arthritis	YES	(NO)	High Blood Pressure	YES	(NO)
Bleeding Disorder	YES	(NO)	Kidney Problems	YES	(NO)
Breast Problems	YES	(NO)	Liver Problems	YES	(NO)
Cancer	YES	(NO)	Abnormal Mammogram	(N/A) YES	NO
Chicken Pox	(YES)	NO	Menopause	(N/A) YES	NO
Colon Disorder	YES	(NO)	Mononucleosis	YES	(NO)
COPD/Emphysema	YES	(NO)	Multiple Sclerosis	YES	(NO)
Depression	YES	(NO)	Osteoporosis	YES	(NO)
Diabetes	YES	(NO)	Pneumonia	YES	(NO)
Epilepsy/Seizures	YES	(NO)	Polio	YES	(NO)
Eye Problems	(YES)	NO	Prostate Problems	YES	(NO)
Gallbladder Disorder	YES	(NO)	Skin Problems	YES	(NO)
Stomach Problems/Ulcer	YES	(NO)	Stroke	YES	(NO)
Gout	YES	(NO)	Suicide Attempt	YES	(NO)
Gynecological Problems	YES	(NO)	Thyroid Problems	YES	(NO)
Sexually Transmitted Disease	YES	(NO)	Other	YES	(NO)

Please list your current medications and dosages. Also list over-the-counter and herbal products you use regularly.

Ibuprofen   *Ben-Gay Balm on knees*

MultiVitamin 1 per day

Acetaminophen

The Diagnosis

During the visit, the clinic nurse records the following information in Mr. Nguyen's chart:

Height	5 ft 4 in.
Weight	165 lb (75 kg)
BP	162/94 mm Hg
Pulse	84 beats/min
RR	20 breaths/min
Temp	98.2°F oral

Presenting Complaint: Patient states he is here to become established as a patient at the center and that he has not had a physical exam in over 10 years. Wife accompanies. He is currently experiencing bilateral knee pain that is affecting his work performance. "I am a building inspector. To check on things, I have to climb up and down ladders, lift things, and crawl around a lot." Has not missed any work but has been using increasing amounts of acetaminophen and ibuprofen "to get through the day." The medications provide only limited relief. States pain occurs daily even if not at work. Describes the pain as "achy" and "dull." Feels best when he is off his feet. Desires pain relief and checkup. Explains that both parents had heart disease. Wife expressing worry that he may be developing heart problems "because he's so tired after work and he gets short of breath easy."

The nurse explains to Mr. Nguyen that he will be seen by the nurse practitioner shortly. She asks Mr. Nguyen if he would like his wife to be present for the exam. He answers yes.

Zach Jackson, MSN, FNP, is on duty at the center today. Zach worked as an RN for more than 10 years in the local emergency department and urgent care clinic. He has been a family nurse practitioner (FNP-BC) for more than 5 years. Zach enters the room and introduces himself to the Nguyen couple. To begin the exam, Zach reviews the information Nam supplied on the admission form, and then asks him about his family history.

Zach: "Are your parents still living?"

Nam: "Yes, they're both alive. My father is 80 years old and my mother is 76."

Zach: "I'd like to hear a little more about your family history. Tell me about your father's cancer. How old was he when he was first diagnosed? Has he had treatment?"

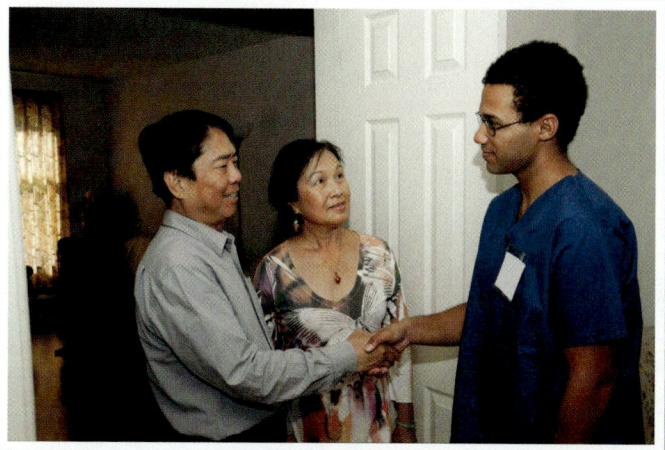

Nam: "He was probably about 60 when he first found out about it. I know he had some kind of surgery and takes medicines but I don't know the details. He seems all right though."

Zach: "Your father also has high blood pressure and heart disease. Please tell me a little more about that."

Nam: "My father and mother both have high blood pressure and heart disease. They both take medicines for their blood pressure. My father had a small heart attack about 10 years ago. My mother has never had a heart attack that I know of, but she sometimes has chest pain."

Jordan: "Your mother also has diabetes?"

Nam: "She's had that for a long time. A lot of people in his family, especially on my father's side, have diabetes but nobody in my mother's family. Yet my mother is the one with the diabetes!"

Yen: "A lot of people in my family have diabetes too. But so far I'm OK, I think."

Zach: "Have you had a health exam lately, Mrs. Nguyen?"

Yen: "Not in about a year, but I'm going to schedule an appointment here."

The Nguyen couple and Zach continue to review the health information. After reviewing the history and discussing current complaints, Zach performs a complete physical exam.

How Nurses Think

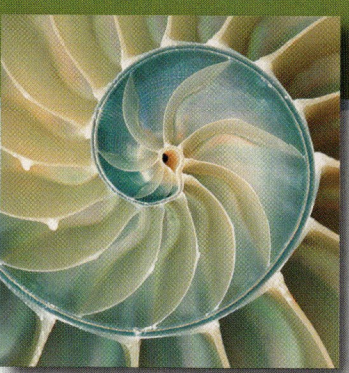

Nursing Past & Present

Learning Outcomes

After completing this chapter, you should be able to:

➤ Describe the role of religion in the development of nursing.

➤ Identify the factors that led to the change of nursing from a vocation of both men and women to a predominantly female profession.

➤ Explain the role of the military in the development of the nursing profession.

➤ Define *nursing* in your own words.

➤ Discuss the transitions that nursing education has undergone in the last century.

➤ Differentiate among the various forms of nursing education.

➤ Explain how nursing practice is regulated.

➤ Give four examples of influential nursing organizations.

➤ Name and recognize the four purposes of nursing care.

➤ Delineate the forces and trends affecting contemporary nursing practice.

If you were assigned readings in the Expanded Discussion on DavisPlus, you should also be able to demonstrate the following outcomes:

➤ Describe the healthcare delivery system in the United States, including sites for care, types of workers, regulation, and financing of healthcare.

➤ Name nine expanded roles for nursing.

➤ Discuss issues related to healthcare reform.

Key Concepts

Nursing

Nursing image

Contemporary nursing education

Contemporary nursing practice

Related Concepts

See the Concept Map at the end of this chapter.

Caring for the Nguyens

This feature allows you to practice the kind of thinking you will use as a full-spectrum nurse. There is usually more than one correct answer to a critical thinking question, so we do not provide answers for these features. It is more important to develop your nursing judgment than to "cover content." Discuss the questions with your peers. If you are still unsure, consult your instructor.

Review the opening scenario in the front of the book. On the preliminary visit of Nam Nguyen at the Family Medicine Center, he is examined by Zach Jackson, MSN, FNP-BC.

A. How would you respond to Nam's concern that he was examined by someone who is "just a nurse"?

B. What factors might be causing Mr. Nguyen to question care by "a male nurse"?

 Go to **Caring for the Nguyens Response Sheet** on *DavisPlus.*

Nurses Make a Difference . . .

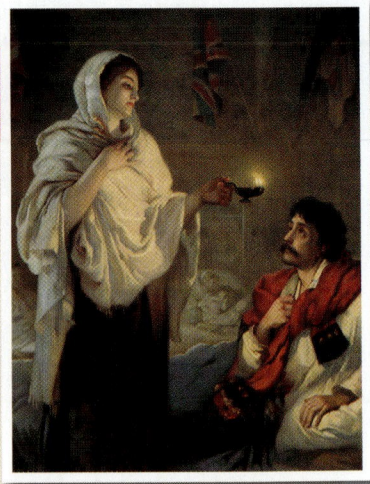

Then & Now

Time: 1854, Üsküdar (now part of Istanbul, Turkey) in the Crimea

The hospital tent is set up away from the battlefield. The injured and dying soldiers are lying on the bare earth, soiled and covered with crusted blood. The rank odor of disease and death are inescapable in the stifling hospital tent. Scanning the scene, Florence Nightingale and her staff of 38 nurses review the environment in the tent, the health problems of the soldiers, and the supplies and equipment they have. First, they open the tent to allow in fresh air. Then they clean the tent, bathe the wounded, and provide clean bedding. They assess and dress the wounds, feed the soldiers a nutritious meal, and comfort those who are dying or are in pain. They offer encouragement and emotional care to the healthier soldiers and help them to write letters home. Within a brief period of time, the mortality rate drops from 47% to 2% and morale improves immeasurably.

Time: 2014, Your Local Hospital

While standing at the bedside mixing an antibiotic solution, Susan listens to the ventilator cycle. She notes that her patient has begun to trigger breaths on his own. In the background she hears the cardiac monitor sounds, which have become more irregular over the past hour. She mentally runs through her patient assessment. "Why is his heart so irritable?" she wonders. She calls the lab for the morning blood work results. When the lab technician e-mails the results, Susan notes that the potassium level is low at 2.9 mEq/L. She notifies the physician of the test results and the cardiac irritability. Susan says, "The patient's potassium is low from the diarrhea he's had since we began the antibiotics." Together they develop a plan to raise the potassium level and check it every 8 hours. Susan administers intravenous (IV) potassium chloride. Several hours later she documents that the *ectopy* (irregular heartbeat) has decreased to less than 2 beats/min.

Time: 2030, A Local Home

Yesterday, Mr. Samuels underwent cardiac surgery. He was discharged home this morning. As a home health nurse, your role is to assess his condition; provide skilled care; teach Mr. Samuels how to care for himself; instruct his family about his care; and coordinate any required additional services. Mrs. Samuels greets you at the front door. She tells you that her husband is in a lot of pain and that the chest drainage system is full. She looks frightened as she says, "When my father had cardiac surgery 25 years ago, he spent 4 days in the hospital. I don't understand why my husband got sent home so quickly." You explain that changes in technology and the healthcare system allow you to take care of clients in the home who would previously have been in the hospital. As you begin your assessments, you tell Mrs. Samuels, "After I've gathered more information, we'll make a plan for his care that will make all of us more comfortable."

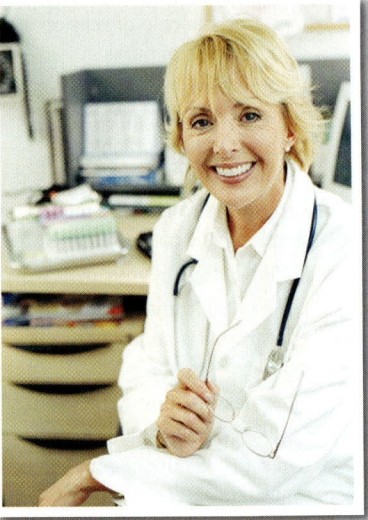

In each of these scenarios, the nurses engaged in *full-spectrum nursing;* that is, they used their minds and their hands to improve the client's comfort and condition. As the scenarios illustrate, nursing roles have changed over time. Yet nursing remains a profession dedicated to care of the client.

ThinkLike a Nurse 1-1

The Quality and Safety Education for Nurses (QSEN) project and the Institute of Medicine (IOM) have identified quality and safety competencies for nurses: (1) patient-centered care, (2) teamwork and collaboration, (3) evidence-based practice, (4) quality improvement, (5) safety, and (6) informatics (Cronenwett, Sherwood, Barnsteiner, et al., 2007). Which of these did Florence Nightingale demonstrate? Explain your thinking.

ABOUT THE KEY CONCEPTS

The overarching concept for this chapter is the definition of *nursing*. As you come to understand other key concepts (i.e., nursing images, contemporary nursing education, and

contemporary nursing practice), you will grasp how the image of nursing and actual nursing practice have changed over time.

NURSING IMAGES THROUGHOUT HISTORY

An understanding of the past can give insight into the present. Throughout history, artwork, television, popular stories, advertisements, and greeting cards have all portrayed nurses in many ways. Whether the images are flattering or demeaning, accurate or inaccurate, they influence how people view nursing. Some of these images may have, in either a positive or negative way, influenced your decision to become a nurse.

Common Images of Nurses

In the next few pages you will see how nursing has been portrayed in art and popular culture at different periods in history, and relate the truth and fiction of those images to the practice of contemporary nursing. This will help you appreciate the rich traditions of nursing and the forces that have shaped nursing as it is today. Pay close attention to the rate of change in recent years, and keep in mind that nursing and healthcare are likely to change even more rapidly in the future.

When you think of nursing, what images do you think of? As you reflect on each of the three scenarios at the opening of this chapter, what pictures come into your mind? Is this the same image you get when you imagine yourself as a nurse? In the following sections we explore four common nursing stereotypes.

The Angel of Mercy

Images of the angel-nurse are usually serene and content, with a halo or other religious symbol. This image grew out of the influence of religion and the risks inherent to the practice of nursing.

Influence of Religion. The strong link between nursing and religious orders can be traced back to ancient cultures. In Egypt, Greece, and Rome, temples were health centers as well as places of worship. Priests and priestesses treated the ill with a combination of physical care, prayer, and magic spells. In Asia, some of the earliest writings about a distinct nursing occupation are included in the Vedas, the ancient sacred books of the Hindu faith (circa 1200 BCE). The nurses included in these texts were always men who were part of a priestly order and who possessed knowledge of the preparation, compounding, and administration of drugs; wisdom; purity; and devotion to the patient. In later centuries, lay deacons and deaconesses in the early Christian church visited the sick in their homes and functioned as nurses until the first hospitals were established in the first century. The oldest continuously existing hospital, Hôtel Dieu, in France, was founded in 542 (Fig. 1-1). In the United States, all training programs for nurses were affiliated with religious orders until well after the Civil War.

Today, many nursing programs, universities, colleges, and healthcare institutions are affiliated with religious groups. Examples include the University of Notre Dame, the Seventh Day Adventist hospital system, and the American Baptist nursing home system.

Effect of the Protestant Reformation. Christianity gradually lost influence in general society over the 15th to

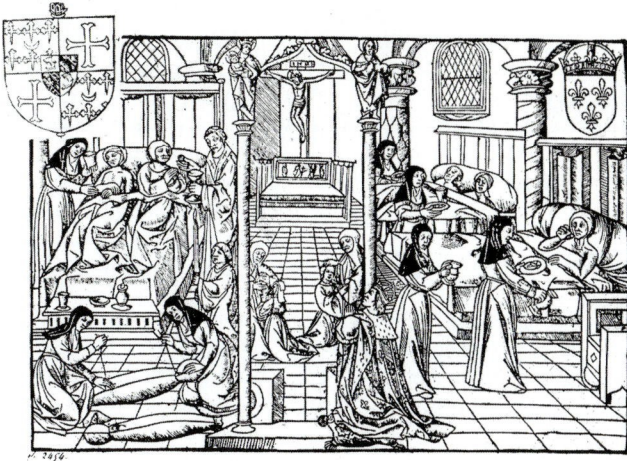

FIGURE 1-1 Hôtel Dieu in France, the oldest continuously existing hospital.

the 19th centuries. Catholic religious orders were often persecuted, and many monasteries were closed during the Protestant Reformation (16th and 17th centuries CE), forcing many nurses to flee in order to avoid imprisonment or death. Medicine in this period moved to the universities, with major advances in theoretical knowledge of anatomy, physiology, and communicable disease. After the 19th century, religious groups gradually regained influence, and many modern nursing programs, universities, colleges, and healthcare institutions are affiliated with religious groups. Although most of these organizations have mission statements that incorporate charitable values, such as compassion and caring, they no longer require religious dedication from their nursing students.

Risks Involved in Patient Care. Another reason for the association between nursing and spirituality is the inherent risks involved in patient care, especially in the recent past. Before the development of microscopes and techniques for culturing microorganisms in the 19th century, people who entered nursing placed themselves at risk for exposure to diseases that were poorly understood and often could not be cured. Even as recently as the 1950s, antibiotics were not readily available, and the chief cause of mortality (death) was infectious disease. Providing care in spite of these risks was considered self-sacrificing, much like the call to serve in religious life.

ThinkLike a Nurse 1-2

Which aspects of the nurse-as-angel concept appeal to you most when you think about the way you will practice nursing? Why?

The Handmaiden

The validity of this image has changed over time. While the nurse's role was initially limited, nurses now collaborate with all members of the healthcare team, planning and providing care not only at the direction of physicians but also along with them. Many activities that nurses now do independently were once performed only by physicians, including taking vital signs, performing physical assessments, and administering IV and other injectable medications (Table 1-1). Nevertheless, while nurses perform these and other critical and complex

Table I-I ➤ Examples of Nursing Activities

DEPENDENT ACTIVITIES	INDEPENDENT ACTIVITIES
Administering prescribed medication	Evaluating the patient's response to medication and withholding the next dose if the patient has a negative reaction
Assisting with a diagnostic test (e.g., opening trays, handing instruments to the physician)	Teaching the patient what to expect from the diagnostic test; preparing the patient for the test (e.g., shaving a site); supporting the patient during the test
Administering IV fluids	Evaluating the patient's response to treatment; monitoring the flow rate; evaluating the site for redness or leakage
Ensuring that the patient receives the prescribed diet	Teaching a pregnant woman about additional nutrients needed in her diet

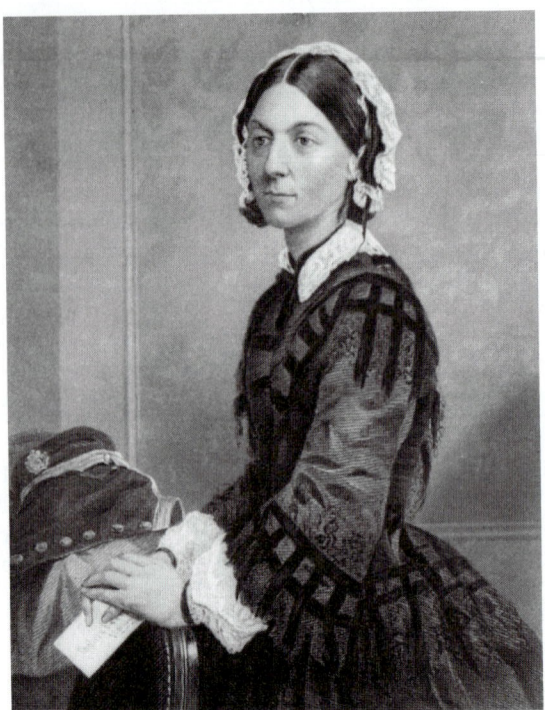

FIGURE 1-2 Florence Nightingale (1820–1910).

tasks, the physician remains the final decision maker for most patient care.

- **Physicians derive much of their power from legal and financial authority.** Early physicians from wealthy and educated classes wrote and lobbied for legislation that awarded them extensive power and ensured control of healthcare. Now it is very difficult to change these laws to accommodate the expanded role of modern nurses (Quadagno, 2004; Rockwell, 1994; Safriet, 1994).
- **Without physicians, the institution does not generate income.** Most patients—or their insurers—directly pay the facility to provide care that is prescribed by the physician. In contrast, nurses, with the exception of advanced care nurses, are often employees of healthcare institutions. Therefore, they are considered an expense because they cannot bill for the services they provide. To learn more about circumstances that have made it difficult to expand the role of nursing,

 Go to Chapter 1, **Reading More About Nursing Past and Present,** on DavisPlus.

- **In the past, not all nurses considered themselves to be subservient to physicians.** The letters and writings of Florence Nightingale (Fig. 1-2), the founder of modern nursing, indicate that she considered nurses the colleagues of physicians rather than their servants. She stated at one time that the standard description of nurses as "devoted and obedient . . . would do well for a porter" and "[i]t might even do well for a horse" (Chambers, 1958, p. 130).

Despite the protests of her wealthy, upper-class family, Nightingale went on to study nursing in Germany at the age of 24. She became a field nurse during the Crimean War, where she became known as "the Lady of the Lamp" because of her nighttime care to the wounded. Upon her return to England, she used her experience in the Crimea to immediately lobby politicians and physicians about the importance of nursing and the need for public health reform. Nightingale's major contributions include the following:

The establishment of nursing as a distinct profession
Introduction of a broad-based liberal education for nurses
Major reform in the delivery of care in hospitals
The introduction of standards to control the spread of disease in hospitals
Major reforms in healthcare for the military

If you would like more information about other historical nursing leaders,

 Go to Chapter 1, **Supplemental Materials: Nursing Leaders,** on DavisPlus.

- **The employment status of most nurses is another factor that must be considered when looking at the validity of the handmaiden image.** As we said earlier, most nurses work for healthcare institutions rather than directly for physicians. If nurses have indeed been handmaidens, perhaps it has been to the institutions that employ them. Nurses are actively working to combat the handmaiden stereotype; for instance, they have formed unions to improve their working conditions and benefits and to advocate for patient safety. The increased number of advance practice nurses and nurse entrepreneurs further rebukes the validity of the handmaiden image. It is interesting that with changes in the healthcare system, more physicians are becoming employees of healthcare institutions as well—and some, like nurses, are forming unions. The increasing costs of healthcare, coupled with decreasing reimbursement for health services, appear to be driving these changes.

ThinkLike a Nurse 1-3

What similarities or differences do you see between the angelic and handmaiden images of nursing?

The Battle-Ax

The image of the nurse as a battle-ax is in direct opposition to the image of the angel of mercy, but these opposing images have coexisted for centuries. Charles Dickens created an early version of the abusive nurse in his 1844 novel *Martin Chuzzlewit*, in the character of Sairey Gamp. Mrs. Gamp personified the view of nurses that many people held at that time: She was corrupt, harsh, and frequently intoxicated. In the 1975 film *One Flew Over the Cuckoo's Nest*, Nurse Ratched personifies the contemporary image of the nurse as the battle-ax or torturer, treating her patients with cruelty and disdain. How did these negative images come about? And why does this image persist? Again, history may provide insight.

Fading Influence of Christianity. Before the 14th century, religious-affiliated nursing orders provided most of the care for the sick. However, as science and philosophy grew more sophisticated and popular, religious orders for nursing became less common, and much of the devotion and knowledge of caring for the sick was lost. Municipal authorities took over hospitals and began to sentence criminals to care for the sick in the hospitals—to assume the nursing role. Forced to care for large numbers of patients without training, supplies, assistance, or time off, these criminals often managed their workload by treating patients harshly and drinking alcohol while on duty. Most patients who entered such hospitals died there. Such practices persisted until the 1860s in Europe and until after the Civil War in the United States. It is no wonder, then, that the battle-ax image of nurses endured so long.

Perception of Nursing Activities. Nurses give injections, clean and dress wounds, draw blood, and start intravenous lines—such activities are performed to improve the patient's health, but they may cause significant pain, contributing to the persistence of the battle-ax image. Unfortunately, the association with pain helps to perpetuate the image of nurses as unfeeling. Aware of the power of this image, nurses on pediatric units typically wear colorful uniforms with child-friendly patterns, such as cartoon characters or cuddly animals, to avoid frightening children who may associate "nurse" with "pain." Providers in many pediatric and outpatient facilities deliver care in street clothes without white lab coats in order to reduce patient anxiety.

The Naughty Nurse

The image of the sexy, risqué nurse arose in the early part of the 20th century with burlesque shows and persists in popular culture today. In many television programs such as *Nightingales*, *M*A*S*H*, and more recently *Grey's Anatomy*, nurses are portrayed as sexy, mindless, irrelevant, or simply potential dates for bright and talented surgeons. Get-well cards often portray nurses in short skirts, fishnet stockings, high heels, and cap, as do paperback novels, comic books, CDs, and other print media. An Internet search yields links to legitimate sites with realistic pictures of nurses, but also a large number of cartoons, greeting cards, and pornographic Web sites featuring women who are supposedly nurses. Their role is implied through props—a nursing cap, a stethoscope, or a uniform—in the background.

Why is this so? What gives this image its power? As trusted health professionals, nurses frequently provide care that involves exposing the patient's body, contact with bare skin, and discussion of intimate aspects of the client's life. In addition, hospitalized patients are in a weakened, vulnerable state, and the nurse may seem quite powerful by contrast. Thus, despite the fact that nurse–patient contact is professional and does not involve sexual intimacy, the "naughty nurse" stereotype may express a forbidden desire for intimate contact with a stranger in a position of power. In addition, the traditionally female nurse's collaboration with traditionally male physicians may reinforce the stereotype of the nurse in a sexual role. The "naughty nurse" stereotype may be popular, but it is not founded on truth.

ThinkLike a Nurse 1-4

- How do the images of the nurse as a battle-ax or sex object affect your view of nursing?
- As a nurse, what can you do to counteract these images?

The Military Image

Nursing imagery is often military, both in the general public and within the profession itself. Throughout the past century, nurses were frequently portrayed in uniform providing support at the battlefield, and nurses are still often characterized as warriors fighting disease. What is the history of these two military images?

Nurses on the Battlefield

Nurses' involvement in the military dates from 27 BCE, as the Roman Empire began to consolidate its dominion. Because the Roman Empire relied on the success of military excursions to extend its domain, the well-being of its soldiers was critical. Thus, one of the great contributions of the Roman Empire was the development of the military hospital and the practice of providing first aid on the battlefield.

During the Middle Ages, the two largest influences on nursing were the military and religion. These two threads fused in the Crusaders, soldiers who went to battle to conquer Islamic lands and spread Christianity throughout the world. Among the Crusaders were **hospitalers,** specialized soldiers who at the end of battle returned to the outposts to care for the sick and injured (Fig. 1-3). The hospitaler order known as

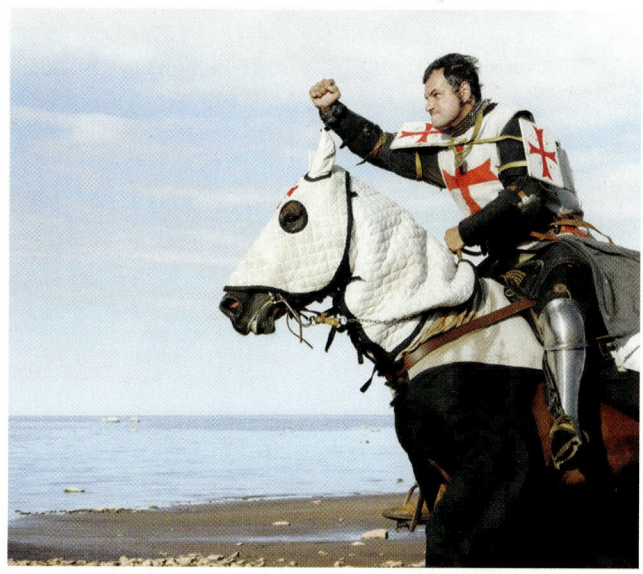

FIGURE 1-3 A hospitaler at the time of the Crusades.

the Knights of St. John of Jerusalem established men's and women's branches throughout Europe—one of which still exists in England as the Order of Malta.

Nursing presence on the battlefield continued during the Civil War. The U.S. government established the Army Nursing Service in 1861, and its role was to organize nurses and hospitals and coordinate supplies for the soldiers. Many trained nurses joined the Army Nursing Service from religious orders. Thousands of laypersons also volunteered, including the following:

- **Clara Barton.** Among the lay nurses was Clara Barton, who organized her own nursing efforts. Rather than providing care in base hospitals, far removed from the battlefield, Barton and her volunteers provided care in tents set up close to the fighting. Barton did not discriminate when giving care, nursing soldiers from both the North and South, black and white. When the war was over, Barton continued this universal care through the establishment of the American Red Cross.
- **Other laypersons.** Other notable figures who served as nurses include Harriet Tubman, who helped slaves escape to freedom on the Underground Railroad; the poet Walt Whitman; the author Louisa May Alcott; and Dorothea Dix, the Union's Superintendent of Female Nurses during the Civil War.

Nurses also served in World War I, World War II, the Korean and Vietnam wars (Fig. 1-4), the Gulf War, and the conflicts in Iraq and Afghanistan. In these wars the nurses were all formally trained. Formal training for nurses became widespread in Europe in the 1860s after the widely publicized success of Nightingale in the Crimea. In the United States the first formal training program was established in 1873.

Nurses Fighting Disease

A second military image portrays nurses as warriors in the fight against disease. This image is common in public awareness campaigns against infectious diseases.

- **Florence Nightingale.** Florence Nightingale's contributions in public health and **epidemiology** (the study of the distribution and origins of disease) were among the first nursing efforts to fight disease. In her *Notes on Hospitals* (1863), Nightingale stated that air, light, nutrition, and adequate ventilation and space assist the patient to recuperate. The hospitals she designed to incorporate these ideas were associated with decreased mortality, decreased length of hospital stay, and decreased rate of **nosocomial infection** (an infection associated with a healthcare facility and now more commonly called healthcare-associated infection).

- **Lillian Wald and Mary Brewster.** Another notable event in the fight against disease occurred in 1893 when Lillian Wald and Mary Brewster founded the Henry Street Settlement in New York to improve the health and social conditions of poor immigrants. This is considered the start of public health nursing in the United States. Since then, nurses have played an important role in improving health and preventing illness by promoting safe drinking water, adequate sewage facilities, and proper sanitation measures in communities.

In spite of the historical association of nursing with the military, currently only a small percentage of licensed U.S. nurses work in the armed services. Similarly, despite the powerful image of the nurse fighting diseases, only approximately 8% of nurses work in community and public health agencies, which includes school and public health departments (Health Resources and Services Administration [HRSA], 2010).

Caucasian Women

Historically, images of nurses have been of Caucasian women. Rarely are the images of various ethnicity or men of any race. To a degree, this reflects reality. About 83% of RNs in the United States are Caucasian, and only about 9% of nurses in the United States are men (HRSA, 2010). Male nurses make up a higher percentage in other countries (12.5% in Great Britain, for example); nevertheless, men are a minority of the total nursing population worldwide (Fig. 1-5) (Pullen, 2006). This is ironic considering that many ancient nursing orders were exclusively male. In early Christianity, deacons provided nursing care to parish men while deaconesses provided care to women, and even today the majority of medics and hospital corpsmen who provide battlefront first aid are men.

The trend in the United States now is toward a slightly more diverse workforce. In 2008, 16.8% of nurses were other than Caucasian—an increase from 12.2% in 2004. The percentage will likely increase, because RNs from racial and ethnic

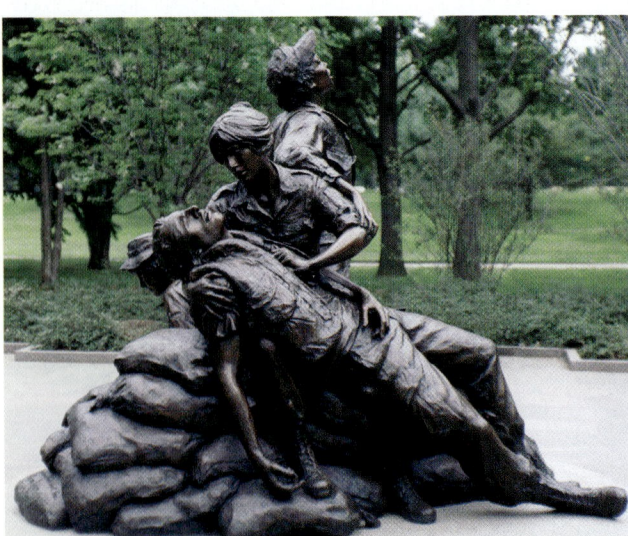

FIGURE 1-4 Women's Memorial for the Vietnam War. (Copyright 1993, Vietnam Women's Memorial Foundation, Inc. Glenna Goodacre, sculptor.)

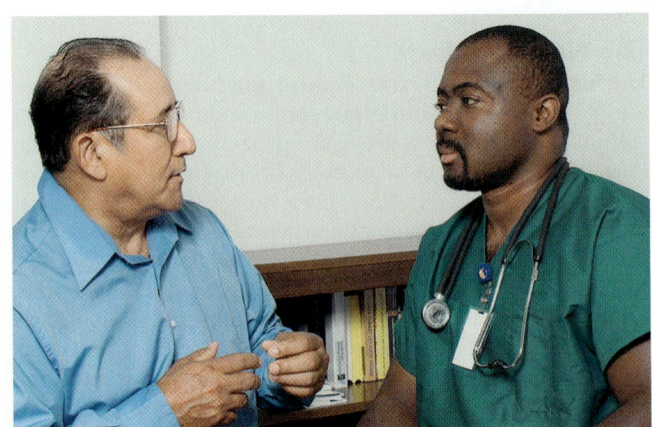

FIGURE 1-5 The roles of men in nursing are now as varied as those for women, and the opportunities for personal and professional fulfillment are as great.

minority groups represent a larger portion of recent nursing school graduates than in earlier years (see Table 1-2).

It is encouraging for diversity that more men are being recruited into nursing. For example, in 2006, 8.3% of nursing students in the United States were men (Pullen, 2006). During 2008–2009 the proportion of men increased to 13.8% (National League for Nursing, n. d.). However, it is important that practicing nurses embrace these changes and welcome others into the field.

ThinkLike a Nurse I-5

In your opinion, what efforts, if any, should nursing organizations take to recruit a more diverse workforce?

Full-Spectrum Nurse

Nurses have often been shown actively caring for the patient—dressing wounds, bathing, giving medications—but the intellectual or thinking side of nursing is rarely portrayed. The angel of mercy and military stereotypes reinforce the idea that nursing is a duty and that nurses are carrying out orders. The naughty nurse, battle-ax, and handmaiden images suggest a woman who is quick to act but may not carefully consider her actions. In reality, a large portion of the nursing role involves thinking.

✚ To be safe providers, nurses must carefully consider their actions and think carefully about the patient, the treatment plan, the healthcare environment, the patient's support system, the nurse's support system, resources, and safety.

Full-spectrum nursing involves clinical judgment, critical thinking, and problem-solving. You will learn more about this in Chapter 2.

Clinical judgment involves observing, comparing, contrasting, and evaluating the client's condition to determine whether change has occurred. It also involves careful consideration of the client's health status in light of what is expected based on the client's condition, medications, and treatment.

These actions are intertwined with the nursing process stages of assessing, diagnosing, and evaluating.

Critical thinking is a reflective thinking process that involves collecting information, analyzing the adequacy and accuracy of the information, and carefully considering options for action. Nurses use critical thinking in every aspect of nursing care. Critical thinking is discussed at length in Chapter 2 and applied in every chapter in this text.

Problem-solving is a process by which nurses consider an issue and attempt to find a satisfactory solution to achieve the best outcomes. You will often use problem-solving in your professional life. The nursing process (see Chapters 2 through 7) is one type of problem-solving process.

ThinkLike a Nurse I-6

In the three scenarios of Nurses Make a Difference . . . Then & Now, what image of nursing predominates: thinking or doing?

CONTEMPORARY NURSING: EDUCATION, REGULATION, AND ORGANIZATION

As a student about to enter your new professional life, you need a realistic understanding of the nature and demands of your chosen career. To help you to better acquaint yourself with nursing today, the remainder of this chapter discusses the current state of nursing, nursing education, and the trends affecting nursing.

How Is Nursing Defined?

As you have seen, there are many perceptions of nursing. These images are only loosely based on fact and sometimes they conflict. They make it difficult for the public to know the reality of nursing—and they are also confusing to nurses and other members of the healthcare team. In addition, the constantly changing nature of nursing, healthcare, and society further complicates the definition of *nursing*. Therefore, it is important for nurses to articulate clearly what nursing is and what nurses do. The following are the views of three important nursing organizations with regard to the question, "What is nursing?"

International Council of Nurses Definition

In 1973 the International Council of Nurses (ICN), an organization representing nurses throughout the world, defined *nursing* according to the beliefs of respected theorist Virginia Henderson:

> *The unique function of the nurse is to assist the individual, sick or well, in the performance of those activities contributing to health or its recovery (or to peaceful death) that he would perform unaided if he had the necessary strength, will or knowledge. (Henderson, 1966, p. 15)*

In the decades since the adoption of this definition, nursing throughout the world has changed. Advances in healthcare have altered the type of care required by clients. To reflect these changes, the ICN has revised its definition of nursing, as follows:

> *Nursing encompasses autonomous and collaborative care of individuals of all ages, families, groups and communities, sick or well and in all settings. Nursing includes the promotion of health, prevention of illness, and the care of ill, disabled and dying people. Advocacy, promotion of a safe environment, research, participation in shaping health policy and in patient and health systems management, and education are also key nursing roles. (International Council of Nurses [ICN], 2007)*

Table I-2 ▶ Racial and Ethnic Distribution Upon Graduation From Initial Nursing Education		
GRADUATION YEAR	**WHITE, NON-HISPANIC**	**NON-WHITE OR HISPANIC**
1980 or earlier	87.7%	12.3%
1981–1985	88.0%	12.0%
1986–1990	82.4%	17.6%
1991–1995	80.5%	19.5%
1996–2000	79.4%	20.6%
2001–2004	78.5%	21.5%
2005–2008	77.5%	22.5%

Source: Compiled from the U. S. Dept. of Health and Human Services, Health Resources and Services Administration (HRSA). (September 2010). *The registered nurse population. Findings from the 2008 National Sample Survey of Registered Nurses.* Retrieved January 6, 2011, from http://bhpr.hrsa.gov/healthworkforce/rnsurvey/2008/nssrn2008.pdf

ThinkLike a Nurse 1-7

Look at the three scenarios of Nurses Make a Difference . . . Then & Now. What nursing actions did the nurses perform that are represented in the International Council of Nurses (ICN) definition of *nursing*?

American Nurses Association Definition

You can see similar changes in the approach of the American Nurses Association (ANA). In 1980, the ANA defined *nursing* as "the diagnosis and treatment of human responses to actual and potential health problems" (p. 2). Attempts to refine this definition have been difficult. Nurses are a heterogeneous group of people with varying skills who perform activities designed to provide care ranging from basic to complex in a growing number of settings. It is very difficult to describe the boundaries of the profession.

In 2010, the ANA acknowledged five characteristics of registered nursing:

1. Nursing practice is individualized.
2. Nurses coordinate care by establishing partnerships (with persons, families, support systems, and other providers).
3. Caring is central to the practice of the registered nurse.
4. Registered nurses use the nursing process to plan and provide individualized care to their healthcare consumers.
5. A strong link exists between the professional work environment and the registered nurse's ability to provide quality health care and achieve optimal outcomes. (pp. 4–5)

The ANA now defines professional nursing as the following:

The protection, promotion, and optimization of health and abilities, prevention of illness and injury, alleviation of suffering through the diagnosis and treatment of human response, and advocacy in the care of individuals, families, communities, and populations. (American Nurses Association [ANA], 2010)

Importance of a Definition

You may wonder why there has been so much emphasis on creating a definition. Nursing organizations and leaders have pushed for accurate definitions to (1) help the public understand the value of nursing, (2) describe what activities and roles belong to nursing versus other health professions, and (3) help students and practicing nurses understand what is expected of them within their role as nurses. Undoubtedly nursing will continue to change as nursing knowledge increases and society changes. Box 1-1 lists several additional definitions of nursing for you to consider.

As a student entering nursing, you can use definitions and descriptions to understand what is expected of you. To aid you in this task, Table 1-3 reviews the essential components of the nursing role. While in the clinical setting, you will observe nurses functioning in each of these capacities. Nursing is a flexible career that requires you to move effortlessly among these various roles to meet the needs of the patient.

KnowledgeCheck 1-1

- What factors make it difficult to define nursing?
- Based on the ICN definition of nursing, what does a nurse do?

Is Nursing a Profession, a Discipline, or an Occupation?

One strategy used to describe a field of work is to categorize it as a profession, a discipline, or an occupation.

BOX 1-1 ■ What Is Nursing?

- I use the word *nursing*, for want of a better. It has been limited to signify little more than the administration of medicines and the application of poultices. It ought to signify the proper use of fresh air, light, warmth, cleanliness, quiet, and the proper choosing and giving of diet—all at the least expense of vital power to the patient (Nightingale, 1876, p. 5).
- Events that give rise to higher degrees of consideration for those who are helpless or oppressed, kindliness and sympathy for the unfortunate and for those who suffer, tolerance for those of differing religion, race, color, etc.—all tend to promote activities like nursing which are primarily humanitarian (Dock & Stewart, 1938, p. 3).
- Nursing has been called the oldest of the arts and the youngest of the professions. As such, it has gone through many stages and has been an integral part of societal movements. Nursing has been involved in the existing culture—shaped by it and yet helping to develop it (Donahue, 1985, p. 3).
- Nurses provide care for people in the midst of health, pain, loss, fear, disfigurement, death, grieving, challenge, growth, birth, and transition on an intimate front-line basis. Expert nurses call this the privileged place of nursing (Benner & Wrubel, 1989, p. xi).
- Nursing: The care and nurturing of healthy and ill people, individually or in groups and communities [Taber's also includes as a part of the definition the ANA "essential features" involving holism, use of subjective and objective data, application of scientific knowledge, and provision of a caring relationship.] (Venes, D., 2009).

Profession. Although the term *profession* is freely used, Starr (1982) said that a group must meet certain criteria to be considered a **profession** (see Table 1-4). Nursing appears to meet all criteria of a profession as defined by Starr.

Discipline. To be considered a **discipline,** a profession must have a domain of knowledge that has both theoretical and practical boundaries. The **theoretical boundaries** of a profession are the questions that arise from clinical practice and are then investigated through research. The **practical boundaries** are the current state of knowledge and research in the field—the facts that dictate safe practice (Meleis, 1991). A case can be made that nursing is both a profession and a discipline:

- It is a scientifically based and self-governed *profession* that focuses on the ethical care of others.
- It is a *discipline*, driven by aspects of theory and practice. It demands mastery of both theoretical knowledge and clinical skills.

Occupation. In spite of meeting criteria for both designations (profession and discipline), nursing is often described as an **occupation,** or job. Unlike physicians, most of whom are in control of their practice environment, working conditions, and schedule, most nurses are hourly wage earners. The employer, not the nurse, decides the conditions of practice and the nature of the work. Nurse practice acts do not prevent nurses from functioning more autonomously, however.

Rather than continuing to develop arguments to "prove" that nursing is a profession, the following actions might do more to improve the status of nursing:

- Standardizing the educational requirements for entry into practice

Table 1-3 ▶ Roles and Functions of the Nurse

ROLE	FUNCTION	EXAMPLES
Direct care provider	Addressing the physical, emotional, social, and spiritual needs of the client	Assessing the client Giving medications Patient teaching
Communicator	Using interpersonal and therapeutic communication skills to address the needs of the client, to facilitate communication in the healthcare team, and to advise the community about health promotion and disease prevention	Counseling a client Discussing unit staffing needs at a meeting Providing pregnancy prevention education at a local school
Client/family educator	Assessing and diagnosing the teaching needs of the client, group, family, or community. Once the diagnosis is made, nurses plan how to meet these needs, implement the teaching plan, and evaluate its effectiveness.	Preoperative teaching Prenatal education for siblings Community classes on nutrition
Client advocate	Supporting clients' right to make healthcare decisions when they are able to voice their opinions and protecting clients from harm when they are unable to make decisions	Helping a client explain to his family that he does not want to have further chemotherapy
Counselor	Using therapeutic communication skills to advise clients about health-related issues	Counseling a client on weight-loss strategies
Change agent	Advocating for change on an individual, family, group, community, or societal level that enhances health. The nurse may use counseling, communication, and educator skills to accomplish this change.	Working to improve the nutritional quality of the lunch program at a preschool
Leader	Inspiring others by setting an example of positive health, assertive communication, and willingness to improve	Florence Nightingale Walt Whitman Harriet Tubman
Manager	Coordinating and managing the activities of all members of the team	Charge nurse on a hospital unit (e.g., assigns patients and work to staff nurses)
Case manager	Coordinating the care delivered to a client	Coordinator of services for clients with tuberculosis
Research consumer	Applying evidence-based practice to provide the most appropriate care, to identify clinical problems that warrant research, and to protect the rights of research subjects	Reading journal articles Attending continuing education; seeking additional education

- Enacting uniform continuing education requirements
- Encouraging the participation of more nurses in professional organizations
- Educating the public about the true nature of nursing practice

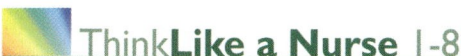 ThinkLike a Nurse 1-8

Evaluate the status of nursing. Is nursing a respected profession? Give examples to support your opinion.

How Do Nurses' Educational Paths Differ?

The transition into the nursing profession involves the concepts of formal and informal processes. **Formal education** consists of completing the initial and continuing education required for licensure. **Informal education** involves a gradual progression in skill and clinical judgment that allows the nurse to advance in the profession.

Formal Education

When the patient calls out "Nurse!" who can respond? To legally use the title *nurse,* a person must be a graduate of an accredited nursing education program and have successfully passed a licensure exam. Students may enter nursing through two paths: as a practical nurse or a registered nurse. Other personnel may respond to the patient's call, but they cannot legally be considered nurses.

Practical and Vocational Nursing Education

Practical nursing education prepares nurses to provide bedside care to clients. Practical nurses are known as licensed practical nurses (LPNs) or licensed vocational nurses (LVNs).

Table 1-4 ➤ Nursing: Is It a Profession?

STARR CRITERION	EXAMPLES IN NURSING
The knowledge of the group must be based on technical and scientific knowledge.	▪ Entry-level nursing education requires coursework in basic and social sciences as well as humanities, arts, and general education. ▪ Nursing education and practice are increasingly based on research from nursing and related fields.
The knowledge and competence of members of the group must be evaluated by a community of peers.	▪ State or provincial regulatory bodies have defined the criteria that nurses must meet to practice, and they monitor members for adherence to standards.
The group must have a service orientation and a code of ethics.	▪ Nursing is clearly focused on providing service to others. ▪ The major professional organizations have developed ethical guidelines to guide the practice of nursing.

In the United States a student who wishes to become an LPN/LVN may attend one of approximately 1,200 approved programs given at technical schools and community colleges. Educational programs for LPN/LVNs offer both classroom and clinical teaching and usually last 1 year. After completing the practical nursing education program, the student must pass the NCLEX-PN® exam. Practical nurses work under the direction of the registered nurse (RN) or the primary care provider.

Registered Nursing Entry Education

Currently, five educational pathways lead to licensure as a registered nurse (RN). Graduates of all these programs must successfully complete the NCLEX-RN® exam to practice as RNs.

▪ **Diploma.** Until the 1960s, diploma programs were the mainstay of nursing education. These programs are usually associated with a hospital. The typical program lasts 3 years and focuses on clinical experience in direct patient care. Since the 1960s the number of diploma programs has steadily decreased. In 2004, only about 4% of nursing schools were diploma programs; in 2008, about 20% of U.S. RNs reported their initial education was in a diploma program (HRSA, 2010).

▪ **Associate degree.** Most associate degree (AD) programs are offered in community colleges. Although the nursing component typically lasts 2 years, students are required to take numerous other courses in liberal arts and the sciences. In 2008, 45% of U.S. RNs reported their initial education was in an AD program (HRSA, 2010). ADN students are prepared to provide direct patient care.

▪ **Baccalaureate degree.** Students in baccalaureate programs pursue a course of study like that of other undergraduate students. The course of study lasts at least eight semesters. Students are prepared to provide direct patient care, to work in community care, to use research, and to enter graduate education (Bureau of Labor Statistics, 2009). In 2008, BSN graduates accounted for 34% of U.S. RNs (HRSA, 2010). Many AD graduates enter RN-to-BSN (or RN "completion") programs to obtain a baccalaureate degree in nursing. The length of time required to complete the BSN varies according to the program and the number of credits each student can transfer.

▪ **Master's entry.** The typical student in these programs has a baccalaureate degree in another field and has entered nursing as a second career. Programs usually are completed in 3 years of full-time study. At the completion, the student is eligible to take the licensing exam and is awarded a master's degree in nursing.

▪ **Doctoral entry.** This is the most unusual entry pathway into nursing. The nursing doctorate (ND) path parallels the pathway through which physicians enter the healthcare field. This entry path has very limited enrollment.

For several decades, nursing leaders have debated about the most appropriate educational pathway for entry into the profession. For an overview of this debate,

 Go to Chapter 1, **Supplemental Materials: Entry-into-Practice Debate,** on *DavisPlus.*

Graduate Nursing Education

Graduate education prepares the RN for advanced practice, expanded roles, or research. **Master's degree programs** prepare RNs to function in a more independent role, for example, as advanced practice nurses (APNs) or educators. Programs typically last 2 years or longer. **Doctoral programs** in nursing offer professional degrees. Typically the student has completed a baccalaureate and master's degree before entry into a doctoral program. Degrees awarded are usually the DNS (doctor of nursing science) or PhD (doctor of philosophy). The DNS program prepares the nurse for advanced clinical practice. The PhD is a research degree. For additional discussion on expanded nurse roles,

 Go to Chapter 1, **Supplemental Materials: Expanded Career Roles,** on *DavisPlus.*

Other Forms of Formal Education

To stay current with advances in healthcare after graduating, you must participate in ongoing education.

▪ **Continuing education** programs are intended to ensure that nurses keep up with current clinical knowledge. These programs are available at work sites, at colleges and universities, through privately operated educational groups, on the Internet, and in professional journals. In 23 states, renewal of the nursing license requires successful completion of a specified number of continuing education courses. When you receive your initial nursing license, your state board of nursing (SBN) will notify you about continuing education requirements, if any. Thereafter, the SBN will notify you of any changes in the requirements—regulations change frequently. For an overview of the continuing education requirements for license renewal in the United States,

 Go to Chapter 1, **Supplemental Materials: Continuing Education Requirements for Nurses,** on *DavisPlus.*

▪ **Inservice education** is another form of ongoing education. It is offered at the work site, and usually does not count

toward meeting the continuing education requirement for license renewal. For instance, inservice education might focus on the use of new equipment or the introduction of new policies in an institution, or it may resemble traditional continuing education programs.

Informal Education

In addition to formal programs of study, education also requires socialization into the profession. **Socialization** is the informal education that occurs as you move into your new profession. It is the knowledge gained from direct experience, observation in the real world, and informal discussion with peers and colleagues. Professional socialization begins when you enter the educational program and continues as you gain expertise throughout your career. Informal education complements formal education to create clinical competence.

Benner's Model

Patricia Benner (1984) described the process by which a nurse acquires clinical skills and judgment. Expertise is not merely demonstration of skilled application of knowledge, but rather a personal integration of knowledge that requires technical skill, thoughtful application, and insight. That is what we mean in this text when we use the term *full-spectrum nursing*. Expertise requires thinking, doing, and caring. Benner's process occurs in stages:

S*tage 1: Novice.* This phase begins with the onset of education. The novice is typically receptive to education and is "learning the rules" of the profession.

Stage 2: Advanced beginner. After considerable exposure to clinical situations, nurses improve in performance and, through repeated experiences or mentoring, begin to recognize the elements of a situation. The nurse functioning at this level begins to use more facts and is more sophisticated with use of the rules. A new graduate usually functions at this level.

Stage 3: Competence. Nurses achieve competence after a few years of practice. Competent performers have gained additional experience and wrestle with more complex concerns. They are able to handle their patient load and prioritize situations. They are also more involved in their caregiving role and may be emotionally involved in the clinical choices made. Although competent nurses manage clinical care with mastery, they often do not fully grasp the overall scope and most important aspects.

Stage 4: Proficient. Proficient nurses are a resource for less experienced nurses. They are able to see the "big picture" and can coordinate services and forecast needs. They are much more flexible and fluent with their role and able to adapt to nuances of various patient situations. Proficient nurses plan intuitively as well as consciously.

Stage 5: Expert. Expert nurses are able to see what needs to be achieved and how to do it. They trust in and use their intuition while operating with a deep understanding of a situation. They have expert skills and are often consulted when others need advice or assistance.

Benner's model deals with the development of clinical wisdom and competence. Nurses do not automatically move through the stages as they gain experience. Instead, this model assumes that, to improve in skill and judgment, you must also be attuned to each clinical situation. This requires an ability to take in information from a variety of sources and to notice subtle variations. Although expertise (stage 5) is a goal, not everyone can achieve this level of skill.

Nursing Organization Guidelines

The ANA and other organizations also help nurses to continue to improve their practice (e.g., by setting standards and articulating nursing values). For example, in the Code for Nurses, the ANA provides guidelines for nurses to conduct themselves in their day-to-day practice. These guidelines describe behaviors and values that help improve practice and participation in the profession. Box 1-2 presents some values and behaviors associated with nursing. See Chapter 42 for further discussion of nursing values and the ANA Code for Nurses.

KnowledgeCheck 1-2

- Compare and contrast formal and informal education.
- Name and describe five educational pathways leading to licensure as an RN.

How Is Nursing Practice Regulated?

Nurse Practice Acts. Nurse practice acts are laws that regulate nursing practice. In the United States, each state enacts its own nurse practice act. The state board of nursing is the agency responsible for regulating nursing practice. Although there are minor variations, each board of nursing is responsible for the following:

- Defining the practice of nursing
- Establishing criteria that allow a person to be considered a registered nurse (RN) or licensed practical or vocational nurse (LPN/LVN)
- Determining activities that are in the scope of practice of nursing: that nurses may perform (and by implication, those they may not); and those that may be performed only by licensed nurses
- Enforcing the rules that govern nursing

To practice nursing, an individual must be licensed as a nurse. Licenses are issued by the state. All states require graduation from an approved nursing program and successful completion of the National Council Licensure Exam (NCLEX®). To receive licensure in another state, the nurse simply applies for reciprocity. For further details about licensing and the regulation of nursing practice, see Chapter 43.

Standards of Practice. Nursing is also guided by **standards of practice,** which "describe a competent level of nursing practice and professional performance common to all registered nurses. . . . They are authoritative statements of the duties that all registered nurses, regardless of role, population, or specialty, are expected to perform competently" (ANA, 2010, p. 2). Standards are used by individual nurses, employers of nurses, professional organizations, and other professions.

As a student of nursing, you may use the ANA standards of nursing practice to get a better understanding of nursing (Table 1-5). Practicing nurses use the standards to judge their

---

BOX 1-2 ■ Nursing Values and Behaviors

- The nurse's primary concern is the good of the patient.
- Nurses ought to be competent.
- Nurses demonstrate a strong commitment to service.
- Nurses believe in the dignity and worth of each person.
- Nurses constantly strive to improve their profession.
- Nurses work collaboratively within the profession.

Table 1-5 ➤ American Nurses Association: Scope and Standards of Clinical Nursing Practice

Standards of Care

Standard 1	Assessment	The registered nurse collects comprehensive data pertinent to the healthcare consumer's health and/or the situation.
Standard 2	Diagnosis	The registered nurse analyzes the assessment data to determine the diagnoses or the issues.
Standard 3	Outcome Identification	The registered nurse identifies expected outcomes for a plan individualized to the healthcare consumer or situation.
Standard 4	Planning	The registered nurse develops a plan that prescribes strategies and alternatives to attain expected outcomes.
Standard 5	Implementation	The registered nurse implements the identified plan.
Standard 5A	Coordination of Care	The registered nurse coordinates care delivery.
Standard 5B	Health Teaching and Health Promotion	The registered nurse employs strategies to promote health and a safe environment.
Standard 5C	Consultation	The graduate-level prepared specialty nurse or advanced practice registered nurse provides consultation to influence the identified plan, enhance the abilities of others, and effect change.
Standard 5D	Prescriptive Authority and Treatment	The advanced practice registered nurse uses prescriptive authority, procedures, referrals, treatments, and therapies in accordance with state and federal laws and regulations.
Standard 6	Evaluation	The registered nurse evaluates progress toward attainment of outcomes.

Standards of Professional Performance

Standard 7	Ethics	The registered nurse practices ethically.
Standard 8	Education	The registered nurse attains knowledge and competence that reflects current nursing practice.
Standard 9	Evidence-Based Practice and Research	The registered nurse integrates evidence and research findings into practice.
Standard 10	Quality of Practice	The registered nurse contributes to quality nursing practice.
Standard 11	Communication	The registered nurse communicates effectively in all areas of practice.
Standard 12	Leadership	The registered nurse demonstrates leadership in the professional practice setting and the profession.
Standard 13	Collaboration	The registered nurse collaborates with healthcare consumer, family, and others in the conduct of nursing practice.
Standard 14	Professional Practice Evaluation	The registered nurse evaluates her or his own nursing practice in relation to professional practice standards and guidelines, relevant statutes, rules, and regulations.
Standard 15	Resource Utilization	The registered nurse utilizes appropriate resources to plan and provide nursing services that are safe, effective, and financially responsible.
Standard 16	Environmental Health	The registered nurse practices in an environmentally safe and healthy manner.

Source: American Nurses Association (2010). *Nursing: Scope and standards of practice* (2nd ed.). Silver Spring, MD: Nursebooks.org.

own performance, develop an improvement plan, and understand what employers expect of them. Employers incorporate the standards into annual evaluation tools at hospitals and health facilities. Professional organizations use the standards to educate the public about nursing, to plan for continuing education programs for nurses, and to guide their efforts at lobbying and other activities that advocate for nurses. Finally, other professions read the standards of practice to examine the boundaries between nursing and other health professions.

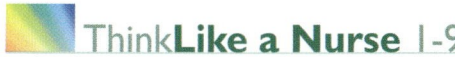 ThinkLike a Nurse 1-9

What additional information have you learned about nursing from your review of the American Nurses Association (ANA) and Canadian Nurses Association (CNA) standards of practice?

What Are Some Important Nursing Organizations?

Numerous organizations are involved in the profession of nursing. Some of the most influential are discussed here.

American and Canadian Nurses Associations

The ANA and the CNA are the official professional organizations for nurses in their respective countries. Both of these organizations were formed in 1911 from an organization previously known as the Nurses' Associated Alumnae of the United States and Canada.

Originally, these organizations focused on establishing standards of nursing to promote high-quality care and work toward licensure as a means of ensuring adherence to the standards. Representatives are elected from the local branches of the state organizations to bring their concerns to the national level. As such, they track healthcare legislation, serve as liaisons with national government representatives to inform them of how current and proposed legislation will affect nursing, and develop and sponsor legislation that will have a positive effect on nursing and on patient care. The ANA publishes educational materials on nursing news, issues, and standards.

National League for Nursing

Originally founded as the American Society of Superintendents of Training Schools for Nurses in 1893, the National League for Nursing (NLN) was the first nursing organization with a goal to establish and maintain a universal standard of education. The NLN sets standards for and evaluates all types of nursing education programs, studies the nursing workforce, lobbies and participates with other major healthcare organizations to set policy for the nursing workforce, aids faculty development, funds research on nursing education, and publishes the journal *Nursing Education Perspectives*.

International Council of Nursing

The International Council of Nursing (ICN) represents nursing on a global level. It is composed of a federation of national nursing organizations from more than 120 nations. The ICN aims to ensure quality nursing care for all, supports global health policies that advance nursing and improve worldwide health, and strives to improve working conditions for nurses throughout the world.

National Student Nurses Association

The National Student Nurses Association (NSNA) represents nursing students in the United States. It is the student counterpart of the ANA. Like the ANA, this association is made up of elected volunteers who advocate on behalf of student nurses. The NSNA sponsors yearly conventions to address student concerns. Local chapters are usually organized at individual schools. The NSNA also publishes *Image*, a journal dedicated to nursing student issues. In Canada, the Canadian University Student Nurses Association serves in the same capacity as the NSNA.

Sigma Theta Tau International

Sigma Theta Tau International (STTI) is the national honor society for nursing. Members are sought from the clinical, educator, and researcher nursing communities as well as from senior-level baccalaureate and graduate programs. The goal of this organization is to foster nursing scholarship, leadership, and research.

Specialty Organizations

Numerous specialty organizations have developed around clinical specialties, group identification, or similarly held values. The following are some examples:

- **Clinical specialty.** Association of Operating Room Nurses (AORN); Association of Nurses in AIDS Care (ANAC); Emergency Nurses Association (ENA)
- **Group identification.** National Organization for Associate Degree Nursing (NOADN), National Association of Hispanic Nurses (NAHN), American Assembly for Men in Nursing (AMN)
- **Similar values.** Nurses Christian Fellowship (NCF), Nursing Ethics Network (NEN)

Web sites of a variety of nursing organizations are identified on Davis*Plus*.

 Go to Chapter 1, **Resources for Caregivers and Health Professionals,** on Davis*Plus.*

CONTEMPORARY NURSING: CARING FOR CLIENTS

Look again at the definitions of *nursing* you have read in this chapter (e.g., Box 1-1). Notice that they all agree that nursing is about caring for clients. Recent studies show that when the percentage of RNs increases in an agency, quality of care rises, death and infection rates drop (Potera, 2007), and length of stay is shorter by at least 30% (Kane, Shamliyan, Mueller, et al., 2007).

Who Are the Recipients of Nursing Care?

The recipients of nursing care may be individuals, groups, families, or communities. They can be referred to as patients, clients, or persons. **Direct care** involves personal interaction between the nurse and clients (e.g., giving medications or teaching a client about a treatment). Nurses deliver **indirect care** when they work on behalf of clients to improve their health status (e.g., restocking a resuscitation cart or arranging unit staffing). A nurse may use independent judgment to determine the care needed or may work under the direct order of a primary care provider.

As a nurse, you should not view patients as passive recipients of care. On the contrary, nurses should actively encourage patients' involvement in decisions about their care, and facilitate their participation as collaborative members of the healthcare team (e.g., by being informed and speaking up about their concerns).

What Are the Purposes of Nursing Care?

Nurses provide care to achieve the goals of health promotion, illness prevention, health restoration, and end-of-life care. Together these aspects of care represent a range of services that cover the health spectrum from complete well-being to death.

Health Promotion

The World Health Organization, in 1948, defined **health** as "a state of complete physical, mental, and social well-being and not merely the absence of disease or infirmity." The definition has not been changed since that time (WHO, 2007). This inclusive definition can be applied to individuals, groups, families, or communities. **Health promotion** activities foster the recipient's highest state of well-being. For example, at the individual level you might counsel a pregnant client about the importance of adequate prenatal nutrition to promote health. Group and family-level health promotion activities might include teaching about nutrition during pregnancy in family education programs. On a community level your activities would be focused on reaching a larger number of people. For example, you could post signs in grocery stores recommending food sources for pregnant women and lobby for the labeling of substances that should be avoided in pregnancy.

Illness Prevention

Illness prevention focuses on avoidance of disease, infection, and other comorbidities. Activities are targeted to decrease the risk of developing an illness or to minimize the risk of exposure to disease. For example, pneumonia affects society's most vulnerable: the very young, the very old, and the very ill. Some nursing activities to decrease the risk of pneumonia include:

- Teaching the importance of hand hygiene to decrease the transmission of infection
- Advocating for and administering pneumonia immunizations to those at high risk

Health Restoration

Health restoration activities foster a return to health for those already ill. To restore health, the nurse provides direct care to ill individuals, groups, families, or communities. Direct care is what most people think of when they envision the nursing role. Recall that health has physical, mental, and social dimensions. When you engage in health-restoration activities, your care should address each of these dimensions, for example:

- Providing hygiene care
- Providing client teaching
- Lobbying for health policy changes to improve access to care

End-of-Life Care

Death is the inevitable destination on the journey of life. Nurses have been active in promoting the respectful care of those who are terminally ill or dying. Nursing activities for the dying are designed to promote comfort, maintain quality of life, provide culturally relevant spiritual care, and ease the emotional burden of death. Nurses work with dying individuals, their family members and support persons, and organizations that focus on the needs of the terminally ill. You will learn more about this in Chapter 17.

KnowledgeCheck 1-3

Recall the last time you had a cold. Identify health-promotion, illness-prevention, and health-restoration activities for individuals, families, groups, and communities in relation to the common cold.

Where Do Nurses Work?

As a nurse you will have the opportunity to work in a variety of settings. During your education you will have assignments in many settings and clinical units that will allow you to see some of the options available to you upon graduation. Approximately 62% of nurses work in hospitals. The remaining 40% work in extended care facilities, ambulatory care, home health settings, public health, or nursing education (HRSA, 2010).

Hospitals. Hospitals provide services to patients who require around-the-clock nursing care. This type of care is frequently referred to as *acute care*. Length of stay is limited to the amount of time that the client requires 24-hour observation.

Extended Care Facilities. These facilities provide care for clients for an extended period of time—usually longer than 1 month. They include nursing homes, skilled nursing facilities (also known as convalescent hospitals), and rehabilitation facilities. The distinction among them is based primarily on whether they provide skilled or custodial care. **Skilled care** includes services of trained professionals that are needed for a limited period of time after an injury or illness. **Custodial care** consists of help with activities of daily living: bathing, dressing, eating, grooming, ambulation, toileting, and other care that people typically do for themselves (e.g., taking medications, monitoring blood glucose levels).

- **A nursing home** provides custodial care for people who cannot live on their own but are not sick enough to require hospitalization. It provides a room, custodial care, and recreation. In the United States approximately 16,000 nursing homes provide care for approximately 1.7 million residents (Centers for Disease Control and Prevention [CDC], n.d.).
- **A skilled nursing facility** primarily provides skilled nursing care for patients who can be expected to improve with treatment. For example, a patient who no longer needs hospitalization may transfer to a skilled nursing facility until she is able to return home.

Ambulatory Care. Ambulatory care is also referred to as *outpatient care*. Clients live at home or in nonhospital settings and come to the site for care. Ambulatory care sites include private health and medical offices; clinics; outpatient therapy centers; and walk-in clinics in shopping centers, pharmacies, and other retail sites. Typically they treat only common ailments and refer complex or serious illnesses to specialized physicians or emergency rooms (Darcé, 2007).

Home Care. Home healthcare is provided to clients who are homebound or unable to get to ambulatory care centers for services. Home care services may also be used when the client or family prefers to receive care in the home—particularly when the client is terminally ill. Home care is also appropriate when a client still requires skilled care but is discharged from the hospital because his reimbursable length-of-stay has expired. Services are usually coordinated by a home health or visiting nurse service and include nursing care as well as various therapies and home assistance programs.

Community Health. Community health deals with care for the community at large. Community health nurses provide services to at-risk populations and devise strategies to improve the health status of the surrounding community. Examples of community health programs include healthcare for the

homeless and school-based programs designed to decrease the incidence of teen pregnancies. Community, public health, and home care are discussed in Chapter 41.

The Healthcare Delivery System

For an expanded discussion of the preceding workplaces and services, as well as the organization and regulation of the healthcare delivery system in the United States,

 Go to Chapter 1, **Healthcare Delivery Systems—Expanded Discussion,** on Davis*Plus.*

QSEN Commission and Quality Improvement

Recall that the Quality and Safety Education for Nurses (QSEN) project and the Institute of Medicine (IOM) have identified quality and safety competencies for nurses. You will find those in the accompanying QSEN box. Your nursing education should enable you to achieve these competencies.

To see the KSAs for the QSEN competencies,

QSEN

What are QSEN Competencies?

Competencies

Patient-Centered Care, Teamwork and Collaboration, Evidence-Based Practice, Quality Improvement, Safety, Informatics

The QSEN (pronounced *cue*-zen) competencies are six areas of expertise nursing students are expected to acquire before graduation. Each competency includes a list of associated knowledge, skills, and attitudes (KSAs) that operationalize the concepts. The six competencies and their definitions are as follow:

- ➤ **Patient-Centered Care**: Recognize the patient or designee as the source of control and [a] full partner [when] providing compassionate and coordinated care based on respect for patient's preferences, values, and needs.
- ➤ **Teamwork and Collaboration:** Function effectively within nursing and inter-professional teams, fostering open communication, mutual respect, and shared decision making to achieve quality patient care.
- ➤ **Evidence-Based Practice:** Integrate best current evidence with clinical expertise and patient/family preferences and values for delivery of optimal HC [healthcare].
- ➤ **Quality Improvement (QI):** Use data to monitor the outcomes of care processes and use improvement methods to design and test changes to continuously improve the quality and safety of HC systems.
- ➤ **Safety**: Minimize risk of harm to patients and providers through both system effectiveness and individual performance.
- ➤ **Informatics:** Use information and technology to communicate, manage knowledge, mitigate error, and support decision-making.

Source: Cronenwett, L, et al (2007). See Appendix A for specific Knowledge, Skills and Attitudes.

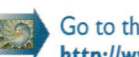 Go to the QSEN web site, at **http://www.qsen.org/ksas_prelicensure.php**

One important QSEN competency is **quality improvement (QI)**. QSEN defines that competence as the ability to "use data to monitor the outcomes of care processes and use improvement methods to design and test changes to continuously improve the quality and safety of healthcare systems" (Cronenwett, Sherwood, Barnsteiner, et al., 2007). For more detailed information about quality improvement programs and processes,

 Go to Chapter 1, **Supplemental Materials: How Do Providers and Facilities Ensure Quality Care,** on Davis*Plus.*

WHAT FACTORS INFLUENCE CONTEMPORARY NURSING PRACTICE?

Contemporary nursing practice is influenced by factors outside the profession in society at large, and factors within nursing and healthcare.

Trends in Society

As you have seen, our historical roots strongly influence current nursing practice and will undoubtedly continue to do so. In addition, nursing is influenced by trends in the economy, the growing number of older adults, increased consumer knowledge, legislation, the women's movement, and collective bargaining.

The National Economy. The economy has a tremendous impact on nursing. In the United States, health insurance coverage is linked to full-time employment with health insurance benefits (although that is changing with recent federal legislation). Thus, when unemployment is high or businesses reduce their employee healthcare benefits, fewer people have insurance. Fearing the high cost of healthcare, many uninsured people delay seeking treatment. The effect is that they are often sicker when they enter the healthcare system. This taxes the system's resources and raises the level of nursing care required.

Another consideration is that the healthcare industry—even in a strong economy—is very expensive to operate. Downturns in the economy affect institutional investments and profits, and the amount of taxes the government can collect; these in turn limit the medications and services that are available in public-supported healthcare programs. Similarly, the salaries of healthcare providers are influenced by national economic trends.

The Growing Proportion of Older Adults in the United States. A larger older adult population creates a need for more medical and nursing care; at the same time, there are fewer younger people to provide care. The growth rate for adults 65 years and older has greatly outpaced the growth of the population of the country as a whole. In 2007, 13% of the total U.S. population was 65 and older. By the year 2030, about one in five people will be age 65 and older, and the oldest old (those 85 years and older) will continue to be the fastest growing part of the population into the next century (Hobbs, 2001; U.S. Census Bureau, 2007). As people age, they tend to need more assistance with activities of daily living, and they experience more acute and chronic illnesses.

Changes in Healthcare Consumers. Historically, patients relied on the knowledge and decision making of the

physician or the healthcare team. Now, however, consumers are demanding greater choice in the decisions that affect their health, including legislation. Patients have access to vast amounts of health and medical information, particularly through the Internet (e.g., through Web sites such as WebMD). Informed consumers tend to be active participants in discussions about their health problems and therapy options. Clients may request their healthcare providers to prescribe specific trade name therapies they have heard about in the media, so nurses need to be prepared to address the truthfulness of the advertisements, present balanced information to clients, and address the appropriateness of the advertised products and services for the individual person's needs.

The Women's Movement. Historically, only unmarried women were allowed to practice nursing. As the women's movement gained momentum, women were no longer forced out of nursing if they chose to have a family. However, the women's movement also opened up more career choices for women, and nursing has become just one of many options as opposed to a preferred career pathway. Also, as you have seen, societal views of nursing as a women's profession influence the decisions of men to enter nursing.

Collective Bargaining. Collective bargaining is a form of negotiating that allows nurses to seek better wages and working conditions as a group rather than individually. A union or organization that represents the nurses usually conducts collective bargaining. Collective bargaining has resulted in significant improvements in wages, benefits, and working conditions for nurses, as well as safer conditions for patients. Not all states have collective bargaining groups for nurses.

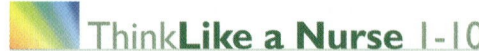 **Think Like a Nurse 1-10**

What effect do you think the women's movement has had on the number of women in the nursing workforce? Speculate also on the ways in which women entering nursing might have been different before and after the women's movement.

Trends in Nursing and Healthcare

In addition to societal factors, trends in nursing and healthcare also affect contemporary practice. We discuss the most significant trends here.

Increased Use of Complementary and Alternative Medicine

Complementary and alternative medicine (CAM) consists of healthcare treatments or services outside the traditional healthcare system. CAM includes homeopathy, naturopathy, chiropractic, and traditional Chinese medicine, as well as specific treatments, such as herbal medications, dietary changes, massage therapy, yoga, aromatherapy, prayer, and hypnotism. The following factors have contributed to this interest in CAM. Many people have turned to CAM as a result of the rising costs of traditional care, concern about the safety of traditional healthcare, distrust of the role of insurance and managed care organizations in determining treatment options, and confusion over changing recommendations (e.g., how often to have a screening exam for breast cancer). In addition, as the population becomes more culturally diverse, there is an accompanying exchange of information about therapies from different cultural traditions. If you want to know more about CAM, see Chapter 46.

 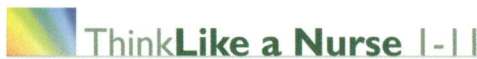 Go to Chapter 46, **Holistic Healing,** on DavisPlus.

Expanded Variety of Settings for Care

Nearly 40% of RNs now work outside the hospital setting, as compared to 20% in 1980 (ANA, 2010; HRSA, 2010; Jonas & Kovner, 2005). As the site of employment shifts away from the hospital, nurses must be prepared to function in these alternative settings. This change requires entry-level education programs to prepare nurses for this type of work (Wilkinson, 1996). In the hospital, nurses have access to support personnel, consultation with other nurses and healthcare providers, ready access to equipment and diagnostic testing services, and increased access to the patient. In outpatient, community, or home settings, nurses must be prepared to function more autonomously and creatively, adapting care to the equipment available at the site.

Think Like a Nurse 1-11

What is your nursing program doing to prepare you to work outside the hospital setting?

Interest in Interprofessional Collaboration

The growing role of nursing outside the hospital, the increasing complexity of care, the limited supply of nurses, and the increased use of technology are changing nursing from a largely supportive role to one of increasing responsibility. More and more, leaders in healthcare are finding interprofessional teamwork to be essential to providing safe, high-quality patient outcomes.

Collaboration is the process of joint decision making among independent parties, involving joint ownership of decisions and collective responsibility for outcomes (Disch, Bellman, & Ingbar, as cited in Sterchi, 2001). However, in a relationship in which there is a power imbalance, true collaboration can occur only if the more powerful parties are willing. Physicians and nurses tend to have different values and to place different emphases on patient care. This may contribute to strained relationships and disagreements about a patient's plan of care, which may lead to undesired outcomes for patients. True collaboration occurs when institutions state it as a goal and give recognition to those who practice it.

Increased Use of Advanced Practice Nurses

The increased use of advanced practice nurses (APNs) has resulted in greater public exposure for nurses. Professional and public reports (e.g., Tourangeau, Doran, Hall, et al., 2007) demonstrate high patient satisfaction with APNs; comparable, and at times superior, patient outcomes over physician-provided care; better understanding of and compliance with treatment regimen; fewer hospitalizations; and greater cost effectiveness when compared with physician providers. This positive exposure has resulted in increased acceptance and support for all nurses.

Increased Use of Nursing Assistive Personnel

Nursing assistive personnel (NAP) are healthcare providers who help nurses and physicians provide patient care. Common NAP roles include nurse aide, assistant, orderly, and technician. NAPs may perform simple nursing tasks (e.g., bathing, taking temperatures, or making beds) under the direction of the licensed nurse. Some institutions even train NAPs for more complex tasks traditionally reserved for licensed nurses

Toward Evidence-Based Practice

Capezuti, E., Wagner, L., Brush, B., et al. (2007). Consequences of an intervention to reduce restrictive siderail use in nursing homes. *Journal of the American Geriatrics Society,* *55*(3), 334–341.

This study of more than 700 nursing home residents at four sites found that routine use of side rails does not reduce the risk of bed-related falls.

Brush, B. L., & Capezuti, E. (2001). Historical analysis of siderail use in American hospitals. *Journal of Nursing Scholarship, 33*(4), 381–385.

This study used social historical research methods to examine the pattern of siderail use, the value attached to side rails, and attitudes about raising side rails over time. Initially siderails were used for temporary protection of confused patients. Siderails on adult beds were rare until the 1930s; nurses used continual watchfulness to ensure patient safety. During the 1930s, recurrent nurse shortages, litigation against hospitals and nurses for fall-related injuries,

and the move away from ward structure toward semiprivate and private rooms all promoted the use of siderails instead of nursing observation. They now have become a permanent fixture of the hospital bed. However, recent research has demonstrated that side rail-induced injuries may occur. In spite of these recent research-based findings, side rail use remains the norm in promoting patient safety.

1. What trends and factors currently affecting nursing might influence whether siderail use will change in the near future?

2. What additional information would you like to know before advocating for a change in siderail use?

 Go to Chapter 1, **Toward Evidence-Based Practice Suggested Responses,** on Davis*Plus.*

(e.g., inserting urinary catheters, giving certain medications). This redistribution of workload has prompted controversy about safety and quality of care.

Although it may seem appropriate to allow the NAP to assume the simple tasks, this distances the licensed nurse from many aspects of direct patient care. The nurse retains ultimate responsibility for the patient, yet may have to base important patient care decisions on information obtained by the NAP. Unfortunately many nurses now in practice were never taught in their formal nursing programs about delegation and supervision, so they are uncertain about what they can safely and legally delegate and how much responsibility they retain. To remedy this problem, nursing schools are now adding coursework on delegation; and textbooks, such as this one, include information about delegation.

Influence of Nurses on Healthcare Policy

Professional nursing organizations are actively involved in local, state, and national politics. Each of the major professional organizations actively lobbies and educates elected and appointed officials about the role of nursing in healthcare. Nursing organizations sponsor legislation that promotes the interest of the profession and supports changes that positively influence health outcomes. Nurse-sponsored legislation has addressed safe staffing in hospitals, needle-exchange programs to decrease the transmission of HIV and other infectious diseases, and funding to increase nursing enrollment during times of nursing shortages.

As individuals, nurses should vote, lobby their elected representatives, and run for political office. Together, nurses represent the largest health professional group; as a voting block, they have strong political power. Many nurses organize local nursing groups to support candidates or legislation, or speak out in the community on health and nursing issues. Nurses are typically trusted and respected political candidates,

running successful campaigns at the local, state, and national level. You should consider all of these political activities as you move into the profession.

Divergence Between High-Tech and High-Touch

Advances in clinical knowledge and technology have contributed to improved care for many patients who are critically ill (e.g., premature newborns and patients with advanced cardiovascular, pulmonary, or renal disease). However, in prolonging life, technology has created numerous legal and ethical dilemmas, particularly about end-of-life care. This trend is in contrast to the concurrent trend toward holism and high-touch therapies, which often avoid technology. One of the challenges in healthcare is integrating these two divergent trends. For an excellent discussion on these colliding values, read *Holistic Health and Healing* by Mary Anne Bright (2002).

 To explore learning resources for this chapter,

 Go to Davis*Plus* at http://www.Davisplus.fadavis.com, **keyword Treas.**
Chapter Resources for Chapter 1:
    Knowledge Check and Think Like a Nurse Response Sheets
    Knowledge Check Answers
    Resources for Caregivers and Health Professionals
    Reading More About Nursing Past & Present (Suggested Readings)
    What Are the Main Points in This Chapter?
NCLEX-Style Review Questions
Chapter Overview Podcasts

Concept Map

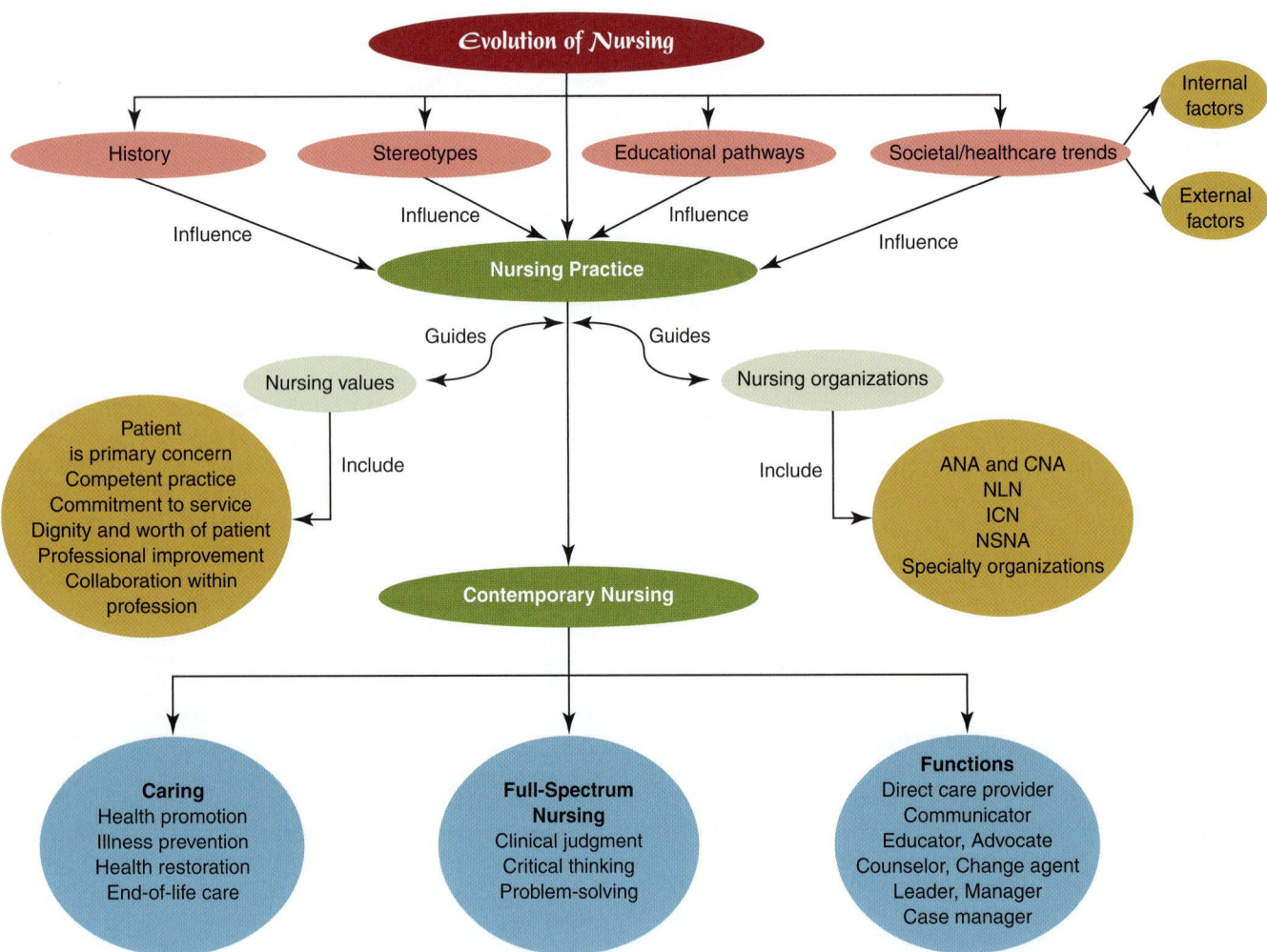

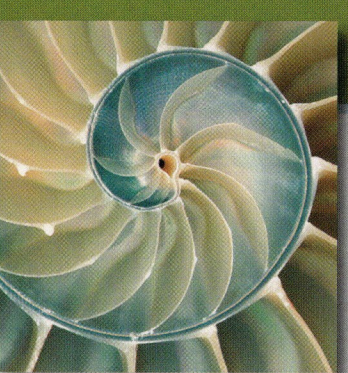

Critical Thinking & the Nursing Process

Learning Outcomes

After completing this chapter, you should be able to:

➤ Give one definition and one example of *critical thinking*.

➤ List at least six critical-thinking skills and attitudes.

➤ Review seven attitudes of the critical thinker.

➤ Explain ways in which nurses use critical thinking.

➤ Describe the six overlapping and interdependent phases of the nursing process.

➤ Explain how critical thinking is used in the nursing process.

➤ Explain what is meant in nursing by the concept of *caring*.

➤ Discuss, and give examples of, the difference between practical/procedural knowledge and theoretical knowledge.

➤ Name and describe the main concepts of the full-spectrum nursing model.

➤ Explain how the key concepts of nursing knowledge, nursing process, and critical thinking work together in full-spectrum nursing.

Key Concepts

Critical thinking
Full-spectrum nursing
Nursing knowledge
Nursing process

Related Concepts

See the Concept Map at the end of this chapter.

Caring for the Nguyens

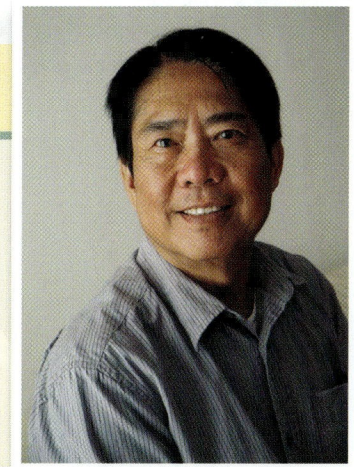

This feature allows you to practice the kind of thinking you will use as a full-spectrum nurse. There is usually more than one correct answer to a critical thinking question, so we do not provide answers for these features. It is more important to develop your nursing judgment than to "cover content." Discuss the questions with your peers. If you are still unsure, consult your instructor.

Review the opening scenario of Nam Nguyen in the front of this book. Imagine you are the clinic nurse at the Family Medicine Center. Based on the information presented in the scenario, work through the following questions:

A. Patient Situation

- Why is Mr. Nguyen at the clinic?
- What are his wife's concerns?
- Are they similar to or different from his?

B. Critical Thinking

- How do I go about getting the data I need? What sources should I use?
- Are my data congruent?
- What is one possible explanation for what is happening in this situation?

(Continued)

Caring for the Nguyens (continued)

C. Nursing Knowledge

- What type of nursing knowledge (theoretical, practical, ethical, or self-knowledge) is needed to answer the following questions?
- What health concerns does Mr. Nguyen have that should be addressed by the healthcare team?
- What is the role of Zach Jackson on the healthcare team?
- What role will you play in the care of Mr. Nguyen?

D. Nursing Process

- In what phase of the nursing process are you engaged when you are asking Mr. Nguyen about the reason for his visit?
- What activities are involved in the diagnosis phase? In planning outcomes? In planning interventions?
- Why would you not, at this point, be using the evaluation phase?

 Go to **Caring for the Nguyens Response Sheet** on DavisPlus.

Explore Your Nursing Role

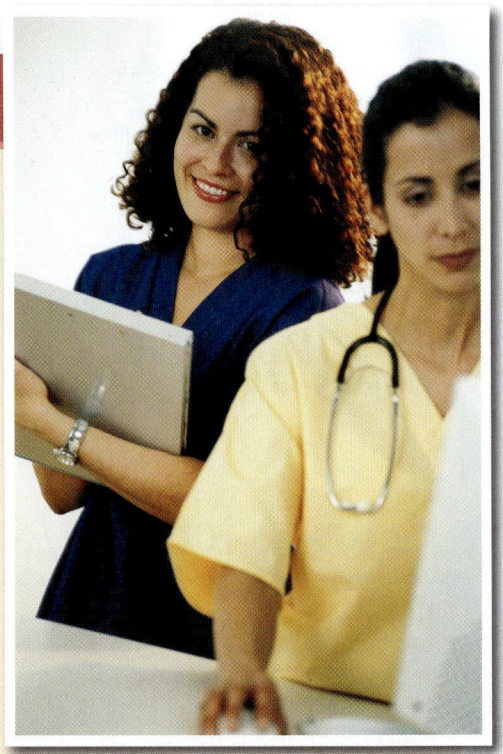

It's a pleasant Saturday afternoon, and you're meeting with an old friend whom you haven't seen in 2 years. She asks, "I hear you've decided to become a nurse. What made you choose that? I don't think I could be around people who are sick and in pain. Hospitals are such sad places."

She listens to your answer with interest. To respond to this statement, you will need to consider your motivation for entering nursing and your beliefs about the profession.

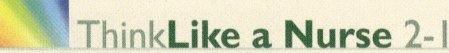 ThinkLike a Nurse 2-1

How would you reply to her question?

ThinkLike a Nurse 2-2

- What factors or persons influenced your decision to be a nurse?
- Have others asked you why you chose to become a nurse? How have the reactions you received before colored your explanation of your career choice?
- What makes this situation similar to or different from your prior experiences?
- What's important in this situation?

- Of the possible answers you are considering, which answer best reflects your true feelings about your career choice? Why are the other answers not appropriate?
- What beliefs and assumptions are coloring your response?

If you are able to answer these questions, then you have used critical thinking to guide your decision making. Critical thinking involves careful consideration of a situation to arrive at a solution, based on analysis of the data. Critical thinking is vital when considering important decisions. It is the kind of thinking you will use as a nurse.

WHAT IS YOUR VIEW OF NURSING?

Chapter 1 introduced you to nursing roles, responsibilities, and activities, and the career of nursing. Throughout this text, you will learn much more. Thus, your view of nursing may change as you progress in your studies. To track your progress, establish a baseline by examining your current view of nursing.

ThinkLike a Nurse 2-3

What is your image of nursing? List at least five attributes a nurse should have, and at least five responsibilities that you consider to be part of nursing.

In the preceding exercise, when you listed some nursing responsibilities, you may have mentioned activities such as "gives medications" or "performs tests and treatments." And you were correct—partially. Much of nursing is about *doing*, and nursing is activity oriented. But don't forget the importance of *caring*. And now more than ever the emphasis is on *thinking*. So, another way to describe nursing is to say that *nursing involves thinking, doing, and caring.*

The scientific basis for patient care changes constantly. Research continually uncovers new information that alters the practice of all healthcare providers. Therefore, you should know up front that you cannot possibly learn everything about healthcare and nursing in nursing school. In fact, to be a safe and competent nurse you must constantly update your knowledge and skills throughout your career. As a lifelong learner, you will need to develop and refine your critical-thinking skills. Critical thinking helps you to know what is important about each patient's situation, when you need more information, and when you need help to make the best decision.

TheoreticalKnowledge
knowing **why**

ABOUT THE KEY CONCEPTS

Keep the key concepts in mind as you read this chapter. They will give you the "hooks" on which you can "hang" the other details in the chapter. As you gain understanding of critical thinking, nursing knowledge, and nursing process, you will begin to see how they all work together in full-spectrum nursing.

WHAT IS CRITICAL THINKING?

If critical thinking is so important, then you might be wondering what exactly it is. One simple definition is that critical thinking is "the art of thinking about your thinking while you are thinking in order to make your thinking better: more clear, more accurate, or more defensible" (Paul, 1990). On closer study, this definition makes an important point. It tells us that we should reflect on the thinking process we are using to figure something out: "Why did I ask those particular questions? Do I have enough information to decide, or have I jumped to a conclusion? Have I considered all the possibilities?"

Box 2-1 provides several definitions of critical thinking, or you may want to use the following more formal definition:

Critical thinking is a combination of reasoned thinking, openness to alternatives, an ability to reflect, and a desire to seek truth.

BOX 2-1 ■ Some Definitions of Critical Thinking

- Critical thinking is the disciplined, intellectual process of applying skillful reasoning as a guide to belief or action (Paul, Ennis, & Norris, 1996).
- Critical thinking is careful and deliberate determination of whether to accept, reject, or suspend judgment (Moore & Parker, 2001).
- Critical thinking is reasonable and reflective thinking focused on deciding what to believe or do (Ennis, 2004).
- In nursing, critical thinking for clinical decision making is the ability to think in a systematic and logical manner with openness to questions and to reflect on the reasoning process used to ensure safe nursing practice and quality care (Heaslip, 1992).
- Critical thinking is disciplined, self-directed, rational thinking that supports what we know and makes clear what we don't know (Wilkinson, 2011).
- The ideal critical thinker is inquisitive, open-minded, flexible, fair-minded, well informed, persistent in seeking the truth, wise in judgments and decision making, logical, and honest with facing personal biases. The critical thinker uses sound reasoning and is willing to consider valid alternatives (American Philosophical Association, 1990).

There are many definitions of critical thinking because it is a complex concept and people think about it in different ways—none of them are wrong. In fact, any situation that requires critical thinking is likely to have more than one right answer. You do not need critical thinking to add 2 + 2 and come up with the answer. However, you do need critical thinking to work through important decisions.

Critical thinking is linked to evidence-based practice, which you will learn more about later in this book. Evidence-based practice is a research-based method for judging nursing interventions. An important aspect of critical thinking is the process of identifying and checking your assumptions—and this is also an important part of the research process.

Critical thinkers are flexible, nonjudgmental, inquisitive, honest, and interested in seeking the truth. They possess intellectual skills that allow them to use their curiosity to their advantage, and they have critical attitudes that motivate them to use those skills responsibly.

What Are Critical-Thinking Skills?

Skills in critical thinking refer to the cognitive (intellectual) processes used in complex thinking operations such as problem-solving and decision making. In this example, the skills are italicized, and the complex thinking processes are in bold type:

When planning nursing care, nurses *gather information* about the client and then **draw tentative conclusions about the meaning of the information** to *identify the client's problems.* Then they *think of several different actions* they might take to help **solve or relieve the problem.**

The following are a few examples of critical-thinking skills:

- Objectively gathering information on a problem or issue
- Recognizing the need for more information
- Evaluating the credibility and usefulness of sources of information

Table 2-1 ➤ Critical-Thinking Model

THINKING PROCESS	DESCRIPTION	QUESTIONS FOR FOCUSING THINKING
Contextual awareness (deciding what to observe and consider)	An awareness of what's happening in the total situation, including values, cultural issues, interpersonal relationships, and environmental influences	■ What is going on in the situation that may influence the outcome? ■ What factors may influence my behavior and that of others in this situation (e.g., culture, roles, relationships, economic status)? ■ What about this situation have I seen before? What is new? ■ Who should be involved in order to improve the outcome? ■ What else was happening at the same time that affected me in this situation? ■ What happened just before this incident that made a difference? ■ What emotional responses influenced how I reacted in this situation? ■ What changes in behavior alerted me that something was wrong?
Inquiry (based on credible sources)	Applying standards of good reasoning to your thinking when analyzing a situation and evaluating your actions	■ How do I go about gathering the information I need? ■ What framework should I use to organize my information? ■ Do I have enough knowledge to decide? If not, what do I need to know? ■ Have I used a valid, reliable source of information (e.g., patient, other professionals, references)? ■ Did I (do I need to) validate the data (e.g., with the client)? ■ What else do I need to know? What information is missing? ■ Are the data accurate? Precise? ■ What's important and what's not important in this situation? ■ Did I consider professional, ethical, and legal standards? ■ Have I jumped to conclusions?
Considering alternatives	Exploring and imagining as many alternatives as you can think of for the situation	■ What is one possible explanation for what is happening or what happened? ■ What are other explanations for what is happening? What is one thing I could do in this situation? ■ What are two more possibilities/alternatives? ■ Are there others who might help me develop more alternatives? ■ Of the possible actions I am considering, which one is most reasonable? Why are the others not as reasonable? ■ Of the possible actions I am considering, which one is most likely to achieve the desired outcomes?
Analyzing assumptions	Recognizing and analyzing assumptions you are making about the situation and examining the beliefs that underlie your choices	■ What have I (or others) taken for granted in this situation? ■ Which beliefs/values are shaping my assumptions? ■ What assumptions contributed to the problem in this situation? ■ What rationale supports my assumptions? ■ How will I know my assumption is correct? ■ What biases do I have that may affect my thinking and my decisions in this situation?
Reflecting skeptically and deciding what to do	Questioning, analyzing, and reflecting on the rationale for your decisions	■ What aspects of this situation require the most careful attention? ■ What else might work in this situation? ■ Am I sure of my interpretation of this situation? ■ Why is (was) it important to intervene?

THINKING PROCESS	DESCRIPTION	QUESTIONS FOR FOCUSING THINKING
Table 2-1 ➤ Critical-Thinking Model—cont'd		
		■ What rationale do I have for my decisions?
		■ In priority order, what should I do in this situation and why?
		■ Having decided what was wrong/happening, what is the best response?
		■ What might I delegate in this situation?
		■ What got me started taking some action?
		■ What priorities were missed?
		■ What was done? Why was it done?
		■ What would I do differently after reflecting on this situation?

Sources: Model based on Brookfield, S. D. (1991). *Developing critical thinkers.* San Francisco: Jossey-Bass; McDonald, M. E. (2002). *Systematic assessment of learning outcomes: Developing multiple-choice exams.* Boston: Jones and Bartlett; Paul, R. W. (1993). *Critical thinking: What every person needs to survive in a rapidly changing world* (3rd ed.). Santa Rosa, CA: Foundation for Critical Thinking; Raingruber, B., & Haffer, A. (2001). *Using your head to land on your feet.* Philadelphia: F.A. Davis; and Wilkinson, J. M. (2011). *Nursing process and critical thinking* (5th ed.). Upper Saddle River, NJ: Prentice Hall.

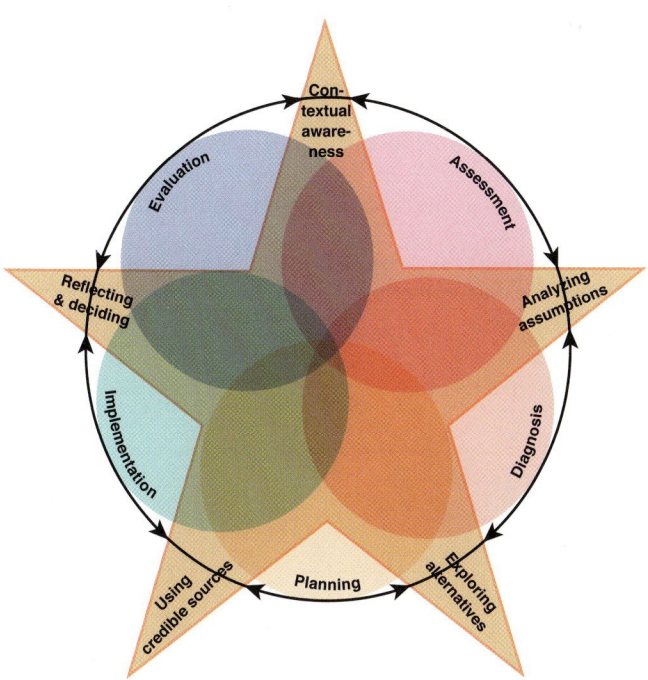

FIGURE 2-1 Model of critical thinking and the nursing process.

your first clinical day so that you will be well prepared and able to function safely?

■ **Contextual Awareness.** One of the first things you need to consider is your usual response to new experiences. How do you react to change? What other tasks or assignments do you have that will dictate the timing of your preparation? Have you had any previous experiences that will aid or hamper you in your preparation? As you consider these questions, you are addressing the star point of *contextual awareness*.

■ **Using Credible Sources.** You need to gather information about the clinical experience. It is important to use *inquiry based on credible sources* as you gather data. For example,

you may want to ask your instructor for guidance on how to best prepare. You may also wish to consult a student who has successfully completed the same course. If you have been assigned to provide care for a client, you need to obtain accurate information about the client. You could use the client's chart and your textbooks to prepare. You should use only knowledgeable, reliable sources of information—for example, nursing texts and nursing journals, not popular (nonscholarly) magazines (such as *Parents* magazine) or certain Internet sites. After you have more information, you should go back and analyze your response to the situation. You may find that you are feeling less anxious already! All of this is a part of inquiry.

■ **Exploring Alternatives and Analyzing Assumptions.** Now that you know something about the clinical experience, you can plan your day. You need to *consider alternatives* and *analyze your assumptions* about the experience. What is expected of you? What do you expect from the experience? How should you approach your client? How will you introduce yourself? What skills do you have? How will you apply them to caring for your client?

■ **Reflecting and Deciding.** After you feel that you have addressed these concerns, you need to quickly review your preparation (reflective skepticism). Have you gathered enough information to feel comfortable in the situation? Have you left anything out? Do you need more information?

This was a demonstration of how you might apply the critical thinking model to a real experience. In this example, you also used theoretical, practical, personal, and ethical knowledge, which are explained in the next section.

WHAT ARE THE DIFFERENT KINDS OF NURSING KNOWLEDGE?

Critical thinking does not occur in a vacuum—you must have something to think about: your knowledge base. Nurses use various kinds of knowledge: theoretical, practical, personal, and ethical. Every chapter of this text is designed to help you gain practical knowledge and theoretical knowledge. Put very

simply, that is knowing what (to do) and knowing how (to do it). In fact, the chapters are organized according to those two types of knowledge.

Theoretical Knowledge. Each chapter begins by presenting theoretical knowledge. **Theoretical knowledge** consists of information, facts, principles, and evidence-based theories in nursing and related disciplines (e.g., physiology and psychology). It includes research findings and rationally constructed explanations of phenomena. You will use it to describe your patients, understand their health status, explain your reasoning for choosing interventions, and predict patient responses to interventions and treatments.

Practical Knowledge. Each chapter then provides the practical knowledge that enables you to apply your theoretical knowledge to caring for patients. **Practical knowledge**—knowing what to do and how to do it—consists of processes (e.g., the decision process and the nursing process) and procedures (e.g., how to give an injection), and is an aspect of nursing expertise.

Self-Knowledge. In addition to theoretical and practical knowledge, nurses use **self-knowledge,** that is, self-understanding. To think critically, you must be aware of your beliefs, values, and cultural and religious biases. This kind of knowledge helps you to find errors in your thinking and enables you to tune in to your patients. You can gain self-knowledge by developing personal awareness—by reflecting (asking yourself), "Why did I do that?" or "How did I come to think that?"

Ethical Knowledge. Finally, nurses use **ethical knowledge,** that is, knowledge of obligation, or right and wrong. Ethical knowledge consists of information about moral principles and processes for making moral decisions. Ethical knowledge helps you to fulfill your ethical obligations to patients and colleagues. Chapter 42 will help expand your ethical knowledge.

KnowledgeCheck 2-2

Think about the preceding discussion of the five points of the critical-thinking model and identify the actions that demonstrate use of each of the four types of knowledge.

PracticalKnowledge
knowing **how**

WHAT IS THE NURSING PROCESS?

The **nursing process** is a systematic problem-solving process that guides all nursing actions. It is the type of thinking and doing nurses use in their practice. In fact, the American Nurses Association (ANA) organizes its standards of care around the nursing process (ANA, 2010).

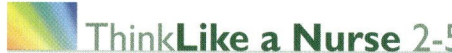 ThinkLike a Nurse 2-5

Practice your critical thinking. What questions should you ask about the last paragraph you have just read? For hints, look at Figure 2-1 and Table 2-1.

When evaluating the last paragraph, you should ask about the credibility of the sources cited, and you should ask yourself whether you have enough information about them to judge their credibility. Do you know what the ANA is?

What they do? Who are their members? What are standards of practice, and who decides what will be included in them? What effect do they have on what you will be doing as a nurse? Those are the kinds of questions you should ask when you see such statements. If you have read Chapter 1, you can probably answer most of these questions. You will see standards of care and practice quoted in other chapters throughout this book, beginning in Chapter 3.

All nurses apply the nursing process, to well and ill clients alike, in many settings (e.g., homes, clinics, hospitals). The purpose of the nursing process is to help the nurse provide goal-directed, client-centered care. The nursing process, like nursing itself, involves both thinking and doing. Nurses must have good psychomotor and interpersonal skills, and they must use a sound knowledge base and good judgment to use the nursing process effectively.

What Are the Phases of the Nursing Process?

The nursing process consists of six phases (or steps): assessment, diagnosis, planning outcomes, planning interventions, implementation, and evaluation (Wilkinson, 2011). A model illustrating these phases is shown in Figure 2-2. Note, though, that experts organize the phases in different ways. Many have a five-step process, combining outcomes and interventions into one planning phase. Some even have a four-step process; they combine assessment and diagnosis into one phase that they call *assessment*. There is no "right" way to do it, and experienced nurses do not use the steps separately anyway. Your text presents them as distinct and separate only to make it easier for you to learn how the process works.

Assessment. Assessment is the first phase of the nursing process: the data-gathering stage. You will obtain information

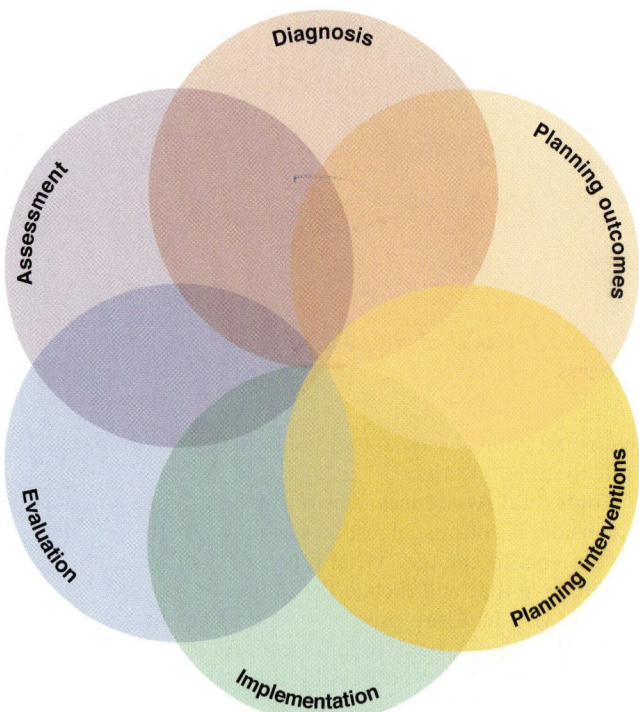

FIGURE 2-2 The phases of the nursing process.

from many sources: the client via history or physical exam, the client record, lab or test results, other health professionals, the client's family or support system, and the professional literature. In this phase, your purpose is to gather data that you will use to draw conclusions about the client's health status.

Diagnosis. This is the second phase of the nursing process. In this step you will identify the client's health needs (usually stated in the form of a problem) based on careful review of your assessment data. You need to analyze all your data, synthesize and cluster information, and hypothesize about your client's health status. The term *diagnosis* has been thought of as being medical, such as a diagnosis of cancer or diabetes. However, nursing diagnoses reflect the client's responses to actual or potential health problems and are different from medical diagnoses, as you will discover in Chapter 4.

Planning. The third and fourth steps of the nursing process both involve planning. Planning can be divided into two phases: planning (predicting) outcomes and planning interventions. The finished product of the planning phases is a holistic nursing care plan, individualized to reflect the client's problems and strengths. A care plan is a written or electronic document containing detailed instructions for a client's nursing care (see Fig. 5-2).

- In the **planning outcomes** step you work with the client to decide goals for your care—that is, the client outcomes you want to achieve through your nursing activities. These outcomes will drive your choice of interventions. The following is an example of an outcome statement you might find in a care plan:

  Nutritional status will improve as evidenced by a weight gain of 3 lb (1.4 kg) by July 1.

  See Chapter 5 for more about goals and outcomes.
- In the **planning interventions** phase you develop a list of possible interventions based on your nursing knowledge and then choose those most likely to help the client to achieve the stated goals. The best interventions are evidence based; that is, supported by sound research. See Chapter 6 for more about interventions.

Implementation. This is the action phase. During implementation, you will carry out or delegate the actions that you previously planned. You may delegate an action to another member of the healthcare team only if it is an action that may safely and legally be carried out by that team member. Delegation is discussed further in Chapter 7. In the implementation phase, you also document your actions and the client's responses to them.

Evaluation. The final phase of the nursing process is evaluation. In this phase, you determine whether the desired outcomes have been achieved, and judge whether your actions have successfully treated or prevented the client's health problems. You then modify the care plan as needed. For example, if a problem has been resolved, you delete it from the care plan; if outcomes have not been achieved, you determine why. It may be that a new intervention is needed. If so, you add it.

Notice that the nursing process is not intended to be *linear* (one step rigidly following another). Instead it is a *cyclical* process that follows a logical progression. You can see that the evaluation step requires you to begin again using all the other steps. You will find that you go back and forth between the steps, especially as you gain nursing experience. In addition to being cyclical, the steps may be *concurrent*. That means that some of the steps may occur at the same time. For example, while inserting a urinary catheter (implementation step), the nurse also observes the urine that returns through the tube (assessment step). You will learn about each nursing process phase in depth in Chapters 3 through 7.

KnowledgeCheck 2-3

- List the six phases of the nursing process.
- In which stage does the nurse collect data?
- Which stage involves problem identification?
- What does the nurse do in the evaluation step?

How Is the Nursing Process Related to Critical Thinking?

Critical thinking and the nursing process are interrelated, but not identical:

- Nurses use critical thinking for decisions unrelated to the nursing process (e.g., to decide how many nurses are needed to staff the unit).
- Some nursing activities (e.g., applying a cardiac monitor, inserting a urinary catheter), although they must be done skillfully, do not require reflective critical thinking.

The nursing process is essentially a problem-solving process. As such, it is one of the *complex critical-thinking skills* (see Box 2-1). Complex thinking skills, such as the nursing process, make use of many different critical-thinking skills (see Table 2-1 and Fig. 2-1). The following sections illustrate how nurses use critical thinking, nursing knowledge, and caring in each phase of the nursing process.

WHAT IS CARING?

Caring involves personal concern for people, events, projects, and things. It allows you to connect with others and to give help as well as receive it. One aspect of self-knowledge is to be aware of what and whom you care about. Knowing what the patient cares about reveals what is stressful for the patient, because only things that matter can create stress. Caring also enables the nurse to notice which interventions are effective.

A caring perspective highlights each person as unique and valued, so caring is always specific and relational for each nurse–person encounter. It is not an abstraction. That is, you don't just care for "suffering humankind," but you respond compassionately to *this* patient's needs right now, in the moment, even if you are busy and tired. Caring involves thinking and acting in ways that preserve human dignity and humanity, and does not treat people as objects. For example, a caring nurse drapes a patient for privacy when inserting a urinary catheter. A caring nurse's actions are never routine or mechanical.

Caring has at least five components:

- *Knowing.* Striving to understand what an event (e.g., an illness) means in the life of the patient
- *Being with.* Being emotionally present for the patient (e.g., making eye contact, actively listening)
- *Doing for.* Doing what the patient would do for himself if he could (e.g., bathing)
- *Enabling.* Supporting the patient through coping with life changes and unfamiliar events, such as hospitalization

- *Maintaining belief.* Having faith in the patient's ability to get through the change or event and to find fulfillment and meaning (Swanson, 1990)

Caring is the central concept in several nursing theories. You will learn more about those theories in Chapter 8.

KnowledgeCheck 2-4

List all the characteristics of caring that you can remember.

WHAT IS FULL-SPECTRUM NURSING?

Full-spectrum nursing is a unique blend of thinking, doing, and caring. It is performed by nurses who fully develop and apply nursing knowledge, critical thinking, and the nursing process to patient situations for the purpose of effecting good outcomes.

What Concepts Are Used in the Full-Spectrum Nursing Model?

When we put concepts (ideas) together to explain something, it is called **a model.** You'll learn more about concepts in Chapter 8; for now, think of them as ideas. The four main concepts that describe full-spectrum nursing are thinking, doing, caring, *and* patient situation (or context) (Table 2-2).

In order to think, you must have something to think about. When nurses think, they use the nursing knowledge that they have stored in their memory. In addition, they think about the patient situation, which they acquire through use of the nursing process. *Situation,* or *context,* refers to the context for care, the patient's environment outside the care setting, relationships, resources available for patient care, and so on. Figure 2-3 is a simple, visual model of full-spectrum nursing. You can see that the concept's full model involves everything you have learned in this chapter: critical thinking, nursing knowledge, and nursing process—but organized under the simple concepts of thinking, doing, caring, and patient situation.

Let's see how the model concepts work together for a full-spectrum nurse. They are all interrelated and overlapping, but we divide them into simple categories to help you understand and remember them. You can see that a full-spectrum nurse needs excellent thinking skills because there is so much to think *about* and so much to do.

KnowledgeCheck 2-5

- What are the four main concepts of the full-spectrum model of nursing?
- Where do the four types of nursing knowledge fit into the full-spectrum model?
- What is the ultimate purpose of full-spectrum nursing?

How Does the Model Work?

The full-spectrum nursing model is used throughout this text, so it is important that you understand how it works. Nurses use critical *thinking* in all steps of the nursing process. They also apply critical thinking to the four kinds of nursing knowledge, and when they are *doing* for the patient. *Caring* motivates and facilitates the thinking and doing. The goal of all this is to have a positive effect on a patient's health outcomes.

The patient situations in Table 2-3 illustrate how the three main concepts of full-spectrum nursing work together. As you read, notice how the concepts overlap. For example, recall that nursing process and problem-solving are themselves complex critical-thinking skills. Also notice how the nurse uses critical thinking with nursing knowledge and the nursing process.

As a full-spectrum nurse, you will apply thinking, doing, and caring to patient situations to help benefit patients and bring about good outcomes.

Table 2-2 ➤ Full-Spectrum Nursing Concepts			
THINKING	**DOING**	**CARING**	**PATIENT SITUATION**
Critical Thinking Enables you to fully use your knowledge and skills	**Practical Knowledge** Skills, procedures, and processes (including the nursing process)	**Self-Knowledge** Awareness of your values, beliefs, and biases	**Patient Data** Physical, psychosocial, spiritual
Theoretical Knowledge Principles, facts, theories; what you have to think *with*	**Nursing Process** *Assessment and Evaluation:* Everything you know about the patient including context	**Ethical Knowledge** Understanding your obligations; sense of right and wrong	**Patient Preferences, Context** Context for care, environment, relationships, culture, resources, supports
	Planning and Implementation: What you do for the patient		

Table 2-3 ➤ Application of the Full-Spectrum Nursing Model

Patient Situation 1. When taking a patient's oral temperature, a nurse sees a glass of ice water on the overbed table. Realizing that a cold drink can reduce the accuracy of the temperature reading, she asks the patient, "How long since you've taken a drink of water?" The nurse is busy and tired, but she returns to take the patient's temperature again at a later time.

THINKING	DOING	CARING
Theoretical Knowledge The nurse realized that a cold drink can lower the temperature reading. The nurse used interviewing principles to get more information from the patient. **Critical Thinking** The nurse recognized relevant information and identified the need for more information. She used the patient's answer to decide what to do. Being aware of context is also critical thinking. The context in this scenario includes ice water within the patient's reach and that the patient was physically capable of reaching it.	**Practical Knowledge** The nurse used a psychomotor skill when she measured the patient's temperature to acquire more patient vital sign data and a communication process to question the patient. **Nursing Process (Assessment)** The nurse observed the glass of ice water on the table. The nurse asked, "How long since you've taken a drink of water?" The nurse also observed the environmental data (e.g., ice water at the bedside). *(Implementation)* The nurse took the patient's temperature.	**Ethical Knowledge** The scenario does not say this, but a caring nurse, even a very busy one, would not be annoyed with the patient for the inconvenience of having to come back again to take the temperature. Self-knowledge might include the nurse's awareness that she is tired and feeling irritable. Ethical knowledge would tell her that she has an obligation to obtain an accurate temperature from the patient, rather than thinking, "Oh, I'll just record the reading a degree or two higher, as it doesn't matter that much."

THINKING	DOING	CARING

Patient Situation 2. Thirty minutes after giving a pain medication, a nurse checks with the patient to see whether the pain has been relieved. The nurse is using the desired outcome ("States pain relief is adequate . . .") as a criterion for evaluating the effectiveness of the nursing activity. The patient says, "I don't think that medicine is helping a bit." On a scale of 1 to 10, the patient reports her pain as 9. The nurse notifies the primary care provider to request an increase in the dosage of pain medication. She then gives the new medication to the patient and, even though it is the end of her shift, she sits with the patient to help him use guided imagery and deep breathing strategies to reduce his pain until the medication takes effect.

THINKING	DOING	CARING
Theoretical Knowledge The nurse had theoretical knowledge of the interval needed for the medication to take effect. She also knew facts and principles about pain rating scales and strategies to relieve pain without medication. **Critical Thinking** Criterion-based evaluation is a critical-thinking skill. The nurse applied knowledge of the medication's action to know when to evaluate the patient's response to it. She realized she needed more data about the patient's pain scale. She was also able to generate more interventions, such as requesting an adjustment in the dosage of medication and using guided imagery and deep breathing.	**Practical Knowledge** The nurse undoubtedly used practical knowledge when administering the medication (e.g., knowledge of how to administer the medication) and helping the patient with guided imagery and deep breathing to distract him from his pain. **Nursing Process (Assessment)** The nurse had apparently previously assessed the patient, identified a nursing diagnosis of Acute Pain, set a desired outcome, implemented an intervention, and then evaluated its effect based on new patient data. She also implemented care when she called the primary provider, administered the medication, and used guided imagery and deep breathing. In addition to data about the pain, you might assume that the nurse knew the following about the context: From the way the goal is stated, we can assume that the patient can speak. The patient is most likely hospitalized because he is not administering his own medication, and the nurse plans to check on him in 30 min. Certainly the nurse had all that contextual information.	**Ethical Knowledge** The nurse served as a patient advocate when she telephoned the care provider for a new prescription. She cared enough about the patient to stay with him and help him reduce the intensity of his pain using nonpharmacological methods until the new medication took effect, even though this meant working late. **Self-Knowledge** Perhaps this nurse values a stoic, "tough it out," response to pain. Knowing this about herself, she could put this aside and see the reality of suffering for the patient and how the experience of pain is individual and personal.

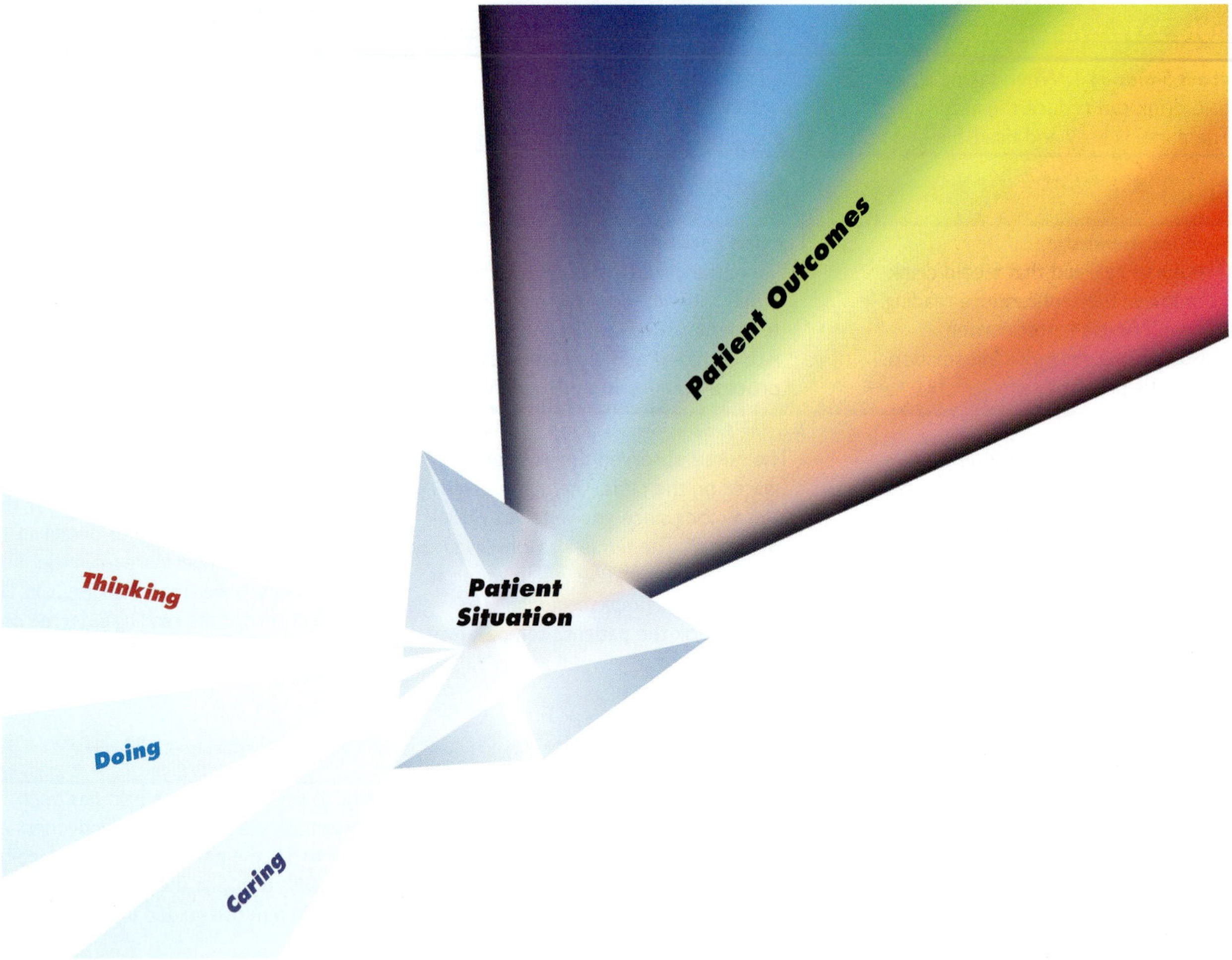

FIGURE 2-3 Model of full-spectrum nursing.

Toward Evidence-Based Practice

Eisenhauer, L.A., Hurley, A. C., & Dolan, N. (2007). Nurses' reported thinking during medication administration. *Journal of Nursing Scholarship, 39*(1), 82–87.

This study used interviews and real-time tape recordings to document 40 nurses' self-reported thinking processes during medication administration. They identified that nurses used judgment in dosage, timing, and selection of specific medications, and that these situations provided the best data about nurses' use of critical thinking. A key element was the nurses' constant professional vigilance to ensure that patients received the correct medications. Researchers concluded that nurses' thinking processes extended beyond following rules and procedures, and were based on patient data and professional knowledge.

1. What examples of full-spectrum nursing can you see in this brief abstract?

2. Based on this abstract, which of the following questions might this study answer satisfactorily for you? Explain your reasoning.
   a. Do nurses use critical thinking in many aspects of patient care?
   b. Do some nurses use critical thinking when administering medications?
   c. Do all nurses use critical thinking when administering medications?
   d. Which of the 40 nurses demonstrated the highest level of critical thinking?

   Go to Chapter 2, **Toward Evidence-Based Practice Suggested Responses,** on Davis*Plus.*

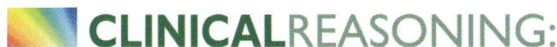 **CLINICAL**REASONING:
Applying the **Full-Spectrum Nursing Model**

Because the following critical thinking activities allow you to practice the kind of thinking you will use as a full-spectrum nurse, they usually have no single right answer. Discuss them with your peers—if you have difficulty with any of the questions, consult your instructor.

PATIENT SITUATION

Mrs. Castillo has late-stage cancer and is not expected to live more than a few months. With chemotherapy, she could live perhaps a year or two more. She cannot decide what to do. She knows that the chemotherapy will have unpleasant side effects, and be very expensive, and she wants to protect her family from the emotional and financial hardships of a lingering illness. She is showing physical signs of anxiety and distress (e.g., increased heart rate, restlessness, tearfulness). You want to provide support for her decision, whatever it may be.

THINKING

1. *Theoretical Knowledge:* What theoretical knowledge do you need to help Mrs. Castillo?
2. *Critical Thinking (Contextual Awareness):* What details in the scenario represent "patient situation" or "context"?

DOING

3. *Practical Knowledge:*
   a. What practical knowledge do you need to help Mrs. Castillo?
   b. Which skills can you already do, and which ones would you need to learn or review before caring for this patient?

CARING

4. *Ethical Knowledge:* Depending on Mrs. Castillo's decision, can you think of one ethical issue that might arise for you or members of her family later on?

 Go To Chapter 2, **Clinical Reasoning: Applying the Full-Spectrum Nursing Model Response Sheet** on *DavisPlus.*

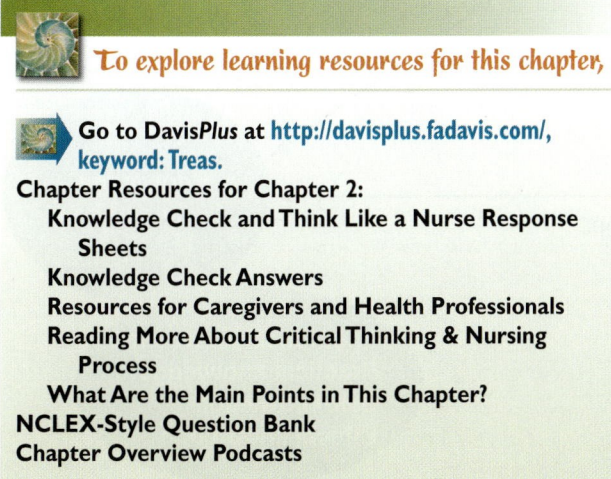

To explore learning resources for this chapter,

Go to Davis*Plus* at http://davisplus.fadavis.com/, **keyword: Treas.**
Chapter Resources for Chapter 2:
    Knowledge Check and Think Like a Nurse Response Sheets
    Knowledge Check Answers
    Resources for Caregivers and Health Professionals
    Reading More About Critical Thinking & Nursing Process
    What Are the Main Points in This Chapter?
NCLEX-Style Question Bank
Chapter Overview Podcasts

Concept Map

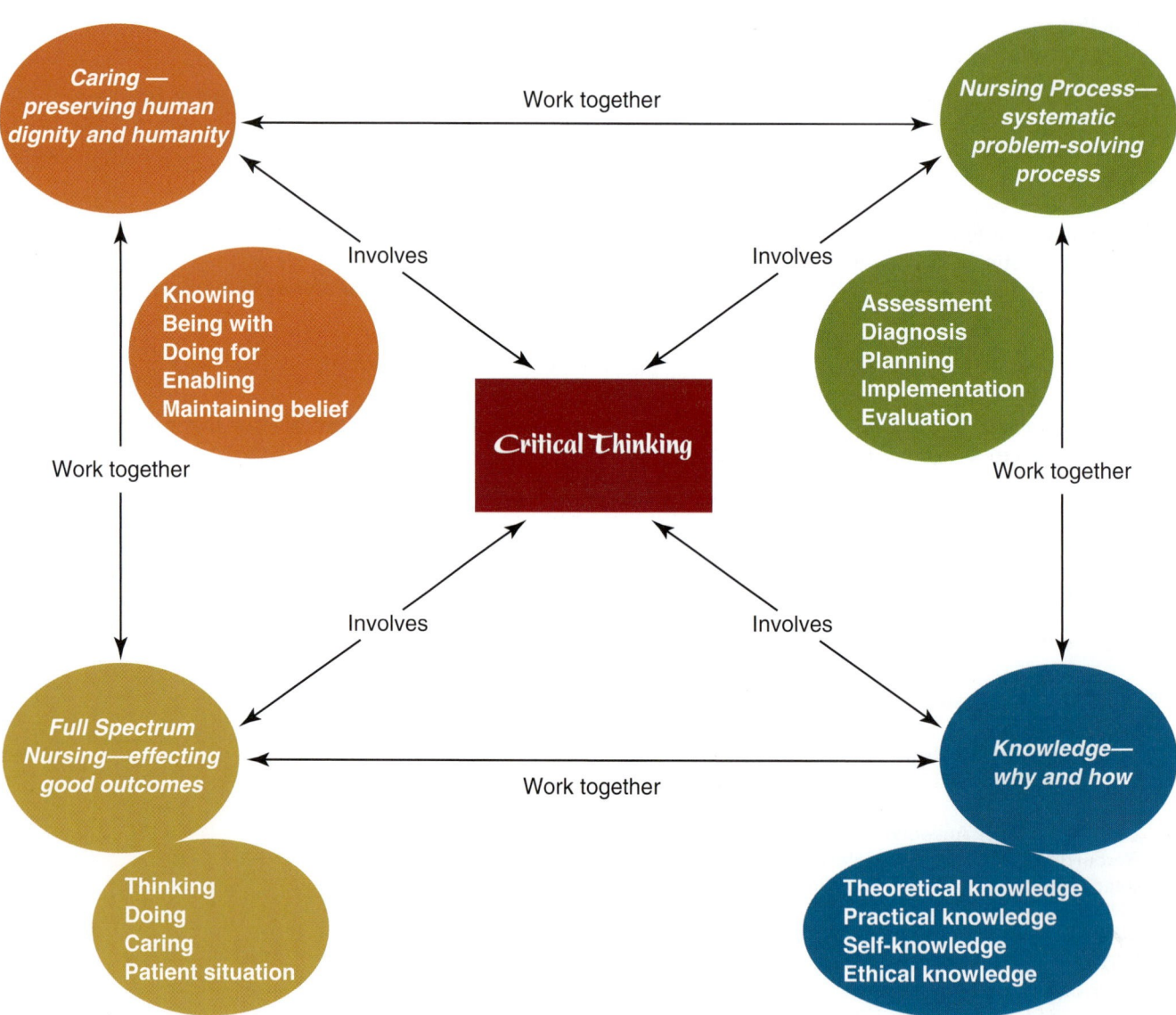

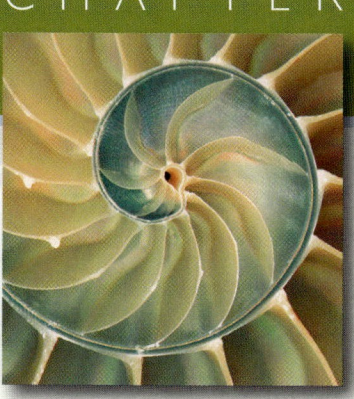

CHAPTER 3

Assessment

Learning Outcomes

After completing this chapter, you should be able to:

➤ Define *nursing assessment,* including the four features common to all its definitions.

➤ Explain how assessment is related to each of the other steps of the nursing process.

➤ State the ANA position on delegating assessment.

➤ Name the requirements of the Joint Commission regarding patient assessment.

➤ Use assessment skills to gather data during a nursing assessment.

➤ Describe initial, ongoing, comprehensive, focused, and special needs assessment and state when or why you would use each.

➤ Explain the importance of discharge planning assessment.

➤ Identify the following types of data: subjective, objective, primary source, and secondary source.

➤ Identify at least four components of a nursing health history and state the purpose of each.

➤ Discuss how to prepare for and conduct an interview.

➤ Compare and contrast open-ended and closed questions.

➤ Describe three circumstances in which you should validate data.

➤ Use nursing frameworks to organize data.

➤ State four guidelines for documenting data.

➤ Compose three questions to use when evaluating the quality of your assessments.

Key Concepts

Assessment

Data

Related Concepts

See the Concept Map at the end of this chapter.

Caring for the Nguyens

This feature allows you to practice the kind of thinking you will use as a full-spectrum nurse. There is usually more than one correct answer to a critical thinking question, so we do not provide answers for these features. It is more important to develop your nursing judgment than to "cover content." Discuss the questions with your peers. If you are still unsure, consult your instructor.

Review the opening scenario of Nam Nguyen in the front of the book. Imagine you are the clinic nurse at the Family Medicine Center. Based on the information in the scenario, work through the following questions:

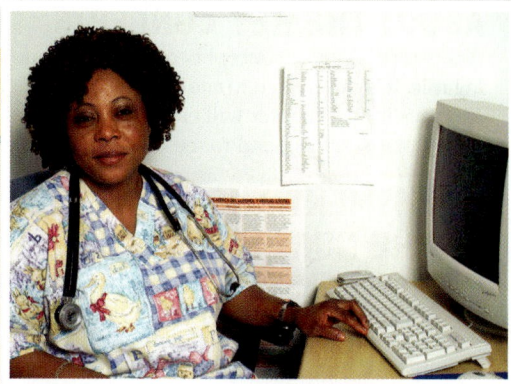

A. What type of assessment, comprehensive or focused, is being performed at this clinic visit? Explain your thinking.

B. Identify the types of data (e.g., subjective/objective, primary/secondary) that have been gathered so far. Give an example of each type.

(Continued)

Caring for the Nguyens (continued)

C. How might you verify data that Mr. Nguyen provided on the intake sheet?

D. Based on what you know about Mr. Nguyen, what follow-up assessments would provide useful data to help with

the care of Mr. Nguyen? Why would you make these assessments?

 Go to **Caring for the Nguyens Response Sheet** on *DavisPlus*.

Meet Your Patient

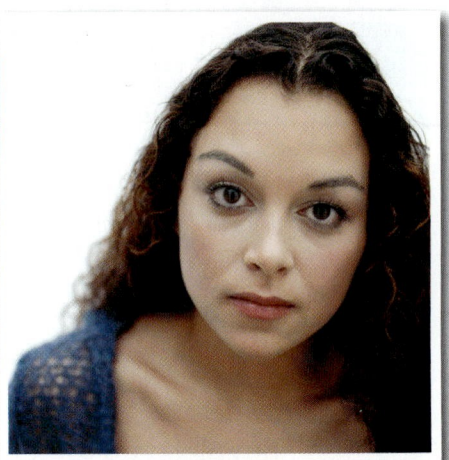

As the intake nurse in a community-based clinic in Miami, Florida, your role is to complete a comprehensive nursing assessment and initiate a plan of care for the clients. Your first client is a 27-year-old single woman, Sami, who is requesting clinic services for her general healthcare needs. Sami is Cuban American and lives alone in a one-bedroom apartment. She works as a fitness trainer at the local YMCA while attending college part-time. Her family lives in Tampa, Florida. Sami's earnings place her at the poverty level. She realizes that she must have access to healthcare to prevent health problems and to detect and receive treatment of illnesses should they arise. You will be asked to apply full-spectrum thinking to Sami's case throughout the chapter as you learn the concepts of assessment.

Theoretical Knowledge
knowing **why**

In this section, you will learn about the role of assessment in the nursing process and collaborative care; about various types of assessment, including comprehensive assessment; and about data.

ABOUT THE KEY CONCEPTS

Assessment is a key concept because it is so integral to the nursing role. It is closely tied to another key concept: data. The related concepts in this chapter will enable you to fully understand the notion of assessment and to see how they all fit together.

ASSESSMENT: THE FIRST STEP OF THE NURSING PROCESS

Assessment is the systematic gathering of information related to the physiological, psychological, sociocultural, developmental, and spiritual status of an individual, group, or community. Although various definitions exist, all definitions of assessment include the following features: collecting data, categorizing data, recording data, and using a systematic and ongoing process.

The purpose of assessment is to obtain data to allow you to help the patient. The nursing interview and the physical assessment findings become a part of the **patient database** (all the pertinent patient data obtained by nurses and other health professionals). You will use the facts, impressions, and contextual information obtained in your assessment to develop a plan of care.

How Is Assessment Related to Other Steps of the Nursing Process?

Assessment is the first phase of the nursing process. Data must be accurate and complete, because the remainder of the nursing process rests on this foundation of data. Assessment is related to other nursing process steps, as follows (Fig. 3-1):

- *Diagnosis*—Assessment provides the data necessary for identifying client problems and strengths.
- *Planning outcomes*—Data about the client's motivation, family, and available resources help you formulate realistic goals.
- *Planning interventions*—Assessment data help you to choose the most effective interventions.
- *Implementation*—As you perform nursing actions, you will also gather data by observing the client's responses to your interventions. For example, while helping a client ambulate, you might observe that the client becomes short of breath. If this is new information, you might then identify a new diagnosis of Activity Intolerance.
- *Evaluation*—After performing interventions for nursing diagnoses, you assess client responses. This *reassessment* provides the basis for changes in the care plan.

How Does Nursing Assessment Fit Into Collaborative Care?

As a nurse, you will focus on your clients' *responses* to illness, which include their physical responses, their understanding of the illness, how the illness affects their lives and their ability to care for themselves, and their emotional responses and concerns. You will also use assessment with healthy clients to help them identify ways to maintain their

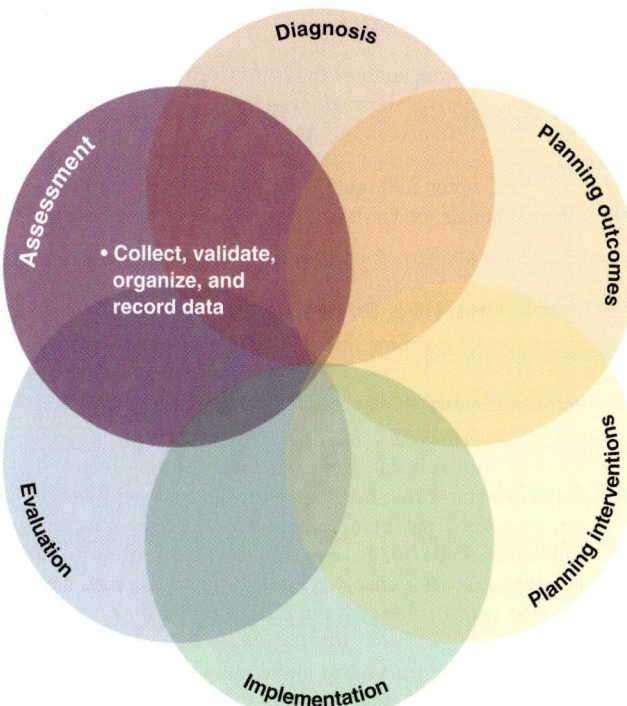

FIGURE 3-1 Nursing process: assessment.

current level of wellness and prevent disease. This is different from medical assessments, which focus on identifying disease.

Other healthcare professionals can access the database created from the nursing assessment findings. In some settings, the nurse reviews the database and delegates or makes referrals to other professionals with expertise in a particular area of healthcare. This helps ensure that clients receive proper care by qualified individuals at the time it is needed.

To illustrate, use Sami's case: Sami has not had a gynecological (female) examination for 5 years. She tells you that her mother has had breast cancer and that her sister is being treated for endometriosis. You first ask whether, because of any religious or other beliefs, Sami would be offended by an open discussion. Then you ask about her sexual activity, assuring her that you will keep all information confidential. As a result of this interview, you encourage Sami to get a women's health examination as soon as possible. She agrees, and you refer her to a women's clinic, where she will be charged according to her ability to pay.

What Do Professional Standards Say About Assessment?

Standards of governmental agencies, professional organizations, and accrediting bodies, such as the following, emphasize that complete, skillful, and timely assessment of all clients is an important skill for nurses in all healthcare settings.

The American Nurses Association (ANA) standards for clinical practice, which apply to professional nurses (registered nurses [RNs]), identify assessment as a professional responsibility (Box 3-1).

Nurse practice acts regulate the practice of nurses in individual states. The National Council of State Boards of Nursing (2011, Article II, Section 2) *Model Nursing Practice Act* also asserts that the scope of nursing includes surveillance and comprehensive assessment of the health status of individuals, families, groups, and communities.

The Joint Commission (2008, Section 1, pp. 171–179) identifies assessment as an essential element of patient care. In agencies in which there is an RN on staff, the RN must assess patients' needs for nursing care within 24 hours of inpatient admission. The Joint Commission standards require agencies to provide evidence that

- Assessments are written, comprehensive, and used to identify and assign priorities for care.
- Agency policy designates (1) when each patient is to be reassessed and (2) which disciplines can make which assessments.
- All patients are assessed for pain (p. 186).

KnowledgeCheck 3-1

- What are the four features common to all definitions of assessment?
- How is a nursing assessment similar to a medical assessment?
- How is it different?

Can I Delegate Assessments?

For data to be reliable, a professional nurse must perform the assessment portion of the nursing process. Nurse aides or other nursing assistive personnel (NAP) and licensed practical nurses (LPNs) may collect patient information such as temperature, height, and weight. However, it is the responsibility of the professional nurse to assign those tasks, validate the data collected, conduct the interview, and complete the physical assessment. The ANA's *Code of Ethics for Nurses*, Provision 4 (2008), states, "The nurse . . . determines the appropriate delegation of tasks consistent with the nurse's obligation to provide optimum patient care." See Chapters 7 in this book and Chapter 45, on *DavisPlus* for a thorough discussion of delegation of tasks to NAPs. The following resources can guide you in deciding which caregivers are qualified to perform parts or all of an assessment:

- *State nurse practice acts.* Each state nurse practice act specifies which portions of the assessment can legally be completed by individuals with different credentials. Look for statements related to delegation. For example, the definitions in the National Council of State boards of Nursing (NCSBN) *Model Nursing Practice Act* (2011) differentiate between assessments by RNs and LPNs/LVNs (Box 3-2).

BOX 3-2 ■ NCSBN Model Nursing Practice Act (2010), Nursing Assessment Definitions

Comprehensive Assessment by the RN

An extensive data collection for individuals, families, groups, and communities:
- Addressing anticipated and emerging changes in conditions in client's health status
- Recognizing alterations to previous client conditions
- Synthesizing the biological, psychological, and social aspects of the client's condition
- Evaluating the impact of nursing care
- Using this broad and complete analysis to make independent decisions and nursing diagnoses
- Planning nursing interventions
- Evaluating need for different interventions
- Communicating the need to communicate and consult with other health team members.

Focused Assessment by the LPN/LVN

An appraisal of an individual's status and situation at hand, contributing to comprehensive assessment by the registered nurse, supporting ongoing data collection, and deciding who needs to be informed of the information and when to inform.

Source: Adapted from the NCSBN Web site (http://www.ncsbn.org) and used by permission from the National Council of State Boards of Nursing (NCSBN) 2010.

- *Agency policies/procedures,* such as how often to change a urinary catheter
- *Accrediting agencies,* such as the Joint Commission
- *The American Nurses Association (ANA) Scope and Standards of Practice* (2010). To access the ANA Web site,

 Go to Chapter 3, **Resources for Caregivers & Health Professionals,** on DavisPlus.

ThinkLike a Nurse 3-1

Think about the following situations, then answer the questions. More than one answer may be acceptable. Compare your ideas with those of other students, and if you have any questions, consult your instructor.

- Suppose you are a nurse in a healthcare setting where the policy states that nursing assistive personnel (NAP) can take vital signs (blood pressure, pulse, temperature, and respirations). You have a patient who is critically ill and whose condition is changing rapidly. Would you measure the vital signs or delegate the task to the NAP? Why or why not?
- Imagine that you are a nurse in the same hospital on a different day. All but one NAP have called in sick today because of an influenza outbreak. This NAP is inexperienced and overwhelmed by her tasks. Would you bathe the patients in your caseload (even though that is usually done by a NAP), or would you ask the NAP to do it? Why or why not?

It is obvious from the previous examples that you must use good judgment when applying standards and policies and deciding when to delegate assessments.

Sources of Data

Subjective data (*covert data, symptoms*) are the information communicated to the nurse by the client, family, or community. Subjective data reveal the perspective of the person giving the data, and include thoughts, feelings, beliefs, and sensations. Thus, subjective data from two different people can vary. For example, people with insomnia often report getting much less sleep than their sleep partner says they do. Subjective data can be used to clarify objective data (e.g., "How did you get this scar?"). Some people (e.g., infants, adults in mental illness) are unable to provide subjective data. Others can give subjective data, but you might question their accuracy. For example, how credible is a diabetic patient's response that she complies with a diabetic diet and medication regimen when her blood sugar level is markedly elevated? What could you do to double-check the subjective data?

Objective data (*overt data, signs*) are gathered through a physical assessment or from laboratory or diagnostic tests. They can be measured or observed by the nurse or other healthcare providers. Examples are vital signs, x-ray results, skin color, and urine output. One use of objective data is to validate (check) subjective data. In the preceding example, if you thought the report of dietary intake and insulin use was inaccurate, you would measure the blood sugar and ask for a dietary journal.

You may also use objective data to verify subjective information that seems accurate. For example, when Sami told you her family and sexual history, you learned that she has significant risk factors for breast and cervical cancer and referred her for a gynecological exam. The results of the breast exam and Pap smear (Papanicolaou test, a smear of cervical cells) provide objective data related to these risk factors.

Primary data are the subjective and objective information obtained from the client: what the client says or what you observe. **Secondary data** are obtained secondhand, for example, from the medical record or from another caregiver. A client's husband may say, "She seems more confused than usual." Or the NAP may report, "Mr. Atlas's heart rate was 100 beats per minute this morning." If you count the heart rate yourself, though, it is primary data. Table 3-1 provides further examples of types and sources of data.

Table 3-1 ▶ Examples of Data Types	
Data Types	
SUBJECTIVE DATA	**OBJECTIVE DATA**
"I have been having a lot of pain in my abdomen."	Suprapubic area firm to light palpation. Lower abdomen semisoft.
"My throat hurts when I swallow."	White patches noted at the back of the throat and tonsillar area reddened and swollen.
"Our children have no place to go after football games. That is why they get into so much trouble."	In a windshield survey, no public facility was open after football games to allow young people to socialize under supervision.
Data Sources	
PRIMARY SOURCE (CLIENT)	**SECONDARY SOURCES (EVERYTHING ELSE)**
Pulse rate 100 beats/min	From chart: WBC count 14,000/mm^3.
States feeling short of breath.	In transfer report, nurse states that the surgical dressing is dry.
Abdomen tender on palpation.	Client's wife states that he has been tired a lot lately.

KnowledgeCheck 3-2

During Sami's appointment at the women's clinic, she has a Pap smear, breast exam, and blood work. She also informs the nurse that her menstrual flow is very heavy and that she experiences severe abdominal cramping. All of these data are added to the database as references for future visits. Sami's Pap smear results and breast exam are normal, but she is moderately anemic (she has a low hemoglobin level). When the nurse sees the lab results, she suspects that the heavy flow may be causing Sami's anemia. According to clinic protocol, she prescribes birth control pills for Sami to control her heavy, painful periods and provide contraception. Ongoing assessment will include visits every 6 months to evaluate her birth control pills and monitor the anemia. State whether the following data are primary or secondary, subjective or objective:

- You see in Sami's health record that her breast exam was normal.

- Sami tells the nurse that she experiences cramping with her menstrual cycle. *For the nurse*, is this primary or secondary, subjective or objective data?
- The nurse tells you that Sami is anemic.
- You check the result of the Pap smear in her electronic health record and see that it is normal.

Types of Assessment

Assessment can be broad and general or very specific. The type of assessment you do depends on the client's status. In acute care settings, such as the emergency department, the assessments are rapid and focused on the presenting problem. In inpatient settings, you may perform an initial comprehensive assessment at admission and other, more focused assessments over time, according to the client's needs.

Initial and Ongoing Assessments

An **initial (admission) assessment** is completed when the client first comes to the healthcare agency. First obtain data related to the person's reason for seeking nursing or medical assistance. Then complete a comprehensive assessment if the client's condition permits. Data gathered from the initial assessment provide guidance for care and determine the need for further assessment. Initial assessment data tend to be static; for example, demographic data (marital status, occupation) are not likely to change often.

Ongoing assessment is performed as needed, at any time after the initial database is completed. Ideally, you will make at least some observations at every contact with a client. You use data from ongoing assessments to identify new problems or to follow up on previously identified problems. In comparison to the initial assessment, ongoing assessment reflects the ever-changing state of the client. For example, vital signs may change rapidly, which is an important indicator of developing or resolving health problems.

Comprehensive Assessments

A **comprehensive assessment** (also called a *global assessment, patient database,* or *nursing database*) provides holistic information about the client's overall health status. It enables you to identify client problems and strengths. You need comprehensive data to enhance your sensitivity to a patient's culture, values, beliefs, and economic situation.

A comprehensive assessment contains both subjective and objective data. Figure 3-2 shows what information is gathered in an initial comprehensive assessment (database) and how it fits into the broad concept of assessment in the nursing process. Whether assessment is initial or ongoing, comprehensive, or focused, you will use the skills of observation, physical examination, and interviewing to collect data. To see a nursing admission data form,

 Go to Chapter 3, Tables, Boxes, Figures: **Nursing Admission Data Form**, on Davis*Plus*.

A comprehensive assessment is organized into three sections: observations, physical examination, and the nursing history (or interview).

Observation refers to the deliberate use of all of your senses to gather and interpret patient and environmental data. All that you see, hear, feel, or smell becomes data in the context of assessment. You should try to use the same sequence of observation at each patient contact. By making systematic observations each time you are with a patient, you

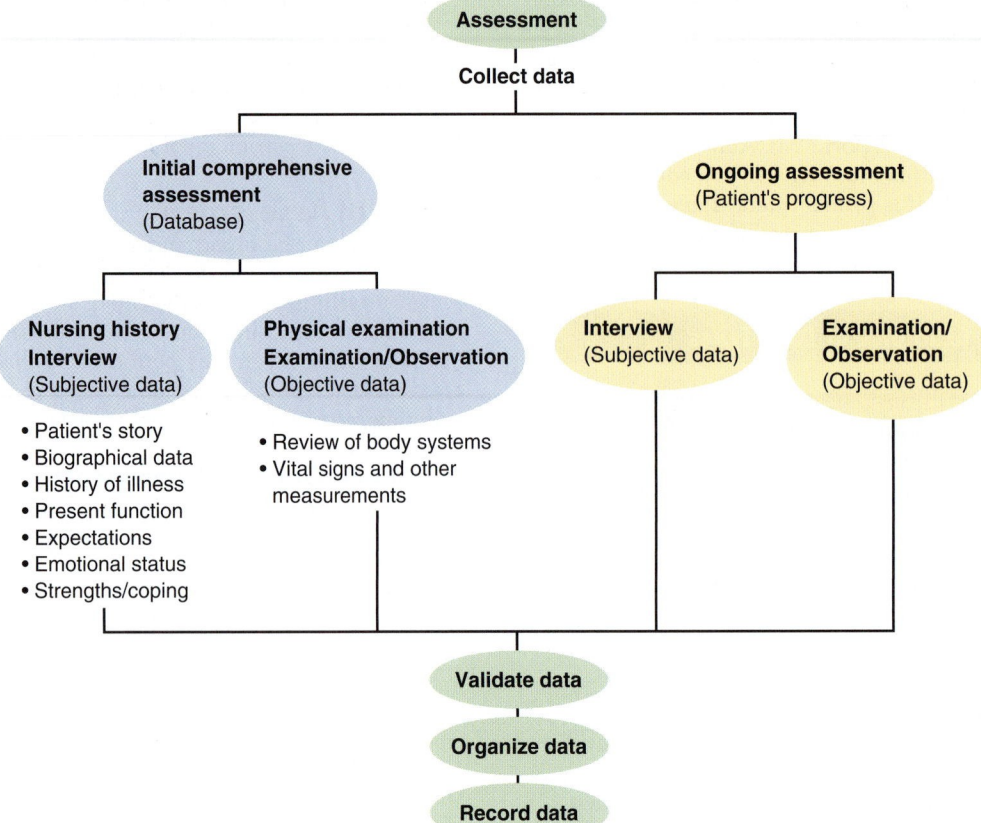

FIGURE 3-2 Overview of assessment content and methods. (*Source*: Wilkinson, J. M. [2011]. *Nursing process and critical thinking* [5th ed.], p. 78. Reprinted by permission of Pearson Education, Inc. Upper Saddle River, NJ.)

are less likely to miss an assessment area. The mnemonic (memory aid) in Box 3-3 may help you.

Physical assessment (or *physical examination*) produces primarily objective data and makes use of the techniques of inspection (visual examination), palpation (touch), percussion (tapping a body surface), direct auscultation (listening with the unaided ear), and indirect auscultation (listening with a stethoscope). All of these are described in detail in Chapter 21.

BOX 3-3 ■ Mnemonic for Systematic Observing

Use the first letter of each word to systematically help you when entering a patient's room.

HELP!!

Help. Observe first signs the patient may need help. Look for signs of distress (e.g., pain, pallor, labored breathing).

Environment and equipment. Next look for safety hazards (spills, equipment cords, sharps). Check to see that all equipment is working: IV line running? Catheter draining?

Look more closely. Examine the patient thoroughly for appearance, breathing, condition of dressings, correct positioning, skin color and condition, odors, condition of linens, and any other clues that might indicate a need for care.

People. Who are the people in the room? Family? Other caregivers? What are they doing?

The Nursing History (Interview). A **nursing interview** is purposeful, structured communication in which you question the patient to gather subjective data for the nursing database. You will learn about the components of a nursing history, and also about interview techniques, in the Practical Knowledge: Knowing How section.

KnowledgeCheck 3-3

Give at least two more examples of data you might obtain with each of your following senses. One example is provided for each.

- Touch (e.g., bladder distention)
- Vision (e.g., facial expression of pain)
- Smell (e.g., fecal odor)
- Hearing (e.g., bowel sounds)

Focused Assessments

A **focused assessment** is performed to obtain data about an actual, potential, or possible problem that has been identified or is suspected. It focuses on a particular topic, body part, or functional ability rather than on overall health status (e.g., a pain assessment or a lifestyle assessment). These specialized assessments add to the database created by the comprehensive initial assessment. An *initial focused assessment* is used to follow up on client-reported symptoms or unusual findings during the first exam (e.g., on admission to a hospital). An *ongoing focused assessment* is used to evaluate the status of existing problems and goals. Consider the following examples:

Initial focused assessment. When the nurse asks Mr. Jacobs why he has come to the clinic today, he replies, "I can't

get rid of this pain in my foot." The nurse asks questions to get in-depth information about this symptom. For example, When did it begin? On a scale of 1 to 10, how severe is it? What makes it worse? What do you do to make it feel better? She also examines the foot for joint mobility, redness, edema, and tenderness to touch.

Ongoing focused assessment. After surgery, Ms. King has a nursing diagnosis of Acute Pain secondary to abdominal incision. The nurse assesses her pain level at least every 2 hours and before and after administering pain medication.

ThinkLike a Nurse 3-2

- Give examples of each type of assessment (initial, ongoing, comprehensive, focused) using patients you have observed or cared for or your own personal experiences as a patient.
- How might age and developmental stage make a difference in your assessment of a patient?
- Suppose you are the triage nurse at the community clinic in the Meet Your Patient scenario. What kind of assessment do you perform at Sami's first visit (initial, ongoing, comprehensive, focused)? What type will the care provider at the women's clinic perform?

Special Needs Assessments

A **special needs assessment** is a type of focused assessment. It provides in-depth information about a particular area of client functioning and often involves using a specially designed form. The Joint Commission requires certain special needs assessments (e.g., of nutrition status and pain) for all clients. In some settings, such as hospice, home health, and rehabilitation settings, other special needs assessments (e.g., of functional abilities) are also required. You should perform a special needs assessment at any time assessment cues suggest risk factors or problems in an area of client functioning.

Teaching Self-Assessment

Self-Care

As you learned in Chapters 1 and 2, it is essential for nurses to provide information that will help clients to care for themselves. One important aspect of self-care is performing regular self-assessments to detect symptoms of disease. Before you begin teaching, make the following assessments:

➤ Readiness and willingness of your client to learn some type of assessment.

➤ Client's current knowledge or understanding of the topic to be discussed.

The following are important assessments that every person needs to know:

➤ Breast self-exam or testicular self-exam—monthly (Note that this is not currently recommended by all care providers or all best practice guidelines.)

➤ Skin assessment—daily but at least weekly

➤ Feet assessment—daily if diabetic or elderly, otherwise weekly

See Chapter 21 for details of these assessments.

Special needs assessments can be quite lengthy; therefore, you need to think carefully about when and how to use them. You need enough data to provide holistic care, but you must balance this need against the need not to intrude on the client's privacy. The data you obtain should enhance the care provided to the client and add to the comprehensive assessment. The following are some special needs assessments:

- **Functional Ability Assessment.** Health problems and normal aging changes often bring a decline in functional status. Functional ability is especially important in discharge planning and home care. Future rehabilitation needs are derived from initial and ongoing functional ability assessments. The Joint Commission (2008) requires a functional ability assessment for all patients "as appropriate." The following three functional assessment tools are commonly used:
  - **The Katz Index of ADL Scale (1963).** This instrument is one of the best for assessing independent performance in very basic areas. It assigns 1 point for independence in each of the following areas: bathing, dressing, toileting, transfer, continence, and feeding (Wallace & Shelkey, 2007). Nurses often use the data to plan staffing and appropriate placement of clients. See Box 3-4 for questions to

BOX 3-4 ■ Questions for Assessing Independence in Activities of Daily Living

Mobility
Does the client require devices (e.g., cane, crutches, walker, wheelchair) for support?

Transfer
Can the client get in and out of bed and in and out of a chair without assistance?
If not, how much help does the client need?
Is the client completely confined to bed?

Bathing
Can the client perform a sponge bath, tub bath, or shower bath with no help?
If not, specifically what assistance does the client need?

Dressing
Can the client get all necessary clothing from drawers and closets and get dressed without help?
If not, specifically what assistance does the client need?

Feeding
Can the client feed self without assistance?
If not, specifically what assistance does the client need (e.g., help with cutting meat)?

Toileting
Can the client go to the bathroom, use the toilet, clean self, and rearrange clothing without help?
If a night bedpan or commode is used, can the client empty and clean it independently?
If the client needs help with these activities, specifically what does it include?

Continence
Does the client independently control urination and bowel movements?
If not, how often is the client incontinent of bladder or bowel?
Does the client require an indwelling urinary catheter?

use when assessing activities of daily living (ADLs). For a link to the Katz scale,

 Go to Chapter 3, **Resources for Caregivers and Health Professionals, Functional Assessment,** on DavisPlus.

- **Lawton Instrumental Activities of Daily Living (IADL) Scale (1969).** This easy-to-use tool is particularly helpful in assessing a person's ability to independently perform the more sophisticated tasks of everyday life, such as shopping. Identifying early functional decline is important for discharge planning. The Lawton scale is especially useful for older adults, who may begin to experience functional decline within 48 hours of hospital admission (Graf, 2008; Lawton & Brody, 1969). The eight activities assessed are the following: using the telephone, getting to places beyond walking distance, shopping for groceries, preparing meals, doing housework or home repairs, doing laundry, taking medications, and managing money. To see and use the Lawton scale,

 Go to Chapter 3, Tables, Boxes, Figures, **ESG Box 3-2: Lawton IADL,** on DavisPlus.

- **The Karnofsky Performance Scale** (Karnofsky & Burchenal, 1949). This tool is used primarily in palliative care settings to assess functional abilities at the end of life. To see this tool,

 Go to Chapter 3, Tables, Boxes, Figures, **ESG Box 3-2: KarnofskyPerformance Scale,** on DavisPlus.

- **Nutritional Assessment.** See Chapter 28 for more information about nutritional assessment.
- **Pain Assessment.** Recall that accrediting agency (e.g., the Joint Commission) standards require you to perform a thorough pain assessment on all patients during initial and ongoing assessments. See Chapter 32 for more information on pain assessments.
- **Cultural Assessment.** For content included in a cultural assessment, see Chapter 15.
- **Spiritual Health Assessment.** See Chapter 16 for detailed information on assessing spiritual health.
- **Psychosocial Assessment.** Perform a focused psychosocial assessment if initial assessment data indicate that social and emotional needs are not being met (e.g., if the client is very anxious or exhibiting symptoms of stress), or if sociocultural factors (e.g., unemployment) present a risk to health. See Chapter 13 for more details.
- **Wellness Assessment.** Health promotion focuses on activities of a well person to achieve a higher level of health. See Chapter 27 for a more detailed discussion of assessing wellness.
- **Family Assessment.** Family assessment is discussed in Chapter 14.
- **Community Assessment.** Community assessment provides information about community demographics, resources, health concerns, points of referral, environmental risks, and community norms and values. See Chapter 41 for more information about community assessment.

 Think**Like a Nurse** 3-3

Based on the data you have so far about Sami, consider the need to perform any of the special-purpose assessments. What is your rationale for using or not using a special needs assessment?

PracticalKnowledge knowing**how**

In this chapter, practical knowledge involves your skill in using structured and unstructured methods of data collection, as well as validating, organizing, and documenting your assessment findings.

WHAT ARE THE COMPONENTS OF A NURSING HEALTH HISTORY?

Suppose that an elderly man has a fractured hip. The physician is interested in the cause of the fracture, the extent of the injury, and any preexisting medical problems that suggest the client is a poor surgical risk. As the nurse, you would also ask about the cause of the injury but you would want to know what effect the injury has on the man's ability to perform his everyday activities. You would also identify supports and strengths to begin planning for his eventual discharge and self-care. So you see, the nursing health history covers some of the same topics as the medical history, but the rationale for the questions is different.

Health history forms vary according to purpose among agencies (e.g., inpatient, clinic, surgery, medical, emergency room), but most include the following subjective information:

- **Biographical Data.** This is relatively unchanging information, such as name, address, age, gender, race, religion, marital status, and occupation. The person's responses to these questions reflect his mental status and ability to communicate.
- **Chief Complaint/Reason for Seeking Healthcare.** This is the client's perception of or reason for seeking medical or nursing advice. From this, you will be able to target your assessment to gather the most relevant and important data. For example, ask, "Tell me why you have come to the hospital today." The client might respond, "I just don't feel right," or "I'm having chest pain." Be sure to document the answer in the client's words, and follow up by asking him specifically what caused him to seek help (e.g., chest pain, a checkup).
- **History of Present Illness.** This is an in-depth exploration of the client's chief complaint. Find out when the illness or problem began, whether the onset was sudden or gradual, how often it occurs, what makes it worse, what the person does to relieve it, how the client's health has changed from his usual status, and what effect the illness has had on his daily life.
- **Client's Perception of Health Status and Expectations for Care.** This includes the client's knowledge about his illness and its potential effects on his life. For example, does a client with arterial insufficiency believe his foot will be "normal" again? What does the client expect will be done for him (e.g., Does he understand that his foot will be amputated)? What does he want the nurses to do to help (e.g., Leave a light on at night, bring his medication)?
- **Past Health History.** Sometimes called the *medical history,* this includes childhood diseases and immunizations, previous hospitalizations, and previous surgeries. The past medical history helps guide your assessment and helps

you to understand some of the data you obtain. For example, if Sami tells you that she had her appendix out when she was 5 years old, you would expect to find a scar on her abdomen.

- **Family Health History.** This includes data on first-degree blood relatives such as mother, father, siblings, and maternal and paternal grandparents. It includes data about diseases they have had, their current state of health and chronic disease, whether or not they are alive, and cause of death if they are not. Risk factors for various illnesses and disorders (e.g., hypertension, allergies) are often tied to multigenerational health problems. The family history may also include a **genogram:** a pictorial tool to display the relationship of family members with pertinent health-related information (see Fig. 14-6 and Box 14-1).
- **Social History.** This includes information about family and other relationships, economic status, occupations, exposure to toxic materials, home and neighborhood conditions, and ethnicity. It also includes data about tobacco, alcohol, and drug use as well as exercise habits.
- **Medication (Nutritional Supplements, Herbs) History and Device Use.** Past and current medication usage may uncover some medical history the client has forgotten to disclose. As you continue with the assessment, you can direct questions toward previous episodes of medical treatment and use of medical devices, such as braces, inhalers, and home oxygen therapy. Also inquire about the use of vitamin and nutritional supplements and alternative-therapy medications such as herbal remedies.

✚ Data about current medications are essential because (1) they may interact with newly prescribed medications and (2) some may affect certain body symptoms, causing abnormalities in your assessment findings (e.g., skin color, laboratory values).

- **Complementary/Alternative Modalities (CAM).** These are therapies used instead of or in addition to the allopathic therapies recommended by physicians—for example, chiropractic care, homeopathy, aromatherapy, music therapy, massage therapy, energy work (therapeutic touch, Reiki), and acupressure or acupuncture. Such therapies can support or interfere with conventional therapies, so this is important information.
- **Review of Body Systems and Associated Functional Abilities.** This review consists of subjective data regarding body systems (e.g., Do you have a productive cough?). It includes functional abilities (e.g., difficulties with dressing, bathing, eating, and elimination). You can obtain this information during the physical assessment as well as in the interview.

ThinkLike a Nurse 3-4

The Quality and Safety Education for Nurses (QSEN) competency of patient-centered care identifies assessment as a necessary skill. The nurse is expected to elicit patient values, preferences, and expressed needs as part of the clinical interview (Cronenwett, Sherwood, Barnsteiner, et al., 2007). Where do you think this type of patient information fits into the preceding components of a nursing health history? Why?

INTERVIEWING PATIENTS

The admission interview is planned, but during ongoing assessment, the interview may be informal, brief, and narrowly focused. This section describes types of interviews and explains how to prepare for, conduct, and close an interview.

Types of Interviews

Interviews may be directive or nondirective. Use **directive interviewing** to obtain factual, easily categorized information (e.g., age, sex), or in an emergency situation. In this type of interview, you control the topics and ask mostly closed questions to obtain specific information. **Closed questions** are those that can be answered with a yes, no, or other short, factual answer. They usually begin with *who, when, where, what, do (did, does),* and *is (are, were).* Closed questions are useful for patients who are very anxious or who have communication difficulties.

When you want to promote communication, build rapport, or help the patient to express feeling, use **nondirective interviewing.** This means that you allow the patient to control the subject matter. Your role is to clarify, summarize, and ask mostly open-ended questions that facilitate thought and communication. **Open-ended questions** specify a topic to be explored, but are phrased broadly to encourage the patient to elaborate. Ask open-ended questions when you want to obtain subjective data.

Directive interviewing is efficient but may cause you to miss topics important to the patient. Nondirective interviewing allows you to find out what is important to the patient, but it is time consuming and can produce much irrelevant data. A successful interview includes both closed and open-ended questions. Use broad, open-ended questions to guide the patient to talk about certain topics. From the answers to the broad questions, you can decide which topics to clarify or follow up with specific and closed questions. Part of the interview with Sami might have gone like this:

NURSE	When was your last physical examination? *(closed question)*
SAMI	I had a female exam about 5 years ago.
NURSE	What problems have you had in that area? *(open-ended question)*
SAMI	None, really.
NURSE	What about other women in your family? *(open-ended question)*
SAMI	Well, my mother had breast cancer about the same time that I went for my checkup. She's OK now though.
NURSE	Go on . . . *(open-ended question)*
SAMI	And my sister has been taking some pills for endometriosis. She hasn't been able to get pregnant because of that.
NURSE	Are you sexually active? *(closed question)*
SAMI	Yes.
NURSE	Tell me about that. *(open-ended question)*

See Table 3-2 for other examples of closed and open-ended questions.

Preparing for the Interview

While they are learning, some students feel uncomfortable interviewing patients. You may have one of the following concerns:

- **You are imposing on the patient, who clearly needs rest more than you need information.** This may be because you believe a "real nurse" has already obtained the information, or because you don't have a clear idea of how the information will be used to help the patient.

Table 3-2 ➤ Examples of Closed and Open-Ended Questions	
CLOSED QUESTIONS	**OPEN-ENDED QUESTIONS**
Are you having any pain?	Tell me about your pain.
Do you ever drink excessively?	Tell me about your alcohol use.
Why did you come to this clinic?	I am glad to see you here today. Could you tell me a little bit about why you decided to come see us?
Do you have any family history of heart disease?	Tell me about your family members and what kind of experiences they may have had with heart disease or problems with circulation.
Are there any parks where you can walk safely?	Tell me about safe places here in your community where you might go to take a walk.

- **The patient won't be receptive to answering personal questions from a stranger (you).** To help set the tone for the interview, be sure to tell your patients that the information given will be kept confidential and that they can refuse to answer any question. Remember that the patient is free to choose what to tell you and what to withhold from you. Also be aware that the patient may have been feeling the need to talk about something, has not known how to bring it up, and is actually relieved that you have introduced the topic.
- **Some of your questions will upset the patient—the person will cry or become angry.** Remember that patients usually feel better after expressing their emotions. Expressions of strong emotion are hard to accept, but you must learn to do it. You will have large gaps in your data if you avoid difficult topics, and your patients will not get the help they need.

  Your interviews will go more smoothly if you take time to prepare yourself, your patient, and the interview space before you begin asking questions.

Prepare Yourself

Use the following guidelines when preparing yourself to interview a patient:

- Be sure you know the purpose of the interview and how the data will be used. As a student, this may simply mean preparing thoroughly for your clinical assignment.
- Read the patient's chart. This will give you an idea of where to start with the interview and keep you from covering topics already assessed by other caregivers. Keep an open mind because if you approach an interview with preconceived ideas, you may overlook important data.
- Form some goals for the interview, and think of some opening questions.
- Schedule some uninterrupted time for the interview. Giving the patient your undivided attention builds rapport and helps him to feel free to share information with you.

- Gather the necessary assessment forms and equipment. You will need a stethoscope, pen, pencil, blood pressure cuff, and thermometer.
- Take a deep breath and compose yourself just before entering the room.

Prepare the Space

Give some thought to the following guidelines for preparing the environment for the interview:

- Provide privacy (e.g., ask visitors to wait outside, shut the door) unless you need information from the visitor. The presence of even a close family member may inhibit the client in some situations.
- If others must be present, keep the focus on the client as much as possible. In some interviews, the client's spouse, family, or partner will offer information that may or may not be pertinent. Focus on the client, but do not ignore the information provided by others.
- Remove distractions (e.g., turn off the television, arrange for someone to watch children, if they are present).
- Position yourself at the same level as your client, even if the client is in bed. Sit down. Do not hover over the bed.

Prepare the Patient

The following actions will encourage your patient to be more receptive to the interview:

- Introduce yourself to the patient and others in the room.
- Call the patient by name; ask what name the patient prefers. Don't use endearing terms such as "grandma," "dear," and "sweetie." You may think you are being friendly or expressing caring, but many people feel belittled by these terms.
- Tell the patient what you will be doing and why. Explain that you will be taking notes and that you will keep all information confidential. Be certain that the patient is comfortable with note taking.
- Assess for and provide comfort (e.g., assess and medicate for pain, offer the bedpan, offer a drink of water).
- Assess for anxiety. Be sure the patient is comfortable emotionally as well as physically. A very anxious person cannot provide good information, so you may need to intervene to relieve anxiety before proceeding.
- Assess readiness to discuss health issues. If the patient indicates that now is not a good time, reschedule (e.g., if the patient has just received some bad news about his condition, he may need some time to process that information before he can concentrate on interview questions).
- Audio or video recording of interviews are only done during research projects, and the researcher must be sure to obtain written permission from the patient by first receiving institutional review board (IRB) approval and using a stamped approval consent form.

Conducting a Patient Interview

Keep the following guidelines and techniques in mind as you are interviewing the patient:

- **Individualize your approach.** Ask yourself, "What approach is best considering the client's age and developmental level?" Respect the generational differences of a person older or younger than you.
- **Be sensitive to cultural differences.** For example, consider the patient's comfort with eye contact and his need for space.
- **Begin with neutral topics.** One example is biographical data (e.g., contact person, occupation). Ask more personal or

sensitive questions after you and the client are more comfortable with each other.

- **Use active listening**. This is the most important interviewing technique. Focus intently on trying to understand what the client is saying, rather than thinking ahead to what your response to the statement will be. Use the mnemonic FOLK:

  Face the patient (either sitting or standing).

  Open, relaxed posture (arms and legs uncrossed).

  Lean toward the patient.

  Keep eye contact.

- **Do not get caught up in note taking.** Excessive writing interferes with eye contact and may inhibit the client's responses, especially when you are discussing personal issues.
- **Pay attention to nonverbal communication.** Body language may signal that the person is tired or in pain but is too polite to say so. If the person is fatigued, you may need to end the interview and finish it at another time.
- **Use open-ended questions.** Use these questions as much as possible because they encourage the client to talk.
- **Avoid asking too many questions.** Asking many questions may make you seem merely curious instead of genuinely interested in the client.
- **Curb your curiosity.** Do not get caught up and sidetracked in the details of the client's response. Focus on the information you need to plan care.
- **Use neutral statements instead of questions.** For example, instead of "How many children do you have?" say, "Tell me about your family."
- **Avoid asking "why."** For example, do not ask, "Why have you stopped taking your pills?" For some people, "why" suggests disapproval and can cause them to become defensive.
- **Do not use healthcare jargon.** For example, say, "I want to take your temperature and blood pressure" instead of "I want to take your vital signs."
- **Do not "talk down" to the client.** For example, don't say, "I need to feel your tummy" when interviewing an adult.
- **Be sure your client understands what he says.** Confirm that clients actually understand the terminology they use. If a client says, "It's the inflammation that causes me the trouble," you might say, "Tell me where the inflammation is and what happens when you have it." People may repeat words they hear from care providers without really knowing what the words mean.
- **Refocus the client as needed.** When a response becomes scattered or does not produce useful information, refocus and redirect. Direct the client to topics that need to be covered (e.g., "We haven't talked about your surgery. What do you expect to happen?").
- **Do not give advice or voice approval or disapproval.** Even if the advice is good (e.g., "You were right to take your pills on time."), it may cause the client to be less open because he knows you are judging him. This can interfere with your ability to gather data.

Closing the Interview

When you are nearly finished with the interview, prepare the patient for closure. Begin by telling her that the interview is nearly finished. Then be sure to also do the following during the closing:

- Summarize the key points of the interview.
- Be sure you have recorded all the important data. Ask the patient, "Is there anything else you would like to tell me?" or "Is there anything else we should talk about?"

- Thank the patient for answering the questions.
- Encourage the patient to keep you informed. For example, you might say, "Please let us know if you think of anything else."
- Tell the patient what to expect next. Let the patient know when you will be leaving, when you will see her again, and what she can expect for the rest of the day (e.g., tests, treatments).
- And finally, ask, "Is there anything I can do for you before I leave?"

KnowledgeCheck 3-4

- What are the 10 components of a nursing history and why are they important? What are two things you should do to prepare yourself before an interview?
- List several things you could do to be sure the client is comfortable before the interview.
- State four guidelines that will help you to obtain complete and accurate data when conducting an interview.

HOW AND WHEN SHOULD I VALIDATE DATA?

Suppose a patient has told you that he has never had high blood pressure (BP), but you obtain an abnormal BP reading of 180/98 mm Hg. What would you do? Would you record the 180/98 mm Hg reading, or would you:

- Ask the patient some more questions? "What do you mean when you say you have never had high blood pressure?" or "What have you been doing in the last 15 minutes?"
- Ask another nurse to double-check your findings?
- Check when the sphygmomanometer was last calibrated?
- Retake the BP using a different sphygmomanometer?
- Compare the reading to previous entries in the chart?
- Check the BP in the patient's other arm?
- Wait a few minutes and take the reading again in the same arm?

All of these are ways to **validate,** or double-check, your data. Validating data helps to ensure that they are accurate, complete, and factual and that you have not jumped to conclusions. If the patient tells you that he was running late and has just jogged the two blocks from the parking lot, you would know that 180/98 mm Hg does not reflect his usual BP and that you need to check it again later.

Not all data must be validated. You can usually assume, for example, that laboratory results are correct and that the patient has given you correct information about data such as height, weight, and birth date. You should validate data under the following circumstances:

- Subjective and objective data do not agree, or do not make sense together.

  Example: In the preceding situation, the subjective data was "never had high BP," but the objective data, BP 180/98 mm Hg, is a high reading.
- The patient's statements differ at different times in the interview.

  Example: A patient tells you he follows a low-cholesterol diet. However, later when describing his usual daily food pattern, he includes eggs for breakfast, a cheese sandwich for lunch, and a hamburger for dinner.
- The data fall far outside normal range.

  Example: A patient has no symptoms of infection or high fever, but you obtain an elevated oral temperature

reading of 106°F (41.1°C). (Ask him if he has just had something warm to drink.)

■ Factors are present that interfere with accurate measurement. *Example*: The patient has very thin arms, and there are no appropriately sized BP cuffs available. Therefore, because the BP will not be accurate, you should measure it again after you can obtain appropriate equipment.

HOW CAN I ORGANIZE DATA?

Professional standards require systematic data collection (see Box 3-1). This means that you collect and record data in predetermined categories, not just at random. Data in most initial (e.g., admission) assessments are automatically categorized by the agency's data-collection form. For ongoing assessments, you may need to provide your own organizing structure, or framework. Because a **framework** represents a particular way of thinking about clients and health, it indicates which information is significant and guides you in deciding which patient data to observe. The major concepts of a model/framework help you to cluster data and find patterns. If you don't understand what a framework is, refer to Chapter 8.

Non-Nursing Models

ANA professional standards state that nursing data collection should be holistic. Many agencies use a **body systems (medical) framework** for at least a section of the assessment form. This model is useful for identifying medical problems, but it needs to be combined with other models (e.g., a nursing model or Maslow's hierarchy of needs) to provide the holistic data you need to identify both nursing and medical problems.

Maslow's hierarchy of needs (Maslow, 1970; Maslow & Lowery, 1998) groups data according to human needs. It states that the basic needs must be met before higher needs can be addressed. Maslow's categories of needs follow, from most basic to highest:

Physiological. Basic survival needs (e.g., oxygen, water, food, and shelter)

Safety and security. The need to be safe and comfortable (e.g., safe from falls and treatment side effects as well as the need for psychological security)

Love and belonging. The need for love and affection (e.g., family, social supports)

Esteem and self-esteem. The need to feel good about oneself (e.g., body image, pride in achievements, admiration from others)

Cognitive. The need for knowledge, understanding, and exploration

Aesthetic. The need for symmetry, order, and beauty

Self-actualization. The need to achieve one's potential; the need for growth and change (e.g., extent to which goals are achieved, role performance)

See Chapter 8 for a more complete discussion of Maslow's model.

Nursing Models

Nurse theorists have developed many different theories and models for thinking about nursing, clients, health, and the environment. Nursing models produce a holistic database that is useful in identifying nursing rather than medical diagnoses. Several nursing theories are described in Chapter 8. Box 3-5 identifies the major concepts of five models frequently used to structure nursing assessments. The concepts are the categories that you would use to gather and cluster data.

HOW SHOULD I DOCUMENT DATA?

The ANA *Scope and Standards of Practice* (2010) and the Joint Commission standards (2008) stress the importance of documenting patient information, including assessment data, in a retrievable format. Accurate, timely, and clear documentation of all assessment findings benefits patients by providing the basis for planning effective nursing care. Furthermore, because the nursing database is a permanent part of the client's record, documentation protects you, the nurse, by establishing that you actually performed the needed assessments. Malpractice suits are not unusual, and

---

Toward Evidence-Based Practice

Jones, A. (2007). Admitting hospital patients: A qualitative study of an everyday nursing task. *Nursing Inquiry, 14*(3), 212–223.

This qualitative study explored the everyday work of hospital nurses. It examined the initial assessment of patients being admitted to the hospital to compare what the nursing literature says about assessment with the assessments the researcher observed in practice. The literature clearly states assessments should be patient centered and that they are the important first step to a therapeutic nurse–patient relationship. The researcher concluded that the actual nursing admission assessments were at odds with recommendations in the literature. The nurses used a routinized, bureaucratic approach to assessment as a means of doing the work faster.

Which of the following inferences can you make? State whether the study summary provides *extensive*, *limited*, or *no* evidence to support each inference.

1. These results occurred because the nurses used a printed form created by the hospital.

2. The nurses did not care about their patients.

3. The nurses were feeling pressured by their workload.

4. The nurses did not know how important the initial assessment is.

5. Nursing practice is not always done according to the literature.

 Go to Chapter 3, **Toward Evidence-Based Practice Suggested Responses,** on Davis*Plus*.

BOX 3-5 ■ Assessment Models: Major Concepts

Gordon's Functional Health Patterns

Describe common patterns of behavior that can be functional or dysfunctional. Gordon intended the model for nursing assessment. The functional health patterns are major model concepts:
- Health perception/health management
- Nutritional/metabolic
- Elimination
- Activity/exercise
- Cognitive/perceptual
- Self-perception/self-concept
- Sleep/rest
- Role/relationship
- Sexual/reproductive
- Coping/stress tolerance
- Value-belief

Source: Adapted from Gordon, M. (1994). *Nursing diagnosis: Process and application* (3rd ed.). St. Louis, MO: Mosby, p. 70.

The NANDA-International Nursing Diagnosis Taxonomy II

Consists of functional patterns and is a modified version of the Gordon model. It is intended as a model for categorizing nursing diagnoses, not as a fully developed theory of nursing. The NANDA-I domains (categories) include the following:

Health Promotion	Sexuality
Nutrition	Coping/Stress Tolerance
Elimination and Exchange	Life Principles
Activity/Rest	Safety/Protection
Perception/Cognition	Comfort
Self-Perception	Growth/Development
Role Relationships	

Source: Adapted from NANDA International. (2009). *NANDA nursing diagnoses: Definitions & classification 2009–2011.* Philadelphia: NANDA International.

The Taxonomy of Nursing Practice (NANDA/NOC/NIC)

Intended as a model for categorizing nursing diagnoses, client outcomes, and nursing interventions. It consists of four domains and 28 classes.

Functional Domain Activity exercise, comfort, growth and development, nutrition, self-care, sexuality, sleep/rest, values/beliefs

Physiological Domain Cardiac function, elimination, fluids and electrolytes, neurocognition, pharmacological function, physical regulation, reproduction, respiratory function, sensation/perception, tissue integrity

Psychosocial Domain Behavior, communication, coping, emotional, knowledge, roles/relationships, self-perception

Environmental Domain Healthcare system, populations, risk management

Source: Dochterman, J. M., & Jones, D. A. (Eds.). (2003). *Unifying nursing languages: The harmonization of NANDA, NIC, and NOC.* Washington, DC: American Nurses Association, NursesBooks.org.

The Roy Adaptation Model

Conceptualizes patients as adapting constantly to internal and external demands within a biological and psychosocial context. Using this model, you would assess the person's ability to achieve balance in the following "adaptive modes":

Activity and rest	Temperature regulation
Nutrition	Regulation of the senses
Elimination	Physical self-concept
Fluid and electrolytes	Personal self-concept
Oxygenation	Role function
Protection	Interdependence

Source: Adapted from Roy, C., & Andrews, H. (1991). *The Roy adaptation model: The definitive statement.* Norwalk, CT: Appleton & Lange, pp. 15–17; and Roy, C., & Andrews, H. (1999). *The Roy adaptation model* (2nd ed.). Norwalk, CT: Appleton and Lange.

Orem's Self-Care Model

Conceptualizes health as the ability to perform self-care. Using this model, you would gather data to identify the following universal self-care deficits that require nursing assistance:
- Maintenance of a sufficient intake of air, water, and food
- Maintenance of a balance between activity and rest
- Maintenance of a balance between time alone and time with others
- Provision of care associated with elimination processes and excrements
- Prevention of hazards to human life, functioning, and well-being
- Promotion of human functioning and development within social groups in accord with human potential, limitations, and desire to be normal (by science, culture, and social values)

Source: Adapted from Orem, D. (1991). *Nursing: Concepts of practice* (4th ed.). St. Louis, MO: Mosby-Year Book, p. 126; and Orem, D. E. (1995). *Nursing: Concepts of practice* (5th ed.). St. Louis, MO: Mosby.

court cases may be presented years after you care for a patient. Your documentation is the only evidence supporting the care that you gave. The assumption in malpractice cases is, "If it isn't documented, it wasn't done."

Guidelines for Recording Assessment Data

Follow these guidelines when recording assessment data:
- *Document as soon as possible* after you perform the assessment.
- *Write neatly, legibly, and in black ink.*
- *Use acronyms sparingly,* using only agency-approved abbreviations.
- *Write the patient's own words, when possible,* in quotation marks. If the comments are too long, summarize what the patient says (e.g., Patient states that he is sleepy).
- *Record only the most important patient words.* If you record everything the patient says, the narrative will probably be too long and contain irrelevant data. For example, write "Patient states, 'I hardly slept at all last night,'" even though what the patient actually said was, "I hardly slept at all last

night. I tossed and turned and people kept waking me up. Then the thunder and lightning came, and then I had to get up to go to the bathroom, and my wife called early this morning."

- *Use concrete, specific information* rather than vague generalities such as *normal, adequate, good,* and *tolerated well.* For example, what does it mean to say, "Patient slept well"? Did she fall asleep easily and sleep for 6 hours? Did she fall asleep with difficulty, but sleep for 8 hours? Did she sleep only 4 hours, but state that she feels well rested? It is much better to write, "Patient fell asleep before 2100 hr and slept until 0600 hr. She states that she woke up only once during the night and feels rested now. Observed sleeping three times during the night."
- *Record cues, not inferences.* **Cues** are what the client says and what you observe. **Inferences** are judgments and interpretations about what the cues mean. In other words, "just the facts, Jack (or Jill)." When recording cues, you do not need to "waffle" with the words *appears* and *seems.* Don't write "incision seems red" or "edges appear separated." For example:

Cues	Inferences
"My head hurts."	Patient has a headache.
Incision red, draining pus	Incision is infected.

Tools for Recording Assessment Data

Each organization has its own forms and formats for documenting initial and ongoing assessments. You will record data on a variety of documents, including nurses' notes and the following:

- *Graphic flow sheet.* Includes vital signs such as blood pressure, pulse, respirations, and temperature so trends over time can be seen clearly (Fig. 3-3).
- *Intake and output (I&O) sheet.* May be on the graphic sheet, as in Figure 3-3, or separate. This form has spaces for all intake: oral, intravenous, and tube feedings. There is also space to record all output: urine, fluid from drainage tubes, wound drainage, and bowel movements.
- *Nursing admission assessment.* Although agency forms differ in organization, all collect similar data as specified by the Joint Commission for standards for initial assessment. To see and use a comprehensive nursing admission data form,

 Go to Chapter 3, Tables, Boxes, Figures: **ESG Figure 3-1, Nursing Admission Data Form**, on *DavisPlus.*

- *Nursing discharge summary.* This may be a part of the initial assessment form because data obtained at admission are used for discharge planning.
- *Special-purpose forms.* Examples are diabetic flow sheets and medication administration forms.
- *Computer documentation.* Initial and ongoing assessment data are many times entered into a computer program for organization, shared communication, and easy retrieval.

REFLECTING CRITICALLY ABOUT ASSESSMENT

After gathering and recording patient data, use critical thinking to help you evaluate the quality of your assessment. See Chapter 2 for a review of critical thinking, as

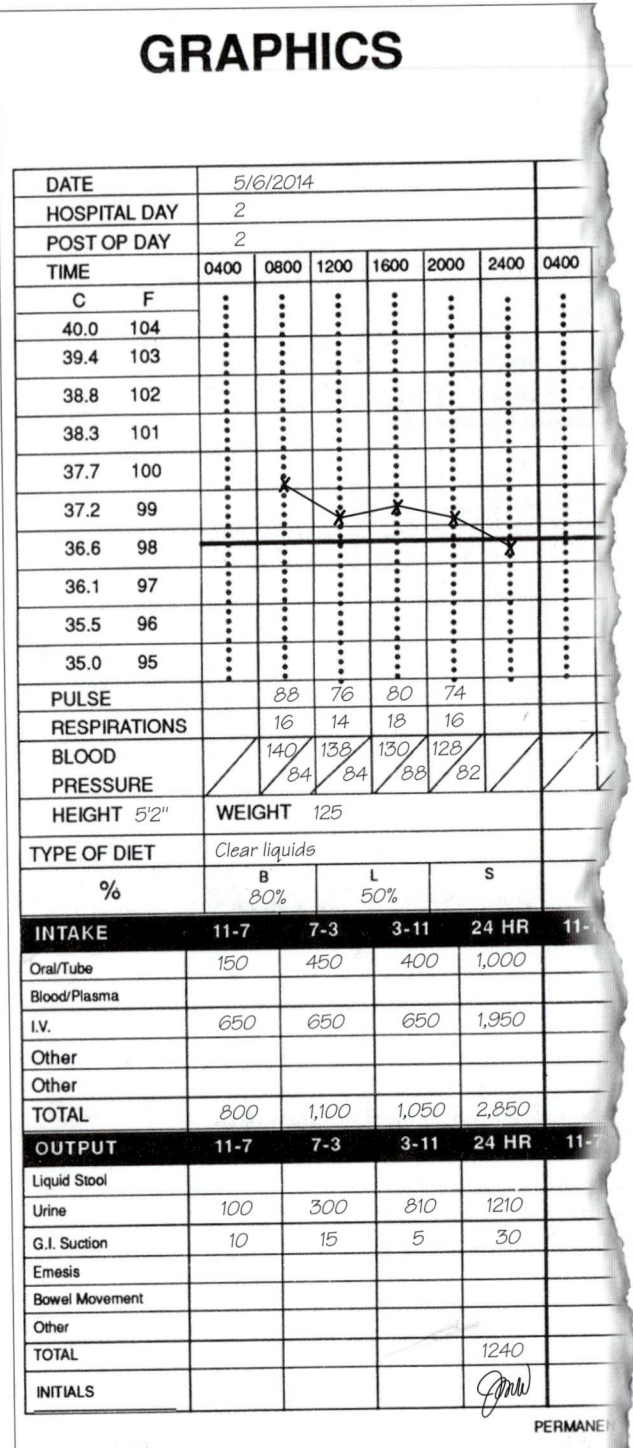

FIGURE 3-3 Graphic flow sheet. (Courtesy of Smith Northview Hospital, Valdosta, GA.)

needed. The following are questions to guide your final judgments about your data:

1. Are my data complete?
   - Have I completed all areas of the assessment form?
   - Is there anything else I need to know to identify or rule out a nursing diagnosis?

- Have I collected holistic data: physical, emotional, interpersonal, spiritual, and cultural?

2. How do I know the data are accurate?

3. Have I recorded data rather than conclusions (cues, not inferences)?

4. Did I validate any data that do not make sense? Do any of the data conflict with other data?

5. Did I record the data in clear, specific terms, using the patient's own words, when possible, for subjective data? Did I avoid vague terms such as "normal," "good," and "slept well"?

6. Have I followed up with in-depth special needs assessments when appropriate?

7. Have I included only relevant data, taking care to protect the client's privacy?

8. The assessment interview:
   - Did I use therapeutic communication during the assessment?
   - Did I avoid asking too many questions and using too many closed questions?
   - How comfortable was I during the interview?
   - What signals did I get from the client in response to my questions? Did I follow up?

9. Physical assessment, observation, and examination:
   - Did I miss something in the environment?
   - How did the client and significant others respond to me verbally and nonverbally?
   - Did I pay attention to detail?
   - Were my assessment techniques performed skillfully (palpation, percussion, auscultation, inspection)?

10. Memory:
   - Did I have to ask questions in the sequence found on the forms?
   - Did I have to depend on the forms for all aspects of the assessment?
   - Did I have to repeat any area of assessment because I could not remember what I saw, heard, smelled, or felt?

If you have followed the recommended processes and reflected critically on your assessment, you should have the data necessary to create a holistic plan of care individualized to meet the client's needs.

If you would like to practice your assessment skills,

 Go to **Interactive Clinical Scenarios**, on Davis*Plus* for this text.

CLINICALREASONING:
Applying the **Full-Spectrum Nursing Model**

Because the following critical thinking activities allow you to practice the kind of thinking you will use as a full-spectrum nurse, they usually have no single right answer. Discuss them with your peers—if you have difficulty with any of the questions, consult your instructor.

PATIENT SITUATION

As the intake nurse in a community-based clinic in Miami, Florida, your role is to complete a comprehensive nursing assessment and initiate a plan of care for the clients. Your first client is a 27-year-old single woman, Sami, who is requesting clinic services for her general healthcare needs. Sami is Cuban American and lives alone in a one-bedroom apartment. She works as a fitness trainer at the local YMCA while attending college part-time. Her family lives in Tampa, Florida. Sami's earnings place her at the poverty level, but she realizes that she must have healthcare to prevent illness and to detect and receive treatment of illnesses should they arise.

THINKING

1. *Theoretical Knowledge:* To care for Sami, what knowledge would you need that you do not already have? List the URL for at least one online, reputable source for this information.
2. *Critical Thinking:* The nurse asks Sami, "If you can't afford healthcare, couldn't you get a roommate to save some money on rent?" What are some critical thinking questions you should ask yourself when reflecting on this question later?

DOING

3. *Practical Knowledge:* What practical knowledge will you, as the nurse, use in this scenario?
4. *Nursing Process:* What kind of assessment will you perform of Sami (e.g., comprehensive, focused, special needs, discharge)?

CARING

5. *Self-Knowledge:* In what ways are you similar to Sami? In what ways are you different?

 Go to Chapter 3, **Clinical Reasoning: Applying the Full-Spectrum Nursing Model-Response Sheet** on Davis*Plus*.

 To explore learning resources for this chapter,

 Go to Davis*Plus* at davisplus.fadavis.com, keyword Treas.
Chapter Resources for Chapter 3:
   Knowledge Check and Think Like a Nurse Response Sheets
   Knowledge Check Answers
   Resources for Caregivers and Health Professionals
   Reading More About Nursing Process: Assessment (Suggested Readings)
   What Are the Main Points in This Chapter?
NCLEX-Style Review Questions
Chapter Overview Podcasts

Concept Map

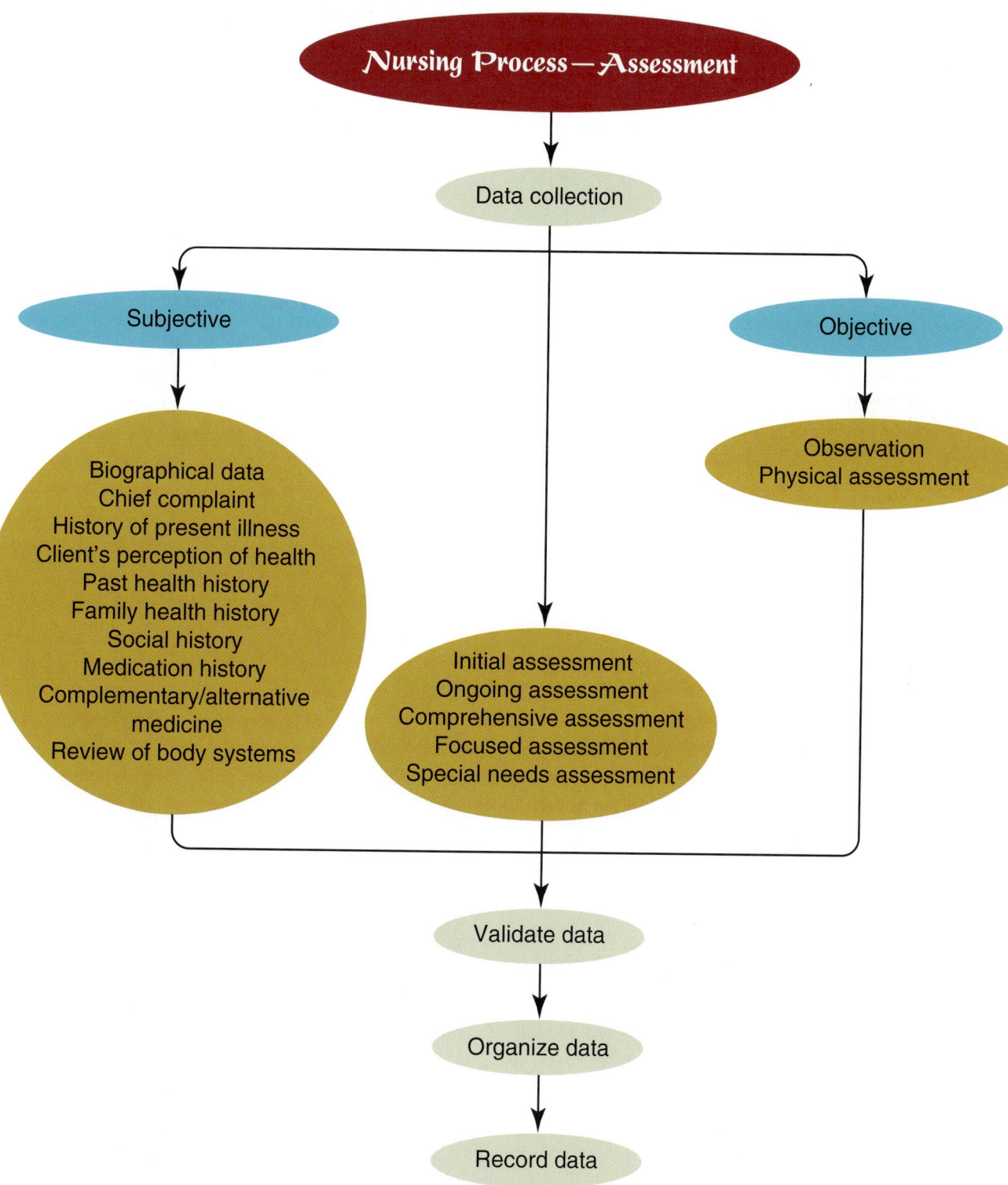

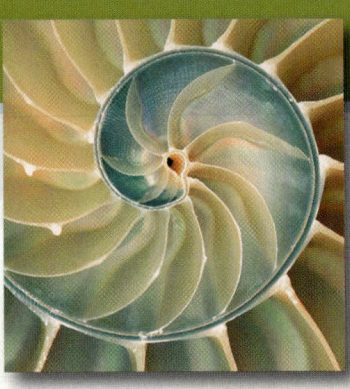

CHAPTER 4

Diagnosis

Learning Outcomes

After completing this chapter, you should be able to:

➤ Define the following terms: *diagnosis, nursing diagnosis, diagnostic reasoning, diagnostic label, defining characteristics, related factors, risk factors,* and *health problem.*

➤ Explain how nursing diagnosis is related to the nursing process.

➤ Differentiate between nursing diagnoses, medical diagnoses, and collaborative problems.

➤ Explain the differences between actual, potential, risk, syndrome, and wellness nursing diagnoses.

➤ Describe the diagnostic process.

➤ Explain why an etiology is always an inference.

➤ Describe at least two frameworks for prioritizing nursing diagnoses.

➤ Describe errors of theoretical and self-knowledge that may occur in diagnostic reasoning.

➤ Use standardized nursing language to write nursing diagnoses.

➤ Use collaborative problem statements appropriately.

➤ Explain the relationship between nursing diagnoses and goals/interventions.

➤ State at least five criteria for judging the quality of a diagnostic statement.

➤ Discuss issues associated with the NANDA-I diagnostic labels and with standardized language.

Key Concepts

Nursing diagnosis
Diagnostic process
Diagnostic format

Related Concepts

See the Concept Map at the end of this chapter.

Caring for the Nguyens

This feature allows you to practice the kind of thinking you will use as a full-spectrum nurse. There is usually more than one correct answer to a critical thinking question, so we do not provide answers for these features. It is more important to develop your nursing judgment than to "cover content." Discuss the questions with your peers. If you are still unsure, consult your instructor.

Review the opening scenario of Nam Nguyen in the front of this book. After the nurse practitioner completed the interview and physical examination of Mr. Nguyen, he listed the following diagnoses on the problem list:

Hypertension
Obesity
Musculoskeletal pain
Tobacco abuse

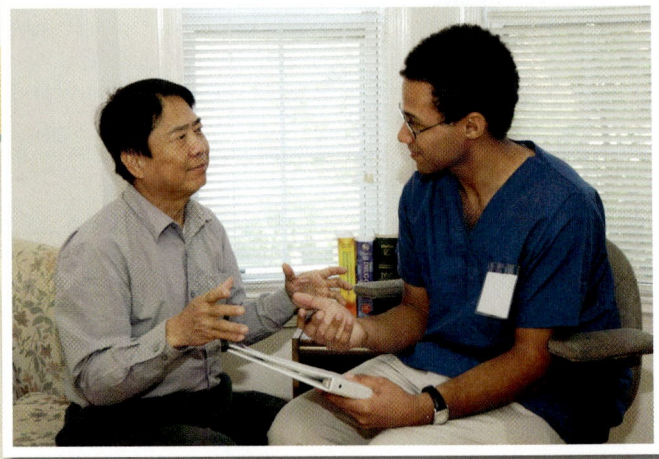

Family history of prostate cancer
Family history of cardiovascular disease
Family history of diabetes mellitus (DM)

Caring for the Nguyens (continued)

A. What type of problem list does this represent? How is it similar to or different from a problem list that you might generate?

B. Based on the data in the scenario, identify at least one actual, one potential, and one wellness diagnosis for Mr. Nguyen. Identify the NANDA-I labels, and describe the cues that support your choices.

C. The nurse has identified a problem of Imbalanced Nutrition: More Than Body Requirements for Mr. Nguyen.

  ■ What information do you need in order to determine the etiology of this problem?

  ■ Because you do not have that information, write a two-part diagnostic statement describing Mr. Nguyen's nutritional status.

D. Now rewrite the nutrition statement as a three-part statement, including the phrase "as evidenced by."

E. The nurse has identified Acute Pain (knees) for Mr. Nguyen. If the pain were caused by a medical condition, osteoarthritis, how would you write a two-part diagnostic statement to describe this health status?

 Go to **Caring for the Nguyens Response Sheet** on DavisPlus.

Meet Your Patient

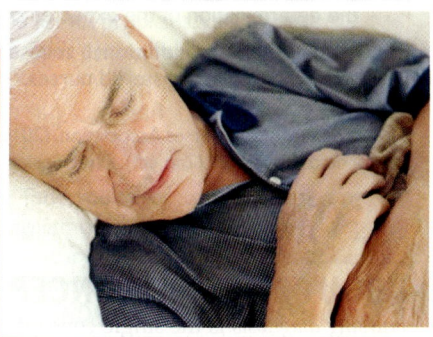

On your unit at an acute care facility, you will be admitting a client, Todd, from the emergency department (ED). Todd's ED nurse telephones you to give a report on his status. Todd's admitting medical diagnosis is chronic renal failure. He is married, 58 years old, employed, and has a longstanding history of type 2 diabetes mellitus (DM). In the past 3 days, he has developed decreased sensation in his bilateral lower extremities with slight mobility impairment.

You still have many questions concerning Todd's immediate and long-term needs. You will need to ask Todd about his medication regimen, his compliance with his diabetes treatment plan, and the extent to which his family is involved. You will also need to find out what laboratory tests have been completed and how severe his renal dysfunction has become. After you obtain necessary data, you need to organize and analyze it to form some initial impressions about what it means. For example:

■ Admitting diagnosis is chronic renal failure; anticipate a problem with fluid balance.
■ Admitted to the hospital and is acutely ill; therefore, he may be anxious and fearful.

■ Decreased sensation in lower extremities; patient may have a mobility and a safety problem.
■ Diabetes; patient is at risk for impaired skin and tissue integrity.
■ Diabetes and renal failure require complex regimens and patient self-care; therefore, it is possible that Todd may not be managing his therapy effectively, because he either is not motivated to do so or he lacks the knowledge he needs to comply with treatment.

When Todd and his family arrive on your unit, you begin gathering additional data. Using your comprehensive data, you then make a list of Todd's health problems, in order of priority. These actions illustrate the diagnosis phase of the nursing process. The purpose of diagnosing is to identify the client's health status, from which you will create an individualized plan of care.

Theoretical Knowledge
knowing **why**

Professional standards of nursing practice, as well as many state nurse practice acts, identify diagnosing as the responsibility of the professional nurse (Box 4-1). Although many nursing activities may be delegated, diagnosing cannot. To meet practice expectations and professional obligations as a registered

nurse (RN), you will assume the role of diagnostician and make clinical judgments. Most state nurse practice acts limit the role of the licensed practical nurse (LPN/LVN) to gathering data that will be analyzed by the RN. However, LPN roles vary among states and agencies, and they are subject to change. Furthermore, LPN and RN roles are becoming more closely linked through statewide career ladder programs. Therefore, all clinicians need to stay current with updates in practice acts and standards.

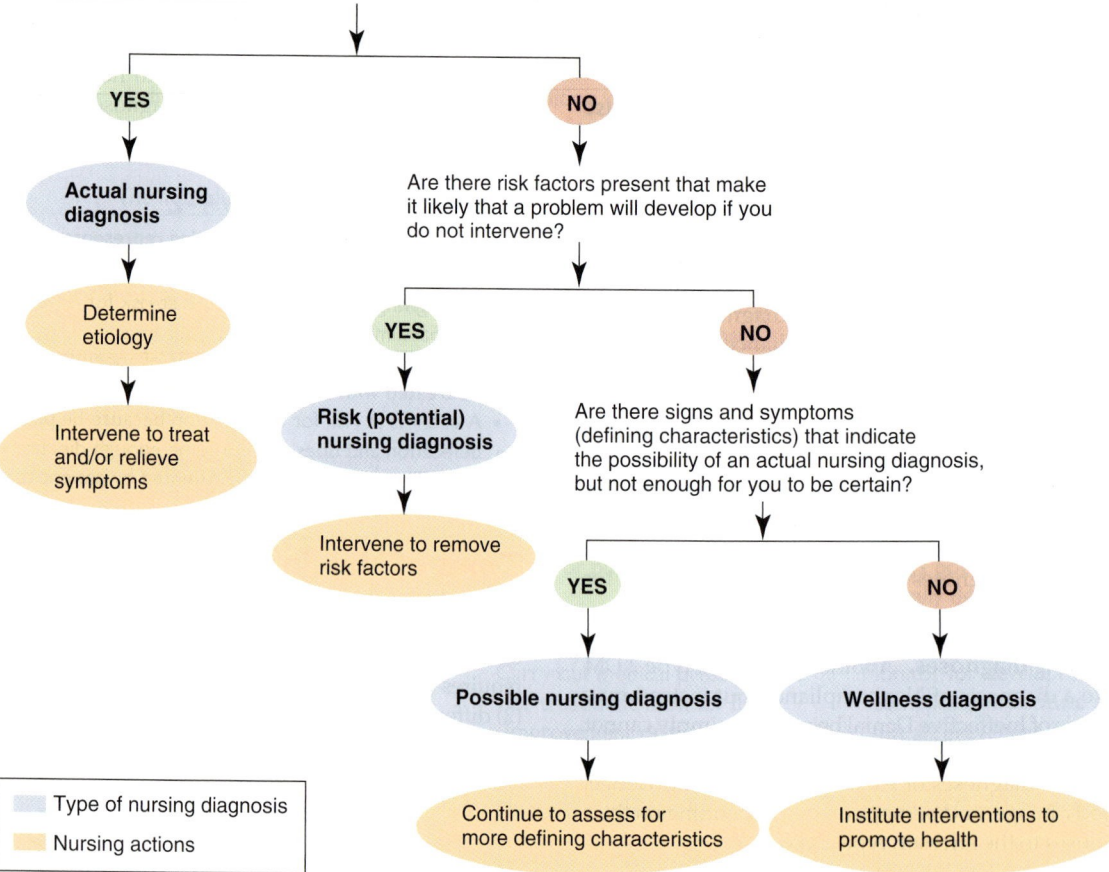

At the time of assessment, does the patient have enough signs and symptoms (defining characteristics) to identify the specific nursing diagnosis?

YES

Actual nursing diagnosis

Determine etiology

Intervene to treat and/or relieve symptoms

NO

Are there risk factors present that make it likely that a problem will develop if you do not intervene?

YES

Risk (potential) nursing diagnosis

Intervene to remove risk factors

NO

Are there signs and symptoms (defining characteristics) that indicate the possibility of an actual nursing diagnosis, but not enough for you to be certain?

YES

Possible nursing diagnosis

Continue to assess for more defining characteristics

NO

Wellness diagnosis

Institute interventions to promote health

Type of nursing diagnosis
Nursing actions

FIGURE 4-4 Algorithm for determining whether a nursing diagnosis is an actual diagnosis, a risk (potential) diagnosis, a possible diagnosis, or a wellness diagnosis.

Actual Nursing Diagnosis: Problem Is Present. An **actual nursing diagnosis** is a problem response that exists at the time of the assessment. You identify it by the signs and symptoms (cues) that are present. Todd (Meet Your Patient) has no actual nursing diagnoses. He may have actual Impaired Walking or perhaps Impaired Physical Mobility, related to his lack of peripheral sensation; however, no signs and symptoms were given in the scenario to support that diagnosis.

Risk Nursing Diagnosis: Problem May Occur. A **risk nursing diagnosis** describes a problem response that is likely to develop in a vulnerable patient if the nurse and patient do not intervene to prevent it. You will identify a risk diagnosis when the patient does not have signs/symptoms of the problem, but does have risk factors present that increase his vulnerability. For example, Todd's loss of lower limb sensation is a risk factor for a diagnosis of Risk for Falls, even though Todd has no symptoms or history of falling.

Use risk nursing diagnoses (also called potential nursing diagnoses) only for patients who have more susceptibility to the problem than others in the same or a comparable setting. For example, all surgical patients have at least some risk for developing infection, so you should not routinely write Risk for Infection on every surgical care plan. You would, instead, write Potential Complication of surgery: infection (incision and systemic). Use the nursing diagnosis Risk for Infection for patients who are *unusually* susceptible to infection (e.g., one who is undernourished or one with a compromised immune system).

Possible Nursing Diagnosis: Problem May Be Present. A **possible nursing diagnosis** exists when your intuition and experience direct you to suspect that a diagnosis is present, but you do not have enough data to support the diagnosis. The main reason for including this type of diagnosis on a care plan is to alert other nurses to continue to collect data to confirm or rule out the problem. Todd (Meet Your Patient) has a symptom of slightly impaired mobility. This could indicate the diagnoses Impaired Physical Mobility, Impaired Walking, or Risk for Falls. You need more data to decide which nursing diagnosis is appropriate, so you might write a nursing diagnosis of Possible Risk for Falls related to decreased sensation in both legs.

Syndrome Nursing Diagnosis: Several Related Problems Are Present. A **syndrome nursing diagnosis** represents a collection of nursing diagnoses that usually occur together. For example, the NANDA-I label Risk for Disuse Syndrome is used to represent all the complications that can occur as a result of immobility (e.g., pressure ulcer, constipation, stasis of pulmonary secretions, thrombosis, body image disturbance).

Wellness Nursing Diagnosis: No Problem Is Present. You will use a **wellness diagnosis** when an individual, group, or community is in transition from one level of wellness to a higher level of wellness. A wellness diagnosis describes health status, but it is not a health problem. For you to make a wellness diagnosis, two conditions must be present: (1) The client's present level of wellness is effective and (2) the client wants to move to a higher level of wellness.

Caring for the Nguyens (continued)

A. What type of problem list does this represent? How is it similar to or different from a problem list that you might generate?

B. Based on the data in the scenario, identify at least one actual, one potential, and one wellness diagnosis for Mr. Nguyen. Identify the NANDA-I labels, and describe the cues that support your choices.

C. The nurse has identified a problem of Imbalanced Nutrition: More Than Body Requirements for Mr. Nguyen.
- What information do you need in order to determine the etiology of this problem?

- Because you do not have that information, write a two-part diagnostic statement describing Mr. Nguyen's nutritional status.

D. Now rewrite the nutrition statement as a three-part statement, including the phrase "as evidenced by."

E. The nurse has identified Acute Pain (knees) for Mr. Nguyen. If the pain were caused by a medical condition, osteoarthritis, how would you write a two-part diagnostic statement to describe this health status?

 Go to **Caring for the Nguyens Response Sheet** on *DavisPlus.*

Meet Your Patient

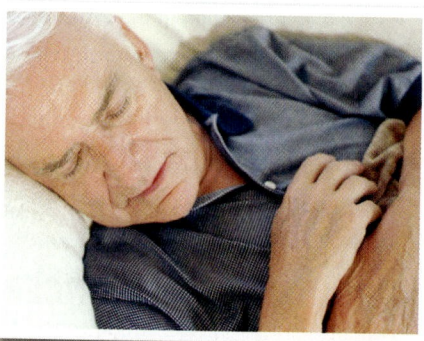

On your unit at an acute care facility, you will be admitting a client, Todd, from the emergency department (ED). Todd's ED nurse telephones you to give a report on his status. Todd's admitting medical diagnosis is chronic renal failure. He is married, 58 years old, employed, and has a longstanding history of type 2 diabetes mellitus (DM). In the past 3 days, he has developed decreased sensation in his bilateral lower extremities with slight mobility impairment.

You still have many questions concerning Todd's immediate and long-term needs. You will need to ask Todd about his medication regimen, his compliance with his diabetes treatment plan, and the extent to which his family is involved. You will also need to find out what laboratory tests have been completed and how severe his renal dysfunction has become. After you obtain necessary data, you need to organize and analyze it to form some initial impressions about what it means. For example:

- Admitting diagnosis is chronic renal failure; anticipate a problem with fluid balance.
- Admitted to the hospital and is acutely ill; therefore, he may be anxious and fearful.

- Decreased sensation in lower extremities; patient may have a mobility and a safety problem.
- Diabetes; patient is at risk for impaired skin and tissue integrity.
- Diabetes and renal failure require complex regimens and patient self-care; therefore, it is possible that Todd may not be managing his therapy effectively, because he either is not motivated to do so or he lacks the knowledge he needs to comply with treatment.

When Todd and his family arrive on your unit, you begin gathering additional data. Using your comprehensive data, you then make a list of Todd's health problems, in order of priority. These actions illustrate the diagnosis phase of the nursing process. The purpose of diagnosing is to identify the client's health status, from which you will create an individualized plan of care.

Theoretical Knowledge
knowing **why**

Professional standards of nursing practice, as well as many state nurse practice acts, identify diagnosing as the responsibility of the professional nurse (Box 4-1). Although many nursing activities may be delegated, diagnosing cannot. To meet practice expectations and professional obligations as a registered

nurse (RN), you will assume the role of diagnostician and make clinical judgments. Most state nurse practice acts limit the role of the licensed practical nurse (LPN/LVN) to gathering data that will be analyzed by the RN. However, LPN roles vary among states and agencies, and they are subject to change. Furthermore, LPN and RN roles are becoming more closely linked through statewide career ladder programs. Therefore, all clinicians need to stay current with updates in practice acts and standards.

BOX 4-1 ■ Professional Standards for Diagnosing

American Nurses Association Standards of Nursing Practice

Standard 2. Diagnosis

The registered nurse analyzes the assessment data to determine the diagnoses or the issues.

Competencies

The registered nurse:
- Derives the diagnoses or issues from assessment data.
- Validates the diagnoses or issues with the healthcare consumer, family, and other healthcare providers when possible and appropriate.
- Identifies actual or potential risks to the healthcare consumer's health and safety or barriers to health, which may include but are not limited to interpersonal, systematic, or environmental circumstances.
- Uses standardized classification systems and clinical decision support tools, when available, in identifying diagnoses.
- Documents diagnoses or issues in a manner that facilitates the determination of the expected outcomes and plan.

Note: There are additional measurement criteria for advanced practice registered nurses.

Source: American Nurses Association. (2010). *Nursing: Scope and standards of practice* (2nd ed.). Silver Spring, MD: Nursebooks.org.

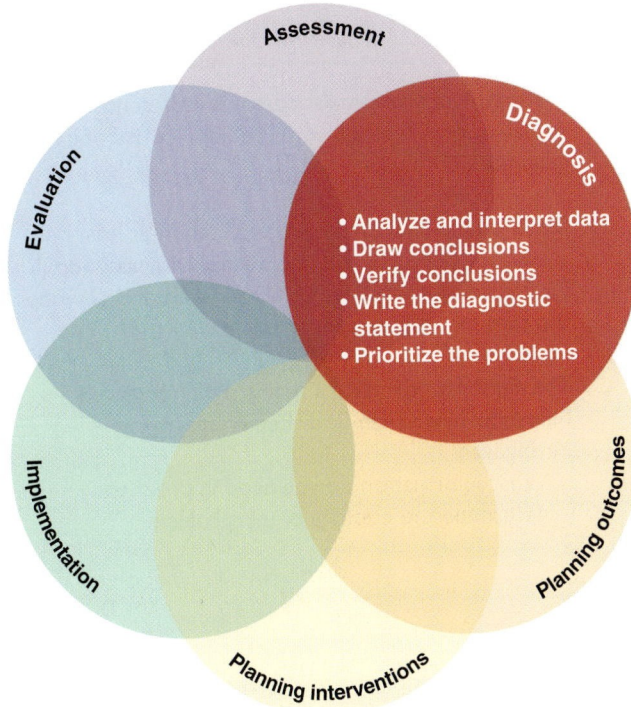

FIGURE 4-1 Nursing diagnosis: Second phase of the nursing process.

ABOUT THE KEY CONCEPTS

Nursing diagnosis is the single concept in this chapter that ties all the other concepts together.

The *diagnostic process* represents the thinking aspect of nursing diagnosis, and the *diagnostic format* is the concrete product.

DIAGNOSIS: THE SECOND STEP OF THE NURSING PROCESS

Diagnosis is the second step of the nursing process. It is the phase in which you analyze the assessment data. Using critical thinking skills, identify patterns in the data and draw conclusions about the client's health status, including strengths, problems, and factors contributing to the problems. As in all phases of the nursing process, involve the patient and family as much as possible.

As you can see in Figure 4-1, diagnosis overlaps with the other nursing process steps. Most nurses actually begin diagnostic reasoning during the assessment phase. For example, you probably formed your initial impressions about Todd while you were still gathering data. On learning the medical diagnosis, chronic renal failure, you would have immediately considered the diagnosis Risk for Imbalanced Fluid Volume, but you would have obtained more data before actually recording that as a nursing diagnosis. So your tentative diagnostic conclusion would actually lead you to collect more data: *Is he still producing urine? What is his oral intake? Does he have edema?* Do you see how you would move back and forth between assessment and diagnosis? The two stages are not separate at all, but we present them that way to make it easier for you to learn.

Diagnosis is critical because it links the assessment step, which precedes it, to all the steps that follow it (Fig. 4-2). Assessment data must be complete and accurate for you to make an accurate nursing diagnosis. Accuracy is essential because the nursing diagnosis is the basis for planning client-centered goals and interventions.

The term **nursing diagnosis** in the nursing literature has the following meanings:
- The second phase of the nursing process
- The reasoning process used in interpreting assessment data
- A formal diagnostic statement of the client's health status, containing both the problem and etiology (factors contributing to the problem)
- The list of standardized terms (labels) used to write diagnostic statements. Those terms are actually problem labels; you must add a second part (etiology) in order to create a complete diagnostic statement.

Table 4-1 summarizes and provides examples of how nursing diagnosis terminology is used in this text.

What Are the Origins of Nursing Diagnoses?

Before the 1950s, nurses assisted physicians by collecting data to help them diagnose and treat disease. Nursing care was thought of as a set of tasks and organized as a list of things to do. The term *nursing diagnosis* was first used in 1953 to differentiate nursing from medicine, when Fry (1953) stated that a nursing diagnosis identifies the client's needs for nursing rather than for medical care. Until the early 1970s, nursing diagnosis was not widely used in nursing practice, but two major events in 1973 spurred change:
- The First Conference on Nursing Diagnosis was held (Gebbie, 1976). A national task force was formed to begin developing a language to describe the health problems treated by nurses.
- The American Nurses Association (ANA) *Scope and Standards of Nursing Practice* included nursing diagnosis as an expectation of professional nurses.

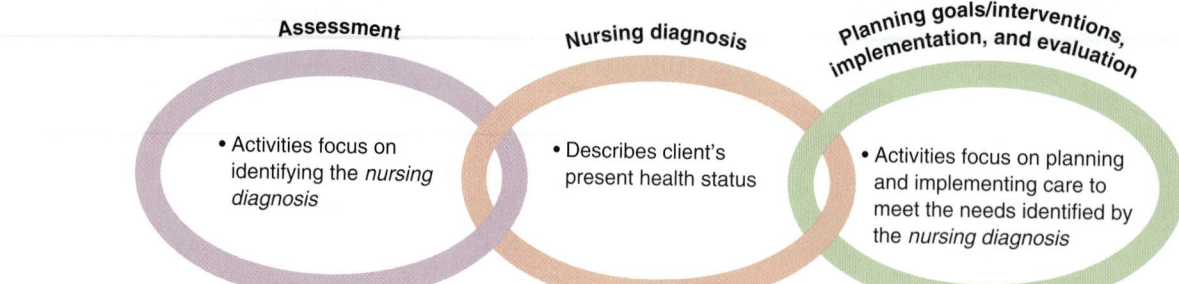

FIGURE 4-2 Diagnosis links the assessment phase to the rest of the nursing process.

Table 4-1 ➤ Nursing Diagnosis Terminology		
TERM AND EXISTING MEANINGS	**TERMINOLOGY USED IN THIS BOOK**	**EXAMPLE**
Diagnosis		
1. The second phase of the nursing process 2. The reasoning process used in identifying patient problems and strengths	1. Diagnosis 2. Diagnostic process, diagnostic reasoning, or diagnosing	With Todd (Meet Your Patient), you used *diagnostic reasoning* to *diagnose* and list his problems. This was the *diagnosis phase* of the nursing process.
Nursing Diagnosis		
1. The end product of the diagnostic reasoning process: a full diagnostic statement describing client health status. It contains both problem and etiology. 2. A standardized problem label from the NANDA-I taxonomy (e.g., Anxiety)	1. Nursing diagnosis, diagnostic statement 2. Label, NANDA-I label, problem label, diagnostic label	For Todd, you might have made a *nursing diagnosis* of Excess Fluid Volume secondary to renal failure. To write that statement, you would have used the *NANDA-I label* Fluid Excess Volume.

In 1980, the ANA published *the ANA Social Policy Statement,* which characterized nursing as "the diagnosis and treatment of human response to actual or potential health problems" (ANA, 1980, p. 2). As a result of this definition and the work of the nursing diagnosis task force, most state nurse practice acts began to designate nursing diagnosis as an exclusive responsibility of registered nurses. Nursing diagnosis is now widely used in nursing education and practice. The formal list of nursing diagnostic labels describes health problems that can be addressed by independent nursing actions and, in that sense, forms the body of knowledge that is unique to nursing.

Since the first conference, the nursing diagnosis group has continued to meet every 2 years. In 1982 it adopted the name North American Nursing Diagnosis Association (NANDA). In 2002, the name was changed to NANDA International (NANDA-I), to reflect its large number of members from countries outside North America. NANDA-I continues to review and refine the diagnostic labels and to discuss new and revised labels at each biannual conference. The diagnoses on the official list are approved for clinical use and further study; the list is not intended to represent a finished product, because many of the diagnoses are only partially substantiated by research. NANDA-I encourages individual nurses and nursing organizations to submit new and revised diagnoses.

KnowledgeCheck 4-1

- Why is the diagnosis step so critical to the other phases of the nursing process?
- Which two nursing organizations have been responsible for making diagnosis a part of the professional nursing role?

What Are Health Problems?

A **health problem** is any condition that requires intervention to promote wellness or to prevent or treat disease or illness. After you identify a health problem, you must decide how to treat it: independently or in collaboration with other health professionals. The answer determines whether it is a nursing diagnosis, a medical diagnosis, or a collaborative problem. See Table 4-2 for a comparison of these problem types.

Recognizing Nursing Diagnoses

A **nursing diagnosis** is a statement of client health status that nurses can identify, prevent, or treat independently. It is stated in terms of **human responses** (reactions) to disease, injury, or other stressors, and it can be either a problem or a strength. Human responses can be physiological, psychological, developmental, sociocultural, or spiritual. For example, Todd's medical diagnosis is chronic renal failure. A *physiological response* to renal failure is Excess Fluid Volume. Admission

Table 4-2 ➤ Comparison of Nursing Diagnoses, Medical Diagnoses, and Collaborative Problems

	NURSING DIAGNOSIS	MEDICAL DIAGNOSIS	COLLABORATIVE PROBLEM
Definition	A clinical judgment about individual, family, or community responses to a health problem	Disease, illness, injury, or condition validated by signs and symptoms and medical diagnostic studies	Certain potential physiological complications that are always associated with a disease, test, or treatment
Focus	The individual/person	Disease, pathology, and medical treatments/procedures	Pathophysiology (complications caused by the disease process)
Characteristics	Holistic; describes physiological, psychological, social, interpersonal, and spiritual responses	Describes disease or pathology; does not consider the broader range of human responses.	Describes potential physiological complications only; not holistic.
Who Diagnoses?	Professional nurse	Physicians, advanced practice nurses, physician's assistants	Nurses
Who Orders Treatment?	Professional nurse, primarily	Physician, advanced practice nurse, physicians' assistants	Physician prescribes primary interventions; however, the nurse can order some as well.
Problem Status	Can be actual, potential, or possible.	Actual or possible (rule out)	Always potential; if the problem actually develops, it is then a medical diagnosis.
Purpose of Nursing Interventions	Treat or prevent the problem; relieve the symptoms.	Carry out medical prescriptions for treatment; monitor for improvement or worsening of the condition.	Monitor for development of the complication; institute some, but not all, preventive interventions.
Example of Diagnostic Statement	Ineffective Denial related to difficulty coping with new diagnosis of "heart attack"	Myocardial infarction	Potential Complication of myocardial infarction: Congestive heart failure
Example of Data to Support the Diagnosis	Waited more than 6 hours before coming to hospital. Minimizes symptoms, refuses pain medications. States, "I've got to get back to work. I can't stay in the hospital." Laughing, joking, saying, "It's nothing."	Cardiac enzyme levels elevated; has had severe chest pain; elevated white blood cell count; electrocardiogram (ECG) and echocardiogram diagnostic of cardiac muscle ischemia	58-year-old man with diagnosis of myocardial infarction (MI); acknowledges chest pain; ECG and lab work diagnostic of MI

to the ED is also a stressor, to which his *psychological response* might be Anxiety or Fear. What other actual or potential responses were identified for Todd in the situation? Take a moment to write them down.

Recall that Todd has decreased sensation in his lower extremities. This is a stressor, to which he has responded with slight impairment of mobility. Perhaps you identified that because of diminished feeling in his feet, Todd might be at risk for falling (safety), impaired skin or tissue integrity, and ineffective management of his therapy. All of these are responses to disease, illness, or stressors. Also note that as well as being a stressor, the decreased sensation in Todd's lower extremities can be considered a physiological response to type 2 DM. Was this response on the list you just made?

ThinkLike a Nurse 4-1

Imagine that you have been in an automobile accident. You have internal injuries and broken bones and will be hospitalized for at least 2 weeks, right before your final exams. What human responses (physical, emotional, interpersonal, social, spiritual) would you have?

In 1990, NANDA-I officially defined *nursing diagnosis* as "a clinical judgment about individual, family, or community responses to actual or potential health problems/life processes. Nursing diagnosis provides the basis for selection of nursing interventions to achieve outcomes for which the nurse is accountable" (NANDA International, 2009, p. 419). This definition emphasizes the clinical judgment aspect of diagnosing.

Recognizing Medical Diagnoses

A **medical diagnosis** describes a disease, illness, or injury. Its purpose is to identify a pathology so that appropriate treatment can be given. A medical diagnosis is more narrowly focused than a nursing diagnosis. Todd has two medical diagnoses: chronic renal failure and type 2 DM.

Except for advanced practice nurses (nurse practitioners), nurses cannot legally diagnose or treat medical problems. Your assessment data will help the medical team to identify disease states and evaluate the effects of medical therapies. For example, if your assessment indicates that a medication does not adequately relieve a patient's pain, you would inform the primary care provider, who would prescribe a different

medication or dosage. You need to know the pathophysiology of the patient's illness to understand and evaluate the effects of medical treatments and to know how to focus your assessments. The following are some differences between medical and nursing diagnoses:

You cannot predict a patient's nursing diagnoses just by knowing his medical diagnosis or pathology. Nursing diagnoses are human responses that are complex and unique to each person. A medical diagnosis, in contrast, remains the same as long as a particular injury or pathology is present. Todd's medical diagnosis of type 2 DM will not change, because the fact that his body cannot use glucose normally will not change. This is not true for his nursing diagnoses. Suppose Todd has a nursing diagnosis of Noncompliance with diabetic diet r/t (related to) lack of knowledge about food groups. If he learned about the foods and began following his diet, this nursing diagnosis would no longer apply. However, he would still have the medical diagnosis of type 2 DM.

A medical diagnosis, disease, or pathological condition can have any number of nursing diagnoses associated with it. For example, in response to his type 2 DM, Todd might have nursing diagnoses of Noncompliance and Risk for Impaired Skin Integrity.

Clients with the same medical diagnosis may have different nursing diagnoses. Another client with type 2 DM may not have a diagnosis of Noncompliance, but instead may have a diagnosis of Ineffective Denial because he simply cannot accept that he truly has diabetes. Other patients with type 2 DM might have diagnoses of Anxiety, Deficient Knowledge, Disturbed Body Image, and perhaps others, depending on their unique responses to the stressor, type 2 DM.

Recognizing Collaborative Problems

Collaborative problems are "certain physiologic complications [of diseases, medical treatments, or diagnostic studies] that nurses monitor to detect onset or changes in status" (Carpenito, 2006, p. 19). They have the following characteristics:

- **All patients who have a certain disease or treatment are at risk for developing the same complications.** The collaborative problems (complications) are determined by the medical diagnosis or pathology. Consider these examples:

  Todd, because he has type 2 DM, has the collaborative problem Potential Complication of type 2 DM: hyperglycemia and/or hypoglycemia. All other patients with type 2 DM also have those potential complications.

  All patients having surgery have the collaborative problem Potential Complication of surgery: infection.

  Use your theoretical knowledge of anatomy, physiology, microbiology, and pathophysiology, and so on as the basis for identifying the complications associated with a particular disease or treatment.

- **A collaborative problem is always a potential problem.** If it becomes *actual*, then it is no longer a collaborative problem, but a medical diagnosis requiring physician interventions. Consider what would be needed if the preceding potential complications became actual problems. Either condition would require medical intervention to prevent serious harm to the patient.

  Actual hyperglycemia (high blood glucose) or actual hypoglycemia (low blood glucose)

  Actual infection of a surgical incision

- **If you can prevent the complication with independent nursing interventions alone, it is not a collaborative problem.** Collaborative problems require both medical and independent nursing interventions to prevent them or to

minimize the complications. The purpose of independent nursing interventions is primarily to monitor for onset of complications, although nurses can provide some independent preventive measures.

See Figure 4-3 for an algorithm to help you differentiate nursing diagnoses from medical diagnoses and collaborative problems.

KnowledgeCheck 4-2

State whether each of the following represents a nursing diagnosis, medical diagnosis, or collaborative problem:

- After giving birth, all women are at risk for developing postpartum hemorrhage.
- A patient has signs and symptoms of appendicitis, which must be treated with surgery and antibiotics.
- A client is at risk for constipation because he postpones defecation and does not consume enough dietary fiber and fluids. The problem can be prevented by patient teaching, which the nurse is licensed to do.

Types of Nursing Diagnoses

The status, or type, of each nursing diagnosis must be determined. Is it an actual or potential problem; a wellness diagnosis; or a syndrome diagnosis? This is important because each status requires (1) different wording in the diagnostic statement and (2) different nursing interventions (Fig. 4-4).

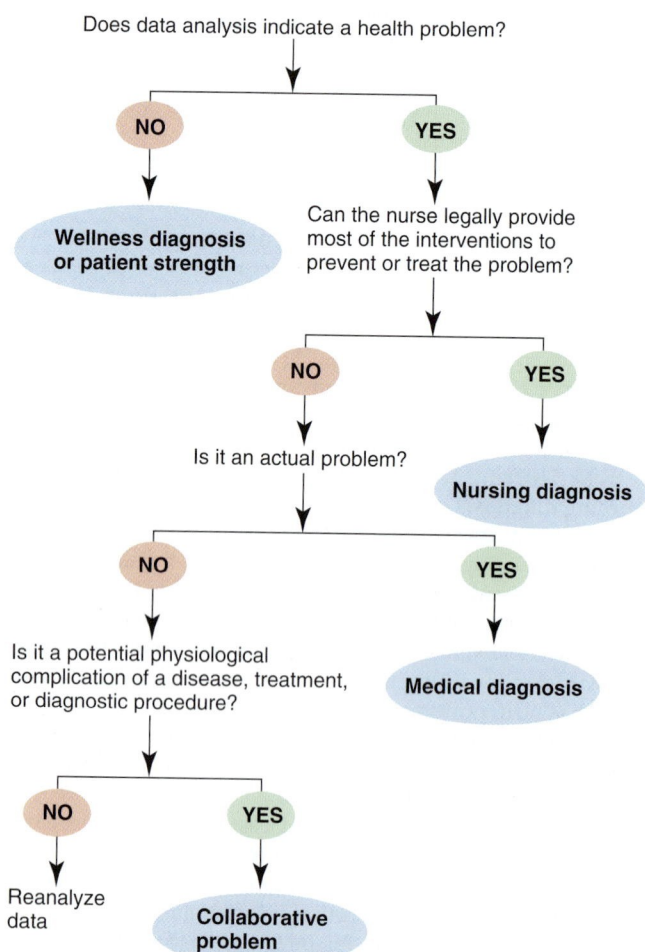

FIGURE 4-3 Algorithm for distinguishing among nursing, medical, and collaborative problems.

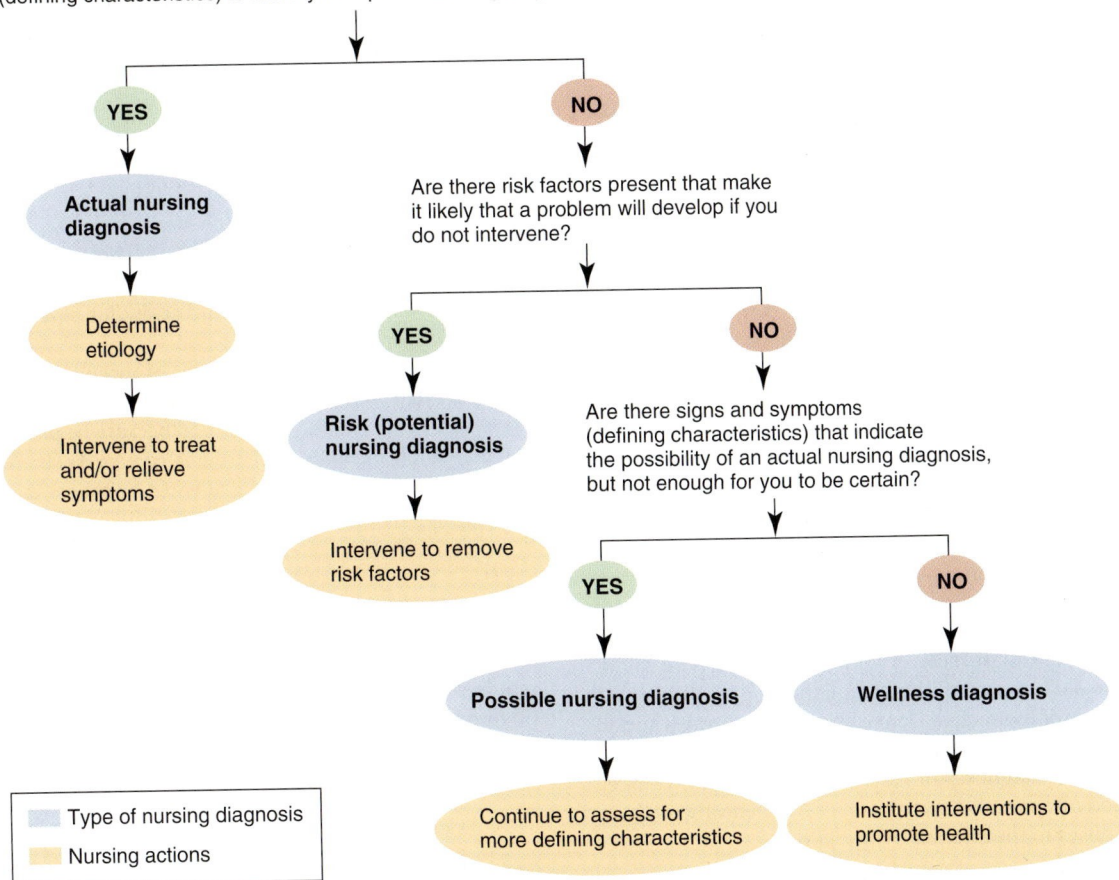

At the time of assessment, does the patient have enough signs and symptoms (defining characteristics) to identify the specific nursing diagnosis?

YES

NO

Actual nursing diagnosis

Are there risk factors present that make it likely that a problem will develop if you do not intervene?

Determine etiology

YES

NO

Intervene to treat and/or relieve symptoms

Risk (potential) nursing diagnosis

Are there signs and symptoms (defining characteristics) that indicate the possibility of an actual nursing diagnosis, but not enough for you to be certain?

Intervene to remove risk factors

YES

NO

Possible nursing diagnosis

Wellness diagnosis

Type of nursing diagnosis

Nursing actions

Continue to assess for more defining characteristics

Institute interventions to promote health

FIGURE 4-4 Algorithm for determining whether a nursing diagnosis is an actual diagnosis, a risk (potential) diagnosis, a possible diagnosis, or a wellness diagnosis.

Actual Nursing Diagnosis: Problem Is Present. An **actual nursing diagnosis** is a problem response that exists at the time of the assessment. You identify it by the signs and symptoms (cues) that are present. Todd (Meet Your Patient) has no actual nursing diagnoses. He may have actual Impaired Walking or perhaps Impaired Physical Mobility, related to his lack of peripheral sensation; however, no signs and symptoms were given in the scenario to support that diagnosis.

Risk Nursing Diagnosis: Problem May Occur. A **risk nursing diagnosis** describes a problem response that is likely to develop in a vulnerable patient if the nurse and patient do not intervene to prevent it. You will identify a risk diagnosis when the patient does not have signs/symptoms of the problem, but does have risk factors present that increase his vulnerability. For example, Todd's loss of lower limb sensation is a risk factor for a diagnosis of Risk for Falls, even though Todd has no symptoms or history of falling.

Use risk nursing diagnoses (also called potential nursing diagnoses) only for patients who have more susceptibility to the problem than others in the same or a comparable setting. For example, all surgical patients have at least some risk for developing infection, so you should not routinely write Risk for Infection on every surgical care plan. You would, instead, write Potential Complication of surgery: infection (incision and systemic). Use the nursing diagnosis Risk for Infection for patients who are *unusually* susceptible to infection (e.g., one who is undernourished or one with a compromised immune system).

Possible Nursing Diagnosis: Problem May Be Present. A **possible nursing diagnosis** exists when your intuition and experience direct you to suspect that a diagnosis is present, but you do not have enough data to support the diagnosis. The main reason for including this type of diagnosis on a care plan is to alert other nurses to continue to collect data to confirm or rule out the problem. Todd (Meet Your Patient) has a symptom of slightly impaired mobility. This could indicate the diagnoses Impaired Physical Mobility, Impaired Walking, or Risk for Falls. You need more data to decide which nursing diagnosis is appropriate, so you might write a nursing diagnosis of Possible Risk for Falls related to decreased sensation in both legs.

Syndrome Nursing Diagnosis: Several Related Problems Are Present. A **syndrome nursing diagnosis** represents a collection of nursing diagnoses that usually occur together. For example, the NANDA-I label Risk for Disuse Syndrome is used to represent all the complications that can occur as a result of immobility (e.g., pressure ulcer, constipation, stasis of pulmonary secretions, thrombosis, body image disturbance).

Wellness Nursing Diagnosis: No Problem Is Present. You will use a **wellness diagnosis** when an individual, group, or community is in transition from one level of wellness to a higher level of wellness. A wellness diagnosis describes health status, but it is not a health problem. For you to make a wellness diagnosis, two conditions must be present: (1) The client's present level of wellness is effective and (2) the client wants to move to a higher level of wellness.

KnowledgeCheck 4-3

- What are the five types of nursing diagnoses?
- What kind of nursing diagnosis is each of the following?
  a. Jane Thomas regularly engages in exercise but tells you she would like to increase her endurance.
  b. Mrs. King has several of the signs and symptoms (defining characteristics) of the nursing diagnosis Ineffective Coping.
  c. Alicia Hernandez seems anxious, but you are not sure. You would like to have more data in order to diagnose or rule out a diagnosis of Anxiety.
  d. Charles Oberfeldt has no symptoms of constipation. However, he reports that he does not include many fiber-rich foods in his diet and drinks few liquids. In addition, he is now fairly inactive because of a back injury. These are all risk factors for a diagnosis of Constipation.

WHAT IS DIAGNOSTIC REASONING?

A comprehensive patient assessment produces a great deal of data. **Diagnostic reasoning** is the thinking process that enables you to make sense of it. This text presents diagnostic reasoning (also referred to as **analysis**) in separate steps so that it is easier to learn, but that is not the way it really occurs (Fig. 4-5). When you first begin to use diagnostic reasoning, follow the steps in the order we present so that you will not miss anything. But just as you move back and forth between assessing and diagnosing, you will soon find yourself moving back and forth among the steps of diagnostic reasoning, skipping steps, returning to previous steps, and doing some steps simultaneously.

In diagnostic reasoning, you will use your critical thinking to analyze and interpret data, draw conclusions about the patient's health status, verify problems with the patient, prioritize the problems, and record the diagnostic statements.

Analyze and Interpret Data

As you analyze and interpret the data, you will gradually narrow the quantity of data you must deal with. But even as you narrow the field of data to the significant points and patterns, you will note the need for new information and further assessments. To analyze and interpret data, follow three steps: (1) identify significant data, (2) cluster cues, and (3) identify data gaps and inconsistencies.

1. Identify Significant Data

Significant data (also called **cues**) are data that influence your conclusions about the client's health status. A cue should alert you to look for other cues that might be related to it (i.e., form a pattern). You may be thinking, "How will I recognize a cue?"

A cue is usually an unhealthy response. One way to recognize cues is to draw on your theoretical knowledge (e.g., of anatomy, physiology, psychology) and compare each piece of data to standards and norms. For example, suppose you have noted that a woman's pulse rate is 110 beats/minute. Is this an unhealthy response—a cue? You would of course use as one standard the average rate (80 beats/min) and normal range (60–100 beats/min) for an adult pulse. But this woman is a long-time cigarette smoker who also drinks coffee and caffeinated energy drinks. These habits increase pulse rate, so 110 beats/minute may be a normal finding for this client. See Box 4-2 for other indications of cues.

KnowledgeCheck 4-4

- What is a cue?
- What are five ways you can recognize a cue?

BOX 4-2 ■ Recognizing Cues

The following may indicate cues:

A deviation from population norms
Example: For a well-conditioned athlete who is not a smoker, a heart rate of 120 beats/min would probably be an unhealthy response (cue). However, remember that, in addition, you must always consider whether the response is normal for the patient or the situation.

Changes in usual health patterns are not explained by developmental or situational changes
Example: What change has Todd (Meet Your Patient) experienced in the 3 days before admission to the ED? Is there any developmental or situational explanation for his decreased sensation and mobility? No. It is an unhealthy response: a cue.

Indications of delayed growth and development
Example: A 17-year-old girl has not yet experienced menses, her breasts are just barely developed, and she has very scant pubic and underarm hair.

Changes in usual behaviors in roles or relationships
Example: During her first year at college, a previously successful student begins to skip classes. She stays up late partying and sleeps most of the day. She no longer keeps in contact with her friends, and despite a previous close relationship with her parents she barely talks to them when they contact her.

Nonproductive or dysfunctional behavior
This may or may not be a change in behavior. It could be a long-standing dysfunctional behavior. *Example:* A man has been abusing alcohol for many years, even though it is causing many problems with his family and job and has begun to damage his liver.

Source: Adapted from Gordon, M. (1994). *Nursing diagnosis: Process and application* (3rd ed.). St. Louis, MO: C.V. Mosby.

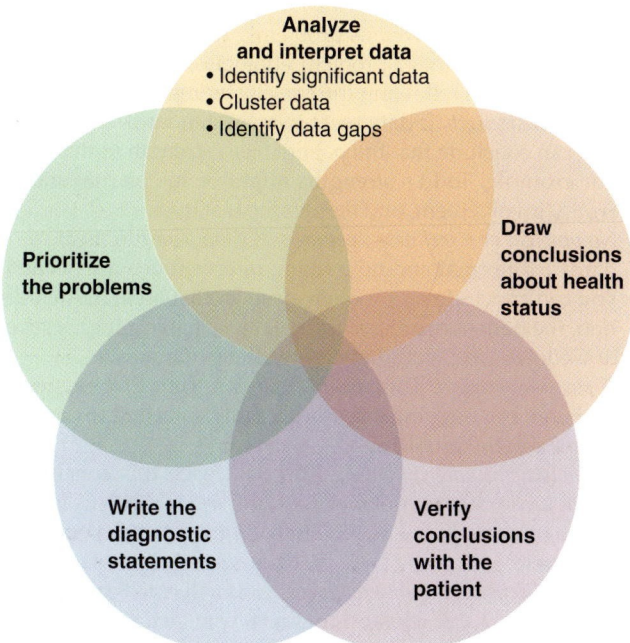

FIGURE 4-5 The diagnostic reasoning process.

Analyze and interpret data
- Identify significant data
- Cluster data
- Identify data gaps

Draw conclusions about health status

Prioritize the problems

Write the diagnostic statements

Verify conclusions with the patient

2. Cluster Cues

A **cluster** is a group of cues that are related to each other in some way. The cluster may suggest a health problem. To help ensure accuracy, you should always derive a nursing diagnosis from data clusters rather than from a single cue.

Consider this example. Alma was transferred to the hospital from a long-term care facility. Because of a CVA (cerebrovascular accident, or stroke), Alma can make sounds but cannot speak; and because of joint contractures, she cannot use her hands and arms. Alma is frequently incontinent of urine, so the nurses have diagnosed Overflow Urinary Incontinence and are resigned to the idea that Alma will not be able to control her urine. Because Alma makes loud vocal noises, they have placed her in a room near the nurses' station. When a nursing student is assigned to care for Alma, the student looks for cues in addition to urinary incontinence. The student notices that urinary incontinence often occurs after Alma's loud vocalizing. She sees a pattern in these cues: urinary incontinence, cannot use hands and arms, and cannot communicate verbally. The student changes the nursing diagnosis to Self-Care Deficit: Toileting related to immobility and inability to communicate the need to void. After the student provides a call device that fits under Alma's arm, Alma is able to press the device and call the nurse when she needs to void. She is no longer incontinent of urine.

ThinkLike a Nurse 4-2

For each of the following cue clusters, decide whether the cues represent a pattern; that is, are all the cues related in some way? If so, explain how they are related. If not, state which cue does not fit. If you do not have enough theoretical knowledge to know for sure, draw on your past experiences and discuss the clusters with other students.

a. Dry skin; abnormal return of skin turgor (more than 4 seconds); thirst; and scanty, dark yellow urine
b. Pain and limited range of motion in knees, uses walker, medical diagnosis of osteoarthritis
c. Has hard, painful bowel movement about every 3 days; does not exercise regularly; eats very little dietary fiber; skin is dry

Clustering data forces you to think about the relationships between the cues. For item (c) in the preceding exercise, you would think, "What might cause hard, painful bowel movements? I know that dietary fiber promotes peristalsis, so lack of fiber might contribute to constipation. And I remember that lack of exercise and dry skin are associated with constipation. However, I don't see how dry skin would be related to constipation."

3. Identify Data Gaps and Inconsistencies

As you cluster and think about relationships among the cues, you will identify the need for data that was not apparent before. In Think Like a Nurse 4-2 item (c), you have enough data to support a diagnosis of Constipation. However, you still need to identify factors contributing to the problem. You have two: lack of dietary fiber and lack of exercise. But you should also ask about other causes of Constipation. Does the patient postpone defecation? Does he have a history of relying on laxatives? How much fluid does the client drink? For example, Todd's (Meet Your Patient) skin is dry. Could that be because he is fluid deficient?

Data Gaps. As another example, look again at Todd's data. Except for medical diagnoses, there are very few data. The following data gaps exist:

- His admitting diagnosis, chronic renal failure, suggests the possibility of fluid imbalance; however, there are no other data to support that. What is his intake? His output? His skin turgor? The appearance of his urine? Does he have edema? Does he complain of thirst? What are his hemoglobin and hematocrit levels?
- Admission to the ED could cause Anxiety. Observe for physical and verbal symptoms of Anxiety.
- Decreased sensation in his lower extremities might create mobility or safety problems. You would need to know the degree of sensation loss and the exact meaning of "slight loss of mobility" to determine whether to focus on the mobility or the safety issue.
- The effect of diabetes on circulation and skin certainly places Todd at risk for skin problems. However, you need more data to determine whether he has any actual skin problems (e.g., presence of sores on his feet).

Inconsistencies. In addition to missing data, look for inconsistencies in the data. Suppose a client tells you, "I really don't eat much. Three meals a day, and I don't snack between meals." However, she is 5 ft tall and weighs 190 lb. This seems inconsistent because your theoretical knowledge tells you that obesity is usually caused by excessive intake of calories. Even though there are many causes a for being overweight, you wonder if someone could be so much overweight without "eating much." In this case, you would need more specific data about what the client actually eats; consider having her keep a food diary of everything she eats for a week or two. What else would you want to know? For example, does she have any medical problems that might cause obesity (e.g., hypothyroidism)? Is there any reason she might not want to tell you the truth about her eating pattern? Does she know the number of calories in various foods? Is she actually aware of how much she is eating? More data will help answer your questions.

Draw Conclusions About Health Status

After clustering cues and collecting any missing data, the next step is to begin drawing conclusions about the patient's health status—strengths as well as problems. You will need to make inferences and identify problem etiologies, as well as decide which one of the following the cue cluster represents:

- *A patient strength.* If data seem to meet standards and norms, you can conclude that the patient has a strength in that area. For example, Todd's strengths might be his marital status, family involvement, and employment status.
- *No problem or a wellness diagnosis.* If data seem to meet standards for normal and no nursing interventions are needed, you can conclude no problem exists in that area. If, in addition, the patient expresses the wish to achieve a higher level of wellness, you would make a wellness diagnosis.
- *A possible problem.* This means there are cues that suggest a problem, but ongoing monitoring will be needed to confirm or rule out the problem.
- *An actual nursing diagnosis.* You will reach this conclusion when a cue cluster contains the signs and symptoms (defining characteristics) of a problem you can treat independently as a nurse.
- *A risk (potential) nursing diagnosis.* You will reach this conclusion when a cue cluster contains risk factors that make nursing interventions necessary to prevent a problem from developing.

- *A collaborative problem.* The client's medical diagnosis or treatment indicates the need to monitor for development of complications and to take some measures to prevent the complication, but you cannot prevent or treat the problem independently.
- *A medical diagnosis.* Nurses are not licensed to make medical diagnoses. If you recognize signs and symptoms suggestive of a medical diagnosis, consult a medical provider for diagnosis and treatment.

1. Make Inferences

Making inferences is a *critical thinking skill.* Recall that cues are facts (or data), whereas inferences are conclusions (judgments, interpretations) that are based on the data. An inference is not a fact, because you cannot directly check its truth or accuracy. For example:

Fact:	Patient is crying. (You can observe that directly.)
	Patient is trembling. (You can observe that directly.)
Inference:	Patient is anxious. (You cannot observe anxiety, but you know that crying and trembling may be signs of anxiety.)

Even though you cannot ever be completely sure that an inference is accurate, it is clear that some inferences are supported by more complete and reliable data than are others. In the preceding example, suppose you said to the patient, "You seem upset. Can you tell me what's going on?" And the patient then replied, "I've never been in the hospital before. So much has been happening, I guess I'm just anxious about everything." Now you have enough data to support your inference, and you can be reasonably sure that it is accurate (valid). But remember, you can't be absolutely certain. For example, although it is unlikely, the patient might not be telling you the truth. Perhaps she is crying because her husband said hurtful things to her, and she is too embarrassed to share that with you. Or perhaps she is a spy and is trying to divert your attention while an accomplice finds the hospital's hidden secrets. Yes, that is far-fetched, but that exaggerated example should convince you that an inference—even one that appears to be more valid than this one—is not a *fact.*

This is an important point in diagnosing. Nursing diagnoses, because they are inferences, are only reasoned judgments about a patient's health status. Try not to think of a diagnosis as being either right or wrong, but instead as more accurate or less accurate. Realize that you can never construct a perfect diagnosis, but strive to make your diagnostic statements as accurate as possible. Incorrect diagnoses can result in ineffective care.

KnowledgeCheck 4-5

- What are the possible conclusions you can draw about a client's health status (e.g., that no problem exists)?
- What is the difference between a cue and an inference?
- How can you be satisfied that you have made a valid inference?

2. Identify Problem Etiologies

An **etiology** consists of the factors that are causing or contributing to the problem. Etiologies may be pathophysiological, treatment related, situational, social, spiritual, maturational, or environmental. It is important to correctly identify the etiology because it directs the nursing interventions. Consider this nursing diagnosis:

Constipation related to inadequate intake of dietary fiber

The etiology suggests that you encourage the client to eat more high-fiber foods. You might also teach the client about foods that are high in fiber. But what if that etiology is incomplete? What if you overlooked the fact that the client does not drink enough fluids? Or that he gets very little exercise? And what if he often postpones defecation because he is a kindergarten teacher in a crowded, bustling classroom, and he simply cannot leave the children unattended except at scheduled times? In that case, your efforts to increase intake of high-fiber foods would probably not help relieve the person's constipation.

To identify the etiology of a health problem, use your theoretical knowledge (e.g., of psychology, physiology, disease processes) and the patient data to answer questions such as the following:

- What factors are known to cause this problem?
- What patient cues are present that may be contributing to this problem?
- How likely is it that these factors are contributing to the problem?
- What past experiences support my judgment that these factors are linked to the problem?
- Are these cues *causing* the problem, or are they merely *symptoms* of the problem?

An etiology is always an inference because you can never actually observe the link between etiology and problem. You can often be certain that the etiological factors are present. For example, in the preceding Constipation diagnosis, you could measure (observe) the person's fiber intake. You could also observe infrequent, hard stools (Constipation). But you cannot observe that the lack of fiber is the cause of the Constipation. You must infer that link based on your knowledge of normal elimination and your experiences with other patients.

ThinkLike a Nurse 4-3

How would your nursing interventions be different for the following diagnoses?

- Constipation related to lack of knowledge about laxative use
- Constipation related to weakened abdominal muscles secondary to long-term immobility

Verify Problems With the Patient

After identifying problems and etiologies, verify them with the patient. A diagnostic statement is an interpretation of the data, and the patient's interpretations may differ from yours. For example, if you have diagnosed Ineffective Breastfeeding related to lack of knowledge about breastfeeding techniques, you might verify it by saying, "It seems to me you are having difficulty breastfeeding your baby because you are not sure how to position him and get him to latch on to your breast. Does this seem accurate to you?" The woman might confirm your diagnosis, or she might say, "No. I *do* know how to do it; I am just tired and a little nervous with you watching me." Think of nursing diagnoses as tentative, and remain open to changing them based on new data or insights from the patient.

Prioritize Problems

Up to this point, the diagnostic process has focused on identifying and validating health problems. However, clients often have more than one problem, so you must use nursing judgment to decide which ones to address first and which can wait until later. This is **prioritizing.** Prioritizing places the problems in order of importance, but it does not mean you must resolve one problem before attending to another.

Problem priority is largely determined by the theoretical framework that you use—for example, whether your criteria are human needs, problem urgency, future consequences, or patient preference.

Maslow's Hierarchy of Human Needs

Even though it is not a nursing framework, many nurses use Maslow's hierarchy to prioritize nursing diagnoses (Fig. 4-6). In Maslow's model, basic needs must be met before a person can focus on higher needs. Maslow (1970) ranks human needs on eight levels, beginning with the most basic needs. Table 4-3 shows examples of nursing diagnoses at various levels of Maslow's hierarchy. For further information on the Maslow theory, see Chapter 8.

 ThinkLike a Nurse 4-4

Prioritize the following nursing diagnosis labels (problems) based on the Maslow framework.

(1) First assign each diagnosis a high, medium, or low priority. Some may have the same priority.

(2) Next rank them in order of importance, with 1 being most important and 5 being least important. Use each number only once.

_____ Ineffective Airway Clearance
_____ Ineffective Breathing Pattern
_____ Diarrhea
_____ Risk for Falls
_____ Impaired Memory

Problem Urgency

If you use problem urgency as your ranking criteria, you would rank the problems according to the degree of threat they pose to the patient's life or to the immediacy with which treatment is needed. Assign:

High priority to problems that are life-threatening (e.g., Ineffective Airway Clearance) or that could have a destructive effect on the client (e.g., substance abuse)

Medium priority to problems that do not pose a direct threat to life, but that may cause destructive physical or emotional changes (e.g., Ineffective Denial, Unilateral Neglect)

Low priority to problems that require minimal supportive nursing intervention (e.g., Risk for Delayed Development, Mild Anxiety)

Future Consequences

When assigning priorities, also consider the possible future effects of a problem. Even if a problem is not life threatening, and even if the patient does not see the problem as a priority, it may result in harmful future consequences for the patient. For example, suppose that Todd (Meet Your Patient) is hospitalized for 5 days and undergoes inpatient dialysis. His physician prescribes a renal diet and insulin (instead of his previous oral medications) to treat the DM. Todd announces that he would like to go home as soon as possible. "I need to get back to my job and my family," he tells you. He resists learning about his medicines and how to administer his insulin. "Just give me a list of my medicines, and I'll take them when I get home," he says. You are aware that his renal failure is secondary to uncontrolled DM and that he was erratic about taking his medication in the past. You suspect that he has not been taking his medicines because he is in denial about his health problems. Clearly his Ineffective Denial may lead to further problems with his treatment plan. You would assign high priority to this problem and address

it before attempting to provide teaching for his nursing diagnosis of Deficient Knowledge (insulin).

Patient Preference

Give high priority to problems the patient thinks are most important, provided that this does not conflict with basic/survival needs or medical treatments. Patients cooperate more fully with interventions they consider important. In addition, they may be more motivated to work on other problems after their own priorities are addressed.

Consider this example. Mr. Amani has had a major surgery within the past 24 hours. His main concern is to obtain pain relief. He refuses to turn, deep-breathe, and cough (TDBC) because it causes pain. However, as his nurse, you realize that these activities are essential for preventing Ineffective Airway Clearance, so you cannot safely support Mr. Amani's priorities. You should of course provide pain medication before helping him TDBC, but it may be impossible for him to be entirely pain free during these activities. You would explain your actions and continue to emphasize the importance of TDBC. When you explain the importance of your priorities, patients often come to agree with them.

Documenting Priorities

You will usually prioritize problems as you are recording them. You can indicate the priority by designating each

FIGURE 4-6 Maslow's Hierarchy of Human Needs can be used for prioritizing problems. Most nursing diagnoses fall at the cognitive and lower levels. (*Source:* Adapted from Maslow, A. (1971). *The farther reaches of human nature.* New York: Viking Press; and Maslow, A., & Lowery, R. [Eds.]. (1998). *Toward a psychology of being* [3rd ed.]. New York: John Wiley & Sons.)

Table 4-3 ➤ Using Maslow's Hierarchy to Prioritize Diagnoses

BASIC NEEDS (MOST BASIC TO HIGHEST LEVEL)	EXAMPLES OF HUMAN NEEDS	EXAMPLES OF NURSING DIAGNOSES
Physiological	Food, air, water, shelter, sleep and rest, elimination, activity, temperature regulation	Imbalanced Nutrition: Less Than Body Requirements Impaired Gas Exchange
Safety and Security	(Includes both physical and psychological safety); law, order, shelter, stability	Risk for Falls Fear Risk for Self-Directed Violence
Love and Belonging	Roles, relationships, the need to give and receive affection, the feeling of belonging	Impaired Social Interaction Ineffective Sexuality Pattern Risk for Impaired Attachment
Self-Esteem	Feelings of confidence, capability, and independence; respect, recognition, and appreciation from others.	Chronic Low Self-Esteem Social Isolation
Cognitive	Knowledge, understanding, exploration	Acute Confusion Impaired Memory Delayed Growth and Development
Aesthetic	Symmetry, order, beauty	It is unusual for nursing diagnoses to fall into this, or the two higher, categories.
Self-Actualization	Personal growth, reaching one's highest potential	
Transcendence	Connecting to something beyond self, helping others reach their potential	Readiness for Enhanced Spirituality Spiritual Distress

Sources: Adapted from Maslow, A. (1971). *The farther reaches of human nature.* New York: Viking Press; and Maslow, A., & Lowery, R. (Eds.). (1998). *Toward a psychology of being* (3rd ed.). New York: John Wiley & Sons.

---

problem as high, medium, or low priority or by ranking all the problems in order from highest to lowest (i.e., 1, 2, 3, 4). For example:

Labeling Each Problem	*Ranking the Problems*
Pain (high)	1—Risk for Falls
Risk for Falls (high)	2—Pain
Chronic Low Self-Esteem (low)	3—Imbalanced (low) Nutrition
Imbalanced Nutrition (medium)	4—Chronic Low Self-Esteem

Notice that risk problems can have a higher priority than actual problems. In this example, it is more urgent to prevent falls than it is to treat low self-esteem.

ThinkLike a Nurse 4-5

Suppose that upon Todd's (Meet Your Patient) transfer from the ED, you made the following nursing diagnoses for him. Using problem urgency as your criterion, assign each of these diagnoses in low, medium, or high priority order. You may not have much theoretical knowledge about type 2 DM and chronic renal disease, but use the information provided in the scenario

and in the etiologies to prioritize as well as you can. Discuss the case with your classmates and your instructor.

- Risk for Imbalanced Fluid Volume secondary to renal failure
- Risk for Falls r/t decreased sensation and mobility in legs
- Anxiety r/t unknown prognosis of renal failure and ED environment
- Deficient Knowledge (renal disease process) r/t new diagnosis of renal involvement r/t type 2 DM

Computer-Assisted Diagnosing

Many institutions use computers for planning and documenting patient care. Some expert (knowledge-based) systems allow you to enter assessment data, and the computer program will generate a list of possible problems. After you choose a problem label, the computer will provide a screen with the definition and defining characteristics of the problem so you can compare them to the actual patient data. After you "accept" the diagnostic label, complete the problem statement by choosing etiologies from the next computer screen. To see examples of such computer screens,

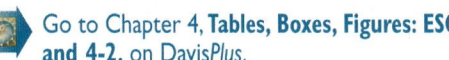

Go to Chapter 4, **Tables, Boxes, Figures: ESG Figures 4-1 and 4-2,** on DavisPlus.

Knowledge**Knowledge**Check 4-6

List the steps in the diagnostic process.

REFLECTING CRITICALLY ON YOUR DIAGNOSTIC REASONING

Diagnostic reasoning is complex and vulnerable to error. After you have your prioritized list of problems, you need to evaluate the list for accuracy. With the implementation of electronic health records, there is an even greater need for accuracy of nursing diagnoses (Lunney, 2008). When diagnosing, apply critical thinking to your theoretical and self-knowledge and to the patient data and situation (recall the full-spectrum nursing model in Chapter 2).

Critical thinking + Knowledge + Data =
Statement of health status

Think About Your Theoretical Knowledge

The better your knowledge base is, the better your diagnostic reasoning will be. Ask yourself the following questions:

- Are my diagnoses based on sound knowledge (e.g., of pathophysiology, psychology, nutrition, and other related disciplines)?
- Do I have sound knowledge about the defining characteristics associated with various nursing diagnoses?
- Do I feel reasonably sure I have interpreted the data correctly?
- Have I identified the problem type correctly—that is, can this problem be treated primarily by nursing interventions?
- Am I qualified to make these diagnoses, or should I ask for consultation (e.g., from a more experienced nurse or other member of the collaborative healthcare team)?

To avoid diagnostic error, build a good knowledge base and learn from your clinical experiences. If you lack knowledge in an area, review the literature. Solid theoretical knowledge will help you (1) to recognize cues and patterns, (2) to associate patterns with the correct problem, (3) give you confidence in your ability to reason, and (4) keep you from relying too much on authority figures (Wilkinson, 2011).

Think About Your Self-Knowledge

Realize that your beliefs, values, and experiences affect your thinking and can be misleading. For example, imagine that a nurse in a labor and delivery unit believes it is important to be strong and uncomplaining, even when experiencing severe pain. When this nurse cares for a woman in early labor who cries out and complains of pain, the nurse sees it as a problem of either Anxiety or Ineffective Coping, not as a problem of Pain. Can you see how that changes the focus of the nurse's care? Ask yourself the following questions (Wilkinson, 2011).

What biases and stereotypes may have influenced my interpretation of the data? A **bias** is the tendency to slant your judgment based on personal opinion or unfounded beliefs, as the nurse did in the preceding example. **Stereotypes** are judgments and expectations about an individual based on the personal beliefs you have about this group (e.g., men are unemotional; Asians are intelligent; teenagers are irresponsible). Referring to patients by their diagnosis or developmental group is a form of stereotyping (e.g., "the elderly man in room 110"; "the broken hip in 288"). You form stereotypes by making flawed assumptions when you have little or no actual experience with a person or group.

Did I rely too much on past experiences? This is like stereotyping in that you draw conclusions about an individual based on what you know about people in similar situations. Consider, for example, a nurse who has cared for many first-time mothers (primiparas) during labor. Many of these women experienced moderate anxiety even during early labor. Now each time the nurse cares for a primipara, she expects to see anxiety, and she tends to identify cue clusters as Anxiety, failing to check for other explanations such as Pain or Deficient Knowledge.

Did I rely too much on the client's medical diagnosis, the setting, or what others say about the client (e.g., "He's angry and uncooperative") instead of on the data? Medical diagnoses and statements from others can help you to think of possible explanations for your data, but they can also bias your thinking and prevent you from gathering your own data. For example, Ms. Grayson has cancer. She returned to the unit last evening after undergoing a total colectomy and colostomy (removal of the colon and creation of an artificial opening for removal of stool). She had expected to undergo only an exploratory laparotomy surgery to evaluate abdominal symptoms. This morning in report, the night shift nurse stated, "Ms. Grayson is aware that she has cancer and is coping well." While bathing Ms. Grayson, you begin to tell her about her colostomy. She seems shocked. "I didn't know they did that! What's wrong with me?" As you answer her questions, you realize that she has been very groggy from the anesthesia and pain medication and does not recall being told about her surgery and cancer.

Think About Your Analysis and Conclusions

After reflecting on your knowledge, think about how you used the diagnostic process. Be sure your analysis of the data was thorough, that you have accurately identified the patient's problems, and that they are logically linked to the etiologies. Review your interactions with the patient: Do the diagnostic statements reflect her perceptions and priorities, or did she give you only the answers she thought you wanted? Use the questions in Box 4-3 to critique your diagnostic process.

KnowledgeCheck 4-7

To help you fix them in your mind, list at least 10 questions to ask yourself when evaluating your diagnostic reasoning. Refer to Box 4-3 if you need help preparing this list.

PracticalKnowledge
knowing **how**

After you have completed the diagnostic reasoning process, the final activity in the diagnosis step is to record the strengths and problem statements. Practical knowledge regarding nursing diagnosis involves selecting the correct standardized problem labels and writing the diagnostic statements.

HOW ARE DIAGNOSTIC STATEMENTS WRITTEN?

This section explains the need for standardized languages, describes the NANDA-I standardized terminology for nursing diagnoses, explains how to choose the correct label, and

BOX 4-3 ■ Critiquing Your Diagnostic Reasoning Process

Data Analysis,

Did you:
- Identify all the significant data (cues)?
- Omit any important cues from the cluster?
- Include unnecessary cues that may have confused your interpretation?
- Try more than one way of grouping the cues?
- Consider the patient's social, cultural, and spiritual beliefs and needs?
- Identify all the data gaps and inconsistencies?

Drawing Inferences and Interpretations of the Data

- Did you consider all the possible explanations for the cue cluster?
- Is this the best explanation for the cue cluster? Remember that a variety of explanations may be possible.
- Did you have enough data to make that inference? If not, suspend judgment until you gather more data.
- Did you look at patterns, not single cues?
- Did you look at behavior over time, not just isolated incidents?
- Did you jump to conclusions? Or did you take the time to carefully analyze and synthesize the data?

Critiquing the Diagnostic Statement (Problem + Etiology)

- Is the diagnosis relevant, and does it reflect the data?
- Does the diagnostic statement give a clear and accurate picture of the patient's problem or strength?

- When identifying the problem and etiology, did you look beyond medical diagnoses and consider human responses?
- Did you consider strengths and wellness diagnoses?
- Can you explain how the etiology relates to the problem—that is, how it would produce the problem response?
- Does the complete list of problems fully describe the patient's overall health status?

Verifying the Diagnosis

- Did the patient verify this diagnosis?
- When you verified the diagnosis, are you certain that the patient understood your description of his health status?
- Did you obtain feedback from the patient, or did you merely assume that the patient agreed?
- Did you keep an open mind, realizing all diagnoses are tentative and subject to change as you acquire more data?

Prioritizing

- Considering the whole situation, what are the most important problems?
- What aspects of the situation require immediate attention?
- Did you consider patient preferences when setting priorities? If not, was there a good reason?

---

describes formats for nursing diagnosis and collaborative problem statements.

Standardized Nursing Languages

In order to communicate, people need a shared language. A **standardized language** is one in which the terms are carefully defined and mean the same thing to all who use them. One example is the periodic table for chemical elements. When a chemist in the United States writes Fe or Zn, all other chemists in the world know that she means iron or zinc. Moreover, they know exactly what is meant by iron and zinc, because each is defined by its own atomic number, atomic mass, number of protons, number of neutrons, and so on. There is no confusion. **Standardized nursing languages** are a comparatively recent attempt to bring such clarity to communication about nursing knowledge and nursing thinking. Nurses need clear, precise, consistent terminology when referring to the same clinical problems and treatments. A standardized language can do the following:

- Support electronic health records
- Define, communicate, and expand nursing knowledge
- Increase visibility and awareness of nursing interventions
- Facilitate research to demonstrate the contribution of nurses to healthcare and influence health policy decisions
- Improve patient care by providing better communication among nurses and other healthcare providers and facilitating the testing of nursing interventions

For a full discussion of the benefits of a standardized nursing language,

 Go to Chapter 4, **Supplemental Materials: Why Do We Need a Standardized Nursing Language?** on Davis*Plus.*

What Is a Taxonomy?

A **taxonomy** is a system for classifying ideas or objects based on characteristics they have in common. Classifications are created and used for various reasons. As mentioned earlier, the periodic table classifies elements according to their atomic mass, number of protons, and so on. Medications are classified in various ways; one way is to classify them according to their use (e.g., analgesics, antibiotics). The following classification systems are widely used in healthcare:

- The American Psychiatric Association (APA) *Diagnostic and Statistical Manual (DSM-IV)* describes mental disorders (e.g., bipolar disorder, schizoaffective disorder) (American Psychiatric Association, 2000).
- The *Manual of the International Classification of Disease and Related Health Problems (ICD-10)* names and classifies medical conditions (World Health Organization [WHO], 1992).
- The *Current Procedural Terminology: CPT 2010*, used for reimbursement of physician services, names and defines medical services and procedures (American Medical Association [AMA], 2010).

The following are classification systems the American Nurses Association (ANA) has recognized for describing nursing diagnoses (some describe outcomes and interventions as well):

- *NANDA International (NANDA-I)*. This is the first nursing taxonomy. It includes approximately 200 diagnostic labels with etiologies, risk factors, and defining characteristics. Most chapters of this textbook use NANDA-I terminology.
- *Clinical Care Classification (CCC)*. Similar to the NANDA-I system; includes nearly 200 labels. Contains interventions as well as nursing diagnoses. The CCC was developed for home health use, but can be used in any setting.

- *Omaha System.* Contains 42 nursing diagnosis concepts (also interventions and outcomes). The Omaha system is primarily for community health use, but can be used in other settings.
- *Perioperative Nursing Data Set (PNDS).* For use in perioperative nursing only. Consists of 64 nursing diagnoses (also includes nursing interventions and patient outcomes). This was the first nursing language developed by a nursing specialty.
- *International Classification for Nursing Practice (ICNP).* Includes diagnoses, outcomes, and nursing actions. The ICNP intends to provide a common language for nurses in various clinical settings worldwide (International Council of Nurses, 2005).

NANDA-I Taxonomy of Diagnostic Terminology

Which of the following could you group together? In what ways are the grouped objects similar?

a five-dollar bill	a penny
weeds (still growing)	new grass
an iron skillet	a needle

You could make these groupings:

A $5 bill and a penny (because they are both money)

A penny, an iron skillet, and a needle (because they are all metal)

A $5 bill, grass, and weeds (because they are all green)

Maybe you thought of even other groupings. Any number of principles can be used to classify things and to organize a taxonomy. The first NANDA taxonomy was simply an alphabetical list. To see that taxonomy,

 Go to **Additional Resources, NANDA-I Nursing Diagnoses, 2012—2014, Alphabetical List,** on Davis*Plus*.

NANDA-I's Taxonomy II (NANDA International, 2012) categorizes nursing diagnoses into 13 domains and 47 classes. A **domain** is an area of activity, study, or interest (e.g., health promotion, nutrition). A **class** is a subdivision of a domain (e.g., health awareness is a class under health promotion; digestion is a class under nutrition). To see and use NANDA-I Taxonomy II,

 Go to Chapter 4, **ESG Box 4-1, NANDA-I. Taxonomy II: Domains, Classes, and Diagnoses (Labels),** on Davis*Plus*.

One strength of the NANDA-I taxonomy is that it has been developed by nurses from administration, education, practice, and research, and from all specialty areas (e.g., maternity, mental health, medical-surgical, community). Because they represent the thinking of a broad spectrum of nurses, the diagnostic labels can be used in any setting or specialty.

What Are the Components of a NANDA-I Nursing Diagnosis?

Each nursing diagnosis in the NANDA-I taxonomy has four parts: label, definition, defining characteristics, and either related or risk factors. You must consider all four parts when formulating a nursing diagnosis.

Diagnostic Label

The **diagnostic label (title** or **name)** is a word or phrase that represents a pattern of related cues and describes a problem or wellness response, such as Disturbed Body Image or Readiness for Enhanced Nutrition. Some labels include descriptors for time, age, and other factors (e.g., acute, deficient, delayed). For the complete list of descriptors for NANDA-I nursing diagnoses, see Box 4-4.

Definition

The **definition** explains the meaning of the label and distinguishes it from similar nursing diagnoses. For example, for a patient with a sleep problem, would you label the problem Sleep Deprivation or Disturbed Sleep Pattern? The following definitions can help you to decide:

Sleep Deprivation: Prolonged periods of time without sleep

Disturbed Sleep Pattern: Time limited disruption of sleep amount and quality

Defining Characteristics

Defining characteristics are the cues (signs and symptoms) that allow you to identify a problem or wellness diagnosis. To use a problem label appropriately, a cluster of defining characteristics must be present in the patient data. For example, you cannot decide to use the label Sleep Deprivation merely by reading the definition. You must be sure the patient actually has some of the defining characteristics for Sleep Deprivation.

Related Factors

Related factors are the cues, conditions, or circumstances that cause, precede, influence, contribute to, or are in some way associated with the problem (label). They can be pathophysiological, psychological, social, treatment-related, situational, maturational, and so on. NANDA-I lists the related factors that are most often associated with each problem label, but keep in mind:

1. *The list is not exhaustive.* Factors other than those listed by NANDA-I could also be associated with the problem. For example, imagine the vast number of factors that might cause someone to have Chronic Low Self-Esteem.
2. *The problem may have more than one related factor.* Human beings are complex, and their problems rarely have one single cause. Nursing diagnoses may have multiple factors as their etiology.
3. *An individual patient will not have all the factors on the list* in the NANDA-I Related Factors for his problem etiology.

Risk Factors

Risk factors are events, circumstances, or conditions that increase the vulnerability of a person or group to a health problem. They can be environmental, physiological, psychological, genetic, or chemical. For example, ignoring the urge to defecate and being pregnant both increase the risk a person will become constipated. The diagnostic statement would be Risk for Constipation r/t pregnancy and habitually ignoring the urge to defecate.

For potential (risk) nursing diagnoses, risk factors function as the defining characteristics. Risk factors must be present to make a potential diagnosis, and they form at least a part of the etiology of the diagnostic statement. If **related factors** are present, an actual, rather than potential, problem exists. To help you remember, as a rule:

Related factors are similar to signs and symptoms (of actual problems)

Risk factors are similar to etiologies (of potential problems)

KnowledgeCheck 4-8

- What are the four parts of a NANDA-I nursing diagnosis?
- What purpose does each part of the nursing diagnosis serve for directing the care of the client?

How Do I Know Which Label to Use?

During the diagnostic process, you will already have determined the general topic of the problem and perhaps even have some tentative problem labels in mind. For the following sections, you will need access to the NANDA-I labels, definitions,

BOX 4-4 ■ Descriptors for NANDA-I Nursing Diagnoses

Some NANDA-I labels may include one or more of these descriptors. You may add descriptors to other labels, if necessary, to clarify the diagnostic statement.

Descriptors for the Subject of the Diagnosis (Axis 2)

Individual: A single human being distinct from others, a person
Family: Two or more people having continuous or sustained relationships, perceiving reciprocal obligations, sensing common meaning, and sharing certain obligations toward others; related by blood or choice
Group: A number of people with shared characteristics
Community: A group of people living in the same locale under the same governance. Examples include neighborhoods and cities.

Descriptors for Judgment (Axis 3)

(Suggested; not limited to the following)
Compromised: Damaged, made vulnerable
Complicated: Intricately involved, complex
Decreased: Lessened (in size, amount, or degree)
Defensive: Used or intended to defend or protect
Deficient: Insufficient, inadequate
Delayed: Late, slow, or postponed
Disabled: Limited, handicapped
Disorganized: Not properly arranged or controlled
Disproportionate: Too large or too small in comparison with a norm
Disturbed: Agitated; interrupted, interfered with
Dysfunctional: Not operating normally
Effective: Producing the intended or desired effect
Enhanced: Improved in quality, value, or extent
Excessive: Greater than necessary or desirable
Imbalanced: Out of proportion or balance

Impaired: Damaged, weakened
Ineffective: Not producing the intended or desired effect
Interrupted: Having its continuity broken
Low: Below the norm
Organized: Properly arranged or controlled
Perceived: Observed through the senses
Readiness for: In a suitable state for an activity or situation
Situational: Related to a particular circumstance

Descriptors for Age (Axis 5)

Fetus, neonate, infant, toddler, preschool child, school-age child, adolescent, adult, older adult

Descriptors for Time (Axis 6)

Acute: Lasting less than 6 months
Chronic: Lasting more than 6 months
Intermittent: Stopping or starting again at intervals, periodic, cyclic
Continuous: Uninterrupted, going on without stop

Descriptors for Status of the Diagnosis (Axis 7)

Actual: Existing in fact or reality, existing at the present time.
Health: Behavior motivated by the desire to increase well-being and actualize human
Promotion: health potential (Pender, Murduagh, & Parsons, 2006, as cited in NANDA-I (2009).
Risk: Vulnerability, especially as a result of exposure to factors that increase the chance of injury or loss
Wellness: The quality or state of being healthy

Source: NANDA International. (2012). *Nursing diagnoses: Definitions and classification 2012–2014.* Ames, IA: Wiley-Blackwell.

and so on, as well as to *Taxonomy II.* You can either use a NANDA-I handbook, a nursing diagnosis handbook; or if you want to print out NANDA-I *Taxonomy II* and use that,

 Go to Chapter 4, **ESG Box 4-1, NANDA-I. Taxonomy II: Domains, Classes, and Diagnoses (Labels)**, on DavisPlus.

1. *First, identify the broad topic (or domain) that seems to fit the cue cluster.* You can look at the NANDA-I taxonomy to see which domain the problem seems to fit. For example, suppose that after further assessment, you find that Todd (Meet Your Patient) has the following defining characteristics:
Intake exceeds output
Oliguria (low volume of urine)
Generalized edema
Recent rapid weight gain
Which of the following NANDA-I domains are suggested by those cues?

Health Promotion	Role Relationships
Nutrition	Self–Perception
Elimination	Activity/Rest

The most logical domains would be Nutrition and Elimination. However, you would need to read the domain definitions in the NANDA-I Taxonomy II and look at the taxonomy classes to be sure.

2. *Narrow your search (to the class or most likely labels).* In the NANDA-I list, read the definitions for the Nutrition and

Elimination domains. Then look at the classes in each. Under Elimination, you will find that Class 1 is Urinary Function. Because Todd has renal failure, you may think that his nursing diagnosis will be found in this class. However, remember that renal failure is a pathology or pathological condition; you are looking for Todd's *responses* to renal failure. On examining the diagnostic labels in the Urinary Function class, you will see none of these represents Todd's defining characteristics.

Next look at the Nutrition domain. You will see the classes Ingestion, Digestion, Absorption, Metabolism, and Hydration. Look at the diagnostic labels listed for the class Hydration. All five of these labels describe fluid balance. You can easily eliminate both risk labels because Todd has an actual problem (he has symptoms). You can eliminate Readiness for Enhanced Fluid Balance because it is a wellness diagnosis. So, you must choose between Deficient Fluid Volume and Excess Fluid Volume. From this point, you simply compare Todd's cue cluster to the defining characteristics and definitions of those two labels and choose the best match.

3. *Using a NANDA-I or other nursing diagnosis handbook, compare definitions and defining characteristics of the diagnostic labels to your cue cluster.* A brief look at the NANDA-I list should convince you that you cannot know exactly what a diagnostic label means from the label name alone. For example, suppose you have a patient who is not sleeping well at night. As a result, she is too tired to

concentrate during the day. Which label would you use to describe this problem: Activity Intolerance, Fatigue, or Acute Confusion? You can answer that question only if you know the definition and defining characteristics of those nursing diagnosis labels.

Not all of the defining characteristics need to be present, but recall that the more data you have when you make an inference, the more certain you can be that your inference is correct.

Examples: NANDA-I lists 14 defining characteristics for Ineffective Thermoregulation, including the following:

1. Fluctuations in body temperature above and below normal range
2. Cyanotic nail beds
3. Pallor
4. Slow capillary refill
5. Tachycardia

You could diagnose Ineffective Thermoregulation on the basis of the first defining characteristic alone, but you might be more certain of your diagnosis if the other cues were also present.

ThinkLike a Nurse 4-6

- In the preceding example, what if the first defining characteristic (temperature fluctuations) was not present and you had only cyanotic nail beds, pallor and slow capillary refill as cues? Could you conclude that Ineffective Thermoregulation is causing those signs? What other explanations might there be for cyanotic nail beds, pallor, and slow capillary refill?
- What if the last defining characteristic was present without the first one? What could cause tachycardia? Do you see the importance of using clusters rather than individual cues?

Components of a Diagnostic Statement

A diagnostic statement consists of a problem and an etiology linked by a connecting phrase.

Problem

The problem describes the client's health status (or a human response to a health problem) and identifies a response that needs to be changed. Use a NANDA-I label when possible. As noted earlier, many NANDA-I labels include a descriptor such as *acute, impaired,* or *deficient.* You will see them arranged in alphabetical lists with the descriptor after the main word (e.g., Physical Mobility, Impaired). However, you should record them as you would say them; for example:

> *Incorrect:* Physical Mobility, Impaired r/t pain in left knee
> *Correct:* Impaired Physical Mobility r/t pain in left knee

Etiology

As discussed earlier, the etiology contains the factors that cause, contribute to, or create a risk for the problem. The etiology may contain several factors, including a NANDA-I label, defining characteristics, related factors, risk factors, or other factors. The etiology will help you to individualize nursing care because etiologies are unique to the individual. For example, suppose two patients have the following nursing diagnoses:

> *John:* Anxiety r/t lack of knowledge of the treatment procedure
> *Janet:* Anxiety r/t prior negative experiences and lack of trust in health professionals

The problem, Anxiety, is defined the same for both patients. They probably share some of the same defining characteristics, and you would use some of the same interventions for both John and Janet. For example, for all anxious patients, regardless of etiology, a calm, reassuring approach is important. However, to prevent the anxiety from recurring, you would need to treat its cause. To relieve John's anxiety, you would teach him what to expect from the impending procedure. But teaching would do nothing to relieve Janet's anxiety. For her, you would need to spend time building a relationship that demonstrates you can be trusted. You would also encourage her to talk about her fears and feelings.

Because the etiology directs the nursing interventions, include only factors that are influenced by nursing interventions. This is why you should not use a medical diagnosis or treatment as an etiology. As an example, there are no independent nursing actions that would change the etiologies in the following diagnosis: Deficient Fluid Volume related to medical order of NPO (nothing by mouth).

Most NANDA-I-related factors are listed in nonspecific terms, so you will usually need to individualize them to reflect each person's unique problem etiology. For example, one of the related factors for Impaired Skin Integrity is "extremes in age." To plan care, you need to know whether this means very old or very young; even better, you should specify the exact age. You would write the diagnostic statement as Impaired Skin Integrity r/t very young age (2 days).

Connecting Phrase (related to)

Most nurses use *related to* (r/t) to connect the problem and etiology, because the phrase *due to* implies a direct causal relationship. Because humans are complex, there are usually many factors that combine to "cause" a problem, so it is nearly impossible to determine an exact cause. In fact, even if you eliminate the etiological factors, the problem might remain. For example, even if Janet begins to trust health professionals, she may become anxious for another reason.

Formats for Diagnostic Statements

A diagnostic statement should describe the client's health status as specifically as possible. The format will vary depending on the type of problem you are describing (Table 4-4).

Basic Two-Part Statement

The two-part statement is used for actual, risk (potential), and possible diagnoses:

Problem	r/t	Etiology
Or		
NANDA-I label	r/t	related factors

For actual diagnoses, the etiology consists of related factors; for risk diagnoses, it consists of risk factors. For example, for a client with excessive vomiting you might write Risk for Deficient Fluid Volume r/t excessive losses through vomiting.

Basic Three-Part Statement

The three-part statement is also called the **PES format** (problem, etiology, and symptom). Some nurses use *AEB (as evidenced by),* whereas others use *AMB (as manifested by).* The following format is used:

> *Problem r/t etiology as manifested by (AMB) signs or symptoms*

This format adds the patient signs or symptoms that led you to make the diagnosis. For example: *Constipation r/t inadequate intake of fluids and fiber-rich foods AMB painful, hard stool and bowel movement every 3 or 4 days.* This is a good method for

Table 4-4 ➤ Examples of Diagnostic Statements

FORMAT	PROBLEM TYPE	PROBLEM (CLIENT RESPONSE; NANDA-I LABEL)	ETIOLOGY (RELATED OR RISK FACTORS)	DEFINING CHARACTERISTICS OR "SECONDARY"
Basic One-Part	Wellness diagnosis	Health-Seeking Behaviors (salt-restricted diet)	None	
	Syndrome diagnosis	Disuse Syndrome	None	
	Very specific label	Death Anxiety	None	
Basic Two-Part	Actual problem	Impaired Social Interaction	r/t self-consciousness following amputation of bilateral lower extremities	
	Potential problem	Risk for Impaired Attachment	r/t separation from infant at birth because of mother's illness	
	Possible problem	Possible Impaired Attachment	r/t separation from infant at birth because of mother's illness	
Basic Three-Part	Actual Problem	Impaired Social Interaction	r/t self-consciousness following amputation of bilateral lower extremities	AEB avoidance of others, social isolation, blaming others for current condition
	Possible Problem	Impaired Social Interaction	r/t self-consciousness following amputation of bilateral lower extremities	AEB blaming others for current condition
Variations	(Specify)	Decisional Conflict (whether to accept chemotherapy)	r/t desire to protect family from financial hardship of a lingering illness	
	Secondary to	Decisional Conflict (whether to accept chemotherapy)	r/t desire to protect family from financial hardship of a lingering illness	Secondary to diagnosis of terminal cancer
	Two-part NANDA-I label	Imbalanced Nutrition: Less Than Body Requirements	r/t loss of appetite from nausea	Secondary to side effects of chemotherapy
	Adding words to the label	Impaired Physical Mobility: Inability to turn self in bed	r/t generalized weakness	Secondary to residual effects of stroke
	Unknown etiology	Parental Role Conflict	r/t unknown etiology or possibly r/t recent divorce	
	Complex etiology	Chronic Low Self-Esteem	r/t complex etiology	
Collaborative Problems	Potential complications of disease, test, or treatment	Potential Complication of preeclampsia: renal failure	None	

AEB = as evidenced by.

students because it helps to ensure that you have enough data to support the problem you have identified.

Although ideally the problem and etiology should thoroughly describe the patient's health status, you can sometimes make the description more clear and useful by including the cues in the statement. However, this method can create a long, unwieldy statement. For example:

Decisional Conflict (whether to accept chemotherapy) r/t desire to protect family from financial hardship of a lingering illness AMB verbalizing uncertainty about what to do and feelings of distress; indecision about having and not having chemotherapy; exhibiting physical signs of anxiety (increased heart rate, restlessness); questioning personal values and beliefs ("I'm not sure what to do. I hate to leave them any sooner than I have to, but I don't want to ruin them financially, either").

For such situations, you can record the cues in the nurses' notes instead of in the diagnostic statement. Another alternative is to list the signs and symptoms below the nursing diagnosis on the care plan instead of including it as part of the statement. For example:

Decisional Conflict (whether to accept chemotherapy) r/t desire to protect family from financial hardship of a lingering illness

Subjective cues: Verbalizes uncertainty about what to do and feelings of distress; vacillates between having and not having chemo; questions personal values and beliefs ("I'm not sure what to do. I hate to leave them any sooner than I have to, but I don't want to ruin them financially, either").
Objective cues: Exhibits physical signs of anxiety (increased heart rate, restlessness)

Obviously you cannot use the PES format for risk nursing diagnoses, because symptoms are not present with risk diagnoses.

One-Part Statement
You can omit the etiology from certain kinds of diagnostic statements:

Syndrome Diagnoses. Recall that a syndrome diagnosis is a label that represents a collection of several nursing diagnoses. A syndrome diagnosis usually does not need an etiology.

Wellness Diagnoses. As a rule, NANDA-I wellness diagnoses are one-part statements beginning with the phrase Readiness for Enhanced (e.g., Readiness for Enhanced Parenting). Because the wellness label does not represent a problem, no etiology (cause) is needed.

Very Specific Labels. A few NANDA-I labels are so specific that they imply the etiology, or the only possible etiology is a medical diagnosis (e.g., Death Anxiety, Latex Allergy Response). For example, for Latex Allergy Response, it would be redundant to write Latex Allergy Response r/t sensitivity to latex. The etiology adds nothing to your understanding of the problem, nor does it suggest interventions different from those suggested by the problem label.

Other Format Variations
The following are some variations of the basic two- and three-part formats.

"Specify"
You will see the word *specify* in some NANDA-I labels, for example, Decisional Conflict (specify). This means that the label is useful only if you describe the problem more specifically; for example, Decisional Conflict (whether to accept chemotherapy) r/t desire to protect family from financial hardship of a lingering illness.

"Secondary to"
When the defining characteristics are vague (e.g., Chronic Pain r/t chronic physical disability) you may need to add a second part to the etiology following the words *secondary to (2°)*. This second part is usually a pathophysiology or disease process (e.g., Chronic Pain r/t chronic physical disability secondary to rheumatoid arthritis). As a rule, you should avoid using pathophysiology or medical diagnoses in the etiology because they cannot be addressed by independent nursing interventions. The words *secondary to* make it clear that the nurse is not ultimately responsible for that part of the etiology. Do not use this phrase routinely. Use it only if it adds to the understanding of your diagnostic statement.

Two-Part NANDA-I Label
Some NANDA-I labels have two parts. The first part describes a general response; the second part, following a colon, makes it more specific, for example, Imbalanced Nutrition: Less Than Body Requirements.

Adding Words to the NANDA-I Label
The problem phrase must describe the client's health status precisely because general categories are not useful for planning nursing care. Therefore, you may create a two-part label because of the need to add words to clarify the NANDA-I label. For example, what do you think the problem label Impaired Physical Mobility means? Does it mean that the patient cannot grasp objects with her hands, or that she cannot walk, or that she cannot move at all? For such labels, you will need to add your own words to the label to make it more descriptive, for example, Impaired Physical mobility: *Inability to turn self in bed* r/t generalized weakness secondary to residual effects of stroke.

Other labels that often need to be clarified include Acute Pain, Chronic Pain, Risk for Infection, and Risk for Injury. Think carefully about whether the clarifying words belong in the problem or the etiology. For example, you may see a pain diagnosis written as Acute Pain r/t surgical incision. However, surgical incision is a medical treatment and should not be used as the etiology. It would be better to write Acute Pain (abdominal incision) r/t turning and moving secondary to abdominal surgery. When adding words, first try to make the statement specific or descriptive by writing a good etiology, using the PES format, or adding *secondary to*. If that does not fully describe the health status, add descriptive words to the problem label.

Unknown Etiology
Sometimes you will be able to identify the patient's problem but not know the etiology. For example, your patient might have defining characteristics for Parental Role Conflict, but you may need more information to determine the cause. Perhaps there is an impending divorce; perhaps she has just had to take on the care of an elderly parent, and so on. In this case, you could write Parental Role Conflict r/t unknown etiology. Later, when you obtain more data, you will be able to complete the etiology. A similar situation exists when you have some, but not enough, information about the etiology. In this case you would write Parental Role Conflict possibly r/t recent divorce.

Complex Etiology
Some problems have too many etiological factors to list, or the etiology is too complex to explain in a brief diagnostic statement. For example, imagine the number of factors that might contribute to problems such as Chronic Low Self-Esteem, Disabled Family Coping, and Adult Failure to Thrive. For such problems you can replace the etiology with the phrase *complex factors* (e.g., Disabled Family Coping r/t complex factors).

Collaborative Problems

A collaborative problem is always a potential problem—a complication of a disease, test, or medical treatment. The disease, test, or treatment is actually the etiology of the problem. Because you cannot treat the etiology with independent nursing interventions, you should not use the problem + etiology format. The focus of your interventions is monitoring for and preventing the complication. The format is shown in the following example:

Potential Complication of thrombophlebitis: Pulmonary embolism

As you can see, the word(s) following the colon represent the problem you are monitoring and trying to prevent.

In actual practice, you would not write an etiology for a collaborative problem. However, as a student, you may wish to do so when it clarifies your diagnostic statement or when it helps to suggest nursing interventions (Wilkinson, 2011). For example, a student statement might be:

Potential Complication of magnesium sulfate therapy: Respiratory depression r/t *increased blood levels of magnesium because of decreased kidney function secondary to preeclampsia (a pregnancy-related disorder with hypertension as a major pathology.)*

In addition to alerting you to monitor for respiratory depression, this statement might help remind you to monitor the serum magnesium level, assess for other data related to kidney function, and monitor blood pressure. Again, as a professional nurse, you would *not* write an etiology.

KnowledgeCheck 4-9

Write an example of each of the following diagnostic statement formats using the listed components—mix and match:

Problem labels: Anxiety, Pain (lower back)
Etiologies: Unknown outcome of surgery; muscle strain and tissue inflammation
Cues: Exhibits physical manifestations of anxiety (e.g., hands shaking); states pain is 9 on a scale of 1 to 10.

- Basic two-part statement
- Basic three-part statement
- Basic two-part statement, using "secondary to" (create your own disease/pathology)
- Statement with unknown etiology
- Possible nursing diagnosis
- Risk nursing diagnosis

How Does the Nursing Diagnosis Relate to Outcomes and Interventions?

As a general rule the problem suggests goals, and the etiology suggests interventions. Keep in mind that there are exceptions, though.

The Problem Suggests Goals

The problem describes a health status that needs to be changed. From the problem, you can determine the patient outcomes to measure this change. Consider the following diagnostic statement: Risk for Impaired Skin Integrity r/t complete immobility 2° spinal cord injury. The goal, or outcome, is the opposite of the unhealthy response: Skin will remain intact and healthy.

The goals then suggest assessments, which are actually a type of nursing intervention. The diagnosis Risk for Impaired Skin Integrity tells you to monitor the patient's skin condition. If the problem is not an accurate statement of health status, then your goals and resulting assessments will be wrong. If you incorrectly identified the previous problem as Impaired Physical Mobility 2° spinal cord injury, then the goal would suggest that you monitor the patient's mobility—which would not improve—and you might miss a developing skin problem.

The Etiology Suggests Interventions

The aim of the nursing interventions is to alter the factors contributing to the problem. In the preceding mobility example, you could not cure the spinal cord injury or restore the patient's ability to move about. However, you could provide some mobility by turning and repositioning the patient frequently. This would help prevent Impaired Skin Integrity.

If the etiology is incorrect or incomplete, it could cause you to omit important nursing interventions. Suppose there are missing etiological factors in the preceding skin diagnosis and it should have read: Risk for Impaired Skin Integrity r/t poor nutritional status and complete immobility 2° spinal cord injury. You can see that interventions to support mobility would not be adequate to prevent Impaired Skin Integrity.

REFLECTING CRITICALLY ABOUT DIAGNOSTIC STATEMENTS

Just as you critiqued your diagnostic reasoning process, you must reflect on the content, format, and meaning of your diagnostic statements. After you have written your diagnostic statements, use the following criteria to judge their quality (Wilkinson, 2011):

1. *In choosing a NANDA-I label, do not rely on the label definition alone.* Always compare patient data to the defining characteristics and the definition.

   Example: The definition for Parental Role Conflict is "parent experience of role confusion and conflict in response to crisis."

   You cannot actually observe role confusion and conflict in a patient; however, the defining characteristics for this label include more specific cues, such as "Reluctant to participate in usual caretaking activities."

2. *Include both problem and etiology, with cause and effect stated correctly.* A quick check of this is to read your statement backward: "Etiology causes problem," and see if it makes sense.

   Correct example:
   Diagnostic statement: Ineffective Breastfeeding r/t Deficient Knowledge (positioning infant at breast)
   Read backward: This statement says that deficient knowledge about positioning the infant at breast "causes" Ineffective Breastfeeding. This makes sense.
   Incorrect example:
   Diagnostic statement: Deficient Knowledge r/t Ineffective Breastfeeding (incorrect positioning infant at breast)
   Read backward: This statement says Ineffective Breastfeeding causes deficient knowledge. This does not make sense.

3. *Be sure the etiology does not merely restate the problem.*

   Incorrect example: Impaired Physical Mobility r/t inability to walk
   Correct example: Impaired Physical Mobility: Inability to walk r/t weakness and pain in legs

   In the incorrect example, inability to walk is not *causing* the Impaired Physical Mobility; it *is* the impaired mobility.

The etiology should state the factors that are causing inability to walk.

4. *Avoid using medical diagnoses and treatments as etiological factors.* The nurse should be able to provide interventions to change or remove the etiological factors. What could the nurse do to change the following etiology?

Incorrect example: Risk for Impaired Skin Integrity (ulcers, infection) r/t diabetes mellitus

The answer, of course, is that the nurse can do nothing to change or get rid of the DM. Try to reword the etiology in terms of something the nurse can change, as follows:

Correct example: Risk for Impaired Skin Integrity (ulcers, infection) r/t lack of knowledge of self-care measures for inspecting feet and trimming toenails

If you cannot reword the etiology in terms of something the nurse can change, you may have identified the problem incorrectly; perhaps it is merely the stimulus for another patient problem that you can address independently. In the following example, Risk for Impaired Skin Integrity is one possible response to the stimulus, Impaired Physical Mobility.

Incorrect example: Impaired Physical Mobility (total) r/t paralysis secondary to high spinal injury
Correct example: Risk for Impaired Skin Integrity (pressure ulcers) r/t Impaired Physical Mobility (total) secondary to high spinal injury

If none of these seem to work, you can resort to using *secondary to* instead of *related to,* as in the following example: Risk for Deficient Fluid Volume secondary to prescribed NPO. This is usually the case if a physician order is written, such as a prescription for NPO.

5. *Write the statement clearly.* The statement should give a clear picture of the client's health status, and other health professionals should be able to understand it readily. Avoid abbreviations and jargon as much as possible. For example, do you know what the first statement below means?

Incorrect example: Imp. Phys. Mobility (inability to get OOB w/o assist.) r/t muscle weakness and pain in LL
Correct example: Impaired Physical Mobility (inability to get out of bed without assistance) r/t muscle weakness and pain in left leg

6. *Write the statement concisely.* A wordy statement is likely to be unclear. The following will help limit statement length:
   - Use the words complex etiology instead of listing numerous etiological factors.
   - If there are numerous signs and symptoms, either do not use PES format, or describe the signs and symptoms in the nurses' notes.

Correct example: Constipation r/t complex factors (see nurses' notes)

7. *Be sure the statement is descriptive and specific.* A vaguely stated problem and/or etiology cannot provide guidance for formulating goals and nursing interventions. Follow this guideline even if it means the statement is not as

concise as you'd like. You can make the NANDA-I labels more specific by doing the following:
   - Being sure to include all appropriate etiological factors
   - Reviewing the label definition. (Do not write the definition, but when you know the meaning of the label, you may find that it is descriptive enough.)
   - Using PES format to add the patient's signs and symptoms
   - Adding qualifying words (e.g., *mild, severe, occasional,* or *constant*) to the label

Example: Severe Neck Pain r/t muscle spasms 2° herniated intervertebral disc

   - Adding *secondary to* to the etiology.

Example: Severe Neck Pain r/t muscle spasms 2° herniated intervertebral disc

   - Adding a colon and descriptors to the label.

Example: Impaired Physical Mobility: Inability to walk r/t weakness and pain in legs

8. *State the problem as a patient response.*
   - A problem is not a patient need. As a rule, avoid using the word *need* in a problem statement. A need may cause a problem, but it is not a human response.

Incorrect example: Needs increased fluids related to . . .
Correct example: Risk for Deficient Fluid Volume, or Deficient Fluid Volume related to. . .
   - A problem is not a medical test, treatment, diagnosis, or equipment.

Incorrect examples	Correct examples
Starting on a diabetic diet	Deficient Knowledge, Ineffective Denial
Foley catheter in place	Risk for Infection, Urinary Retention
Risk for pneumonia	Risk for Ineffective Airway Clearance
Traction to left leg	Impaired Physical Mobility

   - A problem is not a nursing goal, a nursing problem, or a nursing action.

Incorrect examples	Correct examples
Prevent urinary tract infection (nursing goal)	Risk for Urinary Tract Infection
Combative, hits caregivers (nursing problem)	Risk for Other-Directed Violence, Ineffective Coping, Confusion
Provide emotional support (nursing action)	Anxiety, Decisional Conflict, Grieving

9. *Use nonjudgmental language.* If you examine your biases during the diagnostic process, your statements should be neutral. Look for phrases that imply criticism of a patient, for example:

Incorrect: Risk for Infection r/t poor hygiene and housekeeping
Better: Risk for Infection r/t lack of information about sanitation and handwashing

10. *Avoid legally questionable language.* Look for phrases that seem to blame caregivers or patients or that refer negatively to patient care. For example, do not write:

Risk for Falls r/t lack of staff to adequately supervise ambulation

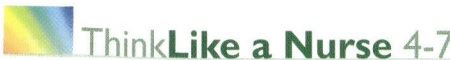
ThinkLike a Nurse 4-7

Rewrite the preceding diagnostic statement so it contains no legally questionable language. Use imaginary etiological factors if you need to.

Critiquing the NANDA-I Taxonomy

Despite their potential benefits, some nurses have criticized the use of standardized language and the NANDA-I taxonomy

in particular. See Box 4-5 for some objections and for responses to counter them. Meanwhile, try not to reject the idea of standardized language just because of a few problematic labels. You do not need to use the official NANDA-I labels exclusively. If you are uncomfortable with a label, change the wording to make it more useful, or write a completely new label. **Key Point:** *Remember, the point of a standardized language is to more clearly communicate the nature of the patient problem in nursing terms.* For a more comprehensive critique of standardized nursing language, and the NANDA-I system in particular,

 Go to Chapter 4, **Supplemental Materials: Critique of NANDA-I Standardized Language,** on Davis*Plus.*

BOX 4-5 ■ Critique of Standardized Nursing Language

1. Criticism: *The labels are hard to use or not useful.*
(1) They are too abstract to be useful (e.g., Impaired Adjustment)
(2) Some labels are merely reworded medical diagnoses (e.g., Decreased Cardiac Output)
(3) Few outside nursing knows what the labels mean (e.g., "Why not just say 'tooth decay' or 'missing teeth' instead of 'Impaired Dentition'?").

Response
(1) These are legitimate concerns, but when you know the label definition, the term is more meaningful, whether it is one you believe is too abstract, too medical, or too obscure.
(2) You can also make the labels more specific and useful by adding meaningful descriptors, etiological factors, and defining characteristics to the diagnostic statement.
(3) Compared to the terminology for describing medical diagnoses, the NANDA-I system is relatively new (recall that it was initiated just over 30 years ago). Only a little more than 30 years ago AIDS was not a medical diagnosis. All classification systems evolve and change, so many of the difficulties with individual labels will be corrected as the terminology is refined.

2. Criticism: *The NANDA-I diagnoses have not been researched.* Historically, this was true.

Response
(1) An elected diagnostic development committee evaluates each submitted diagnosis to determine if it complies

with the criteria for inclusion in the taxonomy. A label can be approved for testing. It must be validated by the literature, preferably research-based, to remain on the approved list.
(2) Research on the labels has been conducted and is continuing. In 1994, a research team at the University of Iowa (the Nursing Diagnosis Extension Classification [NDEC]) began collaborating with NANDA-I to extend and refine the NANDA-I work. They intend to address some of the difficulties with the labels, such as specificity, clinical usefulness, and clinical testing.

3. Criticism: *Using a NANDA-I label to describe health status is "labeling"—it dehumanizes and stereotypes the patient.* The most serious criticisms are leveled by those who say nurses should not use any standardized languages to describe nursing knowledge and nursing work because "we should not label people."

Answer: (1) If this is true, then medical diagnoses would meet the same objection. No one seems to object if a patient is "labeled" with appendicitis or emphysema. (2) This objection ignores the fact that we must name *all* objects and ideas in order to communicate them to other people. (3) Many "labeling" criticisms arise out of disillusionment. It may be that nurses expect too much from nursing diagnoses. Although diagnosis is important, it is, after all, merely a process for identifying, naming, and communicating patient health status. We should not expect it to be the miracle that single-handedly cures all problems of the nursing profession and the patients.

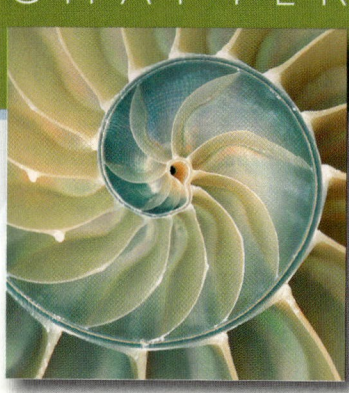

CHAPTER 5

Planning Outcomes

Learning Outcomes

After completing this chapter, you should be able to:

➤ Describe formal, informal, initial, ongoing, and discharge planning.

➤ Identify patients who need a comprehensive, formal discharge plan.

➤ Explain the importance of a written plan of care.

➤ Describe the information contained in a comprehensive nursing care plan.

➤ Compare critical pathways to integrated plans of care (IPOCs) and other standardized care-planning documents.

➤ Discuss the advantages and disadvantages of computerized care planning.

➤ Describe a process for writing an individualized care plan, making use of available standardized care-planning documents.

➤ Define the following terms: *goal, outcome, expected outcome,* and *nursing-sensitive outcome.*

➤ Differentiate between short-term and long-term goals.

➤ Explain how a goal is derived from a nursing diagnosis.

➤ Differentiate between essential and nonessential goals.

➤ Write appropriate goals for actual, risk, and possible nursing diagnoses.

➤ Use standardized terminology to state patient goals.

➤ Write realistic specific, concrete, and observable goals that do not conflict with the medical plan of care and are stated in terms of patient responses/behaviors.

Key Concepts

Goals/Outcomes

Nursing Care Plan

Planning

Related Concepts

See the Concept Map at the end of this chapter.

Caring for the Nguyens

This feature allows you to practice the kind of thinking you will use as a full-spectrum nurse. There is usually more than one correct answer to a critical thinking question, so we do not provide answers for these features. It is more important to develop your nursing judgment than to "cover content." Discuss the questions with your peers. If you are still unsure, consult your instructor.

Review the opening scenario of Nam Nguyen at the front of this book. As the clinic nurse, you have written the following nursing diagnostic statement: Imbalanced Nutrition: More Than Body Requirements related to inappropriate food choices and serving size as evidenced by body mass index (BMI) of 28.5.

Write at least two short-term and two long-term goals for Mr. Nguyen based on this diagnostic statement.

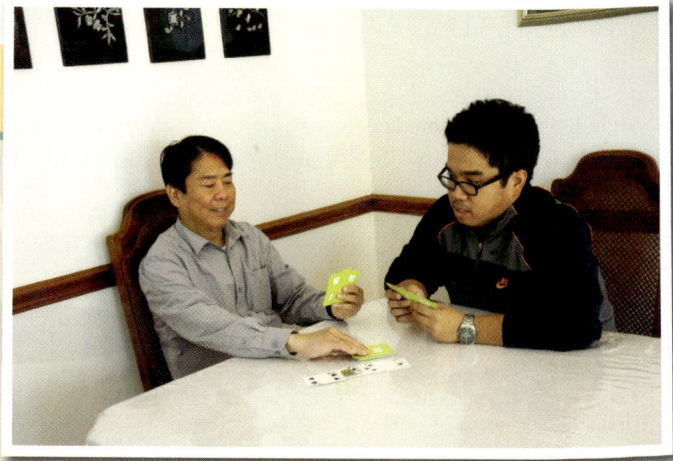

Remember that your goals must be realistic and take into account Mr. Nguyen's other health problems.

 Go to **Caring for the Nguyens Response Sheet** on *DavisPlus.*

Meet Your Patient

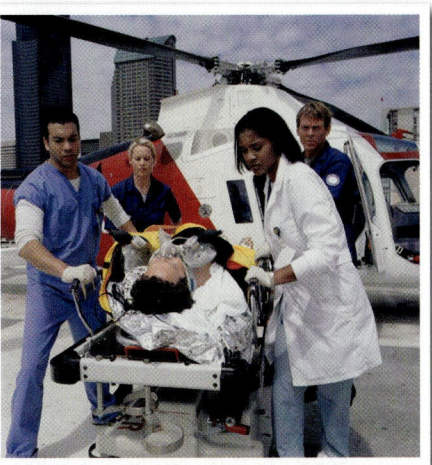

Ben Ivanos has just been admitted to an orthopedic unit after a motorcycle accident. Mr. Ivanos is 24 years old and normally healthy; he takes no medications. He has casts and traction on both legs and a cast on one arm. He is receiving morphine sulfate intravenously via a patient-controlled analgesia (PCA) pump. Imagine that you are an orthopedic nurse and must plan care for Mr. Ivanos. You rank the following nursing diagnoses as highest priority:

1. Acute Pain secondary to musculoskeletal trauma (arms, legs, body) and muscle spasms
2. Risk for Peripheral Neurovascular Dysfunction secondary to casts/traction

You write the following desired outcomes (goals) on the care plan:

Goals for diagnosis 1

Demonstrates correct use of PCA pump.
Rates pain not higher than 4 on a scale of 1 to 10 at all times.

Goals for diagnosis 2

Peripheral pulses palpable
Fingers and toes warm
Fingers and toes without pallor or cyanosis
No edema of fingers and toes
Capillary refill less than 3 seconds

These goals will guide you in choosing nursing interventions for relieving Mr. Ivanos's pain and preventing peripheral neurovascular dysfunction. When the nursing shift changes, the written care plan provides directions for the new caregivers so that they will continue to focus on Mr. Ivanos's most important needs.

Theoretical Knowledge
knowing why

This text separates the process of planning outcomes from the process of planning interventions because, although related, they are distinctly different activities. This chapter (1) describes planning as a general process, (2) explains how to create a nursing care plan, and (3) discusses how to write patient goals/expected outcomes. Chapter 6 explains how to plan nursing interventions and write nursing orders.

ABOUT THE KEY CONCEPTS

To help you understand and remember the content in this chapter, try to organize what you learn under the key concepts of planning, goals and outcomes, and nursing care plans. Planning is the broad umbrella term that covers the rest of the chapter concepts. In this chapter, you will learn how they are all related.

WHAT IS PLANNING?

The professional nurse is responsible for care planning, and cannot delegate it. However, you should be aware that some healthcare facilities list care planning in their job description for licensed practical or vocational nurses. Certainly licensed practical nurses (LPNs/LVNs) can provide valuable input for registered nurses (RNs) who are planning the care. Box 5-1 lists American Nurses Association (ANA) standards that specifically identify planning as the role of the registered nurse.

Planning can be formal or informal. **Formal planning** is conscious and deliberate. It involves decision making, critical thinking, and creativity (Wilkinson, 2011). During the planning phases of the nursing process, you will work with the patient and family to derive desired outcomes from identified patient problems (e.g., nursing diagnoses) and then to identify nursing interventions to help achieve those outcomes. The end product of formal planning is a holistic plan of care that addresses the patient's unique problems and strengths.

Not all plans are written. **Informal planning** occurs while you are performing other nursing process steps. For example, while performing neurovascular checks for Ben Ivanos, you might discover that he is not obtaining adequate pain relief. Reflect on this situation. What would you do? Any response in that scenario would require some planning. For example, you might make a mental note (plan) to notify your patient's prescriber for an increase in the analgesic dose.

How Is Planning Related to Other Steps of the Nursing Process?

Nursing process steps are overlapping and interdependent. To develop a plan of care with realistic goals and effective nursing orders, you must have accurate, complete *assessment* data and correctly identified and prioritized *nursing diagnoses*. The *goals/desired outcomes* flow logically from the nursing diagnoses. By stating what is to be achieved, the goals then suggest nursing interventions (which are written as nursing orders in the *planning interventions* phase). The plan of care is carried out in the *implementation* phase. In the *evaluation* step, the goals/desired outcomes serve as criteria for evaluating whether the nursing care has been effective. Figure 5-1 illustrates the relationship of planning outcomes to the other stages of the nursing process.

Initial and Ongoing Planning

Initial planning begins with the first patient contact. It refers to the development of the initial comprehensive care plan, which should be written as soon as possible after the initial assessment. The nurse who performs the admission

BOX 5-1 ■ American Nurses Association Standards of Nursing Practice for Outcomes and Planning

Standard 3. Outcomes Identification

The registered nurse identifies expected outcomes for a plan individualized to the patient or the situation.

Competencies

The registered nurse:

Involves the healthcare consumer, family, healthcare providers, and others in formulating expected outcomes when possible and appropriate.

Derives culturally appropriate expected outcomes from the diagnoses.

Considers associated risks, benefits, costs, current scientific evidence, expected trajectory of the condition, and clinical expertise when formulating expected outcomes.

Defines expected outcomes in terms of the healthcare consumer, healthcare consumer culture, values, and ethical considerations.

Includes a time estimate for attainment of expected outcomes.

Develops expected outcomes that facilitate continuity of care.

Modifies expected outcomes based on changes in the status of the healthcare consumer or evaluation of the situation.

Documents expected outcomes as measurable goals.

Standard 4. Planning

The registered nurse develops a plan that prescribes strategies and alternatives to attain expected outcomes.

Competencies

The registered nurse:

Develops an individualized plan in partnership with the person, family, and others considering the person's characteristics or situation, including, but not limited to, values, beliefs, spiritual and health practices, preferences, choices, developmental level, coping style, culture and environment, and available technology.

Establishes the plan priorities with the healthcare consumer, family, and others as appropriate.

Includes strategies in the plan that address each of the identified diagnoses or issues. These may include, but are not limited to, strategies for:

- Promotion and restoration of health
- Prevention of illness, injury, and disease
- The alleviation of suffering
- Supportive care for those who are dying

Includes strategies for health and wholeness across the lifespan.

Provides for continuity in the plan.

Considers the economic impact of the plan on the healthcare consumer, family, caregivers, or other affected parties.

Integrates current scientific evidence, trends, and research.

Utilizes the plan to provide direction to other members of the healthcare team.

Explores practice settings and safe space and time for the nurse and the healthcare consumer to explore suggested, potential, and alternative options.

Defines the plan to reflect current statutes, rules and regulations, and standards.

Modifies the plan according to the ongoing assessment of the healthcare consumer's response and other outcome indicators.

Documents the plan in a manner that uses standardized language or recognized terminology.

Note: There are additional standards for advanced practice nurses.

Source: American Nurses Association. (2010). *Nursing: Scope and standards of practice* (2nd ed.). Silver Spring, MD: ANA.

---

assessment has the benefit of personal contact and the best information about the patient. This nurse, ideally, should initiate the care plan.

You may sometimes need to begin care planning even though the initial database is incomplete. For example, the patient may require emergency care before assessment is complete. Or a different patient may need your immediate attention. In such situations, make a preliminary plan with whatever information you have. You can complete and refine the plan when you are able to perform a more detailed assessment.

Ongoing planning refers to changes made in the plan (1) as you evaluate the patient's responses to care, or (2) as you obtain new data and make new nursing diagnoses. For example, nurses discovered that Ben Ivanos (Meet Your Patient) had not slept well on his first night in the hospital. They identified a new nursing diagnosis for him: Disturbed Sleep Pattern r/t unfamiliar environment and pain. They then developed a plan to address this problem. Ongoing planning allows you to decide which problems to focus on each day that you care for the patient.

Discharge Planning

If the recommended length of stay for patients with surgical reduction of fractures is 2 days, then Ben Ivanos will still have casts on his arm and both legs when he leaves the hospital.

Obviously, he will not be able to manage his own activities of daily living (shopping, cooking, bathing, etc.). What questions come to your mind when you think about how he will manage after he leaves the hospital? Take a moment now to jot down your ideas.

You may have thought of some questions: Is there anyone who can help Mr. Ivanos with his personal care? Will he need to go up and down stairs? Who will drive him home from the hospital? Can he be discharged home or will he need to go to a rehabilitation facility? How soon does he need to see his primary care provider again? How will he manage his pain at home; what will he use in place of the PCA narcotics?

Discharge planning is the process of planning for self-care and continuity of care after the patient leaves a healthcare setting. Ben Ivanos's case is not unusual. In the United States, outpatient surgeries and short hospital stays are the norm. Many patients are discharged despite ongoing need for nursing care and complex treatments. This means that nurses must prepare family members to perform tasks such as changing sterile dressings and monitoring intravenous medications. If family members are not available or if skilled nursing care is needed, arrangements must be made for home healthcare or transfer to a skilled nursing or rehabilitation facility. Sometimes a case manager is assigned, but often staff nurses must

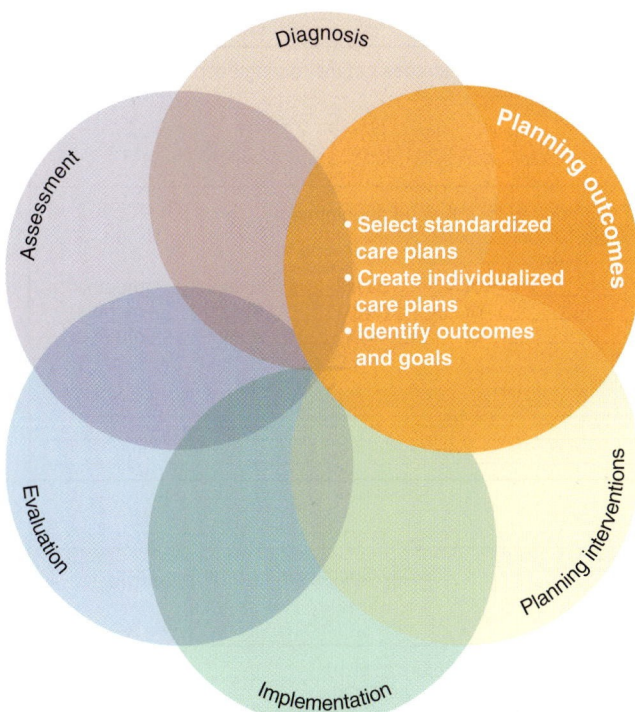

FIGURE 5-1 Nursing process phases: Planning outcomes.

plan and coordinate services. If appropriate services are not provided or if family members perform care incorrectly, the patient may experience delayed recovery or complications that require further treatment or hospital readmission.

To learn more about the process of discharging patients from an institution, refer to the section Maintain Trust During Transitions in Chapter 11. Also see Procedure 11-4, Discharging a Patient from the Healthcare Facility.

Discharge Planning Begins at Initial Assessment

Because patients are in the surgery center or hospital for such a short time, discharge planning must begin at the initial assessment. You will need the following patient data:

- Physical condition and functional and self-care limitations
- Emotional stability and ability to learn
- Financial resources (e.g., personal finances, insurance, community resources such as food stamps, Medicaid)
- Family or other caregivers available
- Caregiving responsibilities the patient may have for others
- Environment, both home and community (e.g., stairs, space for supplies and equipment, availability of transportation to healthcare services)
- Use of community services before admission

Written Discharge Plans

All patients need at least some discharge planning. Sometimes it is enough to include discharge assessments and teaching as nursing orders on the patient's comprehensive care plan. For example, a middle-aged patient who has been hospitalized for deep vein thrombosis (a blood clot in a major vein, usually the lower leg) will be able to care for herself independently when she goes home. For this patient, you could simply write a nursing order to teach her about the side effects of the warfarin (Coumadin), an anticoagulant she will be taking at home. In contrast, you will probably need a written, comprehensive discharge plan if the patient is an older adult or is likely to have

one or more of the following (NSW Department of Health, 2011; Walker, Hogstel, & Curry, 2007):

- Self-care problems
- Lives alone
- Has responsibilities to care for others
- Used community services before admission
- Has a complex treatment regimen
- Takes three or more medications and has had medications changed recently

For an example of a discharge planning form, see Figure 5-2.

Discharge Planning for Older Adults

The percentage of older adults in hospitals is quite high, and they tend to have complex needs when discharged. Therefore, it is especially important to start discharge planning at the initial admission assessment. This means that assessment of functional abilities, cognition, vision, hearing, social support, and psychological well-being must be a part of the initial assessment so that you can identify needed services at discharge. A comprehensive discharge process for older adults should help to achieve the following objectives:

- Maintain functional ability.
- Lengthen the time between rehospitalizations.
- Involve all concerned parties in decision making.
- Improve interagency communication (e.g., hospital to nursing home).
- Emphasize client and family involvement and interdisciplinary collaboration (Walker, Hogstel, & Curry, 2007).

Discharge Planning Requires Collaboration

Comprehensive discharge planning involves collaboration. Ideally, it is done *with*, not *for*, the patient—patient involvement is important for achieving desired outcomes. In addition, a patient's postdischarge needs often call for services from a multidisciplinary team, which may include home care service personnel; private-duty nurses; hospice team; physical therapists; social service professionals; speech, occupational, and hearing therapists; physicians; and members of the patient's family.

KnowledgeCheck 5-1

- What does the nurse do in the planning phases of the nursing process?
- What is the purpose of initial planning? Ongoing planning? Discharge planning?

NURSING CARE PLANS

The **comprehensive nursing care plan** (also called *patient care plan*) is the central source of information needed to guide holistic, goal-oriented care to address each patient's unique needs. It is a document—usually several documents—that specifies dependent, interdependent, and independent nursing actions necessary for care of a specific patient. It usually combines both standardized and individualized approaches to care.

Why Is a Written Nursing Care Plan Important?

A well-written comprehensive care plan benefits the patient and the healthcare institution by doing the following:

- Ensuring that care is complete
- Providing continuity of care
- Promoting deficient use of nursing efforts
- Providing a guide for assessments and charting
- Meeting the requirements of accrediting agencies. (e.g., the Joint Commission)

FOLLOW-UP CARE	When to call the doctor; symptom management (pain, nausea); plan for meeting outcomes not met during hospitalization:

Call your primary physician to find out if an insurance referral form is needed for follow up appointments.
After discharge, you need to call for an appointment to see physician.

Clinic/Physician   Phone #   Date   Time

_____   _____   _____   _____   or _____ days _____ weeks _____ months
_____   _____   _____   _____   or _____ days _____ weeks _____ months
_____   _____   _____   _____   or _____ days _____ weeks _____ months

Plans for follow-up Labs/Tests/Treatments

Date   Time   Test/Treatment   Location   Ordered by

_____ _____ _____ _____ _____
_____ _____ _____ _____ _____
_____ _____ _____ _____ _____

PERSONAL CARE

Bathing: ❏ No restrictions   ❏ Other:

Treatment/Therapy/Wound or Skin Care/ Supplies Needed   2-Day Supply Sent Home ?   ❏ Yes

---

ACTIVITY/ REHAB

❏ No restrictions   ❏ Do not climb stairs   ❏ Drive_____   ❏ Return to Work _____
❏ Do not lift   ❏ May lift up to _____ lbs   ❏ Weight Bearing _____ #   ❏ Other

---

DIET

❏ No restrictions   ❏ Other:

Food/Drug Interactions: ❏ Coumadin   ❏ MAO Inhibitors   ❏ Other:

MEDICAL EQUIPMENT

❏ 2nd pair of TED hose given

COMMUNITY RESOURCES

Referral Resource	Agency	Phone #	
Home IV Therapy	_____	_____	Transportation Arrangements for discharge: ___
Home Health	_____	_____	_____
Home Oxygen	_____	_____	Education/Community Resources:_____
Home PT/OT/Speech	_____	_____	_____
Ask-A-Nurse	_____	816-932-0000	

Preprinted Discharge Instruction Sheet given to patient   ❏ NA   ❏ Yes
   List Instruction Sheets:

I understand these instructions and agree with this plan of care _____
                                                      Patient/SO Signature

---

MULTIDISCIPLINARY DISCHARGE INSTRUCTIONS
Shawnee Mission Medical Center
9100 W. 74th Street
Shawnee Mission, Kansas 66204

Form # 60869 Revised: 4/01 PILOT Page 1 of 2

Source: Courtesy of Shawnee Mission Health System, Shawnee Mission, KS

FIGURE 5-2 Discharge planning form. (*Source:* Courtesy of Shawnee Mission Health System, Shawnee Mission, KS.)

What Information Does a Comprehensive Nursing Care Plan Contain?

Regardless of their format, comprehensive care plans include directions for four different kinds of care and include both medical and nursing interventions:

1. *Basic needs and activities of daily living (ADLs).* This includes the routine assistance that the patient needs with hygiene, nutrition, elimination, and so on.
2. *Medical/multidisciplinary treatment.* Nurses need to know the medical orders for each patient (e.g., prescriptions for IV fluids and medications) and the nursing activities necessary for carrying out those orders.
3. *Nursing diagnoses and collaborative problems.* This section may be referred to as the *nursing diagnosis care plan.* It contains goals and nursing orders for the patient's nursing diagnoses and collaborative problems.
4. *Special discharge needs or teaching needs.* Finally, the plan should contain instructions for formal discharge planning and special teaching if they are needed.

What Documents Make Up a Comprehensive Nursing Care Plan?

You will use a variety of documents to create a care plan. Care plans vary widely in format, appearance, and use. In most healthcare organizations, caregivers use preprinted, standardized plans that can be adapted to meet individual

needs. Figure 5-3 shows the documents that are most commonly included in a comprehensive nursing care plan.

Form for Client Profile and Basic Needs

Some essential client data either do not change or are used or updated often. This includes the client's profile (e.g., age, providers, and so on), basic needs (e.g., for hygiene and elimination), and diagnostic tests and treatments (e.g., laboratory tests, radiology procedures). To provide quick and easy access, such information is usually recorded on a durable, standardized form and not organized according to medical or nursing diagnoses (see Fig. 5-3a). These are often in electronic format, but may be printed on cardstock and kept in a central location. For an example of a printed Kardex,

 Go to Chapter 5, **Tables, Boxes, Figures: ESG Figure 5-1,** on Davis*Plus.*

For clients who require more than routine attention to their basic needs, you may need to write a nursing diagnosis care plan. Examples include a client with no appetite and the nursing diagnosis Imbalanced Nutrition: Less Than Body Requirements, or an immobile client with the diagnosis Risk for Impaired Skin Integrity.

Preprinted, Standardized Plans

As shown in Figure 5-3b, a comprehensive care plan usually includes one or more preprinted, standardized documents. It would be too time consuming to produce a handwritten

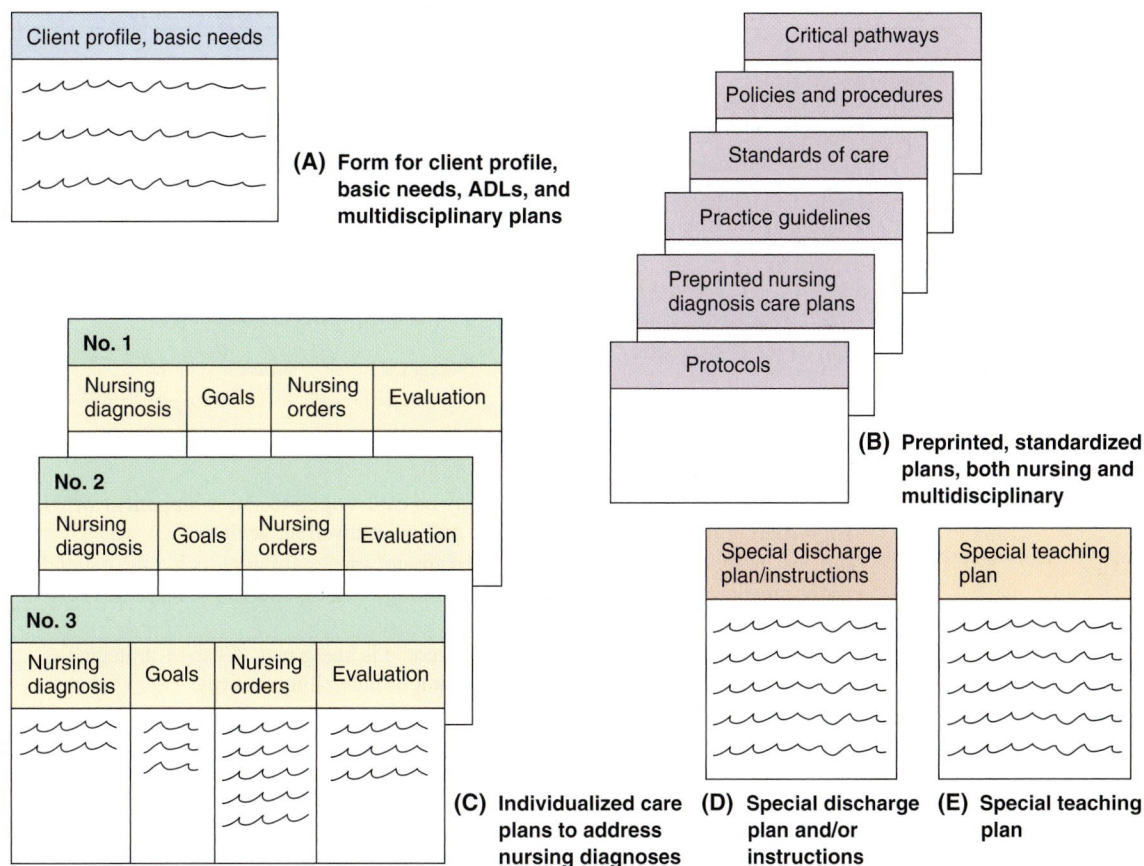

FIGURE 5-3 Components of a nursing care plan. A, Form for client profile, basic needs, ADLs, and multidisciplinary plans. B, Preprinted, standardized plans, both nursing and multidisciplinary. C, Individualized care plans to address nursing diagnoses. D, Special discharge plan and/or instructions. E, Special teaching plan.

complete care plan for every patient. Standardized plans save nursing time, promote consistency of care, and help ensure that nurses do not overlook important interventions. You will find standardized instructions for patient care in a variety of documents. A document may (1) contain nursing or multidisciplinary interventions and (2) prescribe care for one or more nursing diagnoses (e.g., Anxiety) or a disease or medical condition (e.g., pneumonia). The following are examples of standardized, preprinted instructions for care.

Policies and Procedures

Policies and **procedures** are similar to rules and regulations. When a situation occurs frequently or requires a consistent response regardless of who handles it, management develops a policy to govern how it is to be handled. You should consider individual needs and use critical thinking to interpret policies in a caring manner. For example, in some critical care units a patient is allowed one visitor for 10 minutes each hour. Imagine, though, that a patient is expected to die soon, and that his daughter has come from a distant state and brought her three children for one last visit. Would you tell the daughter to take the children in to see their grandfather? Would you insist that

she follow the rule and send them in without her, one at a time over a period of 3 hours?

Protocols

Protocols cover specific actions usually required for a clinical problem unique to a subgroup of patients. For example, not every patient on a medical-surgical unit is at risk for falls, but many are. The nurse would therefore add a falls protocol to the care plan for a patient in that subgroup, such as in Figure 5-4. Protocols may be written for a particular medical diagnosis (e.g., seizure), treatments (e.g., administration of oxytocin to induce labor), or diagnostic tests (e.g., barium enema). They contain both medical and nursing orders. Some include definitions and rationales for interventions.

Unit Standards of Care

Unit standards of care describe the care that nurses are expected to provide for all patients in defined situations (e.g., all women admitted to a labor unit or all patients admitted to a critical care unit). In this way, they are similar to protocols. Unlike protocols, however, they (1) apply to every patient in the defined situation, rather than a subgroup; (2) do not

---

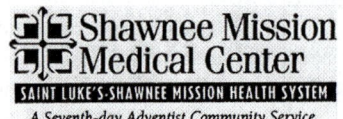

Patient Care Protocol

Title: Fall or Injury/Disruption of Care, Care of the Patient at Risk for   **Effective Date:** 1/9/11

Expected Outcome: The patient at risk for falls will be identified and preventive measures initiated.
                          The patient will not pull out indwelling devices.

Relevant Information: Initiate this protocol for adult patients who have a <u>Conley Fall Scale</u> score of ≥3.

Assessment: 1. The Conley Fall Scale will be administered on admission to adult inpatients. Further assessment
                              will be based on patient population and identified patient need.

Interventions: Make alterations in environment, such as:
  - Avoiding clutter in room.
  - Moving patient closer to Nursing Station if indicated.
  - Making sure call light, telephone and other personal items are within reach

Educate patient and family about:
  - The possibility that family and friends may be called upon to stay with patient with high risk for fall or injury or who attempts to pull out indwelling devices.
  - The possibility that, if the above measures are not successful in reducing the patient's fall risk or preventing attempts to pull out indwelling devices, alternative measures such as the use of restraints may have to be considered.

Evaluation: 1. Evaluate frequently to determine if expected outcome is being met. Change strategies as
                              needed to reduce fall risks or to prevent disruption of indwelling devices.
                          2. **Criteria for initiation of Restraint Protocol:**
  - If interventions have been implemented and patient continues to be at risk of falling or disrupting medical treatment, the protocol <u>Care of the Patient in Restraint for Medical/Surgical Management</u> is initiated.
  - The CRN/Supervisor is notified at the time the restraint is initiated for med/surg management and reviews the need for restraint.

FIGURE 5-4 Portion of patient care protocol for patient at risk for falls. (*Source:* Courtesy of Shawnee Mission Health System, Shawnee Mission, KS 66204.)

become part of the patient's care plan but are kept on file on the unit; and (3) do not usually include specific medical orders. Instead of describing ideal care, standards of care describe the minimum level of care the nurses are expected to achieve given the institution's resources and the client population. Unit standards of care usually are not organized according to nursing diagnoses; and they usually resemble a list of things to do (e.g., complete comprehensive assessment within 2 hours of admission) rather than detailed instructions for care.

ThinkLike a Nurse 5-1

- Think of some other "defined situations" for which unit standards of care might be useful.
- Suggest some more subgroups for which a protocol might be appropriate.

Standardized Nursing Care Plans

Standardized (model) nursing care plans detail the nursing care that is usually needed for a particular nursing diagnosis or for all nursing diagnoses that commonly occur with a medical condition. Figure 5-5 is a standardized care plan for a single nursing diagnosis. Although similar to unit standards of care, model care plans are different in that they usually:

- Provide more detailed interventions. They may add to or delete from unit standards of care.
- Are organized by nursing diagnosis and include specific patient goals and nursing orders.
- Are a part of the patient's comprehensive care plan and become a part of the permanent record.
- Describe ideal rather than minimum nursing care.
- Allow you to incorporate addendum care plans.
- Include checklists, blank lines, or empty spaces so that you can individualize goals and interventions.

Students sometimes purchase model care plan books. You can use them as guides, but be aware that they do not address a client's individual, specific needs. For this reason, they may lead you to focus on the common, predictable problems and overlook an unusual—and perhaps more important—problem the person is experiencing. Beginning with the standardized plan may stifle your creativity. It is best to first use the process for writing a nursing care plan (see What Is the Process for Writing an Individualized Nursing Care Plan? later in this chapter) and then consult the model plan to see whether you have missed anything.

Critical Pathways

Critical pathways are often used in managed care systems. They are outcomes-based, interdisciplinary plans that sequence patient care according to case type. They specify predicted patient outcomes and broad interventions for each day, or in some situations, for each hour (see Table 5-1). They describe the minimal standard of care required to meet the recommended length of stay for patients with a particular condition or *diagnosis-related group* (DRG; e.g., postpartum, myocardial infarction). An agency usually develops critical pathways for its most frequent case types or for situations in which standardized care can produce predictable outcomes. Although critical pathways are developed by a multidisciplinary team, they tend to emphasize medical problems and interventions. To see a full-page critical pathway,

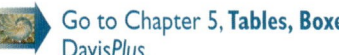 Go to Chapter 5, **Tables, Boxes, Figures: ESG Figure 5-2** on Davis*Plus*.

Integrated Plans of Care

Integrated plans of care (IPOCs) are standardized plans that function as care plans as well as documentation forms. Therefore, there is a different form—or sometimes a different column—for each day of care. Many critical pathways are designed as IPOCs; however, IPOCs do not necessarily (1) organize care according to diagnosis, (2) describe minimal standards of care, or (3) specify a timeline for interventions and outcomes. For an example of an IPOC,

 Go to Chapter 5, **Tables, Boxes, Figures: ESG Figure 5-3**, on Davis*Plus*.

Individualized Nursing Care Plans

Nurses use individualized care plans to address nursing diagnoses unique to a particular client (see Fig. 5-3c). These care plans reflect the independent component of nursing practice, and therefore best demonstrate the nurse's critical thinking and clinical expertise. In addition to including goals and nursing orders that you write specifically for a patient, a complete individualized care plan may contain standardized single-problem care plans (see Fig. 5-5).

Standardized plans do not address unusual problems and may not meet a patient's individual needs. Therefore, you should always adapt standardized plans by adding the necessary nursing diagnoses, goals/outcomes, and nursing orders they do not include. For example, a standardized plan for a client with a myocardial infarction (heart attack) would undoubtedly prescribe care for the nursing diagnosis Pain and for the potential complication of heart failure. However, it might not address the needs of a person who is not complying with treatments because he is in denial about his illness (nursing diagnosis: Ineffective Denial). An individualized plan for resolving the patient's denial would improve the likelihood that the rest of the plan will be successful.

You may sometimes include medical orders in a nursing diagnosis or collaborative problem care plan, especially in a student care plan. For example, for a client with a nursing diagnosis of Deficient Fluid Volume, you might list the medical prescription for intravenously administered fluids in the Nursing Orders column.

Nursing Diagnosis	*Nursing Orders*
Deficient Fluid Volume r/t vomiting and diarrhea	1. Check skin turgor q4hr 2. Medical order: IV normal saline, 150 mL/hr

Special Discharge or Teaching Plans

A nursing plan of care may also contain one or more discharge or teaching plans (see Fig. 5-3d). These are sometimes referred to as *special-purpose* or *addendum* care plans. You can address routine discharge planning and teaching needs by using standardized plans or by including teaching as part of the nursing orders on an individualized care plan. For example, a care plan for the diagnosis Acute Pain might include the nursing order "Teach patient to splint incision when turning in bed." Chapter 26 shows an example of a teaching plan for the diagnosis Deficient Knowledge.

Computer Plans of Care

Many healthcare organizations use electronic health records, including *computer-generated care plans*. The computer stores standardized plans (e.g., for nursing diagnoses, medical diagnoses, or diagnosis-related groups [DRGs]). When you

PATIENT PLAN OF CARE - GENESIS MEDICAL CENTER - Davenport, Iowa

PAIN, ACUTE: Experience of an unpleasant sensory and emotional sensation for a duration of less than 6 months.
SIGNS & SYMPTOMS: Observed or reported (select at least 2)

☐ Change in BP   ☐ Restlessness   ☐ Grimacing   ☐ Crying
☐ Patients self report of pain   ☐ Diaphoresis   ☐ Increased muscle tension   ☐ Change in pulse rate
☐ Change in respiratory pattern   ☐ Whimpering   ☐ Whining

OUTCOME SCORING

RELATED FACTORS	OUTCOMES	ADM				DC	INTERVENTIONS
☐ Physical injuring agent ☐ Psychological injuring agent	[4] Pain control behavior – Recognizes causal factors – Uses non-analgesic relief measures – Uses analgesics appropriately – Reports pain controlled [3] Pain level – Oral/facial expressions of pain – Change in respiratory rate, heart rate BP – Restlessness – Reported pain [3] Comfort level – Reported satisfaction with symptom control – Expressed satisfaction with pain control – Reported physical well-being						☐ Pain management ☐ Analgesic administration ☐ Patient-controlled analgesic (PCA) assistance ☐ Analgesic administration: Intraspinal ☐ Environmental management: comfort ☐ Anxiety reduction ☐ Transcutaneous electrical nerve stimulation (TENS) ☐ Heat/cold application ☐ Distraction ☐ Simple relaxation therapy ☐ Simple massage ☐ Developmental care ☐ Preparatory sensory information ☐ Positioning

Definition of scoring scales	1	2	3	4	5
Pain control — Personal actions to control pain	Never demonstrated	Rarely demonstrated	Sometimes demonstrated	Often demonstrated	Consistently demonstrated
Pain level — Severity of reported pain	Severe	Substantial	Moderate	Slight	None
Comfort level — Extent of physical and psychological ease	None	Limited	Moderate	Substantial	Extensive

Diagnosis _____

Date Initiated _____ RN Initials _____

Date Resolved _____

FIGURE 5-5 Computer printout of standardized care plan for a single nursing diagnosis using standardized language. (*Source:* Adapted from Genesis Medical Center, Davenport, IA 52804. Used with permission.)

Table 5-1 ➤ Portion of Postoperative Critical Pathway for Total Knee Replacement

	POST-OP DAY 1	POST-OP DAY 2
Assessments	■ N&V checks & VS q4hr	■ N&V checks & VS q8hr
	■ Pain	—>
	■ Side effects of opioids	—>
	■ S&S of deep vein thrombosis	—>
	■ Pulse-ox 18 hr if on O_2	■ D/C pulse-ox if O2 D/C
	■ Drsg/wound status q4hr	■ Drsg/wound status q8hr
Tests	■ CBC	—>
		■ INR (if on warfarin)
Medications	■ IV heplock	—>
	■ Anticoagulation	—>
		■ Consider conversion to oral pain meds

Transfer to rehab when:

1. Able to participate in care

2. Tolerating 2 physical therapy sessions

3. Not requiring IV pain medicine

4. Blood values are stable

5. Motivation is commensurate with projected functional status

Discharge to home when:

1. Mobility and ADLs appropriate for degree of assistance at home & home environment

2. Appropriate assistive device and necessary adaptive equipment are used

3. Independent with hip/knee precautions

4. Independent with home exercise program or ongoing PT in the home or outpatient

IF D/C TO HOME, ENSURE APPROPRIATE CONSULTS TO ARRANGE HOME CARE FOLLOW-UP AND EQUIPMENT.

Source: Adapted from Hospital of the University of Pennsylvania, Philadelphia, PA.

---

enter a diagnosis or a desired outcome, the computer generates a list of suggested interventions. You then choose appropriate interventions from the list, individualize by choosing from checklists, or type in your own interventions and strategies.

Computer prompts help ensure that you consider a variety of actions and keep you from overlooking common and important interventions. After the initial learning curve, they also reduce the time spent on paperwork. However, computerized planning requires constant use of a step-by-step thinking process, which may cause a decrease in intuition, insight, ability to care, and nursing expertise (Harris, 1990). You must resist the temptation to accept "one size fits all" solutions. Always look for creative approaches that might be more effective for a particular individual. Think, "What would work for *this* person?"

ESG Figure 5-4 at Davis*Plus* shows a computer screen displaying a care plan for the nursing diagnosis Pain. It lists a patient goal and broadly stated interventions, including assessments and patient education. Most computer programs allow you to print the plan.

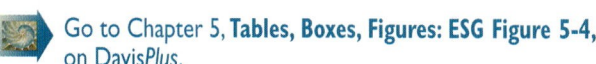 Go to Chapter 5, **Tables, Boxes, Figures: ESG Figure 5-4,** on Davis*Plus.*

KnowledgeCheck 5-2

- In addition to care related to the patient's basic needs, what other types of information does a comprehensive care plan contain?
- How are critical pathways different from other standardized care plans?
- What is the main disadvantage of computerized and standardized care plans?

ThinkLike a Nurse 5-2

Suppose a nurse sees one of your student care plans and says to you, "You're wasting your time writing those things. We never use the nursing process in the real world." Take a few minutes to write down how you might respond.

Student Care Plans

You may have noticed that the care plans you see in clinical settings look different from the ones you create as a part of your clinical preparation. This is because student care plans are a learning activity as well as a plan of care. They are designed to help you learn and apply concepts from the nursing process, physiology, and psychopathology. For this reason,

they may contain more detailed nursing orders as well as other information the instructor may require (e.g., information about lab tests, medications, and assessment data to support the nursing diagnoses). Some instructors may ask you to write rationales and cite references to support them. **Rationales** state the scientific principles or research that supports nursing interventions. Writing rationales helps ensure that you understand the reasons for the interventions—understanding *why* you do *what* you do is one aspect of functioning as a professional. For an example of a student care plan,

 Go to Chapter 5, **Student Care Plan Example,** on Davis*Plus.*

Mind-Mapping Student Care Plans

Mind-mapping is a technique for showing relationships among ideas and concepts in a graphical, or pictorial, way. Mind-mapping is thought to stimulate "whole-brain" and critical thinking, and to foster the development of holistic plans of care (Mueller, Johnston, & Bligh, 2002). A mind-mapped care plan uses shapes and pictures to represent the parts of the nursing process (i.e., assessment data, nursing diagnoses, patient goals, interventions, and evaluation), as well as the patient's pathophysiology, medications, and other pertinent information. Your instructor may ask you to mind-map your care plans, so if you need to learn more about mind-mapping,

 Go to Chapter 5, **Supplemental Materials: Mind-Mapping Student Care Plans,** on Davis*Plus.*

PracticalKnowledge
knowing **how**

WHAT IS THE PROCESS FOR WRITING AN INDIVIDUALIZED NURSING CARE PLAN?

Writing an individualized nursing care plan follows in natural sequence from the assessment and diagnosis phases of the nursing process:

Make a Working Problem List. Earlier in the nursing process, you will already have developed and prioritized a list of the patient's nursing diagnoses, collaborative problems, and strengths. Suppose that, after assessment, you prioritized Ben Ivanos's (Meet Your Patient) problems as follows:

1. Acute Pain secondary to musculoskeletal trauma (arms, legs, body) and muscle spasms
2. Risk for Peripheral Neurovascular Dysfunction secondary to casts/traction
3. Self-Care Deficit (Total) r/t immobility secondary to casts, especially cast on dominant right arm
4. Potential Complication of fracture: Delayed, union, malunion, or nonunion of bone

Decide Which Problems Can Be Managed With Standardized Care Plans or Critical Pathways. What institutional documents are available? Suppose that the hospital unit has a critical pathway for "Patients With Casts and/or Traction." This critical pathway would contain goals and interventions to guide the care for problems 2 and 4, above. It would specify regular neurovascular assessments, for example.

Individualize the Standardized Plan as Needed. Cross out instructions that do not apply to your patient, and add or adapt nursing orders as needed. For example, if the

plan reads, "Perform neurovascular (NV) checks q_____," you would fill in the frequency of the NV checks according to Mr. Ivanos's needs.

Transcribe Medical Orders to Appropriate Documents. For example, you might write the prescriptions for pain medications on a special medication administration record. Details about Mr. Ivanos's traction would probably go on a Kardex or special section of the critical pathway.

Write ADLs and Basic Care Needs in Special Sections of the Kardex, Care Plan, or Computer. For Ben Ivanos, you might note on the Kardex that he requires a complete bed bath and help with eating.

Develop Individualized Care Plans for Problems Not Addressed by Standardized Documents. For Ben Ivanos, you would need to write a plan for problems 1 and 3 above. The critical pathway probably contains some expected outcomes and basic interventions for problem 1, Pain, but you might need to individualize them to make them more effective. If your unit had a Pain protocol, similar to the Falls protocol in Figure 5-4, you would add it to Mr. Ivanos's care plan. If not, you would hand-write goals and interventions for the Pain diagnosis.

Problem 3, Self-Care Deficit, would be partially addressed in the basic care section of Mr. Ivanos's Kardex, but he has special needs. For example, he will need teaching and therapy to increase his ability to care for himself. So you would need to hand-write a plan for this nursing diagnosis.

KnowledgeCheck 5-3

Briefly describe a process for creating a comprehensive, individualized care plan that incorporates collaborative care and standardized planning documents.

PLANNING PATIENT GOALS/OUTCOMES

After assessment and diagnosis, the next step in individualized care planning is to formulate goals for improving or maintaining the patient's health status. **Goals** (also called **expected outcomes, desired outcomes,** or **predicted outcomes**) describe the changes in patient health status that you hope to achieve. **Nurse-sensitive outcomes** are those that can be influenced by nursing interventions. Although critical pathways describe the expected outcomes of multidisciplinary care, they do not provide a way to judge *nursing* effectiveness. The rest of this chapter discusses individualized care planning and nurse-sensitive outcomes.

Goals are important for planning, implementation, and evaluation. The purposes of precise, descriptive, clearly stated goals/expected outcomes are to:

- Provide a guide for selecting nursing interventions by describing what you wish to achieve.
- Motivate the client and the nurse by providing a sense of achievement when the goals are met. This is especially important when the client must make difficult lifestyle changes.
- Form the criteria you will use in the evaluation phase of the nursing process.

Goal/expected outcome formulation is the responsibility of the professional nurse (see Box 5-1). You should involve the client as much as possible in goal setting, because goal achievement is more likely if the client believes the goals are important and realistic. Of course, the client must be alert and independent enough to participate. If physical or mental impairments prevent active participation, the nursing team acts on the client's behalf to develop client-centered goals.

What Do the Terms Goal and Outcome Mean?

Many nurses use the terms *goal* and *outcome* interchangeably. In this text, we usually use the Nursing Outcomes Classification (NOC) terminology: The word *outcome,* used alone, means *any* patient response (positive or negative) to interventions (e.g., the pain could become better or worse; both are outcomes). When referring to desired (positive) patient responses, we use *goals, expected outcomes, desired outcomes,* or *predicted outcomes.* For example:

Outcome	Decision Making
Goals/expected outcomes	Participates in decisions about own care.
	Chooses between two or more alternatives.

Some nurses use the term *goal* to mean a broad, nonspecific statement about the desired results of nursing activities. They use *outcomes* (and other outcome terms such as *expected outcomes*) to mean the more specific, observable responses that you would use to judge whether the goal has been met. When goals are defined in this way, you must include both goals and expected outcomes on the care plan because a broad goal does not provide enough guidance for evaluating patient responses to care. You can combine the broad goal and specific expected outcome into a single statement by writing *as evidenced by,* as in the following example:

Broad statement (goal)	Constipation relieved
Specific expected outcome (evaluation criteria)	Will have soft, formed bowel movement within 24 hours
Combined statement (goal + outcome)	Constipation will be relieved *as evidenced by* soft, formed bowel movement within 24 hours

Use of broad goals on the care plan is optional; however, you *must* include expected outcomes on the care plan.

How Do I Distinguish Between Short-Term and Long-Term Goals?

Short-term goals are those you expect the patient to achieve within a few hours or days. They are important:

- In situations in which the patient may be discharged before you can evaluate progress toward long-term goals (e.g., as in a day surgery).
- For providing positive reinforcement to clients who are working toward long-term goals.

Long-term goals are changes in health status that you wish to achieve over a longer period—perhaps a week, a month, or longer. They describe the optimum level of functioning you expect the patient to achieve, given health status and available resources. Ideally, this is a return to normal functioning, but that is not always possible. See Table 5-2 for a comparison of short-term and long-term goals.

KnowledgeCheck 5-4

Refer to Meet Your Patient, at the beginning of the chapter. State whether each of Mr. Ivanos's goals was a short-term or a long-term goal.

What Are the Components of a Goal Statement?

Every expected outcome/goal statement must have the following parts:

- *Subject.* The subject is understood to be the client, but it can also be a function or part of the client. For example:

[Mrs. Johnson] Will walk to the doorway with the help of one person by 12/13/14.
Lung sounds will be clear to auscultation within 2 days after receiving antibiotics.

Assume that the subject is the client unless otherwise stated. For example, in the first goal, you should not write "Mrs. Johnson." Think, "Client will . . ." to help you phrase the goal statement correctly, but do not write it.

Table 5-2 ▶ Comparison of Short-Term and Long-Term Goals	DEFINITION	SITUATIONS FOR USE	EXAMPLES
Short-Term Goals	■ Can be achieved in a few hours or a few days.	■ Acute care ■ Day surgery ■ Clinics ■ Focus on immediate needs ■ Students ■ Evaluation of progress toward long-term goals	■ Describes pain as <3 on a 1–10 scale within 30 min after receiving analgesic. ■ Limits food intake to 1,500 calories per day.
Long-Term Goals	■ Expected changes that occur over a week, a month, or more ■ Optimum level of functioning given health status and resources	■ Home healthcare ■ Extended-care facilities ■ Rehabilitation centers ■ Chronic illness ■ Conditions that are managed, not cured	■ Infant will double birth weight within 5 mo. ■ Within 3 mo after physical therapy treatments, will dress self except for buttons.

- *Action verb.* Use an action verb to indicate the action that the client will perform: what the client will learn, do, or say (e.g., Will *walk* to the doorway). Use concrete verbs (i.e., describing actions that you can see, hear, smell, feel, or measure), such as the following:

apply	explain	report
choose	eat	select
demonstrate	list	transfer
describe	measure	turn
drink	prepare	verbalize

- *Performance criteria.* These describe the extent to which you expect to see the action or behavior. Write them in concrete, observable terms because they indicate what you need to measure in order to evaluate outcomes. Performance criteria specify:
  (a) How, what, when, or where something is to be done
  (b) Amount, quality, accuracy, speed, distance, and so forth

  The following example specifies the distance the client is expected to walk: [Client] Will walk *to the doorway* with the help of one person by 12/13/14.
- *Target time.* This is the realistic date or time by which the client should achieve the performance or behavior. The target time is the "when" part of the performance criterion: [Client] will walk to the doorway with the help of one person *by 12/13/14.*

  Other examples of target times are *by discharge, within 24 hours, at the next visit, each hour, at all times.* For risk (potential) nursing diagnoses, the desired outcome is that the problem will never occur. You can assume that the desired response should occur "at all times," but you may wish to schedule times for evaluating the outcome. For example:

  Nursing diagnosis: Risk for Constipation r/t inadequate fluid intake
  Expected outcome: Bowel movements will be of normal frequency and consistency.
  Target time: At all times
  Evaluate: Daily
- *Special conditions.* Special conditions describe the amount of assistance or resources needed or the experiences/treatments the client should have to perform the behavior. Include special conditions when it is important for other nurses to know them. For example: [Client] Will walk to the doorway *with the help of one person* by 12/13/14.

KnowledgeCheck 5-5

In the following predicted outcomes, identify the subject, action verb, performance criterion, target time, and special conditions (if any). State which components are assumed, if any.

- Will walk to the doorway with the help of one person by 12/13/13.
- After two teaching sessions, (client) will be able to identify foods to avoid on a low-fat diet by 3/1/13.
- Bowel movements will be soft and formed and of his usual frequency.
- Lungs sound clear to auscultation at all times.

How Do Goals Relate to Nursing Diagnoses?

Expected outcomes are derived directly from the nursing diagnosis. Therefore, they will be appropriate only if you identify the nursing diagnosis correctly. The problem clause (the clause at the left) of a nursing diagnosis describes the response or health status you wish to change. A desired outcome states the *opposite* of the problem and implies this response is what the interventions are intended to achieve (Table 5-3).

ThinkLike a Nurse 5-3

Answer the following questions for Ben Ivanos's (Meet Your Patient) nursing diagnosis of Acute Pain secondary to musculoskeletal trauma (arms, legs, body) and muscle spasms:

- What would be the opposite, healthy response to his problem?
- What changes should you see in appearance, body functions, symptoms, knowledge, and emotions?
- If the problem is prevented or solved, how will Mr. Ivanos look or behave? What will you be able to observe (e.g., see, hear, smell, taste, or touch)?
- What should Mr. Ivanos be able to do to demonstrate a positive change? How well, or how soon, should he be able to do it?

You might have said that the opposite response to pain would be absence of (or relief from) pain, but you couldn't really observe that. "Absence of pain" might serve as a broad goal statement. But how about more specific, observable expected outcomes? How would you know that Mr. Ivanos's pain was relieved? A few specific, observable behaviors that demonstrate absence of pain include the following: Relaxed body posture, states that his pain is relieved, rates pain as less than 3 on a scale of 1 to 10.

Table 5-3 ➤ Comparison of Nursing Diagnoses and Goals

NURSING DIAGNOSIS (PROBLEM SIDE)	GOAL/EXPECTED OUTCOME
Problem response	Opposite of problem response
Present health status	Desired health status
Response that you hope to change	Response that you hope to achieve
Examples:	*Examples:*
Ineffective Airway Clearance ⟶	Lungs clear to auscultation
r/t ineffective cough secondary to incision pain ⟶	Coughs productively

Essential Versus Nonessential Goals

In general, the problem side of the nursing diagnosis suggests the goals, and the etiology suggests nursing interventions. You can also derive some goals from the etiology; however, the **essential patient goals** flow from the problem side of the nursing diagnosis (see the bold print in Table 5-4) because the problem side describes the unhealthy response you intend to change.

Notice in Table 5-4 that the goals derived from the etiology may help resolve the problem, but they could also be achieved without resolution of the problem. Suppose that for a patient with Ineffective Airway Clearance you had written only the goals in regular type. If the patient achieves all three goals, you might discontinue the interventions for Ineffective Airway Clearance. However, the problem might still exist. Even a client who demonstrates all three of those responses might not be coughing productively enough to clear the airways and might still not have clear lung sounds. Always follow this rule:

For every nursing diagnosis, you must state one goal that, if achieved, would demonstrate resolution or improvement of the problem.

Goals for Actual, Risk, and Possible Nursing Diagnoses

You will develop expected outcomes to promote, maintain, or restore health, depending on the status of the nursing diagnosis. See Table 5-5 for explanations and examples. Review Chapter 4 as needed.

Goals for Collaborative Problems

Recall that collaborative problems are physiological complications of diseases (e.g., diabetes) or medical treatments (e.g., cardiac catheterization) that nurses monitor to detect onset or changes in status. The desired outcome is always that the complication will not develop. However, unlike outcomes for nursing diagnoses, these outcomes are not nurse-sensitive; that is, they do not result primarily from nursing interventions. They occur as a result of interventions by several disciplines. Consider the following example:

Collaborative problem: Potential Complication of abdominal surgery: Paralytic ileus (paralysis of the ileum of the small intestine)

Goal: Patient will not develop paralytic ileus

Suppose that 36 hours after the surgery, the patient's bowel sounds are absent, his abdomen is distended and painful, and he begins vomiting. What could the nurse have done to prevent this situation? What can the nurse do to relieve the ileus and bring about return of peristalsis? Very little, actually. The primary interventions are medical and, if there is obstruction, probably surgical. Therefore, it would not be appropriate to include a goal for this problem on a nursing care plan, because that would imply that nurses are primarily accountable for the outcome.

Collaborative goals are appropriate on multidisciplinary care plans and critical pathways. However, all goals on a nursing care plan should be nursing-sensitive goals. For collaborative problems, instead of a patient outcome, instead of patient goals, you might wish to write a *nursing goal,* such as, "Early detection of complication, should it occur." See Table 5-5.

On student care plans, to aid your learning, you can write the symptoms of the complication or the normal physiological response you hope to observe (e.g., Bowel sounds present within 24 hours; no abdominal distention; no vomiting), but these are not appropriate on an institutional care plan.

How Do I Use Standardized Terminology for Outcomes?

In Chapter 4, you learned about the NANDA-I standardized terminology for nursing diagnoses. The ANA has also approved several standardized vocabularies for describing client outcomes. The one used throughout most of this book is the Nursing Outcomes Classification (NOC) (Moorhead, Johnson, Maas, et al., 2008).

The **NOC** is a standardized vocabulary of more than 385 nursing-sensitive outcomes developed by a research team at the University of Iowa. In the NOC vocabulary, an **outcome** is "an individual, family, or community state, behavior, or perception that is measured along a continuum in response to nursing interventions" (Moorhead, Johnson, Maas, et al., 2008, p. 35). Thus, the NOC is versatile because it is appropriate for use in all specialty and practice areas.

Components of a NOC Outcome

Each NOC outcome consists of an outcome label, indicators, and a measurement scale. The **outcome label** (usually referred to as *the outcome*) is broadly stated (e.g., Decision Making,

Table 5-4 ▶ Deriving Goals and Interventions from Nursing Diagnoses

NURSING DIAGNOSIS		GOALS/EXPECTED OUTCOMES		NURSING ACTIVITIES
Problem: *Ineffective Airway* *Clearance*	⟶	**Lungs clear to auscultation** **Coughs productively** **Respirations 12–20 breaths/min** **No pallor or cyanosis**	⟶	Teach deep breathing and coughing Auscultate lungs q4hr Assess respiratory rate, breathing, and skin color q4hr
r/t		**No dyspnea or shortness of breath (SOB)**		
Etiology: *Ineffective cough* *secondary to incisional* *pain*	⟶	Coughs forcefully/effectively Rates pain as <3 on 1–10 scale Splints incision while coughing	⟶	Teach to splint incision while coughing Turn, deep-breathe, and cough (TDBC) hourly Medicate for pain 30 min before TDBC

Table 5-5 ▶ Expected Outcomes for Various Problem Types

TYPE OF PROBLEM	EXAMPLE OF DIAGNOSIS	EXPLANATION OF DIAGNOSIS	PURPOSE OF NURSING INTERVENTIONS	EXAMPLE OF EXPECTED PATIENT OUTCOME
Actual Nursing Diagnosis	Constipation r/t inadequate dietary fiber and fluids	Symptoms of constipation present (e.g., no bowel movement [BM])	Resolution or reduction of problem; prevention of complications	Will have normal, formed BM within 24 hr after receiving stool softener.
Risk (Potential) Nursing Diagnosis	Risk for Constipation r/t inadequate dietary fiber and fluids	Risk factors present (e.g., not drinking enough or eating adequate fiber)	Prevention and early detection problem	Will have bowel function within normal limits for patient (e.g., daily BM with no need for stool softener or laxative).
Possible Nursing Diagnosis	Possible Constipation r/t suspected inadequate intake of dietary fiber and fluids	Not enough data (e.g., no BM for 2 days, but no data on intake or on his usual bowel habits)	Confirm or rule out problem.	No patient goal. The nursing goal is "Confirm or rule out the problem."
Collaborative Problem	Potential Complication of abdominal surgery: ileus	Medical treatment creates risk for complication that is prevented by collaborative care.	Primarily detection; prevention is collaborative.	None. Patient responses depend on collaborative care. The broad nursing goal is early identification of the problem.
Wellness Diagnosis	Readiness for Enhanced Nutrition	Bowel habits and dietary intake within normal limits, but can be improved	Maintain or promote higher level of health.	Reports increased intake of dietary fiber and fluids; reports bowel functioning within normal limits.

Mobility Level). It is a neutral label (a variable), to allow for positive, negative, or no change in patient health status. Because NOC outcomes are linked to NANDA-I nursing diagnoses, you can look up a nursing diagnosis to see the list of outcomes suggested for it (Box 5-2). You can find suggested outcomes for each NANDA-I diagnosis in the NANDA/NIC/NOC "linkages" book (Johnson, Bulechek, Butcher, et al., 2012). You can find Additional Associated Outcomes for each diagnosis in Part IV of the *Nursing Outcomes Classification (NOC)* (Moorhead, Johnson, Maas, et al., 2008).

The **indicators** are the observable behaviors and states that you can use to evaluate patient status. In Table 5-6 the indicators are in the first (left) column. The first one is "Identifies relevant information." This indicator is one sign that Decision Making (the broad outcome) was being achieved. For each outcome, you select the indicators that are appropriate to the patient. You can add to the list of indicators if necessary.

For each outcome, NOC has a 5-point **measurement scale** (the numbers in Table 5-6) for describing patient status for each indicator. As a rule, 1 is least desirable and 5 is most desirable. If you are using NOC, you do not need to write traditional goal statements. You simply write the label, choose the appropriate indicators, and assign a number from the measurement scale. In your initial assessment, you assign the number that represents the patient's present health status. To form the "goal," you

assign the scale number that the patient can realistically achieve after the interventions. Using Table 5-6, you might assign the following numbers:

(NOC Outcome) **Decision Making**
Goals (Indicators + measurement scale)
Identifies relevant information (4, mildly compromised)
Identifies alternatives (4, mildly compromised)
Identifies potential consequences of each alternative (5, not compromised)
For a list of the NOC measurement scales,

 Go to Chapter 5, **Standardized Language Table ESG 5-1,** on DavisPlus.

KnowledgeCheck 5-6

Figure 5-5, a patient plan of care for Acute Pain, uses NOC language.

- What outcomes did the nurse choose for this patient?
- List two indicators for each of the outcomes.
- For which outcome does the nurse expect the highest level of functioning to occur after interventions? (Note that in this care plan the measuring scale has been applied to the outcomes rather than to the indicators.)

BOX 5-2 ■ Outcomes Linked to NANDA-I Diagnosis

Nursing Diagnosis

Situational Low Self-Esteem

Definition

Development of a negative perception of self-worth in response to a current situation (specify)

Suggested Outcomes

Adaptation to Physical Disability
Grief Resolution
Personal Resiliency
Psychosocial Adjustment: Life Change
Self-Esteem

Sources: Johnson, M., Bulechek, G., Butcher, H., et al. (2012). *Nursing diagnoses, outcomes, & interventions: NANDA, NOC, and NIC linkages* (3rd ed.). St. Louis, MO: C.V. Mosby, pp. 377–378; and NANDA International. (2012). *Nursing diagnoses: Definitions & classification 2012–2014.* Ames, IA: Wiley-Blackwell, p. 193.

Additional Associated Outcomes

Abuse Recovery Status
Abuse Recovery: Emotional
Abuse Recovery: Physical
Abuse Recovery: Sexual
Anxiety Level
Body Image
Burn Recovery
Coping
Development: Late Adulthood
Development: Middle Adulthood
Development: Young Adulthood
Fear Level
Fear Level: Child
Neglect Recovery
Personal Autonomy
Role Performance
Stress Level

Source: Moorhead, S., Johnson, M., Maas, M., et al. (2008). *Nursing outcomes classification* (4th ed.). St. Louis, MO: Mosby/Elsevier.

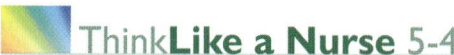

ThinkLike a Nurse 5-4

In Figure 5-5, what do you think the nurse expects to happen? Why do you think she ranked the outcomes this way?

Using NOC With Computerized Care Plans

Standardized language (e.g., NOC) is especially useful in computerized care systems. To see computer screens for locating and choosing NOC outcomes and for choosing NOC indicators, respectively,

 Go to Chapter 5, **Tables, Boxes, Figures: ESG Figures 5-5 and 5-6,** on Davis*Plus.*

In those figures, the nurse chose Circulation Status as a patient outcome, and the program provided the definition and the NOC indicators for that outcome. The nurse would then check the indicators that apply to the patient.

Remember that the computer does not think for you. You are responsible for deciding which outcomes and indicators to use for each patient, and for identifying a target time. Most electronic health records have a screen that allows you to type in your own goals as well.

How Do I Write Goals for Groups?

Home and community health nurses are especially likely to write goals for aggregates (groups), such as families and communities. **Community health goals (public health goals)** are those you would use to specify and evaluate the health of groups, aggregates, or populations. They tend to emphasize health promotion, health maintenance, and disease prevention outcomes. For example, the U.S. Public Health Service (USPHS) has proposed four group goals—the following broad, overarching goals for improving the health of the nation by a target date of 2020 (*Healthy People 2020,* 2010):

- Attain high-quality, longer lives free of preventable disease, disability, injury, and premature death.
- Achieve health equity, eliminate disparities, and improve the health of all groups.
- Create social and physical environments that promote good health for all.
- Promote quality of life, healthy development, and healthy behaviors across all life stages.

NOC currently includes 10 outcomes targeted to Community Health. Two examples are Community Competence and Community Risk Control: Lead Exposure. NOC also has 14 outcomes that describe the health of a family as a unit. Two examples are Family Coping and Family Health Status. NOC outcomes can be used in all settings, including home and community nursing. For further explanation, see Chapter 41. Also, search for Nursing Outcomes Classification on the Web or

 Go to the NOC Web site at http://www.nursing.uiowa.edu/center-for-nursing-classification-and-clinical-effectiveness

The following taxonomies were created specifically for describing family and community outcomes.

The Clinical Care Classification (CCC). The CCC system was developed by Virginia Saba, a nurse researcher, for use in home health nursing. In the CCC, you form goals by adding modifiers to the nursing diagnoses. This system has four nursing diagnoses that are clearly for family units: Family Coping Impairment, Compromised Family Coping, Disabled Family Coping, and Family Processes Alteration.

The CCC includes one diagnosis specifically for communities: Community Coping Impairment. For a complete description of the CCC system,

 Go to the CCC Web site at http://www.sabacare.com

The Omaha System. The Omaha System was developed specifically for community health nursing. In that system, you must label all nursing diagnoses as *individual, family,* or *group.* You can write aggregate outcomes by specifying a *family* or *group* diagnosis and then creating a goal from it, by using terms in a Problem Rating Scale for Outcomes, as in the following example.

Omaha Nursing Diagnosis: Personal Hygiene. Family. Deficit (Actual Problem)

Present status	*Expected outcome*
Minimal knowledge of family personal hygiene	Adequate knowledge of family personal hygiene

Table 5-6 ➤ Example of an NOC Outcome

Decision Making (0906)

Domain—Physiologic Health (II)

Class—Neurocognitive (J)

Scale(s)—Severely compromised to Not compromised

Definition: Ability to make judgments and choose between two or more alternatives

DECISION MAKING	SEVERELY COMPROMISED	SUBSTANTIALLY COMPROMISED	MODERATELY COMPROMISED	MILDLY COMPROMISED	NOT COMPROMISED
Overall Rating					
Identifies relevant information.	1	2	3	4	5
Identifies alternatives.	1	2	3	4	5
Identifies potential consequences of each alternative.	1	2	3	4	5
Identifies needed resources to support each alternative.	1	2	3	4	5
Identifies time frame necessary to support each alternative.	1	2	3	4	5
Identifies sequence necessary to support each alternative.	1	2	3	4	5
Recognizes contradiction with others' desires.	1	2	3	4	5
Acknowledges social context of the situation.	1	2	3	4	5
Acknowledges relevant legal implications.	1	2	3	4	5
Weighs alternatives.	1	2	3	4	5
Chooses among alternatives.	1	2	3	4	5

Source: Moorhead, S., Johnson, M., Maas, M., et al. (2008). *Nursing outcomes classification* (4th ed.). St. Louis, MO: Mosby/Elsevier.

For a complete description of the Omaha System, and to see the Problem Rating Scale for Outcomes,

 Go to the Omaha System Web site at
http://www.omahasystem.org

KnowledgeCheck 5-7

- Which standardized classification system was designed specifically for community health nursing?
- Which standardized classification system was designed specifically for home healthcare?
- Which standardized classification system was designed for use in all areas and specialties of nursing?

How Do I Write Goals for Wellness Diagnoses?

Whether standardized or individualized, expected outcomes for wellness diagnoses describe behaviors or responses that demonstrate health maintenance or achievement of an even higher level of health. For example, "Over the next year, [Mr. Needham] will continue to eat a balanced diet with more emphasis on including whole grains and fiber." By using the highest number (5) on the rating scale, you can use the NOC to write wellness outcomes. For example:

> *Nursing diagnosis:* Readiness for Enhanced Nutrition
> *Expected outcome:* Nutritional Status: (5) Not compromised

In addition, many NOC outcomes can be used to measure health (e.g., Activity Tolerance, Child Development, Growth, Nutritional Status). See Chapter 27 or go to the NOC Web site for a complete list of wellness outcomes.

Outcomes for Special Teaching Plans

As discussed earlier, some patients need a special teaching plan to address learning needs. Expected outcomes are written in the same way as on any other type of care plan, but they are usually called teaching objectives. **Teaching objectives** describe what the patient is to learn and the observable behaviors that will demonstrate learning; they should state whether

learning is to be cognitive, psychomotor, or affective. Consider the following examples:

Cognitive: By May 1, will list four foods to avoid on a low-fat diet.

Affective: By May 1, will verbalize feeling less anger about diet limitations.

Psychomotor: By May 1, will demonstrate how to use grasp extender to obtain food from the top shelf.

For further information about teaching objectives, see Chapter 26.

REFLECTING CRITICALLY ABOUT EXPECTED OUTCOMES/GOALS

After writing the expected outcomes for a client, use the full-spectrum nursing model to help you evaluate their quality. Use the following questions as a guide:

For each nursing diagnosis:

1. *Is there at least one goal that, when met, would demonstrate problem resolution;* that is, does at least one goal flow from the problem clause?

2. *Do the predicted outcomes completely address the nursing diagnosis?* Review Table 5-4.

For each expected outcome:

3. *Is the outcome appropriate for the nursing diagnosis?* If not, a new nursing diagnosis should be written rather than adding a not-quite-related goal to the existing plan.

4. *Is each outcome derived from only one nursing diagnosis?* That is, does it describe only one patient response?
Incorrect: For a diagnosis of Diarrhea: Will have no diarrhea in the next 12 hours, and skin will be intact and without redness in the perianal area.

5. *Is the outcome stated as a patient behavior, not a nurse activity?*
Incorrect (nurse activity): Prevent skin irritation
Correct (patient response): Skin will not show signs of irritation

6. *Is the outcome stated in positive terms?* When you can do so, state what you intend to occur, rather than what should not occur. For example, use "incision dry," rather than "no incision drainage." This is not always possible, especially for potential problems. It is better, for example, to write "No redness" (even though it is negative) than to write "Skin color normal," because "normal" is too vague.

7. *Is the outcome measurable or observable?*
Correct: Explains the actions and side effects of Coumadin, by 8/11/14
Incorrect: Understands the actions and side effects of Coumadin, by 8/11/14

8. *Are the performance criteria specific and concrete?* Avoid words such as *normal, sufficient, enough, more, less, adequate, increased.* Vague words can be interpreted differently by different people.

9. *Does each goal include all the necessary parts?*

10. *Is the expected outcome realistic and achievable by this patient, given the available resources?* Be sure to consider the patient's support system, financial status, available community services, and physical and mental status. Also consider institutional resources.

11. *Does the outcome conflict with the medical or other collaborative treatment plan?* For example, an outcome of "Ambulates to end of hall" would not be compatible with the medical treatment plan for a patient who is sleepy and lethargic from the side effects of medications.

12. *Does the patient, family, or community value the outcome?* The care plan is more likely to be effective if the goal is important to the client. When your goals conflict with the patient's, explore the patient's reasoning. Explain your reasoning and try to find a compromise or an alternative approach.

13. *Does the goal conflict with any religious or cultural values?* When a patient is "noncompliant," the reason may be that she is complying with her cultural beliefs rather than the caregiver's plan of care.

KnowledgeCheck 5-8

List at least eight questions you could use to critically evaluate the quality of your goal/outcome statements.

Toward Evidence-Based Practice

Scherb, C. A., Stevens, M. S., & Busman, C. (2007). Outcomes related to dehydration in the pediatric population. *Journal of Pediatric Nursing, 22*(5), 376–382.

The purpose of this pilot study was to (1) determine whether there was a meaningful difference (in statistical terms) in nursing-sensitive patient outcome ratings from admission to discharge and (2) to describe nursing interventions used for children (younger than age 18 years) admitted with a primary diagnosis of dehydration. During the study period, researchers examined 29 patient care records that were a part of a computerized clinical documentation system in a midwestern hospital. The documentation system used the standardized nursing languages of NANDA-I, NOC, and NIC.

Standardized care plans (also using NANDA-I, NOC, and NIC) were initiated upon a child's admission, and individualized as needed. NOC outcomes were rated upon admission and at discharge. Examples of outcomes on the care plan include Nutritional Status, Fluid Balance, and Urinary Elimination. Of the eight outcomes on the care plan, seven had statistically significant changes (showing the child's improvement).

1. If you had to decide on the basis of this study alone, would you be for or against using standardized nursing languages for documentation and patient care plans in your organization? Explain your reasoning.

 Go to Chapter 5, **Toward Evidence-Based Practice Suggested Responses,** on Davis*Plus.*

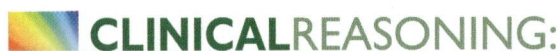

CLINICALREASONING:
Applying the **Full-Spectrum Nursing Model**

Because the following critical thinking activities allow you to practice the kind of thinking you will use as a full-spectrum nurse, they usually have no single right answer. Discuss them with your peers—if you have difficulty with any of the questions, consult your instructor.

PATIENT SITUATION

Ivan Benjamin has just been admitted to an orthopedic unit after an automobile accident. He was driving. Mr. Benjamin is 80 years old and has been living at home. He has these preexisting comorbidities: type 2 diabetes and osteoarthritis. He has casts and traction on both legs and a cast on one arm. He is receiving morphine sulfate intravenously via patient-controlled analgesia (PCA) pump. Imagine that you are an orthopedic nurse and must plan care for Mr. Benjamin. The admitting nurse wrote the following diagnoses and goals on the plan of care.

NURSING DIAGNOSES

1. Acute Pain secondary to musculoskeletal trauma (arms, legs, body) and muscle spasms

2. Risk for Peripheral Neurovascular Dysfunction secondary to casts/traction

GOALS/EXPECTED OUTCOMES

- Demonstrates correct use of PCA pump
- Rates pain not higher than 4 on a scale of 1 to 10 at all times

- Peripheral pulses palpable
- Fingers and toes warm
- Fingers and toes without pallor or cyanosis
- No edema of fingers and toes
- Capillary refill less than 3 sec

THINKING

1. *Theoretical Knowledge:* What general *theoretical knowledge* will you need to care for this patient? Just identify the topics; limit the answer to about 150 words.
2. *Critical Thinking (Considering Alternatives):* Older adults are especially sensitive to certain medications, including morphine sulfate. What is one thing you could do to ensure Mr. Benjamin's safety while managing his acute pain (there are several; think of just one)?
3. *Critical Thinking (Inquiry):* List at least two more things you need to know about Mr. Benjamin in order to begin his discharge planning.

DOING

4. *Practical Knowledge:* What general practical knowledge will you need? What would you do to obtain this knowledge?
5. *Nursing Process:*
   a. *Diagnosis:* What is another nursing diagnosis you might want to assess for Mr. Benjamin?
   b. *Planning Goals:* On the care plan, rewrite the goals/expected outcomes for Acute Pain so that they will have all the required components. Assume that today's date is January 4.

CARING

6. *Self-Knowledge:* What beliefs, values, biases, or emotional responses might interfere with your ability to provide the best care to Mr. Benjamin?

CONTEXT

7. *Think critically about the context.* Is there anything in this situation that you have seen before? Identify any familiar elements. For example, you may have an elderly male relative, even if you have never cared for an 80-year-old patient before.

 Go to Chapter 5, Clinical Reasoning: **Applying the Full-Spectrum Nursing Model Response Sheet** on Davis*Plus*.

To explore learning resources for this chapter,

 Go to Davis*Plus* at http://www.Davisplus.fadavis.com, keyword Treas.

Chapter Resources for Chapter 5:
   Knowledge Check and Think Like a Nurse Response Sheets
   Knowledge Check Answers
   Resources for Caregivers and Health Professionals
   Reading More About Planning Outcomes (Suggested Readings)
   What Are the Main Points in This Chapter?
NCLEX-Style Review Questions
Chapter Overview Podcasts

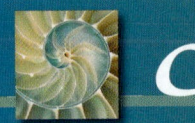 Concept Map

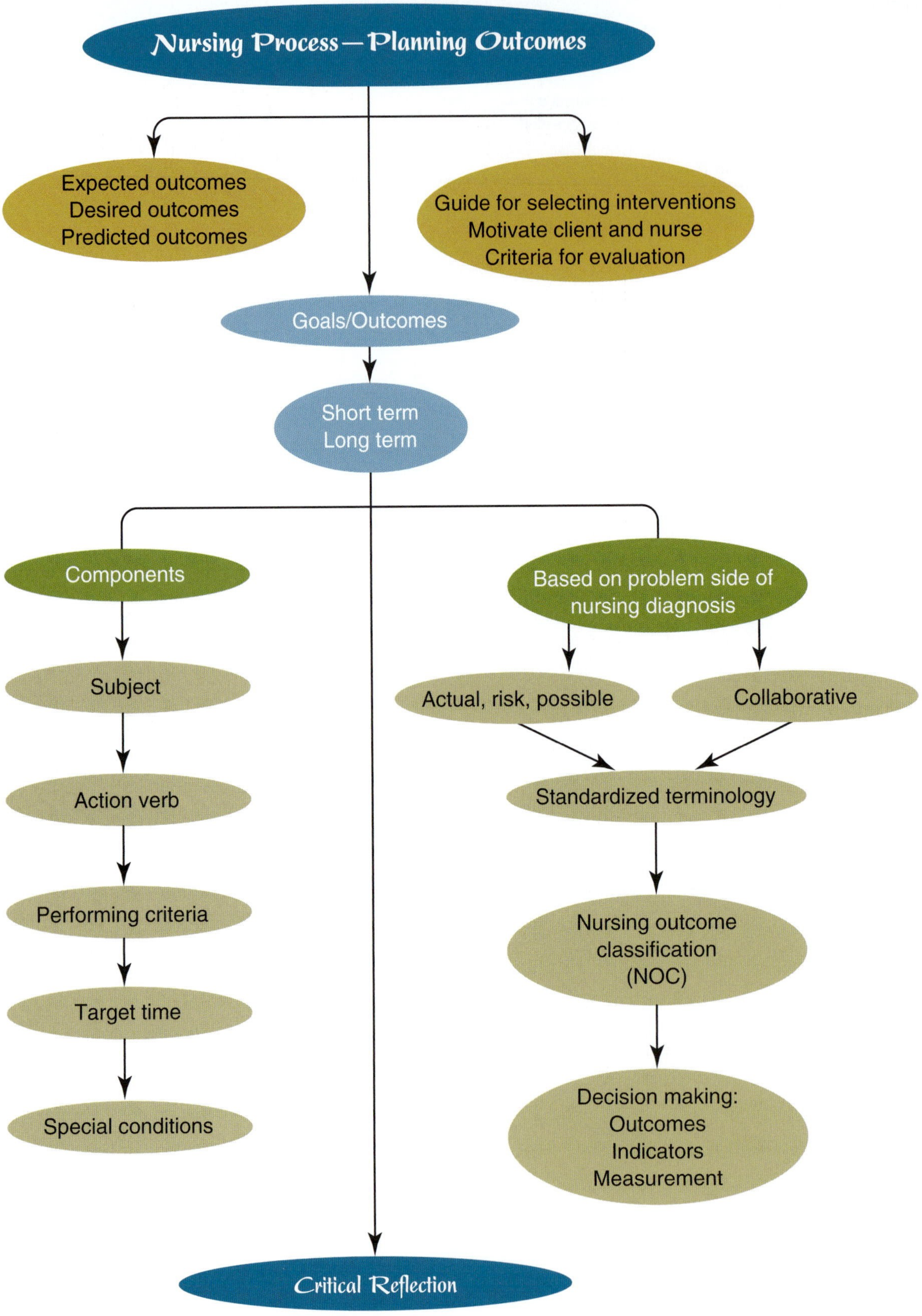

Nursing Process—Planning Outcomes

Expected outcomes
Desired outcomes
Predicted outcomes

Guide for selecting interventions
Motivate client and nurse
Criteria for evaluation

Goals/Outcomes

Short term
Long term

Components

Based on problem side of nursing diagnosis

Subject

Actual, risk, possible

Collaborative

Action verb

Standardized terminology

Performing criteria

Nursing outcome classification (NOC)

Target time

Special conditions

Decision making:
Outcomes
Indicators
Measurement

Critical Reflection

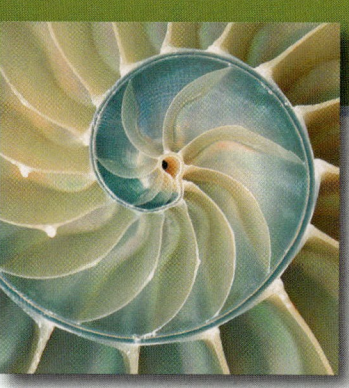

CHAPTER 6

Planning Interventions

Learning Outcomes

After completing this chapter, you should be able to:

➤ Define the term *nursing intervention*.

➤ Compare and contrast independent, dependent, and interdependent (collaborative) nursing interventions.

➤ Explain how theories, research, and evidence-based practice influence the choice of nursing interventions.

➤ Describe a process for generating nursing interventions for a client.

➤ Explain how to use a standardized vocabulary for nursing interventions and activities.

➤ Give one example of a standardized wellness (health promotion)

intervention and one individualized nursing order for performing that intervention.

➤ Give one example of a standardized spirituality intervention and one individualized nursing order for performing that intervention.

➤ Write complete, detailed nursing orders, in correct format, for patients.

➤ Give examples of some questions for reflecting critically about nursing orders you have written.

Key Concepts

Evidence-based practice
Nursing interventions

Related Concepts

See the Concept Map at the end of this chapter.

Caring for the Nguyens

This feature allows you to practice the kind of thinking you will use as a full-spectrum nurse. There is usually more than one correct answer to a critical thinking question, so we do not provide answers for these features. It is more important to develop your nursing judgment than to "cover content." Discuss the questions with your peers. If you are still unsure, consult your instructor.

Recall that you have written the following nursing diagnosis for Mr. Nguyen:

Imbalanced Nutrition: More Than Body Requirements related to inappropriate food choices and serving size, as evidenced by body mass index (BMI) of 28.5.

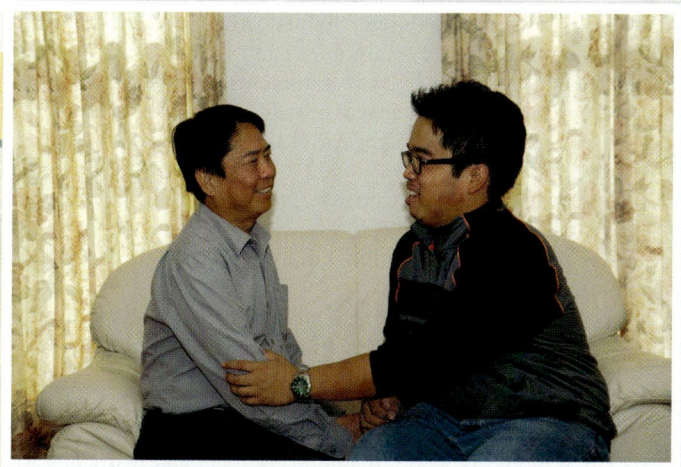

A. Based on the outcomes you wrote in Chapter 5, Planning Outcomes, identify four possible interventions to address the diagnosis and outcomes.

B. Review the interventions, and identify two that would be most appropriate for Mr. Nguyen given all of the information you have about his health status.

C. Write a nursing order for each of the two interventions you identified above.

 Go to **Caring for the Nguyens Response Sheet** on *DavisPlus*.

Meet Your Patient

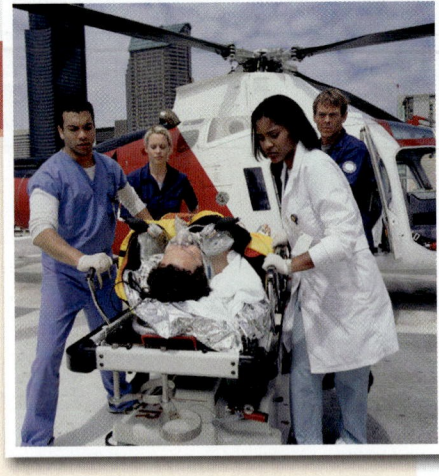

Ben Ivanos, whom you met in Chapter 5, is confined to bed after a motorcycle accident. He has casts and traction for both legs and a cast on one arm. Since admission to the hospital 3 days ago, he has been receiving narcotic analgesics for severe pain. He has a new nursing diagnosis today: Constipation related to immobility and decreased gastrointestinal (GI) motility secondary to narcotic analgesics. The nurse enters the diagnosis into a care-planning program. In addition to a list of suggested assessments, the computer database generates the following list of suggested treatment interventions:

1. Institute a program to establish a regular pattern of bowel movements.
2. Administer laxative or stool softener, as ordered.
3. Administer enema.
4. Remove stool manually.
5. Encourage increased fluid intake, including warm liquids.
6. Instruct on and encourage a high-fiber diet.
7. Encourage a regular program of activity and exercise.
8. Perform manual reduction of rectal prolapse.

Which interventions should the nurse choose? Which can he eliminate, based on the information provided? You may not yet have enough nursing knowledge to be sure about your answers to these questions, but before reading on, try to think it through with the information and life experience available to you.

The nurse eliminated interventions 1, 3, 4, 7, and 8. Take a few moments to see if you can explain the nurse's reasons for deleting these interventions.

Theoretical Knowledge
knowing why

Compare your explanations to the following reasons given by the nurse in the Meet Your Patient scenario. The nurse eliminated intervention:

- **1** because it is useful for patients who are constipated as a result of irregular bowel habits, whereas Mr. Ivanos's problem is caused by immobility and narcotic side effects.
- **3 and 4** because Mr. Ivanos's symptoms did not seem severe enough to warrant an enema or manual removal of stool.
- **7** because it is not practical: Mr. Ivanos cannot exercise in his present condition.
- **8** because it is not relevant: Mr. Ivanos does not have rectal prolapse.

The nurse chose the following interventions to include in the care plan:

- **2** because it directly addresses the problem, Constipation.
- **5 and 6** because they address the etiology of the problem—fluid and fiber soften the stool and help to stimulate bowel activity.

The nurse also reasoned that because narcotics cause constipation, it would be good to administer them less frequently to Mr. Ivanos—if other satisfactory pain-relief measures could be found. So he added the following nursing orders to the care plan:

    Assist to change position every 1–2 hours.
    Encourage distraction (e.g., watching TV, reading, listening to music).
    Assist with relaxation and visualization techniques.
    Obtain medical order for nonnarcotic analgesics to enhance nonpharmacological pain-relief measures.
    Assess effectiveness of nonpharmacological interventions for pain.
    Give prescribed narcotic analgesics if other measures are ineffective.

The nurse knows people are often self-conscious or embarrassed about using a bedpan, especially in the presence of others. So he also added the following to the care plan:

    Encourage Mr. Ivanos to summon the nurse when he feels the urge to defecate (place call light within reach). If he does not, then ask at least every 4 hr whether he needs the bedpan.
    Warm the bedpan and provide privacy: Pull the bed curtain; turn on the TV or radio if he has a roommate; explain that you will leave the room and that he should call when he is ready for you to return; and shut the door.

As you can see, to develop interventions to meet Mr. Ivanos's needs, the nurse needed to do more than just look at a list and follow physician orders. He thought critically about (1) his theoretical knowledge (of narcotics, bowel elimination, and psychological needs), (2) his past experiences with similar patients, and (3) the patient situation (the data about Mr. Ivanos and the factors contributing to his problem). By thinking of interventions to meet the client's specific needs, this nurse may prevent Mr. Ivanos's constipation from worsening. A nurse with less knowledge and experience might have used only the interventions in the computer database, failing to effectively meet the desired outcomes (goals) for Mr. Ivanos.

ABOUT THE KEY CONCEPTS

As you study this chapter, try to think about how related concepts (such as theories, standardized language, nursing orders, and so on) are linked to the key concepts of evidence-based practice and nursing interventions. This should aid in your understanding and retention of chapter material, as well as your ability to use your knowledge in caring for patients.

WHAT ARE NURSING INTERVENTIONS?

Nursing interventions are actions, based on clinical judgment and nursing knowledge, that nurses perform to achieve client outcomes. Interventions are also referred to as *nursing*

actions, measures, strategies, and *activities.* This chapter uses those terms interchangeably except when referring to the Nursing Interventions Classification (NIC) standardized labels (discussed later in the chapter), which are always called *interventions.* Figure 6-1 shows how planning interventions relates to the other phases of the nursing process. No matter what term is used, nursing interventions include a broad range of activities:

- **Direct-care interventions** are performed through interaction with the client(s) (e.g., physical care, emotional support, and patient teaching).
- **Indirect-care interventions** are performed away from the client but on behalf of a client or group of clients (advocacy, managing the environment, consulting with other members of the healthcare team, and making referrals).

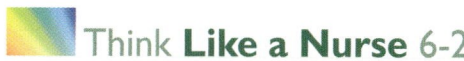

Think **Like a Nurse** 6-1

- Can you think of an example of a direct-care intervention?
- Can you think of an example of an indirect-care intervention?

Nurses work collaboratively with other healthcare providers. Some things you do for patients will require a physician's order; many will not. Sometimes the activities of care providers overlap. For example, physicians, nurses, and respiratory therapists may all measure a client's blood pressure; and a nurse and a dietitian may both teach the client about a diet to help manage hypertension. Interventions may be independent, dependent, or interdependent (collaborative).

Independent Interventions. *Nurse A makes a nursing diagnosis of Anxiety related to deficient knowledge about barium enema; she writes a nursing order to teach the patient what to expect from the upcoming diagnostic test.* This is an **independent intervention**—one that registered nurses are licensed to prescribe, perform, or delegate based on their knowledge and skills. It does not require

a provider's order. Knowing how, when, and why to perform an activity makes the action **autonomous** (independent). As a rule, nurses prescribe and perform independent interventions in response to a nursing diagnosis. As a nurse, you are **accountable** (answerable) for your decisions and actions with regard to nursing diagnoses and independent interventions. If patient teaching did not relieve the patient's anxiety in this example, it might be that the nurse misdiagnosed or chose an ineffective intervention.

Dependent Interventions. *Nurse B reads a prescription in a patient's chart: Give cephalothin sodium (Keflin) 1 g IV [through the intravenous line] before surgery, and then every 6 hours for 24 hours. She prepares and administers the medication.* This is a **dependent intervention**—one that is prescribed by a physician or advanced practice nurse but carried out by the bedside nurse. Dependent interventions are usually orders for diagnostic tests, medications, treatments, IV therapy, diet, and activity. In addition to carrying out medical prescriptions, you will be responsible for assessing the need for the prescription, explaining the activities to the patient, and evaluating the effectiveness of the prescription. For example, after giving the Keflin (an antibiotic), Nurse B observes that the patient has developed a severe rash. Suspecting an allergic reaction, she contacts the prescriber so that the medication can be changed and antibiotic prophylaxis can be continued without danger to the patient.

You may also write nursing orders to individualize a medical order, based on the patient's condition. For example, the provider may prescribe, "Give oral fluids up to 3,000 mL every 24 hours." You might individualize the order to give 1,500 mL on the day shift, 1,000 mL on the evening shift, and 500 mL during the night, so that the patient will not have to be awakened frequently during the night.

Interdependent (Collaborative) Interventions. *Nurse C notes that a client newly diagnosed with diabetes has been seen by a dietitian, who taught and provided materials about a diabetic diet. The nurse observes the client's menu choices. She notes that the client is eating candy brought by visitors. She explains to the client how concentrated sugar affects his diabetes; she also communicates her assessments and teaching to the dietitian.* This is an **interdependent (collaborative) intervention**—one that is carried out in collaboration with other health team members (e.g., physical therapists, physicians).

Think **Like a Nurse** 6-2

- What are some other examples of independent interventions?
- What are some other examples of dependent interventions?
- What are some other examples of interdependent interventions?

HOW DO I DECIDE WHICH INTERVENTIONS TO USE?

To review American Nurses Association (ANA) (2010) standards of care related to planning interventions, refer to Box 5-1, Standard 4. Use the ANA standards to guide you in selecting interventions appropriate for the client's nursing diagnoses (or collaborative problems) and the desired outcomes. In addition to the ANA standards, a variety of theories, nursing research, and the client's problem status will all influence your choice of interventions.

As a nurse, you will be responsible for choosing nursing interventions. You cannot delegate this responsibility to nursing

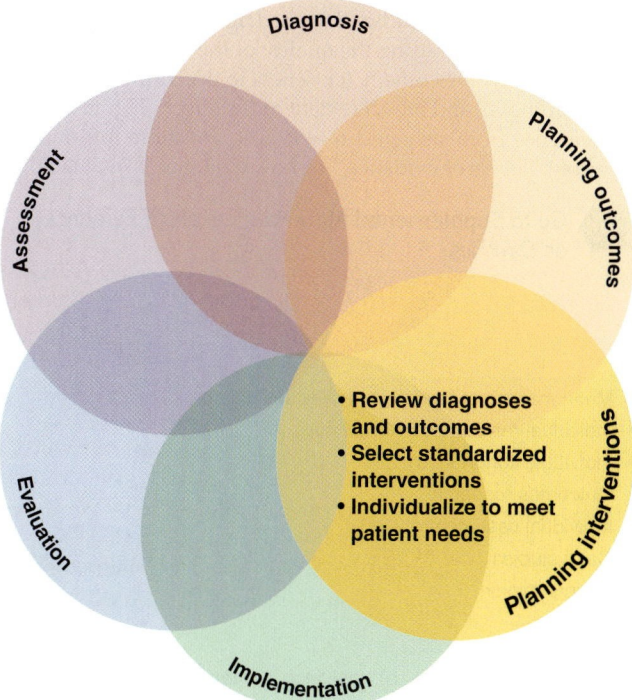

- Review diagnoses and outcomes
- Select standardized interventions
- Individualize to meet patient needs

FIGURE 6-1 Nursing process phase: planning interventions.

assistive personnel. As a rule, licensed practical/vocational nurses (LPN/LVNs) give care according to a plan created by the RN. In many situations, the LPN/LVN contributes to the plan by providing data or by giving feedback about the effectiveness of the interventions. For more information about delegation, see What Should I Know About Delegation and Supervision? in Chapter 7.

How Do Theories Influence My Choice of Interventions?

A **theory** is a set of interrelated concepts (ideas) that describes or explains something—nursing, for example. A theory, like a lens, influences your perspective: what you notice, what you consider to be a problem—and how you define a problem—more or less determine what you choose to do about it. For example, suppose a patient is pale and fidgeting and has sweaty palms and a rapid pulse. If you looked at this person through the lens of psychology theory, your first thought might be that the patient is anxious. Your first intervention would probably be to assess for the cause of his anxiety. If you were using a physiology lens, you might suspect pain. In that case, your first intervention might be to ask the patient if he is having pain. To understand more about nursing theories, see Chapter 8.

How Does Nursing Research Influence My Choice of Interventions?

Although much nursing and medical practice is still based on tradition, experience, and professional opinion, this is not an ideal basis for choosing an intervention. Ideally, a nurse should choose an intervention because of firm evidence that it is the best possible approach for the patient. Such interventions would be those that were developed from a sound body of scientific research.

American Nurses Association (ANA) Standards. Regarding evidence, the ANA Standards of Nursing Practice (2010) state that the registered nurse:

- (Standard 4) Integrates current scientific evidence, trends, and research.
- (Standard 9) Utilizes current evidence-based nursing knowledge, including research findings, to guide practice.

QSEN Competencies. According to the Quality and Safety Education for Nurses (QSEN) group, one competency you should achieve in your nursing program is to differentiate clinical opinion from research and evidence summaries. To see an expanded discussion of this competency,

 Go to **http://www.qsen.org/ksas_prelicensure.php**

Research-based support for an intervention includes single studies, critical pathways and protocols, clinical practice guidelines, systematic reviews of the literature, and evidence reports. In Chapter 8, you will learn how to ask "PICOT" questions that help you use evidence to decide which interventions to use.

Single Studies

It is not difficult to find individual studies that give you an idea of the effectiveness of an intervention. Research reports are available in research journals, and they are often interpreted and published in such widely circulated journals as the *American Journal of Nursing (AJN)*, *Nursing*, and *RN*, as well as online sites. Unfortunately, there may be only one or two studies of an intervention, and they may have included only a small number of patients. Thus, single studies may not be reliable. To see several examples of single intervention studies,

 Go to Chapter 6, **Reading More About Planning Interventions**, on Davis*Plus*.

Critical Pathways and Protocols

Critical pathways (also called *clinical pathways* and *collaborative care plans*) are standardized plans of care for frequently occurring conditions (e.g., total hip replacement) for which similar outcomes and interventions are appropriate for all patients who have the condition. They are tools developed by an organization for its own use and are intended to guide best practice at the local level. However, they may not be based on research, especially if the practitioners who develop them are reluctant to change traditional practices they believe to be effective. Furthermore, issues of cost to the organization influence the decision to include an intervention in the plan of care. Nevertheless, critical pathways have, at the very least, been developed on the basis of expert opinion. So they do provide some guidance for nursing interventions. See Chapter 5 for discussion and examples of critical pathways and protocols.

What Is Evidence-Based Practice?

You can feel more confident about an intervention if several studies have supported it. **Evidence-based practice (EBP)** is an approach that uses firm scientific data rather than anecdote, tradition, intuition, or folklore in making decisions about medical and nursing practice. In nursing it includes blending clinical judgment and expertise with the best available research evidence and patient characteristics and preferences. The goal of evidence-based practice is to identify the most effective and cost-efficient treatments for a particular disease, condition, or problem. Steps in the EBP process include the following:

1. Formulating an answerable question (e.g., a PICOT question) about prevention, diagnosis, prognosis (likely outcome), and interventions
2. Conducting a systematic review of published evidence (research) to find studies that shed light on the desired topic
3. Evaluating or grading the quality of the evidence obtained. Quality involves *validity* (closeness to the truth), *applicability* (usefulness), and *impact* (extent of the effect). Figure 6-2 lists evidence from strongest to weakest. For more information about "levels of evidence," or how evidence is evaluated,

 Go to **Supplemental Materials, Levels of Evidence,** on Davis*Plus*.

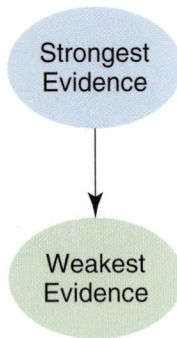

- Meta-analysis of randomized clinical trials
- Individual randomized clinical trials
- Individual cohort study
- Outcomes research
- Individual case-control study
- Case studies
- Expert opinion

Strongest Evidence

Weakest Evidence

FIGURE 6-2 Hierarchy of research evidence. (Source: Courtesy of Fain, J. A. (2008). *Reading, understanding, and applying nursing research: A text and workbook* [3rd ed.]. Philadelphia: F. A. Davis)

4. Compiling and analyzing the data to prepare a structured report of the review
5. Translating the evidence into guidelines for practice
6. Integrating the guidelines and evidence with clinical expertise and the patient's preferences and characteristics

A number of healthcare organizations and groups are devoted to compiling study results that provide evidence to use in formulating guidelines for medical and nursing practice. Online examples include the Joanna Briggs Institute and the Cochrane Database of Systematic Reviews. You will find such compiled information in clinical practice guidelines, evidence reports, and sometimes in local healthcare agency tools (e.g., clinical pathways and protocols). For full discussion on the importance of research and evidence-based nursing practice, see Chapter 8.

Evidence Reports

Evidence reports are state-of-the-art, systematic reviews of clinical topics for the purpose of providing evidence for practice guidelines, quality improvement, quality measures, and insurance coverage decisions (Cronenwett, 2002). Evidence reports are usually developed by scientists rather than by clinicians, patients, and advocacy groups. One source of such reports is the Evidence-Based Practice Center (EPC) Program of the federal Agency for Healthcare Research and Quality (AHRQ). The EPC uses explicit grading systems to review studies and rank the strength of their evidence. For free access to online reviews,

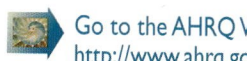 Go to the AHRQ Web site at
http://www.ahrq.gov/clinic/epcindex.htm

Clinical Practice Guidelines

Evidence reports often form the basis for developing clinical practice guidelines. **Clinical practice guidelines** are systematically developed statements to assist practitioners and patients in making decisions about appropriate healthcare for a particular disease or procedure (Institute of Medicine, 1992). Clinical practice guidelines are usually developed by clinicians, patients, and advocacy groups and are published by specialty organizations, universities, and government agencies. The following are examples:

- The Joanna Briggs Institute *Best Practice* information sheet on Topical Skin Care in Aged Care Facilities (JBI, 2007)

- University of Iowa research-based guidelines for care of the elderly (Titler, Mentes, Rakel, et al., 1999)
- National Guideline Clearinghouse, initiative of the Agency for Healthcare Research and Quality (AHRQ), U.S. Department of Health and Human Services, is a comprehensive database of guidelines for health professionals (http://www.guideline.gov/)

Clinical practice guidelines form the basis for nursing interventions. One example of clinical practice guidelines is found in Box 6-1. For years, relying on conventional wisdom and word of mouth, nurses tried to prevent pressure ulcers by writing the nursing order, "Massage skin over bony prominences." They reasoned that because poor circulation can contribute to the formation of pressure ulcers, improving circulation to the area would prevent them. But as you can see in Box 6-1, research-based practice guidelines show that massage may actually be harmful. This report would certainly motivate you, as a full-spectrum nurse, to remove this "standard" intervention from your practice.

KnowledgeCheck 6-1

- Explain how theory influences your choice of nursing interventions.
- Why does a clinical practice guideline provide better support for an intervention than does a single study?
- Why does a clinical practice guideline provide better support for an intervention than does an agency's critical pathway?

How Does Problem Status Influence Nursing Interventions?

Nursing interventions include activities for observation/assessment, prevention, treatment, and health promotion. As you can see in Table 6-1, the status of the problem (i.e., whether it is a collaborative problem or an actual, potential, possible, or wellness nursing diagnosis) determines which types of activities are required (for a review of problem status, see Chapter 4).

A nursing strategy can be a preventive measure in one situation and a treatment in another. For example, you might write the nursing order, "Teach the importance of adequate fluids," to treat a patient with an actual diagnosis of Constipation or to help prevent the problem for a patient with a diagnosis of Risk for Constipation.

BOX 6-1 ■ Portion of a Clinical Practice Guideline on Pressure Ulcer Prevention

Note: This is not the complete practice guideline.

Assessment*

- Use a reliable and standardized tool for doing a risk assessment, such as the Braden Scale.
- Risk assessment documentation on admission to a facility and whenever the client's condition changes and based on patient care setting (e.g., acute care, every 48 hr)

Nursing Care Strategies and Interventions

- ✚ Do not massage bony prominences.

- Use pressure-reducing devices (static air, alternating air, gel, water mattresses). (Evidence Level II)

- Raise heels of bedbound clients off the bed; do not use donut-type devices. (Evidence Level III)
- Avoid hot water and soaps that are drying when bathing elderly. Use body wash and skin protectant. (Evidence Level III)

---

*"Strength of evidence" is an AHRQ ranking (I to VI) of the amount and quality of research supporting the guideline. The best ranking is I.

Source: Agency for Healthcare Research and Quality (AHRQ) (2003; updated 2008). Guideline summary. Preventing pressure ulcers and skin tears. In: *Evidence-based geriatric nursing protocols for best practice.* Retrieved April 10, 2011, from http://www.guideline.gov/content.aspx?id=12262&search=pressure+ulcer#Section442

Table 6-1 ➤ Relationship of Problem Status to Intervention Type

Problem Status	Intervention Type			
	OBSERVATION	**PREVENTION**	**TREATMENT**	**HEALTH PROMOTION**
Actual nursing diagnosis	To detect change in status (improvement, exacerbation of problem)	To help keep the problem from becoming worse	To relieve symptoms and resolve etiologies (contributing factors)	
Potential (risk) nursing diagnosis	To detect (1) progression to an actual problem or (2) an increase or decrease in risk factors	To remove or reduce risk factors in an effort to keep the problem from developing		
Possible nursing diagnosis	To obtain more data to confirm or rule out a suspected nursing diagnosis			
Collaborative problem	To detect onset of a complication for early physician notification	To implement nursing and medical orders to help prevent development of a complication	To implement nursing and medical orders for relieving or eliminating the underlying condition for which complications may develop	
Wellness diagnosis	To assess a client's wellness practices	To prevent specific diseases (e.g., giving immunizations)	Clients usually manage their own wellness treatment	To support a client's health promotion efforts and achieve a higher level of wellness

KnowledgeCheck 6-2

Review problem status (actual, potential, or possible nursing diagnosis; collaborative problem; or wellness diagnosis) in Chapter 4. For which type(s) of problem(s) would you write:

- Nursing orders for observation/assessments?
- Nursing orders for treatments?
- Nursing orders for health promotion interventions?
- Preventive nursing orders?

What Process Can I Use for Generating and Selecting Interventions?

As you can see from the case of Ben Ivanos (Meet Your Patient), there are usually several nursing measures that might be effective for any one problem. The idea, of course, is to select those most likely to achieve the desired goals. In doing that, you must consider the patient's abilities and preferences; the education, experience, and capabilities of the nursing staff; the resources available (e.g., time, equipment); medical orders; evidence base; and institutional policies and procedures. When generating interventions, you will use critical thinking skills. For example, imagine you are caring for a hospice patient who has cancer and is dying. She has told you that she is experiencing significant pain, but also that she

wants to spend her last hours with her husband and two daughters, who are staying with her. Thinking critically, you might reason as follows:

The patient wants to spend quality time with her family before she dies. Because the morphine will make her drowsy, I should find out if she wants me to give a smaller dose, even though it will not provide good pain relief. I have used imagery successfully in similar situations; I might suggest it to this woman as well.

You must always rethink an intervention for each patient. You cannot assume a strategy that was useful in the past will be effective in every situation. A full-spectrum nurse takes such details into account before choosing an intervention. The following sections describe a process that will help you to select the best interventions (Wilkinson, 2011). Begin by reviewing the nursing diagnosis.

Review the Nursing Diagnosis

The etiology of a nursing diagnosis describes the factors that contribute to the unhealthy response. Choose strategies you expect will reduce or remove the etiological factors of actual problems, or that will reduce or remove risk factors for potential problems.

When it is not possible to change the etiology, choose strategies to treat the patient's symptoms (the AMB part of a diagnosis, referred to in Chapter 4). For example, if the cause of pain is a surgical incision, you cannot suddenly "cure" the incision. Your nursing actions should focus on measures to relieve the pain.

You may not always know the etiology of the problem. However, some interventions may relieve a problem regardless of its cause. For example, when a client is anxious, regardless of the cause, it is helpful to approach the patient calmly; and when a client has Constipation, regardless of the cause, it is always appropriate to assess the characteristics of the stool. Consider the nursing diagnosis and interventions for Mr. Ivanos in Figure 6-3.

Obviously, some people with constipation do not have pain. The pain-relief nursing order, which flows from the etiology of the problem, is specific to Mr. Ivanos's needs. Administering a stool softener and laxative, however, is a common strategy for constipation, whatever its cause. As a rule, standardized interventions (care common to all patients with a particular condition) flow from the problem side of a nursing diagnosis; individualized interventions, from the etiology.

 Think **Like a Nurse** 6-3

For the following nursing diagnoses, write one intervention to address the problem and one for the etiology of the problem.

- Ineffective Airway Clearance r/t thick secretions and decreased chest expansion secondary to dehydration and pain
- Self-Care Deficit: Bathing/Hygiene and Dressing/Grooming r/t fatigue secondary to disturbed sleep pattern

Review the Desired Patient Outcomes

Desired outcomes (goals) suggest nursing strategies that are specific to the individual patient. For example, Table 6-2 shows some goals and outcomes for Mr. Ivanos's Constipation

diagnosis. For each goal on the care plan, column 3 answers the question: "What intervention(s) will help to produce this patient response?" As you can see, there may be one or more interventions for each goal, and a single intervention may help to achieve more than one goal. There is no strict one-to-one correspondence between goals and interventions.

Identify Several Interventions or Actions

The next step in choosing interventions is to think of several nursing activities that might achieve the desired outcomes. Don't try to narrow your list at this point; include unusual and creative ideas. You can refer to a standardized list of interventions (e.g., the Nursing Interventions Classification [NIC] list in the **Student Resources** on Davis*Plus*) or choose interventions from standardized care plans and agency protocols. Alternatively, you can generate the interventions yourself, based on your knowledge; experience; and use of nursing texts, journal articles, practice guidelines, and professional nurses. To get started, ask yourself: For this nursing diagnosis, (1) What assessments/observations do I need to make? (2) What do I need to do for the patient? Include both dependent and independent activities as appropriate.

Choose the Best Interventions for the Patient

The best interventions are those you expect to be most effective in helping to achieve client goals. When possible, choose interventions based on research and scientific principles. Use the following critical-thinking questions from the full-spectrum nursing model (in Chapter 2) to help you determine the best actions.

Contextual Awareness

- Is this intervention acceptable to the client (e.g., congruent with the patient's values and wishes)?
- Is this intervention culturally sensitive?
- What is going on in the patient's life (e.g., family, work situation, financial status) that may enhance or interfere with the effectiveness of the intervention?
- What is going on in the patient's health status (e.g., knowledge, abilities, resources, severity of illness) that may enhance or interfere with the effectiveness of the intervention?

Credible Sources

- Have I used valid, reliable sources of information to identify this intervention (e.g., patient, other professionals, references)?
- Did I consider professional, ethical, and legal standards?
- What is the research basis for this intervention, if any?

Considering Alternatives

- Is there adequate rationale for this intervention (e.g., principles, theory, facts)?
- Which action(s) is (are) most reasonable? Why are the others not as reasonable?
- Which action(s) is (are) most likely to achieve stated goals?

Analyzing Assumptions

- What beliefs, values, or biases do I have that may affect my thinking and my choice of interventions?
- Do I feel any discomfort with this intervention?

Reflecting Skeptically

- Are there other interventions I have overlooked?
- What might be the consequences of this intervention?
  - "What will happen if . . . ?"
  - Does it have any potential ill effects? If so, how will we manage them?

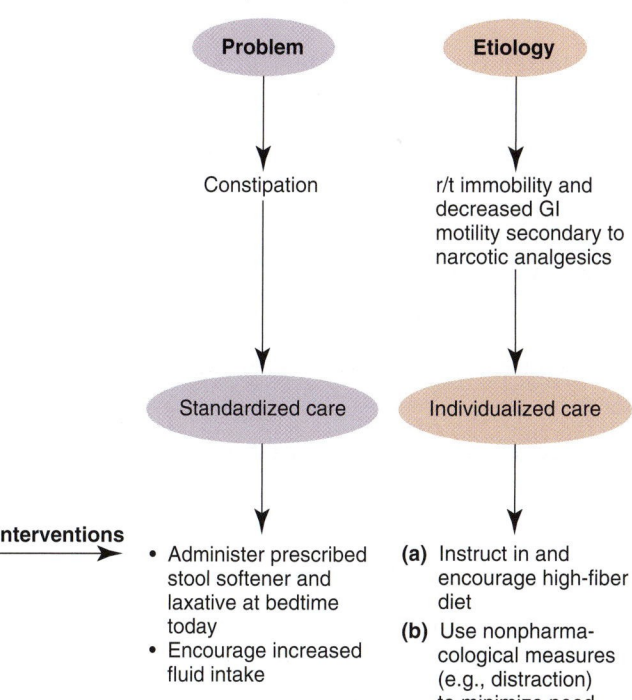

FIGURE 6-3 Nursing interventions flow from the nursing diagnosis.

Table 6-2 ➤ Interventions Flow From Desired Outcomes

GOALS/OUTCOMES	STRATEGIES SUGGESTED BY GOALS	DISCUSSION
1. **Will have bowel movement within 12 hr after receiving stool softener and laxative.**	A. **Administer prescribed stool softener and laxative at bedtime today.**	Strategy A would help to achieve goal 1; but because the effects of these medications are short lived, it would do nothing to achieve goals 2 through 4.
2. Will have daily soft, formed bowel movement during rest of hospital stay.	B. Instruct in and encourage high-fiber diet. C. Encourage increased fluid intake.	Strategies B and C both help to achieve goal 2.
3. <u>Within 24 hr, will need narcotics to manage pain <2/day.</u>	D. <u>Use nonpharmacological measures (e.g., distraction) to minimize need for narcotics.</u>	Strategy D (minimize narcotics) directly addresses goal 3 and indirectly helps to achieve goal 2.
4. *Calls nurse when urge to defecate is felt; does not delay defecation.*	E. *Encourage Mr. Ivanos to summon the nurse when he feels the urge to defecate.* F. *Provide privacy (e.g., pull the bed curtain, turn on the TV, leave room).*	Strategies E and F both directly address goal 4 and indirectly address goal 2.

Note: Dotted lines indicate indirect contribution to goal.

- Is this intervention feasible? For example, is it cost effective? Are the time and personnel available for it? Can the patient or family manage it at home?
- How will the intervention interact with medical orders? For example, you cannot order "elevate head of bed" to facilitate breathing if there is a medical order to keep the patient flat to improve circulation to the neck and head.
- In priority order, what should I do in this situation and why?
- Do I have the knowledge and skills needed for the intervention, or do I need to consult with someone more qualified in this area?
- What might I delegate in this situation?

Individualize Standardized Interventions

Practice guidelines, systematic reviews of the literature, protocols, critical pathways, and even textbooks describe interventions that are appropriate for most people or the average person. However, they cannot take into account all the individual factors that contribute to a problem or that might affect the effectiveness of an intervention. You must always consider how an intervention can be used with a particular person. For example, after Ben Ivanos's nurse decided which of the computer-generated list of interventions to use, he adapted them to fit Ben's unique needs and preferences. Table 6-3 provides examples of standardized and individualized interventions for Mr. Ivanos.

KnowledgeCheck 6-3

Describe a five-step process for generating and choosing nursing interventions.

Computer-Generated Interventions

Most computerized care planning programs will generate a list of suggested interventions when you enter either a problem (nursing diagnosis, medical, collaborative) or an outcome (Fig. 6-4). You then choose the interventions appropriate for the patient (as in the case of Ben Ivanos) or type in nursing actions of your own. Computer prompts provide a wide range of interventions for your consideration. However, you

Table 6-3 ➤ Individualizing Nursing Actions for Ben Ivanos

STANDARDIZED INTERVENTIONS	INDIVIDUALIZED NURSING ORDERS
1. Encourage increased fluid intake.	1. Remind patient to drink a glass of water every hour; also keep ice and tea available at the bedside.
2. Instruct on and encourage a high-fiber diet.	2. Assist with menu choices to obtain more fiber; encourage family to bring salads and fruits from home for snacks.
3. Encourage distraction (e.g., watching TV, reading, listening to music).	3. Provide books from hospital library (he does not enjoy TV); have family bring radio or MP3 player and headphones from home.
4. Give prescribed narcotic analgesics if other measures are ineffective.	4. Give Tylenol #3 every 4 hr if relaxation, visualization, and distraction are not effective. If orally administered Tylenol #3 is not effective, advise patient to administer IV morphine via patient-controlled analgesia pump.

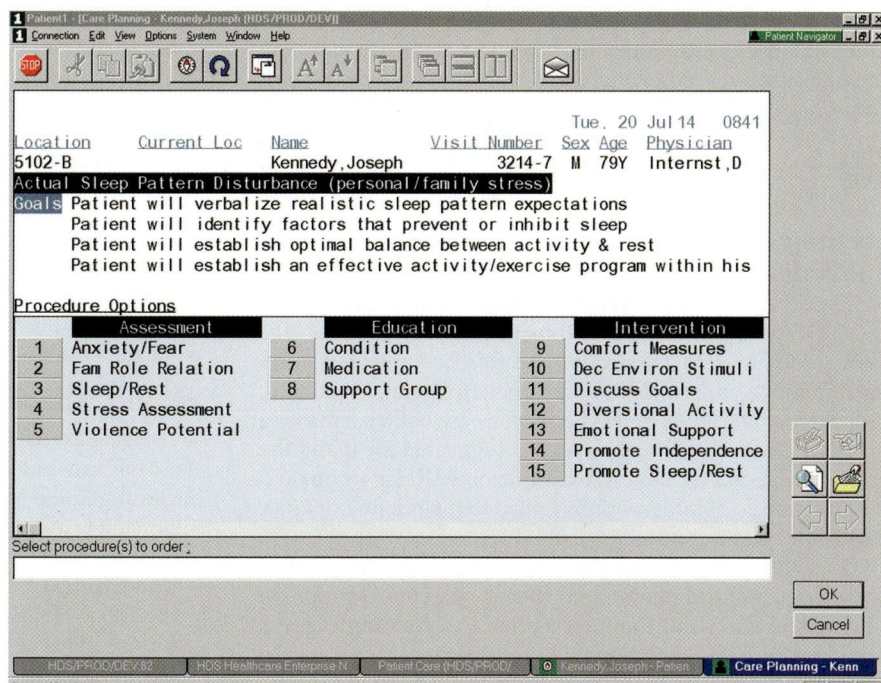

FIGURE 6-4 Computer care planning: When the nurse selects a nursing diagnosis of Sleep Pattern Disturbance, the computer database generates a list of suggested goals and "procedure options" (interventions); the nurse then chooses those best suited for the patient. (Source: Copyright © Ergo Partners, L.C. All rights reserved. Used with permission.)

must resist the temptation to settle for the ready-made solutions. Always look for other, perhaps more effective, strategies based on the patient data. Always think, "Are there other interventions I have overlooked? How should I adapt this for *this* patient?"

To see a computer screen showing how an intervention (Pain Control Techniques Education) is converted to nursing orders,

Go to Chapter 6, **Tables, Boxes, Figures: ESG Figure 6-1,** on Davis*Plus*.

HOW CAN I USE STANDARDIZED LANGUAGE TO PLAN INTERVENTIONS?

As a review before reading this section, you may wish to read the discussion of standardized language in Chapter 4 (NANDA-I for nursing diagnoses) and in Chapter 5 (NOC for patient outcomes).

Recall that standardized nursing terminologies are important for electronic health records (EHR), for research, and for clear, precise, consistent communication among nurses and with other disciplines. The American Nurses Association (ANA, 2006) has recognized 12 standardized vocabularies for recording and tracking the clinical care process. Those most commonly used for describing nursing interventions are the Nursing Interventions Classification (NIC), the Clinical Care Classification (CCC), and the Omaha System. NIC classifies only interventions. The CCC and the Omaha System also include nursing diagnoses and outcomes.

What Is the Nursing Interventions Classification?

Developed by a research team at the University of Iowa, the Nursing Interventions Classification (NIC) was the first comprehensive standardized classification of nursing interventions (McCloskey & Bulechek, 1992). The NIC (Bulechek, Butcher,

& Dochterman, 2008) describes 542 direct- and indirect-care activities performed by nurses. The NIC (pronounced "nick") is versatile—appropriate for use in all specialty and practice areas, including home health and community nursing.

Each NIC intervention consists of a label, a definition, and a list of the specific **activities** nurses perform in carrying out the intervention (Box 6-2). The **label,** usually consisting of two

---

BOX 6-2 ■ NIC Intervention: Bathing

Definition

Cleaning of the body for the purposes of relaxation, cleanliness, and healing

Activities

Assist with chair shower, tub bath, bedside bath, standing shower, or sitz bath, as appropriate or desired.

Wash hair, as needed and desired.

Bathe in water of a comfortable temperature.

Use fun bathing techniques with children (e.g., wash dolls or toys; pretend a boat is a submarine; punch holes in bottom of plastic cup, fill with water, and let it "rain" on child).

Assist with perineal care, as needed.

Assist with hygiene measures (e.g., use of deodorant or perfume).

Administer foot soaks, as needed.

Shave patient, as indicated.

Apply lubricating ointment and cream to dry skin areas.

Offer handwashing after toileting and before meals.

Apply drying powders to deep skin folds.

Monitor skin condition while bathing.

Monitor functional ability while bathing.

Source: Bulechek, B. M., Butcher, H. K., & Dochterman, J. M. (Eds.). (2008). *Nursing interventions classification (NIC)* (5th ed.). St. Louis, MO: C.V. Mosby, p. 153. Used with permission from Elsevier Science.

or three words, is the standardized terminology. The **definition** explains the meaning of the label. You are free to word the activities any way you choose in a care plan or client record. For a complete list of NIC intervention labels and definitions,

 Go to **NIC Interventions** on Davis*Plus*.

Locating Appropriate NIC Interventions and Activities

NIC interventions are linked to NANDA-I nursing diagnoses and NOC outcome labels in a "linkages" book, *NOC and NIC Linkages to NANDA-I and Clinical Conditions,* referred to by most nurses as the NNN linkages book (Johnson, Moorhead, Bulechek, et al., 2012). In this book, you can look up a nursing diagnosis to see the list of outcomes suggested for it and the interventions for achieving each outcome. Refer to Box 6-3 for an example of interventions linked to the nursing diagnosis Risk for Aspiration.

Once you have chosen the interventions (based on your knowledge and judgment), you then choose the appropriate activities to carry out the intervention. As you might guess from looking at Box 6-2, you will probably never need to perform all the activities for a client. Choose the best ones for the situation and individualize them to fit the client and the resources (e.g., supplies, equipment) available.

Using NIC in Computerized Care Plans

Standardized language is especially useful in computerized care systems. For a computer screen with suggested NIC interventions for a NANDA-I nursing diagnosis,

 Go to Chapter 6, **Tables, Boxes, Figures: ESG Figure 6-2,** on Davis*Plus*.

For any NIC intervention, the program will also list the more specific nursing activities, which you can individualize as nursing orders.

 Go to Chapter 6, **Tables, Boxes, Figures: ESG Figure 6-3,** on Davis*Plus*.

Remember that you are responsible for choosing which interventions to use for each patient, when to use them, and which activities to write as specific nursing orders. You can reject *all* of the suggested interventions if they do not fit the patient's unique needs and, in many systems, type or write in your own interventions and activities.

Standardized Languages for Home Health and Community Care

The NIC includes interventions applicable in all settings, including home health and community nursing. However, the following taxonomies were created specifically for community-based practice.

- **The Clinical Care Classification (CCC).** Previously called the *Home Healthcare Classification,* the CCC was developed for use in home healthcare (Saba, 1995, 2006). In addition to terminology for nursing diagnoses and outcomes, the CCC has 198 interventions. For a complete description of the CCC system, see the nursing process section of Chapter 41 and

 Go to the CCC Web site at http://www.sabacare.com

- **The Omaha system.** The Omaha system was developed for community health nurses to use in caring for individuals, families, and **aggregates** (community groups or entire communities) (Martin, 2005). It includes terminology for diagnoses, outcomes, and interventions. For a complete description of the Omaha system, and for NIC community interventions, see the nursing process section of Chapter 41 and

 Go to the Omaha system Web site at http://www.omahasystem.org

KnowledgeCheck 6-4

- Name and describe three standardized intervention vocabularies recognized by the ANA.
- In the NIC system, what is the difference between interventions and activities?

Does Standardized Language Interfere With Holistic Care?

Some nurses have criticized standardized terminologies for focusing on illness and physical interventions. However, NIC, Omaha, and CCC do include interventions to address health promotion and cultural and spiritual needs. If you have a holistic attitude, you will give holistic care. Using a common language should help rather than hinder your choice of interventions. For further discussion of holistic nursing care,

 Go to **Chapter 46, Holistic Healing,** on Davis*Plus*.

The following sections discuss interventions focused on wellness, spiritual needs, and culturally sensitive care.

Wellness Interventions. When you are caring for a healthy client, the client is the primary decision maker. You will function mainly as a teacher and health counselor. Frequently,

---

BOX 6-3 ■ NIC Interventions Linked to NANDA-I Diagnosis, Risk for Aspiration

Aspiration, Risk for

At risk for entry of gastrointestinal secretions, oropharyngeal secretions, solids or fluids, into tracheobronchial passages.

NICs Associated With Prevention of Aspiration

Airway Management	Medication Administration: Oral
Airway Suctioning	Neurological Monitoring
Artificial Airway Management	Positioning
Aspiration Precautions	Postanesthesia Care
Chest Physiotherapy	Respiratory Monitoring
Cough Enhancement	Resuscitation: Neonate
Dementia Management	Risk Identification
Enteral Tube Feeding	Sedation Management
Gastrointestinal Intubation	Self-Care Assistance
	Surveillance
Mechanical Ventilation Management: Invasive	Swallowing Therapy
	Tube Care: Gastrointestinal
Medication Administration: Enteral	Vomiting Management

Source: Johnson, M., Moorhead, S., Bulechek, G., et al. (2012). *NOC and NIC linkages to NANDA-I and clinical conditions* (3rd ed.). St. Louis, MO: C.V. Mosby, p. 250. Used with permission from Elsevier Science.

the nursing orders outline lifestyle modification or behavior changes the client wants to make, along with self-rewards to reinforce the behaviors. For example:

Specific behavior change: I will consume less than 1,400 calories per day for the next week.

Self-reward: I will reward myself with an evening out to hear my favorite band.

The NIC contains most of the wellness interventions you will need. However, they are not all grouped together in one class. Some examples are Decision-Making Support, Exercise Promotion, and Health Screening. For more information on using standardized languages to describe wellness interventions, see Chapter 27.

Spiritual Care Interventions. NIC, CCC, and the Omaha system all include terminology to describe spiritual interventions. The following are just a few examples:

NIC: Spiritual Growth Facilitation, Religious Ritual Enhancement
CCC: Spiritual Care, Coping Skills
Omaha: Spiritual Support, Bereavement Support

Chapter 16 provides full discussion of standardized nursing interventions to address spiritual needs. As you will see, you could also use most of those interventions (e.g., Coping Skills) for other than spiritual problems.

Culturally Sensitive Care. Except for the NIC Culture Brokerage intervention, there are no standardized interventions that are unique to culturally based needs. All standardized interventions will result in culturally sensitive care if they are delivered by a culturally competent nurse.

PracticalKnowledge
knowing **how**

WHAT ARE NURSING ORDERS, AND HOW DO I WRITE THEM?

Nursing orders are instructions that describe how and when nursing interventions are to be implemented. They are usually written on a nursing care plan. Other nurses and nursing assistive personnel (NAP) are responsible and accountable for implementing nursing orders.

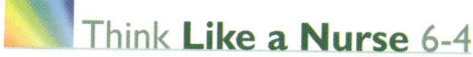
Think **Like a Nurse** 6-4

Suppose you are caring for a patient 24 hours after a major surgery. You see the following order on the nursing care plan: Ambulate 24 hours postoperatively.

- When you care for the patient, how will you go about implementing this nursing order?
- What else do you need to know to effectively carry out this order?

Components of a Nursing Order

Did you have trouble answering the preceding questions? Even experienced nurses would, because this nursing order is incomplete. As you see from this example, nursing orders must be specific and detailed because many caregivers will use the care plan, and they all need to be able to interpret the orders correctly. A well-written nursing order, whether on paper or an electronic care plan, contains the following components:

Date. Indicate the date the order was written. Change the date each time you review or revise the order. Why do you think it is important to have the date?

Complementary & Alternative Modalities (CAM)

Because nursing is a holistic discipline, many nurses are enthusiastic about the techniques and modalities of complementary and alternative care. They believe interventions, such as acupressure, aromatherapy, biofeedback, guided imagery, humor, journaling, music therapy, meditation and relaxation, and therapeutic touch, help them to address the physical, mental, emotional, and spiritual dimensions of care.

Nursing theories and conceptual models of practice (see Chapter 8) and the current standardized language taxonomies support the use of CAM by nurses.
- CAM performed from within a context of a nursing theory takes on meaning as the interventions become part of the purposeful action to achieve goals of care that evolve from the theory.
- CAM performed and documented according to one of the standard taxonomies makes clear that the techniques are appropriate as nursing interventions.

Source: Frisch, N. C. (2001, May 31). Nursing as a context for alternative/complementary modalities. *Online Journal of Issues in Nursing, 6*(2), Manuscript 2, p. 2. http://www.nursingworld.org/MainMenuCategories/ANAMarketplace/ANAPeriodicals/OJIN/TableofContents/Volume62001/No2May01/AlternativeComplementaryModalities.aspx

Subject. Nursing orders are instructions to nurses, so they are written in terms of *nurse* behaviors. Therefore, the subject of the order is "the nurse." Because anyone reading the care plan should understand this, you do not actually need to write "the nurse" in your orders. For each order, think, but do not write, "The nurse will . . ." or "The nurse should. . . ." This will help you to state the order properly so that it doesn't sound like a goal statement. Goals state patient behaviors; nursing orders state nurse behaviors. For example:

Goal/expected Outcome — *Nursing Order*
[Patient] Drinks 100 mL — [Nurse will] Offer 100 mL fluids (water or juice) per hour on the day shift

Action Verb. This tells the nurse what action to take—what to do. Examples of action verbs are *assist, assess, auscultate, bathe, change, demonstrate, explain, give, teach,* and *turn.* The following nursing orders show the action verbs in italics:

Teach the components of a healthy diet, 9/13, day shift.
Offer 100 mL water every hour.
Administer acetaminophen 500 mg orally at least 30 min before dressing change.

Times and Limits. State when (e.g., which shift, what day), how often, and how long the activity is to be done. Consider the unit routines (e.g., visiting hours, mealtimes), the patient's usual rest times, scheduled tests and procedures (e.g., x-ray studies), and treatments (e.g., physical therapy). The following nursing orders show times and limits:

Teach the components of a healthy diet *on 9/13, day shift.*
Offer 100 mL water *every hour between 0700 and 1900.*
Administer acetaminophen 500 mg orally *at least 30 min before dressing change.*

If you omit specific times, such as saying only "day shift," the order may not be followed. It is easy for a nurse to think, "Perhaps someone else will do it (or has done it)."

Signature. The nurse writing the order should sign it. A signature indicates that you accept legal and ethical accountability for your orders and allows others to know whom to contact if they have questions or comments about the order. If interventions are chosen on an electronic care plan, there may not be an actual signature. However, the name of the nurse who chose the intervention should be indicated in some manner.

KnowledgeCheck 6-5

List the five components of a nursing order.

Reflecting Critically About Nursing Orders

After writing the nursing orders, reflect on the interventions you have chosen. If you followed the process in the section What Process Can I Use for Generating and Selecting Interventions? you will already have thought critically and made some considered decisions as you were choosing the interventions and activities. The following are questions to guide your final judgments about the plan of care:

1. *Is the set of orders complete?* That is, do they address all aspects of the problem?
   - Do they address the etiology of the problem?
   - If the etiology cannot be changed, do the orders focus on the symptoms of the problem?

   - Have I considered physical, emotional, interpersonal, spiritual, and cultural needs?
2. *Is each order technically complete?* That is, does it contain all the required components?
3. *Are the orders clear, specific, and precise?* If you have included all the required components, the orders will usually provide specific enough directions (when, how often, etc.) to be useful to other nurses. However, you must avoid vague language. For example, an order to "Offer emotional support" is too general to offer direction for care. One nurse might think this means to ask the client about his family, another might sit quietly with the patient, and still another might use a therapeutic statement such as, "This must be difficult for you." Ask yourself, "Would all nurses interpret this order in the same way? Would they all do the same thing after reading it?"
4. *Is the order individualized for this particular patient?* For example, even if you have written an order to "Offer 100 mL fluids every hr," it is even better if you make a note of the kinds of fluids the patient likes or can tolerate.
5. *Are the orders concise?* Long, complex statements may be unclear. Keep the orders as brief as possible without sacrificing clarity and specificity. If the patient requires complex procedures (e.g., insertion of a urinary catheter), don't write the details of the procedure on the care plan. Simply refer to the source of instructions for the

---

Toward Evidence-Based Practice

Orr, P. M., McGinnis, M. A., Hudson, L. R., et al. (2006). A focused telephonic nursing intervention delivers improved adherence to A1c testing. *Disease Management, 9*(5), 277–283.

This 6-month study investigated whether a focused telephone intervention would improve patient adherence to hemoglobin A1c testing (a test of diabetes control). Subjects were already enrolled in a diabetes disease management program and were receiving various types of phone calls and educational materials. During the study, when a routine call was made to a member of the program, the clinician determined whether the A1c had been tested in the past 6 months. If not, a specific goal was created with the member during the conversation (e.g., "I will make an appointment to follow up on my A1c test"); a copy was mailed to the member. Phone calls were repeated every 2 weeks to check on the person's progress in meeting the goal. Patient records were examined for evidence that an A1c test had been done. At the end of the 6 months, quantitative analysis of data was done. The number of group members who received an A1c test increased significantly, by 12%. Gender did not affect adherence to A1c testing, but age did. The greatest improvement was observed in the 0- to 19-year age group (14.9%), those ages 50 to 59 (12.7%), and those ages 60 to 69 years (13.4%). All other age categories showed increases ranging from 8.1% to 10.6%. Increases in the number of phone calls made to a member were associated with subsequent increases in A1c testing adherence.

Duhamel, F., Dupuis, F., Reidy, M., et al. (2007). A qualitative evaluation of a family nursing intervention. *Clinical Nurse Specialist, 21*(1), 43–49.

In this qualitative study, a clinical nurse specialist met with each of four couples for four 60-minute therapeutic meetings. Meetings were also audiotaped. The patients were retired men with congestive heart failure (CHF), whose wives were their caregivers. Researchers used semistructured interviews before and after the intervention and analyzed them qualitatively. Results showed that both spouses were experiencing a high level of suffering, which was relieved through a family nursing meeting that allowed them to obtain a better understanding of each other's experience.

1. How are these two studies similar? (If you need to do so, read about research in Chapter 8.)

2. Now think about the interventions tested in the two studies. What are their differences?

3. Using these two studies, write two nursing orders for a client who will be discharged tomorrow after being hospitalized for the fourth time for CHF. He will be cared for at home by his wife. (Assume that whatever services you recommend will be available and affordable.)

 Go to Chapter 6, **Toward Evidence-Based Practice—Suggested Responses**, on Davis*Plus*.

procedure: perhaps an agency procedure manual, or a list of instructions to be found at the bedside. You will, however, need to write in the care plan any modifications to a procedure (e.g., "Do not use alcohol; client's skin is very dry").

6. *Which orders have priority?* Which nursing orders must be implemented immediately? Which must be done on this shift? Which must be done today? If possible, write them in priority order. In Chapter 4 you learned about frameworks for prioritizing nursing diagnoses (e.g., Maslow's hierarchy, problem urgency, future consequences, and patient preference). You can use these same frameworks to help you prioritize nursing orders.

If you have followed the recommended processes and reflected critically on your interventions, you should have a holistic plan of care individualized to meet the client's needs.

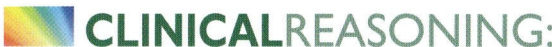

CLINICALREASONING:
Applying the **Full-Spectrum Nursing Model**

Because the following critical thinking activities allow you to practice the kind of thinking you will use as a full-spectrum nurse, they usually have no single right answer. Discuss them with your peers—if you have difficulty with any of the questions, consult your instructor.

PATIENT SITUATION

Mr. Sanborn is a 65-year-old man who has come to the clinic for a complete physical checkup. He has no health complaints and his physical examination is negative except for a few minor changes associated with aging. During the interview, he tells you that he is gay, and that he has had the same partner for 5 years. On further questioning, he reveals that he has had numerous sex partners during his lifetime. He says, "I was wondering if I should be tested for HIV" and "Mike, that's my partner, says I ought to get a flu shot and maybe a hepatitis shot. What do you think?"

THINKING

1. *Theoretical Knowledge:* What principles and concepts do you need to know in order to help Mr. Sanborn today?
2. *Inquiry:* Which of those do you already know enough about, and which ones will you have to study further?

DOING

3. *Practical Knowledge:* What psychomotor and communication skills will you need in order to help Mr. Sanborn?
4. *Nursing Process (Assessment):* What further data do you need about Mr. Sanborn's sexual activity?
5. *Nursing Process (Planning Interventions):* What is one important nursing intervention for today?

CARING

6. *Self-Knowledge:* How do you feel about same-sex relationships? Would you be able to care for Mr. Sanborn effectively?
7. *Ethical Knowledge:* What does the ANA *Nursing Code of Ethics* say about relationships to patients and the nature of patient health problems? To see the *Nursing Code of Ethics,*

 Go to http://www.nursingworld.org/MainMenuCategories/EthicsStandards/CodeofEthicsforNurses/Code-of-Ethics.aspx

 Go To Chapter 6, **Clinical Reasoning: Applying the Full-Spectrum Nursing Model Response Sheet** on *DavisPlus.*

To explore learning resources for this chapter,

Go to Davis*Plus* **at** http://www.Davisplus.fadavis.com, **keyword Treas.**

Chapter Resources for Chapter 6:

    Knowledge Check and Think Like a Nurse Response Sheets

    Knowledge Check Answers

    Resources for Caregivers and Health Professionals

    Reading More About Planning Interventions (Suggested Readings)

    What Are the Main Points in This Chapter?

NCLEX-Style Review Questions

Chapter Overview Podcasts

Concept Map

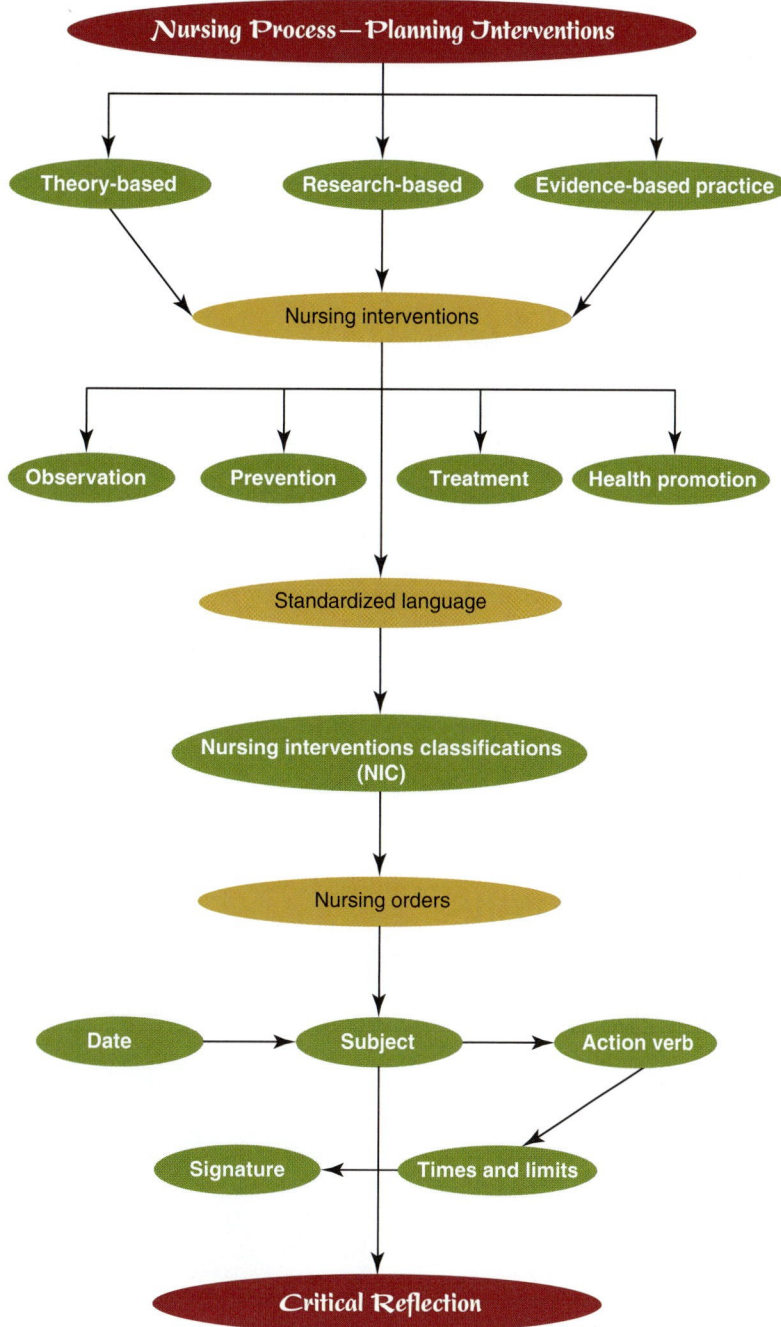

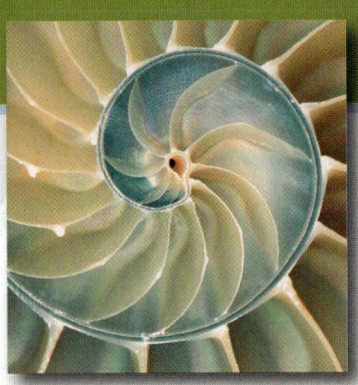

CHAPTER 7

Implementation & Evaluation

Learning Outcomes

After completing this chapter, you should be able to:

➤ Define *implementation*.

➤ State the three broad phases of the implementation process (doing, delegating, recording).

➤ Describe what nurses do in the implementation phase of the nursing process.

➤ Define the terms *delegation* and *supervision*.

➤ Identify and describe the "five rights" of delegation.

➤ Explain how standards and criteria are used in evaluation.

➤ Explain how structure, process, and outcomes evaluation are related.

➤ Distinguish among ongoing, intermittent, and terminal evaluation.

➤ Describe a process for evaluating client health status (outcomes) after interventions.

➤ Describe a process for evaluating the effectiveness of a nursing care plan.

➤ List variables that may influence the effectiveness of a nursing intervention; state which ones the nurse can and cannot control.

➤ Discuss the importance of nurses' involvement in evaluating the quality of care in an organization.

Key Concepts

Evaluation

Implementation

Quality improvement

Related Concepts

See the Concept Map at the end of this chapter.

Caring for the Nguyens

This feature allows you to practice the kind of thinking you will use as a full-spectrum nurse. There is usually more than one correct answer to a critical thinking question, so we do not provide answers for these features. It is more important to develop your nursing judgment than to "cover content." Discuss the questions with your peers. If you are still unsure, consult your instructor.

The following information is recorded on Mr. Nguyen's clinic health record:

9/1/14 Imbalanced Nutrition: More Than Body Requirements related to inappropriate food choices and serving size, as evidenced by BMI of 28.5

Outcome: Will lose 5 lb by 10/15/2014

Interventions:

■ Collect 3-day nutrition history 9/2/2014 through 9/4/2014.

■ Have patient meet with clinic nurse for diet review and nutrition instruction 9/8/2014.

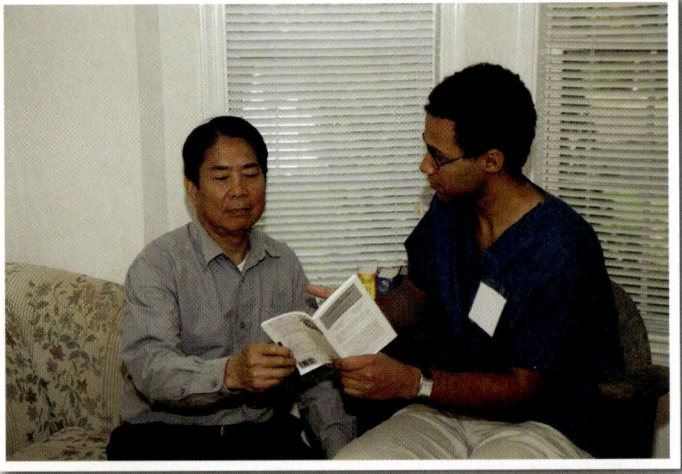

■ Provide sample meal plans at 9/8/2014 instruction.
■ Phone patient 9/22/2014 to discuss nutrition questions and review progress.
■ Have patient return to clinic 10/15/2014 for follow-up visit.

Caring for the Nguyens (continued)

A. What must you do before implementing each nursing intervention?

B. Identify at least two strategies that will help promote Mr. Nguyen's participation in and adherence to the plan.

C. How will you determine whether Mr. Nguyen has met his goal?

 Go to **Caring for the Nguyens Response Sheet** on Davis*Plus*.

Meet Your Patients

Patient 1

Jeannette Wu is a very thin 80-year-old woman who is in the hospital after fracturing her hip. Her hip was surgically repaired 4 days ago, but because of her overall fragile health and some postsurgery confusion, her recovery is slower than usual. One of her nursing diagnoses is Self-Care Deficit (Bathing, Dressing, and Toileting) related to weakness, pain, confusion, and decreased mobility. Her nursing orders (NIC) include Bathing and Self-Care: Activities of Daily Living (ADLs). As the nurse is helping a newly hired nursing assistive personnel (NAP) with Mrs. Wu's bath, she notices a reddened area on Mrs. Wu's sacrum. Realizing that this may be the beginning of a pressure ulcer, the nurse observes carefully and notes a small skin excoriation (abrasion) in the area. She repositions Mrs. Wu to prevent further pressure on her sacrum. After finishing the bath, the nurse records her findings and enters on Mrs. Wu's care plan a nursing diagnosis of Impaired Skin Integrity related to impaired bed mobility and minimal subcutaneous tissue. She writes appropriate nursing orders, including an order to observe skin over bony prominences every 4 hours, and then delegates to the NAP the task of turning and repositioning Mrs. Wu every 2 hours. The nurse also sends a consultation request to a wound care nurse specialist.

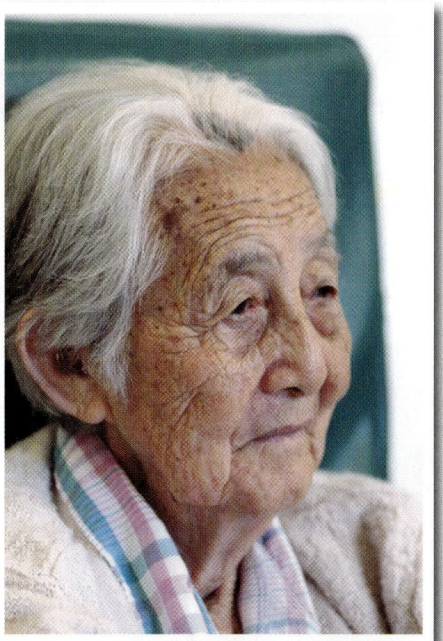

Patient 2

Patsy Jimenez is a healthy 25-year-old woman with no medical problems. She eats a balanced diet but says she does not exercise much. She and the nurse have created a plan to help her increase her physical activity. Ms. Jimenez will try to walk for 30 minutes at least 5 days a week. Each week she is successful, she plans to reward herself with a movie or a milkshake, which she usually avoids because of the fat content. The nurse would prefer that Ms. Jimenez not reward herself with food, but respects the patient's decision and realizes that if it is to serve as motivation, the reward must be something that Ms. Jimenez values.

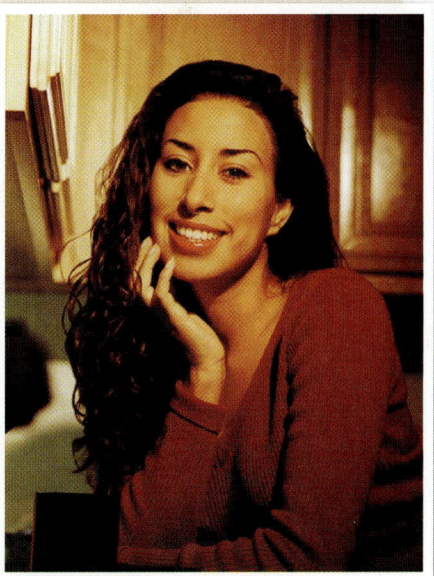

ThinkLike a Nurse 7-1

- For Jeannette Wu, which parts of the scenario illustrate *doing* by the nurse?
- For Jeannette Wu, which parts of the scenario illustrate *thinking* by the nurse?
- For Patsy Jimenez, who will be implementing (carrying out) the plan of care?

ABOUT THE KEY CONCEPTS

As you study this chapter, keep the concepts of implementation, evaluation, and quality improvement in mind. Everything in the chapter will relate to those concepts in some way, and you will also understand how they are related to each other and to your role as a nurse.

IMPLEMENTATION: THE ACTION PHASE OF THE NURSING PROCESS

Implementation involves action. Of course, it involves thinking, but the emphasis is on doing. During **implementation,** you will perform or delegate planned interventions—that is, carry out the care plan. The implementation phase ends when you document the nursing actions; it evolves into evaluation as you document the resulting client responses (Fig. 7-1). In short, implementation is doing, delegating, and documenting. For professional standards relating to implementation, see Box 7-1.

As in all phases of the nursing process, think of the client as a collaborative partner. Encourage the client and family to participate as much as possible in the client's care. When Mrs. Wu is less confused and better able to move about, for example, the nurse will encourage her to help with her own bath. Be aware that clients vary in their ability and desire to participate.

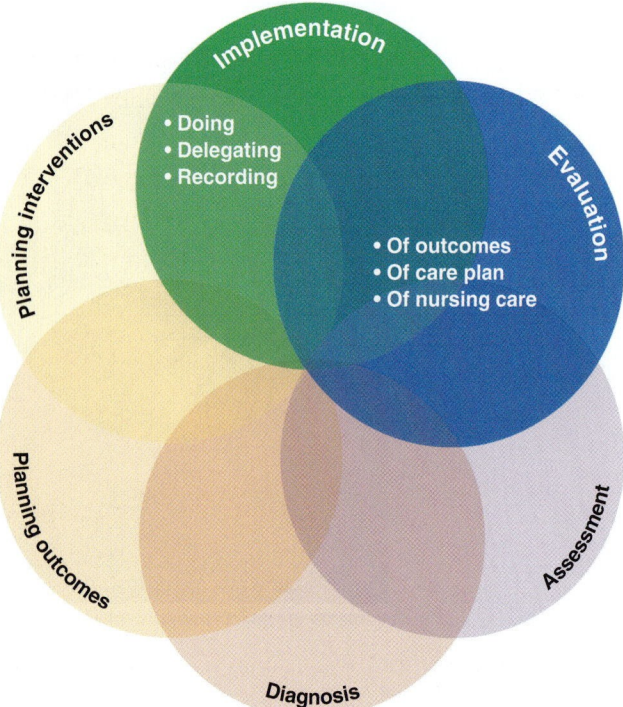

FIGURE 7-1 Nursing process phase: Implementation and evaluation.

In the opening scenarios, Mrs. Wu was able to participate very little, but Patsy Jimenez participated fully.

How Is Implementation Related to Other Steps of the Nursing Process?

Nursing process phases are interdependent (see Fig. 7-1). Without the assessment, diagnosis, and planning steps, implementation would reflect only dependent functions, such as carrying out policies, protocols, and medical prescriptions. The autonomous nursing activities performed during implementation are built on the nurse's reasoning in the previous three steps. Implementation overlaps in some way with every other phase of the nursing process.

Implementation Overlaps with Assessment. Nurses use assessment data to individualize interventions for a specific person rather than just giving "routine care." For example, when implementing a nursing order by taking tea to a patient, you may discover that she prefers it without ice. This information allows you to individualize the nursing order further. Implementation also provides the opportunity to assess your patients at every contact. In Meet Your Patients, what data did the nurse obtain while bathing Mrs. Wu? When performing an ordered ongoing assessment, you are both implementing and assessing. What ongoing assessment was ordered for Mrs. Wu?

Implementation Overlaps with Diagnosis. Nurses use data discovered during implementation to identify new diagnoses or to revise existing ones. What new nursing diagnosis did the nurse make for Mrs. Wu after bathing her?

Implementation Overlaps with Planning Outcomes and Interventions. As you care for a client, you begin to know her better, and her unique needs become more apparent.

Implementation Overlaps with Evaluation. When evaluating patient health status and progress toward goals, you will compare the responses you observe during implementation to the existing goals (which were written in the planning outcomes phase).

Preparing for Implementation

Implementation involves some preparation. Although the care plan will already have been developed in the planning stages of the nursing process, you should do some more planning just before implementing the plan—as explained in the following sections. Notice how important critical thinking and nursing knowledge are to this "doing" phase of the nursing process.

Check Your Knowledge and Abilities

Before beginning a nursing activity, review the care plan and reflect critically on the nursing and medical prescriptions. As a nurse, you are obligated ethically and legally to clarify or question orders that you believe to be unclear, incorrect, or inappropriate. At the same time, you must decide whether you are qualified to carry out the orders. You should ask for help when:

- You do not have the knowledge or skill needed to implement an order (e.g., when administering an unfamiliar medication).
- You cannot perform the activity safely alone (e.g., helping a heavy, weak patient to ambulate).
- Performing the activity alone would cause undue stress for the patient (e.g., giving back care to a patient with multiple fractures).

For a decision tree to help you check whether you are ready to implement care,

Go to Chapter 7, **Resources for Caregivers and Health Professionals,** and follow the link for **Decision Tree,** on Davis*Plus.*

BOX 7-1 ■ ANA Standards of Practice for Implementation

Standard 5. Implementation

The registered nurse implements the identified plan.

Competencies

The registered nurse:
- Partners with the person, family, significant others, and caregivers to implement the plan in a safe, realistic, and timely manner.
- Demonstrates caring behaviors towards healthcare consumers, significant others, and groups of people receiving care.
- Utilizes technology to measure, record, and retrieve healthcare consumer data; implement the nursing process; and enhance nursing practice.
- Utilizes evidence-based interventions and treatments specific to the diagnosis or problem.
- Provides holistic care that addresses the needs of diverse populations across the life span.
- Advocates for health care that is sensitive to the needs of healthcare consumers, with particular emphasis on the needs of diverse populations.
- Applies appropriate knowledge of major health problems and cultural diversity in implementing the plan of care.
- Applies available healthcare technologies to maximize access and optimize outcomes for healthcare consumers.
- Utilizes community resources and systems to implement the plan.
- Collaborates with healthcare providers from diverse backgrounds to implement and integrate the plan.
- Accommodates for different styles of communication used by healthcare consumers, families, and healthcare providers.
- Integrates traditional and complementary healthcare practices as appropriate.
- Implements the plan in a timely manner in accordance with patient safety goals.
- Promotes the healthcare consumer's capacity for the optimal level of participation and problem solving.
- Documents implementation and any modifications, including changes or omissions, of the identified plan.

Standard 5A: Coordination of Care

The registered nurse coordinates care delivery.

Competencies

The registered nurse:
- Organizes the components of the plan.
- Manages a healthcare consumer's care in order to maximize independence and quality of life.

- Assists the healthcare consumer in identifying options for alternative care.
- Communicates with the healthcare consumer, family, and system during transitions in care.
- Advocates for the delivery of dignified and humane care by the interprofessional team.
- Documents the coordination of the care.

Standard 5B: Health Teaching and Health Promotion

The registered nurse employs strategies to promote health and a safe environment.

Competencies

The registered nurse:
- Provides health teaching that addresses such topics as healthy lifestyles, risk-reducing behaviors, developmental needs, activities of daily living, and preventive self-care.
- Uses health promotion and health teaching methods appropriate to the situation and the healthcare consumer's values, beliefs, health practices, developmental level, learning needs, readiness and ability to learn, language preference, spirituality, culture, and socioeconomic status.
- Seeks opportunities for feedback and evaluation of the effectiveness of the strategies used.
- Uses information technologies to communicate health promotion and disease prevention information to the healthcare consumer in a variety of settings.
- Provides healthcare consumers with information about intended effects and potential adverse effects of proposed therapies.

Standard 15. Resource Utilization

The registered nurse utilizes appropriate resources to plan and provide nursing services that are safe, effective, and financially responsible.

Competencies

The registered nurse:
- Delegates elements of care to appropriate healthcare workers in accordance with any applicable legal or policy parameters or principles.
- Modifies practice when necessary to promote positive interaction between healthcare consumers, care providers, and technology.
- Assists the healthcare consumer and family in identifying and securing appropriate services to address needs across the healthcare continuum.

Source: American Nurses Association. (2010). *Nursing: Scope and standards of practice* (2nd ed.). Silver Spring, MD: ANA.

Organize Your Work

Because you will be providing care for more than one patient on each shift, you will need to make a time-sequenced work plan, or worksheet, to prioritize your patient care for the day. Because of the need to control healthcare costs, you must work efficiently. To make the most of every patient contact, think ahead about which interventions you can perform at the same time. Mrs. Wu's nurse performed a skin assessment while she was giving a bed bath. As another example, you might conduct patient teaching while assisting with breathing exercises. Many institutions have forms for this type of scheduling,

or you may need to write your own list of "things to do" in the order you need to do them. For a worksheet you can print and use in clinical,

 Go to Chapter 7, Tables, Boxes, Figures: **ESG Figure 7-1, Worksheet for Organizing Nursing Care,** on DavisPlus.

At first, you may also need to make a time-sequenced list, the size of a 3 × 5 card, to help you organize your day. For example, it might read in part:

0700—Assessments, all patients, begin with Room 310
0730—Ambulation: 315, 318

0800—Change IV, meds 310; check intake
0815—Meds 315, 318, 319; check intake
0845—Toilet and bath, 310

Room numbers take up less space than names on the form, but do not fall into the habit of thinking of your patients by room number or diagnosis. They are people, with names.

Establish Feedback Points

You cannot assume you will be able to carry out a nursing order in exactly the way it was written. For example, suppose the nursing order states, "Help to ambulate in the hall bid." When you help the patient to stand, he becomes pale, dizzy, diaphoretic, and short of breath. Would you still carry out the order? Of course not. You must always be ready to alter the activity on the spot as the patient's responses demand. This means that you must look for **feedback** (how the patient is responding to the activity) as you perform care. In a sense, this is evaluating. However, because it is done before the intervention is complete, we call it *feedback*.

When organizing your work, identify points in each intervention where you want to pause for feedback. For example, if you are assisting with range-of-motion exercises, you might plan to assess for pain during movement of each joint and to assess for activity intolerance after exercising both arms and again after exercising the legs. Feedback is not always verbal; it could be a change in vital signs, skin color, or level of consciousness.

Prepare Supplies and Equipment

Gather all the supplies and equipment you need before you go to the patient's room. This allows you to work efficiently by eliminating the need to go to the supply room for items you have overlooked. Also, it prevents the stress to your patient that occurs when you interrupt a procedure to go get a needed item.

Prepare the Patient

Before performing a nursing activity, identify the patient and reassess him to make sure the activity is still necessary and the patient is physically and psychologically ready for the intervention.

Check Your Assumptions. This is just good critical thinking. Don't assume that an intervention is still needed simply because it is written on the care plan. For example, on postoperative day 6 after Jeannette Wu's surgery, the nursing assistant is preparing to give her a bed bath, as instructed on the care plan (Table 7-1, entry for December 18). However, Mrs. Wu has regained some of her strength and is able to sit in a chair. So the nurse and the assistant agree that, with help, Mrs. Wu can bathe at the sink instead of requiring a complete bed bath.

Assess the Patient's Readiness. To obtain the most benefit from an intervention, a client must be physically and psychologically ready. The hospital's critical pathway for hip fractures recommended a "help bath" on postoperative day 3 for Mrs. Wu. However, her age and physical condition indicated that she needed a complete bed bath on day 3. The nurse did not assume Mrs. Wu was ready to progress just because the critical pathway dictated it. As another example of ensuring readiness: Because her patient was anxious about his test results, a nurse postponed a teaching session until he was feeling calmer.

Explain What You Will Do and What the Patient Will Feel. Clients are not merely passive recipients of your care. Many interventions require their participation or cooperation. Caring nurses take time to explain because it helps to motivate the person and gives him the information he needs to participate. Knowing what to expect helps to relieve anxiety, enables

the person to cope with unpleasant or painful sensations, and promotes a trusting relationship.

Provide Privacy. This helps to assure psychological readiness and respects the patient's dignity.

KnowledgeCheck 7-1

- Why is it important to organize your work before implementing care?
- In addition to organizing your work, what other preparations should you make before implementing care?

ThinkLike a Nurse 7-2

Suppose your patient, Jeannette Wu, has become incontinent of bowel and bladder. Because she already has Impaired Skin Integrity, the physician writes a new order to insert an indwelling urinary catheter (a drainage tube inserted through her urinary meatus into her bladder). Urinary catheterization is a sterile technique. You have practiced this procedure in the skills lab, but you have never actually performed it on a patient.

- As a student, what should you do?
- If you were a licensed nurse, what are some things you could do to ensure that both you and the patient are prepared for the procedure?

Implementing the Plan: Doing or Delegating

After both you and the patient are prepared, it is time to act. Nursing actions include both those you do yourself and those you delegate to others; they may be collaborative, independent, or dependent (see Chapter 6 if you do not recall the meaning of these terms). During implementation, you will coordinate and carry out both the nursing orders on the nursing care plan and the medical orders that relate to the patient's medical treatment.

What Knowledge and Skills Do I Need?

There is almost no limit to the number and kinds of nursing interventions you might perform. The *Nursing Interventions Classification* (Bulechek, Butcher, & Dochterman, 2008), for example, lists 542 broad interventions (e.g., Hypothermia Treatment), each of which includes approximately 15 to 20 specific activities. For example, one activity for Hypothermia Treatment is to "remove cold, wet clothing and replace with warm, dry clothing" (p. 418). During implementation, then, you can expect to use all the types of knowledge presented in Chapter 2: theoretical, practical, personal, and ethical knowledge, as well as knowledge about the patient situation.

You will also use various combinations of cognitive, psychomotor, and interpersonal skills to perform nursing activities (thinking, doing, caring). For example, when you are inserting an IV catheter, you need cognitive knowledge of sterile procedure, interpersonal skills to reassure the patient, and psychomotor skills to apply the tourniquet and insert the IV catheter.

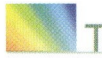
ThinkLike a Nurse 7-3

Use the examples provided in the preceding paragraph to help you write a definition for each of the following terms:

- Cognitive skills
- Psychomotor skills
- Interpersonal skills

Table 7-1 ➤ Portions of the Care Plan for Jeannette Wu

Date: 12/16/14 Care Plan Before Implementation on Post-Op Day 4

NURSING DIAGNOSIS	DESIRED OUTCOMES	NURSING ORDERS	EVALUATION
12/16/14 Self-Care Deficit (Bathing/ Hygiene, Dressing/Grooming, and Toileting) related to weakness, pain, confusion, and decreased mobility	By post-op day 6 (12/18/14) will assist with bath and oral hygiene.	■ Complete bed bath daily in a.m. ■ Give prescribed analgesic ½ hr before bath. ■ Assist with range-of-motion exercises.	

Date: 12/16/14 Care Plan After Implementation on Post-Op Day 4

NURSING DIAGNOSIS	DESIRED OUTCOMES	NURSING ORDERS	EVALUATION
12/16/14 Self-Care Deficit (Bathing/ Hygiene, Dressing/Grooming, and Toileting) related to weakness, pain, confusion, and decreased mobility	By post-op day 6 (12/18/14) will assist with bath and oral hygiene.	■ Complete bed bath daily in a.m. (NAP). ■ Give Tylenol #3, tabs i by mouth, ½ hr before bath. ■ Assist with range-of-motion exercises tid (RN).	12/16/14 Too soon to evaluate.
12/16/14 Impaired skin integrity (sacrum) r/t pressure 2° immobility.	*By 12/23/14, skin healed over sacrum; skin intact and normal color over all bony prominences.*	■ *Turn and reposition q2hr; do not place supine (NAP).* ■ *Observe skin over bony prominences q4hr (RN).*	

Date: 12/18/14 Care Plan After Implementation on Post-Op Day 6

NURSING DIAGNOSIS	DESIRED OUTCOMES	NURSING ORDERS	EVALUATION
12/16/14 Self-Care Deficit (Bathing/ Hygiene, Dressing/Grooming, and Toileting) related to weakness, pain, confusion, and decreased mobility	By post-op day 6 (12/18/14) will assist with bath and oral hygiene.	■ Complete bedbath daily in A.M. ■ *12/18/14 NAP help with bath at sink daily in a.m. Patient can wash hands and face and perform oral hygiene.* ■ Give prescribed analgesic ½ hr before bath. ■ Assist with range-of-motion exercises tid (RN).	*12/18/14 Goal met. Sat in chair for help bath. Performed oral hygiene and washed hands and face.*
12/16/14 Impaired skin integrity (sacrum) r/t pressure 2° immobility.	By 12/23/14, skin healed over sacrum; skin intact and normal color over all bony prominences.	■ Turn and reposition q2hr; do not place supine (NAP). ■ Observe skin over bony prominences q4hr (RN). ■ *12/18/14 Requested foam and fatty mattress pad.* ■ *12/18/14 Refer to nutritionist for evaluation.*	*12/18/14 Skin excoriation over sacrum is larger: now 2 cm × 2 cm, and about ½ cm deep.*

How Can I Promote Client Participation and Adherence?

Different interventions require differing levels of participation. However, even a nurse-initiated intervention, such as inserting a urinary catheter, goes more smoothly if the patient participates at least to the extent of holding still while you perform the procedure. Many interventions (e.g., instituting a low-calorie diet) depend almost entirely on the patient's adhering to the therapy. In the case of Ms. Jimenez, implementation of the intervention (walking for 30 minutes five times a week) depends entirely on the client.

People fail to follow therapeutic regimens for various reasons: lack of understanding, cultural objections, lifestyle difficulties (e.g., no time to exercise), fear of failure, embarrassment, or hesitation to ask questions of a "busy" nurse or physician. You can promote cooperation with treatments and therapies by following these guidelines:

Provide Teaching. Assess the client's understanding of his illness and treatments and provide the necessary information. Keep instructions simple, clear, and as specific as possible. Supply a written copy.

Assess the Client's Supports and Resources. Do not assume that every patient has transportation to the healthcare facility. Even if they wish to follow the therapy, some people do not have enough money for food or medicine; some people cannot read printed instructions; some do not have family or friends to help with their care at home; and so on.

Be Sensitive to the Client's Cultural, Spiritual, and Other Needs. For example, regardless of the need for dietary protein, some people do not like the taste of meat, poultry, or fish; others might have religious or cultural objections to eating these foods. You will need to modify your recommendations to reflect client preferences and beliefs.

Realize and Accept That Some Attitudes Cannot Be Changed. For example, regardless of the effects of obesity on blood pressure, a client will not lose weight simply because you tell him it is important. The client must *want* to lose weight. Information alone will not change a person's behavior.

Determine the Client's Main Concerns. For example, you may be concerned that lack of exercise makes it difficult to regulate a client's blood sugar; the client's main concern may be that exercise makes her joints hurt.

Help the Client Set Realistic Goals. Clients usually more readily accept small, rather than drastic, behavioral or lifestyle changes. Perhaps a client with a child who has asthma cannot even imagine that she could stop smoking. But you may be able to convince her it would be better for her child if she would smoke outdoors rather than in the house or in the car (London, 1998).

Talk Openly and Regularly About Adherence. Let the client know you understand how difficult treatment can be and that others struggle with adherence as well.

What Should I Know About Collaborating and Coordinating Care?

For successful implementation, you need the skills of collaboration and coordination.

Collaboration. As discussed in Chapter 6, **collaboration** simply means working with patients and other caregivers (e.g., physicians, respiratory therapists) to plan, make decisions, or perform interventions. Unlike delegated activities (discussed in the following section) true collaboration requires shared decision making.

According to the Quality and Safety Education for Nurses (QSEN) project, one of the competencies you should acquire in nursing school is the ability to function and collaborate on an interdisciplinary team, as well as with other nurses. This means, in part, that you will learn to be assertive in discussions about patient care. At the same time, you should recognize the differences in authority and power that exist on interdisciplinary teams and choose your communication style carefully, taking that into account (Cronenwett, Sherwood, Barnsteiner, et al., 2007).

Coordination. Coordinating care includes scheduling treatments and activities with other departments (e.g., laboratory, physical therapy, radiology). But it is more than that. In the hospital, nurses are the professionals who have the most frequent and continuous contact with the patient, so they have the most complete picture of the person. Most other caregivers focus on only a very specific aspect of the patient (e.g., breathing, eating, surgical incision). You will be expected to put together the bits and pieces of information (e.g., the patient's response to physical therapy, dietary intake, emotional status, and vital signs) to provide a holistic view of the person. You will need to read the reports of other professionals, help interpret the results for the patient and family, and make rounds with other professionals to be sure that everyone sees the whole picture.

Outside the hospital, the health professional who has the most contact with the client usually assumes the coordination role. For example, if a client is receiving episodic care for ongoing health problems, the primary care provider (e.g., physician or advanced practice nurse) may coordinate care. For a client discharged home after a hip fracture, the physical therapist may coordinate care.

KnowledgeCheck 7-2

- What are some reasons that a client may not follow a recommended treatment regimen?
- List at least four things you could do to promote client participation in care or adherence to recommendations for treatment.

What Should I Know About Delegation and Supervision?

Delegation is the process of directing another person to perform a task or activity; it is a transfer of authority or responsibility. The person delegating retains accountability for the outcome of the activity (American Nurses Association [ANA] and the National Council of State Boards of Nursing [NCSBN], 2006). As a registered nurse, you will frequently delegate patient care activities to licensed vocational (or practical) nurses (LVN/LPNs) and nursing assistive personnel (NAPs), although in some states LVN/LPNs are considered accountable for their actions because they are licensed.

Delegating Is Not the Same as Assigning. You may *assign* tasks to other registered nurses (RNs) (e.g., as a nurse in charge tasks making unit assignments for the day). However, this is not delegation because those RNs are accountable for the outcome of their activities. Remember, you can only delegate *down* in the chain of command.

Understand That You Cannot Delegate Nursing Care Decisions. You can delegate only the responsibility for performing a defined activity in a particular situation. So, even though the nurse has delegated to the NAP the task of turning Mrs. Wu (Meet Your Patients) every 2 hours, it is *the*

nurse who must assess her skin condition and take action if it does not improve.

Use NAPs Appropriately. In some healthcare settings, NAPs are used inappropriately to perform functions that are legally nursing functions (e.g., administering medications) (Dickens, Stubbs, & Haw, 2008). Many nurses are concerned that when there is a nursing shortage, inappropriate delegation is a threat to patient safety. Nurses may find themselves in a difficult position of caring for sicker patients, using new technologies, administering medications, and juggling these activities with overseeing delegated work. According to the ANA, any nursing intervention that requires critical thinking or professional judgment cannot be delegated. However, the ANA takes the position that RN delegation and direction of specific tasks to NAPs in accordance with state nurse practice acts is appropriate, safe, and resource-efficient (ANA, 2007). Standard 15 of the *Nursing: Scope and Standards of Practice* (2nd ed.) (ANA, 2010) states that the registered nurse "delegates elements of care to appropriate healthcare workers in accordance with any applicable legal or policy parameters or principles."

The Five Rights of Delegation

When deciding whether to delegate tasks, you should think critically about the task, the circumstance, the person, the direction or communication, and the supervision and evaluation. For a checklist to help you consider these five critical elements, or "five rights" of delegating, see Box 7-2.

Right Task

The first question to ask is, "Can I delegate this task?" As a rule, you should delegate an activity only if it meets *all* of the following criteria (ANA, 1996; ANA/NCSBN, 2006). The activity:

- Is within your scope of practice to perform and delegate, as defined by your state's nurse practice act.
- Is within the LVN/LPN's or NAP's scope of practice.
- Is in accordance with agency policies, if they exist.
- Is performed according to an established sequence of steps and requires little or no modification from one situation to another.

- Does not require ongoing nursing assessments, interpretation, or decision making.
- Occurs frequently in the daily care of patients on the unit.
- Has reasonably predictable results.
- Does *not* require independent, specialized nursing knowledge, skills, or judgment.
- Is *not* health teaching or counseling.
- Does not endanger a client's life or well-being.

Examples of tasks you might assign to a NAP are bathing a stable patient, ambulating steady patients, obtaining routine vital signs, changing linens, assisting patients with meals, clerical duties, and transporting non-acute patients and specimens.

LPNs can usually provide care to medically stable patients according to an established plan of care; they can give you feedback about patient responses for patients who are expected to respond predictably. Tasks you can usually assign to an LPN include administering some medications (except for IV medications and some controlled substances), starting an IV infusion and administering plain IV solutions, and assisting with identification of blood units for transfusion. You would not assign an LPN to start a blood transfusion, administer chemotherapy, administer or monitor parenteral nutrition, give IV push medications, or create and modify nursing care plans (Ayers & Montgomery, 2008).

Remember that you are assigning staff members to a *task*, not to a patient. You cannot delegate the responsibility for total patient care; and you cannot allow a NAP to delegate care to other NAPs.

Right Circumstance

NAPs are being used in settings in which acuity and technology have increased while length of stay has decreased. This means they are caring for sicker patients. Even tasks such as bathing, feeding, and turning patients may not be appropriate if the patient is seriously ill. Before deciding to delegate, assess your patient to be certain that her needs match the abilities of the NAP or LPN. It is best if the patient is relatively stable (e.g., with a chronic rather than an acute condition) and does not need extensive help with self-care activities. If the client is very

---

BOX 7-2 ■ The Five Rights of Delegation—Checklist

Right Task (*Can I delegate it?*)

The task is:
- Delegable for a specific patient.
- Within the nurse's scope of practice.
- Permitted by the state's nurse practice act.
- Permitted by the agency's policies.

Right Circumstance (*Should I delegate it?*)

Consider patient safety:
- Is patient setting appropriate?
- Are adequate resources available?
- Are there other factors to maintain safety?

Right Person (*Who is best prepared to do it?*)

The right person:
- Is delegating the task (the nurse must be competent to delegate).
- Will be performing the task (the NAP must be competent to do the task).

- Will receive the care (i.e., the severity of the patient's illness is considered).

Right Direction/Communication (*What does the NAP need to know?*)

- The task is described clearly, including its objective, limits, and expectations.
- The delegatee (NAP) understands the communication.

Right Supervision (*How will I follow up?*)

- The nurse monitors, evaluates, and intervenes as needed.
- The nurse obtains feedback from the patient.
- The nurse obtains feedback from the delegatee.

Source: National Council of State Boards of Nursing. (1995). *Delegation: Concepts and decision-making process.* National Council position paper. Chicago: Author.

ill or if the results of the task are unpredictable, the task should probably not be delegated. For a tool to help you make appropriate delegation decisions in the clinical setting,

 Go to Chapter 7, Tables, Boxes, Figures: **ESG Figure 7-2, Delegation Decision-Making Grid,** on *DavisPlus*.

Right Person

You must also be sure that the LPN or NAP is competent to perform the task and that his workload allows time to do the task properly. Take into consideration the person's experience, training, and cultural competence. The following are evidence of competence:

- The facility has documented proof that the person has demonstrated competence.
- The NAP has performed the task often or has worked with patients with similar diagnoses.

If evidence is lacking, you need to establish the NAP's competence. For example, you might observe and evaluate his performance, or you might ask the NAP, "How many times have you done this procedure?" or "Will you need help with this procedure?" Only a registered nurse can evaluate an LPN's or NAP's ability to perform a nursing task.

Right Communication

Right communication means that when you delegate, you should communicate clearly and specifically about each task. You can communicate orally or in writing, but leave no room for misinterpretation.

- **Explain exactly what the task is.** Include what to do and what not to do. For example, "Empty the catheter bag, and measure the amount of urine using the clear, marked plastic container"—not just "Measure the urine."
- **Include specific times and methods for reporting.** For example, "Come tell me the patient's temperature every hour."
- **Explain the purpose or objective of the task.** For example, "Change Mrs. Wu's position every 2 hours to prevent bedsores; she is not able to turn by herself."
- **Describe the expected results or potential complications to expect.** For example, "She will probably cry out when you turn her, but that is more from fear than from pain," or "I have given her medications, so her temperature should be below 100°F by 0900. If not, let me know immediately."
- **Be specific in your instructions.** For example, "Let me know if Mrs. Wu has any red spots or broken skin areas when you turn her"—not "Tell me what her skin looks like."

Right Supervision

Supervision is the process of directing, guiding, and influencing the performance of the delegated task. When you delegate tasks to a NAP or LVN/LPN, you or another RN must be available to answer questions and provide help, if necessary. You are responsible for providing supervision and evaluating the outcomes. This includes the following:

- **Monitoring the NAP/LVN/LPN's work.** You need to be sure the work complies with agency policies and procedures and standards of practice. For example, after the NAP bathes a patient, you could check to see whether the patient is clean; or you might choose to observe for a few minutes while the NAP is working. Make frequent patient rounds and get regular reports from those you have assigned to do tasks.
- **Intervening, if necessary.** Some NAPs receive little training, so you may need to demonstrate some caregiving activities.
- **Obtaining and providing feedback from the worker.** Give positive, as well as negative, feedback often. If performance

is not acceptable, speak privately with the NAP to explain the specific mistakes that were made. Listen to the NAP's view of the situation. For example, there may have been too many tasks to complete in the time allowed.

- **Evaluating client outcomes.** Evaluate both the physical response and the relationship with the NAP. Ask the client for input after the care is given.
- **Ensuring proper documentation.** Some agencies permit NAPs to record vital signs and other patient data. You are responsible for seeing that all necessary data are recorded and that they are accurate.

KnowledgeCheck 7-3

- List the "five rights" of delegation.
- List at least four characteristics of a "right task"—that is, a task that would be acceptable to delegate.
- As an RN, how could you establish that a NAP is competent to perform a task?
- List at least three ways to help ensure that the NAP will understand clearly what she needs to do when you delegate a task.
- List at least three things you should do when providing supervision to an unlicensed caregiver.

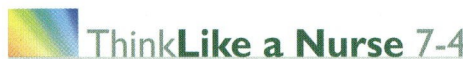 ThinkLike a Nurse 7-4

For your patient, Jeannette Wu:
- Which activity did the nurse delegate to someone else?
- What collaborative activities should the nurse consider?

Documenting: The Final Step of Implementation

After giving care, you will record the nursing activities and the patient's responses. Documentation is a mode of communication among the members of the health team, and it provides the information you need to evaluate the patient's health status and the nursing care plan. For a thorough discussion of documenting, refer to Chapter 18.

Reflecting Critically About Implementation

During the implementation phase, perhaps more than at any other time, nurses combine thinking and doing. You should always be prepared to modify the activity based on the patient's responses. Afterward, when you have some time to reflect, you can think critically about what happened (good or bad) and why. Use the following questions, or refer to the critical thinking model. (See Chapter 2, Table 2-2, if you would like other ideas.)

- What was done? Why was it done? What were the patient's responses?
- Did I forget to do anything?
- What was going on in the situation that may have influenced the outcome?
- What factors influenced my behavior (or others' behavior) in this situation?
- Would the activity have been more successful if I had had more knowledge or skill? If so, why did I not realize that ahead of time, and how can I avoid such lack of insight in the future?
- What assumptions or biases (mine or the patient's) contributed to the problem in this situation?
- Did I communicate clearly to the patient?

Toward Evidence-Based Practice

Read about the following studies, and then answer the questions at the end of the box.

> Standing, T., Anthony, M., & Hertz, J. (2001). Nurses' narratives of outcomes after delegation to unlicensed assistive personnel. *Outcomes Management for Nursing Practice, 5*(1), 18–23.

The authors of this qualitative study analyzed questionnaires and open-ended responses from 148 licensed nurses. Nurses were asked to write two narratives: one to describe a situation in which delegation of a task to a NAP had a positive outcome, and another that had a negative outcome. In addition, phone interviews were conducted with 27 nurses to expand on those findings. Along with the positive reports, the following negative results were also reported:

- Negative outcomes occurred most often because the NAP (1) did not follow directions or agency procedures, or (2) was overconfident (e.g., carried out activities that had not been delegated).
- With regard to the Five Rights of Delegation, deficiencies were most often related to the right communication or right supervision.

> Standing, T., & Anthony, M. K. (2008). Delegation: What it means to acute care nurses. *Applied Nursing Research, 21*(1), 8–14.

The authors of this qualitative study conducted 17 in-depth interviews with acute-care nurses, both novice and experienced, to examine the nature of delegation.

Nurses expressed frustration that they were being held accountable for the NAPs' tasks, while the NAPs themselves were not. Several nurses described NAPs' resentment of RNs. They indicated that the RN–NAP relationship and good communication are at the heart of delegation. The RNs recognized the importance of acknowledging the contribution of the NAP. The RNs pointed out that one negative aspect of delegation is that the NAP sometimes did not perform tasks well, or at all, and sometimes communicated improperly with patients. A positive aspect is that delegation allows the RN time to monitor patient changes, review charts, and focus on more important things. They concluded that nursing education should provide more content on communication and interpersonal relationships.

1. What similarities do you see between the two studies in the authors and the methods?

2. What similarities in results are reported?

3. With your answer to question 2 in mind, what skill do you think you need to learn and practice to prepare for working with and delegating to NAPs?

 Go to Chapter 7, **Toward Evidence-Based Practice Suggested Responses**, on Davis*Plus*.

- Did I convey respect and caring?
- What could I have delegated? What did I delegate that I should *not* have? Why?
- After reflecting on it, what would I do differently in this situation?

Refer to Table 7-2 for examples that demonstrate how the reflection questions might be used in a clinical situation.

EVALUATION: THE FINAL STEP OF THE NURSING PROCESS

Evaluation, the final step of the nursing process, is a planned, ongoing, systematic activity in which you will make judgments about:

- The client's progress toward desired health outcomes.
- The effectiveness of the nursing care plan.
- The quality of nursing care in the healthcare setting.

Evaluation Is Affected By All Other Steps of the Nursing Process. The patient outcomes stated in the *planning outcomes* stage must be concrete, observable, and appropriate for the patient in order to be useful as evaluation criteria. Appropriate outcomes, in turn, depend on complete and accurate *assessment* data and *nursing diagnoses.* You will observe and evaluate client responses during *implementation* in order to make on-the-spot changes in activity. And, of course, *interventions* must be

planned and *implemented* to produce the patient behaviors that you evaluate. Evaluation overlaps greatly with the assessment step—both involve data collection. The difference is in *when you collect* and *how you use* the data.

- *Assessment data* are collected before interventions are performed to determine initial or baseline health status and to make nursing diagnoses.
- *Evaluation data* are collected after interventions are performed to determine whether client goals were achieved.

Evaluation Is an Essential Part of Full-Spectrum Nursing. The following describe several reasons why evaluation is an important part of the nursing role.

- **The patient is the nurse's first priority.** The aim of all nursing activity is to achieve positive outcomes for patients. Evaluation lets you know whether your interventions are helping the patient as intended, and guides your next action. For example, you may need to revise the plan of care if an intervention is unsuccessful or if it is no longer needed.
- **Evaluation helps nurses to conserve scarce resources.** Nurses are in short supply. Therefore, nursing time is precious and must be used wisely. Evaluation allows you to discard interventions that are not working well and focus on more effective ones.
- **Professional standards of practice require evaluation.** For example, see the ANA practice standards in Box 7-3.

Table 7-2 ➤ Examples of Reflecting Critically About Implementation

SITUATION	QUESTION FOR REFLECTION	WHAT MIGHT HAVE HAPPENED?
The nursing order read, "Assist to ambulate to the end of the hall...." However, the patient was able to walk only about half that distance before becoming too weak to stand.	What was going on in the situation that may have influenced the outcome?	Perhaps the patient was weak because he had not slept well the night before, or perhaps he had just had a long, tiring session of physical therapy.
When the patient became too weak to walk, the nurse called for help. Why did she do that instead of helping the patient to sit where he was, or instead of helping him back to the room by herself?	What factors influenced the nurse's behavior in this situation?	Perhaps the patient was very large and the nurse realized she was not strong enough to provide support. Can you think of other reasons that the nurse might have chosen that action?

BOX 7-3 ■ ANA Standards of Practice for Evaluation

Standard 6. Evaluation

The registered nurse evaluates progress toward attainment of outcomes.

Competencies

The registered nurse:

- Conducts a systematic, ongoing, and criterion-based evaluation of the outcomes in relation to the structures and processes prescribed by the plan of care and the indicated timeline.
- Collaborates with the healthcare consumer and others involved in the care or situation in the evaluation process.
- Evaluates, in partnership with the healthcare consumer, the effectiveness of the planned strategies in relation to the healthcare consumer's responses and attainment of the expected outcomes.
- Uses ongoing assessment data to revise the diagnoses, outcomes, the plan, and the implementation, as needed.
- Disseminates the results to the healthcare consumer, family, and others involved, in accordance with federal and state regulations.
- Participates in assessing and assuring the responsible and appropriate use of interventions in order to minimize unwarranted or unwanted treatment and healthcare consumer suffering.
- Documents the results of the evaluation.

Source: American Nurses Association. (2010). *Nursing: Scope and standards of practice* (2nd ed.). Silver Spring, MD: ANA.

- **The ANA Code of Ethics requires evaluation.** "The nurse's primary commitment is to the recipient of nursing and healthcare services—the patient—whether the recipient is an individual, a family, a group, or a community. . . . The nurse has a responsibility to implement and maintain standards of professional nursing practice. The nurse should participate in planning, establishing, implementing, and evaluating review mechanisms designed to safeguard patients and nurses, such as peer review processes or committees, credentialing processes, quality improvement initiatives, and ethics committees" (ANA, 2001, Section 2.1 and Standard 3.4).

- **The Joint Commission and professional standards review organizations (PSROs) require evaluation.** These organizations use outcomes and performance measures to evaluate the quality of care in healthcare institutions. They conceptualize quality of care as the degree to which health services increase the likelihood of desired health outcomes.
- **Evaluation helps ensure nursing's survival.** Linking nursing interventions to achievement of client outcomes demonstrates the value of nursing. In today's competitive healthcare market, that is essential for ensuring continued funding for nursing services, education, and research.
- **Evaluation demonstrates caring and responsibility.** Without evaluation, you would not know whether your care was effective. Examining outcomes implies that you care about how your activities affect your clients.
- **Quality and Safety Education for Nurses (QSEN).** This task force includes quality improvement as one of the competencies to be achieved during your education in nursing.

How Are Standards and Criteria Used in Evaluation?

In a broad sense, evaluation is the systematic process of judging the quality or value of something by comparing it to one or more standards or criteria. In our daily lives, we evaluate many things: a meal, a TV program, an insurance policy we are thinking of buying. However, for formal evaluation, you must decide *in advance* which standards and criteria you will use. As you learned in Chapter 1, **standards** represent expected or accepted levels of performance; they provide a model for what ought to be done. In nursing, standards are used to describe quality nursing care. The ANA's standards of practice are a good example of broadly written standards (see Boxes 7-1 and 7-3).

Notice that each of the ANA standards includes a set of measurement criteria, called *competencies*, to help describe the standard. **Criteria** are measurable or observable characteristics, properties, attributes, or qualities. They describe the specific skills, knowledge, behaviors, and attitudes that are desired or expected. Judges at a diving competition, for example, evaluate a dive by using criteria for difficulty, technique, and style.

The patient goals and outcomes discussed in Chapter 5 are also examples of criteria. As you learned there, these criteria should be concrete and specific enough to serve as guides for collecting evaluation data. In addition, they should be reliable and valid.

Reliability. A criterion is **reliable** if it yields consistent results—that is, the same results every time, regardless of who uses it. For example, suppose you measure a patient's temperature by (1) using an oral thermometer and (2) placing the back of your hand on the patient's forehead. Which method would probably give the same (or nearly same) results every time? As you probably concluded, the oral thermometer is more reliable.

Validity. A criterion is **valid** if it is really measuring what it was intended to measure. For example, fever is often used as a criterion for concluding that a person has an infection. However, if used alone, it is not a valid indicator because (1) other conditions, such as dehydration, can cause a fever and (2) elevated temperature is not present in all infections. Validity of that criterion is increased when you use additional criteria (e.g., elevated white blood cell count, presence of signs of infection such as redness and pus).

ThinkLike a Nurse 7-5

- The outcome "Patient will not complain of pain," by itself is not a valid criterion for measuring pain. Why? What would be a more valid criterion for pain?
- A criterion reads, "Measures client vital signs once per shift, or as ordered." For which of the following standards would it be valid (i.e., which conclusion could you draw if you knew that a nurse measured the vital signs once per shift, or as ordered)?
  Follows unit policies.
  Performs skills accurately.

What Are the Types of Evaluation?

Evaluation is categorized according to (1) what is being evaluated (structures, processes, or outcomes) and (2) frequency and time of evaluation.

Evaluation of Structures, Processes, and Outcomes

Structures, processes, and outcomes all work together to affect care. However, each requires different criteria and methods of evaluation.

Structure evaluation focuses on the setting in which care is provided. It explores the effect of organizational characteristics on the quality of care. It requires standards and data about policies, procedures, fiscal resources, physical facilities and equipment, and number and qualifications of personnel. Examples of criteria for structure evaluation include the following:

At least one RN is present on each unit at all times.
A resuscitation cart is available on each floor.

Process evaluation focuses on the manner in which care is given—the activities performed by nurses (and other personnel). It explores whether the care was relevant to patient needs, appropriate, complete, and timely. Your instructor uses process evaluation to assess your clinical performance. Your clinical evaluation describes what you did and how well you did it. As a rule, it does not describe the *results* of your activities. Examples of criteria for process evaluation include the following:

Protects patient's privacy when performing procedures.
Washes hands before each patient contact.

Outcomes evaluation focuses on observable or measurable changes in the patient's health status that result from the care given. Although structure and process are important to

quality, the most important aspect is improvement in patient health status. The evaluation step of the nursing process uses outcomes evaluation. Examples of outcomes criteria include:

Patient will walk, assisted, to end of hall by postoperative day five.
Patient reports pain less than 4 on a scale of 1 to 10 within 1 hour after analgesic administration.

Outcomes evaluation is also used when evaluating quality of care in an organization. When used for that purpose, the criteria also state the percentage of clients expected to have the outcome when care is satisfactory—as in the following example:

Post-catheterization urinary tract infection does not occur. *Expected compliance: 100%*

This means that the criterion would be met only if no patients developed a urinary tract infection after being catheterized.

Ongoing, Intermittent, and Terminal Evaluation

Evaluation begins as soon as you have completed the first nursing activity and continues during each client contact until all goals are achieved or the client is discharged from nursing care. The client's status determines how often you evaluate. A critically ill patient may need a nurse constantly at the bedside; after a patient undergoes surgery, you may measure vital signs every 15 minutes; as the patient nears discharge, you may evaluate once a day. In long-term care settings, residents often have chronic health problems that require evaluation over an extended period of time. Most care is provided by LVN/LPNs and NAPs, and the RN may participate in weekly care conferences to evaluate the resident's response to the current plan of care.

You will perform **ongoing evaluation** while implementing care, immediately after an intervention, and at each patient contact. In contrast, **intermittent evaluation** is performed at specified times. Both kinds of evaluation enable you to judge the progress toward goal achievement and to modify the care plan as needed. Goals and expected outcomes should designate times for collecting evaluation data. For example:

Will rate pain as <3 on a scale of 1 to 10 *within 1 hr after medication*.
Will lose 1 lb *per week* until weight of 125 lb is achieved.

Terminal evaluation describes the client's health status and progress toward goals at the time of discharge. Most institutions have special discharge forms for terminal evaluation that also include instructions about medications, treatments, and follow-up care.

As in all phases of the nursing process, you should collaborate with the patient and family in evaluation to the extent they are able. As the nurse, you are responsible for drawing evaluative conclusions; however, you should use input from the patient, the family, NAPs, and other caregivers (see Box 7-3).

ThinkLike a Nurse 7-6

For each of the following goals, when or how often should the nurse collect evaluation data?

- Will rate pain as <3 on a scale of 1 to 10 within *1 hr after medication*.
- Will lose 1 lb *per week* until weight of 125 lb is achieved.
- *By the second home visit*, mother will demonstrate proper techniques for breastfeeding.

KnowledgeCheck 7-4

- Explain what is evaluated in each of the following types of evaluation (i.e., the focus of each type of evaluation): structure, process, and outcomes.
- Identify what is evaluated in the list below using the following criteria: structure, process, or outcomes.

    In the Emergency Department, the time from patient sign-in to assessment by a healthcare worker will be less than 15 minutes.

    A fire extinguisher is located in an accessible spot on each unit.

    No patients with indwelling urinary catheters will develop urinary tract infection.
- Define the following: ongoing evaluation, intermittent evaluation, terminal evaluation.

How Do I Evaluate Patient Progress?

Evaluation does not "end" the nursing process. It merely provides the information you need to begin another cycle. After giving care, you compare patient responses to the desired outcomes (goals) and use that information to reflect critically on (1) the care plan and (2) each step of the nursing process as it applies to that patient. When evaluating patient progress, you review the desired outcomes, collect reassessment data, judge whether goals have been met, and record the evaluative statement (Wilkinson, 2011). Figure 7-1 illustrates the relationship of the evaluation phase to the rest of the nursing process.

Review Outcomes

First, review the goals/outcomes on the patient's care plan. The goals and indicators you identified in the planning outcomes phase suggest the kind of assessments you need to make and provide criteria by which to judge the data.

Collect Reassessment Data

Next, assess client responses to the interventions. To minimize confusion, assessments made for the purpose of evaluation are called **reassessments.** Reassessments are always focused assessments (see Chapter 3). As already mentioned, the care plan goals determine the reassessment focus.

- Suppose, for example, that the nursing care plan lists the following goal: "By 8/24/14, will walk, unassisted, to the end of the hall without pallor or shortness of breath." What kind of assessments would you make to know whether this goal has been met?
- Suppose the care plan includes the following goal: "By 8/24/14, will notify nurse as soon as pain begins." How would you obtain the data you need to evaluate this goal?

    For the first example, you would observe the patient's skin color as he walked, observe and count his respirations, and ask him if he felt short of breath at any time. The second example is a little less obvious. If the patient doesn't call you, you cannot assume this means there is no pain. You would need to ask him whether he has had pain (e.g., "I notice that you have not put your call light on. Have you had any pain at all today?"). If the patient does call you, you still cannot assume it is because of pain, or that he called as soon as the pain began. You must question to clarify, for example, "How can I help you?" "Are you in pain?" "When did it start?"

ThinkLike a Nurse 7-7

In the examples in the preceding paragraph, which aspects of critical thinking (in the full-spectrum nursing model in Chapter 2) did you use to decide what data you needed?

Goals can be cognitive, psychomotor, or affective, or they may refer to body appearance and function. The nature of the goal determines the kind of data you need to collect. See Table 7-3 for examples of goal types and the kind of reassessment data they require. As in the assessment phase, you will collect data from the client, family, friends, and health team members, as well as from the client's chart (e.g., laboratory results). The RN is responsible for evaluating goal achievement, even though someone else may have supplied the data.

Judge Goal Achievement

Next, compare the reassessment data with the patient's goals. As always, get the patient's input. Ask her if she thinks the goals have been achieved. Goals or outcomes can be judged to be one of the following:

- *Achieved.* The actual responses are the same as the desired outcome.
- *Partially achieved.* Some, but not all, of the desired behaviors were observed, or the desired response occurs only some of the time (e.g., the desired heart rate is <100 beats/min, a goal that is achieved except for one or two episodes a day, when it is 110 beats/min).
- *Not achieved.* The desired response did not occur (actual outcome does not match desired outcome or goal).

Record the Evaluative Statement

Professional standards require that you record your evaluations. You may write an evaluative summary in the nursing notes or on the care plan, depending on the procedure specified by the institution. An evaluative statement should include:

- The conclusion about whether the goal was achieved
- Reassessment data to support the judgment

An evaluative statement for the pain goal "By 8/24/14 will notify nurse as soon as pain begins" might be the following:

> *8/25/14, 0100. Goal not met. Has not used call light at all this a.m. Restless and grimacing with movement during a.m. care. When asked, described pain as 8 on a scale of 1 to 10.*
> *—J. Hiam, RN*

When using standardized outcomes (e.g., Nursing Outcomes Classification [NOC]) or electronic care plans, your evaluative statements may be different. In the NOC system, each outcome (label) has a scale and indicators (specific patient responses), numbered 1 through 5, which you can use to write goals (see Chapter 5). For example, a patient with a problem of decreased peripheral circulation might have this goal: "Circulation status not compromised." Using standardized language from NOC, you might write a goal (*desired* status) of:

> Goal: *Circulation Status: 5* (5 means "no deviation from normal range" in the NOC scale).

Each of the indicators could also be made into a goal by adding the desired scale numbers, as follows:

> Systolic BP in expected range: 5
> Diastolic BP in expected range: 5
> Mean BP in expected range: 5

Evaluation statements are written exactly the same as goals, but the scale number describes the patient's *actual* status. So, if on reassessment the patient's blood pressure is quite low and he has orthostatic hypotension, the evaluative statement might be:

> Evaluative Statement: *Circulation Status: 3* (3 means "moderately compromised" on this NOC scale)

Figure 7-2 is a computer screen showing the NOC outcome of Acceptance: Health Status. The Initial Scale shows

Table 7-3 ➤ Reassessments for Different Types of Goals

TYPE OF GOAL	INVOLVES	EXAMPLE OF GOALS	REASSESSMENT TECHNIQUES
Cognitive	Increases in patient knowledge	■ By 8/24/14 accurately describes schedule for taking medications. ■ By 8/25/14 correctly describes the procedure for pouring liquid medications.	Ask the person to repeat information or to apply new knowledge (e.g., to describe to you the schedule for taking her medications).
Affective	Changes in feelings, values, beliefs, and attitudes	■ By 8/24/14 expresses positive feelings for the newborn. ■ By 8/24/14 states he is only mildly anxious about changing his own dressing.	Observe client behavior reflecting values and beliefs; talk to the client about feelings and beliefs; observe nonverbal expression of feelings (e.g., laughing, crying).
Psychomotor	Patient's ability to perform skills	■ By 8/24/14 performs own dressing change, using proper aseptic technique. ■ By 8/24/14 measures liquid medication accurately.	Ask the person to demonstrate the new skill (e.g., change a dressing, measure a liquid medication).
Body appearance and function	Changes in body systems and functions	■ Heart rate will be 100 beats/min after ambulation to end of hall. ■ By 8/24/14 can dress self and fasten own zipper.	Observe functioning, examine the body, perform measurements, read laboratory reports (e.g., measure vital signs, observe skin color, assess for pain).

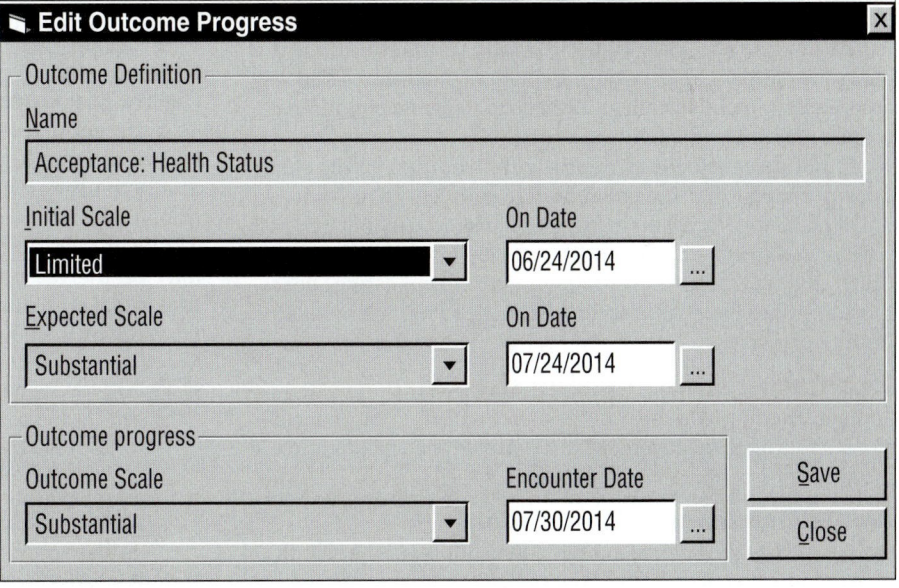

FIGURE 7-2 Computer screen showing outcome progress, using NOC. (*Source: Courtesy of Ergo Partners, L.C., Boulder, CO. Used with permission.*)

Explanation of Figure

Computer field	Nursing process terminology	Represents	Status recorded on computer
Initial scale	Initial assessment	*Actual* status *before* intervention	Limited acceptance of health status
Expected scale	Goal	*Desired* status *after* intervention	Substantial acceptance of health status
Outcome scale	Evaluative statement	*Actual* status *after* intervention	Substantial acceptance of health status

the initial assessment; the Expected Scale is the goal; and the Outcome Scale is the evaluative statement after intervention and reassessment. Did the interventions achieve the desired effect, or not? If you want to see a computer screen showing a NOC outcome definition and indicators,

 Go to Chapter 7, **Tables, Boxes, Figures: ESG Figure 7-3,** on Davis*Plus.*

KnowledgeCheck 7-5

Using the following outcomes and reassessment data, determine whether each goal has been met, partially met, or not met.

Goal: By 8/24/14, will walk, unassisted, to the end of the hall without pallor or shortness of breath.

Reassessment data: 8/24/14. Walked, unassisted, to end of hall; states no shortness of breath, but skin color was noticeably pale.

Goal: By 8/24/14, will walk, unassisted, to the end of the hall without pallor or shortness of breath.

Reassessment data: 8/23/14. Walked, unassisted, to end of hall. Skin color pink; respirations 14 breaths/min; no dyspnea observed; states no shortness of breath.

Goal: By 8/24/14, will walk, unassisted, to the end of the hall without pallor or shortness of breath.

Reassessment data: 8/25/14. Walked halfway to end of hall before becoming pale and short of breath.

How Do I Evaluate Collaborative Problems?

Because collaborative problems are the responsibility of the entire healthcare team, goals for collaborative problems are not included on the nursing care plan, and the evaluation process is slightly different. The desired outcome for all collaborative problems is that no complication will occur. To evaluate, you will compare the reassessment data to established norms (e.g., normal temperature, normal electrocardiogram patter) and determine whether data are within an acceptable range. If the data indicate the client's condition is worsening, notify the medical provider.

If the reassessment data are within normal limits, this does not mean that the collaborative problem is resolved—only that the complication has not occurred. As long as the patient has the medical condition (e.g., myocardial infarction), the collaborative problem (e.g., congestive heart failure) still exists. See Chapter 4 if you need to review collaborative problems.

Evaluating and Revising the Care Plan

After evaluating patient progress, you will use your conclusions about goal achievement to decide whether to continue, modify, or discontinue the care plan.

Relate Outcomes to Interventions

Even when goals have been met, you cannot assume that the nursing interventions caused the patient outcomes. You need to use critical reflection to identify factors that might have supported or interfered with the effectiveness of an intervention. The following are variables that can affect the ability of an intervention to produce the desired outcome:

- The client's ability and motivation to follow directions for treatment
- Availability and support from family and significant others
- Treatments and therapies performed by other healthcare team members

- Client failure to provide complete information during assessment
- Client's lack of experience, knowledge, or ability
- Staffing in the institution (ratio of licensed to unlicensed caregivers; number of patients for whom a nurse is responsible)
- Nurse's physical and mental well-being

Identifying these factors allows you to reinforce or change them. For example, if Jeannette Wu does not achieve a goal of "Intact skin over sacrum" even after being turned every 2 hours by the NAP, you may discover Ms. Wu's skin is more fragile than expected because her hydration and nutrition are not adequate. You could then take measures to support her intake of food and fluids, increasing the effectiveness of the turning intervention. Remember, though, that you cannot control all the variables that might affect the success of an intervention (e.g., the client's lack of experience, staffing in your institution).

Draw Conclusions About Problem Status

Whether you retain or remove a nursing diagnosis from the care plan depends on whether or not goals were met, as follows:

Goals met: If all goals for a nursing diagnosis have been met, you can discontinue the care plan for that diagnosis.

Goals partially met: If some outcomes are met and others not, you may revise the care plan for that problem; or you may continue with the same plan but allow more time for goal achievement.

Goals not met: If goals are not met, you should examine the entire plan and review all steps of the nursing process to decide whether to revise the care plan.

For an example of electronic evaluation of problem status for a client with multiple nursing care needs,

 Go to Chapter 7, **Tables, Boxes, Figures: ESG Figure 7-4,** on Davis*Plus.*

Revise the Care Plan

To decide how to revise the care plan, you must review each step of the nursing process. You cannot just discontinue the ineffective interventions and try new ones. The interventions may not need to be changed at all. When goals have not been met, errors in other steps of the nursing process may be the reason. For a checklist you can print and use to evaluate a care plan and the process by which it was developed (Wilkinson, 2011),

 Go to Chapter 7, **ESG Figure 7-5, Evaluation Checklist,** on Davis*Plus.*

1. *Review of assessment.* Review all initial and ongoing assessment data. Were the data complete, accurate, and validated as needed? All steps of the nursing process depend on complete and accurate data. So if there are errors or omissions, or if there are new data or changes in the client's condition, you may need to revise any or all sections of the care plan (i.e., nursing diagnosis, outcomes, nursing orders).

2. *Review of diagnosis.* Even if there were no assessment errors, you may need to revise or add new nursing diagnoses. Perhaps the nurse who wrote the diagnostic statement did not communicate the patient's condition clearly, or perhaps it was not validated with the patient. Is the diagnosis supported by the data? Has the problem status changed (e.g., from potential to actual or resolved)? Are

problem and etiology logically related? Is the problem specific and individualized to the patient?

3. *Review of planning outcomes.* You will probably need to revise the outcomes if you have added data or revised the nursing diagnosis. If assessment and diagnosis are satisfactory, perhaps the outcomes were unrealistic, written too broadly, or had unrealistic target times. Or perhaps the client's priorities have changed, or the outcomes did not address all aspects of the patient's problem.

4. *Review of planning interventions.* You will probably need to modify nursing orders (a) if you determine that interventions were not effective or (b) if you have revised nursing diagnoses or outcomes. Are the nursing orders clear and specific, and do they address all aspects of the client's health goals? Do the nursing orders include instructions for timing of nursing activities?

5. *Review of implementation.* It could be that goals were not met because of a failure to implement the nursing orders or because of the manner in which they were implemented. For example, the person implementing care may have been tired, in a hurry, or abrupt with the client; or maybe he did not have the necessary knowledge or skills. Get input from the client, significant others, other caregivers, and the client records to find out what went wrong.

6. *Reflecting critically about evaluation.* After evaluating the patient's health status and the nursing care plan, reflect on your thinking during the evaluation process. That's right: Think about your thinking, not just about your actions. The critical thinking model from Chapter 2 suggests some questions you might use for reflection.

Inquiring

Is my evaluation statement clearly stated (goal met or not met, plus supporting data)?

Were my information sources reliable (e.g., was the patient being honest or merely trying to please me)?

Did I jump to conclusions about goal achievement? Do I need any other data to validate my conclusion?

Noticing Context

What was going on either before or during evaluation that might have influenced my ability to gather data or draw conclusions (e.g., Was I in a hurry? Did the patient have visitors in the room?)?

What emotional responses influenced my conclusions about goal achievement (e.g., Would I feel as though I had failed if the goal was not met?)?

Analyzing Assumptions

What biases do I have that may have affected my ability to reassess or evaluate goal achievement?

Reflecting Skeptically

Did I make evaluating a priority? Did I schedule time for it, the same as I do for interventions?

Could I have done it better?

What would I do differently next time?

The most common errors of evaluation are failing to:
- Evaluate systematically.
- Record the results.
- Use the reassessment data to examine and modify the care plan.

Because nurses are action oriented, it is easy for most to make a plan and take action. Most nurses regularly observe the patient's responses to the actions. However, you will need determined effort to make time to observe *regularly and systematically* and *document the patient's responses* to your actions. Only in that way can you be sure the care has met the client's needs.

Evaluating the Quality of Care in a Healthcare Setting

As a nurse, you may be involved in evaluating and improving the overall quality of nursing care in an organization or a geographical area. At a minimum, your documentation will provide data that regulatory agencies (e.g., the Joint Commission, state boards of nursing) use to determine whether nursing care meets nursing standards.

Learning About the Outcomes of Care

Competency: Quality Improvement (Knowledge, Skill, Attitudes)*

All nurses should consider continuous quality improvement (CQI) an essential element of their everyday practice. You are in a unique position to identify problems in the patient populations for which you provide care, but first you must be able to quantify (measure) the outcomes and then determine the cause (or root) of the outcome. For example, suppose you suspect that the incidence of central line infections has increased on your pediatric unit. You have noticed a lot of variation in how different nurses provide central line care. Knowing that variation in treatment often leads to negative variations in outcomes, what data do you need to support your suspicions? What outcome must you measure? What root cause should be assessed (i.e., what nursing practice may be causing the infections)?

If you identified the rate of central line infection as the outcome, and how central line dressing changes are performed on your unit as the nursing practice, you are

correct. Now, how can you obtain data about those two factors? Potential sources in your facility might include databases kept by QI, safety, and/or infection control departments. Some patient care units also track quality measures. The medical records department can develop electronic reports or you can review charts, or collect data prospectively.

Improving the quality of care is possible only with clear measurements. They provide insight into the problem and a baseline against which practice changes can be judged.

Do you see how this box relates to the QSEN competency of QI?

Source: Draper, D., Felland, L., Liebhaber, A., & Melichar, L. (2008)
*For specific Knowledge, Skills, and Attitudes,

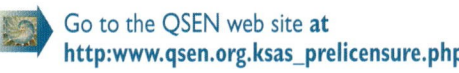
Go to the QSEN web site **at**
http:www.qsen.org.ksas_prelicensure.php

QSEN Competency. Quality improvement is one of the QSEN competencies. That means by the time you graduate, you should be able to "use data to monitor the outcomes of care processes and use improvement methods to design and test changes to continuously improve the quality and safety of healthcare systems (Cronenwett, Sherwood, Barnsteiner, et al., 2007).

Quality Assurance (QA) Programs. These are specially designed programs to promote excellence in nursing. Variations of quality assurance are quality improvement (QI), continuous quality improvement (CQI), total quality management (TQM), and persistent quality improvement (PQI). Whatever the approach, the goal is to evaluate and improve the care provided in an agency or for a group of patients. One hospital reports a reduction in patient falls and medication errors, as well as improvement in nursing documentation after implementation of a QI program chaired by a staff nurse (Johnson, Hallsey, Meredith, et al., 2006).

This chapter has described (1) outcomes evaluation of *client progress* and (2) process evaluation of the *effectiveness of the nursing care plan*. Quality improvement involves evaluation of structures, as well as outcomes and processes. All are important because structures and processes affect patient outcomes. Adequate structures (e.g., staffing, money) and processes (e.g., policies and procedures) do not guarantee desired patient outcomes; however, without them, it is very difficult to obtain good outcomes. For example, a unit could be well staffed (structure) and follow infection-control procedures carefully (process), yet have a higher-than-average rate of urinary tract infections (outcome). The reason may be that most of the patients treated on that unit have compromised immune systems, making them especially susceptible to infection. For more discussion of QSEN and QA/QI evaluation, see Chapter 1 and,

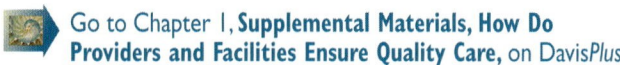

Go to Chapter 1, **Supplemental Materials, How Do Providers and Facilities Ensure Quality Care,** on Davis*Plus.*

CLINICALREASONING:
Applying the **Full-Spectrum Nursing Model**

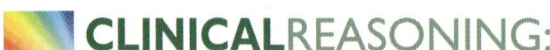

Because the following critical thinking activities allow you to practice the kind of thinking you will use as a full-spectrum nurse, they usually have no single right answer. Discuss them with your peers—if you have difficulty with any of the questions, consult your instructor.

Recall Jeannette Wu, a very thin 80-year-old woman who has just been admitted to a skilled nursing facility after fracturing her hip. Review the Meet Your Patients scenario at the beginning of this chapter to answer the following questions about Mrs. Wu.

THINKING

1. *Theoretical Knowledge:*
   a. What facts and principles do you already know about the causes of pressure ulcers?
   b. Do you have enough information to provide interventions for Mrs. Wu's actual Impaired Skin Integrity? If not, what do you still need to find out?
2. *Critical Thinking (Inquiry):* What resource would be best to use to find out exactly what is meant by Mrs. Wu's diagnosis of Self-Care Deficit? Why?

DOING

3. *Practical Knowledge:* What do you know about positioning patients? How would you explain to the NAP about how to position Mrs. Wu "to prevent further pressure on her sacrum"?
4. *Nursing Process (Evaluation):*
   a. To evaluate Mrs. Wu's Impaired Skin Integrity problem, what reassessments would you make?
   b. To evaluate Mrs. Wu's Self-Care Deficit problem, what reassessments would you make? Who can or should make them? How often, or when, would you reassess?

CARING

5. *Self-Knowledge:* How comfortable would you be caring for Mrs. Wu, who is a frail older adult? What is one problem, not described in the scenario, that might arise?

Go to Chapter 7, **Clinical Reasoning: Applying the Full-Spectrum Nursing Model Response Sheet** on Davis*Plus.*

To explore learning resources for this chapter,

Go to Davis*Plus* at http://www.Davisplus.fadavis.com, **keyword Treas.**

Chapter Resources for Chapter 7

    Knowledge Check and Think Like a Nurse Response Sheets

    Knowledge Check Answers

    Resources for Caregivers and Health Professionals

    Reading More About Implementing & Evaluating (Suggested Readings)

    What Are the Main Points in This Chapter?

NCLEX-Style Review Questions

Chapter Overview Podcasts

Concept Map

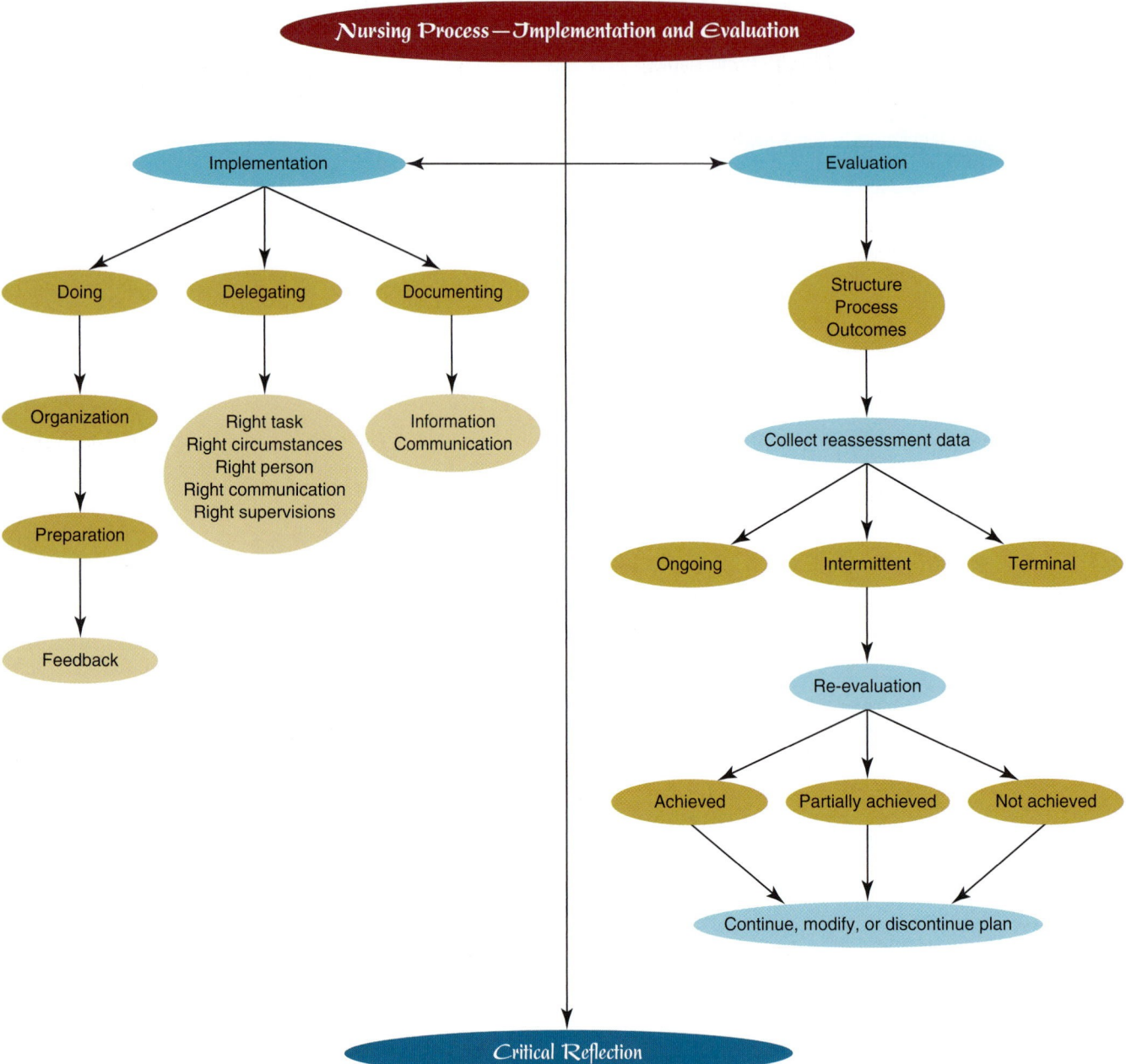

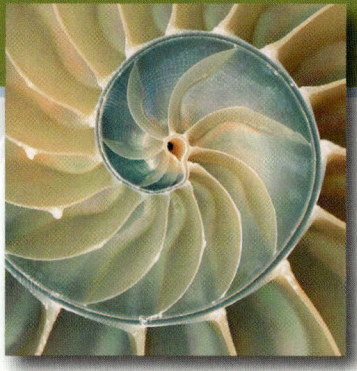

8

Theory, Research, & Evidence-Based Practice

Learning Outcomes

After completing this chapter, you should be able to:

➤ Define *nursing theory*.

➤ List four components of a theory.

➤ Describe how a nursing theory is developed.

➤ List the four essential concepts in a nursing theory.

➤ List three ways that nurses can use nursing theory.

➤ Name three predominant thinkers who proposed theories of caring.

➤ Describe three non-nursing theories and their contributions to nursing.

➤ Describe the significance of evidence-based nursing practice.

➤ Compare and contrast quantitative and qualitative nursing research.

➤ List three components of the research process, and explain their importance.

➤ Name three priorities in the process of protecting research participants.

➤ Describe the PICO method of formulating a question to guide a literature search.

➤ Discuss the process of analytic reading of research reports, and explain their significance to the appraisal of research.

➤ Describe how to use nursing research in nursing practice.

Key Concepts

Evidence-based practice

Nursing research

Nursing theory

Theory

Related Concepts

See the Concept Map at the end of this chapter.

Caring for the Nguyens

This feature allows you to practice the kind of thinking you will use as a full-spectrum nurse. There is usually more than one correct answer to a critical thinking question, so we do not provide answers for these features. It is more important to develop your nursing judgment than to "cover content." Discuss the questions with your peers. If you are still unsure, consult your instructor.

Mr. Nguyen arrives at the clinic for a follow-up visit. As you may recall, he has been diagnosed with hypertension. At a previous visit, you wrote a nursing diagnosis of Imbalanced Nutrition: More Than Body Requirements related to inappropriate food choices and serving size, as evidenced by a body mass index (BMI) of 28.5.

Today you have gathered the following intake data:

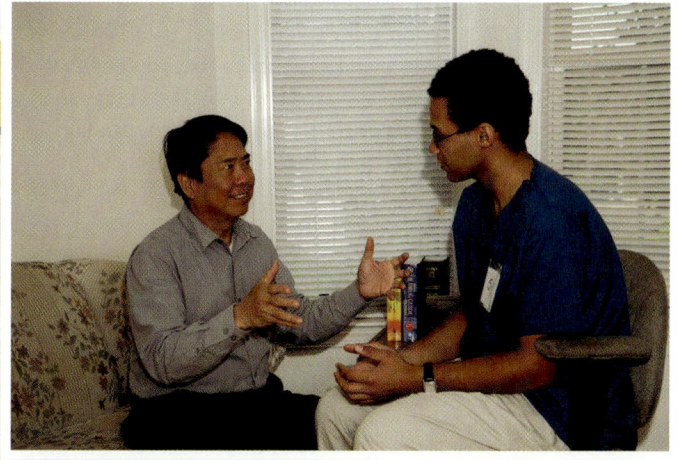

Blood pressure: 174/96 mm Hg
Heart rate: 88 beats/min
Respiratory rate: 18 breaths/min
Temperature: 98.5°F
Weight: 175 lb

(Continued)

Caring for the Nguyens (continued)

A. What observations can you make about today's data in comparison to his initial visit?

B. As part of the treatment plan for Mr. Nguyen, you have been asked to educate him about a diet to assist with weight loss and hypertension management. How would you determine the most appropriate diet to include in your treatment plan?

C. A number of sources recommend the DASH (Dietary Approaches to Stop Hypertension) eating plan. Go to the Internet and search for "Dietary Approaches to Stop Hypertension." Is there sufficient research to support incorporating this information into Mr. Nguyen's treatment plan? If so, describe the research and summarize the DASH eating plan.

 Go to **Caring for the Nguyens Response Sheet** on *DavisPlus*.

Meet Your Patient

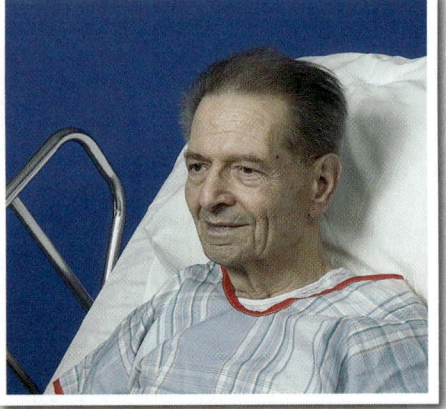

Imagine you are the charge nurse on the night shift at a long-term care facility. You hear the certified nursing assistant (CNA) and another person speaking loudly down the hall. You immediately go to see what has happened. You are surprised and shocked by what you see. An older patient, Mr. Wilkey, is sitting on the bed of another patient, Mrs. Fredrickson, who is crying and shouting, "Get out! Get out!" Mr. Wilkey is tearful and looks frightened. He keeps repeating, "Where is Momma? Where is Momma?" The CNA is visibly upset and is grabbing at Mr. Wilkey in an effort to get him off the bed.

What are you going to do, and why do you think it will help? Don't be concerned if you don't think you know enough to answer this question. Before you read on, try to answer it based on the knowledge and experience that you *do* have.

There are two general ways to approach this problem. One way is to be upset with Mr. Wilkey and escort him from the room immediately, explaining sternly that his behavior is not acceptable and he must stay in his own room. Another possibility is to ask the CNA to calm Mrs. Fredrickson while you talk quietly to Mr. Wilkey and gently guide him out of the room, not rushing him. While you are talking to him, you might ask, "Who is Momma? What does she look like? Do you miss her?" By the time you lead him to his room, you might realize he is exhibiting stage 2 dementia. You infer that he probably woke up scared and confused and began looking for his long-dead mother. Seeing Mrs. Fredrickson, Mr. Wilkey thought he had found his mother and crawled into her bed.

If you chose the first approach in the scenario, you were demonstrating **mechanistic nursing,** which is based on getting tasks done. If you chose the second solution, you based your behavior on **holistic nursing,** which requires meeting the needs of the whole person. This scenario demonstrates the powerful impact of nursing theory and research on your daily practice as a nurse.

Theoretical Knowledge
knowing why

ABOUT THE KEY CONCEPTS

The overall goal of this chapter is that you will understand the concepts of *nursing theory, nursing research,* and *evidence-based practice* well enough to see how they are related and how they form the foundations for patient care.

Think of full-spectrum nursing as a jigsaw puzzle (Fig. 8-1). Initially, a nurse has an idea, which usually comes out of experiences in *practice* (the first puzzle piece). Perhaps the idea is something simple, such as "Why don't I slow down and spend more time with the patients' families? It would really help them if I took more time." After seriously considering the new idea, the nurse may decide the idea is worth investigating with *research* (the second puzzle piece). The research question might be, "How does spending more time with family members affect the quality of care the patient receives?" If the research supported the nurse's idea, she could then use the research findings to develop a *theory* (the third puzzle piece). The nurse might even take the research results to nursing administrators to determine whether the theory could be put into practice in the organization—perhaps as a policy or in a standardized care plan. That would be the beginning of what is called a **clinical practice theory,** a theory that is immediately applicable in the clinical setting.

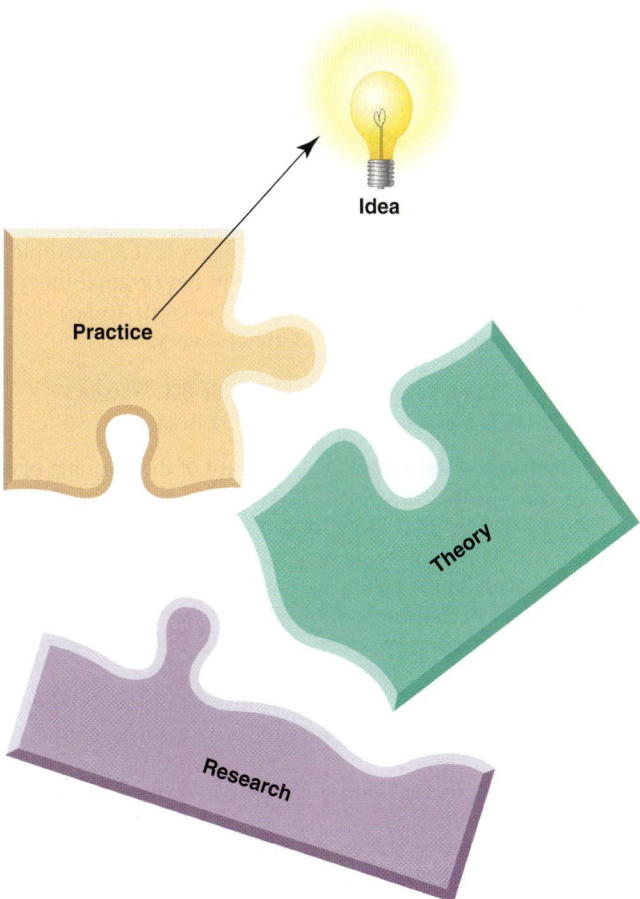

FIGURE 8-1 Practice, theory, and research are interrelated: A nurse has an idea, conducts research to test the idea, and finally develops a theory.

You will also need a grasp of a related concept, *caring*. Although there are several theories that guide nursing practice, this chapter draws heavily on theories of caring to illustrate key points. We believe caring is central to nursing and influences all the actions that nurses take. You may recall that it is an important concept in the full-spectrum model introduced in Chapter 2. You will find other theories that pertain to specific aspects of practice in later chapters. For example, developmental theories are discussed in Chapter 9, theories of self-concept in Chapter 13, and family theories in Chapter 14.

THE IMPORTANCE OF NURSING THEORY AND RESEARCH

Following are three classic examples that demonstrate how important theory and research are to you in your career as a nurse.

The Framingham Studies. The Framingham studies are a longitudinal, multidisciplinary research project (*longitudinal* means done over a long period of time). It consisted of several studies carried out over 50 years (from 1948 to 1998) to identify the health and healthcare practices of one community: Framingham, Massachusetts. The results of the various Framingham studies have influenced healthcare practices for diabetes mellitus, breast cancer, heart disease, osteoarthritis in older adults, and other disease entities. For example, one

commonly accepted practice that came out of the Framingham study is the use of mammography to screen for breast cancer. There was a time when mammography was considered unreliable and unimportant. The Framingham project changed that attitude and, as a result, improved the healthcare of women (National Heart, Lung, and Blood Institute & Boston University [n.d.]).

Watson's Science of Human Caring. Dr. Jean Watson's theory (1988) describes what *caring* means from a nursing perspective. It may not seem that nurses need to be taught how to care, but Dr. Watson and other nursing theorists found that they did. Before the so-called caring theorists, nurses were somewhat mechanistic in the work they did, much like the first alternative for dealing with Mr. Wilkey (Meet Your Patient). A mechanistic nurse has a list of things to do, completes the list, and does nothing more. The "something more" behaviors often are the caring behaviors, such as singing to a frightened child or taking the time to teach a new mother for the second time how to bathe her baby.

This is not to say that nurses didn't care about their patients before Watson. The point is that a *theory* can change the *focus* of nursing. Certainly Nightingale must have cared about the soldiers who were her patients. But what she wrote about and what she taught the nurses was a set of things to do. Nurses were valued for the tasks they performed in patient care. Caring theories demonstrate the value of the non–task-oriented aspects of nursing.

Benner's "Novice to Expert." Dr. Patricia Benner, in the book *From Novice to Expert* (1984), proposed a theory that should be of special interest to you. This theory, which was explained in Chapter 1, describes the progression of a beginning nurse to increasing levels of expertise. You are a **novice**, or a beginning nurse, simply because you are new to the nursing profession. Benner's theory provides the information necessary to understand how you learn and perform your nursing responsibilities. Benner's theory of caring is discussed later in this chapter.

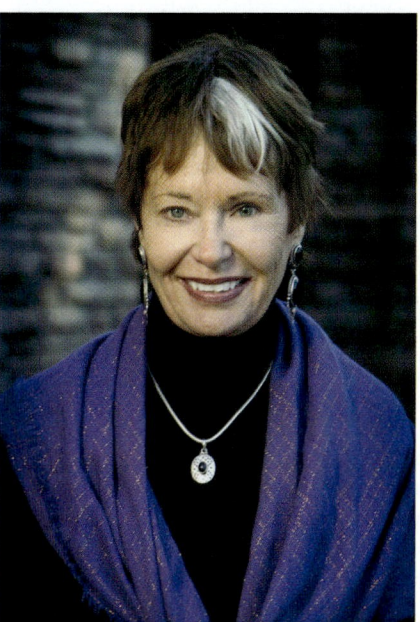

FIGURE 8-2 Dr. Jean Watson, distinguished professor and nursing theorist.

KnowledgeCheck 8-1

- Compare mechanistic and holistic nursing. Select one of these concepts and describe a scenario in which it is used.
- Briefly describe the Framingham studies, and list three diseases for which these studies influenced care.

NURSING THEORIES

Florence Nightingale (1859, 1992) stated that nursing theories describe and explain what is and what is not nursing. That makes them critical for you to learn about. Before focusing on nursing theory, though, you need to learn a little more about theory in general. Exactly what *is* a theory? And how is a theory created?

A **theory** is an organized set of related ideas and concepts that helps us:

- Find meaning in our experiences (such as nursing)
- Organize our thinking around an idea (such as caring)
- Develop new ideas and insights into the work we do.

Put simply, a theory answers the questions *What is this? And how does it work?* Although a theory is based on observations of facts, the theory itself is *not* a fact. A theory is merely a way of viewing phenomena (reality); it defines and illustrates concepts and explains how they are related or linked. Theories can be, and are, changed.

What Are the Components of a Theory?

Theories are made up of assumptions, phenomena, concepts, definitions, and statements (or propositions). You can think of these as the building blocks of a theory.

Assumptions. Ideas that we take for granted are called **assumptions.** In a theory, they are the ideas that the theorist or researcher presumes to be true and does not intend to test with research. For example, Watson assumed nursing had its own professional concepts and that one of them was caring. Assumptions may or may not be stated. For example, most nursing theorists assume but do not state that human beings are complex.

Phenomena. Aspects of reality that you can observe and experience are called **phenomena.** Phenomena are the subject matter of a discipline (in that context, they are often called *phenomena of concern*). Think of phenomena as marking the boundaries (*domain*) of a discipline—making one discipline unique from another. For example, for pharmacists, the phenomena of concern are medications: their chemical composition and their effects on the body. For nurses, the phenomena of concern are human beings and, more specifically, their body-mind-spirit responses to illness and injuries. It may seem a subtle difference, but Watson's theory of caring gave us the words and ideas for describing the nursing phenomena of concern in terms of *human beings in their environments.*

Concepts. A **concept** is a mental image of a phenomenon. It is formed by generalizing an abstract idea from your experiences and observations of events, objects, and properties, and it exists as a symbol (e.g., a word or picture) in your mind. For example, what does the word *fever* bring to mind? From your own experience with fever, you know the subjective feeling that fever produces. You have the theoretical knowledge that it is an elevated body temperature; you know the physiology of temperature regulation, so you know what is going on in the body. You may have the visual image of a thermometer or someone who is warm to the touch and possibly perspiring. The word *fever* is a symbol for all of those ideas and images. It is a concept.

Concepts range from simple to complex and from fairly concrete to very abstract. Simple, concrete concepts are those you can observe directly (e.g., height, weight, gender, body type). More abstract and complex concepts are those you observe indirectly (e.g., hematocrit, brain activity, nutritional status). Abstract concepts are those you must infer from many direct and indirect observations (e.g., self-esteem, wellness).

A theory usually contains several concepts. For example, Watson includes 10 "caring processes" in her original theory (Box 8-1). Each of those is a complex concept. To see how those caring factors have evolved in her theory,

 Go to **Tables, Boxes, Figures: ESG Table 8-1, Watson's Caritas Processes,** in Chapter 8 on DavisPlus.

Definitions. A **definition** is a statement of the meaning of a term or concept that sets forth the concept's characteristics or indicators—that is, the things that allow you to identify the concept. A definition may be general or specific. A **theoretical definition** refers to the conceptual meaning of a term, whereas an **operational definition** specifies how you would observe or measure the concept (e.g., when doing research). For example, for pain:

Theoretical definition: Pain is an unpleasant sensory and emotional experience associated with actual or potential tissue damage.

Operational definition: Pain is the patient's verbal statement that he is in pain.

Statements (Propositions). **Statements,** or **propositions,** systematically describe the linkages and interactions among the concepts of a theory. The statements, taken as a whole, make up the theory. In Maslow's theory, for example, two concepts are *physiological needs* and *self-esteem needs.* An example of a statement in that theory would be: "*Physiological needs* must be met to an acceptable degree before a person can attempt to meet his *self-esteem needs.*"

Theory, Framework, Model, or Paradigm?

In any discussion of nursing knowledge, you may hear the terms *theory, framework, model,* or *paradigm.* It may be difficult to differentiate among these terms because (1) they are so abstract,

---

BOX 8-1 ■ Watson's Ten Caring Processes

1. Forming a humanistic–altruistic system of values
2. Instilling faith and hope
3. Cultivating sensitivity to self and others
4. Forming helping and trusting relationships
5. Conveying and accepting the expression of positive and negative feelings
6. Systematically using the scientific problem-solving method that involves caring process
7. Promoting transpersonal teaching–learning
8. Providing for supportive; protective; and corrective mental, physical, sociocultural, and spiritual environment
9. Assisting with gratification of human needs
10. Sensitivity to existential–phenomenological forces

Source: Watson, J. (1988). *Nursing: Human science and human care. A theory of nursing.* Publication No. 15-2236. New York: National League for Nursing Press.

(2) they are defined differently by theorists, and (3) they are often used interchangeably in general conversation among nurses. As you progress in your career and education, you will need to pay careful attention to the similarities and differences among these terms. The following are some basic definitions:

A **paradigm** is the worldview or ideology of a discipline. It is the broadest, most global conceptual framework of a discipline. For example, the medical paradigm views a person through a lens that focuses on identifying and treating disease. This lens causes you to look in depth at the person's "parts" (e.g., cells, organs). The nursing paradigm views the person through a lens that focuses more broadly on the entire person and how he responds to isolated changes in his cells and organs. Paradigms are not theories; they are just "how we see things."

A **conceptual framework** (also referred to as a *theoretical framework*) is a set of concepts that are related to form a whole or pattern. As a rule, frameworks are not developed using research processes and have not been tested in practice. Frameworks and models are broader and more philosophical than theories. Don't be alarmed if you can't tell the difference between a theory and a theoretical framework. Experts don't always agree, either. Many theorists, for example, classify the early nursing theories (e.g., Orem's self-care deficit theory and others presented in this chapter) as conceptual frameworks; others classify them as theories.

A **model** is a symbolic representation of a framework or concepts—a diagram, graph, picture, drawing, or physical model. The plastic body parts you have seen in anatomy class are models of the real human body; and Figure 8-1 is a model of the relationships between nursing practice, theory, and research. Some models are more complex. A **conceptual model** (often used interchangeably with *conceptual framework*) is a model that is expressed in language—the symbols are words. In one sense, all models are "conceptual" because they all represent ideas. The full-spectrum model (see Fig. 2-3) is a conceptual model or framework.

For now, it is enough for you to remember that:

1. The terms *theory, model,* and *framework* all refer to a group of related concepts.

2. The terms differ in meaning, depending on the extent to which the set of concepts has been used and tested in practice and on the level of detail and organization of the concepts.

3. A theory has a higher level of research, detail, and organization of concepts than do models and frameworks.

KnowledgeCheck 8-2

- Name the five building blocks of a theory.
- How is a *paradigm* different from a *theory*?

How Are Theories Developed?

To begin developing a theory, a nurse has an idea that seems worth exploring through research. As an example, Dr. Jean Watson had an idea about caring behaviors toward patients. Once the idea was clear in her mind, she performed research to see whether her ideas made sense. She validated her ideas to develop her theory. Once she had a research-based theory, she shared it with others, and it changed nursing practice.

Theories are developed through a specific way of thinking called *logical reasoning* (Marriner-Tomey & Raile-Alligood, 2006). Generally, you can think of **reasoning** as connecting ideas in a way that makes sense. The purpose of **logical reasoning** is to develop an argument or statement based on evidence that will result in a logical conclusion. Nursing theories cannot be based on guesswork; they must be developed on a solid foundation of logical reasoning. The most commonly used types of logical reasoning are inductive and deductive reasoning.

Inductive reasoning is often used in the nursing process. If you walk into a person's room and note that the patient has a temperature of 101°F (38°C), a pulse of 104 beats/min, and respiration rate of 20 breaths/min, you could reasonably *induce* (conclude) that the person is ill. Induction moves from the specific to the general. You gathered separate pieces of information, recognized a pattern, and formed a generalization. Remember induction by thinking, "IN-duction: I have specific data 'out there,' and I bring it 'IN' to make the generalization." Refer to Figure 8-3.

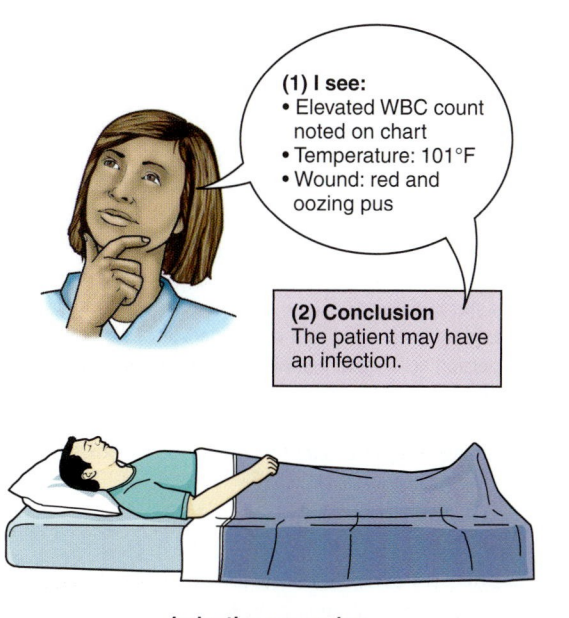

Inductive reasoning

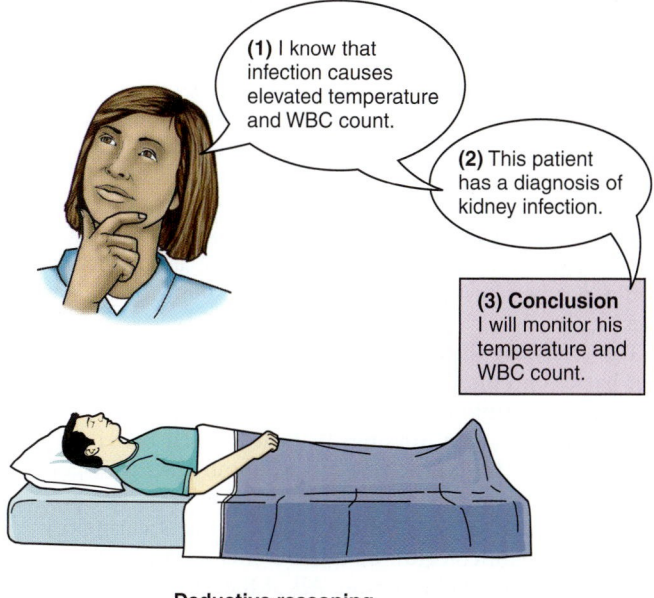

Deductive reasoning

FIGURE 8-3 A comparison of inductive and deductive reasoning. Theorists and nurses in practice use both types of reasoning.

Deductive reasoning is the opposite of inductive reasoning. Deduction starts with a *general premise* and moves to a *specific deduction*. Suppose you receive a call from the emergency department stating they will be admitting a new patient with acute pyelonephritis (kidney infection). Because you know what is involved in the general premise (pyelonephritis), you deduce the patient will probably have an elevated temperature and back pain. You have the "big picture" about what is true in general, and from that you can figure out logically what is likely to be true for a particular individual.

Understanding logical thinking, even on this basic level, will help you understand the thinking that goes into both nursing theory and nursing research.

✚ **Caution:** Induced and deduced conclusions are not facts. They may or may not accurately reflect reality.

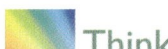 **ThinkLike a Nurse 8-1**

- Your patient is grimacing, groaning, and holding his hands over his abdominal incision. You induce that the patient is having incision pain. How could you be sure your induction is factual (true)?
- Earlier you deduced that your emergency department patient with pyelonephritis will have an elevated temperature and back pain. How confident are you that this is actually so? How could you be more certain your deduction is correct?

The preceding exercise should demonstrate that inductions and deductions are not "facts" or "truth," but rather that they point you in the direction to go in seeking truth (reality). They also allow you to make connections between ideas when you are developing a theory. The more information you have to support your conclusions, the more confident you can be that they are correct.

What Are the Essential Concepts of a Nursing Theory?

Any nursing theory should address four basic concepts: **person, environment, health,** and **nursing** (Yura & Torres, 1975). These concepts are said to represent phenomena of concern for nursing. Notice this further divides the puzzle piece for nursing theory into four more pieces (Fig. 8-4).

A meaningful nursing theory defines these four puzzle pieces and explains how they are related to each other. Consider a theory that does not include the concept of person. Such a theory would not deal with the person's reaction to her health or lack of health. As a result, the person's learning needs, fears, family concerns, or discharge arrangements would not be considered. That sounds quite mechanistic, doesn't it?

The following illustrates how Watson (1988) viewed the four basic concepts. In her science of human caring, she explored the concept of *caring* as it relates to the person, environment, health, and nursing. Watson focused heavily on the *person* and the *nurse*. She talked about the "transpersonal" caring moments that exist between the two. She presented the *environment* as another way to show caring: by keeping it clean, colorful, or quiet or including whatever promotes health for the person. All of the caring behaviors (see Box 8-1) listed in Watson's theory focus on improving the *health* of the person.

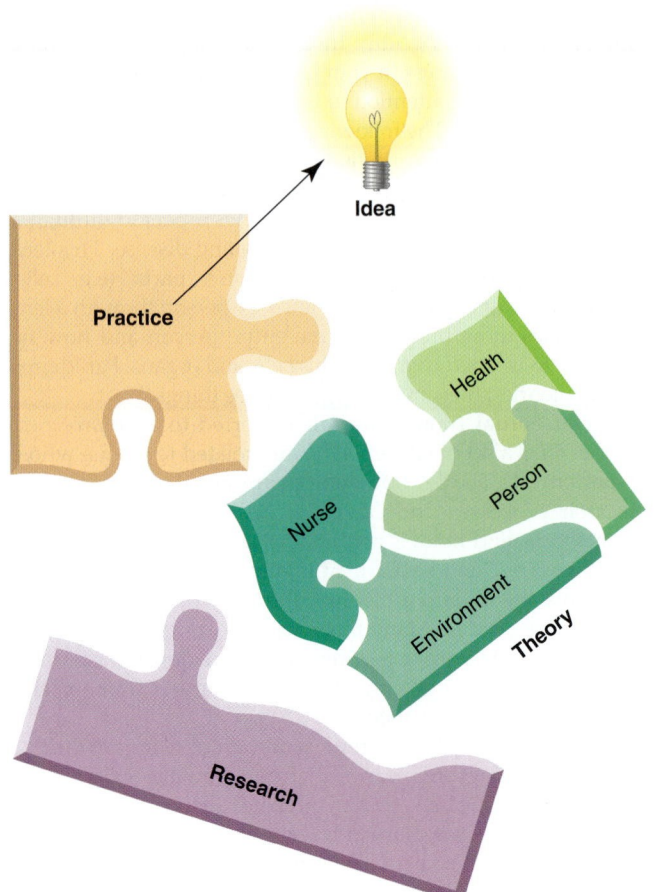

FIGURE 8-4 The four components of a nursing theory are person, nurse, health, and environment.

Observing nursing situations within the framework of the four components of nursing theory will help you understand the importance of each. This is very important because the finished puzzle reflects excellent (full-spectrum) nursing care.

 ThinkLike a Nurse 8-2

Think of an experience you have had in clinical. Perhaps it was taking vital signs or bathing a confused patient. Describe how each of the four components of a nursing theory occurred in your clinical situation. Share your thinking with a classmate or coworker.

- Who was the *person(s)* involved (*person* refers to the patient or resident or the family and support persons)?
- What was the *environment*? A community center? A bathing room in a nursing home? The person's bedside in a hospital?
- What was the *health* condition of the person? For example, was the person seeking information for self-care? Critical? In pain? Ready for discharge?
- How was *nursing* involved? For example, was the nurse compassionate? Angry? Efficient? A novice or an expert?

KnowledgeCheck 8-3

- What are the four essential concepts in a nursing theory?
- What is the title of Dr. Watson's theory?
- Caring processes are critical to her theory. What is the purpose of the caring processes?

How Do Nurses Use Theories?

Nursing theories try to describe, explain, and predict human behavior. The case of Mr. Wilkey (Meet Your Patient) shows how the use of a certain theory could guide the nurse to more compassionate care. Think of a theory as a lens. You can see the stars more clearly if you look at them through a telescope than you can by using binoculars. As another metaphor, the lens of your sunglasses removes glare, allowing you to see more clearly in bright sunlight but decreasing your ability to see in dim light. Theories offer a way of looking at nursing, and in this way they affect your entire perspective. The theory you use influences what you look for, what you notice, what you perceive as a problem, what outcomes you hope to achieve, and what interventions you will choose.

In Nursing Practice

Nursing theories serve as a guide for assessment, problem identification, and choosing nursing interventions. They help nurses communicate to others what it is that makes nurses unique and important to the interdisciplinary team.

Clinical practice theories very specifically guide what you do each day. They are limited in scope—that is, they do not attempt to explain all of nursing. A theory on human interaction directs nurse–client communication; another theory provides a guide for teaching people how to be self-reliant. The following are other examples:

1. Nightingale's theory emphasized the importance of the environment in the care of patients. Her work affected the design and building of hospitals for decades.
2. Dr. Imogene Rigdon developed a theory about bereavement of older women after noticing (and having an idea!) that older women handled grief differently from men and younger women (Rigdon, Clayton, & Dimond, 1987). Hospice organizations all over the country now use this theory to work with older women who have lost a significant other.
3. Nola Pender's theory (Pender, Murdaugh, & Parsons, 2006) on health promotion (see Chapter 27) is the basis for most health promotion teaching done by nurses.
4. Dr. Katharine Kolcaba (1994) developed a theory of holistic comfort in nursing, which provides a more holistic view than earlier theories of pain and anxiety.

In Nursing Education

Some schools of nursing use theories to guide curriculum planning, programs, and projects. These are frequently grand theories, such as Watson's theory of caring or Rogers's science of unitary human beings. A **grand theory** covers broad areas of concern within a discipline. A grand theory is usually abstract and does not outline specific nursing interventions. Instead, it tends to deal with the relationships among nurse, person, health, and environment.

A school using Watson's theory, for example, would include aspects of her theory in each class. A course might even be organized around the caring factors listed in Box 8-1. As another example, an in-service education director in a nursing home may choose a narrower and more specific theory (*midrange* or *practice theory*) of comfort, using it to create policies and procedures and design educational programs.

In Nursing Research

Theories help generate new knowledge by suggesting questions for researchers to study. Researchers also use theories and models as a framework for structuring a study. Theories provide a systematic way to define the questions to study, identify the variables to measure, and interpret the findings. For example, Kolcaba tested her statement that comfort interventions, as defined in her theory, would improve the health of the whole person.

Who Are Some Important Nurse Theorists?

You will need to thoroughly understand the theories you use in practice and the one (or more) used by your school of nursing. As an educated nurse, you should also have at least a nodding acquaintance with the nurse theorists who have influenced nursing practice. The following three theorists are presented in detail because of their historical significance. The description of their theories is simple and applicable to what you do every day as a nurse.

Florence Nightingale

As you learned in Chapter 1, Florence Nightingale revolutionized nursing. When she went to the British military hospital in Scutari during the Crimean War, the soldiers slept on mats on the floor, where rats scampered and raw sewage flowed. Nightingale's "idea" was that *more men would survive if they had a clean and healthy environment and nutritious food (so that the body could heal itself)*. That may not seem remarkable to you, but consider that the germ theory of infectious disease had not yet been identified.

Nightingale also was an outstanding researcher. She stayed awake late at night to keep records of what was happening at the Scutari hospital before and after she introduced her ideas (research). She used her research to develop her theory that a clean environment would improve the health of patients. Because of her theory and research, Nightingale dramatically reduced the death rate of the soldiers and changed the way the entire British Army hospital system was managed (Dossey, 1999). For links to more information about Nightingale,

 Go to Chapter 8, **Resources for Caregivers and Health Professionals,** on Davis*Plus.*

Virginia Henderson

Virginia Henderson began her career as a U.S. Army nurse in 1918. She also became a visiting nurse in New York City and then a teacher of nursing. Her pamphlet, *Basic Principles of Nursing Care,* was published by the International Council of Nursing in 1960 in 20 languages.

While a nursing student at Walter Reed Army Hospital, Henderson began to question the mechanistic nursing care she was taught to give, as well as the fact she was expected to be the physicians' handmaiden. As a teacher of nursing, she came to recognize there was no clear description of the purpose and function of nursing. She was the first nurse to identify that as a concern. Her "idea" was that *nurses deserve to know what it means to be a nurse.*

Henderson's 1966 book, *The Nature of Nursing,* described her theory of nursing's primary, unique function. She identified 14 basic needs that are addressed by nursing care (Box 8-2). Although the simple things on that list are commonplace today, they had not been identified as components of nursing care until Virginia Henderson did so. Henderson's (1966, p. 3) definition of nursing states that "the unique function of the nurse is to assist the individual, sick or well, in the performance of those activities contributing to health or its recovery (or to a peaceful death) that he would perform unaided if he had the necessary strength, will or knowledge. And do this in such a way as to help him gain independence as rapidly as possible."

BOX 8-2 ■ Virginia Henderson's List of Basic Needs

1. Breathe normally.
2. Eat and drink adequately.
3. Eliminate body wastes.
4. Move and maintain desirable posture.
5. Sleep and rest.
6. Select suitable clothes—dress and undress.
7. Maintain body temperature within normal range by adjusting clothing and modifying the environment.
8. Keep the body clean and well groomed, and protect the integument.
9. Avoid dangers in the environment and avoid injuring others.
10. Communicate with others in expressing emotions, needs, fears, or opinions.
11. Worship according to one's faith.
12. Work in such a way that there is a sense of accomplishment.
13. Play or participate in various forms of recreation.
14. Learn, discover, or satisfy the curiosity that leads to normal development and health and use of the available health facilities.

Source: Marriner-Tomey, A., & Raile-Alligood, M. (2006). *Nursing theorists and their work* (6th ed.). St. Louis, MO: C.V. Mosby.

Through her work, Henderson defined what nursing was in the 20th century. If you would like more information on Henderson,

 Go to Chapter 8, **Resources for Caregivers and Health Professionals,** on Davis*Plus.*

Hildegard Peplau

Hildegard E. Peplau was born in 1909 to immigrant parents in Pennsylvania. She was a psychiatric nurse who influenced the advancement of standards in nursing education, promoted self-regulation in nursing through credentialing, and was a strong advocate for advanced nursing practice.

Dr. Peplau's idea was that *health could be improved for psychiatric patients if there were a more effective way to communicate with them.* Again, you may feel this is an unnecessary theory because nurses communicate with patients all the time. But remember in the early 1900s, actually talking to and developing a personal relationship with psychiatric patients simply was not done. Psychiatric patients did not have the benefit of psychotropic drugs currently available to manage their symptoms. They were often agitated and extremely difficult to communicate with.

Peplau's research showed that developing a relationship with psychiatric patients does make their treatment more effective. She developed the theory of interpersonal relations, which focuses on the relationship a nurse has with the patient. This is a theory you use every day without even knowing it existed. For more information on Peplau's theory,

 Go to Chapter 8, **Supplemental Materials: Other Selected Nurse Theorists,** on Davis*Plus.*

The Caring Theorists

It could be argued that the three leading caring theorists in nursing are Dr. Jean Watson, Dr. Patricia Benner, and Dr. Madeleine Leininger. We have been using Watson's ideas to illustrate principles and concepts of theory. In this section, we discuss Benner and Leininger.

Patricia Benner

Caring is the central concept in Benner and Wrubel's *primacy of caring model.* The nurse's caring helps the client cope. Moreover, it offers opportunity for the nurse to connect with others and to receive as well as give help (Benner & Wrubel, 1989). Caring involves personal concern for persons, events, projects, and things. Therefore, it reveals what is stressful for a person (because if something does not matter to a person, it will not create stress) and provides motivation. Caring also makes the nurse notice which interventions are effective. This theory stresses that each person is unique, so that caring is always specific and relational for each nurse–person encounter.

In Chapter 1, we discussed another of Benner's theories. A critical care nurse, she wanted to find out *what makes an expert nurse.* In this case, the idea took the form of a question. An example of an expert nurse, for her, was an intensive care unit (ICU) nurse who knew intuitively when it was time to extubate a critical patient. Benner wanted to know what makes a nurse expert enough to know that and other critical information. She therefore interviewed ICU nurses and, from her data, identified five stages of knowledge development and acquisition of nursing skills. As you may recall, the first level is that of a novice nurse (you). The others are advanced beginner, competent, proficient, and expert nurse (see Chapter 1 if you need to review).

Let's see whether this novice-to-expert theory addresses the four components of a nursing theory. *Person* and *nurse* are very clearly points of focus. Knowing the *nurse's* skill level (novice, advanced beginner, competent, proficient, or expert) provides for an intelligent way to match the nurse's skill with the patient's (*person*) acuity. This is the basis of the theory. The theory also indicates that the nurse contributes to the person's *health* according to her skill level. The *environment* is clearly stated as the ICU. Benner's theory does meet the criteria of the four components of a theory, although some are emphasized more than others. Differences in emphasis are typical of theories, by the way.

Madeleine Leininger

Leininger is the founder of transcultural nursing and was the first nurse in the United States to earn a doctoral degree in cultural and social anthropology. Her theory focuses on caring as **cultural competence** (using knowledge of cultures and of nursing to provide culturally congruent and responsible care). Her idea came from working with children from diverse cultures who were under her care in a psychiatric hospital: *Would psychotherapy for children be more effective if delivered within the framework of the child's culture* (Marriner-Tomey & Raile-Alligood, 2006)?

Leininger performed the research to confirm her idea that culturally competent care made a difference, and then she developed her theory. She followed the pattern of the puzzle pieces referred to throughout this chapter. The *person* in Leininger's theory is an individual with cultural beliefs that are specific to herself and that may differ from the beliefs of others. All human beings can feel concern for others, but ways of caring vary across cultures. The *nurse* is the professional who values the cultural diversity of the person and is willing to make cultural accommodations for the health benefit of the person. This requires specialized cultural knowledge. The *environment* is wherever the *nurse*

and the *person* are together in the healthcare system. *Health* is defined by the *person* and may be culturally specific in its definition. You will learn more about Leininger's theory in Chapter 15.

You may be thinking, "This is all about culture; what does that have to do with caring?" Leininger's theory brings together the cultures of the *person*, the *nurse*, and the *health-care system* (indeed, there is a culture of healthcare, as you will discover in Chapter 15) to improve healthcare delivery and its effectiveness. For example, as a nurse, you may need to welcome the shaman from a Native American tribe who has been asked to perform a sacred dance in the hospital room. This is one way to demonstrate caring and respect for the person who is ill.

A nurse tells this true culture-care story. It is an example of applying a theory directly to the needs of an ill person:

As a young nurse, I was caring for a patient who was a monk. He had just had surgery, and he would not take any pain medication. He wanted to "offer the pain up to God." I believed the patient was jeopardizing his health, yet I did respect his right to live his cultural beliefs. We worked

out a compromise. The monk agreed to take pain medication every 8 hours (instead of the prescribed every 3 to 4 hours), and I made sure to attend to his ambulation, hygiene, and other needs during the times the medication was in effect.

Other Selected Nurse Theorists

You will find a list of selected nurse theorists and a brief description of their theories in Table 8-1. For a more complete discussion of those theories, you could go to the Web sites listed there, and

 Go to Chapter 8, **Supplemental Materials: Other Selected Nurse Theorists,** on Davis*Plus*.

Knowledge Check 8-4

Define in a brief conceptual form or title the nursing theory of each theorist listed below:
- Florence Nightingale
- Virginia Henderson
- Hildegard Peplau

Table 8-1 ➤ Selected Nurse Theorists		
THEORIST	**DATE**	**THEORY**
Peplau, Hildegard E.	1952	Interpersonal relations model: Interpersonal communication can improve mental health.
Henderson, Virginia	1955	14 basic needs addressed by nursing care; definition of nursing; do for the patient what he cannot do for himself.
Abdellah, Faye G.	1960	21 nursing problems; deliver care to the whole person.
Orlando, Ida Jean	1961	Interpersonal process; nursing process theory.
Wiedenbach, Ernestine	1964	The purpose of nursing is to support and meet patients' needs for help. Nursing is a helping art.
Levine, Myra	1967, 1973	Conservation model; designed to promote adaptation of the person while maintaining wholeness, or health.
Johnson, Dorothy	1968, 1980	The behavioral system model: Incorporates five principles of systems thinking to establish a balance or equilibrium (adaptation) in the person. The patient is a behavioral system consisting of subsystems.
Rogers, Martha	1970	The science of unitary human beings focuses on the betterment of humankind through new and innovative modalities. Maintaining an environment free of negative energy is important.
Orem, Dorothea	1971	The self-care deficit nursing theory explains what nursing care is required when people are not able to care for themselves. Goal is to help client attain total self-care.
King, Imogene	1971	First of two theories was the interacting systems framework, designed to explain the organized wholes within which nurses are expected to function, i.e., society, groups, and individuals. The first theory led to the theory of goal attainment, which focuses on mutual goal setting between a nurse and patient and the process for meeting the goals.
Neuman, Betty	1972	Neuman systems model is based on general system theory (a non-nursing theory) and reflects the nature of living organisms as open systems.
Roy, Sr. Callista	1974	Adaptation model was inspired by the strength and resiliency of children. The model relates to the choices that people make as they adapt to illness and wellness.

(Continued)

Table 8-1 ➤ Selected Nurse Theorists—cont'd		
THEORIST	DATE	THEORY
Leininger, Madeleine M.	1978, 1984	Cultural care diversity and universality theory. Caring theory.
Newman, Margaret	1979	Theory of health as expanding consciousness describes nursing intervention as nonintervention, in which the nurse's presence helps patients recognize their own pattern of interacting with the environment.
Watson, Jean	1979	Caring theory. Nursing is an interpersonal process.
Parse, Rosemarie Rizzo	1981	Theory of human becoming focuses on the human–universe–health process and knowledge related to human becoming (or reaching one's potential).
Benner, Patricia, and Wrubel, J.	1989	Primacy of caring model. Caring is central to the model and helps the client cope with stressors of illness.

For more information on these theorists,

 Go to Chapter 8, **Supplemental Materials,** on DavisPlus.

How Do Nurses Use Theories From Other Disciplines?

Theory development is relatively new in nursing. Except for Nightingale (1859, 1992), it was not until the mid-1950s that nursing leaders began to publish their theories about nursing. The profession relied heavily on the theories of other disciplines. Nurses still use knowledge from other disciplines as a part of their scientific knowledge base. The following are a few of the many "borrowed" theories you will use in nursing.

Maslow's Hierarchy of Basic Human Needs

One classic theory still used in most nursing education and practice settings is Maslow's hierarchy of needs (1970). Maslow observed that certain human needs are common to all people, but some needs are more basic than others. The lower-level (e.g., physiological) needs must be met to some degree before the higher needs (e.g., self-esteem) can be achieved (Fig. 8-5). For example, if you sit down to study but the room is cold, you will likely decide to put on a sweater or turn up the heat before opening your books. Nevertheless, a person may consciously choose to ignore a lower-level need in order to achieve a higher need. For example, the first responders at the World Trade Center on September 11, 2001, and volunteer disaster workers in Haiti after the 2010 earthquake ignored their need for safety and security to help others (transcendence of self). In daily life, most people are partially satisfied and partially unsatisfied at each level.

Everyone has a dominant need, but it varies among individuals. For example, a teenager may have a self-esteem need to be accepted by a group. A heroin addict needs to satisfy her cravings for heroin and will not worry much about being accepted by others.

Physiological Needs. Physiological needs, the most basic, are those that must be met to maintain life. They include the needs for food, air, water, temperature regulation, elimination, rest, sex, and physical activity. Most healthy adults meet their physiological needs through self-care. However, many of your nursing interventions will support patients' physiological needs.

Safety and Security Needs. The needs for safety and security are the next priority. Safety and security may refer to either physical or emotional needs. *Physical safety and security*

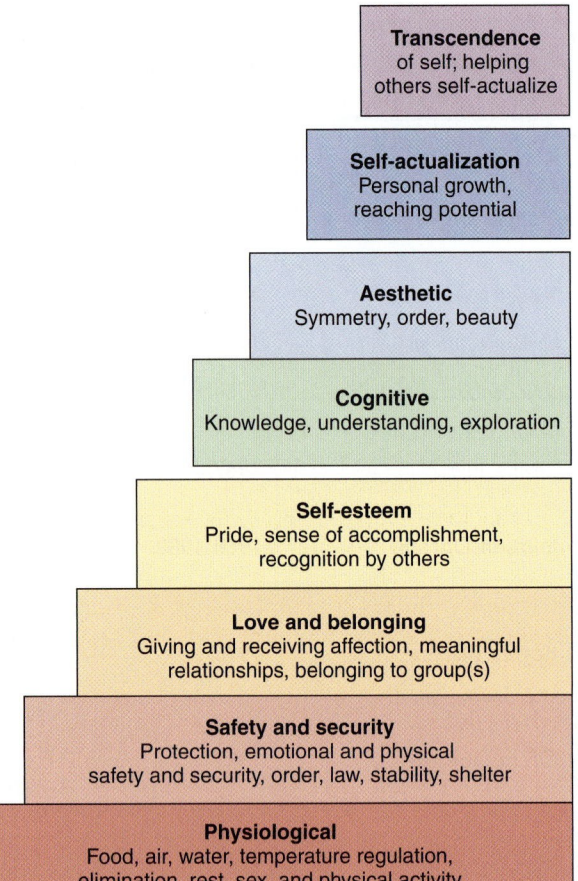

FIGURE 8-5 Maslow's hierarchy of human needs is a theory nurses use every day. (Sources: Adapted from Maslow, A. [1970]. *The farther reaches of human nature.* New York: Viking Press; and Maslow, A., & Lowery, R. [Eds.]. [1998]. *Toward a psychology of being* [3rd ed.]. New York: John Wiley & Sons.)

mean protection from physical harm (e.g., falls, infection, and effects of medications) and having adequate shelter (e.g., housing with sanitation, heat, and safety). *Emotional safety and security* involve freedom from fear and anxiety—feeling safe in the physical environment as well as in relationships.

We need the security of a home and family. If there is an abusive husband, for example, the wife will spend most of her time and energy trying not to trigger episodes of violence or abuse. This leaves little attention for meeting self-esteem and other higher needs.

Love and Belonging Needs. Needs for love and belonging are sometimes called social or affiliation needs. When they dominate, the person strives for meaningful relationships with others. Everyone has a basic need to love and be loved, give and receive affection, and have a feeling of belonging (e.g., in a family, peer group, or community). When these needs are not met, a person may feel isolated and lonely and may withdraw or become demanding and critical.

Self-Esteem Needs. People who have begun to satisfy their need to belong may begin to feel the need for self-esteem. Self-esteem comes through a sense of accomplishment and recognition from others and brings confidence and independence. As we discuss in Chapter 13, illness can affect self-esteem by causing role changes (e.g., inability to perform one's job), or a change of body image (e.g., loss of a body part). When recognition cannot be obtained through positive behaviors, the person may resort to disruptive or irresponsible actions.

Self-Actualization Needs. The highest level on Maslow's original hierarchy, self-actualization refers to the need to reach your full potential and to act unselfishly. At this level, a person develops wisdom and knows what to do in a variety of situations. Maslow studied self-actualized people to develop a list of their characteristics. To see this list,

 Go to Chapter 8, **Tables, Boxes, Figures: ESG Box 8-1,** on *DavisPlus.*

In his later work, Maslow identified two growth needs that must be met before reaching self-actualization (Maslow & Lowery, 1998):

1. *Cognitive needs* to know, understand, and explore
2. *Aesthetic needs* for symmetry, order, and beauty

Transcendence of Self. Later research led Maslow to identify another even higher need (Maslow, 1971): the need for *transcendence of self.* This is the drive to connect to something beyond one's self and to help others realize their potential. Some people include spirituality at this level, which is also the basis for acts of self-sacrifice (e.g., donating a kidney so that another person can live).

Applying Maslow's Theory. The following example illustrates how you might use Maslow's theory when teaching patients. Suppose you have been assigned to teach your patient, Mrs. Gallegos, about her colostomy before her discharge. Because she speaks little English, you put a great deal of effort into obtaining materials in her primary language, and you have arranged for an interpreter in case she has some questions you can't understand or answer. As you walk in the door to begin teaching, you immediately observe that Mrs. Gallegos seems to be in a great deal of pain. What will you do?

Maslow's hierarchy of needs tells you clearly that until the pain (a physiological need) is controlled, Mrs. Gallegos cannot learn. (Maslow considers pursuit of knowledge a self-actualization need.) You arrange for pain medication to be administered and reschedule the teaching session. If you went ahead with the teaching, the experience would be for the sole purpose of crossing it off your list (remember mechanistic nursing?) rather than actually teaching Mrs. Gallegos.

Validation Theory

Validation theory (Feil, 2003) arises from social work and provides for a way to communicate with older people with dementia. The theory asks the caregiver to *go where the demented person is in his own mind.* For example, Mr. Wilkey (Meet Your Patient) is talking about his mother, who has been dead for many years. Learning of his mother's death would be a shocking and traumatic experience, which he would relive each time he heard the news. So instead of telling him that she is dead, you would *go where Mr. Wilkey is in his own mind* by asking him, for example, about the color of his mother's eyes, what songs she sings to him, or other personal questions that will likely stimulate meaningful conversation about his mother.

Stress and Adaptation Theory

Hans Selye (1993) developed the stress and adaptation theory. There are many theories about stress, but Selye's was the forerunner of them all. His theory states that a certain amount of stress is good for people; it keeps them motivated and alert. However, too much stress, called *distress,* results in physiological symptoms and eventual illness. Does that happen to you at the end of the semester when you are distressed over the number of papers due and the difficulty of the tests for which you are studying? Generally the human body will respond to distress with an illness, such as a cold, that will force the body to slow down or simply go to bed. Selye's theory is discussed more in Chapter 12.

Developmental Theories

Developmental theories look at life stages that individuals, groups, families, and communities progress through over time. Several important examples include Erickson's psychosocial developmental theory (discussed in Chapter 9), theories of family development (discussed in Chapters 13 and 14), and Kohlberg's and Gilligan's theories of moral development (discussed in Chapters 9 and 42). These theories are useful in nursing practice because they identify norms and expectations at various stages in development and help you identify activities and interventions that are appropriate for your client.

System Theory

Ludwig von Bertalanffy created system theory in the 1940s (von Bertalanffy, 1976). He intended it to be abstract enough to use for theory and research in any discipline. Today the understanding of systems has evolved to the point that many of the concepts are a part of our everyday language (e.g., healthcare system, body systems, information systems, family systems).

One of the premises of systems theory is that all complex phenomena, regardless of their type, have some principles, laws, and organization in common. A **system** is made up of separate components (or **subsystems**), which constantly interact with each other and with other systems. For example, the cardiovascular and renal systems are subsystems of the body; the cells are subsystems of those systems. All of those systems and subsystems exchange processes and information with each other and with systems outside the body.

A system maintains some organization even though it is constantly facing internal and external changes. All systems have some common elements. The goal (function) of any system is to process **input** (the energy, information, or materials that enter the system) for use within the system or

in the **environment** (everything outside the system) or both. Other common elements include the following:

- **Output** is the product or service that results from the system's throughput. Examples of output are documents, money, nursing diagnoses, and cars.
- **Throughput** consists of the processes the system uses to convert input (raw materials) into output (products). Examples of throughput are thinking, planning, sorting, meeting in groups, sterilizing, hammering, and cutting.
- **Feedback** is information about some aspect of the processing that is used to monitor the system and make its performance more effective (e.g., evaluation in the nursing process: how the patient responded to the interventions).
- **Open systems** exchange information and energy freely with the environment. Open systems are capable of growth, development, and adaptation. Examples of open systems include people, body systems, hospitals, and businesses.
- **Closed systems** have fixed, automatic relationships among their components and little give-and-take with the environment. One example is a rock. A nursing example is a family that is isolated from the community and resists outside influences.

Several nursing theories have been built on system theory, for example, Johnson's (1968, 1980) behavioral system model, King's (1971) interacting systems framework, and the Neuman systems model (Neuman & Young, 1972), to name a few. If you need information about these theorists,

 Go to Chapter 8, **Supplemental Materials: Other Selected Nurse Theorists,** on Davis*Plus*.

KnowledgeCheck 8-5

- Name four theories that nurses "borrow" from other disciplines.
- What are the five original levels of Maslow's basic human needs (not including cognitive needs, aesthetic needs, and transcendence)?

PracticalKnowledge
knowing **how**

Practical knowledge about theory means using theories to guide you in your use of the nursing process. Recall the lens metaphor. In the assessment step of the nursing process, your theory concepts and principles tell you what to assess and provide the rationale for the assessments. Its major concepts serve as categories for organizing the data. In the diagnosis step, your theory guides you in defining patient problems; in fact, it determines whether you will even recognize a cluster of cues as a problem. The theory helps you to generate appropriate, achievable client outcomes; to choose effective nursing interventions; and to provide rationales for your actions.

There is no reason to read about theory unless you can apply the information. To show you how, this section applies caring theory to the planning of nursing interventions. Of course, you can use *any* theory for this purpose. We use caring theory because of the powerful and positive impact it can have on your nursing care. In reading this chapter, you should have become familiar with two well-known caring theories. Test your recall by writing the theorists' names and basic ideas. If you have difficulty, be sure to review the information about caring theorists before proceeding.

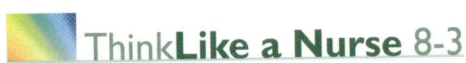

ThinkLike a Nurse 8-3

Write a paragraph describing a clinical experience in which you applied or observed one or both of the caring theories. Record your thinking on a piece of paper, and be prepared to share it with your classmates. You may title it "My Experience in Caring."

Planning Theory-Based Interventions/Implementation

The Nursing Interventions Classification, or NIC (Bulechek, Butcher, & Dochterman, 2008), introduced in Chapter 6, is theory development in an early stage. Each of the standardized intervention labels (e.g., Exercise Promotion, Infection Control) is a concept, and defining or describing concepts is an important step in theory development. In this section, we use nine key concepts of Watson's caring theory to describe how a theory influences your choice of nursing activities and approaches.

1. **Holistic Nursing Care.** Holistic nursing care allows nurses to examine the complete person and his context when making healthcare decisions. It goes beyond just giving the medication or dressing a wound. Physical care is important, but try to see nursing as giving care to the entire person and all that this entails (e.g., family, friends, fears, cultural beliefs).

2. **Honoring Personhood.** The three caring theorists believe the patient is someone who deserves to be honored for individuality in behavior as well as needs. If you accept that belief, you will learn the names of the people in your care and will refer to them by name instead of "Room 331," or "the kidney infection down the hall." Honoring personhood requires you to control the fast pace of nursing and take time with your patients. You need to look at, talk to, and touch the person to understand his personhood.

3. **Transpersonal Caring Moments.** The concept of transpersonal caring is a moral ideal rather than a task-oriented behavior. Such moments occur when an actual caring occasion or caring relationship exists between the nurse and the person. This can be a challenge! The current healthcare environment moves people rapidly through the system. How can you find the time to develop authentic caring relationships? The first step is to make a commitment to be a caring nurse: to go to work with the thought, "Today I will be authentic (genuine, real) with the people in my care." Or you might think, "I will focus on creating transpersonal caring moments instead of rushed and harried interactions." As a student, you might think, "Today I will practice changing dressings or starting intravenous solutions." However, developing the ability to have transpersonal caring moments is just as important. Think back to Mr. Wilkey at the beginning of the chapter. Where did opportunities arise for transpersonal caring moments with him?

4. **Personal Presence.** Another phrase for being authentic and in the moment is *personal presence.* The concept of presence suggests that you, the nurse, are emotionally and physically *with* the person for the time you are there. You are not thinking about a medication you need to give or medical orders you need to get. If the person in the bed is fearful, you should be fully present, recognize the fear, and support the person experiencing it. Your support may take the form of answering simple questions or providing more in-depth

education. It may simply be staying with the person for 2 or 3 minutes while quietly listening and holding her hand. As your psychomotor and nursing process skills become second nature to you, you will find it easier to remain in the moment.

5. **Comfort.** Some nurses think of comfort as the relief of pain, but it is much more. In Kolcaba's (1994) theory, comfort occurs in four contexts: physical, psychospiritual, social, and environmental. For example, is the person comfortable with you as the caregiver? Some women, especially from Middle Eastern or Asian cultures, are uncomfortable with male nurses as their caregivers. You must know and respect the person's cultural values. Other questions to consider for a complex picture of comfort are whether
   - the patient's modesty is being respected
   - there is too much or too little environmental stimuli
   - the room temperature is neither too cold or too warm
   - the patient needs more rest periods in order to heal
   - the patient needs someone to spend a transpersonal caring moment with him so he can express fears and anxiety.

6. **Listening.** Listening requires you to quiet your mind and truly listen with your mind and heart. The caring theorists also talk about listening from within yourself. Some call that *intuition*. Benner believes it is intuition that allows nurses to advance to expert-level practice.

7. **Spiritual Care.** Spiritual care is a critical aspect of holistic nursing care. You need to know what an individual's spiritual needs are and make appropriate plans to meet them. If the person does not want to talk about or deal with her spirituality, you will listen and follow her instructions. However, generally the opposite is true. People who are ill often want to talk about their spiritual needs, but they may be uncomfortable doing so. Helping someone to meet spiritual needs may be as simple as offering to call a clergy member or praying with the person who is sick. Chapter 16 provides more information about spiritual care.

8. **Caring for the Family.** Nurses who base their practice on caring theories recognize the importance of including the family of the person who is receiving care. Nontraditional family structure (e.g., a same-sex couple, a polygamist family) is not a reason to withdraw support, even if it conflicts with your values. What about an older family member with dementia? This person deserves to know what is happening to his loved one even though he most likely will forget the information. If he does forget, patiently repeat what he needs to know. You will find more information about family care in Chapter 14.

9. **Cultural Competence.** This was discussed in the explanation of Leininger's cultural care theory. Also see Chapter 15 if you want more information.

Do you see the value of each of these nine abstract concepts? From them flow very real, concrete nursing actions that make a difference in the lives of patients. Theory is not just "pie in the sky." Understanding nursing theories and applying them throughout your career are essential to full-spectrum nursing care. To perform the essential clinical tasks of nursing within the framework of caring is the highest possible performance of the profession.

KnowledgeCheck 8-6

List and explain three ways to incorporate caring theory into your nursing care.

NURSING RESEARCH

You now have a good beginning (novice) grasp of the concepts in nursing theory. Remember the puzzle pieces (see Fig. 8-2)? A nurse has an idea, does research to determine whether the idea is a valid one, and then develops a nursing theory. It is now time to study the research piece of the puzzle.

TheoreticalKnowledge
knowing **why**

Many people, including some nurses, do not realize that nurses do research. They think of nurses as people who work in hospitals, wear scrubs, and carry a stethoscope in their pocket. Were you aware of the research done in the field of caring before reading this chapter? Most novice nurses would not be. Remember the Framingham studies, which changed medical and nursing practice? Had you heard of that before? To be an effective professional nurse in the 21st century, you need to understand the basic principles of nursing research and their powerful impact on healthcare and the nursing profession. This section of the chapter is designed to show you what research is and how to incorporate it into your practice.

Although there are many definitions of nursing research, this chapter defines **nursing research** as the systematic, objective process of analyzing phenomena of importance to nursing (Nieswiadomy, 2008). Its purpose is to develop knowledge about issues that are important in nursing. Nursing research encompasses all clinical practice arenas, nursing education, and nursing administration.

Nurse researchers currently are making important contributions to the evidence-based practice necessary for professional nursing. Consider this example: When you are in the clinical setting, you will notice that when a nurse discontinues an intravenous (IV) fluid infusion, she sometimes replaces it with a lock, or plug, to maintain a route for IV medications, even though the patient no longer needs the fluids. Not many years ago, she would periodically flush the plug with heparin to keep blood from clotting and blocking the IV catheter. But heparin is a drug, and it has side effects. Nurses and other professionals performed several studies to see whether saline (which has no side effects) would work just as well. Goode and others (1996) performed a meta-analysis of those studies showing that saline was indeed just as effective, and it is now the standard of care in most institutions. (A **meta-analysis** combines and analyzes the data from several different studies.)

Why Should I Learn About Research?

The best reason, of course, is that the ability to read and use nursing research enhances your ability to give quality patient care. Like theory, research affects you every day you are a nurse. Full-spectrum nurses participate in research by doing the following:

- Identifying ideas that should be examined through the research process
- Assisting in, designing, and/or performing research
- Using research as a basis for their practice

In fact, educational and practice standards require that you acquire a degree of research competence.

ANA Standards

The position of the American Nurses Association (ANA) is that all nurses share a commitment to the advancement and ethical conduct of nursing science (ANA, 1994). The following two items from the American Nurses Association (ANA, 2010) standards of practice include the ability to use research in planning care:

Standard 4, Planning—Measurement Criterion: The registered nurse integrates current scientific evidence, trends and research.

Standard 5, Implementation—The registered nurse utilizes evidence-based interventions and treatments specific to the diagnosis or problem.

The ANA Standards of Professional Performance include a separate research standard (Standard 9, Evidence-Based Practice and Research). Four criteria for it follow. The registered nurse:

- Utilizes current evidence-based nursing knowledge, including research findings, to guide practice decisions.
- Incorporates evidence when initiating changes in nursing practice.
- Participates, as appropriate to education level and position, in the formulation of evidence-based practice through research.
- Shares personal or third-party research findings with colleagues and peers.

Educational Competencies

Recall that the Quality and Safety Education for Nurses (QSEN) project has identified quality and safety competencies for nurses. One important competency is evidence based practice: the ability to "integrate the best available current evidence with clinical expertise and patient/family preferences and values for delivery of optimal healthcare" (Cronenwett, Sherwood, Barnsteiner, et al., 2007). To see a description of the knowledge, skills, and attitudes you need for achieving this competency,

 Go to the QSEN web site, at **http://www.qsen.org. ksas_prelicensure.php**

What Is the History of Nursing Research?

The records Florence Nightingale kept while nursing soldiers in the Crimea were the beginning of formalized nursing research. As she developed schools of nursing throughout Britain and the United States, Nightingale urged her students to do clinical research. Yet because she had passed on to them the authoritarian tradition of her time, they were usually not prepared to perform it. Authority-based education does not promote intellectual inquiry or critical thinking, two characteristics essential for research. This is one reason nursing research was slow to develop.

As baccalaureate, master's, and doctoral programs grew, so did the number and quality of research projects nurses performed. Nursing research is now supported by federal funds and private grants, and results are reported in a growing number of nursing (and other) research journals. Nurses present their research at national and international conferences and publish their results in national and international journals. The preparation of doctoral-level nurses with a strong background in research has enhanced the quality and diversity of nursing research.

How Are Priorities for Nursing Research Developed?

Nursing research provides evidence on which to base nursing care. Ideally, all nursing interventions should be validated through research to show their safety and effectiveness.

Professional organizations, such as the ANA and specialty organizations (e.g., the Oncology Nurses Association), have established research priorities that will assist nursing to build a strong knowledge base in areas of importance to society. Brockopp and Hastongs-Tolsma (2003) state that nursing research will continue to be focused on clinical issues. The National Institute of Nursing Research (NINR), a federally funded agency that is a part of the National Institutes of Health (NIH), periodically identifies research themes and priorities for funding (NINR, n. d., 2005, 2010). For more information about nursing research priorities,

 Go to Chapter 8, **Supplemental Materials: What Are the Priorities for Research in the 21st Century?** on Davis*Plus*.

KnowledgeCheck 8-7

- Define *nursing research*.
- According to the text, why has nursing research been slow to develop?

What Educational Preparation Does a Researcher Need?

At each level of educational preparation, nurses function in different roles in the research process.

Associate Degree and Diploma Nursing. At this educational level, there are four research roles you can fulfill. You can (1) be aware of the importance of research to evidence-based practice, (2) help identify problem areas in nursing, (3) help collect data with a more experienced nurse researcher, and (4) use evidence-based practice in planning nursing interventions.

Baccalaureate Degree in Nursing. If you are a baccalaureate-prepared nurse, you should be able to (1) critique research for application to clinical practice, (2) identify nursing research problems and help implement research studies, and (3) apply research findings to establish sound, evidence-based clinical practice.

Master's Degree in Nursing. Nurses with graduate degrees should be able to (1) analyze problems so that appropriately designed research can be used to solve the problem, (2) through clinical expertise, apply evidence-based practice to nursing care situations, (3) provide support to ongoing research projects, and (4) conduct research for the purpose of assuring quality nursing care.

Doctoral Degree in Nursing or Related Field. Doctorally prepared nurses are specifically educated to be nurse researchers. They are qualified to (1) conduct nursing research, (2) serve as leaders in applying research results to the clinical arena, and (3) develop ways to monitor the quality of nursing care being administered by nurses (adapted from ANA, 1981). In addition, they should disseminate their research findings via publications and conferences.

PracticalKnowledge
knowing **how**

No one expects you to have a sophisticated understanding of research at this point in your career. However, you do need some basic practical knowledge, including information about the scientific method, types of research design, the research process, how to find practice-related research articles, how to

identify researchable problems, and how to critique research reports.

How Do We Gain Knowledge?

Recall that in Chapter 2 you learned the different kinds of nursing knowledge: theoretical, practical, ethical, and self-knowledge. There are also various ways to *acquire* knowledge.

Trial and Error Plus Common Sense. Suppose a patient has been medicated but is still in pain. You might try repositioning him. If that doesn't help, you might try distraction, visualization techniques, and perhaps various other measures. If visualization provides some relief, you would probably try that technique first when a similar situation occurs with another patient.

Authority and Tradition. This means to rely on an expert or to do what has always been done. For the patient with unrelieved pain, this would mean you might ask a more experienced nurse what to do. Or you could consult a procedure manual.

Intuition and Inspiration. Intuition is a feeling about something—an inner sense. Nurses say, "I just had a feeling something was wrong with the patient, but I can't explain why." For the patient in pain, you might have a feeling that a complication was developing, that the pain was due to more than just ineffective pain medication. However, as a novice, you should always check with a more experienced nurse before acting on your intuition.

Logical Reasoning. Using your knowledge and the facts available, you form conclusions (refer to the section How Are Theories Developed?). For the patient in pain, you might think, "This man weighs 300 pounds, but I gave him only the standard dose of medication. Probably he needs a higher dose."

Scientific Method. Research uses the scientific method (or scientific inquiry). **Scientific method** is the process in which the researcher, through use of the senses, systematically collects observable, verifiable data to describe, explain, or predict events. The goals of scientific inquiry are to find solutions to problems and to develop explanations of the world (theories). The scientific method has two unique characteristics that the other ways of gaining knowledge do not:

1. *Objectivity*, or *self-correction.* This means the researcher uses techniques to keep her personal beliefs, values, and attitudes separate from the research process.
2. *The use of empirical data.* Researchers use their senses to gather empirical data through observation. They attempt to verify the information gathered through a variety of methods so that the research conclusions are based in reality rather than on the researcher's beliefs, biases, or hunches.

Box 8-3 summarizes the characteristics of the scientific method.

The scientific method makes use of a variety of procedures and study designs intended to help ensure that the data collected will be reliable, relevant, and unbiased. You should recognize the two major categories of research design: *quantitative* and *qualitative.* Each category has within it several specific types of research methodologies; however, for now you need to understand only the basic differences (Table 8-2). For an expanded discussion,

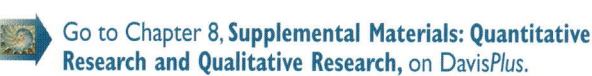

Go to Chapter 8, **Supplemental Materials: Quantitative Research and Qualitative Research,** on DavisPlus.

BOX 8-3 ■ Characteristics of the Scientific Method

Begins with an identified problem or need to be studied.
Uses theories, models, and conceptual themes that have been empirically tested.
Uses systematic, orderly methods to acquire empirical evidence to test theories.
Uses methods of control for ruling out other variables that might affect the relationships among the variables they are studying.
Avoids explanations that cannot be empirically tested.
Prefers to generalize the findings (knowledge) so that they can be applied in cases other than those in the study.
Uses built-in mechanisms for self-correction.

Source: Adapted from Wilson, H. S. (1993). *Introducing research in nursing* (2nd ed.). Redwood City, CA: Addison-Wesley Nursing.

Quantitative Research

The main purpose of **quantitative research** is to gather data from enough **subjects** (people being studied) to be able to generalize the results to a similar population. **Generalizing results** means that you think, "What I found to be so for this sample group of people will probably be the same for all people who are similar" (e.g., "My findings for *this* group of women over age 40 in the United States will probably be useful for *all* women over age 40 in the United States"). In quantitative research, researchers carefully control data collection and are careful to maintain the objectivity of the process. Quantitative data are reported as numbers. The Framingham studies are a classic example of a quantitative study—actually of several quantitative studies. To read more about this landmark research,

Go to http://www.framinghamheartstudy.org/about/index.html and http://www.framingham.com/heart/backgrnd.htm

Another classic example of quantitative nursing research is the Conduct and Utilization of Research in Nursing (CURN) project, which was intended to increase the use of research by direct-care nurses (Horsley, 1983). Many of the protocols (procedures) developed from these studies are used today with some modification. The following are some CURN protocol examples:

Clean intermittent catheterization
Intravenous cannula change
Distress reduction through sensory preparation
Preventing decubitus ulcers

Qualitative Research

Qualitative research focuses on the lived experience of people. The purpose is not to generalize the data, but to share the experience of the person or persons in the study. There is no need for large numbers. A case study of one person can examine the lived experience, for example, of a 19-year-old single mother of triplets or a middle-aged woman with HIV. Qualitative research uses words, quotations from persons interviewed, observations, and other nonnumeric sources of data. The Nun Study, a long-term, multidisciplinary project involving a convent of Catholic nuns in Minnesota, included some qualitative research (e.g., data obtained by interviews

Table 8-2 ➤ Comparison of Quantitative and Qualitative Research

	QUANTITATIVE RESEARCH	QUALITATIVE RESEARCH
Data	Numerical data, e.g., questionnaires, number of incidents, or reactions to a medication	Nonnumerical data; data may consist of words from interviews, observations, written documents, and even art or photos.
Persons Studied	Large numbers of *subjects* so it can be generalized to other similar populations	Often uses small numbers of *participants*; is not designed with the intent to generalize.
Hypothesis	Has a hypothesis.	No hypothesis, because it is the research of the "lived experience" of the person or persons being studied; study may be guided by research questions.
Environment	Can be in a laboratory setting; needs to be a controlled environment.	Is often done in the "natural" setting, i.e., the person's home or work setting.
Analysis	Objective data, tested with statistical methods	Subjective data; identifies themes; sometimes converted to numerical data (e.g., by counting categories).

and reported in the nuns' own words, and samples of writing from the nuns' diaries, reports, and letters). For more information about the Nun Study,

 Go to http://www.nunstudy.org and http://www.msnbc. msn.com/id/22361498/

KnowledgeCheck 8-8

- Define *quantitative research*. Name one study presented as an example in this chapter.
- Define *qualitative research*. Name one study presented as an example in this chapter.

What Are the Phases of the Research Process?

At the novice level, you will be using but not performing research. But in order to evaluate the research you read, you should have a general idea of the steps for conducting valid, reliable research. The research process is a problem-solving process, similar to but not the same as the nursing process. Different study designs require different steps, and you will find some variation in how different authors present the research process steps. However, in general, the steps include the following five phases (Fain, 2009):

1. Select and define the problem.
2. Select a research design.
3. Collect data.
4. Analyze data.
5. Use the research findings.

If you need a more detailed description of those phases,

 Go to Chapter 8, **Supplemental Materials, "What Are the Steps of the Research Process?"** on DavisPlus.

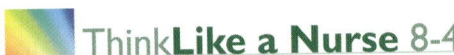 Think**Like a Nurse** 8-4

Take 10 minutes to sit quietly and think about nursing research. Do you have an idea or a problem you would like to see investigated with a research project? If nothing comes to mind quickly, then ponder for a few moments more. Write the information on a sheet of paper. Take the time to do your best

thinking. Then share what you have written with your instructor and other students.

- What would you like to have more information about in nursing? Explain why it is a problem or what brought about your idea.
- If you were the research assistant on a nursing research project on your topic, what one-sentence problem statement would you write regarding your research idea?
- What is the purpose of doing this research project? Why should it be done?

You may struggle with this assignment and wonder about its value to you, yet one of the most important things that nurses do is identify problems. Here is your chance to practice.

What Are the Rights of Research Participants?

Every nurse has a moral and legal responsibility to protect research participants from being harmed during the research process. Although research is crucial to the development of the profession, it should never be held in higher regard than the rights of the individuals being studied.

The current ethical standards for research, from all disciplines, are a direct result of the atrocities committed in the name of research in the German prison camps during World War II. After the trials for war crimes committed at that time, the Nuremberg Code was developed in 1949 to protect research participants from unethical behavior. The Nuremberg Code prompted many other codes and standards for performing ethical research (National Institutes of Health, n. d.). The U.S. government, through the Department of Health and Human Services (DHHS), has a complex set of standards that all researchers must follow.

Informed Consent

As a rule, **informed consent** must be obtained from every participant in a study. Consent is obtained by discussing what is expected of the participant, providing written information on the project to the participant, and obtaining the participant's written consent to be a subject. The following critical concepts are part of the informed consent.

- *Right to not be harmed*. The information given to the participant outlines the safety protocols of the study. If at any time

preliminary data indicate potential harm to the participant, the study must be stopped immediately.

- *Right to full disclosure.* Participants have a right to answers to such questions as: What is the purpose of this research? What risks are there? Are there any benefits? Will I be paid? What happens if I get sick or feel worse? Whom do I contact with questions and concerns?
- *Right to self-determination.* This refers to the right to say no. At any time in a study, the participant has the right to stop participating, for any reason. As the nurse, you are responsible for supporting a participant during the process of withdrawing from a study. Do not allow anyone to coerce the participant into remaining in the study.
- *Rights of privacy and confidentiality.* All research participants have the right to have their identity protected. Generally they are given a code number rather than being identified by name. Once the study is completed and the data are analyzed, the researcher is responsible for protecting the raw data (such as questionnaires and taped interviews).

Institutional Review Boards

The mechanism for overseeing the ethical standards established by the U.S. DHHS is the Institutional Review Board (IRB). Every federally funded hospital, university, or other healthcare facility has an IRB. It consists of healthcare professionals and people from the community who are willing to review and critique research proposals. The two main responsibilities of the IRB are (1) to protect the research participants from harm and (2) to ensure that the research is of value.

KnowledgeCheck 8-9

- List the phases of the research process.
- List four critical concepts that make up informed consent.

How Can I Base My Practice on the Best Evidence?

Recall from Chapter 6 that research provides the data for evidence-based practice. When there is a body of research on a topic, experts and professional groups evaluate the quality of the research reports and translate them into guidelines for practice. In your own evidence-based practice, you should use research findings and practice guidelines when they are available. When they are not, you will need to rely on the research reports themselves. Similar to the phases of research, the following process should assist you in finding the best evidence for your own interventions:

- Identify a clinical problem.
- Formulate a searchable question.
- Search the literature.
- Evaluate the quality of the research you find in the literature.
- Integrate your findings into your practice.

Identify a Clinical Nursing Problem

Even as a novice nurse, you should be prepared to identify clinical problems for research. Identifying a clinical nursing problem comes from being alert and interested in what you are doing each day in your clinical setting. How do you think the tympanic thermometer came into clinical use? Someone became frustrated with the discomfort patients experienced when temperatures were taken rectally. At the same time, there was a great deal of concern over the inaccuracy of axillary temperatures. Someone noticed the problem and wondered, "Is there a better way to do this?"

Common sources of clinical problems are experience, social issues, theories, ideas from others, and the nursing literature (Polit & Beck, 2007). Most of these sources are relevant whether you are identifying a problem for a research study or doing a literature search.

Experience. As you go about your work, you will notice interventions that may not be working or that require a great deal of effort for the minimal good they do. You will wonder, "How could we do this better?" Or you may notice that for clients with a particular health problem, the outcomes are often not good. You will wonder, "How could we improve the care so the patient's health improves?" Other questions might be, "Why do we do this procedure this way? "What do I need to know in order to plan new interventions for patients with this health problem?" If you are curious about why things are done and about what might happen if changes were made, you will find plenty of problems—for example, problems in staffing, equipment, nursing interventions, or coordination among health professionals.

Social Issues. You may be concerned about broader social issues that affect or require nursing care, such as issues of gender equity, sexual harassment, and domestic violence. You may be concerned about patients who do not have access to healthcare or about the health problems of a particular group or subculture.

Theories. Recall that theories must be tested in order to be useful in nursing practice. You might want to suggest research to test a theory you are interested in. If the theory is accurate, what behaviors would you expect to find, or what evidence would you need to support the theory?

Ideas From Others. Your instructor may suggest a topic to research, or perhaps you might brainstorm with nurses or other students. Agencies and organizations that fund research often ask for proposals on certain topics (e.g., the ANA and the National Institute of Nursing Research).

Nursing Literature. Read widely in your field of interest. You may identify clinical problems by reading articles and research reports in nursing journals. This may occur in one of the following ways:

- An article may stimulate your imagination and interest in a topic.
- You may notice a discrepancy in what staff nurses are doing and what the literature recommends.
- You may notice inconsistencies in the findings of two different studies on the same topic.
- You may read a study on a topic of interest to you (e.g., a technique for measuring blood pressure) and wonder whether the results would be the same if the study had been done in a different setting (e.g., a clinic instead of a hospital) or with a different population (e.g., healthy people instead of ill people).

Formulate a Searchable Question

When you have found a topic of interest, the next step is to state it in such a way that you can find it in the vast amount of nursing literature that is published. Stated too broadly, the search may yield thousands of irrelevant results. Stated too narrowly, you may get no results. Using the acronym PICOT enables you to search efficiently. The acronym stands for **P**atient or problem, **I**ntervention, **C**omparison interventions, **O**utcomes, and **T**ime. You may not always need a comparison intervention (C), or a time (T). See Box 8-4.

Search the Literature

Once you have stated your guiding question, the next step is to look for research articles related to the question (or problem statement). You may be thinking, "Where do I look for

BOX 8-4 ■ PICO Questions

	Sample Questions	Example
P—Patient population, or Problem	What is the medical diagnosis, nursing diagnosis, patient problem, symptom, situation, or need that requires an intervention? How would you describe a group of similar patients?	For patients with Impaired Skin Integrity (perineum) related to urinary incontinence
I—Intervention, treatment, cause, contributing factor	Which intervention are you considering? Specifically, what might help the problem (improve the situation, etc.)?	Would applying a barrier cream
C—Comparison intervention	What other interventions are being considered or used?	as compared to washing with soap and water, rinsing well, and air drying after incontinent episodes
O—Outcome	What effect could the intervention realistically have? What do you hope to achieve?	to prevent or achieve less perineal excoriation? Are there any expected undesired effects associated with the intervention?

Sources: University of Southern California, Health Sciences, Los Angeles. Evidence based decision making, asking a good question (PICO). Retrieved from www.usc.edu/hsc/ebnet/ebframe/PICO.htm; Center for Evidence Based Medicine. Asking focused clinical questions. Retrieved from www.cebm.net/index.aspx?o=1036; Sacket, D. L., Richardson, W. S., Rosenberg, W., et al. (1997). Evidence-based medicine: How to practice and teach EBM. New York: Churchill Livingstone; Stilwell, S., Fineout-Overholt, E., Melnyk, G., et al., (2010). Evidence-based practice, step by step: Asking the clinical Question: A key step in evidence-based practice. *American Journal of Nursing, 110*(3): 58-61.

research articles?" As previously stated, evidence reports and practice guidelines may already exist for your clinical problem, so look first for those. If there are none, proceed to search for your topic in research reports in scientific journals.

Indexes and Databases

Obviously you need to go to a library or online and search a database or index for appropriate journal references. A **database** is an electronic bibliographic file that can be accessed either online or on a CD-ROM. The best database for you, as a novice nurse, is the Cumulative Index to Nursing and Allied Health Literature (CINAHL). This is a comprehensive database that includes nearly 3,000 nursing and allied health journals. Generally, you will be able to find in CINAHL whatever you are looking for in clinical nursing. Most university libraries have access to CINAHL and other indexes online. If you are an online user, it will be worth your time to get information from the library about conducting online searches. In the library, you will find the printed version of CINAHL in a set of large books in the reference section.

Once you have access to CINAHL in either format, select words that relate to your topic (e.g., dementia or nursing ethics). The index or database will list journal articles related to the key words. Sometimes you will get a large number of articles (more than 1,000) that contain that word. A PICO question should help you narrow your search, but you may need to ask the librarian for assistance. It is beyond the scope of this chapter to provide detailed instructions for literature searches. For more information about literature databases, see Chapter 44.

KnowledgeCheck 8-10

Where can you go to use CINAHL?

Journals

It also is easy to search in a specific journal for articles. The title of a journal provides clues to the content. The critical care journals will have, obviously, articles about critical care. Oncology, orthopedics, and other specialty journals carry information

specific to their own specialty. Looking for such journals is another way to do a casual search for articles of interest.

You will find the best research articles in refereed journals. **Refereed journals** are scholarly journals (not popular magazines, such as *Today's Parent* or *Time*) in which professionals with expertise in the topic review each article and then recommend whether the article should be published. The easiest way to identify a refereed journal is to see whether it has an extensive editorial board listed in the front of the journal. Refereed journals have a high standard for publication, which makes the information you read more credible (and therefore more useful to your work). Two examples of refereed nursing research journals are *Advances in Nursing Science* and *Nursing Research*. For a more extensive list,

 Go to Chapter 8, **Supplemental Materials: Nursing Research Journals,** on Davis*Plus*.

How can you tell whether the article you retrieve is a research article? Simply look for the steps in the research process described earlier in this chapter. For example, does the article have a problem statement and a purpose? Is there a section on the sample and site of the research? And so on.

If your focus is clinical practice, you should not overlook specialty journals, such as *Geriatric Nursing* or the *Journal of Gerontological Nursing,* if you really want information on, say, older adults with dementia. They are not research journals, but they generally have one or two research articles in each issue. If you do not have a specialty interest, review the *American Journal of Nursing, Nursing,* or *RN* for articles of general interest. Again, remember that it is up to you to identify whether the article is research or another form of information sharing.

Evaluate the Quality of the Research

As mentioned previously, you may be fortunate enough to find clinical practice guidelines related to your topic. If so, the related research has already been evaluated by experts, and

should have a notation about the level of evidence supporting the guideline. For a description of the different levels of evidence described by guidelines panels,

 Go to Chapter 6, **Supplemental Materials, Levels of Evidence,** on *DavisPlus.*

If no practice guidelines are available, you will need to critically appraise the individual research articles you find. You can do this by reading analytically and performing a careful appraisal of the research you read.

Analytical Reading

You cannot expect to do a sophisticated critique of a research report at this stage of your education, or probably even on graduation from your basic education. However, you need to know enough to help you decide which articles are worthy of using in your practice. You will make that decision after you have examined the research to determine whether it is well done and meaningful to your work. Begin this process by learning to read analytically. Wilson (1993, p. 25) says that **analytic reading** occurs when you "begin asking questions of what you are reading so that you can truly understand it." For questions to use when reading analytically, see Box 8-5.

Research Appraisal

Not all research is good research. Some published studies contain serious flaws, and you need to be able to recognize them. An effective strategy for conducting a research appraisal is to read the entire article, using the four questions in Box 8-5 and making notes of questions you have. Then go back and evaluate the article section by section, thinking critically about each (Wilson, 1993).

- *Researcher qualifications* are an easy place to start. Was the researcher qualified as an expert on the study topic? Try to determine whether the author's credentials and background fit with the topic.
- *The title* should be concise and clear. Key words in the title should provide clues to the research topic.
- *The abstract* is a brief (perhaps 500 words) summary of the study. It should be interesting and usually describes at least the purpose, methods, sample, and findings of the study.
- *The introduction* should catch your interest and set the stage for the rest of the report. The introduction may contain the *review of the literature, theoretical (conceptual) framework, assumptions, and limitations.* At this stage of your expertise,

you should primarily check that these are present; however, some explanation follows.

- *Review of the literature* should be thorough and relevant. The references should logically pertain to the study topic and methods and consist primarily of research and theory articles. The references should support the researcher's variable definitions, methodology, and choices of data-collection tools; they should also present background work on the topic being studied.
- *Identify the study assumptions.* Recall that assumptions are beliefs that you "take for granted" as true but that have not been proved. For example, you assume that when people are in bed, they sleep; and you assume that study participants answer truthfully to the researcher's questions. Assumptions should be clearly stated to avoid confusion regarding the study.
- *Limitations of the study.* Every study has limitations or weaknesses. Look for the author to admit the things that could not be controlled. For example, a study may test a population of people that would not generalize to other populations (e.g., testing only Caucasian students instead of testing a variety of students who represent the ethnic diversity of the university).
- *The purpose* should be stated clearly. It should give the reasons for doing the study. Ask these three questions to help you judge it: Will the study (1) solve a problem relevant to nursing, (2) present facts that are useful to nursing, or (3) contribute to nursing knowledge?
- *The problem statement* should be presented early in the report, and it should be researchable; that is, it (1) is stated as a question, (2) involves the relationship between two or more variables, and (3) can be answered by collecting empirical data.
- *Definition of terms* is essential in a formal research report. However, it often is not included in a published article because of the lack of space.
- *The research design* indicates the plan for collecting data. As a novice, you probably cannot judge the adequacy of the design, but you should be sure the researcher names and describes it and discusses its strengths and weakness. The researcher should include an explanation of what was done to enhance the validity and reliability of the study. To oversimplify, **validity** means the study actually measures the concept it claims to measure. **Reliability** refers to the accuracy, consistency, and precision of a measure. That is, if someone else repeated the study using the same design, would they obtain similar results? For example, if you weighed the same item on a scale each day and obtained the same weight each time, you could say that the scale is reliable—but a scale would not give you a valid measure of body fat.
- *Setting, population, and sample.* The researcher should identify the type of setting where the data was collected, describe the population and sample, and state the criteria that were used for choosing study participants. This section may also contain information about how informed consent was obtained.
- *Data-collection methods* answer the basic questions of what, how, who, where, and when. Data-collection instruments are the tools used to gather the data (e.g., questionnaires or a laboratory instrument). The researcher should provide evidence (pilot tests, literature) that the tools used were reliable and valid.
- *Data analysis.* A quantitative report would include statistical analyses of the data. A qualitative report would

---

BOX 8-5 ■ Reading Analytically

When reading analytically, ask yourself the following questions:

1. **What is the book, journal, or article about as a whole?** That is, what is the theme of the article, and how is it developed?
2. **What is being said in detail, and how?** What are the author's main ideas, claims, and arguments? In a research article, you will find this mainly in the abstract and the conclusions.
3. **Is the book, journal, or article true in whole or part?** You must decide this for yourself. The strategies in the section Research Appraisal may help you to determine the truth of a research report.
4. **What of it?** Is it of any significance? Is there any way to use the information to improve patient care, education, or other areas of nursing?

include quotes from the participants. The analyses of both types of data are very specific and beyond the scope of this textbook.

- **Discussion of findings and conclusion** are the sections of a research report that you may find most interesting. They are the "So what was learned?" sections. All findings should be presented in an objective manner, and compared with information found in the literature. The easiest errors for you to recognize with your present knowledge level are that the researcher:
  1. Generalizes beyond the data or the sample. For example, the sample may have been young adult women in a clinic setting, but the researcher might have suggested that the same intervention be used for all women in the clinic, regardless of age.
  2. Does not mention any limitations that might have influenced the results.
  3. Does not present findings in a clear, logical manner (i.e., you have trouble figuring out what the findings actually are).

- **Implications and recommendations** are the final pieces of the research critique. The implications are the "shoulds" of the research. In essence, the researcher says, "Now we know this fact; therefore, nurses should. . . ." For example, the research should be replicated with another population; or the instrument should be revised and retested; or this is how nurses could use the study intervention in their practice.

When you read a research article, examine it for each of the preceding items. Although you have limited knowledge and experience, every time you review an article thoroughly, you will learn more about the research process. As you learn, you will be better able to determine the quality of research you will accept as a basis for changing your nursing practice.

KnowledgeCheck 8-11

- Explain the difference between analytical reading and research appraisal.
- What are the parts of a PICO question?

Integrate the Research into Your Practice

True evidence-based practice requires that after discovering and critiquing the best available evidence, nursing expertise should be applied to see how the recommended interventions fit into the practice setting and whether they are compatible with patient preferences. If the intervention is to involve more than just an individual nurse, nurse managers must consider costs, barriers to change, facilitators for change, and staff education before deciding to implement the clinical practice guideline in their unit or hospital.

Research is more than just an exercise that nurses engage in to earn master's and doctoral degrees. The ultimate reason for conducting research is to establish an evidence-based practice or to gain greater understanding of a phenomenon. This means that nurses in practice have a responsibility for finding and using the research that others do. Remember the discussion of authority-based practice during Florence Nightingale's era? Even in the 21st century, much nursing practice is still based on authority and tradition. That is not acceptable for full-spectrum professional nurses. You must have reasons for what you do. Research can provide those reasons.

Although there are barriers (see Box 8-6), you can use nursing research to enhance your practice by acting on the information in this chapter. Read and talk about research with your colleagues and instructors. Once you have a research-based idea clear in your mind, try it out in your clinical setting (with approval from the nurse manager or instructor). Then discuss it with others. You can learn to read and use research effectively, and then you can motivate others to do the same.

BOX 8-6 ■ Barriers to Using Research

According to Nieswiadomy (2008), there are five reasons nurses *do not* use research as the basis for their practice:
1. Lack of knowledge of nursing research
2. Negative attitudes toward research
3. Inadequate forums for disseminating research
4. Lack of support from the employing institution
5. Study findings that are not ready for the clinical environment

CLINICALREASONING:
Applying the **Full-Spectrum Nursing Model**

Because the following critical thinking activities allow you to practice the kind of thinking you will use as a full-spectrum nurse, they usually have no single right answer. Discuss them with your peers—if you have difficulty with any of the questions, consult your instructor.

PATIENT SITUATION

You are caring for a 90-year-old patient in a long-term care facility. He is completely dependent for activities of daily living. In addition, he has been unresponsive, cannot swallow safely, and for many months has been receiving fluids and nutrition through a feeding tube. His adult grandson has recently discovered a living will, in which the patient had stated that he does not wish to be kept alive by "artificial means, including being tube fed." The grandson, John, insists that the patient's wishes be honored, but the patient's son (Mr. Lee) threatens a lawsuit if the caregivers discontinue the feedings. They argue loudly, and Mr. Lee yells to his son, "You just want him gone because you're in a hurry to get his money! You know you're getting the major part of it."

THINKING

1. *Theoretical Knowledge:* What facts are important to know in order to decide whether to stop the feedings?
2. *Critical Thinking (Analyzing Assumptions):* Without thinking too carefully about it, what is your first thought about what is causing the disagreement between Mr. Lee and his son, John? Examine your assumption. How certain are you it is true? What else might be going on in their lives to cause father and son to disagree on this issue?

DOING

3. *Nursing Process (Assessment):* In order to provide some information about the patient that might be helpful in restoring peace between Mr. Lee and John, what patient assessments should you make?

CARING

4. *Ethical Knowledge:* State one ethical issue involved in this case—or one moral problem that it would be present for you if you were involved in it.

 Go to Chapter 8, **Clinical Reasoning: Applying the Full-Spectrum Nursing Model Answer Sheet** on Davis*Plus*.

 To explore learning resources for this chapter,

Go to DavisPlus at http://davisplus.fadavis.com, **Keyword: Treas.**
Chapter Resources for Chapter 8:
> Knowledge Check and Think Like a Nurse Response Sheets
> Knowledge Check Answers
> Resources for Caregivers and Health Professionals
> Reading More About Theory, Research, & Evidence-Based Practice (Suggested Readings)
> What Are the Main Points in This Chapter?
NCLEX-Style Question Bank
Chapter Overview Podcasts

Concept Map

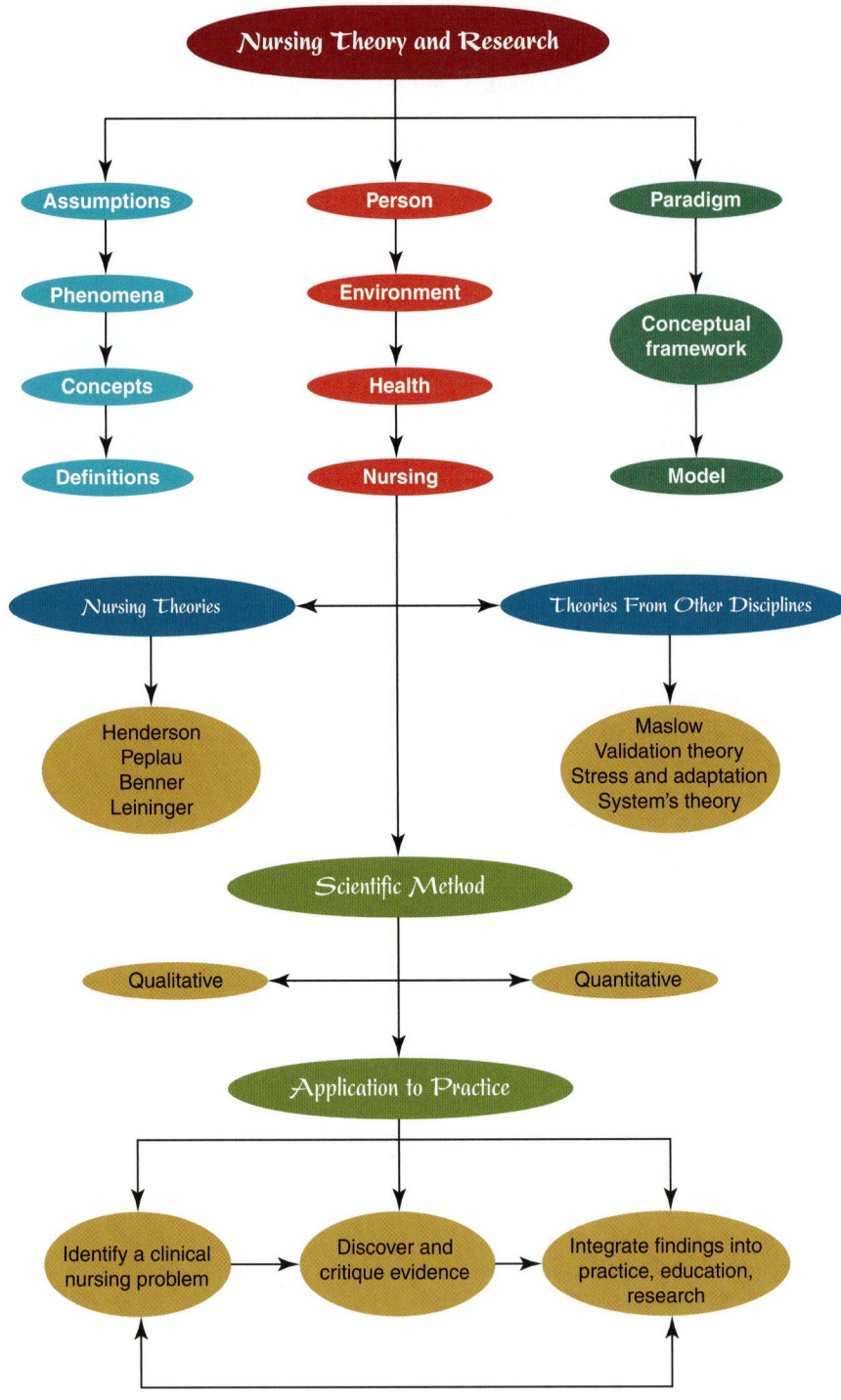

unit 2

Factors Affecting Health

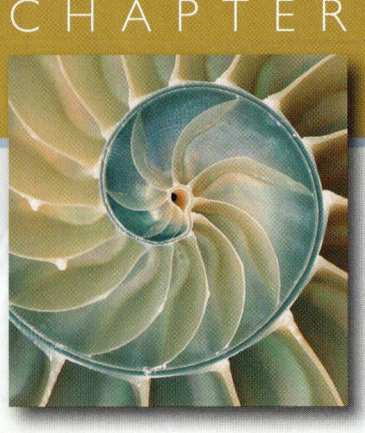
Development: Infancy Through Middle Age

Learning Outcomes

After completing this chapter, you should be able to:

➤ Discuss the principles of growth and development.

➤ Compare and contrast developmental task theory, psychoanalytic theory, cognitive theory, and the psychosocial theory of growth and development.

➤ Outline the major principles involved in moral and spiritual development.

➤ Identify conditions that influence growth and development at all ages.

➤ Discuss the cognitive and psychosocial challenges for each age group, infant through middle age.

➤ Identify common health problems seen in each stage of development.

➤ Describe any special assessments unique to each age group.

➤ Discuss age-appropriate interventions for each age group.

➤ Incorporate developmental principles into nursing care.

Key Concepts

Growth
Development
Stages

Related Concepts

See the Concept Map at the end of this chapter.

Example Problems

Abuse (violence) and neglect
Substance abuse

Caring for the Nguyens

This feature allows you to practice the kind of thinking you will use as a full-spectrum nurse. There is usually more than one correct answer to a critical thinking question, so we do not provide answers for these features. It is more important to develop your nursing judgment than to "cover content." Discuss the questions with your peers. If you are still unsure, consult your instructor.

Review the scenario of Nam Nguyen in the front of this book. Answer the following questions based on that scenario.

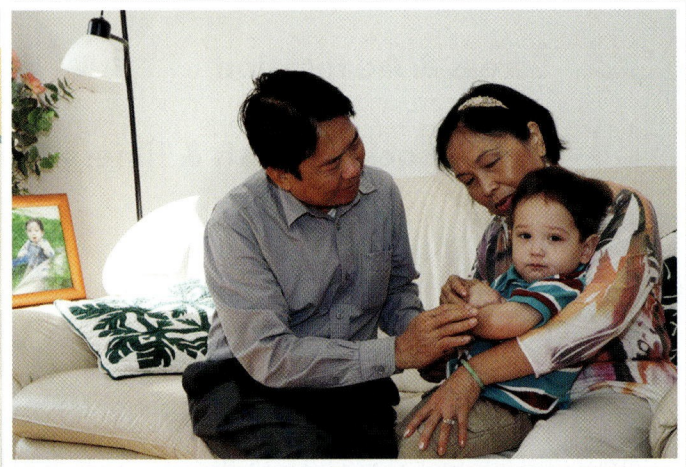

A. Evaluate Mr. Nguyen's physical health status in comparison to what is expected for someone in his age group.

B. Mr. Nguyen and his wife are raising their 3-year-old grandson. What effect might this have on Mr. Nguyen's ability to accomplish his developmental tasks?

 Go to **Caring for the Nguyens Response Sheet** on *DavisPlus.*

Meet Your Patients

At the end of your first clinical day on the pediatric unit, you reflect on your experiences with the patients for whom you provided care. You were assigned to the care of three children who were diagnosed with pneumonia:

- Tamika, a 3-year-old, lives with her grandparents. Her grandmother is present only during afternoon visiting hours because she must care for her husband, who suffers from numerous health problems.
- Miguel, a 2-month-old, lives with his mother. Since his admission yesterday, Miguel's mother has stayed at his bedside and provided most of her son's care.
- Carrie, a 13-year-old, lives with her parents. Both parents are able to visit only during evening visiting hours, when they leave work.

You think back to another clinical day when you were assigned to care for Ms. Lowenstein, a middle-aged patient with pneumonia who lives alone.

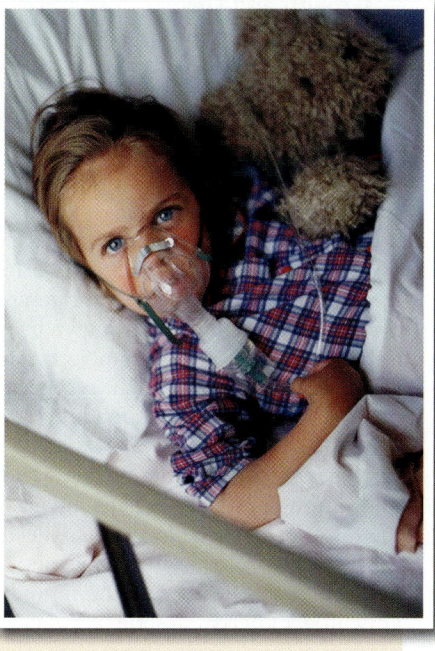

Each of these patients is unique. Although they share the same medical diagnosis, their needs and your nursing care differ dramatically. These differences stem from a variety of factors, one of the most significant of which is each patient's developmental stage. Throughout the life span, human beings are in a constant process of physical, cognitive, and emotional change, whether or not it is visible to the eye.

Theoretical Knowledge
knowing why

In this chapter, we present some principles and theories of growth and development that will serve as the foundation for planning and delivering effective personal care. You will also find a discussion of normal growth and development across the life span, including common health concerns, nursing assessments, and health promotion interventions.

ABOUT THE KEY CONCEPTS

Development refers to the process of adapting to one's body and environment over time, which is enabled by increasing complexity of function and skill progression. A few examples of development are a child who comes to recognize right from wrong, an adolescent who decides on a vocation, and an older adult who recognizes the nearness of death. Growth is the physical aspect of development; the rest is behavioral. **Growth** refers to physical changes that occur over time, such as increases in height, sexual maturation, or gains in weight and muscle tone. As you read this chapter, you will see how the key concept of *stages* is intertwined with the concepts of growth and development.

HOW DOES DEVELOPMENT OCCUR?

What has been the most important force in your becoming the person you are now: characteristics that you inherited from your parents or the environment in which you were raised?

For centuries, scientists have debated the effects of nature versus nurture on growth and development. **Nature** refers to genetic endowment, whereas **nurture** is the influence of the environment on the individual. The birth of a child can be compared to the planting of a tulip. The bulb has all the required factors to produce a beautiful plant, but whether it grows into a flower depends greatly on the environment (e.g., rich soil, sunshine, enough water). A child is similar. The joining of ovum and sperm forms chromosomes that determine appearance, characteristics, and much about how the child will grow and develop. However, environmental factors, such as access to food, love and affection, healthcare, and education, also affect how the child develops and thrives throughout the life span.

Principles of Growth and Development

Important principles of growth and development include the following:

Growth and Development Usually Follow an Orderly, Predictable Pattern. However, the timing, rate of change, and response to change are unique for each individual. For example, all children learn to sit before they walk. One child may learn to sit at 6 months of age and walk at 10 months, whereas another may first sit at 7 months and not walk until 15 months. Each of these children is developing in the same pattern, and both are progressing within a normal time frame. Similarly, menarche in girls follows a series of bodily changes associated with puberty. In one healthy teen, menstruation might begin at age 9; in another, menses might not start until age 15.

Growth and Development Follow a Cephalocaudal Pattern: Beginning at the Head and Progressing Down to the Chest, Trunk, and Lower Extremities. To illustrate cephalocaudal growth, when an infant is born, the head is the largest portion of the body. In the first year, the head, chest, and trunk gain in size, yet the legs remain short. Growth of the legs is readily apparent in the second year. An example of cephalocaudal development is the tendency of infants to use their arms before their legs.

Growth and Development Proceed in a Proximodistal Pattern, Beginning at the Center of the Body and Moving Outward. Proximodistal growth occurs **in utero,** for example, when the baby's central body is formed before the limbs. As an example of proximodistal development, the infant first lifts his head, later pushes up and rolls over. As the infant gains strength and coordination distally, he will crawl and later walk.

Simple Skills Develop Separately and Independently. Later They Are Integrated Into More Complex Skills. Many complex skills actually represent a compilation of simple skills. For example, feeding yourself requires the ability to find your mouth, grasp an object, control movement of that object, coordinate movement of the hand from the plate to the mouth, and swallow solid food.

Each Body System Grows at its Own Rate. This principle is readily apparent in fetal development; however, it applies throughout life. Perhaps the most noticeable example is the onset of puberty. In the years leading up to puberty, the cardiovascular, respiratory, and nervous systems grow and develop dramatically, yet the reproductive system changes very little. **Puberty** is a series of changes that lead to full development of the reproductive system. The hormone changes that occur with puberty also trigger growth in the musculoskeletal system.

Body System Functions Become Increasingly Differentiated Over Time. Have you ever seen a newborn respond to a loud noise? The newborn's startle response involves the whole body. With maturity, the response becomes more focused, for example, covering the ears. An adult is often able to identify the location of the sound and distinguish the origin of the sound.

Theories of Development

Theories of development attempt to explain and describe patterns of development common to all people. Such theories provide an organizing framework to help you understand and plan for the needs of the patients you will encounter, and they provide a basis for nursing interventions and clinical decision making. The needs of a 6-year-old differ greatly from those of a 25-year-old or a 65-year-old, even though they may have the same medical diagnosis or even the same nursing diagnosis (e.g., all may have Constipation or Anxiety). Understanding the tasks associated with a person's developmental stage (1) provides a basis for assessing whether behaviors are as expected or if they need further assessment, and (2) suggests specific ways in which to support and encourage the person's progress through the developmental stage.

Robert Havighurst, Sigmund Freud, Jean Piaget, Erik Erikson, and others have proposed theories to explain life span development. Each theorist has focused on a domain of human nature to examine how humans develop and has divided the life span into stages. Each stage represents a period of time that shares common characteristics. Most theorists have also identified tasks that are usually accomplished in each stage. As with the caring theories discussed in Chapter 8, an understanding of these key developmental theories is essential to full-spectrum nursing practice.

Developmental Task Theory

Robert Havighurst was an educator who theorized that learning is a lifelong process. He believed a person moves through six life stages, each associated with a number of tasks that

must be learned. Havighurst characterizes a **developmental task** as "midway between an individual need and societal demand. It assumes an active learner interacting with an active social environment" (1971, p. vi). Failure to master a task leads to imbalance within the individual, unhappiness, and difficulty mastering future tasks and interacting with others. Table 9-1 presents the tasks associated with each stage of life. It is easy to evaluate a client's completion of Havighurst's broadly written tasks, but the nonspecific time frame limits this theory's usefulness for assessing individuals for appropriate development.

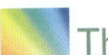

ThinkLike a Nurse 9-1

Which stage in Havighurst's developmental task theory contains the most complex tasks and would be the most difficult to master? Why?

Psychoanalytic Theory

Sigmund Freud was a pioneer in the science of human development. His psychoanalytic theory focuses on the motivation for human behavior and personality development. Freud identified five stages of psychosexual development (Table 9-2). He believed that human development is perpetuated by instinctual drives, such as libido (sexual instinct), aggression, and survival (Sadock & Sadock, 2007). Different drives predominate, depending on the age of the individual. Psychoanalytic theory became the foremost theoretical foundation of early 20th century psychotherapy. However, Freud developed his theory in the Victorian era, when societal norms were very strict. Sexual repression and male dominance over female behavior were the cultural standard. Many of today's social scientists question the relevance of his theory to life in the 21st century.

Freud identified several forces that influence the development of our personality. Each has a unique function. The **id** represents instinctual urges, pleasure, and gratification, such as hunger, procreation, pleasure, and aggression. It is dominant in infants and young children. The **ego** begins to develop around 4 to 6 months of age. It strives to balance what is wanted (id) and what is possible to obtain or achieve. The **superego** is sometimes referred to as our conscience. This force develops in early childhood (ages 5–6). The **unconscious mind** is composed of thoughts and memories that are not readily recalled but unconsciously influence behavior.

In the mid-1950s, Freud's daughter, the psychologist Anna Freud, identified a number of **defense mechanisms,** which she described as thought patterns or behaviors that the ego makes use of in the face of threat to biological or psychological integrity (Townsend, 2009). In other words, defense mechanisms protect us from excess anxiety. For example, after receiving a failing grade in chemistry, a student might refuse to think about it, intellectualize reasons why she failed, blame her teacher, or compensate by emphasizing her A grade in psychology. All people use defense mechanisms to varying degrees. For a comprehensive discussion of defense mechanisms, see Chapter 12 and Table 12-1.

KnowledgeCheck 9-1

- According to Freud, which motivator of personality is based in reality?
- Which is referred to as our conscience?
- What is the purpose of defense mechanisms?

Table 9-1 ➤ Havighurst's Developmental Task Theory

STAGE	TASKS
Infants & Toddlers	**Physical Development** ■ Walking ■ Taking solid foods ■ Talking ■ Controlling bowel and bladder elimination ■ Learning sex differences and acquiring sexual modesty **Cognitive & Social Development** ■ Acquiring psychological stability ■ Forming concepts; learning language ■ Getting ready to read
Preschool and School Age	**Physical Development** ■ Learning physical skills necessary for ordinary games **Cognitive & Social Development** ■ Building wholesome attitudes toward oneself as a growing organism ■ Learning to get along with age-mates ■ Learning masculine or feminine social role ■ Acquiring fundamental skills in reading, writing, and calculating ■ Developing concepts necessary for everyday living ■ Developing a conscience, morality, and a scale of values ■ Achieving personal independence ■ Acquiring attitudes toward social groups and institutions
Adolescents	**Physical Development** ■ Accepting one's physique and using the body effectively **Cognitive & Social Development** ■ Achieving new and more mature relations with age-mates of both sexes ■ Achieving masculine or feminine social role ■ Developing emotional independence from parents and other adults ■ Preparing for future marriage and family life ■ Preparing for a career ■ Acquiring values and an ethical system to guide behavior; developing an ideology ■ Aspiring to and achieving socially responsible behavior
Young Adults	■ Choosing a mate ■ Achieving a masculine or feminine social role ■ Learning to live with a partner ■ Rearing children ■ Managing a home ■ Establishing an occupation ■ Taking on community responsibilities ■ Finding a compatible social group

(Continued)

Table 9-1 ➤ Havighurst's Developmental Task Theory—cont'd	
STAGE	**TASKS**
Middle Adults	**Physical Development** ■ Adjusting to the physiological changes of middle age **Cognitive & Social Development** ■ Assisting teenage children to become responsible and happy adults ■ Achieving adult civic and social responsibility ■ Reaching and maintaining satisfactory performance in one's occupational career ■ Developing adult leisure-time activities ■ Relating oneself to one's spouse as a person
Older Adults	**Physical Development** ■ Adjusting to decreasing physical strength and health **Cognitive & Social Development** ■ Adjusting to retirement ■ Adjusting to a lower income ■ Adjusting to death of a spouse ■ Establishing an open affiliation with one's age group ■ Adopting and adapting flexible social roles ■ Establishing satisfactory physical living arrangements

Adapted from: Havighurst, R. J. (1971). *Developmental tasks and education* (3rd ed.). New York: Longman.

Table 9-2 ➤ Freud's Stages of Psychosexual Development		
AGE	**STAGE**	**DESCRIPTION**
Birth–18 mo	Oral	The infant's primary needs are centered on the oral zone: lips, tongue, mouth. The need for hunger and pleasure are satisfied through the oral zone. Trust is developed through the meeting of needs. When needs are not met, aggression can manifest itself in the form of biting, spitting, or crying.
18 mo–3 yr	Anal	Neuromuscular control over the anal sphincter allows the child to have control over expulsion or retention of feces. This coincides with the child's struggle for separation and independence from caregivers. Successful completion of this stage yields a child who is self-directed, cooperative, and without shame. Conversely, the anal child will exhibit willfulness, stubbornness, and need for orderliness.
3–6 yr	Phallic	The focus is on the genital organs. This coincides with the development of gender identity. Unconscious sexual feelings toward the parent of the opposite sex are common. Children emerge from this stage with a sense of sexual curiosity and a mastery of their instinctual impulses.
6–12 yr	Latency	Ego functioning matures, and sexual urges diminish. The child focuses his energy on same-sex relationships and mastery of his world, including relationships with significant others (teachers, coaches).
13–20 yr	Genital	Puberty causes an intensification of instinctual drives, particularly sexual. The focus of this stage is the resolution of previous conflicts and the development of a mature identity and the ability to form adult relationships.

Cognitive Development Theory

Jean Piaget studied his own children to understand how humans develop **cognitive abilities** (i.e., the ability to think, reason, and use language). According to Piaget, cognitive development requires three core competencies: adaptation, assimilation, and accommodation. **Adaptation** is the ability to adjust to and interact with one's environment. To be able to adapt, one must assimilate and accommodate. **Assimilation** is the integration of new experiences with one's own system of knowledge. **Accommodation** is the change in one's system of knowledge that results from processing new information. For example, an infant is born with an innate ability to suck. Presented with the mother's nipple, the infant is able to assimilate the nipple to the behavior of sucking. If given a bottle, the infant can learn to accommodate the artificial nipple. However, the baby may adapt by accepting the artificial nipple only from the father, crying and fussing if the mother offers a bottle instead of her breast.

According to Piaget, cognitive development occurs from birth through adolescence in a sequence of four stages: sensorimotor, preoperational thought, concrete operations, and formal operations (Table 9-3). A child must complete each stage before moving to the next. The rate at which a child moves through the four stages is determined by inherited intellect and the influence of the environment. Piaget does not address cognitive development after adolescence.

KnowledgeCheck 9-2

- According to Piaget, what core competencies are necessary for cognitive development?
- During which stage is the child the most egocentric?
- When does abstract thinking develop?

Psychosocial Development Theory

In the 1950s Erik Erikson introduced his theory of psychosocial development. Erikson was strongly influenced by Freud but believed that personality continues to evolve throughout the life span as the individual interacts with the social world. He hypothesized that individuals must negotiate eight stages as they progress through the life span. Most individuals successfully move from stage to stage; however, a person can regress during times of stress to earlier stages or be forced to face tasks of later stages because of unforeseen life events, such as terminal illness. Failure to successfully master a stage leads to maladjustment. Erikson's theory is widely used in nursing and healthcare. Below are Erikson's eight stages.

Stage 1: Trust Versus Mistrust (Birth to About 18 Months). The child develops a sense of trust in himself and the external world as a result of having his needs consistently met. This is the beginning of self-confidence. An infant who does not have his needs met develops a sense of mistrust and suspiciousness in others that will affect future interpersonal relationships.

Stage 2: Autonomy Versus Shame and Doubt (About 18 Months to 3 Years). The goal is for the child to develop self-control and independence while maintaining self-esteem. This requires an ability to cooperate and express feelings and thoughts. Failure to successfully negotiate this stage will lead to an adult who lacks self-confidence and feels controlled by others and who may exhibit extreme compliance (self-restraint) or defiance.

Stage 3: Initiative Versus Guilt (3 to 5 Years). The focus of this stage is to develop initiative by gradually assuming responsibility and developing self-discipline. During this stage, the superego (conscience) develops, and the

---

Table 9-3 ▶ Piaget's Stages of Cognitive Development

STAGE	AGE	CHARACTERISTICS OF DEVELOPMENT
Sensorimotor	Birth–2 yr	■ Learns the world through the senses ■ Displays curiosity ■ Shows intentional behavior ■ Begins to see that objects exist apart from self ■ Begins to see objects as separate from self
Preoperational	2–7 yr	■ Uses symbols and language ■ Sees himself as the center of the universe: egocentric ■ Thought based on perception rather than logic
Concrete operations	7–11 yr	■ Operates and reacts to the concrete: What is perceived is actual. ■ Egocentricity diminishes, can see from others' viewpoints ■ Able to use logic and reason in thinking ■ Able to conserve: To see that objects may change but recognizes them as the same (e.g., water may change to ice, or a tower of blocks is the same as a long fence of blocks)
Formal operations	11–adolescence	■ Develops the ability to think abstractly: to reason, deduce, and define concepts in a logical manner ■ Some individuals do not develop the ability to think abstractly.

child learns to manage impulses. Failure to develop initiative leads to guilt, limited creativity, lack of self-confidence, and pessimism.

Stage 4: Industry Versus Inferiority (6 to 11 Years). In this stage, the child learns that recognition comes through achievement and completion of tasks. This success occurs primarily in school. The adult who has not fulfilled the tasks of this stage will demonstrate a sense of inadequacy in all areas of life.

Stage 5: Identity Versus Role Confusion (11 to 21 Years). This stage coincides with puberty. The adolescent develops a sense of self and begins to make decisions about the future. Social groups serve as a place to test out ideas and behaviors. Healthy role models facilitate the development of identity. A person who fails to recognize his abilities and sense of self is unable to experience a solid place in the world. This is manifested by dysfunctional interpersonal relationships and occupational performance. Delinquent and rebellious behavior may be prominent when the task of identity formation is not met.

Stage 6: Intimacy Versus Isolation (21 to 40 Years). Erikson (1963) defined intimacy as "the capacity to commit himself to concrete affiliations and partnerships and to develop the ethical strength to abide by such commitments" (p. 263). Isolation is the avoidance of intimacy. The task at this stage is to develop a commitment to work and relationships. Failure to do so will result in impersonal relationships and difficulty with maintaining a job.

Stage 7: Generativity Versus Stagnation (40 to 65 Years). The goal of this stage is to be creative and productive. Often this is accomplished through work or relationships, such as raising healthy, functional children or contributing to society by developing a distinguished career, for example in nursing. The person who fails to achieve generativity (the desire and motivation to guide the next generation) may manifest stagnation in the form of superficial relationships and self-absorption. Simply having children does not guarantee generativity.

Stage 8: Ego Integrity Versus Despair (Over 65 Years). The task of this stage is the acceptance of one's life, worth, and eventual death. Ego integrity reflects a satisfaction with life and an understanding of one's place in the life cycle. A sense of loss, discomfort with life and aging, and a fear of death are seen in despair.

ThinkLike a Nurse 9-2

Review the case study in the Meet Your Patients section of the chapter. Based on Erikson's psychosocial development theory, what kind of behavior would you anticipate from Carrie?

Moral Development Theory: Kohlberg

Lawrence Kohlberg (1968) developed his theory of moral development by studying the responses to moral dilemmas of 84 boys whose development he followed for a period of 20 years. In this theory, moral reasoning appears to be somewhat age related. According to Kohlberg, moral development is based on one's ability to think at progressively higher levels. Increased maturity provides some degree of higher-level thinking but does not guarantee the ability to function at the highest level. Kohlberg believed that not all people are able to achieve those levels. Kohlberg described the following levels; each has two stages (1968, 1981; Waugh, 1978).

Level I. Preconventional. The person conforms to cultural rules and labels of good and bad but interprets them in terms of punishment and reward or in terms of the physical power of those who enforce the rules. Children ages 4 to 10 years are usually at this level; some adults are, as well.

    Stage 1—punishment–obedience orientation (right action is that which avoids punishment)

    Stage 2—personal interest orientation (right action is that which satisfies personal needs)

Level II. Conventional. The person perceives that meeting the expectations of the family, group, or society is valuable in its own right, regardless of the consequences of the actions. More than just conforming, the person is loyal to the social order and identifies with those involved in it. Others set the standards, but motivation to follow them is internal.

    Stage 3—"good boy–nice girl" orientation (right actions are those that please others)

    Stage 4—law-and-order orientation (right action is following the rules)

Level III. Postconventional, Autonomous, or Principled. The person makes an effort to define moral values and principles that have validity apart from society, groups, or persons in power. At this level it becomes possible for conflict to occur between two socially accepted standards, and the person attempts to decide rationally between them. Both the standards and the decision are internal. Moral principles have validity apart from the authority of groups and persons.

    Stage 5—legalistic, social contract orientation (right action is decided in terms of individual rights and standards agreed upon by the whole society)

    Stage 6—universal ethical principles orientation (right action is determined by conscience and abstract principles such as the Golden Rule)

Kohlberg believed that, even with maturity, not all people are able to achieve level III.

Moral Development Theory: Gilligan

As just noted, all of Kohlberg's research subjects were male. Although Kohlberg claimed that his sequence of stages applies equally to everyone, the validity of his theory for women has been sharply criticized, most prominently by Carol Gilligan (1982, 1993). To address the moral development of women, Gilligan proposed an alternative theory that incorporates the concepts of caring, interpersonal relationships, and responsibility. She described a three-stage approach to moral development.

Stage 1: Caring for Oneself. In this stage, the focus is providing for oneself and surviving. The individual is egocentric in thought and does not consider the needs of others. When concerns about selfishness begin to emerge, the individual is signaling a readiness to move to stage 2.

Stage 2: Caring for Others. At this level, an individual recognizes the importance of relationships with others. The person is willing to make sacrifices to help others, often at the expense of her own needs. When she recognizes the conflict between caring for oneself and caring for others, the individual is ready to move to stage 3.

Stage 3: Caring for Self and Others. This represents the highest stage of moral development. In this stage, care is the focus of decision making. The individual carefully balances her own needs against the needs of others to decide on a course of action.

See Chapter 42 if you would like a fuller discussion of moral development.

Spiritual Development Theory

James Fowler, a minister, defined faith as a universal human concern and as a process of growing in trust. He noticed that his congregants had very different approaches to faith, and the differences depended on their age. Basing his studies on the work of Piaget, Erikson, and Kohlberg, he developed a theory of faith development, which includes a pre-stage (stage 0) and six stages of faith (Fowler, 1981).

Stages 0, 1, and 2 are closely associated with evolving cognitive abilities. In these stages, faith depends largely on the views expressed by the parents, caregivers, and those who have significant influence in the life of the person.

Stage 3 coincides with the ability to use *logic* and *hypothetical thinking* to construct and evaluate ideas. At this point faith is largely a collection of conventional, unexamined beliefs. Fowler's studies demonstrated that approximately one-fourth of all adults function at this level or lower.

Stages 4, 5, and 6 represent increasing levels of refinement of faith. With each increase in level there is decreasing likelihood that an individual can attain this stage of development. Fowler found that the number of people achieving stage 6 was exceedingly rare.

If you would like to see a more thorough description of Fowler's six stages,

 Go to Chapter 9, **Tables, Boxes, Figures; ESG Table 9-1,** on Davis*Plus.*

This rest of this chapter describes the human life span as a series of developmental stages. For each stage, physical development, cognitive and psychosocial development, and common health problems are discussed. To simplify organization, nursing assessments and interventions to promote health are included with the discussion of each stage rather than in a separate practical knowledge section.

THE GESTATIONAL PERIOD: CONCEPTION TO BIRTH

The time between conception and birth is called the **gestational period.** Human gestation (pregnancy) is calculated from the first day of the mother's last menstrual period and lasts approximately 40 weeks, or 280 days. Full discussion of pregnancy and childbirth are beyond the scope of a fundamentals text. If you need more information, refer to a maternal health textbook.

Physical Development During Gestation

Pregnancy is usually divided into three trimesters, each lasting about 13 weeks.

First Trimester. The first 8 weeks is known as the **embryonic phase.** It begins when an egg that has been released from a woman's ovary unites with a sperm cell, usually in one of the woman's fallopian tubes. This is called **fertilization** (or conception). Continual cell division leads to the development of a tiny ball of cells called the **morula,** which travels toward the uterus for a period of about 7 days before implanting as a multicelled **blastocyst** in the woman's uterus. Upon implantation, three primary germ layers begin to differentiate, and the **embryo** begins to resemble a tiny organism with a head and tail. As early as 6 to 7 weeks, the fetal heartbeat can be heard with a fetal ultrasound Doppler. By week 4, the brain, heart, and liver have begun to form, and tiny limb buds are present. By

the end of week 8, all organs are formed, and the embryo is now called a fetus.

Second Trimester. Rapid fetal growth and further development of the body systems characterize the second trimester. At approximately 16 to 20 weeks of pregnancy, the mother can feel her fetus move, a sensation called quickening. At the end of the second trimester, the fetus has all organs and body parts intact that will develop in efficiency during the last trimester. The kidneys are intact, although they do not effectively concentrate urine until later in the third trimester. Even at birth, the kidneys do not function as efficiently as do adult kidneys. The lungs are formed, although they do not contain enough of the substance to keep air sacs open after birth until later in the third trimester.

Third Trimester. In the third trimester, the fetus continues to grow in size and add subcutaneous fat. Body systems mature in preparation for extrauterine life. If born prematurely during this trimester, the newborn may be able to survive with intensive care. By week 37, the fetus is considered full term; birth after 41 weeks is considered post-term.

A normal full-term baby weighs, on average, 5 lb 8 oz to 8 lb 13 oz (2,500 to 4,000 g) and is 20 in. (50 cm) long. If you would like to see a concise timeline of fetal growth,

 Go to Chapter 9, **Tables, Boxes, Figures: ESG Table 9-2,** on Davis*Plus.*

Maternal Changes During Pregnancy

A woman's health during pregnancy is essential for healthy, sustained growth and development of the fetus. It is important for young women to develop good health practices well before conception, including exercise, a balanced diet, smoking cessation, avoidance of alcohol, and regular dental checkups.

The well-being of the growing fetus depends entirely on the health of the placenta for oxygen and nutrition. Therefore, many of the physical changes that the woman experiences during pregnancy are for the purpose of increasing blood flow through the placenta to the baby. The heart of a pregnant woman typically enlarges slightly and the chest wall expands so that respiratory rate and cardiac output increase significantly. In fact, the woman increases her normal blood flow by about 30% by the 35th week of pregnancy.

When conception occurs, menses typically cease. In the first trimester, hormone shifts, primarily in progesterone and estrogen, often cause the pregnant women to experience morning sickness, fullness in the pelvic area, breast enlargement and tenderness, urinary frequency, and fatigue.

During second trimester, the uterus enlarges and hyperpigmentation of the skin occurs, often creating a dark line from the umbilicus to the symphysis pubis and causing the nipples to darken. Cheeks and forehead may also become mottled. The gums may swell and bleed. Mucous membranes in the nose might also swell. The woman begins to feel the fetus moving and may experience mild contractions, called Braxton Hicks.

During third trimester, the breasts begin to produce and secrete colostrum in preparation for lactation. Pressure from the enlarged fetus may cause shortness of breath and urinary frequency. Fetal movement is the predominant feature of the latter period of pregnancy.

Psychosocial challenges during pregnancy involve adjustment to changes in body image, role changes and expectations, concerns about sexuality and whether the partners are sexually satisfied, fears about labor and delivery, concern for the baby's health and safety, planning for care of the child after delivery,

financial pressures, and stresses involving employment during pregnancy. As the birth of a child is a life-changing condition, it is normal for women to feel ambivalent about pregnancy at first, but these feelings usually resolve in the second trimester.

Common Health Problems During Gestation

The uterus is the environment in which the fetus grows. Blood circulating through the placenta carries nutrients and oxygen to the fetus and toxins and metabolic wastes away from the fetus. Other substances also cross the placenta. For example, **teratogens** are substances that interfere with normal growth and development.

✚ Because the brain and other vital organs develop during the first trimester, this is the time when the fetus is most vulnerable to teratogens such as the following:

- Alcohol is a potent teratogen that can cause birth defects, growth retardation, developmental delay, and impaired intellectual development.
- Nicotine interferes with the transport of oxygen to the fetus, contributing to premature birth, low birth weight, and learning disabilities.
- Babies exposed to morphine, heroin, methadone, and other narcotics and street drugs in the uterus suffer from withdrawal at birth. Symptoms include tremors, restlessness, hyperactive reflexes, poor temperature control, vomiting and diarrhea, high-pitched cries, seizures, and sometimes death.
- Cocaine, including crack, and methamphetamines are highly addictive and potentially harmful to the unborn fetus. Infants born to cocaine users and crack users are more likely to suffer from growth retardation and to have sleep disturbances, hyperactive reflexes, irritability, feeding difficulties, attention and behavioral disorders, and learning disabilities at school age. These infants are also more likely to die from **sudden infant death syndrome (SIDS),** the sudden, unexplained death of an infant (discussed in more detail in the next section).

✚ Medications, both prescribed and over the counter, can have teratogenic effects. Examples include the acne medication isotretinoin (Accutane) and tetracycline (Achromycin), phenytoin (Dilantin), and lithium (Lithobid). Pregnant women should check with their primary care provider before taking any medications or herbal remedies

Common Discomforts of Pregnancy

Common discomforts are associated with the physiological changes occurring in the woman's body. In general, they are normal and do not necessarily indicate any underlying problem, and require primarily self-care measures.

- In the first trimester, nausea and vomiting, urinary frequency, fatigue, breast tenderness, increased vaginal discharge, nasal stuffiness, **epistaxis** (nosebleeds) and swelling of nasal mucous membranes, and **ptyalism** (excessive saliva production) may occur.
- In the second and third trimesters, the woman may experience heartburn, ankle edema, varicose veins, flatulence, hemorrhoids, constipation, backache, leg cramps, feeling faint, shortness of breath, difficulty sleeping, round ligament pain (a "grabbing" sensation in the lower abdominal and inguinal area), and carpal tunnel syndrome.

Effects of Maternal Age

The risk for preterm birth and low birth weight is higher for babies born to adolescent mothers. Additionally, the risk of fetal death is higher for teen mothers and mothers over age 40 (Centers for Disease Control and Prevention, 2002). Furthermore, the risk of conceiving a child with Down syndrome (trisomy 21) and other congenital anomalies increases for each year over the age of 35, but dramatically after age 42.

Effects of Maternal Health

Maternal diseases, such as rubella, syphilis, and gonorrhea, although not common, can cause fetal blindness, deafness, or fetal loss. Cytomegalovirus (CMV) is a common viral infection in adults that presents with flu-like symptoms. If the mother acquires CMV during pregnancy, the fetus can suffer intrauterine growth retardation, poor brain growth, enlarged liver (hepatomegaly) with jaundice, irritation of the lung (pneumonitis), and bleeding problems. Toxoplasmosis can be transmitted to the unborn fetus through handling of contaminated cat litter. If the mother experiences an outbreak of genital herpes at the time of delivery, there is risk of passing the virus to the infant. Other diseases, such as maternal diabetes, can result in a low blood sugar after birth and can also have lasting effects on the fetus. Poor glucose control during pregnancy may lead to neural tube and heart defects, as well as **macrosomia** (large body size).

Effects of Maternal Nutrition

Beginning even before pregnancy, maternal nutrition is vital to the fetus. Appropriate, healthy weight management before conception contributes to fetal and maternal health. Appropriate maternal weight gain contributes to appropriate fetal birth weight and reduces the risk of fetal illness and infections. The recommended average weight gain for a pregnancy is 25 to 35 pounds. The expected weight gain is higher for underweight women and lower for overweight women.

✚ Folic acid deficiency in the first weeks of pregnancy—typically before the woman even knows she is pregnant—is a risk factor for neural tube defects, such as spina bifida.

▇ ASSESSMENT

Routine prenatal visits and screenings usually take place monthly until 28 weeks, then every 2 weeks until 36 weeks, then weekly until delivery. In addition to vital signs, weight, fetal heart tones, nutritional status, and other measures of maternal–fetal well-being should be assessed at each visit (see Fig. 9-1).

Screen common discomforts associated with pregnancy, such as nausea, fatigue, and back pain. Preexisting conditions (e.g., diabetes and hypertension) must be carefully monitored during pregnancy. Openly discuss medication use, including over-the-counter drugs (OTCs), the use of alternative therapies, and other substances. Screening is also done for complications of pregnancy, such as the following:

- **Birth defects.** Women who are at higher risk for a fetus with a birth defect are those with advanced maternal age (over age 40), family history of congenital anomalies, maternal diabetes with insulin use, viral infection during pregnancy, and exposure to high levels of radiation. Blood markers and ultrasound screening are done to detect neural tube defects, abdominal wall defects, trisomy 21 (Down syndrome), and trisomy 18. The best time to screen is between 16 and 18 weeks' gestation.

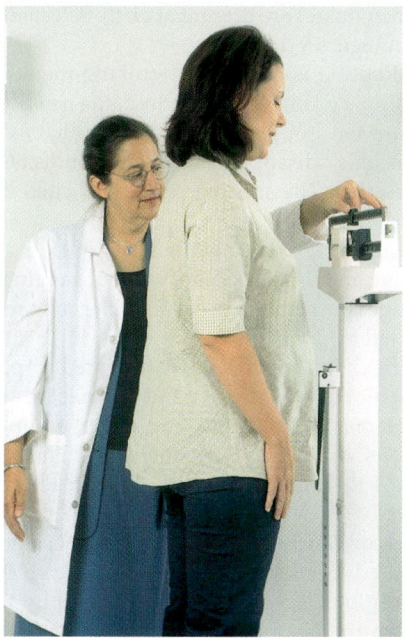

FIGURE 9-1 After establishing a baseline weight in early pregnancy, monitor for appropriate weight gain at each prenatal visit.

- **Gestational diabetes.** Screening for gestational diabetes is most often done between 24 and 28 weeks' gestation, unless there is a history of gestational diabetes with a previous pregnancy.
- **Group B streptococcus.** The Centers for Disease Control and Prevention (CDC), the American Academy of Pediatrics (AAP), and the American College of Obstetricians and Gynecologists (ACOG) recommend that pregnant women be screened for group B streptococcus between 35 and 37 weeks' gestation.

INTERVENTIONS

Key Point. *One of the most important nursing interventions in promoting maternal and fetal health is to facilitate and teach the importance of early and continuing prenatal care.* Early prenatal care makes it possible to identify complications of pregnancy and to prevent some of the effects of maternal diseases such as diabetes. Each prenatal visit is an opportunity for patient education.

Key Point. *Maternal nutrition is important for a healthy baby. The mother's food intake should be well balanced.* The recommended dietary allowances of vitamins and minerals for the pregnant woman range from 25% to 50% higher than for the nonpregnant woman. Pregnant women should increase their caloric intake by 10% to 15%. Inadequate protein affects formation of the placenta and fetal brain development. Increasing folic acid (also called folate) intake to 400 mcg daily reduces the risk of neural tube defects. Women who are of childbearing potential should follow these guidelines daily rather than waiting for pregnancy to occur. This will help achieve a national objective for the year 2020 of reducing the incidence of neural tube defects (U.S. Department of Health and Human Services, 2010). You can find the national goals for 2020 on the Healthy People 2020 Web site:

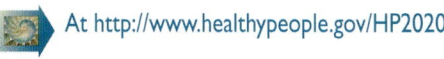 At http://www.healthypeople.gov/HP2020/

Other teaching topics include the following:
> Information regarding sexually transmitted diseases and vaginal infections
> Information about urinary tract infections
> Exercise patterns
> Child care
> Growth and development of the fetus
> Potentially hazardous substances that should be avoided
> Avoiding use of OTC medications without approval from the supervising provider
> Self-care measures for common discomforts of pregnancy
> Danger signs that alert the woman to call her care provider
> Signs of impending labor; when to go to the birthing unit

KnowledgeCheck 9-3

- What are the most common health concerns to monitor in the gestational period?
- Identify at least four important topics for health teaching with the expectant mother.
- Why is early prenatal care so important?

NEONATAL PERIOD: BIRTH TO 28 DAYS

During the neonatal period (the first month of life), the newborn's primary task is to stabilize the body's major organ systems and adapt to life outside the uterus. Behaviors are primarily reflexive.

Physical Development of the Neonate

Growth. The normal full-term newborn weighs between 2,500 and 4,000 g, or 5 lb 8 oz to 8 lb 13 oz. Lower birth weights are seen with prematurity, whereas higher birth weights are associated with gestational diabetes. The neonate measures between 18 and 22 in. (46 and 56 cm) in length (Fig. 9-2), and the arms are slightly longer than the legs.

At birth, the head is one-fourth the total body length, with a head circumference of 33 to 35 cm (13 to 14 in.). For a few days, it may appear asymmetrical because of molding during vaginal birth. The skull consists of six soft bones separated by sutures composed of cartilage (Fig. 9-3), with anterior and posterior **fontanels** (soft spots). These spaces allow room to accommodate the rapid growth of the infant's brain during the first months of life.

Respirations. At birth, the most critical adaptation is the establishment of respirations. Pressure on the baby's chest during vaginal birth helps remove amniotic fluid from the lungs in preparation for breathing. The normal newborn's respirations are irregular, shallow, and 30 to 50 breaths per minute, with brief periods of **periodic breathing** (pauses in breathing).

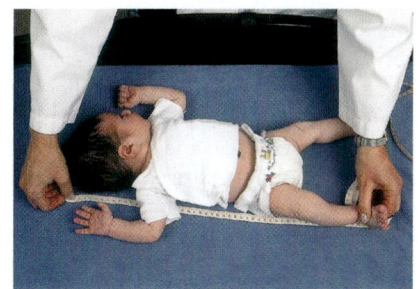

FIGURE 9-2 Measuring the length of a newborn.

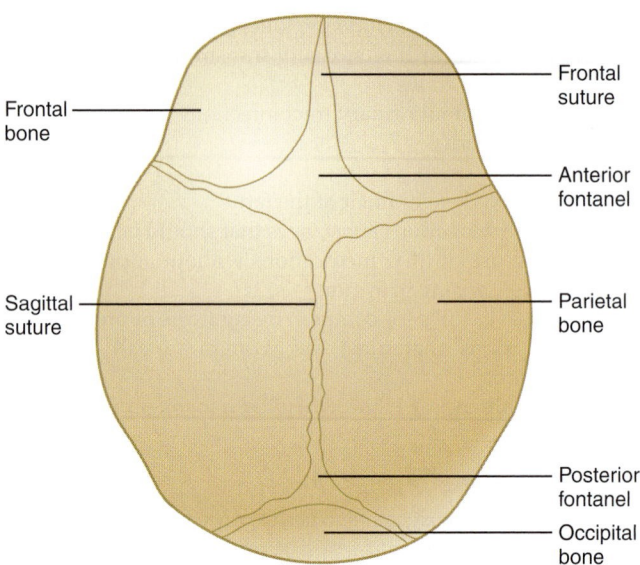

FIGURE 9-3 Sutures and fontanels of the newborn's skull

Cardiovascular System. The cardiovascular system must also adapt to the change from placental blood flow and convert to independent circulation. The average heart rate of a newborn is 120 to 140 beats/min, with slightly lower rates at rest and higher rates with activity or crying. Poor peripheral circulation causes a bluish coloration of the hands and feet; this is normal and usually disappears within a few hours of birth.

Thermoregulation. Thermoregulation is another important new task. The newborn has the capacity to produce adequate heat but cannot protect against heat loss. Heat may be lost by exposure to cool air temperatures, by contact with cooler solid surfaces, or by evaporation of moisture from the skin. The normal newborn's temperature is close to that of an adult. To assist in thermoregulation, it is important to keep the newborn warm and dry, with a cap on his head.

Elimination. At birth, the kidneys produce 15 to 60 mL of urine per kilogram per day. During the first 24 hours, the newborn voids 5 to 25 times. Newborns have limited ability to concentrate urine. At birth, the newborn's lower intestine is filled with **meconium,** a sticky, greenish-black substance formed from amniotic fluid and intestinal secretions. Meconium is usually passed via the rectum within 12 hours of birth, and the stool progressively changes in color to yellow. The full-term infant is able to swallow, digest, metabolize, and absorb proteins and simple carbohydrates. Stomach capacity varies from 30 to 90 mL, depending on the weight of the infant. Normal colonic bacteria are established within a week of birth.

Epidermis and Dermis. The epidermis and dermis are very thin at birth and can be easily damaged. Infants are born with varying degrees of **vernix caseosa,** a cheese-like protective covering for the skin. **Milia,** tiny white spots, may be present on the newborn's face, and the area over the sacrum may show a darkly pigmented area called a **mongolian spot.** All such features disappear spontaneously. **Lanugo** is fine, downy hair that covers the fetus's body but disappears close to term.

Neuromuscular System. The neuromuscular system is not completely developed at birth, but the following **reflexes** (automatic responses) are present at birth. Selected reflexes are illustrated in Figure 9-4.

- **Rooting.** Rooting is elicited by stroking the infant's cheek with the nipple or finger. In response, the newborn turns his head toward the stimulus, opens his mouth, takes hold, and sucks. This reflex disappears by 3 to 4 months of age.
- **Sucking Reflex.** The sucking reflex is elicited by touching the infant's lips.
- **Swallowing Reflex.** The swallowing reflex is coordinated with sucking and usually occurs without gagging, coughing, or vomiting. This response is weak with prematurity or neurological defect.
- **Grasp Reflex.** The grasp reflex is triggered by placing a finger in the palm of the infant's hand (palmar) or at the base of the toes (plantar). The infant's fingers curl around the examiner's fingers, or the toes curl downward. The palmar reflex lessens by 3 to 4 months, and the plantar reflex lessens by 8 months.
- **Tonic Neck or Fencing Reflex.** The tonic neck or fencing reflex is elicited by rotating the infant's head to the left with the left arm and leg extended and the right arm and leg flexed. Turn the head to the right, and the extremities assume the opposite posture. The response disappears by 3 to 4 months.
- **Moro or Startle Reflex.** This reflex is elicited by placing the infant on a flat surface and striking the surface to startle the infant. Symmetrical abduction and extension of the arms are expected as an indicator of overall neurological health. The fingers fan out and form a C with the thumb and forefinger. This response is absent by 6 months.
- **Stepping Reflex.** Elicit the stepping reflex by holding the infant vertically, allowing one foot to touch a surface (e.g., tabletop). The infant will simulate walking by alternating flexion and extension of the feet during the first 3 to 4 weeks of life.
- **Crawling Reflex.** The crawling reflex is noted by placing the infant on her abdomen. The newborn makes crawling movements with her arms and legs. This response should disappear by 6 weeks of age.
- **Babinski Reflex.** The Babinski reflex is elicited by stroking upward along the lateral aspect of the sole. A positive response occurs when the toes hyperextend and the great toe dorsiflexes. An infant who does not respond in this manner should undergo a neurological evaluation. This reflex disappears as the infant begins to walk or between 12 and 18 months.

Cognitive Development of the Neonate

In the first month of life, the neonate responds to stimuli in a reflexive manner. Piaget described this as stage 1 of the *sensorimotor phase.* But despite the newborn's limited voluntary abilities, the sensory functions are well developed.

Vision. At birth, the eyes are treated with antibiotics to prevent blindness caused by gonorrhea. After the ointment has been absorbed, the newborn begins to fixate on an object. During the first few weeks of life, the infant focuses on objects, following from side to side with his gaze. The infant has visual preferences for the human face, black-and-white contrasting patterns, and large objects. Some newborns appear cross-eyed because of undeveloped ocular muscle control; this normally resolves in 3 to 4 months. Eye color varies from dark to slate gray to pale blue. Because the lacrimal apparatus is not fully developed, the newborn does not produce tears until at least week 4 of life.

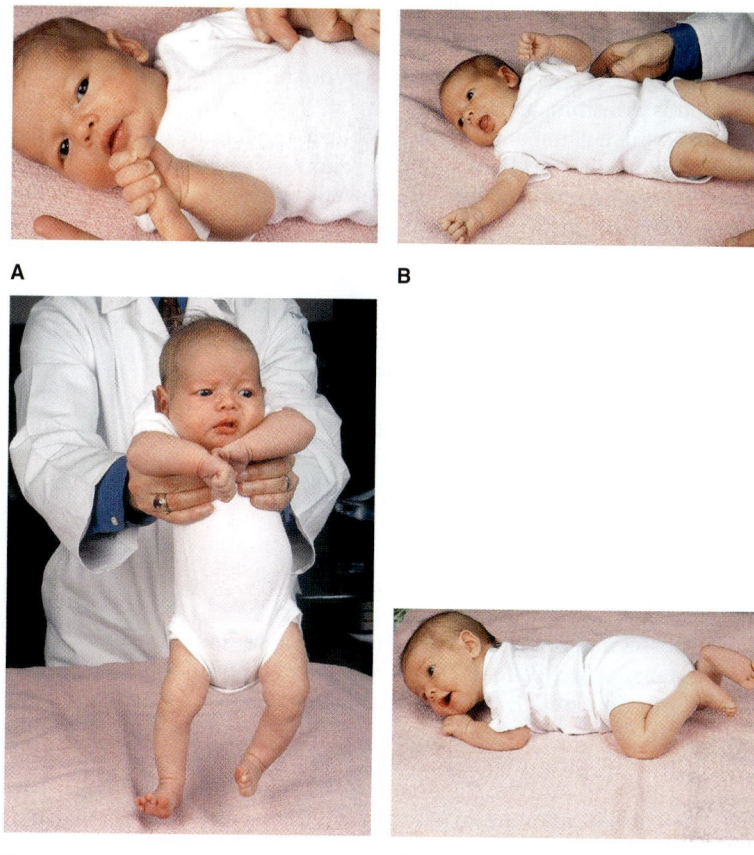

FIGURE 9-4 Several infant reflexes. (A) The palmar grasp reflex. (B) Tonic neck reflex. (C) Stepping reflex. (D) Crawling reflex.

Hearing and Smell. Once the amniotic fluid drains from the ears, hearing is equivalent to that of an adult. Newborns react strongly to pungent odors by turning the head away from a smell and are able to distinguish their own mother's breast milk from that of other women. They will cry for their mother when her breasts are engorged and leaking.

Touch. The newborn has a highly developed sense of touch, and his tactile sensation is surprisingly sophisticated, especially around the mouth, hands, and feet.

Psychosocial Development of the Neonate

The neonate is able to focus on the face of his caregivers. He calms when held or with other pacifying measures, such as a warm blanket, pacifier, and swaddling. Crying is the principal method for communicating a need or displeasure. Sometimes crying occurs simply because the neurological system is immature. Erikson identified the central developmental task of the first 18 months of life as developing a sense of trust. The neonate is completely dependent on her caretakers for all needs. Prompt responses to cries of discomfort create security and trust and promote attachment, emotional bonding between parent and child.

Common Health Problems of the Neonate

Respiratory Distress. Respiratory distress is one of the most serious problems facing newborns. It occurs most commonly in infants born before the lungs mature but can also be caused by aspiration of meconium during the birthing process. Newborns in respiratory distress are typically pale or mottled, with labored respirations, hypothermia, and flaccid muscle tone.

Birth Injuries. Birth injuries may occur at the time of the birthing process. The following are three examples:
- *Caput succedaneum,* edema of the scalp that crosses the suture lines, results from head compression against the cervix during labor. The fluid is reabsorbed in 1 to 3 days.
- *Fracture of the clavicle* occurs with breech presentation or as a result of difficulty delivering a large baby whose shoulder gets stuck behind the mother's pelvic bones. Often no intervention is needed except for careful handling and supporting the affected bone.
- *Birth asphyxia* is a serious and potentially permanent injury resulting from perinatal events, such as a **cord prolapse** (compression of the umbilical cord), placental abruption (bleeding secondary to tear of the placenta), or any other interruption of the blood supply between the baby and placenta or delay in infant respiration after birth.

Congenital Anomalies. Congenital anomalies may be visible at birth or may become apparent in the neonatal period, and treatment, if appropriate, may be initiated. Congenital heart defects, fistulas, and cleft lip and palate are some common birth defects, or the baby may have an inborn metabolic problem.

Infectious Microorganisms. Infectious microorganisms that do not cause illness in older babies can cause sepsis for newborns, especially those born prematurely. Pregnant women should be screened prenatally for sexually transmitted infections, and treatment initiated, if possible. Newborns who may have been exposed to infections during the gestational period should be tested as soon as possible after birth.

Jaundice. Jaundice is another risk for newborns. Within 48 to 72 hours after birth, the newborn's red blood cell (RBC) count normally begins to decrease. One byproduct of RBC destruction is **bilirubin,** a yellowish pigment. If the newborn is not successful in eliminating the excess bilirubin, jaundice develops, giving the newborn's skin a yellowish cast. If the bilirubin level becomes too high, the newborn can suffer neurological consequences as the pigment enters the brain. Sunlight breaks down bilirubin, thus phototherapy is a treatment of choice for jaundice.

Fetal Alcohol Syndrome. Fetal alcohol syndrome is characterized by irregular facial features and cognitive deficits. Newborns of pregnant women addicted to alcohol may show these signs.

Women with Substance Addiction. Newborns born to women who abuse substances during pregnancy are at risk for respiratory distress, behavioral abnormalities, and birth defects, as well as drug withdrawal.

ASSESSMENT

Physical assessment begins at birth. The initial assessment tool is the Apgar scoring system. The score is based on heart rate, respiratory effort, muscle tone, reflex irritability, and skin color (Table 9-4). Each category is scored at 1 and 5 minutes after birth. The 1-minute score indicates how well the baby tolerated the birthing process; the 5-minute score indicates how well the baby is adapting to the new environment. A high score indicates fetal well-being. Prematurity, neuromuscular disease, and maternal sedation during the birthing process are all factors that can lower the Apgar scores.

During the first 24 hours after birth, the infant goes through a transition to extrauterine life. For 6 to 8 hours after birth, the infant alternately cries and appears interested in the environment. The infant then enters the sleep stage, which lasts 2 to 4 hours. The heart and respiratory rates decrease. The infant is in a state of calm. After this restful phase, the infant is alert and responsive. The heart and respiratory rates again increase.

Shortly after birth, newborns are screened for a variety of genetic disorders. Most states require screening for phenylketonuria (PKU) (an inborn error of metabolism), hypothyroidism, galactosemia, and sickle cell disease. You will also need to assess the following parameters:

Vital signs
Elimination after birth (urine and meconium)
Physical assessment for congenital anomalies
Presence or absence of reflexes
Ability to breastfeed or take formula from a bottle
Skin integrity
Parent–infant attachment

INTERVENTIONS

The neonatal period is a time of transition. Feeding concerns and uncertainty about appropriate care are the primary reasons parents seek healthcare advice. Nursing interventions for the neonate are designed to smooth the transition to extrauterine life and help the neonate adjust to his new environment. Activities include the following:

Thoroughly dry the neonate at birth and after bathing to prevent heat loss via evaporation. Also wrap the neonate in blankets, and place her in her mother's arms or in a warmed crib.

- Assist the mother with breastfeeding or formula feeding. Often assistance is needed with the first few feedings as the newborn learns to latch on to the nipple.
- Teach parents the importance of providing warmth, nutrition, and a clean environment to prevent infection.
- Teach the caregivers about expected behavior, including crying, eating, and elimination.

Circumcision is surgical removal of the foreskin of the penis. Many male infants are circumcised a day or two after birth, although there is controversy over risks and benefits. Risks include hemorrhage, infection, and meatal stenosis. Benefits are said to include prevention of penile cancer and cervical cancer in a sexual partner. The main reason most parents elect circumcision for their infant is social—that is, so their child looks like other family members and peers. Parental consent is required for this procedure. Care of the site depends on the procedure used. Whatever the procedure, the nurse should

CATEGORY	0	1	2
Table 9-4 ▶ Apgar Scores			
Breathing effort	Not breathing	Respirations slow (less than 30 breaths/min) or irregular	Infant cries well
Heart rate (by stethoscope)	None	Less than 100 beats/min	Greater than 100 beats/min
Muscle tone	Loose and floppy	Some muscle tone, weak flexion	Active motion, full flexion
Reflex irritability (response to stimulation such as mild pinch)	No reaction	Grimacing	Grimacing and cough, sneeze, or vigorous cry
Skin color	Pale blue	Pink with blue extremities	Entire body is pink

Source: Medline Plus, U.S. National Library of Medicine, National Institutes of Health. (n.d.). *APGAR.* Last updated November 14, 2007. Retrieved March 27, 2011, from http://www.nlm.nih.gov/medlineplus/ency/article/003402.htm#top

observe and teach parents to observe for hemorrhage, swelling, or oozing (signs of infection).

INFANCY: 1 MONTH TO 1 YEAR OF AGE

The remainder of the first year is known as infancy. This is a time associated with dramatic physical changes and acquisition of numerous skills.

Physical Development of the Infant

Growth. During the first year of life, growth is very rapid. The full-term newborn loses approximately 8% to 10% of birth weight in the first days of life but will regain it by 2 weeks of age. The infant gains about 1½ pounds per month for the first 3 months. Birth weight doubles by 5 months of age and triples by 1 year. An infant's length increases approximately 1 inch per month until 6 months of age; it then slows to 1 inch over the next 6 months. Head circumference increases by about 33% in the first year.

Eruption of Primary Teeth. Eruption of teeth varies among children, but there is a distinct, predictable pattern for eruption. The first tooth typically appears between 6 and 8 months of age. First to appear are lower central incisors, followed by the upper central incisors.

Feeding. Infants typically consume about 30 ounces of breast milk or formula per day by 4 months of age. Most infants are physiologically ready to take solid foods between 4 and 6 months of age, but adequate nutrition can be maintained with breast milk or formula for a full year. The choices of when to begin introducing solid foods and what to use are often culturally determined, as is choice of when to wean. Breastfeeding is recommended because it is considered the most complete nutritional source for infants up to 6 months of age. Breastfeeding is accompanied by a lower incidence of food allergies, gastroenteritis, ear infections, and overweight in childhood, adolescence, and adulthood (Waldrop, 2008). In addition, breast milk supplies immunoglobulins that help the infant to resist infection. However, if breastfeeding is not possible or acceptable to the parents, the nurse should support the parents' choice of method.

Sleep Patterns. Sleep patterns vary among infants. Generally, by 3 to 4 months the infant has developed a night pattern of sleeping and can sleep approximately 10 hours. Infants vary in the number and length of naps they take, but the total numbers of hours they sleep per day is about 15.

Motor Development. Motor development follows a predictable pattern. Box 9-1 lists typical milestones.

Cognitive Development of the Infant

Piaget describes the infancy phase of cognitive development as the *sensorimotor phase*. Although the neonate responds in a reflexive manner, the infant makes major strides in motor development and is able to verbally interact with caregivers. Moreover, an infant's visual acuity and color discrimination allow her to see and explore the environment. Hearing is also becoming more discriminating, and infants please themselves by vocalizing with cooing, laughing, and repeating sounds they find pleasurable. By the 12th month, the infant is able to imitate sounds and understand simple words, and may have a vocabulary of four or five simple words, such as "da-da."

At this stage, infants learn by doing. They develop a simple sense of cause and effect, delighting in the fact that squeezing a ball, for example, causes it to squeak, and repeating their experiment over and over again. By 12 months of age, the infant recognizes familiar objects and searches for them when they are out of sight.

BOX 9-1 ■ Milestones of Infants Development

Age	Developmental Milestone
3 mo	Smile
5 mo	Roll from abdomen to back
6 mo	Turn from back to abdomen
7 mo	Most can sit alone
9 mo	Crawl on hands and knees
10 mo	Pincer grasp to pick up food; move from prone to sitting position
11 mo	Walk holding on to furniture ("cruising")
12 mo	Take steps independently; pick up objects and let them go; put objects in a container and take them out; find hidden objects and use objects, such as cups and combs, correctly; respond to simple verbal requests and commands ("Stop"); use simple gestures such as waving bye-bye or shaking their head no, and they may try to imitate adults' words.
	Psychosocial milestones include testing of caregivers to see what response is elicited by crying, refusals, and so on; anxiety with strangers; and strong preference for the primary caregiver (usually the mother).

Psychosocial Development of the Infant

In infancy the central task remains the development of trust. The response of the caregivers in the neonatal phase has set the tone for ongoing interaction between caregivers and child. Continued prompt responses to discomfort, cuddling, and stimulating interaction provide the infant with a sense of trust in the world.

Freud refers to infancy as the *oral stage*. The infant receives pleasure in sucking and learns to quiet himself by oral stimulation such as eating, sucking on a pacifier, or placing his hand in his mouth. At 2 or 3 months of age, infants begin to smile in response to others. At about 9 months they interact more with their environment and socialize with others. They enjoy simple games, such as peek-a-boo and patty-cake.

Common Health Problems of the Infant

Common problems that cause distress for infants and their caregivers include the following.

Crying and Colic

Crying often alarms parents, but it is a form of communication for the infant and a normal infant reaction to discomfort, cold, or hunger. A healthy infant will have "fussy" periods each day that may last up to 1 to 2 hours. Extended crying may be a sign of **colic,** a term used to describe frequent episodes of abdominal pain. The infant is often inconsolable during these episodes. The cause is unknown. Current theories include gulping of air, allergy or intolerance to formula or something that the breastfeeding mother ate, inability to digest the carbohydrates consumed, overstimulation, and parental anxiety. Colic typically disappears at about 3 months of age.

Failure to Thrive

Infants depend on their caregivers for food, water, warmth, comfort, and love. An infant who is deprived of a comforting,

responsive relationship with a mother or caregiver will not thrive even if supplied with adequate nutrition. The infant will fail to gain weight, be unable to meet age-appropriate developmental tasks, be malnourished, and may have difficulty interacting with others. This syndrome, known as **failure to thrive,** is exhibited, for example, in some infants in orphanages. Erikson believed the syndrome was proof of the essential nature of the trust versus mistrust stage. Notice, however, that failure to thrive can also stem from organic causes, such as disease or drug withdrawal.

Dental Caries

Dental caries (tooth decay) can develop even by the end of the first year in infants allowed to sleep with a bottle containing anything other than water. Caries are caused by pooling in the back of the mouth of fluids containing sugar, such as breast milk, formula, or juice. If you need more information about dental problems, see Chapter 24.

Example Problem: Abuse and Neglect

We have chosen abuse and neglect as a classic example of a problem of development because it is a common problem occurring in all developmental stages. You will read about it again and again in sections about other developmental stages, where we discuss how it manifests in those stages and suggest with appropriate nursing interventions.

About 1 in 50 infants in the United States are neglected or abused, according to a recent national study (Brodowski, Nolan, Gaudiosi, et al., 2008). Nearly a third of the infants were 1 week old or younger when the maltreatment was reported. Child abuse may take the form of physical or emotional abuse and neglect or sexual abuse. Abuse more commonly occurs as neglect. Unexplained injuries, neurological defects, seizures, and respiratory difficulty are all overt signs of abuse. **Shaken-baby syndrome** (also known as abusive head trauma), caused by violent shaking of an infant, is a form of abuse that causes severe brain injury but may not produce visible evidence of trauma. It can cause blindness and spinal cord damage, as well as broken bones.

Factors associated with child abuse and neglect include low income status, low maternal education, non-white race, large family size, young maternal age, single-parent household, and parental psychiatric disturbances (Hussey, Chang, & Kotch, 2006; Office on Child Abuse and Neglect (HHS), 2003; Schnitzer & Ewigman, 2005). Household composition is another risk factor: Young children living with unrelated adults, stepparents, or foster parents are at increased risk of fatal injury from maltreatment (Schnitzer & Ewigman, 2008).

Unintentional Injury

Automobile accidents are a major cause of death in infants, often because the child was not properly restrained. Falls, burns, choking, and drowning are other common causes of accidental injury and death in infants. As infants mature, they may attempt to climb from cribs onto chairs or tables, or up or down ungated stairs. Their tendency to explore things with their mouths may lead to choking on small objects, such as bottle caps, buttons, and parts of toys. Rigorous safeguarding of the home environment is critical. Infants should never be left unattended in water, even for a few seconds, no matter how shallow the water. Infants can drown in sinks, shallow baths, and plastic wading pools. Finally, the risk of infant scalding increases when caregivers drink or carry hot foods or fluids while holding the baby, leave hot pots unattended on the stove, or use a water heater set higher than 120°F. If you require more information about infant safety, refer to Chapter 23.

Sudden Infant Death Syndrome (SIDS)

SIDS is the sudden death of a previously healthy infant with no explainable cause. Even postmortem examinations fail to reveal a cause of death. The peak incidence is usually around 3 to 4 months of age, although it may occur up to 12 months of age. An increased incidence is associated with prematurity, low birth weight, male gender, African American race, smoking in the household, swaddling, and putting an infant to sleep in the prone position (Fig. 9-5).

■ ASSESSMENT

The infant typically has regular appointments with the pediatrician or primary care provider until at least 6 months of age. As a rule, visits are timed to coincide with the immunization schedule, at 2, 4, 6, and 12 months. More frequent visits may be required if problems are identified. At each visit, measure the infant's growth and development and compare against standards for height, weight, head circumference, and gross and fine motor skills.

The Denver Developmental Screening Test (Denver II) is a frequently used standardized test to assess development. The Denver II assesses four major areas: personal–social, fine motor skills, language, and gross motor skills. It requires specialized training to administer and evaluate.

You should be aware of factors that increase the risk for child abuse and assess for abuse any time there is an injury that is not well explained by the parent's account of how it occurred. For further discussion about assessing for abuse, see Procedure 9-1.

■ INTERVENTIONS

Nursing interventions for the infant focus on health promotion, safety, and growth and development.

Nutrition. Teach parents about adequate nutrition, adding foods to the diet, and expected elimination patterns. If breastfeeding is not possible, or is not the parents' method of

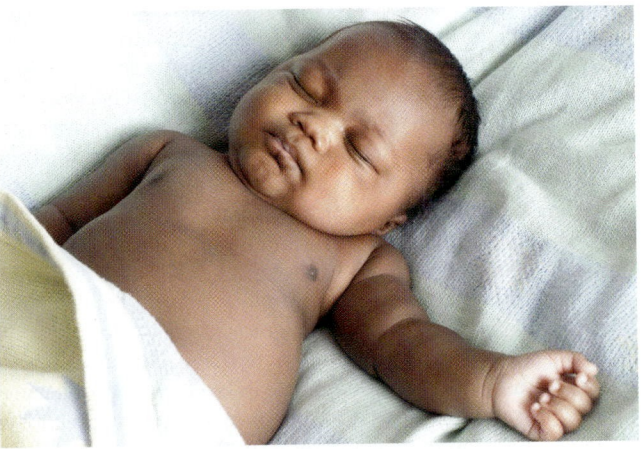

FIGURE 9-5 The Back to Sleep campaign teaches parents to place the infant in the supine position for sleeping.

choice, commercially prepared formulas fortified with vitamins and minerals are acceptable. Cow's milk should not be used during the first year of life because infants have difficulty digesting the fat in it, and it is low in iron.

Colic. Provide information about using warmth, motion, and security to relieve colic. For example, parents might try swaddling the baby, cuddling him close to their body, rocking him, placing him in a "kangaroo" pouch or a backpack, or placing him in a swinging chair.

SIDS. In accordance with recommendations in *Healthy People 2020*, teach parents to place infants on their backs to sleep. Research shows that this greatly decreases the risk for SIDS.

Additional interventions are discussed in Chapter 23.

Car Seats. Stress the importance of car seats. Under federal law, infants must be secured in an approved car seat (in the backseat) every time they are in a vehicle. Because of poorly developed musculoskeletal head support, infants should be placed in a rear-facing position until 2 years of age and until they reach the height and weight recommended by the seat manufacturer (American Academy of Pediatrics, 2011).

For more information about car seat restraints, refer to Chapter 23 and,

 Go to the American Academy of Pediatrics Web site, at http://www.aap.org/healthtopics/carseatsafety.cfm

Immunizations. Immunizations are a major aspect of health promotion for the infant. The infant receives immunizations at 2, 4, 6, and 12 months. Figure 9-6 identifies the optimal immunization schedule for children up to 6 years of age. The CDC is no longer expressing a preference for administering the combined MMRV vaccine rather than two shots (MMR for measles, mumps and rubella, and a separate one for varicella [chicken pox] [CDC, 2011a]).

Unintentional Injury. Stress the importance of constant supervision. As the infant gains greater mobility, potential dangers (e.g., for falls and burns) increase.

Play. Encourage sensory stimulation for the infant through parental interaction and age-appropriate toys.

Interventions for Example Problem: Abuse. Teach parents about the dangers of shaking a baby or picking him up by an arm or leg.

If you suspect abuse, you are legally responsible for reporting your observations. As a beginning student, you may wish to discuss your concerns and findings with your instructor or the nurse assigned to the client before you make a report. Federal funds support a variety of home visit programs directed at high-risk mothers (identified on the basis of risk factors). There is some evidence that they decrease the incidences of child abuse and neglect, but it is not conclusive. Further information on abuse and reporting is included in Chapter 43 and in Procedure 9-1.

Think**Like a Nurse** 9-3

Recall the story of Miguel, a 2-month-old infant, in the Meet Your Patients scenario. How might a prolonged hospitalization affect his growth and development? What nursing actions would you take to offset developmental delays?

Knowledge**Check** 9-4

- Identify at least two reflexes present in the neonate.
- According to Erikson, what is the developmental stage of the infant?
- What teaching guideline is important in reducing the risk of SIDS?

Recommended Immunization Schedule for Persons Aged 0 Through 6 Years—United States • 2011
For those who fall behind or start late, see the catch-up schedule

Vaccine ▼ Age ▶	Birth	1 month	2 months	4 months	6 months	12 months	15 months	18 months	19–23 months	2–3 years	4–6 years	
Hepatitis B	HepB	HepB			HepB							
Rotavirus			RV	RV	RV							
Diphtheria, Tetanus, Pertussis			DTaP	DTaP	DTaP		DTaP				DTaP	Range of recommended ages for all children
Haemophilus influenzae type b			Hib	Hib	Hib	Hib						
Pneumococcal			PCV	PCV	PCV	PCV				PPSV		
Inactivated Poliovirus			IPV	IPV		IPV					IPV	Range of recommended ages for certain high-risk groups
Influenza						Influenza (Yearly)						
Measles, Mumps, Rubella						MMR					MMR	
Varicella						Varicella					Varicella	
Hepatitis A						HepA (2 doses)				HepA Series		
Meningococcal										MCV4		

This schedule includes recommendations in effect as of December 21, 2010. Any dose not administered at the recommended age should be administered at a subsequent visit, when indicated and feasible. The use of a combination vaccine generally is preferred over separate injections of its equivalent component vaccines. Considerations should include provider assessment, patient preference, and the potential for adverse events. Providers should consult the relevant Advisory Committee on Immunization Practices statement for detailed recommendations: **http://www.cdc.gov/vaccines/pubs/acip-list.htm**. Clinically significant adverse events that follow immunization should be reported to the Vaccine Adverse Event Reporting System (VAERS) at **http://www.vaers.hhs.gov** or by telephone, **800-822-7967**. Use of trade names and commercial sources is for identification only and does not imply endorsement by the U.S. Department of Health and Human Services.

FIGURE 9-6 For additional information about vaccines, visit the National Immunization Web site at http://www.cdc.gov/vaccines

TODDLERHOOD: AGES 1 TO 3 YEARS

The toddler period lasts from 12 to 36 months of age. This is a period of increased mobility, independence, and exploration. This is also the time of temper tantrums and negative behavior, stemming from the toddler's desire to gain autonomy.

Physical Development of the Toddler

Compared to that of infants, toddlers' *growth rate* is much slower. The average toddler gains 5 lb (2.3 kg) per year and increases in height by 3 in. (7.6 cm). Length is added mainly in the legs. By the second birthday the typical toddler weighs 27 lb (12.25 kg), is 34 in. (86 cm) tall, and has a head circumference equal to the chest circumference. Between 12 and 18 months, the anterior fontanel closes (see Fig. 9-3).

- *Respirations and heart rate* slow in comparison to infancy, but blood pressure increases.
- *The stomach* increases in size to accommodate larger portions. Toddlers typically eat about six times a day, in relatively small portions, and join the family at mealtimes. Most toddlers enjoy picking up food with their hands to feed themselves.
- *The physical ability to control the anal and urethral sphincters* develops between 18 and 24 months. However, the child is ready to toilet train when she can signal that her diaper is wet or soiled, or is able to say that she would like to go to the potty. This usually occurs at about 18 to 24 months of age, but it is not uncommon for a child to be in diapers until 3 years of age (American Academy of Family Physicians, 2006, updated 2010).
- *Gross motor skills* continue to be refined during toddlerhood. By 10 to 15 months, the toddler can walk using a wide stance. At the age of 24 months, many toddlers can walk up and down stairs one step at a time. At 30 months, he can jump using both feet. Before the age of 3, the toddler can stand on one foot and climb steps alternating feet.
- *Fine motor skills* also continue to be refined. By 1 year, infants can grasp small objects yet are unable to release the object. However, by 15 months the toddler can release objects as well. By 18 months he can throw a ball overhand (Fig. 9-7). The toddler uses his new motor skills and all five senses to explore his environment, and safety continues to be an important concern
- *Visual acuity* improves to 20/40 by the end of the toddler stage, and strabismus (crossed eyes) may still be seen transiently.
- *Hearing* should be fully developed by toddlerhood.

Developmental milestones of toddlerhood are listed in Box 9-2.

Cognitive Development of the Toddler

During toddlerhood the child completes Piaget's *sensorimotor phase* and moves into the *preconceptual phase*. This is a time of rapid language development and increasing curiosity. The toddler is able to name many things and begins to recognize that different objects (such as a ball, a block, and a puzzle) may be named the same thing (toys). This is the beginning of categorization and concept development. In the preconceptual phase, the child abandons trial and error and begins to solve problems by thinking. However, reasoning and judgment lag far behind. This discrepancy places the child at risk for accidents and injuries.

Psychosocial Development of the Toddler

The most important psychosocial developmental task for the toddler is to initiate more independence, control, and autonomy. Erikson refers to this stage as *autonomy versus shame and doubt*. To

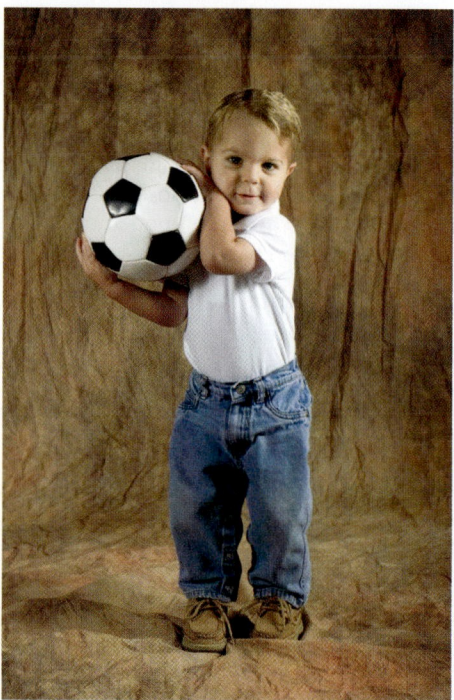

FIGURE 9-7 By 18 mo, the toddler can throw a ball overhand.

BOX 9-2 ■ Milestones of Toddlerhood

- The toddler can ride a tricycle, put simple puzzles together, build a tower of six to eight blocks, turn knobs, and open lids.
- Most toddlers can copy a circle or a vertical line.
- Not only can the toddler find an object that has been hidden in his view, but he can also actively search for and find a hidden object.
- By age 3, most toddlers are toilet trained. However, it is not abnormal for toddlers to continue to experience toileting problems well into the preschool period.
- Most toddlers can play matching games, sorting games, and simple mechanical games.
- Most toddlers have only a limited understanding of jokes and hyperbole; thus, if teased, "That balloon is so big, it might fly away with you," the child may become frightened and try to give the balloon away.
- Many toddlers can speak sentences of four or five words. However, some perfectly healthy toddlers do not yet speak, whereas others can speak in sentences 10 or 11 words in length and even tell complex stories. If the toddler does speak, enunciation is good enough by the end of this period that strangers can usually understand what is said.
- Psychosocial milestones include the following: The toddler tolerates short separations from the primary caregiver, feels possessive of personal property, and openly expresses affection. Most toddlers object vehemently to changes in routine and may suffer regression following a move, change of school, or other upset.
- The toddler imitates adults, peers, and characters seen on television and videos and enjoys pretending to cook, iron, repair something broken, and mimicking other familiar adult tasks.
- In shared play, the toddler can understand the concept of taking turns and wait a short period of time for her turn.

successfully negotiate this stage, the child must learn to see herself as separate from mother, tolerate separation from the parents, withstand delayed gratification, learn to control anal and urinary sphincters, and begin to verbally communicate and interact with others.

Toddlers exert their independence by saying no to parental requests or actions or by "throwing a tantrum" to protest a parental decision they don't like. This behavior is best understood as a necessary attempt to define boundaries and test parental limits; it may be far more challenging to parents who view it as stubbornness or naughtiness. A firm but calm parental response to such "misbehavior" allows toddlers to feel secure while exploring their boundaries.

Freud defined this phase, which coincides with toilet training, as the *anal stage*. To Freud, a successful toilet-training experience accompanied by praise is necessary to becoming a well-functioning adult. Difficulty in this phase would lead to obsessive–compulsive behavior in adulthood. Contemporary theorists find this view somewhat narrow.

Common Health Problems of Toddlers

Unintentional Injury. ✚ Motor vehicle accidents are one of the leading causes of accidental death in this age group. Most deaths are due to improper use of restraints or failure to use them at all.

As toddlers explore their world, accidents happen. Common injuries to toddlers are falls, drowning, burns and scalds, and choking. As toddlers gain increasing mobility, poisoning from household medications and toxic cleansers, as well as access to knives, guns, and other dangers, become concerns. If you are interested in further discussion of safety concerns for toddlers, see Chapter 23.

Infections. The shorter and flatter eustachian tube in infants and toddlers increases their risk for multiple ear infections, which in turn increase the risk for hearing loss. Upper respiratory infections are common among toddlers. They no longer have the passive immunity acquired in utero, and because breastfeeding usually ends before the first birthday, most toddlers no longer receive maternal antibodies in breast milk. Furthermore, as toddlers enter into more public and social settings, they are exposed to more children. Those in day care and those who have school-age siblings are particularly at risk. The most common infections are colds, ear infections, and tonsillitis. Other common infections include parasitic diseases, such as lice and tapeworms.

Infectious Diseases. The CDC (2011a) updated the childhood immunization schedule (see Fig. 9-6) to include the following:

- **Hepatitis B vaccine.** The first dose is given to newborns before leaving the hospital. The second dose should be administered at 1 to 2 months of age, and the third between 6 and 18 months. If hepatitis B vaccine is part of a combination vaccine, a fourth dose is permissible. (Advisory Committee on Immunization Practices, 2008).
- *Haemophilus influenzae* **vaccine.** Annual vaccination is now recommended for all children ages 6 months and older. A trivalent inactivated vaccine or live attenuated vaccine (intranasal influenza vaccine) is indicated for healthy persons ages 2 to 49 years (Advisory Committee on Immunization Practices, 2008).
- **Meningococcal conjugate vaccine.** This vaccine is preferred over the meningococcal polysaccharide vaccine for high-risk children.

- **Td/Tdap.** Tetanus and diphtheria toxoids / tetanus and diphtheria toxoids and acellular pertussis vaccine catch-up schedule requires four doses, with at least 4 weeks between doses 2 and 3, for children who had their first dose before age 12 months (*Morbidity and Mortality Weekly Report*, 2008a).
- **Pneumococcal vaccine.** One dose of pneumococcal conjugate vaccine (PCV) is given to all healthy children ages 24 to 59 months having any incomplete schedule. Administer pneumococcal polysaccharide vaccine (PPV) to children ages 2 years and older with underlying medical conditions (Advisory Committee on Immunization Practices, 2008).
- **Varicella vaccine.** The minimum age is 12 months for the first dose. Second dose is given between 4 and 6 years (Advisory Committee on Immunization Practices, 2008).
- **Hepatitis A vaccine.** The first dose should not be given before 12 months of age. The second dose is given at least 6 months after the first (Advisory Committee on Immunization Practices, 2008).
- **Rotavirus vaccine.** Administer the first dose between 6 to 12 weeks of age. The final dose is given by 32 weeks (Advisory Committee on Immunization Practices, 2008).

Toilet Training. Many parents of toddlers are concerned about what they perceive as delayed toilet training. Physiologically, most children develop sphincter and neurological control by age 2, but more is involved in successful toileting. Children must be able to unfasten their clothing and pull down their pants, use toilet paper effectively, dress again, and wash their hands before complete independence is reached. The child also must be able to sense the need to go to the bathroom, even when preoccupied with play activities, before it is "too late." Accidents are frequent and should be expected.

◼ ASSESSMENT

Toddlers need regular physical examinations. When caring for a toddler, you must be sensitive to the fact that children of this age are generally fearful of strangers. Thus, before assessing the toddler, you will need to establish rapport. To do so, you might engage the child in play—for example, by playing catch with a soft ball or asking the child to introduce you to the stuffed animal he may have brought along. This is a nonthreatening way to assess the toddler's language skills and motor development. Encourage parents to relieve their child's stress and anxiety by holding him during the exam and speaking to him in a calm and reassuring voice.

At each office visit, assess the toddler for height, weight, and growth and development. Evaluate the child's progress against standard growth charts and by comparing his skills against age-appropriate norms. Beginning at age 3, blood pressure should be checked at least once yearly (Uphold & Grahan, 2004).

◼ INTERVENTIONS

✚ **Health Teaching.** Health teaching of safety issues cannot be stressed enough to the parents. Areas of vulnerability are everywhere. Teach parents to childproof the environment. You will need to emphasize that increasing motor skills and dexterity allow the toddler to find many dangers, including stairways, windows, and electrical outlets. To prevent injury or death from such hazards, parents must provide constant supervision. The use of consistent, firm limits helps the toddler remain safe. Parents should also be

vigilant about the toys they buy for their children, in light of recent toy recalls because they contained lead and other toxic substances. Toys should be larger than the diameter of the trachea in order to avoid choking accidents. Plan ahead by teaching parents basic first aid and the choking rescue maneuver (see Chapter 23). Encourage parents to enroll in a basic life support class. You will also find a detailed list of safety measures for toddlers in Chapter 23.

Health Promotion Interventions. Interventions for the toddler include reinforcing at each visit the need for hand-washing, tooth brushing, regular dental exams, and a balanced diet. This is also a time for additional immunizations and boosters (see Fig. 9-6). Children should see a dentist at between 12 and 36 months of age—certainly by age 3, when all teeth have erupted (Uphold & Grahan, 2004).

Methicillin-Resistant Staphylococcus Aureus (MRSA) and Vancomycin-Resistant Enterococci (VRE). These organisms have put a spotlight on the threat posed by drug-resistant bacteria. Teach parents that antibiotics should not be used for simple colds and flu. Explain the importance of taking the entire prescription when an antibiotic is prescribed, even if the child's symptoms resolve. These actions help prevent the development of drug-resistant strains of bacteria. Although this is not specific for MRSA or VRE, also remind parents that many cough and cold medicines marketed to children have not been approved for use in children and that they should be certain that any over-the-counter medicines are truly safe for children.

KnowledgeCheck 9-5

- According to Erikson, what is the developmental stage of the toddler?
- What is the leading cause of accidental death in toddlers?

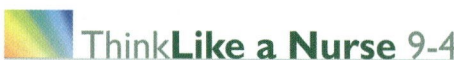

ThinkLike a Nurse 9-4

Recall the story of Tamika, a 3-year-old girl, in the Meet Your Patients scenario. Her grandmother, who is also caring for her ill husband, is raising Tamika. What concerns does that raise about the home environment?

PRESCHOOL STAGE: AGES 4 AND 5 YEARS

The preschooler is growing increasingly verbal and independent and is refining gross and fine motor skills. She is able to maintain separation from parents, use language to communicate needs, control bodily functions, and cooperate with children as well as adults. These skills prepare the child to enter school.

Physical Development of the Preschooler

Growth. By 4 years of age, the average preschooler weighs about 36 lb (16.3 kg) and is 40 in. (1 m) tall. By age 5, the preschooler has gained an additional 5 lb (2.3 kg) and has grown 3 more in. (7.6 cm) in height. The proportions of head to trunk are somewhat closer, and the "pot belly" and exaggerated lumbar curve of toddlerhood gradually disappear. The average pulse rate is 90 to 100 beats/min, and respirations are 22 to 25 per minute.

Sensorimotor Development. The preschooler has mature depth and color perception and 20/20 vision. Hearing is also mature. The preschooler continues to develop eye–hand

coordination. At age 4, the child can hop, skip, and jump on one leg. Improvement in fine motor skills is most evident in artwork. Drawings become much more precise and detailed. The child is becoming independent in the ability to dress. Developmental milestones for preschoolers are listed in Box 9-3.

Cognitive Development of Preschoolers

According to Piaget, the preschooler has entered the phase of *intuitive thought*. She is able to classify objects and continues to form concepts. She continues to use trial and error as a way to solve problems but increasingly uses thought to reason out problems. Verbal skills expand dramatically during this phase, allowing the child to interact with more people. Preschool children are very interested in books, learning to read, and counting.

Preschoolers still lack the ability to reason formally and are unable to understand that two objects that appear different may in fact be the same (e.g., two balls of clay in two different shapes). They have a limited ability to tell time or understand the passage of time, and they may say "yesterday" in describing an event of several months ago. They also retain a strong belief in magic, monsters, and mythic figures, such as Santa Claus. Preschoolers often have irrational fears—for example, of tigers lurking in the basement. Their fascination with powerful figures, such as dinosaurs and superheroes, is one way of coping with their feelings of powerlessness.

Psychosocial Development of Preschoolers

The preschooler is in Erikson's stage of *initiative versus guilt* (Fig. 9-8). This is the stage in which the child develops a conscience and readily recognizes right from wrong. The child

---

BOX 9-3 ■ Milestones of Preschool Development

- By age 5, most children can stand on one foot for 10 sec, skip, jump, hop on one foot or both feet together, climb play structures with ease, repeat simple dance steps, and begin to learn to skate.
- Most preschoolers can copy a triangle, square, and stick figure, print at least some letters, and use a fork and spoon. Most can dress and use the bathroom without assistance.
- Language abilities continue to be variable, but most preschoolers can tell stories, recall parts of a story told to them, and speak in sentences of more than five words. Most can state their name, age, and address, and many can repeat their home phone number. A toddler who is not speaking intelligibly by age 4 requires evaluation.
- Preschoolers can count 10 or more objects, such as buttons or coins, and may be able to name several colors and shapes. They can compare big and small, long and short, and so on and often delight in completing simple mazes and "connect the dots" games.
- Preschoolers become increasingly aware of sex organ differences and curious about sexuality.
- Preschoolers may begin to ask about God, death, how babies are born, and other questions of a philosophical or scientific nature.
- Preschoolers typically can distinguish fantasy from reality and enjoy jokes and simple riddles.
- Psychosocial milestones include assertion of independence; pride in showing off skills, new toys and clothes, and prize possessions to friends; and a strong desire to socialize with peers.

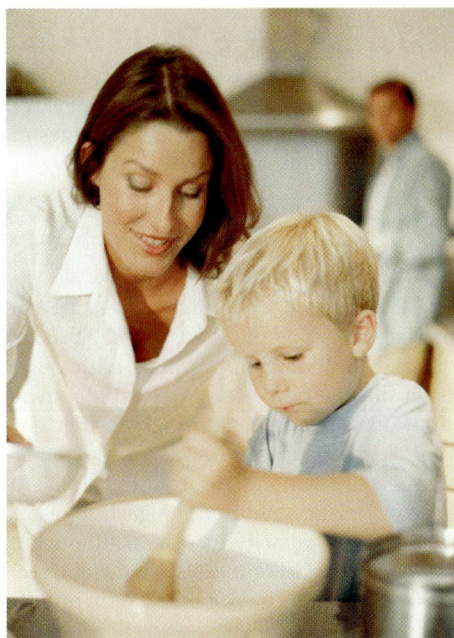

FIGURE 9-8 Preschoolers typically enjoy helping Mother in the kitchen.

becomes socially aware of others and develops the ability to consider other people's viewpoints. At this age, play is often used to teach life experiences.

In this phase, the child begins to fully express his personality and develop a self-concept (see Chapter 13 if you need to learn more about self-concept). He readily expresses likes and dislikes. Encouraging the child to participate in his favorite activities will foster a positive self-concept. Preschool children enjoy playing in small groups and use their language skills to facilitate imaginative play. Often elaborate stories, improvised costumes, and role-playing become part of the play experience. Many preschoolers have a best friend.

Freud identified the preschool years as the *phallic stage* of development. The preschool child is aware of gender differences and often imitates the same-sex parent. The child also develops an attraction to the opposite-sex parent and may feel jealousy toward the same-sex parent.

Common Health Problems of Preschoolers

The preschooler experiences health problems similar to those of the toddler.

Communicable Diseases. Communicable diseases (e.g., respiratory infections, intestinal viruses, and parasitic infections, such as scabies and lice) remain a major health issue, especially as preschoolers expand their social groups and come in contact with more children in play and structured preschool experiences. They interact more with playmates, and are hands-on, so they tend to readily transmit viruses through direct contact and airborne vectors.

Poisoning. ✚ Poisoning remains a significant risk for preschoolers, who often use imitation as a way to learn about new things. This predisposes the child to ingesting substances used by the adults in the house, such as prescription medicines and alcohol, or substances that look similar to these products.

Enuresis. Parents of preschoolers may report a concern about bedwetting (*enuresis*), especially in boys. The causes of enuresis are not fully understood, but it is known that in some children the bladder is simply unable to hold a full night's output of urine until later in childhood, whereas others lack the neurological ability to waken in response to a full bladder. Most cases resolve spontaneously, with only very occasional episodes past age 6. In contrast, daytime wetting or soiling (**encopresis**) requires evaluation.

Example Problem: Child Abuse.

Child abuse can occur at any age. It is often detected in the toddler and preschool period as children come in contact with more people outside the home. Abuse may be physical, emotional, or sexual or due to neglect. Of the confirmed cases of abuse and neglect reported to Child Protective Services, more than half are under the age of 7. Child abuse is not isolated to any one socioeconomic or education level group. The following are a few of the reasons why some people have difficulty meeting the demands of parenthood:

- **Parental characteristics:** Parents who were abused as a child are more likely to abuse their own children, especially when faced with high levels of stress and little support from others. Abuse can occur when parents or caregivers have unrealistic expectations of the child or unmet emotional needs of their own. Immaturity, lack of parenting knowledge, and difficulty in relationships can contribute as well. Depression, anxiety, and other mental health problems are factors for some parents, as are alcohol and drug addiction.
- **Characteristics of the child:** Statistical data indicate that children with a physical or mental disability and those who are born to unmarried parents or who are unwanted are more likely to suffer abuse.
- **Situational characteristics:** Crowded living space, financial difficulty, stresses of child care, employment pressures or unemployment, poor housing, domestic violence in the home, and frequent household moves, are all environmental stressors that can contribute to child abuse. One study found maternal self-report of neglectful behavior to be associated with an increased risk of childhood obesity (Whitaker, Phillips, Orzol, et al., 2007).

For further discussion of child abuse, refer to the preceding section on Infancy, and to Procedure 9-1, Assessing for Abuse.

▬ ASSESSMENT

Assessments for preschoolers should include the following:

Weight and Vital Signs. Gather the data and compare your findings with age-appropriate norms. Body mass index (BMI) should be calculated and plotted at every well-child visit. To obtain information about BMI from the Centers for Disease Control and Prevention Web site,

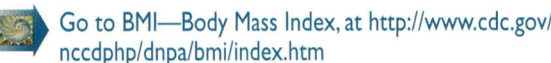 Go to BMI—Body Mass Index, at http://www.cdc.gov/nccdphp/dnpa/bmi/index.htm

Nutrition. The preschool child often has strong food preferences. Assess for food preferences, habits, and amount eaten.

Sleep Habits. Preschoolers are generally very active but require adequate rest. This is also the time when children stop taking afternoon naps. You will need to assess the numbers of hours slept, bedtime rituals, and problems with night awakenings.

Dental Hygiene. During the preschool years, all deciduous teeth have erupted. Therefore, dental hygiene is very important. At each visit, ask the child about tooth-brushing habits. If possible, have the child demonstrate how he brushes. The child should already have made at least one visit to a dentist by age 3.

Safety. ✚ Because the preschool child is mobile and involved in activities such as riding a tricycle, chasing a ball, and crossing streets, accidents increase. Assess for parent and child knowledge of hazards and precautions.

School Readiness. A physical examination is required before the child enters school. This exam should include an assessment for *readiness*—whether the child has acquired skills, such as an ability to converse with adults; follow instructions; hold a pencil; and perform a variety of motor skills, such as jump, hop, and walk a straight line. At the readiness exam, you will also need to review the immunization record. Several boosters and immunizations are due at this time. Any missed immunizations must be administered before the child enters school. To see the CDC Catch-up Immunization Schedule,

 Go to Chapter 9, **Tables, Boxes, Figures, ESG Figure 9-1,** on Davis*Plus.*

Also refer to Common Health Problems of Toddlers, earlier in this chapter.

■ INTERVENTIONS

The preschool child is interactive and curious. Speak directly to the child, and include her in your teaching sessions. Teaching topics include the following:

- *Frequent handwashing to prevent the spread of disease.* Teach the child hand-washing technique, and encourage parents to model frequent handwashing.
- *Proper brushing and flossing of teeth.* At this age, most children still need supervision while brushing their teeth.
- *The essentials of a balanced diet.* Encourage parents to offer a well-balanced diet and to instill healthy eating habits. By the age of 5 most children are willing to try new foods and are better able to sit during an entire meal. Generally, preschoolers eat half the food portion of that of an adult.
- *The importance of adequate rest.* The average preschooler requires at least 12 hours of sleep each night.

✚ *The hazard of stranger danger.* Increasing independence and mobility place the preschool child at risk for abduction. Teach the child to avoid talking to strangers and never to enter a stranger's home or car. This topic is explored in depth once the child is in school.

✚ *The importance of seat belts and car seats.* Current recommendations are to use booster seats for children weighing between 40 and 80 pounds and to continue using the seat until the child is at least 4 feet 9 inches tall.

KnowledgeCheck 9-6

- According to Erikson, what is the developmental stage of the preschooler?
- Identify at least two important assessments to make when providing care to a preschooler.

SCHOOL-AGE: AGES 6 TO 12 YEARS

The school-age child undergoes many changes: The child becomes more independent, places more importance on relationships outside the immediate family, and becomes more confident. Developmental milestones of the school-age period are summarized in Box 9-4.

Physical Development of the School-Age Child

Growth. During the school-age years, the child grows about 2 in. (5 cm) taller and gains 4 to 7 lb (2.3 to 3 kg) per year. The child takes on a slimmer appearance, with longer legs and a lower center of gravity. Muscle mass rapidly increases, and ossification of bones continues throughout this age. Strength and physical abilities rapidly improve, and the child gains more poise and coordination. The brain and skull grow slowly, and facial characteristics mature. The gastrointestinal system matures and stomach capacity increases, although caloric demands decrease. As the immune system develops, the school-age child begins to produce antibodies and antigens. Initially boys and girls vary little in size. Toward the end of this phase, marked differences become apparent. Girls grow rapidly in the latter school-age years, as puberty begins, and experience onset of puberty about 2 years before boys do.

Visual Acuity. Visual acuity improves with age. American Academy of Pediatrics Vision Screening Guidelines specify that all children over age 8 should be able to achieve 20/20 visual acuity using their best eyeglass correction. Younger children should be referred to an ophthalmologist if there is a difference between the right and left eyes of two or more lines on a Snellen chart evaluation (Broderick, 1998).

Dentition. School-age children begin to lose their primary teeth (baby teeth) at about age 6 or 7, and the permanent teeth appear soon after. Their large size in relation to the remaining primary teeth and the child's jaw, as well as the gaps left by teeth not yet replaced, can make even the most beautiful children look somewhat awkward at this stage.

BOX 9-4 ■ Milestones of School-Age Development

- By age 7, most children can tie their own shoelaces; print their names; and perform self-care, such as bathing and feeding themselves. Many can even prepare simple meals.
- By age 8, improved fine motor skills allow the child to begin to write, learn to knit or crochet, and/or take up a musical instrument.
- By age 9, motor development approaches that of an adult.
- School-age children understand the concept of payment for work and the value of money.
- Fears of ghosts and monsters may continue through age 7 but give way to more realistic fears, such as of school failure or divorce of parents, by age 8 or 9.
- By age 6, the child has a vocabulary of 3,000 words and usually can read. By the end of the school-age period, the child can write complex compositions with appropriate grammar, spelling, and accurate description.
- Psychosocial development includes team play, peer friendships, and ability to look beyond family members for social support.

Cognitive Development of the School-Age Child

School-age children use their thought processes to experience actions and events. Piaget describes this as *concrete operations.* Thinking is concrete and systematic, and magical beliefs are gradually replaced with a passion to understand how things really are. The child is also able to see another person's point of view and develops an understanding of relationships. He learns to classify objects according to similarities and enjoys learning by handling and manipulating objects. The child learns to tell time and gains an experiential understanding of the length of days, months, and years. He reads independently and does numerical calculations without representative objects, such as fingers or beads. By the end of the school-age years, the child is able to think through a task and understand it without actually performing the task.

Psychosocial Development of the School-Age Child

Erikson describes this stage as a time of *industry versus inferiority.* In school, the child may be recognized for achievements and accomplishments. Over this stage, she is able to work at more complex projects independently. For the child to progress through this stage, the parent must provide praise for accomplishments. This recognition builds self-confidence. The child will develop a sense of inferiority and lack of self-worth if her accomplishments are met with a negative response.

Peers take on increasing importance, influencing the child's choices of what to eat, wear, and do. Friendships during the school-age years are usually with children of the same gender and may be intense but short-lived (Fig. 9-9). However, some children have one best friend throughout their childhood. In the later school-age years, friendships become more reciprocal with each child recognizing the unique qualities of the other.

Common Health Problems of School-Age Children

School-age children are at risk for problems similar to those of preschoolers, including upper respiratory tract infections, parasitic infections such as scabies and lice, and dental caries. Although violence; bullying; smoking; and experimentation with alcohol, drugs, and sex are more common among adolescents, these problems are also seen toward the end of the school-age years. The presence of a gun in the home significantly increases the risk of accidental death, even in the school-age population.

Childhood Obesity

Obesity among school-age children has become a growing health concern. In 1994, 11% of children ages 6 to 11 were obese (defined as being in the 95th percentile of body mass index); by 2002, that figure had risen to 19%, where it remains (National Center for Health Statistics, n. d., updated 2010). Between 1963 and 2008, obesity rates more than quadrupled among children ages 6 to 11 years. Childhood obesity has reached epidemic proportions, resulting in increased prevalence of obesity-related diseases. Nutrition and lifestyle are primarily responsible for this epidemic. Children spend much less time playing outside than in past generations and more time watching television and playing on computers. Children today eat more fast food, consume bigger portions, and eat fewer vegetables. One-third of people ages 4 to 29 years eat fast food daily (Miller & Silverstein, 2007).

Obesity-related diseases, such as type 2 diabetes mellitus (type 2 DM), hyperlipidemia, and hypertension, have risen in children accordingly. **Type 2 DM** is an endocrine disorder characterized by insulin resistance: Insulin fails to effectively transfer glucose from the bloodstream into the body's cells. The pancreas then attempts to produce more insulin. Eventually, the pancreatic cells lose the ability to secrete adequate levels of insulin, and the person can no longer tolerate normal glucose intake. Treatment involves dietary changes, weight loss, and exercise. Medications are required if these lifestyle changes are not sufficient to control blood sugar.

Childhood Asthma

Asthma, a chronic inflammatory disorder of the airways, affects about 6.8 million children (nearly 10%) in the United States, including 9.3% of children 5 to 10 years of age (CDC, 2006, 2007a). It is the leading cause of school absenteeism due to chronic illness and of childhood emergency department (ED) visits. It accounts for one-third of all pediatric ED visits. Even in children who do not require emergency care, asthma can decrease attention span in school, make participation in school activities difficult, and cause social problems as children are often teased and stigmatized as being "wheezers" or "lazy." Asthma has complex causes, including a strong genetic component, but poverty appears to play at least some role. Recent research has focused on indoor air pollutants, such as dust mites, mouse urine, and the decomposing corpses of cockroaches as significant triggers.

Unintentional Injuries in School-Age Children

School-age children experience fewer injuries than preschoolers because of their increased coordination and improved reasoning abilities. However, falls remain the most common form of nonfatal injury for children ages 6 to 12 years, while the leading cause of unintentional injury death is motor vehicle and traffic injury (54% of the deaths for this group) (Centers for Disease Control, 2005a). School-age children experience a high incidence of fractures, sprains, strains, cuts, and abrasions. Most such injuries related to playground equipment occur at schools and

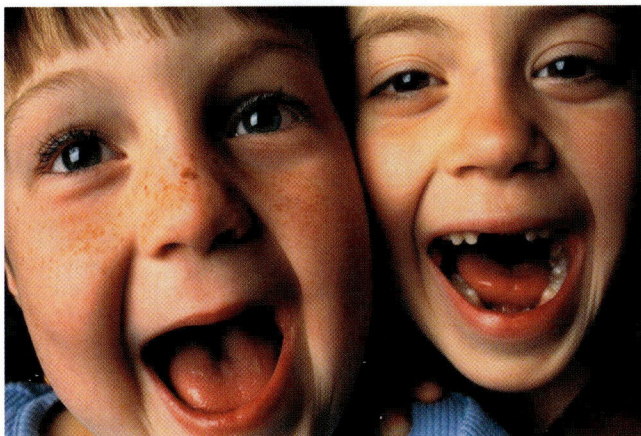

FIGURE 9-9 Same-gender friendships are important to school-age children.

day-care centers. Injuries also occur from riding bicycles on the street, skiing, skateboarding, sledding, and playing sports. If you would like more information about unintentional injuries, see Chapter 23.

ASSESSMENT

The school-age child should have a routine health maintenance visit every 1 or 2 years. Many children participate in sports, so annual physical exams are scheduled for them. Allow time to meet with the child alone as well as time with the caregiver present. School-age children often have questions about puberty and the changes their bodies are undergoing. Private time with the child will allow you to explore these concerns in a private manner.

At each visit, assess the child's vital signs, height, weight, and developmental skills. After weighing the child, correlate your measurements with growth charts. The CDC (n.d.a, updated February 15, 2011) classifies a child as overweight when the BMI reaches the 85th percentile, and obese when the BMI is at or above the 95th percentile. If you want more information about BMI for children,

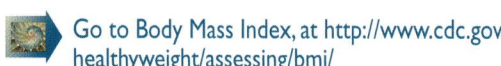 Go to Body Mass Index, at http://www.cdc.gov/ healthyweight/assessing/bmi/

The nursing interview should cover the following topics:

Nutrition. Assess the child's nutrition, including intake of key nutrients such as calcium, vitamin D, and iron.

Allergies. Ask the child whether he ever experiences difficulty breathing or feels too tired to play. Ask about allergy symptoms, including clear nasal discharge, frequent sneezing, or watery eyes. Listen to breath sounds, and observe for allergy symptoms.

Dental Hygiene. Interview the child to determine his knowledge of dental hygiene. Inspect the mouth for secondary teeth eruption according to expected patterns, as well as for tooth decay and gum disease.

Sleep Pattern. Assess the child's sleep pattern. To remain healthy and function well at school, the school-age child needs 9 to 10 hours of sleep each night.

Safety. ✚ Determine the child's awareness of safety. Be sure to assess risk-taking behavior. Has the child tried smoking? Does he have friends who are smoking? What is the child's experience with alcohol and drugs? Has he tried them? What does his peer group think about drinking and drugs? Has he ever been sexually active? Does he have friends who are sexually active? Has the child engaged in fistfights or fights with knives or other weapons? Is there a gun in the home? Does the child have access to it? Although these concerns are seen with greater frequency in adolescence, you should assess for them among school-age children.

Scoliosis Screening. **Scoliosis** is an abnormal spinal curvature that affects primarily females. Screening is done in the preadolescent period, usually in the sixth grade. Refer to an orthopedic surgeon for evaluation and follow-up if an abnormal curvature is discovered.

Immunizations. Review the immunization record. Although immunization against hepatitis B is recommended in infancy, many children skip these immunizations. Several states require students to complete the hepatitis B series prior to entry into seventh grade. The child must begin the series at or before 12 years of age to complete it in time for seventh grade. The CDC (2011a) recommend the following vaccines for school-age children: tetanus, diphtheria, and pertussis booster; human papillomavirus; meningococcal; pneumococcal; influenza; hepatitis A; hepatitis B; inactivated poliovirus; measles, mumps, and rubella; and varicella (Fig. 9-10).

INTERVENTIONS

Since the beginning of the U.S. Department of Health and Human Services' *Healthy People* campaign, the focus of healthcare has shifted toward preventing injury rather than treating

Recommended Immunization Schedule for Persons Aged 7 Through 18 Years—United States • 2011
For those who fall behind or start late, see the schedule below catch-up schedule

Vaccine▼ Age▶	7–10 years	11–12 years	13–18 years	
Tetanus, Diphtheria, Pertussis		Tdap	Tdap	**Range of recommended ages**
Human Papillomavirus		HPV (3 doses)	HPV Series	
Meningococcal	MCV	MCV	MCV	
Influenza	Influenza (Yearly)			**Catch-up immunization**
Pneumococcal	PPSV			
Hepatitis A	HepA Series			
Hepatitis B	HepB Series			**Certain high-risk groups**
Inactivated Poliovirus	IPV Series			
Measles, Mumps, Rubella	MMR Series			
Varicella	Varicella Series			

FIGURE 9-10 Immunizations recommended for children ages 7–18 yr. For additional information, visit the National Immunization Web site at http://www.cdc.gov/vaccines.

illness. Use teaching materials appropriate for school-age children. Your efforts will help promote the national *Healthy People 2020* population objectives.

Teaching for Safety

 To help prevent injury in the school-age child, educate the child and parents on safety and the proper use of equipment and gear. Teach the child and parents to wear seat belts at all times. Encourage parents to be firm about the use of helmets for bicycle safety because head injury is the most common cause of death in this group. Sports injuries are also common. Stress the importance of warming up before playing, using safety equipment that is properly fitted, and avoiding overtraining.

Teaching About Nutrition, Exercise, and Overweight

Encourage children to develop good eating habits by choosing nutritious foods and snacks. For example, encourage them to avoid junk foods, such as sodas, and to choose instead milk, calcium-fortified orange juice, or plain water. Counsel overweight and obese children regarding nutrition for weight loss and the importance of daily physical activity. Refer for further counseling, if indicated. If the diet is severely restrictive, and if it has none of the child's favorite foods, it is likely to fail. Focus on making small but permanent changes.

Recommend that children do 30 to 60 minutes of moderate-intensity exercise 7 days per week (American Academy of Pediatrics, 2006; Miller & Silverstein, 2007). U.S. Department of Health and Human Services (2008) guidelines recommend 1 hour or more of vigorous aerobic physical activity every day.

Explain how important exercise is to weight loss—diet alone will not achieve it for them. Suggest exercise that is not necessarily structured—for example, family walks in the community, bike riding or skateboarding, or swimming in a neighborhood or community pool. Even table tennis requires more activity than watching television. The American Academy of Pediatrics recommends the following:

- Limit TV viewing and video game playing to 2 hours a day.
- Boys should take at least 11,000 steps daily.
- Girls should take at least 13,000 steps daily.

You could suggest that parents buy a pedometer so the child can track the number of steps.

The most effective programs for preventing obesity focus on children, rather than their parents. Teach children about self-regulation of impulse control, decision-making skills, and social competence. However, management of obesity does involve the whole family. A child cannot make lifestyle changes if his environment does not change. Parents can help by modeling healthy eating. Recommend group-based or family-based counseling. Many parents do not perceive that their child is overweight; of course they must come to recognize this if they are to cooperate with needed changes.

Work with the community to involve the schools in obesity prevention. Many schools have removed soda from their campuses and are now offering healthy menus in their cafeterias. In addition, physical education in the schools has been mandated in many states in the United States.

Teaching About Asthma

Teach parents and children about indoor environmental asthma triggers, such as secondhand smoke, dust mites (in mattresses, carpets, and furniture), mold, cockroaches, pets, and nitrogen dioxide (a gas that is a byproduct of indoor fuel-burning appliances such as gas stoves, fireplaces, or wood stoves (U.S. Environmental Protection Agency, last updated October 2010).

Provide and help fill out, as necessary, an asthma action card for the child to carry when away from home. An action plan should include (1) the child's asthma triggers, (2) instructions for asthma medicines, (3) what to do if the child has an attack, (4) when to call the doctor, and (5) emergency telephone numbers. You can obtain a plan form from the U.S. Environmental Protection Agency's Asthma home page,

http://www.epa.gov/asthma/index.html

Teaching About Violence and Risk-Taking Behaviors

The school-age period offers many opportunities to educate children about the hazards of smoking, drinking, and using drugs before they are tempted to try their use. School violence can be addressed through psychological counseling, weapons-screening devices, schoolwide educational programs, and policies calling for the suspension or expulsion of students who are caught intimidating other children or participating in fights on school property.

Helping the Hospitalized Child

Children who are hospitalized report fear of being in an unfamiliar environment, fear of the unknown, and fear of strange professionals. They are afraid of tests and treatments, operations, needles, pain, and dying. They report missing the comforts of home: their mother's cooking, their own room, and so on. They are bothered by separation from family and friends and by loss of control over their personal needs.

You can help them by maximizing their contact with outside friends and school and by minimizing the adverse aspects of the hospital environment. Offer children choices, when possible, to restore some sense of control. For example, they might choose whether to have a tub bath or shower or what they'd prefer to eat for meals. Encourage parents to bring familiar items from home to personalize their space. Involve parents in their care, and provide them accurate information so they can relieve children's anxieties. Finally, help children express their fears and respond to them.

KnowledgeCheck 9-7

- What important physical changes occur in the school-age group?
- According to Piaget, what is the cognitive developmental stage of the school-age child?

ADOLESCENCE: AGES 12 TO 18 YEARS

Adolescence marks the transition from child to adult. **Puberty** refers to the beginning of reproductive abilities. In this period of development, the child experiences progressive physical, cognitive, and psychological change. The major task of the adolescent is to achieve a personal identity and avoid role confusion.

Physical Development of Adolescents

Physical and hormonal changes are readily apparent during the adolescent years. Appropriate intake of calcium and vitamin D is critical in adolescence because of the rapid increase in growth and bone mass.

- Females undergo a growth spurt between 9 and 14 years of age. Height increases 2 to 8 in. (5.1 to 7.6 cm), and weight

gain varies from 15 to 55 lb (6.8 to 24.9 kg). By the onset of menstruation, girls have attained 90% of their adult height.

- Boys undergo a growth spurt between the ages of 10 and 16. Height increases by 4 to 12 in. (10.2 to 30.5 cm), and weight increases by 15 to 65 lb (6.8 to 29.5 kg). Boys continue to grow until 18 to 20 years of age. Bone mass continues to accumulate until about age 20.

In both males and females, the size and strength of the heart, as well as the blood pressure, increase. The pulse rate decreases. Respiratory rate, volume, and capacity reach the adult rates during this time. By the end of the adolescent period, all vital organs reach adult size and blood values are those of the adult.

Onset of Puberty. The onset of puberty varies widely, but the sequences of these changes are standard (Tanner, 1962).

- In females, the time from the first appearance of breast tissue to full sexual maturation is 2 to 6 years. **Menarche** (first menstruation) occurs approximately 2 years after the beginning of puberty. The average age of menarche is 12 years, depending on racial group and body mass.
- The onset of male puberty occurs between 9 and 14 years of age. Throughout puberty, boys become more muscular, the voice deepens, and facial hair begins to grow and coarsen. It may take 2 to 5 years for the genitalia to reach adult size.

In both males and females, hormonal changes are accompanied by increased activity of the sweat (apocrine) glands, and heavy perspiration may occur for the first time. For the same reason, the sebaceous glands become active, and the adolescent may experience acne. For more information about the changes in secondary sexual characteristics associated with puberty for males and females, see the tables in Procedures 21-17 and 21-18, respectively. Developmental milestones of adolescence are summarized in Box 9-5.

Cognitive Development of Adolescents

Piaget refers to adolescence as the period of *formal operations*. The adolescent develops the ability to think abstractly and is receptive to more detailed information. This opens the door to scientific reasoning and logic. She can now imagine what may occur in the future as well as the consequences of her own decisions. Although the adolescent has more refined cognitive abilities, she may still lack judgment and common sense. These develop later through increased life experience.

Psychosocial Development of Adolescents

The major psychosocial task of the adolescent is to develop a *personal identity*. Teenagers shift their emotional attachment away from their parents and create close bonds among their peers (Fig. 9-11). This helps the teenager to further characterize the differences between himself and his parents. The adolescent often takes on a new style of dress, dance, music, or hairstyle. The teenager develops personal values and begins to make choices about career and further education.

One of the strongest needs for teens is to feel accepted within a group of their own choosing. Acceptance onto a sports team, into a club, or into a clique or gang increases the teen's sense of self-esteem. In contrast, unpopular teens feel alienated, resentful, and antagonistic and may react with violence directed at themselves or others (Polan & Taylor, 2007).

By early adolescence, most children have a sense of their emerging sexual orientation. Approximately 4.1% of people between 18 and 44 years of age identify themselves as homosexual or bisexual (CDC, 2005b). A higher percentage report having had same-sex intercourse at least once, but consider themselves heterosexual. Some youth are bisexual—that is, attracted somewhat equally to both males and females.

Common Health Problems of Adolescents

In the United States, 72% of all deaths among young people ages 10 through 24 years result from four causes: motor vehicle crashes (30%), other unintentional injuries (15%), homicide (15%), and suicide (12%). Illnesses are responsible for less than one-fourth of deaths; of those, cancer and heart disease are the most common. Many adolescents engage in behaviors that increase their likelihood of death of injury from these four causes: drinking while driving, carrying a weapon, using alcohol, and using other drugs. In a recent year, 36% of high school students reported having been in a physical fight (Eaton, Kann, Kinchen, et al., 2008).

Example Problem: Substance Abuse

Substance abuse is the regular use of drugs or other substances for purposes other than medical use that causes physical or psychological harm to the person. Substance abuse is a major concern in adolescence because of the physical, mental,

---

BOX 9-5 ■ Milestones of Adolescent Development

- The adolescent reaches adult height and about 90% of peak bone density by the end of this period.
- Menarche occurs by age 14 in most girls, who develop adult primary and secondary sex characteristics by about age 16.
- Boys have developed adult primary and secondary sex characteristics by about age 17 to 19.
- Motor development is equal to that of adults.
- Maturation of the central nervous system allows formal operational thought processes, logic, and abstract reasoning.
- Psychosocial development includes the teen's increasing reliance on peers, ambivalent feelings toward family, anxiety over and/or preoccupation with sex and sexuality, and determination of sexual orientation.

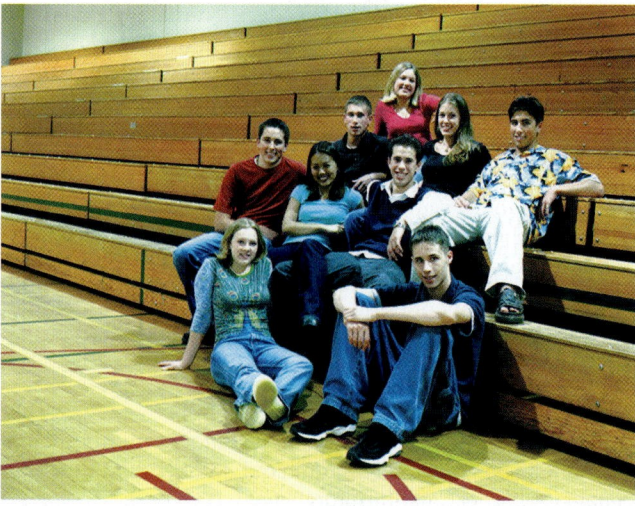

FIGURE 9-11 Teenagers create close bonds among their peers.

and spiritual toll it takes on teens, families, and the community. Substance use is associated with risk-taking behaviors. Car accidents, for instance, are often associated with alcohol or substance abuse.

Alcohol and Other Substances. An adolescent may try alcohol and other drugs out of curiosity or for altering the consciousness to gain a feeling of power, excitement, or confidence. Peer pressure also exerts a powerful influence.

Boys and girls are starting to drink at younger ages. In a recent survey, alcohol use among those ages 12 to 17 years was 15%; youth binge and heavy drinking rates were 9% and 2%, respectively. Three out of four students have consumed more than just a few sips of alcohol by the end of high school. An estimated 11% of those in grades 9 through 12 report having driven a motor vehicle when they had been drinking alcohol (Eaton, Kann, Kinchen, et al., 2008; Substance Abuse and Mental Health Services Administration [SAMHSA], 2009).

Heroin, cocaine, crack, methamphetamine, and the "designer drugs" (ecstasy and others) may be abused, but abuse of over-the-counter and prescription drugs used by the teen's parents, such as OxyContin, is also common.

Tobacco. It is illegal to sell tobacco to minors, yet 9.5% of middle school students and 25.6% of high school students currently use some form of tobacco (American Lung Association, 2010; SAMHSA, 2009), and over 54% say they have tried a cigarette. A majority of these students report that they were not asked to show proof of age when they, themselves, bought cigarettes. Tobacco use is associated with alcohol and illicit drug use; it acts as a "gateway drug" to using illegal drugs. Cigarette use causes an increase in the number and severity of respiratory illness and decreased physical fitness.

Tobacco use primarily begins in early adolescence, frequently by age 14. Smoking during childhood often forms an addiction that persists into adulthood. Once the addiction is formed, it is very difficult to quit. For example, of adolescents who have smoked at least 100 cigarettes in their lifetime, most report that they would like to quit but are not able to do so.

Depression and Suicide

Depression. Depression affects up to 8.3% of adolescents in the United States (About Teen Depression, n. d.), compared to 11% of the adult population. A government survey identifies an even higher percentage: During the 12 months preceding the survey, 28% of students nationwide had felt so sad or hopeless almost every day for more than 2 weeks in a row that they stopped doing some usual activities (Eaton, Kann, Kinchen, et al., 2008). Defining features of depression are the same as for adults, but the way symptoms are expressed varies with the developmental stage. Young adolescents may have difficulty in identifying and describing their emotional or mood states. Instead of saying how bad they feel, they may be irritable or act out by disobeying or misbehaving. They may sulk, be negative or grouchy, feel misunderstood, and get into trouble at school.

Risk factors for adolescent depression include a family history of depression, cigarette smoking, stress, loss of a loved one, breakup of a romantic relationship, learning disorders, attention or behavioral disorders, chronic illnesses (e.g., diabetes), abuse, neglect, or other trauma such as natural disasters. If you would like more information about depression, see Chapter 13.

Suicide. Suicide is the third leading cause of death in teenagers. It is estimated that 6.9% of high school students have attempted suicide (Eaton, Kann, Kinchen, et al., 2008).

Twice as many adolescent girls as boys attempt suicide, but because boys tend to use more lethal methods, such as guns and hanging, they are more likely to die from the attempt. Risk factors include problems at school or in romantic or family relationships, low self-esteem, social isolation, substance abuse, and depression.

Eating Disorders

Although anorexia and bulimia create nutritional problems and manifest as eating disorders, they are psychiatric disorders that require medical and psychiatric intervention.

Anorexia Nervosa. The person with **anorexia nervosa** dramatically restricts food intake and may exercise excessively in an attempt to lose weight. It is the third most common chronic illness among adolescents. It occurs predominately in, but is not limited to, high-achieving adolescent females from upper-middle-class backgrounds. Anorexia is characterized by a distorted body image; often the girl sees herself as fat in spite of being markedly thin. Physical consequences include amenorrhea, bradycardia, low white blood cell count, anemia, infertility, and bone loss. Eating disorders have the highest mortality of any mental illness: 5% to 10% of patients die within 10 years of developing anorexia nervosa (Lippert, Shea, & Seagrave, 2008).

Bulimia. Bulimia is another eating disorder seen in adolescent girls, as well as in boys who participate in sports that require maintenance of a specific weight. **Bulimia** is characterized by binge eating followed by inappropriate mechanisms to remove the food that was consumed (usually inducing vomiting, using laxatives, or excessive exercise). Binge eating may occur every few days or as often as several times a day. People with bulimia frequently experience electrolyte imbalances, decayed teeth from gastric acid exposure, or abdominal pain from gastric overload or laxative use.

Overweight and Obesity

Overweight and obesity continue to be a concern during adolescence. The numbers are staggering. Consider these facts:

- In 1994, 11% of adolescents (ages 12–19) were classified as obese; by 2008, that number had reached 18% (National Center for Health Statistics, n. d., updated 2010); and by 2011, about one in three American children and teens are overweight (American Heart Association, 2011a).
- In the years between 1963 and 2004, obesity rates more than tripled among adolescents.
- Currently in the United States over 30% of children are overweight or obese.

Causes of teen obesity are similar to those of childhood obesity: sedentary lifestyles; eating larger portions; eating fast foods; and substituting high-calorie, nutrient-poor snacks for balanced meals. Even school vending machines contain so-called junk foods such as soda, snack cakes, candy, and chips, although this is changing in some areas. One-third of American children ages 4 to 19 years eat fast food every day. The percentage is undoubtedly higher for adolescents, who eat fewer meals at home and have more freedom to choose their own foods. Food preferences are influenced by television and marketing strategies in other media; on children's television shows, most of the advertising is for foods of poor nutritional value.

Type 2 DM, hypertension, high cholesterol, and heart disease were previously seen predominantly in adults. Now that obesity has become a common problem among youth, these disorders are occurring with increasing frequency in adolescents.

Moreover, overweight children are more likely to be overweight adults.

Risky Sexual Behaviors

Sexual activity is common among teenagers. By age 13, 4% of girls and 10% of boys have had sexual intercourse. This tends to increase with age, with 35% of students (grades 9–12) being sexually active. About 15% of students have had sexual intercourse with four or more persons (Eaton, Kann, Kinchen, et al., 2008).

Condom Use. Almost two-thirds of sexually active high school students report having used a condom at most recent sexual intercourse. Males are more likely to use condoms than are females, and younger teens are more likely to use condoms than are older teens (Eaton, Kann, Kinchen, et al., 2008).

Oral Sex. A fairly recent trend among youth is engaging in oral sex, in the belief that it is not "real sex." In one survey of university students, 62% of females and 56% of males did not believe that oral sex would qualify as sexual intercourse and that it does not take away their virginity. Adolescents almost never use condoms or dental dams when engaging in oral sex (Remez, 2000).

Web-Based Social Networking. A recent study of young men (ages 16–24 years) who have sex with men examined use of the Internet or Web-based social networking sites for meeting sexual partners. Forty-eight percent of the sample had sexual relations with a partner they met online. Of these, only 53% used condoms consistently, and 47% reported having sexual partners more than four years older than themselves. A history of unprotected anal intercourse, multiple anal intercourse partners, and engaging in sexual activity at a sex club or a bathhouse were associated with meeting sexual partners through the Internet. Researchers concluded that young men who have sex with men and who seek partners online also engage in other behaviors that place them at risk for HIV and other sexually transmitted infections (Garofalo, Herrick, Mustanski, et al., 2007).

Sexually Transmitted Infections (STIs). Sexually transmitted infections, including HIV/AIDS, are a major health consequence associated with sexual activity, and especially with unprotected sexual activity. Approximately one in four American teens has an STI. A majority of adolescents believe that sex without a condom is not worth the risk, but most also mistakenly believe that condoms are a foolproof method of preventing STIs and HIV/AIDS. Among adolescents, trichomonal and monilial infections and human papillomavirus are common. Chlamydial infections, syphilis, and herpes simplex type II (genital herpes) occur in both males and females and can have serious complications. As an example, one in four girls ages 15 to 19 years had evidence of or infection with human papillomavirus during 2003 (Gavin, MacKay, Brown, et al., 2009).

AIDS is a major cause of death worldwide, reaching epidemic proportions in some countries. It is transmitted primarily through genital, oral, or anal sexual activities but can be transmitted by other ways as well (e.g., by sharing needles with an infected person). The annual rate of AIDS diagnoses reported among males ages 15 to 19 has nearly doubled in the past 10 years (Gavin, MacKay, Brown, et al., 2009). For more information about STIs, see Chapter 34.

Adolescent Pregnancy. Except for an increase between 2005 and 2007 (Gavin, MacKay, Brown, et al., 2009), teenage birth rates have declined each year since 1991. The 2010 rate of 34.3 births per 1000 teens aged 15 to 19 was the lowest in 70 years (CDC, 2010a). Nevertheless, rates are still high, especially among black and Hispanic teens in the South; and the United States has substantially higher teen pregnancy and birth rates than other industrialized nations (CDC, 2011b, 2012). A similar percentage of teens are sexually active in the United States; however, consistency and effectiveness of condom use are lower.

Adolescents who become pregnant face physiological risks, such as bone density loss and iron-deficiency anemia, the interruption of progress in their own developmental tasks, and loss of educational opportunities. Teen mothers are less likely to complete high school and more likely to live in poverty than are other teens. They are less likely to be married, to receive prenatal care, and gain appropriate weight, and more likely to smoke than are older mothers. This puts them and their babies at higher risk for complications of pregnancy and low-birth-weight infants.

Example Problem: Abuse and Neglect

There is no age limit on abuse and neglect. One study of children age 13 to adulthood reported that more than 9% of the nearly 1,000 subjects had substantiated maltreatment. Maltreatment included sexual abuse, physical abuse, emotional abuse, and neglect. Abuse may be linked to later violent crimes and illicit drug use (Smith, Ireland, & Thornberry, 2005). Adults often ignore symptoms and complaints of adolescent abuse. Young children are perceived as defenseless, but people tend to stereotype adolescents as provoking their own abuse. Fewer than 40% of adolescent maltreatment cases are reported to child protection agencies, compared to 76% of cases involving younger children (McFarlane & Miller, 2005).

ASSESSMENT

A general health examination is recommended every 2 years in the adolescent period. Communicating with persons in this age group can be challenging because adolescents are sometimes rebellious. Attempt to establish rapport, and reassure the teenager that you will maintain confidentiality.

Obtain a Thorough Health History. Obtain information in the following areas:

- *Medications and other drugs.* Be sure to ask about use of prescription and over-the-counter medications as well as recreational drug use. Ask whether the adolescent uses tobacco products; if so, find out what, how much, and for how long.
- *Psychosocial profile.* Obtain a psychosocial profile focusing on health practices and behaviors. A change in academic performance or lack of interest in school may indicate a problem such as depression. Assess the adolescent's ability to cope with stressors.
- *Peer relationships.* Assess the quality of the adolescent's peer relationships, not only to assess risk for social isolation but also to determine risk for school violence and gang-related violence.
- *Nutrition and body image.* Ask questions about body image in relation to the adolescent's nutritional status. Assess both overeating and undereating patterns, as well as intake of key nutrients such as protein, iron, calcium, and vitamin D.
- *Activity and exercise patterns.* If the adolescent engages in activities that increase the risk for injuries, ask about the use of protective equipment, such as helmets, mouth guards, and padding. If the adolescent reports no regular physical

activity, assess his or her understanding of the benefits of exercise.

- *Sleep patterns.* Teens often get little sleep during school days and sleep late on weekends. Ask whether the teen feels refreshed after a night's sleep.

Safety. Determine whether the adolescent wears a seat belt and is aware of the hazards of driving under the influence of drugs and alcohol. Cell phone use for talking and texting is a major hazard while driving. Other distractions, including loud music and other teens in the car, can compete with the attention and focus a teen has for traffic and driving safety.

- *Sexual activity.* Determine whether the adolescent is sexually active. If so, ask about condom use.
- *Review all body systems,* keeping in mind changes or problems that are specific to the adolescent.

General Survey. Complete a general survey after you have gathered the subjective data. Include vital signs, height, and weight. Follow with a head-to-toe physical exam. If you identify any problems in the course of the history and physical examination, actively involve both the adolescent and the parents in a plan of care.

Calculate the BMI using a BMI calculator and BMI-for-age percentiles for children and teens. Adult calculators will not give accurate results for teens. The following are the CDC weight status categories:

Underweight	Less than 5th percentile
Healthy weight	5th to less than 85th percentile
At risk of overweight	85th to less than 95th percentile
Overweight	95th percentile or greater

To use the CDC BMI Percentile Calculator for Child and Teen,

 Go to the CDC Web site at http://apps.nccd.cdc.gov/dnpabmi/

To see the CDC body mass index-for-age percentile charts for girls and boys age 2 to 20,

 Go to Chapter 9, **Tables, Boxes, Figures: ESG Figure 9-2 and ESG Figure 9-3,** respectively, on *DavisPlus,* or go to the CDC Web site.

INTERVENTIONS

When working with adolescents, your goal is to help the adolescent make informed decisions. Avoid scare tactics, and encourage open discussion. Often a teenager will feel more comfortable asking a nurse or other health professional about sensitive topics than asking a parent. Reassure the adolescent that you will maintain confidentiality. However, if there is concern about suicide, explain to the adolescent that you are required to share this information with others. Provide mental health referrals immediately when an adolescent contemplates suicide.

Focus your age-specific interventions on educating the teenager about common health problems and avoidance of injury and disease. Include the following topics in your discussions.

Preventing and Treating Obesity

Help the patient to make small but permanent changes in eating and exercise. These usually work better than a series of extreme short-term diets and exercise plans that cannot be sustained. Gradual weight loss is the healthiest approach.

Even for teens, parental involvement is important—not to police the eating, but to model healthy eating and physical activity.

Calorie Intake. Reducing calorie intake is usually the easiest change to make. As a rule, avoid highly restrictive diets that forbid favorite foods. It is important to encourage strong support from parents and others involved in buying and preparing food and to teach the teen how to choose highly nutritious foods at school. Encourage the adolescent to replace high-fat, high-sugar, junk foods with healthier choices as snacks and to avoid or limit fruit juices and sodas.

Physical Activity. Stress the importance of regular physical activity. Some adolescents may be able to walk to school instead of driving or taking a bus. If this is not practical, try to involve the family in planning regular physical activities—for example, a long walk after dinner. Even mild exercise, such as shooting hoops, swimming, table tennis, or playing catch with a baseball, provides more activity than watching television or playing computer games. You might start with the following goals:

- Limit television and video game use to 1 or 2 hours a day. Discourage use before school, during homework, and late at night. Keep the television off during family mealtimes. Limit viewing of shows or movies containing adult content or violence by using parental controls available on most televisions. Movies and video games are rated based on violence and sexually explicit content.
- Engage in 30 minutes of outdoor activity every day. Some activity is better than none. Work up to an hour a day of more strenuous exercise.

Example Problem: Substance Use Interventions

Discuss with the adolescent the effects of drugs and alcohol and the hazards associated with their use. If your assessment has identified drug or alcohol use, make appropriate referrals.

Explore the hazards of tobacco use and provide information on smoking-cessation programs, if appropriate. More and more teens are using smokeless tobacco products, and some have the mistaken idea that these are safer than smoking. Remind teens that the earlier a person begins smoking, the harder the addiction is to break. Stress the unattractive physical effects, such as bad breath, stained teeth and fingers, and a long-term cough, not to mention the expense and inconvenience of purchasing cigarettes.

Preventing Pregnancy and STIs

Abstinence is the only 100% effective way to prevent pregnancy and STIs. However, if the adolescent is sexually active, explain that using condoms can greatly reduce, although not eliminate, the risk of unwanted pregnancies and STIs. Be sure teens understand that STIs can be transmitted orally and anally, as well as vaginally, so it is important that they use a condom, regardless of the type of sexual activity.

A practice guideline from the American Academy of Pediatrics (AAP) recommends that schools make condoms available for adolescents and, with community involvement, develop a comprehensive sequential sexuality education as a part of a K–12 health education program. It has been shown that making condoms available does not increase the rate of sexual activity (American Academy of Pediatrics, 2005).

Breast and Testicular Self-Exam

Currently there is some controversy about whether we should continue to encourage breast self-examination (BSE). Some studies indicate that it does not reduce death rates from breast

cancer, but others have found that more cancers are discovered and that the cancers detected are smaller in groups who perform BSE (Green & Taplin, 2003; Hackshaw & Paul, 2003). The American Cancer Society (2010) advises that a monthly BSE is optional for women under age 30. BSE is recommended by certain medical groups, such as the American College of Obstetricians and Gynecologists (2009), but not by the U.S. Preventive Services Task Force. Until there is more evidence, it seems reasonable to continue to teach the limitations and benefits of BSE and to teach women how to do it properly. Researchers agree that patients who perform BSE should be trained in proper technique in order to avoid falsely negative findings (American College of Obstetricians and Gynecologists, 2009; Balkaya, Memis, & Demirkiran, 2007; Knutson & Steiner, 2007; Rosolowich, 2006). To see how to perform a BSE, refer to Box 9-6.

Males over the age of 14 should perform a testicular self-examination (TSE) once a month. This is an effective way to become familiar with the body and to detect testicular cancer early, when it is very curable. You should know, however, that the U.S. Preventive Services Task Force (USPSTF) (2004) recommends against routine screening, even though they acknowledge that most testicular cancers are discovered by TSE. They concluded that population outcomes are not sufficiently improved to merit routine TSE. If your patient chooses to perform TSE, advise him to perform the exam after a warm bath or shower (heat relaxes the scrotum, making it easier to find abnormalities). To learn how to perform a TSE, see Box 9-7. If you would like more information about TSE at the Testicular Cancer Resource Center Web site,

 Go to http://tcrc.acor.org/tcexam.html

Immunizations

For adolescents ages 13 to 17, none of the *Healthy People 2010* objectives for vaccinations were met. Fewer than half have current tetanus, diphtheria, and pertussis immunization. About double that number have been vaccinated for hepatitis B, measles, mumps, and rubella. For the recommended immunization schedule for adolescents, see Figure 9-10.

Other Health Promotion Activities

Other nursing activities include promoting adolescent health and safety:

- *Rest.* Explain the importance of adequate rest. Teens need 8 hours of sleep a night for maximum performance in academics and sports.
- *Nutrition.* Stress the importance of adequate nutrition, including intake of 1,300 mg of calcium and 400 IU of vitamin D daily to reach maximum bone density during this critical period of growth. Teach teens how to choose foods that include fruits, vegetables, cereal and grains, lean meats, chicken, fish, and low-fat dairy products and to avoid foods and drinks that are high in sugar, fat, or caffeine.
- *Dental hygiene.* Advise parents that the adolescent should have a preventive dental care visit at least once a year. Teach the teen to brush twice a day with a soft toothbrush and to floss daily.

⊞ Teens should take measures to prevent injury during sports and other activities. Remind teens to wear a seat belt when riding in the car and avoid distractions while driving, such as talking on a cell phone or changing a radio station. Urge them *never* to drink and

---

BOX 9-6 ▪ Breast Self-Examination (BSE)

The best time to examine your breasts is when they are not tender or swollen. Have your technique reviewed periodically by your healthcare professional. It is acceptable to choose not to do BSE or to do to BSE once in a while. Report any changes to your healthcare provider right away.

1. Lie down. Place a pillow under your right shoulder and place your right arm behind your head. *Lying down spreads the breast tissue evenly over the chest wall, making it easier to feel all the tissue.*
2. Using the finger pads (not the tips) of the three middle fingers of your left hand, feel for lumps in the right breast. Use overlapping dime-sized circular motions of the fingers to feel the breast tissue. Move in an up-and-down pattern (see step 4).

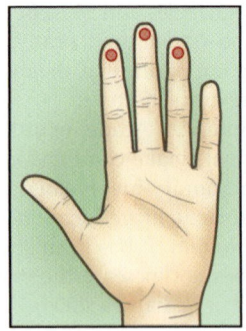 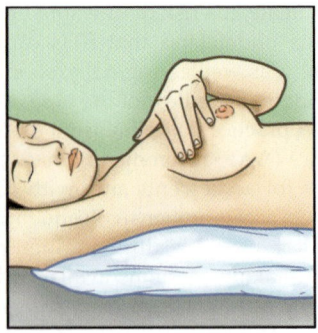

3. Use three different levels of pressure to feel all the breast tissue:
   - Light pressure to feel the tissue closest to the skin

   - Medium pressure to feel a little deeper
   - Firm pressure to feel the tissue closest to the chest and ribs
   Use each pressure level to feel the breast tissue before moving on to the next spot.
4. Start at an imaginary line drawn straight down your side from the underarm. Move across the breast to the middle of the chest bone (sternum), moving in an up-and-down pattern. Check the entire breast area, moving down until you feel only ribs, and moving up to the neck or collarbone (clavicle). Evidence suggests that this vertical (up-and-down) pattern is the most effective way to avoid missing any breast tissue.
5. After completely examining your right breast, put the pillow under your left shoulder and examine your left breast using the same methods.
6. Next, stand in front of a mirror, arms at your sides, and look at each breast. Note the size, shape, contour, and direction of your breasts and nipples.
7. Press your hands firmly on your hips and look at your breasts for any changes in size, shape, contour, or dimpling or redness or scaliness of the nipple or skin.
8. While standing (or sitting) with your arm raised slightly, examine each underarm. If you raise your arm straight up, it tightens the tissue and makes it harder to examine.

Source: Adapted from the American Cancer Society. (n.d.a, last reviewed 2010). "How to Examine Your Breasts." Retrieved March 10, 2011, from htt://www.cancer.org/docroot/CRI/content/CRI_2_6x_How_to_perform_a_breast_self_exam_5.asp

drive. Remind them to wear a helmet and protective gear for activities such as bicycling, in-line skating, and riding a skateboard. Teach the importance of sun safety (e.g., applying a sunscreen of at least SPF 15, avoiding tanning beds, wearing sunglasses when in the sun).

KnowledgeCheck 9-8

- According to Erikson, what is the developmental stage of the adolescent?
- Name two common health problems of adolescents.

 Think**Like a Nurse** 9-5

Recall the story of Carrie, a 13-year-old girl, in the Meet Your Patients scenario. Carrie is hospitalized for pneumonia. What effect might this have on her behavior? As her nurse, how might you intervene?

YOUNG ADULTHOOD: AGES 19 TO 40 YEARS

Young adulthood is the time of transition to independence and responsibility. This transition involves important life events, such as high school graduation, entering college or starting a career, and leaving home. As the young adult leaves home he begins to function independently. The 20s are spent exploring occupations, marriage, or alternative relationships.

BOX 9-7 ■ Testicular Self-Examination (TSE)

This examination is recommended monthly after a warm bath or shower when the scrotal skin is relaxed.
1. Stand in front of the mirror and look for swelling on the skin or scrotum.
2. Using both hands, with the fingers under the scrotum and thumbs on top, gently roll each testicle, feeling for lumps.
3. Palpate the epididymis, a normal cord-like structure on the top and back of each testicle that carries the sperm.

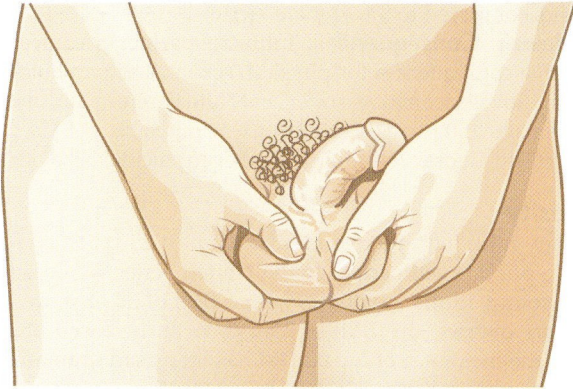

4. Contact your healthcare provider as soon as possible if you palpate a lump or if the area is painful or swollen.

Note: The U.S. Preventive Services Task Force (USPSTF) (2004) recommends against routine screening with TSE. However, from the point of view of the individual patient, because there is no harm in self-examination, and because that is the way most testicular cancers are discovered, we see no reason to discourage it. If a patient chooses to perform TSE, you can teach him this method.

Physical Development of Young Adults

Young adulthood is usually the healthiest stage of a person's life. Maturation of the body systems is complete. Peak bone density is achieved for both females and males by age 25. Vision and hearing are typically acute. For women, the ages between 20 and 30 years are the optimal years for childbearing. For men, male hormone levels that surged in adolescence begin to slowly decrease and stabilize around age 24.

Cognitive Development of Young Adults

Piaget believed that cognitive development terminates in adolescence around age 15. At this point, thought processes and mental abilities are well established. Piaget felt that learning continues throughout life but that patterns of thinking do not alter.

Contemporary psychologists have proposed an additional stage of cognitive development called *post-formal operations.* In the formal operations phase, teenagers are able to think rationally, predict outcomes, and hypothesize about the future. Post-formal operations add a dimension of complexity. In this phase, the young adult is able to accept contradictions and fine points in thinking. For example, the post-formal thinker recognizes that her opinion on a social controversy has aspects of two opposing viewpoints. She sees merit in both parts of the argument and is comfortable with the discrepancy.

Psychosocial Development of Young Adults

Young adults begin to explore options for careers and intimate relationships (Fig. 9-12). They strive to become less dependent and more self-sufficient. Around age 30, most young adults experience a period of self-evaluation. This often results in a job, career, or relationship change.

Erikson describes this period as the stage of *intimacy versus isolation.* Successful completion of this phase requires establishment of lasting friendships and associations. Freud described this phase of life as the *genital stage.* He believed that

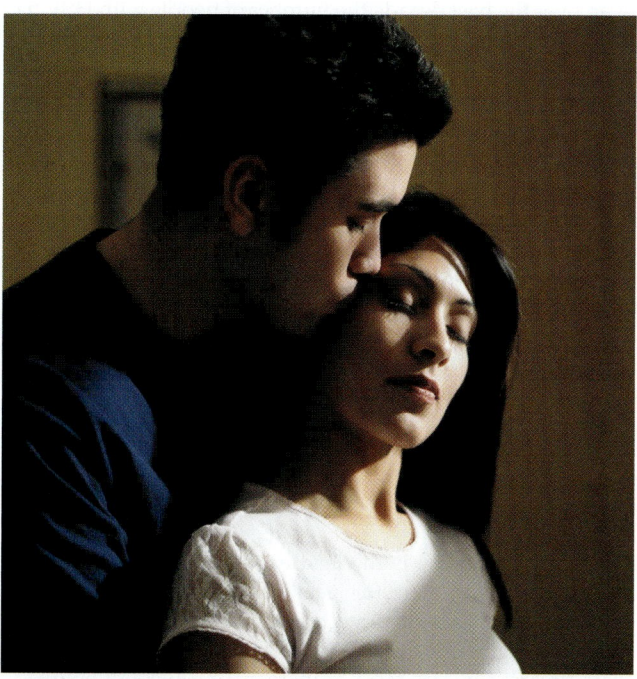

FIGURE 9-12 Young adults learn to develop intimacy.

young adults are instinctively driven to form a sexually intimate relationship.

Common Health Problems of Young Adults

Young adults are generally active and in good physical health. Frequently seen health problems include STIs, unplanned pregnancies, traumatic injury, suicide attempts, substance abuse, domestic violence, obesity, diabetes, and hypertension. In 2006, about one-third of young adults were uninsured.

STIs

Sexual experimentation often continues in this stage. Among adults 15 to 44 years of age, nearly all have had vaginal intercourse and most have had oral sex with an opposite-sex partner. Six percent of men have had oral or anal sex with another man, and 11% of women have had a sexual experience with another woman (Mosher, Chandra, & Jones, 2005).

Chlamydia. Chlamydia is one of the most common STIs among young adults. Individuals are often symptom free, but untreated chlamydia may result in **infertility** (the inability to conceive after 1 year of regular sexual intercourse).

Genital Warts. Genital warts (condyloma acuminata) are also common in both young men and women. This is a typically painless infection, caused by the human papillomavirus (HPV). The warts affect the moist tissues of the genital area; they also grow in the anus and in the mouth and throat of a person who has had oral sexual contact with an infected person. The lesions may be as small as 1 mm in diameter or may multiply into large clusters. The patient may be without symptoms or may have itching and discomfort in the genital area or bleeding with intercourse. Some, but not all, types of HPV have been associated with cervical and other genital cancers.

Genital Herpes. According to a nationally representative study, at least 45 million Americans ages 12 and older have had genital herpes, which is caused by the herpes simplex virus (HSV). After an initial flu-like illness, the virus leaves burning, itchy lesions on the genitals. Some people experience outbreaks as frequently as every month for many years. However, over the past decade the number of people with HSV has decreased. Genital HSV can lead to potentially fatal infections in babies and can increase the susceptibility to HIV infection. Although symptoms vary in severity, genital herpes often causes psychological distress because it cannot be cured and can be transmitted to sexual partners.

AIDS. More than 1 million people in the United States have been diagnosed with acquired immunodeficiency syndrome (AIDS), a fatal infectious disease transmitted via the exchange of body fluids such as blood, semen, and breast milk. One in five persons living with HIV infection is unaware of their infection. The number of men infected with HIV is about three times the number of women: About half of all HIV infections are transmitted by male-to-male sexual contact. In 2005, 15% of new HIV/AIDS diagnoses were among persons age 50 and older (CDC, 2008, 2010b).

Example Problem: Violence, Substance Abuse, and Suicide

Unintentional injury is the leading cause of death in young adults (National Center for Health Statistics, 2009). Suicide, a potential result of untreated depression, is another cause of death among young adults. Roughly 40,000 people a year die from firearm injuries, most of these are suicide and homicide rather than accidental injury. This is a rate of about 1 death per 10,000 people. The male death rate is about 7 times that for females (Heron, Hoyert, Murphy, et al., 2009). Substance abuse is often associated with acts of violence. Drug abuse is commonly thought of as an adolescent problem, but cocaine use is on the rise among young adults with families and careers.

In the young adult years, there is a strong emphasis on getting ahead, establishing a career and family, and becoming independent. These tasks are emotionally difficult. Substance abuse and mental health problems, particularly depression, may result from the tensions that arise.

Example Problem: Intimate Partner Violence

These same stresses may lead to aggression and violence in the family. **Domestic violence** is the abuse of power and control within an intimate relationship, most often between spouses or domestic partners.

Incidence. Surveys typically report that one in three U.S. women are physically assaulted by a spouse or partner at some point in their lives—an estimated 1 to 4 million each year. About half of these incidents result in injury (Moracco, Runyan, Bowling, et al., 2007; Nelson, Nygren, & McInerney, 2004; Thompson, Bonomi, Anderson, et al., 2006; U.S. Department of Justice, 2000). Many victims do not report the abuse, so survey results vary.

Global Problem. Violence against women and girls is a worldwide epidemic. Globally, one in every three women has been assaulted, coerced into sex, or otherwise abused at some point in her life. Most often, the abuser is a family member; more often than not, it is a spouse or domestic partner. Women of all races are equally vulnerable. Females 16 to 24 years of age are the most vulnerable to nonfatal violence.

Risk Factors. Abuse occurs in all ethnic and socioeconomic groups. Factors associated with intimate partner violence include young age, low income status, pregnancy, mental health problems, alcohol or substance abuse by victims or perpetrators, separated or divorced status, and history of childhood sexual or physical abuse (Nelson, Nygren, & McInerney, 2004). Although men are also victims of abuse, the incidence is less than for woman. In the United States, women are 7 to 14 times more likely to be abused than are men. About 31% of female murder victims are killed by an intimate, compared to 3% of male victims.

Health Consequences. Intimate partner violence has negative consequences for physical, sexual, and psychological health. Abuse victims can suffer acute and chronic pain, disability, damage to the eyes, sleep disorders, miscarriage, STIs, poor self-esteem, depression, anxiety, and even suicidal behavior.

Obesity

Obesity rates have increased over the past 25 years, and it is now a public health crisis. In the United States, about one in four young adults are obese, with a BMI of 30 or more, and 27% are overweight (BMI of 25–29). With increased obesity rates, the incidence of type 2 DM has increased dramatically among young adults, as has hypertension. Screening for both diabetes and hypertension is therefore very important in the young adult years, especially for individuals who are overweight or who have a family history of these disorders (National Center for Health Statistics, 2009).

ASSESSMENT

Young adults should have an annual physical examination, including assessment of physical health, mental health, and

lifestyle. For women this should include a pelvic examination. The American Cancer Society recommends a clinical breast examination at least once every 3 years Habits begun in this age period often carry on through life. Be sure to assess nutrition, exercise, sleep, and use of tobacco, alcohol and drugs.

Some clinicians advise men to have a testicular exam routinely until after age 40, but the U.S. Preventive Services Task Force (USPSTF) (2004) no longer recommends it because there is not enough evidence to show that screening reduces the deaths population-wide from testicular cancer. Although the USPSTF acknowledges that most testicular cancers are discovered by TSE, they also do not recommend monthly TSE.

Example Problem: Violence (Screening)

There is no direct evidence that screening for family and intimate partner violence helps decrease disability or premature death, so the USPSTF recommends only that clinicians be alert to physical and behavioral signs and symptoms associated with abuse (USPSTF, 2004). If there is any reason to suspect abuse, conduct a thorough assessment. Many experts recommend asking every woman directly if she has been struck or abused in any way. If you wish to assess for abuse, see Procedure 9-1.

■ INTERVENTIONS

Nursing interventions for the young adult are similar to those for the adolescent. It is important to develop an ongoing relationship with the young adult client. As a newly independent person, the young adult is establishing health patterns, including how she will interact with healthcare providers. Reinforce the teaching that was begun in the earlier age group. Stress the importance of health promotion activities such as annual Papanicolaou (Pap) test (for cervical cancer) for women under age 30.

Breast Self-Examination. Teach BSE if the client chooses to do them (see Box 9-6). Although research has not shown that BSE reduces the number of deaths from breast cancer (National Cancer Institute, 2008), there is the advantage of detecting the cancer early should it occur. Self-exam does not replace screening mammograms, and women younger than 40 who have risk factors for breast cancer should ask their healthcare provider whether they need mammograms. Risk factors include personal and family history of breast cancer, having the first child late in the childbearing cycle, having the first menstrual period before age 12, and certain breast changes (e.g., cells that look abnormal under a microscope). Studies have shown no link between abortion or miscarriage and breast cancer (National Cancer Institute, 2009).

Exercise. Recommend to adults that they engage in 2.5 hours a week of moderate-intensity, or 75 minutes a week of vigorous-intensity, aerobic physical activity. Increasing exercise to 300 minutes a week provides even more health benefits (U.S. Department of Health & Human Services, 2008).

Interventions for Example Problem: Violence

If a patient discloses domestic violence or abuse, act immediately. Ask the patient if she would like you to contact the agency's domestic violence advocate (if there is one). If not, provide contact information for community domestic violence programs. Patients may refuse help the first time it is offered. They are often fearful and isolated and in real danger. Further information on abuse and reporting is included in Chapter 43 and in Procedure 9-1 in this chapter.

KnowledgeCheck 9-9

- According to Erikson, what is the developmental stage of the young adult?
- What is the leading cause of death for this age group?
- What gender-specific assessments should be emphasized with this age group?

MIDDLE ADULTHOOD: AGES 40 TO 64 YEARS

The middle adult years are a time when people realize the difference between their early aspirations and their actual achievements. For families with children, this is often a time when the children mature and leave the home. As a result, many middle adults and their children feel a need to redefine the family roles.

Physical Development of Middle Adults

Physiological changes during the middle adult years include a loss of elasticity of the blood vessels, a loss of muscle tone, a decrease in skin moisture and turgor, graying hair, a decrease in bone mass that causes a slight loss of height, and a decrease in gastrointestinal (GI) motility.

One of the principal changes that women experience in the middle adult years is **menopause,** the cessation of menstrual periods for at least 12 consecutive months. The ovaries no longer produce eggs on a cyclical basis, and reproductive ability is lost. The average age of menopause is 51 years. Although menopause seems to be a clearly defined phenomenon, most women experience a transition that takes place over many years. Perimenopausal symptoms are related to a decline in estrogen levels and may precede menopause by as much as 5 to 7 years. These symptoms include hot flashes, a decrease in breast size, changes in the length of the menstrual cycle and menstrual flow, vaginal dryness, nighttime awakenings, and moodiness.

Hormone replacement therapy (HRT) has been used extensively in the past to treat these symptoms, but findings from the Women's Health Initiative and other studies have raised questions about the safety of hormone therapy to treat a naturally occurring phenomenon. HRT can relieve symptoms such as hot flashes and vaginal dryness. It may also protect against osteoporosis and age-linked eye disease. Some studies show that it may help prevent dementia; others, that it does not. The National Heart, Lung, and Blood Institute (National Institutes of Health, 2008) concludes that the risks of long-term combination hormone (estrogen and progestin) therapy outweigh the benefits for postmenopausal women. Risks include increased risk of heart disease, breast cancer, stroke, and blood clots. Risks and benefits of estrogen-alone therapy are still being debated. Women should be advised to consult their primary care provider about this issue and about certain natural remedies that may provide symptom relief.

Menopause implies the inability to reproduce, although some women do become pregnant after not having menses for a year. Men do not experience such a clear-cut transition, but many men do experience a transitional period known as andropause. **Andropause** is characterized by a decrease in testosterone production, a lower sperm count, and a need for more time to achieve an erection. Andropause does not result in an inability to reproduce but does limit reproductive abilities.

Cognitive Development of Middle Adults

Piaget theorized that the middle adult moves freely between formal operations, concrete operations, and problem-solving as the task demands. The middle adult is able to

reflect on the past and anticipate the future. Creativity may reach its peak during this stage. Memory is intact, but reaction time begins to diminish because of a decrease in nerve impulses.

Psychosocial Development of Middle Adults

Erikson describes middle adulthood as a stage of *generativity versus stagnation*. *Generativity* is the process of guiding the next generation, or improving the whole of society. *Stagnation* occurs when development ceases: A stagnant middle adult cannot guide the next generation or contribute to society. Erikson believes that an inability to meet the developmental tasks of the middle adult years results in lack of preparedness for the final life stage of old age.

Middle adulthood is a time of transition. Middle adults often complain of declining energy and competing demands as they raise children, care for aging parents, and work at the peak of their career (Fig. 9-13). These stressors in combination with visible signs of aging may produce a **midlife crisis**—a recognition that youth is over and that life is limited. Coping skills learned in earlier years are important predictors of how the middle adult reacts to these changes.

Common Health Problems of Middle Adults

In the middle adult years, chronic diseases emerge as a major health problem. The most common chronic diseases are obesity, diabetes, hypertension, cardiovascular disease, and cancer.

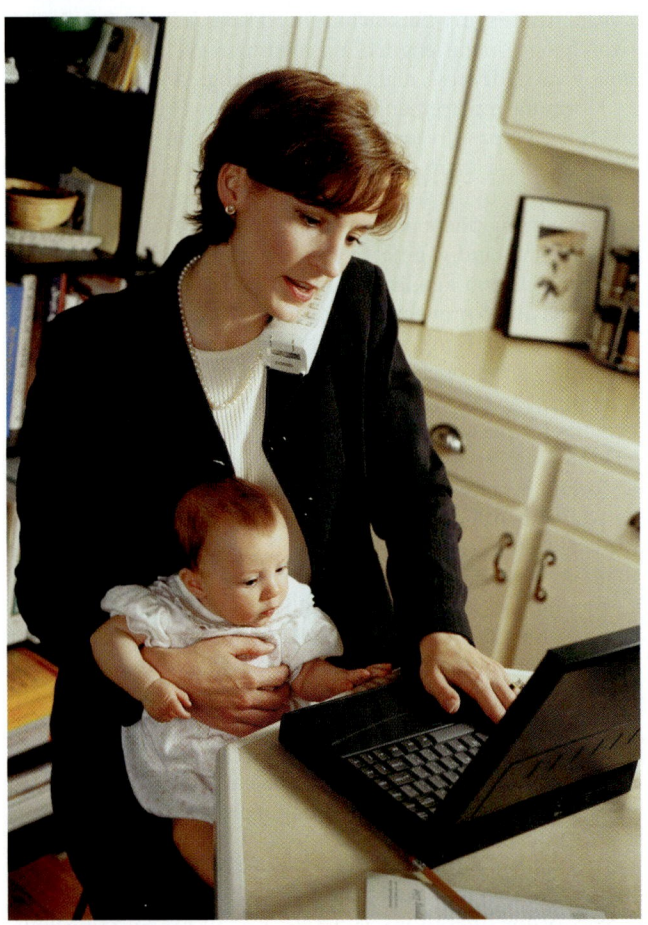

FIGURE 9-13 Middle adulthood is a time of competing demands.

Many interventions for younger age groups are directed at preventing the development of these chronic disorders.

Cancer. Cancer is the second leading cause of death in this age group. The incidence of cancer rises with age, with the majority of cancer diagnoses occurring in the middle and older adult years. Cancers of the lung, breast, colon, prostate, and bladder are among the most common.

Prostate Cancer. A man's risk of prostate cancer increases as he ages. Nearly 65% of prostate cancer cases occur after the age of 65. Several other risk factors increase a man's chances of developing prostate cancer: family history, race (African American men have the highest rate), and possibly diet. There is some evidence that a diet high in animal fat may increase the risk.

Obesity. As we have seen, obesity is a major health problem in all age groups. It often triggers development of type 2 DM; hypertension; joint pain; and cardiovascular diseases, such as coronary artery disease, atherosclerosis, and venous insufficiency. Diet and exercise must be consistently used together to combat obesity. Ironically, obesity leads to a variety of problems that make it even harder to exercise.

Hypertension. Hypertension (high blood pressure) is a complex disorder influenced by age, genetics, diet, exercise, weight, and alcohol and tobacco use. Many hypertension risk factors are under the patient's control—except for age and family history. As the elasticity of the vascular system declines with each passing year, the incidence of hypertension increases. If there is a strong family history of hypertension, the likelihood of needing treatment escalates sharply. Excess weight, sedentary lifestyle, high sodium intake, high fat intake, smoking, and the ingestion of more than 1.5 ounces of alcohol per day all increase the risk of hypertension. For further discussion of hypertension, see Chapter 19.

Cardiovascular Disease. Cardiovascular disease (CVD) is often the end product of poor lifestyle choices. Atherosclerotic plaque develops in the peripheral vascular system, the heart, major vessels, or any combination of these areas. CVD is the result of inadequately treated hypertension, ongoing weight gain or obesity, an aftermath of poorly controlled type 2 DM, and an outcome of a sedentary lifestyle. Smoking and excess alcohol use are additional risk factors, as is long-term hormone replacement therapy for women. CVD is among the leading causes of death in the middle adult years.

Example Problem: Domestic Violence

Domestic violence has negative consequences for physical, sexual, and psychological health. Abuse victims can suffer acute and chronic pain, disability, damage to the eyes, sleep disorders, miscarriage, STIs, poor self-esteem, depression, anxiety, and even suicidal thoughts. Women ages 30 to 49 are the most vulnerable to intimate murder, although younger women are more likely to experience nonfatal violence (Bureau of Justice Statistics, n.d., last reviewed 2011). Also see Common Health Problems of Young Adults, Domestic Violence, preceding.

ASSESSMENT

Middle adults should undergo an annual physical exam. The exam should include the following:
- Vital signs
- Height measurement with comparison to previous height (a screen for osteoporosis)
- Weight and body mass index (BMI) calculation

- Lipid panel screening; total cholesterol, triglycerides, high-density lipoprotein (HDL), low-density lipoprotein (LDL), and ratios
- Blood glucose screening
- Annual clinical breast and pelvic examination for women. There is still controversy about whether to encourage BSE. There is not enough research evidence to support BSE (*The Guide to Clinical Preventive Services*, 2010), but many clinicians believe it to be useful. See Breast and Testicular Self-Exam, in the section on Interventions for adolescents.
- Annual or biannual mammogram for women after age 40 (American Cancer Society, n.d.b). The U.S. Preventive Services Task Force (USPSTF) recommends biannual screening between the ages of 50 and 75 years (National Guideline Clearinghouse, 1998, revised 2012).
- Pap tests to every 2 or 3 years. Women older than age 30 who have had three normal Pap tests for 3 years in a row should ask their healthcare provider if, in their particular case, they may have the tests less frequently.
- Digital rectal exam for prostate evaluation in men should be offered, but not routinely done (American Cancer Society, n.d.b). An enlarged prostate can indicate either benign prostatic hypertrophy or prostate cancer.
- In men, serum prostate-specific antigen (PSA) level is a sensitive indicator of prostate disorders. Recommendations vary. Some caution against routine screening, while others make decisions on an individual basis. The American Cancer Society (n.d.b), says this test should be given beginning at age 45 to men who want to be screened, and at age 40 for those who are at higher risk. The USPSTF recommends that men age 75 and older not be screened for prostate cancer ("Task Force Says," 2008). Medicare does provide coverage for an annual PSA test for all men age 50 and older, but this may change based on the USPSTF recommendations. There is no agreed-upon normal or abnormal PSA level. Many providers are using the following ranges:

    0.0 to 2.5 nanograms per mL—low

    2.5 to 10 ng/mL—slightly to moderately elevated

    10 to 19.9 ng/mL—moderately elevated

    20 n/mL or more—significantly elevated (National Cancer Institute, 2007)
- Annual eye exam; visual changes are common in this age group and include the development of presbyopia (far-sightedness) and the onset of glaucoma and cataracts.
- Sigmoidoscopy or colonoscopy for colon cancer screening at the age of 50; the frequency of repeat exams depends on the findings.
- Stool for occult blood, an annual check for blood in the stool to screen for colon cancer.
- For at-risk women who wish to elect it, a bone density scan (called a DEXA test) at or prior to menopause.

INTERVENTIONS

Care for middle adults focuses on identifying risk factors and promoting a healthy lifestyle. At each annual exam and at periodic health visits, you should discuss the hazards of alcohol and tobacco use, the importance of regular exercise, stress-management techniques, safety, and the benefits of a balanced nutritional intake. You will also need to add teaching topics and interventions if any chronic problem is discovered.

Nutrition. For menopausal women, encourage daily intake of 1,200 mg of calcium and 600 IU of vitamin D, as well as regular weight-bearing exercise, to promote optimum bone density (Institute of Medicine, Food and Nutrition Board, 2010; Office of Dietary Supplements, National Institutes of Health, 2011). There is growing consensus that even this amount may be too low. Many clinicians are prescribing higher doses, especially in cases of known deficiency.

Exercise. Although the usual recommendation is for 60 minutes of exercise daily, and that amount brings the most health benefits, researchers now suggest that even smaller amounts of exercise can improve the quality of life for sedentary, overweight, or obese postmenopausal women. Even 30 minutes a day can improve social functioning and decrease limitations in work and other activities due to physical or emotional problems (American Heart Association, 2011b).

Immunizations. Review the patient's immunization record regularly. Middle adults often require periodic boosters—for example, for tetanus. For clients who have a chronic disease, recommend an annual flu vaccination. Strongly encourage clients with respiratory problems to receive pneumonia vaccination as well.

KnowledgeCheck 9-10

- According to Erikson, what is the developmental stage associated with middle adulthood?
- Identify at least five appropriate topics for health teaching during middle adulthood.

PracticalKnowledge
knowing **how**

This section of the chapter focuses on using standardized nursing language for nursing diagnoses, patient outcomes, and interventions for patients in infancy through middle-adulthood. Specific assessments and interventions were discussed within each of the developmental stages in the Theoretical Knowledge section.

ANALYSIS/DIAGNOSIS

Although most NANDA-I diagnoses can be used for any age group, the following NANDA-I diagnoses focus specifically on growth and development:

    Adult Failure to Thrive

    Delayed Growth and Development

    Risk for Delayed Development

    Risk for Disproportionate Growth

Refer to the four clients in the Meet Your Patients scenario. You would, of course, consider their growth and development needs in your assessments and care. However, they are unlikely to experience any of the four growth and development diagnoses. Short-term illness does not usually lead to delays in growth and development. Growth and development problems are more likely to be caused by family dysfunction, inadequate nutrition, or severe or long-term illness (e.g., Risk for Delayed Development r/t inadequate stimulation secondary to parental substance abuse).

Delayed growth and development may be the defining characteristics (signs and symptoms) of the problem rather than the diagnosis (e.g., Impaired Parenting r/t mother's chronic disability and absent father, as evidenced by height, weight, and verbal skills behind norms for age group).

When used to describe a client's *problem,* the label, Delayed Growth and Development, is too broad to suggest nursing actions. For example, this label is not useful for a mentally handicapped child (e.g., do not write Delayed Growth and Development r/t Down syndrome). Instead, write a nursing diagnosis describing the specific functional task(s) the child cannot perform (e.g., Toileting Self-Care Deficit r/t inability to recognize the urge to void in time to ask for help secondary to Delayed Growth and Development). This label is also not appropriate for a child with failure to thrive. Instead, use one of the family functioning diagnoses (e.g., Impaired Parenting) or Imbalanced Nutrition: Less Than Body Requirements (Wilkinson, 2009, p. 296).

Although there are only four NANDA-I diagnoses that specifically address growth and development, some other NANDA-I diagnoses do address age-specific problems. Because they provide more specific direction for nursing care than the growth and development diagnoses, use these when possible:

Ineffective Infant Feeding Pattern
Interrupted Breastfeeding
Readiness for Enhanced Breastfeeding
Ineffective Breastfeeding
Disorganized Infant Behavior
Risk for Disorganized Infant Behavior
Readiness for Enhanced Organized Infant Behavior
Risk for Impaired Attachment
Impaired Parenting
Readiness for Enhanced Parenting
Risk for Impaired Parenting
Parental Role Conflict

▆ PLANNING OUTCOMES/EVALUATION

NOC outcomes specifically related to growth and development include the following, but many other NOC outcomes may be appropriate depending on the NANDA-I label you use (e.g., Imbalanced Nutrition, Self-Care Deficit).

Child Development: (specify 2 Months, 4 Years, and so on)
Fetal Status: Antepartum
Fetal Status: Intrapartum Growth
Newborn Adaptation
Physical Aging
Physical Maturation: Female
Physical Maturation: Male
Will to Live

Individualized goals/outcome statements for the other NANDA-I growth and development diagnoses might include the following examples:

Diagnosis: Risk for Disproportionate Growth
Goal: The child will continue to gain weight and length as measured at the next well-child checks.

Diagnosis: Risk for Delayed Growth and Development
Goal: The child will continue to gain weight and length and meet developmental milestones as measured at the next well-child check.

▆ PLANNING INTERVENTIONS/IMPLEMENTATION

NIC standardized interventions associated with growth and development diagnoses include the following:

Coping Enhancement
Developmental Care
Hope Instillation
Nutrition Screening
Parent Education: Childrearing Family
Risk Identification
Self-Care Assistance
Self-Responsibility Facilitation
Teaching: Infant Nutrition, Infant Safety, Safe Sex, Sexuality, Toddler Nutrition, Toddler Safety

PUTTING IT ALL TOGETHER

Recall the case of 3-year-old Tamika, who is being raised by her grandmother and has been hospitalized with pneumonia (Meet Your Patients scenario). Imagine that Tamika has been abandoned by her mother, who is addicted to heroin. If you observe that Tamika is small for her size and has not met developmental milestones appropriate for a 3-year-old, you could write the following *diagnostic statement*:

Delayed Growth and Development r/t abandonment by mother, recent change in living status, and gestational heroin exposure as evidenced by underweight status, short stature, limited verbal skills, and onset of walking at 36 months of age

To address Tamika's diagnosis, you might use the following *outcomes*:

NOC outcome: Child Development: 3 Years
Individualized goal: Tamika will achieve growth between the 35th and 65th percentiles for her age group and be able to walk up steps, verbalize with two- to three-word sentences, and eat a variety of foods within 6 months.

Tamika will need care that helps her to catch up developmentally and allows her to establish a strong relationship with her grandmother. Because the grandmother is also caring for her ill husband, you may need to refer this family to community support services for ongoing help.

NIC interventions appropriate for Tamika are as follows:
Developmental Care
Teaching: Toddler Nutrition and Toddler Safety

Specific interventions for Tamika might include therapeutic playing with age-appropriate toys, reading stories, and engaging in conversation, as well as teaching the grandmother about these activities. This family may need counseling to assist with this transition.

CLINICALREASONING:
Applying the **Full-Spectrum Nursing Model**

Because the following critical thinking activities allow you to practice the kind of thinking you will use as a full-spectrum nurse, they usually have no single right answer. Discuss them with your peers—if you have difficulty with any of the questions, consult your instructor.

PATIENT SITUATION

Lani Ettinger is a 30-year-old woman, married, with three school-age children. She has just had a mastectomy (removal of a breast) because her biopsy was positive for cancer. The surgery was uncomplicated, the cancer was removed at an early stage, and she is expected to recover completely. As you are helping her prepare to leave the hospital, she begins crying.

THINKING

1. *Theoretical Knowledge:* What are Havighurst's developmental tasks of young adulthood?
2. *Critical Thinking (Contextual Awareness):* Which of those developmental tasks is/are most likely to be affected by Lani's mastectomy and her emotional reaction to it?

DOING

3. *Nursing Process (Assessment):* When you see that Lani is crying, what do you need to do?

CARING

4. *Self-Knowledge:* Suppose Lani tells you, "My husband has gone to get the car, but when he was here, he didn't want to hug me or kiss me. I asked him if he will still love me and he didn't say anything. He was crying when he left." What would your feelings be about the husband? You do not need to speculate on exactly what he meant; just imagine what your initial feelings would be.

PracticalKnowledge
procedures

If necessary, review the preceding sections concerning child abuse and domestic partner violence. You will find information on elder abuse in Chapter 10; however, the following procedure can be used for patients of all ages.

Keep in mind that if there is an injury, there is the possibility that it was inflicted. The following flow chart and Procedure 9-1 will aid you in identifying cases of abuse.

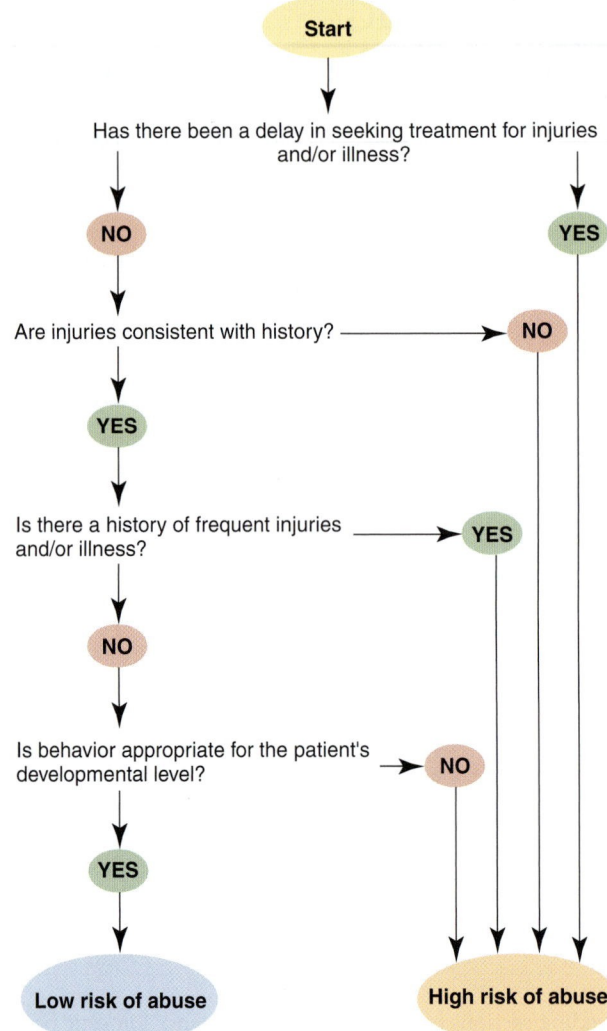

FIGURE 9-14 Possible Abuse Flow Chart.

Procedure 9-1 ■ Assessing for Abuse

➤ For steps to follow in *all* procedures, refer to the Universal Steps for All Procedures found on the page facing the inside back cover of this book.

Critical Aspects

- Assess for abuse any time a child or dependent person has an injury.
- The key to ruling out abuse is to determine whether the injury was intentional or accidental.
- Use a nonjudgmental approach; do not make assumptions.
- Remember, the relationship between the suspected abuser and the victim is complex. Love, fear, self-doubt, anger, guilt, and many other emotions are common and can influence the report of the abuse and details implicating the abuser.
- Obtain a focused health history, assessing for physical, sexual, and psychological abuse and neglect.
- Determine whether the caregiver of the suspected victim has a history of a mental health disorder, such as anxiety, depression, or dysfunctional coping.

- Perform a focused physical assessment; ensure the integrity of evidence that may be needed for criminal prosecution.
- For any sexual examination, always have a witness in the room to protect the patient and the examiner.
- Assess whether the injuries are consistent with the history.
- If appropriate, provide the victim with referrals for help in escaping the abusive situation.
- If appropriate, refer the parent, caregiver, or partner involved in abuse to hotlines or agencies focused on stopping the abuse and protecting the victim.
- Report abuse according to agency, state, and federal guidelines.

Pre-Procedure Assessment

- If you suspect sexual abuse, request a forensic nurse or sexual assault nurse examiner (SANE) be present.

A forensic nurse and SANE are trained to identify findings that indicate abuse, to support the patient, and to handle the evidence to ensure validity in a court of law.

- **Assess for abuse any time a child, dependent person, or spouse has an injury.**

Although there is not a strong base of evidence to support screening, the Joint Commission requires that all patients be screened for abuse and domestic violence.

Delegation

Assessment is a nursing responsibility and cannot be delegated.

➤ When performing the procedure, always identify your patient according to agency policy and be attentive to standard precautions, hand hygiene, patient safety and privacy, body mechanics, and documentation.

➤ Note: Privacy and confidentiality are extremely important for this procedure.

Procedure Steps

1. **Obtain a focused health history.**

   a. **Collect information from the patient and family members or caregivers separately. If more than one caregiver is present, separate them for the interview, as well.**

   An abused person may be afraid to talk with the abuser present. Victims have often been intimidated and will usually support the abuser's version of events. If two adults accompany a child, it may be that one of them is abusing both the partner and the child. To help rule that out, separate the caregivers to be certain that they tell the same story.

   b. **Approach the subject in a non-threatening and caring manner. For example, you might say:**

   "The law requires us to ask about certain injuries. We are not accusing you of anything. I know you care about your child/parent/spouse and want to do everything possible for her health."

   c. **Consider the patient's developmental and cognitive level in assessing whether the story of how the injury occurred is consistent with the injuries.**

   The patient must be developmentally capable of performing an activity in a situation in which an injury occurred. For example, an infant is not likely to have opened a medication bottle and taken pills; and if a child cannot yet walk, it is not likely he reached up to pull a hot pan off the stove.

   d. **Observe whether the patient's behavior is inconsistent with his developmental level.**

   In the presence of the abuser, it is common for the victim to appear passive

and withdrawn and avoid eye contact. The victim may exhibit anxiety or fear; may look to the parent or caregiver before answering questions; may be overly compliant; or may let the abuser answer the questions for him.

   e. **Ask about the injury or incident. Ask detailed questions about how and when the injury occurred or the illness began:**

   "When did this injury happen or when did you first begin to feel ill?" "How did you get this injury?" "What happened to you?" "What have you been doing to treat your symptoms since you first became ill?"

   A delay of treatment of 12 to 18 hours may indicate abuse. If the details of the history of an injury change during the interview, the likelihood of abuse increases.

   f. **Ask about past injuries or incidents: "Have you ever had similar injuries?" "Have you ever required emergency care in the past?"**

   Abusive behavior typically occurs over and over. If an injury is due to abuse, the patient would most likely have experienced abuse in the past and would have evidence of old injuries.

   g. **Ask about the patient's usual diet: "What do you usually eat for breakfast? Lunch? Dinner? What kind of snacks do you have during the day?"**

   Neglect and abuse may be exhibited by an inadequate or inappropriate diet.

   h. **To assess for sexual abuse, ask:**

   If a patient is in a potentially abusive situation, the possibility of sexual abuse must be considered.

   - **Ask directly whether the patient has been touched inappropriately or forced to have sexual relations.**

Question the patient directly so your question will not be misunderstood.

   - **Ask whether the patient has genitourinary symptoms: "Have you had any burning or itching when you urinate? How about any vaginal discharge?"**

   Genitourinary symptoms in a child may indicate sexual abuse or neglect.

   - **Does the child display knowledge or interest in sexual acts inappropriate to his or her age, or even seductive behavior?**

   - **Does the child appear to avoid another person, or display unusual behavior—either very aggressive or very passive?**

   - **Does the victim display destructive behaviors, such as alcohol or drug abuse, self-mutilation, or suicide attempts?**

   - **Is the victim pregnant, particularly if no intimate relationship is known or the victim is very young?**

   i. **To assess for psychological abuse:**

   - **Ask parents or caregivers, "Are there family members or friends who help you with problems?"**

   Isolation is a risk factor for abuse. Parents or caregivers may not have the support they need.

   - **Ask the patient, "Whom do you talk to when you are having problems?"**

   An abuser will try to isolate the victim from family and friends over time. Ask questions to determine the relationship between the victim and family and friends.

(continued on next page)

Procedure 9-1 ■ **Assessing for Abuse** (continued)

■ Ask, "Tell me how you feel about yourself."

An abuser demeans and degrades the victim so that the victim has a low self-worth and feels the "punishment" is deserved; conversely, the victim may desire the attention.

■ Observe if the child acts fearful, shies away from touch, or appears to be afraid to go home.

■ Ask, "Who manages the family finances, and how are decisions made regarding spending?"

An abuser frequently controls all the finances, and restricts the resources of the victim. Abusers typically seek control of victims by fostering dependency and powerlessness.

2. **Perform a focused physical assessment.**

a. If sexual abuse is suspected from the interview, have a forensic nurse or sexual assault nurse examiner (SANE) present if possible.

For any sexual examination, always have a witness in the room to protect the patient and the examiner.

b. Assess the current injury and look for evidence of previous injuries. Look for the following cues:

■ Bruises that form an outline of a hand, cord loop, buckle, or belt

*Injuries of different ages and multiple injuries may show a pattern of abuse. Be careful to assess the bruise accurately. Some home treatments may cause what looks like bruising. For example, **moxibustion** (includes such things as firmly rubbing a warm spoon down the affected area) is used in some Asian cultures.*

■ Injuries that are inconsistent with the history of the injury and are of varying ages (e.g., bruises of different colors, cuts in various stages of healing)

■ Obvious nonaccidental burns, such as burns to both feet and lower legs from immersion in hot water

One method of abuse is to immerse the victim's hands or feet into scalding water. The resulting injury has a well-defined border and usually occurs on both extremities.

■ Circular burns, possibly from cigarettes

Burns at several locations on the body are signs of abuse.

■ Bite marks

■ Oral ecchymosis or injury from forced oral sex

Forced oral sex causes injuries to the mouth.

■ Bruising at the crease above the eyelids, tense fontanel if the victim is an infant, hyphema, subconjunctival hemorrhage or retinal bleeding, detached retina, ruptured tympanic membrane

Injuries to the head are common in abuse. Abusive head trauma (AHT, previously referred to as shaken-baby syndrome) is one of the most common and most serious injuries for a young child.

■ Bleeding or bruising of genitalia, poor sphincter tone, encopresis (poor bowel control) and bruises on inner thighs

■ Positive culture for STI or positive pregnancy test

STI, particularly in a child, can indicate sexual abuse.

■ Bruises on wrists and ankles from being restrained

Abused individuals may be tied or locked in a closet or other small space.

■ Refer to the figure for typical features of injuries that may be nonaccidental:

Injuries to both sides of the body

Injuries in the "triangle of safety": ears, side of face, neck, and top of the shoulders

Injuries to soft tissue ("swimsuit zone" on the trunk, breast, abdomen, genitalia, and buttocks)

Accidental injuries in the triangle of safety are unusual. Accidental injuries are usually over bony prominences rather than soft tissue. ▼

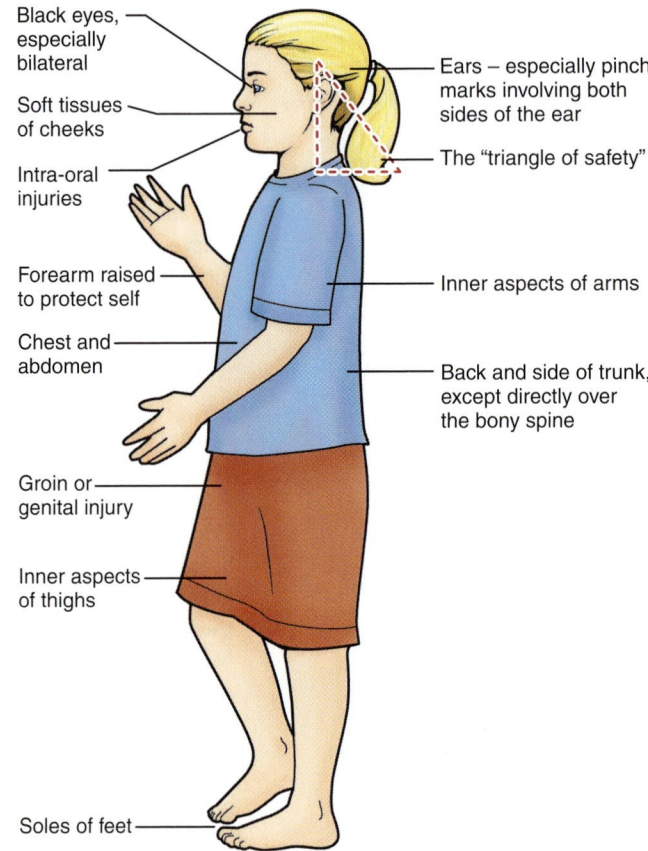

Black eyes, especially bilateral

Soft tissues of cheeks

Intra-oral injuries

Forearm raised to protect self

Chest and abdomen

Groin or genital injury

Inner aspects of thighs

Soles of feet

Ears – especially pinch marks involving both sides of the ear

The "triangle of safety"

Inner aspects of arms

Back and side of trunk, except directly over the bony spine

c. Assess whether injuries are consistent with the history.

If injuries are not consistent with the history, you must assume abuse.

d. Observe for signs of neglect:
- Malnutrition, such as a distended abdomen, or weight markedly below ideal body weight
- Excess body weight for height and age
- Poor hygiene, including oral hygiene
- Ingrown nails
- Untreated sores or pressure sores or other medical conditions
- Matted hair
- Dehydration
- Confusion
- Clothing that is inappropriate for the weather, such as heavy, long-sleeved pants and shirts on hot days
- Periods of time a young child or frail, older adult is left alone without care or supervision

Signs of neglect occur because of long-term starvation or underfeeding, poor personal care, untreated sores or injuries, and inadequate fluid intake. Neglect can also result in childhood obesity as a result of food of poor quality, erratic eating patterns, and poor supervision of the diet.

3. **If the forensic nurse or primary care provider determines** that abuse has occurred, follow legal procedures to ensure that all evidence is secured. If possible, have a forensic nurse and social worker work with the patient.

In situations in which violation of the law has occurred, strict procedures are essential to ensure that your findings can be used in a court of law and to protect yourself against legal liability.

4. **Provide referrals,** if appropriate, for the abused person, partner, family member, or caregiver to obtain assistance in escaping the abusive situation and/or stopping the abuse.

Resources are available to assist the abused individual and to assist the parent or caregiver to stop the abuse. Be aware of local and national resources.

5. **Report concerns** regarding abuse according to agency and state guidelines.

Suspected child and elder abuse must be reported to the appropriate agency, according to federal and state laws. Spousal abuse may be mandatory to report, depending on state law. The Joint Commission requires that all cases of possible abuse or neglect are immediately reported in the hospital.

6. **Treat physical injuries** or refer to the primary care provider for medical care, as needed.

Detection and prevention of abuse require collaborative efforts of the healthcare team.

? What if . . .

- **My patient is a child? Are there any special assessments I should make or actions I should take?**

Follow steps 1 through 6 above, with these modifications:

NOTE: The interview is important in ruling out sexual abuse in children. Physical findings are often absent, even when the perpetrator admits to penetration of the child's genitalia. Most expert interviewers do not interview children younger than 3 years.

a. To assess for sexual abuse, ask whether the patient has been touched inappropriately:
- *Child older than 2:* Ask about being touched in "private parts."
- *Older child:* Ask a question such as, "Sometimes people you know may touch or kiss you in a way that you feel is strange or wrong. Has this ever happened to you?"
- *Adolescent:* Ask, "Sometimes people touch you in ways you feel are wrong. This can be frightening, and it is wrong for people to do that to you. Has this ever happened to you?"

b. Ask the parent or caregiver:
- "Has the child started wetting the bed or soiling himself?"
- "Does the child have fears that seem unreasonable?"

Abuse may result in regression to former behaviors. Symptoms of sexual abuse in children may be general and nonspecific, such as sleep disturbances, bed-wetting, or excessive fears.
- "Has the child been masturbating or sexually acting out with other children?"

A child who is sexually abused may exhibit inappropriate sexual behavior.
- "Has the child ever run away? If she leaves, does she go to somewhere safe?" "Is the child/adolescent sexually active?"

An abused child may have feelings of low self worth and may demonstrate risk-taking behavior, such as running away to places that are unsafe.

c. To assess for psychological abuse, ask the parent or caregiver:
- "Was the child a result of a planned pregnancy? What were the pregnancy, birth, and postpartum period like?"

Risk factors for abuse include an unplanned pregnancy, complications during pregnancy, stressors (e.g., moving, illness, loss of job, divorce), a difficult pregnancy or birth, and lengthy stay in the neonatal intensive care unit.
- "How would you describe the child now?"

An abusive parent may describe the child as a "problem child" who is always doing something wrong. The opposite is sometimes seen, when the child is "perfect."
- "How does the child's behavior compare to that of others in the family?"

Determine whether the parent sees the child differently from siblings. This is a risk factor for abuse.
- "Has the child experienced physical or emotional problems in the past?"

A history of physical or emotional problems may indicate abuse.
- "What are your expectations of the child's behavior (e.g., school performance, following instructions)?"

The expectations of parents or caregivers who are more at risk to abuse a child may be that the

(continued on next page)

Procedure 9–1 ■ **Assessing for Abuse** (continued)

child will "always be a problem" or will be a "perfect" son or daughter.

■ **"What form of discipline works best with the child?"**
Determine whether the parents or caregivers use physical or emotional punishment that may be abusive or disproportionate for the act or situation.

■ **"Do you have any history of depression, anxiety, difficulty coping with situations or everyday life, or other history of mental heath problems?"**
Mental health disorders interfere with a person's ability to perceive others and situations in a realistic and appropriate way. When coping is compromised, the risk for abuse escalates.

d. Perform a physical assessment. Signs of physical abuse and neglect in children include the following:

■ Bruises on head, face, ears, buttocks, and lower back that are inconsistent with the history of the injury and are of varying stages of healing (different colors)

■ Hemorrhage of the eye, detached retina, ruptured eardrum
Bruising may occur in different patterns. Children often have accidental bruises over bony areas, but usually not on the abdomen. Injuries to the head are common in abuse. The abusive head trauma (AHT) syndrome may

cause detached retina(s), hemorrhages, and subdural hematomas.

■ Assess for abdominal pain and other nonspecific complaints.
Abdominal pain may be a symptom of sexual abuse in children. Signs of sexual abuse may be general and nonspecific in children.

? What if . . .

■ **My patient is an older adult? Are there any special assessments I should make or actions I should take?**

a. Ask the patient and caregiver:

■ **"Describe the patient's personal support network. Who visits the patient? How often does the patient have visitors?"**
As in spousal abuse, people who victimize older people often isolate the person from any support network.

■ **"Who is the patient's primary healthcare provider?"**
Multiple healthcare providers, or lack of a provider, can be an indication of abuse. The caregiver may bring the patient to a different physician with each injury or illness to avoid discovery.

■ **"Has the patient ever received the wrong dose of medication?"**
Getting the wrong medication or dosage of medication (especially oversedation) may indicate abuse or inability to provide safe care.

■ **"Who manages the patient's finances?"**
Financial abuse is a fairly common form of abuse in this population. Determine who has control of the older person's finances and makes the decisions regarding spending.

b. Ask the patient:

■ **"Do you feel safe in your home?"**
The patient who is being abused does not feel safe. Keep in mind that abandonment is a form of abuse.

■ **"Tell me about your usual day." "Are you able to take care of yourself?" "Who helps you shower and dress?" or "Do you require help with showering or dressing?" "Who is responsible for grocery shopping and cooking in your home?" "How do you get to your appointments or other places you want or need to go?"**
To determine the patient's usual level of self-care.

c. Observe for signs of self-neglect.

? What if . . .

■ **You feel that you are or the patient is in immediate danger?**

If the patient's or your safety is at risk, immediate intervention is required. You may need to secure the area (e.g., by closing the door), notify the in-house security officer, and then call the police.

Evaluation

■ Determine whether abuse may have occurred.
■ Ensure that appropriate agencies have been notified of the possible abuse.
■ Evaluate whether it is safe to let the patient leave the facility.

Documentation

■ Chart all findings factually—do not add any interpretations. For example:

Don't Chart:

4-year-old boy admitted with immersion burns to both feet extending to midpoint of shins, such as those found in abuse.

Do Chart:

4-year-old boy admitted with second-degree burns to both feet extending to midpoint of shins. Father says, "I put him in the bathtub and didn't realize how hot the water was."

■ Follow legal requirements for documenting possible abuse, including disposition of potential evidence.
■ If possible, include pictures of the injuries in the charting, using a digital camera.
Photos must be saved and stored (or developed, if using film) in-house because of the requirement to protect confidentiality.

Patient Teaching

- Inform the patient, parent, partner, and/or caregiver of local resources for prevention or intervention in situations of child, spousal, or elder abuse.
- Inform the patient that abuse is suspected. Ask for her perceptions of the situation.
- Emphasize to the patient that her safety is the primary concern.

Home Care

- If potential abuse is identified in the home, follow agency and state legal guidelines.
- If the patient's safety is at risk, immediate intervention is required. You may need to notify the police or call an ambulance. Be sure to carry a fully-charged cell phone with you.
- If you believe that you are at risk for harm (common in abusive situations), leave the setting before notifying the police.

Practice Resources

Dembrow, M., Golden, A., Paulk, D., et al. (2007); the Joint Commission (2008); National Guideline Clearinghouse (2007).

 To explore learning resources for this chapter,

 Go to DavisPlus at http://davisplus.fadavis.com/Treas1

Chapter Resources for Chapter 9:
  Knowledge Check and Think Like a Nurse Response Sheets
  Knowledge Check Answers
  Resources for Caregivers and Health Professionals
  Reading More About Development: Infancy Through Middle Age (Suggested Readings)
  What Are the Main Points in This Chapter?
NCLEX-Style Review Questions
Chapter Overview Podcasts

Concept Map

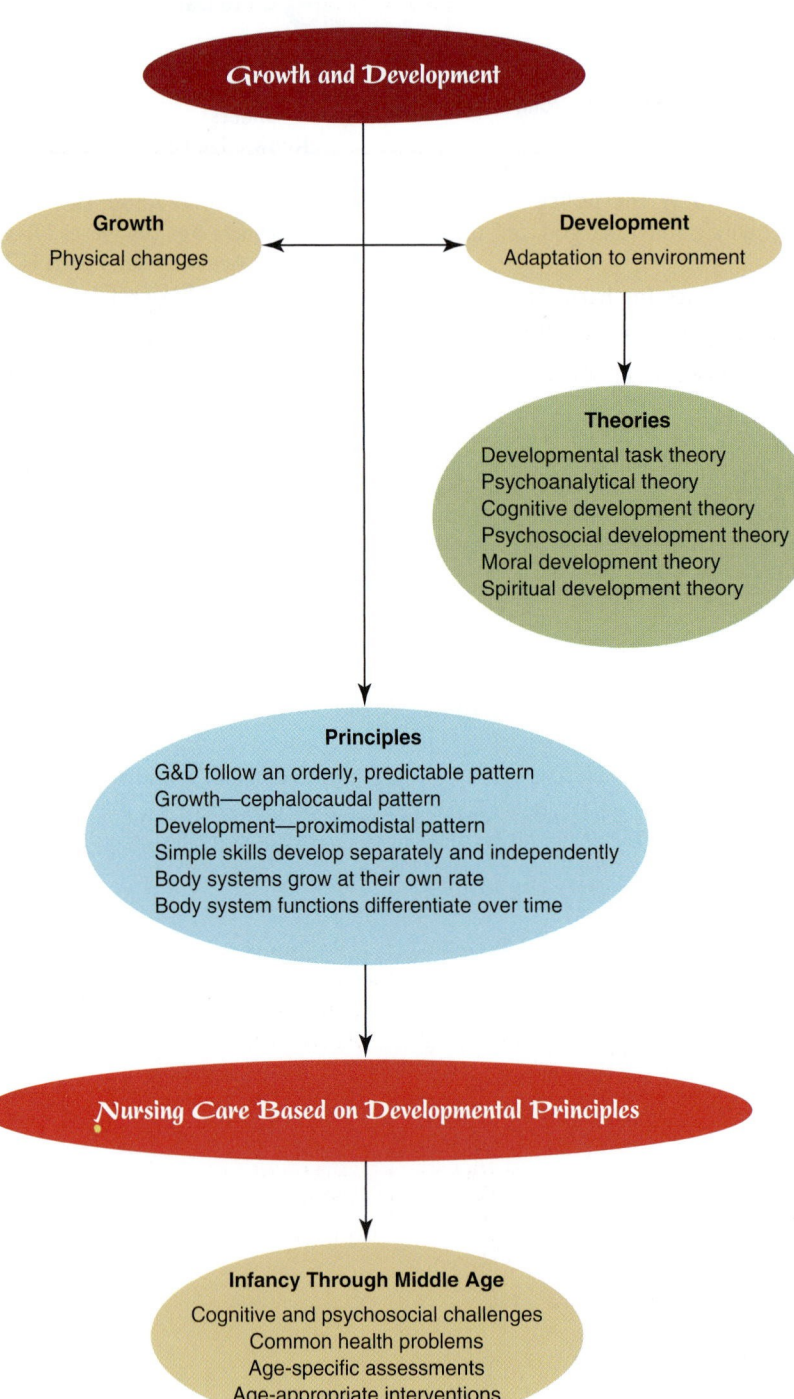

Growth and Development

Growth
Physical changes

Development
Adaptation to environment

Theories
Developmental task theory
Psychoanalytical theory
Cognitive development theory
Psychosocial development theory
Moral development theory
Spiritual development theory

Principles
G&D follow an orderly, predictable pattern
Growth—cephalocaudal pattern
Development—proximodistal pattern
Simple skills develop separately and independently
Body systems grow at their own rate
Body system functions differentiate over time

Nursing Care Based on Developmental Principles

Infancy Through Middle Age
Cognitive and psychosocial challenges
Common health problems
Age-specific assessments
Age-appropriate interventions

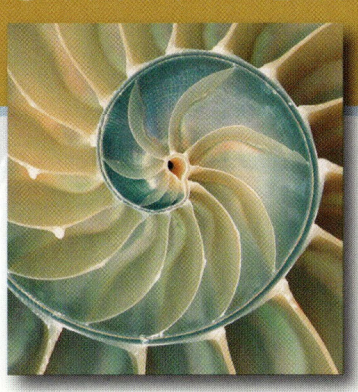

CHAPTER 10

Development: Older Adulthood

Learning Outcomes

After completing this chapter, you should be able to do the following:

➤ Discuss the relationship of life expectancy and livable communities.

➤ Discuss the developmental challenges for each older adult age group.

➤ Identify common health problems seen in each group and for all older adults.

➤ Describe any special assessments unique to each group or older adults.

➤ Discuss age-appropriate interventions for older adults and for each group.

➤ Incorporate developmental principles of aging into nursing care.

Key Concepts

Developmental changes

Functional status

Older adulthood

Related Concepts

See the Concept Map at the end of this chapter.

Example Problems

Dementia

Elder abuse

Frailty

Caring for the Nguyens

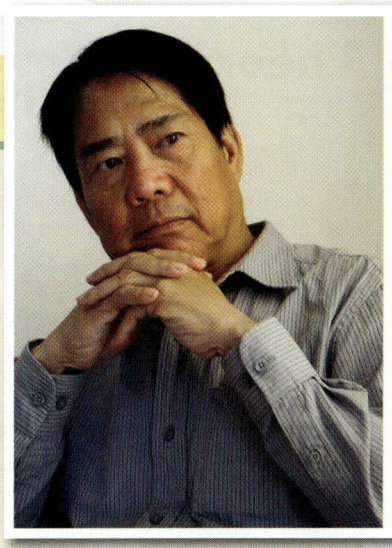

This feature allows you to practice the kind of thinking you will use as a full-spectrum nurse. There is usually more than one correct answer to a critical thinking question, so we do not provide answers for these features. It is more important to develop your nursing judgment than to "cover content." Discuss the questions with your peers. If you are still unsure, consult your instructor.

Nam Nguyen's father, Binh, is 80 years old and has multiple health problems. He has hypertension and heart disease. Although he had surgery for prostate cancer many years ago, the cancer has now metastasized. Because Binh's health was declining rapidly, Nam and Yen moved him and his wife, Mai, into their home last year. Both Nam and his wife work outside the home, so the elderly Mai cares for her husband as best she can during the day. Binh is too weak to get out of bed without help, and his wife is not strong enough to support him. She cooks for him, but he eats only a few bites, then pushes the plate away. Nam telephones today to say, "We can't take care of him safely at home any longer. Can you tell me how to get him admitted to a hospital or a nursing home?"

A. What other ideas do you have for how the Nguyens could care for Binh other than placing him in a hospital or nursing home?

B. Nam's first concern seems to be about getting help for his father. What do you think his next concern will be?

(Continued)

Caring for the Nguyens (continued)

C. What actual data do you have about Binh Nguyen's nutritional status?

D. What else do you need to know to fully assess Binh's nutritional status? If you do not know the answer to this, you might find enough information in the Assessment section of this chapter. If not, refer to Chapter 28.

E. Would you consider Binh Nguyen to be a frail elderly person? Why or why not?

 Go to **Caring for the Nguyens Response Sheet,** on Davis*Plus*.

Meet Your Patient

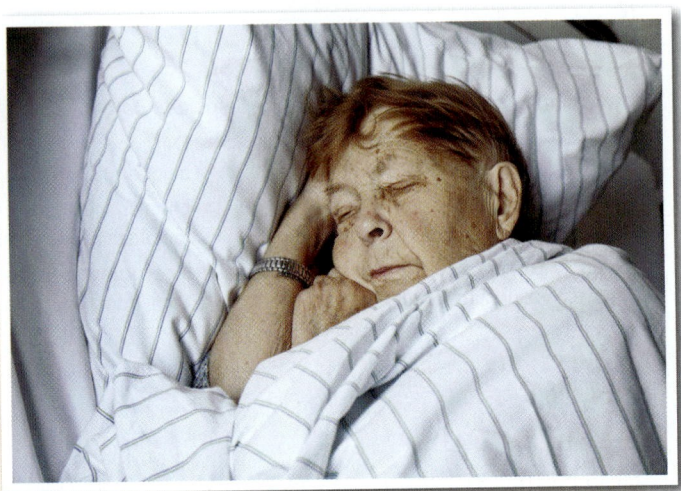

Ethel Higginbotham, an 80-year-old woman, is in the hospital with pneumonia. She lives alone. Her son tells you that she began to lose weight rapidly, complains of no appetite, and became withdrawn after the death of her husband. At a recent visit to her home, he found his mother confused, with a productive cough, and with small open areas on her lower legs. This led to her hospitalization. Even though she is no longer receiving oxygen, you observe that she is very thin and weak, sleeps most of the time, and refuses to eat. "I just want to die," she tells you.

Theoretical Knowledge
knowing how

Why should you learn about older adults? One very important reason is that most of your patients are likely to be older adults. Half of all hospitalized patients are older adults, and because older adults are more likely to have disabilities and chronic health problems, they will likely make up a sizeable number of the patients you see in clinics, home care, and other settings, as well. This chapter presents the most important topics and issues about aging and the development of older adults.

ABOUT THE KEY CONCEPTS

You may have thought of developmental stages as something that applies mostly to children. However, as you learned in Chapter 9, developmental changes occur throughout life, even in older adulthood. You will learn how normal changes, as well as illness, can affect functional status—a major focus in caring for older adults.

PERSPECTIVES ON AGING

Around the world, people in developed countries are living longer and having fewer children. Older adulthood is the fastest growing age group in developed nations. The following statistics illustrate that statement. In 1900, a mere 4.1% of the U.S. population was 65 or over. By 2007, life expectancy had increased, and older adults made up 13% of the population. It is expected that by 2050, one-fifth of the population will be over age 65.

You can understand aging by examining it from different angles. We will discuss the concepts of life expectancy, distribution of age groups, life-span perspective, and percentage of total population. All of these concepts require you to think about numerical descriptions of population characteristics.

Life Expectancy

Life expectancy is one way to view aging. Life expectancy can be calculated in the two following ways: life expectancy at birth, and life expectancy measured at age 65.

- **Life expectancy at birth** has risen dramatically in the United States, as shown by the following two statements:
  In 1900, average life expectancy was 49.2 years.
  In 2005, average life expectancy was 77.8 years.
- **Life expectancy measured at age 65** has risen as the following two statements state:
  In 1900, a 65-year-old person could expect to live 11.9 more years.
  In 2005, a 65-year-old person could expect to live 18.7 more years.

Let's examine what those statements mean. Compare the two statements about the year 2005. They mean that a baby born in 2005 could expect to live for nearly 78 years, whereas a 65-year-old person in 2005 could expect to live another 18.7 years, to almost age 84. Those numbers reflect the average

life expectancy for both sexes and all ethnic/racial groups. However, differences in life expectancy emerge when you examine sex and ethnic group data.

Gender Disparities. For infants born in 2005, the average total life expectancy for females is 80.4 years (*life expectancy at birth*). For males it is only 75 years. This difference is especially noticeable in the 85-plus-year-old population, in which women greatly outnumber men (Kung, Hoyert, Xu, et al., 2008).

Life expectancy measured at age 65 was nearly the same for men and women in 1900; however, women had a lead of about 3 years over men in 2005, narrowing the gap as men age. The longer a man lives, the longer he can expect to live.

Racial Disparities. In 1900, race defined U.S. life expectancy at birth. As of 2005, the picture was less clear. White females continued to have the highest life expectancy at birth but following closely behind were white males and black females. However, the life expectancy of black males at birth in 2005 was a little over 11 years less than white females.

At age 65, white women led life expectancy with 20 years, followed closely by black women at 18.7 and white men at 17.2 years, whereas black men at age 65 had the lowest life expectancy at 15.2. Notice, though, that the gap for ethnicity decreases as a person ages (Kung, Hoyert, Xu, et al., 2008):

- A black baby boy born in 2005 can expect to live to about age 70.
- A black man at age 65 in 2005 can expect to live another 15.2 years, to age 80.

The future population of older adults will be more ethnically and racially diverse, with minority groups (everyone except non-Hispanic, single-race whites) representing 54% of the population in 2050. The non-Hispanic white population—66% of the population in 2008—is projected to decrease and to compose only 46% of the total population in 2050. Latinos are projected to compose 30% of the population and blacks 15% in 2050 (U.S. Census Bureau, 2008).

Migration and Distribution of Age Groups

In addition to life expectancy, in-migration and out-migration within countries and between countries contribute to the distribution of age groups within each country and the median age of a population. For example, between 1995 and 2000, five states had the highest in-migration of newly retired persons: Nevada, Arizona, Florida, North Carolina, and Delaware. By 2020, these five states will begin to face an accelerated growth in the age 85-and-older population. In 2005, the median age (years):

Of the U.S. population	was	36.4
Of the state of Maine	was	41.2
Of the state of Utah	was	28.5

The median age of the population in the United States is increasing:

- In 2005, the median age of the U.S. population was 36.4 years.
- In 2050, the median age of the U.S. population is expected to be 39 years.

KnowledgeCheck 10-1

- About what percentage of people over age 65 live in nursing homes?
- What percentage of people over 85 years old live in nursing homes?
- Who has the longer life expectancy, women or men?

Percentage of Total Population

Yet another way to view aging is by the *percentage of total population* each age group represents. In the United States, older adults composed approximately:

4.1% of the population in 1900
12% of the population in 2005
20% of the population in 2050 (projected by the U.S. Census Bureau, 2008).

Age distribution of a population is often illustrated in a pyramid, with the youngest age group (0–4) at the base and the oldest age group (85+) at the peak, men on the left of the figure and women on the right. The shape of a population pyramid changes to rectangle in developed countries with fewer births and increased life expectancy. To view a population pyramid that illustrates the projected age distribution of the U.S. population in 2025 and 2050, see Figures 10-1 and 10-2, respectively.

Notice also that the percentage for centenarians almost doubles from 2025 to 2050. The Census Bureau reports the following in total number of centenarians (U.S. Census Bureau, 2006, 2008):

79,000 centenarians—actual total number in 2006
600,000 centenarians—projected total number in 2050

ThinkLike a Nurse 10-1

Refer to Figures 10-1 and 10-2.

- In the 85-to-89 age group in the 2025 data, what percentage of the population are men? What percentage are women?
- In the 85-to-89 age group in the 2050 data, what percentage of the population are men? What percentage are women?
- In the 85-to-89 age group, which group increases the most between 2025 and 2050: women or men?

ThinkLike a Nurse 10-2

- What factors do you think account for the overall increase in life expectancy?
- What effect will the distribution of the population by age within your state have on your nursing practice?

Life-Span Perspective

Another way to view aging is from a *life-span perspective*. In this perspective, *genes* inherited at conception, *behaviors* expressed throughout a lifetime, and *environments* within which a person lives, works, and plays interact with each other over time. The cumulative effect of these interactions is seen in older adulthood.

Think of the genetic–behavior–environment interaction as a survival mechanism of aging. Attending to healthy behaviors and avoiding unhealthy behaviors is a lifelong process. Healthy behaviors include, for example, daily exercise and mental stimulation; whereas unhealthy behaviors include tobacco use, poor nutrition, and so on. A lifetime of positive health behaviors interacting with a healthful environment has the potential to shift effects of a harmful genetic trait—that is, a person may have the genetic trait for a particular disease but never show signs of the disease.

Remember the Nun Study discussed in Chapter 8? Some of the nuns demonstrated no symptoms of Alzheimer's disease during their lifetime, yet upon autopsy scientists discovered the typical neurological changes associated with Alzheimer's disease (Snowdon, 2003). The Nun Study results illustrate strong evidence of the power of behaviors

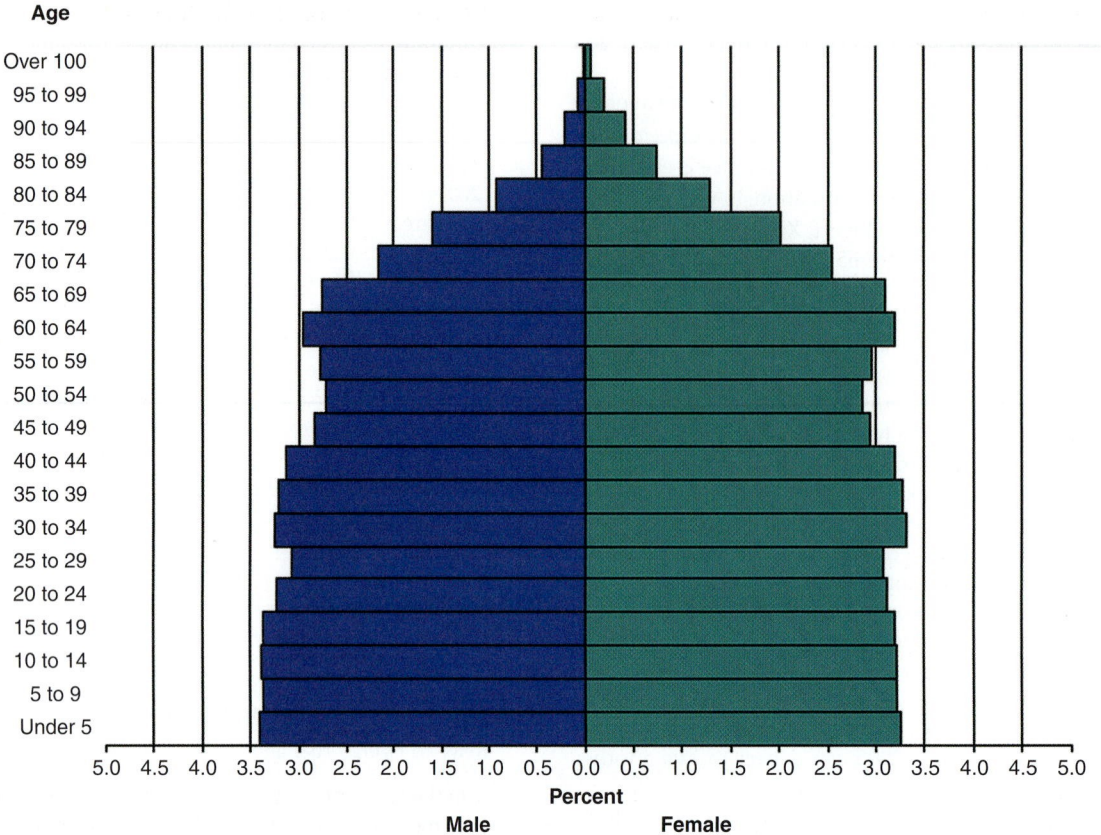

FIGURE 10-1 Projected resident population of the United States as of July 1, 2025, middle series. (Source: U.S. Census Bureau, National population projections III. Population pyramids. Retrieved March 7, 2011, from http://www.census.gov/population/www/projections/natchart.html)

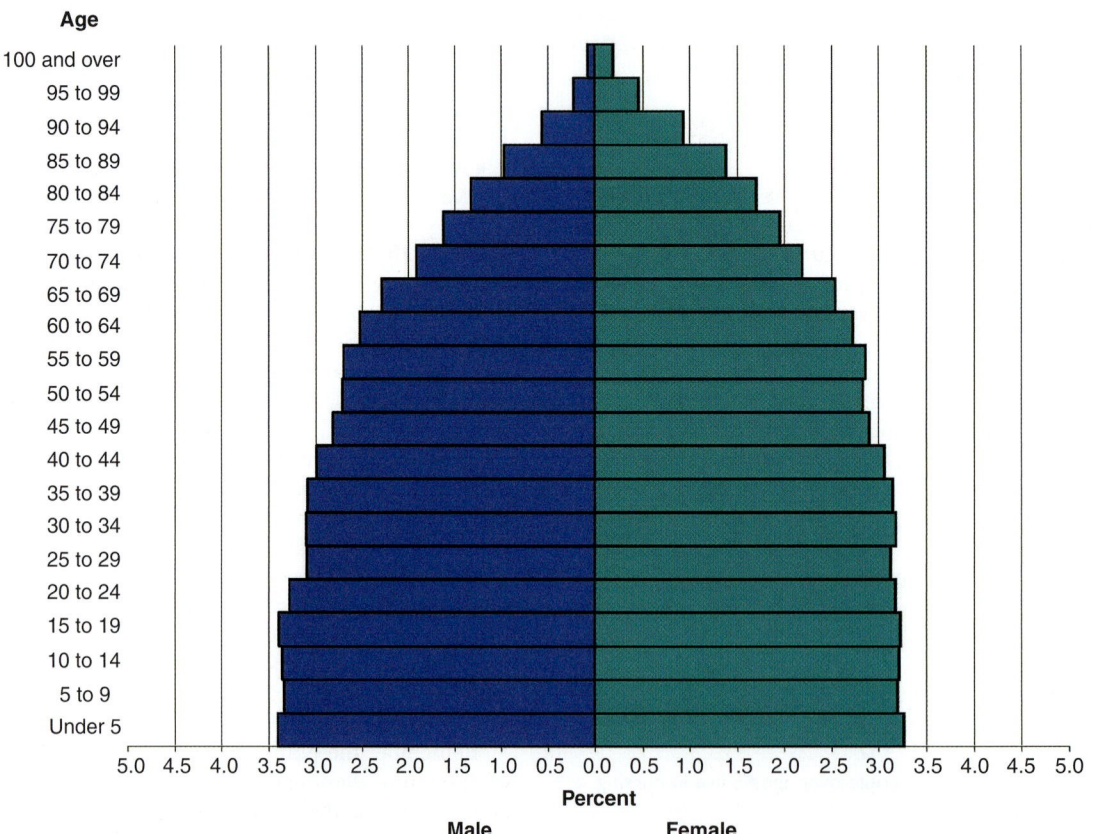

FIGURE 10-2 (NP-P4) Projected resident population of the United States as of July 1, 2050, middle series. (Source: U.S. Census Bureau, National population projections III. Population pyramids. Retrieved March 7, 2011, from http://www.census.gov/population/www/projections/natchart.html)

and the environment over genes resulting in centenarians who are cognitively intact and asymptomatic for Alzheimer's disease.

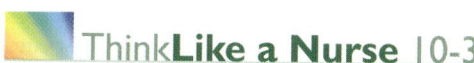

ThinkLike a Nurse 10-3

Plot your birth year on a timeline that extends in 10-year increments through your 65th and 100th year. What is the projected distribution of age and gender when you are an older adult? What genetic, environmental, and behavioral attributes will influence your life expectancy and state of health as an older adult?

AGING IN PLACE AND ALTERNATIVES

Contrary to popular belief, most older adults live independently (Houser, Fox-Grage, & Gibson, 2009). **Aging in place** means that as they age, persons live in their own residences and receive supportive services for their changing needs, rather than moving to another location or type of housing. Aging in place requires an elder-friendly residence and an elder-friendly or livable community that provides maximum accessibility, minimal barriers, and adequate resources and services to maintain independence for as long as possible. The goal of an elder-friendly residence is safe daily interaction with a living environment for persons with normal changes of aging.

Elder-Friendly Residences. Among the considerations for an *elder-friendly residence* are the following:

- Ground-level entry or no-step entry
- One-level living area
- Wide doorways to allow for assistive devices such as walkers and wheelchairs
- Lever-style door and faucet handles for easy grasp
- Grab bars, shower seats, and elevated toilet seat in bathrooms
- Kitchen appliances, cabinets, and surfaces no higher than 48 inches above the floor
- Shelves no more than 10 inches deep, for easy accessibility
- Adequate light in all areas inside and outside the residence
- Walking areas free of clutter, including area rugs.

Elder-Friendly Communities. Livable communities (also referred to as *elder friendly*) "actively involve, value, and support older adults" (Alley, Liebig, Pynoos, et al., 2007, p. 1). To illustrate the need for elder-friendly communities, consider these facts about older adults in 2005 (Houser, Fox-Grage, & Gibson, 2009):

One in three persons age 75+ lived alone

A little over half the persons age 65+ lived at or below 300% of the poverty line (about $30,000 for a single person or $38,000 for a family of two)

Nearly one in five persons age 65+ had a bachelor's degree or higher

12% did not have a vehicle in their household

Many older adults spent at least 30% of their income on housing. This includes:

26% (approximately) of older adults who owned their own homes, and

54% of older adults who were renters

Livable communities offer the following:

- Housing that is affordable and appropriate for all ages
- Supportive services and features
- Dependable and affordable transportation and housing
- Resources that facilitate individual independence and socialization of residents (AARP Public Policy Institute, 2005)

- Affordable and accessible health care
- Safe, low-crime environment
- Community engagement

Naturally Occurring Retirement Communities

When persons "age in place" within a specific apartment building or a community/street of single-family homes, that area is referred to as a *naturally occurring retirement community (NORC)*. Persons within a NORC have aged together. More often than not, they have, over the years, developed access to services needed to maintain the highest quality of life for all within the NORC. When one neighbor needs assistance, others pitch in to help or to obtain help. The U.S. Administration on Aging provides competitive funding to support the development and maintenance of services within a NORC.

Retirement Communities

Some housing developments are planned specifically as retirement communities that provide elder-friendly dwellings and environments for independent living. Typical retirement communities allow older adults to "downsize" into a house that has less than 2,000 square feet in single-level, livable space. Purchase of a home in a retirement community usually includes services such as home maintenance and repair; landscaping; snow, leaf, and trash removal; some home utilities; security; home fire and theft insurance; recreational amenities, such as pool, spa, walking track, and golf and tennis facilities; and planned activities for an annual association fee. They usually have a minimum age restriction of 55, 60, or 62 for either one of the residents in a household or all occupants. However, age restriction may be problematic if grandparents become the primary care providers for a grandchild.

Continuing Care Retirement Communities

Continuing care retirement communities (CCRC), or *life care communities*, offer a wide range of living accommodations from residential living (e.g., cottages, cluster homes, apartments), assisted living, skilled nursing care, rehabilitation, and dementia care on a large campus-like setting. CCRCs also include many amenities, ranging from golf courses, pools, and indoor sport facilities to a full range of hobby and clubrooms and personal services. A CCRC is another example of aging in place, except that an older adult must first move to it. Therefore, in that sense it is not a NORC.

Entrance requirements include physical, mental, and financial health evaluations. Contracts may include lifetime care, time-specified care, or fee-for-service. CCRCs are usually expensive, requiring an entrance fee and monthly fees that may increase with annual cost-of-living estimates. Depending on the contract, monthly fees may cover a set number of meals per month, transportation, housekeeping, unit maintenance, laundry service, health monitoring, some utilities, coordinated social activities, emergency call monitoring, and round-the-clock security.

A health clinic is usually on-site. Healthcare providers may include a registered nurse, nurse practitioner, physician, dentist, and physical therapist. CCRCs vary by their affiliation (e.g., ethnic or religious group, university, corporation) and whether the living space is rented or purchased. University-affiliated CCRCs incorporate all aspects of

academic life into the lives of residents and provide opportunities for cross-generation interactions on the CCRC and university campuses. These interactions are especially important for students interested in careers in gerontology, because they have an opportunity to work or conduct research with CCRC residents in areas that fit their disciplinary focus.

Assisted-Living Facilities

Assisted-living facilities (ALFs) are congregate residential settings that provide or coordinate personal services, 24-hour supervision and assistance (scheduled and unscheduled), activities, and health-related services. ALFs are *not* aging in place environments. State regulations and level of services preclude residents from staying in an ALF when their needs become greater than the resources and services provided. ALFs are designed to:

- minimize the need to move
- accommodate individual residents' changing needs and preferences
- maximize residents' dignity, autonomy, privacy, independence, and safety
- encourage family and community involvement (Assisted Living Quality Coalition, 1998)

There are multiple definitions and goals of ALFs and no common physical size, design, or model. ALFs might be self-standing or housed within a CCRC as one level of housing and service. Each ALF has its own culture, rules, norms, values, and rituals that are created by the residents (Al Omari, Kramer, Hronek, et al., 2005). An ALF may have limitations such as reduced consumer choice, little flexibility, and an illusion of certainty (Zimmerman & Sloane, 2007).

Nursing Care Facilities (Nursing Homes)

Nursing care facilities, or **nursing homes,** provide skilled and unskilled nursing care for older adults and adults with disabilities. To understand the scope of nursing care facilities in the overall picture of aging, consider the following facts. In 2005:

- About 1.5 million residents lived in more than 16,000 U.S. nursing facilities.
- Only 3.3% of persons age 65 and older lived in nursing facilities; however, this rises to 15% for people over 85 years.
- Nearly half of the residents of nursing homes had dementia, and one-fifth had other psychological diagnoses (Houser, Fox-Grage, & Gibson, 2009).
- Women composed nearly 70% of the nursing home population.
- Nearly 75% of residents are age 75 or older; the median age is 83.2 (U.S. Census Bureau, 2007).
- Medicaid is the primary source of payment for most (65%) of the residents; Medicare pays for about 13%, primarily for short stays; and individual long-term care insurance or private sources pay for 22% (Houser, Fox-Grage, & Gibson, 2009).

KnowledgeCheck 10-2

What is the difference between a retirement community and a continuing care retirement community (CCRC)?

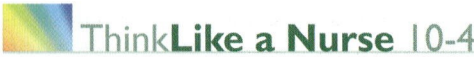

ThinkLike a Nurse 10-4

How elder friendly is the community in which you live?

THEORIES OF AGING

There is no single explanation for how the body ages, but four groups of physiological theories predominate:

Wear-and-Tear Theory. This theory of aging proposes that repeated insults and the accumulation of metabolic wastes eventually cause cells to wear out and cease functioning.

Genetic Theories. Genetic theories of aging propose that cells have a preprogrammed, finite number of cell divisions. Therefore, the time of naturally-occurring death is determined at birth. The genetic messages within the various cells of the body specify how many times the cell can reproduce, thus defining the life of that cell.

Cellular Malfunction. These theories hypothesize that a malfunction in the cell causes changes in cellular DNA, leading to problems with cell replication. The cellular malfunction can be the result of a chemical reaction with the DNA (cross-linking theory), an abundance of free radicals that damage cells and impair their ability to function normally (free-radical theory), or a buildup of toxins over time that cause cell death (toxin theory).

Autoimmune Reaction. This theory hypothesizes that cells change with age. Over time the changes result in the immune system's perceiving some cells as foreign substances and triggering an immune response to destroy the cells.

Despite wide debate of these theories, most scientists consider aging to be a combination of factors, including inherited traits and the cell's response to environmental stressors.

STAGES OF OLDER ADULTHOOD

Older adulthood begins at age 65, according to most references. The stages of older adulthood are typically referred to as the *young-old* (ages 65 to 74), *middle-old* (ages 75 to 84) and *oldest-old* (age 85 and older). The fastest growing segment of older adults is the oldest-old, some of whom are the frail elderly and *centenarians* (people over 100 years old). For more in-depth information about aging and older adults, refer to a life-span development or gerontology resource.

Young-Old: Ages 65 to 74

Physical and psychological adaptations to retirement are paramount in this age group. One key indicator of well-being is use of leisure time. On an average day, young-old persons spend most of their time (55%) watching television; 18% in solitary activities of reading, relaxing, and thinking; 11% socializing and communicating; 4% participating in sports, exercise, and recreation; and the remaining time in other activities, including related travel (Federal Interagency Forum on Aging Related Statistics, 2008).

By the time they reach age 65, many young-old persons are experiencing the effects of chronic illnesses that began in middle adulthood. Also continuing are the effects of lack of time to care for self because of the demands and stressors of work during middle adulthood. Retirement frees up time for the young-old to focus on health-promoting behaviors—to make up for any neglect of their health in earlier years. This can help prevent the decline of health as they age. However, young-old persons face barriers to health, such as the following:

- a lack of supplemental insurance for health screening or physicals that are not covered under Medicare
- perception of self as "getting old"
- changes in physical activity
- being in a deconditioned state by not participating in exercise before retirement. There is some evidence that

the amount of physical activity declines as early as age 63 for some, and by age 70 for most people (Wilson & Palha, 2007).

At retirement, a person's usual social contacts and structure for daily activities may change markedly. A newly retired young-old adult may be searching for new interests outside of the previous work environment. People in this age group may need support for positive retirements, to: identify and overcome barriers to health promotion, evaluate methods for introducing health promotion, making long-term change, and describing short- and long-term benefits of health promotion (Wilson & Palha, 2007).

Middle-Old: Ages 75 to 84

The developmental challenge of middle-old persons is an increasingly solitary, sedentary lifestyle. This age group spends one-fourth of their leisure time in the solitary activities of reading, relaxing, and thinking—more than their younger cohort. They spend only 2% of their time participating in sports, exercise, and recreation—less than their younger cohort (Federal Interagency Forum on Aging Related Statistics, 2008). Without physical activity, the risk of disability associated with chronic conditions increases during the middle-old years.

Adapted physical activity (APA) programs are group exercise programs designed for persons with chronic conditions. APA programs are aimed at correcting sedentary lifestyle and preventing disability secondary to the chronic condition. The focus of APA programs is on functional ability rather than treating existing disability, and they are beneficial throughout the older adult years. Even after critical incidents such as a stroke, APA programs prevent further disability, maximize function, increase quality of life, and curtail the effects of social isolation and depression (Macko, Benvenuti, Stanhope, et al., 2008).

Senior centers are beginning to offer APA programs as they update their programs for the active baby-boomer generation. Some health and fitness facilities may also offer senior health programs and books that illustrate adapted strategies for lifelong walkers and marathon runners. Although physical activity declines in the middle-old group overall, older adults represent the fastest-growing segment of participants in competitive sports, with a rise in the age 80-and-older finishers at road races such as the New York City marathon (Futterman, 2008).

Oldest-Old: Age 85 and Older

The developmental challenges of the oldest-old are sensory impairments, oral health (e.g., edentulism), inadequate nutritional intake, and functional limitations. The following examples are from the Federal Interagency Forum on Aging Related Statistics (2008):

- *Hearing.* Nearly half of older men and more than one-third of older women reported difficulty hearing. This was higher for the 85-plus age group than for the young-old and the middle-old.
- *Vision.* 27% of the 85-plus age group reported trouble seeing.
- *Edentulism.* 32% of those over 85 years old reported **edentulism** (having no natural teeth). This tends to be income related: 39% of older adults below the poverty line reported edentulism, whereas for those above the poverty line, incidence was only 26%.
- *Nutrition.* Edentulism compromises an already inadequate nutritional intake of older adults and fosters a diet of "soft"

foods that may be higher in fats, carbohydrates, and calories. For the oldest-old, this occurs at a time when they need to decrease intake of these foods to combat obesity and counter decreased activity levels.

- *Functional limitations.* Ability to stoop/kneel, reach overhead, walk two or three blocks, and lift 10 pounds are common parameters for determining functional abilities of older adults. Thirty-eight percent of men in the oldest-old group reported they were unable to perform at least one of these activities. More than half of women in that group were unable to perform at least one activity. There were minimal to no differences across ethnic and racial groups.

Centenarians. People age 100 years and older (**centenarians**) are a subgroup of the oldest-old. It appears that surviving to an extreme old age is the result of favorable interactions between genetic composition, environment, and lifestyle (behaviors). The most significant factor may be the presence of a loved one in the life of the older adult. One genetic variation of centenarians has been linked with longevity, but mapping the centenarian genome is essential to determine if they do, in fact, carry a so-called longevity gene (Perls, 2006; Perls, Silver, & Lauerman, 1999). Three prototypes (typical examples) describe centenarians:

Survivors: Persons who had been diagnosed with at least one age-related disease before age 80.

Delayers: Persons in whom no age-related disease had been diagnosed until after age 80

Escapers: Persons without a previous diagnosis of any age-related disease upon reaching their 100th year

Twelve percent of centenarians live independently and 90% are cognitively intact into their 90s. Their commitment to community is also linked to their longevity.

Example Problem: Frail Elderly

As humans age, they are gradually less able to adapt to challenges from internal (disease) and external (injury) environments. *Frailty* was at first used to mean the oldest-old, believing they were the least able to adapt and survive. However, as the oldest-old population increased in number and more is known about their survival, **frailty** has been distinguished in the following ways:

- A set of characteristics, that describes a heightened state of vulnerability for developing adverse health outcomes.
- A multisystem reduction in the person's physiological capacity.
- The point at which the human organism is believed to have its least capacity for survival, and will fail in response to a minor internal or external insult. For example, a frail older adult might die merely as a result of an upper respiratory infection (such as a cold).

KnowledgeCheck 10-3

- Name and give the age ranges for the four stages of older adulthood.
- Name and briefly describe four theories of aging.

DEVELOPMENTAL CHANGES OF OLDER ADULTS

Although not all people age at the same rate, there are predictable patterns of physical, cognitive, and psychosocial change. Older adults also have several, often chronic, health problems in common.

Physical Development of Older Adults

Although aging varies among individuals, patterns of change can be predicted in each body system. Table 10-1 presents an overview of changes seen with aging.

Cognitive Development of Older Adults

Reaction time slows in older adults, and short-term memory declines; it takes longer to respond to a stimulus, and it takes more time to process incoming information. Thus, older adults learn new material more slowly. However, there is no loss of intelligence as a person ages. Loss of short-term memory is more common than loss of long-term memory; thus, older

adults may remember incidents from many years ago but may have trouble recalling what they did earlier in the day.

Physical health problems (e.g., Alzheimer's disease) or medications, not simply aging alone, may affect memory. Other factors that slow memory loss are adequate sleep and rest, a nourishing diet, avoidance of drugs and alcohol, and adequate social stimulation. Research indicates that an active social life with complete engagement and participation in the community delays memory loss with aging (Ertel, Glymour, & Berkman, 2008). Regular mental exercises (e.g., crossword puzzles, conversation) appear to stimulate the brain and enhance memory.

Table 10-1 ➤ Age-Related Changes and Areas for Assessment		
	NORMAL AGING CHANGE	**AREAS FOR ASSESSMENT**
Musculoskeletal	Decreased: muscle strength, body mass, bone mass, joint mobility Increased fat deposit	▪ Activity/exercise tolerance ▪ Joint pain, range of motion ▪ Gait, balance, posture, change in height ▪ Susceptibility to falls ▪ Ability to perform ADLs
Cardiovascular	Decreased cardiac output Increased peripheral resistance, systolic blood pressure	▪ Activity tolerance ▪ Blood pressure ▪ Orthostatic hypotension ▪ Susceptibility to arrhythmia
Respiratory	Decreased elasticity of chest wall, intercostals muscle strength, cough reflex Increased anteroposterior diameter of chest, rigidity of lung tissue	▪ Cough reflex ▪ Use of accessory muscles ▪ Gas exchange ▪ Mouth breathing
Gastrointestinal	Decreased saliva production, GI motility, gastric acid production	▪ Ability to chew ▪ Dentition ▪ Pattern of elimination ▪ Frequency/size of meals
Integument	Decreased skin elasticity, nail growth Increased dryness of skin, thinning of skin layers, nail thickening, hair thinning	▪ Susceptibility to hypo/hyperthermia ▪ Intact skin, bruising ▪ Dry skin ▪ Bathing pattern
Genitourinary	Decreased glomerular filtration rate, blood flow to kidneys, bladder capacity, vaginal lubrication, hardness of erection	▪ Continence ▪ Urgency, frequency, nocturia ▪ Hydration status ▪ Drug levels ▪ Sexual pattern
Nervous	Decreased nerve cells, neurotransmitters, REM sleep, blood flow to CNS	▪ Diminished reflexes ▪ Sleep pattern ▪ Depression

Table 10-1 ➤ Age-Related Changes and Areas for Assessment—cont'd

	NORMAL AGING CHANGE	AREAS FOR ASSESSMENT
Endocrine	Decreased insulin release, thyroid function, estrogen and testosterone	■ Change in weight ■ Libido ■ Energy level
Sensory	Decreased visual acuity (presbyopia, or impaired near vision) and depth perception, tear production, pupil size, accommodation, acuity of smell and taste, hearing of high-frequency sound, sense of balance, changes in pain sensation Increased glare sensitivity, thickening of lens of the eye, changes in pain sensation	■ Adequate lighting ■ Cerumen buildup ■ Home safety ■ Pain sensation ■ Driving ability ■ Environmental stimulation
Cognition	Decreased short-term memory Increased reaction time, information processing time	■ Memory changes ■ Learning barriers ■ Adaptive coping
Personality	Increased cautiousness Retirement, widowhood, grandparenthood	■ Sources of social support ■ Social network

ADLs = activities of daily living; CNS = central nervous system; GI = gastrointestinal; REM = rapid eye movement.

Psychosocial Development of Older Adults

Psychosocial theories of aging attempt to explain the psychological and social adjustment associated with aging.

Disengagement Theory. Cumming and Henry (1961) hypothesized that the older adult and society gradually and mutually withdraw or disengage from each other. Mandatory retirement, chronic illness, the deaths of relatives and friends, poverty, and other factors may contribute to this phenomenon. As a result, interaction between an individual and his world decreases. This decrease allows the individual time for reflection and freedom from societal roles. Power transfers to younger members of society as the older adult withdraws. However, disengagement is not the norm for the current generation of older adults in America, nor is it universally true for cultures that value older adults' advice as essential for family decision making.

Activity Theory. Havighurst's (1963) theory is the counterpart of disengagement theory. Activity theory posits that the individual should stay as active and engaged as possible to enjoy the highest life satisfaction. On retirement, another activity, such as travel, sports, hobbies, or volunteering, replaces time spent at work. The more engaged the older adult is, the greater his life satisfaction will be (Fig. 10-3).

Psychosocial Development Theory. Erikson's (1963) developmental theory identifies *ego integrity versus despair* as the task of the older adult. This stage of development has as its cornerstone the acceptance that one's life has had meaning and that death is a part of the continuum of life. This outlook allows a person to accept the inevitable changes in health and life circumstances. The basic virtue gained at this stage is wisdom. If you would like to see a list of developmental tasks for older adults, refer to Table 9-1, in Chapter 9.

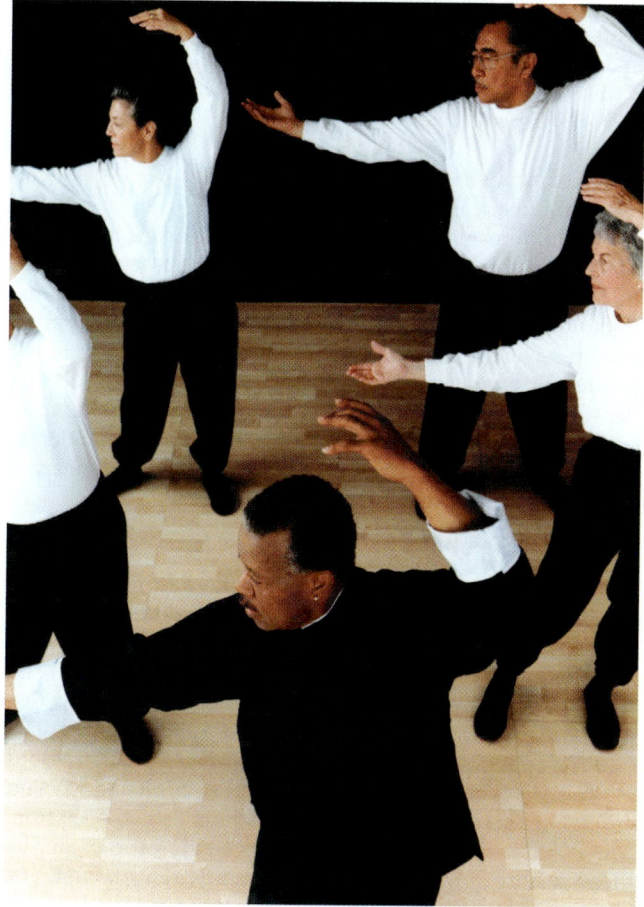

FIGURE 10-3 Many older adults are able to remain active and engaged well into their later years.

Psychosocial changes in this age group are prominent. The older adult must face multiple losses, including the death of a spouse or partner, family members, and friends, as well as challenges to health, independence, and youthful vitality. Loss of independence and the ability to live at home without assistance often have a negative psychological affect on the older adult. Loss is discussed in detail in Chapter 17.

Common Health Problems of Older Adults

The ten leading causes of death for older Americans are as follows (Kung, Hoyert, Xu, et al., 2008):

1. Heart disease
2. Cancer
3. Stroke
4. Chronic lower respiratory diseases
5. Alzheimer's disease
6. Influenza and pneumonia
7. Diabetes mellitus
8. Accidents
9. Kidney disease
10. Septicemia

Six of the seven leading causes of death among older adults are chronic diseases. Heart disease, cancer, stroke, and diabetes are not only among the most common but are also the most costly health conditions. These are long-term illnesses that are rarely cured, but many can be prevented or modified with healthy behavioral interventions. Prevalence of chronic conditions differs by race and ethnicity. For example, consider the different prevalence in diabetes in older adults in 2005–2006 (American Diabetes Association, 2011; Federal Interagency Forum on Aging Related Statistics, 2008):

Non-Hispanic blacks	29%
Hispanics	25%
Non-Hispanic whites	16%
Asian Americans	8.4%

In addition, an estimated 10 million Americans have *osteoporosis*, a loss in bone mineral density that increases the risk of fracture. In advanced cases, bones become so porous that they fracture spontaneously, merely from the stress of bearing a person's weight. The risk increases with age and is much greater for women, in part because of their decreased bone density compared to men, hormonal changes at menopause, and inadequate calcium intake. Cigarette smoking, moderate to heavy alcohol consumption, and lack of weight-bearing exercise also increase risk.

Example Problem: Dementia

Dementia is an irreversible, progressive decline in mental abilities that affects about one in five of adults older than age 70. It is not a normal result of aging. Alzheimer's disease is the primary form and is considered progressive. Increasing age is the greatest known risk factor for Alzheimer's disease. Most persons with the disease are older adults. The odds of developing Alzheimer's disease doubles about every 5 years after age 65. About half the adults age 85 and older have Alzheimer's disease (Alzheimer's Association, 2008). Other dementias may be treatable—for example, those resulting from medication toxicity, sensory deficits, and some physiological problems. It is important to differentiate dementia from acute confusion or delirium that may be precipitated by dehydration, infection, or a medication side effect or overdose. If you need more information about differentiating dementia, delirium, and depression, see Chapter 13.

Polypharmacy

Polypharmacy, the use of multiple medications, is a risk factor for acute confusion, delirium, and depression in older adults (see Chapter 25). The mapping and continued growth in knowledge about the human genome has accelerated the field of **pharmacogenomics** (the discipline that blends pharmacology with genomic capabilities); therefore, the future of drug therapy for older adults will take into consideration DNA variants and individual responses to medical treatments to identify particular subgroups of older adults and develop drugs customized for those subgroups. This technology is expected to increase the efficiency of the drug industry and result in cheaper, more effective drug therapies for older adults.

Depression

Depressive symptoms often accompany physical illness, functional disability, and greater use of healthcare resources. Older women are more likely to report depressive symptoms that are clinically relevant than are older men. In 2004, 17% of older women reported depressive symptoms compared to 11% of older men, numbers that have remained fairly stable for nearly a decade and may be related to appropriate antidepressant drug treatment for older adults (Federal Interagency Forum on Aging Related Statistics, 2008).

Example Problem: Elder Abuse

Elder abuse takes many forms, including the following:
- Battering
- Inappropriate use of drugs and physical restraints
- Force-feeding, physical punishment
- Nonconsensual sexual contact
- Treating an older person like an young child, including infantilizing communication (also referred to as *elderspeak*)
- Giving an older person the "silent treatment"
- Enforced social isolation
- Demeaning an older adult
- Neglect
- Abandonment
- Financial or material exploitation, such as illegal or improper use of an older adult's funds, property, assets, or Social Security checks
- Risk of abuse is higher for women and those with physical and cognitive vulnerabilities (Laumann, Leitsch, & Waite, 2008; Williams, Herman, Gajewski, et al., 2008).

Like domestic violence, elder abuse is seen in all cultures and socioeconomic groups. Risk factors for elder abuse include the following:
- Advanced age
- Physical, functional, or cognitive impairment
- Mental illness, alcoholism, or drug abuse (in elder or caregiver)
- Social isolation or poor social network
- Dependence on others
- Past history of abusive relationships
- Low-income status
- Financial or other family problems (of elder or caregiver)
- Inadequate or unsafe housing

- Depression
- Low self-esteem
- Poor health (of patient or caregiver)
- Caregiver is stressed/frustrated with difficult caregiving tasks

 Suspicion of elder abuse must be reported to adult protection services and/or the authority designated by law in each state to investigate and prosecute elder abuse.

Elder abuse resources include

 The National Center on Elder Abuse (NCEA) (http://www. ncea.aoa.gov) and the Clearinghouse on Abuse and Neglect of the Elderly (CANE) (http://www.cane.udel.edu)

To assess for elder abuse, see the Assessment section and Procedure 9-1.

Ageism

Ageism is age-based discrimination. Negative expectations for older adults can cloud nursing assessments, planning, and interventions. Box 10-1 presents a quiz to test your knowledge of aging. Take the quiz so that you can be prepared to best assist your older adult clients. For answers,

Go to Chapter 10, **Supplemental Materials: Answers to "What's Your Aging IQ?"** on Davis*Plus*.

KnowledgeCheck 10-4

- Name two age-related changes seen in older adults.
- According to Erikson, what is the developmental stage of the older adult?
- What are the top two causes of death among older adults?

PracticalKnowledge
knowing **how**

You would expect differences in functioning in older adults who are relatively healthy and those who have one or more illnesses. You will, of course, base nursing care on individual needs, not on a person's age category. However, in general, you would expect a patient's needs to be different at age 65 than at age 85. Remember, though, that an *individual's* health status and needs are affected by many more variables than just his or her age (e.g., chronic illness, stressors).

This section presents information to use in caring for all older adults: the young-old, the middle-old, the oldest-old, and the frail elderly. In addition to these more general activities, you will find some more specific assessments and interventions under the headings for each of those age groups.

■ ASSESSMENT

Assessment for All Older Adults

Recommend to older adults that they have an annual physical examination. The exam should include the same categories as in middle adulthood, as well as screening for mood, cognition, and ability to perform activities of daily living (ADLs) (e.g., bathing and dressing), and instrumental activities of daily living (IADLs) (e.g., shopping, doing laundry). Table 10-1

BOX 10-1 ■ What's Your Aging IQ?

The following quiz is adapted from one created by the National Institute on Aging to test your knowledge of aging.

1. Which of the following age groups is one of the fastest growing segments of the American population?
   a. Babies and children under age 5
   b. Children age 15 to 19
   c. People over age 85
2. You can be too old to exercise. True/False
3. Diet and exercise reduce the risk for osteoporosis. True/False
4. Heart disease is a much bigger problem for older men than for older women. True/False
5. Screening older people for cancer is not beneficial because they can't be treated. True/False
6. Everybody gets cataracts. True/False
7. People who are older than 80 years should stop driving a car. True/False
8. Most older people are depressed. True/False
9. The older you get, the less you sleep. True/False
10. Everyone becomes confused or forgetful if they live long enough. True/False
11. If your parents had Alzheimer's disease, you will inevitably get it. True/False
12. Older people take more medications than younger people. True/False
13. People should control their weight as they age. True/False
14. People begin to lose interest in sex around age 55. True/False
15. Older adults are not at risk for HIV/AIDS. True/False
16. Families do not take responsibility for care of their older relatives. True/False
17. As your body changes with age, so does your personality. True/False
18. Older people can accept urinary accidents as a fact of life. True/False
19. Falls and injuries "just happen" to older people. True/False
20. "You can't teach an old dog new tricks." True/False
21. Extremes in environmental heat and cold can be especially dangerous for older people. True/False
22. Suicide is most often a risk among teens. True/False

Source: Adapted from U.S. Department of Health and Human Services, Public Health Service, National Institutes of Health. (2003). *What's your aging IQ?* (Reprinted 2006). Retrieved March 26, 2011, from http://www.niapublications.org/tipsheets/pdf/Whats_Your_Aging_IQ.pdf

identifies the areas for physical assessment related to the aging process.

- *Vital signs.* When assessing vital signs, keep in mind that the normal ranges for vital signs are slightly different for older adults (see Chapter 19). The average body temperature, for example, is lower.
- *Height measurement,* with comparison to previous height (a screen for osteoporosis). This begins to be especially important past age 65.
- *Weight and body mass index (BMI) calculation.*
- *Lipid panel screening:* total cholesterol, triglycerides, high-density lipoprotein (HDL), low-density lipoprotein (LDL), and ratios.

- *Blood glucose screening.*
- *Annual clinical breast and pelvic examination* for women aged 40 years and older (American Cancer Society, n.d., last reviewed 2011; American College of Obstetricians and Gynecologists [ACOG], 2011).
- *Breast self-examination (BSE).* There is still controversy about whether to encourage BSE. There is insufficient research evidence to support BSE (National Cancer Institute, 2008; *Guide to Clinical Preventive, 2010–2011,* 2010), but many clinicians believe it to be useful until at least age 85 (American College of Obstetricians and Gynecologists [ACOG], 2011; Flaherty, Morley, Murphy, et al., 2002; Smith, Cokkinides, & Eyre, 2003).
- *Annual or biannual mammogram or thermography* for women over age 65. A woman should have mammograms as long as she is in good health and would be a candidate for treatment. Age alone is not a reason to stop having mammograms (American Cancer Society, 2010 The U.S. Preventive Services Task Force (USPSTF) (2002) does not recommend biannual mammograms after age 74. However, other guidelines recommend them even beyond age 80 or 85 if the woman is in good health (American College of Obstetricians and Gynecologists, 2003, reaffirmed 2006; Flaherty, Morley, Murphy, et al., 2002; Smith, Cokkinides, & Eyre, 2003). Women should be educated on the benefits of mammography and the potential for false-positive results that may be followed by recommendations for further imaging or biopsies that are not actually needed.
- *Pap test.* Some guidelines do not recommend a routine Pap test for women past age 65 (USPSTF, 2003), but the American Cancer Society recommends that they be continued until age 70.
- *Digital rectal exam for colon cancer screening.* The USPSTF recommends against routine screening for those over 75 years of age (USPSTF, 2009a).
- *Digital rectal exam* for colon cancer prostate evaluation in men. An enlarged prostate can indicate either benign prostatic hypertrophy or prostate cancer. The USPSTF (2003) recommends against screening for prostate cancer in men after age 75.
- *Serum prostatic specific antigen (PSA) level* (for men) is a more sensitive indicator of prostate disorders than is the digital rectal exam. Recommendations vary. Some encourage yearly screening for men over age 50; some caution against routine screening, while others make decisions on an individual basis. The USPSTF recommends that men age 75 and older not be screened for prostate cancer ("Task Force Says," 2008; USPSTF, 2003). They concluded that there is a greater chance of harm than health benefits for men age 75 and older. However, at this writing, Medicare does provide coverage for an annual PSA test for all men age 50 and older. Although there is no specific level of normal or abnormal PSA level, many providers are using the following ranges:

  0 to 2.5 nanograms per mL—low

  2.5 to 10 ng/mL—slightly to moderately elevated

  10 to 19.l9 ng/mL—moderately elevated

  20 n/mL or more—significantly elevated (National Cancer Institute, 2007)
- *Eye exam every 2 years* if there are no problems; otherwise annually, particularly if the older adult has chronic conditions such as hypertension, cardiovascular disease, or diabetes. Macular degeneration is a visual problem that may occur in older adults that an eye exam can pick up.

- *Sigmoidoscopy or colonoscopy for colon cancer screening every 10 years* if there are no problems or gastrointestinal problems. Screening CT *colonographies,* or "virtual colonoscopies," are particularly safe for older adults as a noninvasive test that does not require sedation or anesthesia. The American Cancer Society considers CT colonography, as a first-line colon-cancer screening test, to be as effective as the traditional colonoscopy. However, the USPSTF (2009a) recommends against routine colorectal cancer screening for those age 76 years and older.
- *Stool for occult blood,* an annual check for blood in the stool to screen for colon cancer. However the USPSTF (2009a) recommends against routine colorectal cancer screening after age 76.
- *Bone-density scan* for all postmenopausal women, at least by age 60, to determine bone loss. The test is also recommended for older men.

 Think**Like a Nurse** 10-5

To determine whether Mrs. Higginbotham's pneumonia is resolving (Meet Your Patient), you are monitoring her vital signs. Her oral temperature is 98.9°F (37.2°C). What do you need to keep in mind when evaluating the meaning of this reading? Do you think this represents a fever?

Assessing Functional Status

Functional status is the ability to perform self-care and other ADLs and IADLs.

- **Activities of Daily Living.** You can use the Katz Index of Independence in Activities of Daily Living to assess for ADLs. It allows you to rate a client's independence in bathing, dressing, toileting, transferring, continence, and feeding (Katz, Down, Cash, et al., 1970; "Katz Index of Independence," 2007). To use the Katz assessment tool,

 Go to http://consultgerirn.org/uploads/File/trythis/try_this_2.pdf

- **Instrumental Activities of Daily Living. IADLs** are the activities needed to maintain one's immediate environment, for example, shopping, using the telephone, housekeeping, managing money, preparing food, and managing one's medications. Loss of ability to perform IADLs frequently marks a need for assisted living, nursing home placement, or the aid of family or homemaker services to allow an older adult to age in place. For a tool to help you assess IADLs,

 Go to Chapter 3, **Tables, Boxes, Figures: ESG Box 3-1, Patient Assessment Tool, Lawton Instrumental Activities of Daily Living,** on Davis*Plus.*

Assessing for Depression

For more information about depression in older adults, see Chapter 13, Example Problem: Depression, as well as the entire section, Assessment: Depression. To assess for depression, you may wish to use the Geriatric Depression Scale (GDS), a 30-item questionnaire that screens for depression. It is tailored to the concerns that older adults face. To see the Geriatric Depression Scale,

Go to **Resources for Caregivers & Health Professionals,** on Davis*Plus,* and click the links under **Web Sites for Mental Status Exams.**

Assessing Cognitive Status (Example Problem: Dementia)

The Mini Mental State Exam (MMSE) (Folstein, Folstein, & McHugh, 1975) and other similar tools are used to obtain a baseline of cognitive function and to evaluate any interventions. The MMSE assesses various aspects of cognition, including short-term memory. Typically, a score of 25 or under (out of a possible 30) indicates some degree of cognitive impairment. Further work-up would then be required to determine the stability and cause of the impairment.

The "Sweet 16" is a newer cognitive-assessment screening tool consisting of 16 items that test orientation, registration, sustained attention, and short-term memory. It is easy to use and correlates highly with the MMSE. It is useful for identifying problems in thinking, learning, and memory in older adults who might need further evaluation by a specialist (Fong, Jones, Rudolph, et al., 2010).

For a step-by-step procedure for assessing mental status, see Procedure 21-16, Assessing the Sensory-Neurological System. To see the MMSE and the Mini-Cog (a mental status assessment for older adults),

 Go to **Resources for Caregivers & Health Professionals,** on DavisPlus, and click the links under **Web Sites for Mental Status Exams.**

Assessing for Example Problem: Abuse

It is important to assess older adults for abuse any time there is a possibility that an injury may have been inflicted rather than accidental. For a screening tool and a procedure to aid you in assessing for abuse, see Procedure 9-1.

Assessment (Young-Old)

Your assessments of young-old patients should include the following:
- Assess daily routines, social interactions, and short- and long-term goals. This will help determine the degree to which the person has adapted to retirement.
- Determine the level of fitness and the level of effort for physical activity. This and the following point are essential before beginning a program of routine exercise.
- Gain an understanding about how a chronic condition affects the client's ability to do regular physical activities safely.
- Assess the client's barriers to exercise.
- Assess the client's self-confidence in her ability to maintain an exercise program.

Assessment (Middle-Old)

It is critical that you assess the function, support system, social network, and mental health of the middle-old client. Observe for cues to triggers that the client is entering a *spiral of vulnerability*. For example, a decrease in an older adult's mobility and the use of an assistive device such as a cane may indicate prolonged inactivity associated with physiological changes. These may be associated with an unsteady or slow gait and slower response and reaction times—all resulting in deliberate, slow actions. Thus begins a spiral of vulnerability: The older adult may become a victim of abuse, fall, and sustain an injury; the injury may require hospitalization, giving rise to the potential complications of infection and pressure ulcers and the need for rehabilitation. The impact of this spiral of vulnerability is felt in psychological and financial costs to the client and society, as well as loss of client independence. It is easier to intervene and stop the spiral if cues are found early (Fig. 10-4).

Some research indicates that regular mammography or thermography among women over age 80 is associated with diagnosing cancer at an earlier disease stage, and with fewer positive lymph nodes at surgery. However, only about one in five women of this age actually have regular mammograms (Badgwell, Giordano, Duan, et al., 2008).

Assessment (Oldest-Old)

Assessments of physical, psychosocial, and cognitive abilities as well as social engagement and living conditions are crucial for the oldest-old. Psychosocial and environmental factors may be the cues for frailty when subtle physiological changes are not obvious.

Assessment (Frail Elderly)

Assess older adults for risk factors and characteristics associated with frailty. Frail older adults are weak, have little ability for independent living, and often need assistance with ADLs. They may have impaired mental abilities. Most are women, are more than 80 years old, and receive care from an adult child. To be considered frail, a person must have three or more of the following characteristics:
- Low level of physical activity
- Muscle weakness
- Slowed performance
- Fatigue or poor endurance

Recall an earlier discussion of genetic–behavior–environment interaction as a survival mechanism of aging. Psychosocial and behavioral factors, including depression, caregiver problems, and housing conditions, are important to a person's interactions with environment and are believed to predict vulnerability (frailty) and ability to survive (Martin & Brighton,

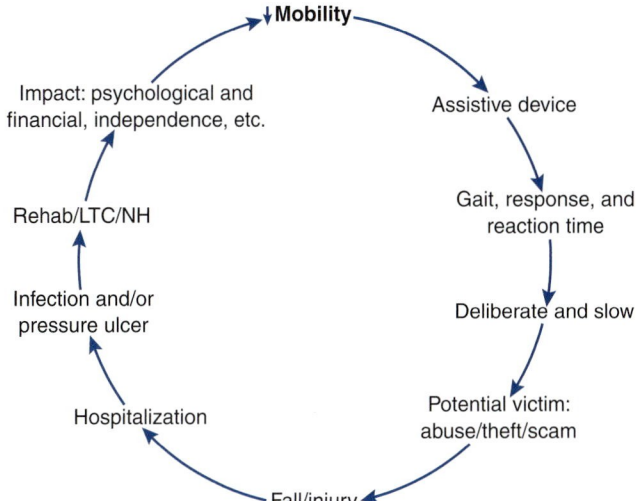

Assessment of the Middle-Old

Spiral of Vulnerability Example

↓Mobility
Assistive device
Gait, response, and reaction time
Deliberate and slow
Potential victim: abuse/theft/scam
Fall/injury
Hospitalization
Infection and/or pressure ulcer
Rehab/LTC/NH
Impact: psychological and financial, independence, etc.

FIGURE 10-4 A seemingly small event for a middle-old adult may trigger a spiral of vulnerability. (Courtesy of V. Rempusheski, PhD.)

2008; Rockwood, 2005; Woodhouse & O'Mahony, 1997). Other risk factors include smoking and being underweight.

ANALYSIS/DIAGNOSIS (ALL OLDER ADULTS)

Although most NANDA-I diagnoses can be used for any age group, the following diagnoses focus specifically on growth and development:

  Adult Failure to Thrive
  Delayed Growth and Development
  Risk for Delayed Development
  Risk for Disproportionate Growth

An understanding of age-related changes can help older adults identify normal changes, adapt their routine, and report alterations in ADLs and IADLs that are outside the expected changes for their age. Many such changes signal conditions that are treatable. Consider these examples:

- Frequent falls and loss of balance are not the result of normal age-related changes but could signal a neuropathology such as Parkinson's disease or early symptoms of dementia and should be reported to a healthcare provider.
- Urinary incontinence is not the result of usual age-related changes. It may signal a urinary tract infection, a prostate problem, excessive urogenital drying, or the need for in-home assistance.

OUTCOMES/EVALUATION (ALL OLDER ADULTS)

Nursing goals for all older adults should be to maintain the person's ability to function independently for as long as possible, arrange for appropriate care, and teach clients and caregivers how and when to call for professional help.

INTERVENTIONS/IMPLEMENTATION

As for all age groups, interventions depend on the nursing diagnoses that you identify for each individual.

Interventions for All Older Adults

Focus on preserving the patient's functional abilities, including both the ability and motivation to function in his environment. Look for simple things you can do to promote better functioning. For example, if the patient cannot see to sort his medications, you might try turning on more lights, or even having a brighter light installed. For all interventions and interactions, always ask yourself, "Does this promote the client's dignity and self-esteem?"

Teach older adults about age-related changes and what these changes mean for their daily routine. For example, age changes affect the speed of processing information, stamina, conditioning, and reflexes. Therefore, when multitasking and performing seemingly non-thinking physical activities, older adults need to be very purposeful in their actions and pay attention to the details of what they are doing (e.g., when multitasking or performing physical activities). Inattention could result in missteps, injury, or exhaustion.

Although the risks of disease and disability increase with age, poor health need not necessarily always occur with aging. Many illnesses and disabilities associated with chronic diseases can be avoided through known prevention measures. Stress to patients the importance of a healthy lifestyle (e.g., healthy eating; regular physical activity; avoiding tobacco use; screening for breast, cervical, and colorectal cancers). Older adults who engage in progressive aerobic training can maintain their independence longer and delay the aging process, perhaps by as much as 10 years (Shephard, 2008).

Health-promotion activities for all older adults include teaching and facilitating immunizations for varicella, influenza, pneumonia, herpes zoster (shingles), and tetanus/diphtheria/pertussis (see Fig.10-5).

Many older adults are Internet savvy. You can empower them by suggesting Web sites offering resources to help them understand and cope with the unknowns of their situation. Some good resources include the following:

  http://www.nihseniorhealth.gov Developed by the National Institute on Aging and the National Library of Medicine, this site provides up-to-date information on a variety of topics such as arthritis, depression, and exercise. It includes videos and quizzes. New topics are added regularly.
  http://www.alz.org/we_can_help_senior_housing_finder.asp The Alzheimer's association designed this site to help families find care for family members with Alzheimer's disease. It is free.
  http://www.lotsahelpinghands.com This is an online service to help family caregivers to organize and communicate with other family members and significant others to coordinate visits and help with meals, transportation, and so on.

Communicating With Older Adults

Many normal changes of aging affect communication with older adults. For example, they tend to process information more slowly, so speak slowly and allow time for the patient to form an answer. Check for sensory deficits at the beginning of your interaction. Until you know there is no hearing deficit, look at the patient as you speak to allow for lipreading. But do not assume that all older adults are deaf or that they do not understand the meaning of your communication. Remember, you need to speak slowly, not loudly.

You will need to rely on body language more than usual. Notice nonverbal communication, such as fidgeting, hand wringing, tearfulness, or quivering lips. Because of memory deficits, some older adults have difficulty finding the words to express what they mean.

Appropriate speech may be accompanied by inappropriate affect. For instance a client may speak coherently and make sense while telling you that she was able to walk to the bathroom today, and then begin crying for no apparent reason. Nevertheless, the information about her ambulation may be credible. Conversely, inappropriate affect and incoherent speech do not always indicate lack of understanding. For example, a client may laugh appropriately at something funny, and not be able to speak clearly or find the words to ask you what time it is.

Be aware that some older adults are confused at one time and not another. A client may begin by giving you credible information, but as the conversation progresses, he may lose track of the topic or talk about something irrelevant. When a client seems confused, use focused assessment to determine his mental status. If you conclude that his communication is unreliable, you can always finish the talk later, when he is less confused.

Recommended Adult Immunization Schedule
UNITED STATES · 2011
Note: These recommendations *must* be read with the footnotes that follow
containing number of doses, intervals between doses, and other important information.

Recommended adult immunization schedule, by vaccine and age group

VACCINE ▼ / AGE GROUP ▶	19–26 years	27–49 years	50–59 years	60–64 years	≥65 years
Influenza*	1 dose annually				
Tetanus, diphtheria, pertussis (Td/Tdap)*	Substitute 1-time dose of Tdap for Td booster; then boost with Td every 10 yrs				Td booster every 10 yrs
Varicella*	2 doses				
Human papillomavirus (HPV)*	3 doses (females)				
Zoster				1 dose	
Measles, mumps, rubella (MMR)*	1 or 2 doses		1 dose		
Pneumococcal (polysaccharide)	1 or 2 doses				1 dose
Meningococcal*	1 or more doses				
Hepatitis A*	2 doses				
Hepatitis B*	3 doses				

*Covered by the Vaccine Injury Compensation Program.

- For all persons in this category who meet the age requirements and who lack evidence of immunity (e.g., lack documentation of vaccination or have no evidence of previous infection)
- Recommended if some other risk factor is present (e.g., based on medical, occupational, lifestyle, or other indications)
- No recommendation

Report all clinically significant postvaccination reactions to the Vaccine Adverse Event Reporting System (VAERS). Reporting forms and instructions on filing a VAERS report are available at http://www.vaers.hhs.gov or by telephone, 800-822-7967.

Information on how to file a Vaccine Injury Compensation Program claim is available at http://www.hrsa.gov/vaccinecompensation or by telephone, 800-338-2382. Information about filing a claim for vaccine injury is available through the U.S. Court of Federal Claims, 717 Madison Place, N.W., Washington, D.C. 20005; telephone, 202-357-6400.

Additional information about the vaccines in this schedule, extent of available data, and contraindications for vaccination also is available at http://www.cdc.gov/vaccines or from the CDC-INFO Contact Center at 800-CDC-INFO (800-232-4636) in English and Spanish, 24 hours a day, 7 days a week.

Use of trade names and commercial sources is for identification only and does not imply endorsement by the U.S. Department of Health and Human Services.

FIGURE 10-5 Recommended U.S. adult immunization schedule, 2011. (*Source:* Centers for Disease Control and Prevention (CDC), Department of Health and Human Services. Retrieved March 8, 2011, from http://www.cdc.gov/vaccines/recs/schedules/downloads/adult/adult-schedule.pdf)

Example Problem: Dementia (Communicating With Persons With Cognitive Deficit)

In addition to the normal changes of aging, many older adults have more severe problems with memory and at least one other cognitive ability (e.g., judgment, thinking, language, or coordination). **Dementia** is an irreversible, progressive decline in mental abilities. People with dementia have difficulty speaking and understanding. In addition to the general approaches for all older adults, the following are some ideas to help you communicate with people with cognitive deficits:

- Use simple, short sentences, containing one idea each: "Where does it hurt" rather than, "Please describe the quality and location of your pain."
- Avoid vague comments (e.g., "I see," "Um-hmm," "Yes, yes, OK.") The patient will not be able to interpret these responses. Instead, echo the patient's comment and state your response directly and simply: "You are hungry. I will bring your lunch."
- If the patient doesn't understand what you say, repeat your words exactly. Under other circumstances, you usually rephrase your sentences when someone doesn't understand, but for patients with dementia, giving new information just adds to their confusion.
- Try to understand that the patient's reality is distorted and he is behaving in the only way he is able. When the patient is conversing superficially and seems comfortable, it may seem he is competent.

Interventions (Young-Old)

Interventions for this age group focus on transitioning to retirement and physical exercise. Providing resources for social and civic engagement will help a new retiree reestablish a satisfying and rewarding retirement.

Teaching and helping the client plan for physical exercise are also important. Research indicates that a sedentary lifestyle increases the risk of aging-related diseases and premature death. Inactivity is thought to influence the aging process. DNA changes occur partly as a result of stress and oxidative damage to cells. By reducing stress, exercise may reduce some of these oxidative changes and the aging process (Cherkas, Hunkin, Kato, et al., 2008). More research is needed.

The U.S. Department of Health and Human Services (2008) recommends the following activities for older adults:

- *Regular aerobic physical activity.* Encourage clients to engage in 150 minutes a week of moderate-intensity aerobic exercise. Alternatively, engage in 75 minutes a week of vigorous-intensity activity. Each episode of activity should last for at least 10 minutes, and the client should spread the exercise throughout the week.
- *Muscle-strengthening activities.* Clients should perform moderate- or high-intensity muscle-strengthening activities on 2 or more days a week. The weight-bearing and toning exercises should involve all major muscle groups.
- *Balance-promoting activities.* These are especially important for older adults at risk for falls.
- *Adapted physical activities.* Encourage older adults with chronic conditions to be as physically active as abilities and conditions allow. Help them to make adaptations that allow them to do so, or refer them to an exercise therapist.

Remind clients that doing some activity at least 3 days a week produces health benefits, reduces risk of injury, and helps avoid excessive fatigue. Of course, more is better. Some practical suggestions for exercising include the following:

- A brisk 15-minute walk twice a day, every day of the week would easily meet the minimum guidelines for aerobic activity.
- Muscle-strengthening activities at least 2 days a week can include use of exercise bands, handheld weights, digging, lifting and carrying as part of gardening, carrying groceries, and some yoga and tai chi exercises.
- Inactive older adults or those with a very low level of fitness should begin with 10 minutes of walking and increase minutes and intensity slowly with subsequent walks.

You can provide support for the client's exercise regimen by suggesting a range of choices and a list of community resources (e.g., parks, organizations, recreation centers). Also, teach the client how to walk, as needed, and safety considerations. Help the young-old adult institute self-monitoring methods to help her see her progress (e.g., a graph, a chart, a step counter), and reinforce personal progress, such as decreased fatigue and weight loss.

Interventions (Middle-Old)

Older adults who have maintained healthy behaviors throughout their lifetimes will remain vital and actively engaged. However, the occurrence of a health crisis and even a short period of restrictive activity will lead to a decreased functional ability and the need for encouragement, support, and a planned program of limited activity progressing to optimal function for clients in this age group.

Interventions (Oldest-Old)

The goal of interventions for the oldest-old is to maximize function and prevent loss of function or disability, thus ensuring independence for as long as possible. Supportive environments and conditions that allow a person to function are vital. Modified adapted activity is especially important for this age group, including walking, flexibility exercises, yoga, tai chi, and water aerobics. Nutrition is an important focus, as well. Whole grains, dark green and orange vegetables and legumes, all types of fruits and vegetables, and fat-free and low-fat dairy products are among the food groups most needing improvement in this age group to combat obesity and inactivity.

Interventions/Implementation (Frail Elderly)

Prevention of frailty and care of the frail elderly are complex and specialized. The following are examples of research that supports some preventive measures that may give you some ideas for positive interventions:

- At least one study suggests that fall-preventive moderate-intensity group exercise programs have positive effects on older adults only *before* frailty occurs. The frail elderly do not appear to benefit (Faber, Bosscher, Paw, et al., 2006).
- One study found that for obese frail older persons, a combination of weight loss and exercise therapy improved their physical status (Villareal, Banks, Sinacore, et al., 2006).
- Maintaining good nutritional status is also thought to be important in preventing or delaying frailty (Bartali, Semba, Frongillo, et al., 2006).
- Sixty-seven frail elders who lived alone were provided Internet access. They maintained physical and cognitive status, whereas the control group declined significantly in both (Tomita, Mann, Stanton, et al., 2007).

Advise caregivers and older adults to take the following measures, thought to prevent or slow the progression of frailty ("Frailty in Older Adults," 2006):

- Engage in daily physical activity to the extent possible: walking and weights to build aerobic fitness, build muscle, and improve joint stiffness and pain.
- Eat a balanced diet, including enough protein, fiber, and fluids.
- Recognize and treat depression and other medical problems.
- Keep the mind active by socializing, working puzzles, reading, or playing games.

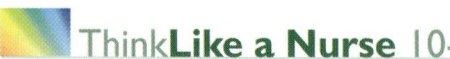

ThinkLike a Nurse 10-6

What factors contribute to a community of functionally active older adults?

PUTTING IT ALL TOGETHER

Recall Ethel Higginbotham, in the Meet Your Patient scenario. She is very thin and frail and refuses to eat. She says, "I just want to die." You might diagnose Ms Higgenbotham with Adult Failure to Thrive. An appropriate *NOC outcome* would be Will to Live. An *individualized goal* might be "Ms. Higginbotham will gain 1 pound and participate in at least one daily group activity by the first of next month." Interventions depend on the diagnosis and its etiology.

Ms. Higginbotham will need care that helps her adjust to widowhood, provides adequate nutrition, and offers activities that provide interaction with others. *NIC interventions* appropriate for Ms. Higginbotham are as follows: Coping Enhancement, Hope Instillation, Self-Care Assistance, Spiritual Support.

Individualized interventions for Ms. Higginbotham include grief counseling, nutritional support, and working with her and her family to determine whether it is appropriate for her to continue to live independently.

As a full-spectrum nurse, you should assess the developmental stage of each of your clients. In maternity and pediatric care, this is a routine part of nursing care. However, growth and development continue to be important throughout the life span. To assess growth and development you must gather data such as the client's age, height and weight, activities the client engages in, and the client's communication skills. You should also perform age-specific assessments, such as those discussed in previous sections.

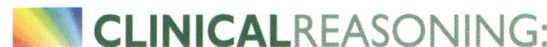 **CLINICAL**REASONING:
Applying the **Full-Spectrum Nursing Model**

Because the following critical thinking activities allow you to practice the kind of thinking you will use as a full-spectrum nurse, they usually have no single right answer. Discuss them with your peers—if you have difficulty with any of the questions, consult your instructor.

PATIENT SITUATION.

Alvin Bell, 82 years old, was just discharged from the hospital following a myocardial infarction (heart attack). On your first home visit to supervise his medication regimen, you notice that the house looks as though it has not been cleaned in weeks. He has what appears to be months' accumulation of newspapers, magazines, and other clutter piled on every flat surface, including the floor. There are dishes piled in the sink, apparently left there before his hospitalization. There is hardly any food in the cupboard; when you weigh Mr. Bell, you see that he has lost 3 pounds in the 3 days he has been home. He admits he has not been eating: "I'm not hungry, and it's too much trouble." As you talk with him, you learn that his wife died of cancer 7 months ago. He says, "I don't know what to do without her. I hate living alone. There doesn't seem to be much reason for going on." Mr. Bell is alert and oriented, but talks and moves very slowly.

THINKING

1. *Theoretical Knowledge:*
   a. What do you know about depression in older adults? Do you have enough knowledge of that topic to be able to assess whether Mr. Bell is depressed? If not, what resources would you use to find out? List specific resources; that is, give the URL, don't just say "the Internet"; give the name or author of the book, not just "my psych-nursing book."
   b. You will also need to know whether it is normal for appetite to decrease in older adults, and what their calorie needs are compared to other age groups. Where can you go to find this information?
2. *Critical Thinking (Considering Alternatives):*
   a. As you survey Mr. Bell's overall situation, what is your first impulse for how to improve his situation? What questions come to you?
   b. What community services might be helpful for Mr. Bell?
   c. How would you handle referrals? Would you leave a list of telephone numbers? Would you call the agencies yourself? Explain your thinking.

DOING

3. *Practical Knowledge:* In your physical examination of Mr. Bell, you find no old or recent bruises or other injuries. However, you wonder if he is suffering neglect or financial abuse. What questions could you ask to find out?

CARING

4. *Self-Knowledge:* Think of one patient you have cared for who has something in common with Mr. Bell. Describe the way(s) in which they are alike.

 Go To Chapter 10, **Clinical Reasoning: Applying the Full-Spectrum Nursing Model Response Sheet,** on *DavisPlus.*

To explore learning resources for this chapter,

Go to Davis*Plus* at http://davisplus.fadavis.com, **keyword Treas**

Chapter Resources for Chapter 10:

> **Knowledge Check and Think Like a Nurse Response Sheets**
>
> **Knowledge Check Answers**
>
> **Resources for Caregivers and Health Professionals**
>
> **Reading More About Development: Older Adults (Suggested Readings)**
>
> **What Are the Main Points in This Chapter?**

NCLEX-Style Review Questions

Chapter Overview Podcasts

Concept Map

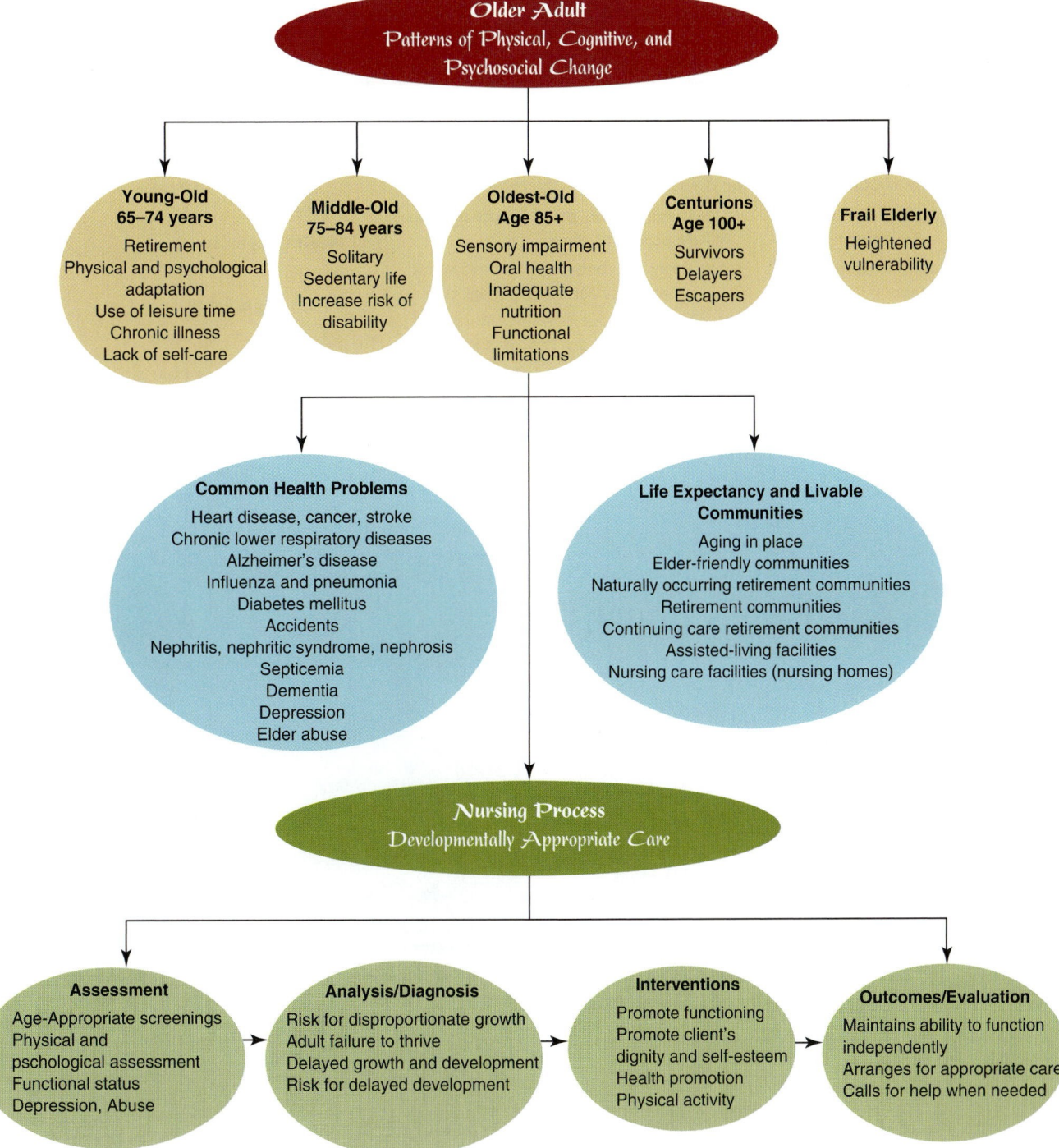

Older Adult
Patterns of Physical, Cognitive, and Psychosocial Change

Young-Old
65–74 years
Retirement
Physical and psychological adaptation
Use of leisure time
Chronic illness
Lack of self-care

Middle-Old
75–84 years
Solitary
Sedentary life
Increase risk of disability

Oldest-Old
Age 85+
Sensory impairment
Oral health
Inadequate nutrition
Functional limitations

Centurions
Age 100+
Survivors
Delayers
Escapers

Frail Elderly
Heightened vulnerability

Common Health Problems
Heart disease, cancer, stroke
Chronic lower respiratory diseases
Alzheimer's disease
Influenza and pneumonia
Diabetes mellitus
Accidents
Nephritis, nephritic syndrome, nephrosis
Septicemia
Dementia
Depression
Elder abuse

Life Expectancy and Livable Communities
Aging in place
Elder-friendly communities
Naturally occurring retirement communities
Retirement communities
Continuing care retirement communities
Assisted-living facilities
Nursing care facilities (nursing homes)

Nursing Process
Developmentally Appropriate Care

Assessment
Age-Appropriate screenings
Physical and pschological assessment
Functional status
Depression, Abuse

Analysis/Diagnosis
Risk for disproportionate growth
Adult failure to thrive
Delayed growth and development
Risk for delayed development

Interventions
Promote functioning
Promote client's dignity and self-esteem
Health promotion
Physical activity

Outcomes/Evaluation
Maintains ability to function independently
Arranges for appropriate care
Calls for help when needed

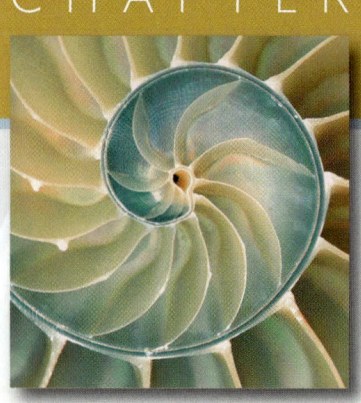

CHAPTER 11

Experiencing Health & Illness

Learning Outcomes

After completing this chapter, you should be able to:

➤ Explore the concepts of health and illness from a holistic perspective.

➤ Compare and contrast three models of health and illness.

➤ Describe the various ways that people experience health and illness.

➤ Identify factors that disrupt health.

➤ Describe the five stages of illness behavior.

➤ Differentiate between acute and chronic illness.

➤ Identify factors that influence individuals' responses to illness.

➤ Apply the concepts presented in this chapter to a variety of patient care situations.

➤ Explain what the concepts in this chapter mean to you as you work toward becoming a full-spectrum nurse.

Key Concepts

Health
Health experience
Illness
Illness experience

Related Concepts

See the Concept Map at the end of this chapter.

Caring for the Nguyens

This feature allows you to practice the kind of thinking you will use as a full-spectrum nurse. There is usually more than one correct answer to a critical thinking question, so we do not provide answers for these features. It is more important to develop your nursing judgment than to "cover content." Discuss the questions with your peers. If you are still unsure, consult your instructor.

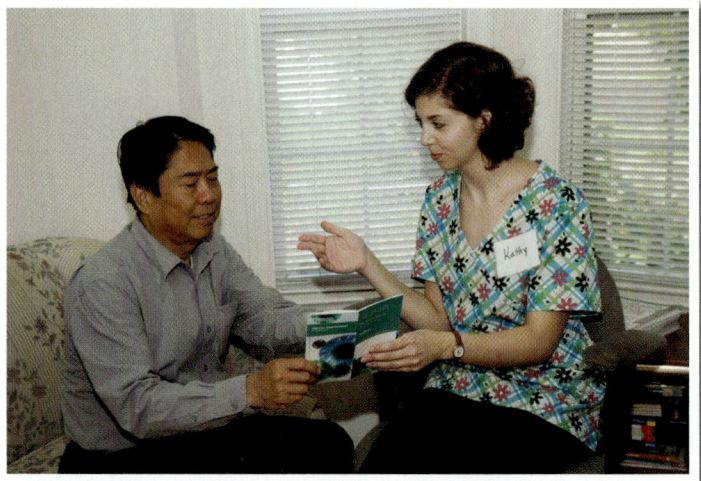

Nam Nguyen has recently been diagnosed with hypertension, obesity, and degenerative joint disease (DJD). He is struggling with these diagnoses. He tells his wife, Yen, "I feel so old now. These are the kind of things my parents are dealing with." At a clinic visit Nam tells you, "It's hard to think of myself as sick. I've been depressed ever since Zach told me about his findings. Now he's asked me to get some lab work. I'm afraid he may find even more problems."

A. Identify the disruptions that Mr. Nguyen must deal with based on these diagnoses. Explain your reasons for choosing these disruptions.

B. How would you evaluate Mr. Nguyen's health status?

C. What kinds of activities could you suggest to Nam to improve his health status?

Caring for the Nguyens (continued)

D. What stage of illness behavior is Mr. Nguyen exhibiting in regard to his recent medical diagnoses? (See The Health–Illness Continuum and Dunn's Health Grid, later in this chapter).

 Go to **Caring for the Nguyens Response Sheet** on *DavisPlus*

Meet Your Patient

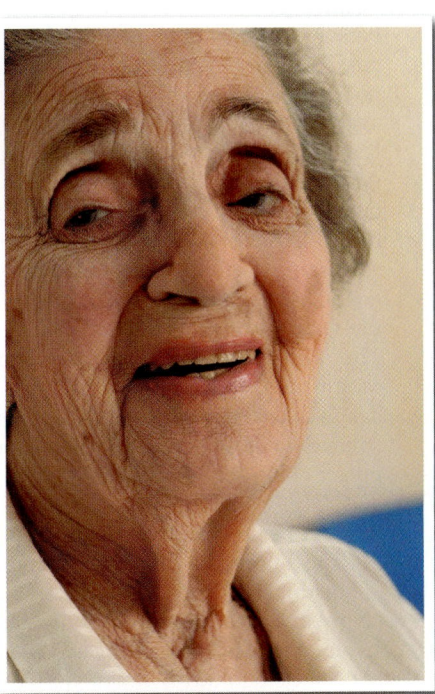

Evelyn is 87 years old and has lived in a long-term care facility for the past 5 years. She suffers from congestive heart failure (CHF), hypertension, diabetes, macular degeneration resulting in near blindness, a severe hearing deficit, urinary incontinence, and immobility resulting from a hip fracture.

Evelyn was married nearly 60 years to Lloyd, who died 6 years ago. They have 5 children, 17 grandchildren, and 14 great-grandchildren. In these past few years, she has experienced the loss of her husband, home, vision, hearing, mobility, and bladder control. Despite these limitations, she keeps current in the lives of all of her extended family and friends.

She is the confidante of the facility staff and knows about their children, their romances, and the gossip around the institution. She is an avid Minnesota Twins fan and also keeps track of the televised high school basketball tournaments. Whenever there is an election, she makes sure that she votes. She "reads" every audio book she can get her hands on. Recently Evelyn was admitted to the hospital in severe CHF. She told her pastor, "I don't want to die yet. I'm having too much fun!"

Evelyn's situation is a far cry from what most people would picture as good health. However, as you consider the ideas of health presented in this chapter, you might conclude that she is a reasonably healthy person from many standpoints.

The goal of this chapter is not so much to help you learn facts about health and illness, but to understand how people experience them. Even the language of the chapter is designed for that purpose. Relax and flow with the chapter. Instead of agonizing over each detail, read it in a way that will help you see the "big picture."

Theoretical Knowledge
knowing why

As a nursing student, you have probably already cared for clients in various stages of health and illness. But have you ever considered what those terms mean? Our understanding of health and illness is influenced by our family, culture, health history, and a host of other factors. As you evolve as a nurse, you'll find that your understanding of these concepts evolves, too. Here we examine some ways that you and your clients might define *health* and *illness* and some ways that full-spectrum nurses have come to understand these terms through their thinking, doing, and caring.

ABOUT THE KEY CONCEPTS

You will need to understand the abstract concepts of health and illness to help you appreciate the experience of health and illness as lived by real, not abstract, people. Strive for an overview of factors that are disruptive to health and factors that nourish health. Understand the subconcepts of hardiness as it relates to patients and of healing presence as it relates to your work as a nurse.

HOW DO WE UNDERSTAND HEALTH AND ILLNESS?

First let's examine the key concept, **health.** What is your image of health? Here are some ideas.

- **The "body beautiful."** Being a "picture of health" can depend on whether you were born in the right era—or in the right country. Styles of beautiful bodies come and go. For instance, much Indian, African, Greek, and European art portrays ideal women as well-rounded creatures. The perfect body view of health also denies the possibility of health to people who use wheelchairs, prosthetics, or even

eyeglasses and hearing aids. Yet many full-spectrum nurses working with disabled clients would indeed describe their clients as healthy.

- **Not having illness.** In describing healthy people, would you disqualify someone with a cold, dandruff, or athlete's foot? What about diabetes, heart disease, or cancer? Doing so would reflect another view of health, that is, not having illness. This view may be unfair because it restricts health only to those who do not have some kind of physical impairment.
- **Something you can buy.** Another popular concept is that health is something you can buy: an exercise bicycle, membership in a health club, medicine, liposuction, gastric bypass, coronary bypasses, and so on. In this view, health does not come from within. It's something "out there" that is available if you have enough money or insurance.
- **Ideal physical and mental well-being.** Health can also be described as an ideal state of physical and mental well-being: something to strive for, but never to attain. Good health is never actually reached, because there is always something more to be achieved. In this view, health is the goal itself, the end instead of one of the means to fulfilling life's purposes.
- **The ability of the soul to cope.** Theologian Jürgen Moltmann (1983) described health in a different way: "True health is the strength to live, the strength to suffer, and the strength to die. Health is not a condition of my body; it is the power of my soul to cope with the varying condition of that body" (p. 142). Similarly, novelist Robert Louis Stevenson wrote of health, "It is not a matter of holding good cards, it's playing a poor hand well." For more traditional definitions of health, refer to Box 11-1.

Now that we've explored some definitions of *health,* let's consider the concept of **illness.** When you think of illness, what comes to mind? If you answered with a list of disorders such as heart disease, diabetes, and schizophrenia, you're not alone. Most people have a medical view of illness as *disease,* which is a pathology affecting an organ or body system. Traditional definitions would also encompass traumatic injury and psychiatric disorders. But is illness merely the sum of these terms?

Nurses Understand Health and Illness as Individual Experiences

If you were the nurse caring for Evelyn in the Meet Your Patient scenario, would you understand health as a perfect body or the absence of disease? Probably not. Nurses understand health and illness as individual experiences, emerging from each patient's unique responses. The person with an illness rarely perceives the experience as a medical diagnosis. Instead, people describe their illness in terms of how it makes them *feel.* Think back to the last time you were ill. How did you feel? Did you feel pain, sadness, fatigue, loss? Did you feel overwhelmed? These responses are disruptions to health and, as such, constitute the lived experience of illness. **Lived experience** is unique to each patient: Just as Evelyn might describe herself as "raring to go," another patient who is 10 years younger and on half as many medications may describe herself as "exhausted all the time" and "just waiting to die." In short, nurses honor the client's understanding of her state of being.

For many years, nurses have recognized that, like Evelyn, some clients strive to maintain a state of optimal health even

---

BOX 11-1 ■ What Do the Experts Say About Health?

The *World Health Organization (WHO)* initially defined health as "a state of complete physical, mental and social well-being and not merely the absence of disease or infirmity" (WHO, 1948).

In 1986 WHO redefined health as "a resource for everyday life, not the objective of living. Health is a positive concept emphasizing social and personal resources, as well as physical capacities" (The Ottawa Charter for Health Promotion, 1986).

- *Traditional Chinese medicine* considers health to be a balance between the opposite energy forces of *yin* and *yang.*
- *Ayurveda,* an ancient Indian medical system, describes health as the trinity of body, mind, and spiritual awareness (Sheinfeld-Gorin & Arnold, 2006).
- *Florence Nightingale* believed that health was prevention of disease through the use of fresh air, pure water, efficient drainage, cleanliness, and light (1859).
- *Nursing theorist Jean Watson* (1979) believes that health implies at least three elements: (1) a high level of overall physical, mental, and social functioning; (2) a general adaptive–maintenance level of daily functioning; and (3) the absence of illness (or the presence of efforts that lead to its absence). Health is a matter of perception. Even a person with a terminal illness may be considered healthy if he has a high level of functioning, is coping with the diagnosis, and is actively making efforts to improve his status.

---

when coping with chronic and even terminal disease. Many experience this state as wellness: "a way of life oriented toward optimal health and well-being in which body, mind, and spirit are integrated by the individual to live more fully within the human and natural community" (Myers, Sweeney, & Witmer, 2000, p. 252). This perspective acknowledges the influence of attitude and lifestyle choices on the client's state of being. It also implies that nursing interventions in support of wellness are important not only for healthy clients, but for those who are experiencing disease, and even those facing death.

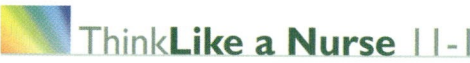

Think**Like a Nurse** 11-1

What qualities are essential to your own personal definition of *health?* How do you define *illness?*

Knowledge**Check** 11-1

- Provide at least two common definitions of *health.*
- Explain how full-spectrum nurses define *health* and *illness.*
- Define *wellness* in your own words.

Nurses Use Conceptual Models to Understand Health and Illness

You can use a variety of models to understand health and illness. Each emphasizes somewhat different aspects of these complex experiences. Nurses have found the following models particularly useful.

The Health–Illness Continuum

Most of us recognize that our health status changes frequently. For example, although today I feel pretty good and yesterday I was exhausted, I believe I was healthy on both of those days. I know that my exhaustion was related to staying up late enjoying the company of good friends. My medical record states that I have diabetes and hypertension, but I keep both diseases in control. I take multiple medications, read food labels, exercise aerobically 5 days a week, and lift weights 3 days a week. Am I healthy, ill, or a health nut?

The preceding example illustrates the complex and dynamic nature of human health. In an effort to describe this complex state, many theorists speak of a **health–illness continuum**, that is, they see health and illness as a graduated spectrum that cannot be divided—except arbitrarily—into parts. A person's position moves back and forth on the continuum with physiological changes, lifestyle choices, and the results of various therapies. As shown in Figure 11-1, the number 1 represents a state of being gravely ill, and 10 represents excellent health, a person in peak form. Notice, however, that a client such as Evelyn (Meet Your Patient) may view herself at various points on this continuum according to how she feels on any particular day. In other words, the continuum is personal and dynamic. Health changes over the course of time.

Dunn's Health Grid

Dunn (1959) created a health grid that plots a person's status on the health–illness continuum against environmental conditions (Fig. 11-2). Many nurses use this grid to help them predict the likelihood that a client will experience a change in health status. For example, Evelyn (Meet Your Patient) has several health problems. On a scale of 1 to 10, an observer who does not know Evelyn well might rate her health as a 3. However, Evelyn has a positive outlook and tells her pastor, "I don't want to die yet. I'm having too much fun!" She also has excellent support from her friends, family, and the facility staff. Clearly, Evelyn is in a favorable environment.

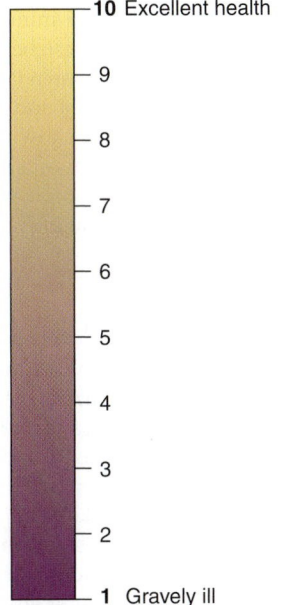

FIGURE 11-1 Over a lifetime, an individual moves up and down on the health–illness continuum.

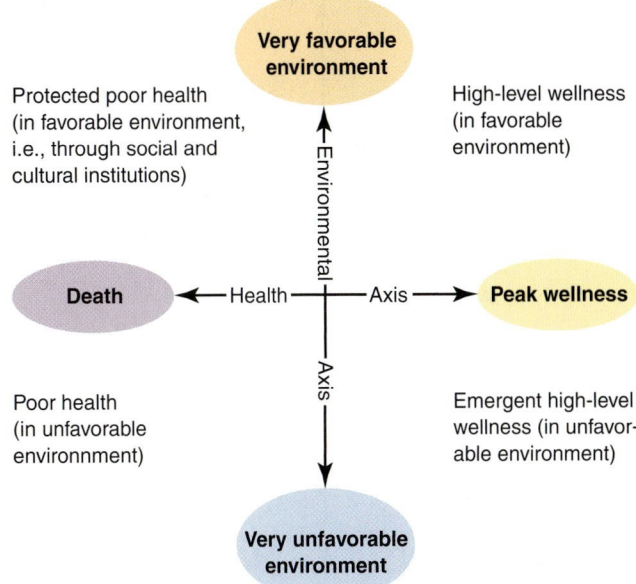

FIGURE 11-2 Dunn's health grid: Health is affected by an individual's status on the health–illness continuum as well as environmental conditions. (*Source:* U.S. Department of Health, Education, and Welfare. Public Health Service. National Office of Vital Statistics.)

This positive setting protects her from harm and provides a good quality of life. On Dunn's grid, Evelyn would probably fall in the area of "protected poor health."

Neuman's Continuum

Nursing theorist Betty Neuman (2002) views health as an expression of living energy available to an individual. The energy is displayed as a continuum with **high energy** (wellness) at one end and **low energy** (illness) at the opposite end (Fig. 11-3). The person is said to have varying levels of energy at various stages of life. When more energy is generated than expended, there is wellness. When more energy is expended than is generated, there is illness—possibly death. Although Evelyn (Meet Your Patient) has several clearly identified health problems, she is engaged in life and active with her family, friends, and long-term care facility staff. We might not all agree on where to place her on Neuman's continuum, but certainly her activity and energy counterbalance her physical frailty.

HOW DO PEOPLE EXPERIENCE HEALTH AND ILLNESS?

In envisioning health and illness as a continuum, full-spectrum nurses promote wellness regardless of the circumstances a client faces now or in the future. This approach requires the holistic understanding that health is multidimensional. The following are some of the many dimensions of health that we experience along the health–illness continuum. An understanding of these dimensions should broaden your concept of health.

Biological Factors

Although biological factors are not entirely within our control, most people consider them when they describe themselves as "well" or "ill." A healthy genetic makeup and freedom from debilitating age-related changes are certainly desired states

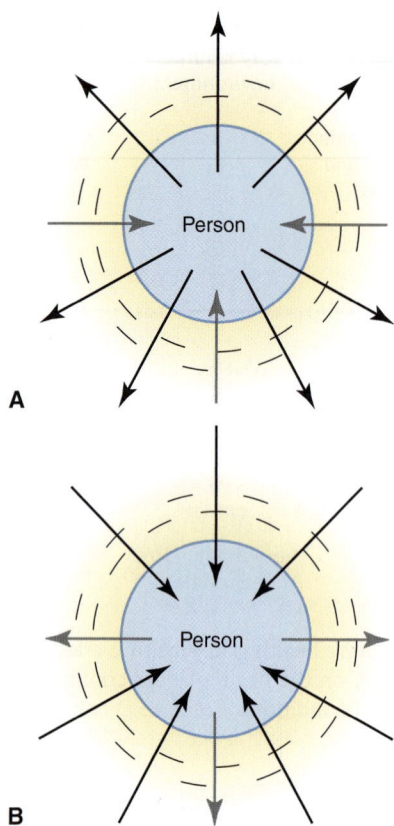

A

B

FIGURE 11-3 Neuman's continuum: A balance of input and output. (A) When energy output exceeds input, illness results. (B) Wellness occurs when more energy is generated than expended. (*Source:* Neuman, B. [1995]. *The Neuman systems model.* In B. Neuman, *The Neuman systems model* [3rd ed.]. East Norwalk, CT: Appleton & Lange, pp. 3–61.)

and, along with gender, they tip the scale toward the wellness end of the health–illness continuum.

Genetic Makeup. For example, the risk of breast cancer increases dramatically in women who have a family history of a mother, sister, or daughter with breast cancer. Recently, a genetic marker for this type of breast cancer has been discovered—that is, some people inherit a tendency to develop breast cancer.

Gender. Many diseases occur more commonly in one gender than in another. For example, rheumatoid arthritis, osteoporosis, and breast cancer are more common in women, whereas ulcers, color blindness, and bladder cancer are more common in men.

Age and Developmental Stage. Age and developmental stage influence the likelihood of becoming ill. Certain health problems can be correlated to developmental stage. For example, more than 75% of new breast cancer cases are diagnosed in women older than age 50. As another example, adolescent boys have much higher rates of head injury and spinal cord injury than the general public because of their tendency toward risk-taking behaviors. For further discussion of growth and development, see Chapters 9 and 10 in this book.

- **Development influences coping ability.** Developmental stage also influences a person's ability to cope with stressors that tend to move him toward the illness end of the continuum. Infants or children who are ill, frightened, or hurt have a limited repertoire of experiences, communication

ability, and understanding to help them in their responses. As we progress through the stages of development, we develop understanding and skills to help us deal with illness.

- **Development influences perceptions.** When disease, loss, or other disruptions occur at a younger age than expected, they change our perception of the event and may present a greater challenge to our coping skills than disruptions that are expected. For example, a child's death may seem more tragic than that of an older adult. It is important, though, not to discount the impact of disruptions that occur during the period of a person's life when they might be expected. For example, the death of a spouse is no less traumatic for an older adult than it would be for a young spouse. Losing someone with whom one has spent most of one's life is an incredible loss, whether or not it is "expected" at that stage of life.

Nutrition

Health requires nourishment, and the most obvious form of nourishment is food. The influence of diet on human health is undeniable: Nutrient-deficiency diseases, such as scurvy and night blindness, are unknown in people who consume a nutritious diet. In addition, many chronic diseases, such as type 2 diabetes mellitus and heart disease, are influenced by our diets, and nutrition appears to play at least a moderate role in a variety of other diseases, such as osteoporosis and some forms of cancer (Thompson & Manore, 2009). As more studies look at the protective properties of some foods (e.g., antioxidants) and the hazards of others (e.g., refined carbohydrates, *trans*-fatty acids), the phrase "You are what you eat" seems more accurate each day. Chapter 28 discusses nutrition in greater detail.

Physical Activity

Healthy people are usually active people. When they are unable to maintain previous levels of activity, they may perceive themselves as less healthy. Studies support the benefit of moderate physical activity in reducing the risk of chronic disease and promoting longevity (Thompson & Manore, 2009). As little as 30 minutes of gardening or 15 minutes of jogging on most days of the week can lead to these benefits. In addition, certain types of exercise have been shown to reduce the risk of specific diseases, such as osteoporosis and heart disease. For example, weight training has been shown to increase bone density and reduce the risk of osteoporosis in women older than age 40, and aerobic activity, such as walking, decreases the risk of heart disease. Physical Activity is discussed more fully in Chapter 33.

Sleep and Rest

Sleep nourishes health. Most of the body's growth hormone, which assists in tissue regeneration, synthesis of bone, and formation of red blood cells, is released during sleep. Sleep is also important to mental health because it provides time for the mind to slow down and rejuvenate. In controlled studies, people kept awake for 24 hours experienced difficulty concentrating and performing routine tasks. With increasing levels of sleep deprivation, sensory deficits and mood disturbances occurred. Outside the laboratory, mild but chronic sleep deprivation is common, particularly among students, mothers of infants and young children, perimenopausal women, and people in pain. Sleep and rest are discussed in more detail in Chapter 35.

Meaningful Work

Many people find that work is a healthy way to cope with stressors. Psychologist Victor Frankl, who survived internment in a Nazi concentration camp, observed in *Man's Search for Meaning* (1959, 1962, 1984, 2004) that engaging in meaningful work promotes health and, even in the midst of horrific stressors, can defend against physical and mental breakdown.

People also experience meaningful work as a dimension of wellness. For many people, volunteering, pursuing hobbies, and engaging in pleasurable activities can be forms of meaningful work. For example, some find that singing, playing a musical instrument, or listening to music is particularly healing. For others, it may be reading, painting, playing basketball, knitting, gardening, hiking in the wilderness, or even shopping. Remember that being healthy is not all about denying yourself the pleasure of ice cream and French fries. Healthful activities can be fun, too. By supporting clients' life work, hobbies, and personal interests, you help them nourish their health in their unique way.

Lifestyle Choices

People who consider themselves healthy are usually those who make healthy lifestyle choices. They are aware of the threats to health created by smoking cigarettes, consuming alcohol, abusing drugs, engaging in unprotected sex, and other risky behaviors. Consider the following examples:

Tobacco. Tobacco use increases recovery time from other illnesses, injuries, and surgery. Smoking also increases the risk of diabetes, infertility, low-birth-weight and preterm babies, and perinatal death.

Alcohol. Studies have indicated that drinking a glass of red wine each day can reduce the risk of heart disease and slow bone loss. In contrast, excessive alcohol consumption damages the brain, liver, pancreas, intestines, and neurological system and can lead to malnutrition. It has also been implicated in several forms of cancer and in fetal alcohol syndrome in newborns. Finally, excessive alcohol consumption is implicated in about half of all motor vehicle accidents, falls, and other injuries.

Other Substances. Abuse of alcohol and illicit drugs leads to a deterioration in health, functioning, and relationships. Even prescription drugs can be abused. Substance abuse is a risk factor in many diseases. For example, people who inject illegal drugs are at increased risk of hepatitis and HIV.

You will learn more about the effects of lifestyle choices on wellness and safety in Chapters 9, 23, and 27.

Personal Relationships

Living in a healthy family is an important dimension of wellness. Moreover, the family influences a person's view of himself as well or ill. Look at Table 11-1. Of the five pairs of families listed there, which family in each pair would you expect to experience a higher level of wellness?

Especially when clients are coping with life-threatening disease, family relationships can provide critical sustenance and preserve optimal wellness during the experience. Weeks before his death from amyotrophic lateral sclerosis (ALS), a neurological disease, sociologist Morrie Schwartz stated, "It's become quite clear to me as I've been sick. If you don't have the support and love and caring and concern that you get from a family, you don't have much at all" (Albom, 1997). You will learn more about the role of family in human health in Chapter 14.

When illness occurs, some people prefer to be totally independent, priding themselves on never asking for or accepting help. But the reality is that during times of disruption, support from others is crucial. Knowing that support is available, and being willing to accept the support, can greatly affect a person's response to disruptions.

Culture

The healthcare culture has traditionally responded to illness with specific therapies aimed at treating a biophysical disorder, whereas nursing, as part of the culture of holism, responds to the physical, emotional, mental, and spiritual dimensions of illness. Culture affects the experience of illness in the following ways:

- **It influences health decisions, behaviors, perceptions, and view of self as well or ill.** This is not to say that individuals can be defined by their culture. Some, either consciously or unconsciously decide to break away from culturally conditioned responses.
- **It influences responses to illness.** Our response to illness is also partly determined by our culture. For example, people who belong to fundamentalist religions may interpret illness as a punishment from God and may bear their symptoms stoically (i.e., hide their symptoms) to try to pay for their sins (retribution). If you need more information about the influence of culture on health and illness, see Chapter 15.

Table 11-1 ➤ Family Personal Relationships

Which Family Would Likely Experience a Higher Level of Wellness?

Family A: Places a high priority on health promotion	OR	**Family B:** Responds to health issues only in times of serious illness
Family C: Encourages adventure and risk-taking	OR	**Family D:** Emphasizes caution in new situations
Family D: Is very open about expressing feelings and disagreements	OR	**Family E:** Squelches personal feelings to avoid conflict in the family
Family F: Views the family as capable and successful	OR	**Family G:** Views them as powerless victims
Family H: Teaches good negotiation skills, builds a network of family support, while encouraging the development of independence	OR	**Family I:** Parents do not have a large repertoire of coping and communication skills to share with their children

Religion and Spirituality

Religion and spirituality are closely tied to culture, and clients' religious beliefs and practices can influence their healthcare choices. For example, some people believe that spiritual beliefs influence the mind–body connection to promote wellness and healing. When healing is not possible because of terminal illness or external circumstances beyond our control, spiritual reserves can help maintain our view of ourselves as "well." You will learn more about the influence of spirituality on health in Chapter 16.

Environmental Factors

The environment can also nourish wellness. For institutionalized clients, establishing a little corner of the room that is uniquely theirs, with photos and other mementos, can be healing. Other clients may be soothed by the quiet of a chapel, a walk in a park, or even a trip to a shopping mall. Spending time in any place where they feel harmony and peace and draw strength can promote clients' health.

On the other hand, environmental pollutants are a common cause of illness. For example, exposure to secondhand smoke causes an estimated 3,400 deaths from lung cancer among American adults each year (Centers for Disease Control and Prevention [CDC], 2010). Carbon monoxide and lead poisoning, molds, radon, chemicals (e.g., insecticides), and other pollutants also cause serious disease. (See Chapter 23 for more information.)

Finances

It is often said that money doesn't buy happiness. Certainly, this is true. However, money does buy access to healthcare and healthcare choices and thus nourishes wellness. In the United States, health insurance is often tied to employment or income level, and health insurance dictates which providers you have access to and what services are available to you. Even in countries with national health programs, such as Canada and some European countries, the standard care available may not include all the services or medications that a person desires. The same is true in the United States, which limits the services available through Medicare and other types of state and national health insurance.

Sometimes healthcare providers wonder why people do not take advantage of services that are available to them. Why do they let things go so long before seeking help—or fail to follow up with recommended treatment plans? A client's apparent lack of concern or lack of compliance to a treatment regimen may be, in reality, a problem of access to healthcare. Any one or more factors may keep individuals and families from getting the help that they need (e.g., distance from the resources, knowledge of available resources, trust in the available resources, and financial status (e.g., to make lifestyle adjustments).

ThinkLike a Nurse 11-2

- In what ways could you improve your eating, exercise, and sleep habits?
- How might a hospitalized patient get away from the hospital routine and find peace and harmony?

WHAT FACTORS DISRUPT HEALTH?

We spend much of our lives trying to maintain good health—eating, sleeping, keeping our bodies at a comfortable temperature—in general, tending to our high-maintenance bodily needs. It's a continual process because of the many disruptions to health we face. Not all of these disruptions are incapacitating, but all challenge our ability to function and enjoy our everyday lives, and they tend to move us toward the illness end of the health–illness continuum. What are **health disruptions**? Let's explore the concept of by learning about some specific examples.

Physical Disease

Disease disrupts our lives in so many ways. It may reduce our ability to perform our life roles or to engage in activities we enjoyed before the illness. Also, the diagnosis of a serious disease may bring shock, fear, anxiety, anger, or grief: Will I become disabled? How will I support my family? What did I do to deserve this? Finally, it may also cause clients to question the meaning and purpose of their lives, to become more inwardly focused, or to embrace life even more fully. When she first learned, of her diagnosis of breast cancer at age 36, Treya Killam Wilber wrote, "Strange things happen to the mind when catastrophe strikes. . . . I was so stunned that it was as if absolutely nothing had happened. A tremendous strength descended on me. . . . I was clear, present, and very determined" (Wilber, 2000).

Injury

Injury can cause the same symptoms and emotions as disease, but perhaps its most disruptive aspect is its suddenness. In *Still Me,* actor Christopher Reeve described his thoughts in the first days after he recovered consciousness following his cervical spinal cord injury: "The thought that kept going through my mind was: 'I've ruined my life, and you only get one.' There's no counter you can go up to and say, 'I dropped my ice cream cone; could I please have another one?'. . . . Why isn't there a higher authority you can go to and say, 'Wait a minute, you didn't mean for this to happen to *me*'" (Reeve, 1998).

Mental Illness

Clients with mental illness and their families experience a level of pain, suffering, and chronic sorrow that is difficult for healthy people to fully appreciate (Godress, Ozgul, Owen, et al., 2005; Kokanovic, Petersen, & Klimidis, 2006). In addition, if the illness affects work ability, they experience loss of income and altered role relationships, accompanied by the costs of various therapies.

Mental illness carries a stigma that has been described as the single most debilitating handicap for people with mental illness (Glod, 1998). This stigmatization can also disrupt the health of family members. For example, an adult sister of a sibling who has schizophrenia stated, "I really feel labeled along with my sister." She reported overhearing a cousin at a family gathering ask, "So where is that crazy Dee? Is she in or out of the hospital again? I hope her sister doesn't catch her craziness" (Glod, 1998). Family members may also live in constant fear that their loved one hurt herself or even commit suicide.

Pain

Whether mild or severe, temporary or long lasting, pain is a disruption. It's not that we can't live with pain—many people do, every day of their lives. However, pain disrupts the smooth operation of our lives; it can change personality, erode coping skills, and interfere with healthy communication. It's hard to concentrate on what we are trying to accomplish when pain is competing for our attention. Pain can interfere in life at all levels, particularly when it is chronic or severe.

Pain that is easily remedied with medications or that is short lived serves only as a minor disruption. However, pain that is all encompassing permeates a person's entire existence. Sometimes that pain is physical, sometimes psychological. One young mother of a profoundly mentally disabled 14-year-old girl spoke of "hurting so bad that my bones hurt."

As we discussed in Chapter 1, some of our nursing interventions inflict pain. We ask patients to turn, deep-breathe, and cough after surgery, even though it hurts—a *lot*! We put needles in them, catheterize them, and get them out of bed when they would rather sleep. We pull off tape. We invade their physical personal space. We ask them questions about personal things, such as their bowel movements. It is a challenge to be a comforting, healing presence when we have to do things that cause discomfort.

Loss

Loss is a disruption that cuts to the core of who we are—whether the loss of a job; the end of a romantic relationship; the death of a loved one; or the loss of youth, beauty, functioning, or identity. Most of us cling to a unique identity, which usually does *not* include gaining weight or getting wrinkles and gray hair, let alone being a patient or losing major bodily functions. The resulting period of significant disintegration may continue until the person either finds a way to cope with the loss or succeeds in reinterpreting the loss in a meaningful way.

Loss of Sense of Self. Many have written about the indignities people suffered in concentration camps, including nakedness, exposure to human excrement, and being treated like children, incapable of thoughtful judgment (Bettelheim, 1979; Frankl, 1959, 1962, 1984, 2004; Valladares, 2001). Those three indignities are crucial threats to a person's sense of self. Sadly, patients in healthcare institutions may also suffer those indignities. Think how patients feel who have to don a hospital gown and allow their body to be exposed for various tests or procedures. One woman who was paralyzed as the result of a lesion on her spine indicated that one of the toughest things she had to deal with was having her daughter give her enemas and clean her up as if she were a baby. As healthcare providers, we may easily forget how humiliating such "routine procedures" may be for the patient. You can help relieve the disruption of disease and injury when you respect patients' dignity, provide for privacy, and allow them to make choices regarding their care.

Permanent Loss. If temporary losses are difficult, what about those that are permanent? C. S. Lewis (1961) wrote about his response to the death of his wife: "I know that the thing I want is exactly the thing I can never get. The old life, the jokes, the drinks, the arguments, the lovemaking, the tiny, heartbreaking commonplace" (p. 22). As nurses, we would like to "fix" everything. Though we can't "fix" the holes that are left when a person suffers a loss, we can be open and sensitive to his heart's cry.

Impending Death

It is easy for most of us to ignore that we all have 100% chance of dying eventually and live as though death were only a remote possibility. Lifton and Olson (1974) state that during middle age, even without the presence of life-threatening illness, people tend to become more aware of the compelling reality of death: "One's life is suddenly felt to be limited. . . . It also becomes apparent that . . . there will not be time for all one's projects" (p. 63).

As a nurse, you will care for clients who are living in disruption of the shadow of death. Some may be aware of their condition; others may choose to deny it, ignore it, or "fight it to the end" by trying a series of conventional and alternative therapies. Caring for dying clients makes us painfully aware of our own frailty and is one of the most difficult experiences you will face as a nurse. Chapter 17 provides further discussion of loss, grieving, and dying.

Competing Demands

Taken independently, the many competing demands of life may be easy to handle. Taken together, the cumulative effect wears us down. In times of illness, the other competing demands continue. Children need to be cared for. Aging parents may need care. Bills still need to be paid. Job responsibilities press in. One man with depression reported, "[T]he whole thing bundled together—one caused the other which caused more and it was just a degenerative loop. . . . [O]ne thing feeds another which feeds another and so forth until you just constantly go down" (Smith, 1992, p. 104).

People May Ignore Health Issues. Sometimes people ignore health issues because the competing demands are too great. Symptoms may even go unnoticed because attention is scattered in so many directions and there is not enough time and energy to research one's symptoms, schedule a doctor's appointment, or follow through with treatments.

Acute vs. Chronic Illness. When an illness is acute, such as a broken bone, the stress is usually bearable because it is usually lasts for a set amount of time. Bettleheim (1979) states, "The worst calamity becomes bearable if one believes its end is in sight" (pp. 3–4). But when the illness is chronic, the competing demands can take a heavy toll. One woman took care of her husband who lived at home, his breathing assisted by a ventilator. She recounted the overwhelming burden she felt when, after 2 years, he was "no better and no worse. This could go on forever!" Although people came in to help, she felt she had to maintain constant alertness in case something went wrong with his ventilator, and she still had to meet many other demands and challenges each day.

As nurses, we sometimes find it easy to criticize how people deal with their situations. But it is so important to realize that the short amount of time that you spend with someone in a hospital or in a home visit is only one tiny fragment of the cumulative experience that patients and their families experience, sometimes unrelentingly for years on end.

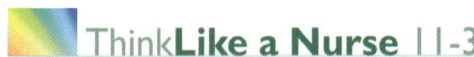

ThinkLike a Nurse 11-3

How might you assist your patient to maintain normalcy in spite of illness?

The Unknown

Even normal life changes present challenges. With some unknowns, there is time to investigate the potential problem and prepare. For example, if an expectant couple learns from an amniocentesis (a prenatal test) that their child has a genetic defect, then during the remaining months of pregnancy they can read about the disorder and meet with other parents who have had children similarly affected. This can help prepare them to anticipate their child's needs. But injuries and illnesses can happen abruptly, with no chance to prepare for new realities. A woman described her experience of finding out she had

cancer of the lung with metastasis: "It was on a . . . Friday—I got to feeling kind of bad—kind of like you had the flu or something, you know? . . . so I went to the doctor. . . . And . . . they started doin' tests on me—all kinds of tests—and found out I had cancer" (Smith, 1992, p. 107).

Imbalance

Our sense of justice tells us that when we are good, good things should happen. When we are bad, bad things should happen. The Buddhist concept of *karma* suggests that there is a fair balance between what one gives to life and what one receives. Thus, when we perceive that life has violated this rule, we experience the violation as a disruption, as in these examples:

- **Death of a child.** Our sense of balance is perhaps most dramatically disturbed by the death of children. Such deaths are sometimes referred to as "out of order" because children (of any age) "should not" die before their parents.
- **Treatment failure.** Balance is also disrupted when patients, expecting that their painful and harrowing treatments "should" help them get better, do not get better. One young woman under treatment for advanced cancer described it like this: "It's just—you've been working hard . . . you're doin' what you're supposed to be doin' and focusing and all this and that—and your body is still not responding" (Smith, 1992, p. 111).

Have you seen the bumper sticker "Life is hard. And then you die"? Cynical perhaps, but most of us realize early in life that as much as we would like for everything to be fair, it is not going to happen. Knowing this intellectually, however, does not necessarily reduce the disruptive effect of the imbalance.

Isolation

How many times have you thought, "No one knows what I'm going through"? A sense of isolation or aloneness seems to accompany suffering. C. S. Lewis (1961) states, "You can't really share someone else's weakness, or fear or pain" (p. 13). The sense of aloneness reported by seriously ill clients is related in part to their actual physical separation from loved ones during treatments, hospitalizations, or clinic visits. But it also stems from their feeling that there is no one who is really "in their world." Having someone physically present does not necessarily remove the sense of aloneness:

> When I lay here it's lonely—very, very lonely. Because [my daughter] can't just sit here and talk to me all the time. She's got wash to do, fold and all that stuff. And then the kids to worry about. . . . The worst thing I've found about this whole disease is the loneliness. . . . Because your family can be with you and if they don't come and sit down and talk to you about different things, you're lonely. It's the loneliness that makes you sad inside. . . . It's like everybody's afraid . . . that maybe they're gonna catch what you got or something. (Smith, 1992)

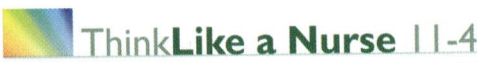

KnowledgeCheck 11-2

Identify at least four factors that disrupt health.

ThinkLike a Nurse 11-4

- What impact do disruptions have on your life?
- How could you apply the information about disruptions to the health of a community? To the health of a nation?

WHY DO PEOPLE EXPERIENCE ILLNESS DIFFERENTLY?

Earlier in this chapter, we mentioned that people vary greatly in terms of their response to life situations. Why is this so? Why do some people react to seemingly insurmountable problems with calmness and grace, while others fall apart over seemingly small disruptions? The human experience is so complex and interactive that is it impossible to make neat little categories that we might add up to determine a score predicting how a person will respond to a given situation. There are several factors, however, that may influence an individual's responses to illness. Focus now on the concepts of illness stage; acute and chronic illness; hardiness; and the intensity, duration, and multiplicity of the disruption.

Stages of Illness Behavior

Illness can be viewed as a social role, in which both the patients and caregivers have duties and expectations that are shaped by the society in which they live. Therefore, how people react to an illness depends in part on their illness stage. Suchman (1972) identified five stages of illness behaviors that people move through as they cope with disruptions to health: experiencing symptoms, sick role behavior, seeking professional care, dependence on others, and recovery.

Experiencing Symptoms. Symptoms are a signal that illness has begun. If the symptoms are recognizable, such as runny nose, sneezing, and a cough, you may identify the problem as a common cold and turn to previously used remedies. Common problems rarely progress beyond this stage. However, if the symptoms are unusual, severe, or overwhelming, you may progress to the next stage.

Sick Role Behavior. When you have identified yourself as ill, you assume the sick role. The sick role relieves you from normal duties, such as work, school, or tasks at home. In Western biomedical culture, the prevailing view is that sick persons are not responsible for their illnesses and that a curative process outside the person is needed to restore wellness. We believe that the sick person has the duty to try to get well, to seek healthcare, and to cooperate with the care providers (Cockerham, 2000). The severity of the symptoms and anticipated length of illness determine whether you will progress further along the stages of illness.

Seeking Professional Care. The next stage is seeking professional care. To reach this stage, you must determine that you are ill and that professional care is required to treat the illness. Persons who seek professional care are asking for validation of their illness, explanations for their symptoms, appropriate treatment, and information about the anticipated length of illness. Healthcare professionals often bypass this stage, relying on themselves to identify and treat the problem. This is not always the best course of action because it is difficult to be objective when examining yourself.

Dependence on Others. When you accept the diagnosis and treatment of the healthcare provider you typically also accept the need to depend on others. The severity of the illness and the type of treatment determine the extent of dependence. This may be limited to listening to the provider's instructions, filling the prescription, and following directions given in the office. However, hospitalization is often associated with dependence on nursing staff and hospital personnel for activities of daily living, medications, and treatments. Some people easily make the transition to dependence; others

remain as independent as possible even in the face of severe illness. Personal characteristics and values play a large role in determining how each of us will respond to the challenges of being dependent.

Recovery. The final stage of illness is called **recovery.** The person gradually resumes independence and returns to normal roles and functioning. In minor illness, this is usually a return to the status quo. Severe illnesses may require a redefinition of optimum function. The greater the change in health status, the more difficult this transition will be. Learning to manage a chronic illness is the equivalent of a cure in an acute illness (Parsons, 1975). Both represent the recovery stage.

The Nature of the Illness

The nature of the illness (e.g., whether the illness is chronic or acute) affects the way persons react to disruptions and respond to illness.

Acute Illness. An **acute illness** occurs suddenly and lasts for a limited amount of time. Acute illnesses, such as a cold, flu, or viral infection, may be minor and require no formal healthcare. More serious acute illness, such as strep throat, may require a visit to a health provider for treatment or even hospitalization or surgery, as in cholecystitis (gallbladder inflammation secondary to gallstone formation) or pyelonephritis (infection of the kidney). Although hospitalization and surgery can be quite traumatic, in each case the person is expected to recover. In acute illness, a person may experience the disruptions of pain, competing demands, and the unknown. However, an end is in sight. Relief is expected.

Chronic Illness. In contrast, **chronic illness** lasts for a long period of time, usually 6 months or more, often for a lifetime. Chronic illness requires the person to make life changes. These changes might be more frequent visits to the clinic or hospital, daily injections, or lifestyle modifications such as a low-fat diet or smoking cessation. Common chronic illnesses include diabetes mellitus, rheumatoid arthritis, and hypertension. Because of the lengthy period of illness, people with chronic disease often experience periods of remission or exacerbation. A **remission** occurs when symptoms are minimal to none. An **exacerbation** ("flare-up") occurs when symptoms intensify. Clients with chronic illness often complain about the unrelenting nature of their health problems. A person with chronic illness may experience virtually all of the disruptions identified earlier. Box 11-2 identifies some interesting facts about chronic conditions.

Hardiness

Why does one client who drinks, smokes, overeats, and avoids exercise live into his 90s, yet another client who "follows all the rules" dies of a sudden heart attack at age 39? Our bodies do not react to the same stressors in the same way. The concept of hardiness may lend insight into this difference. **Hardiness** has been described as developing a very strong positive force to live—and enjoying the fight (Fig. 11-4)!

Will to Live. A man with heart problems said, "I guess everybody that's in the situation, who has to fight to live, and has learned the mental wizardry of it, you know, to make yourself want to live on. But if you want to, you develop this—this very, very strong positive force to make it go" (Smith, 1992, p. 131). Seigel (1986) reported a study by London researchers that revealed a 10-year survival rate of 75% "among cancer patients who reacted to the diagnosis with a 'fighting spirit,'" compared with a 22% survival rate "among those who responded with 'stoic acceptance' or feelings of helplessness or hopelessness" (p. 25).

BOX 11-2 ■ FAQs: Chronic Conditions

- More than 90 million Americans live with chronic conditions.
- Chronic conditions account for about 70% of all deaths in the United States.
- About 80% of older adults have at least one chronic condition; 50% have at least two.
- Approximately 6% of adults older than age 65 have a diagnosable depressive illness.
- The top three risks for functional decline are cognitive impairment, depression, and disease burden.
- The largest declines in functional abilities are associated with these physical conditions: arthritis of the hip or knee; sciatica; and chronic pulmonary diseases.
- Arthritis affects one in five U.S. adults; for more than 40% of those, arthritis limits their activities.
- About 34% of the adult population and 16.9% of children and adolescents ages 2 to 19 years are obese (CDC, 2010 update).
- In a large sample of Medicare beneficiaries, the following were the most frequent chronic physical conditions:

Hypertension (50.5%)	Any cancer (other than skin cancer) (12.7%)
Arthritis of the hip or knee (35.5%)	Emphysema, asthma, or COPD (11.2%)
Arthritis of the hand or wrist (35.5%)	Myocardial infarction (8.8%)
Sciatica (21.0%)	Stroke (5.2%)
"Other" heart conditions (19.3%)	Crohn's disease, ulcerative colitis, or inflammatory bowel disease (4.8%)
Angina pectoris or coronary artery disease (14.1%)	Congestive heart failure (4.6%)
Diabetes (13.7%)	

Sources: CDC, 1998, 2002, 2009, n.d.; Centers for Medicare & Medicaid Services, 2007; Drummond-Dye, 2007; Ellis, Shannon, Cox, et al., 2004; National Institute of Mental Health, 2003; Stuck, Walthert, Nikolaus, et al., 1999.

COPD = chronic obstructive pulmonary disease.

Adapting to Change. Another aspect of hardiness is the willingness to draw on resources within oneself or from others to break out of old patterns of living when life situations change. Some people find it too difficult to make life changes, and they just give up. Hardy individuals are willing to seek out information and take the initiative in dealing with life situations rather than sitting back and letting someone else or a life situation control their lives.

When disruption hits, some people lack the cognitive, communicative, creative, and spiritual resources that would equip them to make it during difficult times. Ironically, other people survive and thrive during times of adversity. Those who see themselves as hardy tend to approach disruptions with an "I can deal with this" attitude.

The Intensity, Duration, and Multiplicity of the Disruption

Everyone has limits. For healthcare providers, too many demands over too long a period of time can lead to *burnout,* a feeling of being overwhelmed and demoralized. For clients and their families, dealing with the cumulative effect of

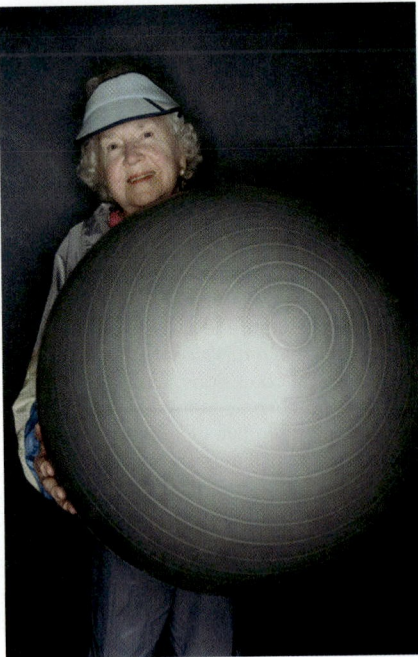

FIGURE 11-4 Hardiness has been described as developing a very strong positive force to live—and enjoying the fight!

illness and other life disruptions can break down what might otherwise be effective coping skills. After reaching a breaking point, their responses may not be typical of what they usually have demonstrated.

KnowledgeCheck 11-3

- Identify the factors that affect how a person responds to the disruptions of illness.
- Define *hardiness*.

PracticalKnowledge
knowing **how**

In the preceding section, you have learned how people experience health, wellness, and illness. In this section, we look at how these concepts can be applied to your nursing practice.

USING THE NURSING PROCESS TO PROMOTE HEALTH

Throughout this textbook, you will learn to use the nursing process to help clients deal with a variety of health problems. But how does the nursing process relate to the broader aspects of health and illness described in this chapter? Overall, it involves helping clients—regardless of the type of health problem—to look within themselves to develop creative ways to deal with the realities they are facing.

Patients may fail to follow a proposed healthcare regimen if healthcare providers develop a plan of care that has no cultural or personal relevance for the patient (or family). Perhaps the plan does not consider the knowledge level of the patient or caregiver; or perhaps it is not feasible in terms of available support, time, energy, finances, or location. Patients may leave a hospital setting *against medical advice* (AMA), thereby endangering their chances of recovery. They may believe the treatment offered them will not help or that the illness is preferable to the proposed treatment. Noncompliance often occurs because the effort, inconvenience, or pain involved with a therapeutic plan of care is too much for them to handle.

Remember that people probably do not refuse to carry out a plan of care simply out of stubbornness, hostility toward healthcare providers, or wanton disregard for their own welfare. The challenge for nurses is to develop an individualized plan of care in collaboration with patients, based on mutual goals and respect.

Toward Evidence-Based Practice

Chan, I. W. S., Lai, J. C. L., & Wong, K. W. N. (2006). Resilience is associated with better recovery in Chinese people diagnosed with coronary heart disease. *Psychology and Health*, 21(3), 335–349.

This study examined the impact of personal resilience (a composite measure of optimism, perceived control, and self-esteem) in 67 Chinese patients in response to an 8-week coronary heart disease rehabilitation program. Results indicated that the patients high in personal resilience achieved better outcomes than those low in personal resilience.

Thompson, C. W., Durrant, L., Barusch, A., & Olson, L. (2006). Fostering coping skills and resilience in home enteral nutrition (HEN) consumers. *Nutrition in Clinical Practice*, 21(6), 557–565.

This qualitative study examined how HEN consumers learned to cope successfully with HEN-related challenges. Researchers interviewed 12 adult HEN consumers who

perceived that they were coping successfully with HEN; they also administered a resilience scale. Results were that these individuals coped successfully by developing an attitude of personal responsibility to accept new life conditions, take charge of their own well-being, seek and accept support, maximize independence and normality, and focus on the positive. In addition, these respondents shared resilient characteristics such as self-efficacy and perseverance.

1. How do the results of these studies apply to the concept of health as presented in this chapter?

2. Can you identify ways in which the methods and findings could be applied to other populations?

 Go to Chapter 11, **Toward Evidence-Based Practice: Suggested Responses,** on Davis*Plus*.

ASSESSMENT

In looking at an individual's health status, physical needs obviously are crucial, but competing issues may be present and cause the client to view the therapeutic interventions as irrelevant or even disruptive. Obtaining data about the psychosocial, emotional, and spiritual aspects of health requires a level of communication that goes beyond a neat list of skills. Communicating genuine care, concern, and sensitivity comes from who you are as a person, not from assuming a professional persona (putting on your "nurse hat").

Settling In. Your initial approach to a patient creates a climate that determines the level of communication that takes place. The patient is probably in a new environment, and your tone, words, and facial expressions can bring comfort and ease. Nurses can find themselves in new situations too, and taking a few moments to settle into the situation can be helpful in establishing a therapeutic relationship and facilitating communication.

Attuning. Being maximally attentive is another key factor in facilitating communication. Most people are hungry for someone to listen to them. So often listeners are so busy thinking about what they want to say that they fail to really listen. Try to focus on what the patient or family has to say instead of thinking ahead to what you want to ask next.

Acceptance. Another vital aspect of communicating is acceptance—acceptance of appearance, lifestyles, ways of coping, and values. You might ask, "How can I be accepting when there are aspects of this person that go against my entire value system?" Accepting is not the same as agreeing with. You can accept people as valued, creative, unique individuals, despite their differences from your own ways of being. This view of acceptance does *not* mean that people should not be held accountable for their actions, for example, in cases of domestic violence and child abuse. It does mean, though, that in your role as a caregiver, you must convey an attitude of accepting the intrinsic value of life—in whatever forms that life takes.

Enjoying. Perhaps even more difficult than accepting is the concept of *enjoying.* You will come into contact with a wide array of individuals, many of whom are different from people you have grown up around and have come to know and enjoy. A challenge for you is to broaden the repertoire of people you enjoy: to see and enjoy commonalities among individuals seemingly so different and to recognize and appreciate the pathos of suffering in the unique experience of each person.

Take Time to Communicate

Settling in, attuning, respecting, and enjoying—certainly this is not a step-by-step process, but each aspect is vital to creating a climate for the openness and communication needed for assessment. You might argue that the healthcare environment does not allow time for such a high level of attentiveness. Consider, though, how much time is spent in delivering nursing care. As a full-spectrum nurse, you will assess patients continually while thinking, doing, and caring for your patients. In fact, the physical contact involved in carrying out nursing procedures seems to break down barriers of communication. Nurses hold a unique opportunity in being with individuals during difficult life situations; indeed, Benner and Wrubel (1989) state that expert nurses call this the "privileged place of nursing" (p. xi).

Identify the Patient's Main Concern

One way to approach assessment, whether in outpatient, acute care, long-term care, or home settings, is to ask the patient, "What is the biggest concern you are dealing with today?" You may have a plan of care that addresses areas that you know to be important, but it may fall far short of meeting your patient's needs if you have not addressed the concern that is fundamental to your patient.

Develop Your Observation Skills

In addition to communicating, developing your observation skills will enable you to assess your patients more fully. Watching your patient's responses to you and your care; observing the presence or absence of visitors and the effect on your patients; and observing signs of religious or cultural practices that have significance all provide important information about your patient's strengths and needs.

ANALYSIS/NURSING DIAGNOSIS

Several of the nursing diagnosis labels identified by NANDA-I relate to health issues discussed in this chapter. Some examples are Anxiety, Caregiver Role Strain, Deficient Knowledge, and Spiritual Distress. An analysis of your assessment data should also provide the information needed to describe related causal factors, such as Spiritual Distress related to fear of impending death or Situational Low Self-esteem related to loss of job secondary to frequent absences for chemotherapy.

KnowledgeCheck 11-4

Compare and contrast attuning, acceptance, and enjoying.

PLANNING OUTCOMES/EVALUATION

Goals and outcomes should be both realistic and valued by the patient and family. When you set goals in the broader dimension of health and illness (as in this chapter), it is harder to be specific in describing expected outcomes and time frames. As a nurse, your role is to help the patient (or family member) envision acceptable outcomes and to set smaller, realistic goals so that the patient recognizes progress. For example, an older woman caring for a spouse with Alzheimer's disease may have a nursing diagnosis of Caregiver Role Strain related to care of spouse with dementia. Together you would establish acceptable goals and break them down into realistic steps. You also would identify outcomes to indicate that the caregiver actually experiences a reduction in strain, such as being able to sleep or having time to pursue meaningful activities.

PLANNING INTERVENTIONS/IMPLEMENTATION

The ideal approach is to draw on patient and family strengths to help achieve the desired outcomes. In the preceding example of the older adult caregiver, you would discuss with her the options available to provide support, but she would identify which options were acceptable to her and her spouse. In the stress of illness, patients and families may not recognize the strengths and creative abilities that they bring to a situation. Part of the art of nursing is to envision strengths and potential in patients and families, just as an artful teacher might recognize a "spark" in a child and encourage that child to learn and grow.

ThinkLike a Nurse 11-5

- How can you use the concepts of health when you are admitting a patient to a hospital setting? To a clinic? To an emergency department? To a rehabilitation or long-term care setting? In initiating home care?

(continued on next page)

- What questions can you ask or what observations can you make to help you gain information about individuals' health strategies, disruptions to health, and factors contributing to their responses to disruptions?
- How would you consider health concepts in planning for patients' discharge from healthcare settings?

How Can I Honor Each Client's Unique Health/Illness Experience?

As a nurse, you can be an instrument of healing in a hurtful world. However, being an instrument of healing does not come automatically with your nursing license. Nor does it allow you the luxury of learning just one approach and applying it to every client. It means you must cultivate a healing presence by listening, being maximally attentive, being aware of your own gifts and limitations of communication, being willing to learn from those in your care, recognizing and respecting others' ways of coping, and enjoying others for who they are.

Patients may be impressed by your skill and knowledge and amazed by the healthcare technology used to diagnose and treat their illnesses. However, what they most often remember, perhaps through the rest of their lives, is that person who connected with them in a very special way. One man, quadriplegic for 26 years following a car accident in his teens, spoke of a senior nursing student who cared for him during his initial hospitalization. He said that after 26 years, he not only still remembered her, but also still could sense the warmth of her caring presence.

During times of vulnerability, people seem acutely atuned to those who are helpful to them and also to those who slight them in hurtful ways, whether intentionally or not. What a challenge this creates for nurses! In this section, we discuss steps you can take to prepare yourself for responding to your clients in ways that are meaningful and healing to them.

Examine Life's Uncertainties

Making health-promoting lifestyle choices is important, but it cannot protect us from risk. Significant life experiences, such as getting married, having children, investing in friendships, venturing into business, and selecting a profession all involve risk. Making a commitment to *anything* is a risk. Each person has a different "risk-comfort range." Some are willing to risk little, have fewer disappointments, and less sparkling achievements. To others, security is not as important, and they are comfortable taking greater risks.

As a nurse, you will face many uncertainties and dilemmas. You will certainly face new experiences and challenges, situations you thought you never would have to deal with. You will observe pain, suffering, and death. You may never understand the apparent unfairness of it all. But often life brings new meaning when it takes a different direction from the one planned. For example, a couple formerly embittered over their third miscarriage found joy in adopting two children with disabilities.

You will also be privileged to witness many joys. Some might even qualify as minor triumphs: a patient taking his first steps after major surgery, a pathology report that isn't as bad as feared, or even a peaceful death that brings closure to a grieving family. As you move from novice to expert, you may find that such witnessing causes you to stop questioning life's uncertainties and instead to start treasuring them.

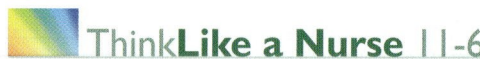

ThinkLike a Nurse 11-6

- What uncertainties have you struggled with?
- What approaches have proven effective for you in dealing with uncertainties?

Envision Wellness for Your Clients and Yourself

Wherever there is a dream, there is someone there to tell you it can't be done, or at least not by you. There is something to be said, however, for "envisioning" wellness for your clients and yourself. Remember Evelyn (Meet Your Patient)? If her nurses had labeled her as debilitated and close to death, how would that have affected her? In contrast, their acceptance of her vision of herself as well and full of life supports her and aids her healing. In the same way, think of how you view your own health. Is the life you envision for yourself characterized by zest and vigor? What are your family relationships like? What are your values? Does your work give meaning and purpose to your life? The wellness that you envision for yourself can be the blueprint for what you want to become. The skeptic in you might say, "What if I do everything that I know to do to maintain a healthy life but I still have a heart attack at 45?" As we have seen, life is full of uncertainties. That does not mean that you have to stop envisioning. Instead, use *flexible envisioning,* adjusting your goals and dreams to each new reality. Health does not mean always getting your first choice. Part of health is being able to dream a new dream, starting over if you need to, but always envisioning that there is something worth striving for.

Establish Trust at Your First Patient Contact

When patients are admitted to a hospital or ambulatory care facility, your role as a full-spectrum nurse is to support them in their transition from wellness to illness, in dealing with the unknown, and in adjusting to a new environment. The relationship and trust you establish in your first contact with patients can go a long way toward relieving their anxiety and preserving the energy needed for healing. Take time to get to know your client. Try to set a tone of caring, respect, and understanding.

You can make the transition smoother for patients if you are prepared. The following activities should be incorporated into your nursing care:
- *Prepare the room.* A room that is prepared for the client conveys a message of acceptance. Room preparation depends on the type of unit or facility, the client's needs, and the anticipated treatment. See Clinical Insight 11-1.
- *Greet the client and family and introduce yourself.* Gather basic information ahead of time, such as name, diagnosis, and anticipated length of stay. Imagine how it might feel if you were a new patient and you heard the staff say, "Who's this? I didn't know we were getting another admit. How am I supposed to take care of this one, too?"

For detailed directions on how to admit a client to a hospital unit, including orienting the client to the room and gathering a health history, see Procedure 11-1.

Provide a Healing Presence

Part of what you do as a healing presence will never show up in a written care plan. However, your healing presence may be the most important aspect of care that you have to offer. A statement by a young woman undergoing

Clinical Insight 11-1 ➤ **Preparing the Room for a Newly Admitted Patient**

Delegation

As a general rule, these tasks can be delegated to nursing assistive personnel (NAPs). The nurse is responsible for evaluating and supervising, as well as for setting up special equipment (although the NAP may obtain it from storage).

Clean the Room

Agencies differ; however, it is common for the housekeeping department to clean the room and change the bed linens when a patient is discharged, so you should find the room ready for your preparations. The rest of these guidelines assume that fact.

Prepare the Bed

- Position the bed according to patient status. If the patient is ambulatory, put the bed in the lowest position and lock the wheels. If the patient will arrive on a stretcher, place the bed at stretcher height.
- If necessary, rearrange the furniture to allow easy access to the bed.
- Fold back the top linens to "open" the bed (see the figure).
  The patient may need to go to bed immediately, so it should be ready when she arrives.

Prepare Routine Supplies

- Most agencies have an admission pack containing a bath basin, soap, lotion, tissues, water pitcher, and drinking glass. Open it and put it in the room.
- Place a hospital gown on the bed and nonslip footwear by the bedside. Patients may choose to wear their own sleep clothing, though.

Prepare Equipment

You will need the following:

- A stethoscope, thermometer, and blood pressure cuff in the room for taking vital signs
- A scale for measuring and weighing the patient
- Bedpan and urinal if the patient is not ambulatory; possibly a bedside commode
- A clean-catch urine specimen container if laboratory work has not already been done
- Set up and check special equipment (e.g., oxygen, suction, cardiac monitor, pulse oximeter, IV pump).

Prepare the Environment

Turn on the lights and adjust the room temperature. Open or close curtains, as needed.

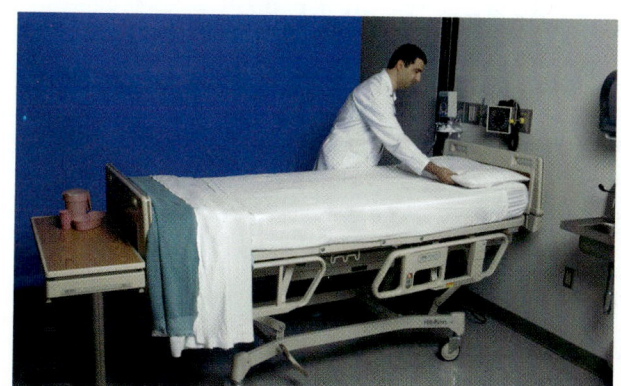

---

chemotherapy illustrates the difference the healing presence of a nurse made:

> The nursing care I got was in response to the physical symptoms I showed. If I was not feeling good, they were sympathetic with me, you know. . . . But it was nothing further than that. There was no exploration of feelings or anything like that.
>
> Some of them were—seemed to be very caring. [One nurse] . . . was just a really nice person. And I remember one time that I was throwing up dreadfully. . . . I rang for her and I said, 'I'm sorry,' and she was almost crying and she said, 'No, I'm sorry you have to do this—you must feel awful.' And she was just very empathetic with it, and I felt like, you know, I wasn't infringing upon her to make her empty my emesis basin or anything like that. (Smith, 1992, pp. 233–234)

Maintain Trust During Transitions

Just as you help patients to transition into illness, your support is important in helping them transition to other units within the agency, other agencies, or home. As discussed in Chapter 5, planning for discharge begins with the admission assessment and continues until the patient is well enough to go home or is transferred to another unit or facility.

Handoffs and Transfers

Patients may transfer from one unit to another when their health status changes. For example, a patient on a general nursing unit may be transferred to an intensive care unit when he develops sepsis (a generalized, systemic infection that is often fatal). Patients may transfer from hospital to a long-term care facility or rehabilitation center when they no longer require an acute care hospital or when their changed health status means that family members will not be able to care for him at home. A patient residing in a long-term care facility may be transferred to a hospital when he becomes acutely ill.

When the patient is transferred, he must adjust to a new environment, new routines, and new caregivers. This is yet another disruption for the patient and family. You can help by ensuring that the transition is smooth and that there is continuity of care. Ensure the patient's comfort and safety, provide for teaching needs, and communicate with the agency or unit sending or receiving the patient. For information on transfer reports, see Chapter 18. Also refer to Procedures 11-2, and 11-3.

Discharge From the Healthcare Facility

As much as patients usually look forward to being discharged, this, too, is a disruption. Patients are discharged when the outcomes of care are met. However, they are often dependent on family members for care and treatments they cannot manage alone. Inability to assume self-care can be stressful and anxiety producing. Successful discharge planning must begin at first patient assessment, on admission to the facility. The same conditions that require a formal discharge plan frequently also indicate the need for referrals for posthospital care in the community. Review Discharge Planning in Chapter 5, as needed.

Procedures for discharge vary among agencies. There may be a discharge planner or case manager to coordinate the transition to another agency or to home, but often you will need to manage the discharge. You can help by communicating and coordinating care and services, and by teaching the patient and caregivers about the continuing care the patient needs (see Figs. 11-5 and 11-6). Also see Procedure 11-4 to learn more about discharging patients from a healthcare facility.

KnowledgeCheck 11-5

Explain how you can promote patient trust during admissions, transfers, and discharges.

Is a Healthy Life Attainable?

The concepts suggested in this chapter for ways to live a healthy life did not come from people who had easy lives. These themes were teased from literature, autobiographies, and interviews with people who were dealing with life situations that would be viewed as difficult from anyone's standpoint. However, in the midst of their circumstances, they were very much involved in *living*. Ripples or even waves of disruption or despair came into their lives, but through it all they evolved an overriding sense of a life worth pursuing. This can be true for you as a nurse and also for those privileged to be under your care.

As a nurse, you offer your personal health and strength to your patients and their families every day. If you barely have enough physical, emotional, and spiritual strength to manage your own stressors, you will not have much available to offer others who are depleted. This is why it is so important for you to nurture yourself in all aspects of your life, to balance learning how to care for others with caring for yourself, to develop yourself as a healing presence in this world.

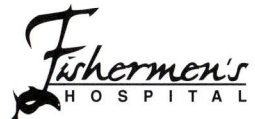

Discharge Assessment/Instructions

Date of Discharge	Time of Discharge	Mode of Discharge ☐ Ambulatory ☐ Wheelchair ☐ Stretcher ☐ Ambulance	Accompanied by:
Belongings sent with patient/family ☐ Yes ☐ No		Personal Medications sent with patient family ☐ Yes ☐ No	
Temp	P	Discharge Destination ☐ Home ☐ AMA ☐ Facility_____ ☐ Home Health	Transfer Information Sent
R	BP		☐ Yes ☐ No

Special Instructions

Patient Assessment and Health Status

	Yes	No		Yes	No		Yes	No
Afebrile	☐	☐	Skin Intact	☐	☐	Hygiene	☐	☐
Able to live independently	☐	☐	Eating Well	☐	☐	Self-Care	☐	☐
Pain Controlled	☐	☐	Adequate Hydration	☐	☐	Assist	☐	☐
Oriented	☐	☐				Total Care	☐	☐
Appropriate Behavior	☐	☐				Adequate Elimination	☐	☐
Functions Independently	☐	☐						

Additional Comments:

Weight monitoring daily   Avoid all tobacco products

Instructions

Diet
☐ No Restrictions

Activity
☐ No Restrictions

Special Equipment/Treatment
☐ No Restrictions

Discharge Medications (Name, Amount, Special Instructions)
☐ No Meds   See Patient Education

Special Instructions/Discharge Summary
Call MD or go to the ER if symptoms worsen

☐ Pt or Caregiver given instructions about and counseled on potential for drug-food interactions

Physician Follow-up Appointment	Outpatient Visit

Referral
☐ None Required

I have received all personal belongings.
I have received a copy and understand the above Instructions.
I have received a copy of the Patient Education form.

_____

Signature/Responsible Party

_____

Physician/Nurse Signature   Date

Patient Identification

0916065

FIGURE 11-5 Discharge assessment/instructions.

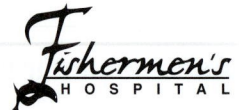

Fishermen's HOSPITAL

3301 Overseas Highway, Marathon, FL 33050 • Ph 305-743-5533 • Fax 305-743-3962

Allergies/Reactions No known drug allergies ☐			IN-PATIENT Circle Y to continue or N to not continue and sign below to authenticate order.			AT DISCHARGE Circle Y to continue at same dose or N to not continue or document any changes in dose.		

MEDICATION NAME (Include Herbal, OTC, Vitamins)	Dose / Route / Freq	Reason Taken	LAST DOSE DATE/TIME	Continue on Admission		Continue at home on same dose		Continue with the following changes:
Patient takes no medication ☐								
				Y	N	Y	N	
				Y	N	Y	N	
				Y	N	Y	N	
				Y	N	Y	N	
				Y	N	Y	N	
				Y	N	Y	N	
				Y	N	Y	N	
				Y	N	Y	N	
				Y	N	Y	N	
				Y	N	Y	N	
				Y	N	Y	N	
				Y	N	Y	N	
				Y	N	Y	N	
				Y	N	Y	N	

Source-of-Medication list *(check all used):*
___ **Bottles/List**
___ **Patient/Family**
___ **Retail pharmacy**_____
_____
___ **MD office records**
___ **Previous discharge medical record**
___ **Medication Administration Record from**_____
___ **Med Reconciliation Form**

Meds:
___ **Sent home with**_____
___ **Removed**
    Sent to Pharmacy for approval

New medications prescribed for patient discharge:		
Meds	Dose / Route / Freq	Reason

ADMITTING NURSE SIGNATURE DATE	DISCHARGE NURSE SIGNATURE DATE

Patient Education Form

Page ____ of ____

FORM N-100, Rev. 12-07   White: Chart   Yellow: Patient

FIGURE 11-6 Patient education form.

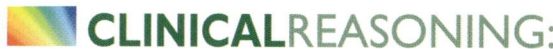 **CLINICAL**REASONING:
Applying the **Full-Spectrum Nursing Model**

Because the following critical thinking activities allow you to practice the kind of thinking you will use as a full-spectrum nurse, they usually have no single right answer. Discuss them with your peers—if you have difficulty with any of the questions, consult your instructor.

PATIENT SITUATION

Recall Evelyn (Meet Your Patient). Evelyn is 87 years old and has lived in a nursing home for the past 5 years. She suffers from CHF, hypertension, diabetes, macular degeneration resulting in near blindness, a severe hearing deficit, urinary incontinence, and immobility resulting from a hip fracture. Despite these limitations, she keeps current in the lives of all of her family members and friends. At the nursing home, staff members confide in Evelyn and she knows about their children, their romances, and the gossip around the nursing home. Whenever there is an election, she makes sure that she gets to vote. She "reads" every audio book she can get her hands on.

Recently Evelyn was admitted to the hospital in severe CHF. When leaving the nursing home, she told her pastor, "I don't want to die yet. I'm having too much fun!" You notice that the papers from the nursing home do not contain an advance directive, and it was not mentioned in their report to you.

THINKING

1. *Critical Thinking (Considering Alternatives):*
   a. What are some possible reasons that that there is no advance directive?
   b. Which of those seems most likely to you?
   c. How might you find out about the status of Evelyn's advance directive?

DOING

2. *Nursing Process (Nursing Diagnosis):* On the care plan from the nursing home, there were two nursing diagnoses:
   - Urge Urinary Incontinence related to difficulty ambulating to bathroom
   - Impaired Skin Integrity related to immobility and incontinence
   Which of these can you remove from the care plan for now? Explain your decision.

CARING

3. *Self-Knowledge:* The next day, despite aggressive treatment, Evelyn's condition worsens. She is not responding to verbal stimuli and her oxygen level is decreasing. There is discussion about putting her on a ventilator.
   a. What would you be feeling?
   b. If Evelyn has an advance directive that says "No ventilator," how would that change your feelings?
   c. If there is an advance directive that says, "Do everything possible to keep me alive," how would that change your feelings?
   Note: We are not asking you what you would do, rather, how you would feel.

 Go To Chapter 11, **Clinical Reasoning: Applying the Full-Spectrum Nursing Model Response Sheet** on Davis*Plus*.

PROCEDURES

The procedures in this chapter are designed to help you admit, transfer, and discharge patients in such a way that you can begin, at first contact, to establish trust.

Procedure 11–1 ■ Admitting a Patient to a Nursing Unit

➤ For steps to follow in all procedures, refer to the Universal Steps for All Procedures found on the page facing the inside back cover of this book.

Equipment

- Identifying armband (if this has not been done in the admissions department)
- Patient's chart, including physician's orders and nursing admission record
- Thermometer, blood pressure cuff, and stethoscope
- Scales for height and weight
- Gown
- Admission pack (e.g., bath basin, water pitcher, soap, comb, toothbrush, mouthwash, and facial tissues)
- Nursing care plan or clinical pathway, if one has already been made
- Hospital brochures, Patient Care Partnership, and other forms
- Admission assessment form

Delegation

A registered nurse is responsible for managing medical orders and assessing the patient's need for nursing care in all settings, although this may vary in some specifics according to hospital policy, the law, and regulations. Most other admission activities can be delegated to a NAP if the patient is stable.

Pre-Procedure Assessments

- Assess for signs of emotional and/or physical distress.
- Assess ability to ambulate and/or move.
- Assess ability to communicate and understand what is occurring.

➤ When performing the procedure, always identify your patient according to agency policy and be attentive to standard precautions, hand hygiene, patient safety and privacy, body mechanics, and documentation.

Procedure Steps

1. **Ensure placement of patient labels** (e.g., on the chart, at the bedside, outside the door).
2. **Introduce yourself to the patient and family.** Explain who you are. Don't be afraid to tell a client that you are a nursing student.
   Many clients are aware that students have more time to spend with them. Talking to the patient and family reassures them and provides information about the patient's level of consciousness and awareness, social relationships, and so on.
3. **Assist the patient into a hospital gown.**
   If the patient is able to stand, assist her into a gown before weighing her to obtain the most accurate weight.
4. **Measure height and weight** while the patient stands on a floor scale, if possible. If she is unable to stand, transfer her into the bed and measure her weight using a bed scale.
   Weigh in the same manner each time to ensure accuracy.

5. **Assist the patient into the bed.**
   Get the patient comfortable before continuing the admission to prevent overtiring her.
6. ✚ **Check the patient's identification band** to ensure the information, including allergies, is correct. Verify this information with the patient or family.

   Questioning the patient about allergies and verifying with the family will ensure that the information is accurate and documented on the wristband and the chart.
7. **Measure vital signs.**
   Measuring the vital signs before completing the rest of the admission ensures that you will be aware of the patient's status. If the vital signs are abnormal, further assess the patient's condition before continuing. Report your findings to the admitting care provider.
8. **Complete the nursing admission assessment,** including health history and physical assessment. Be sure to include the patient's expectations and concerns. For inpatients,

this must be completed within 24 hours after admission. All patients should be screened on admission for risk for pressure ulcers. (Chapter 21 provides a step-by-step approach to physical assessment.)

An admission assessment is needed to identify problems and establish a baseline. The Joint Commission requires that each patient have an admission assessment performed by a registered nurse.

9. ✚ **Check that the list of the patient's current medications** (created in the admitting department) is complete and accurate. Usually the patient's own medications are sent home with the family, or they may be sent to pharmacy for storage.

It is important to know what medications the patient has been taking. The pharmacy will identify medicines from home when necessary. When medications are ordered and given during the patient's stay, they are compared to those on the list so any discrepancies can be resolved.

10. **Orient the client to the room.**
These actions ensure that the patient and family will be able to call for assistance if needed and increase the patient's and family's level of comfort and ability to function in the hospital setting. Remember that one of the disruptions associated with illness is anxiety about the unknown. If you tell your client what to expect, you help to minimize his anxiety.
   a. Make sure that the client knows how to use the bed, the call light, and any equipment that you expect him to use.
   b. Point out the location of personal care items.
   c. Show the client the location of the restroom.
   d. If you will be measuring the client's intake and output, tell him so during your orientation.
      If the client is alert, he may be able to assist you with these measures.

11. **Explain hospital routines,** including use of side rails, meal times, and so on. Answer the patient's and family's questions.
    Hospitalization takes away control of basic decisions. Knowing the routines and available choices increases patient and family comfort.

12. **Verify with the patient that all other admission data on the chart are complete.**
    Basic data such as name, address, marital status, name of admitting physician, admitting diagnosis, consent to treatment, and so on will usually be obtained in the admitting office. However, you will need to be sure all the admitting information is complete, and complete it if it is not.

13. **Ask the patient if he has an advance directive** (e.g., power of attorney or living will). If so, place a copy in the hospital record. If not, explain the purpose of the document and give the patient a form to fill out if he wishes to do so. (See Chapters 17 and 43 if you need more information about advance directives.)
    Advance directives enable patients to indicate their preferences about treatments and prolonging life.

14. **Advise the patient of his privacy rights under HIPAA.** See that he has a written explanation of his privacy rights (see Chapter 43 as needed).

15. **Inventory the patient's belongings.** Encourage the family to take home valuable items and money. If that is not possible, arrange to have valuables placed in the hospital safe. Most agencies require money in excess of $5.00 to be sent home or to the cashier's office.
    Patient belongings, including valuables, are frequently lost during hospitalization. Documenting the disposition of everything ensures being able to return the belongings to the patient upon discharge.

16. **Complete or ensure that all admission orders have been completed** (e.g., laboratory tests, medications, diet and fluid orders).
    Unless it is an unscheduled admission, diagnostic tests are usually completed on an outpatient basis before admission to the hospital. However, there may still be some orders that need to be done immediately, while others can be delayed. Make sure the orders are completed in the most appropriate time frame.

17. **Ensure patient comfort** (e.g., positioning, pain, water at bedside).

18. ✚ **Make one last safety check** (i.e., call light within reach, bed in low position, side rails up as appropriate, equipment functioning properly).

19. **Before leaving, ask if there is anything else you can do** for the patient and family.

20. **Initiate the care plan or clinical pathway.**
    Identifying the patient's priority problems enables the nurse to develop the most appropriate nursing orders.

❓ What if . . .

■ ✚ **The patient may be at risk for falls?**

Perform falls risk assessment as appropriate to the patient, and according to agency policy.
Falls are common in inpatient facilities, especially among older adults. If a patient has falls risk factors, risk reduction measures can be instituted.

■ ✚ **The patient has special care needs?**

When the patient has special needs, such as allergies, a nothing by mouth (NPO) order, or an intake and output order, post patient care reminders at the head of the bed or at the door to remind other care providers.

■ **The patient needs a more in-depth assessment in some areas?**

Perform special needs assessments as relevant to the care and condition of the patient (social situation, nutrition and hydration status, functional abilities, spiritual and cultural variables). If these are warranted, they must be completed within 24 hours after admission or prior to surgery.
In-depth assessment of these topics is not a part of all admission assessments, but should be done if the patient's condition warrants.

■ **The patient has a learning disability?**

If possible, preadmissions should be arranged for the patient and main caregiver. This allows more time to discuss issues of consent, alleviate anxiety, and set up links with a learning disability specialist or social worker. Whether or not this is possible, allow more time for the admission process.
Use short sentences, with one idea at a time.
Include the caregiver in the admission process, but encourage the patient to participate as much as possible.
Document the main caregiver and contact numbers.
Expect the patient to be anxious.
Include special communication and personal needs in the plan of care.
Give the patient hospital information with pictures, such as those given to children, if appropriate for her developmental level.

■ **The patient is an older adult?**

Ask all older adults if they have had any falls in the past year. If they report a fall, observe them as they stand up from a chair without using their arms, walk several paces, and return ("get up and go"). If they are steady, no further assessment is required. If there is unsteadiness or if the person reports more than one fall, further assessment is required.
The incidence and severity of fall-related complications rise steadily after age 60.

(continued on next page)

Procedure 11–1 ■ Admitting a Patient to a Nursing Unit (continued)

Falls rates in nursing homes and hospitals are almost three times the rate for those living at home.

■ **The patient is a child?**

Use a friendly approach.

The first priority is to establish a trusting relationship with the child and parents to help relieve fears and anxiety. Children younger than 3 years may fear being separated *from parents. Older children usually worry more about what is going to happen to them.*

Explain the visiting and rooming-in policies to the parents.

Ask about the child's usual routine (e.g., toileting, bedtime rituals, favorite foods).

Speak to the child directly if she is old enough to understand.

Direct the family to the bathroom, playroom, television, and snack room, if those are available.

Encourage the parents to bring toys and other favorite items from home.

It helps the child feel more comfortable in the unfamiliar surroundings.

Documentation

■ Document all assessment findings on the admission database provided by the institution. If you need an example,

 Go to Chapter 3, **Tables, Boxes, Figures; ESG Figure 3-1: Nursing Admission Data Form,** on Davis*Plus.*

■ Document an admission note and any teaching or other interventions in the nursing notes or flow sheet (according to agency policy).

■ Recall that a discharge plan is created on admission. If you need to see a discharge plan, go to Chapter 5, Discharge Planning Form.

Practice Resources

The American Geriatrics Society, n.d.; The Joint Commission, 2008a.

Procedure 11–2 ■ Transferring a Patient to Another Unit in the Agency

➤ For steps to follow in all procedures, refer to the Universal Steps for All Procedures found on page facing the inside back cover of this book.

Equipment

■ Medical record or chart
■ Care plan
■ Patient's medications
■ Supplies for any ongoing treatments
■ Patient's belongings, clothes, and personal care articles
■ Standardized handoff form, if available
■ A utility cart, if belongings are numerous
■ Wheelchair or transfer cart, if bed is not being moved

Delegation

If the patient's condition allows, you can delegate the physical transfer of the patient and have the NAP move the patient's belongings to the other room. However, as the nurse, you are responsible for obtaining and completing the necessary records, making the final assessment, and gathering and checking the medications. You must also give the handoff report to another nurse.

Pre-Procedure Assessment

■ Make a final, brief focused physical assessment.
■ Assess the patient's mobility and ability to assist.
■ Assess for emotional and/or physical distress (administer medications, as needed).
■ Assess the patient's ability to communicate and understand what is occurring.

➤ When performing the procedure, always identify your patient according to agency policy and be attentive to standard precautions, hand hygiene, patient safety and privacy, body mechanics, and documentation.

Procedure Steps

1. ✚ **Obtain the number of personnel needed to make a safe transfer.**
For efficiency and patient and staff safety.

2. **Gather the patient's medications and label them correctly for the new room.**
Ensures availability of medications when the patient arrives at the new unit; helps prevent medication administration errors.

3. **Notify the receiving unit of the time to expect the transfer; notify other departments** (e.g., dietary, pharmacy, admitting), primary care provider, and family of the transfer.
You need to schedule the transfer with the receiving nurse so he can plan his

work and so you can arrange the transfer time to limit the number of interruptions during the handoff. Limiting interruptions minimizes the possibility of failing to communicate or forgetting information. Other departments must have the transfer data so that services such as meals and physical therapy treatments will not be interrupted. The primary care provider and family, of course, need to know where to find the patient.

4. **Gather the patient's personal belongings, and supplies,** including treatment-related supplies and equipment (e.g., isolation supplies, clean dressings), chart, Kardex, and care plan. Place in a container (e.g., the patient's bath basin) or on a utility cart if necessary.
   Having the supplies and equipment "ready to go" makes the transfer more efficient for you and less stressful for the patient.

5. **Bring the wheelchair or transfer cart to the bedside** and assist the patient to the chair or cart. If using a wheelchair, the patient can hold the pan of supplies; if using a bed or cart, place supplies on the bed.

6. **Take the patient to the new room and give the handoff report.** Follow agency procedure for handoff reports. However, the method chosen should allow both the giver and receiver of patient information the opportunity for questioning.
   a. If you need to review content of an oral handoff report, see

Chapter 18. In general, the report should include name, age, sex, physicians, surgical procedures, medical diagnoses, medications, allergies, laboratory data, special equipment (e.g., oxygen, suction), the patient's current health status, and whether there are advance directives and resuscitation status. Identify the nursing diagnoses and priorities for nursing care.
   b. Consistently use a structured framework or memory aid to guide the handoff process and the oral report.
   The objective of a handoff is to provide accurate information about the patient. The information communicated must be accurate in order to ensure patient safety.

   c. ✚ Be sure to point out to the nurse if patient is taking corticosteroids, anticoagulants, diabetic medications, antibiotics, or narcotic analgesics.

   These medications can have serious side effects and need careful monitoring.

? What if . . .

- **The patient has intravenous (IV) lines and other equipment that cannot be turned off?**

It is common to transfer patients with IV lines. Some wheelchairs are equipped with an IV pole; for others,

you may need to obtain a rolling pole from the unit supply room. The patient may be able to maneuver the rolling pole. Most beds and transfer carts also have portable IV poles, sometimes stored along the underside. Portable oxygen and suction are also available for patients who must have them even during transfer. Be sure to obtain these, set them up, and check their functioning prior to moving the patient from his bed.

- **The patient has too many personal belongings for one person to carry?**

If the patient's condition requires two staff members to transfer, one person can manage the utility cart while the other manages the patient. If only one person can make the actual move, load a utility cart and move all the supplies and belongings to the new room before transferring the patient.

- **The patient is being transferred to the intensive care unit (ICU)?**

If this is an urgent transfer, you may need to notify the receiving nurse and move the patient with his records and medications. Later you can make the other notifications, finish the charting, and move belongings and other supplies. In some ICUs, the family may need to take the patient's personal belongings home.

Evaluation

With the receiving nurse, evaluate the patient's response to the move. The receiving nurse will take vital signs and make a preliminary admission assessment.

Documentation

Just before moving, document as much information as you can, including the patient's status at that time. After handoff,

document the information reported in handoff, the name and title of the person who received the patient, and your report. Sign the note. Some agencies have a standardized form for the transfer note.

Practice Resources

The Joint Commission, 2008a; McFetridge, Gillespie, Goode, et al., 2007.

Procedure 11–3 ■ Transferring a Patient to a Long-Term Care Facility

➤ For steps to follow in all procedures, refer to the Universal Steps for All Procedures found on the page facing the inside back cover of this book.

Equipment

- Health record or chart
- Care plan
- Patient's medications
- Supplies for any ongoing treatments
- Patient's belongings, clothes, and personal care articles
- Standardized transfer form, if available
- A utility cart, if belongings are numerous
- Wheelchair or transfer cart

Delegation

If the patient's condition allows, you can delegate the physical transfer of the patient and have the NAP move the patient's supplies and belongings. However, as the nurse, you are responsible for obtaining and completing the necessary records, making the final assessment, and gathering and checking the medications. You must also give the handoff report to another nurse.

Pre-Procedure Assessment

- Make a final, brief focused physical assessment.
- Assess the patient's mobility and ability to assist.
- Assess for emotional and/or physical distress (administer medications, as needed).
- Assess the patient's ability to communicate and understand what is occurring.

➤ When performing the procedure, always identify your patient according to agency policy and be attentive to standard precautions, hand hygiene, patient safety and privacy, body mechanics, and documentation.

Procedure Steps

1. **Notify the patient and family well in advance** of the upcoming transfer to another facility. Include information about the reasons the patient is being transferred, as well as any alternatives to transfer. You will also need to determine which agency is to arrange transportation for the patient.
Allows them time to adjust emotionally and to make any necessary plans.

2. **Prepare the patient's records.** You may need to send a copy of the patient's health record to the receiving facility. The original remains with the hospital. You will usually also send a copy of the comprehensive nursing assessment and a detailed nursing care plan, as well as prescriptions and cards for future appointments (e.g., with physicians or social workers).
Ensures continuity of care, thus minimizing patient stress.

3. **Gather and pack the patient's personal items and treatment supplies** to send to the long-term care facility with the patient.
Having the supplies and equipment "ready to go" makes the transfer more efficient for you.

4. ✚ **Be certain the medications are labeled correctly.**
Ensures availability and correct administration of medications when the patient arrives at the new facility.

5. **Coordinate the transfer.** Notify the receiving facility of the time to expect the transfer and of any special equipment the patient will need (e.g., IV pole, portable oxygen); notify other hospital departments (e.g., dietary, pharmacy, admitting), primary care provider, and family of the transfer.
You need to schedule the transfer with the receiving agency so they can plan their work and so you can arrange the transfer at a time that will limit the number of interruptions during the transfer. Other in-house departments must have the transfer data so that services such as meals and physical therapy treatments will be discontinued. The primary care provider and family, of course, need to know where to find the patient.

6. **Just before transfer, make your final quick assessment and sign off your charting** (usually there is a preprinted, standardized discharge form for this purpose).
It is important to complete documentation in a timely manner, but it is also important to provide the most recent assessment data to the long-term care facility.

7. **Take the patient off the unit and out of the hospital after you are notified that transportation has arrived** (or delegate this task). Alternatively, a transporter may come to your unit to get the patient.

(*Note:* Some agencies ask you to remove the patient's identification band at time of transfer.)
Keeping the patient on the unit as long as practical helps to minimize his anxiety and fatigue that may occur from a long wait in the hospital lobby.

8. **Give an oral report** to the nurse at the long-term care facility. You will usually give a telephone report unless a nurse comes to your hospital to accompany the patient. The report should include, as appropriate for the care, treatment, and services provided, the following:
   a. The reason the patient is being transferred
   b. The patient's physical and psychosocial status
   c. A summary of care, treatment, and services provided and progress toward outcomes
   d. Referrals, community resources provided to the patient
   A report helps ensure continuity of care and provide a baseline for later changes in the patient's health status.

- ✚ Consistently use a structured framework or memory aid to guide the handoff process and the oral report.
The objective of a handoff report is to provide accurate information about the patient. The information communicated must be accurate in order to ensure patient safety.

- Notify the long-term care agency if the patient is colonized or infected with MRSA or other contagious microorganisms.
So they can arrange for and communicate any special isolation or care activities to their staff. MRSA is a serious problem for long-term care residents

- Be sure to point out to the nurse if patient is taking corticosteroids, anticoagulants, diabetic medications, antibiotics, or narcotic analgesics.
These medications confer particularly high risk of adverse postdischarge drug events, and the long-term care nurses will need to continue careful monitoring.

? What if . . .

- **The patient has IV lines and other equipment that cannot be turned off?**

It is common to transfer patients with IV lines. Some wheelchairs are equipped with an IV pole. If you need to hold the IV bag while taking the patient to the transporting vehicle, always hold the bag well above the patient's chest and arm so that blood does not back up in the tubing. Also, you should notify the long-term care facility so they will have the necessary equipment in the transport vehicle. Portable oxygen and suction are also available for patients who must have them. Usually the receiving facility will bring these, but you need to coordinate that in advance.

- **When you are ready to transfer the patient, her condition worsens and she becomes unstable?**

Perform interventions to stabilize the patient, call for help if needed, and notify the medical provider. Notify the transporter and the long-term care center of the change and postpone the transfer until further medical assessment is done.

Evaluation

The receiving nurse at the long-term care facility will evaluate the patient's response to the move.

Documentation

Just before the transfer, document your final assessment and complete the agency's discharge summary. You will probably put your final nursing note on a transfer or discharge summary, similar to the ones shown in Figures 11-5 and 11-6.

Practice Resources

The Joint Commission, 2008a; McFetridge, Gillespie, Goode, et al., 2007.

Procedure 11–4 ■ Discharging a Patient From the Healthcare Facility

➤ For steps to follow in all procedures, refer to the Universal Steps for All Procedures found on the inside back cover of this book.

Equipment

- Health record or chart
- Patient's medications
- Supplies for any ongoing treatments
- Patient's belongings, clothes, and personal care articles
- Standardized discharge form, if available, with instructions for patient
- A utility cart, if belongings are numerous
- Wheelchair

Delegation

If the patient's condition allows, you can delegate to the NAP such tasks as packing belongings, helping the patient dress, and taking the patient out of the facility. However, as the nurse, you are responsible for obtaining and completing the necessary records, making the final assessment, gathering and checking the medications, and coordinating care.

Pre-Procedure Assessment

- Make a final, brief focused physical assessment.
- Assess the patient's mobility.
- Assess for emotional and/or physical distress.
- Assess the patient's ability to communicate and understand what is occurring.

➤ When performing the procedure, always identify your patient according to agency policy and be attentive to standard precautions, hand hygiene, patient safety and privacy, body mechanics, and documentation.

Procedure Steps

1. **Notify the patient and family as much in advance of the discharge as possible.** This is often done early in the hospital stay.
Allows them time to adjust emotionally and to make any necessary plans.

A Day or Two Before Discharge (Steps 2 and 3)

2. **Make or confirm necessary arrangements.**
   a. Arrange for or help the family arrange for services (e.g., home healthcare, physical therapy, intravenous therapy, social worker) that will be needed at home.

NOTE: To reimburse for home care, insurers require a physician's order for all services, and the patient must meet certain eligibility criteria.

(continued on next page)

Procedure 11–4 ■ Discharging a Patient From the Healthcare Facility (continued)

b. Confirm or arrange for equipment needed in the home (e.g., portable oxygen).

c. Confirm or arrange for transportation.

d. Make necessary referrals (e.g., medical specialists, physical therapists); book appointments, if necessary and if in line with agency policy.

Hospital stays are short, and many patients are still ill enough to require complex treatments and care by family members when they go home.

3. **Communicate and provide teaching to the patient and caregivers.**

Patients who have a clear understanding of their after-hospital care (e.g., medications, follow-up visits) are 30% less likely to visit the emergency department or be readmitted than patients who lack this information (Agency for Healthcare Research and Quality, 2009).

a. Discuss the patient's diagnosis, care needs, and functional abilities with the family/caregiver.

b. Train the patient and caregiver in the use of equipment. Arrange for follow-up evaluation at home to check that equipment is working and being used correctly, and that further training is given if needed.

In the stress of illness and the disruption of transition home, patients may not retain what they are taught in the hospital. Therapies will be ineffective if equipment is used incorrectly, so follow-up is essential to help avoid further illness and hospital readmission.

c. Educate about medication use and side effects.

Medication errors at home are a frequent cause of adverse events and readmissions to the hospital.

d. Ask relatives or the caregiver to bring clothing for the patient to wear home, if needed.

If this was an unplanned admission, the patient may have come in nightwear and a robe.

Day of Discharge (Steps 4 Through 16)

4. **Make and document final assessments.**

a. Assess that the patient's condition remains as expected.

b. Confirm that the patient has house keys, heating is turned on, and food is available.

c. Follow up on diagnostic and laboratory test results.

5. **Bring a wheelchair or other transport device to the bedside.**

6. **Make final notifications.**

a. Contact the family or guardian; confirm transportation.

b. Notify community service agencies and home health nursing of the discharge, as needed.

7. **Gather prescriptions, a list of current medications, any other instruction sheets, and appointment cards;** give to the patient along with the discharge instructions at discharge. Be certain that either the patient or caregiver can read the instructions.

Inadequate literacy has been shown to be a risk factor for readmission.

8. **Gather and pack the patient's personal items and treatment supplies.**

Having the supplies and equipment ready to go makes the transfer more efficient for you and less stressful for the patient and family.

9. ✚ **Prepare the patient's medications.** Be certain the medications are labeled correctly; pack them, and record which medications he is taking home.

This ensures availability and correct administration of medications when the patient arrives home. It also provides a legal record that the patient left with the medications.

10. **Review the following discharge instructions with patient and caregiver** (and provide a written copy to take home).

a. Medication instructions

b. Symptom management and treatments

c. When and with which care provider for the follow-up appointment(s)

d. How to obtain further care, treatment, and services, as needed

e. How and when to call the physician or primary care provider; including signs of a change in condition

f. Whom to contact in an emergency

g. Diet restrictions

h. Maintenance of hydration

i. Activities of daily living, focusing on safety and mobility

Of course, teaching should occur throughout the hospital stay. However, it is important to reinforce with a last-minute summary and written instructions to take home. With the stress of illness and anticipation of discharge, patients may not retain what they are taught.

11. **Address any questions or concerns** of the patient and caregiver.

Improves the ability to transition to home.

12. **Give new prescriptions to the patient, as well as reminder cards** for outpatient appointments (e.g., with social services, physicians).

Ensures continuity of care, thus minimizing patient stress.

13. **Document your final nursing note and complete the discharge summary** (the patient often receives a copy of the summary). The patient needs a copy of (a) his instructions for care at home, which may be called a discharge plan; (b) his discharge summary; and (c) a summary of the progress of his illness and treatment from admission through discharge. Some agencies combine these into one form.

It is important to document the patient's condition at the time he leaves the unit. This provides a baseline for comparison if his condition should deteriorate after discharge.

14. **When you are notified that transportation has arrived,**

accompany the patient off the unit and out of the hospital (or delegate this task).

Keeping the patient on the unit as long as practical helps to minimize the anxiety and fatigue that may occur from a long wait in the hospital lobby while a family member brings a car to the door.

15. **Notify the admissions department of the discharge.** Depending on agency policy, notify the primary care or admitting physician.

This will stop all scheduled services, such as meals, and notify the housekeeping department that the room needs to be cleaned.

16. **Ensure the patient's records are sent to the medical records department.**

Whether paper or electronic, the health record is a legal document and remains permanently in storage in the healthcare institution.

? What if . . .

- ✚ **Near the time of discharge, the patient's condition worsens and he becomes unstable?**

Perform interventions to stabilize the patient, call for help if needed, and notify the provider. Notify the family that discharge will be delayed. Communicate with other hospital departments and community agencies as necessary.

- **The patient is an older adult?**

Allow for more time to dress and leave the hospital.

Allow for more time to communicate, teach, and answer questions.

Obtain feedback to be certain the caregivers have heard and understood instructions.

Consider having a geriatric nurse specialist make follow-up home visits.

Hearing, visual, and mobility deficits become more common with advanced age.

- ✚ **The patient is taking "high-risk" drugs postdischarge?**

Medications with a high risk of postdischarge adverse events include corticosteroids, anticoagulants, diabetic medications, antibiotics, anti-anxiety agents, sedatives, and narcotic analgesics.

Provide teaching for patient, family, and other caregivers throughout the hospital stay. A day or two before discharge, review teaching with patient and family; evaluate their understanding.

On discharge, summarize medication precautions and provide clear written instructions. Be sure the patient and family can read them.

Evaluation

A few weeks after discharge, the facility will contact the patient to evaluate the quality and appropriateness of the discharge process. This may be done by making a home visit, telephoning, or sending a questionnaire. As a nurse, you may or may not be involved in this evaluation. The best evaluation of the multidisciplinary care will be whether the patient must be readmitted to the acute care facility.

Documentation

- For the health record, the primary provider will write a discharge progress note that contains the following information:
  - Reason for hospitalization
  - Significant findings during the stay, including significant changes in status since admission
  - Procedures performed; care, treatment, and services provided during the stay
  - Status of goals for the stay
  - Condition at discharge
- Agency policy determines the format and content of nursing documentation. This is often a combination of a structured discharge form or checklist and a narrative progress note. Regardless of format, you should document the following information:
  - Your final assessment of the patient's health status
  - Information and teaching provided to the patient and caregivers

- Referrals, medications
- How patient left the unit (e.g., in wheelchair) and who accompanied him (e.g., wife, name of staff member)

The Joint Commission recommends standardized formats for documentation.

To see examples of discharge summaries, refer to Figures 11-5 and 11-6

Practice Resources

Agency for Healthcare Research and Quality, 2009; Dudas, 2001; Greenwald, Denham, & Jack, 2007; The Joint Commission, 2008a, 2008b; Naylor, Brooten, Jones, et al., 1994; Phillips, Wright, Kern, et al., 2004; Zwicker, & Picariello, 2003.

To explore learning resources for this chapter,

 Go to DavisPlus at **http://davisplus.fadavis.com/Treas1**

Chapter Resources for Chapter 11:
  Knowledge Check and Think Like a Nurse Response Sheets
  Knowledge Check Answers
  Resources for Caregivers and Health Professionals
  Reading More About Experiencing Health & Illness (suggested readings)
  What Are the Main Points in This Chapter?
NCLEX-Style Review Questions
Chapter Overview Podcasts

Concept Map

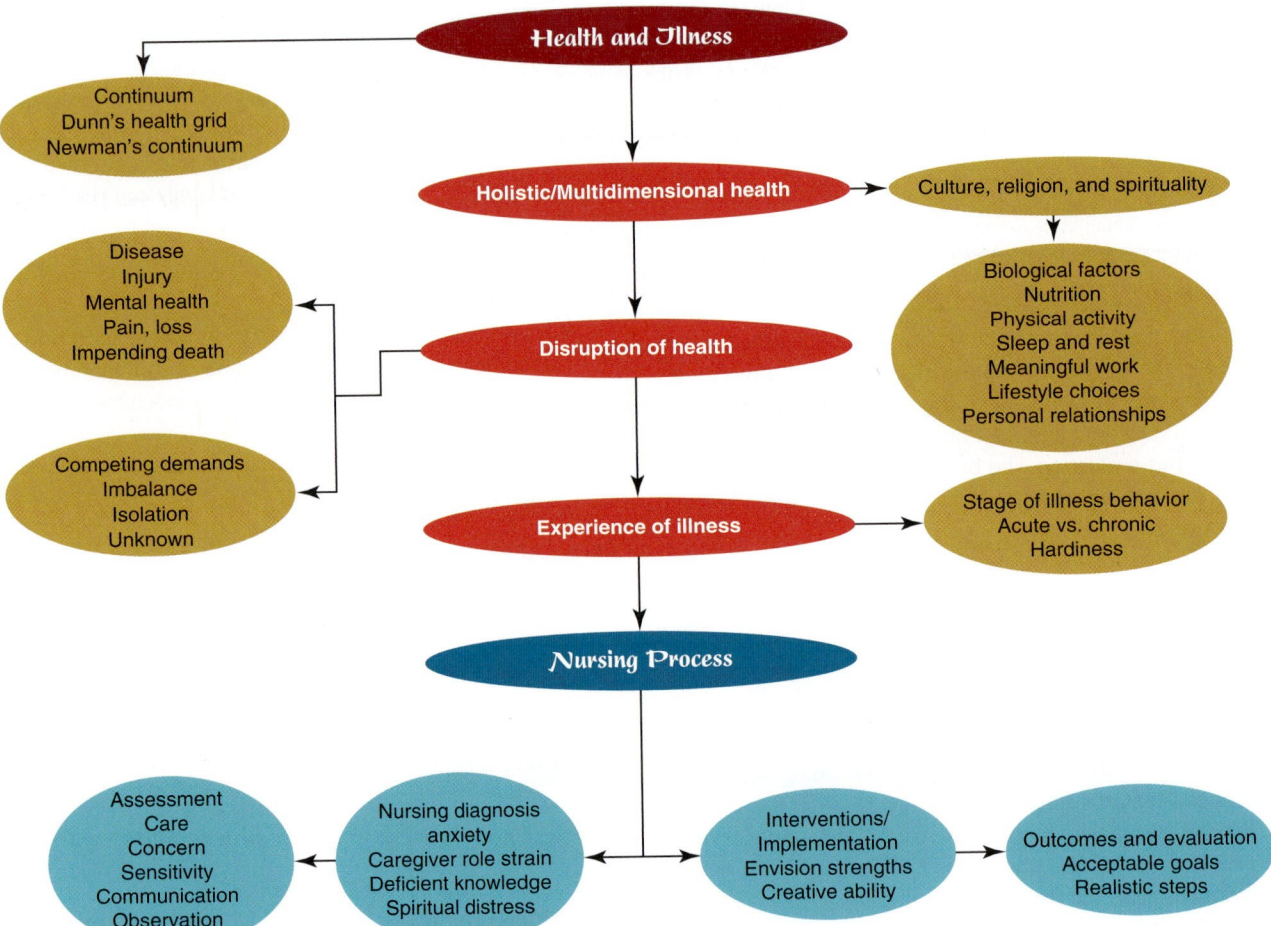

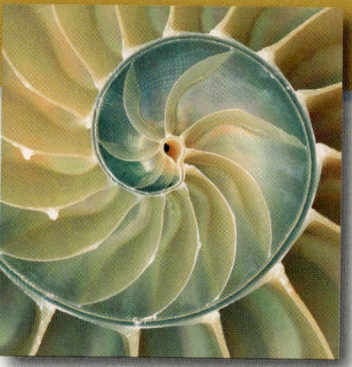

CHAPTER 12

Stress & Adaptation

Learning Outcomes

After completing this chapter, you should be able to:

➤ Define *stress*.

➤ Explain the difference between adaptive and maladaptive coping strategies.

➤ Explain the relationship between stressors, responses, and adaptation.

➤ Describe physical changes occurring during the three stages of Selye's general adaptation syndrome (GAS).

➤ Explain how Selye's local adaptation syndrome (LAS) is different from the GAS.

➤ Discuss the inflammatory response: What triggers it, and what physiological changes occur?

➤ Explain how anxiety, fear, and anger relate to stress.

➤ Provide examples and definitions of specific ego defense mechanisms.

➤ Describe the effects of prolonged stress and unsuccessful adaptation on the various body systems.

➤ Compare and contrast hypochondriasis, somatization, somatoform pain disorder, and malingering.

➤ Compare and contrast crisis and burnout.

➤ State three ways in which you could assess for each of the following: (1) stressors and risk factors, (2) coping methods and adaptation, (3) physiological responses to stress, (4) emotional and behavioral responses to stresses, (5) cognitive responses to stress, and (6) adequacy of support systems.

➤ Describe several interventions or activities for preventing and managing stress.

Key Concepts

Adaptation
Coping
Stress

Related Concepts

See the Concept Map at the end of this chapter.

Caring for the Nguyens

This feature allows you to practice the kind of thinking you will use as a full-spectrum nurse. There is usually more than one correct answer to a critical thinking question, so we do not provide answers for these questions. It is more important to develop your nursing judgment than to "cover content." Discuss the questions with your peers. If you are still unsure, consult your instructor.

After having a comprehensive physical exam at the family health center, Yen Nguyen has been scheduled to have a mammogram and screening laboratory work. When she arrives at the clinic for her mammogram, she tells you she is very nervous. "I have a good friend who just found out she has breast cancer. She's very depressed now. Do I really have to do this test?":

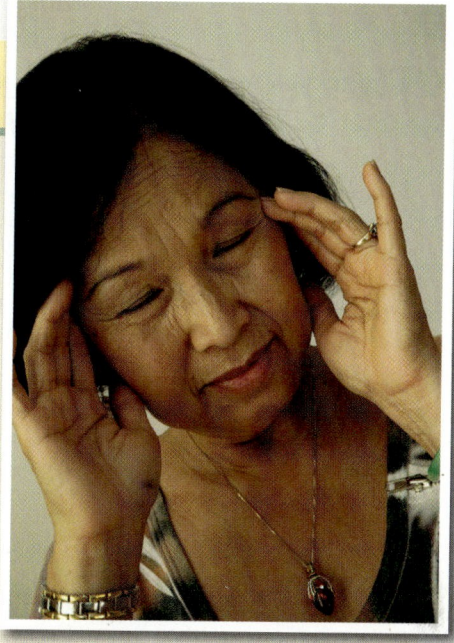

(Continued)

Caring for the Nguyens (continued)

A. What kind of stress is Yen experiencing?

B. Three days later, the radiologist contacts Yen, requesting that she return to the family health center for additional films of the upper outer quadrant of the right breast. "There are some calcifications I want to check out," explains the radiologist.
- What factors might affect Yen's adaptation to this stress?
- Evaluate what you know about Yen's perception of her stress, her overall health status, her support system, and her coping methods.

- What more do you need to know about these topics to fully answer this question?

C. Later, Yen calls the office, frantically explaining that she is very upset about this recent event. She says, "Not knowing is killing me. I'm so nervous I can't stand it! I can't sleep. I can't eat." She asks how she can handle the stress until she comes in for the additional tests next week. What strategies would you recommend to help Yen deal with the stress?

 Go to **Caring for the Nguyens Response Sheet,** on *DavisPlus.*

Meet Your Patients

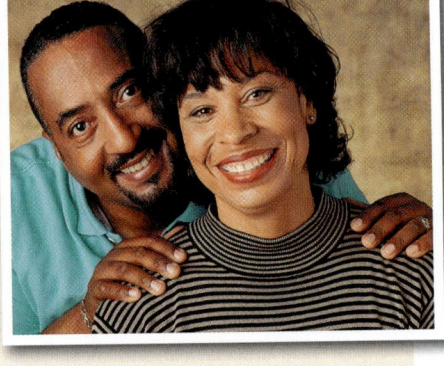

Gloria and her husband, John, live in a residential community from which John commutes to work in a nearby city. Gloria runs an accounting business from their home. They have two teenage boys, who are active in sports, church activities, Boy Scouts, and the school band. The boys need transportation to activities. Gloria and John teach Sunday school and are Boy Scout leaders. Gloria's mother needs knee replacement surgery and cannot take care of Gloria's father, who has early-stage Alzheimer's disease. In addition to her own home responsibilities, Gloria must go to her parents' home to prepare meals and to provide care for them during the day. Gloria's sister comes at 8:00 p.m. to sleep in the parents' home during the night.

Theoretical Knowledge
knowing why

Everyone experiences stress as a part of daily life, but we each perceive and respond to stress in our own unique way. Our responses are holistic—that is, physical, psychological, spiritual, and social. Stress has been directly linked to heart disease, stroke, injury, suicide, and homicide. Indirectly, it is also linked to cancer, chronic liver disease, chronic bronchitis, and emphysema (Quick, Saleh, Sime, et al., 2006). You will encounter many stressful situations in your career, so you must develop healthful ways of responding.

ABOUT THE KEY CONCEPTS

The two overarching concepts for this chapter are stress and adaptation. To help you grasp those concepts, we present definitions and examples, as well as numerous subconcepts that relate to health and illness in various ways. Another important concept is coping. Although we do not define experience for you, all the examples in this chapter are samples of patient experiences. As a nurse, you need to understand stress to help your clients cope effectively and adapt to the stressors of illness and caregiving.

WHAT IS STRESS?

Stress is any disturbance in a person's normal balanced state. A **stressor** is a stimulus that the person perceives as a challenge or threat; it disturbs the person's equilibrium by initiating a physical or emotional response. When stress occurs, it produces voluntary and involuntary **coping responses** aimed at restoring equilibrium (balance, or homeostasis). The changes that take place as a result of stress and coping are called **adaptations.** We can also define *adaptation* as an ongoing effort to maintain external and internal equilibrium, or **homeostasis.**

Stress is not necessarily bad. It can keep you alert and motivate you to function at a higher performance level. For example, when you are preparing for an examination, your desire to succeed can create just enough anxiety to motivate you to study. On the other hand, if you become too anxious, you may be unable to focus on the task or think clearly. **Distress** threatens health, and **eustress** (literally "good stress") is protective. On the Holmes-Rahe Social Readjustment

Scale (1967), for example, marriage and divorce receive similarly high scores.

Types of Stressors

The sources of stress are infinite; however, stressors are commonly categorized in the following ways:

External/Internal. Stressors may be **external** to the person, for example, death of a family member, a hurricane, or even something as simple as excessive heat in a room. Stressors may also be **internal,** for example, diseases, anxiety, nervous anticipation of an event, or negative self-talk.

Developmental/Situational. Developmental stressors are those that can be predicted to occur at various stages of a person's life. For example, most young adults face the stress of leaving home and beginning a career, and many middle-aged adults must adjust to aging parents and accepting their own physical changes. In a sense, developmental stressors may be easier to cope with because they are expected and the person has some time to prepare for them. For theoretical knowledge about developmental stages, refer to the theories of Erikson and Havighurst in Chapter 9. Also see Box 12-1 for examples of developmental stressors.

Situational stressors are unpredictable. For example, you cannot predict if you will experience an automobile accident, a natural disaster, or an illness. Situational stressors can occur at any life stage and can affect infants, children, and adults equally.

Physiological/Psychosocial. Physiological stressors are those that affect body structure or function. You can categorize them as follows; a few examples are given for each category.
- Chemical—environmental toxins, medications, tobacco
- Physical or mechanical—trauma, cold, joint overuse
- Nutritional—vitamin deficiency, high-fat diet
- Biological—viruses, bacteria
- Genetic—inborn errors of metabolism
- Lifestyle—obesity, sedentary lifestyle

Psychosocial stressors are external stressors that arise from work, family dynamics, living situation, social relationships, and other aspects of our daily lives. The Holmes-Rahe Social Readjustment Scale contains examples of psychosocial stressors.

BOX 12-1 ■ Stressors Throughout the Life Span

The following are common developmental stressors. Of course not everyone will experience these stressors.

Childhood

School-age children may also experience stressors at school or among peers; however, children's stressors occur primarily in the home:
- Absence of parental figures
- Failure of parents to meet needs for safety, security, love, and belonging
- Failure of parents to meet basic physiological needs for oxygen, food, elimination, rest, and cleanliness

Adolescence

- Exposure to an expanded environment and a wider circle of friends and acceptance by peers
- Rapid changes in body appearance
- Need for academic achievement, sports performance, or demonstration of other talents
- Peer pressure
- Maintaining self-esteem while searching for identity
- Decisions about the future in the areas of school, work, and relationships
- Conflicts between standards for behavior and the sex drive
- Decisions about and involvement with alcohol and drugs

Young Adult

- Separation from family, starting college or a job
- Making the transition from youth to adult responsibilities
- Preparing for careers: graduation from college, learning a trade
- Establishing career goals and planning how to achieve success and career stability
- Financial stressors around relationships and providing a home for self or family
- Parenting children
- Conflicts between responsibilities for work and family or other relationships

Middle Age

- Concern with career achievement and continuing career challenges
- Continuation of child rearing; marriage of the children; grandparenting
- Changes in appearance and health due to aging
- Dealing with too many responsibilities: e.g., children, work, elderly parents, community activities
- Empty-nest syndrome after the children leave home
- Being "sandwiched" between caring for aging parents as well as children or grandchildren
- "Mid-life crisis" (wanting to escape from one's present life): The person regresses and unrealistically tries to recapture youth, for example, by buying a new sports car that is too small to hold the entire family, making a geographic move, taking an exotic vacation that strains the budget, engaging in an affair, daydreaming excessively about the ideal life in retirement, "partying" and overuse of alcohol and illicit drugs, engaging in "workaholic" behavior. Any one of these behaviors does not necessarily signal mid-life crisis, but they are all examples of behaviors someone might use as an escape.

Older Adults

- Loss of family and friends due to illness or death, resulting in loneliness and isolation
- Changes in physical appearance and functional abilities, including mobility
- Major life changes (e.g., retirement, loss of life partner)
- Health problems (e.g., chronic diseases) with accompanying discomfort or pain
- The cost of healthcare
- Learning to live on a fixed, perhaps inadequate, income
- Adjusting to loss of independence
- Reduction in social status
- Substance and alcohol misuse and abuse is a problem for about 15% of adults older than the age of 50 (Substance Abuse and Mental Health Services Administration, 2007).

The Holmes-Rahe Social Readjustment Scale

This is a way to check your stress level, measured in "life change units." Of course it is not possible to score the exact "amount" of stress. However, this will give you a general idea of your stress level and should provide some insight about the sources of your stress. The following are based on the number of life change units over a 1- to 2-year period:

Over 300 points (major amount of change): 80% chance of major illness

200–299 (Moderate amount of change): 50% chance of major illness

150–199 (Mild amount of change): 33% chance of major illness

0–149 (Insignificant amount of change): Minimal chance of major illness

Of course, your personality and your ability to cope also determine the likelihood of your becoming ill.

Death of spouse	100
Divorce	73
Marital separation	65
Imprisonment	63
Death of a close family member	63
Personal injury or illness	53
Marriage	50
Dismissal from work	47
Marital reconciliation	45
Retirement	45
Change in health of family member	44
Pregnancy	40
Sexual difficulties	39
Gain of new family member	39
Business readjustment	39
Change in financial state	38
Change in number of arguments with spouse	35
Major mortgage	32
Foreclosure of mortgage or loan	30
Change in responsibilities at work	29
Son or daughter leaving home	29
Trouble with in-laws	29
Outstanding personal achievement	28
Spouse begins or stops work	26
Begin or end school	26
Change in living conditions	25
Revision of personal habits	24
Trouble with boss	23
Change in work hours or conditions	20
Change in residence	20
Change in schools	20
Change in recreation	19
Change in church activities	19
Change in social activities	18
Minor mortgage or loan	17
Change in sleeping habits	16
Change in number of family reunions	15
Change in eating habits	15
Vacation	13
Christmas	12
Minor violation of the law	11

KnowledgeCheck 12-1

Refer to the Meet Your Patients scenario, at the beginning of the chapter.

- What are Gloria's stressors? Classify each of them as follows:
  (1) Are they physiological or psychosocial?
  (2) Are they developmental or situational?
- What are John's stressors?

Models of Stress

Some theorists conceptualize stress as a complex, dynamic, and reciprocal transaction between person and environment. Other theorists view stress solely as a stimulus that causes psychological or physiological responses that in turn increase vulnerability to disease. This chapter uses the **response-based model** of Hans Selye (1974, 1976), and our distinction between *stressors* and *stress* stems from this model. Selye found that physical, emotional, psychological, and spiritual stressors, or the anticipation of a stressor (as in anxiety), can initiate non-specific physiological *responses*. Selye defined these responses as stress. For more information about the transaction and stimulus models of stress,

 Go to Chapter 12, **Supplemental Materials: Models of Stress,** on Davis*Plus*.

ThinkLike a Nurse 12-1

- Make a list of your own stressors in the following areas: work, school, family, and living situation.
- What physiological stressors do you have?

HOW DO COPING AND ADAPTATION RELATE TO STRESS?

Coping strategies are the thinking processes and behaviors a person uses to manage stressors. Coping strategies can be adaptive or maladaptive.

Adaptive (effective) coping consists of making healthy choices that reduce the negative effects of stress (e.g., exercising to relieve tension, engaging in a favorite hobby, consulting others for support or advice). Sometimes the difference between effective and ineffective coping is in the degree to which a technique is used (for examples, see Ego Defense Mechanisms later in this chapter).

Maladaptive (ineffective) coping does not promote adaptation. Unhealthful coping choices include overeating, working too much, oversleeping, and substance abuse. Although a maladaptive behavior may temporarily relieve anxiety, it may have other harmful effects. For example, a person who smokes to relieve the tensions of a stressful work situation may experience an immediate decrease in anxiety. However, the person is doing nothing to change or adapt to the stressful situation, and, over time, is increasing her risk of cardiorespiratory disease.

Three Approaches to Coping Are Commonly Used

People use three approaches to cope with stress, at different times and in various combinations:

Altering the Stressor. In some situations, a person takes actions to remove or change the stressor. For example, Gloria (Meet Your Patients) might remove one of her stressors by resigning her position as a Boy Scout leader.

Adapting to the Stressor. It is not always possible to remove or change a stressor. Adapting involves changing one's thoughts or behaviors related to the stressor. Gloria cannot change the fact that her father needs ongoing care and her mother needs surgery, but as she gains experience as a caregiver, she may find easier, more efficient ways to care for her parents. This would give her a little more time to relax or attend to other responsibilities.

Avoiding the Stressor. Sometimes it is healthful to avoid a stressor. For example, you may find that being with a certain person is stressful for you, even though you have tried many times to change the dynamics of the relationship. In that case, it may be best to minimize or end your relationship with the person. In other situations, avoidance may be maladaptive. For example, a woman who discovers a lump in her breast becomes anxious that she may have cancer. She copes with her anxiety by putting it out of her mind and avoids seeking medical care. As a result, if the lump is cancerous, it would not be treated at an early stage.

The Outcome of Stress Is Either Adaptation or Disease

Stress results in either adaptation or disease. Successful adaptation allows for normal growth and development and effective responses to changes and challenges in daily life. The outcome depends on the balance between the strength of the stressors and the effectiveness of the person's coping methods (Fig. 12-1). In the following equation, **E** is the event (stressor), **R** is the person's response (which is determined in part by past experiences, perception of the stressor, and coping methods used), and **O** is the outcome.

E	+	R	=	O
stressful event		response (experience, perception, coping methods)		outcome (adaptation or disease)

Some events produce more stress than others. However, a person with good coping skills can usually adapt to a single stressful event, even a demanding one. But suppose several stressors occur in a short period of time. Gloria (Meet Your Patients) has many stressors, so her coping abilities may be taxed to the limit. When there are many stressors or when stressors continue for a long period of time, adaptation is more likely to fail.

Personal Factors Influence Adaptation

Why do some people succumb to overwhelming stress while others adapt and thrive? Fortunately, successful adaptation does not depend entirely on being able to alter or avoid stressors. Various personal factors also influence the outcome:

Perception of the Stressor. A person's perception may be realistic or exaggerated. Suppose two women with similar coping skills and support systems both must have a mastectomy. Mrs. King thinks, "Yes, I am losing a part of my body, but I am more than just a breast. This will be a difficult adjustment, but I am so grateful to be alive." Mrs. Alan thinks, "I will be so ugly. My husband won't want to touch me. I feel less of a woman now." Which woman do you think is more likely to adapt successfully to this change in her body?

Overall Health Status. On one hand, stressors may actually cause a healthy person to engage in constructive adaptive behaviors that improve health. A person who has just discovered that he has hypertension may react by modifying his diet and exercising to lower his blood pressure and prevent complications. On the other hand, if a person with hypertension also has been coping for years with pain and immobility from arthritis, he may be too overwhelmed and exhausted to take any actions to lower his blood pressure.

Support System. A **support system** may include friends, family, counseling groups, church groups, or other like-minded people who share common interests. A good support system can help a person adapt to stress, provide emotional support, encourage expression of feelings, and help the person solve problems. It may also provide financial and other concrete types of support, such as a place to live, meal preparation, household help, child care, and transportation.

Hardiness. People who thrive despite overwhelming stressors tend to have a quality that has been termed **hardiness.** They maintain three key attitudes that help them weather adversity: commitment, control, and challenge. *Commitment* lets them seek to be involved with ongoing events, rather than feeling isolated. *Control* enables them to struggle and try to influence outcomes instead of becoming passive and feeling powerless. *Challenge* allows them to perceive stressful changes as opportunities for learning (Maddi, 1987, 2002).

Other Personal Factors. Age, developmental level, and life experiences (e.g., learning which coping methods have worked for you) all affect a person's response to stress. For example, infants and the very old may lack physiological reserves to adapt to physical stressors, such as temperature extremes, dehydration, or illness. Even with a positive attitude and good coping skills, excessive amounts of stress can

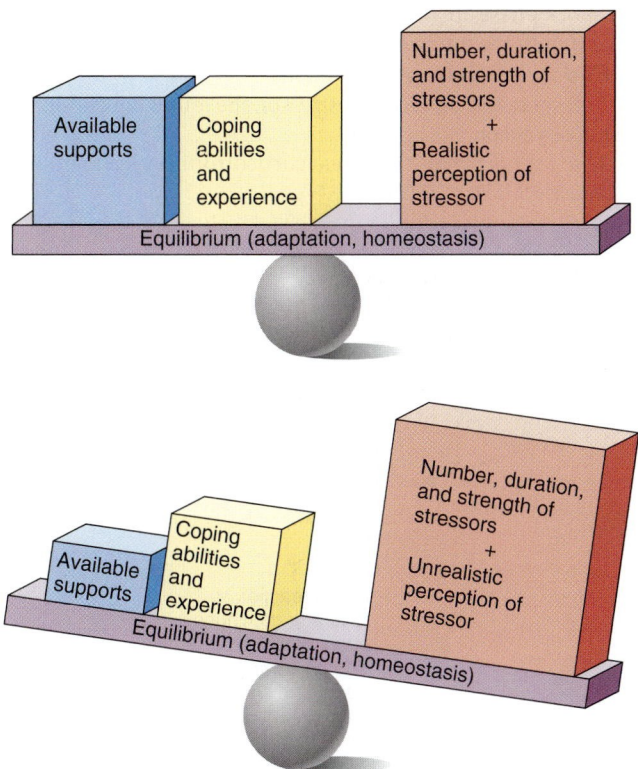

FIGURE 12-1 Adaptation occurs when a person has supports and coping abilities adequate to enable him to deal with the stressors. A realistic perception of the stressful event promotes adaptation, whereas an unrealistic perception makes adaptation more difficult.

lead to maladaptation and disease. Some people succumb to illness after experiencing only a few stressors, whereas others seem to adapt to multiple, intensely difficult stressors. Each person has a different ability to tolerate stress, but everyone has a breaking point at which stress becomes overwhelming.

KnowledgeCheck 12-2

- True or false: The difference between adaptive and maladaptive coping is that maladaptive coping does not relieve stress.
- In addition to avoiding the stressor, what are two other approaches to coping?
- (Complete the sentence.) The outcome of stress (adaptation or disease) depends on the balance among the strength, number, and duration of the stressors and _____.

HOW DO PEOPLE RESPOND TO STRESSORS?

Although Selye's (1974, 1976) response-based model acknowledges physical, emotional, psychological, and spiritual *stressors*, his ideas about responses (*stress*) are primarily physiological. As you know, the body has various mechanisms for regulating its internal environment to maintain a balanced state or **homeostasis**. Selye described the physiological responses to stress as either the general adaptation syndrome (GAS) or the local adaptation syndrome (LAS).

The General Adaptation Syndrome Includes Nonspecific, Systemic Responses

Would you be surprised to know that a near-miss automobile accident and kicking the winning field goal at a football game would both produce the same general body responses? It is true. Regardless of the specific stressor, the responses involve the whole body, especially the autonomic nervous system and the endocrine system. The **general adaptation syndrome (GAS)** is Selye's name for the group of nonspecific responses

that all people share in the face of stressors. The GAS has three stages: (1) the initial alarm stage, (2) resistance (adaptation), and (3) the final stage of either recovery or exhaustion (Fig. 12-2).

Alarm Stage—Fight or Flight

Imagine yourself in this situation: It is dark. You are alone, walking to your car, when you hear footsteps behind you. You stop and look around and see no one. As you begin walking again, the footsteps return. You walk faster; the footsteps are faster. Stop reading, shut your eyes, and use your imagination. How do you feel? Pay attention to your physical and emotional reactions. If you are not feeling a response to this imaginary situation, think back to a time when something similar happened to you—when something frightened you. Is your heart pounding? Are you breathing fast? Is there a flutter in your stomach? What is the physical sensation in your muscles? Do you feel frightened? What are your emotions? Are you straining to hear the footsteps? Do you want to run away, or are you "frozen"? If someone were to walk into the room where you are studying right now, would it startle you?

This scenario should help you to imagine the experience of the alarm stage, during which the body prepares for *fight or flight*. The alarm stage has two phases: shock and countershock. The **shock phase** begins when the cerebral cortex first perceives a stressor and sends out messages to activate the endocrine and sympathetic nervous systems. A surge of epinephrine (adrenaline) and various other hormones prepare the body for fight or flight. The shock phase does not last long—usually less than 24 hours, and sometimes only a minute or two. In the **countershock phase,** all the changes produced in the shock phase are reversed, and the person becomes less able to deal with the immediate threat.

Endocrine System Responses

In response to a perceived stressor, the following endocrine responses occur:

1. The *hypothalamus* releases corticotropin-releasing hormone (CRH).

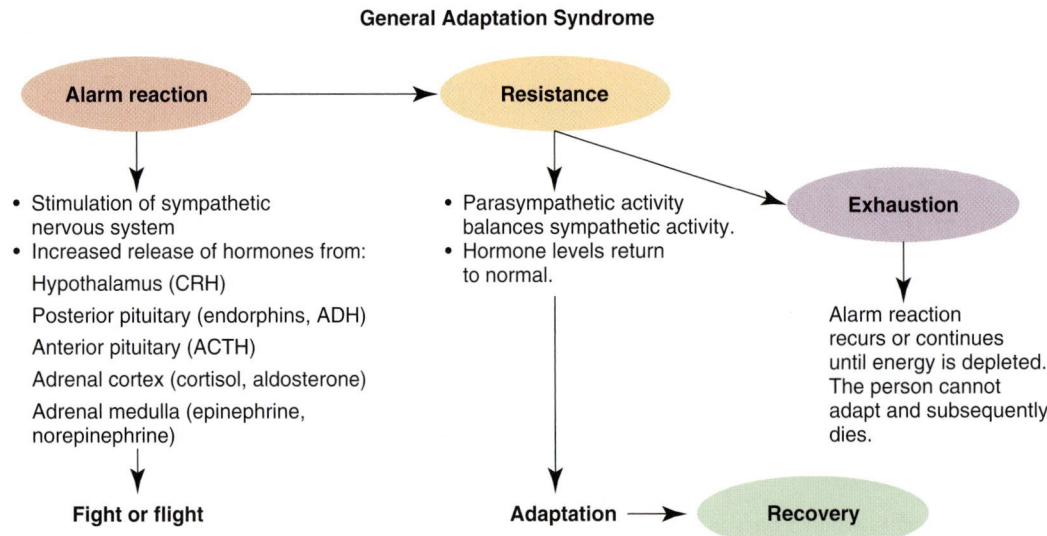

General Adaptation Syndrome

- Alarm reaction → Resistance
- Resistance → Exhaustion
- Resistance → Adaptation

Alarm reaction
- Stimulation of sympathetic nervous system
- Increased release of hormones from:
  Hypothalamus (CRH)
  Posterior pituitary (endorphins, ADH)
  Anterior pituitary (ACTH)
  Adrenal cortex (cortisol, aldosterone)
  Adrenal medulla (epinephrine, norepinephrine)

Fight or flight

Resistance
- Parasympathetic activity balances sympathetic activity.
- Hormone levels return to normal.

Exhaustion
Alarm reaction recurs or continues until energy is depleted. The person cannot adapt and subsequently dies.

Adaptation → Recovery

FIGURE 12-2 The stages of Selye's general adaptation syndrome (GAS) are (1) *alarm* (also called fight or flight); (2) *resistance* (or adaptation), in which the body enacts physical and psychological adaptive mechanisms to maintain homeostasis; and (3) either *recovery* or *exhaustion* (which usually ends in disease or death).

2. *CRH,* together with messages from the cerebral cortex, directs the pituitary gland to release adrenocorticotropic hormone (ACTH) and antidiuretic hormone (ADH).

3. *ACTH* stimulates the adrenal cortex to produce and secrete glucocorticoids (especially cortisol) and mineralocorticoids (especially aldosterone).

   ■ *Cortisol,* in general, has a glucose-sparing effect. It increases the use of fats and proteins for energy and conserves glucose for use by the brain. Cortisol also has an anti-inflammatory effect. See Figure 12-3 for the effects of cortisol during the alarm reaction of the GAS.

   ■ *Aldosterone* promotes fluid retention by causing the kidneys to reabsorb more sodium. In that way, it helps to increase fluid volume and maintain or increase blood pressure.

4. *ADH* also promotes fluid retention by increasing the reabsorption of water by kidney tubules. See Figure 12-4 for the effects of aldosterone and ADH.

5. *Endorphins,* secreted by the hypothalamus and posterior pituitary, act like opiates to produce a sense of well-being and reduce pain.

6. *Thyroid-stimulating hormone (TSH)* is secreted by the pituitary gland to increase the efficiency of cellular metabolism and fat conversion to energy for cell and muscle needs.

Sympathetic Nervous System Responses

The cerebral cortex also sends messages via the hypothalamus to stimulate the sympathetic nervous system. The sympathetic nervous system then stimulates the adrenal glands to secrete adrenaline and norepinephrine, which increase mental alertness. This allows the person to assess the situation and aids in a decision to stand and fight or run away in flight. Adrenaline also increases the ability of the muscles to contract and causes the pupils to dilate, producing greater visual fields. See Figure 12-5 for the effects of adrenaline during the alarm reaction of the GAS.

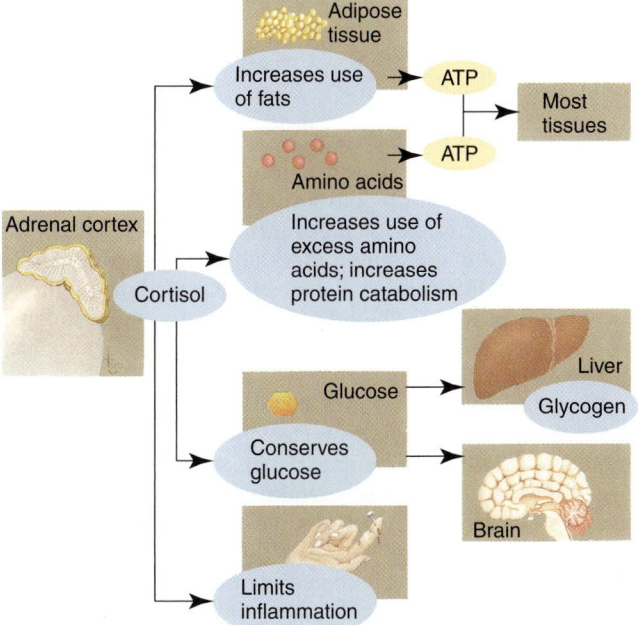

FIGURE 12-3 Functions of cortisol during the alarm stage of the GAS. (From Scanlon, V., & Sanders, T. [2011]. *Essentials of anatomy and physiology* [6th ed.]. Philadelphia: F. A. Davis, p. 241.)

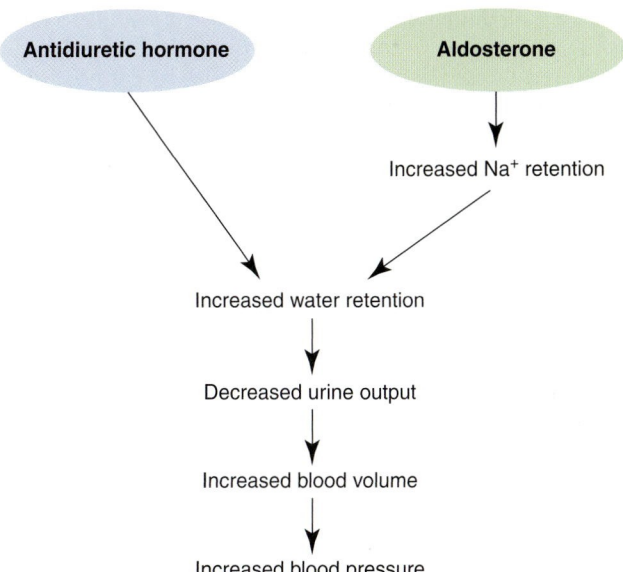

FIGURE 12-4 The release of ADH (from the posterior pituitary gland) and aldosterone (from the adrenal cortex) leads to sodium and water retention, increases blood volume, and increases blood pressure.

Other Body System Responses in the Alarm Stage

The following are some body system responses that occur in the alarm stage as a result of endocrine and sympathetic nervous system activity. Refer to Figures 12-2 through 12-5 to see how these changes are produced.

■ *Cardiovascular system.* The heart rate and contraction force increase. Peripheral and visceral vasoconstriction increases blood flow to vital organs (e.g., brain, lungs) and to muscles preparing for flight. Blood volume and blood pressure also increase, and the blood clots more readily.

■ *Respiratory system.* The bronchioles dilate, thereby increasing the depth of respiration and tidal volume. This makes oxygen available for diffusion to muscle, brain, and cardiac cells.

■ *Metabolism.* The metabolic rate increases. The liver converts more glycogen to glucose (*glycogenolysis*), making it available for energy. Except in the brain, the body uses less glucose for energy. The use of amino acids and the mobilization of fats for energy (*lipolysis*) increase.

■ *Urinary system.* Blood flow to the kidneys decreases, and they retain more sodium and water. The kidneys secrete renin, which produces *angiotensin*. In turn, angiotensin constricts the arterioles and tends to increase blood pressure.

■ *Gastrointestinal system.* Peristalsis and secretions of digestive enzymes decrease. The blood glucose increases to fuel the body with energy needed for fight or flight.

■ *Musculoskeletal system.* Blood vessels dilate, increasing flow of blood (and thus oxygen and energy) to skeletal muscles.

Resistance Stage—Coping With the Stressor

During the second stage of the GAS, **resistance** (or *adaptation*), the body tries to cope, protect itself against the stressor, and maintain homeostasis. Stabilization involves the use of physiological and psychological coping mechanisms. Psychological defense mechanisms for coping are discussed shortly. Physical adaptations help the heart rate, blood pressure, cardiac output, respiratory function, and hormone levels return to normal. If the person adapts successfully or if the stress can be confined to a small area (as in the inflammatory response, also

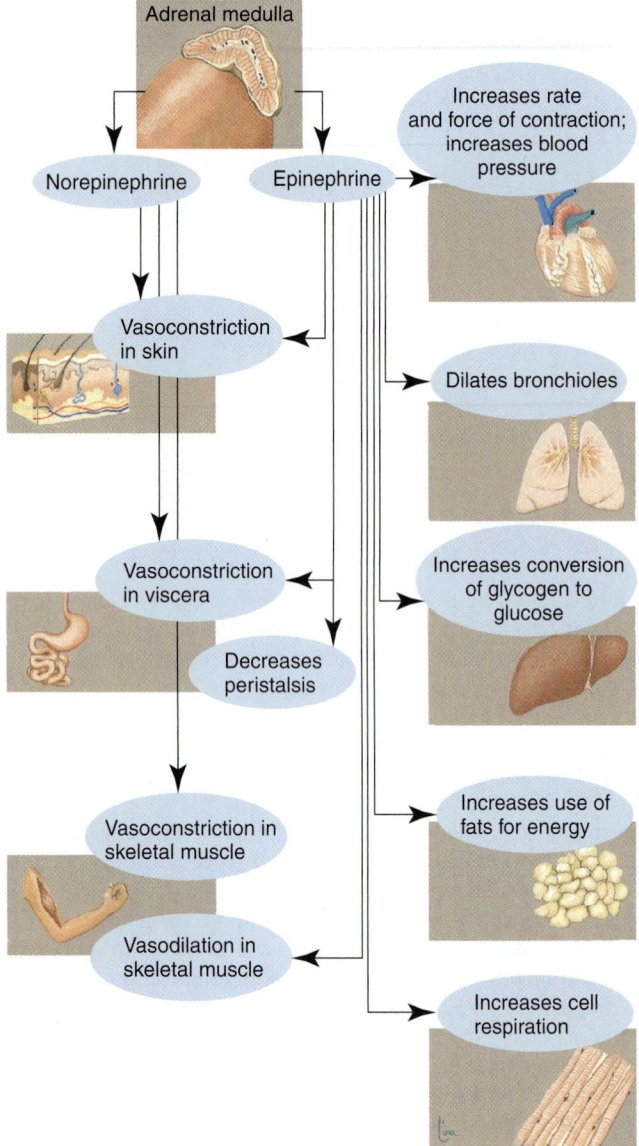

FIGURE 12-5 Functions of epinephrine and norepinephrine during the alarm stage of the GAS. (From Scanlon, V., & Sanders, T. [2011]. *Essentials of anatomy and physiology* [6th ed.]. Philadelphia: F. A. Davis, p. 258.)

discussed shortly), the body regains homeostasis. If the stress is too great (as in serious illness or severe blood loss), defense mechanisms fail, and the person enters the third phase of the GAS.

Exhaustion or Recovery Stage—Final Effort to Adapt

If stress continues and adaptive mechanisms become ineffective or are used up, a person enters the final stage, **exhaustion.** Physiological responses in this stage include vasodilation, decreased blood pressure, and increased pulse and respirations. Physical adaptive resources and energy are depleted. The body is unable to defend itself and cannot maintain resistance against the continuing stressors. Exhaustion usually ends in injury, illness, or death.

In contrast, if adaptation is successful, the final stage is **recovery.** For example, after a miscarriage, a couple participates in a support group and begins to focus more deeply on their

relationship with each other. They are able gradually to resolve their grief.

KnowledgeCheck 12-3

- In general, what is the difference between the alarm stage and the resistance stage of the GAS?
- Name the gland that releases each of the following hormones in response to stress, and name each hormone's function: corticotropin-releasing hormone (CRH), antidiuretic hormone (ADH), adrenocorticotropic hormone (ACTH), aldosterone, cortisol, epinephrine, and norepinephrine.
- In the alarm stage of the GAS, what are the effects of the sympathetic nervous system on each of the following: heart, brain, glycogen stores, and skeletal muscle?
- What is the effect of Selye's resistance stage on the cardiovascular and respiratory systems? On hormone levels?

The Local Adaptation Syndrome Involves Specific Local Responses

Whereas the GAS is a whole-body response to a stressor, the **local adaptation syndrome (LAS)** is a localized body response; that is, it involves only a specific body part, tissue, or organ. It is a short-term attempt to restore homeostasis. As a nurse, the two most common LAS responses you will deal with are the reflex pain response and the inflammatory response. Others include blood clotting and pupil constriction in response to light.

Reflex Pain Response

When you perceive a painful stimulus, especially in one of your limbs, you immediately and unconsciously withdraw from the source of pain. If you've ever accidentally touched a hot stove, you certainly didn't stop to ponder, "Hmmm, I think I will withdraw my hand." You pulled your hand away before you could even think about it. This is a protective **reflex** (an involuntary, predictable response). Pain receptors send sensory impulses to the spinal cord, where they synapse with the spinal motor neurons. The motor impulses travel back to the site of stimulation, causing the flexor muscles in the limb to contract. This is a local, rather than a whole-body, response.

Inflammatory Response

The **inflammatory response** is a local reaction to cell injury, either by pathogens or by physical, chemical, or other agents (Box 12-2). Regardless of the injuring agent (stressor), its mechanisms are the same, and they produce the classic symptoms of inflammation: pain, heat, swelling, redness, and loss of function. The inflammatory process includes a vascular response, a cellular response, formation of exudate, and healing.

Vascular Response. Immediately after injury, blood vessels at the site constrict (narrow) to control bleeding. After the injured cells release histamine, the vessels dilate, increasing blood flow to the area **(hyperemia).** Under the influence of kinins released by the dying cells, the capillaries become more permeable, allowing movement of fluid from capillaries into tissue spaces. The tissue becomes **edematous** (swollen). After **leukocytes** (white blood cells) move into the area, localized blood flow again decreases, to keep them in the area to fight infection.

Cellular Response. Specialized white blood cells **(phagocytes)** migrate to the site of injury and engulf bacteria, other

BOX 12-2 ■ Agents Causing Inflammatory Responses

The following agents stimulate the inflammatory response by causing cell injury:
- Autoimmune disorders
- Antigen–antibody responses
- Body substances (e.g., digestive enzymes leaking into the abdomen; accumulation of uric acid crystals in joints)
- Chemical injury (e.g., acid or alkali burns)
- Ischemia
- Neoplastic growth (i.e., cancer)
- Pathogens (e.g., bacteria, viruses)
- Physical agents:
  Heat or cold
  Radiation
  Electrothermal injury
  Mechanical trauma (e.g., abrasion, contusion, laceration, puncture, incision, fractures, sprains)

foreign material, and damaged cells and destroy them. Sometimes they form a "wall" around an invading pathogen. The accumulation of dead white cells, digested bacteria, and other cell debris in the presence of infection is called *pus.*

Exudate Formation. The fluid and white blood cells that move from the circulation to the site of injury are called **exudate.** The nature and quantity of exudate depend on the severity of injury and the tissues involved. For example, a surgical incision may ooze serosanguineous (clear or pinkish) exudate for a day or two.

Healing. **Healing** is the replacement of tissue by regeneration or repair. **Regeneration** is replacement of the damaged cells with identical or similar cells. However, not all cells can regenerate (e.g., some central nervous system neurons and cardiac muscle cells cannot regenerate). Most injuries heal by **repair,** wherein scar tissue replaces the original tissue. You will find a thorough discussion of wound healing in Chapter 36.

The inflammatory response is adaptive in that it protects the body from infection and promotes healing. However, chronic inflammation, as in arthritis, is itself a stressor.

Do not confuse inflammation with infection. Inflammation is a mechanism for eliminating invading pathogens; therefore, you always see inflammation when there is infection. However, inflammation is stimulated by trauma as well as by pathogens (e.g., swelling of a sprained ankle); thus, it can occur when there is no infection.

KnowledgeCheck 12-4

- What are four characteristics of the local adaptation syndrome (LAS)?
- Name two LAS responses.
- What are the classic symptoms of the inflammatory process?

Psychological Responses to Stress Include Feelings, Thoughts, and Behaviors

Health professionals understand most human health disorders to be *biopsychosocial* in nature (Alford, 2007). This means that we respond and adapt to stress physically, mentally, and behaviorally, and even spiritually.

Psychological responses are both emotional and cognitive, and they include feelings, thoughts, and behaviors (Box 12-3). They may be fleeting, as in a flash of anger that is gone in seconds, or long-term, as in the avoidance of relationships by an adult whose needs for love and security were not met as a child.

As with physical responses, psychological responses can be adaptive or harmful. Consider this example case:

> Both Mr. Laslow and Mr. Harvey have had heart attacks and are both anxious about the future. To relieve his anxiety, Mr. Laslow takes a problem-solving approach, learning about diet, exercise, and lifestyle changes that he must make. Mr. Harvey uses denial; he cannot accept that he has "really" had a heart attack. He says, "I'm not an invalid. I feel fine. I could follow all those rules and still get hit by a truck and die tomorrow." Both of these responses may relieve the person's anxiety. Which one do you think is more adaptive in the long term?

Common emotional responses to stress include anxiety, fear, anger, and depression.

BOX 12-3 ■ Psychological Responses to Stressors

Cognitive Responses

Difficulty concentrating
Poor judgment
Decrease in accuracy (e.g., in counting money)
Forgetfulness
Decreased problem-solving ability
Decreased attention to detail
Difficulty learning
Narrowing of focus
Preoccupation, daydreaming

Emotional Responses

Adjustment disorders
Anger
Anxiety
Depression
Fear
Feelings of inadequacy
Low self-esteem
Irritability
Lack of motivation
Lethargy

Behavioral Responses

Academic difficulties
Aggressiveness
Crying, emotional outbursts
Dependence
Nightmares
Poor job performance
Substance use and abuse
Sleeplessness (or sleeping too much)
Change in eating habits (e.g., loss of appetite, overeating)
Decrease in quality of job performance
Preoccupation (i.e., daydreaming)
Illnesses
Increased absenteeism from work or school
Increased number of accidents
Strained family or social relationships
Avoiding social situations or relationships
Rebellion, acting out

Anxiety and Fear

Anxiety is diffuse and not easily defined. NANDA International (2009, p. 242) defines it as a "vague, uneasy feeling of discomfort or dread accompanied by an autonomic response (the source often nonspecific or unknown to the individual); a feeling of apprehension caused by anticipation of danger. . . ." Notice that the response is not to a danger but to the *anticipation* of danger—to imagining it. An anxious person worries; feels nervous, uneasy, and fearful; may be tearful; and often has physical symptoms, such as nausea, trembling, and sweating.

Fear is an emotion or feeling of apprehension (dread) from an identified danger, threat, or pain. The danger may be real or imagined. Anxiety and fear produce similar responses. However, some experts differentiate them as follows:

- Fear is a cognitive response, whereas anxiety is an emotional response.
- Fear is related to a present event, whereas anxiety is related to a future (or anticipated) event.
- The source of fear is easily identifiable, whereas the source of anxiety may not be identifiable.
- Fear can result from either a physical or a psychological event; anxiety results from psychological conflict rather than physical threat.

Mild to moderate anxiety may be adaptive because it motivates and mobilizes the person to action. However, severe anxiety consumes energy and interferes with the person's ability to focus on and respond to what is really happening. See Chapter 13 for more information on theoretical knowledge of anxiety and fear, including levels of anxiety.

Anxiety and fear initiate the release of epinephrine, which stimulates the sympathetic nervous system and prepares the person for fight or flight. Therefore, living with anxiety can be physically, emotionally, and spiritually exhausting.

 ## ThinkLike a Nurse 12-2

Read the following two scenarios.

1. You are a student assigned to a 6-hour day in the clinical area. Each time you have a clinical day coming up, you feel anticipation and look forward to working in the clinical area. However, you do not know what to expect. You think: "What will my patients be like? How will the day go? Do I know enough to handle it? Do I need to practice any procedures?" It is hard to answer these questions until you are actually on the unit and see your patients.
2. Given the same situation, suppose that when you begin your clinical day, your clinical instructor tells you that he will be in the agency asking questions, supervising, evaluating your performance—and, perhaps from your perspective, making your life miserable.
3. In which situation are you most likely to feel fear rather than anxiety? Explain your reasoning.

Ego defense mechanisms. When faced with a stressful situation, the ego defense systems may kick in to diminish the inner tension associated with the stressors. Just as the body responds physiologically to stressors, it has psychological responses that protect the person from anxiety and assist with adaptation. When used sparingly, and for mild to moderate anxiety, defense mechanisms can be helpful. When overused, however, they become habits that give us the false illusion that we are coping. If psychological defense mechanisms are inadequate to diminish the threat and restore equilibrium, the person may develop an anxiety disorder. Table 12-1 identifies some common psychological defense mechanisms.

Anger and Depression

Anger is a strong, uncomfortable feeling of animosity, hostility, extreme indignation, or displeasure. A person who cannot control stressors may become apprehensive (anxious about what may happen) and respond with anger. Thus, moderate anger is often a first protective response against anxiety. As anxiety increases and the person recognizes fear, he feels more threatened and may resort to bullying behavior to increase the personal feeling of power, control, and self-esteem.

Anger may be expressed in shouting, throwing things, or hitting, or more subtly with sarcastic, caustic remarks. Some people attempt to hide their emotions and soften their hurtful remarks, or make them more socially acceptable, through the use of humor and joking. When anger involves destructive behaviors, such as physical or verbal abuse, it is called **hostility.** When expressed appropriately and clearly (i.e., verbally), anger can be adaptive, because it temporarily releases the person's feelings of tension. When the anger is out in the open, both parties can deal with it. Nevertheless, even verbal expressions of anger can be destructive if the anger persists after the person expresses it.

Depression is sometimes associated with unresolved anger and may result from stress. It is normal to feel depression in response to any loss or a traumatic event, but long-term depression is a reason for concern. See Chapter 13 for more information about anger and depression.

KnowledgeCheck 12-5

- In addition to ego defense mechanisms, name four common emotional responses to stress.
- Explain how mild to moderate anxiety can be adaptive.
- True or false: One difference between anxiety and fear is that the danger in anxiety may be imagined, whereas in fear the danger is real.
- What are ego defense mechanisms?

Spiritual Responses to Stress Are Multifaceted

Spiritual responses—as do all human responses—vary among individuals. Many people depend on a higher power or religious community for support when coping with stress. Some search for a larger meaning in the illness or other stressor. Others may view stress as a test, a punishment, or a challenge.

Spiritual responses to stress are multifaceted. Often, a first response during the alarm stage is to pray or ask for help (e.g., healing, coping). Prayer, meditation, and religious affiliation can also help during the second stage (adaptation). In the final stage, spiritual resources may be exhausted, creating Spiritual Distress, leaving the person feeling abandoned, helpless, and hopeless. If your own spiritual life is healthy, you will be better equipped to support patients who are experiencing spiritual challenges. For more information about spiritual responses to stress, see Chapter 16.

Table 12-1 ➤ Psychological Defense Mechanisms

DEFENSE MECHANISM	EXAMPLES	EXAMPLES AND CONSEQUENCES OF OVERUSE
Avoidance—Unconsciously staying away from events or situations that might open feelings of aggression or anxiety.	"I can't go to the class reunion tonight. I'm too tired; I have to sleep."	The person becomes socially isolated because of the tension he feels when around other people.
Compensation—Making up for a perceived inadequacy by developing or emphasizing some other desirable trait.	A small boy who wants to be on the football team instead becomes a great singer.	Use of drugs or alcohol to gain courage to enter a social situation.
Conversion—Emotional conflict is changed into physical symptoms that have no physical basis. The symptoms often disappear after the threat is over.	Feeling back pain when it is difficult to continue carrying the pressures of life; developing nausea that causes the person to miss a major exam.	Laryngitis, inability to speak on the anniversary of father's death. Continued anxiety can lead to actual physical disorders, such as gastric ulcers.
Denial—Transforming reality by refusing to acknowledge thoughts, feeling, desires, or impulses. This is unconscious; the person is *not* consciously lying. Denial is usually the first defense learned.	A student refuses to acknowledge that he is barely passing anatomy, does not withdraw from the class, and is now failing a nursing course. A person with alcohol dependence states, "I can quit any time I want to."	Overuse can lead to repression and dissociative disorders (e.g., dual personalities, selective amnesia).
Displacement—"Kick the dog." Transferring emotions, ideas, or wishes from one original object or situation to a substitute inappropriate person or object that is perceived to be less powerful or threatening.	Husband loses his job, goes home, and yells at his wife. (This mechanism is rarely adaptive.)	In extreme situations, this mechanism leads to verbal and physical abuse.
Dissociation—Painful events are separated or dissociated from the conscious mind.	A person who was sexually abused as a child describes the events as though they happened to a sibling.	May result in a dissociative disorder, such as multiple personality disorder.
Identification—A person takes on the ideas, personality, or characteristics of another person, especially someone that the person fears or respects.	Children play cowboy, police, fireman, or mommy.	Assumes mannerisms, wears clothing, and arranges hair and physical appearance to match those of the other person.
Intellectualization—Cognitive reasoning is used to block or avoid feelings about a painful incident.	When her husband dies, the wife relieves her pain by thinking, "It's better this way; he was in so much pain." A person says, "I think" rather than, "I feel."	"My husband loves me, but he doesn't like it when another man talks to me; that's why he loses his temper and releases his anger physically by hitting me."
Minimization—Not acknowledging or accepting the significance of one's own behavior, making it less important.	"It doesn't matter how much I drink. I never drive when I'm drinking."	Person engages in unhealthy or antisocial behavior; there is no motivation to change behavior.
Projection—Blaming others. Attributing one's own personality traits, mistakes, emotions, motives, and thoughts to another; "finger pointing."	"The clinical instructor makes me nervous, so I cannot do well." "I forgot to bake cookies because you did not tell me that cookies were due at school today."	Person cannot see his own responsibility for a situation, so he cannot make adaptive behaviors. Person criticizes habits in others that are the same as one's own bad habits.
Rationalization—Use of a logical-sounding excuse to cover up or justify true ideas, actions, or feelings. An attempt to preserve self-respect or approval or to conceal a motive for some action by giving a socially acceptable reason. Similar to intellectualization, but uses faulty logic.	"It was God's will that this happened to me." "If I didn't have to work, I would be a better wife."	This mechanism can lead to self-deception.

(Continued)

Table 12-1 ➤ Psychological Defense Mechanisms—cont'd

DEFENSE MECHANISM	EXAMPLES	EXAMPLES AND CONSEQUENCES OF OVERUSE
Reaction formation—Similar to compensation, except the person develops the exact opposite trait. The person is aware of her feelings but acts in ways opposite to what she is really feeling.	"It's OK that you forgot my birthday" (when it really is not OK).	Overuse can cause failure to resolve internal conflicts.
Regression—Using behavior appropriate in an earlier stage of development to overcome feeling of insecurity in a present situation.	Cooks and eats a comfort food (e.g., hot fudge sundae). A 60-year-old divorcee dresses and acts like a teenager.	Can interfere with perception of reality.
Repression—Unconscious "burying" or "forgetting" of painful thoughts, feelings, memories, ideas; pushing them from a conscious to an unconscious level. It is a step deeper than denial.	Having no memory of sexual abuse by sibling or father. An adolescent forgets to put out the trash because being "bossed" makes him angry, but he feels guilty if he consciously chooses not to do it.	Flashbacks, PTSD, and amnesia
Restitution (*undoing*)—Making amends for a behavior one thinks is unacceptable, to reduce guilt.	Giving a treat to a child who has been punished for wrongdoing.	May send double messages. Relieves the person of the responsibility for honesty about the situation.
Sublimation—Unacceptable drives, traits, or behaviors (often sexual or aggressive) are unconsciously diverted to socially accepted traits.	Anger is expressed by aggression when playing sports. A person who chooses to not have children runs a day-care center.	The "acceptable" behavior might reinforce the negative tendencies, and the person may still show signs of the undesirable trait or behavior. For example, a person indulges in child pornography to obtain sexual gratification.

Adapted from Neeb, K. (2006). *Fundamentals of mental health nursing* (3rd ed.). Philadelphia: F.A. Davis.

PTSD = post-traumatic stress disorder.

COMMON PROBLEMS WHEN ADAPTATION FAILS

Living with continual stress strains adaptive mechanisms. This strain can lead to exhaustion and disease, which in turn can lead to more stress. Once established, this type of positive feedback loop is difficult to break. Three types of disorders that can develop when adaptation fails are stress-induced organic responses, somatoform disorders, and psychological disorders.

Stress-Induced Organic Responses

As a result of repeated central nervous system stimulation and elevation of certain hormones, continual stress brings about long-term changes in various body systems. People who use maladaptive coping strategies (e.g., overeating, substance abuse) create additional stress on the body, further contributing to disease.

Somatoform Disorders

Somatoform disorders are conditions characterized by the presence of physical symptoms with no known organic cause. They are believed to result from unconscious denial, repression, and displacement of anxiety. Certain people seem predisposed to somatoform disorders—for instance, those who suffer from personality disorders and major psychiatric illness; those who do not handle anxiety well; and those who are dependent, emotionally needy, frustrated, and resentful (Neeb, 2006). The physical symptoms allow the person to avoid a situation that, if confronted, would provoke extreme anxiety. The following are examples of somatoform disorders:

- **Hypochondriasis.** The person is preoccupied with the idea that he is or will become seriously ill. The person is abnormally concerned with his health and interprets his real or imagined symptoms unrealistically, fearing that they will get worse or become incurable. The person is not "faking it"; anxiety about his health may trigger the physical sensations.
- **Somatization.** In this disorder, anxiety and emotional turmoil are expressed in physical symptoms, loss of physical function, pain that changes location often, and depression. The patient is unable to control the symptoms and behaviors, and complaints are vague or exaggerated.
- **Pain disorder.** Previously called *somatoform pain disorder,* this is emotional pain that manifests physically. Pain is the

Table 12-2 ► Stress-Induced Organic Responses

BODY SYSTEM	PHYSIOLOGICAL RESPONSE
Cardiovascular system	Continued secretion of epinephrine may cause cardiovascular disorders including angina, myocardial infarction, cardiomegaly, and congestive heart failure, all of which lead to decreased cardiac output. As cardiac output decreases, less oxygen circulates to meet cellular metabolic demands, and the body becomes fatigued. Prolonged secretion of epinephrine and renin result in vasoconstriction, causing hypertension. ADH, aldosterone, ACTH, and cortisol create electrolyte imbalance and retention of sodium and water, thus promoting peripheral edema.
Endocrine system	Continuing high levels of blood glucose and insulin can cause diabetes. Metabolic disorders of hyperthyroidism or hypothyroidism can result as persistent demands for thyroid hormone production cause a rebound failure of the gland. Even prenatal stress can cause adaptive changes in fetal endocrine and metabolic processes that impact later adult health (Sullivan, Hawes, Winchester, et al., 2008).
Immune system	Stress reduces the ability of the body's immune cells to differentiate between self and non-self. Thus, the immune cells begin to attack body tissues, producing autoimmune illness. Common autoimmune illnesses include rheumatoid arthritis, lupus, cancer, and allergies. Research has linked stress to suppression of the immune system and even to viral replication in HIV patients (e.g., Davidson, Kabat-Zinn, Schumacher, et al., 2003; Robinson, Mathews, & Witek-Janusek, 2000).
Gastrointestinal system	The gastrointestinal system may respond to central nervous system stimulation with constipation or diarrhea, gastroesophageal reflux, colitis, or irritable bowel syndrome. Continued secretion of hydrochloric acid produces gastric hyperacidity and erosion of the gastrointestinal tract, especially in the presence of *Helicobacter pylori (H. pylori).*
Musculoskeletal system	Constant readiness for fight or flight produces muscle tension and pain in various body sites. Tension headache and temporomandibular joint pain result from prolonged muscle tension in the head, neck, and spine.
Respiratory system	Epinephrine and circulating hormones dilate the bronchial tubes and increase the rate of respiration. Hyperventilation can produce symptoms of alkalosis, including dizziness, tingling hands and feet, and anxiety. Distress in the respiratory system can exacerbate existing asthma, hay fever, and allergies.

ACTH = adrenocorticotropic hormone; ADH = antidiuretic hormone.

main focus of the person's life. The level of pain the person states is inconsistent with the physical condition—that is, the physical cause is either disproportionate to the pain or cannot be found at all. The pain does not change location.

- **Malingering.** Malingering is different from the other disorders because it is a *conscious* effort to escape unpleasant situations. The patient merely pretends to have the symptoms for personal or tangible gain (e.g., calling in sick because the person does not want to go to work).

KnowledgeCheck 12-6

- Name and describe three stress-induced organic or systemic responses to stress.
- Name and describe at least three somatoform disorders.

Stress-Induced Psychological Responses

Even if coping mechanisms are effective initially, with long-term stress, exhaustion sets in, and the mechanisms begin to fail. The person may then try maladaptive ways to cope. As work and personal relationships deteriorate, the person loses self-esteem. Prolonged stress can eventually result in crisis and burnout (Fig. 12-6). More severe responses include psychiatric illnesses, such as anxiety disorders, clinical depression, and post-traumatic stress disorder (PTSD). Anxiety and

depression are discussed in Chapter 13. We discuss crisis, burnout, and PTSD next.

Crisis. A **crisis** exists when (1) an event in a person's life drastically changes the person's routine and he perceives it as a threat to self, and (2) the person's usual coping methods are ineffective, resulting in high levels of anxiety and inability to function adequately. Such events are usually sudden and unexpected (e.g., serious illness or death of a loved one, serious financial losses, an automobile accident, rape, and natural disasters). Because each person has a different tolerance for stress, an event that creates a crisis for one may be just a minor nuisance for another. Nevertheless, most experts agree that people experiencing crisis go through five phases (Neeb, 2006; Stuart & Sundeen, 2009).

1. *Precrisis.* In response to the event or anxiety, the person uses usual coping strategies, has no symptoms, denies any stress, and may even report a feeling of well-being.
2. *Impact.* In this phase, anxiety and confusion increase. The person may have trouble organizing his or her personal life, and may feel the stress but minimize its severity.
3. *Crisis.* The person experiences more anxiety and tries new ways of coping, such as withdrawal, rationalization, and projection (refer to Table 12-1). The person recognizes the problem but denies that it is out of control.
4. *Adaptive.* The person redefines the threat and perceives the crisis in a realistic way. Rational thinking and positive

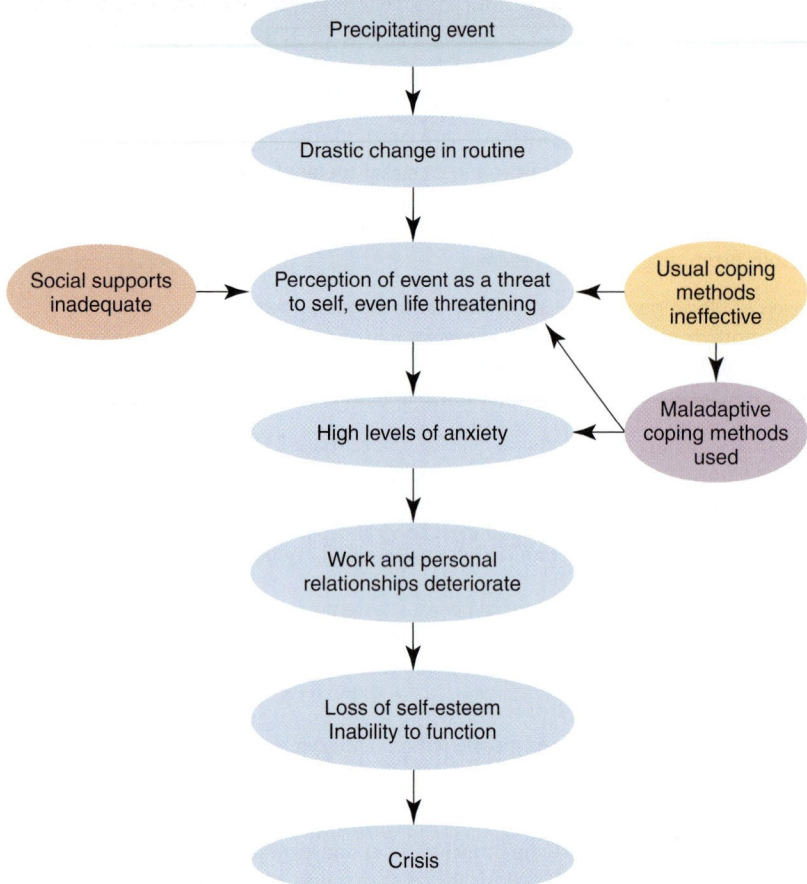

FIGURE 12-6 How a crisis develops.

problem solving helps the person to regain some self-esteem, and begin socializing again. Adaptation is more likely if the person can use effective coping strategies and if situational supports are available.

5. *Postcrisis.* In the aftermath of a crisis, a person may have developed better ways of coping with stress. Or, he or she may be critical, hostile, and depressed, and using maladaptive strategies (e.g., overeating or substance abuse) to deal with what has happened.

People in crisis are at risk for physical and emotional harm, so intervention is essential (see Crisis Intervention later in the chapter).

ThinkLike a Nurse 12-3

Suppose you are the charge nurse on a 30-bed surgical unit. In addition, you must assume care of three more patients because another nurse called in sick. It is a normal, busy day with seven postoperative patients and eight discharges. In addition, a patient went into cardiac arrhythmia and was transferred to the coronary care unit. Because the sick nurse was supposed to work a 12-hour shift and no replacement has been found, you are told you must stay and work 4 hours overtime. You had plans to have dinner with your spouse this evening because it is your anniversary. Now you will surely not be home before 8:00 p.m., and you will be exhausted.

■ What would be the stressors for you in this situation?
■ What thoughts and feelings would you have?
■ What physical responses would you probably notice?

■ What are some psychological responses that you would use to help you adapt and cope with this day?
■ How would you probably react if the same thing were to happen on the following day?

Burnout. Burnout occurs when a person cannot cope effectively with the physical and emotional demands of the workplace. Excessive demands, lack of respect, or little support from an employer or coworkers can serve as a catalyst for burnout. In response, the nurse experiences anger or frustration, feels overwhelmed and helpless, or suffers low self-esteem and depression. Some nurses experience grief, moral distress, and guilt because the situation prevents them from performing as well as they believe they should (Badger, 2008). As a result, a nurse may develop a physical illness or a negative attitude, or may use maladaptive coping techniques such as smoking, substance abuse, or distancing from patients—"going through the motions" but not really interacting with patients in a meaningful way. Many nurses with these feelings may give up and leave nursing. Examples of stressors specific to nursing are listed in Box 12-4. You will find suggestions for preventing burnout later in the chapter.

Post-Traumatic Stress Disorder. Post-traumatic stress disorder (PTSD) is a specific response to a violent, traumatizing event (e.g., earthquake, flood) or to physical or emotional abuse (e.g., rape, torture, war). The victim experiences anxiety and flashbacks that may last for months or years. Other symptoms include social withdrawal, low self-esteem, changes in existing relationships, difficulty forming new relationships, irritability and unexplained angry outbursts, depression, and chemical abuse or dependence. Counseling, special intervention, and

BOX 12-4 ■ Stressors That Can Lead to Burnout

- Dealing with difficult personalities (e.g., patient, supervisors, physicians)
- Working 12-hour shifts with minimal breaks for food, water, or rest
- Frequent rotating shifts that upset the circadian rhythm of the body and lower the immune system response
- Mandatory overtime
- Being "floated" to an unfamiliar unit (e.g., a maternity nurse may be "floated" to an orthopedic unit)
- Workload: low staffing ratio (one nurse to many patients)
- Frustration with patients (e.g., those who do not follow therapeutic routines)
- Need to constantly anticipate patients' needs and cope with the unexpected
- Feeling helpless against a patient's disease process or lack of healing
- Dealing with death and dying
- Lack of rewards (both intrinsic and extrinsic)
- Lack of participation in decision-making
- Inability to delegate responsibilities
- Organizational philosophy that conflicts with personal philosophy

stress management can all help the victim cope with and recover from the impact of the traumatic event (Bisson & Andrew, 2007).

KnowledgeCheck 12-7

Define *crisis*, *burnout*, and *post-traumatic stress disorder*.

PracticalKnowledge
knowing **how**

People under stress may not be thinking clearly or able to communicate effectively; so it is important to intervene to relieve their immediate anxiety as much as possible, demonstrate empathy, and develop rapport before beginning an assessment. Focus the patient by asking short, direct questions and then proceeding to open-ended questions that will provide you with as much information as possible (see Chapter 20 for information on questioning techniques).

ASSESSMENT

Assessment should explore subjective and objective data about the person's stressors, risk factors, coping and

Toward Evidence-Based Practice

Hall, L., Doran, D., & Pink, L. (2008). Outcomes of interventions to improve hospital nursing work environments. *Journal of Nursing Administration, 38(1),* 40–46.

This study evaluated the effects of workplace change interventions on nurse and patient perceptions of work quality and work environment. The intervention was a workplace change designed to improve the availability of resources on patient care units (e.g., improving the linen supply, identifying basic equipment needs). The only statistically significant change after the intervention was that nurses had a more positive perception of work quality and the work environment. Based on data from patients, researchers speculate that nurses' satisfaction with work arrangements can influence patient care.

Hegge, M., & Larson, V. (2008). Stressors and coping strategies of students in accelerated baccalaureate nursing programs. *Nurse Educator, 33(1),* 26–30.

Students in six baccalaureate nursing programs reported their stress level, sources of stress, and coping strategies. Findings indicate that students experienced higher levels and more extended periods of stress than in prior life events. The most helpful coping categories, in order, included seeking social (emotional) support, turning to religion, trying to grow as a person, planning, and acceptance. Students recognized the stress of the nursing program, appraised it in light of previous experience, resolved to meet their academic goals, and used helpful coping strategies to promote positive learning outcomes.

Morgan, P., Fogel, J., Rose, L., et al. (2005). African American couples merging strengths to successfully cope with breast cancer. *Oncology Nursing Forum, 32(5),* 979–987.

This qualitative study examined the process of coping with breast cancer among African American couples. The couples described the importance of combining their strengths and working together as a couple to cope with a breast cancer diagnosis. Authors recommended that nurses use this information to help couples work through a similar experience.

Recall the three approaches to coping and adaptation: altering the stressor, adapting to the stressor, and avoiding the stressor.

1. In which study (or studies) is stress relieved by altering the stressor? Explain your thinking (e.g., what the stressor was and how it was altered).

2. Which study or studies report using support systems to help in adapting to a stressor? Explain your thinking (e.g., what the stressor was and what support system was used).

3. What ideas does each study give you for ways in which you might help Gloria and John (Meet Your Patients).

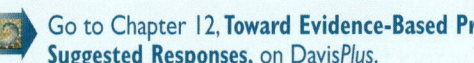 Go to Chapter 12, **Toward Evidence-Based Practice Suggested Responses,** on *DavisPlus*.

adaptation, support systems, and stress responses (psychosocial and physiological).

Assess Stressors, Risk Factors, and Coping and Adaptation

Data about the patient's stressors and risk factors should help you to:

- Determine whether the client has a realistic or an exaggerated perception of the stressors.
- Identify factors that increase risk for future stress.
- Identify interventions to reduce current stress and to provide anticipatory guidance to prevent future stress.

You might begin gathering these data by having the patient complete a stress inventory, such as the Holmes-Rahe Social Readjustment Scale. Then follow up with questions, such as those in the box Assessing for Stress: Questions to Ask. You will also find questions to help you obtain information about patients' coping methods and adaptation in those guidelines.

Assess Responses to Stress

When assessing responses to stress, recall that stress responses are holistic. Therefore, you will need to assess physiological, emotional, cognitive, and behavioral indicators of stress.

Assessing Physiological Responses. Because the GAS is nonspecific, you must obtain data from all body systems (for physical examination techniques, see Chapter 21). A check of vital signs for elevations in pulse, respiration, and blood pressure will indicate whether the fight-or-flight response is present. In your general survey, or overview, of the patient, you should note hygiene, grooming, facial expression, and ability to make eye contact. Box 12-5 summarizes physiological responses that indicate stress. If coping is successful, clinical signs and symptoms of stress may not be present.

Assessing Emotional and Behavioral Responses. Assess for the emotional and behavioral responses to stress that are described in Box 12-3. As the client answers questions, note posture, facial expression, body tension, and other nonverbal behaviors. Also note mood and affect. Does the client seem angry, anxious, or depressed? Check the client's records, and observe for and ask the client about destructive behaviors

(e.g., drug abuse, anger). The client may or may not be aware that the feelings or behaviors are related to stress.

Assessing Cognitive Responses. You can assess the client's cognitive functioning as you assess other functional areas. See Box 12-3 to review examples of cognitive responses. Notice whether the person has difficulty focusing and responding to your questions. When you ask the client to describe and rate the intensity of the stressors, you can begin to assess whether he perceives the stressors realistically or in an exaggerated way. The client's responses concerning any coping strategies will give you an idea of his problem-solving abilities.

Assess Support Systems

Recall that support systems, such as family, friends, and coworkers, are important to the success of a client's coping strategies. Conversely, these people may be affected by the same stressors or by the client's responses to them. For these reasons, you should determine the supports available and their ability to assist the client—that is, do the significant others have the sensitivity and skills to be supportive?

ThinkLike a Nurse 12-4

Review the scenario of Gloria and John (Meet Your Patients). How much does it really tell you about the clients' situation?

- Which aspect of stress do you have the most information about: their stressors, their coping methods and adaptation, their responses to stress, or their support systems?
- What facts do you have about either Gloria's or John's physiological responses to their multiple stressors? What can you infer their responses might be?
- What facts do you have about the clients' emotional and behavioral responses to their stressors?
- What information do you have about how well they are adapting to stress?
- What data do you have about their support systems? What information do you need?

ANALYSIS/NURSING DIAGNOSIS

Stress is nonspecific, so there is almost no limit to the number of nursing diagnoses that could be stress induced. Your theoretical knowledge of the holistic nature of stress should lead you to identify diagnoses in the physical, behavioral, cognitive, emotional, interpersonal, and spiritual domains. The following are some examples.

Physical	Constipation r/t decreased peristalsis secondary to stress
Behavioral	Ineffective Family Therapeutic Regimen Management r/t use of denial as an ego defense mechanism to relieve anxiety
Cognitive	Impaired Memory (short term) r/t overwhelming number and severity of stressors
Emotional	Anxiety r/t uncertainty about the future and ineffectiveness of usual coping mechanisms
Interpersonal	Impaired Parenting r/t maladaptive use of alcohol to cope with recent stress of divorce
Spiritual	Hopelessness r/t perceived lack of support and ability to change the present situation

BOX 12-5 ■ Physiological Responses to Stressors

- Dilated pupils
- Muscle tension
- Stiff neck
- Headaches
- Nail biting
- Skin pallor
- Skin lesions (e.g., eczema)
- Diaphoresis, sweaty palms
- Dry mouth
- Nausea
- Weight or appetite changes
- Increased blood glucose
- Increased heart rate
- Cardiac dysrhythmias
- Hyperventilation
- Chest pain
- Water retention
- Increased urinary frequency or decreased urinary output
- Diarrhea or constipation
- Flatulence

Assessing for Stress: Questions to Ask

1. **Assess stressors and risk factors.** Ask the client to complete a stress inventory, such as the preceding Holmes-Rahe Social Readjustment Scale. Then ask the client the following questions:
   - What is causing the most stress in your life?
   - On a scale of 1 to 10 (1 being "not much" and 10 being "extreme"), rate the stress you are experiencing in each of these areas: work or school, finances, community responsibilities, your health, health of a family member, family relationships, family responsibilities, relationships with friends.
   - How long have you been dealing with the stressful situation(s)?
   - Can you track the accumulation of stress in your life?
   - How long have you been under this stress?
   - Note the client's developmental stage, and determine whether he is functioning as expected for this stage. Review the expanded version in Chapter 9 if you need help in identifying developmental milestones. To help you assess for stressors that can be predicted to occur in each stage, you might ask questions such as the following:

     What challenges do you face as a result of your life and your age?

     Have you had recent life changes?

     Do you anticipate any life changes?

   To review developmental stage changes, refer to Box 12-1, Stressors Throughout the Life Span.

2. **Assess coping methods and adaptation.**
   - What coping strategies have you used previously? What was successful, and what was not successful?
   - Tell me about previous experiences you have had with stressful situations in your life.
   - What do you usually do to handle stressful situations? (If the client needs prompting, you can ask, "Do you cry, get angry, avoid people, talk to family or friends, do physical exercise, pray? Some people laugh or joke, others meditate, others try to control everything, others just work hard and look for a solution. What is your usual response?")
   - How well do these methods usually work for you?
   - What have you been doing to cope with the present situation?
   - How well is that working?
   - During the interview, you should also observe for the use of psychological defense mechanisms.
   - If the patient has not exhibited any defense mechanisms, you could ask about the common ones. For example, "Do you ever cope with a situation by denying it exists or just by trying to put it out of your mind?"
   - Also ask the client about physiological changes and diseases caused by ongoing stress. Check the client's records for a history of somatoform disorders. Ask the client:

     What physical illnesses do you have? How long have you had them?

     What, if any, physical changes have you noticed?

     Do you have other physical conditions, for example, hypertension, cardiac disease, diabetes, arthritis, joint pains, cancer?

3. **Assess physiological responses to stress.**
   The following are examples of questions you should ask:
   - What do you do to stay healthy?
   - Tell me about your health habits.
   - How often do you have a checkup?
   - What are your health concerns?

4. **Assess emotional and behavioral responses to stress.**

   ### Emotional Responses

   Observe for:
   - Anger
   - Anxiety
   - Depression
   - Fear
   - Feelings of inadequacy
   - Low self-esteem
   - Lack of motivation
   - Lethargy

   ### Behavioral Responses

   Observe for:
   - Crying, emotional outburst
   - Dependence
   - Poor job performance
   - Substance use and abuse
   - Sleeplessness or sleeping too much
   - Change in eating habits (e.g., diminished appetite or overeating)
   - Decrease in quality of job performance
   - Preoccupation or distraction
   - Listlessness
   - Increased absenteeism
   - Increased number of accidents
   - Reduced interest in social interactions or relationships
   - Rebellion, acting out

   ### Examples of Assessment Questions

   - Do you smoke?
   - How much alcohol do you drink every day?
   - What do you eat? What is your typical eating pattern?
   - How much fluid do you drink daily?
   - How many hours do you sleep at night? Do you feel rested when you wake up?
   - Do you often wake up very early in the morning and have difficulty getting back to sleep?
   - What prescribed medications, vitamins, over-the-counter medications, or herbs do you take?
   - What regular physical activity or exercise do you engage in?
   - How much time do you spend at work versus at leisure and play?
   - Do you constantly take work home with you? Do you think about work almost all the time?
   - How do you relax?
   - Have you given up activities and relationships you previously enjoyed because you "don't have enough time" or are too tired?
   - How do you express anger?
   - Do you try to be perfect?
   - Would you describe yourself as having the stress-filled lifestyle of a type A personality?
   - How often do you find yourself feeling hopeless? Sad?

5. **Assess cognitive responses to stress.**
   Observe for the following responses when you assess other functional areas:
   - Difficulty concentrating
   - Poor judgment
   - Decrease in accuracy (e.g., in counting money)
   - Forgetfulness
   - Decreased problem-solving ability
   - Decreased attention to detail

(Continued)

Assessing for Stress: Questions to Ask—cont'd

- Difficulty learning
- Narrowing of focus
- Preoccupation, daydreaming
6. **Assess support systems.**
   Ask the following questions:
   - Tell me about your home. Describe your living environment. (Make a home visit if possible, or contact the case manager or social worker to arrange a home evaluation.)

- Who are the persons that provide the most support for you? In what ways do they support you?
- What support is available from family, friends, significant others, community agencies, and clergy that you may not have required until now?
- Do you have or do you seek spiritual support?
- How has your stress affected the family?
- What are your financial resources? What are your financial obligations?

For a more extensive list of stress-related nursing diagnoses you can print out and use within the clinical setting,

 Go to Chapter 12, **Standardized Language: NANDA-I Nursing Diagnoses Associated With Stress,** on Davis*Plus.*

It is important to correctly identify the etiology of the diagnosis so that you can choose interventions to remove or modify the stressor. For example, if you believe a patient's diarrhea is being caused by stress, you would intervene by modifying the stressor, helping the patient to perceive the stressor differently, and so on. If, instead, a gastrointestinal virus were causing the diarrhea, your interventions would not have been helpful.

Knowledge Check 12-8

- How might you identify and assess Gloria and John's stressors (Meet Your Patients)?
- List three questions you could ask to find out how Gloria is coping and adapting to stress.
- List three questions you could ask to assess Gloria's physiological responses to stress. What observations might you also make?
- List three questions you could ask to assess Gloria's emotional and behavioral responses to stress.
- How might you determine whether stress is affecting Gloria's cognitive functioning?
- You know Gloria's sister is providing some support. How could you find out more about the extent of Gloria and John's support system?

◼ PLANNING OUTCOMES/EVALUATION

Individualized goal or outcome statements are also specific to each nursing diagnosis. Broad, general goals for clients experiencing stress are to (1) reduce the strength and duration of the stressor, (2) relieve or remove responses to stress, and (3) use effective coping mechanisms. Examples of specific outcome statements you might write include the following:

- Reports (or physical exam reveals) reduction in physical symptoms of stress.
- Demonstrates less physical tension in facial expression and other muscle groups.
- Verbalizes increased feelings of control in the stressful situation.
- Uses problem-solving and anxiety-reducing techniques.
- Demonstrates relaxation and stress-reducing strategies.

NOC standardized outcomes are outcomes that, if achieved, demonstrate resolution of the problem stated by the nursing diagnosis. For example, if you make a diagnosis of Anxiety related to client's perception that he will not be able to fulfill

family responsibilities, you might use the NOC outcome, Anxiety Control. To use or print a list of NOC outcomes for use with stress diagnoses,

 Go to Chapter 12, **Standardized Language: Standardized Outcomes and Interventions for Stress-Related Nursing Diagnosis,** on Davis*Plus.*

◼ PLANNING INTERVENTIONS/IMPLEMENTATION

NIC standardized interventions for stress may be linked to both the problem and the etiology of the nursing diagnosis. Using the preceding example of Anxiety related to the client's perception that he will not be able to fulfill family responsibilities, some interventions may focus on supporting the client's ability to fulfill family roles (e.g., Caregiver Support); others may focus on general techniques for relieving anxiety, regardless of its cause (e.g., Anxiety Reduction, Calming Technique). To use or print other stress-related NIC interventions,

 Go to Chapter 12, **Standardized Language: Standardized Outcomes and Interventions for Stress-Related Nursing Diagnoses,** on Davis*Plus.*

Specific nursing activities will be individualized on the basis of the patient's needs and the etiologies of the nursing diagnoses. As you implement stress-reduction interventions, it is essential to consider compliance. Will the patient adhere to or cooperate with therapeutic suggestions? Does the person wish to use complementary or alternative care measures? How open is he to deviating from traditional biomedical therapies? Confer and collaborate with patients to determine what will fit most comfortably into their lifestyle. Those are the interventions that will be most effective.

Most stress-relieving interventions work by one or more of the following means:

- Removing or modifying the stressor(s)
- Supporting coping abilities (e.g., changing the person's perception of the stressor)
- Treating the person's responses to stress (e.g., symptoms such as anxiety or diarrhea)

As you read through the following interventions, see whether you can identify the rationale for the action. Look back at the above list if you need to.

Health Promotion Activities

People cannot always control the occurrence of a stressful event, and there are no high-tech treatments for coping with stress. However, a healthy lifestyle can prevent some stressors and improve the ability to cope with others. Chapter 27

provides an in-depth discussion of wellness promotion. The following suggestions are a brief guide to a healthy lifestyle.

Nutrition. **Nutrition** is important for maintaining physical homeostasis and resisting stress. For example, adequate nutrition is essential to maintain the integrity of the immune system; proteins are needed for tissue building and healing. In addition, overweight and malnutrition are stressors that may lead to illness. To summarize, you should advise clients to maintain a normal body weight, eat a balanced diet, and consume alcohol only in moderation. See Chapter 28 if you need detailed information about healthful nutrition.

Exercise. Regular exercise promotes physical homeostasis by improving muscle tone and controlling weight. It also improves the functioning of the heart and lungs and reduces the risk of cardiovascular disease. Exercise also improves emotional homeostasis by promoting relaxation and reducing tension. During exercise, the brain releases **endogenous opioids** (e.g., endorphins), which create a feeling of well-being. To achieve any health benefits, the client needs to exercise for at least 30 minutes at least 5 days of the week. See Chapter 33 for more specific physical activities to manage stress.

Sleep and Rest. Sleep and rest restore energy levels, allow the body to repair itself, and promote mental relaxation. Most people need 7 or 8 hours of sleep a day; however, the amount of sleep varies among individuals. Stress, pain, and illness may interfere with the ability to sleep, so some clients may need help identifying and implementing techniques for relaxing and going to sleep (see Chapter 35 for more information on sleep, as needed).

Leisure Activities. Leisure activities are any activities that provide joy and satisfaction. They may involve physical activity, or they may be sedentary activities, such as reading, painting, and even watching television. Leisure activities are a form of rest and, as such, are restorative.

Time Management. People who manage their time efficiently and organize their life routines feel more in control and, therefore, less stressed. If clients feel overwhelmed, you can help them to prioritize tasks and make "to do" lists. It is also important that they learn to delegate responsibilities and set boundaries on the use of time. For example, a working couple with three children may need to limit the amount of time they spend cooking, reserving meals requiring time-consuming preparation for weekends.

Time management also includes learning to say no. People sometimes try to make everyone happy by agreeing to every request for assistance: from family, friends, and the community. Prompt clients to identify how much they can realistically accomplish—what is essential to do, and what would be nice to do. If you would like more information on time management,

 Go to **Chapter 45, Leadership and Management,** on DavisPlus.

Avoiding Maladaptive Behaviors. Some people use maladaptive behaviors as a response to stress. For others, the behaviors themselves become stressors. Advise clients to avoid the unhealthful behaviors, such as consuming excess caffeine (e.g., coffee, tea, colas), abusing alcohol, smoking or chewing tobacco, using street drugs, abusing prescribed and over-the-counter (nonprescribed) medications, and avoiding social interaction.

KnowledgeCheck 12-9

Name and discuss at least four aspects of a healthful lifestyle that can help prevent or relieve stress.

Relieving Anxiety

Because anxiety is a common response to illness, medical tests, and treatments, you will use anxiety-relief interventions every day of your professional life. For example, when you tell patients what to expect before you perform a procedure or ask them to take deep breaths during a painful treatment, you lessen anxiety. If you have developed a therapeutic, trusting relationship, your very presence will help to ease the patient's anxiety. You will find specific interventions for anxiety in Chapter 13, and many of the interventions in the following sections provide anxiety relief as well. Also see the box Complementary & Alternative Modalities (CAM): Using CAM for Stress Reduction.

Complementary & Alternative Modalities (CAM)

Using CAM for Stress Reduction

Bost, N., & Wallis, M. (2006). The effectiveness of a 15-minute weekly massage in reducing physical and psychological stress in nurses. *Australian Journal of Advanced Nursing, 23*(4), 28–33.

Thirty nurses received a 15-minute back massage once a week; the control group of 30 nurses received no therapy. Physiological stress was measured at weeks 1, 3, and 5 by urinary cortisol and blood pressure readings. Psychological stress levels were measured at weeks 1 and 5 with the State-Trait Anxiety Inventory (STAI). No significant difference in physiological measures was found between the two groups. However, anxiety decreased in the group receiving massage and increased in the control group. The difference was significant. Researchers concluded that massage therapy may be beneficial in reducing nurses' psychological stress.

Keegan, L. (2003). Therapies to reduce stress and anxiety. *Critical Care Nursing Clinics of North America, 15*(3), 321–327.

This article reports on the successful use of alternative and complementary therapies as adjunct therapies to help decrease stress for critical care patients. Therapies included in the report are aromatherapy, hydrotherapy, humor, imagery, massage, music, and relaxation.

Maville, J., Bowen, J., & Genham, G. (2008). Effect of healing touch on stress perception and biological correlates. *Holistic Nursing Practice, 22*(2), 103–110.

The researchers measured heart rate, blood pressure, muscle tension, skin conductance, and skin temperature in healthy adults before, during, and after healing touch treatment. All measures changed except for muscle tension. Results suggested that healing touch treatment is associated with both physiological and psychological relaxation and may be useful as an intervention for stress in healthy adults.

Pemberton, E., & Turpin, P. (2008). The effect of essential oils on work-related stress in intensive care unit nurses. *Holistic Nursing Practice, 22*(2), 97–102.

This small pilot study evaluated the effects of topical essential oils on nurses in intensive care unit settings. Nurses assessed their stress levels on a scale of 1 to 10. The nurses' perceived stress level decreased significantly in the intervention group. Researchers concluded that use of *Lavandula angustifolia* and *Salvia sclaria* in sweet almond oil had a beneficial effect on work-related stress reduction.

Anger Management

Anger is a common response to stress. However, clients usually do not openly say, "I am angry." In fact, they may not even recognize that they are angry. Instead, they engage in angry behaviors. For example, they may become hypercritical of family members or caregivers, become verbally abusive, or become demanding. By now you have probably heard stories from nurses about the client who is "on the call light constantly." Unfortunately, such behaviors often provoke frustration or anger in others—even nurses. Be aware of how you are responding to stressed-out clients. Not only that, but anger also blocks communication and can lead to poor patient care and reduced patient satisfaction. For tips on managing anger, refer to Coping With Violence, in Chapter 23; and Clinical Insight 12-1, Dealing With Angry Patients.

Stress Management Techniques

It is important to teach your clients about relaxation and other **stress management** techniques. Most such techniques focus on discharging tension or simplifying one's life to modify stressors or control stress responses. **Relaxation** is a state of reduced physical and mental arousal. It is an important intervention because it reverses some stress responses. By elongating muscle fibers, relaxation reduces neural impulses sent to the brain and decreases the activity of the brain and other body systems. Blood pressure, heart rate, respiratory rate, and oxygen consumption decrease, while peripheral skin temperatures and brain alpha wave activity increase.

Many of the techniques in this section are CAM therapies that require special training, which are discussed in detail in other chapters. If you would like to have detailed information about CAM and stress management,

 Go to Chapter 46, **Holistic Healing,** on Davis*Plus.*

For 12 weeks of daily suggestions for coping with stress,

 Go to Chapter 12, **Tables, Boxes, Figures: ESG Box 12-1,** on Davis*Plus.*

Exercise. Exercise is used to treat, as well as prevent, stress. It reduces stress because it releases tension held in muscles, improves muscle tone and posture, expresses emotions, and stimulates the secretion of endorphins, thus creating a feeling of well-being and relaxation.

Relaxation Techniques. Relaxation techniques involve teaching the patient to relax individual muscle groups. **Progressive relaxation** in a quiet meditative state or lying in bed, relaxing and contracting muscle groups, is much less traumatic and damaging to fragile joints and muscles than is active

---

Clinical Insight 12-1 ▸ **Dealing With Angry Patients**

- **Be aware of how you are responding to angry patients.** Are you relieving your own stress, or are you relieving the client's stress? *If you respond angrily to relieve your own stress, you may provoke further anger in the patient and even escalate the situation to the point of violence.*

- **Keep reminding yourself not to take anger personally;** remind family members of this as well.

- **Recognize anger and anxiety are normal feelings when facing adversity,** such as a life-threatening or debilitating illness. Do not discount feelings by saying something such as, "Please, don't be so angry," or "You shouldn't talk like that," or, "Everything will be OK. Don't worry."

- **Encourage the client and family to express feelings verbally and appropriately.**

- **Listen instead of defending.** If the patient yells, "Everything about this place stinks!" don't respond with a comment such as, "This hospital is highly rated by The Joint Commission," or, "We really are all trying to do the best we can for you." Instead, say something to encourage the person to express his feelings or give you more information: "You seem really angry; what's going on?" or "Maybe I can help. Tell me a little more about what stinks."

- **Do not take responsibility for the patient's anger.** It is not your fault, so don't apologize (unless you really *do* have something to apologize for). In the preceding

example, for instance, it is not your fault that "the place stinks" or that the patient feels that way. So do *not* say, "I'm sorry we haven't been meeting your expectations."

- **Remain calm.** *This reassures the patient.*

- **Help the patient identify what is causing the anger and try to meet those needs.**

- ✚ **Be alert to your own and to the patient's safety needs.**
  - If the person seems violent, do not allow him to get between you and the door.
  - Be sure you know how to call for help from staff or security personnel if you think you or someone else is in danger.
    Do not wear a stethoscope around your neck, dangling jewelry, or anything a patient might use to hurt you.
    Do not go into a room alone with an angry patient who seems to have a potential for violence.
    Remain at least an arm's length away from an angry and potentially violent patient.
    Do not turn your back on an angry patient.
- **If you believe the patient's anger may escalate to violence, your priority is your own safety and the safety of others in the area.**

Also refer to the NIC intervention, Anger Control Assistance (Bulechek, Butcher, & Dochterman, 2008, pp. 134–135).

exercise. With **passive relaxation,** the person relaxes the muscle groups without first contracting them.

Meditation. Managing stress through meditation involves heightening one's attention or awareness. Regular meditation increases harmony among mind, body, and spirit, thereby reducing anxiety and giving the person control. For a script to lead a client through a guided meditation to reduce stress,

 Go to Chapter 12, **Tables, Boxes, Figures: ESG Box 12-2, Script for Visualization,** on Davis*Plus.*

Visualization or Imagery. Visualization (imagery) techniques are often used to complement the effects of relaxation techniques. They are explained in Chapters 32 in this text. and in Chapter 46, on Davis*Plus.*

Biofeedback. Techniques of biofeedback use electronic instruments to measure neuromuscular and autonomic nervous system activity and provide information about those responses to the person. The immediate feedback helps the person become aware of and learn how to voluntarily control certain physiological responses, such as those produced by stress (Olson, 2003). Biofeedback practitioners require special training, and most are credentialed in biofeedback.

Acupuncture. Acupuncture involves insertion of a needle into "meridian points" to regulate the flow of energy or life force throughout the body. It can modify pain perception and restore normal physiological functions (e.g., decrease the heart rate). Special training is required to use this intervention. If you want more information, see Chapter 32.

Chiropractic Adjustment. Chiropractic adjustment involves manual realignment of the vertebrae. Misalignment of the vertebrae is thought to lead to pain, loss of function, and illness. Realignment is performed to free energy, release muscle tension, and improve body function and health. Chiropractors undergo special education and training before they are qualified to perform adjustments.

Reiki and therapeutic touch. These touch therapies are focused on energy modulation. Healing energy is channeled through a practitioner's hands to improve well-being.

Massage. Through manipulation of the soft tissues, relaxes muscles, massage releases body tension, improves circulation, and allows energy and blood to flow through muscles and soft tissues more readily. See Chapters 32 for more information. For instructions on how to give a back rub, see Procedure 35-1.

Reflexology. Reflexology is the application of pressure to specific points on the feet, hands, or ears; these points are thought to correspond with certain organs of the body. The goal is to relieve blockage, promote the flow of energy, and reduce tension—thus, reflexology may be helpful in treating stress-related illnesses. Reflexology requires special training. The following are simpler activities you can recommend to most clients to aid in relaxation and stress reduction:

Humor. Laughter releases endorphins and relieves feelings of stress (Fig. 12-7). It enhances respiration and circulation, oxygenates the blood, suppresses the stress-related hormones in the brain, and activates the immune system. Some medical centers have begun implementing in-house humor programs (Bennett & Lengacher, 2007; Cousins, 1979; du Pré, 1998; Johnson, 2002).

Listening to Music. Music soothes and relaxes when its vibrations are in harmony with body frequencies. Listening to tranquil music can also relax the mind.

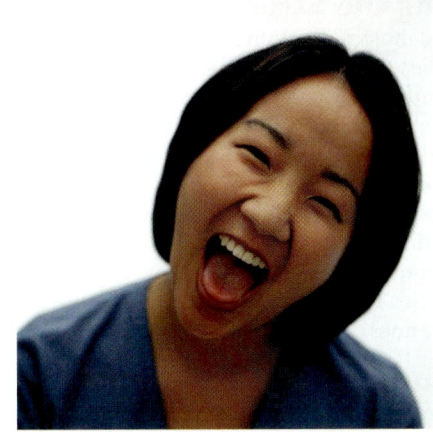

FIGURE 12-7 Laughter releases endorphins and helps relieve stress.

Engaging in Art Activities. Painting, working with clay, and engaging in other art activities help to express emotions and release endorphins.

Dance and Sports. Like other forms of exercise, dance and sports release pent-up physical tension and emotions. Steady-state exercises, such as running or swimming at a consistent pace, offer stress relief in a meditative manner through sustained deep breathing and movement. Physical activity can also enhance self-esteem and help people feel better by the simple act of accomplishing a personal goal.

Journal Writing. Journal writing helps the person to reflect on experiences and express emotions. The venting of emotion that can occur in journal writing often provides insights into causes of stress and ways to modify stressors.

Changing Perception of Stressors or Self

Recall that altering ones perception is one way to improve adaptation to stress. For clients who have an unrealistic perception of the stressor and can imagine only negative outcomes, a technique, called **cognitive restructuring,** may be helpful. With this technique, you help clients to recognize their negative focus and to restructure their thinking in more positive and realistic ways. For example, you might encourage a working mother with demanding family members to take a single positive step, such as saying no to someone at least once a day.

You can also help clients to identify positive aspects of themselves and their coping abilities. This promotes self-esteem and helps them to recognize and use the resources they have for coping with their stressors. **Positive self-talk** is another method for increasing self-esteem. Each time you hear negative self-talk, stop the client, and ask him to rephrase the statement so that it is positive.

Identifying and Using Support Systems

You can facilitate successful adaptation by helping clients to identify and contact people and groups who offer various supports (e.g., listening, encouragement, advice, problem-solving, help with household tasks, financial support). Be aware of the groups available in your community (e.g., Weight Watchers, Alcoholics Anonymous, Parents Without Partners, Reach for Recovery). You may need to teach socialization skills to clients who are socially isolated so that they can begin to build a support system.

Reducing the Stress of Hospitalization

Illness and hospitalization are stressful for patients and their families. In addition to being sick, patients find themselves in unfamiliar surroundings, with little privacy, and a certain loss of control. Promote patient-centered care in the healthcare agency as much as you can. Involving patients and families actively in their care helps them adapt to the stressors of hospitalization. Teach patients what to expect from hospitalization, and give them a few tips to help plan ahead to minimize the stress they experience (see the box Self-Care: Teaching Clients How to Reduce the Stress of Hospitalization).

Providing Spiritual Support

In addition to helping clients obtain spiritual support from church groups and clergy, you can help to strengthen the client spiritually. You may wish to do the following:

Pray for or with clients, if they desire, and if you are comfortable doing so. Prayer can help reduce their feelings of powerlessness and loneliness.

Help clients to define their values and set boundaries that honor themselves and uphold those values.

Teach clients to silently recite an affirming mantra (e.g., on inhalation, say, "I am free." Exhale and say, "Stress, leave me.") or relevant spiritual passages.

For other ways to provide spiritual support, see Chapter 16.

Crisis Intervention

As an entry-level nurse in acute and ambulatory care settings, you are more likely to see patients in the first three phases of crisis and not be present for the adaptive and postcrisis stages.

Crisis centers often rely on telephone counseling (hotlines). If telephone counseling is not adequate, or if observations of the home environment are needed, home visits may be necessary. See Clinical Insight 12-2 for a description of how to intervene when a patient is in crisis.

KnowledgeCheck 12-10

- Describe at least five specific interventions for dealing with an angry person.
- What is cognitive restructuring?
- What is the purpose of positive self-talk?
- List the seven steps of crisis intervention.
- Why is relaxation an important stress intervention?

Stress Management in the Workplace

You will need to pay attention to your feelings, your body, and your personal responses to stress. Do you notice that you are eating more than usual or have lost your appetite? Are you feeling edgy or impatient with family or coworkers, or not sleeping well? Check your body. Do you feel tired or often have headaches or gastrointestinal distress? Are the muscles in your face and shoulders tense? Do you often take work home with you? Are you unable to stop thinking about work, even when you are at home? Do concerns about finances or personal situations consume your thinking and create a sense of doom? If so, you probably need to start managing your stress. You can better manage workplace stress and avoid burnout by following the advice you give your patients. For some tips,

 Go to Chapter 12, **Tables, Boxes, Figures: ESG Box 12-1,** on Davis*Plus.*

Teaching Clients How to Reduce the Stress of Hospitalization

Share the following tips with clients, preferably before hospitalization:

- Bring what you need from home. Make a list of necessities and pack carefully before you go. For example, bring your own soap, toothpaste, lotion, pajamas, and slippers—or your favorite tea bags and sweetener. Having familiar things can make your stay more pleasant for you.
- If you will feel well enough, bring your computer, reading material, crossword puzzles, or whatever you like to do that can help prevent boredom and depression. You might want to bring a few family photos for your nightstand.
- Bring a notepad and pencils so that you can take notes about what your primary care providers tell you (e.g., about diagnostic tests, instructions for care).
- Do *not* bring jewelry, cash, credit cards, or other valuables.
- Do not bring clothing that is not washable or that is uncomfortable or tight.
- Do not allow family or friends to visit if they are ill.
- It helps to ask family or friends to stay at the bedside, particularly when the physician is "making rounds."

They can advocate for you and help you feel confident that everything will go well. You may not feel well enough to ask for what you need, but a family member can do that for you.

- Your family members or friends can also help you interpret and remember information and instructions that you will receive from nurses, physicians, and other care providers. There may be 30 people in your room each day, and when you are ill or taking certain medications, it is hard to keep track of everything.
- Keep a bottle of hand sanitizer by your bed or insist visitors, including family members and care providers, use a hand hygiene product at the door when entering the room, just as you do.
- Know the name of your primary nurse (or nurses) on each shift, and ask as many questions as you need to.
- Even though some things seem to not make sense (e.g., taking your temperature at 3 a.m.), there is likely a medical reason for it. Try to be as patient and cheerful as possible.

Clinical Insight 12-2 ➤ Crisis Intervention Guidelines

For nurses who are at an entry level of practice, the goals of crisis intervention include the following (Brammer & Mac-Donald, 2003; Neeb, 2006):

1. Assess the situation.
   What is the nature of the patient's condition and the severity of the crisis?
2. Ensure safety.
   - Call for help if you are or the patient is in physical danger.
   - Do not leave the patient unless you think you are in imminent danger.
   - First ensure your own safety; then provide for the patient's safety.
3. Defuse the situation.
   - Keep in mind that a person in crisis may not be in control of his actions.
   - Try to calm the person verbally.
   - Attempt physical restraint only as a last resort and only when there is enough help to do it safely for both the staff and the patient.
4. Decrease the person's anxiety.
   - Reassure the person that he is in a safe place and that you are concerned and want to help.
   - Explain gently but firmly that you need his help and cooperation.
   - Help the person to vent feelings of fear, guilt, and anger.

- Use physical contact very cautiously. The person in turmoil may interpret touch as aggression or a sexual approach.

5. Determine the problem.
   - Find out what the patient believes to be the cause of the crisis.
   - Remain calm, and do not pressure the patient to give reasons. Any tension on your part will create further panic in the patient.
6. Decide on the type of help needed.
   - You may be able to calm the person enough for him to understand what just happened, or you may not. Evaluate your ability to calm the patient based on your assessment of his coping skills and resources.
   - Put in place the help needed to restore the person to a minimal level of functioning. This may require long-term treatment. In that case, make the referrals.
7. Return the person to his precrisis level of functioning. This may involve crisis counseling and/or home crisis visits.
   - The goal of crisis counseling is to provide immediate relief, solve the most urgent problems, and give long-term counseling if needed. Crisis centers often rely on telephone counseling (hotlines).
   - If telephone counseling is not adequate or if observations of the home environment are needed, home visits might be necessary.

When stressors arise from the workplace, the following actions are especially important:

- Set realistic expectations of yourself and others. Don't be overcritical; most people, including you, are doing the best they can.
- Ask for help. Seeking the support of others does not indicate weakness or incompetence.
- Offer support to colleagues who need help with tasks or with their feelings. This adds to the overall good feeling on a unit and improves the efficiency of performing many tasks.
- Be proactive about the things you can change and accept the things that you cannot change. Get involved in constructive efforts to change a particular stressor. If you cannot effect the changes, and if you cannot accept things as they are, you may need to think about removing yourself from the situation.
- Join and support professional organizations that address workplace issues (e.g., the National Student Nurses Association [NSNA] and the American Nurses Association [ANA]).
- Strive for balance in these seven key areas: family, financial responsibilities, health, social contributions, career, vocation or education, and spirituality or faith. Focus on

the most important items and task; remember, work affects life, but your life also affects your work.
- Obtain counseling for stress that exceeds your ability to cope.

Making Referrals

This chapter has presented many assessments and interventions for reducing stress. Remember, though, you are not yet an expert nurse and no one, not even an experienced nurse, is an expert in all areas. It is important not to "get in over your head" and attempt to intervene beyond your abilities with clients who are under stress and showing maladaptive coping. You can help by recognizing your limitations and by referring the client to the appropriate professionals as needed (e.g., a spiritual leader, a counselor, a social worker, a practitioner of complementary therapies, a physician, a psychologist, or a psychiatrist).

ThinkLike a Nurse 12-5

Sally is an RN seeking employment at a local nursing home. She left her previous employer because of stress and frustration with agency policy, for which the bottom line was financial gain rather than quality patient care. What can Sally do to help ensure that she will not experience the same problem in the new agency?

CLINICALREASONING:
Applying the **Full-Spectrum Nursing Model**

Because the following critical thinking activities allow you to practice the kind of thinking you will use as a full-spectrum nurse, they usually have no single right answer. Discuss them with your peers—if you have difficulty with any of the questions, consult your instructor.

PATIENT SITUATION

Mrs. Williams is a 76-year-old Indian American woman who was admitted yesterday after suffering a stroke that paralyzed her right side. She has had diabetes and high blood pressure for many years. Since the stroke, she has been unable to speak clearly and becomes frustrated as she attempts to communicate her needs. Her daughter says Mrs. Williams is a proud, independent, and tidy woman who has been living alone since her husband's death last year. Until her stroke, she had been driving her car, cleaning her house, doing her grocery shopping, and maintaining the yard and garden. She wears eyeglasses for reading and driving and has a hearing aid, although she rarely uses it.

THINKING

1. *Theoretical Knowledge:*
   a. What stroke risk factors probably functioned as stressors for Mrs. Williams? (*Hint:* Look up *stroke risk factors* in a medical–surgical nursing or pathophysiology text, or online.)
   b. What are common stressors for patients who must be hospitalized?
2. *Critical Thinking (Contextual Awareness):* Now that Mrs. Williams is in the hospital, what new stressors might she have?

DOING

3. *Practical Knowledge:* What might you advise Mrs. Williams's daughter to do to help her mother adapt more comfortably to the stressors in the hospital?
4. *Nursing Process (Diagnosis):* Based on only the data in the scenario, write one actual nursing diagnosis for Mrs. Williams. Do not use potential diagnoses. Remember, the defining characteristics must be present in the scenario. State the data you would need in order to make the diagnosis more descriptive.

CARING

5. *Self-Knowledge:* Imagine yourself in Mrs. Williams's situation.
   a. What is the one thing that would cause you the most stress? Why would that be the most stressful thing?
   b. What is the single most important thing you would want your nurse to do for you?

 Go To Chapter 12, **Clinical Reasoning: Applying the Full-Spectrum Nursing Model Answer Sheet,** on Davis*Plus*.

 To explore learning resources for this chapter,

 Go to DavisPlus at http://davisplus.fadavis.com/, **keyword: Treas.**

Chapter Resources for Chapter 12:
    Knowledge Check and Think Like a Nurse Response Sheets
    Knowledge Check Answers
    Resources for Caregivers and Health Professionals
    Reading More About the Stress and Adaptation
    Care Planning and Care Mapping Practice Exercises and Answers
    Practice Documentation Exercises and Answers
    What Are the Main Points in This Chapter?
NCLEX-Style Question Bank
Chapter Overview Podcasts
Care Planning and Care Mapping Practice Exercises and Answers
Practice Documentation Exercises and Answers

Concept Map

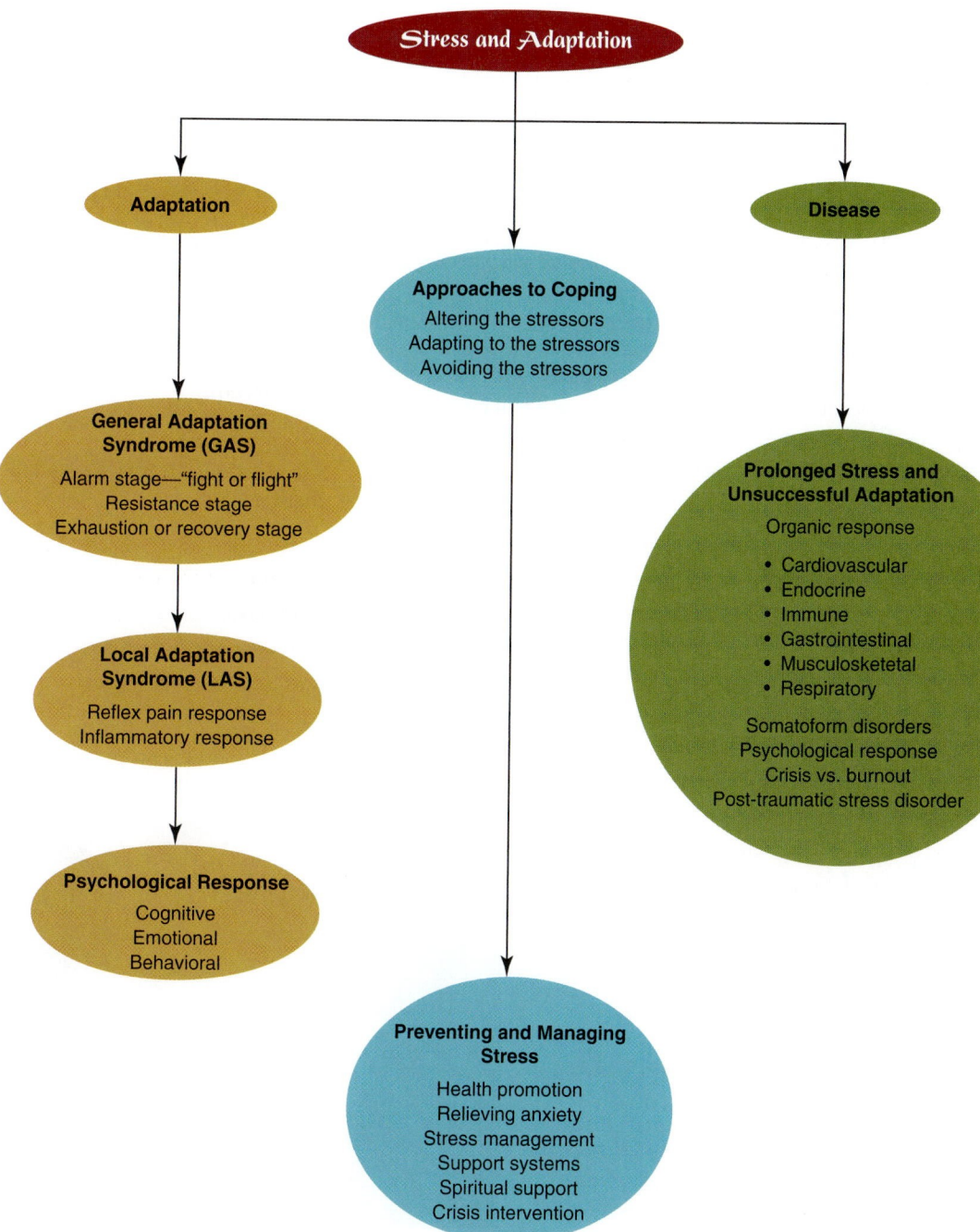

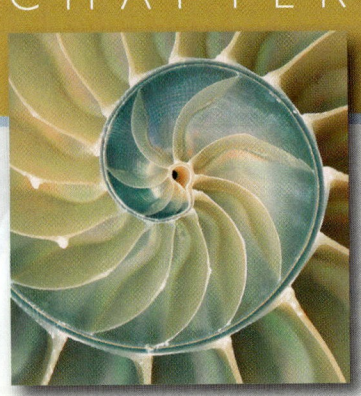

Psychosocial Health & Illness

Learning Outcomes

After completing this chapter, you should be able to:

➤ Explain the relationship of psychosocial factors to overall health and development.

➤ Identify the factors that influence the development and stability of self-concept.

➤ List the four interrelated components of self-concept.

➤ Perform a comprehensive assessment using the domains of self-concept, self-esteem, self-identity, and body image.

➤ Develop a nursing care plan for patients exhibiting disturbances in self-concept and self-esteem.

➤ Identify nursing diagnoses, outcomes, and interventions specific to body image disturbance.

➤ Describe interventions for preventing depersonalization.

➤ List the psychological and physiological effects of anxiety.

➤ Recognize the levels and symptoms of anxiety that are severe enough to merit referral to a mental health professional.

➤ Devise a nursing care plan for the nursing diagnosis of Anxiety.

➤ Differentiate between mild depression and that which should be referred to a mental health professional.

➤ Assess older adults for manifestations of depression.

➤ Plan outcomes and nursing interventions for patients who are depressed.

➤ Plan outcomes and nursing interventions for patients with a diagnosis of Risk for Suicide.

Key Concepts

Anxiety

Depression

Psychosocial health

Self-concept

Self-esteem

Related Concepts

See the **Concept Map** at the end of this chapter.

Example Problems

Anxiety

Depression

Self-Concept Disturbance

Low Self-Esteem

Caring for the Nguyens

This feature allows you to practice the kind of thinking you will use as a full-spectrum nurse. There is usually more than one correct answer to a critical thinking question, so we do not provide answers for these features. It is more important to develop your nursing judgment than to "cover content." Discuss the questions with your peers. If you are still unsure, consult your instructor.

Recall the case of Nam Nguyen. Mr. Nguyen has been diagnosed with hypertension, obesity, and degenerative joint disease. At clinic visits he has made the following comments: "Every time I come in here, I get some new diagnosis. I guess it's amazing I'm not dead yet. I thought I had a lot more time left, but I'm not so sure anymore." When you ask him what his main concerns are, he tells you, "Just take a look at me!

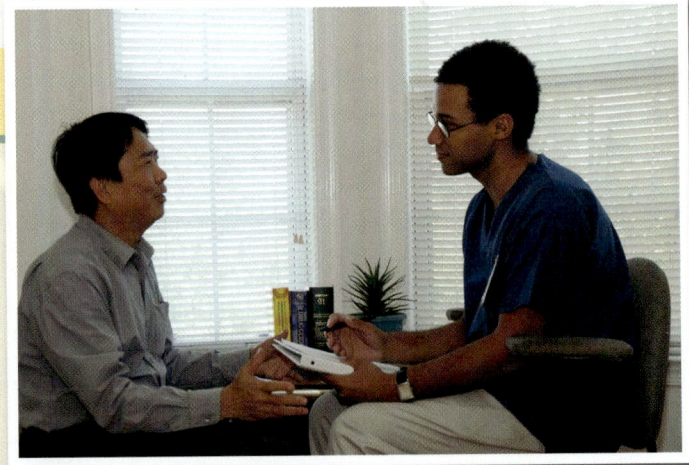

I'm a mess. Nothing is turning out the way I planned. I might as well just die now. It would save my family a lot of grief."

Caring for the Nguyens (continued)

A. What information do you need in order to respond to Mr. Nguyen?

B. How should you respond to Mr. Nguyen?

C. What actions should you take?

D. What conclusions can you make about Mr. Nguyen's self-concept (body image, role performance, personal identity, and self-esteem)? What additional information do you need about his self-concept?

 Go to Chapter 13, **Caring for the Nguyens Response Sheet,** on Davis*Plus*.

Meet Your Patient

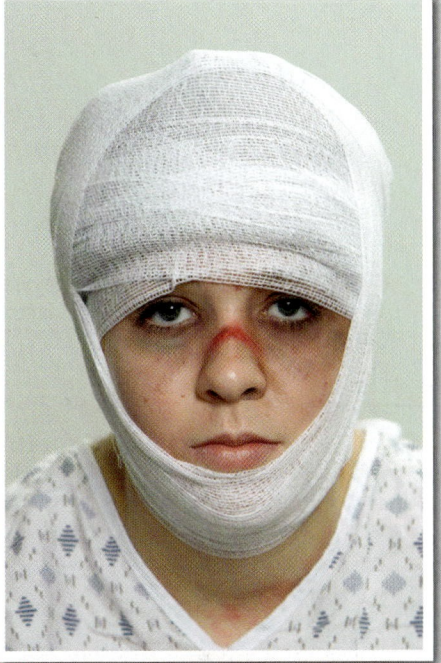

You are caring for a 16-year-old patient named Karli who is suffering from fractures to both arms and several ribs, as well as extensive first- and second-degree burns to 30% of her body, following a motor vehicle accident. Karli was driving her parents' car home from her part-time job when she lost control of the car and crashed into a wall. The car exploded in flames. A passerby quickly reported the accident, and fast action by the emergency response team saved Karli's life.

Karli is suffering from a moderate amount of shock and pain. She alternates among outbursts of anger, self-directed sarcasm, and despondence. She tells you that she cannot understand how the accident happened, that one moment she was adjusting the car radio, and the next moment she awoke in the hospital. Then suddenly she explodes. "It's not fair! I just took my eyes off the road for a second; that's all!" She bursts into tears. Picking at her bandages, she sobs, "No one will ever love me the way I'm going to look. My life is over. I hate myself!" You take her hand. "I used to be pretty," she says, "but now I'll look like a freak! What did I do to deserve this? I know plenty of kids who drive drunk or high all the time. I wasn't doing anything wrong! Why did this happen to me?"

Before reading on, jot down a list of the multiple physical, psychological, and social issues that you would need to consider in developing a comprehensive care plan for Karli. You can revisit your list throughout this chapter to compare your answers.

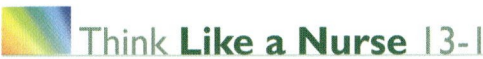 Think **Like a Nurse** 13-1

 Review Chapter 9 as needed.

- What theoretical knowledge about Karli's developmental stage will assist you in determining nursing diagnoses, interventions, and outcomes?
- Considering that Karli will need a significant amount of assistance for activities of daily living (ADLs) because of her fractures and burns, how might you use the time to develop your therapeutic relationship?

ABOUT THE KEY CONCEPTS

This chapter introduces you to the key concepts of psychosocial health, self-concept, anxiety, and depression. As you study the related topics and terms in the chapter, you will gain a more complete understanding of the four key concepts. Conceptual thinking will help you organize the content in your mind so you can remember it longer.

Theoretical Knowledge: knowing **why**

This chapter is designed to help you provide basic psychosocial care for patients in general practice settings.

PSYCHOSOCIAL HEALTH

The interactions of the mind and body are continuous and complex. One of the strengths of nursing is that we can go beyond a *biomedical* (disease-oriented) focus to recognize that patient responses to illness are influenced not only by physical pathology but also by the person's psychosocial health and its relationship to her overall wellness.

The term *psychosocial* encompasses both psychological and social factors: A person's psychological state interacts with his social development and position within society to contribute to his overall—or biopsychosocial—well-being (Fig. 13-1). Figure 13-2 illustrates the interlocking psychosocial influences on health and personal development.

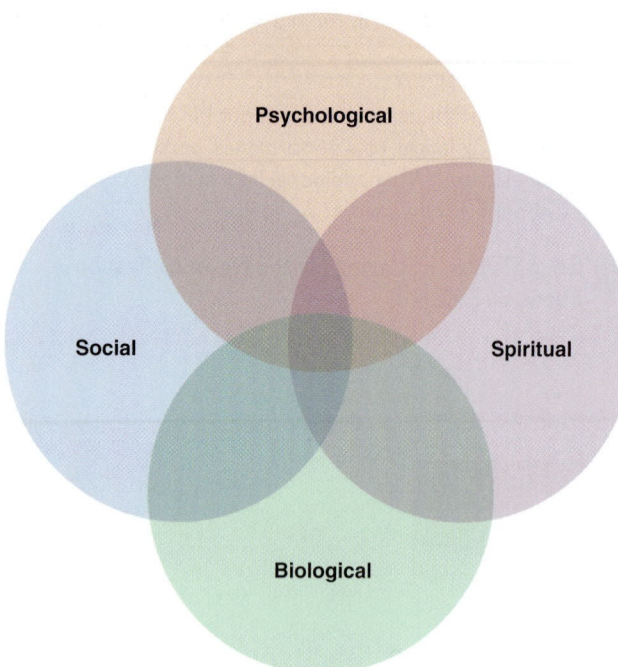

FIGURE 13-1 In the biopsychosocial view of health, biological, psychological, social, and spiritual factors interact to contribute to health.

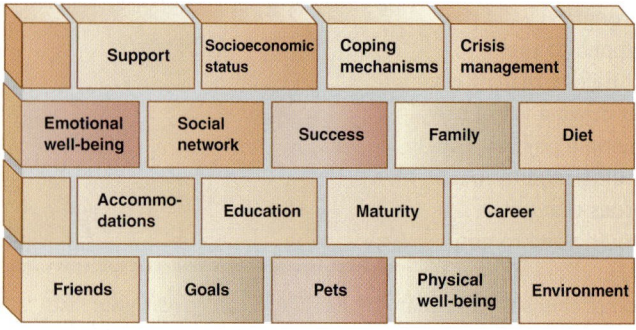

FIGURE 13-2 Interlocking psychosocial influences.

Keep in mind that any human dimension may dominate health needs at a given time. For example, a patient suffering from a severe flare-up of psoriasis (a skin disease characterized by red, scaly patches) may require physiological interventions during the acute stage. He may not be ready to deal with body image issues (psychological dimension) until his skin lesions are better. Remember, though, that your patients' psychosocial needs are just as important as their physical needs (e.g., dietary requirements and pain level).

What Is Psychosocial Theory?

You can think of **psychosocial theory** as a method of understanding people as a combination of psychological and social events. Of the many theories of psychosocial development, the works of the German psychologist Erik Erikson (1902–1994) are foremost. Using Erikson's theory, you can assess for successful completion of developmental tasks. Refer to Chapter 9 for more information about Erikson's theory. For a summary of developmental tasks,

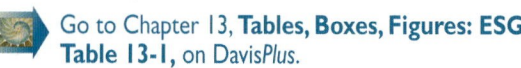

Go to Chapter 13, **Tables, Boxes, Figures: ESG Table 13-1,** on DavisPlus.

Chapter 8 presents another psychosocial theory that is relevant for healthcare providers: psychologist Abraham Maslow's theory of self-actualization and self-transcendence. Maslow (1968) developed a widely accepted hierarchy of human needs and motivations, in which essential needs (e.g., air, water, and food) must be met before higher needs (e.g., learning, creating, understanding, and self-fulfillment). Recall that, in order from most basic to highest need, Maslow's hierarchy includes physiological, safety and security, love and belonging, self-esteem, and self-actualization needs. For more information about psychosocial theories,

 Go to Chapter 13, **Supplemental Materials: Psychosocial Theory,** on DavisPlus.

KnowledgeCheck 13-1

- Why is psychosocial theory relevant to healthcare?
- What does the term *biopsychosocial* mean?
- Explain the implication of Maslow's hierarchy of human needs for working with a homeless man with gangrene.

What Is Self-Concept?

Self-concept is one's overall view of oneself. It is your complete and unique answer to the question "Who do you think you are?" (e.g., "I am a student"; "I am successful and competent"). Self-concept forms out of a person's evaluation of his physical appearance, sexual performance, intellectual abilities, success in the workplace, friendship and approval from others, problem-solving and coping abilities, unique talents, and so on. A person with a healthy self-concept has a mostly positive perception of these evaluations of self.

Self-concept both influences and is influenced by social functioning. For example, in the Meet Your Patient scenario, Karli's self-concept is that she is no longer pretty and that she "looks like a freak." If this self-concept continues, it may cause her to withdraw from social interaction and make it difficult to form new relationships (social functioning). Equally, if others—for example, prospective employers—*do* see her as hideously ugly, she may have difficulty finding a place in society.

The Dynamic Self. The self forms and changes in response to our environment. We discover who we are through a lifelong process of differentiating from and comparing our self to others. As we experience life events, we continually develop our understanding of who we are. Dickstein (1977) called this idea the **dynamic self,** meaning that who we are (the self) is subject to change through social and environmental influence. But if our concept of self is changeable, what factors cause it to change? Can it be harmed, and how? And how does it first develop? These questions are explored next.

How Is Self-Concept Formed?

Humans are not born with a concept of self; rather, it develops during infancy and childhood as the child interacts with family members, peers, and others. The broad steps of self-concept formation are as follows:

Infant—Learning that the physical self is different from the environment: "me; not me."

Child—Internalizing others' attitudes about the self, primarily parents and peers: "Who do *they* say that I am?"

Child and adult—Internalizing standards of society: "How do I compare to others?"

Adult—Self-actualization and self-adjustment: "This *is* who I am and who I will continue to be."

Change occurs gradually, and the steps overlap. Also, the age at which the stages occur varies widely among individuals. For a summary of the growth of self-concept through the various developmental stages,

 Go to Chapter 13, **Tables, Boxes, Figures: ESG Table 13-2,** on Davis*Plus.*

 Think**Like a Nurse** 13-2

- Explain how each of Maslow's five basic needs is related to psychosocial development; that is, how might each of the needs affect psychosocial health if met or not met?
- To what extent do social relationships help or hinder a person in meeting each need?

What Factors Affect a Person's Self-Concept?

Some factors affecting a person's self-concept cannot be changed, for example, gender and developmental level. Others, such as socioeconomic status and family relationships, can be changed to a degree, but are not fully under the person's control—and certainly not during childhood, when the self-concept is forming. Understanding that people may not be able to change such factors may help you provide more sensitive, compassionate care to patients experiencing impaired self-concept.

Gender

Certain aspects of self-concept differ by gender. Some of the differences appear to be related to the role expectations of boys and girls rather than any actual difference in ability. For example,

Girls typically rate teamwork and cooperation as important to their sense of self, whereas most boys place a higher value on individual achievement.

Physical appearance tends to seem more important to girls, and they may be less satisfied and more self-conscious throughout life because of this.

As role expectations and career choices for both men and women expand, these gender-based differences in self-concept may fade.

Developmental Level

As we mature, our self-concept becomes more inner guided. That is, others (e.g., friends, the media) have less influence on our ideas about who we are. We become less likely to view our failures and shortcomings as evidence of worthlessness and more likely to see them as challenges common to humans everywhere.

Family and Peer Relationships

The family strongly influences a child's developing self-concept. As an infant's sense of self-permanence develops and becomes stable, categories of self begin to emerge (Feiring & Taska, as cited in Bracken, 1996). Social identity is first developed by interactions between infants and their parents and broadens in toddlerhood through relationships with immediate and extended family members. For older children, peers become more important than family in this respect.

Internal Influences

Whereas the preceding external influences contribute to the *formation* of our self-concept, internal influences help us to *moderate* it. For example, biochemical brain processes influence perceptual acuity, interpretation abilities, and level of insight and judgment.

- **Internal Locus of Control.** People who allow their inner voice to influence their self-concept have what is called an **internal locus of control.** Such people feel they can exert control over their lives. They take appropriate responsibility for their life experiences and for their responses to them. This enables them to interpret unexpected adverse events (e.g., injuries and illnesses) in a more positive light.
- **External Locus of Control.** In contrast, people who have an **external locus of control** attribute control of their situation to external factors, including other people, institutions, and God. They may feel they lack the ability to change what happens to them.

Knowledge Check 13-2

- When does self-concept become stable?
- What factors have been determined to have an impact on our self-concept?

What Are the Components of Self-Concept?

Self-concept embraces four interrelated subconcepts: body image, role performance, personal identity, and self-esteem.

Body Image

How often do you hear someone say something like the following?

"Look at the muscles on that man. He looks good!"

"Look at her pigging out. She needs that candy like I need a hole in my head."

You probably grew up overhearing similar statements. Such preoccupations with food, weight, and appearance have led to a prejudice against people who do not have perfect bodies. No wonder people engage in unhealthy behaviors in order to be thin or that patients such as Karli have difficulty coping with disfiguring accidents or with surgeries such as limb amputation and mastectomy.

Body image is your mental image of your physical self, including physical appearance and physical functioning. Both cognitive understanding and sensory input influence body image. What we know cognitively is influenced by family, social, ethnic, and cultural norms; education; and exposure to alternative values. For example, the American media portray the ideal male as young, tall, and muscular; nevertheless, many older, short, slender men maintain a positive body image because they understand cognitively that they are in good health, are attractive to their partners, and so on.

Ideal, Perceived, and Actual Body Image. People do not always see their own bodies as objectively as others see them. Some psychological disorders interfere with the ability to interpret sensory data objectively. For example, people with the eating disorders anorexia nervosa and bulimia nervosa see themselves as fat even when their mirror reflects, and other people see, a normal or even an emaciated body. The closer the match between a person's ideal body image and sensory input about his or her body (perceived body image), the more positive the person's body image is likely to be.

For Janalee, thick, luxurious hair is an important component of her ideal body image. Amy hardly thinks about her hair at all; she keeps it very short so that it is easy to care for. Both women have been receiving chemotherapy to treat their cancer, and both are experiencing severe hair loss. Which woman do you think will be more likely to experience body image disturbance because of this?

Appearance and Function Influence Body Image. Not surprisingly, a physical disability, such as blindness, deafness,

or paraplegia, can interfere with the development of a positive body image. Children born with a physical disability have a high incidence of poor self-concept and depression. This is partially due to social values and the child's inability to form adequate social relationships, but it may also relate to the person's perception that he has low social value. In contrast, an attractive appearance and superior functioning, whether in a career, sports, or academics, contribute to a positive body image. But again, cognitive understanding can increase self-concept even in people who are average in appearance or achievement. For instance, people of average appearance who learn to value integrity, honesty, teamwork, and other social values more than physical attractiveness or success in sports are less likely to suffer from body image disturbance.

Gradual Versus Sudden Body Changes. Gradual changes in physical appearance occur naturally throughout life as the body matures and grows old. Most people adapt to such changes relatively easily, partly because their friends and colleagues are aging, too. In contrast, when changes in appearance or functioning occur abruptly (e.g., following an acute illness or an accident, as happened to Karli [Meet Your Patient]), they are much more difficult to accept. Denial, anger, self-hatred, and despair are a few of many reactions that can follow such an abrupt change in body image.

Influence of Body Image on Health. Body image influences health and health behaviors. A negative body image has been associated with the following health problems:

- Depression (McCabe, Ricciardelli, Sitaram, et al., 2006)
- Teen smoking (Clark, Croghan, Reading, et al., 2005; Stice & Shaw, 2003)
- Increased risk for unintended pregnancy and sexually transmitted infections (STIs), including HIV infection (Wingood, DiClemente, Harrington, et al., 2002).

In contrast, a positive body image was found to be a major contributor to overall life happiness, for example in adult women (Stokes & Frederick-Recascino, 2003). There is not yet enough evidence to determine how much of the effect is due to body image alone and how much to body image in combination with other psychosocial issues.

Role Performance

Before you began your nursing program, what were your expectations? What activities did you imagine yourself engaged in, and what behaviors did you think would be expected of you? Together, these expectations make up your conception of the *role* of a nursing student. In addition to being a student, you probably play several other roles, such as parent, sibling, friend, breadwinner, caregiver, volunteer, and so on.

Role performance can be defined as the actions that a person takes and the behaviors that he demonstrates in fulfilling a role. Instead of expectations, role performance is the reality. If you expected that you would sail through your nursing program and instead you find yourself so overwhelmed that lately you have begun to skip classes, then you are experiencing **role strain,** a mismatch between role expectations and role performance. In addition, your ideas about how to perform the nursing student role may be very different from those of your instructors. When that type of mismatch occurs, you are experiencing an **interpersonal role conflict.** Other types of role conflict are also common. For instance, what if you are a single parent and your child's sudden illness causes you to miss a week of classes and clinical days? When two roles make competing demands on an individual, **interrole conflict** occurs.

Personal Identity

How would you describe yourself to others? Make a list of 10 words or short phrases that describe who you are (e.g., student, motorcycle rider, woman). Then list them in order, with the most important one first. Are you happy with your list? Are you satisfied with who you are? Compare your list with a friend's list. Could you identify her based on her list of identifying labels? Could she identify you?

Your **personal identity** is your view of yourself as a unique human being, different and separate from all others. Identity develops over time, beginning in childhood when you identified with your parents, and then later with teachers, peers, and others. Unlike body image, which is expected to change over time, personal identity is relatively constant and consistent. It is culturally determined and learned through socialization.

People with a strong sense of personal identity are less likely to compare themselves to others or to be unduly influenced by them. They tend to appreciate the unique perspective and contributions of others, yet value their own perspectives and contributions. In contrast, people with a weak sense of personal identity have difficulty distinguishing their boundaries from those of others. They may interpret events in the environment personally, or they may interpret their personal experiences as belonging to everyone. For example, a person with a weak personal identity may blame his obesity on his mother because she fed him high-calorie, low-nutrient foods as a child.

Patients may experience an impaired sense of identity when they are challenged by a serious or chronic illness (e.g., cancer, AIDS, or rheumatoid arthritis). They then place too many limitations on their activities or interpret the responses of others in light of their illness. For instance, a woman with osteoporosis (loss of bone density) might say, "I used to enjoy going bird watching, but I don't go anymore because I might trip and fall."

Think**Like a Nurse** 13-3

Think about Karli in the Meet Your Patient scenario. If you asked Karli to list 10 labels to identify herself, what do you think they would be? (You may not have enough information to come up with 10, but think of as many as you can.)

Self-Esteem

Self-esteem is, in the simplest terms, how well a person likes himself. It is the difference between the "ideal self" and "actual self," that is, between "what I think I ought (or want) to be" and "what I really am." The area of overlap in Figure 13-3

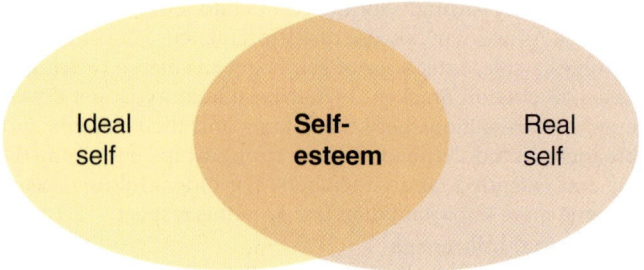

Ideal self: expectations and aspirations; "what I ought to be," "what I wish I were"

Real self: current skills, attributes, and successes; "what I really am"

FIGURE 13-3 Self-esteem is determined by the relationship between an individual's ideal self and real self.

illustrates the extent of self-esteem. The more overlap there is, the higher the self-esteem.

The balance between our self-expectations and our true abilities can be precarious. When we succeed beyond our ambitions, we experience a high sense of self-esteem; but when we aim for an ideal self beyond our capabilities, we risk loss of self-esteem. It is not difficult to imagine how a sudden, disfiguring accident such as Karli's might provoke a crisis in self-esteem, because Karli's ideal self is currently out of her reach. Even mild illnesses and minor setbacks can cause some people to question their self-worth. This is especially true if the problem is interpreted as one incident in a continuing pattern—for example, a couple hoping to become parents who experience a third pregnancy loss.

ThinkLike a Nurse 13-4

What if a person does not have any aspirations to success, but is content to meet each day as a learner, vitalized by her daily discoveries? How do you think a high score on an exam would affect her self-esteem? How do you think a poor score on a clinical skills test would affect her self-esteem?

KnowledgeCheck 13-3

- What four components contribute to an individual's self-concept?
- What is self-esteem?

COMMON PSYCHOSOCIAL PROBLEMS

Think about the advertisements you've seen recently on TV or in newspapers and magazines. How many times do you recall seeing an ad for a medication for anxiety or depression? These two problems are not confined to mental health settings. They are woven into the fabric of our everyday lives. As a nurse, you should be prepared to recognize and provide care for anxious and depressed patients in all practice settings.

Example Problem: Anxiety

I wake up in the middle of the night with a knot in my stomach and thinking about work. I go over and over my day and worry about my decisions and what I should have done instead. I wonder whether I can handle the responsibility. My neck and shoulders are so tense that I get headaches. But when I try to relax and watch TV, I can feel my heart racing, and I feel shaky. I can't concentrate well enough to read.

Anxiety is a common emotional response to a stressor. It is a "vague, uneasy feeling of discomfort or dread (the source often nonspecific or unknown to the individual) accompanied by an autonomic response; a feeling of apprehension caused by anticipation of danger. It is an alerting signal that warns of impending danger and enables the individual to take measures to deal with threat" (NANDA International, 2012, p. 344). An anxious person worries; feels nervous, uneasy, and fearful; may be tearful; and often has physical symptoms such as nausea, trembling, and sweating. Anxiety and fear produce similar responses; however, some experts differentiate them as follows:

Fear is a specific, cognitive response to a known threat. It is related to a present event, either physical *or* psychological.

Anxiety is a vague, emotional response to a known or unknown threat. It is related to anticipation of a future event and is the result of psychological conflict rather than physical threat.

Anxiety is so common that mild anxiety is considered normal and even necessary for our survival. No matter what area of nursing you work in, nearly every patient you meet will have at least some degree of anxiety. Chronic anxiety has been associated with physical problems, such as the risk of heart attack (Moser, 2007; Shen, Avivi, Todaro, et al., 2008).

Patients encounter anxiety-producing situations in healthcare settings because of threats to their basic needs (Stuart & Laraia, 2001). Consider the following examples:

- Physiological—anxiety in anticipation of or in response to a diagnosis of cancer
- Safety and security—an upcoming surgery or diagnostic test, such as cardiac catheterization
- Love and belonging—anxiety over potential or actual loss of a loved one
- Esteem—anxiety over potential or actual loss of ability or appearance
- Self-actualization—anxiety over lack of self-fulfillment

Levels of Anxiety

Anxiety ranges from normal to abnormal, depending on its **intensity** and **duration**—how much anxiety is present and how long it has been present.

- **Normal anxiety** is an essential reaction to a realistic danger or threat to our physical or psychological integrity. In other words, it enables us to survive and, when the threat is no longer present, to move on. For example, anxiety when hiking on a rocky and narrow mountain trail heightens your awareness and quickens your responses, thereby reducing the likelihood of falls.
- **Abnormal anxiety** is out of proportion to the situation and lasts long after the threat is over, perhaps causing the person to alter her lifestyle. For example, after breaking her ankle in a fall down a short flight of stairs, a young woman moves to a ground-floor apartment. Five years later, she still refuses to use stairs.

You should determine a patient's level of anxiety as accurately as possible because each requires different nursing actions. Peplau (1963) described the four levels found in Table 13-1.

Coping with Anxiety

People use a variety of coping behaviors to relieve mild anxiety, such as exercising, talking with others, engaging in pleasurable activities, deep-breathing, or using relaxation programs (Bourne, 2005). Less adaptive behaviors include excessive sleeping, eating, smoking, crying, pacing, fidgeting, drinking, laughing, cursing, nail biting, or finger tapping.

When anxiety is more severe, the person attempts to counteract the anxiety in some way. Each person develops unique patterns of coping with anxiety, called **defense mechanisms,** which are used consciously or unconsciously to relieve the anxiety. Examples of defense mechanisms are **denial** (refusing to acknowledge the existence of a real situation or associated feelings) and **displacement** (transferring feelings from one target to another that seems less threatening—for example, kicking the dog when you are angry at your boss). See Chapter 12 for further discussion of defense mechanisms.

When overused, defense mechanisms can be maladaptive and lead to psychological disorders such as phobias, obsessive–compulsive disorders, and dissociative disorders (e.g., amnesia). Excessive or unrelieved anxiety may also contribute to **psychosis,** which is a loss of ability to differentiate self from non-self or by impaired reality testing (that is, knowing what

Table 13-1 ➤ Levels of Anxiety

	DEFINITION OR DESCRIPTION	SYMPTOMS
Mild Anxiety	This is normal anxiety, experienced in response to the events of day-to-day living. It heightens perception, sharpens the senses, enhances learning, and enables the person to function at his optimal level.	If present, symptoms may include muscle tension, restlessness, irritability, and a sense of unease. The person usually does not experience distress.
Moderate Anxiety	As anxiety increases, the perceptual field narrows, and the person begins to focus on self and the need to relieve his discomfort.	■ Less alert to environmental events. ■ Distracts easily. ■ Shorter attention span. ■ May need help with problem-solving but can attend to his needs with direction. ■ Physical symptoms may include: Increased heart and respiratory rate Increased perspiration Gastric discomfort Increased muscle tension. ■ Rapid, loud, and higher pitched speech.
Severe Anxiety	Perceptual field is so narrow that the person can focus on only one particular detail or may shift focus to many extraneous details. Focus is totally on self and the need to relieve the anxiety.	■ Concentration and attention span are severely limited, so the person has difficulty completing simple tasks. ■ Anxiety prevents problem-solving and learning. ■ May report feelings of dread, confusion, and other unpleasant emotions. ■ Physical symptoms may include headaches, palpitations, tachycardia, insomnia, dizziness, nausea, trembling, hyperventilation, urinary frequency, and diarrhea.
Panic Anxiety	The person becomes unreasonable and irrational and is unable to focus on even one detail in the environment. He may misperceive environmental cues or lose contact with reality (e.g., experience hallucinations or delusions).	■ May react wildly (e.g., shouting, screaming, running about, clinging to something) or withdraw completely. ■ Cannot function or communicate effectively (e.g., may speak incoherently or be unable to speak). ■ May feel terror and impending doom, believe he has a life-threatening illness, or that he is "going crazy." ■ Physical symptoms include dilated pupils, labored breathing, severe trembling, sleeplessness, palpitations, diaphoresis, pallor, and muscular incoordination (Townsend, 2008).

is real and what exists only in one's mind), often accompanied by hallucinations and delusions. Examples of psychotic responses to anxiety include schizophrenia and delusional disorders. These disorders are beyond the scope of this book. If you need more information, refer to a mental health text.

KnowledgeCheck 13-4

■ What is anxiety?
■ When is anxiety a normal response to life?
■ Identify at least three healthcare scenarios that might trigger anxiety in patients.

Example Problem: Depression

Others imply that they know what it is like to be depressed because they have gone through a divorce, lost a job or broken up with someone. But these experiences carry with them feelings. Depression, instead, is flat, hollow, and unendurable.

—Kay Redfield Jamison (1997), An Unquiet Mind: A Memoir of Moods and Madness

The term **depression** is commonly used to describe a feeling of sadness or "the blues." But to psychologists, nurses, and other healthcare professionals, it refers to a specific condition

with characteristic symptoms and often devastating consequences if left untreated (Steptoe, 2007).

Depression occurs in all age groups, even in very young children. It affects about 11% of the adult population in the United States, and is one of the top three risks for functional decline. The incidence is higher in women than in men (Pleis & Lethbridge-Cejku, 2006). See Table 13-2 for common truths and myths about depression.

Criteria established by the American Psychiatric Association (APA) for **major depressive disorder** include the following:

- Depressed mood most of the day nearly every day for at least 2 weeks, typically accompanied by markedly diminished interest or pleasure in activities the person previously enjoyed
- Insomnia or hypersomnia
- Loss of energy
- Feelings of worthlessness
- Diminished ability to concentrate
- Recurrent thoughts of death (APA, 2000)

Unlike the feeling of true sadness, such as might accompany a divorce, death, or other loss, the depressed mood is typically marked by a sense of emptiness. This contributes to the depressed person's tendency to withdraw from social contacts and also explains the characteristically flat affect (Fig. 13-4).

Depression in Older and Middle Adults

Older adults have a slightly higher incidence of depression than does the population as a whole. Of adults ages 65 to 74, 12% reported that they had feelings associated with depression (sadness, hopelessness, worthlessness, and feeling that everything is an effort) "all or most of the time." For adults 75 and older, this was 15%. The incidence is much higher if you count the people who reported having those feelings only "some of the time" (Pleis & Lethbridge-Cejku, 2006, table 14).

We typically think of older adults as being at higher risk for depression because of their many losses and multiple physical illnesses (Stanley, Blair, & Beare, 2005). However, at least one recent large, international study found depression is most common among men and women in their 40s

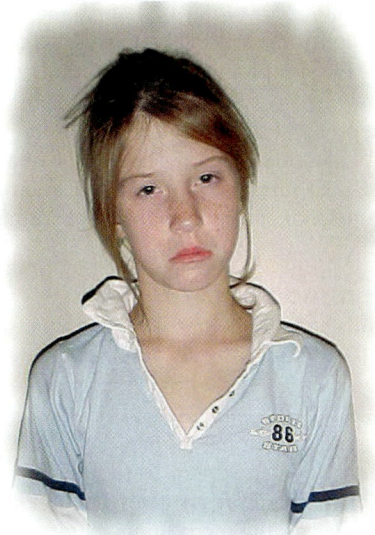

FIGURE 13-4 Depressed affect.

(Blanchflower & Oswald, 2008), and that happiness and sense of well-being reach their lowest in the 40s. This study remains controversial, and more research is needed, but the findings are interesting.

What Causes Depression?

Are our genes responsible for the development of depression? Is depression "anger turned inward"? Depression theories fall into four groupings:

- *Physiological theories* relate depression to biochemical imbalances stemming from hormonal, neurological, or genetic factors.
- *Psychodynamic theories* relate depression to loss, abandonment, and emotional detachment and to diurnal and seasonal mood variations.
- *Cognitive theory* relates depression to negative thinking.
- *Social/environmental theories* relate depression to poor family relationships, difficult interpersonal relationships, and socioeconomic and political factors.

Research has shown that the following factors increase the risk for depression:

Family history of depression
Hormonal or nutritional imbalance
Inability to externalize anger
Low self-esteem
Negative thinking
Learned helplessness and hopelessness
Prior success or failure in coping mechanisms
Traumatic loss
Catastrophic stressors (e.g., unemployment)
Chronic disease
Female sex

What Are the Signs and Symptoms of Depression in Older Adults?

Depression is underdiagnosed and undertreated in older adults. It is difficult to diagnose because in older adults:

- Depression is more likely to be masked rather than exhibited by typical symptoms, such as sadness.
- Symptoms are often physical or expressed as personality changes, such as irritability.

Table 13-2 ➤ Depression: Truths and Myths	
TRUE	**FALSE**
Depressive disorders are more common among women than men (2:1).	"Getting on with life" will cure depression.
Spiritual distress is associated with depression.	Everyone likes to talk about how they feel.
Depression can be defined as a maladaptive emotional response.	Medication is the answer to depression.
Low socioeconomic circumstances and social isolation correlate with depression.	Once depression has been cured, it does not return.

- Depression may occur along with, or be mistaken for, dementia and delirium. In older adults, all three conditions may include the symptoms of confusion, distractibility, and memory loss.
- Some of the physical symptoms of depression (e.g., fatigue, anorexia, constipation, and psychomotor retardation) can be confused with physical illness, medication interactions, substance abuse, or "signs of old age" (Gorman & Sultan, 2008).

How Is Depression Treated?

People who are clinically depressed cannot just snap out of it. If untreated, the symptoms may continue for weeks or even years. The physiological theory of depression predominates in the medical community, and current evidence shows that biochemical processes determine moods, thought, cognition, and perception. Therefore, treatment of serious depression relies more heavily on antidepressant medication than on psychotherapy. However, the medications have a number of unpleasant, and even serious, side effects, and some patients say that they do not effectively elevate their mood. Psychotherapists acknowledge that individual tolerance of symptoms, coping resources, education, and social support networks all have an important effect on outcomes and treatment.

Of course, you will not be conducting psychotherapy with depressed patients in your general practice. However, you *will* care for patients who are taking antidepressant medications and who have situational or even clinical depression. Even without being a psych nurse, there is much you can do to make your care of these patients more effective.

KnowledgeCheck 13-5

- What distinguishes clinical depression from feelings of sadness?
- How might a child manifest depression?
- Why is the nurse–patient (therapeutic) relationship important when caring for depressed individuals?

PracticalKnowledge
knowing **how**

Practical knowledge in this chapter consists of planning, implementing, and evaluating care to promote clients' mental health and provide support when they experience psychosocial and psychological problems. Remember, the physical body is only one dimension of a person. What patients are thinking and feeling may be equally important to their healing process.

As a nurse generalist, your independent role is to assess and document the patient's behavioral state as it relates to his medical–surgical condition, rather than to diagnose and treat mental illnesses. Clients who are anxious, for example, may not understand or recall instructions for self-care; those who are depressed may not have the energy or motivation to follow a medical regimen or keep appointments with their healthcare providers.

NURSING CARE TO PROMOTE PSYCHOSOCIAL HEALTH

Physical illness may be particularly stressful when it occurs in combination with psychosocial issues. For example, think of Karli. Might her condition have been less complicated if (1) she had no disfiguring injuries or (2) if she were an older

adult at a developmental stage when appearance is generally less crucial?

ASSESSMENTS: PSYCHOSOCIAL

No matter what the patient's medical diagnosis, you need to perform accurate and ongoing psychosocial assessments to develop holistic nursing diagnoses and interventions. Most admission assessment forms have a few questions to screen psychosocial status. If any of the answers indicate risk for a problem, you may need to conduct a more comprehensive special needs (or focused) assessment. For an example of a psychosocial assessment tool,

 Go to Chapter 13, **Tables, Boxes, Figures: ESG Figure 13-1,** on Davis*Plus*.

A comprehensive psychosocial assessment should include the following categories:

- Biological details
- Recent life changes or stressors (both positive and negative)
- Lifestyle and social relationships
- History of psychiatric disorders
- Functional abilities (behavioral performance)
- Self-efficacy (the belief that you can influence your own behaviors and outcomes)
- Family relationships
- Social resources and network
- Usual coping mechanisms
- Interpersonal communication
- Understanding about current illness
- Major issues raised by current illness
- Health priorities
- Spirituality (see the HOPE assessment tool in Chapter 16)

Psychosocial information is personal and sometimes sensitive. To encourage patients to share this information, you will need to use good communication skills. For example:

- Be aware of your own biases and discomforts that could influence your assessment.
- Use active listening through eye contact and verbal response. Be sensitive, though—eye contact is uncomfortable for some people.
- Proceed from general details ("How do you get along with your parents?") to the specific ("Does your mother ever hit you?").
- Use an open and positive voice tone, facial expression, and body language (e.g., avoid frowning, criticizing, or expressing shock).
- Keep the focus on the patient.
- Be respectful and sensitive to cultural and gender-specific details.
- Use open-ended questions (questions that cannot be answered with just a yes or no).
- Follow the patient's cues by using reflection and restating.
- Be flexible and use humor as appropriate.
- Provide empathetic feedback and touch as appropriate.

You will learn more about interviewing and communication skills in Chapter 20.

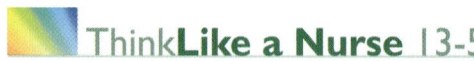 ThinkLike a Nurse 13-5

Psychologically, Karli is worried about the unfairness of her situation, and is probably struggling with body image issues. In addition, what do you think her *social* concerns might be?

ANALYSIS/NURSING DIAGNOSIS: PSYCHOSOCIAL

Psychosocial issues involve nearly all areas of patient functioning, so there is overlap between what we are calling *psychosocial* diagnoses and those used in the rest of the chapter to describe the more specific problems of self-concept, anxiety, and depression. That is, you may use some of these psychosocial diagnoses for clients who have problems of self-concept, anxiety, and depression. It would be impossible to list every possible psychosocial diagnosis; the following are but a few.

- *Family Coping [Compromised and/or Disabled].* A person's usual support (comfort and assistance) from a significant other is either compromised (insufficient or withdrawn) or disabled (competing or maladapted), causing a significant health challenge.
- *Parental Role Conflict.* A parent shows significant role confusion and/or conflict in response to crises.
- *Ineffective Coping.* The patient fails to comprehend and effectively judge stressors, when he perceives incorrect or dangerous life choices as normal, and when there is an inability to use available resources. Inability to identify strengths and resources may be secondary to low self-esteem.
- *Post-Trauma Syndrome.* There is a maladaptive learned response to a traumatic and distressing event.
- *Risk for Loneliness.* The person is separated from persons, culture, objects, or environments to which a person may have ongoing attachments.
- *Social Isolation.* The person experiences significant aloneness that has a negative impact on health, or perceives the isolation as a threat to health.
- *Risk for Other-Directed Violence.* Situations in which a person threatens or uses aggression or violence to harm others. The intention of harm may not be limited to physical harm.

Psychosocial issues can be a problem, a symptom of a problem, or the etiology of a problem. It is important to determine what is cause and what is effect, although this can be hard to unravel at times. As you can see in Table 13-3, what you identify significantly affects your choice of goals and nursing activities.

PLANNING PSYCHOSOCIAL OUTCOMES/EVALUATION

As always, the outcomes you identify will serve as guidelines for ongoing assessment and as criteria for evaluation of your patient's responses to care.

Individualized goal/outcome statements will depend on the nursing diagnoses used, client input, and realistic expectations of what the client can achieve and agrees to. For example, for Compromised or Disabled Family Coping, examples of goal statements are "Involves family members in decision making" and "Expresses feelings and emotions freely." If the nursing diagnosis is Impaired Social Interaction, goal statements may call for the client to develop the skills of "engagement, assertiveness, compromise, confrontation, and consideration."

NOC standardized outcomes. The Psychosocial Health domain of the NOC taxonomy includes approximately 30 outcomes to describe psychological well-being, psychosocial adaptation, self-control, and social interaction. The following are a few examples.

Abusive Behavior Self-Restraint
Coping

Child Adaptation to Hospitalization
Psychosocial Adjustment: Life Change
Role Performance
Social Interaction Skills
Also see

 Chapter 13, **Standardized Language, Psychosocial Outcomes: Examples From NOC Taxonomy,** on Davis*Plus.*

Other NOC domains also include useful psychosocial outcomes. The following are only a few examples (Moorhead, Johnson, Maas, et al., 2008):

Family Coping
Family Functioning
Family Participation in Professional Care
Family Resiliency

PLANNING: PSYCHOSOCIAL INTERVENTIONS/ IMPLEMENTATION

Psychosocial nursing interventions and activities are determined by the nursing diagnoses you identify, especially by the etiologies.

NIC standardized interventions for psychosocial diagnoses are found primarily in the Behavioral and Family domains of the NIC system. The following are some examples from the Behavioral domain:

Anger Control Assistance
Anxiety Reduction
Coping Enhancement
Decision-Making Support
Socialization Enhancement

The following are examples of interventions from the Family domain:

Family Involvement Promotion
Family Support
Family Therapy
Parenting Promotion (Bulechek, Butcher, & Dochterman, 2008)

Specific, individualized nursing activities used to help patients maintain a sense of personhood are discussed in the following section, Preventing Depersonalization. For nursing activities in which the nursing goal is to provide conflict mediation, enhance socialization, or strengthen the family,

 Go to Chapter 13, **Supplemental Materials: Psychosocial Nursing Interventions,** on Davis*Plus.*

Preventing Depersonalization

Illness, and especially hospitalization, can have a depersonalizing effect that alters the self-concept. The ill person may feel that she has become an object to be examined, poked, prodded, and discussed. You can help patients maintain a sense of personhood by using a caring approach:

- Introduce yourself if the patient does not know you.
- Address the patient by her preferred name each time you enter the room, and always speak respectfully.
- Listen actively when the patient speaks.
- Do not talk *about* the patient to others in the room (e.g., do not say, "He seems to be better today, don't you think?"); speak *to* the patient.
- Use eye contact and touch, keeping in mind that people vary in their desire to be touched.

- Always offer an explanation before beginning a procedure, and warn the patient before you touch him ("I'm going to touch your leg now").
- Move, turn, and position the patient gently.
- Provide for privacy when performing procedures or discussing something personal or sensitive.

Nursing Care for Example Problems: Self-Concept Disturbance and Low Self-Esteem

As is true for psychosocial issues, self-concept and self-esteem issues are a part of the holistic care of well and ill patients in all settings.

Table 13-3 ➤ Implications of Identifying a Psychosocial Issue as Problem, Etiology, or Symptom

	AS PROBLEM	AS ETIOLOGY	AS SYMPTOM
Nursing Diagnosis	**Interrupted Family Processes** r/t tumult from parental divorce	Delayed Development r/t lack of stimulation **secondary to Interrupted Family Processes** (parental divorce)	Ineffective Individual Coping (Mother) r/t poor judgment and impaired reality perception, as **manifested by Interrupted Family Processes** and risk-taking behaviors
Sample Goals (based on problem)	**NOC Outcome** Family Functioning	**NOC Outcome** Child Development: 4 years	**NOC Outcomes** Coping, Decision Making, Role Performance, Social Support, Impulse Control
	Goals Members perform expected family roles. Family cares for dependent members.	**Goals** Child demonstrates age-appropriate motor activities. Child uses four- and five-word sentences.	**Goals** Identifies coping strategies that have been effective in the past. Discusses the implications of decision alternatives with family.
Sample Interventions and Activities (based on etiology)	**NIC Interventions** Family Integrity Promotion Family Process Maintenance Normalization Promotion	**NIC Interventions** Developmental Enhancement: Child Parent Education Health Screening	**NIC Interventions** Coping Enhancement Decision-Making Support Impulse Control Training Family Involvement Promotion Support Group Support System Enhancement
	Specific Activities Promote parental involvement in healthcare. Assist the family with skills and education of conflict resolution, coping skills, and problem-solving. Link the individual and family to the appropriate support and education services.	**Specific Activities** Establish time for one-on-one care. Provide for creative play (e.g., clay, blocks, painting). Teach parents appropriate stimulation. Teach parents about developmental milestones and expected behaviors. Assess changes in family processes.	**Specific Activities** Identify and discuss alternative behaviors. Encourage delaying decision making when under stress. Help the mother solve problems constructively. Assist her to evaluate her own behavior. Identify and discuss past successful coping behaviors that she has used.

ASSESSMENT: SELF-CONCEPT AND SELF-ESTEEM

Psychological tests are typically administered by a clinical psychologist or licensed social worker. However, if you were working in a mental health agency, you might collect in-depth information regarding self-concept by using a psychological measurement tool, to be interpreted by a clinical psychologist or licensed social worker.

For an all-purpose assessment you might use screening in any setting, refer to the Focused Assessment box Assessing Self-Concept.

Observe for behaviors and comments specifically associated with low self-esteem. People with low self-esteem tend to avoid eye contact and have a stooped posture. They may move slowly and have poor grooming. Their verbal behaviors include speaking hesitantly; being overly critical of others and of

self ("I never do anything right"); not accepting positive comments about self ("Oh, anybody could have done it"); apologizing frequently, and verbalizing feelings of powerlessness ("Whatever you say is fine with me"; "It doesn't matter what I do; it won't change anything"). To assess specifically for the self-esteem dimension of a person's self-concept, you can use Table 13-4.

If you suspect serious problems with self-concept, document the patient's responses in your nursing notes and refer the patient for appropriate psychological testing.

ThinkLike a Nurse 13-6

In the Meet Your Patient scenario, Karli perceives herself as unlovable "looking this way." You should not assume that you know exactly what Karli means by this. Also from the scenario: "Picking at her bandages, she sobs, 'No one will ever love me the way I'm going to look. My life is over. I hate myself!' You take her hand. 'I used to be pretty,' she says, 'but now I'll look like a freak!'"

- Which of her words do you need to clarify with her?
- What might you say to her to get her to provide more information about the psychosocial meaning of her statement?

ANALYSIS/NURSING DIAGNOSIS: SELF-CONCEPT AND SELF-ESTEEM

Psychosocial and self-concept issues can be a problem, a symptom of a problem, or the etiology of a problem. It is important for you to determine what is cause and what is effect, although this may not always be clear. As you can see in Table 13-3, your analysis significantly affects your choice of goals and nursing activities.

When analyzing data for self-concept problems, keep the following two guidelines in mind:

- *Avoid seeking simplistic cause-and-effect relationships.* Instead, recognize the complexity of human responses. For example, consider the following:

  Molly, a 19-year-old student, has just been admitted to your unit and is presenting with clinical depression and low self-esteem. Is Molly depressed because she has low self-esteem? Or is longstanding low self-esteem causing her to feel depressed? Or are the two interrelated?
- *Avoid confusing low self-concept with clinical emotional and/or behavioral psychiatric diagnoses.* There is no recognized diagnosis describing self-concept disorder in the American Psychiatric Association's *Diagnostic and Statistical Manual of Mental Disorders*, 4th ed., text revision (*DSM-IV-TR*, 2000). Self-concept (particularly self-esteem) plays a secondary role in a number of disorders but is not a primary disorder itself.

Self-Concept or Body Image as a Problem

You can diagnose a body image or self-concept problem when it is the result of a particular condition and might not exist if not for the condition (e.g., a profoundly deaf adolescent develops self-worth problems). The following nursing diagnoses may be useful for patients with either low overall self-concept or difficulties in specific domains of self-concept (e.g., self-esteem):

Chronic Low Self-Esteem. The person expresses ongoing and longstanding overall self-dissatisfaction and negative self-appraisal (i.e., wide differences between "ideal" and

Focused Assessment

Assessing Self-Concept

Assessment Category	Examples of Assessment Questions
Body image	When you look in the mirror, what do you see?
	How do you think others see you?
	How does your current ability to engage in work and leisure activities compare to how you would like to be?
Role performance	What are your three or four major roles (e.g., daughter, student)?
	How successful are you in each of these roles?
	How important is it to you to be successful in each of these roles?
	What is interfering with your ability to perform any of these roles? What can you do about it?
Personal identity	How did you see yourself before your illness/injury/loss?
	How do you see yourself now?
	How would you describe yourself to others?
	What special abilities do you have?
	How do you think others see you?
Self-esteem (also refer to the Assessment box Performing a Self-Esteem Inventory)	How do you feel about yourself?
	What do you like about yourself?
	To what extent do you feel you are in control of your life?
	If you could change one thing about yourself, what would it be?
	Where would you like to be 5 years from now?
	How realistic are your expectations of yourself?
	How do you see your illness/injury/loss in relation to yourself?

Table 13-4 ➤ Performing a Self-Esteem Inventory

Place a check mark in the column that most closely describes the client's answer to each statement. Each check is worth the number of points listed.

	3 OFTEN OR A GREAT DEAL	2 SOME-TIMES	1 SELDOM OR OCCASIONALLY	0 NEVER OR NOT AT ALL
1. I become angry or hurt when criticized.				
2. I am afraid to try new things.				
3. I feel stupid when I make a mistake.				
4. I have difficulty looking people in the eye.				
5. I have difficulty making small talk.				
6. I feel uncomfortable in the presence of strangers.				
7. I am embarrassed when people compliment me.				
8. I am dissatisfied with the way I look.				
9. I am afraid to express my opinions in a group.				
10. I prefer staying home alone rather than participating in group social situations.				
11. I have trouble accepting teasing.				
12. I feel guilty when I say no to people.				
13. I am afraid to make a commitment to a relationship for fear of rejection.				
14. I believe that most people are more competent than I am.				
15. I feel resentment toward people who are attractive and successful.				
16. I have trouble thinking of any positive aspects about my life.				
17. I feel inadequate in the presence of authority figures.				
18. I have trouble making decisions.				
19. I fear the disapproval of others.				
20. I feel tense, stressed out, or "upright."				

Problems with low self-esteem are indicated by items scored with a 3 or by a total score higher than 46.

Source Townsend, M. C. (2009). *Psychiatric mental health nursing Concepts of care* (5tth ed.). Philadelphia: F.A. Davis. p. 248.

"actual" or "perceived" self). *Etiologies* include but are not limited to depression, mismatch in ideal and perceived self, dysfunctional family, anxiety, and failure to adapt to a change in physical appearance or functioning.

Situational Low Self-Esteem. The person exhibits self-disapproval and negative self-evaluations as a specific reaction to loss or change. *Etiologies:* See Chronic Low Self-Esteem, preceding.

Disturbed Personal Identity. The person exhibits negative and incorrect assessment of self-identity and inability to determine boundaries between self and others. *Etiologies* include but are not limited to distorted perceptions of self, such as occur in certain mental illnesses; loss of health, limb, physical appearance, and functioning; or dysfunctional family.

Ineffective Role Performance. A person experiences or perceives difficulty in fulfilling a usual role, or there is a mismatch between role expectations and role performance (either perceived or societal expectations). *Etiologies* include but are not limited to job demands exceeding abilities, inadequate resources or support system, family conflicts, domestic violence, unrealistic role expectations, lack of a role model, substance abuse, cognitive deficits, illness or disease, low self-esteem, pain, fatigue, and cognitive deficits.

Disturbed Body Image. An individual has a confused image of his physical self or negatively evaluates his body or an aspect of it. *Etiologies* include but are not limited to loss of functioning or appearance (e.g., acne, scars, breast removal, amputation), eating disorder, gender conflict, and personality disorder.

ThinkLike a Nurse 13-7

- Refer to Karli in the Meet Your Patient scenario. Look at the preceding five NANDA-I labels for self-concept problems (Chronic Low Self-Esteem, Situational Low Self-Esteem, Disturbed Personal Identity, Ineffective Role Performance, Disturbed Body Image). Which one most clearly applies to Karli? Explain your thinking.
- Write a nursing diagnosis (problem r/t etiology) for the problem you chose.

Self-Concept or Body Image as Etiology

Self-concept problems are an etiology when they precede a condition such as depression and play a central role in the condition (e.g., low self-esteem causing and maintaining depression or leading to an anxiety disorder). The following are examples of nursing diagnoses with self-concept (e.g., self-esteem) as the etiology:

- *Impaired Adjustment*—Use this diagnosis when a patient experiences difficulties adapting perception and evaluation of self after changes in health status.
- *Complicated Grieving*—This diagnosis may develop in anticipation of or following body changes (e.g., hysterectomy) or loss of key roles (e.g., resulting from death of a spouse).
- *Deficient Knowledge.* Lack of knowledge of a healthcare situation may occur because of low self-esteem and lack of confidence in ability to learn or to manage care. Low self-esteem diminishes the motivation to learn.
- *Hopelessness*—May occur because of overwhelming role demands, external locus of control, or lack of confidence in abilities.
- *Impaired Social Interaction*—May occur when the person's low self-esteem and external locus of control cause him to fear criticism or lack of acceptance from others.
- *Ineffective Health Maintenance*—May occur as a result of low self-esteem: not perceiving one's self as capable, or feeling there is no point to making the effort.
- *Sexual Dysfunction* or *Ineffective Sexuality Pattern*—May result from negative body image brought about by changes in body structure or function (e.g., pregnancy, medications, surgery, trauma, diseases such as arthritis, or treatments such as radiation).

PLANNING OUTCOMES/EVALUATION: SELF-CONCEPT AND SELF-ESTEEM

You will choose outcomes based on the client's specific nursing diagnosis. For example:

Nursing Diagnosis: Chronic Low Self-Esteem
NOC Outcome: Quality of Life
Individualized Outcome: Expresses pleasure in participating in activities
Nursing Diagnosis: Disturbed Body Image
NOC Outcome: Body Image
Individualized Outcome: Verbalizes positive aspects of body

To see a more extensive list of *NOC standardized outcomes* and indicators, as well as *individualized goal/outcome statement* examples, for selected self-concept problems,

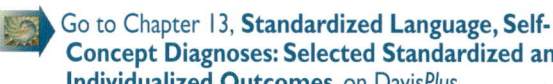

Go to Chapter 13, **Standardized Language, Self-Concept Diagnoses: Selected Standardized and Individualized Outcomes,** on DavisPlus.

When self-concept is the etiology of other problems (e.g., Sexual Dysfunction related to negative body image), choose outcomes based on the problem label (e.g., Sexual Abuse Recovery, Sexual Functioning, Body Image). The overall goal, in all cases, is that the patient's self-concept (or some aspect of it) will improve.

PLANNING INTERVENTIONS/IMPLEMENTATION: SELF-CONCEPT AND SELF-ESTEEM

Common *NIC standardized interventions* for self-concept and self-esteem diagnoses include Anticipatory Guidance, Behavior Modification, Decision-Making Support, and Self-Esteem Enhancement. For a more extensive list, along with examples of nursing activities,

Go to Chapter 13, **Standardized Language, Self-Concept Diagnoses: Selected NIC Interventions and Nursing Activities,** on DavisPlus.

Although not all-inclusive, those examples should give you an idea of the types of care needed to support self-concept.

Specific, individualized, nursing activities used frequently for patients with psychosocial and self-concept diagnoses are discussed in the text that follows. They include supportive measures to promote self-esteem, self-concept, positive body image, and role satisfaction.

Promoting Self-Esteem and Self-Concept

The dependence that often accompanies illness and aging can bring about loss of self-esteem. Although the foundation for self-esteem is laid in childhood and affected by many sociocultural variables, your nursing approach and efforts to preserve self-worth can help enhance a patient's self-esteem.

Identifying Patient Strengths. It is important to help the client identify past achievements and areas of strength. One way to do that is to point out areas of strength that you observe, such as the following:

Emotional strengths might include the ability to express emotions, to "feel" for others.
Relationship strengths include being sensitive to others' needs and being a good listener.
Spiritual strengths may include faith in God and participation in church activities.

Evaluate the client's sense of humor, which can also be a strength—and be sure the client considers special aptitudes, such as cooking, arts and crafts, sports, work, and education.

The following are other nursing actions specific to self-esteem:

- Establish a therapeutic nursing relationship emphasizing trust, consistency, honest communication, and unconditional positive regard.
- Encourage the client to be as independent as possible (e.g., by performing self-care).
- Monitor for and discourage self-criticism and negative self-talk.
- Teach the client to substitute positive self-talk for negative self-talk. For example, the client says, "I know my blood sugar is high, but I can't seem to stay on my diet. I ate way too much again today." You might remind the client that she exercised today and has been following her exercise program religiously. Eventually, she should learn to cue herself.

- Use positive and reaffirming language.
- Be supportive and accepting, but do not invade the client's personal space.
- Help the client develop realistic goals that provide achievable challenges (no-fail situations).
- Encourage the client to take part in activities that offer opportunities for success.
- Role-model communications skills that will help the person develop interpersonal relationships. Provide opportunities for practice.
- Refer to self-help and support groups, as needed.
- When possible, ask the client's advice (e.g., "How do you usually do this dressing change?")
- Point out good health practices and healthy aspects of the client's body functions.
- Refer to the Self-Care box for suggestions about teaching parents about promoting self-esteem in their children.

Promoting Positive Body Image

You can help parents promote a positive body image in their children, and you can help patients develop a different attitude toward their body. (1) Examine your own attitudes about what constitutes a healthy body, and pay attention to the messages you convey to others. (2) Encourage patients to discuss body changes resulting from their illness, surgery, or trauma. (3) Provide the opportunity to interact with people who have had similar body changes. (4) Teach clients the following, some of which are the same as for developing self-concept and self-esteem.

Healthy Does Not Mean Perfect. Help clients to accept that healthy bodies come in a wide range of shapes and sizes. Fashion magazines portray an ideal body that is unrealistic and unhealthy for most people. If they make you feel bad by comparison, don't read them!

Focus on Activity and Healthy Eating. Encourage clients to be active and focus on healthy eating rather than starving and depriving themselves to lose weight.

Don't Make Negative Comments About Your Body. Monitor for negative comments about body functions, weight, or size. Advise the client not to talk negatively about body weight, size, or deformity. Urge clients to be kind to themselves, and point out when they are being unrealistically critical of their body.

Keep a List. Suggest that the client keep a list of things he likes about his body and refer to it when he is feeling down.

Accept Compliments. Provide the client with practice in accepting positive comments about his appearance. Coach his responses as needed (e.g., say, "Thank you" after a compliment).

Challenge Critical Comments. Teach the client to challenge critical comments from others about her appearance.

Surround Yourself With Positive People. Support the client in surrounding herself with positive people who support the changes she is trying to make in her image of her body, and avoid people who are critical.

Use a Counter. Suggest that the client buy a counter and click it each time he makes a deliberate effort to accept positive feedback about his body or engages in positive body behaviors.

To see a care plan and care map for Body Image Disturbance,

 Go to Chapter 13, **Care Plan** and **Care Map,** on Davis*Plus*.

 Think**Like a Nurse** 13-8

- Which of the preceding body image interventions would be most appropriate for Karli's nursing diagnosis?
- For the interventions you did not choose, explain why.

Facilitating Role Enhancement

Sometimes the difficulty with self-concept centers on inability to fulfill one's usual or desired role. Specific actions to enhance role satisfaction include the following:

- Help the client distinguish between ideal and actual role performance.
- Help the person to identify her past, present, and future roles. For older adults, encourage reminiscence.
- Discuss boundaries, expectations, and management defined by lifestyle and family networks.
- Facilitate communication between client and significant other regarding the sharing of role responsibilities to accommodate role changes of the ill person.
- Help the client describe realistic roles and expectations tailored to specific health changes.
- Compare realistic roles to previous and less functional roles.
- Help the client examine the difference between previous roles and current role by providing education and a learning environment that focuses on positive and supportive change.
- Help the client identify and role-play behaviors needed in new roles.

Teaching Parents to Promote Self-Esteem in Children

Demonstrate love and acceptance by:
➤ Spending some one-on-one time with the child as often as possible: reading, playing, or just being together
➤ Being free with touches: a hug, a pat on the back
➤ Refraining from frequent negative criticism
➤ Providing nearly total acceptance of the child

Provide security by:
➤ Having clearly defined limits and consequences for breaking rules
➤ Being firm and consistent in applying the rules
➤ Being sure the rules are reasonable
➤ Allowing some latitude for individual actions within defined limits
➤ Treating the child with respect
➤ Establishing routines, such as bedtime activity, homework before play, dressing for school before breakfast in the morning, and so on
➤ Clearly defining every family member's role

Promote competence by:
➤ Setting realistic expectations about behaviors
➤ Assigning a few chores that are within the child's capability (e.g., picking up toys, making the bed)
➤ Modeling values, such as respect for others, honesty, and responsibility
➤ Providing positive feedback
➤ Helping the child accomplish goals
➤ Providing a stimulating and responsive environment
➤ Providing support in meeting challenges

KnowledgeCheck 13-6

Without looking back at the preceding material, see whether you can do the following:

- List three interventions for preserving self-worth.
- List three interventions for promoting self-esteem.
- List three interventions for fostering positive body image.
- List three interventions for promoting role enhancement.

Nursing Care for Example Problem: Anxiety

In general practice, the focus of nursing care for clients with anxiety is (1) to differentiate between mild anxiety and that which is severe enough to require referral to a mental health professional and (2) to provide interventions to relieve anxiety.

ASSESSMENT: ANXIETY

Your patient assessment should identify the *presence, level,* and *cause* of anxiety. It should include data about the following:

- **Observable behaviors**—poor eye contact, restlessness (e.g., pacing, wringing the hands, fidgeting, shuffling the feet), crying, trembling, rapid speech
- **Cognitive changes**—confusion, difficulty concentrating, forgetfulness

- **Objective physical data**—sweating, rapid pulse and respirations, dilated pupils
- **Subjective data**—shortness of breath, nausea, insomnia, worry

As we have said, most ill patients will have at least some level of anxiety. Anxiety becomes a problem when it escalates to a level that interferes with the ability to meet basic needs. You must determine whether the anxiety is normal and adaptive or whether it is severe enough to require nursing interventions, consultation, or referral to a mental health professional. For a checklist to help you make this determination, refer to the Focused Assessment box, Anxiety Assessment Guide.

✚ Severe Anxiety. If you suspect severe or disabling anxiety, document the patient's responses in your nursing notes, and refer the person to a physician or mental health clinician. Involve a mental health professional immediately (same day) if you discover any of the following:
- Suicidal thoughts and/or plans that make you uncertain of the patient's safety
- Assaultive or homicidal thoughts and/or plans that make you uncertain about the safety of the patient or others
- Loss of touch with reality (psychosis)
- Significant or prolonged inability to work and care for self or family

---

Focused Assessment

Anxiety Assessment Guide

Rating Scale: None = 0, Mild = 1, Moderate = 2, Severe = 3, Disabling (Panic) = 4

Physiological Effects	Rating	Psychological Effects	Rating
Shortness of breath (dyspnea)	____	Depersonalization (unreal)	____
Choking sensation	____	Feeling "on edge"	____
Dry mouth	____	Poor concentration	____
Pounding heart, increased heart rate	____	Poor memory	____
Chest pain	____	Depressed mood	____
Increased sweating and clammy	____	Loss of interest	____
Feeling faint, dizzy, unsteady	____	Restlessness	____
Nausea and abdominal upsets	____	Sense of panic	____
Numbness (pins and needles)	____	Worry, anticipation of the worst	____
Hot/cold flashes	____	Irritability	____
Trembling, shaking	____	Nightmares	____
Muscle tension and aches	____	Feeling of fear and foreboding	____
Exaggerated startle response	____	Excessive apprehension	____
Difficulties in falling asleep and staying asleep	____	Feeling lack of control	____

Assessing Overall Scores

0–28	Mild anxiety
29–56	Moderate anxiety
57–84	Severe anxiety
85–112	Disabling anxiety

Creating a total score from this table can help you assess whether overall anxiety is mild, moderate, severe, or disabling. However, individual physiological or psychological symptoms that are rated as severe (3) or disabling (4) may be more important and relevant to your nursing assessment. For example, your patient's overall or total assessment may be 26 (in the mild range, 0–27) but she has rated "Excessive apprehension" as 4 (disabling).

Physical Assessment. Consider a comprehensive physical assessment for anxious patients, to rule out underlying disease or disorders. For example, a patient who suffers from heart palpitations when anxious may be found to have significant cardiac arrhythmias. Other medical conditions that may mimic anxiety symptoms include hormone imbalance, nutritional deficiencies, electrolyte imbalance, and central nervous system disorders. Most anxious patients, even those with diagnosed obsessive–compulsive disorder or panic attacks, are not admitted to the hospital just for their anxiety. You will encounter them more often in community settings or when they are hospitalized for other illnesses.

ANALYSIS/NURSING DIAGNOSIS: ANXIETY

For severe anxiety (neuroses, psychoses), medical treatment includes anti-anxiety medications and perhaps psychotherapy. The following five NANDA-I labels represent anxiety problems for which nursing interventions may be effective:

- *Anxiety* is a vague, uneasy feeling of discomfort or dread, accompanied by some of the symptoms listed in the preceding Assessment section and box. Anxiety may be unconscious; that is, the patient may not recognize that he is anxious (e.g., "My heart is pounding, and I can't seem to get my breath; what is wrong?").
- *Death Anxiety* is apprehension, worry, or fear related to death or dying.
- *Decisional Conflict* describes a person who is uncertain about what action to take when the choice among the alternatives involves risk, loss, or challenge to personal life values.
- *Fear* is a response to a perceived threat that is consciously recognized as a danger (e.g., "My father died of this same surgery; truly, I'm scared to death"). Fear is difficult to differentiate from Anxiety because many of the symptoms are similar.
- *Ineffective Denial* occurs when the person consciously or unconsciously rejects the knowledge or meaning of an event (e.g., a client having a heart attack says or thinks, "They have made a mistake. It's just sore muscles or pleurisy. I'll go back to work this afternoon.")

Anxiety can be the etiology or a symptom of many other nursing diagnoses, such as Deficient Knowledge, Self-Mutilation, Ineffective Sexuality Pattern, or Insomnia.

KnowledgeCheck 13-7

- List five NANDA-I labels you could use to describe a problem of anxiety.
- List four observations that would alert you that anxiety is severe enough to merit referral to a mental health professional.

PLANNING OUTCOMES/EVALUATION FOR ANXIETY

You will use outcomes developed in the planning stage as criteria for evaluating patient progress and the success of your nursing interventions. Whether anxiety is a symptom, a problem, or the cause or etiology of a problem, one of the desired outcomes is that the anxiety will be relieved.

For selected NOC standardized outcomes and indicators for anxiety-related diagnoses,

 Go to Chapter 13, **Standardized Language, Anxiety-Related Diagnoses: Selected NOC Outcomes and NIC Interventions,** on Davis*Plus.*

Individualized goal/outcome statements should relate the patient's specific nursing diagnosis, stating behaviors that will indicate that the problem is resolving. The following are some examples.

For Anxiety:
Plans coping strategies for anxious situations.
Uses relaxation techniques as required.
Reports absence of physical and psychological manifestations of anxiety.
For Death Anxiety:
Reports feeling less fearful.
Discusses funeral arrangements with family.
For Decisional Conflict:
Identifies relevant information about the decision and its consequences.
Recognizes how various alternatives conflict with others' desires.
For Fear:
Uses effective coping strategies.
Maintains social relationships and control over life.
For Ineffective Denial:
Verbalizes understanding of the complications that may occur if the disease is not treated.
Follows prescribed regimen for treatments and medications.

Think**Like a Nurse** 13-9

 Go to Chapter 13, **Standardized Language, Anxiety-Related Diagnoses: Selected NOC Outcomes and NIC Interventions,** on Davis*Plus.*

Notice that Anxiety Control is listed as a possible outcome for each of the nursing diagnoses. Explain how anxiety relates to each of the diagnoses: Is it a problem, a symptom, or an etiology?

PLANNING INTERVENTIONS/IMPLEMENTATION: ANXIETY

Interventions for anxious clients will depend on the cause of the anxiety; however, for *all* anxious clients, regardless of the etiology, the nursing goals in most situations are to help the client to:

- *Recognize that the client is anxious.* Because the symptoms may be varied, subtle, and physical, a person may demonstrate anxious behaviors without even realizing why he is doing so. Or he may attribute his symptoms to a physical illness.
- *Identify the source of the client's anxiety.* This may require a more extended relationship than you might have with a hospitalized client, because it involves the uncovering of emotional conflicts. Nevertheless, a more permanent relief can be obtained once the client recognizes the conflict and can use his conscious, rational mind to deal with it.
- *Deal with the symptoms of the client's anxiety,* for example, with massage, relaxation techniques, and so forth.

For NIC standardized interventions and selected activities for anxiety-related diagnoses,

Go to Chapter 13, **Standardized Language, Anxiety-Related Diagnoses: Selected NOC Outcomes and NIC Interventions,** on Davis*Plus.*

Specific nursing activities for reducing anxiety include the following:

- Provide a calm and safe environment, including a quiet, reassuring approach to communication and nursing activities. This will help the person remain centered and focused.
- Control the environment by removing anxiety-provoking equipment and people.
- Establish a relationship of trust, caring, and unconditional positive regard (i.e., don't make promises you can't keep; don't make any judgment statements such as, "You ought to . . ." or "You shouldn't . . .").
- Be present and stay with the individual to help allay fears, create trust, and promote safety.
- Help the person identify triggers and situations that create anxiety.
- Use clear and factual knowledge tailored to the individual's circumstances.
- Explain and, if necessary, explore details of all healthcare procedures.
- Develop coping strategies and behavior modification techniques.
- Encourage enjoyable, nonstressful activities to give the person an opportunity to think about something other than the anxiety-producing situation.
- Advise regular physical exercise unless contraindicated by a physical condition.
- Administer and monitor anti-anxiety medication when required.
- Assist the patient in relaxation methods, such as biofeedback, meditation, and therapeutic touch. For specific information about these methods,

 Go to **Chapter 46, Holistic Healing,** on Davis*Plus.*

- In addition, interventions specific for Death Anxiety include the following (also refer to Chapter 17):
  Stay physically close to the patient when he is fearful.
  Obtain spiritual support for the patient and family, as needed.
  Inquire about the patient's and family's specific requests for care.

Nursing Care for Example Problem: Depression

The nurse–patient relationship is vital when you work with a depressed person. Whereas an anxious patient may actively seek your assistance, a depressed person is likely to be apathetic, avoid your approach, or feel unworthy of your time and effort. Establishing a nurse–patient bond requires a specific, empathetic approach involving warmth, acceptance, and understanding (unconditional positive regard) even in the face of an unresponsive, even angry, patient response.

 ASSESSMENT: DEPRESSION

You should be alert for risk factors and signs and symptoms of depression in all healthcare settings. If cues are present, you will need to perform a more thorough screening or comprehensive assessment, such as the Focused Assessment box Depression Assessment Guide: Patient Health Questionnaire (PHQ-9).

Risk Factors Specific to Older Adults. For older adults, risk factors for depression include dementia, cancer, alcohol and substance abuse, stroke, myocardial infarction, functional disability, being widowed, being a caregiver, and social isolation (Kurlowicz, 2008). Presence of risk factors should alert you to the need for a system-specific (or special needs) assessment to determine whether depression is present.

Symptoms of Depression

Because there are so many symptoms of depression, categorizing them may help to you to remember them. Depression is expressed by changes in feelings, cognition, and behaviors, as well as physical symptoms and changes in lifestyle. Symptoms may differ in some ways in children and older adults.

When assessing for depression, observe for symptoms in the following categories:

Feelings. Depression is characterized affectively by a flat affect; difficulty concentrating; and **anhedonia,** a loss of interest or pleasure in previously enjoyable activities (Steptoe, 2007). Finally, the person may feel worthless, guilt ridden, or suicidal. Observe for anger, anxiety, guilt, helplessness, powerlessness, hopelessness, sadness; verbalizing lack of feeling; inability to enjoy previously enjoyable activities; low self-esteem; and worthlessness.

Cognition (Thoughts). The person may be preoccupied with loss (e.g., of job, of function); may experience self-blame, ambivalence, guilt, confusion, inability to make decisions; or blame others. You may observe, or the person may report, slowed thinking, poor concentration, preoccupation with bodily changes, and inability to accept positive comments,

Behavior. The person may be unable to sleep, or sleep too much, dreading the moment when he has to get out of bed and face family members or responsibilities. Some people lose interest in eating and, therefore, lose weight; others eat frequently but without pleasure in an attempt to keep their "emptiness" at bay. Some people become agitated and restless; others experience slowed thinking and lethargy. Many experience fatigue or feelings of exhaustion throughout the day. Depression may be expressed in children by irritability, tantrums, or not eating. Look for persistently sad expression, poor eye contact, tearfulness, regression, restlessness, agitation, psychomotor retardation, withdrawal, poor grooming/hygiene, decreased sexual interest, past or current alcohol or substance abuse, and past history of suicide attempts.

Lifestyle Effects. Social isolation is common. Depression may be masked by attempts to self-medicate with alcohol, over-the-counter drugs, or illegal substances; or by disordered eating, smoking, participation in dangerous sports, or other forms of reckless behavior. In children, depression may manifest in skipping school or difficulty with relationships with others.

Physiological Effects. Like all mental illnesses, depression carries a social stigma; thus, patients who are unwilling to admit—even to themselves—that they might be depressed may present with a physical complaint such as persistent fatigue or a fear of cancer. In such cases, skillful psychosocial assessment is critical. Physical conditions that might accompany depression include dizziness, headache, migraines, joint aches and pains (e.g., back pain), stomach ulcers and digestive upsets, chest pain, lethargy, constipation, sleep deprivation or hypersomnia, fatigue, anorexia or overeating, and weight changes.

Assessing Older Adults: Depression, Dementia, or Delirium?

Delirium, also called *acute confusion,* is an acute and potentially reversible disturbance of consciousness and cognition in response to underlying medical or mental illnesses, drug

Depression Assessment Guide: Patient Health Questionnaire (PHQ-9)

This is a valid and reliable measure of depression developed in 1999 by Pfizer, Inc. It can be self-administered (Kroenke, Spitzer, & Williams, 2001). It may be useful across cultures (Chen, Huang, Chang, et al., 2006).

Over the past 2 weeks, how often have you been bothered by any of the following problems? (Check or circle your answers.)

	Not At All	Several Days	More than Half the Days	Nearly Every Day
1. Little interest or pleasure in doing things	0	1	2	2
2. Feeling down, depressed, or hopeless	0	1	2	3
3. Trouble falling or staying asleep, or sleeping too much	0	1	2	3
4. Feeling tired or having little energy	0	1	2	3
5. Poor appetite or overeating	0	1	2	3
6. Feeling bad about yourself—or that you are a failure or have let yourself or your family down	0	1	2	3
7. Trouble concentrating on things, such as reading the newspaper or watching television	0	1	2	3
8. Moving or speaking so slowly that other people could have noticed. Or the opposite—being so fidgety or restless that you have been moving around a lot more than usual	0	1	2	3
9. Thoughts that you would be better off dead or of hurting yourself in some way	0	1	2	3

ADD COLUMNS [ ] + [ ] + [ ]

TOTAL: [ ]

10. If you checked off any problems, how difficult have these problems made it for you to do your work, take care of things at home, or get along with other people?

Not difficult at all _____

Somewhat difficult _____

Very difficult _____

Extremely difficult _____

(Healthcare professional: For interpretation of TOTAL, please refer to the accompanying score card. *[Note to students: Interpretation requires training. You should report the patient's score to your instructor or your immediate supervising nurse.]*)

Source: Pfizer, Inc. Retrieved from http://www.phqscreeners.com/. Used by permission.

toxicity, and a variety of other causes. **Dementia** is an irreversible decline in mental abilities. It is a permanent progressive decline in cognitive function (APA, 2000). Dementia affects about 22% of adults age 71 years and older. Dementia prevalence increases with age: The rate is about 40% in those older than age 85 (Plassman, Langa, Fisher, et al., 2007). Alzheimer's disease and vascular dementia account for most dementias (53% and 23%, respectively) (Howarth, Health, & Snope, 1999).

Confusion may be present in patients with depression, as well as those who have dementia or delirium. Approximately 10% to 30% of all confusion is reversible (Richardson, 2003).

However, because confusion and cognitive difficulties in older adults are so often caused by dementia, care providers often attribute the patient's confusion to Alzheimer's disease and assume that interventions would be useless (Edwards, 2003). This means that for older adults, depression is underrecognized and undertreated. For a comparison of the symptoms of depression and dementia, refer to the Focused Assessment box Differentiating Depression and Dementia.

The Geriatric Depression Scale is especially useful in screening for depression in older adults. It requires minimal training to use, and will help you decide whether the patient needs further assessment.

Focused Assessment

Differentiating Depression and Dementia

This focused assessment may help you to identify older adults who should be referred for further evaluation to determine whether symptoms are related to depression or dementia. In addition, the Geriatric Depression Rating Scale requires minimal training to use, and will help you decide whether the patient needs further assessment. To use it to screen for depression,

Go to Chapter 13, **Tables, Boxes, Figures, ESG Figure 13-2, Geriatric Depression Rating Scale (Short Form),** on *DavisPlus.*

To determine whether the patient should be referred to a mental health professional, refer to the Focused Assessment box, Identifying Depressed Patients Who Should Be Referred for Evaluation, later in this chapter.

Characteristic	Depression	Dementia
Cause/triggers	Loss (e.g., of spouse, of independence); stress	Physiological causes (e.g., Alzheimer's disease, brain infarcts)
Onset	Acute or chronic; can be related to specific events	Chronic, gradual, and insidious
Course	Varies, depending on cause	Progressive, over a long period of time
Alertness	Usually reduced	Usually normal
Memory	Memory loss and forgetfulness	Recent and remote memory impaired; loss of recent memory is first sign; some loss of common knowledge
Thinking	Inability to concentrate	Difficulty with abstraction and word finding, especially nouns; difficulty with calculations; decreased judgment
Response to questions	Often says, "I don't know."	Answers inappropriately or with "near misses"
Language	Speaks slowly; slow to respond to verbal stimuli	Disoriented, rambling, incoherent; difficulty using nouns
Sleep	Difficulty falling asleep, early morning awakening, much day sleeping	Sleep fragmented; awakens often during night
Reversibility	Potential	Irreversible, progressive

Source: Adapted from Edwards, N. (2003, December). Differentiating the three D's: Delirium, dementia, and depression. *MedSurg Nursing.* Retrieved from http://findarticles.com/p/articles/mi_m0FSS/is_6_12/ai_n18616788

When Should I Refer the Patient to a Mental Health Specialist?

Because depression is so common, many of the patients you see (e.g., medical–surgical, maternity, clinics) will have at least some degree of depression. It will be important for you to differentiate among temporary, situational sadness, low energy, and a psychiatric diagnosis (clinical depression). Figure 13-5 illustrates the continuum of mild to severe depression incorporating aspects of mood, behavior, thoughts, and physical symptoms.

The presence of any of the following should alert you to make a referral. If you suspect severe depression, document the patient's responses in your nursing notes, and refer the patient to a mental health specialist.

- Personal history of recurrent depression or bipolar disorder
- Family history of recurrent depression or bipolar disorder
- Personal history of recurrence of depression within 1 year after stopping effective treatment
- Episode of major depression before age 20
- Severe, sudden, or life-threatening depressive episode (i.e., suicide attempt)

For three alternative methods you can use to identify patients who should be referred to a mental health specialist for evaluation and/or treatment of depression, refer to the Focused Assessment box Identifying Depressed Patients Who Should Be Referred for Evaluation.

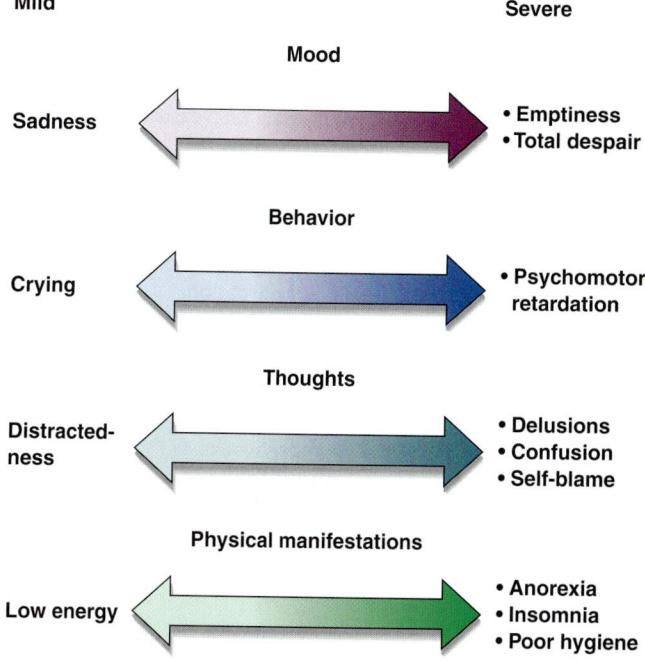

FIGURE 13-5 Depression assessment continuum incorporating mood, behavior, thoughts, and physical state.

✚ If you believe there is a risk for suicide, make the referral immediately (Box 13-1).

ANALYSIS/NURSING DIAGNOSIS: DEPRESSION

Depression is a psychiatric diagnosis, so you will not make that diagnosis. Nevertheless, you will need to describe associated problems that are appropriate for nursing intervention. The NANDA-I taxonomy does not have a specific diagnosis that uses the term *depression;* however, the following nursing diagnoses may be useful in describing the feelings and moods of patients who are depressed:

- *Hopelessness* may apply to a person who is unable to seek or comprehend opportunities, options, and alternatives because of a distressed emotional and unmotivated state. Note that research shows hopelessness to correlate highly with suicide (Cheung, Law, Chan, et al., 2006; Goldston, Reboussin, & Daniel, 2006).

- *Powerlessness* may be diagnosed when a person's perception of control over situations and life events is significantly impaired and externally based.

✚ *Risk for Suicide* must always be considered when a patient is depressed, especially when the person has a history of prior attempts or is verbalizing the desire to die or the intent to kill himself.

Remember that depression can cause a variety of physical and behavioral problems, such as the following nursing diagnoses:

Activity Intolerance	Impaired Social Interaction
Adult Failure to Thrive	Ineffective Health Maintenance
Constipation	Insomnia
Imbalanced Nutrition: Less than Body Requirements	Noncompliance
	Self-Care Deficit (Bathing/ Hygiene, Dressing/Grooming)
Imbalanced Nutrition: More than Body Requirements	Self-Neglect

---

Focused Assessment

Identifying Depressed Patients Who Should Be Referred for Evaluation

Yes/No

One way to identify depression that is more than simple, situational depression is to ask the following two questions. A yes answer merits a referral.

1. "Over the past 2 weeks, have you felt down, depressed, or hopeless?"
2. "Over the past 2 weeks, have you felt little interest or pleasure in doing things?"

Source: U.S. Preventive Services Task Force. (2002). Screening for depression: Recommendations and rationale. *Annals of Internal Medicine, 136*(10), 760–764.

SIGECAPS

Another method is to use the mnemonic SIGECAPS, a concise version of the *DSM-IV-TR* diagnostic criteria. Ask the patient if he has experienced, for 2 or more weeks:

Sleep increase/decrease
Interest in formerly compelling or pleasurable activities diminished
Guilt, low self-esteem
Energy poor
Concentration poor
Appetite increase/decrease
Psychomotor agitation or retardation
Suicidal ideation

Both of the following require referral for evaluation and treatment:

Major depression = depressed mood or interest *plus* 4 SIGECAPS for 2 or more weeks
Mild depression (mood disorder) = depressed mood or interest *plus* 3 SIGECAPS most days for 2 or more years

Source: Brigham and Women's Hospital. (2001).

IN SAD CAGES

Some people prefer a mnemonic from an older source, IN SAD CAGES, which you would use in essentially the same way. Ask the patient if he has experienced, for 2 or more weeks:

Interest reduced
Negative thoughts
Sleep disturbance
Appetite change
Decreased confidence or self-esteem
Concentration reduced
Affect blunt or flat
Guilt
Energy reduced
Suicidal ideas

The original reference does not include a suggested total that requires referral. However, you can assume that the more symptoms, the more severe the depression. We suggest the following:

IN (reduced interest and negative thoughts or depressed mood) *plus* 4 of the other **SAD CAGES** requires referral.

Do not try to differentiate mild and major depression with this method.

Adapted from Rund, D.A., & Hutzler, J. C. (1983). *Emergency psychiatry.* St. Louis, MO: C.V. Mosby, p. 144.

BOX 13-1 ■ Cues Indicating a Possible Risk Factor for Suicide

Risk Factors

- Alcohol substance abuse
- Family history of mental disorders or substance abuse
- Family history of suicide
- Guns in the home
- Family violence, including physical or sexual abuse
- A significant medical illness, such as cancer or chronic pain
- Compulsive gambling
- Recent losses: Physical, financial, personal
- Age, gender, race (elderly or young adult, unmarried, white, male, living alone)
- Recent discharge from an inpatient psychiatry unit

Warning Signs

 Patients with risk factors who exhibit any of the following warning signs clearly raise a red flag and merit immediate referral.

- Withdrawal from social contact
- Desire to be left alone
- Preoccupation with death and dying, or violence
- Risky or self-destructive behavior, such as drug use or unsafe driving
- Changes in routine, sleeping patterns
- Changes in eating habits
- Giving away belongings or getting affairs in order
- Personality changes, such as becoming very outgoing after being shy
- Saying goodbye to people as if they won't be seen again
- Talking about suicide (e.g., "I'm going to kill myself," I wish I were dead," or "I wish I hadn't been born")

Source: Maybury, B. C. (2008). Suicide prevention: Every nurse's responsibility. *Nurse.com,* March 22, 2012. Retrieved from http://news.nurse.com/apps/pbcs.dll/article?AID=200880305017

The diagnoses of *Situational* and *Chronic Low Self-Esteem* are also useful because depressed clients often experience low self-esteem. These diagnoses were presented in the preceding Analysis/Nursing Diagnosis: Self-Concept and Self-Esteem section in this chapter.

PLANNING OUTCOMES/EVALUATION: DEPRESSION

You will use outcomes developed in the planning stage as criteria for evaluating the patient's progress and the success of your nursing interventions.

For selected NOC standardized outcomes and indicators for depression-related diagnoses,

 Go to Chapter 13, **Standardized Language, Depression-Related Diagnoses: Selected NOC Outcomes and NIC Interventions,** on Davis*Plus*.

Individualized goal/outcome statements should relate to the patient's specific nursing diagnosis, stating behaviors that will indicate that the problem is resolving. The following are some examples:

For Depressed Mood:
Affect is appropriate to the situation.
Reports feeling less sadness and depression.

Interacts willingly and appropriately with others.
Eats a well-balanced diet to prevent weight loss.
Bathes, washes and combs hair, dresses—maintains grooming and hygiene.
For Hopelessness:
Expresses positive belief in self, others, and meaning of life.
Demonstrates interest in life/activity.
Maintains spiritual belief system or religious affiliation.
For Powerlessness:
Participates in healthcare decisions to the extent possible.
Sets realistic goals for self.
For Risk for Suicide:
Verbalizes any suicidal ideas to staff.
Trusts staff enough to disclose any specific plans for suicide.

PLANNING INTERVENTIONS/IMPLEMENTATION: DEPRESSION

For *NIC standardized interventions and selected activities* for depression-related diagnoses,

Go to Chapter 13, **Standardized Language, Depression-Related Diagnoses: Selected NOC Outcomes and NIC Interventions,** on Davis*Plus*.

Individualized nursing activities for depression-related diagnoses focus on altering the problem etiologies and relieving symptoms of depression. In general, care of the depressed person involves (1) developing a therapeutic relationship through effective communication and (2) promoting nutrition, exercise, and personal hygiene.

- Use therapeutic communication:
  Be honest and open.
  Be patient.
  Be consistent.
  Do not use false reassurance ("You'll feel better soon").
  Avoid phrases such as "Cheer up" or "Think how lucky you are to have a good family."
  Do make comments such as, "I like the way you look in that dress."
  Do not be overly cheerful.
  Encourage the client to express feelings, including anger.
  Be accepting and nonjudgmental when the client expresses feelings.
  Encourage communication that explores reality, grief, and personal loss.
- Promote activity. Activities in small groups can help build self-esteem.
- Promote and teach good nutrition and hydration.
- Provide support as needed for self-care and decision making, while promoting as much independence as possible.
- Assess for and provide information about use of complementary and alternative therapies for depression (see the Complementary and Alternative Modalities (CAM) box).

Monitor for suicide risk. Ask directly, "Have you thought about harming yourself? If so, what do you plan to do?"

- Institute measures to build self-esteem (see Promoting Self-Esteem and Self-Concept in this chapter).
- Provide information on support and educational groups.
- Encourage the person to maintain his religious affiliations.

Complementary and Alternative Modalities (CAM)

Many people use herbal therapies to relieve symptoms of anxiety and depression. Patients may self-treat, or CAM practitioners may prescribe herbal therapies. You should assess for CAM use to be sure that the method is not contraindicated and that the patient has informed the primary care provider about its use.

DEPRESSION

CAM	Active Ingredients	Side Effects	Contraindications	Patient Teaching
Ginkgo biloba	Ginkgetin, ginkgolic acid, ascorbic acid, flavonols, sterols	Nausea, vomiting, diarrhea (usually mild) Headache	Pregnant or breastfeeding Children Patients using anticoagulants (use with caution) Patients with peptic ulcer disease	Can take 6–8 weeks for patient to feel any better. Mixing with some fruits and nuts could produce poison ivy–like reaction.
Ginseng	Ginsenosides, beta-elemene, sterols, flavonoids, peptides, vitamins B_1, B_2, B_{12}, nicotinic acid, fats, minerals, enzymes	(many) Nausea Vomiting Diarrhea Chest pain Headache Nosebleeds Palpitations Nervousness Insomnia	Cardiovascular disease Hypertension Hypotension Diabetes Pregnancy or breastfeeding Patients with active bleeding Anticoagulants Antiplatelet medications	There are many kinds of ginseng; patient should research the specific type he is using. ✚ Discourage use by patients who are anticoagulated, or who have hypertension or diabetes.
Kava	Kava pyrones, pipermethystine	Visual disturbances Changes in reflexes and judgment Decreased platelet and lymphocyte counts Hepatotoxicity	Pregnancy Breastfeeding Use of alcohol, alprazolam, or central nervous system (CNS) depressants	May experience symptom relief within 1 week. Significant adverse reactions may occur. Kava enhances the effects of alcohol and CNS medications. Because of liver toxicity, the CDC has cautioned consumers against using kava (CDC, 2002). Its use is severely limited and regulated in Australia (Therapeutic Goods Administration, 2005).
St. John's wort	Tannin, naphthodianthrones, flavonoids, bioflavonoids, phloroglucinols	Dry mouth Constipation GI upset Sleep disturbances Restlessness Photosensitivity Interferes with digoxin and indinavir	Pregnancy or lactation Children Use of monoamine oxidase inhibitors (MAOIs), selective serotonin reuptake inhibitors (SSRIs), alcohol, or OTC cold and flu medications	Teach contraindications and side effects. Patients who are depressed should not take this herb without medical supervision
S-Adenosyl methionine (SAMe)	Amino acid and ATP, which are produced naturally in the body and are now being reproduced artificially as well	Few side effects Gastric upset Hypomania (in patients with bipolar disorder) Anxiety (in patients with depression) Headache		Patients with bipolar disorder should not use this supplement unless under direct supervision of their physician. Use enteric-coated forms to decrease gastric irritation.

Anxiety

Kava	See Depression, preceding. Not recommended for use.			

Source: Adapted from Hulisz, D. T. (2008). Top herbal products: Efficacy and safety concerns. *Medscape Nurses.* ©2007. Retrieved March 20, 2012, from http://www.medscape.org/viewprogram/8494; and Neeb, K. (2001). *Fundamentals of mental health nursing* (2nd ed.). Philadelphia: F. A. Davis, pp. 365–378.

Nursing Interventions for Older Adults

Remember that depression is not a normal part of aging. As mentioned previously, it is important to identify depression in older adults and not mistake it for dementia or so-called signs of old age.

Team Communication. If you identify signs of depression, be certain to communicate that to other members of the staff and to the primary care provider. You and the other nurses may be the only ones who have repeated contact with the patient, so you may be able to observe cues that are missed by other providers.

Medications. Because metabolism changes with aging, the risk of adverse medication effects is high for older adults. Closely supervise patients being treated with antidepressants because severe side effects are possible. When a patient is admitted to a hospital there is a risk that self-administered medications may be overlooked. If one of those medications is an antidepressant, missed doses combined with a physical illness may cause depression symptoms to worsen.

Reminiscence. Use life review and reminiscence as an intervention. Encourage the patient to talk about significant positive and negative experiences that have occurred during her life.

Suicide Risk. Keep in mind that depression is a significant predictor of suicide in older adults. As an example, the suicide rate among white men age 85 and older is almost double that of the U.S. general population (National Institute of Mental Health, 2008). Older adults often succeed in their suicide attempts. To illustrate: Among adults older than age 65 years, there is one suicide for every four attempts; among young adults, there is one suicide for every 100 to 200 attempts (Goldsmith, Pellmar, Kleinman, et al., as cited in Centers for Disease Control and Prevention [CDC], 2007).

Professional Help. Encourage the patient to seek professional help. Older adults are likely to try to handle it themselves, or even not think of depression as a health problem. Many think that it is normal to be depressed as they grow older.

Suicide Prevention Interventions

It is not only patients on psychiatric units who commit suicide. They may be the same patients you care for on a medical–surgical unit or in their homes. Illnesses such as advanced cancer and AIDS are often accompanied by uncontrolled pain and delirium. Because of the suffering and dependency they cause, they are associated with higher suicide rates.

Your most important intervention is assessment. Be alert for risk factors and warning signs that may indicate the possibility of suicide (see Box 13-1). Remember that about 80% of those who attempt suicide give some prior verbal or indirect cues.

- Evaluate the patient's medications (e.g., certain antihypertensive agents, steroids, cancer chemotherapeutic agents, amphotericin-B can cause depression).
- If risk factors are present, put them prominently on the care plan and report them to other caregivers.
- Do not avoid the patient because you fear saying the wrong thing. Talking about suicide does not increase the risk.
- Be aware of your personal feelings and anxieties regarding suicide.
- If the patient mentions suicide specifically, be direct. Ask whether he is having thoughts of harming himself.
- If he answers yes, do not leave him. Have someone contact his primary care provider so that a psychiatric consult can be ordered, and possibly transfer to a psychiatric unit if the patient is physically stable.
- Ask if the patient has a plan for suicide, and if so, what it is.
- Remove items that might be used for self-harm, for example, razor blades and other sharp objects, shoelaces, belts, intravenous tubing, telephone cords, pills, and glasses. Search the room and the bathroom.
- Make sure the windows cannot be opened.
- Follow agency policy for continuous monitoring, moving to a room close to the nurses' station, and so on (Gorman & Sultan, 2008; Maybury, 2008).
- Most of all, never attempt to work with a suicidal patient by yourself. Involve other members of the team immediately.

Toward Evidence-Based Practice

(Study A) Smalbrugge, M., Pot, A. M., Jongenelis, L., et al. (2006). The impact of depression and anxiety on well being, disability and use of healthcare services in nursing home patients. *International Journal of Geriatric Psychiatry, 21*(4), 325–332.

Researchers studied 350 elderly patients from 14 nursing homes in the Netherlands to determine the impact of depression and anxiety on well-being, disability, and their use of healthcare services (e.g., the amount of assistance they needed with ADLs). They found depression and/or anxiety was associated significantly with less well-being, but not with more disability. They were also associated with increased use of healthcare services: more need for assistance with ADLs, more consultation of medical specialists, a higher mean number of medications, and more use of antidepressants.

(Study B) Wilkinson, S. M., Love, S. B., Westcombe, A. M., et al. (2007). Effectiveness of aromatherapy massage in the management of anxiety and depression in patients with cancer: A multicenter randomized controlled trial. *Journal of Clinical Oncology, 25*(5), 532–538

Researchers studied 288 cancer patients who were referred to complementary therapy services with clinical anxiety and/or depression. Patients were randomly assigned to a course of aromatherapy massage or usual supportive care alone to determine the effectiveness of supplementing usual supportive care with aromatherapy massage. The researchers concluded that aromatherapy massage does not appear to significantly relieve cancer patients' anxiety and/or depression in the long term, but is associated with clinically important benefit up to 2 weeks after the intervention.

(Continued)

Toward Evidence-Based Practice—cont'd

(Study C) Sendelbach, S. E., Halm, M. A., Doran, K. A., et al. (2006). Effects of music therapy on physiological and psychological outcomes for patients undergoing cardiac surgery. *Journal of Cardiovascular Nursing, 21*(3), 194–200.

This study compared the effects of music therapy versus a quiet, uninterrupted rest period on pain intensity, anxiety, physiological parameters, and opioid consumption after cardiac surgery. A total of 86 patients recovering from cardiac surgery were randomly assigned to receive either 20 minutes of rest in bed (control) or 20 minutes of music. Researchers found that patients who listened to music experienced a significant reduction in anxiety, but that there was no effect on blood pressure, heart rate, or use of opioids.

1. To help you with your analysis for the following questions, complete this table.

	STUDY A	STUDY B	STUDY C
Intervention			
Type of patient			
Result/conclusion			

2. Which of the studies tested an intervention?

3. Which of the interventions was most successful in relieving anxiety? Explain your thinking.

4. Think about the study that did not test an intervention. What, if anything, is its value to nurses or patients?

 Go to Chapter 13, **Toward Evidence-Based Practice: Suggested Responses,** on Davis*Plus.*

▭ CLINICAL REASONING:
Applying the **Full-Spectrum Nursing Model**

Because the following critical thinking activities allow you to practice the kind of thinking you will use as a full-spectrum nurse, they usually have no single right answer. Discuss them with your peers—if you have difficulty with any of the questions, consult your instructor.

PATIENT SITUATION

Matthew has been admitted to the emergency department with extensive wounds to both forearms, including tendon and vascular damage, from a suicide attempt. Matthew seems very quiet, almost withdrawn, and answers most of your questions in monosyllables.

Matthew reports the following: He is the third child in a family of five. Matthew's middle-class parents are now retired, and his brothers and sisters are scattered across the country in various large cities. Although Matthew claims his schooling years were unremarkable, he recalls several occasions when he was bullied and physically beaten by gangs of older adolescents.

Matthew further states that he graduated from Harvard Law School and became vice president of an influential law firm. Despite his apparent success in life, he has continually questioned his self-worth since childhood. Plagued by worries and depression that have increased over the past few years, he says he wrote a note indicating that he now realizes what a failure he is and proceeded to slash both of his forearms with a sharp razor.

Matthew reports that he has not been eating much, feels tired all the time, and has no interest in going outside the house. He says, "I just don't feel like doing anything; I just want to sleep all the time."

THINKING

1. *Theoretical Knowledge:* Using just the information you have in the Patient Situation, use the SIGECAPS method to assess Matthew's level of depression (see the Focused Assessment box, Identifying Depressed Patients Who Should Be Referred for Evaluation). You will need to assume that he is reporting what he has experienced in the past 2 weeks (unless he is obviously referring to the more distant past).

2. *Critical Thinking (Inquiry):* What items of the SIGECAPS cannot be completed with the information in the Patient Situation? What do you need to ask Matthew to complete them?

DOING

3. *Nursing Process (Interventions):* Based on your SIGECAPS data, what do you need to do right away (or be certain it was done in the emergency department)?

CARING

4. *Self-Knowledge:* What do you have in common with Matthew that might help you to empathize with him?
5. *Ethical Knowledge:* Try to put aside your own beliefs now, and answer the following questions from the perspective of (a) Matthew and (b) one of your nursing colleagues on the unit.
   a. Give one reason to support Matthew's claim that he has a right to commit suicide if his despair is too deep to bear.
   b. Give one reason to support a colleague's claim that he does not have a right to commit suicide, no matter how he feels.

 Go To Chapter 13, **Clinical Reasoning: Applying the Full-Spectrum Nursing Model Response Sheet** on Davis*Plus*.

 To explore learning resources for this chapter,

 Go to Davis*Plus* at http://davisplus.fadavis.com/Treas1

Chapter Resources for Chapter 13:
Knowledge Check and Think Like a Nurse Response Sheets
Knowledge Check Answers
Resources for Caregivers and Health Professionals
Reading More About Psychosocial Health and Illness
What Are the Main Points in This Chapter?
NCLEX-Style Review Questions
Chapter Overview Podcasts

Concept Map

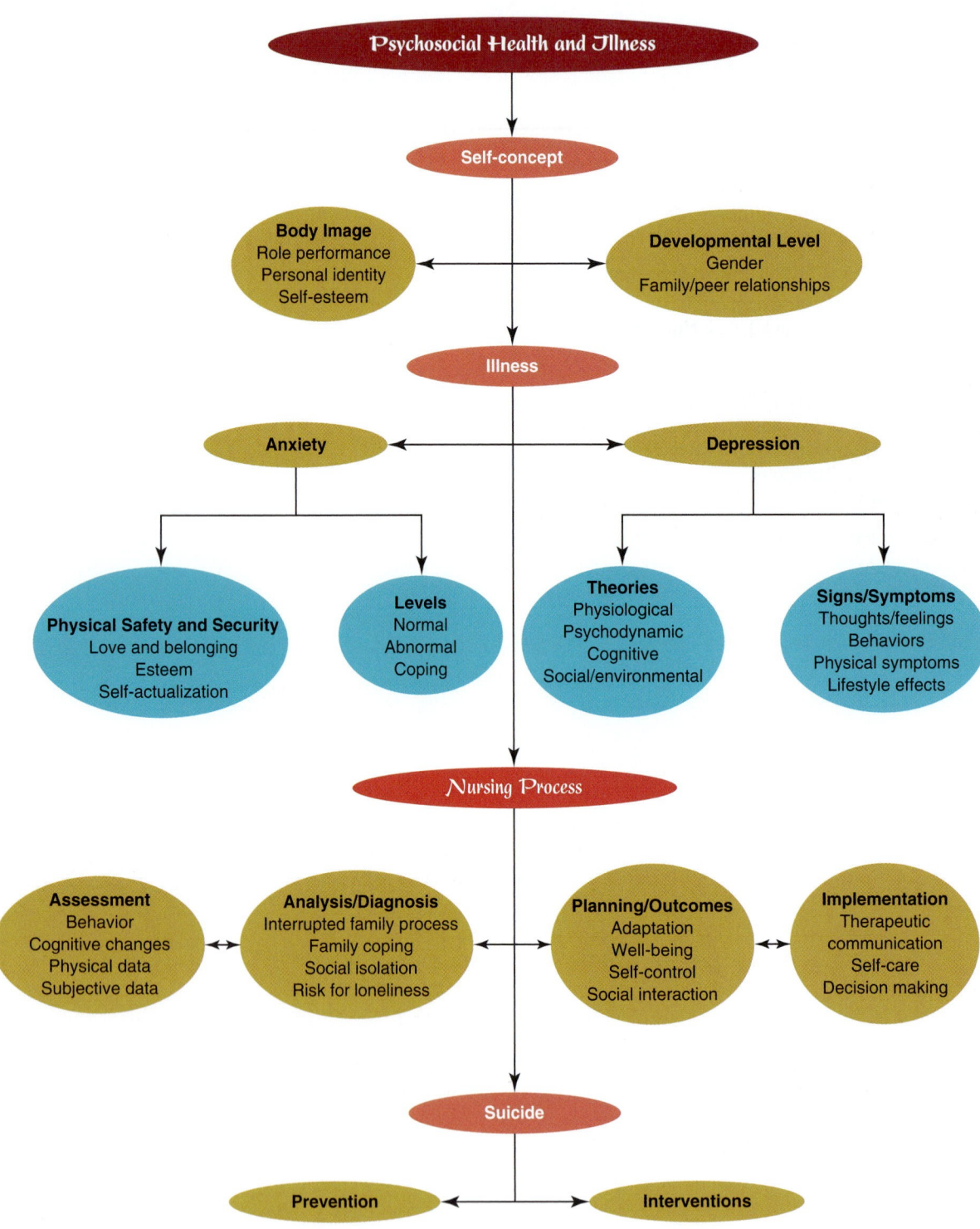

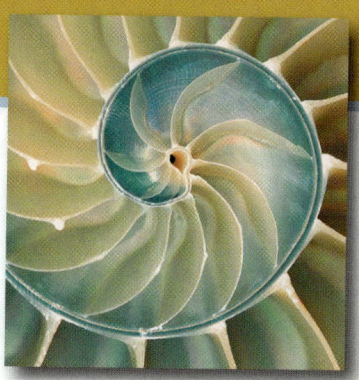

CHAPTER 14

Family

Learning Outcomes

After completing this chapter, you should be able to:

➤ Distinguish among different family structures.

➤ Describe approaches to working with various types of families to provide optimal care to both well and ill clients.

➤ Explain how family theories provide a framework to understand family functioning.

➤ Identify family risk factors in five different stages of the family life span.

➤ Discuss ways in which economic factors influence nursing practice, family care, and access to services.

➤ Present ways chronic, life-threatening illness can affect families.

➤ Identify populations most at risk for homelessness.

➤ Demonstrate an understanding of family violence.

➤ Conduct a family assessment.

➤ Identify common health beliefs and communication patterns among families.

➤ Identify nursing interventions appropriate when a family member is ill.

➤ Review how risk factors, such as illness and death, substance abuse, violence, mental health disorders, financial hardship, unemployment, and other issues, can change a family's structure, communication, and coping strategies.

➤ Discuss the sandwich generation and assessment and intervention strategies for caregiver burnout.

Key Concepts

Family
Family nursing

Related Concepts

See the Concept Map at the end of this chapter.

Example problems

Caregiver role strain

Caring for the Nguyens

This feature allows you to practice the kind of thinking you will use as a full-spectrum nurse. There is usually more than one correct answer to a critical thinking question, so we do not provide answers for these features. It is more important to develop your nursing judgment than to "cover content." Discuss the questions with your peers. If you are still unsure, consult your instructor.

Kim Phan, 3 years old, is the first grandchild for Nam and Yen Nguyen. Until recently, Kim lived with his mother, Trinh Nguyen, the Nguyen's daughter. Trinh was diagnosed with schizophrenia at age 18, but initially was functioning adequately on her medications. However, her condition has been worsening and for the past year she has not been taking her medications. When Trinh became unable to care for Kim, Nam and Yen assumed the child's care. Trinh rarely visits Kim. Nam and Yen convinced Trinh to obtain residential care at a mental health facility. Nam tells you at a clinic visit that he wishes his family were "normal."

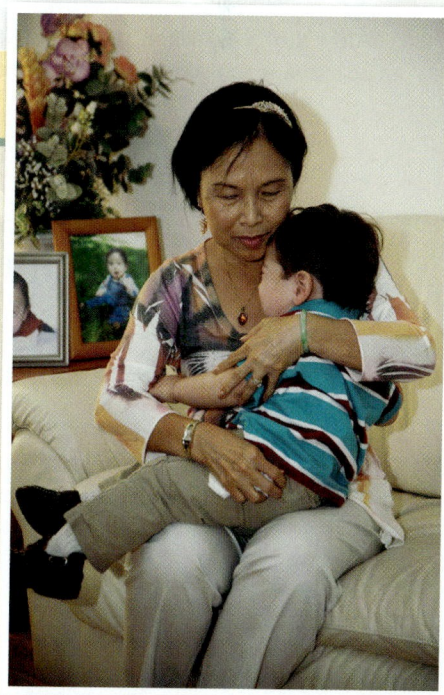

(Continued)

Caring for the Nguyens (continued)

A. What do you need to clarify about Nam's statement about his family?

B. What do *you* think Nam means by a "normal" family?

C. How would you respond to Nam's comments?

D. What effect might this new family structure have on Nam's and Yen's health?

E. How might you promote family functioning for the Nguyens? What assessments should you make? What interventions should you consider?

F. What personal values or biases do you have that may affect your ability to care for the Nguyens?

➤ Go to **Caring for the Nguyens Response Sheet** on Davis*Plus*.

Meet Your Patient

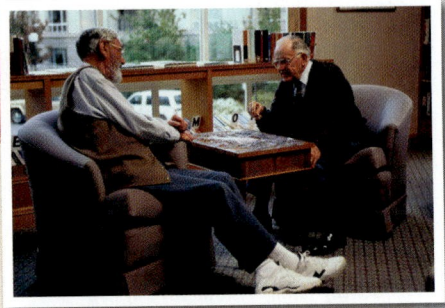

J. B. is an 80-year-old man who is hospitalized for end-stage renal disease. His wife died four years ago. His remaining family includes two married daughters and four grandchildren. J. B. has several siblings, but they live far away and phone or visit only rarely.

J. B. has lived in the same neighborhood for more than 55 years. When he and his wife, Pamela, first moved into the neighborhood, they lived across the street from Mike and Lena. The two families socialized and enjoyed many holidays and festivities together. After the children were grown, the two couples moved into a townhouse near the center of town. They lived next door to each other and continued to spend time together.

After both wives died, J. B. and Mike decided to share an apartment to reduce living expenses. They also wanted the security, support, and companionship that occurs with having a housemate. J. B. subscribes to the local paper, and Mike gets a national paper. They read both papers together over breakfast. They have season tickets to the baseball games and watch sports together on TV. "Thank goodness we have each other," says Mike. Mike comes to the hospital every morning. He brings both papers and breakfast muffins for J. B., himself, and the nurses. He spends the day at the hospital and leaves shortly after dinner.

Theoretical Knowledge
knowing **why**

ABOUT THE KEY CONCEPTS

This chapter is about contemporary families and how they differ from those of the past. As you study the chapter, you will begin to see how family, family nursing, and related concepts apply to the characters in the Meet Your Patient scenario. The key concepts are the basis of the theoretical knowledge to which you will apply the nursing process and your nursing judgment, as you learn to meet the challenges of family health as a full-spectrum nurse.

WHAT IS A FAMILY?

Traditionally, people have thought of a family as consisting of a husband, wife, and children. However, as lifestyles have changed, the concept of family has become broader. The U.S. Census Bureau defines the family household as two or more people related by birth, marriage, or adoption (2009). We describe **family** as two or more individuals who provide physical, emotional, economic, or spiritual support while maintaining involvement in each other's lives. They may or may not be related by blood. Most often, people who consider themselves to be family live in the same household; however, adult children living apart from their parents may continue to define themselves as belonging to one family, which may also include siblings, aunts, uncles, or cousins. In short, families come in many forms, living arrangements, and emotional connections.

Changes in Family Structures

Changes in the living arrangements of families in the United States have resulted from a combination of factors, including an aging population, increasing average age at first marriage, high divorce rates, improvements in the health and financial status of the older population, and changing residential preferences. For instance, traditional family households were the norm 30 years ago (81%), whereas in 2007 the percentage

dropped to 68%. The percentage of people living alone rose from 17% to 27% in the last three decades, with more being women than men (U.S. Census Bureau, 2009).

Traditional Families. In the past, the majority of American families consisted of married couples with at least one child, a husband in the labor force, and a wife not employed outside the home. The U.S. Census Bureau 2007 population survey (2009) estimates that 22.5% of American households consist of married couples with children as compared to 40.3% 30 years prior.

The percentage of children under age 28 living in two-parent homes varies by race:

- Asian—86%
- White, non-Hispanic—77%
- Hispanic—68%
- Black—40%

Nearly 1 out of 4 of children living with a grandparent had no parent present (U.S. Census Bureau, 2009).

Adults Who Are Married but Do Not Have Children. This group was once only a small percentage of American society. It now accounts for more than a quarter of households ((U.S. Census Bureau, 2009).

Dual-Earner Families. A dual-earner family is one in which both parents are in the work force. In contrast to past family structures, nearly two out of three children younger than age 6 live in a dual-earner family (U.S. Census Bureau, 2008).

Single-Parent Families. Single-parent families result from divorce, from the death of a partner, or when partners choose not to marry or live together. They make up more than one-fourth of all families with children. This proportion has nearly tripled since 1960. Most single-parent families are headed by women; however, the number of men raising children without a spouse has increased in recent years. The percentage of single-parent households in the United States varies among geographic areas and ethnic groups. Younger children were more likely to live with one parent than older children (10% of children less than 1 year of age versus 1% of those between 12 and 17 years) (U. S. Census Bureau, 2009).

Blended and Stepfamilies. Single parents commonly remarry to form new family units, such as **stepfamilies** (in which a single parent marries someone who may or may not have children), and **blended families** (in which two single parents marry and raise their children together). Commonly, biological parents who are not living together in the child's home alternate the responsibilities.

Extended Families. In many cultural groups, it is common for extended family members (e.g., grandparents, aunts, uncles, cousins) to live within a single dwelling and be considered immediate family. For example, in the Meet Your Patient scenario, although J. B.'s siblings are members of his extended family, they do not live with him, and he would not consider them part of his immediate family. The growing number of older adults has created the **sandwich generation** (Schwartz, 1979), in which middle-aged adults who still have children at home must care for aging parents and often share their household with them. Trends show more grandparent(s) are raising their grandchildren when the parent(s) are unable to do so because of situations like unemployment, divorce, imprisonment, substance abuse, or serious physical or mental illness. The U.S. Census Bureau reports 6.5 million children are raised in grandparent homes.

Other Family Structures. In addition to families bound by marriage and bloodlines, other family types exist, such as *heterosexual individuals* who may reside in a common household, or *gay and lesbian couples with or without children.* Although *individuals or couples who adopt children* are not biologically related, nonetheless they are very much a family as they are emotionally attached and participate in the children's care and in the experiences in each other's lives. **Cohabiting adults** choose to live together but not marry or live together as a "trial run" prior to marriage. Cohabiting couples who marry have a higher rate of separation than their counterparts who do not live together before marriage.

Recall that a family is a group of individuals who provide support and assistance to each other. In the Meet Your Patient scenario, although J. B. and Mike are not blood relatives, they provide strong support for each other. Many refer to this type of bond as **kith,** persons with a kinship bond. For some people, this bond is stronger than bloodline bonds.

Approaches to Family Nursing

Family nursing refers to nursing care that is holistically focused on the whole family as well as to individual members (Fig. 14-1). Knowing the family unit is affected by acute or chronic illness, hospitalization, or healthcare interventions, the nurse best cares for the family by involving them inpatient care decisions. For J. B. (Meet Your Patient), the nurses would support Mike's daily visits, and Mike is listed on the Health Insurance Portability and Accountability Act (HIPAA) form for communication of patient information. The staff would involve Mike and J. B.'s adult children in his care, discharge planning, and follow-up care at home. They would also teach

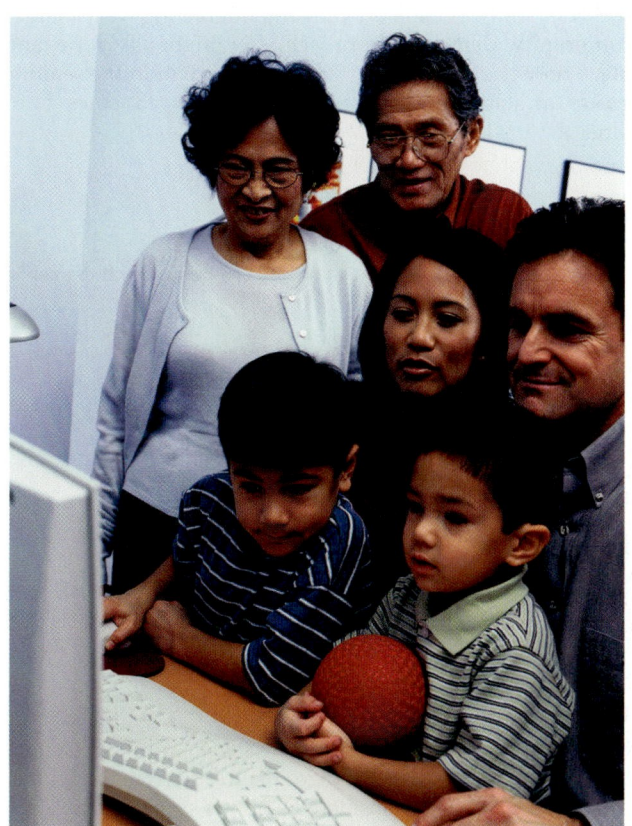

FIGURE 14-1 *Family nursing* refers to nursing care that is holistically directed toward the whole family as well as to individual members.

Mike about J. B.'s medications and treatments so that he can assist J. B. in his activities of daily living (ADLs).

Three perspectives on family nursing include the family as (1) context, (2) unit of care, and (3) system. Family nursing is a specialty; to work with the family as a unit of care or as a system, you may need additional preparation. However, as a graduate nurse, you should be prepared to work with the **family as the context for care** of an individual person. Your focus in this approach is on one individual (the one who is ill); from this perspective, you view the family as either a resource or a stressor to your patient. Using this approach, you would recognize the importance of J. B.'s friend and housemate, Mike, who is his most important source of support. Before discharging J. B., you would ask him, "Will Mike or your daughters be able to help you when you go home?"

A slightly more complex approach views the **family as the unit of care.** Wellness of each member is critical to promoting family health. In this approach, you view the family as the sum of all individual members and provide assessment and care for all family members; however, you might direct interventions to individual family members rather than the family as a whole. For example, you might provide teaching about nutrition and physical activity to all family members to promote their health. Or, to use our earlier example, you might check Mike's blood pressure when he visits J. B.

The third perspective is the **family as a system.** In this approach, you focus on the family as a whole and as an interactional system. Using this perspective, you direct your assessment and intervention to communications and interactions between family members. The systems approach sees the family as embedded in and interacting with a larger community. Using this approach, you might ask, for example, "How has your family's relationship within the seniors' group at your townhouse complex changed since your illness?"

KnowledgeCheck 14-1

- Name at least three types of family structure.
- What are two topics that the nurse can discuss with the family as a unit?

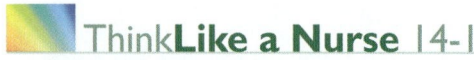

ThinkLike a Nurse 14-1

- How can you promote family cohesion for a family whose members live great distances from each other?

WHAT THEORIES ARE USEFUL FOR FAMILY CARE?

Several theories have been proposed to help us understand family functioning. Four such theories are general systems theory, structural–functional theories, family interactional theory, and developmental theory.

General Systems Theory

General systems theory (see Chapter 8) focuses on interactions between systems and the changes that result from these interactions. The family is considered an open system because the members are interdependent; they function as individuals but also as a family unit as a whole, maintaining balance from within and by the outside environment. Interaction can occur between members of the family or between multiple families.

Healthy families strive to maintain a balance between external stress and internal relationships. Changes in the behaviors or attitudes of an individual member affect the family unit, and changes in family structure and functioning affect individual members. It may help to think of a system as a mobile; if one piece of the mobile is moved, the whole mobile is set in motion.

Other systems surround the family unit (e.g., the community, the city, the state, the healthcare system). Because these systems are broader than the family, they are referred to as **suprasystems.** Smaller components that fit within the family system (e.g., the mother, the marital couple) may be viewed as **subsystems.** Each subsystem has a particular function. For example, one family member might be viewed as the decision maker, another as the peacekeeper, another as the worker, and another as the disciplinarian for the children.

Structural–Functional Theories

Structural–functional family theories are based on the developmental theories of Freud, Erikson, and Havighurst (see Chapter 9 for review) and include the concepts of family roles and interactions. According to Parsons and Bales (1955), the structural–functional approach includes the following assumptions:

- A family is a social system with functional requirements.
- A family is a small group possessing certain features common to small groups.
- The family accomplishes functions that serve both the individual and society.
- Individuals act according to internalized norms that are learned through socialization.

Although they view the family as a social system, structural–functional theories, unlike systems theory, focus on *outcome* rather than process; that is, you would use this theory to assess how well the family functions, both internally among family members and externally with outside systems. Examples of family functions include socialization of children; meeting the physical, financial, and emotional needs of family members; caring for older members; and being productive members of society.

Family Interactional Theory

Family interactional theory views the family as a unit of interacting personalities (Hill & Hansen, 1960). The major emphasis is on family roles. This approach to understanding families deemphasizes the influence of the external world on what occurs within the family. Nurses working from an interactional perspective focus family healthcare on the interaction and communication between family members; their roles and power; family coping; and relationships with other people outside the direct family unit.

Developmental Theories

Developmental theories focus on the stage of family development. Theorists typically identify eight stages in the family life cycle according to the ages of the children and parents: beginning family, childbearing family, family with preschool children, family with school-age children, family with teenagers and young adults, family launching young adults, postparental family, and aging family. Each stage is associated with developmental tasks the family needs to achieve. Most family development theories do not identify stages and tasks for families who remain childless throughout their lives.

Table 14-1 ▶ Family Development

STAGES	TASKS	CHILDREN'S AGES (IF ANY) (APPROXIMATE)
Beginning family	■ Relinquishing the family of origin as the major emotional and economic resource ■ Gaining a sense of autonomy and independence ■ Making the relationship/marriage work; investment in spouse as the major emotional resource ■ Finding a place in the kin network of each partner ■ Exploring options for career development ■ Deciding whether to have children	None
Childbearing family	■ Achieving pregnancy and birth ■ Adjusting to life changes after birth and to the infant's needs ■ Determining ways to meet all members' needs ■ Renegotiating marriage ■ Increasing contact with extended family	Newborn to 2 yr
"No longer newlyweds" (without children)	■ Establishing a sense of the permanence of the relationship ■ Establishing long-term residency ■ Being involved in the community/promoting the well-being of the community	Not applicable
Family with preschool children	■ Adjusting to increased costs associated with family life ■ Socializing the preschoolers ■ Coping with loss of parental energy and privacy	3–5 yr
Mature family (without children)	■ Renegotiating relationship on basis of more maturity ■ Adjusting to changing levels of responsibility in work and community ■ If not done already, achieving financial security	Not applicable
Family with school-age children	■ Adjusting to the needs and demands of growing children ■ Promoting joint decision making among parents and children ■ Encouraging and supporting educational and school-related activities	6–12 yr
Family with teenagers and young adults	■ Maintaining open communication among family members ■ Reinforcing ethical and moral values ■ For teens, balancing independence with parental rules	13–20 yr
Family launching young adults	■ Maintaining support to young adults as they leave the security of family ■ Rediscovering marriage	18–30 yr
Postparental family	■ Preparing for retirement ■ Adjusting to children's moving into new phases of adulthood, marriage or other relationship, and childbearing and to becoming a grandparent	Adult
Middle-aged couple (without children)	■ Accepting that it may be too late to reconsider childbearing or childrearing ■ Reaching the peak of a career or realizing that the peak may not occur ■ Planning for retirement	None

(Continued)

Table 14-1 ➤ Family Development—cont'd		
STAGES	**TASKS**	**CHILDREN'S AGES (IF ANY) (APPROXIMATE)**
Aging family (applies to family without children)	■ Adjusting to retirement and changes associated with aging ■ Adjusting to the loss of a spouse and friendships	Adult *(or none)*

Adapted from Friedman, M. M. (2003). *Family nursing: Theory and practice* (5th ed.). Norwalk, CT: Appleton & Lange; Friedman, M. M., Bowden, V. R., & Jones, E. G. (2003). *Family nursing: Research, theory, and practice* (5th ed.). Upper Saddle River, NJ: Prentice Hall; Hanson, S. M. (2005). *Family health care nursing: Theory, practice, and research* (3rd ed.). Philadelphia: F.A. Davis; and McGoldrick, M., & Carter, E. (1985). The stages of the family life cycle. In J. Henslin (Ed.), *Marriage and family in a changing society*. New York: Free Press.

Generally, the stages follow one another in a linear progression; however, some families may be in more than one stage at a time or may revert to previous stages. This overlap or reversion is most common in families that have children spaced far apart, in blended families, and in stepfamilies. See Chapters 9 and 10 for developmental theories applicable to individual family members.

KnowledgeCheck 14-2

- Which type of theory focuses on interactions among families, family members, and groups in the environment?
- What is the name of the theory that views families as a social system with a focus on outcomes?
- What are some examples of family functions as defined by structural–functional theories?

ThinkLike a Nurse 14-2

- Using systems theory, you could view J. B., his siblings, his children, and his grandchildren as a system. Refer to the section on family structures—how would you categorize this family structurally?
- Again using systems theory, what or who are the subsystems in the family system described in the preceding question?
- Considering J. B. alone, at what developmental stage is his "family"?

WHAT ARE SOME FAMILY HEALTH RISK FACTORS?

Many health risk factors are the same for families as for individuals, and they are similar across age groups and family types. For a more complete discussion of this topic,

 Go to Chapter 14, **Supplemental Materials: What Are Some Family Health Risk Factors?** on Davis*Plus*.

For specific topics related to families, also see Chapters 9 and 10 covering growth and development, Chapter 12 on stress and adaptation, Chapter 20 about communicating, and Chapter 26 on teaching clients.

Childless and Childbearing Couples

Adapting to new roles within the home creates stress for newly married couples; couples who are trying to become pregnant; and new parents who are inexperienced in the challenges and responsibilities of raising a healthy, happy, and safe child (Fig. 14-2). Use of maladaptive coping mechanisms

can lead to health problems, such as the misuse of alcohol. This creates risk for self-injury and liver disease, and the family can suffer from neglect, family violence, and addiction. In addition, childbearing couples face health risks related to pregnancy and birth, including the risk of miscarriage, congenital malformations and genetic defects, and risk to the health and safety of the mother and fetus during and after the labor and birth process.

Families With Young Children

Finding safe, nurturing, and affordable child care can be a major source of family stress for parents working outside the home. Common parenting concerns center around children's development, socialization, education, discipline, nutrition,

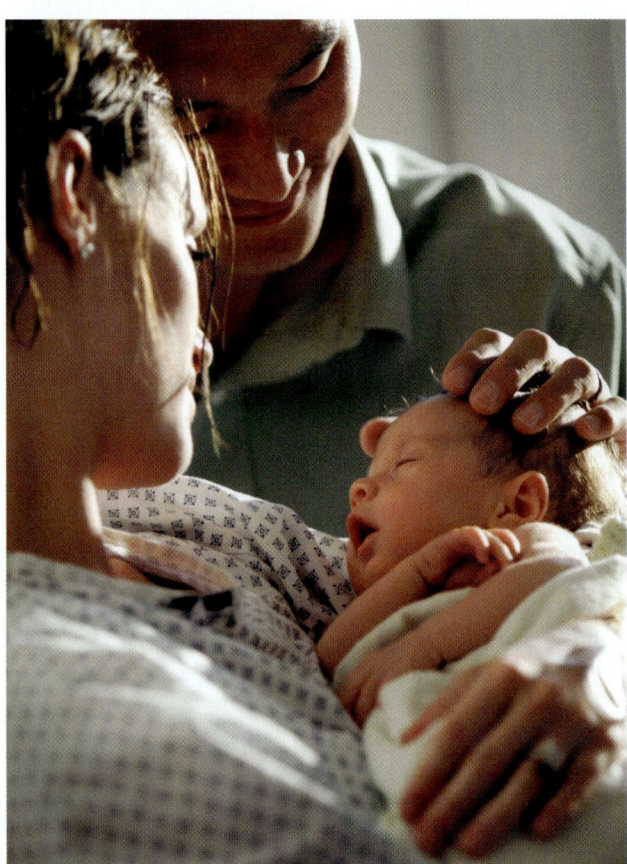

FIGURE 14-2 Newly married couples, couples who are trying to become pregnant, and new parents are vulnerable to stress as they adapt to new roles.

sleeping, toileting, and safety as well as the financial burden of quality care. In addition, the demands of work and childrearing limit the time available to nurture the couple's relationship, increasing risk for marital discord.

Injuries and illness create risks to family health. To reduce the risk for serious infectious diseases (e.g., mumps or hepatitis B), parents need to be aware of the importance of adhering to the recommended childhood immunization schedule. For families who live with a chronic illness, such as asthma or type 1 diabetes, or a developmental or learning disability, such as autism, the stress related to compromised health, educational struggles, financial burdens, and even day-to-day living can become overwhelming.

Families With Adolescents

Families with adolescents are often concerned about teen risk-taking behaviors. Adolescents may participate in risky behaviors to impress peers, to feel cool or important, or to experience a feeling of power. Developmentally, adolescents typically do not feel the threat of real danger. Some specific risk-taking behaviors include using tobacco, alcohol, and other illicit drugs; extreme stunts or dares; rebelling against authority; and sexual promiscuity.

At the same time, these families may be dealing with aging parents or grandparents (Fig. 14-3). Families may become "sandwiched" between the needs of the growing adolescents and the needs of grandparents. Women are particularly at risk for stress in these situations because they are usually the ones who provide the additional care for older relatives.

Families With Young Adults

Young adults commonly move out of the parental home as their school years end, taking on full-time jobs for the first time. This is a time when many marry and begin childbearing and rearing.

Some young adults confront such problems as tight finances, unrealistic expectations for meaningful work and

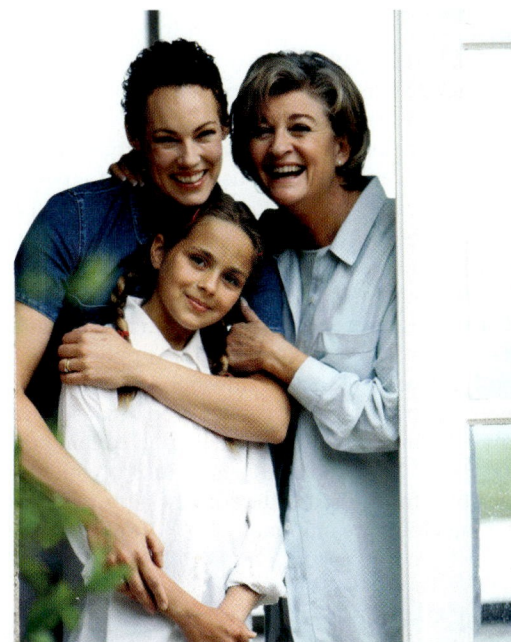

FIGURE 14-3 In families with adolescents or young adults, parents may become "sandwiched" between the needs of the growing adolescents and the needs of their own parents.

personal relationships, travel, and the responsibility for maintaining property. Financial strain might cause a young adult, alone or with newly formed family, to move back in with his parent(s) until he can become fiscally stable. This return to the nest, although sensible, can nonetheless be a stress on the family. Role strain and poor communication are common. Although young adults returning to the home of origin can represent a new opportunity for family attachment, the presence of another person in the household is certain to change family dynamics in one way or another.

At this age, not every transition is a permanent accomplishment or marker of social success. Newfound autonomy and independence are exhilarating for some and anxiety provoking for others. The boundary between adolescence and adulthood is blurred by societal forces (e.g., a contracting economy, changing labor force expectations, and expanding opportunities for women). As this continues, roles within the family will evolve and families will need to find healthy ways to adapt.

Families With Middle-Aged Adults

During the middle years many middle-aged adults examine their life goals and life accomplishments. This is a time of coping with aging and the empty nest; this can be a satisfying time of role fulfillment, career success, financial security, and social comfort. The quality of the spousal relationship might take on a new importance. The middle adult may experience a new sense of freedom and need for self-exploration and personal growth. Without the time demands of raising children, adults have more time available to pursue other personal interests or career paths.

The middle years can also be a time of self-doubt triggered by the changes of aging, menopause, empty nest, care or death of parents, or change in career life or relationships, all of which can cause emotional strain. Some people suffer a **mid-life crisis,** which is a period of intense questioning about the meaning and direction in life, asking what brings personal fulfillment. Adults battling mid-life crisis might display signs of depression, anxiety, or rebellion against the life as they've known it.

The effects of long-standing unhealthy behaviors often become apparent in middle adulthood. For example, people who have used tobacco for many years may now begin to notice an increase in cough and chest congestion; those who have consumed high-fat diets may develop high blood pressure or elevated cholesterol levels. Remember, individual health affects family health.

Families With Older Adults

Falls and trauma are a common health risk for families with older adults. For more information about this, see Chapters 10 and 23.

Older adults are at risk for social isolation and loneliness because of the loss of relationships and changing family dynamics that occur with aging. The death of a spouse, sibling, friend, or other loved one can deeply affect an elderly person's quality of life, affecting clarity of thinking and causing illness or problems with emotional well-being. At the same time, retired individuals deal with the loss of daily contact with colleagues in the workplace and, for some, a reduced sense of responsibility or purpose. Friends and family can be a significant source of support (Fig. 14-4), but functional losses may cause the person to limit physical activity, volunteer work, church attendance, and other social activities.

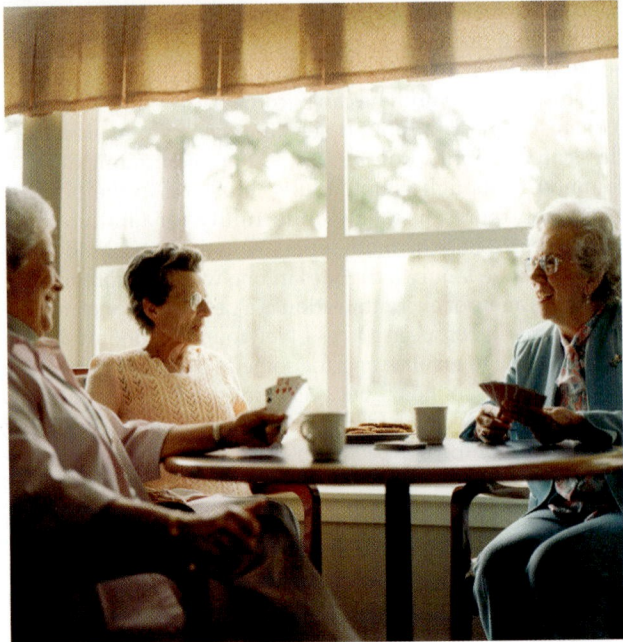

FIGURE 14-4 Friends play an important role in the support system of older people.

Maintaining good nutrition and hydration becomes more difficult as a person ages, particularly for the frail elderly. The following are situations that may compromise the nutrition of older adults:

- Forgetting to eat (especially those who live alone)
- Inadequate or unreliable transportation to shop for food
- Lack of money to buy food
- Physical changes that alter taste (e.g., reduced sensitivity in the taste buds and less saliva for taste and swallowing)
- Loss of appetite
- Poorly fitting dentures

For more information about nutrition, see Chapter 28.

Forgetfulness and confusion can pose risks to safety for older adults, particularly for those living alone or with other aging adults whose mental status is compromised. When older adults, and especially the frail elderly, lose their ability to reason, they are vulnerable to physical harm. The demands of keeping the aging adult safe can lead to caregiver role strain and family stress.

It is easy to understand from the above scenarios the cascading effect that one deficit, such as lack of transportation, can have on the health of an older adult and her family. Some families may need to know there are community resources available to provide help (e.g., Meals on Wheels, home health aides).

ThinkLike a Nurse 14-3

- What developmental stage is your family in? How do you know?
- What basic attitudes, values, or beliefs influenced you in your childhood family?
- How were decisions made in your childhood family? Were people's feelings and individuals' needs considered?
- Can you remember good times and laughter that bonded you together as a family? In your present family life, how often do you laugh together?
- In the Meet Your Patient scenario, what health risks do J. B. and Mike face, considering their age and health?

WHAT ARE SOME CHALLENGES TO FAMILY HEALTH?

We have already mentioned the effect of some demographic changes, such as an aging population, on families. This section examines other regional and national trends that present challenges to family health.

Poverty and Unemployment

When the economy takes a downturn, families may struggle to provide for basic needs (e.g., food and shelter) and healthcare. In 2005 in the United States, 46.6 million people did not have health insurance (U.S. Census Bureau, 2006). Approximately one of every seven pregnant women in the United States failed to obtain first-trimester prenatal care. Nearly half of these women gave as their reason lack of money or insurance to pay for the visits. Teenage pregnancy is yet another factor that is strongly associated with poverty and unemployment (Centers for Disease Control and Prevention [CDC], 2010).

Families in all socioeconomic levels can experience difficulties in an economic downturn, but particularly those with low reserves. In a sluggish economy, nonessential jobs may be eliminated and many sectors of business and service suffer. This means not only that family income is compromised, but also, on a more global level, that fewer workers are paying taxes and government programs supporting families in need may be underfunded. Although some people find creative solutions to family poverty (e.g., a woman who is laid off assumes child care for another family whose members remain employed), many families experience extreme hardships when the economy is suffering.

KnowledgeCheck 14-3

- Which socioeconomic group of families is hardest hit during poor economic periods?
- How are middle-income families affected by poor economic times?

Infectious Diseases

Family health may be affected by any number of new or resistant pathogens, such as severe acute respiratory syndrome (SARS), methicillin-resistant staphylococcal aureus (MRSA), West Nile virus, HIV, and H1N1 virus. The H1N1 virus that struck in 2009, also called swine flu, is a relatively new pandemic virus, causing illness in humans, especially young children, pregnant women, people 65 years and older, and those with certain chronic diseases.

In recent years, diseases once managed with immunization or antibiotics are making a comeback, such as polio, mumps, smallpox, and tuberculosis. Some infections previously believed to have been eradicated have reemerged because of failure to comply with immunization guidelines in certain populations. As a result, **herd immunity** is reduced, which is a group's protection from disease that occurs because a large proportion of the group are immune.

KnowledgeCheck 14-4

- What age and gender groups are experiencing the fastest rate of growth in new HIV cases?
- Name two previously eradicated diseases that have again become a threat.

Chronic Illness and Disability

Chronic illness and disability profoundly change the way families function. Family members' roles evolve over time, especially that of the caregiver. Many people with chronic illness and disability require assistance with ADLs, such as getting around the home, feeding, bathing, dressing, toileting, and getting in and out of a chair or bed. Many are not able to work or generate family income, often creating financial strain or poverty. Long-term illness and disability cause mental, emotional, or physical limitations that affect family communication patterns. In addition, relationships within the family may be difficult due to caregiver strain and issues related to dependency. Long-term care of a family member may increase the risk for abuse and neglect, including maltreatment of frail elderly family members.

The Americans With Disabilities Act of 1990 (ADA) defines **disability** as a substantial limitation in a major life activity. Individuals 15 years and older are determined as having a disability if they meet criteria involving mobility, self-care, physical or sensory limitations, inability to work inside or outside the home, mental or emotional condition that interferes with everyday activities, and receipt of federal benefits based on inability to work. In the United States in 2006:

- 15% of people living within the community reported one or more disabilities. Of these there were slightly more females than males.
- The prevalence of disability was lowest for people ages 16 to 20 (6.9%) and highest for those age 75 and older (52.6%).
- The poverty rate of working-age people with disabilities was 25.3%.
- Among the six types of disabilities, one-third were people with mental disability while the lowest group was those with sensory disability (23.3%) (Rehabilitation and Training Research Center on Disability Demographics Statistics, 2007).

Homelessness

Homelessness is a growing problem in many U.S. cities, not only for individuals but for also for families. Many homeless people sleep on the streets, although others live temporarily with relatives or in community shelters for the homeless. Homelessness is far more complex than lack of housing. This problem might be explained by a number of factors, such as financial crises, socially dysfunctional relationships, unemployment, lack of job skills, substance abuse, healthcare expenses, or the inability or lack of desire to live within the socially accepted norms of society. In the United States, deep poverty and homelessness often result from mental illness, disability, or misfortune.

Homeless families are often socially isolated. Seeking food and shelter requires a majority of the family's time and effort, threatening family relationships and the long-term physical and emotional health of family members. Many homeless children do not attend school, and those who do tend to perform poorly. Often, homeless families do not seek care for significant health problems, primarily because they do not know how to access the healthcare system and qualify for healthcare services.

Single women, members of minority groups, and single-parent families are particularly vulnerable to homelessness and poverty (Fig. 14-5). It is not uncommon for divorced women to end up with less income than their ex-husbands. In addition, some women also might have sole custody of their children, which creates additional expenses. In many states, social services departments are underfunded, and

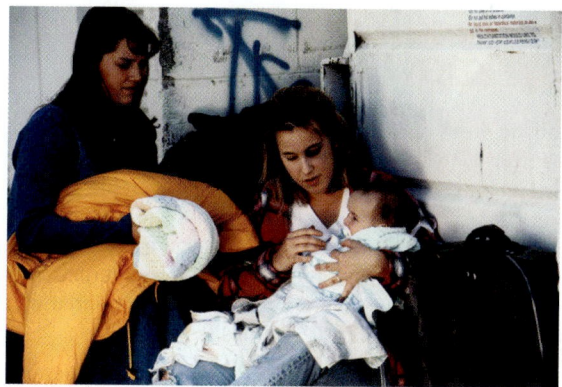

FIGURE 14-5 Many homeless people are single women and children.

they are unable to enforce the law for biological fathers struggling to pay child support while keeping up with their own living expenses.

Violence and Neglect Within Families

Domestic violence—including physical, emotional, and sexual abuse—occurs throughout all strata of our society and among all racial, social, and economic groups. As many as one in every four women will be a victim of violence during her lifetime, and more than 3 million children each year are reported to child protective services agencies as alleged abuse victims. More than 500,000 children in the United States are seriously injured each year by various forms of maltreatment. The U.S. Census Bureau (2006) reports cases of substantiated child abuse and neglect have increased 113% between 1990 and 2005. Children age 3 and younger are the most frequent victims of child fatalities. These children are the most vulnerable for many reasons, including their dependency, small size, and inability to defend themselves.

Any type of violence is likely to have long-lasting effects on the victims and on the family. It may result in the disintegration of the family relationships and structure (e.g., sending the children to foster care, escaping to a battered women's shelter, living with others). Health issues related to domestic violence include physical injury from the assault itself, as well as chronic health problems that emerge either as a complication of traumatic injury or as a physical response to the ongoing stress from violence or neglect. Families experiencing domestic violence have more unintended pregnancies, miscarriages, abortions, and low-birth-weight babies. They also have more sexually transmitted infections (STIs) and higher rates of depression, post-traumatic stress disorder (PTSD), substance abuse, and suicide. Even though the emotional and physical pain may stop when the victim leaves the family environment, often there are long-term effects involving emotional injury, marred self-esteem, or poor quality relationships. Victims of family violence learn patterns of ineffective coping that can be repeated in successive generations.

KnowledgeCheck 14-5

- Name two causes of homelessness.
- Name two groups of individuals who are vulnerable to homelessness.
- Name two types of violence.
- Describe the effects of family violence that generally endure after the physical injury has healed.

PracticalKnowledge
knowing **how**

A holistic view of family health integrates the biological, social, cultural, and spiritual aspects of life and refers to individual members as well as the whole family. Nurses play a vital role in promoting family wellness across the life span. When working with families, you will encourage them to take responsibility for their own family health. Your interactions with families can empower them to practice behaviors that will aid in healing and maintaining good health.

▌ ASSESSMENT

Health assessment for the family is similar to that for individuals. Ensuring family privacy is essential for obtaining an accurate and comprehensive family health assessment. Gather all essential assessment information for each family member. (See Chapter 21 for additional information on physical assessment.) In addition to the individual factors, assess the health of the family unit. For an example of a family assessment form used by a community health agency,

 Go to Chapter 14, **Tables, Boxes, Figures: ESG Figure 14-1,** on Davis*Plus.*

For a description of a family assessment, refer to the Focused Assessment box, Conducting a Family Assessment.

The following sections discuss in more detail the assessment of family health beliefs, communication patterns, coping processes, and caregiver role strain.

Assessing the Family's Health History

The family history can provide clues about a person's health and susceptibility for disease. Genetic linkages have been discovered for common, complex diseases, such as breast cancer, Alzheimer's' disease, diabetes, macular degeneration, seizures, inflammatory bowel disease, lupus, and heart disease, to name a few.

Genomics is the study of human genes and their function, including the interactions among other genes and the environment—it is about the interplay between a person's genetic makeup and food and environmental toxins, lifestyle, and stress. You can use genomics to personalize a patient's plan of care by doing the following:

- Identifying at-risk individuals for certain conditions to provide more effective preventative care
- More accurately detecting illness, even before symptoms appear
- Tailoring healthcare to the individual, instead of using a trial-and-error approach
- Evaluating a person's response to the care, considering multiple factors

Genomics helps us understand how people respond differently to particular drugs and medical treatments. For example, one client with a genetic predisposition for high cholesterol can benefit from a change in diet and exercise to decrease the

---

Focused Assessment

Conducting a Family Assessment

In general, a family assessment should include the following:

Identifying data	Include such information as name, address, phone number, cultural/ethnic background, religious identification, and social affiliation.
Family composition	For each member of the family, include gender, age, relationship, date and place of birth, occupation, and education.
Family history and developmental stage	This refers to the stages and developmental tasks in Table 14-1.
Environmental data	Include a description of the home, neighborhood, and larger community, as well as the family's social supports and transactions with the community.
Family structure	In addition to identifying the structural type (e.g., traditional nuclear, single-parent), assess:
	➤ Communication patterns: Functional and dysfunctional patterns; the manner in which emotions are expressed, and contextual variables that affect communication
	➤ Power and role structures (e.g., How are family decisions made? What are the roles of each member? Have there been changes in these?)
	➤ Family values (e.g., What are their values? What are their priorities? How do they compare to the values of their cultural group? Are there value conflicts in the family?)
Family functions	Assess the effectiveness of the family's:
	➤ Nurturing (e.g., Are the members close? Are they separate or connected?)
	➤ Socialization and child-rearing (e.g., Who is the socializing agent(s) for the children? What are their child-rearing practices? Are needs for play being met?)
Health beliefs, values, and behaviors	How do they define health and illness? What are their dietary, sleep, physical, and drug habits? What are their dental and medical health practices, including physicals, eye exams, immunizations, etc.? Do they have access to health services?
Family stressors and coping	What are their stressors (e.g., financial, family communication or relationships, neighbors, holidays, children's behavior)? What successful coping strategies have they used? What dysfunctional strategies?
Abuse and violence within the family	Because of the prevalence of abuse and because families are likely to be ashamed to discuss it, you should assess every family to see if any abuse or neglect is occurring. For detailed guidelines, go to Procedure 9–1, Assessing for Abuse.

likelihood that the genetic risk will be expressed. Another person may not respond to lifestyle measures and require cholesterol-reducing drugs.

When assessing the family history, you can use a pictorial tool, called a **genogram,** to display the relationship of family members with pertinent health-related information (Fig. 14-6). This type of family tree can provide a quick and useful context in which to evaluate an individual's health risks.

To construct a genogram, you will note the causes of death, genetically linked diseases, and other important health problems. Use a three-generation (or more) genogram to also show environmental (e.g., toxin) and mental health issues (e.g., depression, alcohol abuse, suicide), occupational diseases (e.g., asbestos), infections (e.g., MRSA), and obesity among family members. When developing a genogram, use symbols and abbreviations to denote family members, including a key for interpretation (Box 14-1).

Assessing the Family's Health Beliefs

Health beliefs can vary widely among families and among individuals within families. The differences can be especially great among different generations of a family (e.g., between grandparents and their grandchildren). Some common health beliefs are expressed in adages, such as "Feed a cold, starve a fever." Some families may have an intense skepticism or mistrust of medical care and hospitals and may seek treatment only when absolutely necessary (e.g., when the pain becomes unbearable). Many of these beliefs are passed on from generation to generation.

Even if one family member does not share all of the beliefs of the family, you need to be aware of the family's beliefs because they may influence the individual's decision making. To illustrate this point, consider a family caring for a frail elderly member who is confused and immobile. One family member

> ### BOX 14-1 ■ Family History by Listing Family Members
>
> The following history is for a 37-year-old female patient:
> Patient: Age 37, alive and well
> Spouse: Age 40, divorced, alcoholism
> Daughter: Age 12, alive and well
> Son: Age 8, alive and well
> Brother: Age 32, alive and well
> Sister: Age 30, alive and well
> Father: Age 66, hypertension (HTN)
> Mother: Age 60, mitral valve prolapse (MVP)
> Paternal aunt: Age 65, breast cancer
> Maternal uncle: Age 62, HTN
> Maternal uncle: Deceased age 28, tuberculosis (TB)
> Maternal aunt: Age 64, MVP
> Maternal aunt: Age 58, HTN
> Maternal aunt: Deceased age 9, ruptured appendix
> Paternal grandfather: Deceased age 68, cancer
> Paternal grandmother: Age 80, HTN
> Maternal grandmother: Age 77, HTN, breast cancer
> Maternal grandfather: Deceased age 70, cardiovascular disease (CVD)

believes quality of life issues are more important than quantity. Yet another family member who is giving care disagrees fundamentally with this belief and supports the right of the older adult to receive whatever care is needed for physical safety, emotional fulfillment, and spiritual well-being for any length of time. In this situation, the family is at risk for interpersonal conflict, impaired communication, and caregiver strain. If you would like more information on health beliefs, see Chapter 41.

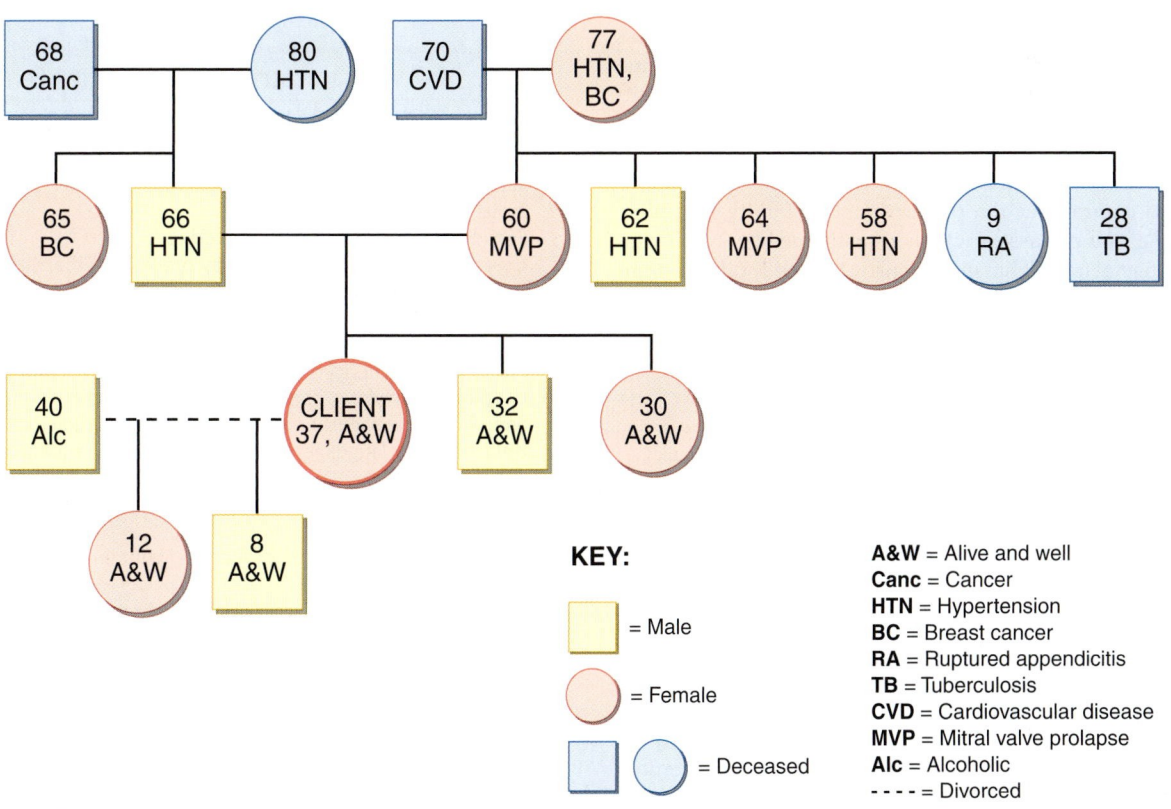

FIGURE 14-6 Family history by genogram.

ThinkLike a Nurse 14-4

- As a nurse, how can you promote overall wellness in a family with a critically ill member?
- What health beliefs would you want to ask J. B.'s (Meet Your Patient) family about?

Assessing the Family's Communication Patterns

To assess family communication patterns, you will need to interview the family and also carefully observe the interactions between family members. Try to uncover the following information:

- Who is the primary decision maker in the family?
- How are family decisions made: by one individual or by family conference?
- What is the most frequent type of communication among family members?

Do not rely solely on the information provided by the family members during the interview process. Family members who participate in dysfunctional communication patterns may not come to scheduled family meetings and may not be present during the initial interview. In addition, when relationships among family members are strained or dysfunctional, individuals may distort the information they provide about a home situation or another family member. Families usually want to "put on the best face" for healthcare providers, so they may be careful to give socially desirable responses. Carefully observe the words people use and other cues involved in communication, such as body language, direct eye contact, and other nonverbal expressions, particularly among family members.

Assessing the Family's Coping Processes

The physiological manifestations of stress (e.g., anxiety, increased pulse rate) may decrease the effectiveness of interventions and negatively affect a client's health. Family members who are not coping effectively may cause the client to become stressed or anxious or have problems sleeping. Assessing family coping is a first step to helping the family develop more effective coping patterns. Observe for physical indications of stress, anxiety, or loss of sleep in the client as well as relationships and communication patterns among family members. As a nurse, you can assess whether family members are irritable and snap at (speak harshly or curtly to) one another. For inpatients, notice who is visiting. Family members who are not coping well may avoid coming to visit the patient, so this may be an indicator of who is coping and who is not.

KnowledgeCheck 14-6

- Why is it important for you to ask about family health beliefs?
- What factors may impede a family's ability to cope with an individual's illness?

Assessing for Example Problem: Caregiver Role Strain

Conflicts between caregiving and other responsibilities can produce tremendous family stress. The physical, emotional, and time demands involved in caring for family members who are chronically ill, disabled, or frail can create difficulties among family members. Relationships can be compromised. Financial stress can also be a factor in family functioning. When these stressors add up, family caregivers might suffer from what NANDA-I terms **Caregiver Role Strain.** This is present when a person has difficulty in performing adequately in the family caregiver role.

To assess for caregiver burnout, observe for dysfunctional communication, such as abusive language and aggression. Look for physical injury to the patient, which may occur when caregivers are overwhelmed and overstressed. Conversely, you might see the caregiver withdrawing emotionally, which could result in emotional neglect and isolation. Caregivers experiencing role strain might exhibit emotional distress, including depressive symptoms and apathy.

▇ ANALYSIS/NURSING DIAGNOSIS

Recall that in the diagnostic process you must analyze the data for cues (data that deviate from norms). Therefore, you should be familiar with the characteristics of a healthy family (refer to Box 14-2) so that you can use them as your basis for comparison. For individual family members, of course, any NANDA-I diagnosis may be appropriate for describing a client's health status. Family diagnoses, however, are meant to describe the health status of the family as a whole. The following are examples:

Caregiver Role Strain (actual and risk for)
Family Coping: Compromised
Family Coping: Disabled
Dysfunctional Family Processes
Impaired Home Maintenance
Impaired Parenting (actual and risk for)
Ineffective Family Therapeutic Regimen Management
Ineffective Role Performance
Interrupted Family Processes
Readiness for Enhanced Family Coping
Readiness for Enhanced Parenting
Relocation Stress Syndrome
Risk for Impaired Attachment
Social Isolation

BOX 14-2 ▪ Characteristics of a Healthy Family

A healthy family requires more than merely the absence of family dysfunction or disease in an individual member. Characteristics of a healthy family are listed as follows:
State of family well-being
Sense of belonging and connectedness
Clear boundaries between family members where the responsibilities of adults are clear and separate from responsibilities of growing children
Sense of trust and respect
Honesty and freedom of expression, including different opinions or viewpoints
Spending time together, sharing rituals and traditions
Relaxed body language, physical touch, and frequent eye contact
Flexibility: adaptability and ability to deal with stress, openness to change
Commitment: working together to maintain the family
Spiritual well-being
Respect for privacy of individual members
Balance of giving and receiving
Positive, effective communication
Accountability, including acceptance when mistakes are made
Appreciation and affection for each other
Responding to the needs and interests of all members
Health-promoting lifestyle of individual members

PLANNING OUTCOMES AND EVALUATION

Individualized goals/outcome statements you might write for a family include the following examples, which represent some of the traits of healthy families in Box 14-2.

Affirms and supports each member.
Teaches respect for others within and outside the family.
Demonstrates a sense of humor and plays together.
Observes rituals and traditions (e.g., celebrates birthdays).
Respects the privacy of each member.
Communicates effectively and openly.

NOC outcomes specifically for families as units are found in the NOC domain Family Health, which includes the classes Family Coping, Family Health Status, Family Integrity, and Parenting Performance. Outcomes from other domains may apply as well, depending on the nursing diagnosis you have made. For a list of NOC outcomes in the Family Health domain, and for Caregiver Role Strain,

 Go to Chapter 14, **Standardized Language: NOC Family Health Outcomes, and NOC Outcomes and NIC Interventions for Caregiver Role Strain,** on DavisPlus.

Remember that the outcomes you develop for the care plan serve as the criteria for evaluating your patient's responses to nursing interventions.

PLANNING INTERVENTIONS/IMPLEMENTATION

Individualized nursing actions you might use with families include the following examples (other interventions are described in succeeding sections):

- Collaborate with family in problem-solving and decision making.
- Refer the family to support groups composed of other families dealing with similar problems.
- Monitor current family relationships.
- Assist with family with conflict resolution.
- Encourage family to maintain positive relationships.

- Establish trusting relationship with family members.
- Counsel family members on additional effective coping skills for their own use.
- Refer for family therapy, as indicated.
- Tell family members it is safe and acceptable to use typical expression of affection when in a hospital setting.

NIC interventions for families as units are found in the NIC domain Family Integrity Promotion, which includes the classes for the Childbearing Family. Interventions from other domains may apply as well, depending on the nursing diagnosis you have made. For NIC family interventions you can print out to use in the clinical setting,

 Go to Chapter 14, **Standardized Language: NIC Family Interventions,** on DavisPlus.

Promoting Family Wellness

Encouraging families to value and incorporate health promotion into their lifestyles will also affect the health of individual members. Health-promotion behaviors are typically learned within the family. You can promote family wellness by addressing both individual and family needs. It is important to identify both strengths and basic weaknesses of the family to adequately meet healthcare needs.

Involving the family in each phase of the nursing process promotes positive health outcomes and helps establish trust between the family and the nurse. Wellness interventions may include contracting, health teaching, anticipatory guidance, and promoting family cohesion during a crisis (e.g., hospitalization of a family member). For specific health promotion activities, see Chapter 27.

Interventions When a Family Member Is Ill

When a family member is ill or hospitalized, the other family members experience a range of emotions—especially when the illness is severe or of sudden onset. Family members may display signs of stress in a variety of ways, for example, by

Toward Evidence-Based Practice

Huges, M. E., Waite, L. J., LaPierre, T. A., et al. (2007). All in the family: The impact of caring for grandchildren on grandparents' health. *Journals of Gerontology Series B: Psychological Sciences and Social Sciences, 62,* S108–S119.

Researchers were interested in knowing what effects on the physical and psychological health occur among older adults when caring for grandchildren. Using a sample of 12,872 grandparents ages 50 through 80, they examined the relationship between various types of grandchild care and health of the grandparents. Researchers found no evidence to suggest that caring for grandchildren has dramatic and widespread negative effects on grandparents' health and mental well-being. In fact, the study actually revealed higher-level physical health and emotional benefits to grandmothers who babysit. However, there was a small number of grandparents whose health might have been

compromised by having children in the home, likely due to infections. The findings were different when the parents are absent or minimally involved with childrearing. When parental involvement was low, grandmothers are more likely to experience poor health behaviors, depression, and lower self-rating of overall health.

1. Based on this research, if you were the nurse, what kinds of information would you want to gather from families where grandparents provided custodial care to grandchildren?

2. What ways can you think of to support grandparents who assume major roles in raising grandchildren?

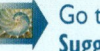 Go to Chapter 14, **Toward Evidence-Based Practice Suggested Responses,** on DavisPlus.

arguing with each other or with healthcare providers, by insisting on immediate care for their loved one, by avoiding the client's room, or by frequently asking that information be repeated. These are normal reactions; do not take them personally.

The patient and family need to understand the medical diagnosis, the plan of care, and what the recovery process will be like. In addition, it is often the nurse who provides extensive discharge instructions to the client and family before they leave the hospital. For interventions to help family members manage stress when a family member is ill, see Box 14-3.

Interventions for Example Problem: Caregiver Role Strain

Interventions specific to caregiver role strain center include the following:

Assessing the caregiver for degree of impaired functioning (e.g., difficult sleeping, weight loss)

Assessing for safety issues that exist for the care receiver

Identifying causes of caregiver strain (e.g., lack of knowledge, frail client with around-the-clock care needs, complex treatments, or conflicts between caregiver and care receiver)

Helping the caregiver to identify and express feelings, including negative ones (e.g., by use of statements such as "This must be hard for you" or "I hear you saying you feel angry and confused")

Supporting the caregiver's ability to manage the situation (e.g., by helping identify community supports, finding someone to share housekeeping activities)

Providing information about and demonstrating caregiving skills and techniques (e.g., dealing with the care receiver's pain)

For a list of NIC interventions for Caregiver Role Strain,

 Go to Chapter 14, **Standardized Language: NOC Outcomes and NIC Interventions for Caregiver Role Strain** on *DavisPlus*

BOX 14-3 ■ Interventions to Help Family Coping With Hospitalization

- Provide written materials explaining the client's diagnosis or condition.
- Actively involve the family in team meetings.
- Promptly follow up with family concerns or questions.
- Encourage the family to go home and rest.
- Encourage the family to call for updates when they cannot be present.
- Suggest ideas for stress-reducing activities (e.g., walking, meditating).
- Inform the family about on-site availability of a chaplain or chapel.
- Encourage the family to participate in care activities as appropriate.
- Keep the family informed of the client's progress.
- Help the family to identify sources of stress and develop strategies to work through and dissolve the root cause.
- Provide anticipatory guidance regarding outcome and expectations for discharge.

Interventions When There Is a Death in the Family

Death of a close family member is one of the most devastating life experiences. A family needs sensitive and compassionate care during this time, and such care is an appropriate focus for family-centered nursing. Interventions include facilitating the grieving process, encouraging communication, providing spiritual support, and providing compassionate care of the body after death. For more in-depth information about care of the family of a dying patient, see Chapter 17.

CLINICALREASONING:
Applying the Full-Spectrum Nursing Model

Because the following critical thinking activities allow you to practice the kind of thinking you will use as a full-spectrum nurse, they usually have no single right answer. Discuss them with your peers—if you have difficulty with any of the questions, consult your instructor.

PATIENT SITUATION

Sandra Jackson is the 22-year-old single mother of an 18-month-old child. Sandra has type 1 diabetes mellitus. Sugar control has been brittle at times, primarily during times of stress and illness. Sandra lives with her mother, two younger sisters, and a brother. At times her boyfriend will stay in the home, depending on the status of their relationship. Sandra works part-time at a retail chain, struggling to meet the financial responsibilities of raising a child. She is showing physical signs of depression and distress (e.g., apathy, anorexia, excessive sleeping, and episodes of crying). Sandra says to you during your home visit, "Something is really wrong with me. I can't snap out of this feeling of darkness. Life is too hard for me and is nothing but pain. I can't take it anymore and want it to be over." You believe she needs immediate mental health support.

THINKING

1. *Theoretical Knowledge:*
   a. What facts and principles do you already know about stress and depression?
   b. How does the emotional well-being of one family member affect others living in the home and the family as a whole?
2. *Critical Thinking (Inquiry):*
   a. What are some factors in Sandra's life possibly contributing to her feelings of hopelessness and thoughts of self-harm?
   b. Name at least three nursing diagnoses that would best suit Sandra's health needs.

DOING

3. *Practical Knowledge:* Based on the knowledge you have about stress and depression, how would you explain to the family about how to support Sandra?
4. *Nursing Process (Evaluation):* What measures would you define to determine whether your nursing plan of care was effective?

CARING

5. *Self-Knowledge:* How comfortable would you be in caring for a patient who is at risk for self-injury? What is one problem not described in the scenario that could possibly arise?
6. *Ethical Knowledge:* What ethical concerns might you have for a woman with a young child who is at risk for self-injury but yet has no financial resources to cover expenses of mental healthcare?

 To explore learning resources for this chapter,

 Go to DavisPlus at http://davisplus.fadavis.com/, keyword: Treas.

Chapter Resources for Chapter 14:
   Knowledge Checks and Think Like a Nurse Response Sheets
   Knowledge Check Answers
   Resources for Caregivers and Health Professionals
   Reading More About Family
   What Are the Main Points in This Chapter?
NCLEX-Style Review Questions
Podcast: Chapter Overview

Concept Map

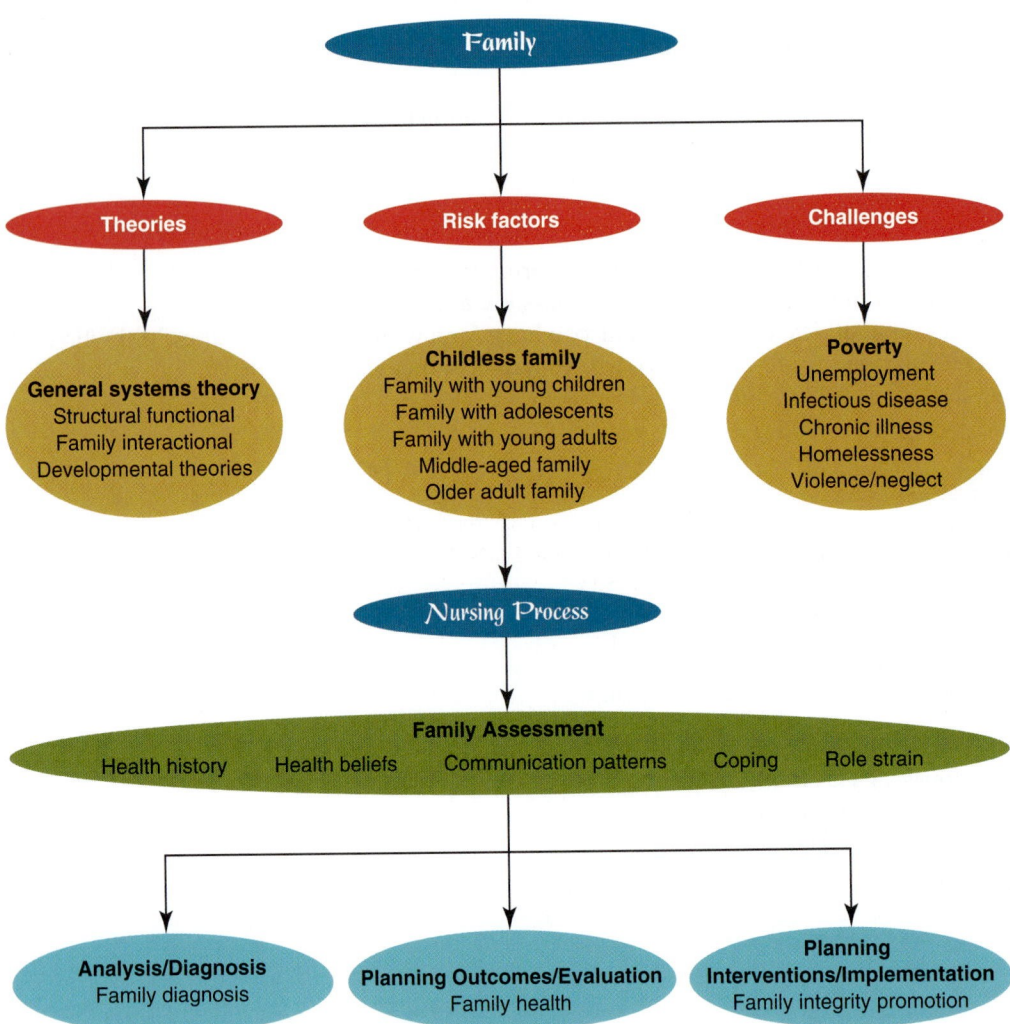

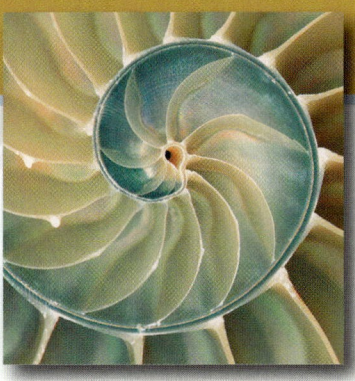

CHAPTER 15

Culture & Ethnicity

Learning Outcomes

After completing this chapter you should be able to:

➤ Explain why cultural competence is important for nurses.

➤ Explain what is meant by *culture* and *acculturation.*

➤ Discuss concepts pertaining to cultural diversity in nursing.

➤ Identify vulnerable populations in the United States.

➤ Define and give an example of *culture universals* and of *culture specifics.*

➤ Differentiate between cultural archetypes and cultural stereotypes.

➤ Describe the culture of the North American healthcare system, including professional subcultures.

➤ Identify the phenomena of culture, including how they can affect the nursing care needs of clients and families.

➤ Discuss the differing views of culturally diverse clients, including biomedical, holistic, and alternative health systems, such as folk medicine.

➤ Explain guidelines for performing a transcultural assessment, including a cultural assessment model.

➤ Recognize the cultural implications inherent in nursing diagnoses.

➤ Describe nursing strategies that promote delivery of culturally competent care to clients and their families.

Key Concepts

Culture

Cultural competence

Related Concepts

See the Concept Map at the end of this chapter.

Caring for the Nguyens

This feature allows you to practice the kind of thinking you will use as a full-spectrum nurse. There is usually more than one correct answer to a critical thinking question, so we do not provide answers for these features. It is more important to develop your nursing judgment than to "cover content." Discuss the questions with your peers. If you are still unsure, consult your instructor.

Review the initial assessment of Nam Nguyen in the front of the book.

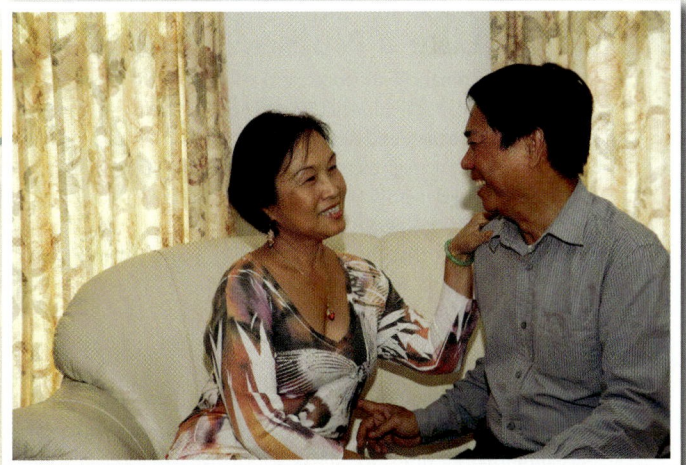

A. How might the Nguyens' cultural heritage affect their health beliefs?

B. What factors would you want to consider when performing a cultural assessment of the Nguyen family?

 Go to **Caring for the Nguyens Response Sheet** on *DavisPlus.*

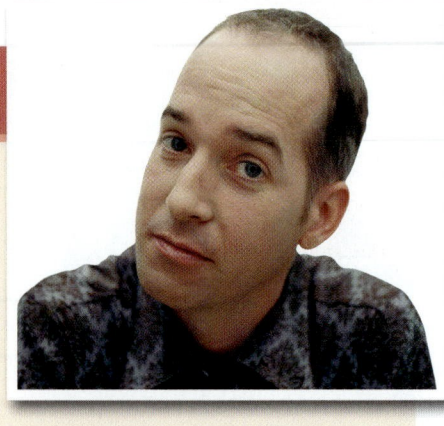

Meet Your Patients

Your clinical assignment is to spend the day in a walk-in clinic with a primary care provider. Your initial job is to greet the clients and help them complete a health history form. These are the patients you see that day:

- Romano Salvatore points to his head and moans. When you ask him what is wrong, he makes a gesture to convey to you that he does not understand what you are saying. He speaks a foreign language that sounds to you like Italian.
- Rosanna is a frantic young mother, carrying her son, José, 4 years old. José is crying and coughing. Rosanna informs you that José complains of a sore throat and has a fever. She tells you she has been to her *curandero,* but José is not getting any better. You notice that José is wearing a heavy coat and knit hat although it is quite warm outside. When you question Rosanna about the child's clothing,

she says that José is cold.
- Lee Chan, an elderly Chinese American man, is accompanied by eight family members. Because the waiting area is small, all except his daughter Kim are asked to wait outside. Mr. Chan is quiet and does not make eye contact with you. His daughter explains that her father has stomach cancer and is in a lot of pain because of disharmony. When you ask Mr. Chan to rate his pain, he just shakes his head and looks away. Would you wonder what *disharmony* means?

Theoretical Knowledge
knowing **why**

Try to answer the following questions about the patients you have just met. You may not have the theoretical knowledge to answer them all—you will acquire that in this chapter—but do your best based on the background you now have.

ThinkLike a Nurse 15-1

- Think about Romano Salvatore.
  If you could speak Italian, what would you ask him?
- Think about Rosanna and her child.
  One question that might spring immediately to your mind is, "What is a *curandero?*" How would you find out this information?
  Why do you think that the child is dressed more warmly than you would expect for the weather?
- Think about Mr. Chan and his family.
  How would you feel about so many of his family members coming with Mr. Chan to the clinic?
  Why do you think he is not looking at or speaking to you?
  How could you communicate with Mr. Chan? Would you assume that he does not speak your language? Explain your reasoning.

ABOUT THE KEY CONCEPTS

The overarching concepts for this chapter are culture and cultural competence. The concept of cultural competence will clarify why the concept of culture is important for nurses to understand. Related concepts, such as assimilation and culture universals, will broaden your understanding of the two key concepts. When you have studied the chapter, you should be able to see how all these concepts are linked to one another.

WHY LEARN ABOUT CULTURE?

The following are some reasons for nurses to learn about culture and cultural competence.

The Population Is Diverse. In your practice you will almost certainly care for patients who are not from your culture. The United States is a multicultural society—that is, made up of many cultures. For the past 20 years, we have seen increasing immigration from Asian and Spanish-speaking nations. In 2007, the U.S. Census Bureau classified 66% of the population as non-Hispanic white. However, in the United States, what were previously referred to as *minority groups* will, when taken together, soon make up a majority. The number and variety of different cultural and ethnic groups has also increased. Figure 15-1 illustrates the change in racial and ethnic makeup expected in the United States by 2050.

ThinkLike a Nurse 15-2

- With what cultural groups do you identify?
- In the neighborhood where you live, identify the cultural or ethnic groups that are different from your own. How many are there?
- In the school you are now attending, how many different cultural or ethnic groups are represented? What are they?

Health Disparities Exist Among Racial and Ethnic Groups. A *Healthy People 2020* overarching goal is to eliminate disparities among racial and ethnic groups and improve the health of all groups (*Healthy People 2020,* n.d.). One disparity is that minority groups experience higher rates of illness and death and, in general, poorer health status compared with the white, non-Hispanic population. For example, in nursing homes, use of physical restraints is higher among Hispanics and Asian/Pacific Islanders than it is among non-Hispanic whites (Agency for Healthcare Research and Quality, 2007, p. 67). If you are interested in learning more about health disparities,

**Racial and Ethnic Makeup
2008 and 2050**

		2008	2050
White (not hispanic)		66%	46%
Hispanic		15%	30%
African American		14%	15%
Asian		5%	9%
All other races		1.6%	2%

Racial and ethnic makeup, 2008

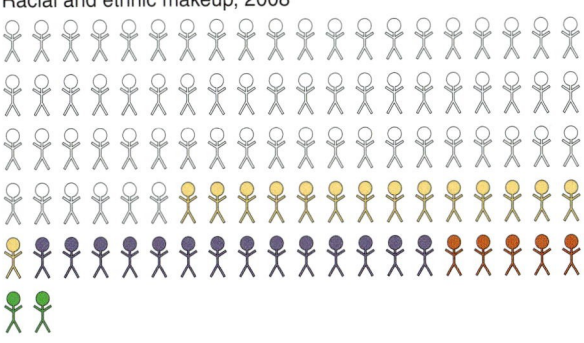

Racial and ethnic makeup, 2050

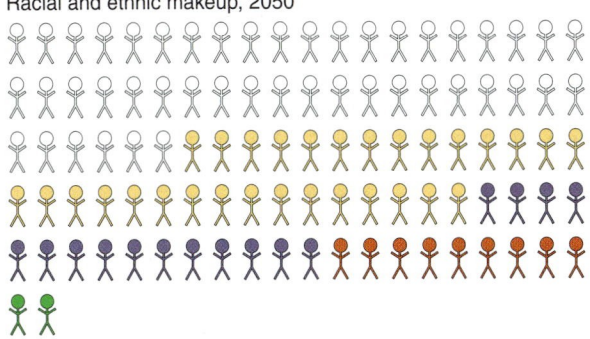

FIGURE 15-1 Racial and ethnic makeup in the United States: 2008 and 2050. (*Sources:* Adapted from Hanson, S. [2001]. *Family health care nursing: Theory, practice, and research* [2nd ed.]. Philadelphia: F. A. Davis, p. 39; U. S. Census Bureau, [n.d.b; 2004]. Retrieved from http://www.census.gov/population/international/

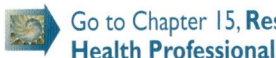 Go to Chapter 15, **Resources for Caregivers and Health Professionals,** on Davis*Plus.*

Nursing Is Challenged to Provide Culturally Competent Care. In North America the healthcare culture reflects the historically dominant, or European-American, culture. However, nurses care for patients from many races and cultures. Care that is appropriate for the dominant cultural group may be ineffective and inappropriate for people who have a different cultural heritage. Of course, it is impossible to know about every culture, but it is important to learn about the ones you will encounter most often in your practice. A good understanding of culture and ethnicity will help you in providing direct care, as well as in teaching, supervising, and modeling culturally competent care for others.

KnowledgeCheck 15-1

- What do recent demographic trends in North America indicate?
- Why should nurses know more about the culture and ethnicity of clients?

WHAT IS MEANT BY CULTURE?

To provide care in a culturally diverse population, you need to understand the concept of *culture.* We know that culture is both *universal* (everyone has it) and *dynamic* (active). Put simply, **culture** is what people in a group have in common, but it changes over time. Purnell and Paulanka (2008) define culture as "the totality of socially transmitted behavior patterns, arts, beliefs, values, customs, lifeways, and all other products of human work and thought characteristics of a population of people that guides their worldview and decision making" (p. 404). For other definitions of culture,

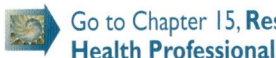 Go to Chapter 15, **Supplemental Materials: Definitions of Culture,** on Davis*Plus.*

Characteristics of Culture

When you are trying to determine what is meant by *culture* or *cultural,* keep in mind the following characteristics:

- **Cultural beliefs provide identity and a sense of belonging** for a culture's members as long as they do not conflict with the dominant culture and continue to satisfy its members.
- **Cultures consist of common beliefs and practices.** Most members of a culture share the same beliefs, traditions, customs, and practices as long as they continue to be adaptive and satisfy the members' needs. Some members of the group may deviate from cultural norms, but for a norm to be considered cultural, many members must follow it.
- **Culture exists at many levels.** Culture exists in both the material (art, writings, dress, or artifacts) and the nonmaterial (customs, traditions, language, beliefs, and practices). See Figure 15-2.

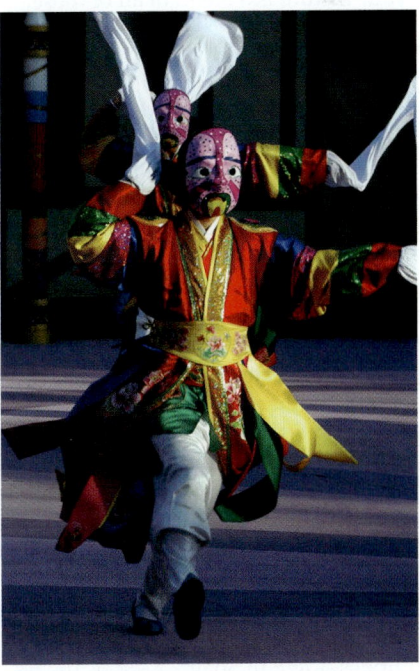

FIGURE 15-2 Traditional lunar New Year dancer in South Korea.

Other characteristics of culture are that it is:

- **Learned and taught.** Cultural values, beliefs, and traditions are passed down from generation to generation. Learning occurs through life experiences shared with other members of the culture, either formally (e.g., in schools) or informally (e.g., in families). Some generations totally adopt the values, beliefs, and traditions of their elders; others partially accept the teachings; and some generations move strongly away from them.
- **Dynamic and adaptive.** Cultural customs, beliefs, and practices change over time and at different rates. Cultural change occurs with adaptation in response to the environment.
- **Complex.** Reread the Purnell and Paulanka (2008) definition of *culture* to review the many aspects of it. Cultural assumptions and habits are unconscious and thus may be difficult for members of the culture to explain to others or to identify as different from another culture.
- **Diverse.** Culture demonstrates the variety that exists among groups and among members of a particular group.
- **All-encompassing.** Culture can influence everything its members think and do.

 Think**Like a Nurse** 15-3

Figure 15-2 depicts an example of ways in which members of particular cultural groups express their cultural uniqueness in dance. Can you think of other ways that people express their culture?

Ethnicity, Race, and Religion

People sometimes use the terms *culture, ethnicity,* and *race* interchangeably, but in fact they have separate, specific meanings. Distinctions between culture, ethnicity, race, and religion might seem confusing, but think of it this way: You are a member of the subculture of nursing, but you are also a member of an ethnic group (e.g., Portuguese Americans from the Azores), a racial group (e.g., white), and a religion (e.g., Roman Catholicism), each with its own sets of beliefs and values. So, your culture is a blend of all of those.

Ethnicity

Ethnicity is similar to *culture* in that it refers to groups whose members share a common social and cultural heritage that is passed down from generation to generation. Ethnicity is also similar to *subculture,* in that the members of an **ethnic group** have some characteristics in common (e.g., race, ancestry, physical characteristics, geographic region, lifestyle, religion) that are not shared or understood by outsiders. Examples of ethnic groups include French Canadians, Roman Catholics, Hmongs, and Latinos.

Ethnicity may include race, but it is not the same as race. To demonstrate, the U.S. Census Bureau (2010a) has numerous categories for *race* (see the next section). In addition, it identifies two categories for *ethnicity:* (1) Hispanic, Latino, or Spanish and (2) *Not* Hispanic, Latino, or Spanish.

- **Hispanic** Americans are people who originally came from any Spanish-speaking country (e.g., Mexico, Spain). More than 60% of the Hispanic population in the United States are of Mexican origin.
- **Latino,** strictly speaking, refers only to people from Central or South America.
- **Spanish** implies origin in Spain.

If you know a client's country of origin, it is more accurate to use it when referring to the client's ethnicity (e.g., Mexican American, Colombian American) than to use either of the terms *Hispanic, Latino,* or *Spanish.*

Race

Unlike ethnicity, race is strictly related to biology. **Race** refers to the grouping of people based on biological similarities, such as skin color, blood type, or bone structure (Purnell & Paulanka, 2008). The terms *race* and *ethnicity* overlap somewhat, because race can be a characteristic of a specific ethnic group. The U.S. Census Bureau now divides the population into the following lengthy list of racial categories (U.S. Census Bureau, 2010a). People of Hispanic, Latino, or Spanish origin may be of any race, because the U.S. Census Bureau does not include Hispanic/Latino/Spanish as a race, but as a sociocultural category. The census form list is as follows:

- White
- Black, African American, or Negro
- American Indian or Alaska Native
- Asian Categories
- Native Hawaiian
- Pacific Islander Categories

Remember, those are U.S. Census Bureau terms. The census questions ask people to choose the race with which they identify.

For definitions of these categories and an expanded list of the Asian, Pacific Islander, and Hispanic/Latino/Spanish categories,

 Go to the link for **ESG Fig. 15-5 2010 U.S. Census Questionnaire Reference Book,** on Davis*Plus*

Can you determine a person's race by his appearance? Frequently you cannot. So, is race determined by heredity? What race is someone whose father is black and whose mother is white? Historically, most North Americans would say that the person is black. In some other countries (e.g., most of South America), though, that same person would be categorized as white. Although we commonly think of race as being based on biological characteristics, many, including the U.S. Census Bureau, believe that race is socially rather than biologically determined. As a culturally sensitive nurse, you will ask people what race they identify with and what name they prefer to use for it. For more information on race as a social construct,

 Go to Chapter 15, **Supplemental Materials: Race as a Social Construct,** on Davis*Plus.*

Key Point: *We all tend to group and categorize data to make it meaningful and useful, but we must be careful to avoid using these categories as the basis for interacting with people or providing care.*

Religion

Religion may be confused with ethnicity because people within an ethnic group may share the same religion. For example, the Jewish culture overlaps with Jewish faith community. **Religion** refers to an ordered system of beliefs regarding the cause, nature, and purpose of the universe, especially the beliefs related to the worship of a God or gods (Andrews & Boyle, 2007). In many cultures, religion is a high priority.

Knowledge Check 15-2

- Define *culture.*
- Give an example of each: ethnic group, race, religion.
- How does culture provide identity for an individual?
- Give an example of acculturation.

Concepts Related to Culture

The term **bicultural** describes a person who identifies with two cultures and integrates some of the values and lifestyles of each into his life. The person uses more of one cultural base over another when situations call for it. Consider a Jewish man who marries an Italian Catholic woman. Their bicultural children may choose to follow Jewish tradition while still holding some of the values and beliefs of their Italian heritage. A bicultural person may experience divided loyalties.

In this chapter, **multicultural** refers to many cultures and is used to describe groups rather than individuals. Many regions of the United States are multicultural, meaning that the region is populated by individuals from many different cultural groups. The same can be said about workplace settings. Remember that culture does not always refer to the ethnicity of a group. Think of a hospital: Caregivers may be members of various ethnic, racial, and religious groups, and the nurses, physicians, physical therapists, and students each make up a different subculture. A hospital is thus a multicultural setting.

Socialization, Acculturation, and Assimilation

Socialization is the process of learning to become a member of a society or a group. A person becomes socialized by learning social rules and roles; by learning behaviors, norms, and values; and by perceptions of others in the same group or role. Families, schools, churches, peer groups, and the media are agents of socialization and foster the development of a culture and its members' identification with it.

Immigrants (new members of a group or country) assume the characteristics of the new culture through a learning process called **acculturation.** A person who is acculturated accepts both his own and the new culture, adopting elements of each. Many experts theorize that it takes several years, perhaps three generations, for an immigrant group to become acculturated.

Cultural assimilation occurs when the new members gradually learn and take on the essential values, beliefs, and behaviors of the dominant culture. Assimilation is complete when the newcomer is fully merged into the dominant cultural group. A person becomes assimilated by, for example, learning to speak the dominant language; marrying a member from the new (host) culture; and making close, personal relationships with members of the new group.

Dominant Cultures, Subcultures, and Minority Groups

What do you think is the dominant culture of the United States? If you said white or Caucasian or European American, you would be only partially correct. The ancestors of most white Americans emigrated from Europe, and many were of Protestant or other Christian religions. We can then say that the dominant culture in the United States and Canada is white Anglo-Saxon Christian of European descent. A **dominant culture** is the group that has the most authority or power to control values and reward or punish behaviors. It is usually, but not always, the largest group.

Because the white culture has been dominant in North America, most white people have been around others similar to themselves. When asked about their culture, they may even say, "I don't think I have one." They have not been aware of their culture because they did not see it in contrast to other ways of being. Or, if they did see differences, they assumed

their ways were the norm and that everyone else was culturally different.

Ethnocentrism is the tendency to think that your own group (cultural, professional, ethnic, or social) is superior to others and to view behaviors and beliefs that differ greatly from your own as somehow wrong, strange, or unenlightened. The tendency to ethnocentrism exists in all groups, not just in the dominant culture.

Subcultures are groups within a larger culture or social system that have some characteristics (e.g., values, behaviors, ancestry, ways of living) that are different from those of the dominant culture. People in subcultures have had different experiences from those in the dominant group because of status, residence, gender, sexual orientation, ethnic background, education, or other factors that unify the group (Purnell & Paulanka, 2008). You may be able to recognize subcultures by their speech patterns, dress, gestures, eating habits, lifestyles, and so on. Some examples of subcultures are street gangs, physicians, nurses, women, older adults, persons with disabilities, gays and lesbians, people of Appalachian heritage, rural Midwesterners, and people who abuse certain drugs.

Minority groups are also made up of individuals who share race, religion, or ethnic heritage; however, a minority group has fewer members than the majority group. Depending on the type of group, they may or may not share beliefs, practices, or physical characteristics. The term *minority* is sometimes used to refer to a group of people who receive different and unequal treatment from others in society. Some consider it an offensive term because it suggests inferiority and marginalization.

Vulnerable Populations as Subcultures. Vulnerable populations are groups that are more likely to develop health problems and experience poorer outcomes because of limited access to care, high-risk behaviors, and/or multiple and cumulative stressors. Examples include people who are homeless (Fig. 15-3), poor, or mentally ill; people with

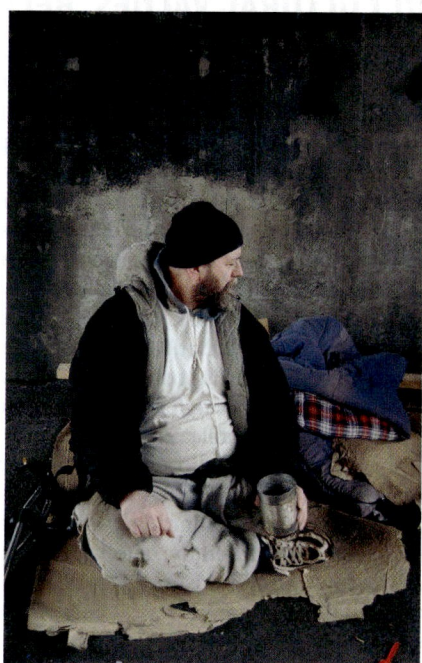

FIGURE 15-3 A homeless man sits on his cardboard, begging for spare change.

differences from those norms (e.g., African Americans metabolize antihypertensives differently from European Americans). The following are a few examples of biological variations:

- African American and Caucasian men are on average about 3.5 inches taller than Asian American men, and 2 inches taller than Mexican American men.
- African Americans have a higher incidence of hypertension and sickle cell anemia.
- Asian Americans tend to experience more gastrointestinal side effects from opiates, even though the analgesic effect is less.

For more information about biological variations and about biological susceptibility to diseases,

 Go to Chapter 15, **Tables, Boxes, Figures: ESG Box 15-1, Biological Variations** and **Supplemental Materials: Disease Risks for Each of the Major Cultural Groups of the United States**, respectively, on Davis*Plus*.

Other Culture Specifics. The following may also be culture specifics. The first two (religion/philosophy and education) vary among subcultures in the United States. The other three (technology, politics/law, and the economy) exert broader effects that can be seen among different countries, but less so among subcultures within a country.

- **Religion and Philosophy.** A person's religion may determine what healthcare is acceptable to him (e.g., blood transfusions, abortion).
- **Education.** Education influences the perception of wellness and illness, the knowledge and understanding of options that are available for healthcare, and the person's expectations for care.
- **Technology.** The availability of supplies and equipment determines what is used in the healthcare setting and what comes to be culturally expected. Nurses in most of North America, for example, assume they will have bed linens, water, electricity, necessary medications, electrocardiography, and x-ray imaging. In many parts of the world, however, these items are not available.
- **Politics and the Law.** Governmental policies affect healthcare. They determine what practitioners will be available and what programs will be funded. For example, the federal government helps fund Medicare, which provides basic medical insurance for people age 65 and older, but Medicare limits the frequency and types of treatment for which it will pay. The legal system defines roles, functions, and standards of health professionals.
- **Economy.** The condition of the economy directly affects the availability of funds for publicly funded services. It also affects the individual's ability to pay for healthcare.

For more information about each of these dimensions of culture,

 Go to Chapter 15, **Tables, Boxes, Figures: ESG Table 15-1, Culture Specifics Affecting Health**, on Davis*Plus*.

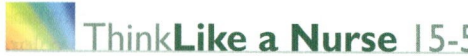 Think**Like a Nurse** 15-5

Consider this example: Mrs. Miyagi, a Japanese American, has been admitted to your care from the postanesthesia care unit (PACU), having undergone a major surgical procedure. She refuses pain medicine, although to you she appears to be in pain.

As the hours pass, Mrs. Miyagi continues to refuse the pain medication, so eventually the nurses stop asking.

- Do you assume that she is experiencing no pain?
- Are you or the other nurses stereotyping her for her cultural response to pain?
- What would you do?

Knowledge Check 15-3

- Explain the difference between an archetype and a stereotype.
- Identify at least six culture specifics affecting health.
- How could you use this information about culture specifics to provide better care to your clients?

WHAT IS THE "CULTURE OF HEALTHCARE"?

In any culture, two healthcare systems usually exist side by side: indigenous and professional (Leininger & McFarland, 2002). Each has its own culture.

The Indigenous Healthcare System

The **indigenous healthcare system** consists of *folk medicine* and *traditional healing methods,* which may also include over-the-counter (OTC) and self-treatment remedies. Different groups have different folk practices (Table 15-1), but all cultural groups probably use the professional healthcare system to at least some degree.

The Professional Healthcare System

In contrast, the **professional healthcare system** is run by professional healthcare providers who have been formally educated and trained for their appropriate roles and responsibilities. In North America, professional healthcare is dominated by the **biomedical healthcare system,** which combines Western biomedical beliefs with traditional North American values of self-reliance, individualism, and aggressive action. This system is also known as Western medicine and allopathic medicine. Table 15-2 summarizes the norms of the North American professional healthcare system.

The professional healthcare system also includes practitioners formally trained in alternative healthcare, such as diet therapy, mind–body control methods, therapeutic touch, acupressure, reflexology, naturopathy, kinesiology, and chiropractic. If you would like more information about alternative healthcare,

 Go to **Chapter 46, Holistic Healing,** on Davis*Plus*.

Sometimes conflicts arise: The professional provider may view the indigenous beliefs and practices as uncivilized and based on the supernatural, and believers in indigenous methods may view the professional healthcare culture with distrust. This type of thinking benefits no one. As a nurse, you should become aware of and understand a variety of health beliefs and practices so that you can better meet the needs of your clients.

Health Belief Systems. To provide culturally competent care, you need to know how people in various cultural groups understand life processes, how they define health and illness, and what they believe to be the causes of illness (American Nurses Association [ANA], 1991). Generally speaking, people follow one of three major health belief

Table 15-1 ➤ Folk Healers and Practices

FOLK HEALERS	FOLK PRACTICES	FOLK HEALERS	FOLK PRACTICES
White, European American		**African American**	
Nurse	Medicines (OTC and prescribed)	"Old lady" healers	Herbs
Physician	Therapeutic or modified diets	Spiritualist	Oils and poultices
Chiropractor	Exercise	*Hougan,* or voodoo priest or priestess	Talismans and amulets (worn or carried to ward off evil)
Acupuncturist	Religious healing rituals (including prayer)		Religious rituals ("laying on of hands")
Massage therapist	Sleep	**Native American, Eskimo, and Aleut**	
Physical therapist	Cleanliness	*Shaman*	Herbs, incantations, and prayers
Occupational therapist	Amulets	Crystal gazer	Rituals and healing ceremonies
Respiratory therapist	Herbal therapy	Hand trembler	Blessed medicine bundles or other dried plants or flowers, or burning of dried plants
	Naturopathy	Medicine woman or man	
	Massage		Stargazing and sand painting
	Spinal adjustment		
	Aromatherapy		
Hispanic		**Asian and Pacific Islander**	
Curandero/curandera	"Hot" and "cold" therapies	Herbalist	"Hot" and "cold" foods
Espiritualista (spiritualist)	Medals and amulets	Acupuncturist	Herbs
Partera	Prayers	Physician	Meditation
Yerbero (herbalist)	Herbs and herbal teas	Priest	Acupuncture (inserting needles into meridians or life energy pathways)
Sabador	Massage		Acupressure
	Jewelry to ward off the "Evil Eye"		Energy (Qi) to restore yin, yang balance

Sources: Adapted from Andrews, M. M., & Boyle, J. S. (2007). *Transcultural concepts in nursing care* (5th ed.). Philadelphia: Lippincott Williams & Wilkins; Giger, J., & Davidhizar, R. (2008). *Transcultural nursing: Assessment and intervention* (5th ed.). St. Louis, MO: C.V. Mosby; Purnell, L., & Paulanka, B. (2008). *Transcultural healthcare: A culturally competent approach* (3rd ed.). Philadelphia: F.A. Davis; and Spector, R. (2004). *Cultural diversity in health and illness* (6th ed.). Upper Saddle River, NJ: Prentice-Hall.

OTC = over the counter.

systems: scientific, magico-religious, or holistic (Andrews & Boyle, 2007). You are already familiar with the **scientific** or **biomedical health system.** Belief in supernatural (mystical) forces dominates the **magico-religious system,** which is considered "alternative" or "indigenous" in the United States. One example is voodoo, which is practiced in some developing nations in Africa, Latin America, and the Caribbean, and which considers the lion a spiritual symbol (Fig. 15-5). The **holistic belief system** can be similar to magico-religious, but it focuses more on the need for harmony and balance of the body with nature.

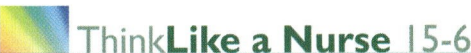

ThinkLike a Nurse 15-6

- What do you do to keep yourself healthy?
- What do you do to treat minor illnesses when you do not want to see a healthcare provider?

What Are Health and Illness Practices? In addition to knowing the values and beliefs of different cultures, you need to know what people in various cultural groups do themselves to maintain wellness. Think about Mr. Chan (Meet Your Patients). If he or his daughter asked for a Buddhist priest to come to his room and perform a ceremony to restore his harmony, do you

Table 15-2 ⮞ Summary of Cultural Norms of the North American Healthcare System	
NORM	**EXAMPLES**
Beliefs and Values	Standardized definitions of *health* and *illness*
	Significance of technology
	Reliance on the biomedical system
	Desire to conquer disease
	Defines *health* as absence or minimization of disease
Practices	Maintaining health and preventing disease through practices such as immunizations and avoidance of stress
	Annual physical examinations and diagnostic tests
Habits	Hand washing
	Use of jargon (e.g., "take your vitals")
	Use of problem-solving methods
Likes	Punctuality
	Neatness and organization
	Compliance (e.g., with medical "orders")
	Documentation
Dislikes	Tardiness
	Disorganization
	Messiness, lack of cleanliness
Customs	Use of procedures (e.g., circumcision, last rites) surrounding birth and death
	Professional respect and observance of hierarchy found in autocratic and bureaucratic systems
	Adherence to a set of ethical standards and codes of conduct
Rituals	Annual physical examination
	The surgical procedure

Sources: Adapted from Giger, J., & Davidhizar, R. (2008). *Transcultural nursing: Assessment and intervention* (5th ed.). St. Louis, MO: C.V. Mosby; Leppa, C. (2000). Transcultural communication within the health care subculture. In J. Luckmann (ed.), *Transcultural communication in health care.* Clifton Park, NY: Thomson Delmar Learning, pp. 74–83; Munoz, C. & Luckmann, J. (2004). *Transcultural communication in healthcare.* Clifton Park, NY: Thomson Delmar; Purnell, L., & Paulanka, B. (2007). *Transcultural healthcare: A culturally competent approach* (3rd ed.). Philadelphia: F.A. Davis; and Spector, R. (2004). *Cultural diversity in health and illness* (6th ed.). Upper Saddle River, NJ: Prentice-Hall.

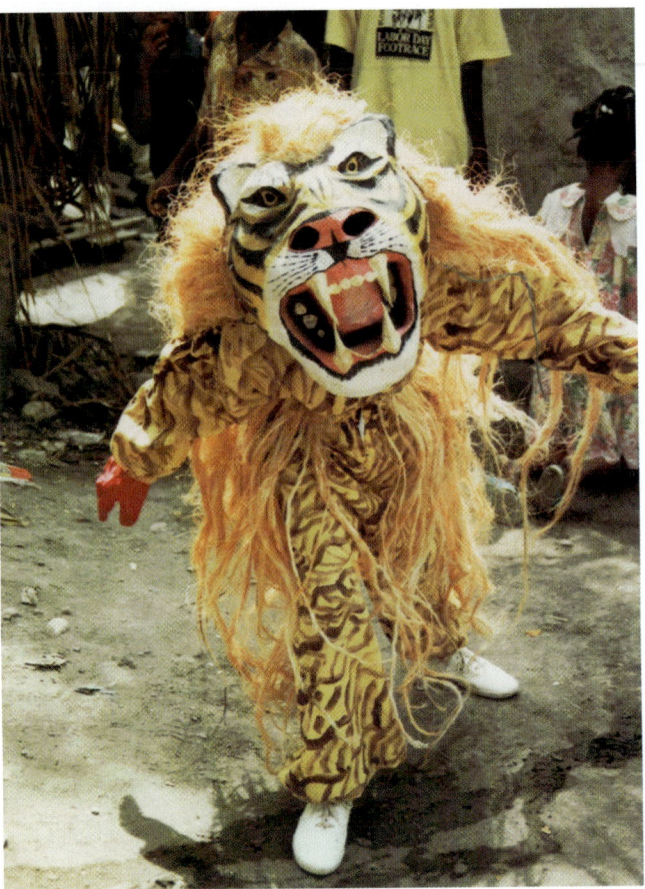

FIGURE 15-5 Voodoo is an example of a magico-religious belief system. Here, a Haitian man is costumed for carnival as the spirit of the lion.

KnowledgeCheck 15-4

- List three types of alternative healthcare that are delivered by formally trained practitioners as a part of the professional healthcare system.
- What are magico-religious belief systems?
- As a nurse, in which of the following cultural health practices would you support your client: efficacious, neutral, dysfunctional, uncertain? Why?
- Refer to the Meet Your Patients feature. Identify an efficacious practice.

ThinkLike a Nurse 15-7

- What aspects of the indigenous and professional systems have you used for yourself or your family? Give examples.

Nursing and Other Professional Subcultures

Members of the biomedical healthcare system in the United States belong to a culture with its own set of norms. That culture can be further divided into subcultures, such as those of physicians, nurses, or respiratory therapists. Nursing is the largest subculture within the healthcare culture. Leininger (1978) defines the **culture of nursing** as the learned and transmitted lifeways, values, symbols, patterns, and normative practices of members of the nursing profession that are not the same as those of the mainstream culture. The nursing subculture's beliefs and values have been formed in part by the society at large, which historically has been dominated by

think this ceremony would be harmful or helpful to him? Would you support or discourage this? As you think about those questions, keep in mind that cultural health practices can be helpful, harmful, or neutral—and sometimes you will be uncertain as to which. We discuss this in more detail in the section, How Should I Respond to a Client's Cultural Health Practices?

white Anglo-Saxon Protestants. Nursing values include, in addition to those listed in Table 15-2, the following:

- Silent suffering as a response to pain
- Objective reporting and description of pain, but not an emotional response
- Use of the nursing process
- Nursing autonomy
- Caring

In this book, we add *knowledge* and *critical thinking* to the list of nursing values. Although these values may not be consistently rewarded in practice, we believe that a steadily increasing number of nurses realize their importance—that nursing is "knowledge work" and that the nurse's knowledge and thinking are of paramount importance to the well-being of patients.

As you become more socialized into the nursing culture, you should continue to examine professional values to see how strongly you identify with them and how they affect your work with patients. You must be careful not to lose the ability to understand health and illness from the patient's point of view. Review the case of Rosanna and José (Meet Your Patients). After a positive strep test, the primary care provider prescribes an antibiotic for José's fever and sore throat. You observe that Rosanna does not seem to be happy with the medicine, so you stress to her the importance of buying the medicine right away to make him better. On her way out of the clinic, Rosanna throws the prescription in the trash. Why do you think she threw away the prescription? If you have difficulty thinking of possible answers to the question, see Table 15-3.

Some people of Mexican heritage believe that illness is caused by the body's imbalance of "hot" and "cold" (not related to temperature). The scenario doesn't tell you for sure, but it could be that Rosanna did not believe that the medication would help her son, so she decided not to spend money on it. This problem might have been prevented if you or the primary care provider had assessed Rosanna's health beliefs and practices and involved her in José's care by discussing treatment options with her. For example, if she considered his ear infection to be "hot," then the provider might have been able to explain that the prescribed medication would get rid of the heat and pain that José is experiencing—or perhaps find another medication that Rosanna would consider to be "cold."

This is an example of what can happen when healthcare providers are so rigidly grounded in the beliefs of the professional healthcare culture that they fail to recognize and understand the health beliefs and practices of their clients. As you may guess, this way of practicing is a barrier to culturally competent care.

Knowledge Check 15-5

How do the cultural norms of the North American healthcare system differ from those of other cultural groups? Refer to Tables 15-2 and 15-3 in this chapter as needed.

Traditional and Alternative Healing

You need to know how healers from various cultures cure and care for members of their group (ANA, 1997). All cultures think of their healthcare system and beliefs as "traditional"; however, we use *traditional* in this chapter to refer to alternative beliefs, those that are not of the Western, North American, biomedical, or professional healthcare systems (previously discussed). You have already learned about different *healthcare beliefs and practices* that clients may have (e.g., biomedical or scientific, holistic, magico-religious). The following section focuses on the types of *healing systems* that are used in different cultures.

Folk Medicine

When you feel as if you're getting a cold or the flu, what do you do? If you said that you take aspirin or vitamin C or eat chicken soup, then you are practicing folk medicine. You most likely do what your mother or some other relative did for you in similar situations. In North America there is a pill for almost everything; virtually everyone self-medicates with over-the-counter medicines (e.g., creams, salves, liquids). For many cultures, folk medicine involves natural medicines, such as herbs, plants, minerals, and animal substances. Magico-religious folk medicine involves the use of charms, holy words, rituals, and holy actions for preventing and treating illnesses (Spector, 2004).

Folk medicine is defined as the beliefs and practices that the members of a cultural group follow when they are ill, as opposed to more conventional (i.e., biomedical or professional) standards (Andrews & Boyle, 2007). All cultures throughout the world use folk medicine. Knowledge of these treatments is passed down from generation to generation by oral, and sometimes written, tradition. Folk medicine includes both self-treatment and use of folk healers.

Why would someone want to see a folk healer rather than a professional healthcare provider? In the dominant North American culture, the folk healer *is* the professional healthcare provider (i.e., the nurse practitioner, physician, certified nurse midwife, and so on). People of other cultures may seek out folk healers because they speak their native language, share their values and beliefs, charge less money, are readily available, or visit the sick at home. If people perceive that the professional healing system cannot meet their needs, they are likely to seek care from the folk healers within their cultures and avoid the professional system. Table 15-1 identifies folk healers of various cultures and their practices.

Complementary and Alternative Medicine

Complementary medicine is the use of rigorously tested therapies *to complement* those of conventional medicine (Andrews & Boyle, 2007). Examples include chiropractic care, biofeedback, and the use of certain supplements. In contrast, **alternative medicine** is defined as therapies used *instead of* conventional (i.e., biomedical) medicine, and whose reliability has not been validated through clinical testing in the United States. Examples of alternative therapies include iridology, aromatherapy, and magnet therapy.

Some complementary and alternative modalities (CAMs) are derived from the ancient and indigenous healthcare systems of people of other countries, such as traditional Chinese medicine (TCM), and **ayurveda,** the traditional healthcare system of India. Certain CAMs require a healer specially trained in their use (e.g., chiropractic, reflexology, massage therapy). If you would like to read a more thorough discussion of CAMs,

 Go to **Chapter 46, Holistic Healing,** on Davis*Plus*.

Knowledge Check 15-6

- What is folk medicine?
- What are some common folk medicine practices?
- Why might members of some cultural groups seek out the local folk healer rather than the conventional healthcare provider?

WHAT IS CULTURALLY COMPETENT CARE?

The terms *cultural awareness, cultural sensitivity,* and *cultural competence* are often used interchangeably; however, they are not the same. **Cultural awareness** refers to an appreciation of the

Table 15-3 ➤ Values and Health and Illness Beliefs and Practices for Selected Ethnocultural Groups in North America

GROUP	DOMINANT VALUES	HEALTH AND ILLNESS BELIEFS	HEALTH AND ILLNESS PRACTICES
Native American	Bonding to family or group Acceptance of nature (Mother Earth) Tradition Sharing Belief in a spiritual power Respect of elders	Health means living in harmony with nature. Surviving under difficult circumstances Body treated with respect Illness is associated with disharmony or evil spirits. Illness is caused by an action that should not have been performed.	Rituals and ceremonies Chanting Purification Meditation Herbs
Asian and Pacific Islander	Extended family Respect for elders Group orientation Subordination to authority Conformity Self-respect and self-control Love of the land	Health is a state of physical and spiritual harmony. Illness is disharmony of basic principles: *yin* and *yang*.	Acupuncture Amulets Moxibustion Meditation Herbs
Black or African American	Family bonding Group identification Matrifocal Spiritual orientation Present-oriented	Health is harmony with nature (mind, body, and spirit). Illness is due to disharmony or failure to eat proper foods.	Prayer Laying on of hands Magic rituals Voodoo Herbs
Hispanic or Latino	Extended family Group emphasis Fatalistic Faith and spirituality	Health is good luck or a reward for good behavior, a gift from God. Illness is body imbalance (hot or cold, wet or dry) or punishment.	Prayer Belief in miracles Wearing of religious metals or amulets Religious relics in home Herbs and spices Rituals "Hot" and "cold" therapy
White or European American	Independence Individuality Wealth Comfort Cleanliness Achievement Youth and beauty	Health is a state of physical and emotional well-being. Illness is contagion or contamination that is hereditary, psychosomatic, or supernatural	Biomedical care Home remedies Religious traditions Diet and exercise

Sources: Adapted from Giger, J., & Davidhizar, R. (2008). *Transcultural nursing: Assessment and intervention* (5th ed.). St. Louis, MO: C.V. Mosby; Munoz, C., & Luckmann, J. (2004). *Transcultural communication in healthcare.* Clifton Park, NY: Thomson Delmar; Spector, R. (2004). *Cultural diversity in health and illness* (6th ed.). Upper Saddle River, NJ: Prentice-Hall; Andrews, M., & Boyle, J. (1999). *Transcultural concepts in nursing care* (3rd ed.). Philadelphia: Lippincott; and Purnell, L., & Paulanka, B. (2008). *Transcultural healthcare: A culturally competent approach* (3rd ed.). Philadelphia: F.A. Davis.

Note: Most people in North America use a combination of biomedical and traditional (specific to their culture) healthcare practices.

external signs of diversity, whereas **cultural sensitivity** has more to do with personal attitudes and being careful not to say or do something that might be offensive to someone from a different culture. **Cultural competence** is achieved on a continuum ranging from incompetent to competent (Purnell & Paulanka, 2008, p. 6). It is a developmental process. As you become more aware of and sensitive to the needs of individuals from various ethnocultural groups, you will move forward on the journey toward cultural competence: being able to use knowledge and sensitivity in practice. The following are some ideas from nursing organizations and theorists about cultural competence.

American Nurses Association

The American Nurses Association's (ANA) *Nursing: Scope and Standards of Practice* (2010) states that the registered nurse should provide holistic care that addresses the needs of diverse populations. This includes providing cultural assessments and formulating individualized and culturally appropriated expected outcomes and nursing interventions.

Quality and Safety Education for Nurses (QSEN)

Several of the QSEN competencies also speak to culturally competent care. For example, the patient-centered care competency says the graduate nurse should be prepared to (1) provide patient-centered care with sensitivity and respect for the diversity of human experience; (2) seek learning opportunities with patients who represent all aspects of human diversity; and (3) recognize personally held attitudes about working with patients from different ethnic, cultural, and social backgrounds (Cronenwett, Sherwood, Barnsteiner, et al., 2007).

Campinha-Bacote

The culturally competent model of care views cultural competence as a process, not an end point. The nurse must see himself as *becoming* culturally competent, rather than *being* culturally competent. The model identifies five components of cultural competence, using the mnemonic ASKED (Campinha-Bacote, 2003):

- *Awareness* is similar to cultural sensitivity in other models. Take an honest look at your personal biases and prejudices toward cultural groups other than your own.
- *Skills* refers to your ability to conduct with sensitivity a cultural assessment and a culturally based physical assessment.
- *Knowledge* pertains to the information that you have about cultural worldviews and theories. You need to know what the patient's view of the world is in order to understand it and work competently with the patient.
- *Encounters* means that it takes practice to become culturally competent. You need as many face-to-face encounters as possible with patients from diverse cultural backgrounds.
- *Desire* suggests that you must *want* to be culturally competent. If there is no genuine desire, you will not be likely to seek out cultural encounters, or work to obtain cultural knowledge and skills.

Purnell and Paulanka

The Purnell model for cultural competence stresses teamwork in providing culturally sensitive and competent care (Purnell, 2000, 2002; Purnell & Paulanka, 2008). In the context of nursing, Purnell's model (Purnell & Paulanka, 2008, p. 404) defines **cultural competence** as "having the knowledge, abilities, and skills to deliver care congruent with the client's cultural beliefs

and practices." The model identifies the following levels of cultural competence. Think about the meaning of the level names.

Unconsciously incompetent
Consciously incompetent
Consciously competent
Unconsciously competent

Increasing one's consciousness of cultural diversity improves the possibilities for healthcare practitioners to provide culturally competent care. If you would like to see the Purnell model for cultural competence,

 Go to Chapter 15, **ESG Figure 15-1,** on Davis*Plus.*

Leininger

Although Madeline Leininger does not use the term *cultural competence,* her theory fits with that concept (Leininger, 2007; Leininger & McFarland, 2006). The goal of her theory is to guide research that will assist nurses to provide *culturally congruent care* using her three modes of nursing care actions and decisions (to be explained later in the chapter). Nurses can achieve this goal by:

- Discovering cultural care and caring beliefs, values, and practices
- Analyzing the similarities and differences of these beliefs among the different cultures

For more information on Leininger's theory of culture care diversity and universality,

 Go to Chapter 15, **Supplemental Materials: Leininger's Theory,** and **Tables, Boxes, Figures: ESG Figure 15-2,** on Davis*Plus.*

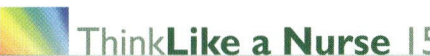 Think**Like a Nurse** 15-8

What kind of knowledge do you need to become culturally competent (theoretical, practical, self, ethical)? Explain your answer. See Chapter 2 to review types of knowledge, if necessary.

WHAT ARE SOME BARRIERS TO CULTURALLY COMPETENT CARE?

Your ability to provide culturally competent care may be hampered by various beliefs, attitudes, and language barriers. People have a tendency to be biased toward their own culture (ethnocentrism), believing that their own beliefs and values are right and that those of other cultures are wrong (or at least bizarre). If you take this attitude, your patient may feel that you disapprove of him or, at the least, you don't understand or respect him. **Bias** is one-sidedness: a tendency to "lean" a certain way, a lack of impartiality. A **cultural stereotype** is the unsubstantiated belief that all people of a certain racial or ethnic group are alike in certain respects. A stereotype may be positive or negative. **Prejudice** refers to negative attitudes toward other people based on faulty and rigid stereotypes about race, gender, sexual orientation, and so on.

Whereas prejudice refers to people's attitudes, the term **discrimination** refers to the behavior manifestations of that prejudice. For example, before the 1960s many U.S. hospitals refused treatment to African Americans. Slightly more subtle discrimination against minority groups still exists in housing, banking, and the job market.

Racism

Racism is a form of prejudice and discrimination based on the belief that (1) race is the principal determining factor of human traits and capabilities, and (2) that racial differences produce an inherent superiority (or inferiority). The word *race*

evokes powerful emotional responses for people who feel that they or their ancestors have been oppressed or exploited, and equally for those who deny such a responsibility. In the United States, the history of discrimination against non-whites has created a focus on differences and racial divisiveness. As a nurse, you must recognize that unconscious racism can play a major role in your ability to communicate with people of other races.

Sexism

Sexism is the assumption that members of one sex are superior to those of the other sex. For example, women have been viewed as more emotional and less rational than men; and assertiveness, considered a positive trait in men, may be seen as pushiness or aggressiveness in women. Men, too, experience sexism. Male nurses must combat the kind of sexism that asserts that it is unnatural for men to engage in caring behaviors. Some female nurses may not accept their male colleagues, and some patients—both male and female—may object to their care, at least initially.

Male chauvinism (assumption of male superiority) is common in many cultures and in healthcare settings. It may be overt or subtle. In the wider society, for example, men may receive higher pay for performing the same work as a woman. When you have the opportunity to do so, observe a conversation between a male nurse and a male physician. You may note that commonly the male nurse communicates more directly and uses more eye contact than female nurses do with this same physician. We are not assuming that all physicians (or nurses) are chauvinistic; we are simply stating that you will probably be able to observe this kind of interchange among some professionals. In all settings, the assumption of equality, by either party, changes the way people communicate.

Language Barriers

According to the U.S. Census Bureau, nearly 47 million U.S. residents (about 1 in 5) speak a language other than English at home. In some areas, 90 percent of the people who live there do not speak English at home. Many others speak English poorly (About.com., 2012; StateMaster.com, 2003-2012a,b). A language barrier will obviously affect your ability to communicate with clients. Language barriers can involve foreign languages, dialects, regionalisms (words or pronunciation particular to a specific region), street talk, and jargon.

Street Talk, Slang, and Jargon. These can be as challenging as a foreign language. Their meaning changes, and not everyone has the same interpretations. For example, the word *bad* can mean "bad" or "good." Ebonics (also called African American Vernacular English, or AAVE) is a type of English that has, in the past, been spoken primarily by African Americans, but many youth of other races, enamored of hip-hop culture, now embrace Ebonics as a way to connect with the street culture. Likewise, not everyone understands the abbreviations used in texting.

Healthcare Jargon. Words or expressions used by a subculture, including medicine, are called **jargon.** In healthcare, we use our peculiar terminology and abbreviations so often that we may forget that our clients do not understand them. For example, you may frighten some patients if you say to them, "I'm going to take your vitals" before assessing their blood pressure. Many patients will not know what you mean if you ask, "Have you voided today?" Even worse, patients may hesitate to ask for clarification because they don't like admitting that they don't understand a certain word.

Other Barriers

Lack of knowledge about the cultural and ethnic values, beliefs, and behaviors of people within their community is not unusual among healthcare providers. It can cause them to misinterpret a client's behaviors. *Emotional responses,* such as fear and distrust (both yours and the client's), can arise when members of different cultural groups meet. If you are aware that this may happen, you may be able to avoid this barrier and communicate with your clients effectively. Self-knowledge is essential in removing barriers.

KnowledgeCheck 15-7

- Define *cultural competence.*
- How do the barriers of ethnocentricism and language impede nursing care of diverse populations?

PracticalKnowledge
knowing **how**

Each phase of the nursing process presents an opportunity to provide culturally sensitive, congruent, and competent care.

■ ASSESSMENT

Various regulating bodies (e.g., The Joint Commission and the Office of Minority Health) require healthcare organizations to integrate cultural data into a patient's health records. Cultural assessment consists of an interview and a physical assessment. When you perform a cultural assessment, you should gather data directly from your client, but if this is not possible you may ask for help from a friend or family member of the client. When you need to use an interpreter, even if it must be a family member, be aware of confidentiality (private information) issues.

The Health History

Regardless of the patient's cultural group, it is important for you to establish rapport before beginning data collection—especially for sensitive or personal information. To encourage clients to talk about themselves, you must convey empathy, show respect, establish trust, listen actively, and provide appropriate feedback (Munoz & Luckmann, 2004). Ask open-ended questions when beginning a cultural assessment.

✚ Always ask clients about their use of alternative medicine and folk remedies so that their effects on traditional biomedical medications and treatments can be evaluated. Some remedies may interfere with traditional treatments; others can be dangerous. Many people use folk remedies, but they may be reluctant to tell you so because they fear ridicule or at least disapproval.

You will not need to perform an in-depth cultural assessment on every client, but you will need to recognize situations in which this is needed. The Focused Assessment box Obtaining Minimum Cultural Information provides a list of questions to help you obtain the minimum information recommended by Lipson and Meleis (1985).

Physical Assessment

Physical assessment may reveal biocultural variations. To assess and evaluate clients accurately, you need to know the normal physiological variations among healthy members of

Toward Evidence-Based Practice

Hagman, L. W. (2004). New Mexico nurses' cultural self-efficacy: A pilot study. *Journal of Cultural Diversity, 11*(4), 146–149.

This study administered a written questionnaire to 15 registered nurses caring for multiethnic patients in New Mexico. They found that the nurses were moderately confident with their cultural knowledge and skills. Because of the small sample, no conclusions could be drawn from the study. Researchers recommended larger, more rigorous studies.

Jackson, A. K. (2007). Cultural competence in health visiting practice: A baseline survey. *Community Practitioner, 80*(2), 17–22.

The researcher administered a survey to explore the beliefs, knowledge, and practice in cultural competence of health visitors working in a county in England. Half the respondents were members of a minority ethnic community, most of Caribbean origin. Results showed a significant difference in respondents' abilities to meet the needs of minority ethnic communities as opposed to those of the white population. They identified language and culture, but not racism, as barriers to culturally competent care. The study concluded that there is a need for cultural competence training.

Broome, B. (2006). Culture 101. *Urologic Nursing, 26*(6), 486–489.

This author states that America is a mix of cultures, ethnic groups, and races; therefore, healthcare providers need to

become more culturally sensitive and competent. She states further that one of the many challenges confronting urologic nurses is learning how culture can influence a patient's response to health and illness.

Suppose you are a nurse on a urology unit that serves mainly European Americans, Mexican Americans, and patients of Caribbean origin. You are trying to answer this question: Would knowledge of patients' cultural values and practices enable nurses on our unit to provide care that better meets the needs of our patients, for example, by improving their compliance with treatment regimens? You are looking for the best available research evidence to support your practice. Answer the following questions:

1. Thinking of the PICO question format (refer to Chapter 8 if you need to review), who in your question would be represented by P?

2. Again using PICO, what is represented by I?

3. There is no C in the question. What is represented by O?

4. Which of the three articles cited provides the best evidence to help answer your question?

 Go to Chapter 15, **Toward Evidence-Based Practice: Suggested Responses,** on Davis*Plus*.

---

selected populations—for example, body proportions, vital signs, general appearance, skin, musculoskeletal system, illness, and laboratory values.

Assessing the Skin. You will need to know about biocultural variations in skin because of the importance of assessing for pallor, cyanosis, jaundice, erythema, rashes, and petechiae, which may be more difficult to evaluate in dark-skinned persons. Darker skin challenges you to be more observant when assessing skin color changes. The following are some helpful suggestions:

- Obtain a baseline skin color by asking a family member or someone who knows the patient well.
- To assess for oxygenation and cyanosis in dark-skinned patients, examine the sclera, buccal mucosa, tongue, lips, nailbeds, palms of the hands, and soles of the feet.
- To assess for jaundice in Asians, examine the sclera.
  For more information about assessing the skin, see Chapter 21.

Assessing for Pain. Culture influences the patient's responses to pain. Because pain and comfort are subjective, you need to quantify them as objectively as possible by using a pain measurement scale. Regardless of the literature descriptions of cultural responses, it is essential to investigate the meaning of pain to each individual and what each views as acceptable ways to express or cope with pain. The following are some common cultural responses to pain:

- May tolerate a great deal of pain—African American, Filipino heritage

- Stoic acceptance; may not complain of pain or ask for interventions—Filipino, Irish, Japanese, Navajo heritage
- Express pain openly, verbally—Arabs (with family members; less so with health professionals), Italian, Jewish, Puerto Rican heritage

If you need a more comprehensive description of cultural responses to pain,

 Go to Chapter 15, **Tables, Boxes, Figures: ESG Box 15-2, Assessing Pain Perception in Selected Cultural Groups,** on Davis*Plus*.

Cultural Assessment Models and Tools

Some agencies have special tools for in-depth cultural assessments. If yours does not, you can structure your assessments using any culture model, such as the following examples:

- Purnell Model for Cultural Competence (2002)
- Andrews and Boyle Transcultural Nursing Assessment Guide (2007)
- Spector's Heritage Assessment Model (2004). Instead of assessing culture specifics, this tool assesses heritage consistency: the degree to which a person's lifestyle reflects his traditional culture (country of origin, race, or ethnic group). This assessment tool also reveals the degree to which the client still identifies with his cultural origins.
- Giger and Davidhizar's Transcultural Assessment Model (2008)

Assessment: Obtaining Minimum Cultural Information

You will not need to perform an in-depth cultural assessment on every patient, but you will need to recognize situations in which this is needed. Lipson and Meleis (1985) suggest that the following minimum information is important:

> ➤ Begin the interview with open-ended questions, such as the following:
> I would like to know more about your family.
> Who will be able to help you when you go home?
> What do you do to help keep yourself well?

> ➤ When you and the client are comfortable, be sure to ask a question such as, "What concerns you the most about your illness and treatment?" This allows you to focus on the individual rather than just on his culture.

Language(s) spoken; proficiency in the language of the host country

> ➤ What language(s) do you speak?
> ➤ Are you comfortable speaking [English], or would you like to have an interpreter?

Length of time client has been here; where client was raised

> ➤ Where were you raised?
> ➤ How long have you lived here?

Ethnic affiliation and identity

> ➤ With what racial and ethnic group(s) do you identify?
> ➤ How closely do you identify with the values of those groups?

Usual religious practices

> ➤ What religion do you practice, if any?
> ➤ Are there any special rituals or practices you want us to be aware of?

Nonverbal communication style

> ➤ You will need to observe the patient and draw on your theoretical knowledge of the patient's cultural group for this information.

Family roles, primary decision maker

> ➤ Who is in your family?
> ➤ What is your role in your family?
> ➤ Who makes most of the decisions?
> ➤ How are decisions made in your family?
> ➤ Whom should I talk to for decisions about your healthcare?

Social support in the new country

> ➤ Do you have family and friends here?
> ➤ Whom can you go to when you need help?
> ➤ Where do you work?
> ➤ Will you need any help with your healthcare expenses?

Practice Resources
Giger & Davidhizar, 2008; Lipson & Meleis, 1985; Spector, 2004; Suzuki & Ponterotto, 2007.

For an example of a focused cultural assessment, see the Focused Assessment box Performing a Focused Cultural Assessment.

For more information about the preceding cultural assessment models,

 Go to Chapter 15, **Tables, Boxes, Figures: ESG Figures 15-3 and 15-4,** and **ESG Boxes 15-3 and 15-4,** on Davis*Plus.*

ANALYSIS/NURSING DIAGNOSIS

There are no NANDA-I diagnoses that specifically address culture. However, cultural factors can be the etiology of various problems. Any of the NANDA-I diagnostic labels can be used for patients of any culture, provided that the defining characteristics are present. Some possible examples include the following:

- **Risk for Imbalanced Nutrition: Less Than Body Requirements** might apply to a patient who is hospitalized and cannot obtain foods prepared in the traditional manner of his ethnic group.
- **Powerlessness** might occur when the patient is unable to make healthcare personnel understand the importance of his religious and dietary beliefs.
- **Impaired Verbal Communication** is sometimes used for patients who do not speak or understand the nurse's language. However, this diagnosis is of questionable value in such circumstances. In a classic study, Geissler (1991) found that Impaired Verbal Communication related more to cultural differences between the patient and healthcare provider than it did to the patient's inability to communicate. The patient and nurse are equally "verbally impaired"; that is, communication is as much a problem for the nurse as for the patient. It is probably better to use Impaired Verbal Communication as the etiology of other diagnoses, such as Ineffective Therapeutic Regimen Management.

- **Noncompliance** can be used for clients and/or caregivers who do not follow a health-promoting or therapeutic plan the healthcare provider believes they agreed to. This may occur because the plan did not fit with the client's perception of the cause of his illness. As another example:

Suppose that a 60-year-old woman who works as a hotel housekeeper is repeatedly admitted to your hospital for uncontrolled hypertension. You determine that she does not take her medication, and you diagnose Noncompliance (failure to take prescribed medication). But do you know that an antihypertensive medication can cost more than $100 for a month's supply? Perhaps your patient is raising her grandchildren and paying for shelter, utilities, food, and clothing uses up her entire income.

You must use this diagnostic label with care. Geissler (1991) also found that additional defining characteristics are needed before Noncompliance can be appropriately applied to clients not of the dominant U.S. culture. In fact, Geissler suggests that nurses use the term *Nonadherence* instead of *Noncompliance.*

The preceding example illustrates the concern that standardized nursing diagnoses are not culturally sensitive; that is, they may not apply accurately to patients who are not from the dominant culture. Nursing diagnoses should describe responses that *patients* see as problematic. A nurse and patient

Focused Assessment

Performing a Focused Cultural Assessment

Assess information listed in the following categories.

CULTURAL UNIQUENESS
➤ Cultural and ethnic identification
➤ Place of birth
➤ Time in country

COMMUNICATION
➤ Voice quality
➤ Pronunciation and enunciation
➤ Use of silence
➤ Use of nonverbal communication
➤ Touch
➤ Spoken language

SPACE
➤ Degree of comfort
➤ Distance in conversations
➤ Definition of space
➤ Body movement

SOCIAL ORGANIZATION
➤ Normal state of health
➤ Marital status
➤ Number of children
➤ Parents living or deceased
➤ Friends
➤ Work
➤ Leisure

TIME
➤ Orientation to time
➤ View of time
➤ Physiochemical reaction to time

ENVIRONMENTAL CONTROL
➤ Locus of control
➤ Value orientation
➤ Health and illness beliefs

BIOLOGICAL VARIATIONS
➤ Physical assessment (including body structure, skin color, skin discoloration, hair color and distribution, other visible physical characteristics, weight, height, lab variances)
➤ Susceptibility to illness
➤ Nutritional preferences
➤ Psychological characteristics

OTHER
In addition, obtain information about the following:
➤ Educational experiences (formal and informal)
➤ Family patterns of healthcare
➤ Family role and function
➤ Healthcare beliefs and practices (folk and professional)
➤ Religious practices
➤ Social networks
➤ Values orientation

Adapted from Giger, J. N., & Davidhizar, R. E. (2008). *Transcultural nursing: Assessment and intervention* (5th ed.). St. Louis, MO: C.V. Mosby.

who are from different cultures will likely have different perceptions of health and illness. This can lead to misdiagnosis. The nurse may either diagnose a problem that doesn't exist for the patient or diagnose a real problem but fail to describe it accurately (Wilkinson, 2011).

The following are a few NANDA-I nursing diagnoses that could be interpreted differently by people from different cultures. Undoubtedly there are others.

Acute Pain	Effective Breastfeeding
Anxiety	Impaired Social Interaction
Chronic Pain	Ineffective Coping
Decisional Conflict	Ineffective Role Performance

The point is to use all labels carefully and to validate nursing diagnoses with the patient to be sure that the statement describes her health status as *she* sees it.

■ PLANNING OUTCOMES/EVALUATION

The outcomes you choose (whether standardized or individualized) depend on the nursing diagnoses you have identified. If the diagnoses are culturally sensitive, the outcomes should be as well. However, you must involve the patient in order to be certain. For example, suppose your patient is dying. Both you and the patient agree that her diagnosis is Acute Pain, but your goals may be different. You might want the patient to be free from pain. However, the patient's goal may be to stay alert enough to interact with her family, even if it means she must endure some pain. When your cultures differ, it is even more important to validate the goals with the patient. Some individualized goal/outcome statements associated with cultural differences might include the following:

- Agrees to take prescribed analgesic (pain medication) before bedtime and after family leaves for the evening.
- Talks to her spiritual adviser about the possibility of surgery conflicting with her religious beliefs.
- Freely shares information about folk practices and over-the-counter medications with the primary care provider.

■ PLANNING INTERVENTIONS/IMPLEMENTATION

When planning care for your clients, information about their cultural values, beliefs, and practices will help you identify interventions that will support these practices and incorporate them into their care as much as possible (Wilkinson, 2011). For example, when you are teaching about a specific treatment regimen ordered by the primary care provider, you should find out whether it conflicts with any of the patient's folk beliefs or alternative treatments so you can suggest any necessary modifications. Remember also to identify educational methods that are most appropriate for your client's needs (e.g., translated materials and/or diagrams) and to make community referrals as necessary.

NIC standardized interventions related to culture include the following:

Active Listening (for Impaired Verbal Communication)
Family Involvement Promotion (for Readiness for Enhanced Family Coping)
Self-Responsibility Facilitation (for Powerlessness)
Culture Brokerage (for Noncompliance)

Culture Brokerage is defined as "the deliberate use of culturally competent strategies to bridge or mediate between the patient's culture and the biomedical healthcare system" (Bulechek, Butcher, & Dochterman, 2008, p. 245).

Individualized nursing activities and focused assessments are important for all patients. However, patients from different cultural and ethnic groups may have unique needs that can be met by some of the activities included in the following discussion regarding culturally competent care.

KnowledgeCheck 15-8

- Describe, in general, how the nursing process can help you provide culturally competent care.
- How can nursing diagnoses cause bias in the planning of care for patients from different cultures?

How Should I Respond to a Client's Cultural Health Practices?

Theorists describe different situations in which nursing decisions and actions are needed regarding a client's cultural health practices (Giger & Davidhizar, 2008; Leininger, 1991; Leininger & McFarland, 2006):

The Practice Is Efficacious (Helpful). You should encourage practices that will likely improve his health. Help the client preserve cultural values related to health. For example, encourage the family to bring ethnic foods that are appropriate for the client's prescribed diet.

The Practice Is Neutral (Neither Helpful nor Harmful). There should be no harm in allowing a patient to continue a neutral health practice. For example, people of Arab heritage associate good health with eating properly and fasting to cure disease. Some may treat illness with prayers or simple foods such as dates, honey, salt, and olive oil (Purnell & Paulanka, 2008). You would not want to interfere with these neutral practices.

The Effects Are Uncertain (Unknown by You). You can neither encourage nor discourage these practices until you obtain more information about them. Do this as soon as possible.

The Practice Is Dysfunctional (Harmful). Discourage folk practices that may cause harm. In such instances, you should support and enable the client to adapt to biomedical therapies or to negotiate with health professionals to achieve satisfying outcomes.

- **Negotiation** acknowledges the gap between the nurse's and client's perspectives. You must negotiate when folk or traditional practices might be harmful to the client.

    Example: Negotiating with the client to continue seeing the curandero, but to come to the clinic every 6 weeks to have his blood pressure checked. If the client refuses all biomedical or nursing interventions, the only avenue still open is to continue monitoring the client to identify changes in his health status. If a health crisis occurs, it may be possible to renegotiate the care.

- **Repatterning/Restructuring** occurs when you attempt to change your actions or the client's lifestyle (Leininger, 1991; Leininger & McFarland, 2006). You would support and encourage the client to greatly modify his behaviors and to adopt new, different, and beneficial health behaviors, while still respecting his cultural values and beliefs.

    Example 1: When the client absolutely refuses to take the prescribed pain medication, the nurse uses massage, distraction, and other nonpharmacological techniques to help relieve his pain (change in nurse's actions).

    Example 2: A client refuses to see a biomedical doctor for her family's needs. However, when the folk healer is unsuccessful in treating her child's illness and the child becomes critically ill, the nurse convinces the client to bring the child to the emergency department (modification of the client's behaviors).

How Do I Communicate With Clients Who Speak a Different Language?

Communicating with clients who do not speak your language can be especially challenging. The best way to provide culturally competent care to such clients is to use a professional medical interpreter. An **interpreter** is specially trained to provide the meaning behind the words, whereas a **translator** just restates the words from one language to another. An interpreter can serve as a cultural broker by conveying the client's responses to questions and by providing general information about the client's culture. Family and friends should not be used as interpreters except on request by the patient (see the CLAS discussion, following).

Culturally and Linguistically Appropriate Services (CLAS) Standards

You should be aware of the standards issued by the U.S. Office of Minority Health (OMH) National Standards for Culturally and Linguistically Appropriate Services (CLAS) in Healthcare. The **CLAS guidelines** require healthcare organizations receiving federal funding to provide language assistance services, including bilingual staff and interpreter services, at no cost to the patient. They must also provide materials and signs in the languages of the commonly encountered groups in their service area (U.S. Department of Health and Human Services, Office of Minority Health, 2001). If you are interested in reading a complete listing of the CLAS standards,

 Go to Chapter 15, **Supplemental Materials: CLAS Standards,** on Davis*Plus.*

Using an Interpreter

Whether you use an interpreter or a translator the following suggestions should be helpful.

- Because of confidentiality issues, avoid asking a family member, especially a child or spouse, to act as an interpreter.
- Avoid using an interpreter who is socially or politically incompatible with the client (e.g., you would not ask an Israeli to interpret for a Palestinian).
- Be aware of gender and age differences. (It usually is preferable to have an interpreter of the same gender as the client.)
- Have the interpreter spend some time alone with the patient.
- Ask the interpreter to interpret the words used by the healthcare provider as closely as possible, except where literal translation might be offensive or misunderstood. In such cases, an interpreter (as compared to a translator) would provide the meaning of your words in terms acceptable to the client.
- Do not use metaphors ("happy as a clam") or medical jargon.
- Observe nonverbal communication (e.g., body language) when the client is listening and talking to the interpreter.
- Address your questions to the client, not the interpreter.
- Maintain eye contact with both the client and interpreter.
- Speak slowly and distinctly, facing the client; do not speak loudly.
- Ask one question at a time; allow time for interpretation and response from the client before asking another question.
- Use active rather than passive voice (e.g., say, "The doctor will see you tomorrow" rather than "You will be seen by the doctor tomorrow.")
- Be aware that many clients can understand more English words than they can express.
- Have health education materials translated into the client's language, or have an interpreter audiotape or videotape instructions.

If there is no one available to interpret for you, in addition to the strategies listed above, the following guidelines should facilitate communication (Munoz & Luckmann, 2004; U.S. Department of Health and Human Services, 2001; Purnell & Paulanka, 2008).

- Greet the client with respect. Greet the person formally, using Mr., Ms., and so forth, until given permission to do otherwise. People in some groups consider it disrespectful to use a person's first name.
- Identify the client's primary language, and use any words that you are familiar with in her language to show that you are trying to communicate.
- If appropriate, use a third language that both of you speak. For example, some Vietnamese and some Cambodians speak French.
- Speak slowly and clearly, using simple sentences to talk about one question or need at a time.
- Use gestures to help convey meaning.
- Restate in different words, if needed.
- Use pictures or diagrams.
- Be aware that some clients may answer yes even if they don't understand what you have said.

Other Strategies

There are several strategies for you to consider and many resources to help you develop strategies specific to various cultural groups (Box 15-1). Consider the following as you move forward on your journey toward cultural competence:

- Consider each client as a unique individual, influenced but not defined by his culture.
- Understand your own cultural values and practices and appreciate how they may differ from those held by people of other cultures.

- Recognize your own biases about people and groups, and consider how they may affect the care you provide.
- Learn as much as you can about the cultural groups in your community and work area.
- Make an effort to incorporate beliefs and practices from various cultures into your nursing care and teaching materials.
- Encourage helpful or neutral cultural practices, and discourage those that are dysfunctional (harmful).
- Suggest alternatives to harmful practices.
- Accommodate cultural dietary practices when possible. For inpatients, some dietary departments can make special foods, and you can encourage families to bring food from home. In all situations, help patients and families adapt cultural foods to therapeutic diets.
- Respect your clients regardless of cultural background, and never force, pressure, manipulate, or coerce them to participate in care that conflicts with their values and beliefs.
- Advocate for all of your clients, but especially for those not from the dominant culture.
- Consider the cultural role of the family member who makes the primary decisions. To ignore this person is to doom your interventions to failure.
- Work with the folk medicine practitioner in the interest of the client.
- Learn from your mistakes, and don't make them again.

This is by no means an exhaustive list. Most likely, you can think of other strategies. It will help if you are aware of your own cultural heritage. Also, appreciate that the client is unique: influenced, but not defined by his culture. Learn about the client's cultural group and incorporate the client's cultural values and behaviors into the care plan.

BOX 15-1 ■ Being Considerate of Cultural Specifics

Consider verbal and nonverbal communication.

- Know, or find out, whether touch (e.g., a handshake) is expected or prohibited.
- Know, or find out, whether eye contact is expected or avoided. Avoiding eye contact, for some, is a sign of respect.
- Ask the client how he wishes to be addressed.
- Know, or find out, the ways people welcome each other.
- Modify communication approaches to meet cultural needs.
- Be considerate of a client's reluctance to talk when the subject involves sexual matters.
- Understand that respect for the client and communicated needs are central to the therapeutic relationship.
- Use validating techniques in communication.

Consider the person's need for personal space.

- Know the person's cultural and religious customs regarding touching and contact.
- Know the usual comfortable distance for conversing in the client's culture.

Consider body language.

- Gestures that are acceptable in one culture may be taboo in another. Know what is acceptable to the client.
- Be aware that smiling does not universally indicate friendliness.

Consider time orientation.

- Tell clients when you are coming, and be on time.
- Avoid surprise visits.
- Share your own expectations about time.
- Ask clients what they expect regarding time, appointments, and so on.
- Be sure you know the times for and meanings of the client's religious and ethnic holidays.

Consider social organization.

- Know which person in the family is the leader or decision maker.
- Know what dates are important and whether gifts are expected or not.
- Know how special events, such as births and funerals, are celebrated, whether certain colors have meaning, and what the expected rituals are.

Consider the person's perspective on environmental control.

- Find out what the client's health traditions and practices are.
- Know whether the person believes she has any ability to "change things."
- Know the general influence of the culture on perception and tolerance of pain.
- Know what foods are forbidden, what foods may or may not be eaten together, and what and how utensils are used.

KnowledgeCheck 15-9

- List five factors to consider when communicating with clients from different cultures.
- List five factors to consider when communicating with a client using an interpreter.
- List five factors to consider when communicating with a client who does not speak your language, when an interpreter is not available.

How Can I Become Culturally Competent?

Of course you can't become culturally competent just by reading. Theoretical knowledge can increase your awareness and appreciation of cultural differences. But you can achieve cultural competence only if you are motivated to do so, and even then only by interacting with people from cultures different from your own. Carballeira (1997) sums up this process with the LIVE and LEARN model for culturally competent family services:

Like		Listen
Inquire		Evaluate
Visit	and	Acknowledge
Experience		Recommend
		Negotiate

Summary. If there were only one single intervention you could choose in the service of cultural competence, you should routinely ask patients what matters most to them in their illness and treatment. No matter how busy, every nurse can find time to do that. You can then use that information to think through the patient's specific needs for care.

CLINICALREASONING:
Applying the **Full-Spectrum Nursing Model**

Because the following critical thinking activities allow you to practice the kind of thinking you will use as a full-spectrum nurse, they usually have no single right answer. Discuss them with your peers—if you have difficulty with any of the questions, consult your instructor.

PATIENT SITUATION

Mrs. Vasquez, a 70-year-old Mexican American woman, has diabetes mellitus and has come to the hospital because of a sore on her lower leg that will not heal. Mrs. Vasquez, a widow, cares for herself at home. She speaks only broken English and has some difficulty understanding your questions. After great effort on your part, you determine that she has missed her last appointment with her diabetes specialist because she has no transportation, so she has just been putting a dressing on the sore. Mrs. Vasquez tells you that she loves to see her grandchildren, who visit often, and that she enjoys cooking and eating Mexican food. She also says that she believes she is sick because she has not pleased God. However, God is a source of comfort and assurance to her. She prays a lot and often has rosary beads in her hand.

THINKING

1. *Theoretical Knowledge (Recall of Facts and Principles):* List six important culture specifics.
2. *Critical Thinking (Application of Knowledge):* Based on your theoretical knowledge, what are your expectations about communicating with Mrs. Vasquez?
3. *Critical Thinking (Compare and Contrast):* Compare your expectations to the actual data you have about her ability to communicate.

DOING

4. *Nursing Process (Assessment):* What are some pertinent cultural data that you should assess for Mrs. Vasquez?
5. *Nursing Process (Analysis/Diagnosis):* Which nursing diagnosis do you think would be best for planning Mrs. Vasquez's care? (Recall that the etiology should suggest your nursing interventions, and the diagnostic label should suggest the expected patient outcome.) Explain your reasoning.
   - Noncompliance (with clinic appointments) r/t lack of transportation
   - Impaired Skin Integrity r/t self-treatment of ulcer
   - Noncompliance (with clinic appointments) r/t beliefs about God and illness

CARING

6. *Self-Knowledge:* What areas of commonality do you have with Mrs. Vasquez, around which you might form a caring relationship?
7. *Self-Knowledge:* Do you agree with Mrs. Vasquez that illness may be caused by displeasing God?
8. *Ethical Knowledge:* Suppose you do not agree with Mrs. Vasquez that she is ill because she has displeased God. Discuss whether you would explain to her that this is most likely not true and then teach her about the cause of diabetic ulcers.

To explore learning resources for this chapter,

Go to Davis*Plus* at http://davisplus.fadavis.com, keyword Treas

Chapter Resources for Chapter 15:
- Knowledge Check and Think Like a Nurse Response Sheets
- Knowledge Check Answers
- Resources for Caregivers and Health Professionals
- Reading More About Culture & Ethnicity (suggested readings)
- What Are the Main Points in This Chapter?

NCLEX-Style Review Questions

Chapter Overview Podcasts

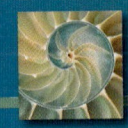

Concept Map

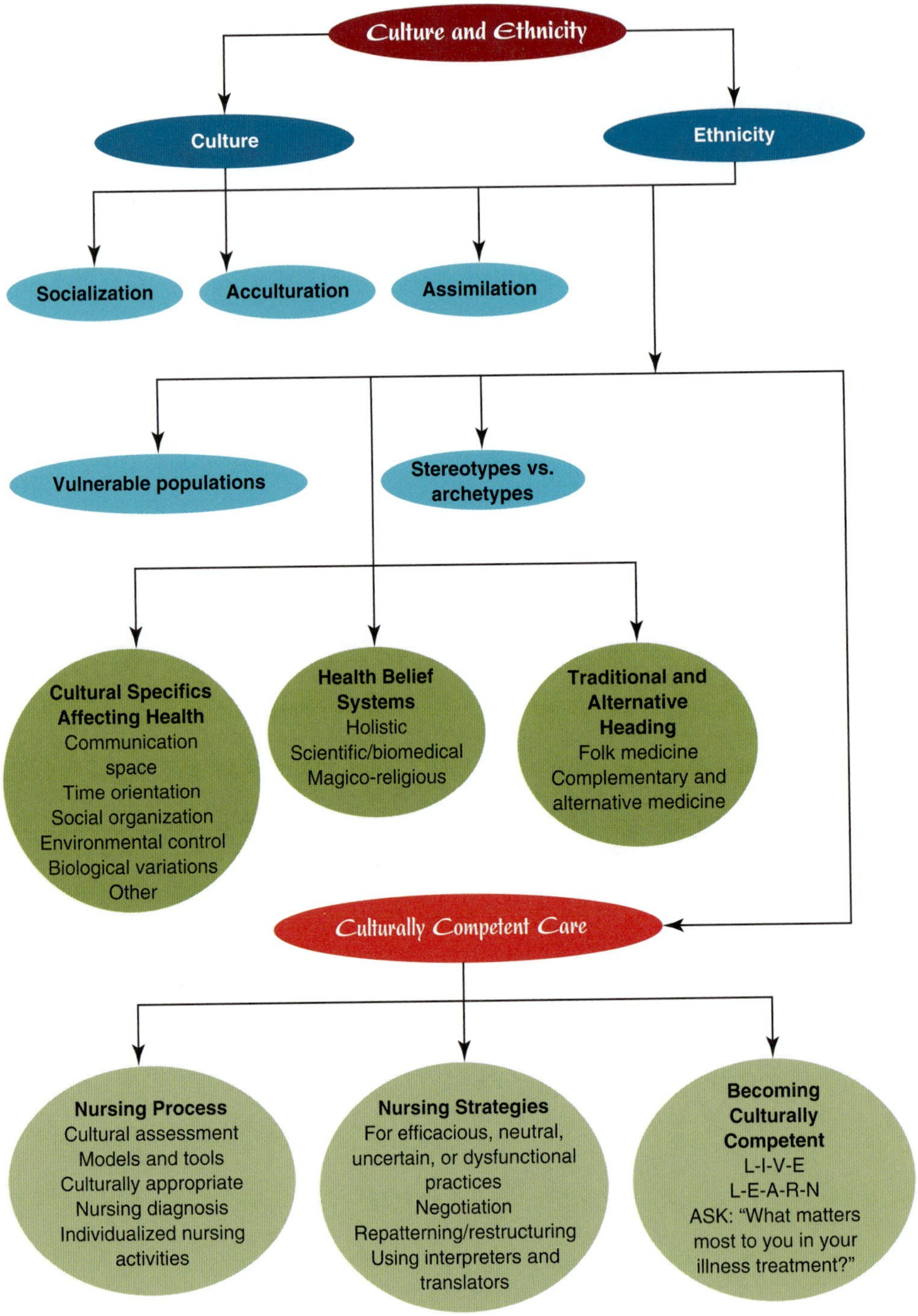

Culture and Ethnicity

Culture

Ethnicity

Socialization

Acculturation

Assimilation

Vulnerable populations

Stereotypes vs. archetypes

Cultural Specifics Affecting Health
Communication
space
Time orientation
Social organization
Environmental control
Biological variations
Other

Health Belief Systems
Holistic
Scientific/biomedical
Magico-religious

Traditional and Alternative Heading
Folk medicine
Complementary and alternative medicine

Culturally Competent Care

Nursing Process
Cultural assessment
Models and tools
Culturally appropriate
Nursing diagnosis
Individualized nursing
activities

Nursing Strategies
For efficacious, neutral,
uncertain, or dysfunctional
practices
Negotiation
Repatterning/restructuring
Using interpreters and
translators

Becoming Culturally Competent
L-I-V-E
L-E-A-R-N
ASK: "What matters
most to you in your
illness treatment?"

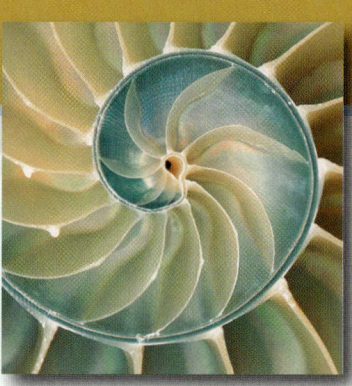

CHAPTER 16

Spirituality

Learning Outcomes

After completing this chapter, you should be able to:

➤ Describe the differences and similarities between religion and spirituality.

➤ Discuss what is meant by spirituality.

➤ For each of the religions briefly covered in this chapter, describe its major beliefs and their implications for nursing care.

➤ Identify five barriers to spiritual care.

➤ Perform a spiritual assessment.

➤ Recognize the differences between spiritual care diagnoses and those that

may serve as etiologies of other nursing diagnoses.

➤ Plan nursing interventions based on the data obtained in a spiritual assessment.

➤ Examine your own level of comfort in terms of performing spiritual interventions.

➤ Describe collaborative efforts to ensure the spiritual care of the patient or family.

Key Concepts

Spirituality

Religion

Spiritual care

Related Concepts

See the Concept Map at the end of this chapter.

Caring for the Nguyens

This feature allows you to practice the kind of thinking you will use as a full-spectrum nurse. There is usually more than one correct answer to a critical thinking question, so we do not provide answers for these features. It is more important to develop your nursing judgment than to "cover content." Discuss the questions with your peers. If you are still unsure, consult your instructor.

Kim Phan is the 3-year-old grandson of Nam and Yen Nguyen. The Nguyens are both practicing Catholics. Kim's mother, Trinh, is the Nguyens' daughter. Trinh feels that Catholicism is "a waste of time" and does not attend church. Kim has had no formal religious experiences or training.

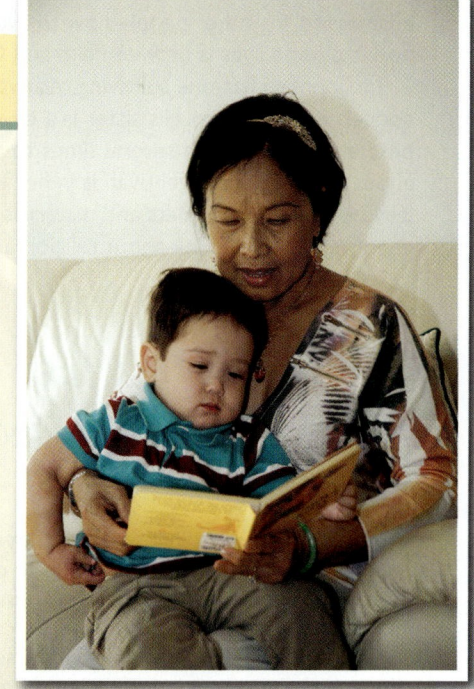

A. At a clinic visit, Nam asks you what you think about keeping religion away from a child. How would you respond?

B. Mr. Nguyen explains his views on the situation: "If anything were to happen to him, he would go to hell. I think we should take him to church and get him baptized

(Continued)

337

Caring for the Nguyens (continued)

right away. I don't know how anyone can live like that. He has no connection to God." Do you agree with this statement? Explain your views.

C. Nam asks you to pray for Kim and his mother. How would you feel about this situation? What would you say to Nam?

 Go to **Caring for the Nguyens Response Sheet** on *DavisPlus.*

Meet Your Patient

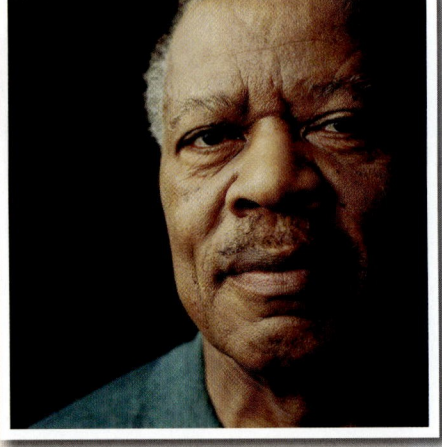

Charles Johnson is a 75-year-old African American man with newly diagnosed lung cancer. His physicians want to start chemotherapy to try to increase his life span. He is unsure whether he wants to have chemotherapy.

Mr. Johnson was brought up in the Baptist Church but has fallen away from his faith over the years. He began smoking at age 15, and has been a heavy drinker all of his adult life. As a young man, he became alienated from churchgoing. He explains that "church folk are all a bunch of hypocrites. I choose not to be a part of any of that." Nevertheless, he says that he tries to be kind to and tolerant of others. "I've messed up my life, so I figure I don't have any business telling other people how to live. I just figure that how a person lives is between him and God."

Mr. Johnson has one surviving relative, a sister, who is concerned about him. His sister is a devout Jehovah's Witness, and she has tried several times to talk to Mr. Johnson about how important Jehovah is in her life. She continually leaves religious pamphlets and materials in his mailbox to encourage him to think about religion again.

Mr. Johnson's wife divorced him 20 years ago because of his drinking behaviors. He has alienated his two middle-aged children, a son and a daughter, so he rarely sees his two grandchildren. He lives alone, is retired, and is having some trouble making ends meet financially. He has one avid hobby: He loves to go out in a boat and fish all day with his buddy, Jim.

- Mr. Johnson clearly has some physical and psychosocial difficulties. Can you identify them?
- Assess Mr. Johnson's support system. Whom can he rely on for help?
- How might you help Mr. Johnson to add some spiritual supports to his available resources?

Theoretical Knowledge
knowing **why**

Spirituality in nursing has multiple layers. The following layers of competing concerns can lead to confusion and frustration in providing spiritual care and, in some cases, cause nurses to avoid spiritual care altogether.

Spirituality of the Nurse. Each nurse has her own spirituality, which serves as part of the guiding framework for her practice.

Spirituality of the Patient and Family. Patients and families understand spirituality in a variety of ways. Their spirituality may be deeply ingrained in religious understandings, or it may be separate from formal religion.

Effects of Nursing Education. Many schools of nursing teach spiritual care interventions while emphasizing

a philosophy of not imposing one's religious beliefs on patients.

Demands of Nursing Practice. In addition, nursing practice settings provide multiple levels of care, which impose time constraints on what you can address in day-to-day activities.

This chapter presents a holistic interpretation of spirituality—one that views spirituality as a component of every person's life. It also encourages you to engage your own spirituality to improve your patients' health and wholeness. It should help you to answer some of the questions posed for Mr. Johnson.

ABOUT THE KEY CONCEPTS

As you study this chapter, try to relate what you are reading to the key concepts of spirituality and religion, and try to understand how those two concepts relate to each other. Doing so will provide a foundation on which you can work with the concept of spiritual care. It is that concept that links you to your patients.

HISTORY OF SPIRITUALITY IN NURSING

Through the ages, nurses and other caregivers have demonstrated deep concern for the spiritual as well as the physical and psychological needs of those who are sick and infirm.

In the pre-Christian era, caring for the sick was an expression of the values of hospitality and charity. People prayed to the god(s) for healing and as an adjunct for primitive medical procedures.

In the early Christian era, nursing the sick was honored and respected because it was one of Jesus Christ's primary teachings, as well as a vital component of loving one's neighbor. Gradually, religious communities of women and men in the 4th through 12th centuries combined the healing arts with religious care.

During the post-Reformation period (the 1700s and later) in Europe, nursing orders flourished, among them the Sisters of Mercy and the Kaiserswerth Deaconesses (Donahue, 1985). Florence Nightingale trained at the Deaconess school and clinic in Kaiserswerth, as well as under the Daughters of Charity of St. Vincent de Paul in France. For Nightingale, spirituality was at the very heart of human nature and thus was fundamental to healing. She instilled this idea in her nurses, particularly during their missions in the Crimea (McDonald, 2007; Macrae, 1995).

By the mid-20th century, nursing in the United States had begun to see spiritual care as less important. As science continued to develop, and as more nurses studied in universities, the spiritual underpinnings of nursing were replaced by what could be seen and tested by the scientific method. Only recently has nursing (and the broader health community) reclaimed spirituality as a vital part of its identity and recognized its power to influence health.

Today, professional standards of care make clear that patients' spiritual needs are a nursing concern. The Joint Commission (2008) has established standards for spiritual care. In addition, the American Nurses Association's (ANA) *Nursing: Scope and Standards of Practice* (2010) states that nurses should consider each patient's lifestyle, value system, and religious beliefs in planning care; and that nursing care measures should enable the patient to live with as much physical, emotional, social, and spiritual well-being as possible.

WHAT ARE RELIGION AND SPIRITUALITY?

Although there is overlap, spirituality and religion differ in several important ways (Table 16-1). One way to distinguish religion from spirituality is to think of religion as a map and spirituality as a journey. We begin by exploring the map.

What Is Religion?

You may use a map to get to a certain location. The "map" of religion (1) tells you what to believe and what values are essential; and (2) provides codes of conduct that integrate beliefs and values into a way of living. The map itself may be in the form of a religious tradition (e.g., Christianity) or denomination (e.g., Baptist), which provides an identity and a lens for reading the world. The rituals, symbols, sacraments, and holy writings associated with religions serve as bases of authority and provide diverse ways to transcend the physical and access the divine (e.g., God). Regardless of their differences, many of the world religions have the following in common:

- **Theology**—that is, discussions and theories related to God and God's relation to the world
- Sacred writings that are regarded as authoritative
- Notion of created order and purpose
- Definition of *human being* that includes important life events
- Notion of sin (primarily in Western religions)
- Explanation of the origin of evil and the nature of suffering
- Conception of either salvation (in Judeo-Christian religions) or enlightenment (in Eastern religions)
- **Eschatology,** or doctrines about the human soul and its relation to death, judgment, and eternal life (primarily a Western concept)
- Explanation of the nature of reality, the higher self or soul, the relationship between humans and the divine, and the purpose of human existence

What Is Spirituality?

If religion is the map, spirituality is the day-to-day, moment-by-moment journey in life and living. Like a journey, spirituality takes place over time. Many life events that prompt spiritual

Table 16-1 ▶ Comparison of Religion and Spirituality	
RELIGION (THE MAP)	**SPIRITUALITY (THE JOURNEY)**
A "roadmap" that defines beliefs, values, and code(s) of conduct and ethics	One's journey through life; a personal quest to define meaning, fulfillment, and satisfaction in life; a will to live; a belief in self
A tradition or system of worship that provides rituals, answers, norms, and connection with God	A dynamic relationship with that which transcends; a capacity to know and be known (a sense of openness, expectation); connectedness with self, others, nature, and a higher power (Cavendish, Konecny, Mitzeliotis, et al., 2003); belief in a divine being, or infinite source of energy (Beckman, Boxley-Harges, Bruick-Sorge, et al., 2007).
The roadmap and tradition define: ■ What is to be believed ■ How beliefs affect life ■ Self-image and identity	A lifelong process of growth (which may involve joy and/or struggle); a constant process of taking in truth and then adding individual insight to arrive at a way of perceiving and acting in the world
Issues: Faith, belief, trust, the nature of good and evil, the meaning of suffering, judgment, or enlightenment	Issues: Faith, hope, love

growth are fulfilling and joyful, but growth often results from painful life events that cause great internal upheaval, struggle, and challenge.

You can think of spirituality as an accumulation of life experiences and insights (i.e., in terms of finding meaning, value, and purpose in life). They may agree or conflict with traditional religious values and cultural teachings. For example, an American raised in the Episcopal Church, after studying a variety of religions and traveling in Asia for several years, may develop a spirituality that is both universal and highly individual and may feel at home in any place of worship in the world.

Like religion, spirituality allows various ways and means to experience the divine in our daily lives, or simply to be still and introspective. For centuries, Eastern traditions have emphasized that spirituality is awareness, paying attention, and being "sensitive to reality" (Krishnamurti, 1989). Life is a process of recognizing an active Spirit in the world, and of learning about ourselves and others in new and profound ways. We can engage the Spirit through such sources as nature, animals, leisure, creativity, and service (Brussat & Brussat, 1996).

It is critical for you to recognize and respect the different ways that patients understand religion and spirituality. You need to understand that most people are fairly comfortable with their beliefs (or lack thereof) and that, in providing spiritual care, your primary goal is to support their healing, not convert them to a different view. You must also be able to recognize situations when patients may be experiencing spiritual distress and may need referral to professionals with more specialized training than you have. These aspects of spiritual care are discussed later in this chapter.

KnowledgeCheck 16-1

- Regardless of their differences, what do many world religions have in common?
- Which can be compared to a journey: religion or spirituality?
- True or false: Both religion and spirituality allow a person various ways to access the divine.
- What is Mr. Johnson's religion (Meet Your Patient)?
- What is his sister's religion?

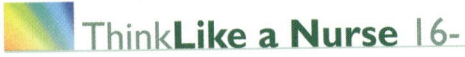 ## ThinkLike a Nurse 16-1

What do you know, or what can you speculate, about Mr. Johnson's (Meet Your Patient) spirituality?

What Are the Core Issues of Spirituality?

As just discussed, spirituality has many dimensions. We limit discussion here to three core issues. In the New Testament of the Bible, the Apostle Paul identified "three things that last": faith, hope, and love. Following in this tradition, a contemporary manual for nursing care of the dying (Aspen Reference Group, 2002) identifies this same trio as the three core "issues" of spirituality.

Faith

Faith is our ongoing effort to make sense of our lives and purpose for being. Like spirituality itself, faith represents a set of beliefs developed over time, through events that cause us to suffer and those that enable us to rejoice. People who are experiencing the *joys of faith* exhibit a sense of self, as well as insights into their gifts and talents.

Faith struggles are common among people who experience illness and significant loss. People experiencing faith struggles might feel anger, guilt, self-judgment, and worthlessness.

C. S. Lewis, a devout Christian, reveals that after the death of his wife, his grief caused him to doubt whether God exists at all, or if so, whether He is perhaps a "Cosmic Sadist" (1961, p. 35) who deliberately tortures us. Finally, Lewis came to understand that such shattering experiences are "one of the marks of His presence" (Lewis, 1961, p. 76).

Hope

Hope includes our basic human needs to achieve, create, and shape something of our life that will endure. If faith is expressed in terms of belief, then hope is rooted in purpose—Who am I? What is my purpose? Why have I been created? People who are confronting a debilitating or terminal illness often lose hope. After suffering a near-fatal spinal cord injury, actor Christopher Reeve experienced such a struggle, yet he wrote in an essay on hope: "Hope . . . is different from optimism or wishful thinking. When we have hope, we discover powers within ourselves we may have never known—the power to make sacrifices, to endure, to heal, and to love" (Reeve, 2002, p. 176).

Love

Although it is better defined as willing the good of another, many people think of love as a trade: we extend our love because we hope to find that love returned in some way. But relationships can be a source of pain. Even when our love is shared, we must inevitably face separation at our death or the death of our loved ones. Thus, while active loving in human relationships opens us up to joy and can give life, meaning, and purpose; it also carries with it the certainty of heartbreak.

Illness and sudden injury commonly prompt such struggles with love. For example, when a man with a debilitating disease loses his ability to work and requires increasing levels of caregiving, he may experience himself as a burden and question whether his loved ones would be better off if he were to die. When patients question the presence of unconditional love in their lives, family members may be invaluable in reminding them of their inner integrity and worth. Reeve stated that the most powerful words his wife spoke to him in the first days after his injury, "the words that saved my life," were, "You're still you. And I love you" (Reeve, 1998, p. 32).

Cures, Miracles, and Spiritual Healing

The patient or family may request a prayer asking God for a cure when your expertise tells you that all curative measures have been exhausted. Certainly you should not say that a cure is impossible. But it is equally important to avoid exposing the patient and family to false hope. In such cases, it may be possible for you, as care provider and companion on the spiritual journey, to reframe the situation. Perhaps healing does not necessarily have to imply the elimination of all types of suffering or of the disease. Rather, it may mean a transformation in a patient's thinking or feeling when that patient has become receptive to the workings of the spirit. In such instances, healing does indeed take place, and the person may experience a miracle.

A **miracle** is anything that allows for the presence of the transcendent (e.g., God, a higher being, the experience of one's angel, or any connection with the divine). It is an event that excites wonder and in which we see God at work in our ordinary day-to-day lives (Macquarrie, 1977), but it does not necessarily involve a physical cure. We typically think of miracles as events that break with the natural order of things (e.g., a blind person suddenly can see, with no treatment or explanation); however, miracles more commonly proceed according to natural law. What makes events miracles is the

fact that they far exceed our expectations. For instance, an elderly woman, bitter for decades over the death of her daughter during childhood, "feels" her daughter's presence and dies in peace. Miracles are spiritual phenomena. As such, they are mysterious; they are difficult to define and comprehend. In one sense, they can be viewed as perfectly ordinary events; in another, they are extraordinary, for they allow the patient to see and know God is present despite illness or other adversity (Macquarrie, 1977).

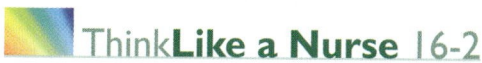

ThinkLike a Nurse 16-2

Faith is a constant search for comprehension and meaning. What are some of your struggles with faith, and what are some of the joys of your faith?

HOW MIGHT SPIRITUAL BELIEFS AFFECT HEALTH?

Although the preceding sections discussed religion and spirituality as two separate concepts, current research into their influence on health tend to combine the two into one: namely, religion. Most studies have measured both religion and spirituality in terms of *religious involvement*. They tend to use broad measures, such as self-reports of one's own religiousness, denominational affiliation, church attendance or membership, membership in the clergy, and dietary and social habits (e.g., "On a scale of 1 to 5, how religious are you?" "How often do you attend church?") Despite such limitations, findings have been surprisingly positive in terms of predicting health outcomes. There is a growing body of literature that investigates the effects of religion on heart disease, cholesterol, hypertension, cancer, mortality, and health behaviors.

- One study found that people who score higher on measures of religious involvement live longer than those with lower religious involvement (McCollough, Hoyt, Larson, et al., 2000).
- Likewise, the literature suggests that even simplistic measures regarding religion and spirituality (e.g., religious affiliation or church attendance) are significant predictors of health outcomes, including increased pain tolerance and decreased depression and anxiety (Harrison, Edwards, Koenig, et al., 2005; Koenig, McCollough, & Larson, 2001).

In all of these, the variables studied tend to be broadly stated and nonspecific and thus do not allow for researchers to examine whether there might be potential harmful effects of religion.

Although the research suggests that religion has a positive influence on healthcare outcomes, it does not yet answer *how* or *why* religion has this effect. However, there is growing awareness that religion and spirituality involve cognitive, emotional, behavioral, interpersonal, and physiological dimensions. For a description of recent research testing more specific variables (e.g., religion as a factor to live a healthy lifestyle),

 Go to Chapter 16, **Supplemental Materials: Religion and Health: Recent Research,** on Davis*Plus*.

KnowledgeCheck 16-2

What are some of the ways that religion might positively influence health?

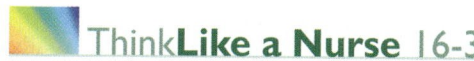

ThinkLike a Nurse 16-3

- How might religion negatively influence health?
- Has there been a pivotal moment in your life, a moment of crisis or despair that eventually provided an opportunity for spiritual growth?

MAJOR RELIGIONS: WHAT SHOULD I KNOW?

The more you know about the differences and similarities among the world's major religions, the more you will be able to offer comprehensive and compassionate care to patients. Of course, learning about other religions requires you to be open and nonjudgmental. When you care for a patient from a known church background, you will need to think about how the person's beliefs affect her ideas of health, healing, hospitalization, and the experience of dying. To help you make these connections, the following brief descriptions of several of the world's major religious traditions provide you with several different worldviews. To learn about their influence on end-of-life care, see Chapter 17. For more detailed information about each religion, and for information about Baha'i, Sikhism, and Rastafarianism,

 Go to Chapter 16, **Supplemental Materials: Major Religions: What Should I Know?** and **Reading More About Spirituality,** on Davis*Plus*.

Judaism

Judaism is one of the Western world's oldest religions and the foundation on which Christianity and Islam were built. The Jewish law is set down in the collective writings of the Torah. Judaism is based on the worship of one God (monotheism), obeying the Ten Commandments, and practicing charity and tolerance toward others. The degree to which Jews celebrate rituals and holy days depends on whether the person identifies with the Orthodox, Liberal, Conservative, or Reconstructionist beliefs (Oxtoby & Segal, 2007; Pawlikowski, 1990).

Jews celebrate the Sabbath from sunset on Friday to sunset Saturday evening. For Orthodox Jews, work is prohibited on the Sabbath. This includes writing, traveling, and switching on lights and appliances. During Passover (in March or April), some Jewish patients may require special foods, dinnerware, and utensils. The Day of Atonement, or Yom Kippur (in September or October), is the holiest day of the Jewish calendar. It is a special day of fasting, but fasting is not required if it would be a danger to the patient. A Jewish patient will normally wish to keep that day to pray and rest. For Orthodox patients, you might offer alternatives to oral medication (e.g., injections or suppositories).

Conservative Jews observe strict dietary laws: Only kosher foods are accepted. **Kosher foods** have been prepared under strict guidelines concerning the slaughter of animals and do not contain pork, certain types of seafood, or combinations of dairy and meat. If possible, consult a rabbi or dietitian who is knowledgeable about Jewish dietary laws for assistance in planning dietary and activity modifications.

Orthodox Jewish women prefer to have their bodies and limbs covered. They may also prefer to keep their hair covered with a scarf and often wear a wig. Orthodox men keep their head covered with a hat or skullcap *(kappel)*. Some Orthodox Jewish sects forbid contraception unless the

woman's health is at risk. Nearly all Jewish boys are circumcised, usually 8 days after birth. Orthodox Judaism usually forbids organ transplants, but opinions vary and decisions may rest with the rabbinic authority.

Christianity

Although rituals and practices vary among denominations, Christians are collectively known for their belief in Jesus Christ and their use of the sacred text, the Bible, which includes the Judaic Old Testament and the New Testament on the life and teachings of Jesus. There are many denominations within Christianity, including Roman Catholicism (with allegiance to the pope in Rome), Orthodoxy (with allegiance to the patriarch of Constantinople), Protestant denominations (e.g., Lutheran, Baptist, United Methodist), and others (e.g., Jehovah's Witnesses, Church of the Latter Day Saints, Christian Science). For the most part, Christians hold that Jesus' death atoned for the sins of men and women, providing a way to experience the forgiveness of God and to gain eternal life.

Many denominations practice baptism, so when infants or children are very ill, baptism should be offered. Christians usually have no special dietary requirements, although some choose to abstain from eating meat on Fridays and/or during Lent. Some Christians may wish to **fast** (abstain from food) before receiving Holy Communion. Some (depending on the denomination) abstain from alcohol.

Family planning varies within Christianity. Some denominations allow artificial birth control methods; others do not. Most denominations do not object to natural family planning methods (e.g., rhythm), blood transfusion, or organ transplantation.

Roman Catholicism. In Roman Catholicism, the **sacraments** are a means to obtain grace. A Roman Catholic who is seriously ill might wish to receive the sacrament of *anointing the sick*. This sacrament, once known as the last rites, can be repeated if the person recovers and then becomes ill at a later time. Only a priest can hear the *sacrament of reconciliation* (confession), during which God, through the agency of the priest, grants forgiveness for past sins. The *Eucharist* (communion bread), consecrated at the *mass* (a religious service), may be brought to hospitalized patients by a priest, deacon, or designated lay Eucharistic minister. Other denominations within Christianity (e.g., Episcopalians and Lutherans) observe certain sacraments as well, although the meaning and details of the rituals may vary.

Christian Science. The Christian Science faith is a unique form of Christianity. Established in the United States in 1879, Christian Science teaches reliance on God, rather than on medicine or surgery, for healing. Therefore, you might encounter followers as patients only after accidents or because of family or legal pressures.

Christian Scientists do not use alcohol and tobacco; strict Christian Scientists may not drink tea or coffee. Adults will probably not accept a blood transfusion, but parents usually consent to transfusion and other medical care for their child if doctors consider it essential or the law requires them to do so. Adults will not usually consent to donate or receive organs.

Jehovah's Witnesses. Jehovah's Witnesses try to live according to the commands of God as written in both the Old and New Testaments of the Bible. They will accept most medical treatments, but they believe that taking blood into one's body is morally wrong. Their interpretation of this means that they will not allow transfusions of whole blood or its components. Their faith also does not permit donation or receipt of an organ through which blood flows. If blood is not involved (e.g.,

corneal transplants) they may accept transplantation. This belief means that meat is not acceptable if an animal has been strangled or shot and not bled properly. Some Jehovah's Witness do not eat meat at all. They do not celebrate birthdays or holidays, except for the anniversary of the death of Christ. The date of that anniversary varies from year to year. Jehovah's Witnesses abstain from tobacco and other recreational drugs. They may drink alcohol but do not condone drunkenness.

Mormonism. The Mormon Church is also known as the Church of Jesus Christ of Latter-Day Saints. Mormons believe in Jesus and one God; however, they adhere to a more recently revealed sacred writing, the Book of Mormon. Mormons follow a strict health code, known as the Word of Wisdom, which advises healthful living and prohibits the use of tea, coffee, alcohol, and tobacco. Some Mormons (both men and women) wear a sacred undergarment that they remove only for hygiene purposes. Nurses may also remove it before surgery, but it must at all times be considered intensely private and be treated with respect (Keddington, 2007).

Seventh Day Adventism. The Seventh Day Adventist Church is distinguished mostly by observance of Saturday, the original seventh day of the Judeo-Christian week, as the Sabbath, a day of rest and worship. To keep the Sabbath holy, Adventists do no secular work or unnecessary business on Saturday. The church also emphasizes diet, health, and culturally conservative principles (e.g., many Adventists are opposed to body piercing and tattoos. Some even refrain from wearing jewelry). Adventists usually practice communion, which begins with a foot-washing ceremony, four times a year. Regarding dietary practices, the church recommends vegetarianism and adherence to the kosher laws in the Old Testament of the Bible. This includes abstinence from pork, shellfish, and other "unclean" foods. However, most Adventists do eat meat. Most do not use alcohol, tobacco, illegal drugs, and beverages containing caffeine.

Although the church is generally anti-abortion, in cases of serious dilemmas (e.g., threat to the woman's life or pregnancy resulting from rape or incest), women are counseled to make their own decisions. The Adventist church is officially against active euthanasia but permits a passive form through withdrawal of medical support to allow the patient to die. Birth control is permitted for married couples.

Islam

The word *Islam* means submission. In particular, a Muslim is one who submits to Allah (God). The principal book of authority in Islam, the Koran (Qu'ran), is the result of a vision received by Muhammad, the founder of Islam, in the early 7th century CE. Islam teaches that all faiths have essentially one common message: There is a supreme being whose sovereignty is acknowledged in worship and whose teaching and commandments must be obeyed.

Muslims are forbidden to eat pork. They may eat other meat, but it has to be *halal* meat, that is, killed in a special manner stated in Islamic law. Fish and eggs are allowed, but not if they are cooked near pork or non-halal meat. During the month of Ramadan, a Muslim fasts between sunrise and sunset; however, those who are sick are not expected to fast. Essential drugs and medicines are allowed at all hours during Ramadan.

Muslims always wash their hands before eating. Patients prefer to wash in free-flowing water, so tub baths are considered unhygienic. If a shower is not available, provide a pitcher to use in the bath.

Women prefer to be treated by female staff. Some women may refuse vaginal examination by a male nurse or physician

because they are forbidden to expose their bodies to or be touched by any man other than their husband. Women may wear a locket containing religious writing around the neck in a small leather bag. These are kept for protection and strength, so you should never remove them.

There is no specific religious rule prohibiting blood transfusion or organ transplantation; however, strict Muslims will not usually agree to organ transplants. Orthodox Muslims do not approve of contraception; however, individuals vary widely in their practices. Abortion is frowned on but may be tolerated for medical reasons.

Hinduism

Hinduism, which many religious scholars believe is the oldest major religion still practiced today, does not embrace a single body of beliefs and practices. It maintains that no one manifestation of God can possibly capture the limitless nature of God. Thus, Hindus may worship several or even hundreds of gods and goddesses. Even elements in the natural world, such as rivers, fire, and so forth, are considered aspects of God. Sacred Hindu texts include the *Vedas*, the *Bhagavad Gita* (Song of the Blessed One), and the *Ramayana*, the story of the life of the god Rama. Despite commonly held beliefs and texts, Hindu religious practices vary a great deal, depending on areas of origin.

Hindus practice **ayurvedic medicine,** which encompasses all aspects of life, including diet, sleep, elimination, and hygiene. Some believe in the medicinal properties of "hot" and "cold" foods—"hot" and "cold" having nothing to do with either temperature or spicy qualities. Although some Hindus will eat eggs and even chicken, most are lactovegetarians, consuming milk but no eggs. Fasting, which may mean eating only "pure" foods such as fruit or yogurt, is common during major festivals but is not expected of the sick. Tobacco and alcohol may or may not be accepted.

Hindus prefer to wash in free-flowing water (e.g., a shower instead of a tub bath). If a shower is not available, provide a jug of water for the person to use in the bath. Women are modest and usually prefer to be treated by female medical staff. Jewelry often has a religious or cultural significance. Some Hindus wear "sacred thread" around the body or wrist. Do not remove or cut this thread without permission from the patient or next of kin. There is no religious objection to contraception, blood transfusion, or organ donation, as a rule.

Buddhism

The Buddha, or the "Awakened One," is revered not as a god but as an example of a way of life (Fig. 16-1). He was born into a royal family in 624 BCE in a part of northern India that is now in Nepal, gained enlightenment at the age of 35, and then began to teach others how to attain liberation from suffering, not only for themselves but also for others. One of the Buddha's core teachings is that suffering can be ended by following the eightfold path: right understanding, right intention, right speech, right action, right livelihood, right effort, right mindfulness, and right contemplation (Bodhi, 2007; Knierim, 2008). **Nirvana,** similar to the Christian concept of heaven, can be attained only through an absence of desire, the achievement of perfection, and the lack of a unique identity.

Many Buddhists follow a vegetarian diet; in some cases, the diet may include both milk and eggs. Fasting customs vary by tradition. Buddhists accept contraception but typically condemn abortion and active euthanasia. They will usually accept blood transfusion and organ transplantation.

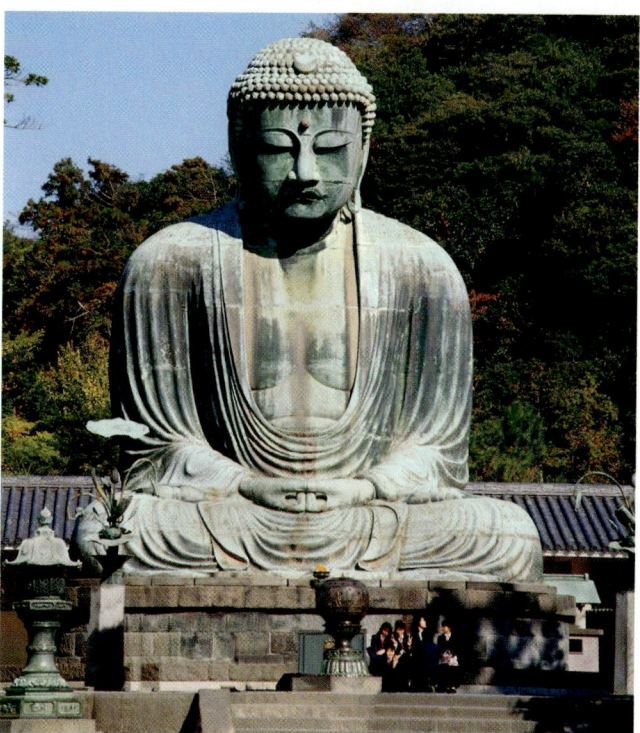

FIGURE 16-1 The Buddha is revered as an example of a way of life.

Native American Religions

There are more than 400 federally recognized Native American nations or tribes in the United States. Although each has its own traditions and cultural heritage, some general beliefs underlie the more specific tribal ideas (Fig. 16-2). Earth is considered to be a living organism, the body of a higher individual, and humankind has an intimate relation with this organism through nature. When Earth is harmed, humankind is harmed, and vice versa. The land belongs to life, life belongs to the land, and the land belongs to itself (Boyd, 1974).

Health is a state of harmony with nature. Whenever disharmony exists, disease or illness can occur. The traditional healer is the medicine man or woman who is wise in the interrelationships of land, humankind, and the universe. Many Native Americans believe that the treatments they receive from their traditional healers are far better than those rendered by the dominant healthcare establishment, which often treats Native Americans with scorn or disrespect.

You should know that note taking by the professional is forbidden; when you take a history or perform an exam, you must rely on your memory to record findings later. Native Americans tend to converse in a low tone of voice and may maintain long periods of silence. Be sure the setting is quiet enough to allow you to hear the patient because it is impolite to indicate that you did not hear the communications.

KnowledgeCheck 16-3

- Which major religion believes in the anointing of the sick or dying?
- Which denomination or religion does not believe in blood transfusions?
- In terms of Native American beliefs and healthcare, who is the traditional healer or the person to be consulted in the event of illness?
- True or false: Most Hindus are vegetarian.

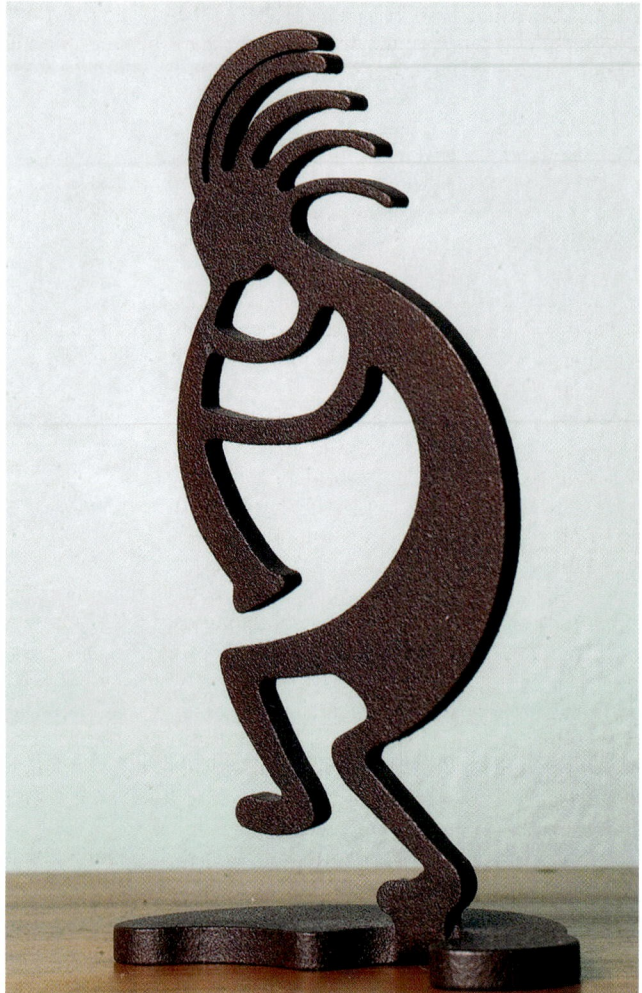

FIGURE 16-2 Kokopelli, the humpbacked flute player, has been a sacred figure to Native Americans of the Southwest for thousands of years. He is a legendary symbol of fertility who brought well-being to the people.

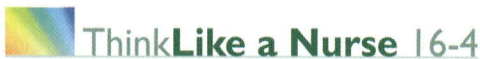

ThinkLike a Nurse 16-4

What are some of the ways that world religions might influence nursing care?

Self-Knowledge: What Every Nurse Should Know

As you have seen, your patients' spiritual and religious backgrounds may be diverse and may involve ways of thinking and doing that seem strange to you or that you do not fully understand. Before trying to understand your patients' religious experience, you must give considerable thought to your own spiritual journey. Attaining self-knowledge is an important aspect of becoming a full-spectrum nurse. This section may be of help to you in that regard.

What Are Your Personal Biases?

We each have our own perspectives and biases. We tend to view the world through lenses we acquired in childhood, adolescence, and early adulthood. In addition, our religious education is sometimes taught with a certain sense of one-up-manship; that is, we are taught that our religious beliefs and practices are superior to all others. When you view your own experience as the norm or as the preferred way of organizing the world, you tend to limit the range of care you provide to the patient who believes differently. Spiritual care demands an open manner of thinking that invites rather than excludes.

ThinkLike a Nurse 16-5

Consider the following examples. For each person, what moral/spiritual judgments must the nurse be careful *not* to make?

- A nurse is caring for a gay man who is hospitalized with end-stage AIDS.
- A woman has come to the clinic to be treated for gonorrhea (a sexually transmitted disease). She says she has had at least six sexual partners this year.
- A man comes to the emergency department (ED) at least once a month to ask for morphine to treat his back pain. He is known to abuse drugs and to visit other EDs for the same purpose.

If you are aware of your biases, it will be easier to avoid abuses of spiritual care, such as the following:

- **Attempting to convert others to your beliefs.** For example, if a patient is near death, he and his family might be offended if their nurse inquires whether they are saved Christians. Remain focused on the patient's need to talk about meaning, salvation, or other end-of-life issues. As another example, notice that Mr. Johnson's sister (Meet Your Patient) seems very close to imposing her religion on him. She may alienate him further if he perceives that he is being pushed.
- **Trying to be all things to all people,** regardless of their background or the extent of spiritual care needed. Clearly, there are times when you should refer to others with more knowledge and experience in religion and spirituality, with the patient's permission, of course. In addition, whenever a patient requests the services of a rabbi, priest, or other spiritual adviser, you should relay that request to the agency's chaplain so that all disciplines remain informed.

In summary, to work effectively with a diverse population, you must first obtain a greater degree of self-knowledge by (1) being open to the many possibilities for diverse thinking, (2) welcoming challenging experiences that allow for personal growth, and (3) taking time to think about how your actions and biases might affect the care of others. The more you know about yourself, the more effectively you care for others.

What Are Some Barriers to Spiritual Care?

Although most nurses would acknowledge that patients have a spiritual dimension, few actually identify spiritual problems or provide spiritual interventions. This may be a result of economic constraints, poor staffing, and high-tech care, which force nurses to focus on physical needs to the exclusion of spiritual needs (Cavendish, Konecny, Mitzeliotis, et al., 2003). You may judge these nurses less harshly after you understand more about the barriers to spiritual interventions by nurses.

Lack of General Awareness of Spirituality

One study of oncology nurses found that more than half incorrectly identified the patient's religion and that only 16% incorporated any kind of spiritual assessment into their care (Sodestrom & Martin, 1987). Highfield's (1992) study confirms the incidence of inaccurate spiritual assessment by nurses. A greater awareness of spirituality in general will help you tune into the spiritual needs of patients and improve your comfort in communicating about spiritual matters.

Lack of Awareness of Your Own Spiritual Belief System

To feel comfortable making spiritual interventions, you will need more than just theoretical knowledge. You will need introspection and an awareness of your own spiritual journey to integrate the spiritual domain into patient care. Lane (1987) identifies three steps in the spiritual growth of nurses:

1. Developing a "greater awareness of the spirit within self" in order to be a better listener for the patient
2. Opening the self by being totally present with the patient
3. Allowing the patient to share his feelings and emotions without reserve

Activities to heighten your awareness of your own spirituality, gain a broader view of spirituality, and increase sensitivity to others' spiritual needs include the following (Beckman, Boxley-Harges, Bruick-Sorge, et al., 2007):

- Increase your knowledge about spirituality.
- Develop your critical and reflective thinking abilities.
- Explore your own spirituality (e.g., reflection, discussing with others). One technique is to write your own epitaph: one or two lines summing up how you would like to be remembered.
- Reflect on your thoughts and feelings about end-of-life issues. Imagine you have only a few weeks to live; think how you would feel.
- Reflect on your personal experience with grief and loss. For example, what is the first death you can remember? What were your feelings at the time? How do you usually cope with loss? What actions by others comforted you?

Find ways to take care of and nurture your own spiritual needs; otherwise, providing spiritual care can be emotionally draining.

Differences in Spirituality Between Nurse and Patient

Patients and nurses can be at different levels in terms of spirituality, whether or not your beliefs are similar. When a patient's spiritual beliefs are different from your own, you must be careful not to impose your beliefs on the patient or discount the importance of the patient's beliefs and rituals. When the patient's views are similar to yours, take care not to make false assumptions about his spiritual needs. Just because you agree on some things does not mean you will have the same views or needs in all areas of spirituality or religion.

Think **Like a Nurse** 16-6

- How does your religion or spirituality differ from Mr. Johnson's (Meet Your Patient)?
- How is it similar?
- Can you think of problems these differences and similarities could cause you in caring for him?

Fear That Your Knowledge Base Is Insufficient

Nurses sometimes avoid giving spiritual care because they believe they lack knowledge of spirituality or of the patient's religion. This is a realistic concern. In several studies, nurses were found to be unsure of what constituted spiritual problems and spiritual interventions (Sodestrom & Martin, 1987; Ryan, 1992). In some cases they did not identify the spiritual dimension of care, or they took religious aspects into account but did not place them into a broader spiritual perspective. Highfield and Cason (1983) found that oncology nurses placed greater emphasis on physical and psychosocial nursing care and that they frequently did not identify the patient's spiritual

needs. Spiritual care has never been more welcomed by patients. You can provide truly holistic care for the patient when you address spiritual needs in a plan of care.

Fear of Where Spiritual Discussions May Lead

Many nurses fear that inquiring into the spiritual domain might cause harm to the patient. For example, what if a patient asks you, "Do you believe active euthanasia is morally wrong? Would it jeopardize my salvation?" Here are some fears that may arise:

- You may not feel prepared to answer the questions.
- You might have an answer based on your personal religious beliefs but fear the patient may think you are imposing your beliefs on him.
- You might wonder whether communicating your own beliefs (e.g., if you favor active euthanasia) might jeopardize the patient's spiritual life if your ideas turn out to be "wrong."

The following ideas may help counter your fears. Most important, the patient's addressing this concern with you indicates that you are open to the spiritual domain of care. Second, the patient in this example is concerned with issues related to euthanasia. This could lead to discussions about the patient's fears of pain, dependence, being a burden on family members, and dying alone. Third, this is an area for which you should seek collaboration with a chaplain, who is more prepared to deal with specific religious issues. You should realize that being open to the spiritual realm and assessing the patient's need for spiritual intervention does not mean that you must be a chaplain or have the extraordinary ability to deal with all spiritual or religious questions or requests. The Practical Knowledge section will provide a more detailed understanding of your role in spiritual care.

Knowledge Check 16-4

- What qualities can you demonstrate that may help you improve the quality of spiritual care you provide?
- What common barriers to spiritual interventions do nurses encounter?
- True or false: No matter how nonjudgmental and open we may think ourselves to be, we all carry our own unique biases and prejudices that have the potential to affect patient care.

Think **Like a Nurse** 16-7

- What are some of the possible abuses of spiritual care provided by nurses?
- What are some ways that you can develop a greater awareness of the "spirit within the self"?
- Discuss ways that nurses (and patients, for that matter) can nurture their own spiritual needs.

Practical Knowledge
knowing **how**

Most hospital admission forms include a place to record the patient's religious preferences, and most nursing assessment forms include more specific questions such as, "What religious rituals do you practice?" Unfortunately, some nurses believe that by completing such forms, they have addressed the patient's spiritual needs. They may be relieved because they don't feel competent to deal any further with spirituality or because they are afraid to be perceived as imposing their own religion on the

patient. However, armed with your basic theoretical knowledge of spirituality and your growing spiritual self-knowledge, you should be able to provide compassionate, caring support.

To see a care plan and care map for a client with Spiritual Distress,

 Go to Student Resources, **Care Plan** and **Care Map** on Davis*Plus*.

ASSESSMENT

People of the same religion often vary greatly in the degree to which they follow religious practices. It is not enough to fill in the Religion blank on an assessment form; you must assess each person individually to determine religious needs and practices. Given the time constraints of the admission process, stresses involved with the patient's introduction to a healthcare setting, and the multiple people involved, it is difficult to obtain meaningful information on initial assessment. For this reason, you may need to limit initial data to the patient's church preference, name of clergy, whom to call in case of emergency, dietary requirements, and any religious implications for medical care (e.g., refusal of organ transplants or blood transfusion). Over time, as you have more contact with the patient and family, trust will develop, and you will be able to obtain more sensitive, complex, and meaningful information.

Sources of Spiritual Data

You can acquire information about a patient's spirituality from a variety of sources other than interviews.

■ **Patient's environment.** Observe the patient's environment for hints about her spirituality (e.g., pictures of family and/or pets, the presence of sacred texts or reading materials, articles used in worship [a crucifix, rosary beads, religious medals, statues], or copies of church bulletins/sermon tapes).

■ **Patient's questions.** The patient may ask questions that are indicative of spiritual comfort, longing, or distress. For example, the patient may ask if you attend a religious service or worship and pray regularly; and if so, whether it provides you with a sense of comfort and meaning.

■ **Patient's behaviors, moods, and feelings.** Emotional behavior gives a clear and certain indication that the patient is struggling with issues that have spiritual overtones. These warrant further assessment and nursing intervention. For example, a patient may ask you if you have ever really felt guilty about something you did as a child.

■ **Nonverbal communication.** Body language may indicate hopeful or distressing times. For example, you may observe a patient praying. Or when asking about spirituality, you may see the patient rolling his eyes, shaking his head, and demonstrating muscle tension.

Spiritual Assessment Tools

Some healthcare agencies have focused spiritual assessment tools tailored to their particular setting. Several others have been developed.

HOPE. One easy-to-use screening method is made up of the HOPE questions (see the Focused Assessment box, The HOPE Approach to Spiritual Assessment: Examples of Questions). The questions have not been validated by research, but they do allow for an open-ended exploration of spiritual resources and concerns (Gowri & Hight, 2001).

SPIRIT. Highfield (2000) has proposed a comprehensive method of spiritual assessment. It involves an interview that is concerned with six key areas designated by the acronym SPIRIT. Refer to the Focused Assessment box, S-P-I-R-I-T Assessment.

Focused Assessment

The HOPE Approach to Spiritual Assessment: Examples of Questions

Mnemonic	Examples of Questions
H—Hope sources: meaning, comfort, strength, peace, love, and connection	What are your sources of internal support?
	What do you hold on to, to get you through difficult times?
	For some people, religious or spiritual beliefs are a source of comfort in dealing with life's ups and downs. Is this true for you?
O—Organized religion	Do you belong to a religious or spiritual community? Does it help you?
	How important is this to you?
	What aspects of your religion are helpful to you?
P—Personal spirituality/ Practices	Do you believe in God? What is your relationship with God?
	Do you have personal spiritual beliefs that are not a part of organized religion? If so, what are they?
	What aspects of your spirituality are most helpful to you (e.g., meditation, prayer, reading scripture, listening to music, nature)?
E—Effects on medical care and end-of-life issues	Has your illness affected your relationship with God? Or to do the things that usually help you spiritually?
	Are you concerned about conflicts between your beliefs and your healthcare treatment plan?
	Do you have any dietary restrictions or other practices I should know about in planning your care?
	Would you like to speak to a clinical chaplain (or community spiritual leader)?

Source: Based on Gowri, A., & Hight, E. (2001). Spirituality and medical practice: Using the HOPE questions as a practical tool for spiritual assessment. *American Family Physician, 63,* 36–41.

S-P-I-R-I-T Assessment

➤ When assessing the following key areas, obtain information from the patient when possible.

➤ For an emergency admission or if the patient cannot give information, consult the next of kin or a designated power of attorney (DPOA) as soon as possible for information.

S—Spiritual/religious belief system

Religion, tradition, sect, or denominational affiliation

Text/writing(s) that provides source of authority and codes for behavior

Name and phone number of supporting or affiliated church, synagogue, temple, or other place of worship

Past experience with a belief system (positive or negative)

Beliefs related to health, illness, healthcare, healthcare providers, Western medicine, adjuvant therapies, herbal or natural healing methods or techniques

Beliefs about suffering, terminal or chronic illness, advanced directives, autopsy, organ donation

Stigmas related to illness, if applicable

P—Personal spirituality

Individual beliefs and practices of affiliation that the patient or family accepts and attempts to follow (may be directly or indirectly related to above assessment areas)

Individual beliefs that may differ or even be contrary to affiliation beliefs

Whether spirituality is a part of personal experience of religion or a separate entity

Level of comfort discussing spirituality

Whether personal spirituality is viewed positively or negatively at the present time

I—Integration within a spiritual community

Name and title of religious or spiritual leader or authority figure(s)

Names and titles of religious groups that may need to be contacted: prayer group leader, prayer chain support person, shaman, medicine man or woman, men's or women's group within denomination

Role of patient or individual in any of above named groups

R—Ritualized practices and restrictions

Activities that patient or family's faith encourages or forbids

Needs for modesty and covering of body parts or appendages

Any special beliefs or needs in relation to drawing blood or to laboratory tests or procedures

Dietary needs and restrictions: food preferences, preparation of foods, and location of food preparation areas

Gender-specific roles and responsibilities of care providers

Prayer needs and restrictions: Who delivers and offers such practices?

Articles or other materials needed for worship, devotion, or prayer (rosaries, prayer beads, prayer books, religious tracts, Bibles, crosses, prayer shawls or cloths)

I—Implications for medical care

Beliefs and practices that healthcare providers should remember while providing care

Specific medications that may not be administered and withheld; implications for pain control

Specific medical procedures or products that may not be administered (abortion, blood products)

Communication patterns and needs for effective care delivery: Who makes decisions? What is the role of parents or guardians when children or other vulnerable populations are the recipients of care? Does the guardian reflect the beliefs of patient, if these are known?

T—Terminal events planning

Wishes for advance directives (cardiopulmonary resuscitation, intubation, ventilator assist, feeding tubes)

Wishes for transplantation or organ donation

Need for religious services (last rites, ministries of healing, baptism, initiation, confession, communion)

Clergy or ministry groups to be contacted and when

Ideas of an afterlife

Treatment of the body at the time of death

Funeral planning

Source: Adapted from Highfield, M. E. F. (2000). Providing spiritual care to patients with cancer. *Clinical Journal of Oncology Nursing, 4*(3), 115–120.

JAREL. The JAREL spiritual well-being scale was developed and is commonly used by nurses to assess the spiritual well-being of older adults (Hungelmann, Kenkel-Rossi, Klassen, et al., 1996). Cutting across religious and atheistic belief systems, it assesses three key dimensions: (1) faith/belief, (2) life/self-responsibility, and (3) life satisfaction/self-actualization.

You can use the SPIRIT model with the JAREL tool presented in ESG Figure 16-1 and the combined assessment tool and plan of care presented in ESG Figure 16-2. To find these tools,

 Go to Chapter 16, **Tables, Boxes, Figures: ESG Figures 16-1 and 16-2,** on Davis*Plus.*

KnowledgeCheck 16-5

What are the six areas for spiritual assessment summarized in Highfield's (2000) acronym SPIRIT?

 ## ThinkLike a Nurse 16-8

Complete the SPIRIT assessment on yourself. Discuss it with your classmates.

■ ANALYSIS/NURSING DIAGNOSIS

When analyzing spiritual assessment data, consider the person's developmental stage. People progress through stages of spiritual development in much the same way that they develop

physically and cognitively. Spiritual behaviors that seem problematic in one stage may not be so in an earlier stage. To review spiritual development, refer to Chapters 9 and 10.

Spirituality Diagnoses

Box 16-1 contains NANDA-I diagnostic labels that specifically deal with religion and spirituality. The following are examples of full diagnostic statements you might write for spiritual problems:

- **Spiritual Distress** related to overwhelming anxiety associated with the need to have a surgical procedure that is not accepted by her religion
- **Risk for Spiritual Distress** related to unremitting pain and loss of hope for relief, as manifested by patient's question about the usefulness of prayer ("God has forgotten about me")

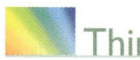

ThinkLike a Nurse 16-9

- Which of these nursing diagnoses would you use for Mr. Johnson (Meet Your Patient): Spiritual Distress, Risk for Spiritual Distress, or Readiness for Enhanced Spiritual Well-Being? Why?

A Non–NANDA-I Diagnosis. Millspaugh (2005) has suggested Spiritual Pain as a diagnosis. When a person experiences a combination of awareness of death, loss of relationships, loss of self, loss of purpose, and loss of control, Spiritual Pain may occur. However, this combination of negative experiences can be balanced by having a life-affirming and transcending purpose and an internal sense of control. The presence and quality of Spiritual Pain is determined by the degree to which the person is experiencing each component, and by the relationship of the components to each other. See Figure 16-3.

Spirituality as Etiology

In the spiritual realm, it is difficult sometimes to determine what is the problem and what is the etiology. Does the patient experience Spiritual Distress because of pain and hopelessness? Or did the patient first lose faith in God, which led to hopelessness and anxiety? Either way, spiritual support is needed.

Several of the NANDA-I diagnoses can relate to spirituality as problem, etiology, or symptom. Examples include Anxiety, Chronic Sorrow, Death Anxiety, Decisional Conflict, Hopelessness, Interrupted Family Processes, Noncompliance, Powerlessness, and Social Isolation. Non–NANDA-I etiologies include anger or resentment; feelings of guilt, shame, inadequacy, abandonment, or distrust; depression or sadness; and the inability to find meaning in life. The

---

BOX 16-1 ■ NANDA-I Spirituality Diagnoses

Moral Distress	Experienced when the person makes an ethical or moral decision, but then is unable to carry out the chosen action. Defining characteristics include anguish, powerlessness, guilt, frustration, anxiety, self-doubt, and fear over the inability to act on the moral choice.
Impaired Religiosity	Difficulty in exercising or impaired ability to exercise reliance on beliefs or to participate in rituals of a faith tradition (e.g., go to church, take communion).
Readiness for Enhanced Religiosity	The ability to increase reliance on religious beliefs and/or participate in rituals of a particular faith tradition. The patient is not experiencing a problem, but wishes to make a satisfactory situation even better.
Readiness for Enhanced Spiritual Well-Being	Describes healthy spirituality. "Ability to experience and integrate meaning and purpose in life through connectedness with self, others, art, music, literature, nature, and/or a power greater than oneself that can be strengthened" (NANDA-I, 2012, p. 394). It is the opposite of Spiritual Distress, so you will see positive expressions of faith, hope, love, courage, acceptance, and peace; healthy connections with others and with art, music, literature, and nature; and prayer and other expressions of a connection with a power higher than oneself.
Risk for Impaired Religiosity	Occurs when risk factors are present, but symptoms are not. Risk factors may be categorized as developmental, environmental, physical, psychological, sociocultural, or spiritual. Specific examples include life transitions, lack of transportation, pain, depression, social isolation, and suffering.
Risk for Spiritual Distress	Related to unremitting pain and loss of hope for relief, as manifested by patient's question about the usefulness of prayer ("God has forgotten about me.")
Spiritual Distress	"Impaired ability to experience and integrate meaning and purpose in life through a person's connectedness with self, others, art, music, literature, nature, or a power greater than oneself" (NANDA-I, 2009, p. 301). Defining characteristics (signs and symptoms) of this diagnosis include the following: ■ *Connections with self:* Expressing a lack of hope, love, courage, acceptance, or peace; a lack of meaning and purpose in life; inability to forgive self; feelings of anger or guilt ■ *Connections with others:* Refusing to see clergy; refusing to interact with family or friends; reporting lack of support system; expressions of alienation ■ *Connections with art, music, literature, nature:* No interest in nature, decrease in previous interest in music, writing, art, no interest in spiritual reading ■ *Connections with power greater than self:* Inability to pray, inability or refusal to participate in religious activities, feelings of abandonment by God or other deity, expressions of anger toward God or other deity, requests to see a religious leader, sudden changes in spiritual practices (increased or decreased)

Source: Adapted from NANDA-I. (2012). *Nursing diagnoses: Definitions and classification 2012–2014.* Ames, IA: Wiley-Blackwell.

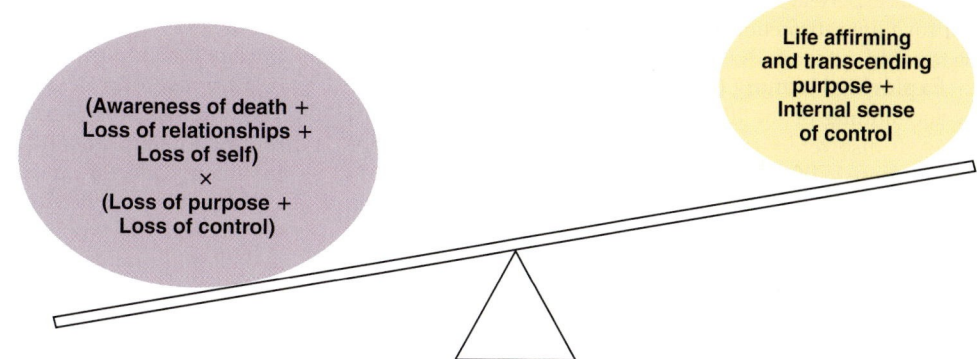

FIGURE 16-3 Components of spiritual pain. *(Based on:* Millspaugh, C. D. [2005]. Assessment and response to spiritual pain: Part II. *Journal of Palliative Medicine,* 8[6], 1110–1117.)

following are examples of diagnostic statements with spiritual etiologies:

Anxiety related to inability to reconcile decision to use birth control with religious proscriptions

Decisional Conflict related to confusion about the religious implications of the decision to forgo heroic treatment measures

Noncompliance (with treatment regimen) related to the belief that the illness is "God's will" and that healing will occur (without treatment) for the same reason.

KnowledgeCheck 16-6

Consider the following statement: A nursing diagnosis that reflects either an actual or a potential problem may reflect religious and/or spiritual dimensions of the human condition.

- Is this statement true?
- Would it be true for a *physical* diagnosis (e.g., Disturbed Sleep Pattern)? Explain your thinking.

PLANNING OUTCOMES/EVALUATION

The outcomes you establish in the planning stage of the nursing process serve as the criteria for evaluation of the patient's progress and the success of the nursing interventions.

NOC standardized outcomes associated with spirituality diagnoses include, but are not limited to, the following: Anxiety Level, Comfortable Death, Comfort Status: Psychospiritual, Dignified Life Closure, Hope, Loneliness Severity, Personal Resiliency, Personal Well-Being, Quality of Life, Spiritual Health, and Will to Live (Moorhead, Johnson, Maas, et al., 2008).

Individualized goals/outcome statements you might write for spiritual diagnoses include the following:

- **For Risk for Spiritual Distress**—Exhibits no signs or symptoms of spiritual distress (e.g., finds meaning in life, expresses hope and faith, follows usual religious practices).
- **For Spiritual Distress**—Returns to previous state of spiritual well-being and comfort (e.g., expresses a sense of peace, asks to see religious adviser).
- **For Readiness for Enhanced Spiritual Well-Being**—Experiences a higher level of connectedness with self, others, higher power, and/or nature.

PLANNING INTERVENTIONS/IMPLEMENTATION

Spiritual interventions are those used to treat and prevent spiritual problems related to the patient's illness. You will direct some nursing activities to resolving the problem, others at removing the etiology, and still others at relieving symptoms. You will, of course, base your nursing activities on the patient's symptoms and the problem etiologies. However, there are some nursing interventions that address spiritual problems in general.

Standardized (NIC) Spirituality Interventions

A few Nursing Interventions Classification (NIC) standardized interventions to promote spirituality are discussed in the following section. The evidence base for these is specific to older adults; however, they would seem to be indicated for other age groups, as well. To see other NIC interventions and selected activities for the spirituality and religiosity diagnoses shown in Box 16-1,

 Go to Chapter 16, **Standardized Language, Using Selected NIC Interventions and Activities to Support Spirituality,** on Davis*Plus.*

When you are performing interventions of a spiritual nature, remember that you absolutely must follow the patient's lead and be caring and respectful without inserting your own beliefs into the conversation. Choose your language carefully—words such as *saved, repentance,* and so on, which may be a part of everyday conversation for people who follow some religions, may cause some patients to feel pressured or uncomfortable. Try to mirror, and not go beyond, the patient's religious terminology. It requires knowledge, skill, and practice to provide religious support without imposing your own beliefs. The safest course of action, of course, is to offer to contact a chaplain for the patient. However, patients cannot always—or may not always want to—wait for a chaplain.

Active Listening (NIC)

The Active Listening intervention allows the nurse to establish a trusting relationship and to hear, understand, and interpret what the client is saying. Listening actively involves four NIC interventions, and one nonstandardized activity.

Presence (NIC). *Presence* means to be with patient and family in meaningful ways. This requires not only your actual presence at the bedside but also being open to issues and concerns of the patient and allowing the patient to lead discussions rather than setting the agenda or controlling the conversation. It involves sincere communication and being fully available to the client, and might include listening to the patient's "stories" about his illness.

Touch (NIC). Caring touch, such as hand holding or touching an arm or shoulder, can facilitate communication. It conveys concern, comfort, and acceptance, especially during

stressful experiences. At least one study has shown touch to improve life satisfaction and faith. Some people prefer not to be touched, so carefully observe the patient's responses.

Exploring Meaning (non-NIC). *Meaning* refers to a clear understanding of the illness or loss (e.g., loss of independence). It also refers to the concepts of finding significance and purpose in life, or a sense of personal worthiness. You can facilitate the patient's search for meaning by asking probing questions, providing explanations, and reframing maladaptive interpretations of life events.

Reminiscence Therapy (NIC). *Reminiscence* is the recalling and sharing with another person past life events. It promotes meaning making by rethinking and clarifying previous experiences. As the patient reminisces, he may make spiritual links by expressing personal beliefs that helped him live through difficult life events. This intervention is more effective within a long-term relationship.

Spiritual Support (NIC)

NIC defines Spiritual Support as "assisting the patient to feel balance and connection with a greater power" (Bulechek, Butcher, & Dochterman, 2008, p. 674). Effective Spiritual Support is based on a focused spiritual assessment, including the person's belief system. It may include assisting with forgiveness, encouraging hope, praying, and reading scriptures or other texts the patient requests.

Forgiveness Facilitation (NIC). Forgiveness is the act of pardoning or being pardoned for an offense, debt, or obligation. Letting go of the resentment felt for another promotes constructive changes in a person's life; a sense of renewal; and reconciliation with God, church, and one's inner being. To provide this intervention, you must first assess the patient's needs for reconciliation with self, others, and God. If, like Mr. Johnson (Meet Your Patient), the person has lost contact with family members because of disagreements, you could collaborate with the social worker and chaplain about ways to facilitate a meeting.

Forgiveness is one aspect of love. People have a spiritual need to forgive others and to be forgiven. When a person cannot forgive others, it separates him from them and interferes with giving and receiving love. When a person cannot forgive himself, he may feel the pain of shame, guilt, and anger.

Sometimes, a person may be hurting because he wants forgiveness from someone he has wronged or from God. Many people interpret illness as punishment for sins.

Some find it difficult to seek forgiveness and to believe that they have been forgiven, but this is important to achieving spiritual peace. You can help by listening when the person expresses self-doubt or guilt, providing guidance, praying with the patient if the patient asks you to, asking him if he is ready to forgive someone else, or offering to contact his chosen spiritual leader if intensive spiritual support is needed.

Hope Inspiration (NIC). Hope is a subjective state of confidence in the possibility of a better future. It includes a positive orientation, faith, and will to live. **Hopelessness** is a state in which the person perceives limited or no alternatives or personal choices. To intervene effectively, it is important to know the source of the person's hope and the factors underlying the feelings of hopelessness. As a nurse, you can encourage spiritual growth, which is thought to facilitate hope, and you can refer your patient to a support group to help in stress reduction, coping, and hope.

Prayer (non-NIC). Prayer is an integral component of almost every religion. A recent study found that about one-third of U.S. adults use prayer for health concerns; 69% found it "very helpful" (McCaffrey, Eisenberg, Legedza, et al., 2004). The numbers are even higher for older adults, 84% of whom reported using prayer as a form of complementary healing treatment, and 96% using it to cope with stress (Dunn & Horgas, 2000). So, it is quite possible that a patient or a family member may ask you to pray for him or with him.

It is important to distinguish between *praying with* and *praying for*. If the patient asks you to pray *with* him, you must determine whether he simply wants you to be present while he or another person leads the prayer. Ask whether he wants you to begin the prayer or whether he wants to begin the prayer. If a patient asks you to pray *for* him, assess what it is that he wants you to pray for. Often the patient is merely asking you to pray for him on your own time, as frequently as your schedule allows.

Regardless of the situation, if you feel comfortable doing so, then you should enter the experience of prayer with confidence; after all, the patient or family member has asked you to be present because he feels at ease with you and trusts in your abilities. However, if you feel at all uncomfortable about offering prayer, then you should state those feelings and offer to find someone who is comfortable with prayer. For example, you might say either of the following to the patient or family, "Thank you for asking me to pray with you; there is another nurse on the floor who is better at this than I am. May I have your permission to seek that person out for you?" Or, you might reply as follows: "I am confident that the chaplain can help you in many ways with your request. May I make a referral to the chaplain for you?"

Prayer has a variety of purposes, expressions, and meanings to patients and their families, as well as to nurses themselves. For many people, prayer provides for periods of intimacy with God, reveals the presence and love of God, and serves as a powerful source of comfort and hope. For those who embrace the power and influence of prayer, it supports their spiritual journeys and may help them experience forgiveness, love, hope, trust, and meaning. Symbolically, a nurse engaged in prayer manifests the reality of God's presence with that patient.

You can support patients' prayer needs by offering to pray, meditate, or read spiritual text with them, or by providing literature, music, or other items the patient uses in prayer. If you wish to pray with a patient, you may wish to follow these guidelines:

- Ask how the patient prefers to address the divine (e.g., God, Allah, Divine Mother).
- Before beginning, ask the patient whether any rituals or religious items are necessary.
- Always feel free to pray or not to pray.
- Know that there are appropriate times and places for the offering of prayer (e.g., it may make people uncomfortable in a crowded waiting room).
- If a patient asks for prayer, you might ask what he would like you to especially address in the prayer. If he tells you, be sure to focus your prayer around the request.
- It is always good to include in the prayer a request for God's help and direction for the patient's healthcare team.
- Once the prayer is over, thank the patient for asking you to participate.

Complementary & Alternative Modalities (CAM)

Intercessory Prayer

Many people pray when they are ill, and prayer seems to have positive effects. But what about the effects of *intercessory prayer*—the prayers of people for *others* who are ill? How useful is intercessory prayer? The following studies, except for Harris, Gowda, Kilb, and colleagues (1999) and Matthews, Marlowe, and MacNutt (2000), provide little support for the use of intercessory prayer as a CAM. However, this is not an exhaustive list of studies of intercessory prayer, and research is ongoing.

➤ **Matthews, Conti, & Sireci (2001).** For 95 adult hemodialysis subjects with end-stage renal disease, this study found no appreciable improvement in physiological and psychological well-being.

➤ **Palmer, Katerndahl, & Morgan-Kidd (2004).** Researchers studied 86 community-dwelling persons, ages 18 to 88 years. Intercessory prayer was used for 1 month to intervene with a life concern or problem that the participant disclosed at the beginning. No effect on problem resolution was found. However, prayer did effectively reduce the subject's level of concern, but only if the subject initially believed that the problem could be resolved. Also, better physical functioning was observed among those who had a high level of belief in prayer.

➤ **Roberts, Ahmed, & Hall (2000).** In a study performed in the United Kingdom, no evidence was found that intercessory prayer affected the numbers of people dying from leukemia or heart disease. Nor did it decrease the odds of a poor outcome for people with heart problems.

➤ **Harris, Gowda, Kilb, et al. (1999).** Remote, intercessory prayer was associated with reduced overall adverse events and shorter length of stay for hospitalized cardiac patients when used as an adjunct to standard medical care.

➤ **Matthews, Marlowe, & MacNutt (2000).** In patients with rheumatoid arthritis, 6 hours of direct-contact intercessory prayer produced overall improvement during a 1-year follow-up. However, there were no additional effects from the supplemental, distant intercessory prayers.

➤ **Benson, Dusek, Sherwood, et al. (2006).** In patients recovering after coronary artery bypass graft (CABG) surgery, this study found that intercessory prayer itself had no effect on complication-free recovery from CABG, but certainty of receiving intercessory prayer was associated with a higher incidence of complications.

For a more in-depth discussion of these guidelines,

 Go to **ESG Box 16-1, Praying With Patients,** on *DavisPlus.*

Other Nursing Activities

Spiritual care involves you in relationships with people who have come face to face with a significant life event that calls forth a new sense of meaning and purpose. Specific nursing activities, to be individualized to each client's needs, are discussed in the text that follows.

▪ **Make Referrals When Needed.** There are times when you should refer a patient to others with more knowledge and experience in religion and spirituality. For example, a patient may be experiencing Spiritual Distress because he believes he needs forgiveness for a past act, or a patient may refuse medical treatment because she thinks her church would not approve. For hospitalized and hospice patients, you can usually ask the chaplain's office to refer the patient and family to clergy or religious counselors in the community. If you are working in a home or community setting, look in the telephone or other directory for local churches. Priests, ministers, rabbis, and other spiritual advisers are all resources for you and the patient.

▪ **Encourage expression of feelings.** The best way to do this is simply to ask the patient how he is feeling or what he thinks about a particular situation.

▪ **Help the patient identify feelings of guilt.** You might ask the following after a patient has voiced a concern: "How do you feel about that?" or "You seem to feel bad about saying/doing that."

Complementary & Alternative Modalities (CAM)

Spiritual Care

Spiritual interventions, especially prayer, are a frequently used CAM:

➤ A recent study found that 63% of adult patients with cancer used at least one CAM therapy, which they all believed helped to improve their quality of life by helping them to cope with stress, obtain a sense of control, and decrease the discomforts of treatments and illness (Sparber, Bauer, Curt, et al., 2000).

➤ In this same study, the CAMs most often used were spiritual, relaxation, imagery, exercise, lifestyle, diet, and nutritional supplementation (Sparber, Bauer, Curt, et al., 2000).

➤ McCaffrey, Eisenberg, Legedza, and colleagues (2004) found that 35% of respondents used prayer for health concerns and reported high levels of perceived helpfulness.

➤ Keegan (2000) found prayer to be the CAM most frequently practiced by both Mexican and Anglo Americans.

➤ Dunn and Horgas (2000) found that 96% of community-dwelling elders use prayer to cope with stress and that 84% used prayer as a form of CAM.

➤ At least one study (le Gallez, Dimmock, & Bird, 2000) found spiritual healing to be ineffective in achieving improved laboratory parameters or clinical symptoms (e.g., pain) in patients with rheumatoid arthritis.

- **Help significant others understand the patient's feelings and needs.** Encourage family members to talk with the patient or simply to have a seat at the bedside. Periods of silence often lead into the most therapeutic of discussions.
- **Maximize the patient's comfort.** This is one of the most important spiritual activities a nurse can perform. A patient cannot think about spiritual issues when suffering physical pain or discomfort.
- **Listen to the patient's stories.** These tell the life history surrounding the person's illness.
- **Assess the patient's needs for reconciliation.** This may include reconciliation with self, others, and God. If, like Mr. Johnson (Meet Your Patient), the patient has lost contact with family members because of disagreements related to past events, you could collaborate with the social worker and chaplain about ways to facilitate a meeting.
- **Explore with the client the possible meanings of** *healing,* *miracle,* **and** *cure.* Refer to the discussion of miracles earlier in this chapter.
- **Collaborate with the dietary department.** Provide foods compatible with the person's religious needs. Encourage family members to bring foods from home, as appropriate.
- **Respect the patient's dress (and other) requirements as determined by his religion.** This may include wearing religious icons, jewelry, or special clothes.

- **Do not make assumptions about the patient's and family's beliefs.** When a patient dies, for example, a seemingly harmless statement such as "He's gone to a better place" assumes the family believes in an afterlife. If they ask, you can briefly share your beliefs, but reflect their questions back to them (e.g., "Tell me what you think happens after death").

KnowledgeCheck 16-7

- What is prayer?
- What are the "uses" of prayer by its believers?
- When a patient asks you to pray for him, what might be your most effective first response?

ThinkLike a Nurse 16-10

A patient dying of lung cancer asks you to pray with him early one morning. You agree and ask him what he would like you to pray for. He responds, "That I may be cured of my cancer and go back home." He is on oxygen therapy, has pain medications given as prescribed, and is in a room by himself. Construct a prayer that might be meaningful and helpful.

Return to the scenario for Charles Johnson (Meet Your Patient). See whether you can answer the three questions more completely now than when you began reading the chapter.

Toward Evidence-Based Practice

Consider the results and/or conclusions from the following studies.

Westlake, C., & Dracup, K. (2001). Role of spirituality in adjustment of patients with advanced heart failure. *Progress in Cardiovascular Nursing,* 16(3), 119–125.

Patients described a process wherein spirituality contributed to their adjustment to advanced heart failure. The process involved regret over past behaviors, the search for meaning in the illness, and the search for hope for the future.

Thomson, J. E. (2000). The place of spiritual well-being in hospice patients' overall quality of life. *Hospital Journal,* 15(2), 13–27.

This study found spiritual well-being to be an important contributor to overall quality of life for hospice patients.

Beery, T., Baas, L., Fowler, C., & Allen G. (2002). Spirituality in persons with heart failure. *Journal of Holistic Nursing,* 20(1), 5–25.

The combined spirituality scores predicted 24% of the variance in total quality of life for people with heart failure being treated medically or via transplant.

Tuck, I., McCain, N., & Elswick, R. (2001). Spirituality and psychosocial factors in persons living with HIV. *Journal of Advanced Nursing,* 33(6), 776–783.

Studying patients with HIV, researchers found spirituality (as measured by a subscale called "existential well-being")

was positively related to the patients' quality of life, social support, and effective coping strategies. It was negatively related to perceived stress, uncertainty, psychological distress, and emotional-focused coping.

Bradley, D. (1995). Religious involvement and social resources: Evidence from the data set "Americans' Changing Lives." *Journal for the Scientific Study of Religion,* 34(2), 259–267. (Abstract obtained from International Center for the Integration of Health and Spirituality.)

This research found that frequent attendance at religious services was strongly associated with the extent of a person's social support network.

Touhy, T. A. (2001). Nurturing hope and spirituality in the nursing home. *Holistic Nursing Practice,* 15(4), 45–56.

This study found that spirituality was the only factor of those studied that contributed significantly to hope in institutionalized elders.

Oxman, T., Freeman, D., & Mannheimer, E. (1995). Lack of social participation or religious strength or comfort as risk factors for death after cardiac surgery in the elderly. *Psychosomatic Medicine,* 57, 5–15. (Abstract obtained from International Center for the Integration of Health and Spirituality.)

Researchers found that religious faith was the most consistent indicator of survival after heart surgery in older patients.

Toward Evidence-Based Practice—cont'd

Those without religious faith had almost three times the risk of death; moreover, the more religious the patient, the greater the protective effect the study found.

Koenig, H. G., et al. (1998). The relationship between religious activities and blood pressure in older adults. *International Journal of Psychology in Medicine, 28(2), 189–213.*

This study found that older adults who both attended religious services at least once a week *and* prayed or studied the Bible at least daily had consistently lower blood pressure. The study also found that people who tuned in to religious TV or radio shows regularly actually had higher blood pressure than those who were less frequent viewers or listeners.

1. For which of the following do these studies, taken as a whole, provide the stronger support? Explain your reasoning.

   a. Spirituality has a positive effect on physical factors.
   b. Spirituality has a positive effect on psychosocial or emotional factors.

2. Suppose you are a nursing home administrator in an institution where the focus is almost entirely on physical care. You are thinking about a program to teach and encourage your staff to integrate spiritual interventions into their care. Evaluate the findings from each of the studies to see how useful it would be in supporting your idea. Explain your thinking.

 Go to Chapter 16, **Toward Evidence-Based Practice Suggested Responses,** on *DavisPlus.*

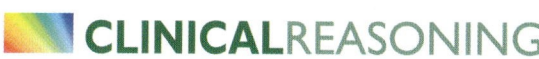

CLINICALREASONING:
Applying the **Full-Spectrum Nursing Model**

Because the following critical thinking activities allow you to practice the kind of thinking you will use as a full-spectrum nurse, they usually have no single right answer. Discuss them with your peers—if you have difficulty with any of the questions, consult your instructor.

PATIENT SITUATION

Recall from the Meet Your Patient scenario that Charles Johnson is a 75-year-old African American man with newly diagnosed lung cancer. His physicians want to start chemotherapy to try to increase his life span. He is unsure whether he wants to have chemotherapy. Review the scenario and refer to it as needed in answering the following questions.

THINKING

1. *Theoretical Knowledge (Recall of Facts and Principles):* Define *forgiveness,* and explain the benefits of forgiving self and others.
2. *Critical Thinking (Application of Knowledge):* Based on your theoretical knowledge about forgiveness, with whom might Mr. Johnson need to reconcile? Why do you think so?

DOING

3. *Practical Knowledge (HOPE Assessment):* Use the HOPE Assessment box (The HOPE Approach to Spiritual Assessment: Examples of Questions) and enter Mr. Johnson's data. Identify sections for which you need additional data.

CARING

4. *Self-Knowledge:* How is your religious background similar to or different from Mr. Johnson's?
5. *Self-Knowledge:* (a) How would you feel if Mr. Johnson said to you, "Church folk are all a bunch of hypocrites, if you ask me. I choose not to be a part of any of that"? (b) How would you respond?
6. *Ethical Knowledge:* Imagine that Mr. Johnson's sister comes to visit and leaves some religious pamphlets on a chair, where he will not see them before she leaves. What would you do?

 Go To Chapter 16, **Clinical Reasoning: Applying the Full-Spectrum Nursing Model Response Sheet,** on *DavisPlus.*

To explore learning resources for this chapter,

 Go to Davis*Plus* at http://davisplus.fadavis.com/Treas1

Chapter Resources for Chapter 16:

Knowledge Check and Think Like a Nurse Response
  Sheets

Knowledge Check Answers

Resources for Caregivers and Health Professionals

Reading More About Spirituality (suggested readings)

What Are the Main Points in This Chapter?

NCLEX-Style Review Questions

Chapter Overview Podcasts

Concept Map

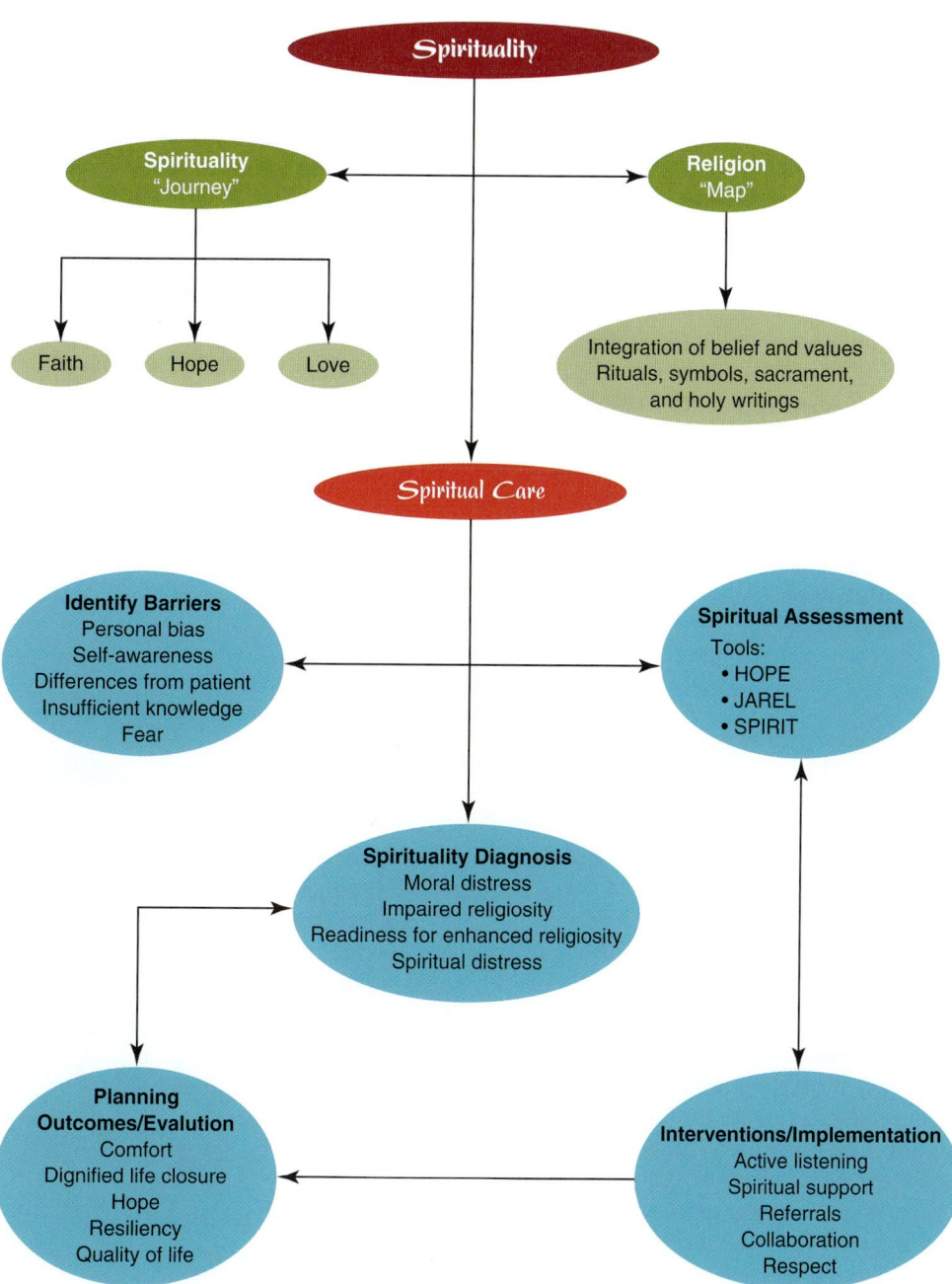

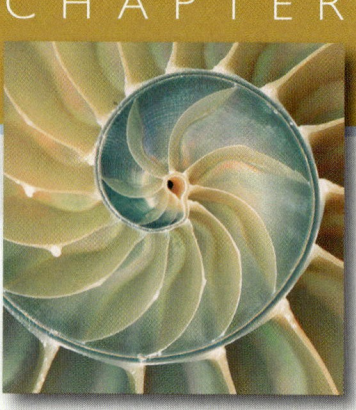

Loss, Grief, & Dying

Learning Outcomes

After completing this chapter, you should be able to:

➤ Name and describe at least four types of loss.

➤ Identify the stages of grief as described by Engel, Worden, Rando, and Bowlby.

➤ Compare and contrast four types of grief.

➤ List and discuss at least five factors that affect grieving.

➤ Define *death* according to the Uniform Determination of Death Act.

➤ Give a definition of *higher-brain death*.

➤ Create a time line of the dying process, indicating the physiological signs and symptoms common to each stage.

➤ List and describe the Kübler-Ross stages of dying and grief.

➤ Define *end-of-life care, hospice care,* and *palliative care.*

➤ Assess, diagnose, plan, and implement care of dying patients and their families.

➤ Describe the responsibilities of the nurse regarding postmortem care.

➤ Identify nursing interventions to help clients who are grieving.

Key Concepts

Loss

Grief

Death/dying

End-of-life Care

Related Concepts

See the Concept Map at the end of this chapter.

Caring for the Nguyens

This feature allows you to practice the kind of thinking you will use as a full-spectrum nurse. There is usually more than one correct answer to a critical thinking question, so we do not provide answers for these features. It is more important to develop your nursing judgment than to "cover content." Discuss the questions with your peers. If you are still unsure, consult your instructor.

At a clinic visit, Nam Nguyen tells you that his father's health is declining rapidly. Mr. Nguyen tells you, "I thought he was doing okay. I knew he had surgery for his prostate, so I thought it was all over. Lately he's been having lots of low back and hip pain. So my mom begged him to go to the doctor, and he told him he has cancer all over." Nam shakes his head and looks away from you. You notice tears in his eyes. As you talk with him, he tells you that his family has avoided discussions about serious illness and death. "It just never got discussed. The whole idea made my parents

uncomfortable. When my father got sick the first time, he refused to discuss it. 'I'm going to get better. Don't even think about it,' he would say." Now Nam feels the need to discuss this situation with his parents but doesn't know how to bring up the topic. He asks for your advice.

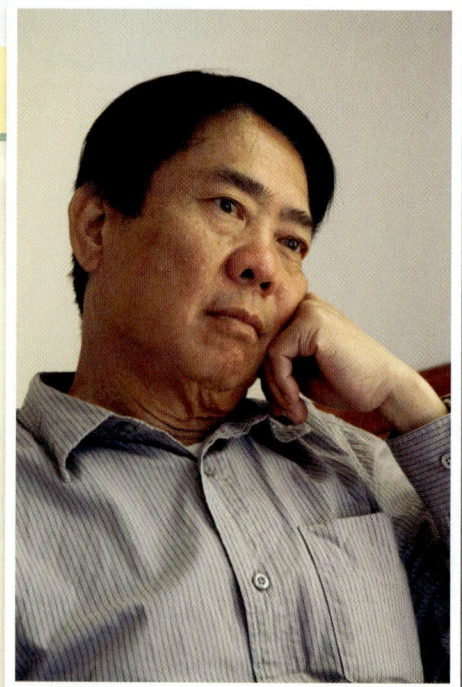

Caring for the Nguyens (continued)

A. What would you think and feel when you see Nam's tears and when he asks for this advice?

B. What would you advise Mr. Nguyen?

C. What type of grief is Mr. Nguyen experiencing?

D. Examine the factors that affect grief. Apply these factors to Nam's situation. You will need to review the family history included in the introduction to the Nguyens (in the front of this book) to fully answer this question. Indicate whether the information for any of the factors to be evaluated is insufficient.

 Go to **Caring for the Nguyens Response Sheet** on *DavisPlus.*

Meet Your Patient

Thomas Manning is a 47-year-old man who is in the oncology unit with end-stage cancer of the pancreas. He is married and has three children, ages 18, 15, and 13. His oldest daughter has been away at college for only 6 months. Mr. Manning's father died 3 months ago from complications of alcoholism, and his mother has been withdrawn and grieving. His wife, Mary, tells you that Thomas "just wants to die" and does not want anyone trying to revive him or "jumping on his chest" if he dies. Mary is distressed and wants him to "keep fighting."

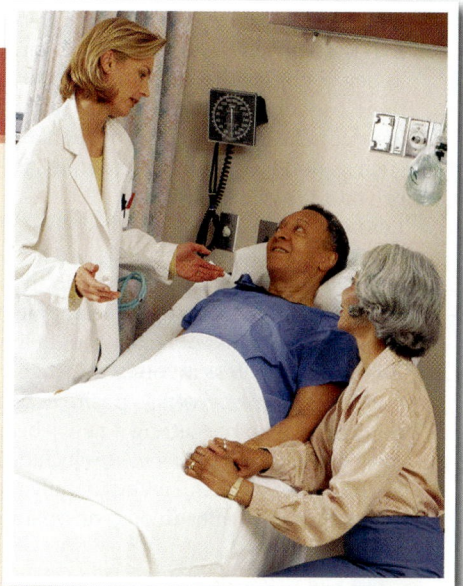

Theoretical Knowledge
knowing **why**

Throughout your nursing career, you will care for patients coping with loss—of youth, beauty, previous health, functioning, or quality of life. Many of your patients, like Thomas Manning, will be confronting their own approaching death, while family members will be facing loss of their loved one. As their nurse, you can help these people cope with their losses and grieve in a way that is healing, even transformative. But to do so, you need to know how to assess each patient's response to loss, plan appropriate outcomes, and intervene with skill and compassion. As a foundation, you must understand your own feelings and attitudes about loss, grief, and dying. We encourage you to increase your self- knowledge as you work through this chapter.

ABOUT THE KEY CONCEPTS

In order to provide care for patients experiencing loss, you will need to understand the key concepts of loss, grief, death and dying, and end-of-life care. Related concepts, such as stages of death, depression, and grief education, will expand the way you think about the key concepts. As you study the chapter, think often about how all the specific "parts and pieces" are related to the key concepts.

WHAT IS LOSS?

What is the first thing that comes to mind when you think of *loss*? Many people think of losing a loved one through death. Loss, however, is a daily occurrence. Our losses begin at birth when we lose the warmth and security of the womb, and end with the ultimate loss, the death of self. **Loss** can be defined as the undesired change or removal of a valued object, person, or situation.

Can you think of the first time you experienced a loss and what that felt like? What other losses have you undergone as you matured? For losses that are common at different developmental stages,

 Go to Chapter 17, **Tables, Boxes, Figures: ESG Table 17-1,** on *DavisPlus.*

Whenever there is change, there is loss. Because we experience many changes throughout life, we also experience much loss. Loss can be categorized in the following ways:

- *Actual versus perceived loss.* **Actual loss** includes the death of a loved one (or relationship), theft, deterioration, destruction, and natural disaster. Actual loss can be identified by others, not just by the person experiencing it (e.g., hair loss during chemotherapy). In contrast, **perceived loss** is internal; it is identified only by the person experiencing it (e.g., a woman diagnosed with a sexually transmitted infection may perceive herself as having lost her purity).
- *Physical loss versus psychological loss.* **Physical loss** includes (1) injuries (e.g., a limb amputation), (2) removal of an organ (e.g., hysterectomy), and (3) loss of function (e.g., loss of mobility). **Psychological losses** challenge our belief system. They are commonly seen in the areas of sexuality, control, fairness, meaning, and trust. Some losses are mixed. For example, after removal of a prostate gland, a man may feel both the physical and psychological loss of sexuality.
- *External versus internal loss.* **External losses** are actual losses of objects that are important to the person because of their cost or sentimental value (e.g., jewelry, pets). These losses can be brought about by theft, destruction, or disasters such as floods and fire. **Internal loss** is another term for perceived or psychological loss.
- *Loss of aspects of self* includes physical losses such as body organs, limbs, body functions, and body disfigurement. Psychological and perceived losses in this category include aspects of one's personality, developmental change (as in the aging process), loss of hopes and dreams, and loss of faith.
- *Environmental loss* involves a change in the familiar, even if the change is perceived as positive. Examples include moving to a new home, getting a new job, and going to college.
- *Loss of significant relationships* includes, but is not limited to, actual loss of spouses, siblings, family members, or significant others through death, divorce, or separation (e.g., during war).

Think**Like a Nurse** 17-1

- Which kinds of loss do you think Thomas Manning (Meet Your Patient) is experiencing?
- Why is it important to recognize loss?

WHAT IS GRIEF?

Whenever there is significant loss, there is grieving. Grieving requires energy, so it can interfere with health and delay healing. However, grieving is positive in the sense that it is essential to psychological healing after a loss. Consider the following losses and the different reactions of the women involved:

Both Mrs. Smith and Mrs. Jones have lost a dog. Mrs. Smith's son left his dog with her when he went away to college last year. It has died of old age. Mrs. Jones's dog has been with her for 10 years and has been her only companion since her husband died 5 years ago. Her dog was killed by a car today as they were on their morning walk. Which woman do you think will grieve her loss more? Why? Discuss this situation with a classmate. Do you both have the same opinion about this?

It is really impossible to decide who would feel "more" grief. The intensity of the grief depends on the meaning the person attaches to the loss. Both women probably felt sad. However, the meaning of and attachment to the dog are different for each one. You might have thought Mrs. Smith's loss was minor; however, her dog was owned by her son and may

have represented him in her mind. Mrs. Jones's dog was a companion and a protector and may have represented security and friendship. Each woman must grieve what the loss represents to her. This is true for everyone, whether the losses are actual or perceived, physical or psychological.

Grief is the physical, psychological, and spiritual responses to a loss. **Mourning** consists of actions associated with grief (e.g., wailing, wearing black clothing). These processes are normal and natural responses to a loss. The mourning and adjustment time after a loss is the period of **bereavement**. Although each person may express grief differently, some aspects of grief are shared by almost everyone.

Knowledge**Check** 17-1

What types of losses commonly occur in our lives?

Stages of Grief

There is no single, correct way to grieve, nor do people move neatly from one stage or step of grief to the next. Rather, grieving is a fluid, ongoing process. There is constant movement among stages, including recurrences of phases the bereaved person thought were resolved. The following are four major stage theorists in the field (also see Table 17-1).

George L. Engel (1961). Engel believed that uncomplicated grief has a clear onset and a predictable course, modified mainly by the abruptness and significance of the loss and how well prepared the bereaved person was. Uncomplicated grief is universal and does not require treatment.

John Bowlby (1982). Drawing on attachment theory, Bowlby suggested that grief occurs when the bereaved learn that the object of their attachment is lost. Some experts assert that Bowlby's theory does not take into account the individual nature of grief and that it implies loved ones can be replaced. Nevertheless, our understanding of grief is broadened by his idea that grief is a mature way of dealing with loss of attachment. He also provides a slightly different perspective on the stages of grief.

Theresa Rando (1984, 1986, 1993, 2000). Rando identified three processes of grieving (Table 17-1). Rando's (1984) stages are commonly described as the six *R*s of grieving:

1. *R*ecognizing the loss (awareness)
2. *R*eacting to the separation (feeling the emotions)
3. *R*ecollecting memories of the deceased (remembering, reliving)
4. *R*elinquishing the old attachment (new ways of living without the deceased)
5. *R*eadjusting to the new environment (new coping skills)
6. *R*einvesting self (energy once turned inward on grief begins to be focused outward again).

William Worden (2002). Worden described the tasks that a grieving person must achieve. They progress from an initial numbness or denial through experiencing and working through pain and grief and eventually moving on with life.

Think**Like a Nurse** 17-2

What are some of the similarities you see in the four theories described?

Grieving as Reconstructing Meaning

Some theorists are moving away from stage models of grieving toward the idea of grieving as a process of reconstructing meaning. For example, Florczak (2008) believes that the

Table 17-1 ▶ Theories of Grief: A Comparison

STAGES	DESCRIPTION
George Engel (1961)—Three Stages of Grief	
Shock and disbelief	Initial phase. The sufferer denies the loss in an attempt to protect himself against the shock of reality.
Developing awareness of the loss	The sufferer experiences painful feelings of sadness, guilt, shame, helplessness, hopelessness, loss, and emptiness. The person may lose interest in usual activities and experience impaired work performance. She may also experience loss of appetite, sleep disturbances, and even physical symptoms of pain or other discomfort.
Restitution and recovery	The final phase, which is prolonged and gradual. The person carries on the work of mourning and overcomes the trauma of the loss, and a state of health and well-being is reestablished.
John Bowlby (1982)—Phases of Grief	
Shock and numbness	Initial stage, in which the person experiences disorientation and feelings of helplessness.
Yearning and searching	The grieving person yearns to be reconnected with the deceased and searches for connections.
Disorganization and despair	The permanence of the loss becomes real. The person feels the pain and emotions of grief to their fullest and feels there is no hope of reconnection.
Reorganization	Adjusting to life without the deceased (or lost object); developing new coping skills
Theresa Rando (1984, 1986, 1993, 2000)—Three Processes of Grieving	
Avoidance	Includes shock, disbelief, denial, anger, and bargaining.
Confrontation	The person actually begins to face the loss; a very emotional and upsetting time, when the person feels the grief most acutely.
Accommodation	The person begins to live with the loss, feel better, and resume some routine activities.
William Worden (2002)—Four Tasks of Grieving	
Accepting the reality of the loss	*Realizing that the loved one (or object) is gone.* In the hours and days after a significant loss, the grieving person typically feels numb and unable to accept the fact of the loss. This numbness is thought to be a helpful form of denial, which allows the person to "take in" only what the psyche is capable of handling at that time. So, the task of realizing the loved one or object is gone may take several days or, in the case of a sudden death, weeks.
Working through the pain and grief	*Feelings and emotions that surface are intense and can change rapidly.* This makes the person feel "out of control." People in this stage may say they feel as if they are "going crazy." This is usually the longest phase for two reasons. First, because none of us likes to be in pain, we become expert at finding ways not to feel it. We overeat, overmedicate, overwork, and drink to excess to avoid feeling the pain, and we thereby prolong the process of grief. Second, caring people do not like to see their loved ones in pain, so they make attempts to remove the pain (e.g., by distraction) rather than letting the person experience it. Like avoidance, this well-meaning behavior also prolongs the process.
Adjusting to the environment in which the deceased is missing	*Adjusting to the environment without the deceased.* This may mean performing alone activities and tasks, such as going for walks or shopping, that were once shared. Or it may include taking on roles and responsibilities that the deceased previously held. Such experiences can be extremely sad, frustrating and challenging, or very rewarding. However, once the person has established the new pattern, he or she typically feels satisfaction and increased self-esteem.
Emotionally relocating the deceased and moving on with life	*Investing emotional energy.* Initially all energy is focused on the deceased: thinking about the person, talking about him/her, reliving memories, and so on. It is nearly impossible to think of anything else. Concentration is difficult, so the grieving person finds it hard to engage in activities such as reading. When the person's energy begins to flow toward others or to different or former interests (e.g., working, socializing), the healing process is in progress.

Sources: Engel, G. L. (1961). Is grief a disease? A challenge for medical research. *Psychosomatic Medicine, XXIII*(1), 18–22; Worden, J. W. (2002). *Grief counseling and grief therapy: A handbook for the mental health practitioner* (3rd ed.). New York: Springer; Rando, T. (1984). *Grief, dying and death: Clinical interventions for caregivers.* Champaign, IL: Research Press; and Bowlby, J. (1982). *Attachment and loss.* 3 vols. New York: Basic Books.

After the patient dies, there is follow-up bereavement care for the families.

Although you may think of hospice as "home" care, hospice is a *way* of caring rather than a setting. Some hospitals are able to devote some inpatient beds to hospice care, and free-standing hospices also exist. The purpose of admitting a patient is to provide a family with some respite for a period of time or to stabilize a patient who requires symptom management, or to care for a patient who is in the end stage of a disease (e.g., AIDS or cancer) and needs a level of expert care that family members cannot provide at home.

Legal and Ethical Considerations at End of Life

The technology of life support makes it possible to prolong bodily functions almost indefinitely, leaving patients and families struggling to decide whether prolonging life is appropriate. More and more clients depend on nurses for education regarding patient rights and choices surrounding end-of-life care. Each situation is unique, and you should be able to explore with clients the various options available. See Chapters 42 and 43, for more information about the ethical and legal aspects of each of the following topics.

Respecting Patient and Family Needs

Competency: **Patient-Centered Care (Skills, Attitudes)***

Karen Litvak is a 64-year-old woman who has lived her entire life with her mother, who is 86 years old. The mother is hospitalized with pneumonia. Karen spends each day at her side. "I don't know how to help her," Karen says to the nurse, "she always took care of me."

One afternoon, Karen's mother stopped breathing. A code was called and doctors, nurses and therapists ran into the room and began aggressive CPR. Karen stood out of the way but did not leave the room. The Chaplin asked her to come out into the hallway with him, but she refused. The Chaplin continued to urge her until she said forcefully "No, I want to stay." Karen looked to the nurses, who nodded yes, she could stay.

The resuscitation efforts were not successful. The nurses asked Karen if she would like to come closer while they cleaned her mother. Karen talked about her mother as the nurses washed the mother's face and hands, put a clean hospital gown on her and folded a clean sheet up to her waist. Karen thanked the nurses and turned to go. The nurses asked her where she would go and if she had anyone to stay with her. She said she had a sister and would stay with her for a while.

Think about it: Patient-centered care means showing respect for the patient's significant other's values and needs and the diversity of human experience.

➤ Should the nurses have allowed the daughter to stay during CPR? Why or why not?

➤ How did the nurses show respect for Karen?

➤ How would you describe the daughter's values and needs?
   *For specific Knowledge, Skills, and Attitudes,

 Go to the QSEN web site at http:www.qsen.org. ksas_prelicensure.php

---

Advance Directives

An **advance directive** is a group of instructions (written or oral) stating a person's wishes relative to his healthcare if he were unable to make that decision. An ordinary power of attorney does not give another person the right to make healthcare decisions for the patient.

The **Patient Self-Determination Act (PSDA),** passed by Congress in 1990, requires that all healthcare providers who receive Medicare funds (e.g., hospitals, home care agencies, hospices, nursing homes) must educate staff and patients and provide an opportunity for all patients to complete an advance directive. The Joint Commission (2008) also requires institutions to address the wishes of the patient regarding end-of-life decisions. State laws regarding advance directives vary. It is important for you to understand the regulations of your own state as well as federal laws and the policies of your institution. Advance directives are of different types and serve different purposes.

- A **living will** is a document prepared by a competent person giving instructions regarding medical care if that person becomes unable to make decisions. The document provides specific instructions about the kinds of healthcare the person would wish or would wish *not* to have in particular situations. For example, it might specify that no artificial food or fluids be administered.

- A **durable power of attorney (DPOA),** or **healthcare proxy,** exists when a competent person names another individual to make decisions regarding his healthcare choices under certain conditions (e.g., irreversible coma, terminal illness) when he is unable to do so. These instructions are usually written and should include specific instructions about the patient's wishes regarding hydration, feeding tubes, medication, resuscitation, and mechanical ventilation. The document must be witnessed by two persons and can be changed or canceled at any time by the patient. For an example of an advance directive,

 Go to Chapter 17, **Tables, Boxes, Figures: ESG Figure 17-1,** on Davis*Plus.*

For details of the Patient Self-Determination Act,

 Go to Chapter 17, **Supplemental Materials: Patient Self-Determination Act,** on Davis*Plus.*

Some people fear that once an advance directive is signed, no further care will be provided. Explain to families and patients that this is not true; instead, the directive is intended to make sure they will get however much or little care *they* wish. Remind people that everyone should have an advance directive and that they should not wait until they become ill to prepare one. Such explanations are independent nursing activities, for which you are responsible.

Orders for DNAR

A **DNAR order** is an order *not* to attempt resuscitation of the patient in the event of a cardiac or respiratory failure. The American Heart Association (AHA) is now using the term *DNAR (do not attempt resuscitation)* instead of *DNR (do not resuscitate).* You must pay careful attention to these orders, agency policies, and any advance directives, so you will be prepared should one of your patients

suffer a cardiac arrest. For an example of a DNAR (DNR) order,

 Go to Chapter 17, **Tables, Boxes, Figures: ESG Figure 17-2, Do Not Resuscitate Orders,** on Davis*Plus*.

In many healthcare settings, cardiopulmonary resuscitation (CPR) is performed almost automatically. This practice may be slowly changing, however. It is interesting that the AHA, which has for so long focused on preserving life, has in its more recent publications begun to point out that it is not always appropriate to use CPR. For example, some of their instructor's materials stress that asystole (no cardiac activity) is usually a confirmation of death rather than a rhythm requiring treatment.

Carefully explain to patients and families what CPR involves and what their options are. They have the right to refuse CPR and may request DNAR orders; the physician cannot legally write a DNAR order if the patient or family does not wish it. The American Nurses Association (ANA, 2004) recommendations regarding DNAR are summarized in Box 17-3. For a complete list of the ANA recommendations,

 Go to Chapter 17, **Tables, Boxes, Figures: ESG Box 17-2,** on Davis*Plus*.

There is growing evidence that strategies such as formal and informal family meetings, daily team consensus processes, palliative care team case finding, and ethics consultation improve communication about end-of-life decisions (Boyle, Miller, & Forbes-Thompson, 2005).

Assisted Suicide and Euthanasia

Assisted suicide means that the patient is physically capable of ending his own life, has expressed the intention to do so, and has turned to the healthcare provider merely to supply the means. The ANA (1994a, 1994b) believes that "the nurse should not participate in active euthanasia (and assisted suicide) because such an act is in direct violation of the Code for Nurses and the ethical traditions of the profession. Nurses have an obligation to provide timely, humane, comprehensive, and compassionate end-of-life care."

The term **euthanasia** comes from the Greek word *euthanatos*, which means "good death." It refers to the deliberate ending of a life of someone suffering from a terminal or incurable illness. **Active euthanasia** occurs as a result of a direct action. Active euthanasia goes a step further than assisted suicide. In assisted suicide, the person assisting makes available the means for the person to take his own life (e.g., medications); in active euthanasia, the assistant also serves as the direct agent of death (e.g., administers the medication).

Passive euthanasia occurs as a result of a *lack* of action (e.g., withholding medications or food necessary to sustain life). Honoring the refusal of treatments that a patient does not desire, that are burdensome, or that will not benefit the patient is not generally considered passive euthanasia and can be ethically and legally permissible. For more information about the ethical and legal issues surrounding euthanasia, see Chapters 42 and 43, respectively.

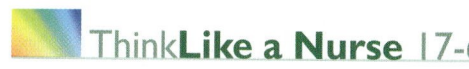 Think**Like a Nurse** 17-6

What are your feelings about assisted suicide and euthanasia? Focus on your feelings, not on principles, explanations, and rationales.

Autopsy

An autopsy is a medical examination of the body to determine the cause of death. Autopsies also provide relevant data about disease processes and causes. The pathologist carefully examines the entire body, removes body organs, and extracts sample tissues for further examination. The organs are then replaced in the body, and the body cavities are closed with sutures. An autopsy requires signed permission from the next of kin, except in cases in which autopsy is required by law (e.g., deaths that are suspicious or unwitnessed).

Organ Donation

Currently all 50 states have adopted some form of the Uniform Anatomical Gift Act (UAGA) for organ donation. A revision of the UAGA was proposed in 2006. About half the states have already adopted the 2006 UAGA, and it has been introduced in the legislation of several others. However, there are some ethical concerns that the new UAGA might override an individual's advance directives or result in people becoming donors or kept on life support against their or their family's wishes. In general, the 2006 UAGA states the following:

- As a rule, general donors must be older than age 18 or be an emancipated minor.
- Next of kin can donate organs when a person dies, unless there was a known objection by the person.
- Relatives cannot revoke a person's donation, even after his death.

BOX 17-3 ■ Highlights of ANA Recommendations Concerning DNAR

- The competent patient's choices have highest priority when there is conflict.
- When the patient is not competent, give highest priority to advance directives or the surrogate decision makers.
- DNAR orders should be discussed explicitly with the patient and significant others.
- DNAR orders must be documented, reviewed, and updated.
- DNAR does *not* mean "discontinue care"!
- Nurses should be aware of and have an active role in developing DNAR policies in the institutions where they work; they should participate in interdisciplinary mechanisms for resolving disputes among patients, families, and healthcare practitioners concerning DNAR orders.
- Nurses have a duty to educate patients and families about technologies and termination of treatment decisions, and to encourage them to think about end-of-life preferences and make their wishes known in advance.
- Nurses have a duty to communicate relevant information and to advocate for a patient's end-of-life preferences to be honored.

Source: Adapted from American Nurses Association (ANA). (2004). Position statement: Nursing care and do-not-resuscitate decisions. Washington, DC: Author. Retrieved February 2, 2011, from http://www.nursingworld.org/MainMenuCategories/EthicsStandards/Ethics-Position-Statements/Copy%20of%20dnr0414405.aspx

- The person making the gift can amend or revoke it at any time before death.
- Time of death must be determined by a physician who is not involved in any transplantation (Kurtz, Strong, & Gerasimow, 2007; Verheijde, Rady, & McGregor, 2007).

To see the UAGA major provisions in greater detail,

 Go To Chapter 17, **Tables, Boxes, Figures: ESG Box 17-3, Major Provisions of the Uniform Anatomical Gift Act,** on Davis*Plus.*

Even though donor cards (Fig. 17-2) are legal in all states, many institutions will not procure organs from the deceased if there is strong family objection. Therefore, if a patient is planning to donate organs or tissues, be sure that he discusses these wishes with family members. If death is imminent, a healthcare team member (physician or nurse) should ask whether the patient has agreed to be an organ donor. In many institutions, a transplant coordinator contacts the family and makes the request for organ and tissue donation.

KnowledgeCheck 17-3

- What are advance directives?
- What is the ANA position on assisted suicide?

PracticalKnowledge
knowing **how**

ASSESSMENT

When a patient is dying or has experienced a loss, you must carefully assess the patient and significant others for the

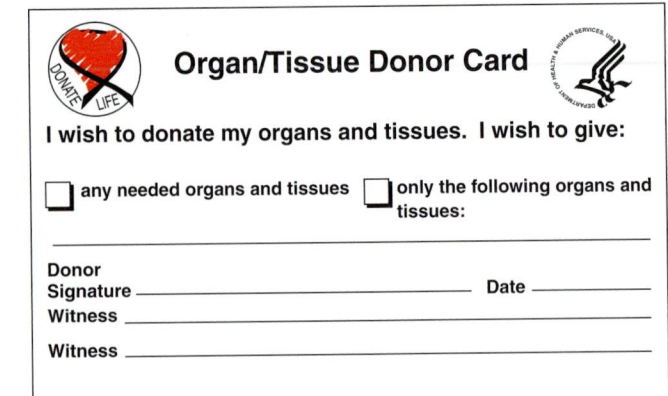

FIGURE 17-2 Example of an organ donor card. (*Source:* U.S. Department of Health and Human Services. Retrieved from http://dying.about.com/od/livingafteradeath/ss/organdonate_3.htm

common grief reactions listed in the Focused Assessment box, Assessing Grief and Loss. Other important areas to assess include knowledge base, history of loss, coping patterns and abilities, meaning of the loss or illness, and support systems. For dying patients, you should also make the following assessments:

- When the client and family are ready, encourage them to talk about the client's intentions for burial or cremation or tasks that the client would like taken care of (e.g., giving away valuables, calling family members).
- Determine whether the dying client has a living will or advance directives.
- Discuss with client and family the possibility of organ donation, if appropriate for the client's circumstances.

Focused Assessment

Assessing Grief and Loss

1. Assess the patient and significant others for common grief reactions.

Physical	Emotional	Behaviors	Cognition
Loss of appetite	Anger	Forgetfulness	Decreased concentration
Weight loss/gain	Sadness	Withdrawal	Forgetfulness
Fatigue	Guilt	Insomnia or too much sleep	Impaired judgment
Decreased libido	Relief	Dreaming of deceased	Obsessive thoughts of the deceased or lost object
Decrease in immune system	Shock	Verbalizing the loss	
Decreased energy	Numbness	Crying	Preoccupation
Possibly physical symptoms, such as headache or stomach pain	Loneliness	Loss of productivity at work or school	Confusion
	Fear		Questioning spiritual beliefs
	Anxiety		Searching to understand
	Powerlessness		Searching for purpose and meaning
	Helplessness		
	Depression		

2. Assess knowledge base of patient and significant others.

a. Can they make informed decisions about healthcare choices? You might ask the following questions:
  ➤ Tell me what you understand about your illness.
  ➤ Are there any questions about your illness that you'd like me to answer?

➤ What are your options for treatment?
➤ Do you know how to reach your provider if you have questions about your care?

b. What and how much do the patient and family want to know? (*Some people wish to have all the details of their condition and care. For others, the details cause anxiety.*)

Organ/Tissue Donor Card

I wish to donate my organs and tissues. I wish to give:

☐ any needed organs and tissues   ☐ only the following organs and tissues:

_____

Donor
Signature _____   Date _____
Witness _____
Witness _____

Focused Assessment

Assessing Grief and Loss—cont'd

3. **Assess the history of loss.** Determine whether the patient or family has sustained recent losses or major changes (e.g., death, moving, divorce, retirement). Ask questions such as the following:
   ➤ Have you had any recent changes in your life?
   ➤ Tell me about your family.
   ➤ Are your parents still living?
   ➤ What previous experiences have you had with the loss of someone you loved (or with this condition)?

4. **Assess coping abilities and support systems.** (The way individuals have coped in the past will affect how they cope with dying or with their current loss. It may also be therapeutic for them to identify their resources and supports.)
   Some coping assessment questions include the following:
   ➤ What do you do to help you reduce stress?
   ➤ Do you have family/friends you can talk with?
   ➤ What would you say is your greatest support when going through difficult times?
   ➤ Tell me about a previous loss and what you did to cope with it.
   ➤ Are you using any community resources to help you get through this? Do you know what they are?

5. **Assess the meaning of the loss or illness.** Be alert for statements such as the following, which may indicate the patient or family is struggling to find meaning in their suffering:
   ➤ I'm being punished.
   ➤ She doesn't deserve this.
   ➤ Why is this happening to me?

6. **Differentiate between grief and depressive disorder.**
   a. Symptoms common to both grief and depressive disorder: sadness, insomnia, poor appetite, and weight loss. (Feelings of sadness and depression are a normal part of grief, provided the depression does not linger too long.)
   b. Symptoms that indicate grief, but not depression: For example, the person may feel relatively better in certain situations, for example, when she is with friends and family. However, triggers, such as the deceased person's birthday, an anniversary, or holidays, cause the feelings to resurface more strongly.
   c. Symptoms that indicate depressive disorder (Ferszt & Leveillee, 2006):
      ➤ The depression is more pervasive. That is, the person rarely gets any relief from the symptoms.
      ➤ Feelings of guilt not related to the loved one's death
      ➤ Thoughts about own death or of suicide (other than feeling the person would be better off dead now that the loved one is gone)
      ➤ Preoccupation with own "worthlessness"
      ➤ Sluggishness
      ➤ Hesitant and confused speech
      ➤ Prolonged and marked difficulty in carrying out activities of daily living
      ➤ Hallucinations, other than thinking he hears the voice of or sees the deceased person

7. **Perform a physical assessment.**
   Look for signs of increased stress, such as tension, forgetfulness, distraction, increased or decreased appetite and sleep, weight gain or loss, fatigue, and decreased self-care (e.g., deficient hygiene). (A thorough physical examination adds data to help you determine how well the patient is coping with the loss or illness.

8. **Perform a cultural and spiritual assessment.**
   a. Assess the patient's and family's religious beliefs, any spiritual needs they may have (e.g., forgiveness, hope, meaning, love), and cultural influences that may affect the way they cope.
   b. Do not assume that a person adheres closely to the dominant values of his religious or cultural group. Always assess. For example, ask, "To what religious and ethnic groups do you belong?" and "How closely do you identify with those groups?"
      See Chapters 15 and 16 for details of cultural and spiritual assessment, if you need them.

9. **Perform these specific assessments for dying patients.**
   For dying patients, in addition to the other assessments in this box, you should also assess the following:
   a. When the patient and family are ready, encourage them to talk about what the patient might want for burial or cremation or whether there are tasks that the person would like taken care of (e.g., giving away valuables, calling family members).
   b. Determine whether the dying person has a living will or advance directives.
   c. Discuss with the patient and family the possibility of organ donation if appropriate for the patient's circumstances.
   d. Observe for physical changes indicating the approach of death:
      1 to 3 months before death: beginning withdrawal from others, increased sleep, decreased appetite, difficulty digesting food, prefers liquids. (Anorexia may be protective, as the resulting ketosis can diminish pain and increase the person's sense of well-being.)
      1 to 2 weeks before death: Cardiovascular deterioration brings decreased blood pressure, pulse and respiration changes (decreased or increased), a yellowish pallor to the skin, extreme pallor of extremities. Observe for temperature fluctuations, increased perspiration, brief periods of apnea during sleep, rattling breathing sounds caused by congestion, nonproductive cough.
      Days to hours before death: possibly a brief surge of energy and mental clarity, with a desire to eat and talk with family members
      ➤ Dehydration, difficulty swallowing, decreasing blood volume, blood pressure, weak pulse
      ➤ Mucous membranes dry and tacky; cracked lips. (Dehydration during the last hours of dying is thought to not cause distress, and perhaps to stimulate endorphin release [Emanuel, Ferris, von Gunten, et al., 2008]).

(Continued)

Assessing Grief and Loss—cont'd

➤ Sagging of tongue and soft palate, diminished gag reflex, secretions accumulating in the oropharynx and/or bronchi

➤ Shallow, rapid, or irregular breathing; respiratory congestion; Cheyne-Stokes respirations; apnea of 10 to 30 seconds; "death rattle." (**Cheyne-Stokes respiration** is a cyclic pattern consisting of a 10- to 60-second period of apnea and then a gradual increase in depth and rate of respirations. Respirations gradually become slow and shallow, and then the cycle begins again with apnea.)

➤ Decreased peripheral circulation, increased perspiration, "clammy" skin; extremities cool and mottled; dependent body parts darker than the rest of the body

➤ Decreased urinary output, concentrated and foul-smelling urine, secondary to decreased circulation and kidney function

➤ Slack facial muscles ("drooping")

➤ Retained feces; bowel and bladder incontinence (due to decreased peristalsis and relaxation of sphincters)

➤ Blurred vision; eyes open but unseeing

➤ Restlessness or agitation (Assess for impacted stool, distended bladder, pain, medications, cerebral hypoxia, unresolved emotional or spiritual issues.)

➤ Decreased communication, quiet, withdrawal. Some become more coherent and energized for a time (Pitorak, 2003).

➤ Fatigue

Moments before death: Does not respond to touch or sound; cannot be awakened. There may be a short series of long-spaced breaths before breathing stops entirely and the heart stops beating (Karnes, 1995). Auscultate to determine whether apical pulse and respirations are absent.

Is It Grief or Depression?

When performing a focused assessment for grief or loss, you will need to distinguish between grief and depression. Sadness and depression are an integral part of grief. However, depression that lingers beyond what is expected may be a sign that the stress of grieving has triggered a major depressive episode (Ferszt & Leveillee, 2006). Although grief and depression have several symptoms in common (e.g., sadness, insomnia, poor appetite, and weight loss), grief tends to come and go—to be set off, for example, by a holiday. To differentiate them, and for guidelines to follow when assessing dying and grieving patients, use the Focused Assessment box, Assessing Grief and Loss.

KnowledgeCheck 17-4

What assessments should you make for your terminally ill patient and his or her family?

ANALYSIS/DIAGNOSIS

When you are analyzing patient data, keep in mind that most grief is normal, not complicated or dysfunctional. You must determine whether loss and grieving are the problem or the etiology, because the etiology influences your interventions. Also note that the same diagnoses can be used in the context of death, dying, grief, or loss, so they are discussed together in the next sections.

Loss and Grieving as a Problem. Various nursing diagnoses may be appropriate for a person who is dying or grieving. The two most obvious ones are Grieving and Complicated Grieving. Do not use a Complicated Grieving diagnosis for every person who is grieving a loss. **Complicated Grieving** is unusual in some way and is characterized by functional impairment and intense emotion. The pain and grief are disabling, or the grieving continues over a very long time (perhaps years). The person may deny or have difficulty expressing feelings of loss or may experience physical symptoms as a result of suppressing feelings.

Other diagnoses may include Ineffective Denial, Hopelessness, Powerlessness, Chronic Sorrow, Spiritual Distress, Self-Care Deficit, Constipation, and many other physiological diagnoses. To see the defining characteristics of NANDA-I diagnoses representing emotional responses to loss or impending death,

 Go to Chapter 17, **Standardized Language, NOC Outcomes and NIC Interventions for Loss and Grieving Diagnoses,** on Davis*Plus.*

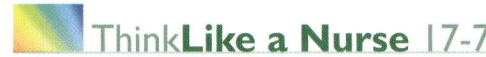 Think**Like a Nurse** 17-7

Refer to the table in **Standardized Language, NOC Outcomes and NIC Interventions** mentioned in the preceding reference. Answer the questions in the table. Also refer to a nursing diagnosis handbook and NIC and NOC manuals, if you need to.

Loss and Grieving as Etiology. Loss, grief, and dying are an etiology when they create problems in other areas of patient or family function. The following are examples of such nursing diagnoses:

▪ Acute or Chronic Low Self-Esteem related to (r/t) inability to change the event for self or significant other; or related to dying while having "unfinished business"

▪ Anxiety r/t possible inability to cope with the loss; or related to unknown outcome of situation

▪ Death Anxiety (or Fear) r/t impending death

▪ Decisional Conflict r/t end-of-life treatment measures (e.g., concern about the expense of "useless" procedures or their effect on the family; knowledge that the treatment may lengthen life but decrease the quality of life)

▪ Deficient Knowledge r/t the new experience of caring for a terminally ill person

▪ Fatigue r/t demands of caring for a dying loved one

▪ Spiritual Distress r/t loss of trust in a loving God

PLANNING OUTCOMES/EVALUATION

Encourage the patient and family to play an active role in planning care. Involving family members helps facilitate their acceptance of the diagnosis and may put the patient more at ease. Questions such as the following will help to elicit the patient's goals for end of life (Matzo, Sherman, Sheehan, et al., 2003):

- What do you still want to accomplish or do?
- What are the things you wish you could still do?
- If you have pain, what would be an acceptable level for you, on a 0 to 10 scale?
- Where do you want to spend the rest of your life? Where are you most comfortable?
- If spiritual peace is important to you, what would help you achieve it?

NOC standardized outcomes are determined by the diagnostic label you use. For examples,

 Go to Chapter 17, **Standardized Language, NOC Outcomes and NIC Interventions for Loss and Grieving Diagnoses,** on *DavisPlus.*

Individualized goals/outcome statements you might write for a grieving or dying person include the following examples. The patient and/or family will:

1. Communicate openly among themselves and with healthcare providers (e.g., express fear, concerns, pain).
2. Obtain satisfactory pain relief and symptom management.
3. Use all resources available to assist with coping.
4. Exercise control in the management of care to the extent possible.

As always, you will use the goals set in the planning stage as criteria for evaluating the patient's or family's health status.

KnowledgeCheck 17-5

- List three nursing diagnosis labels you might consider when dying or grieving is the primary problem.
- List three nursing diagnoses labels that might occur as a result of dying or grieving.

PLANNING INTERVENTIONS/IMPLEMENTATION

NIC standardized interventions associated with death, dying, and bereavement are found in

 Chapter 17, **Standardized Language, NOC Outcomes and NIC Interventions for Loss and Grieving Diagnoses,** on *DavisPlus.*

Specific nursing activities are determined by the nursing diagnosis, especially by the etiology. Your ability to help someone who is grieving or dying is largely determined by your attitude. A compassionate approach is essential but challenging. Watching patients struggle with pain, loss, grief, and death may stir

our own deepest doubts and fears, and we may reject the challenge to respond from the heart. We may be aware that employers usually reward nurses for what they *do* rather than who they *are* as people, so it is easy to rationalize that we have other tasks to accomplish that may be equally important. When we do that, we ignore the real gift we may have to offer the suffering patient: our willingness to "walk the walk" with them, if even for just a short time. Full-spectrum blend thinking, doing, and caring with compassion in ministering to those who are suffering.

Some important nursing interventions, including therapeutic communication, facilitating grief work, helping families, and specific activities involved in care of the dying person are discussed in the following sections. Also see the Nursing Care Plan and Care Map for Grieving.

Therapeutic Communication

It is critical to build a trusting relationship with the dying or grieving patient and significant others. Perhaps most important is to listen to the dying patient and to be alert for and respond to nonverbal cues. Encourage patients and family members to express their feelings, and reassure them that their feelings are normal and not "wrong." In discussions about DNAR or withholding or withdrawing treatments, it is important to find out why the patient is seeking that option: Does she wish to avoid suffering, or does she fear being a burden to loved ones?

Physicians and nurses should always work to improve their communication skills because they are essential for achieving better outcomes at end of life (Boyle, Miller, & Forbes-Thompson, 2005). See Box 17-4 for some barriers to end-of-life communication. For tips on communicating with people who are dying or bereaved, see Clinical Insight 17-1. If you need more information on communication and therapeutic relationships, refer to Chapter 20.

BOX 17-4 ■ Barriers to End-of-Life Communication

- Fear of one's own mortality
- Unresolved personal grief issues (e.g., the loss of one's own parent)
- Lack of experience with death and dying
- Fear of expressing emotion (i.e., crying)
- Fear of not knowing the answer to a question
- Not knowing whether to give an honest (and possibly unwelcome) answer to a question
- Not understanding the family's culture
- Keeping physical distance (e.g., standing away from the person or avoiding eye contact)
- Insensitivity: interrupting communication, patronizing, giving false reassurance

Source: Matzo, M., Shermann, D., Sheehan, D., et al. (2003). Teaching strategies from the ELNEC curriculum. *Nursing Education Perspectives, 21*(1), 176–183.

Nursing Care Plan

Client Data

Wilma Peterson is caring for her son, Henry, who has AIDS. Henry is 20 years old; his older brother, William, died at home of AIDS-related pneumonia 2 years earlier at age 24. William had left home at 18 to live in Miami and returned to his home in rural Alabama when he became too ill to manage on his own. Henry stayed home to help his mother care for William and learned he was HIV-positive just before his brother died. Henry did not tell his mother of his diagnosis until he was hospitalized for the first time with cytomegalovirus (CMV) infection. Since then, he has not followed nutritional and medical advice and has continued to stay out late and party when he feels well enough. His health has steadily declined.

You are participating in a special Caring for the Caregiver program set up by the public health nurse in your community. In this program, registered nurses visit primary caregivers to assess their needs and offer support services as needed. Your client is Wilma Peterson.

Ms. Peterson is initially cordial when you visit but tells you, "This is a mother's responsibility. I don't stop being his mother because he's grown up. I'm always his mama." As your discussion continues, Ms. Peterson wistfully talks about when William and Henry were boys. She says, "I didn't really understand this awful disease until William got so sick. Now, I look at Henry and I know what's waiting for him. I know we are going to lose him. Sad . . . just so sad. . . ." Her voice trails off as tears well in her eyes.

Nursing Diagnosis

Grieving related to the client's anticipating the loss of a second son, as evidenced by her previous experience caring for her other son who died at home of AIDS and by the client's stating, "I know what's waiting for him."

NOC Outcomes	Individualized Goals / Expected Outcomes
Family Coping (NOC 2600) Psychosocial Adjustment: Life Change (NOC 1305)	(Short-term goals) At the end of the initial home visit, Ms. Peterson will: 1. Identify community resources available to help her care for Henry at home during acute illnesses. 2. Begin to feel comfortable discussing her concerns with the nurse. (Long-term goals) Within 6 weeks, Ms. Peterson will: 1. Explore activities she would like to participate in once she is no longer caring for Henry. 2. Talk with Henry to learn what type of funeral he would like.

Nursing Interventions and Activities*	Rationales
NIC Interventions Anticipatory Guidance (NIC 5210) Coping Enhancement (NIC 5230) Grief Work Facilitation (NIC 5290) **Nursing Activities** 1. Encourage Ms. Peterson to talk about her experiences caring for William before he died. 2. Ask her to relate similarities and differences between care for William and care for Henry.	 1. Grieving often occurs in the context of repeated caregiving (Boyle, Bunting, Hodnicki, et al., 2001) or in situations in which the caregiver has other types of previous experience with the same or a similar terminal illness. 2. Asking the client to discuss previous experiences allows the nurse to validate the nursing diagnosis (O'Connor & Lunney, 1998).

*Interventions are only a sample of those linked to this diagnosis by NIC. Activities should be individualized for each client.

Nursing Care Plan (continued)

Nursing Interventions and Activities* | Rationales

3. Ask Ms. Peterson to describe the elements of Henry's care and to identify which she considers to be the most important.

3. Clients are holistic and consider more than just medical treatment in the care of a family member. Their actions are often based on cultural and religious beliefs and their own previous experiences instead of a medically based care plan. Clients may operate on a different, parallel track from that of the healthcare providers (Boyle, Bunting, Hodnicki, et al., 2001). By asking what Ms. Peterson does and how she prioritizes Henry's care, the nurse can learn from the client rather than making assumptions based on the healthcare perspective. By showing respect for her experience as a caregiver, the nurse can build a stronger relationship with Ms. Peterson, which will facilitate future nursing interventions and anticipatory guidance.

4. Talk with Ms. Peterson to find out what community resources she used when she cared for William and whether she has accessed them now that she is caring for Henry.

4. Isolation and loneliness are risk factors for sole caregivers at home. By assessing community resources, the nurse can determine whether Ms. Peterson is "connected" or isolating herself. Isolation puts her at risk for Complicated Grieving (O'Connor & Lunney, 1998). Many community resources provide a sense of belonging and enhance and support coping strategies as well.

5. Promote shared decision making if this is acceptable to Henry Peterson.

5. Informing both Ms. Peterson and Henry about the disease, prognosis, treatment, and comfort options allows them to retain some control over their lives together (Teno, Casey, Welch, et al., 2001). Henry's permission must be obtained to preserve his autonomy.

6. Provide nonjudgmental emotional support to Ms. Peterson, and support healthy coping activities she is using.

6. Establishing a comfortable and emotionally safe environment will allow Ms. Peterson to share her concerns without fear of being judged because of her son's diagnosis (Boyle, Bunting, Hodnicki, et al., 2001).

Evaluation

Review the initial short-term outcomes and goals. Reassess your client to determine whether the goals are achieved in the stated time frame. In this case, long-term goals will fluctuate based on the progression of Henry's illness. The following occurred as the care plan was implemented:

- Ms. Peterson cried as she described the deterioration in William's health before he died. She worries that Henry will suffer and does not want him to lose his dignity the way she believes William did.
- Ms. Peterson's greatest concern is that Henry is not eating enough. Much of her self-value as a mother arises from her ability to prepare homemade meals to feed her family, and Henry doesn't have much appetite. This is very distressing to her.
- She has not contacted community agencies. She is holding off, hoping Henry will not be "so sick for so long. With these new drugs, he can get better."
- She remains involved in her church, which is the same one she attended as a little girl. However, she will not tell her church group that Henry has AIDS. "They talk too much," she says. Instead, she says he has leukemia.

Only one short-term goal is met at this visit—establishing a comfort level between the client and the nurse. Ms. Peterson has not identified community resources related to caring for Henry at this time.

Plan for Further Evaluation

Additional supportive visits will be needed to help Ms. Peterson understand that contacting community agencies does not mean Henry will die sooner; at this time, denying the need for community help is an important coping mechanism for Ms. Peterson and is not affecting her ability to care for her son. If his condition worsens, this issue will need to be addressed promptly.

References

Boyle, J. S., Bunting, S. M., Hodnicki, D. R., et al. (2001); Bulechek, G., Butcher, H., & Dochterman, J. M. (2008); Johnson, M., Bulechek, G., Butcher, H., et al. (2006);
Moorhead, S. Johnson, M., Maas, M., et al. (2008); O'Connor, L., & Lunney, M. (1998); (2008).
Teno, J. M., Casey, V. A., Welch, L. C., et al. (2001).

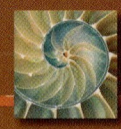

Care Map

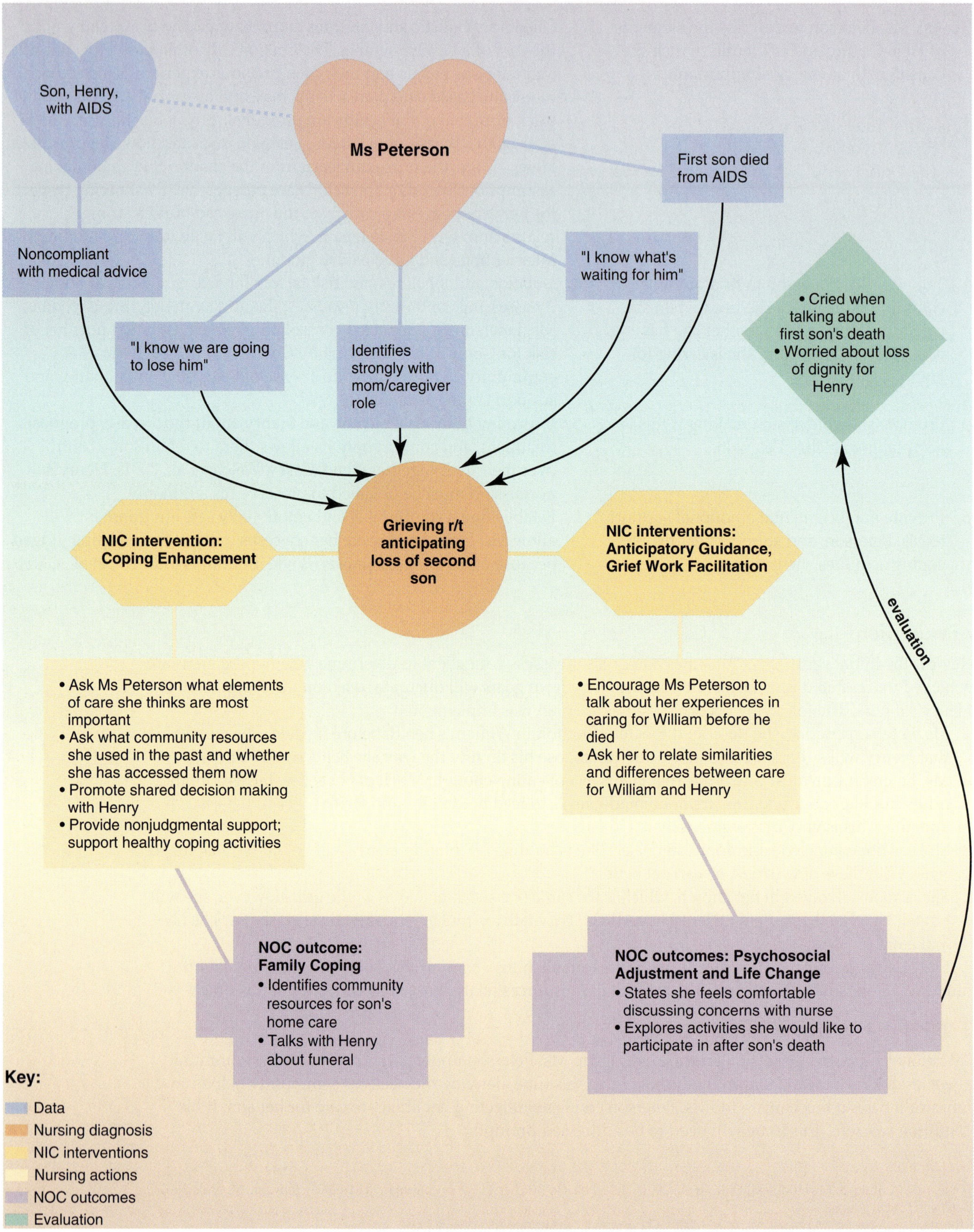

Son, Henry, with AIDS

Ms Peterson

First son died from AIDS

Noncompliant with medical advice

"I know what's waiting for him"

• Cried when talking about first son's death
• Worried about loss of dignity for Henry

"I know we are going to lose him"

Identifies strongly with mom/caregiver role

Grieving r/t anticipating loss of second son

NIC intervention: Coping Enhancement

NIC interventions: Anticipatory Guidance, Grief Work Facilitation

evaluation

• Ask Ms Peterson what elements of care she thinks are most important
• Ask what community resources she used in the past and whether she has accessed them now
• Promote shared decision making with Henry
• Provide nonjudgmental support; support healthy coping activities

• Encourage Ms Peterson to talk about her experiences in caring for William before he died
• Ask her to relate similarities and differences between care for William and Henry

NOC outcome: Family Coping
• Identifies community resources for son's home care
• Talks with Henry about funeral

NOC outcomes: Psychosocial Adjustment and Life Change
• States she feels comfortable discussing concerns with nurse
• Explores activities she would like to participate in after son's death

Key:
Data
Nursing diagnosis
NIC interventions
Nursing actions
NOC outcomes
Evaluation

Clinical Insight 17-1 ➤ Communicating With People Who Are Grieving

Perfect your listening skills. Listen for what is *not* said as well as what is said.

Be alert for and respond to nonverbal cues with appropriate touch and eye contact. A smile, a gentle touch, sitting with a patient, and eye contact all relay a message of genuine care and concern. You may not need to say very much at all.

Encourage and accept expressions of feelings.

- Receiving expressions of intense feelings (e.g., anger and guilt) may be painful for you. It may help to remember that it is therapeutic for people to express their feelings.
- You don't need to change the person's feelings or make them better. As much as we would like to do this, it is not possible.
- You do need to validate the person's feelings (e.g., "It is normal to feel that way; it is OK").

Reassure the person that it is not "wrong" to feel anger, guilt, relief, or other feelings she may believe to be unacceptable. A dying patient might say, "I know it's awful, but I feel so angry with God for giving me this disease." Or a bereaved spouse might admit, "I shouldn't feel this way, but I'm relieved that it's finally over." Patients need to hear you say that their feelings are not "wrong" or "bad" and that they are going through a normal process.

Increase your self-awareness. Become more conscious of your own attitudes and feelings regarding death and dying. *If you are comfortable with your perspective, you will be able to hear patients' expressions of anger, guilt, frustration, fear, and loneliness more comfortably.*

Continue to communicate with dying patients even if they are in a coma. Encourage family members to do so as well.

- Talk to the patient. Tell him what is going on around him, what care you are providing, and when you or others enter or are about to leave the room. *Research indicates that patients continue to hear even though they cannot respond, sometimes up to the moment of death.*
- Avoid discussing the dying person as though he were not present.

Practice Resources

Eisenhandler, 2004; Emanuel, Ferris, von Gunten, et al., 2008; The Joint Commission, 2008; Kruse, 2004; Traylor, Hayslip, Kaminski, et al., 2003.

Facilitating Grief Work

Whatever the type of loss, you can help people work through their grief by encouraging them to express their feelings, recall memories, and find meaning in their lives. Later in this chapter, we discuss interventions specifically for helping families after the death of a loved one. This section focuses more generally on grieving *any* loss.

Expressing Feelings. It is the family, not just an individual patient, who is grieving a death or other loss. In order for people to deal with grief in a healthy way, they need to communicate their feelings. Sometimes people are uncomfortable with expressing their feelings and hold them in. Such reserve will interfere with their grief resolution, so you may have to facilitate the process. Therapeutic communication will be needed (see Chapter 20 as needed). The following are some ways to facilitate expression of feelings:

- Encourage questions, and respond to them within a reasonable time.
- Sit beside the head of the bed; do not appear rushed.
- When you observe the patient or family member expressing feelings, either verbally or nonverbally, encourage them to continue.
- Expect and accept a wide range of feelings, including anger, fear, and loneliness.
- Ask, "How can I help?" "What do you need?" "What would you like for me to do?"
- Ask yourself what you would do if this were your family member.
- Do not compare another person's loss to your own experience. For example, avoid comments such as, "I know how you feel." Instead, say, "Tell me how you feel."

Recalling Memories. Grieving patients and family members may need to recall memories, both good and difficult.

One way to encourage recall is to go through photo albums with them and ask questions about the people in the pictures. Also look for objects of sentiment (e.g., a family heirloom) in the environment and ask the dying or bereaved person to share their significance.

Finding Meaning. Another way to facilitate grief work is to help the patient or family find meaning in their lives or in their past. Talking through this meaning is a healthy way to cope. Facilitating life review is one technique to help the patient and/or family recognize the unique contributions this person has made to family, friends, and society. You can begin by asking about the various aspects of the patient's life, commenting on pictures in the room, or picking up on verbal cues that are expressed.

Bibliotherapy. **Bibliotherapy** is a counseling technique used when grief therapy is indicated. It uses guided reading of self-help literature or fiction to increase client awareness and understanding and promote healing. Poems, novels, and essays can help produce new insights, either as the client retells the story or is guided to discuss his feelings and thoughts about the characters in the story (Briggs & Pehrsson, 2008).

ThinkLike a Nurse 17-8

- What would you say to Mrs. Manning (Meet Your Patient) if you walked into a room and found her sitting in a chair and softly weeping while Mr. Manning sleeps?
- What response would you make when Mr. Manning waves his hand in the air and says, "I'm not taking any more of those damn pills" as you bring him his medications?
- A young woman approaches you in the hall and says, "I want to visit Mom and stay with her, but I just can't stand to see her like that. I feel guilty for wanting to leave." What would be your therapeutic response?

Helping Families of Dying Patients

When a patient is dying, it is especially important to view the family as your unit of care. If the patient is unresponsive, you may find yourself spending most of your care time with the family. This time should be used to provide education, support, and a listening ear. Observing their loved one dying can leave family members feeling confused, angry, helpless, and even devastated; thus, sensitive and compassionate care during this time is essential. You can use the interventions in the preceding sections as you help family members understand that what they see may be very different from what the patient is experiencing. For more specific interventions for helping families of dying patients, see Clinical Insight 17-2.

KnowledgeCheck 17-6

- Describe four ways to facilitate the grief work of a grieving or dying person.
- List two specific interventions for helping grieving families.

Caring for the Dying Person

Most hospitals have an interdisciplinary team to provide holistic care to dying patients and their families. This team may be made up of a physician, nurse, social worker, pastoral care worker, dietitian, physical therapist (and sometimes occupational and speech therapists), and volunteers. Care addresses physiological, psychological, social, sexual, and spiritual needs.

Clinical Insight 17-2 ➤ Helping Families of Dying Patients

View the family as your unit of care. *Family members often rate communication with clinicians as one of their most important needs.*

Provide information, support, and a listening ear. Include specific facts about the patient's condition and prognosis and whom to call about changes in condition.

Communicate medical updates daily. *Information can relieve anxiety and is useful to the family when making decisions.*

Encourage family members to help with care if they are able. Instruct and supervise as appropriate. If family members are not physically or emotionally able to provide care, accept that. *This helps meet their need to be useful, promotes family ties, and makes the patient more comfortable.*

Encourage family members to ask questions. *They may hesitate to do so for various reasons (e.g., may not want to interrupt busy care providers).*

Listen actively to the patient's and family's concerns. Make eye content; clarify when you don't understand. *This helps you avoid misinterpreting the family's concerns and needs.*

Help the family to understand the goals of care and solve problems when needed.

Follow up with other healthcare team members promptly if the family has questions that are outside your scope of practice.

Arrange for a formal multidisciplinary meeting with the family soon after the patient's admission, if possible. Discussions should cover personal, cultural, and religious traditions (e.g., how prayers are to be conducted, how the body is to be handled after death).

Encourage the family to visit the hospital chapel and to speak with a chaplain or with their own spiritual adviser.

Provide anticipatory guidance regarding the stages of loss and grief, *so that they will know what to expect after their loved one dies.*

Acknowledge the family's feelings and the loss they are experiencing. *Many times family members begin the grieving process before the loved one dies.*

Help the family members explore past coping mechanisms; reinforce successful past coping mechanisms.

Refer for ethics consultation if decision making may become a problem.

Remind family members and significant others to take care of themselves.
- Many times they need "permission" to go to eat or to go home and rest.
- If the patient is near death and family and friends do not want to leave the patient's side, make them as comfortable as possible.
- Provide comfortable chairs, coffee, and snacks (according to organizational policy), and be alert for other needs they may have. *Watching a loved one die is a difficult experience. A sensitive, caring nurse can make it a little easier.*

Teach the family what to expect with regard to medications, treatments, and signs of approaching death. *If family members know what is normal, they will be less likely to panic or fear the inevitable.*

As physical signs of death become apparent, keep the family informed. You may say something such as, "Her blood pressure is becoming difficult to hear. That is one of the signs that she is closer to death." Help the family to understand what the patient is experiencing, as this may be very different from what they are seeing.

Reassure families of patients who become withdrawn near the time of death that this does not mean the patient is rejecting them, but only that his body is conserving energy and that he has come to terms with dying and letting go of his connections with life.

When approaching death is apparent, ask family members directly, "Do you want to be present while he is dying?" Tell them what to expect, if they do not know.

When an expected death occurs, shift the focus of your care to the family and those who were caregivers.

Practice Resources
Ahrens, Yancey, & Kollef, 2003; Boyle, Miller, & Forbes-Thompson, 2005; Emanuel, Ferris, von Gunten, et al., 2008; Hudson, 2006; The Joint Commission, 2008; von Gunten, Ferris, & Emanuel, 2000.

Meeting Physiological Needs

Active dying usually occurs over a period of 10 to 14 days (although it can take as little as 24 hours). The phrase *the final hours* refers to the last 4 to 48 hours of life, in which failure of body systems results in death (Pitorak, 2003). In the last hours of life, most patients need skilled care around the clock. Physiological needs during this time include mobility, oxygenation, safety, nutrition, fluids, elimination, personal hygiene, and control of pain and symptoms (nausea, vomiting). See the Focused Assessment box, Assessing Grief and Loss, and the previous discussion of the physiological stages of dying to review signs of impending death. For specific interventions and guidelines to use when caring for a dying patient, see Clinical Insight 17-3.

Meeting Psychological Needs

When a patient is terminally ill, the primary provider is usually responsible for deciding what and how much to tell the person. Ideally, everyone involved with the patient should have input into this decision, and should know exactly what the patient and family have been told. Most patients want to know their prognosis as soon as possible so that they can put personal affairs in order, share their feelings with family members, and come to terms with their life and death. A systematic review of research suggests that efforts to shield patients from the reality of their situation usually creates greater difficulties for them instead of protecting them (Hancock, Clayton, Parker, et al., 2007). A "conspiracy of silence" causes fear, anxiety, and confusion, and it denies people the opportunity to make needed life adaptations. However, culture may determine which family members are to be informed and how much, if any, information is given to the patient. Also, many patients realize without being told that they are dying. For specific interventions to help meet the psychological needs of dying patients, refer to Clinical Insight 17-4.

KnowledgeCheck 17-7

- Describe six nursing interventions to use in meeting the physiological needs of a dying person.
- Describe six nursing interventions to use in meeting the psychological needs of a dying person.
- What should be the focus of your interventions when the patient is very near death?

Clinical Insight 17-3 ▸ Caring for the Dying Person: Meeting Physiological Needs

Encourage the patient to be as independent as possible, *so that she will maintain a sense of control.*

Provide adequate pain control. *This can be a major issue for patients and caregivers. In fact, dying patients are often more concerned about pain and loss of control than about dying itself. Pain is difficult to assess in semiconscious or unconscious patients.* See Chapter 32 if you need more information about pain management.

- Dispel the myths about pain medication (e.g., addiction, overdose). Effective pain control medications exist and can be administered by various routes. Assure the patient and family that analgesics will not be addictive in this situation.
- Respect the patient's informed decision to refuse pain medications. For example, a patient may prefer to endure pain in order to be awake and alert when his family is at the bedside.
- Follow one of the common pain protocols to ensure that pain is controlled.
- Administer pain medication on a regular schedule instead of waiting until the patient asks (prn).
- Teach and perform nonpharmacological pain relief measures when you judge they may be helpful (e.g., meditation, heat/cold therapies, massage, distraction, imagery, deep-breathing, and herbal-scented lotions). It may be soothing to play soft music, add "white noise," or turn off the television.
- Patients who are near death may moan or grunt as they breathe; this does not necessarily indicate pain. Be sure that families understand this. When accompanied by agitation and restlessness, these symptoms may indicate terminal delirium, which may require medications for control.

Monitor the patient's energy level. *Fatigue is a normal part of the dying process. Most dying patients sleep much of the time.*

- Perform hygiene and other activities of daily living, if the patient tires easily or lacks the energy to care for herself.
- Remove environmental stressors that interfere with sleep (e.g., noise, too much light, a room that is too hot or too cold).
- Identify psychosocial stressors (e.g., depression, anxiety, fear) that may keep the patient awake (see Clinical Insight 17-4).

Maintain skin integrity. During the final hours of life, the goal changes from preserving skin integrity to providing comfort. Realize that during this time even excellent care may not prevent skin breakdown.

- Turn the patient frequently unless contraindicated. Refer to the pain control interventions above.
- Assess for increased diaphoresis and/or incontinence.
- Maintain adequate nutrition.

If the patient is comatose or unconscious, provide special care for the eyes so they do not become too dry. Many agencies use a form of artificial tears for this purpose.

If the patient is not able to take fluids, wet the lips and mouth frequently with cool water or with a prepared product *to prevent dryness and cracking of lips and mucous membranes of the nose, mouth, and eyes. There is some evidence that glycerin swabs dry the mucous membranes and should not be used.*

Provide artificial hydration (unless the patient has an advance directive requesting no artificial hydration) per nasogastric (NG) or IV route. *IV fluids can cause edema, nausea, and even pain in a patient who is actively dying.*

(Continued)

Clinical Insight 17-3 ▶ Caring for the Dying Person: Meeting Physiological Needs—cont'd

Dehydration is thought to not cause distress during the last hours, and may even be protective (Emanuel, Ferris, von Gunten, et al., 2008).

Take the vital signs often, unless contraindicated; observe for decreased level of consciousness and pallor.

Assess and provide interventions for constipation, urinary retention, and incontinence. *Constipation may be associated with decreased fluid intake, inactivity, weakness, hypercalcemia, hyperkalemia, and lack of privacy. It can contribute to pain, nausea, vomiting, and anorexia, so intervention is an important comfort measure. Incontinence may occur because of fatigue and loss of sphincter control, and can be distressing to patients and family members.*

- Administer laxatives, stool softeners, and lubricants for constipation.
- Catheterize the patient if he is unable to void and the bladder becomes distended.
- Use pads for incontinence, but change them frequently to prevent skin breakdown and, near the end, to promote comfort.
- Use a rectal tube if diarrhea is severe.

Intervene for death rattle if it occurs and if it is distressing to the family.

- Turn the patient on his side, and elevate the head of the bed.
- Administer antispasmodic and anticholinergic medications if necessary.

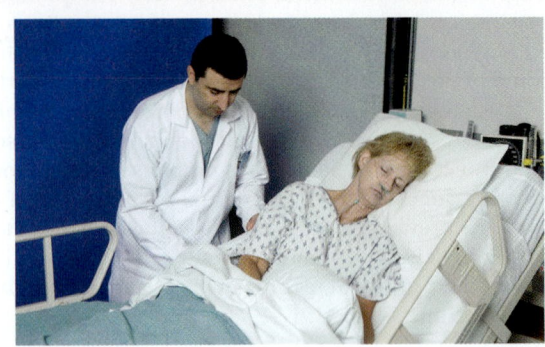

Provide medication for other symptoms, such as nausea and breathlessness.

Continue to speak to the patient as if he can hear.

Do not talk about the patient to others in his presence. Assume the unconscious patient hears everything. *The patient is usually able to hear even after he can no longer respond to sounds and other stimuli.*

Document changes in vital signs and level of consciousness. Record intake and output, noting changes. Document the times of cardiac arrest and cessation of respirations.

Practice Resources

American Nurses Association, 2003; Emanuel, Ferris, von Gunten, et al., 2005; Harvey, 2001; The Joint Commission, 2008; Qaseem, Snow, Shekelle, et al., 2008.

Clinical Insight 17-4 ▶ Caring for the Dying Person: Meeting Psychological Needs

Patients experience many emotions at end of life, including anger, sadness, depression, fear, relief, loneliness, and grief. At this time, communication and support are most helpful. Discussing concerns and issues is a viable means of coping.

If there is an advance directive or living will, locate the documents. Review the documents to be certain you understand the patient's wishes. If you have not already done so, notify all relevant health professionals of the existence of these documents.

Answer all questions honestly.

Explain all care and treatments even if the patient is unconscious. *He may still be able to hear.*

Realize that the patient may feel that he is losing control.

- Help the person recognize what he does have control over.
- Include the patient in care decisions as much as he is able.

Attend to social needs. Some patients may simply need to keep the bonds with family members and friends intact. For other patients, this may be a time to reestablish or mend relationships.

- Notify family members when the patient wishes to see them.
- Allow the patient and family to discuss death at their own pace.
- Offer to contact a chaplain or other spiritual leader if the patient chooses.
- Pray with the patient if he requests it and you are comfortable doing so. *Relationships are a priority at this time.*

Encourage the patient to express feelings. Be prepared to accept a wide range of feelings, including anger, hopelessness, loneliness, and depression.

Early in the dying process, assess the sources of financial support for the patient and family. *Finances may be a concern and may place an additional burden on the family; the patient may feel he is a burden to care for.*

Be aware of sexual needs. Provide realistic information about these issues. For example, suggest ways that a

Clinical Insight 17-4 ➤ Caring for the Dying Person: Meeting Psychological Needs—cont'd

couple can be close and affectionate at this time. Be aware that expressions of sexuality may change as a person becomes closer to death. *Some people may feel it is not right to have sexual feelings when the person they love is dying. Others may be afraid of harming the patient if they are sexually intimate.*

When the patient is very near death, focus on relieving symptoms (e.g., pain, nausea) and emotional distress.

If the person can communicate, ask about immediate concerns:
- Are you in pain? Are you comfortable?
- What are you afraid of now?
- What can we do to help you go peacefully?
- Who do you want in the room with you right now?

If the patient asks whether he is dying, be honest.

If the patient cannot communicate, ask the family what the patient would want. Ask the person most likely to know.

When the patient is very near death, it may be helpful to say something such as, "Your family will be fine" rather than, "It is OK for you to go now." Be aware that some people seem to wait to die until after a significant date (e.g., birthday, anniversary) has passed. Others wait for family to gather, whereas others wait until loved ones leave so they will not upset the family by dying in their presence.

Practice Resources

Duffy, Jackson, Schim, et al., 2006); Emanuel, Ferris, von Gunten, et al., 2008; Hancock, Clayton, Parker, et al., 2007; The Joint Commission, 2008; National Guideline Clearinghouse, 2006; Pitorak, 2003.

Toward Evidence-Based Practice

Hancock, K., Claton, J. M., Parker, S. M., et al. (2007). Truth-telling in discussing prognosis in advanced life-limiting illnesses: A systematic review. *Palliative Medicine, 21, 507–517.*

This was a systematic review of 46 studies related to truth-telling in discussing prognosis with patients with progressive, advanced life-limiting illnesses and their caregivers. Results included the following:
- Many health professionals expressed discomfort at having to inform the patient and family of limited life expectancy.
- The majority of health professionals thought that patients and their caregivers should be told the truth about the prognosis.
- Nevertheless, many either avoid discussing the topic or withhold information.
- Reasons for not telling the truth include perceived lack of training, stress, no time to attend to the patient's

emotional needs, fear of a negative effect on the patient, uncertainty about the prognosis, requests from family members to withhold information, and a feeling of inadequacy because further curative treatment was not available.
- Studies suggested that patients can discuss this topic without it having a negative impact on them.

1. Based on this systematic review, do you think health professionals should inform patients when they have an advanced life-limiting (terminal) illness? Explain your thinking.

2. Health professionals feared a negative effect on patients of telling them the truth about their condition. What sorts of negative effects do you think they might be anticipating?

 Go to Chapter 17, **Toward Evidence-Based Practice Suggested Responses,** on Davis*Plus.*

Addressing Spiritual Needs

When a person is terminally ill, his spirituality may become very important as he searches for meaning in the illness and suffering. The person may be looking for forgiveness and/or acceptance or be reaching out to feel connected. Ways to address this need include (but are not limited to) empathetic listening, contacting pastoral care or clergy if the patient asks for this service, special rituals, praying with the patient, music, meditation, or special readings.

Information about specific religious practices may help you provide appropriate interventions at end of life. For example, after the death of an Orthodox Jewish patient, you should handle the body as little as possible if you are not Jewish. Remember,

though, that there are wide individual differences and that you must assess each patient and family to determine how closely they adhere to the rituals of their religion. Review Chapters 15 and 16, as needed. For detailed information about a variety of religious practices surrounding death,

 Go to Chapter 17, **Supplemental Materials: Addressing Spiritual Needs,** on Davis*Plus.*

Addressing Cultural Needs

A recent study found the following end-of-life concerns were important to people regardless of their culture or gender: comfort, physician communication, having responsibilities taken

care of, hope and optimism, and honoring spiritual beliefs. Most groups also were concerned about love and compassion, being cared for, expressing feelings, fixing relationships, saying goodbye, having choices, making plans, not being in pain, and being "ready to go" (Duffy, Jackson, Schim, et al., 2006).

There is some overlap between religious and cultural practices. For example, most cultural groups engage in some type of religious ceremony that helps the bereaved begin the grieving process. Nevertheless, some death rituals and expressions of grief may be culture based but not necessarily involve religion. For example:

- Some cultures may emphasize keeping emotions more subdued and limiting expressions of grief to private settings, whereas others measure the value of the deceased by the amount of wailing and crying.
- Blacks and Hispanics may be less inclined to withdraw life-sustaining treatment or to use a hospice, whereas Arab Muslims may be reluctant to prolong life unnecessarily (Duffy, Jackson, Schim, et al., 2006).

Despite the commonalities among groups, there are some culture-specific differences. To provide culturally sensitive care at end of life, you will need some information about specific cultural practices surrounding death. For this information,

 Go to Chapter 17, **Supplemental Materials: Addressing Cultural Needs,** on Davis*Plus.*

As with spiritual care, remember that you cannot assume that a person follows the practices of her cultural group; you must assess to be sure.

Providing Postmortem Care

Postmortem care includes care of the patient's body after death and fulfilling any legal obligations. **Rigor mortis** (the stiffening of the body after death) is caused by contraction of the muscles from a lack of adenosine triphosphate (ATP). It occurs about 2 to 4 hours after death. Rigor mortis begins in the involuntary muscles (e.g., the heart). It appears next in the head, neck, and trunk, and finally in the extremities. It disappears about 96 hours after death. **Algor mortis** occurs when the blood stops circulating. The body temperature drops about 1.88°F (1°C) per hour until it reaches room temperature. The dependent parts of the body appear bluish and mottled because when the blood stops circulating, the red blood cells break down, releasing hemoglobin. This is called **livor mortis.**

Ideally, you will have already established a relationship with the family and will have begun to facilitate their grieving during the patient's dying period. And you will have prepared them as the death becomes imminent. For specific guidelines for care of the body and other immediate postmortem interventions to support family members, see Clinical Insight 17-5.

Clinical Insight 17-5 ➤ **Providing Postmortem Care**

Supporting the Family

- **At the moment of death, do not interrupt or intrude on the family.** Wait quietly and observe. If they would feel more comfortable being alone with the patient, leave the room. Give them as much time as they need. When they move away from the body, or have expressed their last good-byes, then it is time to assess the patient and report the lack of vital signs.
- **Immediately after death, express sympathy to the family.** This is very important. Make a simple statement, such as, "I am sorry for your loss." Avoid statements that interpret the situation for the family, such as, "It's God's will." Also avoid attempts to relieve the family members' grief, for example, "It will get better in time," or "You still have your son."
- **If the family wishes to be alone with the body,** straighten the bedcovers and make the patient look as natural as possible.
- **Be accepting of family members' behavior at this time,** no matter how strange it may seem to you. A family might want to take a picture, or the spouse may lie down beside the deceased person.
- **If no family members are present, identify the next of kin** and be sure the family is informed of the patient's death.
- **If family members arrive after the death, offer to take them to the bedside.**

- **If family members wish to be involved in postmortem care,** encourage them to do so. This can facilitate their grieving process.
- **Take care to present the patient's body in a way that is appropriate for the family** (i.e., remove any tubes, IV lines, and so on, according to the institution's policy) and have the patient positioned in a way that appears comforting (e.g., bed covers pulled up, hands at the side).
- **Ask whether each family member wishes to spend time alone with the deceased person,** and arrange for them to do so. Never remove the body until the family is ready.
- **Ask, "How can I help?" "What do you need?" "What would you like for me to do?"**
- **Locate personal effects and give them to the family/next of kin.** If you can't remove a ring, wrap it with gauze, tape it in place, and tie the gauze to the wrist to prevent subsequent loss.

Legal Responsibilities

- **Notify the primary provider of the death.** Usually the physician must pronounce death; however, in some areas a coroner or a nurse may also perform this task.
- **The person who pronounces death must sign the death certificate.** In some agencies, the nurse is responsible for checking to see that it has been signed.

Clinical Insight 17-5 ▸ Providing Postmortem Care—cont'd

- **If the patient is donating organs,** review and make any necessary arrangements.
- **If an autopsy is to be performed,** as a rule, the physician (or other person designated by the institution) is responsible for obtaining signed permission from the next of kin.

Care of the Body

- **Follow agency policies, and respect cultural and spiritual preferences.**
- **Wash the body if there has been any incontinence or drainage.** Place absorbent (e.g., "ABD") pads between the buttocks to absorb rectal drainage. In some cultures, the body is not washed, or family members arrange to have someone special do it; therefore, ask the family before performing this task.
- **Dress the body in a clean gown, comb the hair, and straighten the bed linens.**
- **Place the body supine in a natural position.**
  - Place the dentures in the mouth before rigor mortis occurs.
  - Close the eyes and mouth before rigor mortis occurs. Close the eyes by gently pressing on the lids with your fingertips. If they do not stay closed, place a moist compress on the eyelids for a few minutes and then try to close them again.
  - Tie a strip of soft gauze (e.g., Kling) under the chin and around the head if your institution requires it (not all do). Alternatively, you can place a folded towel under the chin to keep the jaw closed. *This keeps the mouth set in a natural position in case there is a viewing later.*
  - Place a pillow under the head and shoulders *to prevent blood from settling there and causing discoloration.*
- **Be sure that dressings are clean, and unless an autopsy is to be done, remove all tubes and drains.** Be careful when removing tape or dressings. Apply small adhesive bandages to puncture sites. *After death, the skin loses its elasticity and can be torn easily.*

- **If the family asks about the coldness and color of the body,** explain to them about algor mortis and livor mortis.
- **After the family has spent time with the body, arrange to have it sent to the morgue,** where either an autopsy will be performed, or, if not, the funeral home in charge of arrangements will arrive to transport the body.
  - Pad the wrists and ankles to prevent bruising; tie them together with gauze.
  - Wrap the body in a shroud or body wrap for transfer to the morgue.
  - If no relatives were present to receive patient belongings, bag them, label the bag, and send with the patient to the morgue.
  - If possible, close doors to adjoining rooms before transport.
- **Make sure there are identification tags, and hazard labels on the body, on the shroud or body bag, and on the patient's possessions.** Follow agency policy for number and location of tags. They will usually include the patient's name, room and bed numbers, date and time of death, and the physician's name. *Misidentification can create legal problems, for example, if the body is prepared incorrectly for a funeral.*
- **Follow institutional policy if the patient has died of a communicable disease.** By law, there are special preparations to perform in such cases.
- **Handle the body with dignity.**
- **Documentation varies among healthcare facilities.** However, you will almost always document the time that you noted absence of heartbeat and respirations, any auxiliary equipment (e.g., mechanical ventilator) still present, the disposition of the patient's possessions (especially money and jewelry), and the date and time the body is transported to the morgue or funeral home.

Practice Resources

College of American Pathologists, 2007; Harvey, 2001; The Joint Commission, 2008.

KnowledgeCheck 17-8

- Why is it important to position the body with a pillow under the head and shoulders soon after death?
- Why is it important to close the eyes and mouth of the deceased and position the body within at least 2 to 4 hours after death?

Providing Grief Education

Sometime after the immediate postmortem period, explain the stages of grief and point out that it takes months or even years to resolve. Explain that grief may become more intense on the anniversary of the death (or other loss) and on significant dates (e.g., birthdays).

Recall that once the bereaved person accepts that the loss is real, his feelings may be so intense that he may wonder if he is

losing his sanity. The grieving person may be fatigued from not sleeping, may be disoriented or unable to concentrate, and so on; and he may be concerned about what such symptoms mean. Reassure the person that such responses are expected and that there is no single right way to grieve (Egan & Arnold, 2003). Also assure him that although the grief process takes time, the symptoms won't last forever.

Helping Children Deal With Loss

Some families may need information about helping children deal with grief, especially when there is a death in the family. You may need to explain that children perceive death differently from adults. See the accompanying Self-Care box for teaching surviving relatives how to help children deal with grief.

Helping Children Deal With Loss

Teach surviving relatives the following:

➤ If a child is frightened about attending a funeral, do not force him to go. It is important, however, to include the child in some service or observance, such as lighting a candle, saying a prayer, or visiting the gravesite, at a later time.

➤ Spend as much time as possible with the child, making it clear that the child has permission to show her feelings openly or freely.

➤ Assure the child that he was in no way responsible for the death.

➤ The following signs may indicate the need for professional help, especially if they are prolonged:

An extended period of loss of interest in daily activities and events

Inability to sleep

Loss of appetite

Fear of being alone

Regression

Repeated statements about wanting to join the dead person

Withdrawal from friends

Refusal to attend school

Sharp drop in school performance.

Taking Care of Yourself

When caring for dying patients, you will confront your own feelings of mortality. It is important to understand your own attitudes, fears, and beliefs concerning death, so think about these in advance, before you encounter dying patients.

This will enable you to deal in a more healthy way with patients and their families. In addition, suppressing feelings associated with death of patients can take a heavy toll on you emotionally.

When you become involved with people at such an intimate time in their lives, you become connected to them. There is nothing wrong with this emotional involvement; it helps you to be effective in your work. Caring for the dying can be very rewarding, but it is emotionally draining. To be effective in your practice, you must learn to care for yourself as well.

- Recognize that your feelings of grief and loss are normal.
- Talk with other colleagues about your feelings. Nurses are known for being able to take care of everyone but themselves! Don't hesitate to ask for what you need.
- Do not be afraid to confront grief. Some nurses feel they have to be strong and deny their feelings. They overwork and take care of others. If you use this approach, the feelings will accumulate and begin to wear you down physically and emotionally.
- If you wish, it is appropriate for you to attend calling hours and/or funeral services when one of your patients dies. This helps you diffuse some of your feelings of loss. It also is meaningful to family members to know that you took the time to remember them and their loved one.
- Learn how to get support for yourself and how to support your colleagues when they experience the death of a patient. One idea is a nurses' support group, or grief team, that meets regularly to talk about the feelings and to remember those who have died. If you want a facilitator, pastoral care workers and social workers may be available for these services.
- Do some nice things for yourself on a regular basis (e.g., a quiet bubble bath, a massage, a sports event). Try to set aside a special spot in your home that is only for relaxation; decorate it with items that help you focus on peaceful thoughts (e.g., candles, pictures, religious objects).

CLINICAL REASONING:
Applying the Full-Spectrum Nursing Model

Because the following critical thinking activities allow you to practice the kind of thinking you will use as a full-spectrum nurse, they usually have no single right answer. Discuss them with your peers—if you have difficulty with any of the questions, consult your instructor.

PATIENT SITUATION

Marie is 84 years old and has had a right-sided cerebrovascular accident (CVA, or stroke). Doctors say she is unlikely to regain much physical function, if she even awakens from the coma. She was alert and active before her stroke and was able to maintain her independence with the help of a home health aide, who assisted her with activities of daily living (ADLs) and meal preparation three times a week. Kelly and Dan, her children, have met with the physician, who tells them that Marie's chance of survival is slim. He wants to put a feeding tube into Marie and has asked whether they want Marie to be resuscitated in case of cardiac or respiratory arrest. Kelly wants to do what is best for her mother, but she feels that Marie would not want to be kept alive in the condition she is in. She is also concerned about putting her through uncomfortable procedures if there is no chance of recovery. Her brother, Dan, thinks Marie should have the feeding tube. Kelly asks to speak with you and wants to know the best thing to do for her mother.

THINKING

1. *Theoretical Knowledge (Recall of Facts and Principles):* If Kelly and Dan agree that they do not want Marie to be resuscitated, the physician will complete a DNAR order. What do the letters *DNAR* represent?

2. *Critical Thinking (Problem-Solving):* At this stage of your education, you probably need more information about CVAs and tube feedings. Write a PICO question that you could use to search the literature for information about these two topics and how they are related. See Chapter 8 if you need to review PICO questions.

DOING

3. *Practical Knowledge (Nursing Diagnosis):* Write a possible nursing diagnosis to describe Kelly's situation.
4. *Practical Knowledge (Basic Skills):* If Kelly and Dan agree to tube feedings for Marie, as her nurse, what basic nursing skills will you need to perform? How will you learn to perform these skills, if you do not already know how to do them?

CARING

5. *Ethical Knowledge:* How do you think the situation came to this? What might Kelly, Dan, and Marie have done before the stroke to prevent this confusion and indecision?
6. *Self-Knowledge:* What are your responsibilities in this situation? What could you do to help Kelly and Dan?

 Go To Chapter 17, **Clinical Reasoning: Applying the Full-Spectrum Nursing Model Response Sheet,** on Davis*Plus.*

 To explore learning resources for this chapter,

 Go to Davis*Plus* at http://davisplus.fadavis.com, keyword: Treas.

Chapter Resources for Chapter 17:
    Knowledge Check and Think Like a Nurse Response Sheets
    Knowledge Check Answers
    Resources for Caregivers and Health Professionals
    Reading More About Loss, Grief, & Dying (suggested readings)
    What Are the Main Points in This Chapter?
NCLEX-Style Review Questions
Chapter Overview Podcasts

Concept Map

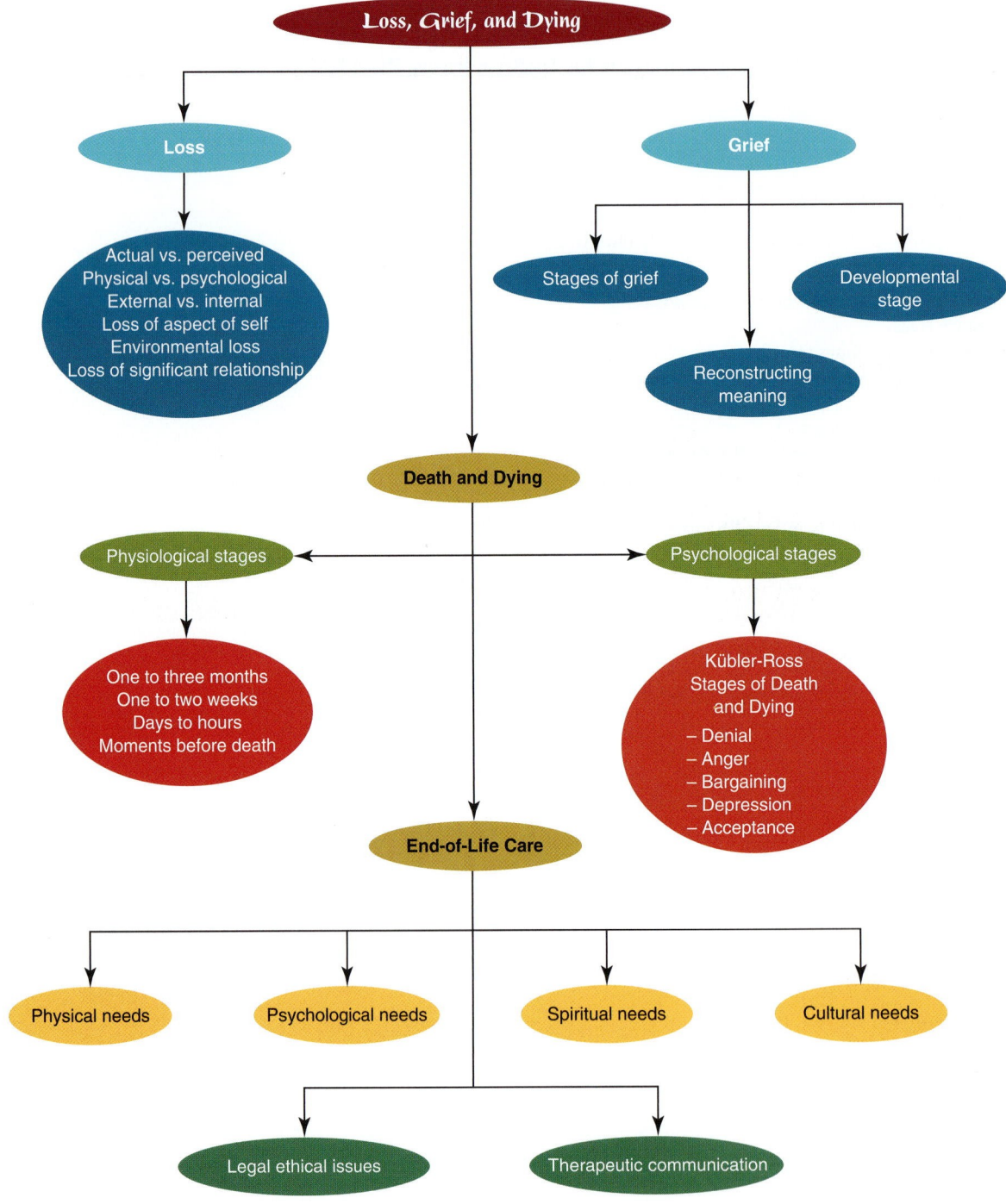

Essential Nursing Interventions

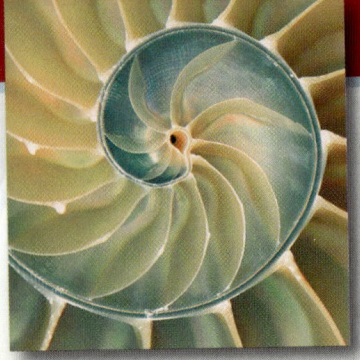

CHAPTER 18

Documenting & Reporting

Learning Outcomes

After completing this chapter you should be able to:

➤ Explain the purposes of documentation.

➤ Compare and contrast the differences between electronic and written documentation.

➤ Identify a variety of charting formats and their purposes.

➤ Use paper and electronic documentation in the clinical setting.

➤ Describe guidelines for documentation.

➤ Identify approved abbreviations to use in charting.

➤ Follow documentation guidelines to accurately record patient health status, nursing interventions, and patient outcomes.

➤ Discuss the key elements of giving an oral patient report.

➤ Explain the process for verifying or questioning a medical order.

Key Concepts

Documentation

Oral reporting

Related Concepts

See the Concept Map at the end of this chapter.

Caring for the Nguyens

This feature allows you to practice the kind of thinking you will use as a full-spectrum nurse. There is usually more than one correct answer to a critical thinking question, so we do not provide answers for these questions. It is more important to develop your nursing judgment than to "cover content." Discuss the questions with your peers. If you are still unsure, consult your instructor.

Yen Nguyen arrives at the Family Medicine Clinic complaining of pain and drainage from her right eye. She requests an appointment. As part of your clinical experience working as a triage nurse at the clinic, you must evaluate the patient's status and determine whether she needs to be seen today. Below is your conversation with Mrs. Nguyen.

Mrs. Nguyen: I don't have an appointment, but I need to see someone today. My husband is a patient here. I have an appointment in 2 weeks for a physical, but I've never been here before. I just can't wait 2 weeks.

You: What seems to be the problem?

Mrs. Nguyen: My eye is killing me. My right one. It burns and stings, and there's all this nasty gunk coming out. I think I need some medicine for it.

You: Tell me a little more about this problem. When did this start?

Mrs. Nguyen: I woke up yesterday with a painful, itchy eye. I used some saline drops, but the eye seems to be worse. I work at a preschool, and they won't let me work unless I take care of this. I also think I need to be checked for other things. I haven't had an appointment in a long time. I suppose I just need some

(Continued)

Caring for the Nguyens (continued)

tests. My husband just found out he had high blood pressure, but I don't think I do. I guess I'm not old enough. I'm 55, but my mother got high blood pressure when she was 70.

As she is talking, you notice a large amount of thick, yellow-green drainage in the corner of her right eye and the eye is reddened. She is rubbing this eye vigorously and

dabbing at it with a tissue. The skin is puffy around the eye as well. Her left eye is slightly red, but there is no drainage.

Her vital signs are as follows: blood pressure, 132/76 mm Hg; heart rate, 88 beats/min; respirations, 18 breaths/min; and temperature 98.9°F (37.2°C). Based on your brief assessment, you ask the receptionist to give Mrs. Nguyen an urgent appointment.

A. Make two charting entries to describe the above events. First make a brief narrative note.

B. Next, construct a SOAPIER note. Be sure to follow charting guidelines when you prepare your note.

 Go to Chapter 18, **Caring for the Nguyens Response Sheet,** on Davis*Plus.*

Meet Your Patient

Steven Stellanski is a 16-year-old male who has just been released from the post-anesthesia care unit (PACU) after an emergency appendectomy. You are to admit him to your unit. Steven is groggy but moaning in pain. "Help me, help me," he whispers. He is holding his abdomen and grimacing. The PACU nurse tells you that Steven has Down syndrome and functions at a school-age level.

Steven's vital signs are as follows: tympanic membrane temperature 99.9°F (37.7°C); pulse, 104 beats/min; respirations, 24 breaths/min; and blood pressure 104/68 mm Hg. An intravenous (IV) bag of lactated Ringer's solution is infusing at 125 mL/hr. The dressing on Steven's right lower

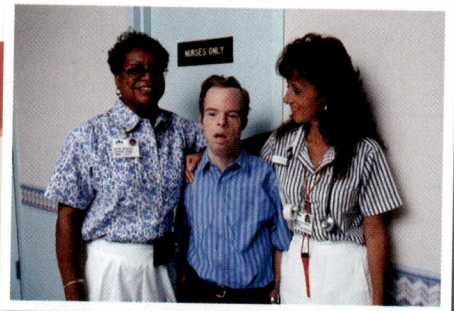

abdomen is dry and intact. An indwelling catheter is draining pale yellow urine.

The postoperative prescriptions for Steven call for starting a patient-controlled analgesia pump that will deliver morphine sulfate at 1 mg every 15 minutes, up to 4 mg per hour. He is to remain NPO (nothing by mouth) for now. The dressing is to be changed tomorrow morning and the nurses are to institute progressive ambulation as tolerated.

Theoretical Knowledge
knowing why

When you imagine yourself working as a nurse, what do you think of? Most people picture themselves at the bedside working with patients. When you look at ads for nursing jobs, they often show a nurse hanging an IV bag or listening to heart sounds. Photos rarely show the nurse charting or reporting care. Yet healthcare professionals rely on these two methods of communication to coordinate patient care. In this chapter, we discuss paper, electronic, and oral communication.

ABOUT THE KEY CONCEPTS

Documentation and oral reporting are the two broad concepts to which all other concepts in this chapter are linked. As you read, think, "What does this have to do with documentation?" and "How does this relate to oral reporting?"

DOCUMENTATION

Documentation is the act of recording patient status and care in written or electronic form, or in a combination of the two forms. Documentation is not just "writing nursing notes"; rather, it is the act of making a written record. The terms *documenting, recording,* and *charting* are often used to mean the same thing. Oral communication about a patient's status is called **reporting**—that is discussed later in this chapter.

Historically, the collection of documentation, orders, and other care information for a patient had been called the **medical record** or **chart**. However, with the present emphasis on health promotion, the medical record is now more commonly referred to as the **health record**. A patient's health record permanently documents the following:

- Care, in chronological order, provided by all healthcare providers
- The patient's responses to interventions and treatments

- Important facts about the client's health history, including past and present illnesses, examinations, tests, treatments, and outcomes

As a nurse, you are responsible for managing and implementing the interdisciplinary plan of care. That responsibility includes documenting the care provided and the progress made toward goals. Research shows that nurses routinely spend 15% to 25% (up to 2 hr) of their workday documenting the care they give, and in some cases considerably more.

How Do Healthcare Providers Use Documentation?

Clear, complete, and accurate documentation in a client health record serves a variety of purposes.

- **Communication.** One important function is communication. Members of the multidisciplinary team use the health record to communicate about the patient's status and care. For example, if it is not possible to speak directly to the respiratory therapist on your shift, you can at least review the progress notes. Documentation enables healthcare professionals to plan and evaluate treatment and monitor health status over time.
- **Legal Record.** The health record will be scrutinized by legal experts if a dispute about a client's care arises. In court, the health record is legal evidence of the care given to a client, and is used to judge whether the interventions were timely and appropriate.
- **Continuity of Care.** For example, if you are concerned that the patient is at high risk for developing an infection, you can include a nursing diagnosis of Risk for Infection on the written or electronic interdisciplinary plan of care. You would then initiate nursing orders for other nurses to regularly observe for and document signs of infection.
- **Quality Improvement.** Healthcare organizations and other agencies perform **manual chart audits** (directed reviews of client medical records) of written documentation. In electronic health record (EHR) systems, reports are run to analyze large amounts of data. Results are used to identify ways to improve care, decrease length of stay, control costs, and so on.

Documentation is also required in order for institutions to be reimbursed by third-party payers, and to determine whether a patient's medical treatments and interventions were necessary and appropriate (called **utilization review**). Other uses of EHRs are for education and research.

    Professional Standards. The American Nurses Association's (ANA) *Nursing: Scope and Standards of Practice* (2010) includes documentation in many of its standards. If you want to know which specific standards include documentation,

 Go to Chapter 18, **Tables, Boxes, Figures: ESG Box 18-1, ANA Standards of Practice Referring to Documentation,** on Davis*Plus.*

Why Are Standardized Nursing Languages Important?

Nurses have long understood the need for a standardized vocabulary for describing what nurses do and the outcomes that result. As healthcare costs escalated, it became necessary to measure nursing's contribution to care and demonstrate the value of nursing. Standardized nursing terminology helps do that by making nursing care and its effect on patient outcomes more visible in patient records.

    The ANA (2010) has recommended that documentation systems such as NANDA International (NANDA-I), Nursing

Interventions Classification (NIC), and Nursing Outcomes Classification (NOC) use ANA-recognized terminology. Standardized terminologies allow researchers to retrieve nursing data for aggregation and analysis. Through the use of standardized languages in nursing documentation, a standard for evidence-based nursing care delivery has now been established. This is a step toward closing the gap between what research shows to be the best nursing practices and the interventions nurses actually use in practice.

    Standardized languages are especially important in EHR systems because computers require standardized information that can be converted to numerical codes. Several standardized nursing language models have been created and are used in nursing documentation, for example, NANDA-I, NIC, and NOC. To review using standardized nursing language models in your own practice, see the standardized language sections in Chapters 4, 5, and 6.

How Are Health Records Systems Organized?

A **health records system** is the overall process by which all patient records are created, stored, and retrieved in an organization. In a sense, it consists of all the EHRs in an organization. Each healthcare agency determines the health record system that is used (e.g., source oriented, problem oriented, or charting by exception). The nursing leaders in each organization usually determine the documentation forms that nurses will use within the records system.

Source-Oriented Record Systems

In a **source-oriented system,** members of each discipline record their findings in a separately labeled section of the chart. In paper records, nurses chart in the nurses' notes section as well as in the graphic data section. A typical source-oriented record includes the following sections:

- *Admission data*—demographic information, insurance data, contact information
- *Advance directive*—information on client's wishes for the extent of care and medical support that should be given in the event of a life-threatening event
- *History and physical*—a detailed summary of the current health problem; past medical, surgical and social history; medications taken; allergies; review of systems; and physical examination data
- *Physician's orders*—orders for medications, treatments, and activities
- *Progress notes*—chronological charting by healthcare team members including patient exams, problem identification, and patient's response to therapy
- *Diagnostic studies*—reports detailing the findings of tests that have been performed, such as x-ray exam, ultrasound, or pulmonary function tests
- *Laboratory data*—a compilation or results from diagnostic test results
- *Nurses' notes*—documentation of patient care and response to treatment recorded by nurses (usually chronological)
- *Graphic data*—numerical data collected over time and displayed visually to allow analysis of trends. Examples include intake and output records; vital sign flow sheets; rating scales; and checklists regarding patient activity, dietary intake, and activities of daily living (ADLs).
- *Rehabilitation and therapy notes*—chronological charting by therapists about assessments, the treatment plan, and patient response to therapy; usually includes physical therapy, occupational therapy, and respiratory therapy

- *Discharge planning*—includes data from utilization review, case managers, or discharge planners on anticipated client needs after discharge

Advantages. In source-oriented records, you can easily find the care provided by each discipline.

Disadvantages. A drawback of this system is that data may be fragmented and scattered throughout the patient's record. You need to review all sections of the chart to fully understand the client's condition and care. It is especially difficult with source-oriented records to track the treatments and client outcomes associated with a particular problem. For example, suppose a client with congestive heart failure (CHF) is retaining fluids, causing her to be short of breath on exertion. To find the interventions for the problem, you would need to look (1) in the primary care providers' (PCP) orders to see whether cardiac drugs or diuretics were prescribed to help with the fluid retention; (2) in the respiratory therapist's notes for breathing treatments and the client's response; and (3) in the nursing notes to see whether the client is being positioned with the head of the bed elevated to facilitate breathing. To see whether the medications were effective, you would need to read the nurse's notes about the client's responses to activity, the PCP progress notes, and the respiratory therapist's notes.

Problem-Oriented Record Systems

Problem-oriented records (PORs) are organized around the patient's problems. There are no separate sections for each discipline. The POR consists of four parts: database, problem list, plan of care, and progress notes.

- The **database** consists of many parts: demographic data, the history and physical, nursing assessment data, and family and social history. As the patient's condition changes, the database is updated to reflect the patient's current status.
- The **problem list** is a concise listing of problems that have been identified from the database. Once a problem is resolved, a notation is made on the problem list. If a problem changes or is redefined, the problem list is updated to reflect the change. See Figure 18-1 for an example of a problem list.
- The **plan of care** includes the primary care provider's orders and the nursing care plan for addressing the identified problems. Other disciplines may also contribute to the plan.

- **Progress notes** are organized according to the problem list. Each discipline charts on shared notes. Charting is labeled according to problem number.

Advantages. First, there is a common problem list that includes input from all disciplines. Second, it is easy to monitor the patient's progress because each problem is readily identified in the notes. Third, each discipline has ready access to the findings of the other members of the health team, which may encourage greater collaboration.

Disadvantages. To work well, the POR system requires a cooperative spirit among health providers as well as diligence in maintaining a current database and problem list.

Charting by Exception

Charting by exception (CBE) is more than a format; it is a system of charting in which only significant findings or exceptions to standards and norms of care are charted. To use the CBE system effectively, you must know and adhere to professional, legal, and organizational guidelines for nursing assessments and interventions.

CBE uses preprinted flow sheets to document most aspects of care. CBE assumes that unless a separate entry is made (an *exception*) all standards have been met and the patient has responded normally. Normal responses for various assessments are defined on the form, sometimes on the back of the form. CBE flow sheets vary by specialty, and, in some cases, even by diagnosis. Each flow sheet has entries for expected aspects of care.

Advantages. CBE reduces the amount of time spent on documentation, reduces repetitive charting of routine care, provides a record that is easily read and understood, and clearly highlights any variations from the expected plan of care. In many organizations, CBE records are kept at the bedside, which promotes timely documentation.

Disadvantages. Inadvertent omissions are the main problem associated with CBE. Omissions may result from disagreement over what constitutes a significant variation. Critics of CBE believe it (1) requires nurses to be overly familiar with the organization's documentation standards and policies; (2) makes it difficult to capture the skilled judgment of nurses; and (3) reduces care to such rote repetitions that you may forget to chart an exception to the established standards. Documentation must be time-sensitive, and under this system, false documentation can be created by assuming that care has been done when it has not.

On the following page is an example of what part of a CBE flow sheet for your patient, Steven Stellanski (Meet Your Patient), might look like. Notice in the first section, the day-shift nurse merely initials that she has made an assessment or taken one of the listed actions at each of the designated times.

Notice also the second half of the table (with the check marks) is a summary for the day shift. This is where the nurse describes and discusses any of the significant findings noted at the individual assessment times.

Electronic Health Record (EHR) Systems

The EHR consists of records that are entered via computer. EHRs typically combine source-oriented and problem-oriented record styles, although the source-oriented system is most common. For example, a client's EHR often contains orders; clinical documentation; laboratory and other test and procedure results; an interdisciplinary plan of care (IPOC); a problem and diagnosis list; and progress notes entered by physicians, nurses, respiratory therapists, and other professional providers.

Problem number	Date entered	Date resolved	Client problem
1	4/10/13	4/11/13	Abdominal pain (unknown etiology) Redefined 4/11/13
1A	4/11/13		Appendicitis resulting in emergency appendectomy
1B	4/11/13		Acute pain r/t abdominal incision 2 appendectomy
2	4/10/13		Down syndrome — functions at school-age level
3	4/11/13		Risk for constipation r/t opioid use for pain control and h/o appendicitis

FIGURE 18-1 A problem list for Steven Stellanski (Meet Your Patient). Note that problem 1 has been redefined now that the cause of Steven's pain has been determined. Note also that the list contains both medical and nursing diagnoses.

DATE: 04/11/13				
HOUR	**0800**	**0900**	**1000**	**1100**
Activity				
Bedrest		LP		
Ambulate	LP*			
Sleeping				
BRP				
HOB elevated	LP	LP		

	DAY	**EVENING**	**NIGHT**
Neurological	√	3	
Cardiovascular	√	3	
Pulmonary	√	3	
Gastrointestinal	√	*	Vomited 3×1, 100 mL clear yellow fluid at 0730. Given Compazine 1 mg IV with relief.

√ = normal findings * = significant finding.

Figure 18-2 shows a section of an electronic form for recording intake and output in source-oriented format. Figure 18-3 shows an electronic IPOC in problem-oriented format. As you can see in Figure 18-2, the input and output (I&O) screen records numerical data. It also allows the nurse to add brief narrative comments in each field. The IPOC can be updated at the times specified by the organization and the I&O data can be entered at any time. Both exist within the same electronic records system.

Advantages of Electronic Records Systems

EHRs have the following advantages:

Enhanced communication and collaboration among healthcare providers

Improved access to information:

Multiple healthcare providers can access the same information at the same time.

Authorized persons can access information remotely (e.g., from a patient's home).

EHRs can integrate client information between multiple departments so that one area can immediately see information from another. For example, when the laboratory enters a critical result, such as a clotting time, you do not need to wait for the lab to phone or to send a paper result to the nursing unit.

- **Time savings:**

Nurses spend up to 25% less time documenting.

Information is stored and retrieved quickly and easily.

Reports can be created quickly because of the computer's ability to aggregate data (e.g., a 24-hr graph of the patient's vital signs).

Repetition and duplication are reduced.

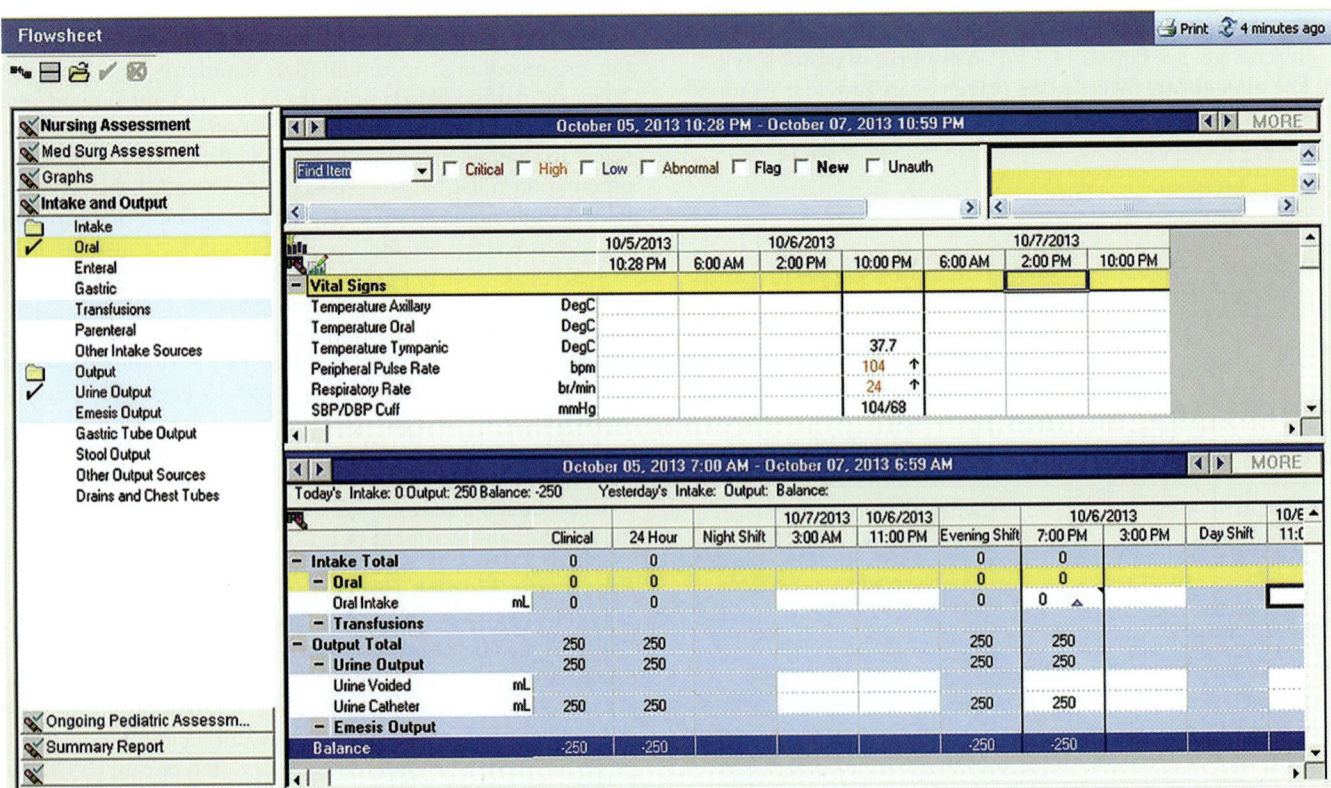

FIGURE 18-2 An electronic intake and output (I&O) entry form. (Courtesy of Cerner Corporation, Kansas City, MO.)

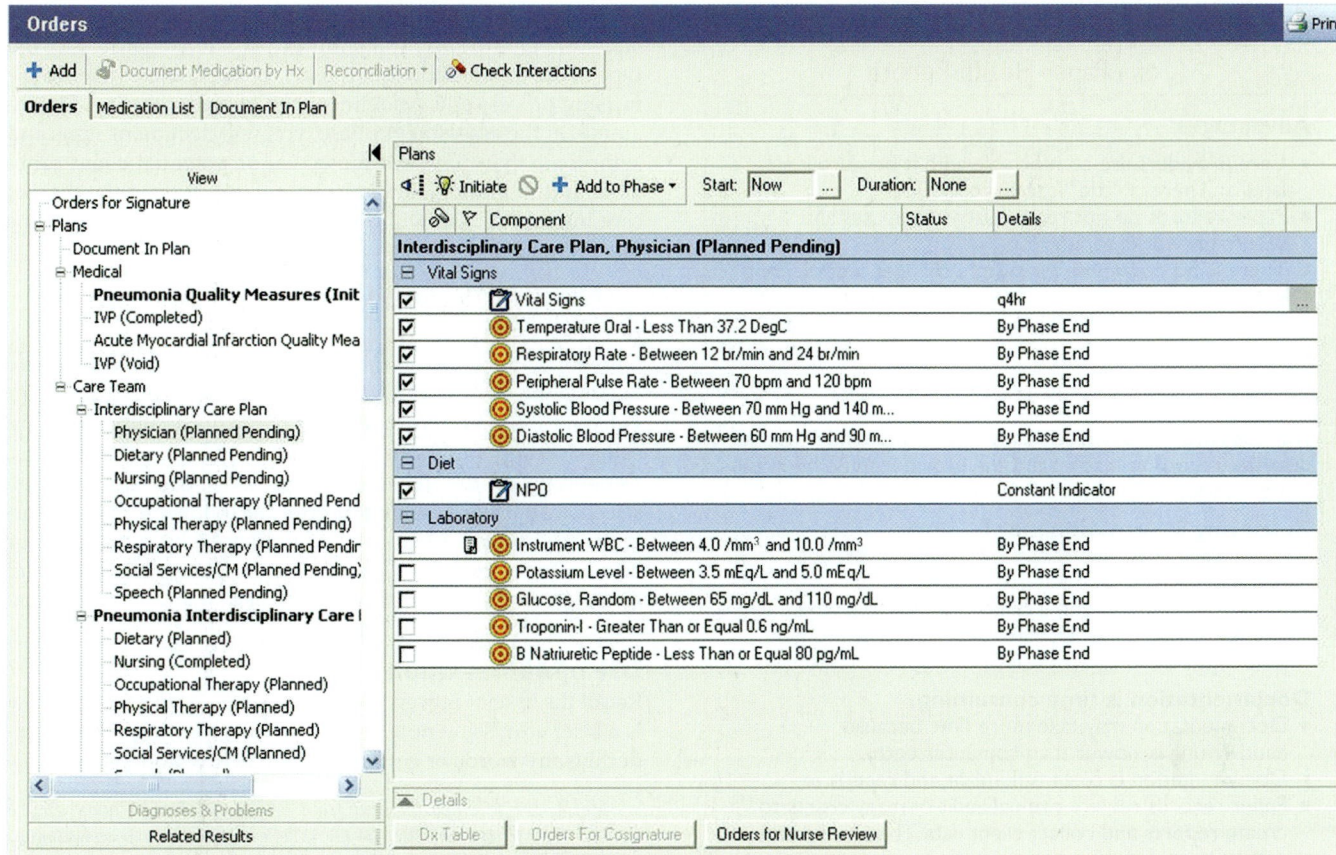

FIGURE 18-3 A portion of an electronic interdisciplinary plan of care (IPOC) form. (Courtesy of Cerner Corporation, Kansas City, MO.)

- **Improved quality of care:**
  The system can use protocols to automatically enter orders based on the client's condition. For example, some EHR systems will automatically enter an order to observe and document risk of falls more often when a patient's "falls score" exceeds a certain level.

  Embedded protocols enhance caregiver knowledge and the ability to follow clinical practice guidelines. For example, suppose there is a medical prescription to administer insulin on the basis of a patient's blood glucose results. In some EHR systems, the nurse can activate an immediate link to the tables of information needed to decide how much insulin to give to the patient.

  Medical errors are minimized by alerts that are automatically displayed when a care provider takes an action that could be harmful (e.g., when a provider prescribes a drug to which a patient is allergic).

  Data can be analyzed when collected, making immediate nursing decision making possible.

  EHRs facilitate evidence-based practice by making it possible to analyze thousands of records in ways that cannot be done with paper forms. With this aggregated data, nursing practice can be compared across populations and geographic locations to support nursing decisions and guide professional and organization quality improvement.

- **Information is private and safe:**
  Information is permanently stored and not likely to be lost.
  Confidentiality of client information is enhanced in several ways: tracking everyone who accesses the chart, proper security clearances, unique passwords, restricted access,

and using screen protectors that require a person to be directly in front of the screen to read it.

Disadvantages of Electronic Health Records

The following are disadvantages of EHRs:

- **Expense:** Electronic documentation systems are expensive.
- **Downtime:** Downtime processes must be in place for times when parts of the EHR are not available (e.g., because of power outages, severe weather, and system upgrades).
- **Difficulties associated with change:**
  Learning to use some documentation systems can be challenging and time consuming.
  Some healthcare providers see no reason to change and resist changing to EHR. Or they don't want to take the time to learn a new system, or have difficulty doing so.
  It is not always easy to capture narrative nursing content from paper documentation into an electronic format.
  Some EHRs are not user friendly (e.g., difficult to quickly find information needed to make care decisions).
  Some systems do not control redundancy well, requiring caregivers to ask the patient for the same information over and over in various sections of the EHR. This can be frustrating for users.
- **Lack of integration:** Most EHRs are not integrated across the different departments: Sometimes a person with a legitimate reason to enter the chart cannot see every part of it from where he is located. For example, you may not be able to access a patient's lab results from the nurses' desk, but must wait for the lab to send a report.

See Box 18-1 for advantages and disadvantages of paper health records.

BOX 18-1 ■ Advantages and Disadvantages of a Paper Health Record

Advantages

- Care providers are comfortable with it because it is familiar. There is little "learning curve."
- Paper records do not require large databases and secure networks to function.
- There is no downtime for system changes, weather, and so on.
- It is relatively inexpensive to create new forms and update old ones.

Disadvantages

Access may be delayed. Only one care provider can access the record at a time; and the provider must be in the same location as the chart.

Retrieving information may be slow.
- Healthcare providers may need to search through multiple pages to find needed information.
- Specific documentation is difficult to retrieve when needed, especially when files are archived in another part of the building.

Documentation is time consuming.
- Documentation may take more time because handwriting is slower than computer entry.
- Documentation is often redundant and repetitive.
- Paper records require manual audit of many charts to create reports and collect client data. This is time and resource intensive.

There is a relatively high risk for patient care error.
- Narrative documents are hard to read if the handwriting is illegible or messy. This means nurses have to take time from patient care to contact providers to clarify handwritten prescriptions.
- Papers can be lost from the chart or damaged, leading to duplicate assessments or medication errors.
- There is much inconsistency in how the same client information is documented, even within the same organization. Often, standardized terminology is not used.

Storage of paper records is expensive.

Confidentiality is difficult to protect. There is no way to know who may have access to the paper health record without proper authorization.

KnowledgeCheck 18-1

- Identify the purposes of the client health record.
- What are the key differences in the organization of source-oriented records, PORs, electronic documentation systems, and CBE systems?
- What are three advantages of paper health records?
- What are three advantages of EHRs?

Documentation and the Nursing Process

The goal of all nursing documentation is a clear, concise representation of the client's healthcare experience that is easily accessible and understood by all members of the healthcare team. Effective documentation allows you to help clients to make sound health decisions. It also enables use of current and consistent data, problem statements, diagnoses, goals, and strategies to support continuity of care. Regardless of the type of documentation that is used, you will use or refer to the nursing process as a guideline when you are charting. For example, in the assessment phase, you will document signs and symptoms that may indicate actual or potential client problems. In the implementation phase, after putting the plan of care into effect, you will document the specific interventions that were used.

What Are Some Common Formats for Nursing Progress Notes?

Nursing documentation can take many forms, including paper documents, computerized electronic documents, audio or video files, e-mails, faxes, scanned paper documents, electronically stored photographs, x-ray findings, and other images. Depending on the documentation model your organization selects, you may use one or more of the following charting formats. Choice of format is also influenced by whether your nursing documentation is written on paper, captured and stored electronically, or in a blend of the two. In all formats, you must learn to use abbreviations appropriately.

Use of Abbreviations

Recall the case of Steven Stellanski (Meet Your Patient). Below is a brief admission note using narrative charting format. Underline any words or entries that you do not understand:

4/11/13 Pt received on unit from PACU. VSS. TM temp 99.9°F (37.7°C), P 104, and BP 104.68. LOC unstable. Arouses when name called but quickly drifts off to sleep. PERRLA. Moaning, grimacing, holding abd, whispers "Help me. Help me." LR at 125 mL/hr infusing in R forearm. Urinary catheter in place, draining pale yellow urine. Drsg dry & intact. Morphine sulfate PCA ordered. Will initiate. ——————— Ray Allenby, RN.

You can see from this entry that nurses use many abbreviations in their paper record charting. Every healthcare institution has a list of abbreviations that may and may not be used in documentation. Be sure to consult your organization's list before you chart. For a list of commonly used abbreviations in healthcare, see Box 18-2. For abbreviations to use when giving medications, see Chapter 25.

The Joint Commission (2008a, 2010) mandates that healthcare organizations not use the following abbreviations. This is referred to as the "do not use" list.

- "U" or "u" for unit
- "IU" for International Unit
- Q.D., QD, q.d., qd (daily)
- Q.O.D., QOD, q.o.d., qod (every other day)
- Trailing zero (X.0 mg) and lack of leading zero (.X mg)
- MS, MSO4, and MgSO4—could mean morphine sulfate or magnesium sulfate.

The following abbreviations and symbols are under serious consideration for inclusion on The Joint Commission's "do not use" list in the future. Some institutions have already stopped using them:

- The symbols ">" and "<" (write "greater than" or "less than")
- All abbreviations for drug names (write drug names in full)
- Apothecary units (use metric units instead)
- The symbol "@" (write "at" or "each")
- The abbreviation "cc" (write "mL" or "milliliters")
- The abbreviation "μg" (write "mcg" or "micrograms")

BOX 18-2 ■ Abbreviations Commonly Used in Healthcare*

Abbreviation	Meaning	Abbreviation	Meaning
ADLs	Activities of daily living	ht	Height
ad lib	As desired, if the patient desires	HTN	Hypertension
AKA	Above-knee amputation	hyper	Above or high
Amb	Ambulation, ambulatory	hypo	Below or low
Amt	Amount	ICU	Intensive care unit
ASAP	As soon as possible	I&O	Intake and output
bid	Twice a day	Isol	Isolation
BM	Bowel movement	IV	Intravenous
BR	Bedrest	IVP	Intravenous push (caution: do not use to mean "IV piggyback")
BRP	Bathroom privileges		
BSC	Bedside commode	L	Liter
$\bar{c}$	With	lb	Pound
c	Calories	LMP	Last menstrual period
Cath	Catheter	LPN	Licensed practical nurse
CBC	Complete blood count	LVN	Licensed vocational nurse
CCU	Critical care unit or coronary care unit	mcg	Microgram
		MD	Medical doctor
c/o	Complaint of	med	Medication
CO_2	Carbon dioxide	mg	Milligram
CPR	Cardiopulmonary resuscitation	mL	Milliliter
CVA	Cerebrovascular accident (stroke)	MN	Midnight
D&C	Dilation and curettage	NAS	No added salt
DM	Diabetes mellitus	N/V/D	Nausea, vomiting, diarrhea
dsg or drsg	Dressing	NKA or NKDA	No known allergies or no known drug allergies
DX or Dx	Diagnosis		
EBL	Estimated blood loss	NG	Nasogastric
ECG/EKG	Electrocardiogram	NGT	Nasogastric tube
ED/ER	Emergency department, emergency room	noc	At night
		NPO	Nothing by mouth
EEG	Electroencephalogram	O_2	Oxygen
EENT	Eyes, ears, nose, throat	OB	Obstetrics
ETOH	Alcohol	OOB	Out of bed
F	Female	OPD	Outpatient department
FBS	Fasting blood sugar	ortho	Orthopedics
Ft	Foot	OR	Operating room
Fx	Fracture	os	Mouth, opening
GI	Gastrointestinal	OT	Occupational therapy
gtt(s)	Drop(s)	oz	Ounce
GU	Genitourinary	pc	After meals
GYN	Gynecology	PCA	Patient-controlled analgesia
HA	Headache	PO	By mouth
HMO	Health maintenance organization	P, $\bar{p}$	After
h/o	History of	PPBS	Postprandial blood sugar
hob or HOB	Head of bed	prn	As needed
HOH	Hard of hearing	Pt	Patient
H&P	History and physical	PT	Physical therapy
hr	Hour	q	Every

(Continued)

BOX 18-2 ■ Abbreviations Commonly Used in Healthcare*—cont'd

Abbreviation	Meaning	Abbreviation	Meaning
qam	Every morning	TB	Tuberculosis
qh	Every hour	TO	Telephone order
qid	Four times a day	TPR	Temperature, pulse, respirations
RN	Registered nurse		
RX or Rx	Treatment or prescription	tid	Three times a day
$\bar{s}$	Without	VO	Verbal order
SCD	Sequential compression device	VS	Vital signs
SOB	Short of breath	WBC	White blood count
$\bar{ss}$	One-half	w/c	Wheelchair
SSE	Soapsuds enema	WNL	Within normal limits
STAT	Immediately	wt	Weight
STI or STD	Sexually transmitted infection or sexually transmitted disease		

*Key Point: *Abbreviations vary among healthcare agencies. Furthermore, they change often because of changes in regulating agency (e.g., The Joint Commission) guidelines. Therefore, you will need to be familiar with the abbreviations in the agency in which you work.*

Narrative Format

Narrative format is used with written source-oriented and problem-oriented charts. The **narrative chart entry** tells the story of the patient's experience in a chronological format (i.e., in the order that it happens). The goal is to track the client's changing health status and progress toward goals. Narrative charting is especially useful when attempting to construct a time line of events, such as a cardiac arrest or other emergency situations.

Problem–Intervention–Evaluation (PIE)

The problem–intervention–evaluation (PIE) system organizes information according to the patient's problems and requires keeping a daily assessment record and progress notes. This eliminates the need for a separate care plan and provides a nursing-focused rather than medical-focused record.

Problem: Use data from your original assessment to identify appropriate nursing diagnoses.

Intervention: Document the nursing actions you take for each nursing diagnosis.

Evaluation: Document the patient's response to interventions and treatments.

Problems are identified from the admission assessment. Subsequent entries begin with identification of the problem number. This type of charting establishes an ongoing care plan. A PIE charting entry for Steven Stellanski might look like this:

4/11/13   1630

P: 1B

I: Pt .1 mg doses up to 4 mg morphine/hr. Pt groggy yet c/o pain. Has not triggered PCA independently. Rates pain as 8 on scale of 1–10. PCA use reviewed with pt. Demonstrated use $\bar{c}$ 1st dose at 1615.

E: Pt still moaning & grimacing. Has not initiated another dose via PCA. 2nd dose given as additional demo. Will reevaluate in 1 hr. May need continuous infusion if pt unable to use to control pain. ——————Ron Allen, RN

SOAP/SOAPIE/SOAPIER

The SOAP format is often used to write nursing and other progress notes. It can be used in source-oriented, problem-oriented, and electronic health records. The acronyms SOAP, SOAPIE, and SOAPIER are explained below.

- *Subjective data*—What the patient or family members tell you about the client's signs and symptoms and the reason they are seeking healthcare. Typically this is documented by quoting the actual words said.
- *Objective data*—Factual, measurable clinical findings such as vital signs, test results, and quality of breath sounds.
- *Assessment*—Conclusions drawn from the subjective and objective data, usually patient problems or nursing diagnoses. SOAP terminology is different from nursing process terminology. In the nursing process chapters (3 through 7) we refer to conclusions about data as inferences or problems, and state that assessment does *not* include conclusions about data. When using SOAP, you *should* document your conclusions under *A*.
- *Plan*: Short-term and long-term goals and strategies that will be used to relieve the patient's problems.
- *Interventions*: Actions of the healthcare team that are performed to achieve expected outcomes.
- *Evaluation*: An analysis of the effectiveness of interventions.
- *Revision*: Changes made to the original care plan.

Recall that a POR is organized according to specific patient problems, and has five components: database, problem list, initial plan, progress notes, and a discharge summary. You will refer to and use the following four parts when charting in SOAP format.

Problem List. This numbered list of the patient's current problems in chronological order is compiled so that you can refer to the number when entering your notes.

Initial Plan. This includes expected outcomes and plans for further care interventions and teaching. There is only one initial plan; you update and change the plan in subsequent progress notes.

Progress Notes. This is where you record the SOAP(IER) information. As a rule, you enter a note for each current problem every 24 hours or when the patient's condition changes.

Discharge Summary. At discharge, each problem on the list is addressed and a notation made about whether it was resolved. Unresolved problems, with plans for each, are included when communicating with the patient, other facilities, and home health agencies.

Following is an example of SOAP progress notes using the admission data of Steven Stellanski (Meet Your Patient). In the previous section, these same data were used to create a narrative note. Notice that the data are similar, but the narrative note is organized by data source. Steven's SOAPIER charting entry related to his postoperative nausea and pain could look like this:

4/11/13	0830	#1 – Nausea related to anesthesia
		S – Pt states "I feel sick to my stomach. Help me."
		O – Pt vomited 100 mL clear, light yellow fluid.
		A – Pt is nauseated secondary to anesthesia.
		P – Monitor nausea and give antiemetic as needed.
		I – Pt given Compazine 1 mg IV at 0830.
	0900	E – Pt states he feels less sick to his stomach. ————Ron Allen, RN
4/11/13	0830	#1B – Acute pain related to abdominal incision 2° appendectomy
		S – States, "help me, help me." Moaning and grimacing.
		O – Moaning and grimacing; holding abd. Drsg dry & intact. BP 104/68 mm Hg, P 104 beats/min, Resp 24 breaths/min, and TM temp 99.9°F. PERRLA.
		A – Postoperative pain
		P – Give analgesic as needed.
		I – Morphine PCA initiated at 0835. Pt. instructed in use. 1st dose (1 mg) administered as demonstration.
	0900	E – Still moaning & grimacing even after 2nd dose given as additional demo. Still has not initiated additional PCA dose.————Ron Allen, RN
	0930	R – Still no pain relief; still has not used PCA independently. Discussed w/ Dr. Jadu. Continuous infusion begun at 2 mg/hr. Will supplement up to 4 mg/hr prn. Ron Allen, RN

Focus Charting®

The term *focus* is used to encourage you to view the client's status from a positive perspective rather than the negative focus in problem charting. **Focus Charting®** uses assessment data to evaluate client care concerns, problems, or strengths. It also identifies necessary revisions to the care plan as you document each entry.

The focus is often a nursing diagnosis (e.g., Ineffective Breathing Pattern), a sign or symptom (e.g., shortness of breath), a client behavior (e.g., inability to follow inhaler instructions), a special need (e.g., non-English-speaking), an acute change in condition (e.g., sudden appearance of chest pain), or a significant event (e.g., surgery). Focus Charting® works well in acute care settings and in areas in which the same care and procedures are repeated frequently.

The first column contains the time and date. The second column identifies the focus or problem addressed in the note. The third column contains charting in a DAR format. DAR is an acronym for *data*, *action*, and *response*.

Data. Subjective and objective information that supports the focus. This section reflects the assessment phase of the nursing process and includes other data, such as laboratory results or other diagnostic testing.

Action. Interventions performed, such as administering medications or making calls to the primary provider. This section reflects the planning and implementation phases of the nursing process.

Response. The patient's response to your interventions. This section reflects the evaluation phase of the nursing process.

The following is an example of a Focus® note.

4/11/13 1800	Focus: Developmental delay	D: 16 y.o. rec'd on unit at 1600 from PACU post-appendectomy. Pt w/ Down syndrome. Morphine PCA initiated. Pt unable to use PCA to control pain. Continuous infusion at 2 mg/hr begun at 1745. PERRLA. Alert, drifting in & out of sleep. PACU RNM reports pt functions at school-age level.
		A: Will discuss pt status w/parents and adjust plan of care accordingly. ———— Ron Allen, RN
1830		R: Met w/ parents, who report that pt has significant developmental delays & needs supervision w/ all ADLs. Pt comfortable on 2 mg/hr infusion of morphine. Use of PCA for supplementary pain control reviewed with parents. Parents demonstrated understanding and that they will assist pt w/ PCA if add'l meds are needed ————Ron Allen, RN

FACT System

Noted for its individual elements, the FACT documentation model incorporates many CBE principles and includes four key elements:

*F*low sheets individualized to specific services

*A*ssessment features standardized with baseline parameters

*C*oncise, integrated progress notes and flow sheets documenting the client's condition and responses

*T*imely entries documented when care is given

FACT documentation includes only exceptions to the norm or significant information about the patient. It eliminates the need to chart normal findings. The following is a FACT example for Steven Stellanski.

DATE/TIME	04/12/13 0900	04/12/13 1330
Neurological Alert and oriented to time, place, and person. PERRLA. Symmetry of strength in extremities. No difficulty with coordination. Behavior appropriate to situation. Sensation intact without numbness or paresthesias.	√	√
Orient patient		
Refer to neurological flow sheet		
Pain No report of pain. If present, include pain scale intensity choice by patient (0–10) with location, description, duration, radiation, precipitating and alleviating factors.	Abdominal incision pain – score 10	√
Location	RLQ	
Description	Dull, constant	
Relief measures	Percocet 1 tablet by mouth	
Pain relief: Y = yes / N = no	Y	
Cardiovascular Apical pulse 60 to 100. S_1 and S_2 present. Regular rhythm. Peripheral pulses (radial, pedal) present bilaterally. No edema or calf tenderness. Extremities pink, warm, moveable within patient's ROM.	√	√
IV Solution and Rate	D5½ NS at 125 mL/hr	D5½ NS at 125 mL/hr

Electronic Entry

Electronic clinical information systems are being used more and more frequently. The streamlined electronic processes make documentation more accurate and efficient, and reduce the risk of human error. This frees you to do the expert work that only nurses can do.

Electronic documentation requires a shift in how you document your work. EHRs force change from paper to electronic documentation, change in where documentation is done (e.g., at the bedside using a portable wireless device vs. at the nursing station), and change in decision-making processes (immediate vs. gradual).

Electronic documentation forms and flow sheets (such as Fig. 18-2) already include the information that your organization has decided is important to document. Reminders to document specific kinds of information, such as overdue medications and overdue nursing interventions, display automatically to help prevent late or omitted care. Also, the extensive use of clearly named data entry fields, drop-down menus, check boxes, and specially created templates allows you to enter your nursing documentation quickly and efficiently, usually with minimal keyboard typing.

Depending on the EHR system used, progress notes may be documented electronically in prebuilt note formats in various prebuilt charting forms. In some electronic systems, you may still need to write progress notes on lined paper, in narrative, SOAP, PIE, POC, Focus®, or FACT formats.

Transitioning from paper to electronic documentation can be challenging. It usually takes a few days to know where to document your nursing care and feel confident that you haven't overlooked anything. However, EHR software is becoming more logical and user friendly. Many organizations have printed information, classes, and Web-based tutorials that provide information about electronic charting. Take advantage of opportunities to build your knowledge when they arise.

KnowledgeCheck 18-2

Summarize the characteristics, advantages, and disadvantages of each of the different kinds of nursing documentation formats (narrative, PIE, SOAP, Focus®, CBE, FACT, and electronic entry).

ThinkLike a Nurse 18-1

Compare the documentation examples (narrative, PIE, SOAP, Focus®, CBE, FACT, and electronic documentation). If you have had experience with charting in the clinical setting, apply this experience as well. With which charting format do you feel most comfortable? Why?

What Forms Do Nurses Use to Document Nursing Care?

Documentation forms vary by purpose, institution, and unit. However, regardless of the system or forms used, nursing documentation reflects the nursing process. You record assessments, diagnoses, planning, implementation (what you actually did), and evaluation of client responses. This section discusses the most commonly used paper and electronic documentation forms that are used in addition to the nursing progress notes discussed in the preceding sections.

Nursing Admission Data Forms

A separate nursing admission form or a combined interdisciplinary form is completed at the time the patient enters the healthcare system. Figure 18-4 shows an example of a screen from an electronic nursing admission data form. For examples of a paper admission form,

 Go to Chapter 3, **Tables, Boxes, Figures: ESG Figure 3-1, Nursing Admission Data Form,** on Davis*Plus,* and to Chapter 18, **Tables, Boxes, Figures: ESG Figure 18-1, Adult Inpatient Admission Assessment,** on Davis*Plus.*

You will use admission forms in all settings, for example, in ambulatory clinics and long-term care facilities. An ambulatory care admission form includes demographic data, allergy information, current medications, family health data, social history, and the client's past medical history. The form completed by Nam Nguyen at his first clinic visit is an example of an ambulatory care admission form. To see Mr. Nguyen's completed form, see Meet the Nguyens at the beginning of the book.

Discharge Summary

Discharge data are obtained with the admission assessment, but are often recorded on a separate form. Discharge needs should be evaluated when the patient first enters a healthcare facility, especially in acute-care facilities. Ask yourself what this patient would need if he were to go home in the next few days. For example, would he need help with food preparation? Does he understand how to use his medicines?

A **discharge summary** is the last entry made in the paper chart. In the electronic chart, the discharge summary can be begun any time after admission and revised throughout the hospitalization. A summary is completed when the patient is transferred within the same organization, transferred to another facility, or discharged to home. The discharge summary may be a multidisciplinary document or each discipline may write a separate summary. The forms are different in each organization, but they contain similar data. For an example of an electronic discharge summary, see Figure 18-5. For paper discharge forms, see Figures 11-5 and 11-6.

As you can see in Figure 18-5, there is a drop-down menu in which the Nursing Discharge Note is located. It is important to clearly document the patient's condition on discharge because the discharge summary serves as baseline data for the healthcare professionals who will follow up on the patient after discharge.

Flow Sheets and Graphic Records

You will use flow sheets and graphic records to document assessments and care that are performed frequently, on a recurring schedule, or as a part of unit routines. For example, most hospital units require that vital signs be taken every 8 hours for all patients. How often you perform and document care activities depends on your patient's condition and the unit policy. In the first hour after surgery, for example, you would probably record vital signs every 15 minutes, and after that, every hour for 4 hours.

The simplest paper forms are organized with time in columns across the top and the activities or patient assessment parameters in rows down the side. On electronic forms, the areas (fields) to enter the time and activities are arranged close together. Flow sheets and graphic records allow you to see patterns of change in patient status. For instance, you may view a

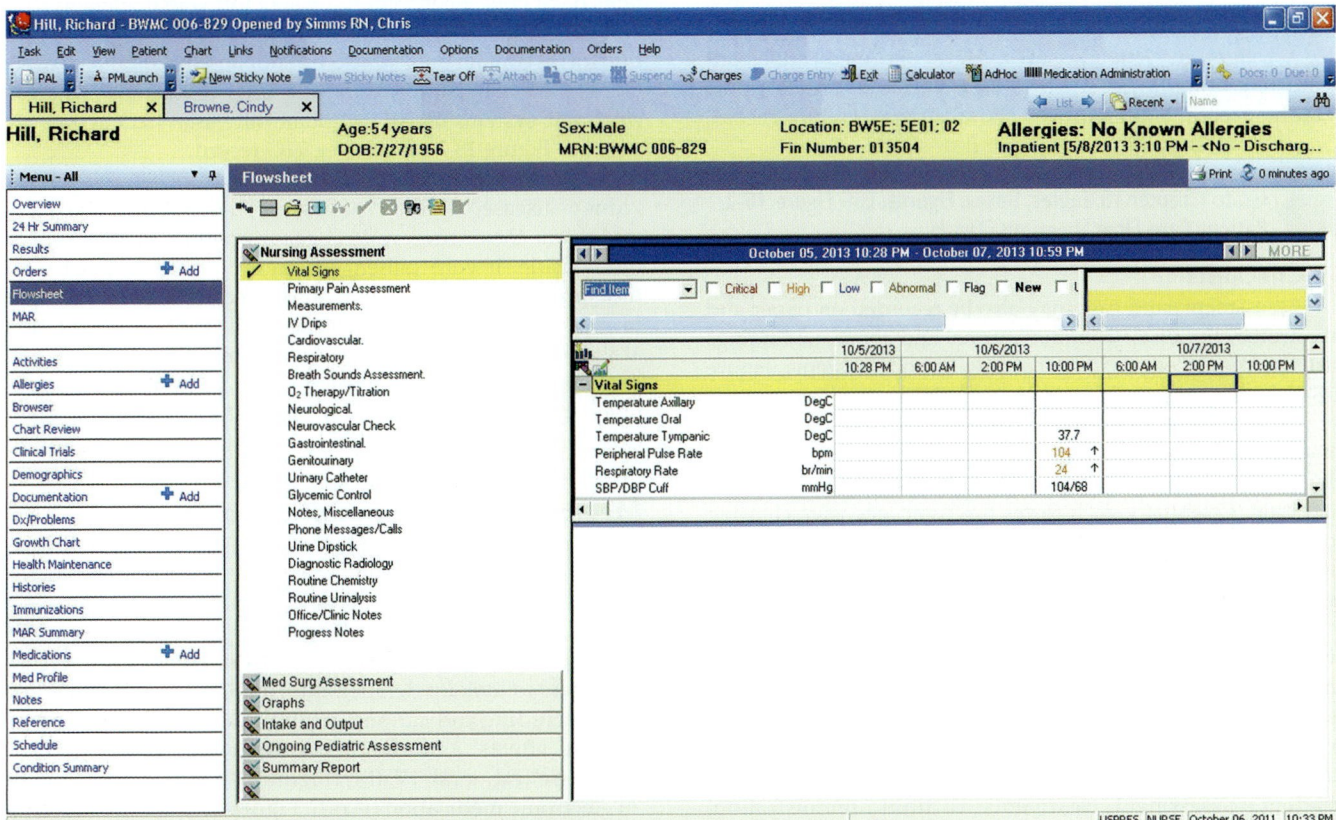

FIGURE 18-4 Adult admission history electronic screen. (Courtesy of Cerner Corporation, Kansas City, MO.)

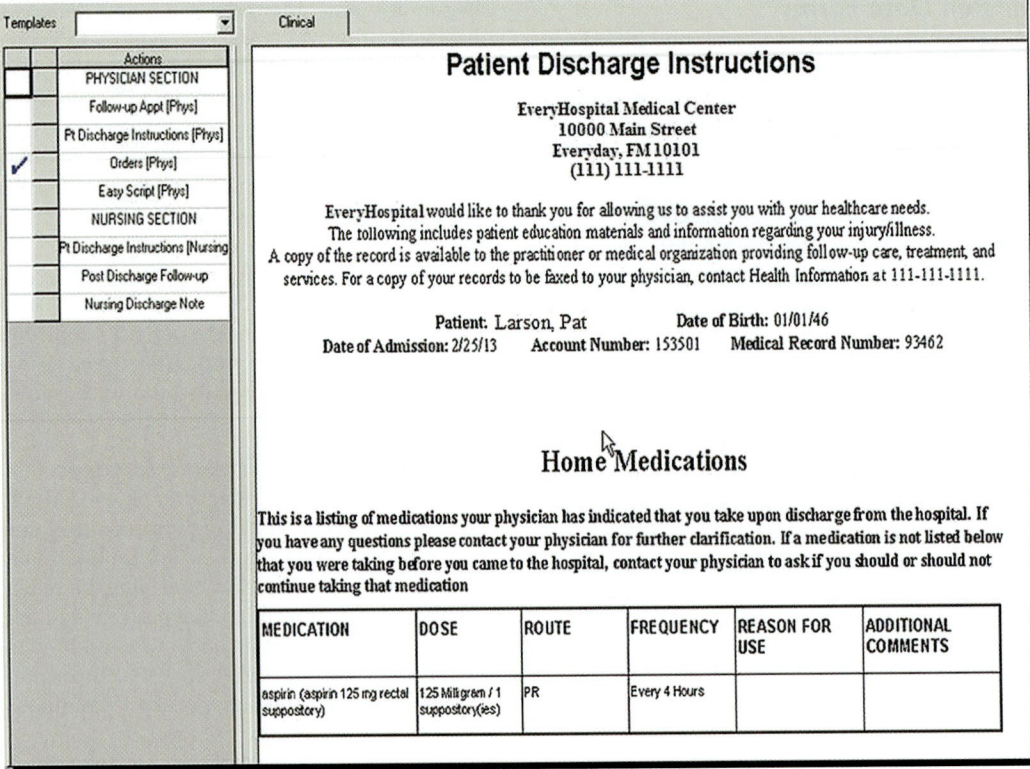

FIGURE 18-5 A portion of an electronic discharge planning form. (Courtesy of Cerner Corporation, Kansas City, MO.)

steady increase in the line representing a patient's blood pressure compared to his pain score on an electronically generated graph. On a paper form, you may scan across a row to see that your patient has not had a bowel movement for several days. Other types of information recorded on flow sheets include I&O, weight, hygiene measures, ADLs, and medications administered. Figure 18-2 shows an example of an electronic graphic record, and Figure 3-3 shows a paper graphic record. To see a nursing assessment paper flow sheet,

 Go to Chapter 18, **Tables, Boxes, Figures: ESG Figure 18-2, Patient Care Flow Sheet,** on DavisPlus.

Checklists

Assessments and care may also be recorded on paper and electronic checklists. Common normal and abnormal findings are commonly organized according to body systems. Figure 18-6 shows an example of a paper checklist.

Using a paper form, the nurse checks the box that reflects the current assessment findings. Some checklists include nursing actions, such as wound care, treatments, or IV fluid administration. Essentially such forms are comprehensive charting documents (e.g., ESG Fig. 18-2). Exceptions, patient care activities, and patient responses are recorded in the narrative note section of the paper form.

Using an electronic field-based checklist, the nurse enters values or text in the appropriate fields and saves the documentation. Electronic flow sheets typically contain content similar to that on paper checklists, but also include a greater range of potential documentation areas that can be opened as needed. This allows for a more comprehensive record of a patient's assessment, treatments, IV fluid administration, and many other parameters.

Intake and Output Records

You will sometimes use separate I&O paper records to document data about the patient's fluid balance. Electronic systems have flow sheet sections or I&O forms to document I&O and save it into the patient's EHR. Usually these documentation forms contain data totaled by shift and by 24-hour periods (see Fig. 18-2). Paper forms must be totaled manually, whereas electronic systems usually automatically total I&O figures for you. See Figure 18-7 for a paper I&O record.

I&O records are particularly important for clients who have kidney disease, CHF, or pulmonary edema, or who have undergone major surgery. I&O paper graphics may be kept at the bedside. If your patient or family is able to assist with measuring his I&O, teach him how to record data on the paper form. You might also complete electronic I&O documentation at the bedside using a portable computer. When appropriate, patients can still track their own intake and output on paper, but you will need to enter the patient's I&O data into the EHR. Chapter 30 provides detailed information about monitoring intake and output.

Medication Administration Records

Medication administration records (MARs) contain information about the medications that have been prescribed for the client. The information and format of MARs vary by setting, with significant differences between outpatient and inpatient facilities. Some electronic MARs allow care providers to look up detailed information about the medication, including indications, contraindications, expected or adverse effects, and standard dosages for the prescribed drug type (e.g., oral, IV, IM). Figure 18-8 shows a portion of an electronic medication record. Figure 25-6 shows an example of a paper MAR.

DATE   /   /

PHYSICAL ASSESSMENT - SHIFT _____

NEURO

LOC	ORIENTATION	SPEECH
❑ ALERT	❑ X3 ❑ FOR AGE	❑ APPROPRIATE
❑ SEDATED	❑ PERSON	❑ APHASIA
❑ LETHARGIC	❑ PLACE	❑ SLURRED
❑ UNRESPONSIVE	❑ TIME	❑ RAMBLING

SENSATION	FONTANELS	
❑ INTACT	❑ FLAT	❑ NA
❑ NUMBNESS	❑ SUNKEN	
❑ TINGLING	❑ BULGING	

CARDIOVASCULAR

RHYTHM	PULSE	EDEMA	CAP. REFILL
❑ REGULAR	❑ STRONG	❑ ABSENT	❑ < 3 SEC.
❑ IRREGULAR	❑ WEAK	❑ _____	❑ > 3 SEC.
❑ MURMUR			

MONITOR RHYTHM

RESPIRATORY

EFFORT		BREATH LU LL SOUNDS RU RL	
❑ NORMAL	❑ DYSPNEA ❑❑	CLEAR	❑❑
❑ LABORED	❑ COUGH ❑❑	CRACKLES	❑❑
❑ NASAL FLARING	❑ SPUTUM ❑❑	RHONCHI	❑❑
❑ RETRACTIONS	❑ CRYING ❑❑	WHEEZING	❑❑
❑ IRREGULAR		DIMINISHED	❑❑
		ABSENT	❑❑

GASTROINTESTINAL

ABDOMEN		
❑ FLAT	❑ FIRM	❑ NAUSEA
❑ ROUNDED	❑ TENDER	❑ VOMITING
❑ DISTENDED	❑ NON-TENDER	
❑ SOFT		
❑ GIRTH_____ CM		

BOWEL SOUNDS	STOOL	
❑ ACTIVE	❑ REGULAR	LAST BM
❑ ABSENT	❑ CONSTIPATED	
❑ HYPER	❑ DIARRHEA	_____
❑ HYPO	❑ INCONTINENT	

SUCTION
❑ INTERMITTANT   ❑ CONSTANT   ❑ CLAMPED
❑ FEEDING TUBE   ❑ PATENT
❑ NG   ❑ PLACEMENT ✔
DRNG COLOR:

GU

URINE	❑ CATHETER
❑ CLEAR, YELLOW / AMBER ❑ QS	❑ PAIN
❑ OTHER _____ ❑ FREQUENT	
❑ RETENTION ❑ INCONTINENT	

MUSCULOSKELETAL

MOBILITY	MUSCLE TONE	ROM
❑ NORMAL	❑ GOOD	❑ FULL
❑ ASSIST X _____	❑ OTHER	❑ LIMITED
❑ AMBULATORY		
❑ BED REST		
❑ OTHER	❑ P.T. CONSULT	

SKIN

CONDITION	TURGOR	MUCOUS MEM
❑ WARM, DRY INTACT	❑ ADEQUATE	❑ MOIST
❑ BREAKDOWN	❑ DECREASED	❑ DRY

COLOR ❑ NORMAL
❑ PALE ❑ CYANOTIC ❑ FLUSHED ❑ _____

WOUND/INCISION/ DRESSING

LOCATION/CONDITION/DRAINAGE	HEALING NO S/S INFECTION
_____	❑
_____	❑
_____	❑

TUBES/DRAINS

LOCATION/CONDITION/DRAINAGE	GRAVITY	SUCTION
_____	❑	❑
_____	❑	❑
_____	❑	❑

IV'S

IV SITE / CONDITION	PATENT, NO REDNESS OR SWELLING	PUMP
_____	❑	❑
_____	❑	❑
_____	❑	❑

NURSING ASSESSMENT   PATIENT NAME

PAIN
❑ ABSENT   PAIN SCALE _____
❑ PRESENT   LOCATION _____
❑ CONTROLLED

PSYCHOSOCIAL

EYE CONTACT ❑ YES ❑ NO		
❑ APPROPRIATE	❑ RESTLESS	❑ COMBATIVE
❑ FLAT AFFECT	❑ AGITATED	❑ BELLIGERENT
❑ UNCOOPERATIVE	❑ CRYING	❑ ODOR
❑ ANXIOUS	❑ SUBSTANCE USE	

DISCHARGE

DISCHARGE PLAN
❑ NA	❑ ONGOING	❑ COMPLETED
❑ D.P. CONSULT	❑ O.T CONSULT	❑ H.H. CONSULT

EQUIPMENT

❑ BED ALARM	❑ CARDIAC MONITOR
❑ CPM	❑ FEEDING PUMP
❑ IV PUMP X_____	❑ K - PAD
❑ OXIMETER	❑ PCA PUMP
❑ PASSPORT	❑ POLAR ICE
❑ SUCTION	❑ TELEMETRY
❑ _____	❑ _____
❑ _____	❑ _____

SIGN

SIGNATURE X_____ TIME_____
REASSESSED BY X_____ TIME_____

OBSERVATION / INTERVENTION / EVALUATION
(TIME & INITIAL ENTRIES)

PHYSICAL ASSESSMENT - SHIFT _____

NEURO

LOC	ORIENTATION	SPEECH
❑ ALERT	❑ X3 ❑ FOR AGE	❑ APPROPRIATE
❑ SEDATED	❑ PERSON	❑ APHASIA
❑ LETHARGIC	❑ PLACE	❑ SLURRED
❑ UNRESPONSIVE	❑ TIME	❑ RAMBLING

SENSATION	FONTANELS	
❑ INTACT	❑ FLAT	❑ NA
❑ NUMBNESS	❑ SUNKEN	
❑ TINGLING	❑ BULGING	

CARDIOVASCULAR

RHYTHM	PULSE	EDEMA	CAP. REFILL
❑ REGULAR	❑ STRONG	❑ ABSENT	❑ < 3 SEC.
❑ IRREGULAR	❑ WEAK	❑ _____	❑ > 3 SEC.
❑ MURMUR			

MONITOR RHYTHM

RESPIRATORY

EFFORT		BREATH LU LL SOUNDS RU RL	
❑ NORMAL	❑ DYSPNEA ❑❑	CLEAR	❑❑
❑ LABORED	❑ COUGH ❑❑	CRACKLES	❑❑
❑ NASAL FLARING	❑ SPUTUM ❑❑	RHONCHI	❑❑
❑ RETRACTIONS	❑ CRYING ❑❑	WHEEZING	❑❑
❑ IRREGULAR		DIMINISHED	❑❑
		ABSENT	❑❑

GASTROINTESTINAL

ABDOMEN		
❑ FLAT	❑ FIRM	❑ NAUSEA
❑ ROUNDED	❑ TENDER	❑ VOMITING
❑ DISTENDED	❑ NON-TENDER	
❑ SOFT		
❑ GIRTH_____ CM		

BOWEL SOUNDS	STOOL	
❑ ACTIVE	❑ REGULAR	LAST BM
❑ ABSENT	❑ CONSTIPATED	
❑ HYPER	❑ DIARRHEA	
❑ HYPO	❑ INCONTINENT	

SUCTION
❑ INTERMITTANT   ❑ CONSTANT   ❑ CLAMPED
❑ FEEDING TUBE   ❑ PATENT
❑ NG   ❑ PLACEMENT
DRNG COLOR:

GU

URINE	❑ CATHETER
❑ CLEAR, YELLOW / AMBER ❑ QS	❑ PAIN
❑ OTHER _____ ❑ FREQUENT	
❑ RETENTION ❑ INCONTINENT	

MUSCULOSKELETAL

MOBILITY	MUSCLE TONE	ROM
❑ NORMAL	❑ GOOD	❑ FULL
❑ ASSIST X _____	❑ OTHER	❑ LIMITED
❑ AMBULATORY		
❑ BED REST		
❑ OTHER	❑ P.T. CONSULT	

SKIN

CONDITION	TURGOR	MUCOUS MEM
❑ WARM, DRY INTACT	❑ ADEQUATE	❑ MOIST
❑ BREAKDOWN	❑ DECREASED	❑ DRY

COLOR ❑ NORMAL
❑ PALE ❑ CYANOTIC ❑ FLUSHED ❑ _____

WOUND/INCISION/ DRESSING

LOCATION/CONDITION/DRAINAGE	HEALING NO S/S INFECTION
_____	❑
_____	❑
_____	❑

TUBES/DRAINS

LOCATION/CONDITION/DRAINAGE	GRAVITY	SUCTION
_____	❑	❑
_____	❑	❑
_____	❑	❑

IV'S

IV SITE / CONDITION	PATENT, NO REDNESS OR SWELLING	PUMP
_____	❑	❑
_____	❑	❑
_____	❑	❑

FIGURE 18-6 A portion of a nursing assessment checklist.

INTAKE AND OUTPUT SHEET

DATE	Time	INTAKE						OUTPUT						SIGNATURE OF NURSE
		ORAL	IV	IV MED	BLOOD PRODUCT	OTHER	TOTAL	URINE	EMESIS	STOOL	SUCTION	OTHER	TOTAL	
	6 A.M.-2 P.M.													
	2 P.M.-10 P.M.													
	10 P.M.-6 A.M.													
	TOTAL													
	6 A.M.-2 P.M.													
	2 P.M.-10 P.M.													
	10 P.M.-6 A.M.													
	TOTAL													

FIGURE 18-7 Nurses use I&O records to record data about the patient's fluid status.

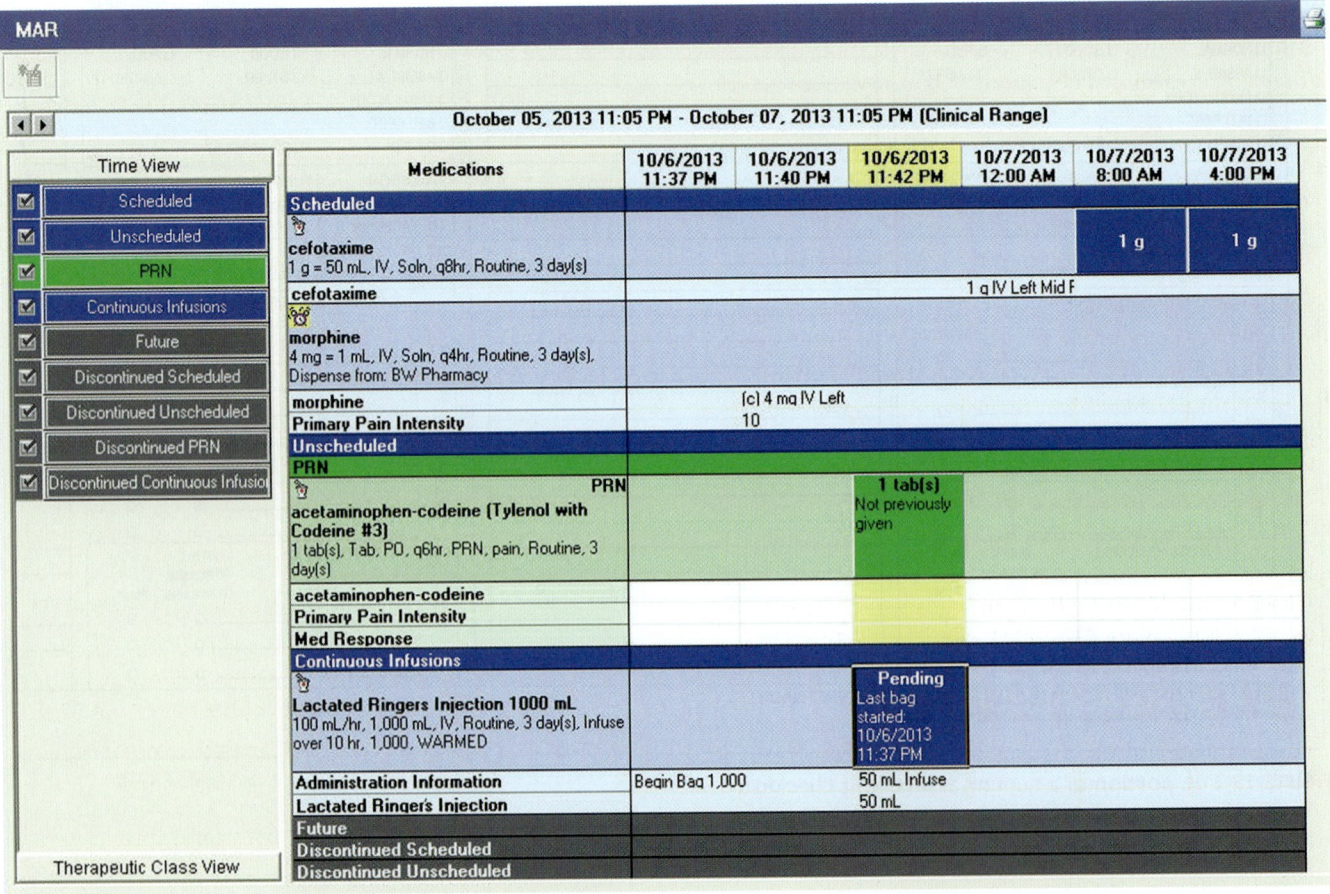

FIGURE 18-8 A portion of an electronic medication administration record. (Courtesy of Cerner Corporation, Kansas City, MO.)

On the MAR, you will document medications according to the times they are given: scheduled, unscheduled, continuous, prn, STAT, and so on.

- **Scheduled medications** are medications that are to be given on a regularly scheduled basis.
- **Unscheduled medications** are medications that are to be given on call at the appropriate time. An example of an unscheduled medication is a preoperative medication to be given right before the patient goes to the operating room.
- **Continuous infusions** are IV fluids that are running consistently unless stopped for a blood transfusion or to give an IV medication that is not compatible with the IV fluid running.
- The abbreviation **prn** stands for the Latin term *pro re nata*, or "as needed." Prn medications are given only when the patient meets certain conditions that are set when the prn medication is prescribed. Typical prn medications include those used for pain, fever, mild discomfort, nausea, and constipation. You administer a prn medication when you assess that the patient needs it or when the patient requests it.
- A **STAT** medication is given immediately and only once.
- A **single-order** medication is given once at a specified time, not necessarily immediately.

For scheduled medications, you may only have to initial and make a check mark in the column with times preprinted at the top. In circumstances such as the following you will usually need to record additional information on the MAR and sometimes even in the progress notes.

- **Injections.** If you administer an injection, you must chart the site of administration. This documentation protects the patient from repeated injections in the same location.
- **Assessment required before administration.** Some medications require you to make a specific assessment before administering the drug to ensure that it is safe to give it. For example, according to most protocols, you should not give digoxin (a cardiac medication) if the heart rate is below 60 beats/min. You should hold it and notify the prescriber. Blood pressure and pain medications, insulin, and anticoagulants also require assessments before administration. You will need to document the assessment data on the paper MAR or into the electronic MAR, along with the time of administration and other required information (see Chapter 25).

✚ **Drug allergies.** Drug allergies are always noted on the MAR, whether paper or electronic. This makes them easily visible for caregivers who are prescribing and administering medication. If the patient has an allergic reaction to a medicine, be sure to document this response on the MAR; make note of this change in the nurses' notes or in the appropriate electronic form. Of course you would notify the prescriber; however, that is reporting, not recording. Reporting is discussed later in this chapter.

- **STAT, prn, unscheduled, and single-order medications.** Chart on the MAR the time the medication is given. On a paper MAR, make a narrative note that documents your assessment findings and the patient's response to the medication. On an electronic MAR, enter the time of administration and the patient's response to the medication. If necessary, you can also add an electronic comment that briefly describes your assessment findings. Some documented data, such as the pain score before administration of an analgesic, may automatically migrate from other documentation sources to become visible on the MAR.

✚ You may occasionally see a prn order that provides a *range* of medication to be given based on your assessment of the patient, for example, "Titrate morphine 2 mg IV every 1–2 hours to achieve pain control." In the electronic MAR system, medication range orders (e.g., 1 to 2 mg) are difficult to order, so The Joint Commission and most agency protocols no longer allow dosage range orders.

- **Patient Refusal.** If the patient refuses a medication, note the refusal on the paper or electronic MAR. Your organization's policy will determine how this is recorded. On paper, you might draw a circle around the scheduled time of administration. When documenting electronically, you can click on an option offered in the MAR, such as Not Given, and then select *Patient Refused* from a drop-down field listing multiple reasons that a medication is not given.
- **Omitted Medication or Delayed Administration.** If the patient is not available or is experiencing health changes that require immediate interventions, it may be necessary to withhold a medication or delay its administration. On the paper MAR, you may find a boxed section at the bottom of the MAR with a code to indicate why the medication was withheld or given at a different time. Circle the scheduled time and fill in the symbol. You will also have to document the omission or delay in your nurses' notes. In the electronic MAR, it is often possible to reschedule administration times for a single dose or permanently going forward, or to document that a medication could not be given at the scheduled time and will be skipped.

MARs for Inpatient Facilities

If you work in an inpatient facility, you will be responsible for administering the patient's medications unless a medication requires special certifications to administer (e.g., anesthesia or chemotherapy). An inpatient medication record not only contains a list of medications ordered, but also tracks medication administration and usage for the agency. For a comparison of the content of inpatient and outpatient MARs, see Table 18-1.

Table 18-1 ▶ Comparison of Content of MARs for Inpatient and Outpatient Facilities	
INPATIENT MARS	**OUTPATIENT MARS**
■ Drug name	■ Drug name
■ Dosage	■ Dosage
■ Route of administration	■ Route of administration
■ Frequency	■ Number of pills, patches, and so on, to be dispensed at each prescription refill
■ Duration	
■ Scheduled times of administration	■ Number of refills ordered
■ Charting of medication	■ Directions for using the medication, including frequency and duration
■ Administration	
■ Signatures (written or electronic) of nurses administering medication	■ Historical information about prescriptions, pharmacies used, and refills authorized

MARs for Outpatient Facilities

Outpatient facilities include clinics, primary care offices, and treatment facilities. Because patients do not stay at the facility, usually the medication record primarily contains information about how the patient is to use the medications ordered. Patients retain responsibility for administering their own medications either independently or with the help of family or caregivers.

Kardex® or Patient Care Summary

As discussed in Chapter 5, the Kardex® is a special paper form or folding card that briefly summarizes a patient's status and plan of care. Paper Kardex® and electronic patient care summaries typically pull patient data from multiple areas of the health record (medical and nursing diagnoses, orders, treatments, results). Figure 18-9 is an example of an electronic patient care summary screen. To see a paper Kardex®,

 Go to Chapter 5, **Tables, Boxes, Figures: ESG Figure 5-1,** on DavisPlus.

Paper Kardex® are usually kept together in a portable file in a central location in the nurses' station to allow all team members access to patients' summary information. Each patient has a separate electronic summary screen. All authorized members of the care team can access the electronic care summary at the same time, whether they are away from the patient or even outside the organization in a remote location, depending on the institution's permission for access. The paper Kardex® and the electronic care summary are not a permanent part of the patient's health record.

Integrated Plan of Care

IPOCs are a combined charting and care plan form. They are customized to fit common patient situations in a unit. An IPOC maps out, day by day, the patient goals, outcomes, interventions, and treatments for a specific diagnosis or condition from admission to discharge. Lab work, diagnostic testing, medications, and therapies are all included in the pathway as well as standardized interventions captured in the plan. IPOCs help administrators predict length of stay, monitor costs of care, and can assist with staffing. They can also reduce duplicate charting by more than one nurse, increase team effort, and enhance the nurse's teaching about what the patient can expect during the hospital stay. Figure 18-3 shows an example of an electronic IPOC. For examples of complete printed IPOCs,

 Go to Chapter 18, **Tables, Boxes, Figures: ESG Figure 18-3, An example of an Integrated Plan of Care (IPOC),** on DavisPlus.

Occurrence Reports

An **occurrence report**, or *incident report*, is a formal record of an unusual occurrence or accident. This is an organizational report and is not part of the client's health record. Paper occurrence forms and electronic occurrence forms completed online on the organization's secure internal network are both used to track problems and identify areas for quality improvement and to create safer processes and procedures for clients and staff. The following are examples of events requiring an occurrence report:

- Patient fall or other injury
- Medication error
- Incorrect implementation of a prescribed treatment
- Needlestick injury or other injury to staff
- Loss of patient belongings
- Injury of a visitor
- Unsafe staffing situation
- Lack of availability of essential patient care supplies
- Inadequate response to emergency situation

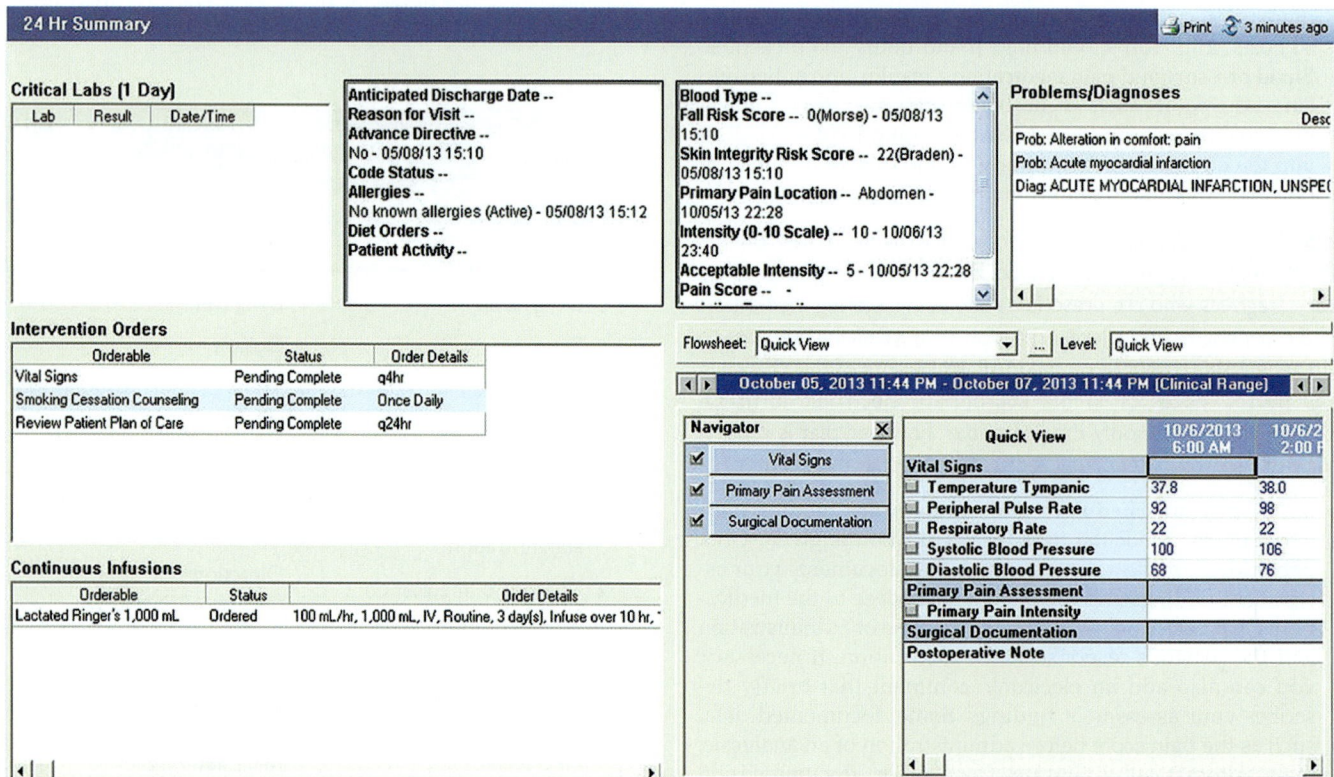

FIGURE 18-9 A portion of an electronic patient care summary screen. (Courtesy of Cerner Corporation, Kansas City, MO.)

You should report all errors, even if there was no adverse impact on the client. When completing an occurrence form, be sure to clearly identify the client, date, time, and location. Briefly describe the incident in objective terms. Quote the client or persons involved if possible. Avoid drawing conclusions or placing blame. Identify any witnesses to the event and any equipment involved.

Although you would document in the paper nurses' notes or in the client's EHR that a fall, medication error, or similar incident occurred, you usually do not mention the occurrence report itself (e.g., do not chart "occurrence report completed"). However, you must follow agency policy for documenting reportable incidents. Remember, the nurses' notes or EHR reflect the client's response to the plan of care. Chapter 43 provides additional information on occurrence reports.

What Is Unique About Documentation in Home Healthcare?

Although you will perform many of the same assessments and interventions in home care that you do in other areas of healthcare, the documentation is unique. The Centers for Medicare & Medicaid Services (CMS) guidelines govern home healthcare documentation. Among the requirements for care are (1) certification of homebound status, (2) a plan of care, and (3) ongoing assessment of the need for skilled care.

The most commonly used paper home health documentation form is known as OASIS—the Outcome and Assessment Information Set. Because of a federal government mandate that Medicare providers convert to electronic e-prescribing, home health is now moving toward electronic documentation. Many home health nurses use laptop computers to retrieve patient data and record progress notes in the home. The computer also allows the nurse to conveniently order supplies needed for home care and to coordinate scheduling of follow-up visits.

In home care, a monthly summary describing the patient's status and ongoing needs is required. The patient's primary care provider signs this form, which is submitted for reimbursement. Chapter 41 provides further information about home care.

Whether your home health documentation is done on paper or electronically, the following will be included:

- Your assessment highlighting changes in the client's condition
- Interventions performed (wound care, dressing changes, teaching, etc.)
- The client's response to interventions
- Any interaction or teaching that you conducted with caregivers
- Any interaction with the patient's primary care provider
  If you would like to see an OASIS form,

 Go to Chapter 18, **Tables, Boxes, Figures: ESG Figure 18-4, Outcome and Assessment Information Set (OASIS),** on Davis*Plus.*

 Think**Like a Nurse** 18-2

Why do you think it is essential to document homebound status and the ongoing need for skilled care?

What Is Unique About Documentation in Long-Term Care?

Documentation requirements for long-term care depend on the level of care the client requires. All clients in long-term care facilities must have a comprehensive assessment at admission.

Federal law requires that a resident be evaluated using the Minimum Data Set for Resident Assessment and Care Screening (MDS) within 14 days of admission. The MDS must be updated every 3 months and with any significant change in client condition. For an example of an MDS form,

 Go to Chapter 18, **Tables, Boxes, Figures: ESG Figure 18-5, Minimum Data Set (MDS),** on Davis*Plus.*

Legal requirements to protect older adults mandate that you report changes in a client's condition to the primary care provider as well as the client's family. Document your reports in narrative notes on paper or in the appropriate areas of electronic forms. If you are caring for a client receiving Medicare-reimbursed services, such as IV therapy, wound care, or rehabilitation services, documentation is required with each shift. In addition, a summary written by a nurse must be recorded weekly. The weekly summary for adult clients must include the following:

- A summary of the client's condition
- An evaluation of the client's ability to perform ADLs
- The client's level of consciousness and mood
- Hydration and nutrition status
- Response to medications
- Any treatments provided
- Safety measures (e.g., bed rails, bed alarm, wander guard)

Long-term care facilities also provide intermediate-care services for clients who need assistance with medications, nutrition, and ADLs. These clients require a nursing care summary every 2 weeks. For a nursing assessment flow sheet used in long-term care,

 Go to Chapter 18, **Tables, Boxes, Figures: ESG Figure 18-6, A Flow Sheet Used in Long-Term Care,** on Davis*Plus.*

Knowledge Check 18-3

- How do home care and long-term care documentation differ from hospital-based documentation?

 Think**Like a Nurse** 18-3

Why do long-term care clients require less frequent charting than clients in acute care settings?

The Transition to Electronic Health Records

Although nursing documentation has evolved over time, there was little change in the ways that nurses recorded data until the late 20th century, when computers and digital electronic forms began to be widely used in healthcare organizations. Healthcare organizations were slow to adopt EHR because of the high cost to buy, customize, and maintain systems and the cost and time involved in training personnel to use a new electronic system.

In 2007, only 11% of community hospitals had fully implemented EHRs, more than half of hospitals reported "partial" implementation, and about one-third indicated no initiation of EHRs (AMNews, 2007). However by 2011, more than half of office-based physicians reported using full or partial EHR systems (Hing, Burt, & Woodwell, 2006; Jamoom, Beatty, Bercovitz, et al., 2012). The shift to EHR is expected to continue and accelerate as the population continues to become

increasingly computer literate. The move to EHRs may occur even faster if the federal government continues its support in the massive task of making all health records standardized and electronic. For more discussion of the shift to EHRs,

 Go to Chapter 18, **Supplemental Materials,** on DavisPlus.

As a nurse, you will almost certainly need to have computer skills. You will play a crucial role in the development and evaluation of effective EHR systems that make sense to nurses. You may even participate directly in the design–implementation–redesign cycle of the EHR system in your organization.

Whether you document in the client's room, in the hallway or at nurses' station, or on a mobile or handheld device, EHRs promote efficient use of nurses' time, improve interdisciplinary collaboration, streamline processes, make procedures more accurate and efficient, and ensure improved patient safety and care outcomes.

KnowledgeCheck 18-4

- Identify at least five types of paper documentation forms.
- What should you document after administering a prn medication?
- What are some reasons for the slow adoption of electronic documentation and EHRs in the United States?
- What is the purpose of an occurrence report?
- Identify the following abbreviations:

abd	OOB
BRP	pc
DM	prn
fx	STD
NKDA	tid
q	LUQ

ORAL REPORTING

The purpose of giving an oral report is to maintain continuity of care. The oral report provides an opportunity for professional communication that assists in organizing your work, and also for learning, building team relationships, and collaborating to improve patient care. Whether the source of the information shared is from a written report form, a paper Kardex®, or a summary view in the EHR, the quality of the report you give and receive influences how you and others plan the day's (or night's) work. Restrict your oral reports to patient-focused discussion and limit unimportant details and social conversation.

How Do I Give a Handoff Report?

The purpose of a **handoff report** (sometimes called a *change-of-shift report* or *handover report*) is to alert the next caregiver about the client's status or recent changes in the client's condition and to discuss planned activities, tests, procedures, or concerns that require follow-up. A handoff report may be given at the bedside or in a conference room using paper notes or a mobile or desktop EHR device.

Handoff reports are usually given orally. As a student nurse, you will receive reports from either the nurse completing the shift or from the nurse assigned to the patient during the shift you will be working. Report any changes to the nurse assigned to the patient during your shift, and always give a report before leaving the unit.

- A **bedside report,** sometimes known as "walking rounds," allows you to observe important aspects of care, such as patient appearance, IV pumps, and wounds. With a bedside report, the outgoing nurse can introduce you to the patient and you can begin your assessment. If the patient is alert, give him the opportunity to participate in the report and ask questions. Although this type of report is time consuming, it encourages continuity of care, team collaboration, and patient/family communication.
- A **face-to-face oral report** may involve only the outgoing and oncoming nurse or may include the entire oncoming shift. When given in a conference room, an oral report does not let you directly observe the patient, but it is time efficient and still allows interaction between nurses.
- An **audio-recorded report** is a convenient way to transmit information. The outgoing nurse audio-records a report on her patients. This method can be time consuming. The main difficulty, though, is that an audio-recorded report does not allow you to ask questions about the patient. Occasionally, the audio quality is poor and the report is not clear. If the outgoing nurse has already left the unit, it may be impossible for you to speak directly with him. If you have questions, you must then phone the nurse or rely on his written notes if you are unable to speak with the nurse directly. Few agencies use audio-recorded handoff reports because The Joint Commission (2008b) recommends using a method that allows for questioning between the giver and receiver of the information.

Standardized Report Formats. No matter where or how the handoff report is given, you should use a standardized approach. The **PACE** format is one example of a standardized approach to handoffs, and was developed specifically for that purpose. The mnemonic stands for **P**atient/**P**roblem, **A**ssessment/**A**ctions, **C**ontinuing/**C**hanges, and **E**valuation (Schroeder, 2006).

The **SBAR** (**S**ituation-**B**ackground-**A**ssessment-**R**ecommendation) is an easy-to-remember, concrete acronym useful for framing any conversation. Because nurses and physicians communicate in very different ways, SBAR is useful for interdisciplinary communication, especially critical situations requiring a clinician's immediate attention and action. SBAR allows for an easy and focused way to set expectations for what will be communicated and how between members of the team. The SBAR technique can be adapted for handoff reports, see the guidelines in Box 18-3. For additional information about communicating with SBAR and PACE, see Clinical Insight 20-3, Communicating With SBAR.

Regardless of the format used, to prepare to give a handoff report, you need to collect the following information:

- Client progress made during your shift
- Therapies and treatments administered
- Teaching done
- Consultations done or planned with other disciplines
- Status of identified desired outcomes
- Any changes in client status
- Progress made on discharge planning

KnowledgeCheck 18-5

- What data should be included in a handoff report?
- What are the types of handoff reports?

What Is a Transfer Report?

Transfer reports are given when a patient is transferred from unit to unit or from facility to facility. For information to include in an oral transfer report, see Box 18-3. If the

BOX 18-3 ■ Giving Oral Reports

1. **For all types of report formats:**
   Remember the acronym CUBAN (Currie, 2002): **C**onfidential, **U**ninterrupted, **B**rief, **A**ccurate, **N**amed nurse
2. **Use a Standardized Format.** The following are examples.

PACE

Patient/Problem—Include patient's name, room number, diagnosis, reason for admission, and recent procedures. State the present problem. Briefly summarize medical history relevant to the current problem.

Assessment/Actions—Nursing assessments and interventions directed to the problem, including teaching done and status of discharge planning

Continuing/Changes—Continuing needs and potential changes include the following:
- Patient care and treatments that must be monitored on other shifts (e.g., dressing changes)
- Changes in the patient's condition or the care plan, recent or anticipated (e.g., new orders, changes in discharge date)

Evaluation—Evaluation of responses to nursing and medical interventions, progress toward goals, and effectiveness of the plan

3. **Include the following content.**
In a handoff report:
- Patient's name, age, and room number
- Patient's admitting diagnosis—one or several may exist
- Patient's relevant past medical history
- Treatments that the patient has received during this admission, such as surgery, line placements, breathing treatments
- Upcoming diagnostic tests, surgeries, or treatments
- Patient restrictions, such as diet, bedrest, isolation, activity limits
- Plan of care, such as IV therapy, pain management, current medications, wound care, and patient or family concerns
- Significant assessment findings from the previous shifts
In a transfer report:
- Your name, facility, and phone number
- Patient's name, age, gender, and admitting and current diagnoses
- Patient's physician(s), if still following patient

- Procedures or surgeries performed
- Current medications and last date/time each was taken
- Patient status at present as well as progression since admission
- Last set of vital signs, plus any pertinent trends since admission
- Tubes in the patient, such as IVs, catheters, drainage tubes, along with the intake and output of each tube or drain
- Presence of wounds or open areas of the skin plus current interventions for each
- Names and contact numbers for family and significant others
- Special directives, such as code status, preferred intensity of care, or isolation required
- Reason the patient is being transferred

4. **When your report is finished:**
- Ask the receiving nurse if he has any questions.
- Get the nurse's full name, and then record it plus the transfer date and time in your transfer documentation.

SBAR
Identify yourself, the patient, and the agency.

Situation—"Here's the situation: . . ."

Background—"The supporting background information is . . ."

Assessment—"My assessment of the situation is that . . ."

Recommendation—"I recommend that you . . ."

For additional information about SBAR, see Clinical Insight 20-3, in Chapter 20

References

Haig, K., Sutton, S., & Whittington, J. (2006). SBAR: A shared mental model for improving communication between clinicians. *Joint Commission Journal of Quality and Patient Safety, 32*(3), 167–175.

Kaiser Permanente of Colorado. (n.d.). SBAR technique for communication. Institute for Healthcare Improvement. Retrieved March 30, 2012, from http://www.ihi.org/knowledge/Pages/Tools/SBARTechniqueforCommunicationASituationalBriefingModel.aspx

Schroeder, S. (2006). Picking up the PACE: A new template for shift report. *Nursing 2006, 36*(10), 22–23.

---

patient is being transported to another unit in the same facility, you will need to transport a paper chart with the patient. If both organizations are using an EHR documentation system, then the receiving unit will access the client record electronically. Detailed information about the patient's health history can be communicated between healthcare professionals or transmitted before transfer. Your organization will have a policy on what is to be copied and how materials should be transmitted to the receiving facility. For a review of transfers and discharges, see Chapter 11 and Procedures 11-2, 11-3, and 11-4.

How Do I Receive and Document Verbal and Telephone Orders?

✚ Although licensed nurses may find it necessary to accept verbal or telephone orders on occasion, such orders increase the risk of hearing or recording the order incorrectly. The Joint Commission says that to best avoid the dangers you should "verify the complete order or test result by having the person receiving the information record and 'read-back' the complete order or test result" (The Joint Commission, 2008a).

Telephone Orders

Telephone orders can lead to error because of differences in pronunciation, dialect, or accent; background noise; and unfamiliar terminology. Taking a telephone order may be acceptable when there has been a sudden change for the worse in your patient's condition and the client's primary care provider is not in the hospital, or does not have access to placing orders electronically outside the hospital. Verbal or telephone orders are also acceptable in a life-threatening emergency, but you must apply the "read-back" safeguard. Faxes and e-mail have reduced the need for telephone orders; however, the need for them may never disappear entirely. For guidelines to use when taking telephone orders, refer to Clinical Insight 18-1.

QSEN

Handoff Reporting: Decreasing Communication Errors

Competencies: Safety (Knowledge, Skills, and Attitudes); Teamwork and Collaboration (Knowledge, Skills, and Attitudes)*

Think about the number of patient handoffs per day among nurses and other professionals (e.g., physicians). Then consider the risk to patient safety that can be caused by miscommunication.

➤ Actual errors that have occurred because of poor *physician handoff reporting* include amputating the wrong leg, removing a healthy adrenal gland, failing to obtain serial sodium levels from a patient with diabetes insipidus (DI), failing to act on stroke symptoms, and failing to correct electrolyte imbalances. All of these errors resulted in death or permanent brain damage.

➤ Potential harm in *nursing shift change handoffs* include delays in initiating critical medications or obtaining specimens; failing to initiate new treatments, communicate change in patient status, or report critical lab results; repeating outdated information; and many other possibilities.

Factors contributing to poor-quality handoffs include lack of a standardized protocol or form, reliance on memory, lack of experience, and lack of dedicated time for reporting.

Collaborate with others in your facility to suggest the following strategies for improving quality of care, teamwork, and patient safety:

➤ Standardize the information to be conveyed but customize reports to avoid giving too much or too little information.

➤ Use a structured communication technique such as SBAR.

➤ Include "if . . . then" statements for current problems (e.g., *if* the glucose level is still elevated *then* call physician for insulin prescriptions).

➤ Develop an electronic form or other tool to reinforce transfer of knowledge and responsibility.

➤ Conduct training sessions to lessen the chance of reporting errors.

 *For specific Knowledge, Skills, and Attitudes,

 Go to the QSEN web site at http:www.qsen.org.ksas_prelicensure.php

Sources: Collins, Stein, Vawdrey, et al., 2011; Kitch, Cooper, Zapol, et al., 2008; Riesenberg, Leisch, & Cunningham, 2010.

✚ *Clinical Insight 18-1* ➤ Receiving Telephone and Verbal Orders

You should accept verbal and telephone prescriptions (orders) only in specific situations when the primary care provider is not able to write or enter the prescriptions personally.

■ If possible, have a second nurse listen to the order to verify its accuracy.

■ Write or enter the order electronically only if you heard it yourself; no third-party involvement is acceptable.

■ Repeat the prescription even if you believe you have clearly understood it. Spell unfamiliar names to be sure the spelling is correct.

■ Pronounce digits of numbers separately. For example, instead of "seventeen," say "one, seven." Mishearing a number can lead to a serious error in medication dosage.

■ Make sure the order makes sense in light of the patient's current status.

■ Transcribe the prescription directly into the chart as quickly as possible. Writing it on a piece of paper, then copying it again onto a paper order sheet introduces an additional chance of error. If entering the prescription electronically, it's best to have the EHR's order entry area open and begin entering the order as the prescriber is dictating it to you.

■ Write the order while the prescriber remains on the telephone or in the building so that you can ask any necessary questions immediately without the need for a return call.

■ When writing the order onto a paper order sheet, first document the date and time. Next write the text of the order. Following the text of the order, depending on how you received the order write "TO" (telephone order) or "VO" (verbal order), followed by the ordering provider's name and then your name. The following is an example of a telephone order:

12/17/13 0815—Morphine 2 mg IV push ×1 for pain now. ——————————————————

———————————TO Dr. Clayton Kent/Sarah Hogan, RN

■ If entering the prescription electronically, indicate during order entry that it was given verbally or over the telephone, the date and time the order was given, and then search for and select the prescriber's name. Click "sign" or whatever option in your EHR indicates the order is signed and is now active.

■ Be sure you have the phone number so that you can reach the provider if future questions arise.

■ The physician, physician assistant, or nurse practitioner must countersign all verbal and telephone orders within 24 hours.

References

The Joint Commission, 2008b, 2010.

Verbal Orders

Verbal orders are spoken directions for patient care given to you in person, usually during an emergency. Providers should never use verbal orders (prescriptions) as a routine method of communicating orders. When recording a verbal order, include the date, time, and the written text of the order or the electronic entry. If you are writing the prescription on an order sheet, the indicator VO, designating verbal orders, is then followed by the provider's name and your name. If you are entering the prescription electronically, then it will be designated as a verbal order and be routed to the selected physician for co-signature. Follow The Joint Commission safety guidelines, above and see Clinical Insight 18-1 for guidelines.

KnowledgeCheck18-6

- What important factors should you document when receiving a telephone order?
- What is the purpose of a verbal order? When should it be used?

How Do I Question an Order?

If you feel uncertain about a prescription, you must question it. As a student, you will first want to discuss your concerns with your clinical instructor or the nurse you are working with during your clinical time. Remember, the goal is to provide safe care. If you have concerns, do not remain quiet—act on them.

As a nurse, you will follow your organization's policy for clarifying orders. If a prescription is written illegibly on a paper order sheet or is entered into the EHR missing details or order components, contact the provider directly to seek clarification. If you believe a prescription is inappropriate or unsafe, you are legally and ethically required to question it. Generally, you should contact the provider who wrote the order. If the provider leaves the order as-is and you still don't feel comfortable with it, or believe there is an error, you may refuse to carry it out. Inform your chain of command at your organization about your refusal. Usually the person you will speak with is the charge nurse, who may then contact the nurse manager or nursing supervisor. The nature of the order will determine how this situation is handled.

As a new nurse, you may feel uncomfortable about questioning an order. Even experienced nurses sometimes feel uneasy with this challenge. If you are uncertain how to proceed, you can discuss your concerns with your colleagues, the charge nurse, or the supervisor before contacting the provider. Your efforts to clarify orders help to protect your patient. If you do refuse to follow an order, you must document your refusal and the actions you took to clarify the order.

PracticalKnowledge
knowing how

To document care effectively, you need to be familiar with the forms and requirements of your institution. Chart routine nursing actions (e.g., skin care) on the designated paper or electronic flow sheets or forms; and chart your assessments,

interventions, and patient responses to care in the format approved by your organization.

Home-care, hospitals, and long-term care facilities have specific guidelines for the frequency of charting and the type of data that must be recorded. Clinic and office settings also have requirements that must be met so that services can be reimbursed. Familiarize yourself with the requirements in your work setting.

Remember that the patient's health record is permanent and that information contained in the chart is confidential. As a student, you are granted access to client's charts for educational purposes. You have a duty to keep the information private and confidential. As a student, in most cases you will be asked to use only the client's initials on school assignments. Health Insurance Portability and Accountability Act (HIPAA) regulations affect access, storage, transfer, and discussion of patient information. For more information about privacy, confidentiality, and HIPAA, refer to Chapters 42 and 43.

GUIDELINES FOR DOCUMENTING CARE

For a brief set of documentation tips, see Box 18-4. The following section provides detailed documentation guidelines, including when to document, what to document, and how to document (i.e., the quality of the documentation). For additional guidelines specific to paper health records and for EHRs, refer to Clinical Insights 18-2 and 18-3, respectively.

When to Document

Whether you are documenting on paper or in an EHR, documentation begins at the start of your shift in a hospital or long-term care facility, or when you first encounter the client during a home visit or at an outpatient facility.

After Care or Assessment. Chart as soon as possible after you give care or make an observation. The longer you wait, the less you will recall.

Beginning of Shift. Begin charting at the beginning of your shift or work time.

As needed. Document narrative notes often enough to clearly describe what your client is experiencing, including responses to interventions and treatments.

Chronologically, to Communicate Changing Status. On paper, document specific times in chronological order. (Most EHRs automatically insert the current date and time when forms are opened, although those dates and times can be changed if necessary before signing the form.)

Never Chart Ahead (before performing an intervention). It is impossible to be sure that what you expect to happen will actually happen. Charting ahead threatens the record's credibility.

BOX 18-4 ■ Documentation ABCs

Accurate	**E**asy to read
Bias free	**F**actual
Complete	**G**rammatical
Detailed	**H**armless (legally)

Avoid "Block" Charting, such as "From 1300 to 1500." Each entry between 1300 and 1500 needs to be made individually.

Late Entries, Paper. Add late entries to the first available line. Record the time and date you are charting, but in the body of the entry clearly designate that this is a late entry. If you know legal action is pending, do not place a late note in the health record without notifying the nurse manager or risk management officer first. It is a criminal offense to alter a patient record after the organization's approved time limit for doing so has passed.

Late Entries, EHR. Open the appropriate form and change the automatically generated current date/time to the date/time that your care was actually done; then sign.

What to Document

Document the condition of your patient when you first observed him. Was he awake? Was he in bed? Did he have any complaints? What did you do? As your shift or visit progressed, you performed your assessment and nursing interventions. What were your findings? Did any abnormalities exist? Finally, what was the patient's response to your intervention? Did any changes from the initial assessment occur? Also document the following:

- **Your Interventions, the Patient's Responses and Progress Toward Goals.** This is often done on the interdisciplinary plan of care.
- **Any Significant Events or Changes in Condition.** When possible, quote the patient's interpretation of the event or change.
- **Details About the Client's Condition.** When possible, give specific examples. Descriptive details allow caregivers to better grasp your patient's individual needs.
- **Interventions.** If you chart a symptom, also chart your interventions. For example, if you chart "c/o pain," without also documenting what you did about it and how the patient responded, it may appear that you did not respond to the patient's needs.
- **Informed Consent.** signed the consent. The physician conducting the procedure is legally responsible for discussing the procedure and its risks and benefits. For further discussion on informed consent, see Chapters 42 and 43.
- **Patient Teaching.**
- **Attempts You Have Made to Contact the Primary Care Provider** about the patient's condition or attempts to clarify orders. If you are unable to make contact with the provider, document any contact with your charge nurse, nurse manager, supervisor, medical director, and hospital administrator.
- **Patient Leaving the Facility Against Medical Advice (AMA).** Chart the patient's condition, any explanations of risks and consequences given to the patient, the patient's destination (if known), and your notification of the patient's care providers. Many facilities have specific forms for AMA departures. If possible, use the designated form. If the form is hard-copy paper, have the patient sign the form before leaving.
- **The Patient's Refusal of Treatment.**
- **Spiritual or Other Concerns** expressed by the patient and/or family. Document your interventions.

How to Document

The following suggestions will help you improve the quality of your documentation.

- **Record Data Accurately.**
- **Use Neutral, Nonjudgmental Language.** Avoid labeling patients or members on the care team. Do not chart personal opinion or judgments, such as "Patient obnoxious and refuses prescribed medication." Also avoid documenting judgments about decisions made by members of the team.
- **Avoid Vague, Subjective Words Such as** *Good, Average,* or *Normal.* Such terms do not clearly define the status of the client.
- **Use Only the Abbreviations Authorized by Your Organization.** See Box 18-2.
- **Use Correct Spelling and Grammar.** Incorrect spelling may raise questions about what you are attempting to communicate. Incorrect grammar implies carelessness on your part and creates a question of your competence if your chart is reviewed.
- **Date and Time All Your Notes (Paper or Electronic) Accurately.** To avoid confusion between a.m. and p.m., many organizations use a 24-hour clock or military time. The day begins at 0001, which is equivalent to 12:01 a.m., and ends at 2400 (12 midnight). After 12 noon, just add 12 to the p.m. time (e.g., 1:30 p.m. + 12 = 1330 in military time). See Figure 18-10.
- **Use of Restraints.** Most facilities have a separate form that allows you to document the reason for restraint use, the type of restraint, and frequent checks of the patient. The primary care provider must place a signed order for restraints in the chart or in the EHR. Restraint orders must be reordered inside a specific time frame set by the organization or the restraints are discontinued (see Chapter 23).
- **Occurrences Such as Falls and Medication Errors.** Chart your findings accurately and objectively, and fill out a separate occurrence form. Do not make reference to the occurrence form anywhere in your charting.
- **Complete Data About Medications.** When the MAR is on paper, include the date, time given, medication given, and

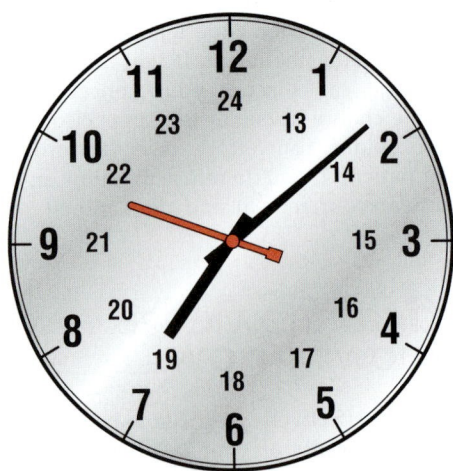

FIGURE 18-10 Many healthcare facilities use the 24-hour clock.

your initials. If the MAR is electronic, ensure the date, time, and medication given are accurate, then sign electronically that the administration was accomplished successfully.

- **Unscheduled, prn, IV Infusions, and STAT Medications.** Chart on the paper or electronic MAR. Include any comments regarding the medication in your narrative charting or insert a comment in your electronic charting. Certain prn medications require that a follow-up response be documented within a specific period of time after administration, usually 15 to 30 minutes after the medication is given.
- **Think About What You Say.** Remember that the patient's record is permanent and that the information is confidential.
- **Do Not Assume That Everything You See Already Documented Is Correct,** especially if your patient's condition makes the prior documentation illogical or unlikely. Be sure to question this with the appropriate persons, preferably the person who originally made the entry.
- **Chart Your Own Nursing Actions.** Never allow anyone to chart for you.
- **Do Not Document Others' Actions** as though you had performed them.
- **If You Need to Document the Actions of Someone Else, Be Sure to Designate That Clearly.** For example, if the nursing assistive personnel (NAP) helps the patient ambulate, do not chart "Patient ambulated to bathroom." Instead, chart "J. Scott, NAP, assisted patient to bathroom." If you are documenting electronically, you can indicate another person performed the action in an added comment, or by searching for and selecting the other care provider in the appropriate field, then signing.
- **Don't Chart What Someone Else Said, Heard, Felt, or Smelled Unless the Information Is Critical.** If it is, then use quotations and attribute the remarks to the person who made them. For example, "Wife stated, 'My husband told me that he is in a lot of pain, but does not want to bother the nurses.'"

KnowledgeCheck18-7

- What aspects of care should be documented?
- When should care be documented?
- How is documentation on paper different from documentation in an EHR or on an electronic digital form?

ThinkLike a Nurse 18-4

You are caring for two clients on a medical–surgical unit. One of your clients is short of breath and complaining of chest pain. Your other client is recovering from abdominal surgery. He is alert, stable, and free from pain at this time. After stabilizing your first client, you realize you are 45 minutes late administering a medication to the abdominal surgery patient. You are not sure how to proceed.

- What theoretical knowledge do you need?
- You give the medicine as soon as you can (60 min late). How and when should you chart the medication administered?
- If you had been aware that you were going to be late with the medication, what might you have done to be sure it was given on time?

Can I Delegate Charting?

In some facilities, each member of the team is responsible for documenting her part in the care of the client. Nursing assistants or other NAPs often chart ADLs, activity, and I&O on graphic records. You are responsible for documenting the nursing care you provide. Never chart the actions of others as though you performed them. If an action is crucial to a chain of events, you may document that action, referring clearly to the

---

Clinical Insight 18-2 ▶ Guidelines for Documenting in the Paper Health Record

- **Before you begin writing:**
  Keep patient paper records in designated areas to which only healthcare providers have access.
  Recognize good forms. Paper documentation forms must be efficient, comprehensive, and reasonable, and should prompt nurses to document appropriately.
  Ensure that you have the correct form (e.g., I&O sheet, graphic record).
  Check that the chart and documentation forms are clearly marked with the patient's name and identification number.
- **Write legibly, neatly, in an organized manner.** This enables others to read your entries when making clinical decisions. Sloppy or illegible handwriting creates errors or at least leads to poor communication.
- **Always use black ink** for handwritten notes (some agencies do permit blue ink). Inks other than black or blue are not legible when a chart is photocopied. Do not use green or red pen. Remember, the chart is a legal document.
- **Do not leave blank lines in the narrative notes.** If you need to leave space for clarity, draw a straight line through the area and begin on the next line. Open areas leave an opportunity for later tampering.
- **Draw a line through the incorrect charting and initial it.** Never use a correction fluid, "scribble over," or otherwise cover up written notes.
- **Sign all your paper charting entries with your first name, last name, and professional credentials,** such as Judy Long, RN.
- **Use only abbreviations that are approved by your organization.** Don't write in "shorthand" or your own abbreviated symbols.
- **Do not provide written or verbal patient information to anyone not involved in the direct care of the patient,** unless the patient has consented to allow that person access.

Clinical Insight 18-3 ➤ **Guidelines for Documenting in the Electronic Health Record**

Well-designed nursing documentation forms and systems help you organize your work, manage your care plans, track client diagnoses and outcomes, and support decision making by all members of the healthcare team. Initial reluctance to use EHRs usually decreases quickly as nurses become more comfortable using them (Moody, Slocomb, Berg, et al., 2004). To ensure that your documentation in the EHR is most efficient and effective, keep the following in mind:

What Skills Do I Need?

- You must have basic computer, mouse, and software skills to document effectively in the EHR.
- If you are uneasy or more stressed using computers or unfamiliar with the software, it may take you longer to make the transition to documenting in the EHR.
- Help keep patient rooms clutter free so that you have a place to use a portable computer in the room for direct charting.

What Is Unique About Entering the Data?

- *Before opening charting forms,* ensure that the patient's name, patient identification number, and any other unique health record identifiers are correct.
- *If your EHR allows you to save partially completed documentation* before signing it, ensure that you do complete the documentation and sign it as quickly as possible. In most EHR systems, saved documentation is not seen by others until it is signed.
- *Electronic forms and flow sheets are often built in a format similar to a checklist.* This can make it more difficult to capture detailed patient changes and findings.
- *If you make an error, it can be corrected* (e.g., if you make entries on the wrong chart or enter and sign the wrong information). The entry can never be completely deleted; however, only the corrected information will be visible to anyone viewing the chart.

What Happens If the Computer Doesn't Work?

EHR systems can have periodic downtimes due to scheduled maintenance or network or interface problems. Client care does not stop, so you need to know the processes and procedures to follow when the EHR is offline and inaccessible. Follow organization policies regarding the amount of time the EHR needs to be "down" before you begin documenting on paper form.

How Do I Maintain Confidentiality and Data Security?

- *Do not leave the computer unattended after you have logged on.* When moving away from the open EHR, close the screen and temporarily or permanently log off to ensure confidentiality and privacy. Most computer stations will automatically log off after a specified period of inactivity. This helps keep unauthorized viewers from having access to patient information.
- *Some computer screens are equipped with privacy filters to* protect patient information from the view of unauthorized viewers.
- *Create a secure password*—not something obvious, such as your birth date, Social Security number, or family members' names. Instead, you might choose a password that is at least six characters long and includes at least one capital letter (if the system is case sensitive), one number, and (if allowed by the system) one symbol. The system you are using will determine the specifications.
- *Change your password at regular intervals* even if your organization does not require it. Some systems will lock you out of the system if your password is not changed as required.
- *Do not share your personal username or password* with anyone. You are responsible for the data recorded and saved using your electronic identity. If someone else enters data or accesses charts under your identity, you will be held responsible for those actions if the patient initiates legal action.
- *Do not leave a portable device (e.g., a laptop or PDA) unattended in a public location,* such as on a countertop in the nurses' station. This increases the possibility of theft or unauthorized access to secured patient information.
- *Never access client health records that you have no professional reason to view.* This is a severe breach of client privacy rules. Some states have or are planning harsher penalties for these privacy violations.
- *Become familiar with your organization's policies* regarding network and patient health record information security and confidentiality.

person who did the action. For example, "Became dizzy; assisted to chair by Nora Roverdale, NAP."

KnowledgeCheck 18-8

- Can charting be delegated?
- You are a student nurse on a medical–surgical unit. You review your client's chart and notice that the physician entered prescriptions that do not appear to be appropriate for your client. The physician is still in the area. How would you handle this situation?

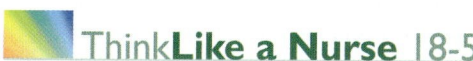

ThinkLike a Nurse 18-5

You note that your client with asthma is having increasing difficulty breathing. You call the physician, who gives you a telephone order for an asthma medication, and then hangs up. When you enter the order electronically as a verbal order, you find out the medication is a nonformulary medication that your pharmacy does not carry.

- Is this an acceptable reason to take a verbal order?
- The physician becomes irritated when you call back and says, "I prescribed what I wanted." How would you handle this situation?
- You entered the order electronically after the physician hung up. How could this situation have been avoided?

Toward Evidence-Based Practice

Smith, K., Smith, V., Krugman, M., et al. (2005). Evaluating the impact of computerized clinical documentation. *CIN: Computers, Informatics, Nursing, 23*(3), 132–138.

A computerized system for planning and documenting patient care was initiated, using the framework of Nursing Interventions Classification (NIC) and Nursing Outcomes Classification (NOC) standardized languages. The software includes both order entry and a charting application. Staff surveys, observations, and chart audits were conducted before and after the computerized system was implemented. Data demonstrated that after the new system was implemented (1) staff attitudes toward computers were less positive, (2) the time required for charting was unchanged, and (3) nurses' charting entries were more complete and comprehensive.

Kossman, S., & Scheidenhelm, S. (2008). Nurses' perceptions of the impact of electronic health records on work and patient outcomes. *CIN: Computers, Informatics, Nursing, 26*(2), 69–77.

This study addressed nurses' use of EHRs and their views of the impact of EHRs on job performance and patient outcomes. Questionnaires, interviews, and observation data from 46 nurses in medical–surgical and intensive care units at two community hospitals were collected and analyzed. Results indicated that nurses (1) preferred EHR to paper charts and were comfortable with technology; (2) thought use of EHR impaired critical thinking, decreased interdisciplinary communication, and created a high demand on work time (73% reported spending at least half their shift using the records); (3) believed that EHR improved organization, efficiency, and information access; and (4) thought the use of EHR enabled them to provide safer care but decreased the quality of care.

1. Refer to the section Advantages of Electronic Health Records. Compare the advantages of the EHR in that section to the findings in the above studies. Which EHR advantage is *not* supported by either of these studies? What is the statement in each study that conflicts with the advantages discussed in that section?

2. Which study disagrees with the statement that EHR improves communication between healthcare providers? What does the study say about that?

 Go to Chapter 18, **Toward Evidence-Based Practice—Suggested Responses,** on *DavisPlus.*

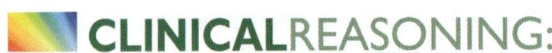 **CLINICAL**REASONING:
Applying the **Full-Spectrum Nursing Model**

Because the following critical thinking activities allow you to practice the kind of thinking you will use as a full-spectrum nurse, they usually have no single right answer. Discuss them with your peers—if you have difficulty with any of the questions, consult your instructor,

PATIENT SITUATION

Ellen is 85 years old and has sustained a right-sided cerebrovascular accident (CVA, or stroke). Doctors say she is unlikely to regain much physical function, if she even awakens from the coma. Her children, Mary and Dale, have met with the physician, who tells them that Ellen is not likely to survive. The physician wants to insert a feeding tube and has asked whether they want Ellen to be resuscitated in case of cardiac or respiratory arrest. Mary tells you she wants to do what is best for her mother, but she feels that Ellen would not want to be kept alive in the condition she is in. She is also concerned about putting her through uncomfortable procedures if there is no chance of recovery. Her brother, Dale, says, "Mom needs the feeding tube. I can't sit and watch her starve to death. As long as she's alive, there's hope."

THINKING

1. *Theoretical Knowledge (Recall of Facts and Principles):* You plan to use the Focus Charting® format to document this interaction.
   a. Write the focus for this note.
   b. What does the acronym *DAR* stand for?
2. *Critical Thinking (Contextual Awareness):*
   a. What aspects of this situation have you experienced or observed before in your role as a caregiver?
   b. How might those past experiences affect your perception in this situation?

DOING

3. *Practical Knowledge (Handoff Report):* Ellen's last name is Smith; assume her children are also named Smith. Ellen is in room 820. Using the PACE format, what would you say to the oncoming nurse during handoff report? You will be able to address only a small amount of physiological information because the scenario does not provide it.

CARING

4. *Self-Knowledge:* In what way(s) can you identify with any of the people involved in this scenario?

 Go To Chapter 18, **Clinical Reasoning: Applying the Full-Spectrum Nursing Model Response Sheet,** on Davis*Plus.*

 To explore learning resources for this chapter,

Concept Map

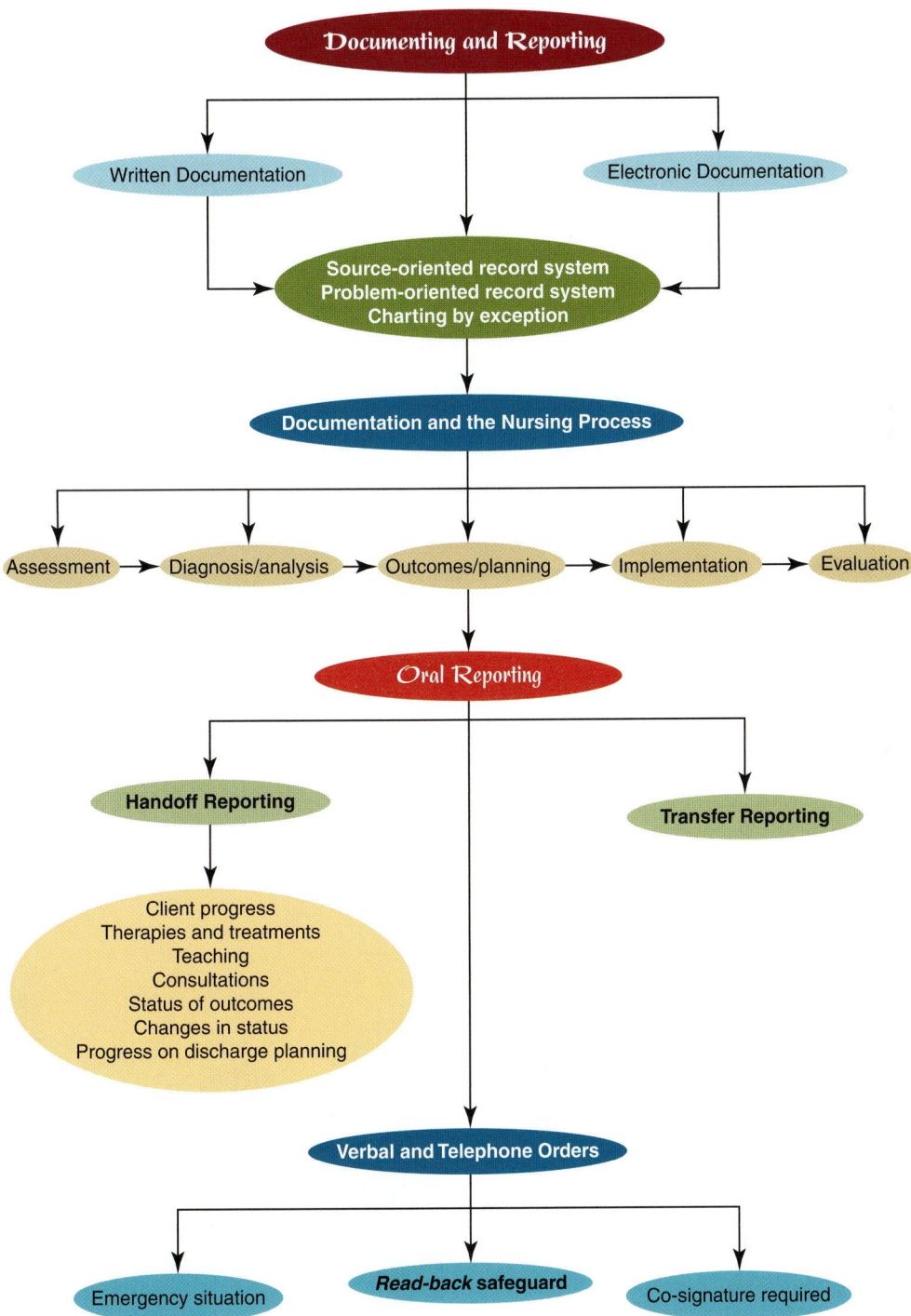

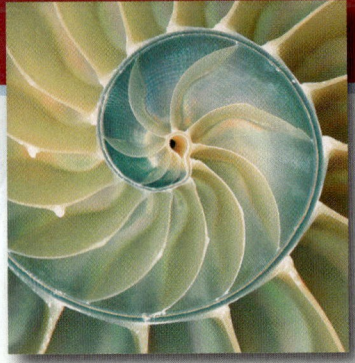

CHAPTER 19

Vital Signs

Learning Outcomes

After completing this chapter, you should be able to:

➤ Describe the physiological processes involved in regulating body temperature, pulse, respirations, and blood pressure.

➤ Convert between the Fahrenheit and centigrade temperature scales.

➤ For different patient situations, choose the best procedure for measuring temperature, pulse, respiration, and blood pressure, including site and equipment.

➤ Discuss the concept of a "normal" temperature.

➤ Describe nursing interventions for the patient with temperature alterations.

➤ Given a client's age, differentiate between normal vital signs findings and those that should be referred to the primary healthcare provider.

➤ State at least one nursing diagnosis that might be used to describe a problem for each of the vital signs: temperature, pulse, respirations, and blood pressure.

➤ Define *arterial oxygen saturation, hypoxia, hyperventilation,* and *hypoventilation.*

➤ Discuss nursing interventions for the client with impaired respiratory status.

➤ State the normal temperature, pulse, respiration, and blood pressure ranges for the average adult.

➤ Explain why it is important to interpret a client's blood pressure pattern rather than relying on a single reading.

➤ Discuss the importance of cuff size when obtaining a blood pressure reading.

➤ Define *hypotension, hypertension, essential hypertension,* and *secondary hypertension.*

➤ Identify nursing interventions for the client with hypertension.

➤ Demonstrate correct technique for measuring temperature, pulse, respiration and blood pressure.

Key Concepts

Vital signs

Thermoregulation

Perfusion (pulse, blood pressure)

Oxygenation (respirations)

Related Concepts

See the Concept Map at the end of this chapter.

Example Problems

Pyrexia (fever)

Hyperthermia

Hypothermia

Hypertension

Hypotension

Caring for the Nguyens

This feature allows you to practice the kind of thinking you will use as a full-spectrum nurse. There is usually more than one correct answer to a critical thinking question, so we do not provide answers for these features. It is more important to develop your nursing judgment than to "cover content." Discuss the questions with your peers. If you are still unsure, consult your instructor.

Recall that on Nam Nguyen's preliminary visit to the Family Medicine Center, his blood pressure (BP) was 162/94 mm Hg. On subsequent visits, his BP was 168/100 and 174/96 mm Hg, and he was continuing to gain weight. Mr. Nguyen was diagnosed with hypertension and

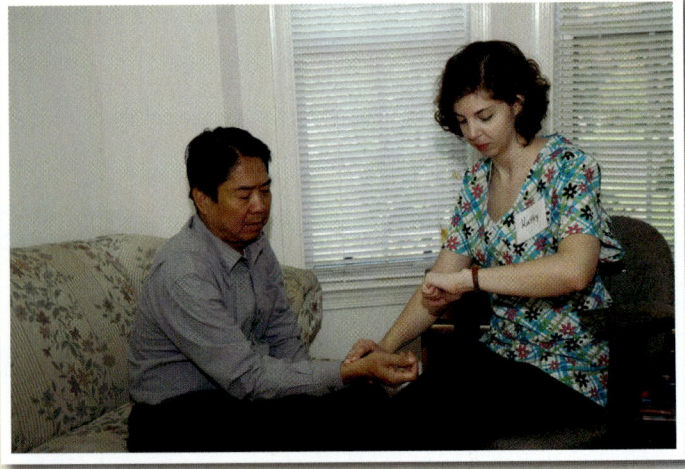

Caring for the Nyugens (continued)

prescribed an antihypertension medication to be taken each morning. This morning Mr. Nguyen has come to the clinic for follow-up. The following information is gathered as he checks in for his visit.

VS: BP, 168/92 mm Hg; pulse, 80 beats/min; respirations, 20 breaths/min; temperature, 98.4°F (36.9°C)
Weight: 180 lb (82 kg)

Review the preliminary data and the preceding information to answer the following questions:

A. What patterns do you see in the data?

B. Do you have enough information to draw any conclusions? If not, what other information should you gather?

C. Identify three alternatives that may explain what is happening with Mr. Nguyen's vital signs.

D. How could you determine which of these alternatives provides the best explanation of what is happening?

E. Why is it important to intervene in this situation?

 Go to **Caring for the Nguyens Response Sheet** on *DavisPlus*.

Meet Your Patients

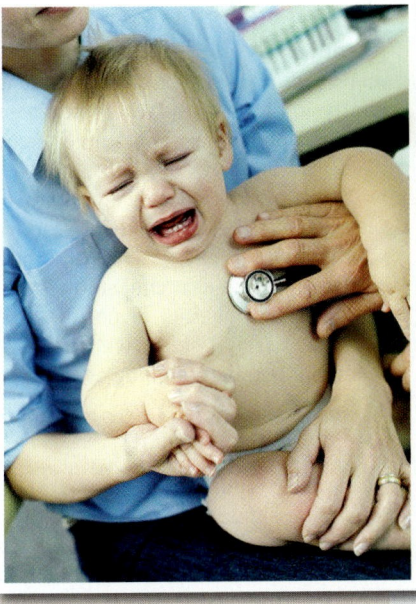

Your instructor has scheduled a clinical day at a local community health fair. Students will be available to answer health-related questions; administer flu vaccines; check blood sugar levels; and measure temperature, pulse, respirations, and blood pressure. You have been asked to check vital signs.

- **Rosemary.** The first person who arrives at the booth is Rosemary, a young mother, with Jason, her 2-year-old son. She tells you he has been eating poorly and is very irritable. The child's skin is warm and dry, and he is flushed. Rosemary explains that she does not have a thermometer, and she would like you to take her son's temperature. Jason's axillary temperature is 101.8°F (38.8°C). Now it is time to think like a nurse! What could this temperature reading mean? What, if any, additional data should you collect? How will you explain your findings to Rosemary? What action would you advise Rosemary to take? You may not yet have all the theoretical knowledge you need to answer these questions, but try to do so anyway, based on your present knowledge base and your life experiences.
- **Ms. Sharma.** The next person to arrive at the booth is Ms. Sharma, an active 80-year-old woman who works part time in a local literacy program and walks 3 miles four times per week. Ms. Sharma notes that she has "lost a little pep. I don't feel sick, but I'm tired lately." Her pulse is difficult to feel. The rhythm is irregular, and some beats are strong while others are weak. What might this finding mean? What questions do you have

for Ms. Sharma? What, if any, additional data should you collect? How will you explain your findings to Ms. Sharma? What action would you advise her to take?
- **Mr. Jackson.** As Mr. Jackson sits down next to you, you notice he is short of breath. His respiratory rate is 28 breaths/min, and he appears to be struggling to breathe. What do you think this respiratory rate means? What should be your next action? What would you say to Mr. Jackson?
- **Lucas.** The next client to arrive is Lucas, a 35-year-old accountant who works in a nearby office building. Lucas tells you he has been under a lot of stress and is worried about his blood pressure. You measure his blood pressure as 150/98 mm Hg. Is this an acceptable blood pressure? What does this reading mean? What should you discuss with Lucas? What advice should you offer?

You will gain the theoretical knowledge that you need to answer the preceding questions as you work through this chapter and learn more about vital signs.

ABOUT THE KEY CONCEPTS

All of the content in this chapter pertains to the concept vital signs. The key concepts of thermoregulation, perfusion, and oxygenation pertain to specific vital signs you will learn about (temperature, pulse, respirations, and blood pressure). A grasp of these underlying concepts will help you understand and remember the rationale for what you do when measuring vital signs.

WHAT ARE VITAL SIGNS?

The term **vital signs (VS)** suggests assessment of vital or critical physiological functions. Variations in temperature, pulse, respirations, or blood pressure are indicators of a person's state of health and function of the body systems. Therefore, these four measurements are among the most frequent assessments you will make as a nurse. Because of the importance of each of the vital signs, you must be very accurate in your measurements and recordings. This chapter explains the meaning of each of the vital signs and how to assess them.

Do not become complacent when a client's vital signs are within normal limits. Although stable vital signs *indicate* physiological well-being, they do not *guarantee* it. For example, vital signs may sometimes remain stable even when there is moderately large blood loss. Evaluate the vital signs in the context of your overall assessment of the client.

Other Vital Signs. A fifth vital sign, a measure of *pain*, has recently been proposed. See Chapter 32. Some experts recommend *pulse oximetry* be added to the four traditional measures of physiological status when accurate monitoring are essential. Pulse oximetry is a technique for assessing oxygenation and is discussed later in this chapter. Also, although it does not fit with the traditional concept, some researchers suggest that *smoking status* be considered a VS during the initial patient encounter (Vital Signs, 1999). Still others recommend including *emotional distress* as a vital sign. Rather than being overly concerned about whether or not these parameters should be referred to as vital signs, we recommend that nurses include them in all of their ongoing assessments of patients.

When Should I Measure a Patient's Vital Signs?

In the Meet Your Patients scenario, clients asked you to take their vital signs. However, in many clinical settings you and other care providers will determine how often to measure and record VS. In general, the frequency depends on the patient's condition and the events taking place. The following are common occasions for assessing vital signs:

- On admission to the hospital
- For inpatients, at the beginning of a shift
- At a visit to the healthcare provider's office or clinic
- Before, during, and after surgery or certain procedures
- To monitor the effects of certain medications or activities
- Whenever the patient's condition changes

Although there has been little research to support the ideal frequency for assessing vital signs, agency policies usually require that nurses monitor and record vital signs regularly. The frequency varies by setting and situation. Below are commonly used frequencies:

- In the hospital: once every 4 to 8 hours
- In the home health setting: at each visit
- In the clinic: at each visit
- In skilled nursing facilities, also known as convalescent hospitals: weekly to monthly

It is up to the nurse to decide whether vital signs need to be monitored more often than the primary care provider has prescribed. Initially, you will measure VS to establish the patient's baseline.

Key Point: *A baseline is important because (1) a change in vital signs may be caused by a disease state, the effect of therapies, or merely by changes in activity and environment; and (2) there are normal variations in vital signs among individuals.*

Table 19-1 shows average or normal findings for adults, but it is important to remember that each person has his or her own baseline for "normal." If a patient's vital signs vary from established norms, compare the finding to that person's baseline to determine the degree and severity of the variation. When a client's VS vary from their baseline, assess and document them more frequently, perhaps every 5 to 15 minutes. As a beginning practitioner, you should validate your clinical assessments with a more experienced nurse.

How Do I Document Vital Signs?

Most agencies have special flow sheets for documenting vital signs. If the VS are not within normal limits, you will also document them in the nurses' notes, along with any associated symptoms (e.g., cyanosis [blue-gray skin] with abnormal respirations). Document any interventions as well (e.g., elevating

Table 19-1 ➤ Vital Signs: Average Normal Findings for Adults	
Mean Adult Temperature	
Oral	98°F (36.7°C)*
Rectal	98.6°F (37°C)*
Pulse	
Normal range	60–100 beats/min
Average	80 beats/min
Respirations	
Normal range	12–20 breaths/min
Blood Pressure	
Normal range	100–119 mm Hg systolic and 60–80 mm Hg diastolic
Prehypertensive	120–139 mm Hg systolic and 80–89 mm Hg diastolic
Average	110/70 mm Hg (the middle of the "normal" range) (Joint National Committee on Prevention, Detection, Evaluation, and Treatment of High Blood Pressure, 2003)

*This is revised downward from the traditional norms to reflect more recent research (Mackowiak, Wasserman, & Levine, 1992) and a systematic review of the literature (Sund-Levander, Forsberg, & Wahren, 2002). The systematic review reported the following mean normal temperatures: Oral 97.3°F (36.3°C), Rectal 98.3°F (36.9°C). The traditional Wunderlich (1871) average normal temperature is 98.6°F (37.0°C) to 99.5°F (37.5°C), depending on measurement site.

the head of the bed when the patient has shortness of breath). For an example of a graphic flow sheet for recording vital signs, see Figure 19-1.

BODY TEMPERATURE

Body temperature is the degree of heat maintained by the body. It is the difference between heat produced by the body and heat lost to the environment. Because this is a chapter about skills, the focus is on body temperature. However, your theoretical knowledge must include the concept of thermoregulation in order to assess and support regulation of body temperature at a professional level. You will also need to know the normal temperature range, how heat is produced by and lost from the body, and factors that influence body temperature.

Theoretical Knowledge
knowing why

What Is a Normal Temperature?

No single number can be considered "normal," because baseline body temperature varies among individuals as a result of differences in metabolism. For example, older adults tend to have lower body temperatures, and pregnant women run higher baseline body temperatures. Furthermore, each person's temperature fluctuates with age, exercise, and environmental conditions. However, the body does function optimally within a narrow temperature range (Table 19-1).

There is little definitive evidence about what, exactly, is a normal temperature. You may see different values in the many sources you read. However, we can conclude that, based on available research, the traditionally used 98.6°F (37°C) for an average normal reading is too high. A systematic review of the literature found a mean normal adult oral temperature of 97.3°F (36.3°C) (Sund-Levander, Forsberg, & Wahren, 2002). For age-related variations for all vital signs, including temperature,

 Go to Chapter 19, **Tables, Boxes, Figures: ESG Table 19-1, Comparison of Normal Vital Signs for Various Ages,** on Davis*Plus*.

An adult's normal internal temperature, called the **core temperature,** ranges from about 97°F to 100.8°F (36.1°C to 38.2°C). See Figure 19-2. Most research and clinical practice situations do not report core body temperature because it is not convenient to measure. The core temperature is typically 1°F to 2°F (0.6°C to 1.2°C) higher than surface (skin) temperature. Rectal and tympanic membrane measurements are used to represent core temperatures; oral and axillary measurements reflect surface temperatures.

Temporary, slight variations of temperature above or below normal usually are not significant. Greater variations indicate a disturbance of function in some system or region of the body. However, the degree of temperature elevation does not always indicate the seriousness of the underlying disease or condition. For example, some acute, even fatal, infections may cause only a mild temperature elevation. However, a continuous

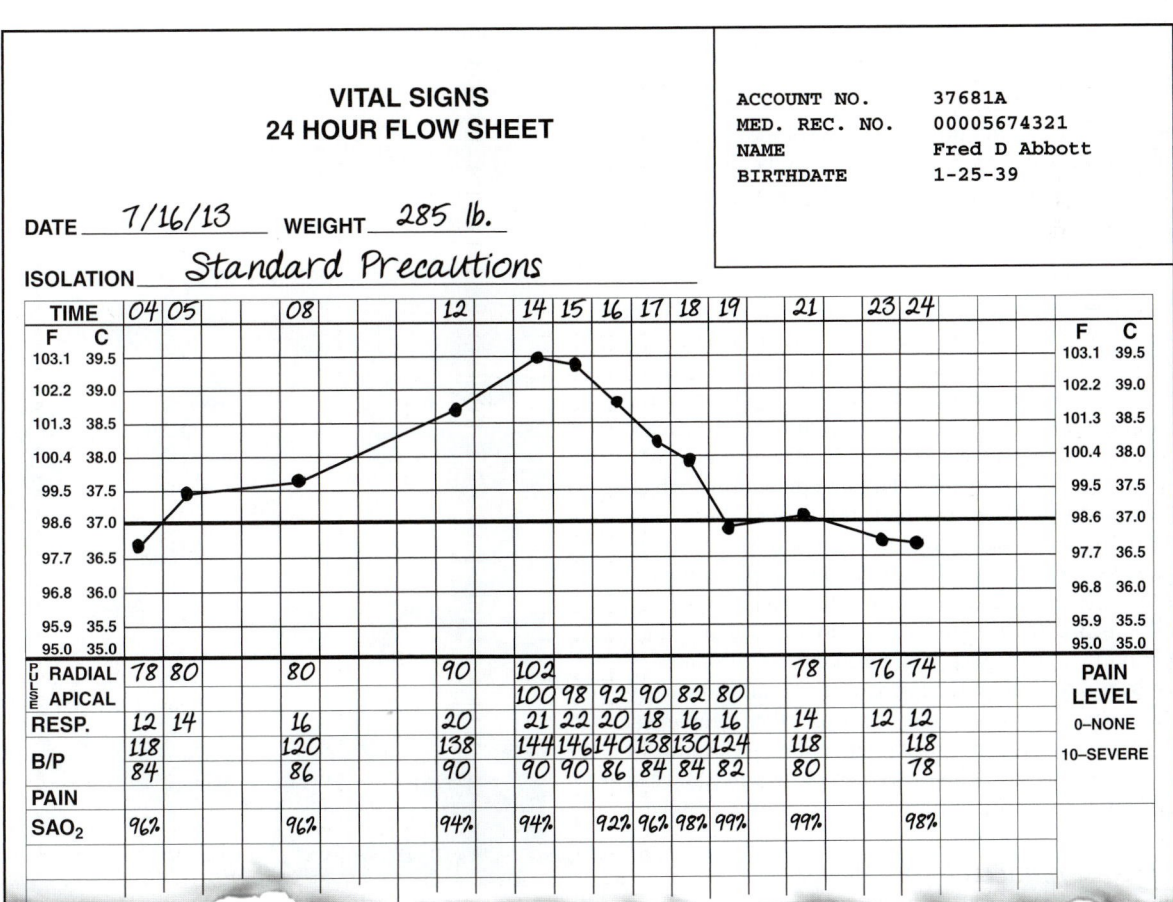

FIGURE 19-1 Graphic flow sheet for recording vital signs.

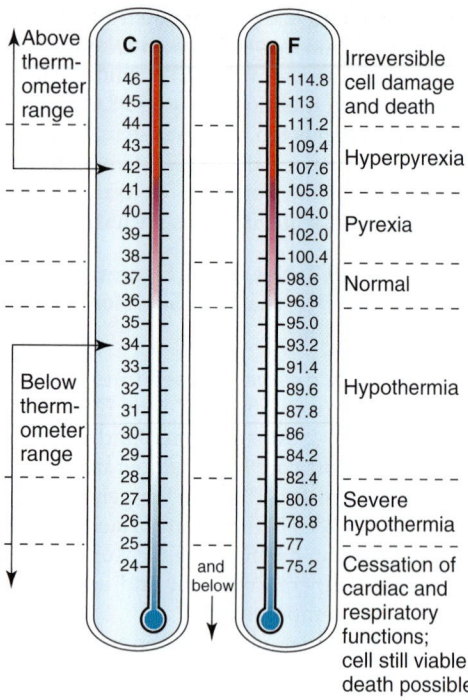

FIGURE 19-2 Ranges of normal and altered body temperatures.

elevation, even if slight, is cause for concern and indicates a need for further evaluation.

What Is Thermoregulation?

Thermoregulation is the process of maintaining a stable temperature. To keep the body temperature constant, the body must balance heat production and heat loss. This balance is controlled by the hypothalamus, located between the cerebral hemispheres of the brain. Similar to a thermostat, the hypothalamus recognizes even small changes in body temperature that are sent to it by sensory receptors in the skin.

Decreasing the Body Temperature. When heat sensors in the hypothalamus are stimulated, they send out impulses to mechanisms that inhibit heat production and activate sweating and peripheral vasodilation to cool the body. Vasodilation diverts core-warmed blood to the body surface, where heat can be transferred to the surrounding environment.

Increasing the Body Temperature. When sensors in the hypothalamus detect cold, they send out impulses to increase heat production and reduce heat loss. To produce heat, the body responds by shivering and releasing epinephrine, which increase metabolism. Two mechanisms reduce heat loss: (1) **Vasoconstriction** (narrowing of the blood vessels) conserves heat by shunting blood away from the periphery (where heat is lost) to the core of the body, where the blood is warmed; and (2) **piloerection** (hairs standing on end) also occurs, but it is not an important heat-conserving mechanism in humans.

Behavioral Control of Temperature. In addition, body temperature is under our voluntary control. When people feel cool, they can turn up the thermostat, put on more clothing, or move to a warmer place. When they feel too warm, they can turn on an air conditioner, remove some clothing, or take a cool shower.

How Is Heat Produced in the Body?

The body produces heat through the interaction of three factors: metabolism, the movement of skeletal muscles, and nonshivering thermogenesis.

Metabolism. **Metabolism** is the sum of all physical and chemical processes that take place in the body. Metabolism uses energy and generates heat. The **basal metabolic rate (BMR)** is the amount of energy required to maintain the body at rest. Body size, lean muscle mass, and numerous hormones influence BMR. For example, when the thyroxine level is low (hypothyroidism), less heat is produced, and clients commonly report feeling cold. Epinephrine and norepinephrine, produced from stimulation of the sympathetic nervous system, increase BMR and heat production.

Skeletal Muscle Movement. Skeletal muscles need fuel to function. The breakdown (catabolism) of fats and carbohydrates in muscle produces energy and heat. It requires very little muscle activity to sit and read this text. However, if you were to go for a run, you would use more skeletal muscles. After your run, your body temperature would be higher, perhaps as high as 101°F to 104°F (38.3°C to 40°C). In contrast, if you were to go outside without a coat when the temperature was 35°F (1.6°C), you would begin to feel cold. Your hypothalamus would sense a drop in body temperature and you would begin shivering. This mechanism is so efficient that body heat production can rise to about four times the normal rate in just a few minutes.

Nonshivering Thermogenesis. Nonshivering thermogenesis is the metabolism of brown fat to produce heat. It is used by infants because they cannot produce heat through shivering, as do adults and children. This mechanism disappears in the first few months after birth.

How Is Heat Exchanged Between the Body and the Environment?

Heat moves from an area of higher to an area of lower temperature; that is, cool air and objects "pick up" heat from warmer ones. The mechanisms that effect the exchange of heat between the body and the environment are radiation, convection, evaporation, and conduction (Fig. 19-3).

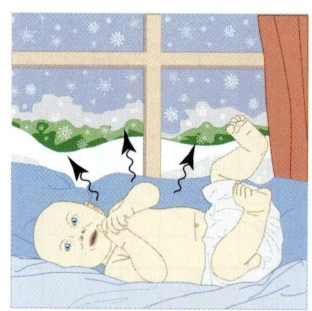
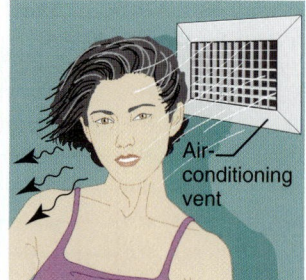
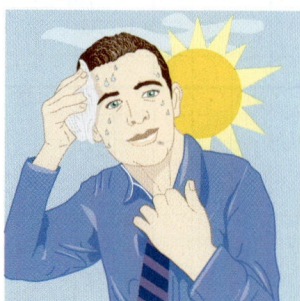
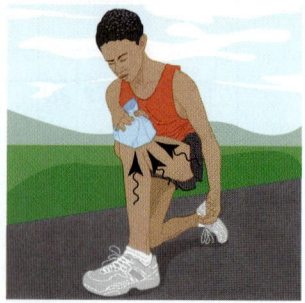

Air-conditioning vent

FIGURE 19-3 Mechanisms of heat exchange with the environment: Radiation, convection, evaporation, and conduction.

Radiation is the loss of heat through electromagnetic waves emitting from surfaces that are warmer than the surrounding air. If the uncovered skin is warmer than the air, the body loses heat through the skin. This is why a cool room warms by radiation when it is filled with many people. In contrast, a person can acquire heat by turning on a heat lamp or being in the sunlight. Radiation accounts for almost 50% of body heat loss.

Convection is the transfer of heat through currents of air or water. Nurses use this principle to intentionally effect changes in a patient's body temperature. Immersion in a warm bath may raise body temperature for a hypothermic client. In contrast, the currents of cool air produced by a fan can help reduce a fever. Together, the processes of convection and conduction account for approximately 15% to 20% of all heat loss to the environment.

Evaporation occurs when water is converted to vapor and lost from the skin (as perspiration) or the mucous membranes (through the breath). Evaporation causes cooling. Water loss by evaporation is called **insensible loss.** Evaporation is affected by the relative **humidity** (moisture in the environment). If the air already contains much humidity, then less moisture evaporates from the skin and less cooling occurs.

Conduction is the process whereby heat is transferred from a warm to a cool surface by direct contact. Suppose that a patient's temperature is 98.6°F (37°C) while he is fully dressed in the examination room. If he is dressed in a thin hospital gown and lying on a cool metal radiology table, his temperature would drop, perhaps as much as a full degree Fahrenheit in the first hour.

What Factors Influence Body Temperature?

The following are some examples of factors involved in the delicate balance of body temperature:

Developmental Level. Infants and older adults are most susceptible to the effects of environmental temperature extremes. Infants lose approximately 30% of their body heat through the head, which is proportionally larger than the rest of the body compared to adults. This places them at increased risk for decreased body temperature. Body temperature begins to stabilize during early childhood and remains relatively stable until older adulthood.

Older adults have difficulty maintaining body heat because of slower metabolism, decreased vasomotor control, and loss of subcutaneous tissue. The average normal temperature for older adults (65 years of age and older) is about 95°F to 96.8°F (35°C to 36°C). Temperatures are lower for very old adults. In a recent study, older adults (average age 80.7 yr) had mean body temperatures ranging from 94°F (34.4°C) to 99.6°F (37.6°C), but few ever reached 98.6°F (37°C) (Gomolin, Aung, Wolf-Klein, et al., 2005). For a comparison of normal VS for various ages,

 Go to Chapter 19, **Tables, Boxes, Figures: ESG Table 19-1, Comparison of Normal Vital Signs for Various Ages,** on *DavisPlus.*

Environment. The environment strongly influences body temperature. For example, warm room temperatures, high humidity, or hot baths can increase body temperature. Very high external temperatures can produce high internal temperatures, causing heat stroke. In contrast, cold environments, especially with strong air currents, can lower body temperatures and, in severe cases, lead to hypothermia.

Gender. A woman's body temperature varies (as much as 1°F, or 0.6°C) with her menstrual cycle and pregnancy due to fluctuation of progesterone levels. Hormonal fluctuations during menopause, when menses stop, often cause temperature fluctuations commonly known as *hot flashes*, which can produce episodes of intense body heat and sweating. At least one study has found differences in the range of normal body temperatures for women and men. However, further studies are needed to confirm these differences (Sund-Levander, Forsberg, & Wahren, 2002).

Exercise. Because it increases metabolism, hard work or strenuous exercise can increase body core temperature to 101°F to 104°F (38.3°C to 40°C).

Emotions and Stress. Emotional stress, excitement, anxiety, and nervousness stimulate the sympathetic nervous system, causing production of epinephrine and norepinephrine, which trigger an increase in the metabolic rate.

Circadian Rhythm. **Circadian rhythm** is a cyclical repetition of certain physiological processes (e.g., changes in temperature and blood pressure) that occurs every 24 hours. Temperature fluctuates 1°F to 2°F (0.6°C to 1.2°C) over the course of 24 hours. It is usually lowest in the early morning hours and highest in late afternoon or early evening.

ThinkLike a Nurse 19-1

- You notice the following temperature readings in your client's chart:
  0400: 97.4°F
  0800: 97.9°F
  1200: 98.4°F
  1600: 99.6°F
  2000: 100.9°F
- You are working the night shift. When you assess the client's temperature at midnight, it is 101.2°F. What do you notice about the pattern of the temperature readings?
  What is important in this scenario?
  As a nursing student, what should you do?

KnowledgeCheck 19-1

- Which age groups are most susceptible to thermoregulation problems, and why?
- List five factors that affect body temperature.
- What are the compensatory mechanisms for decreasing body temperature?
- What are the compensatory mechanisms for increasing body temperature?

Example Problem: Fever (Pyrexia)

Fever, or **pyrexia,** is a temperature above the person's usual range of normal. Traditionally we have thought of fever as an oral temperature higher than 100°F (37.8°C), or a rectal temperature of 101°F (38.3°C) in an adult. But remember that many people, especially older adults, have lower normal body temperatures and that a person's normal body temperature changes by as much as 1°F (0.6°C) throughout the day. So it is likely that many people experience fever at a temperature lower than our traditional definition. A person with a fever is said to be **febrile;** one without fever is **afebrile.** A single high reading may not indicate fever. You need several readings at different times of the day, as well as the person's usual normal reading.

A moderate fever (up to 103°F, or 39.5°C) may be uncomfortable, and it may signal an underlying problem (e.g.,

influenza or other infection). However, the fever itself does not pose a threat to most clients and is the body's natural defense against infection. Higher fevers can damage body cells and cause delirium and seizures. **Hyperpyrexia** is fever above 105.8°F (41.0°C). Hyperpyrexia is dangerous and requires intervention.

Fever occurs in response to **pyrogens** (fever-producing substances). When bacteria or other foreign substances invade the body, they stimulate **phagocytes** (specialized white blood cells), which ingest the invaders and secrete pyrogens (e.g., interleukin-1). Pyrogens induce secretion of **prostaglandins** (substances that reset the hypothalamic thermostat at a higher temperature). The reset value is called the **set point.** The body's heat-regulating mechanisms then act to bring the core temperature up to this new setting. When the stressor is removed, the set point resets at normal.

Fever occurs in three phases:

1. *Initial phase (febrile episode or onset):* The period when body temperature is rising but has not yet reached the new set point. The onset of fever may be sudden or gradual, depending on the condition causing it. The person usually feels chilly and generally uncomfortable and may shiver.

2. *Second phase (course):* The period when body temperature reaches its maximum (set point) and remains fairly constant at the new higher level. The person is flushed and feels warm and dry during this phase, which may last from a few days to a few weeks.

3. *Third phase (defervescence or crisis):* The period when the temperature returns to normal. The person feels warm and appears flushed in response to vasodilation. Diaphoresis occurs, which assists with heat loss by evaporation. This phase is commonly referred to as the fever's "breaking."

There are four types of fever:

- **Intermittent fever:** Temperature alternates regularly between periods of fever and periods of normal or below-normal temperature without pharmacological intervention; or the temperature returns to normal at least once every 24 hours.
- **Remittent fever:** Fluctuations in temperature (greater than 3.6°F, or 2°C), all above normal, during a 24-hour period.
- **Constant (sustained) fever:** Temperature may fluctuate slightly (less than 1°F, or 0.55°C) but is always above normal.
- **Relapsing (or recurrent) fever:** Short periods of fever alternating with periods of normal temperatures, each lasting 1 to 2 days.

At some time in your life, you most likely have taken acetaminophen (Tylenol) or ibuprofen (Advil, Motrin) for a fever. Can you think of a reason why it may not always be a good idea to take these drugs at the first signs of a fever? Why should you think carefully before administering **antipyretic** (fever-reducing) medications to a client?

The answer is that fever, up to a point, is beneficial. High temperatures (up to 102.2°F, or 39°C) enhance the immune response because they (1) kill or inhibit the growth of many microorganisms; (2) enhance phagocytosis; (3) cause the breakdown of lysosomes and self-destruction of virally infected cells; and (4) cause the release of interferon, a substance that protects cells from viral infection.

This does not mean that you should *never* administer, or take, antipyretic medications. They may be needed to keep the temperature from becoming dangerously high. Temperatures of 105.8°F (41.0°C) and above can damage cells throughout the body, especially in the brain, causing agitation, confusion,

stupor, or coma. Vascular collapse may follow, producing cerebral edema, shock, and death. Death usually results if body temperature becomes higher than 109°F to 112°F (43°C to 44°C) (McCance & Huether, 2006). Note that certain patients (e.g., those with epilepsy) are especially sensitive to even slight temperature elevations, so antipyretics might be used at the first sign of temperature elevation.

Example Problem: Hyperthermia (Heat Stroke)

Hyperthermia, like hyperpyrexia (fever), is a body temperature above normal. However, in hyperthermia, the elevated body temperature is higher than the set point. The hypothalamic regulation of body temperature is overwhelmed and does not reset the set point as it does in fever. Hyperthermia occurs because the body cannot promote heat loss fast enough to balance heat production or high environmental temperatures. **Heat exhaustion** and **heat stroke** are common examples. With overexposure to high temperatures and inadequate fluid replacement, the body loses the ability to sweat and is unable to cool down.

Heat Exhaustion may occur with a core temperature of 98.6°F to 103°F (37°C to 39.4°C). Warning signs of heat exhaustion vary, but may include weakness, nausea, vomiting, syncope, tachycardia, tachypnea, muscle aches, headache, diaphoresis (heavy sweating), and flushed skin.

Heat Stroke occurs when the body's temperature regulation fails, usually when the hyperthermia progresses to a temperature above 103°F (39.4°C). Symptoms include rapid, strong pulse; throbbing headache; delirium; confusion; impaired judgment; lethargy; red, hot, dry skin; dizziness; seizures; and coma. Temperatures of 106°F (41.1°C) and higher may be reached. If emergency treatment is not given, heat stroke can result in death.

Example Problem: Hypothermia

The Centers for Disease Control and Prevention (CDC) define *hypothermia* as an abnormally low core temperature, less than 95°F (less than 35°C). You must know the person's usual normal range of temperature because some people, especially older adults, have a normal temperature of less than 95°F. As the body temperature drops, metabolic processes slow. Prolonged exposure to the cold is no longer correctable by shivering and may prove fatal.

Hypothermia may be associated with extended exposure to cold, such as during surgery, extreme weather conditions, immersion in cold water, or lack of shelter and clothing. Hypothermia is sometimes deliberately induced under close monitoring to decrease the need for oxygen in body tissues (e.g., during cardiac or neurological surgery).

Early Signs of Hypothermia include shivering, cyanosis of lips and fingers, and poor coordination. The person first feels cold, then may feel some pain in the extremities. As body temperature continues to fall, the person experiences mental impairment, confusion, disorientation, slowing of the heart rate and respirations, and inability to take precautions from the cold.

Severe Hypothermia occurs when the body temperature drops below 82.4°F (28°C). The person becomes unconscious and stops shivering. The pulse and respirations are irregular and difficult to detect. Although survival has been known to occur at a core temperature of 60.8°F (16°C), death usually results when body temperature falls below 70°F to 75°F (21°C to 24°C).

Practical Knowledge
knowing **how**

Now that you understand the concept of thermoregulation, you are ready to gain the practical knowledge of how to assess and support a patient's body temperature.

ASSESSMENT

In our daily routines, we commonly assess temperature by touch. For example, when you remove a blanket from a warming unit, you can feel that it is warm; however, you probably could not pinpoint the exact temperature of the blanket. The same is true of body temperature. Although some research has shown that people can use simple touch to detect fever, they cannot differentiate *degrees* of fever. Because vital signs are used as indicators of a client's health status, it is essential to have an accurate measure. To see the sequence of steps to take when measuring a patient's temperature, refer to Procedure 19-1.

Temperature Measurement Scales: Fahrenheit and Centigrade

Two scales are used for recording temperature: Fahrenheit and centigrade (or Celsius), a metric scale. Most people in the United States are familiar with the Fahrenheit scale; however, some healthcare agencies use centigrade. Electronic and tympanic membrane thermometers can usually measure temperature in either scale; often all you need to do is to flip a switch. Glass thermometers read only one scale (Fig. 19-4), so you may need to convert a reading from one scale to the other. For a

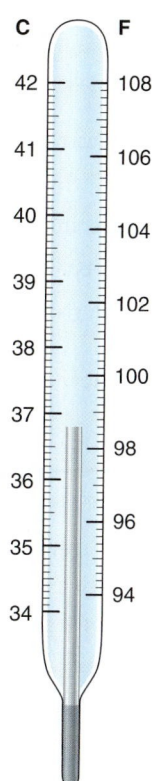

FIGURE 19-4 Some thermometers are available with degree markings in Fahrenheit or centigrade. *Left,* Centigrade scale. *Right,* Fahrenheit scale.

chart you can print and use to convert between Fahrenheit and centigrade readings in the clinical setting,

 Go to Chapter 19, **Tables, Boxes, Figures: ESG Table 19-2, Centigrade-Fahrenheit Conversion Chart,** on Davis*Plus.*

If for some reason you find yourself without access to a conversion chart, you may need to convert mathematically. To convert from Fahrenheit to centigrade, subtract 32 from the Fahrenheit temperature and multiply by 5/9. For example:

A client has a temperature of 102°F. What is his temperature as measured in centigrade?

$$(102 - 32) \times 5/9 = (70 \times 5) \div 9 = 39°C$$

To convert a centigrade reading to Fahrenheit, multiply the centigrade temperature by 9/5, and add 32. As a cross-check we can verify the preceding example:

Client temperature = 39°C

$$(39 \times 9/5) + 32 = (351 \div 5) + 32 = 102°F$$

What Equipment Do I Need?

Nurses measure temperature with various kinds of thermometers. Each type has advantages and disadvantages, so you need to think critically about the type of thermometer best suited for each patient situation. See Table 19-2 for a summary of the advantages and disadvantages of various types of thermometers.

Glass Thermometers. Historically, the thermometer was a glass, mercury-filled tube marked in degrees Fahrenheit or centigrade and read visually. Because of the dangers of exposure to mercury (e.g., when thermometers break), the U.S. Environmental Protection Agency (EPA) and the American Hospital Association now advise against use of equipment containing mercury (U.S. Environmental Protection Agency, 2001). Because they can break, glass thermometers also pose a risk for cuts from the glass.

Electronic digital thermometers have replaced glass thermometers in most healthcare agencies. Glass thermometers containing other liquids, such as alcohol or gallium–indium–tin (galinstan), are available and some agencies still use them.

Electronic Thermometers. An electronic thermometer is a rechargeable unit consisting of an electronic probe attached to a portable unit by a thin wire. A beep sounds when the peak temperature is reached. Disposable plastic sheaths are used to cover the probe. To prevent transmission of infection, discard the sheath after each use. Most units have a separate probe for rectal and oral temperatures, color-coded red and blue, respectively, to be certain the correct probe is used.

Electronic Infrared Thermometers. The electronic infrared thermometer is a rechargeable unit that contains a sensor that detects heat in the form of infrared energy given off by the body, for example, at the tympanic membrane or at the temporal artery. The thermometer does not actually touch the tympanic membrane. A beep sounds when the peak temperature is reached.

Disposable Chemical Thermometers. A disposable chemical thermometer is a thin plastic strip, patch, or tape containing a matrix of chemicals that change color at a designated body temperature. Most are used once for an oral or axillary reading, then disposed of. Disposable thermometers are useful in the home and for patients in protective isolation.

Table 19-2 ➤ Advantages and Disadvantages of Various Thermometers

ADVANTAGES	DISADVANTAGES
Glass Thermometer	
■ Flexibility of use: Can be used for measuring oral, rectal, or axillary temperature. ■ Inexpensive initial cost ■ Accuracy, as indicated by several studies ■ Easily disinfected	✚ Do not use glass thermometers containing mercury. If you find one, recommend that it be replaced immediately. ■ Easily broken, so there is ongoing cost of replacement and risk for injury. For this reason, glass is not recommended. ■ Slow: It takes 3–8 min to obtain an accurate reading, depending on the site. ■ Difficult for some people to read accurately
Electronic Thermometer	
■ Flexibility of use: Can be used for measuring oral, rectal, or axillary temperature. ■ Ease of use ■ Rapid measurement: It takes 2–60 sec to obtain reading, depending on the unit.	■ Expensive initial cost ■ Requires regular inspection and maintenance to ensure accuracy. ■ Data are conflicting regarding their accuracy compared to other types of thermometers. ■ Needs to be kept charged.
Electronic With Infrared Sensor	
■ Ease of use ■ Rapid measurement: It takes 2–5 sec to measure the temperature. ■ May be the most cost-effective method because of time and labor savings from their rapid reading capabilities. ■ Low rate of operator error	■ Expensive initial cost. ■ Less accurate than electronic or glass thermometers when used for tympanic membrane temperatures, as some studies indicate. ■ Requires regular inspection and maintenance to ensure accuracy. ■ Batteries require recharging.
Disposable Chemical Thermometer	
■ Easy to use; requires no special training. ■ Equally as accurate as the electronic thermometer. ■ Less expensive than purchasing supplies for and maintaining an electronic thermometer. ■ Because it is disposable, it may prevent spread of infection among patients. ■ Recommended for measuring axillary temperature among pediatric patients over the age of 2 years. (Cincinnati Children's Hospital Medical Center, 2011).	■ Less accurate/reliable than glass thermometers ■ The skin must be dry ■ Indicates only body surface temperature; does not reflect core. ■ Guidelines presently recommend only for pediatric patients. ■ Associated with more errors than glass thermometers

Recent guidelines conclude that measurements done on children are as accurate as those done with electronic thermometers (Cincinnati Children's Hospital Medical Center, 2011). Although there is some conflicting research, disposable chemical thermometers are associated with more errors than glass thermometers. They are also thought to overestimate or underestimate true readings for adults.

Other Types of Thermometers. For special uses, devices have been created to take measurements from the nasopharynx, the pulmonary artery, the bladder, and the skin. A wireless intestinal temperature monitoring system in the form of a pill and an external receiver is sometimes used, for example, during cardiac surgery. Infrared devices have also been used to take thermal measurements of skin surface temperature.

What Sites Should I Use?

Temperatures in the pulmonary artery, esophagus, and bladder accurately measure core temperature. These sites are used in surgery and intensive care, but they are invasive, expensive, and impractical for most clinical settings. Pulmonary artery temperature is considered the gold standard to which other sites are compared. A device is placed in the pulmonary artery, and readings are continuously displayed on a monitor.

The usual sites for intermittent measurements are the mouth, rectum, axillae, tympanic membrane, and skin over

the temporal artery. These sites allow the thermometer to contact body tissues that are well supplied with blood vessels. This is essential for accurate measurement. Each site has advantages and disadvantages, so you must choose the safest, most accurate, and most reliable site for each client (Table 19-3).

Temperature readings vary depending on the site used. Research on site differences is conflicting; however, from lowest to highest readings, the sites are generally thought to be as follows: axillary, oral, tympanic membrane, rectal, and temporal artery. For oral, axillary, and rectal temperatures, there is an approximately 0.8°F or 0.4°C difference between each site and the next higher one. For convenience, nurses tend to round the fraction up to a full 1°F (0.5°C). For example, an axillary temperature of 98.1°F is

Table 19-3 ➤ Disadvantages and Contraindications of Various Sites for Measuring Temperature

ADVANTAGES	DISADVANTAGES	CONTRAINDICATIONS
Site: Temporal Artery		
■ Most accurate representation of core temperature ■ Fast. Most scanners provide a reading in about 3 sec. ■ No discomfort is associated with the procedure. ■ Safe. Can be used even for those who cannot follow instructions (e.g., infants). ■ Less prone to error than tympanic thermometer	■ Requires special scanning thermometer. ■ Any covering—hat, hair, etc.— prevents heat from dissipating and causes the reading to be falsely high. This is also true for the side of the head lying on a pillow	
Site: Rectal		
■ Accurately represents core (internal) body temperature. ■ Use for clients who are unable to follow directions for oral temperature monitoring, or in situations where accuracy is crucial.	■ Most clients find this method objectionable or embarrassing. ■ ✚ Not recommended as the first choice of site because of the risk for injury to the rectal mucosa. ■ Requires special positioning of the client. ■ Does not reflect changes in core temperature as rapidly as the oral method. ■ Presence of stool may cause inaccurate reading.	■ ✚ Clients who may be injured by the method (e.g., clients who have a rectal disease, severe diarrhea, or rectal surgery; newborns, whose rectal mucosa is fragile) ■ Because it can slow the heart rate by stimulating the vagus nerve, this method is sometimes contraindicated for clients with cardiac surgery and some heart conditions. ■ Clients with hemorrhoids ■ Immunosuppressed clients or those with clotting disorders
Site: Oral		
■ Simple, convenient ■ Comfortable for most patients ■ Safe for adults and for children who are old enough to follow simple directions	■ ✚ Glass thermometers can break if bitten. ■ Slow; requires up to 8 min to ensure an accurate reading (if glass thermometer used). ■ Patient must keep her mouth closed for several minutes (glass thermometers). ■ Eating, drinking (e.g., ice water, hot tea), and smoking in the 30 minutes before measurement affect the accuracy of the reading. ■ Bradypnea may create false temperature elevations.	■ ✚ Clients who cannot cooperate with the instructions or who might be injured (e.g., infants and small children; patients who have had oral surgery, breathe through the mouth, have chills, or are confused or unconscious)

(Continued)

Table 19-3 ➤ Disadvantages and Contraindications of Various Sites for Measuring Temperature—cont'd

ADVANTAGES	DISADVANTAGES	CONTRAINDICATIONS
Site: Axillary		
▪ Safe ▪ Easy to use ▪ Can be used for children and for uncooperative or unconscious clients. ▪ Recommended over rectal site for routine measurements	▪ Not reflective of core temperature ▪ Considered one of the least accurate sites ▪ Diaphoresis (sweating) can affect the reading. ▪ Thermometer may need to be left in place for a long time (8 min if glass is used).	▪ Clients who are perspiring heavily ▪ Does not accurately diagnose fever. If fever is suspected, confirm with measurement from another route.
Site: Tympanic Membrane		
▪ Fast (2–5 sec) ▪ Can be used for children and for uncooperative or unconscious clients.	▪ Requires a special thermometer, a relatively expensive initial purchase ▪ More variable than oral and rectal sites: ▪ Must be carefully positioned to ensure accuracy; prone to caregiver measurement errors. ▪ Presence of cerumen (earwax) may affect accuracy. ▪ Significant differences have been found between readings in left and right ear of same patient. ▪ Risk of injury to tympanic membrane if not positioned carefully to avoid touching it. ▪ May be uncomfortable for the client. ▪ Chemical thermometers (skin temperatures) have been found to be more accurate and reliable than tympanic membrane instruments. ▪ Hearing aids must be removed.	▪ ✚ Clients who have had recent ear surgery ▪ Contraindicated in the presence of ear infection
Site: Skin (e.g., forehead)		
▪ Safe, convenient ▪ Easy to use for nonprofessionals ▪ Can be used when other sites are contraindicated. ▪ Inexpensive (chemical paper or tape is used)	▪ Forehead skin temperature is generally 2°–4°F (1°–2°C) less than core temperature; if marked deviations in skin temperatures are detected, the readings must be confirmed via a more reliable route.	▪ Should not be used when accurate, reliable readings are required (e.g., in the presence of hypothermia or heatstroke). ▪ However, at least one study has shown skin temperatures to be accurate and reliable when obtained with an infrared skin thermometer (DeCurtis, Calzolari, Marciano, et al., 2008).

similar to an oral reading of 99.1°F or a rectal reading of 100.1°F. Use this *only* to help you understand your patient's data.

✚ You cannot reliably convert temperatures mathematically between sites. When you measure a temperature, record the value you obtain and the site used.

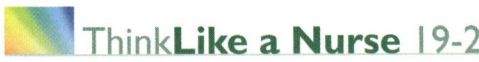

ThinkLike a Nurse 19-2

▪ Convert the following temperatures and analyze the readings. What might they mean?
a. 38.5°C _____ °F
b. 96.5°F _____ °C
c. 37.0°C _____ °F

- Rank the expected early evening temperatures of the following individuals from lowest to highest.
  - a. A 22-year-old college athlete
  - b. A 5-year-old kindergarten student
  - c. An 88-year-old nursing home resident

ANALYSIS/NURSING DIAGNOSIS

Fever and hypothermia may be medical diagnoses, nursing diagnoses, or symptoms of other problems. The following nursing diagnoses may be used when they are considered to be a *client problem* and not just a symptom of an illness or other problem (e.g., fever may be a symptom of problems such as Deficient Fluid Volume, or dehydration). Notice that the nursing diagnosis of Hyperthermia can be used both for temperature elevation from fever (hyperpyrexia) and from heat exhaustion (hyperthermia).

- *Hyperthermia* is diagnosed when a person's body temperature is above normal. Defining characteristics are convulsions, flushed skin, tachycardia, tachypnea, and warmth to touch.
- *Hypothermia* is diagnosed when a person's body temperature is below normal range. Defining characteristics include cool skin, cyanotic nailbeds, elevated blood pressure, pallor, piloerection, shivering, slow capillary refill, and tachycardia.
- *Ineffective Thermoregulation* applies when a person's temperature fluctuates above and below the normal range.
- *Risk for Imbalanced Body Temperature* is used when the temperature is normal but the client is at risk for failure to maintain body temperature within the normal range (e.g., newborns and the frail elderly). As you can see, this diagnosis can also apply to risk for either hypothermia or fever.

PLANNING OUTCOMES/EVALUATION

NOC standardized outcomes for NANDA-I diagnoses pertaining to body temperature include Thermoregulation, Thermoregulation: Newborn, and Vital Signs. For other NOC outcomes you might use for alterations in temperature regulation,

 Go to Chapter 19, **Standardized Language: NOC Outcomes and NIC Interventions Associated With Abnormal Vital Signs**, on Davis*Plus.*

Individualized goals/outcome statements you might write for a client with Hyperthermia include the following:
- Oral temperature of less than 97.6°F (less than 36.4°C) (client's usual normal temperature)
- No clinical signs of fever present (e.g., no chills or flushing)
- Pulse and respiratory rates within normal range for patient
  For a client with Hypothermia, the following are examples of goal statements.
- Oral temperature less than 97.6°F (less than 36.4°C) (client's usual normal temperature)
- No clinical signs of Hypothermia present (e.g., no disorientation, no decrease in urine output)
- Pulse and respiratory rates within normal range
  Use the goals set in the planning outcomes stage to evaluate client responses to interventions.

PLANNING INTERVENTIONS/IMPLEMENTATION

Overall care of the patient depends on the cause of the fever or hypothermia, and on specific prescriptions from the primary provider. Nevertheless, there are nursing interventions and activities that address fever and hypothermia, regardless of the cause.

Interventions for Example Problem: Hyperthermia

NIC standardized interventions for Hyperthermia and Ineffective Thermoregulation include Fever Treatment, Malignant Hyperthermia Precautions, Newborn Care, Temperature Regulation, Temperature Regulation: Intraoperative, and Vital Signs Monitoring. For other NIC labels you might use,

 Go to Chapter 19, **Standardized Language: NOC Outcomes and NIC Interventions Associated With Abnormal Vital Signs**, on Davis*Plus.*

Specific nursing activities for clients with fever and/or nursing diagnoses of Hyperthermia or Ineffective Thermoregulation include the following:

Provide Focused Assessments such as the following:
- *Help determine the cause of the fever.* For example, you may collect specimens for culture.
- *Monitor the temperature and other VS at least every 2 hours,* and more often if the temperature is rising rapidly or if the clinical symptoms are changing. Recall that the increased metabolism accompanying a fever also increases the pulse and respirations. If you suspect fever, it is wise to take a rectal reading with a different type of thermometer for comparison. Obtain an oral reading if the rectal site is contraindicated.
- *Observe for the clinical signs that accompany a fever.* Symptoms vary, depending on the phase of the fever. The characteristic symptoms include flushed face; dry, hot skin; eyes that appear bright and somewhat apprehensive; rapid, shallow respirations; increased heart rate; unusual thirst; loss of appetite; headache; and complaints of nausea. If the fever is extreme, urine may be concentrated and decreased in volume. Seizures, confusion, or delirium can also be associated with very high fevers.

Provide Collaborative Care to Treat the Underlying Cause of the Fever (e.g., antibiotics).

Provide Oral or Intravenous Fluids to replace fluids lost through diaphoresis.

Use Nonpharmacological Measures to Reduce Fever. The following measures are likely to produce shivering, which produces heat; therefore, they can actually raise instead of lower the patient's temperature. When using these measures, be careful not to cause your patient to shiver.
  Cooling blankets that circulate water
  Alcohol or tepid baths
  Cloth-covered ice packs or cool washcloths to the groin, neck, or axillae. Avoid prolonged use.
  Circulating fan in the room
  Instructing the client to use minimal bed covers

Provide Nutritional Support. Food is essential to meet the increased energy needs created by the high metabolic rate accompanying fever. However, lack of appetite is common with a fever, so food must be made appealing to the patient.

Provide Special Mouth Care. Apply a water-soluble lip lubricant. Lips may become dry and cracked, the tongue may be swollen, and sores may be present.

Keep Clothing and Bed Linens Dry to promote comfort and help prevent chilling. Diaphoresis occurs during defervescence.

Provide Emergency Treatment, If Necessary. Heat stroke is a medical emergency because death can occur rapidly. Cooling blankets or cool water baths can be used successfully if the surface temperature is not lowered too

quickly. Rapid lowering of the surface temperature causes vasoconstriction, which delays core cooling.

Provide Patient Teaching for caregivers and older adults.

- Teach emergency treatment for hyperthermia and hyperpyrexia at home: Immediately move the person to a shady area if he is outdoors. Cool the victim by placing him in a tub of cool water or a cool shower, or sponging with cool water.
- Advise older adults to stay in air-conditioned buildings when the outside temperature is extremely high and to take cool baths and showers, limit physical activity, and drink plenty of nonalcoholic and noncaffeinated fluids.
- Advise family to check on elderly neighbors and family members at least twice a day, and make sure they have an electric fan.

Interventions for Example Problem: Hypothermia

NIC standardized interventions recommended for Hypothermia and Ineffective Thermoregulation include Hypothermia Treatment, Newborn Care, Temperature Regulation, Temperature Regulation: Intraoperative, and Vital Signs Monitoring. For other NIC labels,

 Go to Chapter 19, **Standardized Language: NOC Outcomes and NIC Interventions Associated with Abnormal Vital Signs,** on *DavisPlus*.

Specific nursing activities include the following:

- Provide warm, dry clothing, warm blankets, and a warm environment. For mild cases of Hypothermia, this may be enough to restore normal temperature.
- For patients with a temperature below 86°F (30°C), also use warmed intravenous fluids, heating pads or eating blankets, and/or warm baths.
- Give warm, sweet drinks if the person is conscious.

- ✚ Rewarm a patient who is severely hypothermic gradually to prevent complications, such as shock or dysrhythmias (abnormal heartbeats) and to ensure core, as well as surface, warming.
  - *Don't* use electric blankets. Vasoconstricted skin burns easily.
  - *Don't* apply pulse oximetry probes to a vasoconstricted finger.

- Focused assessments include the following:
  Monitor the temperature and other VS frequently. Hypothermia causes vasoconstriction, coagulation in the microcirculation, and tissue ischemia (lack of oxygen). In the heart, this can lead to dysrhythmias.
- Observe for the following symptoms of hypothermia:
  Body temperature less than 95°F (less than 35°C)
  Decreased or irregular pulse, respirations, and blood pressure
  A subjective feeling of being cold
  Severe shivering (only initially)
  Pale, cool, shiny skin
  Decreased urine output
  Disorientation and/or drowsiness

Think Like a Nurse 19-3

Recall the clients in the Meet Your Patients scenario. Two-year-old Jason's axillary temperature was 101.8°F (38.8°C) and his skin was warm, dry, and flushed. His mother told you that he had been eating poorly and was very irritable.

- What changes in behavior alert you that something is wrong?
- Do you have enough theoretical knowledge or patient information to know what is going on?
- What, if any, additional information about the patient situation do you need?

Toward Evidence-Based Practice

Lawson, L., Bridges, E. J., Ballou, I., et al. (2007). Accuracy and precision of noninvasive temperature measurement in adult intensive care patients. *American Journal of Critical Care, 16*(5), 485–496.

Over a period of 6 months, researchers took repeated measurements at various sites, including the gold standard pulmonary artery catheter, from 60 adults with cardiopulmonary disease in intensive care. They found oral and temporal artery measurements to be the most accurate and precise. Axillary measurements were less accurate, and otic (ear) measurements were the least accurate and precise.

Robinson, J. L., Jou, H., & Spady, D. W. (2005). Accuracy of parents in measuring body temperature with a tympanic thermometer. *BMC Family Practice, 6*(1), 3.

Parents and then nurses measured the temperatures of 60 children with a tympanic thermometer designed for home use. Nurses also measured the temperatures with

a model of tympanic thermometer commonly used in hospitals. The readings done by parents were significantly different from the readings by nurses using the hospital thermometer a majority of the time, and parents failed to detect fever about 25% of the time.

Heusch, A. I., & McCarthy, P. W. (2005). The patient: A novel source of error in clinical temperature measurement using infrared aural thermometry. *Journal of Alternative & Complementary Medicine, 11*(3), 473–476.

Researchers used an infrared tympanic thermometer to measure the temperatures of 132 subjects, ages 18 to 48 years, who were asymptomatic with no known pathological problems. Temperatures were measured in both ears. There was a significant difference in the temperature in the left compared with the right ear. Also, at temperatures below 36.7°C (98°F), the left ear registered a lower temperature than did the right. At temperatures above 36.7°C (98°F), the left ear registered a higher temperature than did

Toward Evidence-Based Practice—cont'd

the right ear. Researchers suggested that averaging the temperature taken in both ears might increase the reliability of infrared tympanic thermometers.

Farnell, S., Maxwell, L., Tan, S., et al. (2005). Temperature measurement: Comparison of non-invasive methods used in adult critical care. *Journal of Clinical Nursing, 14*(5), 632–639.

Researchers took 160 sets of temperature measurements from 25 adult intensive care patients, using a chemical (Tempa·DOT™) and a tympanic thermometer. Patients' temperatures were also being measured with the gold standard pulmonary artery catheter. They found the chemical thermometer to be more accurate and reliable than the tympanic thermometer. However, compared with the pulmonary artery catheter, both methods were associated with erroneous readings.

1. Make a table containing the following:

   a. The name of the first researcher listed (e.g., Lawson)

   b. The number and type of subjects in the study

   c. What each study found about *tympanic* temperature measurements

2. Imagine that you are managing a residential long-term care facility that has recently purchased new tympanic thermometers to replace the old mercury-in-glass thermometers. In this facility, VS are routinely taken by nursing assistive personnel (NAPs). What implications do these four studies have for actions you might need to take? What, in general terms, do you plan to do, and why?

 Go to Chapter 19, **Toward Evidence-Based Practice: Suggested Responses,** on Davis*Plus.*

Care**Planning** & **Mapping**Practice

For Care Planning & Care Mapping practice,

 Go to Chapter Resources, **Care Planning & Care Mapping Practice,** on Davis*Plus.*

PULSE

The concept **perfusion** refers to the continuous supply of oxygenated blood to all body cells. The **pulse** is the rhythmic expansion of an artery produced when a bolus of oxygenated blood is forced into it by contraction of the heart. How do you think the pulse is related to perfusion?

Theoretical Knowledge
knowing **why**

To understand the concept of perfusion and to assess and support a client's perfusion, you will need to know the normal pulse range, how the pulse is produced and regulated, and factors that influence pulse rate. An important reason to assess the pulse is to identify when more advanced monitoring is required. When the heart rate is of concern, you will most likely use a cardiac monitor to determine not only the rate, but also the rhythm and intensity of the pulse.

How Does the Body Produce and Regulate the Pulse?

The pulse wave begins when the left heart ventricle contracts and ends when it relaxes. Each contraction forces blood into the already filled aorta, increasing pressure within the arterial system. The intermittent pressure and expansion of the arteries causes the blood to move along in a wavelike motion toward the capillaries. You can palpate a light tap at the peak of the wave, when the artery expands. The trough (low point) of a pulse wave occurs when the artery contracts to push the blood along its way. The peak of the wave corresponds to **systole**, or the contraction of the heart; the trough corresponds to **diastole,** or the resting phase of the heart.

Stroke volume is the quantity of blood forced out by each contraction of the left ventricle. You will not usually know your patient's actual stroke volume, though it averages 70 mL in most healthy adults. If stroke volume decreases (as in a large blood loss, or *hemorrhage*), the body tries to maintain the same cardiac output by increasing the pulse rate. The **cardiac output** is the total quantity of blood pumped per minute. It is expressed in liters per minute and calculated as follows:

$$\text{Cardiac output} = \text{stroke volume} \times \text{pulse (heart) rate}$$

For a person with a pulse of 80 beats/min and an average stroke volume (70 mL), the cardiac output would be about 5,600 mL (or 5.6 L) per minute.

The autonomic nervous system regulates the heart rate. Sympathetic stimulation increases the heart rate (and thus the cardiac output); parasympathetic stimulation decreases it. We discuss this in more detail in Chapter 38.

What Factors Influence the Pulse Rate?

In a healthy adult, the peripheral pulse rate is the same as the heart rate. Therefore, taking the pulse is a quick and simple way to assess the condition of the heart, blood vessels, and circulation. The pulse changes in response to changes in the volume of blood pumped through the heart, variations in heart rate, changes in the elasticity of the arterial walls, or any condition that interferes with heart function. Because the heart and blood vessels are regulated by the nervous system, conditions that interfere with normal functioning of the nervous system also affect the pulse. Other factors that may cause variations in pulse rate, rhythm, or quality include the following:

- *Developmental level.* Newborns have a rapid pulse rate. The rate stabilizes in childhood and gradually slows through old age.
- *Gender.* In general, adult women have a slightly higher pulse rate than do adult men.

- *Exercise.* Muscle activity normally increases the pulse rate. After exercise, a well-conditioned heart returns to normal more quickly than does a nonconditioned heart. Also, people who are well conditioned have lower heart rates, both before and during exercise, than do those who are not.
- *Food.* Ingestion of a meal causes a slight increase in pulse rate for several hours.
- *Stress.* Stress triggers the fight-or-flight sympathetic nervous system response, which increases both pulse rate and strength of the heart contractions (stroke volume).
- *Fever.* The pulse rate tends to increase about 10 beats/min for each degree Fahrenheit of temperature elevation. The reasons are that (1) the metabolic rate increases and (2) the body attempts to compensate for the decrease in blood pressure produced by the peripheral vasodilation that occurs with fever.
- *Disease.* Diseases, such as heart disease, hyperthyroidism, respiratory diseases, and infections, are generally associated with increased pulse rates. Hypothyroidism is associated with decreased pulse rates.
- *Blood loss.* Small blood loss is generally well tolerated and produces only a temporary increase in pulse rate. Theoretically, a large blood loss stimulates the sympathetic nervous system, bringing about an increase in pulse rate to compensate for the decreased blood volume. However, some studies suggest that VS are limited in their ability to detect large blood losses; and stable pulse and blood pressure alone do not ensure that there has been no blood loss.
- *Position changes.* Standing and sitting positions generally cause a temporary increase in pulse rate as a result of blood pooling in the veins of the feet and legs. This decreases blood return to the heart, decreasing blood pressure and subsequently increasing heart rate.
- *Medications.* Stimulant drugs (e.g., epinephrine) increase pulse rate. Cardiotonics (e.g., digitalis) and opioids (e.g., narcotic analgesics) or sedative drugs decrease pulse rate.

PracticalKnowledge
knowing **how**

Now that you understand some of the processes and factors that produce and affect the pulse, you are ready to learn how to assess and support this aspect of physical functioning.

ASSESSMENT

Assess the pulse by **palpation** (feeling) or **auscultation** (listening with a stethoscope). To palpate the pulse, select the pulse site and lightly compress the client's artery against the underlying bone with the index and middle finger of one of your hands. When a client's pulse is difficult to palpate, you may need to use a Doppler device, which has an ultrasound transducer that transmits the pulse sounds to an audio unit. For a summary of the steps for assessing a client's peripheral pulse, see Procedure 19-2.

What Equipment Do I Need?

To count the pulse, you need a watch or clock with a second hand or digital display. To auscultate the pulse, you will use a stethoscope. The stethoscope does not magnify sounds, but rather blocks out noise so that you can hear blood pressure and other faint sounds. A **stethoscope** consists of a sound-transmitting device (bell and diaphragm) that is attached to earpieces by rubber tubing and hollow metal tubes (Fig. 19-5). With the earpieces in place, you can use the bell to hear low-frequency sounds (e.g., certain heart sounds). Use the diaphragm to assess high-frequency sounds (e.g., lung sounds).

Stethoscopes can be either single lumen or double lumen. A single-lumen stethoscope has one tube connected to the chestpiece; a double-lumen stethoscope has two tubes attached to the chestpiece. Double-lumen stethoscopes are more sensitive than single-lumen instruments.

Most stethoscopes come with soft earpieces that help seal your ear canal to block room noise from interfering with the sound. Stethoscopes have varying lengths of tubing. Short tubing requires you to be close to the patient and to bend

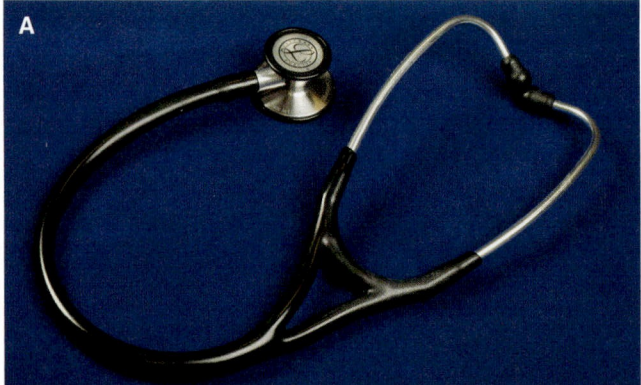

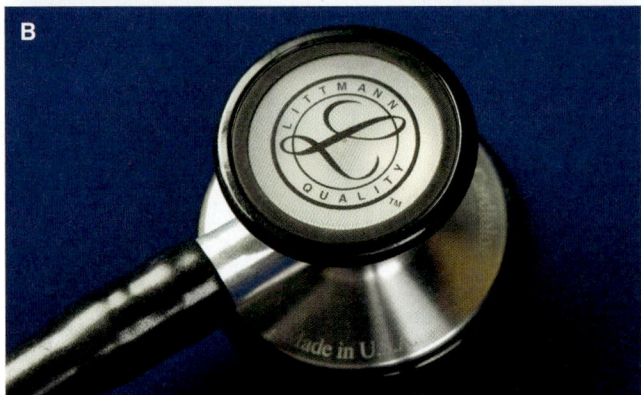

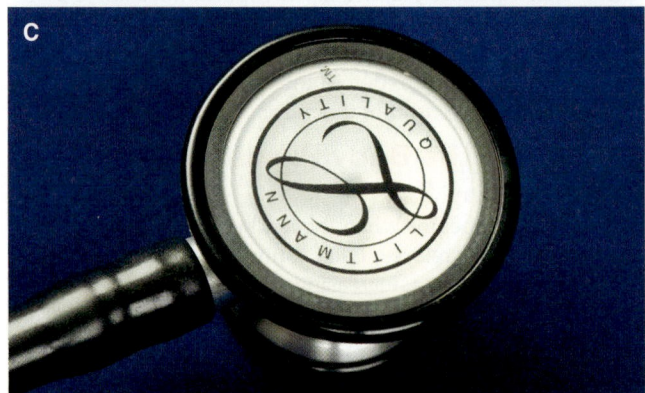

FIGURE 19-5 **(A)** A stethoscope. **(B)** The bell, for low-frequency sounds. **(C)** The diaphragm, for high-frequency sounds.

more, but the sound may be a bit better than with longer tubing, which is more likely to rub against the body or clothing. Some stethoscopes are made to work effectively through clothing; however, unless you know you are using that type you should place the instrument directly on the skin. Digital stethoscopes are also available, to provide sound clarity in noisy environments and with obese patients, as well as for care providers with impaired hearing.

Cleaning the Stethoscope. To prevent cross-contamination, always clean your stethoscope before and after using it to examine a patient. Use a 70% alcohol or benzalkonium chloride wipe. Most stethoscopes are colonized by bacteria, although only a small percentage are pathogenic. Cleaning can reduce the bacterial count by 94% to 100% (CDC, 2008; Kennedy, Dreimanis, Beckingham, et al., 2003; Rutala & Weber, 2004). Antimicrobial stethoscope covers have been developed to prevent surface contamination; however, their effectiveness is still in question. A few agencies have wall-mounted "single-swipe" sterilizers for sterilizing stethoscopes.

➕ For safety reasons, you should not wear a stethoscope around your neck.

What Sites Should I Use?

Nurses assess the pulse at the apex of the heart **(apical pulse)** or at a place where an artery can be pressed by the fingers against a bone **(peripheral pulses).** Peripheral sites are shown in Figure 19-6.

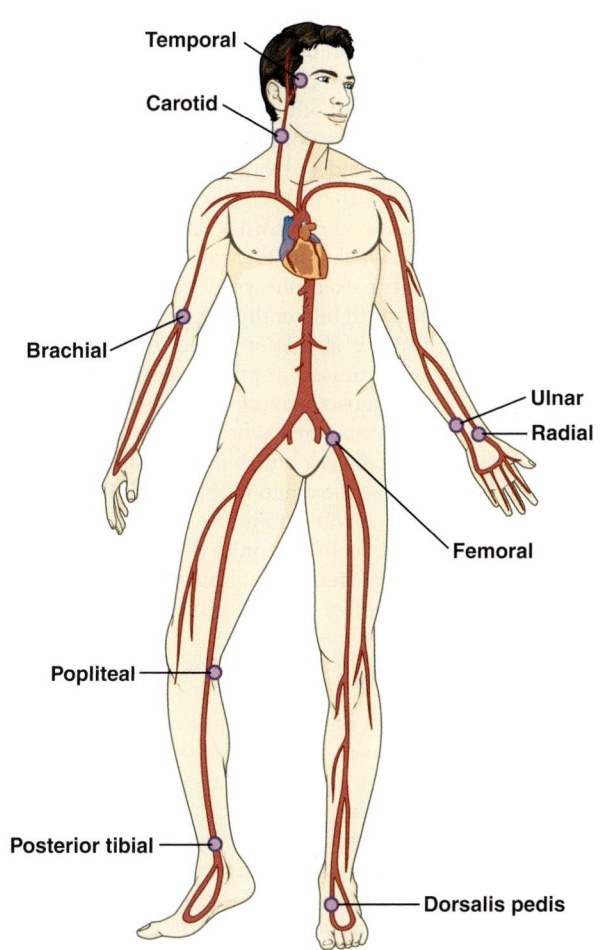

Temporal
Carotid
Brachial
Ulnar
Radial
Femoral
Popliteal
Posterior tibial
Dorsalis pedis

FIGURE 19-6 Sites commonly used for assessing a pulse.

The choice of pulse site depends on the reason for assessing the pulse and/or the accessibility of a site. To measure a peripheral pulse, you would, for example, use the:

- *Radial artery*—for routine assessment of vital signs. This is the most commonly used site because it is easily found and readily accessible.
- *Brachial artery*—when performing cardiopulmonary resuscitation (CPR) of infants.
- *Carotid artery*—when performing CPR of inpatient adults and for assessing circulation to the brain.

➕ Palpate only one side of the neck at a time to avoid interrupting circulation to the head. Palpate lightly so that you don't occlude the artery; don't massage the area because that can decrease the heart rate and blood pressure. Laypersons should not check the carotid pulse.

- *Temporal artery*—when assessing circulation to the head or when other sites are not easily accessible.
- *Dorsalis pedis* (also called *pedal pulse*) and *posterior tibial arteries* for assessing peripheral circulation (feet and legs).
- *Femoral artery* to determine circulation to the legs, in cases of cardiac arrest, and for children.
- *Popliteal artery* for assessing circulation to the lower leg.

🌈 ThinkLike a Nurse 19-4

- If you obtain a very slow radial pulse, how might you check to be sure your count is accurate?
- What kind of nursing knowledge does this require (i.e., theoretical, practical, self, or ethical)?

When Should I Take an Apical Pulse? The apical pulse reading is the most accurate of the pulses. In a healthy person, the apical and peripheral pulses should be about the same rate. However, in some cardiovascular conditions, they can differ. If the heartbeat is weak, for example, some beats may be too weak to feel in a peripheral site. In this case, you would obtain a lower count for the radial than for the apical pulse. The apical pulse most accurately reflects the heart rate. Use the apical site when:

- The radial pulse is weak or irregular.
- The rate is less than 60 beats/min or greater than 100 beats/min.
- The patient is taking cardiac medications (e.g., digitalis).
- The patient is an infant or is a child up to age 3 (because peripheral pulses may be difficult to palpate).

To assess the apical pulse, auscultate and count the number of heartbeats at the apex of the heart. For an adult, this site is on the anterior chest at 3 inches (8 cm) or less to the left of the sternum, at the 4th, 5th, or 6th intercostal space at the midclavicular line. For children, the location is different, depending on age (Fig. 19-7). You will hear two sounds, "lub" and "dub," as the heart valves close. Count each pair of sounds ("lub-dub") as one heartbeat. For step-by-step instructions, refer to Procedure 19-3.

When Should I Take an Apical–Radial Pulse? You will sometimes need to obtain a radial and apical pulse reading at the same time to assess for heart function or the presence of heart irregularities. A difference between the two counts (pulse deficit) indicates that not all apex beats are being transmitted or felt at the radial artery. As you are listening at the apical site, you will hear a beat without feeling a pulse at the radial artery. You should report pulse deficits promptly to the primary care provider. See Procedure 19-4.

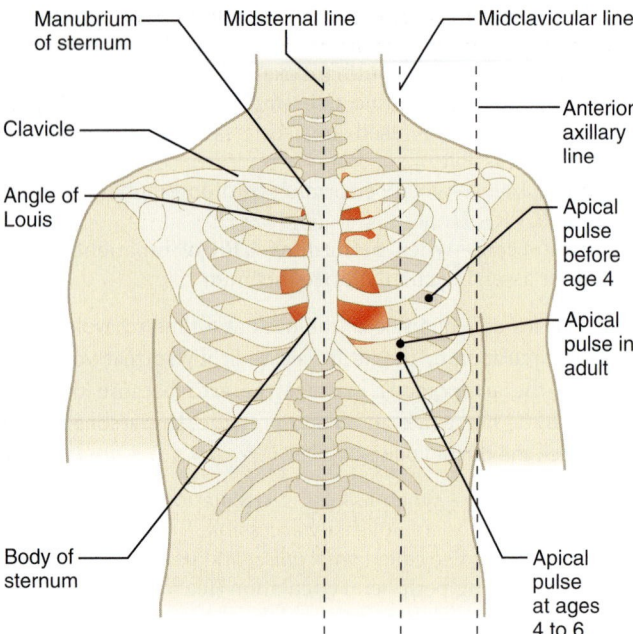

FIGURE 19-7 Location of apical pulse for adults and children.

KnowledgeCheck 19-2

For each of the following, would you expect the pulse rate to be greater or less than the normal adult rate of 80 beats/min?

- A healthy, professional tennis player
- A newborn infant
- An adolescent who has just finished running track
- A client who has just undergone a painful procedure
- A client with a fever
- An accident victim who is hemorrhaging
- A 90-year-old man

What Data Should I Collect?

You will need data about three characteristics of the patient's pulse: rate, rhythm, and quality.

Pulse Rate

To assess the pulse **rate,** count the number of beats per minute while palpating or auscultating. Begin the count with one, rather than zero (Hwu, Coates, & Lin, 2000). For normal, healthy adults with a regular heart rhythm, count the pulse for 15 seconds and multiply the result by 4. Research is conflicting, but some studies indicate that a 30-second count is more accurate; however, there is little research related to measurement of pulses. If the pulse is irregular or slow, always count for one full minute.

The normal range for healthy young and middle-aged adults is 60 to 100 beats/min, with an average rate of 70 to 80 beats/min. Table 19-1 identifies average pulse rates for adults. For average pulse rates for other age groups,

 Go to Chapter 19, **Tables, Boxes, Figures: ESG Table 19-1, Comparison of Normal Vital Signs for Various Ages,** on DavisPlus.

Rates below 60 beats/min are known as **bradycardia** (*brady* = slow, *cardia* = heart). Rates over 100 beats/min are known as **tachycardia** (*tachy* = rapid, *cardia* = heart).

Pulse Rhythm

The intervals between heartbeats establish a pattern known as the **rhythm.** Normally, the heart beats at regular intervals, much like a metronome. When the intervals between beats vary enough to be noticeable, the rhythm is abnormal (**dysrhythmia).** Abnormal rhythms may be single beats that occur too early or too late, or a group of irregular beats that form a pattern. When assessing an irregular pulse, it is important to determine whether the beat is *regularly irregular* (an irregular rhythm that forms a pattern) or *irregularly irregular* (an unpredictable rhythm). To make this distinction, you must count the rate for a full minute. An irregular heart rhythm can be very serious and may require additional assessment by **electrocardiogram (ECG),** a procedure that traces the electrical pattern of the heart.

Pulse Quality

The **quality** of the pulse is assessed by determining the pulse volume and bilateral (both sides) equality of pulses. **Pulse volume** refers to the amount of force produced by the blood pulsing through the arteries. Normally, the pulse volume for each beat is the same. The following terminology refers to pulse volume; numbers are assigned on a scale of 0 to 3.

   0—Absent: Pulse cannot be felt.
   1—Weak (thready): Pulse is barely felt and can be easily obliterated by pressing with the fingers.
   2—Normal quality: Pulse is easily palpated, not weak or bounding.
   3—Bounding or full: Pulse is easily felt with little pressure; not easily obliterated.

Bilateral equality is useful in determining whether the blood flow to a body part is adequate. Assess bilateral equality by comparing the pulses on both sides of the body for equal volume. For example, if you are concerned about the circulation to the left hand, assess both the right and left radial arteries to determine whether the volume is the same. If the pulses feel the same, they are said to be *equal in strength bilaterally.* If one pulse is stronger than the other, then the pulses are *unequal bilaterally.* You would record, "Radial pulses unequal in strength bilaterally; weaker in left arm." Or you might use a pulse volume scale. For example, you could record, "Radial pulses unequal in strength bilaterally; Right 2, Left 1."

If a peripheral pulse is absent or weak, it may be because the circulation is compromised in that extremity. If this is the case, then pallor or cyanosis may be present. **Pallor** refers to the paleness of skin in one area when compared to another part of the body. **Cyanosis** is a bluish or grayish discoloration of the skin due to deficient oxygen in the blood. For example, when circulation to the lower extremities is compromised, the feet often appear pale in comparison to the trunk or arms, the dorsalis pedis and/or posterior tibial pulses may be weak or absent, and the feet may feel cool to the touch.

ANALYSIS/NURSING DIAGNOSIS

An abnormal pulse may present as weak, thready, bounding, irregular, or absent. Pulse changes are symptoms, not problems. Therefore, nursing diagnoses are useful for describing the condition that is *causing* the pulse changes. By itself, a change in pulse (e.g., weak and thready) is not adequate to support the following diagnoses. Other symptoms must also be present.

- **Ineffective Tissue Perfusion (Peripheral)** can be used when a pulse is absent or weak and cool, pale skin is present.
- **Risk for Impaired Skin Integrity** and **Risk for Impaired Tissue Integrity** may be used as secondary diagnoses when

Ineffective Tissue Perfusion is present. If tissue is not adequately perfused, tissue ischemia and *necrosis* (death of tissue) may occur.

- **Deficient Fluid Volume** may cause the pulse to be weak and thready.
- **Excess Fluid Volume** may cause the pulse to be bounding and full.
- **Decreased Cardiac Output** may cause tachycardia, bradycardia, or changes in pulse volume.

PLANNING OUTCOMES/EVALUATION

NOC standardized outcomes include the following:

- Vital Signs Status is the only outcome that directly pertains to assessing the pulse.
- Other outcomes depend on the nursing diagnosis causing the pulse changes. For example, Ineffective Peripheral Tissue Perfusion can be monitored with the NOC label of Circulation Status.

Some *individualized goal/outcome statements* you might write for pulse status follow:

- Apical pulse will be 60 to 80 beats/min when at rest.
- Pedal pulses will be 80 to 100 beats/min, 2 (on a scale of 0 to 3), and equal bilaterally.

 Think**Like a Nurse** 19-5

Did you notice that the pulse rates in the preceding two goals are not the same as the full normal range shown in Table 19-1? What do you think might be a reason for this?

PLANNING INTERVENTIONS/IMPLEMENTATION

NIC standardized interventions include the following:

- Dysrhythmia Management, which applies to monitoring an abnormal pulse
- Vital Signs Monitoring, which may be used for general evaluation of clients who do not have an identified problem with the pulse

Specific nursing activities and focused assessments for a patient with a dysrhythmia depend on the cause of the problem and on specific orders from the physician. For example, a client with a pulse rate of 50 beats/min is usually considered to have bradycardia. However, such a slow resting heart rate would be perfectly normal for a well-trained athlete. Some dysrhythmias are *benign;* that is, they are not dangerous to the client, and they require no interventions. Nursing strategies that address dysrhythmias, regardless of cause, include the following:

- *Closely monitor the patient's VS.* A reduced heart rate may alter blood pressure and tissue perfusion. The extent of intervention depends on the effect of the dysrhythmia on the client's other vital signs.
- *Monitor the patient's activity tolerance.* Degree of activity, orientation, and level of fatigue while the dysrhythmia is present are indicators of the patient's ability to tolerate the dysrhythmia.
- *Collect and assess laboratory data as prescribed.* Cardiac function depends on normal electrolyte balance, particularly potassium, calcium, and magnesium levels. If a client is receiving medications that affect cardiac rhythm, serum levels of these medications must be checked periodically.

- *Help determine the cause of the dysrhythmia.* Determine when the client experiences the dysrhythmia. Are there precipitating or alleviating factors?
- *Administer antidysrhythmic medications* (if prescribed) at regular intervals to control the heart rhythm.
- *Provide emotional support.* The client experiencing a dysrhythmia may be frightened by the experience. Explain all procedures to the client, and maintain a calm presence. Family members may also be frightened. Be sure to include them in your explanations and teaching.

 Think**Like a Nurse** 19-6

- Which of the following findings should be referred to the primary healthcare provider so that an ECG can be ordered? Why?
  Patient A, who has a radial pulse of 100 beats/min, regular, and equal bilaterally
  Patient B, who has a regular apical pulse of 100 beats/min
  Patient C, who has a very irregular apical pulse of 78 beats/min
- Recall the clients in the Meet Your Patients scenario.
  Ms. Sharma is an active 80-year-old woman who works part time and exercises four times per week. She is complaining of feeling tired. You find that her pulse is irregular and uneven.
  What other patient data do you need to know? How would you go about getting this additional information?
  What actions should you consider taking while meeting with Ms. Sharma?
  What theoretical knowledge (rationale) supports your beliefs and actions?

RESPIRATION

Respiration is the exchange of oxygen and carbon dioxide in the body. The process of respiration has two aspects: mechanical and chemical.

Mechanical. The mechanical aspects of respirations involve the active movement of air into and out of the respiratory system. This is known as **pulmonary ventilation** or, more commonly, *breathing.*

Chemical. The chemical aspects of respiration include the following:

- **External respiration**—The exchange of oxygen and carbon dioxide between the alveoli and the pulmonary blood supply
- **Gas transport**—The transport of these gases throughout the body
- **Internal respiration**—The exchange of these gases between the capillaries and body tissue cells

This chapter focuses on the mechanical aspects of respiration. Chapter 37 explores gas exchange and transport throughout the body. For an animated visual explanation of respiration,

 Go to **Animations: Cardiovascular/Pulmonary Animations, Carbon Dioxide/Oxygen Transport,** on the Davis*Plus* Web site.

Theoretical Knowledge
knowing why

To assess and support clients' respirations, you will need to know the normal range of respiratory rates, how respiration is regulated, the mechanics of breathing, and factors that affect respiration.

How Does the Body Regulate Respiration?

Special respiratory centers in the medulla oblongata and pons of the brain, along with nerve fibers of the autonomic nervous system, regulate breathing in response to minute changes in the concentrations of oxygen (O_2) and carbon dioxide (CO_2) in the arterial blood. The primary stimulus for breathing is the level of CO_2 tension in the blood.

- **Central chemoreceptors,** located in the respiratory centers, are sensitive to CO_2 and hydrogen ion (pH) concentrations. Minor increases in either stimulate respirations.
- When the partial pressure of oxygen in arterial blood (PaO_2) falls below normal, **peripheral chemoreceptors** in the carotid and aortic bodies stimulate respirations. The PaO_2 is normally between 80 and 100.

Usually breathing is an involuntary action that requires little effort. However, it is possible to exert conscious control over respiration (e.g., a young child holding his breath during a temper tantrum; a person holding her breath when swimming).

What Are the Mechanics of Breathing?

Pulmonary ventilation depends on changes in the capacity of the chest cavity (Fig. 19-8). In response to impulses sent from the respiratory center along the phrenic nerve, the thoracic muscles and the diaphragm contract. The ribs move upward from midline 0.5 to 1 inch (1.2 to 2.5 cm), the diaphragm moves downward and out about 0.4 inch (1 cm), and the abdominal organs move downward and forward, expanding the thorax in all directions. As expansion causes airway pressure to decrease below atmospheric pressure, air moves into and expands the lungs. This stage of respiration (drawing air into the lungs) is termed **inspiration.**

When the diaphragm and thoracic muscles relax, the chest cavity decreases in size, and the lungs recoil, forcing air from the lungs until the pressure within the lungs again reaches atmospheric pressure. This stage, which involves the expulsion of air from the lungs, is called **expiration.** Expiration is passive and normally takes 2 to 3 seconds compared to 1 to 1.5 seconds for inspiration. During normal breathing, the chest wall and abdomen gently rise and fall.

Knowledge Check 19-3

- Which two gases are exchanged through respiration?
- Which respiratory process involves the movement of air into and out of the lungs?
- What is external respiration?
- What is the primary stimulus for breathing?
- What mechanical forces allow the lungs to expand?

What Factors Influence Respiration?

To interpret the meaning of your clients' respiratory data, you need to be aware of factors that influence breathing.

- *Developmental level.* A newborn's respiratory rate usually ranges from 40 to 60 breaths/min. However, some references give an upper limit of 90 breaths/min so long as it is for a short period of time (transient tachypnea). The rate gradually decreases until it reaches the normal adult rate of 12 to 20 breaths per minute. The respiratory rate decreases slightly in older adults.
- *Exercise.* Muscular activity causes a temporary increase in respiratory rate and depth so as to increase oxygen availability to the tissues and to rid the body of excess carbon dioxide.
- *Pain.* Acute pain causes an increase in respiratory rate but a decrease in depth.
- *Stress.* Psychological stress, such as anxiety or fear, may markedly influence respiration as a result of sympathetic stimulation. The most common change is an increase in rate.
- *Smoking.* Chronic smoking increases resting respiratory rate as a result of changes in airway compliance (elasticity).
- *Fever.* When heart rate increases because of fever, respiratory rate also increases. For every 1°F (0.6°C) the temperature rises, the respiratory rate may increase up to 4 breaths/min.
- *Hemoglobin.* Respiratory rate and depth increase as a result of anemia (reduced hemoglobin), sickle cell anemia (abnormally shaped red blood cells), and high altitudes. When hemoglobin is decreased or abnormal, the rate and depth of respirations, as well as the heart rate, may increase to maintain adequate tissue oxygenation. High altitudes inhibit the binding of oxygen to hemoglobin and trigger similar compensation efforts.
- *Disease.* The rate of breathing may be increased or decreased by various diseases. For example, brainstem injuries and increased intracranial pressure may interfere with the respiratory center, inhibiting respirations or altering respiratory rhythm.
- *Medications.* Central nervous system depressants, such as morphine or general anesthetics, cause slower, deeper respirations. Caffeine and atropine can cause shallow, fast breathing.

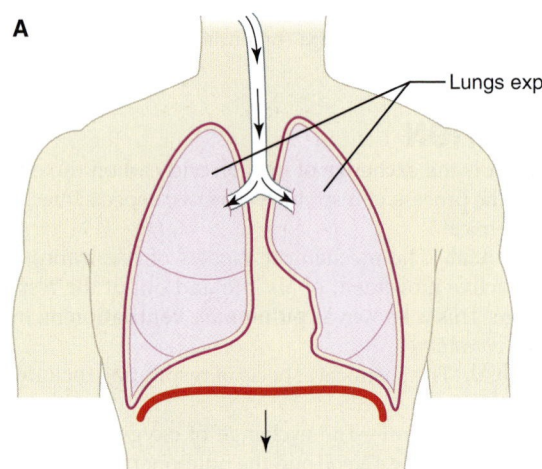

A

Lungs expand

During inspiration (diaphragm contracting)

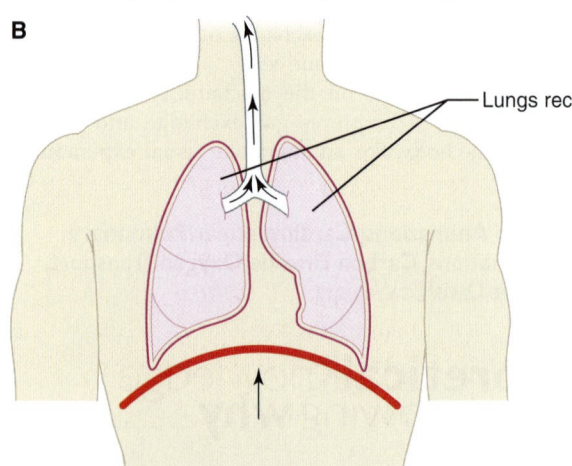

B

Lungs recoil

During expiration (diaphragm relaxing)

FIGURE 19-8 Changes in thoracic cavity during inspiration and expiration. (A) During inspiration. (B) During expiration.

- *Position.* Standing up maximizes respiratory depth; lying flat reduces respiratory depth. Slumping (sitting with shoulders forward, and the back curved in a C shape) prevents chest expansion, which impedes breathing.

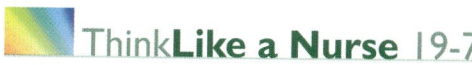

ThinkLike a Nurse 19-7

Consider the following patient situations. What effect would they have on respirations?

- A client with four fractured ribs
- A woman who is 9 months pregnant
- A young child excited at her birthday party
- An adult who has consumed alcoholic beverages

PracticalKnowledge
knowing **how**

Although the adequacy of external and internal respiration are assessed in various ways, it is pulmonary ventilation (breathing) that you assess as a vital sign. Accurate assessment of respirations depends on your ability to recognize normal breathing, abnormal breathing, and factors that affect breathing. This chapter discusses only assessment of respirations. For nursing diagnoses, outcomes, and interventions for respiratory problems, see Chapter 37.

■ ASSESSMENT

Because people can control their breathing rate, it is best to count respirations when the client is unaware of what you are doing. One way to do this is to palpate and count the radial pulse, and then count the respirations before removing your fingers from the client's wrist. To learn this skill, see Procedure 19-5.

What Equipment Do I Need?

The only equipment you need for measuring respiratory rate is a watch with a second hand or digital display. You will need a stethoscope if you auscultate respirations. Many electronic thermometers have counter displays and signals that indicate 15-, 30-, and 60-second time intervals for counting respirations.

What Data Should I Obtain?

In addition to measuring the respiratory rate, you will also observe indicators of overall respiratory function, including depth, rhythm, effort, and others. For additional information on respiratory assessment, see Chapter 21 and Procedure 21-12.

Respiratory Rate

The **respiratory rate** is the number of times a person breathes (or completes a cycle of inhalation and exhalation) within one full minute. You can easily count and observe respirations by:

- Placing your hand on the client's chest (palpating) or observing (inspecting) the number of times the client's chest or abdomen rises (inspiration) and falls (expiration)
- Placing your stethoscope on the client's chest (auscultation) and counting the number of inhalation and exhalation cycles

   For a new patient or when you need to ensure accuracy, you must count for 60 seconds (Vital Signs, 1999). In some situations, for example, for a patient you know well and for whom respiratory rate is not directly relevant to the assessment, you may count for only 30 seconds and multiply by 2. If respirations vary from normal, you should count for one minute by auscultation. A patient's respiratory rate normally varies. Normal adult respirations are identified in Table 19-1. For normal respiratory rates at other developmental stages,

Go to Chapter 19, **Tables, Boxes, Figures: ESG Table 19-1, Comparison of Normal Vital Signs for Various Ages,** on *DavisPlus.*

   Respiratory rate is a measure of the client's general condition, but rate alone is not a good indicator of the adequacy of respiration. You must also assess other characteristics of the respirations. If oxygenation must be carefully monitored, use a pulse oximeter (see Chapter 37 and Procedure 37-2).

   A person can tolerate **apnea,** cessation of breathing, for only a few minutes. If apnea continues for more than 4 to 6 minutes, brain damage and even death can occur. See Table 19-4 for terminology to describe respiratory rhythms.

Respiratory Depth

Tidal volume is the amount of air taken in on inspiration—about 300 to 500 mL for a healthy adult. Specialized equipment is required to measure tidal volume. However, you can estimate the adequacy of tidal volume by observing the depth of a client's respirations. This is a subjective evaluation of how much or how little the chest or abdomen rises during breathing. Respiratory depth is described as *deep* (taking in a very large volume of air and fully expanding one's chest or abdomen), *shallow* (when the chest barely rises and is difficult to observe), or *normal* (between shallow and deep).

Respiratory Rhythm

Rhythm is assessed simply as *regular* or *irregular.* Generally, the period between each respiratory cycle is the same, and there is a regular breathing pattern (see Table 19-4). Infant breathing rhythms are more likely to be irregular than adult rhythms. An abnormal breathing pattern may indicate other healthcare problems and deserves further assessment. Two abnormal breathing patterns, Cheyne–Stokes and Biot's breathing, are discussed in Chapter 37.

Respiratory Effort

Respiratory effort refers to the degree of work required to breathe. Normal breathing is effortless. When diseases such as asthma or pneumonia are present, the person must work harder to breathe. Increased effort with breathing is called **dyspnea,** or labored breathing. It is uncomfortable for the client and frequently produces fatigue and fear. **Orthopnea** is difficulty or inability to breathe when in a horizontal position. You will observe this in some clients with respiratory or cardiac conditions.

Breath Sounds

You will use a stethoscope to listen for breath sounds. Normal respirations are quiet. Abnormal (adventitious) sounds include the following.

- **Wheezes** are high-pitched, continuous musical sounds, usually heard on expiration. They are caused by narrowing of the airways. Wheezes can often be heard without a stethoscope.
- **Rhonchi** are low-pitched, continuous gurgling sounds caused by secretions in the large airways. They often clear with coughing.
- **Crackles** are caused by fluid in the alveoli. They are discontinuous sounds usually heard on inspiration, but they may be heard throughout the respiratory cycle. They may be high-pitched, popping sounds or low-pitched, bubbling sounds, and they have been described as being similar to the sound made by rubbing strands of hair together with the fingertips.

Table 19-4 ➤ Respiratory Rates and Rhythms

TYPE	DESCRIPTION	ILLUSTRATION
Eupnea	Normal respirations, with equal rate and depth, 12–20 breaths/min	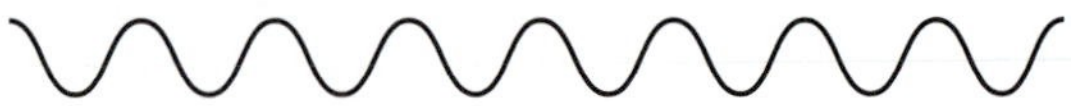
Bradypnea	Slow respirations, <10 breaths/min	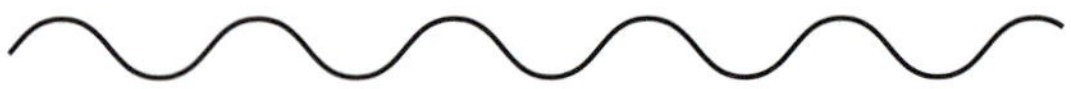
Tachypnea	Fast respirations, >24 breaths/min, usually shallow	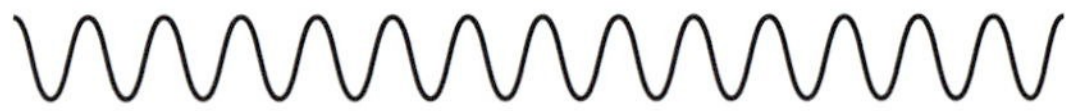
Kussmaul's Respirations	Respirations that are regular but abnormally deep and increased in rate	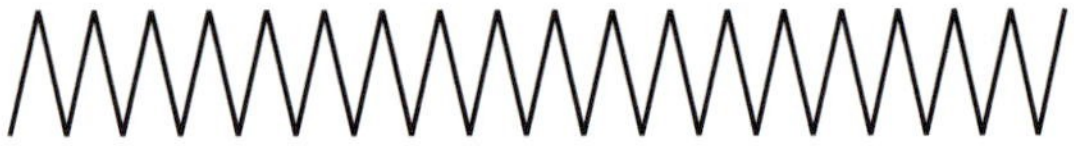
Biot's Respirations	Irregular respirations of variable depth (usually shallow), alternating with periods of apnea (absence of breathing)	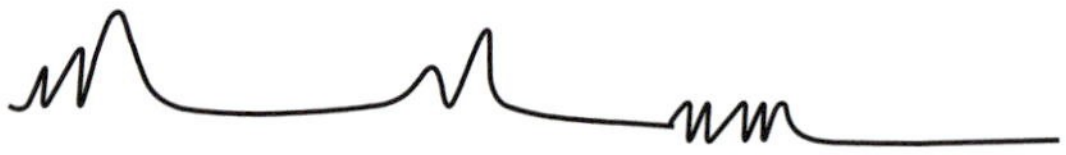
Cheyne–Stokes Respirations	Gradual increase in depth of respirations, followed by gradual decrease and then a period of apnea	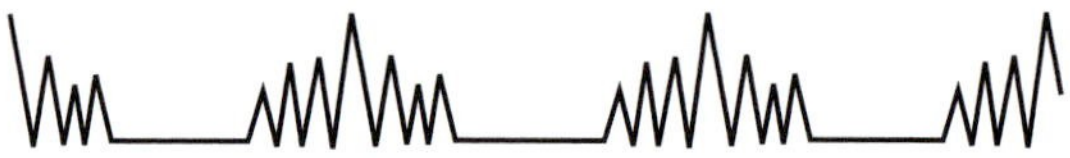
Apnea	Absence of breathing	

- **Stridor** is a piercing, high-pitched sound that is heard without a stethoscope, primarily during inspiration, in infants who are experiencing respiratory distress or in someone with an obstructed airway.
- **Stertor** refers to labored breathing that produces a snoring sound, common with mouth breathing due to nasal congestion. The "death rattle" is a type of stertorous breathing.
  See Chapter 21 for further discussion of abnormal breath sounds. To listen to normal and abnormal breath sounds,

Go to **Sounds: Breath Sounds,** in the Student Resources; also see **Chapter 19, Resources for Caregivers & Health Professionals** on DavisPlus.

Chest and Abdomen Movement
The chest or abdomen normally rises with inspiration and falls with expiration in a gentle and rhythmic pattern. When a person is having difficulty moving air into or out of the lungs, respiratory patterns change. **Intercostal retraction** refers to the visible sinking of tissues around and between the ribs that occurs when the person must use additional effort to breathe. **Substernal retraction** exists when tissues are drawn in beneath the sternum (breastbone), and **suprasternal retraction** exists when tissues are drawn in above the clavicle (shoulder girdle).

Associated Clinical Signs
When you assess respiration, it is important to assess for clinical signs of oxygenation and perfusion. Signs of **hypoxia** (inadequate cellular oxygenation) include pallor or cyanosis, restlessness, apprehension, confusion, dizziness, fatigue, decreased level of consciousness, tachycardia, tachypnea, and changes in blood pressure. When evaluating cyanosis, the tongue and oral mucosa are the best indicators of hypoxia. Cyanosis of the nails, lips, and skin may be caused by hypoxia, but may also be related to cold or reduced circulation in that area. Chronic hypoxia causes **clubbing** (loss of the nail angle) of the fingers.

A **cough** is a forceful or violent expulsion of air during expiration. Coughs may be *constant* (occurring frequently and consistently) or *intermittent* (occurring occasionally). If secretions are expectorated (coughed up), the cough is *productive*. If no secretions are produced, the cough is *nonproductive* or *dry*. A *hacking cough* is a series of dry coughs that occur together, whereas a *whooping cough* is a sudden, periodic cough that ends with a whooping sound on inspiration. Coughs may be symptoms of allergic reactions, lung disease, respiratory infection, or heart conditions.

KnowledgeCheck 19-4
- How can you estimate a client's tidal volume?
- What is the range of normal for an adult's respiratory rate?
- Besides the rate, what other characteristics of a client's respirations should you observe?
- What are some common clinical signs associated with poor oxygenation?

Arterial Oxygen Saturation
The rate, quality, and depth of the respirations are indicators of the general health of the respiratory system. However, they do not measure the amounts of oxygen and carbon dioxide present in the blood—information that is essential for evaluating

the effectiveness of respiratory effort. Two methods exist to measure O_2 and CO_2 blood levels. One method is invasive; the other is not.

- **Arterial blood gas (ABG) sampling** directly measures the partial pressures of the gases in the arterial blood: O_2 and CO_2 and blood pH. This method requires the puncture of an artery followed by laboratory testing of the sample. It provides comprehensive data, but it is invasive, painful, time consuming, and relatively expensive. If you need more information about this diagnostic test, consult a medical–surgical nursing or laboratory tests text.

- **Pulse oximetry** is a noninvasive method of monitoring oxygenation with a device that measures **oxygen saturation** (an indication of the oxygen being carried by hemoglobin in the arterial blood). The oximeter emits light, and a photosensor placed on the client's finger or earlobe measures the light passing through the site and calculates a pulse saturation (SpO_2) that is a good estimate of arterial oxygen saturation. The only risk in pulse oximetry is that clinicians may become overdependent on it or trust erroneous readings. Do not neglect the other aspects of holistic respiratory assessment. In many situations oxygen saturation is monitored routinely along with the other vital signs. For a procedure for applying a pulse oximeter, see Procedure 37-2.

ThinkLike a Nurse 19-8

- Mrs. Dowell has smoked two packs of cigarettes per day for 45 years. She has recently been diagnosed with pneumonia—an infection of the lungs. What VS assessments would be important for Mrs. Dowell, and why?
- Recall the clients in the Meet Your Patients scenario. Mr. Jackson is short of breath and struggling to breathe. His respiratory rate is 28 breaths/min. What else do you need to know about the patient situation? What is important and what is not important in this scenario? What is probably least important?

What Are Some Alterations in Respiration?

As noted earlier, *hypoxia* refers to inadequate cellular oxygenation. It results from decreased oxygen intake, decreased ability of tissues to remove oxygen from blood, impaired ventilation or perfusion, impaired gas exchange between the blood and alveoli, or inadequate levels of hemoglobin.

Hyperventilation occurs when rapid and deep breathing result in excess loss of CO_2 (*hypocapnia*). A client who is hyperventilating may complain of feeling lightheaded and tingly. Causes of hyperventilation include anxiety, infection, shock, hypoxia, drugs (e.g., aspirin, amphetamines), diabetes mellitus, or acid–base imbalance.

Hypoventilation occurs when the rate and depth of respirations are decreased and CO_2 is retained or alveolar ventilation is compromised. Hypoventilation may be related to chronic obstructive pulmonary disease (COPD), general anesthesia, impending respiratory failure, or other conditions that result in decreased respirations.

BLOOD PRESSURE

Blood pressure (BP), an important indicator of overall cardiovascular health, is the pressure of the blood as it is forced against arterial walls during cardiac contraction. **Systolic pressure** is the peak pressure exerted against arterial walls as the ventricles contract and eject blood. **Diastolic pressure** is the minimum pressure exerted against arterial walls,

between cardiac contractions when the heart is at rest. Adequate blood pressure is essential for healthy tissue perfusion.

Blood pressure is measured in millimeters of mercury (mm Hg) and is recorded as systolic pressure over diastolic pressure (e.g., 110/74 mm Hg). The pulse that can be palpated to determine heart rate is due to the difference between the systolic and diastolic pressures. This difference is known as the **pulse pressure.** The pulse pressure for a BP of 120/80 mm Hg is 40 mm Hg. The pulse pressure is an indication of the volume output of the left ventricle. Generally, the pulse pressure should be no greater than one-third of the systolic pressure, as in the example of a BP of 120/80 mm Hg, with a pulse pressure of 40 ($1/3 \times 120 = 40$).

KnowledgeCheck 19-5

- For a client whose BP is 150/80 mm Hg, what is the pulse pressure?
- Is that normal? If so, explain. If not, what should the pulse pressure be?

TheoreticalKnowledge knowing why

To assess and support clients' blood pressure, you will need to know what constitutes a normal reading for a client, how the body regulates blood pressure, and what factors affect the blood pressure.

What Is a Normal Blood Pressure Reading?

For many years, a BP of less than 120 to 129 mm Hg systolic and less than 80 to 84 diastolic was considered "optimal" for adults; and up to 130 systolic and 85 diastolic was considered "normal" for adults. More recently, an expert panel has classified "normal" as systolic BP below 120 and diastolic BP below 80—that is, less than 120/80 mm Hg (Joint National Committee on Prevention, Detection, Evaluation, and Treatment of High Blood Pressure, 2004). See Table 19-5.

How Does the Body Regulate Blood Pressure?

Blood pressure regulation is a highly complex process. It is influenced by three factors: cardiac function, peripheral vascular resistance, and blood volume. The body constantly regulates and adjusts arterial pressure to supply blood to body tissues via perfusion of the capillary beds. For in-depth discussion, see Chapter 37.

Cardiac Function

Recall that *cardiac output* is the volume of blood pumped by the heart per minute, and that it reflects the functioning of the heart. An increase in cardiac output causes an increase in BP; a decrease in cardiac output causes a decrease in BP (if all other factors remain the same). A change in either stroke volume or heart rate alters cardiac output.

Conditions that *increase* cardiac output by increasing stroke volume include the following:

- Increased blood volume (e.g., as occurs during pregnancy).
- More forceful contraction of the ventricles (e.g., as occurs during exercise).

Table 19-5 ➤ Classification of Adult Blood Pressure*

CATEGORY	SYSTOLIC (MM HG)		DIASTOLIC (MM HG)	FOLLOW-UP
Normal	<120	and	<80	Encourage lifestyle modification if there are risk factors. Recheck in 1–2 yr or sooner if there are risk factors.
Prehypertension	120–139	or	80–89	Encourage lifestyle changes; recheck in 1 yr or sooner if indicated. Antihypertensives are prescribed only with compelling indications, such as renal disease.
Stage I Hypertension	140–159	or	90–99	Encourage lifestyle modification. Follow up with primary care provider in 1–2 mo. (Most patients will be started on thiazide-type diuretics.)
Stage II Hypertension	≥160	or	≥100	Encourage lifestyle modification. Refer for care within 1 wk, or immediately if warranted. (Most patients will be given a two-drug combination therapy, e.g., thiazide-type diuretics with angiotensin-converting enzyme [ACE] inhibitors.)

Source: Data from the Joint National Committee on Prevention, Detection, Evaluation, and Treatment of High Blood Pressure. (2004). *JNC 7 Complete Report. The seventh report of the Joint National Committee on Prevention, Detection, Evaluation, and Treatment of High Blood Pressure.* Bethesda, MD: National Institutes of Health. Retrieved February 22, 2011, from http://www.nhlbi.nih.gov/guidelines/hypertension/index.htm

*For adults age 18 and older, based on the average of two or more readings taken at each of two or more visits after an initial screening.

Conditions that *decrease* cardiac output by decreasing stroke volume include the following:

- Dehydration
- Active bleeding
- Damage to the heart (as seen after myocardial infarction, or heart attack)
- A very rapid heart rate. Up to a point, an increase in heart rate increases cardiac output. However, a very rapid heart rate limits the time allotted for the ventricles to fill, resulting in decreased stroke volume and, ultimately, decreased cardiac output.

Peripheral Resistance

Peripheral resistance refers to arterial and capillary resistance to blood flow as a result of friction between blood and the vessel walls. Increased peripheral resistance creates a temporary increase in BP. The amount of friction or resistance depends on blood **viscosity** (thickness), arterial size, and arterial **compliance** (elasticity). The walls of the veins are thin and very distensible, so they have little influence on peripheral resistance and BP.

Blood Viscosity. Blood viscosity influences the ease with which blood flows through the vessels. Viscosity is determined by the **hematocrit** (the percentage of red blood cells in plasma). Any disorder that increases hematocrit (e.g., dehydration) increases blood viscosity and, therefore, BP. Conversely, a low hematocrit, as seen in anemia, lowers viscosity and may reduce BP.

Arterial Size. The smaller the radius of a blood vessel, the more resistance it offers to blood flow. Constricted arteries prevent the free flow of blood and, subsequently, increase BP. Dilated arteries allow unrestricted flow of blood, thereby reducing blood pressure. The sympathetic nervous system controls vasoconstriction and vasodilation.

Arterial Compliance. Arteries with good elasticity can distend and recoil easily and adequately. When age- or disease-related changes in arterial structure cause a loss of elasticity, peripheral resistance, and possibly BP, increase. **Arteriosclerosis** (hardening of the arteries) is a common contributor to increased BP in middle-aged and older adults.

Blood Volume

The normal volume of blood in the body is about 5 liters (5,000 mL). A significant volume decrease, as occurs with hemorrhage or other fluid losses, reduces vascular volume, and BP falls. When vascular volume is increased above the norm, as occurs with renal (kidney) failure and fluid retention, BP increases.

What Factors Influence Blood Pressure?

Blood pressure normally changes from minute to minute with changes in activity or changes in body position. Therefore, you must establish BP *patterns* rather than relying on individual BP readings when determining whether a client's BP is normal or abnormal. This is even more important for older adults because their BP tends to fluctuate even more. The following are some factors that affect the BP:

Developmental Stage. An average newborn has a systolic BP of about 40 mm Hg. It increases gradually throughout childhood. A child or adolescent's BP depends on body size; a smaller child or adolescent has a lower blood pressure than does a larger child. Both systolic and diastolic BP continue to increase with age as a result of decreased arterial compliance. For BP normal ranges for different age groups,

 Go to Chapter 19, **Tables, Boxes, Figures: ESG Table 19-1, Comparison of Normal Vital Signs for Various Ages,** on Davis*Plus.*

Gender. The average BP for men is slightly higher than that for women of comparable age. After menopause, a woman's BP tends to increase, possibly due to a decrease in estrogen.

Family History. A family history of hypertension markedly increases the likelihood of an individual's developing hypertension.

Lifestyle. Increased sodium consumption, smoking, and consumption of three or more alcoholic drinks per day have been shown to elevate BP. Caffeine may raise BP for a short while after ingestion, but it has no long-term effect on the BP.

Exercise. Physical fitness has been shown to reduce BP in many individuals. However, muscular exertion temporarily increases BP as a result of increased heart rate and cardiac output. You should, therefore, wait about 30 minutes before you assess the BP of someone who has been physically active.

Body Position. BP is higher when a person is standing than when she is sitting or lying down. Readings are higher if taken with the client's arm above heart level or if the arm is unsupported at the client's side. Seated readings are higher if the client's feet are dangling rather than resting on the floor or if the legs are crossed at the knees.

Stress. Fear, worry, excitement, and other stressors cause BP to rise sharply because of sympathetic nervous system stimulation (fight-or-flight response). One example of this is "white-coat hypertension." This occurs when a patient's BP is elevated in the physician's office or clinic—a situation in which he is likely to experience stress—but not at other times. However, white-coat hypertension may indicate what happens during other times of stress, so if it is consistently displayed, treatment may be indicated.

Pain. Pain often causes the BP to increase. However, severe or prolonged pain can significantly decrease BP.

Race. African Americans have a higher rate of hypertension than do European Americans, and they have a higher incidence of complications and hypertension-related deaths (McCance & Heuther, 2006).

Obesity. As a rule, obesity increases BP. This increase is related to the additional vascular supply required to perfuse the large body mass and the resultant increase in peripheral resistance.

Diurnal Variations. Generally, BP varies according to the person's daily schedules and routines. BP is lower while the person is sleeping and when he first gets up, rising during the day and dropping again toward bedtime.

Medications. Many medications alter BP. This effect may be intended, as with antihypertensive medications, or unintended, such as the drop in BP that often results when a client receives pain medication. Many over-the-counter preparations, herbal products, and illicit drugs can affect BP.

Diseases. Diseases that affect the circulatory system or any of the major organs of the body (e.g., the kidneys) may affect BP.

ThinkLike a Nurse 19-9

- Evaluate the following adult blood pressures. Are they high, low, or normal?
  116/90 mm Hg
  80/50 mm Hg
  184/102 mm Hg
  140/90 mm Hg
  40/0 mm Hg
- What theoretical knowledge did you use in evaluating the blood pressures?

PracticalKnowledge
knowing **how**

Now that you understand how blood pressure is maintained and regulated, you are ready to learn the practical knowledge of how to assess and support this aspect of physical functioning.

ASSESSMENT

Blood pressure may be assessed directly or indirectly.

Direct Method. In the *direct method*, a catheter is threaded into an artery under sterile conditions and attached to tubing that is connected to an electronic monitoring system. The pressure is constantly displayed as a waveform on the monitor screen. Although the direct method of measuring BP is very accurate, its use is confined to critical care areas and surgery because of the risk of sudden arterial blood loss.

Indirect Method. Usually, you will measure BP via the *indirect*, or *noninvasive, method*. This is an accurate estimate of arterial BP that can be performed in any clinical or community setting. For a procedure for noninvasive blood pressure monitoring, see Procedure 19-6. For an animated visual explanation of blood pressure readings,

 Go to **Animations Library: Reading Blood Pressure,** on the Davis*Plus* Web site.

What Equipment Do I Need?

You will need a stethoscope, a blood pressure cuff and sphygmomanometer, or an electronic blood pressure monitor to assess blood pressure. Electronic monitoring is gradually replacing the stethoscope and sphygmomanometer in inpatient settings. A common stethoscope and sphygmomanometer are sufficient to hear most clients' blood pressures. When blood pressure is weak, ultrasonic stethoscopes are useful for magnifying sound waves occurring during systole.

Evidence-based guidelines suggest that using the bell of the stethoscope enables you to hear blood pressure sounds more accurately, especially at diastolic pressures (Perloff, Grim, Flack, et al., 1993; Vital Signs, 1999). However, most people use the diaphragm because it is easily placed and because some stethoscopes do not have a bell (see Fig. 19-5). The key to clarity of sound is to use a high-quality stethoscope with short tubing (Pickering, Hall, Appel, et al, 2005).

A **sphygmomanometer** consists of a vinyl or cloth cuff, a pressure bulb with a regulating valve, and a manometer (Fig. 19-9). Blood pressure cuffs contain an inflatable rubber bladder. The cuff is attached to a gauge or manometer and a valved pressure bulb that inflates the bladder (Fig. 19-10). Cuffs can be placed on either the upper arm or midthigh and are supplied in various sizes.

Sphygmomanometers are either aneroid or mercury.
- **Aneroid** manometers have dials that register BP by pointers attached to a spring.
- **Mercury** manometers measure BP using a calibrated upright tube containing mercury (see Fig. 19-9, top). As the bladder of the cuff is inflated, the pressure pushes the column of mercury up the tube. The column of mercury falls as the cuff is deflated. They are easier to maintain and more accurate than are aneroid manometers, which require frequent calibration. However, mercury manometers pose a health hazard if the mercury tube is broken. The American Hospital Association and the EPA recommended that the healthcare industry eliminate mercury-containing waste by the year 2005 (U.S. Environmental Protection Agency, 2001). This would include phasing out mercury manometers, and most agencies have done that.
- **Electronic blood pressure monitors** use either microphones to sense sounds or sensors that detect pressure waves as blood flows through arteries (Fig. 19-9, bottom). They can be set to monitor and record BP at timed intervals and do not require the use of a stethoscope. They measure systolic, diastolic, and mean arterial pressures. Electronic monitors are useful when

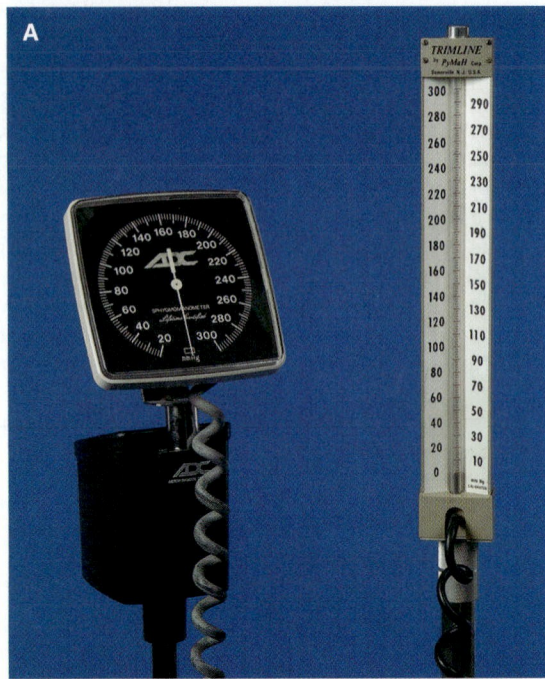

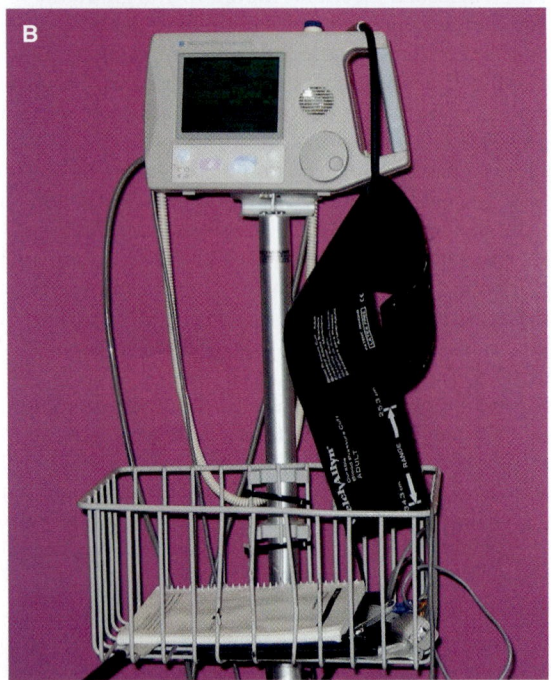

FIGURE 19-9 Types of manometers: *top left*, aneroid; *top right*, mercury; *bottom*, electronic.

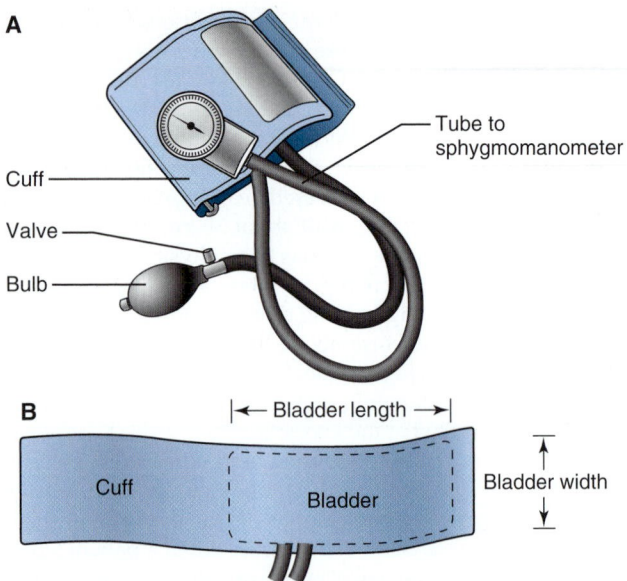

FIGURE 19-10 (A) Parts of the blood pressure cuff. (B) Placement of bladder within the cuff.

you must monitor BP frequently (e.g., during surgery or when a client is critically ill). However, some evidence suggests that they may be less accurate than auscultated blood pressures, so you should auscultate a baseline BP before initiating automatic monitoring (Pickering, Hall, Appel, et al., 2005).

- Many clients use a version of the electronic BP monitor in their homes. These devices can be purchased in grocery stores and pharmacies. They are useful for screening, but clients should seek follow-up care when readings are not within their normal range. The accompanying Home Care box identifies teaching topics for clients using electronic BP monitors.

Cuff Size. As shown in Figure 19-10, the width of the bladder of a properly fitting cuff will cover approximately two-thirds

of the length of the upper arm (or other extremity) for an adult, and the entire upper arm for a child (National Heart, Lung, and Blood Institute, 1996, 2007). Alternatively, you can check that (1) the cuff width is 40% of the arm circumference and (2) the length of the bladder encircles 80% of the arm in adults (Perloff, Grim, Flack, et al., 1993; Pickering, Hall, Appel, et al., 2005).

Using a cuff or bladder of the incorrect size can result in a measurement error of as much as 30 mm Hg. If the cuff is too narrow, your reading will be too high; if it is too wide, the reading will be too low. Although cuffs are manufactured in various sizes, in practice you will probably have access to only two or three different adult sizes. If you must use a cuff of the improper size, (1) it is better to use one that is too large than one that is too small, and (2) be sure to document the cuff size along with the BP reading. Refer to Figure 19-11 and Tables 19-6 for information about cuff sizes in centimeters. Also refer to Clinical Insight 19-1.

Which Site Should I Use?

You usually use the *brachial artery* for assessing BP. However, the condition of the client's arm as well as other factors can interfere with accurate BP measurement. Avoid assessing blood pressure in an arm that has an intravenous access device, renal dialysis fistula, or skin graft; that is paralyzed, diseased, or has extensive trauma; that has a cast or dressings; or that is on the same side of breast or shoulder surgery. In these and similar instances, you can use the forearm, thigh, or calf. Systolic pressure may be 20 to 30 mm Hg higher in the lower extremities than in the arms, but diastolic pressures are similar. Also, forearm and upper arm readings may not be interchangeable. Document the site used.

Auscultating Blood Pressure

Blood pressure can be measured indirectly by auscultation or palpation. The preferred, and most commonly used, method is auscultation; however, palpation is useful in certain situations. When auscultating BP, place your stethoscope over an

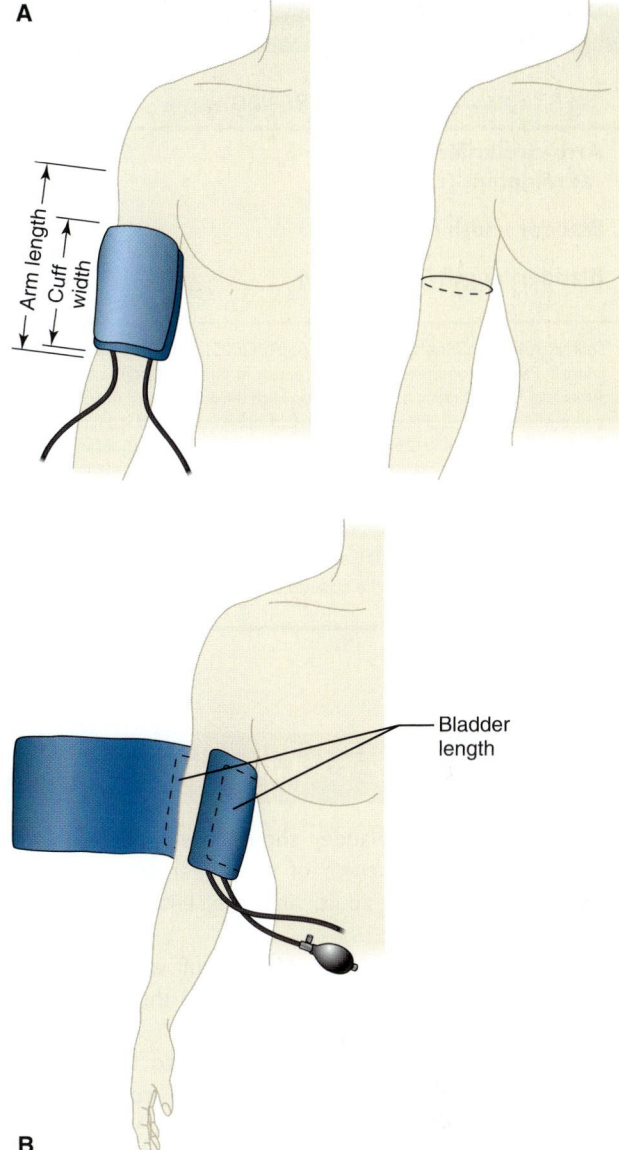

Home Care

Teaching Your Client Self-Monitoring of Blood Pressure

Various models of common, acceptable BP devices are available for self-monitoring using the upper arm (finger monitors are inaccurate).

➤ With a portable home device, the client simply pushes a button, and the cuff inflates and deflates automatically. The device provides an electronic digital readout of the BP. Because these devices are sensitive, arm movement or improper cuff placement can cause inaccurate readings. These devices must be recalibrated at least every 6 to 12 months.

➤ Some grocery stores, fitness clubs, and other public places have stationary automatic BP devices for public use. The person places his arm in the cuff, which fits over his clothing. The machine gives a visual display of the BP reading. The accuracy of these machines varies.

Benefits of Self-Monitoring

➤ May detect high BP in those who have not previously had a problem (screening).

➤ Allows for observation of the BP *pattern* in those with high normal BP, rather than a one-time office reading.

➤ Distinguishes white-coat hypertension from actual hypertension.

➤ For clients with hypertension, self-monitoring increases participation in treatment and may improve compliance with treatment.

Disadvantages of Self-Monitoring

➤ Possible incorrect use of the BP device.

➤ Needless anxiety over a single elevated reading.

➤ Clients with hypertension may make adjustments to their medications based on the BP readings without consulting their care provider.

Nursing Implications

➤ Teach proper use of the self-measurement devices.

➤ Periodically evaluate the client's technique.

➤ Teach the meaning of BP readings and the need to look for patterns from multiple readings, not just a single reading.

➤ Explain the need for calibration of the home-monitoring device at least once a year (American Heart Association, n.d.a).

➤ Have the client bring the home-monitoring device to clinical visits so that readings can be compared with simultaneously recorded auscultatory readings.

➤ Teach the client to have abnormally high or low readings (occurring on more than one occasion) rechecked by a healthcare provider. Home readings of 135/85 mm Hg or higher should be considered elevated.

➤ Advise the client to keep a written record of BP readings, including the date and time for each, and bring it to each clinic or office visit.

FIGURE 19-11 Determining correct BP cuff size. (A) The cuff width should be two-thirds of the length of the upper arm, or should encircle 40% of the arm. (B) The length of the bladder should encircle 80% of the upper arm.

artery, inflate the cuff, and listen for sounds as you deflate the cuff.

As you *inflate* the cuff, the artery is occluded as the pressure of the cuff exceeds the pressure in the artery. At that point, blood flow through the artery is halted, and no sound can be heard. As you *deflate* the cuff, blood begins to flow rapidly through the partially open artery, producing turbulence that you will hear through the stethoscope as a tapping sound.

▪ *The first sound* you hear when the cuff is slowly deflated is the systolic pressure.

▪ *The disappearance of sound* identifies the diastolic BP. When the artery is no longer compressed, blood flows freely, and no sound is heard.

The sounds you listen for when you assess BP are called **Korotkoff sounds.** These sounds, described by Russian neurologist Nicolai Korotkoff in 1906, are used to describe the sounds of blood pulsating through arteries (Fig. 19-12).

1st sound—Systolic BP. As you deflate the BP cuff, you will initially hear a sound that occurs during systole. It is a tapping sound that corresponds to the pulse.

2nd sound—Occurs as you further deflate the cuff. It is a soft, swishing sound caused by blood turbulence.

Table 19-6 ➤ Blood Pressure Cuffs: Acceptable Bladder Sizes*

CUFF TYPE———>	NEWBORN	INFANT	CHILD	SMALL ADULT	ADULT	LARGE ADULT	ADULT THIGH
Arm circumference at midpoint (cm)**	<6	6–15	16–21	22–26	27–34	35–44	45–52
Bladder width (cm)	3	5	8	12	16	16	16
Bladder length (cm)	6	15	21	22	30	36	42

Sources: American Heart Association (AHA). (2005). AHA scientific statement. Recommendations for blood pressure measurement in humans and experimental animals. Part 1: Blood pressure measurement in humans: A statement for professionals from the subcommittee of professional and public education of the American Heart Association Council on High Blood Pressure Research. *Hypertension, 45,* 142. Retrieved February 10, 2011, from http://hyper.ahajournals.org/cgi/content/full/45/1/142; Perloff, D., Grim, C., Flack, J., et al. (1993). Human blood pressure determination by sphygmomanometry. AHA Medical/Scientific Statement, Product Code: 88:2460–2467. Dallas: American Heart Association; and Pickering, T., Hall, J., Appel, L., et al. (2005). Recommendations for blood pressure measurement in humans and experimental animals: Part 1: Blood pressure measurement in humans: A statement for professionals from the subcommittee of Professional and Public Education of the American Heart Association Council on High Blood Pressure Research. *Hypertension, 45*(1): 142–161.

*The National Heart, Lung, and Blood Institute states that, practically speaking, "correct cuff size equals the largest cuff that will fit on the upper arm with room below for the stethoscope head" (2007).

**Arm circumference is half the distance from the acromion to the olecranon process. If correct size not available, use next larger (rather than smaller) size.

Clinical Insight 19-1 ➤ Choosing a Blood Pressure Cuff Size

- The *width* of the bladder should cover approximately two-thirds of the *length* of the upper arm (or other extremity) for an adult, and the entire upper arm for a child.
- Another method for sizing: (1) the cuff width should be 40% of the arm circumference, and (2) the *length* of the bladder should encircle 80% of the arm.
- Perhaps the easiest sizing method is to measure *arm circumference* and follow this guideline from Pickering, Hall, Appel, and colleagues (2005):

For arm circumference	Cuff should be
22–26 cm ($8\frac{1}{2} \times 10\frac{1}{4}$ in.)	"small adult" size: 12 × 22 cm ($4\frac{3}{4} \times 8\frac{3}{4}$ in.)
27–34 cm ($10\frac{1}{2} \times 13\frac{1}{2}$ in.)	"adult" size: 16 × 30 cm ($6\frac{1}{4} \times 11\frac{3}{4}$ in.)
35–44 cm ($13\frac{3}{4} \times 17\frac{1}{4}$ in.)	"large adult" size: 16 × 36 cm ($6\frac{1}{4} \times 14\frac{1}{4}$ in.)
45–52 cm ($17\frac{3}{4} \times 10\frac{1}{2}$ in.)	"adult thigh" size: 16 × 42 cm ($6\frac{1}{4} \times 16\frac{5}{8}$ in.)

Practice Resources

Pickering, Hall, Appel, et al., 2005.

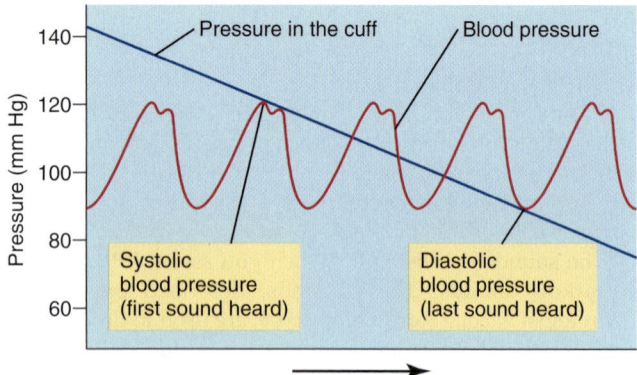

FIGURE 19-12 Relationship of blood pressure to changes in cuff pressure and the first and fifth Korotkoff sounds (BP 120/80).

3rd sound—Begins midway through the BP and is a sharp, rhythmic tapping sound.

4th sound—Like the third sound, but softer and fading.

5th sound—Diastolic BP. Silence; it corresponds with diastole.

You will not always be able to identify each of the five sounds. In some clients the sounds are distinct, but in others you will note little difference between beginning and ending sounds. To hear these sounds,

 Go to **Sounds: Blood Pressure Sounds,** in the Student Resources; also go to **Chapter 19, Resources for Caregivers and Health Professionals, Sounds,** on Davis*Plus.*

Palpating Blood Pressure

When the BP is difficult to hear (e.g., in shock or other conditions that compromise circulation) you can use palpation alone. You can usually palpate only the systolic BP, because diastolic pressure is difficult to feel.

Using Palpation With Auscultation

You should use palpation with auscultation for calculating the proper cuff inflation pressure before auscultating the BP and for detecting an auscultatory gap, to be discussed shortly.

Calculating Proper Inflation Pressure. The first time you measure a client's BP, you do not know what the systolic BP will be. Should you pump the cuff to 200 mm Hg just to be sure you don't miss the first sound? The answer is NO. If you overinflate the cuff, the patient will feel discomfort. However, if you underinflate it (e.g., stop inflating at 110 mm Hg), you may miss the first sound and obtain an incorrect reading. For a method that allows you to estimate the systolic BP and ensure that you inflate the cuff to the proper level, refer to steps 7 and 8 in Procedure 19-6.

Recognizing an Auscultatory Gap. If the client has hypertension, as you auscultate the BP during deflation of the cuff you may note the loss of sounds for as much as 30 mm Hg, followed by the return of sound. This loss and later return of sound is referred to as an *auscultatory gap*. Palpating first and then auscultating (as described in the preceding paragraph and in Procedure 19-6) ensures that you will not miss the isolated first sound. You should record the range of pressures in which the gap occurs (e.g., BP left arm, sitting, 170/90 with an auscultatory gap from 170 to 140). Failure to recognize an auscultatory gap can result in a serious misreading of the systolic BP. For tips that will help ensure the validity of your BP measurements, see Clinical Insight 19-2.

KnowledgeCheck 19-6

- Which of the Korotkoff sounds would you record as the systolic pressure?
- Which of the Korotkoff sounds would you record as the diastolic pressure?
- A nurse is auscultating a BP. He hears the first sound at 170 mm Hg. The sound disappears immediately. At 150 mm Hg, the sound appears again and continues until there is silence at 80 mm Hg. The pressures were taken in the client's right arm while the client was lying down.
  - How should the nurse record these pressures?
  - How do you explain what happened?

◼ ANALYSIS/NURSING DIAGNOSIS

Hypotension and hypertension are medical diagnoses or, more commonly, symptoms rather than nursing diagnoses. However, they may be the etiology of nursing diagnoses—for example, Risk for Falls related to orthostatic hypotension.

Example Problem: Hypotension

Hypotension is diagnosed when systolic blood pressure is less than 100 mm Hg. A low blood pressure is usually not considered a problem. However, further evaluation is always called for if:

- The client is also experiencing dizziness, fatigue, concentration problems, activity intolerance, or shortness of breath.
- The low blood pressure is of sudden onset.

Hemorrhage and heart failure are two causes of hypotension. Very low BP (hypovolemic shock) is a medical emergency. If you need more information on hypovolemic shock, consult a medical–surgical nursing text.

Orthostatic, or **postural, hypotension** occurs when a person's BP drops suddenly on moving from a lying position to a sitting or standing position. Orthostatic hypotension is defined as a decrease of 10 mm Hg in standing blood pressure when associated with dizziness and/or fainting (Joint National Committee, 2004). Postural hypotension results from peripheral vasodilation without a compensatory increase in cardiac output. It is most likely to occur in older adults, pregnant women, clients on prolonged bedrest, and clients with decreased blood volume (e.g., from dehydration or recent blood loss).

The following are examples of nursing diagnoses with hypotension as the etiology.

- Risk for Falls related to dizziness secondary to postural hypotension

---

Clinical Insight 19-2 ➤ **Taking an Accurate Blood Pressure**

To improve your technique and accuracy of measurement, use the following tips in addition to Procedure 19-6.

- Explain the procedure, particularly on admission or when changing the routine, to reduce patient anxiety.
- Wait 30 minutes before assessing BP after client has ingested caffeine or smoked.
- Do not assess BP while the client is in pain.
- Apply the cuff over bare skin, if possible. Controversy surrounds this issue, so follow the manufacturer's instructions. Advise clients who are home monitoring to apply the cuff over bare skin.
- Instruct the client not to talk during BP measurement, and you should not talk as well.
- Keep environmental noise and client movement to a minimum.
- Hold the stethoscope lightly but completely against the skin; do not put your thumb on top of the bell or diaphragm. Try not to allow the tubing to brush against your clothing or the bed.

- Do not be influenced by the client's previous BP measurements.
- Use the same limb for each measurement, unless you are comparing arms or averaging readings from both arms.
- For the initial reading, measure the BP in both arms and use the arm with the higher reading for subsequent measurements.
- If you obtain an elevated reading, confirm in the other arm.
- Do not draw conclusions based on one reading. Take two or more readings, at least 2 to 5 minutes apart, and average them. If the readings differ by more than 5 mm Hg, obtain and average additional readings.

Practice Resources

Joint National Committee on Prevention, Detection, Evaluation, and Treatment of High Blood Pressure, 2004; Ma, Sabin, & Dawes, 2008; McKay, 2008.

■ Fear of falling related to fainting secondary to postural hypotension

Example Problem: Hypertension?

A transient elevation in BP is a normal response to physiological or psychological stress (e.g., after eating, after exercise). **Prehypertension** is a BP reading of 120 to 139 mm Hg systolic or 80 to 89 mm Hg diastolic, obtained with two readings taken 6 minutes apart, with the patient sitting. **Hypertension** is a persistently higher than normal BP. It is diagnosed when BP is above 140 mm Hg systolic or above 90 mm Hg diastolic on two or more separate occasions. Physiologically, hypertension is related to thickening of the arterial walls and decreased elasticity of the arteries.

Hypertension is a major cause of illness and death in the United States. It increases the stress on the heart and blood vessels, and if untreated, it may lead to heart attack, heart failure, peripheral vascular disease, kidney damage, or stroke. The severity of the disorder is directly related to the degree of elevation; however, the latest guidelines (Joint National Committee, 2004) recommend that even prehypertension be treated by lifestyle modifications to prevent coronary artery disease. The diagnosis of hypertension is often delayed because symptoms are mild or absent. Those who experience symptoms may complain of early morning suboccipital headaches, fatigue, and visual changes.

Primary, or **essential, hypertension** is diagnosed when there is no known cause for the BP elevation. Essential hypertension accounts for at least 90% of all cases of hypertension. Although no single cause is identified, family history, age, race, obesity, diet, heavy alcohol consumption, smoking history, high cholesterol levels, and stress all contribute to the development of essential hypertension.

Secondary hypertension occurs when there is a clearly identified cause for the persistent rise in BP. A variety of renal and endocrine disorders may lead to secondary hypertension. Several prescription and nonprescription drugs can also cause BP elevation (e.g., nonsteroidal anti-inflammatory drugs [NSAIDs], oral contraceptives, some decongestants, and adrenal steroid hormones). Nicotine and caffeine cause transient BP increases. Other causes of hypertension include use of cocaine, amphetamines, and other illicit drugs, as well as chronic overuse of alcohol. Treatment is directed at eliminating the underlying cause.

Hypertension is not a nursing diagnosis; it is a medical diagnosis. However, there are nursing diagnoses associated with it, as in the following examples:

■ Risk for Decreased Cardiac Output occurs as a response to hypertension (i.e., hypertension is the etiology of this nursing diagnosis). As blood pressure rises, peripheral resistance increases. Over time the heart is unable to compensate, and cardiac output declines.

■ Some nursing diagnoses may be the contributing factors for hypertension, for example,

Imbalanced Nutrition: More than Body Requirements may be used if obesity (more than 20% above ideal body weight) is a factor in a patient's hypertension.

Imbalanced Nutrition: More than Body Requirements (for salt) could be used for a client whose high dietary sodium intake is contributing to hypertension.

■ Hypertension may be a defining characteristic (symptom) of some nursing diagnoses, for example, Anxiety and Pain may cause an increase in BP.

■ Hypertension may create the need for a diagnosis of Deficient Knowledge related to the need to make lifestyle changes.

You may need goals for overall blood pressure monitoring, but more likely you will use them for problems related to hypotension and hypertension.

Outcomes for Example Problem: Hypotension

The *NOC outcomes and goals* you use depend on the nursing diagnosis (the problem caused by the hypotension). For Risk for Falls, you might use NOC's Falls Occurrence. You might write *an individualized goal* such as, "Patient will have no falls while walking."

Outcomes for Example Problem: Hypertension

The NOC standardized outcome for assessing the blood pressure is Vital Signs Status. If it becomes necessary to monitor cardiac output, you could use the labels of Cardiac Pump Effectiveness and Circulation Status.

Individualized goals/outcome statements are developed from the nursing diagnosis. For example, for Decreased Cardiac Output, goals might be, "BP will be at least 110/80," and "Extremities will be warm to the touch with quick capillary refill." If the nursing diagnosis were Imbalanced Nutrition: More Than Body Requirements, the desired outcomes would address the target weight for the client and the ideal number of calories to be consumed.

PLANNING INTERVENTIONS/IMPLEMENTATION

NIC standardized interventions for monitoring VS include the following:

Vital Signs Monitoring applies to monitoring an abnormal blood pressure.

Hemodynamic Regulation would be used to evaluate Decreased Cardiac Output.

Interventions for Example Problem: Hypotension

NIC standardized interventions will be determined by the nursing diagnosis you use. For example, for Risk for Falls related to orthostatic hypotension, you might use the following: Fall Prevention; Self-Care Assistance: Transfer; and Surveillance: Safety.

Specific nursing activities, regardless of the nursing diagnosis used, must address the etiology, for example, the orthostatic hypotension. When you detect orthostatic hypotension:

1. Help the client lie down, and then notify the physician or nurse in charge.
2. Next, obtain *orthostatic vital signs*—that is, take the pulse and BP with the client supine, sitting, and standing. Take each reading 1 to 3 minutes after the client changes position.
3. When documenting orthostatic vital signs, record the client's position in addition to the pulse and BP measurements (e.g., supine P = 80, BP = 150/90; sitting P = 84, BP = 140/84; standing P = 90, BP = 104/60).

Interventions for Example Problem: Hypertension

Specific nursing activities for the patient with hypertension depend on whether hypertension is primary or secondary and on specific prescriptions from the primary provider. Nursing activities and focused assessments that address hypertension, regardless of its cause, include the following:

Perform focused assessments:

Monitor all VS. An elevated BP may affect the client's other VS. Watch for increases in pulse and respiratory rate.

Monitor the patient's activity tolerance. The patient's degree of involvement in care, orientation, and level of fatigue while experiencing hypertension are all important indicators of decreased cardiac output.

Accurately measure intake and output. If intake is appreciably greater than output, the increased blood volume will cause the BP to rise further. Pay attention to free fluids as well as fluid in food sources. Also monitor for edema, which is an indicator of fluid retention.

Weigh the client regularly. Weight loss of as little as 10 pounds (4.5 kg) lowers BP in many overweight persons with hypertension. Weight gain may signal poor compliance with the treatment plan and/or indicate fluid retention.

Collect and assess laboratory data as ordered. Blood urea nitrogen (BUN), creatinine, electrolytes, hemoglobin, hematocrit, and lipid levels must all be assessed regularly.

- Administer antihypertensive medications (as prescribed).
- For self-monitoring of BP, see Home Care: Teaching Your Client Self-Monitoring of Blood Pressure. One study has found that self-monitoring data better predicted clinical outcomes than single office measurements.
- For client teaching regarding hypertension, see Self-Care: Teaching Your Client About Hypertension.
- Teach stress management and relaxation techniques. Such training has been effective in helping older adults with systolic hypertension to eliminate at least one antihypertensive drug and reduce their BP to target levels.
- Teach and encourage self-management of behaviors; provide positive feedback when the patient makes lifestyle changes.

KnowledgeCheck 19-7

- Which of the patients with the following BP has hypertension?
  150/80 mm Hg on two separate occasions
  180/100 mm Hg on one occasion
  138/88 mm Hg on two occasions

- Which of the following client(s) has/have *primary* hypertension?
  Client A, who is obese and has a high sodium intake
  Client B, who is in renal failure
  Client C, who has hypertension induced by pregnancy
  Client D, who has a family history of hypertension

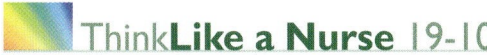

ThinkLike a Nurse 19-10

Recall the clients in the Meet Your Patients scenario. Lucas is 35 years old. He has been under a lot of stress. His blood pressure is 150/98 mm Hg.

- To evaluate his BP, what else do you need to know about Lucas's situation (the context)?
- What possible actions should you consider while meeting with Lucas?
- What is the theoretical knowledge (rationale) to support your decisions?

PUTTING IT ALL TOGETHER

In the hospital setting, you will usually take a complete set of VS on patients at regular intervals. In ambulatory care settings, the VS you measure may vary according to the client's chief complaint. Regardless of setting, you will need to use clinical judgment about which VS to measure and how often to measure them.

Evaluating Vital Signs

You should evaluate the client's VS on the basis of known norms as well as the particular client's trends. Suppose your client's BP has consistently been 150 to 160/90 over the past 3 days. This afternoon his BP is 108/60. Although this BP is theoretically normal, it is significantly different from his norm. Therefore, you must evaluate the cause of the change. Has there been a change in the other VS? Has there been a change in the client's medications or condition? How does the client feel? Has his activity level been altered by the change in BP? This change

---

Self-Care

Teaching Your Client about Hypertension

Teach the Client and Family about Lifestyle Changes for Preventing and Managing Hypertension.

➤ Limit salt intake to 1 teaspoon per day (2,400 mg of sodium).

➤ Consume a diet high in potassium (e.g., fresh fruits and vegetables, such as bananas, potatoes, yogurt, and acorn squash).

➤ Consume a diet high in calcium (e.g., milk and milk products, sardines, molasses, tofu).

➤ Limit alcohol intake to 1 or 2 drinks per day for men; 1 for women. (One drink is a can of beer, one jigger of liquor, or a glass of wine. Wine is preferred.)

➤ Maintain ideal body weight; lose weight if overweight.

➤ For overall cardiovascular health, reduce saturated fat and cholesterol intake.

➤ Eliminate smoking.

➤ Engage in aerobic exercise (30 to 45 min, several days a week, or a total of 150 min per week).

➤ Try to reduce stress and stressful situations.

➤ Teach the client that even one lifestyle change has effects similar to treatment with a single antihypertensive drug. More than one change has an even more positive effect on the BP.

Teach the Need for Follow-up Assessments.

➤ **If BP is less than 120/80**, recheck at each healthcare encounter or at least every 2 years.

➤ **If BP is greater than 120 mm Hg systolic or greater than 80 mm Hg diastolic**, review lifestyle modifications and consult the primary health provider within 1 to 2 months.

➤ **If BP is greater than 140 mm Hg systolic or greater than 90 mm Hg diastolic**, review lifestyle modifications and schedule follow up with a healthcare provider within 1 to 2 months.

➤ **If BP is 160 mm Hg systolic or higher, or 100 mm Hg diastolic or higher**, consult the primary care provider within 1 week, or immediately if the clinical situation warrants.

➤ When readings are obtained by self-monitoring, reduce all numbers in the three preceding items by about 5 mm Hg (e.g., a BP greater than 115 mm Hg systolic or greater than 75 mm Hg diastolic would merit lifestyle modifications and consultation with the primary health provider) (National Guideline Clearinghouse, 2007).

may be positive or negative. You must put all the VS and other clinical signs together to determine your course of action.

A high fever can cause BP to drop precipitously. Suppose this client's temperature is 103.5°F (39.7°C). In that case, in addition to his drop in BP, you should also anticipate a rise in pulse and respiratory rate. What should you do? Your action depends on the client's condition and the context. What else is going on in the situation? If medication for the fever has been prescribed for the client, you would administer the medication and evaluate the VS again at frequent intervals. If the VS do not improve, you would then notify the primary care provider.

Now change the context slightly. Add to your preceding data that the client has undergone a surgical procedure and is not taking any antibiotics. Now what should you do? If your answer is to notify the primary care provider, you are correct. Always evaluate all the VS as a unit. A sudden change in the client's condition requires you to thoroughly assess the client and report your findings to the primary care provider.

A change in a client's VS may also be a positive sign. For instance, if the client has been in severe pain for 3 days and has finally obtained pain relief, a decrease in BP probably indicates that the current medication regimen has provided better control of the pain. You would still need to monitor the VS at more frequent intervals, however, to ensure that the BP does not continue to fall.

Delegating Vital Signs

In many healthcare settings, several providers interact with the clients. VS may be obtained by unlicensed personnel. However, if you are working in a team nursing model as the registered nurse (RN), you are responsible for reviewing and interpreting the findings of all NAPs. This includes evaluating the technique of NAPs and the accuracy of their measurements. The professional nurse *never* relinquishes the responsibility for interpretation of VS trends and decisions based on abnormal VS findings. As a student nurse, you are responsible for functioning within your scope of knowledge. If you are unsure how to interpret the meaning of a patient's VS, you must discuss the findings with your instructor and/or the nurse assigned to care for your client. Even though you are participating in the client's care, the assigned nurse maintains responsibility for client oversight.

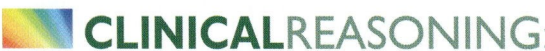

CLINICALREASONING:
Applying the **Full-Spectrum Nursing Model**

Because the following critical thinking activities allow you to practice the kind of thinking you will use as a full-spectrum nurse, they usually have no single right answer. Discuss them with your peers—if you have difficulty with any of the questions, consult your instructor.

PATIENT SITUATION

A patient in the critical care unit had a stable pulse and BP for the first few days. He has become more ill and now his pulse and BP are weak and difficult to palpate. His last BP reading was abnormally low, so it must be monitored frequently. He is receiving intravenous fluids in both arms.

THINKING

1. *Critical Thinking (Reflecting and Deciding What to Do):* Which of the patient's vital signs (temperature, pulse, respirations [TPR], and BP) might you be able to delegate to a NAP?

DOING

2. *Practical Knowledge:* How would you take the patient's blood pressure? Be specific: (a) What site would you use? (b) What equipment would you use?
3. *Nursing Process (Assessment):*
   a. Will you need to validate any of the vital signs you obtain? If so, why?
   b. How could you validate those vital signs?

CARING

4. Assume that you are very busy. How would you demonstrate caring to this patient while you are assessing his vital signs (the ones you did not delegate to a NAP)?

 Go To Chapter 19, **Clinical Reasoning: Applying the Full-Spectrum Nursing Model Response Sheet,** on DavisPlus.

PracticalKnowledge
procedures

Use the Procedures, Clinical Insights, and tables in this section when assessing your patients' vital signs.

Procedure 19–1 ■ Assessing Body Temperature

➤ For steps to follow in *all* procedures, refer to the Universal Steps for All Procedures found on the page facing the inside back cover.

Equipment

- Thermometer (An oral thermometer generally has a blue tip. A rectal thermometer generally has a red tip.)
- ✚ Glass-and-mercury thermometers should not be used in any healthcare setting, but because many people still use them at home, we include them in this procedure. They should be used with disposable covers, and cleaned and sterilized regularly according to the manufacturer's instructions.
- Thermometer cover, if needed
- Procedure gloves, if taking a rectal temperature or if there is risk of contact with body fluids (e.g., saliva)
- Water-soluble lubricant, if taking a rectal temperature
- Towel, if needed, for taking an axillary temperature
- Tissues

Delegation

You can delegate temperature measurement to a NAP if you conclude that the patient's condition and the NAP's skills allow. Perform the pre-procedure assessments, and inform the NAP of the route and type of thermometer used. Explain any special considerations (e.g., be sure the patient has not had anything to eat or drink in the last 20 to 30 min) and inform the NAP if the patient is confused. Ask the NAP to record and report the temperature to you, and to report immediately if the temperature is elevated (e.g., greater than 100°F [37.8°C]).

Pre-Procedure Assessments

- Determine the site that is most appropriate for the patient. Consider patient comfort, safety, and accuracy. For example, do not use the oral route for patients who are unable to hold the thermometer properly, for children or others who cannot follow instructions (e.g., unconscious patients), or for patients who use "mouth breathing."
- For an oral temperature: Determine how long it has been since the patient smoked, had anything to eat or drink, or chewed gum.
  Smoking, eating, drinking, and chewing gum can all affect an oral reading. If any of these have occurred, wait 20 to 30 minutes before taking an oral temperature.
- Assess for any contraindications to using the site you have chosen. For example:
  Tympanic: Assess for impacted earwax or hearing aid.
  Rectal: Check the client record for diarrhea or impacted stool.
  Axillary: Check the client record for presence of fever or hypothermia.
  Skin: Assess for the presence of conditions that require a very precise, reliable reading (e.g., fever, hypothermia).
  Some conditions increase the risk for patient injury; others contribute to inaccurate, unreliable temperature measurement.
- What were the previous recordings, if any?
  Noting changes over time is important in all patient assessments.
- Assess for clinical signs and symptoms of temperature alterations.

Procedure 19–1A ■ Taking an Axillary Temperature

➤ When performing the procedure, always identify your patient according to agency policy and be attentive to standard precautions, hand hygiene, patient safety and privacy, body mechanics, and documentation.

Procedure Steps

1. **Slide the thermometer into a protective sheath** (depending on type of thermometer).
   A protective sheath provides a barrier to prevent transmission of organisms.
2. **Dry the patient's axilla**, as needed.
   Moisture from perspiration alters the temperature reading.
3. **Position the patient and the thermometer.**
   a. Assist the patient to a supine or sitting position.

b. Place the thermometer tip in the middle of the axilla.
c. Position the patient's upper arm down, with the lower arm across the chest.
   Puts the thermometer in close proximity to the axillary blood vessels, allowing it to better reflect the core temperature. ➤

4. **Hold the thermometer in place for the recommended time.**
   a. Leave an electronic probe in place until it beeps.

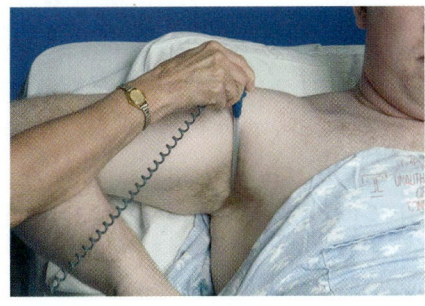

b. If you must use a glass thermometer in place for 8 minutes, or according to agency policy (usually 5 min for children).

(continued on next page)

Procedure 19–1 ■ Assessing Body Temperature (continued)

Study findings differ for accuracy of temperature measurements at the axillary site. Follow agency policy.

5. Remove the thermometer and discard the thermometer cover. If there is no cover, wipe the thermometer with a tissue.

Removes any moisture that may have accumulated in 8 minutes' time.

6. Read the temperature.
a. Electronic thermometer: Read the digital display.
b. Glass thermometer: Hold at eye level, and rotate it until the

markings are clear. Avoid using glass, if possible.

7. Clean and replace the thermometer in the storage base, following agency policy.
Prevents microbial growth on thermometers and recharges the battery.

Procedure 19–1B ■ Taking an Oral Temperature

➤ When performing the procedure, always identify your patient according to agency policy and be attentive to standard precautions, hand hygiene, patient safety and privacy, body mechanics, and documentation.

Procedure Steps

1. If you must use a glass thermometer, shake down the liquid if necessary.
a. Stand in an open area away from tables and other objects.
Prevents thermometer breakage.
b. Hold the end opposite the bulb between your thumb and forefinger, and snap your wrist downward.
c. Shake the thermometer until the reading is less than 96°F (36°C).
The reading must be lower than the anticipated temperature measurement.

2. Slide the thermometer into a protective sheath.
Provides a barrier to prevent transmission of microorganisms.

3. Place the thermometer tip under the tongue in the posterior sublingual pocket (right or left of frenulum).
Puts the tip in close proximity to the major blood vessels under the tongue, allowing the thermometer to reflect the core temperature. ➤

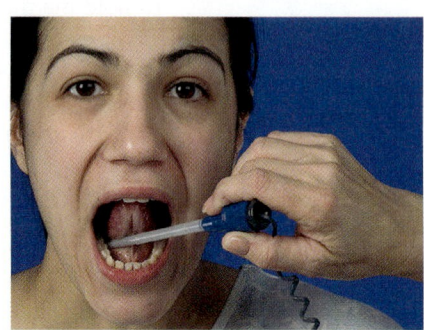

4. Have the patient close his lips around the thermometer, cautioning him not to bite down on it.
Protects the thermometer from exposure to the air, which could alter the reading. Biting may break a glass thermometer, injuring the mouth.

5. Leave the thermometer in place for the recommended time.
a. Glass thermometer: 5 to 8 minutes
b. Electronic (digital) thermometer: Until it beeps
c. According to agency policy
Research findings differ on the optimal time for measuring an oral temperature; follow agency policy.

6. Remove the thermometer; discard the cover. If there is no cover, wipe the thermometer with a tissue.
Wiping removes mucus that can make the markings on a glass thermometer difficult to read.

7. Read the temperature.
a. Glass thermometer: Position the thermometer at eye level, and rotate it until the markings are clear. ▼

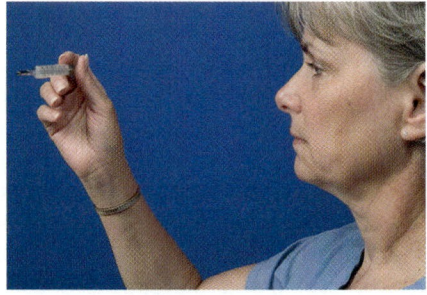

b. Electronic thermometer: Read the digital display.

8. Clean and replace the thermometer. Follow agency policy.
Prevents microbial growth and recharges battery of electronic thermometers.

Procedure 19–1C ■ Taking a Rectal Temperature

➤ When performing the procedure, always identify your patient according to agency policy and be attentive to standard precautions, hand hygiene, patient safety and privacy, body mechanics, and documentation.

➤ *Note:* This procedure primarily describes use of an electronic (digital) thermometer.

Procedure Steps

1. Slide the thermometer into a protective sheath.
A protective sheath provides a barrier to prevent transmission of microorganisms.

2. Position an adult patient in Sims' position (on the side with the knees flexed); place a child in

the prone position. Drape the patient so that only the anal area is exposed. You can lay a small child face down across your lap or a parent's lap.
Flexing the knees helps relax the muscles to ease insertion and aid in visualization. Draping provides privacy and decreases embarrassment. ➤

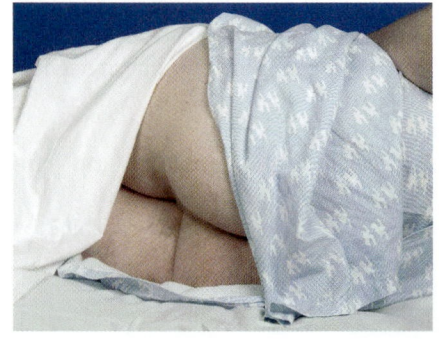

3. **Lubricate the tip of the thermometer** by squeezing water-soluble lubricant onto a tissue and then applying it to the thermometer. *Prevents injury to the rectal mucosa and eases insertion. Inserting the thermometer into the lubricant container would contaminate contents of the container.*

4. **Don a procedure glove on your dominant hand**, or on both hands if necessary.

5. **With your nondominant hand, separate the patient's buttocks** to visualize the anus.

6. **Gently insert the thermometer** approximately:
   Adult: 1 to 1.5 in. (2.5 to 3.7 cm)
   Child: 0.9 in. (2.5 cm)
   Infant: 0.5 in. (1.5 cm)

The thermometer must be placed past the rectal sphincter.

a. Have the patient take a deep breath. Insert the thermometer as he exhales. *Helps relax the anal sphincter.*

b. If you feel resistance, do not use force.

Inserting the thermometer too far or forcing against resistance may injure the rectal mucosa.

7. **Hold the thermometer in place until it beeps.** (If you must use a glass thermometer, hold the thermometer 3 to 5 min.)

The thermometer must be held in place to prevent inadvertent injury to the patient. An electronic thermometer will beep when a constant temperature is reached. Research differs on the optimal time for measuring a rectal temperature; follow agency policy.

8. **Remove the thermometer, discard the cover, and read the digital display.**

9. **Remove the procedure glove(s) and discard in a biohazards container.**

10. **Follow agency policy for cleaning and storing thermometers.** *Prevents microbial growth on thermometers and recharges electronic thermometer battery.*

Procedure 19-1D ■ Taking a Temporal Artery Temperature

➤ When performing the procedure, always identify your patient according to agency policy and be attentive to standard precautions, hand hygiene, patient safety and privacy, body mechanics, and documentation.

Procedure Steps

➤ *Note:* If the patient has been lying down, do not measure the temperature on the side that was lying on the pillow. Do not measure if a cap or hair has been covering the area over the temporal artery.

These can prevent heat dissipation and produce a falsely high reading.

1. **Remove the protective cap** from the instrument; **clean the lens/probe** according to the manufacturer's instructions.

2. **Place the probe flat on the center of the forehead**, midway between the eyebrow and the hairline. ▼

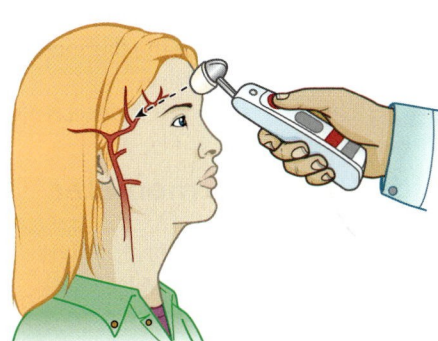

3. **Press and hold the button while you stroke the thermometer medially to laterally across the forehead**; keep the lens/probe flat and in contact with the skin, and slide in a reasonably straight line until you reach the hairline. ▼

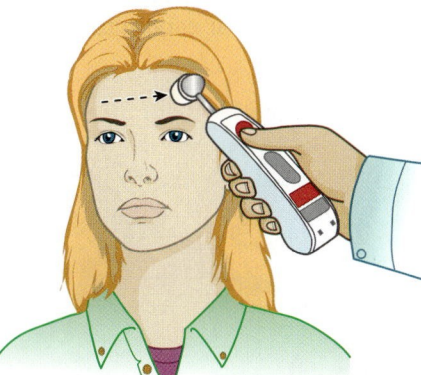

4. **Still holding the button, touch the thermometer lens/probe behind the ear lobe**, in the soft depression below the mastoid.

This step is necessary for an accurate reading if there is any moisture at all on the patient's forehead. ➤

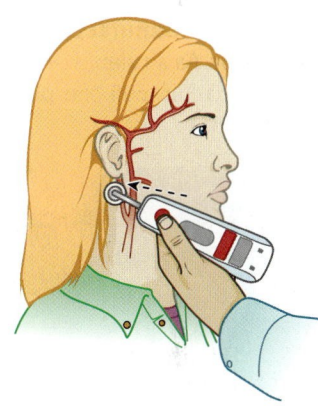

5. **Release the button for the temperature reading.** ▼

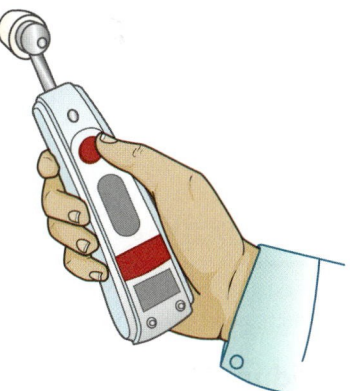

(continued on next page)

Procedure 19-1 ■ **Assessing Body Temperature** (continued)

Procedure 19-1E ■ **Taking a Tympanic Membrane Temperature**

➤ When performing the procedure, always identify your patient according to agency policy and be attentive to standard precautions, hand hygiene, patient safety and privacy, body mechanics, and documentation.

Procedure Steps

1. **Make sure the thermometer lens is intact and clean.**
   Ensures an accurate reading.
2. **Place a disposable cover tightly over the lens**, making sure the clear film is smooth across the lens.
   Ensures an accurate reading and prevents cross-contamination.
3. **Position the patient's head to one side**. If you are right-handed, try to use the right ear; if you are left-handed, use the left ear.
   Allows you to better visualize the ear canal.
4. **Straighten the ear canal, or follow the manufacturer's instructions.** As a rule:
   a. For an adult, pull the pinna up and back. ▼

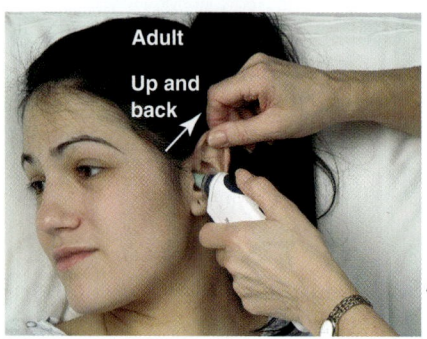

   b. For a child, pull the pinna down and back. ➤

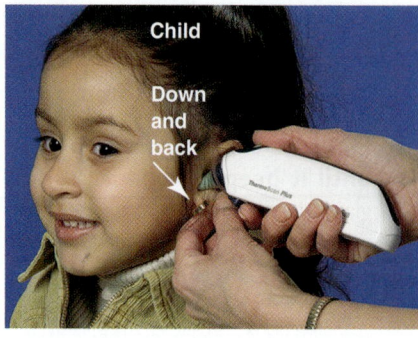

Some tympanic thermometers require you to straighten the ear canal; others do not. Some instruct, for adults, to pull the ear up, backward, and slightly away from the head. Some models instruct, for a child, to pull the pinna straight back instead of down and back. The external auditory canal is curved upward in children younger than 3 years of age. In an adult, it is a slightly S-shaped structure.

5. **Insert the probe into the ear canal** gently and firmly, directing it toward the tympanic membrane and inserting far enough to seal the opening. ▼

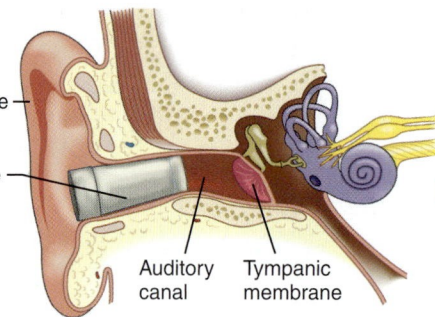

Auricle —
Probe tip —
Auditory canal   Tympanic membrane

Creates a seal to obtain an accurate reading without causing trauma to the ear canal.

6. **For some thermometer models, rotate the probe handle toward the jaw**. Follow the manufacturer's instructions; not all models require this.
   Aims the lens toward the tympanic membrane.
7. **Take the measurement.**
   a. Press and release the button to obtain the reading.
   b. Follow the instructions for the specific tympanic thermometer being used.
   Some tympanic thermometers record the reading immediately; for some you must wait for about 3 seconds.
8. **When you hear a beep and the display flashes, remove the thermometer.** Note the reading in the display window.
9. **Repeat the measurement in the other ear.**
   A study of 132 adults found significant differences in temperature in the left compared with the right ear. In addition, the left ear tended to register a lower temperature than the right ear at temperatures below 36.7°C (98.1°F) and a higher temperature above 36.7°C (Heusch & McCarthy, 2005).
10. **Discard the probe cover** (usually you will press an "eject" button to do this), and replace the thermometer in its charging base.
    Recharges the battery and protects the instrument.

Procedure 19-1F ■ **Taking a Skin Temperature Using a Chemical Strip Thermometer**

➤ When performing the procedure, always identify your patient according to agency policy and be attentive to standard precautions, hand hygiene, patient safety and privacy, body mechanics, and documentation.

Procedure Steps

➤ *Note:* If the temperature is not within the normal range, retake it with an electronic or other thermometer.

1. **Place the thermometer strip (paper or tape) on the patient's skin**, generally on the forehead or abdomen.
   The thermometer strip must be in contact with the skin to work properly. ➤

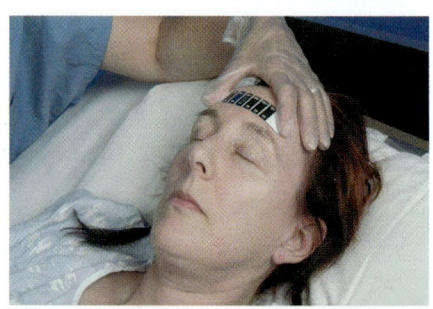

2. **Leave the thermometer strip in place 15 to 60 seconds (or as the manufacturer directs).**
3. **Observe for color changes.**
   Chemical strips have indicators that change colors to indicate temperature changes.
4. **Read the temperature before removing the strip from the patient's skin.**
   Ensures the most accurate reading.
5. **Remove and discard the thermometer strip.**

? What if . . .

- **The patient's temperature is not within normal range?**

Identify whether the temperature reading indicates hypothermia, fever, or hyperthermia (e.g., heat stroke).
Perform other assessments to determine the cause or severity of the findings.
Assess for clinical signs to confirm an abnormal temperature reading.
Institute interventions to raise or lower temperature, as appropriate.
Provide comfort measures (e.g., change linens if they are wet from diaphoresis).

Clean the thermometer before and after using with soap and water or approved solution; rinse.
Use disposable covers, if available.
When reading the thermometer, hold it at eye level and rotate it until the markings are clear and easy to read.
Handle carefully and store in an appropriate container to avoid breakage.

- **You are using a glass thermometer?**

Be sure it does not contain mercury
Before and after using, shake down the thermometer as needed.

Evaluation

- Compare to normal range for developmental stage, site used, and client's baseline data.
- Look for trends to identify potential concerns.
- Notify the appropriate healthcare professional of abnormal findings.

Patient Teaching

- Inform the patient of the temperature reading.
- Explain the significance of the temperature reading and any interventions that may be needed.

Home Care

Clients commonly use chemical strip (disposable), glass, or tympanic membrane thermometers at home. Teach the following points:

Do not use an oral thermometer to take a rectal temperature. Use a specially shaped, more rounded, rectal thermometer to avoid injury to the rectum.

Do not use glass-and-mercury thermometers. If you discover a glass-and-mercury thermometer, urge the client to replace it with a safer instrument. Arrange for an exchange if there is a procedure for this in your agency or community.
Glass-and-mercury thermometers carry the risk of breakage, cuts, and exposure to toxic mercury.

- If you obtain a high or low reading using a chemical strip or tympanic thermometer, retake the temperature using a glass or digital thermometer.
- Teach the same procedures you have learned for measuring temperature. Observe as the client takes a temperature to ensure correct technique.
- Clients often use the oral site. Remind them to not drink, eat, or smoke for 30 minutes before taking the temperature.
  Reinforce the following points about care of reusable thermometers:
- If you use the same thermometer for more than one person, use disposable covers, if possible; clean the thermometer well between uses.

- If the person has an infection or communicable illness, soak the thermometer in 70% isopropyl alcohol between uses.
- Clean the thermometer after each use, even if it is used for only one person. Wash with soap and water, rinse with cold water, dry well, and store in a clean, dry container.
- If you store a thermometer in alcohol, rinse it with cold water before taking the temperature.
- Do not use the same thermometer for both oral and rectal temperatures.

Documentation

You will usually record temperature on a graphic flow sheet (see Figure 19-1). In some situations (e.g., a fever), you may need to write a nurse's note. If so, follow these suggestions:
- Document the temperature, indicating the route of measurement, according to agency policy.
- Document supporting findings, such as "Skin is hot and dry" and state whether the temperature reading is consistent with the client's condition.

Practice Resources
Gyi, 2007; Heusch, & McCarthy, 2005; Lockwood, Conroy-Hiller, & Page, 2004; Quatrara, Coffman, Jenkins, et al., 2007; Rabinowitz, Cookson, Wasserman, et al., 1996; Robinson, Jou, & Spady, 2005; Therapeutic Research Center, 2007; "Vital Signs," 1999.

Thinking About the Procedure

 Go to the **Fundamentals of Nursing Skills Videos, Temperature: Axillary.**

1. Why did the nurse use the blue thermometer probe instead of the red one?
2. What did the nurse do to ensure that the thermometer probe was in good contact with the axillary skin?

 For suggested responses, go to Chapter 19, **Thinking About the Procedure Suggested Responses,** on Davis*Plus* at http://davisplus.fadavis.com, keyword: Treas.

Procedure 19-2 ■ Assessing Peripheral Pulses

➤ For steps to follow in *all* procedures, refer to the Universal Steps for All Procedures found on the page facing the inside back cover.

Equipment
- Watch with a second hand or digital readout
- Pen, pencil, and flow sheet or personal digital assistant (PDA)

Delegation
You can delegate measurement of pulses to the NAP if you conclude that the patient's condition and the NAP's skills allow. For example, if pedal circulation is critical and you suspect it may be difficult to palpate, you should not delegate assessment of the pedal pulse. If you do delegate, perform the pre-procedure assessments, and tell the NAP which site to use. Inform the NAP of any special considerations (e.g., to note what the patient's activity has been just before taking the pulse). Ask the NAP to record and report the pulse to you and to report immediately if it is outside normal limits (you must specify what is "normal" for each patient).

Pre-Procedure Assessments
- Determine why assessment of pulses is indicated.
  Conditions requiring an assessment of pulses include blood loss, cardiac or respiratory disease, diabetes mellitus, and other conditions that affect oxygenation.
- Assess factors that may alter the pulse, such as activity and medications. If the client has been active recently, wait 5 to 10 minutes before measuring.
  Activity increases the pulse rate; increased intracranial pressure decreases the rate; medications such as digoxin decrease the rate; other medications, such as albuterol, increase the pulse rate.

Procedure 19-2A ■ Assessing the Radial Pulse

➤ When performing the procedure, always identify your patient according to agency policy and be attentive to standard precautions, hand hygiene, patient safety and privacy, body mechanics, and documentation.

Procedure Steps

1. **With the patient sitting or supine, flex the patient's arm, and place the patient's forearm across his chest.**

2. **Palpate the radial artery.**
   The radial site is the most frequently used to calculate the patient's heart rate because it is generally the easiest site to use.
   a. Place the pads of your index or middle fingers (or both) in the groove on the thumb side of the patient's wrist, over the radial artery.
   b. Press lightly but firmly until you are able to feel the radial pulse. Start with light pressure to prevent occluding the pulse, and gradually increase the pressure until you feel the pulse.
   The fingertips are the most sensitive parts of the hand to palpate arterial pulsations. Avoid using the thumb, because it has its own pulsation and may interfere with the accuracy of your count. ➤

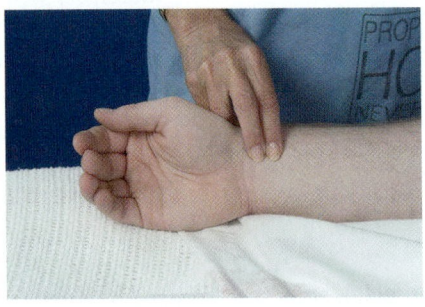

3. **Note the rhythm and quality of the pulse.** Note whether the thrust of the pulse against your fingertips is bounding, strong, weak, or thready.
   The rhythm and quality of the pulse are a reflection of the patient's cardiac output. The strength of the pulse reflects the volume of the blood that is ejected against the arterial wall with each contraction of the heart. An irregular or weak pulse indicates decreased cardiac output. A bounding pulse indicates increased cardiac output.

4. **Count the pulse:**
   a. Count for 60 seconds the first time you take a patient's pulse. After that, you can count a pulse with a regular rhythm for 15 seconds and multiply by 4, or count for 30 seconds and multiply by 2 to get the beats per minute. If you do not know the patient well, count for 1 full minute to be certain to detect any irregularities. Also see step 4c rationale, below.
   b. Begin timing with the count of 1—starting with the first beat that you feel.
   c. Count an irregular pulse for 1 full minute (60 sec).
   Research is conflicting. Some studies indicate that a 60-second count is most accurate; others say that accuracy is not affected by a 30-second, or even a 15-second, count if the pulse is regular. You must count an irregular pulse for 1 full minute to be accurate.

5. **For an admission assessment or peripheral vascular check,** palpate the radial pulses on both wrists simultaneously.
   a. Note any difference in the quality of the pulse between arms. Is the pulse on one side weaker than that on the other?
   Palpating simultaneously enables the recognition of small differences in the peripheral circulation.

Procedure 19-2B ■ Assessing the Brachial Pulse

➤ When performing the procedure, always identify your patient according to agency policy and be attentive to standard precautions, hand hygiene, patient safety and privacy, body mechanics, and documentation.

Procedure Steps

1. **Palpate the brachial artery.**
   a. Using firm pressure, press in the inner aspect of the antecubital fossa until you palpate the brachial artery.
   b. If you have difficulty palpating the pulse, ask the patient to pronate the forearm (i.e., turn the palm of the hand downward).

This brings the brachial artery over a bony prominence and makes the pulse easier to feel. ▼

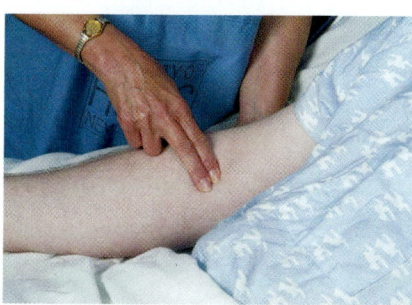

2. **Assess pulse rate, rhythm, and quality, and assess bilaterally.**
   The brachial pulse is used most frequently to assess blood pressure and during CPR in an infant.

Procedure 19-2C ■ Assessing the Carotid Pulse

➤ When performing the procedure, always identify your patient according to agency policy and be attentive to standard precautions, hand hygiene, patient safety and privacy, body mechanics, and documentation.

✚ **Caution!** Do not palpate the carotid pulse except during cardiopulmonary resuscitation in an adult, and in certain situations to assess for circulation to the head. Pressure on the carotid (especially in older adults) can stimulate the vagus nerve, causing the pulse and blood pressure to drop suddenly, and perhaps fainting or circulatory arrest. It can also decrease circulation to the brain.

Procedure Steps

1. **Palpate the carotid artery lightly.** Place your fingers on the patient's trachea, and slide them to the side into the groove between the trachea and the sternocleidomastoid muscle.

   ✚ NEVER compress the carotid artery on both sides of the neck at the same time.

   See the preceding Caution! ➤
2. **Assess the rate, rhythm, and quality, and compare bilaterally.**

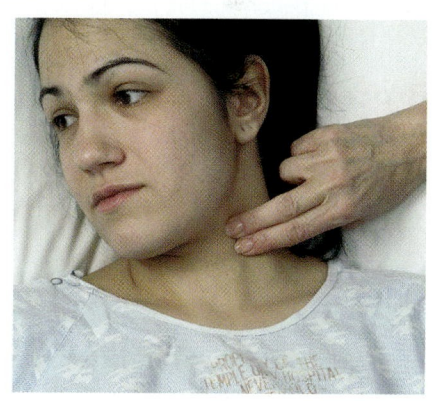

Procedure 19-2D ■ Assessing the Dorsalis Pedis Pulse

➤ When performing the procedure, always identify your patient according to agency policy and be attentive to standard precautions, hand hygiene, patient safety and privacy, body mechanics, and documentation.

Procedure Steps

1. **Palpate the dorsalis pedis pulse.**
   a. Run your fingers up the groove between the great and first toes to the top of the foot.
   b. Palpate very lightly.
   The dorsalis pedis pulse is easily obliterated, so use very light pressure.
2. **Assess pulse rate, rhythm, and quality, and assess bilaterally.** ➤

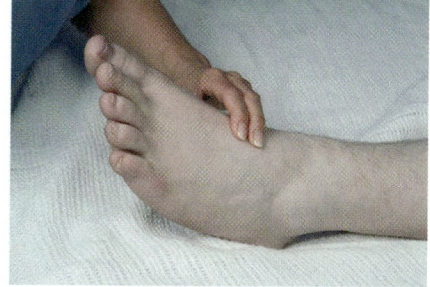

3. **If you are unable to palpate the dorsalis pedis pulse, use a Doppler ultrasound device** to listen for the pulse.

(continued on next page)

Procedure 19-2 ■ **Assessing Peripheral Pulses** (continued)

Procedure 19-2E ■ **Assessing the Femoral Pulse**

> ➤ When performing the procedure, always identify your patient according to agency policy and be attentive to standard precautions, hand hygiene, patient safety and privacy, body mechanics, and documentation.

Procedure Steps

1. **Palpate the femoral pulse** by pressing deeply in the groin midway between the anterosuperior iliac spine and the symphysis pubis.
   The femoral artery lies very deep and requires significant pressure to palpate. You may need to use both hands to feel the pulse on an adult. ➤

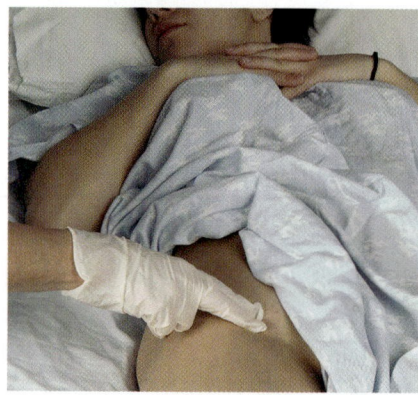

2. **Assess pulse rate, rhythm, and quality, and assess bilaterally.**
   The femoral pulse is used to determine the presence of a pulse during CPR and to assess circulation to the leg.

Procedure 19-2F ■ **Assessing the Posterior Tibial Pulse**

> ➤ When performing the procedure, always identify your patient according to agency policy and be attentive to standard precautions, hand hygiene, patient safety and privacy, body mechanics, and documentation.

Procedure Steps

1. **Palpate the posterior tibial pulse** by pressing on the inner (medial) side of the ankle below the medial malleolus.
   The posterior tibial pulse is usually palpated easily, but it may be deeper in some people. Therefore, press down moderately and then increase pressure until you feel the pulse. It is relatively easy to obliterate. ➤

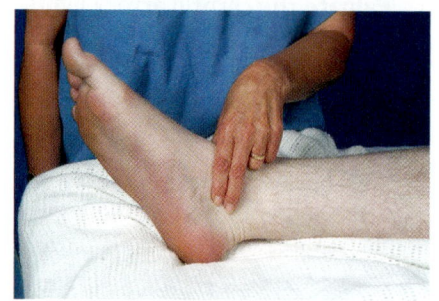

2. **Assess pulse rate, rhythm, and quality, and assess bilaterally.**
   The posterior tibial pulse is used to assess circulation to the lower extremity; it is assessed along with the dorsalis pedis pulse.

Procedure 19-2G ■ **Assessing the Popliteal Pulse**

> ➤ When performing the procedure, always identify your patient according to agency policy and be attentive to standard precautions, hand hygiene, patient safety and privacy, body mechanics, and documentation.

Procedure Steps

1. **Palpate the popliteal pulse** by pressing behind the knee in the middle of the popliteal fossa.
   The popliteal pulse can be difficult to feel. It is used only when specifically indicated because of absence of pedal pulses or for taking a thigh blood pressure. ➤

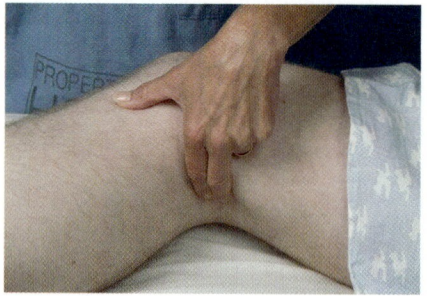

2. **Assess pulse rate, rhythm, and quality, and assess bilaterally.**

Procedure 19-2H ■ **Assessing the Temporal Pulse**

➤ When performing the procedure, always identify your patient according to agency policy and be attentive to standard precautions, hand hygiene, patient safety and privacy, body mechanics, and documentation.

Procedure Steps

1. **Palpate the temporal pulse** by pressing lightly lateral (outside area) and superior to (above) the eye. ▼

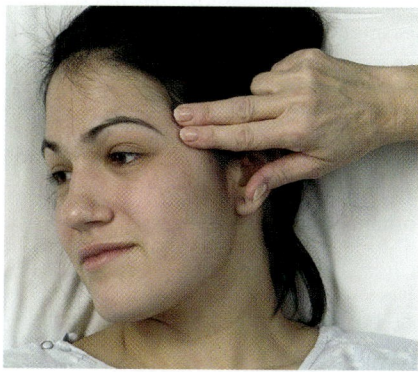

2. **Assess pulse rate, rhythm, and quality, and assess bilaterally.**
   The temporal pulse is easily accessible and is used frequently in infants.

? What if . . .

■ **The patient is an infant or a child younger than age 3 years?**

Auscultate an apical pulse rate.
Rates are faster and small arteries more difficult to feel in a child or infant.

If a parent is present, encourage the parent to hold the child to reduce anxiety.
Fear increases the pulse rate.

■ **The patient is an older adult?**

Have the patient at rest for 15 to 20 minutes after activity and before assessing the pulse.
The pulse tends to return to baseline more slowly in older adults.

If the pulse is fast, take repeated measures; if a pattern of fast rate emerges, note this for the primary care provider for further evaluation.
An elevated heart rate is related to increased mortality in older adult women, so it is a simple index of general health status.

■ **The pulse is faint or weak?**

Use a Doppler ultrasound device to detect blood flow.
Lack of pulses indicates inadequate circulation to the lower extremities. If you cannot feel the pulse, you must determine whether the pulse is absent or whether you are having difficulty feeling. To draw

the conclusion that the pulse is "absent," you must use a Doppler.

Apply transmission gel to the end of the probe. Do not use water-soluble lubricant as a substitute for transmission gel.

Place the probe lightly on the skin over the artery you are using.

Turn on the instrument and set the volume control to the lowest setting.

Tilting the probe to a 45° angle to the artery, move the probe slowly in a circular motion to locate the signal (a rhythmic hissing noise). Count for 60 sec.
Avoids distorting the signal.

When you are finished, wipe the gel off the patient's skin. Clean the probe with soapy water or an antiseptic solution. Do not immerse the probe or bump it against anything hard.
Clean the probe to prevent cross-contamination to other patients. Probes are fragile and may malfunction if bumped against a hard surface.

Evaluation

Especially if pedal pulses are decreased, observe for other indications of inadequate circulation, such as cool skin, decreased capillary refill, and bluish or ashen skin tone. You must provide supporting evidence if you chart that pedal pulses are decreased or absent. The complete absence of a pulse requires immediate intervention.

Patient Teaching

■ Teach the patient about the significance of any abnormalities in pulse rate or rhythm.
■ Explain any interventions that may be needed.

Home Care

Assess the skill level of the person who will be assessing the client's peripheral pulses in the home, and provide instruction if necessary.

Documentation

Usually you will document routine VS, including pulse, on a flow sheet or graphic. If you record it in a nurse's note, document the pulse rate, rhythm, quality, and site (e.g., "radial pulse 64 beats/min, regular, and strong bilaterally").

Practice Resources

Best practices: Evidence-based nursing procedures, 2007; Gyi, 2007; Lockwood, Conroy-Hiller, & Page, 2004; Perk, Stessman, Ginsberg, et al., 2003; Trim, 2005; Vital Signs, 1999.

Thinking about the Procedure

 Go to the **Fundamentals of Nursing Skills Videos, Pulse: Carotid.**

1. Why do you think the nurse might be assessing this patient's carotid pulse?
2. What two landmarks does the nurse use to locate the carotid artery?

 For suggested responses, go to Chapter 19, **Thinking About the Procedure Suggested Responses,** on *DavisPlus.*

Procedure 19-3 ■ Assessing the Apical Pulse

➤ For steps to follow in *all* procedures, refer to the Universal Steps for All Procedures found on the page facing the inside back cover.

Equipment

Watch with a second hand or second readout
Stethoscope
Alcohol wipes (to clean stethoscope)

Delegation

You can delegate measurement of the apical pulse to the NAP if you conclude that the patient's condition and the NAP's skills allow. First perform the following assessments. Then inform the NAP of any special considerations (e.g., to note what the patient's activity has been just before taking the pulse, or to mark the time exactly so you can compare it to the patient's ECG). Ask the NAP to record and report the pulse to you, and to report immediately if it is outside normal limits (you must specify what is "normal" for each patient).

Pre-Procedure Assessments

■ Determine why assessment of the apical pulse is indicated. *Conditions that require assessment of the apical pulse include digitalis therapy, blood loss, cardiac or respiratory disease, or other conditions that affect oxygenation status.*

■ Assess factors that may alter the pulse, such as activity and medications. If the client has been recently active, wait 10 to 15 minutes before obtaining a measurement.

➤ When performing the procedure, always identify your patient according to agency policy and be attentive to standard precautions, hand hygiene, patient safety and privacy, body mechanics, and documentation.

Procedure Steps

1. **With the client supine or sitting, expose the left side of the chest**, but only as much as necessary.
   Prevents distortion of sound from the patient's gown rubbing on the stethoscope, while also protecting the patient's privacy. ▼

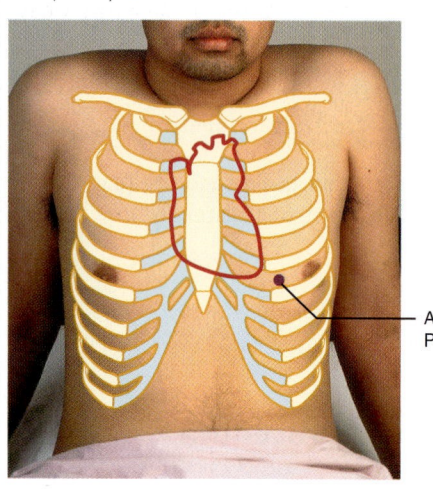

Apex, PMI

2. **Wipe the stethoscope with a 70% alcohol or benzalkonium chloride wipe before and after examining the patient.**
   Cleaning can reduce the bacterial count by up to 100%.

3. **Palpate the 5th intercostal space at the midclavicular line** for the apical pulse.
   The left ventricle of the heart and the point of maximum impulse (PMI) lie in this area. The apical pulse is generally best heard at the PMI, over the apex of the heart.

   a. To locate the 5th intercostal space, slide your finger down from the sternal notch to the angle of Louis (the bump where the manubrium and sternum meet).
   b. Slide your finger over to the left sternal border to the 2nd intercostal space.
   c. Now place your index or ring finger (depending on which hand you use) in the 2nd intercostal space, and count down to the 5th intercostal space by placing a finger in each of the spaces.
   d. Slide over to the midclavicular line, keeping your finger in the 5th intercostal space.

4. **Palpate the apical pulse.**
   a. The palpated apical pulse is also called the PMI.
   b. The pulse area should be about the size of a quarter, without lifts or heaves.
   A larger than normal pulsation may indicate ventricular hypertrophy.

5. **Warm the stethoscope in your hand for 10 seconds. Then place the diaphragm over the PMI, and listen to the normal S_1 and S_2 heart sounds (lub-dub).**
   A cold stethoscope placed on the skin may startle the patient and increase the
heart rate. Heart sounds result when blood moves through the valves of the heart. The first heart sound is louder at the apical area and should be audible when the pulse is auscultated.

 Go to the sound file, **Heart Sounds**, in **Student Resources**, on Davis*Plus*.

6. **Count the apical heart rate for 1 full minute.**
   Ensures accuracy. Because the apical heart rate is needed as an assessment measure for the administration of some medications (e.g., digoxin), accuracy is essential. Some cardiac conditions cause either slow or irregular rates, both of which must be counted for 1 full minute to ensure accuracy.

? What if . . .

■ **The apical rate is less than 60 beats/min?**

   ➤ *Note:* You may also see "bpm" as an abbreviation for "beats per minute.")
   If the patient is taking cardiac medications, withhold them and consult with a physician about whether to adjust dosage.
   Certain cardiac medications (e.g., digoxin) are given to slow the heart rate;

bradycardia may indicate that blood levels are too high.
Assess for chest pain, dizziness, dyspnea. *May indicate decreased cardiac output.*

■ **The apical rate is greater than 100 beats/min?**
Obtain a complete set of vital signs.

Assess for pain, anxiety, fever, dehydration, decreased oxygenation, hypotension, and decreased exercise.
These factors may increase pulse rate.

Evaluation
- Are the findings within normal limits?
- Are there other factors supporting the findings?
- What are the trends over time?
- Is the skin pink, warm, and dry?
- Is there any cyanosis?

Patient Teaching
- Teach the patient about the significance of any abnormalities in the pulse rate or rhythm.
- Explain any interventions that may be necessary.

Home Care
- Assess the skill level of the person who will be assessing the client's apical pulse in the home, and provide instruction if necessary.
- Teach the home caregiver when to hold medications and/or to call primary care provider (e.g., to hold the digitalis if the rate is less than 60 beats/min, or lower than the patient's baseline).
- Before leaving the home, clean the stethoscope with detergent or disinfectant, when possible, or place it in a plastic bag for transporting to the reprocessing location.
- If the patient has a multidrug-resistant organism infection, reusable equipment such as stethoscopes should remain in the home. If the stethoscope cannot remain in the home, clean and disinfect it before leaving the home, using a low- to intermediate-level disinfectant. If this is not practical, place the stethoscope in a plastic bag and transport it to another site for cleaning and disinfection.

Documentation
Document the pulse rate, rhythm, and site.

Sample Nurse's Note:

9/05/15	0900	Apical pulse rate 64, regular and

strong. ————————————————————Janice Jonas, RN

Practice Resources
Best practices, 2007; CDC, 2008; Gyi, 2007; Hwu, Coates, & Lin, 2000; Lockwood, Conroy-Hiller, & Page, 2004; Siegel, Rhinehart, Jackson, et al., 2006; Vital Signs, 1999.

Thinking About the Procedure

Go to the **Fundamentals of Nursing Skills Videos, Pulse: Apical.**

1. How does the nurse position the patient in the video?
2. How is this the same as or different from the position described for this procedure in this textbook?
3. Can you think of any reasons why the nurse in the video may have positioned her client in this manner?

For suggested responses, go to Chapter 19, **Thinking About the Procedure Suggested Responses,** on Davis*Plus.*

Procedure 19-4 ■ Assessing for an Apical–Radial Pulse Deficit

➤ For steps to follow in *all* procedures, refer to the Universal Steps for All Procedures found on the page facing the inside back cover.

Equipment
- Watch or clock with a second hand or second readout
- Procedure gloves, if indicated
- Stethoscope
- Alcohol wipes to clean the stethoscope

Delegation
Instead of delegating measurement of an apical–radial pulse to a NAP, you would most likely ask the NAP to assist you in this procedure because it is best performed by two persons working together.

Pre-Procedure Assessments
- Determine why assessment of pulse deficit is indicated.
  Conditions that require assessment of pulse deficit include digitalis therapy, blood loss, cardiac or respiratory disease, and other conditions that affect oxygenation status.
- Assess factors that may alter the pulse, such as activity and medications.

(continued on next page)

Procedure 19-4 ■ **Assessing for an Apical–Radial Pulse Deficit** (continued)

➤ When performing the procedure, always identify your patient according to agency policy and be attentive to standard precautions, hand hygiene, patient safety and privacy, body mechanics, and documentation.

Procedure Steps

1. **Wipe the stethoscope with a 70% alcohol or benzalkonium chloride wipe before and after examining the patient.**
   Cleaning can reduce the bacterial count by up to 100% and prevent the transmission of microbes.

2. **Expose the left side of the patient's chest**, minimizing patient exposure.
   Prevents distortion of sound from the patient's gown rubbing on the stethoscope and protects privacy.

3. **If two nurses are performing the procedure, place the watch so that the second hand is visible to both nurses.**
   Using one watch increases accuracy of counts.

4. **Nurse 1 palpates the 5th intercostal space at the midclavicular line for the apical pulse, and holds the diaphragm of the stethoscope in place, using firm pressure.**
   Aids in hearing high-pitched sounds and ensures good contact between the diaphragm of the stethoscope and the skin. ➤

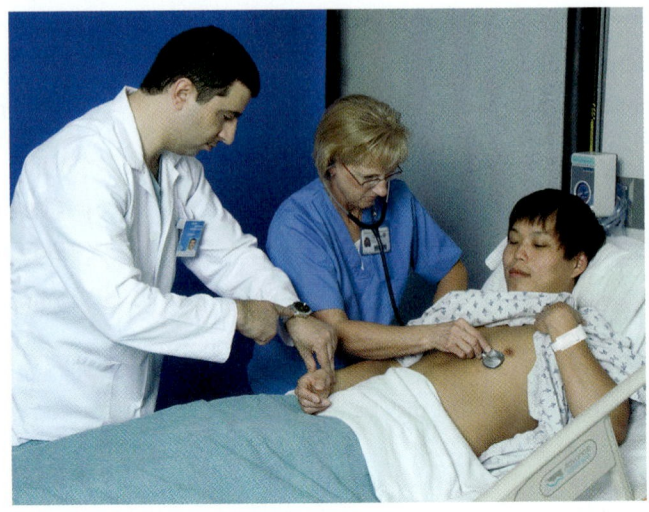

5. **Nurse 2 palpates the radial pulse and assesses rate, rhythm, and quality.**

6. **Nurse 2 says, "Start" when ready to begin and "Stop" when finished. Both nurses count the pulse simultaneously for 1 full minute.**
   Count simultaneously to ensure accuracy. Counting for 1 full minute is necessary for an accurate assessment of any discrepancies that may exist between the two sites.

7. **To obtain pulse deficit, subtract the radial rate from the apical rate.**

   Apical Rate – Radial Rate = Pulse Deficit

   Atrial and ventricular dysrhythmias may cause beats that do not perfuse, so although you hear an apical heart beat, you do not feel a peripheral pulse. The pulse deficit is the number of heartbeats that do not perfuse.

? What if . . .

■ **There is not another nurse available to assist?**

Hold the stethoscope in place with the one hand while palpating the radial pulse with the hand wearing the watch. *Even if you cannot manage to count both rates, you should be able to feel any differences between the apical and radial pulses.*

■ **There has been an increase in pulse deficit since the last measurement?**

An increase in pulse deficit means that the patient's cardiac output has decreased.

Evaluation

■ Identify the presence of an apical-pulse deficit, and compare to previous findings.
■ Assess other measures of cardiopulmonary status to identify a decline in the patient's condition
■ Look for trends.
   The presence of any apical–radial pulse deficit is abnormal.

Patient Teaching

■ Teach the patient about the significance of an apical–radial pulse deficit.
■ Explain any necessary interventions.

Home Care

■ Assess the skill level of the person(s) who will be measuring the client's apical–radial pulse deficit in the home, and provide instruction if necessary.
■ Before leaving the home, clean the stethoscope as described in the Home Care section of Procedure 19-3.

Documentation

■ Document the apical–radial pulse deficit.

Sample Nurse's Note:

09/05/15   0900   *Apical-radial pulse deficit is*
4 beats/min. ————————————Jon Albertson, RN

Practice Resources

Best practices, 2007; CDC, 2008; Jevon, Ewens, & Lowe, 2000; Gyi, 2007; Lockwood, Conroy-Hiller, & Page, 2004; Siegel, Rhinehart, Jackson, et al. 2006; Vital Signs, 1999.

Thinking About the Procedure

 Go to the **Fundamentals of Nursing Skills Videos, Pulse Deficit: Apical–Radial.**

1. Use the visual (non-narrated) video. How did the nurses show respect for the patient's personhood?

2. What safety measures did they demonstrate?
3. At the end of the procedure, what would you assume they did that was not shown on camera?

 For suggested responses, go to Chapter 19, **Thinking About the Procedure Suggested Responses,** on *DavisPlus.*

Procedure 19–5 ■ Assessing Respirations

➤ For steps to follow in *all* procedures, refer to the Universal Steps for All Procedures found on the page facing the inside back cover.

➤ *Note:* To listen to breath sounds,

 Go to **Sound Files: Breath Sounds,** in the **Student Resources,** on DavisPlus.

they are not within the normal range for this patient (specify the range).

Equipment

■ A watch with a second hand (or a wall clock)

Delegation

You can delegate the counting of respirations to the NAP if you conclude that the patient's condition and the NAP's skills allow. Perform the pre-procedure assessments, and inform the NAP of any special considerations (e.g., the need to keep the patient in a certain position). Ask the NAP to record and report the respirations to you, and to report immediately if

Pre-Procedure Assessments

■ Observe for signs of respiratory distress—breathing faster or slower than normal, gasping breaths, confusion, circumoral (around the month) cyanosis.
  Signs of hypoxemia may indicate that the patient is not adequately oxygenated.
■ Determine the baseline respiratory rate and character of respirations.
■ Assess for factors that may affect the respiratory rate (e.g., pain, activity, fever, respiratory disorders).

➤ When performing the procedure, always identify your patient according to agency policy and be attentive to standard precautions, hand hygiene, patient safety and privacy, body mechanics, and documentation.

Procedure Steps

1. **Position the patient.**
   With the patient in a sitting position (preferably), flex the patient's arm, and place her forearm across her chest.
   Aids in counting the patient's pulse rate by making the rise and fall of the chest more discernible and by making the patient less aware that you are measuring the respiratory rate. The patient's awareness might alter the respiratory rate and/or pattern because respirations are partially under voluntary control. ➤

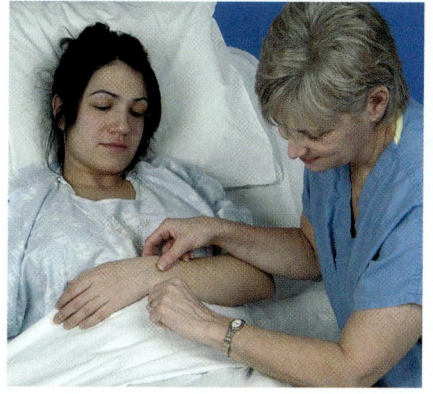

2. **Palpate and count the radial pulse; remember that number.**

Then, keeping your hand on the patient's wrist, count the respirations.
Allows you to count the respirations unobtrusively.

3. **Observe the respiratory rate, rhythm, and depth.**
   a. Rate: Normal for patient's age, fast (tachypnea), or slow (bradypnea)
   b. Rhythm: Regular or irregular
   c. Depth: Normal, shallow, or deep (e.g., Kussmaul's)
   All of these characteristics are necessary to evaluate respiratory status. Different pathologies affect each of these characteristics differently.

(continued on next page)

Procedure 19–5 ▪ **Assessing Respirations** (continued)

4. Count the number of breaths per minute. Begin timing the respirations with a count of 1, not 0, the same as with pulse measurement.

  a. If the respiratory rhythm is regular, count the rate (one inhalation and one exhalation is one respiration) for 30 seconds, and multiply by 2.

  b. If the rhythm is irregular, count the rate for 1 full minute (60 sec). Variations in rhythm may cause an inaccurate rate when counted for less than 1 minute.

? What if . . .

▪ **The patient is an infant?**

Place your hand on the abdomen to assess the respiratory rate. For infants, auscultate breath sounds with a stethoscope.

Infants and young children breathe rapidly and are abdominal breathers, so it is difficult to see each and every rise and fall of the abdomen. Using a stethoscope increases the accuracy of the count, as well as providing information about the breath sounds.

For infants and very young children, count for 1 full minute.

Infants and young children have irregular respirations. Counting for 1 full minute provides a more accurate rate for irregular respirations.

▪ **The patient is receiving oxygen therapy, or requires careful assessment of respiratory status?**

Apply a pulse oximeter (see Procedure 37-2, Monitoring Pulse Oximetry).

Evidence suggests that pulse oximetry is useful for detecting deterioration of physiological function that might otherwise be missed (e.g., during the perioperative period or in seriously ill patients).

Evaluation

▪ Compare the respiratory rate and rhythm with previous readings.

▪ Note other vital signs, especially temperature.

▪ Look for trends, and note whether the respiratory rate and rhythm are changing in conjunction with changes in the other vital signs.

If the patient has an elevated temperature, the respiratory rate will increase. Corresponding elevation in pulse with respiratory rate may indicate hypoxemia. If respirations are not within normal parameters, assess oxygenation with a pulse oximeter.

Patient Teaching

▪ Teach the patient about factors that affect respiratory status, such as smoking and activity.

Home Care

▪ Assess the skill level of the person(s) who will be measuring the client's respiratory rate in the home, and provide instruction as needed.

Documentation

You will document routine VS (including respirations) on a graphic or flow sheet. When a nurse's note is needed, follow these guidelines.

▪ Document the respiratory rate and rhythm.

▪ Document that respirations are either labored or unlabored; if labored, describe in what way (e.g., intercostal retractions, use of accessory muscles, nasal flaring).

Practice Resources

CDC, 2008; Gyi, 2007; Lockwood, Conroy-Hiller, & Page, 2004; "Vital Signs," 1999.

Thinking About the Procedure

 Go to the **Fundamentals of Nursing Skills Videos, Respirations.**

1. Write an example of a nursing note describing Mr. Johnson's respiratory status. Assume that his rate is 12 breaths/min (it may be difficult to count in the video). What else can you observe?

 For suggested responses, go to Chapter 19, **Thinking About the Procedure Suggested Responses,** on Davis*Plus.*

Procedure 19-6 ■ Measuring Blood Pressure

➤ *Note: For steps to follow in* all *procedures, refer to the Universal Steps for All Procedures found on the page facing the inside back cover.*

Equipment

■ Stethoscope

■ ✚ *Note:* Do not wear a stethoscope around your neck. It may become entangled in intravenous and other lines. There is also a risk that a confused or delirious patient could use it to harm you. In addition, wearing a stethoscope can be a source of cross-contamination.

■ 70% alcohol or benzalkonium chloride wipes.
■ Sphygmomanometer with a cuff of the appropriate size. Refer to Figure 19-10, Table 19-6, and Clinical Insight 19-1. *Using a cuff that is too small will result in a false-high reading; using a cuff that is too large will result in a false-low reading.*
  ➤ *Note:* This procedure describes the use of an aneroid manometer or an electronic measuring device.

Delegation

You can delegate measurement of BP to the NAP if you conclude that the patient's condition and the NAP's skills allow. Perform the pre-procedure assessments, and inform the NAP of the site (e.g., radial, brachial) to use. Inform the NAP of any special considerations (e.g., not to place a BP cuff on the same side as the site of a mastectomy). Ask the NAP to record and report the BP to you, and to report immediately if it is outside normal limits (you must specify what is "normal" for each patient). Tell the NAP that if BP is elevated, to note which arm, the patient's position during measurement, and activity immediately preceding the measurement.

Pre-Procedure Assessments

■ Check for factors or activities that may alter the readings. *Caffeine, smoking, exercise, and stress can all elevate the BP. Be certain the patient has been lying or sitting for at least 5 minutes (30 min after strenuous exercise) and is relaxed.*
■ Check the previous recording, if any. *Noting changes over time is important. Because BP changes constantly and because so many factors affect it, you cannot draw conclusions from a single measurement.*
  ➤ *Note:* To improve the accuracy of your readings, also refer to Clinical Insights 19-1 and 19-2.

➤ When performing the procedure, always identify your patient according to agency policy and be attentive to standard precautions, hand hygiene, patient safety and privacy, body mechanics, and documentation.

Procedure Steps

1. **Clean the stethoscope before and after the procedure.**
   Although only a small percentage of microorganisms are pathogenic, cleaning can reduce the bacterial count by 94% to 100%.
2. **Position the patient comfortably,** ensuring that:
   a. The legs are uncrossed, the back is supported, and the feet are resting on the floor (if the patient is sitting in a chair), or that the patient is supine.
      This position allows for the most accurate reading. Crossing the legs may elevate the BP reading.
   b. The measurement arm is being supported at heart level, slightly flexed, with the palm facing upward.
      The blood pressure will be lower if the arm is above the heart and higher if the arm is below the heart or not supported.

3. **Fully expose the arm, being careful that clothing is not tight.** Remove clothing rather than rolling up a sleeve.
   Clothing that is tight enough to restrict blood flow will alter the reading.
4. **Place the cuff on the upper arm.**
   a. Wrap the cuff snugly.
   b. Ensure that the cuff is totally deflated, and palpate the brachial artery.
   c. Place the bottom edge of the cuff approximately 1 in. (2.5 cm) above the antecubital space.
   d. Place the center of the cuff bladder directly over the brachial artery (the center is often indicated with an arrow on the BP cuff).
      The center of the cuff bladder needs to be directly over the brachial artery to obtain an accurate reading. Loose application of the cuff results in overestimation of the pressure. ➤

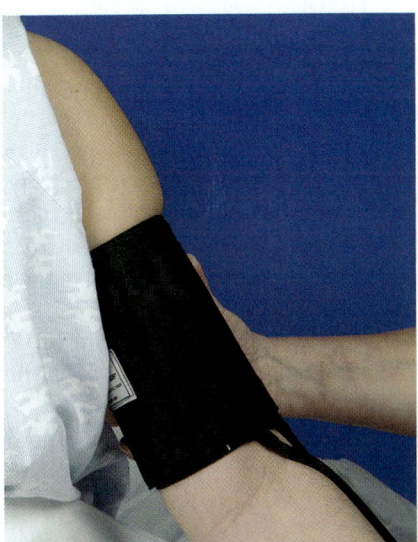

5. **Place the stethoscope earpieces in your ears, pointing slightly forward.**
   Directs sound into the ear canal, making the sounds more audible.
6. **Palpate the brachial artery on the arm with the cuff.** (Use the radial artery for this step if you prefer.)

(continued on next page)

Procedure 19-6 ■ **Measuring Blood Pressure** (continued)

7. Inflate the cuff, as follows:

a. Close the sphygmomanometer valve and inflate the cuff rapidly to about 80 mm Hg.

b. Then palpate the pulse while you continue inflating in 10 mm Hg increments until you no longer feel the pulse.

c. Note the pressure at which the pulse disappears.

d. Go to step 8 or the variation, as you prefer.

These steps ensure that the cuff is inflated higher than the systolic BP. If the patient has an auscultatory gap, the systolic pressure can be mistakenly identified as lower than it actually is. Palpation is particularly important if the baseline systolic BP is unknown or if the patient is hypertensive.

8. Continue inflating the cuff to a pressure that is 20 to 30 mm Hg above the level at which the pulse disappeared.

Helps ensure that you will not miss an auscultatory gap or a faint first sound.

Variation in Cuff Inflation Technique

■ Do not continue palpating after the pulse disappears; instead, deflate the cuff rapidly.

■ Wait 2 minutes, then place the stethoscope over the brachial artery and inflate the cuff to a pressure that is 20 to 30 mm Hg above the palpated level.

■ Continue with steps 9 and 10.

9. Place the stethoscope over the brachial artery as follows: ▼

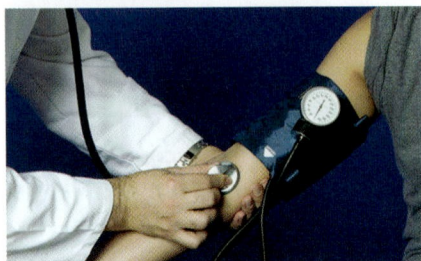

a. Be certain that the stethoscope tubing is not touching anything and that the diaphragm is not tucked under the edge of the cuff.

When the tubing rubs against clothing, for example, it produces artifact

sounds that make it difficult to hear the BP sounds. Placing the bell or diaphragm under the cuff can partially occlude the brachial artery, delaying the appearance of the Korotkoff sounds.

b. Using the bell will enable you to hear BP sounds more accurately, especially at diastolic pressures. However, most people use the diaphragm because it is easily placed and because some stethoscopes do not have a bell.

10. Deflate the cuff slowly (2 to 3 mm Hg per second or per beat), listening for the Korotkoff sounds as you deflate.

Deflating the cuff too slowly increases patient discomfort and may alter the reading. Deflating the cuff too fast may cause errors in hearing the Korotkoff sounds.

a. Note the point on the manometer at which you hear the first sound. This is the systolic BP. (If you are using an electronic BP device, read the digital screen when the numbers appear. Follow the manufacturer's instructions.)

The first Korotkoff sound is the systolic pressure.

b. Continue deflating the cuff, and note the level at which the sounds become muffled and disappear. The diastolic pressure is the point at which the sound disappears.

The fifth Korotkoff sound (the disappearance of sound) is the diastolic BP in adults. The fourth Korotkoff sound (the muffling of sounds) is the diastolic BP in children. The American Heart Association (AHA) recommends recording the first sound, muffling, and last sound in children younger than 13 years, pregnant women, and people with high cardiac output or peripheral vasoconstriction.

11. If you need to repeat the measurement, deflate the cuff completely, and wait 2 minutes before reinflating it.

Prevents venous congestion and false high readings.

? What if . . .

■ **You cannot feel the brachial pulse?**

While supporting the arm at the elbow, have the patient pronate her forearm. *This moves the brachial artery more over a bony prominence, making the pulsation easier to feel.*

■ **You have difficulty hearing BP sounds for many patients?**

You may need a stethoscope with a built-in amplifier.

■ **You are not certain of the systolic reading when you begin to deflate the cuff?**

Do not stop cuff deflation to recheck the systolic reading. Deflate the cuff completely and wait 1 to 3 minutes before taking another measurement. *Stopping deflation and retaking the BP too soon can lead to a muffling of the Korotkoff sounds and inaccurate results.*

■ **You must use a mercury manometer?**

If you must use a mercury manometer, be certain the meniscus of the mercury is at eye level when taking the reading.

✚ Take care not to bump equipment against the glass cover over the column of mercury. *Because mercury is a health hazard, always use an aneroid manometer or an electronic BP device if one is available.*

■ **You are using an automatic blood pressure device?**

Follow the same guidelines as for a manual BP (e.g., cuff size and placement, patient position).

Turn on the machine; be sure the cuff is deflated.

Apply the cuff.

Press the button to start the measurement.

At the tone, read the digital measurement.

■ **You do not have a cuff size to fit the upper arm?**

Use the forearm, thigh, or calf. See **Procedure Variations A, B, and C,** respectively.

- **The patient requires contact or isolation precautions?**

Follow agency guidelines for equipment (e.g., stethoscope, BP cuff). Generally, the equipment remains in the room with the patient; otherwise it must be disinfected before leaving the room. For information about contact precautions and protective isolation, see Chapter 22.

Procedure Variation A.
Measuring Blood Pressure in the Forearm

- Place a properly sized cuff on the forearm, midway between the elbow and the wrist. Auscultate over the radial artery.
- Note that a forearm reading is not interchangeable with an upper arm reading.

Procedure Variation B.
Measuring Blood Pressure in the Thigh

- Use the thigh or the calf if the cuff will not fit either the upper or lower arm.
  - ➤ Note: The thigh systolic measure may be 20 to 30 mm Hg higher than an arm BP reading. The diastolic reading is generally comparable.
- Place the patient in a prone position. If patient cannot be prone, place supine with knee slightly bent.
- Choose the correct cuff size. Wrap the cuff snugly around the thigh so that the lower edge of the cuff is approximately 1 in. (2.5 cm) above the popliteal fossa and the center of the cuff bladder is positioned directly over the popliteal artery (often indicated with an arrow on the blood pressure cuff).
- Palpate and auscultate over the popliteal artery. ▼

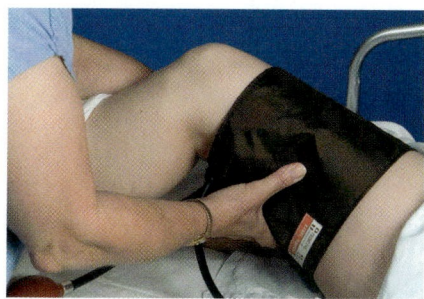

Procedure Variation C.
Measuring Blood Pressure in the Calf

- Use the thigh or the calf if the cuff will not fit either the upper or lower arm.

- Place the patient supine.
- Choose the correct size cuff. Wrap the cuff snugly around the calf so that the lower edge of the cuff is approximately 2.5 cm above the malleoli or ankle.
- Place the stethoscope over either the dorsalis pedis or the posterior tibial artery. Calf BP measurements are not equivalent to upper arm measurements in adults; they tend produce a higher systolic BP.

Procedure Variation D.
Palpating the Blood Pressure

- Apply the cuff, and palpate for the radial or brachial pulse.
- Begin to inflate the cuff. When you can no longer feel the pulse, inflate the cuff about 30 mm Hg more.
- As you release the valve and slowly deflate the cuff, note the reading on the manometer at which you once again feel the pulse.
- Record the palpated blood pressure according to the way it was assessed (e.g., "Palpated, low Fowler's, left arm 86/——" [or "86 systolic"]).

Evaluation

- Compare the BP reading with previous readings.
- Look for trends. Is the BP slowly decreasing (e.g., impending shock) or slowly increasing (e.g., hypervolemia)?
- Look for a corresponding change in pulse rate, indicating potential hypoxemia.
- If this is the first BP measurement for the client, check readings in both arms.
  A difference of 10 mm Hg or less is normal.
- Report any significant changes in the BP reading.

Patient Teaching

Teach the patient about:
- Normal BP values (keep in mind that prehypertension is diagnosed at a lower level when using self-monitored readings).
- Significance of the BP reading.
- Further follow-up that may be necessary.

Home Care

- The AHA and other guidelines recommend self-monitoring of BP at home.
- Assess the skill level of the person(s) who will be measuring the patient's BP in the home, and provide instruction if necessary.

- If possible, use the same equipment each time to prevent false changes in measurement.
- Assess whether self-monitoring is causing the client to be anxious.
  Some clients do become overly anxious when they know they must monitor their BP, or when they obtain a high reading. Self-monitoring should not be used if it produces too much anxiety; this raises the BP even more.
- Teach clients not to change their medication dosage without consulting their primary provider when their BP goes up or down.

- ✚ Before leaving the home, clean the stethoscope and sphygmomanometer with detergent or disinfectant, when possible; or place them in a plastic bag for transporting to the reprocessing location.

- ✚ If the client has an infection with a multidrug-resistant organism, reusable equipment such as stethoscopes should remain in the home. If the stethoscope and sphygmomanometer cannot remain in the home, clean and disinfect them before leaving the home, using a low- to intermediate-level disinfectant. If this is not practical, place them in a plastic bag and transport them to another site for cleaning and disinfection.

- Also see the Home Care box.

(continued on next page)

Procedure 19-6 ■ Measuring Blood Pressure (continued)

Documentation

- You will usually document BP on a flow sheet.
- Document the blood pressure systolic/diastolic readings (e.g., 130/80).
- If you hear the 4th Korotkoff sound or muffling, document systolic/muffling/diastolic (e.g., 130/80/70).
- If you hear an auscultatory gap, document "systolic/diastolic with an auscultatory gap from . . ." For example, "170/90 with an auscultatory gap from 170 to 140 mm Hg."
- Follow agency policy regarding the recording of muffled sounds.
- If you chose an alternate site, document the site used and the reason for not using the upper arm.

Practice Resources

American Association of Critical-Care Nurses, 2010; American Heart Association. n.d.; British Hypertension Society, Hypertension Influence Team, 2006; CDC, 2008; Gyi, 2007; Joint National Committee on Prevention, Detection, Evaluation, and Treatment of High Blood Pressure, 2004; Lockwood, Conroy-Hiller, & Page, 2004; Rhinehart, 2001; Pickering, Hall, Appel, et al., 2005; Siegel, Rhinehart, Jackson, et al., 2006; Vital Signs, 1999.

Thinking About the Procedure

 Go to the **Fundamentals of Nursing Skills Videos, Blood Pressure: Manual and Automatic.**

1. At the beginning of the procedure, using the manual method (with an aneroid manometer), the nurse places her left hand on the patient's legs for a moment. Why did she do that?
2. What size cuff did the nurse use?
3. When using the automatic device, how many times did the nurse press on the machine? For what reasons did she do so?

 For suggested responses, go to Chapter 19, **Thinking About the Procedure Suggested Responses,** on *DavisPlus*.

 To explore learning resources for this chapter,

 Go to DavisPlus at http://davisplus.fadavis.com/Treas1

Chapter Resources for Chapter 19:
 Knowledge Check and Think Like a Nurse Response Sheets
 Knowledge Check Answers
 Resources for Caregivers and Health Professionals
 Reading More About Vital Signs (Suggested Readings)
 What Are the Main Points in This Chapter?
NCLEX-Style Review Questions
Chapter Overview Podcasts

Concept Map

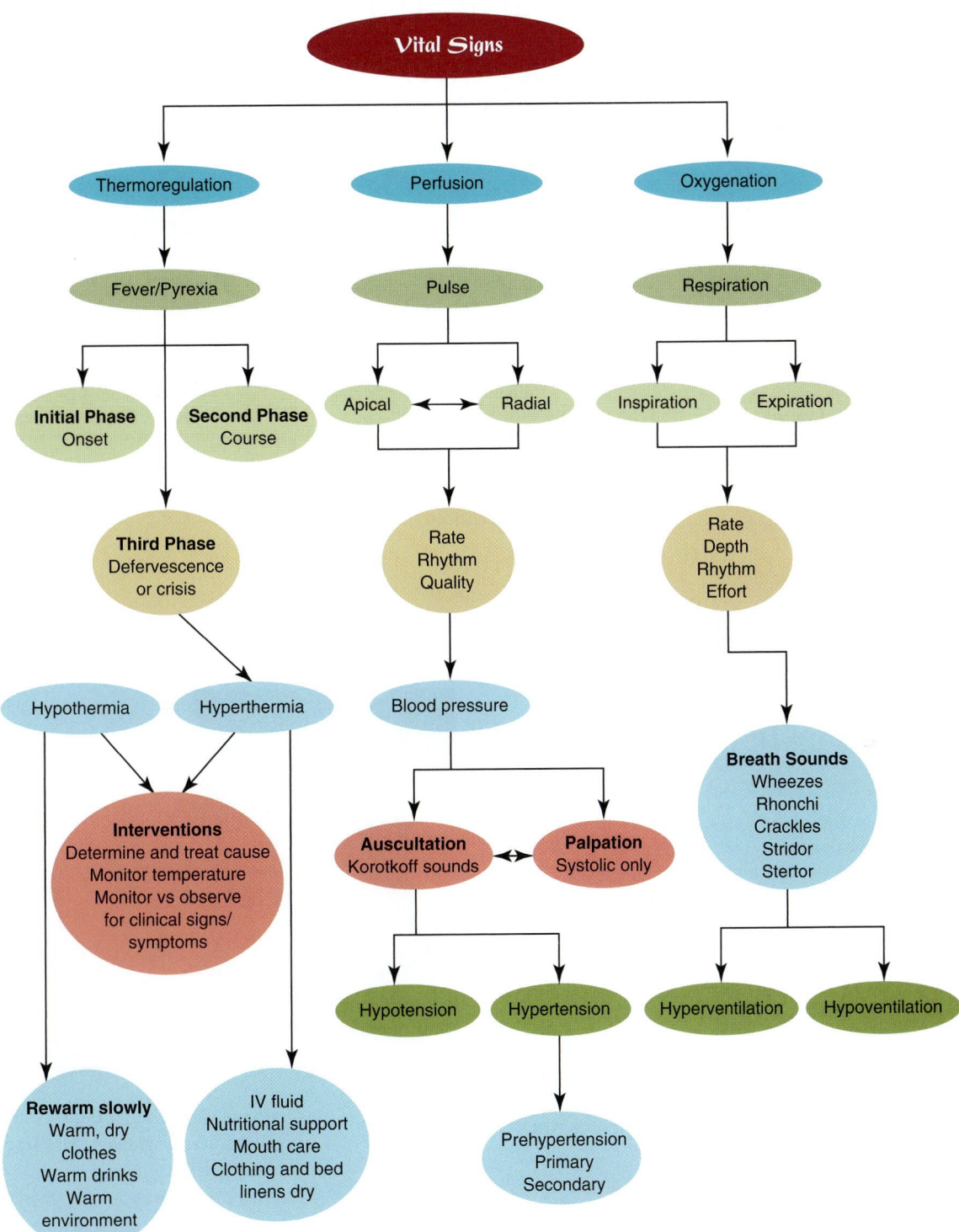

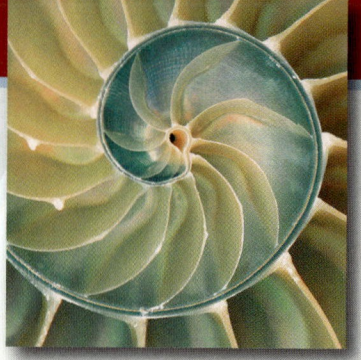

CHAPTER 20

Communicating & Therapeutic Relationships

Learning Outcomes

After completing this chapter, you should be able to:

➤ Define *communication*.

➤ Identify the three basic levels of communication.

➤ Discuss the elements of the communication process.

➤ List the characteristics of verbal and nonverbal communication.

➤ Analyze factors that influence the communication process.

➤ Describe the elements of collaborative professional communication.

➤ Describe the role of communication in each of the four phases of the therapeutic relationship.

➤ Compare and contrast techniques that enhance communication to techniques that hinder communication.

➤ Communicate with clients with impaired hearing, speech, or cognition.

➤ Communicate with clients whose culture or language is different from yours.

➤ Write a nursing care plan for a client experiencing impaired communication.

Key Concepts

Communication
Communication techniques
Therapeutic relationships

Related Concepts

See the Concept Map at the end of this chapter.

Caring for the Nguyens

This feature allows you to practice the kind of thinking you will use as a full-spectrum nurse. There is usually more than one correct answer to a critical thinking question, so we do not provide answers for these features. It is more important to develop your nursing judgment than to "cover content." Discuss the questions with your peers. If you are still unsure, consult your instructor.

Below is a transcript of an interaction that occurred during Nam Nguyen's first visit to the family healthcare clinic. As you may recall, Zach Jackson is a family nurse practitioner who is examining Nam Nguyen. Analyze the interaction. Identify open-ended and closed questions and therapeutic communication techniques. Comment on responses that Zach might have improved on.

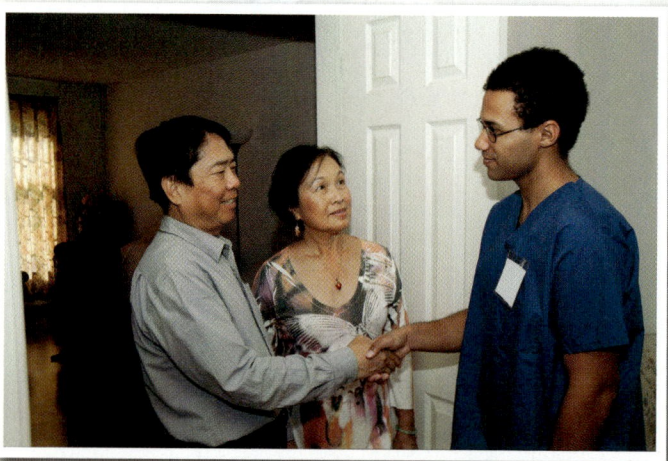

Zach: "Are your parents still living?"
Nam: "Yes, they're both alive. My father is 80 years old and my mother is 76."
Zach: "I'd like to hear a little more about your family history. Tell me about your father's cancer. How old was he when he was first diagnosed? Has he had treatment?"
Nam: "He was probably about 60 when he first found out about it. I know he had some kind of surgery and takes medicines, but I don't know the details. He seems all right though."

(Continued)

Caring for the Nyugens (continued)

Zach: "Your father also has high blood pressure and heart disease. Please tell me a little more about that."

Nam: "My father and mother both have high blood pressure and heart disease. They both take medicines for their blood pressure. My father had a small heart attack about 10 years ago. My mother has never had a heart attack that I know of, but she sometimes has chest pain."

Zach: "Your mother also has diabetes?"

Nam: "She's had that for a long time. A lot of people in my family, especially on my father's side, have diabetes but nobody in my mother's family. Yet my mother is the one with the diabetes!"

Yen: "A lot of people in my family have diabetes, too. But so far I'm OK, I think.

Zach: "Have you had a health exam lately, Mrs. Nguyen?"

Yen: "Not in about a year, but I'm going to schedule an appointment here."

Go to **Caring for the Nguyens Response Sheet** on *DavisPlus*.

Meet Your Patient

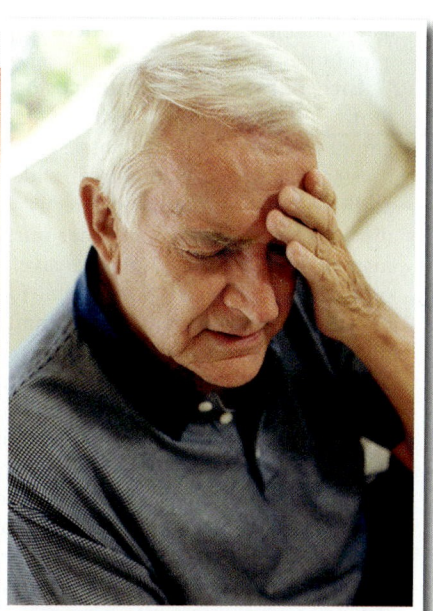

You have been assigned to care for John Barker, a 56-year-old man admitted to the hospital with bleeding in the lower gastrointestinal (GI) tract. When you approach Mr. Barker to introduce yourself, you find him in his room with his wife at the bedside. They are holding hands, and clearly both have been crying. You begin by saying, "Good afternoon, Mr. Barker, I am a nursing student from the nearby university. I've been assigned to care for you tomorrow." Mr. Barker swallows hard and says, "I don't think you'll be able to do anything for me!" His wife says, "Don't take it personally. It's not a good time right now. Please just leave us alone."

You leave the room, unsure how to respond. When you go to the unit station to review the chart, the charge nurse says, "Oh my! You've been assigned to him? I hope you've got a lot of experience." As you review the chart, you realize that Mr. Barker was just informed that he has metastatic colon cancer and probably has only a few months to live.

Theoretical Knowledge knowing why

As a resource to you while you are learning what it means to care for patients in difficult situations such as Mr. Barker's, you might look to the following professional and regulatory agencies that stress the importance of good communication:

Quality and Safety Education for Nurses (QSEN). To provide for patient safety, nurses need to effectively communicate their concerns about hazards and errors to patients, families, and the healthcare team (Cronenwett, Sherwood, Barnsteiner, et al., 2007).

- **The Joint Commission (2011). The Joint Commission National Patient Safety Goal 2** aims to improve patient safety by improving communication among caregivers.

- **The Joint Commission (2008).** Performance standards state that patients have the right to receive effective, understandable information.

ABOUT THE KEY CONCEPTS

In this chapter you will learn how communication techniques link to the concept of communication, and how they both help you to form therapeutic relationships. With an understanding of these and the related concepts, you will be able to communicate more effectively with patients, families, and members of the healthcare team.

WHAT IS COMMUNICATION?

Communication is a dynamic, reciprocal process of sending and receiving messages. The messages may be verbal, nonverbal, or both, and they may involve two or more people. As such, communication forms the basis for sharing

meaning, expressing needs, and building effective working relationships among individuals, families, and the health-care team.

Communication is more than the act of talking and listening (Box 20-1). It is a basic function of human life. From the first cry of a newborn to the whisper of a patient who is dying, the primary purpose of communication is to share information and obtain a response.

Communication Occurs on Three Levels

When we think about communication, we usually imagine a dialogue between two individuals. But communication actually occurs on any of three levels.

Intrapersonal Communication is conscious internal dialogue, sometimes known as self-talk. Constructive affirmations, or positive self-talk (e.g., "This will work! I can do it"), promote success in a task. In contrast, negative self-talk (e.g., "I can't do this, it is too difficult") may adversely affect a person's ability to complete a task. Nurses often engage in intrapersonal communication. For example, if you enter a room and notice that your patient is pale, diaphoretic (perspiring profusely), and moaning, you may ask yourself, "What's happened? This client appears to be in a lot of pain."

Interpersonal Communication occurs between two or more people. Nurses use interpersonal communication to gather information during assessment, to teach about health issues, to explain care, and to provide comfort and support. In addition to communicating directly with clients, professional nurses communicate with other nurses and healthcare team members to provide comprehensive care for clients. Because professional nurses are accountable for appropriate delegation of activities, they must also communicate effectively with nursing assistive personnel (NAP).

Group Communication is interaction occurring among more than two people. *Small-group communication* occurs when you engage in an exchange of ideas with two or more individuals at the same time. Examples of small-group communication include staff meetings, committee meetings, educational groups, self-help groups, and family teaching sessions. Working with groups requires effective communication skills and a basic understanding of group processes—discussed later in the chapter.

Public speaking is a unique form of group communication. Generally, the speaker addresses a large group (but it may be only a few people) with varying degrees of interaction. Nurses engage in public speaking to educate groups of people about health issues, to lobby for health legislation, and to address colleagues at professional conferences.

BOX 20-1 ■ What Is Communication?

Communication is . . .
- Sharing or transmitting thoughts or feelings
- A way to meet physical, psychosocial, emotional, and spiritual needs
- A process—the act of sending, receiving, interpreting, and reacting to a message
- Content—the actual subject matter, words, gestures, and substance of the message

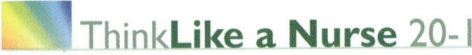

KnowledgeCheck 20-1

- What is the purpose of communication?
- Describe the three levels of communication.
- What level of communication was used in the Meet Your Patient scenario?

ThinkLike a Nurse 20-1

Evaluate your own skills with the three levels of communication.

Communication Involves Content

Communication has two major components: content and process. The **content** of communication is the actual subject matter, words, gestures, and substance of the message. It is the message that everyone can hear or see. For example, suppose your client said, "I slept through lunch." This statement is open to interpretation. It does not tell you whether he thinks this is a good thing because he wanted or needed rest, or a bad thing because he is so exhausted, or a complaint about the staff because they did not wake him for lunch, or an apology and request for a late lunch. As you can see, the words are just a part of communication. You must also consider the process.

Communication Is a Process

Process refers to the act of sending, receiving, interpreting, and reacting to a message. Figure 20-1 illustrates the relationship among the following five elements of the communication process.

- The **sender** begins the conversation to deliver a message (content) to another person. The sender, also called the *source* or the *encoder,* uses verbal and nonverbal methods to transmit the message.
- **Encoding** refers to the process of selecting the words, gestures, tone of voice, signs, and symbols used to transmit the message. For example, as a beginning nursing student, you might feel anxious about caring for Mr. Barker (Meet Your Patient). How could you communicate your concerns to your instructor? You might directly state, "It makes me nervous to be assigned to him." You might avoid eye contact with your instructor and tell her, "I'm going to need some help today." Both styles communicate your anxiety, but they are encoded differently.
- The **message** is the verbal and/or nonverbal information the sender communicates. It might be content of a conversation, a speech, a gesture, a letter, and so forth. Effective messages are complete, clear, concise, organized, timely, and expressed in a manner that the receiver can understand. The message must be appropriate for the situation and for the developmental level of the person receiving the message.
- The **channel** is the medium used to send the message. Face-to-face communication is a commonly used channel. Nurses frequently use touch as a nonverbal way to communicate caring and concern. Other channels include written pamphlets, audiovisual aids, recordings, telephone and text messages, and the Internet. When choosing the best channel for communicating, consider the type of message, its purpose, and the size of the audience.
- The **receiver** is the observer, listener, and interpreter of the message. Interpretation, also called **decoding,** refers to relating the message to your past experiences to determine the

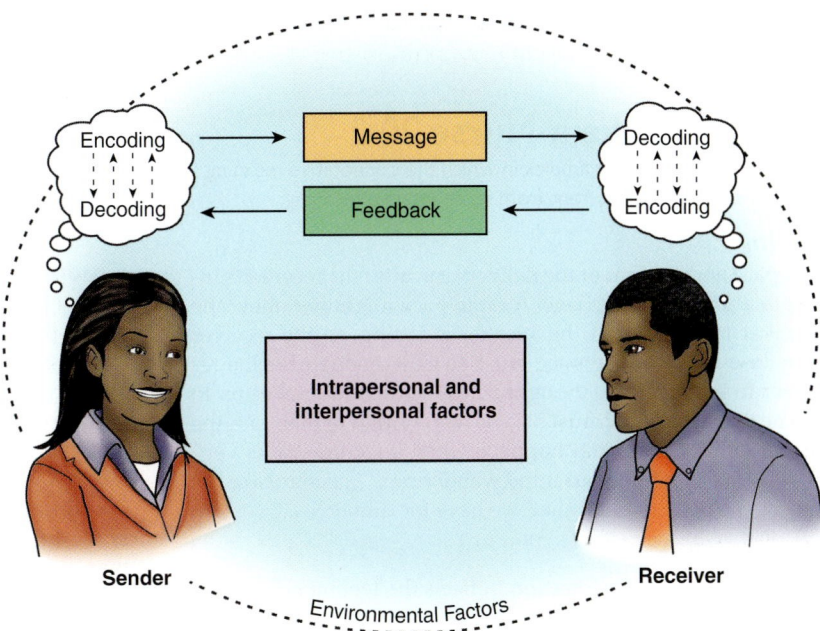

FIGURE 20-1 Communication: A sender encodes and transmits a message to a receiver, who decodes it and transmits feedback.

sender's meaning. The receiver uses visual, auditory, and tactile senses to decode the message. If the decoded meaning matches the intended meaning, then the message was effective. However, messages are sometimes misinterpreted, especially when the receiver is not physically or emotionally ready to receive the message. For example, if you approached your instructor to discuss your concerns about your patient when she was assisting with an emergency, she might be unable to receive your message.

- **Feedback** may be verbal, nonverbal, or both. Once the receiver has received and interpreted the message, he may be stimulated to respond by providing feedback to the sender. Feedback validates that the receiver received the message and understood it as the sender intended. Verifying the message avoids confusion.

KnowledgeCheck 20-2

Using the Meet Your Patient scenario, identify at least one sender, one message, one receiver, one channel, and one example of feedback.

Verbal Communication

People send and receive messages both verbally and nonverbally. The two forms of communication occur spontaneously and simultaneously. **Verbal communication** is the use of spoken and written words to send a message. It is influenced by educational background, culture, language, age, and past experiences. Verbal communication is generally a conscious act in which the sender is able to select the most effective words to communicate a message. When delivering a verbal message, your goal is for the receiver to understand both your words and your meaning. Keep in mind the many factors, following, that affect how a message is received.

Vocabulary

Healthcare workers have a large vocabulary of technical terms and jargon. However, laypersons are often unfamiliar with the language of healthcare and find its use intimidating

or at best, puzzling. Consider the following example, in which a nurse says:

> You are scheduled for surgery tomorrow. You need to be NPO after 2400. I'll be in to prep the op site at about 8. You'll need to void before your pre-med. After that we'll move you to a gurney and transfer you to the holding area.

Do you think most clients would understand this message? Do *you* understand all the words? How much better it would be if the nurse had said:

> Your surgery will be tomorrow morning. You will not be able to eat or drink anything after midnight. I'll come in about 8 in the morning to clean your hip and get it ready for your surgery. Then you'll need to urinate before I give you some medicine to relax you. After that, we'll put you on a cart and roll you up to the operating area.

Use medical terms only when you are certain that the listener will understand them. When encoding a message, consider the receiver's age, knowledge, education, and any cultural differences, including primary language spoken. (These factors are discussed shortly.)

Denotative and Connotative Meaning

Denotation is the literal (dictionary) meaning of a word. **Connotation** is the implied or emotional meaning of the word. Consider the following examples:

A mother says to her infant, "Don't cry, Baby."
A 40-year-old man says to his nurse, "Would you rub my back, Baby?"
A 10-year-old boy says to another boy, "You're a baby!"

The denotative meaning of *baby* is a very young child who is not yet able to walk. However, the connotative meaning is different in each example. In the first example, the connotative meaning is the same as the denotative meaning. In the second example, the nurse might interpret it as a sexist remark; and in the last example, the 10-year-old boy undoubtedly meant *baby* as an insult. As you can see, words are often value laden or

biased. Use terms that provide clear, objective data and are not open for misinterpretation.

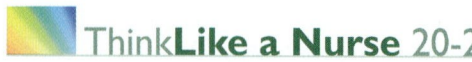

ThinkLike a Nurse 20-2

Think of two other examples in which the connotative meaning of a word may be different from its denotative meaning.

Pacing

The pace and rhythm of the delivery can alter the receiver's interpretation of the message. A rapid pace might not allow the receiver to track what the speaker is saying, so the receiver may lose interest. The pace must be slow enough for the receiver to interpret one thought before the sender moves on to the next thought, but must also be fast enough to maintain the listener's interest. What happens when a lecturer talks very slowly? Do you find your mind wandering? "I need to take the dog to the vet. . . . What shall we have for dinner? . . ."

Intonation

"Tone of voice," or **intonation**, reflects the feeling behind the words. We get a sense of a person's intonation by listening to the *pitch* (high or low), *cadence* (rising and falling of the pitch), and *volume* (soft or loud). For example, experiment with the variety of ways you might say, "Your test results are in."

Pitch, cadence, and volume can either reinforce or contradict the message while conveying various emotions. People tend to tune out when someone speaks in a monotone (does not vary the pitch, cadence, and volume). Before presenting lengthy information, whether to an individual or to a group, experiment with pitch, cadence, and volume to ensure that the listener remains engaged with your topic.

When electronic messaging is used, the receiver does not have the advantage of intonation or body language. This may lead to miscommunication. People sometimes insert *emoticons* (symbols such as "smiley faces") or uppercase to provide cues to the emotional tone of a message.

Clarity and Brevity

Clarity in communication requires that you select words that convey the intended meaning and that you make sure your spoken words and the nonverbal language send the same message. You can achieve brevity by using the fewest words possible. A conversation that is clear and brief holds the interest of all parties and effectively conveys the intended messages.

Timing and Relevance

Timing is crucial. Before starting a conversation, assess your client. A person who is distracted by pain, hunger, or other physiological needs will not receive the message as you intended it. Similarly, a client attempting to cope with stressors, such as limited finances, an upcoming surgery, or a terminal diagnosis, may be unable to listen effectively. Consider the following principles of timing and relevance.

Consider the Presence of Others. Asking a client about a personal issue in a public place may inhibit his response. You will receive a different response if you ask the same question in a more private setting. In contrast, if you are instructing a client about a recommended diet, be sure that the person who is responsible for shopping and cooking is also present. If your client does neither in his household, he may pay little attention to your instruction—it will not be relevant to him.

Communication Is Effective When Both Parties Value the Interaction and Find the Discussion Relevant. To teach your client about his medicines, begin by reminding him of the purpose of the discussion: "I'm going to teach you how to take this medication so that it effectively controls your pain."

The Interaction Must Allow Time for Response. A rapid flow of questions or one-sided conversations inhibit interaction.

Credibility

Clients judge the **credibility** (or believability) of the message on the trustworthiness of the sender. Your credibility depends on a pattern of honest, factual, and timely response to patient concerns, as well as congruence between your verbal and nonverbal communication.

Give Information Only If You Are Certain of the Facts. As a nurse, you will be called on to provide information on a wide range of topics. A response such as "I don't know, but I'll find out and let you know" is far more credible than an incorrect answer or guess.

Never Lie to or Mislead the Patient. Lying can take many forms, but it always destroys trust. If you tell the patient you will be right back with pain medication but forget to return until she reminds you an hour later, she may doubt your credibility.

If a Situation Makes You Uncomfortable, It Is Better to Acknowledge Your Discomfort Than to Risk Loss of Credibility. For example, you may feel uncomfortable talking to Mr. Barker (Meet Your Patient) about his recent diagnosis. You may be tempted to say, "Maybe the test results are wrong," or "The time line is just a guess. I think you can beat this." This approach avoids uncomfortable discussion and may make the patient feel better temporarily. However, a more honest approach would be to tell Mr. Barker that you would like him to meet with a counselor or hospital chaplain.

To Be Credible, Your Nonverbal Communication Must Match Your Spoken Words. For example, if your client asks you if his wound is "ugly," he will pay attention to your facial expressions as well as your spoken response. If you respond that "The wound looks good," but frown or fail to make eye contact, the client will most likely believe that you are not being completely honest. This may jeopardize future interactions.

Humor

Laughter can create physiological changes that contribute to well-being and provide an emotional release. However, use humor cautiously. Humor is highly subjective and personal; it also depends on cultural norms. Use humor cautiously, and never direct humor at the client, disease process, or treatment team. Misused humor can have a negative effect on self-esteem, self-confidence, or the client's confidence in the treatment team. As an example of appropriate use of humor, imagine that you notice that an older patient thoroughly enjoys visits from his young grandchildren. You might consider sharing with him an amusing story about your own children.

Nonverbal Communication

Nonverbal communication (or body language) is the exchange of messages without the use of words. Verbal communication is a highly conscious activity; nonverbal communication occurs on a more unconscious level. Because nonverbal language emerges from how the sender is feeling, it more accurately conveys the true meaning of a message. It may thereby reinforce or contradict the spoken message.

Your patient's body language, including posture and eye gaze, can tell you how he is coping with what he is hearing and how he is processing the information. When speaking to your patient who is sitting or lying in bed, it is helpful to crouch or kneel down to be at eye level, rather than speaking from an elevated, standing position. This can put him at ease and help form a genuine connection. Eye contact, common language, and face-to-face interactions are certainly important; however, genuine empathy and warmth are the most powerful in making a connection with your patient and fostering good communication. For example, Mr. Barker (Meet Your Patient) uses few words. However, he is tearful and distressed. That body language gives you valuable insight into how he is adjusting to the news of his cancer. Let's look at some nonverbal messages.

Facial Expression

Expressions of the face and especially the eyes are some of the most obvious forms of nonverbal communication. Facial expressions communicate joy, anger, sadness, concern, or fear. Raised eyebrows, staring, squinting, or darting eyes all convey meaning.

The interpretation of many facial expressions is culturally dependent. For example, downcast eyes may indicate sadness, poor self-esteem, a desire to avoid the conversation, respect, powerlessness, or submissive behavior. In Western cultures, eye contact usually indicates an interest in the conversation and a willingness to communicate; however, in Eastern cultures, the amount of eye contact considered acceptable varies. Chapter 15 discusses cultural variations.

A mismatch between your verbal message and facial expression may cause the client to doubt your credibility (Fig. 20-2). For example, suppose that a patient states, "I just had my pain pill. Why is my pain still so bad?" You answer, "The medication should take effect within a few more minutes. If it doesn't, call me." Imagine what different effects this reply would have if you were smiling, frowning, raising one eyebrow, or avoiding eye contact.

Posture and Gait

Body position, gait, and posture offer clues to a person's attitudes, emotions, physical well-being, and self-concept. When you see someone with an erect posture, head held high, and a quick gait, what do you think? In Western culture, these are nonverbal indicators of health and a sense of self-assuredness. In contrast, a slow, shuffling gait may signify someone who is ill, is depressed, or has poor self-esteem.

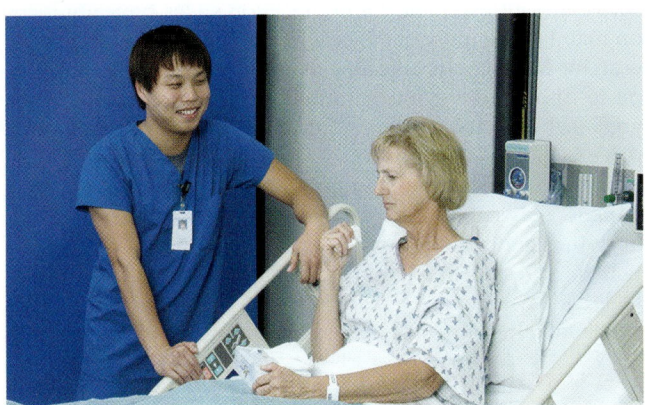

FIGURE 20-2 The nurse's facial expression is not appropriate because the patient appears to be in distress.

Personal Appearance

Clothing and personal appearance provide clues to a person's feelings, socioeconomic status, culture, and religion. A person who is ill, tired, or depressed may lack energy for hygiene and grooming. Lack of attention to personal appearance is especially significant in a person who typically engages in meticulous grooming. As with all nonverbal data, you need to investigate the meaning of personal appearance to avoid drawing erroneous conclusions.

Dress and accessories are powerful cultural clues. Does the patient dress in a style that differs from local custom? Are pieces of jewelry or religious medallions visible? These are clues to the patient's values as well as the patient's socioeconomic status, livelihood, and religion, for instance. Pay attention to these clues, but do not make assumptions from them. A person who wears an elaborate religious medal may like the ornamentation but not espouse the beliefs that are attached to the symbol.

Have you thought about what your own personal appearance conveys to your patients and colleagues? As a nurse, you must also consider how patients perceive you and whether your appearance helps or hinders your patient relationships. Issues of safety and cleanliness are also essential for nurses, when choosing clothing, hairstyles, and body adornment (e.g., jewelry, nail polish, tattoos, body piercings). The traditional white nursing uniform has been almost completely replaced by "scrub clothes" of various colors, which makes it difficult for patients to differentiate nurses from the rest of the healthcare team. To counteract this, some agencies are assigning colors for various workers (e.g., blue for physicians, purple for nurses).

Gestures

Hand and body gestures emphasize and clarify the spoken word. They are good indicators of the feeling tone behind the conversation. Imagine that your client says, "I'm OK." What might it mean if he accompanies his statement with raised arms? What might it mean if, instead, he lowers his head to his hands?

Gestures vary among individuals and cultures, so use them with caution. For example, consider the gesture of a V made with the second and third fingers of the hand. To some people, this is a peace sign; to others, it is a victory sign; and still others may attach no meaning to it at all. Gestures can help you communicate with individuals with impaired verbal communication.

Touch

Touch can convey affection, caring, concern, and encouragement. However, you must use it with conscious awareness of the situation, environment, culture, and receptivity of the patient. Avoid using touch when dealing with someone who is angry or mentally disturbed because the touch may be misinterpreted (e.g., as a sign of aggression or sexual attraction).

See Clinical Insight 20-1 for examples of therapeutic nonverbal behaviors and how patients may interpret them.

KnowledgeCheck 20-3

- Identify the components of verbal and nonverbal communication.
- What action should you take when there is a discrepancy between the client's spoken word and nonverbal body language?

Clinical Insight 20-1 ➤ **Enhancing Communication Through Nonverbal Behaviors**

Nonverbal Behaviors	Interpretation
Direct eye contact	Demonstrates interest and attention. Consider the client's cultural heritage when determining how much eye contact is appropriate.
Concerned facial expression	Lends credibility, if congruent with conversation.
Leaning forward	Shows interest in the conversation.
Personal space	Maintaining a distance of 18 inches to 4 feet allows most clients to feel comfortable during the interaction. Adjust the distance within that range based on the client's preference.
Professional appearance	Gives people an impression of how you may act in your role as a healthcare provider.
Sitting down to talk	Communicates willingness to listen and a sense of not wanting to rush the interaction with the client.
Touch	Conveys caring and concern when used appropriately.

ThinkLike a Nurse 20-3

- Observe an interaction between family members or your fellow students. Look for congruence between verbal and nonverbal communication. Strategize what you would say to validate the intended meaning when the two modes of communication are not in agreement.
- Recall the brief interaction with the charge nurse in the Meet Your Patient scenario. What might you say or do in response?

WHAT FACTORS AFFECT COMMUNICATION?

The following is a discussion of the major factors, in addition to verbal and nonverbal language, that affect communication.

Environment

Communication is most successful in an environment that is quiet, private, free of unpleasant smells, and at a comfortable temperature. As you become accustomed to noise and distractions in the healthcare setting, you may not even notice them. Be sensitive to how the environment is affecting your client. Background noise is distracting, interferes with hearing, and can create confusion. Being around others in pain or distress creates anxiety and fear; lack of privacy may cause embarrassment. All of those feelings may prevent your patient from sharing personal information or understanding your communication.

Think creatively to secure the most comfortable environment possible. Hospital chapels, foyers, and activity rooms may be ideal locations for conversation. To discuss private matters, consider talking with the patient in a conference room rather than a shared room. If none of these is possible, at least close privacy curtains and turn off the radio or television.

Developmental Variations

Physical and cognitive development, language skills, level of education, and maturity influence the communication process. Thus, you will need to modify your communication strategies to communicate effectively, respectfully, and compassionately with patients at all developmental stages. For detailed information on expectations for each developmental stage, see Chapters 9 and 10.

- *Infants and young toddlers* with limited language skills communicate nonverbally. Your response may combine verbal and nonverbal communication. For example, if a hospitalized 1-year-old cries out for his mother, you might cuddle the child with his favorite toy and explain that "Mama will be back very soon."
- *Older toddlers and preschoolers* have more verbal ability. Although they may prefer to have a parent present, they are likely to talk with you and answer questions.
- *School-age children* are usually comfortable interacting verbally. Pay attention to their vocabulary as they speak, and be sure to match it as closely as possible, using words and phrasing that the child will understand. By the time children reach adolescence, most can process abstract concepts. As a result, they are usually able to understand disease processes, treatments, and other health issues. Bear in mind that children with chronic health problems, who have required frequent interventions, are often more knowledgeable than would be expected for their age.
- *Older adults* may be affected by sensory alterations, such as hearing loss or vision changes, or any of a variety of healthcare problems that affect cognition and expression. Communication strategies for these situations are discussed in Planning Interventions/Implementation later in this chapter.

Gender

Males and females communicate differently and may interpret the same communication differently. Women often communicate to form connections and establish relationships (Tannen, 2001). In contrast, male communication styles typically focus on maintaining independence and favorable positions in a hierarchy. Male communication tends to be purpose driven—more about conveying information and accomplishing a goal—whereas female communication tends to be relationally driven.

Gender differences are important because male and female patients may communicate their needs very differently. Similarly, the gender of the nurse may affect the response to the patient's requests. For example, a female patient might state, "I feel so lousy today." A female nurse may interpret this as a desire to talk. In contrast, a male nurse may discuss pain control.

Personal Space

People vary in the amount of physical space they prefer when communicating. The distance they maintain between one another is influenced by the relationship of the individuals,

the nature of the conversation, the setting, and cultural influences (Fig. 20-3). Also see Chapter 15 for cultural preferences for personal space. Hall (1992) describes four distinct distances for communication: intimate, personal, social, and public distance.

Intimate Distance is the area immediately surrounding people that they define as their private space. People prefer to maintain intimate distance between themselves and others during conversations. In Western cultures, intimate distance is typically within 18 inches of the other person. Within this distance, people can easily interpret facial expression, maintain eye contact, and hear each other speaking at a low volume. As a nurse, you invade a client's personal space to perform assessments and procedures, or even while using touch to offer support. This may make some clients uncomfortable. Before providing nursing interventions in the client's intimate distance, discuss what you are about to do. It is best to ask the client's permission, even for gentle touch, if you are in the slightest doubt about his receptivity.

Personal Distance is from 18 inches to 4 feet. Your interactions with clients and healthcare team members will commonly occur in this range. This distance facilitates sharing of feelings or personal thoughts and is appropriate to maintain when communicating caring or concern.

Social Distance is a distance of 4 to 12 feet. It is used in more formal interaction or when communicating with a group of individuals. At this distance, individuals are not within range to be physically touched. The volume of the spoken words may be loud enough for others to overhear, so people share personal feelings and thoughts less often at this distance. For example, if you stand by a client's door and ask how she is feeling, you will likely receive a more impersonal response than if you were to ask the same question at her bedside.

Public Distance is considered to be beyond 12 feet. This distance requires loud and clear enunciation for communication. Public speakers and large educational groups use this form of personal space. This distance is characterized by a lack of individuality and a greater focus on the group or community.

Territoriality

Territoriality refers to the space and things that an individual identifies as his own. In a hospital setting, many clients consider everything within the curtain boundary to be their territory. Clients may be offended if you change, rearrange, or interfere with this personal space by moving furniture, discarding objects, or borrowing items from the room, even if they are institutional property. Be aware of this and request permission to move things your client's territory. Also recognize that hospitalized clients are not in their "home" territory and are therefore likely to be less at ease during interactions.

Sociocultural Factors

Culture and socioeconomic status strongly influence communication. Facial expressions, nonverbal communication, and even the selection of whom to interact with are affected. For example, in some cultures it would be unacceptable for a male nurse to address and provide care to a female patient.

Social status also plays a role in communication. Have you ever been present while a physician explained a treatment plan to a patient? Often the client asks no questions or nods approval; and waits until the physician leaves to ask you questions or express concerns. This may be because many clients perceive less social distance between themselves and the nurse. Social distance can also play a role in how health professionals view clients. For example, you may see impoverished clients being treated differently than affluent members of the community; although this is obviously not an example you will want to follow.

Roles and Relationships

Think of the way you interact with your instructor. Compare this with the way you interact with your classmates. What are the differences? The roles and relationships of the sender and receiver affect the choice of vocabulary, tone of voice, use of gestures, and distance associated with the communication.

Many patients have stereotyped notions about nurses. Some may view you as an authority figure. Others may perceive nursing as a lowly occupation and limit conversation with you to matters of comfort and hygiene. Still others become confused by the fact that many healthcare workers, such as medical assistants and NAPs, call themselves nurses in spite of the fact that they cannot legally use the title. If you are working with NAPs or other team members, be sure to clarify their roles with the patient so he can communicate his questions and concerns to the appropriate care provider.

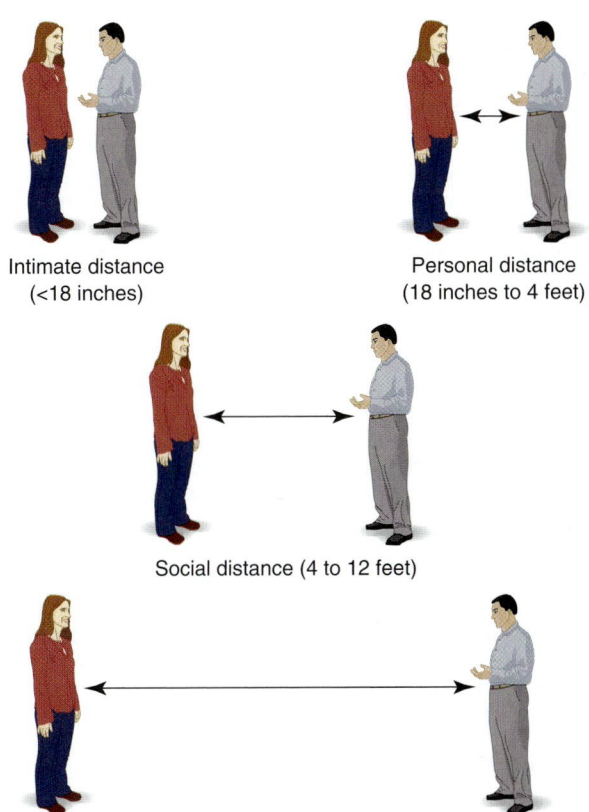

Intimate distance
(<18 inches)

Personal distance
(18 inches to 4 feet)

Social distance (4 to 12 feet)

Public distance (12 feet)

FIGURE 20-3 The distance that individuals engaged in communication maintain between one another is influenced by their relationship, the nature of the conversation, the setting, and cultural influences.

KnowledgeCheck 20-4

- What are the major factors that affect communication?
- In what distance(s) do most nurse–client interactions occur?

WHAT IS COLLABORATIVE PROFESSIONAL COMMUNICATION?

Communication is essential to collaborative practice. As a member of the healthcare team, you need to communicate effectively with nurses, physicians, and health professionals from other disciplines. Each of you shares the common goal of providing optimal patient care. This goal should guide the manner in which you communicate—at the bedside, at the nurse's station, in care conferences, or via the patient record. Nurses also communicate with peers and colleagues in order to contribute to their professional development. See Box 20-2 for statements from professional organizations about collaborative communication.

Think of communication styles as a continuum from passive through assertive to aggressive. A **passive approach** avoids conflict and allows others to take the lead. It tends to be submissive, helpless, indecisive, apologetic, or whining. "Whatever you want. I'll just sit here and wait for you to decide what you're going to do" is an example of a passive approach. In contrast, an **aggressive approach** forces others to lose. The goal is to win and be in control (e.g., "My way is the correct way. You don't know

what you're talking about"). Aggressive communication can also be bossy, arrogant, opinionated, sarcastic, manipulative, intolerant, or overbearing.

Why might you adopt a **nonassertive style?** When speaking to physicians, some nurses still communicate their needs in a style that assures physicians that they are not telling them what to do (e.g., "Do you think Mrs. King's heart rate is a little fast today?" instead of "Mrs. King's heart rate was 120 at 8 a.m."). This has been referred to as the *doctor–nurse game* (Stein, Watts, & Howell, 1990). Such unclear, indirect communication contributes to errors and poor patient outcomes.

Communicating Assertively

To advocate for clients, question care decisions, and discuss errors or poor clinical judgment with coworkers, you will need to communicate assertively. **Assertive communication** is the expression of a wide range of positive and negative thoughts and feelings in a style that is direct, open, honest, spontaneous, responsible, and nonjudgmental. Assertiveness recognizes your rights while still respecting the rights of others. It allows you to take responsibility for your own thoughts and actions without blaming others, encourages feedback, and enables you to find mutually satisfying

---

BOX 20-2 ■ Collaborative Professional Communication

American Nurses Association (ANA) (2010)

Standards of professional performance stress the importance of communication to collegiality and collaboration. The following are some of the competencies for these three standards. The registered nurse:

Standard 11. Communication

- Assesses communication format preferences of healthcare consumers, families, and colleagues.
- Assesses his or her own communication skills in encounters with healthcare consumers, families, and colleagues.
- Seeks continuous improvement of communication and conflict resolution skills.
- Conveys information to healthcare consumers, families, the interprofessional team, and others in communication formats that promote accuracy.
- Questions the rationale supporting care processes and decisions when they do not appear to be in the best interest of the patient.
- Discloses observations or concerns related to hazards and errors in care or the practice environment to the appropriate level.
- Maintains communication with other providers to minimize risks associated with transfers and transition in care delivery.
- Contributes her or his own professional perspective in discussion with the interprofessional team.

Standard 12. Leadership

- Develops communication and conflict resolution skills.
- Communicates effectively with the healthcare consumer and colleagues.

Standard 13. Collaboration

- Communicates effectively with the healthcare consumer, the family, and healthcare providers regarding healthcare consumer care and the nurse's role in the provision of care.

- Applies group process and negotiation techniques with healthcare consumers and colleagues.

Standard 14. Professional Practice Evaluation

- Provides peers with formal or informal constructive feedback regarding their practice or role performance.

American Association of Critical-Care Nurses (AACN)

Skilled communication is necessary to a healthy work environment. Nurses must be proficient in communication skills. Critical elements of communication include the following:
- Focusing on finding solutions and achieving desirable outcomes
- Seeking to protect and advance collaborative relationships among colleagues
- Inviting and hearing all relevant perspectives
- Striving for goodwill and mutual respect
- Building consensus and arriving at common understanding
- Achieving congruence between words and actions, and holding others accountable for doing so
- Developing proficiency with communication technologies (2005)

Quality and Safety Education for Nurses (QSEN)

Communication is essential for teamwork and collaboration. On graduation from nursing school, you should be able to analyze differences in others' communication style preferences and describe the impact of your own communication style on others (Cronenwett, Sherwood, Barnsteiner, et al., 2007).

The Joint Commission (2006)

The 2006 National Patient Safety Goals added Goal 2E, recommending a standardized approach to "hand off" communications, including an opportunity to ask and respond to questions. The broad Goal 2 calls for improving the effectiveness of communication among caregivers.

solutions to conflict by confronting people constructively. To communicate assertively, you should do the following:

- *Question care decisions openly and honestly.* Refuse to play the doctor–nurse game. Avoid beginning your statements with self-effacing statements that fail to take credit for your contributions (e.g., "You may disagree with this, but . . ."). Be frank, but be flexible and open minded.
- *Use "I" statements.* An "I" statement should include the elements of behavior (or facts), feeling, and effect (on you). For example, instead of saying, "Why haven't you ordered Mrs. Johnson's pain medications yet?" you might say, "I telephoned you this morning about Mrs. Johnson's lack of pain relief, but I don't see a change in her analgesic order. I am concerned about her discomfort and the effect it may have on her willingness to ambulate."
- *Focus on the issue, not the participants.* For example, say, "I think this approach might be the best, but I'd like to hear your thoughts."
- *Use effective nonverbal language.* Your body and verbal language should be congruent. Eye contact demonstrates interest and shows sincerity. Use a calm, well-modulated voice tone, and add appropriate gestures for emphasis.
- *Don't invite negative responses.* For example, say, "I would really appreciate it if you could help me weigh Mr. Max on the bed scale," rather than, "Can you help me weigh him?"
- *Use "fogging" to help you accept criticism without becoming anxious or defensive.* Acknowledge that there may be some truth to it, but remain the judge of your own action. Suppose Mrs. Johnson's physician says, "Are you playing pharmacist today?" You might respond, "I may not know everything there is to know about analgesics. However, Mrs. Johnson needs pain relief and I need your help prescribing pain medication."
- *Use negative inquiry.* You might choose, in the preceding situation, to use negative inquiry. You would reply, "So you believe that I do not have adequate knowledge to discuss Mrs. Johnson's pain control?"
- *Strive for a workable compromise,* but not if it affects patient well-being or your feelings of self-respect. Suppose an administrator comes to a patient's room while you are inserting a nasogastric tube and says, "I need to see you right now. Come to the desk immediately." An example of a workable compromise would be to say, "I understand that you need to talk to me right away, and I need to finish what I am doing. So what about meeting you at the desk as soon as I finish, in about 10 minutes?"

It may help to practice ahead of time how you want to look and sound before attempting assertive communication. Assertiveness is a learned skill and role-playing with a colleague can build your confidence. For a summary of assertive communication techniques, refer to Clinical Insight 20-2.

Using the SBAR Model

Using a standard framework helps you to convey key information clearly and concisely, thus improving interdisciplinary communication and patient outcomes. The SBAR model is designed to overcome differences in nurse-physician communication styles. For a summary this model and the meaning of "SBAR," see Clinical Insight 20-3.

Clinical Insight 20-2 ➤ Assertive Communication

- Maintain eye contact, as culturally appropriate.
- Speak clearly and firmly.
- Project a clear tone of voice.
- Communicate self-confidently.
- Maintain professional composure.
- Communicate in a positive manner.
- Refrain from sarcasm.
- Ensure congruence between verbal and nonverbal messages.
- Guide the direction of the discussion.
- Use "I" statements.
- Focus on the issues.
- Do not invite negative responses.
- Avoid self-effacing statements.

Clinical Insight 20-3 ➤ Communicating With SBAR*

Situation	In 10 seconds, identify yourself and the patient and describe the present situation that prompted you to call. State
	  ■ your name
	  ■ your unit
	  ■ the patient's name and room number
	  ■ the problem

Background	Give other information pertinent to the situation—not the patient's entire history since admission, but circumstances leading up to the situation (e.g., medications, lab results, current symptoms).
Assessment	State the problem and what you think is causing it. This is an inference rather than traditional data collection.
Recommendation	State what you think will correct the problem, or what you need from the physician.

*If you need other information about SBAR, see Chapter 18.

Practice Resources

Beyea, 2004; Carroll, 2003; Haig, Sutton, & Whittington, 2006; Pope, Rodzen, & Spross, 2008.

If you need other information about giving a verbal report, also see Chapter 18.

WHAT IS THE ROLE OF COMMUNICATION IN THERAPEUTIC RELATIONSHIPS?

A **therapeutic relationship** focuses on improving the health of the client, whether an individual or community. **Therapeutic communication** is client-centered communication directed at achieving client goals. It is used to establish the therapeutic relationship, provide and obtain healthcare information, and express interest and concern for the client and family.

Communication Is Essential to All Phases of the Therapeutic Relationship

The therapeutic relationship consists of four phases. As you read about each phase, notice the fundamental role of client-focused communication.

Pre-interaction Phase. The **pre-interaction phase** occurs before you meet the client. Pre-interaction involves gathering information about the client, but the nurse and client do not communicate directly. As a student, you initiate this phase as you prepare for clinical days. The client also experiences a pre-interaction phase, which begins when she identifies the need for healthcare. This can be an anxious time for the client.

Orientation Phase. The **orientation** phase begins when you meet the client. For Mr. Barker (Meet Your Patient), it began when you approached him to introduce yourself. The goal of the orientation phase is to establish rapport and trust. Orientation begins with introductions, followed by an initial exchange of information, such as the client's reason for the visit or chief concerns. Orientation ends when the relationship has been defined. Ideally there is time at the beginning to exchange pleasantries and develop a level of comfort, but in some clinical situations, such as during an emergency, this phase is very brief or omitted altogether.

Working Phase. The bulk of therapeutic communication occurs in the **working phase,** the active part of the relationship. During this phase, the nurse communicates caring, the patient expresses thoughts and feelings, mutual respect is maintained, and honest verbal and nonverbal expression occurs. Key communication goals are to assist the client to clarify feelings and concerns. A professional relationship is courteous, trustworthy, and confidential, and accomplished by active listening and other techniques of therapeutic communication presented later in this chapter.

Termination Phase. The conclusion of the relationship marks the **termination phase,** whether at the end of the nurse's shift or on the client's discharge from the unit, facility, or service. Reviewing and summarizing help to bring the relationship to a comfortable conclusion. If communication has been effective, the termination phase prepares the nurse and client for future interactions. Unsuccessful communication may affect the client's health outcomes or understanding of his disease process, as well as affect the nurse's job satisfaction.

ThinkLike a Nurse 20-4

Recall the scenario of Mr. Barker (Meet Your Patient).
- What phase of the therapeutic relationship is illustrated in the scenario?
- How might the interaction between you and Mr. Barker change if it occurred in a different phase of the therapeutic relationship?
- What could you have done differently?

Therapeutic Communication Has Five Key Characteristics

The therapeutic relationship requires conscious use of your knowledge and skills to effect change in the patient. This is often called the *therapeutic use of self.* Five qualities characterize communication in the therapeutic relationship: empathy, respect, genuineness, concreteness, and confrontation.

Therapeutic use of self requires practice so that you will be able to recognize boundaries and to keep the focus on the patient rather than on your own feelings and experiences. For more information about that, follow the link for Reading More About Communication at the end of this chapter.

Empathy. Empathy is the desire to understand and be sensitive to the feelings, beliefs, and situation of another person. Empathy requires you to be willing to adapt your style, tone, vocabulary, and behavior to create the best approach for each client situation. It is relatively easy to have empathy for people who are like you and who are likeable. It is more difficult to connect with people you see as difficult or different. To empathize with a client, you must look beyond outward appearance or behavior and put yourself, mentally and emotionally, in the client's place. The empathy with which you care for your patient, deliver difficult news, or guide him through complex decisions can make an enormous difference to that patient's and family's experience and adaptation to illness.

Respect. In the therapeutic relationship, you communicate respect by valuing the client and being flexible to meet the client's needs. Making even minor adjustments, such as delaying breakfast for an hour to allow the client to sleep, communicates that you respect the client's wishes. Most healthcare experiences strip the client of power—clothes are removed, roles are discontinued, people are separated from loved ones and familiar surroundings, and schedules are altered. When a relationship is grounded in respect, both parties maintain power and self-esteem. You show your respect for clients in the way you address them, the words and intonation that you choose, and in your acknowledgment of their strengths and needs.

Genuineness. When interviewing clients, we expect them to respond truthfully. Similarly, clients have a right to expect truthful responses from healthcare providers. **Genuineness** is the ability to respond honestly. If you are unable to answer a client's question, do not offer guesses. Be honest. Tell the client you need assistance before you can answer the question. Genuineness also involves willingness to self-evaluate. How well did I communicate? Did I handle that situation appropriately? How could I improve my communication?

Concreteness and Confrontation. In a therapeutic relationship, you must offer understandable responses to a client's questions and concerns. To do so requires you to express in concrete, specific terms what you mean. The message must be constructed and delivered in a manner that is suitable for the client. Conversely, if your client is unable to express his thoughts clearly, you must be willing to confront him to request clarification. Similarly, you must be willing to be confronted if you are unclear.

Communication Is Important in Group Helping Relationships

Nurses frequently communicate with groups. Group communication occurs when you interact with a family, a community, or a committee. Groups can enhance problem-solving and creativity, generate understanding and support, enhance morale, and provide affiliation. However *group think,* a pattern of communication in which consensus overrides creativity in

BOX 20-3 ■ Skills Needed in a Therapeutic Relationship

The ability to do the following:
- Appreciate experiences and beliefs that differ from your own.
- Recognize and interpret verbal and nonverbal messages.
- Guide the interaction to accomplish goals.
- Determine whether communication is taking place.
- Speak when appropriate and remain silent when appropriate.
- Adapt to the pace, tone, and vocabulary of the client.
- Evaluate your own participation in an interaction.

problem-solving, can emerge, particularly in cohesive groups or those with unbalanced power structure.

Task Groups. Task groups are formed to address a task or fulfill a need. Members are chosen based on ability to complete the task. Other times members are selected for reasons of convenience, such as availability, interest, or political agenda, rather than for the skills needed to accomplish the goal of the group. Short-term groups disband once the task is completed. Short-term groups might include a task force to address holiday scheduling or a panel to critique response to a disaster drill. Because the group members' time together is limited, the focus of communication is on the task at hand. Often, time to develop rapport or relationships is limited. Direct verbal communication with congruent nonverbal communication allows the group to function most effectively.

Ongoing Groups. Ongoing groups address issues that are recurrent. Committees are a form of an ongoing task group. Common ongoing committees in healthcare organizations include quality assurance, infection control, and discharge planning. A committee has a leader or chairperson that may be elected from within or appointed. Members have designated roles within the group (e.g., recorder, time keeper). In small groups, all members have an opportunity to communicate their opinions. In larger groups, patterns of communication form; some members voice their opinion regularly, whereas others are often silent. When not all members speak, it is essential to examine nonverbal behavior to determine whether the nonspeaking members are in agreement.

Self-Help Groups. **Self-help groups** are voluntary organizations composed of individuals with a common need. Members who have met the goals of the group often run meetings. Alcoholics Anonymous may be the most widely recognized self-help group. Other well-known self-help groups include Weight Watchers, Narcotics Anonymous, and Reach for Recovery (for women with breast cancer). Nurses may be members, facilitators, or consultants for self-help groups. Members are encouraged to share experiences and seek help from other members of the group. The facilitator, usually chosen by the members, may serve as a leader of the group or coordinate room arrangements and schedules but acts as a member during sessions. Self-help groups may have face-to-face meetings, participate in Internet chat groups, or communicate via newsletters. Communication of shared interests is the link that holds these groups together.

Therapy Groups. Therapy groups are formed to help individual members cope with issues, improve relationships, or address stress. They may be ongoing or have a designated length of operation. Community, public health, and psychiatric nurses sometimes facilitate therapy groups. Group facilitators arrange the time and place that the group meets and

often introduce topics for discussion. Many groups are organized around themes, such as coping with divorce, loss of a spouse, or motherhood. These groups are also called *self-awareness* or *growth groups*.

Work-Related Social Support Groups. Work-related social support groups help members of a profession cope with the stress associated with their work. The helping professions can be emotionally draining. Social support groups provide an opportunity to share concerns and offer mutual support through formal meetings with a facilitator or informal drop-in events. Formation of a group does not guarantee its success. To be successful, a group must have characteristics that allow the group to function and achieve its goals (Box 20-4).

KnowledgeCheck 20-5

- Identify and describe the phases of the therapeutic relationship.
- What are the five characteristics of therapeutic communication?
- Describe the difference between a task group and a self-help group.
- Compare and contrast the role of a therapy group with a work-related support group.

ThinkLike a Nurse 20-5

Review the local newspaper, phone book, hospital bulletin board, the Internet, and school intranet. Identify at least three group helping experiences available. How might you learn more about these organizations? How would you determine whether they are resources that you might make available to your patients?

PracticalKnowledge knowing how

Therapeutic communication is used throughout the nursing process. In the next few sections we explore communication problems as well as therapeutic interventions.

■ ASSESSMENT

Assessment is essential to effective communication. You should assess for factors that alter a client's ability to receive, process, or transmit information, such as the following:

- *Language barrier.* If you were unable to speak or read the language spoken by people around you, how would you communicate that you were nauseated or in pain? How would you tell them when the symptom started or what

BOX 20-4 ■ Characteristics of a Successful Group

A successful group includes the following:
- Clearly defined purpose
- Shared set of guidelines under which the group functions
- Sense of shared responsibility
- Shared leadership
- Mutual trust
- Comfort among members
- Climate that is cohesive but does not stifle individuality
- Members who are willing to share feelings, concerns, or beliefs
- Flexibility to change what is not working

QSEN

Limits and Boundaries of Therapeutic Relationships

Competency: Patient-Centered Care (Knowledge, Skill)*

Boundaries are important psychological tools that define personal space and allow people to communicate comfortably. This box illustrates the effects of boundaries on the competency, Patient-Centered Care.

Professional relationships have stricter boundaries than o personal relationships: Questions and comments that friends can make to each other may be inappropriate between colleagues or a client. Also, boundaries between patients and healthcare providers are unequal and not always clear. Patients are asked intimate details of their lives, often physically exposed, and often dependent on the care provider. Consider how these factors make patients vulnerable. What Knowledge and Skills must a nurse possess to develop trust-based therapeutic relationships with patients and their families? What can the nurse do help patients maintain their dignity?

The National Council of State Boards of Nursing (NCSBN) recommends that in developing professional, therapeutic boundaries, nurses:

➤ Show respect for human dignity.

➤ Avoid personal gratification at the client's expense.

➤ Avoid interfering in the patient's personal relationships.

➤ Promote patient autonomy and self-determination.

➤ Understand that the nurse–patient relationship is based on trust.

Behaviors that suggest you might have boundary issues include (1) thinking about the patient while away from work; (2) socializing with the patient outside of work; (3) disclosing personal information to the patient; and (4) engaging in physical contact or flirting, including through texting or online messaging.

Nurses have a moral duty to protect patients from inappropriate relationships. If you observe these behaviors in yourself or a colleague, discuss it with your supervisor. Patient-centered care is possible only when patients and their families feel safe.

*For specific Knowledge, Skills, and Attitudes

 Go to the QSEN web site at http:www.qsen.org. ksas_prelicensure.php

Sources: Hall, 2011; Holder, & Schenthal, 2007; National Council of State Boards of Nursing, 2007.

---

makes it worse? Also consider your client's education and literacy. You cannot assume that everyone has an extensive vocabulary, nor that they can read and write.

- *Cognitive skills.* Difficulty understanding or engaging in communication may signal cognitive impairment. Developmental delays and pathology or injury of the central nervous system affect receptive and expressive language and cognitive skills.
- *Sensory perceptual alterations.* Assess hearing and vision. Assess for **aphasia** (a difficulty expressing or interpreting messages that may develop after cerebrovascular accident [stroke] or neurological disease).
- *Physiological barriers.* Barriers, such as respiratory problems, loose-fitting dentures, or cleft palate, may interfere with speaking.

◼ ANALYSIS/NURSING DIAGNOSIS

Communication can be the problem or the etiology of a nursing diagnosis. The following NANDA-I diagnosis labels describe communication problems. Note that communication problems may involve the inability to receive, interpret, or express spoken, written, and nonverbal messages.

- *Readiness for Enhanced Communication* is appropriate when the client expresses willingness to enhance communication that is already effective.
- *Impaired Verbal Communication* is an appropriate diagnosis if the client has (1) expressive aphasia or a physiological problem such as dyspnea, stuttering, or laryngeal cancer that impairs the ability to speak; or (2) receptive aphasia or sensory deficits that impair the ability to receive messages.

- *Impaired Communication* is the preferred diagnosis if the client is unfamiliar with the dominant language or has some other difficulty receiving and sending messages. Note that this is not a NANDA-I label.

Etiologies of Communication Diagnoses

Your assessment data will help you determine whether communication impairment is the primary problem or whether it is a result of other health problems. Some nursing diagnoses may cause or contribute to communication problems. For example:

- Clients with Acute or Chronic Confusion often have difficulty expressing or receiving verbal and nonverbal messages. Confusion may be related to physical or mental health problems, or may be a side effect of medications or sleep deprivation.
- Mental health problems can also lead to communication problems. For example, Anxiety impairs the ability to deliver and receive messages, and Chronic or Situational Low Self-Esteem often results in limited interaction with others.

Communication as Etiology of Other Nursing Diagnoses

Impaired Verbal Communication may be the etiology of other nursing diagnoses, for example:

- Anxiety r/t inability to communicate needs
- Social Isolation r/t difficulty maintaining relationships secondary to Impaired Verbal Communication
- Impaired Social Interaction r/t inability to carry on conversation

Communication

A focused assessment should identify factors that alter a patient's ability to receive, understand, and transmit verbal and nonverbal messages.

Medications

Is the patient taking medications that might interfere with speech, cognition, or level of consciousness?

Language barriers

➤ What is the patient's primary language?
➤ Does the patient have sufficient command of the dominant language?
➤ Is an interpreter (foreign language or sign language) required?
➤ Can the patient read and write? At what level and in what language?

Cognitive function

➤ What is the patient's level of consciousness?
➤ Is there short-term or long-term memory loss, or both?
➤ Is intellectual function at, below, or above expectations for age?
➤ Can the patient read simple instructions?
➤ Can the patient follow simple spoken instructions?
➤ Can the patient understand a yes or no choice?
➤ Are there symptoms or a diagnosis of mental illness or dementia?
➤ If the patient is unconscious, are there nonverbal responses that indicate that he can hear you (e.g., blinking, moving the head, squeezing your hand)?

Hearing

➤ Ask the patient, and observe, whether there are hearing problems.
➤ Is the patient wearing a hearing aid? If so, is it working properly? Does the patient appear to be reading your lips?
➤ Is the patient trying to use sign language to communicate?

➤ Refer to Chapter 21 for tests of hearing (e.g., ticking watch).

Vision

➤ Is the patient wearing glasses or contact lenses?
➤ Is the patient able to see adequately?
➤ Refer to Chapter 21 for vision tests.
   Also see **Brief Physical Assessment,** Skills Videos to Accompany Fundamentals of Nursing.

Aphasia

➤ Is there a history of stroke, or a diagnosis of aphasia?
➤ Is there receptive aphasia (inability to receive or interpret verbal or nonverbal messages)?
➤ Is there expressive aphasia (inability to express verbal or nonverbal messages)?

Physiological barriers

Does the patient have conditions that cause difficulty speaking, such as
➤ Dyspnea?
➤ Artificial airway?
➤ Oral problems, such as poorly fitted dentures?
➤ Cleft palate or other structural problems?

Communication style

➤ Is it difficult to understand what the patient says (e.g., slurring words, stuttering, inability to pronounce certain sounds)?
➤ Does the patient speak readily, or refuse to speak?
➤ Does the patient speak slowly or rapidly; spontaneously or hesitantly?
➤ Is the vocabulary adequate for the purpose needed?
➤ Has the vocabulary changed from the person's normal vocabulary?

Other

➤ Are verbal and nonverbal communication congruent?

■ Chronic Low Self-Esteem r/t fear of conversing with others secondary to stuttering

PLANNING OUTCOMES/EVALUATION

Individualized client outcomes and goals depend on the nursing diagnosis you identify. For example, for Impaired Verbal Communication, you might write the following desired outcomes. The client:
■ Uses alternative methods of communication (e.g., writing, picture board, gestures) effectively (specify time frame).
■ Demonstrates minimal frustration with communication difficulties (specify time frame).
■ Communicates effectively using a translator or interpreter.
■ Interprets messages accurately, as evidenced by appropriate verbal or nonverbal feedback.

For *NOC standardized outcomes* associated with Impaired Verbal Communication,

 Go to Chapter 20, **Standardized Language: Selected NOC Outcomes and NIC Interventions for Impaired Verbal Communication,** on DavisPlus.

Using NOC indicators with those outcomes, you can develop goals for clients' communication problems.

PLANNING INTERVENTIONS/IMPLEMENTATION

Specific nursing activities for communication problems depend on the etiology of the problem and on the goals selected. The focus of nursing interventions is to facilitate communication and to resolve or reduce the factors interfering with it.

For *NIC standardized interventions* and selected nursing activities for Impaired Verbal Communication,

 Go to Chapter 20, **Standardized Language: Selected NOC Outcomes and NIC Interventions for Impaired Verbal Communication,** on Davis*Plus.*

Enhancing Therapeutic Communication

The following are techniques and activities you can implement immediately to improve your communication with patients and others.

Active Listening

At first glance, the term *active listening* appears to be an oxymoron. People often think of listening as a passive activity. If you have ever been in a one-sided conversation, you are certainly aware that listening can be passive. In contrast, an active listener uses all senses to focus on the sender's message, gives undivided attention, and allows the sender the opportunity to complete comments without interruption. To listen actively, pay attention to verbal and nonverbal communication and look for congruence. If a message is unclear, seek clarification through use of probing questions or reflective comments, such as "Tell me more," or "When you say . . . what do you mean?"

You can demonstrate active listening by facing your client, making eye contact, and focusing the conversation on issues of importance to the client. Taking notes during a conversation distracts you from active listening. If you must take notes, record only key words to stimulate your memory at another time. Active listening behaviors convey caring, signal a willingness to listen, and provide a comfortable environment for the client to share his concerns.

Failure to listen to your client will result in missed messages or misinterpretation. Consider the following example:

Patient: I guess I'm going to have surgery tomorrow.
Nurse: [*Checking the IV fluids and hanging a medication.*] Uh-huh.
Patient: The surgeon says I'll be in intensive care for a few days.
Nurse: [*Looking at the drainage in the urine collection bag.*] OK. Your urine looks good.
Patient: I guess this is pretty risky surgery.
Nurse: [*Recording on the flow sheet.*] Yep.

How do you think the patient must feel in this situation? The patient is clearly expressing concern about his upcoming surgery and seems to want to talk about it with the nurse. However, the nurse is busy with a variety of tasks and is not paying attention to the conversation. Undoubtedly the patient will continue to feel anxious. In fact, his unsuccessful attempts to communicate may even increase his anxiety. If the nurse were listening, this would be an excellent opportunity to discuss the patient's concerns, provide preoperative teaching, and help the patient ease his anxiety.

Establishing Trust

Mutual trust is an essential component of both professional and therapeutic communication because it facilitates disclosure and honesty. As you and the client establish trust, the client can more easily relay information and share feelings. To establish trust, always greet the client by name, listen actively, respond honestly to the client's concerns, and provide care competently and consistently.

Being Assertive

An assertive person is one who is confident and comfortable and remains in charge of steering the course of the conversation. Assertive communication enables you to deal directly with stressful interpersonal communication, for example, with a client who needs to make some lifestyle changes. An assertive nurse also serves as a role model for the client. The therapeutic relationship is a safe place for clients to practice being assertive and to receive feedback about their communication. As needed, review assertiveness and collaborative professional communication, earlier in this chapter.

Restating, Clarifying, and Validating Messages

Restating means using your own words to summarize the message you received from the client. This demonstrates concern, active listening, and understanding of what the patient has said. Below is an example:

Client: I'm so worried about this diabetes. I have young kids. I want to see them grow up. Every diabetic I've known has died young.
Nurse: Diabetes is a serious disease. I understand your worry about its effects on you. However, we want to focus on becoming well controlled so that you can avoid complications.

Clarifying messages helps ensure that you have accurately interpreted the information. For instance, you might state, "I'm not sure what you mean when you say you're so worried about your diabetes." Or, "When you say you're worried, what do you mean?"

To **validate** the message, ask the client whether you are making a correct interpretation: "When you say you're worried about your diabetes, do you mean you are afraid you will die soon?" These techniques help to identify client concerns and focus communication. They are especially helpful if the client is unclear or vague with a message.

Interpreting Body Language and Sharing Observations

Be attentive to what the patient says and how she says it. Note the tone of voice, rate of speech, distance, eye movement, facial expressions, and gestures. Look for congruence between the spoken message and the nonverbal message. If there is inconsistency, share your observations with the patient. You can share your observations by describing the patient's body language or tone of voice. For example, you might state, "I know you said you feel well, but your voice and hands are trembling. How can I help you?" Or more simply, "You're frowning. Has something upset you?"

Exploring Issues

Ask open-ended questions to obtain a clear understanding of an issue and follow your client's thoughts (see Chapter 3). Probing comments such as "Tell me more" encourage your client to share information.

Using Silence

Learn to be comfortable with silence. When you remain attentive, silence demonstrates acceptance and allows clients to compose their thoughts and provide further information. It is especially effective if your client is emotionally upset.

Process Recordings

A strategy commonly used to improve therapeutic communication skills is called **process recording.** In process recording, two people converse while a third records the conversation. Afterward, the participants analyze the interaction. Audio

recording effectively captures the words and intonation of the conversation, but it must be supplemented by notes taken on nonverbal communication. Videotaping allows participants to examine both verbal and nonverbal communication. As you examine an interaction, look for the five qualities just discussed. Box 20-3 identifies skills associated with these qualities. Later, the chapter presents specific strategies for enhancing communication, as well as barriers to therapeutic communication. Look for these techniques and barriers in any conversation that you analyze.

Summarizing the Conversation

At the end of the conversation, summarize what you have heard. For example, you might say, "Today we talked about diet, exercise, and medications for high blood pressure. Your job now is to review the handouts and start taking your medication every morning. I'll see you in 2 weeks when you return for your follow-up visit." Summarizing demonstrates active listening and allows the client to clarify any misunderstandings.

Barriers to Therapeutic Communication

As you learn to communicate therapeutically, you may find yourself thinking, doing, or saying things that seem to close down your conversation. If so, acknowledge your error and return to therapeutic patterns. The following sections describe the most common barriers to therapeutic communication.

Asking Too Many Questions

Asking questions at the appropriate time is important. However, asking too many questions, especially closed questions (requiring only a yes or no answer), can make clients feel that they are being interrogated. Excessive questioning may suggest insensitivity or lack of respect to the client's issues, as in the following dialogue:

Patient:	I feel lousy today.
Nurse:	Didn't you sleep well?
Patient:	No, hardly at all.
Nurse:	Did you take anything to help you sleep?
Patient:	No.
Nurse:	Do you think you should have taken something?
Patient:	I guess.
Nurse:	Why didn't you tell the night nurse you needed something?
Patient:	I don't know.

As you can see, this approach controls the range and nature of responses that the client provides. In contrast, open-ended questions stimulate conversation and exploration.

Toward Evidence-Based Practice

Ammentorp, J., Sabroe, S., Kofoed, P. E., et al. (2007). The effect of training in communication skills on medical doctors' and nurses' self-efficacy: A randomized controlled trial. *Patient Education and Counseling, 66*(3), 270–277.

This research investigated the effect of communication skills training on doctors' and nurses' self-efficacy. (Self-efficacy is the extent to which you believe that you are capable of performing actions that influence events and outcomes, for example patient outcomes.) One group of clinicians received a 5-day communication course; the control group did not. Clinicians who participated in the communication course improved their self-efficacy for specific communication tasks by up to 37%. The improvements remained constant for the following 6 months. Researchers concluded that communication skills training can improve clinicians' evaluation of their ability to perform a specific communication task.

Edwards, N., Peterson, W. E., & Davies, B. L. (2006). Evaluation of a multiple component intervention to support the implementation of a "therapeutic relationships" best practice guideline on nurses' communication skills. *Patient Education and Counseling, 63*(1–2), 3–11.

Researchers tested an intervention to assist nurses to implement the best practice guideline of the Registered Nurses' Association of Ontario for establishing therapeutic relationships. They read client scenarios aloud and asked nurses to respond verbally as though they were interacting with the client. They measured the frequency and quality of nurses' active listening, initiating, and assertiveness skills

before and after implementation of the guideline. After implementation of the guideline, they found a significant decrease in the number of active listening skills used, but a significant improvement in the quality of active listening and initiating skills. They also found increased frequency of initiating skills. They concluded that nurses demonstrated improvements in select communication skills.

1. Which of the following statements is well supported by the evidence in the first report (Ammentorp, Sabroe, Kofoed, et al., 2007)?
   a. Communication courses for healthcare professionals should be at least 5 days long.
   b. If you personally took a 5-day communication course, you would have more faith in your ability to perform specific communication tasks.
   c. People who take a communication course can expect that they will feel more comfortable about performing certain communication tasks.
   d. People who take a communication course can expect some improvement in their ability to perform specific communication tasks.

2. Suppose you are an in-service educator in a hospital. You have decided to institute a hospital education program to train nurses in a few specific communication skills. Use the above studies to provide rationale for your decision. Write a brief statement explaining why your decision is reasonable.

 Go to Chapter 20, **Toward Evidence-Based Practice Suggested Responses,** on DavisPlus.

Contrast the preceding conversation with the conversation below.

Patient: I feel lousy today.

Nurse: Lousy? Tell me more.

Patient: Well, my back and neck hurt, and I hardly slept at all. I thought it would go away, but I just lay in bed last night worrying.

Nurse: What kind of things are you worrying about?

Patient: I'm worried about . . .

In the second conversation, the nurse asked open-ended questions. These prompts encouraged the patient to discuss his concerns.

Fire-Hosing Information

Sometimes a healthcare provider might meet with a patient or family and deliver an overwhelming amount of information. The patient or family members might understand what the provider said, but afterward remember only a fraction of it. Or they might feel stunned, confused, intimidated, and helpless. Instead, engage your patient in a *dialogue* in which you give important information while your patient shares his own concerns and questions. You can then ask him how he understands what has been shared and clarify when needed.

Asking Why

In many health situations, we want to learn why a patient acted or responded as he did. However, directly asking for reasons suggests criticism to some people. If you ask, "Why did you stop taking your medication?" the patient may become defensive and stop talking. A more subtle approach is usually more comfortable for the patient. You might ask, "What concerns do you have about your medicines?" or "Tell me more about your experience with the medicines." Both of these approaches will help you gather more information about the client's concerns, without suggesting criticism. Review the first dialogue in the previous section, Asking Too Many Questions, for another example of the effect of *why* questions. How do you think this patient felt?

Changing the Subject Inappropriately

Abruptly changing the topic of discussion makes you seem uninterested. This often occurs when the nurse is intent on one issue and the client is focused on another. For example, imagine that you want to tell the patient about a change in the scheduling for a diagnostic test before you forget. As you enter the room, your patient says, "I am having a lot of pain in my knee today." This situation requires you to address the patient's concern first and postpone discussing the schedule change until the patient can be receptive to the information. In an ongoing dialogue, changing the subject can stop the flow of conversation cold. Both patients and nurses sometime use this tactic to avoid discussing sensitive topics. The following is an example:

Nurse: This must be a tough time for you. Your wife is very sick. How are you handling this?

Patient's husband: Yes, it's tough, but I went out to a movie last night. Have you seen that new movie with the avatars? The special effects . . .

Your relationship with the patient's husband and the facts of the patient's situation determine whether you would redirect this conversation back to the original subject or allow him to wander. You may choose to give the husband more time to be comfortable with you before approaching this topic again.

Failing to Probe

Failing to probe can result in incomplete assessment and affect the quality of your care. A thorough assessment requires you to explore issues in detail. Review the following conversations:

Patient: I'm having a lot of discomfort in my back.

Nurse: How much does it hurt?

Patient: Quite a bit. I had trouble sleeping last night.

Nurse: I'll get you something for pain.

Compare that conversation with the next example, in which the nurse gathers additional data:

Patient: I'm having a lot of discomfort in my back.

Nurse: Tell me about the discomfort.

Patient: It hurts a lot. I had trouble sleeping last night.

Nurse: When did you first notice this pain?

Patient: It started in the middle of the night.

Nurse: What does it feel like?

Patient: I feel sore. I'd like to turn over to my side, but I can't because of this heavy cast.

Nurse: Let me help you turn. [*Assists patient to turn and uses pillows to hold the patient on her side*]

Patient: Oh, that feels better!

Nurse: How is the discomfort now?

Patient: It's pretty much gone.

Nurse: I'm glad you're feeling better. Would you like something for pain as well?

Patient: I think I'm OK now.

In the second example, the nurse followed her original question with additional probing questions. A few additional questions helped clarify what the patient needed and led to immediate comfort.

Expressing Approval or Disapproval

You should exercise caution when expressing approval or disapproval in the nurse–patient relationship. Although it may seem supportive, expressing approval can inhibit further sharing—it puts you in the position of being the judge of what is "right." This often prompts the patient to continue to seek approval. He thinks, "I'd better be careful; she may not approve of the next thing I was going to tell her. She expects me to be *this* way." Consider instead offering recommendations and allowing the patient to choose. Read the following exchange:

Patient: I've decided I'm going to have the surgery.

Nurse: That's great. I think you made the right choice.

Compare that conversation with the following example:

Patient: I've decided I'm going to have the surgery.

Nurse: Tell me about your decision.

Patient: Well, my shoulder has been bothering me for several months now. I know I said I wanted to put off surgery, but I think I'll have a faster recovery if I just get the surgery done now.

Nurse: So your choices are to do a trial of physical therapy and anti-inflammatory medicines, to try a steroid injection, or to have surgery.

Patient: Right. But there's a good chance I'll still need surgery even if I try the therapy or medicines. The only thing that will actually fix the problem is surgery. The others don't guarantee improvement.

Can you see how different the conversation becomes if the nurse does not express approval? By allowing the patient to discuss the choices, the nurse has empowered the patient to make his own healthcare decisions.

Offering Advice

Offering an opinion is rarely helpful. Avoid statements such as "If I were you . . ." or "You should . . ." These statements impose your opinion on your clients. In effect, your statements function as approval if they agree with the client's thoughts or disapproval if they do not. As with other forms of approval or disapproval, conversation halts. If the client asks, "What should I do?" help clarify the options, and provide her with information about the choices. Giving the client your solution negates the client's opportunity to participate as a mutual partner in the decision-making process.

Providing False Reassurance

Providing reassurance helps to ease concern, offers comfort, and communicates empathy. So it is an appropriate and therapeutic action—if the reassurance is warranted. For example, consider the client who presents to the emergency department (ED) for treatment of an acute episode of asthma. Because anxiety exacerbates asthma, it is certainly therapeutic to reassure the client that he will be cared for promptly and effectively. In contrast, false reassurance is a barrier to therapeutic communication. When clients or family members ask for information or tell you that they are worried, it is easy to reassure them that everything will be fine. However, such responses are uninformed and inaccurate and may feel dismissive—even condescending—to the receiver. Examine the following scenario:

> You are a nurse working at the triage station in the local ED. Your role is to evaluate the condition and prioritize the care of all clients presenting for treatment. An ambulance arrives with a man complaining of severe chest pain. He is ashen and short of breath. He tells you his pain is "crushing." Suspecting a heart attack, you immediately move him to the critical care bay of the ED and request urgent evaluation. Several minutes later his wife arrives by private car and approaches the triage station. She anxiously asks, "How is my husband?" How would you respond?

It may be tempting to offer a response such as this: "Don't worry, everything will be all right." But do you really know that will be the case? A better approach is to provide accurate information: "I had him immediately taken in for treatment. I'll get you in to see him as soon as I can. Please have a seat, and I'll check on him." This comment is accurate, calming, and avoids misleading the person.

Stereotyping

As discussed in Chapter 15, racial, cultural, religious, age-related, or gender stereotypes distort assessment and prevent you from recognizing the patient's uniqueness. Examples of statements reflecting a stereotype include the following: "He's old, he won't remember anything you tell him," and "Men are always the biggest wimps about pain." Such comments may shut down communication and escalate tension. Avoid their use with patients and colleagues.

Stereotypes may be blatant or subtle. Blatant examples, such as those above, are easily recognized and may create an intense reaction. Subtle stereotypes, however, may be equally disruptive to care and include the following:

- Believing a patient will be calm and know what to expect because he has had previous hospitalizations for the same diagnosis, has had previous surgeries or other procedures, or was given information about his condition.
- Assuming patients will understand their healthcare because of their educational level or work experience (e.g., expecting that a physician who has suffered a heart attack needs no explanation of her care.)
- Expecting all patients with the same surgery or diagnosis to experience similar responses.

Using Patronizing Language

Patronizing language communicates superiority or disapproval. Statements such as "You know better than that" are patronizing and offensive to the client. Condescending approaches, such as "You should have used the call button before you got up. You're lucky you didn't hurt yourself" do not communicate respect for the client.

Have you heard staff call clients "Sweetie," "Dearie," or "Mama"? The term **elderspeak** describes ways that healthcare workers may unintentionally show disrespect to elderly patients by using such phrases and speaking to them in a loud, high-pitched, slow, repetitive, child-like voice. Staff may also alter pronouns, saying, for example, "Are we ready for our bath?" Although the intent is to communicate caring, patients may be offended because it sounds as though you are speaking to a child. Research indicates mentally competent nursing home residents are irritated by elderspeak, and that people with moderate Alzheimer's disease become more agitated and resistant to care if they are addressed in this manner (Williams, Herman, Gajewski, et al., 2009).

When you first meet your client, use a formal title—Mr., Ms., and so on. This conveys respect, which is essential to a successful therapeutic relationship. In the orientation phase of the relationship, ask your patient how he would prefer to be addressed. If the patient is unable to respond, ask family members how to address the patient.

KnowledgeCheck 20-6

Identify at least five barriers to communication.

Enhancing Communication With Clients From Another Culture

The way you address your patient will vary depending on the culture he is from. In the United States, France, and many other countries, people use a formal salutation (Mr., Mrs., Ms., Dr.). The given name (personal name) precedes the surname. Other countries, such as Korea and China, go by surname, followed by first name. Other times people from another culture adapt their name to fit within the culture in which they are living. Be sensitive to the practices of your patient and ask his preference.

Healthcare facilities should provide interpretation (including translation) services as necessary (The Joint Commission, 2008, p. 156). Many health facilities have in-house translation services available for communication with non-English-speaking patients. Translators may also be available through telephone contact; a few are linked via computer to a healthcare interpreter network to enable video teleconferencing. Use relatives as translators only if there are no other options. It is often culturally unacceptable to have family members ask personal questions. As a result, translations may be altered or questions remain unasked. See Chapter 15 for additional information on the use of translators.

Spanish-speakers currently constitute 1 in 10 U.S. households, so it is not unusual to encounter patients who speak only Spanish. If you do not speak Spanish, most computers have programs for crudely translating English and Spanish terms; however, it is good to learn a few key words to help you communicate until a translator arrives. For a list of a few useful Spanish terms and for guidelines for communicating with clients from other cultures, see Clinical Insight 20-4.

Clinical Insight 20-4 ▶ Communicating With Clients From Another Culture

General Guidelines

- Most important: Be aware of your own cultural beliefs and attitudes.
- Learn about other cultures, especially those in your area.
- Convey empathy and show respect.
- Be certain the communication strategies you usually use are culturally appropriate for the individual.
  Is direct eye contact viewed as aggressive or impolite?
  How much space should you keep between yourself and the patient?
- Use touch cautiously. In some cultures, it is inappropriate to touch certain parts of the body.
- Proceed slowly. Rushing may cause the patient to be more anxious, and is offensive to some.
- Smile and be polite, but not overfriendly or casual. Use the patient's title and last name when introducing yourself.
- Use short words and sentences. Don't give too much information in one sentence.
- Present one idea at a time.
- Provide written teaching materials.

If There Is a Language Barrier

- Written information provided must be appropriate to the population served and the language of the patient (The Joint Commission, 2008, p. 156).
- Use a trained medical interpreter, if possible.
- To review guidelines for communicating with clients who speak a different language, refer to How Do I Communicate With Clients Who Speak a Different Language? in Chapter 15 of this book.

  Some medical dictionaries (e.g., *Taber's Cyclopedic Medical Dictionary*, 2009) have a comprehensive list of English–Spanish phrases.

  The following are some useful Spanish words and phrases.

ENGLISH	SPANISH	ENGLISH	SPANISH
How do you feel?	¿Como se siente?	Cough	Tosa
Good	Bien	Open your mouth	Abra la boca
Bad	Mal	Take a deep breath	Respire profundamente
Have you any difficulty breathing?	¿Tiene dificultad al respirar?	You may eat	Puede comer
Are you thirsty?	¿Tiene sed?	Tea	Té
Have you any pain?	¿Tiene dolor?	Coffee	Café
Show me where	Enséñeme dónde	I will give you something for	Le dare algo para eso
Is it worse now?	¿Está peor ahora?	A pill	Una píldora

Spanish Patient-Education Materials

The following U.S. government sites offer free, reliable patient-education materials in Spanish:

- **http://www.fda.gov/ForConsumers/ByAudience/ForWomen/FreePublications/ucm116729.htm**
  "Spanish Publications." The Food and Drug Administration (FDA). U.S. Department of Health & Human Services. (Easy to read.)
- **http://www.ahrq.gov/consumer/espanoix.htm**
  "Spanish Information." Agency for Healthcare Research and Quality (AHRQ), U.S. Department of Health & Human Services. (Topics such as how to prevent medical errors, having surgery, and choosing a health plan.)
- **http://www.cdc.gov/spanish/**
  Patient and provider education materials. Centers for Disease Control and Prevention.

- **http://www.usa.gov/gobiernousa/Temas/Salud-Nutricion-Seguridad.shtml**
  "Health, Nutrition, and Safety." U.S. General Services Administration, FirstGov.gov site. (Basic health topics, community health services, food safety, and so on.)
- **http://www.nlm.nih.gov/medlineplus/spanish/healthtopics.html**
  "Health Topics." MedlinePlus, U.S. National Library of Medicine, National Institutes of Health, Department of Health and Human Services. (Health information sorted by body location and systems, disorders, demographic groups, and so on.)
  For other online resources:

 Go to Chapter 20, **Resources for Caregivers & Health Professionals,** on Davis*Plus*.

Enhancing Communication With Clients Who Have Impaired Hearing or Speech

For guidelines to help you communicate with clients who have speech, visual, or hearing deficits, respectively, take a look at Clinical Insight 20-5. Also see Clinical Insight 31-2: Communicating with Visually Impaired Clients, and Clinical Insight 31-3: Communicating with Hearing-Impaired Clients.

Enhancing Communication With Clients With Impaired Cognition or Reduced Level of Consciousness

Communicating with cognitively impaired clients can be difficult, time consuming, and frustrating for even the most experienced healthcare provider. Make every effort to communicate regardless of whether the client can understand you. For guidelines to help you communicate with clients with impaired cognition or consciousness, see Clinical Insight 20-6.

Clinical Insight 20-5 ➤ Communicating With Clients Who Have Impaired Speech

Healthcare agencies should address the communication needs of those with vision, speech, hearing, language, and cognitive impairments (The Joint Commission, 2008, p. 156).
- Nonverbal communication is the key to communication with clients with impaired speech.
- Ask the client to use hand gestures and a picture board, as appropriate.
- Solicit family assistance in understanding the client's speech.

- Provide a comfortable environment for the client to practice speaking.
- Be positive and patient.
- Although the client may have difficulty speaking, you should continue to speak and explain all procedures.
- A referral to a speech pathologist may be necessary.

Practice Resources

Adams-Wendling & Pimple, 2007.

Clinical Insight 20-6 ➤ Communicating With Clients Who Have Impaired Cognition or Consciousness

Clients Who Are Cognitively Impaired

Always try to communicate.	Make every effort to communicate, even if you think that the client cannot understand you.
Don't rush the client.	Provide adequate time to allow the client to communicate. He needs time to respond to your questions or commands.
Use multiple communication modalities.	Provide verbal and written discharge instructions. Review the instructions several times with the client before discharge, and include family members in the teaching.
Provide reminders.	Use memory aids, schedules, and reminder notices to reinforce information.
Orient the client.	Verbally orient to time, person, and place, and provide visual orientation materials, such as a calendar or schedule.
Stimulate memory.	If the client loses his place in the conversation, stimulate memory by repeating his last expressed thought. For instance, you might say, "We were talking about your back pain. Tell me more about your back pain."
Use short sentences.	Use short sentences, containing a single thought, such as "Are you hungry?" Avoid complex statements. You could say "You look hungry. Would you like a sandwich or a milk shake, or can you hold off until dinner?"
Ask "yes/no" questions.	Ask direct questions that require only a yes or no answer. ("Are you hungry?")
Limit choices.	Limit choices to avoid confusing or frustrating the patient.
Be concrete and specific.	Do not use vague comments to indicate that you are listening. The client may be unable to interpret comments, such as "I see." Instead, repeat the client's words and directly state your response. "You are cold. I will bring you a blanket."
Avoid slang and jargon.	The client may not understand. For instance, if you say to your patient. "Are you cool?", she might think you mean body temperature when you might actually mean, "Are you feeling OK?"
Use gestures.	Model desired behaviors. You might say, "Brush your teeth now," and then enact brushing your teeth.

(Continued)

Clinical Insight 20-6 ➤ **Communicating With Clients Who Have Impaired Cognition or Consciousness—cont'd**

Don't assume.	Bear in mind that the client cannot behave differently and that he may be confused about reality. When the person is talking about superficial, routine matters, he may seem more competent than he is.
For clients with expressive difficulties:	■ If you are sure of the word the person is trying to say, repeat it. Don't guess, though.
	■ Pay close attention to nonverbal communication.
	■ Assess for and anticipate unmet needs, such as hunger, thirst, and pain.
	■ Respond to the emotion, not the words.
	■ Do not reprimand the patient if she curses or is aggressive.

Patients Who Are Unconscious

■ Touch and speak to unconscious or sedated patients, and advise them of care that you are providing. Although the patient may not be able to respond, she may be able to hear your comments.

■ Consult with previous caregivers or the family to determine what the patient responds to.

■ Begin each interaction by identifying yourself and calling the patient by name.

■ Speak calmly and slowly.

■ Explain all healthcare procedures.

■ Provide soothing music and periods of rest.

Practice Resources

Jayasekara, 2009; Miller, 2008.

CLINICALREASONING:
Applying the **Full-Spectrum Nursing Model**

Because the following critical thinking activities allow you to practice the kind of thinking you will use as a full-spectrum nurse, they usually have no single right answer. Discuss them with your peers—if you have difficulty with any of the questions, consult your instructor.

Choose *two* of the following communication techniques and plan to consciously use them with your next patient. Use the following thinking, doing, and caring questions to reflect on your interaction.

Active listening
Communicating assertively using "I"
    statements
Restating a message
Clarifying messages

Validating messages
Sharing observations about body language
Asking open-ended questions
Using silence
Summarizing the conversation

THINKING

1. *Critical Thinking (Contextual Awareness):* Before you have the conversation, make a note of what is going on in the situation (e.g., values, environment, culture) that might influence the effectiveness of the two techniques you will be using.

DOING

2. *Nursing Process (Assessment):* Before using the two techniques, assess for factors that might affect the patient's ability to communicate. Make a note of them.
3. *Nursing Process (Implementation):* As soon as possible after using the techniques, record the conversations. Try to remember the exact words.
4. *Nursing Process (Evaluation):* Evaluate your ability to use the two techniques you chose.
   a. Did you use them at an appropriate time in the conversation: for example, as an appropriate response to something the patient said?
   b. What effect did your communication have on the interaction? How did the patient respond to what you said?
   c. Do you think your communication was therapeutic for the patient?

CARING

5. *Self-Knowledge:*
   a. What were your thoughts and feelings before, during, and after the interaction?
   b. In what way has your comfort level with these two techniques changed?
   c. Describe the type of patient or situation in which you would be the least confident in your ability to communicate therapeutically.

 Go To Chapter 20, **Clinical Reasoning: Applying the Full-Spectrum Nursing Model Answer Sheet** on Davis*Plus.*

 To explore learning resources for this chapter,

 Go to Davis*Plus* at http://davisplus.fadavis.com, keyword: Treas.

Chapter Resources for Chapter 20:
   Knowledge Check and Think Like a Nurse Response Sheets
   Knowledge Check Answers
   Resources for Caregivers and Health Professionals
   Reading More About Communication & Therapeutic Relationships (Suggested Readings)
   What Are the Main Points in This Chapter?
NCLEX-Style Review Questions
Chapter Overview Podcasts
   Note: For a complete bibliography,

 Go to **Student Resources: Bibliography,** on Davis*Plus.*

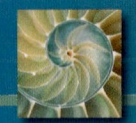

Concept Map

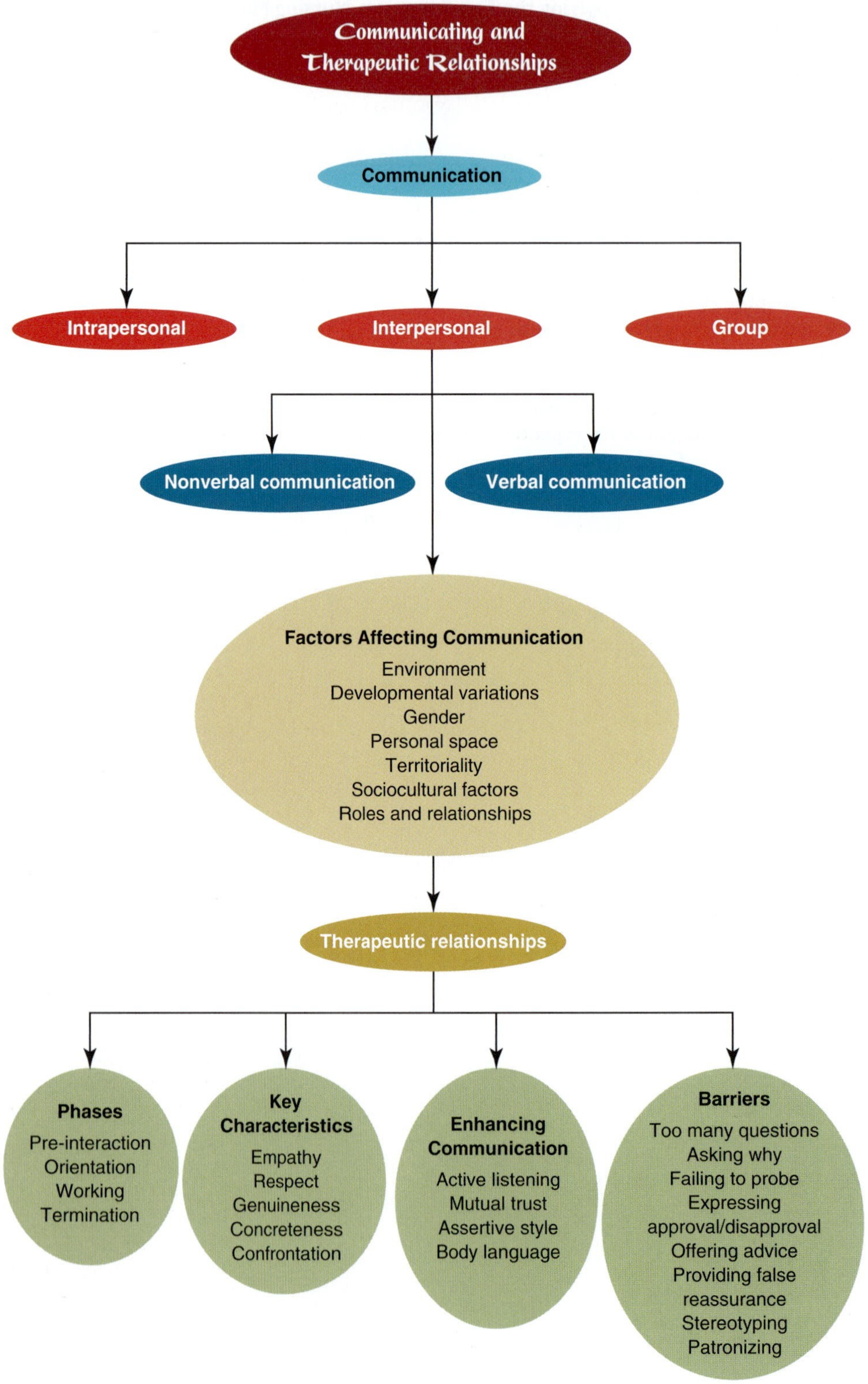

Communicating and Therapeutic Relationships

Communication

Intrapersonal

Interpersonal

Group

Nonverbal communication

Verbal communication

Factors Affecting Communication
Environment
Developmental variations
Gender
Personal space
Territoriality
Sociocultural factors
Roles and relationships

Therapeutic relationships

Phases
Pre-interaction
Orientation
Working
Termination

Key Characteristics
Empathy
Respect
Genuineness
Concreteness
Confrontation

Enhancing Communication
Active listening
Mutual trust
Assertive style
Body language

Barriers
Too many questions
Asking why
Failing to probe
Expressing approval/disapproval
Offering advice
Providing false reassurance
Stereotyping
Patronizing

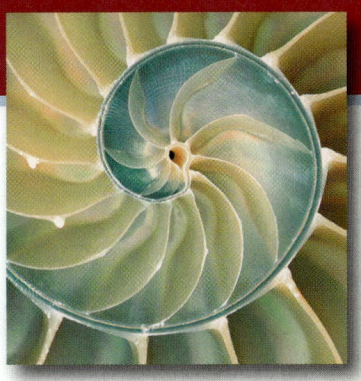

CHAPTER 21

Physical Assessment

Learning Outcomes

After completing this chapter, you should be able to:

➤ Identify the purposes and components of a physical examination.

➤ Discuss the differences among comprehensive, focused, and ongoing physical examinations.

➤ Describe how to prepare for a physical examination.

➤ Demonstrate the skills used in physical examination.

➤ Explain adaptations that may be required when you examine clients of various ages.

➤ Identify the components of the general survey.

➤ Conduct a full physical examination of a client.

➤ Discuss the expected findings of a physical examination.

➤ Document the findings of a physical examination.

➤ Perform a brief bedside physical examination.

Key Concepts

Health assessment

Nursing assessment

Physical assessment

Related Concepts

See the Concept Map at the end of this chapter.

Caring for the Nguyens

This feature allows you to practice the kind of thinking you will use as full-spectrum nurse. There is usually more than one correct answer to a critical thinking question, so we do not provide answers for these features. It is more important to develop your nursing judgment than to "cover content." Discuss the questions with your peers. If you are still unsure, consult your instructor.

Nam Nguyen has come to the family health center for a scheduled comprehensive physical exam. As you recall, he has previously been seen and evaluated by Zach Jackson, RN, FNP, and has medical diagnoses of hypertension, degenerative joint disease, obesity, and heavy tobacco use. During an earlier visit, Zach instructed Mr. Nguyen about a low-salt, low-fat diet and advised him to lose weight and quit smoking. Zach also ordered lab work to establish a baseline for wellness and detect abnormalities that might indicate illness. At today's visit, Zach also reviews Mr. Nguyen's lab results with him. After Nam's appointment, his wife, Yen Nguyen, will also have a comprehensive exam. Review the results of Mr. Nguyen's lab work that follow.

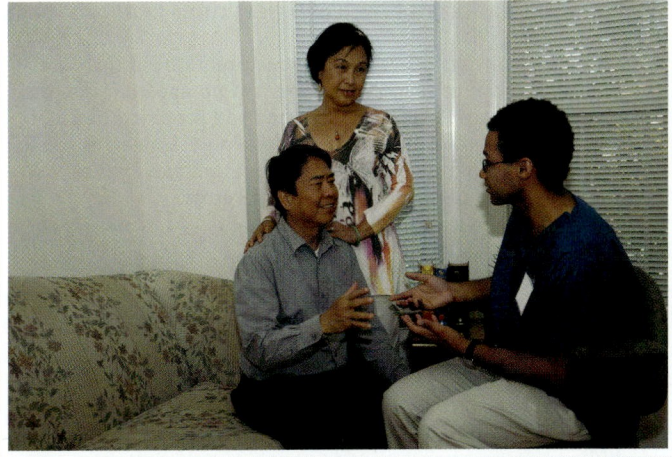

After Zach completes Nam's physical exam, he records the data. Review Zach's charting entry, following. Recall that Zach is an advanced practice nurse and has performed a comprehensive physical assessment. Therefore, this examination and charting entry are more extensive than what would be expected of a staff nurse. Keep in mind that you should use only abbreviations on your clinical agency's approved list.

If you cannot answer these questions now, try again after you have studied this chapter.

(Continued)

Caring for the Nguyens (continued)

A. Discuss how each of the following would differ from the examination Zach Jackson conducted and what would be expected if:
- A registered nurse conducted the exam.
- A nursing student performed the exam.

B. Review Zach's documentation of the exam. Identify the abnormal findings.

C. Review the laboratory work. Identify the abnormal findings.

D. What conclusions, if any, can you draw from these findings? What actions should you consider based on these conclusions?

E. Identify at least two nursing diagnoses based on these findings.

F. Zach Jackson has identified a problem of Imbalanced Nutrition: More Than Body Requirements for Mr. Nguyen.
- What information do you need to determine the etiology of this problem?

- Because you do not have that information, write a two-part diagnostic statement describing Mr. Nguyen's nutritional status.

G. Now rewrite the nutrition statement as a three-part statement, using "as evidenced by."

H. Zach Jackson has identified the diagnosis Acute Pain (knees) for Mr. Nguyen. If the pain is caused by a medical condition, osteoarthritis, how would you write a two-part diagnostic statement to describe this health status?

I. How would the examination of Yen Nguyen differ from the exam Nam experienced?

J. How would the examination of Kim Phan, Nam's 3-year-old grandson, differ?

K. If you were responsible for examining Nam Nguyen, what aspects of the exam would you find most challenging? Explain why.

 Go to **Caring for the Nguyens Response Sheet** on *DavisPlus*.

Documentation of Physical Assessment Findings for Nam Nguyen

General Survey. 66-year-old moderately obese man presents to the clinic for a physical exam in no apparent distress. Pt. appears stated age; is well dressed and groomed; and alert and oriented to time, place, and person. Speech is clear, response and affect appropriate. Moves all extremities well, gait steady and balanced. Smells of cigarettes.

Height	5 ft 4 in.
Weight	185 lb (84 kg)
BP	166/100 mm Hg
Pulse	88 beats/min
RR	22 breaths/min
Temp	98.5°F (36.9°C), oral
BMI	33

Integumentary. Skin even in color, warm & dry, good turgor, no suspicious lesions. Well healed scar in right inguinal area. Hair clean, coarse, evenly distributed. Some graying. Nails pink, brisk capillary refill, no clubbing.

Head & Neck. Normocephalic, erect, midline. Scalp mobile, no lesions, tenderness, or masses. Facial features symmetrical. Thyroid gland symmetrical and not enlarged; cervical lymph nodes not palpable or tender.

Eyes. Snellen = right eye 20/100, left eye 20/100, both eyes 20/100. Color vision intact. Difficulty noted with near vision. Visual fields normal by confrontation. Extraocular movements intact. PERRLA at 3 mm by direct and consensual. Eyes clear and bright, + blink, no lid lag or abnormalities. Anterior chamber clear. Cornea & iris intact. Sclera white, conjunctiva clear. Lacrimal glands and ducts nontender. + red reflex bilateral, discs flat with sharp margins, vessels intact, retina & macula even in color.

Ears, Nose, & Throat. Skin intact, no masses, lesions, or discharge. Position WNL. External ears nontender to palpation. + whisper test. Weber—no lateralization. External canals clear without redness, swelling, lesions, or discharge. Tympanic membranes intact, light reflex and bony landmarks visible; frontal and maxillary sinuses nontender. Nares patent, able to distinguish familiar odors, mucosa pink, no discharge, septum intact with no deviation.

Mouth. Lips, oral mucosa, gingivae pink with no lesions. All teeth present and in good repair. Pharynx pink, tonsils absent, palate intact. Symmetrical rise of the uvula, + gag and swallow reflex. Tongue smooth, pink, symmetrical, mobile, without lesions, taste intact (correctly identified sweet, salty, and sour).

Respiratory. Respirations 22 breaths/min and unlabored. Trachea midline, AP less than transverse chest diameter. Chest expansion symmetrical. No tenderness, scars, masses, or lesions. Diaphragmatic excursion 5 cm. Lungs clear to auscultation.

Cardiovascular. PMI @ MCL at 5th ICS, P 85, regular, no murmurs, gallops, or thrills present; pulses +2, no bruits or thrills, no varicosities; jugular venous pulsation 2 cm at 45°. Carotids without bruits.

Breasts. Symmetrical. No masses, lymphadenopathy, or discharge.

Abdomen. Abdomen soft, rounded; no masses or pulsations. Surgical scar right inguinal area. +bowel sounds, +tympany throughout.

Musculoskeletal. Normal spinal curvature. Joints and muscles symmetrical, no deformity. +Bilateral knee pain (right more than left). Full ROM in upper and lower extremities; +5 muscle strength; moderate crepitus right knee.

Documentation of Physical Assessment Findings for Nam Nguyen—cont'd

Neurological. Awake; alert; and oriented to time, place, and person. CN I–XII intact. Gait steady and coordinated; negative Romberg; unable to do deep knee bends due to pain. Point-point localization; superficial and deep sensation intact; +2 deep tendon reflexes.

Genitourinary. Circumcised male; penis nontender, no masses, urethral meatus midline, no discharge; testicles descended bilaterally, nontender, inguinal and femoral canals free of masses, prostate small, smooth, mobile, nontender. Rectal wall smooth, no masses, stool hemoccult negative.

Laboratory Data for Nam Nguyen

Name: Nam Nguyen **DOB:** 7/12/50
Acct#: K00205412 Family Medicine Center, Z. Jackson

Test	Result	Reference Range*
CBC/Differential		
WBC	5.6 x 10^3/mm³	5–10 x 10^3/mm³
Hemoglobin	14.8 g/dL	M: 14–18 g/dL F: 12–16 g/dL
Hematocrit	45.1%	M: 42–52% F: 37–47%
RBC count	5.1 million/mm³	M: 4.7–5.14 million/mm³ F: 4.2–4.87 million/mm³
MCV	84 mm³	85–95 mm³
MCH	29 pg	28–32 pg
MCHC	34%	33–35%
Neutrophils	57%	59%
Lymphocytes	30%	34%
Monocytes	5%	4%
Eosinophils	2.5%	2.7%
Basophils	0.7%	0.5%
Platelet count	197,000/mm³	150,000–400,000/mm³

Test	Result	Reference Range*
Comprehensive Metabolic Panel		
Sodium	138 mEq/L	135–145 mEq/L
Potassium	4.3 mEq/L	3.5–5.0 mEq/L
Chloride	101 mEq/L	97–107 mEq/L
Carbon dioxide	27 mEq/L	23–29 mEq/L
BUN	16 mg/dL	10–31 mg/dL
Creatinine	0.8 mg/dL	M: 0.6–1.2 mg/dL F: 0.5–1.1 mg/dL
Glucose	156 mg/dL	75–110 mg/dL
Albumin	4.0 g/dL	19–60 years: 3.2–4.8 g/dL
Total protein	7.2 g/dL	6.8–8.0 g/dL
ALT (alanine aminotransferase, also called SGPT)	18 units/L	M: 10–40 units/L F: 7–35 units/L
ALP (alkaline phosphatase)	43 units/L	M: 35–142 units/L F: 25–125 units/L
AST (aspartate aminotranspeptidase, also called SGOT)	26 units/L	M: 19–48 units/L F: 9–36 units/L
Bilirubin, total	0.7 mg/dL	0.3–1.2 mg/dL
Calcium	8.5 mg/dL	8.2–10.2 mg/dL

Test	Result	Reference Range*	
Lipid Panel**			
Total cholesterol	201 mg/dL	<200 200–239 >240	-Desirable -Borderline high -High
LDL cholesterol (Primary target of therapy)	140 mg/dL	<100 mg/dL 100–129 mg/dL 130–159 160–189 >190	-Optimal -Near optimal/ above optimal -Borderline high -High -Very high
HDL cholesterol	34 mg/dL	<40	-Low
Triglycerides	196 mg/dL		

**To interpret lipid panel results, follow the most recent guidelines of the National Cholesterol Education Program (NCEP) Expert Panel on Detection, Evaluation, and Blood Cholesterol in Adults available at www.nhlbi.nih.gov/guidelines/cholesterol/atglance.pdf. The reference range figures in this table will undoubtedly be revised (and lowered) by NCEP in the near future.

Also, the norms for an individual patient's lipid panel depend on the calculation of risk factors. Nam is hypertensive, is obese, and has an elevated blood sugar. His norms reflect high risk for coronary heart disease; they would be about <160 for total cholesterol, <100 for triglycerides, <100 for LDL, and >45 for HDL.

Test	Result	Reference Range*
Urinalysis		
Appearance	Clear	Clear
Color	Amber	Light yellow to amber
Odor	Aromatic	None–aromatic
pH	6.0	5.0–9.0
Specific gravity	1.012	1.001–1.035
Leukocyte esterase	Negative	Negative
Nitrites	Negative	Negative
Ketones	Negative	Negative
Protein	5 mg/dL	<20 mg/dL
Crystals	None	In acid urine: uric acid, calcium oxalate, amorphous urates In alkaline urine: triple phosphate, calcium phosphate, ammonium biurate, calcium carbonate, amorphous phosphates
Casts	None	None, except rare hyaline
Glucose	Negative	Negative
WBC	1/hpf	<5/hpf
RBC	1/hpf	<5/hpf
PSA (prostate-specific antigen)	2.8 ng/mL	<4 ng/mL
Fecal occult blood screen		
Sample #1 — negative		
Sample #2 — negative		
Sample #3 — negative		

*For most studies, each laboratory establishes its own reference range.

TheoreticalKnowledge
knowing **why**

In this chapter, theoretical knowledge consists mostly of information about the key concepts and about preparing yourself and the client for the examination, and about modifying your assessments for different age groups.

ABOUT THE KEY CONCEPTS

Health assessment is a comprehensive assessment of the physical, mental, spiritual, socioeconomic, and cultural status of an individual, group, or community. **Nursing assessments** focus on the client's functional abilities and physical responses to illness and other stressors. In contrast, medical assessments focus on disease and pathology. As a nurse practitioner, Zach Jackson combines the nursing and medical approaches.

We usually think of **physical examination,** or **physical assessment,** as the techniques used to gather objective data about the body. However, you will also ask questions to obtain subjective data about each body system or area. This may be done in a separate nursing interview (a nursing history) or as you perform the physical examination. Both the interview and the exam require tact and sensitivity.

WHAT ARE THE PURPOSES OF A PHYSICAL EXAMINATION?

A physical examination is performed for any of several reasons:
- *To obtain baseline data* about physical status and functional abilities to serve as a comparison as the patient's health status changes.
- *To identify nursing diagnoses, collaborative problems, and wellness diagnoses,* to form the basis for the plan of care.
- *To monitor the status of a previously identified problem.* For example, Mr. Nguyen has already begun treatment for hypertension. Today's examination will be linked to the lab results to further explore the status of his hypertension.
- *To screen for health problems.* Regular checkups can help to identify health problems at early stages. Because Mr. Nguyen has an enlarged prostate, a prostate-specific antigen (PSA) test was done to screen for prostate cancer.

The type of physical examination you perform will depend on the client's health status, the nature of the client encounter, and the setting. For example, at an outpatient appointment for an annual physical, on a client's admission to an inpatient setting, or at the initial home health visit, you would perform a **comprehensive physical assessment,** which includes a health history interview and a complete head-to-toe examination of every body system.

In an emergency situation, your assessment will be rapid and focused on the presenting problem. A **focused physical assessment** pertains to a particular topic, body part, or functional ability rather than overall health status, and it adds to the database created by the comprehensive assessment. A **system-specific assessment** is a focused assessment limited to one body system (e.g., the lungs, the peripheral circulation). The following are examples of focused and system-specific physical assessments, respectively:
- Assessing bowel sounds when a client has abdominal pain
- Listening to breath sounds, counting respirations, and obtaining pulse oximetry readings to assess a patient's respiratory status

Ongoing assessment is performed as needed, after the initial database is completed, and, ideally, at every interaction with the patient. For example, on a medical–surgical unit, each nurse who provides care to a client conducts a brief ongoing assessment to determine changes in the client's status. For more details on the types of assessment, see Chapter 3. To learn how to perform a brief bedside assessment, see Procedure 21-20.

How Do I Prepare to Perform a Physical Examination?

You should develop a systematic approach and follow the same order each time you perform a physical exam. This will help you recall the steps and include all the important data. A **head-to-toe approach** starts at the head and neck and progresses down the body, examining the feet last. A **body systems approach** examines each system in a predetermined order (e.g., musculoskeletal, cardiovascular, neurological). Whatever the approach, prepare yourself, the environment, and the client before you begin.

Prepare Yourself

Preparing for a physical examination requires theoretical knowledge of anatomy and physiology, examination equipment and techniques, therapeutic communication, and documentation. Self-knowledge is also important. How comfortable are you when performing an examination? What skills do you need to review or practice? Will you need assistance to perform some aspects of the exam? Will you need help documenting your findings? Honestly evaluate your strengths as well as areas that need improvement. Be sure to seek help from your instructor, an experienced nurse, fellow students, or other healthcare providers as needed.

Before approaching the patient, familiarize yourself with his situation. What are the patient's main health concerns? What is the purpose of your exam? For instance, if you are doing a focused assessment of a client's wound, you will need to learn about the wound being examined. Is there a dressing over the wound? What supplies will you need to remove and replace the dressing? Has the patient required pain medication before exams in the past? Reviewing previous findings helps you work efficiently and to formulate any questions you might want to ask the patient.

Finally, unless this is an initial assessment, review the nursing plan of care and keep it in mind as you examine the patient. Your assessment data may lead to modification or updating of the care plan.

Prepare the Environment

Physical examination requires you to observe and touch the client's body, so privacy is essential. You will need a room with curtains or a door to shield the client from view. For additional privacy, drape your client and uncover only the area you are examining. For convenience you may use bed linens and/or a gown to drape. Disposable paper drapes are also available.

Because you will need to hear the patient and listen to a variety of sounds during the exam, turn off the television, radio, or other media. You will need good lighting to observe subtle changes in skin and body contours. Adjust the temperature of the room according to patient comfort.

Determine the instruments and equipment you will need (see Box 21-1). Take everything you need so that you will not have to leave the client to obtain supplies.

BOX 21-1 ■ Equipment Needed for Physical Examination: Usual Equipment for Ongoing Assessment

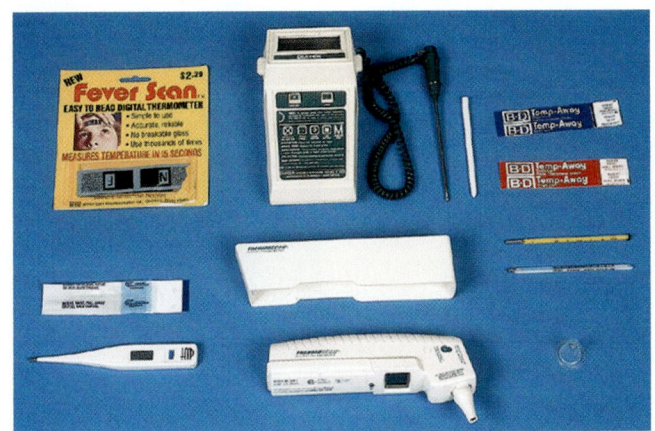

Thermometer (for measuring temperature)

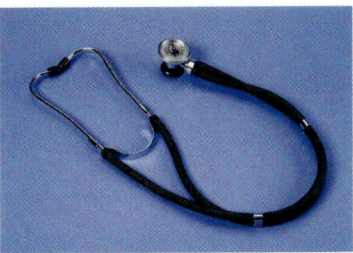

Stethoscope (for measuring blood pressure and listening to heart, lung, and bowel sounds)

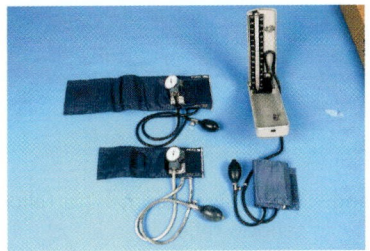

Sphygmomanometer (for measuring blood pressure)

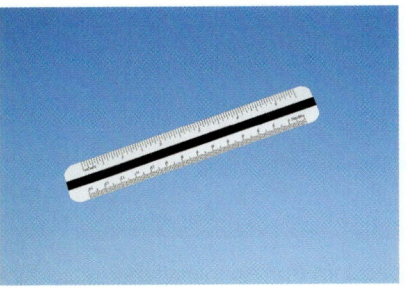

Pocket ruler (to measure size or distance)

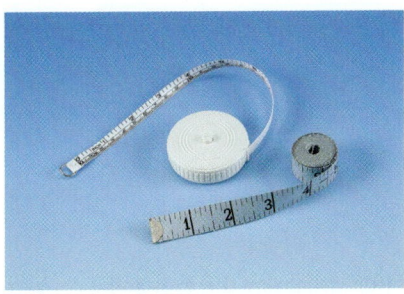

Tape measure (to measure circumference and length)

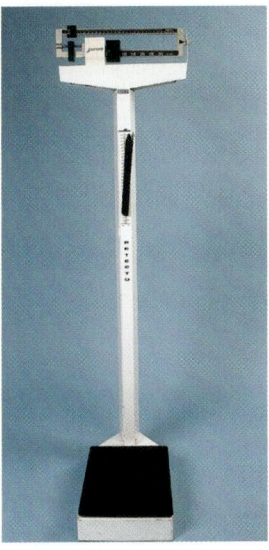

Scale (to measure weight and height)

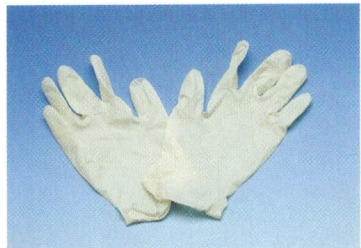

Gloves (to wear if there is any possible exposure to blood or body fluids)

(Continued)

BOX 21-1 ■ Equipment Needed for Physical Examination: Usual Equipment for Ongoing Assessment—cont'd

Additional Equipment for a Comprehensive Assessment

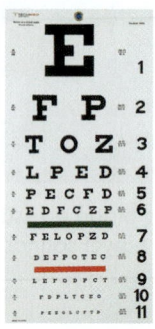

Snellen acuity chart (for screening vision)

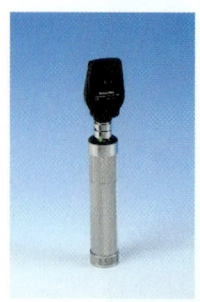

Ophthalmoscope (for inspection of the internal structures of the eye)

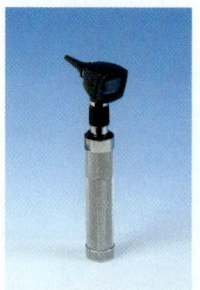

Otoscope (for examining the external auditory canal and tympanic membrane)

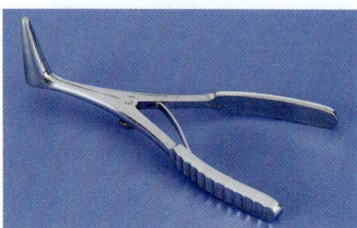

Nasal speculum (for examining the nasal turbinates)

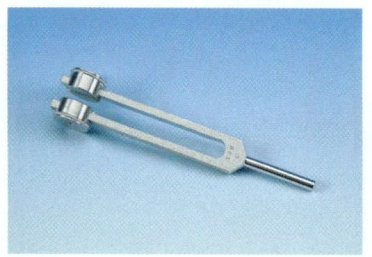

Tuning fork (for auditory screening and assessment of vibratory sensation during the neurological exam)

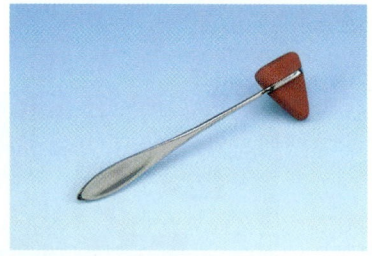

Percussion hammer (for eliciting deep tendon reflexes)

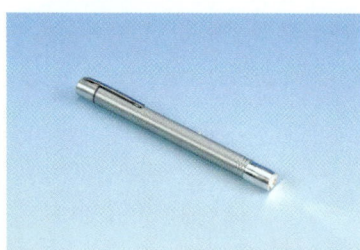

Penlight (for visualizing the eyes and inside of mouth, or highlighting a skin lesion)

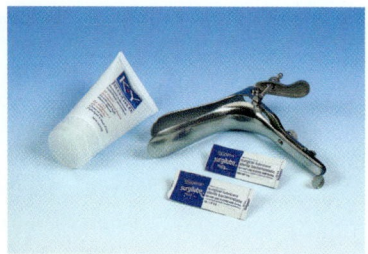

Vaginal speculum and lubricant (for examining the female pelvis; lubricant is also used for rectal exams)

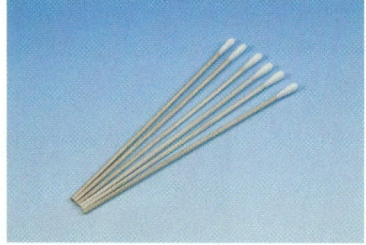

Cotton-tipped applicators (for obtaining specimens)

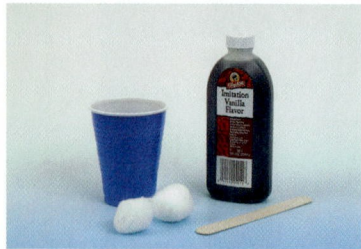

Cotton balls, tongue depressor, strong-smelling substance, a glass of water (for testing various cranial nerves)

Prepare the Client

In most clinical settings, you must examine a client often to evaluate a changing status, and timing will be decided by the client's condition rather than by convenience. However, when possible, select a time when the client is comfortable and receptive to the exam. Avoid conducting the exam when the client is in pain or is hungry, tired, anxious, or unwilling to cooperate in the assessment.

Take the time to establish rapport with the client, to help him relax and cooperate fully in the assessment. Introduce yourself, ask the client how he wishes to be addressed, and explain what you will be doing. Ask the client to void before the examination; this promotes relaxation and also makes it easier to palpate the abdomen. Always alert the client before touching him. For example, before you start to palpate the neck for lymph nodes, say, "I'm going to feel your neck now." Proper positioning during the exam also promotes comfort (see the following section). Pay attention to the pace of your exam, being careful not to prolong it and tire the client.

Consider developmental and cultural differences. For example, some clients may wish to have a family member present during an exam; some may require a same-sex clinician. If you and the client do not speak the same language, arrange to have an interpreter present.

KnowledgeCheck 21-1

- What are the purposes of a physical examination?
- Describe how you would prepare for a physical exam.

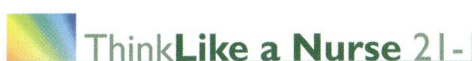

ThinkLike a Nurse 21-1

- The nurse conducts a physical assessment for Nam and Yen Nguyen (see Caring for the Nguyens) at an outpatient clinic. Discuss the differences between their planned experience and a focused physical exam of a hospital inpatient.
- Identify a plan to practice and improve your assessment skills.

How Do I Position the Client for a Physical Examination?

The client will need to assume a variety of positions during a comprehensive physical examination. To begin the examination, seat the client on the side of the bed or examination table. Face the client, and establish eye contact. This helps to build rapport and put the client at ease. If your client is unable to sit, assist him to a position on his back with the head of the bed elevated. An upright position allows the client to expand his lungs fully and is useful for assessing vital signs, the head and neck, the heart and lungs, the back, and the upper extremities. As you place your client in positions that allow you to best observe each body system, be alert to special needs that call for you to modify the position. For example, a patient with a cervical spine problem

would need a neck roll when lying supine. Table 21-1 illustrates and describes the major positions you will need to use.

KnowledgeCheck 21-2

Identify the best positions for examining the lungs, heart, pulses, and abdomen.

What Techniques Do I Need to Perform a Physical Examination?

The skills used in physical examination include inspection, palpation, percussion, auscultation, and sometimes olfaction. You will use these skills in that order except when performing an abdominal assessment, in which case you will perform auscultation before percussion and palpation to avoid disturbing the abdominal sounds.

Inspection is the use of sight to gather data. You begin to use inspection the moment you meet the client and continue as you observe the person's gait, personal hygiene, affect, and behavior during the general survey. You will also use inspection as you evaluate each body system. Adequate lighting and proper positioning aid inspection. The otoscope, ophthalmoscope, and penlight also enhance your inspection abilities.

Palpation is the use of touch to gather data. Use palpation to assess temperature; skin texture; moisture; anatomical landmarks; and such abnormalities as edema, masses, or areas of tenderness. As you begin and move through the assessment of each body system, always inform the client that you are about to touch him, and use a gentle approach. Be certain your hands are warm. Begin with light pressure to detect surface characteristics. Then move to deep palpation to assess the underlying structures. Examine last any areas of discomfort or sensitivity. Following is a list of the most common palpation techniques, using different parts of the hand.

- *Fingertips:* Use for fine tactile discrimination, including assessment of skin texture, swelling, and specific locations of pulsations and masses.
- *Dorsum of hand:* Use for temperature determination.
- *Palmar surface of hand:* Use for locating general area of pulsations.
- *Grasping with fingers and thumb:* Use to detect the position, shape, and consistency of a mass.

Percussion is tapping your fingers on the skin using short strokes. Tapping produces vibrations, and the resulting sound allows you to determine location, size, and density of underlying structures. Percussion is especially useful when assessing the abdomen and lungs. Percussion takes practice. To learn more about percussion, see Clinical Insight 21-1. A quiet environment allows you to perceive the subtle differences in percussion notes. To learn terminology for the notes you may hear when assessing your clients,

 Go to **Sound Files: Percussion Notes** on *DavisPlus.*

Table 21-1 ➤ Positioning the Client

POSITION AND DESCRIPTION	COMMENTS
Standing	
Upright posture with both feet flat on the floor.	Use to examine the musculoskeletal and neurological systems and to assess gait and cerebellar function. Clients who are weak or who have poor balance may not be able to assume this position.
Sitting	
Sitting upright at side of bed or exam table 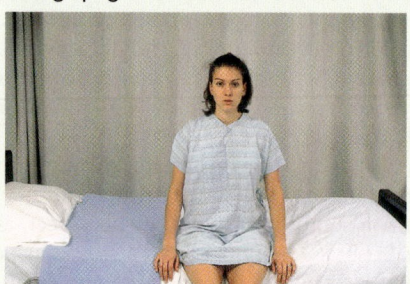	Use to assess vital signs, head and neck, chest, cardiovascular system, and breasts. If your client is weak, he may need assistance to maintain this position.
Supine	
(Including Fowler's and semi-Fowler's positions). Lying flat on the back with arms and legs fully extended 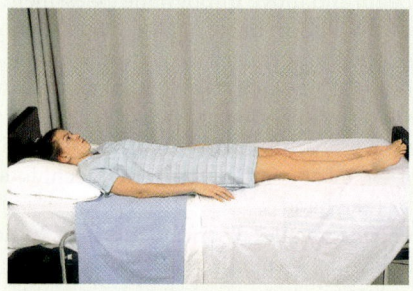	Use to assess the abdomen, breasts, extremities, and pulses. If your client becomes short of breath, raise the head of the bed (HOB). In **Fowler's position**, the head is elevated 60°. In **semi-Fowler's position**, the head is elevated only 30°–45°.
Dorsal Recumbent	
Supine with knees flexed 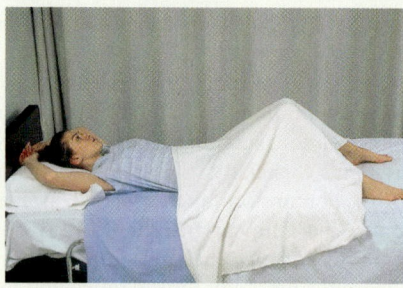	Use for abdominal assessment if your client has abdominal or pelvic pain. Flexing the knees promotes relaxation of the abdominal muscles.
Lithotomy	
Dorsal recumbent position at end of table with feet in stirrups, legs flexed, and widely open 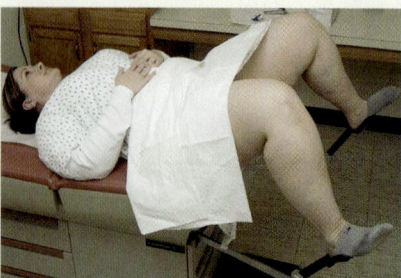	Use for a female pelvic exam; provides maximum exposure of genitals. Older patients may need support to assume and maintain this position. The patient's legs are exposed here to illustrate position. To see a privacy drape, refer to Procedure 22-4.

Table 21-1 ▶ Positioning the Client—cont'd

POSITION AND DESCRIPTION	COMMENTS
Sims'	
Flexion of the hip and knees in a side-lying position 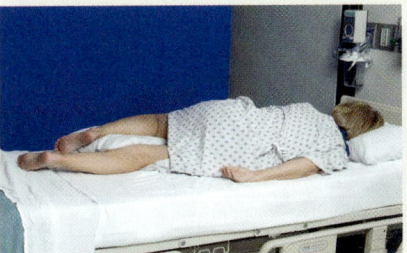	Use to examine the rectal area. Use for a female pelvic exam if the patient is unable to assume the lithotomy position. Do not use if the client has had total hip replacement.
Prone	
Lying on stomach (A small pillow under the abdomen makes this position more comfortable.) 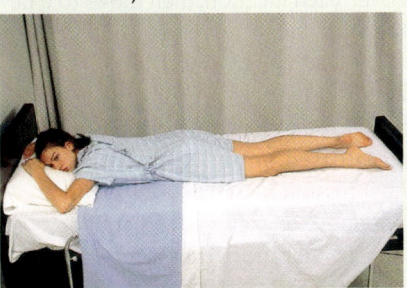	Use to examine the musculoskeletal system, especially hip extension; may also be used to examine the back and buttocks. May be difficult to assume by clients with respiratory problems.
Lateral Recumbent	
Lying on the side in a straight line 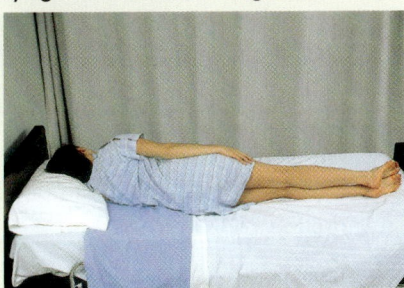	Left lateral recumbent is used to evaluate heart murmur or during a thorough cardiovascular assessment. This position brings the heart closer to the chest wall. If the client cannot assume this position, listen to the heart with the client seated and bending forward.
Knee–Chest	
On hands and knees with head down and buttocks elevated 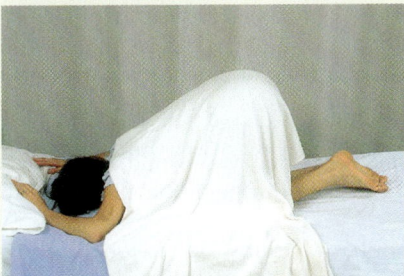	Provides good visualization for examining the rectal area. However, it is not used often because it is embarrassing and uncomfortable for the client.

Clinical Insight 21-1 ➤ **Performing Percussion**

Direct Percussion

Tap lightly with the pads of the fingers directly on the skin.

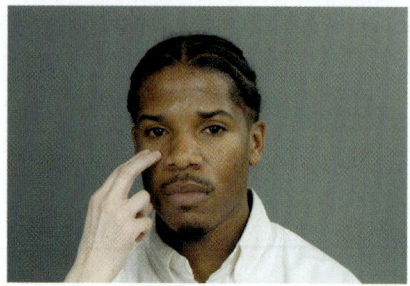

Direct percussion over the sinuses.

Indirect Percussion

- Keep your fingernails short.
- Strive for a quiet environment: Turn off all entertainment media and music, shut the door, and so on. This allows you to better perceive the subtle differences in percussion notes.
- One hand is considered the stationary hand; the other is the striking hand.
- Hyperextend the middle finger of your stationary hand, and place its distal portion firmly against the client's skin over the area you wish to percuss.
- Lift the rest of your fingers off the patient's skin. Prevents dampening the sounds produced.
- Be sure both of your hands are relaxed to best perform the technique. Stiff hands will not effectively produce the percussion sounds for assessment.

- Use the middle finger of your dominant hand as the striking finger **(plexor),** and tap the distal portion of the middle finger of the stationary hand using a quick motion from your wrist.

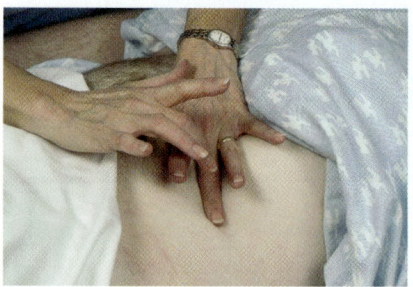

Indirect percussion.

- Use enough force to elicit a clear sound.
- Percuss two times over each location, then move to a new body location and repeat.

Describing Sounds

Use the terms in the following list to describe the sounds you hear. The terms are based on the components of the sounds produced by percussion.

- *Amplitude*—The loudness or softness of a sound
- *Pitch*—The number of vibrations per second; can be either high or low in nature
- *Quality*—A distinctiveness about the sound produced
- *Duration*—How long the sound lingers

Percussion Notes

SOUND	AMPLITUDE	PITCH	QUALITY	DURATION	EXAMPLE
Resonant	Medium-loud	Low	Hollow	Medium	Normal lung
Hyperresonant	Louder	Lower	Booming	Longer	Hyperinflated lung (as in emphysema)
Dull	Soft	High	Muffled thud	Short	Liver/spleen
Flat	Very soft	High	Absolute dullness	Very short	Thigh or tumor
Tympany	Loud	High	Musical	Longest	Gastric air bubble, intestinal air

Auscultation is the use of hearing to gather data. Direct auscultation is listening without using an instrument. If you have heard wheezing or chest congestion without the use of a stethoscope, you have already performed direct auscultation. Indirect auscultation is listening with the help of a stethoscope. The stethoscope has two end pieces, the diaphragm and the bell. To improve your skill in indirect auscultation, see Clinical Insight 21-2.

Olfaction is the use of the sense of smell to gather data. Some clinicians may not consider this a formal assessment skill; however, you will certainly use this skill in the clinical setting. Olfaction adds information to the data you collect through the other techniques. Consider these examples:

- If a client is slurring his words, you will want to look for data that reveal the cause of the problem. Slurred speech

might be caused by a stroke or by sedative medications. However, if the client smells of alcohol you would first investigate recent alcohol use as a probable cause for the slurred words.

- If an older client smells of urine, you would want to assess for problems with leakage of urine or inability to perform self-care.
- If the client's breath has a "fruity" or "acetone" odor, you would suspect ketoacidosis (which may accompany diabetes). You would know to assess the urine for ketones and contact the primary care provider if necessary. You would also ask the client about dietary patterns, because a high-protein, high-fat, low-carbohydrate diet can cause a buildup of ketones in the blood.

Clinical Insight 21-2 ➤ Performing Auscultation

- Provide a quiet environment to facilitate auscultation.

- ✚ Clean your stethoscope with a 70% alcohol or benzalkonium chloride wipe before and after using it to examine a patient. Most stethoscopes are colonized by bacteria, although only a small percentage are pathogenic. Cleaning can reduce the bacterial count by 94% to 100%.

- Use the diaphragm to listen to high-pitched sounds that normally occur in the heart, lungs, and abdomen. Press the diaphragm hard enough to produce an obvious ring on the patient's skin.

- Use the bell to hear low-pitched sounds, such as extra heart sounds (murmurs) or turbulent blood flow (bruits). Apply the bell lightly with just enough pressure to produce an air seal with its full rim.

- Place the earpieces facing forward. Seals the ear canal and improves detection of sounds.

- Warm the stethoscope before you place it on the client's skin.

- Place the stethoscope directly on the client's skin. Do not listen through clothing. Clothing can create artifact or reduce the quality of auscultation.

- If body hair prevents good contact with the skin, dampen the hair before you listen.

- Close your eyes as you listen through the stethoscope. This helps improve your focus.

- Concentrate on one sound at a time. Do not try to evaluate breath and heart sounds at the same time. Improves the quality of the data.

Practice Resources

Centers for Disease Control and Prevention (CDC), 2008; Kennedy, Dreimanis, Beckingham, et al., 2003; Rutala & Weber, 2004.

KnowledgeCheck 21-3

- Identify five physical assessment skills.
- In what order are these skills performed?

ThinkLike a Nurse 21-2

Think about olfaction as an assessment technique. Give two or three additional examples of data you might collect through the use of smell.

How Do I Modify Assessment for Different Age Groups?

The basic techniques of physical assessment remain the same for all age groups. However, your approach will vary according to the developmental stage of your patient.

Infants. Use the assessment as an opportunity to teach the parent about normal growth and development. Infants usually feel most secure if a parent holds them during the examination, either against the chest or, for older infants who can sit without support, on the parent's lap. Otherwise, position an infant on a padded examination table.

✚ If there are siderails, raise them to prevent falls. Do not leave the infant's side or turn your back on the infant.

Toddlers. Toddlers can be challenging to examine. They are interested in exploring the environment, but they also like to stay close by a parent, often in the parent's lap. Because they may be fearful of invasive procedures, such as examination of the oral cavity or inner ear, perform these procedures last. Most toddlers enjoy making choices, so use this characteristic to promote the toddler's cooperation. For example, you might provide a choice by saying, "Should I listen to your chest first, or should we see how much you weigh?" Allow the child to show you his developmental skills. If he needs assistance to remove clothing, have the parent help, and observe how the parent and child interact. Always praise the toddler for his abilities and cooperation. This sets the stage for positive feelings about healthcare.

Preschoolers. Preschool children are developing initiative and, as a result, usually cooperate with an examination. However, children of this age have fantasies and fears that may arise during the examination. For example, they may object to a noninvasive procedure because they believe it will cause pain or injury, or they may refuse to step on the scale because to them it resembles a monster. In such cases, it may be helpful to demonstrate the procedure on a doll or have the parent step on the scale before you approach the child.

Allow the preschool child to sit in a parent's lap if she wishes. By age 5, most children will be comfortable enough to lie on the examination table if a parent is present. Let the child help with the exam. For example, have her hold equipment or remember her height and weight. Give reassurance as you go through the examination, for example, "Your lungs sound very healthy." Always compliment the child on her cooperation.

School-Age Children. The school-age child has a rapidly expanding vocabulary and usually seeks approval of parents, teachers, and healthcare providers. Develop rapport by asking the child about his favorite school or play activities. Allow the child to undress himself and get up and down from the exam table. Demonstrate your equipment before you use it. The school-age child will be interested in how his body works, so use this opportunity for teaching.

Adolescents. The adolescent is self-conscious and introspective and may wish to be examined without parents or siblings present, at least during the more personal aspects of the exam. Offer the adolescent this choice. Adolescents often worry about the "normalcy" of their changing bodies and appreciate respect for their privacy. Be certain to discuss the normal physiological changes that accompany puberty. If you need to review those changes, refer to Chapter 9.

Adolescent behavior may be strongly influenced by peer values, so emphasize lifestyle habits that promote wellness, including a healthful diet; adequate rest and exercise; and avoidance of tobacco, alcohol, and other drugs. Also discuss sexually transmitted infections and cancer, particularly

testicular cancer and human papillomavirus. The first pelvic examination and breast examination usually begin in the teen years. Because suicide is the third leading cause of death among adolescents, you should also use this opportunity to screen for depression and suicide risk (see Chapter 13 for a review of depression and suicide).

Young and Middle Adults. Most young and middle adults are able to cooperate during a physical examination and do not require a modified approach. Modifications may be required if the client has acute or chronic illness or cannot understand or follow instructions.

Older Adults. Older adults are adjusting to changes in physical abilities and health. As part of a comprehensive exam, assess the client's support system and ability to perform activities of daily living. Observe your client's energy level during the physical examination and provide rest periods if needed. If the client tires easily, arrange the exam sequence to limit position changes. Also be aware that stiff muscles and arthritic joints may make it impossible for the client to assume certain positions. Older adults may have impaired vision or hearing, so you may need to adapt your techniques to compensate for this. Obtain feedback to be sure the patient is seeing and hearing you adequately.

The acronym SPICES will help you to remember common problems of older adults that require nursing intervention (Fulmer, 1991, 2007) and to focus your assessment as you perform a comprehensive physical examination:

S—Sleep disorders
P—Problems with eating or feeding
I—Incontinence
C—Confusion
E—Evidence of falls
S—Skin breakdown

KnowledgeCheck 21-4

What exam modifications, based on developmental stage, should you consider for the following clients (Caring for the Nguyens)
▪ Nam Nguyen?
▪ Nam's 3-year-old grandson, Kim Phan?
▪ Nam's elderly mother, Mai Nguyen?

The remainder of the chapter discusses each of the components of a comprehensive physical examination. As you perform your physical assessments, you may wish to refer to laboratory tests associated with each of the systems you are assessing. You can find some normal lab values in the Laboratory Data for Nam Nguyen (Reference Ranges) at the beginning of this chapter. For a list of various laboratory tests,

 Go to Chapter 21, **Supplemental Materials: Laboratory and Diagnostic Tests by System,** on *DavisPlus.*

THE GENERAL SURVEY

The general survey is your overall impression of the client. It begins at first contact and continues throughout the exam. When you discover a deviation from normal in the general survey, you will explore it further during focused assessment of that body system. For example, if on meeting the patient you notice a drooping eyelid (ptosis) on one side of her face, you will keep that in mind as you perform the neurological assessment. Ptosis may be caused by a stroke or neurological injury. For a step-by-step approach, see Procedure 21-1. The following are aspects of the general survey.

Appearance and Behavior

Observe the client's general characteristics. Are his speech and behavior appropriate for his developmental stage? Look for indications of his mood and mental status—for instance, does he make eye contact with you? Notice any signs of distress, either physical or emotional. Observe the condition of your client's face, and note the quality of the visible skin; for example, excessive wrinkling of the skin from sun exposure, tobacco use, or illness may make the client appear older than his stated age. Be sure to consider cultural background, because this may influence your findings and interpretation.

Body Type and Posture

Next, observe your client's body size, build, and gait. As you introduce yourself and greet him, assess his muscle strength, mobility, and skin temperature and texture. Does he use a cane or other assistive device? Posture is a clue about overall health status. A slumped position may indicate fatigue, depression, osteoporosis, or pain. If your client is immobile, observe his ability to move from side to side and change positions in the bed. An unsteady gait may be associated with joint, muscle, or neurological disorders. Focused assessments in the remainder of the exam will help to reveal the exact meaning of such cues.

Speech

As you speak with the client and ask health-related questions, look for clues offered by his speech.
▪ Inappropriate or illogical responses may be associated with psychiatric disorders.
▪ Difficulty speaking or changes in voice quality may indicate a neurological problem.
▪ Rapid speech may be a sign of anxiety, hyperactivity, or use of stimulants.
▪ Hoarseness could indicate inflammation in the throat from infection, overuse, a foreign body, or perhaps a tumor or other obstructive material.
▪ Slow speech may be due to depression, sedation from medications, or neurological disorders.
▪ Vocabulary and sentence structure provide information about the client's educational level and comfort with the language.
▪ A foreign accent with hesitancy and/or sparse verbalization may signal a language barrier and a need for an interpreter.

Dress, Grooming, and Hygiene

A client's ability to dress and perform personal hygiene is affected by physical and emotional well-being. An unkempt appearance may reflect chronic pain, fatigue, depression, or low self-esteem. Poor hygiene may indicate a self-care deficit or physical or mental origin, or lack of easily accessible bathroom facilities.

Mental State

Mental state includes level of consciousness and capacity to interact. If the client has an altered mental status, ask a family member about the onset of the change. Keep in mind that many medications, especially in older adults, may contribute to confusion or other changes in mental status.
▪ Bizarre responses may signal a psychiatric problem.
▪ Lethargy may be due to medications; depression; or a neurological, thyroid, liver, kidney, or cardiovascular disorder.
▪ Confusion and irritability may indicate hypoxia or medication side effects.
▪ Inability to provide a health history or to recall information may indicate a neurological disorder.

Vital Signs

You should assess vital signs as a part of the general survey and with subsequent assessments. Analyze for trends. See Chapter 19 for a complete discussion of vital signs, if needed.

Height and Weight

Height and weight provide valuable information about your client's growth and development, nutritional status, overall general health, and risk for various diseases such as diabetes and heart disease. These data are important for proper dosing of medication. For adults who can stand, measure height and weight using a platform scale with a sliding ruler (Fig. 21-1). When possible, the client should wear minimal clothing (gown) and no shoes. If the client cannot stand safely, use a bed scale. To measure an infant's length, use a stationary measure, such as the marked side of an infant scale. Because children have frequent changes in growth, their measurements are documented on growth charts for easy monitoring and comparison to age- and gender-related standards. For growth charts for males and females from birth to 20 years of age,

 Go to Chapter 21, **Supplemental Materials: Growth Charts,** on Davis*Plus*.

Body mass index (BMI) evaluates the relationship between height and weight. You can calculate the BMI for adults using a BMI calculator or table (see Procedure 21-1). Because the proportion of fat to muscle affects BMI calculation, the BMI is not useful for athletes (who have a larger proportion of muscle, which is denser than fat mass), for pregnant and lactating women (who have a larger blood and tissue volume), for growing children, or for frail and sedentary older adults.

Once you have completed your general survey of the client, you can begin to focus on each body system. Whether you are doing a complete or focused physical assessment, remember that all body systems are interrelated. A problem in one system may affect or be affected by other systems.

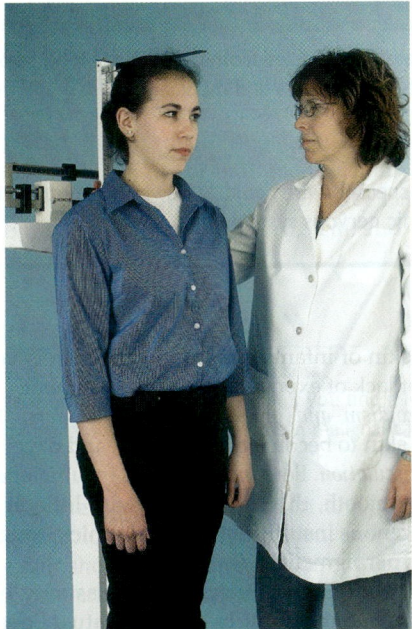

FIGURE 21-1 For adults, measure height with the client's back to the platform scale.

THE INTEGUMENTARY SYSTEM

The integumentary system consists of the skin, hair, and nails. In a comprehensive exam, you assess this system briefly in the general survey, and then in greater detail as you move to examine other areas of the body. This allows the client to remain draped as long as possible.

The Skin

To perform a skin assessment, observe skin color, lesions, and other characteristics. Also notice unusual odors. An unpleasant body odor may be a sign of poor hygiene, the presence of a wound, or underlying disease. Excessive sweating may be related to activity (e.g., if the client has just finished exercising), thyroid problems, or overactive sweat glands. An odor of urine or stool may indicate a nursing diagnosis of Self-Care Deficit or Bowel or Urinary Incontinence. For step-by-step instructions, see Procedure 21-2.

Skin Color

Skin color varies according to age and race, although each person's skin color is fairly uniform. Exposed areas, such as the hands, face, and neck, are often darker than unexposed areas, whereas the palms, soles, and nailbeds are lighter than the rest of the skin. In people with dark skin, the lips are also usually lighter than surrounding skin. Variations in skin color commonly seen in neonates and infants include the following:

- **Mongolian spots** are benign, blue-black birthmarks that occur on the lower back and buttocks of African American, Hispanic, Native American, and Asian babies. They are due to pigmented cells in the deeper areas of skin. Most fade by age 2 but can persist until early adolescence.
- **Capillary hemangiomas,** sometimes known as "stork bites," are small, irregular pink-red areas that are often seen around the face and nape of the neck in newborns. They typically disappear in infancy although can persist until age 5.
- **Café-au-lait spots** are light brown birthmarks that can occur anywhere on the body. The name of these birthmarks is French for "coffee with milk" because of their light-brown color. Most often café-au-lait spots are not associated with medical problems, although they can sometimes signal a genetic disorder. Table 21-2 discusses the significance of other skin color variations that may be seen in clients of any age.

Skin Characteristics

As does color, the temperature, texture, and turgor of the skin offer clues to the client's health status. Although it is not technically a skin characteristic, you should also check for edema while you are assessing the skin.

Skin Temperature. Use the dorsum of the hand or fingers to assess skin temperature. Compare the temperature of the hands with that of the feet, and compare the right side of the body with the left. The skin should feel warm, but keep in mind that the temperature should be consistent with the room temperature and the patient's activity level. Be sure to check the temperature of the skin over any area of erythema. Erythema accompanied by warmth may indicate infection or inflammatory changes.

If the patient's skin feels excessively warm, validate your data: Check her temperature to determine whether she has a fever. Hyperthyroidism stimulates the metabolism and may also elevate skin temperature. Excessive coolness may be due

Nail Shape

A change in nail shape may indicate underlying disease. The typical nail plate angle is 160°. Clubbing, in which the nail plate angle is 180° or more, is associated with long-term hypoxic states, such as occurs with chronic lung disease (see Procedure 21-4). Spoon-shaped nails may result from iron deficiency.

Nail Texture

Nails are normally smooth in texture. You may see the following indications of problems:

- Thickened nails may result from poor circulation.
- A thick nail with yellowing is an indication of fungal infection known as *onychomycosis*.
- Brittle nails are seen with hyperthyroidism, malnutrition, calcium and iron deficiencies, and repeated use of harsh nail products.
- Soft, boggy nails are seen with poor oxygenation.

The tissue surrounding the nail should be smooth epidermis. Chronic nail-picking results in callus formation around the nail. Occasionally the surrounding skin becomes inflamed. This condition, known as **paronychia,** is painful and may require drainage if infection is present.

 ThinkLike a Nurse 21-3

You are caring for a woman who has no hair on her head. How might you determine the cause of her hair loss? What other assessments should you perform?

THE HEAD

Assessment of the head is often referred to by the acronym HEENT: **H**ead, **E**yes, **E**ars, **N**ose, and **T**hroat. You will use all the assessment techniques—inspection, palpation, percussion, and auscultation—in the HEENT exam.

The Skull and Face

Taking individual variation into account, on inspection the skull should be rounded and the face symmetrical in appearance and movement. Inspect head size; if it seems unusual, measure it.

- A large head in an adolescent or adult may be associated with **acromegaly,** a disorder associated with excess growth hormone. Head size is familial, as well.
- **Microcephaly,** an abnormally small head size, is seen in clients with certain types of mental retardation.
- In infants, abnormal shape or flattening of the skull may result from trauma during a vaginal birth or placing the baby in the same position for several hours every day.
- In infants and children, a head that is growing disproportionally faster than the body may be a sign of **hydrocephalus** (an accumulation of excessive cerebrospinal fluid).
- Asymmetry may be the result of trauma, surgery, neuromuscular disorder, paralysis, or congenital deformity.
- Facial appearance that is inconsistent with gender, age, or racial/ethnic group may indicate an inherited or chronic disorder, such as Graves' disease, hypothyroidism with myxedema, or Cushing's syndrome.

The skull should be smooth and symmetrical to palpation. Contour abnormalities, bulging, or tenderness result from trauma, congenital anomalies, or surgery. Irregular jaw movement or cracking of the jaw may indicate **TMJ (temporomandibular joint) syndrome.** To learn how to assess the skull and face and to view some facial abnormalities, see Procedure 21-5.

The Eyes

In examining the eyes, you will inspect and palpate the external eye structures, assess vision, and examine the internal eye structures. For step-by-step instructions, see Procedure 21-6. For convenience, you may wish to perform some cranial nerve testing along with the eye exam (e.g., corneal reflex, pupillary reaction, accommodation, and extraocular movements). For instructions on performing a cranial nerve examination, see Procedure 21-16.

External Structures of the Eye

To review the structure of the external eye, see Figure 21-2. Normal eyelid margins are moist and pink with short lashes that are evenly spaced and curl outward. The lower eyelid margin appears at the bottom edge of the iris, and the upper eyelid covers half the upper iris. The conjunctiva is smooth, glistening, and peach in color, with minimal blood vessels present. There should be no pallor, dryness, or edema.

Eyelids. The following are common abnormal findings on the eyelids:

- Crusting, scales, or swelling of the lid is associated with infection of the eyelids or eyelashes.
- A **pterygium** is a growth or thickening of conjunctiva from the inner canthus toward the iris.
- **Ectropion,** an everted eyelid, is commonly seen in older adults secondary to loss of skin tone. It can lead to excessive dryness of the eyes.
- **Entropion,** an inverted eyelid, can lead to corneal damage.
- **Ptosis,** or drooping of the lid, may be seen in clients who have experienced a stroke (cerebrovascular accident [CVA]) or Bell's palsy (paralysis of the facial nerve, see Procedure 21-5). For ptosis and other eye abnormalities, refer to Procedure 21-6.

Sclera and Conjunctiva. Numerous disorders may affect the sclera and conjunctiva, including infection, allergies, injuries, and liver disorders. For example, yellow (**icteric**) sclera may be seen with an elevated bilirubin. Blood visible in the sclera is known as a **subconjunctival hemorrhage** and may be related to trauma or hypertension.

Lens and Cornea. The lens and the **cornea,** or outermost layer of the eyeball, should be transparent, smooth, and moist. Lens opacities, known as **cataracts,** are frequently seen in older

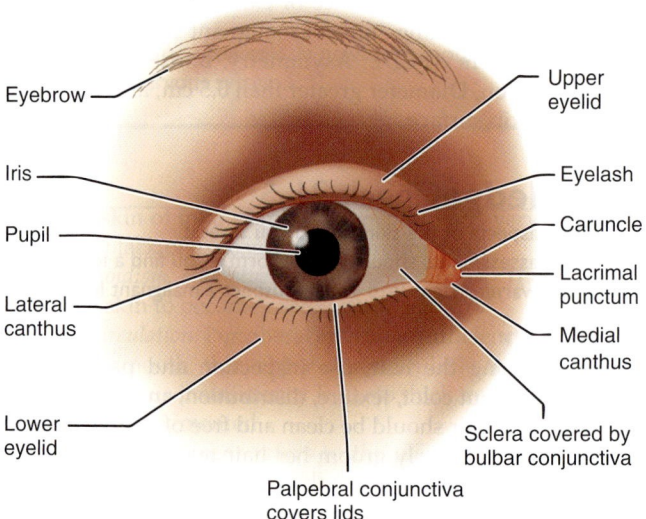

FIGURE 21-2 The external eye and eyelid.

adults and may impair vision. Roughness or irregularity of the cornea is seen with trauma or a corneal abrasion.

Pupils. The **pupils** should be uniform in color, equal in size, and round. They should **accommodate** equally, that is, the pupils constrict and the eyes converge (cross) as a person attempts to focus on an object moving toward him. This is typically charted as PERRLA: **P**upils **E**qual, **R**ound, **R**eactive to **L**ight and **A**ccommodation. The following are common pupillary abnormalities:

- Sluggish accommodation may be caused by anticholinergic drugs or advanced age.
- Failure of one or both pupils to accommodate may reflect a cranial nerve III problem or **exophthalmos** (associated with hyperthyroidism). Congenital cataracts, although rare, may be seen in infants and are checked during an eye exam using the "red reflex."
- Cloudy pupils, a finding related to cataracts, are commonly seen in older adults.
- **Mydriasis** (enlarged pupils) may be seen with glaucoma, an increase in intraocular pressure. Many medications affect pupil size. Medications called *mydriatics* are used to dilate the pupil to allow better visualization of the internal eye during examination.
- **Miosis** (constricted pupils) often results from medications to treat glaucoma.
- **Anisocoria** (unequal pupils) may be seen with central nervous system disorders such as stroke, head trauma, or cranial nerve injuries. In some individuals, anisocoria may be normal.

Visual Acuity

Visual acuity is a measure of the eye's ability to detect the details of an image. When testing visual acuity, you will assess distant, near, peripheral, and color vision. Nurses usually perform screening tests of visual acuity. Other testing is performed by nurses in advanced or specialty practice or by an optometrist or ophthalmologist as needed.

Distance Vision

Use the Snellen chart from a distance of 20 feet to assess distance vision. Assess each eye separately, and then assess both eyes together. Normal vision is a measure of clear vision at 20 feet (20/20) in the right eye, left eye, and both eyes. If a patient hesitates when reporting the letters or symbols he sees on the chart, document "with hesitation." If he misses one or two items in a line, record the number of items missed.

Myopia, or diminished distant vision, is associated with a smaller fraction. For example, 20/100 vision means that to see text a person with normal vision can read at 100 feet, the client has to stand just 20 feet from the Snellen chart. A child's distance vision does not reach 20/20 until around 6 or 7 years of age.

Near Vision

Test near vision by having the client read newsprint from a distance of 35.5 cm (14 in.). A client with normal near vision will be able to read the newsprint without hesitation with either eye and both eyes. With **hyperopia,** or diminished near vision, the client must hold the paper more than 35.5 cm (14 in.) away. As we age, the lens of the eye naturally loses some ability to accommodate to near objects. In clients older than 45 years of age, diminished near vision is known as **presbyopia.**

Color Vision

Color vision is the ability to detect color. **Color blindness** may be genetically inherited (usually seen in males), or it may result from macular degeneration or other diseases that affect the cones of the eye. Use the color bars at the base of the Snellen chart to test color vision. *Ishihara cards* (see Procedure 21-6) are specialized cards that enable thorough testing for color blindness. They contain embedded figures within a field of color. A person with normal color vision will be able to successfully identify the figures in the cards or the bars on the base of the Snellen chart; one who is color blind will not.

Visual Field

Visual field is the area the eye is able to observe. It is related to peripheral vision and extraocular muscle (EOM) function. Visual field abnormalities may be caused by problems with cranial nerves III, IV, and VI or with the retina. Poorly controlled diabetes, cataracts, macular degeneration, and advanced glaucoma are other disorders that limit the visual field. **Peripheral vision** describes the boundaries of the visual field while the eye is in a fixed position. The common phrase "I see you out of the corner of my eye" refers to peripheral vision.

The **EOMs** control the movement of the eye and eyelids and allow you to track movement. Three cranial nerves (CN) innervate the EOM. They are CN III (oculomotor), CN IV (trochlear), and CN VI (abducens). CN III also works together with CN II (optic) to control the pupillary reaction to light. Figure 21-3 illustrates the eye positions affected by the EOM and the corresponding cranial nerves.

Strabismus (crossed eye) is a condition in which one or both eyes deviate from the object they are looking at. It is normal during the first 1 or 2 months of life. After that, it may be caused by weak intraocular muscles or a lesion on the oculomotor nerve. Constant strabismus of one eye may result in **amblyopia** ("lazy eye"), in which the brain does not fully acknowledge the images seen by the amblyopic eye. This creates reduced vision in that eye, not correctable by glasses or contact lenses.

Internal Structures of the Eye

Use an ophthalmoscope to visualize the internal structures of the eye (the optic disc, physiological cup, retinal vessels, retinal background, and macula). This is an advanced assessment technique; however, advanced practice nurses and registered nurses (RNs) on specialty units do perform it with training. This technique provides information about certain diseases that affect the eye, such as hypertension and diabetes.

KnowledgeCheck 21-6

- What are the major components of an eye assessment?
- Identify the cranial nerves involved with eye movement and function.

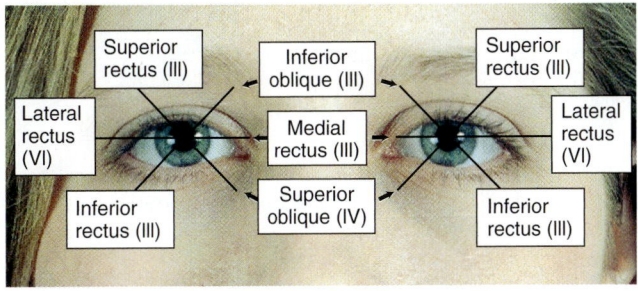

FIGURE 21-3 Cranial nerves and the extraocular muscles.

The Ears and Hearing

The ears are involved in both hearing and equilibrium. The **external ear** collects and conveys sound waves to the middle ear. It protects the middle ear from environmental factors such as humidity and temperature and prevents entry of foreign matter. The **middle ear** contains the tympanic membrane and cavity, the eustachian tube, and the **ossicles** (the small bones of the middle ear: the malleus, incus, and stapes). The middle ear conducts sound waves to the inner ear. The **inner ear** is responsible for hearing and equilibrium. Figure 21-4 illustrates the structures of the ear.

For procedure steps and guidelines for using the otoscope and tuning fork to examine the ears, see Procedure 21-7. As with the eyes, nurses are usually responsible only for screening and making referrals. However, in some settings nurses perform advanced assessments.

Examining the External and Middle Ear

On inspection, the ears should be of equal size and similar appearance. Normally the pinna is level with the corner of the eye and within a 10° angle of vertical position. Altered placement of the ear may be a sign of hearing deficit or genetic disorders, including Down syndrome. There should be no lesions or drainage. Bloody drainage may result from trauma. Purulent drainage may be seen with infection.

On palpation, a painful auricle or tragus may be associated with **otitis externa** (an outer ear infection), whereas tenderness behind the ear is seen with **otitis media** (a middle ear infection).

As you begin the otoscopic examination, you may notice that the external auditory canal contains **cerumen** (wax), which protects the middle ear from excessive drying. However, it should not completely obstruct the ear canal. Cerumen may be black, dark red, yellowish, or brown in color and waxy, flaky, soft, or hard, with no odor; all are normal variations. Be careful as you manipulate the otoscope, because the inner two-thirds of the canal can be tender with the pressure and manipulation of the otoscope head.

Normally the **tympanic membrane (TM)** is pearly gray, shiny, and translucent. The structures of the middle ear should be visible through the membrane. Changes in its appearance arise from abnormalities such as otitis media (which causes a red, bulging TM) and the presence of pressure equalization tubes in young clients with chronic ear infections.

Assessing Hearing

To assess hearing, you will need a quiet room and a tuning fork. Gross hearing ability includes the ability to hear both high- and low-pitched tones. A client who hears low tones will be able to hear and repeat words whispered from 1 to 2 feet behind him. The client can hear high tones if he is able to hear a watch ticking at 5 in. (12 to 13 cm) from each ear.

The Weber and Rinne Tests

Hearing involves transmission of sound vibrations and generation of nerve impulses along CN VIII. The **Weber test** assesses both aspects. When you place a vibrating tuning fork on the center of the client's head, he should be able to sense the vibration equally in both ears. Record a positive Weber test if the vibration is louder in one ear.

If the Weber test is positive, you will need to perform the Rinne test to assess the type of hearing problem. The **Rinne test** also uses a tuning fork to compare air conduction (AC) and bone conduction (BC). Normally AC is twice as long as BC. For step-by-step instructions for performing the Weber and Rinne tests, see Procedure 21-7.

The Romberg Test

Along with the cerebellum and midbrain, vestibular cells in the ear are responsible for maintaining equilibrium. To assess equilibrium, perform the Romberg test. The client should be able to stand with feet together and eyes closed, and maintain balance with minimal swaying. Swaying and moving (positive Romberg) may indicate a vestibular or cerebellar disorder. You may prefer to perform the Romberg test with examination of the neurological system instead of with the ears.

Knowledge Check 21-7

Your client has a negative Weber test. What further testing is required?

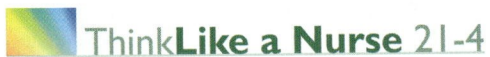

ThinkLike a Nurse 21-4

What type of symptoms would you expect a client to be experiencing if he had a positive Romberg test?

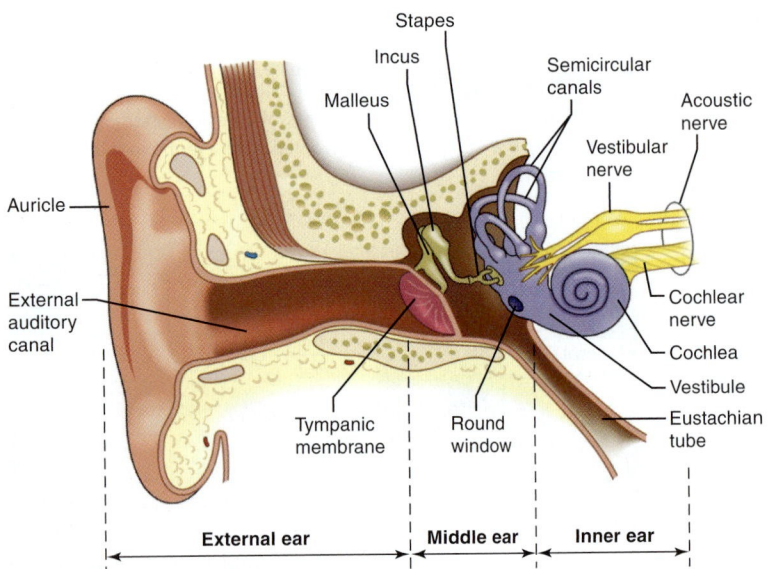

FIGURE 21-4 Cross section of the ear.

The Nose

The nose and sinuses are part of the respiratory system and are the organs of smell. Vaporized molecules sniffed into the upper nasal cavities trigger receptors that generate impulses along the olfactory nerve (CN I) that travel to olfactory centers in the temporal lobes. The sense of smell diminishes in older adults because of a gradual decrease in and atrophy of the olfactory nerve fibers. To identify the paranasal sinuses and for a procedure for assessing the nose and sinuses, see Procedure 21-8.

The Mouth and Oropharynx

The structures of the mouth include the lips, tongue, teeth, **gingiva** (gums), uvula, hard and soft palate, and salivary glands and ducts. On external inspection, the mouth and lips should be symmetrical and without lesions, swelling, or drooping. For an illustration of structures of the mouth and for instructions on examining the mouth and oropharynx, see Procedure 21-9.

The Lips, Buccal Mucosa, and Gingiva

The lips, **buccal mucosa** (mucous membrane of the cheeks), and gums should be smooth, moist, and pink in color. Increased pigmentation (e.g., bluish or dark patches) occurs in dark-skinned clients. No lesions should be present. Be sure to ask your client about use of tobacco, either smoked or chewed. Both forms of tobacco are associated with increased risk for oral cancer. The following are abnormal findings:

- Pallor may indicate anemia or inadequate oxygenation.
- **Gingivitis** is a sign of periodontal disease. You will see red, swollen, or spongy, bleeding gingiva and receding gumlines. The gums may be tender.
- **Parotitis** is an inflammation of the parotid salivary gland.
- **Stomatitis** is inflammation of the oral mucosa.
- **Leukoplakia** (thick, elevated white patches) that do not scrape off may be precancerous lesions; white, curdy patches that scrape off and bleed indicate **thrush** (a fungal infection).
- Redness or abrasions of the gingiva may be caused by poorly fitted dentures.
- **Aphthous ulcers** are small, painful vesicles with a reddened periphery and a white or pale-yellow base. **Canker sores** are a benign type of aphthous ulcer believed to be caused by viral infection, allergies, stress, or trauma. So-called major aphthous ulcers may be caused by herpes simplex virus, human immunodeficiency virus, and bacterial infections.

The Teeth

The teeth should be fixed to the gum and without obvious debris or darkening that may indicate caries. Tooth decay and periodontal (gum) disease are common. Poor oral hygiene is a major contributing factor for both. As you examine the mouth and teeth, talk to the patient about his oral care. Recommend toothbrushing after each meal, daily flossing, and dental checkups every 6 months. See Chapter 24 for a more complete discussion of oral hygiene and prevention of periodontal disease.

The Tongue

When inspecting the mouth, carefully examine all aspects of the tongue: dorsal, ventral, and lateral. The **tongue** should be moist, symmetrical, slightly rough, smooth, pink, and freely movable. The following are abnormal findings:

- Deviation from the midline, which may be caused by damage to the hypoglossal nerve (CN XII)
- Limited mobility of the tongue
- **Glossitis** (inflammation of the tongue)

- A dry, furry tongue, which is associated with dehydration
- A black, "hairy" tongue, which is associated with fungal infections
- Absence of papillae, reddened mucosa, and ulcerations, which may indicate allergy, inflammation, or infection
- Swelling, nodules, or ulcers
- A smooth, red tongue, which may occur in clients who have a deficiency of iron, vitamin B_{12}, or vitamin B_3

The Hard and Soft Palates and Oropharynx

The hard palate, soft palate, and oropharynx should be pink, moist, and intact. If the tonsils are present, they should be symmetrical, small in size, and free of exudate in a healthy person. The uvula is midline and should rise on **phonation** (vocalization).

THE NECK

The neck has components of the musculoskeletal, neurological, vascular, respiratory, endocrine, and lymphatic systems. The sternocleidomastoid and trapezius muscles form the landmarks of the neck, known as the **anterior and posterior triangles.** The symmetrical neck muscles center and coordinate movement of the head. Asymmetrical head position may result from damage to the muscles, swelling, or masses. Painful or erratic movement may be due to a benign condition, such as muscle spasm, or to significant problems, including meningitis, neurological injuries, or chronic arthritis.

The trachea, thyroid gland, anterior cervical nodes, and carotid arteries are positioned in the anterior triangle; the posterior cervical nodes are in the posterior triangle. You will palpate the tracheal rings and the cricoid and thyroid cartilage in the midline of the anterior neck. To see instructions for assessing the neck and illustrations of structures of the neck, consult Procedure 21-10.

The Thyroid Gland

Normally the thyroid is smooth, firm, and nontender. It is often nonpalpable. However, thyroid abnormalities are common. An enlarged thyroid may be associated with either hypothyroidism or hyperthyroidism. Thyroid tenderness usually results from inflammation. Thyroid masses may be malignant but are usually benign.

The Cervical Lymph Nodes

The cervical lymph nodes occur in three chains (see Procedure 21-10, step 2). The anterior chain is in the anterior triangle, the posterior chain in the posterior triangle. There is a deep cervical chain under the sternocleidomastoid muscle. The lymph nodes are generally not palpable, although occasionally nodes can be felt, especially in young children. Normal nodes are small, mobile, soft, and nontender. You should describe enlarged nodes (greater than 1 cm in diameter) according to their location, size, shape, consistency, mobility, and tenderness. Enlarged or tender nodes may be caused by infection, malignancy, and other diseases.

Think**Like a Nurse** 21-5

A client complains of sore throat, fever, chills, and runny nose. What assessments should you perform?

THE BREASTS AND AXILLAE

The breasts consist of glandular, adipose, and connective tissue; smooth muscle; and nerves. The functions of the female breast are sexual stimulation and milk production for

nourishing offspring. Breast size and shape vary among women, and commonly one breast is slightly larger than the other. At puberty, the ovaries produce estrogen and progesterone, which stimulate the breasts to develop. The menstrual cycle, pregnancy, and breastfeeding also enlarge breast tissue. Although breasts are thought of as female organs, men also have breasts. However, because of limited estrogen and progesterone levels, normal male breasts develop only minimally.

Breast tissue and lymph drainage for the breast extend up into the axilla. The majority of breast tumors are found in the tail of Spence, in the axilla. A breast exam therefore always includes an exam of the axillae. Many women have breast reconstruction, either after breast removal due to cancer or breast augmentation for cosmetic reasons. These women should not omit breast examination, and it is performed in exactly the same way as for natural breasts.

Breast Self-Examination. Currently there is controversy about whether we should continue to encourage breast self-examination (BSE) (Tarrant, 2006). The American College of Obstetricians and Gynecologists (ACOG) guidelines recommend that breast self-awareness should be encouraged and that this can include breast self-examination. Some studies report increased rates of cancer discovery and earlier detection in groups who perform BSE; however others indicate that it does not reduce death rates from breast cancer (ACOG, 2011; Green & Taplin, 2003; Hackshaw & Paul, 2003; Kösters & Gøtzsche, 2003; Weiss, 2003). Until there is more evidence, it seems reasonable to continue to use BSE as a screening tool along with the recommended mammograms. Researchers agree patients who perform BSE should be trained to use proper technique in order to avoid false negative findings (ACOG, 2009a; American Cancer Society, 2010, 2011; Balkaya, Memis, & Demirkiran, 2007; Knutson & Steiner, 2007; Rosolowich, 2006). You should perform a breast exam for the woman if she cannot do it herself, and demonstrate the procedure as part of client teaching for self-care.

Clinical Breast Examination. Clinical breast exams should be done annually for women aged 40 and older, and every 1 to 3 years for women ages 20 to 39 (ACOG, 2011). Guidelines vary as to the age at which women should start having clinical breast exams (CBE) and mammograms to screen for breast cancer. For a step-by-step guide to examining the breasts and axillae, see Procedure 21-11.

Mammography and Thermography. Annual or biennial mammograms or breast thermography most commonly begin after age 40, or at a younger age and more often for those at high risk. ACOG recommends annual mammograms (ACOG, 2011; American Cancer Society, 2010, 2011). Evidence presently does not support the need for a CBE if a mammogram is done ([USPSTS], 2009a).

ThinkLike a Nurse 21-6

What strategies might encourage more women to regularly perform breast self-examination, if your agency has decided to promote that measure?

THE CHEST AND LUNGS

The chest, or thorax, is the bony cage that protects the heart, lungs, and great vessels. The ribs, sternum, and vertebrae form the chest. Be systematic in your assessment: Always assess the areas of the chest and lungs in the same order. To learn how to assess the chest and lungs, see Procedure 21-12.

Chest Landmarks

Before beginning the thoracic exam, review the following important landmarks that will help you visualize the underlying structures and perform an accurate assessment:

- Identify positions vertically on the anterior chest in relation to the ribs. For example, the space between the 5th and 6th ribs is known as the 5th intercostal space (5th ICS). You can easily palpate the ribs and count the spaces if you remember that the 1st rib is tucked up next to the clavicle (Fig. 21-5).
- On the posterior chest, identify positions vertically in relation to the vertebra (Fig. 21-6). The prominent vertebra at the base of the neck is the 7th cervical vertebra (C7). The next one down is T1 (1st thoracic). Counting down to about T9 should be adequate.
- Use a series of imaginary vertical lines to further aid in identifying locations. Figure 21-7 illustrates the location of these lines. Use them with the rib spaces to describe locations on

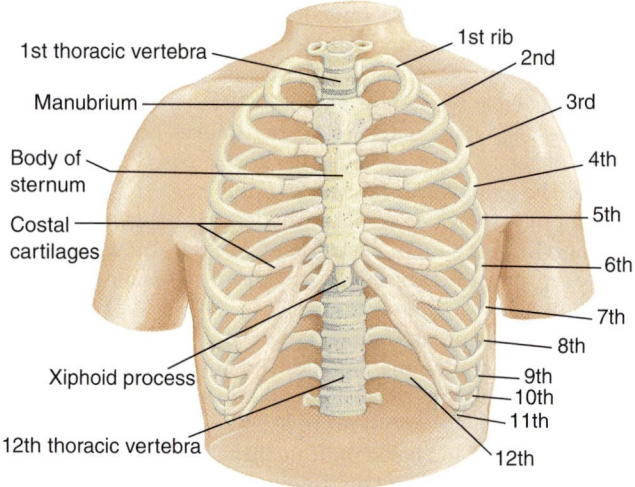

FIGURE 21-5 The anterior thoracic cage and the bony landmarks.

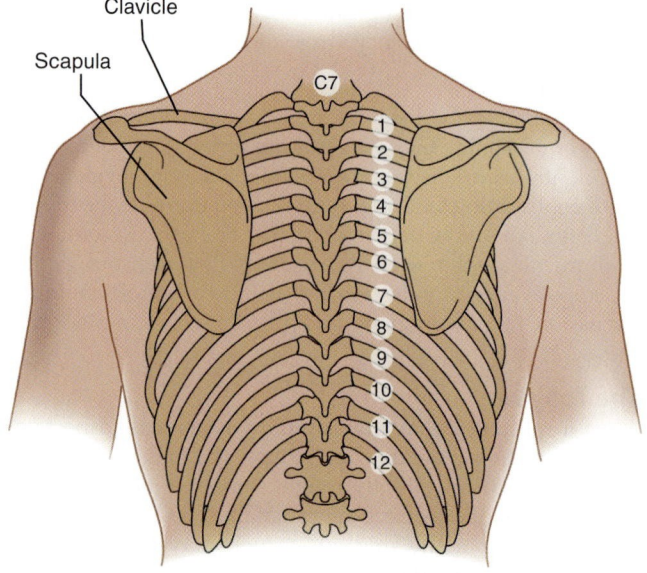

FIGURE 21-6 The vertebrae are the landmarks on the posterior chest.

the anterior chest (Fig. 21-7A). For instance, the apex of the heart is usually located in the 5th intercostal space at left midclavicular line (5th ICS MCL).

- Use imaginary lines on the lateral and posterior chest as well (see Fig. 21-7B and C). Notice that the anterior axillary line can be used to locate sounds on both the anterior and lateral chest.

Chest Shape and Size

The normal adult chest is symmetrical and rises and falls with respirations. The chest diameter expands up to 3 in. (7.6 cm) with deep inspiration. The anteroposterior diameter of the chest is half the size of the lateral diameter (written as AP: Lateral = 1:2). The slope of the ribs is less than 90°. In young children, the chest is apple shaped. Musculoskeletal changes associated with aging result in a gradual increase in the anteroposterior diameter. This change is also seen, regardless of age, in clients who have chronic obstructive pulmonary disease (COPD), a disorder associated with long-term smoking. Procedure 21-12 contains an illustration of the normal chest ratio and the barrel chest appearance that develops with COPD, in which the anteroposterior and lateral diameters may be equal.

Spinal alterations, such as **kyphosis** (excessive curvature of the thoracic spine) and **scoliosis** (lateral curvature of the spine) alter the shape of the thoracic cage. Osteoporosis, a common disorder associated with aging, is associated with increased porosity of the vertebrae. As a result, vertebrae may compress or collapse, shortening the length of the spine and pushing the ribs forward and downward.

Breath Sounds

Listen to breath sounds in a quiet room by auscultating one full respiratory cycle at each site. Directly apply the stethoscope to the client's skin. Compare breath sounds bilaterally. Three types of breath sounds are heard (Fig. 21-8):

- **Bronchial breath sounds** are loud, high-pitched, tubular sounds; expiration is of longer duration than inspiration. Air moving through the trachea produces these sounds, which you will hear best over the trachea on the anterior chest and below the nape of the neck on the posterior chest.
- **Bronchovesicular breath sounds** are medium pitched with an equal inspiratory and expiratory phase. Air moving through the large airways of the bronchi produces these sounds, which are best heard over the 1st and 2nd ICS adjacent to the sternum on the anterior chest and between the scapulae on the posterior chest.
- **Vesicular breath sounds** are soft, low-pitched, breezy sounds with a lengthy inspiratory phase and a short expiratory phase. Air moving through the smaller airways produces these sounds, which are best heard over the lung fields.

Breath sounds that differ from those above are abnormal.

- **Diminished breath sounds** are heard with poor inspiratory effort, in the very muscular or obese, or with restricted airflow.
- **Misplaced breath sounds** (e.g., bronchial breath sounds heard over the lung fields) indicate constriction of flow.
- **Adventitious breath sounds,** such as wheezes, rhonchi, and rales, are sounds heard over normal breath sounds. If an abnormal sound is heard, have the client cough and listen again.
- Other abnormal findings include **bronchophony, whispered pectoriloquy,** and **egophony.** These are abnormal voice sounds that result from consolidation of lung tissue.

To find a discussion of these sounds and to listen to normal and adventitious breath sounds,

 Go to Chapter 21, **Supplemental Materials: Abnormal Vocal Sounds,** and **Sound Files: Breath Sounds,** on Davis*Plus*.

For more information about the respiratory system, see Chapter 37. For a table describing abnormal lung sounds and the procedure for performing a respiratory assessment, see Procedure 21-12.

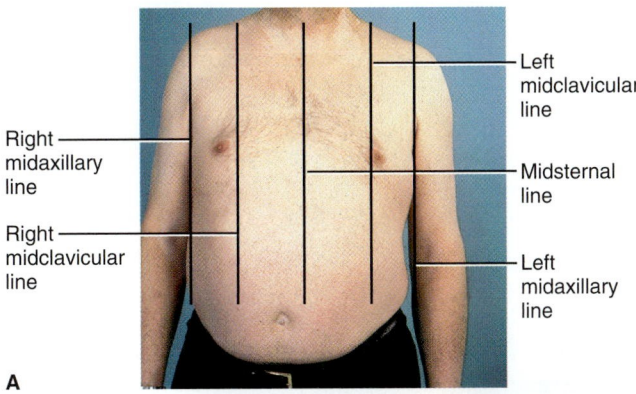

A

Right midaxillary line
Right midclavicular line
Left midclavicular line
Midsternal line
Left midaxillary line

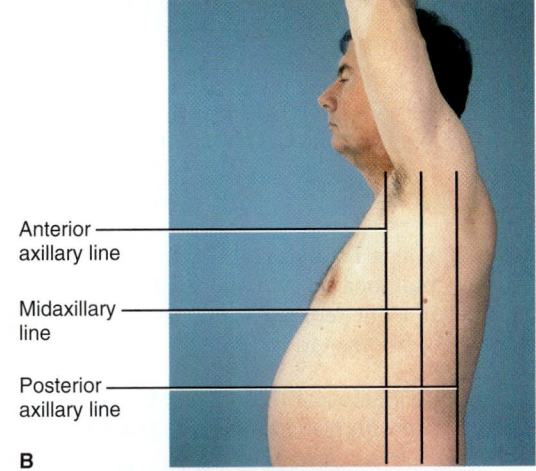

B

Anterior axillary line
Midaxillary line
Posterior axillary line

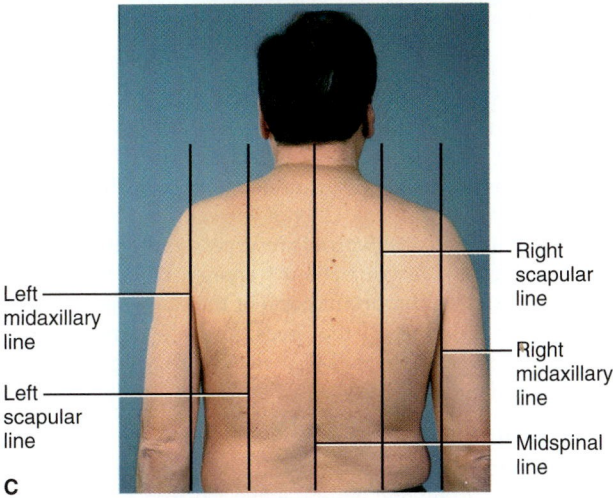

C

Left midaxillary line
Left scapular line
Right scapular line
Right midaxillary line
Midspinal line

FIGURE 21-7 A. A series of imaginary vertical lines is used to describe locations on the chest. B. Lateral chest landmarks. C. Landmark lines on the posterior chest.

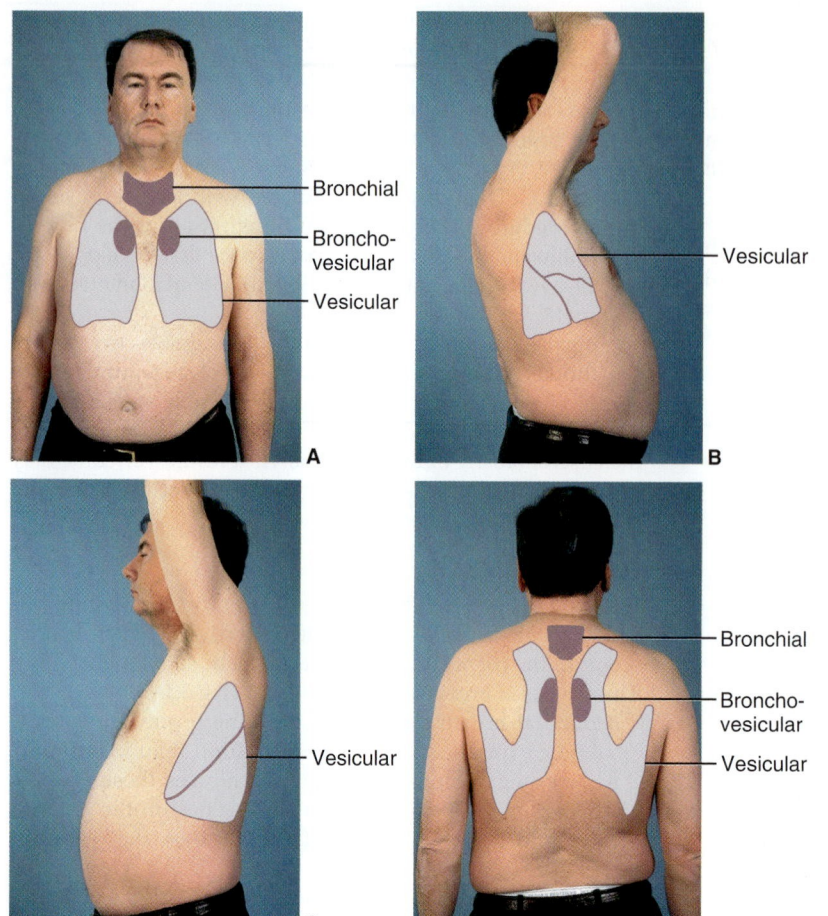

A — Bronchial
Broncho-vesicular
Vesicular

B — Vesicular

C — Vesicular

D — Bronchial
Broncho-vesicular
Vesicular

FIGURE 21-8 Normal breath sounds. A. Anterior. B. Right lateral. C. Left lateral. D. Posterior.

KnowledgeCheck 21-8

- List and describe the location of the horizontal and vertical landmarks of the anterior chest.
- List and describe the location of the horizontal and vertical landmarks of the posterior chest.
- List and describe the location of the vertical landmarks of the lateral chest.

THE CARDIOVASCULAR SYSTEM

The cardiovascular system consists of the heart and the blood vessels. The heart is a muscle that pumps blood throughout the body. In a healthy adult, it is about the size of a clenched fist. The blood vessels, which make up the vascular system, have two main networks: the pulmonary circulation and the systemic circulation. See Chapter 38 if you need to review the anatomy of the cardiovascular system.

Oxygen-depleted blood circulates from the heart into the lungs, where it is oxygenated, then back to the heart. This system is known as the **pulmonary circulation.** From the heart, the blood enters the **systemic circulation.** The left ventricle is the largest chamber of the heart. It pumps blood into the systemic circulation via the arterial system. The arteries subdivide many times, becoming smaller and smaller until they separate, in the tissues and organs, into capillaries. It is at the capillary level that oxygen is delivered to the tissues. The venous system collects the oxygen-depleted blood and returns it to the right atrium of the heart to begin the circuit again. **Coronary circulation,** which circulates blood through

the heart itself, is a part of the systemic circulation. For further discussion on pulmonary circulation and oxygenation, see Chapter 38. For animated presentations of the circulatory system and oxygen transport,

 Go to Student Resources, **Animations: Blood Flow** and **Carbon Dioxide/Oxygen Transport,** on Davis*Plus.*

For a complete step-by-step procedure for assessing the heart and vascular system, refer to Procedure 21-13.

The Heart

The heart is positioned at an angle on the left side of the chest in the 3rd, 4th, and 5th intercostal spaces (ICS). To facilitate auscultation of specific heart sounds, perform the cardiac assessment with the client in three positions: sitting, supine, and left lateral recumbent. Clients with chronic heart or lung problems may have little cardiac reserve, so minimize position changes to conserve your client's energy. Be systematic. To keep from missing important parts of the exam, always listen in the same order to all the areas. To help minimize your client's anxiety, explain that it always takes time to examine the heart and circulatory system.

The Cardiac Cycle

During a cardiac cycle, the atria and ventricles alternately contract and relax to fill and empty; while the atria are contracting (emptying), the ventricles are relaxing (filling), and vice versa. **Systole** refers to the contraction, or emptying, of the ventricles. **Diastole** refers to the relaxation, or filling, phase of the ventricles.

Inspecting and Palpating the Heart

Begin your assessment of the heart with the client sitting. Observe the **precordium,** the area of the chest over the heart, for visible pulsations. A small pulsation at the 5th ICS midclavicular line, also known as the **point of maximal impulse (PMI),** is normal. Other visible pulsations on the precordium, known as **heaves** or **lifts,** are associated with an enlarged ventricle.

Also palpate for vibrations. A **thrill** is a vibration or pulsation palpated in any area except the PMI. A thrill is associated with abnormal blood flow and usually has an accompanying **murmur** (additional heart sound).

Auscultating the Heart

Auscultate to establish cardiac rate and rhythm and to identify normal and abnormal heart sounds. A quiet room is essential. You can hear heart sounds from any location on the anterior chest wall. However, the four sites located over the heart valves are the preferred listening areas. Table 21-3 describes these locations; they are also shown in Procedure 21-13, step 8.

Auscultate in an orderly fashion. Start at the aortic area, and move gradually through each landmark. The following is a mnemonic you may use to recall the order of the heart sound landmarks:

*A*unt	Aortic
*P*olly	Pulmonic
*T*akes	Tricuspid
*M*eds	Mitral

Listen carefully at each site to each component of the heart sounds.

First Heart Sound. The first heart sound (S_1, or "lub") results from the closure of the valves between the atria and ventricles. S_1 ("lub") is a dull, low-pitched sound, loudest over the mitral and tricuspid areas. S_1 marks the beginning of systole.

Second Heart Sound. The second heart sound (S_2, or "dub") corresponds to closure of the semilunar valves (between the ventricles and the great arteries exiting the heart). "Dub" is higher in pitch and shorter than the S_1 "lub." The S_2 is loudest at the aortic and pulmonic areas. S_2 marks the beginning of diastole. Normally, the mitral and tricuspid valves and the aortic and pulmonic valves close within a fraction of a second from each other. This near-simultaneous closure results in a singular S_1 and S_2 sound. However, a split sound may occur, at either S_1 or S_2, if there is a delay in closure of one of the valves.

Third Heart Sound. A third heart sound (S_3), heard immediately after S_2, has a gallop cadence that follows the rhythm of the word "KenTUCKy." It is best heard at the apical

site with the client lying on his left side. An S_3 is normal in young children and adolescents when they are sitting or lying, but it disappears when they stand or sit up. It is also a normal variant in the third trimester of pregnancy. In adults, an S_3 that does not disappear with position change is abnormal and represents heart failure or volume overload.

Fourth Heart Sound. A fourth heart sound (S_4), heard immediately before S_1, has a rhythm that follows the word "FLOrida." S_4 is best heard at the apical site, using the bell of the stethoscope, with the client lying on his left side. An S_4 is normal in athletes and some older clients. It may also be heard in adults with coronary artery disease, hypertension, and pulmonic stenosis. To listen to heart sounds,

 Go to **Sound Files: Heart Sounds,** on *DavisPlus.*

Murmurs. **Murmurs** are additional sounds produced by turbulent flow through the heart. Some murmurs are innocent, but others represent pathology such as alteration in valve structure. Identifying and classifying a murmur are advanced skills that require practice. To learn more about assessing murmurs, see, Procedure 21-13. Also,

 Go to Chapter 21, **Supplemental Materials: Heart Murmurs, and Tables, Boxes, Figures: ESG Table 21-1,** on *DavisPlus.*

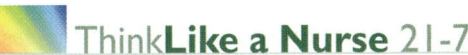 Think**Like a Nurse** 21-7

What findings would you anticipate when assessing Mr. Nguyen's thorax (Caring for the Nguyens)?

The Vascular System

The vascular system is a network of arteries and veins that transport oxygen, carbon dioxide, and nutrients to the cells of the body. Arteries carry blood away from the heart: The pulmonary arteries carry oxygen-depleted blood from the right ventricle to the lungs, whereas the systemic arteries carry oxygenated blood from the left ventricle to the body periphery. Veins carry blood toward the heart: The pulmonary veins transport oxygenated blood from the lungs to the left atrium, whereas the systemic veins return oxygen-depleted blood from the periphery to the right atrium of the heart.

The Central Vessels

The carotid arteries and internal jugular veins run alongside the sternocleidomastoid muscle on both sides of the neck (see Procedure 21-13 for illustrations). These central vessels provide circulation to the brain.

The Carotid Arteries

Because the carotid arteries are large and close to the heart, you can easily feel a pulse over the carotid artery even when it is difficult to palpate a peripheral pulse.

➕ Never palpate both carotid arteries at the same time because bilateral pressure may impair cerebral blood flow. Palpate very lightly and avoid massaging the carotid artery, because pressure on the carotids will cause the pulse rate to drop, and can even lead to cardiac arrest. As a general rule, avoid palpating the carotids except during cardiopulmonary resuscitation or when it is necessary to assess them for a specific reason (such as in a comprehensive physical exam, or when an underlying pathology makes it necessary to establish that circulation to the head is adequate).

Table 21-3 ▶ Locations for Assessing the Heart		
TITLE	**STRUCTURE ASSESSED**	**LOCATION**
Base Right	Aortic valve	2nd ICS right sternal border
Base Left	Pulmonic valve	2nd ICS left sternal border
Left Lateral	Tricuspid valve	4th ICS left sternal border
Apex	Mitral valve	5th ICS MCL

Turbulent blood flow through the carotid artery produces a whooshing sound known as a **bruit,** which you can auscultate using a stethoscope. Bruits are common among older adults. The following conditions cause turbulence: **carotid stenosis** (narrowing from plaque), increased cardiac output secondary to fluid overload, use of stimulants, or hyperthyroidism. If you hear a bruit, lightly palpate the neck for thrills (pulsations or vibrations), which further confirm turbulent flow.

The Jugular Veins

The jugular veins return blood from the brain to the superior vena cava. The external jugular veins are superficial; the internal jugular veins are deep. Normally the jugular veins are flat when the client is in an upright position and distend when the client lies flat. Jugular venous distention (JVD) is seen when the right side of the heart is congested due to inadequate pump function. The best position for assessment of JVD is semi-Fowler's (30° to 45° angle).

The Peripheral Vessels

If you were to lay out all the blood vessels in the peripheral system of an average sized person, you would find more than 60,000 miles of arteries, arterioles, capillaries, and venules. The peripheral vessels supply blood to all the body cells. The **arteries** are a high-pressure system with several palpable pulse sites. The **veins** are a low-pressure system with valves to prevent backflow due to gravity. The veins return blood to the heart via the continuing pressure from the arterial system and pumping action of the adjacent skeletal muscles. You will assess the peripheral vascular system by:

- *Measuring the blood pressure* (see Chapter 19). Usually you will measure the blood pressure at the start of the exam as part of the general survey.
- *Palpating the peripheral pulses* (see Chapter 19). Weak, absent, or asymmetrical pulses may indicate partial or complete occlusion of the artery. Other signs of arterial occlusion include pain, pallor, cool temperature, paresthesia, or paralysis.
- *Inspecting and performing tests for adequate perfusion.*

The data you obtain when inspecting and palpating the integumentary system provide some information about peripheral tissue perfusion. Recall that when an area is not adequately oxygenated, the skin may be pale, cyanotic, cool, and shiny; hair growth may be sparse, and there may be clubbing of the nails. Inadequate tissue oxygenation may be a result of chronic pulmonary problems; however, it can also result from impaired central or peripheral circulation.

Also inspect the veins for signs of distention. Superficial spiderlike veins, especially on the lower extremities, may occur with normal aging. Ropelike distended veins, or **varicosities,**

may be painful. If a client has varicosities, assess for valve competence using the manual compression test discussed in step 11 of Procedure 21-13.

KnowledgeCheck 21-9

Identify the precautions to take when evaluating the carotid arteries.

THE ABDOMEN

The method most commonly used to identify the location of assessment findings is the four-quadrant method, which divides the abdomen into four sections by "drawing" a line vertically from the xiphoid process to the symphysis pubis and a horizontal line at the level of the umbilicus (see Procedure 21-14, step 4). For the rarely used nine-region method,

 Go to Chapter 21, **Tables, Boxes, Figures: ESG Table 21-2** and **ESG Figure 21-1,** on Davis*Plus.*

Examination of the abdomen differs in sequence from all other body systems. Percussion and palpation stimulate the bowel and may alter bowel sounds. Therefore, you should inspect and auscultate before performing percussion and palpation. To promote comfort during the assessment, ask the client to empty his bladder before the examination. Have the client assume a supine position with flexed knees. This relaxes the abdominal muscles and is usually the most comfortable position. If the client has a painful area, examine that area last to minimize discomfort during the rest of the exam.

Inspecting the Abdomen

The skin over the abdomen is usually paler than that over other parts of the body. The abdomen should be symmetrical with a rounded contour and sunken umbilicus. See Figure 21-9 for normal variations in abdominal shape. You may be able to see peristalsis and aortic pulsations on a very thin client, but in most clients usually you will see no movement. In clients with abdominal distention, the skin will appear taut. Distention may be normal, as with pregnancy, or it may be due to gas or fluid retention or to bowel obstruction.

Auscultating the Abdomen

Proceed in an organized manner, listening in several areas in all four quadrants. Use the same pattern for every examination so that it becomes a habit.

First Auscultate Bowel Sounds. Bowel sounds are high-pitched, irregular gurgles or clicks lasting one to several seconds and occurring every 5 to 15 seconds (or 5 to 30 times

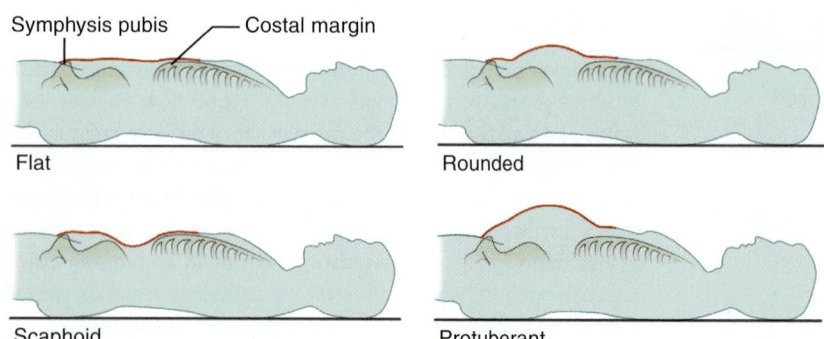

FIGURE 21-9 Normal variations in abdominal contour.

Symphysis pubis — Costal margin

Flat

Rounded

Scaphoid

Protuberant

per min) in the average adult. If the client has a nasogastric (NG) tube that is attached to suction, discontinue the suction or clamp off the tube while listening for bowel sounds. Otherwise, you may mistake the sound of suction in the stomach for bowel sounds. Abnormal bowel sounds are described in Procedure 21-14.

To hear some bowel sounds,

 Go to **Sound Files: Bowel Sounds,** on Davis*Plus*.

Next Auscultate the Major Arteries. Major arterial vessels lie in the abdomen below the intestines. Listen over the aorta and the renal iliac and femoral arteries for the presence of bruits.

Percussing the Abdomen

Use indirect percussion to assess for fluid, air, organs, or masses. Normally there is generalized tympany over the bowels (due to the presence of gas) and the abdomen is nontender, soft, and without masses. You will hear dullness when percussing organs, masses, or fluids. Some practitioners include percussion of the kidney with the abdominal examination.

Palpating the Abdomen

For information about palpating the abdomen, see Procedure 21-14. Palpation of the liver and spleen is an advanced technique not usually performed by staff nurses, except perhaps in some specialty areas.

KnowledgeCheck 21-10
- What strategies can you use to make the client more comfortable during an abdominal assessment?
- Identify the sequence of assessment for the abdominal exam.

THE MUSCULOSKELETAL SYSTEM

The musculoskeletal system consists of bones, muscles, and joints. Bone is complex living tissue that responds to nutrition, stress, and illness. The bones include *long bones,* such as the humerus and tibia; *flat bones,* such as the sternum and ribs; and *irregular bones,* such as the vertebrae and pelvis. Tendons, ligaments, and cartilage serve as connecting structures. **Bursae,** small disc-shaped, fluid-filled sacs, act as cushions to reduce friction between the joint and the tendons that cross over the joint (Fig. 21-10). The musculoskeletal system provides shape and support to the body, allows movement, protects internal organs, produces red blood cells in the bone marrow, and stores calcium and phosphorus. Assessment of the musculoskeletal system includes evaluation of the client's posture, gait, bone structure, muscle function, and joint mobility. The procedure is described in Procedure 21-15.

Body Shape and Symmetry

To assess bone structure, examine body shape and symmetry. Major deformities in bone structure affect posture and gait. The client should be able to stand upright with the neck and head midline. There are four normal curvatures of the spine. The cervical and lumbar curves are concave, and the thoracic and sacral are convex. Commonly seen abnormalities include kyphosis (accentuated thoracic curve), scoliosis (lateral S deviation of the spine), and lordosis (accentuated lumbar curve) (see Procedure 21-15).

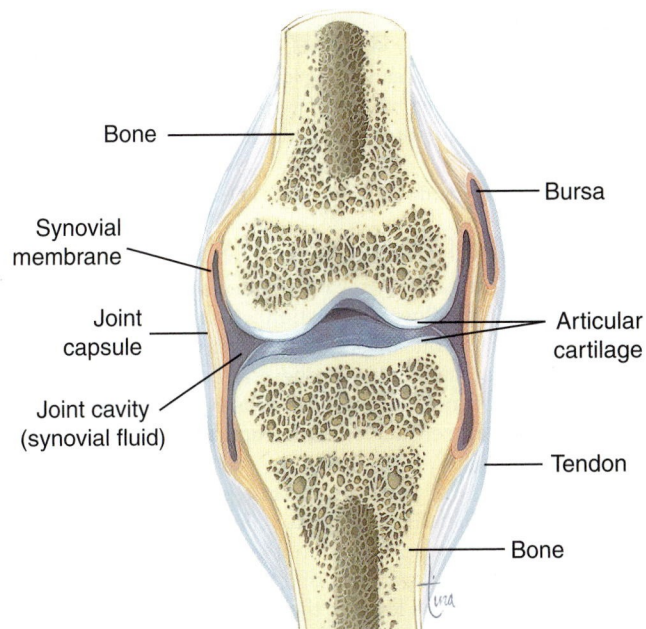

FIGURE 21-10 Many synovial joints have bursae that act as cushions against friction.

Balance, Coordination, and Movement

Walking is a complex task involving balance, coordination, and movement. Pay attention to the *base of support* and *stride* as the client walks. A wide base of support or shortened stride may indicate a balance problem. If the client has an altered gait, try to identify the specific portion of the gait that is abnormal. Abnormal gait may be caused by muscle hypertonicity (e.g., from stroke or brain tumor), lumbar disc problems, muscle atrophy, nerve damage, Parkinson's disease, cerebral palsy, multiple sclerosis, or spinal tumors. If you need additional information on gait, see Chapter 33 and the illustrations in Procedure 21-15. Tests for *balance, movement,* and *coordination* are also explained in Procedure 21-15.

As you perform each assessment, pay attention to the client's stability and level of comfort. Do not attempt movements that may produce pain or cause the client to fall. For example, recall that Mr. Nguyen (Caring for the Nguyens) has bilateral knee pain. Before asking him to perform deep knee bends or hop in place, you would want to assess his pain and its triggers.

Joint Mobility and Muscle Function

Any joint deformity requires investigation. Color changes in a joint indicate inflammation or infection. If you see erythema or swelling, investigate further by feeling for warmth. Determine any effect the deformity has on function.

Joints should move freely and without pain or **crepitus** (clicking or grating at a joint). To assess function, test range of motion (ROM) and muscle strength. **Active ROM** requires the client to move the joint through its full ROM. **Passive ROM** is used when the client is unable to exercise each joint independently. Instead, you support the body and move each joint through its ROM. Assess **muscle strength** along with movement by asking the patient to perform ROM while you apply resistance to the part being moved. For more information about the musculoskeletal system, see Chapter 33.

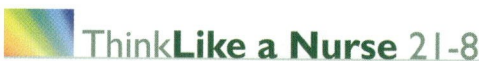

ThinkLike a Nurse 21-8

As you recall, Mr. Nguyen (Caring for the Nguyens) is moderately obese and has been having pain in both of his knees.

- What history questions would you ask him to assess his knee pain?
- What would you do to examine his knees?

THE NEUROLOGICAL SYSTEM

The neurological system controls or affects the function of all body systems and allows interaction with the external world. Its work is carried out through the transmission of chemical and electrical signals between the brain and the rest of the body. The basic functions of the nervous system are cognition, emotion, memory, sensation and perception, and regulation of homeostasis.

A comprehensive neurological assessment takes hours to complete and is usually reserved for clients with symptoms of neurological problems. As a staff nurse in general practice, you usually perform only portions of a neurological exam. In the next few sections, we look at the components of a focused neurological exam. Also see Procedure 21-16.

Developmental Considerations

When interpreting a neurological exam, consider the following developmental changes and modifications:

Infants. Reflexes present at birth include rooting, sucking, palmar grasp, tonic neck reflex (fencing), and Moro. These reflexes disappear during infancy. With neurological injury, as may occur with stroke or trauma, these reflexes may return, indicating severe problems. To review these reflexes, see Chapter 9.

Young Children. Because language skills and motor development are age-dependent, the Denver II is used as a neurological screening test for young children. The Denver II examines motor, language, and coordination skills. Chapter 9 provides additional information on the Denver II. For toddlers and older children, you can usually perform a comprehensive neurological exam with age-appropriate modifications. For example, when testing for smell use materials that a young child knows, such as bananas or apples.

Older Adults. In those of advanced age, you will commonly observe slower reaction time, a decreased ability for rapid problem solving, and slower voluntary movement. The number of functioning neurons decreases. However, intelligence, memory, and discrimination do not change with normal aging. Neurological deficits in older adults are usually the result of adverse effects of medications, nutritional deficits, dehydration, cardiovascular changes that alter cerebral blood flow, diabetes, degenerative neurological conditions (e.g., Parkinson's disease or Alzheimer's disease), alcohol or drug use, depression, or abuse.

Cerebral Function

Cerebral function refers to the client's intellectual and behavioral functioning. It includes level of consciousness, orientation, mental status and cognitive function, and communication.

Level of Consciousness

Level of consciousness (LOC) includes arousal and orientation. Arousal may range from alert to deeply comatose. Arousal is classified based on the type of stimuli (auditory, tactile, or painful) required to produce a response from the client. An alert client responds to *auditory stimuli* (e.g., verbal communication or noise). Remember, if your client does not speak your language he may not respond to questions or commands. If the client does not respond to auditory stimuli, try *tactile stimuli* (touch). Be aware that many clients who have hearing deficits lip-read to compensate. If you catch the client's attention by touching her hand, she may be able to respond to the combined auditory and visual stimuli. If still no response is obtained, use *painful stimuli* (see Procedure 21-16, step 2). Clients who respond to painful stimuli withdraw when pressure is applied.

Document LOC by describing the client's response or using the Glasgow Coma Scale (GCS) to grade eye, motor, and verbal responses. The GCS evaluates eye opening, motor responses, and verbal responses. Its limitations are that it relies heavily on vision and verbal interaction, and does not evaluate brainstem reflexes. A systematic review of evidence suggests that best practice should include use of the GCS plus other evaluation of brainstem reflexes, eye examination, vital signs, and respiratory assessment. A new tool, the Full Outline of UnResponsiveness (FOUR), provides additional information beyond that of the GCS. Both scales are included at the end of Procedure 21-16.

If you are not using the GCS, use the following terms to describe LOC:

- **Alert**–Follows commands in a timely fashion.
- **Lethargic**–Appears drowsy, easily drifts off to sleep.
- **Stuporous**–Requires vigorous stimulation before responding.
- **Comatose**–Does not respond to verbal or painful stimuli.

Although these terms are widely used, a thorough description is preferable. Look at the following two chart entries:

Pt. lethargic.

Pt. responds to repeated tactile and verbal stimulation. Quickly drifts off to sleep if stimulation is discontinued.

As you can see, the second charting entry provides significantly more information than the first.

Orientation

Orientation refers to the client's awareness of time, place, and person. **Time orientation** includes awareness of the year, date, and time of day. Older adults who become disoriented to time usually think it is an earlier date. If a client offers a bizarre time or futuristic date, consider psychiatric concerns as the cause of disorientation. Hospitalized patients are subjected to lights and noise around the clock; are roused in the middle of night for medications or time-sensitive treatments; and are given anesthesia and pain medications that alter their sense of awareness, so they easily become disoriented to time.

Orientation to place involves awareness of surroundings. The patient should know that he is, for example, in the hospital and not in church. Patients who have been moved (e.g., from the emergency department to a ward bed) may not recall their room number but are easily reoriented.

Orientation to person involves recognition of familiar persons and self-identity. The client should be able to state her name or identify people in photographs at the bedside. Because a client may meet many health professionals during a hospitalization, she may not be able to recall your name unless you have had repeated encounters with her.

Mental Status and Cognitive Function

Mental status and cognitive function include behavior, appearance, response to stimuli, speech, memory, communication, and judgment. By this point in the exam, you would have already

interviewed the client and talked with him while performing the exam, so you would have a good deal of information about his mental status and cognitive function. You would have already assessed posture, gait, motor movements, dress, and hygiene through the general survey and the musculoskeletal exam; and you would be aware of the client's mood based on his tone of voice, actions, and statements.

Many clinicians choose to screen for mental status and cognitive function by working questions into the interaction with the client as they assess other body systems. This type of informal assessment is not only more natural for the client, but it is more accurate. If you choose this method, observe for clarity of thought, appropriate content, concentration, memory, and ability to perform abstract reasoning. Normal findings include the ability to express and explain realistic thoughts with clear speech; speak with a smooth, natural pattern; follow multistep directions; listen; answer questions; and recall significant past events.

Cranial Nerve Function

Cranial nerve assessment is a key component of the neurological exam. The cranial nerves control a variety of sensory and motor functions (Table 21-4 and Fig. 21-11).

Reflex Function

Deep tendon reflexes (DTRs) are automatic responses that do not require conscious thought from the brain. A reflex produces a rapid, involuntary response that occurs at the level of the spinal cord (see Procedure 21-16, step 23, for an illustration). Because the brain is not involved, muscle response is instantaneous. Intact sensory and motor systems are required for a normal reflex response. Each DTR corresponds to a certain level

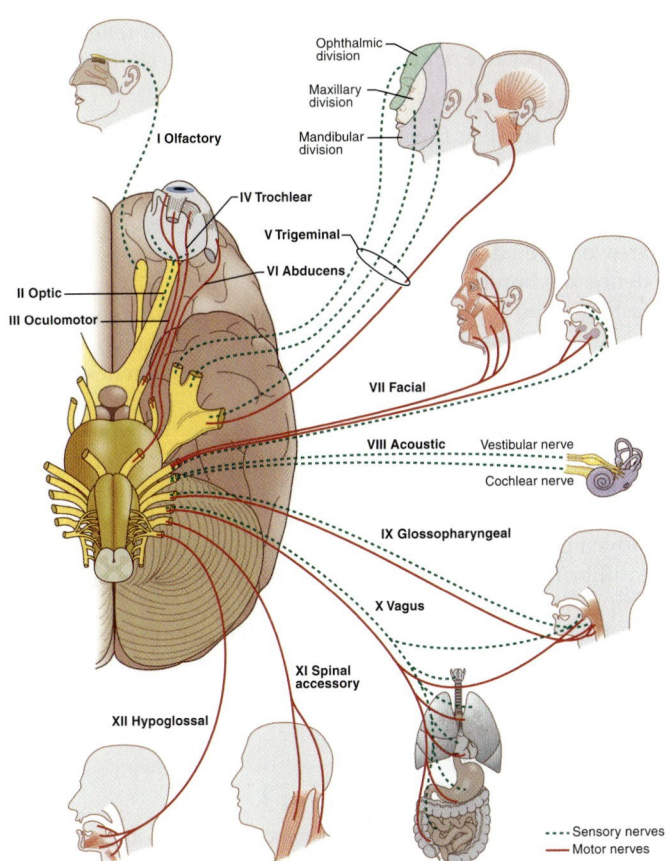

FIGURE 21-11 Origin of cranial nerves.

Table 21-4		Cranial Nerves
CRANIAL NERVE NUMBER & NAME	**TYPE OF NERVE**	**FUNCTION OF NERVE**
I. Olfactory	Sensory	Smell
II. Optic	Sensory	Visual acuity, visual fields, and ocular fundi
III. Oculomotor	Motor	EOM, pupil constriction
IV. Trochlear	Motor	EOM
V. Trigeminal: 3 branches	Sensory and motor	Corneal reflex; scalp, teeth, and facial sensation; and jaw movement
VI. Abducens	Motor	EOM
VII. Facial	Motor and sensory	Facial movement, sense of taste
VIII. Auditory	Sensory	Hearing and equilibrium
IX. Glossopharyngeal	Motor and sensory	Swallowing, gag response, tongue movement, taste, secretion of saliva
X. Vagus	Motor and sensory	Sensation of pharynx and larynx; motor activity of swallowing and vocal cords; sensory in cardiac, respiratory, and blood pressure reflexes; peristalsis; digestive secretions
XI. Spinal accessory	Motor	Head movement and shoulder elevation; motor to larynx (speaking)
XII. Hypoglossal	Motor	Tongue movement

of the cord and is graded on a scale. Superficial reflexes are graded as positive or negative (see Procedure 21-16).

Sensory Function

To assess sensory function, ask the client to keep his eyes closed as you apply various stimuli. Ask him to indicate when he feels a sensation. Vary your location and approach so that you test sensation, not pattern recognition. If you notice an area of altered sensation, systematically assess the area to define the border of the change. Usually you will limit your testing to the upper and lower extremities and the trunk. If the client has known or suspected deficits, you should test at numerous other sites. For techniques for assessing reflexes and sensory function, see Procedure 21-16.

The neurological system coordinates the function of the skeleton and muscles. Motor pathways transmit information between the brain and muscles and the muscles control movement of the skeleton. The cerebellum helps coordinate muscle movement, regulate muscle tone, and maintain posture and equilibrium. The cerebellum is also largely responsible for proprioception, or body positioning. Disorders of motor and cerebellar function result in pain or problems with movement, gait, or posture. Thus, when you assess the musculoskeletal system, you also assess the motor functions of the neurological system.

KnowledgeCheck 21-11

- Identify and describe the components assessed in the neurological exam.
- What approach to assessment should you take if:
  Your client has no neurological problems but you are performing a comprehensive exam?
  Your client is hospitalized for a documented cerebrovascular accident?
  Your client has been admitted with an acute head injury and the extent of neurological injury is unknown?

THE GENITOURINARY SYSTEM

In most practice settings, nurses assess only the patient's external genitalia and inguinal lymph nodes. Nurse practitioners and physicians perform comprehensive examinations of the female and male reproductive and urinary systems, as do nurses working in specialty areas. However, even as a novice nurse you may assist with exams or just be present as a witness or to provide emotional support to the client.

Because a genitourinary (GU) assessment focuses on sexual and reproductive function, it might be embarrassing or uncomfortable for many people. As a result, the assessment requires a competent, professional approach. Your confidence and ease with these topics will help the client to feel more relaxed.

The Male Genitourinary System

The male genitourinary system includes the reproductive system and the urinary system. A complete examination includes assessment of the external genitalia, evaluation for hernias, and a rectal exam for prostate screening. The penis and scrotum are examined by inspection and palpation. You will assess some of the urinary system organs when examining the back (kidneys, ureters) and the abdomen (bladder); the prostate gland is palpated during the exam of the rectum and anus (discussed later in this chapter). For steps to follow in examining the male genitourinary system, and for illustrations, see Procedure 21-17.

Recently, as a result of the scarcity of clear, scientific evidence, the American Academy of Pediatrics no longer recommends **circumcision** (excision of the foreskin of the penis) as a routine practice. However, circumcision is tied to some religious and cultural beliefs (e.g., among Jews and Muslims), so it is still common.

A **hernia** is a protrusion of the intestine (or other organ) through the wall that contains it. In men, this is most likely to be a protrusion of the intestine either through the abdominal wall **(direct hernia)** or into the inguinal canal and possibly into the scrotum **(indirect hernia).** A hernia may be a small protrusion or it may cause pain and distention as a loop of bowel extends into the scrotum. An **umbilical hernia** (fairly common in infants) is an outward bulging due to delayed closure around a small muscle around the umbilicus (belly button). For an illustration of an umbilical hernia, see Procedure 21-14.

KnowledgeCheck 21-12

- What assessment techniques are used when examining the male genitourinary system?
- What is the most common hernia occurring in men?

The Female Genitourinary System

You may be called upon to assist with a comprehensive examination. For a procedure for inspecting external female genitalia and palpating inguinal lymph nodes, see Procedure 21-18.

External Examination

For adolescents and young women who are not sexually active, an external GU examination includes the inspection of the amount and distribution of pubic hair, the skin of the pubic area, and the external genitalia; and palpation of the inguinal lymph nodes.

Internal Examination

Women who are sexually active; who have abnormal findings on external examination; who have abdominal, pelvic, or genitourinary complaints; or who are on hormone therapy require an internal genital examination. The exam includes the following:

- Palpation of Bartholin's glands and Skene's ducts (see Procedure 21-18)
- Assessment of vaginal muscle tone and pelvic musculature
- Speculum examination
- **Bimanual examination,** wherein the examiner palpates the cervix, uterus, and adnexal tissues with the use of one or two fingers within the vagina and the other hand on the outside to help bring the inner structures toward the two hands.

Pap Smear. Routine annual Papanicolaou tests (Pap smears) to screen for cervical and uterine cancer are recommended for women by age 21, and for younger women who are sexually active. Women age 30 or older should follow the advice of their provider about spacing out Pap tests to every 2 or 3 years. Women older than age 65 are not usually routinely screened unless they are at high risk. Of course those with certain vulnerabilities (e.g., weakened immune system, HIV-positive) should have a Pap test every year (Agency for Healthcare Research and Quality [AHRQ], n.d.; American Cancer Society, 2010; National Guideline Clearinghouse, 2005, revised 2011). National screening guidelines vary, and they change frequently.

Additional cultures or screens may be done if there is unusual discharge or risk of sexually transmitted infection. A **speculum examination** is performed to collect specimens and assess the cervix. You will need to gather equipment, explain to the client what will happen, prepare the client, assist the client and examiner during the procedure, assist the client after the procedure, and document your findings.

To learn about assisting with a speculum exam, see Clinical Insight 21-3.

KnowledgeCheck 21-13

What are the responsibilities of the nurse during an internal exam of the female genitourinary system?

Clinical Insight 21-3 ➤ Assisting With a Speculum Exam

Equipment

- Patient drape
- Nonsterile gloves
- Vaginal speculum (see accompanying figure)
  The speculum may be plastic or metal.
  The size of the speculum depends on the patient's history. Use a small speculum for a woman who has never been sexually active or an older woman who is not sexually active.
  If a culture or a Pap smear is to be obtained, lubricate the speculum with warm water. Otherwise, use a water-soluble lubricant.
- Lubricant
- Pap smear slide, spatula, brush, or specimen broom and container with solution
- Fixative, if the smear technique is used
- Genital culture supplies
- Additional light source

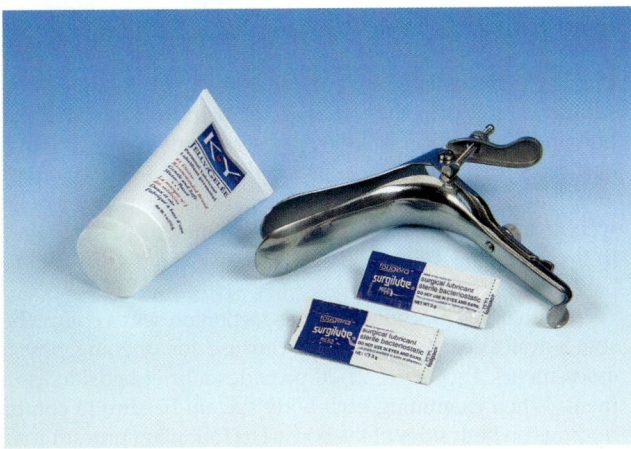

Equipment. A vaginal speculum.

Preparing the Patient

- Explain to the patient that an internal examination of her vagina and pelvic organs will be performed. The examination usually takes only a few minutes, and although it might not be comfortable it should not be painful.
- Have the woman urinate before the examination if needed. Emptying the bladder helps the patient to feel more comfortable during the exam.
- Provide privacy and keep the patient warm during the procedure.
- Assist the woman to the lithotomy position, and cover her with a drape.

Inserting the Speculum

The speculum is inserted into the vagina to visualize the cervix (see accompanying figure). Once the speculum is inserted, you may need to adjust the light source for the examiner.

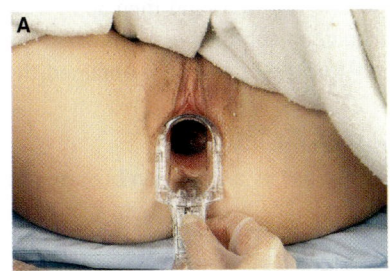

A. A vaginal speculum examination. Placement of the speculum in the vagina.

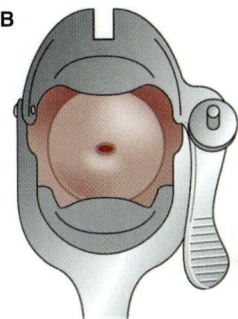

B. View through the speculum.

Collecting Specimens

If a routine screening for cervical and uterine cancer is being done, a specimen will be collected. Additional cultures or screens may be required if there is unusual discharge or risk of sexually transmitted infection. Genital cultures are endocervical smears.

Pap Smear Procedure

Most commonly, the examiner inserts a small brush through the cervical os and rotates it to obtain cells from within the cervical canal (endocervical smear). The brush is then rolled onto the slide.

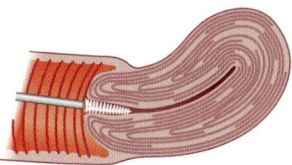

Using a specimen broom to obtain endocervical cells.

(Continued)

Clinical Insight 21-3 ➤ Assisting With a Speculum Exam—cont'd

A second specimen may be obtained by lightly scraping the cervix with a wooden spatula to obtain cells from the ectocervix (the lowest portion of the cervix that protrudes into the vagina).

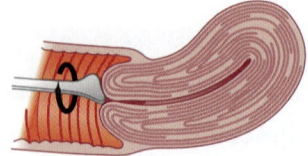

Using a spatula to obtain ectocervical cells.

The spatula is then smeared on the slide. Some examiners use both specimen sources and then apply a fixative, usually a spray or liquid, on top of the specimen to preserve it for examination. After the samples are obtained, the speculum is removed.

Pap Smear, Alternative Method

■ The examiner inserts a specimen broom into the cervical os and rotates it. The broom is then inserted into a fixative solution and rotated to disperse cells into the solution. This technique is gaining popularity because it is considered

more sensitive for detection of cervical changes. After the samples are obtained, the speculum is removed.

Bimanual Exam

After removing the speculum, the examiner inserts lubricated gloved fingers into the vagina while pressing down on the lower abdomen and suprapubic area. This is known as a **bimanual exam.** It is used to assess the consistency of the cervix; the size of the uterus; and to detect tenderness over the ovaries, fallopian tubes, or with movement of the cervix.

Post-Procedure

■ Assist the woman to a sitting position at the end of the exam.
■ You may need to assist the woman with perineal care.
■ If there is any bleeding or discharge, provide a perineal pad.
■ Document the date and time of the procedure, the name of the examiner, the patient's tolerance of the procedure, and any nursing assessments or interventions performed.

Practice Resources
ACOG, 2009b.

The Anus, Rectum, and Prostate

Examining the rectum and anus is the last aspect of a comprehensive examination. For the female client, this exam is usually performed at the end of a bimanual pelvic examination while the client is still in the lithotomy position. Usually a male client assumes the Sims' position, and you perform the exam after completing your examination of the genitals. For a step-by-step procedure, see Procedure 21-19.

Inspect the anus and rectum for skin condition and hemorrhoids and palpate for muscle tone, masses, and tenderness. Skin irritation and erythema are common in clients who have diarrhea and infants and toddlers who wear diapers. **Hemorrhoids** (dilated, usually painful, anal vessels) may be seen in clients with a history of constipation. Many women develop hemorrhoids with pregnancy and childbirth.

A comprehensive examination for a man should include a digital rectal examination to assess for prostate enlargement. An enlarged prostate may indicate benign enlargement of the prostate, which is common in men older than age 50; or it may indicate prostatitis. A hard nodule or multiple nodules may indicate prostate cancer.

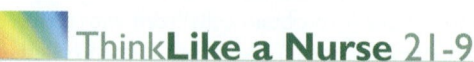

ThinkLike a Nurse 21-9

How will examination of the rectum and anus differ for Nam and Yen Nguyen (Caring for the Nguyens)?

PracticalKnowledge procedures

The RN is responsible for patient assessment. As the RN, you should (1) perform the initial assessment to establish a baseline and (2) perform follow-up assessments for any changes. You can instruct nursing assistive personnel (NAPs) to report any changes to you. You can delegate assessment of height, weight, and vital signs to the NAP. You may want to obtain the first set of vital signs yourself, because they will serve as a baseline.

Together, the procedures in this section present a comprehensive physical examination you can use for ongoing physical assessments. Procedure 21-20 provides a brief bedside assessment. When examining each body system be sure to compare findings on both sides of the body. The following procedures are described mainly for adult patients. To review ways in which to adapt your examination to people of different ages, see the earlier section How Do I Modify Assessment for Different Age Groups?

Procedure 21–1 ■ Performing the General Survey

➤ For steps to follow in *all* procedures, refer to the Universal Steps for All Procedures found on the page facing the inside back cover.

Positioning

- Have the client seated as you begin the examination (on an exam table or on the side of the bed).
- If the client is unable to sit, use Fowler's or semi-Fowler's position.

Focused History Questions

- How are you feeling today?
- (If the client is an outpatient) What brings you to the clinic today?
- Are you in any discomfort or pain?
- Have you had any hospitalizations or surgeries?
- What medicines do you take? That includes prescribed as well as over-the-counter drugs.
- How much alcohol do you drink per day? Do you smoke cigarettes? If so, how many per day and for how long? Do you use drugs for non-medical purposes?
- Do you use any herbal products or natural remedies?
- Do you have any difficulty falling asleep or staying asleep? This is a common problem for perimenopausal women and older adults.

Developmental Modifications for Infants and Children

- Encourage the parents to be present for the examination. Position an infant on a padded examination table or held against the parent's chest.
  Infants and toddlers usually feel most secure if a parent is present.
- Offer toddlers choices. Involve the parent in the exam. Praise the toddler for cooperation.
- Allow the preschool child to sit in the parent's lap if she wishes. Let the child help with the exam. Give

reassurance as you proceed. Compliment the child on her cooperation.
  Preschoolers often are fearful of body injury and invasive procedures.
- Support the school-age child's independence. Develop rapport by asking the child about his teacher or favorite school and play activities. Allow the child to undress himself and get up and down from the exam table. Demonstrate and let the child touch your equipment before you use it.
  Equipment will seem less threatening to the child if she touches it. It is unlikely that the child would break the equipment.
- Adolescents should be examined without parents or siblings present unless they request otherwise. Provide privacy.
  Adolescents tend to be self-conscious and introspective.

Developmental Modifications for Older Adults

- Observe the older adult's energy level during the physical examination, and provide rest periods if needed. If the client tires easily, arrange the exam sequence to limit position changes.
- Allow extra time to interview and examine older adults.
- Be aware that stiff muscles and arthritic joints may make it impossible for older adults to assume certain positions.
- Be alert for hearing and vision deficits in older adults, and adapt your interview techniques accordingly (e.g., elicit feedback to be sure the client has heard you correctly).
- Assess the older adult's functional status. You can use the Lawton Instrumental Activities of Daily Living (IADL) (see Chapter 3).
- Work the SPICES assessment into the examination of various body systems: **S**leep disorders, **P**roblems eating or feeding, **I**ncontinence, **C**onfusion, **E**vidence of falls, **S**kin breakdown.

➤ When performing the procedure, always identify your patient according to agency policy and be attentive to standard precautions, hand hygiene, patient safety and privacy, body mechanics, and documentation.

Procedure Steps

1. **Identify signs of distress** (e.g., pain, fear, or anxiety). If signs of distress are present, perform a focused assessment, and address the immediate problem.

2. **Observe apparent age, sex, and race.** Ask the patient, "What racial or ethnic group do you identify with?" Ask yourself,
   - Is apparent age consistent with biological age?
   - Are there cultural or gender-related factors that influence the exam or findings?

Expected and Abnormal Findings

Expected findings: The client is in no apparent distress. The client appears relaxed, with no evidence of pain, fear, or anxiety.

Abnormal findings: Pain, grimacing, breathing problems, skin color changes

Expected findings: Client appears his stated age. Makes eye contact consistent with his cultural norms. Is reasonably comfortable with being examined.

(continued on next page)

Procedure 21–1 ■ Performing the General Survey (continued)

3. **Note facial characteristics**, including facial expression, symmetry of facial features, and the condition and color of the skin. Ask yourself,
   - What is the client's face telling me?
   - Is the facial expression appropriate to the situation?
   - Are facial features symmetrical (palpebral fissure and nasolabial folds)?
   - Are there any changes in condition or color of skin?
   - Does the client maintain eye contact?

   Expected findings: Face is symmetrical; visible skin is intact without excessive wrinkling, discoloration, or deformity.

4. **Note body type and posture.** Greet the client with a handshake. Be aware that shaking hands is not acceptable in all cultures.
   Allows you to assess muscle strength and surface skin characteristics while at the same time conveying that you care.
   Ask yourself:
   - Is the body build stocky, slender, average, obese, or **cachectic** (very thin, wasted appearance)?
   - Are the body parts proportional to the client's overall size?
   - Does the client have abnormal fat distribution?
   - Does the client assume a specific position for comfort (e.g., sitting versus supine)?

   Expected findings: Posture is upright, and body appears proportionate. Grip is strong.

5. **Observe gait, and note any abnormal movements.** If the client has Impaired Bed Mobility, determine ability to move and amount of assistance needed. Ask yourself,
   - Does the client move in a coordinated manner?
   - Are there any obvious gait problems?
   - Does the client walk with a wide base of support or short stride length?
   - Does the client use assistive devices?
   - Are there any abnormal or spastic movements?

   Expected findings: Movements are coordinated; gait is steady; does not use assistive devices.

   Abnormal findings: Unstable or shuffling gait; spastic movements, stiff movements

6. **Listen to your client's speech pattern, pace, quality, tone, vocabulary, and sentence structure.** Ask yourself,
   - Are the responses appropriate?
   - Is there any difficulty with speech?
   - Does the client's tone of voice match her statements

   Expected findings: Client responds appropriately to questions. Tone of voice matches responses. Speech is clear, evenly paced, and rises and falls based on content.

   Abnormal findings: Rapid speech, slow speech, slurred speech

7. **Assess mental state and affect.**
   a. Determine level of consciousness.
   b. Determine orientation to time, place, and person.

   Ask yourself,
   - If the client is disoriented, does he reorient easily?
   - What is the client's mood? Is it appropriate for the situation?

   Expected findings: Awake, alert, and oriented to time, place, person, and self. Mood is appropriate for the situation.

   Abnormal findings: Confusion and irritability, inability to recall information or provide history, lethargy and somnolence, bizarre responses

■ Many medical conditions and medications can affect mental status. If you note any abnormal findings: during the general survey, be sure to focus on them when you assess mental status during the sensori–neurological examination.

8. **Observe dress, grooming, and hygiene.** Ask yourself,
   ■ Is the client appropriately and neatly dressed?
   ■ Is the client well groomed?
   ■ Are there any unusual odors?

Expected findings: Client is dressed appropriately for the climate. Skin is clean, and clothing is in good repair. No noticeable odor.

Abnormal findings: Poor hygiene, dirty skin or nails, uncombed hair, visible soiling of clothing, mismatched or wrinkled clothing, objectionable odor

9. **Measure vital signs:** blood pressure, temperature, radial pulse, respiratory rate. If your initial observations and interview indicate that the client is in pain, perform a pain assessment, as well (see Chapter 32.)

Expected findings:

BP: <120/80 mm Hg

Temperature: 97.3°F–98.6°F (36.3°C–37°C) oral

Pulse: 60–100 beats/min, regular, and easily palpated

Respiratory rate: 12–20 breaths/min, regular and even

Abnormal findings: See Chapter 19.

10. **Measure height and weight.**
    a. For adults: Calculate BMI, or use the accompanying table.

    $$\frac{\text{Wt (lb)} \times 703}{\text{Ht (in.)}^2} = \text{BMI}$$

    b. For children: Plot height and weight on growth chart.

Developmental Modifications
Infants and children
■ Weigh infants without clothing; weigh older children in their underwear.
■ For infants and children younger than age 2 yr, position supine to measure height; be sure knees are extended.
■ For infants and children younger than age 2 yr, also measure head circumference.

Expected findings: For adults: BMI is 18.5–24.9.

For children: Height and weight are consistent with previous trend on growth chart.

Abnormal findings:
BMI < 18.5 = underweight
BMI 25–29.9 = overweight
BMI ≥ 30 = obese
BMI 30–34.9 Level I Moderate obesity
BMI 35–39.9 Level II Severe obesity
BMI > 40 Level III Morbid obesity

? **What if . . .**

■ **There is an apparent language barrier?**

Obtain an interpreter; and refer to Clinical Insight 20-4, in Chapter 20 of this book.

Use this table to find body mass index, based on height and weight, or use a BMI calculator such as the ones found at http://www.nhlbisupport.com/bmi/bmicalc.htm and http://www.cdc.gov/nccdphp/dnpa/bmi/adult_BMI/english_bmi_calculator/bmi_calculator.htm ▼

(continued on next page)

Procedure 21–1 ■ Performing the General Survey (continued)

Weight (lb)

Height (ft/in)	120	130	140	150	160	170	180	190	200	210	220	230	240	250	260	270	280	290	300	310	320	330
4'5"	30	33	35	38	40	43	45	48	50	53	55	58	60	63	65	68	70	73	75	78	80	83
4'6"	29	31	34	36	39	41	43	46	48	51	53	56	58	60	63	65	68	70	72	75	77	80
4'7"	28	30	33	35	37	40	42	44	47	49	51	54	56	58	61	63	65	68	70	72	75	77
4'8"	27	29	31	34	36	38	40	43	45	47	49	52	54	56	58	61	63	65	67	70	72	74
4'9"	26	28	30	33	35	37	39	41	43	46	48	50	52	54	56	59	61	63	65	67	69	72
4'10"	25	27	29	31	34	36	38	40	42	44	46	48	50	52	54	57	59	61	63	65	67	69
4'11"	24	26	28	30	32	34	36	38	40	43	45	47	49	51	53	55	57	59	61	63	65	67
5'0"	23	25	27	29	31	33	35	37	39	41	43	45	47	49	51	53	55	57	59	61	63	65
5'1"	23	25	27	28	30	32	34	36	38	40	42	44	45	47	49	51	53	55	57	59	61	62
5'2"	22	24	26	27	29	31	33	35	37	38	40	42	44	46	48	49	51	53	55	57	59	60
5'3"	21	23	25	27	28	30	32	34	36	37	39	41	43	44	46	48	50	51	53	55	57	59
5'4"	21	22	24	26	28	29	31	33	34	36	38	40	41	43	45	46	48	50	52	53	55	57
5'5"	20	22	23	25	27	28	30	32	33	35	38	38	40	42	43	45	47	48	50	52	53	55
5'6"	19	21	23	24	26	27	29	31	32	34	36	37	39	40	42	44	45	47	49	50	52	53
5'7"	19	20	22	24	25	27	28	30	31	33	35	36	38	39	41	42	44	46	47	49	50	52
5'8"	18	20	21	23	24	26	27	29	30	32	34	35	37	38	40	41	43	44	46	47	49	50
5'9"	18	19	21	22	24	25	27	28	30	31	33	34	36	37	38	40	41	43	44	46	47	49
5'10"	17	19	20	22	23	24	26	27	29	30	32	33	35	36	37	39	40	42	43	45	46	47
5'11"	17	18	20	21	22	24	25	27	28	29	31	32	34	35	36	38	39	41	42	43	45	46
6'	16	18	19	20	22	23	24	26	27	29	30	31	33	34	35	37	38	39	41	42	43	45
6'1"	16	17	19	20	21	22	24	25	26	28	29	30	32	33	34	36	37	38	40	41	42	44
6'2"	15	17	18	19	21	22	23	24	26	27	28	30	31	32	33	35	36	37	39	40	41	42
6'3"	15	16	18	19	20	21	23	24	25	26	28	29	30	31	33	34	35	36	38	39	40	41
6'4"	15	16	17	18	20	21	22	23	24	26	27	28	29	30	32	33	34	35	37	38	39	40
6'5"	14	15	17	18	19	20	21	23	24	25	26	27	29	30	31	32	33	34	36	37	38	39
6'6"	14	15	16	17	19	20	21	22	23	24	25	27	28	29	30	31	32	34	35	36	37	38
6'7"	14	15	16	17	18	19	20	21	23	24	25	26	27	28	29	30	32	33	34	35	36	37
6'8"	13	14	15	17	18	19	20	21	22	23	24	25	26	28	29	30	31	32	33	34	35	36
6'9"	13	14	15	16	17	18	19	20	21	23	24	25	26	27	28	29	30	31	32	33	34	35
6'10"	13	14	15	16	17	18	19	20	21	22	23	24	25	26	27	28	29	30	31	32	34	35

Less risk → More risk

Documentation

- Document BP as right or left arm, and note the patient's position: sitting, standing, or lying.
- Document temperature measurement route: oral, rectal, or tympanic membrane.
- For children, document height and weight on a growth chart.

Go to Chapter 21, **Supplemental Materials: Growth Charts,** on DavisPlus.

- If you need more information about documenting, see Caring for the Nguyens at the beginning of the chapter. Also see Chapter 19 for documenting vital signs on a graphic flowsheet.

Practice Resources

Management of Overweight and Obesity Working Group, 2006; National Heart Lung and Blood Institute, n.d.

Procedure 21-2 ■ Assessing the Skin

➤ For steps to follow in *all* procedures, refer to the Universal Steps for All Procedures found on the page facing the inside back cover.

Equipment

- Nonlatex gloves (if exposure to body fluids is a possibility)
- Flexible transparent ruler—to measure lesions
- Penlight—to provide adequate lighting to unexposed areas
- Magnifier—for better visualization of lesions
- Pen and record form

Focused History Questions

Ask the patient about the history or presence of any:
- Rashes
- History of allergies
- Areas of skin that have changed color
- Skin lesions

- Skin with rough or unusual texture
- Skin that is always warm or cool, regardless of room temperature

Developmental Modifications for Older Adults

- Assess the level of risk for pressure ulcers. For assessment tools (Braden scale, Norton scale), go to Chapter 36 in this textbook.

  As adults age, the subcutaneous tissue layer thins. The dermal layer loses elasticity as a result of changes in collagen fibers; and the strong bond between the epidermal and dermal layers decreases. These changes make the skin prone to breakdown.

➤ When performing the procedure, always identify your patient according to agency policy and be attentive to standard precautions, hand hygiene, patient safety and privacy, body mechanics, and documentation.

Procedure Steps

1. **Inspect skin color, including mucous membranes, tongue, and conjunctiva.**

   To assess color changes of exposed and unexposed areas. Color changes and odors may indicate underlying disease and should be fully investigated.

   a. Provide good lighting.
   b. In dark-skinned clients, look for color changes in the conjunctiva or oral mucosa, tongue, lips, nailbeds, palms of the hands, and soles of the feet.

      Skin color varies widely among individuals by age and ethnicity, but in each individual, skin color is fairly uniform over his body. ▼

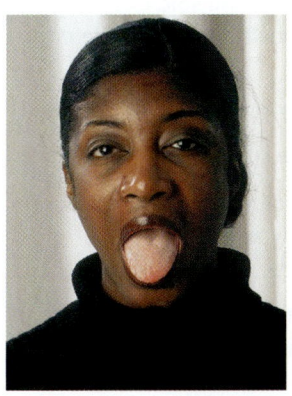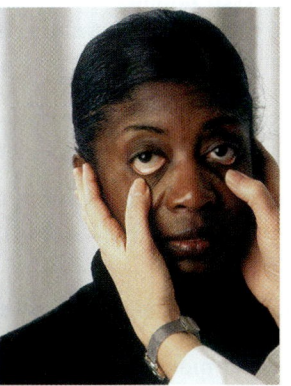

   c. Note any unusual odors.
   d. To assess for cyanosis, be sure to examine the tongue.

      Exposure to cold causes the lips to turn blue, but not the tongue. Cyanosis affects the color of the skin, mucous membrane, and tongue.

Expected and Abnormal Findings

Expected findings: Skin color is uniform, with darker exposed areas. Mucous membranes and conjunctiva are pink and moist. No unusual odors.

Developmental Variations

Newborns—May be jaundiced for a few weeks. Blue-black mongolian spots and pink-red capillary hemangiomas are common and fade with time.

Older adults—May have thin, translucent skin and wrinkles due to loss of elasticity. Fragile skin is not uncommon among lighter skinned, older adults.

Abnormal findings: Pallor, jaundice, cyanosis, erythema, hyperpigmentation, hypopigmentation. If there are abnormal findings, ask the patient (or someone who knows him well) about the baseline skin color.

(continued on next page)

Procedure 21–2 ■ Assessing the Skin (continued)

2. Palpate skin for temperature.
  a. Wear procedure gloves and discard after examining any open areas of the skin.
  b. Use dorsal aspect of hand or fingers.
  c. Compare bilaterally.
  The dorsa of the hands and the fingers are most sensitive to temperature variations.

Expected findings: Skin is warm; temperature is the same bilaterally.

Abnormal findings: Local area(s) that are warmer or cooler than the rest of the skin; generalized temperature increase or decrease. If the skin is excessively warm, assess for fever. Localized warmth with erythema can indicate an infection. Cool skin might be a sign of compromised circulation or dehydration, particularly in the older adult.

3. Palpate skin for turgor. Test an unexposed area, such as the area below the clavicle, inner thigh, sternum, or forehead, by gently pinching up the skin, noting its return when you release it.

Developmental Modifications
Infants—Check skin turgor on the abdomen.
Older adults—Check skin turgor over the sternum or clavicle. ▼

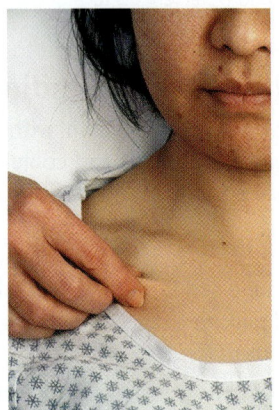

Expected findings: Skin returns immediately to its original position.

Developmental Variations
Older adults have decreased skin turgor due to decreased elasticity.

Abnormal findings: Decreased or increased turgor. *Tenting (decreased turgor):* Skin takes several seconds to return to original position. *Decreased turgor (tenting) is seen with dehydration or normal aging. It predisposes the patient to skin breakdown.*

Increased turgor: Skin tension does not allow the skin to be pinched up.

4. Palpate the skin for texture.
  Texture varies, depending on the area being assessed and the age of the client

Expected findings: Skin is smooth and soft. Exposed areas and extens.or surfaces (e.g., elbows and knees) are drier and coarser than other areas.

Developmental Variations
Infants and young children—Have smooth skin.

Abnormal findings: Coarse, thick, rough, or dry skin; very smooth, thin, fine-textured, shiny skin

5. Palpate skin for moisture (hydration). Use the dorsum of your hand.

Expected findings: Skin is warm and dry.

Developmental Variations
Older adults—Skin may be dry and flaky because of decreased activity of sebaceous and sweat glands.

Adolescents—May have skin that is oilier than normal.

Abnormal findings: Increased moisture (skin feels damp, visible diaphoresis); decreased moisture (skin feels dry)

6. Inspect for edema.
  a. Press firmly with your fingertip for 5 sec over a bony area, such as the tibia.
  b. Release your finger, and observe the skin for the reaction.
  c. If edema is present, note the location, degree, and type of swelling. For example, if you observe edema in the lower leg, how far up the leg does it extend?

Expected findings: No edema. Normally there will be no evidence of the pressure once you release your finger. If pitting edema is present, you will see a depression in the skin.

Grading System

Trace: Minimal depression with pressure.

+1: 2-mm depression; rapid return of skin to position.

+2: 4-mm depression that disappears in 10–15 sec.

+3: 6-mm depression that lasts 1–2 min. Area appears swollen.

+4: 8-mm depression that persists for 2–3 min. Area is grossly edematous.

Abnormal findings: Edema is an abnormal finding.

7. Identify any skin lesions.
  a. Inspect and palpate lesions.
  b. When you notice bruises, be alert for signs of abuse (see Chapter 9).
  c. Ask the client: "Do you have any new moles or other lesions? Has there been any change in existing moles/lesions?"
  d. Assess for malignant lesions using ABCDE:
    A. (asymmetry)
    B. (irregular borders)
    C. (color variations)
    D. (diameter: 0.5 cm)
    E. (elevation).

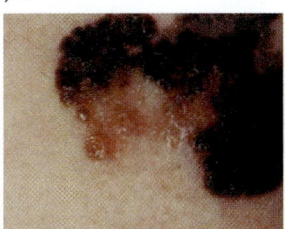

Malignant melanoma

Expected findings: No lesions are present.

Normal variations include moles, freckles, birthmarks, striae (in pregnant women or clients who have lost much weight), and wrinkles.

Developmental Variations

Newborns—**Milia** (tiny collections of sebum, usually on the face) are common.

Adolescents—Acne is a common, abnormal finding among adolescents.

Adults—**Acrochordons** (skin tags) may be seen around the neck, axillae, skinfolds, or areas where clothing rubs.

Older adults—Flat beige or brown macules are common on exposed skin areas.

Abnormal findings: See the table Describing Skin Lesions following this procedure. Also,

Go to Chapter 21, **Tables, Boxes, Figures: ESG Table 21-3, Abnormal Atlas: Skin Lesions,** on *DavisPlus.*

Describing Lesions

When you observe a lesion, evaluate and describe the following:
- **Size.** Measure the length, width, and depth of the lesion.
- **Shape and pattern.** Describe the *shape* of individual lesions. If there are clusters or groups, describe the *pattern.* Is it linear or circular? Are the *borders* distinct, or do they run together? Is the border smooth or irregular?
- **Color.** Describe the color of the lesion, and determine whether there is any variation of color within the lesion.
- **Distribution.** Are the lesions distributed over the entire body? Are they confined to a specific region? What parts of the body are affected?
- **Texture.** The texture (e.g., smooth, rough, scaly) of a lesion helps with classification.
- **Surface relationship.** To assess surface relationship, you will need to palpate the lesion. Is it flat, raised, or depressed? Is it firmly attached to the surrounding skin or mobile?
- **Exudate.** Examine the lesion(s) for signs of drainage. Describe the color, appearance, amount, and odor of drainage, if present.

- **Tenderness, pain, or itching.** Press on the lesion, and determine the patient's reaction. Does touching the lesion cause pain or discomfort?

Patient Teaching

Teach the patient the signs and symptoms of skin cancer, the importance of the skin exam, and preventive measures.

Home Care

- Assess the skill level of the caregiver. Instruct the caregiver in the importance of skin assessment and measures to prevent skin breakdown.
- Be alert for lesions (e.g., burns, bruises) that may signal physical abuse. For more signs of abuse, refer to Procedure 9-1.

Documentation

- If lesions are present, describe the history: onset, duration, associated or aggravating factors (e.g., itching), factors that relieve symptoms, treatments that have been used, and responses to treatment.

(continued on next page)

Procedure 21–2 ■ **Assessing the Skin** (continued)

- Sketch the location of skin lesions on body diagrams, if available (see example below); or sketch a body if necessary. ▼

Practice Resources

Yifan Xue, 2007.

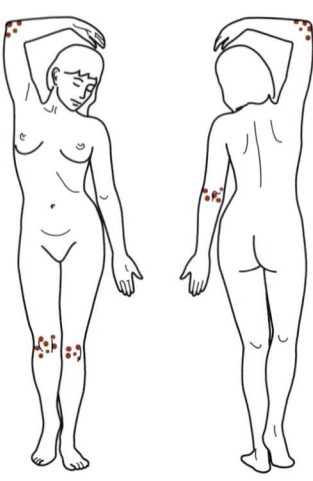

Describing Skin Lesions		
PRIMARY LESIONS		
Types		**Description**
Macule (nonpalpable, < 1 cm) 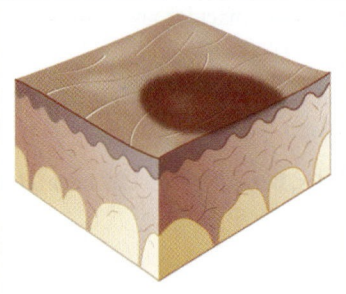	Macule (nonpalpable, < 1 cm) 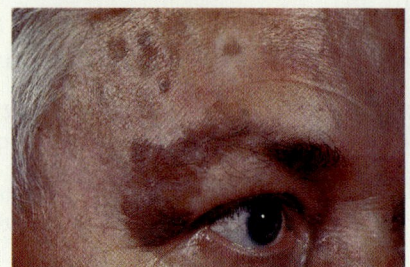	Flat and colored. Examples: freckle, petechiae, birthmark, mongolian spot
Papule (palpable), < 1 cm; plaque, > 1 cm 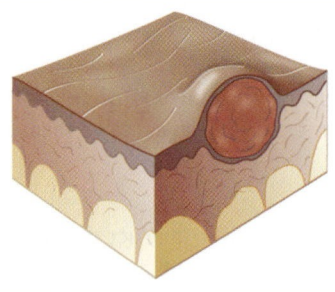	Papules (seborrheic keratosis) 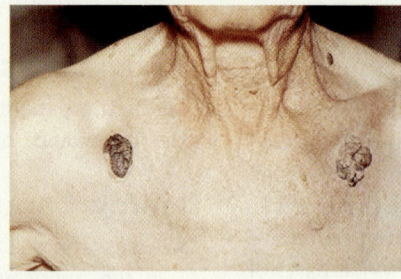	Elevated and raised, but superficial. Examples: mole, psoriasis

Describing Skin Lesions—cont'd

PRIMARY LESIONS

Types		Description
Vesicle (palpable), < 1 cm; bulla, > 1 cm 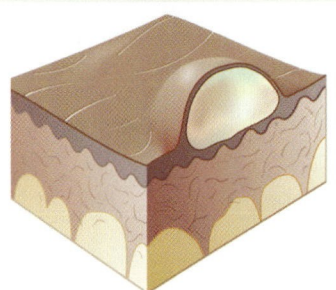	Vesicles (blisters) 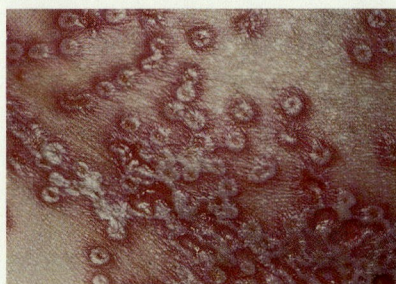 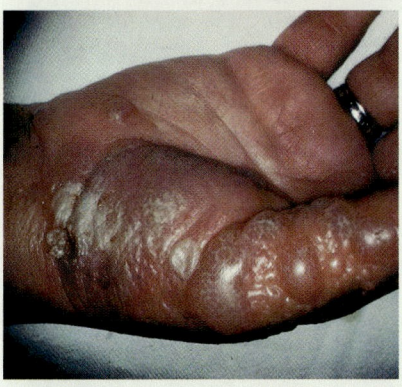	Elevated and filled with serous fluid. Examples: blister, herpes simplex
Cyst (palpable), < 2 cm 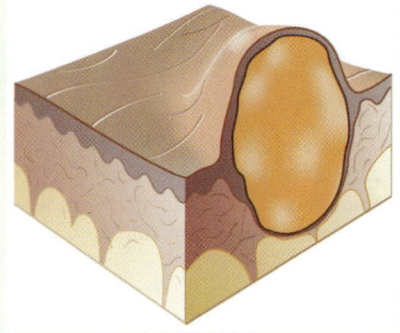	Keratogenous cyst 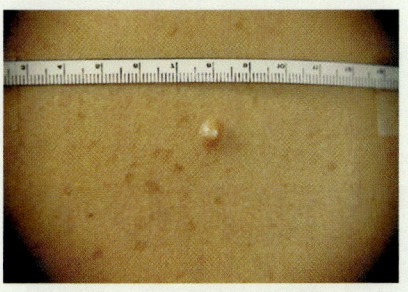	Palpable, fluid filled, and encapsulated. If not fluid filled, called a *nodule*
Pustule (palpable) 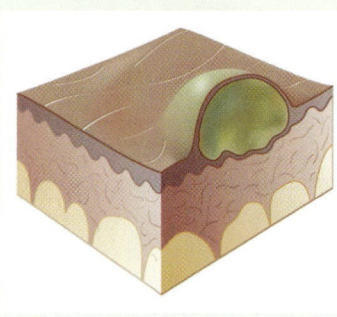	Pustules (acne) 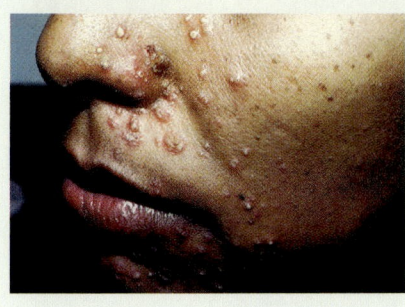	Elevated and filled with pus. Examples: acne, folliculitis, impetigo

(continued on next page)

Procedure 21–2 ■ Assessing the Skin (continued)

Describing Skin Lesions—cont'd

PRIMARY LESIONS

Types		Description
	Nodule (palpable) 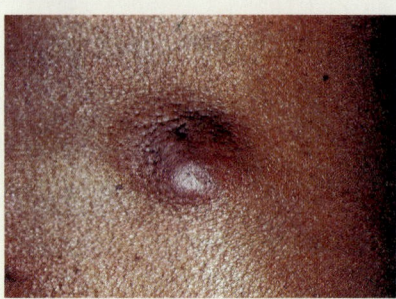	Elevated, solid, and firm, with depth into dermis. Examples: wart, lipoma (fatty cyst)
Wheal 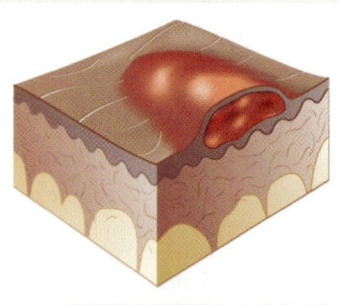	Hive 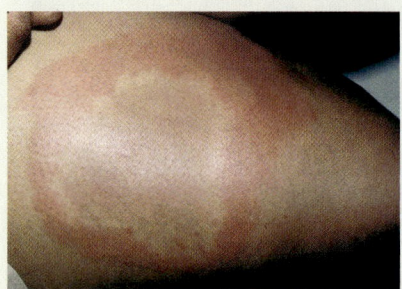	Elevated, superficial, with localized edema. Examples: insect bites, hives

SECONDARY LESIONS

Types		Description
Excoriation 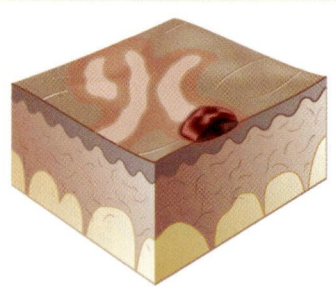	Excoriation from pruritus 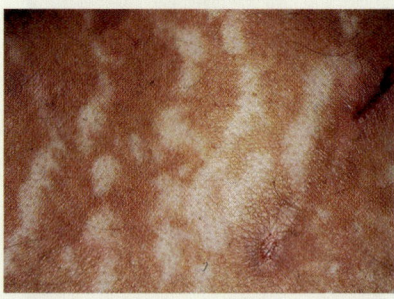	Abrasion or loss of skin that does not extend beyond the superficial epidermis. Examples: scratches, stasis dermatitis, atopic dermatitis
Erosion 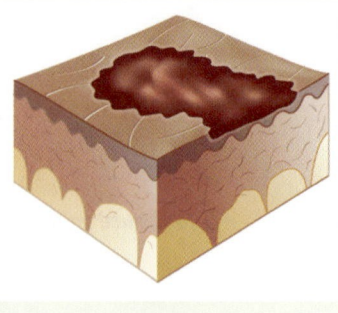	Erosions 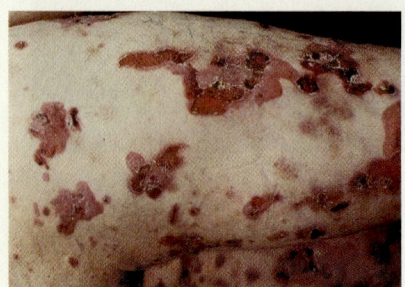	Loss of superficial epidermis, usually secondary to rupture of a blister. Examples: abrasions and impetigo

Describing Skin Lesions—cont'd

SECONDARY LESIONS

Types		Description
Fissure 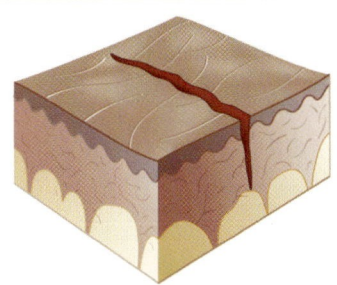	Cheilitis 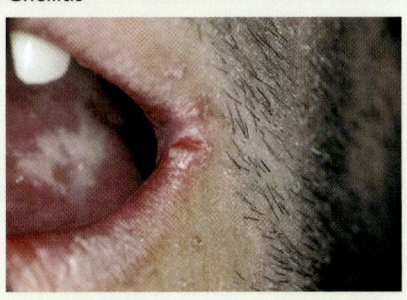	Linear break in the skin ("crack"); may extend to the dermis. Examples: athlete's foot, cheilitis
Ulcer 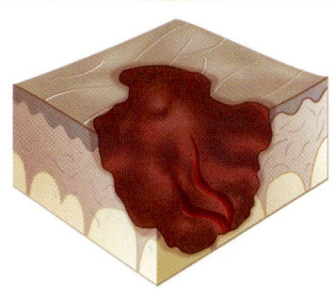	Stasis ulcer 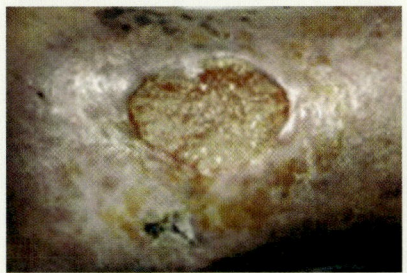	Irregularly shaped with loss of tissue. Graded based on depth and tissue involvement. Examples: pressure ulcers, stasis ulcers
Crust 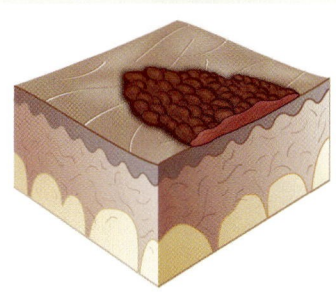	Crust 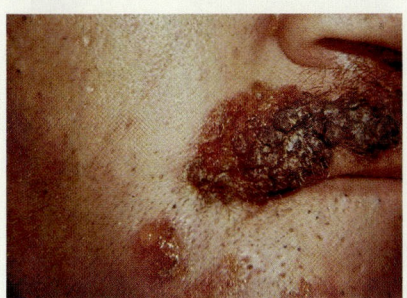	Elevated, rough texture with dried exudate. Examples: impetigo, herpes simplex
Scales 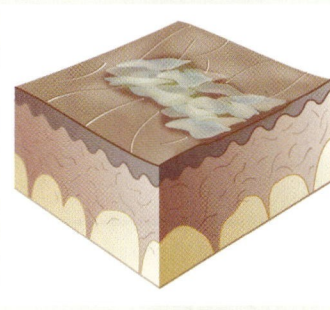	Psoriasis 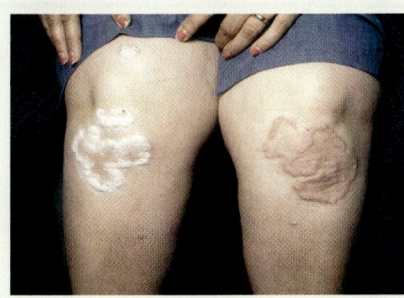	White to tan flaking, dead skin cells; may be adherent or loose. Examples: psoriasis and dandruff

(continued on next page)

Procedure 21–2 ■ **Assessing the Skin** (continued)

Describing Skin Lesions—cont'd		
SECONDARY LESIONS		
Types		**Description**
Scar		Fibrous tissue at site of injury, trauma, or surgery. Examples: surgical site, trauma site
Keloid	Keloids	Raised and irregular scar due to excess collagen formation. Examples: surgical scars, ear piercing

Practice Resources

Yifan Xue (2007).

Procedure 21-3 ■ **Assessing the Hair**

➤ For steps to follow in *all* procedures, refer to the Universal Steps for All Procedures found on the page facing the inside back cover.

Equipment

- Nonlatex procedure gloves (if exposure to body fluids is a possibility)
- Pen and record form

Focused History Questions

- Have you had any changes in hair texture?
- Have you had any hair loss?
- Do you use dyes or chemical treatments for curling or straightening?

➤ When performing the procedure, always identify your patient according to agency policy and be attentive to standard precautions, hand hygiene, patient safety and privacy, body mechanics, and documentation.

Procedure Steps

1. Inspect the hair and scalp. Check the color, quantity, and distribution of the hair and the condition of the scalp. Note the presence of lesions or pediculosis.

Sex, genetics, and age affect hair distribution on the head, legs extremities, pubis, and axillae. With aging, melanocyte function declines and sebaceous gland function decreases.

Expected and Abnormal Findings

Expected findings: The hair is evenly distributed on the scalp, and fine body hair is present over the body. The hair is clean and free of debris or pediculosis.

Developmental Variations

Infants—May have very little scalp hair.

Adolescents—May have oily hair. Puberty marks the onset of pubic hair growth and increased hair growth.

Older adults—Scalp, axillary, leg, and pubic hair may be dry and thin; hair of the ears, nostrils, and eyebrows may become coarse.

Abnormal findings: Generalized hair loss not attributed to genetics or aging; patchy hair loss; **hirsutism** (excess facial or trunk hair). Also,

 Go to Chapter 21, **Tables, Boxes, Figures: ESG Table 21-3, Abnormal Atlas: Hair,** on Davis*Plus*.

2. Palpate the texture of the hair.

Expected findings: Hair texture varies (fine, medium, coarse) depending on genetics and treatments.

Abnormal findings: Very dry, coarse hair; very fine, silky hair

3. Palpate the scalp for mobility and tenderness.

Expected findings: Scalp is smooth, firm, symmetrical, nontender, and without lesions

Abnormal findings: Tenderness, lesions.

Patient Teaching

If indicated, teach the patient to check for head lice, and provide preventive measures.

Documentation

If you need more information about documenting, review Caring for the Nguyens, including the box Documentation of Physical Assessment Findings for Nam Nguyen.

Procedure 21–4 ■ Assessing the Nails

➤ For steps to follow in *all* procedures, refer to the Universal Steps for All Procedures found on the page facing the inside back cover.

Equipment

- Nonlatex gloves (if exposure to body fluids is a possibility)
- Pen and record form

Focused History Questions

- Have you had any recent changes in the way your nails grow or look?
- Have you had any recent trauma to your nails?
- Do you use acrylic nails?
- Do you have any medical problems, such as peripheral vascular disease or diabetes?

(continued on next page)

Procedure 21–4 ■ Assessing the Nails (continued)

> ➤ When performing the procedure, always identify your patient according to agency policy and be attentive to standard precautions, hand hygiene, patient safety and privacy, body mechanics, and documentation.

Procedure Steps

1. Inspect nails.
- Check nails for color, condition, texture, and shape.
- Examine nails on both hands and feet. However, for efficiency you may defer examination of the toenails until the assessment of peripheral circulation.▼

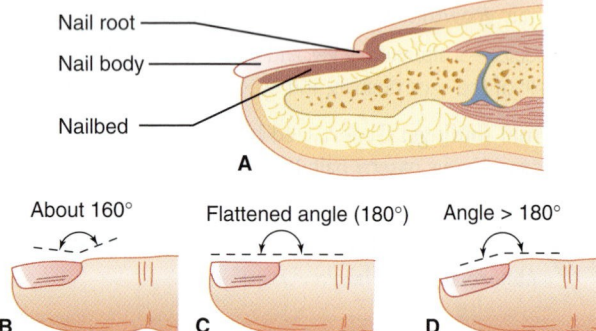

Nail root
Nail body
Nailbed

A

About 160°   Flattened angle (180°)   Angle > 180°

B   **C**   **D**

2. Inspect and palpate for texture.
Grooves or lines in the nails provide information about nutrition and health problems.

3. Assess capillary refill: Briefly press the tip of the nail with firm, steady pressure; then release and observe for changes in color.
This test assesses circulatory adequacy rather than the nails themselves. However, circulatory insufficiency affects the nails and nailbeds. It is convenient to perform the assessment at this point in the exam. ▼

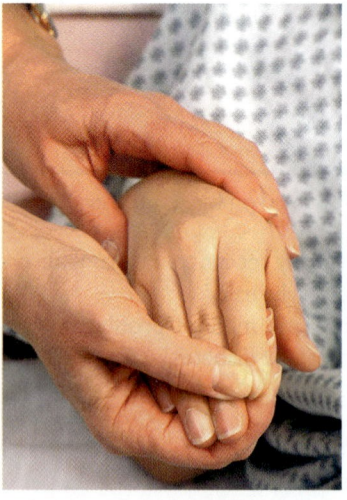

Expected and Abnormal Findings

Expected findings: Healthy nailbeds are level, firm, and similar to the color of the skin. The shape is convex, with a nail plate angle of about 160°.

Developmental Variations

Newborns—Have very thin nails.

Children—May bite their nails. Most children outgrow this habit.

Older adults—Nails grow more slowly, become thicker, and tend to split.

Abnormal findings: Yellow, blue, or black discoloration. White spots may indicate zinc deficiency. Spoon-shaped (concave) nails are associated with iron deficiency.

Expected findings: Nails are smooth and uniform in texture.

Abnormal findings: Thickened, brittle, or soft nails; nails with deep vertical grooves

Expected findings: Normal capillary refill is less than 2 to 3 sec.

Developmental Variations

Older adults—Capillary refill time (CRT) is slower.

Males—CRT faster than in women

Environment—CRT is slower in a cool environment.

Abnormal findings: Delayed capillary refill. Also,

 Go to Chapter 21, **Tables, Boxes, Figures: ESG Table 21-3, Abnormal Atlas: Nail Appearance,** on Davis*Plus.*

Documentation

- If you need more information about documenting, review Caring for the Nguyens, including the box Documentation of Physical Assessment Findings for Nam Nguyen.

Practice Resources

Anderson, Kelly, Kerr, et al., 2008.

Procedure 21–5 ■ Assessing the Head and Face

➤ For steps to follow in *all* procedures, refer to the Universal Steps for All Procedures found on the page facing the inside back cover.

Equipment

- Nonlatex gloves (if exposure to body fluids is a possibility)
- Penlight (to transilluminate the sinuses)
- Pen and record form

Positioning

Preferably, the client should be sitting, if possible.

Focused History Questions

- Have you had any recent headaches?
- Have you ever had a head injury or loss of consciousness?
- Have you ever had a seizure?
- Do you have jaw or facial pain?

➤ When performing the procedure, always identify your patient according to agency policy and be attentive to standard precautions, hand hygiene, patient safety and privacy, body mechanics, and documentation.

Procedure Steps

1. **Inspect the head: Check for size, shape, symmetry, and position.**

Developmental Modifications
Newborns and infants—Assess and transilluminate fontanels, and measure head circumference.

Expected and Abnormal Findings

Expected findings: There is wide variation in head size and shape, although the shape should be symmetrical and rounded. The head should be erect, midline, and proportional to the body size based on age.

Developmental Variations
Newborns and infants—Cranial bones are not fused at birth, and head shape may reflect normal pressure or trauma during vaginal birth for several weeks. The anterior fontanel ("soft spot") fuses at about 18 mo; the posterior, at about 8 wk. Infants normally cannot hold their head up until about 6 mo of age.

Abnormal findings: Larger or smaller than expected size for age, asymmetry of skull

2. **Inspect the face.** Note the client's facial expression. Ask yourself:
   - Are the facial features symmetrical?
   - Are there any abnormal facial movements?
   - Are there any visible lesions or abnormal hair distribution?

Helpful hint: Look for symmetry in the palpebral fissures and the nasolabial folds. ▼

Expected findings: Facial expression is appropriate for the situation. No visible lesions. Facial features and movement are symmetrical.

Abnormal findings: Facial appearance inconsistent with sex, age, or racial/ethnic group; asymmetry of facial features or facial movement ▼

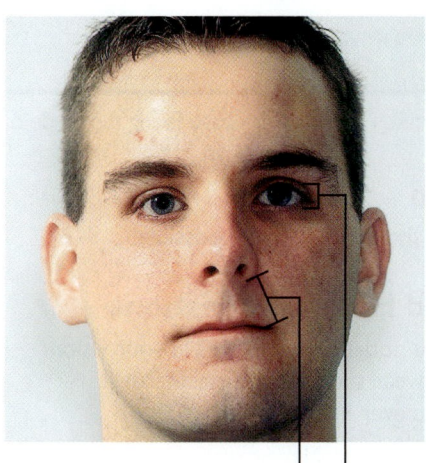

Nasolabial fold
Palpebral fissure

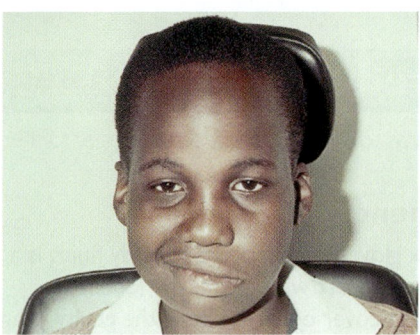

Bell's palsy

(continued on next page)

Procedure 21–5 ■ Assessing the Head and Face (continued)

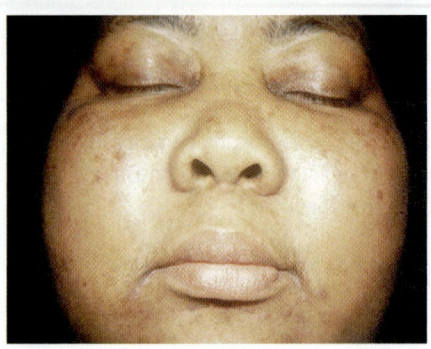

Cushing's syndrome

3. Palpate the head. Check for masses, tenderness, and scalp mobility.

Developmental Modifications
Newborns and infants—Palpate anterior and posterior fontanels.

Expected findings: The head should be relatively smooth, with no tenderness or lesions.

Abnormal findings: Contour abnormalities (e.g., indentations, "bumps")

4. Palpate the face for symmetry, tenderness, muscle tone, and TMJ function. ▼

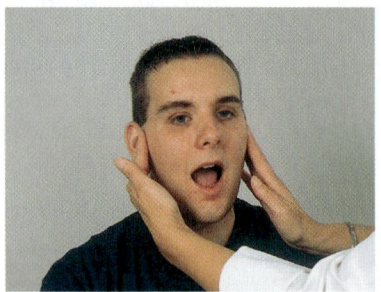

Expected findings: Smooth, symmetrical movement with no pain, crepitus, or clicking of the jaw

Abnormal findings: Irregular or uneven movement of the jaw; pain or popping with movement

Documentation

- If you need more information about documenting, review Caring for the Nguyens, including the box Documentation of Physical Assessment Findings for Nam Nguyen.

Procedure 21–6 ■ Assessing the Eyes

➤ For steps to follow in *all* procedures, refer to the Universal Steps for All Procedures found on the page facing the inside back cover.

Equipment
- Nonlatex gloves—if exposure to body fluids is a possibility
- Visual acuity chart with color bars (Snellen)
- A card—to cover one eye during the acuity exam
- Penlight
- Cotton ball and cotton-tipped applicator
- Ophthalmoscope
- Pen and form

Position
The client should be sitting, if possible.

Focused History Questions
- Have you noticed any changes in your vision?
- Do you wear glasses or contact lenses?
- Have you ever had an eye injury?

- Have you ever had an eye infection or stye?
- Do you have problems with excessive tearing or dry eyes?
- Have you ever had eye surgery?
- Have you ever experienced blurred vision?
- Do you have difficulty with nighttime vision?
- Do you ever see halos of light, spots or floaters, or flashes of light?

- Do you have a history of eye problems, such as glaucoma, or medical problems, such as diabetes or hypertension?
- When was your last eye exam?
- Do you use any prescription or over-the-counter eye medications?

➤ When performing the procedure, always identify your patient according to agency policy and be attentive to standard precautions, hand hygiene, patient safety and privacy, body mechanics, and documentation.

Procedure Steps

1. **Test distance vision.**
   - Depending on patient's age and literacy level, use the Snellen standard eye chart or Snellen E chart (for those who cannot read). Picture charts are available for preschoolers.
   - If the client wears corrective lenses, they should be worn during a test.
     a. Have the patient sit or stand 6 m (20 ft) from the chart. With a card, cover the eye not being tested; ask the patient to read the smallest line of print that he can distinguish. Consider a line to be read correctly if the client makes no more than two mistakes in that line.
     b. Test the opposite eye.
     c. Test both eyes together.
     d. At the end of each line of the Snellen chart is a fraction—the top line is 20/200. After each test, record the resulting fraction: the number at the end of the smallest line the patient could read with no more than two errors. ▼

Expected and Abnormal Findings

Expected findings: Expect 20/20 vision in the right eye, left eye, and both eyes. The top number of the fraction indicates the distance the person was standing from the chart; the bottom number is the distance from which a person with normal vision would be able to read the chart.

Developmental Variations

Children—Distance vision does not reach 20/20 until around age 6 or 7 yr.

Middle adults—At about middle age, the lens of the eye begins to lose some ability to accommodate to near objects.

Abnormal findings: A smaller fraction (e.g., 20/100) indicates diminished distant vision or myopia. A larger fraction (e.g., 20/15) indicates diminished near vision, called hyperopia.

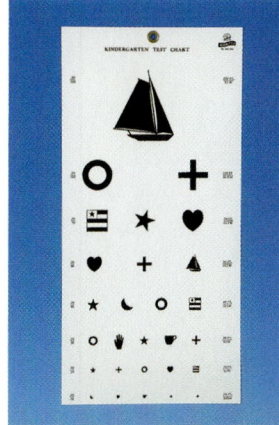
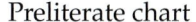

Preliterate chart

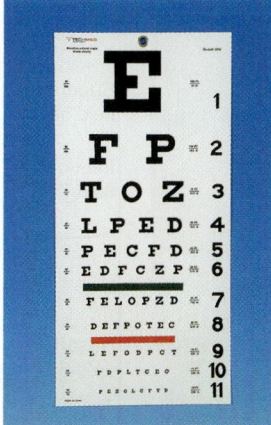

Snellen standard chart

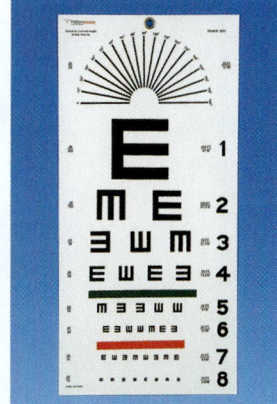

Snellen E chart

2. **Test near vision.** Test the client's ability to read newsprint at a distance of 35.5 cm (14 in.) from the eyes. Use print-sized pictures if the patient is unable to read.

Expected findings: The client reads newsprint at a distance of 35.5 cm (14 in.).

Abnormal findings: The need to hold the print at a greater distance indicates hyperopia or presbyopia.

(continued on next page)

Procedure 21–6 ■ **Assessing the Eyes** (continued)

3. Test color vision.
  a. Have the patient differentiate patterns of colors on color cards or identify the color bars on the Snellen eye chart.
  b. Inability to distinguish colors requires a thorough evaluation using the Ishihara cards to determine the scope of the color deficit. ▼

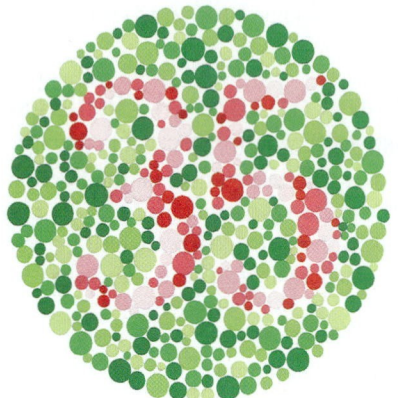

Expected findings: Color vision is intact.

Developmental Variations

Older adults—Experience some decline in color vision, especially in the ability to see purples and pastels.

Abnormal findings: Inability to distinguish colors

---

4. Test peripheral vision.
  a. Seat the client 60–90 cm (2–3 ft) from you.
  b. Have client cover one eye and fix the gaze straight ahead while you bring an object in from the periphery to the center of the visual fields. Be sure to begin by holding the object well outside the range of normal peripheral vision. Instruct the client to identify when the object becomes visible.
  c. Repeat this in each of the four visual fields, moving clockwise

Expected findings: Expect no deficits in the visual fields.

Abnormal findings: Loss of peripheral vision. Report gross deficits to an ophthalmologist for further assessment.▼

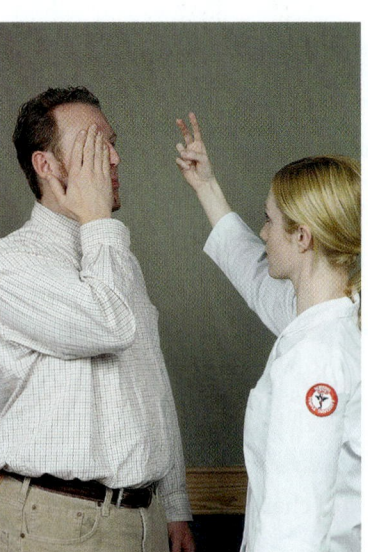

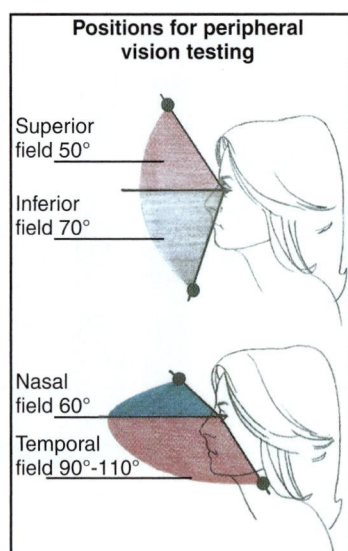

Positions for peripheral vision testing

Superior field 50°

Inferior field 70°

Nasal field 60°

Temporal field 90°-110°

Step 4

5. Assess extraocular movements.

a. Inspect the eyes for parallel alignment.

b. Test the corneal light reflex by shining a penlight at the bridge of the nose. Note where the light reflects on the cornea of each eye.

c. Test the six cardinal fields of gaze. Stand in front of the patient, and have the patient follow an object through the six cardinal fields without moving his head. ▼

a. **Expected findings:** The eyes should be in parallel alignment.

b. **Expected findings:** Corneal light reflex appears at the same position in each eye.

Abnormal findings: An asymmetrical corneal light reflex may indicate weak extraocular muscles or strabismus.

c. **Expected findings:** The eyes move through all six gaze positions.

Abnormal findings: Inability to move through all gaze positions.

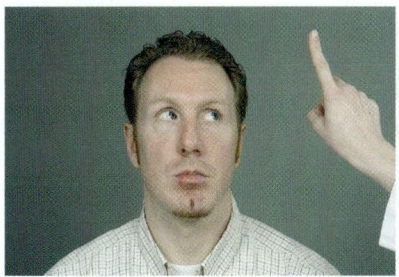

Up left

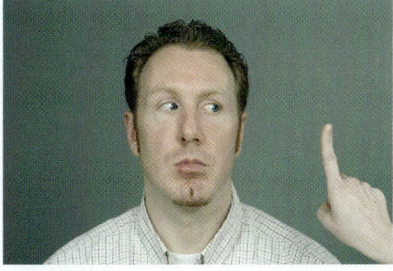

Side left

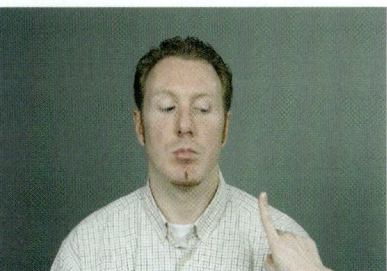

Down left

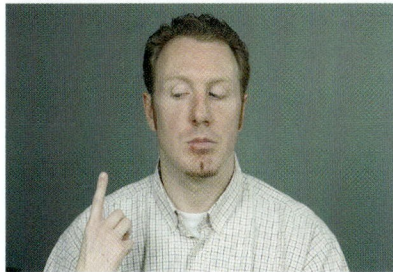

Down right

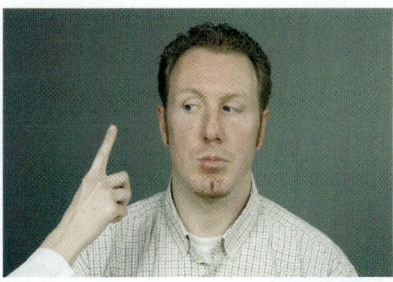

Side right

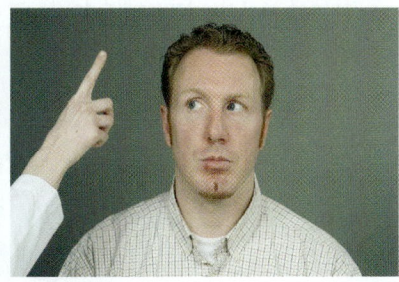

Up right

d. Perform the cover/uncover test. Cover one eye and have the patient gaze at a distant object. Uncover the eye. Repeat on the opposite side.

d. **Expected findings:** The gaze should be steady when the eye is covered and uncovered.

Abnormal findings: A shift in gaze indicates weak eye muscles.

6. Inspect the external structures.

a. **General appearance:** Check the color and alignment of the eyes.

a. **Expected Findings:** Eyes clear, bright, and in parallel alignment.

Developmental Variations

Older adults—A decrease in periorbital fat may give the eyeballs a sunken appearance.

Abnormal findings: Glazed eyes may indicate a febrile state.

b. **Inspect the eyelids.** Note the presence of any lesions, edema, or lid lag.

 Go to Chapter Resources, Chapter 21, **ESG Table 21-3, Abnormal Atlas,** on Davis*Plus*.

b. **Expected Findings:** No lesions present; lids move freely. Upper eyelid covers half of the upper iris.

Developmental Variations

Older adults—The lower lids may sag; skinfolds are prominent in the upper lids.

Abnormal findings: Asymmetry of lids may result from CN III damage or from a stroke. Lesions may be benign (e.g., a stye) or pathological (e.g., basal cell carcinoma).

(continued on next page)

Procedure 21–6 ■ Assessing the Eyes (continued)

c. **Inspect the eyelashes.** Note symmetry and distribution.

c. **Expected findings:** Eyelashes are evenly distributed and curve outward. No crustations or infestations are present.

Abnormal findings: Inflammation of the eyelids, which may be caused by infection; inverted eyelashes (entropion); everted eyelashes (ectropion); visible sclera between the iris and upper lid

d. **Inspect the lacrimal ducts and glands.** Note any edema, excessive tearing, or drainage.

d. **Expected findings:** No periorbital edema or lesions are present. No drainage

Abnormal findings: Swelling, redness, drainage, or tenderness

e. **Inspect the conjunctivae.** Note the color, moisture, and contour of the conjunctivae.
   (1) The palpebral conjunctivae cover the lids. To assess, have the patient look up as you place a cotton-tipped applicator on the upper lid, gently grasp the upper lid and lashes, and evert the lid over the cotton-tipped applicator.
   (2) The bulbar conjunctiva covers the eyeball. To assess, pull the lower lid down. ▼

e. **Expected Findings:** The palpebral conjunctivae are smooth, glistening, and peach in color. Minimal blood vessels are present. The bulbar conjunctivae are clear with few underlying blood vessels and white sclera visible.

Developmental Variations

Older adults—The conjunctivae may be pale or have a slightly yellow tint due to fat deposits.

Abnormal findings: Pallor, dryness, edema; pterygium; subconjunctival hemorrhage

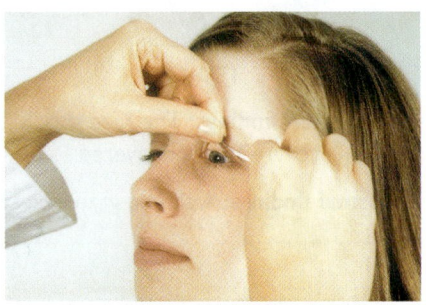

Examining the palpebral conjunctiva.

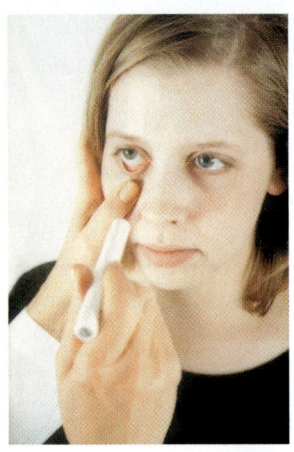

Examining the bulbar conjunctiva

f. **Inspect the sclera.** Note the color of the sclera and whether lesions are present.

f. **Expected Findings:** The sclera should be smooth, white, and glistening. Dark-skinned patients may have a yellowish cast to the peripheral sclera or small brown spots more centrally.

Abnormal findings: Yellow (icteric) sclera

g. **Inspect the cornea and lens.** As the client looks straight ahead, shine a penlight at an angle to the eye, and move it across the corneal surface. Note the color and whether any lesions are present.

g. **Expected Findings:** The cornea and lens are clear, smooth, and glistening.

Developmental Variations

Older adults—Arcus senilis is a normal variant.

Abnormal findings: Lens opacities (cataracts); roughness or irregularity of the cornea

h. **Test the corneal reflex.** Touch the cornea with a wisp of sterile cotton, or use a needleless syringe to shoot a small amount of air over the cornea.

➕ NOTE: *This is not routinely performed on conscious patients. A conscious person can blink intentionally, so there is no need. In addition, there is a slight risk of corneal abrasion from cotton.*

i. **Inspect the iris and pupils.** Note the **color, size, shape, and sym**metry.

j. **Test pupillary reaction.** In a dimly lighted room, have the patient look straight ahead. Bring a penlight in from the side, and shine the light onto one eye. Note the reaction, equality, and speed of response of both eyes. For example, when you shine a light onto the right eye, the right pupil reaction is direct; the left eye is consensual. Repeat the test on the opposite eye. ▼

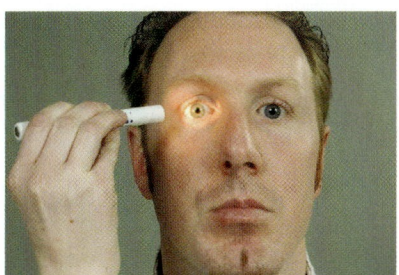

Testing pupillary reaction to light

k. **Test pupil accommodation.** Have the patient look straight ahead and focus on an object about 30 cm (12 in.) from his face. Slowly bring the object in toward the patient's eyes. Note pupil size and location.

l. **Inspect the anterior chamber.** Shine a penlight across the eye from the side as the patient looks straight ahead. Observe color, size, shape, and symmetry.

h. **Expected Findings:** Blink reflex is prompt.

Abnormal findings: Failure to blink may result from neurosensory deficits.

i. **Expected Findings:** The iris is blue, green, brown, or a combination of these colors; its shape is circular. The pupils are round and of equal size. Unequal pupils (anisocoria) can be a normal variation if the difference is less than 0.5 mm.

Developmental Variations

Older adults—Pigment degeneration may cause the iris to be pale with brownish discolorations.

Abnormal findings: Damage to one eye may cause the iris to be a different color. Absence of part or all of the iris is a congenital problem. Unequal pupils may result from CN III damage, brain herniation, or increased intracranial pressure.

j. **Expected Findings:** Normal direct and consensual response to light is brisk, with equal constriction of both pupils.

Developmental Variations

Older adults—Pupil reaction may be slower but should be symmetrical.

Abnormal findings: Sluggish or fixed pupils may result from CN II damage or brain injury. Absence of consensual response may result from nerve compression or anoxia.

k. **Expected Findings:** The pupils constrict and the eyes cross as a person attempts to focus on a near object.

Developmental Variations

Older adults—Accommodation may be slow.

Abnormal findings: One or both pupils fail to accommodate, or they accommodate slowly.

l. **Expected Findings:** The chamber should be clear and symmetrically curved.

Abnormal findings: Blood or pus in the chamber. Also see Abnormal Atlas: Eyes at the end of this chapter.

(continued on next page)

Procedure 21–6 ■ **Assessing the Eyes** (continued)

7. **Palpate the external structures**.
   a. Gently palpate the globe (eyeball) with your fingertips on the upper lids over the sclera. Note the consistency and any tenderness.
   b. Palpate the lacrimal glands and ducts by palpating below the eyebrow and below the inner canthus of the eye. Note tenderness and excessive tearing or discharge. ▼

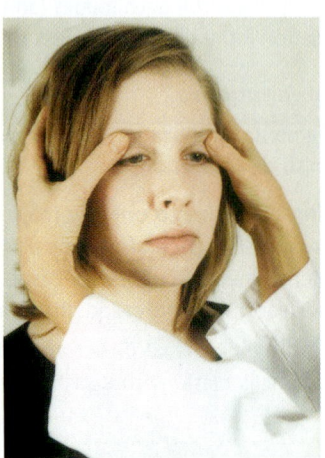

Expected Findings: The globe is firm and nontender. Lacrimal glands are nonpalpable; no tenderness is present.

Abnormal findings: Firm or tender globe; swelling and tenderness over the lacrimal glands. Also,

 Go to Chapter 21, **Tables, Boxes, Figures: ESG Table 21-3,** on Davis*Plus.*

8. **Assess the internal structures via ophthalmoscopy**. This is an advanced physical assessment technique.
   a. Darken the room.
   b. Stand about 1 ft from the patient at a 15° lateral angle.
   c. Dial the lens wheel to zero with your index finger. Hold the ophthalmoscope to your brow.
   d. Have the patient look straight ahead while you shine the light on one pupil and identify the red light reflex. ▼

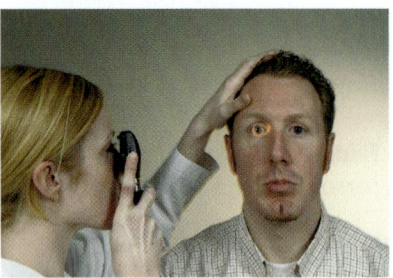

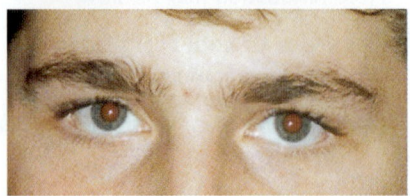

   e. Once you identify the red light reflex, move in closer to within a few inches of the eye and observe the internal structures of the eye. Adjust the lens wheel to focus as

Expected Findings: A positive red light reflex. On internal examination, the optic disk is round with sharp margins. There are no opacities and the cup:disk ratio is 1:2. The disk is yellow with a white cup.

Abnormal findings: Any findings not consistent with the above should be reported promptly.

needed. Use your right eye to examine the patient's right eye, and your left eye to examine the patient's left eye. ▼

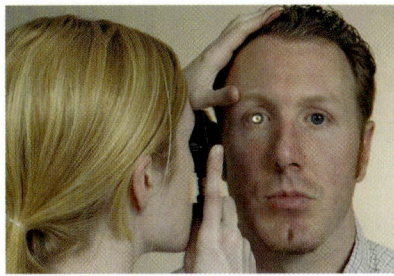

Examining internal structures of the eye

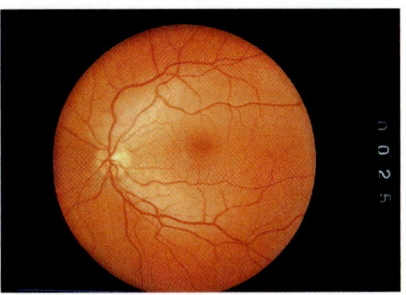

Normal fundus

f. Repeat for the opposite eye.

Patient Teaching

Teach the patient the importance of routine eye examinations.

Documentation

- If you need more information about documenting, review Caring for the Nguyens, including the box Documentation of Physical Assessment Findings for Nam Nguyen

Procedure 21-7 ■ Assessing the Ears and Hearing

➤ For steps to follow in *all* procedures, refer to the Universal Steps for All Procedures found on the page facing the inside back cover.

Equipment

- Nonlatex gloves (if exposure to body fluids is a possibility)
- Tuning fork
- Watch that ticks (or a similar device)
- Otoscope with pneumatic tube
- Pen and record form

Position

Have the patient seated, if possible.

Focused History Questions

- Do you have any hearing problems?
- Have you ever had ringing in your ears?
- Have you had any changes in your hearing?
- Do you have any ear drainage? If yes, how much and what color?
- Do you have any ear pain?
- Do you have any balance problems, dizziness, or vertigo?
- Do you have a history of head trauma?
- Are you exposed to noise pollution at work or in your home environment?

➤ When performing the procedure, always identify your patient according to agency policy and be attentive to standard precautions, hand hygiene, patient safety and privacy, body mechanics, and documentation.

Procedure Steps

1. **Inspect the external ear.**
   a. Check the placement and angle of attachment of the ear. ▼

Expected and Abnormal Findings

a. **Expected findings:** The normal angle of attachment is 10°.

Abnormal findings: High or low placement of the ear may be a sign of hearing deficit or genetic problems.

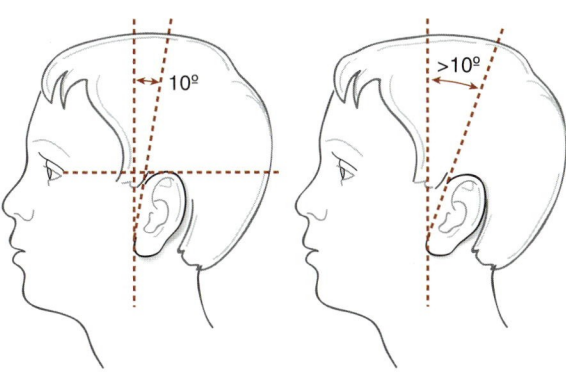

Normal ear attachment   Deviated alignment

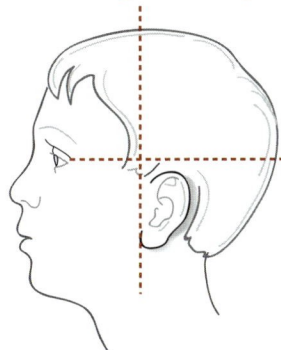

Low-set ear attachment

(continued on next page)

Procedure 21-7 ■ Assessing the Ears and Hearing (continued)

b. Note the shape, size, and symmetry of the ears. ▼

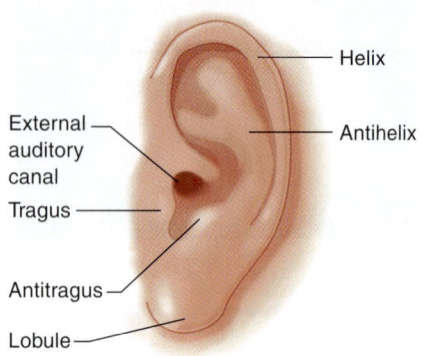

Helix

External auditory canal

Antihelix

Tragus

Antitragus

Lobule

b. **Expected findings:** The helix, antihelix, antitragus, tragus, and lobule are present. The ears are 4–10 cm in length and symmetrical in size and shape.

Developmental Variations

Older adults—The ear changes shape as the lobe elongates.

Abnormal findings: Absence of any of the landmarks may indicate a hearing deficit. Ears that are less than 4 cm long or greater 10 cm long may indicate a genetic disorder.

c. Observe the color of the ear.

c. **Expected Findings:** Color is consistent with skin color.

Abnormal findings: Redness may indicate inflammation or infection.

d. Observe the condition of the skin; observe for drainage and visible lesions.

d. **Expected findings:** Skin is intact with no drainage or lesions. Piercings may be present.

Developmental Variations

Older adults—May have coarse hair on the helix, antihelix, and tragus; skin may be dry.

Abnormal findings: Bloody or purulent drainage; lesions. The ears are a common location for skin cancer.

2. **Palpate the external structures of the ear.** Note the consistency of the skin, the presence of lesions, and any signs of tenderness.

Expected findings: Skin is soft, pliable, and nontender. No nodules or lesions are present.

Abnormal findings: Tenderness is often associated with infection.

3. **Perform an otoscopic exam.**
   This is an advanced physical assessment technique.
   a. Use a speculum with the largest diameter and shortest length that the ear canal can accommodate. 4 mm is a common size for adults.
   b. Have the patient tilt his head to the side not being examined.
   c. For adults, grasp the pinna and gently pull upward and back. For a child, position the pinna down and back.
      It positions the ear canal with more direct alignment, allowing for improved visualization.
   d. Insert the speculum no further than halfway into the ear canal. As you advance the speculum, examine the canal for redness, open areas, drainage, foreign objects, and so on. ▼

3. **Expected findings:** The ear canal is light in color and patent, with a small amount of yellow cerumen (color may vary). Tympanic membrane (TM) is shiny and pearly gray with a cone of reflective light on the nasal aspect that would be 7 o'clock in the left ear and 5 o'clock in the right ear. Bony landmarks are visible. The TM is mobile. No bulging or retraction of the TM. ▼

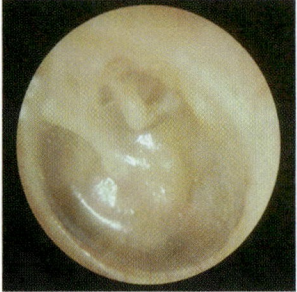

Normal TM left ear

Developmental Variations

Older adults—May have dry earwax. The TM is translucent, and the light reflex may be diminished.

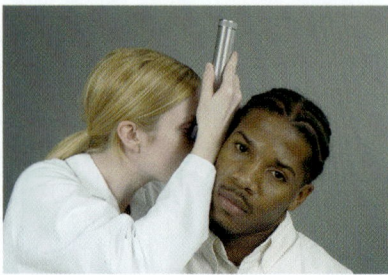

Otoscope insertion with handle up

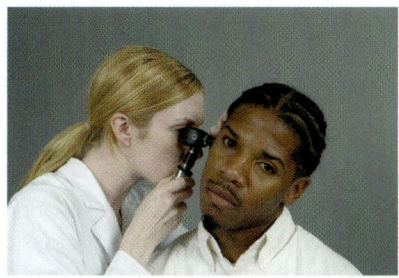

Otoscope insertion with handle down

f. Look through the magnifying lens.
(1) Observe the ear canal.
(2) Observe the TM.
g Test the mobility of the TM by using the otoscope's pneumatic tube to gently "puff" air into the external ear canal while observing movement of the cone of light.

NOTE: The ears are mirror images, with the cone of light at 7 o'clock in the left ear and 5 o'clock in the right ear.

Developmental Modifications

Children—Many young children fear the otoscopic examination. Demonstrating the procedure on a parent or a doll may relieve their anxiety.

h. Carefully remove the otoscope from the ear canal, being careful not to traumatize the delicate tissue.

Abnormal findings: Excessive wax may occlude the canal. TM that is red, with a distorted light reflex, suggests otitis media. A change in the position or shape of the cone of light reflex indicates an imbalance in middle ear pressure. ▼

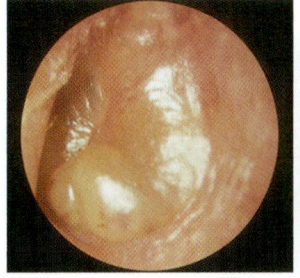

Otitis media

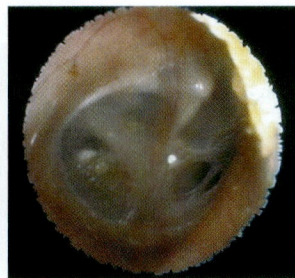

Perforated TM

---

4. **Test gross hearing.**
a. Stand 1–2 ft behind the patient. Have the patient cover one ear as you whisper some words. Repeat on the other side. Have the patient repeat the words she heard.
A test of hearing also indicates cranial nerve XIII is intact.
b. Have the patient occlude one ear. Hold a ticking watch next to the patient's unobstructed ear. Slowly move it away until the patient says she can no longer hear the sound. Repeat for the opposite ear.

Developmental Modifications

Infants—For infants younger than age 3 mo, loudly clap your hands behind the infant and observe whether he startles. After age 3 mo, the infant should turn his head or eyes toward a sound, for example, when the parent stands behind the infant and calls his name.

Expected findings: The patient is able to hear you whisper on both sides. The patient hears the watch at a distance of about 12 to 13 cm (5 in.).

Developmental Variations

Older adults—Often have a generalized loss of hearing. It first occurs in the high-frequency sounds (*f, s, sh,* and *ph*) and then progresses to include all frequencies.

Abnormal findings: Problems with the whisper test indicate low-tone hearing loss. Problems with the watch-tick test indicate a high-pitch deficit.

(continued on next page)

Procedure 21-7 ■ Assessing the Ears and Hearing (continued)

5. Perform the Weber test: Place a vibrating tuning fork on top of the patient's head. Ask the patient whether the sound is the same in both ears or louder in one ear. ▼

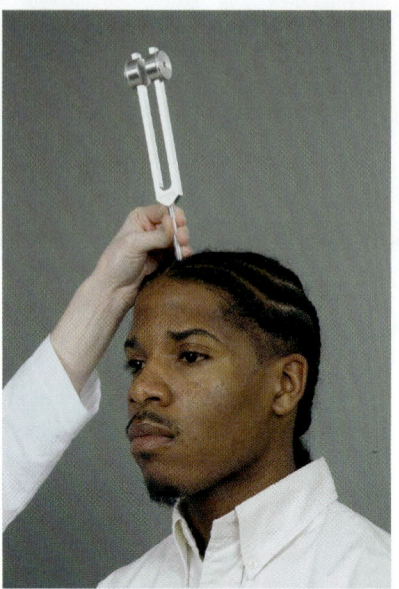

Weber test

Expected findings: The patient hears the sound equally in both ears.

Abnormal findings: Sound is louder in one ear.

- If there is a conductive hearing loss, the vibration will be louder in the impaired ear. Conductive hearing loss may be caused by external or middle ear problems, such as infection, blockage of the canal by cerumen, or trauma to the TM.
- If there is a sensorineural hearing loss, the sound will be louder in the unaffected ear. Sensorineural loss may result from inner ear problems or from some medications.

---

6. If the Weber test is positive: Perform the Rinne test.
   a. Strike a tuning fork on the table. While it is still vibrating, place it on the patient's mastoid process.
      Tests bone conduction of sound.
   b. Measure the elapsed time in seconds that the patient hears the vibration.
   c. Move the tuning fork to 2.5 cm (1 in.) in front of the ear, and measure the elapsed time until the patient can no longer hear the vibration.
      Tests air conduction of sound.
   d. Repeat for the opposite ear. ▼

Expected findings: Normally, sound transmission through air (step 6c) is twice as long as transmission through bone (step 6b); that is, $AC = 2 \times BC$.

The ratio of air conduction (AC) to bone conduction (BC) is similar in both ears.

Abnormal findings:

- Conductive loss: $AC < 2 \times BC$.
- Sensorineural loss: AC is $> BC$ but not $2 \times$ longer; or the patient is unable to hear the tuning fork through BC.
- A difference between ears indicates unilateral hearing loss.
- Inability to hear the tuning fork through BC indicates sensorineural hearing loss.

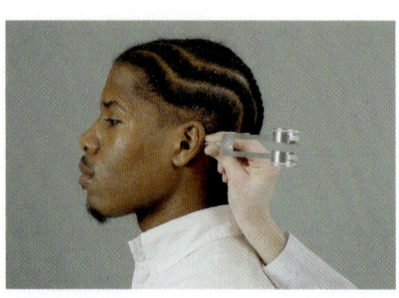

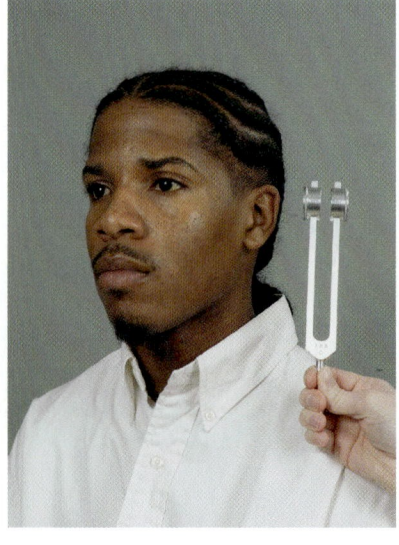

7. **Perform the Romberg test:** Have the patient stand with feet together, hands at side, with eyes opened and then with eyes closed. Note the patient's ability to maintain balance.

✚ Stand nearby in case the client loses his balance.

The Romberg tests for balance. Strictly speaking, it does not assess the ears, but the vestibular nerve and other parts of the central nervous system. Therefore, you may prefer to perform the test during the neurological exam.

Expected findings: The patient maintains balance with minimal sway.

Abnormal findings: Positive Romberg (swaying) is seen with vestibular and cerebellar disorders.

Patient Teaching

Teach the patient the importance of routine hearing examinations.

Documentation

- If you need more information about documenting, review Caring for the Nguyens, including the box Documentation of Physical Assessment Findings for Nam Nguyen.

Procedure 21–8 ■ Assessing the Nose and Sinuses

➤ For steps to follow in *all* procedures, refer to the Universal Steps for All Procedures found on the page facing the inside back cover.

Equipment

- Nonlatex procedure gloves (if exposure to body fluids is a possibility)
- Penlight
- Nasal speculum or otoscope with a wide-tipped speculum
- Pen and record form

Position

Have the patient seated, if possible.

Focused History Questions

- Do you have any nasal congestion?
- Do you have a history of nose or sinus problems?
- Do you have problems with seasonal or environmental allergies?
- Do you have a history of sinus headaches?
- Do you experience nosebleeds (*epistaxis*)?
- Have you ever broken your nose?
- Have you had any changes in your sense of smell?
- Do you use nasal sprays or allergy medications?

➤ When performing the procedure, always identify your patient according to agency policy and be attentive to standard precautions, hand hygiene, patient safety and privacy, body mechanics, and documentation.

Procedure Steps

1. **Position the client for the exam.**

2. **Inspect the external nose.** Note the position, shape, and size. Observe for discharge and flaring.

3. **Check for patency of the nasal passages.** Ask the patient to close his mouth, hold one naris closed, and breathe through the other naris. Repeat with the opposite naris.

Expected and Abnormal Findings

Expected findings: The nose is midline and symmetrical. No discharge or flaring

Abnormal findings: Asymmetry suggests congenital deformity or trauma. Flaring suggests respiratory distress (especially in infants, who cannot breathe through the mouth). Clear drainage suggests allergy; yellow or green drainage suggests upper respiratory infection; bloody drainage may result from trauma, hypertension, or a bleeding disorder.

Expected findings: The client breathes freely through both nares.

(continued on next page)

Procedure 21-8 ■ **Assessing the Nose and Sinuses** (continued)

4. Inspect the internal structures.

   a. Use a nasal speculum or an otoscope with a large speculum (or a penlight with a speculum) to assess the internal structures.

   b. Tilt the patient's head back to facilitate speculum insertion and visualization.

   c. Brace your index finger against the patient's nose as you insert the speculum.

   d. Insert the speculum about 1 cm into the nares. Use the other hand to position the client's head and to hold the penlight if you do not have a lighted scope. ▼

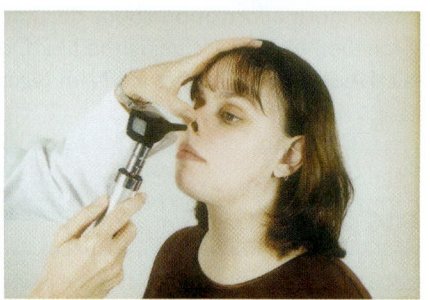

   e. Observe the nasal mucosa for color, edema, lesions, erosion or ulceration, blood, and discharge. Inspect the septum for position and intactness.

   f. Check for sense of smell using commonly recognized objects, such as a lemon or vanilla. Do not use a noxious odor. You can defer this test until the sensorineurological part of the exam if you choose, but keep the same order for every exam.

   Cranial nerve I is intact when the patient shows an ability to detect odor.

Developmental Modifications

Infants and children—You will not need a speculum to examine internal structures. Push the tip of the nose upward with your thumb, and direct a penlight into the nares.

5. Transilluminate the frontal and maxillary sinuses.
First, darken the room.

   a. *Frontal sinuses:* Shine a penlight or the otoscope with speculum below the eyebrow on each side. ▼

Expected findings: Nasal mucosa is pink and moist. Septum is intact and midline. No lesions

Abnormal findings: Deviated septum; polyps. Pale boggy mucosa is seen with allergies; bright red mucosa is associated with rhinitis, sinusitis, and cocaine use. Clustered vesicles suggest herpes infection. Erosion of nasal mucosa should signal you to investigate further for other signs or history of crack/cocaine use. Blood in the nasal passage indicates trauma, nosebleeds, or polyps. ▼

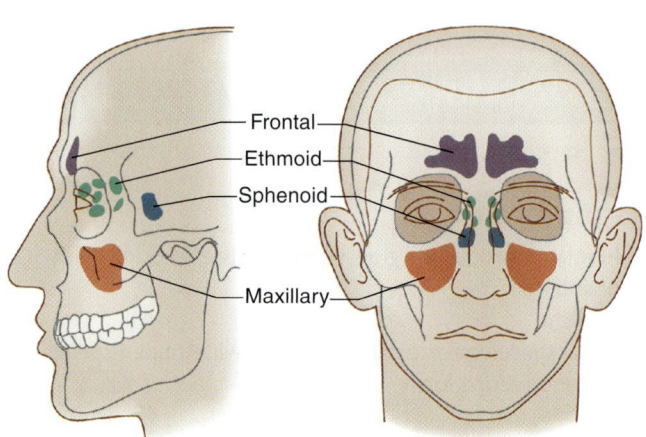

Paranasal sinuses: frontal, ethmoid, sphenoid, and maxillary.

   a. **Expected findings:** A red glow is seen above the eyebrow, indicating that the frontal sinus is patent.

b. *Maxillary sinuses:* Place the light source below the eyes and above the cheeks. Look for a glow of red light at the roof of the mouth through the client's open mouth. ▼

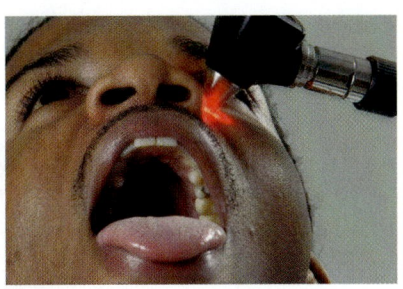

b. A red glow may be (but is not always) seen in the roof of the mouth, indicating that the maxillary sinus is patent.

Abnormal findings: Absence of transillumination may result from mucosal thickening or sinusitis.

---

6. **Palpate the external structures.**

Expected findings: No tenderness, lesions, or deformity

---

7. **Palpate the frontal and maxillary sinuses.**

Expected findings: No tenderness

Abnormal findings: Tenderness may indicate infectious or allergic sinusitis.

Documentation

- If you need more information about documenting, review Caring for the Nguyens, including the box Documentation of Physical Assessment Findings for Nam Nguyen.

Procedure 21–9 ■ Assessing the Mouth and Oropharynx

➤ For steps to follow in *all* procedures, refer to the Universal Steps for All Procedures found on the page facing the inside back cover.

Equipment
- Nonlatex procedure gloves
- Penlight
- Tongue blade
- Small gauze pad
- Pen and record form

Position
Have the patient seated, if possible.

Focused History Questions
- Do you have any problems with your mouth or teeth?
- When was your last dental exam?
- Do you have any discomfort in your mouth or throat?
- Have you had any recent changes in your mouth or teeth?
- How often do you brush your teeth? Floss?
- Do you smoke or chew tobacco?
- Do you have any sores or irritation in your mouth? If so, when did you first notice this?

➤ When performing the procedure, always identify your patient according to agency policy and be attentive to standard precautions, hand hygiene, patient safety and privacy, body mechanics, and documentation.

Procedure Steps
1. **Inspect the mouth externally.** Locate the placement of the lips and their color and condition. Ask the client to purse his lips.

Expected and Abnormal Outcomes
Expected findings: The lips are midline, symmetrical, moist, and intact with no lesions. Coloring is consistent with ethnic group/race. The client can purse his lips.

Abnormal findings: Asymmetry (may be due to congenital deformity, trauma, paralysis, or surgical alteration); pallor; cyanosis; redness; inability to purse lips (may indicate facial nerve damage); lesions (may be caused by bacteria, viruses, or trauma)

(continued on next page)

Procedure 21–9 ■ Assessing the Mouth and Oropharynx (continued)

2. **Note the color and condition of the oral mucosa and gums.**
   a. Don procedure gloves. Inspect and palpate the lower lip. Pull the lower lip away from the teeth, and inspect the inner side of the lip. Palpate any lesions for size, mobility, and tenderness.
   b. Inspect the buccal mucosa, top to bottom and back to front. ▼

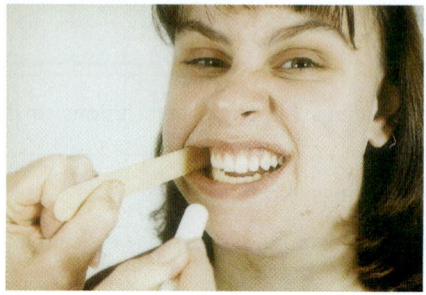

Inspecting the buccal mucosa

   ■ Ask the client to open his mouth. Use a tongue depressor to retract the cheek, then shine a penlight onto the mucosa.
   ■ Using a tongue blade and penlight, inspect the Stensen's duct openings to the parotid glands.
   ■ Finally, palpate inside each cheek by placing a finger inside and thumb outside. Grasping the cheek between them, move the finger about. Repeat on both sides.
   c. As you are inspecting the buccal mucosa, also examine the gums. Check for color, bleeding, edema, retraction, and lesions. Press gum tissue gently with gloved finger or tongue blade to assess firmness.

Expected findings: Oral mucosa is pink, moist, and intact; no lesions. Gingiva is consistent in color with the other mucosae and is intact, with no bleeding. Buccal mucosa is pink and moist, with no lesions. Mucosa is darker in dark-skinned clients. ▼

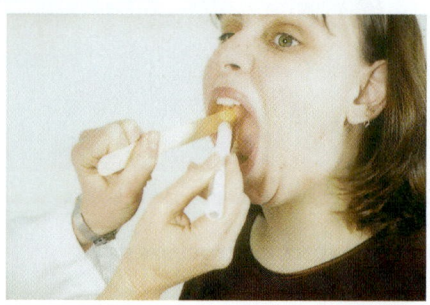

Developmental Variations

Older adults—Mucosa is drier than in young adults because of decreased salivary gland activity; brownish pigmentation of gums may be seen, especially in dark-skinned people.

Abnormal findings: Receding gums, sponginess, bleeding, inflammatory changes, gingival hyperplasia, ulcerations, or other lesions ▼

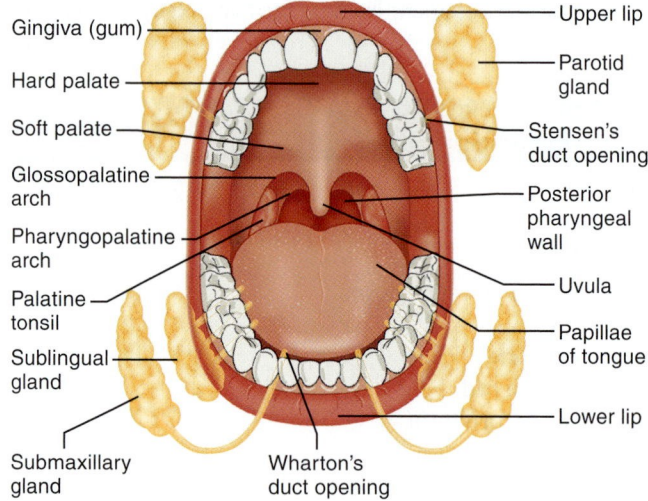

Gingiva (gum)
Hard palate
Soft palate
Glossopalatine arch
Pharyngopalatine arch
Palatine tonsil
Sublingual gland
Submaxillary gland
Wharton's duct opening
Upper lip
Parotid gland
Stensen's duct opening
Posterior pharyngeal wall
Uvula
Papillae of tongue
Lower lip

Structures of the mouth and oropharynx

3. **Inspect the teeth.** You can do this while you are inspecting the oral mucosa and gums, in step
   a. Observe the number, color, and condition of the teeth. Note the occlusion ("bite") and any loose teeth.
   b. If the client wears dentures, ask her to remove them. Inspect for cracked or worn areas; assess the fit. ➤

Expected findings: Most adults have 28 teeth, or 32 if the wisdom teeth have erupted. Children have 20 teeth. The teeth should be white, in good repair, with no caries and good occlusion. The top front teeth should slightly override the lower ones.

Developmental Variations

Older adults—May have receding gums, so teeth appear longer. Teeth may be chipped, eroded, or stained.

Abnormal findings: Missing or poorly anchored teeth, misalignment, and brown or black enamel (indicative of

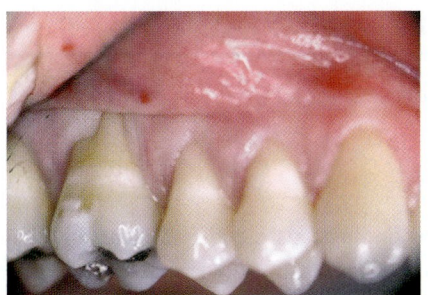

Gingival recession

dental caries or staining, e.g., from taking tetracycline). White spots may indicate excessive fluoride intake.

Also,

 Go to Chapter 21, **Tables, Boxes, Figures: ESG Table 21-3,** on Davis*Plus*.

4. **Inspect the tongue and the floor of the mouth.**
   a. Ask the client to "stick out" his tongue. Examine the upper surface for its color, texture, position, and mobility.
   b. Ask the client to roll his tongue upward and move it side to side.
   c. Have the client place the tip of his tongue on the roof of his mouth, as far back as possible. Using the penlight, inspect the underside of the tongue, the frenulum (which fastens the tongue to the floor of the mouth, in the center), and the floor of the mouth.
   d. Inspect the two Wharton's duct openings to the submaxillary glands, on either side of the frenulum.
   e. Use a tongue blade or gloved finger to move the tongue aside and examine the lateral aspects of the tongue and the floor of the mouth bilaterally. Use caution when placing your finger into the mouth of a noncompliant client. ▼

Expected findings: Tongue is moist, and the coloring is consistent with the client's race. Mucosa has no lesions or discoloration. Papillae are intact. Tongue is midline with full mobility. The base of the tongue is smooth with prominent veins. No tenderness; no palpable nodules. A geographic tongue is a common normal variant.

Developmental Variations

Older adults—May have varicosities under the tongue.

Abnormal findings: Red, smooth, or painful tongue; inflamed mucosa or ducts; tongue that is not midline or has restricted mobility; ulcerations of the tongue or the floor of the mouth (e.g., from trauma, viral infection, or cancerous changes); white plaque or black, hairy tongue (fungal infection)

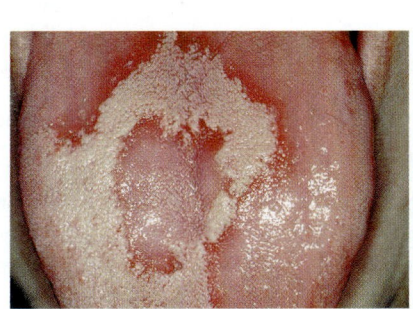

Geographic tongue

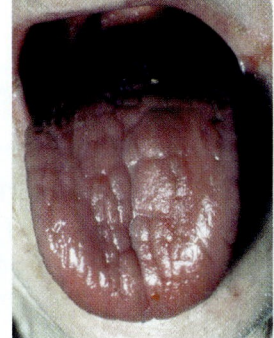

Red, beefy tongue

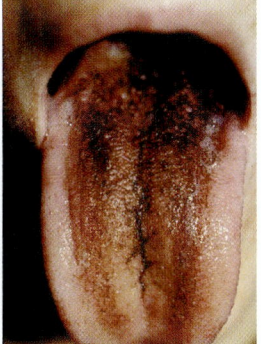

Black, hairy tongue

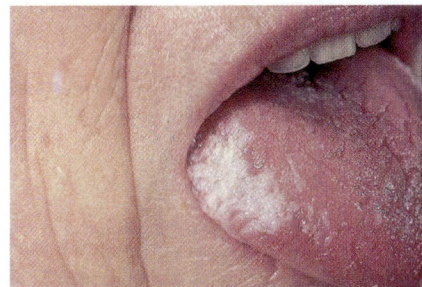

Leukoplakia

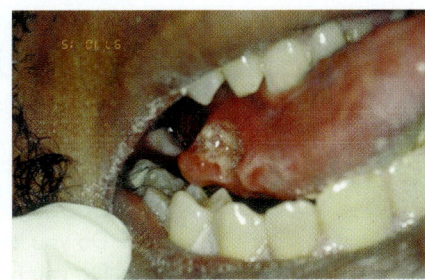

Cancer of the tongue

(continued on next page)

Procedure 21–9 ■ **Assessing the Mouth and Oropharynx** (continued)

5. Palpate the tongue and floor of the mouth. Stabilize the tongue by grasping it with a gauze pad. Palpate top, bottom, and sides with your other index finger.

---

6. Inspect the oropharynx (hard/soft palate, tonsils, and uvula). Note the color, shape, texture, and condition.
   a. Have the client tilt his head back and open his mouth as widely as possible. Depress the tongue with a tongue blade, and shine a penlight on the areas to be inspected.
   b. To inspect the uvula, ask the client to say, "Ah," and watch the uvula as the soft palate rises.
   c. Inspect the oropharynx by depressing one side of the tongue at a time, about halfway back on the tongue.
   d. Note the size and color of the tonsils; note any discharge, redness, swelling, or lesions.
   e. Look and palpate for cleft palate, especially in infants.

Expected findings: Hard and soft palate are pink and smooth. Uvula is midline and rises symmetrically. Tonsils are pink, symmetrical, and without lesions or exudate.

Developmental Variations

Children—Until about age 12, the tonsils may extend beyond the palatine arch.

Abnormal findings: Redness, edema, lesions, plaques, drainage; yellow or greenish streaks on the posterior wall of pharynx (indicate postnasal drainage); tonsils that are red, edematous, or enlarged or have white or pale patches of exudates. Asymmetrical rise of the uvula may indicate a problem with CN IX or X.

---

7. Test the gag reflex by touching the back of the soft palate with a tongue blade.

Expected findings: Positive gag reflex is present.

Developmental Variations

Older adults—May have a slightly slower gag *response.*

Abnormal findings: Absence of a gag reflex is seen with extreme sedation, head injury, or damage to CN IX and X. Inability to articulate the specified words indicates CN XII is not intact.

---

8. Ask the client to repeat the following words: *Light, tight, dynamite.* Again, you may defer this test to the sensorineurological portion of the exam if you choose.

Patient Teaching

Instruct the patient in the importance of dental care and the need for regular checkups.

Documentation

- If you need information about documenting your findings, review Caring for the Nguyens, including the box Documentation of Physical Assessment Findings for Nam Nguyen.

Procedure 21–10 ■ **Assessing the Neck**

➤ For steps to follow in *all* procedures, refer to the Universal Steps for All Procedures found on the page facing the inside back cover.

Equipment

- Stethoscope and antiseptic wipe
- Pen and record form

Position

- Have the client seated, if possible.
- For infants and children, use a supine position.

Focused History Questions

- Do you have any difficulty swallowing?
- Do you have any neck pain or stiffness?
- Do you have any neck masses or lumps?
- Do you have any history of thyroid disease?
- Do you have any difficulty swallowing?

➤ When performing the procedure, always identify your patient according to agency policy and be attentive to standard precautions, hand hygiene, patient safety and privacy, body mechanics, and documentation.

Procedure Steps

1. **Inspect the neck.** Note symmetry, ROM, and the condition of the skin.
   a. Inspect the neck in a neutral position.
   b. Inspect the neck when it is hyperextended.
   c. Inspect the neck when the patient swallows water.

2. **Palpate the cervical lymph nodes.** Note the size, shape, symmetry, consistency, mobility, tenderness, and temperature of any palpable nodes.
   a. Use light palpation with one or two fingerpads in a circular movement.
   b. Palpate the cervical nodes in the following order:
      (1) *Preauricular*—in front of the ear
      (2) *Posterior auricular*—behind the ear
      (3) *Tonsilar*—at the angle of the jaw
      (4) *Submandibular*—halfway up the lower jaw
      (5) *Submental*—under the tip of the chin
      (6) *Occipital*—at the base of the skull in the occipital area
      (7) *Superficial cervical*—below the tonsilar node over the sternocleidomastoid muscle
      (8) *Deep cervical*—under the sternocleidomastoid muscle
      (9) *Posterior cervical*—in posterior triangle along trapezius muscle
      (10) *Supraclavicular*—above the clavicle
   c. Use the same sequence every time so that the steps will become automatic and you will not omit any area.

3. **Palpate the thyroid.**

To use the posterior approach:
   a. Stand behind the client, and ask her to flex her neck slightly forward and to the left.
   b. Position your thumbs on the nape of the client's neck.
   c. Using the fingers of your left hand, locate the cricoid cartilage, which is located below the thyroid cartilage. Push the trachea slightly to the left with your right hand as you palpate just below the cricoid cartilage and between the trachea and sternocleidomastoid muscle.▼

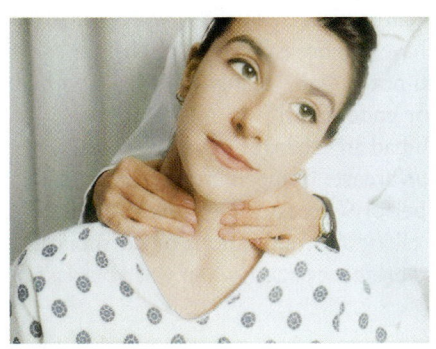

Expected and Abnormal Findings

Expected findings: Neck is erect, midline, and symmetrical with full ROM. No masses are present; skin is intact. Larynx and trachea rise with swallowing. Thyroid is not visible.

Abnormal findings: Swollen lymph nodes may be visible. An enlarged thyroid may be visible in the lower half of the neck.

Expected findings: Lymph nodes are supple and nontender; no masses are palpable. ▼

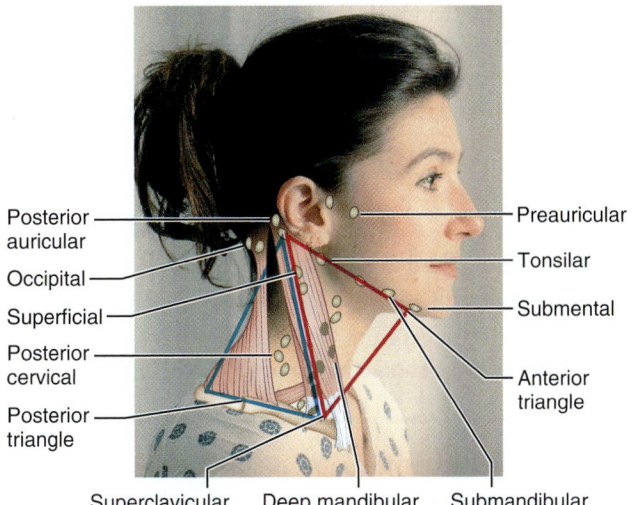

Abnormal findings: Lymphadenopathy (palpable nodes 1 cm or greater). Immobile nodes may indicate malignancy, inflammation, or infection in the area they drain.

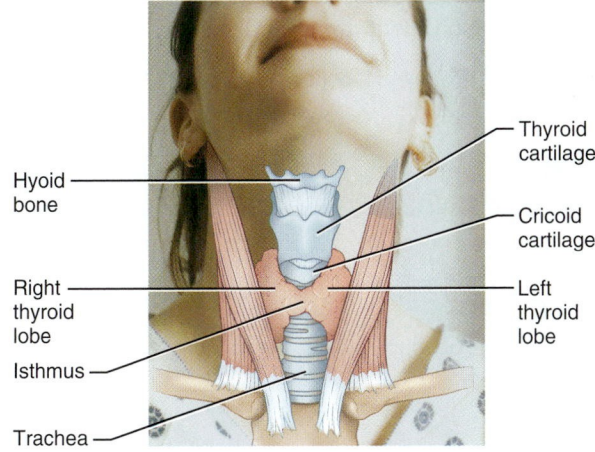

(continued on next page)

Procedure 21–10 ■ **Assessing the Neck** (continued)

d. Ask your client to swallow (give her small sips of water if necessary), and feel for the thyroid gland as it rises up.

e. Reverse and repeat the same steps to palpate the tright thyroid lobe (use the fingers of your left hand to displace the trachea to the right, while using the fingers of your right hand to palpate the thyroid to the right of the trachea).

To use the anterior approach:

f. Stand in front of the client, and ask her to flex her neck slightly forward and in the direction you intend to palpate.

g. Place your hands on the neck, and apply gentle pressure to one side of the trachea while palpating the opposite side of the neck for the thyroid as the client swallows.

h. Reverse and repeat the same steps on the opposite side.

Expected findings: The thyroid is generally nonpalpable. If some tissue is palpable, the consistency is firm and smooth. There is no nodularity, enlargement, or tenderness.

Abnormal findings: An enlarged thyroid may signify a tumor or goiter. A tender thyroid is associated with inflammation.

? **What if . . .**

■ **The thyroid gland is enlarged or there is a mass?**

Auscultate the thyroid for bruits using the bell portion of the stethoscope. Ask the client to hold her breath as you auscultate. There should be no bruits.

Patient Teaching

Teach the patient how to perform a "neck check"—self-check the thyroid with a glass of water and a handheld mirror. Tell the patient, "Hold the mirror in your hand and focus on your neck just below the Adam's apple and above your collarbone. Tip your head back, take a drink of water, and swallow. As you swallow look at your neck. Check for any bulges in this area as you swallow." To download neck check instructions, and for more information about thyroid health,

 Go to http://thyroid.about.com/

Documentation

■ If you need information about documenting your findings, review Caring for the Nguyens, including the box Documentation of Physical Assessment Findings for Nam Nguyen.

Procedure 21–11 ■ **Assessing the Breasts and Axillae**

➤ For steps to follow in *all* procedures, refer to the Universal Steps for All Procedures found on the page facing the inside back cover.

Equipment

■ Nonlatex procedure gloves, if exposure to body fluids is possible
■ Glass slide
■ Culturette
■ Pen and record form

Positioning

The patient must assume several positions during breast examination (see step 1).

Focused History Questions

■ Do you have a lump or thickening in your underarm or breasts that persists throughout your menstrual cycle?
■ Do you have any breast pain or discharge?
■ Have you noticed any changes in the skin on your breasts, nipples, or underarms?
■ Have you had any changes in your nipples?
■ Have your breasts changed in size, shape, or contour?
■ Do you perform breast self-examination (BSE)?
■ Are you taking any medications or hormones?
■ If you are premenopausal, when was your last period?

➤ When performing the procedure, always identify your patient according to agency policy and be attentive to standard precautions, hand hygiene, patient safety and privacy, body mechanics, and documentation.

Procedure Steps

1. **Inspect the breasts.** Note size, shape, symmetry, and color. Inspect with the client in each of the following positions:
   a. Sitting or standing with arms at her side
   b. Sitting or standing with arms raised slightly but not over her head
      Aids in detecting dimpling or retraction of breast tissue
   c. Seated or standing with her hands pressed on her hips
      Aids in detecting dimpling or retraction of breast tissue
   d. With the client leaning forward
      Helpful when examining large, pendulous breasts
   e. With the client supine with a pillow under the shoulder of the breast being examined
      Helps spread the breast tissue over the chest wall

Expected and Abnormal Findings

Expected findings: The breasts are symmetrical; however, the dominant side may be more developed, resulting in a slightly asymmetrical appearance. Skin color is lighter than exposed areas, and there are no lesions, redness, or edema. Texture is smooth, with no dimpling or retraction. Striae are a normal variation.

Developmental Variations

Newborns—You may see breast enlargement and watery, white discharge from the nipples during the first 2 wk of life.

Children—Breasts typically begin to develop at about age 13 yr; the breasts may not develop at equal rates.

Pregnancy—Breast size increases; areolae and nipples darken; superficial veins become prominent; stretch marks may be present; colostrum (a thick, yellow precursor to breast milk) can sometimes be expressed as early as the second trimester.

Older adults—Breasts lose firmness and become flaccid and pendulous.

Abnormal findings:

- Asymmetry warrants further investigation.
- Swelling or erythema may be seen in infection (mastitis).
- **Peau d'orange** (dimpled skin texture) skin changes may be seen with lymphatic obstruction that is present in some forms of breast cancer.
- Puckering, lesions, and retraction may also be seen with breast cancer.
- **Gynecomastia** (enlargement of breasts in males) may indicate hormone imbalance.

2. **Inspect the nipples and areolae.** Note color, shape, and symmetry. Observe for any discharge.

Expected findings: The areolae and nipples are darker in color than breast tissue. Nipples are everted and point in the same direction. No discharge is present, except in newborns and during pregnancy and lactation. No lesions or erosion is present.

Abnormal findings:

- Nipple discoloration that is not associated with pregnancy
- Nipples pointing in different directions. Such findings warrant follow-up as a potential sign of an underlying mass.
- Flat or inverted nipples, which are caused by shortening of the mammary ducts. May make breastfeeding difficult.
- Any nipple discharge not associated with newborns, pregnancy, or breastfeeding requires a thorough evaluation
- Cracks and nipple redness, which may occur with breastfeeding

(continued on next page)

Procedure 21–11 ■ Assessing the Breasts and Axillae (continued)

3. Inspect the axillae. Note the color, condition of the skin, and hair distribution.

Expected findings: Skin is intact with no lesions or rashes. Presence of hair depends on the age of the client and personal preference. Axillary hair develops with puberty. Some women may choose to shave the hair, whereas others will allow it to grow.

Abnormal findings: Rashes, redness, or unusual pigmentation may indicate infection or allergy to deodorants. Dark-pigmented, velvety skin may be seen with *acanthous nigricans,* a condition associated with obesity and type 2 diabetes mellitus.

4. Palpate the breasts, wearing procedure gloves if necessary. Using the fingerpads of your three middle fingers, make small circles with light, medium, and deep pressure. Begin at an imaginary line drawn straight down the side from the underarm; move across the breast to the middle of the sternum. Check the entire breast area, moving down until you feel only ribs and up to the clavicle. Follow one of the following three patterns (evidence suggests the vertical strip method is best).

a. *Vertical strip method:* Start at the sternal edge, and palpate the breast in parallel lines until you reach the midaxillary line. Go up one area and down the adjacent strip (like "mowing the grass"). ▼

Expected findings: Breasts are soft and nontender with no lesions or masses. Consistency depends on age; premenopausal women have firm and elastic tissue, whereas postmenopausal women have softer tissue that may be stringy or cordlike.

Abnormal findings: Breast lumps or masses may be benign or malignant and require follow-up.

Technique Hints
- Do not remove your fingers from the skin surface once you have begun palpating. Move from area to area by sliding the fingers along the skin.
- Most breast lesions in women are found in the upper outer quadrant.
- Most breast cancer in men occurs in the areola.

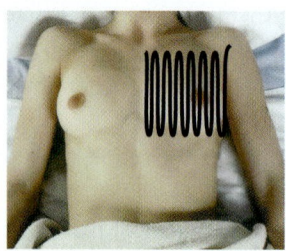

Vertical strip method

b. *Pie wedge method:* This method examines the breast in wedges. Move from one wedge to the next. ➤

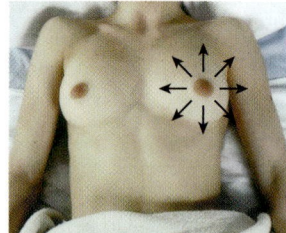

Pie wedge method

c. *Concentric circles method:* Start at the outermost area of the breast at the 12 o'clock position. Move clockwise in concentric, ever smaller, circles. ➤

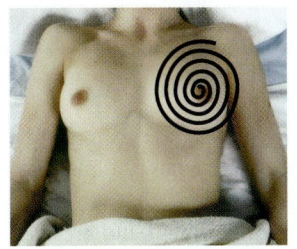

Concentric circle method

---

5. Palpate the nipples and areolae.
   a. If the woman is supine, place a small pillow or folded towel under the shoulder of the breast you are examining.
   b. Squeeze the nipple gently between your thumb and finger to check for discharge.
   c. Note tissue elasticity and tenderness.

Expected findings: Nipples are elastic and nontender. No discharge is present.

Abnormal findings: Loss of elasticity may indicate underlying malignancy. Bloody, purulent discharge may indicate infection. Other forms of drainage may indicate malignancy. Nipple tenderness is normal when establishing breastfeeding.

---

6. Palpate the axillae and clavicular lymph nodes.
   a. Have the woman sitting with her arms at her sides or supine.
   b. Using your fingerpads, move your fingers in circular fashion.
   - *Central nodes:* located high in the midaxillary region
   - *Anterior pectoral nodes:* located on the lower border of the pectoralis major in the anterior axillary fold
   - *Lateral brachial nodes:* located high in the axilla on the inner aspect of the humerus
   - *Posterior subscapular nodes:* located high in the axilla on the lateral scapular border
   - *Epitrochlear nodes:* located above the elbow
   - *Infraclavicular nodes:* located below the clavicle
   - *Supraclavicular nodes:* located above the clavicle

Expected findings: Nodes are nonpalpable.

Abnormal findings: Palpable nodes may be seen with infection or malignancy. Enlarged lymph nodes caused by infection are tender. ▼

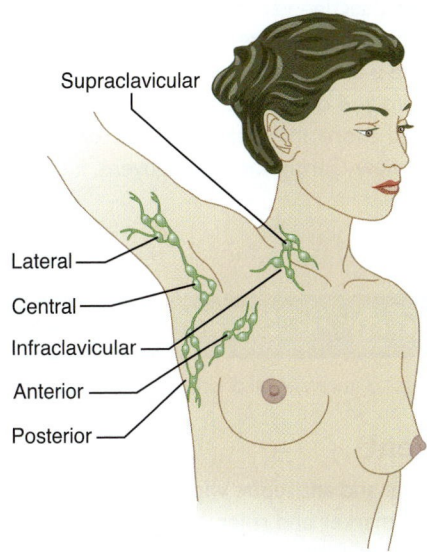

Location of normal lymph nodes

? What if . . .

- **There is a nipple discharge?**

If there is nipple discharge in a woman who is not pregnant or breastfeeding, obtain a specimen by placing a glass slide up to the breast to capture a drop of discharge. Transport the slide to the laboratory as soon as possible. If there is ample discharge, obtain a swab of the discharge with a culturette.

Procedure 21–11 ■ Assessing the Breasts and Axillae (continued)

Patient Teaching

Instruct the patient in BSE and recommendations for mammograms and clinical breast examinations. The American Cancer Society (2010) recommends that women ages 40 and older have a screening mammogram and a clinical breast examination (CBE) every year (other guidelines recommend every 2 years); and that women ages 20 to 30 have a CBE every 3 years. They advise that a monthly BSE is optional. Stress that BSE does not replace the need for mammograms and CBE. This issue remains controversial. There is evidence that BSE does not decrease the death rate from breast cancer; but there is also evidence that BSE, done correctly, does help women to reduce their individual risk and find cancer at earlier stages, when cure rates are higher. BSE is recommended by certain medical groups, such as ACOG (2009a), but not by the U.S. Preventive Services Task Force.

Documentation

- If you palpate a mass or lump, document its size, shape, symmetry, mobility, tenderness, and skin color changes. To ➤ document the location, divide the breast into four quadrants by intersecting vertical and horizontal lines. With the nipple as the center, locate the mass or lump as though the breast were a clock; state the distance in centimeters from the nipple (e.g., 4 o'clock, 2.5 cm from nipple).
- If you need more information about documenting your findings, review Caring for the Nguyens, including the box

Documentation of Physical Assessment Findings for Nam Nguyen.

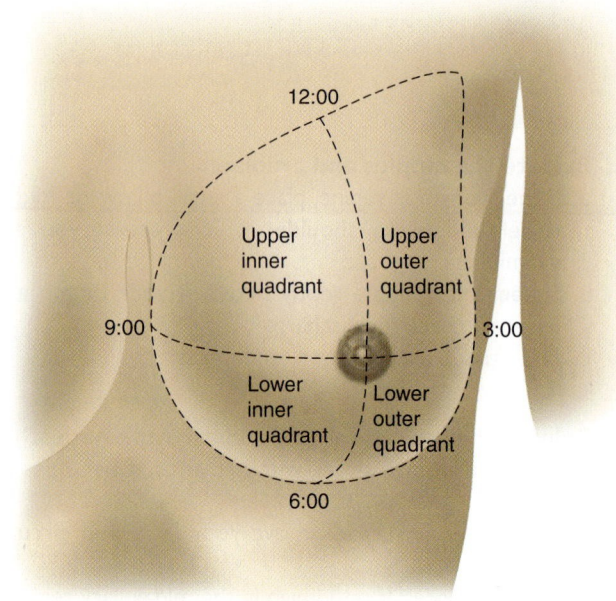

Practice Resources

ACOG, 2010a; American Cancer Society, 2010; Green, & Taplin, 2003; Hackshaw, & Paul, 2003.

Procedure 21–12 ■ Assessing the Chest and Lungs

➤ For steps to follow in *all* procedures, refer to the Universal Steps for All Procedures found on the page facing the inside back cover.

Equipment

- Stethoscope and antiseptic wipe
- Felt-tipped marker and ruler
- Pen and record form

Position

- Have the client sitting, if possible, and leaning forward for the posterior approach.
  If the client is unable to sit up, findings will be distorted.
- If the client is lying down, findings are more evident on the dependent side; help her change positions so that you can assess with each side dependent.

Focused History Questions

- Do you have fatigue or activity intolerance?
- Do you have any current respiratory problems?
- Have you had any recent respiratory problems?
- Do you have a cough?
- Do you have any difficulty breathing?
- What, if anything, causes you to be short of breath?
- Have you had any chest pain?
- Do you have a history of allergies or asthma?
- Do you smoke? If so, how much and for how long?
- If you smoke, have you tried to quit? Would you like to quit?
- Are you exposed to air pollutants at home or at work?

➤ When performing the procedure, always identify your patient according to agency policy and be attentive to standard precautions, hand hygiene, patient safety and privacy, body mechanics, and documentation.

Procedure Steps

1. **Count the respiratory rate, and observe the rhythm and depth; observe the symmetry of chest and respiratory movements.** (See Chapter 19 if you need more information about counting respirations.)

Expected and Abnormal Findings

Expected findings:

- Respirations are quiet with a regular rhythm and depth.
- Chest movement is symmetrical.
- Respiratory rate is 12–20 breaths/min for adults.

Developmental Variations

Infants and children—The normal respiratory rate varies by age. A newborn may have a respiratory rate of 40–90 breaths/min. The rate gradually declines as the child matures. Newborns breathe abdominally, so you will see little chest movement.

Older adults—Rate changes very little; however, respirations decrease in depth as muscles become weakened.

Abnormal findings:

- Chest asymmetry may be seen with musculoskeletal disorders of the spine, such as kyphosis or scoliosis.
- Asymmetrical chest movement during breathing is seen in rib fractures, pneumothorax, and atelectasis; affected chest area may not move at all with respiration.
- Sternal and intercostal retractions are seen with hypoxia, respiratory distress, and airway obstruction.
- Respiratory rate may be increased with activity, smoking, fever, pain, or anemia.

2. **Inspect the chest.**
   a. Inspect the anteroposterior (AP): lateral ratio. ▼

a. **Expected findings:** The normal adult AP: lateral ratio is 1:2.

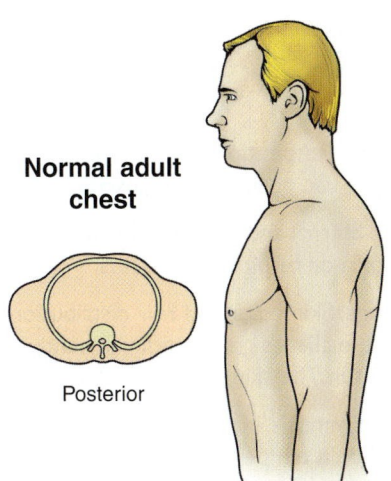

Normal adult chest

Posterior

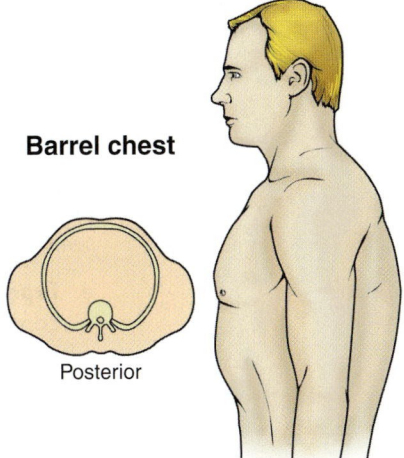

Barrel chest

Posterior

Developmental Variations

Infants—AP is equal to the lateral diameter

Older adults—Kyphosis, osteoporosis, and COPD change the size and shape of the chest; weakening thoracic and diaphragm muscles allow the chest to widen and become more barrel shaped.

Abnormal findings: AP:lateral ratio is increased dramatically in COPD (barrel chest).

(continued on next page)

Procedure 21–12 ■ Assessing the Chest and Lungs (continued)

b. Inspect the costal angle. ▼

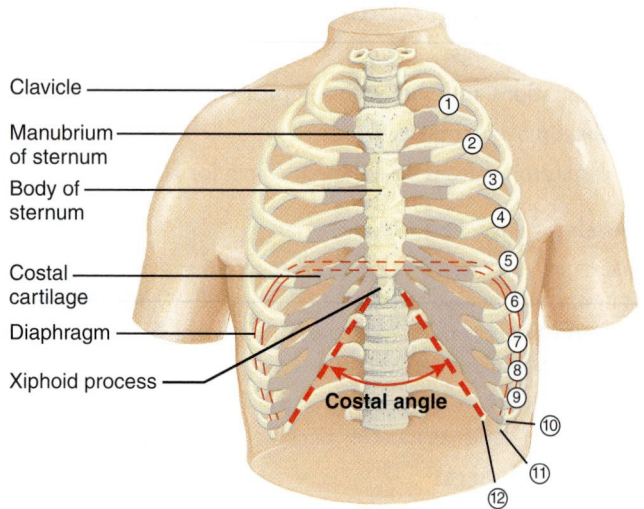

Clavicle

Manubrium of sternum

Body of sternum

Costal cartilage

Diaphragm

Xiphoid process

Costal angle

① ② ③ ④ ⑤ ⑥ ⑦ ⑧ ⑨ ⑩ ⑪ ⑫

c. Identify any spinal deformities.

d. Observe the effort required to breathe.

e. Note the color and condition of skin.

b. **Expected findings:** The costal angle is < 90°.

Abnormal findings: Costal angle is > 90° in COPD.

c. **Expected findings:** The spine is straight without lateral curvatures or deformity.

Abnormal findings: Scoliosis is a lateral curvature of the spine. Kyphosis is excessive thoracic curvature. ▼

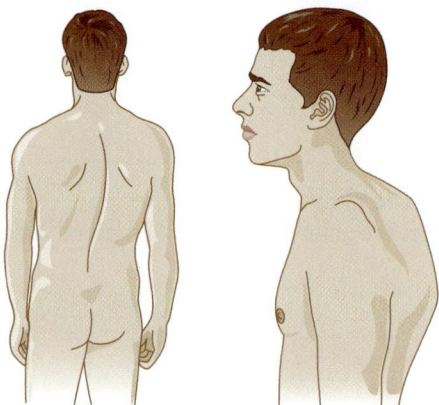

d. **Expected findings:** Respirations appear effortless. There is no retraction or use of accessory muscles.

Abnormal findings: Sternal and intercostal retractions are seen in severe hypoxia or respiratory distress.

e. **Expected findings:** Skin color and hair distribution are consistent with the client's gender, ethnicity, and exposure to the sun. The skin is intact with no scars.

Abnormal findings: Cyanosis of the chest wall (due to extreme hypoxia or cold temperature).

3. **Palpate the trachea.** Place your fingers and thumb on either side of the trachea and note its position. (In a comprehensive exam, you may have already done this with the neck examination.)

Expected findings: Trachea is in the midline.

Abnormal findings: Tracheal deviation may occur from a mass in the neck (e.g., thyroid enlargement) or from excess pressure in the lungs (e.g., tension pneumothorax).

Developmental Modifications

Infants—Neck is short, so it may not be possible to palpate the trachea.

4. Palpate the chest.
- Observe for tenderness, masses, or **crepitus** (crackling skin due to air in the subcutaneous tissue).
- Palpate the anterior, posterior, and lateral chest by placing your hands on the chest wall.

Expected findings: The chest is nontender. No masses or crepitus is present.

Abnormal findings: Pain in the chest wall may be due to fracture, inflammation, or trauma. Crepitus results from air leaking into the subcutaneous tissue. It is most likely to occur around wounds, central IV line sites, chest tubes, or a tracheostomy.

---

5. Palpate chest excursion (expandability).
a. Place your hands at the base of the client's chest with fingers spread and thumbs about 5 cm (2 in.) apart (at the costal margin anteriorly and at the 8th to 10th rib posteriorly).
b. Press your thumbs toward the client's spine to create a small skinfold between them.
c. Have the client take a deep breath, and feel for chest expansion. This may be performed on the anterior or posterior portion of the chest, or both. ▼

Expected findings: Chest excursion is symmetrical on the anterior and posterior aspect of the chest (you should feel equal pressure on your hands; thumbs should move apart equal distances).

Abnormal findings: Limited chest excursion may occur with shallow breathing, restrictive clothing, or restrictive airway disease. Asymmetrical excursion may result from airway obstruction, pleural effusion, or pneumothorax.

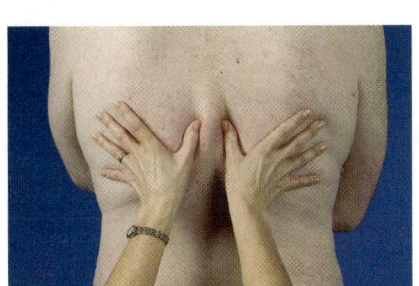

---

6. Follow the same pattern and sequence for palpating fremitus, percussing, and auscultating the chest. See the accompanying diagram. ▼

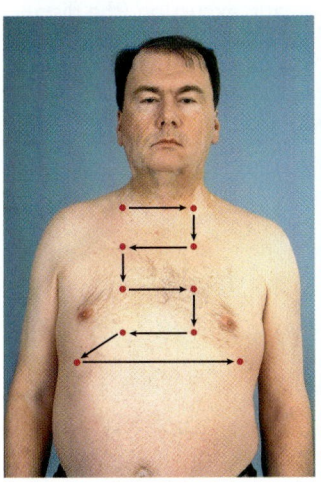 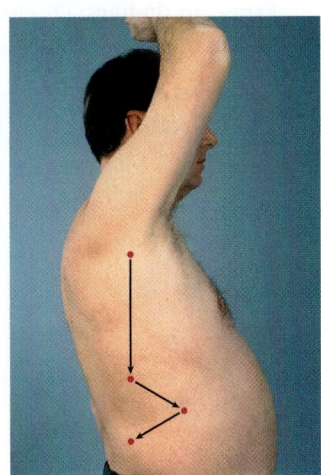 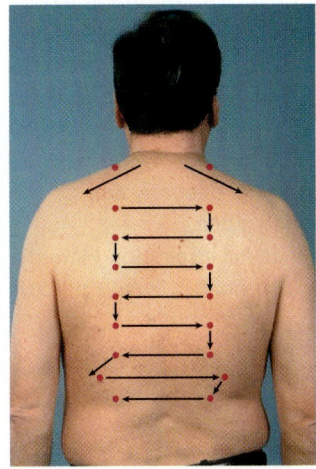

Percussion and auscultation sites

---

7. Palpate the chest for tactile fremitus.
a. Use the palmar surface of your hands, but raise the fingers off the client's chest so that you palpate with the bony metacarpophalangeal joints of your hands.
Bony prominences are best for detecting vibrations.

Expected findings: Tactile fremitus is equal bilaterally on the anterior and posterior chest; it is diminished at midthorax. Fremitus is normally diminished if the chest wall is very thick or the voice very soft.

(continued on next page)

Procedure 21-12 ■ Assessing the Chest and Lungs (continued)

b. Palpate for vibrations as the client says, "Ninety-nine." ▼

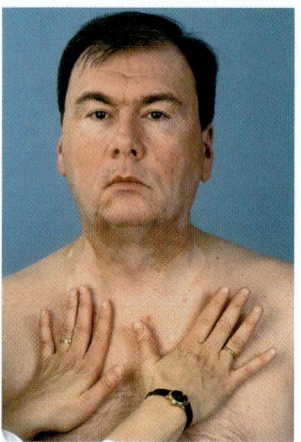

Developmental Modifications

Infants—Place your hand over the chest while the infant is crying.

Developmental Variations

Children and thin adults—May have increased fremitus.

Abnormal findings: Increased fremitus occurs with conditions that cause fluid in the lungs (e.g., pulmonary edema). Decreased or absent fremitus occurs when there is decreased air movement or tissue consolidation (e.g., emphysema, asthma).

---

8. Percuss the chest.

a. Percuss over the intercostal spaces rather than over the ribs.
   Percussion over bone produces less resonance.

b. Use the indirect percussion method on the anterior, posterior, and lateral chest, following the diagram in step 6. Compare the right side to the left side.

Expected findings:

- The anterior chest is resonant to the 2nd ICS on the left and to the 4th ICS on the right.
- The lateral chest is resonant to the 8th ICS.
- The posterior chest is resonant to T12.

Abnormal findings: Dullness is heard with fluid or masses in the lungs. Hyperresonance is heard with air trapping that occurs with emphysema.

---

9. Percuss the posterior chest for diaphragmatic excursion.

a. Percuss the level of the diaphragm on full expiration. Have the client exhale completely and hold his breath while you percuss (beginning just below the scapula) from resonance over the lung downward toward the diaphragm. The sound will become dull at the diaphragm. Mark the area with a pen.

b. Percuss the diaphragm level on full inspiration. Have the client take a deep breath and hold it as you percuss again. Mark the location.

c. Measure the distance between the two marks. ▼

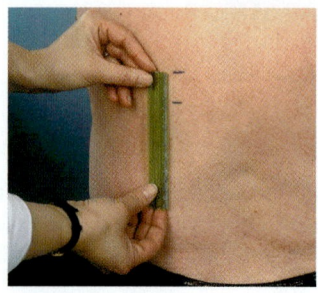

Expected findings: Diaphragmatic excursion (the distance between the two marks) is normally 3–6 cm.

Abnormal findings: Decreased excursion may indicate paralysis, atelectasis, or COPD with overinflated lungs.

10. Auscultate the chest.
  a. Follow the pattern in step 6.
  b. Use the diaphragm of the stethoscope.
  c. Have the client take slow, deep breaths through his mouth as you listen at each site through one full respiratory cycle.

For lung sounds, refer to the tables at the end of this procedure. Also, to listen to some lung sounds,

 Go to **Sound Files: Lung Sounds,** on *DavisPlus.*

Expected findings: No abnormal or adventitious sounds are heard. Lung fields are clear to auscultation. *Bronchial* breath sounds are heard over the trachea. *Bronchovesicular* breath sounds are heard over the sternum anteriorly and between the scapulae posteriorly. *Vesicular* breath sounds are heard over most of the lung fields.

Developmental Variations

Infants—Breath sounds are louder than in adults.

Abnormal findings: Crackles or rales, rhonchi, wheezing, stridor, friction rub, grunting

11. Auscultate for abnormal voice sounds if there is evidence of lung congestion. Follow the pattern in step 6.
  a. Assess for bronchophony by having the client say, "1, 2, 3" as you listen over the lung fields.
  b. Assess for egophony by having your client say "eee" as you listen over the lung fields.
  c. Assess for whispered pectoriloquy by having your client whisper, "One, two, three" as you listen over the lung fields.

Expected findings: No abnormal voice sounds are heard.

Abnormal findings:

  a. **Bronchophony** is present if the words are clearly heard over the lungs.
  b. **Egophony** is present if the sound you hear is "ay".
  c. **Whispered pectoriloquy** is present if you hear "One, two, three" clearly.

Patient Teaching

Instruct the patient about the dangers of tobacco use, especially smoking; exposure to air pollutants and environmental pollutants, such as radon or asbestos; and the signs and symptoms of lung cancer.

Home Care

- Instruct clients or caregivers to identify any pollutant within the home that may cause respiratory problems, such as radon, dirty heating/air-conditioning systems, or mold.

- Instruct caregivers or patients with allergies and/or asthma to eliminate potential allergens, such as cigarette smoke, dust, feathers, and pet dander.

Documentation

- If you need information about documenting your findings, review Caring for the Nguyens, including the box Documentation of Physical Assessment Findings for Nam Nguyen.

Normal Lung Sounds			
NORMAL SOUNDS	**LOCATION**	**DESCRIPTION**	**ILLUSTRATION**
Bronchial or tubular	Heard over the trachea	Blowing, hollow sounds; inspiration is shorter than expiration and lower pitched.	Inspiration / Expiration "Inspiration" and "Expiration"
Bronchovesicular	Heard over the 1st and 2nd ICS anteriorly and over the scapula posteriorly	Medium-pitched, medium intensity, blowing sounds; inspiration and expiration are equal length and similar pitch	Inspiration / Expiration "Inspiration" and "Expiration"

(continued on next page)

Procedure 21–12 ■ Assessing the Chest and Lungs (continued)

Normal Lung Sounds—cont'd

NORMAL SOUNDS	LOCATION	DESCRIPTION	ILLUSTRATION
Vesicular	Heard over the lung periphery	Soft, low-pitched sounds; inspiration is longer, louder, and higher-pitched than expiration	"Inspiration" and "Expiration"

Abnormal Lung Sounds

ABNORMAL LUNG SOUNDS	CAUSE	CHARACTERISTICS	EXAMPLES
Crackles (sometimes called rales)	Air bubbling through moisture in the alveoli	Bubbling, crackling, popping. Soft, high-pitched, and very brief sounds, usually heard during inspiration	Pneumonia Congestive heart failure (CHF) Bronchitis Emphysema
Rhonchi	Mucus secretions in the large airways	Course, snoring, continuous low-pitched sounds heard during inspiration and expiration. May clear with coughing.	Bronchitis Emphysema Narrowed airways Fibrotic lungs
Wheezes	Narrowing of small airways by spasm, inflammation, mucus, or tumor	High-pitched musical or squeaking sounds heard during inspiration or expiration	Acute asthma Emphysema
Stridor*	Partial upper airway obstruction or tracheal or laryngeal spasm	High-pitched, continuous honking sounds heard throughout the respiratory cycle but most prominent on inspiration	Acute respiratory distress Foreign body in airway Epiglottitis
Friction rub	Rubbing together of inflamed pleural layers	A high-pitched grating or rubbing sound that may be heard throughout the respiratory cycle. Loudest over lower lateral anterior surface.	Pleuritis
Grunting	Retention of air in the lungs	A high-pitched tubular sound heard on expiration	Emphysema

*Patients with stridor need immediate medical evaluation.

Procedure 21-13 ■ Assessing the Heart and Vascular System

> ➤ For steps to follow in *all* procedures, refer to the Universal Steps for All Procedures found on the page facing the inside back cover.

Equipment

- Combination stethoscope with bell and diaphragm
- Alcohol or other antiseptic wipe
- Two rulers
- Pen and record form

➕ Clean stethoscope and rulers before and after using unless they are only used for one patient.

Position

Place the client in three positions: sitting, supine, and left lateral (to facilitate hearing specific sounds).

Focused History Questions

- Have you experienced any fatigue or activity intolerance?
- Do you have a history of high blood pressure or stroke?
- Have you ever passed out or felt light-headed?
- Do you have any problems with your heart or circulation?
- Do you ever experience chest pain? If so, describe the circumstances that triggered the pain.
- What was the pain like? What did you do to relieve it?
- Do you ever experience palpitations or a rapid heart beat?
- Do you ever feel short of breath?
- Do you ever get swelling in your feet?
- What medications are you taking?

> ➤ When performing the procedure, always identify your patient according to agency policy and be attentive to standard precautions, hand hygiene, patient safety and privacy, body mechanics, and documentation.

Procedure Steps

1. **Inspect the neck.**
   a. With the patient supine, inspect the carotid and jugular venous system in the neck for pulsations.

   b. Assess jugular flow: Compress the jugular vein below the jaw. The vein collapses, and the jugular wave is more prominent at the supraclavicular area.
   The jugular venous pulse is easily obliterated with gentle pressure.

   c. Assess jugular filling: Compress the jugular above the clavicle. The vein distends and the jugular wave disappears.

Expected and Abnormal Findings

Expected findings: Carotid pulsation is easily visible. A slight pulsation in the supraclavicular area or suprasternal notch indicates jugular venous pressure. The pulsation should be easily obliterated when you apply pressure to the area.

Abnormal findings: Significant jugular vein distention suggests right-sided heart failure. ▼

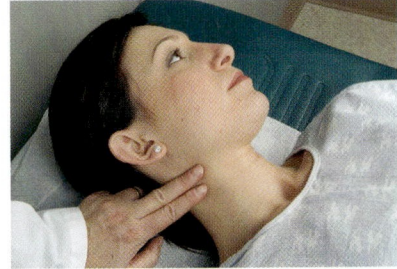

Assessing jugular flow

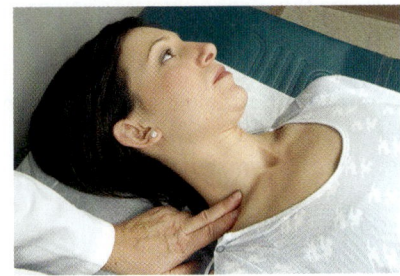

Assessing jugular filling

2. **Measure jugular venous pressure (JVP).**
   a. Elevate the head of the bed to a 45° angle.
   b. Identify the highest point of visible internal jugular filling.
   c. Place a ruler vertically at the sternal angle (where the clavicles meet).

Expected findings: Normal jugular venous pressure is less than 3 cm.

Abnormal findings: Elevated JVP (in CHF or constricted flow into the right side of the heart); low JVP (in hypovolemia)

(continued on next page)

Procedure 21–13 ■ **Assessing the Heart and Vascular System** (continued)

d. Place another ruler horizontally at the highest point of the venous wave.

e. Measure the distance in centimeters vertically from the chest wall. ▼

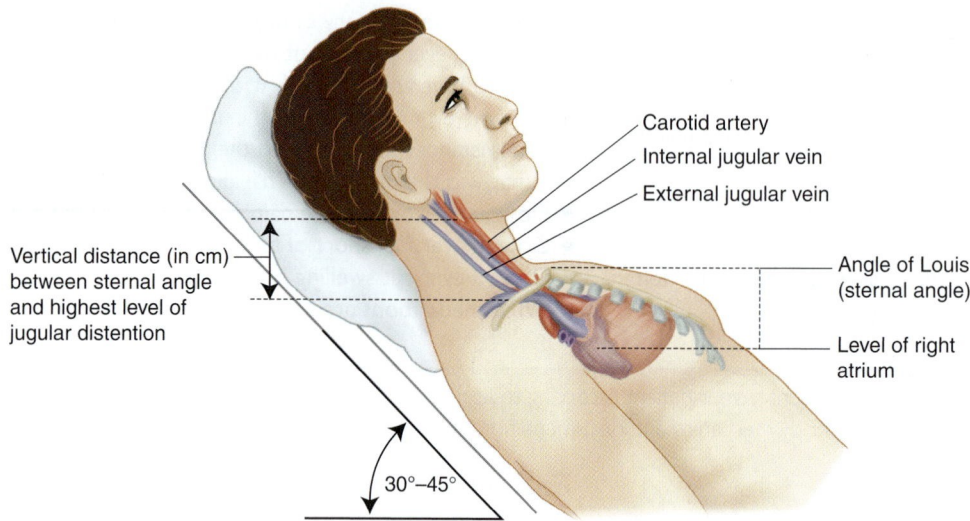

Carotid artery
Internal jugular vein
External jugular vein

Vertical distance (in cm) between sternal angle and highest level of jugular distention

Angle of Louis (sternal angle)

Level of right atrium

30°–45°

---

3. Inspect the precordium for pulsations. (Position the patient supine with tangential lighting.)

Expected findings: Visible pulsation at the point of maximal impulse (PMI, the 5th ICS in the midclavicular line)

Developmental Modifications

Children—Look for the PMI more medially and at about the 4th ICS in children younger than age 8.

Developmental Variations

In thin adults and children, a pulsation may also be visible over the base of the heart.

Abnormal findings: A pulsation (a heave or lift) displaced toward the axillary line indicates left ventricular hypertrophy. Pulsations to the right of the sternum may indicate an aortic aneurysm.

---

4. Very gently palpate the carotid arteries.
   a. Palpate each side separately.
      Bilateral pressure may impair cerebral blood flow.
   b. Avoid massaging the carotid artery as you palpate.
      Increased pressure on the carotid will lead to a drop in the heart rate and blood pressure.
   c. Note the rate, rhythm, amplitude, and symmetry of the pulse.
   d. Note the contour, symmetry, and elasticity of the arteries.
   e. Note any thrills.

Expected findings:
   ■ Rhythm is regular with 2 amplitude.
   ■ Contour: There should be a smooth upstroke with less acute descent.
   ■ Symmetry: Pulses are equal bilaterally.
   ■ Elasticity: Carotids are soft and pliable.

Developmental Variations

Pulse rate is age dependent.

Older adults—The carotids may be stiff and cordlike.

Abnormal findings: A thrill indicates turbulent flow.

---

5. Palpate the precordium.
   a. For this part of the examination, have the patient sit up and lean forward. If lying down, have him turn to the left side.
   b. Palpate in all five areas: apex, left lateral sternal border, epigastric area, base left, and base right.
   c. Feel for pulsations, lifts, heaves, and thrills.
      Brings the apex of the heart closer to the chest wall.

Expected findings: PMI is palpable at the apex over a 1- to 2-cm area. Slight pulsation from the abdominal aorta may be felt at the epigastric area. No pulsations, lifts, heaves, or thrills are palpable.

Abnormal findings: A pulsation, lift, or heave may be seen with left ventricular hypertrophy. A *lift* is a pulsation that is forceful enough to seem to lift the examiners fingers with

Helpful hint: Perform cardiac palpation and auscultation from the patient's right side, whenever possible.
This allows you to stretch the stethoscope during auscultation so that you minimize interference and "static."

---

6. **Auscultate the carotids.**
   a. Place the bell portion of the stethoscope over the carotid artery to listen for bruits.
      Bruits are low-pitched sounds, best heard by the bell portion.
   b. Have the patient hold his breath as you listen.
      Breath sounds over the trachea are loud and could interfere with the ability to hear a bruit.

---

7. **Auscultate the jugular veins.**
   a. Place the bell portion of the stethoscope lightly over the jugular veins to listen for a low-pitched venous hum.
   b. Have the patient hold his breath as you listen.

---

8. **Auscultate the precordium.** To review heart sounds,

    Go to **Sounds: Heart Sounds,** on DavisPlus.

   - Ask the patient to sit upright and lean forward a bit.
     This will position the heart closer to the chest wall for clearer auscultation.
   - Listen for the S_1, S_2, S_3, and S_4 sounds.
   - Listen for murmurs.
   - Listen with both the bell and the diaphragm at the sites in the following figure:
     These sites are located along the pathway the blood takes as it flows through the atria, ventricles, and valves of the heart.

---

palpation. A **heave** is a pulsation that feels rolling under your fingers. A **thrill** indicates turbulent flow and feels like a vibration over the PMI.

Expected findings: No audible bruit is present.

Developmental Variations

Children—Bruit may be heard because of a high-output state.

Abnormal findings: In adults, a bruit suggests carotid stenosis.

Expected findings: No venous hum is audible.

Developmental Variations

Children—A venous hum may be heard. This is a benign condition whereby, blood travels to the brain and back down again to the heart, causing the vein walls to vibrate.

Expected findings: No extra sounds are heard. No murmurs, clicks, or rubs are present.

Developmental Variations

Infants—You may hear a split S_2 when the child takes a deep breath.

Children—The chest wall is thinner, so heart sounds are louder than in adults.

Older adults—An S_4 sound is considered normal; extra systoles per minute are considered normal. ▼

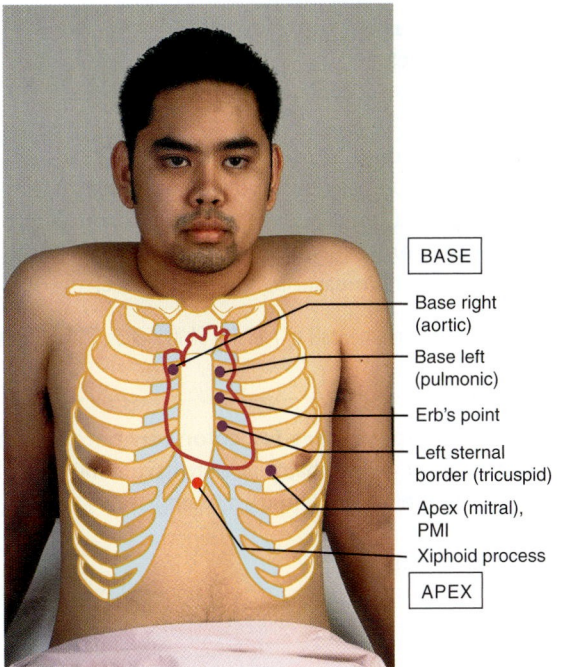

BASE
- Base right (aortic)
- Base left (pulmonic)
- Erb's point
- Left sternal border (tricuspid)
- Apex (mitral), PMI
- Xiphoid process
APEX

Cardiac auscultation sites

(continued on next page)

Procedure 21–13 ■ Assessing the Heart and Vascular System (continued)

a. *Base right (aortic valve)*. Locate the angle of Louis. (It is the prominence on the sternum, two to three fingerbreadths below the suprasternal notch.) Slide your fingers laterally until you feel the 2nd ICS.
The right 2nd ICS is the best place to auscultate the aortic valve.

a. **Expected findings:** $S_1 < S_2$

b. *Base left (pulmonic valve)*. Locate the angle of Louis (the prominence on the sternum, two to three fingerbreadths below the clavicular notch). Slide your fingers laterally until you feel the 2nd ICS.
The left 2nd ICS is the best place to auscultate the pulmonic valve.

b. **Expected findings:** $S_1 < S_2$

c. *Apex (mitral valve)*. You may be able to locate the apex by observing the pulsation at the PMI. It is at the 5th ICS in the midclavicular line.

c. **Expected findings:** $S_1 > S_2$

Developmental Variations

Children—You will hear S_3 at the apex in about 30% of children.

d. *Left lateral sternal border (LLSB) (tricuspid valve)*. From the apex, *slide* your finger up to the 4th ICS, then move close to the sternum.

d. **Expected findings:** $S_1 \geq S_2$. You may hear a split S_1.

Abnormal findings: Extra sounds (S_3 or S_4), murmurs, clicks, or rubs. NOTE: A diastolic murmur or a murmur greater than grade 3/6 is never innocent. Also, *in infants*, a split S_2 sound during normal respirations may indicate an atrial–septal defect.

Assessing Murmurs

Auscultating murmurs is an advanced technique that requires practice and experience. However, if you hear a murmur, assess its:
- Location
- Quality
- Frequency (high, medium, or low pitch)
- Intensity (loudness)
- Timing (in relation to S_1 and S_2)
- Duration
- Configuration (constant or crescendo/decrescendo)
- Radiation (can you hear this in other locations?)
- Respiratory variation (does it change with breathing?)

If you need more information about assessing apical and peripheral pulses and measuring blood pressure,

 Go to the *Fundamentals of Nursing Skills Videos*, **Vital Signs.**

Classifying Murmurs

Grade
$1/6$ Very faint, comes and goes
$2/6$ Quiet, but heard immediately
$3/6$ Moderately loud
$4/6$ Loud, associated with a thrill
$5/6$ Heard with stethoscope half off the chest wall; thrill present
$6/6$ Heard with stethoscope entirely off the chest wall; thrill present

For a description of murmurs,

 Go to Chapter 21, **Tables, Boxes, Figures: ESG Table 21-1,** on *DavisPlus*.

---

9. **Inspect the periphery for color, temperature, and edema.** (You will probably already have done this when examining the integumentary system.)

Expected findings: Skin is warm. No edema is present. Color is appropriate for race.

Abnormal findings: Pallor, cyanosis, coolness, shininess, sparse hair growth, and clubbing of the nails (may indicate pulmonary oxygenation problems or impaired central or peripheral circulation).

10. **Palpate the peripheral pulses:** radial, brachial, femoral, popliteal, dorsalis pedis, and posterior tibial.
    a. Using the distal pads of your second and third fingers, firmly palpate pulses.
    b. Palpate firmly but not so hard that you occlude the artery.
    c. If you have trouble finding a pulse, vary your pressure, feeling carefully at the correct anatomical location.
    d. Assess pulses for rate, rhythm, equality, amplitude, and elasticity.
    e. Describe pulse amplitude on a scale of 0–4:
       0 = absent, not palpable
       1 = weak, barely palpable, easily obliterated by the finger
       2 = normal, obliterated by strong finger pressure
       3 = full, increased, not easily obliterated
       4 = bounding, forceful, obliterated only by strong finger pressure

Expected findings: All pulses are regular, strong, and equal bilaterally. Pulse amplitude is +2.

Developmental Variations

Older adults—Arterial pulses may be difficult to palpate because of decreased arterial perfusion.

Abnormal findings: Weak, absent, or asymmetrical pulses may indicate partial or complete occlusion of the artery. Other signs of arterial occlusion include pain, pallor, cool temperature, paresthesia, or paralysis.

---

11. **Inspect the venous system.** If a client has varicosities, assess for valve competence with the **manual compression test.**
    a. With the client standing, compress the distal portion of the vein.
    b. Still holding the distal portion, compress the proximal portion.

Expected findings: Veins are not distended. Superficial spiderlike veins, especially on the lower extremities, may occur with normal aging.

If the valves are competent, you will not feel backflow. If the valves are incompetent, you will feel a wave pulsation with your lower hand as a result of backflow when you press on the proximal segment of the veins.

Developmental Variations

Older adults—*Often have peripheral edema as a result of chronic venous insufficiency.*

Abnormal findings: Ropelike, distended, tortuous, or painful veins **(varicosities)**

NOTE: See More Extensive Tests for Abnormal Findings at the end of this procedure.

? What if . . .

- **The patient is obese and heart sounds are difficult to hear?**

The larger the body mass over the heart, the more difficult it is to hear heart sounds clearly. However, it may help to have the patient sit upright and lean forward as you auscultate.

- **Findings from inspecting and palpating peripheral pulses are abnormal?**

If inspection or palpation findings are abnormal, perform the following more extensive tests.

Patient Teaching

Instruct the patient in the risk factors of heart disease and stroke and in the signs and symptoms of heart disease.

Documentation

- If you need information about documenting your findings, review Caring for the Nguyens, including the box Documentation of Physical Assessment Findings for Nam Nguyen.

(continued on next page)

Procedure 21–13 ■ **Assessing the Heart and Vascular System** (continued)

More Extensive Tests for Abnormal Findings

TESTS	EXPECTED FINDINGS
1. *Perform the capillary refill test* anywhere you note signs of diminished blood flow. a. Press the skin with sufficient pressure to produce blanching. b. Release the pressure and observe the return of color.	Color returns in less than 3 sec.
2. *Perform Allen's test* to assess abnormal pulse findings and arterial flow in the hands. a. Have the client form a tight fist with one hand. b. With her fist still clenched, compress her radial and ulnar arteries. c. Ask the client to open her hand; observe for pallor. d. Release the ulnar artery and watch for natural color to return. e. Then repeat the process, but release the radial artery	In a healthy individual skin color returns rapidly with each maneuver. Failure to return to normal color indicates impaired flow through the open artery. Normally pallor resolves in 3–5 sec.
3. *Check the ankle–brachial index (ABI)* to assess circulatory impairment of the feet. a. Use a Doppler (handheld ultrasonic device) to measure blood pressure at the posterior tibialis or dorsalis pedis pulse sites. b. Compare that pressure with blood pressure obtained over the brachial artery. c. To calculate the ABI, divide the systolic pressure at the ankle by the systolic pressure at the brachial site.	Normally ankle pressure is higher than brachial pressure. The following is a summary of ABI findings: Normal: 1 or greater Minimal disease: 0.8–0.95 Moderate disease: 0.8–0.4 Severe disease: 0.4–0 *Example:* If the systolic pressure at the ankle is 75 and at the brachial artery is 100, the ABI is 75/100, or 0.75. This indicates moderate peripheral vascular disease.
4. *Perform the color change test* to assess arterial circulation in the legs. a. While the client is lying supine, elevate the legs to increase venous return. b. Have the client quickly move to a sitting position with the feet dangling.	Normal color should return to the feet in less than 10 sec. Pallor with the legs elevated and dependent rubor (reddish-purple color) are signs of arterial insufficiency.

Procedure 21–14 ■ **Assessing the Abdomen**

➤ For steps to follow in *all* procedures, refer to the Universal Steps for All Procedures found on the page facing the inside back cover.

Equipment

- Stethoscope and antiseptic wipe
- Felt-tipped marker
- Tape measure and ruler
- Penlight or examination light
- Pen and record form

✚ Clean stethoscope and other equipment before and after using unless they are only used for one patient.

Position

Begin with the client supine, arms at sides, with small pillows under the head and knees.
Relaxes the abdominal muscles.

Focused History Questions

- What types of foods do you typically eat?
- Are there any foods that you cannot eat? If so, why?
- How many cups of coffee, tea, cola, or caffeinated beverages do you drink per day?
- Do you smoke? If so, how much and at what age did you start?
- Do you drink alcohol? If so, how many drinks per day? Per week?
- Do you use any drug for non-medical purposes?
- Do you have any abdominal pain?
- How often do you have a bowel movement (BM)?
- Have you noticed any changes in your BMs?
- Are you having any problems with constipation, diarrhea, or getting to the bathroom in time to use the toilet?

- Have you ever seen blood in your stool or noticed blood when you wipe after a BM?
- Have you ever had black, tarry stools?
- How often do you use antacids, laxatives, enemas, aspirin, or anti-inflammatory medicines, such as naproxen (Anaprox) or ibuprofen (Motrin)?
- What home remedy, herbal, or over-the-counter medicines do you use?
- What prescription medicines do you use?
- Have you ever been immunized for hepatitis?
- Have you ever had a blood transfusion?
- What is your occupation?
- Have you ever been diagnosed with an ulcer, hemorrhoids, hernia, bowel problem, cancer, hepatitis, liver problems, cirrhosis, or appendicitis?
- Have you ever had abdominal surgery? If so, when, what type, and what if any follow-up was done for the problem?

- Do you have any family history of abdominal problems, such as ulcers, gallbladder disease, bowel disease, or cancer?
- Do you ever have trouble with:
Swallowing?
Heartburn?
Nausea?
Vomiting?
Diarrhea?
Bloating?
Excess gas?
Yellowing of the skin?

Developmental Modifications

For older adults, recall that "Problems with eating" is a part of the SPICES assessment. Ask clients, for example:

- Do you have difficulty chewing or swallowing your food?
- How is your appetite?
- Are you able to shop for and prepare your food?

> ➤ When performing the procedure, always identify your patient according to agency policy and be attentive to standard precautions, hand hygiene, patient safety and privacy, body mechanics, and documentation.

Procedure Steps

1. Have the client void before the exam.
Empties the bladder so that you do not mistake a full bladder for a mass.

2. Position the client supine with the knees slightly flexed.
Relaxes the abdominal muscles.

3. Inspect the abdomen.
   a. Observe the size, symmetry, and contour of the abdomen.
   (1) Stand at the client's side and view across the abdomen.
   (2) If distention is present, use a tape measure to measure girth at the level of the umbilicus.
   (3) Have the client raise his head and check for bulges.
   Accentuates hernia, if present.

   b. Observe the condition of skin and skin color. Look for lesions, scars, striae, superficial veins, and hair distribution (if you have not already done this in your examination of the integumentary system).

Expected and Abnormal Findings

a. **Expected findings:** Abdomen is flat, slightly rounded, scaphoid (concave), or slightly protuberant; sides are symmetrical. No visible masses or distention are present.

Developmental Variations

Infants and toddlers—Protuberant abdomen is normal.

Abnormal findings: Tumors, cysts, bowel obstruction, or scoliosis may cause asymmetry.

b. **Expected findings:** Skin color is consistent with ethnicity but is usually lighter in color than exposed areas. No lesions are present. Hair distribution is appropriate for age and gender. Striae, superficial veins, and scars are common variations.

Abnormal findings:
- Skin color changes may be associated with bruising, internal bleeding, or jaundice.
- Striae occur after periods of rapid growth or weight gain. Pink striae are new. Older striae are silver-white in color.
- Dilated veins are associated with liver disease and obstruction of the vena cava.

(continued on next page)

Procedure 21–14 ■ **Assessing the Abdomen** (continued)

c. Note abdominal movements.

c. **Expected findings:** On a thin client, peristalsis and aortic pulsations may be visible. Men tend to use their abdominal muscles for breathing.

Developmental Variations

Infants and children—Peristaltic waves are often visible. Abdominal breathing is common in infants and young children.

Older adults—Abdomen may be more rounded because of decreased muscle tone.

Abnormal findings:
- Persitaltic waves may be seen if there is intestinal obstruction.
- Abnormal respiratory movements may be seen with respiratory distress.
- Pulsations (in other than a thin client) may indicate an aortic aneurysm.

d. Note the position, contour, and color of the umbilicus. ▼

d. **Expected findings:** Umbilicus is inverted and in the midline. No discoloration or discharge is present.

Abnormal findings: Protrusion of the umbilicus may result from a hernia or underlying mass. ▼

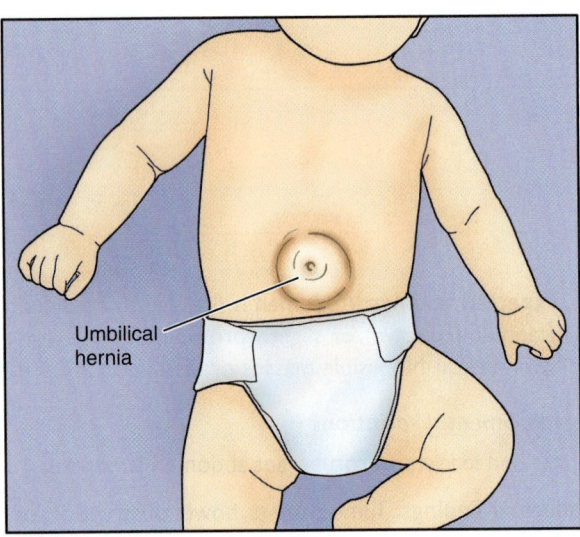

Umbilical hernia

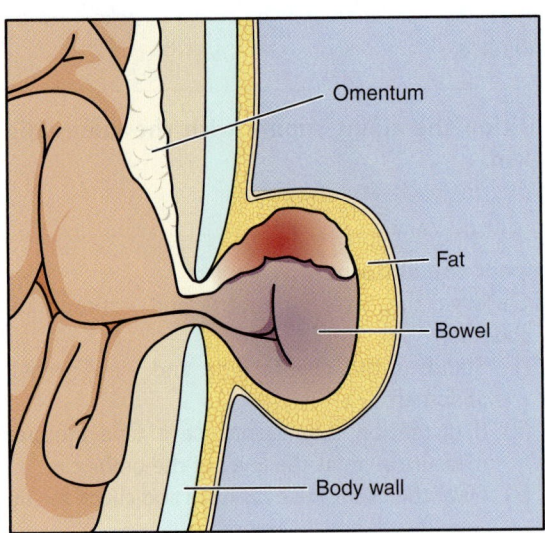

Omentum

Fat

Bowel

Body wall

4. **Auscultate the abdomen.**

To hear a sample of bowel sounds,

 Go to **Sound Files: Bowel Sounds,** on Davis*Plus.*

a. Ask the client when he last ate.
Bowel sounds are loudest 5 or 6 hr after the person eats, when the small intestine contents empty through the ileocecal valve into the large intestine. They also increase immediately after eating.

b. Listen for bowel sounds.
   (1) Using the stethoscope diaphragm, listen in several areas in all four quadrants (see the figure).
   The diaphragm of the stethoscope is used because bowel sounds are high-pitched.
   (2) If bowel sounds are infrequent or difficult to hear, listen to the right of the umbilicus over the ileocecal valve.
   (3) Listen for 5 min before concluding that bowel sounds are absent.
c. Use the stethoscope bell to listen for bruits over the aorta and the renal, femoral, and iliac arteries. ▼

b. **Expected findings:** Audible bowel sounds, occurring every 5–15 sec or 5–30 times per min in a healthy adult.

Abnormal findings:
- *Hyperperistalsis* (hyperactive bowel sounds): > two or three sounds per sec or > 30 bowel sounds per min; loud, rushing sounds
- *Hypoperistalsis:* < 5 sounds per min; faint sounds
- *Absent* bowel sounds: none after listening for 5 min

c. **Expected findings:** No audible bruits are present.

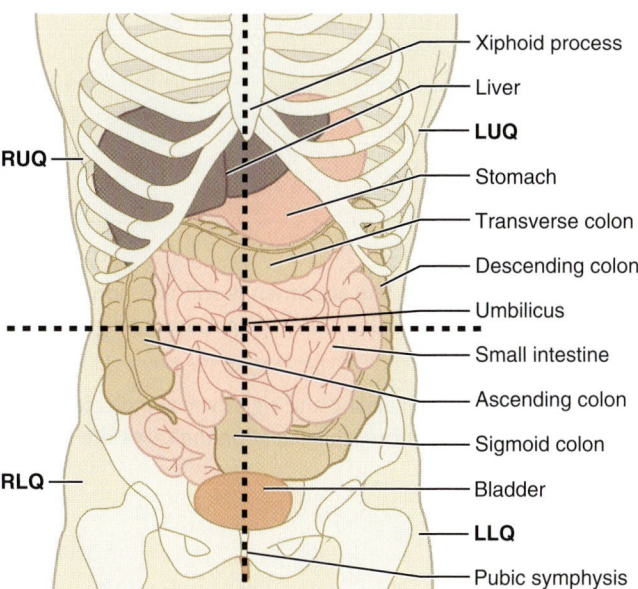

The four abdominal quadrants

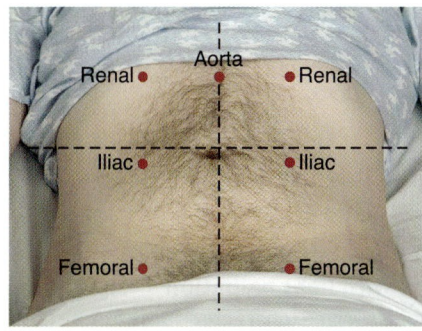

Abnormal findings: A bruit is abnormal and may indicate an aneurysm or altered blood flow.

5. Percuss the abdomen. (See Clinical Insight 21-1.)
   a. Use indirect percussion to assess at multiple sites in all four quadrants.
   b. Estimate organ size by noting the change in sounds as you percuss over the liver, spleen, and bladder. ▼

Expected findings: Tympany, with dullness over organs or fluid, is present. No tenderness

Abnormal findings: Extremely high-pitched tympanic sounds are heard with distention. Extensive dullness indicates organ enlargement or underlying mass.

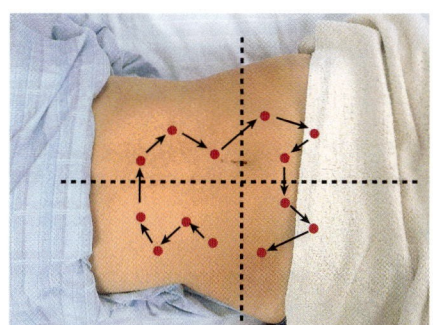

(continued on next page)

Procedure 21–14 ■ **Assessing the Abdomen** (continued)

6. Using fist or blunt percussion, percuss the cos-tovertebral angle (where the end of the rib cage meets the spine) bilaterally to assess for kidney tenderness. ▼

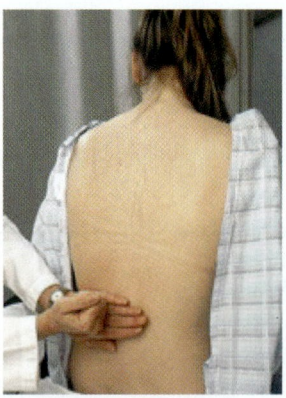

Expected findings: No costovertebral angle tenderness is present.

Abnormal findings: Pain or tenderness is associated with kidney infection or musculoskeletal problems.

---

7. Palpate the abdomen.
   a. **Begin with light palpation** throughout the abdomen. Identify surface characteristics, tenderness, muscular resistance, and turgor. If the client is having pain in one area of the abdomen, palpate that area last.

   A guarding response to pain from palpation can interfere with your assessment of the other areas.

   (1) Using your fingertips, press down 1–2 cm in a rotating motion.
   (2) Lift your fingers and move to the next site.
   (3) Palpate the entire abdomen if possible.
   (4) Proceed in an organized fashion through all quadrants, using the same sequence in every examination.
   (5) Observe for grimacing, guarding, or verbal statements of tenderness or pain.

a. **Expected findings:** The abdomen is soft and nontender, with no masses. Muscles are easily palpated; no guarding is present.

Abnormal findings: Guarding and rigidity may indicate peritonitis. Tenderness on light palpation indicates the need for further evaluation.

Developmental Modifications

Encourage a child to place her hand lightly over yours as you palpate.

✚ Caution: Do not palpate the abdomen if the client has a Wilms' tumor, a large diffuse pulsation, or a history of organ transplant.

   b. **Use deep palpation** to palpate organs and masses. See the table Deep Palpation Techniques at the end of this procedure.

b. Tenderness may be noted in a normal adult near the xiphoid process and over the cecum and sigmoid colon.

Developmental Variations

Older adults—May have a higher pain threshold, so they may not react to palpation even if there is an abnormality in the abdomen.

Abnormal findings: A mass indicates the need for further evaluation.

   c. **Palpate the liver.**
   (1) Stand at the client's right side.
   (2) Place your right hand at the client's right midclavic-ular line under the costal margin, parallel to the right costal.

c. **Expected findings:** The liver is not normally palpable unless the client is very thin. If it is palpable, the edge should be smooth and nontender.

(3) Place your left hand under the client's back at the lower (11th to 12th) ribs, and press upward. This elevates the liver toward the abdominal wall.

(4) Ask the client to inhale and deeply exhale while you press in and up, gently but deeply, with your right fingers.

Alternative approach: Hooking technique. Place your hands over the right costal margin, and hook your fingers over the edge. Have the client take a deep breath, and feel for the liver's edge as the liver drops down on inspiration and then rises up over your fingers during expiration. ▼

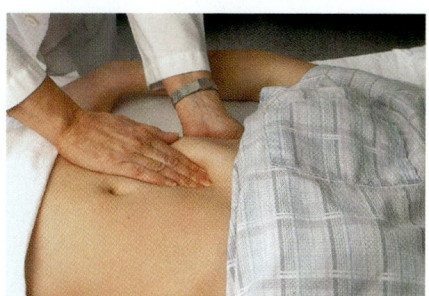

Developmental Variations

Children—Liver is relatively large and can be palpated 1–2 cm (0.5–1 in.) below the right costal margin.

Abnormal findings: Palpation below the costal margin indicates liver enlargement.

d. Palpate the Spleen

(1) Stand at the client's right side.

(2) Reach across the client to place your left hand under the costovertebral angle, and pull upward to move the spleen anteriorly.

(3) Place your right hand under the left anterior costal margin, and have the client take a deep breath.

(4) During exhalation, press your hands together (inward) to try to palpate the spleen. ▼

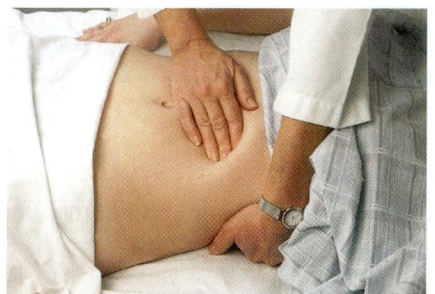

d. Expected findings: The spleen is not normally palpable.

Abnormal findings: Splenic enlargement or tenderness may result from infection, enlargement, trauma, or cancer.

? What if . . .

- **The patient is ticklish or guarding when you palpate the abdomen?**

Distract the person by giving her a task, such as "Count aloud to 10" or "Count backward from 100." Alternatively, have the client place her hand on her abdomen; place your hand on hers and begin light palpation. When she begins to feel more relaxed, slip your hand underneath hers and continue.

- **The patient complains of abdominal pain?**

Check for rebound tenderness: Place your hand perpendicular to the abdomen. Press firmly and slowly then release quickly. *If pain increases when you remove your hand, this indicates peritoneal irritation. Rebound tenderness in the right lower quadrant may be a sign of appendicitis.*

Patient Teaching

Instruct the patient in the importance of proper diet, the signs and symptoms of colorectal cancer, and the importance of screening colonoscopy.

Documentation

- If you need more information about documenting your findings, review Caring for the Nguyens, including the box Documentation of Physical Assessment Findings for Nam Nguyen.

(continued on next page)

Procedure 21–14 ■ **Assessing the Abdomen** (continued)

Deep Palpation Techniques

DEEP PALPATION: ONE-HANDED TECHNIQUE	DEEP PALPATION: BIMANUAL TECHNIQUE
■ Using your fingertips, press down 4–6 cm in a dipping motion. ■ Proceed in an organized fashion through all four quadrants.	■ This technique is useful when palpating a large abdomen. ■ Place your nondominant hand on your dominant hand. ■ Depress your hands 4–6 cm (1.5–2 in.) in a dipping motion. ■ Proceed in an organized fashion through all four quadrants.

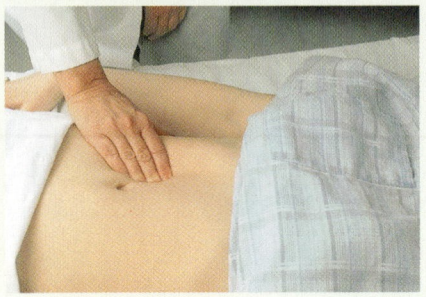

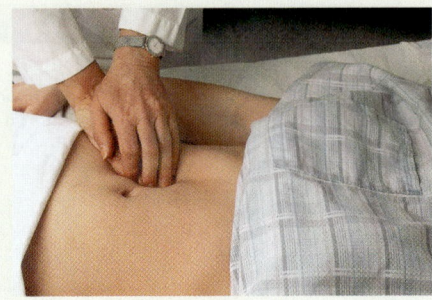

❔ What if . . .

■ **You palpate a mass?**

Have the client tighten her abdominal muscles.

If the mass is in the abdominal wall, it will become easier to palpate. If it is deep in the abdomen, it will be difficult to palpate.

Procedure 21–15 ■ **Assessing the Musculoskeletal System**

➤ For steps to follow in *all* procedures, refer to the Universal Steps for All Procedures found on the page facing the inside back cover.

Equipment

■ Tape measure
■ Goniometer
■ Pen and record form

Developmental Modifications

For older adults, recall that "Problems with falls" is a part of the SPICES assessment. If your facility has a falls assessment tool, perform that focused assessment.

Focused History Questions

■ Do you have any difficulty with coordination (e.g., folding clothes, brushing your teeth)?
■ Do you now have, or have you ever had, musculoskeletal problems, pain, or disease? If so, what medications or treatments are you using?
■ Have you ever injured your bones or joints?
■ Do your joints, muscles, or bones limit your activities?
■ Do you lose your balance or fall?
■ Do you have any occupational hazards that could affect your muscles and joints?

➤ When performing the procedure, always identify your patient according to agency policy and be attentive to standard precautions, hand hygiene, patient safety and privacy, body mechanics, and documentation.

Procedure Steps

1. **Assess posture.**
   a. Note the body and head position.

   b. Check the alignment and symmetry of the shoulders, scapula, and iliac crests. Inspect from the front, back, and side.

Expected and Abnormal Findings

a. **Expected findings:** Posture is erect, with the head in the midline.

b. **Expected findings:** The shoulders, scapula, and iliac crests are symmetrical.

Developmental Modifications

Newborns—Palpate clavicles for fractures that may have occurred at birth. Check for congenital hip dysplasia (dislocation) by examining for asymmetry of the gluteal folds or shortening of the femur.

c. Assess the spinal curvature by:
   (1) Observing the client's profile while he is standing erect.
   (2) Having the client bend forward at the waist with arms hanging free at the sides.

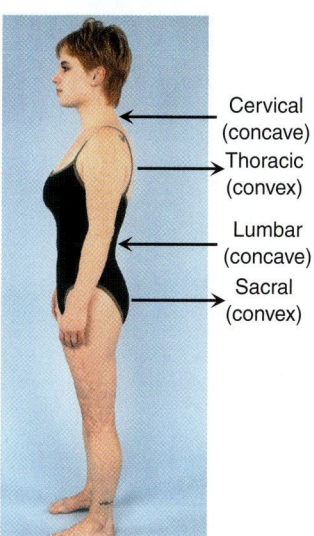
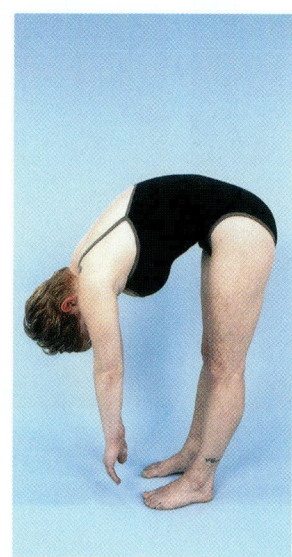

Cervical (concave)
Thoracic (convex)
Lumbar (concave)
Sacral (convex)

Assessing for normal curves   Assessing for kyphosis and scoliosis

d. Have the client stand upright with the feet together. Note the position of the knees. ▼

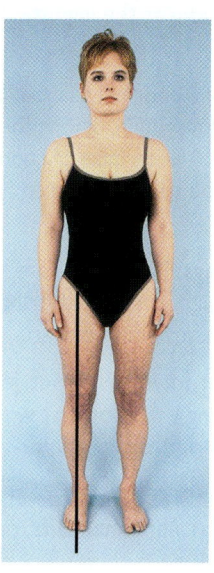

c. **Expected findings:** Cervical and lumbar curves are concave; thoracic and sacral curves are convex.

Developmental Variations

Children—**Lordosis** (exaggerated lumbar curve) is normal before age 5.

Abnormal findings: Kyphosis, scoliosis, lordosis. Also,

Go to Chapter 21, **Tables, Boxes, Figures: ESG Table 21-3,** on Davis*Plus.*

d. **Expected findings:** Patella is in the midline on an imaginary line drawn from the anterior superior iliac crest to the feet.

Developmental Variations

Children—**Genu varum** (bowlegs) is normal for 1 year after a child begins to walk.

(continued on next page)

Procedure 21–15 ■ Assessing the Musculoskeletal System (continued)

Abnormal Spinal Curvature ▼

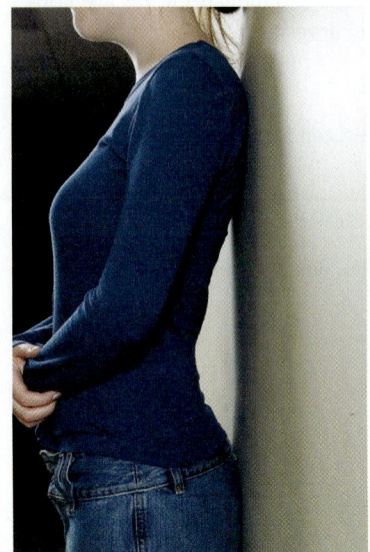

Lordosis

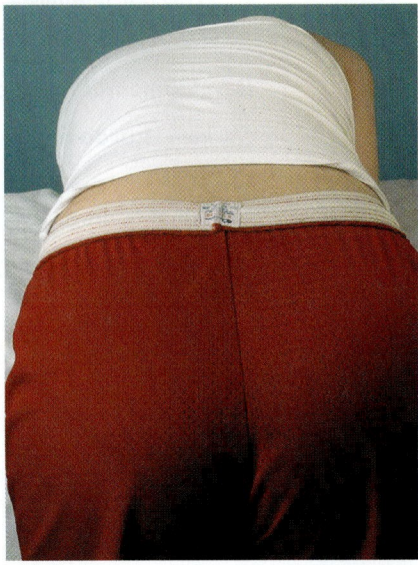

Scoliosis

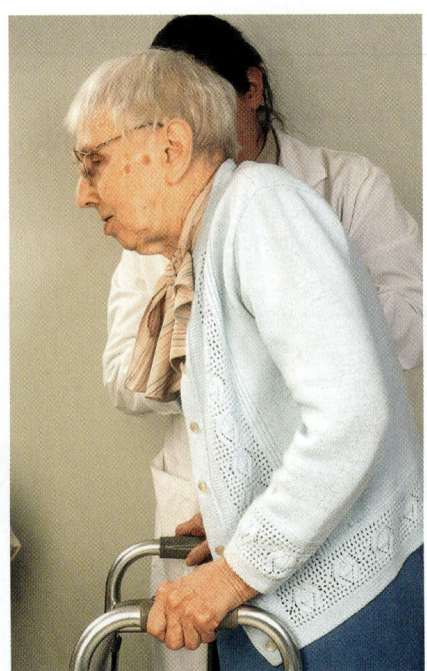

Kyphosis

2. **Assess gait by observing the client walking.**

Developmental Modifications

Children—Observe them at play.

a. Pay attention to the base of support (distance between the feet) and stride length (distance between each step).

a. **Expected findings:** Average base of support for an adult is 5–10 cm (2–4 in.). Average stride length is 30–35 cm (12–14 in.); the longer the legs, the longer the stride length.

Abnormal findings: Abnormal gait can be caused by muscle weakness, joint stiffness, pain, deformities, and central nervous system dysfunction. A wide base of support and shortened stride length reflect a balance problem, placing the client at risk for falls.

b. Observe the phases of the gait.

b. **Expected findings:** Movements are smooth and coordinated, weight is evenly distributed, arms swing in opposition, and toes point forward.

Abnormal findings: Toeing in or out, jerky or shuffling movements, touching the floor first with the toe rather than the heel, arms held out to the side or front. Also,

Go to Chapter 21, **Tables, Boxes, Figures: ESG Table 21-3, Abnormal Atlas: Abnormal Gaits,** on Davis*Plus*.

Stance Phase ▼

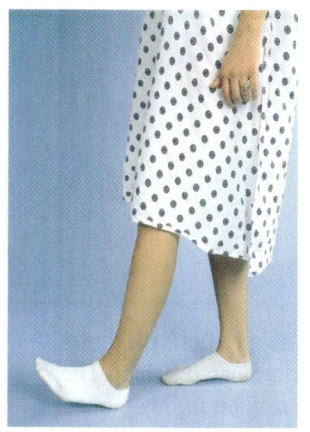 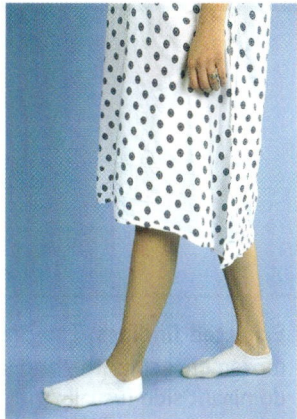 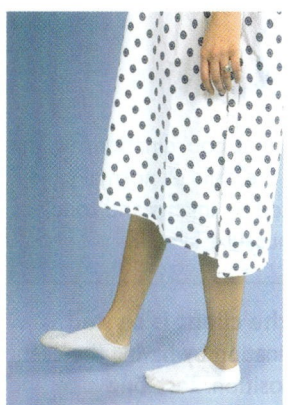 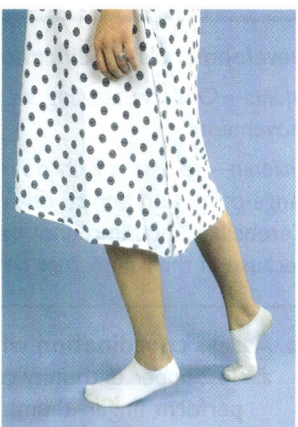

Heel strike   Foot flat   Midstance   Push-off

Swing Phase ▼

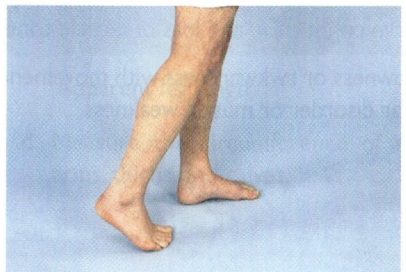 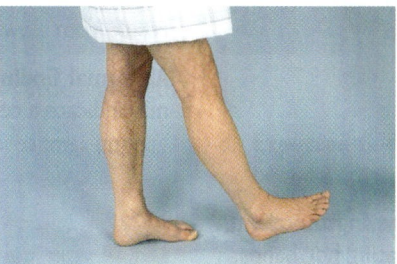 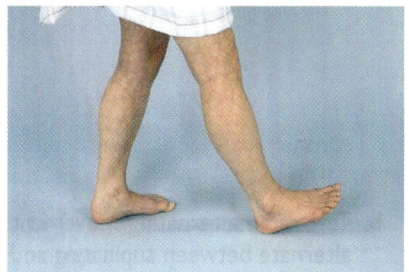

Accelerate   Swing-thru   Decelerate

3. Assess balance. ▼

✚ If the client's balance was unsteady when walking, do not complete this portion of the exam. Proceed only if the gait is steady; stand nearby in case the client loses his balance.

a. Have the client tandem walk heel-to-toe.
b. Have the client walk alternately on heels and toes.
c. Ask the client to do a deep knee bend.
d. Ask the client to hop in place on each foot several times.
e. Perform the Romberg test (if you did not already do so when examining the ears): Have the client stand with feet together and eyes open. Then have him close his eyes and stand still.

Expected findings: The client is able to perform each of these maneuvers smoothly. The Romberg test (see Procedure 21-7) is negative—the client is able to maintain balance with minimal sway with eyes open and closed.

Developmental Variations

Infants—Should be able to sit alone by age 8 mo.

Abnormal findings: Balance problems may indicate a cerebellar disorder, an inner ear problem, or muscle weakness.

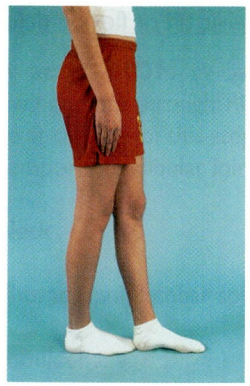 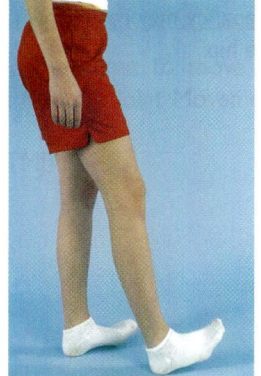 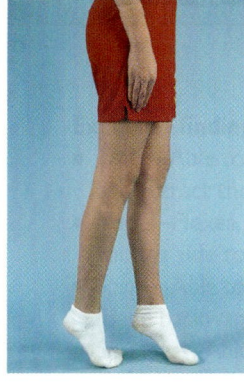

Walking heel-to-toe   Walking on heels   Walking on toes

(continued on next page)

Procedure 21–15 ■ Assessing the Musculoskeletal System (continued)

Muscle Strength Rating Scale

RATING	CRITERIA	CLASSIFICATION
5	Active motion against full resistance	Normal
4	Active motion against some resistance	Slight weakness
3	Active motion against gravity	Weakness
2	Passive ROM	Poor ROM
1	Slight flicker of contraction	Severe weakness
0	No muscular contraction	Paralysis

? What if . . .

■ **The client cannot move the limb?**

Put the joint through passive range of motion.

■ **There is limited ROM in a joint?**

Use a goniometer to measure the limited motion in degrees. Place the goniometer over the joint, matching the angle of the joint.

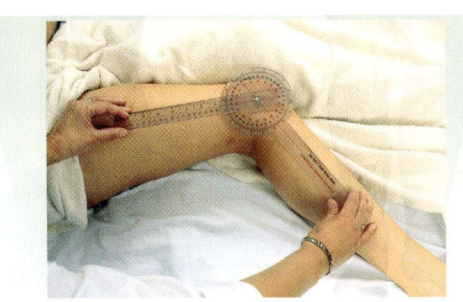

Using a goniometer

Documentation

■ If you need information about documenting your findings, review Caring for the Nguyens, including the box Documentation of Physical Assessment Findings for Nam Nguyen.

Procedure 21–16 ■ Assessing the Sensory–Neurological System

➤ For steps to follow in *all* procedures, refer to the Universal Steps for All Procedures found on the page facing the inside back cover.

➤ *NOTE:* This procedure provides guidelines for performing a comprehensive neurological exam. Steps 1–10 assess cognitive status, and the box at the end of the procedure contains questions that are useful for screening cognitive status.

Equipment

■ Pen and record form
■ Wisp of cotton
■ Sharp object, such as a toothpick or sterile needle
■ Objects to touch, such as a coin, button, or key
■ Something fragrant, such as coffee or rubbing alcohol
■ Something to taste, such as sugar, salt, or lemon
■ Tongue blade
■ Two test tubes
■ Reflex hammer
■ Ophthalmoscope

Developmental Modifications for Children

■ For children younger than age 5 years, use the Denver Developmental Screening Test II to assess neurological and motor function.

■ Check the child's ability to understand and follow instructions.

Developmental Modifications for Older Adults

■ You may need to perform the sensory–neurological exam over several sessions. The full exam is lengthy, and older adults fatigue easily. If the client seems to be getting tired, stop the test and finish at a later time.

Focused History Questions

■ Do you have any neurological ("nerve") problems?
■ Have you ever had head trauma, loss of consciousness, dizziness, headaches, or seizures?
■ Do you have memory problems, forgetfulness, or inability to concentrate?

- Have you noticed any changes in your ability to see, smell, taste, hear, feel, or maintain balance?
- Do you have any weakness, numbness, or paralysis?
- Do you have any problems performing activities of daily living (ADLs)?
- Do you have any problems walking?

- Do you have mood problems or depression?
- Do you use alcohol or drugs for non-medical purposes? If so, how much and how often?
- Have you ever been treated for neurological or psychiatric problems?
- Do you have a history of hypertension, diabetes, stroke, or circulation problems?

> ➤ When performing the procedure, always identify your patient according to agency policy and be attentive to standard precautions, hand hygiene, patient safety and privacy, body mechanics, and documentation.

Procedure Steps

Expected and Abnormal Findings

1. Assess behavior. Note the client's facial expression, posture, affect, and grooming.

Expected findings: The client is well groomed, with an erect posture, pleasant facial expression, and appropriate affect.

Abnormal findings: Inappropriate behavior may result from neurological or psychological problems, as well as from a variety of medications, alcohol, and street drugs.

2. Determine level of arousal (LOA):
   a. Note the client's response to **verbal stimuli.**
   b. If the client does not respond to verbal stimuli, try **tactile stimulation:** Gently shake the client's shoulder.
   c. If the client does not respond to tactile stimuli, try **painful stimuli:** Squeeze the trapezius muscle, rub the sternum, apply pressure on the mandible at the angle of the jaw, or apply pressure over the "moon" of the nail.

The Glasgow Coma Scale and the FOUR Scale at the end of this procedure provide standard references for assessing LOA for a patient with head injury.

Expected findings: The patient is awake and alert and readily responds to verbal stimuli.

Abnormal findings: Lethargy, stupor, or coma may result from trauma, neurological disorder, hypoxia, or chemical substances

✚ A changing level of arousal (along forgetfulness, restlessness, or sudden quietness) is one of the earliest indicators of increased intracranial pressure, which can be life threatening.

3. Determine the level of orientation.

   a. *Orientation to time:* Ask the client to state the year, date, and time of day.

   b. *Orientation to place:* Ask the client to state where he is (i.e., city, state, where he lives).

   c. *Orientation to person:* Ask the names of family members. Ask, "Do you know who I am?" If the client cannot answer these questions, ask him to state his name. *Self-identity remains intact the longest.*

Expected findings: The client is awake, alert (see step 2), and oriented to time, place, and person (AAO × 3).

   a. Hospitalized patients commonly lose track of date and time of day, but they easily reorient. As a rule, they should at least know the year.

   b. Interpret data carefully. In some situations (e.g., after an automobile accident away from home), the patient may know he is in the hospital but not know which hospital or which city.

   c. Patient should know you are a healthcare worker, but not necessarily your name.

Developmental Variations

Older adults—The stress of an unfamiliar situation can create confusion in an older adult.

Abnormal findings: Disorientation may result from physical or psychological problems. Bizarre responses are usually associated with psychiatric problems.

(continued on next page)

Procedure 21–16 ■ **Assessing the Sensory–Neurological System** (continued)

4. Assess memory.

a. *Assess immediate memory* by asking the client to repeat a series of three numbers that you speak slowly (e.g., 1, 5, 8). Gradually increase the length of the series until the client cannot repeat the series correctly. Record the length of the last correct series (e.g., "Successfully repeats a series of 7 numbers correctly.")

b. *Repeat the test*, beginning with a series of three numbers, but ask the client to repeat them back to you in reverse order.

c. *Assess recent memory* by naming three items (e.g., "mirror, truck," and "the letter *X*") and asking the client to recall them later during the exam. Alternatively, you can ask questions such as, "How did you get to the hospital? What did you have for breakfast?" However, you will need to verify the patient's answers.

d. *Assess remote memory* by asking the client his birth date or the date of a major historical event.

Developmental Modifications

Children—Assess memory by using names of toys (e.g., truck, ball, puzzle), names of people in his family, or names of familiar cartoon characters.

Expected findings: Immediate, recent, and remote memories are intact. Average series recall is 5–8 numbers in sequence and 4–6 numbers in reverse order.

Developmental Variations

Children—Number of objects recalled is usually fewer than the child's age in years.

Older adults—Loss of immediate and recent memory is common; long-term memory is usually not impaired.

Abnormal findings: Memory problems may be benign or may signal underlying neurological problems. Temporary memory loss may occur after trauma.

5. Assess mathematical and calculation skills.

a. Have the client solve a simple mathematical problem, such as 3 + 3.

b. If he is able to solve that problem, present a more complex example, yet simple enough that regardless of math skills the client could still determine the appropriate response, such as, "If you have $3 and you buy an item for $2, how much money will you have left?"

c. To assess both calculation skills and attention span, ask the client to count backwards from 100.

d. A more difficult test is to have the client perform serial threes or serial sevens. Ask him to begin at 100 and keep subtracting 3 (or 7).

Consider the person's language, education, and culture in deciding whether this test is appropriate for him.

Expected findings: Mathematical and calculation ability is appropriate for the patient's age, education level, and language ability. The average adult can solve simple mathematical problems and can complete serial sevens in about 90 sec with three or fewer errors.

Abnormal findings: Inability to calculate at a level appropriate for age and educational level may indicate neurological impairment or developmental delay.

6. Assess general knowledge.

■ You can ask questions directly or work this into the overall interaction with the client.

■ Ask the client how many days in the week or months in the year.

Expected findings: Vocabulary and general knowledge are intact.

7. Evaluate thought processes. Assess throughout the exam. Notice attention span, logic of speech, ability to stay focused, and appropriateness of responses.

Expected findings: Thought processes are clear, client responds appropriately, and speech is coherent and logical.

Abnormal findings: Alteration in thought processes may be due to physical disorders, such as dementia; psychiatric disorders, such as psychosis; or alcohol and drugs.

8. **Assess abstract thinking.** Ask the client to interpret a maxim (or saying), such as "A penny saved is a penny earned" or "A rolling stone gathers no moss."

Expected findings: Abstract thinking is intact.

Abnormal findings: Inability to think abstractly is associated with dementia, delirium, mental retardation, and psychosis.

Developmental Modifications

Children—The ability to think abstractly does not develop until the late school-age years or adolescence. To assess a child under the age of 12, ask her to describe things that are like and unlike a named object (e.g., "Tell me something that is like a cup.")

9. **Assess judgment.** Ask the client to respond to a hypothetical situation, such as, "If you were walking down the street and saw smoke and flame coming from a house, what would you do?"

Expected findings: Judgment is intact.

Abnormal findings: Impaired judgment may be associated with dementia, psychosis, or substance abuse.

10. **Assess communication ability.**
    a. **Listen to the client's speech.** Note the rate, flow, choice of vocabulary, and enunciation.

    a. **Expected findings:** Speech flows easily, and patient enunciates clearly. Vocabulary is consistent with the client's age, education, and language fluency.

    Abnormal findings: Problems with flow (e.g., halting speech, stuttering, very rapid speech, slurred words) may be due to language problems, nervousness, anxiety, or neurological problems.

    b. **Test spontaneous speech:** Show the client a picture, and have him describe it.

    b. **Expected findings:** Spontaneous speech is intact.

    Abnormal findings: Impaired spontaneous speech is associated with cognitive impairment.

    c. **Test motor speech** by having the client say "Do, re, mi, fa, so, la, ti, do." Assess ability to swallow. Observe for clarity of speech, facial mobility, drooling, and oral hypotonia. Ask the client to repeat a short phrase 2 or 3 times and observe for lack of coordination.

    c. **Expected findings:** Motor speech is intact.

    Abnormal findings: Impaired motor speech is associated with problems with CN XII or with coordination of speech muscles.

    d. **Test automatic speech** by having the client recite the days of the week.

    d. **Expected findings:** Automatic speech is intact.

    Abnormal findings: Cognitive impairment or memory problems cause difficulty with automatic speech.

    e. **Test sound recognition** by having the client identify a familiar sound, such as clapping hands.

    e. **Expected findings:** Sound recognition is intact

    Abnormal findings:

    f. **Test auditory–verbal comprehension** by asking the client to follow simple directions (e.g., "Point to your nose; rub your left elbow.")

    f. **Expected findings:** Auditory–verbal comprehension is intact.

    Abnormal findings: Temporal lobe problems affect reception. Frontal lobe problems affect expression.

    g. **Test visual recognition** by pointing to objects and asking the client to identify them.

    g. **Expected findings:** Visual recognition is intact.

    Abnormal findings: Impaired visual recognition indicates parieto–occipital lobe problems.

    h. **Test visual–verbal comprehension** by having the client read a sentence and explain its meaning.

    h. **Expected findings:** Visual-verbal comprehension is intact.

    Abnormal findings: Impaired visual-verbal comprehension indicates cognitive impairment.

(continued on next page)

Procedure 21–16 ■ Assessing the Sensory–Neurological System (continued)

i. **Test writing** by having the client write her name and address.

i. **Expected findings:** Writing ability is intact.

j. **Test ability to copy figures** by having the client copy a circle, letter X, square, triangle, and star.

j. **Expected findings:** The client is able to copy figures.

---

11. Test cranial nerve I—olfactory nerve

NOTE: You can assess CN I with your examination of the nose and sinuses (see Procedure 21-8).

a. Before testing, check the patency of the nostrils by gently occluding each nostril and having the client sniff.

b. Have the client occlude one nostril and hold an aromatic substance (e.g., lemon, coffee, vanilla, alcohol) under the nostril.

c. Repeat with a different substance under the other nostril. ➤

Expected findings: The client can identify the substances.

Developmental Variations

Older adults—May have a decreased sense of smell.

Abnormal findings: Anosmia is the loss of the sense of smell. It may be genetic, related to chronic nose or sinus problems, heavy tobacco use, snorting cocaine, or zinc deficiency.

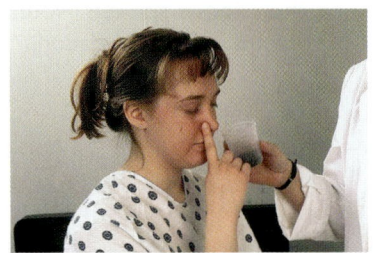

Developmental Modifications

Children—Select a substance that you are certain the child is familiar with (e.g., peanut butter).

---

12. Test cranial nerve II—optic nerve.

NOTE: You can assess CN II with your examination of the eyes (see Procedure 21-6).

a. Test visual acuity by asking the client to identify the smallest print readable on the Snellen chart.

Developmental Modifications

Use picture chart for small children, Snellen E for school-age children.

b. Identify visual field by having the client describe the boundaries of the visual field while her eye is in a fixed position.

c. Perform a fundoscopic exam (see Procedure 21-6).

a. **Expected findings:** Visual acuity is 20/20 in the right eye, left eye, and both eyes.

Abnormal findings: Many visual deficits are correctable with eyeglasses or contact lenses. They are not necessarily caused by optic nerve damage.

b. **Expected findings:** Peripheral vision range is approximately 50° in the superior field, 70° in the inferior field, 60° in the nasal field, and 90°–110° in the temporal field.

c. **Expected findings:** Disc margins are sharply demarcated. The cup is half the size of the disc or less.

Abnormal findings: CN II deficits may be due to tumor or CVA.

13. Test cranial nerves III, IV, and VI—oculomotor, trochlear, and abducens nerves.

a. Test EOMs by having the client move the eyes through the six cardinal fields of gaze while holding her head steady. ▼

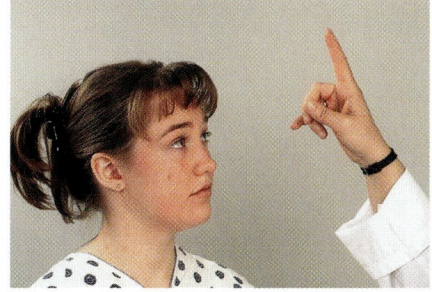

b. Test pupillary reaction to light and accommodation.

NOTE: See Procedure 21-6 for further details on each of these tests.

Expected findings: Client can move her eyes through the six cardinal fields of gaze. Pupils are equal in size and react to light and accommodation.

Abnormal findings: Changes in intracranial pressure (ICP) may affect EOMs and pupillary reaction.

---

14. Test cranial nerve V—trigeminal nerve.

a. Test motor function by having the client move his jaw from side to side, clenching his jaw, and biting down on a tongue blade.

NOTE: You can assess this function in your examination of the mouth and oropharynx (see Procedure 21-9).

b. Test sensory function by having the client close her eyes and identify when you are touching her face at the forehead, cheeks, and chin bilaterally—first with your finger and then repeat with a toothpick.

c. Test the corneal reflex by touching the cornea with a wisp of cotton or puffing air from a syringe over the cornea.

✚ The corneal reflex is not usually tested on a conscious person because the procedure is unpleasant and a corneal abrasion can occur. A conscious person can blink intentionally, so there is no need to stimulate the blink

NOTE: You can assess the corneal reflex in your examination of the eyes (see Procedure 21-6).

Expected findings: The client is able to perform all motor functions and can perceive light touch and superficial pain bilaterally; corneal reflex is intact.

Abnormal findings: Inability to perceive light touch and superficial pain may indicate peripheral nerve damage. An absent corneal reflex is an ominous neurological sign.

---

15. Test cranial nerve VII—facial nerve.

a. Test motor function by having the client make faces, such as smile, frown, or whistle.

NOTE: You can assess this function in your examination of the head and face (see Procedure 21-5).

b. Test taste on the anterior portion of the tongue by placing sweet (sugar), salty (salt), or sour (lemon) substance on the tip of the tongue. Do not test taste by using pungent, bitter, or markedly unpleasant flavors.

NOTE: You can assess this function in your examination of the mouth and oropharynx (see Procedure 21-9).

Expected findings: The client is able to perform all movements and can distinguish sweet, salty, and sour tastes.

Developmental Variations

Older adults—Have decreased taste sensation, especially sweet and salty, due to taste bud atrophy and diminished sense of smell.

Abnormal findings: Asymmetrical movement may be seen with nerve damage from a CVA or Bell's palsy. Impaired taste may be associated with nerve damage, chemotherapy, or radiation to the face or neck.

(continued on next page)

Procedure 21–16 ■ Assessing the Sensory–Neurological System (continued)

16. Test cranial nerve VIII—acoustic nerve.

NOTE: You can assess this function in your examination of the ears (see Procedure 21-7).

a. Perform watch-tick test for hearing by holding a watch close to the client's ear.

b. Perform Weber and Rinne tests to assess air and bone conduction.

c. Test balance with the Romberg test, if it has not already been performed.

See Procedures 21-7 and 21-15 for further details on these tests.

Developmental Modifications

Children—Romberg test is appropriate only after age 3.

Expected findings: Hearing is intact. Romberg test is negative.

Abnormal findings: Hearing loss, loss of balance, or vertigo may result from acoustic nerve damage.

---

17. Test cranial nerves IX and X—glossopharyngeal and vagus nerves.

a. Observe ability to talk, swallow, and cough.

b. Test motor function by asking the client to say, "Ah" while you depress a tongue blade and observe the soft palate and uvula.

c. Test sensory function by taking a tongue blade and gently touching the back of the pharynx to induce a gag reflex.

d. Test taste (sweet, salty, and sour) on the posterior portion of the tongue. Avoid bitter or repulsive tasting substances.

Expected findings: Swallow and cough reflex are intact. Speech is clear. The uvula and soft palate rise symmetrically, and the gag reflex is intact. Taste on the posterior tongue is intact.

Developmental Variations

Older adults—Have decreased taste sensation, especially sweet and salty, due to atrophy of the taste buds and a diminished sense of smell.

Abnormal findings: Damage to CN IX and X impairs swallowing. Damage to CN X changes voice quality.

---

18. Test cranial nerve XI—accessory nerve.

NOTE: You can assess this motor nerve function with your examination of the musculoskeletal system (see Procedure 21-15).

a. Place your hands on the client's shoulder, and have the client shrug his shoulders against resistance. ▼

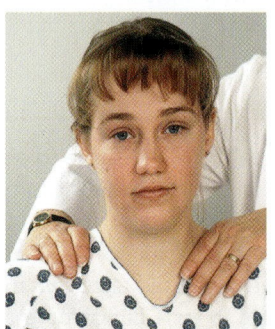

b. Have the client turn his head from side to side against resistance.

Expected findings: Movement is symmetrical and pain free. Full ROM of the neck with 5 strength.

Abnormal findings: Asymmetrical movement, pain, or absent movement indicates CN XI disorders.

19. Test cranial nerve XII—hypoglossal nerve.
  a. Ask the client to say, "d, l, n, t."
  b. Have the client protrude the tongue and move it from side to side.

Expected findings: The client can articulate the sounds and move the tongue easily.

Abnormal findings: Tongue paralysis

20. Test superficial sensations.
- Begin with the most peripheral part when testing the limbs (e.g., test the foot before the leg).
  If the client can feel sensation in the most peripheral part, you can assume the sensory nerve is intact to that point.
- If the client does not perceive the touch in an area, determine the boundaries of the dysfunction by testing at about every inch (2.5 cm). Sketch the area of sensory loss.
- Wait about 2 sec before moving to each site.
  Wait so that you can be sure that the patient is perceiving each stimulus separately.
  a. *Light touch:* With the patient's eyes closed, brush a cotton wisp on various areas of the body, comparing sides. Ask the client to say, "Now," when he feels your touch and to point to the spot you are touching.
  b. *Pain:* With the patient's eyes closed, use a toothpick (or sterile needle) with dull and sharp ends. Touch various areas of the body (except the face), and have the patient identify whether the sensation is dull or sharp. Alternate the dull and sharp ends as you move from spot to spot. Compare sides of the body.
  c. *Temperature sensation:* Test only if the patient's perception of pain is abnormal. Use test tubes filled with hot and cold water. Touch the tube to various areas of the body, comparing sides; have the client say "Hot," "Cold," or "Don't know."
  If pain sensation is intact, temperature will be, too, because sensations for pain and temperature are transmitted along the same tracts.

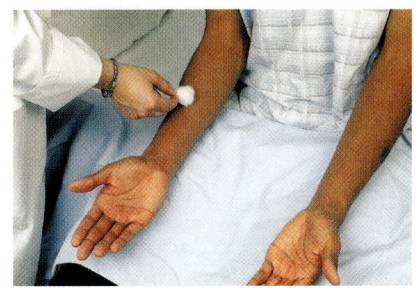

a. **Expected findings:** Able to identify areas of light touch.

Abnormal findings: Diminished sensation or areas of absent perception

b. **Expected findings:** The client is able to identify the areas stimulated and the type of sensation.

Abnormal findings:
- **Hyperalgia:** increased pain sensation
- **Analgesia:** no pain sensation
- **Paresthesia:** numbness and tingling

Developmental Variations

Older adults—May have a decreased perception of temperature and deep pain.

21. Test deep sensations.
  a. *Assess vibratory sensation* by placing a vibrating tuning fork on a metatarsal joint and distal interphalangeal joint. Have the patient identify when she feels the vibration and when it stops. ▼

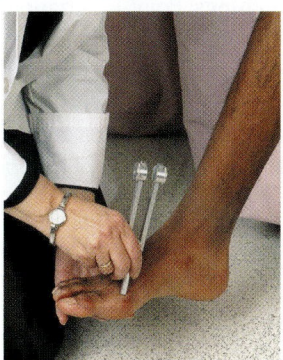

a. **Expected findings:** Vibratory sense is intact bilaterally in the upper and lower extremities.

Abnormal findings: Diminished or absent vibration sense is seen with peripheral nerve damage from vascular disease, diabetes, alcoholism, or damage to the posterior column of the spinal cord.

(continued on next page)

Procedure 21–16 ■ Assessing the Sensory–Neurological System (continued)

b. *Test kinesthetic sensation* (position sense) by holding the client's finger or toe on the sides and moving it up or down. Keeping her eyes closed, have the client identify the direction of the movement. ▼

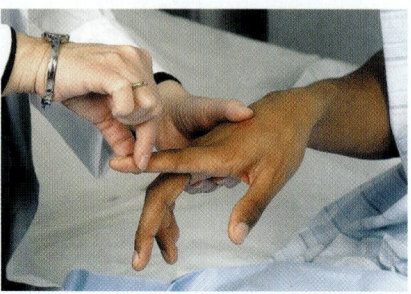

b. Expected findings: Position sense is intact bilaterally in the upper and lower extremities.

Developmental Variations

Older adults—May lose position sense in the great toes.

Abnormal findings: Diminished or absent position sense indicates nerve or spinal cord damage.

22. Test discriminatory sensations.

a. *Assess stereognosis* by placing a familiar object (e.g., a coin or a button) in the palm of the client's hand and having her identify it.

b. *Assess graphesthesia* by drawing a number or letter in the palm of your patient's hand and having the patient identify what was drawn.

c. *Test two-point discrimination* with toothpicks. Have the patient close her eyes. Touch her on the finger with two toothpicks simultaneously. Gradually move the points together, and have the patient say, "One," or "Two," each time you move the toothpicks. Document distance and location at which she can no longer feel two separate points. ▼

d. *Test point localization* by having the patient close his eyes while you touch him. Have him point to the area you touched. Repeat on both sides and the upper and lower extremities.

e. *Test sensory extinction* by simultaneously touching the patient on both sides (e.g., on both hands, both knees, both arms). Have the patient identify where he was touched.

Developmental Modifications

Older adults—May need more time to respond to a stimulus, as reaction time may be slower.

a. Expected findings: Stereognosis is intact bilaterally.

b. Expected findings: Graphesthesia is intact bilaterally.

c. Expected findings: Discriminates between two points on fingertips no more than 0.5 cm apart.

d. Expected findings: Point localization is intact bilaterally in the upper and lower extremities.

e. Expected findings: Extinction is intact: Client should feel the sensation on both sides of his body.

Abnormal findings: Abnormalities in any of the discriminatory sensation tests may indicate a lesion or disorder of the sensory cortex or disorder of the posterior column of the spinal cord.

23. **Test deep tendon reflexes.**
Use the accompanying scale to grade responses.

Deep Tendon Reflex Grading Scale

   0 No response detected
+1 Diminished response
+2 Response normal
+3 Response somewhat stronger than normal
+4 Response hyperactive with **clonus** (involuntary contractions that continue after the first contraction is elicited by the hammer)

a. *Biceps reflex* (spinal cord level C5 and C6). Rest the patient's elbow in your nondominant hand, with your thumb over the biceps tendon. Strike the percussion hammer to your thumb. ▼

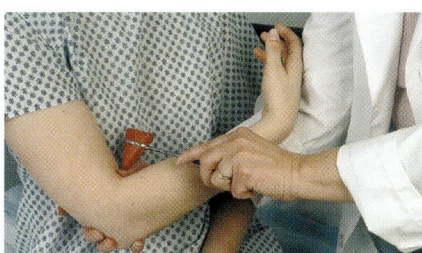

b. *Triceps reflex* (spinal cord level C7 and C8). Abduct the patient's arm at the shoulder, and flex it at the elbow. Support the upper arm with your nondominant hand, letting the forearm hang loosely. Strike the triceps tendon about 2.5–5 cm (1–2 in.) above the olecranon process. ▼

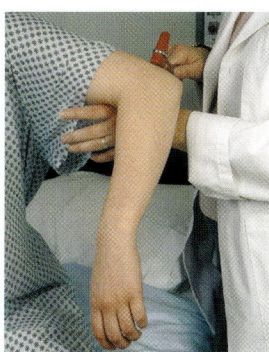

c. *Brachioradialis reflex* (spinal cord level C3 and C6). Rest the client's arm on her leg. Strike with the percussion hammer 2.5–5 cm (1–2 in.) above the bony prominence of the wrist on the thumb side. ▼

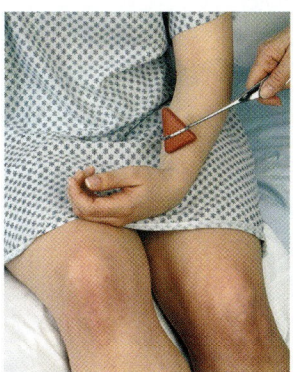

Developmental Variations

Older adults—Reflex responses may not be as strong as in young adults. Reaction time is slower as well.

a. **Expected Findings:** +2 response: You can feel the biceps contract with your thumb; slight flexion of the elbow.

b. **Expected Findings:** +2 response: Contraction of triceps with slight extension at elbow

c. **Expected Findings:** +2 response: Flexion at elbow and supination of forearm

(continued on next page)

Procedure 21–16 ■ **Assessing the Sensory–Neurological System** (continued)

d. *Patellar reflex* (spinal cord level L2, L3, and L4). Have the client sit with her legs dangling. Strike the tendon directly below the patella. ▼

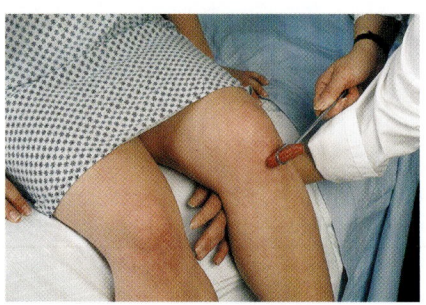

d. **Expected Findings:** +2 response: Contraction of quadriceps with extension of leg

e. *Achilles reflex* (spinal cord level S1, S2). Have the patient lie supine or sit with her legs dangling. Hold the patient's foot slightly dorsiflexed, and strike the Achilles tendon about 5 cm (2 in.) above the heel with the percussion hammer. ▼

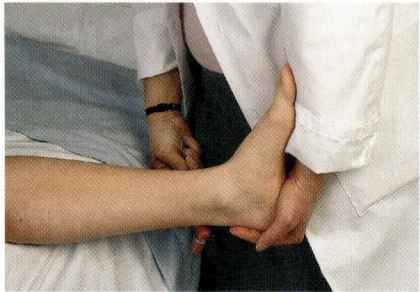

e. **Expected Findings:** +2 response: Plantar flexion of foot.

Developmental Modifications

Newborns—test the following reflexes:

- **Rooting reflex**—Stroke the cheek; the head should turn to the side you touched.
- **Palmar grasp**—Place one finger in the baby's hand; his fingers should curl around your finger.
- **Tonic neck reflex**—Position the baby supine; turn his head to one side. The arm and leg on that side should extend, and those on the other side will flex.

Developmental Variations

Older adults—May lose this reflex.

Abnormal findings:

- Absent or diminished responses are seen with degenerative disease, nerve damage, or lower motor neuron disease.
- Hyperactive reflexes are seen with spinal cord injuries and upper motor neuron disease.
- Rooting, palmar grasp, and tonic neck reflexes present after age 6 mo.

24. Test superficial reflexes.

Plantar reflex (Babinski's response): With your thumbnail or pointed object, stroke the sole of the client's foot in an arc from the lateral heel to medially across the ball of the foot. Record response as negative (normal) or positive (abnormal). ▼

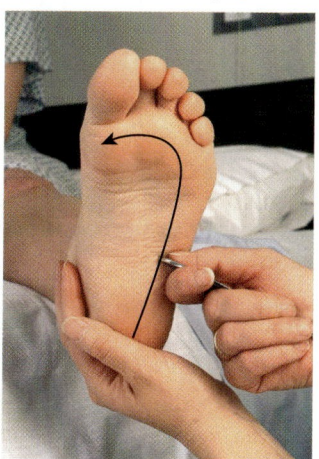

Expected findings: Babinski's response is negative: All the toes curl downward or there is no response

Infants and children—Positive Babinski's is normal until age 2 yr or until the child begins walking.

Abnormal findings: A positive Babinski's response: dorsiflexion of the great toe and fanning of the other toes. Seen with drug or alcohol intoxication or upper motor neuron disease

Developmental Modifications

Older adults—This reflex may be difficult to elicit.

25. Mental status screening.

The following questions may be used for a rapid evaluation of cognitive status. You may have already assessed for some aspects of mental status (e.g., orientation to time).

Questions for Evaluating Cognitive Status

This complete set of questions is included so that you can use them for a mental status exam that is not part of a comprehensive assessment. In a comprehensive assessment, do not repeat questions you have already covered in other portions of the assessment.

QUESTION	FUNCTION ASSESSED
What is today's date?	Orientation to time
What time is it?	Orientation to time
Where are you?	Orientation to place
What is the reason for your visit? (If the patient is hospitalized, modify the question: Why are you in the hospital?)	Communication, vocabulary, thought processes, recent memory
Ask the patient to count backward from 100.	Word comprehension, abstract reasoning
Ask the patient to name several objects that you point to. Be sure to use common objects such as a pen, shoe, or window.	Vocabulary, general knowledge, and word comprehension
Write a brief command, such as "Clap your hands," on a slip of paper. Hand the paper to the patient and ask him to follow the instructions.	Reading comprehension
Ask the patient to write the names of his family members, along with their relationship to him.	Writing, thought processes, memory, sound recognition
Ask the patient to name three things that begin with the letter *D*.	Auditory comprehension, thought processes
Ask the patient to draw a circle, square, and triangle next to each other on a sheet of paper.	Word comprehension, mathematical and calculation skills, communication (naming)

Difficulty with any of these questions requires further evaluation.

(continued on next page)

Procedure 21–16 ■ Assessing the Sensory–Neurological System (continued)

What if . . .

■ **The patient is an older adult?**

For a mental-status exam for older adults,

 Go to the link to the Mini-Cog exam in Chapter 21, **Resources for Caregivers & Health Professionals, Web Sites for Mental Status Exams,** on Davis*Plus.*

You should also assess older adults for dementia, which is characterized by these four features:
■ Mental status change of sudden onset, or fluctuating course
■ Difficulty focusing attention, distractible

■ Disorganized, illogical thinking
■ Increased or decreased level of consciousness (e.g., hyperalert, lethargic)

Delirium occurs in 15% to 60% of older hospitalized patients. You should assess them frequently to facilitate prompt identification and management of delirium.

For a reliable tool for assessing confusion and dementia in older adults,

 Go to the link for **The Confusion Assessment Method Instrument** in Chapter 21, **Resources for Caregivers & Health Professionals, Web Sites for Mental Status Exams,** on Davis*Plus.*

Home Care

Instruct caregivers in home safety if the client has cerebral function deficits or sensory or motor deficits.

Documentation

■ If you need information about documenting your findings, review Caring for the Nguyens, including the box Documentation of Physical Assessment Findings for Nam Nguyen.

Glasgow Coma Scale

EYE RESPONSE	SCORE	MOTOR RESPONSE	SCORE	VERBAL RESPONSE	SCORE
Opens spontaneously	4	Obeys verbal commands for movement	6	Oriented and converses	5
Opens to verbal commands	3	Reacts purposefully to localized pain	5	Disoriented but converses	4
Opens to pain	2	Withdraws in response to pain (generalized body response)	4	Uses inappropriate words	3
No response	1	Assumes flexor posture (decorticate posturing—arms flexed to chest, hands clenched and internally rotated) in response to pain. *Indicates problem is at or above the brainstem*	3	Makes incomprehensible sounds	2
				No response	1
		Assumes extensor posture (decerebrate posturing—arms extended, hands clenched and hyperpronated); Indicates problem at the brainstem level	2		
		No response	1		
Totals	_____		_____		_____

Full Outline of UnResponsiveness (FOUR)

Eye Response
4—Eyelids open or opened, tracing, or blinking on command
3—Eyelids open but not tracking
2—Eyelids closed but open to loud voice
1—Eyelids closed but open to pain
0—Eyelids remain closed with pain

Motor Response
4—Thumbs-up, fist, or peace sign
3—Localizing to pain
2—Flexion response to pain
1—Extension response to pain
0—No response to pain or generalized myoclonus status

Brainstem Reflexes
4—Pupil and corneal reflexes present
3—One pupil wide and fixed
2—Pupil or corneal reflexes absent
1—Pupil and corneal reflexes absent
0—Absent pupil, corneal, and cough reflexes

Respirations
4—Not intubated, regular breathing pattern
3—Not intubated, Cheyne-Stokes breathing pattern
2—Not intubated, irregular breathing
1—Respirations greater than ventilator rate
0—respirations at ventilator rate or apnea

Note: Education is necessary to use this scale properly.
To see how to use it,

Go to Mayo Clinic Proceedings, Wolf, Wijdicks, Bamlet, et al., 2007. Further validation of the FOUR Score Coma Scale by intensive care nurses, figure 1, at http://www.mayoclinicproceedings.com/content/82/4/435/F1.large.jpg

Sources: Rauen, C.A., Chulay, M., Bridges, E., et al. (2008). Seven evidence-based practice habits: Putting some sacred cows out to pasture. *Critical Care Nurse, 28*(2), 98–124; and Wijdicks, E. F. M., Bamlet, W. R., Maramattom, B.V., et al. (2005). Further validation of the FOUR Score coma scale by intensive care nurses. *Annals of Neurology, 58*(4), 585–593.

Procedure 21–17 ■ Assessing the Male Genitourinary System

➤ For steps to follow in *all* procedures, refer to the Universal Steps for All Procedures found on the page facing the inside back cover.

Equipment
- Nonlatex procedure gloves
- Penlight
- Pen and record form

Developmental Modifications for Children
- Obtain the parent's permission to perform this assessment.
- Explain to the child what you are going to do, and expect some resistance or embarrassment.
  Children are taught not to let strangers touch their genitals, and many children are modest.

Developmental Modifications for Older Adults
- Assess for incontinence.
  Incontinence is one of the elements of the SPICES assessment model for older adults.

Focused History Questions
- Have you noticed any redness, swelling, discharge, or odor in your genital area?
- Have you noticed asymmetry, lumps, or masses in your genitals? If so, describe them, and show me where they are.
- Have you ever been told you have a hernia?
- Have you ever had trauma to your genitals?
- Are you having any problems urinating?
- Are you sexually active? If not, have you ever been?
- Do you have sex with men, women, or both?
- What types of sexual activity do you engage in? Oral, anal, genital?
- Do you have more than one partner? How many partners have you had in the past 6 months?
- Do you use birth control? If so, what type and how often?
- Have you ever been treated for a sexually transmitted infection (STI)? If so, what type?
- Are you concerned about STIs or HIV?
- Do you take any precautions to avoid infections?
- Do you have any concerns about your sexual function?
- Do you have any difficulty achieving or maintaining an erection?
- Have you been taught to examine your testicles?
  In spite of the low prevalence of testicular cancer, men should be aware that a lump in the testicle, feeling of heaviness or swelling in the scrotum could be a sign of testicular cancer and should report these findings to his healthcare provider immediately (American Cancer Society, 2010).
- How often do you do testicular self-examination?
- Have you had any surgery of your reproductive tract?

(continued on next page)

Procedure 21–17 ■ Assessing the Male Genitourinary System (continued)

➤ When performing the procedure, always identify your patient according to agency policy and be attentive to standard precautions, hand hygiene, patient safety and privacy, body mechanics, and documentation.

Procedure Steps

1. Instruct the client to empty his bladder and undress to expose the groin area.

2. Have the patient stand while you sit at eye level to the genitalia; alternatively, the patient can lie supine on the exam table with his legs slightly apart.

3. Inspect the external genitalia.
  a. **Hair.** Note the hair distribution pattern and condition of pubic hair. See the table discussing Tanner staging at the end of this procedure.
  The appearance of the external genitalia depends on the client's developmental stage.
  b. **Skin.** Inspect the condition of the skin of the penis. Observe for the presence or absence of the foreskin. Note the position of the urethral meatus and any lesions or discharge.

  c. **Scrotum.** Observe the condition, size, position, and symmetry of the scrotal sacs.

  d. **Inguinal area.** Note the condition of the inguinal areas. Look for swelling or bulges. The best way to do this is to have the client bear down while you palpate the inguinal canal.

4. Palpate the penis.
  a. With a gloved hand, use your thumb and fingers to palpate the shaft of the penis. Note consistency, tenderness, masses, or nodules.
  b. Retract the foreskin if present.

Expected and Abnormal Findings

a. **Expected findings:** Hair distribution is triangular and appropriate for age. No pediculosis is present.

Abnormal findings: Sparse or absent hair may result from genetic factors, aging, or local or systemic disease.

b. **Expected findings:** Skin is intact with no lesions or discharge. Color is consistent with ethnicity. The urethral meatus is midline. The foreskin may be absent (circumcised); if present, it covers the glans and easily retracts.

Developmental Variations:

Infants—Foreskin is difficult to retract in the uncircumcised male until about age 3 mo.

Older adults—Penis and testes decrease in size.

Abnormal findings: Ulcerations or lesions (may be seen with a number of STIs, such as genital warts and genital herpes); **phimosis** (foreskin cannot be retracted and becomes swollen)

c. **Expected findings:** The skin should be free of lesions, nodules, swelling, rash, and erythema. The skin is rugated and deeper in color than the rest of the body. Size and shape vary greatly. The left scrotal sac is usually lower than the right.

Abnormal findings: A rash may be caused by **tinea cruris,** a fungal infection often called "jock itch." Swelling may indicate hernia, tumor, or infection.

d. **Expected findings:** The inguinal area should be free of swelling or bulges.

Abnormal findings: A bulge may indicate a hernia or enlarged lymph node.

Expected findings: The penis is nontender with no masses or nodules. Pulsations are present on the dorsal side. The foreskin, if present, easily retracts.

Abnormal findings: Inability to palpate a pulse may indicate vascular insufficiency; difficulty retracting the foreskin or problems with its return to position need further evaluation.

5. Palpate the scrotum, testes, and epididymis.

a. Don a procedure glove and use your thumb and fingers to palpate. ▼

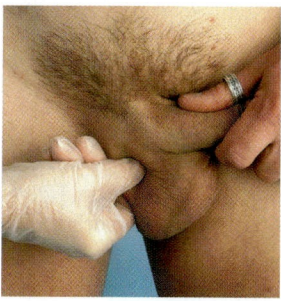

b. Note size, shape, consistency, mobility, masses, nodules, or tenderness.

c. Transilluminate any lumps, nodules, or edematous areas by shining a penlight over the area in a darkened room. ▼

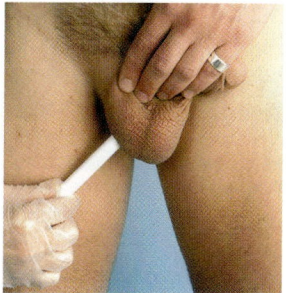

Expected findings: The scrotal skin is rough but without lesions. Each testicular sac contains a testicle and epididymis. The testes are rubbery, round, movable, and smooth. They are sensitive to pressure but nontender. The epididymis is comma shaped. The spermatic cord is smooth and round. There is no swelling or nodules. The left scrotal sac is usually lower than the right.

Abnormal findings:

- A unilateral mass
- Painless intratesticular masses may represent testicular cancer.
- A testicle that is swollen or tender may indicate infection or torsion.

6. Palpate the inguinal and femoral area for hernias.

a. Assess for inguinal hernias with a gloved hand. Have the patient hold his penis to one side. Place your index inger in the client's scrotal sac above the testicle, and invaginate the skin. Follow the spermatic cord until you reach a slit-like opening (Hesselbach's triangle). Ask the client to cough or bear down as you feel for bulges.

b. Palpate for femoral hernias by palpating below the femoral artery while having the client cough or bear down. ▼

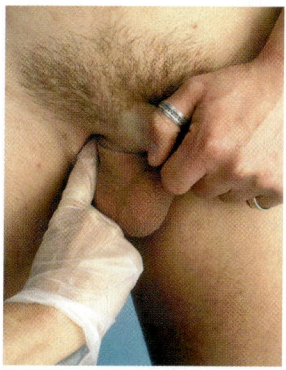

Expected findings: No bulges or palpable masses are present in the inguinal or femoral area.

Abnormal findings: A bulge or mass often represents a hernia.

Direct hernia: protrusion through the abdominal wall.

Indirect hernia: protrusion into the inguinal canal or into the scrotum.

(continued on next page)

Procedure 21–17 ■ Assessing the Male Genitourinary System (continued)

7. Palpate the lymph nodes in the groin area and the vertical chain over the inner aspect of the thigh.

Expected findings: Nodes should be < 1 cm in size and freely mobile.

Abnormal findings: Enlarged or tender lymph nodes may indicate local or systemic disease.

Also,

 Go to Chapter 21, **Tables, Boxes, Figures: ESG Table 21-3, Abnormal Atlas: Male Genitourinary System,** on DavisPlus.

Documentation

■ If you need more information about documenting your findings, review Caring for the Nguyens, including the box Documentation of Physical Assessment Findings for Nam Nguyen.

Tanner Staging			
STAGE	**PUBIC HAIR**	**PENIS**	**TESTES AND SCROTUM**
Stage 1: Preadolescent	No pubic hair except for fine body hair similar to that on abdomen	Same size and proportions as in childhood	Same size and proportions as in childhood
Stage 2	Sparse growth of long, slightly pigmented, downy hair, straight or only slightly curled, chiefly at base of penis	Slight or no enlargement	Testes larger, scrotum larger, somewhat reddened and altered in texture
Stage 3	Darker, coarser, curlier hair spreading sparsely over pubic symphysis	Larger, especially in length	Further enlarged
Stage 4	Coarse and curly hair, as in adult; area covered greater than in stage 3 but not as great as in adult	Further enlarged in length and breadth, with development of glans	Further enlarged; scrotal skin darkened

Tanner Staging—cont'd			
STAGE	**PUBIC HAIR**	**PENIS**	**TESTES AND SCROTUM**
Stage 5 Adult	Hair same as adult in quantity and quality, spreading to medial surfaces of thighs but not up over abdomen	Adult in size and shape	Adult in size and shape

Adapted from: Tanner, J. (1962). Growth at adolescence (2nd ed.). Oxford: Blackwell Scientific.

Procedure 21–18 ■ Assessing the Female Genitourinary System

➤ For steps to follow in *all* procedures, refer to the Universal Steps for All Procedures found on the page facing the inside back cover.

Equipment

- Patient drape
- Additional light source
- Nonlatex procedure gloves (if exposure to body fluids is a possibility)
- Pen and record form

Positioning

Place patient in the lithotomy position, if possible.

Developmental Modifications for Older Adults

- Assess for incontinence.
  Incontinence is one of the elements of the SPICES assessment model for older adults.
- Older women may have arthritis, which, along with muscle weakness, may make it difficult for them to assume the lithotomy position. You may need to use Sims' position and/or provide support for them to maintain a position.

Developmental Modifications for Children

- Obtain parental permission for this examination.
- Explain to the child what you are going to do, and expect some resistance or embarrassment.
  Children are taught to not let strangers touch their genitals, and many children are modest.
- Do not perform internal assessment of an adolescent unless the girl is sexually active.

Focused History Questions

- Are you having any problems urinating?
- Have you noticed any redness, swelling, discharge, or odor in your genital area?
- Have you ever been told you have a hernia?
- Have you ever had trauma to your genitals?
- Are you sexually active? If not, have you ever been?
- Do you have sex with men, women, or both?
- What types of sexual activity do you engage in? Oral, anal, or genital?
- How many partners do you currently have?
- How many partners have you had in the past 6 months?
- Do you use birth control? If so, what kind and how often?
- Have you ever been treated for a sexually transmitted infection (STI)? If so, what type?
- Are you concerned about STIs or HIV?
- Do you take any precautions to avoid infection?
- Do you have any concerns about your sexual function?
- Have you had any surgery of your reproductive tract?
- When was your last menstrual period?
- How often are your periods?
- Do you have any problems with your periods, such as cramping, breast pain, or heavy flow?
- How often do you have a gynecological health exam?
- When was your last Pap smear?
- Have you ever had an abnormal Pap smear? If so, how was it treated?
- How many times have you been pregnant?
- How many children do you have?
- Have you ever had a miscarriage? An abortion?

(continued on next page)

Procedure 21–18 ■ Assessing the Female Genitourinary System (continued)

➤ When performing the procedure, always identify your patient according to agency policy and be attentive to standard precautions, hand hygiene, patient safety and privacy, body mechanics, and documentation.

Procedure Steps

1. **Inspect the external genitalia.**

   a. Note the hair distribution pattern and the condition of pubic hair. See the table Maturation Status in Females at the end of this procedure.

   The appearance of the external genitalia depends on the developmental stage of the client.

   b. **Inspect the condition of the skin of the mons pubis and labia.** Observe for color, condition, lesions, and discharge.

Expected and Abnormal Findings

a. **Expected Findings:** Hair distribution in the pubic region is inverse triangular. Some hair may extend onto her abdomen and upper thighs. Hair distribution is appropriate for age. No pediculosis pubis (pubic lice).

Abnormal findings: Sparse or absent hair (may result from genetic factors, aging, or local or systemic disease); lice, **nits** (white lice eggs), or flecks of dried blood on the skin.

b. **Expected findings:** Skin is intact with no lesions or discharge. Labia majora and minora are symmetrical, with smooth to moderate wrinkling. Skin color is consistent with ethnicity. No ecchymosis, excoriation, nodules, edema, rash, or lesions are present.

Developmental Variations

Older adults—Labia and vulva are atrophied.

Abnormal findings: Ulcerations or lesions may occur with a number of STIs.

2. **Inspect the clitoris, urethral meatus, and vaginal introitus.**

   a. Wearing gloves, use your thumb and index finger to separate the labia and expose the clitoris. Observe the clitoris for size and position. ▼

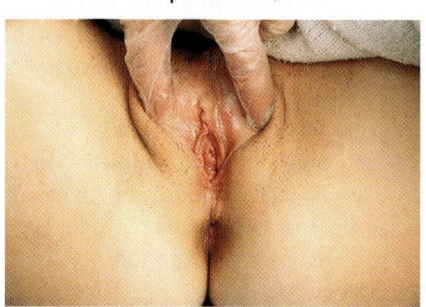

   b. With the labia separated, observe the urethral meatus and vaginal introitus. Observe for color, size, and presence of discharge or lesions.

   c. Have the client bear down while you observe the introitus.

a. **Expected findings:** The clitoris is about 2 cm long and 0.5 cm in diameter. No redness or lesions are present.

Abnormal findings: Enlargement of the clitoris may result from androgen excess or swelling related to trauma. Absence of the clitoris, along with parts of the labia, is seen with female circumcision.

b. **Expected findings:** The urethral meatus is slit-like; midline; and free of discharge, lesions, swelling, or erythema. The mucosa of the introitus is pink and moist. Some clear to white discharge may be present and is odor free.

c. **Expected findings:** The introitus is patent, and there is no bulging or discomfort with bearing down.

Abnormal findings: Discharge, redness, or swelling may result from infection. Pale and dry mucosa may result from aging or use of topical steroids. Bulging may indicate prolapse of the uterus, bladder, or rectum.

3. Palpate Bartholin's glands, the urethral glands, and Skene's ducts.
   a. Lubricate the index and middle fingers of your dominant hand with water-soluble lubricant.
   b. To palpate Bartholin's glands, insert your lubricated fingers into the vaginal introitus, and palpate the lower portion of the labia bilaterally between your thumb and fingers. ▼

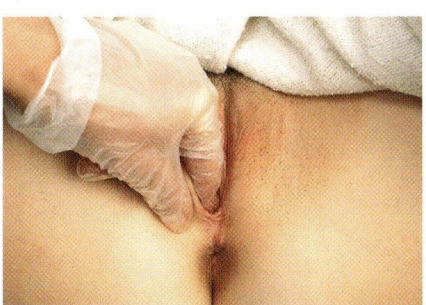

   c. To palpate Skene's ducts, rotate your internal fingers upward, and palpate the labium bilaterally. ▼

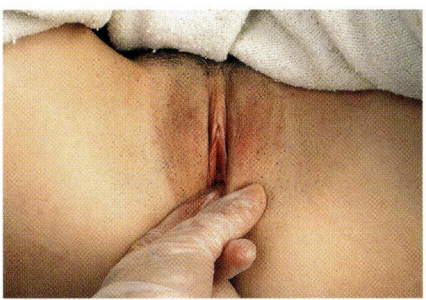

   d. To milk the urethra, apply pressure with your index finger on the anterior vaginal wall, and observe for urethral discharge. Culture any discharge you see.

Expected findings: No swelling, masses, or tenderness of the glands is/are present. There is no urethral discharge. The labia are uniform in texture, and there is no discharge or pain with palpation. The perineum is smooth and firm in **nulliparous** women (women who have had no children), thinner in **parous** women (women who have had children).

Abnormal findings: Pain or discharge from the glands may indicate infection. Fissures or tears in the perineum are painful and require treatment.

---

4. Assess vaginal muscle tone and pelvic musculature.
   a. Insert two gloved fingers into the vagina.
   b. Ask the woman to constrict her vaginal muscles and then to bear down as though she were having a bowel movement.

Expected findings: Muscle tone should be strong in women who have never given birth. With increasing **parity** (number of births), pelvic muscle tone diminishes. Diminished tone may also result from injury, age, or medication. No bulges should be noted.

---

5. Palpate the inguinal and femoral area for hernias.

Expected findings: No bulges or palpable masses are present in the inguinal or femoral area.

---

6. Palpate the lymph nodes in the groin area and the vertical chain over the inner aspect of the thigh.

Expected findings: Nodes should be < 1 cm in size and freely mobile.

Abnormal findings: Enlarged or tender lymph nodes may indicate local or systemic disease. Also,

 Go to Chapter 21, **Tables, Boxes, Figures: ESG Table 21-3, Abnormal Atlas: Female Genitourinary System,** on Davis*Plus*.

Documentation

- If you need more information about documenting your findings, review Caring for the Nguyens, including the box, Documentation of Physical Assessment Findings for Nam Nguyen.

(continued on next page)

Procedure 21–18 ■ Assessing the Female Genitourinary System (continued)

Maturation Status in Females

STAGE OF DEVELOPMENT	BREASTS	PUBIC HAIR
Stage 1. Prepuberty	Elevation of papilla.	No pubic hair except for fine body hair similar to hair on abdomen.
Stage 2	Breast bud. Elevation of breast and nipple and increased diameter of areola.	Sparse growth of long, slightly pigmented, downy hair, straight or only slightly curled, mostly along labia.
Stage 3	Areola deepens in color and enlarges further. Glandular tissue begins to develop beneath areola.	Hair becomes darker, coarser, and curlier and spreads sparsely over pubic symphysis.
Stage 4	Areola appears as a mound; breast appears as a mound; papilla and areola form a secondary mound.	Pubic hair is coarse and curly as in adults. It covers more area than in stage 3, but does not extend to the medial thighs.

Maturation Status in Females—cont'd		
STAGE OF DEVELOPMENT	**BREASTS**	**PUBIC HAIR**
Stage 5. Adult	Mature breast. Areola recesses to general contour of breast; nipple projects forward.	Quality and quantity are consistent with adult pubic hair distribution and spread over medial surfaces of thighs but not over abdomen.

Adapted from: Tanner, J. (1962). *Growth at adolescence* (2nd ed.). Oxford: Blackwell Scientific.

Procedure 21–19 ■ Assessing the Anus and Rectum

➤ For steps to follow in *all* procedures, refer to the Universal Steps for All Procedures found on the page facing the inside back cover.

Equipment
- Water-soluble lubricant
- Hemoccult test
- Nonlatex procedure gloves
- Pen and record form

Developmental Modification for Infants and Children
You will not usually perform a rectal exam on infants and children.

Focused History Questions
- Do you have any pain or discomfort around your anus?
- Do you ever have difficulty passing stool?
- Have you ever noticed blood on your stool or when you wipe?
- Do you have or have you ever been told you have hemorrhoids?
- For men, have you ever had a prostate exam or a prostate-specific antigen (PSA) blood test? If so, what were the results?

➤ When performing the procedure, always identify your patient according to agency policy and be attentive to standard precautions, hand hygiene, patient safety and privacy, and body mechanics.

Procedure Steps
1. **Inspect the anus.** Note the condition of the skin and the presence of any lesions.

Expected and Abnormal Findings
Expected findings: Anal area is intact, with no inflammation or lesions. Anus is a darker color than surrounding tissue.

Abnormal findings:
- A fissure or tear may be due to trauma, severe constipation, or an abscess.
- External hemorrhoids or skin tags may be visible.

2. **Palpate the anus and rectum.**
   a. For women, change gloves to prevent cross-contamination. Insert a lubricated index finger gently into the rectum. Palpate the rectal wall, noting masses or tenderness.

Expected findings: Good sphincter tone. Rectum is nontender. No palpable masses or hard stool. The stool is brown and negative for occult blood.

(continued on next page)

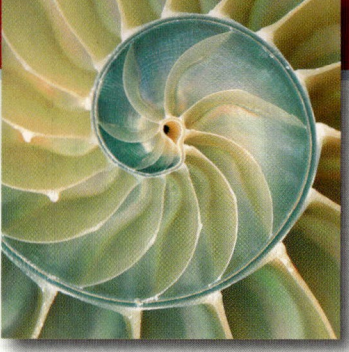

CHAPTER 22

Infection Prevention & Control

Learning Outcomes

After completing this chapter, you should be able to:

➤ Discuss the six links in the chain of infection.

➤ Describe the stages of a typical infectious process.

➤ Describe processes involved in the body's primary, secondary, and tertiary defenses.

➤ Identify activities that promote immune function.

➤ Discuss the factors that place an individual at increased risk for infection.

➤ Explain why it is important to be aware of emerging infectious diseases.

➤ Explain why multiple-drug-resistant pathogens are of special concern in healthcare.

➤ Use standard precautions to prevent transmission of infection through blood and body fluids.

➤ Describe additional precautions that must be taken when there is concern about contact, droplet, or airborne disease transmission.

➤ Compare and contrast methods of preventing infection by breaking the chain of infection.

➤ Implement measures to prevent healthcare-related infections.

➤ Use medical asepsis when providing care to clients.

➤ Discuss infection prevention and control measures in the home and community.

➤ Implement sterile technique in selected patient-care activities.

➤ Discuss the nurse's role in recognizing, preventing, and helping to contain the spread of a biological epidemic.

Key Concepts

Infection

Medical asepsis

Surgical asepsis

Body defenses

Infection prevention and control

Related Concepts

See the Concept Map at the end of this chapter.

Example Problems

Drug-Resistant Pathogens

Caring for the Nguyens

This feature allows you to practice the kind of thinking you will use as a full-spectrum nurse. There is usually more than one correct answer to a critical thinking question, so we do not provide answers for these features. It is more important to develop your nursing judgment than to "cover content." Discuss the questions with your peers. If you are still unsure, consult your instructor.

Mrs. Nguyen works as a preschool teacher in her community. Kim, her grandchild, has been attending the preschool since he came to live with his grandparents. Mrs. Nguyen tells you at a recent visit to the clinic that Kim has had "a lot of problems with colds and a runny nose since he started preschool."

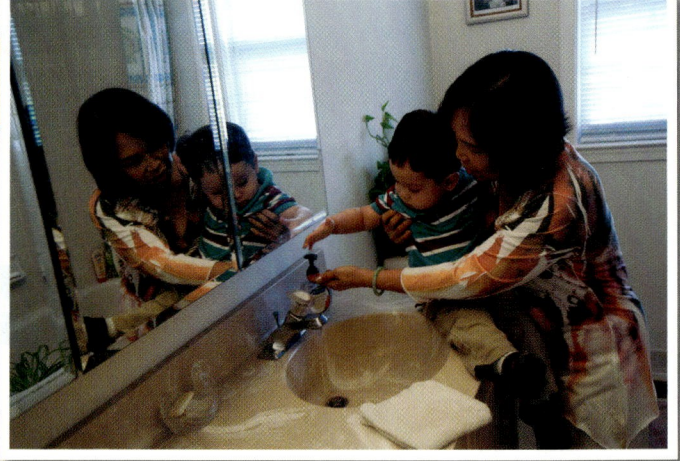

Caring for the Nguyens (continued)

A. Based on your theoretical knowledge of asepsis and immunity, what is the most likely explanation for Kim's symptoms?

B. Do you have enough patient data to make any conclusions? If not, what other information should you gather?

C. Identify three alternatives that may explain what is happening.

D. What strategies could you recommend that Mrs. Nguyen implement at the preschool to help limit the number of infections? Identify at least two strategies.

 Go to **Caring for the Nguyens Response Sheet** on *DavisPlus*.

Meet Your Nursing Role Model

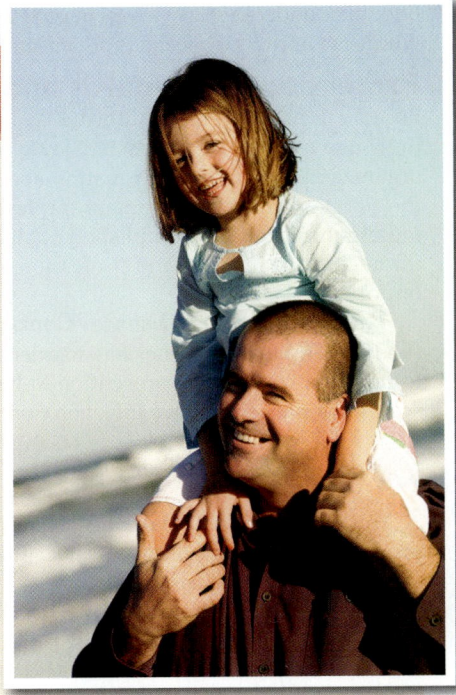

Stephanie Sergi is the 7-year-old daughter of Jason Sergi. Jason works as a nurse on a busy labor and delivery unit in a major medical center. One night at the dinner table, Stephanie asks, "Daddy, what was the most important thing you did at work today?" Jason takes a few minutes to consider his reply. Finally Jason answers, "I washed my hands—a lot."

Jason tells his daughter that he also assisted in the birth of five infants, resuscitated one of the infants who was initially struggling for breath, and identified several problems that prevented complications or even death of mothers in labor. "Daddy, I don't understand why you think washing your hands was so important," Stephanie protested. "Look at all the *really* important things you did today!"

As you read this chapter, think back to Jason's discussion with his daughter. Perhaps you will someday say the same thing to your child or anyone who asks about your day.

Theoretical Knowledge
knowing **why**

Theoretical knowledge about infections continues to grow. New infectious microorganisms are being discovered, and researchers are currently investigating the role of viruses in the development of cancer and other diseases. For example, virally induced cancers include Hodgkin's disease, Kaposi's sarcoma, and cervical cancer. Other research is investigating the role that certain species of bacteria play in producing heart disease (e.g., Spahr, Klein, Khuseyinova, et al., 2006).

ABOUT THE KEY CONCEPTS

A grasp of the broad concept of infection will enable you to promote biological safety for your clients, using infection prevention and control activities. Those activities include medical and surgical asepsis and interventions to support patients' body defenses.

WHY MUST NURSES KNOW ABOUT INFECTION PROCESSES?

The goals of infection prevention and control discussed in this section are to:
- Protect patients from healthcare-related and other infections.
- Meet professional standards and guidelines.
- Protect yourself from diseases. You must know how to avoid contact with infectious material and exposure to diseases such as hepatitis B and C, and drug-resistant tuberculosis, as well as the many common illness-producing microorganisms you will encounter.
- Help lower the cost of healthcare. In hospitals alone, healthcare-associated infections add billions of dollars annually in healthcare costs.

In this chapter, you will learn how infections occur and about measures to prevent them. We will discuss healthcare-associated infections and related professional standards and guidelines.

Healthcare-Associated Infections

Healthcare-associated infection (HAI) refers to infections associated with healthcare given in any setting (e.g., hospitals, home care, long-term care, and ambulatory settings). The older term, **nosocomial** infection, refers more specifically to hospital-acquired infections. HAIs aggravate existing illness and lengthen recovery time. They are the leading complication of hospital care and one of the 10 leading causes of death in the United States (Agency for Healthcare Research and Quality, 2009; Klevens, Morrison, Nadle, et al., 2007; Siegel, Rhinehart, Jackson, et al., 2007). You may be surprised at these facts. After all, the healthcare system is supposed to cure, not harm, people. But when people come to hospitals (and other facilities) for care, they come into contact with many care providers and patients who can transmit pathogens to them. Ill patients are vulnerable to infection, and they are a source of infection for others. In addition, they undergo many invasive procedures (e.g., injections), which can introduce infectious organisms into their bodies.

Professional Standards and Guidelines

Because HAIs increase healthcare costs and patient suffering, many states have enacted laws requiring healthcare organizations to make information about HAIs available to the public. Various government, professional, and accrediting organizations have published quality-control guidelines for healthcare agencies and professionals. The following are important examples:

The Centers for Disease Control and Prevention (CDC). This federal agency has an extensive Web site devoted to infection control and prevention in healthcare settings. To access this site and retrieve Infection Control Guidelines,

 Go to http://www.cdc.gov/hai/

You will find many of your healthcare facility's policies and procedures to be based on the CDC guidelines. Among the CDC goals for healthcare are to:

- Reduce catheter-associated adverse events [e.g., infections] by 50% . . . in healthcare settings.
- Reduce targeted antimicrobial-resistant bacterial infections by 50% . . . preventing transmission in healthcare settings.

The Agency for Healthcare Research and Quality (AHRQ). Web site features links to information, tools, and resources on HAIs for both healthcare providers and consumers. It also highlights AHRQ-funded research and initiatives to reduce HAIs. To access this site,

 Go to http://www.ahrq.gov/qual/hais.htm

The Joint Commission. This is a quality oversight agency. Their standards of performance include extensive criteria describing what healthcare organizations must do to minimize the risks of infection. In addition, Goal 7 of their National Patient Safety Goals for 2011 is to "reduce the risk of health care associated infections" (The Joint Commission, 2010). They include strategies for healthcare providers to prevent infection in inpatient and community-based settings. To read these initiatives,

 Go to http://www.jointcommission.org/assets/1/6/2011_NPSGs_HAP.pdf

Quality and Safety Education for Nurses (QSEN). This is a group of educators that was formed to identify the competencies necessary to improve the quality and safety of nurses' places of work. Safety is one of the six competencies you should have on completing your nursing education. Although QSEN does not specifically say so, you should assume safety includes being safe from infection. For example, you should be able to:

- Demonstrate knowledge of basic scientific methods and processes [e.g., infectious process, inflammatory process].
- Minimize risk of harm to patients and providers [e.g., infectious diseases] through both system effectiveness and individual performance.
- Demonstrate effective use of technology and standardized practice [e.g., CDC guidelines for infection control] that support safety and quality.

To access the QSEN Web site and see the other competencies,

 Go to http://www.qsen.org

American Nurses Association (ANA). Using the same broad understanding as for the QSEN competencies, you should assume that the following examples criteria from Standard 5 of the ANA *Nursing: Scope & Standards of Practice* (2010) apply to infection prevention and control:

- Partners with the person/family/significant others/caregiver to implement the plan in a safe and timely manner.
- Implements the plan in a timely manner in accordance with the patient safety goals.

HOW DOES INFECTION OCCUR?

Imagine that your clinical instructor alerts you to an outbreak of infectious disease in the hospital where you have your assignment. The hospital census is currently more than 200 patients. So far, 14 have become infected, and one has died. Would that prompt you to wonder how infections are spread and why they seem to affect some people more than others?

Infections Develop in Response to a Chain of Factors

The process by which infections spread is commonly referred to as the **chain of infection.** It is made up of six links (described below), all of which must be present for the infection to be transmitted from one individual to another (Fig. 22-1). Later in the chapter we discuss how to interrupt the chain to limit the spread of infection. For information about common disease-producing microorganisms and their transmission,

 Go to Chapter 22, **Tables, Boxes, Figures: ESG Table 22-1, Common Pathogens,** on Davis*Plus.*

Infectious Agent

Some microorganisms live on or in the human body without causing harm. For instance, the *Staphylococcus* bacteria growing on human skin are usually harmless. Other microorganisms are beneficial or even essential for human health and well-being. They are referred to as **normal flora.** Normal flora in the intestine aid in digestion; synthesize vitamin K; and release vitamin B_{12}, thiamine, and riboflavin when they die. In addition, they limit the growth of harmful bacteria by competing with them for available nutrients.

There are two types of normal flora: transient and resident. **Transient flora** are normal microbes that a person picks up by coming in contact with objects or another person (e.g., when you touch a soiled dressing). You can remove these with handwashing. **Resident flora** live and multiply harmlessly deep in skin layers. They are permanent inhabitants of the skin, and cannot usually be removed with routine handwashing.

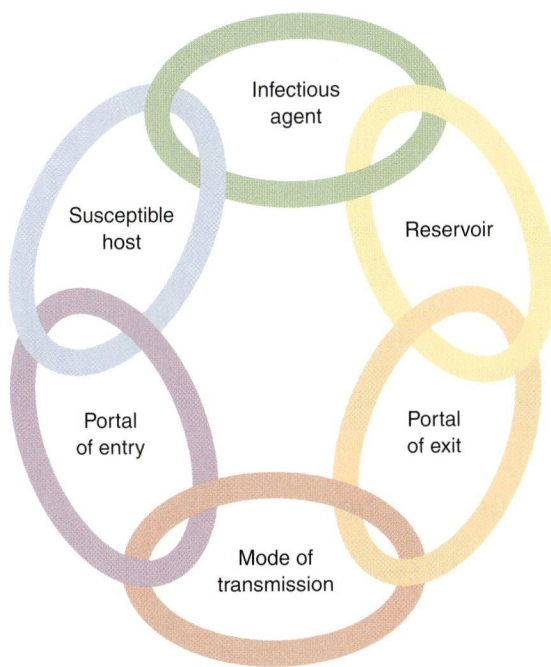

FIGURE 22-1 All six links in the chain of infection must be present for infection to be transmitted from one person to another.

Pathogens are microorganisms capable of causing disease. In fact, the precise accepted definition of the term **infection** is successful invasion of and multiplication in the body by a pathogen). The largest groups of pathogenic microorganisms are bacteria, viruses, and fungi (which include yeasts and molds). Less common pathogens are protozoa, **helminths** (commonly called worms), and **prions**, which are infectious protein particles that cause certain neurological diseases. In addition, normal flora may become pathogenic when a patient is especially vulnerable to disease, or if they enter the deep tissues or body regions they do not normally inhabit. For instance, rupture of the bowel through trauma or disease allows intestinal microbes to enter the abdominal cavity or bloodstream, where they cause infection.

Once a pathogen gains entry into a host, four factors determine whether the person develops infection:

- **Virulence** of the organism (its power to cause disease)
- Ability of the organism to survive in the host environment
- Number of organisms (the greater the number, the more likely they are to cause disease)
- Ability of the host's defenses to prevent infection

Reservoir

A **reservoir** is a source of infection: a place where pathogens survive and multiply. The human body is the most common reservoir for pathogens. Animals and insects are other living reservoirs. Nonliving reservoirs include soil, water, food, and environmental surfaces. Examples include contaminated water, garbage, soiled diapers, and wound dressings. In healthcare facilities, many surfaces act as reservoirs. Microorganisms have mass, and they eventually fall to the floor or onto bedside tables, chairs, or equipment. Other surfaces, such as sinks, toilets, bed rails, and bed linens, may also become reservoirs because of their proximity to patients, family members, and healthcare providers harboring pathogens.

Some people, called **carriers,** are capable of defending themselves from active disease but harbor the pathogenic organisms within their bodies. They have no symptoms, yet they serve as reservoirs and can pass the disease to others.

Most pathogens prefer a warm, moist, dark environment. To live and thrive in humans, microbes must be able to use the body's precise balance of food, moisture, nutrients, electrolytes, pH, temperature, and light. Food, water, and soil that provide these conditions may serve as nonliving reservoirs, as well.

Nutrients. Bacteria can rapidly multiply in food left at room temperature. For example, the bacteria *Salmonella enteritidis*, which causes salmonellosis ("food poisoning"), can multiply in raw and undercooked meat and eggs. To prevent the growth of pathogens, many foods are cooked at high temperatures and stored in a cool environment to limit the growth of pathogenic microbes. Another way to inhibit bacterial growth is by using highly concentrated solutes, such as salting meat and the preserving with pectin in fruit jellies, jams, and preserves.

Moisture. Pathogens require moisture for survival, for example, the moist environment of wounds, the genitourinary tract, and the throat and airways. However, the spores formed by some bacteria allow them to live without water (e.g., the *Bacillus* and *Clostridium* species, both of which cause food-borne disease).

Temperature. For most pathogens, the ideal temperature is 95°F (35°C). Environments that are either too hot or too cold for a particular species will slow its growth or even kill the entire population. In part, the microbes that are pathogenic to humans are so because they thrive at about the same temperature as the human body. Thus, the body produces a fever in response to infection to inhibit and even kill invading pathogens.

Oxygen. Many bacteria and most protozoa and fungi are **aerobic.** That is, they must have oxygen to live and grow. For example, the yeast *Candida albicans* causes infections in the oral mucosa ("thrush") and the vaginal mucosa. **Anaerobic organisms** do not require oxygen for growth and may even be killed in its presence. One example is *Clostridium tetani,* a spore-forming bacterium, which causes tetanus when a spore enters the body through an open wound.

pH and Electrolytes. To live in humans, pathogens need the body's precise balance of moisture, sugars, pH (acidity), and electrolytes. Most prefer a pH range of 5 to 8. Therefore, they cannot survive in the highly acidic environment of the stomach. When patients take antacids, stomach pH increases (acidity decreases) and removes this defense. The organisms multiply and can then cause infection in other systems, such as the lungs. Microbes that have a higher or lower pH and electrolyte concentration than the human body are not pathogenic to human beings. That's why, for example, the bacteria that thrive in the Great Salt Lake would not cause infection on your skin.

Light. Microbes grow best in dark environments (e.g., inside the body, deep in wounds, and under dressings). Ultraviolet light is sometimes used to remove pathogens such as *Staphylococcus, Salmonella,* and viruses from surgical instruments and other objects. It is also used to disinfect drinking water in developing countries to prevent diseases such as cholera and typhoid fever.

KnowledgeCheck 22-1

- What is a pathogen?
- What is the role of normal flora?
- Identify at least five reservoirs of infection.

Portal of Exit

A contained reservoir is only a potential source of infection. For infection to spread, a pathogen must exit the reservoir. In the case of human or animal reservoirs, the most frequent **portal of exit** is through body fluids, including blood, mucus, saliva, breast milk, urine, feces, vomitus, semen, or other secretions. The body's natural response to foreign materials, including pathogens, is to try to expel them. If you have a pathogen in the respiratory system, you cough and sneeze. If it is in the gastrointestinal system, you vomit or experience intestinal cramping and diarrhea. Microbes responsible for sexually transmitted infections can exit via semen, vaginal secretions, or blood that is present during sex.

Cuts, bites, and abrasions also provide an exit for body fluid. Blood and pus seeping from a wound help transport pathogens away from the broken skin but become a portal by which infection may be transmitted to others. In healthcare-related infections, puncture sites, drainage tubes, feeding tubes, and intravenous lines commonly serve as routes for pathogens to exit the body.

Mode of Transmission

Contact, either direct or indirect, is the most frequent **mode of transmission** of infection. **Direct contact** between two people usually involves touching, kissing, or sexual intercourse. Animals commonly transmit infection via scratching and biting as well. **Indirect contact** involves contact with a **fomite,** a contaminated object that transfers a pathogen. For example, suppose that while you are charting you begin to sneeze or cough. If you cover your nose and mouth with your hand and then resume charting, you may transmit pathogens to the pen, paper, and chart (or keyboard). Shoes, eyeglasses, stethoscopes, and other items we wear also commonly serve as fomites, as do contaminated needles. Some microbes can live only a few seconds on fomites; others can live for years. It depends on the type of microorganism and the environment.

Droplet transmission occurs when the pathogen travels in water droplets expelled as an infected person exhales, coughs, sneezes, or talks. It may also occur during suctioning and oral care. The usual method of transmission is for the droplet to be inhaled or enter the eye of a susceptible person. Although droplets can travel only a few feet from the infectious person, within that distance they may readily contaminate fomites that then transmit the organism by contact.

Airborne transmission occurs with much smaller organisms that can float considerable distances on air currents. Airborne pathogens can travel through heating and air conditioning systems to infect large numbers of people. Sweeping a floor or shaking out contaminated bed linens can stir up airborne microorganisms and launch them on air currents—think of a flying magic carpet (of pathogens). The agents of measles and tuberculosis, as well as many fungal infections, are commonly transmitted in this manner.

A **vector** is an organism that carries a pathogen to a susceptible host, typically by biting or stinging, creating another portal of entry into the body. The mosquito is a common vector for diseases, including malaria, yellow fever, and the West Nile virus. Ticks, fleas, mites, and other insects also carry various diseases.

Portal of Entry

Pathogens can enter the body through various **portals of entry.** Normal body openings, such as the conjunctiva of the eye, the nares (nostrils), mouth, urethra, vagina, and anus are potential portals of entry, as are abnormal openings, such as cuts, scrapes, and surgical incisions. Vectors, such as mosquitoes, create portals of entry when they bite through the skin. In healthcare settings, common portals of entry include wounds, surgical sites, and insertion sites for tubes or needles.

Susceptible Host

A **susceptible** (or compromised) **host** is a person who is at risk for infection because of inadequate defenses against the invading pathogen. Various factors can increase susceptibility to infection, among them: age (the very young or very old), compromised immune system (as in those receiving immune suppression for organ transplantation or treatment of cancer or chronic illness), and immune deficiency conditions (e.g., HIV, leukemia).

KnowledgeCheck 22-2

- Identify the six links in the chain of infection.
- What kinds of microbes favor the human body as a reservoir of infection?

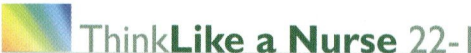 **ThinkLike a Nurse** 22-1

You are working as a nurse on a medical–surgical unit. What roles might you play in the chain of infection?

Infections Can Be Classified by Location and Duration

Infections are classified according to their location in the body, whether it is the patient's first infection, where it was acquired, and how long it lasts.

Local or Systemic. Some infections cause harm in a limited region of the body, such as the upper respiratory tract, the urethra, or a single bone or joint. Such infections are said to be **local.** In contrast, **systemic** infections occur when pathogens invade the blood or lymph and spread throughout the body. **Bacteremia** is the clinical presence of bacteria in the blood, whereas **septicemia** is symptomatic systemic infection spread via the blood.

Primary or Secondary. A **primary infection** is the first infection that occurs in a patient. Especially in immunocompromised patients, one or more **secondary infections** may follow a primary infection. For example, a frail client infected with pneumonia may develop herpes zoster (shingles), a viral infection related to past infection with varicella, secondary to the stress of illness.

Exogenous or Endogenous. Healthcare providers need to determine the source of pathogens in a patient infected while he is in the facility. In **exogenous healthcare-related infections,** the pathogen is acquired from the healthcare environment. In **endogenous healthcare-related infections,** the pathogen arises from the patient's normal flora, when some form of treatment (e.g., chemotherapy or antibiotics) causes the normally harmless microbe to multiply and cause infection. For example, candidal vaginitis (yeast infection) may develop in a client receiving antibiotics after surgery.

Acute or Chronic. Infections that have a rapid onset but last only a short time (e.g., the common cold) are said to be **acute.** In contrast, **chronic infections** (e.g., an abscess) develop slowly and last for weeks, months, or even years. Some chronic infections, such as relapsing fever, recur after periods of remission. **Latent infections** cause no symptoms for long periods of time, even decades. Tuberculosis and human

immunodeficiency virus (HIV) are examples. HIV typically causes an initial, brief illness that is then followed by about 10 years of latency before the patient begins to experience symptoms of AIDS.

Infections Follow Predictable Stages

Many infections follow a fairly predictable course of events, although the precise duration and intensity of symptoms in each stage vary from one individual to another:

- **Incubation** is the stage between successful invasion of the pathogen into the body and the first appearance of symptoms. In this stage, the person does not suspect that he has been infected but may be capable of infecting others. This stage may last only a day, as with the influenza virus, or as long as several months or even years, as with tuberculosis.
- The **prodromal stage** is characterized by the first appearance of vague symptoms. For example, a person infected with a cold virus may experience a mild throat irritation. Not all infections have a prodromal stage.
- **Illness** is the stage marked by the appearance of the signs and symptoms characteristic of the disease. If the patient's immune defenses and medical treatments (if any) are ineffective, this stage can end in the death of the patient.
- **Decline** is the stage during which the patient's immune defenses, along with any medical therapies, successfully reduce the number of pathogenic microbes. As a result, the signs and symptoms of the infection begin to fade.
- **Convalescence** is characterized by tissue repair and a return to health as the remaining number of microorganisms approaches zero. Convalescence may require only a day or two or, for severe infections, as long as a year or more.

Why Must Nurses Be Aware of Emerging Pathogens and Diseases?

Continental and intercontinental travel allow for many ways of spreading emerging diseases. Infected travelers serve as reservoirs for pathogens. The close quarters and recirculated air systems in airplanes provide an ideal environment for the transmission of airborne pathogens and for both direct and indirect contact contamination between passengers. Air travel also enables a person to infect many people headed for widespread locations, often even before the reservoir person shows symptoms of the disease. The 2003 severe acute respiratory syndrome (SARS) outbreak is a good example of flight travel as a means of transmission: A Chinese physician unknowingly infected at least a dozen guests at a hotel in Hong Kong where he was staying; the guests then flew to Vietnam, Singapore, and Canada, prompting outbreaks in those countries.

An **epidemic** is an outbreak of a disease that suddenly affects a large group of people in a geographic region (e.g., a city or state) or in a defined population group (e.g., children, healthcare workers). A **pandemic** is an exceptionally widespread epidemic—that is, one that affects a large number of people in an entire country or worldwide. Examples of pandemics are H1N1 influenza ("swine flu") and malaria. You should also know the term **emerging infectious disease.** Although there are various definitions, you can think of emerging infectious diseases as:

- Newly identified diseases caused by an unrecognized microorganism (e.g., the virus causing AIDS was unknown before 1980) or by a known organism (e.g., *Streptococcus* infection causing toxic shock syndrome).
- Diseases occurring in new geographic areas (e.g., West Nile virus in the Western hemisphere) or settings (e.g., *Clostridium*

difficile was primarily a hospital-acquired infection and now occurs in the community).

- Microorganisms in animals that extend their host range to begin infecting humans (e.g., avian influenza, or "bird flu," and later the H1N1 virus from swine).
- Microbes that evolve to become more virulent (e.g., a strain of *Escherichia coli*, which now causes severe illness).
- Known diseases that dramatically increase in incidence (e.g., mumps and pertussis, also known as whooping cough).
- Organisms that are deliberately altered for bioterrorism (e.g., the contamination of some mail in the United States with *Bacillus anthracis* [anthrax] in 2001).
- Most emerging pathogens are viruses. For a brief discussion of some important emerging infections,

 Go to Chapter 22, **Supplemental Materials: Emerging Infectious Diseases,** and **Reading More About Infection Prevention & Control,** on Davis*Plus.*

Cooperative efforts among many disciplines and organizations worldwide are required to limit the spread of infectious diseases. To this end, the World Health Organization (WHO) has chosen as the first "global patient safety challenge" the reduction of healthcare-associated infection (WHO, 2008). Also, The Joint Commission (2008a) requires hospitals to have an emergency management plan for responding to large numbers of infectious patients who might need to be treated as a result of an epidemic.

Example Problem: Drug-Resistant Pathogens

Some microorganisms, mostly bacteria, have mutated to develop resistance to one or more classes of antimicrobial drugs. These organisms are said to be **drug-resistant or multidrug-resistant.** Today antibiotic resistance is one of the most significant challenges in treating patients with severe infectious diseases. During the last several decades, the prevalence of multidrug-resistant organisms (MDROs) in U.S. hospitals and medical centers has increased steadily. MDROs are a serious problem because options for treating MDRO infections are limited. Furthermore, they are associated with serious illness, increased mortality, and increased hospital lengths of stay and costs.

A variety of risk factors are associated with MDRO infections (CDC, n.d.a, last modified 2010). Among them are the following:

- Severe illness.
- Previous exposure to antimicrobial agents (e.g., antibiotics).
- Underlying diseases or conditions that make it difficult for the person to fight infection (in particular, chronic renal disease, insulin-dependent diabetes mellitus, peripheral vascular disease, dermatitis, skin lesions).
- Invasive procedures and devices, such as dialysis, urinary catheterization, and intravenous lines.
- Repeated contact with the healthcare system, especially acute care facilities and intensive care units (where infection rates tend to be highest).
- Advanced age.

MDROs are transmitted by the same routes as other microorganisms. A major factor, though, is transmission in healthcare settings via the hands of healthcare workers, especially for methicillin-resistant *Staphylococcus aureus* (MRSA), *Clostridium difficile,* and vancomycin-resistant enterococci (VRE), which are summarized below. Other significant MDROs include multidrug-resistant tuberculosis (MDR-TB),

penicillin-resistant *Streptococcus pneumoniae,* multidrug-resistant *E. coli,* and *Klebsiella pneumoniae.* If you need more information about diseases caused by those seven organisms, consult a medical–surgical textbook or,

 Go to Chapter 22, **Supplemental Materials: What Are Drug-Resistant Pathogens?** on Davis*Plus.*

- **Methicillin-Resistant** *Staphylococcus aureus* **(MRSA).** More than a million hospitalized patients acquire MRSA infection each year in the United States (Association for Professionals in Infection Control and Epidemiology [APIC], 2010; Elixhauser & Steiner, 2007); it can be fatal. The organism is spread by skin-to-skin contact and by living in crowded conditions. Control of MRSA has become a national priority.
- **Vancomycin-Resistant** *Enterococci* **(VRE).** Most VRE infections occur in hospitals. Their spread is attributed to failure to follow infection control measures (Rice, 2001). Risk factors include previous long-term antibiotic treatment, weakened immune system, surgical procedures, long-term devices (e.g., urinary catheters), or colonization with VRE (CDC, 2008).
- *Clostridium difficile.* The elderly and people who have had prolonged treatment with antibiotics are at greater risk for this disease. The bacteria are found in the feces. *C. difficile* thrives in unsanitary hospital environments and spores can survive for days on inanimate objects such as doorknobs and toilet seats.

 Think**Like a Nurse** 22-2

- Why are emerging infections of special concern in healthcare?
- Why are multidrug-resistant organisms (MDROs) of special concern in healthcare?

WHAT ARE THE BODY'S DEFENSES AGAINST INFECTION?

The human body has three "lines of defense" against infectious disease:

- Certain anatomical features limit the entry of pathogens.
- Protective biochemical processes fight pathogens that do enter.
- The presence of pathogens activates immune responses against specific, recognized invaders.

The first two lines of defense are nonspecific; that is, they have no means of adapting their response to each specific invader. Instead, they act in precisely the same way against any and all intruders, from a simple cold virus to deadly fungal spores.

Primary Defenses

The "soldiers" in the first line of defense are the structural barriers of the human body. These **primary defenses** prevent organisms from entering the body. The normal flora of the body provide one such defense. Any treatment that disturbs the balance between the normal flora and other microorganisms can increase the risk of developing disease. For example, when broad-spectrum antibiotics are used to treat infection, they may eliminate normal flora in addition to those causing the infection. This allows other kinds of pathogens to multiply, producing a **superinfection.** Other primary defenses are as follows:

- *Skin.* Intact, healthy skin prevents entry of many pathogens. Normal skin flora inhibit multiplication of other organisms that land on the skin.

- *The respiratory tree.* The nares, trachea, and bronchi are covered with mucous membranes that trap pathogens. The nose contains hairs that filter the upper airway; the nasal passages, sinuses, trachea, and larger bronchi are lined with **cilia**, tiny hairlike cells that sweep microorganisms upward from the lower airways. Coughing and sneezing forcefully expel organisms from the respiratory tract.
- *Eyes.* The lacrimal glands produce tears that contain lysozyme, an antimicrobial enzyme. The tears help wash infective organisms from the eyes.
- *The mouth.* The mouth normally has a large number of pathogenic microorganisms, but saliva, like tears, contains lysozyme and continually washes microbes from the teeth and gums. The rich blood supply of the mouth swiftly transports defensive blood cells (discussed later in this section) that keep the microorganisms in check. In addition, normal flora of the mouth compete for nutrition with invading organisms, thereby limiting the number of pathogens.
- *The gastrointestinal tract.* Many pathogens are destroyed in its acidic environment of the stomach. Those that successfully enter the small intestine face the antimicrobial action of bile. Simple peristalsis, as well as diarrhea and vomiting, remove pathogens that invade the gastrointestinal tract. In addition, normal flora in the intestine secrete antibacterial substances.
- *The genitourinary tract.* The epithelial cells lining the mucous membranes of the urethra, vagina, and anus secrete mucus, which adheres to pathogens to promote their excretion through urine and stool. Urine itself is highly acidic and contains lysozyme (an antibacterial enzyme). In addition the high acidity and normal flora of the vagina keep pathogens in check.

Secondary Defenses

Pathogens that dodge the primary defenses and gain entry into the body begin to release wastes and secretions and to cause the breakdown of cells and tissues. The presence of such chemicals activates a set of **secondary defenses.**

Phagocytosis. The process by which **phagocytes** (specialized white blood cells [WBCs]) engulf and destroy pathogens directly is called **phagocytosis.** Phagocytic WBCs include neutrophils, monocytes, and eosinophils. Table 22-1 summarizes the types of WBCs and their roles in defending against infection.

Complement Cascade. The complement cascade is a process by which a set of blood proteins, called *complement,* triggers the release of chemicals that attack the cell membranes of pathogens, causing them to rupture. Complement also signals basophils (WBCs), to release histamine, which prompts inflammation.

Inflammation. The inflammatory process begins when histamine and other chemicals are released either from damaged cells, or from basophils being activated by complement. With inflammation, blood vessels dilate and become more permeable, which increases the flow of phagocytes, antimicrobial chemicals, oxygen, and nutrients to the affected area. The classic signs and symptoms of inflammation are localized warmth and erythema (redness), which develop as blood flow is increased. In addition, fluid leaking from the more permeable blood vessels accumulates in the surrounding tissue, causing edema, which in turn prompts pain as pressure is exerted on nerve endings.

Fever. Fever is a rise in core body temperature that increases metabolism, inhibits multiplication of pathogens, and triggers specific immune responses (discussed shortly). Believing that low-grade fevers are a necessary natural

Table 22-1 ➤ Types and Functions of White Blood Cells

TYPE	FUNCTION
Granular WBCs	
Basophils: 0.5%–1% of total WBCs	Release histamine and heparin granules as part of the inflammatory response. Percentage normal during infections.
Eosinophils: 1%–3% of total WBCs	Bind to helminthes and release toxins to destroy them; mediate allergic reactions; have limited role in phagocytosis. Percentage increases in parasitic infections.
Neutrophils: 55%–70% of total WBCs	Phagocytize pathogens
Agranular WBCs	
Lymphocytes: 20%–35% of total WBCs	T cells—responsible for cell-mediated immunity; recognize, attack, and destroy antigens.
	B cells—responsible for humoral immunity; produce immunoglobulins to attack and destroy antigens. Percentage of total lymphocytes increases in viral infection and chronic bacterial infection; decreases in sepsis.
Monocytes: 3%–8% of total WBCs	Able to phagocytize directly as well as to differentiate into macrophages, which help clean up damaged tissue, infection, and cellular debris. Percentage increases in tuberculosis, protozoal, and rickettsial infections.

Note: Laboratory values alone are not adequate for diagnosing infection. Presence of clinical signs (e.g., fever, pus, swelling) must be assessed.

defense mechanism, many clinicians do not treat a fever unless it's greater than 102°F (38.9°C).

Tertiary Defenses

Why is it that people who recover from an infectious disease such as measles or chickenpox never get the disease again, even if they are repeatedly exposed to the virus? The answer lies in **specific immunity:** the process by which the body's immune cells "learn" to recognize and destroy pathogens they have encountered before.

The cells involved in specific immunity are the **lymphocytes,** WBCs produced from stem cells in the red bone marrow. *B lymphocytes,* or *B cells,* grow to maturity in the bone marrow, whereas *T lymphocytes,* or *T cells,* mature in the thymus. After maturing, most B cells and T cells travel to the lymph nodes, spleen, and other sites of lymphatic tissue. Some circulate in blood and lymph. From all of these locations, lymphocytes seek out foreign cells and other matter to target for destruction. Lymphocytes recognize foreign substances by the molecules present on their surfaces. These

molecules that trigger a specific immune response are called **antigens.** The two types of specific immunity involving B cells and T cells are discussed next.

Humoral Immunity

The humoral immune response acts directly against antigens. In response to the presence of antigens, macrophages and a class of T cells called *helper T cells* stimulate B cells to become plasma cells and produce **antibodies,** also called **immunoglobulins (Ig).** Antibodies are proteins with a base region and two arms (somewhat like the letter *Y*). They bind to target antigens and destroy them by any of the following methods (Fig. 22-2):

- *Phagocytosis.* Antibodies signal leukocytes (macrophages and neutrophils) to phagocytize the pathogens to which the antibodies are bound.
- *Neutralization.* By binding to a pathogen's attachment sites, antibodies disable the pathogens' machinery for adhering to and invading body cells. Thus, the pathogens are effectively neutralized.
- *Agglutination.* Antibodies have two attachment sites; therefore, each antibody can attach to two pathogenic cells in a population. This quality causes the pathogens to clump together (agglutinate), reducing their activity and increasing the likelihood that the group will be detected and phagocytized by leukocytes.
- *Activation of complement and inflammation.* Antibodies trigger the complement cascade and stimulate the release of inflammatory chemicals to destroy the antigen.

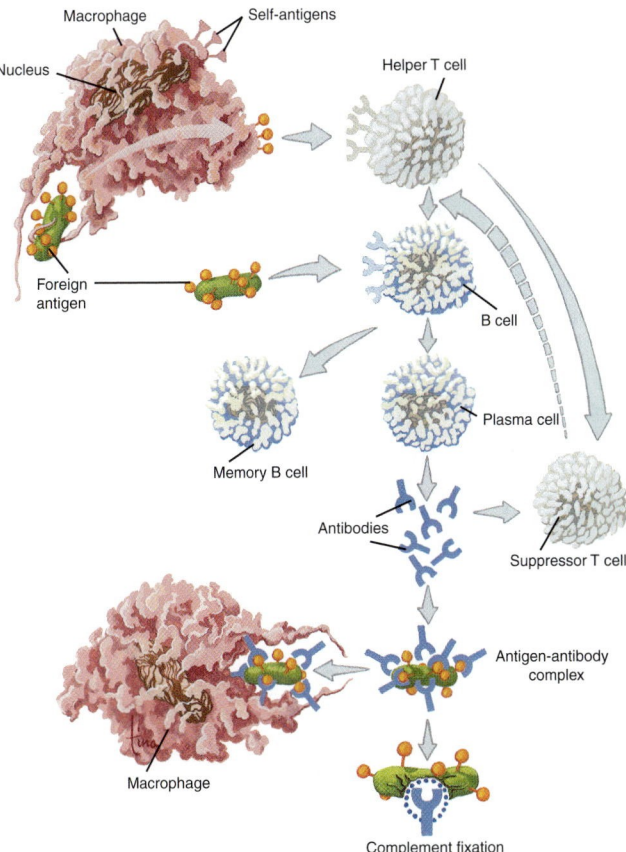

FIGURE 22-2 The humoral immune response produces antibodies to destroy antigens.

Five classes of antibodies, or immunoglobulins (Igs), are secreted by B lymphocytes. They are usually written as IgM, IgG, IgA, IgD, and IgE.

- IgM is the first antibody to appear when an antigen is encountered for the first time.
- IgG is the most common immunoglobulin in the body. It takes at least 10 days for IgG to be produced in response to an initial infection. IgG is the only immunoglobulin that can cross the placenta to provide temporary immunity to the fetus/infant. Small amounts are also found in breast milk.
- IgE is the immunoglobulin primarily responsible for the allergic response.
- IgD antibodies form on the surface of B cells and trap potential pathogens.
- IgA antibodies are secreted by mucous membranes around body openings, in the intestines, respiratory and urinary tracts, saliva, tears, and in breast milk. IgA provides additional immune protection by secreting around the body openings.

For more information about the five classes of antibodies,

 Go to Chapter 22, **Supplemental Materials: Humoral Immunity,** on Davis*Plus.*

Cell-Mediated Immunity

Whereas the humoral immune response acts directly against antigenic cells, the cell-mediated immune response destroys microorganisms (usually viruses). Four types of T cells are responsible for the cell-mediated immune response:

- *Cytotoxic (killer) T cells* directly attack and kill pathogens and infected body cells.
- *Helper T cells* help regulate the action of cytotoxic T cells, as well as that of B cells in humoral responses.
- *Memory T cells.* The first time an antigen invades the body, T cells form that respond to that specific antigen. The memory T cells are able to increase the speed and amount of the T-cell response with subsequent invasions by that antigen.
- *Suppressor T cells* are thought to stop the immune response when the infection has been contained.

KnowledgeCheck 22-3

- Identify and describe the purpose of the body's three major lines of defense against infection.
- Mr. Jefferson has an acute infection. If lab work reveals that IgM, but not IgG, is present in his blood, what can you conclude about this infection?

WHAT FACTORS INCREASE HOST SUSCEPTIBILITY?

Anything that weakens the defenses makes a person more susceptible to infection. In addition, any factors that increase the person's exposure to pathogens, such as working at a day-care center or being a nurse, increase the risk for infection. Some common factors are discussed below.

Developmental Stage. Young children are vulnerable because their immune systems are immature and they have had limited exposure to pathogens. Children frequently begin to have more infections when they start interacting with people outside their family (e.g., when they begin day care or start school). This is a natural process known as acquiring **active immunity.** Older adults are also susceptible hosts because the immune response declines with aging. Skin, a primary defense, becomes less elastic and more prone to breakdown with aging. Elders also tend to be less active, and their nutrition may be inadequate.

Breaks in the First Line of Defense. A break in the skin, whether caused by a surgical procedure, skin breakdown, an insect bite, or insertion of an intravenous device, creates a portal of entry for infectious microorganisms.

Illness or Injury. Recuperation from infection or injury limits the physical resources available to combat a new pathogen.

Tobacco Use. Smoking is a major risk factor for pulmonary infections. Smoking interferes with normal respiratory functioning, including the ability to move the chest, cough, sneeze, or have full air exchange. Chemicals in tobacco paralyze cilia; thus, secretions pool in the lower airways, creating a hospitable environment for bacterial growth. People exposed chronically to secondhand smoke (e.g., bartenders, children of smokers) are also at increased risk for infection.

Substance Abuse. Alcohol curbs hunger. As a result, many chronic alcohol users do not consume an adequate diet. Alcohol is also toxic to the liver and to the cells lining the intestinal mucosa. Inhaled substances, such as marijuana and cocaine, affect respiratory cilia in a manner similar to tobacco. Any substances that affect orientation and energy level will diminish food intake, activity, rest, and hygiene—factors that support host defenses. Injecting substances leads to breaks in skin integrity, further increasing the risk of infection.

Multiple Sexual Partners. The more sexual partners a person has, the higher his risk of acquiring a sexually transmitted infection (STI).

Environmental Factors. Increased exposure to pathogens in one's work situation (e.g., kindergarten teacher, healthcare worker), living situation (e.g., nursing home, parents with young children who are in preschool), and other environmental factors increase one's risk for infection.

Chronic Disease. Many chronic diseases diminish the body's ability to fight infection. Diseases that impair peripheral circulation, such as uncontrolled hypertension (high blood pressure) and diabetes mellitus, make the patient prone to infection in the extremities. Poor circulation prevents antibodies and T cells from reaching the pathogens and damages tissue, making it easier for pathogens to enter and thrive. Leukemia, a form of cancer of the blood, increases the production of abnormal white blood cells, but these cells are ineffective in combating infection. Because HIV infects T cells, patients with AIDS have a reduced ability to fight off secondary infections.

Medications. Some medications are given for the purpose of reducing the immune response, for example, to patients receiving organ or tissue transplants. For most patients, though, decreased immunity is an unwanted side effect of treatment. Even common medications, such as nonsteroidal anti-inflammatory agents (NSAIDs) (e.g., ibuprofen), decrease the immune response. As a side effect, some medications, such as chemotherapeutic agents, decrease the production of white blood cells or cause the cells produced to be abnormal. Even antibiotics can increase the risk for infection. For example, an antibiotic given for a respiratory infection may cause a vaginal yeast infection because it destroys colonies of normal vaginal flora, allowing the harmful microbes to thrive. These are considered **superinfections** (opportunistic growth of harmful transient pathogens that are normally kept in check), and some can be extremely challenging to treat.

Nursing and Medical Procedures. Several procedures are associated with an increased risk of infection. For example, urinary catheterization may injure the fragile urethral mucosa, provide a direct pathway for pathogens into the bladder, and prevent the normal flushing of the urethra. Also, an IV line inserted to infuse an antibiotic may serve as a portal of entry for pathogens.

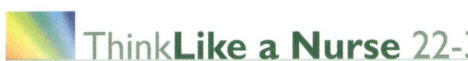

KnowledgeCheck 22-4

What factors increase a client's risk for infection?

ThinkLike a Nurse 22-3

- Consider your current lifestyle. How would you evaluate your ability to support your body's defenses?
- Recall the scenario of Jason Sergi, the labor and delivery nurse, and his daughter (Meet Your Nursing Role Model). Why did Jason say that handwashing was the most important thing he did at work that day? Explain your answer by referring to all of the links in the chain of infection.

PracticalKnowledge
knowing how

As a nurse you will have direct contact with patients who are infected with a variety of pathogens or who are at increased risk for infection. The remainder of this chapter provides practical information for preventing infection in your clients and for caring for clients with infection.

ASSESSMENT

Some elements of the nursing history and physical assessment focus specifically on the risk factors and symptoms of infection.

Nursing History

To elicit information related to infection, ask the client about the following:

- Any exposure to pathogens in the environment, including at work, recent or international travel, contact with people who are ill, and unprotected sexual behavior

- If the patient is febrile, ask "Have you recently traveled outside the country?"
- Any unusual foods or products ingested
- Past and present disease or injury history
- Medications, over-the-counter preparations, herbal products, alcohol intake, and any substances currently in use
- Current level of stress
- Immunization history
- Symptoms of illness

Physical Assessment

Observe the patient's general appearance: Does he seem fatigued? Is he diaphoretic (perspiring profusely)? Is he wrapped in blankets or complaining of feeling chilled? Does the patient appear well nourished? Are the mucous membranes dry?

Physical assessment includes a thorough examination of the skin. Check turgor (elasticity). Look for signs of local infection evidenced by pain, redness, swelling, and warmth. Note the presence or absence of rashes, along with any breaks or reddened areas of the skin. Patients with poor peripheral circulation often have various skin discolorations, rather than signs of inflammation, when experiencing an infection.

Swollen lymph nodes indicate the possible presence of an infection in the area that drains into the nodes. Elevated temperature and pulse rate are classic signs of an infection.

The presence of one infection does not eliminate the risk for an additional infection. For example, a patient being treated with IV medications for a wound infection is at risk for infection at the IV site, as well as for a superinfection or an infection related to insufficient immunizations.

For a list of tests commonly used to evaluate evidence of or risk for infection, see the accompanying Diagnostic Testing box. Each specific test should be evaluated based on the patient's condition, age, and coexisting conditions.

Common Tests for Evaluating the Presence of or Risk for Infection

TEST	DESCRIPTION
White blood cell (WBC) count with differential	A breakdown of the number and types of WBCs; normal WBC count is 5,000–10,000/mm^3.
Blood cultures	A sample of blood placed on culture media and evaluated for growth of pathogens. Normally, should show no growth of infectious microorganisms.
Urine cultures	Urine is normally sterile with no microorganism growth.
Throat cultures, wound cultures	Presence of microorganisms is normal, but there should be no growth of infectious microorganisms. To yield the most reliable results, blood cultures should be obtained from peripheral sites, using venipuncture by trained phlebotomists, unless a culture is specifically ordered from a central catheter or peripherally inserted central catheter.
Disease titers	Blood tests for specific disease immunity (e.g., to rubella)
Panels to evaluate specific disease exposure	Blood tests to evaluate exposure to specific diseases (e.g., HIV, hepatitis)
Immunoglobulin (IgG, IgM) levels	Blood tests to evaluate humoral immunity status
C-reactive protein (CRP)	A blood test to measure inflammatory change or bacterial infection
Agglutinins, warm or cold	Used to diagnose atypical infections by detecting antigens in the blood
Erythrocyte (red blood cell) sedimentation rate (ESR or sed rate)	A measure of inflammatory changes. Sed rate increases with inflammation. Normally it is at 15 mm/hr for men and < 20 mm/hr for women.
Iron level	Normally 60–90 g/100 mg. Lower in chronic infection.

Diagnostic Testing

ANALYSIS/NURSING DIAGNOSIS

The following two NANDA-I diagnoses directly pertain to infection:

Readiness for Enhanced Immunization Status. This is a wellness diagnosis, used to describe a person who is already following the local, national, and/or international standards of immunization, but who wants to enhance behavior to prevent infectious disease, and learn more about providers of immunizations, possible problems associated with immunizations, knowledge of standards, and record keeping.

Risk for Infection. Virtually all patients in a healthcare setting are at risk for being infected due to exposure to pathogens in the environment. Use this diagnosis only for patients who are at higher than usual risk (e.g., those with poor nutritional status) and who need nursing interventions to help prevent infection. Do not use it for the generic assessments you do routinely for all patients (e.g., assessing temperature, routine examination of surgical incision). Examples of appropriate use of this diagnosis include the following:

- Risk for Infection r/t altered immune response secondary to corticosteroid therapy
- Risk for Infection r/t impaired skin integrity and poor nutritional status. (Patients with *actual* infection are managed collaboratively with the healthcare team.)

Infection may be a medical diagnosis or the etiology of other nursing diagnoses, such as Fatigue, Risk for Imbalanced Body Temperature, or Pain. Patients with infection may experience other health problems due to their infected status. For example:

- Social Isolation r/t communicable disease (e.g., tuberculosis [TB])
- Deficient Diversional Activity r/t inability to leave room secondary to protective isolation

Other diagnostic statements may apply, depending upon the patient's condition, treatment ordered, and the patient's response to illness. For a care plan and care map for Risk for Infection,

 Go to Chapter 22, **Care Plan** and **Care Map**, on DavisPlus.

PLANNING OUTCOMES/EVALUATION

For NOC standardized outcomes for Risk for Infection,

 Go to Chapter 22, **Standardized Language,** on DavisPlus.

Individualized goals/outcomes statements depend on the specific nursing diagnosis and etiology. For example, for an undernourished woman, if the nursing diagnosis is Risk for Infection r/t intravenous puncture site and inadequate nutrition, an appropriate goal would be the following:

Patient will show no signs of localized infection at the infusion site, as evidenced by the absence of swelling, redness, excessive warmth, pain, or drainage.

You will evaluate the nursing care plan by examining the extent to which such goals have been met.

PLANNING INTERVENTIONS/IMPLEMENTATION

When caring for a patient at risk for infection, nursing activities are aimed at breaking the chain of infection at every possible link. Some of the most common reasons that patients are diagnosed with Risk for Infection are: exposure to pathogens, bypass of their normal defense mechanisms, increased physiological stress, or inadequate immune response. Direct nursing care toward these concerns, and provide the following broad interventions:

- Reduce exposure to pathogens through the use of aseptic technique (discussed shortly).
- Maintain skin integrity and support natural defenses against infection.
- Reduce stress.
- Promote immune function through collaborative care.
- Provide supportive measures to decrease the length of time that a patient needs invasive devices, such as intravenous lines and urinary catheters.

For NIC standardized interventions for Risk for Infection:

 Go to Chapter 22, **Standardized Language,** on DavisPlus.

Specific nursing activities will be based on the unique situation of the client, as described in the etiology of the diagnostic statement. For example:

- For clients who have had surgery and general anesthesia or who are at risk for pneumonia, promote coughing and deep breathing on a regular basis.
- For clients being mechanically ventilated, provide special oral care designed to prevent ventilator-associated pneumonia. (See the accompanying QSEN box for an example.)
- For clients who are at risk for disease based on age, debilitated state, congregate living arrangement, or employment in healthcare facilities, facilitate participation in vaccination programs, which can help them acquire immunity from some communicable diseases.
- Community health nurses can limit disease transmission through surveillance of the community, tracking of disease patterns, and initiation of prompt treatment.
- For clients who have breaks in the skin or incision sites, provide regular assessment for infection status and follow appropriate medical or surgical asepsis guidelines.
- For all clients at risk for infection, provide care that is based on principles of medical asepsis.

Other preventive nursing activities are discussed in the following sections. They include providing client teaching, supporting host defenses, and practicing medical and surgical asepsis.

Teaching Infection Prevention

Clients and caregivers in their own homes are usually at less risk for infection than they are in the hospital. The client and home caregiver share the same potential pathogens and antibodies, and there is limited exposure to others with illness. Nevertheless, to protect their own health and the health of others, clients need to understand basic principles of medical asepsis, personal hygiene, and infection control. You should also teach them to recognize signs and symptoms of infection; and for those who have an infection, help them to understand that particular organism and disease process. For information about teaching infection control in the home and community, see the Home Care box Preventing Infection in the Home and Community. To help clients avoid acquiring or spreading community-acquired MRSA (CA-MRSA), see the Self-Care box Teaching Your Patient About Preventing the Spread of CA-MRSA.

QSEN

Successful QI Project: Improving the Rate of Ventilator-Associated Pneumonia (VAP)

Competency: Quality Improvement (Knowledge, Skills, Attitudes)*

You and your colleagues have the opportunity to become partners in improving the quality of patient care. Think about the following project and consider what Knowledge, Skills, and Attitudes were required for its success.

Nurses and physicians at the Mercy Medical Center Critical Care Unit in Springfield, Maine, wanted to decrease their rate of ventilator-associated pneumonia (VAP). They collected data to establish the existing rate, which was 12.6 cases per 1,000 ventilator days. Then they developed an intervention: Nurses provided oral care with cetylpyridinium chloride (Oral-B) using a suction toothbrush every 4 hours. After that, they cleaned the patient's mouth with a hydrogen peroxide treated suction swab, performed deep oropharyngeal suctioning, and applied mouth moisturizer. The result? Incidence of VAP declined 72%, and after changing the tooth cleanser to chlorhexidine gluconate, VAP declined by an impressive 90%!

Time Frame	Intervention	Cases/1,000 Vent Days	% of Decline
2004	Usual care	12.6	
5/2005–12/2005	Oral care protocol introduced	4.12	67%
2006	Oral care protocol maintained	3.57	72%
2007	Oral care protocol maintained; tooth cleanser changed to chlorhexidine gluconate (Peridex)	1.3	90%

➤ What QSEN Knowledge and Attitudes did nurses and team members need before changing the care of patients on ventilators?

➤ How is choosing a meaningful and measurable outcome an essential Skill for effective quality improvement interventions? Is the outcome a direct result of the care?

➤ What is your attitude about the significance of the team's work? How will the team's efforts affect patients?

Source: Hutchins K., Karras, G., Erwin, J., et al. (2009).
*For specific Knowledge, Skills, and Attitudes,

 Go to the QSEN web site at http:www.qsen.org. ksas_prelicensure.php

---

Home Care

Preventing Infection in the Home and Community

➤ To disinfect the home environment, mix a solution of 1 part regular-strength bleach to 50 parts water. The mixture may be stored for a month in an opaque container.

✚ NEVER mix the solution with other household cleaners.

➤ Procedures performed using sterile technique in the hospital (e.g., urinary catheterization) are often performed by clean procedure in the home.

➤ Healthcare workers can carry pathogens into the home and should use caution to avoid infecting the client.

➤ If the client or family member is capable and willing to perform the required treatment, provide the necessary teaching. The client will have less exposure to pathogens than he would if a healthcare provider comes to provide care.

➤ Assess for subtle signs of infection: temperature increase, fatigue, lymph gland enlargement, delayed healing of wounds, fever, chills, or drainage.

➤ Instruct clients and family members in the signs and symptoms of infection and how and when to contact their primary care provider to report these findings.

➤ Advise those planning international travel to get vaccinations before departing, especially for travel to sub-Saharan Africa, South-Central Asia, or Latin America, where they may contract malaria, dengue, rickettsiosis, and influenza.

➤ Teach clients and family members the following basic hygiene and infection prevention measures in the home:
Always wash hands before preparing food, before eating, and before putting the hands near the face, and after going to the bathroom or blowing the nose.
Keep the home environment clean.
Prepare and store food safely (see Chapter 23).
Do not share personal care items (e.g., towels, washcloths, toothbrushes, combs).
Washing dishware and eating utensils in a dishwasher with hot water and detergents is sufficient decontamination

➤ Teach clients and family members actions they can take to help prevent infection when they are outside the home, for example:
Wash hands and do not touch surfaces in a public bathroom.
Carry and use antibacterial hand gel as needed while in public places.
Use a wet-wipe on the receiver and mouthpiece of public phones before making a call.
Wash hands upon returning home (e.g., from shopping).
Ask healthcare providers to wash their hands before touching you, if they have not done so.
Use tongs, not fingers, to get food from serving trays in grocery stores and restaurants.
Ask for clean silverware or napkins if an item is dropped on the floor in a restaurant.

➤ For additional information on home care practices, see Chapter 41.

Self-Care

Teaching Your Patient About Preventing the Spread of CA-MRSA

As measures to prevent community-acquired MRSA, everyone should:

➤ Take antibiotics as prescribed. Take *all* the medication, or as recommended.
➤ Contact your healthcare provider if the infection doesn't improve after a few days of taking an antibiotic.
➤ Never use antibiotics prescribed for someone else; do not give your medication to others.
➤ Follow your healthcare provider's recommendations for influenza and pneumonia vaccinations. Preventing respiratory infections decreases antibiotic use.
➤ Make sure your healthcare providers clean their hands before they touch you. This is one of the most important infection prevention and control measures.
➤ Wash your hands often with soap and water. Wash for 15 to 30 seconds, or as long as it takes to sing the "Happy Birthday" song.
➤ Use alcohol-based hand sanitizer if soap and water are not available or hands are not visibly soiled. Sanitizer should contain at least 60% alcohol.
➤ Avoid sharing personal items (e.g., towels, makeup, combs, clothing).
➤ Pay attention to symptoms that may indicate an infection (e.g., drainage or inflammation of a wound), and contact your healthcare provider immediately.
➤ Cough and sneeze into your elbow and wash your hands after using a tissue.

Clients who have MRSA on their skin or who are infected with MRSA should be taught to:

➤ Keep all sores and cuts clean and covered with bandages.
➤ When changing a bandage:
  Don't touch the sore with your bare hands. Wear gloves.
  Immediately discard the soiled bandage and gloves in a plastic bag where no one else can touch them.
  Wash your hands after removing the gloves.
➤ Avoid touching other people's cuts or bandages.
➤ Avoid close-contact activities until your skin infection is healed, unless you can ensure that your sore will not come in contact with another person (e.g., if your sore can be well covered by a bandage and clothing).
➤ Shower daily, using antibacterial soap if your healthcare provider advises it.
➤ Wash your clothing, towels, and bedding separately from other family members' items. Use warm or hot water and bleach, if possible. Use warm or hot setting on the dryer.
➤ Wash exercise clothes after each use.

Sources: Adapted from CDC. (n.d.d, last updated June 2009). Antibiotic resistance questions & answers. Retrieved March 24, 2011, from http://www.cdc.gov/getsmart/antibiotic-use/anitbiotic-resistance-faqs.html#h; Holcomb, S. (2008). MRSA infections. *Nursing 2008, 38*(6), 33; and Leung-Chen, P. (2008). Emerging infections. Everybody's crying MRSA. *American Journal of Nursing, 108*(8), 29–31.

Wellness Promotion to Support Host Defenses

Efforts to promote wellness help break the chain of infection by strengthening a person's defenses against pathogens. Lifestyle factors that promote host defenses are healthful nutrition, adequate hygiene, rest and exercise, stress reduction, and immunizations.

Nutrition. An acute infection depletes the body's nutritional stores. Therefore, it is important to monitor and support client nutrition, including protein, vitamins, minerals, and water. Nutrients are required to replace lost stores, to maintain production of white blood cells, and to repair damaged tissues. Fever and increased mucus secretions, which are common defenses against infection, increase water loss. Additional water is needed to supplement the lost fluid and to support the increased metabolic rate that occurs with a fever. Chapter 28 further discusses the importance of adequate nutrition.

Hygiene. Good hygiene is crucial for maintaining intact skin, a primary host defense. Encourage frequent handwashing, as well as regular showering or bathing, to decrease the bacterial count on the skin. However, be aware that overzealous cleanliness diminishes the skin's natural oils and may lead to cracking of the skin. Chapter 24 focuses on the importance of hygiene for health. Also see the Home Care box.

Rest and Sleep. Rest and sleep conserve energy needed for healing. Sleep needs vary, and there is really no "correct" amount or pattern of sleep. However, sleep of 6 to 9 hours per night is considered fully restorative for most people.

Exercise and Activity. Research demonstrates that exercise is just as important as rest and sleep. Too little activity causes circulation to slow and the lungs to supply less oxygen. Excessive exercise leads to fatigue and joint injury. Chapters 33 and 35 provide in-depth discussion on activity, exercise, rest, and sleep.

Stress Reduction. Whether physical or mental, stress decreases the body's immune defenses. Numerous studies demonstrate a correlation between stress and disease (Cousins, 1979; Franco, de Barros, Nogueira-Martins, et al., 2003; Schneider, Alexander, Staggers, et al., 2005). Laughing, in contrast, increases oxygenation, promotes body movement, and increases immune responses. See Chapter 12 if you want further details on the effects of stress.

Immunizations. Immunization via vaccination can protect against several infectious diseases (e.g., measles, mumps, and other childhood diseases; pneumonia, influenza, smallpox, and shingles). Unfortunately, some pathogens, such as the virus that causes the common cold, mutate too rapidly for an immunization to be developed. Encourage clients to follow recommendations for immunizations. For most diseases, at least 85% of the population must be immunized in order to protect the entire population from the disease. If you need specific recommended immunizations throughout the life span and their role in health promotion, see Chapter 9 for various age groups, Figures 9-6 and 9-10; and Chapter 10 and Figure 10-5, for older adults. Also,

 Go to Chapter 9, **Tables, Boxes, Figures: ESG Figure 9-1,** on Davis*Plus*.

KnowledgeCheck 22-5

What actions improve host ability to prevent infection?

PRACTICING MEDICAL ASEPSIS

Asepsis is a term that means absence of contamination by disease-causing microorganisms. **Medical asepsis** ("clean technique") refers to procedures that decrease the potential for the spread of infections. You probably already practice medical asepsis in other settings without realizing it. For example, at home you wash your hands before and after handling foods. Before chopping food, you make sure the cutting board and utensils you use are clean. After using it, you wash the board with hot, soapy water. In the healthcare setting, medical asepsis includes hand hygiene, environmental cleanliness, standard precautions, and protective isolation. The effectiveness of these measures, and the patient's safety, depend on nurses' rigorously and consistently following the principles of asepsis.

✚ When you are hurrying, you may be tempted to take shortcuts or forget to follow a guideline. Remember: You are putting your patient, and possibly yourself, at risk for an infection that could cause serious illness. Assume every patient is potentially infected or colonized with an organism that could be transmitted to others.

Maintaining Clean Hands

Hand hygiene is the single most important activity for preventing and controlling infection. The WHO (2008) has chosen as the first "global patient safety challenge" the reduction of healthcare-associated infection, with the theme "clean care is safer care." They have made hand hygiene the cornerstone strategy because it is simple, standardized, low-cost, and based on solid scientific evidence.

Although you may think you already know how to wash your hands, remember that in healthcare settings you are coming in contact with pathogens that are potentially dangerous to you and your patients. Decisions about the type of hand hygiene to use, how long to wash, when to wash, and so on are based on the amount of contact you have with patients or contaminated objects, as well as the patient's infection status and susceptibility to infection. For specific details and guidelines to use when making handwashing decisions, see Clinical Insight 22-1. For a step-by-step hand hygiene procedure, see Procedure 22-1. Handwashing involves five key factors: time, water, soap, friction, and drying. Both the Clinical Insight and the Procedure follow the CDC recommendations for these factors (Boyce & Pittet [CDC], 2002).

Despite the importance of clean hands in preventing transmission of infection, research demonstrates that clinical staff do not consistently observe hand hygiene guidelines (Pratt, Pellowe, Wilson, et al., 2007). In 2008, Medicare has stopped paying for patient complications arising from certain hospital-acquired infections, which in many cases result from poor handwashing. You can help improve clinical practice by serving as a role model for good hand hygiene.

Maintaining a Clean Environment

A clean environment includes the surfaces in a patient's room, as well as supplies, equipment, and other objects brought into the room. An object is said to be contaminated if it becomes unclean—that is, if you suspect it may contain pathogens. The floor, soiled dressings, used tissues, sinks, commodes, and bedpans are other examples of contaminated items. Agency policies determine whether a reusable item is cleaned, disinfected, or sterilized, based on how the item is used.

Cleaning

Cleaning is the removal of visible soil (organic and inorganic) from objects and surfaces. It is usually accomplished manually or mechanically using water with detergents or enzymatic products. A goal of medical asepsis is to keep all public and patient-care areas within the facility clean and free from dust, debris, and contamination. Any spilled liquids, dirty surfaces, or potentially contaminated areas should be cleaned immediately. In your home, you use hot water and general cleaning supplies. However, healthcare facilities use special techniques and cleaning solutions formulated to inhibit microbial growth. Items must be cleaned thoroughly before they can be disinfected or sterilized.

Disinfecting

Disinfection removes virtually all pathogens on inanimate objects by physical or chemical means, including steam, gas, chemicals, and ultraviolet light. Disinfection reduces microbial populations, but it does not guarantee that all pathogens are eliminated, because certain viruses, other pathogenic microbes, and spores can remain (Bauman, Machunis-Masuoka, & Tizard, 2006). Chemical germicides can achieve three levels of disinfection. *High-level disinfection* kills all organisms except high levels of bacterial spores. *Intermediate-level disinfection* kills bacteria, mycobacteria, and most viruses. *Low-level disinfection* kills some viruses and bacteria. Disinfection is used for semicritical and noncritical items:

- **Semicritical items** are those that contact mucous membranes or nonintact skin. This category includes reusable devices, such as flexible endoscopes, and respiratory therapy and anesthesia equipment, for example. They must be free of all microorganisms except bacterial spores, so they must at least be disinfected, and sometimes sterilized.
- **Noncritical items** are supplies and equipment that come in contact with intact skin but not mucous membranes. They do not carry a high risk of infection transmission, and they can be decontaminated where they are used. Examples of noncritical patient-care items are bedpans, stethoscopes, and blood pressure cuffs. Examples of noncritical environmental surfaces include floors, food utensils, bed linens, and bed rails (CDC, 2008). Disinfection is adequate for noncritical items.

Sterilizing

Sterilization is the elimination of all microorganisms (except prions) in or on an object. The major sterilizing methods used in hospitals are (1) autoclaving with moist heat, (2) ethylene oxide gas, and (3) dry heat. Sterilization is used when absolute purity of an object or surface is critical.

- **Critical items** are ones that pose a high risk for infection if they are contaminated with any microorganism. Critical items include those that enter the vascular system or sterile tissue, or those items through which blood flows. Examples are intravenous catheters, needles for injections, urinary catheters, surgical instruments, some wound dressings, and chest tubes.

If you need more specific information on methods for disinfection and sterilization of patient-care items and environmental surfaces,

Go to Chapter 22, **Tables, Boxes, Figures: ESG Table 22-3, Methods for Disinfection and Sterilization of Patient-Care Items and Surfaces,** on Davis*Plus*.

Specially trained personnel carry out disinfection and sterilization in most agencies. As a nurse, you must be familiar with the agency's policies and procedures for cleaning, handling, and transporting items to be disinfected and sterilized, and for working collaboratively with other departments (e.g., the housekeeping department) to keep the patient-care area as clean and free of clutter as possible. Levels of disinfection and sterilization may differ in home care because clients and caregivers share the same potential pathogens and antibodies, and there is limited exposure to others with illness and to care providers carrying unusual pathogens.

For more specific information about maintaining a clean environment in institutional and home care, see Clinical Insight 22-2.

Clinical Insight 22-1 ▶ **Guidelines for Hand Hygiene**

When to Wash

- When hands are visibly dirty or soiled with blood or body fluids
- When arriving on and leaving the patient-care unit
- Before direct contact with a patient, even if you intend to wear procedure gloves
- Before donning and after removing gloves (either procedure or sterile)
- When gloves are changed during a procedure.
- After contact with a patient's intact skin (e.g., when taking a blood pressure)
- After contact with body fluids, mucous membranes, nonintact skin, and wound dressings even if hands are not visibly soiled
- When moving from a contaminated body site to a clean body site during patient care
- Before and after contact with objects and equipment in the patient's immediate vicinity
- Before and after touching any area on your face and hair

What to Use

Iodine compounds are also effective, but usually too *irritating for regular hand hygiene.*

- Use alcohol-based hand rub (at least 60% alcohol) for routine hand hygiene and if hands are not visibly soiled.
- Use soap and water when hands are dirty or visibly soiled.
- Use soap and water after using a restroom.

➕ Use soap and water if there is potential for exposure to *Bacillus anthracis* (or other spore-producing bacteria such as *C. difficile*). Alcohol-based solutions are not effective against spores.

- Use warm, not hot, water.
- Use disposable paper towels.
- If you are interested in a comparison of the effectiveness of various hand-hygiene antiseptic agents,

Go to Chapter 22, **Tables, Boxes, Figures: ESG Table 22-2, Antimicrobial Spectrum and Characteristics of Hand-Hygiene Antiseptic Agents,** on Davis*Plus*.

How to Wash

Refer to Procedure 22-1.

Fingernails

- Do not wear artificial nails or extenders when caring for patients at high risk (e.g., in intensive care and oncology units).
- The 2007 epic2 guidelines in the United Kingdom recommend artificial nails and extenders not be worn at all (Pratt, Pellowe, Wilson, et al., 2007). The CDC's position is that although studies provide evidence that wearing artificial nails poses an infection hazard, additional studies are warranted.
- It is best to not wear nail polish because it chips easily and can harbor microorganisms.
- Keep nail tips less than 1/4 inch long. Some researchers suggest nail tip length not more than 2 mm (not past the tips of the fingers). Longer nails are associated with increased microbial carriage on the hands.

Jewelry

- We recommend that you not wear a watch or rings in the clinical setting, especially rings with stones.
- The CDC has stated jewelry is still an unresolved issue. They noted that hand contamination with pathogens increased when nurses wear rings, but that no studies have related that practice to the transmission of pathogens to patients. However, the epic2 guidelines advise against wearing wrist and hand jewelry.
- If your agency permits you to wear jewelry, clean it thoroughly and often.

Practice Resources

Boyce, & Pittet, 2002; Pratt, Pellowe, Wilson, et al., 2007; Rupp, Fitzgerald, Puumala, et al., 2008; Siegel, Rhinehart, Jackson, et al., 2007.

Clinical Insight 22-2 ➤ Providing a Clean Patient Environment

Use the following guidelines along with standard precautions for all patients.

Supplies and Equipment

- Do not stock rooms with unnecessary supplies.
- Consider supplies brought into a patient's room contaminated. Do not return them to the linen or supply cart; instead, handle them according to agency policy.
- Consider contaminated any items brought from the patient's home, gifts from visitors, and so forth.
- Mobile computing devices should be cleaned (e.g., pagers, smartphones, point-of-care keyboards, and medication administration devices). However, most hospitals lack infection prevention policies for mobile devices. Be sure to wash your hands after using such a device.

Often, electronic devices cannot be decontaminated without damage; in that case, only hand hygiene can protect you and the patient from these vectors.

- Clean stethoscopes with alcohol before use on a patient. Disposable stethoscopes are commercially available, but not commonly seen in healthcare agencies.

Stethoscopes are often contaminated with *S. aureus.*

- Clean reusable equipment that is soiled with blood or body fluids according to agency policy—typically, cleaning then autoclaving or using ethylene oxide gas or dry heat.
- Do not reuse equipment for the care of another patient until it has been cleaned and reprocessed appropriately.
- Dispose of single-use equipment soiled with blood or body fluids in appropriate biohazard containers.
- Wear gloves when handling visibly contaminated equipment. Perform hand hygiene.

Linens

- Carefully handle contaminated linens to prevent skin and mucous membrane exposure, contamination of clothing, and transfer of microorganisms to other patients or the environment.

Linens may harbor microorganisms that may transfer to your clothing, open skin, or mucous membranes, which could then be carried to other clients or environment.

- Bag and remove soiled linens from the room immediately.

Uniforms and Lab Coats

- Do not wear a uniform (e.g., scrubs) or a lab coat for more than one day without laundering.

Care provider clothing is often contaminated as care providers move from patient to patient. The traditional white lab coats are being banned in some hospitals because they are a vehicle for dangerous pathogens. Although contaminated clothing has not been implicated directly, the potential exists for it to transfer pathogens to patients (CDC, 2008).

- If you wash your uniforms at home, they require only washing with warm or hot water and detergent (except in the case of possible exposure to multidrug-resistant organisms, for which you should add bleach).

Spills and Waste

- Empty and clean bedpans, urinals, and emesis basins immediately after use.
- Place soiled dressings, drains, and so forth in appropriate waterproof bags for disposal, not in an open trashcan.
- Wipe up small spills from tabletops and floors. Notify the housekeeping or environmental services department for large spills.

Needles and Sharps

✚ Do not recap, bend, break, or hand-manipulate used needles. If recapping is necessary, use a one-handed scoop technique. Place used sharps in puncture-resistant containers.

Practice Resources

Carling, Parry, & Von Beheren, for the Healthcare Environmental Hygiene Study Group, 2008; CDC, 2008; Davidson & Malkary, 2008; Perry, Marshall, & Jones, 2001; Siegel, Rhinehart, Jackson, et al., 2007.

CDC Guidelines for Preventing Transmission of Pathogens

In addition to handwashing and maintaining a clean environment, you should follow other precautions to protect yourself and your patients. CDC guidelines provide for two tiers of protection.

- **Standard precautions,** the first tier of protection, apply to care of all patients.
- **Transmission-based precautions,** the second tier of protection, outline precautions to be taken based on the mode of transmission of the infection (Siegel, Rhinehart, Jackson, et al.,

2007). Recall from the discussion on the chain of infection that pathogens may be transmitted by contact, droplet, or air. Each mode of transmission requires a different approach to prevent infection. For all transmission-based precautions, institute measures to counteract adverse effects of isolation on patients (i.e., anxiety, depression, perceptions of stigma, reduced contact with staff, and increases in preventable adverse events).

- Table 22-2 provides a comparison of standard and transmission-based precautions. For detailed guidelines to aid you in following both types of precautions, refer to Clinical Insights 22-3 and 22-4.

Table 22-2 ➤ Comparison of CDC Standard and Transmission-Based Precautions

STANDARD PRECAUTIONS	TRANSMISSION-BASED PRECAUTIONS
"Tier One" Precautions	"Tier Two" Precautions
Use with all clients, in all settings, regardless of suspected or confirmed presence of infection	Use for patients known or suspected to be infected or colonized with infectious agents.
Principle: All blood, body fluids, secretions, excretions except sweat, nonintact skin, and mucous membranes may contain pathogens.	*Principle:* Routes of transmission for some microorganisms are not completely interrupted using standard precautions alone. Used *in addition to* standard precautions.
Include: Hand hygiene; use of gloves, gown, mask, eye protection, or face shield (depending on expected exposure); and safe injection practices	**Three categories of precautions:** *Contact Precautions*—For organisms spread by direct contact with the patient or his environment. This is the most common form of transmission.
Added for protection of patients more than of healthcare personnel: Safe injection practices, respiratory hygiene and cough etiquette, and wearing a mask when performing special lumbar puncture procedures	*Droplet Precautions*—For pathogens spread through close respiratory or mucous membrane contact with respiratory secretions (e.g., sneezing, coughing, talking); pathogens that do not remain infectious over long distances.
Standard precautions do not completely protect against microorganisms spread by contact, droplets, or through the air.	*Airborne Precautions*—For pathogens that are very small and remain infectious over long distances when suspended in the air; and easily transmitted through air currents (e.g., fanning linens, ventilating systems).

Source: Siegel, J. D., Rhinehart, E., Jackson, M., et al. (2007). *2007 Guideline for isolation precautions: Preventing transmission of infectious agents in the healthcare setting.* Retrieved March 11, 2011, from http://www.cdc.gov/ncidod/dhqp/pdf/guidelines/Isolation2007.pdf

Clinical Insight 22-3 ➤ Following CDC Standard (Tier 1) Precautions

When to Use: Standard precautions (Tier 1) apply to all clients and should be used whenever there is a possibility of coming in contact with blood, body fluids (except sweat), excretions and secretions, mucous membranes, and breaks in the skin.

Standard precautions are designed to protect you from exposure to potential pathogens, to decrease the likelihood that you will transmit pathogens among patients, and to protect the patient from microorganisms that you may carry.

TIER 1 COMPONENT	RECOMMENDATIONS
Hand Hygiene	**Refer to Clinical Insight 22-1 for details.**
Respiratory Hygiene/Cough Etiquette for Patients	▪ Instruct symptomatic persons to cover mouth/nose when sneezing/coughing. ▪ Provide and use tissues and dispose in a no-touch receptacle. ▪ Perform hand hygiene after soiling hands with respiratory secretions or after using a tissue or covering the mouth/nose. ▪ Wear a surgical mask if tolerated or do not come within 3 ft of another person if possible. Some patients may not be able to tolerate the decreased oxygen that is available when breathing room air through a mask.
Masks and Eye Protection (for the Nurse)	▪ Wear a mask and eye protection or a face shield to protect mucous membranes of the eyes, nose, and mouth during patient-care activities that are likely to generate splashes or sprays of blood, body fluids, secretions, and excretions. Barrier protection helps keep microorganisms from accidentally entering your mucous membranes, eyes, nose, or mouth.

Clinical Insight 22-3 ➤ **Following CDC Standard (Tier 1) Precautions—cont'd**

TIER 1 COMPONENT	RECOMMENDATIONS
Patient Placement	■ Place in a single-patient room if the patient is at increased risk of transmitting or acquiring infection, does not maintain appropriate hygiene, is likely to contaminate the environment, or is at increased risk of developing adverse outcome following infection.
Gowns	■ Wear a clean, nonsterile, nonpermeable gown during procedures and activities when you anticipate contact of clothing or exposed skin with blood or body fluids, secretions, and excretions (e.g., when there is a risk of spray or splash onto clothing). ■ Promptly remove the gown once it is soiled. Avoid contaminating clothing when removing the gown. ■ Wash hands after removing the gown. ■ See Procedure 22-2, Donning and Removing PPE.
✚ **Needles and Sharps**	■ Never recap, bend, or break used needles, or otherwise manipulate them using both hands, nor use any other technique that involves directing the point of a needle toward any part of the body. Instead, use either a one-handed "scoop" technique or a mechanical device designed for holding the needle sheath (see Procedure 25-10, Recapping Needles . . .). ■ Use safety features (e.g., retractable needle) when available. ■ Place sharps (e.g., scalpels, needles, etc.) in puncture-resistant containers for disposal.
Patient Resuscitation	■ Use one-way valve mouthpieces, resuscitation bags, or other ventilation devices as an alternative to mouth-to-mouth resuscitation methods in situations when the need for resuscitation is predictable. To prevent contact between rescuer's and client's mucous membranes and airflow, preventing transmission of microorganisms.
Soiled Patient-Care Equipment, Environment, Textiles, & Laundry	■ See Clinical Insight 22-2 for details. ■ Wear gloves if the equipment or laundry is visibly contaminated. ■ Handle equipment, textiles, and laundry in a manner to prevent transfer of microorganisms to others and the environment. ■ Perform hand hygiene. ■ Develop procedures for routine care, cleaning, and disinfection of environmental surfaces, especially frequently touched surfaces in patient-care areas.
Gloves	**When to Wear** ■ If you have an area of irritation or a break in the skin, wear gloves or apply an occlusive dressing during patient contact. ■ Wear gloves when contact with blood or other potentially infectious materials, mucous membranes, and nonintact skin could occur. **When to Remove or Change** ■ Remove gloves immediately after caring for a patient. Avoid touching clean items, environmental surfaces, or another patient. ■ Do not wear the same gloves for care of more than one patient; do not wash gloves and reuse gloves between patient contact. Research shows that washing and reusing gloves between patient contacts results in increased bacterial counts on the hands. ■ Change gloves during patient care if moving from a contaminated body site to a clean. ■ Change gloves between tasks or procedures on the same patient if you have made contact with material that may contain a high concentration of microorganisms.

(Continued)

Clinical Insight 22-3 ► Following CDC Standard (Tier 1) Precautions—cont'd

TIER 1 COMPONENT	RECOMMENDATIONS
	Use and Storage ■ When preparing for a procedure, first collect equipment and place at the bedside ready for use; then wash your hands and put on gloves just before performing the procedure. Donning gloves ahead of time allows them to become contaminated before the procedure. ■ Do not carry gloves in your pocket. Keep them in their original box and remove them when and where required. ■ Do not store gloves on top of trash containers or on windowsills. ■ Wash or disinfect your hands, regardless of whether gloves are being initially donned or are being changed. Gloves are not completely impermeable to microorganisms; furthermore, they may leak or tear. Hands can be easily contaminated when removing gloves, as well.

For a comparison of glove materials (latex, nitrile, vinyl, and polyethylene),

 Go to Chapter 22, **Tables, Boxes, Figures: ESG Table 22-4, Comparison of Glove Materials,** on *DavisPlus*.

Practice Resources

Best practices: Evidence-based nursing procedures, 2007; Boyce, & Pittet, 2002; Occupational Safety & Health Administration, U.S. Department of Labor, n.d.; Pratt, Pellowe, Wilson, et al., 2007; Siegel, Rhinehart, Jackson, et al., 2007; U.S. Department of Labor, n.d.).

Clinical Insight 22-4 ► Following Transmission-Based (Tier 2) Precautions

Note: Refer to Clinical Insight 22-3 if you need to review standard precautions.

    When to Use: Use transmission-based (Tier 2) precautions when the routes of transmission are not completely interrupted using Standard Precautions alone. Pathogens may be transmitted by contact, droplet, or air. Each mode of transmission requires a different approach to prevent infection, and has a different set of precautions. For some diseases, you may need to use more than one of the categories.

Contact Precautions

Follow all standard precautions.

When to Use: Use contact precautions when direct contact with the patient or the patient's environment can lead to spread of the pathogen. This is the most common form of transmission. Draining wounds, dressings, patient supplies, and secretions are sources of infection. Indirect contact, or contact with fomites, can also transmit pathogens that spread by this method.

Patient Placement and Transport
■ Ideally, consult with an infection preventionist for patient placement.
■ Place in a private room, if available. Private room provides the most effective protection.
■ If no private room is available, place patient in a room with a patient with an active infection caused by the same organism and no other infections.
■ When transporting the patient, ensure that infected or colonized areas of the body are contained and covered.
■ *Ambulatory care:* Place the patient in an exam room or cubicle as soon as possible.

Personal Protective Equipment (PPE)
■ Wear clean nonsterile gloves when touching the patient's intact skin. Don gloves on entry to the room.
■ Wear a clean gown if you anticipate your clothing may contact the patient or any contaminated items in the room.
■ Remove PPE and observe hand hygiene before leaving the room. Take care that your skin and clothing do not contact environmental surfaces on the way out of the room.

Clinical Insight 22-4 ▶ **Following Transmission-Based (Tier 2) Precautions—cont'd**

Equipment, Supplies, and Environment
- Keep contact precaution supplies just outside the patient's room on a cart.
- Double bag all linen and trash (or use a single waterproof bag), and clearly mark them contaminated.
- Use disposable equipment (e.g., blood pressure cuffs) if possible; otherwise, clean and disinfect the equipment per institutional policy before removing them from the room and before use on another patient.
- Ensure that the patient room is cleaned and disinfected at least daily.
- *Home care:* Limit the amount of nondisposable equipment brought into the home. If possible, leave the equipment in the home until discharge from home care.
- *Home care:* If equipment cannot remain in the home, clean and disinfect items before taking them from the home, or place them in a plastic bag for transport to a reprocessing area.

Other
- Follow any additional precautions specific to the microorganism.
- Discontinue contact precautions after signs and symptoms have resolved or according to pathogen-specific recommendations.

Droplet Precautions
Follow all standard precautions.
Follow all contact precautions.

When to Use: Use droplet precautions when the pathogen can be spread via moist, large droplets (e.g., sneezing, coughing, talking). Droplets can spread infection by direct contact with mucous membranes or through indirect contact, for example, suctioning or touching a bedside table that was contaminated with moist droplets and then rubbing your eyes.

Patient Placement and Transport
- If no private room is available and the patient must be placed with patients who have a different infection, ensure that the patients are physically separated by more than 3 ft. Keep the privacy curtain closed. This minimizes contact between patients. Ideally, consult with an infection preventionist for patient placement. A private room provides the most effective protection.
- Limit transport outside the room to medically necessary purposes; if transport is necessary, the patient should wear a mask. The transporter is not required to mask.

Personal Protective Equipment
- Keep droplet precaution supplies just outside the patient's room on a cart.
- Wear a mask when working within 3 ft of the patient. Don the mask on entry into the room. Whether to wear goggles is an unresolved issue. Follow agency policy.
- Change PPE and perform hand hygiene between contact with patients in the same room, regardless of whether one or both patients are on droplet precautions.

Other
- Instruct patients to observe respiratory hygiene/cough etiquette.
- Discontinue droplet precautions after signs and symptoms have resolved or according to pathogen-specific recommendations.

Airborne Precautions
Follow all standard precautions.
Follow all contact precautions.

When to Use: Use airborne precautions to control the spread of infections that are transmitted person-to-person on air currents. These include tuberculosis, varicella (chickenpox), SARS, and rubeola (measles). Pathogens spread by this method are very small and can be easily transmitted through ventilating systems as well as by any activities that stir the air, such as fanning sheets, shaking out towels, or sweeping the floor.

Patient Placement and Transport
- Place the patient in an airborne infection isolation room (AIIR)—one with negative pressure that discharges and exchanges the air outside or through a high-efficiency particulate air (HEPA) filtration system. Monitor air pressure daily (usually this is via an electronic device with an alarm).
- If such a room is not available, transfer the patient to a facility where one is available.

(Continued)

Clinical Insight 22-4 ➤ Following Transmission-Based (Tier 2) Precautions—cont'd

- Keep the room door closed when not required for entry and exit. To maintain the negative pressure and contain the airborne organisms.
- In the event of an outbreak involving large numbers of patients who require airborne precautions, consult with infection preventionists for patient placement.
- Limit transport of the patient outside the room to medically necessary purposes. If transport is necessary, cover any infectious skin lesions and have the patient wear a mask. The transporter is not required to mask if the patient is wearing a mask and infectious skin lesions are covered. Notify the receiving department. The receiving department can then take airborne precautions.
- *Ambulatory care:* Triage and identify patients with suspected airborne precautions upon entry to the agency. Place the patient in an AIIR as soon as possible. If one is not available, place a mask on the patient and place him in an exam room. Do not reuse the room for at least an hour after the patient leaves it.

Personal Protective Equipment

- Keep airborne isolation supplies just outside the patient's room on a cart.
- Don a mask on entering the room. Wear a special, fit-tested, approved mask (e.g., N95 respirator) if the patient is suspected of having pulmonary tuberculosis or smallpox.
- Remove your respirator/mask outside the room after closing the door. If the respirator is not disposable, clean and store according to the manufacturer's instructions.
- When using a respirator mask, check the seal. Hold your hands over the respirator and exhale. If you feel air around your nose, adjust the nosepiece; if you feel air at the edges, adjust the straps.
- When the patient has rubeola, varicella (chickenpox), or disseminated zoster, the CDC makes no recommendation about use of PPE if, based on your history of vaccination or disease, you think you are presumed immune to the disease.
- If the patient has or is suspected of having rubeola or varicella, only immune caregivers should provide care. Immune caregivers do not need to wear masks.

Other

- Discontinue airborne precautions according to pathogen-specific recommendations of the CDC.
- Tape a waterproof bag to the bedside. Doing so facilitates proper disposal of tissues.

Practice Resources

American Heart Association, 2008; *Best practices: Evidence-based nursing procedures,* 2007; Pratt, Pellowe, Wilson, et al., 2007; Siegel, Rhinehart, Jackson, et al., 2007; U.S. Department of Labor, n.d.a.

Personal Protective Equipment. The CDC recommends and the United States Occupational Safety and Health Administration requires employers to provide personal protective equipment (PPE) for healthcare workers (e.g., gloves, gowns, face masks, and eye protection [Fig. 22-3]) (U.S. Department of Labor, n.d.a). This equipment is to be used in standard precautions as well as transmission-based precautions. Figure 22-4 shows a disposable N-95 respirator mask. To learn how to don and remove PPE, refer to Procedures 22-2 and 22-3.

KnowledgeCheck 22-6

Under what circumstances are standard precautions used?

Interventions for Example Problem: Preventing MDROs

Evidence suggests that MDROs are carried from one person to another via the hands of healthcare personnel. To prevent

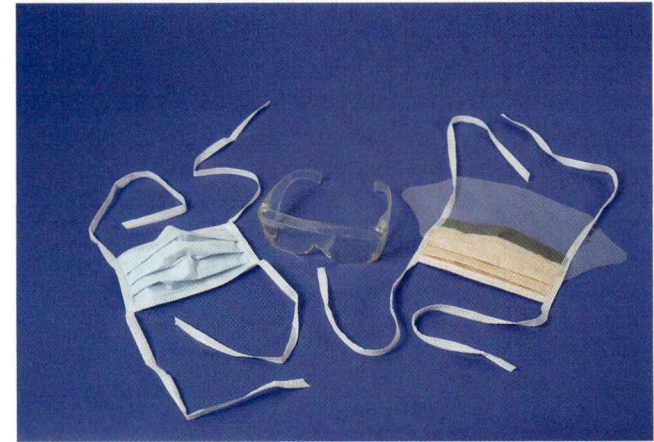

FIGURE 22-3 Several types of face masks and eye shields are available.

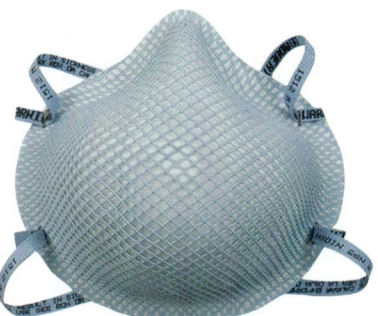

FIGURE 22-4 A disposable N-95 respirator mask, for airborne precautions. *(Courtesy of Moldex-Metric, Inc., Culver City, CA, http://www.moldex.com)*

MDROs, you must adhere strictly to published recommendations for hand hygiene, glove use, and isolation precautions as well as for performing invasive procedures such as intravenous and urinary catheterization and care of central venous ports. Agencies should place infected patients in private rooms and require care providers to wear gowns and masks and use antiseptic/disinfectant for handwashing. For actions you can take to help prevent MDROs, see Clinical Insight 22-5.

For an optional CDC podcast on community associated MRSA risk factors and prevention strategies, as well as for associated Web sites,

 Go to Chapter 22, **Resources for Caregivers and Health Professionals,** on DavisPlus.

Also refer to the Home Care box and the Self-Care box Teaching Your Patient About Preventing the Spread of CA-MRSA in this chapter. For extensive information about monitoring MDROs, consult a medical–surgical or infectious diseases textbook. For CDC guidelines for MRDO prevention and control,

 Go to http://www.cdc.gov/hicpac/mdro/mdro_4.html

"Protective Environment" in Special Situations

Patients who are immunosuppressed (e.g., receiving chemotherapy) are sometimes placed in a special form of isolation, called *protective isolation* or *reverse isolation*. However, the CDC states that standard and transmission-based precautions are adequate protection for most of those patients. They recommend a "protective environment" only for a special class of stem cell–transplant patients, who are neutropenic (have a low white blood cell count) secondary to chemotherapy. Most of the recommendations are engineering and environmental services rather than nursing measures. If you are interested in, or have a need to, learn the details of maintaining a protective environment,

 Go to Chapter 22, **ESG Clinical Insight 22-1, Maintaining a "Protective Environment" in Special Situations,** on DavisPlus.

Patients with compromised immunity are more likely to become infected by pathogens harbored in their own bodies

than from pathogens transmitted by other people (Siegel, Rhinehart, Jackson, et al., 2007). Therefore, except for the special situations described above, standard and transmission-based precautions should protect even unusually vulnerable patients from organisms brought in by healthcare workers and visitors

Nevertheless, in practice you may see what has been called **protective isolation** being used for clients with low WBC counts, clients undergoing chemotherapy, or clients with large open wounds or weak immune systems. Protective isolation usually includes following standard precautions; placing the patient in a private room; restricting visitors; wearing a mask, gown, and gloves for patient care; and special cleaning or disposal of the patient's equipment and supplies. Some units, such as neonatal intensive care units, burn units, and labor and delivery suites, may follow some aspects of protective isolation all the time.

Control of Potentially Contaminated Equipment and Supplies

Whenever possible, use disposable equipment in an isolation room. Nondisposable equipment and supplies require special handling.

- **Protective Isolation.** If a client is in protective isolation, be sure that equipment has been disinfected *before* it is taken into the room. Take linen and dishes directly to the protective isolation room, and hand them to someone wearing the required protective garb.
- **Transmission-Based Isolation.** If the client is in transmission-based isolation, disinfect the equipment *on removal* from the room. When removing linen or nondisposable items from a room with contact, droplet, or airborne isolation, place them in special isolation bags.

Disposing of Used Isolation Supplies. Place contaminated disposable equipment and materials containing body fluids in special isolation bags. This process requires two healthcare workers. The worker inside the room wears protective clothing and handles only contaminated items. The second worker stands at the door and holds the isolation bag open. The first worker places items inside the bag without touching the outside of the bag. If the bag contains linens, the isolation bag is closed and placed in a laundry hamper. Securely close the isolation trash bag, and place it in a special isolation trash container. Special disposal methods are used to prevent these objects from going into a landfill, where they could become a reservoir of infection. Because this trash is much more expensive to process, take care to put only contaminated materials in the contaminated trash.

Sharps Disposal. Always place disposable needles, syringes, and other sharp items, such as broken glass, in special disposable sharps containers immediately after their use. Never recap a contaminated needle. Refer to Chapters 23 and 25 if you need further information on preventing needlestick injuries.

Laboratory Specimens. Laboratory specimens contain blood and body fluids and are always considered contaminated. Label the specimen container in a clean area before taking it to the patient. Have the specimen collected by a healthcare worker wearing appropriate protective clothing. Once the specimen is collected, place it in a special transport bag. Do not allow the outside of the bag to touch any contaminated item, including your gloves.

Clinical Insight 22-5 ► **Preventing Multidrug-Resistant Organism Infections (MDROs)**

Note: Refer to Clinical Insights 22-1, 22-2, 22-3, and 22-4. Those instructions are also followed in preventing the transmission of MDROs. ✚ Preventing MDROs requires instituting some measures over and above the other precautions, but does not replace them.

Note: The CDC recommends that hospitals try to reduce infection rates by improving hygiene and standard precautions, and to resort to special measures, such as screening all high-risk patients, only if other methods fail.

General Recommendations

- **Perform meticulous hand hygiene, for all patient care.**
- **Observe standard precautions for *all* patients.** See Clinical Insight 22-2. Standard precautions, including hand hygiene, are absolutely essential in preventing spread of infection. There is some evidence that standard precautions alone may be as effective as isolating MRSA patients in private rooms and wearing PPE (Halcomb, Griffiths, & Fernandez, 2008a). However, most studies reporting successful MDRO control used a combination of several control measures.
- **Observe (or modify) contact precautions routinely for patients infected or colonized with target MDROs.** Usually this continues until the patient has a negative culture for the organism. The type of organism and extent of disease it causes vary by population and institution. Approaches to prevention and control must be tailored to the needs of individual institutions and populations.
  - *MRSA:* Prevention is a national priority. The organism can survive on hands, clothing, environmental surfaces, and equipment, so healthcare institutions are targeting it with staff education, aggressive handwashing, increased use of protective gloves and gowns, and targeted screening (Klevens, Morrison, Nadle, et al., 2007).
  - *C. difficile.* Prevention focuses on the following: Contact precautions for patients with diarrhea Accurate patient identification Consistent hand hygiene, using soap and water rather than alcohol-based handrubs (for mechanical removal of spores)

Patient Placement and Transport

- Observing contact precautions, assign the infected patient to a single room, if available. Give highest priority to those having conditions that may lead to transmission of infection (e.g., uncontained secretions or excretions, inability to follow cough hygiene).
- If no single room is available, place with a patient with the same MDRO.

Personal Protective Equipment

- Use masks according to standard precautions when performing splash-generating procedures (e.g., wound irrigation). Masks are not recommended for routine care (e.g., upon room entry).
- Use gloves and gowns according to standard precautions.
- *Home care and ambulatory care:* Follow standard precautions for PPE.

Equipment, Supplies, and Environment

- Ensure that patient rooms are cleaned well and often. Disinfect high-touch surfaces (e.g., bed rails, door knobs, bedside commodes) in the room.
- Dedicate noncritical equipment (e.g., stethoscope, blood pressure cuff) to use on individual patients colonized or infected with MDROs.
- Follow standard precautions for handling linens and eating utensils.
- *For C. difficile:* Use a bleach-containing disinfectant for environmental disinfection.
- *Home care:* Limit the amount of patient-care equipment brought into the homes of patients infected or colonized with MDROs. See Contact Precautions in Clinical Insight 22-4 to review this.

Other

- Actively observe for symptoms of infections, such as MRSA. Some institutions require screening cultures at admission, or on admission to certain units (e.g., intensive care).
- Be aware of and practice preventive measures, such as:
  - Use intravenous and urinary catheters only when essential, and with scrupulous sterile technique.
  - Special measures to prevent lower respiratory tract infection in intubated patients
  - Judiciously select and use antimicrobials.

If Further Measures Are Needed

Note: If MDROs continue to be a problem in spite of diligent infection control measures, your agency might consider intensifying infection control practices. For example:

- Donning gowns and gloves before or upon entry to the patient's room
- Assigning the same personnel to the care of MDRO patients only
- Stopping new admissions to the unit or facility
- Obtaining environmental cultures
- Screening high-risk patients on admission

Practice Resources

Association for Professionals in Infection Control and Epidemiology (APIC), 2010; Calfee, Salgado, Classen, et al., 2008; Halcomb, Griffiths, & Fernandez, 2008; Institute for Healthcare Improvement, 2006; Siegel, Rhinehart, Jackson, et al., 2007.

For specific guidelines on care of contaminated equipment and supplies, refer to Clinical Insights 22-2, 22-3, and 22-4, as needed.

Supporting the Psychological Needs of Patients in Isolation

Keep in mind that it is the disease that is being isolated, *not* the person who has the disease. Patients who are in isolation continue to have a need for human contact. In fact, isolation may produce anxiety and increase the desire for human contact. Search for ways to reassure and maintain contact with the patient in protective isolation. Possible solutions include the following:

- When wearing the required protective equipment, touch the patient.
- Organize the time you spend in the patient's room to include time for discussion about how the client is coping with isolation.

- If the patient is in droplet isolation, remember that the danger area is 3 feet from the patient. You can go to the door of the room and speak to the patient without a mask.
- Reassure the patient that precautions are temporary.
- Explain that the precautions and the PPE protect you and the patient, as well as family members and other patients.

KnowledgeCheck 22-7

- If you needed to disinfect a sink in a client's home, what would you use?
- List at least three actions clients can take to help avoid infection when they are out in the community.

PRACTICING SURGICAL ASEPSIS

Sterile means without life. If an object is sterile, it contains no life and therefore no infectious organisms. The exception is *prions*, the protein particles that cause severe neurological

---

Toward Evidence-Based Practice

Siegel, J. H., & Korniewicz, D. M. (2007). **Keeping patients safe: An interventional hand hygiene study at an oncology center.** *Clinical Journal of Oncology Nursing, 11*(5), 643–646.

The purpose of this study was to investigate whether the introduction of a handheld sanitizer spray improved hand hygiene compliance of healthcare workers at an oncology center. Subjects included 25 licensed and 22 unlicensed healthcare professionals. Researchers assessed hand hygiene before and after routine clinical procedures. Participants were observed for 2 weeks before and then for 14 weeks after introduction of the handheld sanitizer spray. Baseline compliance rates were 53% before the sanitizer spray and 49% after it was introduced.

Raskind, C. H., Worley, S., Vinski, J., & Goldfarb, J. (2007). **Hand hygiene compliance rates after an educational intervention in a neonatal intensive care unit.** *Infection Control & Hospital Epidemiology, 28*(9), 1096–1098.

This observational study assessed the impact of a staff education program to promote hand hygiene. Observations were made before and after the education program. Before the education program, hand hygiene compliance was 89%; 1 month after the education program it increased to 100%. At 3 months, though, the rate decreased to the baseline 89%.

Gammon, J., Morgan-Samuel, H., & Gould, D. (2008). **A review of the evidence for suboptimal compliance of healthcare practitioners to standard/universal infection control precautions.** *Journal of Clinical Nursing, 17*(2), 157–167.

Internationally standard/universal precautions are regarded as fundamental in infection control and prevention. These researchers examined findings from international research about the extent to which practitioners comply with infection control precautions. They used 37 different studies. They concluded that compliance to infection control precautions is internationally suboptimal, and that compliance does improve after an intervention (e.g., education program). They stated that research fails to indicate whether after a period of time the compliance returns to the prestudy norm.

Ganczak, M., & Szych, Z. (2007). **Surgical nurses and compliance with personal protective equipment.** *Journal of Hospital Infection, 66*(4), 346–351.

A total of 601 surgical nurses from 18 randomly selected hospitals in Poland were surveyed using a confidential questionnaire. They found that compliance with PPE varied considerably. Eighty-three percent used gloves, but only 9% used eyewear, and only 5% routinely used gloves, masks, protective eyewear, and gowns when in contact with potentially infective material. They found higher compliance among those with previous training in infection control or experience of caring for an HIV patient. The most commonly stated reasons for noncompliance (each at about 30%) were nonavailability of PPE, conviction that the patient was not infected, and belief that following the recommended practices interfered with providing good patient care. Researchers recommended wider training in and evaluation of infection control.

1. From these abstracts, what do you know about the subjects in the studies?

2. In what way(s) does the Gammon study support the other three studies? Where is the support lacking?

 Go to Chapter 22, **Toward Evidence-Based Practice Suggested Responses,** on DavisPlus.

degeneration in animals and humans, such as in bovine spongiform encephalopathy (BSE, also known as mad cow disease) in cattle and Creutzfeldt–Jakob disease (CJD) in humans. Inanimate objects, such as surgical equipment, gauze dressings, or wound irrigation fluid may be sterilized. However, humans will always have microorganisms in and on their bodies; and researchers have not yet determined what types of techniques, if any, can destroy prions.

Surgical asepsis, or **sterile technique,** requires creation of a sterile environment and use of sterile equipment. It differs from medical asepsis in that it is more complex and it is not necessary to use it with all patients. Sterilization can be accomplished through the use of special gases or high heat. Surgical equipment and implanted devices are examples of materials that must be sterilized. If you need more information about sterilization processes,

 Go to Chapter 22, **Tables, Boxes, Figures: ESG Table 22-3, Methods for Disinfection and Sterlization of Patient-Care items and Surfaces,** on Davis*Plus.*

To create a sterile area, environmental services personnel perform extensive cleaning using special solutions and procedures. All health personnel working in the area must wear appropriate surgical attire and perform a surgical hand scrub.

Levels of Asepsis. Recent guidelines suggest using modified sterile technique for many bedside procedures that have traditionally used sterile technique. (e.g., tracheostomy care and wound care). The following summarizes the practical differences in sterile, modified sterile, and clean techniques:

- **Sterile technique** is the use of sterile gloves and sterile supplies (e.g., drapes, bandages, instruments, water)
- **Modified sterile technique** is use of nonsterile procedure gloves with sterile supplies.
- **Clean technique** is use of clean hands or nonsterile gloves and clean, rather than sterile, supplies (e.g., tap water).

Performing a Surgical Scrub

A **surgical scrub** is a modification of the handwashing procedure described earlier (see Table 22-3 for a comparison). It traditionally involves an extended scrub of the hands using a sponge, nail cleaner, and a bactericidal scrubbing agent. A newer method uses a brushless scrub, using a bactericidal scrubbing agent. All methods require a prewash before the surgical scrub. For a description of the steps involved, refer to Procedures 22-4 and 22-5.

Donning Surgical Attire

Burn units, labor and birth units, and some surgical wards, intensive care units, nurseries, and oncology wards require surgical attire for patient caregiving. In each of these units, nurses care for clients who are at increased risk for infection or are undergoing an invasive procedure that places them at increased risk. The goal on all of these units is to protect patients from infection transmitted by healthcare workers.

All personnel on these units don *clean,* not sterile, surgical attire, or scrub suits, when they arrive on the unit. These scrub suits should not be worn outside the unit. If you must transport a patient to another area or leave the unit to gather supplies, wear a covering over the scrub suit. Remove the covering on your return to the unit. Additional precautions may include a disposable hat to cover the hair, shoe coverings, and face masks.

Table 22-3 ➤ A Comparison of Hand Hygiene and Surgical Scrub		
	HAND HYGIENE	**SURGICAL SCRUB**
No visible soil	Use alcohol-based hand rub or soap (plain or antimicrobial) and water.	1. Perform a handwash with soap and water. 2. Then perform the surgical scrub using either an FDA-approved antimicrobial scrub product or an antiseptic hand rub that is FDA-approved for surgical hand asepsis.
Hands visibly soiled	Wash with soap (plain or antimicrobial) and water.	Surgical scrub steps remain the same, even with visible soil.

Sources: The Association of periOperative Registered Nurses (AORN). Recommended Practices Committee. (2004). *Recommended practices for surgical hand: Antisepsis/hand scrubs.* AORN *Journal, 79*(2), 416–431; Boyce, J. M., & Pittet, D. (2002, October 25). Guideline for hand hygiene in health-care settings. Recommendations of the Healthcare Infection Control Practices Advisory Committee, & the HICPAC/SHEA/APIC/IDSA Hand Hygiene Task Force. *Morbidity and Mortality Weekly Report, 51*(RR16), 1–44; Pratt, R. J., Pellowe, C. M., Wilson, J. A., et al. (2007). Epic2: National evidence-based guidelines for preventing healthcare-associated infections in NHS hospitals in England. *Journal of Hospital Infection, 65*(Supplement 1), S1–64.

Personnel engaged in surgery or certain invasive procedures must dress in *sterile* surgical attire. As a beginning student, you will soon find yourself in such a situation. Initially your role will be limited to observation, but you will need to be prepared for these experiences.

First you will change into a scrub suit, apply shoe coverings, and put on a disposable hat; wash your hands and apply a face mask. If there is potential for spray of fluids, wear a face mask with an eye shield. Be sure to adjust the mask so that it is comfortable to breathe through. Once you have adjusted the mask, perform the surgical scrub. If a surgical gown is required, don it after the hand scrub.

If you are applying full surgical attire, you will need to apply gloves using a closed method, after you have put on your gown. Once you don sterile gloves, you may touch only sterile items. To learn how to don sterile gloves and gown using the closed method, see Procedure 22-6.

You will often wear sterile gloves for procedures that do not require full surgical attire. For this, you will use the open method of gloving. Some key points are to open the glove packaging slowly, avoid fanning the wrapping or touching the gloves, and put the first glove on your dominant hand. A general rule to consider when applying the second glove is to touch glove-to-glove and skin-to-skin. The already-gloved hand may touch any of the sterile surfaces of the second glove. The second hand may touch only the inside of the glove—the portion that will have contact with the skin. For complete instructions for open-method sterile gloving, refer to Procedure 22-7.

Using Sterile Technique in Nursing Care

Healthcare providers use sterile technique to perform a variety of procedures. Some of the procedures require full surgical attire (e.g., inserting a central venous catheter); others do not. Some examples of procedures that use both sterile technique and principles of medical asepsis are administering an injection, starting an IV line, and performing a sterile dressing change. To clarify, when administering an injection, you prepare the patient, cleanse the injection site, and remove the needle cap using standard precautions; you do not don sterile gloves. However, for the rest of the procedure you observe sterile technique by taking care not to touch or otherwise contaminate the exposed sterile needle.

Before performing a sterile procedure, determine what supplies you will need and whether you will need assistance. If the patient is unable to maintain a position required for the procedure, you will need a helper to hold the patient during the procedure. Wash your hands before gathering materials from the sterile supply area, and then gather the other required supplies and equipment. Check the expiration date on each package. Check the package to make sure it is intact. If it has paper or cloth wrapping, be sure there are no indications that it has ever been wet. For guidelines related to sterile technique and preparing and maintaining sterile fields, see Clinical Insight 22-6.

Preparing and Maintaining Sterile Fields. There are some variations in how you might set up sterile fields.

Clinical Insight 22-6 ➤ **Guidelines for Preparing and Maintaining Sterile Fields**

For steps in setting up a sterile field and adding supplies and solutions, see Procedure 22-7.

Tip: Sterile touches sterile. Unsterile touches unsterile.

Setting Up the Field

- Close doors and limit the number of people in the area when setting up a sterile field. Air currents can carry dust and microorganisms.
- Prepare a sterile field as close as possible to the time of use. To minimize the opportunity for contamination via air currents.
- You may establish a sterile field by using a sterile drape or by using the inner side of a sterile package wrapping. Touch the inside of the wrapper only after you don sterile gloves.
- When you are placing a sterile drape, protect your gloved hands by cuffing the drape over your hands.

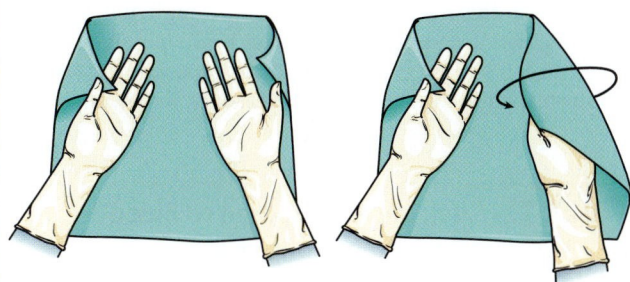

Protecting gloved hands.

What Areas Are Considered Sterile?

- A sterile field is sterile only on the horizontal plane (e.g., the draped table top). Consider nonsterile any material that drapes over the horizontal plane.
- Consider a 1-inch margin around the border of a sterile drape unsterile even if it remains on a horizontal surface. Because it is in contact with contaminated surfaces.
- If you are wearing sterile attire, consider only the front of your body from the chest to the level of the sterile field to be sterile, nothing else.
- Sleeve cuffs are considered unsterile when your hands

pass beyond the cuff (cuffs are sterile if you don gloves using the closed method).

Keeping the Field Sterile

- No one in unsterile garb should come near a sterile field. They should remain at least 1 foot away.
- Remain at least 1 foot away from nonsterile areas if you are wearing sterile garb.
- Never turn your back to a sterile field. A sterile field or open sterile items must be kept in constant view. You are responsible for monitoring and maintaining the sterility. If you cannot see the field, you do not know if it has become contaminated.
- Keep conversation to a minimum around the sterile field. To reduce the spread of droplets from the mouth.
- Avoid reaching over a sterile field even if you are in sterile garb.
- Handle sterile equipment only if you are wearing sterile gloves.
- Limit the amount of time a sterile field remains set up in advance of a procedure
- Sterile liquids must be contained in sterile bowls on the field or the sterile drape must be nonpermeable in order to avoid wicking. Liquid can act as a wick and contaminate a field.

Adding Sterile Items

- Only sterile items can be placed on a sterile field.
- Immediately before adding items to a sterile field, inspect them for proper packaging, integrity, and inclusion of a sterilization indicator.
- Never assume an item is sterile. If there is any doubt about its sterility, consider it contaminated.
- All items applied to a sterile field must be sterilized in an approved manner.

Practice Resources

The Association of periOperative Registered Nurses (AORN), 2006.

Sometimes it is as simple as opening a package of supplies wrapped in a sterile disposable cover. At other times, you may work with a larger, reusable or disposable sterile drape (wrapped in an outer wrapping). In that situation, you open the outer wrapping, then pick up the sterile drape grasping only the corners, and allow it to fall open to create a sterile field, perhaps to entirely cover a table surface or to create a sterile field on the patient's bed. To learn a procedure for maintaining a sterile field, as well as adding supplies and sterile liquids to it, see Procedure 22-8A.

Adding Supplies to a Sterile Field. Some supplies (e.g., urinary catheter kits) are packaged a wrapper that can form a sterile field. The outside of these packages is considered clean, and the inside is sterile. You must open these packages in a way that does not contaminate the inside of the wrapping. Be cautious when adding supplies to a sterile field. If they are light and small, gently add them to the sterile field by separating the package flaps and allowing them to fall onto the field. If the object is large, such as an irrigation bowl, slowly unwrap the packaging and, grasping it through the outside wrapper, place the bowl on the field. If any object falls only partly on the field, it is no longer sterile. For detailed instructions on how to add supplies to a sterile field, see Procedure 22-8B.

Adding Sterile Solutions to a Sterile Field. Add sterile liquids to a sterile field by slowly pouring them into a container on the field. Some sterile drapes contain an impermeable membrane between layers. This membrane serves as a barrier to moisture and prevents wicking. With this type of drape, you may pour sterile liquid directly on gauze pads on the field. Pour only an amount of liquid that is sufficient to make the gauze pads damp. Excess fluid may run off the field, causing the field to become contaminated—a wet field is not sterile because it does not provide a barrier to microorganisms on the unsterile surface under the drape. For step-by-step instruction in how to add sterile solutions to a sterile field, refer to Procedure 22-8C.

KnowledgeCheck 22-8

- When will you need to don sterile gloves using the closed method?
- True or false: Some procedures require both standard precautions and sterile technique.
- What part(s) of a sterile field are considered to be unsterile?

INFECTION CONTROL AND PREVENTION FOR HEALTHCARE WORKERS

It is critical that you learn how to protect yourself from infections—not only to avoid personal illness, but also to avoid becoming a reservoir for infection. Nurses and other patient-care workers are at increased risk of acquiring infections because they come in contact with a large number and variety of pathogens. Skin and mucous membrane contact and puncture wounds often serve as portals of entry.

Nursing assistive personnel (NAP), ancillary personnel, housekeeping and maintenance workers, visitors, volunteers, and family are often present on nursing units. You need to protect them and yourself from potential hazardous exposure as well as from microorganisms brought into the unit. As a nurse, you need to monitor other healthcare workers, patients, and visitors for breaks in infection control and prevention.

What Role Does the Infection Preventionist Nurse Play?

The task of the infection prevention nurse is to minimize the number of infections in the healthcare facility. Because it is not possible to provide absolute protection all the time, the nurse must balance the risks for infection with the costs of protective measures and the benefits of various strategies. Infection preventionists must keep current with information about pathogens, antibiotic resistance, and infection control. The nurse also functions as an epidemiologist, tracking down the source of HAIs and strengthening measures to prevent their recurrence. Finally, all members of the infection prevention team enforce compliance with federal, state, and local regulations related to infection control and prevention.

What Should I Do If I Am Exposed to Bloodborne Pathogens?

Exposure to blood, body secretions, or body tissues containing blood or secretions requires immediate action. See Box 22-1 for complete instructions. The first step is to minimize the exposure by washing the area thoroughly. Then notify the appropriate people, complete an injury report, and seek medical attention.

Anyone exposed to bloodborne pathogens should have baseline lab work done to check for hepatitis and HIV. If the patient source is known, the infection preventionist will arrange to have the patient tested. Subsequent testing and possible preventive treatment are based on the type of exposure and what is known about the source and the injured person. To limit risks from the exposure, the infection prevention team will provide counseling and recommendations as soon as possible after the event. Chapters 23 and 25 present information on preventing needlestick injuries.

How Can I Minimize the Effects of Bioterrorism and Epidemics?

In 2001, anthrax spores were sent through the U.S. mail. This incident brought new attention to the possibility of biological agents being used as weapons, especially by terrorists. **Bioterrorism** is the intentional release, or threatened release,

---

BOX 22-1 ■ If You Are Exposed to Blood or Other Body Fluids

If you are stuck by a needle or other sharp, or get blood or other potentially infectious materials in your eyes, nose, mouth, or on broken skin:

1. Immediately flood the exposed area with water and clean any wound with soap and water or a skin disinfectant if available.
2. Report the exposure immediately to the appropriate person in the agency. If you are a student, also report immediately to your instructor.
3. Seek immediate medical attention. Consent to testing and follow-up treatment as advised.
4. Complete an incident or injury report.
5. Attend counseling sessions provided by the agency.

Source: Bloodborne pathogens and needlestick prevention. Post-exposure evaluation. (n.d.). Occupational Safety & Health Administration. U.S. Department of Labor. Retrieved from http://www.osha.gov/SLTC/bloodbornepathogens/postexposure.html

of disease-producing organisms or substances for the purpose of causing death, illness, harm, economic damage, or fear. Six diseases with recognized bioterrorism potential are anthrax, botulism, pneumonic plague, smallpox, viral hemorrhagic fevers, and tularemia. The U.S. government has recently funded development of drugs to treat three of these diseases (anthrax, plague, and tularemia).

Recognize an Outbreak

Should a biological event occur, either as a result of bioterrorism or a naturally occurring epidemic, a key factor in minimizing its effects is the ability to quickly recognize unusual disease patterns and detect the presence of infectious diseases. Some electronic patient record systems include special pattern identification programs. The use of these systems supplements, but does not replace, clinical observation skills. Nurses need to assess not only the individual patient's condition, but also clusters of symptoms. Hospital, emergency department, and clinic nurses are in key positions to recognize outbreaks because they see patients from multiple primary care providers. Nurses must keep the following questions in mind:

- Am I seeing an unexpected number of infectious diseases, or diseases possibly caused by infectious organisms?
- Am I seeing similar cases that are not responding to medical treatment?
- Are healthcare workers who come in contact with infectious patients becoming ill?

Notify the Safety Officer

After identifying a suspicious pattern, you should notify the institution's interventionist or safety officer as soon as possible. Appropriate cultures will be needed, and the federal and state health departments should be notified. If the infectious organism is unknown, samples must be preserved for future analysis.

Institute Appropriate Level of Standard Precautions

In the event of an epidemic, the essential principles of hand hygiene and standard precautions will be the core of your infection prevention and control measures. Patients with similar symptoms should be cared for by a minimum number of healthcare personnel, and those personnel must use appropriate isolation precautions. If the etiology and transmission route of the causative organism are unknown, standard, contact, and airborne precautions should be implemented as needed. The Occupational Safety and Health Administration (OSHA) (n.d.) defines types of personal protective equipment and situations in which you are required to wear it.

Prepare Clients for a Pandemic

Teach clients that preparing for pandemic disease is similar to preparing for other general kinds of emergency preparedness, such as power outages and natural disasters (see the accompanying Self-Care box, Teaching Your Patient About Preparing for a Pandemic Disease Outbreak).

Self-Care

Teaching Your Patient About Preparing for a Pandemic Disease Outbreak

- ➤ Make a preparedness plan with your family and others in the community (e.g., school, business, church groups). Help organize local response planning and be available to help if there is an outbreak. Participate in emergency planning at work and get training if it is available.
- ➤ Talk with family members about what will be needed to care for them in your home if someone becomes ill.
- ➤ Expect that usual community services may be disrupted—for example, banks, stores, post offices, and even hospitals and public buildings may be closed
- ➤ Store a 2-week supply of bottled water and food. Keep extra nonperishable foods. Examples of food and nonperishables include the following:
  Ready-to-eat canned meats (e.g., ham, tuna)
  Canned fruits, vegetables, beans, soups
  Protein or fruit bars
  Dry cereals
  Peanut butter or nuts
  Dried fruit
  Crackers
  Canned juices
  Canned baby food and formula
  Pet food
- ➤ Periodically check your regular prescription drugs to keep a continuous supply on hand.
- ➤ Have nonprescription drugs and health supplies on hand. Examples include:
  Medical supplies, such as blood-pressure and glucose monitors
  Medicines for fever (e.g., acetaminophen, ibuprofen)
  Thermometer
  Soap and water or alcohol-based (60%–95%) handwash
  Antidiarrheal medication

  Vitamins
  Fluids with electrolytes
- ➤ Keep a 2-week supply of other emergency supplies on hand, such as a flashlight, batteries, portable radio, manual can opener, trash bags, tissues, toilet paper, and disposable diapers.
- ➤ Keep your family's health information up to date, organized, and accessible.
- ➤ Make sure you have more than one method to communicate (e.g., telephone and e-mail) and that you can get information from the outside world (including by battery-powered radio).
- ➤ Be sure everyone on the family washes hands frequently and properly and covers coughs and sneezes with tissues.
- ➤ Teach family members to stay away from others as much as possible if they are sick. Stay home from work and school if sick.
- ➤ Get an annual seasonal influenza vaccination.
- ➤ Explore the possibility of working by telecommuting during a pandemic to avoid unnecessary exposure.

Sources: Davey, V. (2007). Disaster care. Questions and answers on pandemic influenza. *American Journal of Nursing, 107*(7), 50–57; Emergency preparedness & response: Emergency preparedness and you (n.d.). Centers for Disease Control and Prevention. Retrieved March 27, 2011, from http://emergency.cdc.gov/preparedness/; New York State Department of Health. (2011). Emergency preparedness. Retrieved March 27, 2011, from http://www.health.state.ny.us/environmental/emergency/; U.S. Department of Health & Human Services. (n.d.). Flu pandemics. Retrieved March 27, 2011, from http://www.flu.gov/individualfamily/about/pandemic/index.html; U.S. Department of Homeland Security. (2010). Make a plan. Retrieved August 8, 2008, from http://www.ready.gov/america/makeaplan/index.html; and Veneema, T. G., & Töke, J. (2006). Early detection and surveillance for biopreparedness and emerging infectious diseases. *Online Journal of Issues in Nursing, 11*(1).

SUMMARY

After studying this chapter, you should be armed with the basic concepts and skills you need to protect yourself and your clients from infection. However, knowledge and skill are not enough. Research continues to show that healthcare professionals too often fail to comply with guidelines for infection prevention, especially the simple measures such as hand hygiene and standard precautions. Your role as a nurse is to integrate the best current evidence with your clinical expertise and, through your own individual performance, to minimize harm to patients and others. This includes using technology and standardized practices that support patient safety and quality.

 Wash your hands! Follow standard precautions!

If you would like to know more about pathogens,

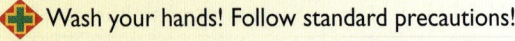 Go to **Student Resources: A Brief Introduction to Microbiology,** on DavisPlus.

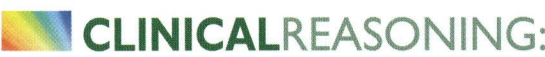

CLINICALREASONING:
Applying the **Full-Spectrum Nursing Model**

Because the following critical thinking activities allow you to practice the kind of thinking you will use as a full-spectrum nurse, they usually have no single right answer. Discuss them with your peers—if you have difficulty with any of the questions, consult your instructor.

PATIENT SITUATION

Mr. Long, a frail elderly man, is in the hospital because he has become dehydrated and needs supportive care. The nurse administered intravenous fluids. Mr. Long also has a fairly large decubitus ulcer (bedsore), which was cultured recently and found to be infected with *Staphylococcus aureus*. The nurse wore gloves to treat the ulcer. While doing so, she noticed that the IV was infusing too fast and, without thinking, regulated the IV without removing her soiled gloves. The next nurse to regulate the IV did so with her bare hands, and then, without realizing it, rubbed her neck. Later, the nurse developed a boil on her neck, which was infected with *S. aureus*.

THINKING

1. *Theoretical Knowledge:*
   a. What are the six links in the chain of infection?
   b. Why do you think the *S. aureus* was able to thrive in Mr. Long's decubitus ulcer?
   c. What are the three modes of transmission of microorganisms? Which one is the most frequent mode of transmission?
2. *Critical Thinking (Reflecting):*
   a. What was the reservoir for the *S. aureus*?
   b. What was the exit from Mr. Long?
   c. What was (were) the fomite(s) for transmission to the nurse?
   d. What was the portal of entry into the nurse?

DOING

3. *Nursing Process (Implementation):* In addition to wearing gloves, what other PPE (if any) does the nurse need if she is performing decubitus care and changing Mr. Long's bed linens?

CARING

4. *Self-Knowledge and Ethical Knowledge:* Think of one instance in the clinical setting in which you did *not* follow standard precautions. Why do you think that happened?

 Go to Chapter 22, **Clinical Reasoning: Applying the Full-Spectrum Nursing Model Response Sheet,** on DavisPlus.

Practical Knowledge procedures

As a nurse, you play a vital role in preventing transmission of infection. Most infection control measures are independent nursing activities. You do not need a medical prescription for them. You do need theoretical knowledge and scrupulous medical and surgical asepsis technique. The procedures in this section, as well as the Clinical Insights in preceding sections, provide the guidance you will need to perform this important role.

Procedure 22-1 ■ Hand Hygiene

➤ For steps to follow in *all* procedures, refer to the Universal Steps for All Procedures found on the page facing the inside back cover. For this procedure, also refer to Clinical Insight 22-1 as needed.

Equipment

- Liquid soap (antimicrobial) or alcohol-based handrub
- Paper towels
- Warm, running water
- Hand moisturizer (optional)

Pre-Procedure Assessments

- Check your hands for breaks in the skin.
  Breaks in the skin provide a route for microbial entry.

- Inspect the condition of your nails.
  Nails should be no longer than $1/4$ inch from the fingertips.
  Do not wear artificial nails or extensions.
  Nail polish should not be chipped.
  Preferably, do not use polish.
  Research indicates the area under the nails, artificial nails/ extensions, and chipped polish act as reservoirs for microorganisms.

Procedure 22-1A ■ Using Soap and Water

➤ When performing the procedure, always identify your patient according to agency policy and be attentive to standard precautions, hand hygiene, patient safety and privacy, body mechanics, and documentation.

Procedure Steps

1. **Bare your hands and forearms.** Push your sleeves above your wrists, and remove your wristwatch and rings.
   Moist clothing facilitates transfer of microorganisms; jewelry harbors bacteria and creates a moist area on the skin, which facilitates bacterial growth.

2. **Turn on water**—warm, not hot.
   Warm running water opens pores to aid in removing microorganisms without removing excess skin oils. It also reduces chapping. Hot water increases the potential for skin breakdown.

3. **Wet your hands and wrists.** Keep your hands below your wrists and forearms.
   The hands are considered more contaminated than the wrists and arms, so prevent water from running from your "dirty" hands onto your "clean" wrists and forearms.
   a. Avoid splashing water onto clothing.
   b. Avoid touching the inside of the sink.

Microorganisms travel in moisture. The inside of the sink is considered contaminated. ▼

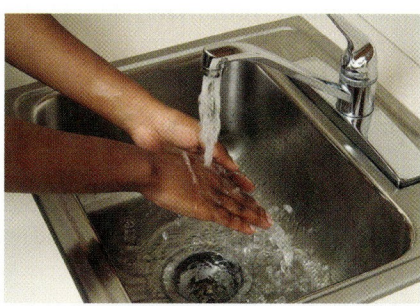

4. **Apply 3 to 5 mL of liquid soap,** (typically 3 to 4 pumps using a soap dispenser). Rub the soap over all surfaces of your hands.
   Provides enough soap to completely cover the hands for maximum effectiveness to remove transient microorganisms.

5. **Vigorously rub your hands together for at least 15 seconds,** lathering all surfaces, interlacing fingers, rubbing around each finger and thumb, rubbing the backs and palms of the hands in a circular motion. ▼

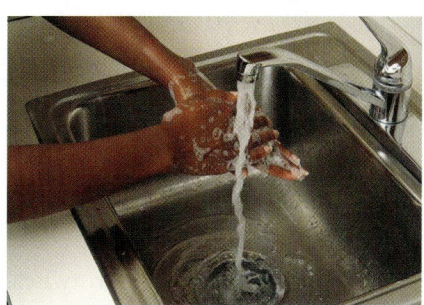

Washing for at least 15 seconds is required for mechanical removal of microorganisms and to give antimicrobial products adequate contact with the skin surfaces to be effective. Attention to all areas of the hands is essential; research indicates areas of the hands most often missed are the thumb, the wrist, and areas between the fingers.

6. **Clean under your fingernails,** if needed, using a disposable nail cleaner.
   Areas under the nails harbor high concentrations of microorganisms.

(continued on next page)

Procedure 22-1 ■ **Hand Hygiene** (continued)

Procedure 22-1A ■ **Using Soap and Water**

7. Rinse your hands thoroughly. Keep your hands below your wrists and forearms.

Rinsing from wrist to fingertips mechanically washes away debris and microorganisms to flow into the sink and not back up the hand and arm.

8. Dry your hands thoroughly, moving from your fingers up to your forearms and blotting with paper towel.

Move from the area you wish to keep cleanest (hands). Blotting decreases skin irritation.

9. Turn off the faucet with a dry paper towel. Do not handle the paper towel with the opposite hand. ➤

Prevents contamination of hands from the faucet. The paper towel has had contact with the contaminated faucet and may transfer microorganisms to your freshly washed hand. Many pathogens can live on environmental surfaces, such as faucets and countertops.

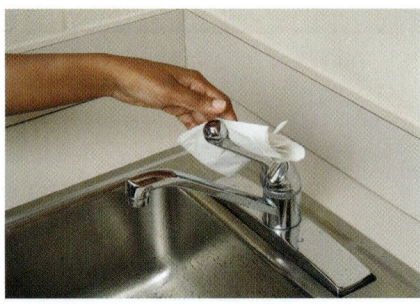

10. Apply a hand moisturizer at least twice daily; use hand care products recommended by infection preventionists.

Hand moisturizer is recommended to prevent skin from drying, which may lead to skin damage and increase the risk for transmission of infection. Petroleum-based products compromise latex gloves, resulting in permeability. Anionic-based moisturizers can neutralize the residual effects of chlorhexidine gluconate and chloroxylenol.

Procedure 22-1B ■ **Using Alcohol-Based Handrubs**

➤ When performing the procedure, always identify your patient according to agency policy and be attentive to standard precautions, hand hygiene, patient safety and privacy, body mechanics, and documentation.

Procedure Steps

1. Use alcohol-based handrubs when hands are not visibly soiled and when certain pathogens are suspected.

Antiseptic solutions are not effective when organic material or dirt from hands is present. Alcohol handrubs cannot remove spores, and therefore should not be used for hand hygiene when Clostridium difficile or Bacillus anthracis is suspected of being present.

2. Bare your hands and forearms. Push your sleeves above your wrists. Remove your jewelry and wristwatch.

3. Apply a sufficient quantity (at least 3 mL) of antiseptic solution to cover the hands and wrists.

All surfaces must be covered with sufficient product to effectively remove microorganisms.

4. Vigorously rub antiseptic solution into your hand for 15 to 30 seconds (or as long as it takes to sing "Happy Birthday" if no clock is available). Cover all surfaces of the hands: interlacing fingers, rubbing around each finger and thumb, and rubbing the backs and palms of the hands in a circular motion, including

under the nails, until the solution is completely dry.

Fifteen to 30 seconds is recommended by the Centers for Disease Control and Prevention (CDC) for effective disinfection by alcohol handrubs ▼

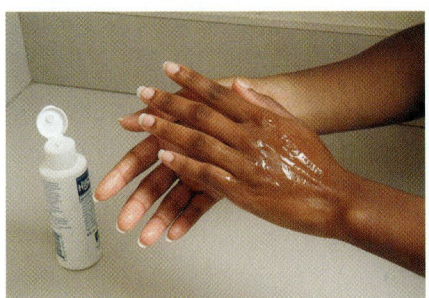

Evaluation

Hands are free of handrub and dry.

Documentation

Hand hygiene is a responsibility of all healthcare providers. It does not require documentation.

Practice Resources

Association of periOperative Registered Nurses, 2004; Boyce, & Pittet, 2002; Larson, Girard, Pessoa-Silva, et al., 2006; Pratt, Pellowe, Wilson, et al., 2007; Siegel, Rhinehart, Jackson, et al., 2007.

Thinking About the Procedure

 Go to the *Fundamentals of Nursing Skills Videos*, **Asepsis: Handwashing.**

1. How does the nurse clean her fingernails?
2. Does the nurse turn off the faucet with a paper towel? What is the reason for what she does?

 For suggested responses, go to Chapter 22, **Thinking About the Procedure Suggested Responses,** on DavisPlus.

Procedure 22-2 ■ Donning Personal Protective Equipment (PPE)

➤ For steps to follow in *all* procedures, refer to the Universal Steps for All Procedures found on the page facing the inside back cover.

Equipment

Following CDC recommendations, you will usually use some combination of gloves, gown, mask, and eye protection; depending on the organism and level of precaution. In certain situations, you may need hair covers and shoe covers (e.g., when full barrier precautions are needed).

- Disposable gloves of the proper size
- Disposable isolation gown

- Face mask (or N-95 respirator mask, as indicated)
- Face shield or goggles
- Hair cover (if needed)
- Shoe covers (if needed)

➤ When performing the procedure, always identify your patient according to agency policy and be attentive to standard precautions, hand hygiene, patient safety and privacy, body mechanics, and documentation.

Procedure Steps

1. **Assess the need for PPE**. If you need more information about choosing PPE, refer to Clinical Insights 22-3, 22-4, and 22-5.

   a. **Gloves:** When you may be exposed to any body secretions directly or indirectly

   Gloves provide a barrier against body fluids. All patients are considered potentially infected per Standard Precautions.

   b. **Gowns:** When your uniform (e.g., scrubs) may become exposed to potentially infective secretions (e.g., excessive wound drainage, fecal incontinence, or other discharges from the body; or when fluids may be splashed [as in eye irrigation]).

   c. **Face mask:** To prevent transmission of pathogens spread through close respiratory (3 ft or less) or mucous membrane contact with respiratory secretions

   Surgical masks provide a barrier to large-particle droplets (> 5 microns in diameter).

   d. **Face shield or eye goggles:** When splashing might occur and fluids enter your eyes (e.g., blood splashes, respiratory droplets, or wound débridement). To protect the entire facial area, wear a face shield (for maximum protection, it should protect the crown and chin and wrap around the face to the ear).

   Helps prevent pathogens from entering the conjunctiva directly or indirectly.

   e. **N-95 respirator:** When caring for clients infected with airborne organisms (< 5 microns) such as the tuberculosis bacillus.

   This device prevents the airborne transmission of the tuberculosis bacterium. The respirator mask in Figure 22-4 is disposable; others are reusable.

   f. **Hair covers:** When there is a potential for spraying or splashing of body fluids

   Although not included in the CDC report (Siegel, Rhinehart, Jackson, et al., 2007), agency policy may advise hair covers in certain situations.

   g. **Shoe covers:** When there is a potential for contamination of shoes with body fluids

   The floor (and anything in contact with it) is considered contaminated. Although not in the CDC report (Siegel, Rhinehart, Jackson, et al., 2007), agency policy may require shoe covers in certain situations. Furthermore, certain categories of pathogens require full protective gear, and in those circumstances shoe covers are necessary. Wear shoe covers to protect against exposure to airborne organisms or contact with a contaminated environment and as a part of full barrier precautions (e.g., when the patient has hemorrhagic disease or severe acute respiratory syndrome [SARS]).

2. **Determine the availability of appropriate personal protective equipment**. Do not substitute a patient gown for a disposable isolation or protective gown.

   Isolation gowns must be made of moisture-repelling materials to prevent contamination of underlying clothing and skin.

3. **Don the isolation gown.**

   While donning PPE, the goal is to not contaminate the PPE.

   a. Pick up the gown by the shoulders, allowing the gown to fall open without touching the floor or other surfaces.

   Avoids contaminating the gown with environmental pathogens. ▼

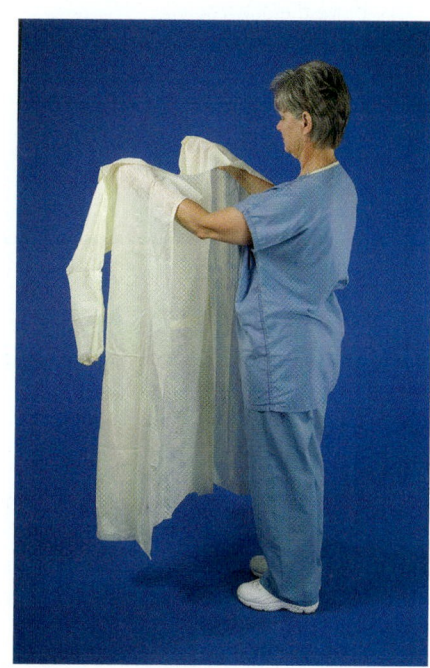

(continued on next page)

Procedure 22-2 ■ **Donning Personal Protective Equipment (PPE)** (continued)

b. Slip your arms into the sleeves. ▼

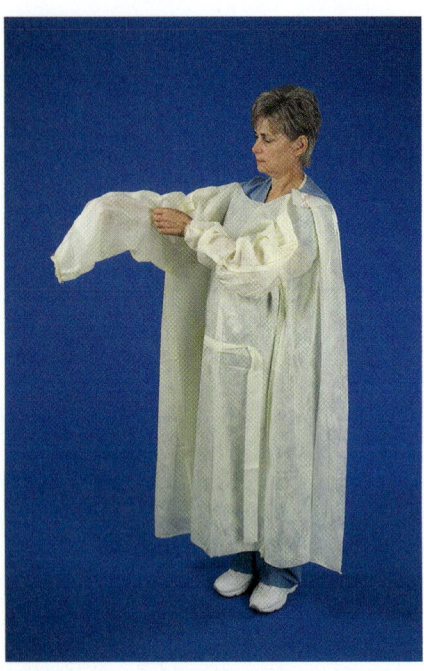

c. Fasten ties at the neck.
d. Position the gown so that it covers the back, and fasten the ties at the waist. Do not bring ties around to the front of the gown.
   The front of the gown is considered contaminated after you enter the patient's room. If the ties are at the front of the gown, they will be contaminated, making it difficult to remove the gown safely.
e. If the gown does not completely cover your clothing in the back, wear two gowns. Put on the first gown so that the opening is in the front, and then place the second gown over the first, so that the opening is in the back.

4. **Don the face mask or N-95 respirator.**
   a. Determine how the mask is secured. Identify the top edge of the mask by locating the thin metal strip (nosepiece) that goes over the bridge of the nose.
      Surgical masks may be secured by ties at the back of the head and neck, loops around the ears, or elastic bands.
   b. Place the mask over your nose, mouth, and chin. Press the flexible metal strip so that it conforms to the bridge of your nose.
      The mask must fit snugly to your face for maximum barrier protection. Correct positioning will also keep your glasses or goggles from fogging. ▼

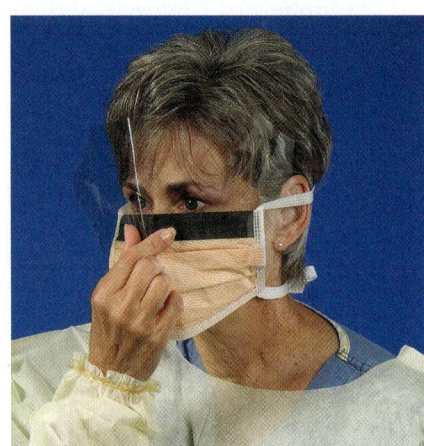

   c. Tie the upper ties to the back of your head and the lower ties to the back of your neck or slip the loops around your ears or place the elastic bands as with the ties.

   d. Place the lower edge of the mask below your chin, and tie the lower ties.
      Covering the nose and mouth creates a barrier to prevent droplet pathogens from entering through the nasal and oral mucous membranes or the respiratory system.

5. **Don the face shield or goggles.**
   a. *Face shield:* Place the shield over your eyes, adjust the metal strip over the bridge of your nose, and tuck the lower edge below your chin. Secure the straps behind your head.
   b. *Safety glasses or goggles:* Set them over the top edge of the mask.
6. **Don hair cover, if indicated.**
7. **Don shoe covers, if indicated.**
8. **Don gloves.**
   a. Select nonsterile disposable gloves of the appropriate size.
      The correct size will prevent gloves from falling off or ripping while you are working with the client.
   b. If you are wearing a gown, make sure that the glove cuff extends over the cuff of the gown. If skin is visible between the gown and the glove, tape the glove cuff to the gown cuff, covering all visible skin.
      To provide complete protection of hands and wrists, no skin should be visible between the glove and gown.

Patient Teaching

Answer questions the patient may have and educate about the need for PPE, his disease process, and the purpose of isolation.

Home Care

■ Identify the type of PPE needed, and ensure that the necessary supplies are available.
■ Develop a plan with the client and family for using and disposing of personal protective equipment and contaminated items.

■ Teach family members to don PPE as needed.
■ Obtain referral for a home health agency to provide support.

Documentation

The use of personal protective equipment is generally assumed and does not require documentation.

Practice Resources

Minnesota Department of Health, n.d.; Siegel, Rhinehart, Jackson, et al., 2007.

Thinking About the Procedure

 Go to the *Fundamentals of Nursing Skills Videos,* **Asepsis: Personal Protective Equipment, Donning.**

1. When donning PPE, what does the nurse do that indicates that she thinks splashing may occur during her care of the patient?

 For suggested responses, go to Chapter 22, **Thinking About the Procedure Suggested Responses,** on *DavisPlus.*

Procedure 22-3 ■ Removing Personal Protective Equipment (PPE)

➤ For steps to follow in *all* procedures, refer to the Universal Steps for All Procedures found on the page facing inside back cover. For this procedure, also refer to Clinical Insights 22-2 and 22-3 if you need more information.

Procedure Steps

1. **Remove gloves first** (unless the gown ties in front; in that case, see "What if . . .").
   Gloves are the most contaminated PPE and must be removed first to avoid contamination of clean areas of the PPE during removal.
   a. Remove the first glove by grasping the outside cuff of the glove with the opposite gloved hand and pulling downward so that the glove turns inside out. Do not touch the skin of your wrist or hand with your gloved hand.
   The outside of both gloves are contaminated. To prevent contamination of your skin, touch only the outside (contaminated) surface of first glove to outside (contaminated) surface of second glove. "Dirty touches dirty" and "clean touches clean." ▼

   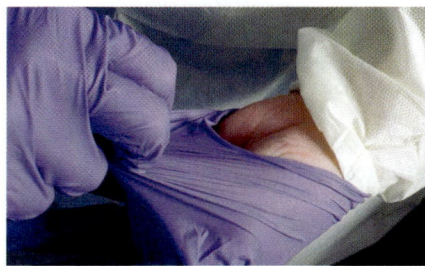

   b. Hold the removed glove in the palm of your gloved hand. Slip two ungloved fingers inside the cuff of the remaining glove. Pull the glove off, inside out, over the glove that hand is holding.

The inside of the gloves are considered "clean" because they have not been in contact with client or contaminated surfaces. Therefore, you can touch the insides with your bare hands. ▼

   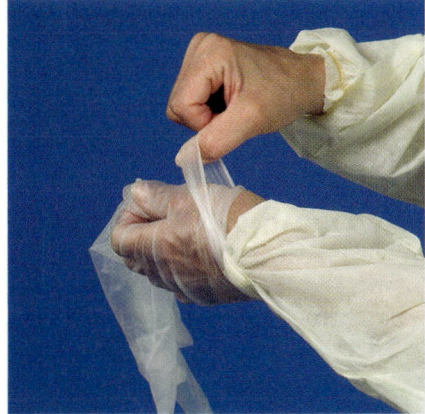

   c. Hold gloves away from your body and dispose of them in a designated waste receptacle.

2. **Remove the gown:**
   a. Release the waist ties and the neck ties of the gown, bending slightly forward to allow the gown to fall forward.
   The ties and the inside area of the gown are considered clean. Gown front and sleeves are contaminated. Allowing the gown to fall forward exposes the clean area for the hands to grasp more readily.
   b. Slip your hands inside the neck and peel the gown away from the shoulders. Reach inside to pull off

the cuff and remove your arm from the sleeve. Repeat the maneuver to remove the second sleeve. Do not touch the front of the gown, even if it is not visibly soiled.
The inside of the gown is clean and will not contaminate your hands. The front of the gown and the sleeves are considered contaminated. ▼

   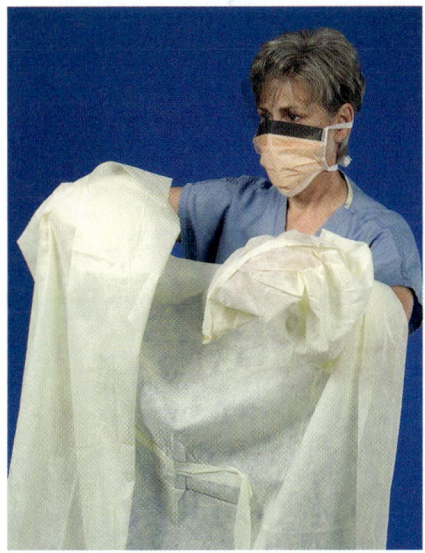

3. **Roll up and dispose of the gown.** Fold the gown so the inside of the gown is to the outside. Holding the gown away from your uniform, roll it up with the contaminated front and sleeves in the center, and place in the designated waste receptacle.
   The inside of the gown is considered clean. Folding the gown prevents

(continued on next page)

Procedure 22-3 ■ Removing Personal Protective Equipment (PPE) (continued)

contamination of your hands, the clothing, and the environment. ▼

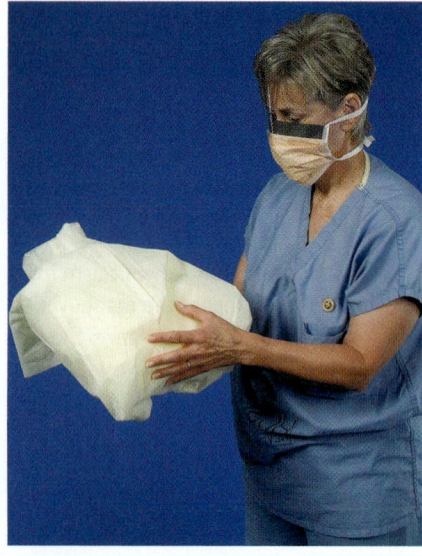

4. **Remove goggles** (if wearing them). Grasp only the earpieces (or head band) of the goggles and pull off the face. Place in the receptacle provided for disinfection if the goggles are not disposable.
   Earpieces are considered clean. Some goggles are cleaned and reused.

5. **Remove your mask or face shield** (if wearing one). Untie the lower ties first. Untie the upper ties next, being careful not to let go of the ties. Touch only the ties; do not touch the front of the mask. Dispose of the mask by holding on to the ties and placing it in a designated waste receptacle.
   Ties are considered clean. The front of the mask is potentially contaminated; touching it would contaminate your bare hands.

6. **Remove your hair covering**, if you are wearing one. Slip your bare fingers under the edge of the hair cover, being careful not to touch the outside of it. Lift it up and away from your hair. Touching only the inside of it, place it in a designated waste receptacle.
   The inside of the hair covering is considered clean, so you may touch it with your bare hands.

7. **Remove shoe covers**, if wearing them. Be careful to touch only the insides of the covers.

8. **Perform hand hygiene before leaving the room.**
   Wash your hands after all patient contact even if gloves are worn to prevent contamination.

9. **Close the door.**
   Keeping the door closed contains contaminants and makes precautionary signage more visible.

What if . . .

■ **The gown is tied in front?**

This would be an unusual circumstance, but if that occurs, you must untie the front gown ties before removing your gloves; then remove the gloves and untie any back ties (e.g., at the neck). Because the front of the gown (including a front tie) is considered contaminated, once you remove your gloves, you could not use your bare hands to untie a front tie.

■ **You are wearing two gowns (top one tied in back, inner one tied in front)?**

Remove gloves; untie waist ties of outer gown, remove the gown and fold it inside out. Remove the inner gown by untying it in front. Fold inner gown inside out. Take off goggles and face mask or shield.

Patient Teaching

See Procedure 22-2.

Home Care

See Procedure 22-2.

Documentation

The removal of personal protective equipment is generally assumed and does not require documentation.

Practice Resources

Siegel, Rhinehart, Jackson, et al., 2007; U.S. Department of Labor, n.d.a & b.

Thinking About the Procedure

Go to the *Fundamentals of Nursing Skills Videos,* **Asepsis: Personal Protective Equipment, Removing.**

1. When removing her gloves, how does the nurse protect her hands from contamination?

For suggested responses, go to Chapter 22, **Thinking About the Procedure Suggested Responses,** on *DavisPlus.*

Procedure 22-4 ■ Surgical Handwashing: Traditional Method

➤ For steps to follow in *all* procedures, refer to the Universal Steps for All Procedures found on the page facing the inside back cover. For this procedure, also refer to Clinical Insights 22-2 and 22-3 if you need more information.

Equipment

- Antimicrobial soap (60% to 95% alcohol, or other FDA-approved for surgical hand asepsis)
- Soft, nonabrasive scrub sponge
- Disposable single-use nail cleaner
- Deep sink with foot or knee controls
- Surgical shoe covers, cap, and face mask
- Sterile gloves of the correct size
- Surgical pack containing a sterile towel

➤ When performing the procedure, always identify your patient according to agency policy and be attentive to standard precautions, hand hygiene, patient safety and privacy, body mechanics, and documentation.

Procedure Steps

1. **Determine the agency policy** for the duration of the surgical scrub and the type of cleansing agent used. *The type of cleansing agent determines how long to scrub. Typically, an alcohol-based antimicrobial soap requires 2 to 6 minutes.*

2. **Avoid chipped polish or artificial nails.** Trim so nails do not extend beyond fingertips. Remove rings, watches, and bracelets. Preferably, do not wear nail polish. *Rings are a substantial risk factor for harboring moisture and gram-negative bacilli and S. aureus; and artificial nails and chipped polish are more likely to carry gram-negative pathogens, including Pseudomonas, because water collects between the artificial and real nails.*

3. **Put on surgical shoe covers, cap, and face mask before the surgical scrub.**

4. **Determine that sterile gloves, gown, and towel are set up for use after the scrub.** *To maintain sterility, the sterile towel, gown, and gloves must be ready for use immediately after you scrub. If you need to gather supplies after the scrub, you will need to start the scrub procedure over again.*

5. **Perform a prewash** before the surgical scrub (see Procedure 22-1). *The prewash removes any visible soil, reduces the number of microorganisms on your skin, and allows you to begin the surgical scrub with clean hands.*

6. **Remove debris from underneath your fingernails** using a single-use nail file under running water. *Decreases the number of microorganisms.*

7. **To begin the surgical scrub, turn on the water, using the knee or foot controls** or motion sensors. Adjust the temperature so that the water is warm. *Hot water removes the skin's protective oils. Knee and foot controls help to prevent contamination of the hands. You cannot touch any unsterile surfaces once you begin the surgical handwash.* ▼

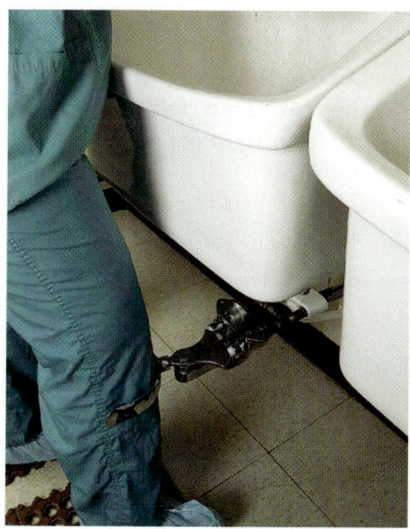

8. **Wet your hands and forearms from elbows to fingertips**, keeping hands above elbows and away from your body. If using a scrub sponge, wet the sponge. *Prevents water running down from your "dirty" elbows and forearm over "clean" rinsed hands.*

9. **Apply a liberal amount of antimicrobial soap onto your hands and the sponge;** lather well to 2 inches above the elbow. Do not touch the inside of the sink with your fingers, hands, or elbows. Avoid splashing your surgical attire. *Scrub brushes are harsh on the skin. Soft, nonabrasive sponges are recommended instead. Antimicrobial soap reduces the number of microorganisms.*

10. **Using a circular motion, scrub all the surfaces of one hand and arm.** Start at the fingers. Scrub at least 10 strokes each on nail, all four sides of each finger, hands, and arms. When scrubbing the arm, use 10 strokes each for the lower, middle, and upper areas of the forearm. Keep your hands higher than your elbows. ▼

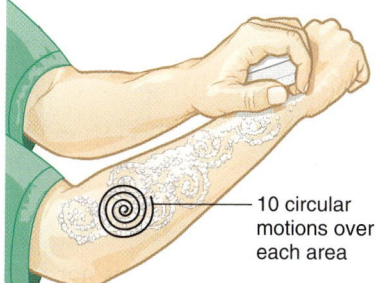

10 circular motions over each area

11. **Rinse the brush, and reapply antimicrobial soap.** Repeat the scrub on the second hand and arm. Normally the scrub takes at least 2 to 6 minutes. *The purpose of the scrub is to decrease the number of microorganisms on the hands. The length of the scrub depends on the time needed for the particular scrub agent to be effective.*

(continued on next page)

Procedure 22-4 ■ Surgical Handwashing: Traditional Method (continued)

12. Rinse your hands and arms, keeping your fingertips higher than your elbows. ▼

Avoids contamination of hands from water runoff.

15. Grasp the sterile towel, and back away from sterile field. ▼

17. Use one end of the towel to dry one hand and arm. Use the opposite end to dry the other hand and arm. Be certain your skin is thoroughly dry before donning sterile gloves.

Dry skin prevents maceration and allows gloves to go on much more easily. Use a separate section of the towel to prevent rewetting the skin.

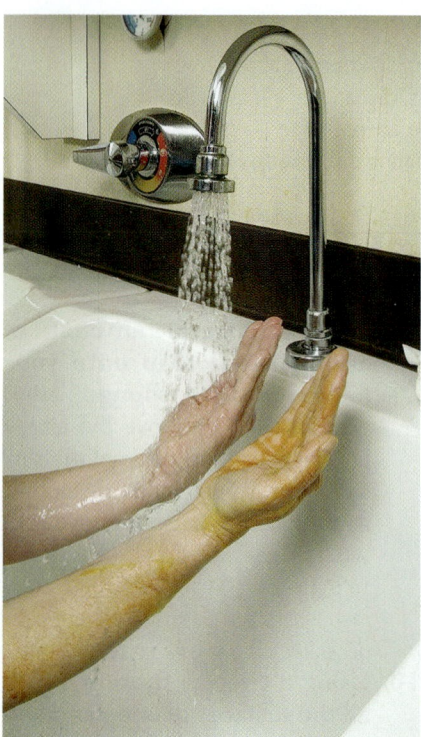

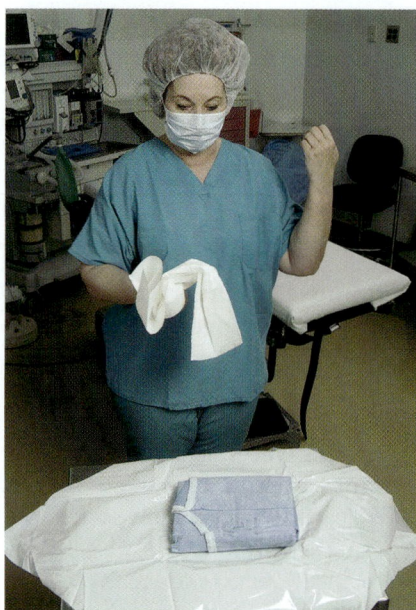

13. Repeat steps 8 through 12 if directed to do so by the soap manufacturer or agency policy.

14. Move to the area with the sterile towel and gown, keeping your arms flexed and your hands held higher than your elbows and away from your body.

Backing away keeps the sterile field dry and prevents you from inadvertently brushing against the table, which would contaminate the field. Never turn your back on a sterile field.

16. Lean forward slightly, and allow the towel to fall open, being careful not to let it touch your clothing.

The towel would be contaminated if it brushed against your uniform.

? What if . . .

■ **The agency uses an alcohol-based surgical hand-scrub product?**

a. Perform steps 1 through 6. Omit steps 7 through 17.

b. Using the indicated amount of handrub, rub all surfaces of the hands, including the nails and up the arm to 2 inches above the elbow, according to the manufacturer's recommendations and agency policy.

Many different products are on the market. Be careful to follow the manufacturer's guidelines for use for maximum effectiveness.

c. Allow the handrub to dry completely before you don sterile gloves.

Patient Teaching

If the patient is able to observe the procedure, explain the purpose of the surgical scrub and sterility.

Documentation

A surgical hand scrub does not require documentation. Instead, chart the procedure (or surgery) and how the patient tolerated it.

Practice Resources

The Association of periOperative Registered Nurses (AORN). Recommended Practices Committee, 2004; Boyce & Pittet, 2002; Siegel, Rhinehart, Jackson, et al., 2007.

Procedure 22-5 ■ Surgical Handwashing: Brushless System

➤ For steps to follow in *all* procedures, refer to the Universal Steps for All Procedures found on the page facing the inside back cover. For this procedure, also refer to Clinical Insights 22-2, 22-3 if you need more information.

Equipment

- Antimicrobial soap (60% to 95% alcohol, or other FDA-approved for surgical hand asepsis)
- Disposable single-use nail cleaner
- Deep sink with foot or knee controls
- Surgical shoe covers, cap, and face mask
- Sterile gloves of the correct size
- Surgical pack containing a sterile towel

➤ When performing the procedure, always identify your patient according to agency policy and be attentive to standard precautions, hand hygiene, patient safety and privacy, body mechanics, and documentation.

Procedure Steps

1. **Determine agency policy** for duration of the surgical scrub and the type of cleansing product to be used.
   Policies vary from institution to institution, although all should be based on sound principles for infection control designed in accordance with CDC guidelines. The type of cleansing agent determines how long to scrub. Typically, alcohol-based handrub is rubbed onto hands and arms until dry.

2. **Before starting the surgical scrub**, gather supplies and set up sterile gloves, gown, and towel for use after the scrub.
   To maintain sterility of the hands after the scrub, the sterile gloves, gown, and towel must be ready before washing.

3. **Observe recommended hygiene.**
   a. Avoid wearing artificial nails and extenders and chipped polish; nails should not extend beyond the end of the fingers. Preferably, do not wear nail polish.
   The AORN and CDC recommend avoiding these when in direct contact with patients or in high-risk situations, such as the perioperative setting or among those receiving immunosuppressant therapy. Individuals wearing artificial nails have been shown to harbor more pathogenic organisms in the subungual area than those with natural nails, particularly gram-negative bacilli, especially Pseudomonas, and various strains of yeast. Long nails can tear gloves.
   b. Remove rings, watches, and bracelets before starting the surgical scrub.

   Hand jewelry can prevent the handrub from reaching all skin areas and increase the spread of potential pathogens. Risk of infection from microorganisms increases exponentially in relation to the number of rings worn.

4. **Don shoe covers, a cap, and a mask.** Tuck hair completely under the cap.
   Masks filter out possible airborne pathogens carried in the nose or mouth, preventing contamination of sterile areas. Covering the hair reduces the transmission of pathogenic organisms that adhere to the hair shaft or scalp, which is a warm, moist environment for organisms.

5. **Perform a prewash before the surgical scrub.** Use a pick and running water to remove dirt and debris from under the nails; discard.
   The prewash removes any visible soil, reduces the number of microorganisms on your skin, and allows you to begin the surgical scrub with clean hands. The area under the nails harbors dirt, debris, and microorganisms.

6. **Turn on the water, using the knee or foot controls or motion controls.** The temperature usually adjusts automatically in a surgical scrub sink.
   Water temperature that is too hot can cause injury to the skin, making it prone to disruption in integrity. In addition, it can remove the skin's normal flora and natural oil, which has a protectant effect.

7. **Wet hands and forearms from the fingertips to elbows**, keeping hands above the elbows and away from the body at all times.
   Prevents water running down from your elbows and forearm over washed and rinsed hands.

8. **Dispense a palmful of antibacterial soap into your dominant hand**. Insert the fingertips of your nondominant hand into the soap using a twisting motion to apply the product to the fingertips and nails. Then rub the hands together to distribute the soap over the hands. ▼

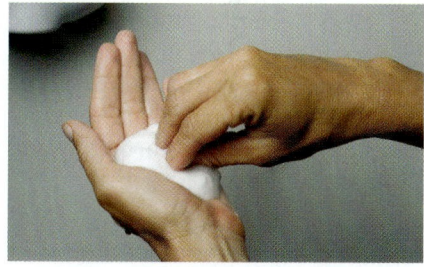

9. **Vigorously rub all surfaces of your nondominant hand and fingers**, adding water as needed. Be sure to rub each digit on all sides. Do not touch the inside of the sink during the cleansing procedure.
   Complete contact and friction are necessary for removal of microorganisms adherent to the skin's surface. The inside of the sink is considered contaminated with microbes and should be avoided. Incidental contact necessitates repeating the cleansing procedure.

10. **Rub the hands together** and cleanse the back side of the hand and the lower third of your nondominant arm (nearest the wrist).
    Although the palmar surface carries more organisms than the back side of the hands and arms, this area, nonetheless, should be cleansed thoroughly to reduce microbial colonization.

11. **Rinse using deep basin sink with knee-, foot-, or motion-operated controls.**

(continued on next page)

Procedure 22-5 ■ **Surgical Handwashing: Brushless System** (continued)

Improved adherence to sterile technique commonly results from use of motion- or foot/knee-operated or motion controls for faucets.

12. **Repeat the hand cleansing and rinsing process** on the dominant hand and forearm.

13. **Rinse and dispense soap into hands each time when cleansing a new area.** Be sure the soap dispenser is not blocked.

    A blocked dispenser can prevent dispensing the proper amount of product needed for reducing bacterial colonization. Many products are available for the brushless surgical scrub procedure. Adhere to the manufacturer's guidelines for use.

14. **Cleanse the remaining two-thirds of the nondominant arm** to 2 inches above the elbow. Cover every aspect of the middle and upper third of the forearm.

15. **Repeat the wrist-to-elbow scrub on the dominant arm.**

16. **Rinse each arm thoroughly and independently.**

17. **Repeat all the scrub steps (8 through 16), stopping before the elbow.** The scrub is complete after cleansing every aspect of the hands and forearms for 3 full minutes. *The CDC promotes a 2- to 3-minute scrub time using an antiseptic detergent in order to achieve maximal microbicidal activity while avoiding irritant contact dermatitis. Reduced time required to perform the surgical scrub often results in increased compliance with the prescribed technique.*

18. **Move to the area with the sterile towel and** gown, keeping the arms flexed and hands held higher than the elbows away from the body. *This position prevents water running down from your elbows and forearm over rinsed hands.*

19. **Grasp the sterile towel, and back away from the sterile field.** Lean forward slightly, and allow the towel to fall open, being careful not to let it touch clothing or gown. *This motion is performed to maintain a dry sterile field and prevent inadvertent brushing against the table and*

contaminating the field. Do not turn your back on any sterile field.

20. **Use one end of the towel to dry one hand and arm.** Dry the other hand and arm with the opposite end of the towel. *Use of a separate section of the towel guards against inadvertently rewetting the skin or contaminating an already clean area.*

21. **Allow time for the skin to dry thoroughly** before donning sterile gloves. *Dry skin prevents maceration and allows the gloves to go on more easily. Moisture left on the skin can be a source of further microbial contamination.*

22. **Once the brushless scrub is complete, keep your hands in front of your body and above the waist.** It may be necessary to enter backward through the door of the surgical suite. *These actions help prevent contamination of the hands and forearms when moving from the scrub sink to the sterile table.*

Documentation

A brushless surgical hand scrub does not require documentation in the patient's medical record, although there may be a checklist. However, you must adhere to the institution's policy for performing the technique.

Patient Teaching

If the patient is able to observe the procedure, explain the purpose of a diligent approach to surgical scrub for promoting a low-risk environment for infection.

Home Care

Sinks in the home environment typically do not have knee- or foot-operated controls or motion-sensor on/off devices. Therefore, when scrubbing for a sterile procedure in the home, contact with the faucet handles is performed with barrier objects (e.g., a paper towel or a sterile towel for a sterile scrub) between the clean hands and the environmental surface.

Practice Resources

Association of periOperative Registered Nurses (AORN). Recommended Practices Committee, 2004; Centers for Disease Control and Prevention, 2002.

Thinking About the Procedure

 Go to the *Fundamentals of Nursing Skills Videos,* **Asepsis: Surgical Handwashing, Brushless System.**

1. The nurse does not dry her hands before she leaves the sink area. Why?
2. How did she dry her hands to keep them surgically clean?

 For suggested responses, go to Chapter 22, **Thinking About the Procedure Suggested Responses,** on Davis*Plus.*

Procedure 22-6 ■ Sterile Gown and Gloves (Closed Method)

➤ For steps to follow in *all* procedures, refer to the Universal Steps for All Procedures found on the page facing the inside back cover. For this procedure, also refer to Clinical Insights 22-2, and 22-3, if you need more information.

Equipment

■ Sterile gloves of the correct size

■ Sterile gown

(These should be lying on a sterile field. If they are not, you will need to create a sterile field to place them on.)

➤ When performing the procedure, always identify your patient according to agency policy and be attentive to standard precautions, hand hygiene, patient safety and privacy, body mechanics, and documentation.

Procedure Steps

1. **Grasp the gown at the neckline. Hold the gown up and allow it to fall open** as you step back from the table. Be careful not to allow the gown to come into contact with nonsterile areas while you are lifting it off the table and opening it. ▼

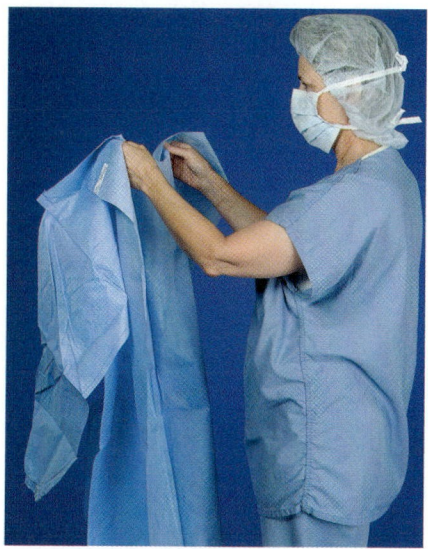

The gown will be contaminated if it touches unsterile objects.

2. **Slide both arms into the sleeves,** but do not extend your hands through the cuffs.

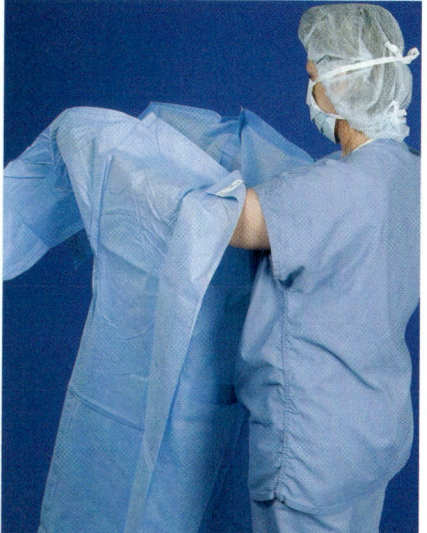

3. **Keep the sleeves of the gown above waist level.**
   Hands will contaminate the sleeve edge if allowed to pass through the cuff.

4. **Have a coworker stand behind you and pull the shoulders of the gown up and tie the neck tie** (this will be the circulating nurse, if you are in the operating room). The coworker touches only the inside of the gown while pulling it up.
   Touching only the inside prevents contamination of the gown with the nurse's hands.

5. **Don sterile gloves using the closed method.**
   a. Open the sterile glove wrapper, keeping your fingers inside the sleeve of the gown. The outer wrapper has already been discarded.
   b. **Glove the dominant hand:**
      (1) With your nondominant hand, keeping your hands inside the

gown sleeves, grasp the cuff of the glove for your dominant hand. Turn your dominant hand palm up.
Keeping the hand inside the cuff ensures that you are making contact with the sterile gown; sterile is touching sterile.

   (2) Lay the glove on the dominant gown cuff, thumb side down with the glove opening pointed toward the fingers, and thumb of glove positioned over the thumb-side of the hand. ▼

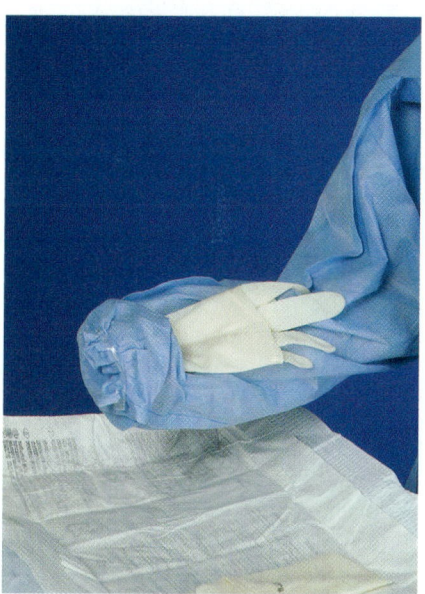

   (3) Keeping your nondominant hand inside the sleeve, grasp the upper side of the glove cuff and stretch the glove cuff up over the gown cuff. ▼

(continued on next page)

Procedure 22-6 ■ Sterile Gown and Gloves (Closed Method) (continued)

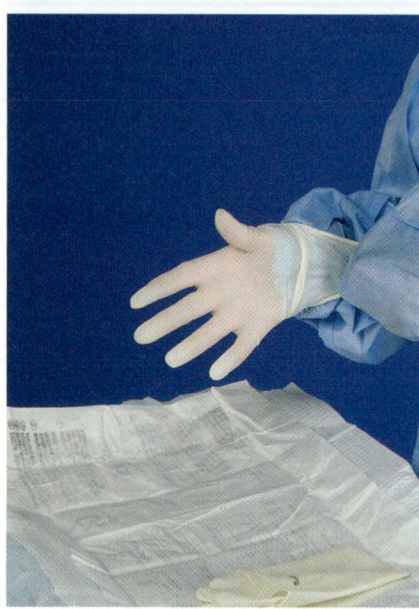

(4) Pull the sleeve of your gown up to pull the glove cuff over the wrist and move your fingers into the glove fingers.

c. **Glove the nondominant hand.**

(1) Place the fingers of your gloved hand under the cuff of the second glove. Lay the glove on the forearm of your nondominant hand. Grasp

and anchor the inside glove cuff with your nondominant hand through the gown, being careful to keep fingers inside the gown.

(2) With your dominant hand, pull the glove cuff over the cuff of the gown as you move your fingers into the glove. ▼

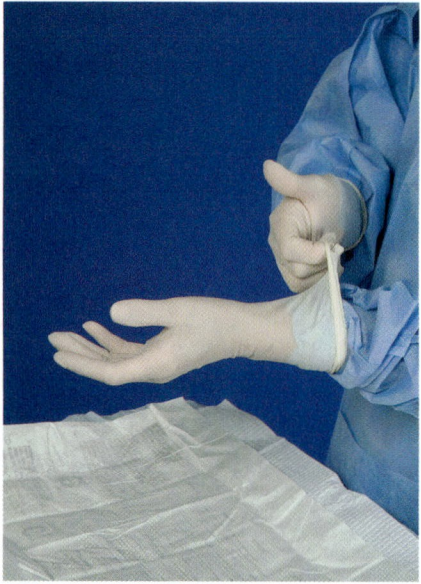

d. **Adjust the fingers in both gloves** so the excess glove is pulled over the fingertips.

Maintains sterility of the gown and gloves by maintaining a closed system. The final adjustment of the gloves is done when both gloves are in place, to prevent contaminating the gloves.

6. **Grasp the waist tie on the gown, and hand the tie to the circulating nurse** or a coworker who is wearing a hair cover and mask. Your coworker will grab the tie with sterile forceps.

The tie is considered sterile. You will need help pulling it around you. A coworker can help you. Using sterile forceps keeps the tie sterile.

7. **Make a three-quarter turn, and receive the tie from your coworker.**

Because only areas within your field of vision are considered sterile, a coworker must pull the waist tie around you.

8. **Secure the waist tie.**

Ensures that the gown is secured and will not expose clothing to a sterile field.

Patient Teaching

If the patient is alert during the procedure, explain:
- The need for the sterile procedure
- Why he must not touch the drapes
- Why he must not move or talk once the drapes are in place
- Any special precautions during the procedure

Documentation

- Donning sterile gown and gloves does not require documentation.
- You will need to chart the procedure performed and how the patient tolerated it.
- In the operating room, the circulating nurse charts about the surgery and the patient's response.

? What if . . .

- **Your hand inadvertently comes through the cuff opening when putting on the gown?**

  Change gowns. The cuff would have been contaminated and would then contaminate your glove.

Practice Resources

The Association of periOperative Registered Nurses (AORN), 2005a, 2005b, 2006; Centers for Disease Control and Prevention, 2002.

Thinking About the Procedure

 Go to the *Fundamentals of Nursing Skills Videos*, **Asepsis: Sterile Gown and Gloves, Closed Method.**

1. In the early part of the procedure, a nurse in white is touching the surgical nurse with her hands. Is this an error? Why or why not?
2. After the surgical nurse has gloved, she hands her gown ties to an unsterile coworker. This person does *not* take the tie with a forceps as the textbook procedure (above) instructs. Why, in this instance, is that acceptable?

 For suggested responses, go to Chapter 22, **Thinking About the Procedure Suggested Responses,** on *DavisPlus*.

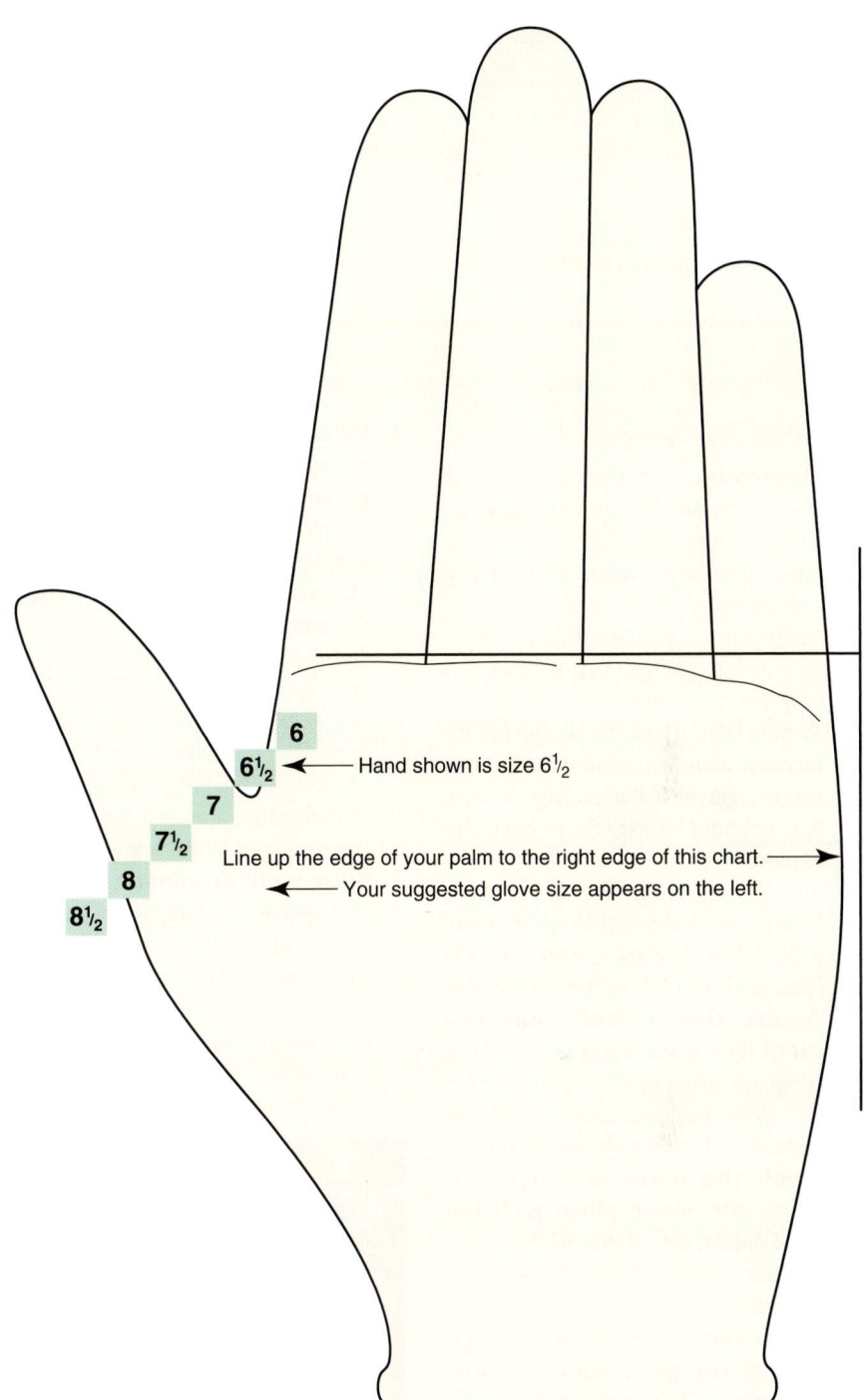

6

$6^{1}/_{2}$ ← Hand shown is size $6^{1}/_{2}$

7

$7^{1}/_{2}$

Line up the edge of your palm to the right edge of this chart. →

8

← Your suggested glove size appears on the left.

$8^{1}/_{2}$

Sterile glove sizes. This can help you determine the proper size glove you need for your hand.

Procedure 22-7 ■ Sterile Gloves (Open Method)

➤ For steps to follow in *all* procedures, refer to the Universal Steps for All Procedures found on the page facing the inside back cover. For this procedure, also refer to Clinical Insights 22-2, 22-3, and 22-6 if you need more information.

Equipment

■ Sterile gloves of the correct size

➤ When performing the procedure, always identify your patient according to agency policy and be attentive to standard precautions, hand hygiene, patient safety and privacy, body mechanics, and documentation.

Procedure Steps

1. **Determine the correct size of sterile gloves.** The gloves should be snug, but not tight.

   Gloves that are too loose are more easily contaminated and make handling equipment or supplies difficult. Gloves that are too tight are uncomfortable and may tear during use.

2. **Assess the glove package** for intactness and expiration date. Do not use the gloves if the package is torn, has become moist, or is past the expiration date.

   Torn packaging may allow the gloves to become contaminated. Moisture allows wicking and may cause contamination. Past-date gloves are not considered sterile.

3. **Assess the patient's environment** for a space that is clean and has adequate space to allow you to open the glove package. Don the gloves without touching a nonsterile item.

4. **Open the outer wrapper, and place the inner glove package on a clean, dry surface.**

   Prevents contamination of the gloves inside the package.

5. **Open the inner glove package so that the glove cuffs are closest to you.** Be careful to fully open the flaps of the package so that they do not fold back over and contaminate the gloves.

   The outer 1-inch border of the glove package is considered contaminated. ▼

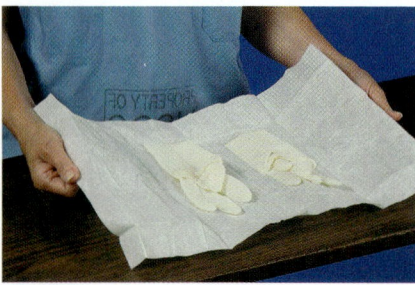

6. **With your nondominant hand, grasp the inner surface of the glove for the dominant hand.** Lift the glove up and away from the table, keeping it away from your body. Take care to not touch anything else on the sterile field.

   The inside of the glove is not considered sterile because it is in contact with your skin. Lifting the glove up and away from the table prevents you from accidentally touching the table or your clothing while donning the glove and thereby contaminating the glove.

7. **Slide your dominant hand into the glove,** keeping your hand and fingers above your waist and away from your body.

   The area below the waistline is considered contaminated. Keeping gloves away from your body prevents accidental contamination. ▼

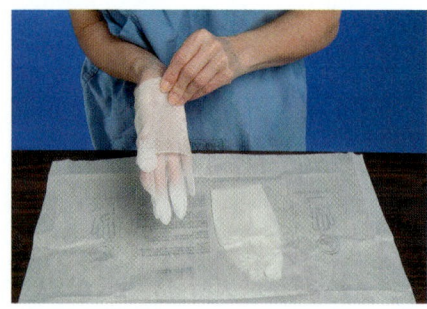

8. **Slide your gloved fingers under the cuff of the remaining glove,** keeping your gloved thumb well away from your ungloved hand. Lift the glove up and away from the table and away from your body.

   The outside of the glove is sterile and may be touched with your sterile gloved hand. ➤

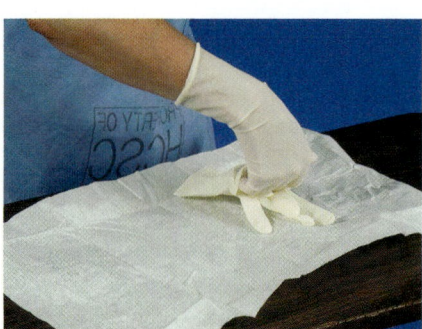

9. **With gloved fingers still under the cuff, slide your nondominant hand into the glove and pull it on,** being careful to avoid contact with your gloved hand, especially the thumb. ▼

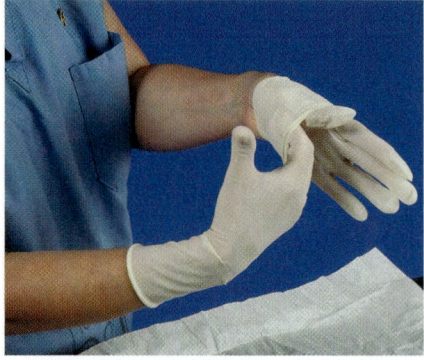

10. **Adjust both gloves to fit your fingers.** If necessary, pull the fingers of the gloves down so that no excess is at the fingertips.

    Adjusting your gloves after both have been donned decreases the risk of contamination and allows for greater dexterity during the procedure.

11. **Keep your hands between shoulder and waist level in front of you.**

    Keeps the gloves within your field of vision to avoid contamination.

    NOTE: To remove soiled gloves after the procedure, refer to Procedure 22-3.

Patient Teaching

Explain why sterile gloves are needed for the procedure.

Home Care

- Many home care procedures are clean rather than sterile. The client is in his own environment and not surrounded by other patients, who may serve as hosts for infection.
- You may need to teach caregivers how to apply sterile gloves for some procedures. No modifications are required. Demonstrate the procedure, and have the caregiver do a return demonstration.

Documentation

- No special documentation is needed for sterile gloving.
- Chart the procedure you performed and the patient's response to the procedure.

Practice Resources

The Association of periOperative Registered Nurses (AORN), 2005a, 2006.

Thinking About the Procedure

 Go to the *Fundamentals of Nursing Skills Videos,* **Asepsis: Sterile Gloves (Open Method).**

1. At the beginning of the procedure, the nurse opens the outer (clear plastic) glove package and turns the inner (white paper) package out on a table top. Does this break sterile technique? Why or why not?
2. There is no break in sterility, but at one point in the procedure, the nurse almost contaminates a glove. What happened?

 For suggested responses, go to Chapter 22, **Thinking About the Procedure Suggested Responses,** on Davis*Plus.*

Procedure 22-8 ■ Sterile Fields

➤ For steps to follow in *all* procedures, refer to the Universal Steps for All Procedures found on the inside back cover. For this procedure, also refer to Clinical Insights 22-2, 22-3, and 22-6 if you need more information.

Equipment

- Package of sterile supplies required for the procedure
- Sterile gloves of the correct size

Procedure 22-8A ■ Setting Up a Sterile Field

➤ When performing the procedure, always identify your patient according to agency policy and be attentive to standard precautions, hand hygiene, patient safety and privacy, body mechanics, and documentation.

Procedure Steps

1. **Assess the sterility of all packages and equipment.** Check to make sure the packaging is intact and the expiration dates have not passed.
   Only sterile items should enter a sterile field. Any compromise in packaging means that the item is assumed not to be sterile.

2. **Arrange the environment** for performing the sterile procedure.
   a. Clean off the surface you will use to set up the sterile field.
      Inadequate space causes inadvertent contamination during sterile procedures.
   b. Position the patient as needed for the procedure.
      Allows you to immediately proceed with the planned procedure. Once the sterile field is established, air

movement can create contamination of the sterile items.

Procedure Variation. Using Sterile Packaged Equipment

3. **Place the sterile package on a clean, dry surface.**
   Prevents contamination of the sterile item. If a surface is damp, strike-through of moisture may occur, making the item unsterile. ▼

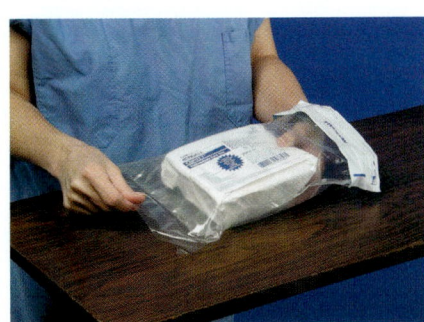

4. **Open the flap away from you first.**
   To prevent passing an unsterile arm over the sterile items. ▼

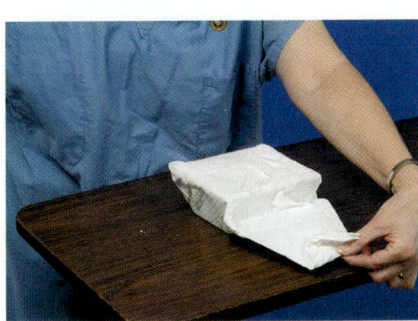

(continued on next page)

Procedure 22-8 ■ Sterile Fields (continued)

5. Open the side flaps.▼

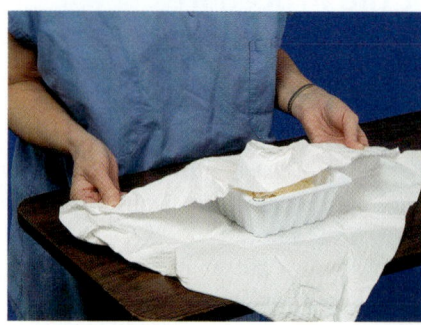

6. Pull the final flap toward you. The wrapper is now the sterile field. The area 1 inch from the edge of the wrapper and 1 inch from the table edge is considered unsterile. Do not readjust the sterile area after the package has been opened.

Only the horizontal surface of the draped area is considered sterile. Any part of the sterile wrapper that falls below the level of the sterile area (e.g., top of the table) is considered unsterile. If you move the field after opening, the field shifts and places unsterile areas of the wrapper on the surface.

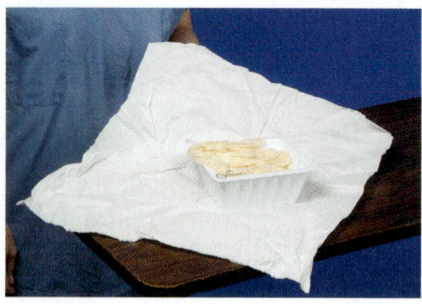

Procedure Variation. Opening a Fabric- or Paper-Wrapped Sterile Package

7. Check and remove the chemical indicator strip.

The indicator tape per manufacturer or institution confirms that the package was sterilized. The pack usually is also dated.

8. Remove the outer wrapper, and place the inner wrapped package on a clean, dry surface.

The outer wrapper is not considered sterile and is discarded.

9. Open the inner wrapper following the same technique described in steps 3 through 6.

Procedure Variation. Using a Sterile Drape

Omit steps 3 through 9.

10. Place the package on a clean, dry surface. Hold the edge of the package flap down toward the table, grasp the top edge of the package, and peel back.

The sterile drape is inside the outer wrapper. This maneuver opens the package without contaminating the sterile drape.▼

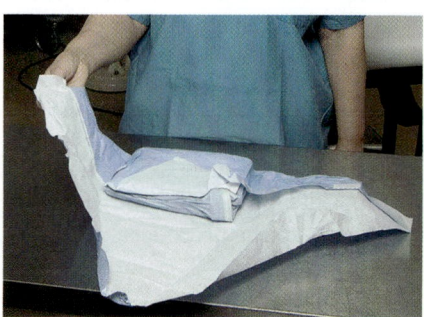

11. Pick up the sterile drape by the corner. Allow the drape to fall open, away from your body and away from unsterile surfaces. Place it on a clean, dry surface by touching only the edge of the drape. Avoid fanning the drape.

A 1-inch border around the sterile drape is considered unsterile.

Procedure 22-8B ■ Adding Supplies to a Sterile Field

➤ When performing the procedure, always identify your patient according to agency policy and be attentive to standard precautions, hand hygiene, patient safety and privacy, body mechanics, and documentation.

Procedure Steps.

1. Hold the sterile package in your dominant hand. Grasping the corner of the wrapper, peel each corner back with your nondominant hand.

The inside of the wrapper is sterile and will be used as a barrier when placing the sterile item onto a sterile field.

2. Holding the contents several inches above the field, allow the supplies to drop onto the field inside the 1-inch border of the sterile field. Do not let your arms pass over the sterile field.

By holding the package upside down, you ensure that the sterile part of the package is facing the sterile field and that you deposit the item onto the sterile field.▼

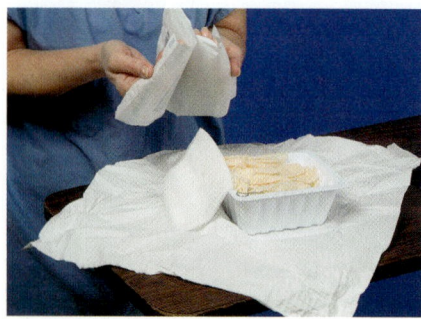

3. Dispose of the wrapper, and continue opening any needed supplies for the procedure.

Once sterile gloves are on, you will not be able to add items without contaminating the gloves.

Procedure 22-8C ■ **Adding Sterile Solutions to a Sterile Field**

➤ When performing the procedure, always identify your patient according to agency policy and be attentive to standard precautions, hand hygiene, patient safety and privacy, body mechanics, and documentation.

Procedure Steps

1. **Use a sterile bowl or receptacle** if the sterile field is fabric or at risk for strike-through.
   - You may add a sterile bowl to the field by unwrapping (as discussed above) and holding the bowl through the sterile wrapper as you place it near the edge of the sterile field. The sterile bowl may also be placed next to the sterile field.
   - If you place the sterile bowl on the field, place it near the edge so that you can pour the sterile solution from the back of the sterile field. This prevents you from reaching over and thereby contaminating the field.

2. **Check that the sterile solution is correct**, and confirm that the expiration date has not passed and that the solution and concentration are correct and have not expired.

3. **Remove the cap off the solution bottle** by lifting it directly up and throw it away.
   The edge of the container is considered contaminated after the contents have been poured and the sterility of the contents cannot be ensured if the cap is replaced.

4. **Hold the bottle 4 to 6 inches above the bowl and pour** the needed amount of the solution into the bowl.
   Prevents you from inadvertently touching the sterile bowl with the bottle and thereby, contaminating the bowl. Limited height reduces the risk of splashing, which strikes through and contaminates a cloth or permeable sterile field. A disposable sterile drape generally has a plastic membrane in the middle to prevent strike-through. ▼

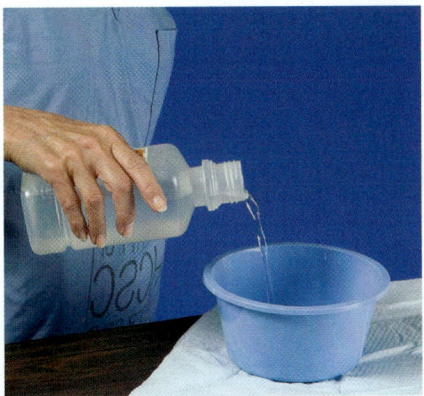

5. **Discard the remaining solution.**
   Reusing open containers may cause contamination due to drops contacting the unsterile areas and running back over the container opening.

6. **Before donning sterile gloves to perform the procedure**, double-check that all supplies have been added to the field. Do not leave the sterile field unattended. Do not turn your back to the sterile field.
   If a sterile item is out of your field of vision, it is no longer considered sterile because airborne particles, insects, or liquids could contaminate the field.

Home Care

- Most sterile procedures in the home are done by visiting nurses.
- Procedures performed by clients or family members are usually clean rather than sterile.

Documentation

- You will not usually document the actual setting up of the sterile field.
- Document the procedure, your assessment of the patient's tolerance for the procedure, and your assessment of the area being treated by the procedure.

Practice Resources

The Association of periOperative Registered Nurses (AORN), 2006.

Thinking About the Procedure

 Go to the *Fundamentals of Nursing Skills Videos,* **Asepsis: Sterile Fields.**

1. When opening the large sterile bowl, what is the first thing the nurse does to ensure sterility?

2. What does the nurse do with the cap and the bottle of solution after she pours from it into the sterile bowl? Why does she not set it beside the sterile bowl?

 For suggested responses, go to Chapter 22, **Thinking About the Procedure Suggested Responses,** on Davis*Plus*.

 To explore learning resources for this chapter,

 Go to Davis*Plus* at http://davisplus.fadavis.com/, keyword Treas:
Chapter Resources for Chapter 22:
   Knowledge Check and Think Like a Nurse Response Sheets
   Knowledge Check Answers
   Resources for Caregivers and Health Professionals
   Reading More About Infection Control & Prevention (Suggested Readings)
   What Are the Main Points in This Chapter?
NCLEX-Style Review Questions
Chapter Overview Podcasts

Concept Map

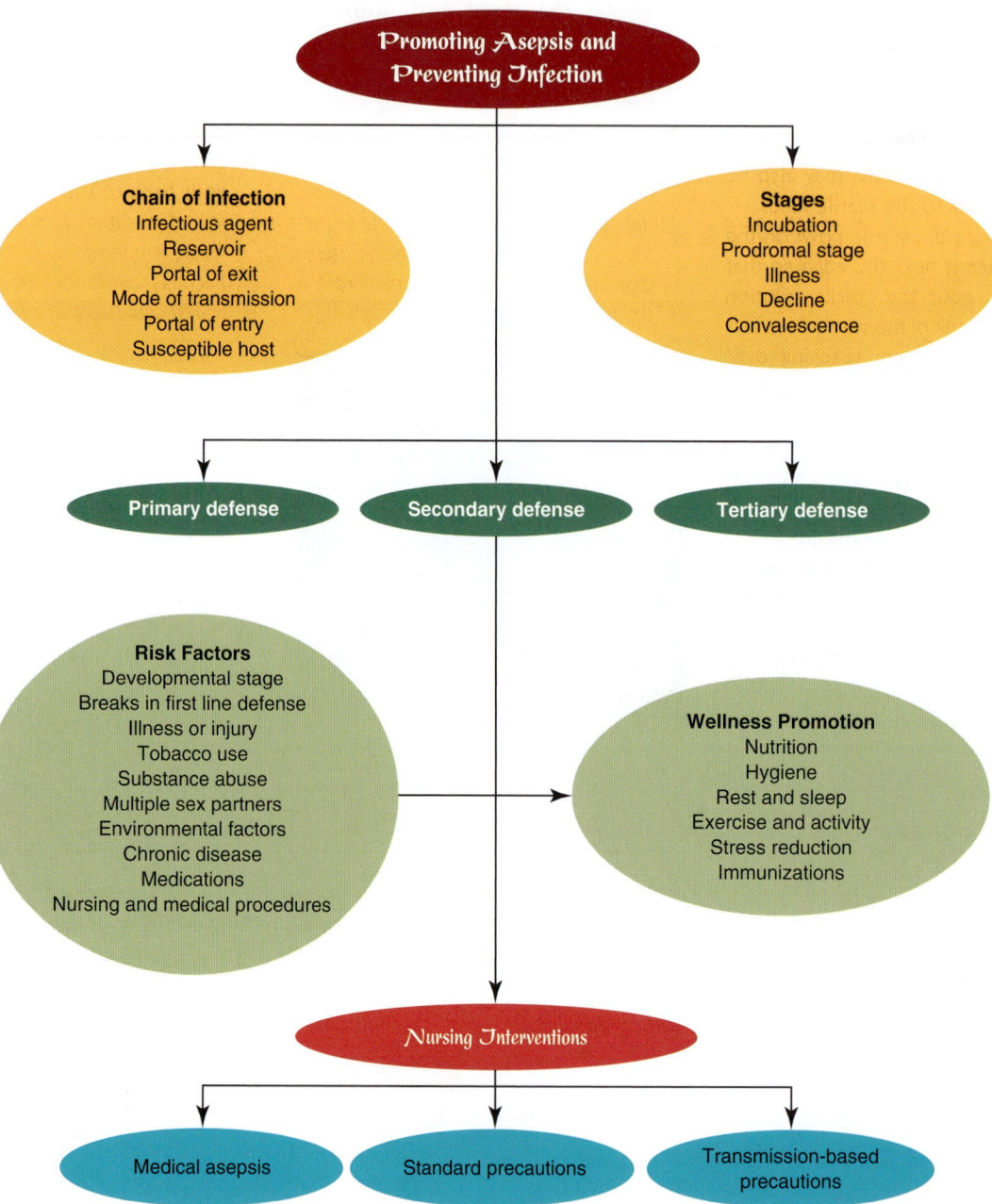

Promoting Asepsis and Preventing Infection

Chain of Infection
Infectious agent
Reservoir
Portal of exit
Mode of transmission
Portal of entry
Susceptible host

Stages
Incubation
Prodromal stage
Illness
Decline
Convalescence

Primary defense   Secondary defense   Tertiary defense

Risk Factors
Developmental stage
Breaks in first line defense
Illness or injury
Tobacco use
Substance abuse
Multiple sex partners
Environmental factors
Chronic disease
Medications
Nursing and medical procedures

Wellness Promotion
Nutrition
Hygiene
Rest and sleep
Exercise and activity
Stress reduction
Immunizations

Nursing Interventions

Medical asepsis   Standard precautions   Transmission-based precautions

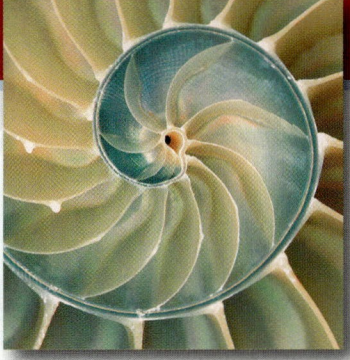

CHAPTER 23

Safety

Learning Outcomes

After completing this chapter, you should be able to:

➤ List the three leading causes of accidental death in the United States.

➤ Discuss developmental and individual factors that create safety risks.

➤ Identify at least five safety hazards in the home environment and interventions to prevent injury from them.

➤ Discuss the steps to follow when you suspect that a client has ingested a poisonous substance.

➤ Describe the choking rescue maneuver, and identify instances when it is appropriate to use it.

➤ Describe the four main physical hazards that are found in the community and interventions to prevent injury from them.

➤ Describe and give examples of hazards encountered in the healthcare agency.

➤ Identify four interventions to prevent falls in the healthcare agency.

➤ Discuss when it is appropriate to use siderails in the healthcare agency.

➤ Properly apply restraints and discuss measures to prevent injury in clients who are restrained.

➤ Discuss at least one data collection instrument that is used to assess risk for falls.

➤ Formulate a nursing diagnosis in relation to preventing injury in the environment.

➤ Write an individualized goal for clients with a nursing diagnosis of Risk for Falls.

Key Concepts

Safety

Related Concepts

See the Concept Map at the end of this chapter.

Example Problem

Falls

Caring for the Nguyens

This feature allows you to practice the kind of thinking you will use as a full-spectrum nurse. There is usually more than one correct answer to a critical thinking question, so we do not provide answers for these features. It is more important to develop your nursing judgment than to "cover content." Discuss the questions with your peers. If you are still unsure, consult your instructor.

Refer to the database for Nam Nguyen in the front of this book. Use full-spectrum thinking to identify safety hazards for Mr. Nguyen, his 3-year-old grandchild (Kim Phan, who lives with him), and his widowed mother, Mai Nguyen, who lives alone.

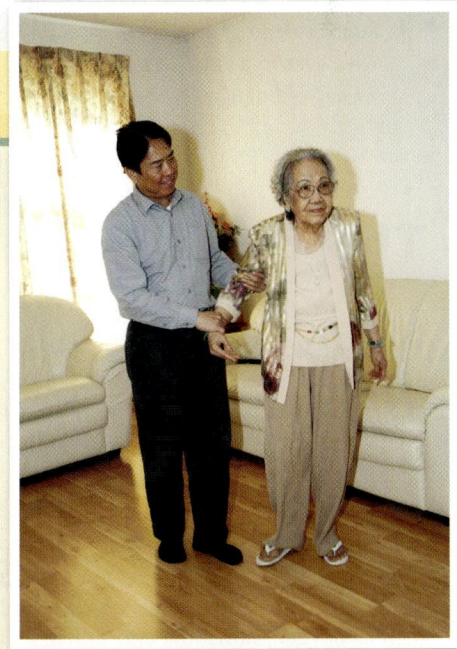

(Continued)

Caring for the Nguyens (continued)

A. Without even using any patient data from the database (except ages), what theoretical knowledge do you have that will help you to identify risks that commonly occur in the developmental stages represented by these three clients?
Mr. Nguyen
Mr. Nguyen's 3-year-old grandchild, Kim
Mr. Nguyen's widowed mother, Mai

B. From Mr. Nguyen's database, what data can you put with your theoretical knowledge to identify the most likely safety risks for him? What are those risks?

C. From the risks and possible risks you have identified, for which one do you definitely need more data before deciding whether it increases his risk for accidents?

That is, which piece of data is especially vague? What do you need to find out?

D. You know the theoretical (or possible) risks for Mr. Nguyen's mother. What data do you need in order to determine her *actual* safety risks?

E. What, if any, data do you have that would help you to identify any *actual* safety risks for Mr. Nguyen's grandchild? What, if any, are those risks?

F. What would you want to assess at the child's preschool to be sure that safety measures exist for preventing falls?

 Go to **Caring for the Nguyens Response Sheet** on Davis*Plus*.

Meet Your Patients

■ Alvin Lin is a 79-year-old man who was just transferred from a long-term care facility to your medical unit. His admitting diagnosis is dehydration and pneumonia. In the handoff report you were told that he had rested well during the night and was alert and oriented. When you enter his room, he is confused and does not know where he is. He is becoming combative and is trying to get out of bed. How should you respond to the situation?

■ Suppose you are a nurse making a home visit to Teresa, who lives in a rural area. Teresa is 20 years old and has a 2-year-old daughter. She is also responsible for caring for

her elderly grandmother, who is recovering from a hip fracture. Teresa states that it is getting more difficult to keep up with her toddler, who is "into everything," and to care for the needs of her grandmother. Her grandmother has a fear of falling and is reluctant to do anything for herself.

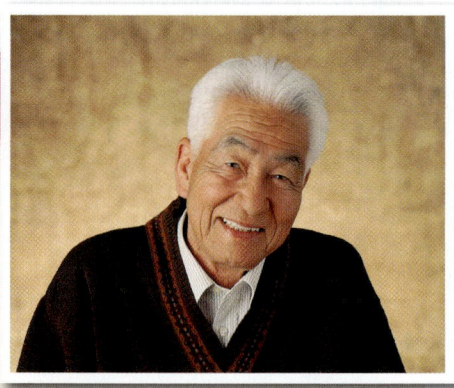

Theoretical Knowledge
knowing why

This chapter will increase your ability to recognize safety hazards in the home, community, and healthcare facility, and to plan interventions that promote safety for clients of all ages, such as the two in Meet Your Patients. Many accidental injuries can be prevented by being aware of hazards and taking reasonable precautions.

ABOUT THE KEY CONCEPTS

Safety is a basic human need, second only to survival needs such as oxygen, nutrition, and fluids. As a nurse, the concept of safety is fundamental to the care of your clients. You must also be concerned with your own safety and the safety of other care providers. In this chapter, we consider the concept of safety in the home, the community, and the healthcare facility.

IMPORTANCE OF SAFETY

According to the National Safety Council (NSC), accidents, or unintentional injuries, are the fifth leading cause of deaths in the United States. An estimated 118,000 people die each year as a result of accidents (NSC, 2011). Expressed another way, one person dies from an accident every 5 minutes. Motor vehicle accidents continue to be the number one cause of unintentional death, followed by poisonings, falls, choking, fires, and drowning. Of course, the death rate is not the only noteworthy number: In 2008, approximately 26 million people received injuries that disabled them beyond the day of injury (NSC, 2010).

Many healthcare organizations are campaigning for safer patient care in an effort to reduce the cost of healthcare and the burden of suffering. The following are examples:

■ **The Joint Commission,** the accrediting body for healthcare facilities, each year publishes National Patient Safety Goals. For example, in 2011 the goals include improving the

accuracy of patient identification, improving the safety of medication use, reducing the risk of healthcare associated infections, and preventing mistakes in surgery.

- **Institute of Medicine's (IOM)** report *To Err Is Human: Building a Safer Health System* brought public attention to patient safety. It stated that it is simply not acceptable for patients to be harmed by the same healthcare system that is supposed to offer healing and comfort. The report identified six major aims that can raise the quality of healthcare. Safety is among these aims (Committee on Quality of Health Care in America, 1999).

- The **American Nurses Association's (ANA)** *ANA's Health System Reform Agenda* (2008a) recommends six major public policy changes that can raise the quality of healthcare. Quality Aim 1 is safe healthcare.

- **Quality and Safety Education for Nurses (QSEN),** a task force to improve nursing education, identified and described six competencies that all nursing students should have by graduation. Safety is one of those competencies (Cronenwett, Sherwood, Barnsteiner, et al., 2007). For a list of the essential features that demonstrate the safety competence,

 Go to Chapter 23, **Tables, Boxes, Figures: ESG Table 23-1, QSEN Safety Competency,** on Davis*Plus*.

- **Medicare** has identified "never events" or hospital-acquired conditions (HAC): costly errors that cause serious injury or death, and that are mostly preventable. Included in the list of never events are injuries from falls, burns, restraints, or bedrails. Medicare will no longer pay institutions for care required to treat the effects of such errors (Centers for Medicare & Medicaid Services, 2006a, 2008).

WHAT FACTORS AFFECT SAFETY?

To promote client safety, you will need theoretical knowledge about developmental stages and individual risk factors that affect clients' ability to avoid accidental injury. This chapter discusses specific risk factors and describes hazards in three environments: the home, the community, and the healthcare agency.

Developmental Factors

The type and incidence of accidents vary among age groups. You will find interventions for all age groups integrated into the topics throughout this chapter. Keep in mind that the descriptions given for each age group are characteristics common to most people in that group. However, individuals progress through developmental stages at their own pace, so there will always be some people who do not fit the group description closely. For supplemental discussion of safety needs during different developmental stages, see Chapters 9 and 10.

Infant/Toddler. Motor vehicle accidents are the leading cause of death for children ages 1 to 3, followed by drowning. Falls, choking, sudden infant death syndrome (SIDS), and ingesting poisons are other critical safety concerns. Infants and toddlers are completely dependent on others for their care. They have the ability to walk and manipulate objects before they have the judgment to recognize dangers such as falling. In addition, infants and toddlers are curious and tend to explore the environment by putting objects in their mouth. This is why the incidence of choking is highest

between 6 months and 3 years of age. (National Center for Injury Prevention and Control, Centers for Disease Control and Prevention [CDC], 2006).

Preschooler. Motor vehicle injuries are a major cause of accidental death, along with drowning, fires, and poisoning. Falls are the primary cause of nonfatal injuries. After age 3 years, children are a little less prone to falls because their gross and fine motor skills, coordination, and balance have improved. However, the extension of play to the outside environment (e.g., playgrounds, pools, front yards) creates additional safety concerns. Adult supervision continues to be essential.

School-Age Child. Motor vehicles continue to be the leading cause of accidental death in this age group. The leading cause of nonfatal injury is falls. School-age children have developed more refined muscle coordination and control, and their decision-making skills have improved. However, because they become more involved in activities outside the home, bone and muscle injuries are common. Injuries are often related to sports, skateboarding, bicycle riding, and playground injuries. Most school-age children are less fearful than are toddlers, and are ready to try any new skill with or without practice or training. Exposure to the wider school and neighborhood environment also increases the risk for injury inflicted by people outside the home (e.g., abduction).

Adolescent. The leading cause of death in this group is motor vehicle accidents, followed by homicide—both frequently associated with alcohol and drug use. Sports and recreational injuries, including diving and drowning incidents are also common, especially when drinking and drug use are involved. Peak physical, sensory, and psychomotor abilities give teenagers a feeling of strength and confidence, yet they lack the wisdom and judgment of adults. This, along with feelings of being indestructible, makes them more likely to participate in risk-taking behavior, and, in turn, more prone to injury.

Adult. Among people 35 to 54 years old, unintentional poisoning causes more deaths than motor vehicle accidents (Centers for Disease Control and Prevention [CDC], 2010a). Workplace injury may also be a significant concern. Other injuries to adults are related to lifestyle (e.g., excessive alcohol use), stress, carelessness, abuse, and decline in strength and stamina. For many, work and family responsibilities often leave little time for regular physical activity, increasing the risk of musculoskeletal injury in the so-called weekend athlete.

Older Adult. Although many older adults have intact senses that enable them to continue to enjoy life as they age, physiological changes do occur (e.g., reduced muscle strength and joint mobility; slowing of reflexes; decreased ability to respond to multiple stimuli; and sensory losses, particularly hearing and vision). These changes increase the older adult's risk for falls, burns, car accidents, and other injury. Falls are the most common cause of accidental death for adults age 65 and older (CDC, n.d.c).

Individual Risk Factors

In addition to developmental stage, individual factors also influence a person's risk for unintentional injury. These include lifestyle, cognitive awareness, sensoriperceptual status, ability to communicate, mobility status, physical and emotional health, and awareness of safety measures. Table 23-1 summarizes individual risk factors.

Table 23-1 ➤ Individual Risk Factors for Injury	
RISK FACTORS	**BEHAVIOR MANIFESTATION**
Lifestyle	Smoking, alcohol abuse, risk-taking behaviors
Cognitive awareness	Confusion due to stress and loss of short-term memory
Sensory and perceptual status	Loss of senses (e.g., vision, hearing, pain), which provide first line of defense
Impaired communication	Language barriers and hearing and speech impairment related to disease processes
Impaired mobility	Impaired strength with accompanying problems in mobility, balance, and endurance
Physical and emotional well-being	Reduced physical stamina and depression, with feelings of loss of control and helplessness
Safety awareness	Reduced cognitive awareness (e.g., of older adult) and immature development of the child

KnowledgeCheck 23-1

- What are some important developmental considerations when providing a safe environment for a preschool child?
- What is the main cause of injuries during the adolescent period?
- What are some ways that the aging process makes the older adult more prone to injury?
- Based on your theoretical knowledge and the scant patient data you have, why do you think Teresa's toddler (Meet Your Patients) is at risk for accidents? What about Teresa's grandmother?

WHAT SAFETY HAZARDS ARE IN THE HOME?

What safety issues in the home environment would you need to assess with regard to Teresa's toddler and grandmother (Meet Your Patients)? If you cannot answer this question, you should be able to do so after reading this section, which provides an overview of safety hazards in the home.

Except for motor vehicle accidents, most fatal accidents occur in the home. The leading causes of death in the home are poisonings, falls, fires and burns, and choking. For children, maternal depression, lack of parental social support, and domestic conflict are associated with less safe homes (Rhodes & Iwashyna, 2007).

Poisoning

Poisoning death rates have more than tripled in the past 20 years. Although young children are frequent victims, the increase has been mainly among adults. In many cases, the person does not die but becomes ill or suffers other effects. Poisoning exposure accounts for about 2,000 emergency department visits per day (CDC, 2010b). Most poisoning

of young children occurs because of improper storage of household chemicals, medicines and vitamins, and cosmetics. Box 23-1 lists poisonous agents commonly ingested by children.

The use of lead in paint was banned in 1978, but lead-based paint can still be found in older homes and in toys produced in some foreign countries. Some soil (which young children often put in their mouth) contains high lead content. In the United States, poor, urban, and immigrant populations are at higher risk for lead exposure than are other groups.

Older children and adolescents may attempt suicide by overdosing with medicines or be poisoned accidentally when experimenting with recreational or prescription drugs intended for adults. In adults, most poisonings occur as a result of illegal drug use or misuse or abuse of prescription drugs, especially narcotic medications, tranquilizers, and antidepressants.

Treatment choice depends on the poison ingested. For most poisonings, the most effective intervention is professional administration of activated charcoal orally or via gastric tube. However, charcoal is not effective for ethanol, alkali, iron, boric acid, lithium, methanol, or cyanide. Depending on the situation, other options for medical treatment include gastric lavage, dialysis, administration of antidotes, and forced diuresis. For a list of medical treatments for commonly ingested poisons,

 Go to Chapter 23, **Tables, Boxes, Figures: ESG Table 23-2, Sources and Medical Treatment for Commonly Ingested Poisons**, on DavisPlus.

✚ Never induce vomiting when the ingested material is acidic or caustic to the esophagus. Although the American Academy of Pediatrics no longer recommends inducing emesis (e.g., with syrup of ipecac), some practitioners may still do so. The National Poison Control Center does not support the routine stocking of ipecac in households with young children. They state that it should be given only on specific recommendation from a poison center or qualified medical personnel (American Association of Poison Control Centers, n.d.a).

BOX 23-1 ■ Poisonous Agents Commonly Ingested by Children

- Household cleansers, including oven cleaner, drain cleaner, toilet bowl cleaner, and furniture polish
- Medicines, including cough and cold preparations, vitamins, pain medications, antidepressants, anticonvulsants, and iron tablets, which to children may look like candies
- Indoor houseplants, including poinsettia, Dieffenbachia, philodendron, and many others
- Cosmetics, hair relaxer, nail products, mouthwash
- Pesticides
- Kerosene, gasoline, lighter fluid, paint thinner, lamp oil, antifreeze, windshield washer fluid, lighter fluid, and other chemicals
- Alcoholic beverages
- Wild plants and mushrooms
- Pesticides, rodent poisons

Carbon Monoxide Exposure

Carbon monoxide (CO) is a colorless, tasteless, odorless toxic gas. Exposure can cause headaches, weakness, nausea, and vomiting; prolonged exposure leads to seizures, dysrhythmias, unconsciousness, brain damage, and death. Each year in the United States, CO poisoning causes approximately 500 unintentional deaths (King & Bailey, 2007). It accounts for a majority of deaths at the scene of fires, and is also a relatively common method of suicide. Many CO deaths occur during cold weather among older adults and the poor who seek nonconventional heat sources (e.g., gas ranges and ovens) to stay warm.

Scalds and Burns

The following are common causes of scalds and burns:

- *Scald injuries* (e.g., from hot water, steam, or grease) are the most common cause of burns in children younger than age 3. Scalding burns (especially on both feet or both hands) and cigarette burns in children and vulnerable older adults should always prompt you to assess for abuse. To assess for abuse, refer to Procedure 9-1.
- *Warming food or formula in the microwave* may cause the food to become hotter than intended, leading to burns in infants and young children.
- *Sunburn* can cause a first- or second-degree burn
- *Contact burns* may occur from contact with metal surfaces and vinyl seats when cars are parked in the sun. The risk of contact burns in all age groups is greater in the presence of heating devices such as kerosene heaters, wood-burning stoves, and home sauna heating elements. People may use these as heat sources when they cannot afford the cost of traditional furnace fuels.
- *Chemical agents*, such as acid, alkali, or other organic compounds, can also cause localized burns.

Fires

Home fires are a major cause of death and injury. Older adults and children under age 5 have the greatest risk of fire death. Most *fatal* home fires occur while people are asleep, and most fire-related deaths occur from smoke inhalation. The following are common causes of fire in the home:

- *Cooking fires* are the number one cause of home fires and home fire injuries.
- *Smoking* (e.g., cigarettes) is the leading cause of fatal home fires, but during the winter months *heating equipment* is equally responsible.
- *Home oxygen administration equipment* is also a hazard. In 75% of the home fires involving oxygen, smoking materials are the ignition source; cooking and candles are other common factors. When more oxygen is in the air, items such as hair, plastic, skin oils, clothing, and furniture catch fire at lower temperatures. Any fire that starts will burn hotter and faster. Other causes of fire include unsupervised children playing with matches, improper use of candles, and faulty wiring.

Example Problem: Falls

Falls are the third leading cause of injury-related deaths—the leading cause for older adults. An average of 4 in 100 people experience a nonfatal fall for which they seek medical advice. The rate triples for adults older than 75 years (Adams, Barnes, & Vickerie, 2007). More than half of all falls occur in the home, and about 80% of home falls involve people age 65 years and older. Health issues that increase the risk for falls include poor vision, hypotension (low blood pressure), a history of falls, dizziness, pain, alcohol use, cognitive impairment, polypharmacy, arthritis, gait or balance deficits, and age greater than 80 years (Akyol, 2007; Kenny, Rubenstein, Martin, et al., 2001).

Firearm Injuries

Gun ownership is a controversial issue. Some people keep guns in the home for protection and/or recreation (e.g., hunting, target shooting). However, guns are a source of unintentional injury and death. Gun safety and security are especially important when there are children or someone with a substance abuse problem in the home. Household access to firearms has been implicated as a risk factor for youth suicide and domestic homicide, as well as unintentional injury (Hizel, Ozcebe, Sanli, et al., 2008). Because of the frequency and severity of unintentional firearm injuries involving children, the American Academy of Pediatrics and other groups have mounted efforts to educate parents about firearm safety.

ThinkLike a Nurse 23-1

- What are some initial questions you might ask Teresa regarding the home environment?
- What are some basic interventions you might suggest to Teresa to help child-proof her home? To answer this question, you will need to recall information about:
  Safety hazards that we encounter in the home
  Developmental and lifestyle factors that affect safety
  Specific nursing activities that can be used to prevent accidents or injuries related to the environmental hazards (e.g., firearms)\

Suffocation/Asphyxiation

Suffocation by smothering is the leading cause of death for infants younger than 1 year. Suffocation may be caused by drowning, choking on a foreign object, or inhaling gas or smoke. Drowning is an important cause of accidental death in children age 1 to 18 years. Food items, including hot dogs, raw vegetables, popcorn, hard candies, nuts, and grapes, are responsible for most nonfatal choking incidents. Nonfood items, such as latex balloons and plastic bags, cause the majority of suffocation deaths in young children. Suffocation of infants is often related to bed or crib hazards, such as excess bedding or pillows, or toys hung from long ribbons inside the infant's crib. Infants can become entangled in cords from window blinds or in the ribbon or string used to hang a pacifier around an infant's neck.

KnowledgeCheck 23-2

- What are the most common poisonous agents ingested by children?
- Name one source of CO (carbon monoxide) poisoning.

Take-Home Toxins

Take-home toxins are hazardous substances transported from the workplace to the home. The National Institute for Occupational Safety and Health (NIOSH) reports that pathogenic microorganisms, asbestos, lead, mercury, arsenic, pesticides, caustic farm products, and dozens of other agents cause significant morbidity and mortality in workers' homes (NIOSH, 2003, 2004). These toxins are most likely transported to workers' homes on the workers themselves,

on their clothing, or on objects brought from the workplace. In the home, contamination occurs via any of three sources:

- Direct skin-to-skin contact, or direct contact with contaminated clothing
- Arthropod vectors, such as ticks that are responsible for Lyme disease
- Transmission on dust particles that are inhaled (e.g., anthrax spores, arsenic in mine and smelter dust)

WHAT SAFETY HAZARDS ARE IN THE COMMUNITY?

Hazardous agents in the community are a major contributor to illness, disability, and death worldwide. This section discusses four major hazards: motor vehicle accidents, pathogens, pollution, and electrical storms.

Motor Vehicle Accidents

As mentioned in the beginning of the chapter, motor vehicle accidents (MVAs) are the leading cause of accidental death in American adults and children older than 1 year. They account for about 34% of all accidental deaths (CDC, n.d.b). Failure to use seat belts and proper child car seats continues to be the major contributing factor. Severe injuries and death also occur from air bag deployment when young children are improperly placed in the front passenger seat. Many of the fatal MVAs during adolescence involve abuse of alcohol or other substances (CDC, 2007, 2010c; Miniño, Heron, Murphy, et al., 2007). The risk of being injured or killed in a car crash increases for older adult drivers. Every day, on average, 500 people over age 65 are injured in an automobile accident.

Pathogens

A **pathogen** is any microorganism capable of causing an illness. Pathogens can enter the body through several sources in the environment: food, vectors (e.g., mosquitoes and other insects; rodents and other animals), and unclean water.

Food-Borne Pathogens

Food poisoning is a nonspecific term that describes illness caused by ingesting bacteria and other microorganisms, or their toxins, in food. Improper food storage and preparation are a major cause of food poisoning. Raw foods, such as raw meat, poultry, eggs, shellfish, raw fruits and vegetables, and unpasteurized milk and fruit juice, are commonly associated with food-borne illness. Poisonous chemicals in the environment, such as mercury, arsenic, zinc, and potassium chlorate, may also contaminate foods. Education is an important intervention for preventing food poisoning. See the section Food Safety under the heading Intervention: Teaching for Safety Self-Care later in the chapter.

Vector-Borne Pathogens

Vectors are organisms that transmit pathogenic bacteria, viruses, and protozoa from one host to another. The following are examples:

Mosquitoes. The severity of the reaction to a mosquito bite depends on the degree of allergy to the mosquito's saliva. In addition to the discomfort caused by bites, infected mosquitoes can transmit diseases such as West Nile virus and malaria. They can also transmit parasites to domestic animals (e.g., canine heartworm, equine encephalitis).

Other Insects. Other insects, such as roaches, fleas, sand flies, lice, and ticks (which are, technically, arachnids and not insects) can also transmit serious diseases and produce a wide variety of allergens. Allergic sensitivity to cockroaches, for example, is a predictive factor for asthma severity (Lopes, Miranda, & Sarinho, 2006).

Animals. Rodents and other animals can also act as vectors and allergens. For example, rabies can be spread through the bite of a rabid animal, some fungal diseases can spread via the inhalation of bird droppings, and mouse proteins have been implicated in occurrence of asthma. Structural defects in a building (e.g., roofs and walls) permit entry of birds, rodents, and other small animals, and dead spaces in walls permit their circulation among apartments in multiunit dwellings (Berg, McConnell, Milam, et al., 2008; Krieger & Higgins, 2002).

Water-Borne Pathogens

Sanitation refers to measures to promote and establish favorable health conditions, especially those related to the community's water supply. People who live in substandard housing may not have safe drinking water, hot water for washing, or adequate methods of waste disposal. People in rural areas often depend on private wells, which may not be adequately maintained and tested for pathogens such as *Giardia lamblia, Cryptosporidium,* and *Escherichia coli.* These are primarily community health problems.

Pollution

Pollution is any harmful chemical or waste material discharged into the air, water, or soil. Examples of pollutants are gaseous fumes, asbestos, carbon monoxide, and cigarette smoke. Each year Americans generate millions of tons of waste in their homes and communities (U.S. Environmental Protection Agency [EPA], 2008).

Air Pollution. Motor vehicle emissions are a major cause of *outdoor air pollution* in the United States. Other toxic outdoor air pollutants include asbestos; toluene; metals such as mercury, chromium, and lead compounds; and other emissions from sources such as factories and power plants. *Indoor pollutants* include radon; carbon monoxide; and allergens from dust mites, cockroaches, mold, rodents, and pets. Passive exposure to tobacco smoke is associated with respiratory disease and cancer; and environmental air pollution is linked to cardiovascular disease and respiratory viral infection (Ciencewicki & Jaspers, 2007; National Cancer Institute, n.d.; Walker & Mouton, 2008; U.S. Department of Health and Human Services, 2006).

Water Contamination. Contamination in lakes, rivers, and streams ultimately affects both recreation and food production. Pollution occurs when inadequately treated or inappropriate quantities of human, industrial, or agricultural wastes are released into the water systems. If the pollution is severe enough, the water may become unsafe for human consumption.

Noise. Substantial exposure to noise is associated with various adverse health effects, including hearing loss, stress, elevated blood pressure, and loss of sleep. Noise is pervasive in our society—for example, from road traffic, jet planes, garbage trucks, construction equipment, lawn mowers, and loud music. People who live or work near major roads, bus depots, airports, and trucking routes are at greater risk, as are those in certain work environments (e.g., railroad workers).

Soil. Improper waste disposal and excessive use of pesticides can contaminate soil. Agricultural, industrial, and manufacturing processes create solid and toxic waste. Animal, radioactive, and medical wastes pose special problems. Household products, such as paints, cleaners, oils,

batteries, and pesticides, contain corrosive or toxic ingredients that contaminate the environment when disposed of improperly (e.g., in household trash or poured down the drain, on the ground, or into storm sewers).

Electrical Storms

According to the National Weather Service, deaths from lightning strikes lead all other categories of storm-related fatalities, exceeded in some years only by floods (Cooper & Kulkarni, 2011). Weather conditions play a major role in outdoor recreation programming. It is important for professionals, participants, and outdoor recreation providers to understand severe weather conditions, specifically thunderstorms and lightning, and the dangers associated with them.

KnowledgeCheck 23-3

- What are the major causes of injuries from MVAs (motor-vehicle-related accidents)?
- List at least three tips for preventing food poisoning.
- List three sources of noise pollution.

 ThinkLike a Nurse 23-2

Identify an environmental problem in your neighborhood. What are some possible solutions?

WHAT SAFETY HAZARDS ARE IN THE HEALTHCARE FACILITY?

As many as 98,000 people die from medical injuries each year in U.S. hospitals ("Overview of the 100,000 Lives Campaign," n.d.). Several characteristics of healthcare facilities pose safety hazards for residents and workers. We have already discussed the hazard of infection in Chapter 22. Box 23-2 lists The Joint Commission's National Patient Safety Goals for 2011, which

---

BOX 23-2 ■ The Joint Commission 2011 Patient Safety Goals

Goal 1. Improve the accuracy of patient identification.
Goal 2. Improve effectiveness of communication among caregivers.
Goal 3. Improve the safety of using medications (including anticoagulants).
Goal 7. Reduce the risk of healthcare associated infections (including hand hygiene, multidrug-resistant organisms, central-line bloodstream infections, and surgical site infections).
Goal 8. Accurately and completely reconcile medications across the continuum of care.
Goal 15. The organization identifies safety risks inherent in its patient population.
Universal Protocol: The organization meets the expectations of the Universal Protocol. (This is a preprocedure verification process to make sure that all documents, information, and equipment are available, and that the correct procedure is performed on the correct person and site.)

Source: Adapted from The Joint Commission. (2011). The Joint Commission: Accreditation program, Hospital. National patient safety goals (effective January 1, 2011). Retrieved May 9, 2011, from http://www.jointcommission.org/assets/1/6/2011_NPSGs_HAP.pdf

---

should give you an idea of the types of accidents that occur in healthcare agencies. If you would like to see a full explanation of the patient safety goals,

 Go to The Joint Commission Web site in Chapter 23, **Resources for Caregivers and Health Professionals, Web Sites,** on DavisPlus.

What Are Never Events?

Never events are healthcare-acquired complications that can cause serious injury or death to a patient, and should *never* happen in a hospital. The list of never events has been expanded over time to mean events that are clearly identifiable and measurable, serious, and usually prevented. You can gain insight into healthcare facility hazards by examining the following list of never events identified by the Centers for Medicare & Medicaid Services (2008). Be aware that this list may grow and change more over time.

- Foreign object (such as a sponge) left in patients after surgery
- Air embolism
- Administering the wrong type of blood
- Severe pressure ulcers
- Falls and trauma
- Infections associated with urinary catheters
- Infections associated with intravenous catheters
- Symptoms resulting from poorly controlled blood sugar levels
- Surgical site infections following certain elective procedures (e.g., certain orthopedic surgeries, bariatric surgery for obesity)
- Deep vein thrombosis or pulmonary embolism following total knee and total hip replacement procedures.

The Institute for Healthcare Improvement (IHI), an independent, not-for-profit organization, has launched the 100,000 Lives Campaign to recommend healthcare changes to reduce morbidity and death in American healthcare. To read the entire list of recommendations,

 Go to Chapter 23, **Tables, Boxes, and Figures: ESG Box 23-1, The 100,000 Lives Campaign,** on DavisPlus.

 ThinkLike a Nurse 23-3

Many never events can be reduced by good nursing care. By preventing complications and maximizing reimbursement, nurses can prove their value to an organization and make the case for better staffing. Over which of the never events do you think nurses have the most control? Explain your thinking.

Example Problem: Falls

Although most falls occur in the home, they are a major concern in healthcare facilities, as well. Falls are by far the most common incident reported in hospitals and long-term care facilities, occurring at one for every 2,000 patient stays (CDC, n.d.c; Centers for Medicare & Medicaid Services, 2006a, 2008). Infants and older adults are especially at risk for injury from falls. Many patients have risk factors, such as poor vision, cognitive impairment, difficulty with walking or balance, orthostatic hypotension, weakness or dizziness from disease or therapy, and drowsiness from medications. Many cases involve falling from a bed, and falls occur more frequently on nights, weekends, and holidays. Most agencies have established procedures and safety features to prevent falls.

Equipment-Related Accidents

Equipment-related accidents usually occur because of equipment malfunction or improper use, for example, when suction devices and infusion pumps are not working properly, oxygen cylinders are transported incorrectly, or wheelchairs and beds are not locked during transfer activities.

Fires and Electrical Hazards

Because most institutions promote a smoke-free environment, fire in a healthcare agency is more often related to anesthesia or improperly grounded or malfunctioning electrical equipment. Nevertheless, patients and visitors do break the rules, so smoking cannot be discounted as a hazard. Most healthcare agencies have policies for preventing electrical hazards.

When a fire occurs in a public building, an announcement is made over the communication system. Often, words such as "Code Red" or "Code Yellow" are used in an effort to prevent panic among patients and visitors. Depending on the situation, the announcement may ask visitors to leave the building.

> ✚ All personnel must know the fire escape route and follow hospital policy regarding fires. If you discover a fire, your first instinct may be to contain or put out the fire. Fight that instinct! Your first action is to rescue the patient—that is, move the patient(s) away from the area. Only then should you sound the alarm and attempt to confine the fire.

Restraints

A **restraint** is a device or method used for the purpose of restricting a patient's freedom of movement or access to his body, with or without his permission. The most obvious form of restraint is the use of physical force by another person. A restraint may also be (1) a mechanical device, material, or equipment, such as a cloth vest or siderails; or (2) a chemical restraint (medication) given to control disruptive behavior, for example, sedatives and psychotropic agents.

- Devices such as casts and traction are not considered restraints (Centers for Medicare & Medicaid Services, 2006b; The Joint Commission, 2008).
- Physical holding of a patient is not always considered restraint. Sometimes it is necessary to use devices or methods that involve the physical holding of a patient for routine physical examinations or tests.

Restraints are classified according to the reason for their use: medical–surgical restraints or behavior management restraints. Medicare has specific guidelines for each circumstance. Guidelines are more restrictive when restraints are used for behavior management.

As a safety measure, nurses traditionally restrained highly dependent older adults, patients with poor mobility, those with impaired cognitive status, and others they judged to be at risk for falls. However, they have found that restraints make care more time consuming and do not reduce falls. Restraints are themselves a safety hazard, and actually increase the likelihood of injury. A restrained person has a natural tendency to struggle and try to remove the restraint and, as a result, can become entangled, suffer nerve damage, circulatory impairment, and even suffocation. Restraint-imposed immobility can cause pressure ulcers, contractures, loss of strength, and other hazards of immobility. Emotionally, the person may suffer anger, fear, humiliation, and diminished self-esteem.

Avoid Restraints When Possible

Research indicates that less restraint use saves time and money, and reduces patient injuries (leBel & Goldstein, 2005; Tilly & Reed, 2008). For those reasons, healthcare facilities are trying to achieve restraint-free environments. When the decision is made to avoid restraints, it is essential to provide alternatives for keeping the patient safe. Multiple approaches are needed, including careful and ongoing assessment and surveillance; finding ways to communicate with the patient; and tailoring exercise programs, medication reviews, and environmental modifications to the needs of individual patients.

To provide the safest possible care environment, The Joint Commission encourages healthcare facilities to do the following:

- Promote among all direct-care staff a commitment to reduce the use of restraints and seclusion.
- Educate caregivers before they take part in any restraint-related activity.
- Document restraint episodes specifically, in detail.
- Maintain one-on-one viewing of patients in restraint and seclusion.
- Include staff members when deciding whether to explore new technology that is considered a safe alternative to traditional restraint devices.
- Budget for an adequate number of qualified staff to attend to patients.

Restraint Is Sometimes Necessary

Guidelines are slightly different depending on whether restraints are used to directly support medical healing or for a behavioral health reason (e.g., when a patient is irrational and pulling out his IV lines). Use restraints only as a last resort. As much as possible, use technology (such as bed alarms) and better anticipation of patient needs instead of restraints.

> ✚ If you must use restraints, Medicare, The Joint Commission, and other regulators require that restraints be medically prescribed and that you first try all less restrictive interventions.

Do Not Depend on Siderails

Based on the Centers for Medicare & Medicaid Services (CMS) standards, siderails can be viewed as a restraint. A full-length siderail is a restraint when it is used to prevent the patient from getting out of bed regardless of whether he is able to do so safely. A half- or quarter-length upper siderail can be an aid to independence if it is used by the patient for the purpose of getting into and out of bed. Similarly, split rails are not considered restraints if a client requests them in order to feel more secure (Talerico & Capezuti, 2001).

Remember that older or cognitively impaired adults may regard siderails as a barrier rather than as a reminder that they need assistance. Several studies have shown that siderails may lead to serious falls and injuries. These findings have led healthcare providers to reevaluate the use of restraints and to recommend that siderails not be used routinely (Brush & Capezuti, 2001; Capezuti, Wagner, Brush, et al., 2007; Evans & Cotter, 2008).

KnowledgeCheck 23-4

- What is a typical cause of fire in healthcare facilities?
- What measures should you take, and in what order, if a fire occurs in the hospital?

Mercury Exposure

Mercury is a heavy, odorless, silver-white liquid metal. Mercury can be inhaled, ingested, or absorbed through the skin. It accumulates in muscle tissue and can cause renal and neurological disorders, especially in fetuses and neonates. It is toxic in both acute and chronic exposure. Because of its shiny color and ability to form beads or balls, mercury is appealing to curious children. See Table 23-2 for potential health effects.

Products containing mercury include thermometers, thermostats, batteries, fluorescent light bulbs, blood pressure devices, and electrical equipment and switches. For more information about products and devices that may contain mercury,

 Go to Chapter 23, **Tables, Boxes, Figures: ESG Box 23-2, Products and Devices that May Contain Mercury,** on *DavisPlus*.

In 1998, the American Hospital Association (AHA) and the EPA launched a program to eliminate mercury-containing waste in the healthcare industry and prevent it from entering the environment via incinerators, landfills, and wastewater. Mercury thermometers are no longer being made in the United States. However, some people may still have them in their homes. Most, but not all, healthcare facilities have eliminated mercury thermometers and sphygmomanometers. You can help prevent mercury poisoning by taking an active role in eliminating mercury-containing items from your workplace. Some hospitals conduct thermometer exchanges, providing free or low-cost nonmercury thermometers to anyone who brings in a mercury thermometer.

Table 23-2 ▶ Potential Health Effects of Mercury

PRIMARY ROUTE	POTENTIAL HEALTH EFFECTS
Acute Effects	
Toxicity	Symptoms of chills, nausea, malaise, chest tightness and pain, dyspnea, coughing, stomatitis, gingivitis, excess salivation, and diarrhea. High levels can cause severe respiratory irritation, digestive disturbances, and severe renal damage.
Inhalation	Respiratory damage, wakefulness, muscle weakness, anorexia, headache, ringing in the ears, chest pain, inflammation of the mouth, and pneumonitis
Eye	Irritation and corrosion
Skin	Irritation and allergic dermatitis
Ingestion	Intestinal obstruction
Chronic Effects	
Primarily central nervous system	Numbness or tingling of the hands, lips, and feet; behavior and personality changes
Other	Fatigue, weakness, anorexia, weight loss, and gastrointestinal disturbances

Healthcare facilities must have policies and procedures for hazardous waste spills. These are required by The Joint Commission and federal agencies such as the EPA and the Occupational Safety and Health Administration (OSHA). You are not likely to encounter mercury exposure in acute care and ambulatory agencies.

Biological Hazards

As a nurse, you will place a high priority on the biological safety of patients. Institutionalized patients are at especially high risk from infectious microorganisms, some of which are highly resistant to antibiotics. To learn about or review healthcare-related infections, asepsis, and infection control, refer to Chapter 22.

Hazards to Healthcare Workers

Nursing is an active profession, and workplace injuries are all too common. Nurses sometimes hesitate to report they have been injured because they fear being labeled a complainer or troublemaker, or being denied opportunities for promotion and other consequences. However, OSHA requires that employers show employees how to report a workplace injury and prohibits discrimination against employees who make such reports. If you are injured, report it. By doing so, you help (1) pinpoint trends and areas of need in safety, and (2) ensure you will receive necessary treatment and follow-up. Common accidents include back injuries, needlestick injuries, radiation injury, and violence.

Back Injury

Nursing personnel are consistently listed in the top 10 occupations for work-related musculoskeletal disorders (MSDs). Most often the MSD involves the shoulders and back (Bureau of Labor Statistics, 2006). The ANA reports that 52% of nurses report chronic back pain (ANA, 2003, 2008b), likely because many nursing tasks require bending and twisting of the torso, activities that can cause injury when the nurse does not use correct body mechanics. Among the most stressful activities are transferring patients (e.g., from toilet to chair), weighing patients, lifting a patient in bed, repositioning patients in beds or chairs, and changing bed linens.

In 2003, the ANA launched the "Handle With Care" campaign, in which they recommended that nurses use assistive equipment and devices for such patient-handling activities in order to prevent injury to themselves and patients. The ANA states that manual patient handling should be used only in exceptional situations when it cannot be avoided. For those situations, you can reduce your risk to some degree by using appropriate body mechanics. Refer to Chapter 33 for information about body mechanics and how to safely lift and move patients. For more information about ANA's campaign to prevent musculoskeletal injuries,

 Go to the ANA's Safe Patient Handling Web site, at http://www.anasafepatienthandling.org/default.aspx; also see Chapter 23, **Resources for Caregivers and Health Professionals,** on DavisPlus.

Needlestick Injury

Healthcare workers, mostly nurses and housekeeping staff, suffer up to 1 million injuries per year from needles and other sharps, putting them at risk for infectious diseases, such as hepatitis B and AIDS. A federal Needlestick Safety and Prevention Act and OSHA standards require employers to maintain a log of sharps injuries and to purchase needleless systems and safer medical and needle devices. Needlestick

injury rates declined by more than 36% during the 3-year period following passage of that law. Nevertheless, a recent survey found that 26% of nurses still report having had at least one injury from a sharp, usually a needle, contaminated with a patient's blood (Delahanty & Myers, 2007). Some employers still have not complied completely with OSHA regulations. For discussion on how to handle needles safely, refer to Procedure 25-10, Recapping Sterile Needles With One-Handed Technique. For other suggestions about how you can prevent needlestick injuries, see Clinical Insight 23-1.

Radiation Injury

Radiation is the process of emitting radiant energy in the form of waves or particles. Ionizing radiation is used in computerized tomography (CT scans) in diagnostic radiology, linear accelerators in radiotherapy, and positron emission tomography (PET scans) in nuclear medicine. Patients are deliberately exposed to radiation during diagnostic tests and certain medical treatments. Healthcare workers who care for these patients are unavoidably exposed to small doses of radiation.

Take precautions to avoid excessive radiation exposure for the patient and yourself during x-ray procedures. Follow the principles of time, distance, and shielding when caring for a patient who is being treated with an internal radioactive implant:

- Organize nursing care to limit the amount of time with the patient.
- Perform near the patient only the nursing care that is absolutely necessary.
- Wear protective shielding (e.g., a lead apron), if available, and wear a film badge if you deliver care that exposes you to radiation regularly. The film badge will indicate any radiation exposure.

Clinical Insight 23-1 ► **Preventing Needlestick Injury**

✚ Use needleless systems (e.g., retractable needles) when possible. More than 80% of needlestick injuries can be prevented with the use of safe needle devices (ANA, 2002).

Before beginning a procedure:

- Provide adequate lighting and space to perform the procedure.
- Place the sharps container near the work area, if it is moveable.
- Obtain assistance if there is a risk that the patient may be uncooperative, combative, or confused.
- Inform the patient about the procedure and explain the importance of avoiding any sudden movement.

During the procedure:

- Be sure you can see the sharps container at all times.
- When handling a sharp, be aware of other persons in the immediate area.
- Do not hand-pass exposed sharps from one person to another.
- When using a safety needle, observe for audio or visual cues that the feature has engaged.

Handling needles:

- Do not shear or break contaminated needles.
- Avoid recapping, bending, or removing contaminated needles and other sharps unless there is no feasible alternative.
- When you must recap a sterile needle, use a mechanical recapping device or a modified "scoop" technique (see Procedure 25-10).
- Never carry syringes in your uniform pocket.

Sharps containers:

- Keep puncture-proof needle disposal containers in every room.
- Place sharps containers at eye level; do not overfill the container.

- Make sure the container is large enough to hold the entire sharps device.
- Dispose of sharps immediately. Do not wait until you have finished the procedure.
- Inspect sharps and waste containers for protruding sharps. If found, notify safety personnel for removal of the hazard.

If your agency does not use needleless systems or protective devices, you should do the following:

- Explain the OSHA Bloodborne Pathogens Standard (BPS) to your employer, including the need to provide needleless systems or protective devices for blood products and parenteral medication administration.

 Refer your employer to the **OSHA Web site** at http://www.osha.gov/needlesticks/needlefaq.html

- OSHA requires worker involvement in evaluating, selecting, and implementing the use of safer needle products; volunteer to serve on that committee.
- Ask your agency for a copy of their exposure control plan, which is required by the BPS for monitoring compliance with the new law.
- Keep a record of needlestick injuries on your unit and of "near-misses" (e.g., overfilled sharps containers, sharps left on bed or overbed table).
- Submit written concerns to your employer.
- If your employer refuses to purchase safety devices, you may want to file an OSHA complaint. If you do, refer to Chapter 42's section on whistleblowing. Complaints can be filed anonymously.
- For complaint filing,

 Go to http://www.osha.gov/as/opa/worker/complain.html

Sources: Adapted from ANA, 2002; NIOSH, n.d.; U.S. Department of Labor, Occupational Safety and Health Administration, 2001; Wilburn, 2004.

Violence

Hospital security may not be sufficient to protect you from injury if violence breaks out among patients, visitors, and/or staff. This is especially true in the emergency department (ED), which has 24-hour accessibility and may sometimes be crowded and chaotic. Under the stress of an acute illness, patients and family members alike may become anxious and angry and act out in ways that are unpredictable and atypical for them.

Violence typically begins with anxiety and escalates in stages through verbal aggression and then physical aggression. If you can relieve a patient's anxiety, you may be able to halt the progression to physical violence. Certain emotional and physical conditions increase the risk for patient aggression (refer to Practical Knowledge, Assessing the Risk for Violence).

Gang activity, which is widespread in U.S. cities, is another potential source of violence. As gangs spread, so does the likelihood that gang members will be treated in the ED or admitted to the hospital (Grossman, 2003).

KnowledgeCheck 23-5

- What measures can healthcare workers use to reduce exposure to radiation?
- What safety measures help reduce equipment-related injuries in the healthcare facility?
- As a nurse, what can you do to help prevent injuring your back?

PracticalKnowledge
knowing **how**

This section provides focused assessments for certain safety risks, general interventions for addressing patient safety, and specific nursing interventions for safety hazards discussed in the preceding Theoretical Knowledge section.

◼ ASSESSMENT

It is important to assess the client's immediate environment, developmental stage, and individual risk factors. The following will help you to perform focused assessments for falls risk, home safety, and risk for violence.

Assessments for Example Problem: Falls

Assess all inpatients for falls risk when they are admitted to the healthcare setting. For clients at risk for falls, repeat the risk assessment every 8 hours, and monitor the patient more frequently. Also identify medications that increase the risk for falling (e.g., opioid analgesics, sedatives, and antihypertensives). Most institutions have policies, guidelines, and special forms for assessing risk for falls.

Morse Fall Scale

The Morse Fall Scale uses the following questions to assess a person's risk for falls:

1. Does the patient have a history of falling?
2. Does the person have more than one medical diagnosis?
3. Does the person use ambulatory aids, such as crutches or a walker?
4. Does the person have an IV line or a saline lock?
5. Is the person's gait normal or stooped or otherwise impaired?
6. What is the person's mental status (e.g., disoriented, forgetful)?

You can easily score, tally, and record those six variables on the patient's chart. The risk of falling varies greatly with different patient populations, different times of day, and different stages of the patient's illness. Age alone is not a predictor of falls, but the items scored by the scale are more common in older adults (Morse, 2001). Ideally, the Morse Fall Scale should be calibrated for each particular unit so that fall prevention strategies are targeted to those most at risk. Institutions implementing the Morse Scale should train personnel in the proper use of the scale (Morse, 1997, 2009). To see the complete Morse Fall Scale,

 Go to Chapter 23, **Tables, Boxes, Figures: ESG Figure 23-1**, on Davis*Plus*.

Assessing Older Adults for Falls

For a flowchart summarizing falls assessment for older adults, refer to Figure 23-1. At least once a year, ask the older adult (or caregivers) about falls.

Get Up and Go Test. The purpose of the Get Up and Go test is to identify those at risk for falls and those who need more evaluation. Perform the following assessments if the patient reports having had even a single fall or if you observe any difficulty with ambulation,

- **Initial Check.** The Get Up and Go test is simple. Seat the patient in a chair and observe as he follows these instructions:
  1. Stand up without using your arms for support as you rise and stand.
  2. Walk several paces, turn, and return to the chair.
  3. Sit back in the chair without using your arms for support.
     Those who can do this with steadiness need no further assessment. If the person is unsteady or has difficulty performing this test, perform the follow-up assessment below.
- **Follow-Up Assessment.** Ask the person to follow these instructions:
  1. Sit.
  2. Stand without using your arms for support.
  3. Close your eyes for a few seconds while standing in place.
  4. Stand with your eyes closed while I push gently on your chest (sternum).
  5. Walk a short distance (specify) and come to a complete stop.
  6. Turn around and return to the chair.
  7. Sit in the chair without using your arms for support.

Comprehensive Fall Evaluation. In any of the following situations, you should refer the patient to a practitioner with advanced skills and experience for a comprehensive fall evaluation:

- The patient is seeking care because of a fall.
- The patient or family reports recurrent falls in the past year.
- The patient's gait or balance is abnormal.

In addition, primary care providers should annually perform a Timed Up & Go test for fall risk assessment for all patients over age 65. This is a version of the Get Up and Go test, in which the patient is asked to get up and walk 8 feet in 8.5 seconds or less. (AHI of Indiana, n.d.; American Academy of Neurology, 2008a, 2008b; Hendrich, 2007; Kenny, Rubenstein, Martin, et al., 2001).

Assessing for Home Safety

As you know, many accidents occur in the home (e.g., fire, poisoning). Everyone should take a few minutes to check for environmental safety hazards.

- A **home safety checklist** is a convenient way for clients to identify potential hazards. For an extensive checklist you can print and use in a home assessment,

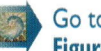 Go to Chapter 23, **Tables, Boxes, and Figures: ESG Figure 23-2, Home Safety Checklist,** on Davis*Plus*.

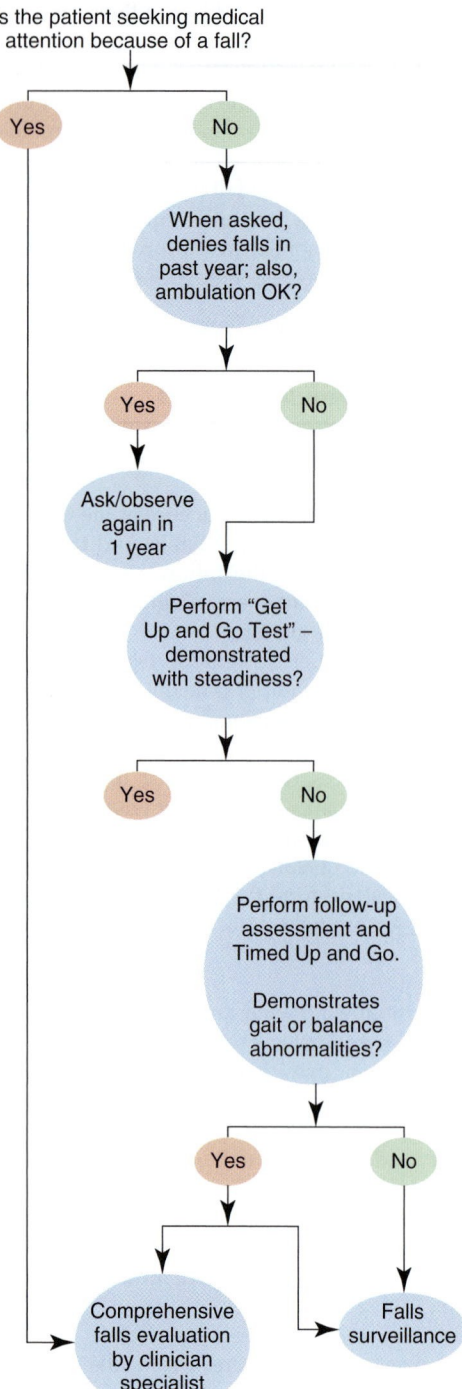

FIGURE 23-1 Falls assessment flowchart.

- **The safety assessment scale (SAS)** is an objective way to evaluate the dangers incurred by people with memory and cognitive deficits who live alone at home. You can use the short version of the SAS (Fig. 23-2) to assess the individual's risk status and decide whether she should have an in-depth evaluation. In addition to assessing risk for injury, this scale evaluates whether the cognitively impaired person is capable of cooking, taking medications independently, shopping, and performing other activities of daily living (ADLs).

Assessing for Violence

You can be prepared to intervene and perhaps even prevent violence if you recognize risk factors and early warning signs (Flores, 2008).

1. Assess for factors that increase the risk for aggression:
   - Mental disorders, such as dementia, delirium, schizophrenia, and bipolar disorder
   - Being under the influence of alcohol or other drugs
   - Withdrawal from alcohol or other drugs
   - History of violence
   - Clinical conditions such as high fever, epilepsy, head trauma, and hypoglycemia
2. Assess for signs of anxiety:
   - Agitation and restlessness
   - Pacing
   - Talking loudly, speaking rapidly
   - Gesturing widely
   - Be alert for verbal aggression, such as threats, sarcasm, and swearing.

Knowledge Check 23-6

- Which assessment tool would you use for a slightly confused home care client to assess her ability to safely live alone and perform activities of daily living?
- List the six risk factors that are assessed on the Morse Fall Scale.
- How should you screen older adults to see if they need a comprehensive falls evaluation?

ANALYSIS/NURSING DIAGNOSIS

How would your interventions differ for each the following two nursing diagnoses?

Risk for Falls r/t poor vision secondary to cataracts
Risk for Falls r/t to muscle weakness, joint instability, and poor sense of balance

The nursing diagnoses listed above illustrate that problem etiologies are important because they affect your choice of interventions. Etiologies may include environmental hazards as well as the developmental and individual risk factors discussed in the preceding sections. Keep in mind that you must state *specific* etiologies for each individual—not just general ones such as "environmental hazards." For example:

Correct: Risk for Falls r/t cluttered home environment and joint instability
Incorrect: Risk for Falls r/t environmental and physical factors
For NANDA-I labels to use in describing safety problems,

 Go to Chapter 23, **Standardized Language: NANDA-I Diagnoses and NOC Outcomes for Safety Problems,** on Davis*Plus.*

Use the diagnosis Risk for Injury only when the risk cannot be described by one of the more specific nursing diagnoses.

PLANNING OUTCOMES/EVALUATION

The *NOC standardized outcomes* you use will depend on the nursing diagnosis. For some examples (e.g., Abuse Protection, Fall Prevention Behavior),

 Go to Chapter 23, **Standardized Language: NANDA-I Diagnoses and NOC Outcomes for Safety Problems,** on Davis*Plus.*

Name _____

CLSC CÔTE-DES-NEIGES

S.A.S. | **SAFETY ASSESSMENT SCALE**

CAREGIVER AND LIVING ENVIRONMENT (1)

a) This person lives on her own.   Yes [1]   No [0] _____ _____

b) This person is alone at home.
Always [4]   Most of the time [3]   Occasionally [2]   Never [1] _____

SMOKING (2)

This person leaves cigarette bum marks on the floor, furniture or clothing..
Yes [1]   No [0] _____

FIRE AND BURNS (3)

a) The stove on/off buttons are located...
on the front of the stove [1]   on the top of the stove [2]
behind the hotplates [3] _____

b) This person is capable of turning on the stove him/herself
Yes [1]   No [0]   Doesn't know [1] _____

c) This person cooks his/her own food.
Always [4]   Most of the time [3]   Occasionally [2]   Never [1] _____

d) This person forgets a pan on the stove.
Very often [4]   Often [3]   Sometimes [2]   Never [1] _____

e) The heating system uses...
electricity [1]   natural gas [2]   wood [3] _____

NUTRITION (4)

a) This person receives meals-on-wheels or other prepared meals.
More than once a day [1]   Once a day [2]
A few times a week (2 to 6 times a week) [3]   Once a week or less [4] _____

b) This person's meals contain foods from different food groups
(dairy products, meat or fish, cereals, fruit and vegetables).
Always [1]   Most of the time [2]   Occasionally [3]   Never [4] _____

FOOD POISONING AND TOXIC SUBSTANCES (5)

This person can tell the difference between food that is fresh and food
that is spoiled.   Yes [0]   No [1] _____

MEDICATION AND HEALTH PROBLEMS (6)

a) This person takes, on a regular basis...*
1 to 3 medications [2]   4 to 6 medications [3]
7 medications or more [4]   Does not take any medication [1]
*prescribed medications only _____

b) This person takes medication to help him/her sleep or relax.
Yes [1]   No [0] _____

c) Does this person suffer from any physical health problem?
None [1]   Minor [2]   Moderate [3]   Severe [4] _____

d) This person accepts treatment for his/her physical health problems.
Yes [0]   No [1]   Does not apply [0] _____

WANDERING AND ADAPTATION TO CHANGING TEMPERATURE (7)

a) This person gets lost in familiar surroundings.
Very often [4]   Often [3]   Sometimes [2]   Never [1] _____

b) Has this person ever gotten lost?   Yes [1]   No [0] _____

c) Can this person find his/her way home?   Yes [0]   No [1] _____

d) Does this person dress appropriately according
to the changing temperature, both indoors and outdoors?
Yes [0]   No [1] _____

An Affiliated University Centre
Affiliated with McGill University

Assessed by _____

SCORE

‾‾‾
47

Source: Dr. Louise Poulin de Courval ©CLSC Côte-des-Neiges. Used with permission.

FIGURE 23-2 Safety assessment scale (SAS).

Individualized goals/outcome statements you might write for a client's safety diagnoses include the following:

- The child will be free of injury.
- (Client) will experience no physical injury due to environmental hazards.
- Falls will not occur.
- Family members will describe their planned escape routes in case of fire.

PLANNING INTERVENTIONS/IMPLEMENTATION

NIC standardized interventions will be determined by the nursing diagnosis you use. To see the more than 50 interventions in the NIC Safety domain (category) (e.g., First Aid, Sports-Injury Prevention: Youth), and some interventions from other NIC domains that are applicable to safety needs,

 Go to Chapter 23, **Standardized Language: Examples of NIC Interventions Related to Safety,** on Davis*Plus.*

General Interventions Related to Safety

Specific nursing activities are designed to monitor and manipulate the physical environment to promote safety in all types of settings and circumstances. The following are some general activities that provide an overview of your role in patient safety:

- Assess and continually monitor the safety needs of patients, based on their level of physical and cognitive function and past history of behavior.
- Assess and continually monitor safety hazards in the environment (i.e., physical, biological, and chemical).
- Remove hazards from the environment, when possible.
- Provide clients with emergency phone numbers.
- Modify the environment to minimize hazards and risk.
- Teach clients about specific safety measures.
- If an accident or injury occurs in the healthcare setting, file an incident report according to agency policy. See Chapter 18 for more information on this topic.
- Urge patients to be active members of the healthcare team (Box 23-3).

The QSEN Safety Competency should also help you to understand your role in keeping patients safe. To review the knowledge, skills and attitudes necessary for that competency,

 Go to Chapter 23, **Tables, Boxes, Figures: ESG Table 23-1, QSEN Safety Competency,** on Davis*Plus.*

Home Care Safety Interventions

Specific interventions follow for promoting safety related to particular hazards in home care. After a brief discussion, you will find a series of boxes containing specific home safety interventions.

Prevent Poisoning in the Home

Nursing interventions focus on teaching parents how to child-proof the home and what to do if someone ingests a poisonous substance. All homes should be equipped to handle an emergency if poisoning occurs. Teach parents to keep the telephone number for the nearest poison control center (PCC) easily accessible. The national number is (800) 222-1222; they will connect you to a local PCC. Teach parents if they suspect a child has ingested a poisonous substance, it is crucial to obtain help immediately so there is less time for the substance to enter the child's system. Call 911 or the local emergency

---

number right away. Even if the person is having no symptoms, call the PCC as soon as possible.

If there are no young children in the home, advise families with older adults to prevent accidental overdose or misuse of prescribed medications by using a medication organizer that may be filled once a week by the patient or family member. For steps to prevent poisoning, see the Home Care box Preventing Poisoning in the Home. For actions to take if poisoning occurs at home,

 Go to Chapter 23, **Tables, Boxes, Figures: ESG Box 23-3, Home Care: If Poisoning Occurs at Home,** on Davis*Plus.*

Prevent Carbon Monoxide Poisoning

If carbon monoxide (CO) intoxication is suspected, the person should be treated with 100% humidified oxygen. A simple blood test may be done to confirm CO levels in the blood. Nursing interventions include teaching prevention measures, such as the following:

- Buy, install, and maintain a home CO detector.
- Ensure that gas or wood-burning appliances are adequately vented to the outside.
- Repair rust holes or defects in vehicles that could allow exhaust fumes to enter the passenger compartment.
- Never use a kerosene heater, gas oven, or gas range to heat a house, even for a short time.

Home Care

Preventing Poisoning in the Home

Young children will eat and drink almost anything. Most victims of accidental poisoning are children younger than the age of 5. Tips to prevent poisoning include the following:

Careful Words and Actions

- Never leave a small child unattended near household cleaning supplies or medicines, even for a moment. If you must answer the phone or doorbell, take the child with you.
- Children act fast; it takes only a moment for them to swallow something.
- Avoid taking medicines in front of children; children tend to imitate adults.
- Never call medicines or vitamins "candy." Instead, use the correct name (e.g., "cough medicine").

Careful Storage

- Store medicines or household chemicals on high shelves or in locked cabinets and drawers. Never leave them on kitchen or bathroom counters.
- Store all household chemicals away from food.
- Keep medicines and household chemicals in their original containers. Leave the original labels on. Especially do not store chemicals in containers that normally hold food.
- Use child-resistant packaging for medicines and household chemicals. Close the container securely after each use.
- Do not assume your child is safe around substances in child-resistant containers; research has shown that many toddlers and preschoolers can open them.

Careful Disposal

- Teach clients to take advantage of any community programs that take back unwanted medications for safe disposal (e.g., call the local trash service or a local pharmacy for options in your area).

- Teach clients how to safely dispose of outdated prescription medications:
  Crush the medication or add water to dissolve it.
  Mix the drugs with an undesirable substance such as kitty litter or used cooking grease to make it less desirable for pets and children to eat.
  Place the mixture in an empty can or resealable bag and put it in the trash.
  Remove all identifying information from prescription labels before throwing containers in the trash or recycling them.
  It is no longer considered safe to dispose of drugs down the toilet or sink. Wastewater treatment plants are not fully designed to deal with medications, and small amounts have shown up in surface waters. Although there is no evidence of harm to humans or the environment, the long-term effects on people, animals, and the environment are unknown.

Careful Environment Checks

- Before purchasing a houseplant, verify that it is nontoxic.
- Examples of toxic plants are rhododendron, philodendron, English ivy, holly, mistletoe, and lily of the valley.
- Find out whether any plants growing in your yard are poisonous, and, if so, remove them.
- Teach children that they must never eat berries, wild mushrooms, or other edible-looking plants in yards, fields, and forests.
- A wide variety of plants can cause illness and even death in young children.
- Warn parents to keep children from chewing on windowsills, and so on, and to carefully clean up flakes of paint. Advocate for clients who need to have lead-based paint replaced in their homes.
- Lead-based paint can still be found in older homes, and some soil contains a high lead content. Young children often put dirt in their mouths and chew on furniture and windowsills, especially when they are teething.

- Never operate gasoline-powered engines (e.g., automobiles, generators, lawn mowers) near open doors or windows or in confined spaces, such as garages or basements.
- Never burn charcoal inside a home, cabin, recreational vehicle, or tent—not even in a fireplace.

Prevent Home Fires

Nursing interventions include teaching families how to prevent fires and measures to take should a fire occur. Stress the following measures:

Have a Warning System. Have working smoke alarms and change batteries every six months or more often. Keep a phone near the bed or chair for people who have limited mobility.

Have an Escape Plan. Develop a home fire escape plan and practice it at least twice a year. Keep a rope or other type of ladder for escape from rooms above ground level. Have a fire extinguisher in the home, and know where it is located and how to use it. Check fire extinguishers regularly and replace them when they become outdated.

Have a Preventive Frame of Mind. When decorating Christmas trees and the exterior of your home, always use

fire-safe lights. Do not leave old light sets hung on the outside of your home year after year. Always unplug Christmas tree lights before leaving home, and remove the Christmas tree from the home when it becomes dry. Other cautions include the following:

- Never leave burning candles unattended. Do not use candles near curtains or other flammable materials.
- With charcoal grills, use only charcoal starter fluids designed for barbecue grills.
- With gas grills, be sure that the hose connection is tight, and check hoses for leaks.
- Store flammable materials (e.g., oil-soaked rags) in appropriate containers (e.g., metal container with a tight lid.
- Do not smoke, especially in bed—and especially in a home where oxygen is in use.
- Never use an open flame when oxygen is in use.

Promote Electrical Safety in the Home. Make sure electrical outlets have covers. Routinely inspect electrical appliances for damaged cords; replace frayed cords. Do not place electrical cords under carpets, and make sure cords do not hang off of tables and countertops.

QSEN

Creating a Culture of Safety—cont'd

to determine what systems need to be in place to build the culture of safety. Some critical features include the following:

➤ All levels of leadership make safety a visible priority and take actions that promote safety. *Why is leadership important in changing culture?*

➤ All staff members providing care are formally encouraged to communicate their concerns to the team. *Why do you think nurses or junior doctors might not communicate concerns?*

➤ All information needed to appropriately manage the patient across shifts, units, facilities or after other handoffs is available at all times. *What types of errors can occur during handoffs?*

➤ Facility adopts a nonpunitive response to error and uses strategies such as root cause analysis to identify system issues. *What effect might a punitive culture have on error reporting?*

➤ Facility recognizes both individual and system causes of error but emphasizes a systems approach to error reduction. *Describe one system that can break down and make error more likely.*

➤ Each person providing care acknowledges own potential for error and values own role in preventing errors. *What can you do to help prevent errors?*

_____

Sources: Institute of Medicine (IOM). (2001, 2011).

*For specific Knowledge, Skills, and Attitudes,

 Go to the QSEN web site at http:www.qsen.org.ksas_prelicensure.php

CLINICALREASONING
Applying the **Full-Spectrum Nursing Model**

Because the following critical thinking activities allow you to practice the kind of thinking you will use as a full-spectrum nurse, they usually have no single right answer. Discuss them with your peers—if you have difficulty with any of the questions, consult your instructor.

PATIENT SITUATION

Recall your patient, Alvin Lin, from Meet Your Patients. Mr. Lin, is a 79-year-old man who was just transferred from a long-term care facility to your medical unit. His admitting diagnosis is dehydration and pneumonia. In the handoff report you were told he had rested well during the night and was alert and oriented. When you enter his room, he is confused and does not know where he is. He is becoming combative and is trying to get out of bed.

THINKING

1. *Theoretical Knowledge:*
   a. What is the pathophysiology of pneumonia?
   b. When the oxygen level of the blood falls, what is the effect on the central nervous system? If you do not know the answer to this question, consult a reliable reference.
   c. What are the defining characteristics for the NANDA-I diagnosis, Deficient Fluid Volume?
2. *Critical Thinking (Considering Alternatives):*
   a. Which of the three defining characteristics (in 1c) may increase Mr. Lin's risk for falls? Why?
   b. What else may be increasing his confusion and his risk for falls?

DOING

3. *Practical Knowledge:* Suppose you have tried all the less restrictive restraints, but Mr. Lin still attempts to get out of bed. He has even pulled out his intravenous line. You decide you must apply restraints to keep him safely in bed. You have called the physician, but he has not returned your call. You cannot wait any longer because you have other patients who need you, and yet you must stay with Mr. Lin to keep him from falling. What should you do right now?
4. *Nursing Process (Diagnosis):* Which nursing diagnosis seems more useful to you in planning care for Mr. Lin?
   a. Confusion related to disease process
   b. Risk for Falls related to confusion and possibly r/t weakness

CARING

5. *Self-Knowledge:*
   a. Do you think having a restraint-free facility is a valuable goal, or not? Explain your thinking.
   b. How did you come to believe that?

6. *Ethical Knowledge*: Suppose Mr. Lin is too confused to give consent for restraints, and you cannot reach his family by telephone. How can you justify applying restraints, and what must you do later to follow up?

 Go To Chapter 23, **Clinical Reasoning: Applying the Full-Spectrum Nursing Model Response Sheet,** on *DavisPlus.*

PracticalKnowledge
procedures

Procedure 23–1 ■ **Using a Bed Monitoring Device**

➤ For steps to follow in *all* procedures, refer to the Universal Steps for All Procedures found on the page facing the inside back cover.

Equipment

Bed or chair exit monitoring device

There are at least four types of notification systems that may be used to warn caregivers that a patient is leaving a bed or chair: (1) pressure sensitive, (2) posture indicators, (3) motion sensors, and (4) pull-cord and combination alarms.

Delegation

As the nurse, you must determine whether a monitoring device is needed. You must also select the appropriate device and provide ongoing evaluation of its effectiveness. You may delegate to a nursing assistive personnel (NAP) the installation of the device, after verifying the NAP has the necessary knowledge and skill.

Pre-Procedure Assessments

Assess for intrinsic factors that increase the risk for falls:
- Older than age 75
- History of a recent fall or fear of falling
- Bowel and bladder incontinence (particularly urge bladder incontinence)
- Cognitive impairment
- Mood changes, lability

- Dizziness
- Functional impairment
- Medications (especially new medications or changes in regimen)
- Other medical problems (diseases such as dementia, hip fracture, type 2 diabetes, Parkinson's disease, arthritis, and depression)

Assess for extrinsic environmental factors that increase the risk of falling:
- Use of an assistive device
- Equipment in the room
- Wet or uneven floors
- The use of physical restraints
- Inappropriate footwear
- Poor lighting
- Lack of grab rails and bars in the bathroom
- Furniture and adaptive aids that are in disrepair or unstable (e.g., bed rails, IV poles)
- Clothing that may cause tripping

Identify factors that increase risk for more severe injury in the case of a fall. These include use of anticoagulants (e.g., Coumadin, Plavix or aspirin) and osteoporosis. Check the alarm on the monitoring device to ensure that it is working properly.

➤ When performing the procedure, always identify your patient according to agency policy and be attentive to standard precautions, hand hygiene, patient safety and privacy, body mechanics, and documentation.

Procedure Steps

1. **Apply the device.**

Bed or Chair Monitor

Place sensor pads under the patient's buttocks.

The sensor will alarm when the patient attempts to get out of the bed or chair; it alarms when there is no weight on it for

more than a few seconds. Many electronic beds have bed exit and patient position monitors for which you must select the desired alarm sensitivity. For example, you may set the system to alarm when the patient exits the bed, when the patient attempts to exit the bed, or even when the patient moves in the bed. ➤

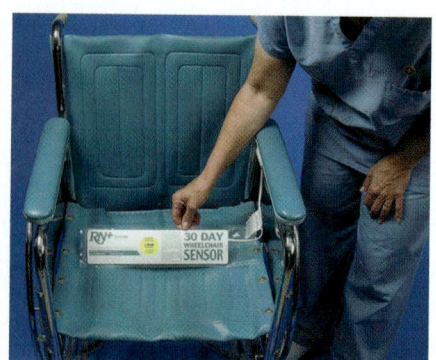

(continued on next page)

Procedure 23–1 ■ **Using a Bed Monitoring Device** (continued)

Leg Sensors

Place sensors on the patient's thigh.

The alarm will sound when the leg assumes a near-vertical position. ▼

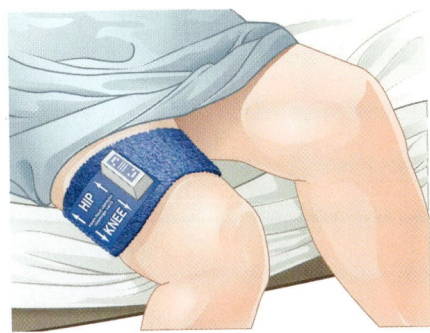

Infrared Beam Detector

Attach next to the bed or on the wall.

Cord-Activated Sensor

Attach one end of the cord (clip) to the patient's garment. Attach the other end to the control unit. The cord should be long enough to allow moderate movements, but short enough to prevent false alarms. Be sure the cord is free to pull straight out from the monitor and is not blocked by pillows, bedding, or bedrails.

The alarm is activated when the patient's movement causes the cord to be detached from the control unit. Some patients will deactivate the alarms, including removing the alarms clipped to their garments.

2. **Connect the control unit to the sensor pad.**

Bed or Chair Monitor

Mount the control unit on the bed or chair.

Leg Sensor

Mount the control unit directly on the leg sensor.

Infrared System

Mount the control unit next to the bed or on the wall.

Cord-Activated System

Mount the control unit next to the bed or on the wall.

3. **Connect the control unit to the nurse call system**, if possible.

   Allows for a quicker response; however, not all call systems will accommodate this.

4. **Disconnect or turn off the alarm before assisting the patient out of the bed or chair.**

   Prevents false alarms. Some systems have a standby setting to allow the alarm to be temporarily suspended.

5. **Reactivate the alarm after assisting the patient back to the bed or chair.**

   Helps improve the timeliness of staff response, which may prevent patient falls.

6. **Be sure the patient can reach the nurse call light.**

Evaluation

- Assess the sensitivity of the monitoring device, and adjust as needed to ensure that the alarm is activated if the patient tries to get out of the bed or chair.
- Continue to assess fall risk per agency policy and as indicated by the patient's physical and/or mental status.
- In the event of a fall, perform a post-fall assessment to identify possible causes. Monitor patients closely for 48 hours after a fall.

Patient Teaching

- Explain to the patient and family that a bed or chair exit monitoring device alerts the staff when the patient tries to get out of the chair or bed.
- Explain that the purpose of the device is to help prevent falls using the least restrictive method possible. This will reassure the patient and family.
- Explain to the patient that she will need to call for assistance when she wants to get up.

  Calling for assistance will prevent the alarm from sounding. Summoning for help can prevent the patient from falling.

Documentation

- Document the initial sensor placement, including type of sensor used and the location of placement.
- After documenting initial placement, follow agency policy for documenting the use of bed exit monitor. Usually, the minimum documentation for exit monitors is every 8 hours.
- Place the patient on fall risk precautions according to agency policy.
- Document on the fall risk assessment sheet, restraint flow sheet, and nursing notes according to agency policy.

Sample documentation:

9/06/14, 1230.   Continues to be confused and to stand up without assistance. Wheelchair exit alarm placed on wheelchair and monitoring clip attached to back of client's gown. Notified client's daughter, June Kennedy, via telephone. Daughter agreed the exit alarm would help keep her father from falling. —————————————— Mary Clinton, RN

Practice Resources

Gray-Micelli, 2008; Park & Tang, 2007.

Thinking About the Procedure

 Go to the *Fundamentals of Nursing Skills Videos*, **Safety: Ambulatory Alarm—Bed and Chair.**

1. Where and how does the nurse attach the bed monitoring device control unit?
2. Where does the nurse put the sensor?

 For suggested responses, go to Chapter 23, **Thinking About the Procedure Suggested Responses,** on Davis*Plus*.

Procedure 23–2 ■ Using Restraints

➤ For steps to follow in *all* procedures, refer to the Universal Steps for All Procedures found on the page facing the inside back cover.

➤ *Caution:* This procedure describes Medicare standards, but state and agency policies may be more restrictive.

Equipment

- Restraint of the appropriate size: belt, vest, wrist or ankle, or mitt
- Soft gauze or cotton padding for bony prominences

Delegation

As the nurse, you must determine whether restraints are needed in each specific situation. You must also select the least restrictive type of restraints, evaluate their effectiveness, and continue to assess for complications that may occur. You may delegate to the NAP the application and periodic removal of ordered restraints, after verifying that the NAP has the knowledge and skill to do so.

Pre-Procedure Assessments

- Assess the patient's risk for falls, including mobility status and level of awareness.
- Assess for need for restraints: The immediate physical safety of the patient, a staff member, or others is threatened.
  If a patient must be temporarily restrained so that a procedure may be performed, this is not considered restraint.
- Determine that all less restrictive interventions have been tried unsuccessfully.
- Identify the appropriate restraint:
  - Should be the least restrictive possible.
  - Does not interfere with care or exacerbate patient's medical condition.
  - Does not pose a safety risk to the patient.
  - Can be changed easily to keep it clean.

➤ When performing the procedure, always identify your patient according to agency policy and be attentive to standard precautions, hand hygiene, patient safety and privacy, body mechanics, and documentation.

Procedure Steps

1. **Determine whether dangerous behaviors continue** despite attempts to eliminate causal factors using less restrictive interventions.
2. **Obtain a physician's prescription for restraint**, including type of restraint, indications for use, site of restraint application, and duration. Determine if the restraint is being used for medical–surgical or behavioral reasons.
   Federal and state regulations and laws permit healthcare facilities to use restraints only when they are medically needed. Restraints can be used only with an order from a physician or advanced practice nurse. The order must be for a specified and limited time. When the restraint prescription expires (maximum 24 hr), physician assessment and a new prescription are needed. No "standing orders" or "as needed" orders for physical restraint are allowed.
3. **Notify the family of the change in patient status and the need for restraints.** Obtain patient and family consent when clinically feasible.

Patients have the right to refuse treatment. Consent may not be necessary if there is an immediate threat to patient safety; however, as a rule, the family must be notified of the use of restraints if the patient has cognitive impairment. Many times family members prefer to sit with the patient as an alternative to restraint.

4. **Pad bony prominences and apply the appropriately sized restraint**, using appropriate knotting techniques.

   ✚ Use a quick-release knot, such as the half-bow, when tying restraints to the bed frame or wheelchair. Do not tie restraints to the siderails.

   A quick-release knot is used to prevent patient injury and for ease in caring for the patient. Tie the knot on an immovable part of the bed to prevent injuring the patient if the siderails or head of bed are lowered. A quick-release knot will not tighten or slip when the patient moves about, but unties quickly when you pull on the loose end.

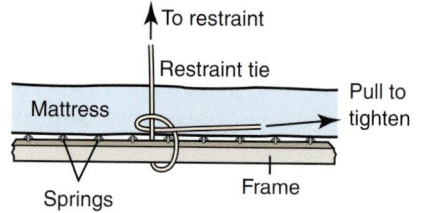

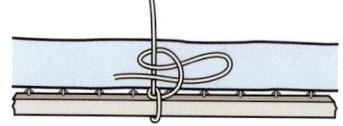

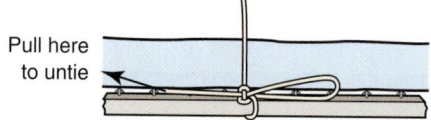

Belt Restraint

   a. Place the belt restraint at the patient's waist, removing any wrinkles.
   b. Make sure that the belt is snug but does not constrict the patient's waist.
   c. Some belts have a key-locked buckle to prevent slipping.

(continued on next page)

Procedure 23–2 ■ Using Restraints (continued)

A belt restraint is used mainly to prevent a patient from falling when getting up from a chair or wheelchair and may be used to remind a patient not to get out of bed unassisted. ▼

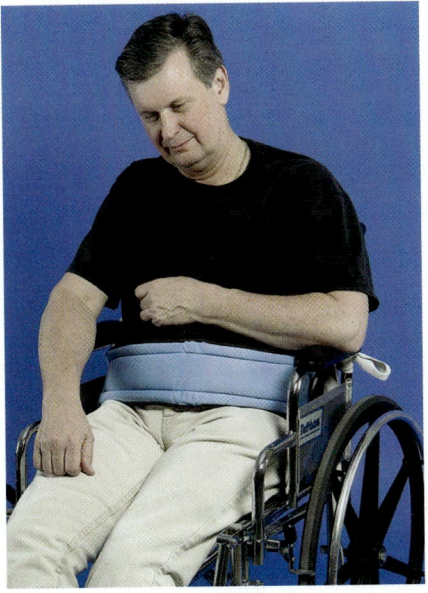

Vest or Jacket Restraint

a. Place the patient in the vest restraint. A zipper-style vest is preferred.

A vest restraint with a rear zipper is less likely to accidentally strangle the patient.

b. Attach the vest straps to the bed or wheelchair.

A vest restraint is used mainly to prevent a patient from falling out of a chair or wheelchair and sometimes to prevent a patient from getting out of bed unassisted. ▼

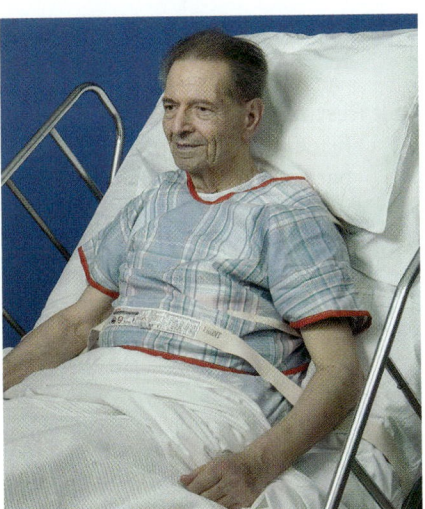

Wrist or Ankle Restraint

a. Apply the padded portion of the wrist or ankle restraint around the patient's wrist or ankle.

b. Make the restraint snug enough to prevent the patient from being able to slip it off, but not tight enough to impair circulation.

c. Attach the restraint strap to the bed frame. Do not attach to bed rails.

A wrist restraint is used mainly to prevent an agitated patient from pulling at tubes, such as IV sites and nasogastric tubes. ▼

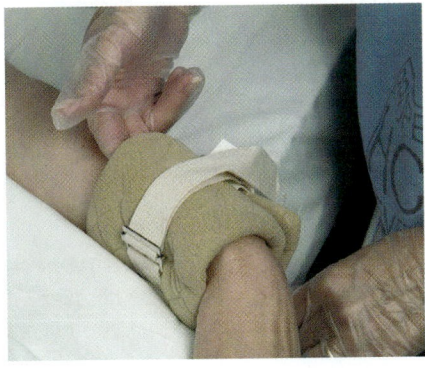

Mitt Restraint

a. Place patient's hand in the mitt restraint, ensuring that fingers are slightly flexed in the mitt.

b. Attach restraint strap to the bed frame if necessary.

A mitt restraint is used mainly to prevent a patient from pulling at tubes, such as IV sites and nasogastric tubes. Mitt restraints limit the use of the fingers, which may be enough to prevent the patient from grasping the tube. If this is the case, mitts that are not tied to the bed frame are the least restrictive restraint. ▼

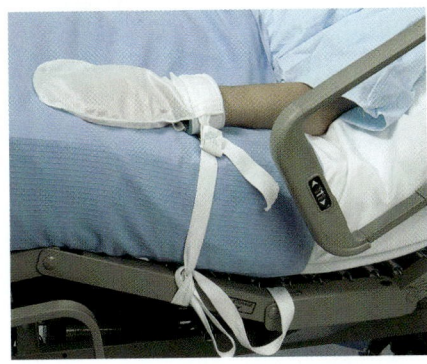

Enclosed Bed

a. Place patient in the bed and zip all sides. Be sure zippers are completely closed and zipper tabs are positioned in the upper aspects of the net panels out of the patient's reach.

b. Adhere to the manufacturer's minimum height and weight recommendations.

c. Never leave the bed in the high position with the patient unattended.

An enclosed bed is a canopy-like padded bed that is used mainly to keep a patient from wandering or from falling out of bed. The bed has nylon netting on all four sides, with zippered panels that can be opened to provide care. The patient has full freedom of movement and access to all parts of his body. Patients in enclosed beds have a higher risk of becoming entrapped between the bed rails and the mattress, risking suffocation. The dangers are greater for smaller patients and when the bed is left in a high position.

5. **Adjust the restraint to maintain good body alignment, comfort, and safety.** You should be able to slide two fingers under a wrist or ankle restraint.

The restraint should be snug enough to prevent it from slipping off, but not tight enough to impair circulation.

6. ✚ **Release restraints at least every 2 hours to provide skin care, passive and active range of motion, ambulation, toileting, hydration, and nutrition. Assess for the continued need for restraint.**

Prevents impaired circulation and injury. Medicare- and Medicaid-certified healthcare agencies must ensure that a patient's abilities do not decline unless the decline cannot be avoided because of the patient's medical condition. Patients often lose the ability to bathe, dress, walk, toilet, eat, and communicate when they are regularly restrained. If restraints are necessary, they must be used in a way that does not cause these losses.

7. Place the patient on fall risk precautions according to agency policy.
Patients who are restrained have a higher incidence of falls.

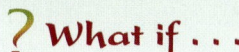 **What if . . .**

■ **I must apply a restraint in an emergency, for the safety of the patient or others?**

In such an emergency, an RN may initiate a restraint. When you apply restraint in an emergency, obtain the order as the restraint is being applied, or as quickly as possible afterward.

Evaluation

■ Assess the initial restraint placement, circulation, and skin integrity. Observe for pallor, cyanosis, and coolness of extremities when extremities are restrained.
■ Check the restraint every 30 minutes (more often for a behavioral restraint).
■ Release the restraint to assess circulation, the patient's response to the intervention, and the need for continuing the use of the restraint every 2 hours; remove it when it is no longer needed.
Ensures that the restraint is still functioning as intended. Monitoring and reassessment are critical components of caring for patients in physical restraints. Frequency of monitoring is determined by the type of restraint (behavioral vs. medical–surgical). Patients in behavioral restraints require more frequent monitoring and in some circumstances require continual observation.
■ Check every 24 hours to see that the restraint prescription has been renewed.
■ Remove the restraint as soon as possible.
■ Modify the plan of care to reflect the application of restraints and the plan for monitoring.

Patient Teaching

■ Explain to the patient and family the need for the restraints.
■ Explain that the restraints will be removed as soon as possible.

Home Care

■ The same guidelines apply to clients in the home.
■ Evaluate caregivers' knowledge and skill in using restraints, and provide teaching as needed (e.g., regarding padding bony prominences and the need to periodically release restraints).
■ If an enclosed bed is used in the home, instruct the caregiver in safe use.

Documentation

Document the following:
■ All nursing interventions that were done to eliminate the need for the restraint (e.g., moving patient closer to the nurses' station, asking a family member to remain with the patient, reorienting the patient)

■ Reasons for placing the restraint (e.g., patient behaviors)
■ The initial restraint placement, location, circulation, and skin integrity
■ The teaching session with the patient and family members
■ Circulation checks, range of motion, and restraint removal per agency protocol
■ Entries on fall risk assessment sheet, restraint flowsheet, and nursing notes according to agency policy

Practice Resources

American Nurses Association, 2001; Centers for Medicare & Medicaid Services, 2006b.

Thinking About the Procedure

 Go to the *Fundamentals of Nursing Skills Videos,* **Safety: Vest Restraints.**

1. What type of restraint did the nurse use?
2. After putting the restraint on the patient, where did the nurse tie the restraint straps?

 For suggested responses, go to Chapter 23, **Thinking About the Procedure Suggested Responses,** on *DavisPlus*

 To explore learning resources for this chapter,

 Go to DavisPlus at http://www.Davisplus.fadavis.com, **keyword Treas.**
Chapter Resources for Chapter 23:
　Knowledge Check and Think Like a Nurse Response Sheets
　Knowledge Check Answers
　Resources for Caregivers and Health Professionals
　Reading More About Safety (Suggested Readings)
　What Are the Main Points in This Chapter?
NCLEX-Style Review Questions
Chapter Overview Podcasts

Concept Map

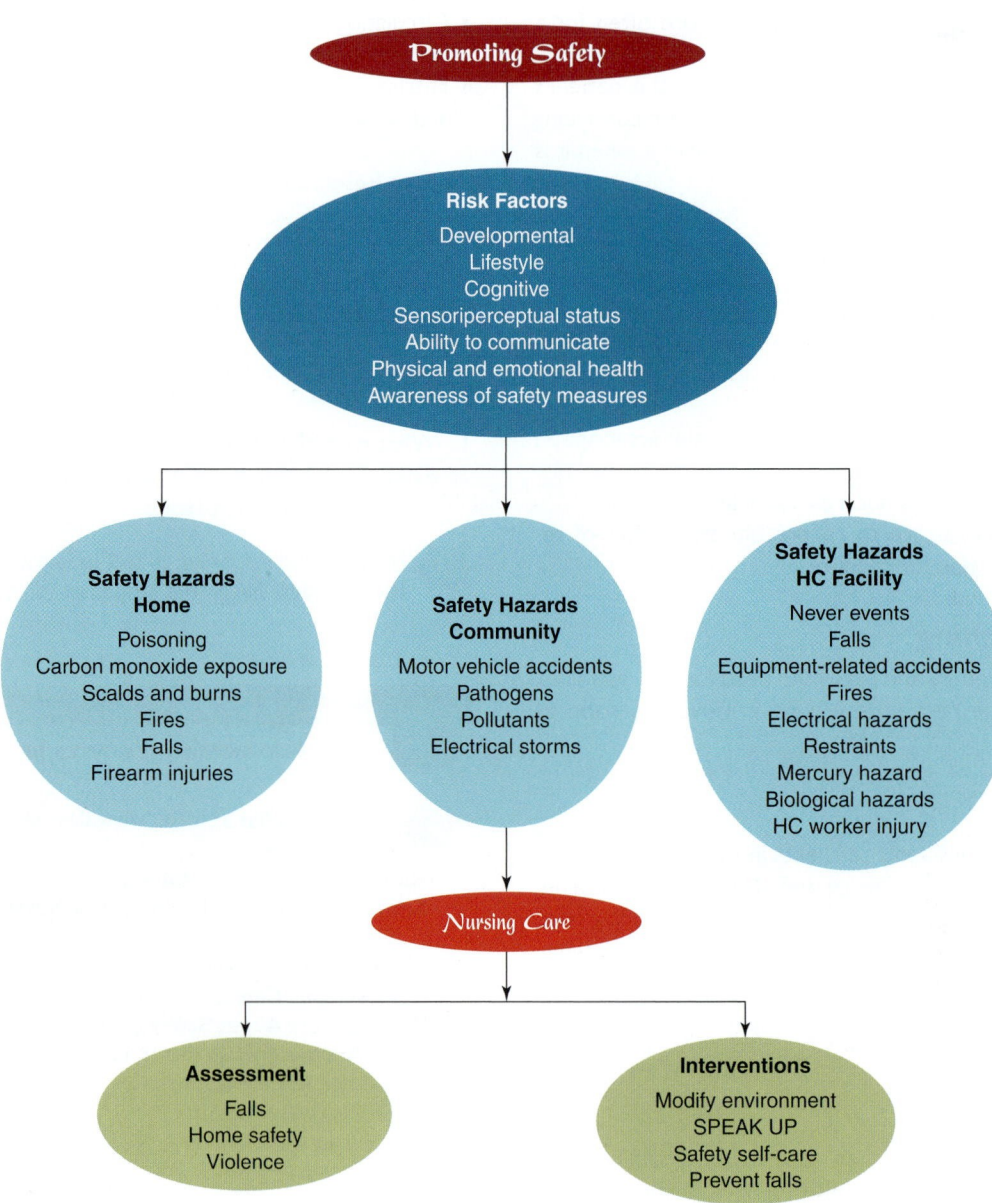

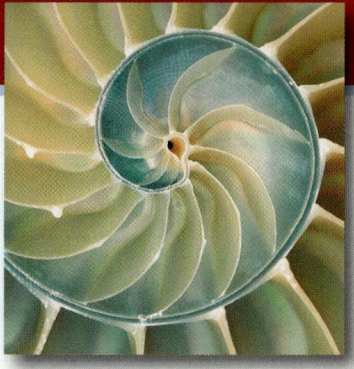

CHAPTER 24

Hygiene

Learning Outcomes

After completing this chapter, you should be able to:

- ➤ Explain how personal hygiene relates to health and well-being.
- ➤ Identify factors influencing personal hygiene practices.
- ➤ Discuss delegation of hygiene activities to nursing assistive personnel (NAPs).
- ➤ Discuss the nurse's role in determining a client's self-care ability.
- ➤ Identify nursing diagnoses related to self-care ability and hygiene practices.
- ➤ Describe routine assessments to make when providing hygiene care of the skin, feet, nails, mouth, hair, eyes, ears, and nose.

- ➤ Describe the following types of baths: complete, assist, partial, towel, bag, shower, tub, and therapeutic.
- ➤ Apply the nursing process to common hygiene-related problems of the skin, feet, nails, mouth, hair, eyes, ears, and nose.
- ➤ Demonstrate nursing skills to promote patient hygiene, such as bathing, foot care, and bed making.
- ➤ Demonstrate care of the eyes, ears, and teeth, including glasses, contacts, hearing aids, and dentures.
- ➤ Discuss the relationship between a patient's overall well-being and the immediate environment.

Key Concepts

Activities of daily living
Hygiene
Self-care ability

Related Concepts

See the Concept Map at the end of this chapter.

Caring for the Nguyens

This feature allows you to practice the kind of thinking you will use as a full-spectrum nurse. There is usually more than one correct answer to a critical thinking question, so we do not provide answers for these features. It is more important to develop your nursing judgment than to "cover content." Discuss the questions with your peers. If you are still unsure, consult your instructor.

Yen Nguyen works as a preschool teacher. She schedules a clinic visit to discuss a variety of concerns. For each of the concerns she mentions, answer the following four questions:

1. What theoretical knowledge do you need?
2. Where could you find it?

3. What, if any, additional patient information do you need?
4. How would you respond to Mrs. Nguyen's concerns?

A. Yen tells you that her skin is very dry and irritated.

B. Yen tells you that several of the children at the preschool have recently been diagnosed with head lice. She would like to know how to assess for pediculosis.

C. Yen tells you that her 3-year-old grandson, Kim, frequently refuses to bathe. She asks for advice on how to handle this.

 Go to **Caring for the Nguyens Response Sheet** on *DavisPlus.*

Meet Your Patients

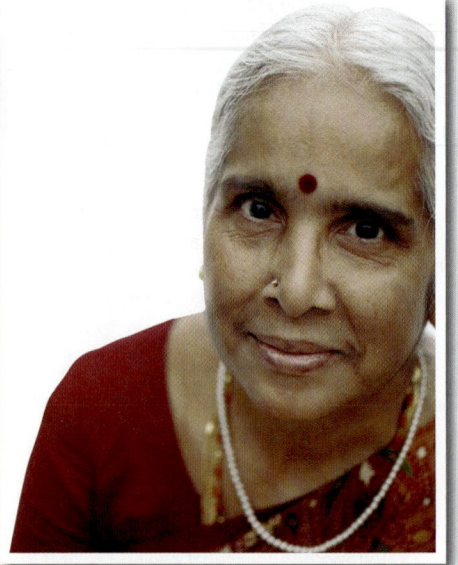

You and a nursing assistive personnel (NAP) are to assist the following patients with their hygiene.

The first patient is Mrs. Williams, a 76-year-old woman of Indian heritage who was admitted yesterday after suffering a stroke that paralyzed her right side. Since the stroke, she has been unable to speak clearly and becomes frustrated as she attempts to communicate her needs. Her daughter says Mrs. Williams is a proud, independent, and tidy woman who has been living alone and caring for herself independently since her husband's death last year, even maintaining the yard and garden. She wears eyeglasses for reading and driving and has a hearing aid.

Your second patient is Mr. Gold, a 68-year-old Orthodox Jewish man admitted last week after a massive heart attack. Although his eyes are open, he does not respond to external stimuli. Because of Impaired Swallowing, Mr. Gold is unable to take food or fluid orally. A feeding tube was placed to ensure adequate nutrition and hydration. His oral mucous membranes and lips are dry and crusty. He is incontinent of urine and stool. Mr. Gold's son, Ira, tells you that throughout his life Mr. Gold adhered to Orthodox Jewish law and requests that, in honor of his father, certain aspects of these laws be included in the care plan.

Think about the following questions now, then again after you have read the chapter. What immediate concerns come to your mind about each of these patients? How will you ensure that their hygiene needs are met? Are there any safety issues? Which parts of their hygiene care can you delegate, if any?

Theoretical Knowledge
knowing **why**

This chapter provides the theoretical knowledge you need to answer the preceding questions, as well as others that will arise as you care for patients. It begins first with an explanation of the concepts of hygiene, activities of daily living, and self-care.

ABOUT THE KEY CONCEPTS

Hygiene is the broadest of the key concepts because everything in the chapter is related to hygiene. However, the concepts of activities of daily living and self-care ability must also be considered key concepts because every aspect of hygiene must include consideration of these two ideas. That is, you need to know the patient's ability to perform an activity of daily living in order to know how to give appropriate hygiene care (e.g., can he wash his entire body, or just his hands and face?)

HYGIENE AND SELF-CARE

Hygiene describes activities involved in maintaining personal cleanliness and grooming. **Activities of daily living (ADLs),** such as taking a bath or shower or brushing teeth, promote comfort, improve self-image, and decrease infection and disease. Healthy people perform their own personal hygiene; however, some patients need assistance because of illness or injury. As a nurse, you are responsible for providing the necessary assistance and, at the same time, encouraging as much self-care as possible to promote activity, independence, and self-esteem.

What Factors Influence Hygiene Practices?

Every patient is unique, so personal hygiene practices vary greatly. To reflect caring, respect and accommodate each person's preferences and differences whenever possible.

Personal Preferences. Some people prefer a shower, others a bath. One person may shower in the morning to wake up and feel clean for the day, whereas another bathes in the evening to relax before going to sleep. Choice of soaps and shampoos varies as well.

Culture and Religion or Spirituality. Cultural and family values and beliefs about hygiene form the foundation for our beliefs as adults. Generally, people in North America consider brushing the teeth, daily bathing, and use of deodorant necessary to eliminate body odors. However, people in some cultures may find a weekly bath sufficient. Religious or spiritual beliefs can also influence hygiene practices. For example, Orthodox Judaism prohibits receiving personal care from a member of the opposite sex.

Economic Status or Living Environment. Inadequate bathing facilities or lack of money for hygiene supplies (e.g., lack of access to running water or soap) can influence how often a person bathes. People living in poverty must focus on meeting basic needs for food and shelter before they can spend money and energy on hygiene.

Developmental Level. Parents and other caregivers perform hygiene care for infants and young children. Older children learn practices that become habits, such as brushing and flossing the teeth. As older children begin to perform their own hygiene independently, they are influenced by the media and societal norms. For example, some preteens may bathe only under parental duress, but teenagers, who are typically

very self-conscious, may begin to take several showers a day. Many teenagers have oily skin and can tolerate frequent bathing, but as we age, the oil-producing sebaceous glands become less active. Older adults may find it necessary to bathe only every 2 or 3 days, use less soap, and increase the use of skin moisturizers.

Knowledge and Cognitive Levels. Not everyone has the knowledge needed to make appropriate decisions. For example, some people may not know the importance of flossing their teeth. Or, some women may not be aware of the importance of cleansing the perineum from front to back after using the toilet. Patient teaching is an important part of your hygiene care because most people will, eventually, take care of their own personal hygiene.

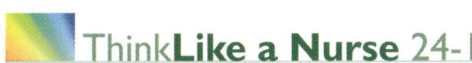

ThinkLike a Nurse 24-1

Think about Mrs. Williams and Mr. Gold (Meet Your Patients). After reviewing each of the factors presented, determine the following for each patient.

- Which factor(s) will have the most influence on the hygiene practices of this patient?
- Why do you think so?
- How will this factor affect the individual plan of care?

PracticalKnowledge
knowing **how**

This section of the chapter will assist you to assess for and promote self-care abilities and to plan care for patients with Self-Care Deficits. Plan hygiene care around the patient's needs, not facility routines or staff convenience.

ASSESSMENT (SELF-CARE)

Assess your patient's functional status regularly. This enables you to identify the need to modify the care plan and set achievable goals for self-care. Focus on the patient's *ability* to perform hygiene measures and the need for assistance, not necessarily on the *quality* of these measures. Use the following guidelines when assessing self-care abilities for hygiene care. If you would like to have a focused hygiene assessment guide that includes assessment of the skin, feet, nails, oral cavity, hair, and eyes,

 Go to Chapter 24, **Tables, Boxes, Figures: ESG Assessment Box, Assessment Guidelines: Hygiene,** on Davis*Plus*.

For thorough assessment of those body systems, you can also refer to physical assessment Procedures 21-2, 21-3, 21-4, 21-6, and 21-9.

Assess Independence in Activities of Daily Living

Consult with the patient to assess his willingness and ability to perform ADLs. The Katz Index of Independence in Activities of Daily Living (ADL) is used extensively to assess functional abilities in activities of daily living (bathing/hygiene, dressing/grooming, feeding, toileting) (Katz, Down, Cash, et al., 1970). To use the Katz ADL Index,

 Go to Chapter 24, **Tables, Boxes, Figures: ESG Table 24-1,** on Davis*Plus*, or go directly to http://consultgerirn.org/uploads/File/trythis/try_this_2.pdf

Assess Overall Self-Care Abilities

To describe a patient's self-care abilities, use a standardized functional status rating scale (see Box 24-1), if one is available. Begin your assessment of self-care ability by conducting an initial interview with the patient and/or family, which includes the following:

- **Obtain a health history.** Identify underlying illness, injury, or disease that might contribute to a self-care deficit or affect tolerance of hygiene procedures. *Cognitive impairment,* such as is found in patients with dementia, delirium, stroke, or traumatic brain injury, may make it impossible for the person to determine the need for hygiene, much less know how to accomplish related tasks. *Depression, psychoses,* or *delusions* may cause a profound lack of energy or motivation, causing patients to have poor hygiene and dress inappropriately for the situation.
- **Assess cognitive ability and physical functioning.** Determine overall grooming and cleanliness, level of consciousness, short- and long-term memory, ability to follow instructions, range of motion, mobility, level of knowledge, and energy level.
- **Assess for sensory disturbances.** Assess for auditory, visual, tactile, or olfactory disturbances that interfere with the ability to perform hygiene care safely and independently. For example, a person who has decreased tactile sensation (sense of touch) may be at risk for burns because he is not able to feel the temperature of the bath water.
- **Assess mobility.** Limited mobility (e.g., from IV lines, joint and muscle problems) makes it difficult to perform hygiene activities such as bathing.
- **Assess pain.** Pain and analgesic side effects can severely limit the ability and motivation to perform ADLs.
- **Assess for other factors.** Identify other factors (e.g., cultural, religious) that may influence hygiene practices and preferences.
- **Determine preferences and practices.** Identify the patient's previous hygiene measures, normal routines, preferences, need for assistive devices, or any other existing problem areas.

KnowledgeCheck 24-1

- What are the benefits of personal hygiene?
- Why should you respect and accommodate your patients' hygiene preferences?
- Identify two economic or living environmental factors that may influence how frequently a person bathes.
- Identify one example of a cognitive impairment that may make independent initiation of grooming impossible.
- Why may people experiencing depression neglect their grooming and hygiene?

BOX 24-1 ■ Functional Level Classification

Level

If the patient is not completely independent with self-care, identify one of the following functional levels.
1. Requires use of equipment or devices.
2. Requires help from another person(s) for assistance, supervision, teaching.
3. Requires help from another person(s) and equipment or device.
4. Dependent; does not participate in self-care bathing or hygiene.

Source: Gordon, M. (2006). *Manual of nursing diagnosis* (11th ed.). Sudbury, MA: Jones and Bartlett, p. 175.

ThinkLike a Nurse 24-2

Answer the following questions for Mrs. Williams (Meet Your Patients).

- What factor(s) may interfere with Mrs. Williams's self-care ability?
- How can you ensure maximum independence with hygiene for her?
- How might you encourage her to strive toward optimal functioning?

ANALYSIS/NURSING DIAGNOSIS (SELF-CARE)

When a person is unable to perform one or more ADLs, a self-care deficit exists. NANDA International (NANDA-I) self-care diagnoses related to hygiene are Bathing, Dressing, Toileting, and Feeding; and sometimes Self-Neglect (2009). Except for Feeding Self-Care Deficit, which is included in Chapter 28, you can find definitions and defining characteristics for each diagnosis if you

 Go to Chapter 24, **Standardized Language: NANDA-I Diagnoses to Describe** Self-Care Abilities, on DavisPlus.

Common etiologies for self-care diagnoses include such factors as fatigue, environmental barriers, and pain. For a more extensive list of etiologies, see the preceding Theoretical Knowledge section on Hygiene and Self Care. Also,

 Go to Chapter 24, **Standardized Language: Common Etiologies for Self-Care Diagnoses,** on DavisPlus.

When writing self-care diagnoses, classify the patient's functional level if you have access to a standardized scale, such as the one found in Box 24-1. Otherwise, use descriptive terms such as mild, moderate, severe, and total. The following are examples of diagnostic statements you might write:

Using a scale: Bathing Self-Care Deficit **(2)** related to severe knee pain secondary to degenerative joint disease

Using descriptive words: Toileting Self-Care Deficit **(severe)** related to inability to walk to the bathroom secondary to muscle weakness

ThinkLike a Nurse 24-3

- Which of the preceding NANDA-I self-care diagnoses apply to Mrs. Williams and Mr. Gold (Meet Your Patients)?
- Explain the reasoning for your choices.
- For each patient, what are the related factors for his or her Self-Care Deficit?
- Write a self-care diagnostic statement for Mrs. Williams and Mr. Gold.

PLANNING OUTCOMES/EVALUATION (SELF-CARE)

To access a bathing and hygiene plan of care and care map,

 Go to Chapter 24, **Care Plan: Bathing Self-Care Deficit,** and **Care Map,** on DavisPlus.

The NOC standardized outcome Self-Care: Activities of Daily Living (ADLs) is appropriate for all of the Self-Care Deficit diagnoses. For outcomes for more specific diagnoses,

 Go to Chapter 24, **Standardized Language: Selected Standardized Outcomes and Interventions for Self-Care Deficit Diagnoses,** on DavisPlus.

Individualized goals/outcome statements you might write for Self-Care Deficits include the following examples:

- Verbalizes satisfaction with body cleanliness and oral hygiene after A.M. care.
- Accepts assistance with ADLs or total care, if needed.
- By October 4, will complete bath independently, except for back and feet, after nurse provides equipment and assists patient to the bathroom.

You will use the outcomes developed in the planning outcomes phase of the nursing process as the criteria for evaluating patient responses to self-care interventions.

PLANNING INTERVENTIONS/IMPLEMENTATION (SELF-CARE)

Although cleanliness can contribute to well-being, comfort, and health, it can also be stressful—for example, to critically ill patients, the frail elderly, and those with dementia. Adverse events may include decreased oxygenation or ventilation, hypertension, hypotension, intracranial hypertension, or even cardiorespiratory arrest (Robles, Corcoles, Torres, et al., 2002). This does not mean you should avoid hygiene care for such patients, but you may need to modify it and evaluate patient responses constantly as you work. For example, you might provide care in small segments, allowing the patient to rest after brushing his teeth.

Even when a patient needs assistance with hygiene measures, the overall goal is to promote eventual self-care. Of course, critically ill patients need rest, so you will not push them to perform at their highest level of function. If the patient is able to perform self-care, you might sometimes need to allow him to rest while you perform part of the care, for example, washing his feet and legs.

For *NIC standardized interventions* for Self-Care Deficit diagnoses,

 Go to Chapter 24, **Standardized Language: Selected Standardized Outcomes and Interventions for Self-Care Deficit Diagnoses,** on DavisPlus.

Individualized interventions depend on the extent of the client's Self-Care Deficit, as well as the etiology of the problem. The following are some examples:

- Demonstrate the use of assistive devices (e.g., to help patient grasp and pull on socks).
- Use Velcro fasteners instead of buttons and zippers.
- Allow sufficient time for all ADLs to prevent fatigue and frustration.
- Offer pain medication before ADLs.

You will find a thorough discussion of specific hygiene-care activities (e.g., care of the skin, oral hygiene) in the remainder of this chapter.

Types of Scheduled Hygiene Care

The following types of scheduled hygiene care are provided in most inpatient facilities (e.g., hospitals and long-term care settings). Although they are scheduled routinely, you should individualize these activities and involve the patient as much as possible.

Hourly rounding, also referred to as *comfort rounds* or *safety rounds,* consists of seeing the patient every hour, on schedule. They are done to offer help with self-care needs such as pain relief, positioning, and toileting. Hourly rounding improves patient safety and greatly reduces call light use.

Early morning care is provided soon after the patient awakens. It includes preparing the patient for breakfast or

other activities, such as diagnostic tests. As needed, provide comfort measures and assist with toileting, washing the face and hands, and giving mouth care.

A.M. (morning) care is hygiene care that occurs after breakfast. Depending on the patient's self-care ability, assist with toileting, bathing, oral hygiene, skin care, hair care (including shaving if needed), dressing, and positioning or helping the patient transfer to a chair. Also change or straighten bed linens, according to agency policy, and tidy the room.

P.M. (afternoon) care consists of preparing patients to receive visitors or afternoon rest. You may assist nonambulatory patients with toileting, handwashing, and oral care; straighten bed linens; reposition the patient; and offer other comfort measures (e.g., pain medications).

H.S. (hour of sleep) care is given before the patient goes to sleep. Offer the same care as given in the afternoon, adding a back massage to help relax the patient. Also place within easy reach the call light, water glass, urinal, or anything else the patient may need during the night. Turn off lights and TV, and close the door before leaving the room (according to patient needs and preferences). For a back-massage procedure, see Procedure 35-1.

Delegating Hygiene Care

In many institutions, NAPs perform most of the hygiene care. However, you will need to carefully assess patients to ensure that it is safe to delegate their care. If the patient is unstable or the NAP is inexperienced or unfamiliar with the patient's limitations, you must assist or perform the care yourself. Read "What Should I Know About Delegation and Supervision?" in Chapter 7 for a review of making delegation decisions.

Before assigning a NAP to assist with a bath, shower, or toileting, give instructions about the following:

- Patient's limitations and restrictions, and the amount of assistance necessary
- Use of any assistive devices (e.g., cane, walker, or gait belt)
- Specific safety precautions to follow (e.g., use of gait belt or shower chair)
- Any obstacles present, such as drainage tubes, catheters, IV tubing, or bandages, and how to maintain them during bathing or toileting
- Observations to make during the procedure (e.g., skin condition; presence of any lesions; areas of special concern over bony prominences and under abdominal folds and breasts; presence, appearance, and amount of urine or stool, or the need to collect a specimen). Explain why the observations are important.

Remember, as the professional nurse, you are responsible for making assessments and determining the meaning of the data reported to you by the NAP. Assisting with or supervising care (especially a bath) is an excellent opportunity for you to assess the patient's level of consciousness, short- and long-term memory, ability to follow instructions, range of motion, skin condition, activity tolerance, and overall self-care ability.

 Think Like a Nurse 24-4

Think of Mrs. Williams (Meet Your Patients). You have delegated her bathing and oral hygiene to a NAP.

- What information do you need to share with the NAP about this patient's needs, limitations, or preferences?
- What, if any, specific observations will you ask the NAP to make for Mrs. Williams?
- What, if any, specific observations will *you* need to make for Mrs. Williams?

- What action will you take if you determine that the patient's needs and preferences were not met by the NAP?

CARE OF THE SKIN

The preceding sections introduced you to the broad topic of hygiene and activities of daily living. The rest of the chapter will deal with specific topics, such as care of the skin.

Theoretical Knowledge
knowing **why**

To assist patients with skin care, you must have theoretical knowledge about personal hygiene measures and the structure and function of the **integument** (skin).

Anatomy and Physiology of the Skin

The **integumentary system** consists of the skin, the subcutaneous layer directly under the skin, the hair, nails, and the sweat and sebaceous glands. The skin has two distinct layers, the epidermis and the dermis (see Fig. 36-1, in Chapter 36). The **epidermis** (the thicker, outer layer) consists of stratified squamous epithelial tissue composed of keratinized (dead) cells, which are fused to make the skin waterproof. The **epidermis** continually sheds (desquamates) and is completely replaced every 3 to 4 weeks. The epidermis contains melanin, a pigment that provides protection against the ultraviolet rays of the sun and that, together with circulating blood, gives skin its color. The **dermis** (the thinner, second layer) contains blood and lymphatic vessels, nerves, bases of hair follicles, and sebaceous and sweat glands.

Functions of the Skin

The skin has the following five main functions.

1. *Protection.* Intact skin is the body's first line of defense against bacteria and other microorganisms that can enter the body and cause infection. It also provides a barrier to protect underlying tissues from thermal, chemical, and mechanical injury. **Sebaceous glands** secrete an oily substance called *sebum,* which helps to waterproof and lubricate the skin and decrease bacterial growth.
2. *Sensation.* The skin contains sensory organs or receptors for heat, cold, pressure, touch, and pain.
3. *Regulation.* The skin helps maintain fluid and electrolyte balance by preventing the escape of excess water and electrolytes from the body. It helps to regulate body temperature through the processes of dilating and constricting blood vessels and activating or inactivating sweat glands located in the skin. **Sweat glands,** concentrated in the axillae and external genitalia, excrete water in the form of perspiration; evaporation produces a cooling effect on the skin.
4. *Secretion/excretion.* The sweat glands secrete fatty acids and proteins and excrete nitrogenous wastes (*urea*), sodium chloride, and water in perspiration.
5. *Vitamin D formation.* The skin contains a form of cholesterol that is changed to vitamin D on exposure to ultraviolet light from the sun.

See Chapter 36 for more information about the structure and functions of the skin.

Factors Affecting the Skin

In addition to a person's hygiene practices, health status and developmental stage also affect skin condition.

Health Status

Anything that interferes with the hydration, circulation, and nutrition of the skin creates a risk to skin integrity. As you read each of the following factors, think whether it would be present for Mr. Gold (Meet Your Patients).

- **Dampness.** Excessive perspiration (e.g., in fever and certain illnesses) and incontinence of urine or bowel cause the skin to become damp. The skin then breaks down more easily, especially in the skinfolds. This is called **maceration.**
- **Dehydration.** Fluid loss (e.g., from vomiting, diarrhea, or fever) and insufficient fluid intake can cause dehydration. This causes the skin to become dry and to crack easily.
- **Nutritional Status.** People who are very thin or very obese are more likely to experience skin irritation and injury. *Morbid obesity* makes it physically difficult to reach and clean all areas of the body, and can lead to development of odor and fungal conditions.
- **Insufficient Circulation.** Immobility, vascular disease, and overall inadequate nutritional status compromise circulation. This predisposes the patient to local tissue death and ulceration when skin cells do not receive enough oxygen.
- **Skin Diseases.** Skin diseases such as impetigo (a bacterial infection of the skin) and systemic diseases, such as measles and chickenpox, cause lesions that create discomfort and require special hygiene care.
- **Jaundice.** Certain diseases cause a yellow skin discoloration caused by accumulation of bile pigments in the skin. Jaundice causes the skin to be itchy and dry.
- **Lifestyle and Personal Choices.** Some people damage their skin by exposure to ultraviolet rays because they want to be tan. Some use sunscreen; some do not. As another example, many people have skin tattoos or piercings, creating the risk for systemic and local infection and scarring.

Developmental Stage

Infants have fragile, easily injured skin. As a child matures, the skin becomes more resistant to injury and infection, but children need adults to provide or supervise the cleanliness of their skin. In adolescence, the sebaceous glands enlarge, and secretions increase. The skin becomes oily and susceptible to acne.

With aging, the skin changes in numerous visible ways, increasing the older adult's risk for skin problems, such as pressure ulcers and reduced ability to heal. Refer to Table 24-1 for a description of normal skin changes in older adults.

KnowledgeCheck 24-2

- What are five functions of the skin?
- How does the skin help regulate body temperature?
- What changes take place in the skin as a person ages?

PracticalKnowledge
knowing **how**

ASSESSMENT (SKIN)

Assisting with a bath provides an excellent opportunity to assess the patient's skin. Although you can instruct a NAP to report her observations of the patient's skin, you are ultimately responsible for making the assessments. Patients may be sensitive about skin problems or poor hygiene practices,

---

Table 24-1 ➤ **Normal Skin Changes in Older Adults**

STRUCTURE	CHANGE IN STRUCTURE AND ACTIVITY	CLINICAL EFFECTS
Epidermis	Thinner; decreased rate of cell turnover	Skin appears pale and somewhat translucent; slower healing.
Subcutaneous tissues	Thinner and more fragile, less fat	Decreased protection of bony prominences and thermoregulation
Collagen and elastin fibers in the dermis	Weaken and become less elastic	Skin becomes wrinkled.
Sebaceous and sweat glands	Activity decreases.	Skin becomes dry, scaly, and itchy. Temperature regulation in hot weather becomes more difficult.
Hormones (estrogen and progesterone)	Production decreases.	Contributes to drying and thinning of the skin.
Skin	Vascularity decreases.	Skin becomes cool and pale.
Hair follicles	Diminish in number and activity.	Hair becomes thin, grows more slowly.
Melanocytes (pigment cells)	Numbers decrease.	Hair turns gray or white; skin may become unevenly pigmented.
Nails	Thicken; become softer; growth rate diminishes.	Nails tear easily.
Skin growths	Become more common (e.g., warts, "liver spots," "age spots")	Most are caused by years of sun exposure; most are harmless (except for skin cancers, which are fairly common but not normal changes).

so as you direct your questions to the patient, do so in a nonjudgmental, respectful manner. Protect the patient's privacy by closing the curtain and exposing only the area being bathed or examined. Be mindful of the room temperature, and try to reduce drafts to avoid chilling the patient.

In your assessment, observe for the following changes in skin color:

- **Pallor** in a light-skinned person may appear as pale skin without underlying pink tones. In a dark-skinned person, observe for an ashen gray or yellow color.
- **Erythema** is redness of the skin. It is related to vasodilation and inflammation. It is difficult to see in dark-skinned people, so you may discover it by palpating the skin for areas of increased warmth.
- **Jaundice,** a yellow discoloration of the skin, occurs in patients with impaired liver function. It is best seen in the sclerae of the eyes.
- **Cyanosis,** a bluish coloring of the skin, is caused by decreased peripheral circulation or decreased oxygenation of the blood. It may be related to cardiac, pulmonary, or peripheral vascular problems (e.g., arteriosclerosis). In dark-skinned patients, you can best see cyanosis by examining the conjunctivae, tongue, buccal mucosa, and palms and soles for a dull dark color.

For a thorough discussion of skin assessment, including how to describe and document your observations, see Chapter 21. However, as you provide skin hygiene you should routinely make the observations found in the accompanying Focused Assessment box.

KnowledgeCheck 24-3

- True or False: The professional nurse is responsible for making assessments.
- True or False: Assisting with the bath is an excellent time to assess the patient.

Hygiene-Focused Skin Assessment

Focused Assessment

Subjective Data

Ask the patient about the following:

➤ Usual bathing and skin care practices and preferences
➤ Past and current skin problems, including their effects on the patient's life
➤ Prescription and over-the-counter (OTC) or herbal remedies used to treat any skin problems
➤ Allergic skin reactions to food, medications, plants, skin care products, or other substances
➤ History of diseases or other factors that are known to cause skin problems, for example, decreased mobility, decreased circulation, incontinence, inadequate nutrition, or deficient knowledge

Objective Data

➤ Inspect each area of the skin in an orderly, head-to-toe manner, noting overall cleanliness, condition, color, texture, turgor, hydration, and temperature.
➤ Look for rashes, lumps, lesions, and cracking.
➤ Observe for drainage from wounds or around tubes.
➤ Observe for four significant color changes: pallor, erythema, jaundice, and cyanosis.

- To inspect for pallor in a dark-skinned person, which areas would you assess for an ashen gray or yellow color?
- What is the term that means "a bluish color of the skin"?
- Name two causes of erythema.
- Where can you best see jaundice?

ANALYSIS/NURSING DIAGNOSIS (SKIN)

You should be familiar with the following common skin problems and observe for them as you give skin care:

- **Pruritus** (itching) may lead to scratching and breaks in the skin.
- **Dry skin** tends to crack, burn, or itch.
- **Maceration** is softening of the skin from prolonged moisture (e.g., urinary incontinence). It makes the epidermis more susceptible to injury.
- **Excoriation** is a loss of the superficial layers of the skin caused, for example, by scratching and by the digestive enzymes in feces.
- **Abrasion,** a rubbing away of the epidermal layer of the skin, especially over bony areas or prominences, is often caused by friction or shearing forces that occur when a patient moves or is moved in bed.
- **Pressure ulcers** (decubitus ulcers) are lesions caused by tissue compression and inadequate perfusion. See Chapter 36.
- **Acne** is an inflammation of the sebaceous glands that is common among adolescents and young adults.
- **Burns** are a type of traumatic injury caused by thermal, electrical, chemical, or radioactive agents.

To see illustrations of most of those skin problems, see Procedure 21-2 and

 Go to Chapter 21, **Tables, Boxes, Figures: ESG Table 21-3, Abnormal Atlas,** on DavisPlus.

Impaired Skin Integrity as the Problem. When you wish to focus on prevention or treatment of the *skin condition,* use the following diagnostic labels NANDA-I (2012):

- **Risk for Impaired Skin Integrity.** *Definition:* At risk for skin being adversely altered.
  Risk factors: NANDA-I lists about 20 specific risk factors (e.g., radiation, obesity). It may be easier for you to remember the general conditions that affect the skin: dampness, dehydration, inadequate circulation, nutritional status (thin or obese), skin diseases, systemic diseases, and jaundice.
  Example: Risk for Impaired Skin Integrity related to immobility secondary to casts and traction
- **Impaired Skin Integrity.** *Definition:* Altered epidermis or dermis.
  Defining characteristics: Invasion of body structures, destruction of skin layers (dermis), disruption of skin surface (epidermis).
  Example: Impaired Skin Integrity related to skin fragility secondary to severe peripheral edema

Impaired Skin Integrity as the Etiology. Impaired Skin Integrity may be the etiology of other nursing diagnoses. Certain skin problems place the patient at risk for infection by causing cracks or breaks in the skin. Others may contribute to discomfort and low self-esteem. The following are examples:

Risk for Infection related to skin lacerations and abrasions
Situational Low Self-Esteem related to appearance and self-consciousness about skin lesions secondary to severe eczema

ThinkLike a Nurse 24-5

- Why are Mrs. Williams and Mr. Gold (Meet Your Patients) at risk for Impaired Skin Integrity?
- What are the specific kinds of skin integrity problems that pose an increased risk to both patients?

PLANNING OUTCOMES/EVALUATION (SKIN)

For *NOC standardized outcomes* for problems of the skin, feet, nails, mouth, teeth, hair, eyes, ears, and nose,

   Go to Chapter 24, **Standardized Language: Selected NOC Outcomes and NIC Interventions for Hygiene Problems,** on Davis*Plus.*

Two examples of NOC outcomes are Tissue Integrity: Skin and Mucous Membranes, and Self-Care: Oral Hygiene.

Individualized goals/outcome statements you might write for a patient with skin problems include the following:
- Skin will remain intact and free of secretions.
- Skin will remain free of lesions.
- The patient will follow a regimen to improve skin dryness.

PLANNING INTERVENTIONS/IMPLEMENTATION (SKIN)

For *NIC standardized interventions* for skin integrity and skin care,

   Go to Chapter 24, **Standardized Language: NOC Outcomes and NIC Interventions for Hygiene Problems,** on Davis*Plus.*

Individualized nursing activities for patients with Impaired Skin Integrity include bathing and massage. You will usually delegate patient bathing to NAPs (see Fig. 24-1). Therefore, your most important interventions may be to be certain that the patient actually gets a satisfactory bath.

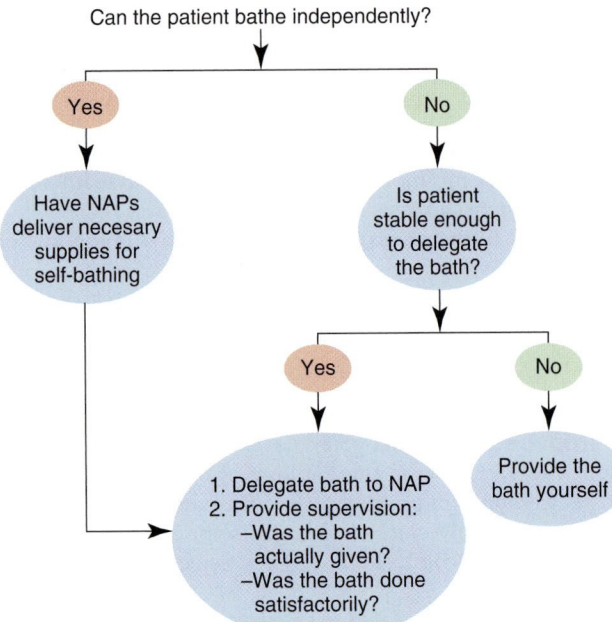

FIGURE 24-1 The RN should assess the patient, delegate bathing as appropriate, and provide supervision.

Bathing. Bathing serves three purposes: health, social interaction, and pleasure or relaxation. Bathing removes perspiration and bacteria from the skin surface, helping to prevent body odor. The warmth from the bath solution and the friction of bathing dilate the blood vessels near the surface of the skin, increasing the circulation. Bathing stimulates depth of respirations and provides sensory input. It can also be a time to strengthen the nurse–patient relationship, promote relaxation and comfort, enhance well-being, and improve self-image.

Back Massage. Regardless of the type of bath used, when possible end the bath with a back massage to provide relaxation and stimulate circulation. As with all procedures, be sure there are no contraindications to massage (e.g., fractured ribs, burns, recent heart surgery). To learn a procedure for giving a back massage, see Procedure 35-1.

Caveat for all Baths

New guidelines express concern about bacterial contamination from reusable basins and biofilm in water pipes and faucets. They vary, but most recommendations are to use disposable basins, use sterile or distilled water instead of tap water, use pH-balanced cleansers, and to bathe daily with chlorhexidine gluconate (CHG) solution. **Guidelines are changing; be alert for practice changes.**

Choosing the Type of Bath to Meet Patient Needs

The type of bath you give depends on your nursing judgment; the patient's preference, self-care ability, and endurance; and the medical plan of care. **Assist bath** is a term commonly used to indicate that the nurse helps the patient with areas that may be difficult to reach, such as the back, feet, and legs. If a complete bath would be stressful to the patient, you may sometimes give a **partial bath;** that is, you will cleanse only the areas that may cause odor or discomfort, such as the axillae and perineum. The following sections discuss other types of baths in detail.

Traditional Baths and Modified Bed Baths

A **bed bath** is for patients who must remain in bed but who are able to bathe themselves. You will assist by placing the bath supplies on the bedside stand or overbed table. Provide privacy, and place the call device within reach. If the patient cannot bathe all areas of his body, complete the bath for him. A **complete bed bath** means you will wash the patient's entire body without assistance from the patient. For complete instructions, see Procedure 24-1. The following are three types of bed bath:

- A **towel bath** is one in which you place a large towel and a bath blanket in a plastic bag, saturate them with a warmed, commercially prepared mixture, and use them to bathe the patient. Because the solution dries rapidly, there is no need to towel-dry the patient. Patients find towel baths satisfactory, and some agencies prefer towel baths because they take less time than a traditional bed bath. This is a preferred method for patients who have mild to moderate Impaired Skin Integrity or Activity Intolerance and for patients with dementia (e.g., Alzheimer's disease). See Procedure 24-2.
- A **bag bath** is one in which you use 8 to 10 washcloths instead of a towel and bath blanket. They are warmed, and each part of the patient's body is cleansed with a fresh cloth.
- A **packaged bath** refers to a set of commercially prepared and packaged, premoistened, disposable washcloths that are warmed and used in the same way as a bag bath. Be certain

the patient knows what they are for and how to use them. See Procedure 24-3. Recent studies and guidelines suggest that prepackaged baths instead of the traditional bath basin and water should be used to help prevent healthcare-acquired infections (American Association of Critical Care Nurses, 2013; Johnson, Lineweaver, & Maze, 2009; Larson, Ciliberti, Chandler, et al., 2004; Vernon, Hayden, Trick, et al., 2006).

 Think**Like a Nurse** 24-6

Suppose you have been providing towel baths to a patient who has mild dementia. One day a visiting family member says, "My father tells me that he has not had a bath all week. What's going on here?" What would you do? How could you help to prevent this misunderstanding in the future?

Showers and Tub Baths

Most ambulatory patients prefer a shower. It is a time-saver and refreshing as well as cleansing. Some clients can manage a shower mostly on their own. For complete information, refer to Clinical Insight 24-1.

If a client is ambulatory but requires much assistance with bathing (e.g., because of pain and stiffness in the hands and arms) you may prefer a tub bath. It will be easier for you to wash and rinse the patient, and you will not get as wet as with a shower. Immersion also helps to soak areas that are crusty, scaly, or soiled and relaxes stiff, sore muscles and joints.

Clinical Insight 24-1 ➤ **Assisting With a Shower or Tub Bath**

- Assess the patient's self-care abilities: sensorimotor, musculoskeletal, and cognitive function; activity tolerance; level of knowledge.
- Ensure that the patient has the necessary supplies (e.g., soap, washcloth, towel, clean gown).
- Hang a sign on the door to ensure privacy.
- Help wash and dry any areas that the patient cannot reach (e.g., feet, back).

✚ Assist the patient to the shower or bathroom as needed.

- Ensure that there is a nonskid surface or mat in the shower or tub.
- For patients who have impaired mobility or activity intolerance, use a shower chair in the shower or tub.
- Be sure that the shower or tub is clean and safe. Most hospitals and long-term care facilities have grab bars and handrails in the bathrooms.
- To avoid burns, verify water temperature for clients with impaired cognition or decreased sensory perception. Water should be 110°F to 115°F (43°C to 46°C).
- Provide a call device for the patient to obtain help if needed; point out the emergency call device in the bathroom (usually it is a red button or cord on the wall).

Home Care

✚ Encourage clients and families to install hand bars on the sides of the bathtub and on the wall next to the tub. Most hospitals and long-term care facilities have grab bars and handrails in the bathrooms, but these may need to be installed in the home.

- Advise parents never to leave a child alone in the tub or shower and to have a way to unlock the bathroom door from outside the room.
- Advise older adults or those who are ill not to lock the bathroom door while bathing so that help can be summoned if needed (e.g., if they become faint or fall).
- Help families to obtain benches for transferring into the bathtub, or use a plastic chair in the shower.

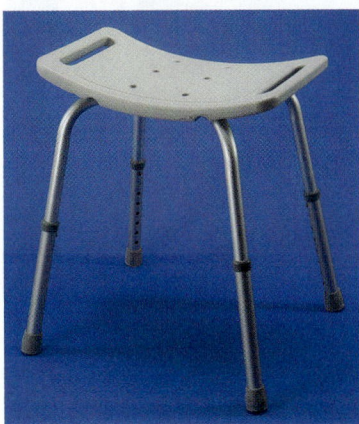

Shower chair

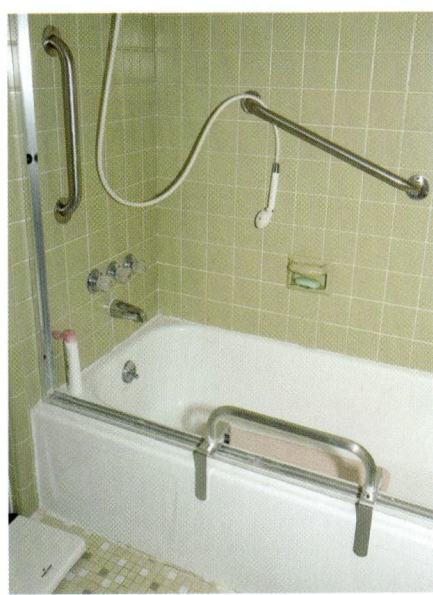

Bathtub with handrail and grab bars

Some patients need assistance getting into and out of a tub. Some kneel or squat first and then sit in the tub. For completely dependent patients, specially designed tubs reduce the need to lift patients into and out of the tub. You can also use a hydraulic lift and a regular tub (Fig. 24-2).

Therapeutic Bath

The primary care provider may prescribe **therapeutic baths** for some patients. It is your responsibility to add the medically ordered substance, ensure prescribed temperature, assist the patient into the tub, and clean the tub at the end of the bath. Oatmeal or coal tar baths are examples of therapeutic baths that are used to treat specific skin conditions, such as chickenpox lesions or psoriasis. A warm sitz bath, using a disposable small tub, is another example; it helps to cleanse and soothe inflamed perineal, vaginal, or rectal, tissues.

Perineal Care

The **perineum** (the area between the anus and vulva in a female, or the anus and scrotum in a male) is a dark, warm, moist area that supports bacterial growth. Perineal care promotes comfort and prevents odor, skin excoriation, and infection. You will usually give perineal care (including the external genitalia) along with a complete bed bath. Give perineal care more frequently if the patient is incontinent of urine or feces or has drainage from the area.

Because of personal, cultural, or religious beliefs, some patients may wish to have a same-sex caregiver provide the bath. Whether you and the patient are of the same or opposite sex, perineal care may at first be embarrassing for you both. Perform care in a professional manner, and provide privacy (e.g., shut the door, pull bed curtains, drape properly). A matter-of-fact, sensitive approach puts most patients at ease. For complete information about providing perineal care, refer to Procedure 24-4.

KnowledgeCheck 24-4

- What causes body odor?
- What is the best intervention to rid the skin of body odor?
- What is the rationale for providing perineal care?
- How can you protect patient privacy during perineal care?

ThinkLike a Nurse 24-7

- Which of your patients (Meet Your Patients) will require nurse-assisted perineal care? Explain your reasoning.
- Which patient, if you are a woman, is most likely to be embarrassed by perineal care? Explain your reasoning.
- If you need more theoretical knowledge to answer these questions, what is it? Where could you find the information?

Bathing Patients With Dementia

Bathing should be a pleasant experience, not a stressful one. But patients with dementia tend to become agitated when told it is time to bathe, and often yell, scream, pinch, or hit their caregivers (Rasin & Barrick, 2004). The reason for agitation is usually that they experience pain, cold, fear, and loss of control. When you meet the patient's comfort needs (e.g., by adjusting the water temperature or taking special care when washing arthritic joints), the patient becomes less agitated and aggressive behavior declines significantly.

Nurses and NAPs sometimes focus, mistakenly, on the need to give a daily tub bath or shower. You can significantly reduce aggressive behaviors by giving a towel bath or bag bath instead (Rasin & Barrick, 2004). Despite the common myths about bathing, keep in mind that:

- It does not take a large amount of water (e.g., a shower) to get a person clean.
- The bath does not have to be performed at the same time every day, nor in the way "we have always done it here."

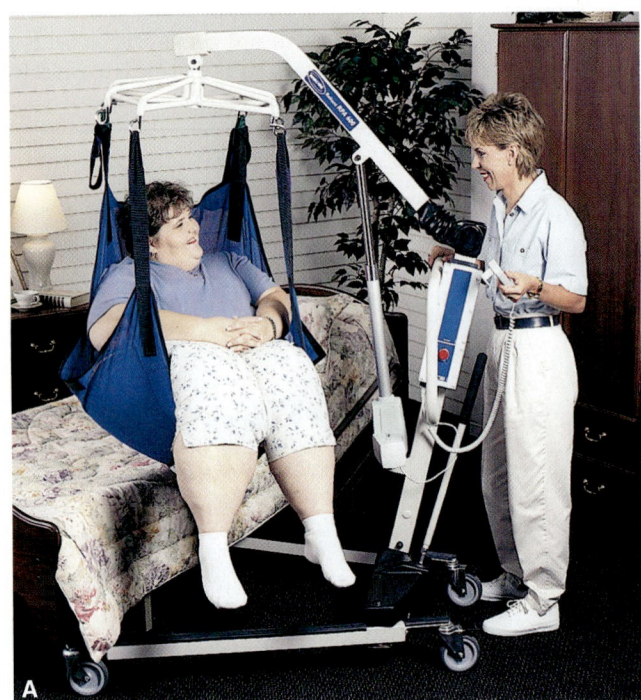

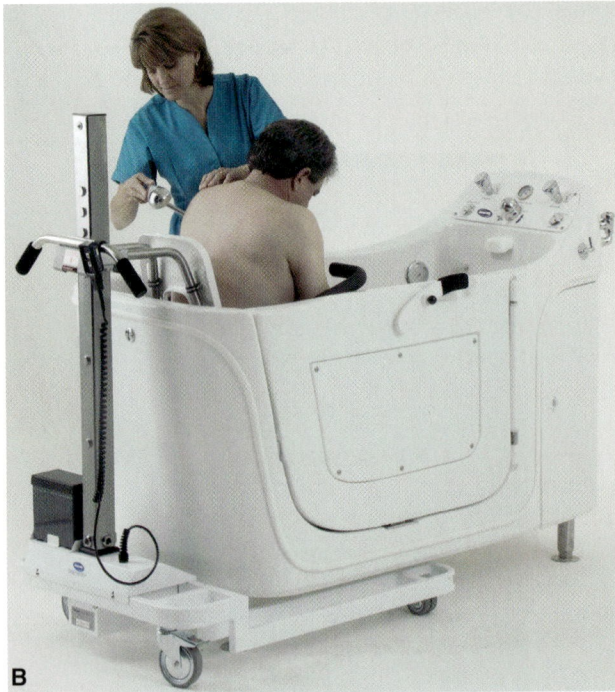

FIGURE 24-2 A. A hydraulic lift allows you to transport a patient to a bath or shower. B. A tub with a side-opening door enables patients to safely and easily enter the tub.
(Courtesy of Carroll Health Care, London, Ontario, Canada.)

You can educate families that showers and tub baths are not the only ways to get clean.

- The patient will not be at more risk for skin problems or infections if a towel bath is used.
- It is not necessary to bathe a person who is resisting. You can adapt the approach, method, and time.
- Patients who are forced to bathe do not "just forget about it"; many stay upset and agitated for hours.

For more discussion of bathing myths and for instructions about providing a towel bath for a person with dementia, see Clinical Insight 24-2.

Bathing Morbidly Obese Patients

Obesity is traditionally defined as 20% to 40% above ones ideal weight. A person is considered severely, or **morbidly,** obese when he is 100% over ideal weight. For the morbidly obese person, thorough skin assessment is essential, but difficult. Be sure to obtain adequate assistance to reposition the patient during the skin exam, so that you do not miss any areas. Pay special attention to skinfolds. Refer to Table 24-2 for etiologies of skin problems in morbidly obese clients, and for interventions to use when providing skin care for them. Teach these interventions to NAPs and to patients who bathe independently.

Bathing Older Adults

For older adults, especially the bed-bound and frail elderly, you must provide proper skin care and bathing techniques to prevent skin breakdown. At the same time, you should promote comfort and encourage independence in ADLs. Goals are to prevent drying of and injury to the skin. Bag baths adequately address the problems of skin itching and irritation, improve skin integrity, and are far less distressing to frail older adults (Lentz, 2003). Other interventions include avoiding use of soap, cleaning the skin immediately after soiling, and applying skin moisturizer. For further guidelines, see Procedure 24-1.

KnowledgeCheck 24-5

- A nurse has given a bath in which he washed a bedridden patient's entire body without assistance from the patient. What is the term for this bath?

- What are the advantages of a towel or bag bath?
- For which type of bath will you most likely have a medical prescription?

ThinkLike a Nurse 24-8

- Which type of bath would be most appropriate for each of your patients (Meet Your Patients)? Provide rationales for your choices.

CARE OF THE FEET

Foot care is a necessary part of hygiene and essential at any age for tissue health, proper posture, and ambulation.

TheoreticalKnowledge
knowing **why**

When providing foot care, you will need theoretical knowledge about the structure of the feet, life span variations, and common foot problems. The feet provide support for the weight of the entire body and absorb a significant amount of shock during walking. Their musculoskeletal structure is complex, consisting of 26 bones and many muscles, tendons, and ligaments. The feet can be affected by congenital malformations, injuries, improper footwear, and medical conditions.

Developmental Variations. Foot problems tend to increase with aging. Because of diseases such as arteriosclerosis and peripheral vascular insufficiency, older adults often have decreased circulation to the lower extremities. This increases their risk for foot ulcers and infection. The incidence of diabetes is high among older adults, further increasing the risk for infection secondary to delayed healing. In addition, the skin becomes dry predisposing the skin to cracking.

Common Foot Problems. More than 43 million people in the United States have foot abnormalities (e.g., pain, deformity, and disability). Many of these problems are the result of improperly fitting shoes.

- A **corn** is a cone-shaped thickening of the epidermis caused by continuous pressure (e.g., from improperly fitting shoes)

Clinical Insight 24-2 ▶ Bathing a Patient With Dementia

- Focus on the patient, not the task; provide choices.
- Distract with food or by playing relaxing music.
- Use a gentler type of shower head for rinsing. A strong spray may frighten the patient.
- Avoid sensory overload: Turn down lights, warm the room, play soft music, speak calmly. People with dementia have trouble processing information. Overloading the senses may trigger aggression.
- Ensure continuity of care. The patient can build a relationship with the caregiver and reduce fear.
- Encourage the patient to wash her own face if able. Makes her feel like an active participant, preserves some independence.
- Bathe at a regular time—preferably the same time as when the patient bathed at home.

- Explain the procedure simply, using short sentences.
- Provide privacy. Patients with dementia do not necessarily lose their modesty and sense of privacy.
- Let the patient know before you touch her or spray her with water. Sudden actions are often frightening to patients with dementia.
- Do not rush. The patient will feel the tension and may become agitated.
- Be creative; try bathing one part of the body each day.
- Teach techniques to caregivers at home (e.g., being flexible with time, using a towel bath, etc.)
- Also refer to the What if . . .? section of Procedure 24-1.

Table 24-2 ➤ Skin Care for Morbidly Obese Clients

PROBLEM AND ETIOLOGY	INTERVENTIONS
Hygiene	
Morbidly obese clients find it physically difficult to reach all areas of the body. In addition, they may have limited mobility. Inability to maintain good hygiene may lead to odor and fungal infections.	Ask how the patient handles skin care at home. Use the same adaptations, if possible. Provide a trapeze to assist the patient to lift and reach difficult areas. Provide a handheld shower and long-handled brushes. Experts vary on the use of soap. Certainly the skin should be rinsed and dried well.
Moisture	
Skin in skinfolds stays damp because perspiration cannot evaporate. Moisture contributes to the development of fungal and other skin infections.	Use moisture barrier creams, particularly in skinfolds and the perineal area. Use fans, if permitted. Change linens often. Manage incontinence. If fungal infections occur, you may need a medical prescription for antifungal powders, sprays, cream, or ointment.
Pressure	
Pressure can be caused by limited mobility, by skinfolds where skin rubs on skin, by tight clothing, catheters, and so on.	Reposition the patient frequently to redistribute the pressure of the skinfolds. Reposition catheters and tubes often; use tube holders to prevent rubbing. Separate the skinfolds with towels.
Shear and Friction	
The patient is at risk for friction and shearing injury from pulling skin across the linens when moving in the bed and chair.	The ANA's position is that you should use specialized lifts and other equipment to move patients safely and avoid injury to yourself (de Castro, 2004). If, in an emergency, you must move the patient, obtain sufficient help to avoid pulling the skin across the sheet or other surfaces. Do not use sheepskins. Use a waterproof and breathable mattress cover. Keep linens wrinkle free. Provide a trapeze.
Nutrition	
Morbidly obese patients may have poor nutritional status because of lifestyle factors (e.g., fast-food intake and other poor dietary habits) and lack of exercise or mobility.	Recommend evaluation by a nutritionist. Monitor blood sugar. Encourage adequate protein intake.

Source: Adapted from Rose, M., & Drake, D. (2008). Best practices for skin care of the morbidly obese. *Bariatric Nursing and Surgical Patient Care, 3*(2), 129–134.

over bony prominences, such as the toe joints. Corns are often painful.

- **Calluses** are usually found over bony prominences in the weight-bearing part of the foot: the heels, soles, or plantar surfaces of the feet. They are similar to corns but cover a wider area and are not painful.
- **Tinea pedis,** or athlete's foot, is a fungal infection of the skin. It is aggravated by moisture accumulation in unventilated shoes. Symptoms include itching and burning skin with blisters,

scaling, and cracking, especially between the toes. Athlete's foot may be contracted by walking barefoot in public showers.

- An **ingrown toenail** may result from improperly trimming the toenails and wearing poorly fitting shoes. The toenail grows inward into the soft tissues around it and the tissue at the nail border becomes swollen, inflamed, and painful. The nail may need to be surgically removed.
- **Foot odor** is produced when microorganisms growing on the feet interact with perspiration. The warm, moist environment

created by shoes encourages both perspiration and bacterial growth.

- **Plantar warts** are painful growths caused by a virus. They may occur on any part of the sole of the foot but often develop under pressure points, such as the heel or ball of the foot.
- **Pressure ulcers** are lesions caused by unrelieved pressure that impairs the circulation; this usually occurs over a bony prominence. In patients confined to bed, the back of the heels, the ankles, and the great toes are common locations; pressure ulcers do, of course, occur over other bony prominences.
- A **bunion** (hallux valgus) is a progressive disorder that begins the enlargement of the first metatarsal joint at the base of the great toe and then progresses to leaning of the big toe, gradually changing the angle of the bones. A characteristic bump occurs slowly and continues to become increasingly prominent with aging. Tight-fitting shoes (particularly with high heels) are thought to be the cause of bunions in the large majority of patients. Genetics also play a role, as do some diseases, such as arthritis. For optional illustrations and more information about bunions,

 Go to the URL of the American College of Foot and Ankle Surgeons, at the link provided in Chapter 24, **Resources for Caregivers and Health Professionals,** on Davis*Plus.*

Practical Knowledge
knowing **how**

The nursing focus for foot care is on prevention and early identification of problems. For associated *NOC standardized outcomes* and *NIC interventions* for patients with common foot problems,

 Go to Chapter 24, **Standardized Language: Selected NOC Outcomes and NIC Interventions for Hygiene Problems,** on Davis*Plus.*

ASSESSMENT (FEET)

Careful assessment of the feet allows for early detection of common foot problems. This chapter describes routine observations that you can make when giving foot care. For a thorough discussion of foot assessment, see Chapter 21 and the Pre-Procedure Assessments in Procedure 24-5. For specific questions to ask,

 Go to Chapter 24, **Tables, Boxes, Figures: ESG Assessment Box, Assessment Guidelines: Hygiene,** on Davis*Plus.*

The color and temperature of the feet provide data about circulation and oxygenation. For example, cold, dusky, or pale feet may indicate impaired circulation or tissue perfusion secondary to peripheral vascular disease.

ANALYSIS/NURSING DIAGNOSIS (FEET)

The following are examples of nursing diagnoses associated with the feet:
- Impaired Skin (or Tissue) Integrity (feet) r/t mechanical pressure from wearing shoes that do not fit properly

- Risk for Impaired Skin Integrity (feet) r/t (1) decreased sensation secondary to diabetes mellitus and (2) decreased circulation to the feet secondary to arteriosclerosis
- Impaired Walking r/t foot pain secondary to arthritis
- Risk for Injury (to feet) r/t deficient knowledge of foot hygiene

PLANNING OUTCOMES/EVALUATION (FEET)

NOC outcomes for foot care are the same as for other areas of the body, as they relate to circulation, infection, tissue integrity, wound healing. For example, Tissue Integrity: Skin and Mucous Membranes is useful for any area of the body.

Individualized goals/outcome statements you might write for a patient with foot problems include the following:
- Demonstrates proper cleansing, rinsing, and drying of the feet.
- Avoids trimming calluses.
- Wears shoes that fit properly.
- Inspects feet regularly.

PLANNING INTERVENTIONS/IMPLEMENTATION (FEET)

Examples of *NIC standardized interventions* include Foot Care, Skin Surveillance, and Circulatory Care: Arterial Insufficiency.

Individualized nursing activities related to care of the feet are those that prevent infection, odor, and trauma to the soft tissues of the feet. While performing foot care, teach the patient about self-care measures for care of the feet (see the Self-Care box Teaching Your Client About Foot Care). To learn how to administer foot care, see Procedure 24-5.

Diabetic Foot Care. Because of impaired circulation, delayed healing, and increased risk for infection, people who have diabetes are at high risk for problems with their feet. If they have neuropathy, they may not experience pain with a foot injury, so treatment may be delayed. If untreated, a seemingly minor foot lesion can progress to gangrene and require amputation. The instructions in the Self-Care box Teaching Your Client About Foot Care are especially important for people with diabetes, as well as for those with impaired peripheral circulation.

Knowledge Check 24-6
- What are some causes of ingrown toenails?
- What is the cause of foot odor?
- Why should you *not* apply lotion between the toes?

CARE OF THE NAILS
The nails are part of the integumentary system. They are composed of epithelial tissue. Healthy nailbeds are usually clean, pink, smooth, convex, and evenly curved. Present at birth, the nails change very little throughout life; however, as one ages, nails thicken, become ridged, and may yellow or become concave in shape. Other changes are caused by certain pathological conditions. For example, trauma to the nail can lead to nail bruising or falling out; and inadequate diet or metabolic changes can cause the nails to become brittle. Also, patients with diabetes mellitus are much more prone to infection and must be vigilant about toenail care.

Teaching Your Client About Foot Care

Use the time during foot care to teach your client the following self-care activities. Most people should follow these measures; they are especially important for people who have diabetes or poor peripheral circulation.

Daily Foot Inspection

> Inspect the feet daily, using a mirror to view all surfaces. Check between the toes for cracks or redness. Look for calluses, blisters, wounds and lesions, or dry areas. If you cannot check your own feet, have someone else do it.

Hygiene for Feet and Nails

> Wash, rinse, and dry the feet well.
> Avoid soaking the feet if you are diabetic, or if there is decreased circulation to the feet.
> Apply a water-soluble lotion to feet, but do not use lotion between the toes, because it may cause maceration.
> Use an antifungal powder, if necessary, for athlete's foot.
> Do not cut or file callused areas.
> Cut and file toenails straight across. Do not use a razor blade on the nails or feet.

Shoes and Stockings

> Wear cotton or wool socks, which absorb perspiration.
> Wear well-fitted, sturdy shoes with nonskid soles and arch support. Natural materials, such as canvas and leather, are best because they allow air to circulate and perspiration to evaporate. Shoes should allow $^1/_2$ to $^3/_4$ inch of toe room.
> Avoid open-toed shoes, sandals, high heels, and thongs. They do not protect the feet.
> Before putting on shoes, check for foreign objects; check that the inside of the shoe is smooth.

Protecting the Feet

> Avoid measures that impair circulation to the feet, such as wearing tight garters or knee stockings, or crossing the legs.
> Do not go barefoot, even when getting out of bed at night. Wear slippers.
> Do not put tape or OTC corn medicines or pads or other medications (e.g., hydrogen peroxide) on the feet.
> Do not smoke. This further decreases circulation to the feet.

Seek Medical Attention for the Following:

> Pain in the feet or legs. This may be a sign of loss of circulation, serious infection, or nerve damage (neuropathy).
> Wounds or ulcers on the feet, especially if they don't seem to be healing.
> A cut to the feet or lower legs that extends deep into the skin and bleeds significantly.
> Cuts or cracks in the feet.
> Generalized redness or red streaks surrounding a wound or ulcer on the feet or lower legs. This might be a sign of infection of the tissue (cellulitis).
> Fever greater than 101°F (38.5°C).
> Confusion. This can be a sign that a wound infection has entered the bloodstream (septicemia). A change in mental status might indicate low blood sugar, which occurs with serious infection, or if the patient is diabetic.
> If you have diabetes, have your feet checked regularly by a professional.
> Seek professional help for foot problems, such as numbness or tingling, decrease in sensation, cold skin temperature, corns, ingrown toenails, and for trimming very thick nails—especially if you have diabetes.

For NANDA-I diagnoses, *NOC standardized outcomes,* and *NIC interventions* for patients with common nail problems,

 Go to Chapter 24, **Standardized Language: Selected NOC Outcomes and NIC Interventions for Hygiene Problems,** on Davis*Plus.*

ASSESSMENT (NAILS)

When assessing the nails, you should obtain subjective data about the patient's usual nail care practices, any history of nail problems, and their treatments. To obtain objective data, inspect the nails for shape, contour, and cleanliness. Look for redness or swelling of the skin around the nails, and observe whether they are neatly manicured and trimmed appropriately, straight across. Unclean or rough fingernails may scratch or abrade the skin and create a risk for infection. Other nail changes may reflect an underlying disease process. In addition, the area under the nail can harbor dirt and bacteria, which can be another source for transmitting microbes. If you want to print out more information about physical assessment of the nails, see Chapter 21, and

 Go to Chapter 24, **Tables, Boxes, Figures: ESG Assessment Box, Assessment Guidelines: Hygiene,** on Davis*Plus.*

ANALYSIS/NURSING DIAGNOSIS (NAILS)

There are no NANDA-I labels to describe nail problems. However, the following are examples of nursing diagnoses related to nail care:

- Risk for Impaired Tissue Integrity related to ingrown nails secondary to trimming too close to the cuticle
- Risk for Infection related to loss of skin integrity secondary to hangnails, cracked cuticles, or trauma from using sharp scissors or nail clippers

PLANNING OUTCOMES/EVALUATION (NAILS)

There are no *NOC outcomes* that relate especially to nail care, but you can use outcomes that relate more generally to circulation, infection, tissue integrity, wound healing.

Individualized goals/outcome statements you might write for a patient with problems associated with nail care may include the following:

- Demonstrates proper care of the nails.
- Trims fingernails with supervision.

- Seeks care of a **podiatrist** (physician who specializes in foot care) for toenail care.

PLANNING INTERVENTIONS/IMPLEMENTATION (NAILS)

Examples of *NOC standardized interventions* for nail care include Nail Care and Self-Care Assistance.

Individualized nursing activities related to proper care of the nails include the following:
- Teaching for self-care (see the Self-Care box Teaching Your Client About Nail Care)
- Providing nail care for dependent patients (the procedure for care of the fingernails is the same as for care of the toenails). Also see Procedure 24-5.

KnowledgeCheck 24-7

- True or False: Healthy nails are usually clean, smooth, and convexly curved.
- List at least three nail changes that occur with aging.
- List at least four things you should teach clients about self-care of their nails.

ORAL HYGIENE

To maintain the integrity of the mucous membranes, teeth, and gums, and to prevent tooth loss and gum disease, it is important to have (1) routine dental checkups, (2) adequate nutrition, and (3) daily mouth care (oral hygiene). Mouth care removes food particles and secretions. In addition, a clean mouth helps to promote a better appetite. It also reduces the incidence of healthcare-acquired pneumonia in older adults and critically ill patients in acute care settings.

TheoreticalKnowledge
knowing **why**

Digestion of food begins in the mouth (oral cavity). The tongue and teeth begin digestion by breaking up food and mixing it with saliva. Front teeth, also called **incisors,** are for biting and tearing while the teeth in the back of the mouth, known as **molars,** are used for chewing. Saliva, produced by three pairs of salivary glands in the mouth, also acts as a mechanical cleaner of the mouth. The structures of the mouth pertinent to oral hygiene include the tongue, **gingiva** (gums), and teeth.

Developmental Variations

The first set of teeth **(deciduous teeth)** erupts between ages 6 months and 2 years. By age 2, a child usually has 20 teeth. Between ages 6 and 12 years, the deciduous teeth loosen, fall out, and are eventually replaced with 32 permanent teeth (Fig. 24-3). **Wisdom teeth** are the very back molars on either side of each jawbone.

The tooth surface wears away with aging and the gums may begin to recede, resulting in bone and tooth loss and necessitating the use of dentures (false teeth). Other changes that may occur with aging are a brownish pigmentation of the gums and dryness of the oral mucosa, which is caused by decreased saliva production.

Risk Factors for Oral Problems

Oral health is influenced by heredity, nutrition, and oral hygiene. Therefore, any condition that prevents good oral hygiene can lead to oral problems. Risk factors include the following:
- *History of periodontal disease*
- *Lack of money or insurance* for dental care
- *Pregnancy.* Increased estrogen during pregnancy increases the vascularity of the gingiva, so the gums may bleed easily and become puffy and tender. Good hygiene is needed to prevent infection.
- *Poor nutrition or eating habits.* Adequate intake of calcium, phosphorus, and vitamin D is essential for healthy teeth and gums. Excessive intake of refined sugars leads to dental decay. One example of this is **baby-bottle tooth decay,** which occurs when parents put an infant or toddler to bed with a bottle or sippy cup of milk, fruit juice, or other

Teaching Your Client About Nail Care

Self-Care

- ➤ Inspect the nails daily.
- ➤ Trim nails with a nail clipper. (People with diabetes or circulatory problems should file only, because cutting poses a risk for injury to the tissues.)
- ➤ File the nails straight across, rounding the corners slightly to prevent scratching. Do not cut deeply into the lateral corners because this may cause ingrown nails.
- ➤ Remove hangnails by carefully removing them with cuticle clipper.
- ➤ Clean under the nails with an orangewood stick or other blunt instrument.
- ➤ Push back the cuticles gently.
- ➤ Use a moisturizing lotion to soften cuticles.
- ➤ Avoid biting nails.
- ➤ Consult a podiatrist for ingrown toenails or other nail problems.
- ➤ Recommend to patients with diabetes, circulatory insufficiency, or nail problems that they seek nail care from a podiatrist.

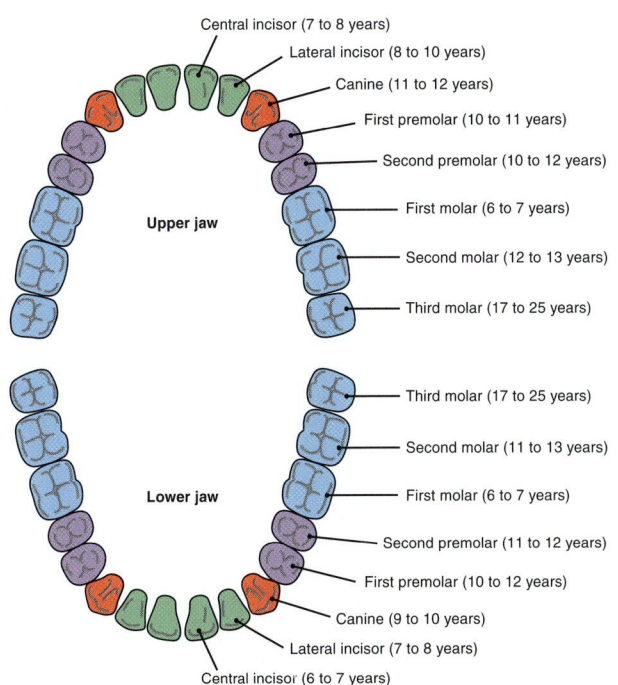

FIGURE 24-3 Most adults have 32 permanent teeth. (Courtesy of P. Dillon [2007]. Nursing Health Assessment [2nd ed.]. Philadelphia: F. A. Davis.)

Labels for Figure 24-3:
Central incisor (7 to 8 years)
Lateral incisor (8 to 10 years)
Canine (11 to 12 years)
First premolar (10 to 11 years)
Second premolar (10 to 12 years)
First molar (6 to 7 years)
Second molar (12 to 13 years)
Third molar (17 to 25 years)
Upper jaw
Third molar (17 to 25 years)
Second molar (11 to 13 years)
First molar (6 to 7 years)
Second premolar (11 to 12 years)
First premolar (10 to 12 years)
Canine (9 to 10 years)
Lateral incisor (7 to 8 years)
Central incisor (6 to 7 years)
Lower jaw

sugary beverages. Carbohydrates in the fluid cause demineralization of the tooth enamel, leading to major decay.

- *Medications.* The anticonvulsant phenytoin (Dilantin) causes gingival **hyperplasia** (excessive growth of cells). Other medications (e.g., diuretics) cause dryness of the mouth.
- *Medical treatments.* Medical treatments affecting the oral cavity include the following:

  Jaw surgery, which requires scrupulous oral hygiene to prevent infection

  Radiation treatments of the head and neck, which can permanently damage the salivary glands.

  Oxygen therapy, which dries the oral mucosa

- *Any situation that causes dry mouth* predisposes to cracking of the mucosa, including heavy cigarette smoking, excessive alcohol use, inadequate fluid intake (e.g., being NPO), dehydration, and mouth breathing
- *Compromised self-care abilities* may be caused by:

  Decreased level of consciousness (e.g., a person who is comatose or heavily sedated).

  Serious illness or injury, weakness, activity intolerance, or paralysis

  Cognitive impairment (e.g., developmental delay, dementia)

  Depression

  Lack of knowledge or motivation to perform self-care

KnowledgeCheck 24-8

- How do the teeth aid in digesting food?
- How many deciduous teeth does a child usually have?
- List at least three factors that cause dry mouth.
- List at least two medications or medical treatments that can cause oral problems.
- Name four situations that can compromise self-care ability for oral hygiene.

ThinkLike a Nurse 24-9

- For which of your patients, Mrs. Williams or Mr. Gold, does the scenario provide *actual data* to indicate that the patient is at risk for oral problems? What are the data?
- Why is the patient's nursing diagnosis Risk for Impaired Oral Mucous Membrane instead of Impaired Oral Mucous Membrane?

Common Problems of the Mouth

Dental **caries** (cavities) and periodontal disease are the two most frequent problems affecting the teeth. They are discussed here along with other common mouth problems:

Halitosis. Also known as bad breath, halitosis results from poor oral hygiene, eating certain foods (e.g., garlic, onions), tobacco use, dental caries, infections, or even systemic diseases, such as uncontrolled diabetes or liver disease.

Dental Caries. Failure to remove plaque is the primary cause of dental caries. **Plaque,** an invisible, destructive bacterial film that builds up on the teeth, eventually leads to destruction of the tooth enamel. Untreated plaque can result in tooth loss. The plaque builds up with dead bacteria and forms hard deposits at the gumlines **(tartar).** The tartar causes deterioration of the supporting structures that hold the teeth in the gums and also attacks the bone tissue, causing the teeth to become loose. Other factors that contribute to the formation of cavities include excessive intake of refined sugars, a lack of brushing and flossing, and infrequent visits to the dentist.

Gingivitis. Inflammation of the gum tissue surrounding the teeth is known as **gingivitis.** If untreated, it may progress to periodontal disease.

Periodontal Disease (Pyorrhea). The major cause of tooth loss in adults 35 years and older is periodontal disease, or **pyorrhea.** It is an inflammation characterized by bleeding and receding gums and destruction of the surrounding bone structure. The patient experiences halitosis and complains of a bad taste in the mouth. When pyorrhea is advanced, the gums become infected, and the teeth loosen and may fall out or need to be removed.

Stomatitis. An inflammation of the oral mucosa, **stomatitis** has numerous causes, including bacteria, mechanical trauma, irritants, nutritional deficiencies, and systemic infection. Symptoms may include pain, halitosis, and increased salivation.

Glossitis. An inflammation of the tongue, **glossitis** is caused by deficiencies of vitamin B_{12}, folic acid, and iron.

Cheilosis. A cracking and/or ulceration of the lips, **cheilosis** forms reddened fissures at the angles of the mouth. It is usually caused by vitamin B–complex deficiencies.

Oral Malignancies. Teach patients to see a dentist immediately if any of the following are present in the mouth: lumps, ulcers, white or red patches, bleeding, pain, persistent sores, or numbness. Oral malignancies must be detected as early as possible.

KnowledgeCheck 24-9

- Identify and define several causes of halitosis.
- What are the two most common problems affecting the teeth?
- What is the end result of severe periodontal disease?

PracticalKnowledge
knowing **how**

You should assess the patient's oral cavity when performing or assisting with oral hygiene. This is particularly important for older adults because of the association between oral health and systemic disease.

For *NANDA-I diagnoses, NOC standardized outcomes,* and *NIC interventions* for patients with problems of the mouth,

 Go to Chapter 24, **Standardized Language: Selected NOC Outcomes and NIC Interventions for Hygiene Problems,** on Davis*Plus.*

■ ASSESSMENT (ORAL CAVITY)

You might begin your subjective assessment by asking the patient about his usual hygiene practices. You should also interview the patient or examine his records for the risk factors for oral problems discussed in the preceding section (e.g., history of oral problems, nutritional status, access to dental care, medications such as anticonvulsants or diuretics, radiation therapy). Ask about tobacco and alcohol use.

As part of your objective assessment, inspect the lips, oral mucosa, gums, and tongue. Mucosa and gums should be pink and moist without lesions or bleeding. Look for loose, missing, or decaying teeth; tartar; and stomatitis; and note any unusual odors or halitosis. Check to be sure the tongue is normal in color and without lesions.

The Kayser–Jones Brief Oral Health Status Examination (BOHSE) is used to assess the oral cavity of older adults. It was specifically designed for nursing home residents, with both normal and impaired cognitive functioning, and can be used by a variety of nursing personnel. The tool assigns a numerical

rating to findings for items such as lips, tongue, tissue inside the mouth, gums, saliva, and condition of natural teeth. For a copy of the BOHSE assessment,

 Go to Chapter 24, **Tables, Boxes, Figures: ESG Table 24-2,** on Davis*Plus.*

To learn more about physical assessment of the oral cavity, refer to Chapter 21. Also,

 Go to Chapter 24, **Tables, Boxes, Figures: ESG Assessment Box, Assessment Guidelines: Hygiene,** on Davis*Plus.*

ANALYSIS/NURSING DIAGNOSIS (ORAL CAVITY)

In addition to Self-Care Deficit, discussed in the first part of the chapter, the following are examples of nursing diagnoses that may be useful in describing problems of the mouth:

- Risk for Infection related to mouth lesions
- Impaired Dentition (caries) related to inability to afford dental care
- Impaired Oral Mucous Membrane related to inability to manage mouth care secondary to impaired mobility
   Oral and dental problems can be the etiology of other nursing diagnoses, for example:
- Deficient Knowledge related to lack of interest in learning about oral hygiene
- Imbalanced Nutrition related to lack of teeth for mastication
- Pain related to mouth lesions

PLANNING OUTCOMES/EVALUATION (ORAL CAVITY)

NOC standardized outcomes for oral problems include Oral Hygiene, Self-Care: Oral Hygiene, and Knowledge: Health Behavior.

Individualized goals/outcome statements you might write for mouth problems include the following examples:

- Oral mucous membranes will remain pink, moist, and intact.
- Demonstrates correct technique for brushing and flossing.
- Makes preventive dental visits every 6 months.

PLANNING INTERVENTIONS/IMPLEMENTATION (ORAL CAVITY)

For some clients, you may need only to provide the necessary supplies for mouth care. For others, you will need to assist with or completely provide care as often as necessary to keep the mouth clean and moist. Rinsing with mouthwash is not a substitute for a thorough cleaning of the teeth and mouth.

NIC standardized interventions for mouth care include Oral Health Maintenance, Self-Care Assistance, and Teaching: Individual.

Individualized nursing activities related to oral hygiene include teaching for self-care (see the Self-Care box Teaching Your Client About Oral Hygiene) and assisting with and providing oral hygiene for dependent patients.

Denture Care

A patient may have a complete set of removable dentures or just an upper or lower plate. A **bridge,** or partial plate, consists of one or more artificial teeth. A bridge may be permanently fastened to other teeth, or it may be removable. Artificial teeth are fitted to the individual and should not be used by anyone

else. If the person leaves the prosthesis out of his mouth for long periods, the shape of the gums will change, and it will no longer fit properly. Poorly fitted or loose dentures can lead to chewing difficulties and even nutritional deficiencies. The nurse's role is to ensure cleanliness by teaching for self-care (see the Self-Care box Teaching Your Client About Oral Hygiene) or to provide denture care for dependent clients. For further information, refer to Procedure 24-7.

Oral Care for Critically Ill Patients

Patients in long-term care settings and critically ill patients in acute care settings are at high risk for healthcare-associated pneumonia. This is especially true for those dependent on a ventilator. Ventilator-associated pneumonia (VAP) is the most common hospital-acquired infection among critically ill patients. A simple and inexpensive way to reduce the risk of pneumonia for these patients is to keep their teeth clean, thus reducing the number of bacteria that cause pneumonia (American Association of Critical-Care Nurses [AACN], 2007). The regimen includes the following:

- Brush the teeth twice a day.
- Use a soft toothbrush.
- Moisturize oral mucosa and lips every 2 to 4 hours.
- Use a chlorhexidine gluconate (0.12%) rinse twice a day during the perioperative period for adult patients who undergo cardiac surgery.
- Use mouthwash inside the mouth twice a day for adult patients who are on a ventilator.

Oral Care for Unconscious Patients

Oral care for unconscious patients is particularly important because they often breathe through the mouth. If the patient is receiving oxygen per cannula or has a nasogastric (NG) or feeding tube inserted, the mucous membranes become even drier.

An unconscious patient often responds to oral stimulation by biting down, so use a padded tongue blade instead of your fingers to hold the mouth open. Also use a padded tongue blade when providing oral care for a patient with seizures to avoid the patient biting you.

Follow agency practices for the type and frequency of special mouth care. Some patients may need it every hour or two. You may use commercially packaged applicators or foam swabs to clean the mouth. However, do not use lemon-glycerine swabs because they are drying to the mucosa and may causes changes in tooth enamel. Likewise, do not use hydrogen peroxide because it is irritating to oral mucosa and may alter the balance of normal flora of the mouth. To learn more about how to provide oral care for unconscious patients, see Procedure 24-8.

Oral Care for Patients With Dementia

Poor oral health and dental pain impact on general well-being—specifically, on the ability to eat, type of diet, weight, speech, hydration, appearance, and social interactions. This is especially true for older adults with dementia who also have many oral diseases and dental problems. Dental disease and pain may be the source of some of the behavior problems in this population. Because it is a challenge to provide oral hygiene for patients with dementia, staff sometimes neglect care. Residents may be uncooperative: refusing care, refusing to open the mouth, biting the toothbrush, and so on. Research is needed to identify the best interventions (Joanna Briggs Institute, 2004).

Teaching Your Client About Oral Hygiene

Measures to promote oral health and prevent periodontal disease and caries include the following:

Preventing Caries and Periodontal Disease

➤ Eliminate between-meal snacks with high sugar content (ice cream, soft drinks, candy, gum, jams and jellies).
➤ Include in the diet cleansing, fibrous foods, such as raw fruits and vegetables.
➤ Include an adequate intake of calcium; phosphorus; and vitamins A, C, and D.
➤ Have regular dental checkups every 6 months.
➤ Brush teeth with a soft brush and toothpaste after each meal and at bedtime (some dentists say twice a day). Bacteria do the most damage to the teeth in the first 24 hours after eating.
➤ Floss between the teeth daily to remove food debris and stimulate the blood flow to the gingiva.
➤ Use a fluoride toothpaste to strengthen tooth enamel.
➤ You can make your own cleanser by combining one part baking soda with two parts salt.
➤ Follow the dentist's recommendations for topical applications of fluoride.

Brushing and Flossing

➤ Make sure the brush is small enough to reach all teeth. If it is too firm, it can injure enamel and gum tissue.
➤ Electric toothbrushes are effective; however, you should consult your dentist about using water-spray units, because they can force debris into pockets of the gums.
➤ Brush at a 45° angle, from the gum to the tooth crown, using small circular or vibrating motions.
➤ When flossing (1) wrap one end of the floss around each of your middle fingers. (2) Hold about 1 to 2 inches of floss tightly between the fingers. (3) Insert floss between the teeth by gently moving it back and forth; do not force it. (4) Floss adjacent sides of both teeth to the gum tissue, but not into the gum, because you may injure the tissue. (5) Use a fresh section of floss when it becomes soiled or frayed. (6) Rinse your mouth well when you are finished. A variety of convenient flossing devices are available as an alternative to this method.

Oral Hygiene for Children

➤ Begin oral hygiene when the first tooth erupts. Use a washcloth, cotton ball, or gauze pad moistened with water.
➤ Do not put a child to bed with a bottle or sippy cup. Milk, juice, or any other liquid with sugar can lead to dental caries in the young child when the liquid sits on the teeth at night or during naps.
➤ Begin brushing the child's teeth with a soft toothbrush when she is about 18 months old. Start first using water only. Later, switch to a fluoride-containing toothpaste.
➤ Follow your dentist's instructions for giving a fluoride supplement.
➤ Schedule a visit to the dentist when all 20 deciduous teeth have erupted.
➤ See your dentist if you notice any problems, such as chipping, redness or swelling, caries, or misalignment.
➤ For school-age children, parents may need to supervise mouth care to be sure it is done adequately.

Care of Dentures

➤ If you have dentures or other removable prostheses ("bridges"), wear them. If you do not, the gums are likely to shrink, and you will have further gum loss.
➤ Clean dentures and bridges at least once a day, preferably after each meal.
➤ Remove dentures from the mouth to clean them.
➤ Use regular toothpaste or special denture-cleaning compounds.
➤ Do not use hot water on dentures; it may damage them.
➤ If the dentures have metal parts, do not soak them overnight in cleaning solutions.
➤ Store dentures in a denture cup, in water, to prevent drying. Do not wrap them in tissues because they may accidentally be thrown away.
➤ Clean dentures over a plastic pan or towel in the sink. They are fragile and may break if dropped.

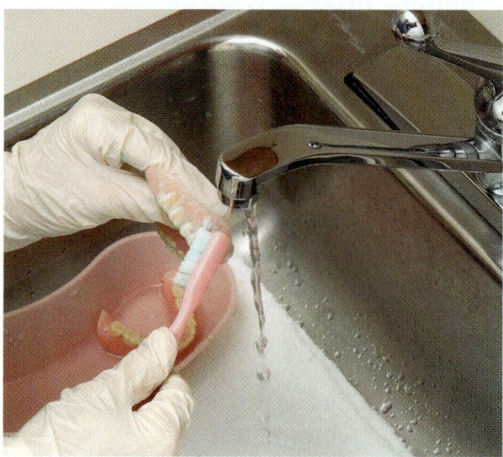

Dentures must be cleaned thoroughly as a part of daily oral hygiene.

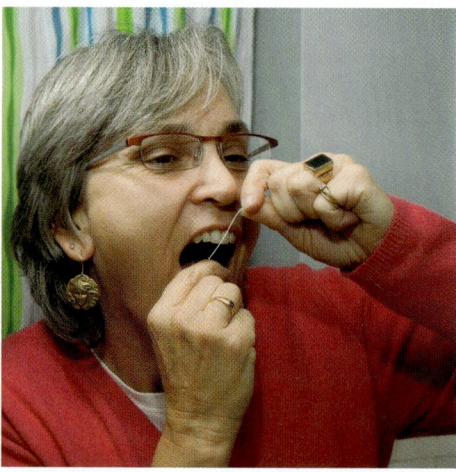

Flossing between the teeth is an essential part of oral hygiene.

Toward Evidence-Based Practice

American Association of Critical-Care Nurses (AACN). (2007). AACN practice alert. Oral care in the critically ill. Retrieved December 18, 2008, from http://classic.aacn.org/AACN/practiceAlert.nsf/Files/OC/$file/Oral%20Care%20in%20the%20Critically%20Ill%20.pdf

This evidence report reviewed 14 references and graded the evidence for the conclusions they drew. They used a scale of I to VI, with Level VI being the strongest support and Level I being the weakest (manufacturer's recommendations only). The following are two AACN recommendations for oral care in the critically ill:

- Use oral chlorhexidine gluconate (0.12%) rinse twice a day for adult patients undergoing cardiac surgery; not routinely for all patients. (Level V)
- Brush teeth, gums, and tongue at least twice a day. (Level II)

Sona, C., Zack, J., Schallom, M., et al. (2008, Nov. 17). The impact of a simple, low-cost oral care protocol on ventilator-associated pneumonia rates in a surgical intensive care unit. *Journal of Intensive Care Medicine.* Abstract retrieved December 22, 2008, from http://www.ncbi.nlm.nih.gov/pubmed/19017665

Researchers examined the effects of an oral care protocol on VAP rates on ventilator patients in a surgical intensive care unit. The protocol included brushing the teeth twice daily with a fluoride toothpaste and brush and applying chlorhexidine gluconate (0.12%) twice daily. They concluded that the oral care protocol led to a significantly decreased risk of acquiring VAP in surgical intensive care patients.

Watando, A., Ebihara, S., Ebihara, T., et al. (2004). Daily oral care and cough reflex sensitivity in elderly nursing home patients. *Chest, 126*(4), 1066–1070.

These researchers explored the effects of intensive oral care on improvement of cough reflex sensitivity in elderly nursing home residents. Caregivers cleaned the subjects' teeth after every meal for 1 month; a control group of patients cleaned their own teeth after every meal. No special paste or solution was used. The intervention significantly improved cough reflex sensitivity in the intervention group. Therefore, researchers concluded that intensive oral care may reduce the incidence of pneumonia by improving cough reflex sensitivity in elderly nursing home residents.

1. Suppose you are a critical-care nurse, using the AACN Practice Alert guidelines. For which of the two AACN recommendations would you most want to have further research evidence?

2. Which of the two studies above provide additional support for that guideline? Explain your thinking.

3. How are the patients in the two studies alike or different from the patients for whom the AACN Practice Alert was designed?

 Go to Chapter 24, **Toward Evidence-Based Practice Suggested Responses,** on DavisPlus.

Meanwhile, for experts' suggestions for ways to provide oral care to patients with dementia, see the What if . . .? section in Procedure 24-6.

KnowledgeCheck 24-10

How would you position Mr. Gold (Meet Your Patients) to perform his oral hygiene?

CARE OF THE HAIR

Hair is an accessory structure of the skin. The hair helps to maintain body temperature, serves as a receptor for tactile sensation, and influences a person's self-image. **Vellus hair** is the short, fine hair present over much of the body. **Terminal hair,** which is coarser, darker, and longer, is found on the scalp, eyebrows, axillae, perineum, and legs. Sebaceous glands at the base of the hair follicle secrete sebum, or oil, to lubricate hair and scalp. The condition of the hair is a measure of a person's overall health. See Chapter 21 for more information about changes in hair that occur through the life span and as a result of illness.

For *NOC standardized outcomes* and *NIC standardized interventions* for patients with problems related to care of the hair,

 Go to Chapter 24, **Standardized Language: Selected NOC Outcomes and NIC Interventions for Hygiene Problems,** on DavisPlus.

ASSESSMENT (HAIR)

For the purposes of hygiene, you will need information about the patient's history of hair problems or current conditions needing treatment (e.g., pediculosis), diseases or therapy that affect the hair (e.g., chemotherapy), and factors influencing the patient's ability to manage her hair and scalp care (e.g., Impaired Mobility). Ask the patient about special products she uses and about her preference for styling her hair. Inspect the condition and cleanliness of the hair, and inspect the scalp for dandruff, lesions, and so forth. For more complete information about assessing the hair, see Chapter 21. Also,

 Go to Chapter 24, **Tables, Boxes, Figures: ESG Assessment Box, Assessment Guidelines: Hygiene,** on DavisPlus.

ANALYSIS/NURSING DIAGNOSIS (HAIR)

Common problems associated with the hair and scalp include the following (also see Chapter 21):
- **Dandruff** is a condition in which there is excessive shedding of the epidermal layer of the scalp. Primary symptoms include itching and flaking of the scalp, which may be caused by fungal infection.
- **Pediculosis** is an infestation of head lice. Though frequently associated with poor hygiene practices, it knows

no socioeconomic boundaries. Head lice spread through sharing of combs, brushes, hair ornaments, hats, and caps.

- **Alopecia,** or hair loss, can be very stressful and affect self-image. Abnormal hair loss, which may be gradual or sudden, can be caused by an autoimmune disorder, hormonal imbalance, thyroid disease, stress, fever, certain medications, or chemotherapy.

There are no NANDA-I labels that apply specifically to the hair. When the difficulty lies with self-care ability, you can, of course, use Dressing Self-Care Deficit and Bathing Self-Care Deficit. Examples of other nursing diagnoses that may apply include the following:

- Risk for Impaired Skin Integrity related to secretions on the scalp
- Situational Low Self-Esteem related to alopecia secondary to chemotherapy

KnowledgeCheck 24-11

- List at least four assessments you should make of a patient's hair.
- What is pediculosis?
- What is alopecia?

PLANNING OUTCOMES/EVALUATION (HAIR)

As always, select outcomes based on the client's nursing diagnoses. *Individualized goals/outcome statements* you might write for a patient with problems related to the hair include the following:

- Scalp and hair are clean.
- By 9/18, brushes own hair.
- Hair and scalp are free from infestation, infection, irritation, or dryness.
- Verbalizes improved comfort and self-esteem.

PLANNING INTERVENTIONS/IMPLEMENTATION (HAIR)

Individualized nursing activities related to the care of the hair include daily brushing and combing of the hair, shampooing, and, for men, shaving and beard care.

Hair Care

Brush the hair daily to remove tangles, massage the scalp, stimulate the circulation, and distribute oil down the hair shaft. Use a stiff-bristled brush, but be sure the bristles are not sharp enough to injure the patient's scalp. Likewise, a comb with broken or uneven teeth or one that is too fine can break or snarl the hair or scrape the scalp. Comb tightly curled hair with a wide-toothed comb or pick. Encourage patients to brush and comb their own hair, if they are able to do so. Encouraging family members to assist with hair care will involve them in the patient's care and reduce feelings of helplessness. Do not cut a patient's hair unless he or she consents to the haircut.

Shampooing the Hair. Shampooing cleans the hair and scalp. It is soothing and relaxing to many patients. Hair can be shampooed while the person is in the shower, standing or sitting over a sink, or in bed. Protect the patient's eyes with a dry washcloth, and make sure the water temperature is appropriate for the patient. For patients who are unable to tolerate a standard shampoo procedure, you can use a dry

shampoo as an alternative. However, it is not as effective as shampooing with water. Commercially prepared shampoo caps are available and have, in most institutions, replaced the dry shampoo method. For more information, refer to Procedure 24-9.

Hair Care for African Americans Hair care is equally important for all patients, so if a patient's hair requires special care, you must learn how to do it. The hair of African Americans varies in texture from some other ethnicities—it may be long or short, straight or kinky, thick or thin. Worn naturally, very curly hair can easily become entangled or matted, and it tends to be fragile and easily broken. The scalp also tends to be dry. The hair requires careful handling, especially if it has been chemically straightened, relaxed, or curled.

Shampoo and groom the hair according to the person's preference. In general, though, you should comb and brush the hair daily and apply a light oil to the scalp (e.g., mineral oil or a light moisturizing cream). Ask a family member to bring from home the product the patient prefers to use. Do not apply chemical relaxers to a patient's hair. Only a licensed beautician should do this.

Beard and Mustache Care

Beards and mustaches tend to collect food particles. They should be washed daily during a bath or shower and combed and trimmed as necessary. Do not shave a patient's mustache or beard without permission to do so. For details of beard and mustache care, see Procedure 24-10.

Shaving

Depending on the culture, shaving is an important part of grooming and helps patients feel better about their appearance. Many men shave their facial hair every day. Women may shave to remove axillary and leg hair. If the patient has a bleeding disorder or is taking anticoagulant medication, you should use an electric razor. For important points about shaving, see Procedure 24-11.

Some dark-haired men (e.g., African Americans and Mediterraneans) have tightly curled facial hair, which curls back into the skin when shaved. An inflammatory reaction may occur, resulting in the formation of papules and pustules. In such cases, the man may wish to use a **depilatory** (hair-removing agent) instead of shaving. If you apply a depilatory, be sure to keep the chemical from contacting the patient's eyes, nose, mouth, and ears. Do not use a straight or safety razor to remove the depilatory, because it will irritate the skin. Some men with this condition prefer to grow a beard, especially when they are ill and unable to care for themselves.

CARE OF THE EYES

Usually you will not need to provide special hygiene care for the eyes. The eyelids and lashes keep dust and debris from entering the eyes, and tears continually cleanse and lubricate them. When necessary, you may gently cleanse the eyes, from the inner to the outer canthus, with a moistened washcloth (without soap). If there is drainage or crusting, use a different cloth for each eye to prevent cross-contamination.

ASSESSMENT (EYES)

When performing hygiene care, inspect the eyes for redness, lesions, swelling, crusting, excessive tearing, or discharge. Also check the color of the conjunctivae. You should also ask

the patient or check his records to see whether he wears glasses or contact lenses. If the patient wears glasses, ask when he uses them (e.g., for reading, for driving), and ask how well he sees without them. If the patient wears contact lenses, determine the following:

- The type of lens (hard, soft, long wearing, disposable)
- How often he wears them (daily, occasionally) and for how long at a time
- Whether they are worn during sleep
- History of or current problems with lens usage (e.g., cleaning, removal)
- Usual practices for cleaning and storage
- History of or current problems with the eyes (e.g., redness, tearing, irritation, dryness, or "scratchy feeling")

These should be adequate data for hygiene care. However, it is not a complete eye assessment. For detailed information about assessing the eyes, see Chapter 21.

ANALYSIS/NURSING DIAGNOSIS (EYES)

Other than Bathing Self-Care Deficit, there is only one NANDA-I label specific to the eyes: Disturbed Sensory Perception: Visual. This label is of limited use for hygiene care. Other diagnoses that might occur include the following:

- Risk for Infection related to improper handwashing and improper lens cleaning
- Risk for Injury (to eyes) related to wearing lenses longer than recommended

PLANNING OUTCOMES/EVALUATION (EYES)

The only *NOC standardized outcome* specific to the eyes is Sensory Function: Vision. Its use is limited with regard to hygiene care; instead, you would use it if the client has a diagnosis of Disturbed Sensory Perception: Visual.

Individualized goals you might write for eye care include these examples:

- Demonstrates proper cleaning and storage of contact lenses.
- Eyes appear clean and without redness or drainage.

PLANNING INTERVENTIONS/IMPLEMENTATION (EYES)

For *NIC standardized interventions* related to eye care,

 Go to Chapter 24, **Standardized Language: Selected NOC Outcomes and NIC Interventions for Hygiene Problems,** on Davis*Plus.*

Individualized nursing activities related to the care of the eyes include providing eye care to unconscious clients, caring for eyeglasses and contact lenses, and caring for artificial eyes.

Eye Care for the Unconscious Client

Having lost the blink (corneal) reflex, comatose or critically ill patients need more frequent eye care (every 2 to 4 hr). Keep their eyes lubricated with saline or artificial tears to protect them from corneal abrasions and drying. You may also need to use a protective eye shield to keep the patient's eyes closed. Instill eye ointment or drops in the lower lids as prescribed.

To review a procedure for administering ophthalmic medications, refer to Procedure 25-2.

Caring for Eyeglasses and Contact Lenses

Eyeglasses need to be cleaned at least once a day. Using warm water and a soft cloth, clean gently to prevent scratching of the lens. Ask the patient whether the lenses require a special cleaning solution; some patients bring their own. Label each patient's glasses, and store them in a safe place within the patient's reach, preferably in a glasses case in the drawer of the bedside table. They are expensive, so take care that they are not lost or damaged.

An alternative to glasses, contact lenses are plastic discs worn on the cornea over the pupil. They float on the tears of the eye and stay in place because of surface tension. The cornea is nourished mainly by oxygen from the atmosphere and from tears, so in order to ensure an optimal supply of oxygen, contact lenses must be removed periodically. Wearing time varies from daily wear to up to around 30 days, depending on the type of lens. If you want more information about several different types of contact lenses:

 Go to Chapter 24, **Supplemental Materials: Types of Contact Lenses,** on Davis*Plus.*

People usually care for their own contact lenses. Contact lens users must be careful to keep them free of microorganisms that could cause eye infections and to be careful to avoid eye irritation. Teach cleaning and disinfecting measures to clients as needed (see the Self-Care box Teaching Clients About Cleaning and Storing Contact Lenses), and follow those measures when you must care for a client's lenses. If you need to remove a patient's lenses during an emergency, follow universal precautions and handle the lenses as you would any other valuable patient property.

Never use your fingernails to remove a lens, as you may scratch the eye or damage the lens. For more detailed instructions see Procedure 24-12.

Caring for Artificial Eyes

An artificial eye is made to look like a natural eye. It can be made of glass or plastic. Some artificial eyes are permanently implanted in the socket, but others must be removed daily for cleaning of the prosthesis and the eye socket. If the patient is not able to perform his own eye care, ask about and follow his usual routines, when possible. For details about removing, cleaning, and replacing an artificial eye, see Figure 24-4 and Procedure 24-15.

Knowledge Check 24-12

- True or False: Eyes should be cleansed from the outer to the inner canthus.
- How can a contact lens wearer help prevent eye infections?
- After you have cleaned a prosthetic eye, should you dry it before reinserting it, or leave it wet?

CARE OF THE EARS

Healthy ears require minimal care. However, you will need to help patients who have limited self-care abilities and teach others about self-care. For example, **cerumen** (wax) impaction is a common cause of functional hearing loss, especially in older adults. People sometimes believe that hearing loss is a normal

Teaching Clients About Cleaning and Storing Contact Lenses

> Cleaning and disinfecting procedures and solutions vary among manufacturers. Depending on the type of lens, use saline solutions or special rinsing and soaking solutions.

> Use a special container for the lenses, with a cup labeled for the left and right lens. Some lenses are stored in a solution; others are stored dry. Follow manufacturer's instructions.

> Always wash your hands before touching the eyes or the lenses.

> Be careful not to allow the lenses to come in contact with soaps, hair sprays, or cosmetics.

> Do not wear soft lenses while using eye drops or ointment (wait 1 hr after using drops and at least 4 hr for ointment).

> Be aware of the risk for eye irritation when in the presence of smoke or chemical vapors.

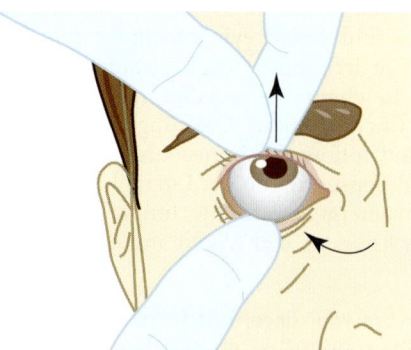

FIGURE 24-4 To remove a prosthetic eye, apply pressure just below the eye.

part of aging and fail to seek treatment. Encourage them to see their primary care provider whenever hearing loss occurs.

✚ Teach patients to avoid using rigid objects such as bobby pins or toothpicks to clean their ears. Such instruments can traumatize the ear canal and may rupture the **tympanic membrane** (eardrum). Likewise, never use cotton-tipped applicators; they will push the cerumen further into the ear, causing a blockage.

For dependent patients, assess for drainage, excess cerumen, and hearing loss during the bath. Clean the auricle, and remove wax from the canal with the tip of the moistened washcloth. If cleansing with a washcloth does not effectively remove excess wax buildup, obtain a prescription for **cerumenolytic** drops and water irrigation. You can delegate ear cleaning and hearing aid care to the NAP if you are sure that the NAP knows how to perform these tasks. See Chapter 31 for information about ear irrigations.

Care of Hearing Aids. A hearing aid is a battery-powered device that amplifies sound. Three types of hearing aids are shown in Figure 24-5. Also, some patients wear a hearing aid in

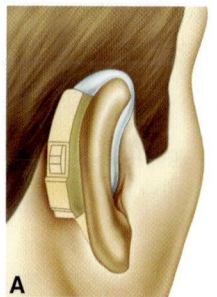 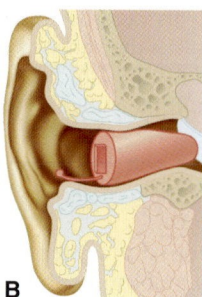 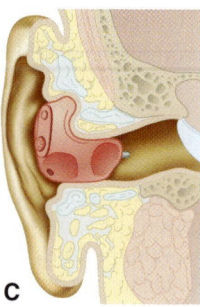

A   **B**   **C**

FIGURE 24-5 Hearing aids. A, The postaural (behind-the-ear) aid is the most widely used. A plastic tube connects it to an earmold. B, An in-the-canal aid is the least visible. C, The in-the-ear aid is made in one piece; all components are in the earmold.

the temple pieces of their eyeglasses. People with severe hearing loss may wear a body hearing aid that clips onto the clothing or a harness-type carrier that connects by a cord to the earpiece. Digital hearing aids are rapidly replacing the analog models.

Hearing aids are expensive and often essential to the patient, so handle and store them properly. They require regular cleaning and replacement of batteries. Even with good care, they usually need to be replaced every 5 to 10 years, and ear molds usually need adjustment more often than that. Never place a hearing aid in water. Additionally, humidity can reduce their effectiveness. To learn how to remove, clean, and replace a hearing aid, refer to Procedure 24-16.

CARE OF THE NOSE

Usually the nose requires no special care. Have the patient remove excess secretions by gently blowing into a tissue with both nostrils open. Holding one nostril shut can force secretions into the eustachian tubes. In debilitated or unconscious patients, dried secretions can interfere with respirations. Remove secretions by gently inserting a moistened cotton-tipped applicator into the nostrils. Occasionally you may need to instill saline into the nares and suction secretions to keep the airway patent. If the patient has an NG tube, the constant pressure on the skin may cause breakdown. Provide special skin care and a lubricant at the point where the tube touches the nares.

THE CLIENT'S ENVIRONMENT

A comfortable environment contributes to the client's well-being. It is your responsibility, as a nurse, to see that the bedside unit and surroundings are clean, safe, and comfortable.

ASSESSMENT (SCANNING THE ENVIRONMENT)

Each time you enter a patient's room, you should scan the environment to see whether you need to make adjustments to ensure patient safety and comfort:

- Is the room temperature comfortable?
- Are the siderails up, when indicated?
- Is the bed in low position, and the wheels locked?
- Are bed linens clean and free of wrinkles?
- Is the patient's call device within reach?
- Is the overbed table clean and uncluttered?
- Is there uncluttered walking space?
- Are there unpleasant odors?

Each time you leave the room, ask, "What else can I do for you?" This ensures that you have not overlooked anything.

PLANNING INTERVENTIONS/IMPLEMENTATION (THE ENVIRONMENT)

Adequate ventilation; proper room temperature; low noise level; and neat, clean surroundings are important to ensure the patient's comfort.

Promoting Ventilation

Body secretions such as urine, feces, vomitus, or draining wounds cause odors in both inpatient facilities and the home. Odors can be offensive, and patients often feel embarrassed by them, so work quickly to free the environment of any sources of odors. Cleanliness is the best way to prevent odors. Other suggestions include the following:

- Provide good ventilation, if this is under your control. For example, open a window or use a fan.
- Empty urinals, bedpans, or emesis basins promptly.
- Dispose of soiled dressings or other malodorous items in appropriate containers, and immediately remove them from the room.
- Unless contraindicated by the patient's illness, you can use a room deodorizer to help eliminate odors.
- Most institutions ban smoking in patient rooms, in part because of the odor.

Controlling Room Temperature

Although preferences may vary, a room temperature between 68°F and 74°F (20°C and 23°C) is usually comfortable for most patients. Those who are very ill, very young, or very old may need a higher than normal room temperature. If there is no thermostat in the room, you may need to provide blankets, open a window, provide a fan, and so on to adjust the room temperature.

Limiting Noise

People who are ill are often sensitive to environmental noises, such as an ice machine, suction equipment, paging systems, loud talking, and laughter. In addition, sleeping in a new and strange environment or in the presence of pain may be difficult. Make it a priority to control noise. Keep unnecessary conversations to a minimum, and speak quietly. Some hospitals have instituted a "quiet hour" each day to promote better rest. Others have installed decibel meters to help nurses be mindful of noise escalation during activity in the nurses' station.

Standard Bedside Equipment

In a hospital, standard bedside equipment usually includes a bed, bedside stand (end table), overbed table, and one or two chairs. The wall unit may consist of a call light, oxygen, suction and electrical outlets, and light fixtures and switches. The patient's personal items are usually kept in the bedside stand. Therefore, you should request permission from the patient before opening the stand. A disposable washbasin, bedpan, and urinal may also be kept in the lower cabinet of this stand.

Hospital Beds

Hospitalized patients spend a significant amount of time in bed. Hospital beds can be uncomfortable and may contribute to restlessness and poor sleep. Memory foam and moisture control mattresses are available and provide more comfort. However, they are expensive and not used routinely. Hospital beds are generally standard in size and higher and narrower than a home bed. This allows you to reach the patient more easily and safely.

Hospital beds are usually electronically controlled, so the patient and nurse can raise and lower the head and foot separately by the push of a button (see Fig. 24-6 for bed positions).

✚ Patient safety is your priority, so although you should raise the entire bed to a working level that is comfortable for you, be sure to place the bed in the lowest position before leaving the bedside. Long-term care settings usually have low beds to make it easier for ambulatory patients to transfer into and out of bed. As a part of the admission procedure, you will teach patients how to use the bed controls.

Patients may use siderails when moving into and out of bed. Siderails may help to prevent falls for patients with decreased consciousness. However, siderails are considered a passive restraint and may pose risk to a patient with a cognitive impairment. See Chapter 23 for additional information about the safe use of siderails and other equipment.

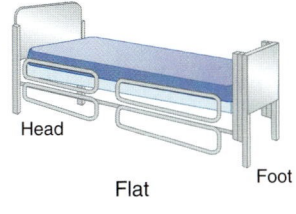

Flat

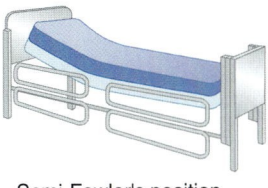

Semi-Fowler's position (30° angle)

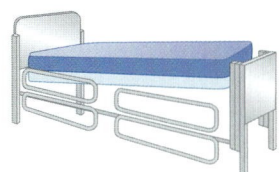

Trendelenburg's position

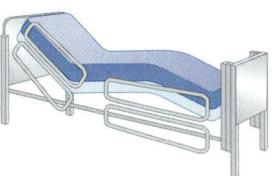

Fowler's position (45° angle)

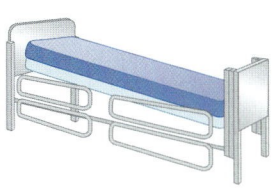

Reverse Trendelenburg's position

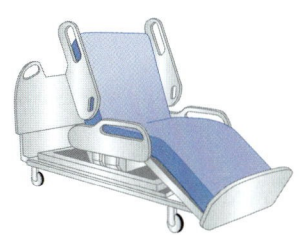

Sitting position (special wound-care beds; also adjust to standing postion)

FIGURE 24-6 Hospital beds adjust to several positions.

✚ Always be sure to lock the wheels on a hospital bed when it is stationary. For example, an unlocked bed could roll out from under an ambulatory patient who is moving from the bed to a chair. Ensure that the wheels are locked when you are helping the patient to a sitting position on the side of the bed or assisting with a transfer to a chair or stretcher.

Mattresses and Linens

Mattresses are usually firm and covered in a water-repellant material that resists staining and soiling and may be easily wiped down with a germicidal cleaner. A variety of special therapeutic mattresses are available to help reduce the effects of pressure over the bony prominences (e.g., sacrum, heels). See Chapter 36 for further discussion of special mattresses.

Using a mattress cover and/or pad promotes patient comfort and prevents soiling of the mattress. Plastic covers, however, do not allow moisture to escape, and contribute to skin maceration for patients who are incontinent or diaphoretic. If a plastic surface lies directly under the sheet, you should place a cloth or other absorbent pad between the patient and the sheet. Other linens include drawsheets, washable incontinence pads, pillowcases, blankets, bedspreads, and gowns.

Bed Making

Clean, wrinkle-free bed linens help promote comfort and a sense of well-being. In contrast, wrinkled and soiled linen can contribute to skin breakdown and pressure areas. Linens are generally changed daily after the bath and when soiled. If patients are up and about during the day, such as on a rehabilitation unit, beds are made daily, but bed linen may be changed weekly or only when soiled. If the patient is immobile or on bedrest, the bed is made while the patient occupies it. You or the NAP may make an unoccupied bed or an occupied bed. For more information about bed making, see Procedures 24-13 and 24-14.

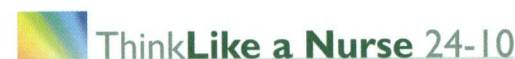 ThinkLike a Nurse 24-10

For which of your patients (Meet Your Patients) will you most surely need to make an occupied bed? Why?

CLINICALREASONING:
Applying the **Full-Spectrum Nursing Model**

Because the following critical thinking activities allow you to practice the kind of thinking you will use as a full-spectrum nurse, they usually have no single right answer. Discuss them with your peers—if you have difficulty with any of the questions, consult your instructor.

PATIENT SITUATION

Alice Baker is a frail elderly woman, 93 years old, who lives in a nursing home. She has almost total Self-Care Deficit related to her weakness, painful joints, and dementia. Her mental and physical conditions are not likely to improve. Imagine that your charge nurse has instructed you to provide a complete bed bath and other hygiene care for Ms. Baker. When you enter her room with bath supplies and say, "Good morning, Ms. Baker, it's time for your bath," she screams, "Go away from me. I just had a bath. I don't want a bath." You discuss this with the charge nurse, who says, "She has not had a bath, and she needs one today. You will need to do it whether she likes it or not." You tend to agree that Ms. Baker needs a bath because her clothing and linens have food stains, and she smells of urine and perspiration.

THINKING

1. *Theoretical Knowledge:*
    a. What benefits does a bath have for Ms. Baker?
    b. What are the disadvantages of bathing a patient with dementia who is resisting the bath?
2. *Critical Thinking (Considering Alternatives, Deciding What to Do):*
    a. What do you think Ms. Baker is feeling and experiencing, and how does that help you know what to do?
    b. What are some alternatives to a complete bed bath that would achieve the same purposes?

DOING

3. *Practical Knowledge:* Imagine that you have, indeed, decided that Ms. Baker needs a bath. Which type of bath you will give her? What supplies will you need, and where will you find them in the clinical agency you have attended most recently?

CARING

4. *Self-Knowledge:* What is your greatest concern about bathing Ms. Baker; what is the cause of your concern?

 Go To Chapter 24, **Clinical Reasoning: Applying the Full-Spectrum Nursing Model Response Sheet,** on DavisPlus.

Practical Knowledge procedures

The following procedures provide the practical knowledge you will need to assist patients with personal cleanliness and grooming.

Procedure 24-1 ■ Bathing: Providing a Complete Bed Bath

➤ For steps to follow in *all* procedures, refer to the Universal Steps for All Procedures found on the page facing the inside back cover.

✚ **Practice Alert!** Avoid traditional basin baths. This procedure is modified for use when a patient refuses a prepackaged product or when there is generalized gross soiling.

Equipment

- Disposable basin for water
- Bath blanket, bath towels (2) and washcloths
- Clean patient gown (with shoulder snaps or Velcro closures if the patient has an IV line)
- Clean bed linen
- No-rinse pH-balanced cleanser
- Orangewood stick
- Deodorant, lotion, and/or powder as needed
- Procedure gloves (for anal and perineal care)
- Bedpan or urinal
- Laundry bag
- Sterile or distilled water, if possible

Delegation

You can delegate this procedure to the NAP if the patient's condition and the NAP's skills allow. Perform the pre-procedure assessments, and inform the NAP of the specific type of bath (e.g., basin, bag bath) and the amount of help the patient needs. Inform the NAP of any special considerations, such as IV lines or drains. Ask the NAP to report the patient's skin condition, level of self-care, and ability to tolerate the procedure.

Pre-Procedure Assessments

- Assess mobility, activity tolerance, type of bath needed, and ability to perform bathing self-care.
  A patient who has decreased activity tolerance or mobility (e.g., chest pain or shortness of breath) may have limited ability to bathe. Having the patient assist as much as possible increases mobility and sense of control.
- Check for positioning or activity restrictions (e.g., maintaining hip abduction following a total hip replacement).
- Determine the number of people you need to safely bathe and reposition the patient.
  Helps prevent injury to the patient or the nurse.
- Assess for personal and cultural issues that may be of concern to the patient regarding the bath.
  Bathing may conflict with the patient's sense of privacy or modesty.
- Assess for specific patient needs and preferences, such as special soaps or lotions and extra washcloths or towels.
  Advanced age, the presence of skin conditions, or skin breakdown may require special soaps and/or lotions. Incontinence or drainage may require additional washcloths, towels, and precautions. Meeting patient preferences helps prevent depersonalization and promotes patient cooperation with the procedure.

➤ When performing the procedure, always identify your patient according to agency policy and be attentive to standard precautions, hand hygiene, patient safety and privacy, body mechanics, and documentation.

➤ *Note:* You may need to adapt the bathing order and other steps to meet individual needs.

Procedure Steps

1. **Provide for patient privacy and comfort.**
   a. Close the door or privacy curtains, adjust room temperature, and assist the patient with elimination as needed.
   b. Ask the patient and family if they wish family members to assist with the bath.
   Assisting the patient with elimination before beginning the bath helps
prevent interruptions during the procedure. Bathing practices differ among cultures and individuals, but are often private. The patient or family may wish to have a family member assist with the bath, or the patient may prefer that they leave the room.

2. ✚ Fill the basin with warm water (approximately 105°F, or 41°C). Check the temperature with a thermometer or your hand. If possible,
ask the patient to test the water temperature.

Use water that is comfortable for the patient. Hot water removes protective skin oils and can injure the patient. If the water is too cool, the patient may become chilled.

3. **Adjust the bed to working height**, lower the siderail nearest you, and position the patient supine close to the side of bed you will be working on.

(continued on next page)

Procedure 24-1 ■ Bathing: Providing a Complete Bed Bath (continued)

✚ **Raise the siderail before you leave that side of the bed.**

Prevents patient falls and keeps you from having to lean over the patient or reach across the siderail, which can cause back strain or injury.

4. **Remove the bedspread**, and **spread the bath blanket** over the top sheet; then ask the patient to hold the bath blanket in place while you remove the top sheet.

Protects modesty and prevents chilling. If no bath blanket is available, you can use the top sheet in its place. However, if the sheet becomes wet, it may chill the patient. ▼

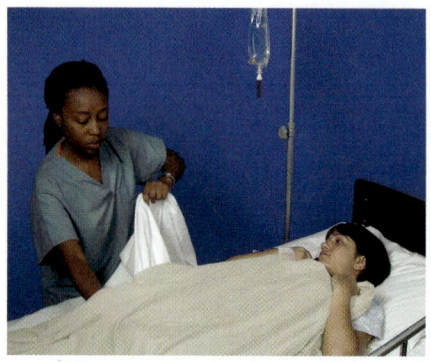

NOTE: *Before proceeding to the next step, assist the patient with oral hygiene. See Procedures 24-6 and 24-7, as needed.*

5. **Remove the patient's gown**, keeping the patient covered with the bath blanket. During the bath, expose just the part of the body you are bathing.

Maintains the patient's modesty and prevents chilling.

Patient With an IV Line

If the patient is wearing a gown that does not have snap-open sleeves:

  a. Remove the gown first from the arm without the IV.
  b. Lower the IV container, and pass the gown over the tubing and the container, keeping the container above the level of the patient's arm.

  Keeps blood from backing up into the IV line.

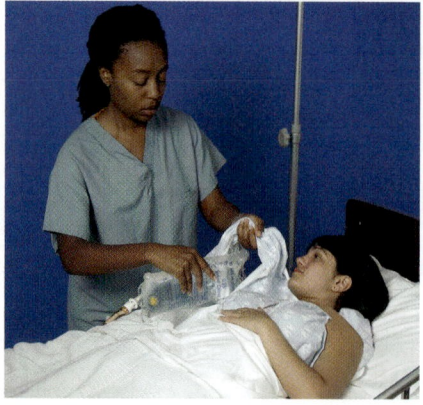

  c. ✚ *Never* disconnect the IV tubing; this breaks the sterile system and provides a portal of entry for pathogens.

  d. Rehang the container; check the flow rate.

  Manipulating the IV equipment may have changed the flow rate.

  e. After the bath, replace the gown by threading the IV equipment from inside the arm of the gown and onto the affected arm. Then place the unaffected arm through the other gown sleeve.

6. **Don procedure gloves** if exposure to body fluids is likely or if either you or the patient has any breaks in the skin.

Follows universal precautions; helps prevent transfer of microorganisms.

7. **Wash the patient's face, neck, and ears.**

  a. Fold the washcloth around the hand to make a mitt, tucking in loose corners.

  Keeps loose ends from dragging across the skin. This is uncomfortable because loose ends cool quickly.

  b. Wet the washcloth and wring out excess water. You may wash the face without cleanser if the skin is dry or if the patient prefers.

  c. Use a different corner of the washcloth (without soap) to gently wipe each eyelid outward from the inner canthus.

  Soap is irritating to the eyes and drying to the skin. A major principle is

cleaning from "clean to dirty" to prevent contamination of a cleaner area. The inner canthus is considered the cleanest area. Prevents moving debris toward the nasolacrimal duct, which is located near the inner canthus. ▼

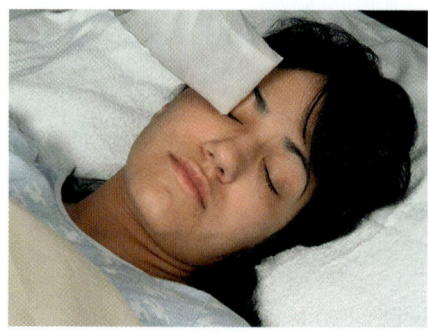

  d. Wash the rest of the patient's face, neck, and ears.

  Move sequentially through the bath to make it less tiring for the patient and more efficient for the nurse.

  e. Rinse as needed, and pat face and neck dry.

  A no-rinse cleanser is preferred. Pat instead of rubbing to avoid irritation.

8. **Wash the patient's arms and chest.**

  a. Rinse and wring out the washcloth.

  Rinse the washcloth frequently to ensure that it is clean and warm.

  b. Fold the bath blanket off one arm at a time, and place a folded bath towel under the arm. Beginning with the patient's far arm, support the arm, and wash the arm from the hands upward using long strokes.

  The folded towel keeps the bottom sheet from getting wet and cold. Long strokes increase circulation in the extremity. Washing from distal to proximal increases venous return from the periphery. Lifting the arm provides range of motion to preserve joint mobility.

  c. Continue to support the arm while washing the axilla.

  A sprain, subluxation, or dislocation of the joint can occur when an

extremity is not properly supported, especially in older adults.

d. Rinse as needed, and pat the arms dry.

Preserves skin integrity by preventing the drying effect of the cleanser.

e. Apply deodorant and/or powder if desired.

Follow patient preferences whenever possible to increase feelings of comfort.

f. Place the basin of water on the towel. Place the patient's hand in the water. Wash and dry. Clean under the nails with an orangewood stick as needed.

Soaking the hand helps with cleaning under the fingernails and promotes comfort.

g. Repeat the preceding steps 8a–f for the arm nearest you.

h. Cover the patient's chest with a bath towel, and lower the bath blanket to the patient's waist.

Maintains patient warmth and modesty.

i. Wash the chest. For women, gently lift each breast to wash the skinfold if needed. Keep the chest covered between the wash and rinse.

Skinfolds are a source of odor and can become reddened and irritated because of skin-to-skin irritation and dampness from perspiration.

j. Pat the chest dry. Cover with a bath towel.

9. **Wash the abdomen, legs, and feet.**

a. Fold the bath blanket down to the perineal area, and cover the chest with a bath towel.

b. Wash the abdomen, including the umbilical area; pat dry. Pay special attention to any skinfolds.

Helps promote cleanliness and drying and prevents irritation. Perspiration and bath water do not evaporate well from skinfolds, predisposing skinfolds to maceration.

c. Cover the abdomen and chest with the bath blanket.

Prevents chilling.

d. Uncover one leg at a time, beginning with the leg farthest from

you. Place the bath towel under the leg.

Keeps the sheet dry; prevents chilling.

e. Place the basin of water on the towel. Supporting the ankle and heel with your hand, and the leg on your arm, help the patient bend his leg and place his foot in the basin of water to soak.

Support reduces strain on joints. Soaking allows for better cleansing of the foot, especially the toes and nails, and increases patient comfort.

f. Wash the leg from distal to proximal with long, gentle strokes. Rinse and pat the leg dry.

✚ Do not massage the calves of the legs.

Washing from distal to proximal may help to promote venous return. If a venous thrombus is present, massaging might dislodge the clot and cause an embolus. ▼

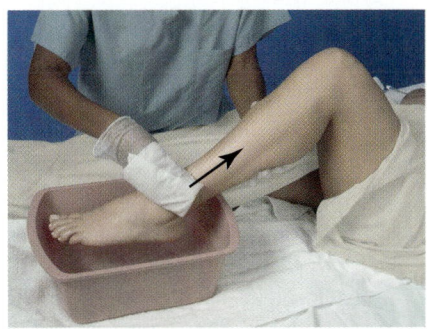

g. Thoroughly wash the foot and toes. Pat the foot dry; dry well between the toes. Apply lotion as needed, but not between the toes.

Disease processes frequently decrease circulation to the feet and lower legs, increasing the likelihood that minor skin irritations may become more severe. Leaving damp areas between the toes can lead to skin breakdown.

h. Repeat the procedure on the other leg.

10. **Wash the back and buttocks.**

a. Position the patient on his side with his back facing you, or in the prone position. Make sure the siderail on the far side of the bed, facing the patient, is still up.

Provides for clear visualization of back and access to the area.

b. Exposing only the back and buttocks, place the bath towel under the back and buttocks. Wash the back first and then the buttocks. Pat dry, paying particular attention to gluteal folds. Observe for redness and skin breakdown in the sacral area.

Maintains the principle of "clean to dirty." The sacral area is a common site of pressure sores. Bath towel keeps bottom sheet from getting wet and cold. ▼

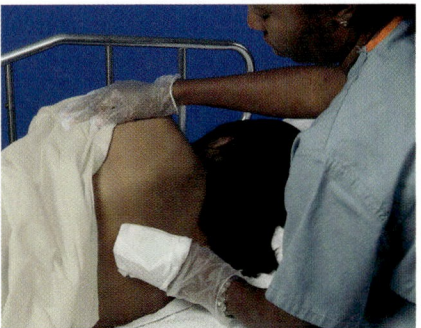

c. Unless contraindicated, give the patient a back rub, applying lotion to the back and buttocks (see Chapter 35, Procedure 35-1: Giving a Back Massage).

Stimulates circulation and maintains the health of the skin. Because the patient is in bed, he is at risk for skin irritation and breakdown from immobility and friction. A back rub may be contraindicated for patients with musculoskeletal injuries or cardiovascular disease.

d. Don procedure gloves if you have not already done so and remove any fecal matter with tissues before washing the rectal area with the washcloth. Wash from front to back.

Washing the rectal area at this time removes the need for the patient to turn to his side again and helps prevent soiling clean linen when changing the linen in an occupied bed. Fecal matter usually contains microorganisms. Washing from front to back helps

(continued on next page)

Procedure 24-1 ■ Bathing: Providing a Complete Bed Bath (continued)

prevent transferring bacteria from the rectum to the vagina and urethra. ▼

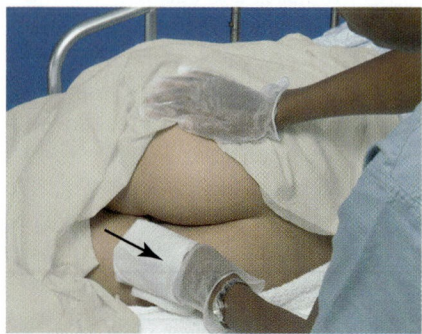

e. Discard the soiled washcloth, and change the bathwater. Wash and wipe out the basin before refilling it. Cover any soiled linen before repositioning the patient.

f. Remove soiled gloves and wash hands or use an alcohol-based hand rub. Don new procedure gloves before providing perineal care.

Prevents transferring microorganisms from anal to genital area—cleansing the gluteal and anal areas contaminates the washcloth, towel, and water. Maintains standard precautions during the bath and prevents soiling of clean linens during bed change and cross contamination to other body sites.

11. **Wash the perineal area.** See Procedure 24-4 as needed.

12. **After providing perineal care, reposition and cover the patient with the bath blanket.** Remove soiled gloves and wash hands or use alcohol-based handrub. Help the patient put on a clean gown, and attend to other hygiene needs (e.g., hair grooming).

Prevents contaminating clean linen with soiled gloves. Ensures proper body position and warmth.

13. **Change the bed linen** as needed, including soiled linen or linen that became damp during the bath. See Procedure 24-13 or 24-14.

Ensures patient safety, comfort, and privacy.

14. **Dispose of the bath basin.**

A recent study concluded that bath basins are a reservoir for bacteria and may be a source of healthcare-associated infections. (Johnson, Lineweaver, & Maze, 2009). The AACN (2013) recommends using disposable basins, stored in central storage.

? What if . . .

■ **You are bathing the patient without assistance, or you are not tall enough to comfortably reach across the patient?**

These situations put you at risk for back strain. Thus, you may want to bathe one side of the body—that is, the right arm, trunk, right leg—and then move to the other side of the bed to bathe the opposite side of the body (instead of the order given in steps 8 and 9). Move the patient close to you before beginning the bath.

■ **You are bathing a patient in leg traction?**

You may decide to bathe the arms and trunk first. Then have the patient sit forward so that you can cleanse his back. Next have the patient lift up slightly so that you can wash his buttocks. Finally, wash the lower extremities.

■ **You are bathing a patient with dementia?**

Use your knowledge of the person's bathing practices and preferences to determine a time of day and a routine the person will accept. Keep stimulation to a minimum. Turn on some calming music, speak softly and reassuringly, and don't rush. Keep the patient warm. If the patient becomes agitated and you cannot calm him, do not force him to bathe. A towel bath is preferred if the patient will agree to it (Procedure 24-2). Also refer to Clinical Insight 24-2.

Many steps in the bathing process may be misinterpreted or stressful for the

person with dementia and may present in the appearance of disruptive or agitated behaviors. If forced to bathe, the patient may be upset for hours. Towel baths are effective hygiene measures.

■ **Your patient becomes agitated and uncooperative during the bath?**

Speak calmly and softly. Give the patient a few minutes to calm down. Discontinue the bath if the patient remains upset.

Your patient is an older adult?

a. Administer a bag bath with no-rinse skin cleanser, if possible.
   These help prevent skin dryness.

b. If you use a tub bath use warm, not hot, water.
   Prevents burns (older adults may have decreased sensation in their extremities).

c. Clean the tub well after each use *to prevent infection.*

d. Use antibacterial cleanser or a mild soap substitute. If you must use soap, it should be perfume-free and rich in moisture. If you use soap, rinse the skin well.

e. Pat the skin dry; do not rub.

f. Apply a moisturizer immediately after drying, while there is still moisture in the skin. Wash your hands before applying the moisturizer.

g. Cleanse the skin immediately after every incident of soiling (e.g., after a bowel movement).
   Prevents maceration and irritation from enzyme activity.

h. Some clinicians recommend bathing older adults every other day instead of daily, and it is generally agreed that they should not bathe more than once a day unless soiling occurs.

Evaluation

- Assess how well the patient tolerated the procedure. Was there any discomfort, shortness of breath, and so on?
- Observe the patient's mobility, both range of motion and ease of movement.
- Note the skin condition, including redness and other abnormal findings, especially in skinfolds.
- Ask the patient whether he is comfortable and satisfied.
- If someone other than the nurse performs the procedure, the nurse must still evaluate the care to be certain that it was done and performed satisfactorily.

Patient Teaching

- Discuss the need for activity (e.g., moving about in bed) and the hazards of immobility.
- Discuss usual skin care and how to increase the health of the skin.
- Demonstrate bathing procedure to family or other caregivers.

Home Care

NOTE: Many of the following apply to older adults and others with self-care deficits.

- Evaluate the home for bathing safety considerations (not limited to bed bath), such as the following:
  - Safety bars in the bathroom?
  - A safe water supply for bathing?
  - Bathing supplies that are available and accessible?
  - Nonskid mat or abrasive strips for shower or tub?
  - Stool for shower; transfer bench or stool for getting into the tub?
  - Hand-held shower spray?
  - Long-handled brush or sponge?
- Assess the client's ability to help with the bath or to bathe independently.
- Ask how the client usually bathes (e.g., shower, at the sink). Follow the client's preference as much as possible.
- Ask what supplies the client usually uses, and ask where they are stored. You will need to adapt the procedure depending on the available equipment and supplies.
- Suggest the use of large plastic trash bags or a shower curtain to protect the mattress during a bed bath.
- Instruct caregivers to wear gloves when handling linens that are soiled with blood or other body fluids. Linens should be washed in cold water, separately from other household laundry, and then washed again, using hot water, detergent, and bleach.

  Hot water coagulates proteins in the blood and makes it more difficult to remove. Detergent and bleach are used to destroy pathogens.

Documentation

Chart the type of bath given, how much patient was able to help with the bath, how well the patient tolerated the procedure, the patient's mobility, and any abnormal findings. Hygiene care is charted on checklists and flow sheets in most agencies.

Practice Resources

American Association of Critical Care Nurses, 2013; Downey & Lloyd, 2008; Dunn, Thiru-Chelvam, & Beck, 2002; Flori, 2007; George, & Naik, 2006; Haas, & Larson, 2008; Johnson, Lineweaver, & Maze, 2009; Kovach & Meyer-Arnold, 1997; O'Flynn, 2007; Siegel, Rhinehart, Jackson, et al., 2007; Stern, 2007.

Thinking About the Procedure

 Go to the *Fundamentals of Nursing Skills Videos*, **Hygiene: Bed Bath, Oral Hygiene, Foot Care, and Back Massage.**

1. After the patient performs oral hygiene, how many basins of water does the nurse fill for the bath? Why?
2. How did the nurse check the temperature of the water?

 For suggested responses, go to Chapter 24, **Thinking About the Procedure Suggested Responses,** on Davis*Plus*.

Procedure 24-2 ■ Bathing: Providing a Towel Bath

> For steps to follow in *all* procedures, refer to the Universal Steps for All Procedures found on the page facing the inside back cover.

> Note: Because the towel bath is a variation of the bed bath, only the steps differing from a bed bath are listed.

Equipment

- Large plastic bag containing a bath blanket (or a very large towel, about 3 ft × 6 ft), one standard bath towel, and two or three washcloths
- Dry bath blankets (two or more) and dry bath towels
- Pitcher and approximately 2 qt (2,000 mL) of warm water (105°F [41°C]). Use distilled or sterile water if available and agency policy allows.
- 30 mL of no-rinse liquid cleanser or commercial solution of soap, moisturizer, and disinfectant
- Other supplies for a bed bath; see Procedure 24-1.

Delegation

You can delegate this procedure to the NAP if the patient's condition and the NAP's skills allow. Perform the pre-procedure assessments, and inform the NAP of the amount of help the patient needs and any special considerations, such as IV lines and drains. Ask the NAP to report the patient's skin condition, level of self-care, and ability to tolerate the procedure.

(continued on next page)

Procedure 24-2 ■ Bathing: Providing a Towel Bath (continued)

Pre-Procedure Assessments

- Assess mobility and activity tolerance to determine whether the patient will be able to assist with the bath, whether a bag bath is appropriate, and the amount of help you will need.

A patient with decreased activity tolerance or mobility (e.g., because of chest pain or shortness of breath with exertion) may have limited ability to assist with the bath. For severely compromised patients, having two nurses give the bath will make the procedure quicker and less demanding on the patient.

➤ When performing the procedure, always identify your patient according to agency policy and be attentive to standard precautions, hand hygiene, patient safety and privacy, body mechanics, and documentation.

Procedure Steps

1. **Prepare the towel bag.**
   a. Prefold the bath blanket.
      Allows for organized application and ease of handling the blanket.
   b. Fill a large pitcher with about 2,000 mL of warm distilled or sterile water (approximately 105°F [41°C]).
      The amount of water varies depending on the size of the bath blanket and bath towel. Use enough water to saturate them. Hot water can injure the patient and removes more of the skin's protective oils, but if the water is too cool, the patient may become chilled.
   c. Add 30 mL no-rinse soap solution to the water according to the manufacturer's instructions.
      Adding a prescribed amount of solution before pouring water into the bag prevents excessive sudsing.
   d. Pour the solution into the bag, over the bath blanket and bath towel, to ensure even distribution.
2. **If you do not plan to change the linen**, work one dry bath blanket under the patient.
   Protects the linen and provides warmth.
3. **Spread a dry bath blanket over the patient**; remove the patient's clothing, working underneath the blanket.
   Protects privacy and prevents chilling.
4. **Replace the dry blanket** with the wet blanket:
   a. Take the wet bath blanket or towel out of the bag, squeezing out excess water so that it does not drip.
   b. Push the dry bath blanket down to the patient's waist, and place the wet bath blanket on the patient's chest.

   c. Continue to unfold the wet bath blanket until it covers the patient, pushing the dry bath blanket out of the way as you do so.
      The wet bath blanket will feel warm and relaxing. You will use the dry bath blanket to dry the patient.
   d. If necessary, place yet another dry blanket on top of the wet one.
      This helps hold in the warmth if the patient is chilling or the room is cool.
5. **Bathe the patient**, beginning at the feet and working toward the head.
   a. Keeping the patient covered, use the wet bath blanket to wash the legs, abdomen, and chest.
   b. As you work, replace the wet bath blanket with the dry one.
      Keeps the patient from chilling. ▼

   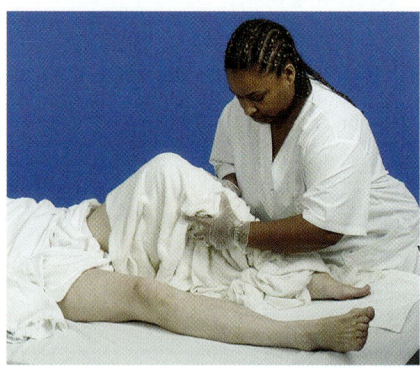

   c. Fold the wet bath blanket as each area is bathed, allowing only clean surfaces to contact clean surfaces.
      Prevents contamination of the clean side of the wet bath blanket.
   d. Use one of the wet washcloths to wash the patient's face, neck, and ears.
      Notice that this varies from the order of most baths, which proceed from head to toe. However, this is the most efficient way to accomplish a towel bath. It does not compromise the clean-to-dirty principle because the

   legs, abdomen, and chest are usually equally "clean," and you are washing those before the back, buttocks, and perineum.
6. **Don procedure gloves**. Roll the client to one side, unfold the wet bath towel so the clean surface covers the patient, and use the wet bath towel to wash the back and then the buttocks.
7. **Change procedure gloves and wash your hands.** Wash the perineal area with a washcloth. See Procedure 24-4, as needed.
8. **Finish the bath** as in Procedure 24-1. Follow patient preferences whenever possible to increase feelings of comfort.
9. **Change linen as needed**, including soiled linen or linen that became damp during the bath. You will almost certainly need to change the linen if you have not padded the bottom sheet well before the bath.
   Ensures patient safety and comfort. Because the bath is finished rapidly, there is no need to pad the bottom sheet if you know that you will have time to change the linens after the bath.

? What if . . .

- **Your patient becomes agitated and uncooperative during the bath?**

   Speak calmly and softly. Give the patient a few minutes to calm down. Discontinue the bath if the patient remains upset.

Practice Resources

AACN, 2013; Downey & Lloyd, 2008; Flori, 2007; Joanna Briggs Institute, 2007.

Procedure 24-3 ■ **Bathing: Providing a Packaged Bath**

➤ For steps to follow in *all* procedures, refer to the Universal Steps for All Procedures found on the page facing the inside back cover.

Equipment
- Packaged disposable washcloths (e.g., Comfort Bath)

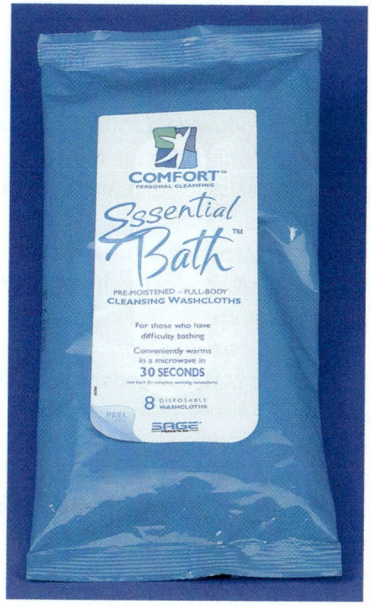

- Lotion, deodorant, and/or powder as needed
- Clean patient gown (with shoulder snaps or Velcro closures if the patient has an IV line)
- Clean linen
- Procedure gloves
- Plastic trash bag for used cloths and other disposable soiled items

Delegation
You can delegate this procedure to the NAP if the patient's condition and the NAP's skills allow. Perform the pre-procedure assessments, and inform the NAP of the amount of help the patient needs and of any special considerations, such as IV lines or drains. Ask the NAP to report the skin condition, level of self-care, and ability to tolerate the procedure.

Pre-Procedure Assessments
Assessments are the same as in Procedure 24-1, Bathing: Providing a Complete Bed Bath.

➤ When performing the procedure, always identify your patient according to agency policy and be attentive to standard precautions, hand hygiene, patient safety and privacy, body mechanics, and documentation.

Procedure Steps

1. **Peel open the label** on the commercial bath without completely removing it.
   Allows for steam to escape as contents heat without spilling the contents.
2. **Warm the solution:**
   Helps prevent chilling the patient.

If Using a Microwave

➕ Heat the package in the microwave for no longer than 1 minute. The temperature of the contents should be approximately 105°F (41°C). This step is controversial. Some references suggest, for safety, using the commercial bag bath at room temperature.

If Using a Warmer Unit
You do not need step 2 because the bags are always warm.

3. **Prepare the patient for the bath** as described in Procedure 24-1.
4. **Using one washcloth for each body area,** wash the patient

following the sequence in Procedure 24-1. Or follow the manufacturer's recommended sequence for the number of washcloths in the bag.
5. **Allow body areas to air dry;** do not rinse.
   Prevents the emollient and surfactant skin protectants from being removed.
6. **Discard each washcloth after use.**
   Ensures following the "clean to dirty" principle.
7. **Help patient don a clean gown.**

❓ What if . . .

- **A commercial bag bath is not available?**
  You can make your own bag bath. The washcloths can be prepared ahead of time and kept in a warming unit if one is available. But do not store for longer than 24 hours, to prevent bacterial growth.
  a. Place eight washcloths in a large self-locking plastic bag.

b. Mix an emollient or a no-rinse surfactant with warm water, and pour over the washcloths in the bag.
c. If the water is not warm enough (105°F [41°C]), warm in a microwave oven for 1 to 2 minutes. Check the temperature of the washcloths before using.
d. Use one cloth for each of the following areas: face, back, chest, right arm, left arm, right leg, left leg, perineum.
e. Put used washcloths in the laundry for future use.

For Evaluation, Documentation, and Patient Teaching, see Procedure 24-1: Bathing: Providing a Complete Bed Bath.

Practice Resources
AACN, 2013; Birch & Coggins, 2003; Chu, 2004; Joanna Briggs Institute, 2007; Larson, Ciliberti, Chantler, et al., 2004.

Procedure 24-4 ■ Providing Perineal Care

➤ For steps to follow in *all* procedures, refer to the Universal Steps for All Procedures found on the page facing the inside back cover.

Equipment

- Procedure gloves
- Disposable basin or perineal wash bottle
- Waterproof pad
- Bedpan or disposable sitz tub (optional)
- Bath towel and washcloth
- Toilet paper
- Cleansing solution
- Perineal ointment or lotion, if needed

Delegation

You can delegate perineal care to the NAP if the patient's condition and the NAP's skills allow. Perform the pre-procedure assessments, and inform the NAP of the amount of help the patient needs and any special considerations (e.g., presence of a urinary catheter, vaginal drainage). Ask the NAP to report the condition of the patient's perineum (skin, drainage), level of self-care, and ability to tolerate the procedure.

Pre-Procedure Assessments

- Assess mobility and activity tolerance.
  Determine whether the patient will be able to assist with the perineal care. Doing as much self-care as possible increases the patient's sense of independence and maintains modesty.
- Check for positioning or activity restrictions, such as maintaining hip abduction following a total hip replacement.
  Prevents injuring the patient during the procedure.
- Assess for psychosocial issues that may concern the patient regarding perineal care.
  You must consider cultural norms to ensure that the perineal care is appropriate for the patient. For example, in some cultures a woman would find it completely unacceptable for a male nurse to perform her perineal care (pericare).
- Assess for any specific patient needs for perineal care.
  For example, if there are lesions or skin breakdown, you may need to use special soaps and/or lotions. Incontinence or drainage requires assessment and follow-up to prevent Impaired Skin Integrity.
- Assess for the presence of a urinary drainage catheter, perineal surgery, or lesions.
  You may need to adapt the procedure to clean around an indwelling urinary catheter or surgical incisions.

➤ When performing the procedure, always identify your patient according to agency policy and be attentive to standard precautions, hand hygiene, patient safety and privacy, body mechanics, and documentation.

Procedure Steps

1. **Adjust the room temperature,** and assist with elimination as needed.
   Assisting the patient with elimination before perineal care helps prevent interruptions during the procedure and allows for thorough cleansing. Adjusting room temperature prevents chilling.

2. ✚ **Fill the basin or perineal wash bottle** with warm water (approximately 105°F [41°C]). Use distilled or sterile water, if available and in accord with agency policy.

   Hot water can injure the skin, and cool water can cause chilling. Use water that is comfortable for the patient.

3. **Wash the perineal area.**
   a. Position the patient on her back (supine). Place waterproof pads under the patient if they are not already in place. You may wish to

place the patient on a bedpan or disposable sitz tub, especially if the perineum is grossly soiled.
   Placing the patient on a bedpan raises the hips to increase visualization and allows for more thorough cleansing. A bedpan also allows for using additional water when needed.
   b. Wear procedure gloves (and other protective wear as needed) when providing perineal care. Wear a procedure gown and goggles if you are concerned about splashing (e.g., if the patient is confused and may be unable to follow instructions).
   When providing perineal care there is a possibility of coming in contact with urine, vaginal secretions, or fecal material.
   c. Drape the patient to protect privacy.

For Female Patients
- Drape the bath blanket so that one point faces the patient's head (drape it in the shape of a diamond).
- Take one of the side points of the diamond, and wrap it around the patient's leg. Anchor the end of the blanket under the patient's foot.
- Repeat on the other leg with other point of the diamond. ▼

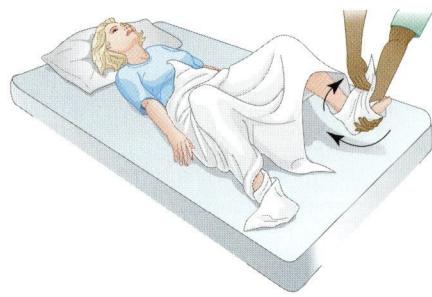

- Fold the center lower point of the diamond up to expose the patient's perineum.

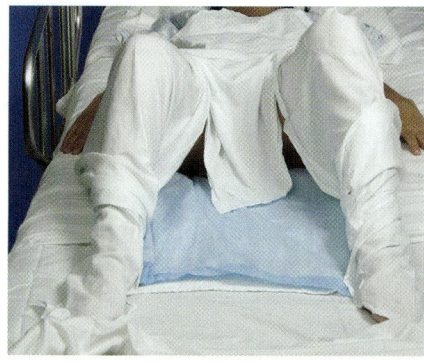

This draping technique covers the patient as much as possible, which helps maintain privacy and prevents chilling during the procedure. The patient can also relax her legs against the bath blanket.

For Male Patients

- Place the bath blanket over the patient's chest.
- Fold the bed linens down to expose only the patient's groin.
  - d. Remove any fecal material with toilet paper.
    Prevents contamination of the perineum with feces, which can lead to bladder or incisional infections. If you are providing perineal care as part of giving a bed bath, you will have cleaned the anal area when the patient was in the lateral position.
  - e. Moisten the washcloth with the water in the basin, or spray the perineum with the perineal wash bottle.
    Moistens the area or washcloth thoroughly to ensure adequate cleansing.
  - f. Wash the perineum.

Female Patient

Wash the perineum from front to back, using a clean portion of the washcloth for each stroke. Cleanse the labial folds and around the urinary catheter, if one is in place.

Prevents contaminating the urethra with fecal material. Any fecal particles that are left can cause skin breakdown due to enzyme activity, and may increase the risk of a urinary tract infection because of the presence of Escherichia coli in the feces.

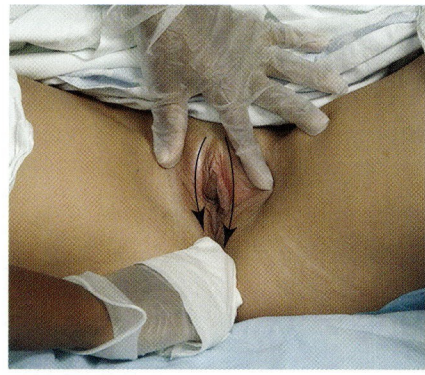

Male Patient

Retract the foreskin, if present, and gently cleanse the head of the penis using a circular motion. Replace the foreskin, and finish washing the shaft of the penis, using firm strokes. Then wash the scrotum, using a clean portion of the washcloth with each stroke. Handle the scrotum with care, because the area is sensitive.

To adequately clean the head of the penis in an uncircumcised male, you must retract the foreskin. After cleaning, replace the foreskin to prevent constriction and edema of the penis.

Firm strokes may help to prevent an erection. Using a clean portion of the washcloth for each wipe prevents fecal contamination of the urethra and perineum. ▼

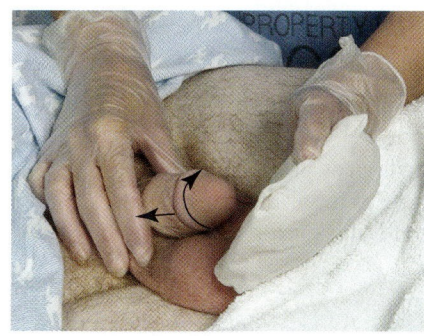

- g. In both males and females, cleanse the skinfolds of the groin area thoroughly. Examine the skin creases for redness or excoriation.
  Detects and prevents excoriation in skinfold areas, where moisture accumulates.
4. **Rinse, if not using no-rinse cleanser, and pat dry.**
  Prevents skin injury secondary to maceration. If you are using perineal wash solution, rinsing is not required.

5. **If perineal care is not being done as part of the bath,** also clean the anal area. Ask the patient to turn to the side, and wash, rinse, and dry the buttocks and anal area as needed.
   Fecal contamination of the perineum can lead to urinary tract infections and skin irritation. Therefore, the anal area is cleansed last.
6. **Apply skin protectants** as needed. Powder only if the patient requests it.
   If urinary or fecal incontinence is present, skin barriers may be used to prevent urine, feces, or other drainage from contacting the skin. This helps prevent skin breakdown. For female patients, powder is a medium for bacterial growth. In the presence of moisture, it also creates a paste, which irritates the skin.
7. **If the patient has an indwelling catheter** and if agency policy requires special catheter care, you will usually provide the care at this point. Don clean gloves before providing catheter care, and follow the agency's procedure. For more information about catheter care, see Caring for a Patient With an Indwelling Catheter, in Chapter 30.
8. **Reposition and cover** the patient with the bath blanket. Remove soiled gloves, discarding appropriately.
   Prevents contaminating clean linen with soiled gloves.
9. **Change linen as needed,** including soiled linen or linen that became damp during perineal care.
   Ensures patient safety, comfort, and privacy.

? What if . . .

- **The patient is unable to control bowels and/or bladder?**

Gently cleanse and dry the perineal/perigenital area after each incontinence/soiling and apply a moisture barrier according to agency protocols.
Minimizing contact with irritants such as moisture, urine, and stool can help prevent incontinence-associated dermatitis.
Use a spray, no-rinse cleanser and soft wipes.

(continued on next page)

Procedure 24-4 ■ Providing Perineal Care (continued)

These help prevent irritation from friction, and reduce drying effects on the skin.
Follow agency policy and use skin assessment tools (some geared particularly to perineal skin):
- Assess for signs of secondary infection in addition to irritation and report as needed.

- Consider bowel and bladder retraining and scheduling to reduce frequency of incontinence.

- **The patient is postpartum?**
Educate the patient about perineal care. Include the importance of handwashing before and after cleansing the perineum, measures to keep the perineum clean, frequent changing of sanitary pads, and checking for signs and symptoms of abnormal lochia. If the patient had an episiotomy, laceration, or tear, also teach management of discomfort and signs of wound infection.

Evaluation

- Assess the patient's responses to the procedure. Was there any discomfort?
- Observe for difficulty with movement or range of motion during the procedure.
- Note the condition of the skin, including redness and other abnormal findings.
- Ask the patient whether she feels comfortable now.

Patient Teaching

- Discuss adaptations to perineal care. For example, if the area is tender wash the area with warm water after going to the bathroom, instead of using toilet paper; or use a skin protectant on the area.
- Review the importance of handwashing after elimination.
- If appropriate, teach the caregiver how to provide perineal care, including the principle of cleaning front to back ("clean to dirty"). Stress the importance of wearing gloves and washing hands.
- Advise women not to douche because it disturbs the balance of normal vaginal flora and can irritate or injure mucosal cells.
- Explain that scented and deodorant feminine hygiene products are not necessary for cleanliness and may even be harmful. Plain soap and water are the most effective means of odor control.

Home Care

- Evaluate the ability of the client or caregiver to provide perineal care.
- Determine the availability of supplies needed for perineal care.

- You will need to adapt the procedure depending on the available equipment and supplies. Major issues involved in perineal care in the home are the lack of clean water and/or linens. In some instances, you may need to use bottled water or boil water for the procedure. A preferred option is to use prepackaged moistened towelettes (e.g., Comfort Bath towelettes). These products may be heated in a water bath or microwave oven.

Documentation

Usually perineal care is part of routine hygiene care and is charted on a flow sheet. If you need to write a narrative note, chart that perineal care was given, any patient responses to the procedure, and the condition of the perineal area.

Practice Resources

Bliss, Zehrer, Savik, et al., 2006; Gray, Bliss, Doughty, et al., 2007; National Collaborating Centre for Primary Care, 2006; Siegel, Rhinehart, Jackson, et al., 2007; Warshaw, Nix, Kula, et al., 2002.

Thinking About the Procedure

Go to the *Fundamentals of Nursing Skills Videos*, **Perineal Care: Female, and Perineal Care: Male.**

1. In the skill Perineal Care: Female, do you think this patient is incontinent of urine or feces? Why or why not?
2. In the skill Perineal Care: Male, what did the nurse use to protect the patient's privacy before beginning the procedure?

For suggested responses, go to Chapter 24, **Thinking About the Procedure Suggested Responses,** on Davis*Plus.*

Procedure 24-5 ■ Providing Foot Care

➤ For steps to follow in *all* procedures, refer to the Universal Steps for All Procedures found on the page facing the inside back cover.

Equipment

- Procedure gloves (if there are open lesions)
- Pillow (if procedure is done with the patient in bed)
- Disposable basin for water (consult agency policy)
- Liquid no-rinse soap

- Bath towel and washcloth
- Waterproof pad
- Orangewood stick
- Toenail clippers and nail file
- Lotion or prescribed ointment or cream

Delegation

You can delegate foot care to the NAP if the patient's condition and the NAP's skills allow. For example, as a rule you should not delegate care if the patient has impaired peripheral circulation or foot ulcers. Perform the pre-procedure assessments, and inform the NAP of the amount of help the patient needs and any special considerations (e.g., ability to sit in a chair). Ask the NAP to report the condition of the patient's skin and nails, level of self-care, and ability to tolerate the procedure.

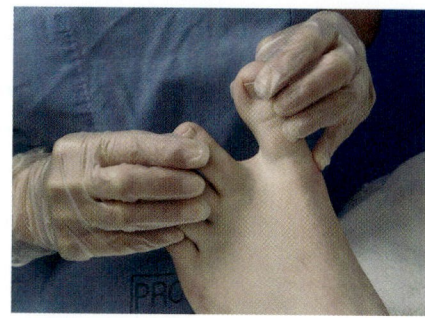

Pre-Procedure Assessments

- As you assess the feet and toenails, compare findings for both feet.
- Assess bilateral dorsalis pedis pulses, capillary refill, skin color, and warmth. Palpate pulses at the same time bilaterally to determine whether one side is weaker than the other.
  Decreased circulation to the feet increases the risk for tissue injury and infection. A variety of diseases can cause poor circulation. For example, cardiac or renal disease may cause pedal edema, which impairs circulation to the skin, and diabetes causes vascular changes leading to poor circulation to the lower extremities.
- Assess for diseases (e.g., diabetes mellitus and peripheral vascular disease) that create risks for foot problems.
- Thoroughly assess all areas of the feet for skin integrity, edema, condition of toenails, and any abnormalities. Check carefully between the toes for cracks or fungal infection.
  Decreased circulation in the feet commonly causes such problems as thickened toenails, dry skin, and increased risk of infection. Changes in vision and mobility can increase the risk for injuries to the feet. Patients with diabetes also may have neuropathy, which prevents them from knowing when they have injured their feet. Identifying abnormalities enables you to provide interventions to help prevent potential problems.

- Check institutional policy to verify whether a nurse is allowed to trim nails. Obtain a primary provider's prescription for trimming the patient's nails, if necessary.
  Patients who have diabetes or impaired circulation to the lower extremities require a prescription for trimming their nails. Refer the patient to a podiatrist if the circulation is severely compromised or if edema would make the procedure difficult.
- Assess the patient's usual footwear.
  Improperly fitting shoes, especially if they are too tight, are a common cause of foot problems (e.g., bunions, ingrown toenails).
- Assess the patient's self-care ability to provide foot care. Evaluate the need for a referral. Determine whether the patient has the necessary vision and mobility to be able to provide his own foot care.
- Assess the patient's knowledge about foot care, including usual foot care practices.

  ✚ Identify potential deficits in understanding that may require additional teaching or referral to a podiatrist, general practice physician, or advanced practice nurse. Many home remedies for foot problems can damage the tissue. For example, corn pads can increase pressure on the tissue, compromising circulation and causing local tissue ischemia. Cutting the sides of the toenails can lead to ingrown toenails.

➤ When performing the procedure, always identify your patient according to agency policy and be attentive to standard precautions, hand hygiene, patient safety and privacy, body mechanics, and documentation.

Procedure Steps

1. **Wear procedure gloves** and other protective wear as needed when providing foot care.
   Follows standard precautions. The heel is a common place for skin breakdown, so use gloves if you are unable to see the area without lifting the foot. If the patient has significant drainage to the area, such as a draining wound, you may need to wear a protective gown.
2. **Ask the patient to sit in a chair** with a waterproof pad or bath towel under the feet, if possible. If the

patient is unable to sit in a chair, place him in semi-Fowler's position in bed; place a pillow under his knees.
It is easier to perform the procedure with the patient in a chair. The pillow supports the knee joints and prevents muscle fatigue.

3. ✚ **Fill the basin halfway** with warm water (approximately 105°F to 110°F [40°C to 43°C]). Use distilled or sterile water, if possible.
   Hot water can injure the skin. Warm water promotes circulation. Filling the basin halfway prevents spilling when the patient places his foot in the water.

4. **Help the patient place one foot in the water,** first checking with the patient that the temperature is comfortable.
   a. If the patient is in a chair, place the basin on the floor (on the waterproof pad).
   b. If the patient is in bed, place the basin near the foot of the bed on the waterproof pad; pad the basin with a towel.
   The waterproof pad keeps the bed dry. Padding the basin prevents pressure on the back of the leg, which could cause discomfort and interfere with circulation.

(continued on next page)

Procedure 24-5 ■ Providing Foot Care (continued)

5. **Allow the foot to soak** for 5 to 20 minutes, depending on the patient's tolerance and the condition of his feet. ✚ Soaking is not recommended for patients with diabetes or peripheral vascular disease (PVD).

   Soaking softens the skin and helps relax the patient. For patients who have diabetes or PVD, soaking is not recommended because it may remove natural oils and cause cracking of the skin, and may cause burns even if the water is at the recommended temperature.

6. **Clean the foot** with mild (preferably no-rinse) soap.

   Removes loose debris. No-rinse soaps do not dry the skin. ▼

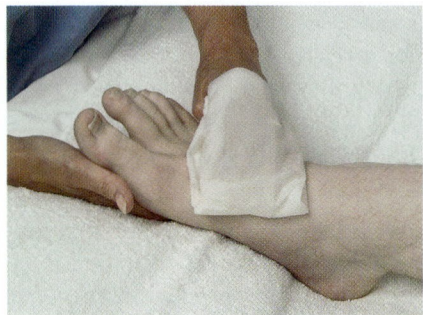

7. **Clean under the nails** with the orangewood stick while the foot is still in the water.

   Water softens the nails and makes cleaning easier.

8. **Rinse if needed.** Remove the foot from the water, and dry it gently and thoroughly.

   Remaining moisture, especially between the toes, can cause maceration and promotes development of fungal infections.

9. **Change the water,** if necessary.

   Ensures proper temperature.

10. **Soak the opposite foot** while performing steps 11 through 14 for the first (clean) foot.

    Saves time.

11. **Gently push the cuticles back** with the orangewood stick or towel.

    Increases cuticle health. Do not damage the cuticle; doing so can increase the risk of infection.

12. **Trim the nails straight across** with toenail clippers, if not contraindicated by the patient's condition and if permitted by agency policy. Note whether the nail has cut into the skin of the toe being trimmed or the adjacent toes. If the nails are brittle or thick, allow the foot to soak for 10 to 20 minutes before trimming.

    Trimming straight across prevents ingrown toenails. Early recognition and treatment of problems will prevent further complications, such as infection. ▼

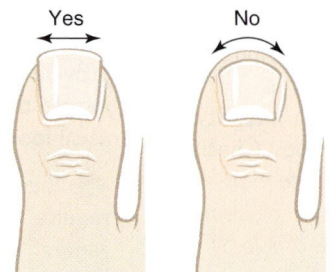

Yes   No

13. **File the nails** with an emery board.

    Smoothes the edges to prevent scratching the skin with the toenails.

14. **Apply cream, lotion,** or foot powder lightly to the feet and toes.

    Cream hydrates the skin; however, excess cream can cause maceration. Foot powder absorbs moisture and functions as a nonirritating deodorant for patients whose feet perspire heavily.

15. **Repeat steps 11 through 14** with the second foot.

16. **Check the patient's footwear** for rough edges that may injure feet.

? What if . . .

- **My patient has Impaired Bed Mobility?**

  Apply protective devices (e.g., lamb's wool) as needed.

- **My patient has an injury, lesions, or pain?**

  You may need to use a bed cradle to keep the pressure of the bedding off the patient's feet. Refer to Chapter 36 for other measures to preserve skin integrity.

- **My patient has diabetes mellitus?**

  In addition to controlling blood glucose levels, adhering to a specific foot care plan is essential for people with diabetes. Include the following in your teaching:
  - The importance of inspecting the feet daily
  - Ways to protect the feet (e.g., by wearing shoes when out of bed)
  - Potential complications involving the feet
  - Management of symptoms
  - When to seek advice from a healthcare professional
  - What to include in the foot care regimen (apply moisturizing lotion on tops and bottoms of feet but not between toes)—and what not to do (cut corns and calluses, use topical corn removers, or soak the feet)
  - Elderly patients with diabetes are especially at risk for developing foot-related complications. Visual changes and loss of flexibility could make it challenging to bend and visualize the feet. Plastic mirrors may be helpful in this regard.

  Early detection and treatment of problems can minimize foot-related complications.

Evaluation

- Observe that feet are clean, smooth, and intact; nails are trimmed and smooth; skin is pink and warm.
- Be sure that foot problems are identified and interventions provided.
- Ask the patient to demonstrate or describe correct foot care.

Patient Teaching

Refer to the Self-Care box Teaching Your Client About Foot Care, earlier in this chapter.

Home Care

The procedure does not vary in the home. The nurse must:
- Work with the client and care provider to determine the availability of supplies needed for foot care (e.g., clean water).

- Identify home care practices, and teach the client and/or caregiver proper foot care techniques. Influencing older adults can be especially difficult if they have usual routines, such as walking barefoot, that put them at risk for injury. For clients with diabetes, the biggest risk to foot health is inadequate regulation of their blood glucose levels.

Documentation

In most agencies you will not document routine foot care (except, perhaps, on a checklist) unless there are problems. If you do document, chart that foot care was given, and chart assessment findings.

Practice Resources

National Collaborating Centre for Primary Care, 2004; Plummer & Albert, 2008; Siegel, Rhinehart, Jackson, et al., 2007.

Thinking About the Procedure

 Go to the *Fundamentals of Nursing Skills Videos,* **Bed Bath, Oral Hygiene, Foot Care, and Back Massage.**

1. The nurse performs foot care near the end of this procedure. Which step was mentioned by the narrator but not demonstrated on the video?
   a. Dry well between the toes.
   b. Trim the nails straight across.
   c. Push the cuticles back with an orangewood stick.
   d. Soak the patient's foot.
   e. Apply lotion to the foot.
   f. File the nails with an emery board.

 For suggested responses, go to Chapter 24, **Thinking About the Procedure Suggested Responses,** on Davis*Plus.*

Procedure 24-6 ■ Brushing and Flossing the Teeth

➤ For steps to follow in *all* procedures, refer to the Universal Steps for All Procedures found on the page facing the inside back cover.

Equipment

- Toothbrush or sponge toothettes
- Toothpaste
- Dental floss (two pieces, each about 10 in. long) and floss holder (optional)
- Tonsil-tip suction connected to suction source (if aspiration is a concern)
- Emesis basin
- Towel
- Glass of water
- Mouthwash and/or lip moisturizer, if desired
- Procedure gloves; mask and goggles if splashing may occur

Delegation

You can delegate oral hygiene to the NAP if the patient's condition and the NAP's skills allow. Perform the pre-procedure assessments, and inform the NAP of the specific type of oral care and the amount of help the patient needs. Ask the NAP to report the condition of the patient's mouth, level of self-care, and ability to tolerate the procedure.

Pre-Procedure Assessments

- Assess the patient's ability to assist with oral care.
  Having the patient assist whenever possible promotes independence and supports a positive self-image.
- Determine whether the patient has dentures, bridgework, or partial plates.
  Determines how you will provide oral care.
- Assess general oral health, including the gag reflex and the condition of the teeth, gums, and mucous membranes. If a patient has dentures, examine the mouth with and without the dentures.
  If the patient has a hypoactive or absent gag reflex, you will need a suction setup to prevent aspiration. Inflammation or lesions in the mouth increase the risk of infection and may make eating difficult or painful, leading to malnutrition. Poorly fitting dentures can cause irritation of the gums.
- Assess the patient's usual oral care, including cultural practices.
  Helps determine the type of oral care you will provide and identifies areas of patient teaching needed.

➤ When performing the procedure, always identify your patient according to agency policy and be attentive to standard precautions, hand hygiene, patient safety and privacy, body mechanics, and documentation.

Procedure Steps

1. **Position the patient** in a high-Fowler's position or in a chair, if possible. If the head of the bed cannot be elevated, position the patient on her side.
   Prevents aspiration and makes the procedure easier.

2. **Set up suction,** if needed: Attach suction tubing and tonsil-tip suction; check suction.
   Suctioning equipment may be needed to prevent aspiration of secretions during the procedure.

3. **If the patient is able to perform self-care:**
   a. Arrange supplies within the patient's reach.
      Promotes the patient's ability to do self-care and therefore independence.
   b. Assist with brushing and flossing as needed.
      Ensures that the teeth are thoroughly cleaned.

(continued on next page)

Procedure 24-6 ■ Brushing and Flossing the Teeth (continued)

For nurse-administered brushing and flossing:

4. **Place the towel across the patient's chest.**
   Prevents getting the patient's gown or linen wet during the procedure.

5. **Don procedure gloves.** Wear gown and goggles if splashing might occur, such as with a confused patient.
   Follows standard precautions.

6. **Adjust the bed to working height**; lower the siderail nearest you.
   Prevents you from needing to lean over the patient or reach across the siderail, possibly causing back strain or injury.

7. **Moisten a small, soft toothbrush,** and apply a small amount of toothpaste.
   A small toothbrush fits more easily into the mouth and reaches more areas. The soft bristles can be used to brush the tongue and also the gums if the patient is edentulous. Excess toothpaste does not increase the cleaning, and toothpaste residue has a drying effect on the mucosa. Moistening the toothbrush increases patient comfort because patients frequently have dry mouths.

8. **Place, hold, or ask the patient to hold** the emesis basis under the chin.
   Collects oral secretions and protects clothing and linens.

9. **Brush the teeth,** holding the bristles at a 45° angle to the gumline.
   a. Using short circular motions, gently brush the inner and outer surfaces of the teeth, from the gumline to the crown of each tooth.
   b. Brush the biting surface of the back teeth by holding the brush bristles straight up and down to the teeth and brushing back and forth.
   This is the most effective technique for removing all food particles and plaque from the teeth and gums. Removing debris and subsequent plaque helps to decrease microbial colonization.
   c. If the patient is frail, perform oral suctioning when fluid accumulates in the mouth.
   Prevents choking and aspiration.

10. **Gently brush the patient's tongue.**
    Removes coating and accumulated debris that can be a reservoir for bacteria. Brush gently to prevent gagging or vomiting. ▼

Brush teeth, holding bristles at a 45° angle to the gumline. Using short circular motions, gently brush the inner and outer surfaces of the teeth, including the gumline.

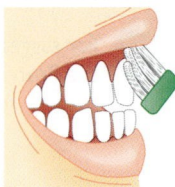

Clean front teeth.

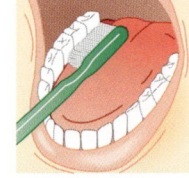

Clean both inner and outer surfaces of the teeth.

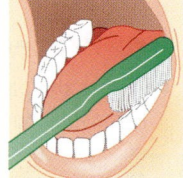

Brush the biting surfaces of the back teeth with the brush bristles straight up and down.

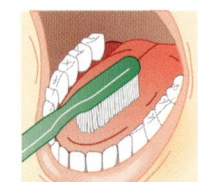

Brush the surface of the tongue.

---

11. **Floss the teeth.** Grasp dental floss in both hands, or use a floss holder. ▼

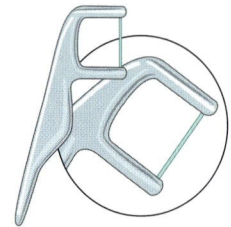

   a. **If you are not using a floss holder.** Wrap one end of the floss around the middle finger of each hand. ▼

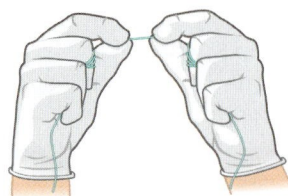

   b. Stretch the floss between your thumbs and index fingers, and move the floss up and down against each tooth. ➤

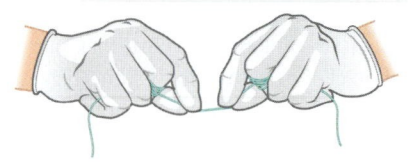

c. **Floss between and around all teeth.** ▼

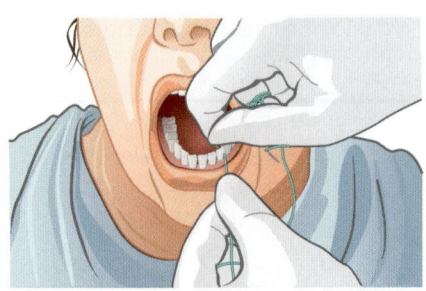

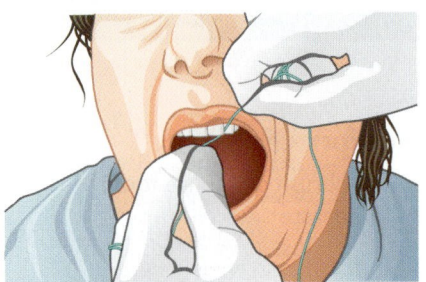

Moving the floss up and down instead of back and forth prevents damaging the gums.

12. **Assist the patient in rinsing** his mouth, suctioning as needed. Or, ask the patient to rinse vigorously and spit the water into the emesis basin.
    Removes food particles from mouth. Suction if the patient has a decreased or absent gag reflex.

13. **Offer a mild or dilute mouthwash,** and apply lip moisturizer, if desired.
    Prevents irritation of the mucous membranes. Apply lip moisturizer for dry lips, for unconscious patients, or those on a ventilator, or per patient preference.

14. **Reposition the patient** as needed and return the bed to the low position.
    Ensures patient comfort and safety.

? What if . . .

- **Your patient has an excessively dry oral cavity?**

  You may need to use a saliva substitute. *Aging, adverse medication effects, and illness often lead to decreased salivary production.*

■ **Your patient has viscous (thick) mucus?**

Use appropriately diluted sodium bicarbonate to dissolve viscous mucus.

■ ✚ **Your patient has a high risk of gum bleeding (e.g., such as associated with thrombocytopenia), has painful mouth lesions, or toothbrushing is otherwise contraindicated?**

You may use foam or cotton mouth swabs instead of a toothbrush. Do not use glycerin swabs, lemon glycerin swabs, or gauze squares. Use normal saline mouthwash.

Foam swabs are less effective in removing debris and plaque, so it is best to brush when not contraindicated. Lemon glycerin swabs are drying to the mucosa may cause decalcification of tooth enamel. Mouthwashes may be painful.

■ **Your patient has dementia or is uncooperative and agitated for other reasons?**

Use behavior management strategies such as the following:

Older adults with dementia frequently accumulate greater amounts of plaque and calculus, exhibit a higher incidence of periodontal gingival bleeding, and demonstrate a greater prevalence of denture-related oral mucosal lesions, yet they often resist oral care.

■ Provide oral hygiene at the same time every day, not necessarily at bathing time.
■ Use as many staff members as necessary.
■ Give care in a quiet, distraction-free environment. Keep stimulation to a minimum; turn on some calming music.

■ Speak softly; give one-step directions in short, simple sentences.
■ Use a relaxed, slow approach; be sure your facial expression does not reflect tension.
■ Give reassuring body contact and use gentle touch.
Promotes trust. Quick or forceful touch may frighten the patient.
■ Provide diversion.
Occupies the patient's hands and prevents "grabbing."

■ ✚ Never place your fingers between the teeth.

■ Try placing a spare toothbrush or a rolled facecloth in the patient's hands while you provide oral care. *Minimizes "grabbing."*
■ Use the "hand over hand" technique to gently guide the patient's own hand.
■ Try starting the task (e.g., brushing), then having the resident help finish it.
■ If the procedure is not going well, find another caregiver to come in and attempt the task.
■ Use modified equipment and aids, if available (e.g., mouth props, backward-bent and suction toothbrushes).

■ **Your patient is on a ventilator, is a frail older adult, or has undergone cardiac surgery?**

Be certain the teeth are brushed twice a day.
In addition to brushing, use moisturizer on lips and oral mucosa every 2 to 4 hours.
Apply a 0.12% chlorhexidine gluconate solution twice daily to complement oral care.

■ **Your patient is receiving chemotherapy?**

Stress the importance of good oral hygiene, including brushing the teeth after meals and before going to bed. *Chemotherapy can cause neutropenia (reduced white blood cell count), predisposing the patient to infections. The oral cavity is a common site for infections in patients with neutropenia.*
Routine rinses of mouthwashes with chlorhexidine are not recommended. Instead, use a bland rinse of diluted salt and/or sodium bicarbonate. Patients should swish for a minimum of 30 seconds and then expectorate the residue.
Chlorhexidine products have not proved superior to bland rinses in preventing or reducing either chemotherapy/radiation-induced mucositis or yeast colonization. In addition, chlorhexidine products may contain alcohol, cause discomfort, alter taste sensations, and stain teeth. Bland rinses containing 1 teaspoon of salt or sodium bicarbonate per pint of water reduce the acidity of oral secretions, lessen mucus accumulation, and discourage yeast colonization.
An antifungal agent or a multiagent rinse (sometimes labeled "magic" or "miracle" rinse) may be used, followed by a short NPO period of 30 to 60 minutes. If other mouthwashes or rinses are also being used, allow 30 minutes to pass between their use and the use of an antifungal agent.

✚ *Multiagent rinses typically contain lidocaine. The resulting numbing effect may pose risks for a biting injury or aspiration. These rinses can neutralize antifungal agents.*

Evaluation

■ Inspect the teeth, gums, and mucous membranes to verify that they are free of food particles.
■ Inspect for abnormalities, such as bleeding, that may have been stimulated by the brushing or flossing.
■ Observe for patient discomfort or gagging during the procedure.
■ If the procedure was performed by the NAP, the nurse should still evaluate the care. This includes physical assessment of the oral cavity as well as objective and subjective findings related to the patient's tolerance of and satisfaction with the care.

Patient Teaching

■ Discuss the importance of daily oral care.
■ Review any areas of brushing or flossing that the patient has not been performing adequately.
■ Discuss any problems that need further follow-up, such as inflammation, bleeding, dryness, caries, missing teeth, or broken or missing dentures.

(continued on next page)

Procedure 24-6 ■ **Brushing and Flossing the Teeth** (continued)

Home Care

The procedure does not vary in the home. The issues are that the nurse must:

■ Work with the client and care provider to determine supplies needed for the home.

■ Determine whether suction is needed (e.g., if the client is unconscious or has a decreased gag reflex). Explain to the client and/or caregiver how to obtain a portable suction unit.

■ Demonstrate how to position the client and perform the procedure if the height of the bed is not adjustable or if both sides of the bed are not accessible.

Documentation

Document that oral care was given, the patient's response, appearance of teeth and mucous membranes, any abnormal findings, and nursing interventions. Oral care is usually charted on a flow sheet.

Practice Resources

American Association of Critical-Care Nurses (AACN), 2007; Berry, 2007; Chalmers, 2005; Coughlan & Healy, 2008; Harris, Eilers, Harriman, 2008; Joanna Briggs Institute, 2004; Watando, Ebihara, Ebihara, et al., 2004.

Thinking About the Procedure (Procedures 24-1 through 24-6)

 Go to the *Fundamentals of Nursing Skills Videos*, **Bed Bath, Oral Hygiene, Foot Care, and Back Massage.**

1. How does the nurse protect the patient's gown during oral hygiene?
2. What does the nurse do after the patient uses the mouthwash?

 For suggested responses, go to Chapter 24, **Thinking About the Procedure Suggested Responses,** on Davis*Plus*.

Procedure 24-7 ■ **Providing Denture Care**

➤ For steps to follow in *all* procedures, refer to the Universal Steps for All Procedures found on the page facing the inside back cover.

Equipment

■ See Procedure 24-6: Brushing and Flossing the Teeth.
■ Denture cup

Delegation

You can delegate denture care to the NAP if the patient's condition and the NAP's skills allow. Perform the pre-procedure assessments, and inform the NAP of the specific care and the amount of help the patient needs. Ask the NAP to report the condition of the patient's mouth and dentures, level of self-care, and ability to tolerate the procedure.

Pre-Procedure Assessments

See Procedure 24-6: Brushing and Flossing the Teeth.

➤ When performing the procedure, always identify your patient according to agency policy and be attentive to standard precautions, hand hygiene, patient safety and privacy, body mechanics, and documentation.

Procedure Steps

1. **Don gloves, and remove dentures** (if the client cannot do so).

   a. *Upper denture:* With a gauze pad, grasp the denture with your thumb and forefinger, and move it gently up and down. Tilt the denture slightly to one side to remove it, without stretching the lips. Place the denture in the denture cup.

   The gauze gives you a better grip. Breaking the seal on the top dentures can be difficult; movement breaks the suction. Always place

   dentures in a denture cup as soon as you remove them to prevent accidental breakage. ▼

   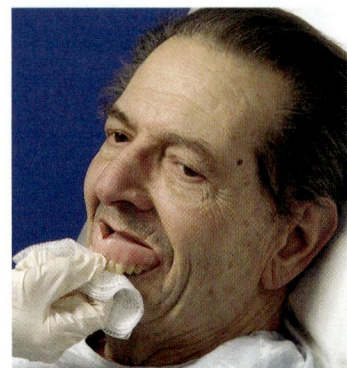

   b. *Lower denture:* Use your thumbs to push up gently on the denture at the gumline to release from the lower jaw. Grasp the denture with your thumb and forefinger, and tilt it to remove it from the patient's mouth. Place the denture in the denture cup.

   A gauze pad is not usually needed to grasp the lower dentures; however, you can use one if the dentures are difficult to grasp. Pushing up on the dentures breaks the seal. Rotating

the dentures is necessary to remove the dentures from the patient's mouth. ▼

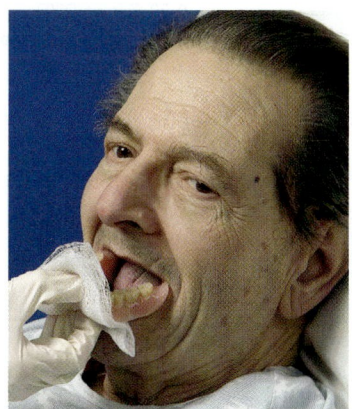

2. **Place the towel in the sink, and cleanse the dentures** under cool running water.

   Heat can damage some dentures. The towel helps prevent the dentures from breaking if they are dropped. Dentures are expensive and usually not reimbursed by insurance.

   a. Apply a small amount of special denture paste to a soft-bristled toothbrush.

      Denture paste assists in cleaning. Toothpaste and stiff-bristled brushes may be too abrasive for dentures. However, follow the patient's preference in use of denture cleaner. Some patients prefer to soak their dentures in a cleanser overnight. If dentures have been soaking, rinse them well before placing them in the patient's mouth.

   b. Brush all surfaces of each denture.

      Loosens all food particles and any old denture adhesive.

   c. Rinse thoroughly with cool water.

      Removes loosened particles and the cleaning agent. Do not use hot water with dentures, because hot water can make the denture material sticky.

   NOTE: You can soak stained dentures in a commercial cleaner, following the manufacturer's instructions. Do not soak the denture overnight if the appliance has metal parts.

Soaking can cause corrosion of the metal parts.

3. **Inspect dentures** for rough, worn, or sharp edges.

   These can irritate the tongue, gums, or oral mucous membranes.

4. **Inspect the mouth** under the dentures for redness, irritation, lesions, or infection.

   If present, refer to a dentist to check the fit of the dentures or to make needed repairs.

5. **Apply denture adhesive** as needed (ask the patient whether he uses denture adhesive).

   Adhesives are needed to "seal" some dentures and prevent slipping and irritation of the gums.

6. **Moisten the top denture**, if it is dry. Then insert the top denture, at a slight tilt, and press it up against the roof of the mouth.

   Moistening the dentures eases insertion. You can tell when you have securely seated the dentures by checking to feel for any slippage or to confirm that the dentures stay in place. Because the top denture is larger, it is removed first and inserted first for ease of insertion.

7. **Moisten the bottom denture**, if it is dry. Then insert bottom denture, rotating it as you put it in the patient's mouth.

   Because it is smaller, the bottom denture is inserted after the top one. ▼

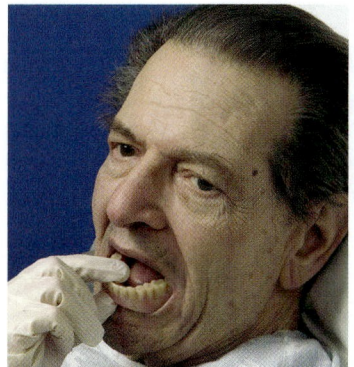

8. **Ask the patient** whether the dentures are comfortable.

   Ensures that the dentures are properly placed.

9. **If the patient does not wish to wear the dentures,** cover them with water in a clean denture container with a lid. Label the container with the patient's name and the agency identifying number. Place the container in a bedside drawer rather than on top of bedside table for safekeeping.

   Drying can cause dentures to warp. Having the denture out of the mouth for several hours a day relieves pressure on the oral tissues, allows saliva to clean the tissues, and helps to minimize gingival irritation.

10. **Offer mouthwash**.

? What if . . .

■ **The patient develops Candida-related denture stomatitis?**

Follow agency protocols. Microwave disinfection of complete dentures has been documented as an effective treatment of *Candida*-related denture stomatitis and can reduce the recurrence of infections.

Denture stomatitis ranges in severity. Treatment includes good oral and denture hygiene and administration of antifungal agents. Recurrence of infection after treatment can be due to colonization of Candida on the dentures.

(continued on next page)

Procedure 24-7 ■ **Providing Denture Care** (continued)

Evaluation

- See Procedure 24-6: Brushing and Flossing the Teeth.
- Check to see that dentures are comfortable and fit properly.

Other

For Documentation, Patient Teaching, and Home Care, see Procedure 24-6: Brushing and Flossing the Teeth.

Practice Resources

Neppelenbroek, Pavarina, Spolidorio, et al., 2008; Pappas, Rex, Sobel, et al., 2004; Siegel, Rhinehart, Jackson, et al., 2007.

Thinking About the Procedure

 Go to the *Fundamentals of Nursing Skills Videos*, **Oral Hygiene: Denture Care.**

1. In the video, how does the NAP protect the dentures from breakage?
2. What did the NAP do to check whether the dentures were securely seated?

 For suggested responses, go to Chapter 24, **Thinking About the Procedure Suggested Responses,** on Davis*Plus.*

Procedure 24-8 ■ **Providing Oral Care for an Unconscious Patient**

➤ For steps to follow in *all* procedures, refer to the Universal Steps for All Procedures found on the page facing the inside back cover.

Equipment

- Toothbrush with soft bristles or sponge oral swabs
- Toothpaste
- Denture cup, if the patient has dentures
- 4 in. × 4 in. gauze pad to remove dentures if present
- Tonsil-tip suction connected to suction source (you may use a product that combines the toothbrush or oral swab with the suction device)
- Tongue blade (padded) or bite-block
- Towel
- Waterproof linen protector
- Emesis basin
- Water-soluble lip moisturizer
- Procedure gloves and goggles

Delegation

As a rule, you should not delegate oral hygiene for an unconscious patient to a NAP. However, in some situations it may be acceptable—for example, when the NAP has a great deal of experience caring for unconscious patients and when the NAP's ability to perform oral hygiene safely for them is documented. Perform the pre-procedure assessments, and inform the NAP of any special considerations for care (e.g., if the patient must have the head of the bed elevated to facilitate breathing). Ask the NAP to report the condition of the patient's mouth and his ability to tolerate the procedure (e.g., ask the NAP to take vital signs before and after the procedure, or to note the oxygen saturation if it is being monitored).

Pre-Procedure Assessments

- Determine whether the patient has dentures or partial plates.
  The presence of these appliances determines how you will provide oral care. You may leave dentures out for an unconscious patient to decrease the risk that they will be damaged or block the airway. However, when possible, keep the dentures in place to help ensure they will fit adequately later. Remove partial plates in an unconscious patient to prevent the plate from causing aspiration or damage to the mouth if it becomes loosened.
- Assess the patient's gag reflex.
  If the patient has an intact gag reflex, the risk of aspiration is lower.
- Assess the patient's general oral health, including the condition of the teeth and gums, and hydration of the mucous membranes. If the patient has dentures, examine the mouth with and without the dentures.
  Unconscious patients tend to breathe through the mouth, so oral mucosa are often dry. Because the oral mucosa act as a

barrier against microorganisms, inflammation or lesions in the mouth increase the risk for infection. The lips, gums, and mucous membranes should be pink, moist, and intact. The teeth should be intact and clean. The condition of the mouth determines what you will use to provide oral care. Assess the fit of dentures and the condition of the skin under the dentures to determine whether the fit is proper and whether any irritation is present.

➤ When performing the procedure, always identify your patient according to agency policy and be attentive to standard precautions, hand hygiene, patient safety and privacy, body mechanics, and documentation.

Procedure Steps

1. ✚ **Position the patient** in a side-lying position, with head turned to the side and, if possible, with the head of the bed down.
   Secretions will pool in the dependent side of the mouth. This position helps prevent aspiration and facilitates the removal of secretions by gravity.

2. **Don procedure gloves and eye goggles.**
   Follows standard precautions. Eye protection is needed when suctioning because of the risk of splashing.

3. **Place a waterproof pad** and then a towel under the patient's cheek and chin.
   To absorb water and keep the bed linens dry.

4. **Set up suction:** Attach suction tubing and tonsil-tip suction; check suction.
   Suctioning helps ensure that the patient does not aspirate oral secretions during mouth care.

5. **Brush the patient's teeth.**
   a. Use a padded tongue blade or bite-block, as needed, to hold the patient's mouth open.
   A padded tongue blade or bite-block is used to hold the mouth open so you can visualize and reach the different areas of the mouth without injuring the oral mucosa. It also keeps the patient from biting the nurse's fingers. ▼

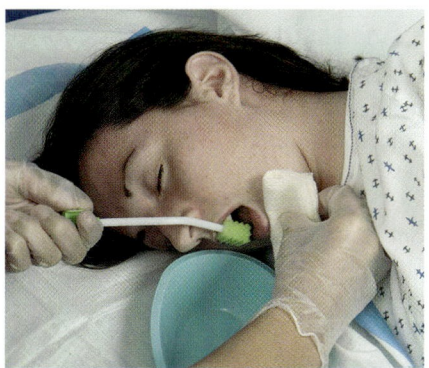

   b. Place an emesis basin under the patient's cheek.
   Catches the secretions draining from the patient's mouth.
   c. Moisten the toothbrush, and apply a small amount of toothpaste.
   Excessive toothpaste does not increase the cleaning. Brushing the teeth with a soft-bristled brush stimulates the mucosa, which increases the health of the gums.
   d. Brush the teeth, holding the bristles at a 45° angle to the gumline.
      (1) Using short circular motions, gently brush the inner and outer surfaces of the teeth, including the gumline.
      (2) Brush the biting surface of the back teeth by holding the brush bristles straight up and down to the teeth and brushing back and forth.
      (3) Brush the patient's tongue.
      This is the most effective technique for removing plaque and debris from the teeth and gums. The tongue can be a reservoir for bacteria.
   e. ✚ **Perform oral suctioning** when fluid accumulates in the mouth.
   Removing fluid prevents choking and aspiration.
   f. Draw about 10 mL of water or mouthwash (e.g., dilute hydrogen peroxide) into a syringe; eject it gently into the side of the mouth. Allow the fluid to drain out into the basin, or suction as needed.
   Removes any toothpaste residue, which may have a drying effect. Remove all fluid from the mouth to prevent aspiration into the lungs. Use a minimal amount of solution to prevent aspiration.

6. **Provide denture care,** as needed. See Procedure 24-7: Providing Denture Care.

7. **Clean the tissues in the oral cavity** according to agency policy. Use foam swabs or a moistened gauze square wrapped around a tongue blade. Use a clean swab for each area of the mouth: cheeks, tongue, roof of the mouth, and so on.
   Oral tissues may be dry and sticky from mouth breathing. Using separate swabs prevents transfer of microorganisms from one area to another.

8. **Remove the basin, dry the patient's face** and mouth, and apply water-soluble lip moisturizer.
   ✚ *Petroleum-based lip moisturizers (e.g., mineral oil, petroleum jelly) are not recommended because of the possibility of aspiration, which might cause pneumonia. Never use petroleum-based jelly for patients receiving oxygen therapy; it can cause burns.*

9. **Remove the waterproof pad** and towel; turn off suction equipment; discard gloves and used supplies.

10. **Reposition the patient** as needed.
    Maintains good body alignment.

11. **Cleanse and store reusable oral hygiene tools** in clean containers, separate from other articles of personal hygiene.
    Prevents possible contamination from the environment and other personal hygiene tools.

? What if . . .

■ **You are providing oral care to a patient receiving mechanical ventilation?**

Provide oral cleansing, including subglottic suctioning, at least every 2 hours and prn. Brush the teeth at least twice a day.
Keeping the oral cavity clean and clear of secretions has been proven to decrease the incidence of ventilator associated

(continued on next page)

Procedure 24–8 ■ **Providing Oral Care for an Unconscious Patient** (continued)

pneumonia (VAP). Pooled oral secretions become rapidly colonized with pathogens that contribute to VAP.

Avoid tap water. Use normal saline or a half strength solution of saline for oral rinses.

Studies show hospital plumbing and tap water are often colonized with microbial organisms.

Apply a 0.12% chlorhexidine gluconate solution twice daily to complement oral care.

■ **It is difficult to floss the patient's teeth, or the patient doesn't tolerate flossing?**

Handheld interdental tools may be used instead of floss. These devices are special small brushes, picks, or sticks.

Toothbrush bristles can't reach between teeth to dislodge food particles and bacteria. Interdental cleaners can be as effective as floss in keeping these areas clean.

■ **Oral tissues are dry and sticky?**

Use appropriately diluted sodium bicarbonate to dissolve viscous mucus.

Evaluation

■ Inspect the teeth, gums, and mucous membranes for cleanliness.
■ Observe the oral mucosa and gums for hydration, inflammation, bleeding, or infection.
■ Observe the patient's overall responses to the procedure (e.g., gagging, coughing, vital signs, skin color).

Patient Teaching

■ Discuss with family members any problems that need further follow-up.
■ Teach oral hygiene measures, as needed.

Home Care

The procedure steps do not vary in the home.
■ Work with the client and caregiver to determine supplies needed for the home.
■ Determine whether suction is needed, and explain to caregivers how to obtain a portable suction unit.
■ Demonstrate how to position the client and perform the procedure if the height of the bed is not adjustable or if both sides of the bed are not accessible.

Documentation

Document that oral care was given, any abnormal findings, and nursing interventions. Typically, though, oral care is documented on a checklist or flow sheet.

Thinking About the Procedure

 Go to the *Fundamentals of Nursing Skills Videos*, **Oral Hygiene: Unconscious Patient.**

1. What protective gear does the nurse use?
2. How does the nurse protect the bed linens?
3. Why did the nurse not use the padded tongue blade?

 For suggested responses, go to Chapter 24, **Thinking About the Procedure Suggested Responses,** on Davis*Plus*.

Practice Resources

American Association of Critical-Care Nurses (AACN), 2007; American Dental Association, n.d.; Berry & Davidson, 2007; Cason, Tyner, Saunders, et al., 2007; Human & Bell, 2007; Slot, Dörfer, & Van der Weijden, 2008.

Procedure 24-9 ■ **Shampooing the Hair**

➤ For steps to follow in *all* procedures, refer to the Universal Steps for All Procedures found on the page facing the inside back cover.

Delegation

You can delegate this procedure to the NAP if the patient's condition and the NAP's skills allow. Perform the pre-procedure assessments, and inform the NAP of the amount of help and the specific type of procedure needed (e.g., in bed, at sink, disposable shampoo equipment). Inform the NAP of any special considerations, such as positions the patient cannot assume or presence of scalp lesions. Ask the NAP to report the condition of the patient's scalp and hair, level of self-care, and ability to tolerate the procedure.

Pre-Procedure Assessments

■ Assess for contraindications to a shampoo (e.g., scalp sutures or limited head or neck movement). A rinse-free shampoo would be more appropriate in these cases.
■ Determine the patient's ability to assist with the procedure.
  Promotes independence and provides active range of motion.
■ Assess the condition of the hair and scalp. Note any dryness or irritation.
  Dry and brittle hair may indicate hypothyroidism or malnutrition and may require special shampoos or conditioners.
■ Determine the need for special hair care products.
  Dandruff, lice, and dry hair are examples of conditions that require medicated shampoos or conditioners.
■ Ask the patient how she normally cares for her hair.

Procedure 24-9A ■ Shampooing the Hair for a Patient on Bedrest

➤ When performing the procedure, always identify your patient according to agency policy and be attentive to standard precautions, hand hygiene, patient safety and privacy, body mechanics, and documentation.

Equipment

- Shampoo; conditioner is optional
- Shampoo tray or commercial system, if available
- Washbasin, plastic pail, small easy to handle plastic container
- Towels (2), washcloth, bath blanket
- Waterproof pads or plastic trash bag
- Brush and comb
- Procedure gloves, if indicated by the presence of lesions or infestation
- Hair dryer

Procedure Steps

1. **If lesions or infestation are present, don procedure gloves.**
   Observes standard precautions.

2. **Unless contraindicated** (e.g., by a neck condition), lower the head of the bed, take the pillow from under the patient's neck, and place it under her shoulders.
   Hyperextends the neck and helps keep water from the patient's eyes.

3. **Place the waterproof pad** or plastic trash bag under patient's shoulders, and cover with towels. A commercial system will have a drain hose to use.
   Protects the bed from getting wet.

4. **Collect warm, not hot, water** in a container and bring to the bedside.

5. **Place the shampoo tray** under the patient's shoulders (or head, depending on the type of tray). If you are using a hard plastic tray, pad the neck area with a towel. An inflatable shampoo tray needs minimal padding, but you will need to inflate it before beginning the procedure, either by mouth or with an air pump.
   Protects the patient from lying on a hard surface and prevents water from leaking out onto the bed.

6. **Ensure that the tray will drain** into the washbasin or plastic pail.
   Helps keep the bed and floor dry.

7. **Fold the top linens down** to the patient's waist, and cover her upper body with a bath blanket.
   Keeps the linen dry; keeps the patient warm.

8. **Work your fingers through the patient's hair,** or comb the hair to remove tangles prior to washing.
   It is easier to remove tangles from dry hair. Note that very tangled or matted

hair may sometimes indicate a lice infestation.

9. **Wash the hair.**
   - Wet the hair, pouring warm water from the pitcher. Do not get water in the person's eyes or ears.
   - Next, apply shampoo and lather well, working from the scalp out and from the front to the back of the head.
   - Gently lift the patient's head to rub the back of the head.

10. **Rinse** thoroughly.
    Shampoo is drying if left in the hair. ▼

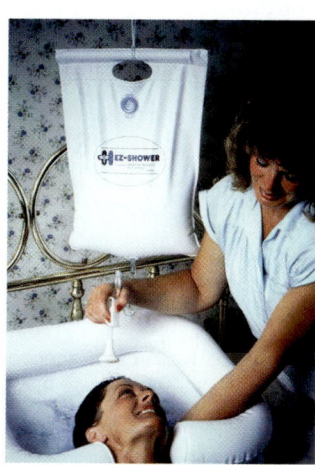

11. **Apply conditioner to the hair,** if desired. Conditioner should be used for patients with hair that tangles easily, such as dry, long, curly, or kinky hair. Rinse if needed. Leave-in conditioner can be used and is recommended for curly hair.

12. **Remove the tray,** and blot-dry the hair with the towel. Do not use circular motions to dry the hair.
    Circular motions increase tangles.

13. **Comb or brush the hair** to remove tangles, starting at the ends and working toward the scalp.

Prevents excessive pulling on the patient's hair, which may cause breakage.

14. **Dry hair** with a hair dryer at a medium temperature, if desired.
    Use a medium temperature to prevent burning the patient.

15. **When you are finished,** be sure that the patient's clothing and bed linens are dry. Wash the shampoo tray and the brushes and combs.

Procedure Variation: Shampooing the Hair of African American Clients

16. **If the hair is in cornrows or braids,** do not take out the braids to wash the hair. You may need to apply a cloth or net cap to the head prior to shampooing.

17. **Handle the patient's hair very gently,** being careful not to pull on the hair.
    Many African Americans have fragile hair that breaks easily. Because it is fragile, apply moisturizer, if needed, to untangle the hair.

18. **When shampooing,** thread your fingers through the hair from the scalp out to the ends. Do not massage the hair in circular motions.

19. **Rinse thoroughly,** then apply a conditioner on the hair if the hair is dry and fragile.
    A leave-in conditioner helps minimize tangles and breakage.

20. **Comb through the hair.**
    a. Use a wide-toothed comb or hair pick on the patient's hair. Do not use a brush or fine-toothed comb.

(continued on next page)

Procedure 24-9 ■ **Shampooing the Hair** (continued)

b. Part the hair into four sections, and begin combing near the ends of the hair, working through each section.

c. Use additional moisturizer to help soften and ease combing.
Never pull on the hair, because it will break easily.

21. **Apply a natural oil to the hair**, if desired. Examples of natural oils are coconut, sweet almond, shea butter, and avocado. Many commercial products use these oils.
Mineral oil and petroleum jelly tend to clog pores and damage the hair, so use

them only if the patient still prefers them after receiving this information.

22. **Let the hair air-dry** if possible.
Prevents the hair from becoming frizzy. A high temperature, such as from a hair dryer, will also damage the hair.

Procedure 24-9B ■ **Shampooing the Hair Using Rinse-Free Shampoo**

> ➤ When performing the procedure, always identify your patient according to agency policy and be attentive to standard precautions, hand hygiene, patient safety and privacy, body mechanics, and documentation.

Equipment

■ Rinse-free shampoo (no water is needed); conditioner is optional

■ Bath towel
■ Brush or hair pick and comb
■ Procedure gloves (if scalp lesion or infestation present)

Procedure Steps

1. Elevate the head of the bed, if possible,.
Makes it easier to maintain good body mechanics during the procedure.

2. **Place a protective pad** or bath towel under the patient's shoulders.
Prevents the linen from getting wet.

3. **Don procedure gloves** if lesions or infestations are present.
Helps prevent transmission of disease.

4. **Work your fingers through the hair**, or comb the hair to remove tangles before washing. If the patient has her hair in small braids, do not take out the braids to wash the hair.

5. **Apply rinse-free shampoo.** Apply enough shampoo to thoroughly wet the hair. One application is usually sufficient to clean the hair.

6. **Work the shampoo through the hair**, from scalp down to ends.
Helps prevent pulling on and damaging the hair.

7. **Dry the hair** with a bath towel.
Removes the shampoo. Leaves the hair feeling clean and soft.

Procedure 24-9C ■ **Shampooing the Hair Using Rinse-Free Shampoo Cap**

> ➤ When performing the procedure, always identify your patient according to agency policy and be attentive to standard precautions, hand hygiene, patient safety and privacy, body mechanics, and documentation.

Procedure Steps

1. **Warm the shampoo cap** using a water bath or microwave according to package instructions. Be careful to not overheat. Check the temperature before placing on the patient's head to prevent burns.
A commercial no-rinse shampoo cap is a microwavable cap that contains a no-rinse shampoo and conditioner. Different products are available. Be sure to follow the directions on the package.

2. **Place the cap** on the patient's hair, and gently massage.

3. **Remove the cap**, and towel-dry the patient's hair.

Removes the shampoo and excess water.

4. **Complete hair care** according to the patient's needs (see Procedure 24-9A, steps 12–15, preceding).

? **What if . . .**

■ **You discover head lice or nits as you begin the shampoo?**

Stop the procedure. Discuss your findings with the patient and offer reassurance. Leave the patient in a position of comfort and safety. Perform hand hygiene. Report the findings and obtain a prescription for a medicated shampoo.

■ **You do not have a shampoo tray?**

Improvise by using a new bedpan, and reserve it only for washing the hair. Pad it liberally with towels.

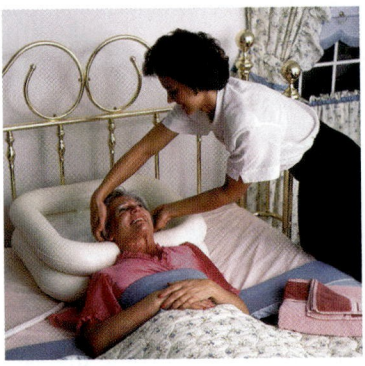

Evaluation

- Observe that the hair is clean, dry, and free of tangles.
- Observe for patient discomfort or fatigue during the procedure.
- Ask the patient how the hair and scalp feel.

Patient Teaching

- Advise patients with coarse hair to wash it less frequently (every 3 to 7 days, depending on dryness). Leave-in conditioners are often recommended for dry, curly, or kinky hair.
- Discuss potential adaptations in washing hair. Products such as rinse-free shampoos or a shampoo tray can make shampooing easier to accomplish for a bedridden patient.

Home Care

- Determine how and where the client usually washes her hair.
- If the client is confined to bed, work with the caregiver to develop a effective plan for washing the client's hair. For example, if a shampoo tray is not available, you can make one by using a plastic garbage bag and pillows or rolled towels.
- Rinse-free products or the inflatable shampoo tray may be good choices for the client.
- If the client cannot afford the adaptive equipment needed, refer the caregiver to the local resources, such as senior services.
- If the client is ambulatory, recommend a shower stool. The stool needs to fit into the shower or bathtub securely, without wobbling, to prevent the client from falling.

- If the client has only a bathtub, an adaptor for the faucet can be used to attach a hand-held showerhead. Using a shower stool will make the procedure easier.

Documentation

Chart that hair was shampooed, the condition of the hair and scalp, and the patient's responses to the procedure.

Practice Resources

EZ-Shampoo Instructions for Use, 2005; Thompson Healthcare, Inc., 2008. (Caveat: These are not research articles; they are manufacturers' recommendations.)

Thinking About the Procedure

 Go to the *Fundamentals of Nursing Skills Videos,* **Hygiene: Shampoo Hair in Bed.**

1. This nurse did not have a commercial tray available. What did she use to position the patient for the shampoo, and how did she place it?
2. What did the nurse use as a substitute for a shampoo tray?
3. Specifically, how did the nurse wet the patient's hair?

 For suggested responses, go to Chapter 24, **Thinking About the Procedure Suggested Responses,** on Davis*Plus.*

Procedure 24-10 ■ Providing Beard and Mustache Care

➤ For steps to follow in *all* procedures, refer to the Universal Steps for All Procedures found on the page facing the inside back cover.

Equipment

- Scissors or beard trimmer
- Wide-toothed comb
- Mild shampoo; conditioner for coarse and/or dry hair
- Basin
- Bath towel
- Procedure gloves (if skin nicks occur, contact with blood may occur)

Delegation

You can delegate beard and mustache care to the NAP if the patient's condition and the NAP's skills allow. Perform the pre-procedure assessments, and inform the NAP of the amount of help and specific type of care needed (e.g., in bed, at sink, safety razor, electric razor). Inform the NAP of any

special considerations, such as skin irritation or activity intolerance. Ask the NAP to report the condition of the patient's skin and beard, level of self-care, and ability to tolerate the procedure

Pre-Procedure Assessments

- Ask the patient or family about preferences for beard and mustache care.
  Beards and mustaches may have personal and/or cultural meaning. Men in some cultures never cut or trim their beards. Some patients use a comb and scissors to do a slight trim of their beard and/or mustache, whereas others use a beard trimmer for a closer trim.
- Assess the patient's skin and hair condition.
  Determine whether the skin has any reddened or dry areas and whether skin treatments are needed.

(continued on next page)

Procedure 24–10 ■ Providing Beard and Mustache Care (continued)

➤ When performing the procedure, always identify your patient according to agency policy and be attentive to standard precautions, hand hygiene, patient safety and privacy, body mechanics, and documentation.

Procedure Steps

1. **Drape the towel around** the patient's shoulders.
   Protects the patient's clothing from falling pieces of hair and water from shampooing the beard or mustache.
2. **Trim the beard and mustache** when they are dry.
   The beard and mustache are often shorter when dry. If they are cut when wet, they may be shorter than desired after they dry.

Using a Comb and Scissors

   a. Comb through the beard, and cut the hair on the outside of the comb. Be conservative; cutting too little is better than cutting too much.
   Trimming too much off the beard can be upsetting for the patient, whereas if you cut too little, you can always trim off more.
   b. Trim from the front of the ear to the chin on one side, and repeat on the other.
   Keeps the beard equal on both sides of the face.

Using a Beard Trimmer

   c. Select the trimming guide to the correct length. Adjust the guide to a longer length rather than a shorter length.
   Ensures that you do not cut the beard too short.
   d. Trim from the front of the ear to the chin on one side, and repeat on the other.

3. **Trimming the mustache:**
   a. Comb the mustache straight down.
   Cuts the length equally so that the mustache is just above the upper lip.
   b. Using either scissors or a beard trimmer, start in the middle, and trim toward one side of the mouth and then toward the other. Do not trim the top of the mustache.
   Trimming from the center out toward each side helps you cut both sides equally.

4. **Define the beard line** by one of the following methods:
   a. Using either the scissors or a beard trimmer, trim the line of the beard so that it is well defined. Trim very little to ensure that you only define the beard and do not change the length. ➤

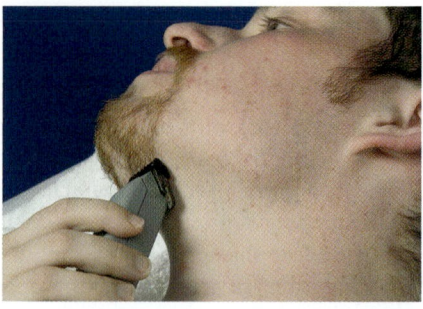

   b. Shave the neck to define the beard line, particularly for short beards.
5. **Apply procedure gloves**, if needed, and shampoo the beard and mustache using warm water and a mild shampoo.
   The skin under a beard or mustache can be tender, so treat it gently. Follow standard precautions, because it is possible to nick the skin and cause bleeding.
6. **Rinse well, and pat and wipe the beard and mustache dry with the towel.**
   Any shampoo left can irritate the skin, as can rubbing motions with the towel.
7. **Apply conditioner,** if desired.
8. **Comb the beard and mustache** with a wide-toothed comb or a brush.
   Do not use a fine-toothed comb, because it will pull the hair.

Evaluation

- Make sure that the beard and mustache are trimmed to the desired length and are clean.
- Verify that skin problems are identified and treatment initiated.

Home Care

No adaptations are required in the home. The patient's usual supplies are sufficient, as a rule.

Documentation

Chart that beard and mustache were trimmed and shampooed; chart the condition of the skin.

Practice Resources

Procter & Gamble, 2008. (Caveat: This is not an evidence-based practice article. It is a manufacturer's recommendation.)

Procedure 24–11 ■ Shaving a Patient

➤ For steps to follow in *all* procedures, refer to the Universal Steps for All Procedures found on the page facing the inside back cover.

Equipment

- Safety razor or electric razor
- Shaving cream or soap; after-shave lotion, if desired
- Shaving brush, if desired
- Warm water
- Face towel and bath towel
- Procedure gloves

Delegation

You can delegate shaving to the NAP if the patient's condition and the NAP's skills allow. Perform the pre-procedure assessments, and inform the NAP of the amount of help and specific type of care needed (e.g., safety or electric razor, in bed, or at the sink) the patient needs. Inform the NAP of any special

considerations, such as skin irritation or activity intolerance. Ask the NAP to report the condition of the patient's skin, level of self-care, his ability to tolerate the procedure.

Pre-Procedure Assessments

- Determine how much assistance the patient needs.
  Aids you in promoting as much independence possible.

- ✚ Assess the patient's skin and hair condition for redness, skin lesions, or moles.
  Identify skin problems and determine whether skin treatments are needed or the procedure must be modified. To prevent abrading the skin, do not shave any areas that have skin lesions or moles.

- Assess the patient's usual shaving method, including use of electric razor or safety razor.
  When possible, follow the patient's routine. The patient may or may not use shaving cream or shaving soap, shaving brush, and after-shave lotion.

- ✚ Check for any contraindications to shaving, such as an increased risk of infection or bleeding (e.g., because of neutropenia, thrombocytopenia, or the administration of anticoagulants, such as warfarin or heparin).

➤ When performing the procedure, always identify your patient according to agency policy and be attentive to standard precautions, hand hygiene, patient safety and privacy, body mechanics, and documentation.

Procedure Steps

1. **Don gloves.**
   To prevent exposure to blood if skin is nicked or scratched.

2. **Place a warm, damp face towel** on the patient's face for 1 to 3 minutes.
   Opens the pores and softens the beard to prevent pulling. Do not use hot water, because it will dehydrate the skin and can burn sensitive skin.

3. **Apply shaving lotion** to the face with your fingers or a shaving brush. Lather well for 1 to 2 minutes.
   Helps to further soften the beard. Do not use shaving creams that contain numbing agents, because they close the pores and stiffen the beard.

4. **Shave the patient.**
   a. Pull skin taut with your nondominant hand, and gently pull the razor across the skin. If you are using a safety razor, hold the blade at a 45° angle to the skin.
   b. Shave the face and neck in the same direction of hair growth (the direction is not the same for all people). Using short strokes, start shaving at the sideburns, and work down to the chin on each side and then the neck.
   c. Last, shave the chin and upper lip.
   Usually the hair on the face grows down toward the chin and, on the neck it grows up toward the chin. The hair is generally thickest on the chin and upper lip, so shaving them last allows more time for the shaving cream to soften the hair. Shave in the same direction in which the hair is growing to prevent skin irritation. ▼

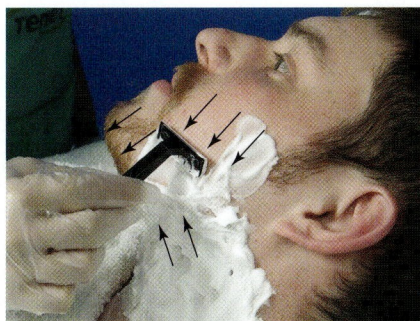

5. **Rinse the razor** frequently while you are shaving.
   Avoids clogging the blade.

6. **When you are finished shaving,** rinse the patient's face with cool water, and gently pat it dry.
   Cool water helps close the pores. Pat dry, do not rub, to prevent irritating the skin.

7. **Apply after-shave lotion,** if desired.
   After-shave lotions that contain alcohol are not recommended, because alcohol stings and dries out the skin. A moisturizer is recommended.

8. **Dispose of the single-use razor** in the sharps container.
   Prevents cutting injury to others.

Multiuse Razor

Shake the razor to remove excess moisture. Do not bang the razor against objects or dry with a towel. Store the razor in a covered container.
Banging or wiping the razor edge will dull the razor and may damage the holding mechanism. A covered container protects others from a cutting injury.

? What if . . .

- **Your patient has a condition that predisposes him to bleeding (e.g., thrombocytopenia) or infection (e.g., neutropenia)?**

  Such patients must be shaved carefully using an electric razor, if at all.
  A razor scratch or cut causes a break in skin integrity, providing a portal of entry for pathogens. This could be especially serious for a patient whose defenses against infection are compromised. For a patient with a delayed clotting time, a cut could cause excessive blood loss.

(continued on next page)

Procedure 24–11 ■ **Shaving a Patient** (continued)

Evaluation

- Inspect the patient's face closeness of the shave, as well as for nicks or cuts.
- If the procedure was performed by the NAP, ask the patient about his satisfaction with and tolerance of the care.

Patient Teaching

Teach patients about changes that need to be made in their shaving technique as a result of changes in health status. For example, a patient who has begun taking anticoagulants may need to change from a blade to an electric razor because of an increased risk of bleeding.

Home Care

The procedure does not vary in the home. The nurse must:
- Determine the availability of supplies

- Assess the client's or caregiver's ability to perform the procedure.

Documentation

Chart that the patient was shaved and the condition of the skin. There will probably be a flow sheet or checklist for this information.

Practice Resources

Coughlan & Healy, 2008; Procter & Gamble, 2008. (Caveat: Of the two resources, only Coughlan & Healy's paper is an evidence-based resource. Procter & Gamble's are manufacturer's instructions.)

Procedure 24–12 ■ **Removing and Caring for Contact Lenses**

➤ For steps to follow in *all* procedures, refer to the Universal Steps for All Procedures found on the page facing the inside back cover.

Equipment

- Contact lens wetting solution
- Contact lens soaking solution
- Sterile saline (optional)
- Contact lens case
- Contact lens remover (optional)
- Procedure gloves

Delegation

You can delegate this procedure if the patient's condition and the NAP's skills permit. For example, if the patient is unconscious, you must determine whether contact lenses are present, and you should not delegate their removal.

Pre-Procedure Assessments

- Determine whether the patient is wearing contact lenses. If the patient is unconscious, examine the eyes for the presence of contact lenses by shining a penlight across the eye. You should be able to see the edge of the lens.
  Some lenses are larger than others, so examine the surface of the cornea carefully.
- Determine the type of contact lenses in place.
  Hard lenses are smaller than soft lenses. Each type of contact lens has different care requirements. Hard lenses can be worn for only up to 18 hours. Rigid gas-permeable (RGP) lenses may be worn overnight or for about 7 days, depending on the kind. Soft contacts are used for either short or longer periods.
- Ask the patient whether he is able to remove his contact lenses.

➤ When performing the procedure, always identify your patient according to agency policy and be attentive to standard precautions, hand hygiene, patient safety and privacy, body mechanics, and documentation.

➤ *Note:* It is difficult to remove a contact lens when wearing procedure gloves. For hard lenses, you can use a suction cup device if one is available. ✚ If you must use ungloved hands (e.g., in an emergency situation), it is extremely important to wash your hands thoroughly before and after the procedure. *Do not use* your fingernails.

➤ *Note:* Lens cases are marked L and R to indicate left and right lenses. Clean, rinse, and place the lens you remove first into its designated cup before removing the second lens.

Procedure Steps

1. **Perform hand hygiene** and don gloves.
2. **Instill one to two drops of contact lens wetting solution** to moisten the lenses.
   Aids in lens removal.

3. **Remove the lenses.**

Hard or Gas-Permeable Contact Lens

   a. ***Alternative 1:*** If the lens is not centered over the cornea, place your finger on the patient's lower eyelid, and apply gentle pressure to

move the lens into position. Place your index finger at the outer corner of the eye, and gently pull sideways toward the ear; position your other hand below the eye to "catch" the lens. Ask the patient to blink. As the skin tightens and the

palpebral fissure narrows, the lids catch on the edge of the lens and pop it out. ▼

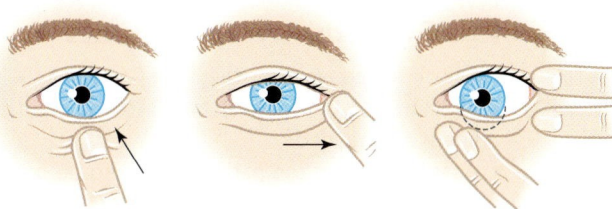

b. **Alternative 2:** Use a small suction cup contact lens remover. Gently press the suction cup end of the remover onto the contact lens, and lift straight up off the eye.

c. **Alternative 3:** Gently pull the top eyelid up and the lower lid down beyond the top and bottom edges of the lens. Then gently press the lower eyelid up against the bottom of the lens. When the lens is slightly tipped, move the eyelids together. This should cause the lens to slide out. ▼

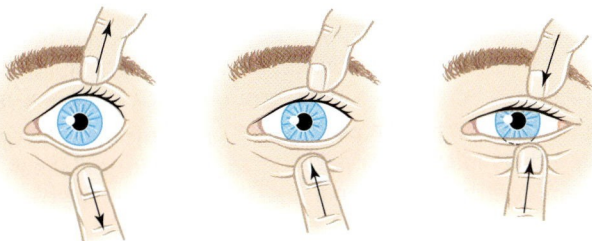

Soft Contact Lens

d. Hold the eye open with your non-dominant hand.
Allows you to visualize the contact lens.

e. Gently place the tip of your index finger on the contact lens, and slide it down off the pupil to the white area of the eye.
To prevent potential damage to the eye, do not pinch a lens directly over the pupil. ▼

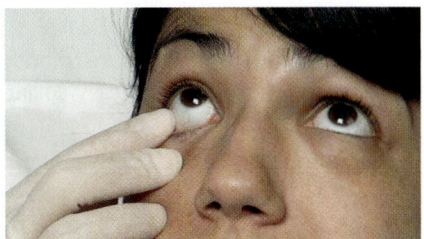

f. Using your thumb and index finger pads, gently pinch the lens, and lift it straight up off the eye. If the edges stick together moisten with a few drops of wetting solution. Rub gently until edges separate.
A soft contact lens is very flexible and pinches easily.

4. **Clean the lens** according to the instructions on the cleaning solution bottle. If there is no lens cleaner, use sterile saline. Be careful not to tear soft lenses.

5. **Rinse the lenses** with contact lens solution or sterile saline.
Removes any particles from the lenses.

6. **Place the lenses** in a contact lens case containing soaking solution or sterile saline (see note above regarding lens cases).
Prevents bacterial growth on the contacts and keeps the lenses from drying out.

Evaluation

Examine the eyes for redness or irritation.

Patient Teaching

- Review with the patient and/or family the importance of keeping the contact lenses clean and moist.
- If hard contact lenses are used, they must be removed at bedtime to prevent hypoxia of the cornea.

Documentation

Chart that contacts were removed, what type of lenses they are, what solution they are stored in, and the condition of patient's eyes.

Practice Resources

Bausch & Lomb, 2008, 2009; Holman, Roberts, & Nicol, 2005; Massachusetts Eye and Ear Infirmary, n.d..

Procedure 24-13 ■ Making an Unoccupied Bed

➤ For steps to follow in *all* procedures, refer to the Universal Steps for All Procedures found on the page facing the inside back cover.

Equipment

- Bottom and top sheets, possibly drawsheet
- Pillowcase for each of the pillows
- Linen bag or hamper
- Procedure gloves (if exposure to body fluids is possible)
- Moisture-proof gown (if heavy soiling of linens with body fluids is possible).

Delegation

You can delegate this procedure to the NAP. You are responsible for supervising to ensure that the procedure is performed correctly.

Pre-Procedure Assessments

- Check to see whether the linen (including the mattress pad, blanket, and bedspread) needs to be changed, and what linens are needed.
- Assess whether the patient is able to be out of bed during the linen change.
- Assess for drainage or incontinence to determine whether personal protective equipment, such as procedure gloves and gown, is needed.

➤ When performing the procedure, always identify your patient according to agency policy and be attentive to standard precautions, hand hygiene, patient safety and privacy, body mechanics, and documentation.

➤ *Note:* This procedure describes bed making by one person. It is more efficient for two people to work together on opposite sides of the bed.

Procedure Steps

1. **Assist the patient to a chair.** Provide a robe and/or blanket if needed. *Ensures that the patient is comfortable and will be warm enough during the bed change.*

2. **Prepare the environment:** Position the bed flat, raise to appropriate working height, put on the brakes, and lower the siderails. Move the overbed table and other furniture, as needed. Place the linen bag or hamper conveniently near the bed. *Maintains good body mechanics and prevents back strain during the procedure. Remove obstacles to allow easy access to the bed. Place all items so you can work efficiently, saving time and energy.*

3. **Don protective gloves** and other gear if necessary. Loosen all the bedding. *This observes Standard Precautions and reduces the risk of contaminating your clothing.*

4. **If the blanket or bedspread is clean,** fold it and place it on a clean area (e.g., on the back of a chair). *Do not place on another patient's bed or furniture. Reuse the blanket and/or bedspread if it is not soiled. Placing the item on a clean area prevents cross-contamination.*

5. **Remove the bottom and top sheet,** drawsheet, and pillowcases.
   a. Do not shake the linens.
      Minimizes dispersal of dust, skin cells, and microorganisms into the environment.
   b. Holding the items away from your body, place them in a laundry bag or hamper. Place the pillows on a clean area (e.g., on a chair).
      Hold dirty linen away from your uniform to prevent contamination. ▼

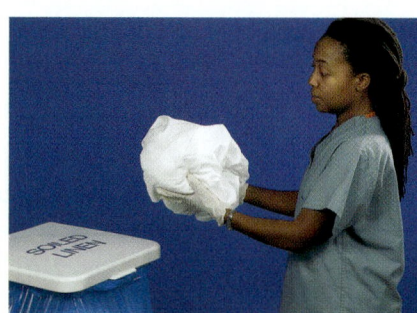

6. **Working on one side of bed,** to save steps:

Contour-Bottom Sheet
   a. Fit the contour-bottom sheet on one side of the bed, and smooth it out over half the mattress.

Flat-Bottom Sheet
   b. Fold the flat-bottom sheet lengthwise with the center crease in the middle of bed and unfold with the rough side facing down.
   c. Position the bottom sheet so that approximately 10 inches hang over at the top and sides. The hem of the bottom sheet should be just even with the bottom edge of mattress.
   d. Tuck in the sheet, mitering the sheet at the top corner (see step 11).
      When using a flat bottom sheet, having extra sheet at the top helps keep it in place when the head of the bed is raised and lowered. Unfold the sheet rather than shake or fan to reduce dispersing microorganisms into the air. The sheet will not be long enough to tuck in at the bottom.

7. **Place the drawsheet** with the center fold in the middle of the mattress and unfold. Tuck the side in under the mattress, and smooth out over half of the mattress.
   Ensures that all wrinkles are out of the bottom sheet and drawsheet. ▼

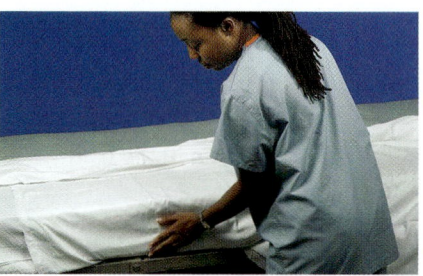

8. **Go to the other side of the bed**, straighten the linen, and finish tucking in the bottom sheet and drawsheet.

   a. Make the drawsheet tight, and smooth any wrinkles in the bottom sheet and drawsheet.

   b. If desired, place a waterproof pad on or under the drawsheet.

      Pulling the drawsheet tight helps prevent wrinkles from developing under the patient when she moves around in bed. ▼

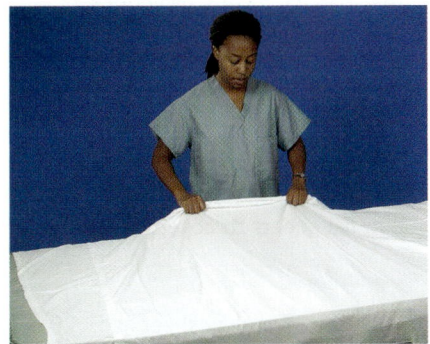

9. **Place the top sheet and bedspread** along one side of the mattress. Center the top sheet and bedspread, so that when you straighten them from the other side of the bed, they fall equally over each side of the bed.

   Putting the linens on one side of the bed at a time saves steps.

10. **At the foot of the bed,** make a small pleat in the top sheet and bedspread.

    Prevents the top covers from placing pressure on the patient's toes. ▼

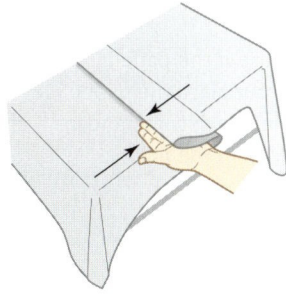

11. **Tuck in the top sheet** and bedspread at the same time, mitering the corners.

    a. Tuck in the sheet and bedspread at the bottom of the mattress.

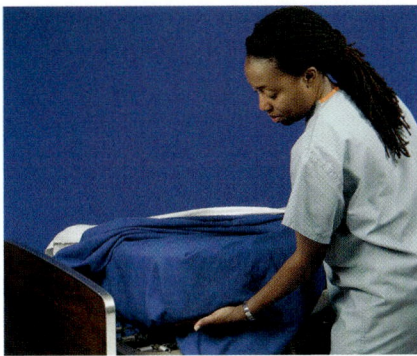

   b. Bring the edge of sheet and the bedspread up to make a right angle. ▼

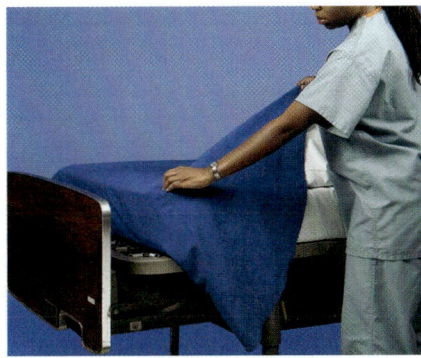

   c. Tuck the lower edge of sheet and bedspread under the mattress.

      Mitered corners help secure the linen at the foot of the bed. ▼

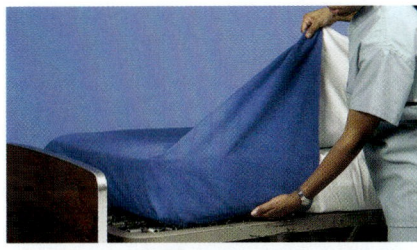

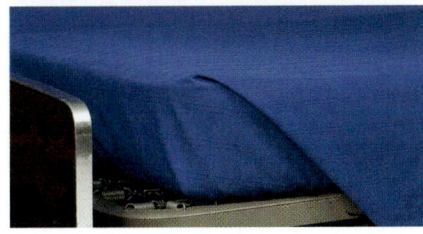

12. **Move to the other side of the bed,** smooth top linens, and repeat step 11. At the head of the bed, fold the edge of sheet down over the bedspread.

Prevents the bedspread from rubbing against the patient's skin. ▼

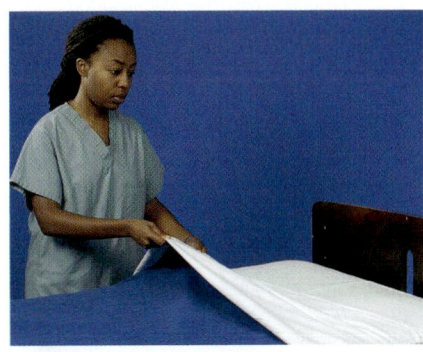

13. **Fanfold the top sheet** and bedspread back to the foot of the bed.

    Makes it easier for the patient to get into bed. ▼

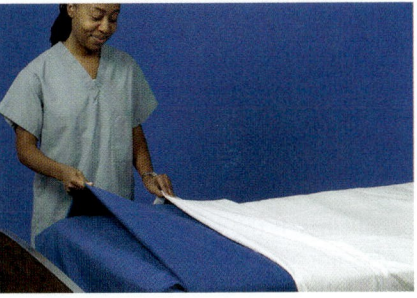

14. **Change pillowcases**.

    a. Turn the pillowcase wrong side out.

    b. Grasp the middle of the closed end of the pillowcase.

    c. Reaching through the pillowcase, grasp the end of the pillow. ▼

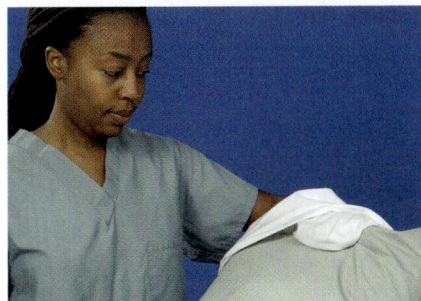

   d. Continuing to grasp the end of the pillow, pull the pillowcase down over the pillow.

(continued on next page)

Procedure 24-13 ■ Making an Unoccupied Bed (continued)

Do not hold the pillow under your arm or chin to put on pillowcase because contamination can occur.

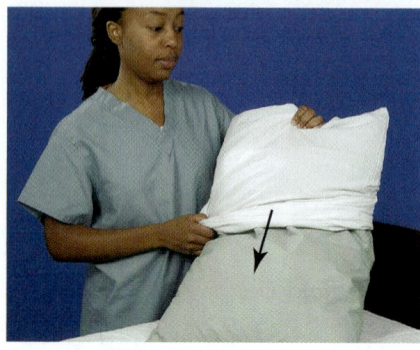

15. Assist the patient back to bed, return the bed to the low position, place the call signal within reach, and place the bedside table and overbed table so that they are accessible to the patient.
Provides for patient comfort and safety.

? What if . . .

■ **The linens have been contaminated by body fluids?**

Follow recommended infection control procedures for laundering of linens (e.g., wear procedure gloves, place linen in moisture-proof bags).

■ **The mattress has become contaminated by body fluids?**

Follow agency policies for cleaning the mattress before putting on clean linens. This often involves notifying another department, such as housekeeping or environmental services, whose members are trained in this procedure.

■ **The patient has a specialty bed or specialty mattress?**

Several products are available with specific criteria to match patients' needs in terms of comfort, prevention or treatment of pressure ulcers, and movement (e.g., specialty beds designed for bariatric patients). Follow the manufacturer's directions (e.g., a recommendation for a specific mattress may be to use only one layer of sheet over the mattress for maximum benefit). If you find the sheets are not large enough to accommodate a specialized mattress, you may need to use two flat sheets to cover it.

Home Care

The only adaptations at home depend on the type of bed the patient has. If the height of the bed is not adjustable or the bed is not accessible from both sides, the procedure may be more difficult.

Documentation

Linen changes are generally recorded on a checklist, if at all. Additional charting would need to be done only if something abnormal occurred, for example, "The drawsheet had a 20-cm circular area of serosanguineous drainage."

Practice Resources

Bloomfield, Pegram, & Jones, 2008; Sehulster & Chinn, 2003; Shiomori, Miyamoto, Makishima, et al., 2002; Siegel, Rhinehart, Jackson, et al., 2007.

Procedure 24-14 ■ Making an Occupied Bed

➤ For steps to follow in *all* procedures, refer to the Universal Steps for All Procedures found on the page facing the inside back cover.

Equipment

- Bottom and top sheets; drawsheet
- Pillowcase for each of the pillows
- Bath blanket (as needed)
- Linen bag or hamper
- Procedure gloves (if exposure to body fluids is possible)
- Moisture-proof gown (if heavy soiling of linens with body fluids is possible)

Delegation

You can delegate this procedure if the patient's condition and the NAP's skills permit. For example, if the patient is very ill, in pain, or requires two people for turning and repositioning, you should assist with or perform the linen change yourself.

➤ When performing the procedure, always identify your patient according to agency policy and be attentive to standard precautions, hand hygiene, patient safety and privacy, body mechanics, and documentation.

➤ *Note:* If linen change is done at the same time as the bed bath, some of these steps will vary.

Pre-Procedure Assessments

- Determine the patient's ability to assist with the procedure and whether additional help or assistive devices are needed.

- Make other assessments listed in Procedure 24-13.

Procedure Steps

1. **Prepare the environment:** Move the overbed table and other furniture, as needed, to allow access to the bed. Place the linen bag or hamper conveniently near the bed.
   To allow easy access to the bed and enable you to work efficiently, saving time and energy.

2. **Don protective gloves** and other gear if necessary.
   This observes standard precautions and reduces the risk of contaminating your clothing.

3. **Position the bed flat** if possible, and raise it to working height. Lower the siderail nearest you.
   Maintains good body mechanics and prevents back strain during the procedure. Having the head of the bed flat makes it easier to smooth the bottom sheet. To prevent the patient from falling out of bed, lower the siderails only on the side where you are standing.

4. **Disconnect the call device,** and remove the patient's personal items from the bed.
   Prevents items from getting lost.

5. **Check that no tubes** (e.g., IV, NG) are entangled in the bed linens.
   Prevents dislodging tubes accidentally.

6. **If the blanket or bedspread is clean,** fold it and place it on a clean area (e.g., the back of a chair); do not place it on another patient's bed or furniture.
   Reusing the blanket and/or bedspread if it is not soiled conserves resources.

7. **Cover the patient with a bath blanket,** if available, or leave the top sheet over the patient.
   Prevents chilling and preserves modesty.

8. **Slide the patient to the far side** of bed and place him in a side-lying position, facing the siderail. Place a pillow under his head. If needed for support, place a pillow between the patient and the siderail.
   Placing the patient close to the siderail will allow you to place the clean linen over a larger area. Patients who cannot maintain the side-lying position should have a pillow placed between their chest and the siderail to prevent them from rolling into the siderail.

9. **Roll or tightly fanfold** the soiled linens toward the patient's back. Tuck the roll slightly under the patient. Cover any moist areas with a waterproof pad.
   Cover any moist areas to prevent contact with the clean linen or patient. ▼

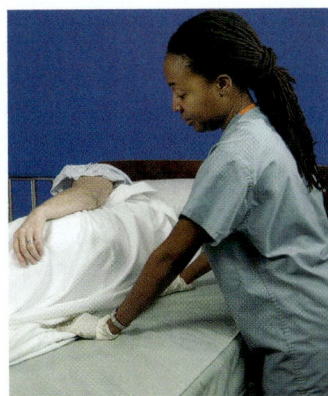

10. **Remove soiled gloves** and don clean gloves.

11. **Place the clean bottom sheet** and drawsheet (or pad) on the near side of the mattress, with the center vertical fold at the center of the bed. Fanfold the half of the clean linen that is to be used on the far side, folding it as close to the patient as possible and tucking it under the dirty linen. Tuck the lower edges of clean linen under the mattress. Smooth out all wrinkles.
    Wrinkles under the patient can cause skin irritation. ▼

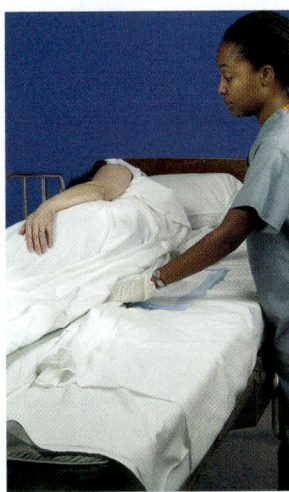

12. **Roll the patient over the clean and dirty linen,** turning him toward you. Explain to him that he will be rolling over a "lump," and then gently

pull the patient toward you so that he rolls onto the clean linen.

13. **Raise the siderail** on the clean side of the bed.
    Prevents the patient from falling.

14. **Move the pillows to the clean side.** Position the patient comfortably on his side, near the siderail.
    Always ensure patient comfort and safety before going to the other side of the bed.

15. **Go to the opposite side of bed,** and lower the rail. Pull the soiled linen from under the clean linen, and place it in laundry bag or hamper. Never place linen on the floor.
    Prevents cross-contamination. ▼

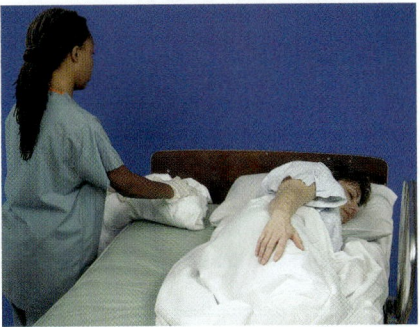

16. **Remove soiled gloves and don clean gloves.** Pull clean linens through, and tuck them in. Pull taut, starting with the middle section.
    Taut linens ensure that no wrinkles will be under the patient. ▼

17. **Assist the patient to a supine position** close to center of the mattress, then turn to face the bed rail. ▼

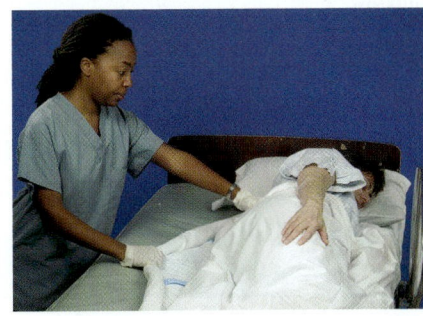

18. **Place the top sheet** and bedspread along one side of the mattress, and continue making the bed as in Procedure 24-13, steps 9 through 14, *except* remove the bath blanket from under the top linens before tucking them in.

(continued on next page)

Procedure 24-14 ■ Making an Occupied Bed (continued)

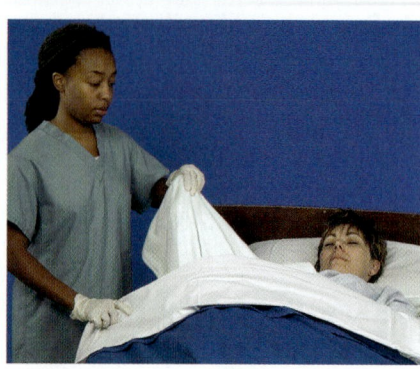

19. Return the bed to the low position, raise the siderails, and attach the call light within patient's reach. Position the bedside table and overbed table within patient's reach. *Ensures patient safety and comfort.*

? What if . . .

■ **You are making the bed with a patient in leg traction?**

It may be easier to make the bed from top to bottom, as follows:

- Loosen all bed linens and bring the dirty linens from the top of the bed to hip area. Put the clean bottom sheet on the top corners of the mattress, bring down to hip level and tuck under the dirty linen. Cover any moist areas with a waterproof pad.
- Ask the patient to grasp the trapeze and raise his buttocks. If the patient is unable to raise his buttocks, use an assistive device per agency policy.
- Bring the dirty bottom sheet along with the clean bottom sheet toward the foot of the bed. Remove dirty linen and place in the laundry bag.
- Tuck the clean sheet under the mattress. Cover with the top sheet. To accommodate traction equipment, do not tuck in the top sheet.

■ **You need to move or reposition a patient in bed who is not able to assist or is obese?**

✚ Before making the occupied bed, assess the patient's ability to move. Use assistive equipment such as friction reducing devices, mechanical lifts, air-powered mattresses, and/or lateral transfer devices.

These are essential tools in preventing work-related injuries. You should limit the need to use your own strength while lifting, turning, or repositioning the patient in bed because of the stress placed on the weaker muscles in the arms and shoulders.

Follow agency policies and use patient-moving devices appropriately.
Many healthcare facilities have adopted safe lifting and patient handling policies as a means to protect both the patient and the healthcare worker.

Evaluation

■ Assess how well the patient tolerated the procedure. Was there any discomfort, shortness of breath, and so on?
■ Ask the patient whether he feels comfortable.

Home Care

The only adaptations at home depend on the type of bed the client has. If the height of the bed is not adjustable or the bed is not accessible from both sides, the procedure may be more difficult.

Documentation

Linen changes are usually recorded on a checklist. Additional charting needs to be done only if something abnormal occurred.

Practice Resources

Bloomfield, Pegram, & Jones, 2008; Collins, Nelson, & Sublet, 2006; Nelson, Lloyd, Menzel, et al., 2003; Nelson, Pragala, & Menzel, 2003; Siegel, Rhinehart, Jackson, et al., 2007; Trinkoff, Brady, & Nielsen, 2003.

Thinking About the Procedure

➤ Go to the *Fundamentals of Nursing Skills Videos,* **Linen Change: Occupied Bed.**

1. Where has the nurse placed the clean linen?
2. What did the nurse do to protect the patient's privacy?

➤ For suggested responses, go to Chapter 24, **Thinking About the Procedure Suggested Responses,** on Davis*Plus.*

Procedure 24-15 ■ Caring for Artificial Eyes

➤ For steps to follow in *all* procedures, refer to the Universal Steps for All Procedures found on the page facing the inside back cover.

Equipment

■ Procedure gloves
■ Normal saline solution
■ Labeled container filled with saline or tap water
■ Cotton balls

Delegation

You can delegate this procedure to the NAP if the patient's condition and the NAP's skills allow. Perform the pre-procedure

assessments, and inform the NAP of any special considerations. Ask the NAP to report the patient's ability to tolerate the procedure.

Pre-Procedure Assessments

Assess the patient's activity tolerance and whether you will need another caregiver to assist.

➤ When performing the procedure, always identify your patient according to agency policy and be attentive to standard precautions, hand hygiene, patient safety and privacy, body mechanics, and documentation

Procedure Steps

1. **Wash hands and don gloves.**
2. **Position the patient lying down.**
   If you accidentally drop the eye when removing it, it will fall onto the bed instead of the floor.
3. **To remove the artificial eye**:
   a. Raise the upper eyelid with your nondominant hand, and depress the lower lid with your dominant hand.
   b. Apply slight pressure below the eye to release the suction holding it in place.
   c. Catch the eye in the palm of your dominant hand.

   d. Alternatively, you can use a small bulb syringe, place it directly on the eye, and squeeze to create suction and lift the eye straight up from the socket. (See Fig. 24-4.)
4. **Clean the eye with saline**, and store it in a labeled container filled with saline or tap water.
   Do not use solvents, disinfectants, or alcohol.
   These chemicals may irritate the socket or damage the artificial eye.
5. **Wipe the edge of the patient's eye** socket with a moistened cotton ball, wiping from outer canthus toward the nose.

6. **Inspect the socket** for redness, swelling, or drainage.
   Irritation or infection can occur if debris has entered the socket.
7. **To reinsert the eye**:
   a. Remove the prosthetic eye from the container, but do not dry it.
   b. Hold the eye between your thumb and the index finger of your dominant hand.
   c. With your nondominant hand, pull down on the lower lid while lifting the upper lid, and guide the eye into the socket.
   The prosthesis will slide into place more easily when it is wet.

Evaluation

- Observe that the eye has been placed correctly in the socket.
- Ask the patient how the eye area feels.
- Observe the eye area for redness or irritation.

Patient Teaching

- Advise the patient to periodically inspect the eye area.
- Review the importance of hand hygiene and proper handling of the eye.
- If the eye wearer experiences dryness or irritation, a lubricant made for ocular prosthetics can be used.
- If the eye needs to be cleaned but not removed, wipe from outer canthus toward the nose.
  Wiping outward may dislodge the prosthesis.
- Encourage the patient to sleep in the prosthesis at night and remove it every 1 to 3 weeks for cleaning (follow prosthesis specialist's advice). Some patients do find that it is necessary to remove and clean the prosthesis every day.
  Frequent removal can irritate the lining of the socket and increase the amount of discharge produced by the eye socket.

- The eye should be professionally polished every 6 to 12 months. Symptoms that may indicate the need for a polish are: irritated or itchy lids, increased drainage or discomfort, or changes in the appearance of the artificial eye.

Home Care

- In the home care setting, determine how the client usually performs eye care.
- Discuss ways to promote the safety of the artificial eye.
- Work with the client or caregiver to develop a plan of care for cleaning the eye and care of the area associated with the socket.

Documentation

Chart that the artificial eye was cleansed, the condition of the socket, care given to the area around the socket, and the patient's responses to the procedure.

Practice Resources

Erikson Labs Northwest, n.d.; Hospital Info, 2010; Peters, 2010.

Procedure 24-16 ■ Caring for Hearing Aids

➤ For steps to follow in *all* procedures, refer to the Universal Steps for All Procedures found on the page facing the inside back cover.

Equipment

- Face cloth, dry towel
- Damp cloth
- Cotton applicators
- Wax-loop and wax brush, if available
- Pipe cleaner or toothpick, if wax-loop and wax brush unavailable

- Procedure gloves (to prevent contact with earwax or ear drainage)

Delegation

You can delegate hearing aid care to the NAP if the patient's condition and the NAP's skills allow. Perform the pre-procedure assessments, and inform the NAP of the specific

(continued on next page)

Procedure 24-16 ■ Caring for Hearing Aids (continued)

type of care needed (e.g., type of hearing aid), and the amount of help the patient needs. Inform the NAP of any special considerations, such as skin irritation or usual volume setting. Ask the NAP to report the condition of the patient's ear, level of self-care, his ability to tolerate the procedure, and his ability to hear in a normal conversation.

■ Determine the type of hearing aid in use. The three common types of hearing aids are (1) postaural hearing aid, (2) in-the-canal hearing aid, and (3) in-the-ear hearing aid. *The cleaning procedure varies according to the type of hearing aid. (See Fig. 24-6.)*

■ Assess the patient's ear and outer canal for redness, skin lesions, earwax buildup, or drainage. *To identify skin problems and determine whether any symptoms of infection exist. Earwax buildup increases with age and does not necessarily indicate a health problem.*

Pre-Procedure Assessments

■ Determine how much assistance the patient needs. *Aids you in promoting independence as much as possible.*

➤ When performing the procedure, always identify your patient according to agency policy and be attentive to standard precautions, hand hygiene, patient safety and privacy, body mechanics, and documentation.

Procedure Steps

1. **Don gloves**. *The hearing aid may contain earwax buildup or drainage.*

2. **Place a towel on a nearby table or flat surface.** *The towel helps prevent the hearing aid from breaking if it is accidentally dropped. Hearing aids are expensive.*

3. **To remove the hearing aid:**
   a. Turn the hearing aid off by applying slight pressure against the volume control wheel and turning it backward (away from the nose). *Stops the hearing aid from whistling.*
   b. Rotate the earmold slightly forward (toward the nose), and gently pull it out. Do not pull on the battery door or the volume wheel. *Pulling on the battery door or the volume wheel may damage the faceplate.*
   c. Place the hearing aid on the towel. *Prevents the hearing aid from rolling off the table or banging against the table.*

4. **Clean the hearing aid.**
   a. Wipe all external surfaces with a damp cloth.
   b. Clean the canal portion of the hearing aid using the wax-loop and wax brush, cotton-tipped applicator, pipe cleaner, or toothpick. Clean the top portion only. Do not insert anything into the hearing aid itself. *Poking utensils into any part of the hearing aid except for the canal portion may damage the hearing aid.*

Detachable Earmold
■ Disconnect the earmold, and soak it in soapy water. Rinse and dry well, and then reattach it. Do not use alcohol. Never immerse a hearing aid in water, only the earmold. *Detaching an earmold that is glued or fastened by a small metal ring will break the hearing aid. Alcohol will damage the earmold material.*

■ Check the hearing aid and any tubing for cracks and loose connections. *A damaged hearing aid will be less effective and may cause injury to the ear. Early detection of hearing aid damage may allow for repair rather than replacement of the device.*

5. **Cleanse the outer ear** using the corner of a washcloth or a cotton-tipped applicator. Inspect these areas for redness, abrasions, swelling, drainage, or other irregularities. *Poorly fitting or improperly positioned hearing aids may cause trauma to the ear.*

6. **Insert the hearing aid.**
   a. Check that the battery is functioning. Hold the hearing aid in your hand. Close the battery compartment door if open. Turn the power on, turn the volume high, and listen for a whistling sound. *Whistling indicates proper power level and functioning of the battery.*
   b. Set the volume control to Off. *Prevents whistling during insertion and prevents from a sudden, loud noise.*
   c. Handle the hearing aid by the edges using your thumb and forefinger. *Prevents whistling during insertion.*

   d. Holding the hearing aid in your dominant hand, use your non-dominant hand to gently pull the ear up and back. *Opens the ear canal slightly for an easier insertion and better fit.*
   e. Insert the canal portion of the hearing aid into the ear. Apply slight pressure and gently rotate the hearing aid back and forth until the canal portion rests flat in the ear. *Allows a better fit and prevents hearing aid from falling out.*

Inserting a Postaural Hearing Aid
Insert the earmold first and then place the earmold over the ear.

Inserting an In-the-Canal Hearing Aid
Insert with the volume control at the top. The canal should be facing away from your hand.

Inserting an In-the-Ear Hearing Aid
Insert with the volume control at the bottom.

7. **Turn the hearing aid on** and adjust the volume by turning the volume control wheel toward the nose. Set the volume control as low as possible. *Normal setting requires a one-third to two-thirds turn of the volume control wheel. A noisier environment requires less volume, or one-fourth turn.*

8. **Protect the hearing aid** from curling irons, hair dryers, hair spray and other hair products. *Heat and moist aerosols will damage the hearing aid.*

Procedure Variation: Storing the Hearing Aid

9. **Open the battery compartment** and place the hearing aid in a closed container labeled with the patient's name.

   Saves battery power and allows any moisture to evaporate. Protects the hearing aid from accidental damage or loss.

10. **If the hearing aid is to be kept stored** and not worn for a week or more, remove the battery completely.

    Prevents battery acid from leaking and damaging the hearing aid.

11. **Store the hearing aid** in a cool, dry place, preferably in the bedside drawer. Keep the hearing aid away from children and pets.

    Moisture and heat will damage the hearing aid. Hearing aids and containers are easily lost. A child may choke on the hearing aid. Dogs and cats are attracted to the whistling noise and odor of the hearing aid and sometimes attempt to eat the device.

Procedure Variation: Replacing the Battery

12. **Use your finger** to swing the battery door open. Never force the door.

13. **Peel the tab off the new battery.**

14. **Hold the battery with the positive. (+) side up** and slide it into the door, not into the hearing aid itself.

15. **Gently close the battery door.** Never force the door.

16. **Dispose of the old battery** in the regular trash.

Guidelines for Care of the Batteries

- Always dispose of old batteries. Do not throw into a fire.
  Minimizes damage from leaking battery acid and prevents mistaking fresh battery for used battery. Heat and fire may cause the battery to explode.
- Store batteries in a cool, dry place. Do not place zinc-air batteries in the refrigerator.
  Heat shortens the life of the battery. Cold batteries warming to room temperature are exposed to condensation and subsequent corrosion.
- Do not store batteries near coins or other metals.
  Contact with other metals can short-circuit the batteries.
- Do not remove the tab from the battery until the battery is ready for use.
  The tab keeps air out of the battery. Once the tab is removed, the battery is activated. Early removal decreases the life of the battery.
- ✚ Keep batteries away from children, confused adults, and pets.
  Minimizes accidental swallowing.

? What if . . .

- **The hearing aid becomes wet?**

  If the hearing aid becomes exposed to moisture, dry it as much as possible.

Remove the battery and throw it away. Keep the battery door open. Place the hearing aid in its container and allow it to dry overnight. Do not place a new battery in the hearing aid until the next morning.
Moisture will cause the battery to corrode.

- **The patient wears bilateral hearing aids?**

  Be sure to identify which hearing aid is for the left ear and which hearing aid is for the right ear. Most hearing aids have a color marking for easy identification: red = right ear and blue = left ear.
  Attempting to force a hearing aid into the wrong ear may cause trauma to the ear.

- **The patient continues to have hearing difficulties despite hearing aids?**

  Hearing aids will not restore full hearing. General tips when communicating with a person with a hearing deficit are listed in Clinical Insight 31-3, Communicating With Clients Who Have Impaired Hearing.
  Hearing aids will not block out background noise. A clear, distinct, low-pitched voice helps the client to understand what is being said.

Evaluation

- Assess how well the patient tolerated the procedure. Was there any discomfort, difficulty with insertion, and so on?
- Note the condition of the patient's skin, including pain, redness and abnormal discharge.
- Note the condition of the hearing aid itself.
- Assess the patient's ability to hear normal speaking voices.
- Ask the patient whether he feels comfortable and hears satisfactorily.

Patient Teaching

- Discuss the importance of daily hearing aid care.
- Review any areas of care that the patient has not been performing adequately.

- Discuss any problems that need further follow-up, such as earwax build up, faulty or broken hearing aid, or ill-fitting hearing aid.

Home Care

The procedure does not vary in the home. The issues are that the nurse must:

- Work with the patient and care provider to determine supplies needed for the home.
- Determine whether further knowledge is required (e.g., if the patient must expose hearing aids to prevailing weather conditions, uses a telephone extensively, must make several adaptations from quiet to noisy environments throughout the day).

(continued on next page)

Procedure 24–16 ■ **Caring for Hearing Aids** (continued)

■ Provide a list of available resources (e.g., AARP, National Institutes of Health, Better Hearing Institute).

Documentation

Chart that the patient is wearing a hearing aid, the condition of the ear, and the ability to hear. There will probably be a flow sheet or checklist for this information.

Practice Resources

Department of Veteran Affairs, n.d.; National Institute on Deafness and Other Communication Disorders, 2007; U.S. Food and Drug Administration, 2009.

To explore learning resources for this chapter,

Go to Davis*Plus* at http://davisplus.fadavis.com/, keyword Treas.

Chapter Resources for Chapter 24:
    Knowledge Check and Think Like a Nurse Response Sheets
    Knowledge Check Answers
    Resources for Caregivers and Health Professionals
    Reading More About Hygiene (Suggested Readings)
    What Are the Main Points in This Chapter?
NCLEX-Style Review Questions
Chapter Overview Podcasts

Concept Map

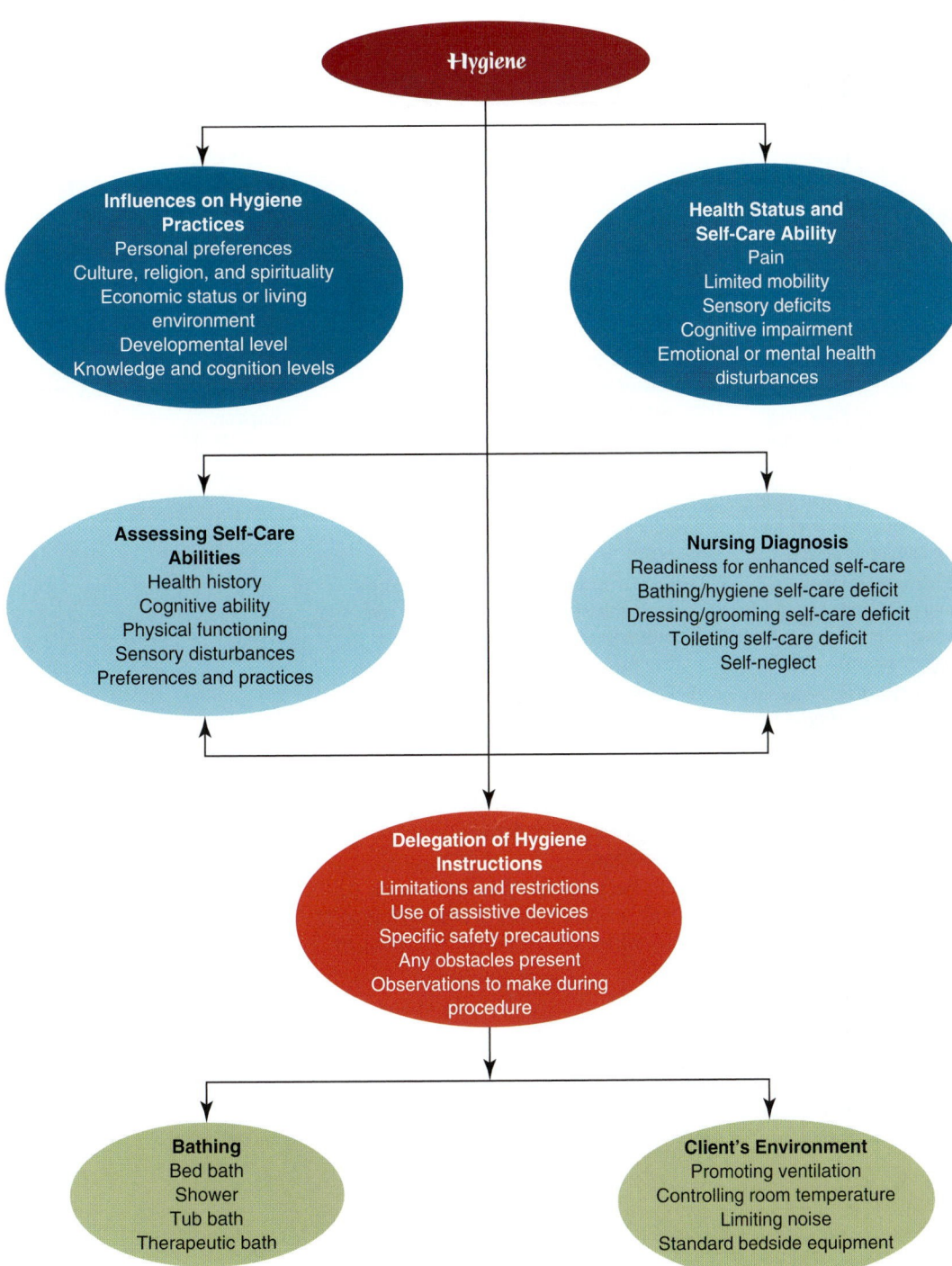

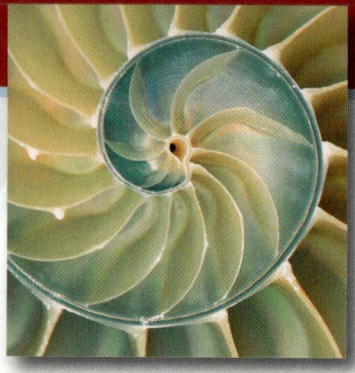

CHAPTER 25

Medicating Patients

Learning Outcomes

After completing this chapter, you should be able to:

➤ Name at least five sources of medication information.

➤ Distinguish among various nomenclature systems for naming and classifying drugs.

➤ Discuss the concepts and processes of pharmacokinetics, including drug absorption, distribution, metabolism, and excretion.

➤ Define *onset, peak,* and *duration of drug action; therapeutic level, peak level,* and *trough level;* and *biological half-life.*

➤ Compare and contrast primary, secondary, cumulative, and side effects; and adverse, toxic, allergic, anaphylactic, and idiosyncratic reactions.

➤ Define *drug-drug interaction, antagonistic drug relationship, synergistic drug relationship, drug incompatibility,* and *medication contraindications.*

➤ Correctly calculate drug dosages, including (1) conversion among the metric, apothecary, and household measurement systems and (2) working with units and milliequivalents (mEq).

➤ List the types of medication prescriptions, including the methods for communicating them.

➤ Discuss the agencies and legislation that help to ensure drug quality and safety.

➤ Describe nursing assessment before, during, and following the administration of a drug.

➤ Plan care for clients with problems of Risk for Injury and Noncompliance related to medications.

➤ Administer medications using the "three checks" and "rights of medication."

➤ Describe appropriate steps you would take if communicating a medication error.

➤ Demonstrate the correct procedure for administering medications by the oral, enteral, inhalant, and parenteral routes.

➤ Demonstrate the intramuscular injection procedure at the following sites: ventrogluteal, deltoid, and vastus lateralis.

➤ Explain why the dorsogluteal site is no longer recommended for intramuscular injections.

➤ List five steps you can incorporate in your practice to ensure safe medication administration and prevent a medication error.

Key Concepts

Medication administration

Medication safety

Pharmacology

Related Concepts

See the Concept Map at the end of this chapter.

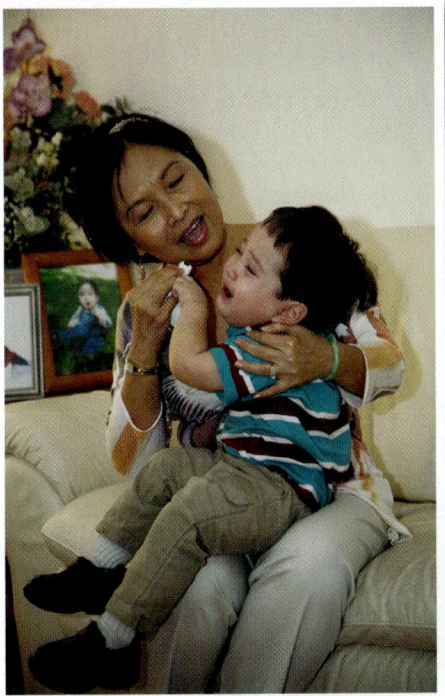

Caring for the Nguyens

This feature allows you to practice the kind of thinking you will use as a full-spectrum nurse. There is usually more than one correct answer to a critical-thinking question, so we do not provide answers for these features. It is more important to develop your nursing judgment than to "cover content." Discuss the questions with your peers. If you are still unsure, consult your instructor.

Kim Phan, the 3-year-old grandson of Nam and Yen Nguyen, has been tired and observed to be sitting down a great deal at preschool. Last week, he developed coughing, wheezing, shortness of breath, nasal congestion, and extreme fatigue. The pediatrician at the Family Medicine Center diagnosed asthma. He prescribed a 5-day tapering course of prednisone, a leukotriene inhibitor (Singulair) 4 mg orally daily at bedtime, and periodic treatments with albuterol through a home nebulizer system.

Nam's mother, Mai Nguyen, became very upset when she saw the bottle of prednisone elixir. She was even more upset when she learned that Kim received an injection of the medicine in the office. She advised Yen not to give Kim the medicine because, she said, it causes weak bones and stunts growth. Yen has called the clinic asking for advice on how to handle this problem.

A. What theoretical knowledge do you need to answer these concerns?

B. What are some reliable sources where you might find this information?

C. What explanation could you offer to Yen to explain the safety of the prednisone prescription? You will need to use a variety of references to answer this question.

D. Yen asks you to explain why Kim received both a shot and pills. How would you respond?

E. Why is Kim receiving a leukotriene inhibitor (Singulair) orally and albuterol by nebulizer? Look up the medications, and use your knowledge of different routes of administration.

 Go to **Caring for the Nguyens Response Sheet** on *DavisPlus.*

Meet Your Patients

You are scheduled to administer medications to five patients on the medical–surgical unit today. You will be administering medications unsupervised for the first time. Your clinical instructor will be available as a resource. Your patients are:

- Margaret Marks, an 82-year-old woman who has a fractured hip and experiences periods of confusion
- Cary Pearson, a 70-year-old man with feeding and swallowing difficulties who receives his medications through a gastrostomy tube
- Cyndi Early, a 32-year-old woman with diabetes who is scheduled for surgery at 1000 today
- James Bigler, a 44-year-old man who has had a repair of a compound fracture of the right arm and is receiving intravenous fluids and medications

- Rebecca Jones, an 84-year-old woman with compression fractures of two lumbar vertebrae resulting from a fall at a nursing home.

You have reviewed your assignment but are unsure of where to begin. Should you visit your patients first and perform an assessment? Should you review the charts first? What should you do with the medication administration records (MARs)? There are so many questions running through your head, and you are a little nervous being on your own. Perhaps you could

(Continued)

Meet Your Patients (continued)

use the model of full-spectrum nursing (Chapter 2) to focus your thinking. In general, any time you give a medication, you will need to incorporate the following:

1. *Theoretical Knowledge:* Find out about the actions and expected effects of the medications you are to give.
2. *Patient Situation:* Assess the health status (e.g., disease process) of each patient as it relates to his medications.
3. *Critical Thinking:* Why is the drug being given? Is there anything about the patient's physiology that may alter

his responses to the drug? Do you need to modify the administration procedure in any way?
4. *Practical Knowledge:* Be sure that you know the procedures for administering each medication safely.

By the time you complete this chapter, you will have the information you need to make those kinds of judgments. Remember that while you are a student, your instructor and the staff nurses will be there for support.

Theoretical Knowledge
knowing **why**

Pharmacology is the science of drug effects. It deals with all drugs used in society, legal and illegal, prescription and non-prescription, and "street" drugs. Because of their potential for harm as well as benefit, you should thoroughly understand the medications you administer.

ABOUT THE KEY CONCEPTS

The broadest concept identified in this chapter is medication administration. The concept of medication safety is intimately related to it. In order to administer medications without causing harm to patients, you will need theoretical knowledge of pharmacology (another key concept), as well as practical knowledge about safe procedures. You will identify many related concepts as you read this chapter (e.g., pharmacodynamics, pharmacokinetics). Try to understand how they relate to the three key concepts. If you can organize information this way in your mind, you are likely to remember it better.

HOW ARE DRUGS NAMED AND CLASSIFIED?

A **drug** is a chemical that interacts with a living organism and alters its activity. In healthcare, drugs are used in diagnosing, treating, or preventing a disease or other medical condition. The term is used interchangeably with *medication*, although some people may think the term *drug* refers to an illegal substance.

Drug Names

A drug may have multiple names. The **chemical name,** rarely used in nursing practice, is the exact description of the drug's chemical composition and molecular structure. For example, *2-(p-isobutylphenyl) propionic acid* is the chemical name of the anti-inflammatory drug ibuprofen. When the developing manufacturer is ready to market a drug, the United States Adopted Name Council (USAN Council) assigns the **generic (nonproprietary) name.** This is usually similar to the chemical name, but it is in a simpler format. The generic name is also the **official name** that is listed in publications such as the *United States Pharmacopeia (USP)* and *National Formulary (NF)*. For example, *ibuprofen* is both a generic and an official name. When the drug is marketed, the manufacturer sells it under a **brand (trade** or **proprietary) name.** The brand name is easily recognized because it begins with a capital letter and sometimes has

a registration mark (®) following the name. Different manufacturers of the same medication may give the medication different brand names. For example, Advil, Nuprin, and Motrin are all brand names for ibuprofen.

Prescription drugs require a written order from a healthcare provider (e.g., physician or advanced practice nurse) who is licensed by the state to prescribe or dispense drugs. **Nonprescription,** or **over-the-counter (OTC),** drugs may be purchased without an order and are assumed to be safe for the general population if consumers follow the manufacturer's directions. Some drugs are nonprescription at low doses but require a prescription for the consumer to purchase in a higher dose. For example, naproxen sodium 200 mg is sold over the counter as Aleve, whereas naproxen 500 mg is sold as Naprosyn and requires a prescription. Some drugs once available only by prescription may become OTC, such as with loratadine (Claritin).

Drug Classifications

It is not realistic to know everything about every drug, so "looking it up" must become second nature. If you learn the common characteristics for a drug classification, then when you encounter a new drug, you will be able to associate it with its classification and make inferences about its basic characteristics.

- By usage—why the drug is used
- By body system—where the drug works
- By chemical or pharmacological class—what the drug is made of

To see an explanation and examples of those classifications methods,

 Go to Chapter 25, **Tables, Boxes, Figures: ESG Table 25-1, Drug Classification System,** on Davis*Plus*.

A drug can be placed in more than one category in a classification system. Classified by usage, for example, ibuprofen (Motrin) can be an analgesic, anti-inflammatory, and an antipyretic agent. A drug can act on more than one body system, as well; in fact, most do. For example, diazepam (valium) is used for its anti-anxiety effects, but it also decreases the activity of the intestinal system and other smooth muscles.

KnowledgeCheck 25-1

- Name three ways a drug may be classified.
- List at least four ways a drug could be named.

WHAT MECHANISMS PROMOTE DRUG QUALITY AND SAFETY?

Before the 20th century, the United States did not have mechanisms for publishing drug ingredients, regulations to govern the contents of drugs, or limitations regarding drug sales. Now, reliable sources of drug information, state and federal regulations and standards controlling drug administration, and a variety of systems for storing and distributing medications in healthcare agencies all work together to protect consumers.

Drug Listings, Directories, and References

When in doubt, look it up! As a nurse, you are professionally, morally, legally, and personally responsible for every dose of medication you administer. Always use current information when researching a medication.

Pharmacopoeia and Formularies. The *United States Pharmacopoeia (USP)* is the directory of drugs approved by the U.S. Food and Drug Administration (FDA) that lists the physical and chemical composition of each drug. Any drug included in this book has met rigorous standards of quality, strength, and purity and the manufacturer is permitted to use the letters *USP* after the drug name. The *National Formulary (NF)* is another official resource for medication information, as are the *British Pharmacopoeia* and the *Canadian Formulary*.

Physician's Desk Reference (PDR). This book, commercially compiled by the pharmaceutical companies, lists manufacturers' prescribing information and is a standard resource for professionals prescribing and administering medication. The *PDR* does not include nursing interventions but does contain information on dosing, routes of administration, and side effects.

Nursing Drug Handbooks. Available from textbook and other publishers, handbooks serve as a quick resource for information (e.g., dosage, side effects) and nursing interventions associated with a drug.

Pharmacology Texts. A textbook provides more information about physiology and pathophysiology than does the drug formulary or a handbook. It may or may not have detailed information about the specific drug you are giving, but it will include a thorough discussion of the drug's classification.

Electronic and Internet-Based Formularies. The Internet, computer software, and other handheld devices offer convenient access to formulary databases.

Pharmacist. A clinical pharmacist can assist you with medication-related concerns (e.g., dosage calculations, drug compatibility).

Medication Package Inserts. Most medications are packaged with an insert that provides information identical to that found in the drug formulary and specific for that particular drug.

Institutional Medication Policies and Procedures. You should know the policies and protocols for medication administration for each institution in which you practice.

ThinkLike a Nurse 25-1

Mr. Pearson (Meet Your Patients) has a medication, metoprolol (Lopressor), due at 0800. You are not familiar with this medication.

- What do you need to know before giving the drug?
- What resources might you use to learn about this medication?

- Which is the generic and which is the brand name of this medication?
- Select a nursing drug handbook and research this medication. What kinds of information are available to you in the book?
- Now look up the drug in a pharmacology text. How is that information similar to and different from the information in the handbook?

Legal Considerations

In the United States, federal, state, and local laws control drug administration. Standards of nursing care, state nurse practice acts, and organizational policies and procedures define your role and responsibilities in administering medications. You must be familiar with them to know what you can and cannot do. In addition, you must recognize the limits of your own experience, skills, and knowledge.

The U.S. Food and Drug Administration (FDA) of the U.S. Department of Health and Human Services (DHHS) regulates the testing, manufacture, and sale of all medications. This agency also monitors the safety and effectiveness of medications available to consumers. This process helps to ensure that ineffective or unsafe drugs are not marketed; if later found unsafe, they are subject to a recall. However, many medicinal products are *not* regulated by the FDA. For example, herbal remedies and some naturopathic supplements are considered "food products" and are not regulated, yet they are advertised as providing health benefits.

Nurse Practice Acts. In most states, a nurse (other than an advanced practice nurse [APN]) cannot prescribe or administer medications without an authorized provider's (e.g., physician or APN) order. If you give medications without an order/prescription, your state board of nursing could revoke your license to practice nursing.

For a state-by-state summary of scope of practice regulations for licensed practical nurses (LPNs)/licensed vocational nurses (LVNs) administering intravenous (IV) medications,

 Go to Chapter 25, **Tables, Boxes, Figures: ESG Table 25-2, LPNs/LVNs State-by-State Scope of Practice for IV Administration,** on Davis*Plus*.

ThinkLike a Nurse 25-2

Obtain a copy of your nurse practice act for the state in which you work. To find a copy,

 Go to the National Council of State Boards of Nursing Web site at http://www.ncsbn.org/

What does your state's nurse practice act tell you about administering medications?

U.S. Drug Legislation. Various state and federal agencies regulate the manufacture and sale of medications. Each state must conform to the federal regulations. The states may institute additional controls. Local governments may enact regulations for the use of alcohol and tobacco. For a historical list of U.S. laws regulating drug quality and safety,

 Go to Chapter 25, **Tables, Boxes, Figures: ESG Table 25-3, U.S. Legislation for Drug Quality and Safety,** on Davis*Plus*.

Regulation of Controlled Substances. Controlled substances are drugs that have either limited medical use or high potential for abuse or addiction. Under the Controlled Substances Act (CSA) of the Comprehensive Drug Abuse Prevention

and Control Act of 1970, it is illegal to possess a controlled substance without a valid prescription. For a summary of categories of controlled substances,

 Go to Chapter 25, **Tables, Boxes, Figures: ESG Table 25-4, Schedules for Controlled Substances,** on Davis*Plus.*

Controlled substances must be stored, handled, disposed of, and administered according to regulations established by the U.S. Drug Enforcement Agency (DEA). Only prescribers with a *national provider identification number* have the authority to prescribe controlled substances. Controlled substances must be stored in locked drawers within a second locked area. (This process is known as **double locking.**) The facility must also keep a record of every dose administered. A count of all controlled substances is performed at specified times, usually at change of shift. To facilitate counting and tracking inventory, drug manufacturers package many narcotics in sectioned containers, with each tablet separately and consecutively numbered (Fig. 25-1).

 Think Like a Nurse 25-3

Locate the controlled substance area on your nursing unit.
- Is a double-locking system in place?
- Who is responsible for "carrying" the narcotics keys?
- What is done if there is a discrepancy between a narcotic sign-out sheet and the actual number of narcotic doses present?

Systems for Storing and Distributing Medications

Most inpatient healthcare facilities have specific areas designed for preparation of medications. Usually this is a central room ("medication room") or mobile cart. Some nursing units store drugs and supplies in a locked cabinet in or near patient rooms. Whatever the method, all drugs are secured in designated areas accessible only to nurses.

Stock Supply

Medications used most frequently may be kept in **stock supply** (bulk quantity), labeled, and in a central location. For example, acetaminophen elixir and cough syrups may be kept in large multidose bottles from which you measure doses for more than one patient. Stock supplies require you to measure

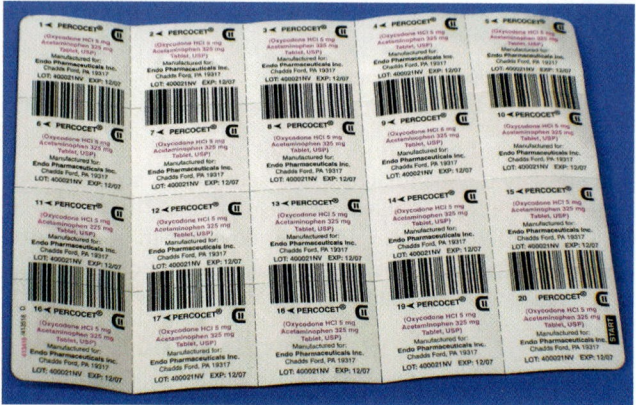

FIGURE 25-1 To facilitate counting, many narcotics are packaged in sectioned containers with each tablet numbered consecutively.

the dose each time a patient needs it, so the potential for measurement error is present each time a dose is prepared. However, a bulk supply of medication is often very cost-effective.

Unit-Dose System

A locked, mobile cart is used, with drawers containing separate compartments for each patient's medications. Extra drawers contain supplies, such as medication cups, syringes, and alcohol swabs. The pharmacy staff refills the drawers each shift or every 24 hours. Limited amounts of **prn** ("give according to patient need") medications and stock medications are also kept in the mobile cart.

A **unit dose** is the prescribed amount of drug the patient receives at a single time. For example, if 800 mg of ibuprofen (Motrin) is prescribed to be given every 8 hours, the unit dose is 800 mg. Each unit dose (usually one tablet) is individually packaged and labeled with drug name, dose, and expiration date. The pharmacist checks each unit dose before sending the drug to the nursing unit, and you will recheck the drug and dose when preparing it for administration. The unit-dose system not only saves nursing time, but also is the safest method because of the double-check system.

Automated Dispensing System

An automated dispensing system is a computerized system similar to a unit-dose system. The locked cart contains all the medications frequently used on a particular nursing unit, and the computer database contains records and counts of the medications, as well as the medication prescriptions for each patient on the unit. Each nurse uses a password to access the machine and enters the data about the needed drug, after which the machine dispenses the medication. The machine tracks dispensed medications for billing and controlled-substances monitoring. The medications are usually packaged in unit doses, but some bulk medications may also be kept on the cart. This method allows for immediate administration of newly prescribed medications, prn medications, controlled substances, and emergency medications because the nurse does not need to wait for the pharmacy to fill a prescription.

Self-Administration

At times while in the hospital, patients may self-administer medications. For example, sublingual nitroglycerin (used for chest pain) is self-administered in the outpatient setting, and some patients can continue self-administration of the drug while in the hospital. The drugs prescribed for self-administration are supplied in individual containers and stored at the bedside. Remind the patient to tell you when he takes the dose. This method promotes independence and allows you to evaluate the patient's ability to manage medications safely and accurately before the patient is discharged. Be sure to check on the policy in your institution; some institutions do not permit patients to administer their own medications.

Knowledge Check 25-2

- What legislation defines controlled substances in the United States?
- How is medication quality managed?

WHAT IS PHARMACOKINETICS?

Pharmacokinetics is a subconcept of pharmacology. It refers to the absorption, distribution, metabolism, and excretion of a drug (Fig. 25-2). These four processes determine the intensity

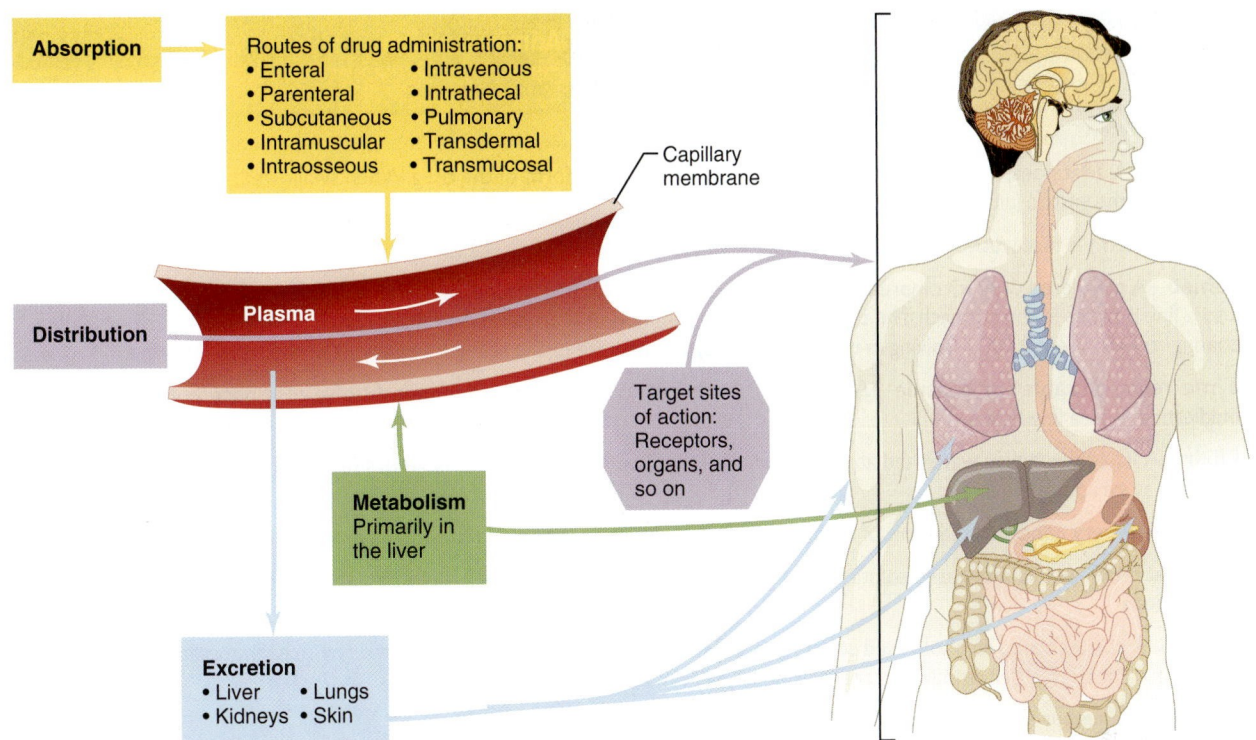

FIGURE 25-2 Pharmacokinetics is the study of drug absorption, distribution, metabolism, and excretion, which determine the intensity and duration of a drug's actions in the body.

and duration of a drug's actions. Each drug has unique pharmacokinetic characteristics. As you study these concepts, think how they relate to each other and to the key concepts, pharmacology and medication administration and safety.

What Factors Affect Drug Absorption?

Absorption refers to the movement of the drug from the site of administration into the bloodstream. The rate of absorption determines when a drug becomes available to exert its action; thus, absorption also influences metabolism and excretion. Absorption depends on the route of administration, form of the drug, drug solubility, effects of pH, blood flow to the area, and body surface area.

Route of Administration

Drugs are given for either local or systemic effect. The **local effects** of a drug occur at the site of application (e.g., certain topical applications of drugs to the skin), so no absorption occurs. When a medication is given for a **systemic effect,** the drug must be absorbed into the bloodstream before it can be distributed to a distant location. A drug may enter the circulation either by injection into a vein or by absorption from other areas into which it has been placed (e.g., muscle, stomach lining, mucous membranes, skin).

Drugs are manufactured for a specific route of administration: oral, sublingual, buccal, inhalant, topical, enteral, and parenteral and are absorbed at different rates depending on the route. The form (preparation) of a drug usually determines its route of administration. Medications are available in a variety of forms (e.g., capsule, elixir).

Table 25-1 summarizes the preparations and the advantages and disadvantages for the various routes of administration. The choice of route is crucial in determining the suitability of the drug for an individual patient. For example, if your patient

is vomiting, an oral drug will not be absorbed effectively in the stomach and would likely be expelled during vomiting. If the patient has diarrhea, rapid motility of the gastrointestinal (GI) tract would decrease absorption.

Solubility of the Drug

Solubility refers to the ability of a medication to be transformed into a liquid form that can be absorbed into the bloodstream. **Enteric-coated** drugs cannot be decomposed by gastric secretions; they dissolve in the small intestine. In this way, the coating delays the action of the medication. It also decreases irritating effects of the medication on the stomach. **Timed-release (sustained-release)** medications are formulated to dissolve slowly, releasing small amounts for absorption over several hours. Oral preparations (e.g., suspension or solutions) must be water soluble and at least partially lipid soluble; they are absorbed faster than tablets or capsules because the medications are already dissolved.

- *Water-soluble drugs.* Drugs must be water soluble in order to dissolve in the (watery) contents of the GI tract.
- *Lipid-soluble drugs.* Lipid solubility depends partly on the drug's chemical structure and partly on the environment at the site of absorption. Lipid-soluble drugs can penetrate lipid-rich cell membranes and enter the cells, whereas water-soluble drugs, such as penicillin, cannot penetrate these areas. That is why a highly fat-soluble drug, such as nitrous oxide, can cross the blood–brain barrier and effect sedation.

Effects of pH and Ionization

The **pH** (relative acidity or alkalinity) of the local environment also affects the absorption of a drug. The acid content of the stomach aids in transporting the medication across the mucous membranes, so *acidic* medications, such as aspirin, are more readily absorbed in the stomach it just seems *basic*

(text continues on page 754)

Table 25-1 ▶ Advantages and Disadvantages of Routes of Administration

ROUTE: ORAL The drug is swallowed and absorbed from the stomach or small intestines.

Preparation Types

- **Capsule**—A gelatinous container that holds the liquid, powder, or oil form of the drug. When swallowed, the gelatin container dissolves in the gastric juices.
- **Pill**—This term is rarely used now. *Tablet* is the preferred term.
- **Tablet**—A powdered drug is compressed into a hard, compact form (e.g., round, oval) that is easy to swallow and then breaks up into a fine powder in the stomach. The tablet is the most common oral preparation. *Enteric-coated tablets* have an acid-insoluble coating to keep them from dissolving in the stomach; they disintegrate in the alkaline secretions of the small intestine.
- **Time-released tablet or capsule**—A tablet or capsule formulated so that it does not dissolve all at once, but gradually releases medication over a few hours
- **Elixir**—A liquid containing water and about 25% alcohol that is sweetened with volatile oils (e.g., aromatic elixir); not as sticky or as sweet as syrups
- **Extract**—A very concentrated form of a drug made from animals or vegetables; may be a syrupy liquid or a powder
- **Fluid extract**—An alcohol-based solution of a drug from a vegetable source (e.g., belladonna); the most concentrated of the fluid preparations
- **Spirits**—A concentrated alcohol-based solution of a volatile (easily evaporated) substance or oil (e.g., ammonia, peppermint oil, orange oil); contains larger amounts of the substance than can be dissolved in water
- **Syrup**—An aqueous solution of sugar, used to disguise unpleasant taste of drugs
- **Tincture**—An alcohol or water-and-alcohol (with a high percentage of alcohol) solution made by extracting potent plants; may also be used externally (e.g., tincture of iodine)
- **Powder**—Finely ground drug(s), usually mixed with a liquid before ingesting; some are used internally, others externally. (Some are mixed with diluents for parenteral injection.)
- **Solution**—Drug(s) dissolved in a liquid carrier. *Aqueous solutions* are medications dissolved in water. (May be used orally, externally, and parenterally.)
- **Suspension**—Drug(s) that are suspended (not completely dissolved) in a liquid. *Aqueous suspensions* are suspended in water. *Never used for IV or intra-arterial routes*

ADVANTAGES	DISADVANTAGES
■ Convenient	■ Unpleasant taste may cause noncompliance.
■ Sterility is not needed for oral use.	■ May irritate gastric mucosa.
■ Economical	■ Patient must be conscious.
■ Noninvasive, low-risk procedure	■ Digestive juices may destroy drug.
■ Easy to administer, good for self-administration	■ Cannot use if patient has nausea and vomiting or decreased gastric motility.
■ Capsule can mask unpleasant taste of a drug.	■ Cannot use if patient has difficulty swallowing.
■ Capsule can be time-release.	■ Potential for aspiration
	■ May be harmful to teeth.
	■ Onset of action is slow.

ROUTE: ENTERAL The drug is given directly into the stomach or intestine (e.g., through a nasogastric or gastrostomy tube).

Preparation Types

Same as for oral medications

ADVANTAGES	DISADVANTAGES
■ Can be used for patients with Impaired Swallowing as an alternative to parenteral administration	■ Not all tablets or capsules can be crushed; medications can clog the NG tube.
	■ NG tube itself presents some risk of aspiration.

Table 25-1 ➤ Advantages and Disadvantages of Routes of Administration—cont'd

ROUTE: SUBLINGUAL (a variation of transmucosal administration)—The drug is held under the tongue and absorbed across the sublingual mucous membrane.

Preparation Types

Lipid-soluble lozenge (troche)—A flat, round preparation that dissolves when held in the mouth. May act locally or be absorbed through mucosa for systemic effect.

Tablet—See oral route.

ADVANTAGES	DISADVANTAGES
■ Used for local or systemic effects	■ May inadvertently be swallowed in the saliva.
■ Convenient	■ Not useful for drugs with unpleasant taste
■ Sterility not needed	■ May irritate the oral mucosa.
■ Quick delivery to general circulation	■ Patient must be conscious.
■ Bypasses stomach and intestines; absorbed directly into bloodstream	■ Useful only for highly lipid-soluble drugs
	■ Patient must hold the drug in place until it is dissolved, which may take a few minutes.
	■ Limited period of effectiveness, requiring frequent redosing

ROUTE: BUCCAL/TRANSMUCOSAL ADMINISTRATION Medication is held against the mucous membrane of cheek until it dissolves.

Preparation Types

Lipid-soluble lozenge or tablet—See oral and sublingual routes.

Spray—Can be dispersed to the nasal or pharyngeal mucosa for rapid absorption.

ADVANTAGES	DISADVANTAGES
■ Same as sublingual	■ Same as sublingual
■ Rapid, convenient, portable	

ROUTE: TOPICAL (SKIN) The drug acts locally or is absorbed directly through skin (transdermal or percutaneous absorption).

Preparation Types

Gel or **jelly**—A clear or translucent semisolid substance that liquefies when applied to the skin

Liniment—An oily liquid to rub into the skin

Lotion—An *emollient* (softening or soothing agent) for use on the skin; may be a clear solution, suspension, or emulsion

Ointment—A semisolid, fatty (usually petroleum jelly or lanolin based) substance for skin or mucous membranes; usually not water soluble

Paste—Similar to an ointment, but thicker and stiffer

Tincture—See oral route.

Transdermal patch—Releases constant, controlled amounts of medication, for systemic effect.

ADVANTAGES	DISADVANTAGES
■ Long-acting systemic effect	■ May cause local irritation, especially if the patient is allergic to latex or tape.
■ Useful if patient is unable to take oral medications	■ Discarded patches may pose danger of poisoning.
■ Acceptable to most patients	■ Leaves residue on skin.
	■ Accurate doses can be difficult to obtain when the drug is in a tube or jar.

Preparation Types

Aerosol spray or foam—A liquid or foam that is sprayed by air pressure onto the skin

Cream—A non-oily, semisolid substance applied to the skin

(Continued)

Table 25-1 ➤ Advantages and Disadvantages of Routes of Administration—cont'd

ADVANTAGES	DISADVANTAGES
▪ Continuous dosing ▪ Sterility is not needed. ▪ For local or systemic effects	▪ Effective only for lipid-soluble drugs and must be specially formulated

ROUTE: TOPICAL: INSTILLATIONS   The drug is placed into a body cavity (e.g., urinary bladder, rectum, vagina, ears, nose, eye).

Preparation Types

Solutions (for nose, ears, and eyes; enemas per rectum)—Drug(s) dissolved in a liquid carrier

Suppositories (for bladder, vagina, rectum)—Drug(s) mixed with a glycerin-gelatin or cocoa butter base and shaped for insertion into the body. They dissolve gradually at body temperature.

Jellies, creams (for vagina and rectum)—See skin route.

ADVANTAGES	DISADVANTAGES
▪ Continuous dosing ▪ Sterility is not needed ▪ Useful if patient is unable to take oral medications ▪ May be used for local or systemic effects	▪ May be embarrassing for the patient. ▪ Drugs may be poorly absorbed from the rectum if stool is present or if the patient defecates before the suppository melts.

ROUTE: TOPICAL: INHALATION   A device (e.g., nebulizer, face mask) breaks the drug into finely dispersed particles, which are breathed into the respiratory passages. Some drugs are intended for local effects in the respiratory passages; others (e.g., anesthetic gases) are for systemic effects, especially in the brain.

Preparation Types

Aerosols—Aerosols are liquids in very fine particles that can be inhaled into the lungs; they are sprayed under air pressure.

Gases—Gas is a basic form of matter (i.e., solid, liquid, and gas). A gas must be kept in a closed container; otherwise, the fast-moving molecules escape into the air. Examples are oxygen, nitrogen, carbon dioxide, and anesthetic gases.

ADVANTAGES	DISADVANTAGES
▪ Quick and efficient local and systemic route through the lungs ▪ May be given to unconscious patient. ▪ Allows continuous dosing, and dosage can be easily modified.	▪ Requires special equipment. ▪ May irritate lung mucosa. ▪ Useful only for drugs that are gases at room temperature. ▪ May have unexpected systemic effect when only local effect is desired.

ROUTE: ALL PARENTERAL ROUTES   Drug taken into the body other than through the digestive system.

Preparation Types

Depends on route.

ADVANTAGES	DISADVANTAGES
Patient may be conscious or unconscious.	▪ Requires sterile procedures. ▪ Poses risk for infection because skin is broken. ▪ Requires skill. ▪ May cause some pain. ▪ Produces anxiety. ▪ More expensive than oral administration

ROUTE: PARENTERAL: INTRAVENOUS   The drug is injected directly into the vein, either by bolus or slow infusion.

Preparation Types

Aqueous solutions—Drug(s) dissolved in water

Table 25-1 ➤ Advantages and Disadvantages of Routes of Administration—cont'd

ADVANTAGES	DISADVANTAGES
■ Rapid effect because absorption is bypassed; therefore, good for emergency situations ■ Patient needs only one needlestick, even for multiple doses.	■ Poses risk of transient drug concentrations if drug is injected too rapidly. ■ Limited to highly soluble medications. ■ Poses risk for sepsis because pathogens may be introduced directly into the bloodstream. ■ The patient must have usable veins. ■ Cost of supplies and medications

ROUTE: PARENTERAL: INTRAMUSCULAR The drug is injected into the muscle mass.

Preparation Types

Primarily aqueous solutions (see intravenous route), although some preparations (e.g., penicillin) are suspensions

ADVANTAGES	DISADVANTAGES
■ Rapid absorption, except for oily preparations or suspensions ■ Allows use of drugs that are not stable in solution. ■ Causes less pain (than do subcutaneous injections) from irritating drugs because they are deep in the muscle. ■ Allows administration of a larger volume than does subcutaneous administration. ■ Allows more rapid absorption than does subcutaneous or oral administration.	■ May cause irritation and local reactions. ■ Poses risk for tissue and nerve damage if site is improperly located. ■ Cannot be used where tissue is damaged (e.g., bruised) or peripheral circulation is decreased.

ROUTE: PARENTERAL: SUBCUTANEOUS The drug is injected into the subcutaneous tissue under the skin

Preparation Types

Primarily solutions—Drugs dissolved in a liquid carrier

ADVANTAGES	DISADVANTAGES
■ Allows faster action than does oral administration. ■ Allows better absorption of lipid-soluble drugs than does intramuscular administration.	■ Only very small amounts can be given. ■ Absorption is relatively slow and often confined to the injected area.

ROUTE: PARENTERAL: INTRADERMAL The drug is injected under the skin, into the dermis. Most commonly used for diagnostic testing or screening or for injecting local anesthetic.

ROUTE: PARENTERAL, OTHER

Preparation Types

Intraspinal—Injection of drug into the spinal canal

Intrathecal—Injection of drug into the subarachnoid space around the spinal cord

Epidural—Injection of drug between the vertebral spines into the extradural space.

Most commonly used for regional anesthesia and pain control.

ADVANTAGES	DISADVANTAGES
■ Most rapid absorption. ■ Highly effective.	■ Some patients may be anxious about administration method. ■ Spinal route can produce hypotension, nausea, urinary retention, or headache.

(alkaline) medications, such as sodium bicarbonate, which are readily absorbed in the more alkaline small intestine.

In solution, some of a drug's molecules are in **ionized** (electrically charged) form, and others are **nonionized** (neutral or noncharged). The ionized molecules are lipid insoluble and thus cannot pass easily through the phospholipid layer of cell membranes. Drug molecules can be converted easily from one form to the other, depending primarily on the pH of the environment. For example, when aspirin is dissolved in the stomach acid, most of its molecules remain nonionized, so they easily pass through the membranes of the gastric mucosa and enter the bloodstream. If the person ingests an antacid before taking aspirin, however, it will likely reduce the effects of the aspirin.

Blood Flow to the Area

Medications are absorbed rapidly in areas where blood flow to the tissue is greatest (e.g., oral mucous membranes). Areas with poor vascular supply (e.g., the skin, scarred areas) experience delayed absorption. Consider the following examples:

- Excessive exercise draws blood away from the stomach and intestines to the muscles. Which route would promote absorption for a person who has just exercised heavily: oral or intramuscular (IM)? Why?
- A person in shock has poor peripheral circulation. Which route would promote faster absorption: intramuscular or intravenous (IV)? Why?

For the first question, the IM route would be better for the person who has recently engaged in heavy activity. This is because medication injected deep into the muscle where there is a rich blood supply would be absorbed more readily; while medication administered orally must first dissolve and be absorbed in the GI tract. For the second question, the IV route would be more efficient for the person with poor circulation because drugs act more rapidly, even in healthy people, when they are injected directly into the bloodstream and do not have to be absorbed.

KnowledgeCheck 25-3

- Define *absorption*.
- How are drugs absorbed?
- What factors affect absorption?

How Are Drugs Distributed Throughout the Body?

Distribution is the transportation of a drug in body fluids (usually the bloodstream) to the various tissues and organs of the body. Because blood goes to all parts of the body, theoretically a drug can produce effects (intended or unintended) anywhere. The rate of distribution depends on adequate local blood flow in the **target area** (the site where the drug effects occur). It is also influenced by the permeability of capillaries to the drug's molecules as well as the protein-binding capacity of the drug. For a visual description,

 Go to Student Resources, **Pharmacokinetic Animation: Medication Absorption, Distribution, Metabolism, and Excretion,** on Davis*Plus*.

Local Blood Flow. The blood supply of the target site affects distribution of a drug. For example, it is difficult to deliver a systemic medication to the skin and toes, where the blood vessels are very small. Factors that cause vasodilation in an area (e.g., application of warmth to an injection site, fever,

and rest) increase circulation to area tissues. Factors that cause vasoconstriction (e.g., shock and chilling of the body) decrease circulation to the target tissue.

Membrane Permeability. Drug molecules must leave the blood and cross capillary membranes to reach their sites of action. The capillary networks in some organs consist of tightly packed endothelial cells that prevent some drugs from crossing them. For example, the blood–brain barrier allows distribution into the brain and cerebrospinal fluid of only those drugs that are (1) lipid soluble (e.g., anesthetics and barbiturates) and (2) not tightly bound to plasma proteins. Many antibiotics are only water soluble, and thus cannot be used to directly treat infections of the central nervous system. This barrier can be bypassed by injecting medications intrathecally (via the spinal canal) into the cerebrospinal fluid.

Protein-Binding Capacity. A drug's tendency to bind to plasma proteins in the blood also affects distribution. For a given amount of a drug, some molecules bind to plasma proteins, and the remainder will be "free." Only free (unbound) drug molecules can produce pharmacological effects because only free molecules can be metabolized or excreted. For example, nearly all acetaminophen (Tylenol) molecules are free in the bloodstream and are therefore pharmacologically active. By contrast, about 99% of the anticoagulant warfarin (Coumadin) is bound in the blood; its effects are produced by only the 1% of warfarin molecules that are free. A drug's tendency to bind to plasma proteins depends mostly on its chemical structure. Some medical conditions also affect protein binding. For example, malnourishment and liver disease reduce the amount of protein (serum albumin) available for binding.

KnowledgeCheck 25-4

- Define *distribution*.
- What factors affect distribution of drugs in the body?

How Are Drugs Metabolized in the Body?

Metabolism (or **biotransformation**) is the chemical inactivation of a drug through its conversion into a more water-soluble compound or into metabolites that can be excreted from the body. Once a medication reaches its site of action, it is metabolized in preparation for excretion.

Metabolism takes place mainly in the liver, but medications can be detoxified also in the kidneys, blood plasma, intestinal mucosa, and lungs. If liver function is impaired (e.g., due to liver disease or aging), the drug will be eliminated more slowly, and toxic levels may accumulate. Disease states also affect drug metabolism. For example, patients with diabetes do not metabolize sugar effectively, so they should not take elixirs, which are high in sugar content.

Oral medications are absorbed from the GI tract and circulate through the liver before they reach the systemic circulation. Many oral medications can be almost completely inactivated in this way. This inactivation is known as the **first-pass effect.** For this reason, oral medications are formulated with a higher concentration of the drug than are parenteral medications. Alternatively, some medications can be given parenterally, allowing the drug to be distributed directly to target sites before it passes through the liver. For example, nitroglycerin undergoes this first-pass effect when taken orally; therefore, it is given sublingually or intravenously so that it bypasses the stomach and liver and reaches therapeutic levels in the blood.

KnowledgeCheck 25-5

- Define *drug metabolism*.
- Where are drugs metabolized?
- What factors affect drug metabolism?

How Are Drugs Excreted From the Body?

A drug continues to act in the body until it is excreted. For **excretion** to occur, drug molecules must be removed from their sites of action and eliminated from the body. Drugs may be metabolized completely, partially, or not at all when they are excreted. The following are common organs of excretion.

Kidneys. The kidneys are the primary site of excretion. Adequate fluid intake facilitates renal excretion. If your patient has decreased renal function (e.g., as indicated by an elevated creatinine level), you should monitor for medication toxicity; if signs of toxicity are present, obtain a prescription for adjusted dosing.

Liver and GI Tract. Some drugs broken down by the liver are excreted into the GI tract and eliminated in the feces. Others (e.g., fat-soluble agents) are reabsorbed by the bloodstream, distributed to the target site, returned to the liver, later excreted by the kidneys. This is called **enterohepatic recirculation.** Anything that increases peristalsis (e.g., diarrhea, laxatives, enemas, chronic bowel disease) accelerates drug excretion via feces. Inactivity, poor diet, and decreased peristalsis delay excretion, increasing the effects of a drug.

Lungs. Most drugs removed by the lungs are not metabolized first. Gases and volatile liquids (e.g., general anesthetics) administered by inhalation usually are removed through exhalation. Other volatile substances, such as ethyl alcohol and paraldehyde, are highly soluble in blood and are excreted in limited amounts by the lungs. Strenuous exercise and deep breathing increase pulmonary blood flow and thereby promote excretion. By contrast, decreased cardiac output (as in shock) and hypoventilation (as can happen when a patient is in pain) prolong the period of time for drug elimination.

Exocrine Glands. Drug excretion through the **exocrine** (sweat and salivary) **glands** is limited. The elimination of metabolites in sweat is frequently responsible for such side effects as dermatitis. Drugs excreted in the saliva are usually swallowed and absorbed as other orally administered agents.

ThinkLike a Nurse 25-4

You are notified of a patient being transferred from the ICU to your unit. The patient is 79-year-old Hattie Banks, admitted 2 days ago to the ICU for digoxin toxicity.

- What theoretical knowledge do you have about the metabolism and excretion of digoxin (Lanoxin)?
- What assessments should you be sure to make for Ms. Banks?

Other Concepts Relevant to Drug Effectiveness

In addition to the processes of absorption, distribution, metabolism, and excretion, you need to understand four other concepts related to a drug's effectiveness: (1) onset, peak, and duration of drug action; (2) therapeutic range; (3) bioavailability of the drug; and (4) concentration of the drug at target sites. As you read about them, try to relate these concepts to the key concepts of medication administration and medication safety.

Onset, Peak, and Duration of Action

The **onset of action** is the time needed for drug concentration to reach a high enough blood level for its effects to appear. This is the **minimum effective concentration.** When the concentration of medication is highest in the blood, the medication has reached its **peak action.** The **duration of action** is that period of time in which the medication has a pharmacological effect (before it is metabolized and excreted) (Fig. 25-3). If the serum level of a medication falls below the minimum effective concentration, then the drug is not effective during that time. If the drug level exceeds the peak level, toxicity occurs.

ThinkLike a Nurse 25-5

Refer to Table 25-1. James Bigler (Meet Your Patients) is having right arm pain and needs relief quickly.

- Would it be better to give him oral acetaminophen with codeine (Tylenol #3) or an IM injection of a similar-strength medication? Why?
- Do you have enough information to be completely sure your choice of route will bring the quickest onset of action? Explain.

Therapeutic Range

Even after absorption stops, distribution, metabolism, and excretion continue. When giving multi-dose medication (e.g., an antibiotic), the goal is to achieve a constant, therapeutic blood level. Because a fraction of the drug is constantly being excreted, repeated doses of the medication are given to achieve and maintain a constant therapeutic concentration.

Therapeutic level is the concentration of a drug in the blood serum that produces the desired effect without toxicity.

Therapeutic range of a drug is a range of therapeutic concentrations. At onset of action, serum drug level is minimal.

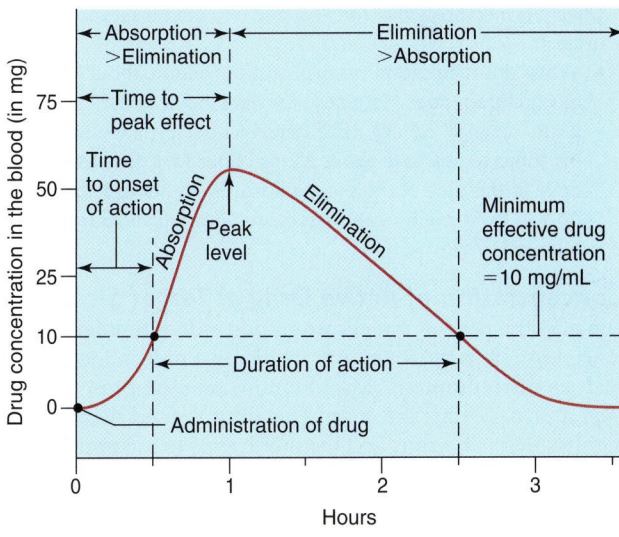

Onset of action = 30 minutes
Peak effect = 1 hour
Duration of action = 2.0 hours

FIGURE 25-3 Once the drug is administered and absorption begins, blood levels begin to rise. When the *minimum effective concentration* is reached, drug effects begin (*onset of action*). *Maximum effect* occurs at peak blood level.

Peak level occurs when the drug is at its highest concentration (when the rate of absorption is equal to the rate of elimination). After that, metabolic and excretory processes begin to remove the drug from the tissues and blood.

Trough level occurs when the drug is at its lowest concentration, right before the next dose is due.

A test called a *peak and trough* helps to ensure the safety and effectiveness of certain drugs. The peak level must be measured when absorption is complete. This, of course, depends on all the factors that affect absorption. The trough level is typically measured about 30 minutes before the next dose of the drug is due. The drug's half-life and the time between doses affect the trough level. You will sometimes need to monitor serum drug levels so the primary care provider can adjust the dose and timing of a medication as needed. For a graphic illustration of peak, trough, and therapeutic levels,

 Go to Chapter 25, **Tables, Boxes, Figures: ESG Figure 25-1,** on Davis*Plus*.

Biological Half-Life

A medication's **biological half-life** is the amount of time it takes for half of the drug to be eliminated. For example, tramadol (Ultram), a narcotic-like pain reliever, has a half-life of approximately 6 hours. This means if you take a 50-mg dose at 0800, by 1400 half of that dose (25 mg) will still be left in your body. In 12 hours, one-fourth of the initial dose (12.5 mg) will be left in your body. Liver and kidney disease, aging, absence of food, and slowed metabolic rate all prolong half-life because of their effects on metabolism and excretion. Drug composition and distribution also affect half-life.

 ThinkLike a Nurse 25-6

Rebecca Jones (Meet Your Patients) received tramadol (Ultram) 50 mg for pain at 0800. The prescription allows her to have the drug every 6 hours. So at 1400, you give her another 50 mg. Ultram is metabolized in the liver and excreted mainly in the urine.

- When this medication reaches onset of action, about how much Ultram does Ms. Jones now have in her body?
- If the "normal" half-life of Ultram is 6 hours, you would expect Ms. Jones to still have about 25 mg of her first dose left in her body at the time of the second dose. Given her age, though, do you think she probably has more or less than 25 mg left at 6 hours? Why?

Concentration of Active Drug at Target Sites

The effectiveness of a medication depends ultimately on its concentration at the intended site. For example, a medication such as nitrofurantoin (Macrodantin) may be prescribed to treat a urinary tract infection. This drug is used because it is highly soluble in urine, and therefore tends to accumulate and concentrate in the bladder and kidneys, where the infection exists.

What Factors Affect Pharmacokinetics?

A drug's pharmacokinetics and therefore its effectiveness and safety, are affected by the following factors:

- **Age.** Infants and young children need smaller doses because of their smaller body mass and immature body systems. Table 25-2 summarizes life-span variations in pharmacokinetics.
- **Body Mass (Weight).** The average adult dose is based on the drug quantity that will produce a particular effect in 50% of

people ages 18 to 65 years and weighing 150 lb. Obviously, a person who is much larger or smaller than this "average" requires an adjusted dose.

- **Sex.** Men and women absorb drugs differently because women usually have lower muscle mass than men, a different hormone profile, and different fat and water distribution.
- **Pregnancy.** Most drugs are contraindicated during pregnancy because of their possible adverse effects on the embryo or fetus. Drugs known to cause developmental defects are called **teratogenic** drugs (e.g., the anticonvulsant phenytoin [Dilantin]).
- **Environment.** Heat and cold affect peripheral circulation. A noisy environment may interfere with a person's response to antianxiety, sedative, or pain medications.
- **Route of Administration.** The route of administration influences the amount of a drug absorbed into the circulatory system and the distribution to the sites of action.
- **Timing of Administration.** The presence or absence of food in the GI tract affects an oral drug's pharmacokinetics. Biorhythms and cycles (e.g., drug-metabolizing enzyme rhythms, blood pressure cycles) also influence drug action.
- **Fluids.** Insufficient fluid intake affects the absorption of solid dosage forms.
- **Pathological States.** Intense pain decreases the effect of opioids; diseases causing circulatory, hepatic, or renal dysfunction interfere with pharmacokinetic processes.
- **Genetic Factors.** Abnormal susceptibility to certain chemicals is genetically determined. Enzyme deficiencies and altered metabolism change a patient's responses to a drug. For example, black people usually respond better to diuretics for blood pressure control than do other racial groups; and people of Asian descent usually metabolize some opioids at a slower rate.
- **Psychological Factors.** Some patients have the same response to a placebo—a pharmacologically inactive substance—as they do to the active drug. If a person has faith that a drug will help him, a *placebo effect* similar to the effect of an active drug may occur. Emotional states, such as anxiety or hostility toward or mistrust of medicine or health personnel can also interfere with a drug's effectiveness.

WHAT IS PHARMACODYNAMICS?

Pharmacodynamics, another subconcept of pharmacology, is the study of how medications achieve their effects at various sites in the body—how specific drug molecules interact with target cells and how biological responses occur. Knowledge of concepts related to pharmacodynamics will help you to administer medications safely and to evaluate patient responses.

What Are Primary Effects?

Primary or **therapeutic effects** of medications are effects that are predicted, intended, and desired. The primary effects, in short, are the reason the drug was prescribed. All other consequences are **secondary effects** (unintended, nontherapeutic). Both primary and secondary effects are dose related, so increasing the dose increases the effects. Medications are given for the following primary effects:

- **Palliative effects** relieve the signs and symptoms of a disease but have no effect on the disease itself. For example, morphine sulfate may be given to a patient with cancer to manage pain, but it does not destroy cancer cells. The goal of palliative therapy is to make the patient as comfortable as possible when treatment options have been exhausted.

Table 25-2 ➤ Drug Therapy Across the Life Span

PHARMACOKINETIC PROCESS	CHILDREN	OLDER ADULTS
Absorption	▪ Exaggerated in infants as a result of lack of gastric acidity and shorter intestines ▪ More complete topical absorption results from a larger body surface and thinner epidermis. ▪ Enteral route is unpredictable. ▪ Decreased muscle tone makes absorption of parenteral drugs unpredictable. ▪ Gastric pH is higher, so that medications absorbed in acid environments are absorbed much more slowly.	▪ Delayed but more complete ▪ Gastric pH is less acidic because of decreased acid production in the stomach. ▪ Decreased gastric pH delays absorption of medications absorbed in acid environments. ▪ Because of decreased intestinal motility, drugs remain in the system longer, allowing for more absorption.
Distribution	▪ Protein binding may be a problem. ▪ Greater chance of toxicity because of low albumin levels. ▪ Water content in the child's body is higher than in adults, so water-soluble drugs are less concentrated in the child and fat-soluble drugs are more highly concentrated.	▪ Low albumin level could create a problem with plasma protein binding. ▪ Increased risk of toxicity due to multiorgan slowdown. ▪ Altered because of less lean mass ▪ Less body water, greater body fat ▪ Dehydration, poor nutrition, and electrolyte imbalances decrease absorption.
Metabolism	▪ Metabolism may be altered because of immature liver. ▪ Best to base dosage on body weight to avoid toxicity.	▪ Presence of diseases may decrease metabolism of the drug. ▪ Changes due to age, higher blood concentration, and less excretion cause greater chances of toxicity. ▪ Some drugs interfere with the liver's ability to metabolize another drug.
Excretion	▪ Excretion is delayed as result of immature kidneys. ▪ Repeat dosing may cause problems.	▪ Decreased glomerular filtration rate inhibits excretion from the kidneys. ▪ Diminished renal function inhibits excretion, thereby increasing the risk of toxicity.

- **Supportive effects** support the integrity of body functions until other medications or treatments can become effective. For a patient with a bacterial infection, you may give acetaminophen (Tylenol) to control fever until blood levels of the prescribed antibiotic are effective in combating the infection causing the fever.
- **Substitutive effects** replace either body fluids or a chemical required by the body for improved functioning. You may, for example, administer insulin to a diabetic patient to replace the insulin no longer produced by the pancreas.
- **Chemotherapeutic effects** destroy disease-producing microorganisms or body cells. Two examples are (1) antibiotics, used to treat infections by killing or limiting the reproduction of certain bacteria and (2) antineoplastic drugs, used to treat cancer by limiting cell reproduction and destroying malignant cells.
- **Restorative effects** return the body to or maintain the body at optimal levels of health. For example, vitamin and

mineral supplements are administered to many patients recovering from surgery.

KnowledgeCheck 25-6

- Name and define the four pharmacokinetic processes.
- How does absorption differ in children and older adults?
- What factors affect excretion?
- You are to administer the following drugs to Cyndi Early (Meet Your Patients): (1) insulin for her diabetes, administered subcutaneously, and (2) morphine to relieve her pain, administered intravenously. For which primary effect is each of these drugs being given?

What Are Secondary Effects?

All medications can cause secondary effects (e.g., side effects, adverse reactions, allergic reactions), which can either be harmless or cause injury and which can sometimes be predicted.

Side Effects

Side effects are unintended, often predictable, physiological effects that are usually well tolerated by patients. They occur at the usual prescribed dose and may be immediate (e.g., dizziness) or delayed (e.g., constipation). For hospitalized patients, you will most often see side effects caused by analgesics, antibiotics, antipsychotics, and sedatives. The most common side effects are nausea, vomiting, diarrhea, dizziness, drowsiness, dry mouth, abdominal distention or distress, and constipation.

If side effects are significant, the medication may be discontinued. For example, lanoxin (Digoxin), which is given to regulate and strengthen the heartbeat, can cause cardiac irregularities, a side effect that can be life threatening. Persistent or undesired side effects may require symptom management with laxatives, antidiarrheals, and antiemetics. For example, levofloxacin (Levaquin), an antibiotic, may cause diarrhea, which is treated with antidiarrheals (e.g., loperamide [Imodium]). Teach your patients what side effects to anticipate with medications and how to manage them.

Adverse Reactions

Adverse reactions are harmful, unintended, usually unpredicted reactions to a drug administered at the normal dosage. They are more severe than side effects and often require discontinuation of the drug.

- When adverse drug reactions (ADRs) are *dose related,* they result from known pharmacological effects of the medication. For example, a diabetic patient treated with insulin may develop very low blood sugar if too much insulin is administered or he doesn't eat.
  - Older adults taking multiple medications are more likely to experience ADRs. Patients seeing multiple providers, who might be prescribing drugs without knowledge of other medications the patient is taking, are at risk for drug incompatibility and ADRs.
  - Age-related changes can alter drug absorption, distribution, metabolism, and excretion, which might lead to accumulation of a drug and potential for ADRs.
  - Older adults and other patients with confusion might not comply with medication regimes as prescribed and take either too much medication, too little, or medication on an erratic schedule, which can lead to ADRs.
- Adverse reactions also occur because of *patient sensitivity,* meaning that the patient is unusually susceptible to the effects of the drug. For example, an older adult with renal impairment would not clear a drug from his system as readily as a healthy adult. Box 25-1 lists patients at high risk for adverse reactions.

The FDA defines **severe adverse reactions** as those that (1) are life threatening; (2) require intervention to prevent permanent impairment or death; or (3) lead to congenital anomaly, disability, hospitalization, or death. Health professionals must document serious adverse reactions according to agency policy and report them to the FDA MedWatch program. To make a report, contact the FDA by calling 1-800-332-1088, or

 Go to the **FDA Medwatch Web site** at http://www.fda.gov/medwatch/

You can also contact the Institute for Safe Medication Practices (ISMP) to report errors, close calls, or hazardous conditions. ISMP guarantees the confidentiality and security of the information received.

BOX 25-1 ■ Risk Factors for Adverse Drug Reactions

- Receiving treatment from two or more providers at the same time
- Concurrent illnesses (e.g., diabetes and renal failure)
- A change in the ability to absorb, metabolize, or excrete a drug (e.g., impaired hepatic or renal function)
- Taking multiple prescription drugs in addition to over-the-counter preparations and herbal remedies and supplements. This is also called polypharmacy
- Taking a drug inconsistently
- Confusion/cognitive impairment
- History of allergies or previous adverse drug reactions
- Long-term use of a drug (may promote accumulation, leading to toxicity)
- Very old or very young age
- Obesity or extreme thinness
- Dehydration or rapid change in hydration status

 Go to https://www.ismp.org/orderforms/reporterrortoismp.asp

Toxic Reactions

Toxic reactions are dangerous, damaging effects to an organ or tissue. They are more severe than adverse reactions, sometimes even causing permanent damage or death. It may help to think of toxicity as poisoning. Antidotes are available for some medications; for example, naloxone (Narcan) is given for opiate toxicity. Toxicity may be caused by any of the following:

- *Overdosing* (administrating a dose that exceeds the prescribed amount). Examples are respiratory depression from excessive morphine and hypoglycemia from too much insulin)
- *Accumulation* of the drug in the tissues (related to long-term use or incomplete metabolism/excretion)
- *Abnormal sensitivity* or allergic response to the drug

Toxic reactions are usually localized, reversible, and immediate. However, they can be:

- Localized to a particular tissue or organ, or they can affect several organ systems.
- Reversible (e.g., tinnitus caused by aspirin) or permanent (e.g., hearing loss caused by aminoglycoside antibiotics).
- Evident soon after administration; although, some toxic reactions take months or even years to develop (e.g., drug-induced cancers).

 Think**Like a Nurse** 25-7

- You have just looked up the antihypertensive drug lisinopril (Zestril) and found the following side effects. What strategy could you use to help you remember all the side effects listed below?

  neutropenia, dizziness, headache, fatigue, depression, somnolence, paresthesia, hypotension, orthostasis, chest pain, nasal congestion, diarrhea, nausea, dyspepsia, impotence, rash, cough, muscle cramps, angioedema, lethargy, hypokalemia, decreased libido

- You have checked the MAR for Margaret Marks (Meet Your Patients) and prepared her next dose of antibiotic for intravenous administration. The MAR also indicates that she is receiving morphine for pain and that her last dose

was given 1 hour ago. When you enter the room, you find her apparently sleeping. You are not able to awaken her to verify her identity. What do you suspect is happening, and how should you respond? (If you need information about antibiotics and morphine, look it up in an appropriate reference.)

Allergic Reactions

In an **allergic reaction,** the immune system identifies a medication as a foreign substance that should be neutralized or destroyed. The patient experiences no problems with the first dose of the medication, but it acts as an antigen, activating the formation of antibodies against the drug. When the drug is again administered, the antigen–antibody-binding complex prompts an allergic reaction.

Allergic reactions range from minor to serious; however, even a small amount of a medication can cause a severe reaction. Urticaria (hives), pruritus (itching), edema of soft tissue and mucosa, and rhinitis (inflammation of the nasal mucosa) usually occur within minutes to 2 weeks after exposure and are considered mild. Such reactions often disappear after the medication is discontinued and the blood level of the drug falls. Medications most frequently implicated in allergic reactions are antibiotics, biological agents, and diagnostic agents. To print out and use a list of specific drugs frequently implicated in allergic reactions,

 Go to Chapter 25, **Tables, Boxes, Figures: ESG Table 25-5, Medications Frequently Triggering Allergic Reactions,** on Davis*Plus.*

An **anaphylactic reaction** is a life-threatening allergic reaction that occurs immediately after administration. Anaphylaxis produces sudden constriction of bronchioles, edema of the larynx and pharynx, severe shortness of breath, wheezing, and severe hypotension (low blood pressure). Immediate treatment includes discontinuing the medication and giving epinephrine, IV fluids, steroids, and antihistamines. Respiratory support (e.g., oxygen, intubation, ventilation) may also be required.

✚ A patient who is allergic to one drug may also be allergic to other medications in the same class. For example, many patients who are allergic to penicillin are also allergic to cephalexin (Keflex), a synthetic penicillin.

✚ People with severe allergic reactions should wear a Medic Alert bracelet (Fig. 25-4) that identifies the person and the allergen, and carry epinephrine for emergency injection.

 Think**Like a Nurse** 25-8

You are administering medications to your assigned patients (Meet Your Patients). What should you do in each of the following situations? Which patient should you attend to first? Explain your thinking.

- Ms. Jones has ibuprofen (Motrin) prescribed for her back pain. She tells you she cannot take this medication because it makes her feel nauseated.
- Mr. Bigler had an open reduction internal fixation of his arm performed yesterday and is receiving an antibiotic, cefazolin (Ancef), 500 mg IV every 8 hours. He has already received three doses of this medication, and you initiated his 0800 dose about 10 minutes ago. He tells you that he thinks his throat is closing shut.

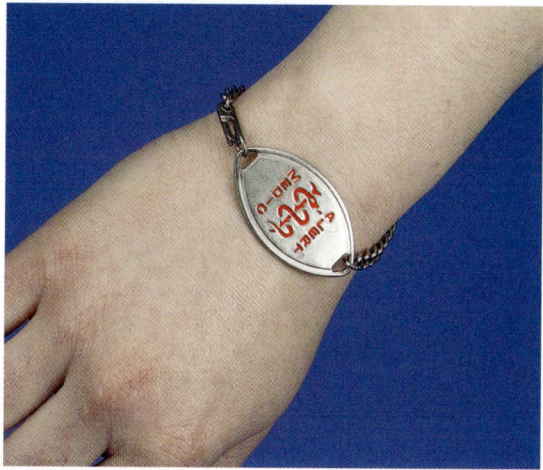

FIGURE 25-4 People with severe allergies to a medication should wear a Medic Alert bracelet.

Idiosyncratic Reactions

An **idiosyncratic** reaction is an unexpected, abnormal, or peculiar response to a medication. Idiosyncratic reactions may take the form of extreme sensitivity to a medication, lack of response, or a paradoxical (opposite of expected) response, such as agitation in response to a sedative.

Cumulative Effect

A **cumulative effect** is the increased response to repeated doses of a drug that occurs when the rate of administration is greater than the rate of metabolism and excretion. This happens when (1) the body cannot metabolize a dose of the medication before the next dose is given, (2) excretion is slowed but absorption is normal or rapid, or (3) absorption is slowed. Unless the dose is changed, the medication accumulates in the system until a toxic level is reached. Opiates and barbiturates are known for their cumulative effects.

Knowledge Check 25-7

- Differentiate between primary and secondary effects of medications.
- List one adverse reaction for each of the following systems: blood, gastrointestinal, neurological, cardiovascular, hepatic, and renal.
- What are some of the symptoms you will see in an anaphylactic reaction?
- What type of patient is most likely to experience an allergic reaction?

How Do Medications Interact?

When one drug alters or modifies the action of another, a **drug interaction** occurs. In an **antagonistic drug relationship,** one drug interferes with the actions of another and decreases the resultant drug effect—that is, the combined effect is less than that of one drug given alone. In a **synergistic drug relationship,** there is an additive effect; that is, the effect of both drugs together is greater than the individual effects. **Drug incompatibilities** occur when multiple drugs are mixed together, causing a chemical deterioration of one or both drugs. The result is an incompatible solution that should not be administered.

You can usually recognize an incompatibility when the mixed solution takes on a changed appearance. However, you should always consult medication resources and compatibility charts *before* mixing medications. Then, after mixing, double-check the medication for changes in appearance.

As a nurse, you must know about drug interactions and monitor your patients for them. The more drugs a patient takes, the higher the risk of a drug interaction. Other variables influence drug interactions: intestinal absorption, competition for protein binding, drug metabolism, renal excretion, and alteration of electrolyte imbalance. Drugs may also interact with certain foods. For example,

High-fat foods and low-fiber foods can delay stomach emptying and drug absorption by up to 2 hours.

Acidic citrus fruits and juices enhance absorption of iron. Some citrus fruits, such as grapefruit, interact with medication in an antagonistic manner.

Carbonated soft drinks can cause medications to dissolve faster, be neutralized, or experience a change in absorption rate in the stomach.

Dairy products taken with an antibiotic, such as tetracycline, decrease the absorption of the drug in the stomach.

To print and use a list of several medications that should be taken with food and those that should be taken on an empty stomach,

 Go to Chapter 25, **Tables, Boxes, Figures: ESG Box 25-1,** on Davis*Plus*.

For a list of common drug-drug and drug-food interactions,

Go to Chapter 25, **Tables, Boxes, Figures: ESG Table 25-6, Drug-Drug and Food-Drug Interactions,** on Davis*Plus*.

Knowledge Check 25-8

- What type of interaction occurs when one drug interferes with the action of another?
- What interactions occur when one drug has an additive effect on another drug?
- What is drug incompatibility?

What Should I Know About Drug Abuse or Misuse?

You should be able to differentiate between tolerance and dependence. **Tolerance** is a decreasing response to repeated doses of a medication. The person then requires more of the drug to achieve the desired effect. In contrast, a person's reliance on, or need for, a drug constitutes **drug dependence.** Dependence leads to compulsive patterns of drug use wherein the user's lifestyle centers on procuring and taking the drug.

Drug misuse is the nonspecific, indiscriminate, or improper use of drugs, including alcohol, OTC, and prescription drugs. In performing self-care, people frequently misuse laxatives, aspirin, acetaminophen, ibuprofen, cough and cold remedies, and sleep-inducing drugs. Older adults are especially prone to misuse of laxatives.

Drug abuse is the inappropriate intake of a substance by amount, type, or situation, continuously or periodically. For example, consuming alcohol at work is considered abuse, but having a glass of wine with dinner is not. Drug abuse may or may not lead to drug dependence. **Illicit drugs,** also known as street drugs, are drugs sold illegally. Many are prescription drugs (e.g., hydrocodone [Oxycontin or Vicodin]) sought for their mood-altering effects. Prescription drugs can be abused when taken for purposes other than medically intended.

HOW DO I MEASURE AND CALCULATE DOSAGE?

Medications are not always available in the exact dosage the patient needs. Therefore, you must be proficient in calculating drug dosages to be sure your patients receive the correct amount of medication.

Medication Measurement Systems

Medications are usually prescribed and measured using the metric system; however, a few are still dispensed using the apothecary and household systems. You will sometimes need to make conversions from one measurement system to another. To learn about how to convert medication doses within one system and between systems,

 Go to Chapter 25, **Supplemental Materials: Measuring and Calculating Dosage,** on Davis*Plus*.

Metric System. The metric system is the preferred system to measure drug dosages because it promotes accuracy by allowing for calculation of small drug dosages. A disadvantage of this system in the United States is that many people outside the healthcare system are not familiar with it.

Apothecary System. The British apothecary system of measurement has been in use in the United States since colonial times. Only a few medications (e.g., aspirin) are measured using this system because it is less convenient and less precise. Apothecary measurements are usually written using Roman numerals, but you may also see them in Arabic numerals. For example, *5 grains* might be written as *grains V* or *gr V.*

 To avoid a dosage error, write out the intended unit of measurement (grains) so gr (grains) is not mistaken for g (grams).

Household System. Because most people are familiar with the household system, it is easier to teach a patient about home medications using this system. However, nurses do not often use it because dosages measured in this system are less precise (e.g., teaspoons, ounces, cup) and can lead to medication dosing error.

Special Measurements: Units and Milliequivalents

Note that units and millequivalents (mEq) *cannot* be directly converted to the apothecary, metric, or household systems.

Units. Insulin, a drug used by diabetics to help control blood sugar, is measured in **units,** with 100 international units (U100) being the standard strength preparation. In this strength, 1 mL of the fluid medication contains 100 units of insulin. Heparin, an anticoagulant, and penicillin are also prescribed in units. The following is a prescription using units: "NPH insulin 14 units subcutaneously every morning."

 Be aware that not all units are the same. For example, 1 mL of heparin does *not* contain 100 units of heparin. You must always read the container label to know the number of units per milliliter.

Milliequivalents (mEq) indicate the strength of the ion concentration in a drug. A milliequivalent is the number of grams of a solid contained in one mL of a solution. Electrolytes, such as potassium chloride (KCl), are measured in mEq. The following is a medication prescriptions using mEq: "D$_5$W 1000 mL with KCl 40 mEq every 8 hours."

Calculating Dosages

You should be able to calculate accurately using several different methods and formulas. Inaccurate calculations result in incorrect dosages and could harm the patient. One easy formula to remember is the following:

$$\frac{\text{Dose on hand}}{\text{Quantity (or volume) on hand}} = \frac{\text{Desired Dose}}{\text{Quantity (or volume) desired}} \quad \text{or} \quad \frac{DH}{QH} = \frac{DD}{X}$$

You must pay attention to both the milligrams (weight of the drug) marked on the medication container and the milliliters (amount of liquid in which the medication is dissolved).

You will sometimes need to make conversions from one measurement system to another. To learn about how to convert medication doses within one system and between systems,

 Go to Chapter 25, **Supplemental Materials: Measuring and Calculating Dosage,** on *DavisPlus.*

If you need help making conversions from one measurement system to another, you should obtain a dosage calculation book and practice the various formulas until you are proficient with conversion.

How Should I Calculate Dosage for a Child?

You must be very careful when calculating medication dosages for children and infants. Most drug references list normal pediatric ranges, which can serve as additional verification.

You should rarely need to calculate a child's dosage on the basis of an adult dose, because medication prescriptions should specify the exact dosage for the individual child. However, you can use either the Body Surface Area (BSA) Formula by using the Nomogram for Children or Clark's Rule for Children to verify the safety of pediatric orders. To find a child's BSA using the nomogram, you must know the child's height and weight. To use a nomogram,

 Go to Chapter 25, **Tables, Boxes, Figures: ESG Figure 25-2,** on *DavisPlus.*

Orders for pediatric dosages are usually either calculated by the prescriber or stated in terms of "milligrams per kilogram of body weight." For example, you might have a prescription for "Erythromycin 30 mg/kg of body weight." You know that 1 kg equals 2.2 lb. If the child weighs 44 lb, then to convert to kilograms you divide 44 by 2.2; the child thus weighs 20 kg. So, 30 mg/kg would be 30 mg × 20, or 600 mg (the dosage for a 20-kg child).

If you want to use Clark's Rule, which is a formula using the child's weight in pounds,

 Go to Chapter 25, **Tables, Boxes, Figures: ESG Box 25-2,** on *DavisPlus.*

For a Web-based dose calculator,

 Go to **Manuel's Web site** at http://www.manuelsweb. com/nrs_calculators.htm

WHAT MUST I KNOW ABOUT MEDICATION PRESCRIPTIONS?

Before administering any medication, you must obtain a **prescription** from the primary care provider and verify that it is complete and legible.

- For inpatients, prescriptions for medications are either entered into an electronic health record for automated dispensing or printed in the medical orders section of the paper chart. This was traditionally referred to as an *order.*
- For outpatients and for medications that will be filled by the patient (instead of the agency pharmacy), the prescription is written on a form similar to Figure 25-5, and given to the patient or family. This is what was traditionally called a *prescription.*

The term *prescription* is now used to refer to both the traditional inpatient *order* and the outpatient *prescription.* A written or printed outpatient medication prescription should contain the following essential elements (Fig. 25-5):

- Patient's full name (some agencies and some states require the address of the patient)
- Name, address, and telephone number of the prescriber, including relevant credentials and legal registration number, such as the National Provider Identification (NPI) in the United States. Providers who are prescribing controlled substances must register with the federal Drug Enforcement Agency (DEA). The prescriber's DEA number must be included on the prescription.
- Date and time prescription was written
- Name of medication
- Dosage (including size, frequency, and number of doses)

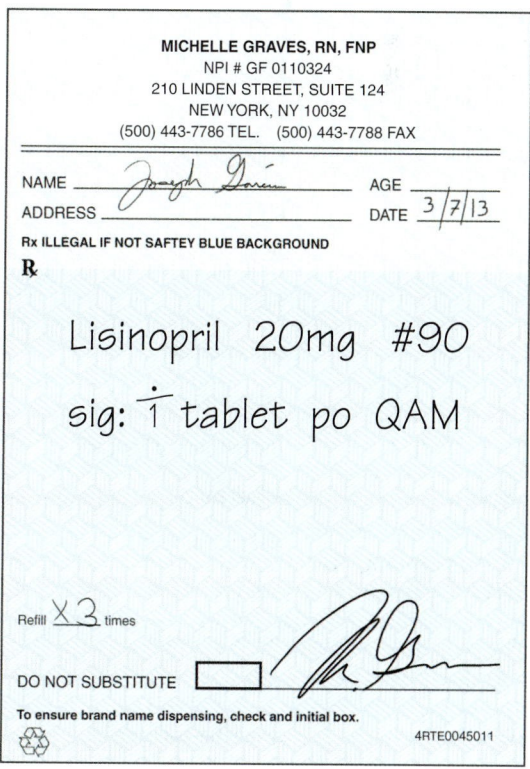

FIGURE 25-5 Example of a prescription.

- Route of administration
- Signature of prescriber

To verify a medication prescription for inpatients, ask yourself the following questions:

Is the prescription legible enough for me to clearly read?

Is the prescribed dose within the normally prescribed dosage range and comparable to previously prescribed dose?

Is the prescribed route appropriate?

Is the drug appropriate for the patient? (For example, you would question an antihypertensive drug to be prescribed for a patient with hypotension.)

Is the patient allergic to the medication prescribed?

Are the administration times appropriate? For example, is an antibiotic prescribed for every 6 hours when the drug formulary indicates it should be taken every 24 hours?

For outpatient prescriptions (to be obtained by the patient):

What are the address, phone number, and National Provider Identification (NPI) of the person prescribing?

Is a DEA number included on prescriptions for controlled substances?

How many doses are there before the prescription needs to be refilled?

How many refills are prescribed?

KnowledgeCheck 25-9

- What are the essential parts of a medication prescription?
- How does an inpatient prescription (order) differ from an outpatient prescription?

What Abbreviations Are Used in Medication Prescriptions?

Because abbreviations can be easily misread, it is better to write words in full, especially when you are working with medications. However, you might still see the following abbreviations (Table 25-3), so you should be familiar with them. Also be sure you are familiar with the list of abbreviations approved for use in your particular agency. Use abbreviations cautiously and avoid using them when possible.

Consult The Joint Commission's official Do Not Use list (see Chapter 18, Use of Abbreviations). You must also know the acceptable abbreviations used in your facility. Also, be familiar with the Institute for Safe Medication Practices List of Error-Prone Abbreviations, Symbols, and Dose Designations in Table 25-4.

Types of Medication Prescriptions

Common types of medication prescriptions are based on the duration, frequency, and/or urgency of the prescription.

- **Standard written prescriptions** apply without a renewal date until the prescriber writes a prescription to alter or

(text continues on page 766)

Table 25-3 ▶ Common Medication-Related Abbreviations

ABBREVIATION	EXPLANATION	ABBREVIATION	EXPLANATION
ac	before meals	pc	after meals
ad lib	as desired	PM	evening
AM	Morning	po or PO	by mouth
bid	twice a day	prn	as needed
c̄	with	qh, qr (q1h, q1hr)	every hour
fl oz	fluid ounce	q2h, q2hr	every 2 hours
g, gm, or GM	gram	q3h, q3hr	every 3 hours
gtt	drop	q4h, q4hr	every 4 hours
h, hr	hour	q6h, q6hr	every 6 hours
IM	intramuscular	qid or QID	four times a day
IV	intravenous	qs	sufficient quantity
IVPB	intravenous piggyback	s̄	without
Kg or kg	kilogram	Stat or STAT	at once
KVO	keep vein open	sup or supp	suppository
L or l	liter	susp	suspension
mEq	milliequivalent	tab	tablet
mL or ml	milliliter	Tbsp	tablespoon
OTC	over-the-counter	Tid or TID	three times a day
oz	ounce	T or tsp	teaspoon

Table 25-4 ➤ Institute for Safe Medication Practices (ISMP) List of Error-Prone Abbreviations, Symbols, and Dose Designations

ABBREVIATIONS	INTENDED MEANING	MISINTERPRETATION AND CORRECTION
μg	Microgram	Mistaken as "mg" *Correction:* Use "mcg."
AD, AS, AU	Right ear, left ear, each ear	Mistaken as OD, OS, OU (right eye, left eye, each eye) *Correction:* Use "right ear," "left ear," or "each ear."
OD, OS, OU	Right eye, left eye, each eye	Mistaken as AD, AS, AU (right ear, left ear, each ear) *Correction:* Use "right eye," "left eye," or "each eye."
BT	Bedtime	Mistaken as BID (twice daily) *Correction:* Use "bedtime."
cc	Cubic centimeters	Mistaken as "u" (units) *Correction:* Use "mL."
D/C	Discharge or discontinue	Premature discontinuation of medications if D/C (intended to mean "discharge") has been misinterpreted as "discontinued" when followed by a list of discharge medications *Correction:* Use "discharge" and "discontinue."
ij	Injection	Mistaken as "IV" or "intrajugular" *Correction:* Use "injection."
IN	Intranasal	Mistaken as "IM" or "IV" *Correction:* Use "intranasal" or "NAS."
HS	Half-strength	Mistaken as bedtime *Correction:* Use "half-strength."
hs	At bedtime, hours of sleep	Mistaken as half-strength *Correction:* Use "bedtime."
IU	International units	Mistaken as IV (intravenous) or 10 (ten) *Correction:* Use "International units."
o.d. or OD	Once daily	Mistaken as "right eye" (OD-oculus dexter), leading to oral liquid medications administered in the eye *Correction:* Use "daily."
OJ	Orange juice	Mistaken as OD or OS (right or left eye); drugs meant to be diluted in orange juice may be given in the eye *Correction:* Use "orange juice."
Per os	By mouth, orally	The "os" can be mistaken as "left eye" (OS-oculus sinister) *Correction:* Use "PO," "by mouth," or "orally."
q.d. or QD	Every day	Mistaken as q.i.d., especially if the period after the "q" or the tail of the "q" is misunderstood as an "i" *Correction:* Use "daily."
qhs	Nightly at bedtime	Mistaken as "qhr" or every hour *Correction:* Use "nightly."
qn	Nightly or at bedtime	Mistaken as "qh" (every hour) *Correction:* Use "nightly" or "at bedtime."

(Continued)

Table 25-4 ➤ Institute for Safe Medication Practices (ISMP) List of Error-Prone Abbreviations, Symbols, and Dose Designations—cont'd

ABBREVIATIONS	INTENDED MEANING	MISINTERPRETATION AND CORRECTION
q.o.d. or QOD	Every other day	Mistaken as "q.d." (daily) or "q.i.d." (four times daily) if the "o" is poorly written *Correction:* Use "every other day."
q1d	Daily	Mistaken as q.i.d. (four times daily) *Correction:* Use "daily."
q6PM, etc.	Every evening at 6 PM	Mistaken as every 6 hours *Correction:* Use "6 PM nightly" or "6 PM daily."
SC, SQ, sub q	Subcutaneous	SC mistaken as SL (sublingual); SQ mistaken as "5 every"; the "q" in "sub q" has been mistaken as "every (e.g., a heparin dose ordered sub q 2 hours before hours before surgery) surgery" misunderstood as every 2 *Correction:* Spell out "subcutaneous."
ss	Sliding scale (insulin)	Mistaken as "55" *Correction:* Spell out "sliding scale"; use "one-half."
SSRI, SSI	Sliding scale regular insulin	Mistaken as selective-serotonin reuptake inhibitor; mistaken as Strong Solution of Iodine (Lugol's) *Correction:* Spell out "sliding scale (insulin)."
i/d	One daily	Mistaken as "tid" *Correction:* Use "1 daily."
TIW or tiw	3 times a week	Mistaken as "3 times a day" or "twice in a week" *Correction:* Use "3 times weekly."
U or u	Unit	Mistaken as the number 0 or 4, causing a 10-fold overdose or greater (e.g., 4U seen as "40" or 4u seen as "44"); mistaken as "cc" so dose given in volume instead of units (e.g., 4u seen as 4cc) *Correction:* Use "unit."

DOSE DESIGNATIONS OR OTHER INFORMATION	INTENDED MEANING	MISINTERPRETATION	CORRECTION
Trailing zero after decimal point (e.g., 1.0 mg)	1 mg	Mistaken as 10 mg if the decimal point is not seen expressed in whole numbers	Do not use trailing zeros for doses.
No leading zero before a decimal dose (e.g., .5 mg)	0.5 mg	Mistaken as 5 mg if the decimal point is not seen	Use zero before a decimal point when the dose is less than a whole unit.
Drug name and drug dose run together (e.g., Inderal 40 mg)	Inderal 40 mg	Mistaken as Inderal 140 mg	Place adequate space between the drug name, dose, and unit of measurement.
Numeric dose and unit of measurement run together (e.g., 10 mg)	10 mg	The "m" can be mistaken for a zero, leading to a 10-fold dosing error	Place adequate space between the drug name, dose, and unit of measurement.
Abbreviations, such as mg or mL with a period following the abbreviation	mg or mL	The period is unnecessary and could be mistaken as the number 1 if written poorly.	Use mg, mL, etc. without a period.

Table 25-4 ➤ Institute for Safe Medication Practices (ISMP) List of Error-Prone Abbreviations, Symbols, and Dose Designations—cont'd

DOSE DESIGNATIONS OR OTHER INFORMATION	INTENDED MEANING	MISINTERPRETATION	CORRECTION
Large doses without properly placed commas (e.g., 100000 units or 1000000 units)	100,000 or 1,000,000 units	100000 has been mistaken for 10,000 or 1,000,000; 1,000,000 has been mistaken for 100,000.	Use commas for dosing units at or above 1,000 or use such words as 100 "thousand" or 1 "million" to improve readability.

DRUG NAME ABBREVIATIONS	INTENDED MEANING	MISINTERPRETATION AND CORRECTION

NOTE: PHARMACIES DO NOT ACCEPT ORDERS FOR ABBREVIATED MEDICATIONS. *ALSO NOTE THAT THE CORRECTIVE ACTION FOR ALL DRUG NAME ABBREVIATION ERRORS IS TO CAREFULLY WRITE OUT THE COMPLETE DRUG NAME.

ARA A	vidarabine	Mistaken as cytarabine (ARA C)
AZR	zidovudine (Retrovir)	Mistaken as azathioprine or aztreonam
CPZ	prochlorperazine (Compazine)	Mistaken as chlorpromazine
DPT	Demerol-Phenergan-Thorazine	Mistaken as diphtheria-pertussis-tetanus
DTO	Diluted tincture of opium, or deodorized tincture of opium (paregoric)	Mistaken as tincture of opium
HCl	hydrochloric acid or hydrochloride	Mistaken as potassium chloride (The "H" is misinterpreted as "K.")
HCT	hydrocortisone	Mistaken as hydrochlorothiazide
HCTZ	hydrochlorothiazide	Mistaken as hydrocortisone (seen as HCT 250 mg)
$MgSO_4$	magnesium sulfate	Mistaken as morphine sulfate
MS, MSO_4	morphine sulfate	Mistaken as magnesium sulfate
MTX	methotrexate	Mistaken as mitoxantrone
PCA	procainamide	Mistaken as patient-controlled analgesia
PTU	propylthiouracil	Mistaken as mercaptopurine
T3	Tylenol with Codeine No. 3	Mistaken as liothyronine
TAC	triamcinolone	Mistaken as tetracaine, adrenaline, cocaine
TNK	TNKase	Mistaken as "TPA"
$ZnSO_4$	zinc sulfate	Mistaken as morphine sulfate

STEMMED DRUG NAMES	INTENDED MEANING	MISINTERPRETATION
"nitro drip"	nitroglycerine infusion	Mistaken as sodium nitroprusside infusion
"Norflox"	norfloxacin	Mistaken as Norflex
"IV Vanc"	intravenous vancomycin	Mistaken as Invanz

SYMBOLS	INTENDED MEANING	MISINTERPRETATION AND CORRECTION
ʒ	dram	Symbol for dram mistaken as "3" *Correction:* Use the metric system.

(Continued)

Table 25-4 ➤ Institute for Safe Medication Practices (ISMP) List of Error-Prone Abbreviations, Symbols, and Dose Designations—cont'd

SYMBOLS	INTENDED MEANING	MISINTERPRETATION AND CORRECTION
ℳ	Minim	Mistaken as "mL" *Correction:* Use the metric system.
x3d	for 3 days	Mistaken as "3 doses" *Correction:* Use "for 3 days."
< and >	greater than and less than	Mistaken as opposite of intended; mistakenly using incorrect symbols *Correction:* Use "greater than" or "less than."
/ (slash mark)	separates two doses or indicates "per"	Mistaken as the number 1 (e.g., "25 units/10 units" misread as "25 units and 110" units *Correction:* Use "per" rather than a slash mark to separate doses.
@	at	Mistaken as "2" *Correction:* Use "at."
&	and	Mistaken as "2" *Correction:* Use "and."
+	plus or and	Mistaken as "4" *Correction:* Use "and" or "plus."
°	Hour	mistaken as zero (e.g., q2° seen as q 20) *Correction:* Use "hr", "h", or "hour."

Source: Institute for Safe Medication Practices. (2004). *IMSP List of Error-Prone Abbreviations, Symbols, and Dose Designations.* Retrieved from http://www.ismp.org/PDF/ErrorProne.pdf

discontinue the medication or indicates on the original prescription a specific stop date. For example, "Give furosemide 20 mg IVP twice a day for 5 days." This type of prescription should be renewed regularly.

- **Automatic stop dates** are protocols that hospitals use for discontinuing medications after a certain length of time. Most narcotic prescriptions are in effect only for 7 days. If the medication is needed after the automatic stop date, the care provider must write another prescription.
- **STAT** prescription means that a single dose of medication is to be given immediately and only once. The word *stat* or *now* should appear in the prescription, for example, "Give furosemide 20 mg IVP STAT," or "Give lorazepam 1 mg IV push now."
- **Single** prescription, or *one-time prescription,* indicates that the medication is to be given only once at a specified time. Preoperative medications, given before surgery or diagnostic procedures or treatments, are an example of a single prescription. For example:

  Versed 25 mg intramuscularly on call for when surgical staff requests premedication to be administered
  Tetanus toxoid 0.5 mL intramuscularly before discharge
- **Standing orders.** When a unit frequently provides care to a standard population of patients—for example, coronary care

patients or knee replacement patients—the primary care provider may develop a set of *standing orders.* These are officially accepted sets of prescriptions to be applied routinely by nurses for the care of patients under certain conditions or under certain circumstances, such as drug allergies or sensitivities. They establish guidelines for treating a particular disease or set of symptoms. For example:

  Coronary care or intensive care units (CCUs or ICUs) may have standing orders for the administration of nitroglycerin for chest pain (e.g., "Give nitroglycerin 0.4 mg sublingually q3–5 min for chest pain, to a maximum of 3 doses in 15 min").
- Many postoperative patients receive a prescribed number of injectable analgesic medications for pain relief. So, for all the postoperative patients on a unit, standing orders would include, "ketorolac 30 mg IV push q12hr for 2 days."
- **prn prescription.** The care provider may prescribe a medication to be given whenever the patient requires (prn). A prn prescription requires the nurse to determine, in collaboration with the patient, when the medication is to be given. The prescription specifies (1) the condition for which the medication is to be given and (2) the minimum time intervals between doses. The medication cannot be given any more frequently than prescribed, even if symptoms persist. Pain medications,

antiemetics (antinausea medications), and laxatives are usually given prn. For example:

Morphine 10 mg intramuscularly q3–4hr prn incisional pain.
Acetaminophen 650 mg PO q4hr prn for temp >101°F.

How Are Medication Prescriptions Communicated?

Medication prescriptions can be communicated in various ways. The nursing implications are slightly different for each. In general, prescribers either write or speak to communicate the intended prescription.

Written Prescriptions. As already discussed, you will find **written prescriptions** either hand written on a prescription form or preprinted standard medication order sheets and protocols. Some agencies accept medication orders or prescriptions transmitted electronically or via facsimile from the prescriber to the nurse, with the original copy provided later. Although this step may save time, the risk of errors is greater because faxed copies may be illegible.

Verbal Prescription. A prescriber may sometimes give a spoken prescription while present with the nurse. This is called a **verbal prescription.** When you receive a verbal prescription, you, as the RN, will write the prescription and sign it with the provider's name followed by your name and credentials. Medication names that sound the same can be confusing and lead to administering the wrong drug (Box 25-2). Repeat the prescription to the provider and spell the medication name to ensure accuracy. Avoid taking verbal prescriptions, and use them only in urgent situations because they increase the risk for miscommunication and errors.

Telephone Prescription. Prescribers may also give medication prescriptions by the telephone. Usually this will be in response to a call you have placed to report a change in the patient's condition or the results of laboratory or other tests. The provider usually must cosign verbal and telephone prescriptions within 24 hours.

What Should I Do if I Think a Prescription Is Incorrect?

As a nurse, you are legally responsible for medications you administer. If you believe a prescription is incorrect, do the following:

- Ask another nurse or physician to check the prescription.
- Look up the medication in a reliable resource (e.g., drug formulary) to verify spelling, usage, dosages, and routes.
- Contact the prescriber for clarifications, concerns, or questions.

- Do not assume you are correctly interpreting the prescription if you have any question at all.

Use your knowledge, common sense, and intuition when administering medications. To avoid errors, you must know and understand the procedures at your facility, be familiar with the medications you give, and always check the prescription. Each agency will have a policy specifying the procedure for checking medication prescriptions. For example, a unit clerk may copy the original prescription onto a medication administration record (MAR), but the nurse must check to be sure the transcription is correct.

ThinkLike a Nurse 25-9

Find the errors in these medication prescriptions. Look the medications up in a drug formulary or nursing drug handbook to check dosages, spelling, and so on.

- Ancef 10 g q6hr IV
- Capatril 25 mg orally twice a day
- Digoxin 0.125 mg daily
- Lasix 400 mg by mouth
- NTG gr 1/150 prn chest pain
- Tylenol orally prn fever

MEDICATION ERRORS

A **medication error** is any preventable event that may cause or lead to inappropriate medication use or harm to a patient. Medication errors occur with surprising frequency. They are among the most common adverse events that occur in hospitalized patients. About one out of five drug doses administered by nurses are in error in some way. The most common errors are confusion caused by similar drug names, lack of knowledge of the drug (e.g., incorrect dosages), and lack of information about the patient (e.g., allergies, lab results). A fairly high percentage of medication errors involve anticoagulants (blood thinners), with nearly 3% of those resulting in patient harm or death (Joanna Briggs Institute, 2005). Box 25-3 describes several causes of medication errors by nurses.

How Can I Avoid Errors?

A variety of system-wide measures help to prevent medication errors in healthcare agencies. The Joint Commission recommends standardizing protocols for prescribing, administering, and documenting medication. Errors can be reduced in the home setting if the patient is prescribed the same dose at home as in the hospital.

To ensure patient safety you need to learn from your mistakes and the mistakes of others. You also need to think defensively. Ask "what if" and "why" questions: "What will happen if I don't do something or if I do something wrong? Why am I hanging this IV or giving this medication?" As a nurse, your critical thinking is the best defense to avoid errors and improve patient care and safety.

For further information about avoiding medication errors, see Ensuring Safe Medication Administration, in the Practical Knowledge section of this chapter.

Error-Prevention Technology

Computers can decrease errors by improving access to information and communication among health professionals. Some healthcare agencies provide nurses with laptops and handheld mobile technologies, allowing them to tap into detailed information about diseases, similar-sounding drugs,

---

BOX 25-2 ■ Medications with Similar-Sounding Names

Alprazolam - lorazepam	NovoLog - Humalog
Baclofen - Bactroban	NovoLog - Novalin R
Cefzil, Keflin - Keflex	Ophthalgan -Auralgan
Celebrex - Celexa, Cerebyx	Percocet - Percodan
Cytoxan - Ciloxan	Phenergan - Phenaphen
Demerol - dicumarol	Procardia - Procardia XL
Digoxin - digitoxin	Quinine - quinidine
Glyburide - glipizide	Ranitidine - amantadine
Humalog - Humulin R	Serzone - Seroquel
Keflex - Kantrex	Taxotere - Taxol
Lamictal - Lamisil	Zantac - Xanax
Lodine - Iodine	Zantac - Zyrtec
Morphine - meperidine	Zostrix - Zestril

BOX 25-3 ■ Why Do Medication Errors Occur?

The following are several factors associated with medication errors:

Lack of Knowledge or Information

- Lack of knowledge of the drug (e.g., incorrect dosages, incorrect mixing, overly rapid infusion, drug interaction, adverse effects) is the most common factor contributing to medication errors.
- Lack of information about the patient (e.g., allergies, other medications, lab results, presence of contraindications) is the second most frequent cause of errors.
- A drug is given by the wrong route.

Faulty Communication

- Written prescription unclear, illegible, or transcribed incorrectly, resulting in giving the wrong drug or dosage (e.g., confusion between drugs with similar names).
- Telephone prescription is taken incorrectly.
- Protocol is not understood or is violated.
- A drug prescription is written on the wrong patient's chart.
- Wrong dosage is prescribed (e.g., by misplacing a zero or decimal point).
- Abbreviations are misunderstood.
- Poor, or no, documentation. For example, administering a medication and failing to record it immediately afterward.

Equipment Errors

- Wrong equipment is used to administer the drug.
- Equipment malfunctions or is not used properly.

Calculation and Measurement Errors

- An error in calculating the dosage is made.
- Confusion about the unit of measurement; for example, a drug is prescribed based on kilograms and dispensed or administered based on pounds (and vice versa).

Other

- Medication is improperly handled or stored.
- Patient's identity is not checked, and the wrong patient receives the medication.
- Lighting is inadequate.
- The nurse is fatigued, distracted, or interrupted.

Sources: Joanna Briggs Institute. (2005). Strategies to reduce medication errors with reference to older adults. *Best Practice,* 9(4), 1–6; and Roy, V., Gupta, P., & Srivastava, S. (2005). Medication errors: Causes & prevention. *Health Administrator, XIX*(1), 60–64.

interactions, and side effects. A variety of error-prevention technologies can reduce the likelihood of medication errors.

Computerized Prescriber Order Entry (CPOE). CPOE helps prevent errors in reading and transcribing orders, particularly when handwritten orders are illegible. Electronic prescribing systems are safer when combined with decision-support tools that automatically alert prescribers to possible interactions, allergies, and other potential problems.

Bar Coding Medications. Especially when combined with CPOE, bar code medication administration, provides a nearly foolproof system for identifying the right patient and transfers data electronically, eliminating the error-prone paper transcription process. When used correctly, bar coding at the unit-dose level helps prevent nurses from selecting an incorrect medication.

Smart Pumps. IV infusion technologies, called smart-pumps, used at the point of care, can help you avoid programming the wrong dose into the pump. If a nurse attempts to program outside dosing limits, the pump halts or triggers an alarm. Once programmed, the delivery rate does not change; if there is a blocked line, an alarm will sound.

Automated Dispensing Units. In the pharmacy, automated dispensing units minimize human handling, which can also reduce error. See QSEN Box for examples of errors that can occur when technologies for administering medication is misused.

QSEN

Understanding the Limitations of Technologies for Medication Safety

**Competencies: Safety (Knowledge); Informatics (Knowledge, Skills, Attitudes)*

It is important for you to understand the limitations of safety-enhancing technologies so that you can apply the technologies correctly (Informatics) and reduce the risk of patient harm (Safety).

Computerized physician order entry (CPOE). CPOE was hailed as the answer to prescribing errors and it has had many positive effects. However, several studies have reported mixed results, one documented 22 new types of errors, and one reported an *increase* in mortality after CPOE implementation. Factors contributing CPOE errors include the following:

➤ "Alert fatigue": the tendency for users to ignore frequent interruptions from warning messages
➤ Rigid programs that take users through multiple unnecessary screens or force unnecessary decisions. These encourage users to bypass decision points.
➤ False sense of security generated by the belief that automated systems prevent errors

Bar-code-assisted medication administration (BCMA). A high rate of false-positive alerts has led to practitioner overrides and work-around actions. Of particular concern is the practice of "back scanning" in which the patient's bar code is scanned *after* medication administration. This greatly increases the risk of error and constitutes negligence.

Smart pump problems. These include software limitations and practitioner misuse (e.g., turning off the pump's dose-checking feature and bypassing alerts). Such actions are ethically and legally indefensible, and do not meet standards of care.

How does Informatics competency relate to the Safety competency? How can you avoid risky behaviors, contribute to the redesign of safety technologies, and put patient safety first when administering medications?

Sources: Amarasingham, R., Plantinga, L., Diener-West, M., et al. (2009); Elias, B. L., & Moss, J.A. (2011); Goedert, J. (2010)); Han, Y.Y., Carcillo, J.A., Venkataraman, S.T. (2005); Poon, E. G., Keohane, C.A., Yoon, C. S., et al (2010); Sittig, D. F., & Singh, H. (2011); Trbovich, P. L., Pinkney, S., Cafazzo, J.A., et al. (2010).
*For specific Knowledge, Skills, and Attitudes,

 Go to the **QSEN** web site at http:www.qsen.org. ksas_prelicensure.php

Pediatric Considerations

Confusion between pounds and kilograms is a source of dosing error. You should weigh patients in kilograms when possible because it is the standard measurement for pediatric prescriptions, medical records, and staff communication. Medication prescriptions should be written with the dose per kilogram of body weight so that the intended dosage can be easily double-checked by nurses and pharmacists. When available, pediatric-specific medication formulations and concentrations are safer than medications dispensed for adults.

What Should I Do if I Commit a Medication Error?

As a nurse, you have a duty to do no harm. With that said, if an error were to occur, even though you might be anxious about having put your patient at risk, and might even be embarrassed to admit that you made a mistake or fear you could lose your job, you must immediately assess the patient's vital signs and physical status. Then follow the guidelines in Clinical Insight 25-1. Check with your institution for agency-specific policy regarding incident reporting.

Although an error does not actually occur until the patient has taken a medication, you may be required to file a report for an averted error (e.g., if you discover that the pharmacy has sent the wrong medication for a patient). Many healthcare facilities are tracking incidents that are near misses. These are errors detected during the checking procedure before drug administration.

Practical Knowledge
knowing **how**

Regardless of the type of medication or the route of administration, when administering a medication you should perform a medication-focused assessment, follow procedures for safe administration, and perform related interventions (e.g., explaining that a certain drug should be taken with food). The remainder of the chapter explains these activities to you. Be

certain to become familiar with the Medication Guidelines: Steps to Follow for All Medications (Regardless of Type or Route) in the Practical Knowledge: Procedures section of this chapter.

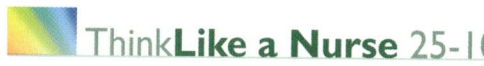

Think**Like a Nurse** 25-10

- Mr. Pearson (Meet Your Patients) refuses to take his 1400 dose of antibiotic, stating that he had just received it. What actions do you take to ensure sound decision making and maintain patient safety?

ASSESSMENT

During your initial patient assessment, you will gather data that you need to administer medications safely. The following are highlights of medication-related assessments.

Before medicating patients:
- Measure vital signs
- Assess whether the patient's general condition is appropriate for the medication
- Evaluate your knowledge of the medication
- Identify biological factors that affect drug metabolism. Also,

 Go to Chapter 15, Tables, Boxes, Figures: ESG Box 15-1: Biological Variations, on Davis*Plus*.

While administering medications, assess the patient's:
- Mental status
- Coordination
- Ability to self-administer the drug
- Swallowing (for oral medications)

After medicating patients, assess for:
- Effectiveness of the drug
- Side effects
- Signs of toxicity or adverse reactions

When taking a medication history, explore the patient's allergy history. Allergic reactions occur with 5% to 10% of all prescriptions; use allergy alert bracelets and stickers; and document allergies in the patient's chart and care plan. You should also ask about the patient's history of illness,

---

Clinical Insight 25-1 ▶ Taking Action After a Medication Error

First check the patient. Take his vital signs, and perform assessments related to the medication that was given.

- If you are unfamiliar with the side effects of the medication, consult a drug reference source.
- Verify that you have made a medication error, and identify the type of error.
- Notify the nurse in charge for guidance if this is your first error.
- Notify the prescriber and follow her orders for intervention.
- Document on the chart that the medication was given, but do not indicate that it was given in error. This alerts anyone reviewing the chart that an error was made.
- Complete an incident report according to the facility's policies. Ask for assistance if you are unfamiliar with the

format or requirement of this form. It is important that the information you provide is factual and accurate.
- Do not document in the patient's chart that an incident report was filed. This alerts anyone reviewing the chart that an error was made and makes the incident report available for legal review in the event of a lawsuit.
- When you are calmer and can think clearly, critically review the error. Identify the influences that led to your making the error. Were you rushed? Did you check the prescription? Did you follow the rights of medication? Whatever the reason, use this situation as a learning experience to improve your practice.

medications, attitudes toward medications, learning needs, and whether the patient (if a woman) is pregnant or breast-feeding. Also check relevant laboratory test results. For more discussion of the components to include in a medication history, and to print out a tool you can use for a full medications history and physical,

 Go to Chapter 25, **Supplemental Materials: Components of a Medication History,** on Davis*Plus*.

The physical examination helps you to identify potential problems and the need for adapting medication administration procedures. For example, you will assess relevant body systems to confirm the need for the drug and provide a baseline for evaluating the patient's responses to it. For oral medications, assess the patient's ability to swallow; for intramuscular medications, assess muscle mass. For more complete information about the physical examination related to medications,

 Go to Chapter 25, **Supplemental Materials: Physical Examination Related to Medications,** on Davis*Plus*.

ANALYSIS/NURSING DIAGNOSIS

The following are some examples of nursing diagnoses associated with patient medications:

Deficient Knowledge related to lack of motivation to learn about medications
Ineffective Self Health Management related to confusion
Risk for Aspiration related to Impaired Swallowing
For examples of other nursing diagnoses,

 Go to Chapter 25, **Standardized Language: Standardized Diagnoses, Outcomes, and Interventions Related to Medication Administration,** on Davis*Plus*.

A few nursing diagnoses represent medication side effects; however, because a wide range of adverse effects is possible, no attempt was made to include them all. The following sections discuss Risk for Injury and Noncompliance.

Risk for Injury

Risk for Injury may be related to polypharmacy and misuse, overuse, or underuse of medications.

Polypharmacy. Many people self-prescribe or rely on OTC medications for relief of symptoms such as insomnia, headaches, joint pains, and indigestion. They may continue taking them in combination with prescribed medications. This practice is called **polypharmacy:** the ingestion of numerous medications in an attempt to treat many conditions simultaneously. Polypharmacy increases the potential for adverse reactions and dangerous drug and food interactions.

Older adults are especially prone to polypharmacy. They typically take several medications prescribed for chronic diseases, and many medicate for symptoms related to the aging process (e.g., constipation). The combination of polypharmacy, increased sensitivity to medications, and declining cognitive and sensory function can be especially dangerous.

Misuse, Overuse, Underuse. Some patients misuse, overuse, underuse, or use drugs inconsistently. They may even use them when contraindicated. For example, prescription medication is misused when a person takes an antibiotic, "feels better" after a few days, and then stops taking the medication or takes it erratically as symptoms come and go.

Such an inconsistent dosage schedule hinders the body's ability to achieve a high enough blood level of the medication to treat the infection or disease. Some drugs, for instance beta blockers, when taken inconsistently can be dangerous or even life threatening.

Noncompliance

Noncompliance (nonadherence) is failure to follow the treatment plan (e.g., not taking a prescribed medication or skipping doses). You cannot assume that the reason a patient is noncompliant is because he hasn't been taught the importance of following the treatment plan. Prescription medications are expensive. Faced with choosing between food and pills, people on a limited budget or without health insurance often simply do not buy the more costly medications, or they may take only partial doses of maintenance medications (e.g., thyroid medications, oral hypoglycemics for diabetes). Some patients, particularly older adults, have visual and motor deficits that limit their ability to read labels and manipulate bottle caps, syringes, and so on. Other reasons for noncompliance include lack of symptoms, inability to tolerate side effects, forgetfulness, and impaired mental capacity. Always investigate the patient's reasons for nonadherence so you can take appropriate actions.

KnowledgeCheck 25-10

- What are the risks involved for patients who engage in polypharmacy?
- List at least three reasons for noncompliance with a medication regimen.

PLANNING OUTCOMES/EVALUATION

NOC standard outcomes depend on the specific nursing diagnoses you choose. For NOC outcomes for selected nursing diagnoses,

 Go to Chapter 25, **Standardized Language: Standardized Diagnoses, Outcomes, and Interventions Related to Medication Administration,** on Davis*Plus*.

Individualized goals/outcome statement you might write for a client should be stated so their achievement reflects resolution of the problem (NANDA-I label). The following are some examples:

After explanation, and within 1 week, describes the expected actions and side effects of his medications.
Self-administers his medications in the correct amounts and on the prescribed schedule.
After demonstration and practice, and within 1 week, correctly draws up and self-administers insulin.

PLANNING INTERVENTIONS/IMPLEMENTATION

NIC standardized interventions depend on the patient's nursing diagnoses, especially on the etiologies.

 Go to Chapter 25, **Standardized Language: Standardized Diagnoses, Outcomes, and Interventions Related to Medication Administration,** on Davis*Plus*.

Specific individualized nursing activities include preparing and administering medications. You will use specific, step-by-step procedures for these activities. However, only the

general principles are presented in this book. Individualized nursing interventions also include activities to address specific nursing diagnoses and, for all patients, the activities to ensure safe administration of medications presented in the remainder of this chapter.

ENSURING SAFE MEDICATION ADMINISTRATION

Medication mistakes are the most common type of healthcare error. Errors include giving the wrong medication or the wrong dose at the wrong time, omitting doses, giving the wrong dose, and giving the dose without authorization.

✚ To prevent making a medication error, you should develop a set routine for administering medications. Learn from your mistakes and the mistakes of others. Many errors occur as a result of interruption or distraction. It is best not to stop what you are doing when preparing or giving medication. You might even wear a bright yellow sash to alert people not to disturb you when preparing or giving medication.

To help prevent errors, perform "three checks" and "rights of medication" when giving medications. Also see Medication Guidelines: Steps to Follow for All Medications (Regardless of Type or Route), in the Practical Knowledge: Procedures section.

Three Checks

Check each medication three times:

1. *BEFORE you pour, mix, or draw up a medication,* check its label against the entry on the MAR. Be sure that the name, route, dose, and time match the MAR entry.
2. *AFTER you prepare the medication,* and before returning the container to the medication cart or discarding anything, check the label against the MAR entry again.
3. *AT THE BEDSIDE, check the medication again* before actually administering it.
   Observing the "three checks" rule will help you to practice the "rights of medication."

Rights of Medication

Following the **rights of medication** means that you will give the (1) right medication to the (2) right patient in the (3) right dose using the (4) right route at the (5) right time with the (6) right documentation of the medication administration. This system helps you to prevent medication errors. Always check the prescription to see whether there have been changes in the medication dosage, route, and so forth—especially after days off, after working a different shift, and after a break. This will help you achieve all of the rights.

Right Drug

Obviously, you must always administer the correct medication. That is one reason for reading each label three times (see the "three checks"). Other ways to ensure giving the correct drug are to:

1. *Think Critically.*
   - If you must take a verbal prescription, always repeat it back to the prescriber to be sure you have heard correctly. Spell the medication name. Many medication names sound the same when you hear but are actually very different drugs (e.g., Isordil, Isuprel).
   - Be familiar with the drugs you administer. If you don't know, look it up.

- Ask yourself if the medication prescription is suitable for the patient's condition. If not, question the prescriber.
- Participate in daily patient rounds so you will be better informed about your patient's plan of care and why the medications are prescribed.

2. *Be aware of the pitfalls in abbreviations, units of measurement, and handwriting.*
   - Double-check all prescriptions transcribed by hand to the MAR.
   - Do not attempt to decipher illegible handwriting or confusing abbreviations. When in doubt, ask the prescriber to clarify.
   - Be alert for names that look very similar (e.g., Keflex and Keflin). It may be impossible to differentiate them when they are handwritten. Do not administer a drug prescribed by a nickname.

3. *Perform the "three checks" of the label against the MAR.*
   - Read the label before and after you prepare the medication, and again at the bedside to verify that you selected the correct product name and strength.
   - Select the prescribed medication from the patient's drug drawer (unless it is a stock drug). Do not "borrow" from another patient's drawer.
   - Do not substitute one medication for another.
   - Even when using unit dose, read the label. Avoid selecting medications based on size and color because many medications are the same size, shape, and color as others.
   - Be alert for similar-looking labels. If you are accustomed to withdrawing oxytocin (given IV to stimulate uterine contractions) from a small vial with a green label, you might be surprised to find that the small green-label vial in your hand is actually hydroxyzine (Vistaril), which would harm the patient if given IV.
   - If a label is hard to read or comes off the container, return the container to the pharmacy. Never give a medication from such a container. Also, do not transfer medications from one pharmacy container to another.

4. *Heparin.* Physically separate the highly concentrated heparin sodium (10,000 units/mL in 1-mL vials) from the more diluted 1 mL vials for flushing heparin locks. There is a risk for fatal hemorrhage if the highly concentrated heparin solution is mistakenly used to flush an IV line. FDA-approved labeling now includes new color and design in order to distinguish various heparin concentrations in the vials. Be extremely careful when administering heparin to infants and children.

Right Dose

The right dose is the dose prescribed for the particular patient. Be sure the dose is within the recommended range for the patient's age, weight, and condition. The following are suggestions for avoiding dose errors:

- Perform the "three checks" of the container against the MAR. If the pharmacist has sent a dose different from the one prescribed, you may need to calculate how much of it to give. It is a good idea to have another nurse check your calculations.
- For IV medications, use smart infusion pumps to help ensure that the correct dose is delivered.

- How you prepare medications can affect the dose. When you must break a tablet, use a knife or a cutting device. If the tablet does not break evenly, you should discard it. When crushing a tablet to mix with liquid or food, clean the crushing device completely before using it to remove any pieces of a previously crushed drug. Clean it after using it, as well.
- Read and write measurements carefully. It is easy to misread "mg" instead of "mL." There is a significant difference between 1 mg and 1 mL of IV morphine, for example.
- Write out "international units" instead of abbreviating as "IU." IU can be confused with IV.
- Know how and when to use a zero. Always write a zero *before* a decimal point. It is easy to mistake .15 for 115 if the decimal point is written large or the 1 is written small (e.g., write "Lanoxin 0.125 mg," not "Lanoxin .125 mg"). Conversely, never write a decimal point and a zero *after* a whole number. The decimal point may be mistaken for a 1 (e.g., write "5 mg," not "5.0 mg").
- Question prescriptions for multiple tablets or vials as a single dose; most doses are one or two tablets or one single-dose vial.
- Question abrupt and excessive increases in dosage; most dosages increase gradually.
- Question prescriptions that are not consistent with the standard (protocol) dosage range for the patient's age, weight, and condition.
- Examine the standards of care and practice in your institution to see if they comply with The Joint Commission's 2011–2012 National Patient Safety Goal 03.05.01 ensuring safe dosing with anticoagulation therapy.

Right Time

Check the prescription against the time to give the drug, and document the exact time of administration on the MAR. Medications are designed to be given at specific times to maintain constant therapeutic blood levels. However, you can give scheduled medications within a "window" of one-half hour before and one-half hour after the scheduled time, as a rule.

"Right time" also includes timing oral medications in relation to meals. Give drugs that are irritating to the stomach (e.g., potassium, aspirin) with food; give drugs that absorb better on an empty stomach (e.g., tetracycline, iron supplement) before meals.

Determine whether your patient is scheduled for any diagnostic procedures, surgery, or blood tests that require him to remain NPO. If so, you may need to hold oral or enteral medications, or have them changed to another route.

✚ If the drug is not charted, never assume that the patient received it as scheduled. If you do, the patient may not receive an essential medication; if you assume it has not been given and give it, the patient may receive an overdose.

Right Route

Recall that drug absorption is highly dependent on the route of administration. The following are suggestions for ensuring the right route:

- Perform the "three checks," and be sure that the drug is in the proper form for the route prescribed, especially for time-released drugs.
- If the prescription does not specify a route, do not guess; clarify with the prescriber. Many medications are available

in multiple forms; others are made for one specific route. For example, cephalexin (Keflex), an antibiotic, comes in capsules, suspensions for oral use, and injectable forms for IM and IV administration. By contrast, the antibiotic penicillin G procaine (Crysticillin) is prepared for IM injection and is *not* to be given intravenously.

- The right route also includes **right site.** If an intramuscular injection is prescribed, be sure the site is appropriate considering the age of the patient (child, adult, elderly) and the medical condition.
- As an additional safety measure, draw up oral liquids only into an oral syringe to avoid inadvertent IV administration.

Right Patient

Just before giving the medication, always double-check the patient's identification (ID) bracelet to ensure that you have the correct patient. The Joint Commission (2011) National Patient Safety Goals recommend using two methods of patient identification, so you should also ask the patient to state his name. It is best to say, "Please tell me your name," because patients with hearing impairment or confusion might respond "yes" incorrectly when asked, for example, "Are you Mary Smith?" Never skip this step, even if you are familiar with the patient. If you are busy and distracted, it is possible to enter the wrong room. Also, patients, especially when they are confused or emotionally disturbed, may move about. You may enter room 214 with a medication for Mr. Jones but discover an entirely different person in Mr. Jones's bed!

Suppose you are taking an oral tablet to a patient's room. He is in the bathroom and says, "Just leave it; I'll take it when I come out." What would you do? If you leave the tablet, how would you know whether he really took it? And what might happen if another, confused patient (or even a visiting child) wandered into the room and took the tablet?

Be alert for patients with the same last names. It is common to have two patients with same or similar last names (e.g., Williamson, Wilkinson, Wilson, Wilkerson). Look for and place special alerts on charts and MARs to call attention to names that look or sound similar.

CPOE and bar code medication administration provides a nearly fool-proof system for identifying the right patient and transfers data electronically. However, you must ensure that order entry is made in the correct patient record.

Right Documentation

Most nurses consider documentation the sixth right. After administering a medication, document it immediately on the patient's MAR, as in Figure 25-6. To see an electronic MAR, go to Chapter 18. Be sure to document the following information:

- Name of medication given
- Dose of medication given
- Route of administration and injection site for parenteral medications
- Date and time administered
- Your name or initials as administering nurse

Most MARs are preprinted with the patient's name, name of the medication, dosage, and route administered (e.g., intramuscular, oral, or intravenous). If so, you need only to write the time you actually gave the medication, initial each medication, and sign the form one time. As for all charting, write legibly in ink.

If for some reason you do not administer a prescribed medication, document that information on the MAR and write a nurse's note explaining why it was not given. Reasons

HOSPITAL MEDICATION ADMINISTRATION RECORD

Codes For Injection Sites

A - Left Anterior Thigh	H - Right Anterior Thigh
B - Left Deltoid	I - Right Deltoid
C - Left Gluteus Medius	J - Right Gluteus Medius
D - Left Lateral Thigh	K - Right Lateral Thigh
E - Left Ventral Gluteus	L - Right Ventral Gluteus
F - Left Lower Quadrant	M - Right Lower Quadrant
G - Left Upper Quadrant	N - Right Upper Quadrant

Mary Smith 086432

age 46   John Miller, M.D.

ALLERGIES: PCN, Sulfa

					4.16.13	4.17.13	4.18.13
4.16.13		Lanoxin 0.25mg po Q D		0900	09 JW		
4.16.13		Rocephin 1 gm IV Q D		1200	1200 JW		
4.16.13		Zinacef 1 gm IV Q 8 hr		0800 ⎫	08 JW		
				1600 ⎬			
				2400 ⎭			

SIGNATURE / SHIFT INDICATES			7-3	JW	
NURSE ADMINISTERING MEDICATIONS			3-11		
J Wilson, RN			11-7		

FIGURE 25-6 After administering a medication, immediately document the date, time, dose, route, and person administering the medication on the MAR.

may include patient refusal, NPO for surgery, tests, or procedures being performed. For example:

06/20/13 0800—Pt NPO for surgery this a.m. 0800 meds held as prescribed. ————————— Janet King, RN

When giving a prn medication, in addition to recording on the MAR, you should write a nursing note documenting your assessment and the time the drug was given. Then, after allowing time for the medication to be absorbed and take effect, evaluate and document the patient's responses. For example:

06/20/13 0800—Pt reports abdominal pain at incision site rated as a #6 on a scale of 1–10. Active bowel sounds auscultated. Resp 16 breaths/minute, HR 88 beats/min, BP 130/84. Denies N/V. Morphine 10 mg given intramuscularly in right vastus lateralis (see MAR). Janet King, RN

06/20/13 0900—States pain relieved; "about 3" (scale of 1–10). Resp 14 breaths/min, HR 68 beats/min. BP 126/80. ————— J. King, RN

You are responsible for documenting the client's responses to all medications, including therapeutic effects, side effects, and unexpected or adverse reactions. Never document a drug before you give it; never document a medication given by someone else; and do not ask someone else to document medications you administer.

Other Rights

In addition to the rights already discussed, patients also have the following rights about medications they receive:

Right Reason. This includes the right to not receive unnecessary medications. For example, a tranquilizer or sleeping pill should be given because the patient is very anxious or cannot sleep, not for the convenience of caregivers who are weary of his incessant demands.

Right to Know. This means that you tell the patient the name of the medication, why it is being given, its actions, and potential side effects.

Right to Refuse. The patient always has the right to refuse a medication regardless of her reasons and regardless of the consequences.

KnowledgeCheck 25-11

- What are the rights of medication?
- Give an example of each one.
- How many times, and when, should you check the medication against the MAR?

ADMINISTERING ORAL MEDICATIONS

The oral route is the one most commonly used for medications. Recall what you already know about oral medications: Where are they absorbed? What are their advantages and disadvantages? What assessments should you make? If you cannot answer these questions, review discussions of drug preparations and routes of administration, and review Table 25-1. For procedural steps for administering various the following types of oral medications, see Procedure 25-1.

Pouring Liquid Medications

Liquid medications are frequently used for children and older adults. They usually come in multidose bottles, so you will need to pour individual doses into a disposable, calibrated

Teaching Your Patient About Self-Medication

➤ Do not take medications prescribed to others, and do not share your medications with others.

➤ Keep a list of your medications, including doses and times taken. Take this list with you when you visit any primary care provider or an emergency department.

➤ If you take a variety of medications, post a list of them in a prominent place that is easy to get to in the event of an emergency.

➤ Wear a medical alert bracelet or necklace if you are a diabetic, take anticoagulants, or have allergies to any medication.

➤ When you are prescribed a new medication, ask why you are taking it, how long you should take it, what side effects you should expect, whether you should take it with food, and whether there are any special precautions.

➤ Take the medication for the prescribed length of time to make certain you receive the full benefit of the drug. For example, some patients may take only part of an expensive antibiotic, hoping to "save it for later." If you do not take the full course of medication, the infection may recur. Antibiotic resistance may develop, leading to "superinfection," such as methicillin-resistant *Staphylococcus aureus* (MRSA).

➤ Be sure to read the label carefully on the bottle each time you take the medication so that you take the correct medication. Many pills look alike.

➤ Take only the amount and dose prescribed. If you have questions, call your prescriber.

➤ To measure liquids, use kitchen measuring spoons rather than tableware, which can vary in volume.

➤ Notify your prescriber if you have any side effects or adverse reactions.

➤ Do not store your medication in a different container from the one it came in. The medication may lose its strength, or you may take the wrong medication.

➤ Store all your medications in a dry place out of the sunlight and away from the heat. If a medication requires a cold storage, be sure you return it to the refrigerator immediately after use.

➤ Check expiration dates, and discard any outdated medications. Do not take expired medications; they may have lost their strength.

➤ Do not place expired medications in the trash within the reach of children. Disposing of expired medications in the sink or toilet is not environmentally sound (e.g., they can appear in the community water supply). Some communities sponsor an "old medications discard day" or provide a place to discard them to avoid contamination. Some local pharmacies may offer medication disposal as a community service.

➤ Use childproof caps if children have access to your medications. If no children are in the home, replace with simple closure cap for elderly patients who might have difficulty opening the containers.

➤ Monitor your prescription amounts, and get refills before you run out. If you get medications by mail, be sure you send for them in plenty of time.

➤ If you become pregnant, notify your primary care provider as soon as possible so your medications can be discontinued or adjusted.

---

cup. When pouring, hold the bottle so the liquid does not run over the label, making it difficult to read.

Buccal and Sublingual Medications

Buccal and sublingual medications, although placed in the mouth, are intended for absorption in the mucous membranes rather than in the GI tract. Some soluble forms of medications and enzyme preparations are administered by this route and are rapidly absorbed, some within seconds. Buccal medications are held in the cheek; sublingual medications are held under the tongue.

Enteral (Nasogastric and Gastrostomy) Medications

For patients who cannot swallow or who have feeding tubes, you can give oral medications through nasogastric (NG), gastrostomy, or jejunal tubes. Observe the following precautions when administering enteral medications:

▪ Do not give hydrophilic medications, such as psyllium (Metamucil), through feeding tubes because they attract water and will solidify in the tube.

▪ Never crush an enteric-coated or extended-release medication.

▪ If the patient is on fluid restriction, use the smallest amount of water possible to dissolve tablets and flush the tube.

For other precautions and procedures related to enteral tubes, see Procedures 28–2, 28-3, and 28-4.

Special Situations

Some oral medications can discolor or damage tooth enamel. Others can have an objectionable taste. Some might be difficult to swallow or cause the patient to gag. The following methods help patients to take medication:

▪ Mix drugs that discolor tooth enamel with liquid, and have the patient drink the solution through a straw and drink water afterward. Unless contraindicated, encourage the patient drink a liberal amount of flavored liquid (e.g., juice) or water to dilute the medication.

▪ Have the patient suck on ice chips for several minutes before taking the medication. Ice numbs the taste buds.

▪ Store the medication in the refrigerator, unless contraindicated. The smell and taste are less objectionable when chilled, especially for oily liquids.

▪ Use a syringe to place the medication on the back of the patient's tongue. There are fewer taste buds there.

▪ Some medications can be constituted with flavored additive to make the elixir more appealing, particularly for children.

▪ Regardless of method, offer oral hygiene immediately after giving the medication.

▪ Some patients have difficulty swallowing medications; they gag, or the pills become "stuck" in their throat. It may help to crush soluble tablets and place them in liquids or in a small amount of applesauce or pudding. As you

know, some forms (e.g., time-released tablets) should *not* be crushed, so check your drug reference sources to be certain.

Do not give oral medications to patients who:

Cannot swallow fluids. The risk for aspiration is too great.

Have nausea or vomiting; the medication would be lost in the emesis.

Are NPO.

Are not coherent or are comatose.

- In the preceding situations, obtain a prescription for an alternative route or, if the patient is NPO, permission to give the medication with small sips of water. To learn more about which medication to take with or without food,

 Go to Chapter 25, **Tables, Boxes, Figures: ESG Box 25-1,** on Davis*Plus*.

KnowledgeCheck 25-12

- Describe two ways to ensure an accurate dosage when pouring liquid medications.
- What instructions should you give to a patient who is taking a sublingual medication?
- Explain the special steps required when administering enteral medications to a patient who is receiving continuous tube feedings.
- Describe three methods for disguising the taste of objectionable tasting drugs.
- For which patients are oral medications contraindicated?

Medicating Children

Giving medication to young children is sometimes difficult because they are not motivated by logic. They do not grasp the cause and effect of "Take this; it will make you feel better." If they do not like the taste, they simply will not swallow the medication. Another challenge is that before age 5 years, children may not be able to swallow tablets and capsules. For these reasons, most oral medications for children are prepared as sweetened and flavored liquids. Chewable tablets are also popular. For very young children and infants, you must take care to prevent choking and aspiration. Parents can often suggest the best methods for getting their child to take medicines. For other parents, you may need to teach techniques for administering medications at home. See the accompanying Self-Care box Teaching Parents About Medicating Children.

Medicating Older Adults

As you already know, because of physiological changes (e.g., diminished liver or renal function) associated with aging, older adults usually require smaller dosages of drugs. In addition, physical responses to some medications are unpredictable. You need to observe carefully for both therapeutic and undesired effects. Other issues include the following:

- **Difficulty Swallowing Medications.** It may help to crush tablets or give drugs in liquid form. Gently massaging the area just below the chin may help to initiate swallowing. Consult an occupational or speech therapist for other strategies.
- **Reduced Thirst.** As the desire to drink liquids decreases with age, the mouth often becomes drier. Some older adults find it difficult to take large pills or tablets.
- **Slow Reflexes and Reasoning Ability.** You may need to allow more time to explain and administer medications to older adults. Keep the instructions simple.
- **Forgetting to Take the Medications.** Impaired memory is more common with age, so clients need simple plans that they can follow at home. A written schedule or a med calendar might help, especially if you plan the drugs to be taken

---

Self-Care

Teaching Parents About Medicating Children

1. Mark each bottle or syringe with medication using a different color of tape or adhesive label. This makes each clearly distinguishable, even though many medication bottles look alike.
2. You can reuse syringes for oral medications until the markings or tape begins to wear off or the plunger becomes difficult to move. Wash syringes with warm soapy water, rinse well, and allow to air dry.
3. Take your time when giving medication, and find a quiet environment. Don't rush the process. It can be frustrating to struggle with a young child who is resisting taking a medication, especially if your time is limited.
4. Give the medication at the same time each day so it becomes a matter of routine. It is easier to remember when a pattern is established.
5. If the child is old enough to understand, warn him when a medication has an unpleasant taste (e.g., "John, this doesn't taste very good, but you can have a big drink of juice as soon as you swallow it."). You may lose his trust if you surprise him with a bad taste.
6. Give the child a frozen fruit bar or frozen flavored ice pop just before the medication. This helps to numb the taste buds to weaken the taste of the medication.

7. To mask bad-tasting medicines, you can crush tablets or empty the contents of a capsule and mix with soft foods, such as applesauce, hot cereal, or pudding. This is helpful for children who might aspirate liquids, as well. (*Caution:* Check with the prescriber before crushing a tablet or emptying a capsule. Some medications should not be crushed.)
8. Do not use essential foods in the child's diet (e.g., milk or orange juice) to mask the taste of medications. The child may later refuse a food he associates with the medicine.
9. ✚ Take care to prevent choking or aspiration. When giving liquids to infants and toddlers, hold the child in a sitting or semi-sitting position. Use a medicine dropper or syringe to place the medication between the gum and cheek. Apply gentle pressure; avoid giving too much medication too fast.
10. Always praise the child after she swallows the medication.

other than at mealtimes and bedtime. Many people take their medication, only to forget shortly thereafter that they did so. Advise the patient to use a divided pill container or a small glass filled with the medications for each dosage time during the day. If the a.m. container is empty, the person will know he has taken the morning drugs.

- **Impaired Visual Acuity.** For patients who cannot see well, write out the home medication schedule in large letters, or ask family members to help. Display the schedule or med calendar in a convenient and highly visible location.
- **Difficulty Opening Containers and Administering Medications.** Because of pain or stiffness in the hands and fingers, and also because of decreased visual acuity, older adults often find it difficult to open containers or to administer their own insulin injections, inhalers, eye medications, and so on. Avoid childproof, safety lids on containers. Older adults are allowed to sign a release with their pharmacy to have the childproof covers removed for easier handling.

✚ **Families** with young children visiting the homes of older adults need to be alert to the risk of accidental ingestion of medication.

- **Lack of Understanding of the Purpose of Medication.** Some older adults accept unquestioningly everything a physician says, but they may not understand what each drug is for. For example, suppose a patient's tranquilizer is not effective. The physician prescribes a new one, but the patient does not understand that he should stop taking the old one, so for a period of time he takes both medications. This type of situation can happen, too, when patients are being treated by more than one provider (e.g., a podiatrist and an internist may both prescribe a medication to treat toenail fungus).
- **Not Seeing the Need for the Medication.** Some patients may think, "I don't feel any better when I take all this stuff," so they simply do not take it. In the hospital, they may refuse to take medications, or they may put the tablets in their mouth but spit them out when you leave the room. You should stay with the patient until you see that he has swallowed the medications.

✚ To reduce medication-related problems for older adults, nurses need to alert the prescriber to impaired visual acuity, memory, dexterity to open medication containers, mobility, and swallowing. Some action steps you can take as a nurse are listed in Box 25-4.

Knowledge Check 25-13

- What is the chief danger when administering oral medications to children?
- How can you help a person who has some difficulty swallowing oral medications?
- Keeping in mind that patients do have the right to refuse medications, how can you be sure that they are actually taking them and not spitting them out after you leave the room?

ADMINISTERING TOPICAL MEDICATIONS

Topical medications are applied directly to a body site or placed in body cavities by irrigation or instillation. They are usually used for their local effects (e.g., zinc oxide ointment to protect the skin against chafing and chapping associated with bowel and bladder incontinence), but some are absorbed

---

BOX 25-4 ■ Reducing Risk for Medication Errors for Older Adults

- Be alert to unnecessary drug therapy. It is not unusual for prescribers to be reluctant to stop a medication or simply forget to do so. The likelihood of a poor outcome increases as the number of drugs prescribed increases.
- Request the indication for use on all medication prescriptions.
- Suggest primary care provider trials of nonpharmacological interventions (such as warm massage and guided imagery) before prescribing medication for new symptoms.
- Consider the "snowball effect." This occurs when symptoms occur as a side effect of prescribed medication, and the care provider then prescribes another drug to deal with the side effect. This results in yet another side effect, another drug, and so on. To interrupt this phenomenon, the prescriber can either discontinue the medication, reduce the dose, or substitute with one the patient tolerates better.
- Verify that the newly prescribed medication does not have documented drug-drug interaction. Check that the prescribed dosage is correct within the desired range.
- When titrating drug doses, start low and go slow. It's best to start with the lowest possible dose when starting a medication because adverse drug effects are dose related and older adults tend to be more sensitive.
- Assess urinary status. Many drugs are cleared through the renal system. Some have toxic effects on the kidneys, particularly for older adults.
- Recommend safer drugs if the prescriber initiates medication associated with adverse outcomes for older adults. The benefit must exceed the risk to the patient (Zwicker and Fulmer, 2008).

---

through the skin and mucous membranes for their systemic effects (e.g., estrogen patches), depending on the drug preparation. Most must be applied to the skin two or three times per day for maximum effect.

Lotions, Creams, and Ointments

Before applying medications to the skin, assess for contraindications, such as skin irritation, open lesions, or hypersensitivity. Use a cotton swab, tongue blade, or gloved finger to apply corticosteroid creams and other topical medications so that your skin does not absorb them. For the step-by-step procedure, see Procedure 25-7A.

Transdermal Medications

Designed to be absorbed through the skin, transdermal medications are prepared as patches made of a special membrane. Patches allow constant, controlled amounts of medications to be released over 24 hours or more, giving a prolonged systemic effect. Examples of drugs administered by patch include nitroglycerin (used to control angina or chest pain), scopolamine (used to treat motion sickness), nicotine (used to control smoking urges), and fentanyl (used to treat chronic pain). Most patches are prepared with the correct dose already applied and should not be cut. Other gel patches can be cut and are self-adherent; lidocaine and diclofenac are two examples. Be sure to check the package insert or ask a pharmacist

about proper handling, application, and disposal of patches. For guidelines, see Procedure 25-7D.

PERFORMING IRRIGATIONS AND INSTILLATIONS

Washing out a body cavity with a steady stream of fluid or water is called **irrigation.** Sterile water, saline, or antiseptic solutions are flushed into the eyes, ears, throat, vagina, rectum, or urinary tract to wash out the cavity. **Instillation** is the insertion of medication into a body cavity (e.g., eye drops) so the medication can be retained or absorbed through that body cavity. Some medications need to remain in the body cavity for a period of time for maximum absorption and effect.

Irrigations and instillations are performed to remove discharge or foreign bodies (e.g., from the eye or ear); to apply heat and cold to an area; to apply medications, such as antiseptics; and to prepare an area for surgery (e.g., an enema for cleansing the bowels). You will usually not use sterile technique unless there are breaks in the skin. Several types of syringes are used for irrigating and instilling medications and fluids. Each is calibrated to allow you to control the amount and speed of solution delivered into the cavity (Fig. 25-7).

Ophthalmic Medications

Ophthalmic ointments or solutions are used for their local effects, for example, to treat eye irritations, infections, and glaucoma or to lubricate the eye. During an eye examination, eye medications may also be used to anesthetize the eye, dilate the pupil, or temporarily stain the cornea to identify abraded areas. Eye irrigation may be performed to remove foreign bodies, secretions, or harmful chemicals.

Ophthalmic medications are packaged in small bottles or tubes that state, *"For ophthalmic use only."* Do not place any medication in the eye unless this statement appears on the container. The **cornea** (the transparent part of the sclera in front of the iris and pupil) is easily injured, so you should not place medications directly onto the eyeball. Take care to not touch the tip of the dropper or tube to the eye or conjunctiva;

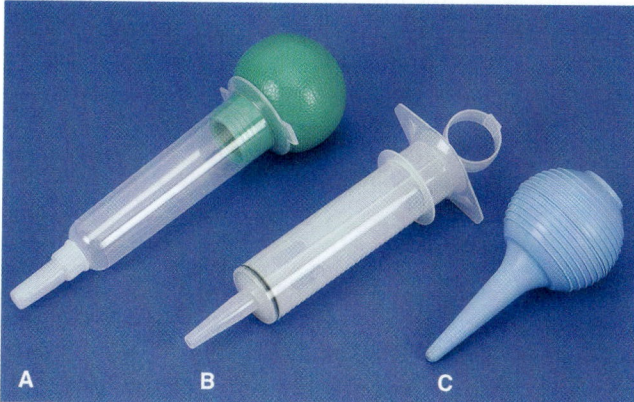

FIGURE 25-7 Syringes for administering enteral medications and performing irrigations and instillations. A, Asepto syringe: Plastic syringe with rubber bulb. B, Toomey (piston) syringe: Calibrated plastic syringe with removable tip that fits into the end of a tube (e.g., urinary catheter or enteral tube). For deep wound irrigation bladder irrigations, and administration of enteral medications. C, Rubber bulb syringe, for ear irrigations.

doing so may lead to bacterial growth on the container or damage the eye.

See Chapters 21 and 31 for information about the structure and function of the eyes and about assessing the eyes. For the step-by-step procedure, see Procedure 25-2.

Otic Medications

Medications or solutions may be dropped into the ear to treat internal and external ear infections, to apply heat to the area, and to soften and remove earwax. Use solutions at room temperature because a solution that is too hot or too cold may cause vertigo, nausea, and pain. You will use clean technique when administering otic medications. However, if the tympanic membrane (eardrum) has been ruptured or if a surgical procedure has been done, you will use sterile technique to help prevent infection. See Chapters 21 and 31 for information about the structure and function of the ear. To learn the skill, see Procedure 25-3.

Nasal Medications

Clients usually self-administer nasal drops and sprays. The most common nasal medications are used to shrink swollen mucous membranes and to loosen secretions and provide drainage for treatment of nasal cavity or sinus infections. Because many nasal medications are available without prescription, caution the patient regarding overuse. Long-term use of decongestants may cause a **rebound effect;** that is, they will be effective immediately after administration, but the nasal congestion often recurs and even increases when the effects of the drug wear off. Frequent use of or swallowing excess decongestant can also cause systemic side effects, such as increased heart rate and increased blood pressure. These effects can be serious in children; saline drops are safer for them. See Chapters 21 and 31 for information about the structure and function of the nose. For complete procedure steps, see Procedure 25-4.

Vaginal Medications

Vaginal medications come in various forms: foams, jellies, liquids (douches), creams, tablets, and suppositories. They may be used for contraception; to destroy bacteria in the vagina before gynecological surgery; to reduce vaginal dryness related to menopause; to treat vaginal itching or infection; or to induce labor. Store suppositories in the refrigerator to keep them firm enough to insert. After insertion, the body temperature causes the suppository to melt. Foams and jellies are inserted using an applicator or inserter. For the complete procedure, see Procedure 25-5.

A **douche** is a vaginal irrigation using low pressure. Vaginal irrigations are used to administer antimicrobial solutions to prevent infection (e.g., before surgery), to remove irritating discharge, and to apply heat or cold (e.g., to reduce inflammation). In the acute care setting, you will usually use sterile supplies. However, this is not usually necessary when the irrigation is self-administered at home because people usually have some resistance to the microorganisms in their daily environment.

✚ Teach women that douching is not necessary for ordinary female hygiene and that it may even be harmful because it disturbs the normal pH and healthy balance of microorganisms in the vagina.

Rectal Medications

Rectal suppositories and liquid instillations **(enemas)** are used to encourage bowel movements or to treat systemic complaints. For example, antiemetic suppositories are often

used to treat nausea. Absorption is slow and erratic because of rectal contents, local drug irritation, and uncertainty of drug retention in the rectum. Other disadvantages include embarrassment to the patient and possible rectal pain if the patient has hemorrhoids. However, the rectal route may provide for higher blood levels of the medication than does the oral route because the venous blood from the rectum does not pass through the liver before entering the general circulation (review the discussion of the first-pass effect in the section "How Are Drugs Metabolized in the Body?", as needed). Rectal administration may be preferred when a drug has an unacceptable taste or odor or when it is not safe to use the oral route, as with a patient who is vomiting or unconscious. As a rule, rectal medications are contraindicated when there is active rectal bleeding. For a procedure for inserting a rectal suppository, see Procedure 25-6; for administering an enema, see Procedure 29-3.

ADMINISTERING RESPIRATORY INHALATIONS

Nebulization is the production of a fine spray, fog, powder, or mist from a liquid drug. The patient inhales the medication mixture by breathing deeply through a mouthpiece attached to the nebulizer. The airways and alveoli are highly vascularized and therefore absorb inhaled medications rapidly.

Types of Nebulizers

The following are four types of devices for achieving nebulization:

- *Atomizers* disperse the medication in the form of large droplets.
- *Aerosol sprayers* suspend the droplets of medication in a gas (e.g., oxygen).
- An *ultrasonic (handheld) nebulizer* mixes a small volume of medication, usually less than 1 mL, with 3 mL of normal saline. The device forces air through the nebulizer and delivers medication and humidity as a fine mist. Because the particles are so small, the mist can be inhaled deep into the lungs.
- A *metered-dose inhaler (MDI)* (Fig. 25-8) is a type of nebulizer that delivers measured doses of a nebulized drug.

No matter which device is used, the smaller the droplets, the farther the medication can be inhaled into the respiratory tract.

Metered-Dose Inhalers

A **metered-dose inhaler (MDI)** is a pressurized container prefilled with several doses of a drug and an eco-friendly substance, called hydrofluoroalkane, or HFA, for propelling the medication forward. The patient inhales while pushing the canister's pump to release a measured dose of medication through a mouthpiece (Fig. 25-8a). Sometimes an extender (spacer) is attached to the mouthpiece to enhance the delivery of medication into the respiratory tract (Fig. 25-8b). Medication is pumped into the extender instead of directly into the patient's mouth. The patient inhales the drug from the chamber.

A **dry powder inhaler (DPI)** is similar to an MDI. The medication is activated by a pump rather than by inhalation. Each powdered dose is in a blister pack that is activated according to the manufacturer's instructions. Once the dose is loaded, the patient simply takes a deep breath. DPIs are not designed to be used with a spacer.

The advantage of MDIs is that high doses of medication can be rapidly instilled in the lungs, producing local effects

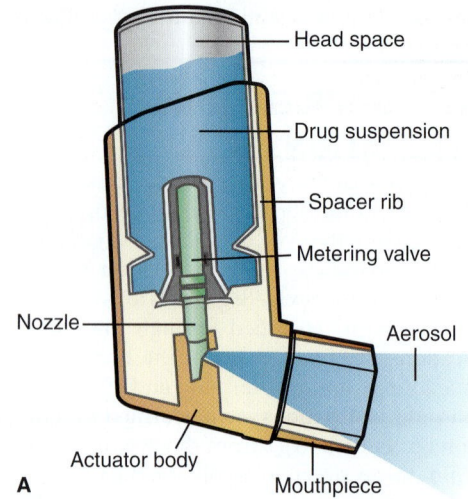

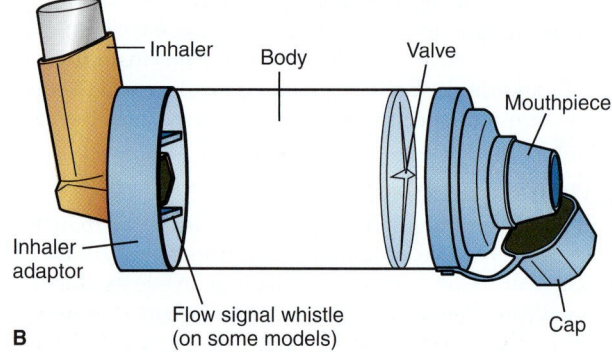

FIGURE 25-8 Inhalers. A, Metered-dose inhaler. B, Inhaler with a spacer.

directly in the airway while avoiding systemic side effects. Disadvantages are the need for manual dexterity, which is often compromised in older adults and young children; skill in coordinating the inhalation of the medication and the pushing of the canister to administer the dose; and the ability to inhale and exhale deeply enough to allow penetration of the medication in the more distal bronchioles.

Patients frequently self-administer inhalations (most often bronchodilators or steroids) using an MDI. You may need to teach your patients how to use the device correctly. Keeping track of how many puffs have been used is problematic for some users, which can lead to a canister being unexpectedly empty when needed. See Procedure 25-8 to learn how to administer a metered-dose inhaler and keep track of the remaining doses.

KnowledgeCheck 25-14

- Why should you use a cotton swab, tongue blade, or gloved finger to apply corticosteroid creams and other topical medications?
- Most of the following routes are used for both local and systemic effects. Which one is used *only* for medications intended for systemic absorption (that is, which one is *not* used for local effects): lotions, creams, ointments, transdermal patches, or irrigations?
- When administering eye drops, how can you prevent injury to the cornea?
- When should you use sterile technique when performing otic instillations?

- What are two of the undesired effects of self-administered nasal decongestants?
- What possible harm can result from vaginal douching?
- When is rectal instillation of a drug preferred over oral administration?
- When, as a rule, are rectal medications contraindicated?
- Define *nebulization*.
- What is the best way to determine if a metered-dose inhaler is empty?

ADMINISTERING PARENTERAL MEDICATIONS

Parenteral medications include those that are injected via the intradermal, subcutaneous, intramuscular, or intravenous routes. Parenteral injections are absorbed faster and more completely than drugs given by other routes; the results are more predictable; and the dosage can be measured more accurately. In addition, they can be used for patients who cannot take oral medications. However, tissue damage may result if the pH, osmotic pressure, or solubility of the medication is not appropriate to the tissue where the medication is given. For example, medications intended for injection into muscle may damage subcutaneous tissue. You must prepare and administer parenteral medications accurately, because the medications, once given, cannot be retrieved. Also see Table 25-1.

Preparing Injectable Medications

When administering injectable medications, you must know about various kinds of needles and syringes. You will need to decide, based on each situation, what size and type of needle and syringe to use. For a summary of the sites and equipment used for parenteral administration,

 Go to Chapter 25, **Tables, Boxes, Figures: ESG Table 25-7, Parenteral Injections: Comparison of Sites and Equipment,** on Davis*Plus*.

Needles

Needles are disposable, stainless steel sheaths that attach to a syringe. Figure 25-9 shows the parts of a needle. Needles are made in various lengths and gauges and with different bevel sizes.

Gauge refers to the inside diameter of the needle lumen. Needle gauges are numbered 14 through 30: the smaller the gauge, the larger the diameter (i.e., a 16-gauge needle has a larger diameter than does a 20-gauge needle). Choose the gauge based on the patient's size and skin condition, the viscosity of medication used, and the speed of administration desired. Smaller needles (25- to 30-gauge) cause less pain and trauma to the tissue, so they are useful for patients who must have frequent or long-term injections (e.g., insulin and

heparin). Larger needles (14- to 18-gauge) are used for blood and more viscous medications, to mix intravenous (IV) medications, or for rapid infusion of IV medications.

Bevel is the slanted tip with a narrow slit. The slant of the tip creates an opening that will close quickly to prevent leakage of medication, blood, and serum. A long bevel tip is sharper and narrower and therefore causes less discomfort during injection. Long bevels are usually used for subcutaneous and intramuscular injections. Short bevels are used for intradermal or IV injections. To see bevel types, refer to the Equipment list in Procedure 25-11.

Needle length is the distance from the tip to the hub (bottom) of the needle. Common needle lengths range from ⅜ of an inch to 3 inches. Use a longer needle for intramuscular injections, and a shorter one for intradermal injections. Vary the length according to the thickness of the patient's muscle and adipose tissue. Although a 1½-inch needle is common for intramuscular injections, you would use a shorter one for a child or a very thin person.

Filter needles and filter straws are used to trap rubber or glass fragments when drawing up a medication from a vial or an ampule. You must replace the filter needle with a regular needle before injecting the medication into the patient or into the IV solution.

Many people (e.g., those who have diabetes) must give themselves repeated injections, perhaps several each day. Supplies for home use are expensive. Insurance may or may not cover the cost, or the person may not have insurance. Therefore, although health professionals and manufacturers recommend that disposable syringes and needles be used only once, some people find it practical to reuse needles and syringes. If they do, you can help them to do it more safely. Refer to Clinical Insight 25-2.

ThinkLike a Nurse 25-11

- You are to give repeated intramuscular injections to a patient who is frail and has very little muscle mass (5 ft, 5 in. tall and weighing 96 lb). You are to give 1 mL of a thin, watery medication. You have these needle sizes available: 16-gauge, 20-gauge, 25-gauge. Which would you use, and why?
- For the same patient, you have needles available in 1-inch and 1½-inch lengths. Which would you use, and why?

Syringes

A syringe consists of a barrel, plunger, and syringe tip (Fig. 25-9). Because injections require strict sterile technique, you may touch the outside of the barrel and end of the plunger but not the inside of the barrel, hub, shaft of the plunger, or needle.

Syringes are usually made of plastic and are disposable. Some have the needle attached; others do not. The syringe tip, either **luer-lock** (twist on) or **non-luer-lock** (slip on), fits into

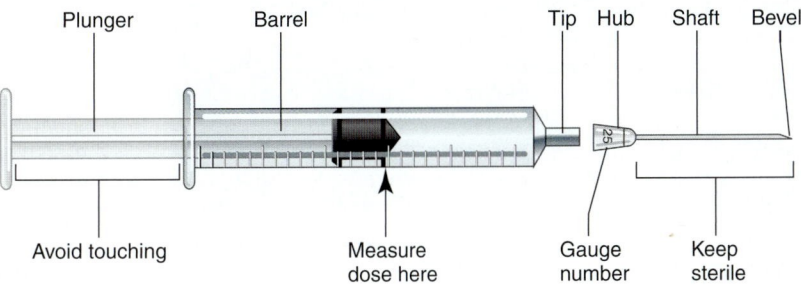

FIGURE 25-9 Parts of a needle and syringe.

Clinical Insight 25-2 ► Reusing Needles and Syringes: Home Care

Assess for the following:

- Assess whether the patient is capable of safely recapping a syringe. This requires adequate vision, manual dexterity, and no obvious tremor.
- Assess for contraindications to needle reuse. Patients with poor personal hygiene, an acute illness, open wounds on the hands, or decreased resistance to infection should not reuse a syringe or needle.

Teach your patient the following:

- Consult your healthcare provider before beginning this practice.
- Recap the needle immediately after use if you plan to use it again.
- To recap a needle, hold the syringe in one hand, rest that arm or hand on a solid surface, and with the other, replace the cap with a straight motion of the thumb. Advise the patient not to guide both the needle and cap to meet in midair, because this frequently results in needlestick injury.
- Discard needles when they become dull. Usually they cannot be used more than 10 times.
- Examine the needle carefully before reusing it. The new 30- and 31-gauge needles can easily be bent at the tip to form a hook, which can lacerate tissue or break off within the skin. Never reuse a needle that is deformed in any way.
- When an injection hurts too much, it means that the silicone coating is wearing off the needle and it's time to discard it.

- Do not reuse a needle if it has come in contact with anything other than the injection site.
- Do not use alcohol to cleanse the needle. Alcohol may remove the silicone coating that makes for less painful skin puncture. It is best to not clean the needle after use; just carefully recap it.
- The syringe and needle may be stored at room temperature. The potential benefits or risks of refrigerating the syringe are unknown.
- Be aware that reusing needles and syringes increases the risk of infection, although most insulin preparations have bacteriostatic additives that inhibit growth of bacteria commonly found on the skin.
- Inspect injection sites for redness or swelling. If these signs are present, do not reuse a needle; consult your healthcare provider.
- Never share syringes or needles with another person. This poses a risk of acquiring a bloodborne viral infection (e.g., hepatitis).
- Dispose of needles safely. Do not bend or break a needle; doing so increases the chance of injury. Use a coffee can or other puncture-proof container with a lid to dispose of needles (see Chapter 23 if you need to review).
- Do not mix insulin types if you reuse needles and syringes. Use one syringe for each insulin type. That means more injections, but certain insulins cannot be mixed without reducing their effectiveness.

---

the needle hub (Fig. 25-10). Syringes are made in various sizes, from 0.5 mL to 60 mL. The larger sizes are used for adding medications to IV solutions and for irrigating wounds. You will usually use a 2-mL or 3-mL syringe for intramuscular injections. Syringes larger than 5 mL are used for IV administration, instillations, and irrigations. Three syringes are shown in

Figure 25-11. For interactive exercises to familiarize yourself with syringe markings,

 Go to **Animations: Syringe Exercises,** on Davis*Plus*.

- **Standard syringes** are supplied in 3-, 5-, and 10-mL sizes. They are commonly supplied without needles or with 18-, 21-, 23-, or 25-gauge needles that are 0.5 to 3 inches long. They are calibrated and marked in 0.1-mL and 1- or 2-mL increments so that drugs can be measured accurately.
- **Tuberculin syringes** have a 1-mL capacity and are calibrated in 0.01-mL increments; they come with a small (usually 25- to 28-) gauge, short (½- to ⅝-in.) needle. Use tuberculin syringes to administer small, precise doses of medication (e.g., when medicating infants or children, for allergy tests, or when administering potentially dangerous medications, such as heparin).
- **Insulin syringes** are calibrated in units and are used to administer insulin. Insulin syringes are marked in 100 units per milliliter. They are made in 0.3-, 0.5-, or 1-mL sizes with very small-gauge needles (26- to 30-gauge).
- **Prefilled unit-dose system**s are reusable syringe holders that hold disposable, single-dose, prefilled medication cartridges. No medication preparation is necessary, but you must check each cartridge and dose carefully because all of the cartridges look alike. You simply insert the cartridge into

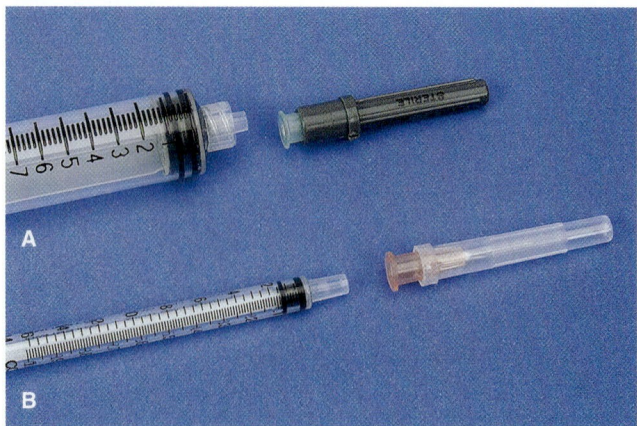

FIGURE 25-10 Syringe tips. A, Luer-lock (twist-on) tip. B, Non-Luer-lock (slip-on) tip.

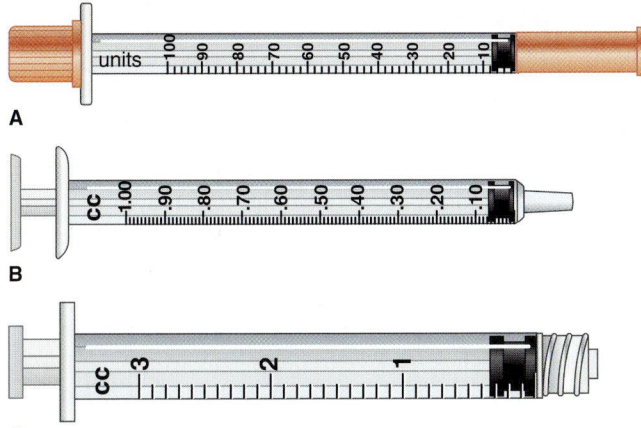

FIGURE 25-11 Syringe types. A, 100-unit insulin syringe marked in units. B, 1-mL tuberculin syringe marked in increments of 0.01 mL. C, 3-mL standard syringe marked in increments of 0.1 mL.

the holder and lock it in place. After administering the medication, dispose of the cartridge; keep the holder for reuse.

- **Disposable prefilled, self-contained systems** are available for hospitals, office practices, nursing homes, and self-administration. The injection plunger is attached to the medication barrel and twists in directly. This ready-to-use syringe reduces the risk of constituting or dosing errors. Because you do not need to remove the cartridge from the holder after using it, the risk of a needlestick injury is reduced (Fig. 25-12). For guidelines for using prefilled syringes, see Clinical Insight 25-3.
- **Safety needles.** Many safety needle devices are available. Examples include a resheathing system with a sliding barrel that shields the needle; syringes with retractable needles that spring back into the barrel of the syringe; and needles with attached covers that reduce the risk of accidental puncture with contaminated needles. Wing-tipped needles are also available for clinical use.

KnowledgeCheck 25-15

- What does the term *parenteral* mean?
- What are two disadvantages of the parenteral route?
- To maintain sterile technique, which part of a syringe must you *not* touch?
- You need to irrigate a wound. Which syringe size would you probably need: 0.5-mL, 3-mL, 5-mL, or 50-mL?
- Which syringe would you use for an intramuscular injection, as a rule: tuberculin, 50-mL, 5-mL, or 3-mL syringe?

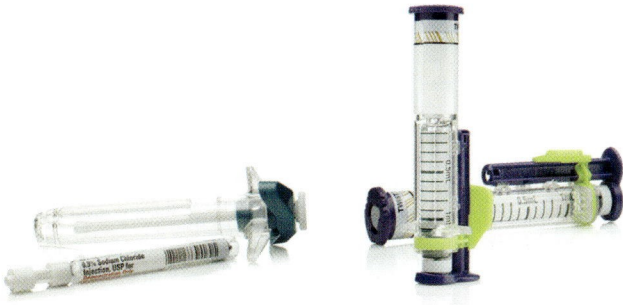

FIGURE 25-12 (*left*) Prefilled unit-dose system. (*right*) Disposable, prefilled, self-contained system.

Drawing Up Medications From an Ampule

An **ampule** is a thin-walled, disposable glass container with a narrow neck that you must snap off to access the medication. To prevent injuries, use an ampule opener to snap the glass (Fig. 25-13). Each ampule holds a single dose of a liquid medication, usually 1 mL to 10 mL, but some hold 50 mL. Because glass fragments may be introduced into the medication, most agencies require you to use a filter needle or filter straw to draw up the medication. Also, see Procedure 25-9A.

Drawing Up Medications From a Vial

A **vial** is a single-dose or multidose plastic or glass container with a rubber stopper that reseals the top after each needle introduction. A plastic or metal cap covers the rubber stopper to protect it until it is used (Fig. 25-14). Because the vial is a closed system, you must inject air into it to withdraw the solution. Otherwise, a vacuum is created in the vial that makes withdrawal difficult. Also see Procedure 25-9B.

Nurses traditionally wipe the rubber stopper with alcohol after removing the cap, even on a single-dose vial; however, there is conflicting scientific justification for this practice as an infection control measure. The practice does remove dust

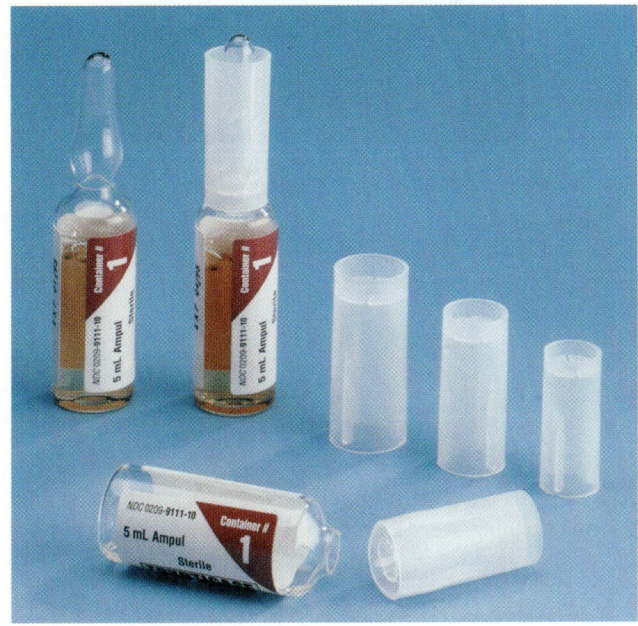

FIGURE 25-13 Safety device for opening glass ampules. (Courtesy of Medi-Dose®, Inc. EPS®, Inc., Ivyland, PA.)

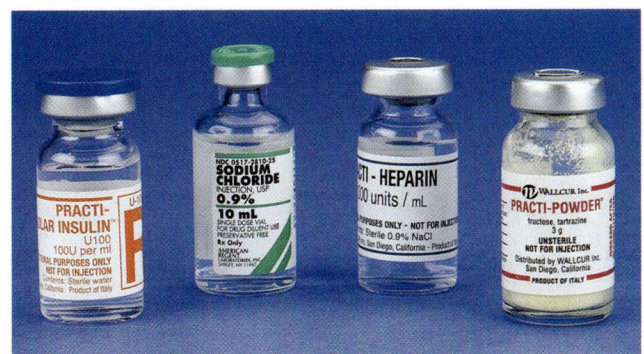

FIGURE 25-14 Vials containing medications.

Clinical Insight 25-3 ▶ **Using Prefilled Unit-Dose Systems**

Prefilled systems are most limited to some office practices and self-administration. They are used infrequently in healthcare facilities, because in some systems, the manipulation required to remove the cartridge from the holder creates a needlestick risk for nurses. Because you may encounter these systems in some clinical sites, we include the technique.

1. Check each medication cartridge and dose carefully, because all of the cartridges look alike.
2. No medication preparation is necessary.
3. Insert the cartridge into the holder.
4. Swing or twist the plunger into place, depending on the type of syringe you use. Lock it securely at the needle end.
5. Attach the plunger, if necessary. (The system may come with plunger attached.)

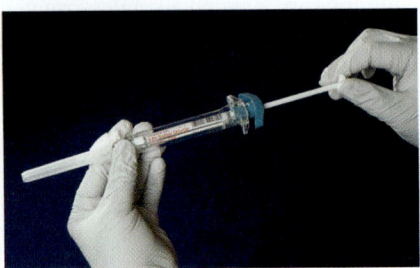

6. Expel air and excess medication.
7. Don gloves.
8. Administer the medication.
9. Dispose of the empty cartridge. Some types are available for reuse.

❓ **What if . . .**

■ **The needle gauge or length is not correct for the patient?**

You can transfer the medication into a regular syringe, maintaining sterile technique. There are two ways you can do it.

Cartridge without removable needle:

1. Pull back on the plunger of the regular syringe and keep a capped, sterile needle ready.

2. Insert the cartridge needle through the open tip of the regular syringe.
3. Eject the medication into the regular syringe.
4. Replace the capped needle onto the regular syringe.
5. Eject the air and check for the correct dosage.

Cartridge with removable needle:

The needle and cap can be removed from some prefilled cartridges, allowing the cartridge to be used as a vial.

This allows you to draw the medications into a different syringe. Do not inject air into a cartridge, because the excess pressure may eject the movable bottom.

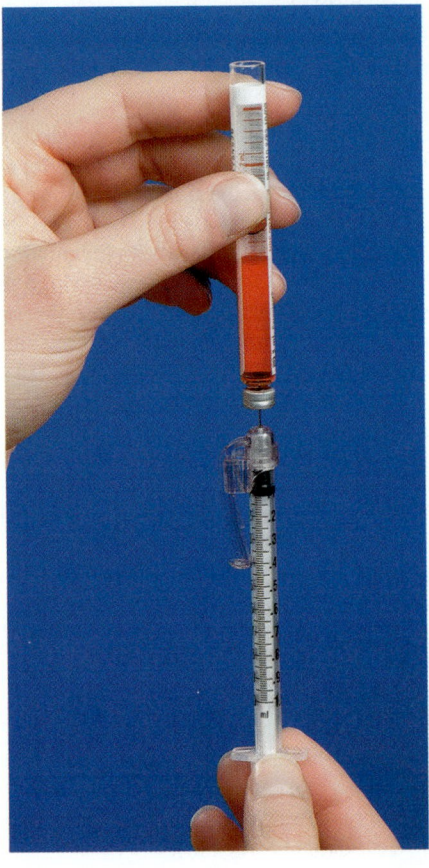

---

and rubber particles from the top of the vial; however, using a filter needle or straw achieves that purpose as well. You will need to follow the policy of the institution in which you work.

Reconstituting Medications

Medications that are not stable in solution are dispensed as powders in vials. You must add a diluent or solvent to the powder to create a solution for injection. The diluent is usually sterile water or saline; however, each packaged vial includes the manufacturer's instructions for the amount and kind of solvent to add. For safety, use a plastic vial access cannula

instead of a needle when possible. For guidelines, refer to Clinical Insight 25-4.

Mixing Medications in the Same Syringe

You can mix two medications in the same syringe (1) if they are compatible, (2) if the total dose is within accepted limits, and, obviously, (3) if they are both to be given by the same route. This technique allows for efficient use of supplies and allows the patient to receive fewer injections.

Medications are *compatible* if they can be mixed without affecting their constituents or actions. Package inserts and medication references usually include compatibility information.

Clinical Insight 25-4 ▸ Reconstituting Medication

1. Remove the caps of both the medication and diluent vials.
2. If a multidose vial is used, scrub the tops of both vials with alcohol wipe or other antiseptic.

To clean the cap of dust and reduce the number of microorganisms.

3. Use a Vial Access Device (VAD), or if agency policy allows, attach a filter needle to the syringe.

To prevent withdrawing glass and rubber particles, which have been found in medications withdrawn from vials and ampules.

4. Draw up the diluent into the syringe:
   a. Draw air into the syringe in a volume equal to the amount of diluent you will be withdrawing.
   b. Insert the safety needle (or VAD) carefully through the center of the rubber cap, and, keeping the bevel of the needle (or cannula) above the diluent, inject the air.

The air prevents negative pressure inside the vial when you withdraw the diluent, allowing you to withdraw the diluent easily. Keeping bevel above diluent helps prevent bubbles.

   c. Withdraw the diluent in the specified amount.
5. Insert the VAD carefully through the center of the rubber cap, and inject the diluent into the medication vial.
6. Mix the medication, taking care not to create bubbles (e.g., roll, do not shake, the vial). If medication does not mix easily, remove the needle or cannula from the vial, and place the syringe and needle on a sterile field (e.g., the wrapper the syringe came in) while you mix more. Alternatively, recap the sterile needle (see Procedure 25-10A).

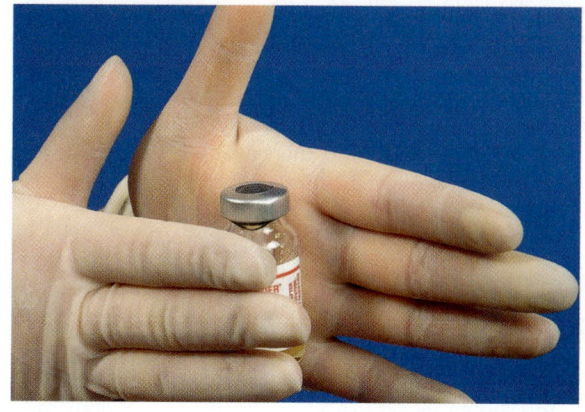

7. Reinsert filter needle or VAD if it was removed), and withdraw the reconstituted medication into the syringe.
8. Remove the filter needle or the cannula from the syringe, and replace it with a sterile needle before measuring the medication.

This ensures that the dose is correct and minimizes discomfort. It also prevents tracking of medication through the tissues; filter needles are usually larger than you will need for an injection. In addition, you should not eject fluid through a filter needle.

9. Hold the syringe vertically, and carefully eject all air from the syringe, but do not eject the medication. Read the dosage.
10. If necessary, hold the syringe horizontally to eject unneeded medication from the syringe to reach the prescribed dose.

✚ Always check the compatibility before mixing medications together. If the contents of the syringe become discolored, there are visible particles in the solution, or there is a change in consistency, do not administer the medications.

When mixing medications in one syringe, you must follow these principles:
- Maintain sterile technique (as with all parenteral medications).
- Do not contaminate one container with medication from the other container. You must use a separate needle to withdraw from each vial (exceptions: when both are single-dose vials, and in the case of different types of insulin).

✚ Never reuse a needle or syringe for drawing up a later dose of medication. A single-use vial contains only one dose of medication. Even if you do not administer the entire dose, the vial should be used only once for one patient, using a sterile needle and sterile syringe.

- Draw the second drug up slowly and carefully. If you draw up too much of the second drug, you must discard the syringe and medication and begin again.

- Ensure the total, final dosage is correct before administering the medication.

For the complete steps of this skill, see Procedure 25-9C.

Accounting for Needle "Dead Space"

Some nurses believe a small amount of the patient's medication remains in the needle when an injection is given. Therefore, they have recommended adding 0.2 mL of air to the syringe after measuring a medication for IM injection. Nurses are not in agreement about the need for adding air and, unfortunately, there is scant research to settle the question. Theoretically, on injection the 0.2 mL of air would clear the needle of medication, ensuring that the patient receives the entire dose. However, because syringes are calibrated to account for medication left in the needle, and because the medication left in the needle after injection is the same amount as before the injection, many believe that air should not be added. We recommend that you add air only in the following situations:

1. *When the medication is irritating to subcutaneous tissues,* add 0.2 mL of air after measuring the proper dose. The air drives the medication deep into the subcutaneous tissue; the air injected into the tissue creates an air lock above the

medication, preventing it from tracking through subcutaneous tissue.

2. *When you change needles after drawing up the medication,* draw up a dose using a filter needle, then replace it with a new needle, the new needle has air in it instead of medication. If you push the plunger until you see a drop of medication at the tip of the needle, you will see that you no longer have a complete dose in the syringe. Pulling in 0.2 mL air before changing the needle and then pushing the plunger until you see a drop of medication at the tip of the new needle will prevent the loss of medication with the needle change (see Clinical Insight 25-5).

Preventing Needlestick Injuries

Workplace injuries occur from needles and other sharps, putting healthcare workers at risk for bloodborne diseases, such as hepatitis B, hepatitis C, and HIV (see Chapter 23). For this reason, safety devices have been designed to reduce the risk of needlestick injuries through blunting, shielding, retracting needles, and needles with attached covers as

---

Clinical Insight 25-5 ➤ Measuring Dosage When Changing Needles

Note: These are not the old "air lock" techniques.

You should always use a filter needle to withdraw medications, if one is available. However, to give the injection, you must use a needle of the correct gauge and length. You must also eject air to measure the medication; however, pushing medication out of the syringe with the filter needle in place could cause the filter to break and release glass (and other) fragments. In the following method, pulling air into the syringe allows for exact dosage when the medication is injected; when ejected, the air will clear the needle so that the patient receives all the medication that is in the syringe.

For a Nonfilter Needle

When drawing medication from a multidose vial, you may sometimes need to use two regular needles. Alternately, you may use a needleless reconstitution device that is designed with a dispensing spike instead of a needle on one end, and a luer-lock port on the other end that attaches to the syringe. You will use one needle (or needless reconstitution device) for drawing up the medication, and the other for injecting the medication into the patient.

1. To draw medication out of a vial, inject air into the air pocket within the vial. Then withdraw the correct amount of medication from the vial using the first needle. Be sure to keep the tip of the needle in the fluid in order to avoid aspirating air bubbles into the syringe.

2. After drawing up the medication dose, tap on the barrel of the syringe to remove air bubbles, if necessary. Then eject the air out of the syringe (keeping the syringe vertical) while retaining the correct amount of medication in the syringe. Check the volume closely at eye level.

3. Remove the first needle and discard it into a needle-safe container. Put on a fresh needle for injection.

4. Pull back on the plunger, and draw an extra 0.2 mL of air to account for the air within the needle.

5. Check the medication dosage. Your plunger should be 0.2 mL more than the ordered dose.

6. When you inject the patient, she will receive the correct dose; the air will drive the medication from the needle into the patient's tissues. This is important when giving irritating medications, such as iron.

This is an air lock.

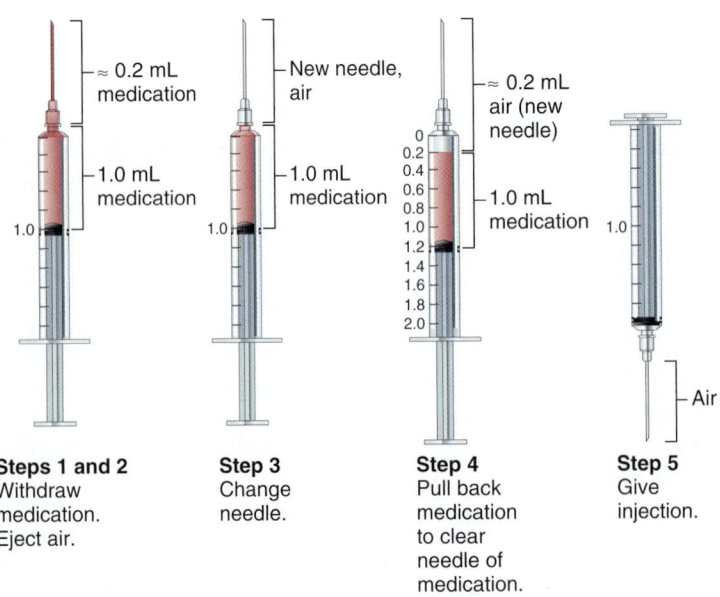

Steps 1 and 2
Withdraw medication. Eject air.

Step 3
Change needle.

Step 4
Pull back medication to clear needle of medication.

Step 5
Give injection.

Clinical Insight 25-5 ➤ Measuring Dosage When Changing Needles—cont'd

For a Filter Needle

Use one filter needle (or filter cannula) and one regular needle.

1. With the filter needle (or cannula), withdraw the exact amount of medication. Eject air bubbles (keeping the syringe vertical) as needed to obtain correct dose.
2. Pull back on the plunger to withdraw all the medication from the filter needle (or filter cannula) into the syringe. Depending on the size of the access cannula, this may be as much as 0.2 mL. It will now appear that you have more than the ordered dose in the syringe (but you do not; the air is taking up some of the space).
3. Change to the needle you are going to use for injection.

4. Hold the syringe vertically, and eject air until you see a drop of medication at the tip of the needle ("drop to the top").
5. Measure the medication. It should be at the correct syringe marking. If it is not, then tip the syringe horizontally, and eject the medication until the dose is correct.
6. When you inject the patient, she will receive the correct dose even though some medication will remain in the needle.
7. If you are giving an irritating medication (e.g., iron) create an air lock by drawing 0.2 mL of air into the syringe before giving the injection.

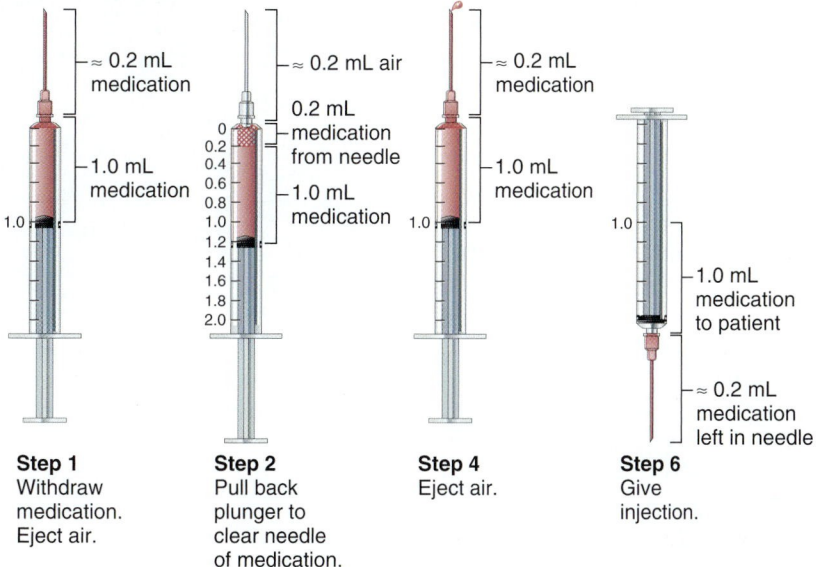

Step 1
Withdraw medication.
Eject air.

Step 2
Pull back plunger to clear needle of medication.

Step 4
Eject air.

Step 6
Give injection.

in Figure 25-15A, B, and C. Figure 25-16 shows a safety syringe with a guard that pulls forward to cover the needle immediately after it is withdrawn from the skin to reduce the risk of accidental punctures with contaminated needles. You then dispose of both needle and sheath in a sharps container. Needles with attached covers reduce the risk of accidental punctures with contaminated needles. Wing-tipped needles are also available in many clinical settings.

The Centers for Disease Control and Prevention (CDC) and the Occupational Safety and Health Administration (OSHA) recommend the use of "needleless" systems. Most systems involve adapters that can be used with regular intravenous tubing and medication vials, permitting access through a valve system without a needle. Figure 25-17 shows three such devices.

Another needle-free system is the jet injection, most often used for immunizations. The jet injectors drive liquid medication into the intradermal, subcutaneous, or intramuscular tissues by creating a narrow stream under high pressure that penetrates the skin. However, local reactions or injury, such as redness, bruising, and pain, occur more often with jet injectors than by use of a needle.

✚ Always dispose of needles, glass, and other sharps in clearly marked, usually red, puncture-proof containers (Fig. 25-18). Never force a needle into an already full container; you may be injured by sharps protruding from the top. Never put a needle or other sharp in a wastebasket, in your pocket, or at the patient's bedside.

For more information about preventing needlestick injury, see Clinical Insight 21-2.

Recapping Contaminated Needles

You should never recap a contaminated needle (e.g., after giving an injection); place it uncapped, needle pointing downward, directly into a sharps disposal container. However, you may occasionally find that you cannot avoid recapping a contaminated needle. The 1991 Bloodborne Pathogens Standard requires bending, recapping, or needle removal using a mechanical device or a one-handed technique (U.S. Department of Health and Human Services [USDHHS], 1991, updated 2008). For step-by-step instructions, see Procedure 25-10.

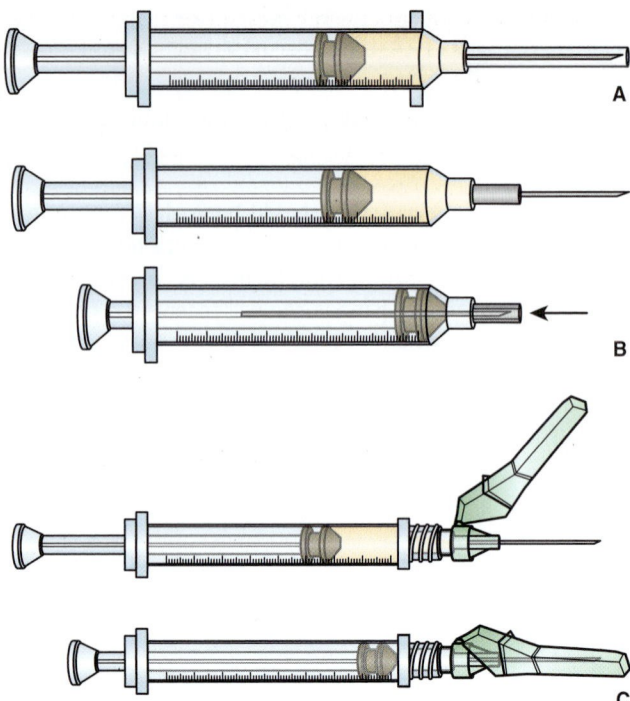

FIGURE 25-15 Needle safety features. A, Self-sheathing safety feature: Sliding needle shields attached to disposable syringes and vacuum tube holders. B, Syringe with retractable needle. C, Needles with covers.

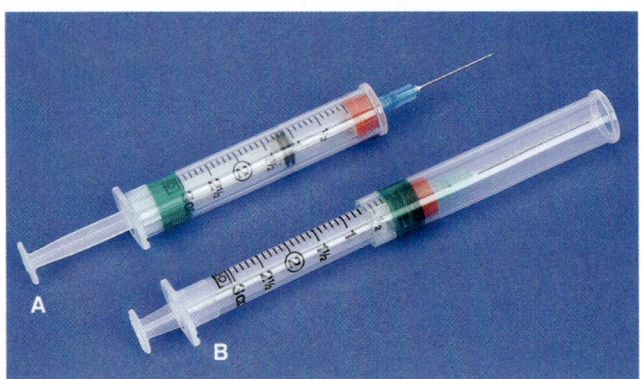

FIGURE 25-16 Safety syringe. A, Needle guard position before injection. B, Needle guard position after injection.

Recapping Sterile Needles

OSHA and the National Institute of Occupational Safety and Health (NIOSH) do not advise against recapping sterile needles (e.g., after drawing up a medication), except to recommend needleless systems and safety systems (NIOSH, n.d.). We suggest that you not use the one-handed "scoop" technique to recap a sterile needle because the risk of contaminating it is high. Consider one of the other methods described in Procedure 25-10.

Administering Parenteral Injections

Parenteral techniques are invasive. They carry the potential for tissue trauma and provide a portal of entry for pathogens through the skin. Therefore, you must maintain strict aseptic (sterile) technique to minimize the risk of infection. When you choose a site for injection, consider the type of medication to

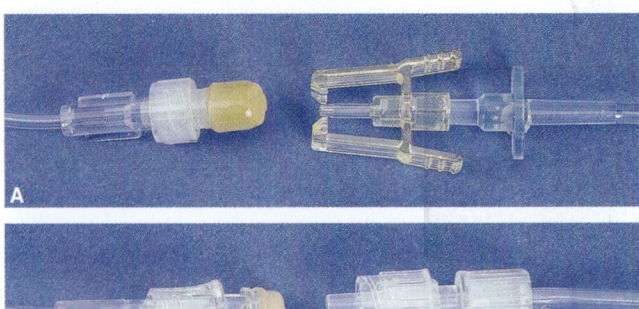
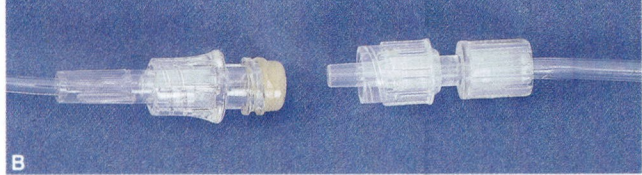
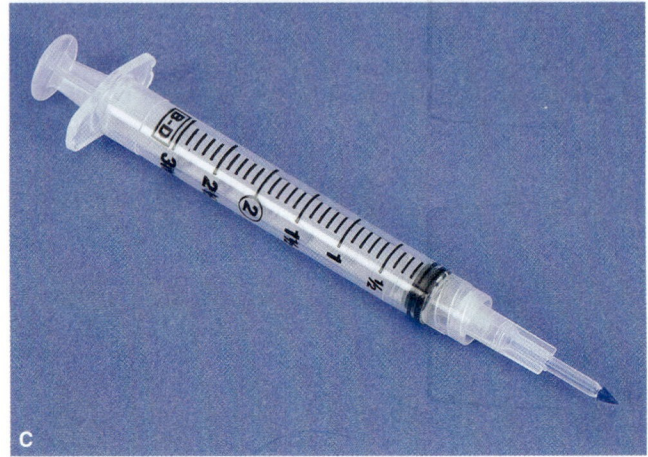

FIGURE 25-17 Needleless systems. A, Lever-lock cannula. B, Threaded lock cannula. C., Blunt-tipped syringe for drawing up medication.

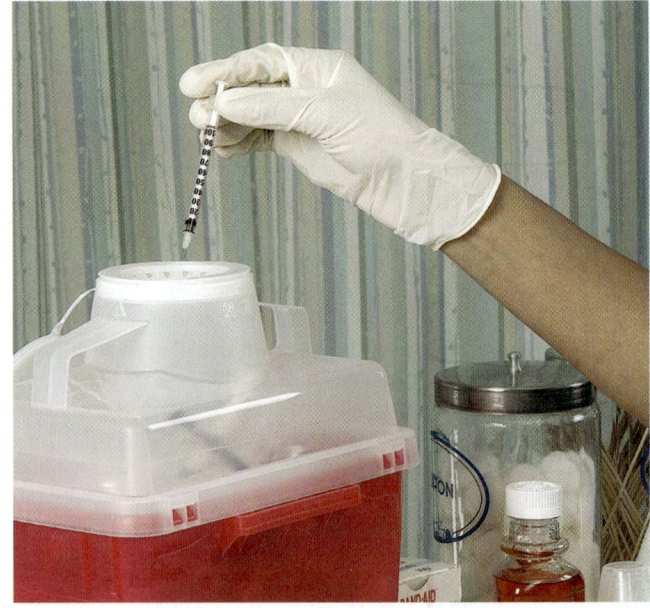

FIGURE 25-18 Disposal system for sharp objects, such as needles and glass. The container must be clearly marked, usually red, and puncture-proof.

be administered, the viscosity of the medication, the volume of the medication, the anatomical landmarks underlying injection sites, and the patient's situation (e.g., the condition of the tissues at the injection site, the accessibility of certain sites).

Your injection technique is critical to patient safety. The following are examples of errors and their consequences:

- Injecting a large volume of medication into a small muscle causes pain and may damage the tissues.
- Injecting into the wrong tissue (e.g., giving an intramuscular medication too shallowly into the subcutaneous tissue) may (1) accelerate or delay the rate of absorption and (2) cause tissue injury and pain.
- Incorrectly locating an injection site may result in bone or nerve injury when you insert the needle.
- An unsteady needle and syringe while injecting the drug could lead to pain and tissue trauma.
- Forgetting to aspirate before injecting risks administration of medication into an artery or vein instead of the muscle. This could result in an adverse, even fatal, effect.

Minimizing Discomfort

The discomfort associated with an injection comes from three sources: the prick of the needle, the pressure of the volume of the drug in the tissues, and chemical irritation caused by some drugs. Fear and anxiety magnify discomfort. Use the following techniques to reduce discomfort:

- Use the smallest needle suited for the site and medication.
- Use two needles when drawing up medications: one to withdraw the medication from the container, and the second one for the injection. If the needle is not free of medication, it may irritate tissues as it is inserted.
- Do not administer too much solution into an injection site. If the total volume is more than the recommended amount, give it in two injections and at two sites.
- For intramuscular injections, help the patient to assume a position that reduces muscle tension.
- For intramuscular injections, use the Z-track technique (see Procedure 25-14B). This prevents leakage of the medication up through the needle track after the needle is withdrawn. The Z-track method is particularly useful when giving medications that irritate or discolor the subcutaneous tissue. It should also be used for elderly patients who have reduced muscle mass.
- Pull the skin taut, and insert the needle quickly to avoid pulling the tissues. Remove the needle quickly and at the same angle you inserted it.
- Steady the syringe with one hand while injecting the medication.
- Inject the medication slowly.
- Distract the patient from the procedure by talking to her.
- Apply gentle pressure (not massage) after injection unless contraindicated.
- Especially with children, acknowledge that they will feel some pain (e.g., "This may hurt a little bit."). If you deny or minimize the pain, the patient might lose trust in you and be even more anxious about future injections.
- After injecting a child, pat or hug him, speak softly to him, and perhaps play with him, so that he does not associate you only with pain.
- Other methods for decreasing pain can be cooling the skin (e.g., applying ice) or flicking or tapping over the injection area before injecting. Both send distracting signals to the brain so that when the needle comes, it can't process the stimulus as easily.

Developmental Considerations

Because older adults may experience muscle atrophy or have decreased muscle mass, you may need to use a shorter needle. Infants and children also require shorter, thinner needles. Also, you should ask a parent or another caregiver to immobilize an infant or young child to prevent injury during the injection.

The preferred intramuscular site for infants is the vastus lateralis muscle, because there are no major nerves or blood vessels in the area and the gluteal muscles have not yet been developed by walking. For children who are walking, the site of choice is the ventrogluteal muscle because the muscle is more developed.

Do not use the dorsogluteal site for patients of any age, including older children and adults.

Intradermal Injections

Intradermal injections are given into the **dermis,** or the layer of the skin located beneath the skin surface. The intradermal route is commonly used for allergy or tuberculosis (TB) testing. Most nurses use the patient's nondominant arm for TB screening and the dominant arm, chest, or upper back for all other tests (Fig. 25-19). Give only small amounts of medication by this route—about 0.1 mL. Use a 1-mL syringe and a short, small (26- to 28-gauge) needle, and insert at an angle of 5° to 15°. For procedure steps, see Procedure 25-11.

Do not apply pressure or massage the injection site, because the capillaries in the dermal tissue will quickly absorb the medication.

Subcutaneous Injections

Subcutaneous (subQ) injections are given into the subcutaneous tissue, the layer of fat located below the dermis and above the muscle tissue. Absorption is slower than it is through the intramuscular route because subcutaneous tissue does not have as rich a blood supply as muscle. However, speed of absorption varies with the subcutaneous site selected. Sites on the abdomen and arms offer fastest absorption; those on the thigh and upper buttocks, the slowest absorption. Medication is absorbed more evenly from the abdomen than from the thighs and buttocks because it is less affected by activity.

You do not need to aspirate for blood return when giving a subcutaneous injection because of the shallow depth of the needle into the subcutaneous layer under the skin. For the full procedure, see Procedure 25-12.

Choosing a Subcutaneous Site

Avoid sites of abnormal subcutaneous tissue, such as areas lying beneath burns, birthmarks, inflamed tissue, or scars. Do not use sites with lesions or sites over bony prominences, large underlying vessels, or nerves. When using the abdominal site,

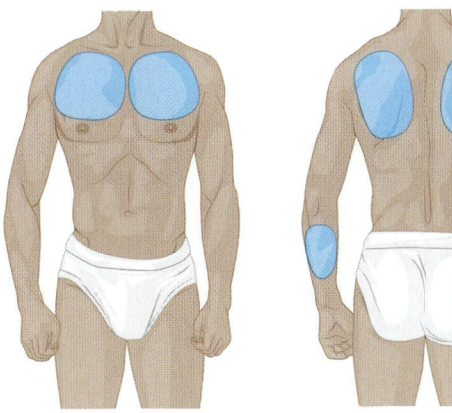

FIGURE 25-19 Sites commonly used for intradermal injection.

Toward Evidence-Based Practice

Zaybak, A., & Khorshid, L. (2008). A study on the effect of the duration of subcutaneous heparin injection on bruising and pain. *Journal of Clinical Nursing, 17*(3), 378–385.

This study was done to learn whether there is a difference in bruising or pain when subcutaneous injections of heparin are given quickly or slowly. Researchers studied 50 patients who required treatment with heparin. Injections on the right abdomen were given over 10 seconds, on the left abdomen, over 30 seconds. Bruising occurred in almost two out of every three (64%) of those who received the rapid injection; however, fewer than half (42%) of the patients bruised after receiving slower injection. Also, the size of the bruising was smaller in the 30-second injection. Pain intensity and pain duration were statistically significantly lower for the slower injection than for the more rapid one.

Chan, H. (2001). Effects of injection duration on site-pain intensity and bruising associated with subcutaneous heparin. *Journal of Clinical Nursing, 25*(6), 882–892.

This study was done to examine the relationship between how quickly a subcutaneous injection is performed and the occurrence of bruising and pain at the injection site. The research involved 34 stroke patients receiving heparin. For each subject, two injection techniques were used: one injection 10 seconds in duration and the other, 30 seconds. Results showed the 30-second duration injection technique resulted in statistically significantly less intense site-pain and fewer and smaller bruises. Researchers concluded that administering a subcutaneous heparin injection over longer duration reduces injection site pain and bruising.

Ipp, M., Taddio, A., Sam, J., et al. (2007). Vaccine-related pain: Randomized controlled trial of two injection techniques. *Archives of Disease in Childhood, 92*(12), 1105–1108.

The aim of this study was to compare pain during immunization using a slow injection versus a rapid technique. One hundred and thirteen healthy infants 4 to 6 months of age receiving routine DPTaP-Hib immunization were studied. One group received the intramuscular dose using a technique with slow aspiration before injection, slow injection, and slow withdrawal. The technique used for infants in the other group involved no aspiration, rapid injection, and rapid withdrawal. Infants receiving the slower injection technique cried twice as often, cried longer, and took more time to have the vaccine injected. Researchers concluded that immunization using a rapid intramuscular injection technique is less painful than a slower technique and should be recommended for routine intramuscular immunization.

1. You are providing care to an older adult patient who is receiving heparin therapy via subcutaneous injection. Based on the preceding studies, would you give subcutaneous doses over 10 seconds or 30 seconds?

2. You are working in a pediatric clinic. You want to administer intramuscular medication and immunizations to children in as pain-free a way as possible. Would you give IM injection slowly or more rapidly? Why would you choose that technique?

3. Why do you think subcutaneous injection might be less painful and produce less bruising when given more slowly even though IM injection using the same technique might be more painful?

 Go to Chapter 25, **Toward Evidence-Based Practice Suggested Responses,** on Davis*Plus*.

---

do not inject any closer than 5 cm (2 in.) from the umbilicus. For repeated injections, each injection should be at least an inch apart. It is important to rotate sites for repeated injections. Using the same spot can cause scarring and hardening of fatty tissue that will interfere with the absorption of medication. See Figure 25-20 for sites to use for subcutaneous injections.

Choosing a Subcutaneous Needle

As a general rule, use a syringe with a short and small needle for subcutaneous injection—that is, long enough to penetrate beyond the skin into the fatty subcutaneous layer and yet not into the muscle. The needle length will vary depending on the amount of adipose the patient has and the type of injection that is needed (e.g., insulin, immunization, or other medication). For most subcutaneous injections, a ⅜- to ⅝-inch needle is preferred. However, shorter needles (e.g., ³⁄₁₆- to ⁵⁄₁₆-inch) are more comfortable for some insulin users.

The **gauge,** or needle thickness, for subcutaneous injection should be small, typically 25- to 27-gauge; however, finer needles are often preferred by insulin users (e.g., 28- to 31-gauge). For children and persons with little or average

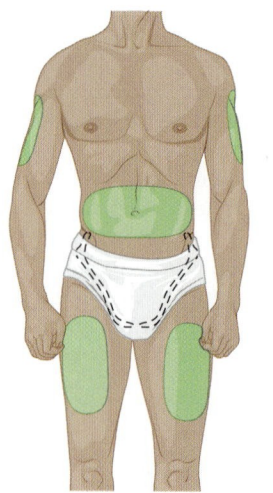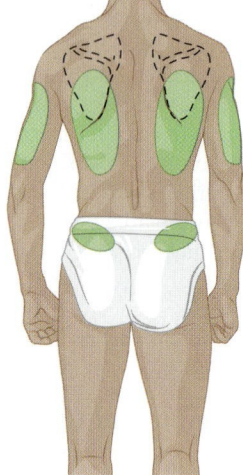

FIGURE 25-20 Sites used for subcutaneous injections.

subcutaneous fat, insert a standard length needle (⅝ in.) at a 45° angle; however, when using a shorter needle, inject at a 90° angle. Obese patients will need a longer needle (e.g., 1 in.) and a 90° angle for injection, and the nurse needs to spread the skin taut rather than pinching. See Figure 25-21.

The medication you are giving influences your choice of syringe. Recall that there are special insulin syringes and that you will use a tuberculin syringe or prefilled cartridge when giving heparin.

 Inject only small amounts (0.5 to 1 mL) of water-soluble medication subcutaneously to avoid creating sterile abscesses (hardened, painful lumps under the skin).

Administering Insulin

Insulin must be administered subcutaneously or intravenously because it is a protein and would be destroyed in the gastrointestinal tract. Insulin is administered using a special insulin syringe. Insulin vials contain 100 units/mL. The prescriber will specify the number of units rather than the number of milliliters or milligrams. Insulin may be prescribed in specific dosages at specific times or on the basis of the patient's blood glucose level before meals. The latter is a **sliding scale,** also called a correction scale. However, the sliding scale is controversial as many studies cite poor glycemic control and deleterious effects with its use. Sliding scale is used less now because basal insulin is available to stabilize blood sugar with fewer fluctuations, and because insulin pumps are in more common use. However, it can be useful when initiating insulin therapy and during times of physical stress such as illness, surgery, and trauma. Be sure to check with your institution regarding the sliding scale.

Categories of Insulin. Understanding the categories of insulin and how they are used for blood sugar control is essential for preventing errors and giving insulin safely.

- **Basal insulin** is given to cover the body's energy needs without taking the diet into account. Common basal insulins are neutral protamine hagedorn (NPH), insulin glargine (Lantus), and insulin detemir (Levemir).
- **Prandial** and **preprandial insulins** are given to prevent high blood sugar after eating a meal. Regular insulin is this type.
- **Correction insulin** is given to reduce an elevated blood sugar level to a normal range. This type of sliding scale blood sugar management is not the best way to manage diabetes because it achieves damage control more than damage prevention.

Using two types of insulin can help keep blood sugar level in a target range. By mixing it in the same insulin syringe, your patient will need only one injection. See Clinical Insight 25-6.

Appearance of Insulin. Regular (unmodified) insulin is rapid acting. It is a clear solution. If a vial of regular insulin is cloudy, you should discard it. Other types of insulin (e.g., Lente, insulin glargine, and NPH) are cloudy because of the addition of proteins, which slow the absorption of the drug, giving the insulin an intermediate to long duration of action. As a rule, remember "clear before cloudy"; that is, draw up the regular (clear) insulin first, and then draw up the modified (cloudy) insulin. Actually, though, you will rarely need to mix insulins because stable premixed insulins are available.

Storing Insulin. The length of time insulin can be stored depends on whether it is refrigerated or stored at room temperature. Check the package insert to know how long the insulin will remain effective after the vial is opened.

Insulin Equipment. Insulin can be administered in a variety of ways.

- **Disposable syringes** for subcutaneous injection are the most common.
- **Automatic injectors** are used by some patients for subcutaneous dosing. By pressing a button on the device, the injector releases the needle into the skin, releasing the insulin dose.
- **Insulin pumps** are becoming more common as a way to maintain glycemic control because of the benefit of fine-tuning the dosing. The pump consists of a tube with a needle on the end of it that is taped to the abdomen, and a computerized device that is worn at the waist. Insulin is received continuously from the pump. A button is pressed at mealtime to release an extra insulin dose.
- **Insulin pen devices** contain a cartridge and disposable needles to deliver certain doses with each injection. Patients who use insulin pens do not have to draw up insulin from a vial.
- **Nondisposable syringes** (glass syringe and metal needle) may be used repeatedly if they are sterilized after each use.
- **Spray injectors** forcefully spray the insulin dose into the skin. This involves a wider area of skin than an injection would.

People with diabetes usually administer their own insulin injections. They should rotate injection sites to promote absorption and minimize tissue damage. Insulin is absorbed at different rates from different parts of the body. For hospitalized patients, you should document site rotation (usually on a diagram of the body) to prevent repeated use of the same site.

To learn more about administering, see

Go to Chapter 25, **Supplemental Materials: Insulin Administration,** on DavisPlus.

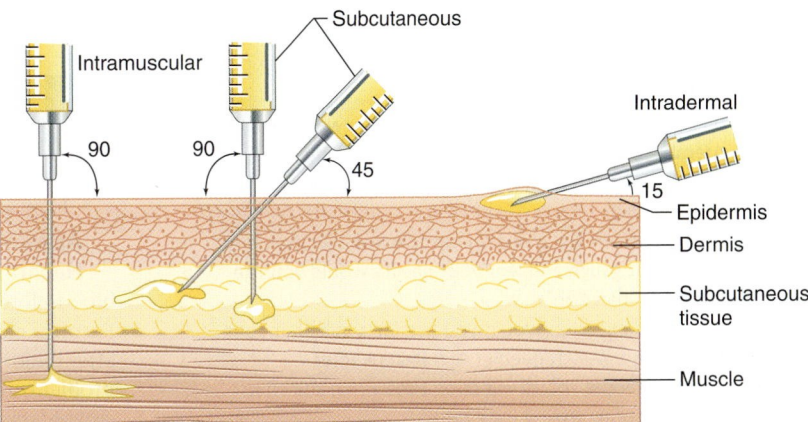

FIGURE 25-21 Standard angles of insertion for intramuscular, subcutaneous, and intradermal injections.

Clinical Insight 25-6 ➤ **Mixing Two Kinds of Insulin in One Syringe**

What You Should Know

- Various combinations of rapid-acting, intermediate-acting, and long-acting insulins may be prescribed. Some can be mixed; some cannot.
- Lente insulins (Lente and Lantus) can be mixed with each other, but not with neutral protamine hagedorn (NPH).
- Although they are compatible, do not mix Lente with regular insulin except for patients who are already controlled on this mixture. Lente will bind with regular insulin, delaying the onset of action.
- A general rule is "clear before cloudy." Regular insulin is clear; all other types are cloudy. Therefore, you would draw up regular insulin into the syringe before Lente or NPH insulin, which are modified. If you draw up a modified type first, the needle may transfer it into the unmodified (regular) vial.

What You Should Do

Follow these steps when drawing up insulin from two vials into one syringe. The procedure assumes you are mixing regular (unmodified) insulin with a modified (e.g., NPH) insulin.

1. Maintain sterile technique throughout.
2. Before preparation, rotate the insulin vials between the palms of your hands for at least 1 minute, and invert them to ensure an adequate concentration. Do not shake the vials because this can create bubbles, which take up space and make it difficult to measure the dose precisely.
3. Scrub vial stoppers with alcohol or other antiseptic (they are usually multidose vials).
4. Using an insulin syringe and needle, inject an amount of air equal to the amount of insulin to be withdrawn from the vial of modified insulin (cloudy vial). Do not allow the needle tip to touch the insulin.
5. Using the same syringe, inject the appropriate amount of air into the vial of regular insulin (clear vial).
6. Do not withdraw the needle; withdraw the correct dose of regular insulin.

7. Remove the syringe from the regular insulin. Eject air, and remove all air bubbles to measure the correct dose.
8. Calculate the total amount on the syringe that the combined types of insulin should measure.
9. Return to the (first) vial of modified insulin (cloudy), and draw the correct dose into the syringe. (For example, if you have 5 units of regular insulin in the syringe and you need 10 units of NPH, the plunger should be at the 15-unit mark when you have drawn up the NPH.)
10. Recall that you have already added air to this vial in a previous step. Draw up the medication slowly and exactly to the total dose, being very careful not to create bubbles and to withdraw only the amount needed. You cannot return any excess to the vial because it is now a mixture of two medications.
11. Administer the insulin mixture within 5 minutes after preparation. Even NPH insulin will bind with regular insulin and delay the onset of its action.

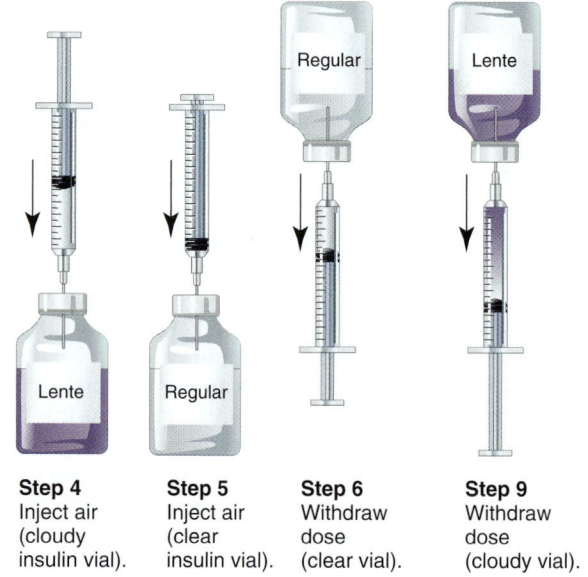

Step 4
Inject air (cloudy insulin vial).

Step 5
Inject air (clear insulin vial).

Step 6
Withdraw dose (clear vial).

Step 9
Withdraw dose (cloudy vial).

Total dose is mixture of clear and cloudy insulins.

KnowledgeCheck 25-16

- List three errors in technique that can occur when giving parenteral injections. State their possible consequences.
- Describe at least four ways to minimize the discomfort of an injection.
- Name two reasons for giving an intradermal injection.
- As a rule, what gauge and length of needle would you use for a subcutaneous injection?
- What angle of injection would you use for a subcutaneous injection using a ⅜-inch needle? A ⅝-inch needle?
- Why should people rotate injection sites when they must have repeated injections over a long time?

ThinkLike a Nurse 25-12

- What do intradermal and subcutaneous injections have in common?
- How are they different?

Administering Heparin

Heparin is a fast-acting medication that interrupts the blood-clotting process. It may be used for patients at risk for harmful clot formation, for example, those who are immobile after major surgery, have undergone vascular surgery, or have problems related to blood clotting, such as cerebrovascular accident (stroke) or myocardial infarction (heart attack). Because

heparin is absorbed poorly from the gastrointestinal tract, it is given intravenously or subcutaneously. If mistakenly given intramuscularly, it will cause hematoma and pain. The dosage is based on the patient's weight and results of blood coagulation studies, so always check laboratory values for coagulation studies before giving.

Give the injection deep into the subcutaneous tissue of the abdomen, at least 5 cm (2 in.) away from the umbilicus. Rotate sites. Because of the anticoagulant properties of heparin, you will need to modify your injection technique. For guidelines to use when injecting anticoagulants subcutaneously, refer to Clinical Insight 25-7.

Intramuscular Injections

Intramuscular (IM) injections (injections into muscle tissue) are absorbed faster than subcutaneous medications because of the rich blood supply in the muscles. Muscles can also tolerate more fluid—you can give as much as 3 or 4 mL of liquid in the large vastus lateralis and ventrogluteal muscles. The smaller the muscle is, the less fluid it can tolerate. For example, you should usually give no more than 0.5 to 1 mL in the average deltoid muscle.

Conventional techniques call for you to aspirate before injecting medication; if there is no blood return, theoretically you are confident that the medication will not be injected into a blood vessel. However, there are not enough scientific studies to confirm that aspiration is a reliable indicator of correct needle placement. Nevertheless, most experts recommend this technique on a theoretical basis to ensure the needle tip is not in a blood vessel.

Choosing an Intramuscular Site

When selecting an IM site, you should look for a site that is
- A safe distance from nerves, large blood vessels, and bones
- Free from injury, abscesses, tenderness, necrosis, abrasion, or other pathology
- Large enough to accommodate the volume of medication to be given

Muscles commonly used are the vastus lateralis, ventrogluteal, and deltoid. Because of their proximity to major nerves and vessels, the rectus femoris and dorsogluteal are no longer recommended sites (Greenway, 2004; Nicholl & Hesby, 2002).

Ventrogluteal Muscle—Site of Choice. Whenever possible, use the ventrogluteal site for intramuscular injections; it is the site of choice for adults and young children who are walking. The ventrogluteal site, located on the lateral hip, involves the gluteus medius and gluteus minimus muscles. Because it is located away from major blood vessels and nerves, it is the safest and least painful site for intramuscular injections. Be aware though, that some medications and immunization, such as those used to treat influenza/pneumonia, are normally given in the deltoid.

When learning to locate this site, many students notice that it feels "hard" when they palpate it. They worry the needle will hit the bone. In part, the muscle feels hard because there is little subcutaneous tissue over it. To reassure yourself it is safe, examine a skeleton model with the muscles attached. Notice the ilium is concave (curves in) and the muscle lies deep down in the "cup" it forms. If you are sure you have located the anterosuperior iliac spine and if you follow the procedure steps, you will not hit a bone. In fact, you are less likely to do so than if you use other sites. For guidelines in locating the ventrogluteal site, refer to Procedure 25-13.

Dorsogluteal Site. The dorsogluteal site consists of the gluteal muscles of the buttocks.

Clinical Insight 25-7 ▶ Administering Anticoagulant Medication Subcutaneously

- Because of the anticoagulant properties of heparin and enoxaparin (Lovenox), you will need to adapt your technique for subcutaneous injections in the following ways:
  - To avoid the loss of drug when using prefilled syringes, do not expel the air bubble from the syringe before the injection.
  - Enoxaparin-prefilled syringes and graduated prefilled syringes are available with a system that shields the needle after injection.
  - Use a ⅜-inch, 25- or 26-gauge needle.
  - After drawing up the correct dose, add 0.2 mL of air to the syringe to ensure that all of the medication is injected into the subcutaneous tissue and is not tracked into the superficial tissue.
  - With your nondominant hand, pinch or spread the skin and insert the needle at a 90° angle, using your dominant hand. If the patient has very little subcutaneous tissue, use a ⅝-inch needle and insert it at a 45° angle. Introduce the whole length of the needle into a skinfold held between the thumb and forefinger; hold the skinfold throughout the injection.
  - Alternate administration among sites on the abdomen. Give the injection subcutaneously deep on the abdomen, at least 2 inches away from the umbilicus.
  - If injecting low-molecular-weight heparin (LMWH [Lovenox]), be sure to alternate between the left and right anterolateral and left and right posterolateral abdominal wall.
  - Do not aspirate before injecting, because doing so can traumatize tissue and cause bruising.
  - Do not massage the site after injecting, because doing so can cause bleeding and bruising. It may also cause the heparin to be absorbed more rapidly than desired.
  - Keep a record of the sites used. Most agencies have a chart of the body on which to record the sites injected.

  ✚ Several mix-ups between heparin and insulin have been reported. To help avoid this (in addition to observing the "3 checks and 6 rights"): (1) Do not store heparin and insulin vials beside each other, (2) have another RN check your preparation before administering IV heparin or insulin, (3) think critically (e.g., ask yourself if giving heparin—or insulin—makes sense given the patient's diagnosis).

✚ Avoid using this site for IM injections because its close proximity to the sciatic nerve and superior gluteal artery, increases the risk of (a) injection into a major blood vessel and (b) damage to the sciatic nerve. Furthermore, the site is difficult to identify accurately in older adults or people with flabby skin.

You may observe some nurses continue to use the dorsogluteal site because they were taught to use it long ago and have not learned how to locate the ventrogluteal site. This gives you the opportunity to improve practice by demonstrating correct technique for locating the preferred site.

Deltoid Site. The deltoid site is located in the middle third of the upper arm. The area has a small muscle mass with little subcutaneous tissue, so medications are absorbed rapidly. This muscle is easily accessible but is not well developed in many older adults; you should use it only for small amounts of up to 1 mL or when other sites are inaccessible. Avoid using the deltoid site in infants; you can use it in children if you are sure the muscle mass is adequate, but the anterolateral thigh is preferred.

The deltoid is small and lies close to the radial nerve and brachial artery. When locating this site, do not merely roll up the sleeve; fully expose the entire upper arm and shoulder. Otherwise, you may miss the muscle mass and injure a nerve or blood vessel. For a guide to locating the deltoid site, see Procedure 25-13.

Vastus Lateralis Site. The vastus lateralis muscle, located in the anterolateral thigh, is the preferred site for young infants, particularly before walking age (CDC, 2002) because it's usually the best developed and contains no large nerves or blood vessels, minimizing the risk for injury. Drugs are rapidly absorbed from this area. Moreover, it can accommodate a larger volume of medication than can the deltoid, and it is not near any major blood vessels or nerves. In addition, this is a convenient location for those who self-administer injections. A disadvantage is that the patient can see you administer the injection, and the psychological effect may create some discomfort. Also, because this muscle is used in walking, an ambulatory patient may notice more residual soreness than in another site.

To relax this muscle for injection, have the patient sit or lie flat with his knee slightly flexed. For children and adult patients with small muscle mass, you should grasp ("pinch up") the body of the muscle during injection to be sure that the medication reaches muscle tissue and the needle does not penetrate to the underlying bone. For a guide to locating the vastus lateralis site, refer to Procedure 25-13.

Rectus Femoris Site. The rectus femoris site, located in the anterior thigh, is no longer recommended for infants and children, although you may rarely use it for adults when rapid absorption is needed or other sites are inaccessible. It is often used by patients who self-administer their intramuscular injections because it is easy for them to reach. A disadvantage is that it is usually painful. Use a shorter needle when injecting this site. For a guide to locating the rectus femoris site, refer to Procedure 25-13.

Choosing an Intramuscular Needle

Although a 1½-inch needle is considered "standard" for intramuscular injections, you should choose the needle gauge and length based on the site, the size of the muscle, the amount of medication to be given, and the amount of adipose tissue over the muscle. In the deltoid muscle, for example, you might use a 23- or 25-gauge, 1-inch needle. But if the solution is viscous, you would need a larger-bore needle (e.g., 20-gauge). For a very thin person, you could use a 1-inch needle, even when injecting into the larger muscles. For an obese person, you might need a needle as long as 3 inches to penetrate adipose tissue and reach the muscle (unfortunately, long needles may not be available in some settings). As a rule, the angle of insertion for an intramuscular injection is 90° (see Fig. 25-21). See Procedure 25-14.

✚ The CDC recommends a 1-inch needle for all thigh intramuscular immunizations in infants ages 1 to 12 months, a 1- to 1¼-inch needle for all thigh intramuscular immunizations in toddlers ages 12 to 24 months, and a ⅝- to 1-inch needle for all deltoid intramuscular vaccinations in children ages 1 to 18 years (Kroger, Atkinson, Marcuse, et al. 2007).

Z-Track Technique

Procedure 25-14B describes the procedure for using the Z-track technique for intramuscular injections. This technique seals the needle track and prevents medication from leaking out of the muscle up through the needle track and into the subcutaneous tissues. You must use this technique for irritating medications, such as iron preparations. The Z-track method is also good for older adults with reduced muscle mass. It is recommended for all intramuscular injections, because it is less painful and helps to prevent irritation of subcutaneous tissues. For this technique, it is best to use the larger muscles: the ventrogluteal and vastus lateralis.

KnowledgeCheck 25-17

- Name three sites for giving intramuscular (IM) injections.
- What is the preferred site for adults? Why?
- From which route is medication absorbed more rapidly: subcutaneous or intramuscular? Why?
- For an "average" adult, what is the standard needle length for IM injections?
- Why is the dorsogluteal site *not* recommended?
- What are the disadvantages of the deltoid site?
- When using the vastus lateralis to give an intramuscular medication to a person with small muscle mass, how can you ensure the medication reaches muscle tissue and the needle does not penetrate to the underlying bone?

Intravenous Medications

Intravenous (IV) medications are given through a catheter, or cannula, inserted into a vein. The onset of medication action takes place within seconds, so IV administration is especially useful in emergencies. However, because an IV drug begins to act immediately, there is no way for you to stop its action if an adverse reaction occurs (unless there is a known antidote). Review Table 25-1 for advantages and disadvantages of using the IV route. IV medications may be administered by a variety of programmable electronic pumps and infusers. These are discussed in Chapter 39.

To prevent complications, when administering IV medications, you should do the following:

- Assess the patient before, during, and after giving the medication.
- Determine the drug is compatible with the fluid that is infusing; consult a pharmacist if necessary.
- Determine the drug is compatible with the plastic IV bag and tubing; you may occasionally need to use a glass IV bottle and special tubing.

- Use sterile technique.
- Administer the medication slowly.
- Observe the patient carefully for signs of adverse reactions.
- Have an antidote on hand if the drug has potentially serious side effects. Be aware, though, that many drugs do not have an antidote.
- Observe the insertion site often, because many IV medications are irritating to the vein and surrounding tissues. Check to be sure the cannula is in the vein before administering a medication, and observe the insertion site frequently. Figure 25-22 provides an example of tissue damage that can occur when certain IV medications escape from the vein into surrounding tissues.

The following sections explain various methods for administering IV medications. You will find the procedures for initiating and maintaining intravenous fluids and using intermittent injection ports in Chapter 39.

Adding Medications to Large-Volume (Primary) Infusions

The safest way to administer a drug intravenously is to mix it into a bag of fluid that is already infusing. This is often normal saline or lactated Ringer's solution or, sometimes, glucose. Vitamins, potassium chloride, oxytocin, and several blood pressure and cardiovascular drugs are commonly given this way. This method is useful when the drug can be infused continuously over a long period of time or when it must be given continuously to achieve the desired effect. The main disadvantage is the danger of infusing too much fluid, especially for children, older adults, and people with cardiac or renal disease. The drug may be premixed with the IV fluid in the pharmacy, or you may need to add a drug to a bag of IV fluids.

A safe method for mixing medication from multidose IV vials while providing sterile air filtration is to use a **reconstitution device**—designed with a sharp, thin, piercing spike to minimize coring and permit easy penetration of rubber top vials. The luer-lock port maintains a secure closure between the device and the syringe. The hinged cap and the sheath over the spike help maintain sterility before use, minimize "touch" contamination, and ensure a closed system for disposal.

A safe method for adding medications to an IV container is to use a **transfer needle** or **cannula**—a blunted plastic needle with a double beveled tip. One end is inserted into the powdered or liquid medication and the other end is inserted into a port of the IV bag. Solution is transferred from the IV bag into the medication vial, which you shake lightly to mix the medication. Then the medication is transferred back into the IV bag for administration.

Refer to Figure 25-23 and Procedure 25-15.

IV Push Medications

IV push (bolus) medications are injected directly into the systemic circulation. Many drugs given by IV push have a package insert that contains specific guidelines for their administration rate (usually between 1 and 10 min). Read the package insert or ask the prescriber how fast the drug can be pushed. Even just a minute can seem like a very long time when you are pushing a medication, so don't guess—look at your watch! Take note that "IV push" does not mean the same thing as "give rapidly." If given too rapidly, IV drugs—particularly potassium—can be quite dangerous. Because you cannot retrieve the medication once it is injected, there is no margin for error. See Procedure 25-16 to learn how to give IV push medications.

Intermittent Infusion

Many medications, such as antibiotics, are administered intravenously by intermittent infusion. Intermittent infusions may be given through the port of a running IV line or, if the patient does not need the IV fluids, through an intermittent injection port, also called a saline or heparin lock (Fig. 25-24).

Most intermittent infusion medications are supplied in bags containing 50 to 250 mL of 5% dextrose in water (D_5W) or normal saline. The drug is given over a period of time, usually 30 to 60 minutes, and at regular intervals (e.g., every 6 hours). The small bag of diluted medication (the "secondary" bag) is attached to the primary IV infusion line for administration. There are two types of setups for intermittent infusion using a primary IV line:

1. A **tandem setup** is connected to the primary IV line at the lower (secondary) port. The medication can be given

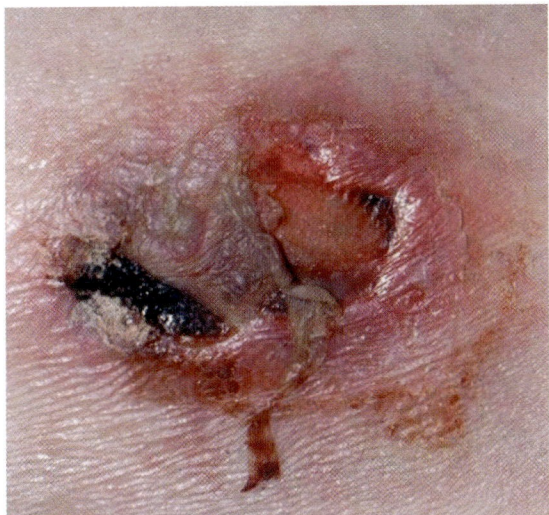

FIGURE 25-22 Tissue and skin injury after intravenous medication leaks into an infiltrated site. (Used by permission of the National Extravasation Information Service [UK]. http://www.extravasation.org.uk)

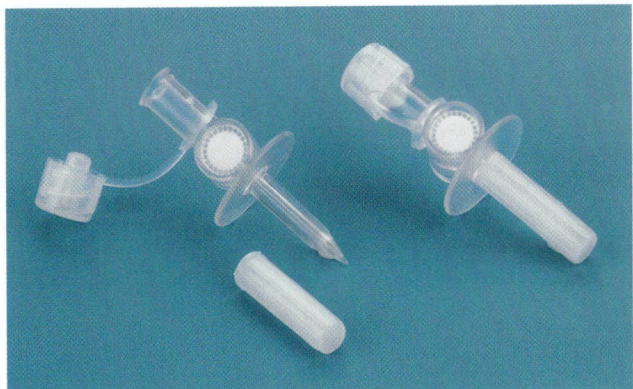

FIGURE 25-23 A reconstitution device is used to add medication from multidose IV vials while providing sterile air filtration. (Courtesy of Medi-Dose® Inc./ EPS® Inc., Ivyland, PA.)

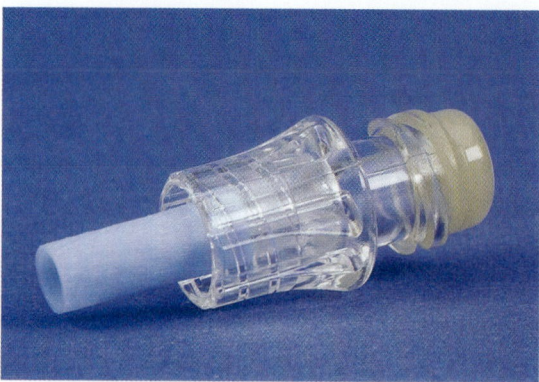

FIGURE 25-24 Intermittent injection port.

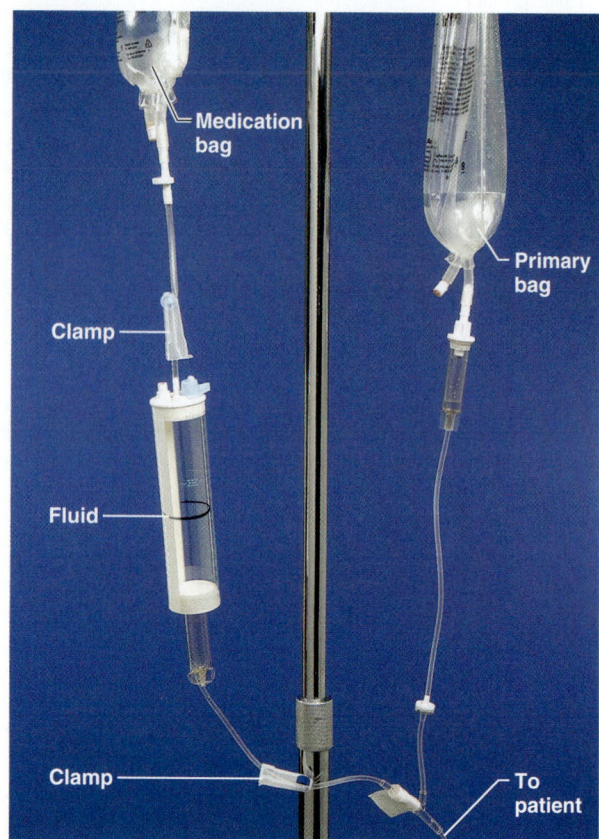

FIGURE 25-25 Volume-control infusion set for intermittent infusion administration; used when the fluid volume is critical and must be carefully monitored.

intermittently or at the same time as the primary IV infusion—both bags can infuse at the same time. See Procedure 25-17C.

2. With an **IV piggyback** setup the smaller (secondary) container is connected to the primary (continuous) infusion line at the upper (primary) port. This setup allows for intermittent use only. See Procedure 25-17B.

Traditionally, the secondary tubing was attached to the primary set tubing by inserting a needle into the port and taping it in place. However, most agencies now use needleless systems (see Fig. 25-17), which use a threaded or lever-type lock to make the connection. In addition to helping prevent needlestick injuries, a needleless system prevents contact contamination at the IV connection site.

Volume-Control Infusion Sets

To effectively control the infusion of smaller amounts of solutions, particularly with pediatric patients, a volume-control infusion set (e.g., Buretrol, Soluset, Volutrol, or Pediatrol) may be used (Fig. 25-25). These are small fluid containers (100 to 150 mL) that are attached directly below the primary fluid container. The medication and the desired amount of IV fluid are added to the volume-control container and administered through the primary line. This system decreases the risk of overhydration because the amount of fluid that can infuse into the patient is limited to the amount that you place in the small container. See Procedure 25-17A.

Central Venous Access Devices

Intravenous medication can be delivered through a central or peripheral vein. The most common reasons for a patient to have a central venous access device (CVAD) are to:

- Give long-term IV therapy
- Provide total parenteral nutrition when the patient cannot eat normally
- Have blood drawn without the trauma and complications of repeated venipuncture
- Be used when peripheral IV placement is difficult

External CVADs can be either tunneled or nontunneled. The *tunneled devices* are surgically implanted peripherally and tunneled to a central vein, typically the superior vena cava. *Nontunneled catheters* are inserted near the destination site. These catheters can be single- or multilumen. This category includes peripherally inserted central catheters (PICCs), which are inserted into the central circulation via a peripheral vein and can remain in place for months. For short-term use, the nontunneled central catheter can be inserted into the jugular, subclavian, or femoral veins.

An **internal, or implantable, port** is a CVAD that can remain in place and be functional for years. Access is gained through the skin via a hollow port with a self-sealing silicone cap. These devices are inserted when long-term IV medication is needed or the medication is too irritating for a peripheral site. See Figure 25-26A for an example of a port for injecting medication into the subclavian vein.

Catheters for central venous delivery can be single- or multilumen (Fig. 25-26B). Although they are more convenient for administering different medications and fluid, some types of multilumen catheters have a higher infection rate than single-lumen catheters. For steps to administer medication through a central venous access device, see procedure 25-18.

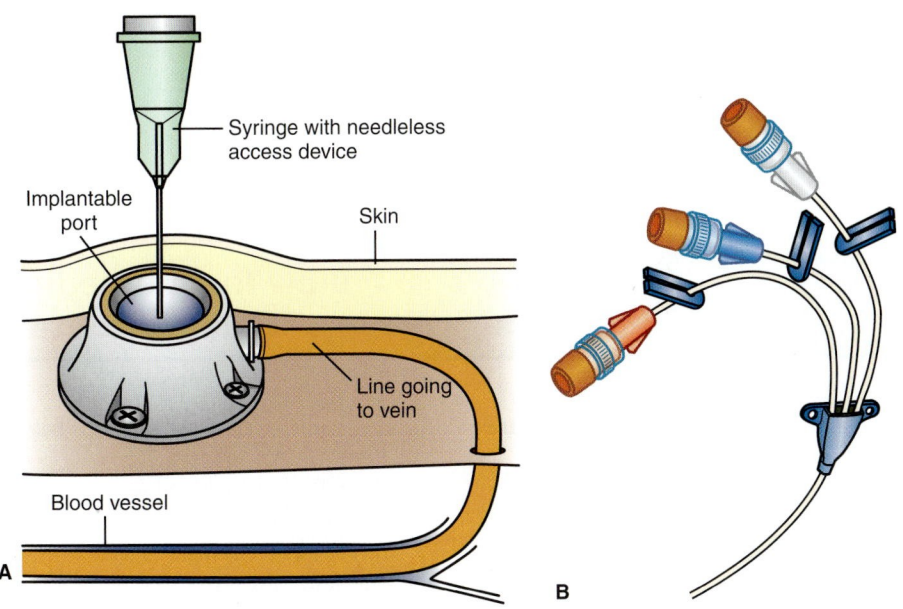

FIGURE 25-26 Central vascular access device: A, Implantable device. B, Multilumen catheter with blunt cannula, split septum, needleless access device.

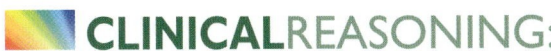

CLINICALREASONING:
Applying the **Full-Spectrum Nursing Model**

Because the following critical thinking activities allow you to practice the kind of thinking you will use as a full-spectrum nurse, they usually have no single right answer. Discuss them with your peers—if you have difficulty with any of the questions, consult your instructor.

PATIENT SITUATION

Leonard LeMonte is a 57-year-old, African American man who has come to his primary care provider because of persistent headaches that increase in intensity as it gets later in the day. His overall health has been good, although he is approximately 50 to 60 pounds overweight. Past medical history is significant for borderline primary hypertension and non-insulin-dependent diabetes, type 2 (diet controlled). Leonard tells you he works in a high-stress environment. He shares great concern with you that he fears losing his job and not being able to pay his bills and meet other financial commitments for his family. Mr. LeMonte tells you he has little time for hobbies or recreational outlets because he works so many hours.

THINKING

1. *Theoretical Knowledge (Facts and Principles):* You see in the chart that the prescriber has been ordering metformin (Glucophage), 1,000 mg daily, to treat Mr. LeMonte's diabetes. By what route is this medication given?
2. *Critical Thinking (Inquiry):* If you did not know the answer to the first question, specifically how did you get that information? State your source.

DOING

3. *Nursing Process (Assessment):* To evaluate Mr. LeMonte's response to his diabetes medication, what questions do you need to ask him?
4. *Practical Knowledge (Skills):* Mr. LeMonte tells you that he forgot to take his Glucophage this morning and also at lunchtime. What should you do?

CARING

5. *Self-Knowledge:* In what areas do you feel compassion for Mr. LeMonte, on which you might build a caring relationship?
6. *Self-Knowledge:* What do you identify as your strength in dealing with Mr. LeMonte's healthcare needs?
7. *Ethical Knowledge:* Mr. LeMonte tells you that he frequently skips doses of his Glucophage because he can't afford the expense. He asks you not to tell his wife about this because he doesn't want her to worry. What will you do?

 Go To Chapter 25, **Clinical Reasoning: Applying the Full-Spectrum Nursing Model Response Sheet,** on Davis*Plus.*

PracticalKnowledge procedures

Procedures in this section will assist you to prepare, measure, and administer various types of medications, to locate injection sites, and to handle needles safely.

Medication Guidelines: ■ Steps to Follow for All Medications (Regardless of Type or Route)

➤ For steps to follow in *all* procedures, refer to the Universal Steps for All Procedures found on the page facing the inside back cover.

➤ Regardless of the type or route of the medication you are giving, you should always follow the steps below.

Delegation

As an RN, you can usually delegate administration of medications (except for intravenous medications [IV]) to an LPN/LVN. You cannot delegate this task to nursing assistive personnel (NAP). You can instruct a NAP in the therapeutic effects and side effects of medications and to report any effects observed.

Nurse practice acts governing medication administration vary from state to state, and policies vary further among healthcare agencies. For example, in some states, in some situations, LPN/LVNs can administer IV medications and specially trained NAPs can administer certain medications (e.g., in long-term care settings). Nevertheless, as the RN you are always responsible for evaluating client responses, which include both therapeutic and side effects.

Pre-Procedure Assessments

- Assess your knowledge of the medication (e.g., drug action, purpose, recommended dosage, time of onset and peak action, common side effects, contraindications, drug interactions, and nursing implications).
- Determine whether the prescribed dosage is appropriate for the patient's age and weight.
  Dosages are generally decreased for children because of both age and weight. Usually dosing for elderly patients is not based

on weight but renal function. Both groups have less efficient liver and renal function, increasing the length of time a drug stays in the body before being excreted.

- Check for any history of allergies to medications or food.
  Some medications (e.g., penicillin and cephalosporin) have cross-sensitivity; that is, a patient with a penicillin allergy is at high risk for also being allergic to cephalosporin. Medications can also have cross-sensitivity with certain foods.
- At least on the first administration, assess the patient's knowledge about the medications being given.
  The patient will be more likely to take the medication correctly if she understands why she is taking the medication.
- Assess for factors that could interfere with drug absorption (e.g., diarrhea, inadequate circulation, impaired liver function, edema, inflammation, or age-related changes, other medications).
- Assess vital signs and check lab studies specific to the medication to determine whether the medication can be safely administered.
  Medications are metabolized more slowly in a person with decreased liver function.
- Assess for any situations in which administering the medication would not be reasonable, (e.g., oral medication prescribed for a patient who is NPO for surgery or a test or who is vomiting).

➤ When performing the procedure, always identify your patient according to agency policy and be attentive to standard precautions, hand hygiene, patient safety and privacy, body mechanics, and documentation.

Procedure Steps

1. **Check the MAR** for the patient's name and identification number, medication, dose, route, time, and drug allergies. The rights of medication administration are: the right patient, right drug, right dose, right route, right time, and right documentation. Initially check the MAR to determine when medications are due (**1st check**).
   Medication prescriptions may change even during your shift; checking the MAR

helps ensure that you do not miss medication changes.

2. **The prescription should include the patient's name, patient identifier, medication name, dose, route, time, and patient allergies.**
   You must clarify any discrepancies before giving the medication.

3. **Follow agency policies** for medication administration, including the time frame for administration. Most agencies allow medications to be given 30 minutes before or 30 minutes after the time indicated

on the MAR. Do not pre-pour medications.
   The time of administration is more important for some medications. For example, if an anti-infective agent is given early or late, a therapeutic blood level may not be maintained.

4. **Wash your hands.**
   Hand hygiene minimizes transmission of microorganisms.

5. **Access the patient's medication drawer,** unlock the medication cart, or log onto the medication dispensing computer. Follow agency policy for obtaining the medication.

6. **If administering a narcotic or barbiturate, obtain the narcotic cabinet key and sign out the medication,** including the patient's name, drug, dose, and other information per agency policy. Note the drug count when removing a narcotic.

   Federal law governs administration of narcotics and barbiturates. All narcotics and barbiturates must be accounted for and witnessed for every shift.

7. **Select the prescribed medication, and compare medication with the MAR** for the first five rights (patient, drug, dose, route, time); check for drug allergies. An inpatient should be wearing an identification band with the drug allergies identified; allergies should be clearly marked in the chart and on the MAR or in the electronic health record (EHR). Question the patient about allergies before giving a newly ordered medication.

   This kind of check ensures that the correct drug is being given to the correct patient at the correct time in the correct dose by the correct route.

8. **Calculate medication dosage.** Double-check it. If you are unable to measure the dose exactly, contact the pharmacist.

9. **Check the expiration date** (on the label or on the box) of all medications.

   A medication that has expired is no longer guaranteed to be effective.

10. **After preparing the medications, do a second check** to verify the correct medication, dose, route, and time **(2nd check).**

    Verifies the first five rights of medication administration.

11. **Lock the medication cart.** Never leave an unlocked medication cart unattended.

    Guards against pilferage and protects children, adults with dementia, or anyone wanting to open the cart.

12. **Administer the medications.**
    a. Take the medication and MAR or handheld portable device with the electronic health record (EHR) into the patient's room.

    You must be able to do the final check in the patient's room and verify that you are administering the correct medication to the correct patient.

    b. Identify the patient carefully using two forms of identification, according to agency policy: checking the identification bracelet, having the patient state her name, comparing the patient to a posted picture of the patient, and checking the patient's date of birth against the MAR.

    Agencies have different means of identifying patients. The Joint Commission requires two forms of identification. ▼

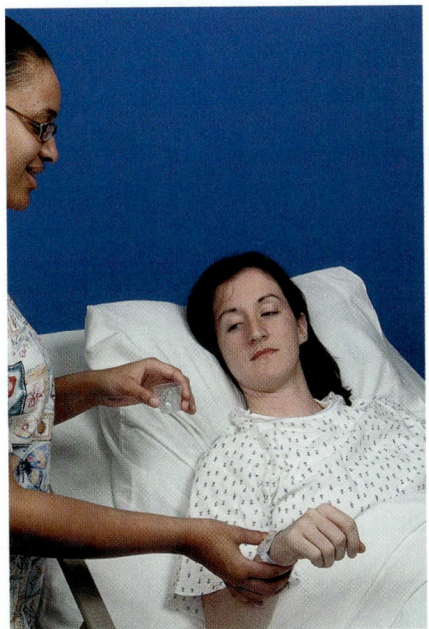

    c. Do a check of the rights of medication for the right patient, right medication, right dose, right route, and right time **(3rd check).**

    Checks for the rights of medication are required for all medications to prevent medication errors.

    d. Perform any assessments needed, such as checking the pulse or blood pressure.

    Some medications can be given only if physical findings or vital signs are within certain parameters. For example, antihypertensive medications may need to be held if the blood pressure is lower than normal.

    e. Explain to the patient that you are there to administer the medication; teach him about the medication.

    Patient teaching increases the patient's understanding of and compliance with treatment. Also, the

    patient may identify potential errors in medication administration.

    f. Administer the medication using appropriate technique (see the procedures for administering medications by the specified route).

    g. Remain with the patient until you are sure that she has taken the medication.

    If you leave a medication at the bedside, someone else (e.g., another patient or a child) might take it, or the patient might discard it.

    h. Document the medication given in the patient's medication record.

    If the documentation is not in the patient's record, there is a risk the dose might be given again in error, presuming a missed dose.

? **What if . . .**

■ **The patient tells you the pill you are ready to give him is a different color than what he normally takes of a certain prescribed medication?**

Determine how and why the tablet is different from what the patient is used to taking. Double-check it to be sure you are giving the correct drug and dosage.

Double-checking whenever you are uncertain about a medication helps prevent medication errors—it is possible you have the wrong drug or dosage.

■ **The label on the medication shows an expiration date that has passed?**

Do not give the medication. Send it back to the pharmacy for reconstitution or replacement.

Expired medication can lose its potency.

■ **The patient refuses to take the prescribed medication?**

Hold the dose and notify the prescriber.

The patient has a right to refuse therapy.

■ **You cannot decipher the prescriber's handwritten medication order?**

Hold the dose and notify the prescriber for clarification. Never administer medication if you are not completely sure what is intended.

(continued on next page)

Medication Guidelines: ■ Steps to Follow for All Medications (Regardless of Type or Route) (continued)

Handwriting that is hard to read is a common cause of preventable error. Electronic prescribing can help to avoid this.

- **Your patient's medication is not available from the pharmacy at the time the dose is due?**

  Do not "borrow" the medication from another patient's supply. Administer

only medication prescribed for that particular patient. Notify the pharmacy of the need to immediately dispense the medication.

Using another patient's medication increases the risk for error because drug dilution or dosage might vary among patients. Or the drug names might be similar

sounding, but in fact they are different medications altogether. Also, other patients' medication may then be missing when their dose is needed. Incidentally, the charges for medication might get mixed up.

Evaluation

- Evaluate the therapeutic effects of the medication. For example, check blood pressure after administering an antihypertensive medication, or check pain level after an analgesic.
- Be alert for any adverse reactions, side effects, or allergic reactions. If present, notify the appropriate care provider.

Patient Teaching

- Describe how the drug is prescribed and when the patient should take the medication.
- Discuss the importance of taking the medication as prescribed.
- Explain the need for any laboratory tests for monitoring the medication, such as tests to measure drug level in the blood, if appropriate.
- Explain the purpose, common side effects, and drug interactions of the medications the patient is taking.
- Teach the patient to observe for side effects that signal the need to contact the prescriber.
- Discuss ways to minimize the side effects of a medication, such as avoiding the sun when taking a medication that causes photosensitivity or rising slowly when taking a medication that causes orthostatic hypotension.
- Discuss potential cultural issues related to taking the medication. An example is the concept of hot and cold conditions and treatments in the Hispanic/Latino culture. If the medication is interpreted as "hot" when the appropriate treatment is "cold," the patient may not take the medication.
- Teach the patient to self-administer medications (e.g., ear drops), as appropriate.

Home Care

- Assess the client's ability to self-administer medications safely.
- Determine the client's financial ability to obtain medications.
- Instruct the client about safe storage of medications.
- Provide instructions for use of each medication.
- Determine whether the client or caregiver has had past problems or present concerns about taking the medications as prescribed.

- If problems have occurred in the past or there are present concerns, discuss possible remedies. For example, you might teach the client or caregiver to use a medication storage container with compartments for the times and days of the week, or setting up a system and a schedule that will work for the patient.

Documentation

- Chart the medication, time, dose, and route given, preadministration assessments, and your signature.
- Do not document before giving the drug; do not document for anyone else; do not ask another nurse to document a drug you have given. Document only *after* administering the medication.
- Chart all therapeutic and adverse effects of the medication. Chart your nursing interventions and teaching potential adverse effects.
- Record the scheduled medications on the MAR. Record prn medications in the nursing notes and in the MAR, including the reason the medication was given and the patient's response to the medication.
- If the patient is unable or refuses to take the medication, document on the MAR that the medication was not administered and the reason, and inform the physician.
- For parenteral medications, chart the site of injection.

Practice Resources

Joanna Briggs Institute, 2005; The Joint Commission, 2006, 2007, 2008; U.S. Food and Drug Administration, Center for Drug Evaluation and Research, 2009.

Thinking About the Procedure

 Go to the *Fundamentals of Nursing Skills Videos,* **Medication Guidelines.**

1. Why should the nurse lock the medication-dispensing unit after the medication dose is administered?
2. What forms of identification did the nurse check to be sure she is giving the drug to the right patient?

 For suggested responses, go to Chapter 25, **Thinking About the Procedure Suggested Responses (Medication Guidelines),** on Davis*Plus.*

Procedure 25-1 ■ Administering Oral Medication

> ➤ For steps to follow in *all* procedures, refer to the Universal Steps for All Procedures found on the page facing the inside back cover.
> Also refer to Medication Guidelines: Steps to Follow for All Medications (Regardless of Type or Route).

Equipment

- Desired liquid for swallowing medications
- Disposable medication cup
- Drinking straw, if needed
- Procedure gloves, if you will need to place a tablet in the patient's mouth
- For enteral medication:
  - Water (for diluting and flushing the feeding tube)
  - 60-mL catheter-tip syringe
  - Clean gloves
- Stethoscope (e.g., *to check the apical pulse before administering some cardiac medications*)

Delegation

As a rule, you can delegate this skill to an LPN/LVN, depending on the medication, but not to a NAP, except under special policies and situations.

Pre-Procedure Assessments

- Assess the patient's condition to determine whether there are contraindications to oral medications or to the specific medication; for example, the patient's ability to swallow. *Impaired swallowing increases the risk for aspiration.*
- Check fluid needs and restrictions. *A prescriber may decide it is medically necessary to administer oral medication to a patient who is NPO. Give additional fluid to a patient with dehydration, and offer only sips for the patient with a fluid restriction.*
- For enteral medications, check that the NG tube is in the stomach and is patent.

> ➤ When performing the procedure, always identify your patient according to agency policy and be attentive to standard precautions, hand hygiene, patient safety and privacy, body mechanics, and documentation.

Procedure Steps

1. **Prepare the medication for administration.**

For Tablet or Capsule

a. If you are pouring from a multi-dose container, do not touch the medication. Pour the tablet into the cap of the bottle, then into the medication cup.

b. If the medication is unit-dose, do not open the package. Place the entire unit-dose package into the cup.

c. Many institutions allow combining all tablets or oral caplets scheduled for the same time for the same patient into the same cup. However, even if the agency protocol permits dispensing from a single container, you will need separate cups for medications that require preadministration assessment (e.g., check the apical pulse rate prior to administering digoxin).
When medications are given at the same time, they can be placed in the same cup. If a medication is held because of a preadministration assess-

ment finding, you can identify it more readily when it has been poured into a separate cup.

d. You may break scored tablets with a knife or a pill cutter if necessary.
Only scored tablets may be broken. Breaking an unscored tablet would deliver an imprecise dose.

e. If a patient has difficulty swallowing, check to see whether the pill can be crushed. If so, use a mortar and pestle to grind it. If the pill is in a unit-dose package, grind the pill while it is still inside the package. Mix the ground pill with a small amount of soft food, such as applesauce or pudding.
Some medications, such as capsules, enteric-coated tablets, and sustained-release formulas, must not be crushed. Crushing such a medication may alter its effectiveness or result in an overdose due to rapid absorption.

For Liquid Medications

f. Check to see whether you must shake the liquid before opening the container.
Some liquids, such as suspensions, will precipitate and need to be

shaken to mix the active ingredient with the suspension liquid.

g. Remove the bottle cap, and place it flat side down on the cart or counter.

h. Hold the bottle with the label in the palm of your hand.
Keeping the label on the upward side of the bottle prevents the liquid from dripping down onto the label and obscuring it. ▼

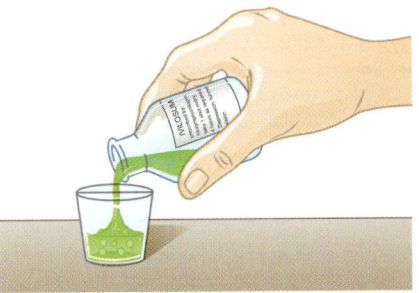

i. Hold or place the plastic medication cup at eye level, and pour the desired amount of medication. Alternatively, place the cup on a level surface, pour the medication, then hold the cup at eye level to read the amount. Read the dose at the lowest part of the concave surface (meniscus).

(continued on next page)

Procedure 25-1 ■ Administering Oral Medication (continued)

Measuring liquids above or below eye level will cause you to read the dose incorrectly and pour too much or too little medication.

j. As you finish pouring medication, slightly twist the bottle to prevent the medication from dripping down the lip of the bottle. If medication does drip down over the lip, wipe the lip with a tissue or paper towel. Wipe only outside the lip of the bottle.

Wiping the outside of the bottle helps prevent contamination, particularly for thicker solution, such as elixir or syrup containing sugar.

2. **Administer the medication.**
   a. Assist the patient to a high-Fowler's position, if possible.
      An upright position prevents choking and facilitates swallowing.
   b. **Powder:** Mix with liquid at the bedside, and give the mixture to the patient to drink.
      Some powders thicken very quickly, so they need to be mixed immediately before administration.
   c. **Lozenge:** Instruct the patient not to chew or swallow it whole.
      Medication is absorbed through the oral mucosa and is generally inactivated by the acidity in the stomach.
   d. **Tablet or capsule:**
      (1) If the patient is able to hold the medication in her hand, place the tablet or medication cup in her hand.

Encourages independence and is easier for the patient.

   (2) Give the patient water or other liquid.
      Liquid moistens the mouth and helps the patient swallow the pill.
   (3) If the patient is unable to hold the tablet, place the medication cup up to her lips, and tip the pill into her mouth.
      Encourage the patient to do as much as possible. Getting the pill to the back of the mouth will assist in swallowing.
   e. **Sublingual medications:** Have the patient place the tablet under the tongue and hold it there until it is completely dissolved.
      Sublingual medications are made to be rapidly absorbed through the oral mucosa. The area under the tongue is very vascular, further speeding absorption. Sublingual medications are inactivated by gastric acid if swallowed. ▼

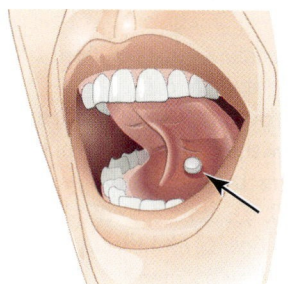

   f. **Buccal medications:** Have the patient place the tablet between the cheek and teeth or tongue.
      Buccal medications act by being absorbed through the oral mucosa or by being dissolved and swallowed in the saliva. ▼

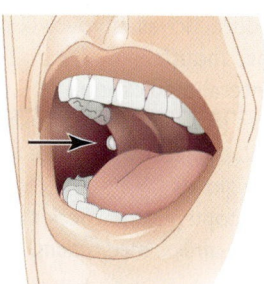

3. **Stay with the patient until all medications have been swallowed or dissolved.**
   Some patients will "chipmunk" the medication in the side of the mouth without swallowing it. Others may spit it out. Staying at the bedside until the patient swallows oral medication ensures that the patient receives the dose.

Procedure 25-1A ■ Administering Medication Through an Enteral Tube

➤ For steps to follow in *all* procedures, refer to the Universal Steps for All Procedures found on the page facing the inside back cover. Also refer to Medication Guidelines: Steps to Follow for All Medications (Regardless of Type or Route).

Preparation

■ If the patient is receiving a continuous tube feeding, disconnect it before giving the medications. Leave the tube clamped for a few minutes after administering the medication, according to agency protocol.

■ If the enteral tube is connected to suction, you will usually discontinue the suction for 20 to 30 minutes after administration, and keep the tube clamped, to allow time for the drug to be absorbed.

➤ When performing the procedure, always identify your patient according to agency policy and be attentive to standad precautions, hand hygiene, patient safety and privacy, body mechanics, and documentation.

➤ *Note:* Follow steps 1a through 1j of Procedure 25-1: Administering Oral Medication. Also, follow precautions for administering enteral medications.

Procedure Steps

1. **Prepare the medication.**
   a. Give the liquid form of medication, if possible. If the solution is hypertonic, be sure to dilute with 10 to 30 mL of sterile water before instilling through a feeding tube.
   Hyperosmolar substances administered too rapidly into the gut can cause bloating, nausea, and osmotic diarrhea.
   b. If pills must be given, verify that the medication can be crushed and given through an enteral tube.
   Some tablets (e.g., sustained-release or enteric-coated tablets) should not be crushed because doing so changes their action.
   c. Crush the tablet and mix it with approximately 20 mL of water or obtain a liquid medication. If you are giving several medications, mix and administer each one separately.
   If you are using a small-bore tube, such as a PEG tube, Keofeed NG feeding tube, or jejunostomy tube, always obtain the liquid form of the medication, because the small-bore tubes clog easily. Ensure that the medication is diluted enough to pass easily through the tube. Instilling drugs one at a time allows you to identify each medication.

2. **Don nonsterile procedure gloves.**
   Gloving maintains standard precautions.

3. **Place patient in a sitting (high-Fowler's) position**, if possible.
   Reduces the risk for aspiration.

4. **For NG tubes, check tube placement** (see Chapter 28, Clinical Insight 28-5) by aspirating stomach contents or measuring the pH of the aspirate, if possible. Other, less accurate, methods are injecting air into the feeding tube and auscultating, or asking the patient to speak.

➕ Never rely on only one bedside method for checking tube placement; use a combination of methods.
NG tubes can become displaced or positioned in the lungs. If medications are given through a misplaced NG tube, the patient may develop aspiration pneumonia.

5. **Check for residual volume** (see Chapter 28, Procedure 28-3).

6. **Flush the tube.** Based on the type of tube, use a piston tip or luer-lock syringe (usually a 30- to 60-mL syringe). Remove the bulb or plunger; attach the barrel to the tube; and pour in 20 to 30 mL of water.
   Flushing ensures patency of the tube and also clears the tube of feeding solution that could clump with medication.

7. **Instill the medication** by depressing the syringe plunger or using the barrel of the syringe as a funnel and pouring in the medication. A smaller tube or thicker medication will require instilling the medication with a 30 to 60 mL syringe, but when larger tubes are used, the medication can be poured. ▼

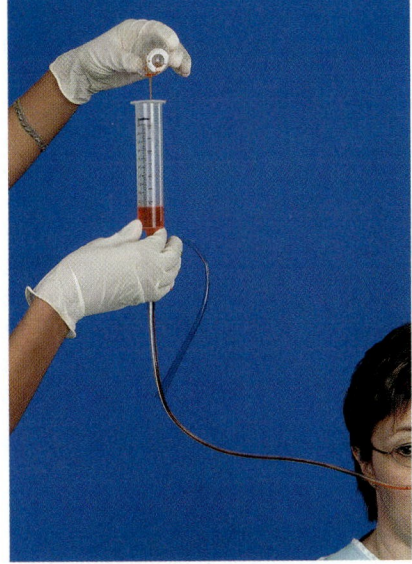

8. **Flush the medication through the tube** by instilling an additional 20 to 30 mL of water.
   Flushing ensures that all the medication has been administered and prevents the tube from clogging.

9. **If there is more than one medication, give each separately, flushing after each.**
   Some medications are less effective when given in combination, or there may be an additive effect if they have similar actions.

10. **Have the patient maintain a sitting position for at least 30 minutes** after you administer the medication.
    Minimizes the risk of aspiration.

? What if . . .

- **My patient is an older adult who is to receive medication through an enteral tube?**

  Check level of consciousness, mentation, or alertness. Check for potential aspiration risk by checking the patient's swallow and gag reflexes.

- **My patient is a child who is to receive medication through an enteral tube?**

  Because of the small size of the feeding tube, only use medications that come in a liquid preparation to prevent occlusion of the tube. Position an infant in a prone or side-lying position, sitting, or reverse Trendelenburg for 30 minutes to 1 hour following medication administration.
  This position facilitates peristalsis and transport of medication through the intestine.

- **The prescribed medication should be given on an empty stomach?**

  Interrupt the feeding 30 minutes before giving the drug. Resume 30 minutes later.
  Waiting to give the medication allows time for the stomach to empty and for drug absorption to occur before the feedings resume.

(continued on next page)

Procedure 25–1 ■ **Administering Oral Medication** (continued)

Evaluation

- For medications administered orally:
  - Note whether the patient has difficulty swallowing, gags, or coughs while swallowing oral medication.
  - Evaluate for gastric discomfort.
  - Assess for any signs of drug allergy or intolerance to the medication.
- For medications administered through a feeding tube, in addition to the preceding assessments, assess that the NG tube is correctly placed and patent before and after administering the medication.

Patient Teaching

- Discuss drug safety measures with the patient, including use of child-safety caps (or using an easy-open cap for an elderly population or with those likely to have difficulty opening containers of this type); keeping the medication in its original container; discarding expired medications; avoiding transferring medication to another container; and carefully reading the label and directions for each medication.
- Discuss the relationship between food and the medication, if needed. For example, is the medication to be taken with food or not? Does taking medication on an empty stomach contribute to nausea or gastric irritation? Does the medication interact with any foods? If you need more information about how drugs interact with food,

 Go to Chapter 25, **Tables, Boxes, Figures: ESG Table 25-6, Drug-Drug and Food-Drug Interactions,** on Davis*Plus.*

For enteral medications:

Cover the preceding topics (for patient teaching about oral medications) plus the following:
- Discuss the importance of upright positioning for 20 to 30 minutes after taking medication through an enteral tube.
- Instruct the patient to immediately notify his healthcare provider if he chokes or has difficulty breathing during or shortly after medication is given by enteral tube. The medication should be stopped immediately and emergency care might be necessary.

Home Care

Advise clients who are receiving enteral medication at home to do the following:
- Notify the healthcare provider: (1) if any of the following lasts for more than a day: diarrhea, constipation, nausea, dark urine, bad-smelling urine, or dry mouth; (2) if the tube becomes clogged or seems to be moving farther out or in; or (3) if the feeding tube falls out or you cannot confirm that the end of the tube is in the stomach.
  To prevent a clogged feeding tube, flush the tube with water each time after giving a medication or feeding.
- If an NG tube remains in place continuously, brush your teeth at least twice daily.
- Clean daily the area where the NG tube goes into the nostrils. Use a cotton-tip applicator moistened with warm water. If your nose becomes sore, you might apply water-soluble lubricant.
- Change the nasal tape every other day or when it is loose.

Documentation

- Often, scheduled medications are recorded only on the MAR.
- Document the drug, dosage, time, route, and your name as the healthcare provider administering the medication.
- Document any suspected drug reaction, intolerance, or patient response to the medication.
- Document on the intake and output record the amount of liquid medication and the water used for swallowing medication. Some patients may be fluid restricted, so all intake should be recorded. Be sure to know what is appropriate in your clinical facility.
  #### *For enteral medications:*
- Document patency, residual volume, and placement of tube.
- Document any difficulty with administering the medications.
- Document on the intake and output record the amount of liquid medication and the water used for flushing. Some physicians order a specific amount of water to flush with each medication administration or feeding. Some healthcare facilities use a protocol amount of water to flush gastrostomy tubes. Be sure to know what is appropriate in your clinical facility.

? What if . . .

- **My patient vomits shortly after taking oral medication?**

  Notify the prescriber for instructions regarding giving the dose again or not.

- **My patient is unable to sit upright to take oral medication?**

  Assist the patient into a side-lying position and offer a straw to take water with pills or tablets.

- **My patient has difficulty drinking from a cup?**

Use a syringe without a needle to place the medication in his mouth. Place the patient in a side-lying or upright position. Place the syringe between the gum and cheek in the back corner of the mouth, and slowly push the plunger to administer the liquid.

- **My patient is NPO or on fluid restriction?**

If the patient is NPO (nothing by mouth), check with the prescriber to determine whether the medication should be given by another route or can be given with small sips of water. If not

NPO, but there is a fluid restriction, consider how much fluid you can give with medication. Use the smallest amount of water needed to swallow or dissolve tablets and to flush enteral tubes.

- **My patient is cognitively impaired?**

  Request the patient open his mouth to see whether he has swallowed the medication; look under the tongue or side pocket near the inside of the cheek.

Practice Resources

Phillips & Nay, 2007, 2008.

Thinking About the Procedure

 Go to the *Fundamentals of Nursing Skills Videos,* **Medication Administration: Oral and Sublingual Medications.**

For suggested responses, go to Chapter 25, **Thinking About the Procedure Suggested Responses,** on Davis*Plus.*

1. How does the nurse dispense the tablet from a multidose container and administer to the patient without having to touch it?

Procedure 25-2 ▪ Administering Ophthalmic Medication

➤ For steps to follow in *all* procedures, refer to the Universal Steps for All Procedures found on the page facing the inside back cover. Also refer to the Medication Guidelines: Steps to Follow for All Medications (Regardless of Type or Route).

Equipment

- Eye drops or ointment
- Tissue

For irrigation, add:

- Prescribed eye irrigation solution (e.g., 500 to 1,000 mL of normal saline or lactated Ringer's solution are commonly used)
- IV tubing or eye irrigation insert, such as the Morgan lens (Follow manufacturer's directions for this specialized equipment.)
- Ocular anesthetic, according to protocol or physician orders
- pH paper
- Basin and towel

Delegation

An RN can usually delegate eye instillations to an LPN/LVN. You usually cannot delegate this task to a NAP unless the NAP has special training for a specific, defined situation (e.g., "medication aides" in some long-term-care settings).

Pre-Procedure Assessment

- Assess the patient's eyes for redness, discharge, or other signs of irritation.
- Determine whether the eyes need to be cleansed before administration of the medication.
  Excess tearing, debris, or excess mucus in the eye could interfere with the effectiveness of the medication.

✚ Check the prescription for where to instill medication. (*Note:* We do not advise using these abbreviations—they have been disallowed by The Joint Commission—but you may still see them written in prescriptions.)
OD = right eye
OS = left eye
OU = both eyes

For irrigations, also assess the following:

- Determine the cause of the eye problem—acid, alkaline, or other chemical burn or body fluid splash; or nonembedded foreign body.
  Irrigations are generally used to remove chemical or physical irritants, but they may be done following surgery or to treat a severe infection. Normal saline (NS) or lactated Ringer's is the solution generally recommended for high-volume eye irrigations because the pH of 6 to 7.5 is closest to the normal tear pH of 7.1. Volumes of 500 to 1,000 mL are generally used.
- Assess the patient's eyes for swelling, redness, drainage, or complaints of pain.
  A baseline assessment is useful for determining the need for and effectiveness of irrigation. Sclera should be smooth, white, and glistening.
- Determine the patient's level of discomfort and ability to cooperate with the procedure.
  Combative or otherwise uncooperative patients refusing instillation of medication can interfere with the safety and efficiency of the procedure. If the patient cannot hold still for the procedure, he may need to be sedated.
- Assess the pain level.
  Debris, chemicals, and some liquids in the eye can be extremely painful. The eye may need to be anesthetized before irrigation or a general systemic pain medication given.

➤ When performing the procedure, always identify your patient according to agency policy and be attentive to standard precautions, hand hygiene, patient safety and privacy, body mechanics, and documentation.

Procedure Steps

1. **Assist the patient to a high-Fowler's position, with head slightly tilted back,** if possible.
   An upright position keeps eye drops in the eye and helps prevent eye drops from draining into lacrimal duct. Do not tilt the head back if the patient has a neck injury or other contraindication.

2. **Don procedure gloves.**
   Complies with standard precautions.

3. **Cleanse the edges of eyelid** from the inner to outer canthus, if needed.
   By following the principle of "clean to dirty," you avoid transferring debris into the nasolacrimal duct.

(continued on next page)

Procedure 25-2 ■ Administering Ophthalmic Medication (continued)

Procedure Variation: Instilling Eye Drops

(Follow steps 1–3.)

4. **Gently rest your dominant hand, with the eyedropper, on the patient's forehead.**

   Stabilizes the hand in the event the patient moves—prevents accidental injury to the eye.

5. With your nondominant hand, **pull the lower lid down to expose the conjunctival sac.**

   Allows visualization of the area where you will administer the medication.

6. **Position the eyedropper about 1.5 to 2.0 cm (½ to ¾ in.) above the patient's eye.** Ask the patient to look up, then drop the prescribed number of drops into the conjunctival sac. Do not let the dropper touch the eye.

   Keeping the dropper away from the globe of the eye reduces the risk of accidental injury to the eye and avoids contamination of the dropper. Having the patient look up helps to decrease the blink reflex. Instilling the eye drops directly onto the cornea could injure the cornea, so drops are instilled into the conjunctival sac. ▼

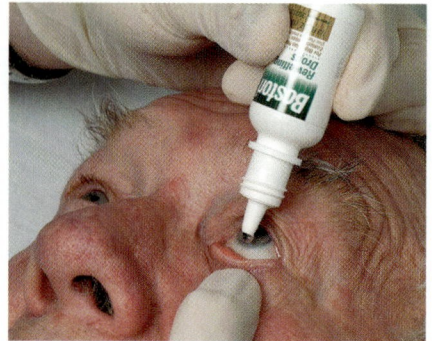

7. Ask the patient to **gently close and move his eyes.**

   Helps to distribute the medication.

8. If the medication has systemic effects, **press gently against the same side of the nose for 1 to 2 minutes to close the lacrimal ducts.**

   Reduces systemic absorption through the lacrimal duct. ▼

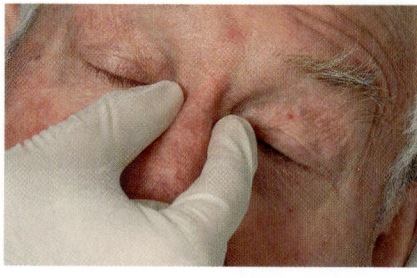

Procedure Variation: Administering Eye Ointment

(Follow steps 1–3).

9. **Gently rest your dominant hand, with the eye ointment, on the patient's forehead.**

   Stabilizing your hand helps to prevent accidental injury to the eye.

10. With your nondominant hand, **pull the lower lid down** to expose the conjunctival sac.

    Allows visualization of area where you will administer the medication.

11. **Ask the patient to look up as you apply a thin strip of ointment**—usually about 2 to 2.5 cm (1 in.)—in the conjunctival sac; twist your wrist to break off the strip of ointment. Do not let the tube touch the eye.

    If the medication ribbon is not broken off, lifting the tube will pull the medication out of the conjunctival sac. ➤

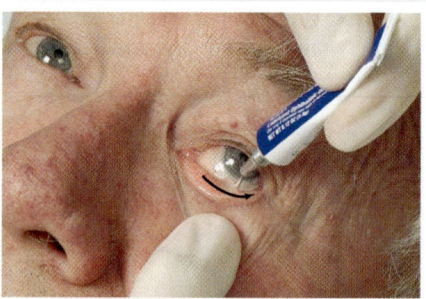

a. Ask the patient to gently close his eyes for 2 to 3 minutes.

   Helps to distribute the medication.

b. Explain to patient that his vision will be blurred for a short amount of time after administration of ointment.

   The viscosity of the ointment can cause blurring.

? What if . . .

■ **My patient is a child who won't open his eye for the application?**

Try distracting the child by turning on the television or offering an age-appropriate toy in view.

Distraction and bribery are effective techniques for coaxing a child when cooperation is essential.

Ask a family member to help you gain cooperation of the child.

It might be fear or mistrust that is causing him to be unwilling to open his eyes.

■ **My patient wears soft contact lenses?**

Have the patient remove contact lenses before administering the medication and wait at least 15 minutes after instilling eye drops before reinserting the lenses.

Procedure 25-2A ■ Irrigating the Eyes

➤ When performing the procedure, always identify your patient according to agency policy and be attentive to standard precautions, hand hygiene, patient safety and privacy, body mechanics, and documentation.

Procedure Steps

1. **Assist the patient to a low-Fowler's position,** with the head tilted toward the affected eye, if possible.

   This position helps to drain the irrigating solution from the eye and

   prevents contamination of the unaffected eye.

2. **Place the towel and basin under the patient's cheek** to absorb the drainage.

   The patient will be more comfortable when he is clean and dry.

3. **Check the pH** by gently touching the pH paper to secretions in the conjunctival sac.

   A litmus test determines the correct irrigating solution and whether the irritant is alkaline or acidic. The normal pH of tears is approximately 7.1.

4. Follow the agency protocol or prescriber's order regarding use of ocular anesthetic drops.

The ocular anesthetic will be washed out by the irrigation fluid, so it needs to be reinstilled every 2 to 3 minutes, or it can be added to the irrigation solution.

5. Connect the solution and tubing, and prime the tubing.

Priming the tubing prevents blowing air across the cornea, which would be uncomfortable.

6. Irrigate the eye.

a. Hold the tubing about 2.5 cm (1 in.) from eye.

A safe distance helps prevent accidental trauma to the eye.

b. Separate the eyelids with your thumb and index finger.

It is easier to irrigate the cornea when the eyelids are separated.

c. Direct the flow of solution over the eye from the inner canthus to the outer canthus.

The inner canthus is considered clean, primarily because of the open duct in this area. Flowing irrigation solution in this manner follows the principle of "clean to dirty." ▼

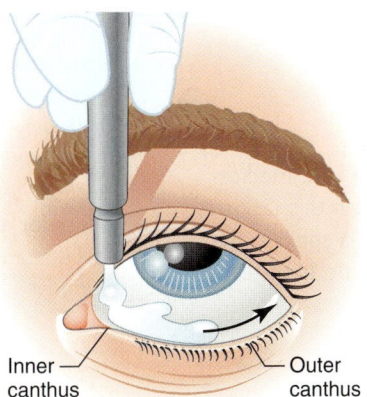

Inner canthus · Outer canthus

7. Recheck pH, and continue to irrigate the eye as needed.

With alkaline or acidic chemical injuries, the pH of the eye needs to be returned to normal as soon as possible to prevent further eye injury.

Evaluation

- Examine the eyes for redness or drainage.
- Observe the patient's ability to follow instructions during the procedure.
- Observe the pain level during the procedure.
- After an irrigation, check for decrease in eye pain.

Patient Teaching

- Discuss how to prevent contaminating eye drops or ointment.
- Teach the best technique for instilling eye drops or ointment.
- If patient needs assistance with instilling drops, discuss use of an eye drop guide.
- Discuss the signs and symptoms with the patient that need to be reported to the physician, including eye pain and increased redness or drainage.

For irrigations:

- Discuss the cause and prevention of eye injuries, including the use of protective goggles.
- Discuss the need for follow-up treatment. If the patient will be instilling eye medications or applying eye patches, ensure that she is able to use the correct technique.

Home Care

If a splash occurs to the eyes in the home, teach the client to immediately flood his eyes with cool water (as follows):

- Hold your eyelids open and put your head under a faucet or pour water from a clean container.
- Roll your eyes as much as possible while running water across your eyes.
- Flood your eyes for at least 20 minutes.
- Get medical help immediately after rinsing your eyes.

Documentation

- *For instillations:* Chart assessment data before, during, and after instillation. Record on the MAR, as for all medications.
- *For irrigations:* Chart the condition of the patient's eyes before the irrigation, including the patient's complaints of pain or burning. Document the eye pH, instillation of anesthetic drops, the type and amount of irrigation fluid used, the eye pH following irrigation, and the patient's response. You also need to record other treatment, such as instillation of lubricating and/or antibiotic ointment and application of eye patches.

Practice Resources

Heller, 2011, updated; Stevens, 2005.

Thinking About the Procedure

 Go to the *Fundamentals of Nursing Skills Videos,* **Medication Administration: Ophthalmic Drops and Ointments.**

1. What does the nurse on the DVD do immediately after instillation of the ophthalmic drops? Why?
2. Which hand does the nurse in the DVD use to hold open the eye and expose the conjunctival sac? Why?

 For suggested responses, go to Chapter 25, **Thinking About the Procedure Suggested Responses,** on Davis*Plus.*

Procedure 25-3 ■ Administering Otic Medication

> ➤ For steps to follow in *all* procedures, refer to the Universal Steps for All Procedures found on the page facing the inside back cover. Also refer to the Medication Guidelines: Steps to Follow for All Medications (Regardless of Type or Route).

Equipment

- Ear drops
- Dropper with flexible rubber tip
- Cotton-tipped applicators
- Cotton ball

Delegation

An RN can usually delegate administration of otic medications to an LPN/LVN. You usually cannot delegate this task to a NAP unless the NAP has special training for a specific, defined situation (e.g., "medication aides" in some long-term care settings in some states).

Pre-Procedure Assessments

- Assess the external ear and canal for erythema, drainage, and cerumen.
  You may need to clean the external ear to remove obstructions so that the medication can be distributed throughout the ear canal. Use the otoscope to evaluate the tympanic membrane if the drainage is bloody or the patient complains of pain or decreased hearing acuity. If the tympanic membrane is ruptured, use sterile technique.
- Assess for any ear pain or hearing impairment.
  Establishes a baseline that can be used to evaluate the effects of treatment.

> ➤ When performing the procedure, always identify your patient according to agency policy and be attentive to standard precautions, hand hygiene, patient safety and privacy, body mechanics, and documentation.

Procedure Steps

1. **Hold the eardrop bottle in your hand to warm it,** or place it in warm water (not hot). Gently shake the bottle before using the drops.
   Warm solution is more comfortable than cool. Also, placing cool solutions in the ear can cause dizziness. Shaking the bottle disperses the medication throughout the solution.

2. **Assist patient to a side-lying position,** with the appropriate ear facing up.
   Facilitates administering drops and prevents drops escaping from the ear.

3. **Clean the external ear** with a cotton-tipped applicator, if necessary.
   Cleaning the ear allows eardrops to reach all areas of the ear canal. Be careful not to push cerumen further into the ear canal.

4. **Fill the dropper** with the correct amount of medication.

5. **For infants and young children, ask a parent or another caregiver to immobilize the child** while you administer the medication.
   Mobilization and restraint reduce the risk for injury for the child who struggles during the procedure.

6. **Straighten the ear canal.**
   a. For a child younger than 3 years old, pull the pinna down and back. ➤

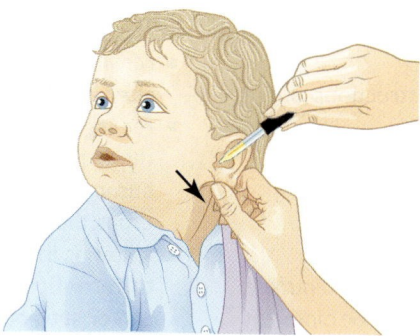

b. For older children and adults, pull the pinna up and back. ▼

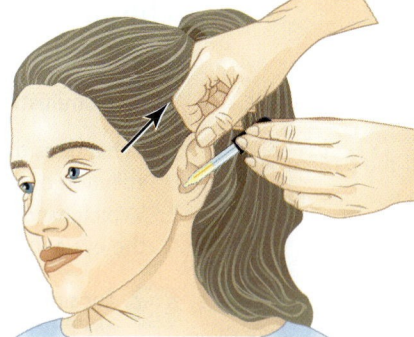

These positions straighten the ear canal for proper channeling of the medication.

7. **Instill the ordered number of drops** along the side of the ear canal, being careful not to touch the end of the dropper to any part of the ear.
   Avoiding contact between the dropper and the ear reduces the risk of contamination of the dropper.

8. **Gently tug on the external ear** after drops are instilled.
   Facilitates flow of medication into the auditory canal.

9. **Instruct the patient to remain on his side** for 5 to 10 minutes.
   Assists in distributing the medication and prevents drops from escaping the ear canal.

10. **Place a cotton ball, or a piece of it, loosely at the opening of the auditory canal** for 15 minutes.
    A cotton ball will absorb excess fluid and keep the medication from flowing out. However, keep in mind that cotton left near an infant can be a choking hazard and must be carefully supervised.

? What if . . .

- **My patient is a child and rolls over so most of the otic medication flows back out of the ear?**

  Estimate the amount of the dosage that was lost. Replace it by repeating the procedure for instillation of the medication, except next time position the child securely until you are confident the medication has had time to penetrate the ear canal.

- **There is too much cerumen (ear wax) in the canal to instill otic drops?**

You can use special drops for softening the cerumen and allow for easier removal. Gentle irrigation with warm saline is effective, unless the person has perforation of the tympanic membrane or myringotomy tubes. You should not use a metal syringe (Pomeroy syringe) for the removal of cerumen because (1) this type of syringe is heavy and difficult to control and (2) it may be associated with a higher risk of perforations of the tympanic membrane because of the pressure exerted. Oral jet irrigators have been associated with some trauma, including tympanic membrane perforation. You should not attempt to remove impaction by "ear candling," which is the application of hot candle wax.

Evaluation

- Assess for discomfort or pain during the procedure and for relief afterward.
- Evaluate for wax buildup, redness, swelling, or drainage.

Documentation

- Assess the amount, color, character, and odor of drainage, if present.
- Note any swelling or redness in the ear canal.
- Document pain or discomfort and hearing loss.

Thinking About the Procedure

Go to the *Fundamentals of Nursing Skills Videos,* **Medication Administration: Otic Medications.**

1. What risk is there to an infant who receives ear drops and has a cotton ball to absorb residual liquid that can flow out of the ear canal?
2. How does the nurse position the ear to instill otic drops?
3. What does the nurse do to aid the drops in draining into the ear canal?

For suggested responses, go to Chapter 25, **Thinking About the Procedure Suggested Responses,** on DavisPlus.

Procedure 25-4 ■ Administering Nasal Medication

➤ For steps to follow in *all* procedures, refer to the Universal Steps for All Procedures found on the page facing the inside back cover. Also refer to the Medication Guidelines: Steps to Follow for All Medications (Regardless of Type or Route).

Equipment

- Medication drops, spray, or aerosol
- Tissues

Delegation

As an RN, you can usually delegate administration of nasal instillations to an LPN/LVN. You usually cannot delegate this task to a NAP.

Pre-Procedure Assessments

- Check for nasal obstruction and congestion.
  Nasal obstruction or congestion could prevent the medication from reaching the nasal mucosa.

Assess nasal discharge for color, consistency, and odor.
  The appearance of drainage is not always diagnostic of infection, especially for people with chronic sinus problems or polyps. Color can be indicative of the body's response to viral, bacterial, and allergic sources.
- Assess nasal mucous membranes for redness, color, moisture, excoriation, or trauma.
  A baseline assessment helps to identify signs of irritation.
  Check the dropper tip to be sure it is not cracked or chipped.
  A cracked or chipped tip might interfere with drawing up the medication and scratch the nasal mucosa.

➤ When performing the procedure, always identify your patient according to agency policy and be attentive to standard precautions, hand hygiene, patient safety and privacy, body mechanics, and documentation.

Procedure Steps

1. **Explain to the patient that the medication may cause some burning,** tingling, or unusual taste.
   The taste of nasal medications can cause patients to become nauseated or vomit. The medication is more likely to cause burning or tingling if the nasal mucosa is inflamed.
2. **Don procedure gloves.**
   Prevents transmission of microorganisms.

3. **Ask the patient to gently blow his nose** and wash his hands afterward.
   Removing nasal discharge allows the medication to come into contact with the mucous membranes without traumatizing already inflamed mucosa.
4. **Position the patient.**
   a. For nasal spray (to medicate frontal sinuses), head down and forward—if the patient can comfortably assume this position, ask

him to lean slightly forward or kneel on the bed with his head down. Administer the medication, and then ask the patient to tilt his head back to medicate the nasal passages. Remember: To spray your nose, look at your toes!
   Radionuclide studies have demonstrated that using nasal drops or sprays with the patient sitting and leaning the head back causes poor

(continued on next page)

Procedure 25-4 ■ Administering Nasal Medication (continued)

distribution of the medications into the nasal complex and sinuses.

b. For drops (to medicate the ethmoid and sphenoid sinuses), assist the patient into a supine position, with his head over the edge of the bed. Support the patient's head. Alternatively, place a towel roll behind the patient's shoulders, and allow the head to drop back. ▼

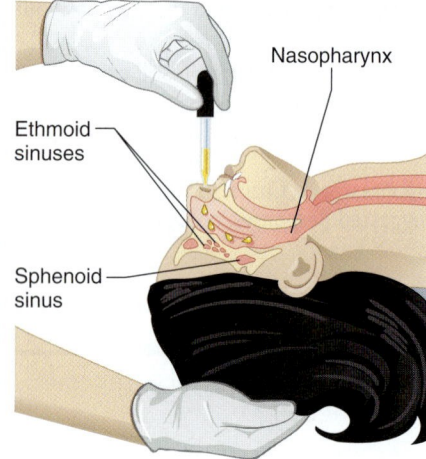

Nasopharynx
Ethmoid sinuses
Sphenoid sinus

These positions help to prevent straining the neck muscles and facilitate distribution of the medication to the ethmoid and sphenoid sinuses.

c. To medicate maxillary sinuses with nasal drops, tilt the head toward the affected side.
Tilting the head promotes gravity to distribute the medication to the frontal sinuses. ➤

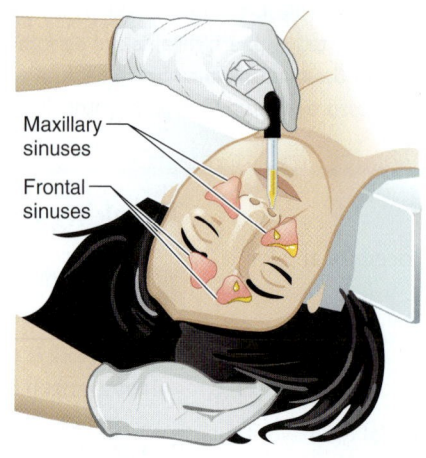

Maxillary sinuses
Frontal sinuses

5. **Ask the patient to exhale and then close one nostril.**
Blocking one nostril provides for deeper inhalation.

6. **Then ask recipient to breathe in deeply through the nose** and while he is breathing in, press down firmly and quickly once on the applicator's shoulder. Ask recipient to breathe out through the mouth. After spray, lean head backward for a few seconds.
Inhaling through the mouth prevents aspiration of the drops into the trachea and bronchi. Touching the dropper to the nostril will contaminate the dropper.

7. **Repeat for the other nostril.**

8. **If nose drops are used, ask the patient to stay in the same position** for 1 to 5 minutes (depending on the manufacturer's guidelines).
Maintaining this position promotes better absorption by using gravity to dis-

perse *the medication throughout the nasal passages and sinuses instead of draining out the nose.*

9. **Instruct the patient to not blow his nose for several minutes.**
If the patient blows his nose, he would expel the medication.

? What if . . .

■ **My patient cannot assume the "head down and forward" position?**

Help him to hold his head upright to administer the drops or spray.

■ **My patient can taste the medicine after it is administered?**

That means his head was not down enough or he did not inhale long enough. Instruct him to put his head back down and sniff again without instilling more medicine.

■ **My patient has an excoriated area on the inside septum?**

Assess further, examining other areas of the nasal mucosa. Determine if the patient has a history of substance abuse. Report the findings to the prescriber before administering nasal medication.

■ **My patient begins to have nosebleeds after using nasal medication?**

First, control the nosebleed. Then hold the medication and notify the prescriber. Assess for other signs of bleeding, bruising, or petechiae.

Evaluation

■ Assess for a reduction of symptoms 15 to 20 minutes after administration.

Patient Teaching

■ Teach the procedure for administering nasal drops or sprays, including proper positioning.
■ Discuss the correct use of the medication and the adverse effects of overusing nasal decongestants.
■ Explain the implications of the color of nasal secretions.

Documentation

■ Chart according to Medication Guidelines: Steps to Follow for All Medication (Regardless of Type or Route). For example, record the administration of the medication on the MAR.
  For nasal instillation, document:
■ Pre-medication assessment
■ Type and amount of solution administered

■ Discomfort the patient experienced during the procedure
■ Patient's report of response to nasal administrations, such as nasal discharge, obstruction of nasal passage, bleeding, or other complication following the procedure

Thinking About the Procedure

 Go to the *Fundamentals of Nursing Skills Videos,* **Medication Administration: Nasal Spray and Drops.**

1. What does the nurse use a small towel for?
2. What position is the patient in when closing a nostril and inhaling deeply?

 For suggested responses, go to Chapter 25, **Thinking About the Procedure Suggested Responses,** on DavisPlus.

Practice Resources

American Academy of Family Physicians, 2004, updated February 2011.

Procedure 25-5 ■ Administering Vaginal Medication

➤ For steps to follow in *all* procedures, refer to the Universal Steps for All Procedures found on the page facing the inside back cover. Also refer to the Medication Guidelines: Steps to Follow for All Medications (Regardless of Type or Route).

Equipment

- Medication: foam, jelly, cream, suppository, douche, or irrigating solution
- Applicator (if indicated)
- Washcloth and warm water for perineal care as needed
- Water-soluble lubricant
- Toilet tissue
- Perineal pad
- Bath blanket
- **For irrigation**: you will also need a waterproof pad, bedpan, vaginal irrigation set (may be disposable; consists of a solution container, nozzle, tubing, and clamp) and IV pole

Delegation

An RN can usually delegate the administration of vaginal medications to an LPN/LVN. You usually cannot delegate this task to a NAP. Nurse practice acts governing medication administration vary from state to state, and policies vary further among healthcare agencies. However, as the RN you are always responsible for evaluating patient responses, both therapeutic effects and side effects. You can instruct a NAP in the therapeutic effect and side effects of medications and to report any effects observed.

Pre-Procedure Assessments

- Assess for vaginal burning, pruritus, and pain.
  A baseline assessment helps to determine the patient's level of comfort and later the effectiveness of treatment. Infections can cause vaginal burning, itching, and pain.
- Inspect the labia and vaginal orifice for redness and lesions.
  This is a good time to assess the perineal area for sign of sexually transmitted infection or other issues requiring healthcare.
- Check for vaginal discharge, including color, amount, consistency, and odor.

➤ When performing the procedure, always identify your patient according to agency policy and be attentive to standard precautions, hand hygiene, patient safety and privacy, body mechanics, and documentation.

Procedure Steps

1. **Ask the patient to void** before you insert the vaginal medication.
   The increased pressure associated with a full bladder could cause discomfort during the instillation of vaginal medications.

2. **Position the patient in a dorsal recumbent or Sims' position**; drape the patient with a bath blanket so that only the perineum is exposed.
   a. *Dorsal recumbent position*—supine with knees flexed and legs rotated outward.
   b. *Sims' position*—semiprone on the left side with the right hip and knee flexed.
   These two positions allow for visualization during administration and promote retention of the medication following administration. Draping respects the patient's modesty.

3. **Prepare the medication.** Remove the wrapper from the suppository and place the suppository on the wrapper or in a medication cup; or fill the applicator according to the manufacturer's instructions. For irrigation, use a warm solution of approximately 105°F (40.5°C).
   Some suppositories come with applicators. Using a warm irrigation solution promotes patient comfort and prevents injury to the vaginal tissue. ▼

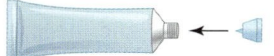

Invert cap and pierce end of medication tube

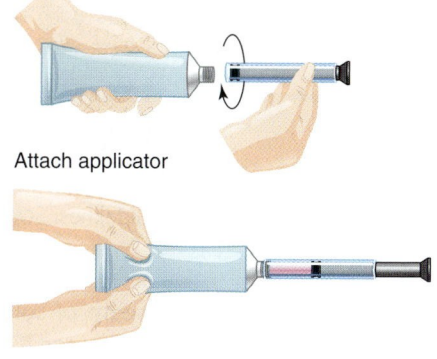

Attach applicator

Squeeze medication into applicator

4. **Don procedure gloves.**
   Prevents contaminating your hands and spreading microorganisms.

5. **Inspect and clean around vaginal orifice.**
   Prevents introduction of microorganisms into the vagina during medication administration.

6. **Administer the medication.**

Suppository
   a. Apply water-soluble lubricant to the rounded end of the suppository and to your gloved index finger on your dominant hand.
      Eases insertion and prevents injury to the vaginal tissue.
   b. Separate the labia with your non-dominant hand.
      Allows visualization of the vaginal orifice.
   c. Insert the suppository as far as possible along the posterior vaginal wall (about 8 cm, or 3 in.) or as far as it will go. If the suppository comes with an applicator, place the suppository in the end of the applicator, insert the applicator into the vagina, and press the plunger.
      The posterior vaginal wall is about 2.5 cm (1 in.) longer than the anterior wall. ▼

(continued on next page)

Procedure 25-5 ■ Administering Vaginal Medication (continued)

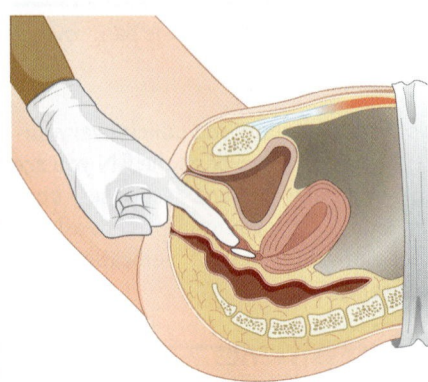

d. Ask the patient to remain in a supine position for 5 to 15 minutes. You may wish to elevate her hips on a pillow.
   Lifting the hips promotes retention and absorption of the medication.

Applicator Insertion of Cream, Foam, or Jelly

e. Separate the labia with your non-dominant hand.

f. Insert the applicator approximately 8 cm (3 in.) into the vagina along the posterior vaginal wall.

g. Depress the plunger on the applicator, emptying the medication into the vagina.

h. Dispose of the applicator, or place it on a paper towel if the applicator is reusable. You will later wash it with soap and water.

i. Instruct the patient to remain in a supine position for 5 to 15 minutes.
   A flat position promotes retention and absorption of the medication.

Irrigation

j. Hang the irrigation solution approximately 30 to 60 cm (1 to 2 ft) above the level of the patient's vagina.
   Makes use of gravity to create enough pressure for continuous irrigation without increasing the pressure so much that it causes the patient discomfort and possibly damages the vaginal tissue. ▼

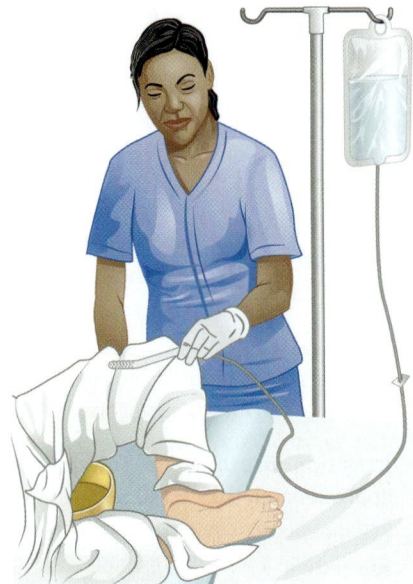

k. Assist the patient into a dorsal recumbent position, and position a waterproof pad and bedpan under her.
   This position is the easiest for performing a vaginal irrigation. Positioning the patient on the bedpan and using a waterproof pad protects the bedding.

l. If using a vaginal irrigation set with tubing, open the clamp to allow the solution to completely fill the tubing.
   Flushing the tubing prevents introducing air into the vagina, which can cause discomfort.

m. Lubricate the end of the irrigation nozzle.
   Lubrication reduces discomfort and irritation to the vaginal mucosa.

n. Insert the nozzle approximately 8 cm (3 in.) into the vagina, directing it toward the sacrum.

o. Start the flow of the irrigation solution, and rotate the nozzle intermittently as solution flows.
   The rotation ensures even distribution of the solution throughout the vagina.

p. After all irrigating solution has been used, remove the nozzle.

q. Assist the patient to a sitting position on the bedpan.
   Promotes removal of all the irrigating solution by gravity.

7. **Cleanse the perineum** with toilet tissue or with warm water and a washcloth. Dry the perineum.
   Drainage could cause skin irritation.

8. Apply a perineal pad if there is excessive drainage.

? What if . . .

■ **The labia are reddened?**

Pour warm water over the labia with an irrigation bottle to soothe irritation and cleanse the area.

Evaluation

■ Assess for complaints of vaginal burning, pruritis, or pain.
■ Assess for purulent vaginal discharge.

Patient Teaching

Discuss with the patient personal hygiene and pericare.

Documentation

■ For vaginal medications, chart according to Medication Guidelines: Steps to Follow for All Medication (Regardless of Type or Route).
■ For vaginal irrigations, chart assessment; the type and amount of solution administered; discomfort the patient experienced during the procedure; and the patient's report of decreased vaginal pain, itching, and/or burning following the procedure.

Procedure 25-6 ■ Inserting a Rectal Suppository

➤ For steps to follow in *all* procedures, refer to the Universal Steps for All Procedures found on the page facing the inside back cover. Also refer to the Medication Guidelines: Steps to Follow for All Medications (Regardless of Type or Route).

Equipment

- Suppository
- Water-soluble lubricant
- Toilet tissue

Delegation

As an RN, you can usually delegate administration of rectal medications to an LPN/LVN. Although in some institutions you can delegate the administration of a glycerine suppository (nonmedicated) to a NAP, you generally cannot delegate administration of rectal medications to a NAP.

Pre-Procedure Assessments

- Determine the presence of contraindications for rectal administration, such as recent rectal surgery, rectal bleeding, or cardiac disease.
- Assess the rectal area for hemorrhoids or irritation.

➤ When performing the procedure, always identify your patient according to agency policy and be attentive to standard precautions, hand hygiene, patient safety and privacy, body mechanics, and documentation.

Procedure Steps

1. **Ask whether the patient needs to defecate** before the suppository insertion.
   Stool in the rectum interferes with insertion of medication against the rectal wall and therefore with retention of the medication.

2. **Don procedure gloves.**
   Gloving prevents exposure to feces and spread of microorganisms; maintains standard precautions.

3. **Assist patient to Sims' position—** lying on the left side with the right hip and knee flexed. Drape the patient, keeping her covered as much as possible.
   Sims' position allows visualization of the anus and promotes retention of the medication because the descending colon is on the left side. It also helps relax the external anal sphincter. Keeping the patient covered prevents chilling and maintains privacy.

4. **For an uncooperative patient, such as a confused patient or a young child**, ask someone to help immobilize the patient while you insert the suppository.
   Helps ensure proper instillation of medication and prevention of injury to the rectal mucosa.

5. **Prepare the suppository:** Remove the wrapper. Using a water-soluble lubricant, lubricate the smooth end of the suppository and the tip of glove on the index finger. If no lubricant is available, apply cool tap water to the anus.

   Lubrication eases insertion and prevents friction damage to the rectal mucosa during insertion.

6. **Explain that there will be a cool feeling from the lubricant** and a feeling of pressure during insertion.
   The patient should not experience severe pain with the insertion of a suppository, but will feel the coolness of the lubricant and pressure as the suppository is inserted past the rectal sphincter.

7. **Using your nondominant hand, separate the buttocks.**
   Separation of the buttocks allows you to visualize the anus.

8. **Ask the adult patient take deep breaths** in and out through the mouth.
   Helps relax the rectal sphincter. Pushing a suppository through a constricted sphincter produces pain.

9. **Insert the suppository:**
   a. Using the index finger of your dominant hand, gently insert the lubricated smooth end first, or follow the manufacturer's instructions.
   Lubrication eases insertion. ▼

   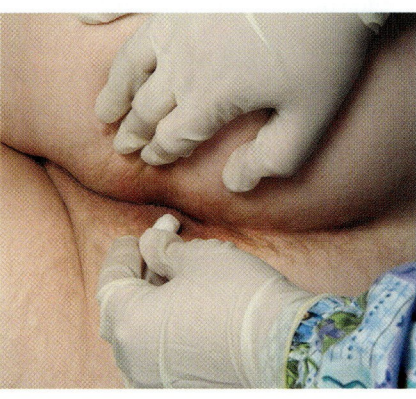

   b. ✚ **Never force the suppository during insertion.**
   Forcing the insertion of the suppository into a fecal mass would affect absorption. Forcing anything into the rectum may cause rectal irritation.

   c. Push the suppository past the internal sphincter and along the rectal wall (½ to 1 in. in infants and 1 to 3 in. in adults).
   The suppository must be in contact with the rectal wall for the medication to be absorbed. Inserting the suppository past the internal sphincter promotes retention. Especially for a child, inserting the suppository too far could damage the rectal mucosa. ▼

   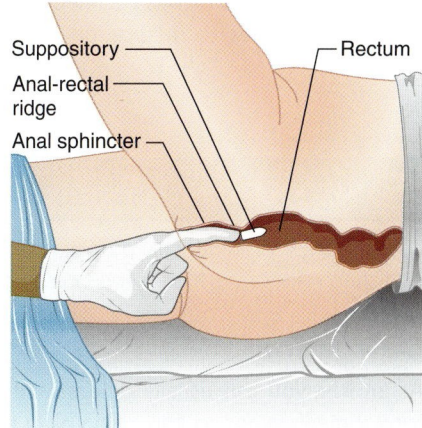

   Suppository — Rectum
   Anal-rectal ridge
   Anal sphincter

10. **Ask the patient to try to retain the suppository** if he is able. If he has difficulty retaining the suppository, hold his buttocks together for a short time.

(continued on next page)

Procedure 25-6 ■ Inserting a Rectal Suppository (continued)

11. Wipe the patient's anus with toilet tissue.
Maintains hygiene and comfort.

12. Explain to the patient the need to remain in the side-lying position for 5 to 10 minutes.
Sim's position promotes retention and absorption of the medication. Explanation promotes compliance.

13. Discard used materials into a biohazard receptacle and wash hands thoroughly.

14. Leave the call device within reach and bedpan handy, if the suppository was a laxative.

In case the patient has a sudden urge to defecate or cannot retain the suppository for the recommended time.

What if . . .

■ **The prescribed dose is only half of the suppository?**

Cut the suppository lengthwise with a clean, single-edge razor blade.

■ **My patient is a child. What is the best way to give a rectal suppository so the child doesn't expel it?**

For pediatric patients, it may be necessary to gently hold the buttocks together for 5 to 10 minutes.

■ **My patient is an older adult. Is there anything special I should know?**

Older adults may have difficulty retaining a suppository because of poor sphincter control. You may need to put the bedpan under the patient while you are inserting the suppository.

Evaluation

■ Assess for pain or burning during insertion of the medication.
■ Determine that the patient retained the suppository for the desired length of time after insertion (reinsertion may be required).
■ Assess for rectal pain, if indicated.

Patient Teaching

Explain that suppositories may take up to 30 minutes to be absorbed, depending on the medication.

Documentation

■ Chart according to Medication Guidelines: Steps to Follow for All Medication (Regardless of Type or Route).
■ Chart the condition of anal tissue if abnormalities are present, any complaints of discomfort that are outside of the expected feelings and experience, and the length of time that the suppository was retained.
■ Chart responses to medication (e.g., symptom relief, side effects).

Practice Resources

American Society of Health-System Pharmacists, Inc., n.d.; Bradshaw, Dip, & Price, 2006.

Thinking About the Procedure

 Go to the *Fundamentals of Nursing Skills Videos,* **Medication Administration: Rectal Suppositories.**

1. How is the patient positioned after insertion of the rectal suppository?
2. Why is he positioned in this manner rather than side lying?

 For suggested responses, go to Chapter 25, **Thinking About the Procedure Suggested Responses,** on Davis*Plus.*

Procedure 25-7 ■ Applying Medication to the Skin

➤ For steps to follow in *all* procedures, refer to the Universal Steps for All Procedures found on the page facing the inside back cover. Also refer to the Medication Guidelines: Steps to Follow for All Medications (Regardless of Type or Route).

Delegation

As an RN, you can usually delegate administration of most topical medications to an LPN/LVN. In many institutions you can delegate the administration of an over-the-counter medication to a NAP. Refer to agency policy regarding administration of topical medication.

Pre-Procedure Assessments

■ Assess for skin irritation, open lesions, areas of hypersensitivity, or other skin abnormality.
■ Determine the presence of contraindications for dermal application; document and report before administering medication.

Procedure 25-7A ■ Applying Topical Lotion, Cream, and Ointment

➤ When performing the procedure, always identify your patient according to agency policy and be attentive to standard precautions, hand hygiene, patient safety and privacy, body mechanics, and documentation.

Procedure Steps

1. **Don clean gloves.**
   Complies with universal precautions and protects your skin from the medication.

2. **Cleanse the skin** with soap and water and pat dry before applying. .
   Clean skin enhances absorption. Moisture on the skin can interfere with adherence of topical ointment, depending on the product used to suspend the medication.

3. **Warm the medication** in your gloved hands.
   This will be more comfortable for the patient and make the preparation easier to apply.

4. **Use gloved hands or an applicator to apply** and spread the medication evenly, following the direction of hair growth when coating the area.

Excessive application may irritate the skin. Gloves protect you from absorbing the medication through your skin. ▼

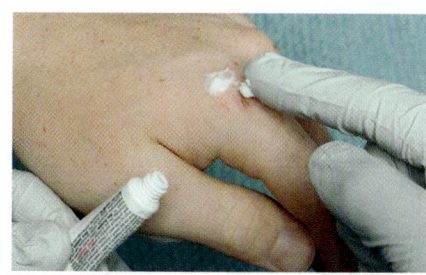

Procedure 25-7B ■ Applying Topical Aerosol Spray

➤ When performing the procedure, always identify your patient according to agency policy and be attentive to standard precautions, hand hygiene, patient safety and privacy, body mechanics, and documentation.

Procedure Steps

1. **Don clean gloves.**
2. **Cleanse the skin** with soap and water and pat dry before applying to enhance absorption.
3. **Shake the container to mix** the contents.
   Active ingredients might not be evenly distributed throughout the aerosolized

suspension and may settle at the bottom of the container.

4. **Hold the container at the distance specified on the label** (usually 6 to 12 in.), and spray over the prescribed area.
   This distance will prevent excess application to a local area.

5. **You will need to hold most containers upright when spraying.** If you are spraying near the patient's head, cover his face with a towel.
   Prevents him from inhaling the spray.

Procedure 25-7C ■ Applying Prescribed Powder

➤ When performing the procedure, always identify your patient according to agency policy and be attentive to standard precautions, hand hygiene, patient safety and privacy, body mechanics, and documentation.

Procedure Steps

1. **Don clean gloves.**
2. **Cleanse the skin** with soap and water and pat dry before applying (to enhance absorption).

Powder applied to a moist surface creates a pasty solution, which is irritating to skin.

3. **Spread apart skinfolds, and apply** a very thin layer to the clean, dry skin.

4. **Be careful that the patient does not inhale the powder.**
   Particulate matter, such as powder, can irritate lung tissue and lead to pneumonitis or other inflammatory processes.

Procedure 25-7D ■ Transdermal Medication

➤ When performing the procedure, always identify your patient according to agency policy and be attentive to standard precautions, hand hygiene, patient safety and privacy, body mechanics, and documentation.

Procedure Steps

1. **Don clean gloves.**
   Complies with universal precautions and protects your skin from the topical medication.

2. **Remove the previous patch,** folding the medicated side to the inside.
   This helps to prevent unintentional contact of the medication on a different area of the patient or another's skin.

3. **Dispose of the old patch carefully** in an appropriate receptacle, keeping it away from children and pets.
   Even a used patch has some active medication on it. Proper disposal is important to prevent medication exposure to others.

4. **Cleanse the skin of traces** of remaining medication. Allow the skin to dry.
   A clean, dry surface optimizes the effectiveness of adherence and penetration of the medication via the skin.

(continued on next page)

Procedure 25-7 ■ **Applying Medication to the Skin** (continued)

5. Remove the patch from its protective covering, and then remove the clear, protective covering without touching the adhesive or the inside surface that contains the medication. ▼

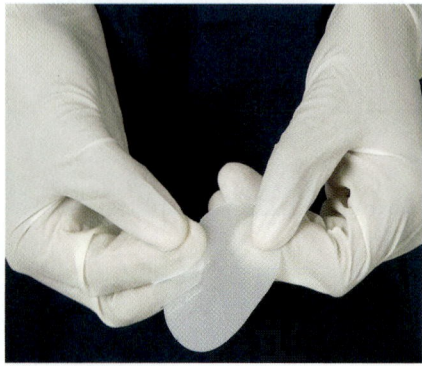

6. Apply the patch to a clean, dry, hairless (or little hair), intact skin area, pressing it down for about 10 seconds with your palm. Be sure the area is free of scars, lesions, and irritation.

A smooth surface maximizes the contact between medication and the skin. Areas of the skin that are disrupted can become irritated by topical medication. Other lesions involving thickened layers of skin should be avoided to avoid compromised absorption.

7. Rotate application sites. Common sites are the trunk, lower abdomen, lower back, and buttocks.

Rotating sites prevents irritation to local areas of the skin

8. Teach the patient to *not* use a heating pad over the area.

Heat can cause some ointments to irritate or even burn the skin.

9. Write the date, the time, and your initials on the new patch.

Complete documentation helps reduce medication errors.

10. Remove gloves and wash your hands again.

11. Observe for local side effects, such as skin irritation, itching, and allergic contact dermatitis.

If an adverse response occurs at the local site, remove the patch, wipe the skin clean, and notify the prescriber.

? What if . . .

■ **The medication is packaged as an ointment form with calibrated paper?**

Wear gloves; apply the ointment in a continuous motion along those marks to measure the required dose. Fold the paper in half to distribute the ointment evenly on the patch.

■ **My patient is a child who does not want the medication to be applied?**

Hold the child securely while medication is applied. Then cover the site with a dressing to keep the child from disrupting the application of medication.

■ **My patient is an older adult and has fragile skin?**

Avoid areas where penetration of the cream or ointment is likely to be reduced or cause irritation. Be gentle with application of anything to the skin and diligent with your assessment of the skin response to medication.

Evaluation

■ Assess for rash, excoriation, hives, redness, swelling, or signs of allergy or skin sensitivity to topical medication.
■ Ask the patient if he feels burning, itching, pain, tenderness, or other sensation to skin where medication was applied.
■ Assess for improvement in the patient's condition.

Patient Teaching

■ Explain that topical medication may take up to 30 minutes to be absorbed, depending on the medication.
■ Tell the patient to never ingest or inhale topical medication.
■ Advise the patient to avoid touching his eyes after handling topical medication.
■ Inform the patient to not use more medicine than prescribed or directed.

Documentation

■ Refer to Medication Guidelines: Steps to Follow for All Medication (Regardless of Type or Route).

■ Record the condition of skin if abnormalities are present and any complaints of discomfort during or after administration.
■ Document responses to medication (e.g., symptom relief, side effects).

Thinking About the Procedure

 Go to the *Fundamentals of Nursing Skills Videos,* **Medication Administration: Transdermal Medications.**

1. Where does the nurse apply the transdermal patch?
2. Why does the nurse apply the medication in this location?

 For suggested responses, go to Chapter 25, **Thinking About the Procedure Suggested Responses,** on Davis*Plus.*

Procedure 25-8 ■ Administering Metered-Dose Inhaler (MDI) Medication

➤ For steps to follow in *all* procedures, refer to the Universal Steps for All Procedures found on the page facing the inside back cover. Also refer to the Medication Guidelines: Steps to Follow for All Medications (Regardless of Type or Route).

Equipment
- Metered-dose inhaler
- Spacer
- Tissues

Pre-Procedure Assessments
Assess the patient's respiratory status before administration of medication to establish a baseline that can be used to evaluate the effects of treatment.

Delegation
An RN can usually delegate administration of MDI medications to an LPN/LVN. You usually cannot delegate this task to a NAP unless the NAP has special training for a specific defined situation (e.g., "medication aides" in some long-term care settings in some states). See the Medication Guidelines at the beginning of the Procedures section.

➤ When performing the procedure, always identify your patient according to agency policy and be attentive to standard precautions, hand hygiene, patient safety and privacy, body mechanics, and documentation.

Procedure Steps

1. **Identify the amount of medication for inhalation remaining** in the canister. Based on the start date and instructions for use, you can determine the number of remaining inhalations. Replace the canister promptly when the canister is nearly empty.
   Historically, patients have been instructed to float the canister in water to determine how much medication remains. However, propellants affect the weight of the canister and may lead to false reassurance that there is medication in an empty container. Some MDI medications are used as rescue agents during asthma attacks or periods of dyspnea. It is important to always have medication available for use.

2. **Assist the patient to a seated position** or high-Fowler's if in bed.
   An upright position helps the patient take a deep inhalation when medication administered.

3. **Ask the patient to rinse out his mouth** and spit the fluid out (not to swallow it).
   This helps to prevent transfer of bacteria from the mouth to the inhaler.

4. **Shake the inhaler.** Remove the mouthpiece cap of the inhaler and insert the mouthpiece into the spacer while holding the canister upright.
   A spacer is the most efficient method to deliver inhaled medications. It should be used if the patient has difficulty coordinating the use of the inhaler, is using a corticosteroid, or if it is prescribed.

Procedure Variation: No Spacer Is Used
If a spacer is not used, place the canister 1 to 2 inches (2.5 to 5.0 cm) from or directly into the mouth.

5. **Remove the cap** from the spacer.

6. **Ask the patient to breathe out** slowly and completely. If a patient is unable to use the MDI independently, time the use of the device with the patient's own respirations.
   Deep breathing helps the patient to time the dose with his natural breathing.

7. **Place the spacer mouthpiece into the patient's mouth** and have him seal his lips around the mouthpiece. Sharply press down on the inhaler canister to discharge one puff of medication into the spacer.
   A good seal allows proper delivery of medication. ▼

8. **Ask the patient to slowly inhale** and then hold his breath for as long as possible. Encourage the patient to hold his breath for 10 seconds if possible.
   When holding his breath the medication can be delivered deep into the lungs.

9. **If a second puff is needed, wait at least 1 minute** before repeating steps 6 through 8.
   Pausing allows the medication to be absorbed and the canister to recharge.

10. **If a corticosteroid inhaler was used,** assist the patient to rinse out his mouth with water and spit out the rinse.
    Prolonged exposure of the oral mucosa to this medication is irritating and can lead to thrush in some patients.

11. **Clear the mouthpiece** with a tissue or moist cloth and replace the cap. Periodically rinse the spacer, mouthpiece, and cap with water.

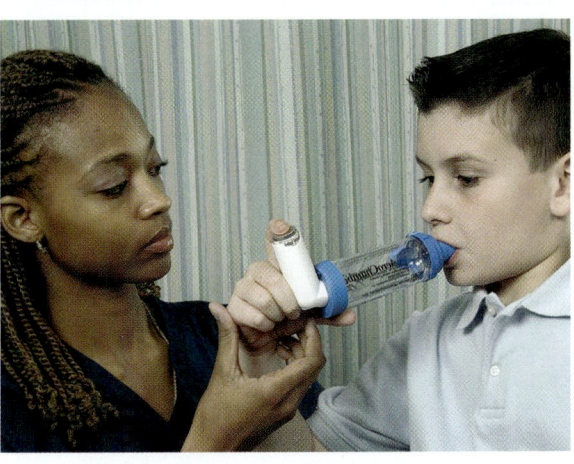

(continued on next page)

Procedure 25–8 ▪ Administering Metered-Dose Inhaler (MDI) Medication (continued)

Proper cleaning of the MDI keeps the dispenser from clogging. The following illustrations summarize the steps for using an MDI. ▼

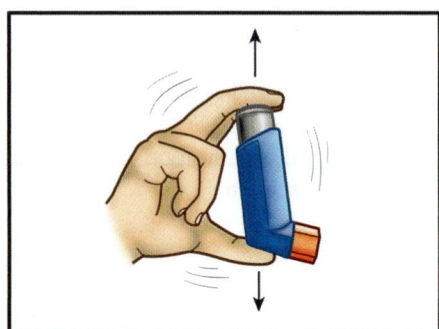

Shake canister.

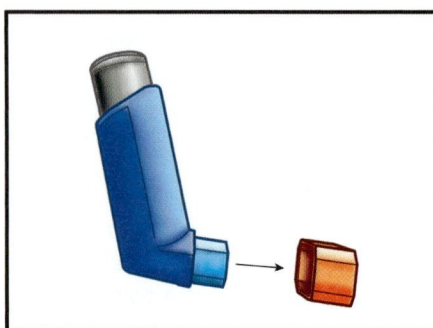

Remove cap. Discharge 2 puffs.

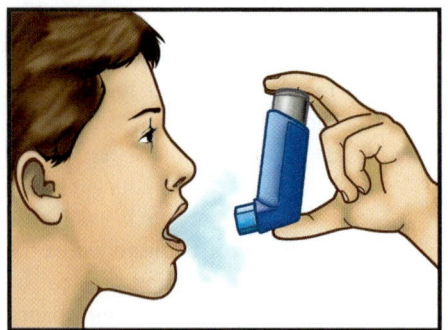

Deep breath out.

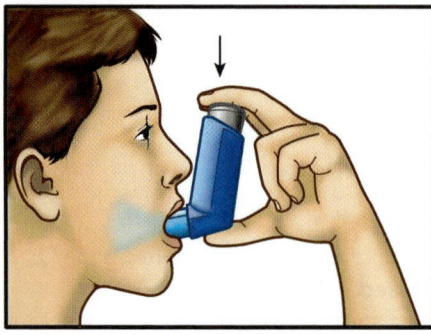

Press top. Inhale med slowly.

Hold breath. Exhale slowly.

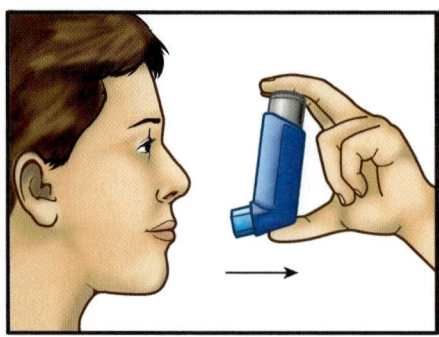

Remove inhaler from mouth.
Wait 1 minute before next puff.

? What if . . .

▪ **Your client is a small child or frail older adult who is unable to assist with taking medication from the inhaler?**

You may need to time discharge of the medication with the client's inspiration if the patient is unable to administer the medication with his own deep breaths.

▪ **Your patient uses an albuterol MDI with chlorofluorocarbon (CFC) as a propellant?**

The FDA ruling, effective December 31, 2008, prohibits use of CFCs in albuterol MDIs. If the patient has an inhaler containing this product, known to be detrimental to the ozone layer, the patient or caregiver can request an alternate prescription.

In addition to the harmful effects of the propellant on the environment, the medication is also likely to be past the expiration date.

Evaluation

Assess for change in respiratory status after medication administration.

Patient Teaching

▪ Explain to the patient when to use the inhaler and what side effects to anticipate.
▪ Teach and demonstrate to patients how to correctly use a spacer and MDI.
▪ Teach patients how to determine if the MDI canister is nearly empty.

▪ Explain that some inhalers are used in combination with others and must be used in correct order to receive the desired effect.
▪ Be aware that many patients who have not been taught to use dry powder inhalers do not get any medication into their lungs.
▪ Errors in using dry powder inhalers increase with age and illness severity. Carefully supervise older adults and very ill patients.

Home Care

General Information to Tell Patients

- Show your healthcare professional how you're using your MDI. If you're having trouble using your MDI, ask for tips or to recommend another device.
- Never puncture or break the canister.
- Do not immerse the MDI in water.
- Keep the MDI where you can get it quickly when needed, but out of children's reach.
- Store the MDI at room temperature. If it gets cold, warm it by rubbing the canister between his palms. Never use anything else to warm it.

Determining the Number of Remaining Doses

- When you begin using a new MDI, write the start date on the canister.
- The only reliable method for determining the number of doses remaining in a canister is to subtract the number of doses used from the number available. Some devices are equipped with counters. Floating MDIs in water is not accurate for assessing remaining doses and often will clog the valve.

Cleaning the MDI

- Clean your apparatus regularly to avoid drug buildup that might keep the medication from reaching the lungs. Specific maintenance procedures may vary with the manufacturer.

- Remove the metal canister that contains the medication by pulling it out.

Documentation

- Refer to Medication Guidelines: Steps to Follow for All Medications (Regardless of Type or Route).
- Document the response to medications.

Thinking About the Procedure

 Go to the *Fundamentals of Nursing Skills Videos*, **Medication Administration: Metered-Dose Inhaler.**

1. What would the nurse do next in the DVD after the dose of medication is completely administered by metered-dose inhaler ?

 For suggested responses, go to Chapter 25, **Thinking About the Procedure Suggested Responses,** on Davis*Plus.*

Practice Resources

American Academy of Family Physicians, 2006; Bollinger, 2005; Brock, Wessell, Williams, et al., 2004; Ram, Brocklebank, White, et al., 2002; U.S. Food and Drug Administration, Center for Evaluation and Research, 2008.

Procedure 25-9 ■ Preparing, Drawing Up, and Mixing Medication

➤ For steps to follow in *all* procedures, refer to the Universal Steps for All Procedures found on the page facing the inside back cover. Also refer to the Medication Guidelines: Steps to Follow for All Medications (Regardless of Type or Route).

Equipment

- Medication vials, ampules, and/or prefilled syringe
- Alcohol prep pad (70% alcohol) or chlorhexidine gluconate (CHG)-alcohol product
- Syringe of the appropriate size for medication volume and viscosity
- Needle of the appropriate size for the site and viscosity to be aspirated through the vial access device (VAD)
- VAD, filter needle, or safety needle.
- Gauze pad or ampule snapper, if you are using ampules ▼

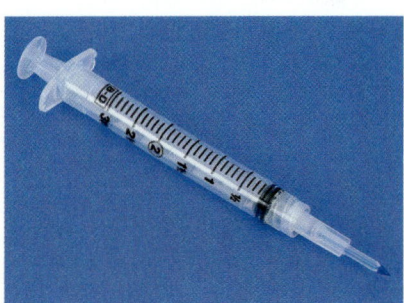

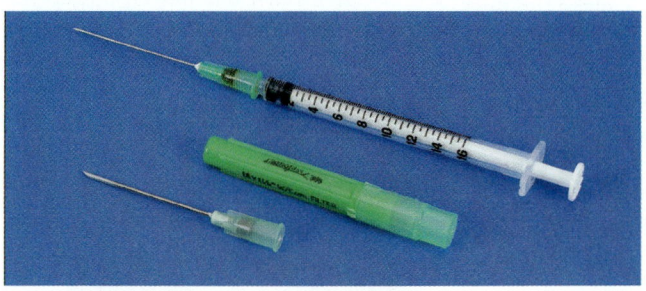

Delegation

An RN can delegate administration of some parenteral medications to an LPN/LVN. You usually cannot delegate this task to a NAP. Nurse practice acts governing medication administration vary from state to state, and policies vary further among healthcare agencies. Nevertheless, as the RN, you are always responsible for supervising and evaluating delegated care. You can instruct a NAP in the therapeutic effects expected from the medication.

(continued on next page)

Procedure 25-9 ■ **Preparing, Drawing Up, and Mixing Medication** (continued)

Pre-Procedure Assessments

- Check the ampule or vial for intactness, cloudiness, particles, and color.
  A change in color, cloudiness, particles, or cracks indicate that the medication is altered or contaminated and should not be used.
- When mixing medications, check the compatibility of the medications.
  Some medications are either chemically or physically incompatible and cannot be mixed. Other medications may be compatible for only 20 to 30 minutes, so they must be given promptly after they are mixed. Although physically incompatible medications can

frequently be identified by a change in appearance, such as precipitation, no such indication exists for chemically incompatible medications.

- Determine the total volume of medications and whether the total volume is appropriate for the administration site.
  Although the reason for mixing medications is to limit the number of injections a patient receives, the total volume of the injections must not be greater than what is appropriate for the site, such as 0.5 to 1 mL for deltoid or 3 to 4 mL for the vastus lateralis or ventrogluteal muscle, depending on muscle size.

Procedure 25-9A ■ **Drawing Up Medication From Ampules**

➤ When performing the procedure, always identify your patient according to agency policy and be attentive to standard precautions, hand hygiene, patient safety and privacy, body mechanics, and documentation.

Procedure Steps

1. With your index finger, **gently flick or tap the top of the ampule** to remove medication trapped in the top of the ampule. An alternate method is to shake the ampule by quickly turning and snapping your wrist, like shaking down a mercury thermometer.
   Medication left in the top of the ampule may lead to administering an inadequate dose. All the medication must be in the bottom of the ampule before you open it.

2. **Wrap a 2 in. x 2 in. gauze pad** (or an unwrapped alcohol wipe) around the neck of the ampule, or slip on an ampule snapper. Snap the top off, breaking it away from you.
   Prevents you from accidentally cutting your fingers or spraying glass fragments toward you. Do not use an opened alcohol wipe to break the ampule, because it is not thick enough to prevent injury. ▼

3. **Attach a filter needle** or filter straw to the syringe. If the syringe has a needle in place, remove both the needle and the cap, and place them on a sterile surface (e.g., a newly unwrapped alcohol pad still in the open wrapper), and attach the filter needle or straw.
   The American Society for Health System Pharmacists recommends filtering solutions drawn up from glass ampules to remove glass particles. Opening a glass ampule produces a spray of tiny glass particles, many of which can enter the ampule and contaminate the contents. The size of the glass particles increases proportionally with the size of the vial.

4. **Withdraw the medication** from the ampule by using one of the following techniques. Be careful not to touch the neck of the ampule with the filter straw or needle while withdrawing medication.
   Touching the neck of the ampule with the needle or straw increases the risk of contamination.

   a. Invert the ampule, place the needle tip in the liquid, and withdraw the prescribed amount of medication. Be careful not to insert needle through the medication into the air at the top of the inverted ampule.
   This method is particularly useful with small ampules. The medication's surface tension prevents the liquid from leaking from the ampule while the ampule is inverted. However, if

you insert the needle too far (into the air pocket above the medication), the medication will run out. ▼

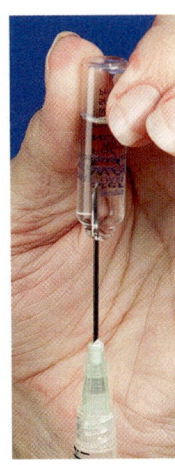

b. Alternatively, tip the ampule, place a filter needle or straw in the liquid, and withdraw all medication. Reposition the ampule so that the needle or straw tip remains in the liquid.
   This method allows you to stabilize the ampule while you withdraw the medication, and may help keep you from contaminating the needle on the edge of the vial opening. ▼

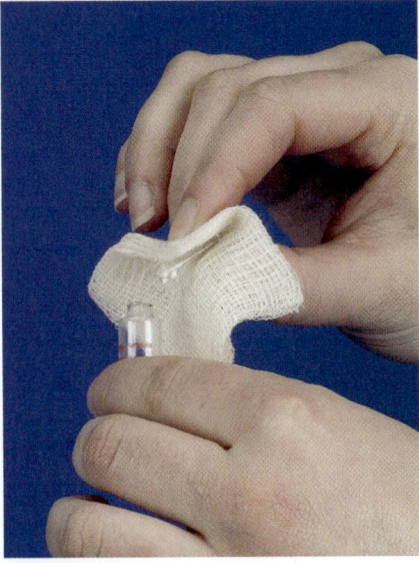

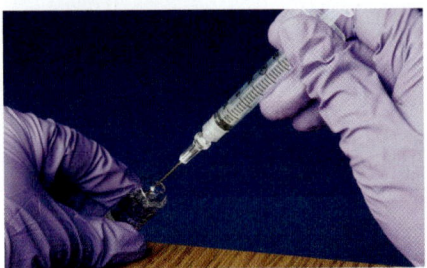

5. **Hold the syringe vertically, and draw 0.2 mL of air** into the syringe (see Clinical Insight 25-5, Measuring Dosage When Changing Needles). Draw up and measure the exact medication dose, plus 0.2 mL of air (the syringe plunger should be at 0.2 mL more than the prescribed dose).

6. **Remove the filter needle** or straw, and reattach the "saved" needle for administering the injection.

7. **Eject the 0.2 mL of air, and read the dose.** After all of the air is ejected, if you need to eject some medication to make the dose correct, tip the syringe horizontally to eject the medication.
Use a filter needle only to withdraw medication; do not eject medication from it. For injection, use a needle of the correct gauge and length. Pushing the medication out of the syringe with the filter needle in place could cause the filter to break and release the glass fragments. Pulling air into the syringe allows for an exact dose when the medication is injected; the air will clear the needle (after the medication) so that the patient receives all the medication that was drawn up in the syringe.

NOTE: This is not the old "air lock" technique; you will eject the air before injecting the medication into the patient.

The syringe must be vertical to eject air; however, if you eject the medication while holding the syringe vertically, the drug will run down the needle and then track through the patient's tissue during the injection.

8. **Alternatively, for a medication that is irritating to tissues,** you can leave the 0.2 mL of air in the syringe for injection. But be sure to account for the air when you read the dose markings on the syringe.
Parenteral iron is an example of medication that is irritating to the tissue.

9. **Dispose of the top and bottom of the ampule** and the filter needle in a sharps container.
Disposal into a puncture-proof container prevents accidental needlestick injury.

Procedure 25-9B ■ Drawing Up Medications From Vials

➤ When performing the procedure, always identify your patient according to agency policy and be attentive to standard precautions, hand hygiene, patient safety and privacy, body mechanics, and documentation.

Procedure Steps

1. **Mix the solution in the vial,** if necessary, by gently rolling the vial between your hands.
Aqueous suspensions will settle to the bottom of the vial, so they need to be mixed. Rolling the vial between your hands will mix the medication without forming air bubbles. Shaking the vial traps air in the medication.

2. **Place the vial on a flat work surface** and thoroughly scrub the rubber top of the vial with an alcohol prep pad or chlorhexidine gluconate (CHG)-alcohol product.
The alcohol prep pad removes dust, grease, and microorganisms.

3. **Uncap the VAD** without touching the needle tip or shaft. If you are using a VAD, attach the device to the syringe, and remove the cap.
VADs can be used only with single-use vials, unless the vial is designed for use with access pins, such as a Life-Shield vial.

4. **Place the needle or VAD cap on a clean surface,** or hold the cap open-side out between two fingers of your nondominant hand.
This method prevents contamination of the cap and the needle during recapping.

5. **Draw air into the syringe** equal to the amount of medication to be withdrawn from the vial.
Injection of air into the vial makes withdrawing the medication easier. For small unit-dose vials, you may not have to instill air prior to withdrawing the medication, but you will need to maintain backward pressure on the plunger until the needle is completely withdrawn. If you release the plunger, the negative pressure in the vial will pull the medication back into the vial.

6. **Insert the needle or VAD** into the vial without coring and while maintaining sterile technique,
   a. Place the tip of the needle or VAD in the middle of the rubber top of the vial, with the bevel up at a 45° to 60° angle. ▼

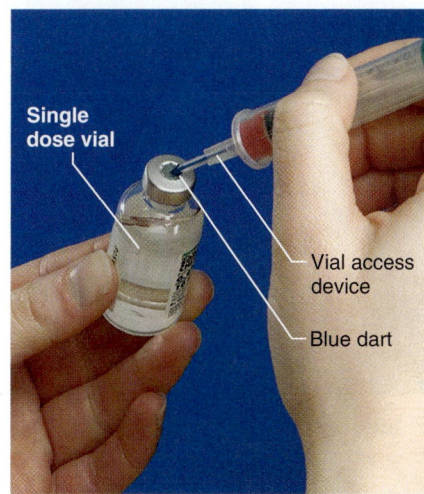

Single dose vial

Vial access device

Blue dart

   b. While pushing the needle or VAD into the rubber top, gradually bring the needle upright to a 90° angle.
   This method helps prevent coring, which occurs when a small piece of the rubber top is trapped inside the needle or VAD during insertion. Coring is more likely to occur with large-gauge needles and VADs.

7. **With the tip of the VAD above the fluid line,** inject the air in the syringe into the air in the vial.
Injecting air into the vial creates positive pressure, making the medication easier to withdraw. Injecting the air into the medication will create air bubbles, which interfere with dosage measurement. ▼

(continued on next page)

Procedure 25-9 ■ Preparing, Drawing Up, and Mixing Medication (continued)

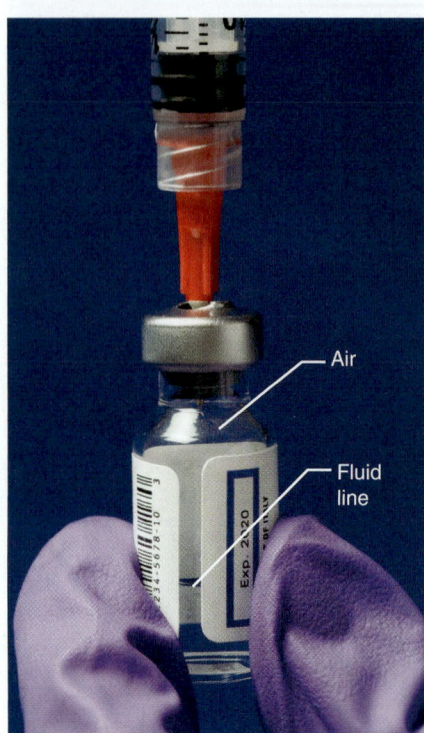

8. Invert the vial, keep the needle or VAD vertical in the medication, and slowly withdraw the medication.

The vial needs to be inverted so that all the medication can be withdrawn. Keeping the needle/VAD in the medication and slowly drawing the medication will help prevent you from drawing excess air into the syringe. ▼

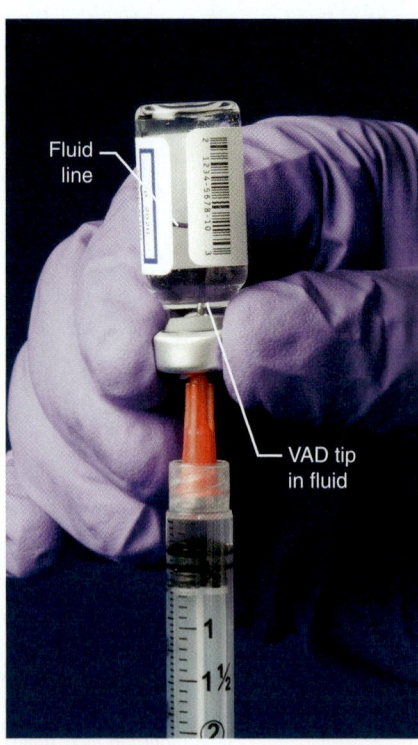

9. Keeping the needle or VAD in the vial, remove any air from the syringe. ▼

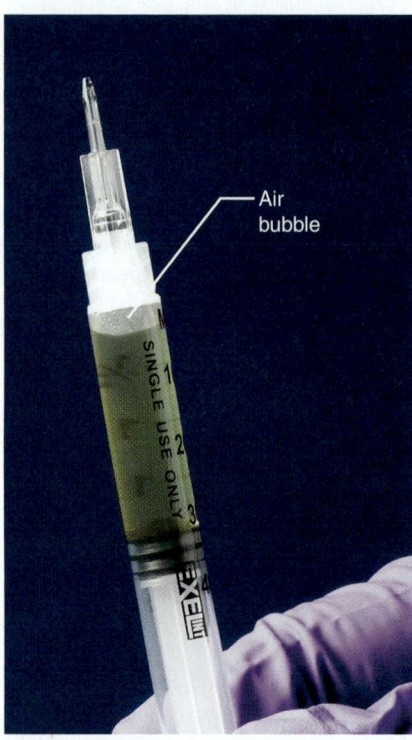

A. **Incorrect**—If syringe is not vertical, air is trapped near the hub.

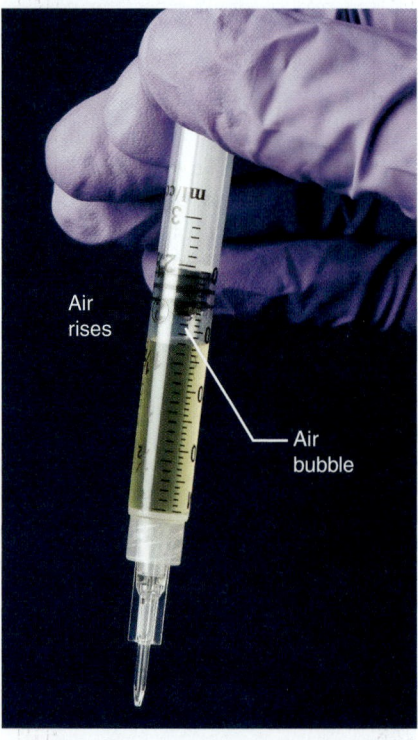

B. **Incorrect**—If tip is down, air is trapped at the plunger.

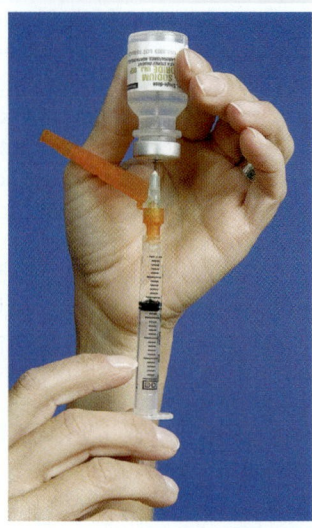

C. **Correct**—Syringe is vertical.

When the VAD is connecting the vial and syringe, a sterile unit is formed. The volume of air in the hub of the syringe and inside the needle/VAD, dead space, will be drawn back into the syringe. Air bubbles alter the dose of medication being administered, so they must be expelled. You can use a pen to tap the syringe if extra force is needed.

a. Carefully stabilize the vial and syringe, and firmly tap the syringe below the air bubbles. When air bubbles are at the hub of the syringe, make sure the syringe is vertical (straight up and down), and push the air back into the vial. *Remember that air rises, so if the syringe is tilted, air will be trapped in it.*

b. Withdraw additional medication, if necessary, to obtain the correct dose.

When working with only one vial, you can withdraw and eject medication into the vial as many times as needed to expel bubbles from the syringe and obtain the correct dose.

10. When the dose is correct, withdraw the needle or VAD from the vial at a 90° angle.

A vertical angle prevents accidental contamination or bending of the needle.

11. Hold the syringe upright at eye level to recheck the medication dose.

Reading the syringe at an angle can result in inaccurate measurement.

12. **Recap the needle or VAD using a needle recapping device** or the one-handed method (see Procedure 25-10).

    Although recapping a sterile needle does not present a threat of bloodborne pathogen exposure, using a mechanical recapping device or the one-handed method helps develop safe habits.

13. **If you are administering an irritating medication or if you used a VAD or filter needle** to draw up medication, change the needle before you inject the medication.

Before changing the needle, draw back on the syringe plunger to remove all medication from dead space in the old needle (or VAD), remove the old needle, and reattach a new one (see Clinical Insight 25-5). Hold the syringe vertically and expel the air; if it is necessary to expel some medication, hold the syringe horizontally to do so.

The difficulty with changing the needles is that you may slightly alter the dose. If you are planning to change the needles, draw slightly more than the ordered dose unless you are combining in one syringe. After changing the needle, remeasure the dose. Holding the syringe horizontally prevents medication from running down the needle and tracking into the patient's skin.*

14. **Dispose of the vial and filter needle(s)** in a sharps container.

    This prevents sharps injury to healthcare workers or others in the vicinity. Proper disposal also reduces the risk of transmitting infectious organisms.

Procedure 25-9C ■ Mixing Medications From Two Vials

➤ First review Medication Guidelines: Steps to Follow for All Medications; Procedure 25-9B (Preparing and Drawing Up Medications From Vials); and Procedure 25-10A (Recapping Contaminated Needles).

➤ When performing the procedure, always identify your patient according to agency policy and be attentive to standard precautions, hand hygiene, patient safety and privacy, body mechanics, and documentation.

Procedure Steps

1. **Scrub the tops of both vials** with an alcohol pad or chlorhexidine gluconate (CHG)-alcohol product. (*Note:* Some experts omit this step for single-dose vials.)

   Not all pharmaceutical companies ensure the sterility of the rubber top on vials, even when they are first opened. However, be aware that once your fingers touch the alcohol pad, it is no longer sterile, either; therefore, you are not sterilizing, but rather cleaning the vial top.

2. **Draw air into the syringe** in the same amount as the total medication doses for both vials (e.g., if the order is for 0.5 mL for vial A and 1 mL for vial B, then draw up 1.5 mL of air). ➤

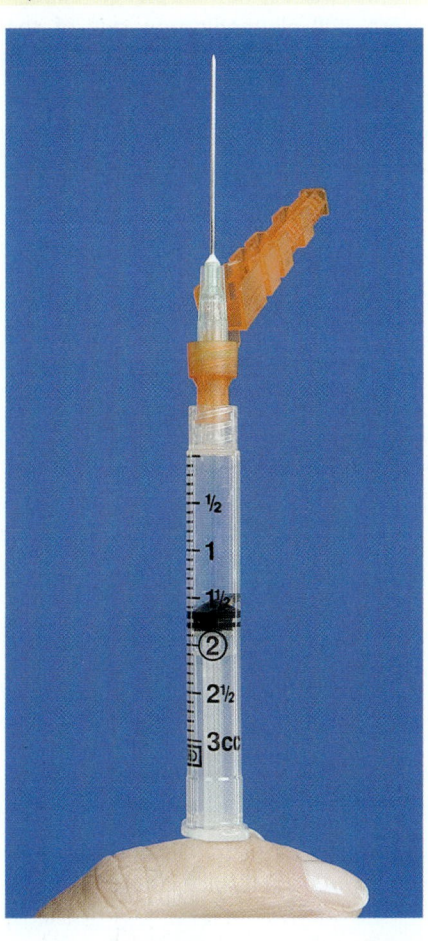

3. **Maintaining sterility, insert the needle (or vial access device [VAD])** into the vial in the middle of the rubber top of the vial with the bevel up at a 45° to 60° angle. While pushing the needle (or VAD) into the rubber top, gradually bring the needle upright to a 90° angle.

   This method helps prevent coring of the rubber top.

4. **Keeping the tip of the safety needle (or VAD) above the medication,** inject an amount of air equal to the volume of drug to be withdrawn from the first vial (e.g., 0.5 mL for vial A in step 2); then inject the rest of the air into the second vial (1.0 mL for vial B). Take care to prevent coring. ▼

(continued on next page)

Procedure 25-9 ■ **Preparing, Drawing Up, and Mixing Medication** (continued)

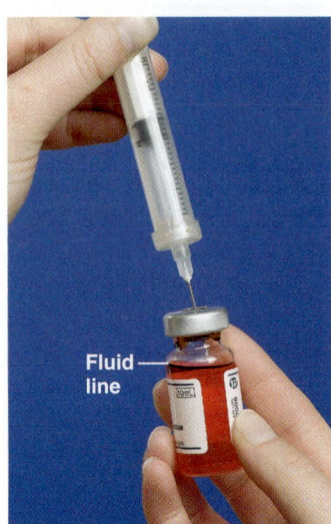

Vial A

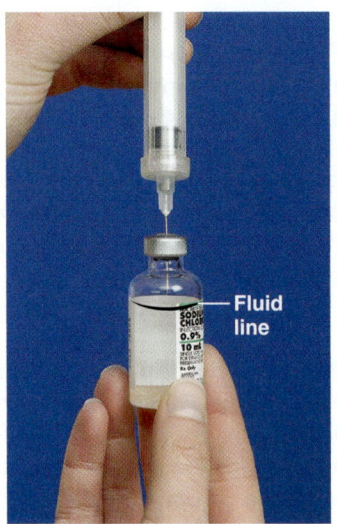

Vial B

Medication is easier to withdraw from a vial with positive pressure. For small unit-dose vials, it may be possible to withdraw the medication without instilling air, but you will need to maintain a slight backward pressure on the plunger until the needle is completely withdrawn. If you release the plunger, the negative pressure in the vial will pull the medication back in. Therefore, it is always safer to instill air.

One Multidose Vial and One Single-Dose Vial

Inject air into the single-dose vial first, and change the needle before injecting air into the multidose vial. You must withdraw medication from the multidose vial before withdrawing from the single-dose vial. However, the needle tip should stay above the medication at all times in steps 3 and 4.

This is an extra precaution to prevent contamination of the multidose vial with medication from the single-dose vial.

Mixing Two Types of Insulin

If you are mixing two types of insulin at step 3, put air into the regular insulin last (see Clinical Insight 25-6 for mixing two types of insulin).

5. **Without removing the needle (or VAD)** from the second vial (B), invert the vial and withdraw the ordered amount of medication. Expel any air bubbles, and measure the dose. Remove the VAD from the vial, then pull back on the plunger enough to pull all medication out of the VAD into the syringe (see Clinical Insight 25-5). Read the dose at eye level. Tip the syringe horizontally if you need to eject any medication.

This allows you to withdraw all the medication. Keeping the needle in the medication and slowly withdrawing will help prevent withdrawing excess air into the syringe and prevent bubbles. ▼

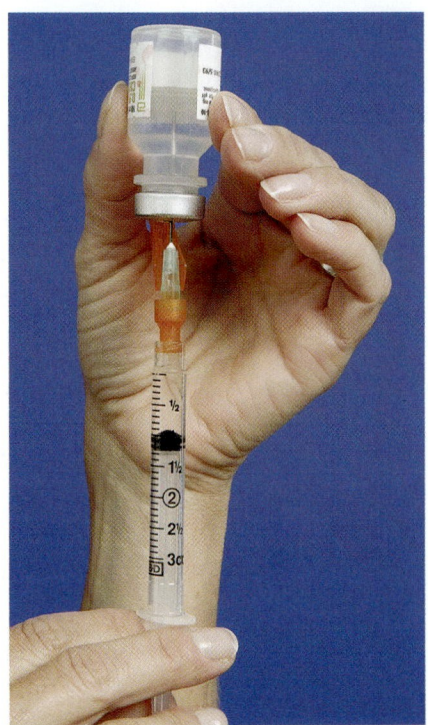

Vial B

6. **Insert the needle or VAD into the first vial (A),** invert, and withdraw the exact ordered amount of medication, holding syringe vertical. When finished, the plunger should be at the line for the total/combined dose for vials A and B. (Using the example in step 2, you would have 1.5 mL of the mixed medications in the syringe.) Be very careful not to withdraw excess medication; keep your index finger or thumb on the flange of the syringe to prevent it being forced back by pressure. If this occurs, you must discard the medication in the syringe and start over.

Because the medications are mixed, withdrawing extra from the second vial makes the entire mixture incorrect. If you eject excess medication from the syringe, you do not know how much of either medication you have ejected; so, even if you have the correct amount of fluid (e.g., 1.5 mL in our example), you would not know how much of that is medication A and how much of it is medication B.

There is no need to change the needle before step 5 because even if one vial is a multidose vial, you would have withdrawn the medication from it first (in step 4). It will not matter if you track medication into the single-dose vial. ▼

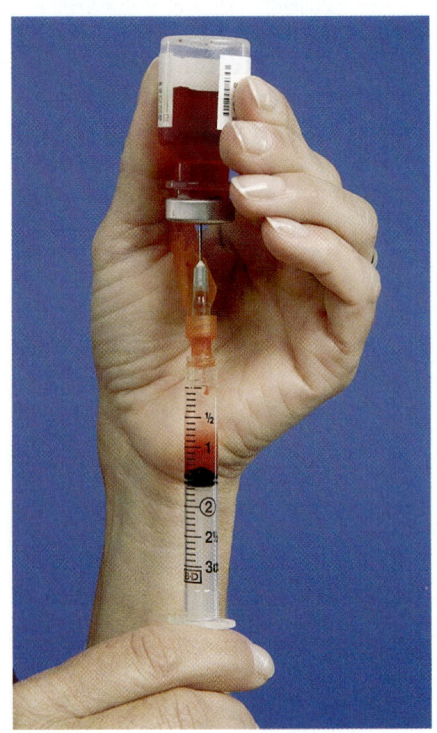

Vial A

7. **Remove the needle or VAD** from the vial, and then recap the needle, using a needle capping device or the one-handed scoop method (see Procedure 25-10, Recapping Needles Using One-Handed Technique).

Although recapping a sterile needle does not present a threat of pathogen exposure, using a mechanical recapping device or the one-handed method helps develop safe habits. We do not recommend using the one-handed scoop for sterile needles; however, this needle will be discarded anyway, so if it is accidentally contaminated with a one-handed scoop, it will not be an error.

8. **Place a new sterile needle on the syringe** for the injection.

Obviously, you must replace a VAD with a needle for injection. In addition, if you used a needle, to withdraw both medications you put it through a rubber vial top at least three times. This dulls the needle. A sharp needle causes less trauma to the patient on injection. A new needle also prevents tracking of the medication through the skin and subcutaneous tissues.

9. **Hold the needle vertically** to expel all air and recheck the dosage (the total for both medications).

Allows for more accurate accounting of the dose.

10. If **you have used a filter needle or VAD**, refer to Clinical Insight 25-5, Measuring Dosage When Changing Needles.

Procedure 25-9D ■ Mixing Medication From One Ampule and One Vial

➤ First review Medication Guidelines: Steps to Follow for All Medications; Procedure 25-9B (Preparing and Drawing Up Medications From Vials); and Procedure 25-10A (Recapping Contaminated Needles).

➤ When performing the procedure, always identify your patient according to agency policy and be attentive to standard precautions, hand hygiene, patient safety and privacy, body mechanics, and documentation.

Procedure Steps

1. **Begin with the vial.** Scrub the stopper of a multidose vial using an alcohol wipe or CHG-alcohol combination product.

   Protects against microbial contamination.

2. **Draw up the same volume of air as the dose of medication ordered** for the vial.

3. **Keeping the tip of the safety needle (or needleless device) above the medication**, inject the amount of air equal to the volume of drug to be withdrawn from the vial. The needle should be injecting air-to-air within the vial.

   Draw from the vial first because you do not need to add air to ampules before drawing up the medication. In addition, if it is a multidose vial, you would contaminate it with the medicine if you withdrew from the ampule first. Injecting air into the vial makes withdrawing the medication easier. For small unit-dose vials, it may be possible to withdraw the medication without instilling air, but you will need to maintain a slight backward pressure on the plunger until the needle is completely withdrawn. If you release the plunger, the negative pressure in the vial will pull the medication back into the vial. Therefore, it is safer always to instill air.

4. **Invert the vial.** Withdraw the prescribed volume of medication, keeping the safety needle tip or VAD in the fluid. See Procedure 25-9B.

5. **Expel any air bubbles and measure the dose** at eye level. Recheck the dosage, and withdraw more or eject the drug as needed.

   This prevents air from entering into the needle or VAD.

6. **After safely recapping the safety needle** or VAD remove it from the syringe. You may place it on an opened, sterile alcohol pad if you need your hands to open the filter needle packaging.

   Keeps the needle sterile, if you are using one; you will reuse it. You would not reuse a VAD from this step on.

7. **Attach a filter needle** or filter straw to the syringe.

   The use of a 5-micrometer (μm) filter minimizes the possibility of withdrawing small glass fragments.

8. **Flick or tap the top of the ampule** (or snap your wrist) to remove medication from the neck of the ampule.

   Flicking the neck of the ampule will help the fluid to drain down into the main part of the ampule, thus, reducing waste.

9. **Open the ampule** by wrapping the neck with a folded gauze pad or an unopened alcohol wipe or use an ampule snapper. Snap open away from you.

   Snapping outward prevents you from accidentally cutting your fingers or spraying glass fragments toward your face. Do not use an opened alcohol wipe to break the ampule, because it is not thick enough to prevent injury.

10. **Withdraw the exact prescribed amount of medication** from the ampule into the syringe (see Procedure 25-9A). Be very careful in drawing up the second medication; if the total amount of the two medications is incorrect, you must discard the syringe contents and start over.

11. **Draw 0.2 mL of air into the syringe.**

   The extra bit of air clears the filter needle (see Clinical Insight 25-5).

12. **Confirm the dose** is correct by holding the syringe vertically and checking the dose at eye level.

   Ensures the total volume in the syringe equals the ordered amount of both medications plus 0.2 mL of air from the needle.

13. **Recap the needle, using a needle capping device** or the one-handed technique recommended in Procedure 25-10.

   Although recapping a sterile needle does not present a threat of pathogen exposure, using a recapping device or the one-handed method helps develop safe habits. Nevertheless, some scoop techniques pose a risk of contaminating the needle, so you must be careful to maintain sterile technique.

14. **Remove the filter needle** or straw and discard it in a sharps container. Replace with a fresh, safety needle for giving the medication to the patient.

(continued on next page)

Procedure 25-9 ■ Preparing, Drawing Up, and Mixing Medication (continued)

This needle-recapping method prevents accidental needlestick injury. You cannot measure the dose accurately with a filter needle. You should not eject medication through the filter needle because of risk of breaking the filter. See Clinical Insight 25-5, Measuring Dosage When Changing Needles.

15. After placing the administration needle on the syringe eject the 0.2 mL of air and check for the correct dose, if there is excess medication in the syringe, you must discard it and start over.

16. Discard used needles and ampules in a puncture-proof sharps container.

Procedure 25-9C ■ Using a Prefilled Cartridge and Single-Dose Vial—For Intravenous Administration

➤ *Note:* It is best to not use this technique with multidose vials because there is a risk of contaminating the multidose vial with the cartridge medication.

➤ *Note:* First review the Medication Guidelines: Steps to Follow for All Medications; Procedure 23-9 (Preparing and Drawing up Medications); and Procedure 25-10A (Recapping Contaminated Needles).

➤ When performing the procedure, always identify your patient according to agency policy and be attentive to standard precautions, hand hygiene, patient safety and privacy, body mechanics, and documentation.

Procedure Steps

1. **Scrub the rubber stopper** of the vial thoroughly with an alcohol prep pad or chlorhexidine-gluconate (CHG)-alcohol-based product.
2. **Assemble the prefilled cartridge** and holder (see Clinical Insight 25-3).
3. **Remove the needle cap** from the prefilled cartridge, expel the air, and measure the correct dose of medication.
   You must confirm that the dose of the first medication is correct before you mix it with the second medication.
4. **Holding the cartridge with the needle up, withdraw an amount of air** equal to the volume of medication you need from the vial.
5. **While continuing to hold the syringe with needle straight up (vertically),** insert the needle into the inverted vial, tip of the needle in the air above the medication, and inject the air into the vial. Maintain pressure on the plunger so that air and/or medication does not flow back into the syringe.
   Injecting air into the vial makes the medication easier to withdraw. ➤

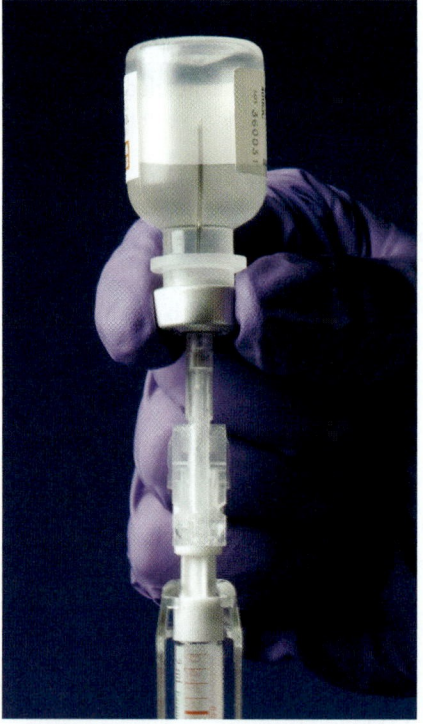

6. **While maintaining pressure on the plunger, pull the needle down into the fluid** and allow the pressure in the vial to push the medication into the syringe. Withdraw the ordered amount of vial medication, being careful not to withdraw any excess.
7. **The pressure will generally push a little less medication than you need,** so carefully withdraw the amount you need for a correct dose—again, do not withdraw any excess.

Withdrawing any excess will result in an altered mixed dose, so you would need to discard the syringe and start over.

8. **Recap the needle (use a one-handed method)** and if possible, remove the needle from the prefilled syringe and replace with an injection cannula for IV administration. For an IM injection, if the prefilled cartridge does not have a safety needle, you would need to transfer the medication to a new syringe and needle for injection.
   VADs and injection cannulas prevent needlestick injury. Unless there is a needle safety device for the prefilled syringe, it is not recommended for IM injections.

? What if . . .

■ **You note particulate matter in the ampule or vial?**

Discard the medication and order a new one.

■ **When withdrawing a second medication from a vial that is to be mixed in one syringe, the medication inadvertently is drawn back into the vial by positive pressure?**

Discard the medication in the syringe and start over.

Documentation

Document on the Medication Administration Record after the medication is administered.

Thinking About the Procedure

 Go to the *Fundamentals of Nursing Skills Videos*, **Medication Administration.**

Drawing Medications: Ampules (Procedure 25-9A)

1. How does the nurse safely open the glass ampule? Why does she do it in this manner?

Drawing Medications: Vials Using Vial Access Device (Procedure 25-9B)

1. After injecting medication into a vial, how does the nurse mix the combined solution?
2. And why does she do it this way?

Drawing Medications: Mixing From Two Vials (Procedure 25-9C)

1. What device does the nurse use to extract liquid medication from a vial?

2. After removing the needle from the second vial and pulling back on the plunger enough to pull all medication out of the needle (or access device) into the syringe, how much medication does the nurse eject to clear the needle?
3. As a last step after two medications are drawn and mixed in one syringe and the air is expelled, what does the nurse do before administering the dose to the patient?

Drawing Medications: Mixing Medication From One Ampule and One Vial (Procedure 25-9D)

1. Why does the nurse insert the needle access device at a 45° angle and then move to 90° angle?
2. How does the nurse get rid of air bubbles in the syringe?

 For suggested responses, go to Chapter 25, **Thinking About the Procedure Suggested Responses,** on Davis*Plus*.

Practice Resource

U.S. Food and Drug Administration, Center for Drug Evaluation and Research, 2008.

Procedure 25-10 ■ Recapping Needles Using One-Handed Technique

➤ For steps to follow in *all* procedures, refer to the Universal Steps for All Procedures found on the page facing the inside back cover.

Equipment

- Mechanical recapping device, if available
- Needle cover
- Safety syringe, if available
- Other supplies depending on the method used.

Delegation

Delegation is not usually an issue because recapping needles is done in conjunction with administering parenteral medications, which you will usually not delegate. If you do delegate administration of parenteral medications to an LPN/LVN, you must supervise and evaluate recapping to ensure that the nurse uses proper technique.

Preparation

- Assess the need to recap the needle.
  Recap a contaminated needle only if doing so is absolutely unavoidable, according to OSHA standards. As a rule, place a contaminated syringe and needle directly into a puncture-proof sharps container, without capping, bending, or breaking the needle.
- Identify whether the needle is sterile or dirty.
  Although a one-handed technique is used to recap both sterile and dirty needles, the goal is different for each. When you use the one-handed method for recapping a sterile needle, it is easy to contaminate the needle without realizing it; so, you should modify

the technique to help prevent that; the primary goal is to "protect" the needle. The danger in recapping a dirty needle is that you will stick yourself with it, exposing yourself to pathogens. The primary goal is to protect yourself.

- Determine the availability of mechanical recapping device or safety syringe.
  Always use a mechanical recapping device or safety syringe, if one is available. ▼

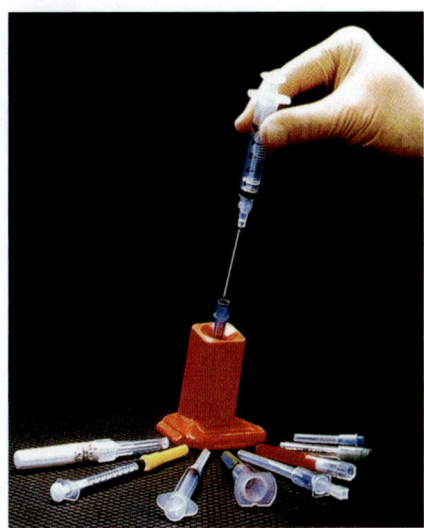

Needle recapping device.

(continued on next page)

Procedure 25–10 ■ Recapping Needles Using One-Handed Technique (continued)

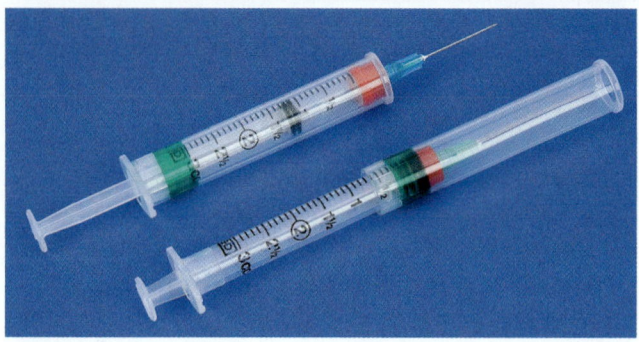

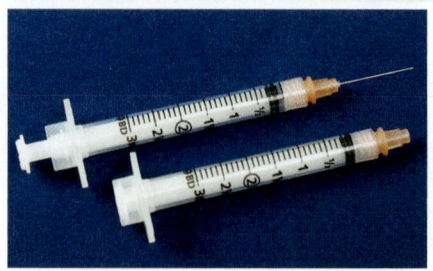

Safety syringe. Top, Before injection.
Bottom, Needle retracted after injection.

Safety syringe. Top, Before injection. Bottom, Cover slides up
after injection.

Procedure 25–10A ■ Recapping Contaminated Needles

➤ When performing the procedure, always identify your patient according to agency policy and be attentive to standard
precautions, hand hygiene, patient safety and privacy, body mechanics, and documentation.

Procedure Steps

1. **If you are using a safety needle,** engage the safety mechanism to cover the needle. (See Equipment.)
   OSHA regulations require the use of safety syringes to prevent needle-stick injuries. You must engage the safety mechanism before placing the needle and syringe into the sharps container.

2. **Alternatively, place the needle cap in mechanical recapping device**, if one is available. (See Equipment.)

3. **If a mechanical recapping device is not available,** use the one-handed scoop method to recap the needle.
   a. Place the needle cover on a flat surface.
      Keeps the needle cover from rolling during the needle capping procedure. ➤

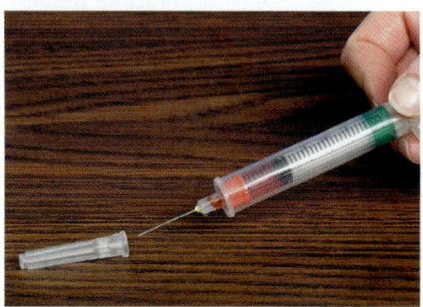

b. Then, holding syringe in your dominant hand, scoop the needle cap onto the needle. Tip the syringe vertically to slip the cover over the needle. Do not hold onto the needle cap with your nondominant hand while scooping. ▼

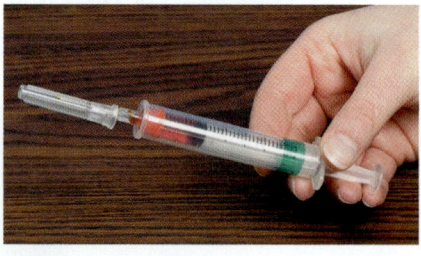

c. Secure the needle cap by grasping it near the hub.
   Prevents an accidental stick if the needle goes through the needle cap. Needles are sharp enough to go through the needle cap if inserted at an angle. ▼

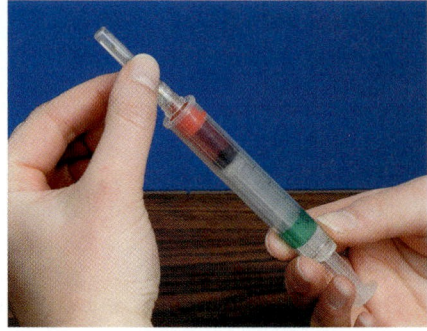

Procedure 25–10B ■ Recapping Sterile Needles

➤ When performing the procedure, always identify your patient according to agency policy and be attentive to standard precautions, hand hygiene, patient safety and privacy, body mechanics, and documentation.

➤ Use one of the following techniques to ensure that you do not contaminate a sterile needle.

➤ If you contaminate the needle, microorganisms will be introduced with the injection.

Procedure Steps

1. **Place the needle cap in a mechanical recapping device**, if one is available.

The device is specially developed to provide safe recapping.

2. **Alternative method:** Place the cap into a small liquid medication cup with the open end facing up. You can then insert the sterile needle into the cap, keeping your free hand well away from the cup.

This step performs the same function as a mechanical recapping device. The needle and cover need to be taller than the cup you are using, so that the open end of the cap protrudes above the cup. ▼

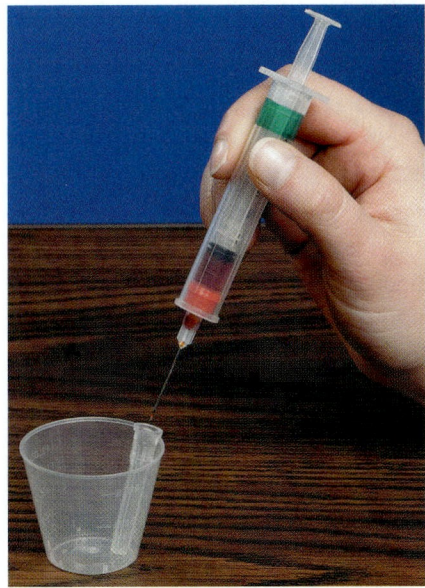

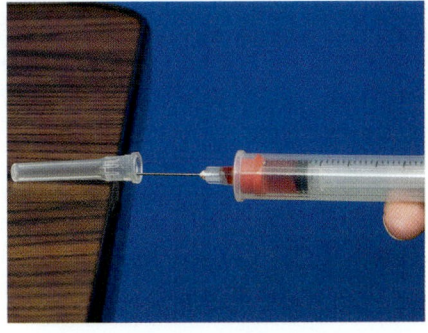

3. **Alternative method:** Place the cap on a clean surface so that the end of the needle cap protrudes over the edge of the counter or shelf, and scoop with the needle; keep your free hand well away from the needle and cap as you are recapping.
This method prevents you from inadvertently hitting an unsterile surface with the needle. ➤

4. **Alternative method:** If the syringe is packaged in a hard plastic tubular container, stand the container on its large end; invert the needle cap; and place it in the top of the hard container. Insert the needle downward into the cap. ▼

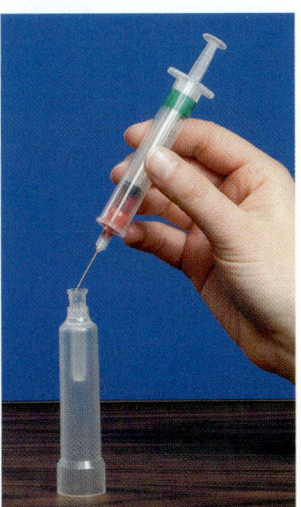

5. **Alternative method:** Place the needle cap on a sterile surface, such as on open alcohol prep pad, and use the one-handed scoop technique. Be very careful to not touch anything with the needle other than the inside of the needle cap.
The alcohol prep pad provides a sterile barrier. Because you must bring the needle parallel to the flat surface, and because the alcohol pad is so small, it is easy to contaminate the needle using this method. ▼

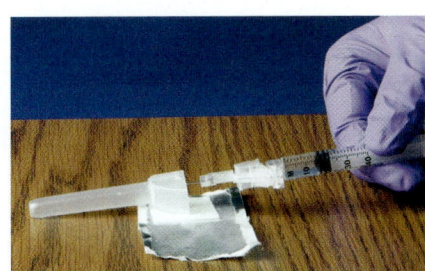

Documentation

No documentation needed for recapping needles.

Practice Resources

U.S. Department of Health and Human Services (USDHHS), National Institute for Occupational Safety and Health (NIOSH), n.d.; U.S. Department of Labor, Occupational Safety & Health Administration (OSHA), 2007; Wilburn, 2004.

Thinking About the Procedure

 Go to the *Fundamentals of Nursing Skills Videos,* **Medication: Parenteral, Recapping Sterile Needles: One-Handed Technique,** and **Recapping Contaminated Needles: One-Handed Technique.**

1. What is the safest method to prevent needlestick injury with a contaminated needle?
2. What are two goals when recapping a sterile needle?
3. If you do not have a safety needle, which method for recapping a sterile needle looks easiest to you?

 For suggested responses, go to Chapter 25, **Thinking About the Procedure Suggested Responses,** on Davis*Plus.*

Procedure 25–11 ■ Administering Intradermal Medication

> ➤ For steps to follow in *all* procedures, refer to the Universal Steps for All Procedures found on the page facing the inside back cover. Also refer to Medication Guidelines: Steps to Follow for All Medications (Regardless of Type or Route).

Equipment

- Alcohol prep pad or chlorhexidine gluconate (CHG)-alcohol product
- 2 in. x 2 in. gauze pad
- Pen (ink or felt)
- 1-mL syringe (tuberculin) with intradermal needle (25- to 28-gauge, ¼- to ⅝-in. with short bevel) ▼

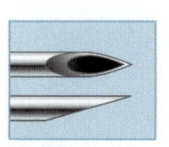 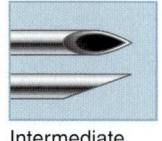 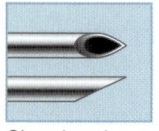

| Regular bevel | Intermediate bevel | Short bevel |

Delegation

As an RN, you can usually delegate administration of parenteral medications to an LPN/LVN. You usually cannot delegate this task to a NAP.

Pre-Procedure Assessments

- Assess for previous reaction to skin testing.
  Some skin tests, such as the tuberculin test, should not be repeated after positive test results.

- Assess for all types of allergies.
- Assess the skin at intradermal sites for bruising, swelling, tenderness, and other abnormalities.
  Do not give intradermal skin tests if skin abnormalities are present. Also avoid giving them in areas where reading the results may be difficult, such as areas of heavy hair growth.

Preparation

- Have appropriate antidotes (usually epinephrine hydrochloride, a bronchodilator, and an antihistamine) readily available before the start of the procedure.
  This is an important consideration because many intradermal injections are used for allergy testing, so the client is at risk for an anaphylactic reaction.
- Know the location of resuscitation equipment (artificial airway, Ambu bag, and code cart)
  Allergic reactions can be fatal.

> ➤ When performing the procedure, always identify your patient according to agency policy and be attentive to standard precautions, hand hygiene, patient safety and privacy, body mechanics, and documentation.

Procedure Steps

1. **Draw up the medication** from the vial (see Procedure 25-9B). The usual dose is 0.01 to 0.1 mL.
   Intradermal sites can accommodate only small volumes of medication.

2. **Select the site for injection.** Usual sites are the ventral surface of the forearm and upper back. The upper chest may also be used. If you need to review site locations, see Figure 25-19.
   Use areas where subcutaneous fat is less likely to interfere with administration and absorption. The forearm is the standard initial starting point because it has the least amount of subcutaneous tissue. The forearm and upper back usually have little hair, permitting easier visualization to interpret results accurately.

3. **Assist the patient to a comfortable position.** If you are using the forearm, instruct her to extend and supinate her arm on a flat surface. If

you are using the upper back, ask the patient to lie prone or lean forward over a table or the back of a chair.
This method stabilizes the injection site. Tension, in general, increases pain perception.

4. **Don procedure gloves.**
   Procedure gloves are not required by OSHA for intradermal injections, but they are recommended by the CDC to prevent accidental exposure to bloodborne pathogens. Remember, gloves cannot prevent needlestick injuries.

5. **Scrub the injection site** with an alcohol prep pad or chlorhexidine gluconate (CHG)-alcohol product pad. Allow the site to dry before administering the injection.
   Scrubbing removes microorganisms, following the principle of "clean to dirty." Allow to dry because alcohol can interfere with the test results if a small amount is introduced during the injection; also, if the

alcohol has not evaporated, it may cause the skin to sting during the injection.

6. **Hold the syringe between the thumb and index finger** of your dominant hand.
   Enables you to administer the solution at the correct angle.

7. **Hold the client's skin taut,** using one of the following methods, with your nondominant hand:
   a. If using the forearm, you may be able to place your hand under the client's arm and pull the skin tight with your thumb and fingers.
   b. Stretch the client's skin between your thumb and index finger.
   c. Pull the client's skin toward the wrist or down with one finger.
   A downward motion while stretching the skin eases needle insertion. Holding the skin taut can be difficult because of the low angle of administration.

8. While holding the client's skin taut with your nondominant hand, **hold the syringe in your dominant hand with the needle bevel up and parallel to the client's skin** at a 5° to 15° angle. Slowly insert the needle. Note that there is some controversy about whether it is better to have the bevel down or bevel up; however, the CDC recommends bevel up.

The low angle of insertion is necessary to place the needle tip in the intradermal layer instead of the subcutaneous tissue. Having the bevel up likely decreases the chance of injecting the medication deeper into the subcutaneous tissue. Patients receiving intradermal injections report bevel up more comfortable. See Figure 25-21.

9. **Advance the needle** approximately 3 mm (⅛ in.) so that the entire bevel is covered. The bevel should be visible just under the skin.
If the entire bevel is not inserted, the solution will leak out of the tissue. If you can see the bevel under the surface of the skin, you can be sure that the bevel is not in the subcutaneous tissue.

10. **Do not aspirate.** Hold the syringe stable with your nondominant hand, and release the tightened skin.

11. **Slowly inject the solution.** You should feel firm resistance. A pale wheal, about 6 to 10 mm (¼ in.) in diameter, will appear over the needle bevel.

The dermis does not have room to absorb the solution, so a wheal forms, stretching the skin. Slow administration gives you time to terminate the injection should a systemic reaction occur. If a bleb (wheal) forms, you have administered the drug properly. The size of the bleb depends on the amount of medication you injected. ▼

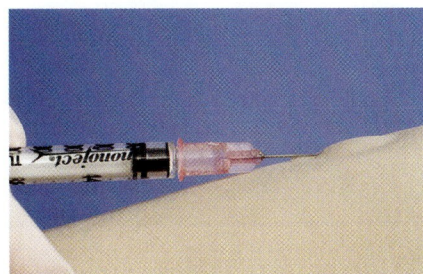

12. **Remove the needle,** engage the safety needle device, and dispose of the needle in a biohazard, puncture-proof container. If there is no safety device, place the uncapped syringe and needle directly in biohazard, puncture-proof container.
Prevents needlestick injuries.

13. **Gently blot any blood** with a dry gauze pad. Do not rub the skin or cover it with an adhesive bandage.
Rubbing may cause the drug to leak out and alter absorption. An adhesive bandage can cause irritation and interfere with the skin test.

14. **With a pen, draw a 1-inch circle** around the bleb/wheal.
Helps you to identify any change in the size of the wheal at a later time.

? What if . . .

- **My patient has a history of a skin reaction to PPD testing?**

Obtain details about the type and severity of the reaction. If the previous reaction involved ulceration at the site, further Mantoux testing is contraindicated. Report this to the prescriber.

- **My patient is pregnant, is receiving chemotherapy, or has severe eczema?**

Defer tuberculosis skin testing and inform the prescriber.

- **My patient received a live vaccine at the time of tuberculosis skin testing?**

Tuberculosis skin testing should be deferred for 1 month after live viral vaccines or other major viral infection.

- **My patient has topical anesthetic cream on the skin?**

Use a site where the topical anesthetic cream was not applied or reschedule tuberculosis skin testing for another date.

Evaluation

- Reassess the client 5 and 15 minutes after administration for allergic reactions that may subsequently occur.
- Read the site within 48 to 72 hours of injection, depending on the test.
- Observe that a wheal (about 6 to 8 mm in diameter) forms at the site and that it gradually disappears.
- Observe for minimal bruising that may develop at the site of injection.

- If the patient has antigens to the injected solution, a histamine response occurs, causing itching, swelling, or irritation. This response generally subsides within a week.
- Discuss the significance of a positive or negative skin test result. Explain that some signs of irritation may occur that do not mean a positive test result.
- Instruct the patient not to scratch, apply lotions or creams, cover the site with a bandage, or scrub the site.
- This might cause irritation and interfere with the test, which may produce false-positive results.

Patient Teaching

- Explain when the patient needs to have the intradermal injection read to determine whether the result is positive or negative.
- Explain that mild itching, swelling, or irritation may occur at the injection site and are normal.

Documentation

- See the information in Medication Guidelines: Steps to Follow for All Medication (Regardless of Type or Route).
- Some medications require documentation of lot numbers (check agency policy).
- Chart when the test is to be read.

(continued on next page)

Procedure 25–11 ■ Administering Intradermal Medication (continued)

Thinking About the Procedure

 Go to the *Fundamentals of Nursing Skills Videos,* **Medication: Parenteral, Intradermal Injection: Locating Sites and Administering.**

1. What site does the nurse in the video use to inject intradermal medication? Why does she choose that location?
2. For intradermal medication administration, what technique for holding the syringe does the nurse in the video use prior to injection?

3. For intradermal medication administration, what size needle will you typically use, excepting insulin?
4. When should you evaluate the site after administering medication intradermally?

 For suggested responses, go to Chapter 25, **Thinking About the Procedure Suggested Responses,** on DavisPlus.

Practice Resources

Howard, Mercer, Nataraj, et al., 1997; National Center for HIV, STD, and TB Prevention, Division of Tuberculosis Elimination, 2008.

Procedure 25–12 ■ Administering Subcutaneous Medication

➤ For steps to follow in *all* procedures, refer to the Universal Steps for All Procedures found on the page facing the inside back cover. Also refer to Medication Guidelines: Steps to Follow for All Medications (Regardless of Type or Route).

Equipment

- Syringe and needle appropriate for volume and site
- Alcohol prep pad or chlorhexidine gluconate (CHG)-alcohol product
- Gauze pad (optional)

Delegation

As an RN, you can usually delegate administration of parenteral medications to an LPN/LVN. You usually cannot delegate this task to a NAP.

Pre-Procedure Assessments

- Check the area for previous injection sites.
  Alternating among the arms, thighs, abdomen, and back changes the absorption rate of the medication. Absorption is fastest from the abdomen, then the arms, and finally the thighs and back. Rotate sites within the same extremity or location, approximately 1 inch from the previous injection. Rotating the site helps prevent the development of lipodystrophy.
- Do focused assessments for the specific medication being administered.
  Insulin—Check capillary blood sugar level, and determine when the patient will be having the next meal; check for signs of hypoglycemia or hyperglycemia.

  Insulin must be balanced with food intake to prevent the patient from developing hypoglycemia or hyperglycemia. Different insulins have specific rates of absorption, peak action, and duration. Some insulins, such as Humalog and regular insulin, are rapid acting. Before you administer rapid-acting insulin, the capillary blood sugar must be within the normal range or above, and the patient must be ready to eat. With Humalog, the patient's food tray should be in front of him before you administer the insulin.

  *Heparin—*Check activated partial thromboplastin time (aPTT) and for signs of bleeding, such as bleeding from gums, IV injection sites, and so on.
  Heparin is an anticoagulant, so the major side effect is bleeding. Check for overt bleeding as well as occult blood loss through the urine and stool. The aPTT will not be monitored as frequently with the low-molecular-weight heparins (LMWHs), because bleeding is less likely to occur.

➤ When performing the procedure, always identify your patient according to agency policy and be attentive to standard precautions, hand hygiene, patient safety and privacy, body mechanics, and documentation.

Procedure Steps

1. **Select an appropriate syringe and needle.**
   a. For insulin administration, you must use an insulin syringe—typically 0.3, 0.5, or 1.0 mL. Most insulin needles are 28- to 31-gauge. Needle length is often

   ³/₁₆ to 1 inch. For more information about giving insulin, see Clinical Insight 25-6.
   Although both insulin and tuberculin (TB) syringes come in a 1-mL size, they are not interchangeable. Insulin syringes are calibrated in units; they have a permanent (non-removable)

   needle and a very small amount of dead space.
   b. For other medications, for volumes less than 1 mL, use a tuberculin (TB) syringe with a 25- to 27-gauge, ³/₈- to ⁵/₈-inch needle.

Because of the small increments on the TB syringe, small doses can be measured more accurately. ▼

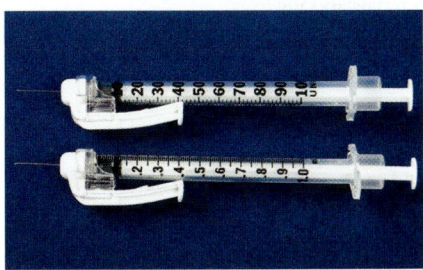

c. For administering a volume of 1 mL, you may use a 3-mL syringe with a 25- to 27-gauge, ⅜- to ⅜-inch needle.
Although you can measure 1 mL with a tuberculin (TB) syringe, it will be difficult to handle the syringe because the plunger will be pulled back as far as it can go. It is easy to pull it inadvertently out of the end of the syringe. Some medications are supplied in prefilled syringes. Examples are enoxaparin sodium (Lovenox) and the other low-molecular-weight heparins (LMWHs). These are usually supplied in unit-dose prefilled glass syringes.

2. **Draw up the medication.** See Procedure 25-9.

3. **Select an injection site** with adequate subcutaneous tissue. If you need to review site locations, see Figure 25-20.
Helps you avoid accidentally injecting into the muscle.

   a. The usual sites are the outer aspect of the upper arms, abdomen (at least 2 in. away from the umbilicus), anterior aspects of the thighs, and high on the buttocks near waist level.
   These areas usually have good circulation and are easily accessible. The buttocks are more convenient when someone is giving the injection other than the patient.

   b. The anterolateral and posterolateral abdomen ("love handles") sites are the only subcutaneous site used for administering heparin or low-molecular-weight heparins (LMWHs). For more information about giving heparin, see Clinical Insight 25-7.
   The tissue 2 inches away from the umbilicus poses less risk of bleeding when an anticoagulant is administered.

   c. Check the site for inflammation, bruising, lumps, or other abnormalities.
   Avoid areas with skin abnormalities, which may alter the absorption rates or increase patient discomfort during the injection.

4. **Position the patient** so that the injection site is accessible and the patient is able to relax the appropriate area.

5. **Don procedure gloves.**
To prevent exposure to bloodborne pathogens. You may prefer to don gloves before step 5; however, you can also do so after step 6 while waiting for the alcohol to dry.

6. **Scrub the injection site** with an alcohol prep pad or chlorhexidine gluconate (CHG)-alcohol product. Allow the site to dry before administering the injection.

7. **Remove the needle cap.**
The needle cap is more difficult to remove when using a one-handed technique.

8. **With your nondominant hand, pinch the tissue at the injection site,** and determine the angle at which to inject the needle. Insert the needle using a 90° angle. If the adipose tissue pinches 2 inches or more (client is obese), use a longer needle and spread the skin taut instead of pinching. See Figure 25-21.
Grasping and lifting the tissue prevents you from accidentally injecting into the muscle. Also, the subcutaneous injection must be given in the fatty tissue and not

into intradermal layer. Traditionally, injections had been using a 45° angle to ensure medication is deposited into the subcutaneous layer.

9. **Holding the syringe between thumb and index finger** of your dominant hand like a pencil or dart, insert the needle at the appropriate angle into the skinfold.
Quickly inserting the needle through the skin minimizes discomfort.

10. Using the thumb or index finger of your dominant hand, press the plunger slowly to inject the medication while stabilizing the syringe with your other hand. Alternatively, after inserting the needle, you can continue to hold the barrel with your dominant hand and use your nondominant hand to depress the plunger.
Slow administration allows the medication to disperse and decreases discomfort. Subcutaneous injections do not need to be aspirated beforehand, because accidental entry into a blood vessel is rare.

11. **Remove the needle** smoothly along the line of insertion.
Prevents pulling against the skin and tissue and thus minimizes discomfort.

12. **Gently wipe the site with gauze** if needed. Do not massage the site unless directed otherwise.
Occasionally there will be blood at the site after the needle is removed. You might have nicked a surface blood vessel when you injected, and blood is following the needle track out to the surface. Massaging or rubbing the site will alter the rate of absorption of the medication.

13. **Engage the needle safety device,** and dispose of the needle in biohazard container. If there is no safety device, place the uncapped syringe and needle directly into a biohazard, puncture-proof container.
A sharps container prevents needlestick injuries.

Evaluation

- Observe for minimal bruising that may develop at the site of injection.
- Reassess the patient for anticipated response and adverse reaction to medication.
  For insulin, observe for signs that patient's blood sugar level has returned to normal and for signs of hypoglycemia.

For heparin, observe that patient has no signs of bleeding. For other medications, observe for side effects.

Patient Teaching

Discuss possible lifestyle adaptations that the patient may need to undertake while receiving the medication, such as diet and exercise recommendations for managing diabetes mellitus.

(continued on next page)

Procedure 25-12 ■ Administering Subcutaneous Medication (continued)

Home Care

- Discuss with the client or caregiver the options for insulin administration to determine the most appropriate choice for the person administering the injections.

  Many options are available, including specially designed syringes that are easier to handle and read, pen injectors, and prefilled syringes.

- In the home environment the client might not routinely use an alcohol wipe to cleanse the site. This is acceptable as long as the skin is clean.

  In the home environment there is less risk for superinfection with resistant strain organisms, and other healthcare-acquired infections.

- Do not encourage reusing needles and syringes. However, if the client or caregiver believes they need to reuse syringes and needles in the home, teach them how to safely do so. Teach them the guidelines in Clinical Insight 25-2.

  Determine whether reusing syringes is appropriate for the patient. Contraindications include inadequate hygiene, immunocompromised status, and difficulty handling equipment to prevent contamination of the needle. The very small insulin needles (30-gauge) bend very easily and are not recommended for reuse.

- Discuss safety concerns regarding subcutaneous medication administration in the home, such as how to dispose of biohazardous wastes correctly and where to obtain a puncture-proof biohazard container.

  The patient or caregiver may use a large plastic bottle or a coffee can. Local regulations regarding disposal must be followed.

- Discuss with the patient the need to rotate sites and reasons for doing so. Recommendation that he give injections due at the same time of the day in the same body location about 1 inch from the previous injection site.

  Repeatedly giving the medication in the same site can cause abnormalities in the tissue and alter absorption rates.

- If the patient is receiving heparin or low-molecular-weight heparins (LMWHs), discuss the need to avoid NSAID medications, such as acetylsalicylic acid (aspirin) and ibuprofen (Motrin, Advil).

  These drugs increase the risk of bleeding.

- For patients receiving heparin or LMWHs, discuss home safety and the need to avoid falls.

  The patient is at risk for bleeding and needs to follow safety guidelines to prevent injury.

Documentation

- Chart according to Medication Guidelines: Steps to Follow for All Medication (Regardless of Type or Route).
- Some agencies have a specific code for documenting subcutaneous injections, which allows exact site documentation on an outline of the body.
- In the nursing notes, document any related patient assessment findings, such as capillary blood sugar, signs of hypoglycemia or hyperglycemia, bruising, and so on.
- Document in the nursing notes as well as MAR any medication that was given prn.

Practice Resources

Chan, 2001; Cocoman, & Barron, 2008; Rowan, 2006; Zaybak & Khorshid, 2008.

Thinking About the Procedure

 Go to the *Fundamentals of Nursing Skills Videos*, **Medication, Parenteral, Subcutaneous Injection: Locating Sites** and **Subcutaneous Injection: Administering.**

1. What are the most common sites for subcutaneous injection? At which site does the nurse demonstrate the procedure?
2. For subcutaneous medication administration, what size needle does the nurse say you will typically use, excepting insulin?

 For suggested responses, go to Chapter 25, **Thinking About the Procedure Suggested Responses,** on Davis*Plus.*

Procedure 25-13 ■ Locating Intramuscular Injection Sites

> ➤ For steps to follow in *all* procedures, refer to the Universal Steps for All Procedures found on the page facing the inside back cover. Also refer to Medication Guidelines: Steps to Follow for All Medications (Regardless of Type or Route).

Delegation

As an RN, you can usually delegate administration of parenteral medications (including locating injection sites) to an LPN/LVN. You usually cannot delegate this task to a NAP. If you delegate the skill, you are responsible for evaluating the LPN/LVN's ability to locate injection sites correctly.

Assessment

- Always palpate the landmarks and the muscle mass to ensure correct placement of the needle. Because patients body shapes differ, the site locations will vary slightly.

Procedure 25-13A ■ Locating the Ventrogluteal Site

➤ When performing the procedure, always identify your patient according to agency policy and be attentive to standard precautions, hand hygiene, patient safety and privacy, body mechanics, and documentation.

Procedure Steps

1. Ask the patient to assume **a side-lying position** with the legs straight, if possible.
This position makes the site easier to locate.

2. **Locate the greater trochanter,** anterior superior iliac spine, and the iliac crest.

3. **Place the palm of your hand on the greater trochanter,** your index finger on the anterior superior iliac spine, and your middle finger pointing toward the iliac crest. (Use your right hand on the patient's left hip; use your left hand on the patient's right hip.) Note that if your hands are very large or very small, the location of the "triangle" will be higher or lower on the hip. Be sure you locate it well in the muscle mass. ➤

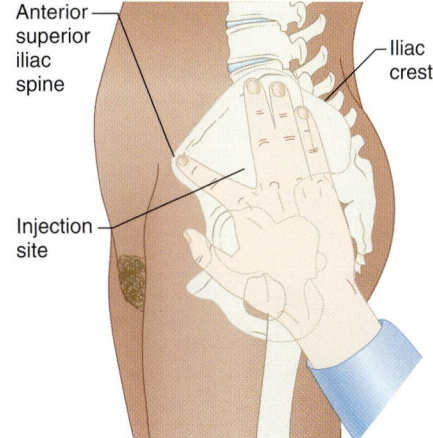

Anterior superior iliac spine — Iliac crest — Injection site

4. **The middle of the triangle between your middle and index fingers is the injection site.**
This is a safe site for IM administration because it is not in close proximity to any major blood vessels or nerves. The landmarks are easy to find. This large muscle

can take volumes up to 5 mL in the average adult. It is safe for patients of all ages and the preferred site for adults and children older than 7 to 12 months (there is some disagreement over the age; always palpate to assess adequacy of muscle mass, regardless of age). ▼

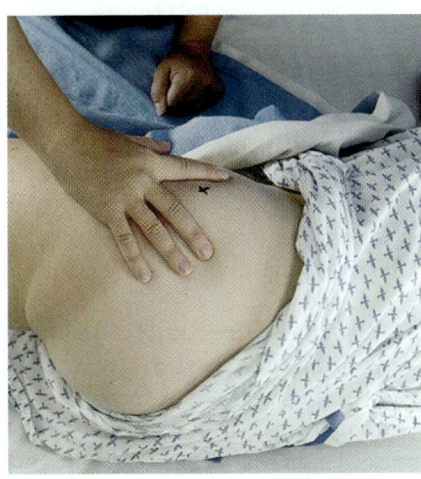

Procedure 25-13B ■ Locating the Deltoid Site

➤ When performing the procedure, always identify your patient according to agency policy and be attentive to standard precautions, hand hygiene, patient safety and privacy, body mechanics, and documentation.

Procedure Steps

1. **Completely expose the patient's upper arm.** Remove the garment; do not just roll up the sleeve.
Incomplete exposure of site and landmarks creates a risk of injecting into other than muscle tissue. This is a small site, and it is easy to make an error in location.

2. a. **Locate the lower edge of the acromion process** (knobby part of shoulder), and go two to three fingerbreadths down (3 to 5 cm). ▼

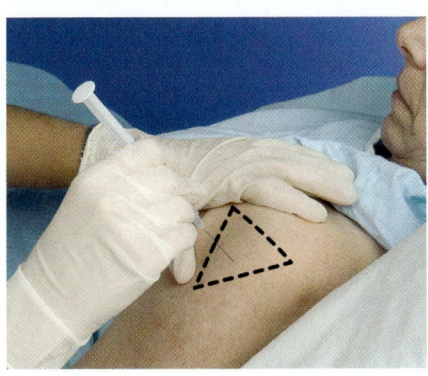

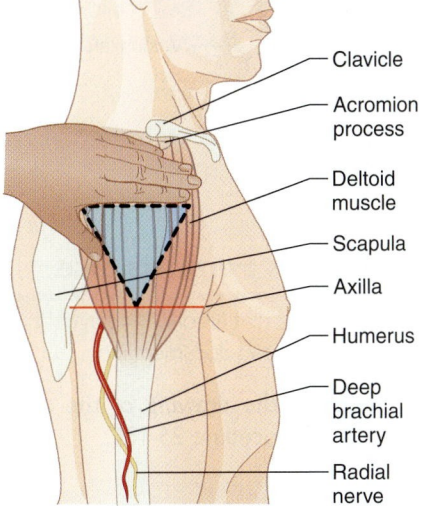

Clavicle — Acromion process — Deltoid muscle — Scapula — Axilla — Humerus — Deep brachial artery — Radial nerve

3. **Draw an imaginary line** from the anterior axillary crease to the posterior axillary crease.

4. **The deltoid site is the resulting inverted triangle.**

5. **An alternative approach** is to place four fingerbreadths across the deltoid muscle, with your top finger on the acromion process. The injection goes three fingerbreadths below the process in the midline of the upper arm.
Locates the appropriate site while avoiding the radial nerve and deep brachial artery. Because it is a fairly small muscle, only 0.5 to 1 mL of medication can be administered.

(continued on next page)

Procedure 25–13 ■ Locating Intramuscular Injection Sites (continued)

Procedure 25-13C ■ Locating the Vastus Lateralis Site

➤ When performing the procedure, always identify your patient according to agency policy and be attentive to standard precautions, hand hygiene, patient safety and privacy, body mechanics, and documentation.

Procedure Steps

1. **Position the patient lying supine or sitting.**
   The patient may perceive the injection as less painful if supine because he cannot see the needle enter his leg. For some people seeing the needle provokes anxiety and intensifies pain.

2. **Locate the greater trochanter** and the lateral femoral condyle.

3. **Place your hands on the thigh**, with one hand against the greater trochanter, and the other edge of hand against the lateral femoral condyle.

4. **Visualize a rectangle between your hands across the anterolateral thigh.** The index fingers of your hands form the smaller ends of the rectangle. The long sides of the rectangle are formed by (a) drawing an imaginary line down the center of the anterior thigh and (b) drawing another line along the side of the leg, halfway between the bed and the front of the thigh. This box marks the middle third of the anterolateral thigh, which is the injection site.
   The rectus femoris lies on the top (or anterior) portion of the thigh and partially covers the edge of the vastus lateralis. Therefore, do not inject too near
   the midline of the anterior thigh. Because it is not near any major blood vessels or nerves, the vastus lateralis site is safe for patients of all ages and recommended site for children younger than age 7 months. ▼

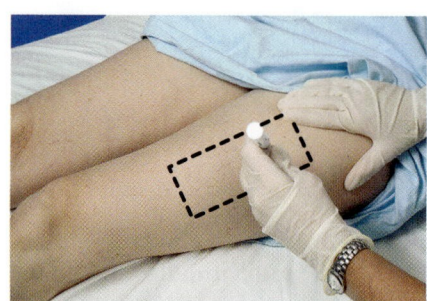

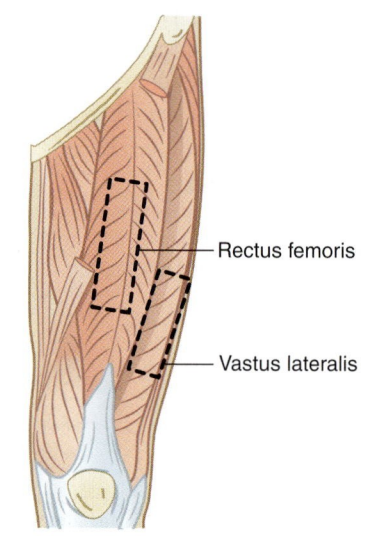

Rectus femoris

Vastus lateralis

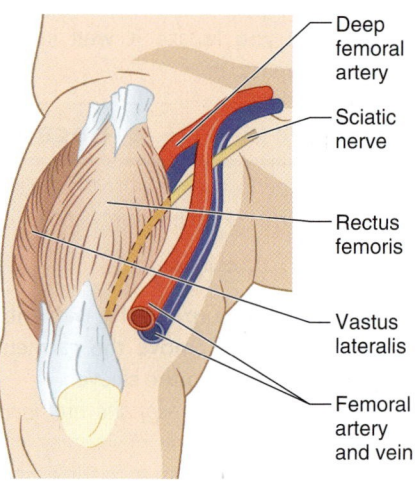

Deep femoral artery

Sciatic nerve

Rectus femoris

Vastus lateralis

Femoral artery and vein

Procedure 25-13D ■ Locating the Rectus Femoris Site

➤ When performing the procedure, always identify your patient according to agency policy and be attentive to standard precautions, hand hygiene, patient safety and privacy, body mechanics, and documentation.

✚ Use this site only if no other sites are accessible and no other medication routes are feasible.

1. Divide the top of the thigh from the groin to the knee into thirds, and identify the middle third.
2. Visualize a rectangle in the middle of the anterior surface of the thigh. This is the location of the injection site.

Refer to the drawing of the adult thigh in Procedure 25-13C.

❓ What if . . .

■ **My patient is a child. What is the best site to give an IM injection?**

Because an infant's muscles are not fully developed, site selection is limited.

For children who are walking, use the ventrogluteal site.
For children who are not yet walking: Do *not* use the ventrogluteal site. Use the vastus lateralis until the gluteal muscles develop further.

Thinking About the Procedure

Go to the *Fundamentals of Nursing Skills Videos,* **Medications: Parenteral, Intramuscular Injections: Locating Sites.**

1. What does the nurse say is the best way to ensure correct hand placement when giving IM injections?

2. Which two sites should be avoided for intramuscular injection?

For suggested responses, go to Chapter 25, **Thinking About the Procedure Suggested Responses,** on *DavisPlus.*

Procedure 25-14 ■ Administering an Intramuscular Injection

➤ For steps to follow in *all* procedures, refer to the Universal Steps for All Procedures found on the page facing the inside back cover. Also refer to Medication Guidelines: Steps to Follow for All Medications (Regardless of Type or Route).

Equipment

- Syringe and needle appropriate for volume and site
- Alcohol prep pad or chlorhexidine gluconate (CHG)-alcohol product
- Gauze pad or adhesive bandage
- Medication
- Procedure gloves
- Biohazard (sharps) container
- Small piece of gauze or cotton ball
- Small adhesive bandage

Delegation

As an RN, you can usually delegate administration of parenteral medications to an LPN/LVN. You cannot delegate this task to a NAP.

Pre-Procedure Assessments

- Identify the site of the previous injection.
- Assess the site for adequate muscle mass, bruises, edema, tenderness, redness, or other abnormalities.
  Muscle mass must be large enough to absorb the amount of medication prescribed. Abnormalities at the site increase patient discomfort and alter the absorption rate of the medication.
- Assess for factors that might affect absorption of the medication, such as decreased intramuscular blood flow, as found in shock or muscle atrophy.
  Decreased peripheral circulation or muscle atrophy decreases the absorption of the medication.

Procedure 25-14A ■ Intramuscular Injection: Traditional Method

➤ When performing the procedure, always identify your patient according to agency policy and be attentive to standard precautions, hand hygiene, patient safety and privacy, body mechanics, and documentation.

Procedure Steps

1. **Select the appropriate syringe and needle.**
   a. The usual syringe size is 1 to 3 mL, depending on volume of medication to be given. For doses less than 1 mL, you can use a tuberculin syringe with an intramuscular needle.
   b. The needle size is usually 21- to 25-gauge, 1½ inch in length for adults (or 1 in. for deltoid site) but a longer needle (3 in.) might be necessary to penetrate the muscle if the patient is obese.
   For IM administration, the needle gauge must be appropriate for the viscosity of the medication, and the needle must be long enough to deliver the medication into the muscle.
   c. Some medications are supplied in prefilled syringes, which are used for administration.

2. **Draw up the medication** (see Procedures 25-9A and 25-9B) or obtain prescribed unit dose and verify medication. If the volume for injection is more than 3 to 5 mL, divide the dose for separate injections.

3. **Don procedure gloves.**
   Procedure gloves are required by OSHA to prevent exposure to bloodborne pathogens. You may prefer to don gloves at step 6, while waiting for the antiseptic to dry.

4. **Using appropriate landmarks,** identify the injection site (see Procedure 25-13). If the client is to receive more than one injection, rotate sites.
   Volumes of 1 to 5 mL may be given, depending on the muscle size (for adults, 0.5 to 1 mL in the deltoid; and typically 1 to 3 mL but up to 5 mL in the vastus lateralis site). If the volume for injection is more than 3 to 5 mL, then divide the
   dose for a separate injection. Rotating sites reduces discomfort and tissue trauma.

5. **Position the patient** so that the injection site is well exposed and the patient is able to relax the appropriate muscles. Be sure the lighting is adequate.
   When the patient's muscles are relaxed (and not tense), it is easier to perform the injection and it helps to decrease patient discomfort during injection. You must be able to fully visualize and safely access the site.
   a. *Deltoid site:* Position the patient with the arm relaxed at the side or resting on a firm surface, and completely expose the upper arm.
   b. *Ventrogluteal site:* Position the patient on the opposite side, with the upper hip and knee slightly flexed.

(continued on next page)

Procedure 25-14 ■ Administering an Intramuscular Injection (continued)

This position causes the trochanter to become more prominent, making it easier to locate the site.

c. *Vastus lateralis:* Position the patient supine or sitting, if the patient prefers.

d. *Rectus femoris:* Position patient supine. Because this site often causes more discomfort than others, use it only if all other sites are inaccessible and no other route is feasible.

e. ✚ *Dorsogluteal:* Do not use this site because the sciatic nerve and major blood vessels are located near this site.

6. **Vigorously scrub the injection site** with a CHG-based antiseptic or an alcohol prep pad. Place the alcohol wipe on the patient's skin outside the injection site, with a corner pointing to the site. Allow the site to dry before administering the injection.
Cleanse to remove microorganisms; follow the principle of "clean to dirty." Leaving the alcohol prep pad on the skin with a corner pointing to the injection site helps identify the location for the injection. If the alcohol has not evaporated, it may cause the skin to sting during injection.

7. **Remove the needle cap.**

8. **With your nondominant hand, spread the skin taut** between your thumb and index finger.

It is quicker, easier, and less painful to insert a needle through the skin that is taut.

9. **After telling the patient what you are going to do** and that he'll feel a prick as you insert the needle, hold the syringe between thumb and fingers of your dominant hand like a pencil or dart and insert the needle at a 90° angle to the skin surface. Insert fully.
Quickly inserting the needle through the skin minimizes discomfort. A 90° angle is needed for the needle to penetrate through the subcutaneous and adipose tissue to the muscle.

10. **Stabilize the syringe** with your nondominant hand.
This prevents the needle from moving around in the tissue, thereby causing discomfort and possible tissue trauma.

11. **Aspirate by pulling back on the plunger** and waiting for 5 to 10 seconds. If you obtain a blood return, remove the needle, discard the syringe, and prepare the medication again. If there is no blood return, continue with step 12.
Aspirating blood indicates that the needle is in a blood vessel. Injecting would result in administering the medication intravenously instead of intramuscularly. If the needle is in a small vessel, it may take a few seconds for the blood to appear in the syringe. There are variations in practice regarding technique for pulling back the plunger to aspirate for blood. Be sure

to check with your instructor or the institution's protocol for the recommended method.

12. **Using the thumb or index finger** of your dominant hand, press the plunger slowly to inject the medication (5 to 10 sec/mL).
Slow administration allows the medication to disperse and decreases discomfort.

13. **Remove the needle** smoothly along the line of insertion and retracting needle carefully.
Removing the needle in this way prevents pulling against the skin and tissue and minimizes discomfort.

14. **Engage the safety needle device,** and dispose of the entire syringe in a biohazard container. If there is no safety device, place the uncapped syringe and needle directly into a biohazard puncture-proof container.
The biohazard sharps container prevents needlestick injuries.

15. **Gently blot the site** with a gauze pad, and apply an adhesive bandage as needed.
Apply pressure to stop the bleeding but do not massage or rub the site after IM injection. This can cause medication to disperse into the subcutaneous tissue where the needle was injected, which might be irritating to the tissue.

16. **Watch for an adverse reaction** at the site for 10 to 30 minutes after the injection.

Procedure 25-14B ■ Intramuscular Injection: Z-Track Method

➤ When performing the procedure, always identify your patient according to agency policy and be attentive to standard precautions, hand hygiene, patient safety and privacy, body mechanics, and documentation.

Procedure Steps

1–7. **Follow Procedure 25-14A,** traditional method, preceding.

8. **With the side of your nondominant hand,** displace the skin away from the injection site, about 2.5 to 3.5 cm (1 to 1.5 in.).
This displaces the skin and subcutaneous tissue over the muscle, so that when it is released after the injection, the medication is sealed in the muscle. ➤

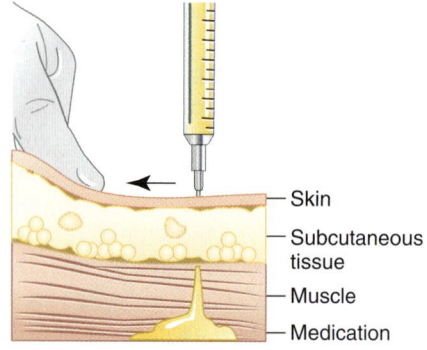

Skin is displaced from the needle after injection.

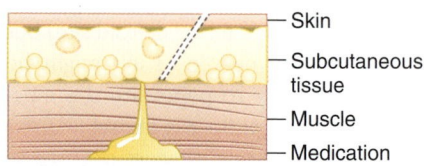

Medication is sealed in the muscle after skin is released.

9. **Holding the syringe between the thumb and fingers** of your dominant hand like a pencil or dart, insert the needle at a 90° angle to the skin surface. Insert fully.

Quickly inserting the needle minimizes discomfort. A 90° angle is needed for the needle to penetrate through the subcutaneous and adipose tissue to the muscle.

10. **Stabilize the syringe** with the thumb and forefinger of your nondominant hand. Keep displacing the skin with your other three fingers.

Stabilizing the needle reduces discomfort and possible tissue injury. You must keep the skin retracted to create a seal after the medication is injected and the skin released.

11. **Aspirate by pulling back slightly** on the plunger for 5 to 10 seconds. If you obtain a blood return, remove the needle, discard the syringe, and prepare the medication again.

Aspirating blood indicates that the needle has penetrated a vein. Continuing could result in administering the medication intravenously instead of intramuscularly. ▼

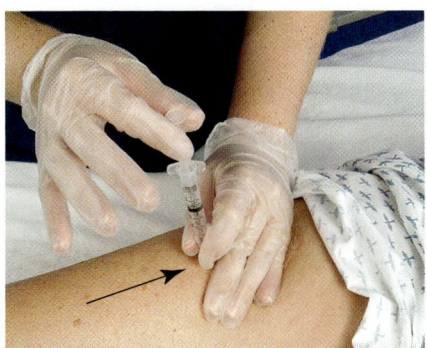

12. **Using the thumb or index finger** of your dominant hand, press the plunger slowly to inject the medication (5 to 10 sec. per mL).

Slow administration allows the medication to disperse and decreases discomfort.

13. **Wait for 10 seconds,** then withdraw the needle smoothly along the line of insertion; then immediately release the skin.

Waiting before removing the needle leaves a zig-zag needle track that traps the medication in the muscle, preventing it from leaking up into the subcutaneous tissue.

14. **Engage the safety needle device,** and dispose of it in a biohazard container. If there is no safety device, place the uncapped syringe and needle directly in a biohazard puncture-proof container.

15. **Hold a cotton ball with light pressure** over the injection site. Do not massage the site. Apply an adhesive bandage if necessary.

Light pressure will stop superficial bleeding at the injection site. Massaging and rubbing can force medication into the subcutaneous tissues.

? What if . . .

- **My patient is unable to cooperate during the procedure?**

  Ask another healthcare provider or family member to help keep the patient from moving during the injection or to help position the patient.

- **My patient is a child; is there anything different about giving an IM injection?**

  - Adapt the procedure to decrease pain: Apply topical anesthetic cream (e.g., EMLA) or a topical cooling spray if time permits. If not, distract the child with conversation, or give him something to do, such as squeeze a hand. Or apply a cold compress over the site.
  - Adapt the way you spread the skin to inject: In infants and small children, grasp the muscle with your thumb and index finger; in obese children, spread the skin and then grasp the muscle.
  - Adapt the medication volume: Inject no more than 1 mL in a single injection, 0.5 mL in a small infant
  - Be aware of the controversy about needle size: The CDC (2007) recommends 1- and 11/4-inch needles for children 1 year old or younger. Follow agency procedures.

- **My patient is an older adult?**

  - Many adults have decreased muscle mass, so use a shorter needle; spread the skin and grasp the muscle to localize and stabilize the site for injection.
  - Older adults tend to bleed from the site after injection because of reduced tissue elasticity. Apply a small pressure bandage if needed.

Evaluation

- Observe for minimal bruising or oozing that may occur at the site of injection.
- Observe for local reactions at site (e.g., pain, swelling, redness).

Home Care

- Discuss safety concerns with administering medication intramuscularly in the home, such as correct disposal of biohazardous wastes and where they can obtain a puncture-proof biohazard container.

  The caregiver or patient can use a large plastic bottle. The local regulations must be followed for disposal.

- Discuss with the client the need to rotate sites.

  Repeatedly giving the medication in the same site can cause abnormalities in the tissue and alter absorption rates.

Documentation

- Document related assessment findings, such as pain level or presence of nausea.
- Unless the medication is prn, you will typically document it only on the MAR.

Practice Resources

Floyd & Meyer, 2007; Kroger, Atkinson, Marcuse, et al., Advisory Committee on Immunization Practices (ACIP) Centers for Disease Control and Prevention, 2006; Nicholl & Hesby, 2002; Nisbet, 2006; Wynaden, Landsborough, McGowan, et al., 2006.

(continued on next page)

Procedure 25–14 ■ Administering an Intramuscular Injection (continued)

Thinking About the Procedure

 Go to the *Fundamentals of Nursing Skills Videos,* **Medication, Parenteral, Intramuscular Injection: Traditional** and **Intramuscular Injection: Z-Track.**

1. How does the nurse mark the site for injection after locating it using landmarks? Do you see any problem with this method?
2. Does the nurse pinch the skin or spread it taut when giving an IM injection using the traditional method?

3. In what instance would you use the Z-track method for administering IM medication?
4. Which IM site does the nurse use to inject medication using the Z-track technique?
5. What hand does the nurse use to inject IM Z-track medication? And what hand does she use to stabilize the syringe?

 For suggested responses, go to Chapter 25, **Thinking About the Procedure Suggested Responses,** on Davis*Plus.*

Procedure 25–15 ■ Adding Medications to Intravenous Fluid

➤ For steps to follow in *all* procedures, refer to the Universal Steps for All Procedures found on the page facing the inside back cover. Also refer to Medication Guidelines: Steps to Follow for All Medications (Regardless of Type or Route).

Equipment

- Prescribed IV solution
- Syringe for measuring medication
- Needleless access device or safety needle (if a VAD is not available)
- Antimicrobial swab
- Label with medication, dose, date, time, and your initials

Delegation

As an RN, you should usually not delegate adding medications to IV fluids to LPN/LVNs. Nurse practice acts governing IV medication administration vary from state to state, and policies can further vary among healthcare agencies regarding which additives may be added by LPN/LVNs. Even if you delegate the skill, as the RN you are always responsible for evaluating the patient's responses, both therapeutic effects and adverse effects.

Pre-Procedure Assessments

- Assess the patency of the IV site.
- Assess the appearance of the IV site.
- Check the medication insert or PDR for appropriate time or rate for infusion and for preparation.

Procedure 25–15A ■ Adding Medication to a New IV Bag or Bottle

➤ When performing the procedure, always identify your patient according to agency policy and be attentive to standard precautions, hand hygiene, patient safety and privacy, body mechanics, and documentation.

Procedure Steps

1. **Determine whether the medication(s) are compatible** with the IV solution and with each other.
   Not all medications or other additives can be mixed with the glucose or saline normally found in the primary IV bag. Multiple additives increase the possibility of incompatibility.
2. **Calculate or verify the amount** of medication to be instilled into the IV solution, and the rate of administration.
   Verifying the dose and the rate of infusion prevents medication errors.

3. **Remove any protective covers**, and inspect the bag or bottle for leaks, tears, or cracks. Inspect the fluid for clarity, color, and presence of any particulate matter. Check the expiration date.
   Double-checking the IV solution reduces the risk of infusing contaminated or expired solutions.
4. **Using the appropriate technique,** draw up the prescribed medication (see Procedures 25-9A and 25-9B, as needed). Alternatively, insert a VAD transfer device into the medication vial.

Medications can come in vials, ampules, or bags.
5. **Scrub all surfaces of the IV additive port** with an alcohol or chlorhexidine gluconate (CHG)-alcohol combination product.
   Diligent scrubbing with antimicrobial products reduces the transmission of microorganisms and helps maintain the sterility of the solution.
6. **Remove the cap from the syringe, insert the needle or the needleless access device into the**

injection port, and inject the medication into the bag, maintaining aseptic technique. ▼

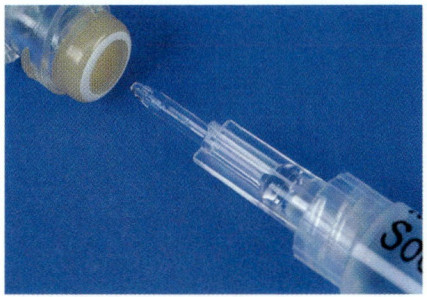

7. **Mix the IV solution and medication** by gently turning the bag from end to end.
   Ensures even distribution of the medication or additive into the solution.

8. **Place a label on the bag** so that it can be read when the bag is hung; include the medication name, dose, route, and your name. Be sure the label does not cover the solution label or volume marks.
   A label informs you of additives to IV solutions. ➤

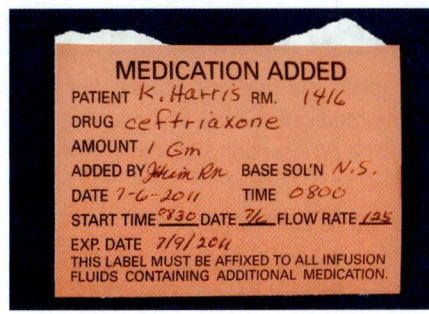

9. **Dispose of used equipment,** syringe, or VAD appropriately.

Procedure 25-15B ■ Adding Medication to a Running IV

➤ When performing the procedure, always identify your patient according to agency policy and be attentive to standard precautions, hand hygiene, patient safety and privacy, body mechanics, and documentation.

Procedure Steps

1. **Determine the compatibility** of the medication being added to the existing solution.
   Not all medications and solutions are compatible.

2. **Note the volume** in the existing IV bag and the amount needed for dilution of medication.
   Adequate solution is needed to dilute the medication.

3. **Clamp the running IV line.**
   Clamping prevents medication from directly infusing into the patient.

4. **Scrub all surfaces of the IV additive port** with the antimicrobial swab (alcohol or chlorhexidine gluconate [CHG]-alcohol combination product).
   Vigorous scrubbing decreases the transmission of microorganisms and maintains the sterility of the solution.

5. **Remove the cap from the syringe,** insert the safety needle or the VAD into the injection port, and inject the medication into the bag, maintaining aseptic technique. ➤

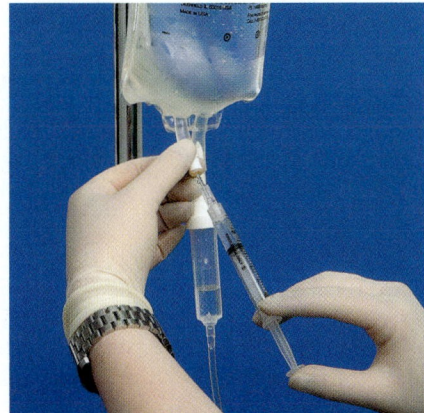

6. **Mix the IV solution and medication** by gently turning the bag from end to end. Keep the bag above the level of the patient's IV insertion site and do not invert the drip chamber.
   Turing the IV bag ensures even distribution of the medication or additive into the solution. Because of gravity, the height of the bag keeps blood from backing up in the IV tubing.

7. **Place the label on the bag** so that it can be read when the bag is hung. Be sure the label does not cover the solution label or volume marks.
   A label provides information regarding additives to IV solutions.

8. **Unclamp the IV line,** and run the IV at the prescribed rate.

9. **Dispose of used equipment,** syringe, needle or VAD appropriately.

? What if . . .

■ **The IV fluid infiltrates into a peripheral site?**

   ■ Discontinue the infusion. Restart the peripheral IV, making sure you have good blood return and the line flushes easily. Some IVs are positional. This means the flow may be partially obstructed when the cannula in the vein lodges against the vein wall. In this case, the rate the IV fluid to be delivered is likely to be compromised.

   ■ If the tissue at the site of infiltration appears to be swollen and tender, you might apply a cool compress to the site. If the infusion contained irritating substances, such as calcium, dopamine, or various chemotherapy agents, you might need to inject antidote medication into the intradermal layer. Call the prescriber for an order, if this is necessary.

Evaluation

■ Check the IV line at least once every hour to ensure that the ordered or calculated rate is maintained.
■ Assess the patient for complaints of pain at the infusion site.

Patient Teaching

■ Discuss reasons the medication is being given intravenously.
■ Let the patient know whether it is a continuous or intermittent infusion.

(continued on next page)

Procedure 25-15 ■ Adding Medications to Intravenous Fluid (continued)

- Explain the need to report immediately any reactions to the medication, such as breathing problems, rashes, or pain at the IV insertion site.

Documentation

- Document information according to Medication Guidelines: Steps to Follow for All Procedures (Regardless of Type or Route).
- If you added medication to an existing IV setup, document related patient assessment findings, such as appearance

of IV site and complaints of pain or discomfort during administration.

- Findings are usually documented on an IV flow record rather than in the nursing notes. Chart a nursing note only if there is something outside of the expected findings (e.g., if the IV has infiltrated).

Practice Resources
Infusion Nurses Society, 2006a, 2006b.

Procedure 25-16 ■ Administering IV Push Medication

➤ For steps to follow in *all* procedures, refer to the Universal Steps for All Procedures found on the page facing the inside back cover. Also refer to Medication Guidelines: Steps to Follow for All Medications (Regardless of Type or Route).

Equipment

- Syringe appropriate for medication volume and the type of line (e.g., peripheral IV, PICC)
- If you are administering through an intermittent device:
  Two 5- to 10-mL syringes, or one 10-mL syringe with 2 to 10 mL of normal saline for flushing the line
  Although either is acceptable, separate syringes pose less risk of contamination.
  Depending on site and facility policy, one 5- to 10-mL syringe containing 2 to 5 mL of heparin flush (or saline) solution
  Agency procedures differ: Some use saline to flush; others use heparin.
- Alcohol prep pad, or CHG-alcohol combination product and gauze pad
- Procedure gloves

Delegation

As an RN, you may, in some situations, be able to delegate administration of parenteral medications to an LPN/LVN. However, this is not a common practice.

Pre-Procedure Assessments

- Check the compatibility of the medication with the existing IV solution, if it is infusing.
  Medications can be physically or chemically incompatible with the IV solution. Physical incompatibility will often be obvious because precipitation may occur. Chemical incompatibility is not obvious and may result in the medication's having a weaker or a stronger effect than anticipated.
- Assess the patency of the IV line.
  If the line is occluded, you will not be able to instill the medication.
- Check the site for redness, swelling, tenderness, and other signs of infiltration or phlebitis.
  Some medications are irritating and may be toxic to the tissue. If the IV line is infiltrated, the medication may leak into the tissue and cause injury. IV medications can also irritate the veins and cause phlebitis. Do not infuse a medication into a compromised site.

Procedure 25-16A ■ Administering IV Push Through an Infusing Primary IV Line

➤ When performing the procedure, always identify your patient according to agency policy and be attentive to standard precautions, hand hygiene, patient safety and privacy, body mechanics, and documentation.

Procedure Steps

1. **Determine how fast the medication** may be administered and whether the medication needs to be diluted for administration. Also, check to be sure the medication is compatible with the solution infusing.
   IV push medications are frequently injected over 1 minute. Some medications

must be administered over a longer time period, and some require diluting before administration. Giving an IV push medication too fast and/or undiluted can result in local or systemic adverse reactions.

2. **Prepare the medication** from a vial or ampule or obtain the prescribed unit dose and verify medication with the order (refer to Procedure 25-9A and Procedure 25-9B).

Dilute as needed. Temporarily pause the infusion pump to administer the medication.

3. **Don procedure gloves.** Thoroughly scrub all surfaces of the injection port closest to the patient with the alcohol prep pad or CHG-alcohol combination product. Use povidone-iodine solution (Betadine) only if the patient is sensitive to the other products.

Follow agency policy. Some facilities require nurses to cleanse the port for 1 minute when accessing venous access devices. Using the port closest to the patient minimizes the distance the medication must travel and gets it into the patient's circulation faster. You must use an injection port, which is self-sealing. If you puncture the plastic IV tubing, it will leak.

4. **Insert the medication syringe** into the injection port. If a needleless system is not available, use a syringe with a safety needle.
   Using a needleless system prevents needle-stick injuries.

5. **Pinch or clamp the IV tubing** between the IV bag and the port.
   Occluding the tubing upline of the port prevents the medication from being injected back toward the IV bag. ▼

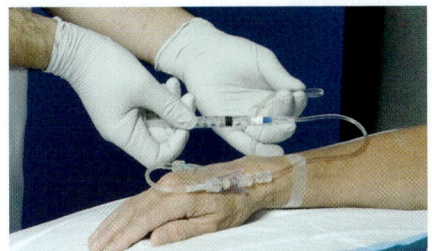

6. **Aspirate by slowly pulling back** on the plunger to check for a blood return.
   (1) A blood return is one indication that the IV catheter is in the vein. An IV site may still be patent if no blood is returned, and an infiltrated IV line may have a blood return. Use the blood return as one indication of patency (Phillips, 2010). (2) Injecting an IV medication into an IV site that is not patent administers the medication into the local tissue at the IV site. Some medications will cause tissue irritation and even necrosis if infused into the subcutaneous tissue. In addition, the patient would not receive the immediate therapeutic benefit from the drug.

7. **If blood is returned,** administer a small increment of the medication while observing for reactions to the medication.
   Slow injection allows you to observe adverse reactions to the medication before all the medication has been injected. Administering IV push medications carries the highest potential risk to the patient because immediate, life-threatening reactions can occur.

8. **Administer another increment** of the medication (you may pinch the tubing while injecting medication and release it when not injecting; this is optional).

9. **Repeat steps 7 and 8** until the medication has been administered over the correct amount of time.
   Medications require different administration times. Follow agency guidelines, physician orders, and pharmaceutical information regarding whether the medication needs to be diluted and the rate of administration.

10. **If you clamped the IV tubing** during the infusion, open it now and reset it to resume at the correct infusion rate.

11. Dispose of used supplies safely and according to agency procedures.

Procedure 25-16B ■ **Administering IV Push Through an Intermittent Device (IV Lock) When No Extension Tubing Is Attached to the Venous Access Device**

➤ When performing the procedure, always identify your patient according to agency policy and be attentive to standard precautions, hand hygiene, patient safety and privacy, body mechanics, and documentation.

Procedure Steps

1. **Check compatibility** of the medication with the existing intravenous solution, if one is infusing. Determine how fast the medication may be administered and whether the medication needs to be diluted for administration.
   IV push medications are frequently injected over 1 minute. Some medications must be administered over a longer time period, and some medications must be diluted before administration. Giving an IV push medication too fast and/or undiluted can result in an adverse local or systemic reaction.

2. **Prepare the medication** from a vial or ampule. Dilute as needed. Refer to Procedures 25-9A and 25-9B.

3. **Select the appropriate size of syringe** for flush solution.
   Smaller syringes exert more pressure against the wall of the IV catheter than do larger syringes. Check with the IV catheter company for specific recommendations, and follow agency policy.

4. **Don procedure gloves.** Thoroughly scrub all surfaces of the injection port closest to the patient with an alcohol prep pad or CHG-alcohol combination product. Use povidone-iodine solution (Betadine) only when the patient cannot tolerate an alcohol-based disinfectant.
   Follow agency policy. Some facilities require nurses to scrub all surfaces of the port with an alcohol-based antimicrobial product for 1 minute when accessing venous access devices. Using the port closest to the patient minimizes the amount of medication in the IV line.

5. **Insert the flush syringe into the injection port.**
   Flushing the line allows you to check for patency before injecting the medication.

6. **Gently aspirate by pulling back** on the plunger to check for a blood return.
   A blood return is an indication that the IV catheter is in the vein. An IV site may still be patent if no blood is returned, and an infiltrated IV may have a blood return. Use the blood return as one indication of patency.

(continued on next page)

Procedure 25-16 ■ **Administering IV Push Medication** (continued)

7. **Administer a flush solution** to clear the line if blood return is obtained. Use a forward pushing motion on the syringe, with a slow, steady injection technique.

   (1) Rapid flushing causes a jet effect that can cause the catheter tip to migrate to other venous locations; this should be avoided. (2) Injecting an IV medication into an IV site that is not patent administers the medication into the local tissue at the IV site. Some medications will cause tissue irritation and even necrosis if infused into the subcutaneous tissue.

8. **Continuing to hold the injection port**; remove the flush syringe; scrub the port with the alcohol prep pad or CHG-alcohol based product. Use povidone-iodine solution (Betadine) only when the patient is sensitive to alcohol-based disinfectants; and attach the medication syringe.

   Cleansing the port reduces the risk of introducing microorganisms into the bloodstream.

9. **Administer the medication** in small increments over the correct time interval.

   For example, if 1 mL of the medication is to be given over 1 minute, inject approximately 0.25 mL every 15 seconds. ▼

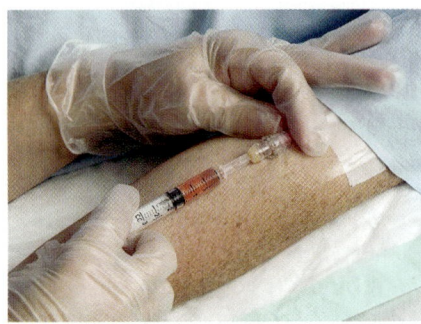

10. **Continuing to hold the injection port**, remove medication syringe, and scrub all surfaces of the port with alcohol prep pad or CHG-alcohol-based product. Attach the flush syringe.

    Vigorous scrubbing reduces the chance of contamination of the port.

11. **Administer the flush solution.**

    Flushing ensures that all the medication has been administered and prevents occlusion of the IV catheter.

12. **Use positive-pressure technique** when removing the syringe by placing your thumb or index finger to avoid movement of the plunger. Follow equipment guidelines; you may not always need to do this.

    This technique prevents blood backflow into the IV catheter, which might cause an occlusion. Follow equipment guidelines because some injection ports maintain positive pressure by removing the syringe and then closing the clamp. ▼

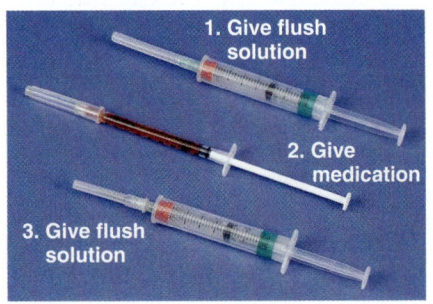

1. Give flush solution
2. Give medication
3. Give flush solution

Procedure 25-16C ■ **Administering IV Push Through an Intermittent Device with IV Extension Tubing**

➤ When performing the procedure, always identify your patient according to agency policy and be attentive to standard precautions, hand hygiene, patient safety and privacy, body mechanics, and documentation.

Procedure Steps

1. **Check the compatibility** of the medication with the existing intravenous solution, if one is infusing. Determine how fast the medication may be administered and whether the medication needs to be diluted for administration.

   IV push medications are frequently injected over 1 minute. Some medications must be administered over a longer time period, and some medications require diluting prior to administration. Giving an IV push medication too fast and/or undiluted can result in a local or systemic adverse reactions.

2. **Prepare the medication** from a vial or ampule. Dilute as needed. Refer to Procedures 25-9A and 25-9B.

   Some medications must be diluted to prevent adverse reactions during administration.

3. **Determine the volume of any extension tubing** attached to the access port.

   The volume of extension sets can be greater than the IV push medication being given. If not accounted for, all the medication may be injected into the patient's bloodstream at once when the second flush solution is given.

4. **Don procedure gloves.**

5. **Scrub all surfaces of the injection port** with an antiseptic wipe.

6. **Administer the flush** after gently pulling back on the plunger to check for a blood return. If blood is not returned, assess patency by administering a small amount of the flush solution

and monitoring for ease of administration, swelling at the IV site, or patient complaint of discomfort at the site.

7. **Again scrub the port.** Attach the medication syringe and inject a volume of medication equal to the volume of the extension set at the same rate as the flush solution.

   This clears the line of saline solution and fills it with medication; it also flushes the IV catheter with saline as the medication pushes the saline through the catheter. When using a 5-mL syringe for peripheral lines and a 10-mL syringe for central lines, administer the flush solution briskly. When you use a smaller syringe, use a slower rate to prevent excess pressure damaging the vein or shearing of the IV cannula. ➤

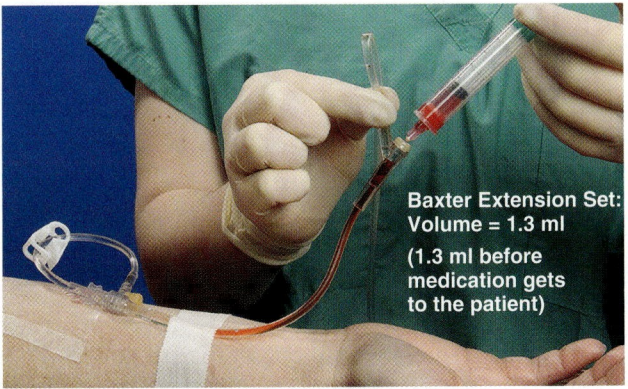

Baxter Extension Set:
Volume = 1.3 ml
(1.3 ml before
medication gets
to the patient)

8. **Using a slow, steady injection technique**, administer the remainder of the medication over the prescribed time interval. Never force the flush solution into the venous access device if you feel resistance. If you feel any resistance when flushing the line, look at the line for a closed clamp or kinked tubing. An inline filter might be clogged. Do not proceed with the medication infusion until you are sure the catheter is still correctly positioned and that the fluid pathway is unobstructed.
Rapid flushing can create a jet effect that can cause the catheter tip to migrate to an unintended venous location.

9. **Continuing to hold the injection connector**, remove the medication syringe, vigorously scrub all surfaces of the injection connector for at least 15 seconds and attach the flush syringe. The only time the catheter hub should be opened is when the needleless connector or primary continuous IV set must be changed (usually at 96-hr intervals).

10. **Administer the same amount of flush solution at the same rate** as the medication, using a slow, steady injection technique. Then administer the remainder of the flush solution. For example, if the extension tubing has a volume of 1.3 mL, give the first 1.3 mL of the flush solution at the same rate as the medication.

At this step, the extension tubing contains all the medication. Administering the flush solution all at once pushes the medication too fast (it will enter the vein all at once). Once you have cleared the medication from the extension tubing and all the medication is already in the vein, then the rate no longer matters as far as the medication is concerned.

11. **Use a slow steady injection pressure** when removing the syringe. Continue to administer the flush solution while withdrawing the syringe cannula from the injection port. Follow equipment instructions regarding the method and order of removing the syringe, closing the clamp, maintaining positive pressure.

12. **Discard the flushing syringe** from the needleless connector into a safety disposal container.

? What if . . .

■ **No blood is returned when I aspirate?**

Do not give IV push medication until you can verify the patency of the IV site. If the patency of the IV site is questionable, restart the IV at another site.
Further assess the patency of the IV line by administering a small amount of the saline flush and monitoring for

ease of administration, swelling at the IV site, or patient complaint of discomfort at the site.
Another technique to determine patency is to lower the IV bag below the level of the IV site—a blood return should occur
If the IV catheter is a small gauge, a blood return may not always be aspirated.

■ **There is resistance when flushing the line?**

Never force the flush solution into the VAD; look for a closed clamp on the catheter or tubing. Or you may check to see if an inline filter is clogged. Do not proceed with the medication infusion until you are sure the catheter is still correctly positioned and that the fluid pathway is unobstructed.

■ **The IV infusing a dextrose solution infiltrates into the surrounding tissue of a peripheral catheter?**

Immediately stop the running fluid and remove the catheter. Initially apply a cool, moist compress to the site and later use heat to promote comfort.
Infiltration can cause tissue injury, inflammation, and edema and may even lead to tissue necrosis and sloughing.

■ Some medications, such as vasopressors (e.g., dopamine), might need intradermal injection of an antidote, such as phentolamine (Regitine), to reverse the effects of extravasation.

■ If the IV fluid contains dextrose at greater than 10% concentration, calcium salts, potassium salts, sodium bicarbonate, blood, and parenteral nutrition, contact the primary care provider, who will likely prescribe injection of hyaluronidase (Amphadase) into the surrounding tissue.

Evaluation

■ Assess the patient for pain or discomfort at the site.

Patient Teaching

■ Discuss why the medication is being administered intravenously.

■ Explain the need to report immediately any reaction to the medication.

Home Care

■ Teach the client and/or caregiver how to care for the IV site, including flushing. Many IV push medications need to be

(continued on next page)

Procedure 25-16 ■ Administering IV Push Medication (continued)

administered by a nurse. However, cost-cutting efforts have led to short hospital stays, and some clients are now being taught to give their own IV antibiotics at home.

- Explain how to identify problems with the IV site, such as infiltration and phlebitis.
- Determine whether the client has adequate facilities for storing the medication, such as refrigeration if needed.
- Discuss safety issues, such as keeping medications and needles and syringes secure and away from children and pets.

Documentation

- Besides charting according to Medication Guidelines: Steps to Follow for All Medications (Regardless of Type or Route), document related patient assessment findings, such as the appearance of the IV site and patient complaints of pain or discomfort during IV administration.
- You will usually document on an IV flow record and/or MAR rather than in the nursing notes. Chart a nursing note only if there is a problem (e.g., if the patient experiences pain when you administer the medication).

Practice Resources

Infusion Nurses Society, 2006a, 2006b; Phillips, 2010.

Thinking About the Procedure

 Go to the *Fundamentals of Nursing Skills Videos*, **Medication, Intravenous: IV Push Through a Primary Line** and **IV Push Through an IV Lock.**

1. When administering an IV push through a primary IV line, what is the technique the nurse uses to ensure the line is patent and the medication doesn't cause an immediate adverse effect?
2. When administering medication by IV push through an intermittent device (IV lock), the nurse aspirates blood back into the extension tubing to check for IV patency. How does she clear the tubing of the blood, and why?

 For suggested responses, go to Chapter 25, **Thinking About the Procedure Suggested Responses,** on *DavisPlus.*

Procedure 25-17 ■ Administering Medications by Intermittent Infusion

➤ For steps to follow in *all* procedures, refer to the Universal Steps for All Procedures found on the page facing the inside back cover. Also refer to Medication Guidelines: Steps to Follow for All Medications (Regardless of Type or Route). For step-by-step instructions in using volume-control devices (pumps), see Procedure 39-9.

Equipment

- Correct size syringe for measuring medication
- Needleless access cannula or safety needle
- Volume-control IV set (e.g., Buretrol, Volutrol, Soluset) or small bag of diluted medication with piggyback or tandem tubing
- Primary IV solution and tubing (unless one is already infusing)
- Antimicrobial swabs
- Labels for the IV tubing and medication administration system

Delegation

Nurse practice acts governing IV medication administration vary from state to state, and policies can further vary among healthcare agencies, regarding which medications or methods of administration the LPN/LVN may perform. You should not delegate this procedure to a NAP.

Pre-Procedure Assessments

- ✚ Check the compatibility of the medication with the IV solution.
  Medications can be physically or chemically incompatible with the IV solution. Physical incompatibility will be obvious if precipitation occurs. Chemical incompatibility is not obvious and may result in the medication's having a weaker or a stronger effect than anticipated.

- Assess the patency of the IV line.
  If the line is occluded, or if the fluid has infiltrated, the medication will not infuse.

- ✚ Check the site for redness, swelling, tenderness, and other signs of infiltration or phlebitis.
  Some medications are irritating to the tissue. If the IV fluid has infiltrated, medication would leak into the tissue and cause injury. IV medications can also irritate the veins and cause phlebitis. Do not infuse a medication into a compromised site.

- Determine the amount of IV solution needed to administer the specific medication.
  Most medications specify (on the order or on the label) specific dilution to prevent potential harm to the patient.

- Determine the time period over which the solution needs to be infused.
  Infusing a medication too slowly may result in an inadequate blood level to achieve therapeutic levels, and infusing a medication too rapidly can cause harm.

- Perform assessments that will provide a basis for evaluating the drug's effectiveness, such as checking blood pressure after administering an antihypertensive agent.

Procedure 25-17A ■ Using a Volume-Control Administration Set

➤ For step-by-step instructions in using volume-control devices (pumps), see Procedure 39-9. If you have not already done so, affix a label to the secondary bag indicating the name and amount of medication, date and time given, and your name or initials.

➤ When performing the procedure, always identify your patient according to agency policy and be attentive to standard precautions, hand hygiene, patient safety and privacy, body mechanics, and documentation.

Procedure Steps

1. **Prepare the volume-control set tubing**.

   a. Close both the upper and lower clamps on the tubing, if they are not already closed.
   Clamping prevents air bubbles from forming in the tubing.

   b. Open the clamp of the air vent on the volume-control chamber.
   Venting allows air to escape so the IV solution can enter the chamber.

   c. Maintaining sterile procedure, attach administration spike of the volume-control set to the primary IV bag.

   d. Fill the volume-control chamber with the desired amount of IV solution by opening the clamp between the IV bag and the volume-control chamber. When the correct amount of solution is in the chamber, close the clamp.
   The drip chamber provides solution for priming the tubing and diluting the IV medication.

   e. Prime the rest of the tubing by opening the clamp below the chamber and running the IV fluid until all the air has been expelled.
   Priming clears the IV tubing of air.

   f. Recheck the amount of fluid in the volume control chamber, and, if needed, add more fluid to the desired amount.
   Priming the tubing alters the volume in the chamber. You must fill to the desired amount.

2. **With an alcohol or chlorhexidine gluconate-alcohol swab**, vigorously scrub all surfaces of the injection port closest to the patient.
   Removes microorganisms and particles from the IV port, which could potentially enter the patient's bloodstream.

3. **Connect the end of the volume-control IV line** to the patient's IV site. Attach it directly to the IV catheter, to the extension tubing, or to the injection port closest to patient.

4. **Scrub the injection port** on the volume-control chamber, attach the medication syringe (preferably with a blunt, needleless device), and inject the medication into the solution in the chamber.

5. **Gently rotate the chamber** to mix the medication in the IV solution.
   Distributes the medication within the IV solution.

6. **Open the lower clamp,** and start the infusion at the correct flow rate.
   Unclamping allows the infusion of the medication. A correct flow rate infuses the medication over the correct amount of time and prevents a toxic reaction to it.

7. **Label the volume-control chamber** with the date, time, medication and doses added, and your initials, according to agency policy.

8. **When the medication has finished infusing**, add a small amount of the primary IV fluid to the chamber, and flush the tubing. For the flush volume, use two times the volume in the dead space of the tubing; check the tubing package for the amount.
   Flushing the line ensures all the medication is given to the patient and does not adhere to the tubing. ▼

9. Dispose of used supplies safely and according to agency procedures.

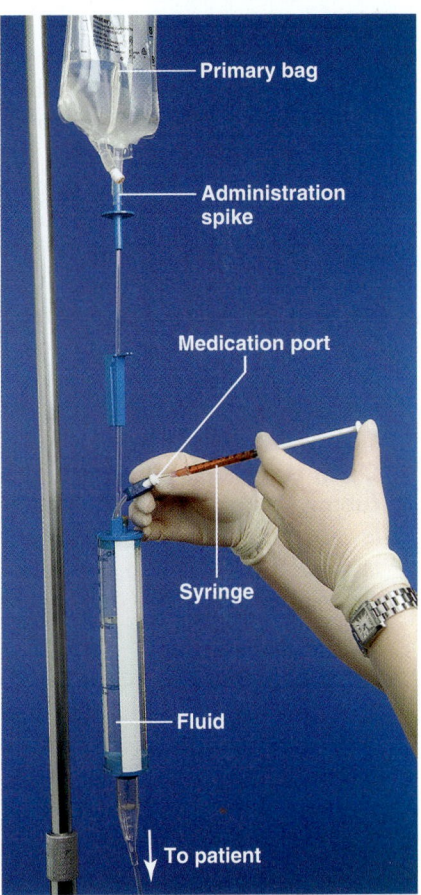

— Primary bag

— Administration spike

— Medication port

— Syringe

— Fluid

↓ To patient

Thinking About the Procedure

 Go to the *Fundamentals of Nursing Skills Videos,* **Medication: Intravenous, Administration Sets: Volume-Control.**

1. When using a volume-control administration set to infuse medication, what does the nurse do to ensure the patient has received the entire medication dose?

 For suggested responses, go to Chapter 25, **Thinking About the Procedure Suggested Responses,** on DavisPlus.

(continued on next page)

Procedure 25-17 ■ Administering Medications by Intermittent Infusion (continued)

Procedure 25-17B ■ Using a Piggyback Administration Set

➤ For step-by-step instructions in using intermittent infusion devices (pumps), see Procedure 39-3. If you have not already done so, affix a label to the secondary bag indicating the name and amount of medication, date and time given, and your name or initials.

➤ When performing the procedure, always identify your patient according to agency policy and be attentive to standard precautions, hand hygiene, patient safety and privacy, body mechanics, and documentation.

Procedure Steps

1. **Draw up the medication**, and inject it into the piggyback solution (see Procedure 25-15).

   This step is not necessary if the medication comes premixed from the pharmacy, which is frequently the case.

2. **Be sure you have the correct tubing.** Attach the piggyback tubing to the medication bag. Do not touch the spike.

   Tubing connects the piggyback to the primary line. Prevents contamination of tubing and solution. Piggyback tubing is short. Tandem tubing is long.

3. **Be sure the slide clamp is closed.** Squeeze the drip chamber, filling it one-third to one-half full.

   Clamping prevents excess air coming into the line when you are priming the tubing.

4. **Open the clamp and prime the tubing,** holding the end of the tubing lower than the bag of fluid. Do not let more than one drop of fluid escape from the end of the tubing. Close the clamp.

"Backflushing" the Piggyback Line

   a. As an alternative, you can clamp the piggyback tubing, scrub all surfaces of the primary "Y" port, and attach the piggyback setup with the needleless system.

   b. Open the clamp on the piggyback tubing, and lower the bag below the primary to prime the piggyback line.

   c. Once the line is primed, clamp the piggyback tubing.

   Priming removes air from the tubing and maintains sterility of the system. Medications are diluted in small amounts of fluid (usually 50 to 100 mL), so you cannot waste any medication. The backflush method ensures you will not do so.

5. **Label the bag with the date,** the medication, the dosage, and your initials. Label the tubing with the time, the date, and your initials.

   Tubing used for intermittent infusions can be used for 48 to 72 hours, depending on facility policy; labeling allows the nurse to know when it must be changed.

6. **Hang the piggyback container** on the IV pole. Lower the primary IV container to hang below the level of the piggyback IV.

   Gravity causes the higher bag (the piggyback IV setup) to flow instead of the primary IV setup. When the piggyback IV solution has infused, the primary IV line will resume infusing.

7. **Open the clamp of the piggyback** line, and regulate the drip rate with the roller clamp on the primary line. Regulate to the prescribed infusion rate for the medication. ▼

Because the piggyback is the only bag running, the primary roller clamp regulates the speed of the piggyback bag.

8. **At the end of the infusion,** clamp the piggyback tubing, and move the primary tubing back to its original height. Use the roller clamp to reset the primary bag to its correct infusion rate.

   This ensures that the primary fluids flow at their ordered rate rather than flowing at the rate the piggyback medication was flowing—which would probably be either faster or slower than the prescribed primary fluid rate.

9. Dispose of used supplies safely and according to agency procedures.

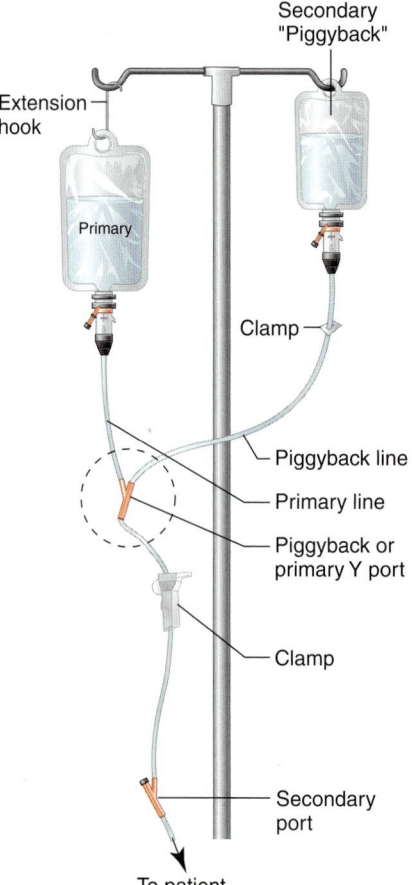

Secondary "Piggyback"

Extension hook

Primary

Clamp

Piggyback line

Primary line

Piggyback or primary Y port

Clamp

Secondary port

To patient

Thinking About the Procedure

 Go to the *Fundamentals of Nursing Skills Videos,* **Medication: Intravenous, Administration Sets: Piggyback.**

 For suggested responses, go to Chapter 25, **Thinking About the Procedure Suggested Responses,** on Davis*Plus.*

1. Which bag is in a higher position? Why?
2. How is the primary bag hung below the level of the piggyback bag?

Procedure 25-17C ■ Using a Tandem Administration Set

➤ For step-by-step instructions in using intermittent infusion devices (pumps), see Procedure 39-3. If you have not already done so, affix a label to the secondary bag indicating the name and amount of medication, date and time given, and your name or initials.

➤ When performing the procedure, always identify your patient according to agency policy and be attentive to standard precautions, hand hygiene, patient safety and privacy, body mechanics, and documentation.

Procedure Steps

1. **Draw up the medication**, and inject it into the tandem solution (see Procedure 25-15A). This step is not necessary if the medication comes premixed from the pharmacy, which is frequently the case.
2. **Be sure you have the correct tubing.** After closing the clamp on the tubing, attach the tandem tubing to the (medication) bag. Do not touch the spike.
   Tubing connects the tandem set to the primary line. Prevents contamination of tubing and solution. Tubing for the tandem set is longer so the bag can be hung for gravity infusion, if a pump is not in use.
3. **Squeeze the drip chamber**, filling it one-third to one-half full.
   Fluid in the drip chamber prevents excess air in line when priming tubing.
4. **Open the clamp and prime the tubing**, holding the end of the tubing lower than the bag of fluid. Do not let more than one drop of fluid escape from the end of the tubing. Close the clamp.

"Backflushing" the Tandem Line

   a. As an alternative, you can clamp the tandem tubing, scrub the tandem port (the one nearest the patient), and attach the tandem tubing with the needleless system.
   b. Open the clamp on the tandem tubing, and lower the bag below the primary line to prime the tandem line.
   c. Once the line is primed, clamp the tubing.
   Priming removes air from the tubing and maintains sterility of the system. Medications are diluted in small

amounts of fluid (usually 50 to 100 mL), so you cannot waste any medication. The backflush method ensures that you will not lose any medication while clearing the line of air.

5. **Label the bag with the date**, the medication, the dosage, and your initials. Label the tubing with the time, the date, and your initials.
   Tubing used for intermittent infusions can be used for 48 to 72 hours, depending on facility policy; allows the nurse to know when it must be changed.
6. **Hang the tandem bag** at the same height as the primary bag. ▼

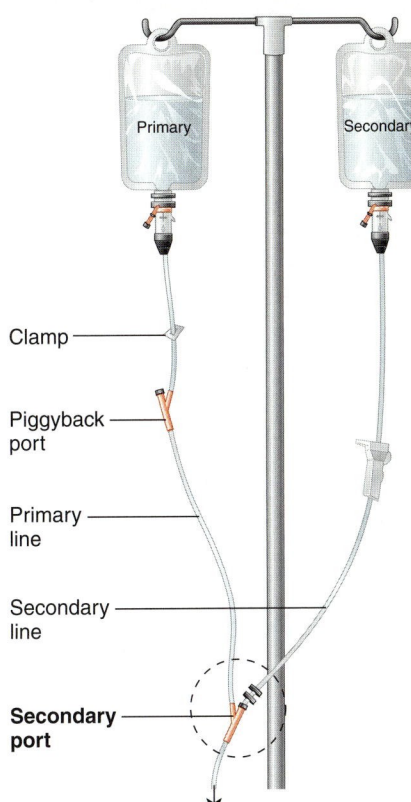

Clamp

Piggyback port

Primary line

Secondary line

Secondary port

To patient

7. **Scrub all surfaces of the lower port** of the primary line with an antimicrobial swab, and connect the tandem tubing to this port with needleless system. (If you backflushed in step 4, the tubing will already be connected.)
   Scrubbing prevents contamination.
8. **When you are using a tandem set**, both the tandem and primary sets run simultaneously. Unclamp the tandem tubing, and regulate the tandem rate at its prescribed infusion rate—the tandem line has its own roller clamp. You also need to verify the primary set flow rate.
   Verifying the medication dosage ensures that the medication is administered at a rate that will provide desired therapeutic effects and reduce possibility of adverse reactions. Infusing the tandem set may change the rate of infusion of the primary set.
9. **At the end of the infusion, clamp** the tandem tubing. The primary bag should continue to flow at its prescribed rate.
10. **Dispose of used supplies safely** and according to agency procedures.

(continued on next page)

Procedure 25–17 ■ Administering Medications by Intermittent Infusion (continued)

Evaluation

- Assess for pain or discomfort at the site.
- Intermittent infusions are generally administered over 15 to 60 minutes; therefore, you need to assess the patient as soon as the medication begins infusing and every 15 to 20 minutes until it is absorbed.

Patient Teaching

- Discuss why the medication is being administered intravenously.
- Explain the need to report immediately any reaction to the medication.

Home Care

- Discuss with the client and/or caregiver how to care for the IV site. Only a nurse should add medications to the IV.
- Explain how to identify problems with the IV site, such as infiltration and phlebitis.
- Assess whether the client has adequate facilities for storing the medication, such as refrigeration if needed.
- Discuss safety issues, such as keeping medications, needles, and syringes secure and away from children and pets.

Documentation

- Chart information according to Medication Guidelines: Steps to Follow for All Medications (Regardless of Type or Route).
- Document related patient assessment findings, such as the appearance of the IV site and patient complaints of pain or discomfort during the administration.

Practice Resource

Infusion Nurses Society, 2006a.

Thinking About the Procedure

 Go to the *Fundamentals of Nursing Skills Videos*, **Medication: Intravenous, Administration Sets: Tandem.**

1. When priming the tubing of a tandem administration set, what does the nurse do with the solution flushed through the line? Why?

 For suggested responses, go to Chapter 25, **Thinking About the Procedure Suggested Responses,** on Davis*Plus.*

Procedure 25–18 ■ Administering Medication Through a Central Venous Access Device

> ➤ For steps to follow in *all* procedures, refer to the Universal Steps for All Procedures found on the page facing the inside back cover. Also refer to Medication Guidelines: Steps to Follow for All Medications (Regardless of Type or Route).

Equipment

- Syringe appropriate for medication volume
- Needleless device or safety syringe with a filter needle for drawing up the medication (you would also need a sterile needle for injection).
- Two syringes for the flush solution
- Saline or heparin flush solution, as prescribed
- Alcohol prep pad or CHG-alcohol combination product and gauze pad
- Procedure gloves

Pre-Procedure Assessment

- Carefully palpate the area around the insertion site through the dressing. If the patient has tenderness, assess for other signs of infection. Check the surrounding catheter insertion site for redness, swelling, warmth, or drainage.
  These can indicate catheter-related infection.
- For all types of CVADs, assess the patient's external chest wall for engorged veins at the surface of the skin. Also check for difficulty moving the neck or jaw, headache, or ear pain.
  These can indicate vein thrombosis.
- Conduct a comprehensive pain assessment, being alert for unusual pain or discomfort.
  Chest discomfort could be associated with the catheter's position in the vein, especially if the line is not in an optimal position.

Procedure Steps

➤ When performing the procedure, always identify your patient according to agency policy and be attentive to standard precautions, hand hygiene, patient safety and privacy, body mechanics, and documentation.

1. Prepare the medication.

a. Check compatibility of the medication with the existing IV solution, if one is infusing.

b. ✚ Verify the medication can safely be administered through a central site. Double check the infusion rate as well.
   Some medication might be incompatible with infusion solution or additives. Because dosage may be different for medications given centrally versus peripherally, and because the medication enters the heart almost instantly, any error is potentially life threatening.

c. Draw up the medication using a needleless device or needle with a filter. Then change to a sterile needle or needleless device for administering the medication.
   Filter needles prevent small particles from entering into the line.

d. Recap needles throughout, using a needle capping device or approved one-handed technique that has a low risk of contaminating the sterile needle (see Procedure 25-10B: Recapping Sterile Needles).
   Recapping prevents needlestick injury and, performed correctly, maintains the sterility of the needle.

e. Dilute the medication, if needed. Fill the medication syringe to the exact volume to be infused; expel excess volume.

f. Label the syringe with the contents, including medication name, dilution, time to be administered, route, name of person constituting the medication.
   Excess volume of medication in the syringe is a risk for inadvertent overdosing.

2. Flush the line.

a. Obtain heparinized or saline solution for flushing the CVAD, following the institution's protocol or as prescribed.
   The usual concentration for heparin is 10 to 100 units/mL of solution for adults. The recommended volume of flush varies by institution. Most facilities recommend 3 to 5 mL of solution to flush the catheter, although some are flushed with 10 mL to flush the line. Some medication might be incompatible with infusion solution or additives. Because dosage may be different for medications given centrally versus peripherally, and because the medication enters the heart almost instantly, any error is potentially life threatening.

✚ Using heparin flush in venous access devices is becoming more controversial because of the potential for heparin-induced thrombocytopenia. Be sure to follow the prescriber's order and the policy of your institution.

b. Before flushing the CVAD, examine the syringe for bubbles. Remove them by flicking the syringe. Eject the bubbles, but be sure you have enough flush solution remaining in the syringe.
   This allows the bubbles to rise to the top. Remove bubbles from the syringe before giving medication through the CVAD port to avoid injecting air into the patient's vein.

c. With clean procedure gloves, using pressure and friction, vigorously scrub all surfaces of the CVAD connectors as well as the luer-locking threads, or the luer lock, including the extension "tail," with an alcohol wipe, CHG-alcohol combination product, or other antimicrobial product for at least 15 seconds. Then let it dry for 15 seconds. Do not touch this connector after cleansing.
   Antimicrobial swabs reduce the risk of line-related infection by decreasing colonization of the port and tubing.

d. Insert the flush syringe at a vertical angle into the port using a needleless system or safety syringe.
   A 90° angle reduces stress on the access port, which may cause shearing or mechanical trauma to the material.

e. Open the clamp between the syringe and the patient.
   The clamp between the access port and the tubing that goes to the patient needs to be patent for medication to be injected through the CVAD.

f. Check for blood return by pulling syringe plunger back.
   Aspiration of blood ensures catheter placement is in the vein (in most cases).

g. Inject saline or heparinized flush solution into the line, per agency protocol or provider's orders. Some catheter types (e.g., Groshong) do not require heparin in the flush solution. Close the clamp.
   Saline or heparin flush is used, depending on the type of CVAD, institutional protocol, and manufacturer's recommendations. If blood is likely to backflow into the line, then heparin might be used in the flush solution in order to reduce the risk of clot formation. Saline is generally indicated when simple clearing of the line is needed. Most often heparin is used for implanted CVAD to reduce the risk of occlusion from a clot forming on the device. Different catheters require different volumes of flush solutions. Some are more prone to clot formation, depending on whether they are open or closed system devices. The initial flush maintains patency of the line and removes any heparin left if the catheter was used previously.

✚ Never force the flush solution into the venous access device if you feel resistance. This risks rupturing the catheter. Look for a closed clamp on the catheter or tubing. Check to see if an inline filter is clogged.

h. Disconnect the flush syringe. If using a needleless connector, do one of the following:

Negative Fluid Displacement Devices
Use a positive-pressure technique:

- For a blunt cannula with split septum, or mechanical valve, withdraw the cannula before the syringe is completely empty, keeping your thumb on the syringe plunger.

(continued on next page)

Procedure 25–18 ■ Administering Medication Through a Central Venous Access Device (continued)

■ For a mechanical valve device with negative displacement, maintain pressure on the syringe plunger, close the clamp on the IV line between the needleless connector and the patient, and then disconnect the syringe.

Positive Fluid Displacement Devices

Do not use a positive-pressure technique.

■ Wait a short time to allow fluid displacement to occur.

■ Disconnect the syringe; then close the clamp.

The positive-pressure technique would keep the internal mechanism from functioning properly.

Neutral Fluid Displacement Devices

Any flushing technique can be used. The clamping and disconnecting sequence does not matter.

The clamping sequence is directly dependent upon the needleless connector being used and is critical for the final locking solution.

   i. After removing the flush syringe from the port, discard it into a safety disposal container.

3. **Administer medication through the CVAD.**

   a. Scrub all surfaces of the needleless connector and extension with an alcohol swab or CHG-alcohol combination product for at least 15 seconds. Allow the port to dry for 15 more seconds.
   Antimicrobial swabs reduce the risk of line-related infection by decreasing colonization of the port and tubing.

   b. Close the clamp to the infusion if a primary IV is running.
   The med could travel back up the line rather than infuse into the patient if the clamp is open.

   c. Inject medication into the port, according to the medication order (infusion time).

Some medication is infused bolus; other medication is given over a period of time.

4. After scrubbing all surfaces of the port again with an alcohol pad or other CHG-alcohol product, administer the second syringe of flush solution.
   The flush prevents incompatible medication or fluid from mixing at later administrations and ensures that all of the medication clears the catheter and enters the bloodstream.

5. **Clamp the tubing** between the syringe and the CVAD port, making sure the tubing is open between the IV fluid and the patient, if there is a running IV.

? What if . . .

■ **My patient is a child; how should I secure the line?**

Dress infants and younger children in a one-piece undershirt that fastens between the legs and tape the line to the shirt, leaving a little bit of slack to allow for movement.

■ **The line does not flush easily?**

Make sure all clamps are unclamped. Check to see if the central line is kinked or twisted.
After straightening lines, attempt to flush the central line again. If the flush solution cannot be injected easily from the syringe into the CVAD, do not force the flush.
Too much flush pressure may dislodge a clot that has formed in the central line.

Check to see if an inline filter is clogged.
Assess the insertion site to see if the stabilization device or dressing may be causing the occlusion.
Try to reposition the patient to lying down and turn to one side.

You might also or have the patient lift his arms above his head and then attempt to flush the central line.
If it is still difficult to flush after repositioning, notify the physician.

■ **The central line inadvertently comes out?**

Hold firm, constant pressure on the site to control bleeding. Have a colleague notify the physician immediately.

■ **The central line is cracked or leaking?**

Close the clamp between the break or leakage in the line and the patient's line insertion site. Wrap an alcohol wipe and gauze around the broken part of the line. Immediately change the tubing.

■ **The clamp on the line is broken?**

Change the tubing. A clamp that works properly is essential for patient safety.

■ **The central line gets caught on or pulled by the patient's clothing?**

Loop the tubing over the dressing and secure with tape.

■ **The patient is short of breath or complains of chest pain?**

Notify the physician immediately. These symptoms could be a sign of fluid overload or other complications, such as a dislodged clot or embolism.

■ **The patient feels pain in the neck or ear on the side where an implantable CVAD is located. Or the patient hears swishing noises or has palpitations?**

Notify the physician immediately. In this case, the implanted device might be dislodged. Placement must be confirmed by x-ray.

Patient Evaluation

■ Monitor for signs of catheter complications (e.g., shortness of breath, chest pain, and palpitations).

■ Monitor for signs of catheter dislodgement (e.g., neck swelling or pain, bleeding at the site or within the line, palpitations, or gurgling noise).

■ Assess for signs of catheter-related infection (e.g., fever, increased WBC count, redness, warmth at the site).

■ Observe for leaking or blood backup at the injection ports, tubing connections, and the site.

■ Observe for bleeding at the CVAD site.

- Assess for sign of allergic response or adverse effects to medication.

Patient Teaching

- Teach patients, families, and caregivers that the overall goal is to maintain a patent CVAD that is free of infection, occlusion, or dislodgement.
- Avoid obtaining blood pressure readings in the arm where a percutaneously inserted central catheter (PICC) line is inserted.
- If a PICC line is in place, do not immerse the arm in water. The patient may shower if the site is covered by an occlusive dressing.
- No activity restrictions are needed for patients with a CVAD.
- Teach signs of catheter complications including line-related infection, thrombosis, and accidental dislodgement.
- Teach signs of catheter dislodgement including pain or swelling in the neck or area near the ear of the affected side of the CVAD. Gurgling sounds might also indicate a problem with the placement of the CVAD.

Home Care

- The goals of home care for clients receiving medication through a CVAD are medication safety and maintaining an infection-free line.
- Candidates for home IV therapy through a CVAD are those who:
  Have a family member or other caregiver who can competently provide or assist with care of the line.
  Have telephone access—either via landline or cell phone.
  Have access to reliable transportation in case of a line-related emergency.
  Ideally, caregivers should be able to read instructions for home care.
- Procedures in the home environment are similar to the hospital setting, except clean technique is used instead of sterile.
- Home health supplies may be different than the ones used in the hospital.
- After discharge, follow-up care in the home environment is important to ensure **safety.**

Documentation

- Document any sign of allergic response to or adverse effects of medication. Document any signs of catheter complications or dislodgement, or signs of catheter-related infection. Record the date and time tubing and port cap are changed. Document all medications infused through the CVAD.

Thinking About the Procedure

 Go to the *Fundamentals of Nursing Skills Videos,* **Medication: Intravenous, Central Venous Access Device: Administering Medications.**

1. What essential action must the nurse do before administering medication through a CVAD?

 For suggested responses, go to Chapter 25, **Thinking About the Procedure Suggested Responses,** on *DavisPlus.*

Practice Resources

Ahlin, Klane-Soderlvist, Brundin, et al., 2006; Infusion Nurses Society, 2006a, 2006b; Hadaway, 2008; National Guideline Clearinghouse, Central Venous Access Device Guideline Panel, 2006.

 To explore learning resources for this chapter,

 Go to DavisPlus at http://davisplus.fadavis.com, **keyword Treas**
Chapter Resources for Chapter 25:
   Knowledge Check and Think Like a Nurse Response Sheets
   Knowledge Check Answers
   Resources for Caregivers and Health Professionals
   Reading More About Medicating Patients (Suggested Readings)
   What Are the Main Points in this Chapter?
NCLEX-Style Review Questions
Chapter Overview Podcasts

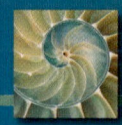

Concept Map

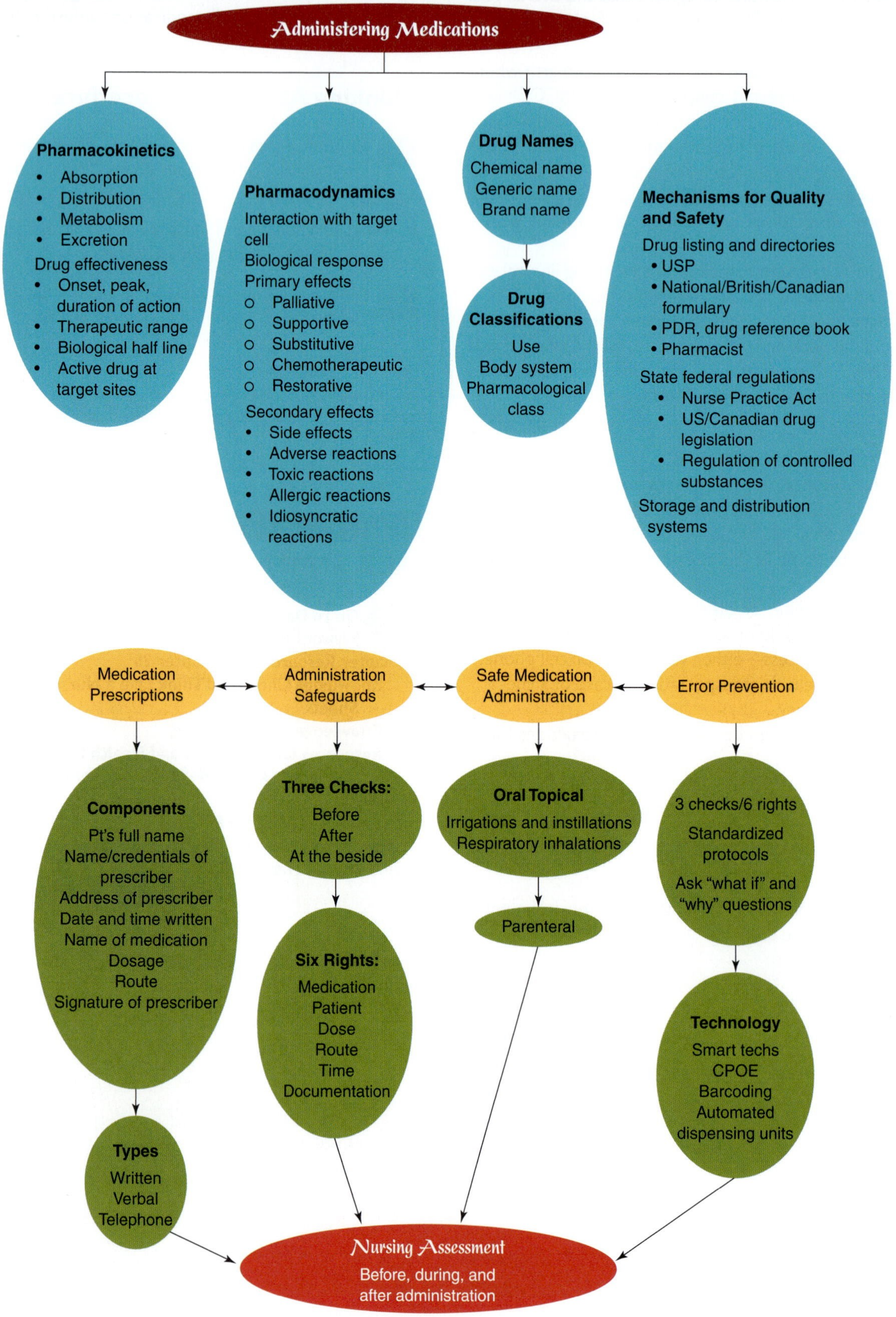

Administering Medications

Pharmacokinetics

- Absorption
- Distribution
- Metabolism
- Excretion

Drug effectiveness
- Onset, peak, duration of action
- Therapeutic range
- Biological half line
- Active drug at target sites

Pharmacodynamics

Interaction with target cell
Biological response
Primary effects
- ○ Palliative
- ○ Supportive
- ○ Substitutive
- ○ Chemotherapeutic
- ○ Restorative

Secondary effects
- Side effects
- Adverse reactions
- Toxic reactions
- Allergic reactions
- Idiosyncratic reactions

Drug Names

Chemical name
Generic name
Brand name

Drug Classifications

Use
Body system
Pharmacological class

Mechanisms for Quality and Safety

Drug listing and directories
- USP
- National/British/Canadian formulary
- PDR, drug reference book
- Pharmacist

State federal regulations
- Nurse Practice Act
- US/Canadian drug legislation
- Regulation of controlled substances

Storage and distribution systems

Medication Prescriptions ↔ **Administration Safeguards** ↔ **Safe Medication Administration** ↔ **Error Prevention**

Components

Pt's full name
Name/credentials of prescriber
Address of prescriber
Date and time written
Name of medication
Dosage
Route
Signature of prescriber

Three Checks:

Before
After
At the beside

Six Rights:

Medication
Patient
Dose
Route
Time
Documentation

Oral Topical

Irrigations and instillations
Respiratory inhalations

Parenteral

3 checks/6 rights

Standardized protocols

Ask "what if" and "why" questions

Technology

Smart techs
CPOE
Barcoding
Automated dispensing units

Types

Written
Verbal
Telephone

Nursing Assessment
Before, during, and after administration

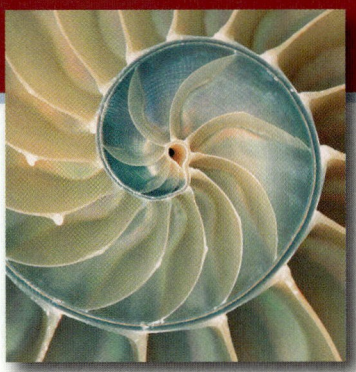

CHAPTER 26

Teaching & Learning

Learning Outcomes

After completing this chapter, you should be able to:

- Present three factors contributing to the expanding role of teaching in professional nursing.
- Describe the concepts of teaching and learning.
- Name, define, and give one example of each of Bloom's three domains of learning.
- Discuss how each of the following factors can affect learning: motivation, readiness, physical condition, emotions, timing, active involvement, feedback, repetition, environment, scheduling of the teaching session, amount and complexity of the content, communication, special needs (e.g., learning disability), developmental stage, culture, and literacy.

- List at least six barriers to teaching and learning.
- Describe some strategies for motivating learners.
- Develop strategies for working with clients with cultural or learning differences.
- Describe the content of a learning assessment.
- Discuss correct and incorrect uses of the nursing diagnosis Deficient Knowledge.
- Develop teaching plans for clients.
- List four methods for evaluating the outcomes of teaching and learning.
- Document teaching content, methods, and patient responses to learning.

Key Concepts

Learning
Health literacy
Learning environment
Teaching

Related Concepts

See the Concept Map at the end of this chapter.

Caring for the Nguyens

This feature allows you to practice the kind of thinking you will use as a full-spectrum nurse. There is usually more than one correct answer to a critical thinking question, so we do not provide answers for these features. It is more important to develop your nursing judgment than to "cover content." Discuss the questions with your peers. If you are still unsure, consult your instructor

Nam Nguyen has medical diagnoses including hypertension, type 2 diabetes mellitus, obesity, and osteoarthritis. There is a positive history of tobacco abuse. Based on the information you know about Nam and his family, consider the following questions:

A. What kinds of information does Nam probably need?

B. What would be the best approach to teach Nam about his healthcare conditions?

(Continued)

Caring for the Nguyens (continued)

C. You have been asked to teach Nam about weight loss. What theoretical knowledge must you have, and where can you obtain it?

D. What patient information do you need to know before planning your teaching?

E. Nam tells you that he feels overwhelmed with his recent diagnoses. He does not believe he can begin a weight loss program or attend any teaching sessions. How might you handle this concern?

F. Nam has been prescribed the following medicines:
Lisinopril 20 mg PO daily
Hydrochlorothiazide 25 mg PO daily
Metformin 500 mg PO bid

G. Devise one or more teaching sessions focused on these medications. You will need to use your pharmacology reference books to devise this plan. As you plan your teaching, recall that Nam is overwhelmed by his recent diagnoses.

 Go to **Caring for the Nguyens Response Sheet** on Davis*Plus*.

Meet Your Patients

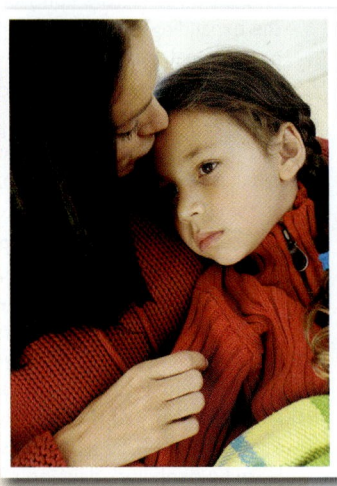

You are the student nurse assigned to Heather, a 20-year-old mother, and her 4-year-old preschooler. They have come to a family practice clinic for a well-child checkup. During the healthcare visit, you notice that the child speaks in one- or two-word phrases. The mother's tone to her daughter is impatient and she repeatedly tells her to "stop using that baby talk." Heather says, "I don't know what I'm doing wrong. All her friends are taller and talking more. She was even small when she was born, so I suppose it's my fault."

Your assessment shows the child is below the 5th percentile for height and weight. What health teaching could you provide that might help resolve this problem? Your nursing instructor tells you to assess for teaching needs and provide anticipatory guidance to the mother. How would you begin to address Heather's learning needs without reinforcing her feelings of self-blame?

Your anticipatory guidance should include information about safety measures for a 4-year-old, nutrition for preschool-age children, and expected growth and development. How can you evaluate whether the teaching has been effective and further promote Heather's retention of this new information?

By the time you finish working through this chapter, you should be able to answer these questions and provide teaching to meet the unique needs of other patients you encounter.

ABOUT THE KEY CONCEPTS

This chapter covers concepts that underlie how people take in and offer information within the healthcare environment. The overarching concepts of **teaching** and **learning** provide a "hook" on which you can hang what you learn about all the other concepts in this chapter. A firm grasp of these (and other) key concepts will allow you to call to mind the information that you will need to apply when teaching patients.

Theoretical Knowledge
knowing why

Nurses have been teaching patients since Florence Nightingale taught about the value of good nutrition, fresh air, exercise, and personal hygiene (Nightingale, [1860] 1992). Since that time, teaching has become progressively more important, due in part to the following:

Patients Participate in Healthcare Decisions. Primary care providers expect patients to take responsibility for their own health; patients and families need information so that they can make *informed* decisions. You can help patients find answers to their questions, discover resources, recognize problems, and develop self-care behaviors.

Hospital Stays are Brief. A great deal of complex care is being given in homes and the community. Patients are often sent home still needing medications, dressing changes, and skilled procedures, such as urinary catheterization. Nurses have a responsibility to teach family members how to provide care and to teach patients to care for themselves as they are able.

Healthcare is Expensive. Patient education can help to decrease the overall cost of healthcare. It does so by helping

to increase patient compliance with medical and nursing regimens, which can shorten hospital stays and decrease frequency of medical treatments and admissions (Bastable, 2008).

The basic purpose of teaching and learning is to provide information that will empower clients and families to (1) perform self-care, and (2) make informed decisions about their healthcare options. Like other interventions, you can use teaching to promote wellness, prevent or limit illness, restore health, adapt to changes in body function, and facilitate coping with stress, illness, and loss.

WHO ARE THE LEARNERS?

As a nurse, your learners are clients, families, and others who care for the client. You will often provide informal, one-on-one teaching while performing other nursing interventions. For example, as you give a medication, you will teach about its therapeutic and side effects. Or you may do more formal teaching to groups of people (e.g., demonstrating a baby bath to a class of expectant parents).

You will find learners wherever you work: hospital, an ambulatory setting, home care, or in the community. As a community health nurse, you would be more likely to teach large groups of people; for example, you might teach a healthy lifestyles class to a group of teens.

As a nurse, you will also be responsible for teaching healthcare workers whom you supervise. For example, you may instruct nursing assistive personnel (NAPs) when you observe an error in technique. Or you may help a new nurse learn to how to use new equipment on the unit. Nurses in practice are also involved in clinical instruction of nursing students, new graduates, and other members of the healthcare team. Most of this teaching may be informal, although you might also present specific topics at unit meetings and conferences. For example, if there is a change in the agency's documentation system, you might teach a class to the nurses on your shift to learn the new system.

WHAT ARE MY TEACHING RESPONSIBILITIES?

Teaching is a major component of clinical practice skills and is an independent nursing function. In many states, nurses' teaching role and responsibility is defined in the Nurse Practice Act.

The American Nurses Association (ANA). The ANA's *Code of Ethics for Nurses With Interpretive Statements* (2001) holds that nurses are responsible for promoting and protecting health, safety, and rights of patients. Patient teaching is essential in fulfilling that responsibility. ANA (2010) Standard 5B states, "The registered nurse employs strategies to promote health and a safe environment." The following are the specific measurement criteria for that standard:

- Provides health teaching that addresses such topics as healthy lifestyles, risk-reducing behaviors, developmental needs, activities of daily living, and preventive self-care.
- Uses health promotion and health teaching methods appropriate to the situation and the healthcare consumer's values, beliefs, health practices, developmental level, learning needs, readiness and ability to learn, language preference, spirituality, culture, and socioeconomic status.
- Seeks opportunities for feedback and evaluation of the effectiveness of the strategies used.

- Uses information technologies to communicate health promotion and disease prevention information to the healthcare consumer in a variety of settings.
- Provides healthcare consumers with information about intended effects and potential adverse effects of proposed therapies.

The Joint Commission. These standards require educators in healthcare organizations to consider the literacy, developmental and physical limitations, financial limitations, language barriers, culture, and religious practices of every patient. Teaching must also include any person who will be responsible for the patient's care (The Joint Commission, 2006).

The American Hospital Association (AHA). The AHA Patient Care Partnership (previously the Patient's Bill of Rights) describes in simple language the right of patients to receive high-quality care. Patient rights include a clean and safe environment; protection of privacy; complete and current information about their diagnosis, treatment, and prognosis; information communicated in ways they can understand; and the right to be informed of hospital policies and practices that relate to them (American Hospital Association [AHA], 2003).

WHAT ARE SOME BASIC LEARNING CONCEPTS AND PRINCIPLES?

The educational process consists of both teaching and learning. **Teaching** is an interactive process that involves planning and implementing instructional activities to meet intended learner outcomes or providing activities that allow the learner to learn (Bastable, 2008). Teachers must have effective communication skills to (1) adequately convey information, (2) assess verbal and nonverbal feedback, and (3) accommodate various learning styles. In patient education, nurses can use teaching, counseling, and behavioral modification together to achieve effective client learning.

Learning is a change in behavior, knowledge, skills, or attitudes. It occurs as a result of planned or spontaneously occurring situations, events, or exposures. *Conscious, goal-oriented learning* is intended and deliberate. It involves motivation to learn. Learning can occur in a rote manner, informally by circumstance, by formal instruction, or by a combination of approaches. It is not enough for the teacher to give the person written or verbal information; information alone will not change behaviors. Box 26-1 summarizes some basic principles of learning and provides a quick check for planning teaching sessions.

For information about learning theories,

 Go to Chapter 26, **Supplemental Materials: Learning Theories,** on Davis*Plus*.

KnowledgeCheck 26-1

- Identify at least three reasons why nurses have a responsibility to teach clients.
- Define *teaching*.
- Define *learning*.

Learning Occurs in Three Domains

People learn in three ways, or *domains:* cognitive, psychomotor, and affective (Bloom & Krathwohl, 1956). You should include each of these domains, involving thinking, doing, and feeling/caring, when writing objectives and planning

BOX 26-1 ■ Five Rights of Teaching

When you are making a teaching plan, you can use this as a checklist to ensure that you consider each of the five "rights" of teaching in the plan.

Right Time

- Is the learner ready, free of pain and anxiety, and motivated?
- Have you and the learner a trusting relationship?
- Have you set aside sufficient time for the teaching session?

Right Context

- Is the environment quiet, free of distractions, and private?
- Is the environment soothing or stimulating, depending on the desired effect?

Right Goal

- Is the learner actively involved in planning the learning objectives?
- Are you and your client both committed to reaching mutually set goals of learning that achieve the desired behavioral changes?
- Are family or friends included in planning so that they can help follow through on behavioral changes?
- Are the learning objectives realistic and valued by the client; do they reflect the client's lifestyle?

Right Content

- Is the content appropriate for the client's needs?
- Is it new information or reinforcement of information that has already been provided?
- Is the content presented at the learner's level?
- Does the content relate to the learner's life experiences or is it otherwise relevant to the learner?

Right Method

- Do the teaching strategies fit the learning style of the learner?
- Do the strategies fit the client's learning ability?
- Are the teaching strategies varied?

teaching and evaluation strategies, which are discussed later in this chapter. Table 26-1 provides examples of client learning in each of the domains. For a more detailed version of this table, which identifies levels of behavior associated with each domain,

 Go to Chapter 26, **Tables, Boxes, Figures: ESG Table 26-1, Bloom's Domains of Learning,** on Davis*Plus*.

Cognitive Learning

Cognitive learning includes storing and recalling information in the brain. Ranging from simple to complex processes, it encompasses six levels of behavior: memorization, recall, comprehension and analysis, synthesis, application, and evaluation of ideas (Table 26-1). Strategies and tools to support teaching cognitive-type content include lectures, reading materials, panel discussions, audiovisual materials, programmed instruction, computer-assisted instruction (CAI), and problem-based learning (e.g., case studies and care plans).

Psychomotor Learning

Psychomotor learning involves learning a skill that requires both mental and physical activity. It requires the learner to

accept and value the skill (the affective domain) as well as know about the skill (the cognitive domain). Strategies and tools used to teach psychomotor skills include demonstration and return demonstration, simulation models, audiovisual materials (e.g., DVDs, streaming video), journaling and self-reflection, and printed materials, especially with photographs and illustrations).

Affective Learning

Affective learning involves changes in feelings, beliefs, attitudes, and values. It is considered the "feeling domain." Levels of affective behavior are shown in Table 26-1. Strategies and tools for promoting affective learning include role modeling, group work, panel discussion, role playing, mentoring, one-to-one counseling and discussion, audiovisual materials (e.g., DVDs, streaming video, interactive computer-based modules, movies), and printed materials.

Krathwohol (2002) adapted Bloom's model describing learning using a more outcomes-based approach, including the following domains:

| Remember | Understand | Apply |
| Analyze | Evaluate | Create |

KnowledgeCheck 26-2

- What are the three domains of learning?
- What strategies and tools are used to promote learning within each of the three domains of learning?
- Give an example of each of the domains of learning.

 ## ThinkLike a Nurse 26-1

By now, you have probably already learned how to assess a patient's blood pressure (BP).

- Think about how you were taught to perform that *skill*. What would have been the best way for *you* to learn to take a BP? To read a book and look at the photos closely? To watch a DVD? To have someone tell you how to do it? To have someone demonstrate the skill? Perform the blood pressure measurement yourself? Some other way?
- Now think about the *principles* involved with BP (e.g., normal ranges, the physiological regulation of the BP). What, for you, would have been the best way to learn the principles? Read a book? Listen to a lecture? Physically obtain a BP reading for a patient? Work a case involving BP? Some other way?
- From your answers to the two preceding questions, what (if anything) can you conclude about different domains of learning and the kinds of activities to use in teaching and learning in each domain?

Many Factors Affect Client Learning

Learning is complex. Many factors can either enhance or interfere with it. An understanding of the following factors will help you to design effective teaching interventions and promote client learning.

Motivation

Motivation is desire from within. It is created by an idea, a physical need, an emotion, or some other kind of force. Without motivation, little learning can occur. Motivation is greatest when clients recognize the need for learning, believe it is possible to improve their health, and are interested in the information they are being given. Think about classes you have taken. Have you studied harder in some

Table 26-1 ➤ Bloom's Domains of Learning

BLOOM'S DOMAIN	EXAMPLES
Cognitive (thinking)	
Includes memorization; recall; comprehension; and ability to analyze, synthesize, apply, and evaluate ideas.	A client is able to report the names and doses of the three medications he is taking.
	A client explains the expected effect of the medication she has been prescribed.
	A client designs a planned schedule for dressing changes for a wound on her leg.
	A client describes how to distinguish between normal inflammation and signs of infection in a wound.
	A client recognizes the need for behavioral changes to decrease the chance of recurrence of infection.
Psychomotor (skills)	
Includes sensory awareness of cues involved in learning as well as imitation and performance of skills and creation of new skills.	A client identifies that he needs to read directions before starting a project.
	A client brings personal equipment to a teaching session.
	A new mother follows the instructor who is demonstrating diapering of her newborn, imitating her movements.
	A new father is observed diapering his newborn after observing a demonstration.
	A client independently changes her complex dressing. The wound heals with no signs of infection.
	A client with limited vision creates a new approach to giving his daily injections.
Affective (feelings)	
Includes receiving and responding to new ideas, demonstrating commitment to or preference for new ideas, and integrating new ideas into a value system.	An adolescent makes eye contact with the nurse as she explains the admission process.
	A client asks questions about what to expect during a procedure he is to undergo.
	A parent of a child who has just been admitted to the hospital expresses commitment to staying with her child after the nurse explains the impact of hospitalization.
	A client who has overcome drug addiction chooses to present his story to high school groups.

Source: Adapted from Bloom, B. S., Mesia, B. B., & Krathwohl, D. R. (1964). Taxonomy of educational objectives (Vol. 1: *The affective domain* and Vol. 2: *The cognitive domain*). New York: David McKay; and Bloom B. S., & Krathwohl, D. R. (1956). Taxonomy of educational objectives: The classification of educational goals. *Handbook I: Cognitive domain.* New York: Longmans, Green.

than in others? What motivated you? Was it because you were intrigued by the information, wanted to earn a good grade or the approval of the instructor, or had other incentives?

Motivation may be based on physical and social needs, the need for task mastery or success, and health beliefs. In your teaching, try to apply the following principles for motivating learners:

- Conveying your interest in and respect for the learner and the learning process helps to motivate the learner.
- Creating a warm, friendly environment can enhance social needs motivation, as can your enthusiasm.
- You can sometimes motivate clients by helping them identify a physical need. For example, Heather (Meet Your Patient) may not be aware that her child is at risk for accidents and injury from home hazards. Helping her to understand the normal behavior of a 4-year-old may help her to see the need for childproofing her home.

- The need for achievement and competence is related to task mastery and self-efficacy. When a person succeeds at a task, he is usually motivated to continue learning. Rewards and incentives can provide this type of motivation.
- The client will be motivated to learn only if she believes that health is important. For example, Heather may understand that a 4-year-old likes to explore and may recognize there are safety hazards in the home; however, she will not be motivated to learn safety measures if her attitude is that "it is no big deal."

Many of the following factors also provide motivation as well as contributing in other ways to learning.

Readiness

Readiness is the demonstration of behaviors that indicate the learner is both *motivated* and *able* to learn *at a specific time.* For instance, a client may not be "ready" for teaching

right before scheduled diagnostic tests or invasive treatments because anxiety makes it difficult to focus on the material. In addition, readiness for learning includes the physical and emotional capacity to take in, process, and recall information.

Physical Condition. Physical factors (e.g., pain, strength, coordination, energy, senses, mobility) and attention contribute to a patient's readiness to learn. You must consider them in your planning. For example:

- Pain interferes with the ability to concentrate on the material the nurse presents.
- The client needs adequate strength, coordination, energy, and mobility to demonstrate psychomotor learning.
- You will need to adapt your teaching and evaluation strategies to accommodate clients with impaired hearing or vision.

Emotions. Emotions are another aspect of readiness. Severe anxiety, stress, or emotional pain interferes with the ability to learn. In addition, the learning itself, and the idea that behaviors must be changed, can create anxiety. However, a mild level of anxiety can enhance learning by providing motivation. For example, a client newly diagnosed with diabetes may not be experiencing physical complications related to the disease, so he may not be interested in learning about diabetes. You may be able to motivate him (i.e., create some anxiety) by pointing out the potential and serious complications (e.g., blindness, kidney damage) of uncontrolled diabetes. Provoke mild anxiety carefully so the client does not interpret your words as a threat, excessive negativity, or preaching.

Timing

You must present information at a time when the learner is open to learning. Timing is therefore related to readiness, and it is important in the following ways, as well.

- People retain information better when they have an opportunity to use it soon after it is presented. For example, a student reads about insulin in her textbook and takes a test on the content 2 weeks later. Another student reads the same information and during the 2 weeks also administers different types of insulin to several patients. The second student will have an advantage at test time.
- For some concepts, the learner might need more time to be able to absorb and apply information, especially when more complex thinking is required.

Active Involvement

Learning is more meaningful when the client is actively engaged in the planning and the learning activities. Learners retain 10% of what they read, but they retain 90% of what they speak and do (London, 1999). Passive listening is not typically as effective for processing and retaining information as activities involving more than one style of learning. For instance, a demonstration with a return demonstration and a patient education brochure is an effective way to teach patients how to perform a new skill. Demonstration is particularly effective for kinesthetic learners (which most adults are). Can you think of other examples of learning that involve multiple senses?

Feedback

Feedback is information about the learner's performance. For example, a test grade is feedback for students, conveying the message, "You need to work on that content some more," or

"You have successfully mastered the lesson." Feedback in the clinical setting or skills lab might be, "You consistently maintained sterile technique."

Positive feedback encourages learners and boosts morale when it comes to tackling difficult content or devoting the time and effort needed to get the most out of the educational process. This is especially critical when significant behavioral changes are required to be a successful learner. Patients, too, tend to respond well to positive interaction while learning. For example, positive feedback reinforces the patient with a new ostomy who successfully changes her appliance or a patient with diabetes who learns to correctly draw up a mixed insulin dose. Sometimes you may need to act like a coach, encouraging the learner with frequent feedback and praise or by suggesting alternatives.

When teaching, you may sometimes need to point out errors, but do so in a positive way when you can. Be careful not to seem judgmental when clients are learning a new skill or are giving home care. Fear of failure or judgment can be a serious barrier to learning at what could be the patient's most teachable moment.

Repetition

The client is more likely to retain information and incorporate it into his life if the content is repeated. Each time the learner hears the information, the likelihood of retention increases. For example, often patients forget what medication is prescribed for certain conditions. Repeating the name of the drug can help patients remember it. This is especially true for learning psychomotor skills. Do you remember the first time you counted a radial pulse? Even that simple skill may have been difficult at first. By now it is probably very easy for you.

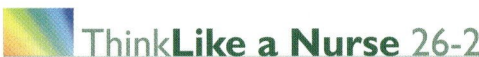

ThinkLike a Nurse 26-2

Use examples from your own experience, if you can. Do not use examples you have read in the preceding sections.

- Give an example to illustrate the importance of relevance in learning.
- Give an example to illustrate the importance of repetition in learning.
- Give an example to illustrate the importance of timing in learning.

Learning Environment

For most people, an ideal learning environment is private, quiet, physically and psychologically comfortable, and free from distractions. However, keep in mind that some learners are best motivated and engaged when teaching occurs in a group situation. Social learners can be distracted from the task when alone in a quiet space.

When you are planning a teaching session, provide good lighting and comfortable seating that is conducive for conversations. Have your teaching materials ready at hand to avoid gaps in the teaching session. If you have an area that is set aside for teaching, try to use inspirational or motivational accessories (e.g., photographs, posters).

A quiet, private space is ideal for teaching, but sometimes there is none available. You can at least try to find a quiet corner, pull the bed curtain shut, close the door, or sit close to the client so that you can talk softly (Fig. 26-1). Make the best of what you have to work with.

Toward Evidence-Based Practice

Caruana, E. (2007, August). Patient information (pre-operative): Knowledge retention. Evidence Summaries—Joanna Briggs Institute. Retrieved from ProQuest Nursing & Allied Health Source database at http://www.joannabriggs.edu.au/pdf/BPISEng_4_6.pdf.

Nineteen scientific trials were analyzed to determine which patient education strategies are most effective in promoting patient knowledge and the use of good technique for self-care activities after surgery. This analysis suggests patient education before surgery is useful for improving patients' knowledge of postoperative treatment and their ability to perform the care needed after surgery. Instruction is likely to be more effective if provided before admission. If done after admission, teaching in a group format is equally as effective as individual instruction. The researchers supported

the use of educational pamphlets to inform patients and improve their skills.

1. What important points does the study pertaining to preoperative teaching make that you could use in your teaching?

2. In the article discussing patient retention of information, why do you think group learning for postoperative care could be an effective approach for patient teaching after admission?

3. Why do you think a patient education pamphlet is important as a teaching aid before admission?

 Go to Chapter 24, **Toward Evidence-Based Practice Suggested Responses**, on Davis*Plus*.

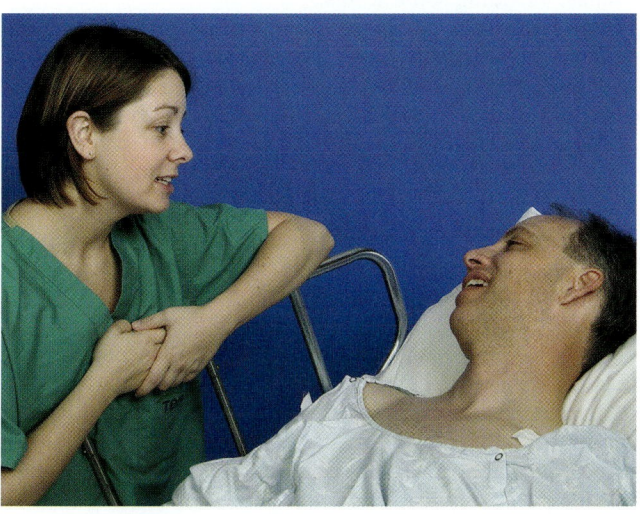

FIGURE 26-1 Sit or stand close to the patient so that you can talk privately.

BOX 26-2 ■ Teachable Moments

A student nurse walks into her patient's room. This week in class she has been studying patient teaching. Her instructor has informed the students that she expects them to incorporate teaching into each clinical day. But the student ponders, "I am way too busy to find time to teach. What am I going to do?" Later in the day, she asks the nurse who is co-assigned to her client for suggestions. The nurse questions the student: "Did you take the patient's blood pressure?" When the student answers that she did, the nurse says, "Did you explain why you were doing that and what the BP readings mean?" Again the student says, "Yes." The nurse asks, "When you gave your patient his medications, did you explain why you are giving each one and the common side effects?" The student says, "Yes," and a light dawns! The student begins to understand that almost every patient contact presents an opportunity for teaching and that teaching can be fit into a short time frame.

Scheduling the Session

Plan for uninterrupted time to allow you to adequately assess and understand the client. The teaching time doesn't need to be long, just uninterrupted. Based on the client's condition (e.g., activity intolerance, attention span, fatigue, pain), shorter teaching sessions may be best for comprehension and retention. Finding suitable time to teach can be a challenge, but a moment can be a teaching session, as shown in Box 26-2.

Amount and Complexity of Content

The more complex or detailed the content is, the more difficult it is for most people to learn and retain, as you probably know from your own learning experiences. For example, imagine teaching parents about the need for isolation precautions for their newborn who has just been diagnosed with a profound immune disorder. In comparison, teaching parents of a healthy newborn about the recommended immunization schedule would be far less challenging.

In addition, the greater the change, the greater the challenge for both teacher and client. For example, a client rehabilitating after a stroke who has to relearn using eating utensils, swallowing, and other basic tasks for daily hygiene and self-care will experience a more intense learning challenge than one who has to learn only a daily schedule for taking medications.

Communication

Communication is central to the teaching and learning process in which teachers and learners communicate information, perceptions, and feelings. Barriers to communication include pain, anxiety, fatigue, illness, hunger, dysfunctional relationships, language differences, vision and hearing impairment, cultural factors, and various environmental issues (e.g., noise and distraction). Attend carefully to verbal and nonverbal feedback that the client gives; it can tell you whether or not the learner is attentive and focusing on the learning activities. For more information about communication, see Chapter 20.

ThinkLike a Nurse 26-3

A client who has a brain injury needs to learn how to administer insulin. Another learner, who must learn to change a wound dressing, has attention deficit-hyperactivity disorder (ADHD).

- How do you think these clients' health status might affect:
    1. Their motivation to learn?
    2. Their ability to be actively involved in the learning?
- What approaches or changes might you need to make in:
    1. The learning environment?
    2. The timing of the teaching session?
    3. The use of repetition?
    4. Your communication?
    5. The amount and complexity of content presented in a session?
    6. Your use of feedback?
    7. The amount of teacher support?

Special Populations

For clients who have special needs (e.g., those with learning disabilities, attention deficit disorder, mental illness, affective or communication disorders, mental illness, or brain injury) you must plan carefully to ensure that you use appropriate strategies to maximize learning. Consider a variety of teaching approaches—one size does not fit all. For example, you may need to use brief, frequent learning sessions or pay special attention to minimizing distracting stimuli in the environment. Or you may need to present information slowly, use repetition, and be satisfied with slower progress. The adaptations you make will depend on the nature of the special need, so if you are not familiar with the patient's condition, you must acquire theoretical knowledge of it. Include a family member, caregiver, or other significant person in the teaching to reinforce the learning and act as a safety net for implementing the information.

Developmental Stage

An understanding of intellectual development will help you to gear your teaching strategies and content to the level of the learner. When teaching psychomotor skills, you will need to assess the person's fine and gross motor development. For example, a young child may not have adequate fine motor skills to complete a skill such as tying shoes without assistance (Fig. 26-2). If you would like to review an

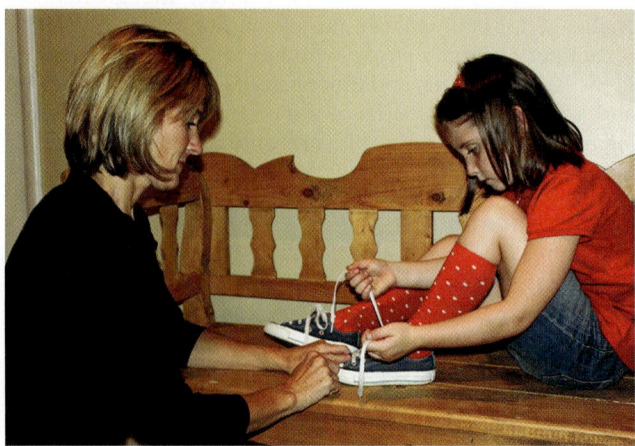

FIGURE 26-2 When teaching psychomotor skills, consider the person's gross and fine motor development.

extensive discussion of intellectual development, including Piaget's theory (1966), refer to Chapter 9.

Stages of Cognitive Development

Piaget identified three stages of cognitive development that are especially important in client teaching in the cognitive domain:

- **The Preoperational Stage** (2 to 7 years old), in which the child begins to acquire language skills and find meaning through use of symbols and pictures.
- **The Stage of Concrete Operations** (7 to 11 years old), in which the child learns best by manipulating concrete, tangible objects and can classify objects in two or more ways (e.g., identify a shape as a triangle and also as green). Logical thinking begins, and the child can understand the relationship between numbers and the idea of reversibility. He also can begin to recognize and adapt to the perspective of others.
- **The Formal Operational Stage** (age 11 years or older), in which the person can use abstract thinking and deductive reasoning. The person can relate general concepts to specific situations, consider alternatives, begin to establish values, and try to find meaning in life. Not everyone reaches this stage, including some adults.

Always assess cognitive development. For clients who have not achieved the stage of formal operations, use examples instead of definitions; use concrete rather than abstract terms.

Teaching Older Adults

When teaching older adults, consider the numerous factors that can adversely affect the teaching. Possible barriers include vision and hearing impairments, illness, pain, reduced social interaction, reduced mobility, medication effects, sensory deficit, sociocultural factors, and a noisy or chaotic environment. Allow extra time for teaching, and stop occasionally for rest periods. Assess for sensory deficits (e.g., hearing and vision) and adapt your style according to any restrictions. Use large print for the visual aids, and repeat information as necessary. Refer to Table 26-2 for some principles that apply specifically to adult learners as well as tips for effectively teaching older adults.

Teaching Children

When you work with children, use strategies to gain trust, reduce their anxiety, promote cooperation, and enhance their emotional readiness to learn. For instance, for a child who needs surgery, schedule a tour of the hospital at least 1 week before the admission date, and introduce the child to staff members and other patients of the same age (if possible). Have the child practice breathing exercises or other aspects of tests or treatments that he will be involved in. With the parents' permission, provide the child with ice cream or other food, game, or material "reward," and give the child a coloring book or other item about the upcoming surgery to take home.

If you are teaching a child in the preoperational stage or an adult with limited cognitive function, you will need to simplify the content and use pictures and concrete examples. For example, there is little point in going into detail with a preschooler regarding the rationale for taking an antibiotic. Instead, tell the child that the medicine will keep her from getting sick; use pictures of a child drinking from a medicine cup, or provide a calendar that the child can mark each time she takes a dose. A reward system is often an effective way of improving compliance.

Table 26-2 ➤ Teaching Adult Learners

CHARACTERISTICS OF ADULT LEARNERS	TIPS FOR TEACHING ADULTS
Attitudes	
Adults are independent and self-directed.	Help them to identify their own learning needs.
Adults must recognize the need to learn before they become willing to learn.	Explain why the information or new skill is important. Be sure to include materials with practical tips and realistic goals for learning.
Some adults may be have trepidation about the learning process because of (1) fear of failure, (2) past unsatisfactory experiences with educational processes, (3) not having participated in formal education for many years, or (4) feeling that "being taught" is for those who don't know.	Present content in a nonthreatening environment, where there is no risk of judgment or embarrassment in front of peers. Offer feedback (evaluation) simply to improve important skills and not for the sake of a grade. Remember the intent of patient education is to improve clinical outcome. Privacy is often necessary.
Adults are more motivated to learn if they think they will be able to use the information or skills immediately.	Plan the teaching session at the time of greatest need. That is, hold the teaching session close to the time the patient will need the information or need to perform a new skill.
Adults prefer to be partners in the learning process—to have some control over what they learn and how they learn it.	Encourage learners to tell you first what they intend to gain from the educational session. Spell out the goals of your session in advance and allow the learner to customize it.
Some adults may feel threatened by the need to learn new information. They may feel, "I've gotten along just fine all these years without needing to know that; why should I learn it now?" Or they may believe that they are "too old to learn." These attitudes may be defenses to avoid failure or to resist change.	Work with the learner to establish the "need to know" at the onset of the program. Involve the learner in defining what he or she intends to gain from the educational session. Reassure the learner about the importance of the information and encourage the learner to tackle a little at a time.
Older adults may be socially less connected and might perceive bias, ageism, or isolation.	As for any group of people, it is essential to honor cultural backgrounds, local customs and practices, and personal preferences.
Experience	
Adults have previous life experiences that can enhance learning.	Relate new content to past experiences and knowledge and have learners use their experiences to solve problems. Encourage older adults to share life experiences.
Messages are best received when they are part of the real-life experience.	In the teacher role, model the message you are conveying to your audience. "Walk the walk" and not just "talk the talk."
Learning Environment	
Many adult learners do well when a hands-on approach is used. Older adults must practice a new skill, or rehearse new information, in order to learn it.	Offer active participation and opportunities for interaction with instructor and other learners. Demonstrations and practical tips are useful for adult learners, particularly older adults.
Many older adult learners need to review new information away from the initial learning environment in order to retain it. It might not be until later that information sinks in.	Use take-home materials, such as colorful posters, table tents, tip sheets, and patient-friendly brochures, to reinforce information.
Older adult learners can be distracted and annoyed by cellular phones and other electronic devices.	Request phones, radios, or other electronic devices are turned off for the educational session. Silence your own phone, as well!
Many older adults were raised in an era when learning occurred primarily through the reading, discussion, and retelling of stories. Technology was not as prevalent as it is today.	Use informal teaching sessions that include storytelling. Tie the patient's past experiences to what you are teaching. To elicit stories, you must be a patient and empathetic listener. Keep your stories short. Ask open-ended questions and be willing to wait for the answer. Convey your genuine interest in your learners before sharing personal stories. Allow more time for older adults, especially those with chronic illness, to tell their own stories.

(Continued)

Table 26-2 ➤ Teaching Adult Learners—cont'd

CHARACTERISTICS OF ADULT LEARNERS	TIPS FOR TEACHING ADULTS
Learning Environment	
Older individuals may bring family members or other caregivers to the teaching session to help interpret or remember information presented. Sometimes the extra people in the room can be noisy and distracting to the patient's learning situation.	If others in the room are distracting, it may be helpful to ask them to minimize their conversations, or in some circumstances to leave the room for a time.
Some older adults learn better when they are not overwhelmed with multiple needs, topics, or skills at one time.	Introduce only a few topics at a time. Usually tackling one to three new topics or skills is enough. Identify what is the most important information for your learner to walk away with. Define those topics and cover them well. Remember, slow and steady wins the race, especially when it comes to learning information that is essential to the patient's health.
Sensory and Physical	
Changes in visual distance, depth, acuity, and light perception occur with aging, thus diminishing the ability to take in information. Older adults experience increased sensitivity to glare and reduced color perception with aging. Processing of sensory information is also slower in the later decades of life.	(1) Avoid colors such as blue, green, and lavender, because they are difficult for older adults to differentiate. (2) Remove physical barriers that could compromise the field of vision, such as projector position, tables, and so on. (3) In teaching materials, choose fonts that are bold, black, and a minimum size of 18-point. Fancy lettering is harder to decipher. (4) A nonglare background without a stylized pattern is easier to see and process than complex designs. (5) For those who cannot read or who have severe visual impairment, consider recording instructional material.
Reduced hearing acuity is common in older adults. Auditory perception for various tones and filtration of extraneous noise also diminish with age.	(1) Speak slowly, using a normal tone of voice. If you must speak more loudly than normal, be careful not to sound demeaning, as though speaking to a child. You don't want learners to perceive annoyance in your tone. (2) Many older adults do some lip-reading, although they may be unaware of it. You can facilitate lip-reading by not distorting your facial features by exaggerated pronunciation. (3) Provide a quiet setting and decrease background noise. Close the door or windows if outside noise interferes with the teaching/learning experience.
Because of some short-term memory loss that occurs with aging, some older adults learn better when they have a source of supplemental information or support.	Reinforce your teaching with follow-up opportunities and connections to the community for information and support in grasping new information or acquiring a new skill.
Older adult learners can be particularly affected by fatigue, illness, medication, pain, stress, and other personal factors.	Be sure to plan the teaching session when the patient is well rested, as pain free as possible, and comfortable.

Cultural Factors

Awareness of norms, values communication, social structure, time orientation, and cultural identification are important in planning teaching (see Chapter 15 to review these concepts). If English is not the client's primary language, you may need to use an interpreter. Cultural sensitivity involves respect for clients' identity and needs, regardless of who they are; where they're from; their speech, age, religion, disability, finances, weight, or social status; or any other aspect that can lead to unfair treatment. Box 26-3 highlights key concepts of teaching with a culturally competent approach.

Health Literacy

Health literacy is the ability to understand basic health information and services needed to make appropriate healthcare decisions (*Healthy People 2020*, 2009). A gap in health literacy results when a healthcare provider uses medical terminology that is unfamiliar or misunderstood by the patient. Limited health literacy is more common among the medically underserved community, minority populations, and older adults, especially for those whose primary language spoken is not English.

Patients with limited health literacy might have difficulty taking medication as prescribed or managing complex or chronic health problems. They are less likely to get cost-saving preventive care, such as flu shots or mammograms, and more likely to seek emergency care and be hospitalized. Older people with limited health literacy, in particular, have a higher risk of mortality and are less likely to comply with medication regimens than those who had a better understanding of medical information (Berkman, Sheridan, Donahue, et al., 2011).

BOX 26-3 ■ Culturally Competent Teaching

- Inquire or observe interactions among family members to decide who is the decision maker and how decisions are made. Include the family in the planning and teaching.
- Assess for customs or taboos that may conflict with the information you plan to present.
- Observe verbal and nonverbal communication patterns.
- Assess whether the family is past, present, or future oriented.
- Determine if the patient and/or family prefers a same-sex nurse to teach a client about personal topics, such as birth control and sexually transmitted infections. Different cultures have different ideas about what is appropriate for discussion between men and women.
- Determine whether the client's values and wishes are in congruence or conflict with the family.
- Respect, accept, and validate the client's beliefs.
- Find sources of information that can help you learn about the culture and its healthcare practices.
- Admit unfamiliarity with the culture, but express willingness to learn.
- Find ways to incorporate the client's current healthcare practices and beliefs into the plan of care unless there is potential for harm.
- Speak slowly and clearly; avoid slurring syllables.
- Do not use slang expressions.
- Use short sentences and concrete rather than abstract words. Present only one idea in each sentence.
- Use pictures and other visual aids to help communicate your meaning.
- Provide teaching materials in the client's language. If you cannot read it, have it translated so that you can judge its appropriateness.
- Avoid using humor; jokes often do not translate well because of connotations, jargon, and culture-specific context.
- Obtain feedback carefully. Do not assume that a client who smiles, nods, and says yes really understands what you are teaching. The client may be embarrassed to ask questions or may feel that it will embarrass you.
- Encourage the client to ask questions; stop often to evaluate client understanding.

BOX 26-4 ■ Promoting Health Literacy With Patients

- Ask questions that involve "how" and "what" rather than "yes" and "no."
- Assist patients in completing forms and/or health histories as needed.
- Organize information so the most important material stands out and is repeated for emphasis and clarity.
- Avoid medical jargon and technical terms.
- Speak using simple words, short sentences, and structuring sentences with active rather than passive voice. For example, instead of saying, "The pill should be taken every 8 hours," say, "Take the pill every 8 hours."
- Use as many drawings and photographs as possible to illustrate your statements.
- For those with Limited English Proficiency (LEP), provide information in primary language or seek an interpreter to translate.

BOX 26-5 ■ Barriers to Effective Teaching and Learning in the Healthcare Environment

Barriers for the Teacher

- Limited time
- Limited opportunity to prepare for teaching
- Lack of space and privacy
- Teaching not seen as a priority (either by the nurse or the organization)
- No third-party reimbursement for teaching
- Frustration with the amount of documentation needed
- Lack of coordination by various healthcare providers

Barriers for the Learner

- Personal stress
- Illness
- Physical condition
- Anxiety
- Low literacy
- A negative environmental influence
- Lack of time to learn
- Overwhelming amount of behavioral change needed
- Lack of support and ongoing positive reinforcement
- Lack of willingness to take responsibility
- The complexity of the healthcare system, which can lead to discouragement or abandonment
- Communication gap resulting from language barrier
- Teaching not adapted to the learner's preferences and learning style
- Provider who uses excessive jargon and technical terminology
- Lack of perceived need for the information taught

In light of the high number of people in the United States who cannot read and/or write English, reading literacy is yet another significant factor in the communication between patients and healthcare providers. Patients who do not read English well would not be as likely to communicate health history to the provider or complete lengthy forms for obtaining healthcare. They might also not be able to grasp information in health-related brochures or printed discharge instructions. To enhance understanding between you and your patients, refer to Box 26-4, which presents tips for promoting health literacy.

Barriers to Teaching and Learning

As you gain experience in teaching, you will learn to recognize the factors we have just discussed (e.g., timing, the environment) and to manipulate those that can be changed to enhance the teaching and learning experience. At the same time, take care to avoid factors that act as outright barriers to teaching/learning (Box 26-5).

KnowledgeCheck 26-3

- List and define six factors that affect the learning process.
- What is one strategy you could use to motivate a client who seems uninterested in learning?
- What are some aspects of the environment that can enhance or interfere with learning?
- What two strategies might you use with a learner functioning with low cognitive ability?

ThinkLike a Nurse 26-4

- List some actions you can take to avoid each of the teaching barriers.
- Give an example of each of the barriers to the learner. For "stress of illness," here is one example: A patient is frightened after having a heart attack, worried about the cost of the medical treatment, and worried about not being able to go to work, so he cannot concentrate on the material being presented to him.

Note: These questions may be difficult, depending on your knowledge and experience. Work with others to answer the questions, as necessary.

PracticalKnowledge
knowing how

The teaching process parallels the nursing process. You will assess learning needs and readiness, make educational diagnoses, write learning objectives, plan and implement teaching strategies, and evaluate client learning. Effective client teaching begins with assessment of learning needs.

ASSESSMENT

A learning assessment will help you to determine the right setting for the teaching, the necessary content to cover, learning goals, and teaching strategies. Your initial assessment consists of general information about the amount of time and resources available for your teaching. Also be clear about your intended audience. For example, with Heather (Meet Your Patient) assess the following:

Learning Needs. To understand her own child's behaviors, Heather needs to learn about normal growth and development and nutritional needs of 4-year-olds. She will need safety and health instructions for the next year because her child may not return for another checkup until age 5.

Client's Knowledge Level. You need to identify Heather's current expectations of her preschooler as well as her understanding of how the child has developed up to this point. You should also find out what Heather knows about preschooler nutrition and language development.

Health Beliefs and Practices. Determine Heather's (and her daughter's) current healthcare practices as well as trust and investment in the healthcare system. For example, what kinds of meals does she offer the preschooler?

Physical Readiness. Is Heather able to sit and listen to the information presented without distraction? You may need to provide appropriate play materials for her preschooler so that she will require less attention from her. Some interruptions are likely, because 4-year-olds have short attention spans. Is Heather too tired to take in information?

Emotional Readiness. In the case of Heather, emotional maturity is a factor in her readiness to learn. Heather has expressed concern that her child is so small, which offers you an opportunity to begin the teaching based on her interest in her child's progress and health. However, she may have trouble focusing on her responses to the care provider during the healthcare visit if her child is restless or if she has limited time for her appointment.

Ability to Learn. During the interview, you can begin to assess Heather's ability to learn, based on her responses to questions. You can also ask about her educational level.

Literacy Level. You might ask Heather to read a short statement or paragraph related to the topic you're teaching Then ask questions to determine if Heather understood the printed information.

Neurosensory Factors. By observing Heather's interactions with her preschooler, you can assess her vision, hearing, and manual dexterity. Observe her response to visual and auditory clues that are given by her child or healthcare providers. Watching her manipulate a pen, pencil, or toy could help you determine manual dexterity.

Learning Styles. Ask Heather how she learns best. Understanding that she probably doesn't have extensive blocks of time or focused attention to read or listen, you might give her single-page handouts, videos, or pamphlets instead of books or more detailed booklets.

For guidelines and questions to ask when conducting a learning assessment, refer to the Focused Assessment box Learning Assessment Guidelines.

ANALYSIS/NURSING DIAGNOSIS

Deficient Knowledge is the most frequently used (and perhaps misused) nursing diagnosis for a teaching plan. It may be either a problem or the etiology of a problem.

Deficient Knowledge as the Primary Problem

You should use Deficient Knowledge only if you believe that the lack of knowledge is the *primary* problem. Use it to describe conditions in which the patient needs new, additional, or extensive knowledge. Identify the specific knowledge deficit as the problem, and follow with the etiology and related signs and symptoms. For example:

> *Deficient Knowledge (diabetic foot care) related to lack of prior experience, as manifested by anxiety and many questions about foot care*

Deficient Knowledge as the Etiology

Deficient Knowledge is probably most effectively used as the etiology of other nursing diagnoses, such as the following:

- Ineffective Health Maintenance related to (r/t) Deficient Knowledge of immunizations
- Risk for Impaired Parenting r/t Deficient Knowledge of child developmental stages and needs for stimulation
- Ineffective Family Therapeutic Regimen Management r/t Deficient Knowledge of the procedure for drawing up and injecting insulin
- Risk for Imbalanced Nutrition: Less Than Body Requirements r/t the pregnant woman's Deficient Knowledge about additional calories and nutrients needed during pregnancy and her fear of "getting fat"

Incorrect Uses of Deficient Knowledge

Beware of routine or premature diagnosing. It is easy to see that a patient lacks information, label it as a Deficient Knowledge problem, and try to solve the problem by giving information—which may not be what the patient needs at all. Always look beyond the knowledge deficit to see what problematic *responses* it produces.

Focused Assessment

Learning Assessment Guidelines

Pre-Assessment

Before assessing the learner, think about the following:

➤ *Time constraints.* How much information do you need to present? How much time do you have to do it?

➤ *Available resources.* What equipment and supplies do you have to work with? Do you have audiovisual equipment? A dry erase board? A copy machine? Books?

Assessing the Learner

You can assess the learner in several ways: through informal conversations, structured interviews, focus groups, questionnaires, tests, observations, and information obtained from the client's chart. You will pick up many cues in your initial comprehensive assessment of the client. A teaching/learning assessment should include the following:

➤ *Intended audience.* Who are you teaching? What is the person's age, occupation, developmental level, and cultural affiliation. Will you be teaching a person or a group?

➤ *Learning needs.* The client's need for information is based on actual or anticipated healthcare or developmental needs. What is the client's medical (or other) problem? What behavioral changes are needed? What self-care knowledge and skills does the client need?

➤ *Client's knowledge level.* Determine what the client already knows so that you can reinforce correct information, correct misinformation, and adapt the teaching plan to the client's learning needs. Ask questions such as, "What do you think caused your health problem? What are your concerns about it? How has the problem affected your usual activities? What are your concerns about treatment [tests, surgery, etc.]?"

➤ *Health beliefs and practices.* Teaching will not be effective unless it falls into the range of beliefs and practices that are acceptable to the client. People are unlikely to incorporate changes that do not fit into their value system. Ask the client to give a general description of her health. Ask, "What do you usually do to stay healthy? What problems do you think you are at risk for? What lifestyle changes would you be willing to make in order to improve your health?"

➤ *Physical readiness.* The client must have adequate concentration, manual dexterity skills, and minimal pain to be able to listen and learn.

➤ *Emotional readiness.* Find out if the client is experiencing anxiety or emotional distress that will interfere with the learning process. Also ask the client whether she would like a family member or friend to be present during the learning.

➤ *Ability to learn.* What are the learner's cognitive and psychomotor developmental level and ability? How does the client learn best (e.g., by memorization or recall, or by problem-solving or applying information)? How well does the client recall previously presented material?

➤ *Health literacy level.* Does the patient have the ability to understand basic health information and services needed to make appropriate health care decisions? Is the information the healthcare provider offers in the patient's primary language? Is the health teaching provided in a format the patient can understand? Is medical jargon or unnecessary technical information used? Can the person read and write?

➤ Adults who have low health literacy may react to learning situations by withdrawal, avoidance, or repeated noncompliance. They may claim that they were too tired, were too busy, or just didn't feel like reading. They may also ask you to read to them with the excuse that their eyes are tired, they are not interested, or they have no energy. They may fail to ask questions or ask for clarification.

➤ *Neurosensory factors.* What is the client's ability to feel, see, hear, and grasp? Does the client have a medical condition that causes neurosensory compromise?

➤ *Learning styles.* Ask the person, "How do you prefer to learn new things? For example, do you prefer to read about them, talk about them, watch a DVD, be shown how to do it, listen to the teacher, or use a computer? Do you like to read? Where do you get information about your health—from the Internet, books, magazines, your family, your healthcare provider? Do you learn best alone or with other people?"

Do not use Deficient Knowledge routinely as a problem label for all patients (Jarrell, Alpers, & Wotring, 2011). There are information needs associated with almost every medical and nursing diagnosis. However, you cannot assume a particular patient needs to be taught that information. For example, a person with a foot ulcer secondary to long-standing diabetes may already know more than you do about foot care. For most nursing diagnoses (e.g., Anxiety, Imbalanced Nutrition), you can merely write a nursing order to provide the informal teaching needed instead of writing a Deficient Knowledge diagnosis.

Do not use Deficient Knowledge for problems involving the client's *ability to learn*. To accurately describe such situations, use non-NANDA-I diagnoses, for example:

- Impaired Ability to Learn r/t fear and anxiety
- Impaired Ability to Learn r/t delayed cognitive development
- Lack of Motivation to Learn r/t feelings of powerlessness

Wellness Diagnoses

Teaching is the primary intervention for wellness diagnoses, such as Effective Breastfeeding, Readiness for Enhanced Communication, and the more than 22 other NANDA-I labels beginning with the phrase "Readiness for Enhanced."

■ PLANNING OUTCOMES

Before making a teaching plan, educators contract with the learner for what they want to accomplish together. **Contractual agreements** are statements of understanding between teacher and learner about how to achieve mutually set goals. The contract usually describes the responsibilities of both teacher and learner, time frame for the teaching, content to be included, and expectations of all participants. Learning contracts increase commitment by the learner

to reach the teaching and behavioral goals. They are usually informal.

Teaching goals are broad in scope and set down what is expected as the final outcome of the teaching and learning process. They should address all three domains of learning. In contrast, **learning objectives** are single, specific, one-dimensional behaviors that must be completed to accomplish the goal. They are short term and ideally are accomplished in one or two sessions. Similar to patient outcomes in the nursing process, learning objectives/goals should include an action verb, an activity that can be measured or observed, the circumstances of the learner's performance, and how learning will be measured. For example:

Goal: Client will demonstrate ability to perform newborn care in 3 days.

Learning Objectives: (1) Client changes infant's diaper, making sure that umbilical cord remains outside the diaper. (2) Client demonstrates bathing baby while maintaining newborn's axillary temperature of greater than 98.5°F (36.9°C).

See Table 26-3 for examples of active verbs for each domain of learning. See Chapter 5 for a review of goals and outcomes.

Table 26-3 ▶	**Active Verbs for Domains of Learning**	
COGNITIVE DOMAIN	**AFFECTIVE DOMAIN**	**PSYCHOMOTOR DOMAIN**
Compare	Cry	Adapt
Define	Choose	Apply
Describe	Defend	Arrange
Design	Discuss	Assemble
Differentiate	Display	Begin
Explain	Form (e.g., an opinion)	Change
Give examples		Construct
Identify	Express	Create
List	Give	Demonstrate
Name	Help	Draw up (e.g., medication)
Plan	Initiate	
State	Justify	Inject (e.g., medication)
Summarize	Relate	Manipulate
	Revise	Move
	Select	Organize
	Share	Show
	Smile	Start
	State a feeling	Take
	Use	Work
	Value	

NOC standardized outcomes for Deficient Knowledge depend on the content that needs to be taught. *Nursing Outcomes Classification (NOC)* (Moorhead, Johnson, Maas, & Swanson, 2008) has identified 42 "Knowledge" outcomes for specific topics, for example, Knowledge: Diabetes Management and Knowledge: Infant Care. To see the complete list of Health Knowledge outcomes,

 Go to Chapter 26, **Standardized Language: NOC Outcomes for Health Knowledge,** on Davis*Plus*.

If you use Deficient Knowledge as the etiology of another diagnosis (e.g., Imbalanced Nutrition) then you would use NOC outcomes linked to that diagnosis (e.g., Knowledge: Diet, or Nutritional Status).

Individualized goals/outcome statements you might write for a client with a diagnosis of Deficient Knowledge include examples such as the following:

- For Deficient Knowledge (Child Physical Safety): After demonstration and explanation, parents will fasten preschooler safely and securely in infant car seat.
- For Deficient Knowledge (Diabetes Management): After reading pamphlets, client will explain the relationship of carbohydrate intake and exercise to blood sugar.

As you can see, choice of outcome is directly related to the area in which the client lacks knowledge or information.

The outcomes you choose depend on whether you have used Deficient Knowledge in the problem clause or the etiology clause of the nursing diagnosis. For example, if your nursing diagnosis for Heather (Meet Your Patient) were Deficient Knowledge (Preschooler Nutrition) related to lack of experience and family support, then one outcome might be, "Heather will plan nutritious meals for her child with a healthy balance of protein, carbohydrates and fats." If, however, your diagnosis for the child were Risk for Impaired Nutrition: Less Than Body Requirements related to the mother's Deficient Knowledge about nutrition, then one outcome might be, "Preschooler will gain weight so that she is in at least the 10th percentile for weight by September of this year."

PLANNING INTERVENTIONS/IMPLEMENTATION

In Chapters 5 and 6, you learned about creating a nursing care plan. For clients and families with learning needs, you will create individualized teaching plans. The teaching plan is often one part of the client's complete nursing care plan.

Creating Teaching Plans

The process of creating a teaching plan differs from that of creating a nursing care plan in two key ways. First, in a teaching plan, the interventions are actually teaching strategies. Second, when planning teaching, you will plan content, sequencing, and the types of instructional materials to be used. Let's apply these aspects of a teaching plan, using Heather (Meet

Your Patient) as an example. You have assessed the need for anticipatory guidance regarding safety for her 4-year-old. Your nursing diagnosis is Deficient Knowledge (safety for a 4-year-old) related to the mother's inexperience.

- *Teaching strategies* are the method used to present content. For Heather, they might include one-to-one instruction and printed information. You must use plain language always. The Joint Commission (2007) recommends "teach back" and "show back" techniques to assess and ensure patient understanding. You may use drawings, models, or devices to demonstrate your teaching message. Always encourage your patients to ask questions to avoid misunderstanding.
- The *content* of your teaching includes the information your learner must understand to reach the desired goal. It can include facts, skills, or emotions. For Heather, the content of your informal teaching might include the following:

Poison control and prevention—Curiosity and lack of ability to understand danger puts the preschooler at greater risk.

Accident prevention—This would include the need for car seats, increased supervision when exploring, and the use of a helmet when the child rides a tricycle.

Risk of choking—Foods that are hard to swallow or chunky (e.g., hot dogs) are a concern for a 4-year-old.

Need for immunizations and physical checkup during the next year.

- *Scheduling and sequencing* refer to how you organize the information, that is, in what order to present the topics. As a general rule, you should present simple topics before those that are complex and nonthreatening topics before more controversial ones. To enhance patients' understanding, you will want to limit the information you present to two or three important points at a time. You must also determine when the teaching session(s) should be scheduled based on the client's and teacher's needs. When extensive content is involved, it is best to schedule a teaching session in advance; the teacher and learner are then committed and prepared for the session. Using small amounts of time can be effective if teaching is brief and organized.

In the example at the beginning of this chapter, you could teach Heather about poison control and accident prevention in the lobby while she and her preschooler are waiting for the child to be examined. During the child's examination, you could review immunizations and the need for an annual checkup. At the end of the examination, when discussing the child's nutrition, you might include a discussion of foods that are a choking hazard, such as a hot dog.

- *Instructional materials* are tools that are used to introduce information and reinforce learning. You might give Heather printed handouts about poison control (including the Poison Control Center [PCC] telephone number) and about accident prevention (e.g., how to properly install a child car seat). The child's immunization record would list current immunizations and the schedule for further immunizations may be printed on it. To involve the child, you might include a coloring book and stickers about one of the topics.

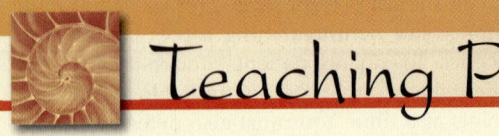

Teaching Plan

Client Data

Emily O'Connor is the advanced practice nurse (APN) in charge of the student health center on campus at State University. A research project by one of her nursing students last semester revealed that only 35% of women surveyed on campus performed monthly breast self-examination (BSE). Emily has decided to teach students and interested campus staff members about the importance of BSE and the proper technique. To reinforce the content information, Ms. O'Connor develops handouts with pictures and charts to make them more visually appealing. She also follows one of the first principles of adult motivation: Provide food, so people who are not a captive audience (as hospitalized patients are) will have an additional reason to attend.

Nursing Diagnosis

Deficient Knowledge (health behaviors) about BSE as evidenced by campus-wide survey results showing that only 35% of women performed monthly BSE.

NOC Outcome

Knowledge: Health Behavior (1805)

NIC Intervention

Teaching: Group (5604)

Teaching Environment

1. Provide an environment conducive to learning. Promote relaxation by making personal introductions and offering refreshments during break time.

   Rationale: When adult learners are in an environment in which they feel comfortable, they are less distracted and more able to learn. Physical and emotional comfort of the participants is important for creating a positive atmosphere for adult learning. The environment influences a learner's interest level and actual motivation to acquire new knowledge (Rankin & Stallings, 2004).

Overall Strategy / Approach

1. Focus on real-world problems.
2. Emphasize application of content to everyday life.
3. Relate content to life experience.
4. Explain how the education will solve a problem.
5. Involve learners in the educational process.
6. Use a variety of methodologies.

   Rationale: Utilizes principles of adult learning. Using a variety of methodologies is important because different people learn in different ways.

Instructional Materials

1. Printed materials (brochures, fact sheets)

   Rationale: Print materials at an appropriate reading level for the target audience allow participants to review information when it is convenient for them. In a study looking at the effectiveness of five different types of media (print paperback booklet, online booklet, spoken audio files, audio with text Web page, and Flash) for improving patient's learning, findings show that although participants preferred multimedia presentations, patients retained information using supplementary materials regardless of form the content was presented in (Bader & Strickman-Stein, 2003).

Instructional Materials

2. Videotape (DVD) of BSE

   Rationale: In a study investigating the effectiveness of videotape for women learning to perform BSE, findings indicate use of an educational videotape increased the frequency of BSE among premenopausal women (Janda, Stanek, Newman, et al., 2002). Another study examining the effectiveness of using DVD to teach clinical skills to medical students found highly significant improvement in outcomes as compared to the group who received instruction through the traditional didactic method (Lee, Boyd, & Stuart, 2007).

Teaching Plan (continued)

Instructional Materials

3. Flash or other interactive multimedia (animation, narration, and text) on computer, to accompany PowerPoint slides.

Rationale: In one study, participants learning about lung cancer received instruction in five forms, and 71% ranked the Flash presentation as their preferred format for learning (Bader & Strickman-Stein, 2003). Women who participated in an interactive multimedia educational program about breast cancer perceived breast cancer to be a more personally important health issue, learned more, and reported less anxiety about cancer screening than did women learning from written materials. It is no longer sufficient to ask the question of whether various forms of educational media are effective but rather look carefully at the quality of the media and software for meeting learners' needs. These researchers have clearly demonstrated that not all multimedia are created equal (Wiljer & Catton, 2003).

Learning Objective	Schedule/ Sequence	Content	Teaching Strategy
By the end of the first educational session, participants will be able to explain why BSE is important.	April 1–8	**1.** Determine date, time, and content of class to be held.	Advertise the educational session by using posters on campus, the campus newspaper, newsletter, and e-mail blasts.
	April 9 6:30–7:00 p.m.	**2.** Social hour. Dessert and beverages. Get acquainted.	
	7:00–7:30 p.m.	**3.** Identify risk factors for breast cancer.	Lecture with slides
		4. Discuss current treatments for breast cancer.	
		5. Describe how BSE helps with early diagnosis, enhancing chances for cure.	
	7:30–7:50 p.m.	**6.** Provide thorough instruction on BSE technique.	Videotaped demonstration of BSE
	7:50–8:00 p.m.	**7.** Promote awareness and incorporate reminders in follow-up contact with participants.	Questions and answers
	8:00–9:00 p.m.	**8.** Provide optional practice and/or online program on BSE.	Set up an online program on three computers for participants to use before and after the formal class hour.

Rationale: Content is based on the Health Belief Model, designed by the U.S. Public Health Service. It identifies four key factors that promote health-seeking behavior (adapted for this setting): (1) Person perceives that she is at risk for disease (breast cancer). (2) Person perceives the disease is harmful and has serious consequences. (3) Person believes the suggested intervention is of value. (4) Person believes treatment (screening) effectiveness is worth overcoming barriers to treatment (screening) (Clarke-Tasker & Wade, 2002; Rankin, Stallings, & London, 2004; The Communication Initiative [TCI], 2003).

Evaluation

Eighteen women attended the session. When Ms. O'Connor began the educational session, participants were seated in chairs facing the front of the room, where the screen was set up for a PowerPoint presentation. She distributed the handout materials and provided a short introduction. Before she began teaching, two women asked questions about breast cancer and screening tests. Three women shared stories about friends and family members who had breast biopsies. One had a question about mammograms. During this discussion, the women turned their chairs to face each other and talked among themselves. When there was a lull in the discussion, one of the participants said she thought she had a lump and was too scared to do anything about it.

(continued)

Teaching Plan (continued)

Ms. O'Connor realized that learning takes place when participants share stories with facilitation by the group leader. Teaching does not have to be led exclusively by the facilitator. Even though she had a teaching plan, she was flexible enough to modify the plan to meet participants' needs. She turned off the projector, turned on the lights, and, instead of lecturing, she shared a personal narrative, imparted information by answering questions, and guided the discussion.

During this process, Ms. O'Connor realized she had made assumptions about the participants' goals for this educational program and their educational needs. She learned that the women who attended came to the program with an understanding of risk factors for breast cancer; they knew that the disease is serious and that interventions are valuable. They wanted to talk about their fears, concerns, and questions; they wanted to separate myths from facts; and they wanted to learn proper technique and how they could remember to do monthly BSE.

After the session, Ms. O'Connor realized that she needed to revise her plan and hold a second session in a week or two. Her assumption that a lack of knowledge was responsible for the low number of women performing BSE was not confirmed by discussion with the women. She developed new goals for the second session:

1. By the end of the educational intervention, participants will do the following:
   a. State that questions about breast cancer have been addressed.
   b. Share strategies for overcoming barriers to performing BSE.
   c. Identify the role anxiety plays as a barrier to BSE.
   d. List steps to follow if a lump or other abnormality is identified.

2. At the 1-year follow-up point, participants will report that they performed monthly BSE in 10 of the last 12 months.

References

Bader & Strickman-Stein, 2003; Clarke-Tasker & Wade, 2002); Janda, Stanek, Newman, et al., 2002; Lee, Boyd, & Stuart, 2007; Rankin, Stallings, & London, 2004; The Communication Initiative (TCI), 2003; Wiljer & Catton, 2003.

Selecting NIC Interventions

NIC standardized interventions related to patient learning depend on the nursing diagnoses you have identified. The *Nursing Interventions Classification (NIC)* (Bulechek, Butcher, & Dochterman, 2008) lists 30 patient education interventions from which to choose, depending on the content being taught. An example is Health Education and Teaching: Disease Process. To see the entire list,

 Go to Chapter 26, **Standardized Language: NIC Interventions for Patient Education,** on Davis*Plus.*

Selecting Specific Teaching Strategies

Nurses use many different approaches for teaching clients in various healthcare settings. Before selecting one, consider the learner's differences, needs, learning style, and advantages and disadvantages of each method.

Lecture

Lecture is a traditional method in which one or more presenters orally share information while learners listen, for example, the nurse teaching a class of expectant parents about childbirth. It can be enhanced by including discussion and question-and-answer periods for clarifying content and by use of computer-projected slide presentation, streaming video, flip charts, transparencies, posters, brochures, models, and other audiovisual formats. Teachers can engage learners with an attention-getting opening and by supporting teaching points with stories, quotes, images, analogies or metaphors, and humor.

Group Discussion

In a group discussion, several participants discuss topics, exchanging information and presenting their points of view. The teacher acts as a facilitator to achieve objectives shared with the group at the beginning of the session. Effective group discussion requires an atmosphere of trust that encourages everyone to participate. Openness to new ideas and confidentiality of the content expressed are essential for participation. One type of group discussion is *brainstorming,* which is a process for generating multiple ideas for solving a problem. Participants suggest a maximum number of ideas and consider a wide array of creative ideas; then they analyze options, identify a best solution, and develop a plan of action.

Demonstration and Return Demonstration

In this method, the teacher explains and demonstrates a skill or task. The learner then demonstrates comprehension by returning the demonstration. Return demonstrations should be scheduled close to the initial teaching of the skill. This format allows for targeted questions and answers and practical matters, rather than theory. This method requires the demonstrator to have specialized expertise if highly technical tasks are involved.

One-on-One Instruction and Mentoring

In one-on-one instruction, generally one teacher presents information to an individual learner. They mutually formulate objectives at the beginning of the session. Often the learner receives printed or audiovisual materials to reinforce the information presented. As a nurse, you will often use this method for patient teaching. Mentoring involves a more personal interaction between teacher and learner, involving not only the exchange of information but also role modeling and problem-solving. It offers an opportunity to directly observe and offer feedback on the learner's performance. Mentoring often involves learners in an authentic clinical setting.

Printed Materials

Printed materials may be available in the form of fact sheets, discharge instructions, printed pamphlets, or detailed booklets. Printed materials for children include storybooks, coloring books, and activity books with mazes and other games. To be sure the clients comprehend the information, you must provide an opportunity for them to ask questions after they have read the materials. You will usually use printed materials to supplement other teaching strategies.

When you are creating your own teaching materials, remember the tips for ensuring readability in the Health Literacy section of this chapter (see Box 26-4). Many standard word processing programs allow you to check the reading level of materials you create. However, keep in mind that health-related information often contains medical terminology, which tends to have words of more syllables. Reading levels computed based on the syllable count can falsely indicate a higher-grade for reading level than what is reflected predominantly in the document. Figure 26-3 is an example of a patient teaching fact sheet written at the level of grade 6.8.

Provide your clients with a take-home summary of the main points you want them most to remember after the teaching session. Having something clients can put their hands on to refer to at a later time can be invaluable for reinforcing important information.

Online Sources of Information

Learners can obtain extensive information and support geared toward the lay public as well as healthcare professionals via the Internet through listserves (subscription electronic mailing lists and credible Web sites) (e.g., Centers for Disease Control and Prevention [CDC], The Joanna Briggs Institute [Best Practice], Hartford Geriatric Nursing Initiative). Electronic learning platforms offer education through multimedia, search engines, electronic libraries,

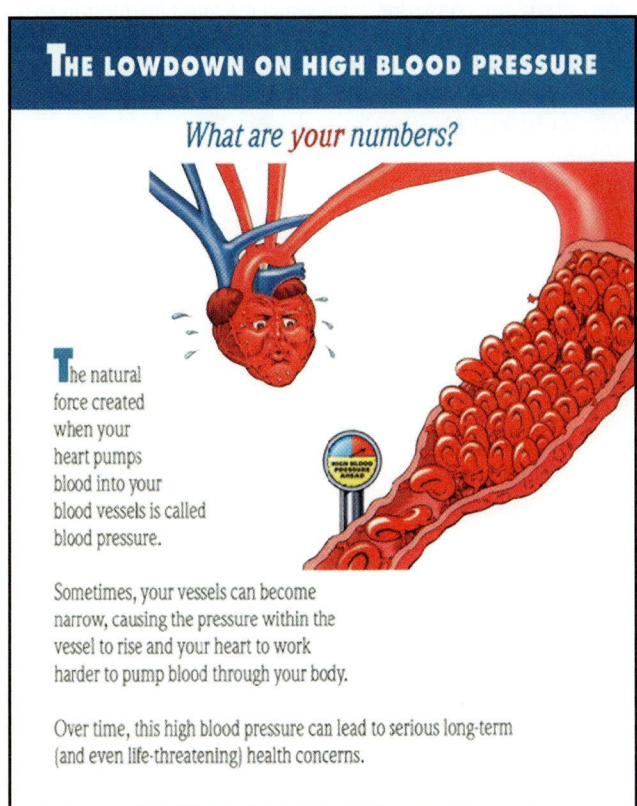

FIGURE 26-3 Reading level of this patient teaching aid is grade 6.8.

content portals, and social networking sites and blogs. Learners can connect with others in similar situations through listserves, which are online communities sharing a common focus or interest. Through listserves and other threaded discussions, participants exchange information; express opinions; offer support; inquire about topics of interest to the greater community; promote special interests; and network with others for personal or professional intent.

Role Modeling

In role modeling, the nurse teaches by example, demonstrating the behaviors and/or attitudes that learners should adopt. Role modeling is even more effective when the teaching point corresponds with the role model's action. Role modeling is integral to mentoring relationships in which patients learn by seeing, hearing, and doing. Be aware that learning occurs unconsciously as well as intentionally. Therefore, you must consider what you are communicating.

Many experienced pediatric nurses find that role modeling using a puppet or a child's own doll or stuffed animal can be helpful in reducing the child's anxiety and enhancing the child's learning. For instance, you can suggest that the child be "the nurse" and "feel Miss Bunny's pulse," or have a puppet "suggest" to a child, "When I get a shot, I say, 'Ouch!' real loud, and then it's all over!"

For more information about other teaching strategies, such as audiovisual materials, simulation (Fig. 26-4), role-playing, role modeling, self-instruction, distance learning, simulation, computer-assisted instruction and online coursework, gaming, case method, and concept mapping,

 Go to Chapter 26, **Supplemental Materials: General Teaching Strategies,** on Davis*Plus.*

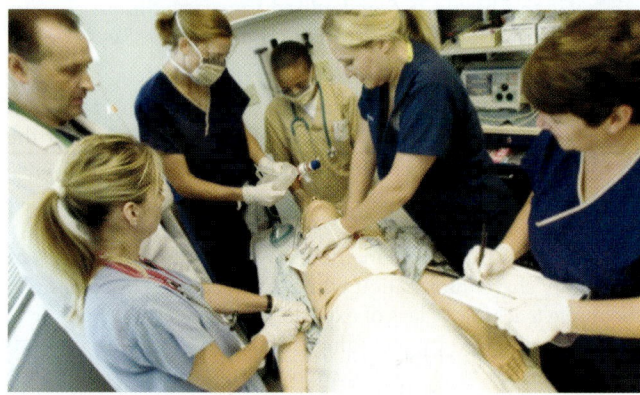

FIGURE 26-4 Simulation mannequins can offer realism and relevance to the educational experience.

Patient Teaching

Teaching Clients Using Lecture

Advantages

A lecture is an efficient and cost-effective way to impart information, especially to large groups. The format is useful for conveying basic concepts and information that serves as the foundation for higher-level, critical thinking later. The presenter can use media-rich formats within the lecture in order to reach learners with auditory and visual learning styles. Lectures may be recorded for future use.

Limitations

Lecture does not allow for individualization of teaching. Didactic learning is a passive-learning technique that for most learners is not suited for optimal retention of information. The lecture may not be geared to the level of the learner. This type of instruction is not effective for teaching in the psychomotor or affective domains. Lectures can lead to oversaturation if too much information is presented in too short a time frame. Boredom is common. This format is not a good strategy for promoting critical thinking. There is little opportunity for assessment of learner comprehension.

Teaching Clients Using Group Discussion

Advantages

Group discussion is learner-centered and effective for teaching in the affective and cognitive domains. Many students enjoy a learning environment with opportunities for interaction with peers. Social involvement can enhance content.

Limitations

May be less effective with large groups. The teacher must be comfortable with less structure and with unpredictable learner responses. Managing group discussion requires good leadership skills of the instructor. Group discussion is not well suited for teaching in the psychomotor domain. The quality of group work can be negatively affected by "group think"—a force that stifles creativity by succumbing to the often subtle pressure of agreeing with the group even though affirmation doesn't reflect the learner's individual opinion. Brainstorming fails when participants are distracted or fail to contribute ideas because of fears of rejection or ridicule by peers. Some might even hold back with brainstorming when anticipating the ideas to be unpopular with the instructor. Individuals who dominate can be equally problematic when crowding out less confident participants. Those who are disruptive or intentionally sabotage the activity can interfere in successful group discussion.

Teaching Clients Using Demonstration and Return Demonstration

Advantages

Demonstration is most effective in teaching psychomotor skills (e.g., use of equipment, self-injection, dressing changes). It can be used in small groups if enough equipment is available. When the task or skill is performed correctly, return demonstration can increase self-confidence.

Limitations

It does not work well with large groups or for those who do not learn best by observing others. This method may not be best suited for participants who learn at different rates; some might need repeated demonstration or slow enactment of steps, while others do not. The method is time-consuming and labor intensive. It involves preparation time to set up equipment. The space must be suitable for the demonstration format.

Teaching Clients Using One-on-One Instruction and Mentoring

Advantages

One-on-one instruction gives the teacher the opportunity to establish a relationship with a learner; convey interest in his learning needs; and tailor the teaching to the learner's needs as the session proceeds. Mentoring allows reluctant learners to more readily ask questions. It enables the teacher to obtain frequent feedback so that material can be repeated and clarified as needed. The method is useful for teaching in all three domains: affective, psychomotor, and cognitive. It provides an opportunity for learners to build skills and problem-solve in situations with expert supervision, guidance, and feedback.

Limitations

One-on-one instruction can be labor intensive and reaches the fewest numbers of learners. It may be overwhelming to learners because of the large quantity of information given in a short period of time, and therefore may not promote retention. One-on-one instruction tends to isolate the learner from others who may share the same learning needs and who could provide support. It can be hampered by personality conflicts. It relies heavily on the instructor, preceptor, or nurse being a good role model and having effective teaching skills.

Teaching Clients Using Printed Materials

Advantages

Printed materials allow for standardized information to be presented to each client, but with some room for individualization. Hard-copy documents are an excellent way to reinforce material taught in lecture, demonstration and return demonstration, or one-to-one instruction. Handouts allow the teacher to cover just the main ideas and high points while using the time more efficiently for face-to-face instruction. Printed materials are portable, so people can read the information when it most convenient.

Limitations

Assumes client literacy, motivation to read the content, organization to keep track of materials, and visual acuity to decipher the print. Materials must be written at a fifth-grade reading level with words that most people understand.

Teaching Clients Using Online Sources of Information

Advantages

The Internet makes a vast amount of information readily available. The easily available health-related information makes it possible for consumers to participate in self-care and make informed decisions. Patients feel empowered when they have access to relevant and understandable information. They often cope better and experience less uncertainty when health information is available.

Limitations

The teacher has little control over the quality of information learners access via the Internet. Before recommending particular Web sites to a patient, you need to read the content yourself to be sure that the information is accurate and the format and reading level are best suited to your patient. See Chapter 44 for information about evaluating materials you obtain from a Web site.

Teaching Clients Using Role Modeling

Advantages

Role modeling allows the learner to identify with the teacher. It can be a subtle but powerful method to increase motivation and ability to perform a desired behavior. It tends to generate high learner interest, and doesn't usually require additional preparation on the part of the role model.

Limitations

Learners need to be aware and receptive to this type of teaching. A role model who does not effectively represent desired behaviors can send the wrong message.

KnowledgeCheck 26-4

- True or false: When a patient has a learning disability, you should use a non-NANDA diagnosis (e.g., Impaired Ability to Learn) to describe the problem.
- True or false: Learning objectives are short-term and, ideally, should be accomplished in one or two teaching sessions.
- List and state the advantages and disadvantages of at least six teaching strategies.

EVALUATION OF LEARNING

As with all nursing interventions, evaluation is central to the educational process—that is, patient learning is an outcome that is achieved or not. Evaluation of the effectiveness of the teaching plan is essential to improving the quality of instruction. You should evaluate the entire nursing process (as you may recall from Chapter 7). Was your assessment adequate, or did you fail to notice that the patient was physically uncomfortable and therefore not ready to learn? Was your nursing diagnosis accurate? Were your learning objectives realistic? When evaluating the teaching, consider the type of strategy you used, the timing of the teaching, the content, the amount of information, and the teaching materials. The client is your best source for feedback. He can tell you whether the materials and methods were helpful, or uninteresting, and so on.

The following methods are commonly used for outcomes evaluation (client learning).

- *Oral questions/interviews/questionnaires/checklists* allow clients to evaluate their own progress and determine future learning needs. You may obtain more information by talking with the client; however, you may obtain more honest responses by using written questions and providing for anonymous completion of the evaluations.
- *Direct observations of client performance* are anecdotal, descriptive notes that you make of the learner's performance. They will help you in providing feedback to the client either to reinforce accurate learning or to correct misinformation.

Provide feedback as soon as possible after you observe performance.

- *Reports and client records* are often helpful. Clients and/or families can keep records of performance and results. You can then evaluate the data and give feedback accordingly. Documentation of performance is best when following criteria or other clear expectations. You can make plans for further teaching when you analyze the data and determine the learners' knowledge deficits.
- *Tests and written exercises* can be used in a formal learning setting to measure retention and progress toward meeting cognitive objectives. This method requires the learner to be actively involved and have adequate literacy skills.

Clients will not remember everything you teach them. That is normal. If you start to question your effectiveness as a teacher, think about one of the courses you took last semester. Did you score 100% on every test? How much of the material presented in that course do you remember now? Repetition, reinforcement, and practice are necessary for retention; and so is information made memorable, relevant, and interesting.

Documentation of Teaching and Learning

As is true for all nursing interventions (as you learned in Chapter 18), it is important to record the responses of the client and family to teaching interventions. Documentation also provides legal evidence that teaching was done and communicates the information to other health professionals. Write objective statements about what was taught and the client skills and behaviors that demonstrate learning. For informal teaching that occurs during other care activities, you may simply record in the nursing notes. For planned teaching that is provided frequently for a particular population of clients, many agencies provide special documentation forms. For an example of a patient education record,

 Go to Chapter 26, **Tables, Boxes, Figures: ESG Figure 26-1, Example of a patient education record,** on *DavisPlus*.

CLINICALREASONING:
Applying the **Full-Spectrum Nursing Model**

Because the following critical thinking activities allow you to practice the kind of thinking you will use as a full-spectrum nurse, they usually have no single right answer. Discuss them with your peers—if you have difficulty with any of the questions, consult your instructor.

PATIENT SITUATION

Katrina Peplowski is a 22-year-old college student from the Ukraine who is transported to the emergency department of a local hospital after passing out in her dorm room. Katrina had been sick with a viral illness and she had a fever for 5 days with nausea, vomiting, and diarrhea. She had been drinking large amounts of Gatorade because of her insatiable thirst, thought to be related to the fever and vomiting. Before the illness, Katrina's friends and family had been commenting about her remarkable weight loss since she started school 2 months earlier in spite of her increased appetite. On arrival to the emergency department, Katrina's blood sugar is 585 mg/dL. She is diagnosed with diabetes mellitus, type 1. After stabilization of her blood sugar with fluid therapy and insulin infusion, Katrina regains consciousness. Although Katrina speaks some English, her proficiency is somewhat limited.

THINKING

1. *Theoretical Knowledge (Recall of Facts and Principles):* As your patient is newly diagnosed with diabetes mellitus, type 1, there are many areas in which Katrina will need healthcare education. List at least six important topics that are relevant to her care.
2. *Critical Thinking (Application of Knowledge):* What considerations do you make as you are devising a teaching plan for Katrina?
3. *Critical Thinking (Synthesis of Knowledge):* What would factors would you consider important for customizing her teaching plan, considering the extent of her ability to communicate?

DOING

4. *Nursing Process (Assessment):* What are some pertinent personal factors that you should assess for Katrina when devising a teaching plan that is best suited to her learning needs?
5. *Nursing Process (Planning):* When setting up a teaching plan involving other members of the healthcare team, how would you plan to optimize Katrina's motivation to learn how to best manage her diabetes after discharge?

CARING

6. *Self-Knowledge:* What areas of commonality do you have with Katrina, around which you might form a caring relationship?
7. *Ethical Knowledge:* Suppose Katrina refuses to receive information from you about diabetes mellitus. She states she is not interested in knowing how to give herself insulin because she doesn't want to give herself injections at home. How should you best respond to Katrina's requests?

 Go To Chapter 26, **Clinical Reasoning: Applying the Full-Spectrum Nursing Model Response Sheet,** on DavisPlus.

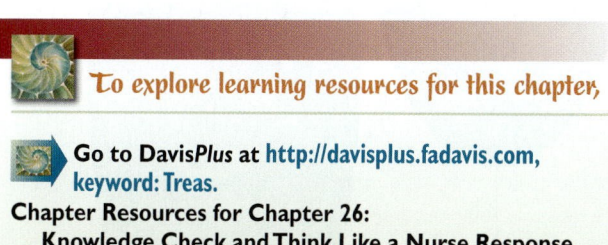

To explore learning resources for this chapter,

Go to DavisPlus at http://davisplus.fadavis.com, **keyword: Treas.**
Chapter Resources for Chapter 26:
  Knowledge Check and Think Like a Nurse Response Sheets
  Knowledge Check Answers
  Resources for Caregivers and Health Professionals
  Reading More About Teaching and Learning (suggested readings)
  What Are the Main Points in This Chapter?
NCLEX-Style Review Questions
  Chapter Overview Podcasts

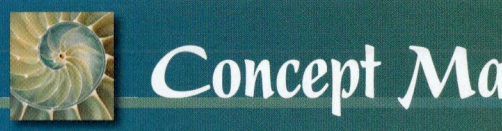

Concept Map

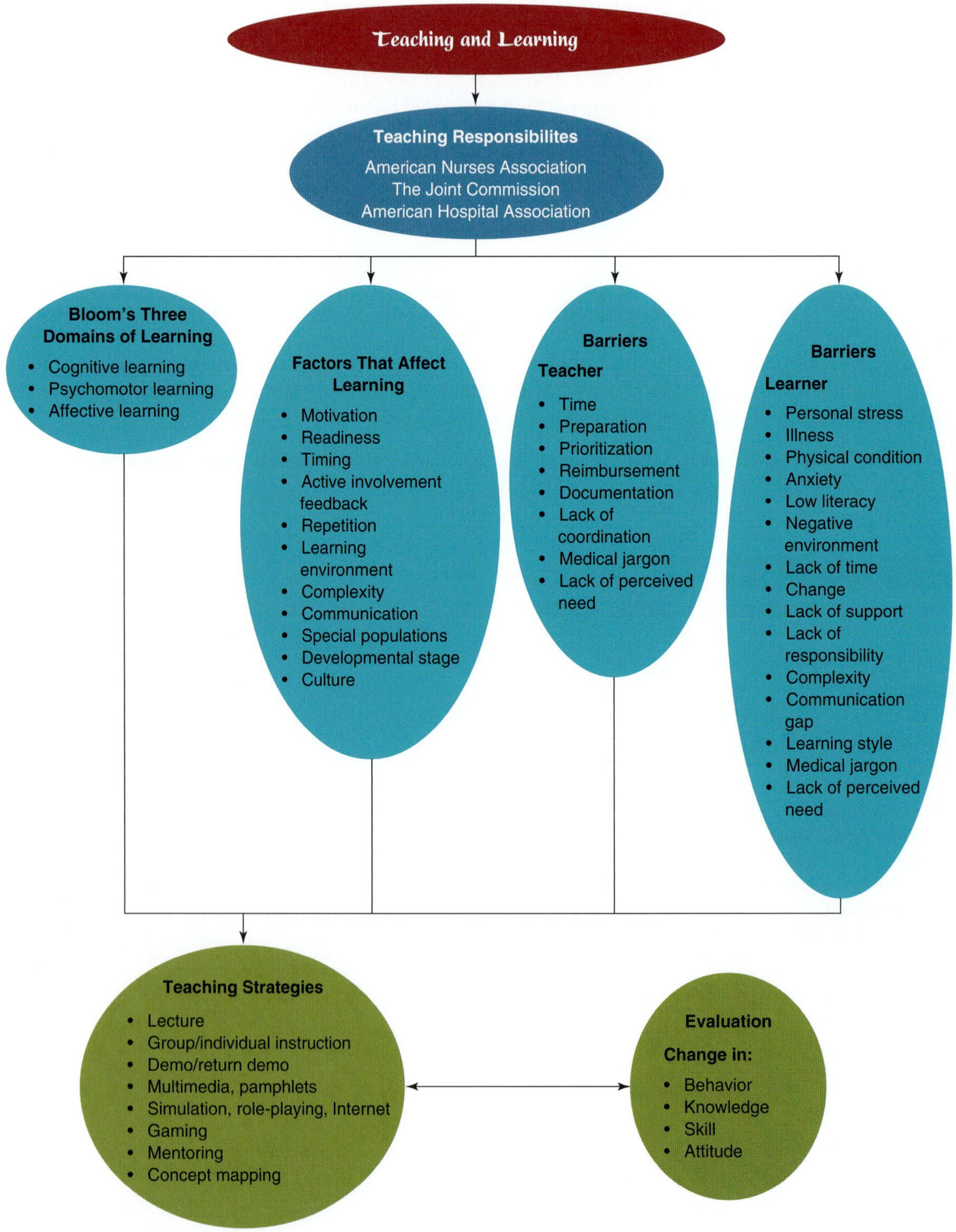

Teaching and Learning

Teaching Responsibilites

American Nurses Association
The Joint Commission
American Hospital Association

Bloom's Three Domains of Learning

- Cognitive learning
- Psychomotor learning
- Affective learning

Factors That Affect Learning

- Motivation
- Readiness
- Timing
- Active involvement feedback
- Repetition
- Learning environment
- Complexity
- Communication
- Special populations
- Developmental stage
- Culture

Barriers

Teacher

- Time
- Preparation
- Prioritization
- Reimbursement
- Documentation
- Lack of coordination
- Medical jargon
- Lack of perceived need

Barriers

Learner

- Personal stress
- Illness
- Physical condition
- Anxiety
- Low literacy
- Negative environment
- Lack of time
- Change
- Lack of support
- Lack of responsibility
- Complexity
- Communication gap
- Learning style
- Medical jargon
- Lack of perceived need

Teaching Strategies

- Lecture
- Group/individual instruction
- Demo/return demo
- Multimedia, pamphlets
- Simulation, role-playing, Internet
- Gaming
- Mentoring
- Concept mapping

Evaluation

Change in:

- Behavior
- Knowledge
- Skill
- Attitude

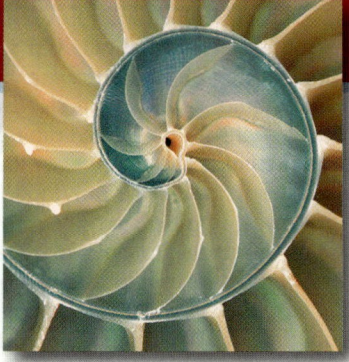

CHAPTER 27

Health Promotion

Learning Outcomes

After completing this chapter, you should be able to:

➤ Define *health, health promotion,* and *health protection.*

➤ Identify health prevention activities and categorize them as primary, secondary, or tertiary levels of prevention.

➤ Discuss the *Healthy People 2020* report in relation to leading causes of death and to health promotion strategies: nutrition, exercise, lifestyles, and environment.

➤ Apply Pender's Health Promotion Model to plan activities designed to change unhealthy behavior.

➤ Identify Prochaska and DiClemente's four stages of change.

➤ Identify specific health promotion strategies (including immunizations and screenings) across the life span.

➤ Discuss nurses' roles in health promotion, and list health promotion activities that a nurse may conduct in acute care facilities, in the workplace, in local communities, and schools.

➤ Identify the areas of assessment in relation to developing a health promotion plan.

➤ Assess a client's cardiorespiratory function, muscle strength and endurance, joint flexibility, and nutrition (body mass index or body fat percentage).

➤ Construct a health promotion plan of care using the nursing process, NANDA-I taxonomy, Nursing Outcomes Classifications, and Nursing Interventions Classifications.

Key Concepts

Health promotion
Health protection
Illness prevention
Wellness

Related Concepts

See the Concept Map at the end of this chapter.

Caring for the Nguyens

This feature allows you to practice the kind of thinking you will use as a full-spectrum nurse. There is usually more than one correct answer to a critical thinking question, so we do not provide answers for these features. It is more important to develop your nursing judgment than to "cover content." Discuss the questions with your peers. If you are still unsure, consult your instructor.

Nam and Yen Nguyen; their 3-year-old grandson, Kim Phan; and Mai Nguyen, Nam's 76-year-old mother, are all patients at the Family Medicine Center. Zach Jackson, the family nurse practitioner at the center, asks you to devise a health promotion program for each member of the family.

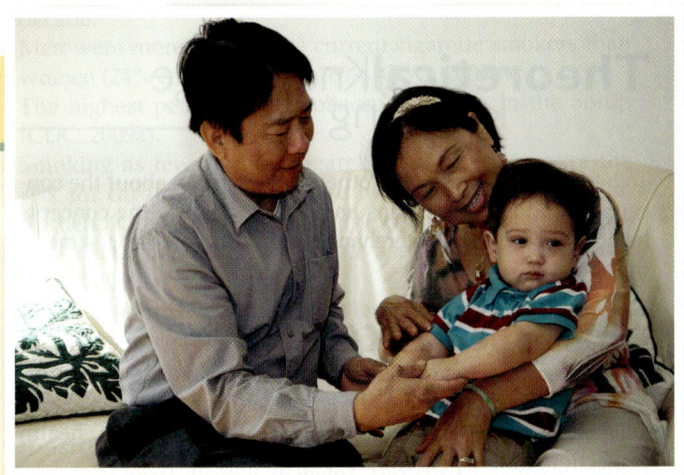

A. What information should you gather before you begin?

B. How might you obtain this information?

(Continued)

only 7.5% of Americans now have five low-risk factors for cardiovascular disease—no tobacco use, normal blood pressure, normal weight, low blood cholesterol, no diabetes, and age younger than 75 years (Ford, van Dam, & Fonarow, 2009).

Sedentary Lifestyle

Exercise reduces the risk of disease and enhances mental and physical health. American adults have made no substantial progress toward achieving recommended levels of physical activity or strength training. Between 2001 and 2008, the percentage of adults 18 years of age and over engaged in regular leisure-time physical activity or strength training activities remained level with approximately one out of every four Americans engaging in no leisure-time physical activity (CDC, 2010).

KnowledgeCheck 27-1

- How does health promotion differ from health protection?
- Which level of prevention is represented by the following activities?

  Mumps, measles, rubella (MMR) vaccination

  Tuberculosis (TB) skin test

  Physical therapy after repair of a hip fracture
- What is the purpose of the *Healthy People 2020* initiative?

Health Promotion Models

A model illustrates a system or framework to help explain what you see in clinical practice. The most common frameworks used for designing health promotion programs are described next.

Pender's Health Promotion Model

Pender's Health Promotion Model (HPM) (Fig. 27-1) identifies three groups of variables that affect health promotion: (1) individual characteristics and experiences, (2) behavior-specific cognitions and affect, and (3) behavioral outcome. The HPM is based on seven assumptions that reflect both nursing and behavioral science perspectives (Pender, Murdaugh, & Parsons, 2006). Two general assumptions concern the interpersonal environment:

1. Health professionals constitute a part of the interpersonal environment, which exerts influence on persons throughout their life span.
2. Self-initiated reconfiguration of person–environment interactive patterns is essential to behavior change.

   The other five assumptions are characteristics of people, whom they assume:

1. Seek to create conditions of living through which they can express their unique human health potential.
2. Have the capacity for reflective self-awareness, including assessment of their own competencies.

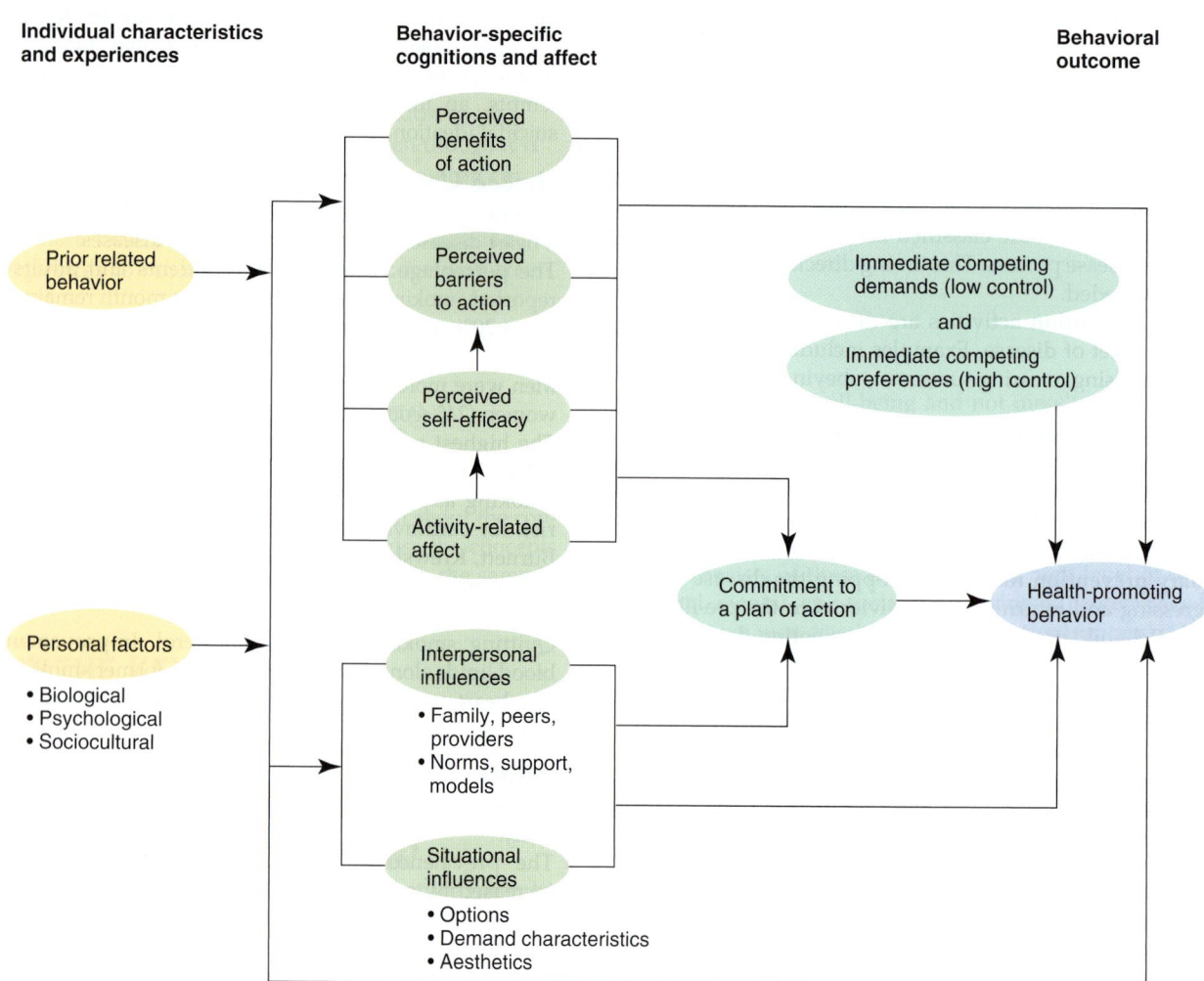

FIGURE 27-1 Pender's Health Promotion Model.

3. Value growth in directions viewed as positive and attempt to achieve a personally acceptable balance between change and stability.
4. Seek to actively regulate their own behavior.
5. Interact with the environment in all their biopsychosocial complexity, progressively transforming the environment and being transformed over time.

Pender's model has been used extensively in several disciplines in research and professional practice focused on health promotion. As a nurse, you should find Pender's focus applicable to your work.

ThinkLike a Nurse 27-1

- How might peers influence health behaviors? At what age might peers have more influence?
- Apply Pender's model to a person trying to lose weight. What might be some perceived barriers (see Fig. 27-1)?

Wheel of Wellness

Several authors have likened the different facets of health to the spokes of a wheel (Hettler, 1984; Myers, Sweeney, & Witmer, 2000; Witmer & Sweeney, 1982). If one of the spokes is weak, the whole wheel is weak. The "spokes" of the health wheel represent the dimensions of health: emotional, intellectual, physical, spiritual, social/family, and occupational (Fig. 27-2). The level of wellness progresses from the center to the outer part of the wheel. The center represents the least amount of wellness, and the outer part represents optimal wellness. If one area of an individual's life is not functioning at optimal level, life will not be as fulfilling as it could be. As a nurse, you should assess each dimension for strengths and weaknesses.

Transtheoretical Model of Change

The transtheoretical model of change (Prochaska & DiClemente, 1982) may serve as a means to alter unhealthy behaviors. Health promotion and protection involve either changing the individual's response to the illness-producing stimuli or changing the environment so that the person will be less likely to encounter

illness-producing stimuli. Either idea involves change. In this model, change occurs in four stages:

Stage 1 Contemplation involves the decision-making process.
Stage 2 Determination is the stage in which the person makes a decision to change a behavior and prepares a plan.
Stage 3 The action stage is the implementation of the plan.
Stage 4 The maintenance stage allows the changed behavior to be reinforced.

Ideally, the stages would progress in the order as listed. Realistically, a person may progress and regress in any of the stages. The change process in persons with some unhealthy habits (e.g., cigarette smoking, substance abuse, and excessive eating) may best be described as a revolving door. An individual may exit at any point as the door goes around. If the exit occurs during or at the end of the maintenance stage, the behavioral change is successful. If the exit occurs before the end of the maintenance stage, relapse will occur, and the individual will return to the previous lifestyle.

Additional stages often precede and follow the change. The **precontemplation stage** precedes the change and identifies those who are not aware of having a particular problem and so are not ready to contemplate change. The **termination stage** completes the maintenance. A person who enters the termination stage has changed the behavior and is not in danger of relapse.

Health Promotion Programs

Health promotion programs help a person advance toward optimal health. In the sections that follow we discuss several types. For further discussion of individual activities that promote health,

 Go to Chapter 27, **Supplemental Materials: Individual Health Promotion Activities,** on DavisPlus.

Disseminating Information. To recognize a problem and understand the options for change, people need information. Information may be disseminated at the individual, group, or community level, as in the following examples:
- Individual level—Teaching a client how to modify his personal dietary intake
- Group level—Classes offered at the local hospital, prenatal education programs, and worksite programs
- Community level—A billboard that presents the dangers of smoking, health blogs on the Internet, and health fairs

Changing Lifestyle and Behavior. These are group-level programs. They focus on such activities as weight loss, smoking cessation, exercise, nutrition, and stress management. These programs usually provide information and offer support. Many times they include a maintenance program to help solidify the change.

Protecting the Environment. The term *environment* refers to air, water, and soil as well as social and political surroundings. Environmental control programs promote health by focusing on air and water quality, toxic waste, healthy homes and communities, infrastructure and surveillance, and global environmental health.

Assessing Wellness and Appraising Health Risk. These programs focus on identifying behaviors that promote health and create the risk for disease. A wellness assessment tends to focus on the healthy behaviors. It supports positive change to improve health. A health risk appraisal identifies risky behaviors that promote disease. These tools are readily available on the Internet, in magazines, and at fitness centers.

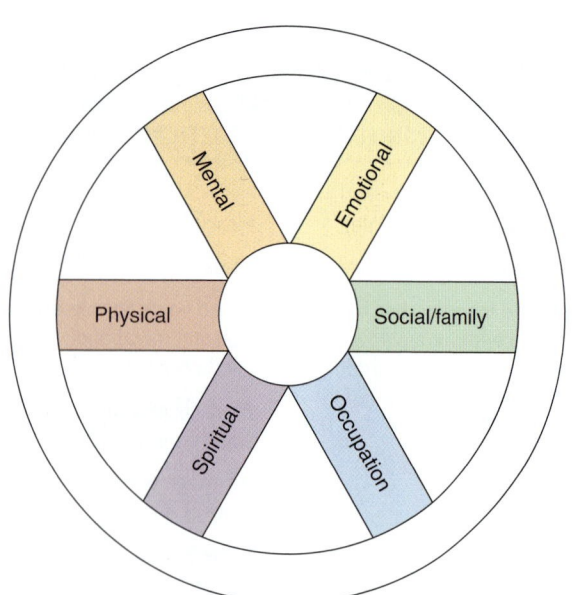

FIGURE 27-2 Wheel of Wellness.

KnowledgeCheck 27-2

- What are the six dimensions of health represented by the spokes on the wellness wheel?
- Identify the stages of change identified by Prochaska and DiClemente.
- Describe the four main types of health promotion programs.

ThinkLike a Nurse 27-2

J.T. drinks a vodka and tonic while eating lunch with his co-workers. He keeps a bottle of vodka in his office desk for use during the day. Later, he stops at a local bar for a drink on the way home. At home, he drinks a six-pack of beer while watching the game. What information do you need to determine which of Prochaska and DiClemente's stages of change he is experiencing? How would you get this information?

Settings for Health Promotion Programs

The most common sites for health promotion programs are health facilities, worksites, and schools. Healthcare settings, such as clinics, physician offices, or hospitals, are natural settings for health promotion. Remember, each interaction between patient and healthcare provider is an opportunity for health promotion. Unfortunately, most interactions focus on the disease process and compliance with treatments. You will need to make a conscious effort to help clients focus on behaviors that prevent illness and promote health.

Nurses work in health clinics within large companies or may be contracted to provide specific health promotion programs, such as smoking cessation, stress management, weight reduction, and fitness training. Employers have found that health programs decrease work-related injuries and sick leave. For instance, Appleton Papers, Inc., is a fictitious example of a company that has an on-site wellness center aimed at reducing musculoskeletal injuries and illness. Staff at the center offer educational programs on topics such as ergonomics, low back injuries, breast cancer awareness, and child car seat safety. There is a fitness center for strength and endurance training. The goal is to decrease injuries, illness, and costs while increasing productivity (Halls & Rhodes, 2002).

Another setting for community health promotion is the local school district. Health learning can begin at an early age,

and nurses and teachers can regularly reinforce healthy behaviors and redirect unhealthy behaviors. Schools provide a setting that allows for continued exposure to information. Interventions may be directed at general health promotion issues, such as physical activity, or they may focus on specific health risks, such as tobacco and alcohol use. Ideally, parents and families are included in the learning. School nurses work closely with teachers and parents to provide health promotion services in the schools.

Health Promotion Throughout the Life Span

Health promotion is a lifelong process that begins at conception. Table 27-1 describes the focus of health promotion programs at each developmental stage, as well the types of screenings recommended for each age group.

PracticalKnowledge knowing how

Pender, Murdaugh, and Parsons (2006) summarized the health promotion process as a series of nine steps that involve the client and the nurse. Notice that many steps of this process are similar to the nursing process:

1. Review and summarize data from assessment.
2. Reinforce the client's strengths and abilities.
3. Identify health goals and related behavioral change options.
4. Identify behavioral or health outcomes that will indicate that the plan has been successful from the client's perspective.
5. Develop a behavior change plan based on the client's preferences, on the stages of change, and on "state-of-the-science" knowledge about effective interventions.
6. Reiterate benefits of change, and identify incentives for change from the client's perspective.
7. Address environmental and interpersonal facilitators and barriers to behavior change.
8. Determine a time frame for implementation.
9. Commit to behavior-change goals, and structure the support needed to accomplish them.

Table 27-1 ➤ Health Promotion Throughout the Life Span

HEALTH PROMOTION FOCUS	HEALTH SCREENINGS	HEALTH PROMOTION FOCUS	HEALTH SCREENINGS
Conception to Birth		**Infancy**	
Education about pregnancy	Alpha-fetoprotein level	Nutrition (breast vs. bottle)	Hearing evaluation
Abstinence from alcohol, cigarettes, and illicit drugs	Screening for gestational diabetes	Introduction of solid foods	Screening for birth defects
Nutrition, including folic acid and iron requirements	Prenatal care	Placing the infant on her back for sleep without a pillow to reduce the risk of sudden infant death syndrome (SIDS)	Blood work to rule out certain metabolic conditions
Exercise to maintain strength and muscle tone and to control weight gain	Abuse	Sensory stimulation	Monthly examinations until at least 6 mo of age
Parenting education	Additional screenings that may be offered:	Safety	After age 6 mo, visits every 2 or 3 mo
	■ Ultrasound	Motor vehicle safety	Growth and development
	■ Amniocentesis	Oral health	Abuse
	■ Chorionic villus sampling		

Table 27-1 ➤ Health Promotion Throughout the Life Span—cont'd

HEALTH PROMOTION FOCUS	HEALTH SCREENINGS	HEALTH PROMOTION FOCUS	HEALTH SCREENINGS
Toddler and Preschool		**Middle Adult**	
Adequate supervision	Annual examinations	Physical activity	Comprehensive exam at least every 3 yr to age 40, yearly after age 40
Safety, including storage of poisons	Growth and development	Safety	
Toilet training	Cognitive skills	Obesity	Blood pressure (BP) screening
Motor vehicle safety	Abuse	Sexuality	
Nutrition	Kindergarten readiness	Lifestyle	Lipid panel
Immunizations		Update of immunizations	Blood glucose
Oral health		Oral health	Stress
Sleep and rest		Substance use and abuse	Mammograms or thermography
School-Age			Digital rectal exam (DRE) for rectal polyps or prostate evaluation in men
Nutrition	Annual examinations		
Physical activity	Growth and development		Prostate-specific antigen (PSA) for men
Safety	Cognitive skills		
Sexuality	Abuse		Annual eye exam
Stranger danger			Sigmoidoscopy or colonoscopy
Oral health			
			Stool for occult blood with comprehensive exam
Adolescence			
Peer pressure	Growth and development		Bone density
Motor vehicle safety	Sexually transmitted infection (STI) screening		Abuse
Safety		**Older Adult**	
Self-esteem	Breast self-exam (BSE) (optional)	Physical activity	Functional skills (activities of daily living [ADLs] and instrumental activities of daily living [IADLs])
Physical activity	Testicular self-exam (TSE) (optional)	Nutrition	
Suicide and depression		Safety	
Firearm safety	Mental health	Obesity	Hearing
Violence	Stress	Sexuality	Falls risk
Sexuality	Alcohol and drug use	Lifestyle	Stress
Substance use and abuse	Abuse	Update of immunizations	Eye exam and glaucoma screen
Limiting sun exposure		Oral health	
Update of immunizations			BP screening
Oral health			Lipid panel
Young Adult			Blood glucose
Physical activity	Comprehensive exam at least every 3 yr		Mammograms and clinical breast exam
Motor vehicle safety			
Safety	Lifestyle		DRE for prostate evaluation in men
Violence	Pap smear		
Sexuality	STI screening		PSA for men who have a life expectancy of at least 10 yr
Substance use and abuse	BSE		
Limiting sun exposure	TSE		Stool for occult blood
Update immunizations	Mental health		Bone density
Oral health	Stress		Follow-up sigmoidoscopy or colonoscopy
	Alcohol and drug use		Mental health
	Abuse		Abuse

ASSESSMENT

A health promotion assessment involves obtaining a health history, physical examination, fitness assessment, lifestyle and risk appraisal, life stress review, analysis of health beliefs, nutritional assessment, and screening activities.

History and Physical Examination

Assessment should begin with a thorough health history, review of body systems, and a physical examination. Ask the client about family history of various health disorders and cause of death of family members. Keep in mind that the accuracy of reporting is higher for relatives without, rather than those affected by, a given disease (Qureshi, Wilson, Santaguida, et al., 2009). Gather the history directly from the client if possible; if not, gather information from the closest caregiver. As always, provide privacy and comfort while conducting the history and exam.

The level of detail of the physical examination depends on the health history. At a minimum, the exam should include vital signs, weight, body mass index (BMI) or waist circumference, auscultation and palpation of the chest and abdomen, inspection of the skin, and palpation of peripheral pulses. The exam may be accompanied by laboratory studies. Recommended lab work depends on the history and exam findings. For most adult clients, screening lab consists of a complete blood count, comprehensive metabolic panel (also known as a chem 20 panel), lipid panel, thyroid function panel, and urinalysis (American College of Sports Medicine [ACSM], 2009). In clients with known cardiac or pulmonary disease, additional disease-specific studies may be performed (e.g., electrocardiogram [ECG], carotid ultrasound, or pulmonary function tests).

Physical Fitness Assessment

Regular physical activity each week, sustained for months and years, can produce long-term health benefits. Regular physical activity is linked with a lower risk for heart disease, stroke, type 2 diabetes, hypertension, high cholesterol, metabolic syndrome, certain types of cancer, and depression. Regular physical activity also prevents weight gain; improves cardiorespiratory and muscular fitness; prevents falls by increasing muscle tone, strength and balance, and promotes better memory and cognition in older adults (ACSM, 2009). A physical fitness assessment includes the following (see the Focused Assessment box Health Promotion: Physical Fitness Assessment):

- *Cardiorespiratory fitness* is reflected in the ability to perform large-muscle, moderate- to high-intensity exercise for prolonged periods of time (ACSM, 2009). There are many different modes of testing, such as field tests (walking or running), treadmills, stationary bicycles, and step testing. Results depend on age and gender.
- *Muscular fitness* refers to both muscle strength and endurance. Muscle strength is a measure of the amount of weight a muscle (or group of muscles) can move at one time. Muscle endurance refers to the ability of a muscle to perform repeated movements.
- *Flexibility* is the ability to move a joint through its range of motion. The most common assessment is to evaluate low back and hip (trunk) flexion.

Focused Assessment

Health Promotion: Physical Fitness Assessment

Cardiorespiratory Fitness

There are many different modes of testing, such as field tests (walking or running), motor-driven treadmills, stationary bicycles, and step testing.

- **Field tests** for running are good for children. A 9-year-old child should be able to complete a 1-mile run in approximately 10 minutes, and a 17-year-old boy should be able to complete a 1-mile run in approximately 7½ minutes (http://www.presidentschallenge.org).

- **The step test** is appropriate for most adults. Using a 12-inch bench, instruct the participant to step up and down at a rate of 24 steps per minute for 3 minutes. At the end of 3 minutes, he should check his heart rate. Stop testing immediately if the participant experiences any chest pain, shortness of breath, or light-headedness. Results depend on age and gender and are available below.

Step Test Evaluation Charts

3-Minute Step Heart Rate Test (Men)

Physical Condition	18–25 yr	26–35 yr	36–45 yr	46–55 yr	56–65 yr	65+ yr
Excellent	<79	<81	<83	<87	<86	<88
Good	79–89	81–89	83–96	87–97	86–97	88–96
Above average	90–99	90–99	97–103	98–105	98–103	97–103
Average	100–105	100–107	104–112	106–116	104–112	104–113
Below average	106–116	108–117	113–119	117–122	113–120	114–120
Poor	117–128	118–128	120–130	123–132	121–129	121–130
Very poor	>128	>128	>130	>132	>129	>130

3-Minute Step Heart Rate Test (Women)

Physical Condition	18–25 yr	26–35 yr	36–45 yr	46–55 yr	56–65 yr	65+ yr
Excellent	<85	<88	<90	<94	<95	<90
Good	85–98	88–99	90–102	94–104	95–104	90–102

Health Promotion: Physical Fitness Assessment—cont'd

Above average	99–108	100–111	103–110	105–115	105–112	103–115
Average	109–117	112–119	111–118	116–120	113–118	116–122
Below average	118–126	120–126	119–128	121–129	119–128	123–128
Poor	127–140	127–138	129–140	130–135	129–139	129–134
Very poor	>140	>138	>140	>135	>139	>134

Muscular Fitness

Muscle strength is recorded as a ratio of weight pushed (or lifted) divided by body weight. For example, a woman weighing 150 pounds who is able to lift 86 pounds will have a ratio of 86 divided by 150, or 0.57.

➤ Instruct the participant warm up and stretch before the test. Weight benches are ideal sites for testing upper body and leg strength.

➤ Compare the ratio obtained to normative standards or to previous personal scores to evaluate improvement.

Muscle endurance is evaluated by the push-up or curl-up (crunch) test. Ask the participant to perform as many push-ups or curl-ups as possible without pausing. The number of repetitions is the score. Once again, compare scores to norms or previous performance.

Flexibility

The sit-and-reach test evaluates low back and hip (trunk) flexion.

➤ Ask the participant sit on a floor mat with legs fully extended and feet flat against a box. Have her extend her arms and hands forward as far as possible and hold for a count of 3.

➤ Using a ruler, measure the distance in inches that the client can reach beyond the proximal edge of the box. If the client cannot reach the edge, measure the distance of the fingertips from the edge, and report it as a negative number.

Norms for trunk flexion vary among men and women. The desired range for men is +1 to +5 inches, and for women it is +2 to +6 inches (Pender, Murdaugh, & Parsons, 2002).

Lifestyle and Risk Appraisal

Lifestyle refers to the manner in which a person conducts his life: physically, emotionally, spiritually, and mentally. Personal habits, recreation, and occupation are part of one's lifestyle. In the context of health and wellness, lifestyle includes all of the activities that promote optimal living, such as taking responsibility for one's health, physical activity, nutrition, interpersonal relations, spiritual growth, and stress management. You can gather this information by interview or by using a variety of questionnaires. A **health risk appraisal (HRA)** is a questionnaire that evaluates risk for disease based on current demographic data, lifestyle, and health behaviors. There are many HRA tools available; many are online. See the Focused Assessment box Lifestyle and Risk Assessment.

Lifestyle and Risk Assessment

The following is an example of an HRA.

Name _____ Age _____ Gender _____

Health View

In general, would you say your present health is?
☐ Excellent   ☐ Good   ☐ Poor
☐ Very good   ☐ Fair

General Practices

1. **Physical activity.** How many days each week do you get at least 30 minutes of physical activity, such as brisk walking, cycling, active gardening, active dance, swimming, jogging, or active sports? _____
2. **Strength exercises.** How many days each week do you do strength-building exercises, such as weight lifting or isometric exercises? _____
3. **Smoking status.** Indicate your present smoking status.
   ☐ Current smoker   ☐ Ex-smoker
   ☐ Nonsmoker, never smoked regularly.

Environmental smoke. Do you live with or work with smokers and breathe second-hand smoke regularly?
☐ Yes   ☐ No
4. **Alcohol.** How many drinks do you typically have on a day you drink? *One drink is a bottle or can of beer (12 oz), a glass of wine or wine cooler (3.5 oz), or a shot glass of liquor (1.5 oz).*
   ☐ Never drink.
   ☐ Have no more than one drink in a day.
   ☐ Have no more than two drinks in a day.
   ☐ Sometimes have three or four drinks in a day.
   ☐ Sometimes have five or more drinks in a day.
5. **Sleep.** How many hours of sleep do you usually get each night? _____

Eating Practices

6. **Breakfast.** How many days each week do you usually eat breakfast (more than just coffee and a roll)? _____
7. **Bread/grains.** How many servings of whole-grain breads and cereals do you eat daily? *One serving =1 slice bread, ½ cup dry cereal, ½ cup cooked oatmeal or other whole-grain cereal or brown rice.* _____

(Continued)

Focused Assessment

Lifestyle and Risk Assessment—cont'd

8. **Fruits and vegetables.** How many servings of fruits and vegetables do you eat daily? *One serving = 1 medium fruit, 6 oz fruit or vegetable juice, 1 cup raw fruit or vegetables, ½ cup cooked fruit or vegetables.* _____

9. **High-fat and high-cholesterol foods.** How often do you eat foods high in saturated fat and cholesterol (e.g., steak, hamburger, hot dog, sausage, bacon, cheese, fried chicken, French fries, ice cream, cheesecake, or other desserts)?
   □ Daily
   □ Eat these foods three or more times a week.
   □ Seldom or never eat these foods.

10. **Nuts/seeds.** How many servings of nuts do you usually eat each week? *One serving = 1 oz or a small handful, or 2 tablespoons of natural nut butter.* _____

11. **Legumes.** How many times a week do you eat legumes (peas, beans, lentils, garbanzos)? *One serving = ½ cup cooked.* _____

12. **Refined foods.** How often do you eat highly refined foods (soda pop, snack foods, chips, refined cereals, pastry, candy)?
   □ Daily
   □ Eat these foods three or more times a week.
   □ Seldom or never eat refined foods.

13. **Weight.** How many pounds have you gained since you were 21 to 24 (enter 0 if you weigh the same, weigh less, or are younger than 21 years). _____

14. **Water intake.** How many glasses (8 oz) of water do you typically drink each day? _____

Mental/Social Health

15. **Happiness.** How happy have you been during the last month?
   □ Very happy
   □ Pretty happy
   □ Not too happy
   □ Very unhappy

16. **Mood/feelings**
   (a) During the past month, have you often been bothered by feeling down, depressed, or hopeless?
      □ Yes   □ No
   (b) During the past month, have you often been bothered by having little interest or pleasure in doing things?
      □ Yes   □ No
   (c) Have your feelings in the past month caused you significant distress or impaired your ability to function socially or at work (or school)?
      □ Yes   □ No

17. **Stress and coping.** How much of the time do you feel stressed out and unable to cope with life?
   □ Seldom or never
   □ Occasionally
   □ Much of the time
   □ Most of the time

Social Support

18. **Support.** Do you have family or friends you can get help from if needed?
   □ Yes   □ No

19. **Social Interaction.** Do you have frequent social contact with family or friends?
   □ Yes   □ No

Community

20. **Community support.** Do you meet regularly with a faith community or other group that gives you support, comfort, meaning, and direction in your life?
   □ Yes   □ No

Safety

21. **Seat belts.** What percentage of the time do you wear seat belts when riding in a car? _____

22. **Smoke alarm.** Do you have a working smoke alarm on each floor of your home, including the area in which you sleep?
   □ Yes   □ No   □ Don't know for sure.

23. **Helmet.** When biking or rollerblading, do you always wear a helmet and protective gear?
   □ Yes   □ No

24. **Substance use and driving.** Do you ever drive soon after drinking alcohol or taking drugs or ride with someone who has been using illicit substances or alcohol?
   □ Yes   □ No

Safer Sex

25. **Practice safer sex.**
   (a) Are you in a monogamous relationship?
      □ Yes   □ No
   (b) Do you always use condoms, or abstain from sexual relations?
      □ Always   □ Don't always practice safer sex

Preventive Exams

26. Do you keep current on recommended preventive exams (see list below) and immunizations?
   □ Yes   □ No   □ Don't know for sure.

Recommended Preventive Exams

➤ Periodic checkup, including blood pressure, height and weight, and cholesterol check as recommended by your doctor.
➤ Pap tests within last 1 to 3 years, for women 18 or older
➤ Mammogram within last 2 years, for women 40 or older
➤ Colorectal cancer screening for all persons 50 or older
➤ Prostate exam, for men 50 or older
➤ Flu and pneumonia immunizations, for everyone 65 or older
   Height _____
   Weight _____
   Blood pressure _____
   Blood cholesterol _____ (mg/dL)

———————————— **Scoring** ————————————

Your score is the number of good health indicators you meet out of the 17 possible listed (below) in this assessment. The higher your score, the healthier your lifestyle. The Average Health Style Score is 9.4

Focused Assessment

Lifestyle and Risk Assessment—cont'd

Health Indicator	Guidelines for Good Health
1. Physical activity	Get 30 or more minutes of physical activity most days of the week.
2. Strength training	Do strength-building exercises at least twice per week.
3. Not smoking	Avoid all tobacco use and frequent exposure to secondhand smoke.
4. Alcohol use	Alcohol is not recommended, but if you drink alcohol, limit to one to two drinks in a day.
5. Adequate rest	Get adequate rest, at least 7 to 8 hours of sleep daily for best health.
6. Breakfast daily	Eat a nutritious breakfast daily for optimal physical and mental performance.
7. Whole grains	Choose whole-grain breads and cereals, at least three or more servings/per day.
8. Fruits and vegetables	Eat at least five servings of fruits and vegetables daily.
9. Fats, cholesterol	Limit high-fat meats, whole milk, and butter. Vegetable oils are healthier than oils from animals.
10. Nuts and legumes	Nuts, such as almonds, contain healthy fats and protect against heart disease. Legumes prevent carbohydrate cravings, prevent metabolic syndrome, provide protein and energy, protect against cancer, and are a source of calcium and other vitamins and minerals.
11. Healthy weight	Maintain a healthy weight by eating well and participating in regular, moderate-intensity physical activity.
12. Mental health	Develop effective coping skills, and maintain a happy, hopeful outlook.
13. Social support	Maintain good social support and frequent contact with family and friends.
14. Community	Participate regularly in a faith community or other group that provides meaning, direction, and support in your life.
15. Safety	Be safety conscious; wear safety belts in the car and helmets when biking.
16. Safer sex	Remain in a monogamous relationship, or always use condoms, or abstain.
17. Regular exams	Get regular exams, including age/gender recommended preventive exams.

Source: Adapted from Hall, D. R. (2004). *Lifestyle check assessment.* Vanderbilt University Health and Wellness. Retrieved on April 30, 2012, from http://healthandwellness.vanderbilt.edu/news/2011/09/the-health-risk-assessment-tool/

ThinkLike a Nurse 27-3

- Evaluate your own compliance with recommended health screenings for your age group. What activities should you incorporate into your own health promotion plan?
- Answer the questions in the Lifestyle and Risk Assessment. How did you score? What additional activities should be added to your health promotion plan?

Life Stress Review

Hans Selye (1976) proposed that stress triggers physiological responses that may, over time, induce illness. Likewise, Richard Rahe (1974) identified some stress-inducing life change events and researched their possible effects on health. He attached numeric values for each change based on the degree of disruption or stress produced by the event. Rahe discovered that a high score on a life-change event scale is associated with a greater likelihood of a negative health change. To see and use a life-change event scale, see the assessment box, Holmes–Rahe Social Readjustment Scale in Chapter 12. Also refer to the Focused Assessment box Life Stress Review.

Other researchers have focused on daily stresses and their effects on actual health or on one's perception of health. Daily stresses involve travel to and from work, taking children to activities, daily chores, waiting in lines at shops, raising teenagers, and traffic jams. Researchers have found these stresses may gradually erode one's coping mechanisms, producing an inability to cope with daily events and an increased likelihood of illness.

Research has also demonstrated that in the face of life events, some people develop hardiness rather than vulnerability

Focused Assessment

Life Stress Review

Daily hassles, life events, and other stressors trigger physiological responses that may, over time, induce illness (Rahe, 1974; Selye, 1976). Refer to the Holmes–Rahe Social Readjustment Scale in Chapter 12. Alternatively, you might want to interview your patient to assess the following:

➤ His belief in his ability to control the experience (e.g., an impending decision, an illness)
➤ How deeply involved he is in the activity that is producing stress (i.e., is it something he can change, or wants to change?)
➤ Whether he is able to view such a change as a challenge to grow

(Maddi, Koshaba, Fazel, et al., 2009). Kobasa (1979) identified hardiness as a quality in which an individual experiences high levels of stress yet does not fall ill (Sinha, 2009). There are three general characteristics of the hardy person:

- **Control**—belief in the ability to control the experience
- **Commitment**—feeling deeply involved in the activity producing stress
- **Challenge**—the ability to view the change as a challenge to grow

These traits are associated with a strong resistance to negative feelings that occur under adverse circumstances (Sinha, 2009). If you need additional information on hardiness, review Chapters 11 and 12.

ThinkLike a Nurse 27-4

- Undoubtedly you are experiencing stress as a student in a nursing program. How would you rate your level of hardiness?
- What statements would demonstrate a hardy personality in each area (commitment, control, challenge)?

Health Beliefs

A health promotion assessment would not be complete without investigating an individual's health beliefs. Health beliefs are embedded in one's culture and personal experiences. Culture consists of characteristics, beliefs, and behaviors of an individual or group (Chapter 15)—all the experiences, biases, beliefs, and rituals. Culture influences beliefs and practices affecting wellness and disease prevention. For example, some people may use certain foods (e.g., garlic to prevent heart disease, orange juice to prevent a cold) or herbs to protect or restore health. It is important for you to respect cultural and religious views regarding health while working with clients to adopt personal health goals.

It will be helpful to know whether health outcomes are a result of actions the person takes, actions of powerful others, or chance. The Multidimensional Health Locus of Control scale (MHLC), developed by Wallston, Wallston, and DeVellis (1978), helps you obtain this information. The MHLC measures the person's perception of the extent of control from each source. The person rates her level of agreement with statements such as "I am in control of my health," "No matter what I do, if I am going to get sick, I will get sick," and "Regarding my health, I can only do what my doctor tells me to do." Identifying a patient's locus of control is of practical importance for several reasons:

- People who feel powerless about preventing illness are least likely to engage in health promotion activities.
- People who respond to direction from respected authorities often prefer a health promotion program that is supervised by a healthcare provider.
- Clients who feel in charge of their own health are the easiest to motivate toward positive change.

For a copy of the MHLC you can print out and use with your patients,

 Go to Chapter 27, **Resources for Caregivers and Health Professionals,** Vanderbilt University Web Site, on Davis*Plus*.

Nutritional Assessment

A nutritional assessment is a key component of an overall wellness assessment. Unhealthy eating habits occur across all ages, ethnicities, and socioeconomic classes. The assessment involves an evaluation of typical eating patterns correlated with physical examination findings and BMI. Body composition is important in identifying health risks. The usual methods for determining body fat composition clinically are by measuring height, weight, circumferences, and skinfolds (Chapter 28).

The pattern of body fat distribution is an important predictor of health risks. People with fat stored around the trunk and abdominal area have a higher incidence of metabolic syndrome, hypertension, hyperlipidemia, heart disease, type 2 diabetes, and premature death than do those who have the fat stored in the extremities. Traditionally, the waist-to-height ratio has been used as a method for determining fat patterns in the body. More recently, the focus has shifted to waist circumference alone. The more fat stored in the abdominal area, the greater the risk for disease (Janssen, Katzmarzyk, & Ross, 2004).

Health Screening Activities

Health screening activities are secondary prevention activities designed to diagnose specific diseases at an early stage so that treatment can begin before there is an opportunity for the disease to spread or become debilitating. Many of these screening activities are part of your usual care. For example, each time you check a client's blood pressure, you are performing a screen for hypertension. Table 27-1 identifies the typical health screening activities with each developmental stage. Box 27-1 provides further information about selected health screening activities.

BOX 27-1 ■ Selected Health Screening Activities

With regard to health screening guidelines, it is important to know the following:

1. Different agencies and groups generate different guidelines for type and frequency of screening. For example, the American Cancer Society (2009c) has different Pap screening recommendations than does the U.S. Preventive Services Task Force; the American Congress of Obstetricians and Gynecologists (ACOG) may have yet another recommendation.
2. Most evidence-based guidelines make use of cost-benefit analysis to arrive at their recommendations.
3. Various third-party payors have different policies regarding the type and frequency of screening for which they will reimburse.
4. Guidelines and recommendations change often.

Clinicians must take all of the foregoing into consideration when they decide which screening tests to offer to their patients.

Lipid screening. Adults age 20 years or older have a fasting lipid panel at least once every 5 years. If total cholesterol is 200 mg/dL or greater—or high-density lipoprotein (HDL) is less than 40 mg/dL—frequent monitoring is required. Overweight children need to receive cholesterol screening, regardless of risk factors for cardiovascular disease (Daniels, Greer, & the Committee on Nutrition, 2008).

Dental health. Clients should have regular dental checkups to detect early signs of oral health problems such as tooth decay, gingivitis (gum disease), and oral cancers.

Colon cancer screening. Both men and women should have a fecal occult blood test every year beginning at age 50 and a screening colonoscopy based on risk factors. If there is a strong family history of colorectal cancer or polyps, screening should begin at an earlier age and be conducted more frequently (American Cancer Society, 2009c).

Breast cancer screening. Breast self-examination (BSE) is an option for women 20 years and older. Women between the ages of 20 and 39 should have a clinical breast examination by a health professional every 3 years. Women age 40 and older should have a screening mammogram and a clinical breast examination by a healthcare professional every year. The clinical breast examination should be scheduled close to and preferably before the scheduled mammogram (American Cancer Society, 2009b, 2009c). Thermal mammography is another method to detect breast cancer without using radiation.

Cervical cancer screening. A Papanicolaou (Pap) smear is used to detect cellular changes in the cervix. Women older than 21 years (or 3 years after first vaginal intercourse) should be screened for cervical cancer every 2 to 3 years.

BOX 27-1 ■ Selected Health Screening Activities—cont'd

Women with risk factors for cervical cancer (e.g., weakened immune system, those who have had abnormal Pap tests) should be screened more frequently. Women age 70 years or older with no abnormal Pap test results in the last 10 years may choose to stop having cervical cancer screening (American Cancer Society, 2009c).

Testicular cancer screening. In spite of the low prevalence of testicular cancer, men should be aware that a lump in the testicle or a feeling of heaviness or swelling in the scrotum could be a sign of testicular cancer and should report these findings to his healthcare provider immediately (American Cancer Society, 2010b).

Prostate screening. Prostate cancer can be detected early with a blood test called the prostate-specific antigen (PSA) test or a digital rectal examination (DRE) by a trained healthcare professional. The American Cancer Society

does not support routine testing for prostate cancer. However, healthcare professionals may consider offering the PSA and DRE yearly to men age 50 years and older at risk for prostate cancer and with at least a 10-year life expectancy—if there are risk factors, testing should begin at age 40 to 45 years (American Cancer Society, 2009c).

Skin screening. During any health assessment or a specialized dermatological exam, a general survey of the skin using the ABCD criteria is a useful approach for assessing for skin malignancy: **A**symmetry, **B**order irregularity, **C**olor variability, **D**iameter greater than 6 mm. Rapidly changing lesions are also associated with an increased risk for cancer. Any suspicious lesions should be biopsied (Agency for Healthcare Research and Quality [AHRQ], 2010; American Cancer Society, 2009a; National Cancer Institute, 2009).

Screening for Breast Cancer. Currently, there is some controversy about whether we should encourage breast self-examination (BSE) (American Academy of Family Physicians [AAFP], 2010). In studies around the world, BSE was found not to reduce mortality due to breast cancer, and may even cause false security and delayed diagnosis when lumps are not detected. Because of the ongoing uncertainty raised by this and other studies and the fact some women do detect lumps that

signal cancer, the American Cancer Society continues to advise women that BSE is an optional screening tool and plays only a small role in finding breast cancer (American Cancer Society, 2009c). However, BSE can be a useful screening strategy when used in combination with regular physical exams and imaging studies. So until evidence is conclusive, it seems reasonable to continue to encourage and teach BSE and to recommend regular clinical breast exams and mammography and thermography.

Toward Evidence-Based Practice

Maddi, S. R., Koshaba, D. M., Fazel, M., et al. (2009, July 1). The personality construct of hardiness, IV. *Journal of Humanistic Psychology, 49*(3), 292–305.

Hardiness is a personality trait involving a blend of commitment, control, and challenge. It is the characteristic of what a person relies on to turn hardship and stressful events into growth opportunities. Researchers studied a large group of college students and found hardiness associated with positive attitudes toward school and instructors. This trait was also linked to students' beliefs in their own inner capabilities and rated higher standards for living. Those rated as hardy expressed satisfaction with life. There was an opposite association of hardiness to depression, anxiety, and hostility.

Tindle, H. A., Chang, Y. F., Kuller, L. H., et al. (2009, August 10). Optimism, cynical hostility, and incident coronary heart disease and mortality in the Women's Health Initiative. *Circulation, 120*(8), 656. Retrieved February 5, 2011, from http://circ.ahajournals.org/cgi/content/abstract/CIRCULATIONAHA.108.827642v1

A large study of nearly 100,000 postmenopausal women compared the incidence of heart disease and cancer between those who showed optimism versus those who displayed cynical, hostile attitudes toward others. Study participants had no known cardiovascular disease or cancer before enrollment in the study. Optimists had lower rates of heart disease (CHD), cancer-related deaths, and total mortality. The most cynical, hostile women had higher rates of CHD and total mortality and cancer-related mortality.

Olson, M. B., Krantz, D. S., Kelsey, S. F., et al. (2005, July–August). Hostility scores are associated with increased risk of cardiovascular events in women undergoing coronary angiography: A report from the NHLBI-Sponsored WISE Study. *Psychosomatic Medicine, 67*(4), 546–552.

The National Heart, Lung, and Blood Institute conducted a large study to look at the occurrence of adverse cardiac events among women with suspected heart attack. They measured cynicism, hostility, and aggression. In the 6-year follow-up period, after accounting for coronary artery disease and other risk factors, researchers found a 35% increased risk of angina, nonfatal myocardial infarction, stroke, and congestive heart failure. This group who suffered adverse cardiovascular events also had poorer survival than those who scored lower on the hostility rating scale.

1. Based on these studies, how might you assess cynicism and hostility in your patient?

2. Why do you think people showing more hostility had poorer survival after suffering a heart-related problem than those rated as hardy?

3. In light of the research examining the impact of attitude on health outcomes, what would you do to promote optimism in your postmenopausal patient preparing for surgery?

 Go to Chapter 27, **Toward Evidence-Based Practice Suggested Responses,** on Davis*Plus*.

Screening for Prostate Cancer. The issue of whether to perform mass prostate-specific antigen (PSA) screening for prostate cancer is also unsettled. The U.S. Preventive Services Task Force concludes that there is not sufficient evidence to recommend for or against routine PSA screening for prostate cancer. However, most experts and organizations agree that the most appropriate candidates for yearly screening are men older than age 50 and younger men who have increased risk factors (National Cancer Institute, 2009).

KnowledgeCheck 27-3

- Identify at least three common sites for health promotion activities.
- What assessments are part of a health promotion assessment?
- What role does stress play in health promotion?

 ThinkLike a Nurse 27-5

Your 55-year-old aunt tells you she hasn't had a physical examination in 20 years. She is a registered nurse. "I don't need one because I feel fine and I can take care of myself." How would you respond?

ANALYSIS/NURSING DIAGNOSIS

Wellness diagnoses are appropriate for health promotion activities. Such diagnoses describe healthy responses in areas where you can intervene to promote growth or maintenance of the healthy response. NANDA International (NANDA-I) defines a wellness diagnosis as describing "human responses to levels of wellness in an individual, family, or community that have a readiness for enhancement" (2009, p. 26). For specific NANDA-I labels that you can use to describe wellness diagnoses,

   Go to Chapter 27, **Standardized Language: Examples of NANDA-I Wellness Diagnoses,** on Davis*Plus*.

New NANDA-I wellness labels are preceded by the phrase "Readiness for Enhanced" and will be one-part statements (e.g., Readiness for Enhanced Parenting) with no etiology. Notice, however, that there are still some wellness labels that have different one-part formats (e.g., Effective Breastfeeding and Health-Promoting Behaviors).

PLANNING OUTCOMES/EVALUATION

NOC standardized outcomes related to health promotion vary depending on the focus area. For example, if the nursing diagnosis is Readiness for Enhanced Nutrition, a NOC outcome might be Nutritional Status. For examples of other NOC wellness outcomes,

   Go to Chapter 27, **Standardized Language: Examples of NOC Standardized Health Promotion Outcomes** on Davis*Plus*.

Individualized goals and outcomes might include losing 20 pounds or exercising for 30 minutes five times per week. The nurse's role in health promotion primarily is to motivate clients and facilitate change. Clients are independently responsible for most of their health promotion activities. You may need to help them identify goals, but it is essential that the goals be the clients', not yours.

You may need aggregate wellness goals for groups as well as individualized goals. Four broad goals for the U.S. population set by the *Healthy People 2020* initiative (U.S. Department of Health and Human Services [USDHHS], 2010, p. 2):

- Attain high-quality, longer lives free of preventable disease, disability, injury, and premature death.
- Achieve health equity, eliminate disparities, and improve the health of all groups.
- Create social and physical environments that promote good health for all.
- Promote healthy development and healthy behaviors across every stage of life.

Interventions to achieve these goals are targeted at the 37 topic areas shown in Box 27-2. Public health agencies at the local, state, and federal levels use these focus areas as a blueprint to design programs aimed at improving the health status of the community (USDHHS, 2010).

To view those objectives,

BOX 27-2 ■ Topics Areas of *Healthy People 2020*

1. Access to health services
2. Adolescent health
3. Arthritis, osteoporosis, and chronic back conditions
4. Blood disorders and blood safety
5. Cancer
6. Chronic kidney disease
7. Diabetes
8. Disability and secondary conditions
9. Early and middle childhood
10. Educational and community-based programs
11. Environmental health
12. Family planning
13. Food safety
14. Genomics
15. Global health
16. Health communication and health information technology (IT)
17. Healthcare-associated infections
18. Hearing and other sensory or communication disorders
19. Heart disease and stroke
20. HIV
21. Immunization and infectious diseases
22. Injury and violence prevention
23. Maternal, infant, and child health
24. Medical product safety
25. Mental health and mental disorders
26. Nutrition and overweight
27. Occupational safety and health
28. Older adults
29. Oral health
30. Physical activity and fitness
31. Public health infrastructure
32. Respiratory diseases
33. Sexually transmitted diseases
34. Social determinants of health
35. Substance abuse
36. Tobacco use
37. Vision

Source: U.S. Department of Health and Human Services, Office of Disease Prevention & Health Promotion and Human Services. (2009, October 30, revised). Proposed *Healthy People 2020 objectives.* Retrieved February 5, 2011, from http://www. healthypeople.gov/hp2020/Objectives/TopicAreas.aspx

Go to the *Healthy People 2020* Web site at http://healthypeople.gov/2020/topicsobjectives2020/pdfs/HP2020objectives.pdf

Whether standardized or individualized, expected outcomes for wellness diagnoses describe behaviors or responses that demonstrate health maintenance or achievement of an even higher level of health. For example, you may write for a patient the following: Over the next year, Mr. Needham will continue to eat a balanced diet, with more emphasis on including whole grains and fiber.

By using the highest number (5) on the rating scale, you can use the NOC to write wellness outcomes. For example:

Nursing diagnosis: Readiness for Enhanced Nutrition
Expected outcome: Nutritional Status: (5) Not compromised

PLANNING INTERVENTIONS/IMPLEMENTATION

Community and public health nurses focus on the problems contributing to disease, such as poor housing conditions, poor sanitation, poor nutrition, poverty, and substance abuse. The wellness focus in acute care is to educate patients about both health and disease.

Once the client identifies his goals, help him to identify the steps that he must take to reach the goals. Recall that change occurs in stages. To create positive change, the client will need to understand the benefits of change, overcome the barriers to change, and make a commitment to follow through on the plan.

For *NIC standardized interventions* for health promotion,

 Go to Chapter 27, **Standardized Language: Selected NIC Wellness Interventions,** on Davis*Plus.*

NIC does not have a special domain, or grouping, for wellness interventions. Instead, they are found throughout all areas of the taxonomy, particularly in the Behavioral, Safety, Family, Health System, and Community domains. Specific nursing activities for health promotion include those in following four subsections. The remainder of the chapter provides some strategies to promote their use.

Nutrition. *Dietary Guidelines for Americans* as well as the Food Guide and MyPlate for Kids (Chapter 28). In short, this means eating a balanced diet and limiting the intake of fats, sugars, and salt.

Exercise. Encourage the development of physical fitness lifestyle habits in people of all ages and abilities. For more information,

 Go to the **President's Challenge** Web site at http://www.presidentschallenge.org

Lifestyle Changes. For healthy living, adults and teens must choose a lifestyle without drugs, including tobacco, and little alcohol. Managing stress is also important.

Sleep. For an expanded discussion of these areas for health promotion,

 Go to Chapter 27, **Supplemental Materials: Individual Health Promotion Activities,** on Davis*Plus.*

Role Modeling

A role model teaches by example, demonstrating the behaviors and/or attitudes to be learned. Models provide inspiration and strategies for health promotion behavior.

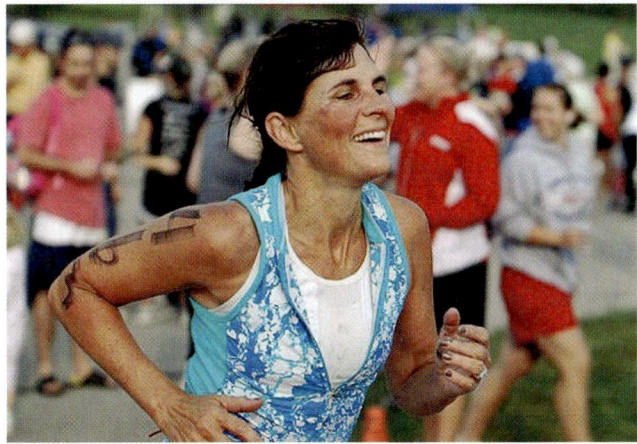

FIGURE 27-3 Vigorous-intensity exercise promotes muscle and bone strength and improves cardiovascular health.

Clients select their own role models, often without making a conscious decision to do so. But it may be helpful for you to facilitate the client's choice. When suggesting a model, consider the client's age, culture, values, and preferred activities. The model should be someone with whom the client identifies. Ideally, the role model should be someone accessible to the client during the early stages of change. This allows for interacting and for exchanging information.

Nurses also serve as role models. As a result, we should provide an example of healthy behaviors. It is difficult to advocate for healthy behavior if you do not follow the behavior that you recommend to clients. Imagine the trust a client loses when he finds out that the nurse who tells him not to smoke cigarettes has a two-pack per day habit. How compelling is a discussion of the importance of weight loss given by an nurse who is obese? To what extent do you role-model healthy behaviors?

Providing Counseling

Counseling is an interpersonal communication process that helps a client to identify problems and make changes. In the context of health promotion, counseling promotes personal growth and helps clients change their lifestyle. Counseling may be formal one-to-one or small-group discussion, or it may be informal discussion with the client at a healthcare encounter. Each meeting with a client is a potential counseling session. In addition to face-to-face contact, counseling may be offered via telephone or even by e-mail.

Individual Counseling

Face-to-face interaction may be helpful when clients are attempting major lifestyle change. In an individual session, you can customize and map out the steps required to meet the client's goals. This may include writing a contract detailing the client's expected behaviors. Print out the contract, and have the client sign it to reinforce his commitment. Suggest that the client post the plan in a location he sees often so that it serves as a frequent reminder.

During counseling sessions, remember to reinforce health-promoting behaviors that have already been established. For example, the client who uses tobacco may eat a balanced diet; reinforce the healthy habit to boost self-esteem. Stress to the client that although the behavior to be changed may be unhealthy, you believe the client can succeed in making the change.

Telephone Counseling

Telephone counseling may be used as a primary counseling approach or as follow-up. Many clients with hectic schedules find it easier to arrange telephone counseling than to schedule a face-to-face interaction. The disadvantage is that telephone counseling does not allow you to detect nonverbal communication.

When using telephone counseling, set goals and map out the strategy for change just as you would in face-to-face counseling. Make sure to inform the client about how and when you can be reached if questions arise. If you are using the telephone for follow-up counseling, it is best to schedule a time to speak. Having an appointment helps keep the patient accountable to the expected behavior and to reinforce the information.

Providing Health Education

Health education may focus on self-care strategies, caregiver concerns, or how to be an effective healthcare consumer. Self-care programs typically cover nutrition, exercise, stress management, or disease prevention. Programs may consist of lectures, printed material, billboards, or posters. For example, the accompanying Self-Care box, Teaching Clients How to Prevent Upper Respiratory Infections, might be reproduced and posted in the lounge, restrooms, or locker areas of a worksite during cold and flu season to decrease absenteeism. Caregiver education programs may teach caregivers how to perform nursing tasks or prevent injuries, or they may provide a list of community resources for respite care. Nurses can teach clients how to be effective healthcare consumers, how to interact with healthcare providers, and how to maneuver through the healthcare system. For a review of teaching and learning, see Chapter 26.

Providing and Facilitating Support for Lifestyle Change

Changing one's lifestyle is difficult. Most clients need support to make the change. You can provide support during your interactions and counseling sessions. You can also help the client to identify available support and resources within the community as well as from family, friends, coworkers, and others.

Group support exists for a variety of lifestyle changes. For example, Weight Watchers® is a group support program for clients who want to lose weight; Alcoholics Anonymous is a group support program for clients who want to become and stay sober; various cancer support groups help clients deal with the common issues and fears associated with dealing with a potentially life-threatening disease. Group support provides clients with a chance to meet people experiencing the same difficulties and perhaps to find a role model. As a nurse, you should be familiar with various programs available in your community and refer clients to them.

KnowledgeCheck 27-4

Identify four strategies to help a client engage in positive lifestyle changes.

Self-Care

Teaching Clients How to Prevent Upper Respiratory Infections

➤ Maintain a healthy lifestyle. That means get adequate sleep, good nutrition, and physical exercise. A balanced diet and physical fitness can boost your immune system to fight infection if it occurs.

➤ Wash your hands often; teach children to do so as well. This helps prevent spread of infection. When using public restrooms, wash your hands. Turn off the faucet with a paper towel. Also use a paper towel to open the door as you leave the room.

➤ Avoid touching your eyes, nose, and mouth because doing so spreads any virus your hands have contacted (e.g., on doorknobs).

➤ Avoid crowds, especially when there is a cold or influenza epidemic.

➤ Throw away tissues as soon as you use them.

➤ When someone in the family has a cold, keep bathrooms and the kitchen very clean and do not drink from the same glass or use the same utensils.

➤ When someone at home or at work has a cold, wipe telephone receivers with soap and water or an antibacterial solution.

➤ If a child has a cold, wash his toys and commonly used items well.

➤ When choosing child care, look for a clean environment; ask what rules are in place concerning keeping the children clean (e.g., washing hands before snack time).

➤ Don't smoke. Cigarette smoke can irritate the respiratory tract, making you more susceptible to colds and illness.

➤ Control stress. People experiencing emotional stress tend to have weakened immunity to fight infection.

➤ Consider taking echinacea or zinc lozenges, although there is no conclusive evidence of their effectiveness (Singh & Das, 2011). Consult your primary healthcare provider.

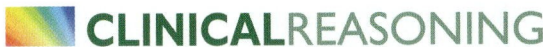 **CLINICAL**REASONING
Applying the **Full-Spectrum Nursing Model**

Because the following critical thinking activities allow you to practice the kind of thinking you will use as a full-spectrum nurse, they usually have no single right answer. Discuss them with your peers—if you have difficulty with any of the questions, consult your instructor.

PATIENT SITUATION

Shandra Shane is a single 37-year-old woman with three children, ages 12, 15, and 17. She is raising the children on her own, although her sister occasionally helps with transportation or advice about disciplining her teenage daughters. Ms. Shane is a night-shift worker at the hospital. Her typical schedule is 3 to 4 hours of sleep in the morning soon after she gets home and then a short nap in the early evening before going back to work. She smokes 1 to 1 1/2 packs of cigarettes per day but tells you she has been trying to smoke less around her children. Her job stress is high, as the hospital is cutting back on the number of staff. Ms. Shane also takes care of her aging mother, who has Alzheimer's and lives with her. Ms. Shane's outlet for stress is going out with friends and drinking beer on the weekend. She is seeking your professional guidance to lose some weight (about 60 pounds) and to feel more energetic.

THINKING

1. *Theoretical Knowledge:*
   List health behaviors that negatively influence health status.
2. *Critical Thinking (Contextual Awareness):*
   What factors in this situation would you consider threatening Ms. Shane's health and could lead to disease later in life?

DOING

3. *Nursing Process (Planning/Intervention):*
   What suggestions might you make about Ms. Shane's diet that could help her to lose weight? Why might these actions be effective for weight loss?
4. *Practical Knowledge:*
   What areas of her daily living other than her diet might you explore further and offer recommendations for improving to promote better health and prevent illness?

CARING

5. *Self-Knowledge:*
   Have you ever been in a situation where you felt stressed, tired, and wanting gratification offered by food, nicotine, or alcohol? Describe your experience.
6. *Ethical:*
   In what ways could you demonstrate genuine caring for Ms. Shane?

 Go to Chapter 27, **Clinical Reasoning: Applying the Full-Spectrum Nursing Model Response Sheet,** on DavisPlus.

 To explore learning resources for this chapter,

 Go to DavisPlus at http://davisplus.fadavis.com, keyword Treas
Chapter Resources for Chapter 27:
   Knowledge Check and Think Like a Nurse Response Sheets
   Knowledge Check Answers
   Resources for Caregivers and Health Professionals
   Reading More About Health Promotion (suggested readings)
   What Are the Main Points in This Chapter?
NCLEX-Style Review Questions
Chapter Overview Podcasts
Care Planning and Care Mapping Practice Exercises

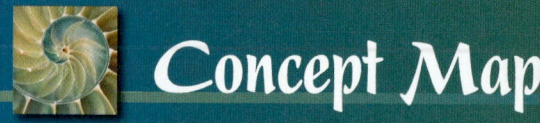

Concept Map

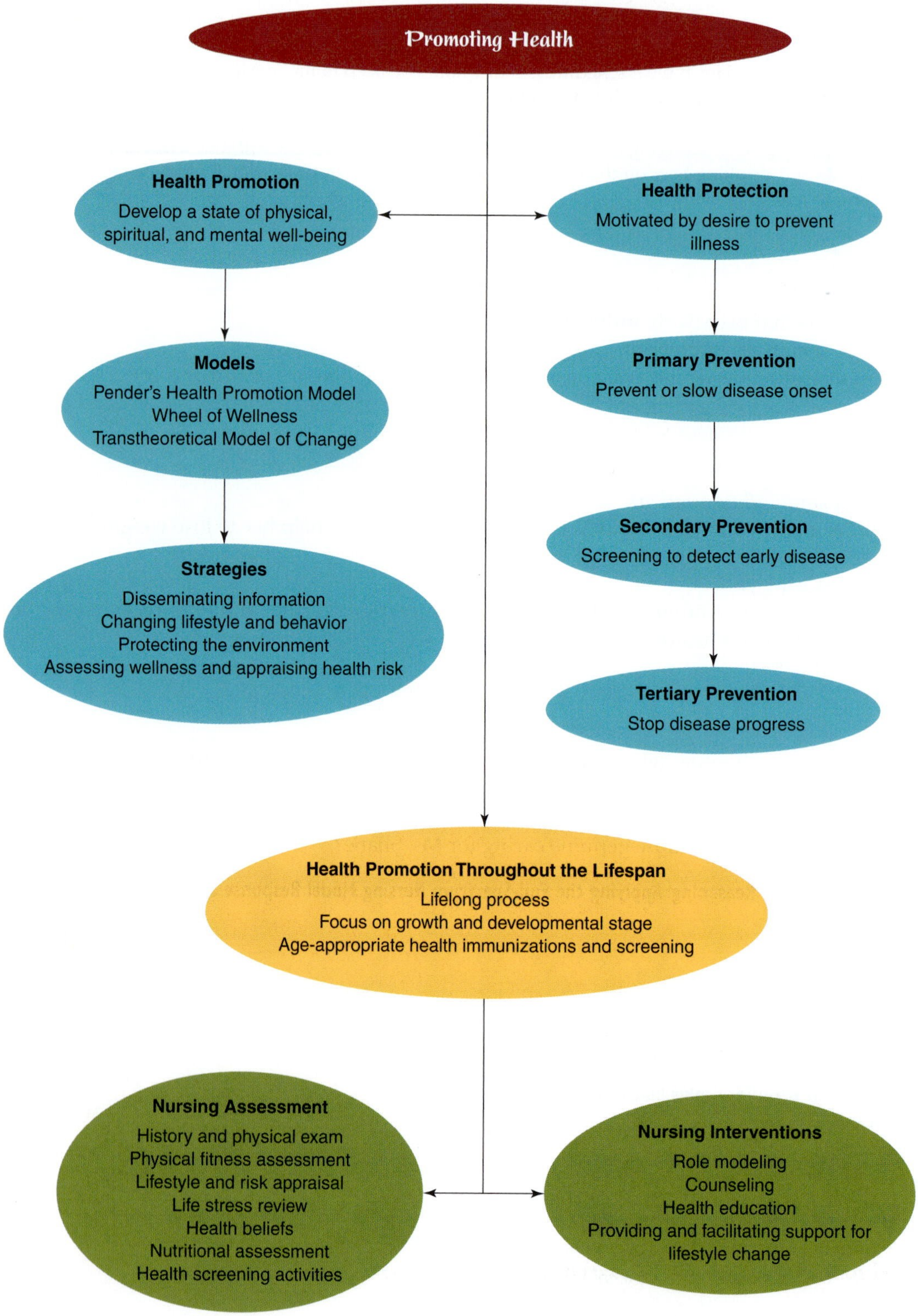

Promoting Health

Health Promotion
Develop a state of physical, spiritual, and mental well-being

Health Protection
Motivated by desire to prevent illness

Models
Pender's Health Promotion Model
Wheel of Wellness
Transtheoretical Model of Change

Primary Prevention
Prevent or slow disease onset

Strategies
Disseminating information
Changing lifestyle and behavior
Protecting the environment
Assessing wellness and appraising health risk

Secondary Prevention
Screening to detect early disease

Tertiary Prevention
Stop disease progress

Health Promotion Throughout the Lifespan
Lifelong process
Focus on growth and developmental stage
Age-appropriate health immunizations and screening

Nursing Assessment
History and physical exam
Physical fitness assessment
Lifestyle and risk appraisal
Life stress review
Health beliefs
Nutritional assessment
Health screening activities

Nursing Interventions
Role modeling
Counseling
Health education
Providing and facilitating support for lifestyle change

Supporting Physiological Function

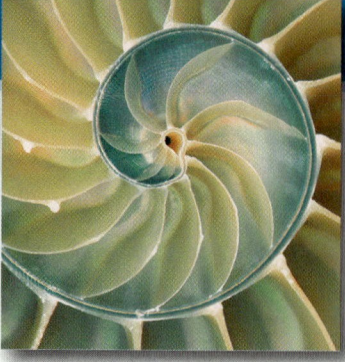

CHAPTER 28

Nutrition

Learning Outcomes

After completing this chapter, you should be able to:

➤ Identify the types, functions, metabolism, and major food sources of (1) the energy nutrients, (2) vitamins, (3) minerals, and (4) water.

➤ Differentiate among the various sources of nutritional information (e.g., USDA dietary guidelines, ChooseMyPlate, DRIs, Nutrition Facts labels).

➤ Calculate a client's basal metabolic rate.

➤ Identify the primary nutritional considerations for various developmental stages.

➤ Discuss how each of the following affects and is affected by nutritional status: lifestyle choices, vegetarianism, dieting for weight loss, culture and religion, disease processes, functional limitations, and special diets.

➤ Describe tools and techniques for gathering subjective data about nutritional status.

➤ Compare the effectiveness of various anthropometric measurements.

➤ Calculate the body mass index for a client.

➤ Explain the significance of body mass index.

➤ List at least five physical assessment findings that indicate nutritional imbalance.

➤ Identify laboratory values that are indicators of nutritional status.

➤ Discuss the need for and advisability of vitamin and mineral supplementation.

➤ Describe nursing interventions for patients with special needs: Impaired Swallowing, NPO, older adults, and Nausea.

➤ Describe techniques for assisting patients with meals.

➤ Identify and discuss six nursing interventions for Imbalanced Nutrition: Less Than Body Requirements and six interventions for Imbalanced Nutrition: More Than Body Requirements.

➤ Safely provide enteral and parenteral nutrition for patients.

Key Concepts

Energy
Metabolism
Nutrition

Example Problems

Overweight and Obesity
Underweight/Undernutrition

Related Concepts

See the Concept Map at the end of this chapter.

Caring for the Nguyens

This feature allows you to practice the kind of thinking you will use as a full-spectrum nurse. There is usually more than one correct answer to a critical thinking question, so we do not provide answers for these features. It is more important to develop your nursing judgment than to "cover content." Discuss the questions with your peers. If you are still unsure, consult your instructor.

Nam Nguyen has been diagnosed with hypertension, type 2 diabetes mellitus, obesity, osteoarthritis, and tobacco abuse. Zach Jackson has advised an 1,800-kcal diabetic diet with no added salt and a brisk daily 30-minute walk. Mr. Nguyen discusses these challenges with his daughter, Trinh.

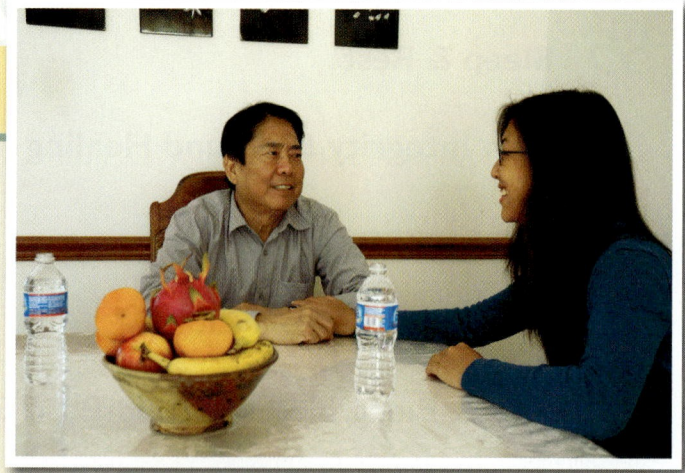

Caring for the Nyugens (continued)

A. Why might Zach have selected this diet plan? Discuss the rationale for each component (i.e., 1,800 kcal, diabetic diet, no added salt).

B. Mr. Nguyen's diet is complex. He tells you he is overwhelmed by the many changes asked of him. How might Zach streamline his instructions about his diet?

C. Nam asks what is the best way for him to monitor his weight loss progress at home and how Zach Jackson will monitor his progress. How would you respond?

D. Identify teaching tools that might help Nam understand his diet.

 Go to **Caring for the Nguyens Response Sheet** on *DavisPlus*.

Meet Your Patients

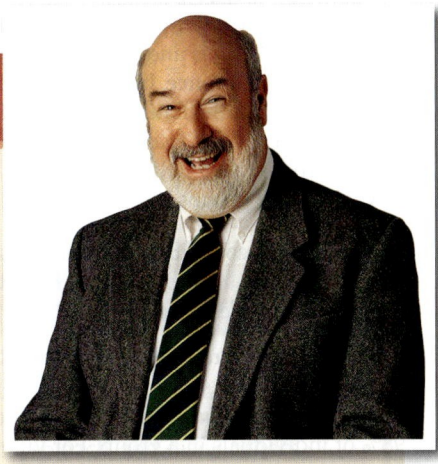

As part of a class assignment, you are to assist a local business with its wellness program. You will be completing health risk appraisals and gathering the following data on each of the employees: height, weight, medical and nutritional history, and lifestyle practices. Today you will screen two employees, and then each will have blood drawn for a complete blood count (CBC), comprehensive metabolic panel, and lipid panel:

- *Isaac Schwartz,* a 65-year-old accountant, works long hours. He describes a sedentary lifestyle, no tobacco use, infrequent alcohol use, no medical problems, and a nutritional history of skipping meals and daily consumption of restaurant food. You measure his height as 69 in. and weight as 245 lb.
- *Sujing Lee,* a 29-year-old project manager, regularly works 65 hours per week. Sujing is 30 weeks pregnant. She does not smoke or drink and has never been hospitalized or had surgery. She has gained a total of 25 lb since becoming pregnant. Her diet consists mainly of traditional Chinese food. She eats three meals a day

and always brings lunch from home. Lately she has felt "tired all the time." At the screening, she weighs 126 lb and measures 63 in. tall.

At the end of your clinical day, you need to compile a report on the clients you have seen. How would you interpret the data on height, weight, and nutrition? What, if any, additional information do you need to help you evaluate their nutritional status? In this chapter, you will read about dietary recommendations, energy balance, and nutritional concerns across the life span. You will gain the theoretical knowledge to answer these questions, as well as practical knowledge about managing nutritional problems.

Theoretical Knowledge
knowing **why**

Organic, natural, low-fat, sugar-free, reduced-calorie, low-sodium, calcium-enriched . . . these are just a few of the hundreds of claims that you find on packaged foods. Television and print ads hype nutritional supplements, weight-loss pills, and new diets, while the media carries conflicting reports on the benefits and dangers of phytochemicals, antioxidants, and *trans*-fatty acids. With so many options and different recommendations about what's healthy or not, it's no wonder that many people are confused about what to eat.

ABOUT THE KEY CONCEPTS

Nutrition is the study of food: how it affects the human body and influences health, and how the body metabolizes food for energy. Good nutrition is essential to wellness, and poor nutrition contributes to disease; so clients need accurate, current, and appropriate nutritional information. Before you can give effective individualized advice, you need to know about the nutrients found in foods. In this chapter you will learn about concepts related to energy, for example, energy balance, nutrients, micronutrients, and factors that influence nutritional status.

sugars) consist of a single unit; **disaccharides** are molecules made up of two saccharides. **Complex carbohydrates** consist of long chains of saccharides, called **polysaccharides. Dietary fiber,** a polysaccharide, is the indigestible "fibrous skeleton" of plant foods. Humans do not have the enzymes to digest fiber; thus, it provides no usable glucose. Carbohydrates perform several functions:

1. *Supply energy for muscle and organ function.* Carbohydrates, which are more easily and quickly digested than proteins and lipids, fuel strenuous short-term skeleton muscle activity and provide nearly all the energy for the brain. Humans store glucose in liver and skeletal muscle tissue as **glycogen.** Glycogen is converted back into glucose to meet energy needs. This process is called **glycogenolysis.**

2. *Spare protein.* If glycogen stores are low (for instance, in a person who is undernourished), physical activity causes the breakdown of body stores of protein **(gluconeogenesis)** and lipids (fats) to use for energy. But when proteins are used for energy, they are not available for their primary functions of tissue growth, maintenance, and repair. Fats are converted directly into an alternative fuel called **ketones;** ketones raise the acidity of the blood and can lead to acid–base imbalance. Fats are used for fuel in persons with diabetes, whose cells cannot use glucose for energy.

3. *Other physiological functions.* Carbohydrates enhance insulin secretion, increase satiety (feeling of fullness and satisfaction), and improve absorption of sodium and excretion of calcium. **Insulin** is a pancreatic hormone that promotes the movement of glucose into the cells for use. To see the basic chemical structure of four types of carbohydrates,

 Go to Chapter 28, **Tables, Boxes, and Figures: ESG Figure 28-1,** on Davis*Plus.*

Proteins

Proteins are complex molecules made up of *amino acids.* Every amino acid consists of a central carbon atom connected to a hydrogen atom, an acid, an *amine* (a region of the molecule containing nitrogen), and a side chain. Just 20 different amino acids are the building blocks of most of the proteins in the human body (Table 28-2). The **essential amino acids** are significant in our diets because the body cannot manufacture them. They must be supplied by food or nutritional supplements. In contrast, the body can synthesize the 10 **nonessential amino acids,** so we do not need to obtain them from food. To see the basic structural formula for an amino acid and a polypeptide,

 Go to Chapter 28, **Tables, Boxes, and Figures: ESG Figure 28-2,** on Davis*Plus.*

For protein synthesis to occur, every amino acid necessary to build that protein must be available. **Complete protein** foods contain all of the essential amino acids necessary for protein synthesis. These usually come from animal sources. **Incomplete protein** foods (e.g., nuts, grains) do not provide all of the essential amino acids. However, by combining two incomplete proteins, a complete protein can be made. For instance, peanut butter on whole-grain bread constitutes a complete protein. Protein complementing allows for a healthful vegetarian diet.

Protein Metabolism and Storage

Although protein digestion begins in the stomach, it occurs mostly in the small intestine, where enzymes break it down into amino acids (see Table 28-1). The body continually breaks down and resynthesizes protein into tissues, adjusting as

Table 28-2 ▶ Amino Acids		
TYPE	**DESCRIPTION**	**EXAMPLES**
Essential	Must be obtained from the diet; cannot be made in the body.	Arginine,* histidine, isoleucine, leucine, lysine, methionine, phenylalanine, threonine, tryptophan, and valine
Nonessential	Easily synthesized by the body.	Alanine, asparagine, aspartic acid, cysteine,** glutamic acid, glutamine, glycine, proline, serine, and tyrosine**

*Considered by some to be "semi-essential" because it cannot be synthesized at a rate that will support growth. Therefore, it is essential for children, but not for most adults.
**Considered conditionally essential. That is, essential in some situations (e.g., in immaturity, during severe stress).
Sources: Guyton, A. C., & Hall, J. E. (2011). *Textbook of medical physiology* (12th ed.), Philadelphia: W. B. Saunders; Lutz, C., & Przytulski, K. (2011). *Nutrition and diet therapy* (5th ed.). Philadelphia: F.A. Davis; Thompson, J., & Manore, M. (2011). *Nutrition: An applied approach* (3rd ed.). San Francisco: Benjamin Cummings; U.S. Department of Agriculture, Food and Nutrition Center (n.d.).

needed to maintain overall protein balance. The body also maintains a balance between tissue protein and plasma protein. When amino acids are catabolized, the nitrogen-containing part is converted to ammonia (NH_3) and excreted in the urine as urea. Therefore, nitrogen balance reflects how well body tissues are being maintained.

Nitrogen balance occurs when intake and output of nitrogen are equal. A **positive nitrogen balance** exists when nitrogen intake exceeds output, making a pool of amino acids available for growth, pregnancy, and tissue maintenance and repair. **Negative nitrogen balance** exists when nitrogen intake is lower than nitrogen loss. This occurs in illness, injury (e.g., burns), and malnutrition.

Functions of Protein

Dietary proteins perform the following functions:

- *Tissue building.* Protein is the structural material of every cell in the body. Except for water, protein makes up the biggest part of the body. It is essential for growth, maintenance, and repair.
- *Metabolism.* Proteins are essential for building body tissue. For example, proteins are precursors to digestive enzymes and hormones (e.g., thyroxine). **Enzymes** facilitate cellular reactions throughout the body. In addition, proteins combine with iron to form hemoglobin, the oxygen carrier in red blood cells.
- *Immune system function.* **Lymphocytes** (specialized white blood cells [WBCs]) and antibodies (components of our immune system that defend against foreign invaders) are proteins.
- *Fluid balance.* Because they attract water, proteins in cells and the bloodstream help regulate fluid balance.

- *Acid–base balance.* Blood proteins function as buffers, helping to regulate acid–base balance.
- *Secondary energy source.* As noted earlier, proteins can be broken down to provide energy when stores of the other energy nutrients are inadequate (Thompson & Manore, 2011).

Protein needs vary according to age, sex, weight, and health. Lean meat is nourishing and healthy as long as it is consumed in modest amounts and is not processed (Honenyard, 2008). Many North Americans eat more protein than they need, especially in the form of meat. There is no health benefit from eating more than the recommended amount of protein. In fact, there may be health risks in eating diets high in animal protein. Animal proteins, high in saturated fat, increase the risk for certain cancers and coronary artery disease.

Lipids

Lipids are organic (carbon-containing) substances that are insoluble in water. They are made up of carbon, hydrogen, and oxygen—the same basic elements that make up carbohydrates. The term *lipid* comes from *lipos,* the Greek word for "fat." Lipids that are solid at room temperature are called *fats,* whereas those that are liquid at room temperature are called *oils.* For example, butter is a fat even when it is melted, because it would be solid at room temperature. You will hear the terms (*lipids* and *fats*) used interchangeably.

People in developed countries typically eat a diet relatively high in fat. In the United States about 45% of our total energy consumption comes from fat. Fat is an essential nutrient, but certain types, when consumed in excess, can also be a health hazard.

Lipid metabolism occurs in the small intestine. Lipids are stored as adipose tissue. Because lipids are insoluble in water, and because blood is primarily water, lipid absorption requires a solvent carrier.

Types and Sources of Lipids

The three types of lipids found in foods are glycerides, sterols, and phospholipids (Box 28-2). **Glycerides** (also called **true fats**) consist of one molecule of glycerol attached to one, two, or three fatty acid chains. *Glycerol* is an alcohol composed of three carbon atoms. *Fatty acids* are long chains of carbon and hydrogen atoms ending in an acid. Most glycerides found in foods are *triglycerides,* which are compounds consisting of a glycerol molecule attached to three fatty acids. To see the basic structural formula for a triglyceride and cholesterol,

 Go to Chapter 28, **Tables, Boxes, and Figures: ESG Figure 28-3,** on Davis*Plus.*

Sterols are lipids, but they are not made of fatty acids. The most important sterol in the body is **cholesterol,** a wax-like substance needed for the formation of cell membranes, vitamin D, estrogen, and testosterone. Cholesterol is synthesized in the liver, and it is also found in animal foods.

Phospholipids (which contain a phosphate group) are soluble in water. They are a key component of **lipoproteins,** which consist of phospholipids and a protein. Because they are water soluble, lipoproteins are the major transport vehicles for lipids in the bloodstream. By "wrapping" triglycerides with water-soluble phosphates and proteins, lipoproteins deliver these substances to body cells.

- **Low-density lipoproteins (LDLs)** transport cholesterol to body cells. Diets high in saturated fats increase LDLs circulating in the bloodstream and may result in fatty deposits on vessel walls, causing cardiovascular disease. As a result, LDL is often known as the "bad cholesterol."
- **High-density lipoproteins (HDLs)** remove cholesterol from the bloodstream, returning it to the liver, where it is used to produce bile; thus, a high blood level of HDL is considered protective against cardiovascular disease. It is often known as the "good cholesterol."

Saturated and Unsaturated Fatty Acids

Fatty acids are classified as saturated, unsaturated, or *trans*-fats (Table 28-3). **Saturation** means that a substance is holding all that it is capable of holding (e.g., think of a wound dressing saturated with blood).

- An **unsaturated fatty acid** is one that is not completely filled with all the hydrogen it can hold. Therefore, it is lighter and less dense. Fats made up primarily of unsaturated fatty acids are called **unsaturated fats.** Molecules of **monounsaturated fats** have one unfilled spot where hydrogen is not attached. **Polyunsaturated fatty acids** contain two or more unfilled spots for hydrogen. At the spot(s) where the molecule does not have a hydrogen attached, it becomes kinked and does not pack together. This is why these fats are liquid at room temperature. Replacing saturated fats in the diet with mono- and polyunsaturated fats reduces the risk of heart disease and stroke. Dietary fat should mainly be polyunsaturated and unsaturated, from food sources, such as fish and nuts.
- **Saturated fatty acids** are those in which every carbon atom is fully bound to (or "saturated" with) hydrogen. The molecules pack tightly together at room temperature and are dense, solid, and heavy. A fat made up mostly of saturated fatty acids is called a **saturated fat.** Animal fats are the primary source of saturated fats in the North American diet; however, many processed foods contain saturated fats.
- *Trans*-**fatty acids** are saturated fats created when food manufacturers add hydrogen to polyunsaturated plant oils, such as corn oil, to break the double carbon bonds and straighten out the molecules. This process solidifies the fat and extends the shelf life of the food. *Trans*-fats are found in margarine and other processed foods containing *hydrogenated vegetable oils.*

Saturated fats and *trans*-fats are the main dietary factors in increasing blood cholesterol levels. They raise LDL cholesterol levels. The FDA mandates that *trans*-fat content be listed on all food labels. Intake of saturated fats and *trans*-fats should be limited.

Essential and Nonessential Fatty Acids

A fatty acid is considered **essential** if (1) the body cannot manufacture it and (2) its absence creates a deficiency disease. The essential fatty acids, **linoleic acid (omega-6)** and **alpha-linolenic acid (omega-3)**, help protect against heart disease. Omega-6 fatty acid is found mainly in polyunsaturated

---

BOX 28-2 ■ Types of Lipids

Glycerol Molecules (bonded to) Fatty Acid Molecules

Glycerides

Monoglycerides	1	1
Diglycerides	1	2
Triglycerides	1	3
Sterols	0	0
Phospholipids	1	2 + a phosphate group

Table 28-3 ➤ Dietary Fats

TYPE OF FAT	SOURCES	EFFECT ON BLOOD CHOLESTEROL
Monounsaturated	Olives; olive oil, canola oil, peanut oil; cashews, almonds, peanuts, and most other nuts; avocados	Lowers LDL and raises HDL.
Polyunsaturated	Corn, soybean, safflower, sesame, sunflower, and cottonseed oils; fish, nuts, and seeds	Lowers LDL and raises HDL.
Saturated	Whole milk, butter, cheese, and ice cream; lard; red meat; chocolate; coconuts, coconut milk, and coconut oil; palm oils; cocoa butter	Raises LDL and HDL.
Trans-fats	Most margarines; vegetable shortening; partially hydrogenated vegetable oil; deep-fried chips; many fast foods (e.g., French fries, donuts); most commercial baked goods	Raises LDL.
Dietary Cholesterol	Foods from animals: meats, egg yolks, dairy products, organ meats (e.g., heart, liver), fish, and poultry	Raises cholesterol.

AMERICAN HEART ASSOCIATION RECOMMENDATIONS

Limit foods high in saturated fat, *trans*-fat, and/or cholesterol. Instead choose foods low in saturated fat, *trans*-fat and cholesterol. Here are some helpful tips (AHA, n.d.[a]):

- Limit intake of whole-milk dairy products, fatty meats, tropical oils, partially hydrogenated vegetable oils, and egg yolks.
- Include a variety of fruits and vegetables in the diet.
- Eat a variety of grain products; include whole grains.
- Eat fish, particularly fatty fish, at least twice a week.
- Include fat-free and low-fat milk products and legumes.
- Choose skinless poultry and lean meats.
- Choose fats and oils with 2 g or less saturated fat per tablespoon (e.g., liquid and tub margarines, canola oil).

vegetable oils, nuts, and seeds. Omega-3 fatty acid can be obtained in adequate amounts by eating fatty fish (e.g., tuna, shellfish) twice a week (American Heart Association, 2008).

Functions of Lipids

Lipids perform the following functions:

1. *Supply essential nutrients.* Food fats supply the essential fatty acids and aid in the absorption of fat-soluble vitamins.
2. *Energy source.* Although carbohydrates are the primary energy source during strenuous physical activity, our bodies burn fat for energy when we are engaging in sustained light activity, when we are at rest, and when glycogen stores are exhausted.
3. *Flavor and satiety.* Lipids give food its creamy taste and texture and promote satiety (the feeling of being "full"). Fats are digested more slowly than carbohydrates, so stomach emptying time is slower.
4. *Other functions.* Body fat provides insulation, protects vital organs, aids in thermoregulation, and enables accurate nerve-impulse transmission. In addition, lipids are a component of every cell membrane and are essential to cell metabolism.
5. *Cholesterol functions.* Cholesterol is a component of every cell in the body, where it lends suppleness and support. It is also an ingredient of bile, which helps digest fats, and serves as a precursor to all steroid hormones, including sex hormones. When lipid metabolism is "disordered," cholesterol contributes to atherosclerosis.

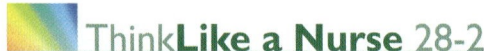

ThinkLike a Nurse 28-2

Review the information you collected on the two employees (Meet Your Patients).

- What conclusions, if any, can you make about their intake of carbohydrates, protein, and fats?
- How might you gather additional data on their intake of the energy nutrients?

WHAT ARE THE MICRONUTRIENTS?

Vitamins and minerals are called **micronutrients** because they are required by the body in only very small amounts. Although they provide no energy, they are critical in regulating a variety of body functions.

Vitamins

Vitamins are organic substances that are necessary for metabolism or preventing a particular deficiency disease. Because the body cannot make vitamins, they must be supplied by the foods we eat. Vitamins are critical in building and maintaining body tissues, supporting our immune system so we can fight disease, and ensuring healthy vision. They also help our bodies to break down and use the energy found in carbohydrates, proteins, and lipids. Vitamins are especially critical during periods of rapid growth, pregnancy, lactation, and healing. Some evidence supports the claim that certain vitamins prevent chronic illness (Institute of Medicine, 2000; Jockers, 2007).

Table 28-4 ➤ Vitamins: Adult Dietary Reference Intakes (DRIs)—cont'd

VITAMIN	FUNCTION	RDA/AI*	SOURCES	EFFECTS OF DEFICIENCY	SYMPTOMS OF EXCESS
B_{12} (cyanocobal-amin)	Metabolic reactions Maintain myelin sheath Hemoglobin synthesis	2.4 mcg/day	Dairy products, meat, poultry, fish, liver, milk, cheese, eggs	Pernicious anemia, irreversible nerve damage, memory loss, dementia	Unlikely; readily excreted
C	Collagen synthesis "Cementing" substance for capillary walls Antioxidant Iron absorption Immune function	*Females:* 75 mg/day *Males (age 19+):* 90 mg/day Additional 35 mg/day for those who smoke	Citrus fruits, tomatoes, potatoes, green vegetables, cauliflower	Anemia, tissue bleeding, easy bone fracture, gingivitis, petechiae, poor wound healing, joint pain, scurvy	Stomach inflammation, diarrhea, oxalate kidney stones

Note: I mcg = 40 International Units (IU).
• Recommended Dietary Allowances (RDAs)—Intake sufficient to meet the needs of 97%–98% of individuals in a group.
• Adequate Intakes (AIs)—Recommended intake believed to cover the needs of all individuals in the group. These are used when RDAs can't be determined.
• Upper Intake Levels (UIs)—The maximum daily intake likely to pose no risk of adverse effects.
†RDAs are usually less than adult values for infants and children, more for pregnant women, and highest for lactating women. RDAs for some vitamins (e.g., vitamin A) are higher for older adults and higher for men than for women.
‡The American Academy of Pediatrics recommends 10 mcg/day of vitamin D for infancy through adolescence (Wagner, Greer, & the Section on Breastfeeding and Committee on Nutrition, 2008). Other clinicians and researchers have suggested that the RDA for adults should be dramatically increased as well, to 20–25 mcg (800–1000 IU) for adults age 50 and older (Jockers, 2007).

 Go to Chapter 28, **Supplemental Materials, Dietary Reference Intakes: Vitamins,** on Davis*Plus.*

Sources: Adapted from National Institutes of Health, Office of Dietary Supplements. *Dietary Reference Intake Levels: Vitamins.* (2011). Retrieved from http://ods.od.nih.gov/Health_information/Dietary_Reference_Intakes.aspx. Complete reports are available at http://fnic.nal.usda.gov/nal_display/index.php? info_center=4&tax_level=3&tax_subject=256&topic_id=1342&level3_id=5140 ; summary tables are available at http://www.iom.edu/Global/ News%20Announcements/~/media/474B28C39EA34C43A60A6D42CCE07427.ashx; Institute of Medicine of the National Academies, Food and Nutrition Board. (2010). DRIs for calcium and Vitamin D. Retrieved on June 16, 2011, from http://iom.edu/Activities/Nutrition/SummaryDRIs/~/media/Files/Activity%20Files/ Nutrition/DRIs/RDA%20and%20AIs_Vitamin%20and%20Elements.pdf; Lutz, C., & Przytulski, K. (2010). Nutrition and diet therapy: Evidence-based applications (4th ed.). Philadelphia: F.A. Davis.

are regularly excreted by the kidneys in the urine. Thus, toxicity is rare except in people with renal disease. However, because excess amounts are excreted, the body cannot store these vitamins, so they need to be consumed every day.

Minerals

Minerals are inorganic elements found in nature. They occur in foods either naturally or as additives, as well as in supplements. **Major minerals (macrominerals)** are minerals that the body needs in amounts of 100 mg/day or greater. **Trace minerals** are essential, but in a lower concentration. In the United States, calcium deficiency is one of the most common mineral deficiencies (Table 28-5).

Minerals assist in fluid regulation, nerve impulse transmission, and energy production; they are essential to the health of bones and blood and help rid the body of by-products of metabolism. Evidence also shows that minerals play key roles in disease prevention and treatment. For example:

1. Adequate *calcium* intake throughout the life span decreases the likelihood of osteoporosis (a condition marked by porous bones). The recommended daily intake of 1,200 mg

for adults age 50 years and older (Lim, Hoeksema, Sherin, ACPM Prevention Practice Committee, 2009; National Guideline Clearinghouse [NGC], 2009; National Institutes of Health, Office of Dietary Supplements, 2011) is difficult to achieve by diet alone.

2. *Iron* deficiency causes anemia, the most common nutritional problem worldwide.

3. *Magnesium* may decrease the risk of hypertension and coronary artery disease in women.

4. *Sodium,* consumed in high amounts (greater than 2,500 mg/ day), increases the risk for high blood pressure, heart attacks, and stroke.

Minerals are absorbed mostly in the small intestine. Salt and potassium are absorbed in the large intestine, however. If the body is deficient in a mineral, it absorbs more; if the body has enough, it absorbs less and excretes more in the feces. Minerals interact with other minerals, vitamins, and other substances to accomplish absorption and metabolism and perform their functions. For example, iron absorption is enhanced in the presence of vitamin C, and vitamin D deficiency inhibits calcium absorption.

Table 28-5 ➤ Minerals: Adult Dietary Reference Intakes*

MINERAL	FUNCTION	RDA[†]	SOURCES	EFFECTS OF DEFICIENCY	SYMPTOMS OF EXCESS
Macrominerals					
Calcium (Ca)	Bone and teeth formation, blood clotting, nerve conduction, muscle contraction, cellular metabolism, heart action	700 mg/day (AI), ages 1–3; 1,000 mg/day (AI) ages 4–8; 1,300 mg/day (AI), ages 9–18; 1,000 mg/day, ages 19–70 (although females 51–70 years need 1,200 mg/day); 1,200 mg/day, age 70 and older.	Dairy products, sardines, green leafy vegetables, broccoli, whole grains, egg yolks, legumes, nuts, fortified products	Bone loss, tetany, rickets, osteoporosis	Kidney stones, constipation, intestinal gas
Magnesium (Mg)	Aids thyroid hormone secretion, maintains normal basal metabolic rate, activates enzymes for carbohydrate and protein metabolism, nerve and muscle function, cardiac function	Females: 310 mg/day (AI), age 19–30 age Males: 400 mg/day (AI), ages 19–30; 420 mg/day, age 31+	Whole grains, nuts, legumes, green leafy vegetables, lima beans, broccoli, squash, potatoes	Tremor, spasm, convulsions, weakness, muscle pain, poor cardiac function	Weakness, nausea, malaise
Phosphorus (P)	Bone and tooth strength, overall metabolism, formation of enzymes, acid–base balance	700 mg/day (AI), age 19+	Dairy products, beef, pork, beans, sardines, eggs, chicken, wheat bran, chocolate	Bone loss, poor growth	Tetany, convulsions
Potassium (K)	Intracellular fluid control, acid–base balance, nerve transmission, muscle contraction, glycogen formation, protein synthesis, energy metabolism, blood pressure regulation	4.7 g/day (AI)	Unprocessed foods, especially fruits, any vegetables, meats, potatoes, avocados, legumes, milk, molasses, shellfish, dates, figs	Muscle weakness (including weakness of heart and respiratory muscles), weak pulse, fatigue, abdominal distention. (Rarely occurs as a result of inadequate dietary intake. More likely due to losses from prolonged vomiting, diarrhea, or some diuretic drugs.)	Cardiac dysrhythmias, cardiac arrest, weakness, abdominal cramps, diarrhea, anxiety, paresthesia
Sodium (Na)	Water balance, acid–base balance, muscle action, nerve transmission, convulsions	1.5 g/day (AI), ages 19–50; 1.3 g/day, age 51–70; 1.2 g/day, age 70+	Table salt (NaCl), milk, meat, eggs, baking soda, baking powder, celery, spinach, carrots, beets	Dizziness, abdominal cramping, nausea, vomiting, diarrhea, tachycardia, convulsions, coma. (Rarely occurs except in heavy exercise and sweating.)	Thirst, fever, dry and sticky tongue and mucous membranes, restlessness, irritability, convulsion

Table 28-5 ▶ Minerals: Adult Dietary Reference Intakes*—cont'd

MINERAL	FUNCTION	RDA†	SOURCES	EFFECTS OF DEFICIENCY	SYMPTOMS OF EXCESS
Trace Minerals					
Copper	Aids in iron metabolism, works with many enzymes in protein metabolism and hormone synthesis	900 mcg/day (AI), age 19+	Liver, seafood, cocoa, legumes, nuts, whole grains	Rarely occurs: anemia, low WBC count, poor growth	Vomiting, nervous system disorders
Fluoride	Increases resistance to dental caries	Females: 3 mg/day (AI), age 14+ Males: 4 mg/day (AI), age 19+	Fluorinated water, toothpaste, dental treatment, seaweed, fish, tea	Increased dental caries	Stomach upset, staining of teeth, bone pain
Iodine	Synthesis of the thyroid hormone, thyroxine	150 mcg/day, age 14+	Iodized salt, salt water fish, dairy products, enriched white bread	Goiter, poor infancy growth, cretinism, hypothyroidism	Skin lesions, thyroid malfunction
Iron	Synthesis of hemoglobin, general metabolism (e.g., of glucose), antibody production, drug detoxification in the liver	Females: 18 mg/day, ages 19–50; 8 mg/day, age 50+ Males: 8 mg/day, age 19+	Meats, eggs, spinach, seafood, broccoli, peas, bran, enriched breads, fortified cereals	Small, pale RBCs, anemia	Hemochromatosis
Zinc	Cofactor for many enzymes involved in growth, insulin storage immunity, alcohol metabolism, sexual development and reproduction	Females: 8 mg/day Males: 11 mg/day	Primarily meats and seafood; also legumes, peas, and whole grains	Skin rash, diarrhea, decreased appetite, hair loss, poor growth and development, poor wound healing	Reduced copper absorption, diarrhea, cramps, depressed immune function

*Dietary Reference Intakes (DRIs) represent:
• Recommended Dietary Allowances (RDAs)—Intake set to meet the needs of 97%–98% of individuals in a group.
• Adequate Intakes (AIs)—Believed to cover the needs of all individuals in the group.
• Upper Intake Levels (UIs)—The maximum daily intake likely to pose no risk of adverse effects.
• Values in table are RDAs unless marked (AI).
†RDAs are usually less than adult values for infants and children, more for pregnant women, and highest for lactating women. RDAs for some minerals are higher for older adults and different for men and women.

 Go to Chapter 28, **Supplemental Materials, Dietary Reference Intakes: Elements; Electrolytes,** on Davis*Plus*.

Sources: Lutz, C., & Przytulski, K. (2011). *Nutrition and diet therapy: Evidence-based applications* (5th ed.). Philadelphia: F.A. Davis; U.S. Department of Agriculture and U.S. Department of Health and Human Services. (2011). *Dietary guidelines for Americans, 2010.* (7th ed.). Washington, DC: U.S. Government Printing Office; and Shaw, A., Fulton, L., Davis, C., et al. (n.d.). *Using the Food Guide Pyramid: A resource for nutrition educators.* U.S. Department of Agriculture Food, Nutrition, and Consumer Services. Retrieved June 7, 2011, from http://www.cnpp.usda.gov/Publications/MyPyramid/OriginalFoodGuidePyramids/FGP/FGPResourceForEducators.pdf#xml=http://65.216.150.153/texis/search/pdfhi.txt?query=SERVING+SIZE&pr=MyPyramid&sufs=2&order=r&cq=&id=4592b7130

WHY IS WATER AN ESSENTIAL NUTRIENT?

Water is made up of hydrogen and oxygen. Water makes up about half of total body weight (55% to 65% in men and 50% to 55% in women). This is because men have greater muscle mass, and muscle contains a relatively large amount of water. Water is distributed in two body compartments. **Intracellular fluid** is the water contained within each living cell. It makes up about 40% of the total body weight. **Extracellular fluid** is external to the cell membrane (e.g., in the fluid portion of blood and lymph and in the gastrointestinal tract); it accounts

for 20% of body weight. Water is critical to the body because its functions are essential to life:

- *Solvent.* Water is the basic solvent for the body's chemical processes.
- *Transport.* Circulating as a component of blood, water serves as a medium for transporting oxygen, nutrients, and metabolic wastes.
- *Body structure and form.* Water "fills in the spaces" in body tissues (e.g., in muscle).
- *Temperature.* Water helps maintain body temperature. When body temperature rises, evaporation of sweat helps cool the body.

The amount of water a person requires varies according to the environmental humidity and temperature, activity level, age, and metabolic needs. The average AI is about 2.7 liters of water per day for adult women and 3.7 liters for men. Eighty percent of those amounts should come from fluids. We also obtain water in the foods we eat (Lutz & Przytulski, 2011).

Overall fluid balance is maintained when fluid intake in liquids, foods, and metabolic reactions matches fluid output through urine, feces, respiration, and sweat. Fluid and electrolyte balance is discussed in Chapter 38.

KnowledgeCheck 28-2

- What is the body's most usable energy source?
- Which nutrient's primary function is growth and repair of tissue?
- Identify five functions of adipose tissue (body fat).
- Which type of vitamin requires daily consumption to maintain appropriate levels?
- What distinguishes a major mineral from a trace mineral?
- Identify at least four functions of water.

WHAT MUST I KNOW ABOUT ENERGY BALANCE?

The energy in carbohydrates, proteins, and lipids is measured in terms of **calories,** or, more precisely, **kilocalories (kcal).** A kcal is the amount of heat required to raise the temperature of 1 kg of water 1° centigrade. To maintain a stable weight, the number of kcal we consume must equal the number of kcal we burn. Any deviation results in weight loss or weight gain. Below is the amount of energy liberated from the metabolism of 1 gram of energy nutrients:

- Carbohydrates = 4 kcal/g
- Protein = 4 kcal/g
- Fat = 9 kcal/g

KnowledgeCheck 28-3

Imagine that you have just eaten a food consisting of 4 grams of protein, 18 grams of carbohydrate, and 1 gram of fat.
- What would your total kcal intake be?
- What percentage of your kcal is from carbohydrates? Protein? Fat?

A diet of too few kcal is likely also to lack essential nutrients. People who are undernourished may experience weakened immunity, stunted growth, and hormonal disruption. Too many kcal can cause obesity, which increases the risk for chronic diseases, such as diabetes, arteriosclerosis, hypertension, hyperlipidemia, and cancers. In determining total energy (kilocalorie) needs, consider two factors: the client's basal metabolic rate and the duration and intensity of daily physical activity.

What Is Basal Metabolic Rate?

The **basal metabolic rate (BMR)** is a measure of the energy used while at rest in a neutral temperature environment—the energy required for vital organs such as the heart, liver, and brain to function. *Direct measurement* of BMR requires use of a calorimeter: an insulated unit that measures temperature changes of water that are produced by exposure to a fasting individual at rest. Although it is very accurate, it is rarely used because most institutions do not have calorimeters and because the test requires a controlled environment and a 12-hour fast. Direct measurement of BMR is used primarily by researchers. *Indirect calculation* of BMR, sometimes called the resting energy expenditure (REE), includes the following:

- Measuring oxygen uptake per unit of time. This can be done in an exercise lab or with portable machines at the bedside. This is most often done for patients in intensive care units. Not all facilities have this capability.
- Serum thyroxine levels (a blood test).
- A formula for calculating BMR when precise measurement is not required (Box 28-3).

What Factors Affect Basal Metabolic Rate?

When interpreting test results, consider the following factors that influence BMR:

- *Body composition.* Lean body tissue has greater metabolic activity than fat and bones. This explains why women, who have on average more adipose tissue than men, also have lower BMRs.
- *Growth periods.* BMR increases during periods of growth, such as the first 5 years of life, adolescence, pregnancy, and lactation.
- *Body temperature.* The BMR increases 7% for each 1°F (0.83°C) rise in body temperature.
- *Environmental temperature.* Cold weather, especially temperatures below freezing, causes a slight rise in the BMR to generate body heat and maintain normal body temperature.
- *Disease processes.* Diseases involving increased cellular activity, such as cancer, anemia, cardiac failure, hypertension, and asthma, result in BMR elevation. For the same reason, systemic injury (e.g., severe burns, traumatic injury) increases BMR.
- *Prolonged physical exertion.* Metabolic demands are also elevated during prolonged physical exertion (e.g., chopping wood, running). See Table 28-6.

How Do I Calculate a Client's Total Energy Needs?

The amount of energy required varies according to the intensity of the activity (Table 28-6). A person's total daily energy requirement is the number of kcal necessary to replace those used for

---

BOX 28-3 ■ Calculating Basal Metabolic Rate (BMR)

Females:	0.9 kcal/kg of body weight per hour
Males:	1.0 kcal/kg body weight per hour
Example:	Isaac Schwartz (Meet Your Patients) weighs 245 lb.
	1 kilogram = 2.2 pounds.
	Divide 245 by 2.2 to convert pounds to kilograms:

$$245 \div 2.2 = 111.3$$

Now complete the calculation:

$$1.0 \times 111.3 \times 24 \text{ hours} = 2671.2$$

Table 28-6 ➤ Energy Expenditures for Various Activities*

INTENSITY LEVEL	LIGHT	LIGHT TO MODERATE	MODERATE	HIGH
Energy Expended	120–150 kcal/hr	150–300 kcal/hr	300–420 kcal/hr	420–700+ kcal/hr
Examples of Activities	Dressing Showering Shaving Rocking Writing Typing Standing	Housework (e.g., sweeping) Light gardening Mowing lawn (motorized) Painting Walking 2–3 mph Bicycling 5½ mph Canoeing 2–3 mph	Digging Mowing lawn (manually) Walking 3½–4 mph Ballet Ballroom dancing Golf (no cart) Tennis (doubles)	Shoveling snow Walking 5 mph Climbing Bicycling 15–25 mph Cross-country skiing Jogging 5 mph or 1 mile in 10 min Swimming Aerobic dancing

*Precise energy use varies with body weight. For example, an individual weighing 200 lb burns about 740 calories per hour during aerobic dance, whereas an individual weighing 125 lb burns about 470 during the same activity.

basic metabolism plus those used in physical activities. The following are simple estimates based on activity level and age:

- Sedentary women and older adults need 1,600 kcal/day.
- Children, teenage girls, active women, and most men need 2,200 kcal/day.
- Teenage boys, active men, and very active women need 2,800 kcal/day.

However, these estimates have limited usefulness. For instance, is a woman who works a desk job but walks for 30 minutes a day sedentary, active, or somewhere in between? To calculate energy use more precisely, you need to know the person's age, weight, and physical activity, including the intensity and duration of the activity (Table 28-7).

Heightened emotional states may also increase energy needs, not because they directly increase metabolic activity, but because they increase muscular activity in the form of muscle tension, restlessness, and agitated movements.

KnowledgeCheck 28-4

You have already calculated the expected BMR for Mr. Schwartz (Meet Your Patients) for a 24-hour period.

- If Mr. Schwartz describes himself as working at a desk 8 to 10 hours per day, lawn mowing manually every other week during the summer, and playing an occasional game of golf, how would you classify his general activity level?

- After interviewing Mr. Schwartz, you estimate his average caloric intake to be approximately 3,000 kcal per day. Determine whether his kcal intake is sufficient or insufficient to maintain his present activity level.

What Are Some Body Weight Standards?

Weight standards have been established to correlate weight with good health and longevity and to help determine a client's ideal body weight. The **general ideal weight guide** uses a formula to determine a reasonable weight based on height:

Men: 106 lb (47.7 kg) for the first 5 ft (150 cm), then add 6 lb/in. (2.7 kg/2.5 cm)

Women: 100 lb (45 kg) for the first 5 ft (150 cm), then add 5 lb/in. (2.25 kg/2.5 cm)

Add 10% for large body frame; subtract 10% for small body frame.

Various **height–weight tables** have been developed over the years. Height–weight tables are based on statistical estimates and often include variations for age, sex, and body frame. To see the World Health Organization (WHO) child growth standards (e.g., length and height-for-age, weight-for-age),

 Go to WHO Child Growth Standards at http://www.who.int/childgrowth/standards/Technical_report.pdf

Table 28-7 ➤ Energy Needs Based on Weight and Activity

For *each pound of body weight*, a person needs the following per day:

ACTIVITY LEVEL	UNDERWEIGHT	NORMAL WEIGHT	OVERWEIGHT
Sedentary	13 kcal	13 kcal	9–11 kcal
Moderately active	18 kcal	16 kcal	13 kcal
Active	18–23 kcal	18 kcal	16 kcal

Use standards and standardized tables with caution because they are based on limited samples and may create unrealistic expectations, especially at the low weight ranges. Consider the following example. You have two male clients; each weighs 200 lb. Mason is 72 in. tall, works out vigorously 5 days per week, and has 18% body fat. Travis is 72 in. tall, rarely exercises, and has 35% body fat. Which of these clients requires more kcal to maintain his present weight? Which of these clients is at lower risk for cardiovascular disease?

If you answered Mason, you are correct. Although both men have the same height and weight, Mason has more lean body mass. He will burn energy more rapidly and be able to eat more without gaining weight. Height–weight tables cannot replace a thorough assessment and analysis of body composition when attempting to determine a client's overall fitness.

Body composition analysis attempts to quantify lean body mass versus percentage body fat. Lean body mass includes muscle, bone, and connective tissue. Lean tissue weighs more than fat; thus, a person who engages in regular weight-bearing exercise and is physically fit may actually weigh more than an individual of similar appearance who is sedentary and unfit. Various methods to assess body composition, known as *anthropometric measurements,* are provided in the Assessment section later in the chapter.

Think**Like a Nurse** 28-3

Examine your dietary intake for the next 3 days to determine how balanced your diet is. Use the form on the Electronic Study Guide and record all intake.

- How does your diet compare to the USDA MyPlate in terms of:
  Servings of bread, cereal, rice, and pasta?_____
  Servings of vegetables? _____
  Servings of fruits? _____
  Servings of milk, yogurt, and cheese? _____
  Servings of meat, poultry, fish, dry beans, eggs, and nuts? _____
  Servings of fats, oils, and sweets? _____
- From what you have learned from this activity, what habits could you change in patterns of eating in order to achieve optimal nutrition?

WHAT FACTORS AFFECT NUTRITION?

Several factors influence nutritional needs and choices. Some can be modified; some cannot. The most influential factors are development, knowledge, lifestyle, culture, disease processes, and functional limitations.

Developmental Stage

At specific developmental stages, nutritional needs and eating patterns vary according to physiological growth, activity level, metabolic processes, disease prevention, and other factors.

Infants to One Year

Humans grow most rapidly during the first year of life. Birth weight doubles by 5 months of age and triples during the first year, and length increases 50%. A baby 20 inches long at birth grows to about 30 inches by age 1 year. Nutritional needs per unit of body weight are greater than at any other time.

Calories and Protein. The infant needs adequate protein for tissue building and enough carbohydrates to furnish energy and "spare" the protein. The period from conception into the second year of life is most critical to brain development. For maximum brain growth, the baby needs optimal

nutrition. Severe protein-calorie deficiency in the last trimester of pregnancy or the first 6 months of life may decrease the number of brain cells by 20%.

Vitamins and Minerals. Fetal iron stores are depleted at 4 to 6 months, so intake of iron becomes important. The infant needs calcium for bone growth and development of teeth, calcium and vitamin C for iron absorption, and vitamin D for calcium regulation.

Fluids. Compared to adults, infants have a higher metabolic rate. They also have greater water loss through the skin, which comprises a greater proportion of the body. These factors, along with immature kidneys, mean that infants need proportionately more fluid than adults. To meet nutritional and fluid needs, the infant requires 1.5 to 2 ounces of breast milk or formula per pound of body weight per day.

Infant Feedings. The only safe choices for meeting fluid and nutrient needs in the first months of life are breast milk and commercially prepared formulas. Breast milk is the ideal food for infants because it is matched to their nutritional requirements. In addition, it enhances maturation of the infant's immune system and provides passive immunity against a number of infections. Breastfed infants also may have a reduced exposure to foreign dietary antigens and a reduced risk of subsequent allergies (Friedman & Zeiger, 2005). They may also have less risk of developing diabetes mellitus later in life (Owen, Martin, Whincup, et al., 2007; Rosenbauer, Herzig, Kaiser, et al., 2007).

When breastfeeding is contraindicated or the mother chooses not to breastfeed, numerous commercial formulas are available. The most commonly used formula is iron-fortified cow's milk available in powder, liquid concentrate, or ready-to-use liquid. Soy-based formulas may be an option for babies who are intolerant or allergic to cow's milk formula or to lactose, a sugar naturally found in cow's milk. For infants who have a milk or soy allergy, protein hydrolysate formulas are easier to digest and are less likely to cause allergic reactions than other types of formula.

✚ Infants younger than 1 year old should not receive cow's milk because it may cause gastrointestinal bleeding and may place too much strain on the infant's kidneys. It also can contribute to iron-deficiency anemia.

✚ Honey and corn syrup should not be used as a source of carbohydrates in preparing infant formula. They are potential sources of botulism toxin, which can be fatal in children younger than 1 year old (Schlenker & Roth, 2006).

At 4 to 6 months, infants may be started on solid foods, beginning with iron-fortified infant rice cereal. They progress to eating table food by 1 year of age. If solid foods are begun too early, they may trigger allergies.

Healthy infants born at term have sufficient iron for their first four months. Iron supplements are usually given beginning at 4 to 6 months (depending on whether breast- or formula-fed), and they may continue after 12 months if iron needs are not being met (American Academy of Pediatrics [AAP], 2010). Fluoride might also be prescribed for infants without a fluoridated water supply.

Toddlers and Preschoolers

Toddlers grow more slowly in comparison to infants, and have fewer energy demands. Toddlers require about 900 to 1,800 kcal and 1,250 mL of fluid per day, depending on body weight. As the gastrointestinal system matures, they are able

to eat most foods and adjust to the adult pattern of three meals a day. By age 3, most children have all of their deciduous teeth and can chew adult food.

 Food should be cut into small pieces to avoid choking in toddlers who sometimes are "too busy" to chew food sufficiently. Sometimes young children "chipmunk" their food and can later choke on it. Do not give food when the child is in a car seat or bouncy chair, where choking is more likely and can occur without a parent noticing.

Toddlers. Toddlers' diets are often deficient in nutrients. One- and 2-year-old children should drink reduced-fat (2%) milk or, in some cases, whole milk to provide adequate essential fatty acids for the still-growing brain. Deficiencies in iron, calcium, and vitamins A and C are also common during this period. Parents need to offer a variety of foods to provide these essential nutrients. This can be a challenge, because toddlers assert their autonomy and manipulate their parents by refusing foods. They may take a long time to eat or refuse to eat at all. Parents should not turn mealtime into a battle of wills or use foods to punish or reward; such reactions may affect the child's attitude toward food or magnify problem behavior related to feeding. To encourage the child to eat, you may offer parents the suggestions in the accompanying Home Care box.

Preschoolers. Preschoolers are similar to toddlers in their growth and nutritional needs; however, their eating patterns typically improve. They begin to form responses to specific foods, such as refusing all green vegetables or drinking less milk. They often refuse casseroles and foods with sauces. They might also eat only one particular food for several days. Because they are active, preschoolers require nutritious between-meal snacks. Lifelong food habits are developed during this stage, so encourage families to widen the variety of foods offered to preschoolers and to investigate the diet provided by their child's day care or preschool. Between ages 2 and 5 fat should provide only about 30% of the child's intake.

Parents and caregivers are the most important influences on the eating habits of children. For tips about how to be a role model for children and set good examples for healthy eating for life,

Go to the **USDA** Web site at http://www.choosemyplate.gov/food-groups/downloads/TenTips/DGTipsheet12BeAHealthyRoleModel.pdf

---

Home Care

Tips for Encouraging Toddlers to Eat

➤ Keep only nutritious foods in the house to avoid battles over nutrient-poor snacks.
➤ Serve foods in a child-friendly way; for example, arrange tortillas, cheese, tomato slices, and beans in a smiling face.
➤ Allow the child to "graze" throughout the day on healthful foods rather than insisting that she sit for formal meals at the table.
➤ Avoid "combined" foods, such as casseroles and stews.
➤ Limit consumption of sweets and snack foods.
➤ Do not use dessert as a reward for eating other foods (e.g., "You can't have cookies until you eat your meat").
➤ Offer healthy foods that are easy to eat (e.g., "finger foods" or those easily chewed).

School-Age Children

In the school-age period, growth and body changes occur gradually. Permanent teeth erupt, and the digestive system matures. School-age children need about 2,400 kcal and 1,750 mL of fluid per day. An adequate supply of vitamins and minerals is critical because the body is still growing and preparing for the demands of adolescence.

Parental control over food intake declines because advertising influences the child's food choices. The child eats away from home and may buy junk food with his lunch money or choose less nutritious foods in the school cafeteria. Even if the child brings lunch from home, he may trade his food or not eat lunch at all. Parents should encourage their children to eat breakfast to provide nutrients and energy to fuel problem-solving skills, memory, and sports and playground activities. Poor eating habits may lead to obesity.

Example Problem: Overweight and Obesity

Thirty-two percent of U.S. children are overweight; 16% are obese; and 11% are extremely obese (Centers for Disease Control and Prevention [CDC], 2008). Leading causes of childhood obesity include the following:

- Routine consumption of high-fat, high-sugar fast foods, nutrient-poor foods, and high-calorie snacks and beverages
- Loss of family mealtime
- Eating in front of a TV, computer, video game
- Lack of regular physical activity to burn the calories consumed (Berkowitz and Borchard, 2009).

Adolescents

Adolescence is a time of dramatic growth and development of the reproductive system. Boys experience an increase in muscle tissue and bone length and density. At menstruation, girls experience fat deposition. The needs of the adolescent body for energy, vitamins, and minerals approach those of the infant. In particular, adolescents need protein, calcium, iron, and B and D vitamins. Boys, in particular, seem to eat constantly. Adolescents have active lifestyles and snack often, preferring ready-to-eat, eat-on-the-run foods, such as chips, pizza, cookies, and fast foods. Unfortunately, most such foods have little nutrient value. Adolescents are responsible for their own food decisions, so the best approach for parents is to keep only healthful snack foods (e.g., cheese, fruit, raw vegetables) in the home and role model a positive attitude towards healthy eating.

Eating disorders are a concern in this group. Most people with eating disorders exhibit their first symptoms before age 20, some as early as age 10. The majority of eating disorder sufferers are female (National Association of Anorexia Nervosa and Associated Disorders, n.d.). Underweight and undernutrition are discussed more in the Practical Knowledge section.

Adults

Young adults continue to require adequate amounts of protein, vitamins, and minerals, but not at the same levels as in adolescence. If adults continue unhealthful behaviors developed in earlier stages, repercussions will begin to show up in adulthood. Calcium, vitamin D, folic acid, and iron continue to be critical, especially in women, for bone and reproductive health. U.S. Preventive Services Task Force (USPSTF) officials recommend that women capable of becoming pregnant should take a daily folic acid supplement of 0.4 mg to 0.8 mg (400 to 800 micrograms [mcg]) to lower the risk for neural tube defects in the fetus (USPSTF, 2009).

The BMR of middle adults decreases, potentially causing weight gain if dietary intake and activity level are unchanged. Individuals may begin to experience chronic illnesses such as diabetes, hypertension, obesity, and hyperlipidemia, often as a result of heredity or poor lifestyle choices. Dietary modification and exercise are essential to control these diseases. Overweight and obesity are discussed as Example Problems in the Practical Knowledge section. For dietary strategies for preventing cancer,

 Go to Chapter 28, **Tables, Boxes, Figures: ESG Box 28-1: Dietary Strategies for Preventing Cancer,** on DavisPlus.

Older Adults

Nutritional needs of older adults vary only slightly from middle adulthood. Lean body mass, physical activity, and BMR decrease, so older adults tend to need fewer kcal; however, they still need the same or higher levels of nutrients. It is not unusual for older adults to lose interest in eating and for the thirst sensation to decrease.

Older adults with chronic diseases may need to adjust to therapeutic diets low in salt, simple sugars, or fat. Unfortunately, the ability to taste and smell diminishes with age, and many clients find these diets unappealing. Other sensory changes, such as diminished vision or hearing, limit mobility and interaction, making it more difficult to purchase and prepare food. Tooth loss and gum disease limit chewing ability, forcing many older adults to eat only soft food. Arthritic hands may create difficulty preparing and eating food, and when they are no longer able to drive, many older adults must rely on local markets, where food choices may be limited and expensive. Other physical problems that may affect nutrition include gastroesophageal reflux, decreased gastric secretions, decreased intestinal peristalsis, and glucose intolerance.

See Table 28-8 for dietary requirements for adults older than 70 years. Notice that the main difference is that older adults require smaller quantities of most foods. In general, they require slightly more of the milk/yogurt/cheese group and slightly less of all other groups, especially the breads/cereal group. Older adults need complex carbohydrates (i.e., fiber) to maintain bowel function. They should be sure to drink at least eight glasses of water or other fluids (e.g., soups) per day and choose primarily green leafy vegetables and brightly colored fruits to help prevent constipation and dehydration. All of this, of course, assumes their medical condition allows this type of diet.

Many older adults may need supplements of calcium, vitamin D, and vitamin B$_{12}$. For example, (1) as bone density decreases, calcium requirements increase, especially in women at risk for *osteoporosis;* and (2) low concentrations of vitamin B$_{12}$ have been linked to cognitive decline in older adults (Clark, Birks, Nexo, et al., 2007).

With advancing age, older adults face many losses. As a result, depression and social isolation are common. Both negatively affect appetite. **Adult failure to thrive** is a complex disorder seen in many institutionalized older adults. It is characterized by weight loss, decreased activity and interaction, and increasing frailty.

Pregnant and Lactating Women

Nutritional requirements increase dramatically during pregnancy as the mother provides for the nutritional needs of the fetus. Folic acid intake is critical in the first trimester of pregnancy (the first 13 weeks) to prevent neural tube defects; a daily supplement of 0.6 to 0.8 mg is recommended during

Table 28-8 ➤ Daily Food Requirements for Adults Older Than Age 70	
FOOD GROUP	**ADULTS ≥ 70 YEARS**
Supplement of calcium, vitamin D, and vitamin B$_{12}$	As prescribed. Not everyone needs supplements. People should consult their healthcare providers.
Fats, oils, and sweets	Use sparingly
Milk, yogurt, and cheese group	3 servings
Meat, poultry, fish, dry beans, eggs, and nuts	2 or more servings
Fruit and vegetable group	Half a plate
Bread, fortified cereals, rice, and pasta group (whole grains and refined grains)	Half a plate
Water equivalents	8 or more servings

Sources: MyPlate for Older Adults (2011). Tufts University, Gerald, J., & Dorothy R. Friedman School of Nutrition Science and Policy. Retrieved from on February 6, 2011, from http://hnrc.tufts.edu/images/MYplate_OlderAdults.pdf; and Russell, R., Rasmussen, H., & Lichtenstein, A. (1999). Modified food guide pyramid for people over seventy years of age. *Journal of Nutrition,* 129(3), 751–753.

pregnancy. Adequate protein and calcium are important for growing muscle, brain, and bone tissues; iron is essential to maintain maternal and fetal blood supplies and stores during pregnancy. It is almost impossible to consume the recommended amount of dietary iron, so supplements are commonly prescribed, as are supplements of folic acid and calcium. Pregnant women need about 300 additional kcal/day in the second and third trimesters of pregnancy.

Women who are breastfeeding need 500 additional kcal per day. They continue to need additional protein and calcium, as well as increased fluid intake to make adequate amounts of breast milk. Needs vary based on the size of the baby and the frequency of breastfeeding. The quantity of the breast milk depends on an adequate supply of fluids and nutrients. However, the nutritional quality of the milk remains the same even if dietary intake is not adequate. For more information on nutrition in pregnancy and lactation, consult a maternal–newborn nursing textbook.

KnowledgeCheck 28-5

- Why is breast milk an ideal food source for infants?
- Why are an infant's nutritional needs per unit of body weight greater than at any other time?
- Why is it sometimes a challenge to meet the nutritional needs of toddlers?
- What is the challenge in meeting the nutritional needs of school-age children?
- Which age group experiences a growth spurt second only to that of infants?
- Why are energy (kcal) requirements less for older adults?

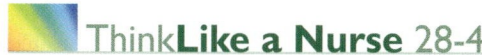

ThinkLike a Nurse 28-4

Make a list of all the food products you have seen advertised on television and in magazines. What implications does this have for the nutritional status of the public?

Lifestyle Choices

Nutrition-related lifestyle choices include the following:

Dietary Patterns. The type of food consumed is as equally important as the amount of food to a person's overall health. Whole foods, such as fresh fruits and vegetables, whole grains, and legumes, promote health, whereas foods high in simple sugars, saturated and *trans*-fats, and sodium increase the risk for health problems.

Cooking Methods. Up to one-half of the water-soluble vitamin content (vitamins B and C) is lost in the cooking water of boiled vegetables. Keeping foods hot longer than 2 hours results in even further loss.

Oral Contraceptive Use. This method of family planning lowers the serum level of vitamin C and several B vitamins. Women with marginal nutrient intake may need vitamin supplements.

Using Food to Cope. If used often, poor coping patterns, such as reacting to stress by skipping meals, binge eating, or consuming too much of a single food (e.g., snack foods, chocolate, or even limited variety of a healthy food item) can result in poor nutrition.

Tobacco Use. Smokers use vitamin C faster than non-smokers. Even children exposed to second-hand smoke tend to have lower plasma levels of ascorbic acid than unexposed children (Aghdassi, Royall, & Allard, 1999; Preston, Rodriguez, Rivera, et al., 2003). If the person cannot quit smoking, a vitamin C supplement may help compensate.

Alcohol. Alcohol contributes to obesity. A 12-oz beer contains 150 calories; a juice-based cocktail contains about 160 calories. This can add many unnecessary calories to the regular diet. In addition, alcohol significantly decreases the rate of fat metabolism. Excessive alcohol use interferes with adequate nutrition by (1) replacing the food in the person's diet, (2) depressing the appetite, (3) decreasing the absorption of nutrients by its toxic effects on intestinal mucosa, and (4) impairing the storage of nutrients. People who use alcohol heavily need multivitamin supplements, especially B vitamins and folic acid.

Caffeine. The most common source of caffeine is coffee—the leading beverage in the United States. Over the years, research reports have claimed a variety of dangers and health benefits for caffeine. Recently a privately funded group (Schardt, 2008) published an analysis of nine scientific reports which state that many of our accepted beliefs about coffee are myths. The group reports that coffee does not create risk for dehydration, heart disease, or cancer, and has little or no role in hypertension. Caffeine may be associated with bone loss; however, its negative effect can be offset by as little as 2 tablespoons of milk. In high doses, caffeine can sometimes cause anxiety and stomach upset. On the positive side, caffeine can enhance mood and mental and physical performance. It aids the ability to burn fat for fuel instead of carbohydrates, and has been linked to a lower risk of Parkinson's disease, type 2 diabetes, stroke, and dementia (Brody, 2008; Schardt, 2008). So it appears that while the evidence is still mixed, caffeinated beverages in moderation are not the villains we once thought.

Vegetarianism

All vegetarian diets exclude red meat and poultry, but beyond this distinction is a wide spectrum of diets. **Semi-vegetarians** are the most inclusive, allowing fish, eggs, and dairy products as well as plant-based foods. **Ovo-lacto vegetarians** are somewhat more strict; they eat eggs and dairy products, but not fish. **Lacto-vegetarians** consume only dairy and plant-based foods. **Vegans** eat only foods of plant origin, and a **fruitarian** diet includes only fruits, nuts, honey, and vegetable oils. Soybeans, soymilk, tofu, and processed protein products can be used by all but fruitarians to enhance the nutritional value of the diet.

People choose vegetarian diets for a number of reasons. As noted in Chapter 16, some religions prohibit consumption of animal flesh or foods of animal origin. Ethical considerations related to humane treatment of animals also cause some people to adopt a vegetarian diet. However, many people adopt a vegetarian diet simply as a health choice, noting the abundant research indicating that vegetarianism reduces the risk of disease and promotes wellness by limiting fat intake.

Although ovo-lacto vegetarians have no higher rate of nutrient deficiencies than the meat-eating population, they must choose foods carefully to include enough of the following nutrients:

- *Vitamin B_{12}* is found only in animal products, such as eggs and milk. Vegans must eat foods fortified with B_{12} or take B_{12} supplements. Long-standing B_{12} deficiency can result in severe and irreversible neurological impairment.
- *Vitamin D* may be inadequately supplied by vegetarian diets, so vitamin D-fortified foods (e.g., soy- and dairy milk are usually vitamin D fortified) or supplements should be included. Adequate sun exposure also helps to compensate for lack of dietary intake.
- *Calcium, iron, and zinc.* Vegans, fruitarians, and others who limit animal foods may need to supplement the diet with calcium, iron, and zinc. This is especially important for bolstering the immune system and growth of children and women who are pregnant or lactating.
  Iron: The iron from plant foods is not absorbed as well as that from animal sources. However, it is easier to absorb dietary iron when it is eaten with foods containing vitamin C, so eating fruit or vegetables containing vitamin C with meals helps to compensate.
  Calcium: Vegans, especially, may find it difficult to obtain enough dietary calcium. It is important to include fortified soymilk and calcium-rich vegetables (e.g., bok choy, broccoli, collards, Chinese cabbage, kale, mustard greens, okra, and fortified tomato juice). Calcium-fortified cereals are also available.
  Zinc: Zinc is readily available from various seed and bean sources, such as pumpkin, sesame, squash, watermelon seeds, wheat, chickpeas (hummus), wheat germ, dark chocolate, and garlic.
- *Protein* may be inadequate, especially in vegan children who do not care for the taste of soymilk, tofu, and other soy-based meat substitutes. For adults, a varied diet that meets normal nutrient and energy needs is also likely to supply adequate amounts of essential amino acids. Complementary proteins should be eaten throughout the day, but careful meal-by-meal balance of amino acids is usually not necessary. Review Table 28-1 and the discussion of complete and incomplete proteins earlier in the chapter.

In addition to following the preceding information, to ensure adequate nutrients it may be wise for vegetarians to consult a

qualified nutrition professional, especially during periods of growth, breastfeeding, pregnancy, or recovery from illness. For recommended servings of vegetarian food groups,

 Go to Chapter 28, **Tables, Boxes, Figures: ESG Table 28-1: Recommended Daily Servings for Vegetarian Meal Planning,** on Davis*Plus*.

As a vegetarian diet can be a healthy option, the USDA also has tips for following a vegetarian diet:

 Go to the **USDA** Web site at http://www.choosemyplate.gov/ food-groups/downloads/TenTips/DGTipsheet8Healthy EatingForVegetarians.pdf

Dieting for Weight Loss

One popular Internet bookseller recently offered no fewer than 36,655 books on weight-loss diets! Many diets, including the *Dietary Approaches to Stop Hypertension* (DASH) diet, the American Heart Association diet, and others, are nutritionally sound, but many others are fad diets, claiming to produce speedy, effortless, almost miraculous weight loss. You can recognize fad diets by the following characteristics. They:

- Promise quick and dramatic weight loss, which is usually achieved only temporarily because it results from loss of body fluids.
- Limit the range of foods from which the dieter can select (e.g., only fruits and vegetables for the first week), leading to an imbalance in nutrients.
- Often recommend purchase of supplements and/or special packaged meals; in many cases, these are brands that they endorse or actually produce.
- Fail to include practical strategies that help dieters permanently change eating and activity patterns.

As soon as they achieve their weight-loss goal, fad dieters typically revert to former eating habits and regain the weight. In contrast, more moderate calorie-restriction diets, such as the American Heart Association diet:

- Describe food selection and preparation tips and other behavior modifications that can lead to slow, sustained weight loss.
- Promote a diet that includes a variety of food choices and a balance of nutrients.
- Encourage physical activity as a cornerstone of weight loss.
- Emphasize self-monitoring, cognitive strategies, and behavior modification.

For more information about reaching a healthy weight,

 Go to the **U.S. Department of Agriculture, ChooseMyPlate. gov, Steps to a Healthier Weight,** Web site at http://www. choosemyplate.gov/weight-management-calories/weight-management.html

Ethnic, Cultural, and Religious Practices

As described in Chapters 15 and 16, religion and culture can have a major impact on diet and lifestyle. The following are examples:

- Language barriers may make it difficult for a client to understand nutritional information. For those patients, simple visual aids may be useful.
- Ethnic/cultural food choices often reflect the foods that were plentiful in the region of origin (e.g., fish in coastal communities, coffee and cocoa beans in equatorial regions), as well as foods that were readily grown in the native soil (e.g., rice in warm wetlands, potatoes in colder climates).

- Other diet choices reflect a concern for food preservation; for instance, people from various geographic regions eat salted meats and dried fruits and cook with fiery spices to combat microbes.
- Certain religions may require fasting or abstaining from certain foods. For example, Roman Catholics fast on Ash Wednesday and Good Friday; kosher dietary laws prohibit eating pork and shellfish.
- The burden of childhood obesity is not spread equally across the U.S. population. For example, obesity has been increasing faster among Mexican American and African American children (National Center for Health Statistics, 2008a).
- Cultural beliefs, perceptions, and attitudes about weight issues may often not match those of health providers. For example, some parents may perceive their children as cute and healthy, even though their body mass index (BMI) indicates they are obese. A slim body is not the ideal in all cultures.

Traditional diets of many cultures are healthful and should not be discouraged; in fact, contemporary adaptations made to these diets may compromise their nutritional quality. For example, the Mediterranean diet, which includes a glass of red wine and is rich in fish, fruits, vegetables, and nuts and low in dairy foods, saturated fats, and red meat, has been linked to decreased risk of death from all causes, including deaths due to cancer and cardiovascular disease in a U.S. population (Mitrou, Kipnis, Thiébaut, et al., 2007).

Disease Processes and Functional Limitations

Chronic diseases (e.g., diabetes mellitus, gastrointestinal disorders) can alter nutrient intake, digestion, absorption, use, and excretion. Any illness, especially when accompanied by fever, increases the need for protein, water, and kcal to meet the demands of increased metabolic rate. Traumatic injury (e.g., burns, surgery) requires extra protein and vitamin C for wound healing and tissue rebuilding. People with long-term insufficient calorie intake (e.g., patients with cancer) also suffer from **protein-calorie malnutrition,** which is characterized by weight loss and muscle and fat wasting. A variety of other physical and psychological disorders and/or their treatments can adversely affect a client's nutrition, for example:

- Reduce appetite
- Limit a person's ability to obtain and prepare food
- Compromise the ability to chew and swallow food
- Stomach and intestinal disorders, increased or decreased peristalsis, diminished secretion or digestive disorders (e.g., lack of lactase needed to digest milk)
- Medications (e.g., laxatives may cause calcium and potassium depletion)

KnowledgeCheck 28-6

- List at least three nutrients that may be more difficult to supply through a vegetarian diet.
- When selecting a program for weight loss, what factors should a person consider?
- Why should you encourage clients from various cultures to follow their traditional diets?
- Describe the effects on nutrition of (1) smoking and (2) heavy alcohol use.

Special Diets

Many people must follow a modified diet to assist in managing their illness. In addition, all inpatients at healthcare facilities must have a diet prescribed by their primary care provider. The following are the most commonly prescribed diets.

Regular Diet

A regular diet, also called the "house diet," is appropriate for clients without special nutritional needs. This diet is a balanced meal plan that supplies 2,000 kcal per day. Many facilities provide vegetarian and ethnic variations (Asian menu, kosher, and so on). Typically, inpatients choose each meal from a list of menu choices.

Have you ever eaten "hospital food"? Or have you heard someone complain that "hospital food is bland and unimaginative"? There is some justification for that complaint. House diets must accommodate the varied tastes of all patients, so they are usually lightly seasoned. Selections are limited to avoid unpopular items (e.g., Brussels sprouts) and restrict fatty, fried, or gas-producing foods, which many patients tolerate poorly. However, you should refrain from making negative comments to patients about the food.

NPO

NPO means no food or fluid (including water) by mouth. This may be ordered before surgery or an invasive procedure to limit the risk of aspiration. Common examples are "NPO after midnight," or "NPO 8 hours prior to procedure." Most well-nourished, well-hydrated patients easily tolerate short-term NPO status. However, no one can tolerate prolonged periods of NPO. Intravenous fluids may be given to provide hydration, and clients who must remain NPO for a lengthy period need enteral (through a stomach tube) or parenteral (IV) nutrition to prevent malnutrition.

Diets Modified by Consistency

Patients undergoing surgery, bowel procedures, or acute illness may, for a short period of time, need a diet modified by consistency (see Table 28-9). Patients with chronic health concerns that affect their ability to chew or swallow (e.g., Impaired Dentition and Impaired Swallowing) may need long-term changes in the consistency of their diet.

Diets Modified for Disease

Some health conditions require modification of dietary intake. The following are the most common diets:

- *Calorie-restricted.* For clients requiring weight reduction
- *Sodium-restricted.* For clients with blood pressure, Meniere's disease (inner ear problem), or fluid balance problems
- *Fat-restricted.* For clients with elevated cholesterol or triglyceride levels; may also be ordered for general weight loss
- *Diabetic.* To manage calories and carbohydrate intake for clients with diabetes mellitus
- *Renal diet.* To manage electrolytes and fluid for clients with renal insufficiency
- *Protein-controlled diet.* To manage liver and kidney disease
- *Antigen-avoidance diets.* For clients allergic to or intolerant of certain foods, such as a gluten-free diet for clients with celiac disease

Table 28-9 ➤ Diets Modified by Consistency		
DIET & DESCRIPTION	**FOODS INCLUDED**	**COMMENTS**
Clear Liquids. Provides fluids to prevent dehydration, and supplies some simple carbohydrates to help meet energy needs.	Water, tea, coffee, broth, clear juice (usually apple, grape, or cranberry juice), popsicles, carbonated beverages, and gelatin.	▪ Does not supply adequate calories, protein, and other nutrients, so timely progression to more nutritious diets is recommended. ▪ If clear liquids are required for more than 3 days, commercial clear liquid supplements are usually prescribed.
Full Liquids. Contains all the liquids included in the clear liquid diet plus any food items that are liquid at room temperature.	Add to clear liquid diet: soups, milk, milk shakes, puddings, custards, juices, some hot cereals, and yogurt.	▪ Difficult to obtain a balanced diet on a full liquid plan; use for a short time only. ▪ If needed for a longer time, a professional dietitian should be involved in planning of the diet. ▪ High-calorie, high-protein supplements are often added.
Mechanical Soft Diet. The diet of choice for people with chewing difficulties resulting from missing teeth, jaw problems, or extensive fatigue.	Add to the full liquid diet: soft vegetables and fruits; chopped, ground, or shredded meat; and breads, pastries, eggs, and cheese. Many food items can be added to this diet by cooking them extensively or blending or grinding to alter their texture.	▪ This diet can supply a full range of nutrients but is quite low in fiber. As a result, constipation is a risk.
Pureed Diet. A pureed diet is a blended diet.	Often liquids are added to the food to create a texture that may be scooped onto serving plates.	

- *Calorie-protein push.* Used when there is a need to heal wounds, maintain or increase weight, or promote growth. If the person cannot consume enough kcal by adding fats and proteins to his regular diet, high-calorie, high-protein supplements may be used.

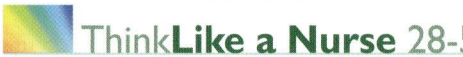 **ThinkLike a Nurse** 28-5

Analyze the following diets. Which nutrients are missing or difficult to obtain from these diets?
- Clear liquid
- Full liquid

PracticalKnowledge
knowing **how**

Good nutrition not only is essential for health, but also is a key aspect of disease management. In the rest of this chapter, we look at assessing nutritional status and diagnosing and planning care for some nutrition problems, such as Impaired Swallowing/NPO status, and Nausea. In addition, we discuss nutritional support for older adults and patients who have the example problems of overweight/obesity and underweight/undernutrition.

Nutrition is a basic human need. But more than a physical necessity, it also has emotional associations. We eat when we are hungry, but we also eat for pleasure because the food tastes good! Food has become a part of most social events and activities. A certain food may symbolize one's cultural or religious affiliation or even be a political statement (e.g., refusal to eat lettuce in support of migrant workers). When supporting patients' nutritional needs, it is wise to keep in mind that food has different meanings to different people. Personal beliefs, habits, and preferences are as important as nutritional knowledge in determining what a person eats.

ASSESSMENT

There are two kinds of nutritional assessment: (1) screening assessments and (2) thorough, focused nutritional assessments. Usually you will perform a screening exam. If you identify nutritional risk factors, you then perform a focused nutritional assessment.

HOW DO I SCREEN CLIENTS FOR NUTRITIONAL PROBLEMS?

Nutritional screening is performed to determine deficiencies or excesses in the diet and to identify risk factors for nutritional problems. The Joint Commission (2008) requires a nutritional screening to be completed within 24 hours of inpatient admission. The degree of screening performed depends on the patient's condition or concerns. **Cursory screening** consists of evaluation of height, weight, and body mass index (BMI) coupled with a brief dietary history. Clients who are found to have risk factors should be evaluated using one of the following screening methods.

- *The subjective global assessment (SGA).* This commonly used screening method makes use of information from the overall medical history and physical examination to evaluate a client's nutritional status. See the accompanying Focused Assessment box Subjective Global Assessment.

- *The Nutrition Screening Initiative (NSI),* developed for older adults, identifies indicators of impaired nutritional status. To see a portion of the NSI, refer to the Focused Assessment box Nutrition Screening Initiative (NSI) for Older Adults. For the entire tool,

 Go to Chapter 28, **Tables, Boxes, Figures: ESG Figure 28-4,** on DavisPlus.

- *The Mini Nutritional Assessment (MNA),* also developed for older adults, can be used with clients of all ages (DiMaria-Ghalili & Guenter, 2008). It is a quick and easy method of identifying clients with nutritional risks or malnutrition. The tool consists of two parts. The first part screens for nutritional risk. The second part is completed only if the person is determined to be at risk. The final score, a total of both parts, determines whether malnutrition exists and requires multidisciplinary follow-up. To see and use the MNA,

 Go to Chapter 28, **Tables, Boxes, Figures: ESG Figure 28-6,** on DavisPlus.

For a tool to use in assessing nutritional status for patients with dementia,

 Go to **Try This, Issue D11.1: Eating and Feeding Issues in Older Adults With Dementia: Part I: Assessment,** at http://www.hartfordign.org/Resources/Try_This_Series/

Focused Assessment

Subjective Global Assessment

In this method, an experienced clinician examines the general medical history and physical examination to evaluate a client's nutritional status. There are six components pertinent to nutritional status:
- *Weight history*—over previous 6 months
- *Dietary history*—including a comparison of usual, recommended, and current intake, as well as changes in eating patterns over the past weeks or months
- *Gastrointestinal symptoms history*—anorexia, nausea, vomiting, and diarrhea
- *Energy level*—including activity level and functional abilities
- *Existing disease*—evaluation of the metabolic demands of any disease states along with acute stressors that may alter those demands
- *Physical examination data*—regarding loss of fat stores, muscle wasting, and the presence of edema and ascites

As a clinician, you would analyze these components to rate the client's nutritional status as normal, mild, moderate, or severe. The effectiveness of this method depends largely on the experience of the clinician (Barone, Milosavljevic, & Gazibarich, 2003; Detsky, McLaughlin, Baker, et al., 1987). For a link to view this tool online and print to use with patients,

 Go to Chapter 28, **Resources for Caregivers and Health Professionals, Subjective Global Assessment,** on DavisPlus.

Focused Assessment

Nutrition Screening Initiative (NSI) for Older Adults: Indications of Impaired Nutritional Status

This portion of the NSI identifies indicators of impaired nutritional status.

MAJOR INDICATORS	MINOR INDICATORS	SYMPTOMS	PHYSICAL SIGNS	LAB VALUES
➤ Significant weight loss over time ➤ Significant high or low weight for height ➤ Significant change in functional status ➤ Significant and inappropriate food intake ➤ Significant reduction in midarm circumference ➤ Significant decrease in skinfold ➤ Osteoporosis or osteomalacia ➤ Folate or vitamin B deficiency	➤ Concurrent syndromes ➤ Alcoholism ➤ Cognitive impairment ➤ Chronic renal insufficiency ➤ Multiple concurrent medications ➤ Malabsorption syndromes	➤ Anorexia, nausea, or dysphagia ➤ Early satiety ➤ Changed bowel habits ➤ Fatigue or apathy ➤ Memory loss	➤ Poor oral or dental status ➤ Dehydration ➤ Poorly healing wounds ➤ Loss of subcutaneous fat or muscle mass ➤ Fluid retention	➤ Reduced levels of serum albumin, transferrin, or prealbumin ➤ Folate deficiency ➤ Iron deficiency ➤ Zinc deficiency ➤ Reduced levels of ascorbic acid

To learn more about the NSI and for tools to use for nutritional screening of older adults,

 Go to Chapter 28, **Tables, Boxes, Figures: ESG Figure 28-4, and ESG Figure 28-5,** on Davis*Plus*.

FOCUSED NUTRITIONAL ASSESSMENT

If screening reveals nutritional problems, perform a focused nutritional assessment to evaluate the client. It is especially important to assess nutritional status in elderly clients carefully to ensure that you detect marginal deficiencies before major problems occur. The nutrition component of the complete physical assessment or any focused nutritional assessment includes both subjective (history) and objective (physical examination) data.

Dietary History

You can obtain a dietary history during any routine assessment. Whether you use a self-administered form or an interview, you will collect general knowledge of the client's basic eating habits, food attitudes and preferences, cultural factors, and use of dietary supplements. A dietary history creates a picture of the client's food habits and eating behaviors. To collect detailed data on what the client is actually eating, ask him to keep a food diary. The following are three types of food diaries:

24-Hour Recall. A 24-hour recall requires the client to name all food eaten within a day. Simply ask questions such as "Yesterday, what did you eat for breakfast/lunch/dinner/snacks?" A 24-hour recall is simple, requires no equipment, and can be used as often as required. However, accuracy of the data may be questionable, because some people have difficulty remembering everything they ate the previous day, and any single day may be atypical. Sometimes, a family member can help the client recall intake more accurately (Garibalia & Forseter, 2008).

Food Frequency Questionnaire. A food frequency questionnaire asks the client to identify the number of times per day, week, or month a particular food group is eaten (e.g., fruits, red meats). You can modify the questions according to the client's specific issues. Food frequency questionnaires provide a more global image of the client's nutritional intake than the 24-hour recall; however, accuracy is still a problem.

Food Record. A food record is the most accurate food diary. It provides information on the quantity as well as the types of foods eaten. You ask the client in advance to keep a record of measured and weighed amounts of all foods he eats in a 3-day period. From the detailed information collected, you can analyze the total kcal and nutrient content for the recorded period. Although the food record provides meaningful results, it requires a high level of cognitive and psychomotor functioning that not all clients have. It also requires commitment to the process for 3 days, which may be difficult for some people.

You may wish to remind some patients there are Web sites and apps that can help them with journaling their diet and tracking nutritional intake, goals, and so on.

Physical Examination

You should correlate physical examination findings with other assessments, such as nutritional and medical history, dietary intake, anthropometric measurements, and laboratory results. Refer to Chapter 21 as needed for a review of physical examination techniques. For guidelines in performing a nutrition-focused physical examination, see the Focused Assessment box Focused Nutritional Assessment.

Assessing Body Composition

When assessing body composition (the proportion of fat in the body), you use **anthropometric measurements.** These are noninvasive physical examination techniques to determine body dimensions such as height and weight. Other examples are discussed in the following sections. Anthropometric measurements are used to assess growth rate in children; to indirectly assess adults' protein and fat stores; and to diagnose overweight, obesity, and underweight. To obtain accurate data, you must use standardized equipment and procedures and compare the data to existing reference standards for men and women. Keep in mind that body weight measurement alone is insufficient.

Focused Nutritional Assessment

If you identify nutritional problems or risks using the screening tools, you should perform a more in-depth nutritional assessment, such as the following.

NUTRITIONAL HISTORY

Item	Components
Demographic data	Name, date, age, sex, date of birth, address, occupation, workplace
Chief complaint	Client's subjective statement of health problem, including onset and duration
Present illness and current health	Detailed data about chief complaint as it relates to nutrition status
	Recent diet changes and reasons
	Recent weight loss or gain and over what period of time
	Usual body weight: 20% above or below desirable weight?
	Change in appetite
	Unusual stress/trauma (surgery, job, family)
	Medications, prescriptions
	Alcohol, nicotine, caffeine consumption
Health history	Previous illnesses, trauma, major dental problems, or issues that could interfere with ability to shop, prepare food, chew, or swallow
	Allergies (i.e., environmental, foods, drugs)
	Eating disorders
	Chronic disease or surgery that affects gastrointestinal tract
	Substance abuse
	Nutritional programs
	Depression
Family health history	Genetic/familial disorders that could affect nutritional status: cardiovascular or gastrointestinal disorders, Crohn's disease, diabetes, cancer, sickle cell anemia, allergies, celiac disease, other food intolerances, obesity
Dietary history	Current food intake pattern using one of the following methods: 24-hour–7-day recall, as appropriate; food frequency questionnaire; food record; and comparison to dietary guidelines and DRIs
	Special dietary considerations, restrictions
	Fad diets
	Vitamin and mineral supplements
	Commercial dietary supplements
	Nonconventional dietary supplements
	Food preferences, dislikes
	Dietary influences from ethnic, cultural, or religious practices
	Counseling needs (based on food knowledge)
Medication history	Recent use of steroids, immunosuppressants, chemotherapy, anticonvulsants, or oral contraceptives

Item	Components
Socioeconomic factors	Adequate food storage, refrigeration, food preparation, payments: Supplemental Security Income (SSI), food stamps, USDA WIC (Women, Infants, and Children) program Who shops for, prepares, and cooks food?
Personal factors	Stress/coping mechanisms, self-concept, social supports
	Daily activity level and exercise regimen

NUTRITION-FOCUSED PHYSICAL EXAMINATION

Correlate the following physical examination findings with the dietary history, screening methods, anthropometric measurements, and laboratory results.

I. The General Survey

Assess vital signs, height, weight, and overall impressions.

➤ *Overall appearance.* Does the client look ill? Does he appear adequately nourished? You will want to investigate any hunches as you move through the physical exam.

➤ *Temperature.* An increase in temperature raises the client's metabolic rate and need for fluid, is a sign of infection, and may decrease the client's appetite.

➤ *Blood pressure (BP) and heart rate* are affected by fluid status. An elevated BP may be related to fluid volume excess; a low BP may be a sign of dehydration. Heart rate usually increases when fluid volume is low.

➤ *Height and weight.* Calculate the body mass index (BMI) on the basis of these measures:

$$\text{BMI} = \text{weight in kilograms} \div (\text{height in meters})^2$$

Note: In adults in long-term care settings or with serious illness, nutritional support should be implemented for those with a BMI less than 21. In this population a BMI of less than 21 is associated with increased mortality (National Guideline Clearinghouse, 2005, updated 2010).

II. Integumentary System

➤ *Skin turgor* is an indicator of fluid status. Poor skin turgor may result from dehydration. Swelling may result from overhydration.

➤ *Skin integrity* reflects overall nutritional status. Poor wound healing may suggest inadequate intake of protein, vitamin C, or zinc. Patients with uncontrolled diabetes often experience slow-healing wounds, especially in the feet and legs.

➤ *Areas of warmth or erythema.* These are signs of inflammation or infection.

➤ *Other nutrition-related skin changes* include red, swollen skin lesions (due to niacin deficiency); excessive bleeding seen as petechiae or ecchymosis (due to vitamin K or C deficiency); and xerosis (dry skin).

➤ *Abnormal nail findings* include spoon-shaped, brittle nails (due to iron deficiency); dull nails with transverse ridge (due to protein deficiency); pale, poor blanching, or mottled nails (due to vitamin A or C deficiency); bruising or bleeding beneath nails (due to protein or caloric deficiency); and splinter hemorrhages (due to vitamin C deficiency).

➤ *Hair* will grow slowly, thin, or break easily if protein is deficient.

Focused Nutritional Assessment—cont'd

III. The Head and Neck

The condition of the mouth, teeth, and gums has a major effect on a client's choice of food, ability to chew, and ability to swallow.

➤ *Facial paralysis or drooping* of one side of the face may be a result of stroke, injury, or nerve irritation, which also affects the ability to chew and swallow (dysphagia).

➤ *Enlarged thyroid gland.* Look for swelling of the thyroid, which may be related to hypothyroid or hyperthyroid states. Both disorders affect metabolic rate and energy requirements.

➤ *Eyes.* Nutritional deficits may cause the eyes to be red and dry and the conjunctiva pale.

➤ *Lips and tongue.* The lips may be chapped, red, or swollen. The tongue may be bright red, purple, or swollen or may have longitudinal furrows.

➤ *Teeth and gums.* Look for cavities, mottled or missing teeth, and for spongy, bleeding, or receding gums.

➤ *Lymph nodes.* Palpate for enlarged or tender lymph nodes under the chin and along the neck. Nodes that are swollen can signal infection, such as a sore throat.

IV. Cardiovascular System

You will have gained initial information about the cardiovascular system by taking the vital signs. As you follow up and listen to the heart and check pulses, you should explore any abnormal vital signs.

➤ *Bounding pulses* are associated with fluid overload, fever, and hypertension.

➤ *Weak, thready pulse* may indicate dehydration, shock, or hypotension.

➤ *Edema in the extremities* may be a sign of fluid overload, inadequate protein stores, or electrolyte imbalance.

V. Abdominal Exam

➤ *Scaphoid or concave abdomen* indicates loss of subcutaneous fat, possibly caused by malnutrition.

➤ *Round or protuberant abdomen* points to obesity due to excess caloric and/or high fat intake.

➤ *Generalized enlarged abdomen* may signify **ascites** (fluid in the abdominal cavity) due to liver malfunction. Ascites results from three mechanisms: abnormal movement of protein and water into the abdomen; sodium and fluid retention; and decreased albumin production in the liver.

➤ *Hyperactive bowel sounds* are heard with gastrointestinal infection, laxative use, and malabsorption disorders.

➤ *Hypoactive bowel sounds* suggest sluggish motility in the GI tract.

VI. Musculoskeletal System

➤ *Thin extremities with excess skinfolds* may indicate muscle atrophy and fat loss related to malnutrition, especially protein and calories. This may also occur as a result of prolonged bed rest and inadequate food intake. Skinfold measurement is also useful in assessing muscle and fat stores.

➤ *Swelling, deformities, or limitation in range of motion* of the joints.

➤ *Kyphosis* of the spine may indicate osteoporosis and possible insufficient calcium intake.

➤ *Joint pain* on palpation or with movement is a sign of arthritis or gout. Arthritis may affect ability to shop for groceries, prepare food to eat, and use utensils for eating and drinking. Gout is often induced by diets high in purines (food substances that break down into uric acid), obesity, and excess alcohol intake.

VII. Neurological System

The neurological examination will give you insight into the client's ability to perform independent tasks.

➤ *Altered level of consciousness or signs of behavioral disturbances and dementia* through general conversation and appropriateness of answers to specific questions.

➤ *Coordination and reflexes*.

➤ *Cognitive deficits or severe psychiatric disorders*. A client with cognitive deficits or severe psychiatric disorders may have difficulty preparing food or judging appropriate nutrient choices.

➤ *Motor or sensory deficits*. Clients with motor or sensory deficits may be unable to purchase, prepare, or eat a variety of foods.

➤ *Confusion, weakness, diminished reflexes, paresthesia, and sensory loss* may be cues to vitamin B deficiencies.

➤ *Tetany or severe and generalized muscle spasm* may indicate calcium or magnesium deficits.

VIII. Signs of Severe Malnutrition?

➤ Symptoms of undernutrition due to insufficient food include reduced physical activity, weight loss, and reduced height.

➤ Children, older adults, and people with chronic illnesses such as cancer, HIV infection, and chronic obstructive pulmonary disease (COPD) are most likely to experience malnutrition.

➤ To assess for malnutrition in children, compare weight, height, and head circumference to the standards (norms) for the child's age. In cases of severe malnutrition, abdominal circumference can signal worsening disease. Other indicators in children include the presence of iron deficiency anemia.

➤ In adolescents, look for a delay of stages of sexual maturation.

Skinfold Measurements

Approximately half of body fat is located subcutaneously. Therefore, skinfold thickness provides an estimate of a person's body fat content. It reveals information about current nutritional status as well as long-term changes in fat stores. Use a caliper to obtain the most accurate measurement. The most reliable location is the triceps for children and women and the subscapular area in men. The combined measurements of triceps skinfold and mid-upper arm circumference yield a better estimate of muscle and fat areas than a single measurement. However, accurate reading can be difficult for those who are obese. See Clinical Insight 28-2.

Clinical Insight 28-2 ➤ **Skinfold Measurement**

- Take measurements directly on the skin, not through clothing.
- Take each reading as soon as the jaws of the caliper come into contact with the skin and the reading has stabilized.
- In each site, take three readings in quick succession, and average the results to the nearest 0.1 mm.
- Add the averages of all skinfold sites to arrive at a total skinfold measurement.
- To determine the percentage body fat, compare the final calculated measurement with the values in the appropriate body fat and skinfold table for the age and gender of the patient.

Measuring Triceps Skinfold

- Locate the midpoint on the posterior side of the dominant upper arm.
- With the client's arm hanging loosely at the side, palpate the measurement site at the midpoint to become familiar with distinguishing muscle from adipose soft tissue.
- From 1 cm above the midpoint, grasp a vertical pinch of skin and only the subcutaneous fat layer between the thumb and index finger. Gently pull the skinfold away from the underlying muscle.
- Place the skinfold caliper at the midpoint, and slowly release the jaw of the caliper while maintaining a grasp of the skinfold.

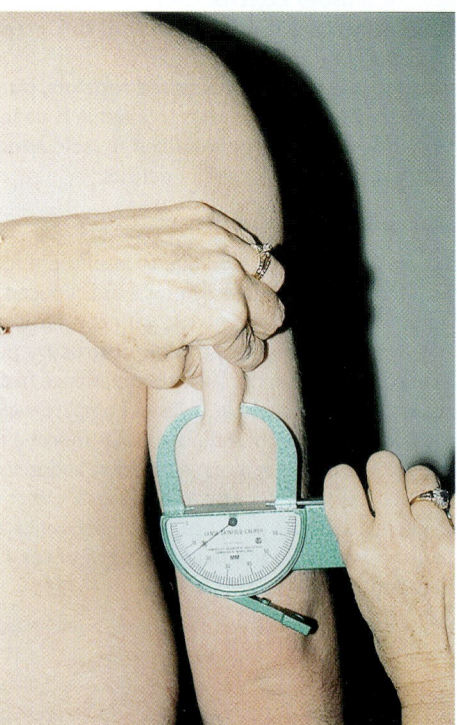

Measuring Subscapular Skinfold

- Follow the same procedure, except measure on the back, just under the shoulder blade. Grasp below the tip of the inferior angle of the scapula 45° to vertical.

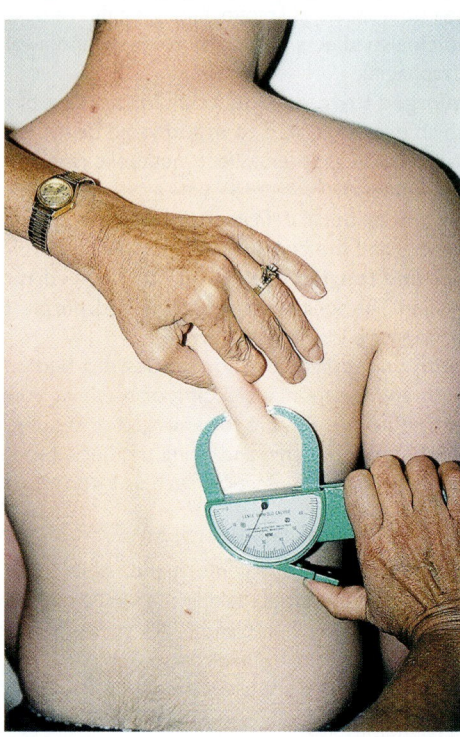

Measuring Biceps Skinfold

- Follow the same procedure, except measure the muscle belly of the biceps. With the patient's arm hanging loosely at the side, grasp the skin and subcutaneous fat layer on the front of the upper arm, over the biceps, about level with the nipple.

Measuring Suprailiac Skinfold

- Follow the same procedure, except measure approximately 1 in. above the hipbone, above the iliac crest in the mid-axillary line.

Calculating Body Mass Index

Calculate the BMI using the following formula:

BMI = weight in kilograms ÷ (height in meters)²

Circumferences

Another method of estimating the percentage of body fat is to use girth, or circumference measurements. *Mid-upper arm circumference* is routinely measured as part of screening. The *abdominal circumference*, measured at the iliac crest, is a simple and inexpensive method to assess body fat distribution. This method is highly accurate and should accompany the BMI measurement for assessment of adiposity. *The waist-to-hip ratio (WHR)* evaluates obesity by assessing abdominal fat. A WHR of greater than 1 in men and greater than 0.8 in women indicates obesity. A high level of abdominal fat is associated with increased risk for hypertension, diabetes, hyperlipidemia, and cardiovascular disease. For specific instructions on measuring mid-upper arm circumference and WHR, see Clinical Insight 28-3.

KnowledgeCheck 28-7

- What are the most reliable locations for skinfold measurement?
- What are the implications of an increased WHR?

Body Mass Index

Body mass index (BMI) is another method of assessing body composition. It can be precisely measured using scanning devices that measure *bioelectrical impedance*—the conduction of a harmless electrical charge through the client's body. Lean tissue readily conducts the charge, whereas adipose tissue does not. However, you will usually roughly estimate BMI by using the calculation formula in Box 28-4. You may also consult tables with precalculated values based on height and weight (National Heart, Lung, and Blood Institute [NHLBI], n.d.). For an example of a height–weight BMI table, see Procedure 21-1: Performing the General Survey. You can also find BMI calculators on the Web. Two reliable examples are at:

 Centers for Disease Control and Prevention, at http://www.cdc.gov/healthyweight/assessing/bmi/adult_bmi/english_bmi_calculator/bmi_calculator.html and **National Heart Lung and Blood Institute,** at http://www.nhlbisupport.com/bmi/bmicalc.htm

The normal BMI for adults ranges from 18.5 to 24.9 (although this may vary slightly among professional organizations). The usefulness of BMI values is limited for athletes because of their highly developed muscle mass, and for pregnant and postpartum women because they have a higher fluid composition. In addition, BMI values have not been specifically calculated for people older than age 65. Despite these limitations, BMI is generally useful in identifying underweight and obese individuals.

KnowledgeCheck 28-8

- What is the most accurate type of food diary?
- Compare and contrast four nutritional screening approaches: cursory screening, subjective global assessment, Mini Nutritional Assessment, and Nutrition Screening Initiative.
- Identify three nutritional risk factors.

Clinical Insight 28-3 ► **Measuring Circumferences to Evaluate Body Composition**

Measuring Mid-Upper Arm Circumference

- Keeping the client's dominant arm parallel to the body, bend the elbow 90°.
- Using a tape measure, measure the distance between the **acromion** (the bony protrusion of the back of the upper shoulder) and the **olecranon process** (tip of the elbow).
- Mark the midpoint between these two landmarks.
- Ask the client to relax the arm, so that it hangs loose and parallel to the body.
- Position the tape around the upper arm at the marked midpoint. Make sure the tape is snug but not so tight as to indent or pinch the skin.
- Record the circumference to the nearest 0.1 cm.

Calculating Waist-to-Hip Ratio (WHR)

- Use a tape measure to measure the circumference of the waist (at the umbilicus with stomach muscles relaxed).
- Use a tape measure to measure the circumference of the hips at their widest point.
- Calculate the waist-to-hip ratio using the following formula:

waist circumference (in.) ÷ hip circumference (in.)

Example: Robert's waist measurement is 32 inches, and his hip measurement is 34 inches. His WHR is 32 ÷ 34 = 0.94.
(Obesity = > 1.0 in males and > 0.8 in females)

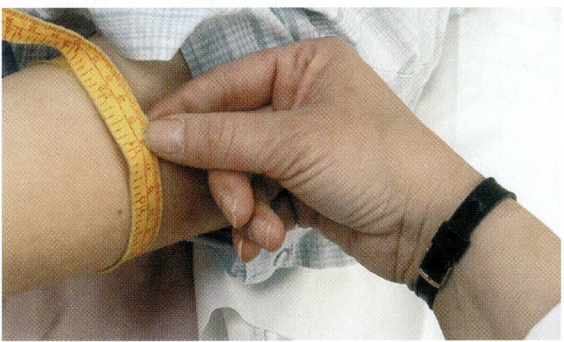

BOX 28-4 ■ Calculating Body Mass Index (BMI)

BMI = weight in kilograms ÷ (height in meters)^2
Example:
Robert weighs 165 lb. Convert his weight to kilograms:
$$165 ÷ 2.2 = 75 \text{ kg}$$
He is 71 inches tall. Convert his height to meters.
$$1 \text{ meter} = 39.37 \text{ inches}$$
Divide 71 inches by 39.37 inches; he is 1.8 meters tall
(rounded off)
$$\text{His BMI is } 75 \text{ kg} ÷ (1.8)^2 = 23$$
The normal BMI for adults ranges from 18.5 to 24.9.

Classification of Body Mass Index Values

Classification	BMI (kg/m^2)
Severely underweight	<16
Moderately underweight	16–16.99
Mild underweight	17–18.49
Underweight	<18.5
Healthy weight	18.5–24.9
Pre-obese	25.0–29.9
Class I obesity	30.0–34.9
Class II obesity	35.0–39.9
Class III obesity	40.0 or higher

Source: Adapted from National Heart Lung and Blood Institute (NHLBI). (1998). Clinical guidelines on the identification, evaluation, and treatment of overweight and obesity in adults: The evidence report. Washington, DC: U.S. Department of Health & Human Services. Retrieved June 18, 2011, from http://www.nhlbi.nih.gov/guidelines/obesity/ob_gdlns.htm; and World Health Organization (2006a). BMI classification. Global database on body mass index. Retrieved June 8, 2011, from http://apps.who.int/bmi/index.jsp?introPage=intro_3.html

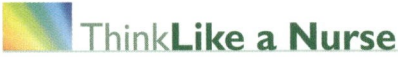

ThinkLike a Nurse 28-6

1. Calculate your waist-to-hip ratio (WHR).
2. Use Box 28-4 to calculate your BMI. Evaluate the result.
   - How useful are these data?
   - Do you feel you need to pursue a program of weight loss? Why or why not?

Imaging Techniques

Imaging techniques are not widely used to evaluate body composition because they are quite expensive to perform. Imaging methods include the following:

- **Dual-Energy X-Ray Absorptiometry (DEXA).** DEXA is used to assess bone mineral content and density. Because lean tissue has different absorptive properties than adipose tissue, this technique shows promise for wider use because it is quick and noninvasive.
- **Computed Tomography (CT).** CT scans measure volume rather than actual body tissue composition. They can provide information about the quantity of adipose tissue, particularly in body cavities.
- **Magnetic Resonance Imaging (MRI).** MRI is an excellent noninvasive method for directly assessing body composition. The cost and availability of the machinery, however, make it impractical for day-to-day evaluation of clients.

Underwater Weighing

Hydrodensitometry, or underwater weighing, is another method of determining body composition. It requires total submersion of the patient in a tank of water. Because fat readily floats, the person's buoyancy will vary depending on his percentage of body fat. This method is considered the gold standard for body composition measures. However, clinical use of this method is limited because it is impractical to use with children, the elderly, or individuals who are severely ill.

KnowledgeCheck 28-9

- Identify at least 10 physical examination findings that would lead you to suspect nutritional problems.
- What factors would lead to poor wound healing?

What Laboratory Values Indicate Nutritional Status?

Various laboratory or biochemical indicators provide information about nutritional status. These include blood glucose, serum protein level and associated indices, total lymphocyte count, and hemoglobin. Norms are given in the Diagnostic Testing box, Tests Reflecting Nutritional Status: Norms.

Blood Glucose

The blood glucose level indicates the amount of fuel available for cellular energy. Levels above normal trigger the release of insulin, which causes the glucose to move into body cells and to be stored in the liver and muscles. A level falling below normal triggers the release of glucagon, leading to the release of glucose from storage.

Hypoglycemia limits the fuel supply to the body, resulting in symptoms ranging from weakness to coma. Hypoglycemia

---

Diagnostic Testing

Tests Reflecting Nutritional Status: Norms

Note: Norms are for adults (ages 19 to 65) unless otherwise noted.

Blood glucose	Less than 70 mg/dL to 100 mg/dL. Capillary blood sugar is frequently assessed at the bedside with a simple fingerstick. Serum blood glucose levels are assessed by drawing a venous blood sample. The level is measured in the laboratory. The American Diabetes Association (2006) recommends for diabetic patients a preprandial plasma glucose level of 70 to 130 mg/dL.
Serum albumin	3.4–4.8 g/dL
Prealbumin	12–42 mg/dL (age 6 yr–adult)
Globulin	2.3–3.4 g/dL
Blood urea nitrogen (BUN)	5–18 mg/dL (children) 8–21 mg/dL (age 14–adult); 10–31 mg/dL (adult older than 90)
Creatinine	0.5–1 mg/dL (female) 0.6–1.2 mg/dL (male)
Hemoglobin	13.2–17.3 g/dL (male) 11.7–15.5 g/dL (female) 12.6–17.4 g/dL (male, older adult) 11.7–16.1 g/dL (female, older adult)

is usually defined as blood glucose of less than 50 mg/dL, but some people may feel symptoms at higher levels. Often the cause is insufficient food intake, excessive physical exertion, or a disproportionate amount of hypoglycemic agents.

Hyperglycemia (blood glucose greater than 109 mg/dL fasting or greater than 126 mg/dL at random) may be a sign of diabetes mellitus, an endocrine problem, which may develop as a result of either insufficient insulin production or resistance to the existing supply of insulin. A high blood glucose level does not mean that there is more fuel available for cellular energy, though. A characteristic of diabetes is that although there is more than enough glucose in the blood, it cannot enter and be used by the cells. Repeated blood glucose measures are required before making a diagnosis of diabetes mellitus because glucose levels may be temporarily elevated as a result of excessive carbohydrate intake or emotional and physical stressors.

A temporary rise in blood sugar may produce weakness or fatigue. Prolonged elevations lead to weight loss, blurred vision, **ketosis** (incomplete metabolism of fat due to inability to use carbohydrates as fuel), renal failure, and **peripheral neuropathy** (damage to nerves due to prolonged exposure to high glucose levels).

Patients with diabetes usually monitor their own blood sugar levels, but you may need to do it for some. Usually this is done by a fingerstick to obtain capillary blood for testing. Some meters can use blood from alternative sites such as upper arm, forearm, base of thumb, or thigh. Other types of monitors are available. For example, one kind uses a disposable sensor placed just under the skin. The sensor communicates with a receiver that reads the levels. Another is a skin-testing device, worn like a watch, pulls tiny amounts of fluid from the skin without puncturing it. For complete fingerstick steps, see Procedure 28-1.

Serum Protein Levels and Indices

Protein molecules dissolve in blood to form plasma proteins. Tissue proteins are a combination of albumin and globulin, so serum protein levels are indicators of protein stores.

- **Albumin** is synthesized in the liver and constitutes 60% of total body protein. Low levels of albumin are associated with malnutrition; malabsorption; acute and chronic liver disease; and repeated loss of protein through burns, wounds, or other sources. The half-life of albumin is 18 to 21 days. As a result, there is a lag in detecting nutritional problems based on serum albumin. Albumin is also affected by fluid status and, therefore, is not an accurate measure in the patient with fluid imbalance. For example, a patient in positive fluid balance (taking in more than excreted) will have a falsely low albumin level.
- **Prealbumin** level fluctuates daily and is considered a better marker of acute change than albumin.
- **Transferrin** is a protein that binds with iron. Because it has a half-life of only 8 to 9 days, it allows for faster detection of protein depletion than does measuring albumin. Transferrin can be measured directly or indirectly (by a total iron-binding capacity test [TIBC]). It also reflects iron status. In a person with iron deficiency, the TIBC will be increased; in a person with anemia, the TIBC will be decreased.

Other markers are used to monitor protein metabolism:

- **Urea** is formed in the liver as an end product of protein metabolism and is excreted through the kidneys. As such, the serum blood urea nitrogen (BUN) level is an indicator of liver and kidney function. An elevated BUN level is seen with impaired kidney function, dehydration, excessive protein breakdown (often seen with diabetes mellitus, hyperthyroidism, or starvation), or excessive dietary protein intake. Low levels are seen with impaired liver function, fluid overload, and low protein intake.
- **Creatinine,** an end product of skeletal muscle metabolism, is excreted through the kidneys and is an excellent indicator of renal function. Increased levels may indicate impaired kidney function or loss of muscle mass.

May I Delegate Nutritional Assessments?

You may safely delegate to nursing assistive personnel (NAPs) the measurement of weight, height, and intake and output; other nursing staff (e.g., licensed practical/vocational nurses) can collect a nutritional history. However, the registered nurse (RN) is responsible for reviewing and interpreting these findings. When delegating these tasks, you must also tell the NAP or LPN how often the measurements are to be made. Review Chapter 7 for making delegation decisions.

KnowledgeCheck 28-10

- What are the likely causes of hyperglycemia?
- Why is it important to identify the serum albumin level?

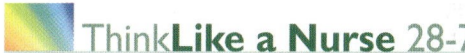

ThinkLike a Nurse 28-7

The Nutrition Screening Initiative (NSI) is completed for a 70-year-old.

- What major indicator on the NSI would indicate impaired nutritional status?
- What minor indicator would you likely see?
- What would malnourishment look like in the adult?
- What type of anthropometric findings would be typical of an older adult with poor nutrition patterns?
- What type of laboratory values would support impaired nutritional status?

ANALYSIS/NURSING DIAGNOSIS

For clients who have no symptoms of or risk factors for nutrition problems, use the diagnostic label Readiness for Enhanced Nutrition. NANDA International (NANDA-I) defines this as "a pattern of nutrient intake that is sufficient for meeting metabolic needs and can be strengthened" (2012, p. 176).

Nutrition as the Problem

You can use the following NANDA-I labels to describe general nutrition problems:

- Adult Failure to Thrive
- Imbalanced Nutrition: Less Than Body Requirements
- Imbalanced Nutrition: More Than Body Requirements
- Risk for Imbalanced Nutrition: More Than Body Requirements
- Self-Care Deficit (Feeding)

As you have learned, nutrition problems have many causes. Etiologies for undernutrition include eating disorders, difficulties with chewing and swallowing, vomiting, alcoholism, food intolerances, metabolic disorders, digestive disorders, and absorption disorders. For overnutrition, etiologies include overeating, lack of exercise, and metabolic or endocrine disorders. The following nursing diagnoses may contribute to nutrition problems: Diarrhea, Impaired Swallowing, Nausea, Noncompliance (with prescribed diet), and Deficient Knowledge (nutrition).

The following is an example of a nutrition nursing diagnosis statement:

Imbalanced Nutrition: Less Than Body Requirements related to difficulty chewing and Impaired Swallowing

Nutrition as the Etiology

Nutritional problems can also be the etiology of problems in other functional areas, for example:

- Ineffective Breastfeeding r/t inadequate milk production 2° insufficient intake of calories and fluids
- Constipation r/t insufficient intake of fluids and fiber
- Diarrhea r/t excessive intake of alcohol and/or sugar
- Risk for Infection r/t inadequate intake of calories and protein
- Impaired (or Risk for Impaired) Skin Integrity r/t inadequate intake of protein and/or vitamin A
- Disturbed Sleep Pattern r/t excessive caffeine intake or to eating fatty and spicy foods near bedtime
- Impaired Social Interaction r/t low self-esteem 2° obesity

PLANNING OUTCOMES/EVALUATION

The overall *Healthy People 2020* nutrition goal for the United States population is to "promote health and reduce chronic disease associated with diet and weight" (U.S. Department of Health and Human Services [USDHHS], 2010a). For specific objectives related to that goal,

 Go to Chapter 28, **Tables, Boxes, Figures: ESG Box 28-2,** on *DavisPlus.*

NOC standardized outcomes directly linked to nutritional problems include the following: Nutritional Status, Nutritional Status: Food and Fluid Intake, Nutritional Status: Nutrient Intake, and Weight Control.

You would choose other NOC outcomes based on the patient's nursing diagnosis. For example, for Situational Low Self-Esteem related to obesity, you might use Self-Esteem; for Noncompliance (prescribed diet), you could use Adherence Behavior, Compliance Behavior, or Treatment Behavior: Illness/Injury.

Individualized goals/outcome statements you might write for a patient with nutrition-related problems include the following:

Loses 1 lb per week until ideal weight is attained.

Follows the prescribed modified diet that, at a minimum, meets the DRIs.

Eats a variety of foods that provide a balanced diet.

PLANNING INTERVENTIONS/IMPLEMENTATION

NIC standardized interventions directly linked to nutrition problems include the broad interventions of Nutrition Management, Nutrition Therapy, Nutritional Counseling, and Nutritional Monitoring. These interventions could probably be used for most nutrition problems, regardless of the etiologies. The other nutrition interventions are grouped under Nutritional Support address specific etiologies (e.g., Swallowing Therapy). To see the entire list,

 Go to Chapter 28, **Standardized Language: NOC Outcomes and NIC Interventions Related to Nutrition,** on *DavisPlus.*

Individualized nursing actions are determined by the patient's nursing diagnosis. They may include, for example, counseling regarding vitamin and mineral supplementation, teaching clients on a limited budget how to buy nutritious foods, supporting special nutritional needs, and assisting clients with meals. These are discussed in the following section.

Vitamin and Mineral Supplementation

Noncredentialed nutrition "experts" recommend, and sell, megadoses of the entire alphabet of vitamin and mineral supplements to prevent cancer and heart attacks, improve your sex life, prevent aging, and work other miracles. However, conservative health professionals may scoff at supplements, insisting that a nutritious diet supplies all the micronutrients you need. Somewhere in the middle, most likely, lies the truth. A growing body of research suggests that certain supplements provide health benefits. Remember, too, that RDAs are for "average" needs. Individual needs for micronutrients vary. During periods of increased nutrient demands, it may be difficult to get enough nutrients from diet alone.

NIC Intervention—Nutritional Counseling

When teaching clients about supplements, keep the following principles in mind:

1. Dietary supplements may be appropriate for people whose diet does not provide the recommended intake of specific vitamins. With a few exceptions, there is little evidence to suggest that people will be harmed by taking vitamin supplements in appropriate amounts (Agency for Healthcare Research and Quality [AHRQ], 2003).
2. Individual needs vary, and those needs should determine the specific nutrients and amounts used. For example:
   - Newborn infants are given a vitamin K injection to prevent hemorrhaging because they do not yet have bacterial flora in the gut to synthesize enough vitamin K.
   - Breastfed infants may need a vitamin D supplement (but not other vitamins) if the mother does not have an adequate diet or if the baby does not receive enough exposure to sunlight. Fetal iron stores are depleted at 4 to 6 months, so breastfed infants also need iron supplementation at that age.
   - Vegetarians who eat little or no animal products may need a vitamin D supplement.
   - Folic acid supplementation is recommended for people taking methotrexate (a drug used to treat certain types of cancer).
   - All women who are capable of becoming pregnant should take a daily folic acid supplement of 400 to 800 mcg, in addition to the naturally occurring folate they eat in foods. Pregnant women need at least 600 mcg daily.
   - Most adults older than 50 years should obtain vitamin B_{12} from fortified foods or supplements.
   - Women age 50 and older should take calcium supplements to prevent osteoporosis; and there is growing evidence that men may need to do so, as well. Adults in the United States do not typically obtain adequate calcium from their diets (Barclay & Lie, 2008). Most calcium supplements come in combination with vitamin D to promote absorption of the calcium.
   - People who do not eat dairy products need supplemental calcium.
3. Food is the best source of nutrients. Supplements do not replace the need to eat a nutritious diet. Vitamins need carbohydrate, protein, and fat to do their work. Specific supplements for certain individual situations are more effective if the person also has an adequate diet.

4. Read supplement labels carefully. They provide information about toxicity levels, dosage, and side effects.
5. Encourage patients to ask their primary care provider's advice before taking vitamins.
6. Advise patients to follow the dosages recommended in the DRIs or RDAs.
7. Be certain that any health claims made for a supplement are based on sound research.
8. The long-term effects of most nutritional supplements have yet to be fully researched.

The same principles apply with regard to mineral supplementation. Supplements of specific minerals may be needed during growth periods (i.e., pregnancy, lactation, and adolescence), but as a rule healthy adults eating balanced diets do not need supplements. People who require mineral supplementation include those who refuse dairy products (and therefore lack calcium), and those with clinical problems such as iron-deficiency anemia, zinc deficiency (e.g., in alcoholism and long-term low-calorie diets), and treatment with certain diuretics (e.g., for hypertension).

Nutritious Foods on a Limited Budget

Hunger and malnutrition are not unusual among the poor in the United States. When your clients cannot afford to buy food, you should teach them about available assistance and make appropriate referrals to programs such as the following:

The Supplemental Nutrition Assistance Program (SNAP). This is the new name for the federal Food Stamp Program. For low-income households, this program issues coupons that can be used to buy food to cover the household's needs.

Commodity Supplemental Food Program. The federal government buys surplus food items to support certain agricultural products. These include both perishable and nonperishable commodities (e.g., peanut butter, cheese, green beans). The foods are made available to low-income pregnant and breastfeeding women, infants, children younger than age 6 years, and older adults at least age 60 years.

Women, Infants, and Children (WIC). This federal program provides free food to low-income women who are pregnant or breastfeeding and to children younger than age 5 years. Typical available foods are milk, eggs, cheese, cereals, juice, and infant formulas. They are intended to supplement the diet with protein, iron, and vitamins. They are not meant to supply all necessary food for the household.

National School Lunch and Breakfast Programs. These federally assisted programs subsidize schools that provide free or reduced-rate breakfasts and/or lunches to low-income children. All students, then, pay slightly less than the full cost of the meal. Lunches must supply about one-third of the child's RDA for energy and nutrients.

NIC Intervention—Teaching: Individual

You can help your clients to use their food dollars creatively by teaching them to follow the suggestions in the Self-Care box, Teaching Your Patients to Buy Nutritious Foods on a Limited Budget.

Supporting Special Nutritional Needs

Patients with special needs (e.g., patients with Impaired Swallowing, patients who are NPO, and older adults) require specific nutrition interventions.

Teaching Your Patients to Buy Nutritious Foods on a Limited Budget

Plan Ahead

➤ Look at the grocery advertisements in the paper or in their fliers, and plan meals around the sale items that are also the most nutrient dense.
➤ Make a list of the foods you need. This will help you to control impulse buying and extra trips to the store.
➤ Avoid eating at fast-food restaurants. Meals are more expensive and less nutritious than those you can prepare at home.
➤ If transportation is not a problem, buy fresh foods at farmers' markets, at consumer co-ops, and from neighbors who have gardens.

Buy Wisely

➤ Buy generic instead of more expensive and widely advertised brands.
➤ Watch for sales of nutrient-dense items. Stock up on and freeze them for later use if you do not need them right away.
➤ Buy in quantity—if it results in real savings and if you can use that amount of food before it spoils.
➤ Limit convenience foods (e.g., frozen dinners); they are expensive and often high in fat and sodium.
➤ Buy foods when they are in season; for example, fresh tomatoes are less expensive, and better tasting, in the summer than in the winter.
➤ Purchase oatmeal and cream of wheat instead of cold, sugared cereals. Buy in bulk rather than single-serving packages, but not so much that food spoils.
➤ Avoid shopping at convenience stores. Items are usually more expensive than in supermarkets.
➤ Buy inexpensive cuts of meat but not high-fat grades; avoid processed lunchmeats and hot dogs.
➤ Buy frozen concentrated fruit juices instead of juice in plastic jugs and cardboard boxes.
➤ Substitute dairy products, beans and lentils, and peanut butter for more expensive meat. Substitute powdered milk for whole milk.
➤ Read the Nutrition Facts panels on prepared foods to be sure you obtain the most nutrition for the money.

Impaired Swallowing

The NANDA-I diagnosis Impaired Swallowing may be caused by mechanical obstruction (e.g., tumor), neuromuscular impairment (e.g., facial paralysis), stroke, cerebral palsy, or a host of other anatomical or physiological defects. Patients with impaired swallowing, or **dysphagia,** are at risk for choking and aspiration. Nutritional support to help your patient feel more comfortable while swallowing and to help mealtime to be safer and more enjoyable, includes activities from the NIC intervention, Swallowing Therapy (Bulechek, Butcher, & Dochterman, 2008, pp. 707–708):

■ Provide/use assistive devices, as appropriate.
■ Avoid use of drinking straws.
■ Assist the patient to position head in forward flexion in preparation for swallowing (chin tuck).
■ Assist patient to place food at the back of the mouth and on the unaffected side.

- Monitor the patient's tongue movements while she is eating.
- Check mouth for pocketing of food after eating.
- Monitor body weight.
- Monitor body hydration (e.g., intake, output, skin turgor, mucous membranes).

In addition, you must also take the following Aspiration Precautions (Bulechek, Butcher, & Dochterman, 2008, p. 145):

- Monitor level of consciousness, cough reflex, gag reflex, and swallowing ability.
- Position the patient upright 90° or as far as possible.
- Keep suction setup available.
- Feed in small amounts.
- Avoid liquids or use of a thickening agent.
- Cut food into small pieces.
- Keep head of bed elevated for 30 to 45 minutes after feeding.

You will sometimes also offer a special dysphagia diet, depending on the degree of difficulty the patient has with swallowing: dysphagia puree, dysphagia mechanically altered, dysphagia advanced, and regular. Liquid diets vary in *viscosity*, or thickness, based on degree of swallowing impairment.

Patients Who Are NPO

Patients who cannot have oral food and fluids need comfort measures. Intravenous fluids for hydration may also include small amounts of glucose, but certainly not enough to meet bodily needs. Provide or assist the patient with oral hygiene. If allowed, provide ice chips, hard candy, chewing gum, or sips of water for rinsing the mouth. Advise family or visitors not to eat or drink around the patient, and try to schedule other activities for the patient at mealtimes.

✚ Remember, too, that remaining NPO for more than 3 days puts the patient at risk for malnutrition.

Patients Who Have Nausea

Nausea can cause vomiting and loss of appetite, leading to Impaired Nutrition. After assessing for the cause of the nausea (e.g., anxiety, pain, constipation, dehydration, post-anesthesia, chemotherapy, pancreatitis), there are things you can do to help the patient feel more comfortable and improve his appetite. The Association of Comprehensive Cancer Centres (Editorial Board Palliative Care, 2006) suggest the following:

- Determine the cause of the nausea.
- Assess for dehydration (you may need to administer parenteral fluid and electrolytes).
- Keep tissues and cool water to rinse the mouth at the bedside.
- Maintain a calm environment.
- Provide cool, fresh air.
- Instruct the patient to wear loose clothing.
- Avoid wearing strong perfumes.
- Immediately remove any food that the patient cannot or will not eat. The sight and smell of food can induce nausea.
- Provide or assist with frequent oral hygiene.
- Ask the patient to sit in an upright position for 30 to 45 minutes after eating, unless contraindicated.
- Provide small, frequent meals; avoid greasy, warm, spicy, or aromatic foods. In some cases cold food is better tolerated. Allow the patient to eat what she finds appetizing and tolerates well.
- Provide cool (not cold or iced) cola to drink.
- Have the patient suck on an ice cube, sorbet, or a piece of frozen fruit (pineapple, kiwi, or apple).

- Recommend a dietary consultation if nausea and vomiting persist.
- For malnourished patients, consult a dietitian. Consider dietary supplements; however, these are often poorly tolerated and may sometimes cause even more nausea.
- When the nausea is related to anxiety, stress, or anticipation of nausea, try certain psychological techniques, such as distraction, relaxation techniques, guided imagery, systematic desensitization, self-hypnosis, biofeedback, and music therapy.
- Administer antiemetics as prescribed or per protocol.

Older Adults

Nutritional problems of older adults are similar to those for adults of all ages, but the incidence of problems may be higher among older adults. The following interventions are appropriate for patients of any age who experience the associated problems.

Self-Care Deficit: Feeding. You will find interventions in the later section, Assisting Patients with Meals.

Loss of Appetite; Diminished Sense of Smell and Taste. Refer to the interventions in the Example Problem: Underweight and Undernutrition, later in this chapter.

Decreased Income. Refer to the Self-Care box Teaching Your Patients to Buy Nutritious Foods on a Limited Budget. In addition, for older adults in the United States, two types of food programs are available for you to recommend. Everyone older than age 60, regardless of income, can eat hot noon meals at a community center (under the Congregate Meals programs). Those who are ill or disabled can receive meals at home under the Home-Delivered Meals Program. Socially needy persons (e.g., those who are homeless) are given priority. These programs are funded by public/private partnerships (e.g., Meals on Wheels).

Nutritional Deficiencies. Advise clients to eat nutrient-dense foods and to eat essential foods first. Because the sense of taste is decreased, older adults may prefer concentrated sweets; and because they may also have a poor appetite, once they eat sweets they may not be hungry enough to eat other foods.

Gastroesophageal Reflux. Advise clients to not eat just before bedtime and to elevate the head of the bed 30° to 40°. It is also important for them to avoid overeating, to avoid bending over, and to take their prescribed medications. They should also avoid fruit juices, fatty foods, chocolate, alcohol, and smoking; all of these stimulate reflux. If overweight, the client with reflux should lose weight.

Decreased Gastric Secretions. People with this problem should eat regularly scheduled meals, chew their food thoroughly, and take prescribed medications. They should be certain to eat foods rich in vitamin D to ensure calcium absorption.

Dry Mouth. This is an age-associated change. Advise clients to avoid caffeine; alcohol; tobacco; and dry, bulky, spicy, salty, or highly acidic foods. Offer sugarless hard candy or chewing gum to stimulate salivation (unless the patient has dementia). Use lip moisturizer and encourage frequent sips of water.

Glucose Intolerance. Obviously, patients with glucose intolerance should avoid concentrated, refined sugars (e.g., candy, ice cream, desserts), unless they have been told to use it to treat hypoglycemia. Complex carbohydrates (e.g., whole-grain cereals, vegetables) are better tolerated. Smaller, more frequent meals may also be necessary.

Decreased Intestinal Peristalsis. To prevent constipation, advise patients to eat a diet high in fiber, including a minimum of five servings of fresh fruits and vegetables every day (prunes and prune juice are often effective); exercise regularly; drink at least eight glasses of water or other fluids per day; and eat meals on a regular schedule.

Avoiding Dementia. At least one study suggests that dementia, especially Alzheimer's disease, is less common among people who eat fruits and vegetables daily, eat fish once a week, and use fats rich in omega-3 fatty acids (e.g., walnut and soy oil) (Barberger-Gateau, Raffaitin, Letenneur, et al., 2007). Of course, this doesn't prove that diet can prevent dementia. It merely suggests there may be a connection. Either way, clients can benefit from this dietary advice.

Nothing by Mouth (NPO) Orders. When older adults must be NPO for tests or procedures, schedule them early in the day to decrease the length of time the patient must be NPO. If testing must be late in the day, ask the primary care provider whether the patient can have an early breakfast.

Assisting Patients With Meals

Some patients are at risk for nutritional deficits as a result of a Self-Care Deficit (Feeding), which may be caused by loss of cognitive, musculoskeletal, or neuromuscular function; weakness; pain; or environmental barriers. Elderly patients, especially, are at risk for undernutrition or malnourishment in inpatient settings. You should institute special nutrition interventions in patients who have one of the following:

- An involuntary weight loss of more than 5% in 30 days or 10% in 180 days.
- Leaving more than one-fourth of their food in the past 7 days or two-thirds of meals (based on a 2000-kcal diet).
- A BMI of 19 or less.

NIC Interventions for this situation are Feeding and Self-Care Assistance: Feeding. Important nursing actions include assisting patients with meals. Other nursing activities include the following:

- Assess for functional deficits that contribute to Self-Care Deficit or Imbalanced Nutrition.
- Monitor intake for nutritional adequacy. Some patients may need liquid oral supplements of protein and calories.
- Collaborate with occupational and physical therapists in planning care.
- See that the patient has protein- and energy-enriched meals.
- Provide mid-afternoon snacks.
- Ensure the nutrition prescribed is actually implemented. Assign someone to be responsible for assisting the patient with meals as necessary. Include this in your instructions to NAPs and other assistive personnel.
- Refer the patient and family to an agency that can help them obtain a home health aide.

For guidelines more specific to assisting with meals, including care of patients with dementia, see Clinical Insight 28-4.

Example Problem: Overweight and Obesity

The BMI is commonly used to define weight status. A client with a BMI greater than 25 but less than 30 is considered **overweight** (or pre-obese). **Obesity** is a BMI of 30 or higher. Something like 32% of noninstitutionalized adults are obese (National Center for Health Statistics, 2008b). Obesity and overweight together affect two-thirds of our adult population, and are associated with several chronic diseases. Therefore, major health agencies consider obesity to be a national epidemic and have issued guidelines encouraging weight reduction. As a nurse, you can assist your clients to achieve and maintain a healthy weight.

Obesity in Older Adults

The proportion of obese adults has doubled in the past 30 years. More than 15% of older adults are obese (Newman, 2009). Obesity is more prevalent among older adults under age 70 and becomes less prevalent with advancing age. Nevertheless, most older adults lead active and healthy lives and are not obese. Furthermore, according to the BMI thresholds set by the WHO, older people considered overweight (rather than obese) are not at a greater mortality risk (Flicker, McCaul, Hankey, et al., 2010). However, according to the BMI thresholds set by the WHO, older people considered to be overweight are not at a greater mortality risk (Flicker, McCaul, Hankey, et al., 2010).

As we age we tend to exercise less, but our eating patterns do not usually change. In addition, aging is associated with hormonal changes and slowing metabolism that cause accumulation of fat (e.g., decreased growth hormone and serum testosterone). Many of the chronic problems associated with aging are made worse by obesity (e.g., respiratory problems, arthritis, cardiovascular disease, cancer, and diabetes).

Interventions are the same as for other groups: dietary modification, exercise, and use of community supports. Older adults may require more assistance improving physical function so they can exercise more. To avoid injuries, exercise should start at low intensity and progress gradually over several months.

ANALYSIS/NURSING DIAGNOSIS (OVERWEIGHT AND OBESITY)

NANDA-I diagnoses define overweight and obesity in the following ways:

- *Imbalanced Nutrition: More Than Body Requirements* is used when a person consumes nutrients in excess of metabolic needs. The defining characteristics are (1) triceps skinfold greater than 15 mm in men and 25 mm in women, or (2) weight 20% over ideal for height and frame.
- *Risk for Imbalanced Nutrition: More Than Body Requirements* identifies the potential for an individual to experience intake of nutrients in excess of metabolic needs.

Etiologies. Etiologies of those NANDA-I diagnoses include the following:

- Consuming more kcal than needed for activity, gender, height, and weight
- Reducing activity level without modifying food intake
- Genetic predisposition to obesity. For example, low BMR and excess adipose tissue distribution are common in certain ethnic groups.
- Ineffective coping mechanisms—for instance, the use of binge eating to reduce anxiety or relieve boredom
- Cultural influences—some cultural norms encourage excess weight, particularly as an indication of wealth.
- Decreased levels of thyroid hormone can lower BMR, causing weight gain.

Clinical Insight 28-4 ➤ Assisting Patients With Meals

General Guidelines

- Recommend having one staff person for every two or three patients who need assistance, allowing about 20 to 30 minutes to feed a patient. Prolonged meal times do not promote appetite; nor does hurrying.
- Feeding assistants should be supervised by an RN or LPN.
- Do not interrupt meals with medications.
- Encourage family members to share mealtimes.
- If the patient's condition allows, encourage him to get out of bed for meals.
- Encourage residents in long-term care settings to eat meals in the dining room instead of in the bedroom (Leydon & Dahl, 2008).

Preparation

- Assess for rituals used before meals (blessings of food, etc.).
- Provide an opportunity for toileting, oral hygiene, and handwashing before meals.
- Assist the patient to eat and drink only as necessary; encourage independence.
- Provide privacy during meals if the patient is embarrassed; to further maintain dignity, use a napkin, not a bib, over the patient's clothes.
- Check for proper fit of dentures.
- Provide music during the meal if the patient wishes.
- Demonstrate the use of assistive devices and alternative methods for eating and drinking.

Assisting the Patient

- If the patient must eat in bed, place the head of the bed at the highest tolerable level, and adjust the overbed table to be in easy reach.
- If the patient can feed himself, prepare the food on the tray for him (e.g., open food containers, cut the meat, peel an orange, open the milk and butter containers, mash food if needed).
- If the client is visually impaired, identify the locations of the meal on the tray based on a clock face (e.g., "The coffee is at 1 o'clock above the plate on the right").

Feeding the Patient

- Feed the patient if she is unable to feed herself.
- Sit down while feeding the patient; do not rush.
- Position yourself so that you can make eye contact.
- Be sure to provide adequate time for her to chew and swallow.
- If possible, ask her what food she would like next.
- Serve one food at a time; serve small amounts.
- Serve finger foods (e.g., fruit, bread) to promote independence.
- Cue older adults whenever possible with words or gestures.

- Have casual conversation with the patient while feeding her to make mealtime more pleasant and relaxed.

After the Meal

- Help the patient to wash hands or use the rest room after the meal.
- Record the amount of food and fluid the patient consumed.
- Document feeding behaviors.
- Document changes in nutritional status.
- Document staffing and staff education, and availability of a supportive interdisciplinary team.

Assisting Older Adults With Dementia

As do all people, older adults with dementia differ in their abilities to eat and communicate. The following are general tips, but you should tailor interventions to each person's specific abilities to achieve the best results. In addition to many of the preceding interventions, try some of the following measures:

- Assess the patient's self-feeding abilities.
- Assess the patient's cognitive limitations and communication abilities.
- Assess for and treat pain.
- Minimize distractions: Turn off the TV; discourage people from entering the room.
- Help the patient to a comfortable chair if possible.
- Assist with oral hygiene and hand hygiene.
- Remove any unnecessary eating utensils; serve only one food at a time.
- Remove items that should not be eaten (e.g., packets of salt or pepper), and hot items that could be spilled.
- Cue the patient verbally to help with self-feeding (e.g., "take a bite," "chew," "swallow").
- Pantomime eating motions so the patient can imitate them.
- Place your hand over the patient's to begin and guide self-feeding (hand-over-hand).
- When assisting, sit at eye level and interact socially with the patient.
- Involve family members if they have assisted with feeding at home.
- Train and supervise NAPs in interacting with and feeding patients with dementia.
- Do not assist too soon—give the patient time to eat independently.
- Do not feed too fast. Feed at a rate that is safe and comfortable for the patient.

References

Amella, 2007; Ebersole, Hess, Touhy, et al., 2009; National Guideline Clearinghouse (NGC); 2003, updated June 2008; National Guideline Clearinghouse, 2001, Reviewed 2006.

- Ineffective Health Maintenance—for example, high-fat diet, inactivity, and avoidance of health assistance
- Impaired Physical Mobility, which limits physical activity and decreases energy expenditure

Overweight and Obesity as Etiology of Other Problems. Being overweight may lead to the development of other nursing diagnoses. Excess weight, and especially obesity, makes activity more difficult; therefore, over time, the person becomes more sedentary, and the body becomes deconditioned (weakened). The following are examples:

- Activity Intolerance r/t deconditioned state secondary to long-term sedentary lifestyle
- Decreased Cardiac Output r/t prolonged deconditioned state
- Constipation r/t inadequate physical activity
- Risk for Injury (and/or Risk for Falls) r/t deconditioned state and generalized weakness
- Social Isolation r/t poor self-image secondary to excess weight

PLANNING OUTCOMES/EVALUATION (OVERWEIGHT AND OBESITY)

A part of your nursing role will be to work with clients to help achieve the *Healthy People 2020* nutrition goals. To review them,

 Go to Chapter 28, **Tables, Boxes, Figures: ESG Box 28-2: Nutrition and Weight Status Objectives From Healthy People 2020,** on DavisPlus.

For *NOC standardized outcomes* for evaluating the outcomes for the example problem Overweight and Obesity,

 Go to Chapter 28, **Standardized Language: NOC Outcomes and NIC Interventions for Adult Failure to Thrive, Overweight/Obesity, and Underweight/Malnutrition.**

Individualized goals/outcome statements include the following examples:

States pertinent factors contributing to weight gain.

Designs dietary modifications to meet individual long-term goal of weight control.

Accomplishes desired weight loss in a reasonable time frame (1 to 2 lb/week).

Incorporates appropriate physical activities requiring energy expenditure into daily life.

PLANNING INTERVENTIONS/IMPLEMENTATION (OVERWEIGHT AND OBESITY)

For the *NIC standardized interventions* for overweight and obese clients,

 Go to Chapter 28, **Standardized Language: NOC Outcomes and NIC Interventions for Adult Failure to Thrive, Overweight/Obesity, and Underweight/Malnutrition,** on DavisPlus.

Individualized nursing activities for clients with the example problem Overweight and Obesity include the following:

- *Weigh the client weekly under the same conditions.* Weekly weights allow the client to monitor his progress and can motivate him to follow the weight-loss regimen.
- *Suggest keeping a food diary for a number of days.* Research suggests that this can double diet weight loss. Analyzing the diary will provide valuable information on intake and circumstances that trigger eating. It may help to identify behavioral or coping issues. Keep in mind that many patients eat less than usual when they are keeping a food diary (Hollis, Gullion, Stevens, et al., Weight Loss Maintenance Trial Research Group, 2008).
- *Educate the client about a healthy diet.* Lifestyle changes must be ongoing to maintain weight loss. For the client, the first step is to learn about a balanced diet and food quality.
- *Encourage the client to eat more fresh fruits and vegetables and fewer fatty foods and sugar-sweetened beverages.*
- *Discuss fat substitutes,* which are available to improve flavor and texture of low-fat foods while reducing total dietary fat. Recall that fats contain 9 kcal per gram, so reducing fat intake is an important part of most weight-loss diets. Fat substitutes are not absorbed; therefore, they contribute few kcal. The American Heart Association (n.d.[b]) states that fat substitutes, used appropriately, can provide flexibility in diet planning. Although the USDA (FDA) considers fat substitutes to be safe, long-term benefits and risks are not yet known. In addition, it is not unusual for people to experience diarrhea and stomach cramps when using fat substitutes.
- *Encourage the client to commit to regular exercise.* Increased physical activity will not only use up excess stores of fat but also increase the body's resting metabolic rate. Individuals should begin gradually with low-impact activities, such as walking for 20 minutes at least four times a week. The American College of Sports Medicine (ACSM) recommends 150 to 250 minutes of exercise per week to prevent weight gain. More than 250 minutes per week are needed to bring about significant weight loss—that is, 50 minutes on 5 days of the week or 40 minutes on 6 days of the week (Donnelly, Blair, Jakicic, et al., 2009). Although increased physical activity aids in weight control, advise your client to set realistic expectations for what exercise can achieve. A recent study concludes that overeating, more than a lack of exercise, is to blame for the American obesity epidemic (Swinburn, Sacks, Lo, et al., 2009).
- *Be encouraging and nonjudgmental,* especially when there are setbacks.
- *Provide weight loss tips* such as those in the Self-Care box Teaching Weight Loss Tips.
- *For children, recommend the 5-2-1-0 program* (Marion County Children's Alliance, n.d.). Children should have the following:
  5 – Servings of fruits and vegetables each day.
  2 – Hours or less of "screen" time per day.
  1 – Hour of physical activity per day.
  0 – Servings of sweetened beverages.
- *For children and adolescents,* weight loss is more effective when it involves the child, the parents, and the community in limiting soda and junk food consumption and limiting hours spent watching television and playing video games (Joanna Briggs Institute; 2007a). Children can be taught to make "best choices" regarding activities and the foods they eat (Speroni, Early, & Atherton, 2007).

To learn more about obesity in adolescents and children,

 Go to Chapter 28, **Reading More About Nutrition,** on DavisPlus.

To see a sample care plan and care map for Imbalanced Nutrition: More Than Body Requirements,

 Go to **Care Plan, Imbalanced Nutrition: More Than Body Requirements, and Care Map, Imbalanced Nutrition: More Than Body Requirements,** on DavisPlus.

Teaching Weight Loss Tips

Getting Ready

Make a commitment.	➤ Promise yourself; promise others. "I will do this."
Set realistic goals.	➤ Aim to lose 1 to 2 lb/wk. To do this you need to burn 500 to 1,000 calories more than you consume. Losing weight faster usually means losing water weight or muscle tissue rather than fat.
	➤ Set "process" rather than "outcome" goals. For example, "I will exercise every day" instead of "I will lose 10 pounds this month." Changing your habits (your "processes") is the key to weight loss.
	➤ Write your goals, your plan for achieving them, and your start date. This makes it reality, not just a thought.
	➤ Review your goals each week. Readjust them as needed. If you are exercising more than you thought, adjust your goal upward, for example.
Plan for setbacks.	➤ Identify situations that might trigger eating or interfere with exercise; plan specific actions you will take to overcome them.

Beginning New Behaviors

Eat healthier foods.	➤ Eat more fruits and vegetables.
	➤ Limit fatty foods and sugar-sweetened beverages.
Get active and stay active.	➤ If you have not been exercising, start slowly.
	➤ Work up to at least 250 min per week to lose weight and maintain the loss.
Get adequate sleep.	➤ For most people, this is 7 to 8 hr a night.
	➤ New research suggests that sleep deprivation can affect levels of the appetite-regulating hormones leptin and ghrelin.
	➤ Sleep loss can affect the type of food you crave. When you are tired you are less able to cope with stress and emotional triggers for eating, and more likely to crave comfort foods such as chocolate and ice cream.

"Sticking with It"

Keep a food diary.	➤ This can double your weight loss.
Decide what and when to eat.	➤ Decide what foods you will eat as well as when you will eat. For example, "I will eat only at the table, 3 meals and 2 snacks daily."
	➤ Make a conscious effort to take small bites and eat slowly.
	➤ Serve your food on small plates.
Shop wisely.	➤ Shop for food on a full stomach.
	➤ Read food labels when purchasing food (for information about calorie and fat content).
Find ways to exercise.	➤ Lay out your exercise clothing ahead of time (e.g., at night if you exercise in the morning).
	➤ Use the stairs instead of the elevator; park in the back of the parking lot, as far from the door as possible.
	➤ Walk or bike to work when possible.
Get emotional support.	➤ Family members can help by not offering you desserts. Weight-loss support groups let you know you are not alone. An exercise partner can help keep you motivated.

Recognize that lifestyle changes must be permanent.
Remember: Healthy eating, physical activity, and sleep are necessities, not luxuries!

Example Problem: Underweight and Undernutrition

A BMI of less than 18.5 is considered underweight (see Box 28-4). For patients in long-term care settings, parameters include one of the following:

1. Involuntary weight loss of more than 5% in 30 days or 10% in 180 days
2. Leaving more than one-quarter of food in the past 7 days or two-thirds of meals based on a 2,000-kcal diet
3. A BMI of 19 or less

For hospitalized patients with serious illness, increased mortality is associated with a BMI of 21 or less (NGC, 2006b).

A person becomes underweight when he consumes fewer kcal than needed based on his activity, sex, height, and weight. Consuming too few kcal may result in serious undernutrition—that is, insufficient intake of protein, fat, vitamins, and minerals. The causes of underweight status may be psychological, social, economic, or physiological (e.g., hospitalization, self-care deficits, illness, eating disorders). A person can also be malnourished with regard to specific nutrients without being underweight.

Severe Malnutrition?

Malnutrition is a condition of impaired development or function caused by a long-term deficiency, excess, or imbalance in energy and/or nutrient intake. Malnutrition caused by deficiency of protein in a diet that is primarily starches is called

kwashiorkor. When protein sources in food are scarce and overall caloric intake is low, **marasmus** occurs, particularly in young children. Severely undernourished people are prone to infections. Symptoms due to insufficient food are reduced physical activity, weight loss, reduced height, abdominal enlargement, and hair loss. Other diseases develop as a result of specific vitamin and mineral deficiency, such as beriberi (neurological deficits), scurvy (delayed wound healing and poor bone growth), and pellagra (diarrhea and dementia). See Tables 28-4 and 28-5 for specific signs of vitamin and mineral excesses and deficits.

Malnutrition is most common in underdeveloped nations and among children, older adults, and people with chronic illnesses such as cancer, HIV, and COPD. Others at risk for malnutrition include those with the following:

- Serum albumin level 3.5 g/dL or less
- Nausea or vomiting lasting 3 days or more
- Clear liquid diet or NPO for 3 days or longer
- Increased nutritional requirements (e.g., wound healing, burns)
- Recent, unplanned loss of 10% or more of patient's usual weight

Eating Disorders

Eating disorders are a growing problem in North America. **Anorexia nervosa** is a psychiatric disorder characterized by self-starvation. **Bulimia nervosa** refers to binge eating (eating an excessive amount of food in a short period of time) followed by self-induced vomiting or laxative abuse to purge food. Although all segments of society are affected, eating disorders are more common in women, and most report the onset of illness before the age of 20. About half of teenage girls either are or think they should be on a diet.

Both anorexia and bulimia can result in hair loss, low blood pressure, generalized weakness, amenorrhea, and cold intolerance. Serious medical complications include osteoporosis and increased risk for fractures; brain damage; decreased resistance to infection; cardiac, renal, liver, and metabolic disorders; and even death. You will need to recognize the early warning signs of eating disorders, such as the behavior changes described in Box 28-5.

ANALYSIS/NURSING DIAGNOSIS (UNDERWEIGHT AND UNDERNUTRITION)

Imbalanced Nutrition: Less Than Body Requirements may be the patient's problem, or it may be the etiology of other nursing diagnoses. The following are examples.

Imbalanced Nutrition: Less Than Body Requirements r/t Impaired Swallowing 2° pain with swallowing

Risk for Disproportionate Growth r/t Imbalanced Nutrition: Less Than Body Requirements 2° anorexia nervosa

For other useful nursing diagnoses and etiologies (e.g., Disturbed Body Image),

 Go to Chapter 28, **Standardized Language: Nursing Diagnoses Associated With Undernutrition,** on DavisPlus.

PLANNING OUTCOMES/EVALUATION (UNDERWEIGHT AND UNDERNUTRITION)

The NOC standardized outcome for assessing weight is Weight Control. If it becomes necessary to monitor nutritional status, you could use the labels of Nutritional Status: Food and Fluid Intake and Nutritional Status: Nutrient Intake.

BOX 28-5 ■ Early Warning Signs of an Eating Disorder

Food Behaviors
- Deliberate self-starvation with weight loss
- Continuous dieting
- Skips meals.
- Takes only tiny portions.
- Will not eat in front of others.
- Always has an excuse not to eat.
- Usually has a diet soda or coffee in hand.
- Eats only food that is low in fat.

Physical Signs
- Excessive facial or body hair (because of inadequate protein in the diet)
- Hair loss
- Abnormal weight loss
- Sensitivity to cold
- Absent or irregular menstruation

Appearance and Body Image Behaviors
- Wears baggy clothes.
- Complains of being fat.
- Obsesses about clothing size.
- Spends lots of time inspecting self in the mirror.

Exercise Behaviors
- Exercises excessively and compulsively.
- May tire easily.
- Pushes self beyond normal expectations.

Social Behaviors
- Tries to please everyone and withdraws if unsuccessful.
- Tries to care for everyone but self.
- Tries to control what and where family eats.
- Relationships tend to be superficial or dependent.

Emotional Behaviors
- Intense fear of gaining weight

Individualized goals/outcome statements include the following:
Progressively gains weight toward desired goal.
Verbalizes willingness to follow diet.
Body mass and weight are within normal limits.
Laboratory values (e.g., albumin, complete blood count [CBC]) are within normal limits.
Recognizes factors contributing to underweight.

PLANNING INTERVENTIONS/IMPLEMENTATION (UNDERWEIGHT AND UNDERNUTRITION)

For the *NIC standardized interventions* for undernutrition,

 Go to Chapter 28, **Standardized Language: NOC Outcomes and NIC Interventions for Adult Failure to Thrive, Overweight/Obesity and Underweight/Malnutrition,** on DavisPlus.

Individualized nursing activities for clients who are underweight or undernourished include the following:
- **Assess for recent changes in physiological status as underlying cause of weight loss or undernourishment** (e.g., pain, fatigue, illness, and immobility).

- **Offer high-calorie and high-protein (nutrient-dense) foods.** Serve these foods when the person is most likely to be hungry. Avoid food with little nutritional value; when intake is limited, it is essential that it not be wasted on empty calories.
- **Consult with a dietitian** about strategies to increase the nutritional content of foods.
- **Weigh the client regularly under the same conditions.** Weigh the client one or two times per week if nutritional status is severely jeopardized to assess the effectiveness of the therapeutic plan.
- **Offer high-protein supplements.** Offer nutritious high-protein supplements between meals to increase intake of protein and kcal. It may be easier for the client to drink a small amount of a supplement than to eat enough food to supply the equivalent nutrients.
- **Suggest community resources** (e.g., Meals on Wheels for clients with Adult Failure to Thrive). Additional assistance may be needed to improve access to food.
- **For eating disorders, see that the client is referred for appropriate counseling** (e.g., dietitian, mental health professional).

The following sections discuss more fully nursing interventions for improving the appetite, as well as alternative feeding methods.

Stimulating the Patient's Appetite

Illness, with its accompanying pain, anxiety, and medications, often causes appetite loss. This is especially true for institutionalized patients, who have little control over food choices and preparation. You will need to make an effort to see that hospitalized patients eat the food that is served. It is not enough merely to order meals and deliver the trays. The following measures may help improve appetite and intake, and subsequently, nutritional status:

- **Offer frequent, small meals.** This helps prevent gastric distention and improves appetite by keeping the patient from being overwhelmed with a large amount of food.
- **Suggest smokers refrain for 1 hour before a meal.**
- **Restrict liquid intake with meals** to prevent gastric distention or feeling full before the patient consumes sufficient nutrients.
- **Keep the patient's environment neat and clean** and free of unpleasant sights, odors, and medical equipment. These often trigger loss of appetite. For example, remove bedpans, urinals, and the emesis basin from the room before mealtimes.
- **Order a late food tray or warm the food** if the patient is not in his room during mealtime.
- **Provide or assist with frequent oral hygiene.**
- **Provide a pleasant eating environment.**
- **Serve foods attractively;** vary textures, colors, and flavors; arrange the tray so the person can easily reach the food.
- **Position** *the person* **comfortably** for mealtime.
- **Find out what the person likes to eat,** and encourage family and friends to bring foods from home.
- **Control pain around the clock,** and avoid painful treatments before meals.
- **If the patient receives a nutritional supplement, delay the meal for at least an hour afterward.**
- **Encourage meals with friends** for those who live alone, or meals at a senior center.
- **Provide nutrient-dense foods** (e.g., add ice cream to appropriate beverages and foods).
- **Arrange for a home health aide** to shop and prepare meals for those who are unable to leave home for groceries, or arrange for Meals on Wheels.

Providing Enteral Nutrition

If a patient cannot meet his nutritional needs through an enhanced diet and measures to stimulate the appetite, you may need to use an alternative feeding method. Feeding can occur through the intestinal tract as enteral nutrition, or intravenously as parenteral nutrition. **Enteral nutrition** (*tube feeding*) refers to the delivery of liquid nutrition into the upper intestinal tract via a tube. Tube feeding may be used in addition to or instead of oral intake. It is the preferred method of feeding for a patient who has a functioning intestinal tract but needs nutritional support (e.g., patients with high metabolic needs, such as those with trauma, burns, or severe malnutrition; neurological disorders that affect swallowing; anorexia nervosa; prematurity; failure to thrive; or specific bowel diseases). Tube feeding may be a short- or long-term therapy.

Enteral feedings are preferred to parenteral (i.e., intravenous) nutrition because they have a lower incidence of sepsis and maintain intestinal structure and function (Kaushik, Pietraszewski, Holst, et al., 2005). However, there are several risks associated with enteral feedings. If enteral formula is aspirated into the lungs, it can lead to infection, pneumonia, abscess formation, adult respiratory distress syndrome (ARDS), and in some cases death. The high glucose content of enteral formulas provides a medium for bacterial growth. Other complications include diarrhea, nausea and vomiting, nasopharyngeal trauma, alterations in drug absorption and metabolism, and various metabolic disturbances. For more about safe use of parental nutrition, see the Quality and Safety Education for Nurses (QSEN) box.

There have been some instances where enteral feedings have been mistakenly connected to intravascular (IV) lines and feeding solutions have been infused into veins. These events, termed "tubing misconnections," are potentially fatal to the patient (The Joint Commission, 2006, 2007; USFDA, 2005). An enteral device manufacturer and a professional organization dedicated to improving patient care by advancing the science and practice of nutrition support therapy have cooperated to develop the "BE A. L. E. R. T." Safety Campaign© to increase the safety of patients on enteral nutrition (see Box 28-6).

Administer feedings at room temperature, and be sure to check the expiration date of any feedings before starting an infusion. For complete instructions on tube feedings, see Procedure 28-3.

Patients may receive enteral or parenteral nutrition in the home as well as in inpatient settings. The Home Care box Home Nutritional Support reviews teaching related to alternative feeding methods in the home. You should review these topics with the patient or caregiver.

Types of Enteric Tubes

Enteric tubes are available in various materials, lengths, diameters, and types. Choose the type of tube you need based on the intended use and the length of time you anticipate it will be left in place. This chapter focuses on the use of enteral tubes as a route for feeding; however, they are inserted for other reasons, as well:

- Lavage of the stomach (e.g., when there is disease, surgery, or bleeding in the GI tract, and in cases of poisoning or medication overdose)
- Collecting a specimen of stomach contents for laboratory tests

QSEN

Safe Use of Parenteral Nutrition

Competency: **Quality Improvement (Knowledge, Skill, Attitudes); Evidenced-Based Practice (Skills, Attitudes); Safety (Knowledge, Skills, and Attitudes)***

Clinicians at Scripps Memorial Hospital (SMH) in La Jolla, California, theorized that their poor processes and variation in methods in use of parenteral nutrition (PN) were producing inconsistent patient outcomes, thus increasing patient risk. The following is a description how they set out to correct this by identifying the root causes of the problems and standardizing care.

▶ **Problems Identified:** Clinicians first organized a multidisciplinary team to collect and analyze data,

develop better practices, and evaluate outcomes. They found several problems: inappropriate use of PN, poor glycemic control in patients on PN, inconsistent and confusing ordering practices, insufficient calorie replacement, and insufficient laboratory monitoring.

▶ **Corrective Interventions** included: Implementing the American Society for Parenteral and Enteral Nutrition's (A.S.P.E.N.) guideline for PN, revising the PN order form, educating physicians and other clinicians, and establishing twice weekly PN rounds. The group measured specific quality indicators before and after implementing the new procedures. The following table shows the top four measures:

Safety Measure	Pre-intervention (2007)	Post intervention (2009)
Compliance with 10 Mandatory Components of a PN Order Form (A.S.P.E.N. guideline)	20%	100%
Appropriate use of parenteral nutrition	60%	97%
Baseline labs ordered before PN starts	30%	80%
Kcal delivered are within 10% of estimated need	54%	85%

▶ **Results/Conclusions:** In addition to improving compliance, the new procedures resulted in significant costs savings.

▶ **Think About It:** Parenteral nutrition is a high-risk treatment associated with serious complications, including death. 1) Do the above measures mean that patient outcomes are improved? 2) In what specific ways does this QI project demonstrate the QSEN competencies of

Quality Improvement, Safety, and Evidenced-Based and Practice? 3) Which specific knowledge, skills, and attitudes does it address?

Source: Boitano, Bojak, McCloskey, McCaul, & McDonough (2010). *For specific Knowledge, Skills, and Attitudes

 Go to the QSEN web site at http://www.qsen.org. ksas_prelicensure.php

---

▪ To prevent nausea, vomiting, and gastric distention postoperatively.

When a nasogastric (or orogastric) tube is placed to empty the stomach (lavage), larger bore, tubes made of polyvinyl chloride (PVC), are used. These are called **Salem** **sump tubes** (Fig. 28-3). A Salem sump tube has a lumen for drainage and one to allow air to enter the stomach. The air port (pigtail) is usually blue. A **Levin tube**, also used for drainage, has a single lumen, with holes in the tip and along the sides.

✚ BOX 28-6 ▪ Be A.L.E.R.T©

To reduce errors and help ensure safe enteral nutrition, use the following mnemonic:

A	**Aseptic** technique.................................	When preparing and delivering enteral formula, practice good hand hygiene; wear gloves when handling feeding tube; avoid touching can tops, container openings, spike, and spike port.
L	**Label** enteral equipment........................	with patient name and room number, formula name and rate, date and time of initiation, and nurse initials.
E	**Elevate** the head of the bed...............	a minimum of 30° for feedings whenever clinically possible; may mitigate risk of reflux and aspiration of gastric content.
R	**Right** patient, **Right** formula, **Right** tube.........	Match formula to patient's feeding order; verify **enteral** tubing set connects formula container to feeding tube.
T	**Trace** all lines and tubing back to patient.........	Avoid misconnections—trace all lines from origin to patient; only enteral-to-enteral connections.

Sources: © 2009 Nestlé HealthCare Nutrition, Inc. The BE A. L. E. R.T. © Poster is a joint effort of the American Society for Parenteral and Enteral Nutrition (A.S.P.E.N.) and Nestlé HealthCare Nutrition, Inc. Retrieved from http://www.nutritioncare.org/WordArea/showcontent. aspx?id52968:AA.S.P.E.N. (2009). Special report: Enteral nutrition practice recommendations. *Journal of Parenteral and Enteral Nutrition.* Retrieved from http://www.nutritioncare.org/wcontent.aspx?id52078.

Clinical Insight 28-5 ➤ Checking Feeding Tube Placement

✚ Always use pH testing in combination with one of the other methods. Aspirate fluid, check the pH, and so on. Tube placement should be verified by x-ray before the initial feeding is given.

Aspirate and Inspect Stomach Contents

- Don procedure gloves. This is a clean, not sterile, technique.
- Just before feeding, draw up 10 to 30 mL of air in a 30- to 60-mL syringe, insert the syringe in the distal end of the feeding tube, and inject air.

To flush out formula, medications, and other substances. This also helps keep a small-bore tube from collapsing when you aspirate.

- With the same syringe, aspirate the air and 20 to 30 mL of stomach or intestinal contents. Use slow, gentle suction—over 3 to 5 minutes if necessary.

It can take a long time to obtain enough fluid, especially from a small-bore tube.

- If you could not aspirate any fluid, inject another 20 mL of air and use a smaller syringe to aspirate again.

Using a small (less than 10 mL) syringe for very small tubes creates less negative pressure and makes it less likely the tube will collapse.

- If you still do not aspirate fluid, repeat the procedure with this variation: Insert air with the large syringe; insert the small syringe into the end of the tubing, and leave it for 15 minutes before aspirating.

To allow fluid to accumulate before aspirating.

- If you are still unsuccessful, reposition the patient and try again after 20 minutes.

Repositioning may move the tube into a place where fluid has pooled.

- Inspect the aspirate. Gastric contents are normally greenish brown and liquid.

Intestinal contents are usually yellow-green because of the influence of bile.

- If the patient is receiving enteral feedings, gastric contents should be curdled and white or a greenish color; intestinal contents will be a more yellow (bile) color with no curdling.
- The colors of gastric and pulmonary secretions are altered by a variety of conditions, so this is not a very reliable method.

Measure the Volume and pH of the Aspirate

- Follow the preceding steps for aspirating stomach contents.
- Measure the residual volume of the aspirate.

Unexpected changes in volume of the aspirate can indicate poor GI motility. Gastric volumes will generally be larger than intestinal or esophageal volumes.

- Measure the pH of the aspirated fluid by using nitrazine paper. See the accompanying figure.

The lower the pH, the more likely that the tube is in the stomach. However, keep the following variables in mind:

- If the client is receiving medications to control stomach acidity (e.g., antacids, H_2 blockers, or proton pump inhibitors), the gastric pH may be as high as 6.
- Intestinal contents usually have a pH of 6 or greater.
- The pH of respiratory secretions is 7 or higher; however, respiratory secretions may occasionally have a pH as low as 6.
- If blood is present, either from epistaxis or from gastric bleeding, the pH of the gastric aspirate will not be helpful, because it will rise to resemble the pH of blood (7.35).
- pH testing is useful only if the fluid you aspirate is acidic, indicating gastric placement.

Because of the action of hydrochloric acid in the stomach, gastric contents measure a pH of 1 to 5.5. If the fluid is alkaline, it might be because the gastric contents are alkaline or because the tip of tube is in the small intestine or the lung. Because such situations occur frequently, even this method should be used in combination with other verification methods (Clarke, Birks, Nexo, et al. 2007; Guedon, 2000; May, 2007; Schmieding, Waldman, and Desaulles, 1997).

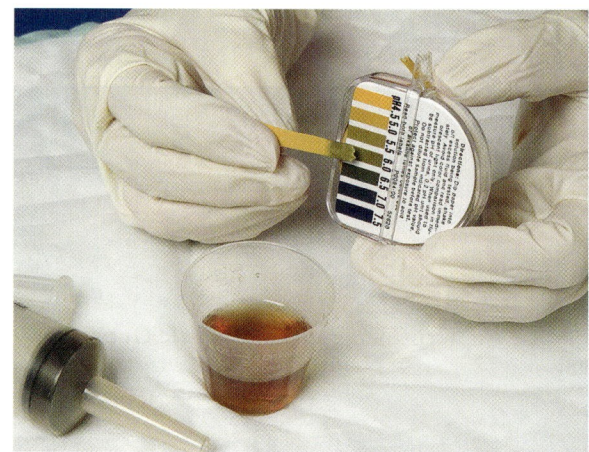

Measure and Observe the Length of the Tube That Extends From the Body

When the tube is inserted, it should be marked with indelible marker where it exits the body (e.g., the naris), and the external length recorded. Compare the external length with previous measurements and with the mark made on the tube when it was inserted. If tube placement does not change, the external length should remain the same.

If the tube is not well secured, it may migrate either up or down, so a consistent measurement of the external tube may help verify tube placement (Peter & Gill, 2009).

Inject Air into the Feeding Tube

Although some professionals still inject air into the feeding tube, this method is the least accurate of the bedside methods. Never rely on this method (or any other bedside method) alone.

Clinical Insight 28-5 ▶ Checking Feeding Tube Placement—cont'd

Because the lungs and stomach lie close together, the sounds created by sending air through the tube can easily be transmitted to nearby areas of the body, causing you to err in determining tube placement.

- Draw 5 to 30 mL of air into a syringe; place the tip of the syringe in the end of the feeding tube.
- Place a stethoscope over the stomach.
- Listen with stethoscope as you inject the air through the tube.

Air injected into the stomach produces a gurgling or whooshing sound in the left upper quadrant. If the tube is in the lungs, you will hear no gurgling.

Observe for respiratory distress.

✚ This method requires monitoring over time to be useful for confirming other methods.

Note cyanosis or difficulty breathing, coughing, or choking.

- The presence of these symptoms is a good indicator that the tube is in the respiratory tract; but keep in mind that the tube could instead be in the stomach and the symptoms caused by something else.
- Absence of symptoms does not necessarily indicate correct placement in the stomach.

The tube might be in the airway and not be causing any respiratory symptoms.

Assess whether the patient can speak

✚ This method requires monitoring over time to be useful for confirming other methods.

Keep in mind that some clients can speak even when the tube is in a lung.

Other bedside verification methods

Capnometry and additional tests of gastric juices may also serve as measures to verify the tube is correctly placed.

- **Capnometry** tests for carbon dioxide (CO_2). The presence of CO_2 with the placement of an NG or NE tube would indicate that the tube has been placed in the respiratory tract. This method is not yet in wide use, and is best used at the time the tube is placed. See the accompanying figure.

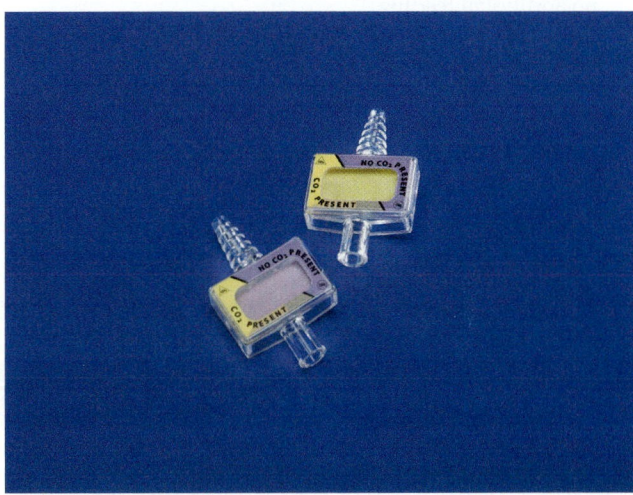

- Measuring bilirubin, trypsin, and pepsin in the aspirate provides a positive determination that the tube is placed in the stomach. Test devices for these three gastric components are not yet commercially available (Elpern, Killeen, Talla, et al., 2007; Peter & Gill, 2009).

BOX 28-7 ■ Types of Enteral Feeding Solutions

- **Basic feeding formulas** are used for clients who have no significant nutritional deficits but are unable to eat or drink sufficiently. They provide 1 kcal/mL of solution, and meet the needs of most clients. A standard formula contains 12%–20% of kcal from protein, 45%–60% of kcal from carbohydrates, and 30%–40% of kcal from fats. They also contain vitamins and minerals. They are usually lactose free and contain complex forms of carbohydrates, fats, and proteins. Therefore, they require digestion and absorption.
- **High-protein formulas** are for clients who have a substantial need for protein, such as those with burns, open wounds, or malnutrition.
- **Elemental formulas** do not contain complex proteins; instead, they contain amino acids or peptides. They are reserved for patients with severe small bowel absorptive dysfunction. These formulas are fiber free and highly osmotic. Their use is controversial.

- **Diabetic formulas** are for clients who require tube feedings to meet nutritional needs but have type 1 or type 2 diabetes mellitus. These formulas control carbohydrate intake.
- **Renal formulas** are for clients who require tube feedings to meet nutritional needs but have renal failure or renal insufficiency as a comorbidity. These formulas limit potassium, sodium, and nitrogen intake.
- **Pulmonary formulas** provide 55% of the calories as fat so that less CO_2 is produced per unit of oxygen consumed. They are used, for example, for patients with lung disease.
- **Fiber-containing formulas.** Because fiber has a potential protective effect for multiple disease states, including diverticulosis, colon cancer, diabetes, and heart disease, fiber-containing formulas may be used for patients in long-term care facilities or patients who require enteral feedings for a prolonged period of time.

participate in activities throughout the day but receives an infusion of enteral formula at night while at rest. Another variant is a 20-hour infusion, during which a 4-hour break allows time for the feeding pump to be disconnected for hygiene and other activities.

Intermittent feedings are given to supplement oral intake or for patients who want greater mobility to take part in activities, such as physical therapy. Feedings are given on a regular or periodic basis several times a day, usually over 30 to 60 minutes. An example of a prescription for a *regular feeding* is, "Give 250 to 500 mL of enteral nutrition every 4 to 6 hours." *Periodic feedings* are often based on oral intake and are considered to be more physiologically similar to normal eating patterns. Consider the following periodic feeding prescription:

If the client consumes 90% to 100% of the ordered diet, give no additional feeding.

> 75% but < 90%, give 100 mL of formula after each meal.

> 50% but < 75%, give 200 mL of formula after each meal.

> 25% but < 50%, give 300 mL of formula after each meal.

0% to 25% of the ordered diet, give 400 mL of formula.

Intermittent feedings are sometimes given by **bolus,** if the patient can tolerate this method. In this method, you use a syringe to deliver 300 to 400 mL of formula through the tube over a 5- to 10-minute period. This is the easiest method to teach family members for home care, and it frees the patient from mechanical devices that limit activity. But because the fluid is given more rapidly by this method, it increases the risk for respiratory aspiration and for stomach distention. You can use it only with gastric tubes, never with intestinal tubes.

Open and Closed Feeding Systems

An **open system** is exposed to the environment. One example is to open cans of formula and use a syringe to inject the formula into the tube; alternatively, you can pour it into a reservoir (e.g., a plastic bag). You should flush and clean the system after each delivery. Most agencies require that an open-system feeding not hang for more than 4 hours.

A **closed system** is a prefilled system (e.g., a bag or a bottle) that functions much like IV fluid. The nurse spikes the container with tubing that is attached to the feeding pump or run through a manually controlled drip chamber. Closed systems decrease the risk of contamination. A prefilled closed-system container can safely hang for 24 to 48 hours if you use sterile technique. You can measure out the specified amount in the drip chamber, allowing the remainder of the container to be used later in the day.

Monitoring Patients Receiving Enteral Nutrition

For patients receiving enteral nutrition, you will need to monitor tube placement, skin condition, laboratory values (especially blood glucose, BUN, and electrolytes), feeding residual, and gastrointestinal status (Clinical Insight 28-6). This will allow you to detect complications that affect metabolism or fluid and electrolyte balance and to assess responses to enteral feeding.

Clinical Insight 28-6 ▶ **Monitoring Patients Receiving Enteral Nutrition**

For patients receiving enteral nutrition, monitor the following:

- **Position of the feeding tube.** Periodically check the placement of the tube. As a rule, check on each shift or at each intermittent feeding. For double-lumen tubes, keep the air vent above the level of the patient's stomach so it will not act as a siphon and leak stomach contents.
- **NG or NE tube insertion site.** An NG or NE tube is secured by adhesive to the nose. Regularly check the skin, gently cleanse the area (with soap and water, as for normal washing; avoid harsh skin cleansers), and retape the tube as needed. Report tissue breakdown, epistaxis (nosebleed), or sinusitis.

These findings may signal a need for insertion of a percutaneous endoscopy gastrostomy (PEG) tube.

- **Gastrostomy tube, PEG/PEJ insertion site.** Inspect the insertion site for erythema or drainage, which are signs of infection. Clean it daily with soap and water.
- **Fluid balance.** Measure all intake and output.
- **Weight.** To assess the adequacy of the feeding, regularly weigh patients receiving enteral nutrition. There is usually a medical prescription for frequency of weighing. Frequent weight checks allow adjustment of the feeding orders to achieve the desired goal.
- **Tube feeding residual volume.** To assess residual volume, aspirate the feeding tube to determine the amount of feeding remaining in the stomach.

If you are able to aspirate a quantity equal to or greater than the formula flow rate for 1 hour (or alternatively, a total of 150 mL), the patient may be receiving too much fluid or may have delayed gastric emptying. However, you should not automatically stop the feeding; if you obtain a single sample of an increased residual volume, recheck it in 1 hour. See Clinical Insight 28-5.

- **Frequency of bowel movements.** Bowel movements should occur regularly.
  - Constipation is usually due to inadequate water or fiber. Some commercial feedings contain fiber. To alleviate constipation, you may add free water and perhaps fiber to the formula.
  - Diarrhea may indicate intolerance of the formula, excessive feeding, or gastrointestinal disease.
- **Bowel sounds.** Check before each feeding, or every 4 to 8 hours for continuous feedings. Peristalsis must be present.
- **Abdominal distention.** Measure abdominal girth daily, at the umbilicus.
- **Serum electrolyte levels.** Monitor regularly (per protocol or prescription).
- **Urine for sugar and acetone.** This is sometimes done as a bedside screen for hyperglycemia. However, treatment is based on blood sugar levels.
- **Skin turgor, hematocrit, and urine specific gravity.**

These are indicators of dehydration and overhydration. Dehydration may occur, for example, if the patient is not consuming enough water, dehydration may occur.

- **Serum blood urea nitrogen (BUN) and sodium levels.** This is especially important for high-protein formulas.

Insufficient fluid intake combined with high protein intake may overload the kidneys so that nitrogenous wastes are not excreted adequately.

Feedings may need to be increased or decreased depending on the patient's changing clinical condition.

 Enteral feeding solutions provide an ideal medium for bacterial growth. Contamination of the feeding can have serious consequences for a patient. To prevent infection in patients receiving enteral feedings, be sure to:

- Check dates on feeding solutions and supplies. Do not use any that are outdated.
- Use sterile equipment and supplies; once you have opened them, handle them as little as possible.
- Disposable feeding equipment is meant for one-time use. Do not wash and reuse.
- Use meticulous hand hygiene; wear nonsterile gloves.
- Replace feeding equipment after 24 hours.
- Store opened feeding solutions in the refrigerator in covered and labeled containers. Allow the solution to return to room temperature before giving it to the patient. Discard after 24 hours. Keep unopened solutions at room temperature.
- Follow agency policy regarding how long a solution may be left hanging. Usually sterile feedings may be hung for up to 24 hours (or unit policy).
- Nonsterile feedings (i.e., reconstituted powder feedings) may hang for up to 4 hours (or unit policy).
- Label the feeding containers with the patient's name and the date and time hung; document the time in the patient record.
- Use sterile water for (1) patients who are immunocompromised, (2) patients receiving jejunal feeds, or (3) initially following a gastrostomy insertion.
- Never allow a feeding to hang below the height of the patient's stomach.
- Do not transfer sterile feedings into a second container.
- Replace the feeding tubes according to the manufacturer's recommendations, or agency policy if that is sooner (Nunwa, 2005).

Removing Feeding Tubes

When a patient's condition has stabilized and she no longer requires enteral nutrition, the feeding tube may be removed. A PEG tube is usually clamped if feedings are no longer required. For a complete set of steps to follow when removing feeding tubes, see Procedure 28-4.

ThinkLike a Nurse 28-8

Your client has dementia and is frequently agitated. She has been progressively losing weight. An interdisciplinary team recommended enteral nutrition due to poor oral intake; however, the client has repeatedly pulled out her NG tube and had an episode of aspiration pneumonia last month. What recommendations might you consider at the next meeting?

Providing Parenteral Nutrition

Parenteral nutrition (PN) is the delivery of nutrition intravenously into a large, central vein. This is the preferred method of feeding for clients who cannot be nourished through the gastrointestinal tract. Some clients (e.g., those with shortened small bowel secondary to injury or disease) who are able to meet some of their nutritional needs may use PN in addition to some oral intake to meet caloric and nutrient needs. Others, such as clients who are severely malnourished, have extensive burns or trauma, or have conditions that require resting the gastrointestinal system, are nourished entirely by PN.

Parenteral Nutrition Solutions. **PN solutions** usually contain a 10% to 70% concentration of dextrose in water (but usually not more than 20%) along with amino acids, and can provide 20 to 30 kcal per kilogram per day, depending on the patient's calculated energy need. Note though that the most common concentrations of glucose provide only 200 kcal per liter. PN also contains vitamins, minerals, and trace elements. Standard PN formulas are available at many healthcare facilities; however, PN can be modified to meet individual needs.

The type of venous access device used to administer PN will depend on the components of the PN and the anticipated duration of PN. Because PN solutions are hypertonic, they should be administered in a large, high-flow vein through a central venous access catheter. The subclavian vein has been the site of choice; however, the jugular vein is preferred for tunneled catheters and implanted ports. Peripherally inserted central catheter (PICC) lines are also used for PN. Whatever the insertion site, all PN catheters must have chest x-ray confirmation that the tip is in the lower portion of the superior vena cava adjacent to the right atrium (see Fig. 28-7) before beginning the first infusion. High blood flow through that vessel causes rapid dilution of the concentrated PN and thereby prevents vessel damage. Some types of PN solutions may be infused via a peripheral vein, but this is not usual.

Lipid Emulsions **Lipid emulsions** contain essential fatty acids, triglycerides, and supplemental kcal. They are administered weekly for patients who rely on PN to prevent essential fatty acid deficiency. They also add calories to the PN mixture so that lower glucose concentrations can be used, thus reducing the risk of glucose fluctuations. Most IV fats are supplied by safflower or soybean oil. They provide 1.1 to 3 kcal/mL.

You may administer lipids at the same time as the PN, through a peripheral line or by Y-connector tubing through a central line. Lipids are also sometimes added to the PN solution (this is called a 3-in-1 admixture), and administered over a 24-hour period. To learn these skills, see Procedures 28-5 and 28-6.

To learn about monitoring and maintenance of patients receiving parenteral nutrition, see Clinical Insight 28-7.

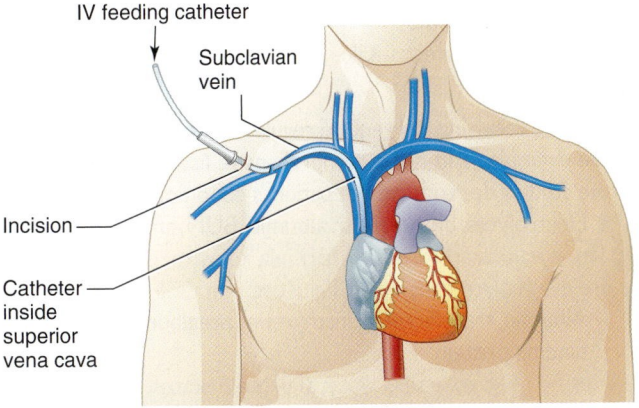

FIGURE 28-7 The subclavian vein is the site of choice for parenteral nutrition.

Clinical Insight 28-7 ➤ Monitoring and Maintenance for Patients Receiving Parenteral Nutrition

Monitoring

For patients receiving PN, you will need to monitor the following:

Catheter insertion site

- Assess catheter insertion site for swelling, redness, drainage, or tenderness.

Signs of infection (and/or phlebitis in PICC lines). The hypertonic PN creates a risk for phlebitis.

- Observe for swelling in the extremity on the same side of catheter insertion.

This is a sign of infiltration or phlebitis.

- Observe for catheter retraction from the vein; observe the length of the catheter from the insertion site to the hub at insertion and periodically.

Supplies and equipment

- Monitor tubing connections to see that they are secure.
- Monitor to see that the dressing is secure and dry.
- Check the rate and amount infused at least hourly.

To ensure the line is patent, the PN is flowing freely, and the pump is functioning properly.

Weight

Regularly weigh the patient (according to medical order or agency policy, but commonly daily or 3 times per wk).
(1) Frequent weight checks allow for assessing the adequacy of the formula and making adjustments as needed to achieve the desired goal. (2) Because of the hypertonicity of the solutions, fluid overload can occur. Rapid weight increase is an indicator.

Glucose

Check blood glucose every 4 to 6 hours until stable, and then at least daily.
The high proportion of glucose in the formulas can cause hyperglycemia, the most common complication of PN. You may need to administer regular insulin according to a sliding scale (or the pharmacist may add it directly to the PN solution). The risk for hyperglycemia is less with 3:1 PN solutions.

Diuresis and dehydration

These can occur if hypertonic dextrose is infused too rapidly.

Intake and output.

To evaluate nutrient intake, fluid balance, and renal function.

Lab values

Patients receiving PN require regular lab studies (the following are examples and not a comprehensive list). The frequency of the studies depends on the patient's condition.

- Electrolytes, blood sugar, albumin, BUN, and creatinine

These values are used for formula adjustment and to evaluate electrolyte balance and glucose metabolism.

- Albumin, transferrin, transthyretin (prealbumin), or retinol-binding protein

May be used to assess visceral protein status.

- 24-hour urine for urine urea nitrogen (weekly)

To assess for nitrogen balance.

- CBC and differential.

To monitor changes in immune function.

- Liver function studies
- Serum zinc
- Plasma urea
- Plasma and urine osmolality
- Blood gases

Symptoms of complications:

- *Electrolyte imbalances:* Symptoms depend on the electrolytes affected. Monitor lab values.
- *Sepsis:* Temperature greater than 100°F (37.8°C) orally, rapid pulse from baseline, chills, hypothermia, edema or erythema of skin, exudate from catheter insertion site, malaise, leukocytosis (increased WBC count), altered level of consciousness.
- *Air embolus:* Cyanosis, tachypnea, hypotension, heart murmur
- *Catheter dislodgement or thrombosis:* Swelling of arm or neck, pain, difficulty flushing catheter, difficulty infusing PN

Nutritional status

- Calculate the daily calorie intake.
- Perform nutritional assessment at 2-week intervals.
- Possibly measure arm circumference and triceps skinfold thickness.
- Most agencies have specialized nutrition teams who will monitor these parameters.

Maintenance

- Change the dressing over the catheter every 24 hours or according to agency policy, or when it becomes wet, soiled, or nonocclusive. Use sterile technique.
- Secure connections with luer-lock connectors; do not use tape.
- Change the filter every 24 hours.
- Do not hang PN bottles for more than 12 hours (some guidelines and agency policies specify 24 hr).

PN solutions are prepared in batches under strict aseptic conditions. Its high nutrient concentration makes PN an excellent feeding alternative; however, it also makes the solution ideal for bacterial growth.

- Use sterile aseptic technique when changing the dressing for a central line, as well as when changing the solution and tubing.
- Do not use the PN infusion line for administering any other medicines or solutions.

To decrease the risk of contamination and infection.

- Infuse PN by pump with a reliable, audible alarm.

To protect against "free flow."

- If an infusion falls behind schedule, do not increase the rate in an attempt to catch up.

This can cause osmotic diuresis and dehydration.

- When PN is discontinued, it may be done gradually (perhaps over as many as 48 hr).

To prevent a sudden drop in blood sugar.

Toward Evidence-Based Practice

Scarmeas, N., Luchsinger, J., Mayeux, R., et al. (2007). **Mediterranean diet and Alzheimer disease mortality.** *Neurology, 69,* 1084–1093.

A Mediterranean diet (MeDi) consists of an average nine servings of fruits and vegetables daily, whole grains, fish once or twice a week, and up to 5 ounces of red wine daily. It limits red meat and avoids *trans*-fats and saturated fats, using instead olive oil for its antioxidant effect and canola oil and nuts to provide omega-3 fatty acids.

Researchers followed 192 community-based individuals diagnosed with Alzheimer's disease (AD) for 4.4 years. 85 of the AD patients died during that period. Researchers concluded that adherence to the MeDi may reduce not only risk for AD but also subsequent disease course: Higher adherence to the MeDi is associated with lower mortality in AD.

Barberger-Gateau, P., Raffaitin, C., Letenneur, L., et al. (2007). **Dietary patterns and risk of dementia.** *Neurology, 69,* 191–193.

This study included 8,085 nondemented participants ages 65 and older in three cities in France. An independent committee validated 281 cases of dementia (including 183 AD). Daily consumption of fruits and vegetables was associated with a decreased risk of all-cause dementia; weekly consumption of fish was associated with a reduced risk of AD, but only among people carrying a high-risk AD gene; regular use of omega-3–rich oils was associated with a decreased risk for all-cause dementia. Researchers concluded that frequent consumption of fruits and vegetables, fish, and omega-3 rich oils may decrease the risk of dementia and AD, especially among those who do not carry the high-risk AD gene.

Vogiatzoglou, A., Refsum, H., Johnston, C., et al. (2008). **Vitamin B$_{12}$ status and rate of brain volume loss in community-dwelling elderly.** *Neurology, 71*(11), 826–832.

This was a 5-year study of 107 community-dwelling elders aged 61 to 87 years with no cognitive impairment at the beginning of the study. They were assessed yearly by magnetic resonance imaging (MRI) scans, cognitive tests, and blood studies. The decrease in brain volume over the 5-year period was greater for those with lower vitamin B$_{12}$ levels. Researchers concluded that low vitamin B$_{12}$ status should be further researched as a cause of brain atrophy and likely cognitive impairment in the elderly.

1. Suppose you are a manager in a long-term care facility that specializes in treating residents with AD. You are planning nutritional interventions for these residents. Which of these three studies is best suited to your patients, and why?

2. How was the cognitive status of the subjects different in all three studies?

3. Based on the third study, for which group would vitamin B$_{12}$ supplementation be most likely to be of benefit? Explain your thinking.
   a. People who have AD and want to extend their life expectancy
   b. Older adults who wish to prevent getting AD
   c. Older adults who want to avoid cognitive impairment from brain changes other than AD.

CLINICALREASONING:
Applying the Full-Spectrum Nursing Model

Because the following critical thinking activities allow you to practice the kind of thinking you will use as a full-spectrum nurse, they usually have no single right answer. Discuss them with your peers—if you have difficulty with any of the questions, consult your instructor.

PATIENT SITUATION

Mrs. Ong is a 75-year-old retired schoolteacher who suffered a stroke 8 months ago. Since leaving the hospital, she has been living in a nursing home. Mrs. Ong has residual weakness on the right side—her dominant side—and has not mastered the use of tableware with her left hand. On admission to the nursing home 7 months ago, she weighed 150 pounds. Today she weighs only 125 pounds. Mrs. Ong refuses to go to the dining room for meals. The NAPs report that she eats a few bites of most foods, but never eats more than half of anything.

THINKING

1. *Theoretical Knowledge*:
   a. Based on Mrs. Ong's gender, age, and activity level, make a rough estimate of the number of kcal/day she needs.
   b. What are two other, more precise, ways you could determine Mrs. Ong's ideal body weight?

2. *Critical Thinking (Considering Alternatives):* What are some possible explanations for why Mrs. Ong is not eating all her food?

DOING

3. *Practical Knowledge:*
   a. Suppose you have decided to use the general ideal weight guide to determine Mrs. Ong's ideal weight. What, specifically, would you need to do? You do not need to actually calculate; just list the action steps.
   b. Suppose you have decided to determine Mrs. Ong's body mass index (BMI). What equipment would you need?
   c. What is the formula for calculating BMI from the height and weight?
4. *Nursing Process (Diagnosis):* Write a nursing diagnosis for Mrs. Ong. Use just the data provided in the situation. Assume her BMI is 20.

CARING

5. *Self-Knowledge:* What would you be feeling if you were in Mrs. Ong's situation?
6. *Ethical Knowledge:* What are one or two things you would do to help Mrs. Ong feel cared for and cared about?

 Go To Chapter 28, **Clinical Reasoning: Applying the Full-Spectrum Nursing Model Response Sheet,** on DavisPlus.

PracticalKnowledge
procedures

To apply concepts that support patient nutrition, you will need to master techniques for assessing nutritional status, feeding patients, administering supplemental feedings, and working with nasogastric and nasoenteric tubes.

Procedure 28–1 ■ Checking Fingerstick (Capillary) Blood Glucose Levels

➤ For steps to follow in *all* procedures, refer to the Universal Steps for All Procedures found on the page facing the inside back cover.

Equipment

- Blood glucose meter
- Test strip
- Sterile lancet (and injector, if available)
- Alcohol (or other antiseptic) pad, if required by policy
- 2 in. × 2 in. gauze pad or cotton ball
- Procedure gloves

✚ Glucometers should be assigned to individual patients. If this is not possible, you must clean and disinfect the device between patients. Injectors, too, should be assigned to individual patients; if possible, use single-use lancets that permanently retract upon puncture. Keep trays or carts with these supplies outside patient rooms. Do not carry supplies in your pocket. If there are unused supplies after the procedure, leave them in the room; do not use them for another patient.
These measures help prevent needlestick injury and transmission of bloodborne pathogens (CDC, 2005).

Delegation

You can delegate this procedure to a licensed practical nurse (LPN) or nursing assistive personnel (NAP) who have been adequately trained in performing the skill if the patient's condition allows. Assess the patient first; if the patient's condition is critical, do not delegate the procedure. Most patients perform this procedure independently at home.

Pre-Procedure Assessments

- Assess the patient's comprehension of the procedure.
  Understanding reduces anxiety and promotes cooperation.
- Assess potential puncture sites for bruising, inflammation, open lesions, poor circulation, or edema.
  Avoid such sites because of risk for infection and inaccurate results.
- Check for factors such as anticoagulant therapy, bleeding disorders, or low platelet count.
  These place the patient at risk for bleeding after skin puncture.

➤ When performing the procedure, always identify your patient according to agency policy and be attentive to standard precautions, hand hygiene, patient safety and privacy, body mechanics, and documentation.

➤ *Note:* The steps of this procedure will vary, depending on the type of glucose meter used.

Procedure Steps

1. **Verify the medical prescription** for frequency and timing of testing.
   A prescription is necessary for testing. Timing and frequency of testing are crucial for accurate insulin dosing.

2. **Ask the patient to wash her hands** with soap and warm water, if able, and to dry completely using a clean towel.
   Reduces the risk for infection and dilates capillaries at the puncture site. Also ensures that the testing site is free of any sugar residue.

3. **Turn on the blood glucose meter.** Calibrate it according to the manufacturer's instructions.
   Calibration readies the meter for testing and checks it for accuracy of the machine.

4. **Check that the strip is the correct type** for the monitor. Check the expiration date on the container of reagent strips. If the strips are expired, replace them.
   Expired strips may alter test results. Different brands of monitors use different kinds of reagent strips.

5. **Don procedure gloves.**
   Gloving protects against exposure to blood.

6. **Remove the reagent strip** from the container and place it into the blood glucose meter. Then tightly seal the container.
   A tight seal protects reagent strips from exposure to air and light.

7. **Select and clean a fingerstick site** with an alcohol (or other antiseptic) pad, according to facility policy. Let it dry thoroughly.
   Helps protect the patient from infection by removing some surface microorganisms. Allowing the alcohol to dry thoroughly will decrease pain of the skin puncture. Using alcohol is controversial, however, because it may interfere with the reagent on the strip, giving a false low reading; it also dries the skin. Follow agency policy and consult practice guidelines periodically.

8. **Use a different site each time** you check the glucose.
   Adult and child: the lateral aspect of a finger (palmar surface, distal phalanx)
   Infant: heel or great toe
   The lateral aspect of the finger contains fewer nerve endings than does the central fingertip, so it hurts less. Capillaries in infants are too small to obtain an adequate blood sample.

9. **Position the finger** (or heel or great toe for an infant) in a dependent position, and massage from the base toward the tip of the finger.
   A dependent position promotes blood flow to the site via gravity and pressure, ensuring an adequate specimen. The massaging action increases blood flow to the tip of the finger, which may prevent the need for repuncture.

10. **Prick the finger** (or other site) with the lancet:

Exposed-Blade Disposable Lancet

   a. Remove the cover from the lancet, if there is a cover.
   b. Place the back of the patient's hand on the table, or otherwise secure the finger (e.g., hold the finger and hand firmly).
   c. Use a darting motion to puncture the site, at a 90° angle to the skin.

Semiautomatic Injector

   d. Engage the sterile injector and remove the cover.
   e. Place the disposable lancet firmly in the end of the injector.
   f. Place the back of the patient's hand on the table, or otherwise secure the finger (e.g., hold the finger and hand firmly).
   g. Position the end of the injector firmly against the skin, perpendicular (at a 90° angle) to the chosen puncture site.
   h. Push the release switch, allowing the needle to pierce the skin.
   Proper positioning and stabilization of the site ensure that the lancet pierces to the correct depth. This prevents patient injury and allows for adequate blood sampling. Patients

tend to pull away as you perform the puncture. ▼

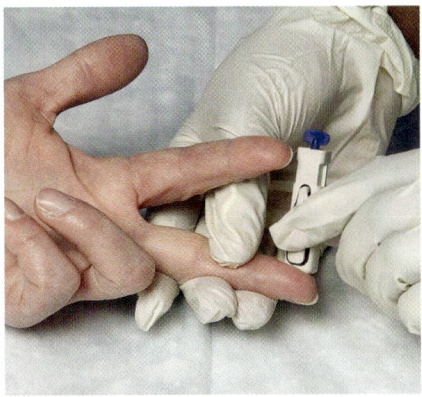

11. **Lightly squeeze the patient's finger** above the puncture site until a drop of blood has collected.
    Squeezing promotes a better blood sample for testing without causing injury to the puncture site.

12. **Wipe away the first drop** with clean gauze and squeeze again to form another droplet.
    The first drop of blood contains more serous fluid and can alter test results.

13. **Place the reagent strip** test patch close to the drop of blood. Allow contact between the drop of blood and the test strip. Do not "smear" the blood over the reagent strip.
    This ensures adequate blood sample for testing. ▼

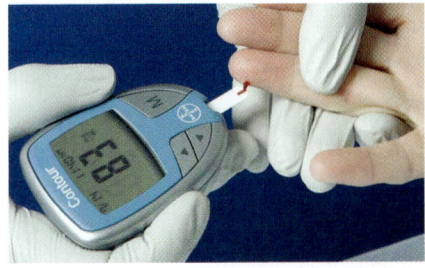

14. **Insert the strip into the meter,** if it is not already inserted (follow the manufacturer's instructions); allow the blood sample to remain in contact with the test strip for the amount of time specified by the manufacturer.
    For some meters you insert the test strip before pricking the finger; with others you put the blood on the reagent strip and then insert the strip

(continued on next page)

Procedure 28–1 ■ Checking Fingerstick (Capillary) Blood Glucose Levels (continued)

into the meter. The blood sample must be on the reagent strip for the specified amount of time to ensure accurate test results.

15. **Using a gauze pad,** gently apply pressure to the puncture site.
    Pressure stops the bleeding by promoting coagulation.

16. **After the meter signals, read** the blood glucose level indicated on the digital display.** ▼

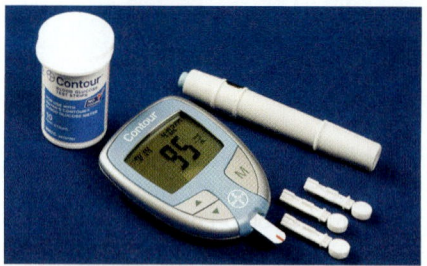

17. Turn off the meter, and dispose of the reagent strip, gauze pad, alcohol pad, and lancet in the proper containers (e.g., a sharps container for the lancet).
    Proper disposal prevents sharps injury and the spread of infection via bloodborne pathogens.

18. **Remove the procedure gloves,** and dispose of them in the proper container. Perform hand hygiene.
    Hand hygiene and gloving reduce the transmission of microbes.

? What if . . .

■ **The patient has poor circulation or is a child or older adult?**

Place a heel warmer or warm cloth on the site for about 10 minutes before obtaining the blood sample. Alternatively, position the patient's hand below the waist for 1 minute.
Capillaries in infants are very small; older adults may have poor peripheral circulation. The warmth may dilate the capillaries, helping you obtain an adequate amount of blood; the dangling of extremities allows blood to pool in the extremity, making it easier for you to obtain the quantity of blood needed.

■ **The patient is taking an anticoagulant such as warfarin sodium (Coumadin)?**

After the procedure, hold pressure for 2 minutes and then apply a pressure bandage if needed. Recheck the site after 5 minutes to make sure bleeding has stopped.

■ **The monitor shows an extremely unusual result or an error message?**

Repeat the process using a different finger or site.

■ **The patient uses a noninvasive method to measure blood glucose?**

A new tool called a continuous blood glucose monitor is now available. It is worn like a wristwatch. Using an electrical current, it pulls fluid from the skin to give a blood glucose reading. It will take readings automatically every 20 minutes for up to 12 hours. Advise the patient to shave his arm if it is very hairy, or the reading may not be accurate. The patient should wear the device for a 3-hour warm-up before taking a reading, and should not bathe or swim during that time.
This does not replace the patient's fingerstick method. Its purpose is to track trends in blood glucose.

Evaluation

- Assess the puncture site for bleeding or bruising.
- Evaluate the patient's understanding of the procedure and the test results.
- Promptly notify the physician of abnormal test results, or administer insulin based on test results, if prescribed.

Patient Teaching

- Explain the procedure, test results, and treatment to the patient.
  Informing the patient allows the patient to participate in his plan of care, and typically increases adherence to the therapeutic regimen.
- If the patient will be performing fingerstick blood glucose testing at home, teach the patient how to perform the procedure. Ask the patient to perform a return demonstration.
- Discuss the importance of maintaining glycemic control.
- Teach the patient to do the following:
  - Read the manufacturer's instructions carefully and call their toll-free number if he has any questions.
  - Always use the test strips that are recommended for the meter.
  - Take your meter to your health provider's office so she can make sure you are measuring your blood sugar correctly.
  - Perform quality control checks (read the instructions) to make sure the meter is measuring accurately.
  - Clean the meter according to the manufacturer's directions. Some meters will give you an electronic alert telling you when to clean them.

Home Care

- Assess the client's ability to perform fingerstick blood glucose monitoring independently.
  A change in the patient's condition may not allow the patient to perform testing. Certain conditions, such as arthritis and limited vision, may limit dexterity.
- Advise the patient about purchasing home glucose monitoring equipment.
- Explain how to dispose of lancets in a labeled, punctureproof container, such as an empty bleach container.
- Instruct caregivers to wear gloves when obtaining a blood sample for glucose monitoring.
- At home, patients do not need to cleanse their fingers with an alcohol wipe before puncturing it. However, they should wash their hands with soap and water and dry well.

Documentation

- Record the fingerstick blood glucose result in the progress notes or special flowsheet, including the date and time the test was performed.
- Note whether the physician was notified and record any treatment given.
- Document patient teaching.
- If the fingerstick is performed in response to patient symptoms, you may need to write a narrative note.

Practice Resources

American Diabetes Association, n.d., 2011; Centers for Disease Control and Prevention, 2005; GlaxoSmithKline, last updated 2008; Glucose monitoring, 2008; U.S. Food and Drug Administration, 2011.

Thinking About the Procedure

 Go to the *Fundamentals of Nursing Skills Videos*, **Nutrition: Blood Glucose Testing (Fingerstick).**

1. When did the nurse don procedure gloves?
2. What is the latest point in the procedure at which the nurse could have donned her gloves?

 For suggested responses, go to Chapter 28, **Thinking About the Procedure Suggested Responses,** on *DavisPlus.*

Procedure 28–2 ■ Inserting Nasogastric and Nasoenteric Tubes

> ➤ For steps to follow in *all* procedures, refer to the Universal Steps for All Procedures found on the page facing the inside back cover.

To watch an animated demonstration of inserting a nasogastric tube,

 Go to **Animations: Inserting a Nasogastric Tube,** on *DavisPlus.*

Equipment

- Nasogastric tube (commonly 16 or 18 Fr for adults, but sometimes smaller) or nasoenteric (small bowel) tube (8 Fr, 10 Fr, or 12 Fr)
- Stylet or guidewire (for small-bore tubes), according to agency policy
- Procedure gloves
- Linen-saver pad or towel
- Water-soluble lubricant
- 50- to 60-mL catheter-tip syringe or bulb syringe for Salem sump tubes; 30-mL luer-lock syringe for small-bore feeding tubes
- Hypoallergenic tape (about 2.5 cm [1 in.] wide) or tube fixation device
- Indelible marker
- Skin adhesive
- Stethoscope
- Emesis basin
- Basin with warm water (for plastic tube) or ice (for rubber tube). Most tubes are plastic.
- Glass of water with a straw
- Penlight
- Tongue blade
- pH test strip
- Tissues
- Safety pin
- Gauze square or small plastic bag
- Rubber band
- Suction equipment (if tube is being connected to suction)

Delegation

This procedure should not be delegated because it requires knowledge of anatomy and physiology and the ability to adapt the procedure based on patient responses. You can, however, delegate associated oral hygiene needs.

Pre-Procedure Assessment

- Verify the medical prescription for type of tube to be placed and whether it is to be attached to suction or drainage.
- Verify the patient's need for NG or NE intubation (e.g., surgery involving the gastrointestinal [GI] tract, impaired swallowing, or decreased level of consciousness).
  NG or NE intubation decreases the risk for aspiration in these patients. In many institutions, only specially trained nurses are allowed to place small bowel feeding tubes.
- Assess each naris for patency, deviated septum, and skin breakdown. Ask the patient to close each nostril alternately and breathe. Select the nostril with the greatest air flow. Ask the patient to blow her nose, if not contraindicated.
  A septal defect or facial fracture may cause obstruction, placing the patient at risk for nasal membrane trauma if insertion is attempted through the affected naris.
- Check medical history for anticoagulant therapy, coagulopathy, nasal trauma, nasal surgery, epistaxis, or deviated septum.
  Patient history may place the patient at risk for injury during NG or NE insertion. Contraindications to NG insertion by a nurse include maxillofacial disorders, surgery, or trauma; esophageal tumors or surgery; laryngectomy; skull fracture; unstable high cervical spinal injuries; and esophageal varices (although these patients may have tubes placed by a medical professional via endoscope or fluoroscope).
- Assess the level of consciousness and ability to follow instructions.
- Assess for a gag reflex, using a tongue blade.
  Absence of gag reflex places the patient at risk for aspiration.

(continued on next page)

Procedure 28–2 ■ Inserting Nasogastric and Nasoenteric Tubes (continued)

➤ When performing the procedure, always identify your patient according to agency policy and be attentive to standard precautions, hand hygiene, patient safety and privacy, body mechanics, and documentation.

Procedure Steps

1. Prepare the tube.

Plastic Tube

Wrap the tube around your index finger and then unwrap it and proceed or place in a basin of warm water for 10 minutes and proceed.

Rubber Tube

Place in a basin of ice for 10 minutes.

Small-Bore Tube

Insert a stylet or guide-wire and secure into position, according to agency policy. (Small-bore tubes may come with the guidewire in them. If so, flush the tube with tap water to lubricate the wire for easy removal. Leave the wire in place until the tube is positioned and its placement has been checked on x-ray film. Once the guidewire is removed, do not reinsert it.) Agency policy determines which nurses are authorized to place small-bore tubes.

Warm water softens a plastic tube, and ice stiffens the rubber tube to make it easier to insert. (Most tubes are polyurethane or silicone-based.) Wrapping a plastic tube around your index finger helps the tube flex into a curve and aids in insertion. A guidewire facilitates passage of small-bore tube but can cause trauma if not secured in a proper position.

2. Assist the patient into a high-Fowler's position with pillow behind the head and shoulders. Raise the bed to a comfortable working level.
This position facilitates tube insertion and prevents aspiration should the patient vomit during tube insertion. Gravity facilitates passage of the tube. Raising the bed reduces strain on the nurse's back.

3. Measure the tube for placement.

Nasogastric Tube

Measure the length of the tube to be inserted by measuring from the tip of the nose to the earlobe, and from the earlobe to the xiphoid process. Mark the length with tape or indelible ink.

This measurement indicates the distance the tube must be inserted to reach the stomach.▼

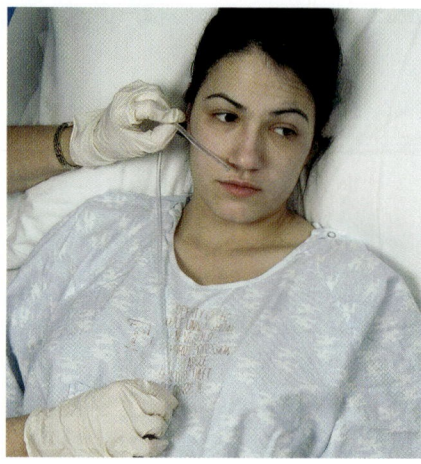

Nasoenteric Tube

Add 8 to 10 cm (3 to 4 in.) to the NG tube measurement, as directed, and mark the tube.

4. Stand on the patient's right side if you are right-handed and on the left side if left-handed. Drape a linen saver pad over the patient's chest, and hand her an emesis basin and facial tissues.
Draping protects the patient's gown from becoming soiled during tube insertion.

5. Prepare the fixation device. Cut a 10-cm (4-in.) piece of hypoallergenic tape if securing tube with tape; split the bottom end lengthwise 2.5 cm (2 in.). If using a commercial feeding tube attachment device, have it ready at this time.
To secure the tube after insertion.

6. Arrange a signal by which the patient can communicate if she wants to stop (e.g., raising her hand).
Relieves anxiety by giving the patient some control over the procedure.

7. Don procedure gloves if you have not already done so.
Reduces the spread of microorganisms.

8. Wrap 10 to 15 cm (5 to 6 in.) of the end of the tube tightly around your index finger, then release.
Forms the tube into a curve that helps it conform more easily to the shape of the nasopharynx.

9. Lubricate the distal 10 cm (4 in.) of the tube with a water-soluble jelly.
Lubrication eases the passage of the tube and prevents injury to the nasal mucosa. Water-soluble lubricant will dissolve if it is aspirated, whereas oil-based lubricants do not dissolve in the respiratory tract and would cause inflammation and blockage of airways if they enter the lungs. Some nurses prefer water as a lubricant because aqueous jelly dries and can block nasal passages, which is irritating to the patient. Some tubes have a surface lubricant and require only that you dip them in room-temperature water.

10. If the patient is awake, alert, and able to swallow, hand her a glass of water with a straw.
Instructing the client to swallow water during insertion eases passage.

11. Instruct the patient to hold her head straight up and extend her neck back against the pillow (slightly hyperextended).

a. Grasp the end of the tube above the lubricant with the curved end pointing downward.

b. Carefully insert the tube along the floor of the nasal passage, on the lateral side, aiming toward the ear.

c. You will feel slight resistance when the tube reaches the nasopharynx; use gentle pressure, but do not force the tube to advance. The patient's eyes may tear; if so, provide tissues.

d. Continue insertion of the tube until just past the nasopharynx by gently rotating the tube toward the client's opposite naris.
Hyperextending the neck straightens the curve where the nasal passage meets the pharynx (nasopharyngeal junction). Gentle insertion prevents trauma to the nasal mucosa. Forcing

against resistance can traumatize the mucosa. Tears are normal. ▼

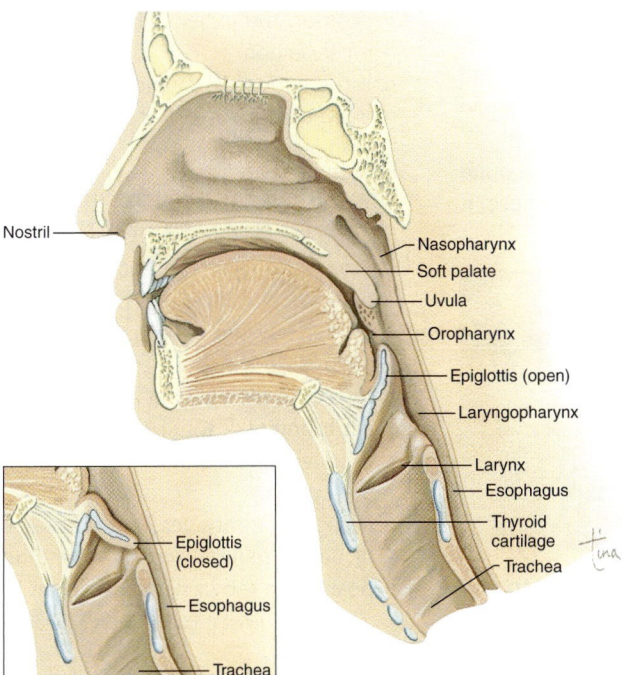

Nostril —
Nasopharynx
Soft palate
Uvula
Oropharynx
Epiglottis (open)
Laryngopharynx
Larynx
Esophagus
Thyroid cartilage
Trachea

Epiglottis (closed)
Esophagus
Trachea

12. **Pause for a moment** to allow the patient to relax, and perhaps use tissues. Explain that the next step requires her to swallow.
   Stopping to relax can give the patient a feeling of control. Also, the rest can reduce gagging.

13. **Instruct the patient to flex** her head toward the chest, take a small sip of water, and swallow.
   This maneuver closes the trachea and opens the esophagus. ▼

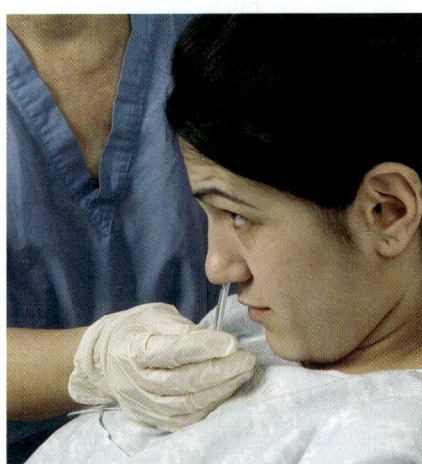

14. **Rotate the tube 180°.**
   Rotation helps to redirect the tube so that it will not enter the patient's mouth.

15. **Direct the patient to sip** and swallow the water as you slowly advance the tube. (If the patient is not allowed water, instruct her to dry swallow or suck air through the straw.) Advance the tube 5 to 10 cm (2 to 4 in.) with each swallow.
   Moving the tube with each swallow uses normal peristaltic movement to help advance the tube into the stomach. Swallowing closes the epiglottis so that the tube cannot advance into the trachea.

16. **Continue advancing the tube** to the desired distance.

17. ✚ **Temporarily secure the tube** with one piece of tape. Then verify tube placement (see Clinical Insight 28-5). Never rely on a single bedside method. You can use a combination of the following methods to verify placement at the bedside; however, radiographic verification is the only reliable method and should be done before medications or fluids are given through the tube for the first time (Rauen, Chulay, Bridges, et al., 2008).

   If you do not secure the tube, at least temporarily, it may move out of position—especially if you are waiting

for placement to be confirmed by x-ray film.

a. Inspect the posterior pharynx for presence of coiled tube.
   Visualization confirms that the tube has gone beyond the oropharynx.

b. Aspirate gently to withdraw stomach contents and measure aspirate pH. Aspirate gently over a period of up to 5 minutes, if necessary, to obtain gastric fluid.
   The pH of stomach contents is normally 1 to 5.5; however, many situations commonly alter the pH of gastric contents, so the usefulness of this method is limited. pH testing is helpful only if the fluid is acidic; if it is alkaline, the gastric contents may have been altered (e.g., by enteral feedings or antacids and other medications), or the tube may be in the lung. This procedure does not reliably confirm gastric placement and should be used in combination with other methods.

c. Take note of the amount, color, and consistency of the aspirate. Gastric aspirates are often white or greenish and may be curdled. Intestinal aspirates will be smaller in quantity, yellowish due to the presence of bile, and not curdled.

d. Inject air into the NG tube and listen with a stethoscope over the stomach. Use this only to confirm other methods; do not use as the primary method of verification because it is the least reliable method.
   If the tube is in the stomach, injecting 5 to 30 mL of air with the syringe should produce a gurgling sound. However, because the lungs and stomach are so close together, a tube inadvertently placed in the respiratory tract or esophagus can transmit a sound similar to that of air in the stomach.

e. Ask the patient to speak.
   If she can do so, the tube is probably in the stomach. Use this only to confirm other methods; it is not reliable enough to use as the primary method of verification.

(continued on next page)

Procedure 28–2 ■ Inserting Nasogastric and Nasoenteric Tubes (continued)

18. **If the tube is not in the stomach**, advance it another 2.5 to 5 cm (2 to 4 in.) and repeat steps 17a through 17e.

19. **After you confirm proper placement**, clamp the end of the tube or connect it to the drainage bag, feeding, or suction machine.

20. **Secure the tube using one of the following methods.**

Securing the Tube With 1-Inch (2.5-cm) Tape

a. Apply skin adhesive to the patient's nose, and allow it to dry.
   A skin adhesive helps the tape to adhere and protects skin from breakdown.

b. Use the 5-cm (2-in.) piece of hypoallergenic tape, split lengthwise for 2.5 cm (1 in.) at one end.
   A split tape can be wrapped around the tube in opposite directions to hold the tube in place more securely.

c. Apply the intact end of tape to the patient's nose.

d. Wrap the split strips around the tube where it exits the nose.

Securing the Tube With ½-Inch Tape

e. Use ½-inch (1.3-cm) tape, 4 inches (10 cm) long. Apply one end of tape to the patient's nose and wrap the other end downward around the tube and then back up to secure on the opposite side of the nose.▼

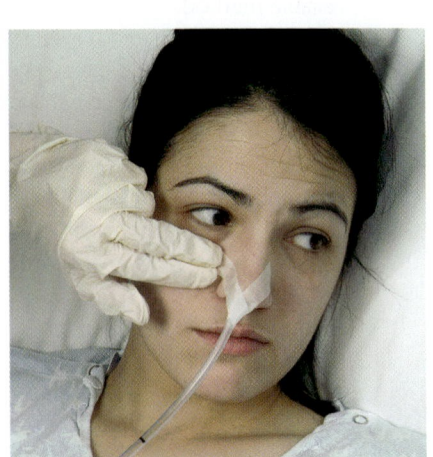

Securing the Tube With a Tube Fixation Device

f. Peel the backing off the pad and place the wide end of the pad over the bridge of the nose.

g. Position the connector around the NG or NE tube where it exits the nose. ▼

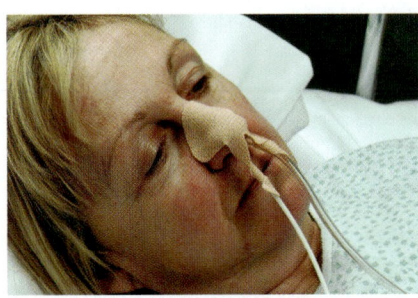

21. **Curve and tape the tube to the patient's cheek** (not necessary with some commercial tube fixation devices).
   Securing the tube to the cheek reduces the tension on the naris.

22. **Fasten the tube to the patient's gown**: Tie a slipknot around the tube with a rubber band. Loop a rubber band in a slipknot near the connection. (Alternatively, wrap a short piece of tape around the tube to form a tab.) Then fasten the rubber band or the tab to the gown with a safety pin (or tape).
   Reduces discomfort produced by the weight of the tube and prevents movement that may cause dislocation of the tube and irritation of the nose.

23. **Elevate the head of the bed 30°** unless contraindicated.

24. **Mark the tube** where it enters the naris with tape, or measure the length from the naris to the connector.
   A marked tube allows you to easily notice whether tube placement has changed.

? What if . . .

■ **The patient is confused, combative, or comatose?**

a. If the patient is comatose, place him into a semi-Fowler's position. Have a coworker use a pillow to help position the patient's head forward for insertion.

b. If the patient is confused and combative, ask a coworker to assist you with insertion.

■ **The patient gags, coughs, or chokes (at steps 11 and 15)?**

a. Stop advancing the tube. Ask the patient to take deep breaths and drink a few sips of water.
   Helps suppress the gag reflex.

b. Instruct the patient to breathe easily and take some sips of water.

c. If coughing continues, pull the tube back slightly.

d. If gagging continues, use a tongue blade and penlight to check the tube position in the back of the throat.
   The tube may be coiled in the back of the throat.

e. Continue to advance the tube to the desired distance.

f. ✚ If the tube is coiled in the back of the throat, the patient coughs excessively during insertion, the tube does not advance with each swallow, or the patient develops respiratory distress (e.g., gasping, coughing, or cyanosis), withdraw the tube completely and allow the patient to rest before reinserting.
   The tube may be in the patient's trachea.

■ **You are unable to obtain an aspirate (at step 17b) when confirming tube placement?**

a. Use a 50-mL syringe and aspirate very slowly over at least 5 minutes.

b. Flush the tube with air, then aspirate.

c. Turn the patient to the left side, wait 20 minutes, then aspirate again.

■ **The prescription states the tube needs to be in the jejunum?**

a. To advance the tube into the jejunum after the tube has been placed in the stomach, position the patient on the right side.
   Positioning on the right side allows gravity to assist tube passage through the pyloric sphincter.

b. Advance the tube 5 to 7.5 cm (2 to 3 in.) hourly, over several hours (up to 24 hr) until radiographic study confirms placement.

Weighted tubes will advance by gravity and peristalsis if a loop of the designated length is made at the entrance to the naris. After reading the initial x-ray, the radiologist or primary physician can provide the measurement needed to advance the tube to the desired position. Note that specially trained nurses usually place these tubes at the bedside.

■ **The procedure is anticipated to cause pain or discomfort?**

Commercial hurricane spray or viscous lidocaine is sometimes used to aid in patient comfort. Some practitioners use them for all NG insertions.

a. You may insert 2% viscous lidocaine into the nasal passage with a syringe before tube placement.

b. Alternatively, you can apply an anesthetic spray to the nasal and oropharyngeal mucosa.

■ **The patient is a child?**

a. Children usually require a tube of a smaller diameter.

b. Encourage parents to comfort infants and children and participate in their care.

c. You may need to apply restraints during insertion.

To prevent dislodging of the tube.

d. Monitor more frequently for complications.

Small children are not able to communicate problems with the tube.

Evaluation

■ Assess how well the patient tolerated the procedure (e.g., discomfort, gagging, coughing?)
■ Note the color, consistency, and pH of NG or NE aspirate.
■ Ask the patient whether she feels comfortable.
■ Assess respiratory status.

Patient Teaching

■ Explain that the sensation of the tube should decrease with time.
■ Explain the importance of immediately reporting tension on the tube or displacement of the tape or fixation device.
■ Discuss the need for frequent mouth care while the tube is in place.

Home Care

■ Assess the client or caregiver's ability to maintain an NG or NE tube at home.
■ Assess the home environment to determine the client's risk for infection.
■ Instruct the client or caregiver about aspirating stomach contents and measuring pH.
■ Teach the client or caregiver how to verify tube placement.
■ Explain to the client or caregiver how to properly secure the NG or NE tube.
■ Reinforce the need for frequent mouth care.

Documentation

Chart the date and time of insertion, size and type of the NG or NE tube and insertion site (which naris), length of tube from tip of the nose to the end of the tube, tolerance of the procedure, any abnormal findings, and methods for confirming NG or NE tube placement. Document description of gastric contents and respiratory status. NG or NE tube insertion is documented in the progress notes and flow sheets in most agencies.

Practice Resources

American Association of Critical-Care Nurses, 2005a, 2005b; Cullen, Taylor, Taylor, et al., 2004; Rauen, Chulay, Bridges, et al., 2008; Shlamovitz, & Shah, 2008; Wiegand, & Carlson, 2005; Wolfe, Fosnocht, & Linscott, 2000.

Thinking About the Procedure

 Go to the *Fundamentals of Nursing Skills Videos*, **Nutrition: Nasogastric Tubes: Inserting and Checking Placement.**

1. What were the patient's responses as the tube advanced down into her throat?
2. What did the nurse do?
3. Why do you think the nurse continued to advance the tube instead of completely withdrawing the tube and starting the procedure all over?

 For suggested responses, go to Chapter 28, **Thinking About the Procedure Suggested Responses,** on Davis*Plus*.

Procedure 28–3 ■ Administering Feedings Through Gastric and Enteric Tubes

➤ For steps to follow in *all* procedures, refer to the Universal Steps for All Procedures found on the page facing the inside back cover.

Equipment

- Prescribed feeding formula at room temperature
- Filtered water or prescribed diluent, if ordered
- Tube feeding administration set and bag
- 60-mL luer-lock or catheter-tip syringe (two needed for syringe feeding)
- Connector to connect administration set to the feeding tube
- Stethoscope
- Enteral feeding infusion pump (if used). Recommended for all continuous feedings.
- IV pole
- Linen-saver pad
- Graduated container
- pH strip
- For gastrostomy and jejunostomy tubes: a small precut gauze dressing

Delegation

You can delegate the procedure to the NAP or LPN if the patient's condition is stable and the NAP's skills allow. You must verify peristalsis, tube placement, and feeding tube patency before the feeding is started. Remind the NAP to position the patient upright and to report patient discomfort and any difficulty with the infusion.

Pre-Procedure Assessment

- Check the chart to determine that tube placement has been confirmed by radiography.
  This is the only reliable method for confirming placement (Rauen, Chulay, Bridges, et al., 2008).
- Check the length of the exposed tube: (1) Compare the length from the naris to the connector recorded after x-ray confirmation of placement; or (2) observe the mark that was made on it where it entered the nostril after insertion.
  These methods help confirm that the tube has not become displaced since radiography. If there is significant change in length, tube position must again be confirmed by radiography.
- Assess fluid status by checking breath sounds, mucous membranes, skin turgor, edema, and intake and output.
  These signs indicate fluid volume excess or insufficiency.
- Obtain baseline weight and laboratory studies.
  Weight change is a sensitive measure reflecting fluid and nutritional status.
- Monitor vital signs before and after feedings.
  Vital signs may vary from baseline due to pain, impaction, or dehydration.
- Auscultate for bowel sounds before each feeding or every 4 to 8 hours for continuous feedings. Also check for distention, nausea, vomiting, and diarrhea.
  These symptoms may indicate intolerance of tube feedings. If GI motility is impaired, feedings accumulate in the stomach along with gastric secretions, predisposing the patient to reflux and aspiration. Some medications (e.g., opioids) also slow gastric emptying.
- Assess frequency of bowel movements.
  Diarrhea may indicate intolerance of the formula, excessive feeding, or gastrointestinal disease.
- Check patient history for food allergies.
  Helps prevent allergic reaction to ingredients in the feeding formula.
- ***For gastrostomy and jejunostomy tubes**:* Assess the exit site at every shift. Report redness or drainage to the physician.
  Leaking of gastric or intestinal contents may cause skin breakdown.

➤ When performing the procedure, always identify your patient according to agency policy and be attentive to standard precautions, hand hygiene, patient safety and privacy, body mechanics, and documentation.

Procedure Steps

1. **Check the medical prescription** for the type of feeding, rate of infusion, and frequency of feeding.
   A medical prescription is required for enteral feedings. Rate and frequency of feeding are crucial for providing adequate nutrition.
2. **Check the expiration date** of the tube feeding formula.
   Expired formula should be discarded.
3. **Prepare the formula.**
   a. Shake the feeding formula well.

Intermittent Feedings

   b. Warm the formula to room temperature.
   Because the formula goes directly into the stomach and is not warmed by the mouth and esophagus, cold formula may cause abdominal cramping and increase the risk for diarrhea.

Continuous Feedings

   c. Keep continuous-feeding formulas cool, but not cold (don't use ice).
   Heat can coagulate some feedings (e.g., those containing egg). Cold feedings may cause vasoconstriction and cramps. Commercially prepared formulas are stored at room temperature.
4. **Prepare the equipment for administration.**

Open System With Feeding Bag

   a. Fill a disposable tube feeding bag with a 4- to 6-hour supply of feeding formula and prime the tubing.
   Limit hang-time to help prevent bacterial growth and prevent air from entering the GI tract.

b. Label the feeding bag with the date, time, formula type, and rate.
Labeling identifies the formula and helps avoid administering formula past the expiration date.

c. Hang the disposable tube-feeding bag on an IV pole.

Open System With Syringe

d. Remove the plunger.

Closed System With Prefilled Bottle With Drip Chamber

e. Attach the administration set to the prefilled bottle of feeding formula, and prime the tubing.

f. Hang the prefilled bottle on an IV pole. A prefilled container can safely hang for 24 to 36 hours (some agencies allow for 48 hours).
Closed systems decrease the risk of contamination and prevents air from entering the GI tract.

5. Elevate the head of the bed at least 30° to 45° unless contraindicated.
A position in which the stomach is higher than the gut reduces the risk for aspiration of gastric contents, a serious risk factor for pneumonia. It also promotes digestion.

6. Place a linen-saver pad under the connection end of the feeding tube. Don procedure gloves. Remove the cap from the end of the feeding tube or disconnect it from the suction equipment.
Draping prevents soiling of the patient's bed linens and gown. Clamping the tube prevents air from entering the stomach or gastric contents from leaking out.

7. ✚ Before the first feeding, tube placement must be verified by radiography. For the first feeding after radiography, you can confirm tube placement by checking the chart for x-ray confirmation and reconfirming at the bedside, using a combination of methods: measuring pH of aspirate, asking the patient to speak, observing for unexpected changes in residual volume, observing whether the external length of the catheter has changed, and using the "whoosh" test. (See Clinical Insight 28-5 for complete instructions.)
Only the x-ray method is reliable for verifying that the tube is in the correct position, so use the other methods in combination to confirm each other.

8. For subsequent feedings, aspirate and measure gastric residual volume. Also use other confirmatory methods, such as pH paper, asking the patient to speak, and so on (see step 7, preceding).

a. Connect the syringe to the proximal end of the feeding tube, slowly draw back on syringe to aspirate contents.

b. Measure the volume of aspirated contents using a syringe (if volume is more than 60 mL, use a graduated container).

c. Reinstill aspirate unless the volume is more than the formula flow rate for 1 hour (or more than 150 mL, or if patient is nauseated). If the residual is too high, see What if . . .?
Allows you to aspirate gastric contents, helps assess gastric emptying, and verifies tube placement. Reinstilling aspirate prevents fluid and electrolyte imbalance. Refer to Clinical Insight 28-5 for more rationale.

Jejunostomy Tube

d. Do not measure residual volume.
Residual volumes evaluate gastric emptying. The feeding is directly into the small intestine (the jejunum), which isn't normally a reservoir; therefore, no residual volume is present in the jejunum. In addition, feedings via small bowel feeding tubes should be administered as a continuous infusion via pump.

e. After initial confirmation by x-ray, check placement using pH indicator strips and measuring length of tube from the naris to the connector.
A pH of 7 to 8 is a normal value for the small bowel.

9. Irrigate the feeding tube with 30 mL of tap water.
Irrigation maintains tube patency.

Procedure Variation A Infusion Pump

10. To begin the feeding, hang the bag on the infusion pump and prime the tubing with supplement (if not already done in step 4).
You can use a pump with a prefilled bag or bottle or an open system with a feeding bag.

11. Thread the bag tubing through the infusion pump according to the manufacturer's instructions. Pinch off the end of the feeding tube.
Pinching the end prevents air from entering the feeding tube. ▼

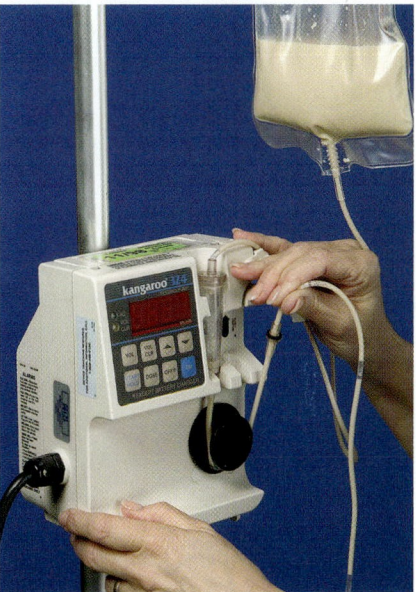

12. If needed, attach a connector to the proximal (open) end of the feeding tube. Connect the distal end of the bag tubing to the connector or directly to the NG or NE tube.

✚ Trace the tubing from the bag back to the patient before starting the feeding.
✚ This ensures that you have not inadvertently hooked the feeding bag to the intravenous line.

13. Turn on the infusion pump. Set the correct infusion rate and volume to be infused.

14. Unclamp the tube and begin the infusion.
An infusion pump delivers continuous tube feeding at the prescribed rate and volume.

Procedure Variation B Open-System Syringe

15. To begin feeding, clamp or pinch off the end of the feeding tube
Prevents air from entering the feeding tube.

(continued on next page)

Procedure 28–3 ■ Administering Feedings Through Gastric and Enteric Tubes (continued)

16. **Attach the syringe** to the proximal end of the feeding tube.

17. **Fill the syringe** with the prescribed amount of formula.

18. **Unclamp the feeding tube**, and elevate the syringe. Do not elevate the syringe more than 18 inches (45 cm) above the insertion site. Allow the feeding to flow slowly.
Gravity allows the formula to flow through the feeding tube. Rate of flow is determined by the height of the syringe. Feeding slowly prevents sudden stomach distention, which can lead to diarrhea, cramping, nausea, and vomiting. ▼

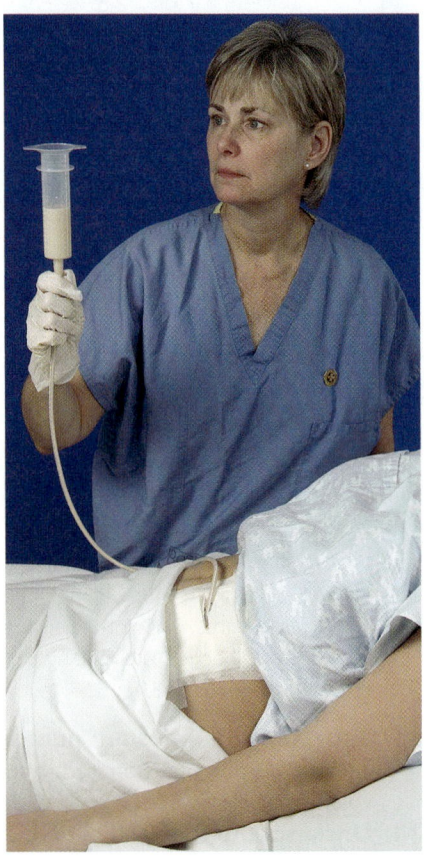

19. **When the syringe is nearly empty**, refill the syringe until the prescribed amount of feeding has been administered.
If the tubing runs dry, air may enter the stomach and cause discomfort associated with gas.

Procedure Variation C Closed System With Prefilled Bottle With Drip Chamber

20. **Pinch off or clamp the end** of the feeding tube.
Prevents air from entering the feeding tube.

21. **Attach administration tubing** to the bottle and prime the tubing, using sterile technique.

22. **Connect the distal end** of the administration tubing to the feeding tube. If needed, first attach a connector to the proximal (open) end of the feeding tube. Trace the tube from the bag back to the patient.

23. **Begin the infusion.**

Step Variation. Infusion Pump

a. Turn on the infusion pump. Set it the correct infusion rate and volume to be infused.

Gravity Drip

b. If your institution uses gravity to infuse prefilled bottles, adjust the drip rate by opening the roller clamp and regulating the flow rate manually.
Ensures administration at the prescribed rate.

24. **When the feeding is infused,** stop the flow, flush the tube, and disconnect the feeding, as in the following variations:
Pinching or clamping the tubing prevents air from entering the feeding tube, and fluid and gas from leaking out. Instilling water helps maintain feeding tube patency and provides the patient with free water to maintain fluid and electrolyte balance.

Infusion Pump

a. Turn off the pump before pinching, then pinch off the proximal end of the feeding tube.

b. Flush feeding tube with the prescribed amount of water (typically 50 to 100 mL).

Open-System Syringe

c. Disconnect the syringe from the feeding tube.

d. Flush the feeding tube with 50 mL of tap water.

Closed System With Prefilled Bottle With Drip Chamber

e. Turn off pump or turn roller clamp off.

f. Disconnect the feeding tube from the administration tubing.

g. Flush the feeding tube with the prescribed amount of water.

Continuous Feeding

h. If administering a continuous feeding, flush the tube with the prescribed amount of water (typically 50 to 100 mL) every 4 to 6 hours.

25. **Cap the proximal end of the feeding tube.**
Prevents spillage of gastric contents and stops air from entering the stomach.

26. **Keep the head of the bed elevated** at least 30° to 45° for 1 hour after administering the tube feeding.
Elevation reduces the risk for aspiration of gastric contents.

27. **Provide or assist with regular oral hygiene** and encourage frequent gargling.
Oral care reduces oropharyngeal discomfort from the tube.

? What if . . .

■ **When checking for residual, the volume is more than the formula flow rate for 1 hour or more than 150 mL?**

Hold the feeding for 1 hour, then recheck the residual. Notify the medical provider if the residual is still elevated. You will likely reinstill the residual very slowly, over a period of time, as the patient tolerates.
High residual volumes indicate delayed gastric emptying.

■ **When checking for residual, none is obtained?**

Use a large syringe and inflate 20 mL of air into the tube; this may move the tube away from the gastric wall or clear the tube of any residual formula, medication, or water.

■ **When irrigating the feeding tube (at step 9), resistance is met? Or**

when instilling the feeding, the fluid does not flow?

- Do not force the solution.
- Do not use any fluid other than water for flushing.
- Check for kinks in tubing and that the pump is working correctly.
- Turn the client onto his left side.
- Remove any enteral feeding solution remaining in the tube. Try instilling 5 mL of warm water into the tube and clamping the tube for 5 minutes. Then apply gentle negative pressure to the tube with a syringe.
- Try flushing with a smaller (e.g., 10 or 20 mL) syringe.
- If these measures fail, the tube may need to be removed and a new one inserted; contact the primary care provider. (*Note:* There are other methods, such as the alkalinized enzyme method; they require a medical prescription.)

Forcing the solution may damage the tube. However, you can use a smaller syringe to exert slightly more pressure.

- **The patient has a cuffed tracheostomy tube?**

Inflate the cuff before administering the feeding, and keep the cuff inflated at for least 15 minutes afterward. *Cuffing helps to prevent aspiration.*

- **During the feeding, the patient vomits or complains of nausea or feeling too full?**

Stop the feeding and assess the patient's condition. Flush the tube, wait an hour, then measure gastric contents and restart the feeding at a slower rate. You may need to obtain a medical order to decrease the volume of the feedings.

- **The patient has a jejunostomy tube?**

Do not instill air into the tube or check for residual before feeding. *The tube is in the jejunum rather than the stomach, and the jejunum isn't normally a reservoir; therefore, no residual volume is present in the jejunum. Gastrostomy and jejunostomy tubes are often placed through the upper abdominal wall; these tubes, of course, cannot inadvertently migrate into the airway. Injecting air into the tube is not necessary and introduces air into the GI tract, causing the patient discomfort from gas.*

Clean the insertion site daily with soap and water. You may apply a small, precut gauze dressing to the site. *Helps prevent bacterial growth; prevents infection.*

Be aware that the delivery rate will likely be slower for jejunostomy tubes because of the loss of the stomach as a reservoir.

Evaluation

- Evaluate the patient's tolerance to the tube feeding; did the patient have any abdominal discomfort, nausea, vomiting, or diarrhea?
- Auscultate bowel sounds and vital signs every 4 hours.
- Check gastric residual volume every 4 hours.
- Monitor intake and output every 8 hours.
- Weigh patient at least 3 times per week.
- Assess the exit site for signs of skin breakdown.
- Assess frequency of bowel movements.
- Check laboratory values to evaluate nutritional status.

Patient Teaching

- Demonstrate the procedure to the patient and caregiver if the patient will be continuing tube feedings at home.
- Explain the importance of flushing the feeding tube with tap water every 4 hours while the patient is awake to maintain tube patency and fluid and electrolyte balance.
- Discuss the importance of remaining upright for at least 1 hour after the feeding.

Home Care

- Provide written instructions.
- Be sure the client has a 7-day supply of enteral feedings.
- Identify with the client the person who will be responsible for care of the enteral tube and administration of feedings at home.
- Explain to the client and caregiver how to measure the prescribed amount of tube feeding formula and water for flushes by using household measuring equipment.
- Explain the importance of washing reusable equipment thoroughly with soap and water to prevent the spread of infection.
- Discuss how and where to purchase and store the formula.

- If home feedings are to be delivered by pump:
  - Facilitate a home care visit to provide training about the feeding pump.
- Arrange for delivery of the feeding pump before discharge (or refer to the appropriate professional for this).
- Ensure that the client has a 7-day supply of disposable feeding sets and 50-mL syringes upon discharge.

Documentation

- Chart the type of tube feeding, rate and volume of infusion, amount of gastric residual volume (if any), and tolerance of procedure.
- Tube feeding intake is documented on the intake and output portion of the flow sheet in most agencies.
- Record all flushes as intake. Subtract any liquids that you aspirate and do not reinstill (e.g., when gastric residual is too high).

Practice Resources

American Association of Critical-Care Nurses, 2005a, 2005b; American Society for Parenteral and Enteral Nutrition (A.S.P.E.N.), 2009a; Cincinnati Children's Hospital Medical Center, 2009; Griffiths, Thompson, Chau, et al., 2006; Metheney, 2006; National Guideline Clearinghouse (NGC), 2006b, 2006c; Rauen, C., Chulay, M., Bridges, E., et al., 2008; Simons and Abdallah, 2012.

Thinking About the Procedure

 Go to the *Fundamentals of Nursing Skills Videos*, **Nutrition: Tube Feeding.**

1. What type of feeding system did the nurse use?
2. What did the nurse do next after turning on the pump and setting the rate?

 For suggested responses, go to Chapter 28, **Thinking About the Procedure Suggested Responses,** on Davis*Plus*.

Procedure 28–4 ■ Removing a Nasogastric or Nasoenteric Tube

> ➤ For steps to follow in *all* procedures, refer to the Universal Steps for All Procedures found on the page facing the inside back cover.

Equipment

- Linen-saver pad
- 60-mL luer-lock or catheter-tip syringe
- Procedure gloves
- Stethoscope
- Disposable plastic bag
- Emesis basin
- Gauze square

Delegation

This procedure should not be delegated to the LPN or NAP.

Pre-Procedure Assessments

- Auscultate the abdomen for the presence of bowel sounds.
  Bowel sounds and flatus confirm peristalsis, which indicates bowel function is present.
- Assess the patient's ability to consume an oral diet.
  Confirms readiness for discontinuing the NG or NE tube.
- Determine how long it has been since the patient's last enteral feeding.
  Wait at least 30 minutes after a feeding to remove the NG tube.

> ➤ When performing the procedure, always identify your patient according to agency policy and be attentive to standard precautions, hand hygiene, patient safety and privacy, body mechanics, and documentation.

Procedure Steps

1. **Check the patient's health record** to confirm removal of the tube. For feeding tubes, make sure tube feeding has been stopped at least 30 minutes before removal.

2. **Assist the patient to a sitting** or high-Fowler's position.
   Proper body alignment facilitates tube removal.

3. **Place the plastic bag and emesis basin** on the bed or within reach. Hand the patient facial tissue. Explain that the procedure may cause some gagging or nasal discomfort, but it will be brief.
   Patients often need to blow their nose after this procedure.

4. **Drape a linen-saver pad or towel** across the patient's chest, and don procedure gloves.
   Draping protects the gown and linens from soiling. Maintains universal precautions.

5. **If you have not already done so,** wash your hands and put on gloves.

6. **If the NG tube is connected** to suction, turn off suction and disconnect the tube.

7. **Stand on the patient's right side** if you are right-handed and left side if left-handed.

8. **Attach the syringe** to the proximal end of the NG or NE tube and flush the tube with 10 mL of water, normal saline, or air.
   Flushing clears the tube of feeding formula or gastric secretions that could cause irritation or be aspirated during tube removal.

9. **Unpin the tube** from the patient's gown, and then untape the tube from the patient's nose. Use an adhesive-remover pad to help loosen the tape as necessary.

10. **Clamp or pinch the end** of the tube in your hand. Hold gauze up to the patient's nose and be ready to grab the tube with the towel in the opposite hand upon removal.
    This prevents gastric fluids from leaking out the end of the tube onto the nurse or patient.

11. **Ask the patient to take a deep breath** and hold it.
    Breath holding closes the epiglottis to prevent aspiration.

12. **Quickly, steadily, and smoothly** withdraw the tube and place it in the plastic bag.
    Rapid removal in one steady motion prevents tissue trauma. The plastic bag acts as a barrier to gastric fluids until the tube can be placed in the trash. Seeing and smelling the tube may cause the patient to become nauseated.

13. **If the patient cannot do so,** clean her nares and provide mouth care. Remove the tape residue from her nose with adhesive remover.
    Promotes patient comfort and prevents infection.

14. **If the NG tube was connected** to suction, measure the drainage and note the character of the content. Dispose of the tube and drainage equipment according to facility policy.
    For patients receiving enteral feedings or gastric suction, record their intake and output. Proper equipment disposal prevents the spread of infection.

15. **Remove and dispose of gloves** in the nearest receptacle.

Evaluation

- Assess the nares for signs of skin breakdown or bleeding.
- Monitor the patient for signs of GI dysfunction, such as food intolerance, nausea, vomiting, and abdominal distention. Auscultate for bowel sounds.
  GI dysfunction could necessitate reinsertion of the tube.
- Monitor intake and output every 8 hours.
- Weigh the patient regularly.
- Check laboratory values to evaluate nutritional status.

Patient Teaching

- Instruct the patient or caregiver on how to remove the feeding tube.
- Explain the importance of reporting nausea, vomiting, food intolerance, or abdominal distention to the physician.
- Explain the importance of and procedure for drinking fluids, if not contraindicated.

Home Care

The procedure does not require special adaptation for home care, except that you might want to place the tube in a plastic zippered storage bag before discarding it in the trash receptacle.

Documentation

- Chart the date and time of removal as well as the patient's tolerance of the procedure.
- Document the amount of drainage if the tube was connected to suction.

- Note any complications following NG or NE tube removal, such as food intolerance, nausea, vomiting, and abdominal distention.

Practice Resources

Best practices, 2007.

Thinking About the Procedure

 Go to the *Fundamentals of Nursing Skills Videos*, **Nutrition, Nasogastric Tubes: Removing.**

1. What was the patient's position for this procedure?
2. What did the nurse use to clear the NG tube before removing it?
3. How did the nurse keep the NG tube out of the patient's sight after removing it?

 For suggested responses, go to Chapter 28, **Thinking About the Procedure Suggested Responses,** on Davis*Plus.*

Procedure 28–5 ■ Administering Parenteral Nutrition

➤ For steps to follow in *all* procedures, refer to the Universal Steps for All Procedures found on the page facing the inside back cover.

Equipment

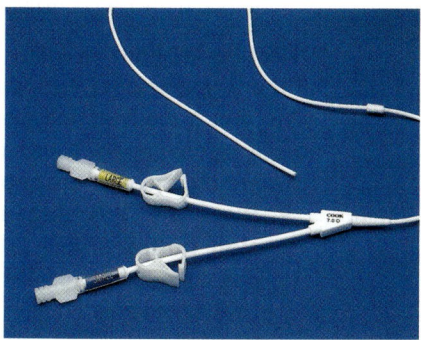

A two-lumen CVC. Note clamps, threaded lumen ends, and color-coded lumens to aid in identification of correct line for PN

- Parenteral nutrition solution
  - Keep the PN refrigerated until 60 minutes before use; do not give cold. Do not hasten warming by placing in a microwave oven or hot water bath.
    Cold solution can cause pain, hypothermia, and venous spasm. Nutrients in PN solution are stable only for this short period of time. Nutrients could precipitate, causing catheter blockage or emboli.
  - Some pharmacies deliver the solution before infusion. Be sure the PN has not been mixed more than 24 hours beforehand. However, in home care you may find that solutions are mixed and delivered weekly.
- Procedure gloves
- Sterile gloves
  Note: If the central line has an injection cap and if IV tubing is connected onto the cap via luer-lock, some agencies do not require gloves.

- Intravenous administration set, extension set if indicated (free of plasticizers, such as DEHP, when fat emulsion is to be infused)
- 0.22-micron filter (1.2-micron filter if solution contains albumin or lipids)
  A 0.22-micron filter will remove most particulates and microorganisms that might have been introduced during mixing, but it is too fine for larger-molecule lipids to infuse properly.
- Time tape
  Even though the PN is delivered by infusion pump, there have been numerous recalls of infusion pumps because of malfunction. This simple tape provides valuable information quickly and is an additional safety measure.
- 70% alcohol pads or chlorhexidine gluconate (CHG)-based pads (e.g., 2% CHG in 70% isopropyl alcohol)
- Infusion pump
- 10-mL syringe and saline
  To check for catheter patency
- Blood glucose testing monitor
- Intake and output record
- Transparent dressing or sterile gauze and tape (if dressing is to be changed)
- Catheter stabilization device (e.g., StatLock)
  These are recommended for all catheters and must be changed with each dressing change.
- If the dressing is to be changed, you also need a transparent dressing or sterile gauze, tape, and a mask.

Delegation

Do not delegate this skill to the LPN or NAP because administration of parenteral nutrition requires advanced assessment and critical thinking skills. The LPN or NAP can

(continued on next page)

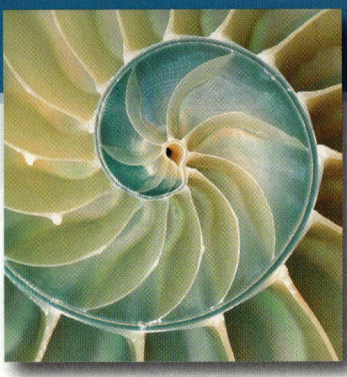

CHAPTER 29

Bowel Elimination

Learning Outcomes

After completing this chapter, you should be able to:

➤ Identify the basic structures and functions of the gastrointestinal system.

➤ Discuss factors that affect bowel elimination.

➤ Describe normal bowel elimination.

➤ Differentiate among the various types of bowel diversions.

➤ Discuss common bowel elimination problems.

➤ Identify appropriate nursing history questions to assess bowel elimination problems.

➤ Perform a physical examination focused on bowel elimination.

➤ List and describe diagnostic tests used to identify bowel elimination problems.

➤ Formulate nursing diagnoses associated with altered bowel elimination.

➤ Describe nursing interventions that promote normal bowel elimination.

➤ Provide care for clients experiencing alterations in bowel elimination.

➤ Discuss nursing care associated with the use of bowel diversions.

Key Concepts

Bowel elimination

Motility

Related Concepts

See the Concept Map at the end of this chapter.

Example Problems

Diarrhea

Constipation and impaction

Bowel incontinence

Caring for the Nguyens

This feature allows you to practice the kind of thinking you will use as a full-spectrum nurse. There is usually more than one correct answer to a critical thinking question, so we do not provide answers for these features. It is more important to develop your nursing judgment than to "cover content." Discuss the questions with your peers. If you are still unsure, consult your instructor.

Yen Nyugen arrives at the family health center for a scheduled appointment, accompanied by her grandson, Kim Phan. Recently, Yen has been constipated and has had several episodes of bleeding with bowel movements (BMs). She has read that a change in bowel habits is a sign of colon cancer and is worried about that. She brought her grandson along because he is also having bowel problems. Kim's bowel habits are erratic. At times he has a soft BM.

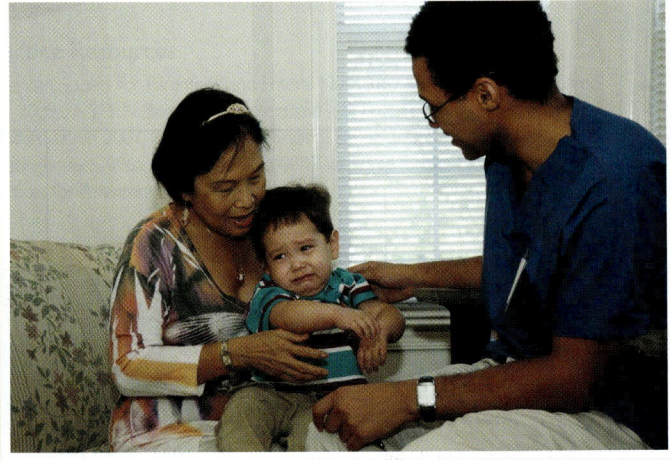

However, he has also had bouts of constipation and diarrhea. Yen would like advice on her grandson's elimination status. As a critical thinker, you will begin by obtaining accurate, credible information.

A. What history questions would be appropriate to ask Yen regarding her bowel concerns? What data do you need? How can you get the data? Are the data accurate? What information is important; what is not? Write some specific questions, just as you would ask them in an interview.

Patient Teaching

- Instruct the patient or caregiver on how to remove the feeding tube.
- Explain the importance of reporting nausea, vomiting, food intolerance, or abdominal distention to the physician.
- Explain the importance of and procedure for drinking fluids, if not contraindicated.

Home Care

The procedure does not require special adaptation for home care, except that you might want to place the tube in a plastic zippered storage bag before discarding it in the trash receptacle.

Documentation

- Chart the date and time of removal as well as the patient's tolerance of the procedure.
- Document the amount of drainage if the tube was connected to suction.

- Note any complications following NG or NE tube removal, such as food intolerance, nausea, vomiting, and abdominal distention.

Practice Resources
Best practices, 2007.

Thinking About the Procedure

 Go to the *Fundamentals of Nursing Skills Videos,* **Nutrition, Nasogastric Tubes: Removing.**

1. What was the patient's position for this procedure?
2. What did the nurse use to clear the NG tube before removing it?
3. How did the nurse keep the NG tube out of the patient's sight after removing it?

 For suggested responses, go to Chapter 28, **Thinking About the Procedure Suggested Responses,** on DavisPlus.

Procedure 28–5 ■ Administering Parenteral Nutrition

➤ For steps to follow in *all* procedures, refer to the Universal Steps for All Procedures found on the page facing the inside back cover.

Equipment

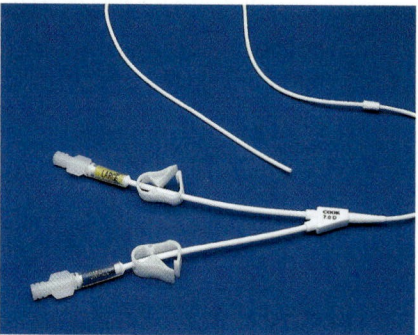

A two-lumen CVC. Note clamps, threaded lumen ends, and color-coded lumens to aid in identification of correct line for PN

- Parenteral nutrition solution
  - Keep the PN refrigerated until 60 minutes before use; do not give cold. Do not hasten warming by placing in a microwave oven or hot water bath.
    Cold solution can cause pain, hypothermia, and venous spasm. Nutrients in PN solution are stable only for this short period of time. Nutrients could precipitate, causing catheter blockage or emboli.
  - Some pharmacies deliver the solution before infusion. Be sure the PN has not been mixed more than 24 hours beforehand. However, in home care you may find that solutions are mixed and delivered weekly.
- Procedure gloves
- Sterile gloves
  Note: If the central line has an injection cap and if IV tubing is connected onto the cap via luer-lock, some agencies do not require gloves.

- Intravenous administration set, extension set if indicated (free of plasticizers, such as DEHP, when fat emulsion is to be infused)
- 0.22-micron filter (1.2-micron filter if solution contains albumin or lipids)
  A 0.22-micron filter will remove most particulates and microorganisms that might have been introduced during mixing, but it is too fine for larger-molecule lipids to infuse properly.
- Time tape
  Even though the PN is delivered by infusion pump, there have been numerous recalls of infusion pumps because of malfunction. This simple tape provides valuable information quickly and is an additional safety measure.
- 70% alcohol pads or chlorhexidine gluconate (CHG)-based pads (e.g., 2% CHG in 70% isopropyl alcohol)
- Infusion pump
- 10-mL syringe and saline
  To check for catheter patency
- Blood glucose testing monitor
- Intake and output record
- Transparent dressing or sterile gauze and tape (if dressing is to be changed)
- Catheter stabilization device (e.g., StatLock)
  These are recommended for all catheters and must be changed with each dressing change.
- If the dressing is to be changed, you also need a transparent dressing or sterile gauze, tape, and a mask.

Delegation

Do not delegate this skill to the LPN or NAP because administration of parenteral nutrition requires advanced assessment and critical thinking skills. The LPN or NAP can

(continued on next page)

Procedure 28–5 ■ **Administering Parenteral Nutrition** (continued)

assist by monitoring vital signs and verifying patient identity with you. Instruct them about complications associated with PN and ask them to inform you of any signs or symptoms or change in the patient's condition.

Pre-Procedure Assessments

- Assess nutrition status and nutritional needs (e.g., daily weights, input and output [I&O], lab results). Patients requiring PN have complex nutritional needs, and actual nutritional status is assessed by a nurse or dietician specializing in nutritional support.
- Check the prescriber's orders for type and concentration of additives in each container and for rate of infusion. (Standardized order forms are recommended by the American Society for Parenteral and Enteral Nutrition.)

- Check the patient's record to confirm that proper CVC tip placement has been established before the initial PN administration.
- Check agency policy.
  A few may require tubing and filter change with every bottle or bag. The CDC recommends changing the PN set every 72 hours and a fat emulsion set at least every 24 hours.
- Check the blood glucose level.
- Assess for apparent patency of the IV site.
  If PN is being administered continuously by pump and the infusion is running and there is no leakage from the insertion, you can begin the first few steps of the procedure. Actual patency is checked at step 14.

➤ When performing the procedure, always identify your patient according to agency policy and be attentive to standard precautions, hand hygiene, patient safety and privacy, body mechanics, and documentation.

Procedure Steps

1. **Gather equipment and place** at the bedside.
   Promotes efficient use of time.

2. ✚ **Identify the patient**, using two identifiers, according to agency policy. Some institutions require, as an extra precaution, that two people identify the patient.
   Multiple patient identifiers help to avoid "wrong-patient" errors. PN solutions are mixed to meet individual needs.

3. **Explain to the patient** the procedure and the rationale for it.
   Respects the patient's right to be informed.

4. **Perform hand hygiene and don procedure gloves.**
   Reduces transmission of infectious microorganisms.

5. **Position the patient supine** in bed.

6. **Obtain and examine the PN container.** Check for leaks, cloudiness, or floating particles. Do not use if any of these are present. Some agencies require that two people examine the solution.

Solutions Containing Lipids (3-in-1 Admixture)

✚ **Do not administer the admixture if it has a brown layer, oil droplets, or oil on the surface. This

indicates that the emulsion has "broken," and the large lipid droplets can cause fat emboli if administered. Also note that this solution requires a 1.2-micron filter.**
To reduce the risk of adverse events such as fat emboli.

7. **Compare the bag to the patient's identification band;** check for correct bag number, expiration date, and additives and their concentration. Compare with the original prescription. Have a coworker verify with you.
   Ensures that the correct solution is administered. Check the expiration date to ensure that the solution will be discarded after that date and time. PN solutions are carefully calculated and prepared using the latest recommendations for sterile compounding of solutions. Therefore, no medications should be added to the bag by the nurse, either before it is hung or while it is infusing.

8. **Connect the IV tubing to the PN solution;** prime the tubing. Note that priming may be done manually now or later (on the pump after the tubing is loaded into the pump), depending on the design of the pump.

   ✚ **Be sure to identify the correct port and IV line.** Trace the PN tubing from the bag to the patient.

   Priming tubing removes air bubbles and prevents air from entering the patient's

bloodstream, possibly causing air embolism. If there is PN already infusing, the old tubing must be removed from the pump and the rate regulated manually for the short period it takes to prime the new administration set.*

IV Tubing Without an Inline Filter
If the IV tubing does not have an inline filter, attach the filter and the extension tubing before priming. Attach the filter as close to the catheter site as possible.

9. **Place the IV tubing in the infusion pump.** (Prime the tubing if not done in step 8.) Set the pump to the prescribed rate.

   ✚ *Administration via pump (preferably volumetric) helps prevent complications associated with too-rapid infusion. PN solutions must be administered by infusion pump with reliable, audible alarms. Catheter tip placement must be confirmed before initial PN administration.*

10. **Identify the correct IV catheter and lumen for the PN.** This is usually a PICC line or a centrally inserted venous line designated solely for PN.
    PN is administered via a central venous catheter (e.g., subclavian catheter, internal jugular, or PICC) whose tip is positioned in the superior vena cava/right atrial juncture. Most guidelines state that a specific intravenous line be reserved for parenteral nutrition and not used for any other purpose. If a single-lumen catheter

is used, it is used only for PN. If a multilumen catheter is used, one lumen will be dedicated for the PN, and blood and other fluids should not be given through that lumen.

11. **Clamp the catheter and the old PN administration set**, if still connected, before disconnecting the tubing.

a. A clamp should be present on the central line catheters with valves built into the catheter itself.

b. As an additional safety measure, instruct the patient to perform the Valsalva maneuver just as you change the tubing (step 14).

c. If Valsalva is contraindicated for a patient, instruct the patient to exhale at a specific time when the lumen is open.

The central line for the PN should already be clamped if no PN is running. If a previous bag is running, always clamp the PN line near the patient before disconnecting. Clamping prevents air from entering the catheter when you open the connection. The Valsalva maneuver increases intrathoracic pressure and creates positive pressure in the central vessels, also helping prevent air embolism.

12. **Remove and discard gloves.** Perform hand hygiene.

In steps 1 through 11, you were observing universal precautions. From this step forward, the emphasis is on preventing the introduction of microorganisms into the catheter lumen or the catheter insertion site.

13. **Don clean gloves (or sterile** gloves, if your agency policy requires them). Disconnect the old administration set. Using an alcohol-chlorhexidine pad or a 70% alcohol pad, thoroughly cleanse all surfaces of the central line injection cap and extension leg (in a needleless system) or the luer-lock, including threads.

Because PN solutions are a good medium for growth of pathogens, and because the IV line enters the central circulation, the risk for sepsis is relatively high.

14. **Determine patency of the line.** Use a 10-mL syringe to aspirate for blood, looking for a brisk return; then

flush with saline. If the PN is running continuously on a pump, there are no occlusion alarms, and the dressing is dry and intact, these are also signs— but not proof—of patency.

When PN is running continuously on a pump, the pump creates a constant fluid flow through the lumen to help keep it patent. There is some controversy about this step. Some experts prefer to aspirate for blood only for the first bag of a continuous infusion, and thereafter to flush without aspirating. As always, follow agency policy.

15. ✚ Attach the infusion tubing to the designated PN port and then turn the luer-lock to secure the connection. "Luer-slip" connections should not be used. Do not use tape. Trace the tubing from the patient back to the PN container to be certain you are using the correct lumen. *Securing the connection with a luer-lock connection prevents separation of the connection and decreases the risk for sepsis or embolism. Tape, even sterile tape, has been found to be a medium for bacterial colonization.*

Previous Infusion Is Still Connected

Be sure the access line and the line to the "old" infusion bag are clamped (step 11). Quickly disconnect from the central line, thoroughly cleanse the port, and connect the new infusion.

16. **Trace the tubing from the bag back to the patient.** Then start the infusion. Check again to make sure the catheter-tubing connection is secure. Infuse at the rate prescribed (depending on the patient's tolerance, PN is usually started at a rate of 40 to 50 mL/hr and then advanced 25 mL/hr every 6 hr).

PN solutions may contain as much as 70% dextrose. A gradual rate increase allows the patient's pancreatic beta cells time to increase their insulin output to handle the increased glucose load. For lower concentrations of dextrose, you can usually run the same rate for the complete 24-hour volume.

17. **Label the tubing** with the date and time of change (if it is new

tubing or if you have changed the tubing).

Labeling allows other nurses to know when tubing is due to be changed and a new solution must be hung.

18. **Remove and discard gloves.** Perform hand hygiene.

? What if . . .

- ✚ **When you flush the catheter (at step 14), you meet resistance?**

Examine the insertion site for leaking fluid or inflammation. Aspirate and try again to flush *gently*. Never forcibly flush against resistance. Reposition the patient and ask him to cough. Roll the patient's shoulder or raise the arm on the same side the catheter is on. If these measures fail, notify the primary care provider.

Occlusion may be caused by a clot; drug precipitation; or catheter migration, kinking, or compression. Forceful flushing may discharge a clot into circulation. Other measures to clear a catheter require a medical order.

- ✚ **The rate falls behind or the pump gives occlusion alarms?**

First check to be sure the pump is turned on, the bag is not empty, and all clamps are fully open. Change the filter if it is clogged. Perform the steps in the preceding item. If those measures do not work, change the pump and send it to biomedical engineering to be checked. Do not attempt to catch up by increasing the rate.

A slow rate may indicate a clogged filter or injection cap, a kinked catheter, or a malfunctioning pump. A clogged filter must be changed; you cannot run the PN without a filter.

- ✚ **The 24-hour total deviates from the prescribed infusion rate by 10% or more?**

Notify the primary provider or nutrition support team.

- ✚ **A PN solution must be discontinued abruptly for any reason?**

Notify the primary provider or nutrition support team. Another solution of 5% or 10% dextrose may be started.

The dextrose solution is started to prevent rebound hypoglycemia. Note that if it is a

(continued on next page)

Procedure 28–5 ■ Administering Parenteral Nutrition (continued)

catheter complication that requires this discontinuation, 10% dextrose is the highest concentration that can be infused through a peripheral vein because infiltrated hyperosmolar fluid causes tissue injury.

■ ✚ **The patient no longer needs parenteral nutrition?**

You may need to decrease the rate gradually, perhaps over 48 hours, before discontinuing the infusion completely. Be sure the patient either receives enteral nutrition or consumes food during the next few hours after stopping PN.
To prevent rebound hypoglycemia

Evaluation

These are post-procedure evaluations. For ongoing monitoring, see Clinical Insight 28-7.

- Assess vital signs, I&O, and weight.
- Observe that the solution is infusing at the prescribed rate.
- Assess patient's tolerance to the infusion (e.g., observe for pulmonary edema; check lab results).
- Observe for skin rashes, flushing, color changes, or other signs of allergic reactions; notify the primary provider. *Note:* These are not common.
- Monitor blood glucose and do not increase the infusion rate until glycemic control is established.

Patient Teaching

- Inform the patient and family of the purpose and duration of the nutritional support.
- Teach them to recognize and report to the nurse symptoms of complications associated with PN.
- Teach the patient that the dressing must remain occlusive, and to notify nurse if it comes loose or gets wet.
- Teach the patient the importance of measures to prevent blood infections.

Home Care

- The home environment must provide dry storage space for supplies, a refrigerator for storing admixtures, a clean low-traffic area for procedure preparation, and electronic outlets for any electronic equipment.
- Teach safe disposal of supplies.
- Provide verbal and written instructions of the procedures; demonstrate and ask for a return demonstration. Role play "what would you do if . . . ?" situations with the patient.
- Clients at home often administer their daily 24-hour total over 12 to 16 hours during the night. This allows them to disconnect from the infusion in the morning, flush the central line, and be free to pursue their usual activities during the day.
- Instruct about solution hang time and management of the access device.
  Depending on the anticipated length of therapy, patients may be sent home with a permanent venous access device.
- Provide 24-hour phone numbers for the primary care provider and home care agency.
- Home PN is less expensive than treatment in the hospital, and in many cases is associated with a lower risk of infection.
- Home nutritional support is usually under the direction of specialized nutrition support teams.

Documentation

- A special form may be used for documenting PN administration.
- Bag number, date and time hung, volume, type of fluid, rate of delivery, additives
- Date and time of dressing or tubing change (if performed)
- Patient's tolerance of procedure
- Pre- and post-administration assessment data, including complications and response to therapy
- Results of fingerstick blood glucose checks
- If insulin is required, type, amount, and route/site administered
- Weight
- I&O

Practice Resources

American Society for Parenteral and Enteral Nutrition (A.S.P.E.N.) Board of Directors, 2009a; A.S.P.E.N. Board of Directors and Task Force on Parenteral Nutrition Standardization, 2007; Infusion Nurses Society, 2006a, 2006b; National Guideline Clearinghouse, 2006a, 2006b, 2008a, 2008b; Task Force for the Revision of Safe Practices for Parenteral Nutrition, 2004.

Procedure 28-6 ■ Administering Lipids

➤ For steps to follow in *all* procedures, refer to the Universal Steps for All Procedures found on the page facing the inside back cover.

➤ *Note:* If administering through a central line, refer to Procedure 28-5 for precautions associated with central lines.

➤ *Note:* This procedure is for administering fat emulsions. If you are administering an admixture with the parenteral nutrition solution, use Procedure 28-5.

Equipment

- Intravenous lipid solution (not refrigerated)
- Special tubing (infusion set) for lipids
  Must be without plasticizers (DEHP). Set should be labeled to that effect.
- Needleless cannula (if using a split septum needleless connector that requires it)
- 70% isopropyl alcohol pads or chlorhexidine gluconate
- Procedure gloves
- Time tape
- Infusion pump
- Intake and output record
- If a filter is a used, it must be a 1.2-micron filter
  Lipid particles are large and will clog a smaller size.

Delegation

Do not delegate this skill to the LPN or NAP because administration of lipids requires advanced assessment and critical thinking skills. The LPN or NAP can assist by monitoring vital signs and verifying patient identity with you. Instruct them about complications associated with lipids and ask them to inform you of any signs or symptoms or change in the patient's condition.

Pre-Procedure Assessments

- Assess for rash; eczema; dry, scaly skin; poor wound healing; and sparse hair.
  These are signs of essential fatty acid deficits.
- Check the history for anemia; coagulation disorders; and abnormal liver, pancreatic, or respiratory function.
  These factors predispose to fat emboli. Your role as a staff nurse is to be certain the PN prescriber is aware of these factors; they do not necessarily contraindicate giving the PN.
- Check peripheral IV site for erythema, infiltration, and patency. Check the central venous access site for erythema or other signs of infection.
- Take baseline vital signs just before infusing the lipids.
  An immediate reaction can occur upon starting the infusion. Note that not all guidelines require this action.

➤ When performing the procedure, always identify your patient according to agency policy and be attentive to standard precautions, hand hygiene, patient safety and privacy, body mechanics, and documentation.

Procedure Steps

1. **Review the prescriber's orders**, identify the patient, and explain the purpose of the procedure.
   Verifying helps to prevent dosage and wrong-patient errors. Explaining respects the patient's right to be informed and encourages cooperation.

2. **Gather equipment** and place at bedside. Adjust lighting as needed.
   Organization promotes efficient use of time.

3. **Perform hand hygiene** and don procedure gloves.
   Hand hygiene and gloving reduces transmission of infectious microorganisms.

4. **Position the patient supine** in bed.

5. **Be certain lipids are not cold**.
   Cold infusion can cause discomfort.

6. **Examine the bottle** for a layer of froth or for separation into fat globules or layers.
   Do not use the lipids if these occur.

7. **Label the bottle** with the patient's name, room number, date, time, rate, and start and stop times. Label the tubing with date and time. *Note:* When lipids are infused with parenteral nutrition, the lipid infusion must be completed within 12 hours.
   Labeling helps ensure that the patient receives the correct infusion.

8. **Compare the lipids bottle** to the patient's wrist band (bag number, expiration date); compare to the original prescription. Have a colleague verify.

9. **Determine patency of the IV line** (see Procedure 28-5).

10. **Cleanse the stopper** on the IV bottle with an antiseptic swab; allow to dry.

11. **Connect the special DEHP-free** lipids-infusion tubing to the bottle, twisting the spike as you insert it. *Note:* You must use new tubing for each bottle.

Twisting the spike helps ensure that particles from the stopper do not fall into the bottle. New tubing reduces the growth of microorganisms (the feeding provides a medium for fungal growth).

12. **Place the primed tubing** in the pump and attach the tubing to the IV catheter lumen.

   ✚ Identify the correct IV line and port for the infusion. Trace the tubing from the bag back to the patient.

   a. Thoroughly scrub the catheter injection port or hub and the luer-lock threads with an antiseptic wipe.
   b. If you are infusing lipids simultaneously with PN, attach the primed lipid tubing to the injection port/hub closest to the patient, below the tubing filter, or through a Y-connection at the catheter hub.
   c. Turn the luer-lock to secure the connection.

(continued on next page)

Procedure 28–6 ■ Administering Lipids (continued)

d. ✚ *Note:* If a previous infusion has been running, clamp the catheter lumen and the old administration set tubing before disconnecting and changing the tubing.

Lipids are compatible with PN and you can piggyback them into the same tubing. However, the lipids must be below the filter because their large particles will not go through a PN filter.

13. **Begin the infusion.** Ideally, infuse slowly at first: 1.0 mL/min for adults and 0.1 mL/min for children (or as prescribed by the physician). Check again to be sure the catheter-tubing connection is secure.

Slow infusion allows time to assess if the patient will have an adverse reaction to the lipids. Nausea, vomiting, and elevated temperature have been reported when lipids are infused quickly.

14. **Take the vital signs now,** then every 10 minutes for 30 minutes. Observe for side effects (e.g., chills, fever, flushing, dyspnea, nausea, vomiting, headache, back pain).

15. **If no reactions occur,** adjust to the prescribed infusion rate and continue monitoring according to your agency's protocol.

16. **Remove gloves and perform hand hygiene.**

17. **When the infusion is finished,** discard the bottle and IV administration set.

Formula contains sugars that are a medium for growth of pathogens.

? What if . . .

- **The entire bottle of lipids is not used?**

Discard partially used bottles.
Prevents contamination.

Evaluation

- If ordered, monitor serum lipids 4 hours after discontinuing the infusion.
- Monitor the IV site for infection, inflammation, and infiltration.
- Monitor for symptoms of fat emboli.
- Monitor the IV line for patency.
- Monitor for allergic reactions (nausea, vomiting, headache, chest pain, back pain, fever).
- Monitor for lipid intolerance (triglyceride levels, liver function tests, hepatosplenomegaly, decreased coagulation, cyanosis, dyspnea).

Patient Teaching

- Inform the patient and family of the purpose and duration of the nutritional support.
- Teach the patient to recognize and report symptoms of complications associated with lipids infusion.

Home Care

- The home environment must provide dry storage space for supplies, a refrigerator for storing solutions, a clean low-traffic area for procedure preparation, and electronic outlets for any electronic equipment.
- Teach safe disposal of supplies.
- Provide verbal and written instructions for the procedures; demonstrate and ask for a return demonstration.
- Instruct about solution hang time and management of the access device.
- Provide 24-hour phone numbers for the primary care provider and home care agency.

Documentation

- A special form may be used for documenting lipids and PN administration.
- Bottle number, date and time hung, volume, type of fluid, and rate of delivery
- Status of dressing, and date and time of dressing or tubing change (if performed)
- Patient's tolerance of the procedure and any problems encountered
- Pre- and post-administration assessment data and blood tests, if any
- Condition of the IV site
- Weight
- I&O

Practice Resources

American Society for Parenteral and Enteral Nutrition (A.S.P.E.N.) Board of Directors, 2009a; A.S.P.E.N. Board of Directors and Task Force on Parenteral Nutrition Standardization, 2007; Infusion Nurses Society, 2006a, 2006b; National Guideline Clearinghouse, 2006a, 2006b, 2008a, 2008b; Task Force for the Revision of Safe Practices for Parenteral Nutrition, 2004.

To explore learning resources for this chapter,

Go to Davis*Plus* at **http://davisplus.fadavis.com,** keyword Treas.

Chapter Resources for Chapter 28:
    Knowledge Check and Think Like a Nurse Response Sheets
    Knowledge Check Answers
    Resources for Caregivers and Health Professionals
    Reading More About Nutrition (suggested readings)
    What Are the Main Points in This Chapter?
NCLEX-Style Review Questions
Chapter Overview Podcasts

Concept Map

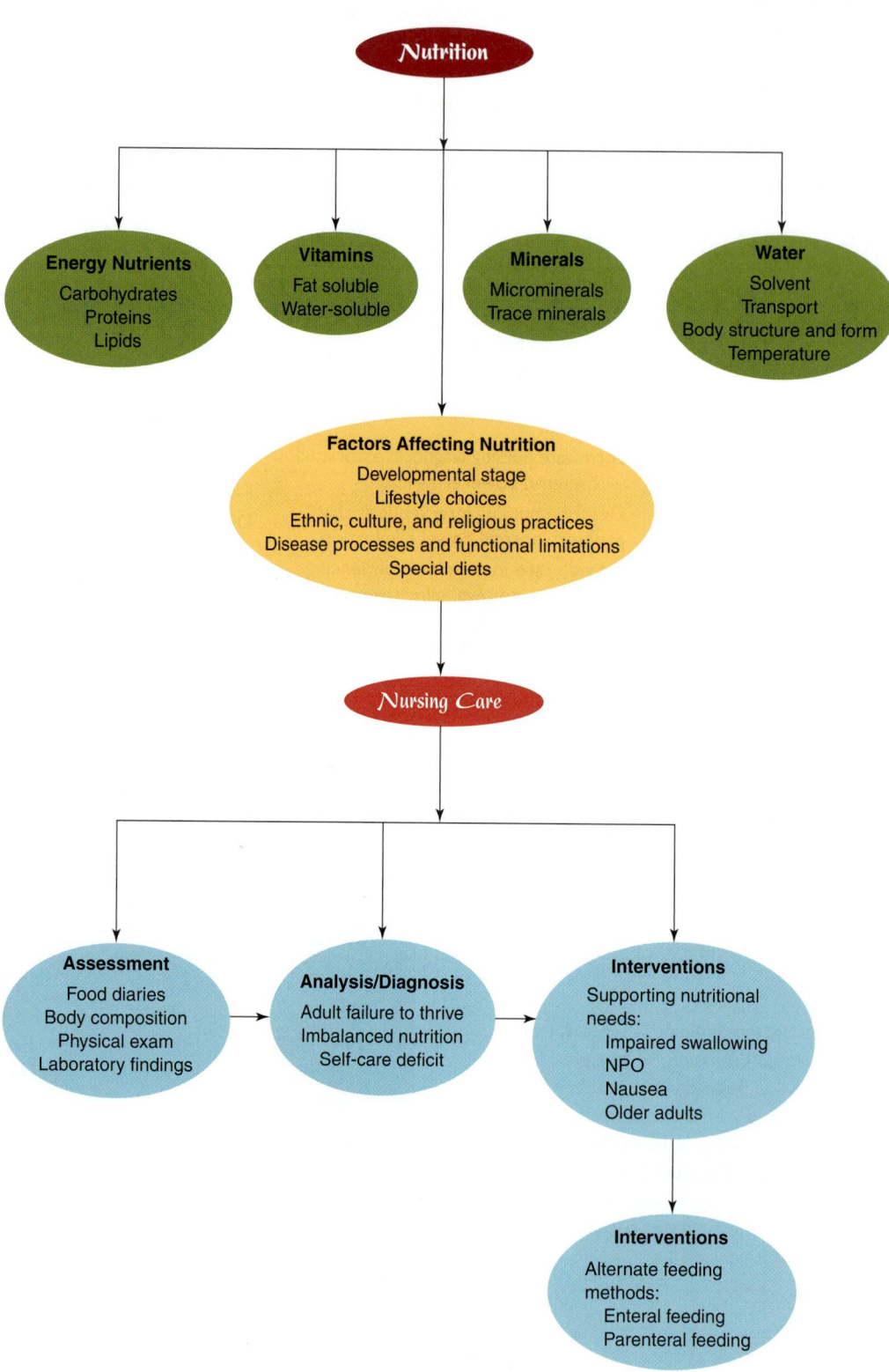

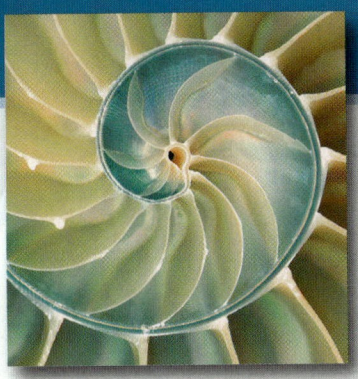

Bowel Elimination

Learning Outcomes

After completing this chapter, you should be able to:

➤ Identify the basic structures and functions of the gastrointestinal system.

➤ Discuss factors that affect bowel elimination.

➤ Describe normal bowel elimination.

➤ Differentiate among the various types of bowel diversions.

➤ Discuss common bowel elimination problems.

➤ Identify appropriate nursing history questions to assess bowel elimination problems.

➤ Perform a physical examination focused on bowel elimination.

➤ List and describe diagnostic tests used to identify bowel elimination problems.

➤ Formulate nursing diagnoses associated with altered bowel elimination.

➤ Describe nursing interventions that promote normal bowel elimination.

➤ Provide care for clients experiencing alterations in bowel elimination.

➤ Discuss nursing care associated with the use of bowel diversions.

Key Concepts

Bowel elimination

Motility

Related Concepts

See the Concept Map at the end of this chapter.

Example Problems

Diarrhea

Constipation and impaction

Bowel incontinence

Caring for the Nguyens

This feature allows you to practice the kind of thinking you will use as a full-spectrum nurse. There is usually more than one correct answer to a critical thinking question, so we do not provide answers for these features. It is more important to develop your nursing judgment than to "cover content." Discuss the questions with your peers. If you are still unsure, consult your instructor.

Yen Nyugen arrives at the family health center for a scheduled appointment, accompanied by her grandson, Kim Phan. Recently, Yen has been constipated and has had several episodes of bleeding with bowel movements (BMs). She has read that a change in bowel habits is a sign of colon cancer and is worried about that. She brought her grandson along because he is also having bowel problems. Kim's bowel habits are erratic. At times he has a soft BM.

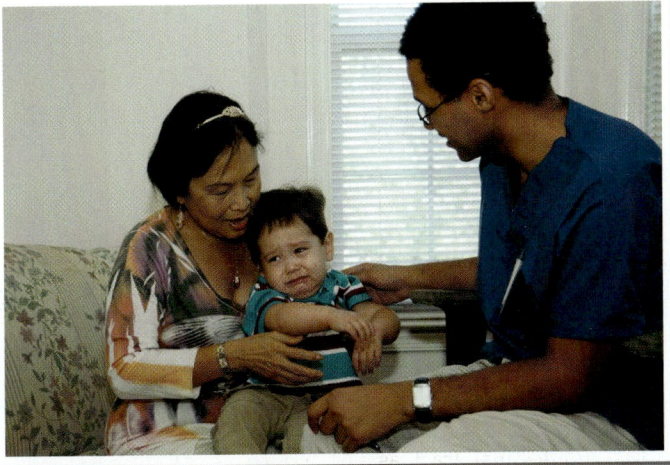

However, he has also had bouts of constipation and diarrhea. Yen would like advice on her grandson's elimination status. As a critical thinker, you will begin by obtaining accurate, credible information.

A. What history questions would be appropriate to ask Yen regarding her bowel concerns? What data do you need? How can you get the data? Are the data accurate? What information is important; what is not? Write some specific questions, just as you would ask them in an interview.

Caring for the Nguyens (continued)

B. What physical assessments would you conduct for Yen to add to, and possibly to validate, your subjective data?

C. Now you must consider the context. What factors must you consider when gathering a history on Kim?

D. The family nurse practitioner (FNP) examines Yen and determines that she has external hemorrhoids that have been bleeding because of recent straining at stool. The FNP prescribes rectal suppositories to decrease the swelling of the hemorrhoids and asks you to teach Yen about necessary lifestyle changes. What additional information will you need to gather to provide this

teaching? Recall that you have already obtained a significant amount of information from the history questions. Again, think about context: Whatever the content of your teaching, Yen will be using that information to care for herself and her grandson in her home.

E. The FNP examines Kim and tells you that the examination is normal. Use your theoretical knowledge of bowel elimination and Kim's developmental stage to think of possible reasons for his erratic bowel pattern.

 Go to **Caring for the Nguyens Response Sheet** on *DavisPlus*.

Meet Your Patient

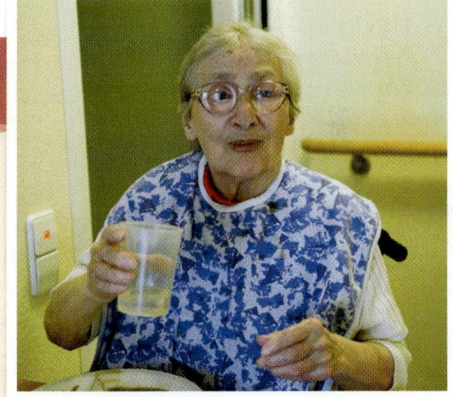

You are assigned to care for Mrs. Zeno, a frail 96-year-old woman who broke her hip last month after a fall at home. Mrs. Zeno was hospitalized for surgical repair of her hip and is now in a skilled nursing facility (SNF) for rehabilitation. The nursing assistive personnel (NAP) informs you that Mrs. Zeno has eaten poorly for the past week, only picking at the food on her meal trays and refusing the protein supplements that were added to her diet. Mrs. Zeno tells you she would like to go home: "I have my routine and the foods I like. I think I'd be better there." As you review the chart in preparation for clinical, you note that she has not had a bowel movement (BM) for 3 days. Her last BM was small and very hard.

What additional assessments should you perform? What, if anything, is of concern about her bowel pattern? What actions should you take with Mrs. Zeno?

In this chapter, you will gain theoretical and practical knowledge to help you answer those questions and provide care for clients with bowel elimination concerns.

Theoretical Knowledge
knowing **why**

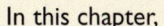

Bowel elimination is a normal process by which we eliminate waste products from our bodies. In this chapter you will come to understand concepts underlying the function of the gastrointestinal tract as well as factors that affect bowel elimination.

ABOUT THE KEY CONCEPTS

Bowel elimination is one of the overarching concepts in this chapter—the "hook" on which you hang your theoretical knowledge. The other key concept, **motility,** helps you to understand how normal elimination occurs and what is occurring in problems such as constipation and diarrhea. Other, more specific, concepts will flesh out your understanding of bowel elimination. For example, when you grasp the concept of bowel diversion, you will see why it is used in various bowel elimination problems. As you study the chapter, identify the concepts and try to understand how they relate to each

other. They will be useful for any medical diagnosis affecting bowel elimination.

WHAT ARE THE ANATOMICAL STRUCTURES OF THE GASTROINTESTINAL TRACT?

The gastrointestinal (GI) tract is a smooth-muscle tube approximately 9 m (30 ft) long for average adult males, running through the body from the mouth to the anus. Its major functions are to digest and absorb the nutrients present in food and to eliminate food waste products as feces. The structures of the GI tract are the mouth, esophagus, stomach, small intestine, large intestine, rectum, and anus (Fig. 29-1).

Mouth

Mechanical digestion begins in the mouth with **mastication,** or chewing. Food is torn into small pieces, mashed, moistened with saliva, and formed into a bolus that is then swallowed into the esophagus. The mouth contains glands that secrete enzymes, such as ptyalin and salivary amylase, which begin the digestion of carbohydrates.

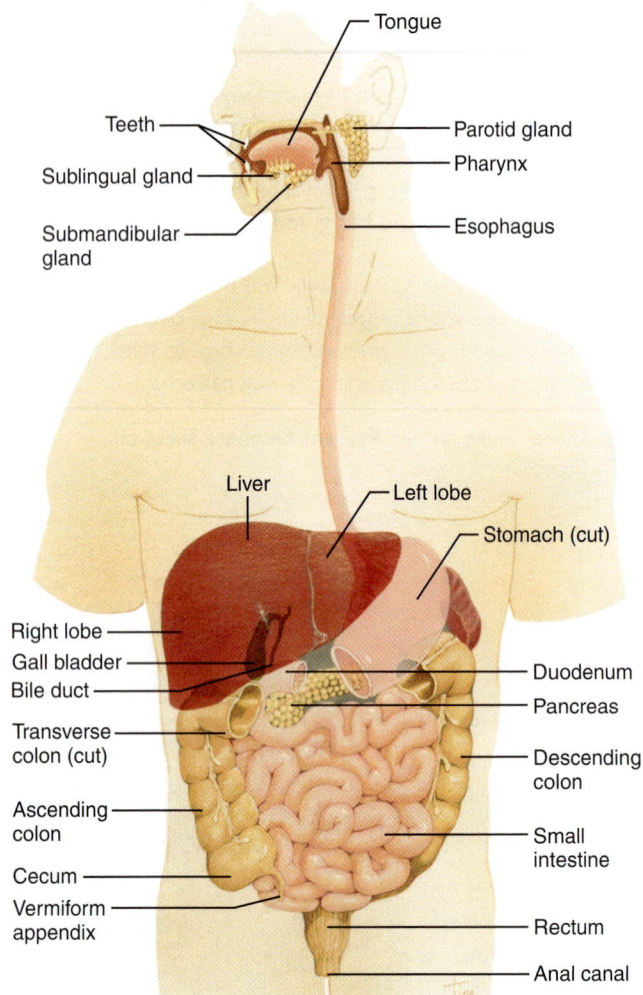

- Tongue
- Teeth
- Sublingual gland
- Submandibular gland
- Parotid gland
- Pharynx
- Esophagus
- Liver
- Left lobe
- Stomach (cut)
- Right lobe
- Gall bladder
- Bile duct
- Transverse colon (cut)
- Ascending colon
- Cecum
- Vermiform appendix
- Duodenum
- Pancreas
- Descending colon
- Small intestine
- Rectum
- Anal canal

FIGURE 29-1 The gastrointestinal tract extends from the mouth to the anus. The major functions of the GI system are to digest and absorb the nutrients in food and to eliminate food waste products as feces. (*Source:* Scanlon, V., & Sanders, T. [2007]. *Essentials of anatomy and physiology* [5th ed.]. Philadelphia: F. A. Davis. Used with permission. p. 371.)

Pharynx

The pharynx is the back part of the throat where food and air pass after chewing. To prevent choking and aspiration, a flap of connective tissue, called the **epiglottis,** closes over the trachea when food is swallowed.

Esophagus

The esophagus is a tube of smooth muscle, which alternately contracts and relaxes in waves of **peristalsis** to push the bolus toward the stomach. The bolus of food travels the length of the esophagus (about 25 cm, or 10 in.) in about 10 seconds. The *cardiac sphincter* (also called the *gastroesophageal sphincter*) then relaxes to allow the food to pass into the stomach. When the cardiac sphincter constricts, it prevents acidic stomach contents from flowing back into the esophagus.

Stomach

The stomach is a J-shaped, distensible sac made of thick, elastic muscle that extends from the esophagus to the small intestine. The stomach stores food while it churns and mixes it, providing further mechanical breakdown. Chemical digestion

continues in the stomach, which secretes hydrochloric acid (HCl), a protein-digesting enzyme called *pepsin,* and *gastric lipase,* an enzyme that begins the digestion of lipids. The stomach lining also secretes a mucous coating that protects the stomach from being corroded by HCl. Food remains in the stomach an average of 4 hours. Food leaves the stomach as a liquid, called **chyme.**

Small Intestine

The small intestine is a folded, twisted, and coiled tube that connects the stomach and the large intestine. About 2.5 cm (1 in.) in diameter and approximately 7 m (22 ft) long in an adult male if fully extended, it occupies most of the abdominal cavity. Most digestion and absorption of food occurs in the small intestine. Chyme travels slowly, by peristalsis, through the small intestine; peristalsis halts periodically to allow for absorption.

The small intestine consists of three segments: the duodenum, jejunum, and ileum.

- The **duodenum** is the first section of the small intestine. It is a C-shaped tube that branches off from the stomach, about 30 to 60 cm (1 to 2 ft) long. The duodenum processes chyme by mixing it and adding enzymes. The bile duct and main pancreatic duct both enter the small intestine at the level of the duodenum, providing bile from the liver and gallbladder to digest lipids and pancreatic enzymes to digest lipids, proteins, and carbohydrates.
- The **jejunum** is the coiled midsection of the small intestine. It is about 1.8 to 2.4 m (6 to 8 ft) long and forms the connection between the duodenum and ileum. Its major function is to absorb carbohydrates and proteins.
- The **ileum** joins the small and large intestine. It is responsible for absorption of fats; bile salts; and some vitamins, minerals, and water. However, nutrients are absorbed mainly in the duodenum and jejunum.

The inner wall of the small intestine is covered by millions of tiny fingerlike projections called **villi** (Fig. 29-2). The villi are covered with even tinier projections, called **microvilli.** The combination of folds, villi, and microvilli increases the surface area of the small intestine greatly, facilitating absorption of nutrients.

Large Intestine

The **large intestine,** also known as the **colon,** is larger in diameter than the small intestine (6.3 cm, or 2.5 in.) but shorter in length—about 1.5 to 1.8 m (5 to 6 ft). It extends from the ileum of the small intestine to the anus. It contains seven segments: the cecum, ascending colon, transverse colon, descending colon, sigmoid colon, rectum, and anus (Fig. 29-3).

Undigested food entering the first portion of the large intestine, the **cecum,** consists mostly of cellulose and water. The connection of the ileum to the cecum is controlled by the **ileocecal valve.** Under most conditions, the valve prevents backflow of chyme from the colon into the small intestine. The **appendix** is a small, finger-like appendage off the cecum. It is believed to be a **vestigial organ**—one whose significance has diminished over time—however, it is lined with lymphatic tissue and may play a role in immune function.

The next three segments, the **ascending, transverse,** and **descending colon,** ring the small intestine. The **sigmoid colon** is a final, small segment of bowel that twists medially and downward to connect with the rectum and anus.

The colon secretes mucus, which facilitates smooth passage of stool, and absorbs water, some vitamins, and minerals.

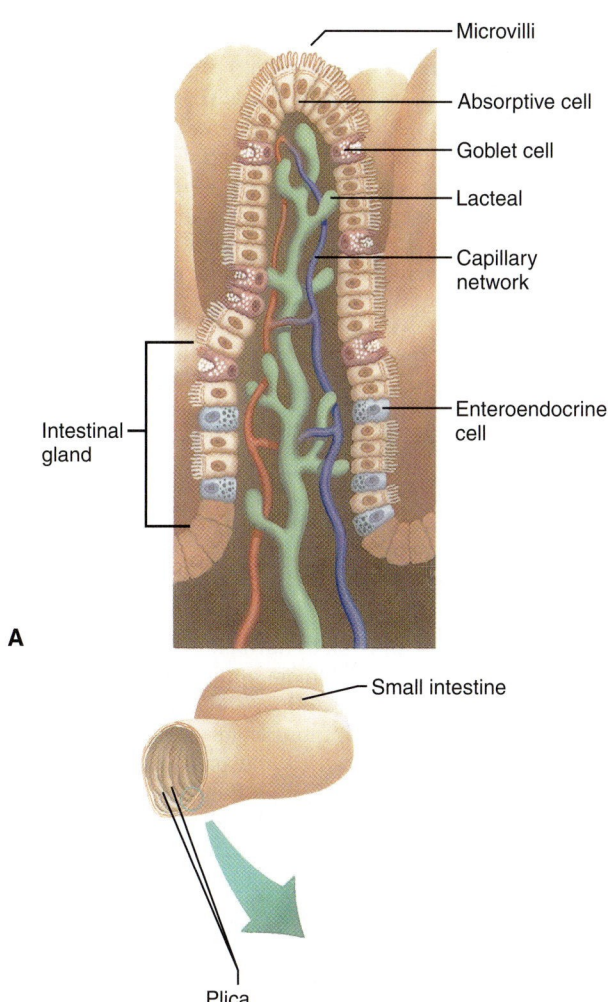

A

B

Plica circulares

FIGURE 29-2 The small intestine is highly folded, providing a vast surface area for absorption of nutrients. The microvilli form a brush border, which is the site of most nutrient absorption. A. Section through the small intestine showing the plica circulares (circular folds) of the mucosa and submucosa. B. Microscopic view of a villus showing the internal structure. (*Source:* Scanlon, V., & Sanders, T. [2007]. *Essentials of anatomy and physiology* [5th ed.]. Philadelphia: F. A. Davis, p. 383. Used with permission.)

Approximately 80% of the fluid that enters the colon is reabsorbed along its passage. Normal flora in the colon aid in the digestive process. These bacteria are responsible for producing vitamin K and several of the B vitamins.

The large intestine has two sets of muscles that give it a puckered appearance. Longitudinal muscles, known as **taenia coli,** run lengthwise along the colon surface. Tension in these muscles gathers up the colon into pouched segments known as **haustra** all along its length (see Fig. 29-3). In addition, the colon wall contains circular muscles that, together with the taenia coli, cause the colon to expand and contract in length and width to achieve haustral churning, peristalsis, and mass peristalsis.

- **Haustral churning** moves digestive contents around within each haustra. This action promotes reabsorption of water.
- **Peristalsis** continues throughout the length of the large intestine, where it propels intestinal contents toward the rectum and anus.
- **Mass peristalsis** is a powerful contraction along a lengthy segment of bowel. It is facilitated by the **gastrocolic reflex,**

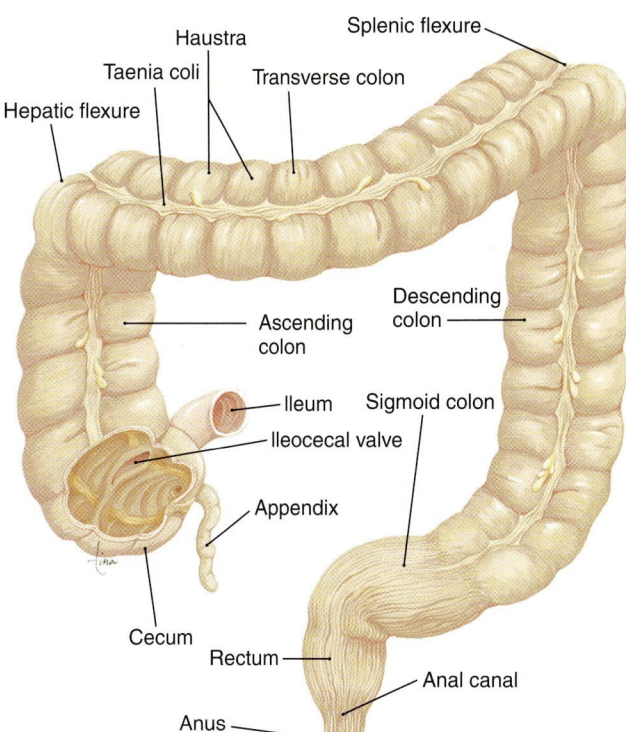

FIGURE 29-3 The large intestine shown in anterior view. The term *flexure* means a turn or bend. (*Source:* Scanlon, V., & Sanders, T. [2007]. *Essentials of anatomy and physiology* [5th ed.]. Philadelphia: F. A. Davis, p. 385. Used with permission.)

which is triggered by food entering the stomach and small intestine. Mass movements usually occur only one to three times each day, and they are responsible for most of the propulsion of the contents in the transverse and sigmoid colon.

Rectum and Anus

The **rectum** is approximately 15 cm (6 in.) long and is continuous with the **anus,** the last 2.5 cm (1 in.) of the colon. A highly vascular folded tube, the rectum is free of waste products until just before defecation.

The anus has two ring-like muscles that function as sphincters. The **internal sphincter** involuntarily relaxes and opens when stool is present in the rectum. The **external sphincter** is under voluntary control. Voluntary relaxation of the external sphincter allows stool to be expelled from the body (Fig. 29-4). The anus is highly vascular. Chronic pressure on the veins within the anal canal, as with prolonged sitting or retained feces, can cause **hemorrhoids** (distended blood vessels within or protruding from the anus).

KnowledgeCheck 29-1

- What are the major functions of the small intestine and large intestine?
- How do the rectum and anus control elimination of feces from the body?

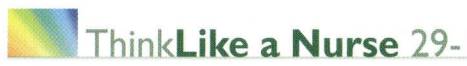 ThinkLike a Nurse 29-1

Based on your knowledge that hemorrhoids are dilated blood vessels in the anal canal, what symptoms would you expect a patient with hemorrhoids to exhibit?

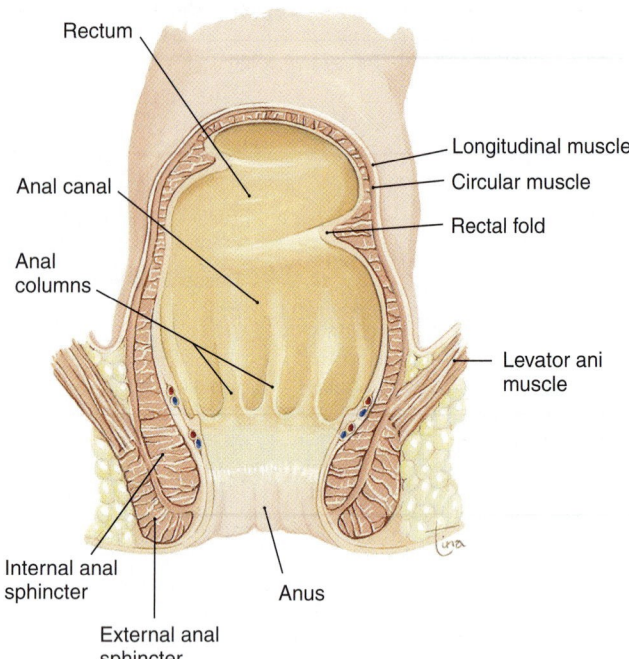

FIGURE 29-4 Internal and external anal sphincters shown in a frontal section through the lower rectum and anal canal. (*Source:* From Scanlon, V., & Sanders, T. [2007]. *Essentials of anatomy and physiology* [5th ed.]. Philadelphia: F. A. Davis, p. 387. Used with permission.)

HOW DOES THE BOWEL ELIMINATE WASTE?

As you have learned, reabsorption of water from chyme in the large intestine produces a semisolid mass known as **feces.** Feces are a mixture of insoluble fiber, undigested food, shed epithelial cells, inorganic material (e.g., calcium and phosphates), bacteria, and water that were not absorbed during passage through the GI tract. Small amounts of fat may be present.

Feces are usually brown because **bile salts,** which aid in the digestion of fat, are excreted in the feces. Bile is normally golden yellow, but the action of bacteria in the GI tract changes the color to brown. Bacteria are also responsible for the odor of feces.

Flatus, or gas, is formed in the digestive process. Some is swallowed air that accompanies the intake of food. A small portion diffuses from blood into the GI tract. However, most of the gas is created by bacterial fermentation in the colon.

The Process of Defecation

The process by which the bowel eliminates waste is called **defecation.** When fecal material reaches the rectum and causes it to distend, (1) stretch receptors are stimulated to start contraction of the sigmoid colon and rectal muscles, and (2) the internal anal sphincter relaxes. At the same time, sensory impulses transmitted to the central nervous system (CNS) produce a conscious urge to defecate. We respond to this signal by voluntarily contracting our diaphragm and abdominal muscles to increase downward pressure, while at the same time relaxing the external anal sphincter. These actions allow feces to be propelled through the anus. If we ignore the signal to defecate, the reflexive contractions ease for a few minutes, until mass peristalsis occurs again.

A person can increase the pressure to expel feces by contracting the abdominal muscles (straining) while maintaining a closed airway (e.g., holding the breath). This is called the **Valsalva maneuver.** Although it assists with the passage of stool, you should caution clients with heart disease, glaucoma, increased intracranial pressure, or a new surgical wound to avoid the Valsalva maneuver because it increases pressure within the abdominal cavity, raises blood pressure, and is associated with an increased risk for cardiac arrhythmias.

Normal Defecation Patterns

Many people avoid the topic of bowel elimination—it is not typically something they chat about with their neighbors. As a result, many patients have unanswered questions about their bowel function and may turn to you for information.

Part of the confusion about bowel function is that there is a wide range of what is considered normal. The frequency of BMs may range from several times per day to once a week. As long as the person passes stools without excessive urgency (needing to rush to the toilet), with minimal effort and no straining, without blood loss, and without the use of laxatives, you can regard bowel function as normal.

Normal stool is a soft, formed semisolid, and approximately 75% water and 25% solid when expelled. If passage through the colon is slowed, more water is reabsorbed from the feces. The stool becomes dry and hard, requiring more effort to pass. If transit time through the colon is faster than normal, less water is reabsorbed, and stools are watery.

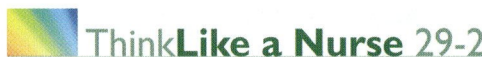

ThinkLike a Nurse 29-2

- Based on your knowledge of normal bowel function, how would you describe Mrs. Zeno's (Meet Your Patient) bowel function? Is it normal or abnormal?
- What additional information, if any, do you need to know to answer this question?

WHAT FACTORS AFFECT BOWEL ELIMINATION?

Each person develops a bowel elimination pattern that is based on several factors, discussed in the sections immediately following.

Developmental Stage

Bowel elimination patterns change gradually and normally throughout the life span.

Infants. During the first few days of life, the term newborn passes meconium through the anus. **Meconium** is green-black, tarry, sticky, and odorless. It is formed by swallowed mucus, hair, and amniotic fluid. Stools transition to a yellow-green color over the next few days. After that, the appearance of the feces depends largely on the type of feeding that the infant receives. Breastfed babies pass golden yellow stools, whereas formula-fed babies pass tan stools. Initially babies defecate frequently, usually after each feeding—especially when they are breastfeeding. The stools tend to be watery while the large intestine is still immature. Normal flora gradually develop in the colon, and stools become firmer and less frequent.

Children. The ability to control defecation typically develops at about age 2 to 3 years. Toilet training requires neural and muscular control as well as conscious effort. The child must be aware of the urge to defecate, be able to maintain closure of the external anal sphincter while getting to the toilet,

and be able to remove clothing. When toddlers become engrossed in play, they sometimes ignore the need to move their bowels, and soiling is common. As children mature, they gradually learn to gain more control over defecation. In fact, school-age children and adolescents often delay defecation until they have come home or have completed an activity.

Adults. The bowel pattern set in childhood normally continues into late adulthood if the client consumes adequate fiber and fluid and engages in regular physical activity. However, peristalsis, intestinal smooth muscle tone, perineal muscle tone, and sphincter control normally decrease with aging. These physiological processes can contribute to constipation among older adults, especially if they decrease their activity and fiber intake.

Personal and Sociocultural Factors

Privacy is important to most people, as is sufficient time to have a bowel movement without feeling the need to hurry. Clients working in fast-paced jobs may have difficulty even consciously recognizing the need to defecate, and some habitually ignore the need, promoting bowel dysfunction. Parents and caregivers of infants and toddlers may postpone their own toileting needs because of fear of leaving the children alone. Some clients are acutely embarrassed by the thought that anyone might realize they are having a bowel movement and will wait until they are entirely alone before even entering the bathroom.

Have you ever heard the following phrase: "He puts his stress in his gut"? Stress has a major influence on motility of the GI tract. It may cause diarrhea or constipation, and it is a primary risk factor in the development of *irritable bowel syndrome*, a disorder associated with bloating, pain, and altered bowel function.

Nutrition, Hydration, and Activity Level

Nutrition, hydration, and activity all affect bowel function.

Foods and Fiber. Regular intake of food promotes peristalsis. People who eat on a regular schedule are likely to develop a regular pattern of defecation, whereas irregular eating contributes to an irregular pattern. Adequate intake of high-fiber promotes peristalsis and defecation. Bulky foods absorb fluids and increase stool mass. The increased mass stretches bowel walls, initiating peristalsis and the defecation reflex. Most people should have at least five servings of high-fiber foods each day. Examples are fresh fruits and berries; dried fruits; vegetables (especially raw); whole-grain cereal products; flaxseed; popcorn; and dried beans, peas, and legumes.

Other foods have specific effects in the bowel. For example, the active bacteria in yogurt stimulate peristalsis, while at the same time promoting healing of intestinal infections. Low-fiber foods, such as pasta and other simple carbohydrates and lean meats, slow peristalsis. Foods like broccoli, onions, and beans lead to excess gas in many people. Spicy foods may also cause gas, as well as more frequent bowel movements.

Dietary Supplements. Dietary supplements can also affect bowel function. For example, calcium supplements may cause constipation, whereas magnesium loosens stools. Supplemental vitamin C softens stools and, in high doses, may cause diarrhea in sensitive clients.

Fluids. A minimum of six to eight 8-ounce glasses (1,500 to 2,000 mL) of fluid per day is required to promote healthful bowel function. Inadequate fluid intake or excessive fluid loss, as in diarrhea or vomiting, slows peristalsis and leads to dry, hard stools that are difficult to pass (Wilson, 2005). Excessive fluid intake (especially beverages with high sugar content) may lead to rapid passage through the colon and soft or watery stools. Different types of fluids have varying effects on sensitive individuals. For instance, consuming large amounts of milk may cause constipation in some people. Coffee promotes peristalsis in many clients and may even cause loose stools in sensitive clients.

Activity. Physical activity seems to stimulate peristalsis and bowel elimination. In addition, sedentary people are likely to have weaker abdominal muscles. Clients with health concerns that limit activity (e.g., shortness of breath, pain, or required bedrest) often experience constipation.

Medications

Many medications may affect peristalsis. All oral medicines have the potential to affect the function of the GI tract. Examples include the following:

- *Antacids,* often used for heartburn, neutralize stomach acid but may slow peristalsis.
- *Aspirin and other nonsteroidal anti-inflammatory drugs (NSAIDs),* such as naproxen and ibuprofen, irritate the stomach. Repeated use can lead to ulceration of the stomach or duodenum.
- *Antibiotics* given to combat infection decrease the normal flora in the colon. The result is often diarrhea. Bacterial populations can be maintained with supplements of probiotics (e.g., acidophilus) or daily consumption of yogurt.
- *Iron,* a common mineral supplement, is available as an over-the-counter (OTC) medication and is often prescribed for the treatment of anemia. Iron has an astringent effect on the bowel and is notorious for causing constipation and changing stool color to black. It also causes nausea when taken when there is no food in the stomach.
- *Pain medications,* particularly opioids (narcotics), slow peristalsis and are associated with a high incidence of constipation.
- *Antimotility drugs,* such as diphenoxylate (Lomotil), may be used to treat diarrhea. They work by slowing peristalsis.
- *Laxatives* are used to treat constipation. In general, laxatives work by stimulating peristalsis (see Box 29-1). They are frequently abused by people who self-medicate with OTC drugs, who may become dependent on them, requiring ever-increasing dosages until the intestine fails to work properly.

Surgery and Procedures

Clients undergoing anesthesia and surgery often experience sluggish bowel elimination. The delay in bowel elimination may be caused by a variety of circumstances:

Anesthesia. General anesthesia (which renders the patient unconscious) and analgesics (administered preoperatively and postoperatively for pain) slow bowel motility. Spinal anesthesia and epidural anesthesia are less likely to cause this effect.

Stress. Regardless of the type of anesthesia, most clients find surgery a stressful event. As you may recall from Chapter 12, if stress activates the general adaptation syndrome (GAS), autonomic nervous system and endocrine responses ensue. Among those responses is a slowing of peristalsis.

Manipulation of the Bowel During Surgery. Abdominal or pelvic surgery in which the bowel is manipulated may result in a **paralytic ileus,** a cessation of bowel peristalsis. Although peristalsis halts, the bowel continues to produce secretions. Without peristalsis, secretions remain stagnant, causing distention and discomfort. To decrease the complications of paralytic ileus, patients who have had bowel surgery typically have a nasogastric (NG) tube with low constant or intermittent suction. The NG tube removes secretions until peristalsis returns. To review insertion of an NG tube or management of a patient with an NG tube, refer to Procedure 28-2.

BOX 29-1 ■ Types of Laxatives

- **Stool softeners** enable moisture and fat to penetrate the stool, thereby softening it and making it easier to pass. Example: docusate sodium. Effectiveness of stool softeners in relieving chronic constipation is being questioned, but they are still in use.
- **Osmotic laxatives** work by drawing water into the bowel from surrounding tissue, resulting in bowel distention. Examples: polyethylene glycol, lactulose.
- **Lubricant laxatives** coat the stool and the GI tract with a thin waterproof layer. Mineral oil is an example. Because the lubricant coats the entire GI tract, it may interfere with the absorption of nutrients.

   ✚ Mineral oil is potentially dangerous in debilitated patients. Inhaled droplets can lead to a form of pneumonia.

- **Stimulant laxatives** are bowel irritants. They irritate the intestinal wall, stimulating intense peristalsis. Examples: senna, bisacodyl, castor oil.
- **Bulking agents** are high in fiber. They must be combined with sufficient fluid intake to be effective. The fiber attracts fluid into the colon, and the increased bulk of the stool stimulates the urge to evacuate. These are considered the safest form of laxative, but may interfere with absorption of some medicines. They are the drug of choice for chronic constipation. Examples: Metamucil, Citrucel, psyllium, FiberCon.
- **Chloride channel activators** increase intestinal fluid and motility to help stool pass.
- **Combination laxatives** are laxatives that contain more than one type of laxative ingredient. The most common type is a combination stimulant laxative and stool softener.

Decreased Mobility. After surgery, patients often experience discomfort that affects mobility. This further hinders GI motility and increases the risk for constipation.

Perineal Surgery. Patients who have had surgical interventions involving the perineal region (e.g., an episiotomy after childbirth) may fear pain or that their sutures will "tear" or "break" during bowel elimination, and therefore they resist the urge to evacuate their bowel.

Anal Sphincter Surgery. Patients who have had surgery that disrupts the anal sphincter may experience uncontrolled drainage after surgery.

Pregnancy

In early pregnancy, many women experience fluid loss due to "morning sickness"—periods of nausea and vomiting. As the pregnancy progresses, the growing uterus crowds and displaces the intestines, and along with the increased level of progesterone, slows intestinal motility. As a result, pregnant women often experience constipation, decreased appetite, and irregular food intake. In addition, the increasing pressure of the uterus and the increased blood volume of normal pregnancy increase the woman's risk for hemorrhoids.

ThinkLike a Nurse 29-3

- Review the case of Mrs. Zeno (Meet Your Patient). What factors may be affecting her bowel elimination?
- What additional information do you need?

Pathological Conditions

Several disorders affect bowel function. Among them are neurological disorders that affect innervation of the lower GI tract, cognitive conditions that limit the ability to sense the urge to defecate, pain or immobility that leads to sluggish peristalsis, and pathological conditions of the GI tract. Constipation and diarrhea are discussed in the Nursing Diagnosis section of the chapter. Other common disorders are food allergies, food intolerances, and diverticulosis.

Food Allergies. The National Institute of Allergy and Infectious Diseases (NIAID) characterizes a **food allergy** as a true immune system reaction prompted by the presence in the body of an allergenic food (NIAID, 2001). Some common food allergens include dairy products, egg whites, shellfish, gluten, peanuts and other nuts, citrus fruits, and soy. Immune responses to foods manifest as a variety of symptoms ranging from a mild rash to anaphylactic shock. Common GI symptoms suggesting food allergy include constipation; diarrhea; a red, blistering rash around the anus; abdominal discomfort; bloating; excessive gas; and intestinal bleeding (Chapman, Bernstein, Lee, et al., 2006).

Food Intolerances. In contrast to a food allergy, **food intolerance** is specifically linked to the GI system. It produces symptoms, such as GI discomfort, pain, gas, bloating, diarrhea, or constipation after the person consumes the food. An example is *lactose intolerance,* a deficiency of the enzyme lactase, which is responsible for the breakdown of milk sugar (lactose). Such symptoms can mimic those of a food allergy, but food intolerances are not caused by immune responses.

Diverticulosis. When the colon must repeatedly move highly compacted fecal material, over time the longitudinal and circular muscles enlarge. This increases force on the mucosal tissues, causing them to "balloon" out between the muscles and to form pouches in which fecal matter becomes trapped. The development of these saclike outpouching of mucosa through the muscle layers of the colon wall is a condition called **diverticulosis.** In some cases, the pouches become infected, a condition called **diverticulitis,** and antibiotics or surgery is required. People whose diets are low in fiber or consist mainly of refined foods are especially at risk for diverticulosis. Obesity and red meat intake are also risk factors (Korzenik, 2008).

KnowledgeCheck 29-2

- What is a normal defecation pattern?
- Identify the factors that affect bowel elimination.

BOWEL CONDITIONS MAY BE TREATED MEDICALLY AND SURGICALLY

As you know, various pathologies affect the GI tract—causing motility changes, inflammation, and so on. Many can be treated with medication (e.g., laxatives, anti-inflammatory drugs). However, some conditions require surgical intervention, such as bowel diversions.

Bowel Diversions

A **bowel diversion** is a surgically created opening for elimination of digestive waste products. The procedure is performed for clients with a variety of conditions, including cancer, ulcerations, trauma, or inadequate blood supply. A client with a bowel diversion does not eliminate via the anus. Instead, the **effluent** (output, fecal material) is expelled through a surgically created opening in the abdominal wall, called a

stoma or **ostomy.** The effluent may range from liquid to solid, depending on the part of the bowel that is being diverted.

Bowel diversions may be temporary or permanent. *Temporary bowel diversions* are common after surgical interventions for benign conditions of the bowel. Once adequate healing has occurred, surgical **reanastomosis** (reconnection) of the bowel is performed, and the patient once again has BMs from the anus. *Permanent bowel diversions* are performed if the bowel is necrotic (dead) or cannot be salvaged because of severe disease or trauma.

Ileostomy

An **ileostomy** brings a portion of the ileum through a surgical opening in the abdomen, bypassing the large intestine entirely. Drainage at this level is liquid and continuous. The patient must wear an ostomy appliance at all times to collect the drainage. Some variations of ileostomy are designed to control drainage more effectively and to cause less body image disturbance. However, many clients are not candidates for these procedures because of their underlying disease. To read about these "continent" ileostomy variations,

 Go to Chapter 29, **Tables, Boxes, Figures: ESG Figure 29-1: Ileostomy Variations,** and **Supplemental Materials: Ileostomy,** on Davis *Plus.*

Colostomy

A **colostomy** is a surgical procedure that brings a portion of the colon through a surgical opening in the abdomen. The location of the colostomy determines the consistency of the feces eliminated, as well as the need to wear an ostomy appliance (Fig. 29-5). The closer the colostomy is to the ascending colon and the ileocecal valve (between the small and large intestine), the more liquid and continuous the drainage will be. In contrast, a colostomy close to the sigmoid colon will produce solid feces. Colostomies near the rectum, such as sigmoid colostomies, can often be controlled by diet and irrigation. As a result, the client may not need to wear an ostomy appliance to collect drainage.

A colostomy created in the transverse colon is usually temporary and may be either a double-barreled or loop colostomy.

- A **double-barreled colostomy** (Fig. 29-5C) has two separate stomas that externalize the bowel on both sides of the portion that has been removed. The proximal stoma is the functioning end that drains fecal material. The distal stoma may drain mucus and is sometimes called a mucous fistula.
- A **loop colostomy** (Fig. 29-6) consists of a segment of bowel brought out to the abdominal wall. The posterior wall of the bowel remains intact, but a plastic rod is wedged under the bowel to keep it from slipping back into the abdomen. The anterior wall is incised, and the mucosal surface is left visible and open to air. It, too, has a functioning proximal end and limited drainage from the distal end.

If you are interested in seeing an animation about colostomies,

 Go to Student Resources, **Animations: Colostomy,** on Davis*Plus.*

KnowledgeCheck 29-3

- What changes in bowel elimination are associated with constipation? With diarrhea?
- Why are bowel diversions performed?
- What determines the nature of the effluent from a bowel diversion?

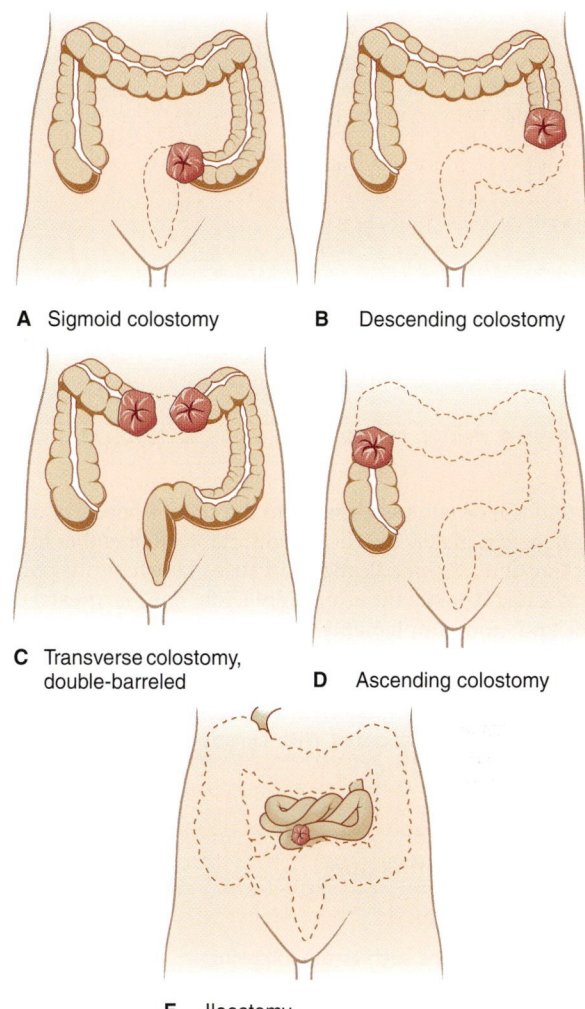

A Sigmoid colostomy   **B** Descending colostomy

C Transverse colostomy, double-barreled   **D** Ascending colostomy

E Ileostomy

FIGURE 29-5 A–E, Location of various bowel diversion ostomies. Shaded areas indicate sections of the bowel that are removed or being "rested." The closer the colostomy is to the ascending colon ("higher"), the more liquid and continuous the drainage will be.

PracticalKnowledge knowing **how**

As a nurse, you will monitor and assist clients with bowel elimination, teach about bowel function, and work collaboratively with the healthcare team to facilitate normal bowel function in well and ill clients. In the remainder of the chapter, we discuss these activities.

ASSESSMENT

To assess bowel elimination, you must obtain a nursing history; perform a physical examination focused on elimination; and review diagnostic and laboratory data.

Focused Nursing History

Because bowel patterns vary, you will need a nursing history to determine what is normal for each client. As you interview clients, pay attention to their reactions to your questions. Many people are embarrassed by discussion about bowel

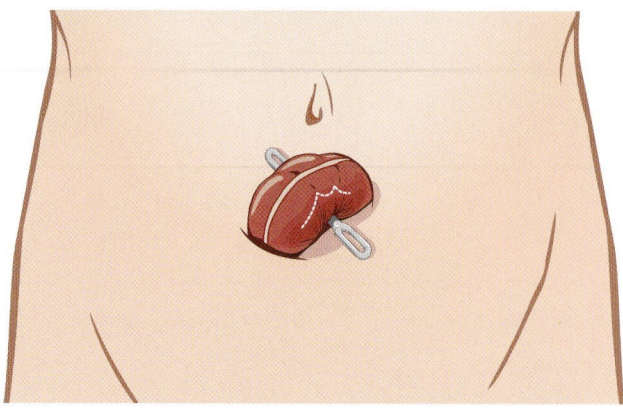

FIGURE 29-6 A loop colostomy.

function. Tailor your assessment to the client's needs, and use language that makes the client comfortable. Remember to ask the client about her medications because many have the potential to cause constipation (e.g., antacids, antidiarrheals, calcium and iron supplements). For examples of medications associated with constipation,

 Go to Chapter 29, **Tables, Boxes, Figures: ESG Box 29-3: Medications Associated With Constipation,** on *DavisPlus*.

For a list of questions that you may use in a focused bowel assessment, see the accompanying Focused Assessment box, Bowel Elimination.

For clients with a bowel diversion, you will also gather data on the client's usual care of the stoma, use of appliances, and adjustment to the ostomy. Table 29-1 describes characteristics of normal and abnormal stool.

Focused Physical Assessment

Physical assessment for bowel elimination includes examination of the abdomen, rectum, and anus. Observe the size, shape, and contour of the abdomen, and listen to bowel sounds. You might also palpate the anus and rectum for the presence of stool or masses. When auscultated,

- *Normal bowel sounds* are high pitched, with approximately 5 to 15 gurgles every minute.
- *Hyperactive bowel sounds* are very high pitched and more frequent than normal. They may occur with small bowel obstruction and inflammatory disorders and may produce diarrhea.
- *Hypoactive bowel sounds* are low pitched, infrequent, and quiet. A decrease in bowel sounds indicates decreased peristalsis, which can result in constipation.
- *Absent bowel sounds.* If after listening for 3 to 5 minutes you hear no bowel sounds, you can describe them as *absent*. Absent bowel sounds indicate a lack of intestinal activity, which may occur after abdominal surgery and indicate a paralytic ileus.

Focused Assessment

Bowel Elimination

Nursing History

Ask questions such as the following:

1. **Normal bowel pattern**
   - How often do you have a bowel movement (BM)?
   - What time of day do you usually have a BM?
   - Do you follow any routines to help you have a BM?
2. **Appearance of stool**
   - How would you describe your stool?
   - What color is your stool?
   - How would you describe the texture of your stool—hard, soft, or watery?
   - What shape is the stool?
   - Have you noticed unusual odor with your stool?
3. **Changes in bowel habits or stool appearance**
   - Have you had any changes in your bowel pattern recently?
   - Have you noticed any changes in the appearance, texture, or odor of your stool?
4. **For clients with a bowel diversion,** you will also gather data on the client's usual care of the stoma, use of appliances, and adjustment to the ostomy.
5. **History of elimination problems**
   - What has been your experience with bowel elimination problems?
   - Have you had any problems with constipation, diarrhea, or severe bloating or gas?
   - Have you ever lost control of your bowels?
   - Have you ever had bowel surgery or diagnostic procedures of the digestive tract?
6. **Use of bowel elimination aids,** including diet, exercise, medications, and remedies
   - What aids, if any, do you use to help you have a BM?
   - What foods help you maintain your bowel pattern?

- What foods do you avoid? What effect do these foods have on you?
- What is your usual fluid intake over the course of a day?
- What is your usual exercise pattern?
- What medications are you taking? Have they had any effect on your bowel elimination pattern?
- What is your current stress level? What effect does stress have on your bowel elimination pattern?

Physical Assessment

Examine the abdomen, rectum, and anus.
- Recall that in abdominal assessment, the order of the exam is inspection, auscultation, percussion, and palpation.
- Observe the size, shape, and contour of the abdomen, and listen to bowel sounds.
- Percuss and palpate the abdomen for tenderness, presence of air or solid, and presence of masses.
- Inspect the anus for signs of hemorrhoids.
- Depending on the policies of your institution as well as your skill with assessment, you might also palpate the anus and rectum for the presence of stool or masses. When listening to bowel sounds, note the presence and timing of the sounds and the presence of any bruits. Note whether bowel sounds are normal, hyperactive, hypoactive, or absent.
- If, after listening for 3 to 5 minutes, you hear no bowel sounds, you can describe them as absent.

    For a complete discussion of physical examination of the abdomen, rectum, and anus, see Procedures 21-14 and 21-19.

Table 29-1 ➤ Normal Characteristics of Feces and Variations

STOOL CHARACTERISTIC	CONDITION	AGE GROUP	DESCRIPTION
Frequency	Normal	Infants*	Bottle-fed—1 to 3 stools/day; Breastfed—4 to 6 stools/day
		Adults	Daily; 2–3 BMs/wk
	Variations (Hypermotility)	Infants*	> 6 stools/day
		Adults	> 3 stools/day
	Variations (Hypomotility)	Infants*	Bottle-fed— < 1 stool every day or 2
			Breastfed— < 1 stool/week
		Adults	< 1 stool/wk
Color	Normal	Infants*	Dark green (1st wk); then yellow
		Adults	Brown
	Variations		*Bile* pigment gives feces its brown color. Infant stools are yellow because of their rapid passage.
			White or clay-colored stool may indicate absence of bile (e.g., as in bile duct obstruction) or use of some antacids.
			Light brown stool may indicate diet high in milk products and low in meat.
			Pale, fatty stool may indicate malabsorption of fat.
			Black, tarry stool (melena) may indicate use of iron medications or upper GI bleeding; eating large quantities of red meat, spinach, and dark green vegetables may cause feces to be almost black.
			Red stool may indicate bleeding in lower intestinal tract or hemorrhoids.
			Stool darkens the longer it is left standing after defecation.
Quantity	Normal	Adults	Approximately 150 g/day
	Variations		Quantity varies with amount of food eaten, from 100 to 400 g per day.
Shape	Normal		Approximately the diameter of the rectum: about 2.5 cm (1 in.) in diameter
	Variations		Narrow, pencil-shaped stool may indicate intestinal obstruction or constriction, or rapid peristalsis.
			Small, marble-shaped stool may indicate slow peristalsis, with longer time in the large intestine.
Consistency	Normal		Formed, soft, moist
	Variations		Consistency is related to gastric motility and is affected by food and fluid intake.
			Hard stool indicates constipation. The more time the stool spends in the large intestine, the more water is reabsorbed, and the harder the stool. May also indicate dehydration.
			Liquid stool may indicate diarrhea; rapid peristalsis (e.g., from infection).
Odor	Normal		Pungent; affected by foods eaten
	Variations		Normal odor is created by putrefaction and fermentation in the lower GI tract. Odor is also influenced by the pH of the stool, which is normally neutral or slightly alkaline.
			Strong, foul odors may indicate blood in the stool, especially in the upper GI tract, or infection.

*All information about infant stool patterns applies after passage of meconium.

For complete details about a focused physical assessment of bowel function, see the Focused Assessment box, Bowel Elimination.

KnowledgeCheck 29-4

- What should you discuss with your client when performing a nursing history focused on bowel elimination?
- Describe the physical assessment you would perform for a client with constipation.

Diagnostic Tests

Several diagnostic tests may be performed to assess for bowel elimination problems (e.g., to screen for colorectal cancer, to diagnose diverticulosis). They may be classified as direct or indirect visualization studies. **Indirect visualization studies** are radiographic views of the lower GI tract. The simplest of the tests is an abdominal flat plate, an anterior to posterior (AP) x-ray view of the abdomen used to detect gallstones, fecal impaction, and distended bowel. **Direct visualization studies** are used for diagnostic and treatment purposes (see the related Diagnostic Testing box). They are invasive procedures and are conducted by a gastroenterologist, who inserts various instruments (e.g., *endoscopes*) to examine the interior of the GI tract. The nurse's role during these studies is to prepare the patient for the test, function as an assistant, and provide aftercare. You might need to assist the patient to the appropriate position, monitor the patient's tolerance of the procedure, provide pain medication or sedation to keep the patient comfortable during the exam, and provide reassurance to the patient as the test proceeds. For nursing care

before, during, and after each of the direct and indirect visualization studies,

 Go to Chapter 29, **Tables, Boxes, Figures: ESG Box 29-1: Diagnostic Testing: Direct Visualization Studies of the Gastrointestinal Tract,** and **ESG Box 29-2: Diagnostic Testing: Indirect Visualization Studies of the Gastrointestinal Tract,** on *DavisPlus.*

 ThinkLike a Nurse 29-4

A client asks you why he must perform a bowel prep with a strong laxative before having a colonoscopy. How might you reply?

Laboratory Studies of Stool

Stool specimens may be analyzed to detect blood, infection, or parasitic infestation. The client must void first and then defecate into a clean, dry bedpan, bedside commode, or a special container (half hat) placed under the toilet seat. A small sample is obtained and sent to the laboratory for analysis or analyzed at the bedside. To obtain a specimen from an infant or young child, you will collect freshly passed feces from a diaper.

Handling Stool Specimens

✚ Wear clean gloves when you handle the container or manipulate stool specimens. Use tongue blades to transfer the stool specimen to the container provided by the lab. Do not contaminate the outside of the specimen container. In most cases you will need approximately 2.5 cm (1 in.) of formed stool or 20 to

---

Diagnostic Testing

Indirect Visualization Studies of the Gastrointestinal Tract

Abdominal Flat Plate

An anterior to posterior (AP) x-ray view of the abdomen is used to detect gallstones, fecal impaction, and distended bowel. This test requires no preparation and no special post-test care.

Barium Enema (BE)

A barium enema is a radiological examination of the rectum, colon, and distal small bowel. The test is especially useful for visualizing polyps, diverticula, and tumors, and may be used to reduce certain obstructions. A rectal tube is inserted into the rectum or an existing ostomy and barium (a contrast medium) is instilled. The patient must retain the barium through several position changes while air is instilled and radiographs are obtained. As a rule, patients are not sedated. The test is invasive, so a signed informed consent is necessary.

Ultrasonography (Ultrasound)

Ultrasonography detects tissue abnormalities such as masses, cysts, edema, or stones. An ultrasound probe, called a transducer, is moved over the skin surface of the abdomen. The probe emits a sound wave that abdominal tissue and organs reflect back based on their density. The sound waves may be transformed into images visible on a computer screen.

Computed Tomography (CT) Scan

Computed tomography (CT) examines body sections from different angles using a narrow x-ray beam. It produces a three-dimensional picture of the area of the body being scanned. This test is useful in diagnosis of many abdominal disorders. A CT scan may be enhanced by injecting contrast dye that allows for improved visualization of circulatory function. The patient needs to lie very still during the procedure.

Magnetic Resonance Imaging (MRI)

Magnetic resonance imaging (MRI) is a test that uses a magnetic field and pulses of radio wave energy to produce cross-sectional images of the organs and structures inside the body. MRIs are very sensitive and may be used to detect edema, hemorrhage, blood flow, infarcts, tumors, and infections in organ structures. MRI utilizes a strong magnetic field and radio waves. It does not use ionizing radiation, so it is free of the hazards of x-rays. When used, the contrast medium is noniodinated, and it is administered intravenously to enhance contrast between normal and abnormal tissues. The patient must lie still in a narrow machine that contains a strong magnet, sometimes for up to an hour.

Source: Van Leeuwen, A., Poelhuis-Leth, D., & Bladh, M. (2011). *Davis's comprehensive handbook of laboratory and diagnostic tests with nursing implications* (4th ed.). Philadelphia: F.A. Davis.

Diagnostic Testing

Direct Visualization Studies of the Gastrointestinal Tract

➤ Because all of the following studies are invasive procedures, you should ensure that the patient has signed an informed consent.

➤ All of the procedures require some degree of advance preparation, such as fasting. Check agency policy, because preparation may vary.

➤ Preparing the patient includes telling him what he will experience and feel during the procedure.

➤ When the patient is sedated (e.g., with midazolam or diazepam), an emergency medical cart ("crash cart") must be in the room during the procedure, and the patient monitored with pulse oximetry.

➤ All of the procedures require teaching for aftercare.

➤ For all tests, explain that rectal bleeding is normal for a few days if polyps were removed or a biopsy was taken.

Esophagogastroduodenoscopy (EGD)

Provides direct visualization of the upper GI system. A *fiberoptic endoscope*, a long flexible tube with a light and lens, is introduced through the mouth and advanced for visualization of the esophagus, stomach, and duodenum. The physician may also perform tissue biopsies or coagulate bleeding sites through the endoscope.

Sigmoidoscopy

Allows visualization of the anal canal, rectum, and sigmoid colon. A rigid metal scope or a flexible fiberoptic scope may be used. The patient is usually not sedated. During the exam, the physician may perform a biopsy, remove polyps (small growths), or coagulate sources of bleeding in the area. A sigmoidoscopy is recommended as a screen for colon cancer for middle and older adults. Subsequent screening depends on the findings of the sigmoidoscopy as well as patient and family history; however, it is commonly done every 5 years.

Fiberoptic Colonoscopy

Provides direct visualization of the rectum, colon, entire large intestine, and distal small bowel. A flexible scope is inserted through the rectum and advanced to the cecum. Colonoscopy is useful in detecting lower GI disease. Many patients and healthcare providers choose a colonoscopy for cancer screening instead of a sigmoidoscopy, because colonoscopy provides greater visualization of the colon. This is the preferred test for clients with suspected problems above the level of the sigmoid colon. It may be done in a clinic or physician's office.

Source: The American Cancer Society. (2011). Detailed guide: Colon and rectum cancer. Last medical review 3/2/11. Retrieved May 9, 2012, from http://www.cancer.org/acs/groups/cid/documents/webcontent/003096-pdf.pdf; and Van Leeuwen, A., Poelhuis-Leth, D., & Bladh, M. (2011). *Davis's comprehensive handbook of laboratory and diagnostic tests with nursing implications* (4th ed.). Philadelphia: F.A. Davis.

---

30 mL of liquid stool. If blood, mucus, or purulent material is present, be sure to include this with the sample. Transport the specimen to the laboratory as soon as possible. If that is not possible, consult the laboratory for appropriate storage. Usually you will need to refrigerate the specimen until it can be received in the lab.

Testing for Fecal Occult Blood

Blood from the GI tract may be visible to the eye or occult (hidden). A fecal occult blood test (FOBT detects blood in the intestines, which is not always visible when passed through the stool from higher up in the intestine. You can perform the test for occult blood at the bedside, although some institutions require that it be done in the laboratory. It requires use of a special reagent that detects the presence of peroxidase, an enzyme present in hemoglobin. Only a small smear of stool is required. For home testing, remind patients to wash their hands before and after collecting stool. For the complete procedure, refer to Procedure 29-1.

Colorectal cancer is the third most common cancer in both women and men. Annual guaiac-based fecal occult blood testing is recommended for all patients age 50 to 75 years and older as one method of screening for colorectal cancer (some guidelines suggest every 2 yr) (American Cancer Society, 2010).

Assessing for Pinworms

Pinworms (an intestinal parasite) are small, white, threadlike worms that live in the cecum. They come to the anal area to deposit eggs during the night and migrate back up through the rectum during the day. In assessing a child, you can spread the buttocks while the child is sleeping and, using a flashlight, examine the anus to see whether any pinworms are visible to the naked eye. You can test for the presence of the eggs with tape. In the morning, as soon as the patient awakens, press clear cellophane tape against the anal opening. Remove the tape immediately, and place it adhesive side down on a slide. Alternatively, or in addition, insert a cotton-tipped swab gently into the rectum for not more than 2.5 cm (1 in.). Smear the specimen on a slide for microscopic inspection for parasites and eggs. The test may need to be repeated on consecutive days.

 Think Like a Nurse 29-5

You are reviewing a client's chart and note that the client was tested for fecal occult blood. The results are as follows:

3/10/14 negative for occult blood
3/11/14 no BM
3/12/14 no BM
3/13/14 no BM
3/14/14 positive for occult blood
3/15/14 negative for occult blood
3/16/14 negative for occult blood

What can you conclude? What questions do these findings raise?

ANALYSIS/NURSING DIAGNOSIS

Common NANDA-I nursing diagnoses related to bowel elimination include the following:

- *Bowel Incontinence* is a change in normal bowel habits characterized by involuntary passage of stool. It is more common among women and older adults. Other risk factors include

neurological diseases, stroke, sphincter damage, and inflammatory bowel disease.

- *Constipation.* Because frequency of bowel elimination varies, constipation is usually defined as a decrease in the frequency of bowel movements resulting in the passage of hard, dry stool. Constipation can be a temporary problem wherein symptoms resolve in a short time. Nearly everyone experiences constipation at some point. *Chronic constipation* typically lasts 3 months or longer and may persist for years. Unrelieved constipation may eventually result in a **fecal impaction,** in which dry, hard stools lodged in the rectum cannot be passed.
- *Risk for Constipation* is an appropriate diagnosis for clients at increased risk because of bedrest, medications such as opioids, or surgery.
- *Perceived Constipation* is an appropriate diagnosis for a client who makes a self-diagnosis of constipation and uses laxatives, suppositories, or enemas to ensure a daily bowel movement.
- *Diarrhea* is the passage of loose, unformed, or watery stools.
- *Dysfunctional Gastrointestinal Motility* is a broad label that encompasses increased, decreased, ineffective, or absent peristaltic activity within the GI system. If you use this label, you need to specify whether the GI motility is increased or decreased.
- *Toileting Self-Care Deficit* is impaired ability to perform or complete own toileting activities.

For definitions and defining characteristics of these diagnoses, consult a nursing diagnosis handbook or

 Go to Chapter 29, **Standardized Language: Nursing Diagnoses Associated With Bowel Elimination,** on Davis*Plus.*

Bowel elimination problems may also form the etiology of other nursing diagnoses and collaborative problems. Examples include the following:

- Social isolation r/t embarrassment secondary to bowel incontinence
- Potential Complication: Electrolyte imbalance secondary to diarrhea. Older adults, very young children, and infants are at especially high risk.
- Impaired Skin Integrity r/t irritating effects of feces secondary to diarrhea
- Anxiety r/t perceived need for a daily bowel movement
- Disturbed Body Image r/t bowel diversion

Think**Like a Nurse** 29-6

- What data do you have about Mrs. Zeno's (Meet Your Patient) bowel function?
- What else would you like to know about her bowel function? What other symptoms often accompany these cues?
- Which NANDA-I nursing diagnosis best describes this cue cluster?
- In addition to this nursing diagnosis, what other data in the scenario might also be contributing to her infrequent BMs?
- From the scenario data, how would you describe the etiology of Mrs. Zeno's problem?
- What questions do you still have about the etiology?

■ PLANNING OUTCOMES/EVALUATION

The general bowel elimination goal is that the patient will have soft, formed bowel movements regularly.

NOC standardized outcomes often used for bowel elimination diagnoses include the following: Bowel Continence, Bowel Elimination, and Tissue Integrity: Skin and Mucous Membranes. For a more comprehensive list of NOC outcomes for various nursing diagnoses,

 Go to Chapter 29, **Standardized Language: Selected Standardized Outcomes and Interventions for Bowel Elimination Diagnoses,** on Davis*Plus.*

When bowel elimination is the etiology, choose outcomes linked to the problem side of the diagnosis. For example, for Impaired Skin Integrity r/t irritating effects of diarrhea stool, the NOC outcomes might fall within Tissue Integrity: Skin and Mucous Membranes.

Individualized goals/outcome statements depend on the nursing diagnosis. Because normal bowel elimination patterns are individualized, regularity is based on the individual's pattern. Examples include the following:

Will resume his normal bowel pattern by (date).

Will discuss his feelings about his colostomy.

■ PLANNING INTERVENTIONS/IMPLEMENTATION

Bowel elimination is a normal physiological function. It is important for you to convey an attitude of acceptance and display professionalism when providing care for patients with bowel elimination problems.

A few examples of *NIC standardized interventions and activities* for patients with bowel elimination problems include: Bowel Incontinence Care, Constipation/Impaction Management, Diarrhea Management, Bowel Management, and Teaching: Individual. For a more comprehensive list of NIC interventions for various nursing diagnoses,

 Go to Chapter 29, **Standardized Language: Selected Standardized Outcomes and Interventions for Bowel Elimination Diagnoses,** on Davis*Plus.*

Specific nursing activities to promote normal bowel function and relieve elimination problems are found in the following sections. Both independent and dependent interventions are discussed.

Promoting Normal or Regular Defecation

Promoting regular defecation entails a number of independent nursing activities. These include providing privacy, positioning, timing, providing hydration and nutrition, promoting exercise, and teaching clients when they should seek medical assistance.

Provide Privacy

Although defecation is a normal physiological function, most patients consider it a very private matter. Taking a matter-of-fact approach confirms to patients that you are comfortable with this aspect of care. Provide privacy for your patient when discussing or providing care related to bowel elimination. When assisting a patient with bowel elimination, excuse visitors from the room, draw the dividing curtains in shared rooms, and close the door. Many patients are embarrassed by the odor of bowel movements and therefore may ignore the urge to defecate. Using an aromatic spray or other odor-reducing product may help to reduce embarrassment.

Nursing Care Plan

Client Data

Olivia Grimaldi, 59 years old, is admitted to the orthopedic unit after having a total knee replacement. She is receiving intravenous opioid analgesics for pain. Mrs. Grimaldi's nurse sits down to talk and complete the nursing admission assessment. The conversation turns to a discussion of bowel habits.

Nurse: Mrs. Grimaldi, we pay special attention to bowel elimination because many people on this unit have problems. How often do you have a bowel movement?

Mrs. G: Not as often as I'd like. I used to be very regular, but lately everything is all mixed up.

Nurse: What has changed? Tell me what's going on.

Mrs. G: Oh, it's so embarrassing. I haven't told anyone about this.

Nurse: When did this problem start?

Mrs. G: Everything started going bad when I fell and landed on this knee a few months ago. Nothing was broken, but the pain has been just awful. I knew I had arthritis, but I never felt anything like this. I couldn't sleep, the pain was so bad. The doctor put me on some pain pills—narcotics—and they helped, but I got so constipated. I started using laxatives to go to the bathroom, but I kept needing to use more and more. Sometimes I would take a laxative and then I would have to get to the bathroom quickly. I had a couple of accidents because I couldn't get to the toilet quickly enough.

Nurse: I think this is something we'll be able to help you with, Mrs. Grimaldi.

The nurse discovers that Mrs. Grimaldi drinks about 32 to 40 ounces of fluid each day and has used several stimulant laxatives and enemas to relieve her constipation. Her mobility has been significantly impaired for the past 2 months.

Nursing Diagnosis

Bowel Incontinence r/t overdistention of the rectum secondary to chronic constipation, as evidenced by client report of constipation when taking opioids and subsequent fecal incontinence with the use of laxatives.

NOC Outcomes	Individualized Goals/Expected Outcomes
Bowel Continence (0500) Bowel Elimination (0501)	*By discharge, Mrs. Grimaldi will:* **1.** Be free from fecal impaction. **2.** Begin to establish a regular pattern of stool evacuation. **3.** Describe four actions she can take to reduce the risk of constipation. *Within 1 month, Mrs. Grimaldi will:* **1.** Control stool passage without any episodes of fecal incontinence.

NIC Interventions

Bowel Management (0430)
Bowel Training (0440)

Nursing Activities	Rationale
1. Conduct a comprehensive assessment of all factors related to fecal incontinence and impaired bowel elimination.	Fecal incontinence has multiple possible causes. The best nursing interventions are those based on client assessment (Norton & Chelvanayagam, 2000). Constipation is attributed to immobility, weak straining ability, use of constipating drugs, neurological disorders, lack of dietary fiber, and poor fluid intake (Scarlett, 2004; Schnelle & Leung, 2004).

Assist With Positioning

An upright seated or squatting position is the most comfortable for defecation and decreases the need to strain. When possible, assist the patient to the bathroom to use the toilet. An alternative is to place a bedside commode next to the bed for patients who are unable to ambulate to the bathroom. A patient who must remain in bed should assume a semi-Fowler's position to use the bedpan. Patients who are unable to assume this position because of surgery, trauma, or other medical conditions must use supine or side-lying positions. These positions are unnatural for bowel elimination and place the patient at risk for constipation.

Raise the siderails or provide an overhead trapeze so that the patient can grip them to maneuver on and off the bedpan. If the patient is very weak, you may need an assistant to help you position him on the bedpan. In addition, you may need to stay with the person while he uses the bedpan to help him maintain his position. For the complete procedure, refer to Procedure 29-2.

Consider the Timing of Defecation

Recall that food entering the duodenum triggers mass peristalsis. As a result, the urge to defecate often occurs after meals. Advise patients not to ignore this urge, because doing so may result in constipation. For patients who are ambulatory, allow some free time after meals to use the restroom. For those who cannot toilet independently, assist them to ambulate to the bathroom or use the bedpan. Discuss with NAPs the need to offer assistance without waiting to be asked, so that patients experience minimal delays.

Support Healthful Intake of Food and Fluids

Teach clients the importance of a balanced diet in promoting soft, formed, regular bowel movements. Encourage a daily intake of 25 to 30 g of fiber to attract water into the stool, and promote peristalsis. The diet should be rich in fresh fruits and vegetables, whole-grain foods, legumes, and water.

Without adequate fluid intake, a high-fiber diet can actually cause constipation. Recommend a minimum intake of 1,500 mL of fluid per day to keep stool soft and aid in production of mucus to lubricate the colon. Ideally, a person should drink eight to ten 8-ounce glasses of fluid daily (2,000 to 2,400 mL). Water is the preferred fluid because soda, coffee, and tea often contain caffeine or additives that promote diuresis. However, because the diuretic effect of these fluids is minimal, they are acceptable for clients who simply will not drink enough plain water.

Also keep in mind that adding fiber does not help to relieve opioid-induced constipation unless the patient's current intake is actually deficient. In fact, excessive fiber might put the patient at risk for bowel obstruction due to the opioid-induced decreased peristalsis, delayed gastric emptying, and prolonged intestinal transit time of the feces (Müller-Lissner, Kamm, Scarpignato, et al., 2005; Yuan, 2005).

Encourage Exercise

Physical activity increases peristalsis and promotes defecation. Encourage patients to exercise three to five times per week and to engage in daily walking or light activity. Assist hospitalized or institutionalized patients to ambulate as soon as their condition permits. Even limited activity, such as getting out of bed or walking 10 feet, decreases the risk for constipation.

Provide range-of-motion (ROM) exercises for patients who must remain on bedrest. Even passive ROM (the joints are moved through ROM by the nurse) promotes peristalsis. Chapter 33 provides additional information about activity and ROM exercises, if you need it.

For clients who can perform them, the following exercises promote abdominal and perineal strength:

- *Thigh strengthening.* Have the client slowly bring one knee up to his chest, briefly hold it, then lower the leg to the bed. Repeat this pattern alternating legs. Encourage the client to perform this exercise several times per hour while he is awake.
- *Abdominal tightening.* Have the client tighten and hold the abdominal muscles for a count of five and then relax. This core exercise works the abdominal muscles used during defecation.

Teach Clients When to See a Primary Care Provider

Obviously many GI symptoms are normal and do not require treatment. For example, everyone has excessive flatus and abdominal distention at some time—perhaps as a result of a high-fat, high-sugar meal. And it is common for bowel movements to occasionally become a little irregular. However, clients need to know when a symptom may be signaling a more serious condition.

✚ Teach clients to see their primary care provider for the following if a symptom lasts longer than 3 weeks or is disabling:
- Blood in the stool (unless they have hemorrhoids and this is not an unusual occurrence for them)
- Severe stomach pain
- Change in bowel habits
- Unintended weight loss
- Constipation is not relieved after trying fiber, fluids, and exercise

KnowledgeCheck 29-5

Identify at least five independent nursing actions that you can take to encourage regular elimination in a well client.

ThinkLike a Nurse 29-7

How could you facilitate regular bowel elimination for Mrs. Zeno (Meet Your Patient)? What information do you need?

Interventions for Example Problem: Diarrhea

Diarrhea may occur as a result of contaminated food, a viral infection, or dietary change, or as a side effect of a medication. Patients with diarrhea are at risk for fluid and electrolyte imbalance, particularly potassium. Ideally, oral liquids replace the lost fluid and potassium. Infants, young children, and the frail elderly are most vulnerable and may require hospitalization and intravenous fluid replacement therapy.

Nursing interventions focus on treating the diarrhea itself, as well as its associated problems (cramping, fluid and electrolyte imbalances, and Impaired Skin Integrity):

Preventive Interventions

Diarrhea can be prevented in the following ways:
- **Teach hand hygiene.** Teach patients to wash their hands often. This helps prevent diarrhea caused by viruses and other pathogens.
- **Provide information about foods that can cause diarrhea.** Highly spiced foods, high-fat foods, greasy snacks, or large quantities of raw fruits and vegetables may cause diarrhea in

some patients. Tell patients to keep track of foods that trigger diarrhea and to eat them in moderation.

Monitoring Interventions

During the diarrhea episode, assess and monitor the following:

- **Monitor stools.** Assess frequency, amount, color, and consistency of stools to determine the severity of the diarrhea.
- **Monitor fluid balance.** Monitor intake and output, body weight, and vital signs to assess hydration. Also assess skin turgor and moistness of mucous membranes.
- **Monitor serum electrolyte levels.**
- **Monitor skin integrity.** Assess the perineal area for alterations in skin integrity. Clients with diarrhea may experience perianal irritation and excoriation.

Treatment Interventions

Treatments include medications, diet modification, and attention to fluid balance and skin integrity.

Medications. Opiates (e.g., paregoric) and opiate derivatives (e.g., loperamide) are the primary antidiarrheal drugs prescribed. Although they slow peristalsis and inhibit diarrhea, they may cause drowsiness; advise patients, especially older adults, to use them with caution. Bismuth subsalicylate (Pepto-Bismol) is a readily available OTC medication that is useful for traveler's diarrhea because it has antimicrobial and antisecretory properties.

Antidiarrheal medications are not recommended for acute diarrhea. In many cases, diarrhea is a response to infection or unusual foods and serves as a mechanism to rid the body of the pathogens or troublesome food. Although antidiarrheal medications are available without a prescription, caution patients to avoid using them unless instructed by their healthcare provider. Medication is usually reserved for use with chronic diarrhea—diarrhea that has persisted for more than 1 month.

Diet and Fluids. During the acute episode, the patient may need to modify his diet to control the diarrhea.

- Teach the patient about, or provide, a clear liquid diet, including electrolyte replacement fluids, (e.g., Pedialyte or sports drinks that have been diluted by 50% or more). Clear broth and gelatin are also good choices.
- Encourage your patient to sip liquids or take ice chips or popsicles often to replace the losses.
- Reduce the amount of fiber in your client's diet by cutting back servings of whole grain bread and fresh fruits and vegetables.
- Limit foods containing caffeine, such as coffee, strong tea, and colas.
- Avoid a sudden large intake of fluid or food when resuming a normal diet, because this may trigger mass peristalsis.
- Several medications, especially antibiotics, may cause diarrhea. A change in medications may be required. Plain yogurt and other probiotic foods consumed daily may help to prevent this response to antibiotics.
- Breastfed infants with acute diarrhea should be continued on breast milk without any need for interruption. In fact, breastfeeding has a well-known protective effect against the development of enteritis, promotes faster recovery, and provides improved nutrition.
- Advise a BRAT diet if a child with diarrhea has an appetite. A BRAT diet consists of bananas, (white) rice, applesauce, and toast. These are easy to digest, provide calories for energy without gastric irritation, and help offset potassium loss. Although developed for pediatric use, the BRAT diet is sometimes used for adults.

Interventions for Example Problem: Constipation

Many of the nursing strategies to prevent and treat constipation are identical to the activities that promote regular bowel elimination.

Short-Term Constipation

Short-term constipation is usually caused by the person's lifestyle. Risk factors include (1) decreased activity or are on bedrest, (2) opioids or other medications that slow peristalsis, and (3) decreased fluid and fiber intake. The following are some interventions:

- Increase the intake of high-fiber foods if intake is inadequate (normal adult Recommended Dietary Allowances/Adequate Intakes [RDA/AI] is 25 to 38 g, depending on age and sex).
- Increase fluid intake.
- Increase physical activity to stimulate peristalsis.
- Provide privacy for using the toilet.
- Assist the patient to a seated or squatting position whenever possible. A semi-Fowler's position is preferred for a client on bedrest.
- Allow the patient uninterrupted time to use the toilet, especially after meals, when mass peristalsis occurs.
- Encourage the patient not to ignore the urge to defecate.
- Assess for complications such as impaction and hemorrhoids.

Chronic Constipation

Chronic constipation may be associated with physiological factors such as dysfunctional intestinal motility, nervous system problems, and dysfunctional anorectal musculature. Chronic constipation causes significant psychological distress and decreased quality of life for many clients, and it may result in complications, which include intestinal impaction, anal fissures, hemorrhoids, volvulus, intestinal obstruction, rectal ulcers, fecal seepage, and bowel perforation. Lifestyle changes and nonprescription medications do not usually adequately treat chronic constipation.

When lifestyle modifications are ineffective in preventing and treating constipation, medications may be given (Box 29-1). Bulking agents are actually fiber in a nonfood source. They are the preferred medications for treating constipation. Many laxatives are readily available without prescription and are used by clients to treat actual or perceived constipation. Habitual laxative use, except for bulking agents, may cause reliance on medications for bowel elimination and, ironically, may lead to further constipation. See the Self-Care box, Teaching Your Patient About Laxative Use for key points to discuss with patients about managing constipation.

Older Adults

Screen older adults for risk factors, including a history of polypharmacy and taking laxatives. Other risk factors include impaired cognitive status, inadequate fluid intake, inadequate dietary fiber, reduced mobility, lack of privacy for toileting, and reliance on others for assistance. These are the same as risk factors for all ages, but they are more likely for older adults. Prevention measures are the same for all ages. However, for those unable to walk or who are restricted to bed, exercises such as trunk rotation, pelvic tilt, and leg lifts may be helpful. For older adults, osmotic laxatives (e.g., milk of magnesia [MOM], Miralax, and lactulose) and bulking agents have been found to be beneficial (Joanna Briggs Institute, 2008).

Teaching Your Patient About Laxative Use

Discuss the following topics with clients who have concerns about the frequency of their bowel movements or ask about laxatives.

1. The frequency of BMs may range from several times per day to once per week. As long as stools are passed without excessive urgency, with minimal effort and no straining, and without the use of laxatives, bowel function may be regarded as normal.
2. To maintain normal bowel function:
   - Eat a well-balanced diet that includes five servings of whole grains, fresh fruits, and vegetables.
   - Drink eight to ten 8-oz. glasses of fluid per day.
   - Engage in daily exercise to stimulate peristalsis.
   - Set aside uninterrupted time after breakfast or dinner for using the toilet.
   - Do not ignore the urge to defecate.
   - Whenever there is a significant or prolonged change in bowel habits, report this to your healthcare provider.
3. If you are experiencing constipation, choose bulking agents, such as Metamucil or psyllium, to treat the problem rather than other over-the-counter laxatives. Be sure to drink plenty of water when using bulking agents.

Managing Fecal Impaction

Fecal impaction is the presence of a hardened fecal mass in the rectum. The impaction often blocks the passage of normal stool and sets up a vicious cycle of furthering hardening. Liquid stool may leak, seeping around the hardened mass, and the patient may report feelings of fullness, bloating, constipation, diminished appetite, and a change in bowel habits. You can detect fecal impaction by digital examination of the rectum. To treat a fecal impaction, you will use enemas or digital removal of stool. Once the impaction has been removed, establish a bowel regimen to prevent recurrence of impactions.

Digital Removal of Stool. If fecal impaction does not respond to use of stool softeners and enemas, you will need to digitally remove feces from the rectum. Digital removal is accomplished by breaking up the hardened mass into pieces and manually extracting the pieces. You may administer an oil-retention enema at least 30 minutes before digital removal to soften the stool and decrease the patient's discomfort during the procedure.

✚ Aside from discomfort, the pressure generated in the rectum may stimulate the vagus nerve, slowing the heart rate. For that reason, you must have a prescription from the primary care provider. For complete steps, see Procedure 29-4.

Administering Enemas

An **enema** is the introduction of solution into the rectum to soften feces, distend the colon, and stimulate peristalsis and evacuation of feces. Some enema solutions are chosen because they irritate the mucosa of the rectum and sigmoid colon and assist with forceful evacuation of stool.

Before administering a prescribed enema, explain the purpose of the enema and what the patient can expect. For example, the patient will probably experience some cramping with a large-volume enema. Reassure the patient that you will be immediately available to help her to the restroom or onto the bedpan.

Responses to an enema are governed by the height of the solution container, the speed of flow, the concentration of the solution, and the resistance of the rectum. Hypotonic and isotonic solutions are easier to retain. Muscle tone and history of constipation or other bowel disorders determine the resistance of the rectum. A client with a long history of constipation is more likely to be able to tolerate a large-volume enema, because the rectum and colon have become distended over time.

Enemas may be classified as cleansing, retention, or return-flow. The primary care provider generally orders the specific type to administer to a patient. To learn the procedure for various types of enemas, see Procedure 29-3.

Cleansing Enemas

Cleansing enemas promote removal of feces from the colon. They may be used to do the following:

- Treat severe constipation or impaction.
- Clear the colon in preparation for visualization procedures, such as colonoscopy.
- Empty the colon when starting a bowel training program.

Cleansing enema solutions include hypotonic solutions and hypertonic solutions. With *hypotonic solutions* (saline, tap water, and soap) you introduce a large volume (500 to 1,000 mL for adults, 100 to 250 mL for infants) of fluid into the rectum. Large-volume solutions may be contraindicated in patients who have weakened intestinal walls.

In contrast, *hypertonic solutions* are usually smaller in volume (70 to 120 mL, or 2.5 to 4 oz, for adults). The hypertonic solution attracts water into the colon, causing distention and stimulating peristalsis and defecation (Table 29-2).

✚ Hypertonic solutions may be contraindicated for patients who tend to retain sodium or water (e.g., those with renal failure and congestive heart failure).

A cleansing enema may be given "high" or "low." A "low" enema is given by standard procedure. A "high" enema attempts to clear as much of the large intestine as possible. With a "high" enema, the client receives initial instillation of the fluid in the left lateral position. The client then moves to the dorsal recumbent position and then the right lateral position for the remainder of the instillation. This turning process allows the fluid to follow the shape of the large intestine.

Retention Enemas

Retention enemas introduce a solution into the colon to be retained for a prolonged period. Consequently the volume is small, usually 90 to 120 mL (3 to 4 oz). The following are the most common forms of retention enemas.

Oil-Retention Enemas. Oil-retention enemas instill 90 to 120 mL of oil into the rectum to soften stool and lubricate the rectum. This type of enema may be used to assist a client to pass hard stool or before digital removal of stool. It may also be used in conjunction with a cleansing enema—at least 1 hour before the cleansing enema.

Carminative Enemas. Carminative enema is a procedure in which 60 to 180 mL (2 to 6 oz) of solution are instilled into the rectum to help expel flatus and relieve bloating and distention. This procedure is used after abdominal or pelvic surgery when peristalsis is slow to return and the client experiences pressure from gas. Solutions may be commercially

Table 29-2 ➤ Solutions Commonly Used in Enemas

SOLUTION	EXAMPLES	ACTION	TIME UNTIL BM	ADVERSE EFFECTS
Hypotonic	500–1,000 mL of tap water	Large volume distends the colon, thereby stimulating peristalsis; water also softens stool.	15 min	Fluid and electrolyte imbalance, especially water intoxication, is possible if enema is not expelled.
Isotonic	500–1,000 mL of normal saline (0.9% NaCl solution)	Large volume distends the colon, thereby stimulating peristalsis; some softening of stool also occurs.	15 min	Fluid and electrolyte imbalance, especially sodium retention
Hypertonic	120–180 mL of sodium phosphate (e.g., Fleet); available as a commercially prepared solution	Attracts water into the colon, thereby causing distention.	Rapid acting: 5–10 min	Sodium retention
Oil	90–120 mL of mineral oil, cottonseed oil, or olive oil; available as a commercially prepared solution	Softens the feces, lubricates the rectum.	Varies widely. An oil-retention enema is often given 1–3 hr before a cleansing enema is administered.	
Soapsuds	Pure castile soap is added to tap water or saline.	Intestinal irritation stimulates peristalsis.	Varies.	Only pure castile soap is safe. Other soaps and detergents can cause bowel inflammation.
Carminative	For example, 1:2:3 "MGW" solution (e.g., 30 mL magnesium, 60 mL glycerin, and 90 mL water)	Provides relief from abdominal distention caused by flatus.		

prepared or prepared on the unit. A common carminative enema is the "MGW" enema: a mixture of magnesium sulfate, glycerin, and water in a ratio of 1:2:3 (e.g., 15 mL of magnesium sulfate, 30 mL of glycerin, and 45 mL of water).

Medicated Enemas. Medicated enemas may be used to instill antibiotics to treat infections in the rectum or anus or to introduce anthelminthic agents for treatment of intestinal worms and parasites.

Nutritive Enemas. Nutritive enemas administer fluid and nutrition through the rectum for patients who are dehydrated and frail. They are most commonly used in hospice care as a means to provide hydration for dying patients.

Return-Flow Enemas

A return-flow enema, known as a *Harris flush*, may be ordered to help a patient expel flatus and relieve abdominal distention (see Procedure 29-3D). For adults, approximately 100 to 200 mL (3 to 7 oz) of tap water or saline is instilled into the rectum. The rectal tube and solution container are then lowered below the level of the rectum to encourage return flow of the solution. This process is repeated several times, or until distention is relieved. If the solution becomes thick, discard it and begin again with new solution.

KnowledgeCheck 29-6

- Identify the types of enemas available for use.
- How do hypotonic and isotonic enemas differ from hypertonic enemas?
- What actions can you take to make the patient more comfortable when he receives an enema?

ThinkLike a Nurse 29-8

Mrs. Zeno (Meet Your Patient) begins to pass liquid stool. What actions should you take? Explain your reasoning.

Managing Flatulence

Recall that flatus is a natural by-product of digestion. When gas is excessive or leads to complaints of abdominal distention, cramping, or discomfort, it is known as **flatulence.** Some people develop flatulence after eating gas-producing foods, such as beans, cabbage, cauliflower, onions, or highly spiced foods. For others, flatulence occurs when fiber intake is increased. Clients with irritable bowel syndrome experience a cluster of symptoms that include flatulence. Constipation is often accompanied by flatulence because digestive by-products undergo prolonged fermentation in the colon.

Use the following interventions to help clients manage flatulence:

- Teach clients to be aware of and avoid foods that trigger flatulence.
- Teach clients to follow self-care strategies (identified earlier) for maintaining regular bowel movements.
- Encourage patients who have had surgery with gaseous anesthesia to ambulate and perform bed exercises to stimulate peristalsis and the passage of gas.
- In severe cases, you may need to insert a rectal tube to aid in the elimination of flatus. To learn the entire procedure, go to Procedure 29-5.

Interventions for Example Problem: Bowel Incontinence

Bowel incontinence (or *fecal incontinence*) is the inability to control the discharge of feces and flatulence. One study suggests that one-third of critically ill patients have fecal incontinence, and it is a leading cause of admission to long-term care facilities in the United States (Beltz, 2006; Landefeld, Bowers, Feld, et al., 2008). Physiological conditions causing bowel incontinence include conditions that affect innervation of the rectum and anus, uncontrolled diarrhea, impaction resulting in leakage of stool, and cognitive or emotional changes that alter perception of the urge to defecate. Bowel incontinence is also created by functional limitations—for example, when a client recognizes the need to have a BM but cannot get to the toilet independently or in time.

Clients with persistent bowel incontinence require special nursing care to prevent Impaired Skin Integrity because of the moisture and the activity of enzymes in the stool. In addition, bowel incontinence may be embarrassing. As clients worry about future episodes, anxiety escalates. Refer to the Nursing Care Plan and Care Map for a patient with fecal incontinence. In general, nursing interventions include the following:

- Monitor the pattern of BMs.
- Provide the bedpan or assist the patient to the bathroom at regular intervals and at times BMs are most likely to occur.
- Change clothing and/or bed linens as soon as possible to prevent skin irritation and embarrassment.
- Provide prompt hygiene care after any episodes of incontinence.
- Monitor skin for evidence of breakdown. Use moisture-barrier cream if redness or irritation is noted. Consider use of a fecal incontinence pouch for skin protection (discussed in a following section).
- Review diet, fluid intake, activity, and medicines. Work with the primary care provider to alter the above factors to encourage regular bowel movements.
- Consider a bowel training program (explained later in the chapter).
- Use containment or indwelling methods to prevent fecal drainage from soiling clothing. Research on patient outcomes of most of these methods is limited.

Toward Evidence-Based Practice

| Baldwin, C., Grant, M., Wendel, C., et al. (2008). Influence of intestinal stoma on spiritual quality of life of U.S. veterans. *Journal of Holistic Nursing, 26*(3), 185–194.

A survey was used to obtain spiritual quality-of-life (QOL) data from male veterans with intestinal ostomies. Researchers used both statistical and qualitative analysis data to explore differences among those with high QOL scores and those with lower QOL scores. Those in the high QOL group expressed more feelings of hope and meaning in life in their narratives. Both the high and low QOL groups reported odor and noise from the ostomy as problematic to church attendance. However, the high QOL group indicated that positive support from church members or clergy was helpful, whereas the low QOL group did not. The high QOL group also reported receiving support through praying, meditating, and attending church or temple.

| Simmons, K., Smith, J., Bobb, K.-A., et al. (2007). Adjustment to colostomy: Stoma acceptance, stoma care self-efficacy and interpersonal relationships. *Journal of Advanced Nursing, 60*(6), 627–635.

Researchers collected data from 51 patients with colostomies. They used questionnaires to measure

acceptance of the stoma, relationship with others, and stoma self-care efficacy 6 months after surgery. Results indicated that these three variables, along with location of the stoma, were strongly associated with adjustment. They concluded that routine care for stoma patients should address psychosocial concerns, with more emphasis on dispelling negative thoughts and encouraging social interaction.

1. Based on these studies, write three nursing interventions you would use to help a patient accept and adapt to a stoma.

2. Suppose you wanted to know whether those interventions would be effective for patients with other medical conditions. For example, would the interventions that help clients adapt to a stoma help other clients to adapt to a different issue? Think of at least two health conditions for which you might want to perform the two studies just described. Explain your thinking.

 Go to Chapter 29, **Toward Evidence-Based Practice Suggested Responses,** on DavisPlus.

Nursing Care Plan

Client Data

Olivia Grimaldi, 59 years old, is admitted to the orthopedic unit after having a total knee replacement. She is receiving intravenous opioid analgesics for pain. Mrs. Grimaldi's nurse sits down to talk and complete the nursing admission assessment. The conversation turns to a discussion of bowel habits.

Nurse: Mrs. Grimaldi, we pay special attention to bowel elimination because many people on this unit have problems. How often do you have a bowel movement?

Mrs. G: Not as often as I'd like. I used to be very regular, but lately everything is all mixed up.

Nurse: What has changed? Tell me what's going on.

Mrs. G: Oh, it's so embarrassing. I haven't told anyone about this.

Nurse: When did this problem start?

Mrs. G: Everything started going bad when I fell and landed on this knee a few months ago. Nothing was broken, but the pain has been just awful. I knew I had arthritis, but I never felt anything like this. I couldn't sleep, the pain was so bad. The doctor put me on some pain pills— narcotics—and they helped, but I got so constipated. I started using laxatives to go to the bathroom, but I kept needing to use more and more. Sometimes I would take a laxative and then I would have to get to the bathroom quickly. I had a couple of accidents because I couldn't get to the toilet quickly enough.

Nurse: I think this is something we'll be able to help you with, Mrs. Grimaldi.

The nurse discovers that Mrs. Grimaldi drinks about 32 to 40 ounces of fluid each day and has used several stimulant laxatives and enemas to relieve her constipation. Her mobility has been significantly impaired for the past 2 months.

Nursing Diagnosis

Bowel Incontinence r/t overdistention of the rectum secondary to chronic constipation, as evidenced by client report of constipation when taking opioids and subsequent fecal incontinence with the use of laxatives.

NOC Outcomes	Individualized Goals/Expected Outcomes
Bowel Continence (0500) Bowel Elimination (0501)	*By discharge, Mrs. Grimaldi will:* 1. Be free from fecal impaction. 2. Begin to establish a regular pattern of stool evacuation. 3. Describe four actions she can take to reduce the risk of constipation. *Within 1 month, Mrs. Grimaldi will:* 1. Control stool passage without any episodes of fecal incontinence.

NIC Interventions

Bowel Management (0430)
Bowel Training (0440)

Nursing Activities	Rationale
1. Conduct a comprehensive assessment of all factors related to fecal incontinence and impaired bowel elimination.	Fecal incontinence has multiple possible causes. The best nursing interventions are those based on client assessment (Norton & Chelvanayagam, 2000). Constipation is attributed to immobility, weak straining ability, use of constipating drugs, neurological disorders, lack of dietary fiber, and poor fluid intake (Scarlett, 2004; Schnelle & Leung, 2004).

Nursing Care Plan (continued)

Nursing Activities	Rationale
2. During physical examination, inspect the perianal skin for possible causes of fecal incontinence or skin irritation resulting from exposure to liquid stool.	Congenital abnormalities and hemorrhoids can lead to incontinence. Skin tags can make cleansing difficult and lead to minor soiling that is difficult to distinguish from actual fecal incontinence (Norton & Chelvanayagam, 2000).
3. Inquire about Mrs. Grimaldi's access to the bathroom and toileting facilities at home and work. Provide regular toileting assistance as long as the client needs it during her hospitalization.	A lack of convenient access to the toilet can precipitate fecal incontinence (Schnelle & Leung, 2004).
4. Work with Mrs. Grimaldi to establish a bowel reeducation program, starting with bowel cleansing.	Cleansing is indicated for any client with rectal impaction or palpable stool in the descending or sigmoid colon. Cleansing with manual disimpaction, laxatives, and/or enema removes any potential blockages to stool elimination (Scarlett, 2004; Schnelle & Leung, 2004).
5. Ensure that Mrs. Grimaldi drinks 30 mL/kg of fluids per day and gradually increase dietary fiber with bran or with bulking agents. Mrs. Grimaldi is drinking only about 1,200 mL of fluid per day. If she weighs 125 lb (56.7 kg), she would need to drink at least 1,700 mL of fluid per day.	Increasing fluid intake may help to normalize stool consistency in clients with constipation who do not have adequate fluid intake (Müller-Lissner, Kamm, Scarpignato, et al., 2005). Increasing dietary fiber improves stool consistency and reduces fecal incontinence (Shakil, Church, & Rao, 2008); however, unless the diet is lacking in fiber, adding fiber does not necessarily alleviate constipation.

Bulk should be added to the diet slowly to reduce the risk of bloating, gas, or diarrhea. Dosing of bulking agents can be increased weekly until desired results are achieved; the results are more important than the amount of fiber ingested. |
| 6. Teach Mrs. Grimaldi about how her body works to produce stool; ways to gently signal the body to defecate; the importance of responding to the urge to defecate; and how immobility, medications, and dehydration can cause constipation. | Gaining knowledge about bodily functions allows clients to be active participants in their care. Addressing causes of constipation can reduce the risk of recurrence (Schnelle & Leung, 2004). |

Evaluation

Review initial outcomes and goals. Reassess daily progress toward stated discharge goals.

The day before Mrs. Grimaldi's discharge, she had no palpable stool on physical exam, and she no longer needed the intravenous analgesics; her patient-controlled analgesia (PCA) pump was discontinued. She was drinking approximately 20 mL/kg per day of fluids, she had begun taking 2 tablespoons of psyllium dissolved in water every morning, and she had a bowel movement each of the previous 2 days with stool of normal consistency for the first time in more than a month. She was able to state the actions she would take at home: Continue the bulk supplements, try to increase her fluid intake to 30 mL/kg per day, use nonconstipating analgesics, and increase her mobility each day. The nurse charted that the goals were met.

References

Bulechek, Butcher, & Dochterman, 2008; Gallagher, O'Mahony, & Quigley, 2008; Ginsberg, Phillips, Wallace, et al., 2007; Moorhead, Johnson, Maas, et al., 2008; Müeller-Lissner, Kamm, Scarpignato, et al., 2005; Norton, & Chelvanayagam, 2000; Norton, 2008; Scarlett, 2004; Schnelle, & Leung, 2004; Shakil, Church, & Rao, 2008.

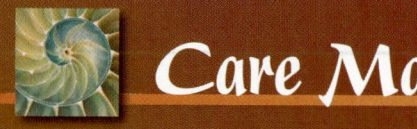

Care Map

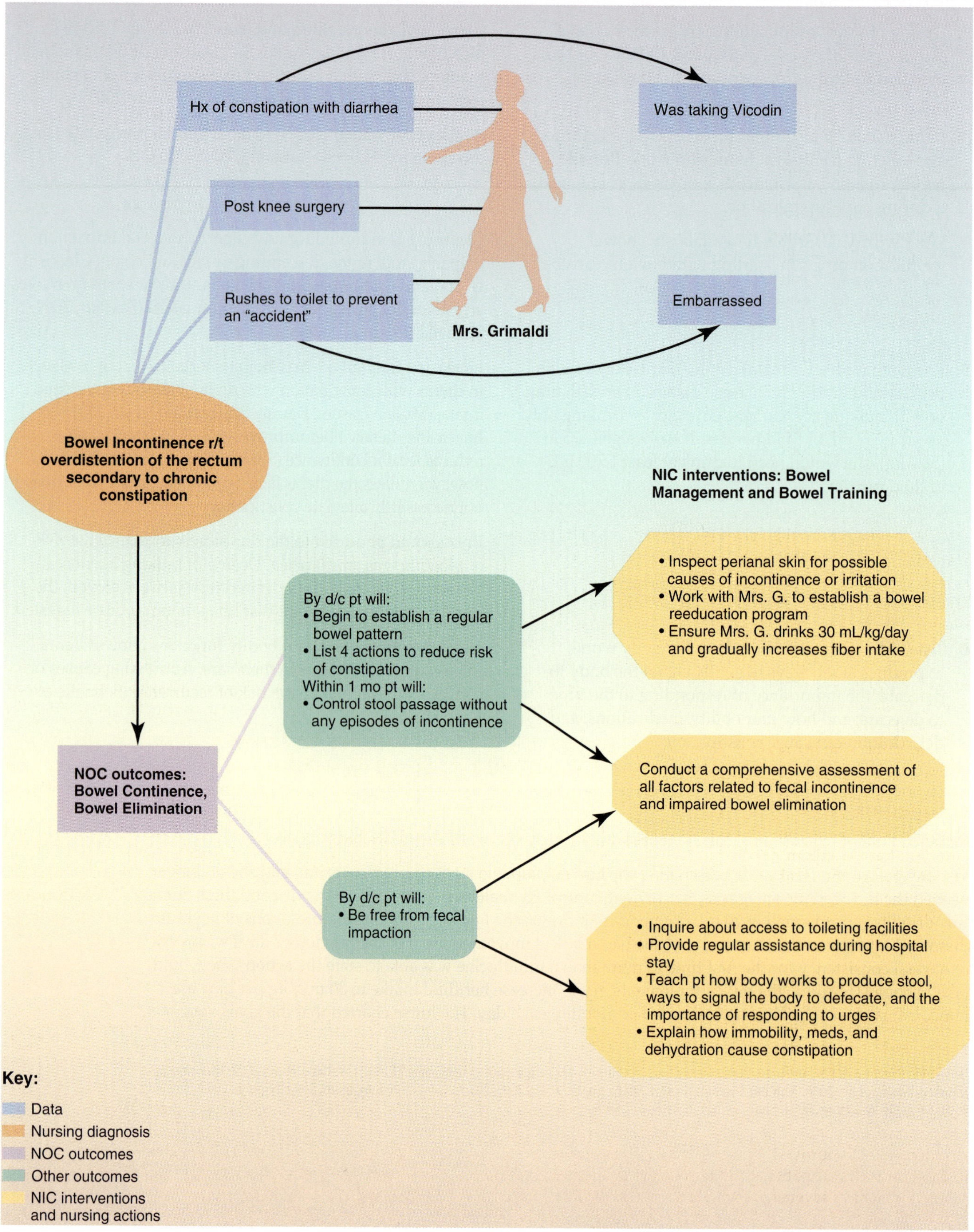

Hx of constipation with diarrhea

Was taking Vicodin

Post knee surgery

Rushes to toilet to prevent an "accident"

Embarrassed

Mrs. Grimaldi

Bowel Incontinence r/t overdistention of the rectum secondary to chronic constipation

NIC interventions: Bowel Management and Bowel Training

By d/c pt will:
- Begin to establish a regular bowel pattern
- List 4 actions to reduce risk of constipation

Within 1 mo pt will:
- Control stool passage without any episodes of incontinence

- Inspect perianal skin for possible causes of incontinence or irritation
- Work with Mrs. G. to establish a bowel reeducation program
- Ensure Mrs. G. drinks 30 mL/kg/day and gradually increases fiber intake

NOC outcomes: Bowel Continence, Bowel Elimination

Conduct a comprehensive assessment of all factors related to fecal incontinence and impaired bowel elimination

By d/c pt will:
- Be free from fecal impaction

- Inquire about access to toileting facilities
- Provide regular assistance during hospital stay
- Teach pt how body works to produce stool, ways to signal the body to defecate, and the importance of responding to urges
- Explain how immobility, meds, and dehydration cause constipation

Key:
- Data
- Nursing diagnosis
- NOC outcomes
- Other outcomes
- NIC interventions and nursing actions

Absorbent Products

You may use absorbent products to prevent fecal drainage from soiling clothing and linens. For small quantities of stool, a long, rectangular pad or a belted absorbent shield can be placed inside clothing. For larger quantities, adult incontinence garments are used. They may pull on like underwear or fasten like a diaper. Moisture-resistant pads placed under the patient help to protect bed linens. When using absorbent products, remember the following important points:

- Never refer to incontinence pads as "diapers" when caring for adults or children who have been toilet trained. This inappropriate reference may cause embarrassment and lower the patient's self-esteem.
- Never place the plastic side of the pad next to the patient's body. This holds moisture next to the skin, which leads to irritation and breakdown.
- Use state-of-the-art skin protection products, such as perineal cleansers and skin barrier products.
- Change the pad as soon as possible after defecation. Keep the skin scrupulously clean.

External Fecal Collection Devices

You may apply an external fecal incontinence pouch to protect perianal skin or to collect large fecal samples. The pouch collects fecal drainage, keeping feces away from the skin. This is a common approach for clients with uncontrolled diarrhea. A variety of pouch systems may be used. Most frequently, a moisture-proof barrier is applied around the anus, and a plastic pouch is secured to the barrier. The equipment may be the same as that used for patients with an ostomy. (Ostomy care is discussed later in the chapter.)

External collection systems can prevent skin breakdown, minimize odor, track output accurately, and enhance patient comfort. However, they are not typically used for patients who are ambulatory, agitated, or active in bed because the device may be dislodged, causing skin breakdown. External systems cannot be used effectively when the patient has Impaired Skin Integrity because they will not seal tightly.

Assess the system regularly to ensure that it has not become dislodged and that no leaks have occurred. Empty the pouch when it is one-third to one-half full to prevent it from getting too heavy. Pay close attention to the perianal skin as you perform your assessment. You may need to use moisture-barrier cream on the surrounding skin. You will usually change the fecal pouch at least every 72 hours and whenever there is evidence of leakage. To learn a procedure for placing both external fecal drainage devices, refer to Procedure 29-6.

Indwelling Fecal Drainage Devices

Indwelling fecal drainage devices are used to collect liquid stool from bedbound, immobilized ill patients. They consist of a soft, latex-free catheter and a collection bag. The tube is inserted and a balloon on the end is filled with saline or water. Internal devices protect perianal skin, protect caregivers from potentially infectious stool, and are thought to decrease urinary tract infections. They are U.S. Food and Drug Administration (FDA) approved, but only for 29 consecutive days, and not for pediatric patients. Other contraindications include patients who have severe hemorrhoids; recent bowel, rectal, or anal surgery or injury; rectal or anal tumors; or stricture or stenosis.

You must follow the manufacturer's recommendations carefully for insertion and maintenance. When the bag is filled, empty or replace it, depending on the type. You must also monitor to confirm placement and may need to irrigate the device. To learn more about placing and caring for a patient with an indwelling fecal drainage device, see Procedure 29-6 and Clinical Insight 29-1.

Bowel Training

A bowel training program assists the patient to have regular, soft, formed stools. It is appropriate for clients who have chronic constipation, impaction, or bowel incontinence. Elements of a bowel training program include the following:

- Plan the program with the patient and caregiver.
- Gradually increase fiber in the diet while monitoring consistency of the stool.
- Increase fluid intake to at least eight glasses of water per day, if not contraindicated.
- Initiate a designated uninterrupted time for defecation: usually after meals, especially in the morning.
- Provide privacy for the patient during the designated time.
- Develop a staged treatment plan if constipation develops. Usually, additional fiber is added as a first measure. A stool softener is next, followed by a suppository such as bisacodyl (Dulcolax).
- Regularly modify the plan based on the patient's response.

KnowledgeCheck 29-7

- What are the major patient care concerns associated with bowel incontinence?
- What are the elements of a bowel training program?

Caring for Patients With Bowel Diversions

Patients experience a variety of reactions to a bowel diversion, and each person has unique physical and psychological needs. Initially you will care for the ostomy, but the goal is for the patient to assume self-care.

Ongoing Assessments

Always begin care with a thorough assessment of the stoma, the stool, and the skin.

- *Stoma.* A healthy stoma (Fig. 29-7) ranges in color from deep pink to brick red, regardless of the patient's skin color, and is shiny and moist. Pallor or a dusky blue color indicates ischemia, and a brown-black color indicates necrosis. Immediately after surgery, the stoma will be swollen and enlarged. As the inflammation subsides and healing occurs, the stoma will shrink. By 6 to 8 weeks, it will be at its permanent size. Stoma size varies according to the size of the person and the part of the bowel that was externalized (Fig. 29-5). An ileostomy stoma is generally smaller than a colostomy stoma. The stoma will protrude above the level of the abdomen by approximately 1.3 to 2.5 cm (0.5 to 1 in.).
- *Output.* Output from an ileostomy stoma is liquid and contains digestive enzymes. An ostomy lower in the GI tract will have more solid output and fewer enzymes. The presence of enzymes in the effluent increases the likelihood of skin breakdown.

Clinical Insight 29-1 ▶ Caring for a Patient With an Indwelling Fecal Drainage Device

A catheter is present in the rectum and is connected to a drainage tube and collection bag.

Nursing Goal 1: Prevent injury to rectal sphincter and/or rectal mucosa.

- Do not add air or fluid to the balloon port of the catheter.
- Check the catheter frequently for kinks or obstructions.
- Monitor for signs of complications and notify the health-care provider immediately if patient experiences rectal pain, rectal bleeding, and abdominal distention or pain.
- Monitor stool for change in consistency (solid or soft-formed stool cannot pass through the catheter and will cause an obstruction).
- How to discontinue the catheter:
  1. Attach a 60-mL syringe to the balloon inflation port and deflate the retention balloon by pulling back on the plunger.
  2. Grasp the catheter as close to the patient as possible and slowly slide it out of the anus.
  3. Dispose of the device accordance to the agency policy for disposal of medical waste.

Nursing Goal 2: Maintain free flow of liquid stool.

- Monitor the patient for changes in stool consistency. If the stool is no longer liquid and flowing, the device must be discontinued.
- Make sure the tubing and bag remain below the level of the patient.
- Irrigate the tube as often as necessary to maintain patency:
  1. Fill a 60-mL syringe with room-temperature tap water.
  2. Attach it to the irrigation port of the catheter and flush by depressing the plunger.

✚ Be sure you are using the irrigation port, NOT the balloon inflation port.

  3. Be sure to subtract the irrigation fluid from the stool volume to maintain an accurate record of intake and output.
- Change the collection bag when it is three-fourths full.
  4. Remove the collection bag from the tubing. Snap the cap onto the used bag and dispose of according to agency policy for medical waste.
  5. Snap new collection bag securely onto the device.

Nursing Goal 3: Prevent transmission of pathogens to others.

- Follow the agency protocol for hand hygiene. Always wear clean procedure gloves when handling the fecal manage-ment device.
- Monitor stool cultures and implement isolation protocols as indicated. If a stool sample is ordered, you may obtain it from the collection bag:
  1. If the collection bag is more than 24 hours old, place a new collection bag before obtaining sample.
  2. Cut the collection bag at the bottom and transfer stool to an appropriate container for transport to the lab.
  3. Apply a new collection bag to the connector at the end of the catheter.

Nursing Goal 4: Maintain perineal skin integrity or prevent wounds from being contaminated by stool.

- Monitor insertion site for leakage and signs of infection.
- If perineal wounds are present, keep clean and dry; notify the primary provider if signs of infection are present.
- Perform perineal care according to agency policy

- *Skin.* Assess the skin surrounding a stoma for signs of irrita-tion, such as redness, tenderness, skin breakdown, and/or drainage.

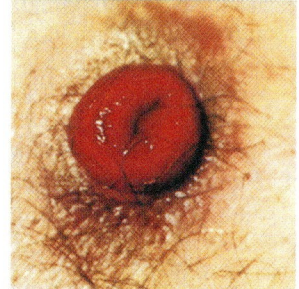

FIGURE 29-7 A healthy stoma is deep pink to brick red and is shiny and moist.

Helping Patients Adapt to the Diversion

Patients experience a variety of reactions to a bowel diversion, and each person has unique needs. Initially you will care for the ostomy, but the goal is to have the patient assume self-care and a normal life. The first step in that direction is for the patient to adjust to the presence of an ostomy. If the patient has been sick before the surgery and the ostomy leads to less pain or discomfort, the transition may be easier. Similarly, patients with continent ostomies may adapt more easily to their stoma.

The following interventions will promote physical and psychological adaptation:
- Be available to discuss the patient's reaction to the stoma. Your attitude and willingness to discuss the patient's body changes will help your patient begin adapting.
- Show acceptance when working with the patient and the stoma.

BOX 29-2 ■ Dietary Changes Associated With an Ostomy

Note: These are only suggestions. Each person must, by trial and error, discover what works best for him.

General Guidelines for Patients

- Initially you may be asked to follow a bland, low-residue or soft diet for a month or two, to prevent obstructions and GI upsets. Advance the diet by adding one new food at a time.
- Eat three or more meals daily at regular times.
- Drink additional fluid to keep well hydrated. Those with colostomies need to compensate for the loss of the large intestine where fluid absorption occurs.
- Avoid chewing gum, as it may cause you to swallow air, causing a noisy stoma.
- Avoid foods that cause gas, odor, blockage, or loose stools. Eventually introduce them into your diet one at a time and be aware of their effects.
- Chew your food well to avoid blockage of the stoma.
- Avoid excessive weight gain.

Foods That May Cause Gas or Odor

Beverages: Alcohol, beer, carbonated beverages
Dairy: Milk, cheese, eggs, and other dairy
Fruits: Melons
Vegetables: Asparagus, beans, broccoli, Brussels sprouts, cabbage, cauliflower, cucumbers, garlic, onions, peas, radishes
Other foods: Fish, cod liver oil, nuts, peanut butter

Foods That May Help Control Gas or Odor

Buttermilk, yogurt
Cranberry juice
Parsley

High-Fiber Foods That May Cause Blockage

You can eat some of these foods (e.g., mushrooms, shrimp) if you cut them into small pieces and chew them very thoroughly. As long as blockage does not occur, these foods should not necessarily be avoided, but used carefully.

- Foods with seeds (e.g., raspberries)
- Foods with tough skins (e.g., corn, dried fruits, pears, tomatoes)
- Mushrooms
- Nuts, popcorn
- Raw or minimally cooked fruits and vegetables (e.g., coleslaw, Chinese stir-fried vegetables, oranges, apple skins)
- Shrimp, lobster
- Stringy foods (e.g., celery, coconut, spinach, bean sprouts, green beans, orange pulp)

Foods That May Cause Loose Stools

Alcohol, beer, caffeine, chocolate, licorice
Milk
Baked beans, cooked cabbage, onions
Bran cereal, whole grains
Highly seasoned foods
Large meals
Prunes, raisins
Raw fruits and vegetables

Note: Never restrict fluids in an effort to control diarrhea.

Foods That May Alleviate Diarrhea

Bananas **R**ice **A**pplesauce **T**oast
Starchy foods (e.g., bread, potatoes)
Cheese and creamy peanut butter

Sources: United Ostomy Associations of America. (2005). *Ostomates food reference chart.* Retrieved from http://www.uoaa.org/ostomy_info/pubs/uoa_diet_nutrition_en.pdf; and Lutz, C., & Przytulski, K. (2006). *Nutrition and diet therapy: Evidence-based applications* (4th ed.). Philadelphia: F. A. Davis.

- Provide adequate ventilation and odor control when assessing the stoma or ostomy appliance.
- Provide ample time to explain stoma care and use of ostomy appliances. For most patients, this is a lifelong task; therefore, patient teaching is essential.
- Teach the client about diet modifications. Ostomy patients no longer have sphincter control, so they may need to modify their diet. Box 29-2 discusses the effects of some foods on a patient with an ostomy.
- Encourage patients to return to their usual activities as much as possible.
- Refer the patient to the local ostomy association, if one is available. Most of the counselors are skillful because they, too, have ostomies. They are able to share practical and personal information based on their own experience with similar challenges. To find the local chapter consult your phone book, or

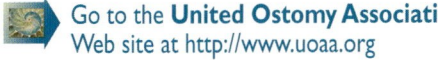 Go to the **United Ostomy Associations of America** Web site at http://www.uoaa.org

With the exception of a temporary double-barreled colostomy, ostomy care is a lifelong task. Patients must learn about appliances, stoma care, and ongoing management of the ostomy. In many hospitals and large communities, you can find an enterostomal therapy nurse to assist patients with their ongoing care and to provide consultation on ostomy appliances.

Caring for the Ostomy

In addition to helping the patient adapt, other nursing interventions include the following:

- Pay close attention to the skin surrounding the stoma. Skin breakdown may lead to infection, pain, and leakage. Use recommended moisture-proof barrier creams and skin care products.
- Monitor the amount and type of drainage from the stoma.
- ✚ Immediately report to the surgeon a stoma that is pale, dusky, or black in color; dry; or with sloughing tissues. These are signs of inadequate blood supply to the portion of intestine that has been externalized.
- Perform colostomy irrigation as needed.

For a full description of the care of an ostomy appliance, including changing, emptying, and irrigating, refer to Procedure 29-7 and Procedure 29-8.

Colostomy Irrigation. Colostomy irrigation may be indicated as an occasional intervention for constipation or in a

select population of patients. Consult with the ostomy nurse and/or physician to see if colostomy irrigation is appropriate for your patient. A stoma above the descending colon usually has liquid output that cannot be controlled. Therefore, it is not irrigated. Patients with an ostomy in the descending or sigmoid colon may use colostomy irrigation as a means to control bowel evacuation and possibly eliminate the need to wear an ostomy pouch. Colostomy irrigation is similar to an enema. After evacuation of the bowel, the client may wear a small

covering over the stoma instead of a pouch. For the complete procedure, see Procedure 29-8.

KnowledgeCheck 29-8

- How can you help a patient adapt psychologically to living with a bowel diversion?
- What does a healthy stoma look like?
- Why is skin care around a stoma so important?

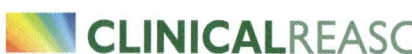 **CLINICAL**REASONING:
Applying the **Full-Spectrum Nursing Model**

Because the following critical thinking activities allow you to practice the kind of thinking you will use as a full-spectrum nurse, they usually have no single right answer. Discuss them with your peers—if you have difficulty with any of the questions, consult your instructor.

PATIENT SITUATION

Lucy Franklin is a frail elderly woman, a long-time resident in a long-term care facility. She can no longer communicate and lies however the NAPs place her in bed, seldom moving. She is very thin, does not eat or drink, and is being fed entirely through a gastrostomy tube. She is incontinent of both stool and urine, and has recently started having copious diarrhea, probably from the tube feedings, but that has not been established definitely. The skin on Lucy's back, buttocks, and perineum is still intact, but it is quite red now. The healthcare team is considering various measures for controlling the diarrhea, but until that can be achieved, nurses want to protect her skin integrity.

THINKING

1. *Theoretical Knowledge:*
   a. Other than tube feedings, what else could be causing Lucy's diarrhea?
   b. In addition to Impaired Skin Integrity, what are some other risks associated with diarrhea?
   c. Why is fecal incontinence, especially with diarrhea, a risk factor for Impaired Skin Integrity?
2. *Critical Thinking:*
   a. *(Contextual Awareness):* What other factors in Lucy's situation do you think might make her even more vulnerable to Impaired Skin Integrity? If you do not yet have the theoretical knowledge you need, draw on your own experiences—and think carefully about everything you know about Lucy.
   b. *(Considering Alternatives):* A fecal incontinence pouch is being discussed as an intervention to preserve Lucy's skin integrity. Do you think it should be an external system or an internal system? Why?

DOING

3. *Practical Knowledge:*
   It has been decided that an external fecal collection system will be used. Describe the steps you will take to apply this system after you have made the necessary assessments.
4. *Nursing Process (Assessments):*
   What ongoing assessments will you need to make after the fecal collection system is applied?

CARING

5. *Self-Knowledge:*
   How comfortable would you be applying Lucy's fecal collection system? What aspects of the situation make you most uncomfortable?

 Go To Chapter 29, **Clinical Reasoning: Applying the Full-Spectrum Nursing Model Response Sheet,** on DavisPlus.

PracticalKnowledge
procedures

The procedures in this chapter will help you to provide care to patients who have problems with bowel elimination.

Procedure 29–1 ■ Testing Stool for Occult Blood

➤ For steps to follow in *all* procedures, refer to the Universal Steps for All Procedures found on the page facing the inside back cover.

➤ *Note:* According to colorectal screening guidelines, for average-risk persons, men and women age 50 or older should be screened with colonoscopy every 10 years. Some healthcare providers recommend all African-Americans to begin screening at age 45. High-risk groups, such as those with personal or strong family history of colorectal cancer or rectal polyps should receive initial screening at a younger age and more often, and should perhaps undergo genetic testing.

Equipment

- Clean gloves
- Tongue blade or other wooden applicator
- Clean, dry collection container to place in the commode, or a clean, dry bedpan
- Facility-specific fecal occult blood test (FOBT) slide or test paper
- Developing solution

Delegation

You can delegate the collection and testing of a stool sample for occult blood to unlicensed assistive personnel (NAP) if the NAP has the necessary skills and the patient's condition is stable. Inform the NAP of any special considerations (e.g., the need to assist the patient with ambulation or the need for a bedpan). Instruct the NAP to inform you if there is visible blood in the stool and to show you the FOBT slide for evaluation of results when the test is complete.

Pre-Procedure Assessment

- Assess the patient's mobility status.
  Determines the patient's ability to participate in stool collection, the need for a bedpan or commode, and so forth.

- Assess the patient's dietary history for the past 24 to 48 hours.
  Some foods, such as red meat, chicken, fish, horseradish, turnips, or raw vegetables, may lead to a false-positive reading. Vitamin C in excess of 250 mg per day can produce a false-negative result (Allison, 2005; American Gastroenterological Association, 2007).

- Assess medication history.
  If the patient is taking medications, such as salicylates, NSAIDs, iron, oxidizing drugs (e.g., iodine salts, boric acid), reserpine, corticosteroids, anticoagulants, colchicines, and high doses of vitamin C, consult with the prescriber. These medications may cause a false-positive reading. If possible, they will be discontinued for 7 days before the test (Atkins, 2008). If the patient must have them, results must be interpreted taking them into consideration.

- Assess for the presence of hemorrhoids.
  Any source of blood may cause a false-positive result for intestinal bleeding.

- If the patient is female, ask whether she is menstruating.

- Ask the patient if she has had any bleeding in the gums or mouth.

- Check the expiration date on the developing solution for the FOBT test slide.

- Assess the patient's or family's understanding of the need for the stool test.
  Provides a baseline for health teaching.

➤ When performing the procedure, always identify your patient according to agency policy and be attentive to standard precautions, hand hygiene, patient safety and privacy, body mechanics, and documentation.

Procedure Steps

1. **Determine whether the test** will be done by the nurse at the point of care (e.g., in the home or at the bedside) or by lab personnel.
   Because of the regulatory and billing practices in some settings, this test may be completed by lab personnel.

2. **Ask the patient to void** before collecting the stool specimen.
   Helps prevent contaminating the stool with urine.

3. **Don procedure gloves** and place a clean, dry container for the stool specimen into the toilet or bedside commode in such a manner that any urine falls into the toilet and the fecal specimen falls into the container. Obtain a clean, dry bedpan for a patient who is immobile.
   Using a sample of stool that comes in contact with either urine or water may produce an inaccurate test result.

4. **Instruct the patient to defecate** into the container, or place the patient on the bedpan. Do not contaminate the specimen with toilet tissue.

5. Once the specimen has been obtained, wash your hands, and **don clean procedure gloves.**
   Prevent the spread of intestinal bacteria.

6. **Be sure you understand** the directions for the testing kit you are using.

This procedure gives instructions for using the FOBT slide method.

7. **Explain the purpose of the test.** Explain to the patient that serial specimens may be needed.
   Testing serial specimens decreases the chances of a false-negative finding.

8. **Open the specimen side** of the FOBT slide. With a tongue depressor or other applicator, collect a small sample of stool and spread it thinly onto one "window" of the FOBT slide.

9. **With a different applicator** or the opposite end of the tongue blade, collect a second small sample of stool from a different location in

(continued on next page)

Procedure 29-1 ■ Testing Stool for Occult Blood (continued)

the large sample. Spread the second sample thinly onto the second "window" of the slide.
Reduces the possibility of a false-negative result. ▼

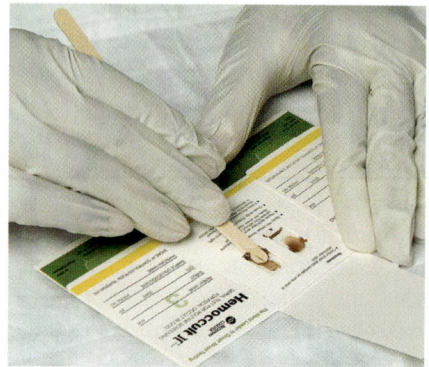

10. **Wrap the tongue depressor** in tissue and a paper towel; place it in a waste receptacle. Do not flush it.
Prevents transfer of microorganisms. Flushing would likely clog the plumbing.

11. **Close the FOBT slide.**
Prevents the transfer of microorganisms from the specimen smears on the slide.

12. **If the test is to be done by laboratory personnel**, transfer the specimen to a clean dry container, being careful not to contaminate the outside of the container with feces. Label the specimen in the presence of the patient according

to agency policy, and place it into the proper receptacle for transportation to the lab.

13. **If you are to perform the test**, turn the slide over, and open the opposite side of the FOBT slide. Place one or two drops of developing solution onto each "window." Follow the directions on the package regarding the number of drops of the developing solution.
Ensures an accurate reading.

Evaluation

- Observe the color of the paper inside the FOBT slide windows for 30 to 60 seconds.
- If the paper turns blue, consider the test for occult blood to be positive.

Patient Teaching

- Inform the patient of the reasons for performing the test.
- Explain the possible implications of a positive occult blood test, if one is obtained.

Home Care

- Determine the client's level of cognition and manual dexterity to assess his ability to follow instructions and physically perform the test.
- Explain necessary dietary and medication restrictions (see the Pre-Procedure Assessment section of this procedure).
- Instruct the client to collect the specimen in a clean, dry container. If an appropriate container is not available, the client may use the toilet.
- If defecating in the toilet, the client should flush it immediately prior to obtaining the sample. If commercial toilet bowl cleaners are in use, remove them from the tank, and flush twice. Then lay rice paper (from the kit) directly on the water; it is okay to get it wet. When using the probe to take the stool sample, take the sample from any area of stool that is above the water line.
- Protect the slide from heat, light, and household chemicals.
- Home collection slides come in a kit, connected together as a set of three. Instruct the client not to tear them apart.

- Emphasize to the client that each sample should be from separate bowel movements on separate days.
- After all three specimens have been collected over the course of at least 3 days, store the slide in a paper envelope to air-dry.
- The client must place the slides in the special mailing pouch that comes with the slides, if they are to be sent back to the lab. The slides should be returned to the care provider or lab no later than 14 days after the first sample was collected.
  For additional instructions,

 Go to the **Hemoccult** Web site at http://www. hemoccultfobt.com

Documentation

- Document the date and time of the specimen collection, both in the patient record and on the specimen container or FOBT kit.
- Note the appearance of the stool (e.g., color, odor) and the presence of blood, mucus, or other abnormal constituents.
- Note any rectal bleeding or discomfort during and after defecation.
- Document the test results on the appropriate agency form.
- Notify the appropriate care provider of the results.

Practice Resources

American Cancer Society, 2010; Foran, Petersen, & Llewandrowski, 2006; Gomella & Haist, n.d.; Institute for Clinical Systems Improvement (ICSI), 2010; The Joint Commission, 2011; Kaiser Permanente Care Management Institute, 2008; Siegel, Rhinehart, Jackson, et al., and the Healthcare Infection Control Practices Advisory Committee, 2007.

Procedure 29-2 ■ Placing and Removing a Bedpan

➤ For steps to follow in *all* procedures, refer to the Universal Steps for All Procedures found on the page facing the inside back cover.

Equipment

- Bedpan
- Two pairs of clean gloves
- Toilet tissue
- Two washcloths, towel, and basin
- Waterproof pad
- Bedpan cover

Delegation

You may delegate the placement and removal of a bedpan to the NAP after ensuring that the NAP has the necessary skills and that the patient's condition is stable. Complete the following assessments, and inform the NAP of any special considerations (e.g., medical or surgical conditions that necessitate the use of a fracture pan, extra care with turning or required positioning based on medical condition).

Pre-Procedure Assessments

- Assess level of consciousness, ability to follow directions, mobility status, and physical status.
  Helps determine the type of bedpan to use and whether one or two persons are needed to complete the procedure.

- Determine the patient's comfort level—note the presence of rectal or abdominal pain, hemorrhoids, or perianal irritation.
  Pain can cause difficulty with positioning and bearing down during defecation. Any unexplained pain should be evaluated by the primary care provider.

- Assess the physical size of the patient and whether the patient can sit up or lie flat when using a bedpan.
  Determines the type of bedpan to use and whether you need additional personnel to assist.

- Identify factors that will necessitate the use of a fracture pan (e.g., a fractured pelvis; total hip replacement; lower back surgery; presence of casts, splints, or braces on lower limbs; or obesity.)

- Auscultate bowel sounds, and palpate for distention if indicated.
  The colon when full with fecal matter is a rounded, firm mass. A smooth, round mass above the symphysis pubis is a distended bladder.

- Review the patient's chart to determine the need to obtain a stool specimen.
  Promotes efficiency by allowing you to obtain a specimen container before placing the patient on the bedpan.

Procedure 29-2A ■ Placing a Bedpan

➤ When performing the procedure, always identify your patient according to agency policy and be attentive to standard precautions, hand hygiene, patient safety and privacy, body mechanics, and documentation.

Procedure Steps

1. **Obtain the necessary supplies**, and take them to the patient's room. Leave clean washcloths, towel, and basin with warm water at the bedside for use during bedpan removal.
   The patient will need to wash her hands after using the bedpan.

2. **If the bedpan is metal**, place it under warm, running water for a few seconds. Then dry it, making sure the bedpan is not too hot.
   A warm bedpan allows the patient to be more comfortable and helps relax the anal sphincter. Most bedpans are made of disposable plastic.

3. **Raise the siderail** on the opposite side from where you are working.
   Prevents patient from falling out of bed and gives the patient something to hold onto while moving around in bed.

4. **Raise the bed to a comfortable height.**
   Allows you to use good body mechanics and prevents muscle strain.

5. **Prepare the patient** by folding down the covers to a point that will allow for placement of the bedpan and yet expose only as much of her body as necessary.
   Privacy facilitates elimination by promoting relaxation.

6. **Wash your hands and don clean procedure gloves.**
   Prevents the spread of microorganisms via contact with urine or feces.

7. **Observe for the presence** of dressings, drains, intravenous fluids, and traction.
   These appliances may hinder the patient from assisting with the procedure and may create the need for assistance from another caregiver.

Procedure Variation For the Patient Able to Move/Turn Independently in Bed

8. **Position the patient.**

Supine Position

a. Lower the head of the bed, placing the patient in a supine position.

b. Ask the patient to lift her hips. The patient may need to raise her knees to a flexed position, place her feet flat on the bed, and push up. You can also assist the patient to raise her hips by sliding a hand under the small of her back.

Semi-Fowler's Position

c. Place the bed in a semi-Fowler's position.

d. Ask the patient to raise her hips by pushing up on raised siderails or by using an overhead trapeze.

(continued on next page)

Procedure 29-2 ■ Placing and Removing a Bedpan (continued)

9 Place the bedpan.

Regular Bedpan

a. Place the bedpan under the patient's buttocks so that the wide, rounded end is toward the back. Do not push the pan under the patient's buttocks.

Fracture Pan

b. When using a fracture pan, place the wide, rounded end toward the front.

10 Instruct or assist the patient to lower her hips onto the bedpan. Move to step 16.

Procedure Variation For the Patient Unable to Move/Turn Independently

11 Ask for help from another healthcare worker if the patient's condition warrants.

12 With the patient in the supine position, lower the head of the bed.

13 Assist the patient to the side-lying position. Use a turn sheet, if necessary.

14 Place the bedpan.

Regular Bedpan

a. Place the bedpan under the patient's buttocks so that the wide, rounded end is toward the back.

Do not push the pan under the patient's buttocks. ▼

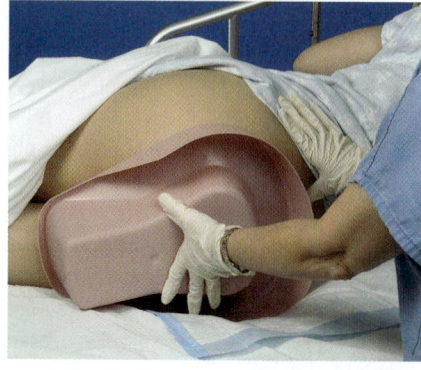

Fracture Pan

b. When using a fracture pan, place the wide, rounded end toward the front. ▼

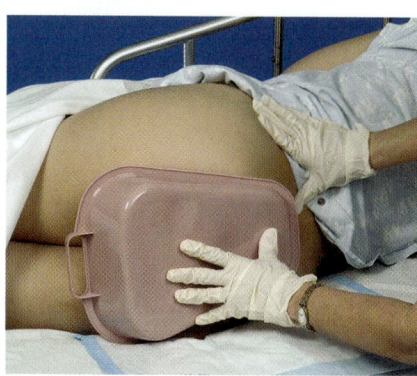

15 Holding the bedpan in place, slowly roll the patient back and onto the bedpan.

16 Replace the covers; raise the head of the bed to a position of comfort for the patient. Place a rolled towel, blanket, or small pillow under the sacrum (lumbar curve of the back). Place the call light and toilet tissue within the patient's reach. Make certain that the bed is returned to its lowest position and that the upper siderails are raised.
Provides privacy, comfort, and safety.

17. Remove your gloves and wash your hands.
Prevents the transmission of intestinal bacteria.

Procedure 29-2B ■ Removing a Bedpan

➤ When performing the procedure, always identify your patient according to agency policy and be attentive to standard precautions, hand hygiene, patient safety and privacy, body mechanics, and documentation.

Procedure Steps

1. Don clean procedure gloves. Wet the washcloths with warm water and place them near the work area.

2. If the patient is immobile, lower the head of the patient's bed. Pull down the covers only as far as needed to remove the bedpan.
Lowering the head of the bed is necessary only if the patient is immobile.

3. Offer the patient toilet paper. Assist patients who are unable to complete this task independently.

4. Ask the patient to raise her hips. Stabilize and remove the bedpan. If the patient is unable to raise

her hips, stabilize the bedpan and assist her to the side-lying position.
Stabilizing the bedpan prevents spillage of urine.

5. Cleanse the buttocks with a warm, wet washcloth. Dry with a towel.
Provides comfort and hygiene and decreases the risk of skin irritation and breakdown.

6. Replace covers, and position the patient for comfort. Offer the patient the second washcloth moistened with warm water to cleanse her hands.
Encourages independence with personal hygiene and decreases transmission of bacteria.

7. Empty the bedpan into the patient's toilet. Measure the output if measuring input and output (I&O) is part of the treatment plan. Clean the bedpan, following facility-specific guidelines.
If there is no toilet in the patient's room, cover the bedpan and carry it to the nearest toilet or soiled utility room for emptying.

8. Remove the soiled gloves and wash your hands.
Prevents transmission of infectious microorganisms.

? What if . . .

■ **Your patient is an older adult**

Offer a bedpan at set intervals, perhaps in conjunction with a turning schedule. For elderly clients with limited mobility you may wish to keep the bedpan readily available.

To minimize episodes of incontinence and/or falls. Trying to get out of bed to use the toilet is a common cause of falls.

Evaluation

■ Assess the amount and characteristics of any urine and/or stool.
■ Observe the skin on the perineum and buttocks for redness and breakdown.

Documentation

■ Document the amount of urine or liquid stool voided if intake and output are being recorded.
■ Note the presence of any unusual characteristics of either stool or urine, and include in the nursing notes. If there are no unusual characteristics, document the passage of stool or urine in the graphic records.

Practice Resources

Ayello & Sibbald, 2008; Balas, Casey, & Happ, 2008; Gray-Micelli, 2008; Siegel, Rhinehart, Jackson, et al., and the Healthcare Infection Control Practices Advisory Committee, 2007.

Thinking About the Procedure

 Go to the *Fundamentals of Nursing Skills Videos,* **Bowel Elimination: Bedpan.**

1. What kind of bedpan did the nurse use: regular bedpan or fracture pan?
2. Describe the method the nurse used to move the patient so she could place the bedpan.

 For suggested responses, go to Chapter 29, **Thinking About the Procedure Suggested Responses,** on *DavisPlus.*

Procedure 29–3 ■ Administering an Enema

➤ For steps to follow in *all* procedures, refer to the Universal Steps for All Procedures found on the page facing the inside back cover.

Equipment

■ Enema administration container, correct enema solution, or prepackaged enema—depends on the type of enema ordered.
  ■ *Enema kit:* This may be a grouping of supplies that includes a small plastic bucket or a 1-liter plastic bag with attached tubing, disposable toweling, lubricant, and castile soap.
  ■ *Prepackaged enema solution:* If a prepackaged enema (e.g., Fleet) is ordered, you may need to obtain the preparation from the pharmacy or central supply department.
■ Washcloths, towels, disposable towelettes, and/or toilet tissue
■ Bath blanket
■ Waterproof pad
■ Bedpan with cover or bedside commode, if needed
■ Water-soluble lubricant
■ Clean procedure gloves
■ IV pole

Delegation

You may delegate this procedure to the NAP if the NAP is trained and the patient is stable. Complete the following assessments, and instruct the NAP about conditions under which the procedure should be stopped (e.g., severe abdominal pain occurs, bleeding is seen, or the patient is unable to retain the solution). Instruct the NAP to report the results of the enema and show you any stool that appears to be abnormal (e.g., containing blood or pus).

Pre-Procedure Assessments

■ Assess for history of bowel disorders (e.g., diverticulitis, ulcerative colitis, recent bowel surgery, abdominal pain, abdominal distention, hemorrhoids).
  Some disorders put the patient at risk for complications, such as mucosal irritation or perforation. Abdominal pain along with hypoactive bowel sounds and distention could indicate a bowel obstruction.
■ Inspect the abdomen for distention.
  Establishes baseline for effectiveness of the enema.
■ Review the patient's chart for the presence of increased intracranial pressure, glaucoma, or recent rectal or prostate surgery.
  These conditions contraindicate an enema.
■ Review lab results, paying particular attention to BUN, creatinine, and electrolytes.
  Hypertonic and hypotonic enemas have been linked to fluid and electrolyte changes. Phosphate enemas (Fleets) have been associated with hyperphosphatemia and hypocalcemia.

(continued on next page)

Procedure 29-3 ■ Administering an Enema (continued)

- Note the date and time of the patient's last bowel movement, recent bowel movement pattern, and bowel sounds.
  Establishes baseline for evaluating bowel function.
- Assess the patient's cognitive level and mobility.
  Determines the patient's ability to follow instructions and the need for placing him on a bedpan for the enema.

- Assess the patient's rectal sphincter control.
  Will determine whether you need to administer the enema with the patient on the bedpan. Also influences the amount of solution to instill.
- Assess for fecal impaction.
  May necessitate the need to obtain a prescription for a different type of enema.

Procedure 29-3A ■ Administering a Cleansing Enema

➤ When performing the procedure, always identify your patient according to agency policy and be attentive to standard precautions, hand hygiene, patient safety and privacy, body mechanics, and documentation.

Procedure Steps

1. **Place the bedpan nearby** or the commode near the bed.
   So you can reach the bedpan during the procedure; or so the patient can easily get to the commode.

2. **Open the enema supplies or kit.** Attach the tubing to the enema pail, if you are using a pail.
   The 1-L enema bag comes with preconnected tubing.

3. **Close the clamp on the tubing,** and fill the container with 500 to 1,000 mL of warm solution. The water temperature should be lukewarm—105°F to 110°F (40°C to 43°C).

   ✚ Check the temperature with a bath thermometer. Never warm the enema solution in a microwave oven.

   a. For infants: Use 50 to 150 mL of solution.
   b. For toddlers: Use 250 to 350 mL of solution.
   c. For school-age children, use 300 to 500 mL of solution.
      Cold solution causes intestinal cramping. Very hot solution can damage the intestinal mucosa. Use the correct amount of solution to decrease the necessity of repeating the procedure.

4. **Add castile soap** (or the soap solution used by your facility) to the fluid at this time if a soapsuds enema has been prescribed.
   Soap causes mucosal irritation, which stimulates peristalsis and defecation.

5. **Hang the container** on the IV pole. Holding the end of the tubing over a sink or waste can, open the clamp and slowly allow the tubing to prime (fill) with solution. Reclamp the tubing when the tubing is filled.
   Expresses air from the tubing. Air introduced into the bowel may cause intestinal distention and discomfort.

6. **Don clean procedure gloves.**
   Prevents the transmission of intestinal bacteria.

7. **Position the patient:** Ask the patient to turn, or assist the patient to turn, to a left side-lying position with the right knee flexed.
   Allows the enema solution to fill the rectum and lower intestine following the natural flow of gravity.
   a. If the patient has shortness of breath associated with a respiratory condition, elevate the head of the bed very slightly. Avoid the semi-Fowler's position.
      The semi-Fowler's position increases the likelihood that gravity will cause the solution to leak out.

   ✚ b. Do not administer the enema with the patient on the toilet.

   The curved rectal tubing can scrape the rectal wall.
   c. If the patient has poor sphincter control, position him on the bedpan in a comfortable dorsal recumbent position.

   He will not be able to retain all of the enema solution.

8. **Place the waterproof pad** under the patient's buttocks or hips.
   Prevents soiling of bed linens.

9. **Drape the patient** with the bath blanket, exposing only the buttocks and rectum. See Procedure 24-4 to review the procedure for draping.
   Promotes patient privacy.

10. **Depending on the patient's** mobility status, place the bedpan flat on the bed, directly beneath the rectum, up against the patient's buttocks.

11. **Lubricate the tip** of the enema tubing generously.
    Allows for ease of insertion, decreases patient discomfort, and helps prevent mucosal irritation.

12. **If necessary, lift the superior buttock** to expose the anus. Slowly and gently insert the tip of the tubing approximately 7 to 10 cm (3 to 4 in.) into the rectum. Have the patient take slow, deep breaths as you complete this step. If the tube does not pass with ease, do not force it. Infuse a small amount of fluid and then try again, inserting the tube slowly.
    Helps the patient to relax, provides additional lubrication, and decreases reflex tightening of the anal sphincter. ➤

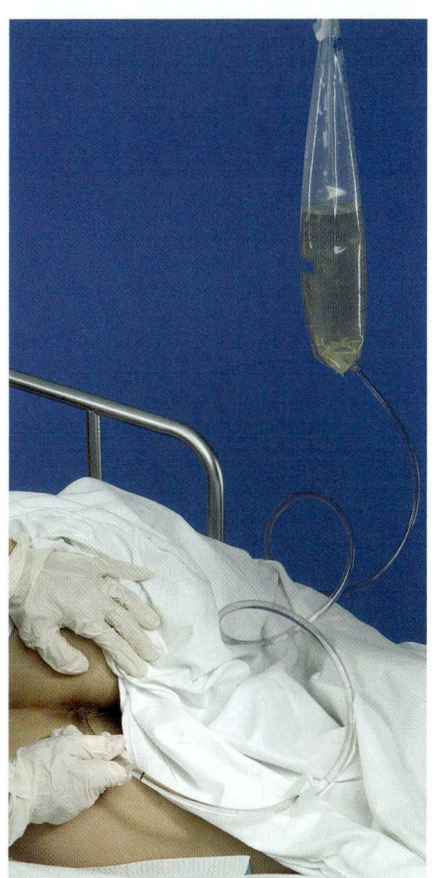

13. **Remove the container from the IV pole**, and hold it at the level of the patient's hips. Unclamp to begin instilling the solution.
Lowering the container slows the force of the instillation, decreasing pressure,
cramping, discomfort, and reflex expulsion of the solution.

14. **Slowly raise the level** of the container, so that it is 30 to 45 cm (12 to 18 in.) above the level of the hips. Adjust the pole and re-hang the container. Continue a slow, steady instillation of the enema solution.
The height of the container determines the speed of the flow. A slow, steady rate of infusion decreases cramping and increases the patient's ability to retain the solution.

15. **Continuously monitor the patient** for pain or discomfort. Assess his ability to retain the solution. If the patient has difficulty with retention, lower the level of the container, stop the flow for 15 to 30 seconds, and then resume the procedure.

    ✚ If the patient feels pain or you meet with resistance at any time during the procedure, stop and consult with the primary care provider.

16. **When the correct amount** of solution has been instilled, clamp the tubing, and slowly remove it from the rectum. If there is stool on the tubing, wrap the end of the tubing in a washcloth or toilet tissue until it can be rinsed or disposed of.
Prevents transmission of pathogens.

17. **Clean the patient's rectal area**, recover the patient, and instruct him to hold the enema solution for approximately 5 to 15 minutes. Place the call light within reach.
Retention of the enema solution will distend the bowel and increase the stimulus to defecate. Leaving the solution in the bowel too long may result in fluid and electrolyte complications. Retaining hypertonic solutions may result in dehydration related to large amounts of fluids moving from the capillary bed into the bowel. Excessive retention of hypotonic solutions may cause fluid overload.

18. **Dispose of the enema supplies** or, if they are reusable, clean and store them in an appropriate location in the patient's room.
Maintains a pleasant environment and helps prevent transfer of pathogens.

19. **Remove your gloves and wash your hands.**

20. **Depending on the patient's mobility** status, assist him onto the bedpan, to the bedside commode, or to the toilet when he feels compelled to defecate. Wash your hands and use clean procedure gloves as necessary.

21. **After the patient has defecated**, inspect the stool for color, consistency, and quantity.

Procedure 29-3B ■ Administering a Prepackaged Enema

➤ When performing the procedure, always identify your patient according to agency policy and be attentive to standard precautions, hand hygiene, patient safety and privacy, body mechanics, and documentation.

Procedure Steps

1. **Open the prepackaged enema.** Remove the plastic cap from the container. The tip of the prepackaged enema container is prelubricated. However, you may need to add extra lubricant.
Extra lubricant decreases discomfort and eases insertion of the tube into the rectum.

2. **Follow steps 6 through 12 of Procedure 29-3A** (regarding gloving, positioning, draping, and inserting the enema tip).

3. **Tilt the container slightly** and slowly roll and squeeze the container until all of the solution is instilled.

Ensures that the container empties completely and that an adequate amount of solution is instilled. ▼

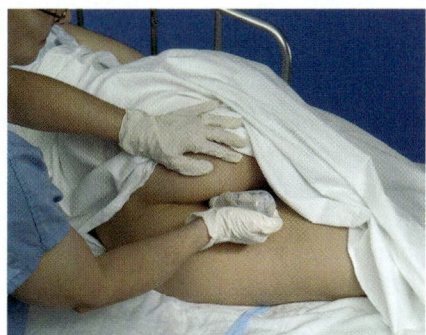

4. **Withdraw the container tip** from the rectum. Wipe the area with a wash-cloth or toilet tissue.
Prevents transmission of pathogens.

5. **Re-cover the patient**, and instruct him to hold the enema solution for approximately 5 to 10 minutes. Place the call light within reach.
Retention of the enema solution will distend the bowel and increase the stimulus to defecate. Retaining the solution for longer than the prescribed time has been associated with dehydration and electrolyte imbalances.

6. **Dispose of the empty container.**
Maintains a pleasant and clean environment.

7. **Follow steps 18 through 20 of Procedure 29-3A** (regarding equipment disposal, assisting the patient, and observations of stool).

(continued on next page)

Procedure 29-3 ■ Administering an Enema (continued)

Procedure 29-3C ■ Administering an Oil-Retention Enema

➤ When performing the procedure, always identify your patient according to agency policy and be attentive to standard precautions, hand hygiene, patient safety and privacy, body mechanics, and documentation.

➤ *Note:* An oil-retention enema may be administered to help a client pass hard stool; it also may be administered before digital removal of stool; or it may be given at least 1 hour before a cleansing enema. See Procedure 29-4 for digital removal of stool.

Procedure Steps

1. **Obtain a commercial oil-retention** enema kit; these kits include a small rectal tube. If a commercial kit is not available, use a small tube and about 90 to 120 mL of the prescribed solution.
   A small tube allows for slower infusion, which minimizes cramping and thereby promotes retention.

2. 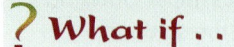 **Warm the oil** to body temperature by running warm tap water over the container. Test a drop on your arm.

   If the oil is too cold, it will cause cramping and expulsion of the oil. If it is too warm, it may injure the patient.

3. **Follow steps 6 through 12 of Procedure 29-3A** (regarding gloving, positioning, draping, and inserting the enema tip).

4. **Instill the oil into the rectum.**
   The oil will soften stool and lubricate the rectum for easier passage of stool.

5. **Withdraw the container tip** from the rectum. Wipe the area with a washcloth or toilet tissue.

6. **Instruct the patient to retain the oil** for at least 30 minutes.

7. **Follow steps 18 through 20 of Procedure 29-3A** (regarding equipment disposal, assisting the patient, and observations of stool).

Procedure 29-3D ■ Administering a Return-Flow Enema

➤ When performing the procedure, always identify your patient according to agency policy and be attentive to standard precautions, hand hygiene, patient safety and privacy, body mechanics, and documentation.

➤ *Note:* A return-flow enema (Harris flush) may be ordered to help a patient expel flatus and relieve abdominal distention.

Procedure Steps

1. **Obtain a rectal tube** and solution container (e.g., bag or canister).

2. **Prepare 100 to 200 mL** (for adults) of tap water or saline.

3. **Follow steps 6 through 12 of Procedure 29-3A** (regarding gloving, positioning, draping, and inserting the enema tip).

4. **Instill all the solution** into the patient's rectum.

5. **Lower the tube and container** below the level of the rectum, and allow the solution to flow back into the container.

6. **Repeat this process** several times, or until the distention is relieved.

7. **Follow steps 18 through 20 of Procedure 29-3A** (regarding equipment disposal, assisting the patient, and observations of stool).

? What if . . .

The solution for a return-flow enema becomes thick with fecal matter?

Discard it and begin again with new solution.

Evaluation

- Observe the amount, color, and consistency of the stool.
- Evaluate the patient's tolerance of the procedure (e.g., amount of cramping, discomfort).
- Determine whether the prescriber's orders require subsequent enema administration.
- Some bowel exams require repeated enemas or enemas administered until the returns are "clear." For the latter, you will need to examine the return and determine whether stool particles are still present. "Clear" does not mean absence of color, but rather absence of stool particles and transparency of the liquid.

Patient Teaching

- Teach the patient that dependence on enemas can disrupt the normal process that stimulates defecation.
- Teach dietary and lifestyle changes that promote regular elimination (e.g., increased fluid intake, diet high in fiber, increased exercise).

Home Care

- Show the patient the box for a prepackaged enema, and instruct him that he may purchase this type of enema at a local grocery or pharmacy.
- Assess the patient's ability to administer his own enema. If you determine that he will be unable to do so, encourage him to seek assistance and instruct the caregiver in the task.
- Teach the patient and caregiver proper handwashing. Encourage them to purchase nonsterile procedure gloves.
  Patients and caregivers may not be aware of the serious infections that can be caused by gram-negative intestinal bacteria.
- If the patient will be attempting to self-administer a cleansing enema, help him determine how and where to hang the container so that it is at the proper height.
- If a soapsuds enema is to be administered in the home setting, teach the patient which household soaps may be substituted for castile soap.
  Some soaps used in the home for cleaning purposes may be too harsh and irritating to the intestinal mucosa.

Documentation

- Document on the nursing notes the type of enema given and, if applicable, the amount of the solution instilled.
- For prepackaged enemas, some facilities require documentation (of the time given and the nurse's initials) on the medication administration record (MAR).
- Document the patient's tolerance of the procedure.
- Document the characteristics and amount of the stool.
- If the prescription is to administer enemas until the returns are clear, document the color of the return solution and the amount of stool seen.

Sample documentation:

*06/04/14   0825   Fleets enema administered
(see MAR). Patient had no cramping; retained enema for
5 minutes. Passed moderate amount of solid, formed,
brown stool with no mucus, but with a streak of blood on
the surface.   — R. Kline, RN*

Thinking About the Procedure

 Go to the *Fundamentals of Nursing Skills Videos,* **Bowel Elimination: Cleansing Enema.**

1. What did the nurse use to drape the patient and protect his privacy?
2. Where was the bag of enema solution when the fluid first began flowing?

 For suggested responses, go to Chapter 29, **Thinking About the Procedure Suggested Responses,** on Davis*Plus.*

Procedure 29–4 ■ Removing Stool Digitally

➤ For steps to follow in *all* procedures, refer to the Universal Steps for All Procedures found on the page facing the inside back cover.

Equipment.

- Two pairs of clean procedure gloves
- Water-soluble lubricant (containing lidocaine, if agency policy permits)
- Bedpan and cover
- Washcloth, soap, and towel or toilet tissue (or moistened towelettes)
- Basin of warm water
- Bath blanket
- Waterproof pad

Delegation

This procedure should not be delegated to a NAP. Ongoing assessment of the patient by the professional nurse is required when stool is manually removed from the rectum. The nurse must monitor the patient for complications, such as bleeding and vagal nerve stimulation. Nursing judgment is necessary in determining the need to halt the procedure.

Pre-Procedure Assessments

- ✚ Assess the patient's baseline vital signs and history of heart disease. Be sure to monitor the patient's pulse before and during the procedure.
  Digital removal of stool can stimulate the vagus nerve, causing bradycardia. Patients who have a history of heart disease or dysrhythmia are at greater risk.
- Assess the patient's white blood cell (WBC) count.
  If the patient has a compromised immune status, evidenced by a low WBC count, you should discuss this procedure with the primary care provider to evaluate the risks and benefits of the procedure.

- Assess the patient's cognitive level and mobility status.
  Determines the patient's ability to follow directions and turn in bed.
- Determine the time of the patient's last bowel movement.
  Infrequent defecation increases the chance that hard stool may form in the rectum.
- Assess the patient for history of fecal impaction.
  Can be a recurrent problem for immobile, disabled, or institutionalized patients.
- Assess stool consistency.
  Patients who are immobilized may become incontinent of watery stool. They may be able to pass small sections of hard stool or small quantities of watery stool. The latter, which may be intermittent or continuous, is a symptom of high colon impaction.
- Determine whether the patient experiences pain on defecation.
  Pain can exacerbate the problem because the patient tends to suppress defecation.
- Assess the patient's pattern of bowel movements, diet, exercise, mobility status, and medications (e.g., iron supplements or narcotic analgesics).
  You should determine whether any of these factors contribute to the problem and then add this information to the nursing care plan to help prevent recurrence.
- Assess bowel sounds and any abdominal distention.
  There can be peristalsis without gastrointestinal patency, which creates distention. Abdominal distention can aggravate constipation.

Guidelines

- Prevention of fecal impaction is the best treatment, but if impaction has occurred, the stool must be removed. The procedure is both painful and embarrassing to your patient.

(continued on next page)

Procedure 29-4 ■ **Removing Stool Digitally** (continued)

- Some practitioners may prescribe an oil-retention enema before the procedure to soften and moisten the stool, making removal easier.
- Also, many advise that you follow digital removal of stool with either an oil-retention and/or tap water enemas.

Enema(s) given after the procedure ensure the evacuation of stool that may not have been reached by digital removal.
- Trim and file your fingernails if they extend past the end of your fingertips.

➤ When performing the procedure, always identify your patient according to agency policy and be attentive to standard precautions, hand hygiene, patient safety and privacy, body mechanics, and documentation.

Procedure Steps

1. **Determine whether lubricant** containing lidocaine is to be used, and obtain the correct lubricant.
   May decrease rectal discomfort for the patient.

2. **Drape the patient** with the bath blanket. Go to Procedure 24-4 to review the procedure for draping. Assist him to turn on his left side, with his right knee flexed toward his head. Place the waterproof pad halfway beneath his left hip.
   Provides privacy and exposes the anus for visualization. The pad protects the bed from being soiled.

3. **Don clean procedure gloves.** Some sources recommend double-gloving.
   Prevents the transmission of intestinal bacteria.

4. **Expose the buttocks.** Place a clean, dry bedpan on the waterproof pad next to the buttocks in line with the rectum.
   The bedpan serves as a receptacle for stool that is removed.

5. **Wet a washcloth,** or have toilet tissue or moist towelettes ready to cleanse the rectal area when you complete the procedure.

6. **Generously lubricate either** the gloved forefinger and/or middle finger on your dominant hand.
   Helps prevent discomfort, pain, and mucosal injury.

7. **Slowly slide one lubricated finger** into the rectum. Observe for perianal irritation.
   The patient may need skin care to reduce pain during additional bowel evacuation. ➤

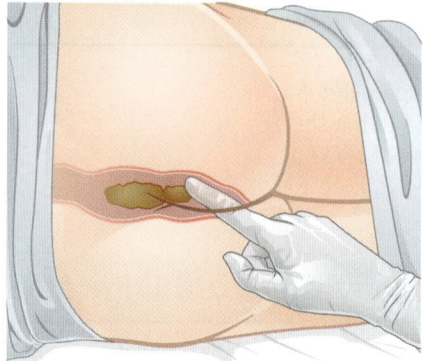

8. **Gently rotate your finger** around the mass and/or into the mass.
   Assists in determining the amount and texture of the fecal bulk.

9. **Begin to break the stool** into smaller pieces. At this point, you may insert a second finger and gently "slice" apart the stool, using a scissoring motion. Remove pieces of stool via the rectum as they become separated, and place them in the bedpan. ▼

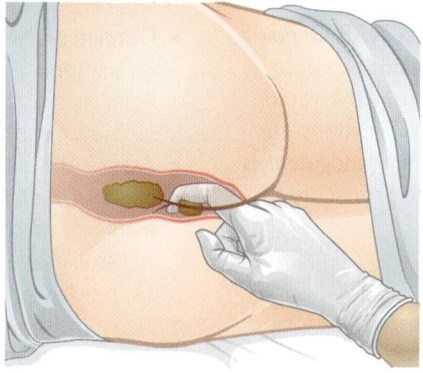

10. **As you proceed, instruct** the patient to take slow, deep breaths.
    Helps the patient to relax his anal sphincter.

11. **Continue to manipulate** and remove pieces of stool, allowing the

patient to rest at intervals. Reapply lubricant (containing lidocaine, if permitted) each time you reinsert your fingers.
Rest periods allow for assessment of and attention to the patient's comfort level and tolerance for the procedure.

12. ✚ **Assess the patient's heart rate at regular intervals.**
    Bradycardia is a sign of vagal stimulation. Stop the procedure if the patient's heart rate falls or the rhythm changes from your initial assessment.
    CAUTION: Some resources suggest that this procedure should be done in small steps (no more than 4 finger insertions in one session), giving a series of suppositories in between stool removal episodes.
    Prevents patient fatigue and pain. Reduces the risk of injury to the rectal tissue and vagal stimulation.

13. **When removal of stool** is complete, cover the bedpan and set it aside. Use a washcloth and/or toilet tissue to cleanse the rectal area.
    Provides personal hygiene and decreases transmission of pathogens.

14. **Assist the patient to return** to a position of comfort. Note the color, amount, and consistency of the stool, and dispose of it properly.

15. **Remove your gloves and wash your hands.**
    Prevents transmission of intestinal pathogens.

? What if . . .

- **The patient is an infant?**
  When treating infants with fecal impactions, avoid enemas and mineral oils. Glycerin suppositories may be used to soften the stool before removal.

Evaluation

- Determine whether evacuation of the retained stool was complete. Perform a rectal exam to assess for presence of stool.
- Reassess vital signs, and compare the results to the initial assessment. Continue to monitor for 1 hour for bradycardia.
- Assess bowel sounds.
- Palpate the abdomen for nontenderness and softness.
- Ask the patient whether he feels relief from rectal pressure or abdominal discomfort.

Patient Teaching

Retained stool is most often the result of poor dietary habits, lack of fluid intake, lack of exercise, inattentiveness to the urge to defecate, and laxative abuse. Focus patient teaching on lifestyle changes that facilitate a regular bowel elimination pattern.

Home Care

Home care should focus on preventing constipation that would require the digital removal of stool. Teach clients about high-fiber foods, adequate water intake, and the importance of exercise. Digital removal of stool may be necessary for some clients as part of a bowel training program (e.g., patients who are paraplegic or quadriplegic). You can teach this procedure to the care provider in the home.

Documentation

- Document the bowel movement on the graphic record.
- Document the procedure and the patient's tolerance for the procedure in the nursing notes.
- Document the patient's pulse rate on the vital signs record.
- Document any unusual characteristics of the stool (e.g., black or green color, blood, or mucus).

Practice Resources

Creason & Sparks, 2000; National Guideline Clearinghouse (NGC), n.d.; Siegel, Rhinehart, Jackson, et al., and the Healthcare Infection Control Practices Advisory Committee, 2007.

Procedure 29-5 ■ Inserting a Rectal Tube

➤ For steps to follow in *all* procedures, refer to the Universal Steps for All Procedures found on the page facing the inside back cover.

Equipment

- 22- to 34-French rectal tube for adults. Choose the size according to the size of the client. For children or petite adults, a smaller size tube (12- to 18-Fr) may be required.
- Water-soluble lubricant
- Procedure gloves
- Toilet paper
- Skin care items (e.g., soap, skin cleanser, water, wipes)
- Collecting device (waterproof pad, graduated cylinder partially filled with water, a urine collection bag nicked at the top to vent)
- Paper tape
- Stool specimen container if needed

Pre-Procedure Assessments

- Obtain baseline vital signs.
- Auscultate bowel sounds; percuss for tympany.
- Observe and palpate the degree of abdominal distention.
- Ask whether the patient is passing any flatus.
- Assess discomfort caused by flatulence.
- Assess the condition of perianal tissues.
- Assess the history of cardiac disease.
  Insertion of a rectal tube can stimulate the vagus nerve, causing bradycardia.

➤ When performing the procedure, always identify your patient according to agency policy and be attentive to standard precautions, hand hygiene, patient safety and privacy, body mechanics, and documentation.

Procedure Steps

1. **Wear procedure gloves.**
   Follows standard precautions.
2. **Ask the patient to lift his hips** or roll from side to side to place a waterproof pad.
   Protects against soiling of linens.
3. **Attach a collecting device** to the end of the rectal tube: Tape a plastic bag or urine collection bag around the distal end of the rectal tube and vent the upper side of the bag; or insert the tube into the specimen container; or place the end of the tube in a graduated container partially filled with water.
   Collects small pieces of stool expelled with flatus. Venting the plastic bag prevents overinflation and bursting the bag. An advantage of using water in the container is that gas generates bubbles, and you will be able to assess the effectiveness of the rectal tube based on the amount of bubbling in the container.
4. **Place patient in the left side-lying** position. Drape for privacy.
   Allows the tube to follow the normal curve of the rectum and sigmoid colon when inserted.
5. **Lubricate the tip of the rectal tube.**
   Prevents trauma to the rectal mucosa.

(continued on next page)

Procedure 29-5 ■ Inserting a Rectal Tube (continued)

6. **Separate the buttocks** and ask the patient to take a deep breath. Gently insert the tube into the rectum. Adults: 10 to 12.5 cm (4 to 5 in.) Children: 5 to 10 cm (2 to 4 in.).
   Deep breaths relax the anal sphincter and ease tube insertion.

7. **For adults, tape the tube in place**; for children, hold it manually.

8. ✚ **Leave the rectal tube in place for 15 to 20 minutes.** If distention persists, you may reinsert the tube every 2 to 3 hours.

Leaving the tube in place for more than 20 minutes may cause pressure necrosis of the mucosa; prolonged stimulation of the anal sphincter may result in loss of the neuromuscular response.

9. **Assist the patient to move** about in bed to promote gas expulsion. A knee–chest position is ideal.
   Because gas is lighter than fluid or solid, the position promotes passage of flatus. Unfortunately, many patients cannot tolerate this position.

10. **Remove the tube**, wipe the patient's buttocks with tissue, and assist to clean the rectal area as needed.
    Prevents transmission of microorganisms from feces; promotes patient comfort and skin integrity.

11. **Dispose of used equipment**; or clean it if it is to be reused. Follow agency procedures for cleaning.

Evaluation

- Evaluate the patient's response to the procedure (e.g., vital signs, fatigue).
- Assess abdominal distention and abdominal comfort.

Patient Teaching

- Teach the patient that chewing gum, sucking on hard candy, using a straw, smoking, and drinking carbonated beverages increase air swallowing and abdominal distention.
- Teach factors that promote normal elimination (e.g., exercise, increased fluid intake, adequate dietary fiber).

Documentation

Record the following:
- Date and time tube inserted
- Size of tube and characteristics of feces collected
- Abdominal distention before and after the procedure
- Pulse and respiratory rates before and after the procedure
- Tolerance of procedure and any complications
- Patient and family teaching

Procedure 29–6 ■ Placing Fecal Drainage Devices

➤ For steps to follow in *all* procedures, refer to the Universal Steps for All Procedures found on the page facing the inside back cover.

Equipment

External Fecal Collection Device

- pH-balanced soap and water or recommended skin cleanser
- Skin protection wipes (e.g., peristomal wipes to protect skin and improve adherence)
- Self-adhesive fecal containment device
- Procedure gloves
- Linen-saver pad
- Scissors

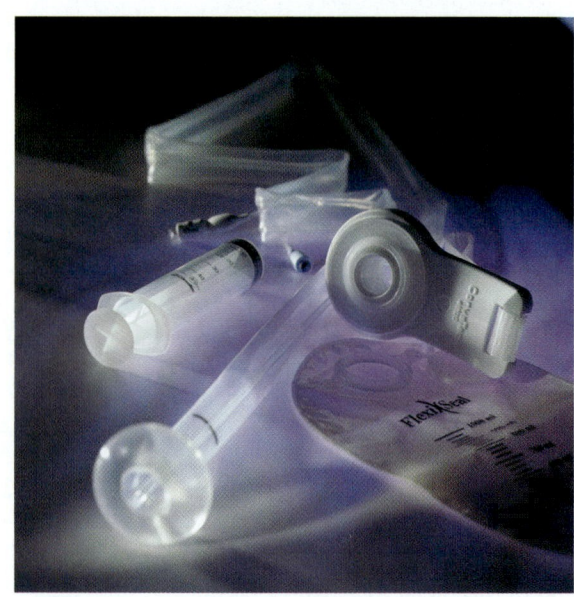

ActiFlo™ indwelling Bowel Catheter System. Courtesy of Hollister Incorporated, Libertyville, IL.

Internal Fecal Collection System

- Fecal device kit: Contains soft silicone catheter tube assembly, a syringe, and a collection bag.
- Water-soluble lubricant
- Approximately 100-mL container of tap water or saline. (Follow the manufacturer's directions for amount and type of solution.)
- 500 mL of lukewarm irrigant (water or saline)
- 60-mL luer-tip syringe and a catheter tip syringe (if not contained in the kit)
- Protective skin-care dressing (e.g., Stomahesive®, DuoDerm®)
- Tape
- Procedure gloves, mask, and goggles
- pH-balanced soap and water or recommended skin cleanser
- Scissors
- Linen-saver pad

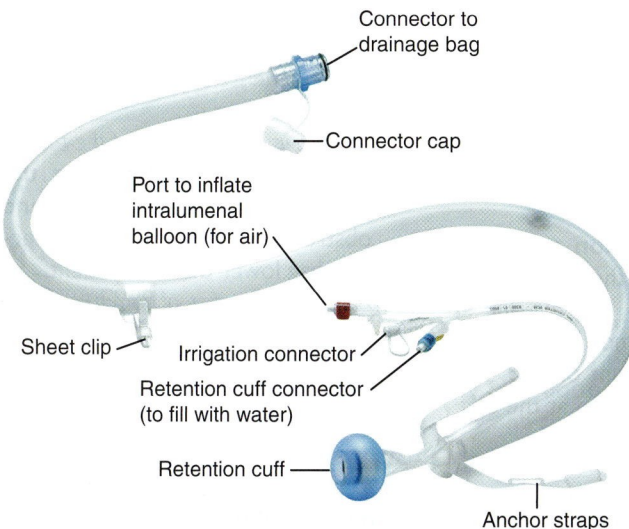

ActiFlo™ indwelling Bowel Catheter System. Courtesy of Hollister Incorporated, Libertyville, IL.

Delegation

Application of an external fecal collection system may be delegated to the NAP. Insertion of a internal fecal collection device is usually performed by a professional nurse, but may be delegated to an LPN depending on agency policy.

Pre-Procedure Assessments

- Assess the patient's bowel patterns.
  Fecal diversion is indicated when the patient is incontinent of liquid or semi-liquid stools (flowing).
- Assess for allergies to silicone. If the patient is sensitive or allergic to any of the materials in the device, it cannot be used.
- Inspect perirectal skin.
  External devices should not be used in patients with impaired skin integrity.

For Indwelling Devices, in Addition:

- Assess whether the patient has had a recent bowel movement.
  Patients who have not had a bowel movement for 2 or more days should be considered as having firm stool and will likely be given a bowel prep or enema before insertion of the indwelling device.
- Check for the presence of any indwelling anal or rectal device (e.g., thermometer for continuous temperature monitoring).
  The treatment plan may need to be changed. If suppositories or enemas are a part of the current treatment plan, collaborate with the prescriber as these medication delivery mechanisms will need to be changed.

- ✚ Identify factors that increase your patient's risk for bleeding, including medications (anticoagulant and/or antiplatelet therapy) and lab results (prothrombin time [PT], partial thromboplastin time [PTT], platelets).
  Patients with an increased risk of bleeding should be monitored carefully.

- ✚ Check the chart for contraindications to an indwelling fecal management system (e.g., proctitis, lacerations, rectal surgery in the past year, large or painful hemorrhoids).
  If your patient has a history of any of these problems, contact the primary care provider immediately. You may elect to use an external device, but an internal fecal catheter is contraindicated.

- ✚ Internal fecal catheters should not be used for children.

Procedure 29-6A ■ Applying an External Fecal Collection System

➤ When performing the procedure, always identify your patient according to agency policy and be attentive to standard precautions, hand hygiene, patient safety and privacy, body mechanics, and documentation.

Procedure Steps

1. **Recruit another nurse or nursing assistant** to help you. Assist the patient to a side-lying position and drape to expose the buttocks.
   For successful application (without leakage) it is best to have one caregiver position the patient and a second person to apply the device.

2. **Don procedure gloves.**
   Observes standard precautions.

3. **Cleanse the perineal area** and dry well. If perianal hair is present, trim it away.
   To obtain a leakproof seal, the device should be attached to clean, dry skin.

4. **Spread the buttocks apart** to expose the rectum. Apply the fecal bag, being careful to place the opening in the bag over the anus and to avoid gaps and creases.
   Careful application helps to obtain a leakproof seal.

5. **Release the buttocks.** Connect the fecal incontinence pouch to a drainage bag. Hang drainage bag below patient.
   To collect and promote gravity drainage of fecal material.

(continued on next page)

Procedure 29-7 ■ Changing an Ostomy Appliance (continued)

skin area and use clinical judgment when changing a pouch. You may delegate to a NAP if it is a preexisting, stable stoma and if you are sure the NAP is qualified to perform the task. If you do delegate this task, instruct the NAP to report any changes or unusual findings (e.g., changes in stoma color, swelling, peristomal redness, excoriation, deviations from expected amount) and color and consistency of drainage from the stoma.

Pre-Procedure Assessments

- Assess the type of stoma (e.g., ileostomy, colostomy, urostomy), number of stomas, and location on the abdomen (e.g., is the stoma near structures that will impact care?).
  Determines the type of pouch or system to use.

- Assess stoma color, shape, size, and/or length of protrusion or retraction; stoma construction (end, loop, double barrel); direction of stoma lumen; and discharge. Does the stoma lie flat or does it protrude?
  The stoma should be moist and red or pink. Alterations in stoma color (purple, black, or blue) may indicate poor circulation and possible necrosis and should be reported to the primary provider. Protruding or retracted stomas will need special adjustments in wafer measurement and placement. It is normal for a new stoma to have yellow or blood-tinged mucus or dried blood on it.

- Assess peristomal skin for redness, rash, irritation, or excoriation. Observe the existing skin barrier and pouch for leakage and length of time in place. You may have to remove the pouch to observe the stoma fully, depending on the type of pouch (i.e., if the pouch is opaque). Notify the provider or an ostomy specialist immediately if you note peristomal skin abnormalities.
  Preserving peristomal skin is critical because skin excoriation may cause an ineffective seal between the wafer and the skin and leakage of effluent. This in turn causes more skin and tissue damage. Leakage may indicate the need for a different type of pouch system or sealant.

- Determine the changing schedule for the pouch.
  Pouches are usually changed every 3 to 5 days, preferably before leakage occurs. Frequency also depends on the type of stoma, the equipment used (e.g., one- or two-piece pouch), the effluent, the patient's preference, and the climate (i.e., pouches are

changed more frequently during the summer). To decrease skin irritation, avoid changing the entire system. In a one-piece or two-piece pouching system, change the skin barrier only every 3 to 7 days, never daily.

- Measure the stoma with each pouching system. Follow the manufacturer's directions and measuring guide for the size of the ostomy pouch and the patient's stoma size.
  Determine the correct size of equipment needed.

- Observe abdominal shape and incision, if present.
  Abdominal shape determines the proper placement of the pouch. Because of stomal and abdominal characteristics, some patients may need convexity in their ostomy pouching system to avoid leakage.

- Assess the patient's willingness to look at the stoma, touch the appliance, and discuss or participate in the task.
  May indicate a readiness or desire to learn.

- Assess the patient's condition and self-care ability. Consider vision, dexterity or mobility, and cognitive ability.

- Auscultate for bowel sounds.
  Determines the presence of peristalsis.

- Observe for effluent from the stoma, and document your findings.
  Change the skin barrier pouch at times of lower fecal output. Avoid changing after meals, when the gastrocolic reflux increases chance of fecal output. Mucous secretion is normal.

- Assess whether a new clamp will be needed or the one on the pouch can be used again. Consult a peristomal nurse or the primary care provider to determine whether an ostomy should be irrigated.

Many patients with left-end colostomies may be safely irrigated as a method of continence management. An ileostomy, however, drains liquid containing high concentrations of sodium, chloride, potassium, magnesium, and bicarbonate.

✚ **Ileostomies should never be irrigated, except in cases of food blockage near the stomal outlet. Only a qualified person, such as an enterostomal therapy nurse, may perform a gentle lavage. For lavage, normal saline is preferred because excessive lavage could lead to a serious fluid and electrolyte imbalance.**

➤ When performing the procedure, always identify your patient according to agency policy and be attentive to standard precautions, hand hygiene, patient safety and privacy, body mechanics, and documentation.

Procedure Steps

1. **Wash your hands and don clean procedure gloves.**
   Prevents transmission of pathogens.

2. **Fold down the bed covers** to expose the ostomy site. Place a clean towel across the patient's abdomen under the existing pouch.
   Helps prevent spilling effluent onto the patient.

3. **Position the patient** so that no skinfolds occur along the line of the stoma.
   Ensures an adequate seal between the wafer and the skin, preventing leakage.

4. **If the present ostomy pouch** is drainable, empty it into the bedpan.
   Pouches should be drained when they are one-third to one-half full because the weight of the contents may dislodge the

skin seal; ostomy drainage is irritating to the skin. The pouch also collects flatus, which needs to be expelled because it can disrupt the skin seal.

   a. To calculate the amount of output in milliliters for an ostomy with a liquid effluent (e.g., ileostomy or urostomy), use a graduated measuring container.

b. For pouches that you open by unrolling them at the bottom, you must remove a clamp to empty the pouch. Save this clamp for reuse.

NOTE: Some pouches cannot be drained.

5. **Using a silicone-based** (hexamethyldisiloxane) adhesive remover, remove the appliance by applying the adhesive remover with one hand as you press the skin away from the wafer barrier with your other hand. Avoid pulling the appliance straight off. Begin at the top and work downward.

Silicone-based adhesive removers are preferred over alcohol- or oil-based products. Pulling the appliance from the skin tends to strip the loosely bound epidermal skin layers, making the skin more susceptible to moisture loss and irritation from effluent. Silicone-based products reduce the bind strength, whereas alcohol dissolves the adhesives; thus, alcohol may cause dryness and irritation. It also causes pain if the skin is not intact. If you use an oil-based solvent, the new pouch will not adhere to the oily skin. ▼

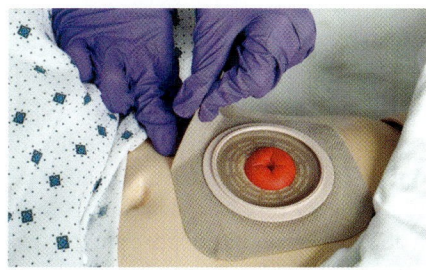

6. **Place the old pouch and wafer** in the plastic bag for disposal. If you were unable to drain the pouch, dispose of it according to agency protocol.
Prevents transmission of infections caused by fecal bacteria.

7. **Inspect the stoma and peristomal** skin area (see Assessment, preceding).

8. **Cleanse the stoma** and surrounding skin using warm water. Allow the area to dry. You may use a skin-cleansing agent with a pH of 5.5 that is designed to both cleanse and moisturize the skin.

Removes old adhesive and any effluent that has leaked. Helps prevent skin irritation and/or breakdown and maintain skin moisture. Select cleansing agents that protect the stratum corneum lipids and proteins.

9. **Measure the size of the stoma.** You can accomplish this in several ways.
   a. Place a standard stoma measuring guide over the stoma.
   b. Reuse a previously cut template.
   c. Measure the stoma from side to side (approximating the circumference).

The stoma may need to be remeasured frequently during the initial postoperative period because the size of the stoma may change as edema subsides. ▼

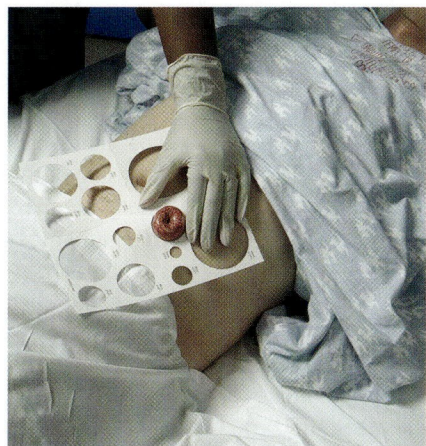

10. **Place a clean 4 in. × 4 in. gauze** pad over the stoma.
Gauze will absorb any leaking effluent, keeping the skin clean and dry during application of the new pouch.

11. **Remove your gloves and wash** your hands.
Decreases the spread of intestinal bacteria.

12. **Trace the size of the opening** obtained in step 9 onto the paper on the back of the new wafer. Cut the opening. The opening in the wafer should be approximately $1/16$ to $1/8$ in. (1.5 to 3 mm) larger than the circumference of the stoma.
Allows for skin movement with activity and prevents impaired circulation to the stoma.

13. **Peel the paper off the wafer.** Some resources suggest first holding the wafer between the palms of your hand to warm the adhesive ring.
Enhances the integrity of the seal by making the ring more "sticky" so that it will bond better with the skin.

NOTE: Some ostomy wafers come with an outer ring of tape attached. Do not remove the backing on this tape until the wafer is securely positioned (see step 16).

14. **Don clean procedure gloves.**

15. **At this time, you may apply** ostomy skin care products per your clinical judgment, hospital protocol, or following the recommendations of the enterostomal therapist (e.g., wipe around stoma with skin prep, apply skin barrier powder or paste, or apply extra adhesive paste).
These products prevent or treat excoriated skin and/or ensure a tight seal between the wafer and the skin.

16. **Remove the gauze.** Center the wafer opening around the stoma, and gently press it down. Press your hand firmly against the newly applied wafer and hold for 30 to 60 seconds. If you are applying a one-piece pouch, make sure the bag is pointed toward the patient's feet. If you have a different type of pouch, see What If at the end of this procedure.
Heat from the hand activates the adhesive ring, making it adhere better thus promoting optimal wear time. Some sources also suggest taping down the edges of the wafer.

17. **Remove your gloves and wash** your hands.

18. **Return the patient** to a comfortable position. Dispose of the used ostomy pouch following your facility's policy for biohazardous waste.

? What if . . .

■ **Your patient has a two-piece pouch?**

After applying the wafer around the stoma with a good seal (Step 16), attach the bag following manufacturer's instructions.

(continued on next page)

Procedure 29-7 ■ **Changing an Ostomy Appliance** (continued)

■ **Your patient's ostomy uses an open-ended pouch?**

After applying the wafer securely around the stoma, fold the end of the pouch over the clamp, and close the clamp, listening for a "click" to ensure that it is secure.

■ **Your patient has poor vision or is blind?**

Patients with poor vision may need to use magnification mirrors and yellow-tinted sunglasses to help reduce glare and

improve contrast when they perform stoma care.

■ **Your patient is immobile?**

Patients with immobility or spinal cord injury may need equipment that has a longer pouch that the patient can easily empty independently when sitting.

■ **Your patient has impaired dexterity?**

Impaired dexterity may warrant the use of a one-piece system or precut pouch

and skin barrier, whereas a two-piece system may be better for patients who need to keep the skin barrier in place for several days and change just the pouch. Patients who are blind can be taught to change their own equipment.

■ **At step 8, you notice that the stoma is bleeding?**

Slight bleeding of the stoma is normal; report excessive bleeding to the primary care provider.

Evaluation

Make the following observations:
■ Characteristics of stoma: color, size, presence of edema, and shape
■ Presence of blisters, redness, or excoriation on peristomal skin
■ Amount and characteristics of effluent: color, odor, consistency
■ Whether the patient expressed a desire to participate in the task
■ Whether the patient demonstrated nonverbal cues that she is ready to learn about the task (e.g., looking at the stoma)

Patient Teaching

Patient teaching is aimed at preparing the patient to complete this skill at home. She (or a caregiver) will need to be instructed in how to complete all the steps of the procedure.

Home Care

■ Assess the patient's self-care ability. Patients with poor vision may need to use magnification mirrors and yellow-tinted sunglasses to help reduce glare and improve contrast when they perform stoma care. Patients who are blind can be taught to change their own equipment.
■ Patients with immobility or spinal cord injury may need equipment that has a longer pouch that the patient can easily empty independently when sitting.
■ Impaired dexterity or vision may warrant the use of a one-piece system or precut pouch and skin barrier, whereas a two-piece system may be better for patients who need to keep the skin barrier in place for several days and change just the pouch.
■ Help the client establish a routine for changing the stoma wafer/pouch. In general, experts recommend changing it twice weekly, or as determined by the physician or ostomy specialist.
■ Change the skin barrier pouch at times of lower effluent output.

■ Avoid changing after meals, when the gastrocolic reflux increases chance of fecal effluent output. Mucous secretion is normal.
■ Advise the client to change the pouch immediately if it begins to leak. *The average wear-time in the United States is 4.5 days for a colostomy and 5 days for an ileostomy or urostomy (Richbourg, Fellows, & Arroyave, 2008).*
■ The client can complete the removal of her pouch and cleansing of the peristomal skin in the shower.
■ The client may need to stand in front of a mirror or sit to change her ostomy appliance if she is unable to view the stoma easily.
■ Teach the client that slight bleeding is normal when the stoma is washed.
■ The client should not use soaps and lotions containing oils. They decrease the adhesiveness of the wafer.
■ The appliance and wafer cannot be flushed down the toilet.
■ Teach the client to report changes in the color or size of the stoma and/or the presence of peristomal irritation or skin breakdown to the primary care provider.
■ Provide information about community support groups.
■ Provide contact information for ostomy supply vendors.

Documentation

Document the following:
■ Your assessment of the stoma and peristomal skin area
■ Patient's tolerance of the procedure
■ Type of appliance used, including the manufacturer and part number
■ Use of any special ostomy skin care products
■ Amount of liquid effluent on the I&O portion of the graphics record
■ Patient teaching and the degree to which the patient participated in the procedure

Practice Resources

Black, 2008; Burch & Sica, 2008; Cronin, 2008; Karadag, Mentex, & Ayaz, 2005; Kent, 2008; Pullen, 2006; Richbourg, Fellows, & Arroyave, 2008; Siegel, Rhinehart, Jackson, et al., and the Healthcare Infection Control Practices Advisory Committee, 2007.

Thinking About the Procedure

 Go to the *Fundamentals of Nursing Skills Videos,* **Bowel Elimination: Colostomy Appliance, Changing.**

1. What did the nurse do to protect the patient's privacy?
2. How did the nurse determine the size of the opening in the new appliance?

3. When applying the new appliance, which direction did the nurse point the drainage end of the pouch: toward the patient's head, left side, right side, feet?

 For suggested responses, go to Chapter 29, **Thinking About the Procedure Suggested Responses,** on Davis*Plus.*

Procedure 29–8 ■ Irrigating a Colostomy

➤ For steps to follow in *all* procedures, refer to the Universal Steps for All Procedures found on the page facing the inside back cover.

Equipment

- Irrigation equipment
  - One-piece system with a fluid container connected to tubing with cone or two-piece system with a container separate from tubing with cone
  - Irrigation sleeve; a sleeve without adhesive backing requires a belt to hold it in place
  - Clamp for a sleeve with an opening at the top
  - Prescribed irrigating solution (usually 500 to 1,000 mL warm tap water, 100°F to 105°F [37.8°C to 40.6°C])
- IV pole or other equipment to hang the irrigation container
- Chair
- Water-soluble lubricant
- Silicone-based adhesive remover
- Skin cleansers and barriers as recommended by your agency
- Toilet tissue
- Washcloth, towel
- Waterproof pad
- Two pairs of clean procedure gloves
- Toilet facilities that include a flushable toilet and a hook or some other device to hold the irrigation container; or bedpan or bedside commode (for patients with impaired mobility)
- New ostomy appliance and skin barrier or stoma cap cover
- Ostomy deodorant (optional)
- Plastic bag for disposal of the used pouch

Delegation

The initial irrigation of a newly created colostomy requires nursing judgment and clinical decision making. Initially, this procedure should not be delegated to the NAP, although in some situations it may be delegated to a licensed practical nurse (LPN), depending on agency policy.

Pre-Procedure Assessments

- Evaluate the defecation pattern (or absence) nature of stool, placement of stoma, abdominal distention, and nutritional pattern.
  Findings may indicate the need to irrigate to stimulate elimination function; consistency of stool varies along the length of the GI tract.
- Assess the type of ostomy.
  Many patients with left-end colostomies may be safely irrigated as a method of continence management. However, do not irrigate an ileostomy.
- Assess the patient's usual bowel pattern.
  The purpose for irrigating a colostomy is to promote a regular pattern for bowel elimination.
- Assess for abdominal distention.
  Report distention to the primary care provider, as it may indicate excess gas or inflammation.
- Assess hydration status.
  The colon may absorb some of the irrigation fluid if the patient is very dehydrated.
- Assess cognitive level and mobility status.
  Determines the necessity for a bedpan or bedside commode. Also determines whether patient teaching will be effective.
- Assess the patient's ability to maintain a sitting position.
- Assess the characteristics of the stoma (See Clinical Insight 28-2).

(continued on next page)

Procedure 29-8 ■ Irrigating a Colostomy (continued)

➤ When performing the procedure, always identify your patient according to agency policy and be attentive to standard precautions, hand hygiene, patient safety and privacy, body mechanics, and documentation.

Procedure Steps

1. **Place the IV pole near** the location of the procedure (e.g., in the bathroom, next to the bedside commode, or next to the bed).
   Allows you to work efficiently.

2. **If possible, assist the patient** to the bathroom or commode. Ask the patient if she prefers to sit directly on the toilet or on a chair in front of it. If the patient must remain in bed, elevate the head of the bed.
   Patients with impaired mobility can sit directly on or in front of the bedside commode, or they may remain in bed in the side-lying position.

3. **Prepare the irrigation container.**
   a. Step 3a. For two-piece systems, connect the tubing to the container. Clamp the tubing. Fill the container with 500 to 1,000 mL of warm tap water.

   ✚ Water that is too cold will cause cramping, nausea, and discomfort. Water that is too hot will damage the intestinal mucosa.

   ➤ Note: Some ostomy resources suggest that using 1,000 mL of water will promote a more effective irrigation of the entire colon and decrease the necessity to irrigate more than once a day.

   b. Prime the tubing. Unclamp the tubing to allow it to fill.
   Removes air from the tubing, preventing gas pains.

4. **Hang the solution container** on the IV pole. Adjust the IV pole so that it reaches the height of the patient's shoulder (approximately 45 cm [18 in.], above the stoma).
   The height of the container regulates the force of the flow.

5. **Wash your hands and don clean procedure gloves.**
   Prevents the transmission of pathogens.

6. **Remove the existing colostomy appliance** (if the patient is wearing one) following the steps in Procedure 29-7. Inspect the stoma and surrounding skin area.

Use of ostomy skin care preparations may be needed when you replace the pouch.

7. **Dispose of the used** colostomy appliance properly. Empty the contents into the bedpan or toilet, and discard the pouch in a moisture-proof (e.g., plastic) bag.
   Prevents transmission of intestinal bacteria.

8. **Assess the characteristics** of the stoma before applying the colostomy irrigation sleeve with an adhesive backing, following the manufacturer's directions.
   - If your patient is sitting on a toilet or bedside commode, then the end of the sleeve should hang down past the patient's pubic area, but not down into the water. Place a waterproof pad under the sleeve over the patient's thighs.
   - If your patient is in bed, place the end of the sleeve into the bedpan.
     Prevents leakage and spilling of irrigation fluid and effluent.

9. **Generously lubricate the cone** at the end of the irrigation tubing with water-soluble lubricant.
   Prevents irritation and damage to the stoma and intestinal lumen.

10. **Open the top of the irrigation sleeve**; insert the cone gently into the colostomy stoma, and hold it solidly in place.
    Gentle insertion prevents damage to the mucosa. ▼

11. **Open the clamp on the tubing,** and slowly begin the flow of water. The fluid should flow for about 10 to 15 minutes or as the patient can tolerate.
    Proceeding slowly allows the patient to adjust to the distention of the bowel.

12. **If the patient complains** of discomfort, stop the flow for 15 to 30 seconds, and ask the patient take deep breaths.
    Allows the patient to rest and adjust to the pressure of solution. Cramping may indicate that the bowel is ready to empty, the water is too cold, the flow is too fast, or the tube contains air.

13. **When the correct amount** of solution has instilled, clamp the tubing, and remove the cone from the stoma.

14. **Wrap the end of the cone** in tissue or paper towel until you can clean or dispose of it properly.
    Prevents transmission of intestinal bacteria.

15. **Close the top of the irrigation sleeve** with a clamp.
    Prevents spillage of irrigation fluid and feces.

16. **Ask the patient to remain sitting** until most of the irrigation fluid and bowel contents have evacuated.
    Alternatively, you can clamp the end of the sleeve and ask the patient to ambulate to stimulate compete

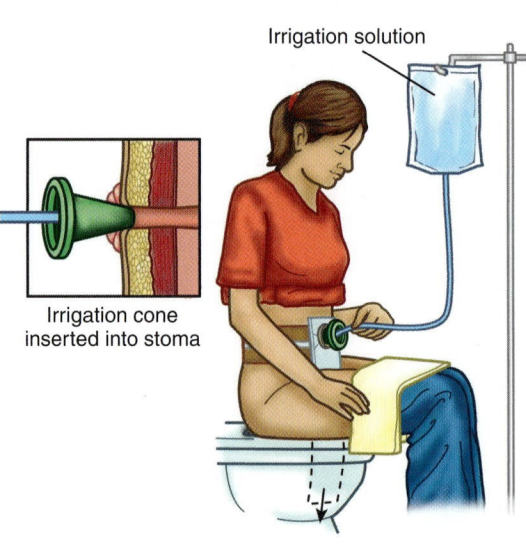

Irrigation solution

Irrigation cone inserted into stoma

evacuation of stool. Massaging the abdomen may also help stimulate return.

This should take about 30 minutes on average. You might wait for about an hour to be certain all the fecal material has been returned.

17. **When evacuation is complete**, open the top clamp, and rinse and remove the irrigation sleeve. Set it aside.

The irrigation sleeve is reusable, but it should be rinsed promptly to make thorough cleansing easier in the following steps.

18. **Cleanse the stoma** and peristomal skin area with a warm washcloth. Prep the skin and apply a new colostomy appliance, if the patient is wearing one, following the steps in Procedure 29-7. Otherwise, cover the stoma with a small gauze bandage.

19. **Clean the irrigation sleeve** with mild soap and water. Allow it to dry. Place the irrigation supplies in the proper place (e.g., in a plastic container or plastic bag).

The irrigation sleeve is reusable, but it must be cleaned well to avoid odors and transmission of pathogens.

20. **Remove your gloves and wash your hands.**
Prevents healthcare-associated infections.

21. **Assist the patient** back to a position of comfort.

? What if . . .

- Your patient has a colostomy sleeve without an adhesive backing?

Place the belt around the patient's waist, and attach the ends to the pouch flange on either side.

Evaluation

Observe the following:

- Characteristics of the stool: color, amount, consistency
- Signs of bleeding from stoma or bowel
- Presence or absence of abdominal distention
- Patient's tolerance of procedure (e.g., cramps, fatigue)
- Patient's ability to participate in the irrigation

Patient Teaching

- Teach the patient the purpose for the procedure.
- Explain that using sufficient fluid will decrease the need for multiple irrigations during the day.
- Teach the steps of the irrigation procedure to prepare the patient to complete the task at home.
- Explain that it takes approximately 6 to 8 weeks to achieve bowel regulation with irrigations.

Home Care

- Help the client determine where this procedure will be completed in the home setting.
- Make sure the client has resources for purchasing the supplies for the irrigation. Provide contact information.
- Help the client locate a place to hang the irrigation container. There may be a hook on the bathroom wall, for instance.
- If the irrigating solution does not flow well, the client should:
- Check the tubing for kinks.
- Change the position of the cone.
- Put the container at a slightly higher level.
- Explain and demonstrate how to care for the irrigation supplies (e.g., how to rinse and clean the sleeve and/or belt, if used).

Documentation

Document:

- Your assessment of the stoma and peristomal area
- The amount of irrigation solution used
- The date and time that you performed the irrigation
- Characteristics of the stool returned in the irrigation fluid
- Patient teaching

Practice Resources

Black, 2008; Burch & Sica, 2008; Cronin, 2008; Karadag, Mentex, & Ayaz, 2005; Kent, 2008; Richbourg, Fellows, & Arroyave, 2008; Siegel, Rhinehart, Jackson, et al., and the Healthcare Infection Control Practices Advisory Committee, 2007.

 To explore learning resources for this chapter,

 Go to Davis*Plus* at http://davisplus.fadavis.com, keyword Treas.

Chapter Resources for Chapter 29:
  Knowledge Check and Think Like a Nurse Response Sheets
  Knowledge Check Answers
  Resources for Caregivers and Health Professionals
  Reading More About Bowel Elimination (Suggested Readings)
  What Are the Main Points in This Chapter?
NCLEX-Style Review Questions
Chapter Overview Podcasts

Concept Map

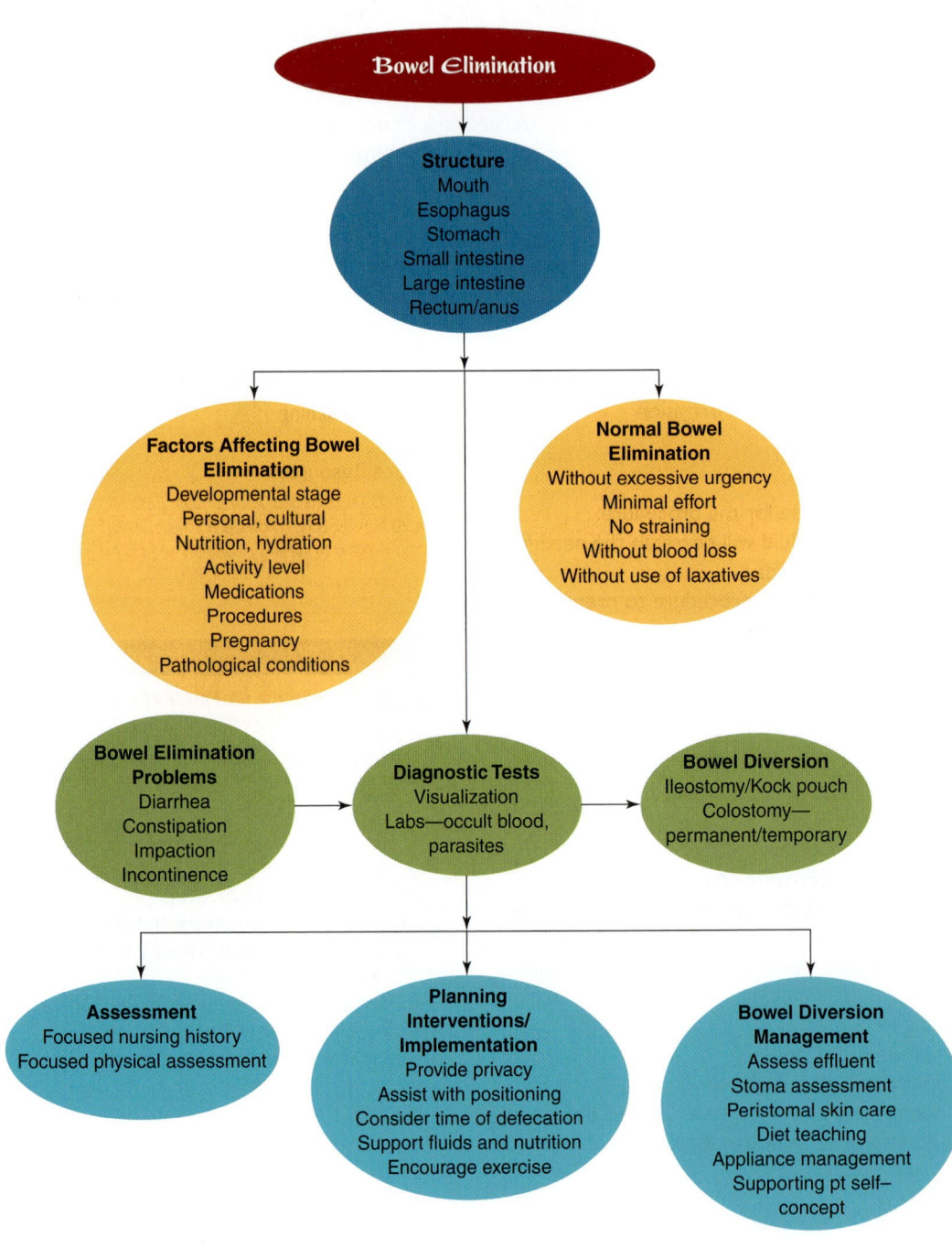

Bowel Elimination

Structure
Mouth
Esophagus
Stomach
Small intestine
Large intestine
Rectum/anus

Factors Affecting Bowel Elimination
Developmental stage
Personal, cultural
Nutrition, hydration
Activity level
Medications
Procedures
Pregnancy
Pathological conditions

Normal Bowel Elimination
Without excessive urgency
Minimal effort
No straining
Without blood loss
Without use of laxatives

Bowel Elimination Problems
Diarrhea
Constipation
Impaction
Incontinence

Diagnostic Tests
Visualization
Labs—occult blood, parasites

Bowel Diversion
Ileostomy/Kock pouch
Colostomy—permanent/temporary

Assessment
Focused nursing history
Focused physical assessment

Planning Interventions/Implementation
Provide privacy
Assist with positioning
Consider time of defecation
Support fluids and nutrition
Encourage exercise

Bowel Diversion Management
Assess effluent
Stoma assessment
Peristomal skin care
Diet teaching
Appliance management
Supporting pt self–concept

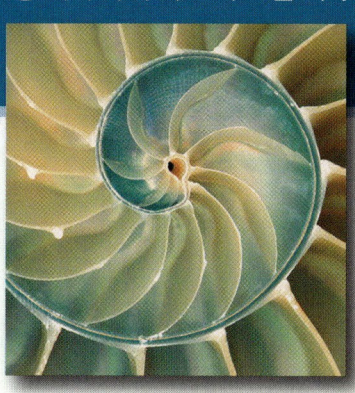

CHAPTER 30

Urinary Elimination

Learning Outcomes

After completing this chapter, you should be able to:

➤ Describe the normal structure and function of the organs in the urinary system.

➤ Describe the processes of urine formation and elimination.

➤ Discuss factors that affect urinary elimination.

➤ Describe the contents of a nursing assessment and physical examination focused on urinary elimination.

➤ Accurately measure urine output.

➤ Describe procedures for collecting various types of urine specimens.

➤ List and describe diagnostic tests used in identifying urinary elimination problems.

➤ Discuss common elimination problems: urinary tract infection, urinary retention, and urinary incontinence.

➤ Identify nursing diagnoses associated with altered urinary elimination.

➤ Describe nursing interventions that promote normal urination.

➤ Provide care for clients experiencing urinary problems.

➤ Perform urinary catheterizations following accepted procedures.

➤ Discuss nursing care appropriate for clients who have a urinary diversion.

Key Concepts

Urinary Elimination

Related Concepts

See the Concept Map at the end of this chapter.

Example Problems

Urinary incontinence

Urinary retention

Urinary tract infections

Caring for the Nguyens

This feature allows you to practice the kind of thinking you will use as a full-spectrum nurse. There is usually more than one correct answer to a critical thinking question, so we do not provide answers for these features. It is more important to develop your nursing judgment than to "cover content." Discuss the questions with your peers. If you are still unsure, consult your instructor.

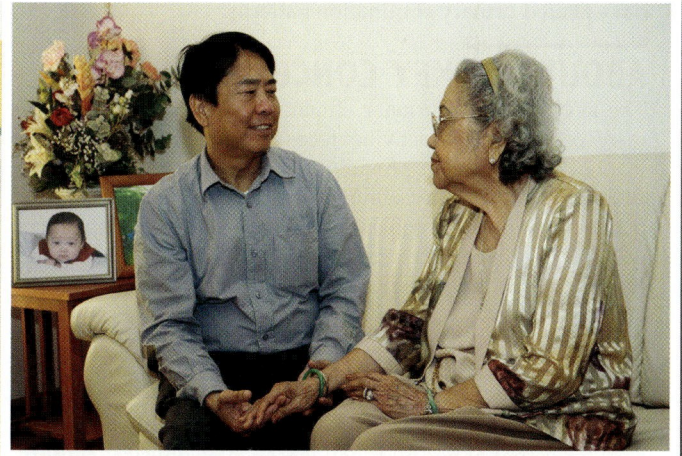

At a recent visit to the Family Health Center, Nam and Yen Nguyen confide that Nam's mother, Mai Nguyen, has had several "accidents." She has denied the problem but Yen tells you that she helped her mother-in-law with laundry recently and many of the clothes smell of urine. They ask you how to approach Mai about this problem.

A. How would you respond?

B. What suggestions, if any, could you make to the Nguyens about treatment for Mai?

C. Yen says that she has been told that surgery is the best form of treatment. She asks you whether this is true. How would you answer her question?

 Go to **Caring for the Nguyen Response Sheet** on *DavisPlus*.

Meet Your Patient

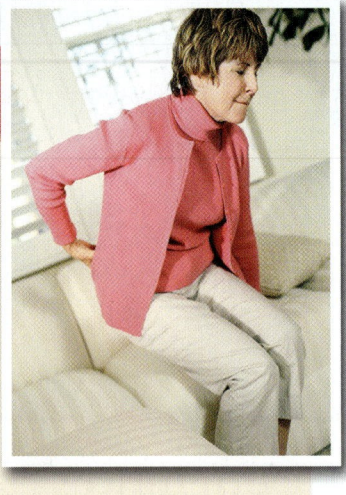

During your assigned clinical experience, you are completing the admission process for Marlena, a 55-year-old woman who is complaining of frequent, painful urination. As you interview her, Marlena becomes embarrassed. "I really don't enjoy talking about this," she admits. When she asks to use the bathroom, you ask her to give you a midstream clean-catch urine sample. She returns with a small specimen of pink-colored, strong-smelling urine. "I have a strong urge to go and then I hardly have any urine. It burns like crazy when I urinate," she reports.

You close the door and interview Marlena in private about her usual urination pattern and current symptoms. Your calm approach and straightforward manner put her at ease. She confides that she is sexually active and that her symptoms began after spending the weekend with her new partner. You take her vital signs: oral temperature 99.4°F (37.4°C), radial pulse 88 beats/min, respiratory rate 20 breaths/min, and blood pressure 108/72 mm Hg.

The emergency department (ED) physician asks you to perform a dipstick urinalysis on the urine sample and to send the urine sample to the lab for culture and sensitivity. He says, "Well, what do you think we need to do next?" How would you answer his question?

As you gain theoretical and practical knowledge of the concepts in this chapter, we will return to this case study to discuss how you might answer the physician's question and support Marlena's recovery. You will also have the opportunity to examine your feelings about giving care that patients may regard as personal or even embarrassing.

Theoretical Knowledge
knowing **why**

A variety of factors play a role in urinary health. You will need theoretical knowledge of the concepts associated with normal physiology of the urinary system, as well as other body systems that influence urinary function. That's why it is vitally important that you take a holistic approach to patients who have altered urinary elimination patterns.

ABOUT THE KEY CONCEPTS

The key concept of urinary elimination is important because many of your nursing activities focus on promoting normal elimination. You will also be providing support for patients who have problems with urinary elimination. In order to best care for patients with urinary problems and provide holistic independent and collaborative interventions for them, you must understand the concepts involved in the formation and elimination of urine.

HOW DOES THE URINARY SYSTEM WORK?

The body removes from food and fluids the nutrients necessary for essential bodily functions, such as physical activity, self-repair, and mental operations. Waste products are left in the blood and in the bowel. The organs of the urinary system that help to excrete wastes and maintain a balance of chemicals and water in the body include the kidneys, ureters, bladder, and urethra (Fig. 30-1).

The Kidneys Filter and Regulate

The kidneys filter metabolic wastes, toxins, excess ions, and water from the bloodstream and excrete them as urine. If kidney function is impaired, these substances reach toxic levels and damage body cells. The kidneys also help to regulate blood

volume, blood pressure, electrolyte levels, and acid–base balance by selectively reabsorbing water and other substances. Secondary functions of the kidneys are to produce erythropoietin, secrete the enzyme renin, and activate vitamin D_3 (calcitriol). The kidneys are located against the posterior abdominal wall

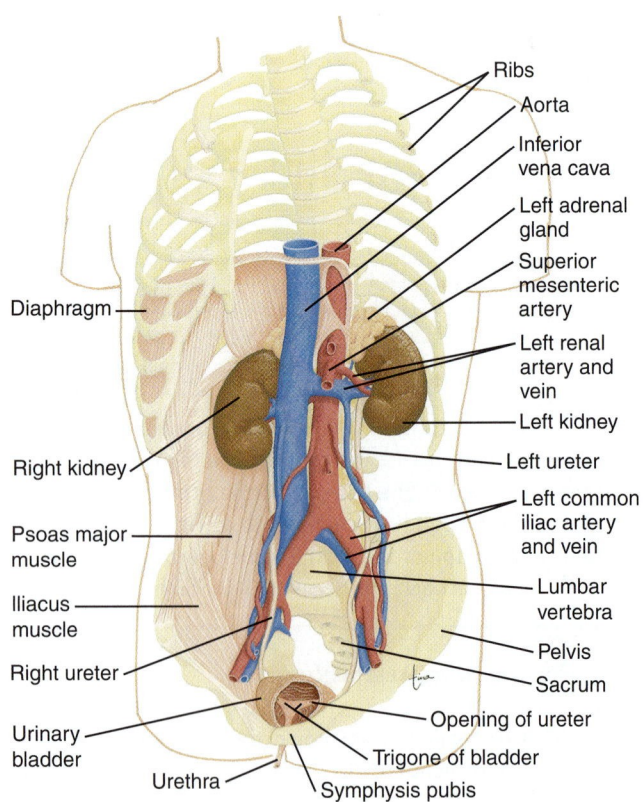

FIGURE 30-1 The organs of the urinary system include the kidneys, ureters, bladder, and urethra.

behind the peritoneum (they are **retroperitoneal).** The average kidney weighs about 5 ounces and is the shape of a kidney bean (see Fig 30-1).

The outer layer, or **cortex,** of the kidney is composed of millions of microscopic functional units, called *nephrons* (Fig 30-2). The inner layer, or **medulla,** consists of 8 to 10 wedge-shaped cones, called the *renal pyramids*. The renal pyramids are made up of bundles of collecting tubules. The innermost area is the **renal pelvis.** Funnel-shaped extensions known as **calyces** (singular: **calyx**) enclose the central portion of each renal pyramid and direct urine into the renal pelvis.

The Nephrons Form Urine

The **nephron** is the basic structural and functional unit of the kidney (see Fig 30-2). There are about 1 million nephrons in each kidney. Each nephron consists of a **Bowman's capsule** (a double-walled hollow capsule) enclosing a **glomerulus** (a knotty ball of capillaries); a series of filtrating tubules; and a collecting duct.

Together, these structures act as a microscopic filter, controlling the excretion and retention of fluids and solutes according to the body's moment-by-moment needs. Urine is formed by filtration, reabsorption, and secretion, as discussed next. For a detailed view of a nephron,

 Go to Chapter 30, **Tables, Boxes, Figures: ESG Figure 30-1,** on Davis*Plus*.

Glomerular Filtration

Figure 30-3 summarizes the process of urine formation. The first step, **filtration,** occurs in the glomeruli. The renal arteries bring blood to the kidneys and into the glomeruli. Blood pressure forces plasma, dissolved substances, and small proteins out of the porous glomeruli into Bowman's capsule to form a liquid called **filtrate.** The **glomerular filtration rate** is the

amount of filtrate formed by the kidneys per minute. Unless the glomerular capillaries are inflamed or damaged, large molecules, such as blood cells and blood proteins, are too large to filter across their walls. Glomerular filtrate resembles blood plasma, except that it contains much less protein and no blood cells.

Renal blood flow progressively decreases with aging, primarily because of changes to the micro blood vessels to the kidney. This decline in glomerular filtration is the most important functional deficit caused by aging (*Merck Manual of Geriatrics*, 2000 [updated 2009]).

To see an animated explanation of the processes of osmosis, diffusion, filtration, and active transport,

 Go to **Animations: Osmosis, Diffusion, Filtration, and Active Transport,** on Davis*Plus*.

Tubular Reabsorption

The filtrate moves from Bowman's capsule into a highly twisted tubule (*proximal convoluted tubule,* Fig. 30-3). As the filtrate journeys through the tubule, 99% is reabsorbed into the peritubular capillaries. Approximately 1% of filtrate returns, as urine, to the *collecting tubule,* which transports it into the ureters. Wastes and toxins that remain in the blood after filtration are actively transported into the filtrate (reabsorbed) in the *distal* and *collecting tubules*. Water and sodium are reabsorbed in these structures when antidiuretic hormone (ADH) and aldosterone are secreted. For an animated explanation of urine formation and elimination,

 Go to **Animations, Urine Formation and Elimination** on Davis*Plus*.

When the amount of fluid in the body decreases (e.g., because of low intake or blood loss), the posterior pituitary gland secretes more ADH. This causes the distal and collecting tubules to reabsorb more water into the blood. At the same time, the adrenal cortex secretes more aldosterone, sodium reabsorption increases, and water follows sodium back into the blood. ADH and aldosterone thus have the effect of maintaining normal blood volume and blood pressure.

When the amount of water in the body increases (e.g., as in ingestion of excessive fluids), ADH is suppressed and the opposite effect occurs. Urine becomes dilute and water continues to be eliminated until its concentration returns to normal (Scanlon & Sanders, 2011).

Tubular Secretion

Some substances are actively secreted from the blood in the peritubular capillaries into the renal filtrate. For example, metabolic waste products, such as ammonia and creatinine, and some medications are secreted into the filtrate and then eliminated in urine. In addition, the kidneys help maintain the normal pH of blood by secreting hydrogen ions (H^+).

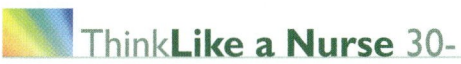 Think**Like a Nurse** 30-1

If a client is suffering from impaired kidney function, what signs and symptoms might you expect to see?

The Ureters Transport Urine

The remaining organs of the urinary system transport or store the urine once it is formed. From the collecting tubules, urine travels into the renal pelvis and enters the ureter. Each kidney has one ureter, approximately 26 to 30 cm (10 to 12 in.) long

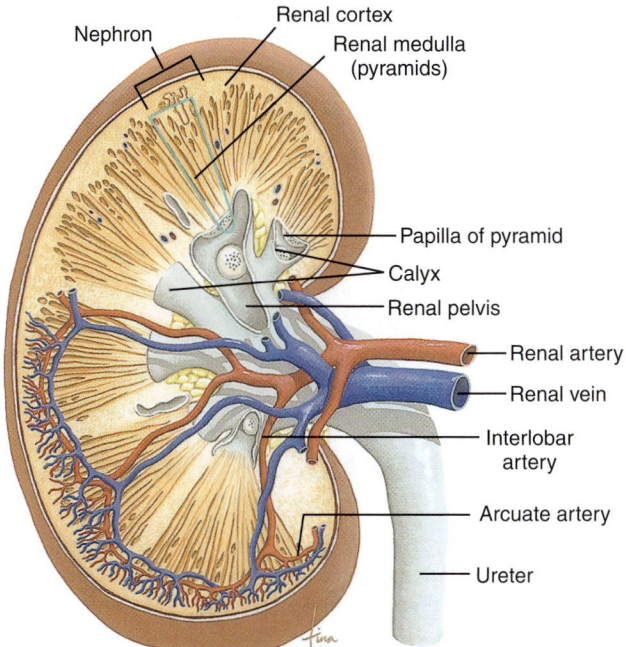

FIGURE 30-2 A cross section of the kidney, showing the renal cortex, medulla, pyramids, and calyces.

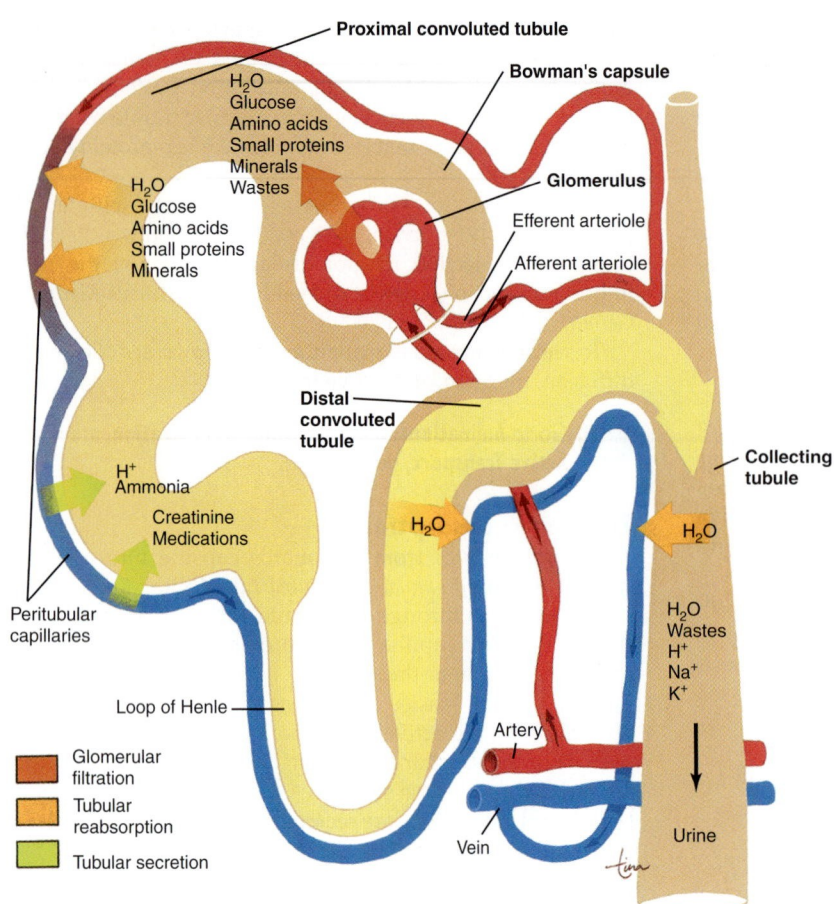

FIGURE 30-3 A schematic representation of the formation of urine.

and 1.25 cm (0.5 in.) in diameter (see Fig. 30-1). The ureters contract in peristaltic waves to move urine toward the bladder. At the opening between the ureter and the bladder is a flap of mucous membrane that acts as a one-way valve, allowing urine to enter the bladder but preventing backflow (**reflux**) into the ureter.

The Urinary Bladder Stores Urine

The urinary bladder (see Fig. 30-1) is a sac-like organ that receives urine from the ureters and stores it until discharged from the body. The wall of the bladder consists of four layers:

- An innermost mucous membrane seals off the remaining layers from exposure to urine.
- A layer of connective tissue supports the mucous membrane.
- Three layers of longitudinal and circular smooth muscle fibers are collectively called the **detrusor muscle.**
- An outermost layer of fibrous connective tissue covers the detrusor layer.

When the bladder is empty, it shrivels and its elastic wall becomes heavily folded. As it receives newly formed urine, it expands and the wall becomes smooth. An average, normal bladder can store 500 mL (1 pint) of urine, but it may distend when needed to a capacity twice that amount. You cannot palpate an empty bladder, but a full or distended bladder extends upward to form a pear shape that you can feel in the suprapubic region.

The Urethra Transports Urine

The urethra transports urine from the bladder to the body's exterior. In women, the urethra is about 3 to 4 cm (1.5 in.) long and is anchored to the anterior wall of the vagina by connective tissue; it opens at the **urinary meatus** between the clitoris and vaginal opening. Because the female urethra is so short, women are especially prone to urinary tract infection from microorganisms residing in the vagina and rectum. In men, the urethra extends about 20 cm (8 in.) from the bladder to the urinary meatus at the distal end of the penis. As it leaves the bladder, the male urethra passes through a surrounding gland known as the **prostate.** In addition to urine, the male urethra also carries semen.

The mucous membrane of the urethra (in both men and women) is continuous with the bladder and the ureters. Therefore, infection in the urethra can easily spread through the bladder and up into the kidneys.

KnowledgeCheck 30-1

- Identify the major structures of the urinary system.
- What are the functions of the kidneys?
- Briefly describe how urine is formed.
- What role do the ureters, bladder, and urethra play in urinary elimination?

HOW DOES URINARY ELIMINATION OCCUR?

Where the bladder connects to the urethra is a thickening of smooth muscle, called the **internal urethral sphincter.** When closed, the internal sphincter keeps urine from entering the urethra. When the bladder contains 200 to 450 mL of urine (50 to 200 mL in children), the distention activates stretch receptors in the bladder wall. The stretch receptors send sensory impulses to the *voiding reflex center* in the spinal cord,

triggering motor impulses that cause the detrusor muscle to contract and the internal sphincter to relax. The internal urethral sphincter is not under voluntary control.

Voiding (also called **urination** or **micturition**) occurs when contraction of the detrusor muscle pushes stored urine through the relaxed internal urethral sphincter into the urethra. This triggers the conscious urge to void. However, voiding may be voluntarily delayed by inhibiting release of an **external urethral sphincter.** When the person is ready to urinate, the brain signals the external sphincter to relax, and urine flows out of the urethra. Further contraction of the detrusor muscle normally forces out any urine remaining in the bladder. After the detrusor muscle relaxes, the bladder begins to fill with urine again.

Voiding and control of urination require that, in addition to normal functioning of the bladder and urethra, the brain, spinal cord, and nerves supplying the bladder and urethra be intact. The person must be aware of the need to urinate and able to respond by either inhibiting the reflex or by going to the toilet.

Normal Urination Patterns

The kidneys produce urine at a rate of about 50 to 60 mL per hour, or 1,500 mL per day. However, output may fluctuate by 1,000 mL to 2,000 mL depending on various factors discussed in the next section. Most people void about five or six times per day, even eight times is normal—typically after awakening, after each meal, and just before bedtime. When fluid intake is increased, urination will be more frequent. Sometimes frequent urination is a sign of other medical problems, such as diabetes or urinary tract infection.

Characteristics of Normal Urine

Specific gravity is a measure of dissolved solutes in a solution. As the concentration of the urine solutes increases, specific gravity increases. The specific gravity of distilled water is 1.000 because there are no dissolved solutes. The normal specific gravity range for urine is 1.002 to 1.028. As fluid intake increases, urine becomes dilute and lighter in color to almost clear as it approaches a specific gravity of 1.000. In contrast, if fluid intake is low or there have been fluid losses, as with diarrhea or vomiting, the urine darkens as the specific gravity rises. Also, see Procedure 30-3B: Measuring Specific Gravity of Urine (Refractometer), at the end of this chapter.

 Think**Like a Nurse** 30-2

- You are admitting a sexually active patient who is complaining of a frequent urge to urinate with burning sensation with urination. Her urine specimen is pink-tinged. How does your patient's urinary elimination pattern differ from normal?
- What would you expect to find if you measured her specific gravity?
- Your patient's symptoms are suggestive of urinary tract infection. How might this be related to the fact that she is sexually active?

WHAT FACTORS AFFECT URINARY ELIMINATION?

Given the complex structure and physiology of the urinary organs, it isn't surprising that many variables affect their function.

Developmental Factors: Infants and Children

A newborn's kidneys produce 15 to 60 mL of urine per kilogram of body weight per day. Newborns do not concentrate urine well and, therefore, may void up to 25 times during the first 24 hours of life. The normal specific gravity of their urine is 1.008. Over the first weeks of life, the urine gradually becomes more concentrated, and the well-hydrated infant produces eight to ten wet diapers a day. Infants do not have voluntary control of voiding because neuromuscular functioning is immature.

The timing of toilet training is highly variable and is influenced by family and culture, as well as the presence of older children who can act as role models. In the United States, most parents begin toilet training when their child is between 18 and 36 months of age. Before toilet training can occur, toddlers must be able to control the external urethral sphincter, sense the urge to void, communicate their need to use the toilet, and remove their clothing. Toddlers usually stay dry in the daytime before they can go without a diaper all night.

Occasional wetting (**enuresis**) is entirely normal in children, even in the early school years, especially when the child is intensely involved in a game, test, or other absorbing activity. Such events should be accepted calmly and not punished. **Nocturnal enuresis,** or nighttime bedwetting, occurs in 15% to 25% of 5-year-old children. By the age of 12 years, 8% of boys and 4% of girls still wet the bed. **Primary nocturnal enuresis** is bedwetting in a child who has not achieved consistent dryness at night. **Secondary enuresis** occurs in a child who has had at least 6 months of nighttime dryness (Thiedke, 2003).

Developmental Factors: Older Adults

The size and functioning of the kidneys begin to decrease at about age 50, and by age 80 only about two-thirds of the functioning nephrons remain. This results in a decline in filtration rate, which affects the ability to dilute and concentrate urine, but does not normally create problems unless an illness alters fluid balance. For example, when older adults lose fluids and electrolytes through vomiting and diarrhea, it is difficult for their kidneys to maintain acid–base and electrolyte balances. Chronic diseases such as arteriosclerosis, common in older adults, can reduce blood flow and impair renal function. Decreased kidney function places older adults at risk for drug toxicity, as well.

The potential volume of the bladder decreases because of a loss of elasticity in the bladder wall; thus, older adults need to urinate more frequently, especially during the night (**nocturnal frequency**). Loss of elasticity and muscle tone also decreases the ability of the bladder to empty completely. Retention of urine after voiding then increases the risk for bladder infections. In women, childbearing may have weakened the pelvic muscles, which can lead to leakage of urine. In older men, the prostate gland may be enlarged, causing urinary frequency and hesitancy. Most older men have some difficulty starting urination or reduced force of the urinary stream, and may experience dribbling.

Personal, Sociocultural, and Environmental Factors

Many people put off voiding while they are working or busy with other activities. Delaying urination promotes urinary stasis and can lead to bladder infections. Other situations can inhibit voiding, as well, such as the following:

- *Anxiety.* A person who is anxious and tense cannot relax the abdominal and perineal muscles and the external urethral sphincter. It is then difficult to void.

- *Lack of time.* Most people find it difficult to void when they feel rushed.
- *Lack of privacy.* Many people require privacy for voiding and if they are in a restaurant or other unfamiliar environment, they may be embarrassed even to ask for directions to a bathroom. Some hospitalized clients may also avoid asking for assistance to the bathroom.
- *Loss of dignity.* In Chapter 11, we talked about the loss of dignity that hospitalized patients experience. Patients who need assistance with toileting may be especially vulnerable to such feelings, especially if they require catheterization or a bedpan.
- *Cultural influences.* Some patients will state personal, cultural, or religious requirements for toileting assistance to be provided by a person of the same gender, or they will wait until a visit from a family member before acknowledging their need for help with voiding.

Nutrition, Hydration, and Activity Level

Substances that contain caffeine, such as coffee, tea, cola, and chocolate, act as diuretics and increase urine production. Consuming large amounts of alcohol impairs the release of antidiuretic hormone (ADH), resulting in increased production of urine. In contrast, a diet high in salt causes water retention and decreases urine production.

The kidneys also conserve water when a person is dehydrated, such as after heavy exercise or when fluid intake is inadequate. This causes the urine to be concentrated and low in volume. During prolonged periods of physical activity, especially in hot weather, the body loses sodium and other electrolytes rapidly through sweat; for this reason, electrolyte replacement beverages may be more beneficial than plain water in helping to prevent dehydration for prolonged or vigorous-intensity activity (Thompson & Manore, 2008). For most adults, pale to clear urine indicates adequate hydration.

KnowledgeCheck 30-2

- What quantity of urine in the bladder will stimulate the urge to void?
- Identify at least three methods for determining whether hydration is adequate and urine output is within normal limits.

Medications

Various medications affect urination. Phenazopyridine hydrochloride (Pyridium), a bladder analgesic, turns the urine a deep orange-red color. *Diuretics,* sometimes called "water pills," treat blood pressure, fluid retention, and edema by increasing elimination of urine. Diuretics are classified as thiazide, potassium-sparing, or loop-acting diuretics (Box 30-1). In contrast, a number of medications have a side effect of urinary retention. They inhibit the free flow of urine due to *anticholinergic effects* (e.g., medications given to relieve bladder spasms). See Box 30-2 for a listing of the most common medications associated with urinary retention.

Still other medications are **nephrotoxic** (damaging to the kidneys). These include some antibiotics, such as gentamicin and amphotericin B (a fungicide), and high doses or long-term use of aspirin and ibuprofen.

Surgery and Anesthesia

Reproductive and urinary tract surgeries can affect urinary solutes, normal urine characteristics, and the ability to pass urine normally. Manipulation of the urinary tract frequently leads to trauma, bleeding, or the introduction of bacteria into a normally sterile tract. Swelling after diagnostic or invasive procedures and childbirth may cause urinary retention.

Surgery in the pubic area, vagina, or rectum is associated with a high incidence of trauma to the urinary organs; lower abdominal swelling; loss of pelvic muscle control; and increased pressure on the kidneys, ureters, or bladder. Surgery on the reproductive organs, such as hysterectomy in women or transurethral resection of the prostate in men, usually requires the use of an indwelling catheter (tube) for draining the bladder postoperatively. The urine may be red or pink tinged after any invasive urinary tract surgery or procedure.

Anesthetic agents can decrease blood pressure and glomerular filtration, thus decreasing urine formation. Spinal anesthesia decreases the patient's awareness of the need to void, which may lead to bladder distention.

Pathological Conditions

Disorders of the urinary system that affect urinary elimination include the following:

- Infection or inflammation of the bladder, ureters, or kidneys
- **Renal calculi** (kidney stones) or tumors, which obstruct the normal flow of urine

---

BOX 30-1 ▪ Common Diuretic Classes

Thiazide Diuretics are used to treat high blood pressure by reducing the amount of sodium and water in the body. They also dilate blood vessels, thereby lowering blood pressure.

Potassium-Sparing Diuretics reduce the amount of water in the body. Unlike other diuretic medicines, these medicines do not cause potassium loss.

Loop-Acting Diuretics cause the kidneys to excrete more urine by reabsorbing less water. This reduces the amount of water in the body and lowers blood pressure.

Medications That Have Significant Interactions With Diuretics include digoxin, antihypertensives, lithium, certain antidepressants (especially with thiazide or loop-acting diuretics), and the immunosuppressant cyclosporine, especially when the patient is taking a potassium-sparing diuretic.

Common Side Effects of Diuretics include weakness, muscle cramps, skin rash, increased sensitivity to sunlight (with thiazide diuretics), dizziness, lightheadedness, joint pain.

BOX 30-2 ▪ Medications Associated With Urinary Retention

Class	Medication
Antihistamines	fexofenadine (Allegra), diphenhydramine (Benadryl), chlorpheniramine (Chlor-Trimeton), cetirizine (Zyrtec)
Anticholinergics/ antispasmodics	hyoscyamine (Levbid), oxybutynin (Ditropan), tolterodine (Detrol), propantheline (Pro-Banthine)
Tricyclic antidepressants	imipramine (Tofranil), amitriptyline (Elavil), nortriptyline (Aventyl)

Source: National Kidney and Urologic Diseases Information Clearinghouse. (2007, updated June 29, 2012). *Retention.* NIH Publication No. 08-6089. Retrieved January 21, 2014. From http://kidney.niddk.nih.gov/kudiseases/pubs/UrinaryRetention/

- In older men, **hypertrophy** (excessive growth) of the prostate gland due to benign or cancerous lesions, which interferes with flow of urine from the bladder into the urethra

Diseases involving other systems can indirectly affect urinary function, for example:

- *Cardiovascular and metabolic disorders* decrease blood flow through the glomeruli and thus impair filtration and urine production.
- *Nervous system* conditions that affect control of the urinary system organs will impair urinary elimination. After a stroke or spinal cord injury, for example, some patients may lose bladder control. **Neurogenic bladder** is an example of impaired neurological function. The person cannot perceive bladder fullness or control the urinary sphincters. The bladder becomes flaccid or spastic, causing frequent involuntary loss of urine.
- *Systemic infection*, especially when accompanied by a high fever, causes the kidneys to reabsorb and retain water.
- *Immobility and impaired communication* may interfere with the ability to get to the bathroom in time or to communicate the need for assistance. This may result in urination in inappropriate settings or at inappropriate times.
- *Cognitive changes* (e.g., brain changes or severe psychiatric conditions) that alter perception of the urge to void or ability to manage activities of daily living may lead to **incontinence** (involuntary loss of urine).

KnowledgeCheck 30-3

- What common medications increase the amount of urine voided?
- What types of medications are associated with urinary retention?
- What types of conditions or surgeries are associated with a high incidence of altered urination?

Example Problem: Urinary Tract Infections

Normally urine is free of bacteria, viruses, and fungi. A urinary tract infection (UTI) occurs when microorganisms, usually *Escherichia coli (E. coli)*, which normally lives harmlessly in the colon, enter the urethra and begin to multiply, overwhelming the normal flora. An infection limited to the urethra is called **urethritis. Cystitis** occurs when bacteria travel up the urethra into the bladder, causing a bladder infection. If not treated promptly, the infection may progress superiorly (upward) to the ureters or kidneys **(pyelonephritis).**

Several biological safeguards are in place in the urinary system to prevent UTIs. One-way valves at the junction of the ureters and bladder help prevent urine from backing up toward the kidneys. In addition, the flow of urine during urination helps wash bacteria out of the body. In men, the prostate gland produces secretions that slow bacterial growth. But despite these safeguards, infections are common.

Risk Factors for Urinary Tract Infection

People who are more prone to UTIs include the following:

- *Sexually active women.* During sexual activity, perineal pathogens may enter the urethra. Because a woman's urethra is short, pathogens, particularly *E. coli,* can gain rapid access to the bladder.
- *Women who use spermicidal contraceptive gel.* Spermicides reduce normal flora in the vagina, allowing pathogens to multiply unrestricted.

- *Older women.* The loss of estrogen associated with menopause leads to drying of the mucosa in the vagina and urethra and a decrease in protective normal flora.
- *Pregnant women.* Some pregnant women are more prone to UTI because of hormonal changes and because of urinary stasis caused by pressure of the uterus on the bladder.
- *Men with an enlarged prostate.* An enlarged prostate may develop as a result of aging or cancerous changes. Pressure from the prostate creates difficulty emptying the bladder, resulting in stagnant urine, which provides a medium for bacterial growth.
- *People with kidney stones.* Kidney stones (*renal calculi*) obstruct the flow of urine, creating stagnation, and irritate the urinary tract as they are passed.
- *Anyone who has an indwelling catheter.* Indwelling catheters pose several risks:

Failing to maintain a closed drainage system increases the risk for infection by allowing bacteria to enter the catheter; the catheter provides a pathway for bacteria to migrate up into the urinary system. (Wong, 1981, updated 2005; Wound, Ostomy, and Continence Nurses Society, 2008).

The catheter irritates the mucosal lining of the urethra, which then creates a portal of entry for microbes. The longer the catheter is indwelling the higher the risk of developing UTI.

The urine collection bag is a reservoir for microorganisms.

- *People who have diabetes mellitus.* Glucose in the urine provides nutrients for bacteria to multiply.
- *Immunocompromised patients.* Susceptible hosts (e.g., neonates, elderly, those receiving immunosuppressive drugs, people with weakened immune system) are less able to maintain a healthy balance of microbes in the urinary tract.
- *People who have a history of UTIs.* Anyone with a previous UTI is more likely to experience a recurrence. This is thought to be related to the absence of certain antigens against bacteria that attach to the lining of the urethra (National Kidney and Urologic Diseases Information Clearinghouse [NKUDIC], 2005).

Recognizing and Treating Urinary Tract Infections

The presence of bacteria in a symptomatic patient is used in the medical diagnosis of UTI. To assist in the diagnosis of UTI, you will need to collect a midstream, clean-catch urine specimen and assess for the following signs and symptoms.

Back pain	Foul-smelling urine
Bladder spasms	Hematuria
Chills	Nausea and vomiting
Dysuria	Pyuria
Edema	Urgency
Fever	Urinary frequency

The classic signs of UTI are urinary white blood cells (WBCs), pyuria, dysuria, urgency, and frequency. Signs of fever, bacteriuria and abnormal blood values do not predict catheter-associated UTIs (Madigan & Neff, 2003). Catheter-associated urinary tract infections are generally assumed to be benign. Such infection in otherwise healthy patients is often asymptomatic and is likely to resolve spontaneously with the removal of the catheter. Occasionally, infection persists and leads to such complications as prostatitis, epididymitis, cystitis, pyelonephritis, and gram-negative bacteremia, particularly in high risk patients (Grabe, Bishop, Bjerklund-Johansen, et al., 2008)

Antibiotics are used to treat UTI. The length and type of treatment depends on the location and severity of infection. In general, a bladder infection may be treated with oral antibiotics for 1 to 5 days. In contrast, pyelonephritis (kidney infection) may require IV antibiotics for several days followed by a course of oral antibiotics. Preventive antibiotic treatment is not recommended for people requiring long-term urinary catheterization (Lo, Nicholle, Classen, et al., 2008; Wooten, Bradley, Cardenas, et al., 2010; Wound, Ostomy, and Continence Nurses Society, 2008). Drug resistance develops easily; therefore, antibiotics are reserved for symptomatic infections (Wilde & Getliffe, 2006).

ThinkLike a Nurse 30-3

In the Meet Your Patient scenario, your patient, Marlena, has a positive urine culture, indicating a urinary tract infection. What additional history questions would you like to ask her?

Example Problem: Urinary Retention

Urinary retention is an inability to empty the bladder completely. Etiologies include obstruction, inflammation and swelling, neurological problems, medications, and anxiety.

Obstruction. Among men, an enlarged prostate is the most common cause of obstruction in the lower urinary tract. Other obstructions include stones lodged in the urethra, strictures or scars from previous injury, tumors or blood clots in the urinary system, and fecal impaction. Impacted stool distends the rectum and causes forward pressure on the urethra, interfering with the flow of urine out of the bladder.

Inflammation and Swelling. Obstruction may also occur as a result of inflammation and swelling, for example, from infection or surgery in the pelvic region. Swelling narrows the diameter of the urethra so that urine cannot flow freely.

Neurological Problems. Recall that voiding requires that the brain, spinal cord, and nerves supplying the bladder and urethra must be intact. Conditions that affect innervation of the bladder include spinal cord tumors or injury, herniated disk, and viral infections involving perineal nerves (e.g., genital herpes).

Medications. Anesthesia and other medications can also cause temporary problems with urination. Box 30-2 provides examples of medications with anticholinergic or alpha-adrenergic effects that may impede urine flow.

Anxiety. Painful urination may produce anxiety and lead to voluntary withholding of urination.

Example Problem: Urinary Incontinence

Urinary incontinence (UI) is a lack of voluntary control over urination. UI affects about two-thirds of older adults, to at least some degree. Women are twice as likely as men to have this condition. Risk factors for incontinence also include neurological disease (e.g., stroke), UTIs, obesity, reduced mobility, and diabetes. It can lead to social isolation, depression, and increased caregiver burden (Dowling-Castronovo & Bradway, 2003, updated 2008). The total number of people affected by incontinence is presumed to be greater than current estimates, in part because healthcare providers often fail to ask specific questions about it. Incontinence affects people of all ages and social and economic levels.

Although incontinence is common, it is not a normal change that occurs with aging. This pervasive myth often leads older adults to avoid seeking treatment. Many people do not mention leakage of urine to healthcare providers because they are embarrassed, believe nothing can be done, or believe it is an inevitable condition of older age. Unfortunately, these views may lead to restriction of activities and ultimately to loneliness, depression, and isolation (Dowling-Castronovo & Bradway, 2003, updated 2008).

In men, UI is most often related to benign prostatic hyperplasia (enlarged prostate) or to prostatectomy. In women, it is often related to childbirth, specifically to vaginal delivery. Other risk factors for UI are perimenopausal status, high body mass index, diabetes, and current cigarette smoking.

Types of Urinary Incontinence

The Agency for Healthcare Research and Quality guidelines (Dowling-Castronovo & Bradway, 2008) identified the following seven types of UI:

- **Urge incontinence** is the involuntary loss of larger amounts of urine accompanied by a strong urge to void. It is often referred to as **overactive bladder.**
- **Stress incontinence** is an involuntary loss of small amounts of urine with increased intra-abdominal pressure. NANDA International (NANDA-I) specifies "loss of less than 50 mL of urine" in the absence of an overactive bladder (2012, p. 196). Etiological factors include pregnancy, childbirth, obesity, chronic constipation, and straining at stool. Activities that produce leakage of urine include exercise, laughing, sneezing, coughing, and lifting.
- **Mixed incontinence** is a combination of urge and stress incontinence.
- **Overflow incontinence** is the loss of urine in combination with a distended bladder. Causes of Overflow Incontinence include fecal impaction, neurological disorders, and enlarged prostate (NANDA-I, 2012).
- **Functional incontinence** is the untimely loss of urine when no urinary or neurological cause is involved. This type of incontinence occurs because of physical disability, immobility, pain, external obstacles, or problems in thinking or communicating that prevent a person from reaching a toilet. NANDA-I (2012, p. 193) defines Functional Incontinence as the "inability of [a] usually continent person to reach the toilet in time to avoid unintentional loss of urine." Etiologies include confusion, disorientation, or mobility problems.
- **Transient incontinence** is a short-term incontinence that is expected to resolve spontaneously. Causes include UTI and medications, especially diuretics.
- **Unconscious (reflex) incontinence** is loss of urine when the person does not realize the bladder is full and has no urge to void. Central nervous system disorders and multisystem problems are common causes. NANDA-I defines Reflex Urinary Incontinence as the "involuntary loss of urine at somewhat predictable intervals when a specific bladder volume is reached" (2012, p. 195). Tissue damage from radiation, cystitis, bladder inflammation, or radical pelvic surgery can also trigger reflex incontinence.

The following are other types of incontinence, not mentioned by the Agency for Health Care Research and Quality (AHRQ):

- **Enuresis,** which tends to be familial, is involuntary urination after about age 5 to 6 years, when control is usually established. Enuresis is *primary* if bladder training was never achieved and *secondary* if control was established and then lost. Enuresis has been associated with stress (e.g., marital discord), UTI, allergies, abnormal electroencephalographic patterns, sleep disorders, hearty laughing, and small bladder capacity; however, the cause is not always apparent.

- **Nocturnal enuresis** (bedwetting) can persist until age 10 or later. If one parent had nighttime bedwetting as a child, there is a high chance the child will also experience it. Most often children outgrow the condition. Only a small percentage of the secondary type is caused by a medical condition, such as UTI, urinary obstruction, diabetes, pressure on the bladder from extreme constipation, or neurological disorders of the spinal cord.

Treatments for Urinary Incontinence

Behavioral interventions, such as timed voiding and Kegel exercises, are the first-line treatment for urinary incontinence. Pelvic floor training should include at least eight contractions, three times a day. Pelvic muscle training should be continued for at least 3 months before moving to more aggressive treatment. The following medical and surgical treatments may be used to manage UI:

- *Medications* include topical estrogen for women who have UI associated with urogenital atrophy, and anticholinergic drugs such as oxybutynin (Ditropan) and tolterodine (Detrol), which inhibit involuntary bladder contractions.
- *Devices*, such as indwelling intravaginal (e.g., pessary) or intraurethral devices to manage urinary incontinence are not used routinely. They are, instead reserved to prevent occasional leakage, for example, during exercise.
- *Sacral nerve stimulation* might be recommended for the treatment of certain types of urinary incontinence in women who have not responded to conservative treatment.
- *Surgical treatments*, such as bladder suspension and prostate resection relieve the pressure of other pelvic organs against the bladder.

Do not use absorbent products, handheld urinals, and other toileting aids to routinely manage urinary incontinence, unless used to supplement other therapy.

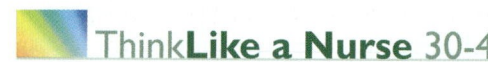

Think**Like a Nurse** 30-4

What types of challenges or problems do you think a patient with a urinary diversion might experience?

PracticalKnowledge
knowing **how**

As a nurse, you will monitor and assist clients with urinary elimination, teach them about bodily functions, and work collaboratively with the healthcare team to facilitate normal urinary function. In the remainder of the chapter, we discuss these activities. Also see the Nursing Care Plan and the Care Map.

ASSESSMENT

To assess urinary elimination, you will use data from the nursing history, physical examination, and diagnostic and laboratory reports.

Nursing History

Because urination patterns vary among individuals, you will need a nursing history to determine what is normal for a particular person. As you interview the client, pay attention to her reaction to your questions. Many people are embarrassed about discussing urination. Tailor your assessment to the client's needs, and use language that makes her comfortable. For specific questions to ask when performing a focused urinary assessment, refer to the Focused Assessment box Urinary Elimination History Questions.

QSEN

Managing Urinary Incontinence

Competency: Patient-Centered Care (Knowledge, Skills, Attitudes); Evidenced-Based Practice (Knowledge, Skills, Attitudes)*

Scenario: Dashondra Simms, RN, lives in a rural area and works in a urology practice. After participating in a radio interview to provide information about urinary incontinence, many women call the urology practice to ask for help. Dashondra asks each woman how she manages her incontinence, where she obtains information, if the condition has changed her quality of life, and if she would be willing to participate in an incontinence support group. Dashondra's notes reveal a population with unmet healthcare needs. To address this, she decides to develop a patient-centered, evidence-based program to increase participants' knowledge and confidence about managing their incontinence.

First, Dashondra accesses The National Guidelines Clearinghouse website to obtain evidence-based guidelines for different incontinence management techniques. She searches databases such as MEDLINE and CINAHL for peer-reviewed studies that identify the psychosocial needs of patients, cultural or ethnic differences in managing incontinence. She also consults colleagues for their opinions.

Dashondra organizes a planning meeting with the women and asks them about the emotional impact of living with

incontinence. The women talk about their feelings of self-worth, dignity, and confidence being affected. Self-image, sexuality, and their sense of freedom also emerged as specific psychosocial issues.

Dashondra asked what would be of value to them in an incontinence self-management program. They identified education about new treatments, a monthly support group meeting, an online forum for members, and telephone or email access to Dashondra as desirable components of the program.

Think about it:

➤ How did Dashondra establish an evidence base for educating group members?

➤ How did she make the intervention patient-centered?

➤ In what ways did Dashondra use information technology to help her design the program?

---

*For specific Skills, and Attitudes

 Go to the QSEN web site at http://www.qsen.org. ksas_prelicensure.php

Resources: Agency for Healthcare Research and Quality (2007); Corna & Cairney (2005); Hayder & Schnepp (2010); Wilson (2004); Schröder, Abrams, Andersson, Artibani, Chapple, Drake, et al. (2009).

Focused Assessment

Urinary Elimination History Questions

Usual Urination Pattern

➤ How often do you urinate?
➤ Do you get up in the middle of the night to urinate?
➤ Do you have difficulty getting to the bathroom in time to urinate?
➤ Do you ever leak urine when you cough, laugh, or exercise?
➤ Do you ever leak urine on the way to the bathroom?
➤ Do you need to use pads or tissue in your underwear to catch urine?
➤ Do you have any difficulty starting to void?

Appearance of Urine

➤ How would you describe your urine?
➤ Have you noticed unusual odor with urination?

Changes in Urination Habits or Urine Appearance

➤ Have you experienced any changes in your voiding pattern recently?
➤ Have you experienced any changes in the appearance or odor of your urine?

History of Urination Problems

➤ What has been your experience with urination problems?
➤ Have you experienced any problems with urinary tract infections or kidney and bladder problems?
➤ Have you ever lost control of your urination?

➤ Have you ever had urinary tract surgery or diagnostic procedures?

Use of Urination Aids

➤ What aids, if any, do you use to help you urinate?
➤ What is your usual fluid intake over the course of a day?
➤ What medications are you taking? Have they had any effect on your urination pattern?

Lifestyle Questions

➤ Where is your bathroom located? Can you get to it easily?
➤ Can you manage your clothing when you go to the bathroom?
➤ How much fluid do you drink each day?
➤ How many caffeinated beverages do you drink?
➤ Do you smoke?
➤ Are you bothered with constipation?
➤ Do you do high-impact exercise (e.g., jogging)?

Presence of Urinary Diversions

➤ Have you ever had surgery of your urinary tract?
➤ If so, what and when?

For Infants and Young Children

➤ Has the child been toilet trained?
➤ What elimination routines have been established?

Physical Assessment

Physical assessment for urinary elimination includes examination of the kidneys, bladder, urethra, and skin surrounding the genitals, as appropriate. For a complete discussion of physical examination of the genitourinary system, see Chapter 21, Procedure 21-17: Assessing the Male Genitourinary System, and Procedure 21–18: Assessing the Female Genitourinary System. Also see the Focused Assessment box, Guidelines for Physical Assessment for Urinary Elimination.

Common Diagnostic Procedures

A variety of diagnostic procedures may be performed on the urinary tract. Many of these procedures are conducted in the operating room, procedures suite, or radiology department. Typically nurses are responsible for preparing the client for the procedure, assisting with specimen collection, delivering aftercare, and sometimes assisting the physician. For a discussion of urinary system studies and the nursing responsibilities associated with them, and for normal values and variations, see the Diagnostic Testing boxes.

Blood Studies

Blood urea nitrogen (BUN) and creatinine levels are commonly measured to assess renal function and hydration. For normal ranges, see the Diagnostic Testing box, Blood Studies: BUN and Creatinine.

Visualization Studies of the Urinary System

The following are commonly used visualization studies. For associated pre- and post-procedure care,

 Go to Chapter 30, **Tables, Boxes, Figures: ESG Box 30-2: Diagnostic Testing: Visualization Studies of the Urinary System**, on Davis*Plus.*

- **Cystoscopy**—Direct visualization of the urethra, bladder, and ureteral orifices by insertion of a scope. May be used to obtain biopsies and treat pathology of visualized areas.
- **Cystometry**—Urodynamic testing of bladder function; measures bladder pressure and volume.
- **Intravenous pyelogram (IVP)**—Uses radiopaque contrast medium to visualize the kidneys, ureters, bladder, and renal pelvis. Evaluates renal function by analyzing flow of contrast over time.
- **Retrograde pyelogram**—Uses radiopaque contrast medium to visualize the renal collecting system. Contrast media is injected via a ureteral catheter inserted through a cystoscope.
- **Ultrasound**—Uses sound waves to produce an image of the organs.
- **Computerized tomography**—Using contrast media, examines body sections from different angles using a narrow x-ray beam to produce a three-dimensional picture of the area of the body being scanned.
- **Renal biopsy**—Removal of a piece of kidney tissue for microscopic evaluation.

Focused Assessment

Guidelines for Physical Assessment for Urinary Elimination

Physical assessment for urinary elimination includes examination of the kidneys, bladder, urethra, and skin surrounding the genitals, as appropriate.

The Kidneys

Technique	Rationale
The **costovertebral (CV) angle** is formed by the junction of the 12th rib and the spine on both sides of the back. Place one palm flat on the CV angle and lightly strike it with the closed fist of the other hand (see the accompanying figure).	You cannot usually palpate the kidneys. Instead, examine them by assessing for costovertebral angle tenderness (CVAT). If kidney inflammation is present, percussion of this angle produces pain.

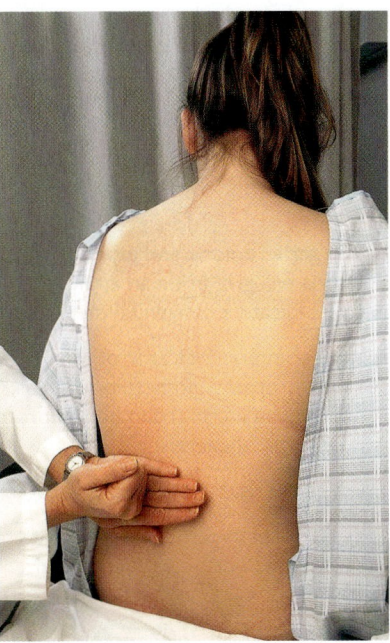

The Bladder

Inspect, palpate, and percuss the lower abdomen. Correlate your findings with data about the client's fluid intake and voiding.

➤ Inspect the lower abdomen.	➤ An empty bladder, or one with limited urine, is small and sits below the symphysis pubis. In contrast, a distended bladder rises above the symphysis pubis. If it is very distended, you may be able to see a rounded swelling above the symphysis pubis.
➤ Lightly palpate the lower abdomen to define the bladder margin. Observe the patient's response to palpation, noting signs of tenderness or discomfort.	➤ An empty bladder, or one with limited urine, will not be palpable.
➤ Percuss the area.	➤ A distended bladder produces a dull sound as opposed to the normal tympanic sound of intestinal air.

The Urethra

➤ Inspect the urethral orifice. Look for erythema, discharge, swelling, or odor.	➤ These are all signs of infection, trauma, or inflammation.

The Perineal Area

➤ Frequently inspect skin color, condition, texture, turgor, and presence of urine or stool.	➤ Clients who have urine leakage or a urinary catheter are at risk for perineal skin problems. Ammonia in the urine may result in skin excoriation, skin breakdown, and subsequent infection. If both urine and stool are present on the skin, the likelihood of skin breakdown increases.

Diagnostic Testing

Urinalysis

Characteristic	Expected Findings	Variations
Color	A freshly voided sample is pale yellow to deep amber.	Urine becomes lighter in color and may even be clear if fluid intake is high or urine output is excessive. Urine becomes dark in color as it becomes more concentrated with decreased fluid intake or excessive fluid loss. Color is also affected by diet and medications.
pH	5.0–9.0, with an average of 6.0	Indicates kidneys' ability to help maintain balanced hydrogen ion concentration in the blood. The pH increases (more alkaline) if the client eats dairy products or citrus fruits or has a vegetarian diet. The pH decreases (more acidic) if the client eats a high-protein diet or consumes cranberry juice.
Specific gravity	1.001–1.035	This is a reflection of the kidney's ability to concentrate urine. Specific gravity rises with limited fluid intake or dehydration. It may also rise with kidney disease. Specific gravity decreases as fluid intake increases.
Clarity	A freshly voided sample should be translucent. If the urine sits for a period of time, it will become cloudy.	Cloudiness in a freshly voided sample indicates the presence of other constituents in the urine. These may include bacteria, red blood cells (RBCs), WBCs, sperm, prostatic fluid, or vaginal discharge.
Odor	Fresh urine is aromatic.	Certain foods, such as garlic, onions, and asparagus, may give urine a distinctive odor. Bacteria will give urine an ammonia-like odor. A sweet syrup odor may indicate a congenital metabolic disorder.
Protein	< 20 mg/dL	Proteinuria is the most common indicator of renal disease. Protein is increased in diabetic nephropathy, glomerulonephritis, nephrosis, and toxemia of pregnancy. May be increased in benign proteinuria secondary to stress or physical exercise.
Glucose	Negative	Glucose is found in the urine with elevated blood sugars and diabetes.
Ketones	Negative	Presence of ketones indicates impaired carbohydrate metabolism. Ketones may be detected with diabetes, fever, fasting, high-protein diets, starvation, vomiting, or the post-anesthesia period.
Hemoglobin	Negative on dipstick If RBCs are assessed via microscopic exam: < 5 per high-power field	Hemoglobin may be detected with infection of the urinary tract, disease of the bladder, glomerulonephritis, pyelonephritis, nephrolithiasis, hemolytic reactions, or trauma. It also may be present in samples from women who are currently menstruating.
Bilirubin	Negative	Increased bilirubin occurs with liver disease.
Urobilinogen	Up to 1 mg/dL	Increased is found in cirrhosis, heart failure, liver disease, infectious mononucleosis, malaria, and pernicious anemia.
Nitrite	Negative	Nitrite is used to test for bacteriuria. Increased in the presence of nitrite-forming bacteria.
Leukocyte esterase	Negative If WBCs are assessed via microscopic exam: < 5 per high-power field	Leukocytes are increased in bacterial infection, calculus formation, fungal or parasitic infection, glomerulonephritis, interstitial nephritis, or tumor.
Renal cells	None seen	Renal cells come from the lining of the collecting ducts. Their presence indicates damage to the tubular network.
Transitional cells	None seen	Transitional cells line the renal pelvis, ureter, bladder, and proximal urethra. Their presence is seen with infection, trauma, and malignancy.
Squamous cells	Rare	Typically insignificant: Squamous cells line the vagina and distal portion of the urethra.

Diagnostic Testing

Urinalysis—cont'd

Characteristic	Expected Findings	Variations
Casts	Rare hyaline; otherwise negative	Large numbers of hyaline casts are seen in renal disease, hypertension, with diuretic use, and fever. Granular casts are seen in renal disease, viral infection, or lead intoxication.
Crystals	Absent in freshly voided sample	Crystals in the urine may indicate an old sample, stone formation in the urinary tract, gout, high dietary intake of oxalates, liver disease, or side effect of chemotherapy.
Bacteria, yeast, parasites	None seen	Microbes in the urine indicate an infection of the urinary tract.

Source: Adapted from Van Leeuwen, A., Poelhuis-Leth, D., & Bladh, M. (2011). *Davis's comprehensive handbook of laboratory and diagnostic tests with nursing implications.* (4th ed.). Philadelphia: F. A. Davis.

KnowledgeCheck 30-4

- What should you discuss with your client when performing a nursing history focused on urinary elimination?
- What are the key elements of a physical assessment for a client with urination problems?

ThinkLike a Nurse 30-5

After gathering a focused nursing history pertaining to urinary elimination, you check your patient's vital signs: oral temperature 99.4°F (37.4°C), radial pulse 88 beats/min, respiratory rate 20 breaths/min, and blood pressure 108/72 mm Hg. What other physical assessment findings might you expect?

Assessing the Urine

In addition to observations already mentioned, assessment of the urine includes measuring urine output and conducting a variety of bedside tests.

Diagnostic Testing

Blood Studies: BUN and Creatinine

Normal Ranges

Blood urea nitrogen (BUN)	8–20 mg/dL
Creatinine	0.5–1.1 mg/dL

Levels may be increased in:
- Renal failure
- Impaired renal perfusion
- Kidney infection or inflammation
- Kidney obstruction
- Dehydration
- Excessive protein intake
- Use of total parenteral nutrition (TPN)

Levels may be decreased in:
- Inadequate protein intake
- Malabsorption syndromes
- Liver disease

Source: Van Leeuwen, A., Poelhuis-Leth, D., & Bladh, M. (2011). *Davis's comprehensive handbook of laboratory and diagnostic tests with nursing implications* (4th ed.). Philadelphia: F. A. Davis.

Measuring Intake and Output

Measuring urine output is part of a comprehensive plan to monitor a client's fluid status. The kidneys produce urine at a rate of approximately 50 to 60 mL per hour (1,500 mL per day). However, urinary output fluctuates depending on the quantity of fluids the patient drinks and on factors, such as the ability of the heart to circulate the blood, adequate kidney functioning, and the ability of the patient to void the urine. Urine output might be low if the person is sweating excessively or has significant vomiting and diarrhea. High fever can also contribute to reduced urine output.

You must know both the intake and the output, as well as relevant physical condition, to interpret the meaning of the patient data. For example, if urine output is low, you cannot assume the patient's kidneys are not working properly. If his intake is also low, he may be dehydrated. But what does it mean if his intake is high and his output low? This could mean his kidneys are not working well. However, it could also mean that his kidneys are producing urine but that he has urinary retention because of something that is obstructing flow.

To measure fluid intake, record all fluids the patient drinks or receives intravenously. Include the following items as fluid intake: oral fluids, semiliquid foods, ice chips, IV fluids, tube feedings, and irrigations instilled and not withdrawn immediately. Fluid output includes the following items: urine output, gastrointestinal fluid loss (e.g., emesis), feces, and drainage (e.g., from suction devices or wounds). Explain to the client, family members, and all caregivers that intake and output (I&O) are being monitored. Posting a sign at the bedside or on the door to the room is a helpful reminder. When possible, have the client assist you with monitoring.

You will usually total the I&O at the end of each shift, as well as for each 24-hour period. In intensive care units, you may measure I&O hourly. Most healthcare facilities have standardized I&O forms. I&O may be recorded on a separate form or be part of a flow sheet. To see examples, see Figure 18-2 and Figure 18-7.

Observe universal precautions when handling urine to prevent exposure to bodily fluids. Always wear disposable procedure gloves, and avoid splashing the urine and contaminating your uniform. The method you use to measure urine is dictated in part by the amount of help the client needs with urination.

Voided Urine. Many ambulatory clients need no assistance with urination. Be sure to inform them you are monitoring

their I&O, and explain how they can help. Place a specimen "hat" (collection container) under the toilet seat to collect urine, or have male clients void into a urinal. Periodically measure the output and empty the urine into the toilet. For clients who can assist with recording the I&O, provide a bedside clipboard.

For the client with mobility problems, use a bedpan or urinal to collect urine output. Use a fracture pan for clients with a fracture of the pelvis, lower back, or legs or for clients who have casts, splints, or braces on their legs. Male clients may void into a urinal while remaining in bed.

See Chapter 29, Procedure 29–2: Placing and Removing a Bedpan. For complete instructions for measuring urine output from a bedpan or urinal, see Procedure 30-1A, at the end of this chapter.

Urine From a Catheter. An indwelling urinary catheter, also known as a Foley or a retention catheter, is a flexible tube that is inserted through the urethra into the bladder (Fig. 30-4). It is held in place by a balloon that is inflated in the bladder above the detrusor muscle. Catheter insertion and ongoing care are discussed in the Planning Interventions/Implementation section of this chapter. You will usually measure urine output from the indwelling catheter at the end of each shift unless otherwise prescribed. Clients who require close monitoring of I&O will have a special collection bag with a measuring chamber. Often this is used to assess hourly urine output. For complete instructions for measuring urine from an indwelling catheter, see Procedure 30-1B, at the end of this chapter.

Obtaining Samples for Urine Studies

Many disorders of the urinary system can be assessed by examining urine. You will perform some of these tests at the bedside. For others, you will collect a specimen that is analyzed in the lab. The various types of urine samples are discussed in the text that follows.

Freshly Voided Specimen

To collect a freshly voided sample, collect the urine in the same manner as when you are measuring I&O. Pour the urine into a specimen container labeled with the patient's name, the date, and the time of collection. Many facilities require packaging the container in a moisture-proof specimen-handling bag. Follow agency policy on additional packaging. Transport the specimen to the lab as soon as possible (according to agency policies). If there is a delay in getting the specimen to the lab, most agencies recommend refrigeration. To learn techniques for obtaining and measuring voided urine specimens, refer to Procedures 30-1 and 30-2, at the end of this chapter.

Clean-Catch Specimen

Many diagnostic tests require a clean-catch urine specimen. The client must cleanse the genitalia before voiding and collect the sample in midstream because the initial flow of urine may contain organisms from the urethral meatus, distal urethra, and perineum. A midstream sample is free of these contaminants. For the complete procedure, see Procedure 30-2A, at the end of this chapter.

Sterile Urine Specimen

A sterile urine specimen aids in determining the presence of a urinary tract infection. You can obtain a sterile urine specimen by inserting a catheter into the bladder or by withdrawing a sample from an indwelling catheter. Do not take the specimen from the collection bag because that urine may be several hours old.

➕ Never disconnect the catheter from the drainage tube to obtain a sample. Interrupting the system creates a portal of entry for pathogens, thereby increasing the risk of contamination. Figure 30-5 illustrates how to obtain a sterile specimen from an indwelling catheter. For a discussion of the steps involved, see Procedure 30-2B, at the end of this chapter.

24-Hour Urine Collection

A 24-hour urine collection, may be prescribed to evaluate some renal disorders by showing kidney function at different times of the day and night. For details about how to collect a 24-hour urine specimen, see Procedure 30-2C, at the end of this chapter.

Routine Urinalysis

A routine urinalysis (UA) is one of the most commonly prescribed laboratory tests. It is used as an overall screening test as well as an aid to diagnosing renal, hepatic, and other diseases. Urinalysis requires a freshly voided sample.

Urinalysis techniques include "dipstick" testing and/or microscopic analysis. Dipstick testing is commonly performed at the bedside; microscopic examination is done in the lab. Box 30-3 contains several terms used to describe urine characteristics and quantity. For the expected findings and common variants of urinalysis, see the preceding Diagnostic Testing box Urinalysis.

Bedside Testing (Dipstick)

Dipstick testing can determine pH and specific gravity and the presence of protein, glucose, ketones, and occult blood in the urine. Commercially prepared kits contain a reagent designed to detect a specific substance (e.g., glucose). The reagent may be a paper test strip, a fluid, or a tablet.

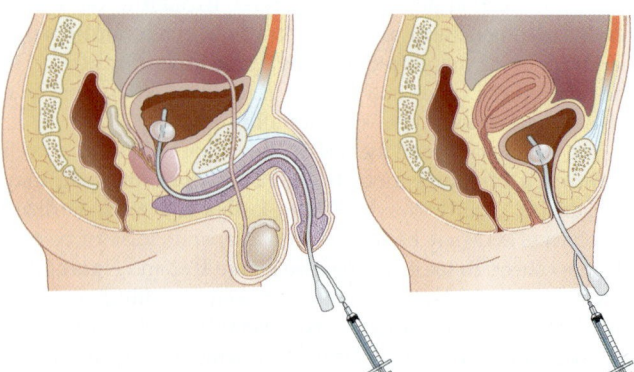

FIGURE 30-4 An indwelling catheter may be used for patients who are unable to void because of inflammation or disease or who require continual observation of urine flow.

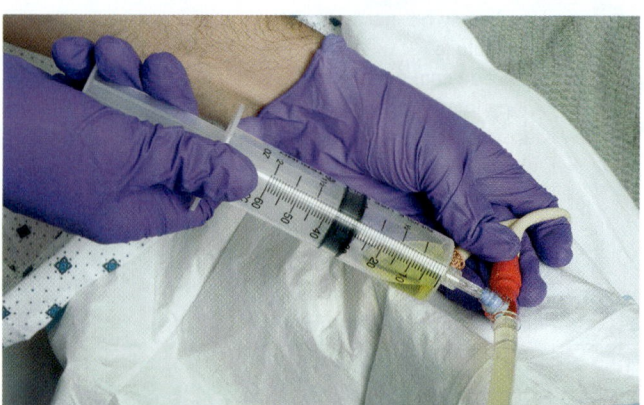

FIGURE 30-5 Inserting a sterile needleless access device and syringe into the specimen port to obtain a sterile specimen from an indwelling catheter.

BOX 30-3 ■ Terms Associated With Urination

Acute renal failure (ARF): An acute rise in the serum creatinine level of 25% or more. May be caused by inadequate blood flow to the kidney, injury to the kidney glomeruli or tubules, or obstruction of kidney outflow.

Anuria: The absence of urine, often associated with kidney failure or congestive heart failure. This term is used when urine output is less than 100 mL in 24 hours.

Dysuria: Painful or difficult urination. May be associated with infection or partial obstruction of the urinary tract as well as medications that trigger urinary retention.

End-stage renal disease (ESRD): A chronic rise in serum creatinine levels associated with loss of kidney function that must be treated with dialysis or transplantation. Also known as chronic renal failure (CRF).

Enuresis: Involuntary loss of urine

Frequency: The need to urinate at short intervals

Hematuria: Blood in the urine. May be due to trauma, kidney stones, infection, or menstruation.

Oliguria: Urine output of less than 400 mL in 24 hours. For pediatric patients, oliguria is < 0.5–1.0 mL/kg per hour.

Nephropathy: A broad term meaning "disease of the kidney."

Nephrotoxic: A substance that damages kidney tissue. Some antibiotics (gentamicin, tobramycin, and amikacin), nonsteroidal anti-inflammatory drugs, lead, and contrast media have the potential to be nephrotoxic.

Nocturia: Frequent urination after going to bed. May be caused by excessive fluid intake as well as a variety of urinary tract and cardiovascular problems.

Nocturnal enuresis: Involuntary loss of urine while asleep

Micturition: To start the stream of urine; to urinate; release urine from the bladder.

Pessary: An incontinence device that is inserted into the vagina to reduce organ prolapse or pressure on the bladder.

Polyuria: Excessive urination. May be caused by excessive hydration, diabetes mellitus, diabetes insipidus, or kidney disease.

Proteinuria: The presence of protein in the urine. May be a sign of infection or kidney disease.

Pyuria: Pus in the urine. May be caused by lesions or infection in the urinary tract.

Urgency: A sudden, almost uncontrollable need to urinate.

When contacted by the urine, a chemical reaction causes a color change that you compare to a color chart (Fig. 30-6). Read the kit label to be certain that you are using the correct reagent and that the kit is not past the expiration date. Follow the manufacturer's directions regarding the amount of urine needed and the time needed for the reagent to develop. For guidelines for dipstick testing and delegation of testing, see Procedure 30-3A, at the end of this chapter.

Specific Gravity

Specific gravity, an indicator of urine concentration, can be measured with a reagent strip. However, when you need to be precise and accurate, you should use a refractometer. Specific gravity is usually tested in the laboratory, but it is a nursing responsibility in some settings. For guidelines when testing urine specific gravity, see Procedure 30-3B.

A **refractometer** measures the extent to which a beam of light changes direction when it passes through the urine (the *refractive*

index). If the concentration of solids is high, the light is refracted more. The method is quick and easy to perform and requires only a few drops of urine. A refractometer (Fig. 30-7) is more precise, requires a much smaller specimen, is more compact, and poses less risk of spills and exposure to bodily fluids than does a urinometer, which for the most part is no longer used.

KnowledgeCheck 30-5

- Explain how to collect a clean-catch urine specimen.
- You are caring for a patient on a hospital unit from 0700 to 1200. Based on the following information, calculate the I&O and comment on your findings.
  Receiving IV fluid at 125 mL/hr
  0800 breakfast—4 oz juice, toast, scrambled eggs, 8 oz coffee
  0930—3 oz water
  0700 to 1200—wound drainage: 360 mL
  0700 to 1200—urine output per indwelling catheter: 180 mL

ThinkLike a Nurse 30-6

- Why do you think the first voided urine is discarded at the start of a 24-hour urine collection?
- Below are the dipstick findings you obtained on your patient's clean-catch specimen.

Feature	Result
pH	8.0
Specific gravity	1.030
Protein	Negative
Glucose	Negative
RBCs	Trace
Nitrite	+1
WBCs	+2
Bilirubin	Negative
Ketones	Negative
Urobilinogen	Negative

a. Identify the abnormal findings.
b. What would you expect the findings of her urine culture and sensitivity to demonstrate?

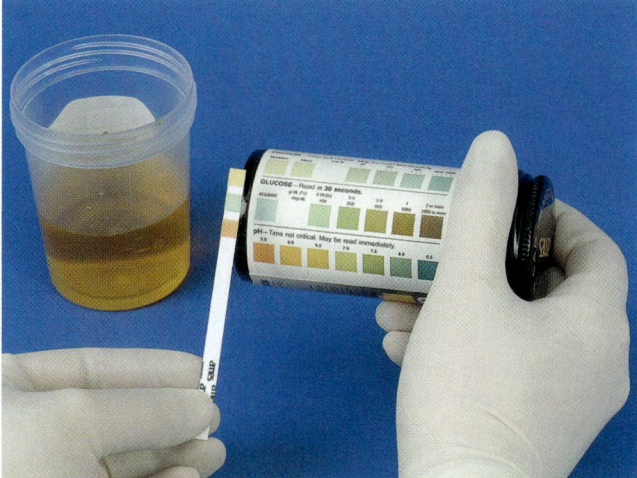

FIGURE 30-6 Commercial testing kits contain a reagent for a specific substance. A chemical reaction with the urine causes a color change that you interpret using a color chart.

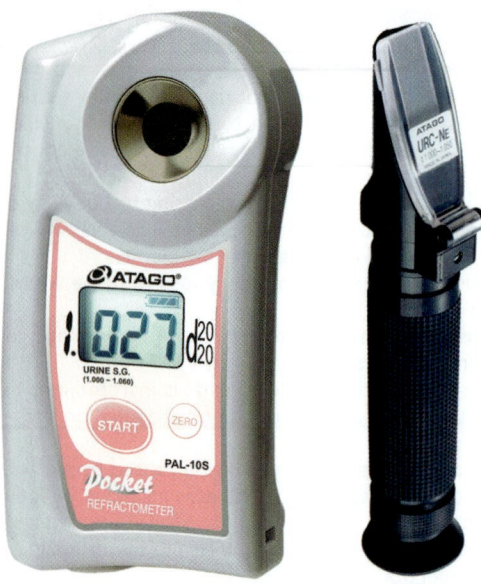

FIGURE 30-7 A refractometer indicates urine concentration by measuring the extent to which a beam of light is refracted ("bent") when passed through the urine. (*Source:* Courtesy of Atago USA, Inc.)

ANALYSIS/NURSING DIAGNOSIS

Urinary elimination problems are described by several nursing and medical diagnoses. NANDA-I diagnoses specific to urinary elimination include the following:

Impaired Urinary Elimination
Urinary Incontinence (Functional, Reflex, Stress, Urge)
Risk for Urge Urinary Incontinence
Urinary Retention
Overflow Urinary Incontinence
Readiness for Enhanced Urinary Elimination
Risk for Infection (Urinary Tract)
Risk for Ineffective Renal Perfusion

Urinary problems may also be the etiology of other nursing diagnoses, such as the following:

Anxiety r/t urinary urgency and recent episode of incontinence
Disturbed Body Image secondary to new urostomy
Acute Pain r/t bladder spasms and urinary tract infection
Social Isolation r/t frequent periods of incontinence
Risk for Imbalanced Fluid Volume
Ineffective Self-Health Management

The rest of this chapter discusses nursing care for common urinary elimination problems, including interventions for the example problems (urinary tract infections, urinary retention, and urinary incontinence).

PLANNING OUTCOMES/EVALUATION

The general goal related to urinary elimination is that patients will comfortably void approximately 1,500 mL of light yellow urine in 24 hours. Because normal urine elimination patterns vary, the frequency and amount of urine are based on the individual's pattern, food and fluid intake, medications, and other factors.

NOC standardized outcomes for urinary problems, regardless of the specific problem, are the following: Kidney Function, Urinary Continence, Urinary Elimination, and Tissue Integrity: Skin & Mucous Membranes (because urinary elimination problems often place the patient at Risk for Impaired Skin Integrity).

Individualized goals/outcome statements you might use to evaluate the effectiveness of interventions for urinary problems include the following:

- Will resume normal urination pattern by (date).
- Will discuss feelings about his urostomy.
- Will have no visible blood in urine after 2 days on antibiotics.
- Responds to the urge to void in a timely manner.
- After voiding, states he feels he has emptied his bladder completely.
- Postvoiding residual volume is < 150 mL.

PLANNING INTERVENTIONS/IMPLEMENTATION

For *NIC standardized interventions* for patients with urinary elimination nursing diagnoses,

 Go to **Standardized Language: NIC Interventions for Urinary Problems,** on Davis*Plus.*

You should select nursing activities to meet individual needs and address problem etiologies.

Specific nursing activities for patients with elimination problems fall into the following categories: promoting normal urination, preventing urinary tract infection, managing urinary retention, managing urinary incontinence, and caring for patients who have urinary diversions. The rest of this chapter discusses those activities.

Promoting Normal Urination

As a nurse, you should have a repertoire of independent nursing activities for promoting normal urination. These include providing privacy, positioning, scheduling toileting routines, providing and monitoring fluid and nutrition, and assisting with hygiene.

Provide Privacy

Although urination is a normal physiological process, most people consider it a private matter. Provide privacy when discussing or providing care related to urination. Excuse visitors from the room, draw the dividing curtains in shared rooms, and close the door to the room. Whenever possible, give the patient time alone to void. Do not, for example, hover outside the bathroom door asking, "Are you OK?" or "Are you finished?" Of course, if the client is weak and frail, you may need to remain with him. Taking a matter-of-fact approach confirms to patients that you are comfortable with this aspect of care.

Assist With Positioning

Most men stand to void and may have difficulty voiding in other positions. Whenever possible, assist the client to the bathroom to use the toilet and allow him to assume his preferred position. Alternatively, provide a bedside commode or urinal for the client to use. To place a urinal, position the patient in a semi-Fowler's position with the legs slightly spread. Place the urinal on the bed between the patient's legs, and insert his penis in the urinal.

Women generally find an upright seated (semi-Fowler's) or squatting position to be the most comfortable position for voiding. If a female patient must remain in bed, provide a bedpan. Raise the siderails or provide an overhead trapeze so that the patient will have grip holds to maneuver herself onto and off the bedpan. If the patient is very weak, you may need an assistant to help you position her on the bedpan, and you may need

to stay with her to help her maintain her position on the bedpan. For the steps involved, see Chapter 29, Procedure 29-2: Placing and Removing a Bedpan.

Facilitate Toileting Routines

Most patients void on awakening, after meals or drinking a large volume of fluid, before bedtime, or during the night for some. Identify your patient's pattern, and stick to it as much as possible. If you anticipate a change in the pattern for elimination, inform the patient. For example, if the patient is to receive a diuretic, explain that he will need to urinate more often. Similarly, if the patient is scheduled for a diagnostic procedure or activity, inform him ahead of time so that he may void before the activity begins.

Provide assistance to all patients who have mobility problems and those who use the bedpan. Discuss with all nursing assistive personnel (NAPs) the need to offer assistance so that patients experience minimal delays.

Promote Adequate Fluids and Nutrition

Adequate hydration promotes urinary tract function and flushes the system of waste products. Unfortunately, many people do not meet the recommended intake. Water is the preferred fluid because soda, coffee, and tea often contain caffeine or additives that may cause diuresis and incontinence. However, the amount of fluid is more important than the type. If the patient will not or cannot drink water, provide the fluid he prefers. Most people should drink eight to ten 8-ounce glasses of fluid daily unless health problems limit the fluid. See Box 30-4 for strategies to increase your patient's fluid intake.

Assist With Hygiene

Urine is irritating to the skin. Therefore, perineal cleansing is an integral part of toileting hygiene. Many ill patients are unable to do this for themselves, so you will need to provide perineal care. If the patient can ambulate to the bathroom, you merely need to assist with her usual cleansing routines. This may include pouring warm soapy water over the genitals while she is seated on the toilet, the bedside commode, or on the bedpan. Be sure to rinse with warm water because soap may be drying to the genital mucosa. Also offer a moist

washcloth or towelette for washing hands after toileting. For further information, see Procedure 24-4: Providing Perineal Care.

KnowledgeCheck 30-6

- Identify activities that promote normal urination patterns.
- Write at least two nursing diagnostic statements for a patient with urinary frequency, burning, urgency, and a fever.

Interventions for Example Problem: Urinary Tract Infection

An important part of UTI treatment is teaching patients how to prevent UTI. The accompanying Self-Care box, Teaching Your Client About Preventing UTI, presents the teaching points that you should include in your sessions with patients at risk for UTI or recovering from a UTI.

Interventions for Example Problem: Managing Urinary Retention

Clients with a mechanical obstruction to urine flow are treated by surgical removal or repair of the obstruction (e.g., resection of the prostate gland, removal of bladder calculi). For clients who have loss of bladder tone, collaboratively you may (1) administer cholinergic medications, such as bethanechol chloride (Urecholine), which promote bladder emptying by stimulating contraction of the detrusor muscle; (2) use **Credé's maneuver** (apply manual pressure over the bladder to promote emptying); or (3) perform

---

BOX 30-4 ■ Strategies to Increase Patients' Fluid Intake

- For patients with limited mobility, keep water or other liquids within easy reach.
- You may need to remind young children or patients with cognitive or psychiatric disorders to drink fluids.
- For patients who have increased fluid needs, provide goals for intake, and remind them to drink frequently.
- Many foods have a high fluid content. If the patient requires additional fluid for hydration, consider adding soup and watery foods, such as watermelon, to the diet. In contrast, if the patient requires fluid restriction, you will have to account for these foods in the fluid balance.
- Try offering liquids through a straw. Patients tend to drink more this way.
- Chilled drinks might be more appealing, particularly if the patient's mouth is dry. Offer beverages with ice if they are to be served cold.
- Provide good mouth care. Patients will often drink more readily if their mouth feels fresh.

Self-Care

Teaching Your Client About Preventing UTI

1. Drink at least 8 to 10 eight-oz. glasses of fluid per day to keep urine dilute and to flush bacteria from the urinary tract. The Institute of Medicine (IOM, 2004) recommends even more, particularly with heat exposure or prolonged exercise. Water is best. Some reports claim a benefit to drinking cranberry juice but this practice is controversial (Kiel & Nashelsky, 2003).
2. Urinate when you first feel the urge. Do not make a habit of postponing urination because bacteria can multiply in stagnant urine.
3. Always wipe from front to back after urination or defecation.
4. Wear cotton underwear, because nylon or other synthetic fabrics prevent evaporation of moisture. Also avoid tight-fitting clothing in the groin area. Bacteria and other microorganisms grow well in a warm, moist environment.
5. Urinate after having intercourse to flush away bacteria that might have entered the urethra.
6. If you have a history of UTI, avoid using a diaphragm, spermicidal contraceptive gel, or unlubricated or spermicidal condoms.
7. If you have a history of UTI, avoid bubble baths and baking-soda baths.
8. Promptly report any symptoms of UTI to your healthcare provider (e.g., urinary frequency, urgency, dysuria, pyuria, fever, chills, bladder spasms, back pain, hematuria, nausea and vomiting, foul-smelling urine).

urinary catheterization. When caring for patients with urinary retention, nurses may do the following:

- Monitor I&O.
- Assess for risk factors for urinary retention (e.g., prostatic hypertrophy, pelvic surgery and medications with anticholinergic side effects, such as diazepam [Valium], some antidepressants, and diphenhydramine [Benadryl]).
- Inspect and palpate for bladder distention.
- Apply heat to the lower abdomen to relax the muscles near where the bladder lies.
- Run water nearby, or place the patient's hands in warm water.
- Pour water over the perineum, or assist the patient to take a warm sitz bath.
- Measure postvoiding residual urine (see the section that follows).
- Advise the patient to contact a medical professional:

    If not previously evaluated for urinary hesitancy, dribbling, or weak urine stream

    For fever, vomiting, side or back pain, shaking chills, or passing little urine for 1 to 2 days

    For blood in the urine, cloudy urine, frequent or urgent need to urinate, or a discharge from the penis or vagina

Urinary Catheterization

Catheterization is the introduction of a pliable tube (catheter) into the bladder to allow drainage of urine. Urinary catheterization is performed to do the following:

- Obtain a sterile urine specimen.
- Drain the bladder for surgical or diagnostic purposes or when emptying is incomplete after urination.
- Prevent or treat bladder overdistention and urinary retention (e.g., after surgery) when other measures fail.
- Measure urine that remains in the bladder after the patient voids. This is commonly referred to as *postvoid residual volume* and is measured as part of the diagnostic workup for a patient with urinary retention or incontinence.

- Protect excoriated skin from contact with urine.
- Reduce the need for unnecessary movement of patients who are near death.

Indwelling urinary catheterization is associated with complications of bacteriuria and urinary tract infection. A catheter provides a connection between the external environment and a normally sterile system. In addition, when the patient has an indwelling catheter, microorganisms are no longer flushed from the urethra through voiding.

In fact, an indwelling urinary catheter is the most common cause of nosocomial infections. To reduce the risk of bacterial contamination, observe strict sterile technique when inserting and caring for a urinary catheter and maintain a closed system (Lo, Nicholle, Classen, et al., 2008).

Catheterization can injure the urethra if the catheter is too large, is forced through strictures, inserted at an incorrect angle, or not well lubricated.

Self-Catheterization

Patients with spinal cord injuries or neurological disorders use intermittent catheterization to drain the bladder and limit the risk of infection. Many actually perform **intermittent self-catheterization,** although caregivers may assist. Although you will use sterile technique for catheterization, most patients who self-catheterize use clean technique. In spite of this difference, intermittent catheterization carries a substantially lower risk of infection than does an indwelling catheter (Clean intermittent self-catheterization 2010, updated; Pilloni, Krhut, Mair, et al., 2005; Ord, Lunn, & Reynard, 2003).

The goals of intermittent self-catheterization are to (1) completely empty the bladder and (2) prevent urinary tract infections. To teach patients the procedure for clean, intermittent self-catheterization, see the Self-Care box Teaching Your Client About Clean, Intermittent Self-Catheterization (CISC).

Toward Evidence-Based Practice

Kessler, T. M., Ryu, G. R., & Burkhard, F. C. (2008). Clean intermittent self-catheterization: A burden for the patient? *Neurourology and Urodynamics, 29*(8). Retrieved June 4, 2011, from http://www3.interscience.wiley.com/journal/121385630/abstract. DOI 10.1002/nau.20610

The aim of this study was to assess patients' perceptions of clean intermittent self-catheterization (CISC) for voiding dysfunction. This study suggests CISC is an easy and painless procedure that did not interfere with daily activities. CISC does not appear to be a burden for the patient and can be a worthwhile approach for patients in the outpatient setting to manage dysfunctional urinary elimination.

1. As a nurse providing home care to a patient with urinary retention, you teach her how to perform clean intermittent self-catheterization (CISC). What information might you convey to maximize the client's receptiveness to performing the procedure?

2. What suggestions might you make for the client performing CISC so that the procedure does not interfere with daily living?

Sublett, C. M. (2008). Adding to the evidence base: A review of two qualitative studies. *Urologic Nursing, 28*(2), 130–131.

Two qualitative studies compared women with urinary incontinence (UI) and healthcare-seeking behavior. Nurses and other practitioners need to be consistently informed that women are choosing to live with UI for many reasons, including lack of knowledge of resources for UI or the fear that providers may not pay attention to them or take their concerns seriously.

1. As a nurse providing care to older adult women, what should you do in your practice to help women with urinary incontinence?

 Go to Chapter 30, **Toward Evidence-Based Practice Suggested Responses,** on Davis*Plus.*

Self-Care

Teaching Your Client About Clean, Intermittent Self-Catheterization (CISC)

In the home setting CISC is a clean procedure rather than a sterile one. In teaching the steps of the procedure, consider the client's physical ability to manipulate the catheter and reach the urethra and manipulate the equipment (e.g., range of motion, fine motor skills, degree of sensation).

➤ Teach the client how to wash her hands before beginning.
➤ The female client must learn how to locate her urethra using a mirror and then by feeling for it at insertion time.
➤ Encourage the client to drink 8 to 10 eight-oz. glasses of fluid without caffeine each day to ensure a quantity of urine adequate to flush the bladder.
➤ Teach the client to report the signs and symptoms of urinary tract infection: burning, frequency, urgency, dull abdominal ache, fever, or malaise; urine that contains sediment or becomes cloudy; or burning on urination or a fever occurs. Older adults may experience confusion before the other signs and symptoms occur.
➤ Advise the client to contact a healthcare provider if there is bleeding, pain, or difficulty inserting the catheter.
➤ Some CISC catheters can be reused; some are disposable.
➤ Catheterize as often as needed—perhaps every 2 to 3 hours at first.
➤ Discard a reusable catheter when it becomes difficult to clean or difficult to insert. A CISC catheter may be reused for 2 to 4 weeks.
➤ Soak the catheter in a white vinegar solution once a week to control odor and remove encrustation or deposits of mucus.

Procedure for Men

1. Try to void before catheterization. If you are unable to void or if the amount is less than 3 oz. (or the amount specified by your healthcare provider), then insert the catheter.
2. Assemble the catheter, lubricant, and drainage receptacle.
3. Thoroughly wash your hands with soap and water; cleanse the penis and the urethral opening.
4. Lubricate the catheter to 6 in. (15 cm).
5. Stand over the toilet or assume a comfortable position (e.g., sitting on the toilet).
6. Hold the penis perpendicular (at a right angle) to the body.
7. Gently insert and advance the catheter.
8. When you meet resistance, at the level of the prostate, take deep breaths to try to relax, and advance the catheter.

9. When urine flow starts, adva (2.5 cm) more; return the pe hold the catheter in place u bladder is empty.
10. Withdraw the catheter sl sure the entire bladder er
11. Wash the catheter with soap and wa Rinse and dry it well. If it is disposable, discard it immediately.
12. Store catheters in a clean, dry, secure place.
13. Record the amount of urine obtained.

Procedure for Women

1. Try to void before catheterization. If you are unable to void or if amount is less than 3 oz. (or the amount specified by your healthcare provider), then insert catheter.
2. Assemble the catheter, lubricant, and drainage receptacle; a good light is important for women.
3. Thoroughly wash hands with soap and water; cleanse the labia and urethra with soap and water or with a moist towelette; rinse. Cleanse and rinse from front to back.
4. Lubricate the catheter to about 1 in. (2.5 cm).
5. Assume a comfortable position. Some women perform CISC standing up with one foot on the toilet.
6. Use a hand mirror to locate the urethral opening, which is between the clitoris and the vagina.
7. Spread the vaginal lips (labia) with the second and fourth fingers; use the middle finger to feel for the urethral opening.
8. Gently insert the catheter into the opening, guiding it upward toward the umbilicus (belly button). This is usually 2 or 3 in. (5 to 8 cm) past the urethral opening.
9. When urine flows, advance the catheter another 1 in. (2.5 cm); hold it in place until the urine stops and the bladder is empty.
10. Withdraw the catheter slowly in small increments; to be sure the entire bladder empties.
11. If the catheter is reusable, wash it with soap and water; rinse and dry it well. If it is disposable, discard it immediately.
12. Store catheters in a clean, dry, secure place.
13. Record the amount of urine obtained.

Source: Clean intermittent self-catheterization (2010, updated).

Types of Urinary Catheters

There are a variety of catheter types and materials to choose from, depending on whether the patient requires catheterization for long-term or short-term use, has product sensitivity, or is at increased risk for infection.

▪ *Silver alloy*–coated catheters were found to reduce infection rates significantly when catheters remained in place for less than 7 days, although they were less effective when used for longer than 1 week (Grabe, Bishop, Bjerklund-Johansen, et al., 2008; Schumm & Lam, 2008). Silver alloy–coated catheters are not routinely used for short-term catheterization (Lo, Nicholle, Classen, et al., 2008) because they are more costly than standard catheters. However, using standard catheters may be a false economy if the patient acquires an infection.

latex is used for short- to medium-term use (...28 days) because the coating reduces friction ...e irritation during insertion and while the catheter ...s in place.

...vinyl chloride (PVC) catheters are designed for long-...m use (up to 6 wk) because they soften and conform to the ...urethra.

- *Silicone or hydrogel-coated* catheters may be used for even longer periods (e.g., up to 3 mo), because these types help prevent encrustation around the urinary meatus and reduce friction with insertion, removal, and while in place (Wilde & Getliffe, 2006).
- A *lubricant and/or antimicrobial coating* is used as a coating on some catheters to help prevent infection.

Always check for latex or Teflon and iodine allergies before performing a catheterization.

Straight Catheter. A **straight catheter** is a single-lumen tube that is inserted for immediate drainage of the bladder (e.g., to obtain a sterile urine specimen, to measure postvoid residual volume, or to relieve temporary bladder distention). After the bladder is empty or the sample obtained, the catheter is removed and the patient resumes voiding independently.

Indwelling Catheter. An **indwelling catheter,** also known as a *Foley* or *retention catheter,* is used for continuous bladder drainage (e.g., when the bladder must be kept empty or when continuous urine measurement is needed). It is usually a double-lumen tube: one lumen is used for urine drainage, and the second lumen is used to inflate a balloon near the tip of the catheter. The inflated balloon holds the catheter in place at the neck of the bladder. The balloon is sized according to the volume of fluid used to inflate it. For most patients you will use a 5-mL balloon; for children, a 3-mL; and for achieving hemostasis after a prostatectomy, a 30-mL balloon. A triple-lumen indwelling catheter is used when the patient requires intermittent or continuous bladder irrigation. Figure 30-8 illustrates the different types of catheters.

Suprapubic Catheter. A **suprapubic catheter** is used for continuous urine drainage when the urethra must be bypassed (e.g., after gynecological surgery or where there is prostatic obstruction). A suprapubic catheter is inserted through an incision above the symphysis pubis (Fig. 30-9). It is often sutured in place but may occasionally be a double-lumen catheter held in place by a balloon.

Catheter Sizing. Catheters are sized by the *diameter* of the lumen; the larger the number, the larger the lumen. For example, 8- and 10-French (Fr) catheters are used for children; they are smaller in diameter than the 14- and 16-Fr catheters typically used for adults. Men usually need a larger size (e.g., 18 Fr) than women. Catheters also come in different *lengths*: A 22-cm catheter is appropriate for women, whereas for men you will need a 40-cm catheter.

Supplies for Urinary Catheterization

The supplies used for inserting a catheter are usually prepackaged. An indwelling catheter kit includes sterile gloves, swabs or cotton balls, a solution for cleansing the urethral meatus, sterile lubricant, a sterile indwelling catheter, a syringe filled with sterile water to inflate the retention balloon, drainage tubing, and a drainage collection bag. Prepackaged kits for straight (single-lumen) catheterization have a drainage basin for collecting urine instead of a drainage collection bag. Both types of kits may also contain a sterile cup for collecting a sterile specimen. Kits contain the most common catheter sizes, usually 12, 14, or 16 Fr. Pediatric kits contain 8- or 10-Fr catheters. The smallest diameter catheter possible that provides proper drainage is recommended to minimize urethral trauma (Lo, Nicholle, Classen, et al., 2008).

KnowledgeCheck 30-7

- Describe the difference between a catheter used for straight catheterization and one used for ongoing drainage.
- Why is intermittent catheterization preferred for patients who must be catheterized over lengthy periods of time?

Urinary Catheter Insertion

To insert a urinary catheter, you will need to gather the appropriate supplies and prepare the patient. Explain to the patient the reason for the catheter insertion, the expected length of time the catheter will be needed, and the sensations he is likely to have. Most patients experience a sensation of pressure and some discomfort (but not pain) when a catheter is inserted. Explain that when the catheter is inserted it may feel as though he is voiding, but the urine is going into the tube, not on the bed. If there is swelling or bleeding in the urinary tract, insertion may be painful.

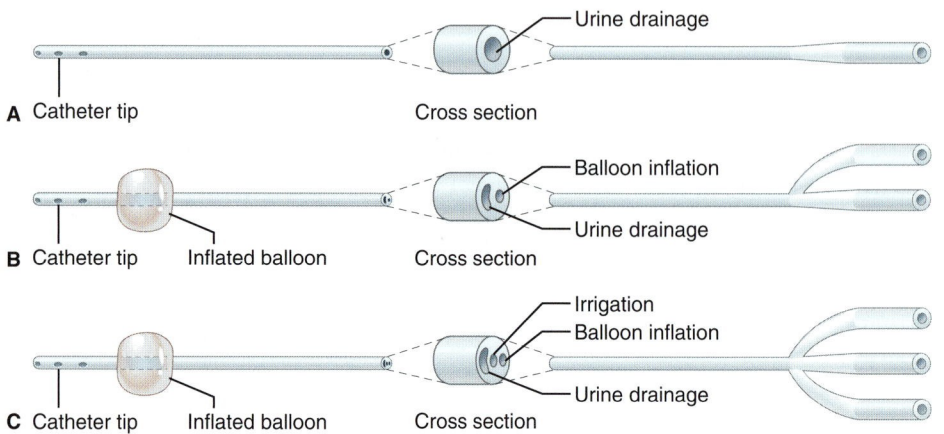

A Catheter tip   Cross section

B Catheter tip   Inflated balloon   Cross section

C Catheter tip   Inflated balloon   Cross section

FIGURE 30-8 Types of catheters. A, A single-lumen catheter is used to obtain a urine sample or immediately drain the bladder. B, A double-lumen catheter is the most commonly used indwelling catheter. C, A triple-lumen catheter is inserted when the patient requires irrigation of the bladder.

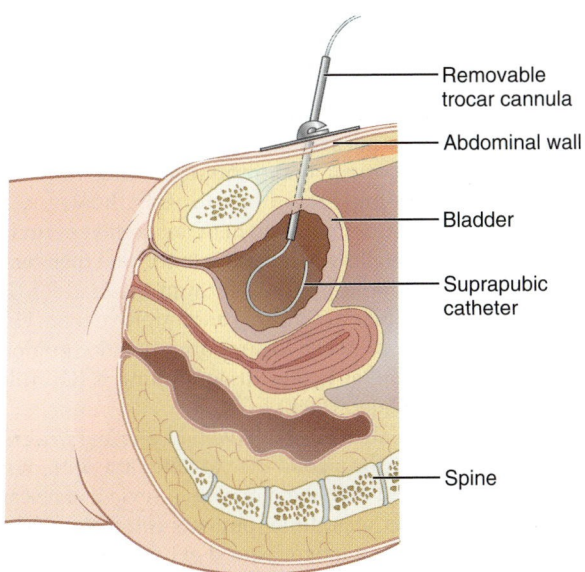

FIGURE 30-9 A suprapubic catheter drains urine from a surgically created opening into the bladder, bypassing the urethra.

Many patients feel embarrassed during this procedure. A professional approach, along with draping and other privacy measures, helps relieve discomfort or distress. As you are draping the patient, offer to answer any further questions he may have.

Use a dorsal recumbent position for women and a supine position for men. For female patients, make sure to lower the knee gatch on the bed so that you can easily visualize the urinary meatus. You may need to place a firm cushion under the patient's buttocks to prevent her sinking into a soft mattress and obscuring visibility of the meatus. For women who are unable to assume a dorsal recumbent position, consider Sims' or a lateral position (Fig. 30-10). To learn how to insert straight and indwelling catheters, see Procedure 30-4, at the end of this chapter.

Caring for the Patient With an Indwelling Catheter

The following are nursing goals when providing care for a patient with an indwelling catheter:

Prevent Urinary Tract Infection

Urinary tract infections (UTIs) are the most common healthcare-associated infection. More than one-third of all UTIs are associated with indwelling urinary catheters. An indwelling catheter is connected to a drainage tube and collection bag, which constitute a closed system.

- ✚ **Do not disconnect the tubing or open the drainage system** (e.g., to obtain specimens). An open system provides a way for pathogens to enter the system and infect the urinary tract.

- Check tubing connections regularly. If the system inadvertently becomes disconnected, wipe the ends of both tubes with antiseptic (e.g., alcohol or chlorhexidine-gluconate-alcohol combination product) before reconnecting them.
- To prevent backflow of stale urine into the bladder, always make sure the collection bag is placed below the level of the bladder. Never place the bag on the bed.
- If the catheter becomes soiled from drainage or feces, cleanse it with mild soap and water; cleaning from the meatus outward. Rinse well and pat dry.
- Empty the collection bag every 8 hours. Avoid touching the spout to any surface.
- Encourage patients with recurrent UTIs to drink cranberry juice. The evidence of effectiveness is scant; however, the hippuric acid in cranberry juice prevents some strains of antibiotic-resistant bacteria from adhering to the walls of the bladder.
- Change the catheter only when necessary. Some agencies have a policy specifying intervals (e.g., weekly). However, this is not advisable because the more often a catheter is changed, the more likely an infection will develop. Change the catheter when any of the following occurs: sediment collects in the catheter; urine does not drain well; the sandy particles that build up inside the drainage tubing cannot be freed by rolling the tubing between your hands.

Prevent Transmission of Infection

When providing catheter care, observe universal precautions. That means to wear gloves when handling the catheter or drainage system and practice hand hygiene before and after providing care to the patient.

Maintain Free Flow of Urine

Free flow of urine prevents backflow of urine into the bladder, which can cause bladder distention and injury. Stasis of urine also provides a medium for growth of microorganisms.

- Make sure the tubing and bag remain below the level of the bladder to prevent backflow. If the bag must be raised at any time, you must clamp the tubing.
- Frequently inspect the tubing for kinks, coils, or compression of the catheter or tubing that may impede flow and cause backup into the bladder.
- If urine is not flowing, check to be sure the patient is not lying on the tubing.
- Do not allow the collection bag to lie on the floor.

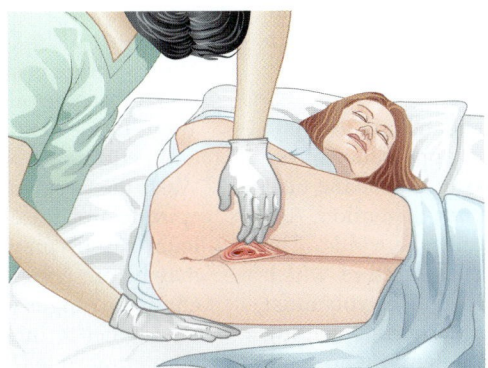
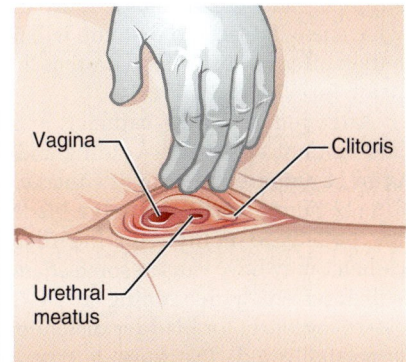

FIGURE 30-10 For women who cannot assume a dorsal recumbent position, you can use the side-lying position and lift the superior buttock to expose the urethral meatus.

Vagina — Clitoris

Urethral meatus

Promote Normal Urine Production

Adequate urine production flushes pathogens out of the bladder, provides natural irrigation of the tubing, and prevents stasis of urine.

- Encourage the patient to drink 8 to 10 eight-ounce glasses (about 3,000 mL) of fluid a day, unless contraindicated by other health problems. For patients unable to take oral liquid, provide an equivalent amount of parenteral or enteral fluids.
- Monitor I&O at least every 8 hours—more often if the patient is experiencing fluid or electrolyte problems
- Observe urine characteristics and color. Report blood, sediment, or evidence of infection to the primary provider.
- Encourage patient activity to the extent possible.

Maintain Skin and Mucosal Integrity

The following will help maintain skin and mucosal integrity:

- Perineal skin and mucosa can be irritated by feces and by movement or encrustation of the catheter. Provide hygiene care after each bowel movement, and more often if there is drainage or excessive sweating.
- Secure the tubing to the leg to prevent traction on the bladder. For men, if the catheter will remain in place long-term, secure the tubing to the abdomen to prevent damage to the penile-scrotal juncture.
- Avoid powders or lotions, as they can irritate the perineal skin.

Bladder Irrigation

You may perform an irrigation to maintain patency of a urinary catheter, to wash out the bladder (e.g., remove blood clots in the bladder after surgery), or to instill medications into the bladder. An *intermittent irrigation* is most commonly used for medication instillation, whereas a *continuous irrigation* is used to maintain patency when blood, clots, or debris is anticipated. Routine intermittent irrigations (e.g., every shift, every week) are sometimes prescribed to ensure patency; however, these should be avoided and irrigation done only as necessary.

A client requiring a continuous irrigation should have a triple-lumen catheter in place: one lumen for injecting water into the balloon when the catheter is inserted, another for the irrigating solution to flow into the bladder, and a third for the solution and urine to flow out of the bladder. ✚ A double-lumen catheter system may need to be opened for irrigation and, therefore, creates a high risk for infection. Although "open" irrigation was used in the past, it is no longer recommended. For complete procedures, see Procedures 30-7A and 30-7B, at the end of this chapter.

Removing an Indwelling Catheter

Removing a urinary catheter is a simple task, but you must monitor patients carefully afterward. Gather the necessary supplies, and tell the patient what you are about to do, what she will feel, and that you will need to monitor her urination after removal. Explain that this procedure is usually painless.

After removing the catheter, note and record the time and amount of the first voiding and the appearance of the urine. Compare the patient's intake to output for the next 8 to 12 hours, and palpate the bladder for distention. Ask the patient to notify you the first time she voids. The catheter may have caused some edema of the urethra, which will interfere with voiding at first. Therefore, you must assess regularly for bladder distention until normal voiding is reestablished. The same is true for patients who have had rectal, perineal, or lower abdominal surgery, which also creates perineal edema.

If a catheter is in place for several weeks and the urine has been draining continuously, the bladder does not stretch and contract as it does in normal voiding. Therefore, the muscle loses tone and the patient may require bladder retraining. Agencies have differing procedures for this; however, one method is to begin clamping the catheter for certain periods of time (e.g., 1 to 4 hr) to allow the bladder to fill, and then releasing the clamp to allow urine to drain from the bladder. This should stimulate the bladder muscle and improve tone. However, there is limited evidence to support a practice guideline for clamping the catheter before discontinuing it (Griffith & Fernandez, 2007, updated 2009).

For hospitalized patients who have had a urinary catheter for a short time, it may be a good idea to time catheter removal for late at night instead of in the morning. A review of research found that when this was done, patients (on average) held urine in the bladder for a longer period of time before voiding in the morning. This led to larger volume for the first void after the catheter was discontinued. Patients with late night catheter removal were discharged sooner and without having to have the urinary catheter reinserted for urine retention (Griffith & Fernandez, 2007, updated 2009).

For guidelines to follow when removing a retention catheter, see Procedure 30-6, at the end of this chapter.

KnowledgeCheck 30-8

- What actions should you take before inserting a catheter?
- When caring for a client with an indwelling catheter, you notice sandy particles around the urethral meatus. What should you do?
- How often should the urine collection bag be emptied?

ThinkLike a Nurse 30-7

You are caring for a patient who had an indwelling catheter removed 12 hours ago. The patient has not voided. What action should you take?

Interventions for Example Problem: Urinary Incontinence

Because urinary incontinence is so prevalent, you are likely to be called on to deal with this problem in your practice. Most incontinence is managed with skin care and behavioral interventions, but medications are sometimes used. For home care interventions, see the Home Care box Managing Incontinence. The other interventions discussed in this section are mainly for inpatients. Also see the Nursing Care Plan and Care Map for Stress Urinary Incontinence.

Perineal Skin Care

Normal urine is acidic. When it remains in contact with the skin, it becomes alkaline, causing dermatitis and skin excoriation. It is essential to keep the skin dry. Change clothing, and bedding as soon as possible after incontinence occurs. Wash the perineum with soap and warm water after each episode and rinse and dry well. Barrier creams (e.g., petroleum-based) may be used for irritated skin; antifungals may be prescribed (e.g., nystatin [Mycostatin]) to prevent or eliminate fungus growth. You may use absorbent products as an adjunct to other control measures, especially for those with intractable UI.

Managing Incontinence

➤ Routinely ask clients and families about incontinence. Patients and families often do not raise the issue. Be direct and ask about continence using simple questions in a way that wouldn't embarrass the patient, such as "Do you wear a pad to keep your clothes dry?" "Do you ever wet your clothing?"

➤ If you determine that the client is incontinent, ask follow-up questions to identify the type of incontinence. For example: "Do you sometimes not make it to the toilet in time?" "Do you ever dribble urine when you sneeze or cough?"

➤ Ask where the toilet is and whether the patient can get there easily.

➤ Encourage use of a bladder diary for at least 3 to 7 days, covering routine day-to-day activities as well as atypical situations.

Teach Danger Signals

➤ Advise patients to contact a healthcare provider if any of the following occur:
  ➤ They have not been previously evaluated for this problem.
  ➤ The urinary stream is weak.
  ➤ There is burning, fever, chills, pain, or passing little urine for 1 to 2 days.
  ➤ Urine is cloudy, unusually foul-smelling.
  ➤ Discharge occurs from the penis or vagina.

Modify the Environment as Needed

➤ Place a commode near where the patient spends most of his time.

➤ In a two-story house with a toilet on only one floor, place a commode on the other floor in the room where the patient spends most of his time. With a written prescription, insurance or government-supported healthcare may reimburse this expense.

➤ For some patients, a commode should be placed by the bedside on a large, absorbent, washable mat (to absorb any urine that leaks).

Recommend Lifestyle Modifications

➤ Advise women who have a BMI > 30 to lose weight. Even a weight loss of 5% to 10% alleviates symptoms and improves quality of life (Finnish Medical Society, 2008).

➤ Because many home caregivers are middle-aged or older women, they may have continence problems of their own. Teach them pelvic muscle exercises and the best techniques for lifting and turning the patient in bed.

➤ Advise the following:
  ➤ Maintain oral fluids to 8 to 10 glasses (3,000 mL) per day, as tolerated.
  ➤ Limit intake of alcohol, artificial sweeteners, spicy foods, and citrus fruits, which may irritate the bladder.
  ➤ Limit caffeine to 100 mg/day. This is about one cup of coffee or two 12-oz. cans of soda. Caffeine is a diuretic and bladder stimulant.
  ➤ Stop smoking (it has been linked to urge UI among men and both stress and urge UI among women).
  ➤ Take prescribed diuretics early in the morning. Taken at night, they can cause nocturia and nocturnal enuresis, leading to interrupted sleep.
  ➤ Avoid constipation. Constipation puts pressure on the bladder.
  ➤ High-impact exercise (e.g., running, jumping rope) is associated with increased stress UI.

Behavioral Interventions

Aggressive nursing intervention can help to improve patients' quality of life, capacity for physical activity, and self-esteem. It can also help to reduce the cost of healthcare. Recent guidelines outline five categories of nonpharmacological treatment options nurses commonly provide independently: lifestyle modification, bladder training, scheduled voiding, pelvic floor muscle rehabilitation, anti-incontinence devices, and supportive interventions (Wyman, 2003). These therapies have been proven to be effective for most patients.

Lifestyle Modification. There are a number of ways to reduce the symptoms of urinary incontinence to recommend to patients. You will find these in the Home Care box Managing Incontinence.

Bladder Training. The goal of bladder training is to enable the patient to hold increasingly greater volumes of urine in the bladder and to increase the interval between voidings. This involves patient teaching, scheduled voiding, and self-monitoring using a voiding diary. In addition to teaching the mechanisms of urination, teach distraction and relaxation strategies to help inhibit the urge to void. For example, instruct the patient to perform serial subtractions or become involved in an activity that requires concentration (e.g., a crossword puzzle) when she feels the urge to void. Other techniques include deep breathing, guided imagery, and performing several pelvic floor contractions to quiet the sensations from the bladder.

Scheduled Voiding. This is a form of bladder training involving timed voiding and habit retraining. The client must be mentally and physically capable of self-toileting. Initially the patient may be scheduled to attempt voiding every 2 hours or even more often. Keep, or have the patient keep, a record of his adherence to the schedule and the number of incontinence episodes. As a pattern develops and the person gains greater control, the length of time between voiding may be increased, usually by 15 to 30 minutes each week. Scheduled voiding is usually combined with other techniques, including lifestyle adjustments and pelvic muscle exercises.

Nursing Care Plan

Client Data

Desmond Washington, a 69-year-old man, comes to the clinic 4 weeks after having a prostatectomy for prostate cancer. He was discharged from the hospital on postoperative day 4 and went home with an indwelling urinary catheter. The catheter was removed at his last visit, 9 days after surgery.

Mr. Washington is meticulously groomed. He is friendly, greeting other patients in the clinic and chatting with the clinic personnel. When his nurse brings him to an examination room and asks how he feels, he says, "I saw the sun come up today. I appreciate that more now. The good Lord has given me a new lease on life, and I intend to use it!" His nurse continues, "That's great, Mr. Washington. How have you been doing since the catheter was removed?" Mr. Washington's smile fades. He lowers his voice and says, "You know, I think that's the worst part of this whole thing. I hate wearing these diapers—they make me feel, well, like an old man. I'm certainly not ready for this."

The nurse continues, "Do you have *any* control of your urine?" Mr. Washington explains, "I may go for hours and stay dry, and then it seems, for no reason, I wet myself. Take yesterday, for example. I was sitting on the sofa watching the ball game when someone came to the door. I got up to answer the door, and all of a sudden, I felt wet. I didn't even have anything to drink so I could make it through the afternoon and stay dry. And if I cough? Forget it. Can something be done so I can hold my urine again?"

Nursing Diagnosis

Stress Urinary Incontinence related to disruption of the urinary sphincter and related pelvic muscles by surgery as evidenced by client report of involuntary loss of urine with increased intra-abdominal pressure.

NOC Outcomes	Individualized Goals/Expected Outcomes
Urinary Continence (0502) Urinary Elimination (0503)	*By the next visit, Mr. Washington will:* **1.** Describe three things he can do that will help regain urinary continence. **2.** Explain three interventions to cope with leaked urine. **3.** Report that he is drinking adequate amounts of fluids during the day.

Nursing Interventions/Activities

NIC Interventions

Urinary Elimination Management (0590)
Urinary Incontinence Care (0610)

Nursing Activities	Rationale
1. Obtain midstream voided urine specimen for urinalysis.	UTI can cause or worsen incontinence (Nazarko, 2008; Urinary Continence Guideline Panel [UCGP], 1992; Wilde & Getliffe, 2006).
2. Identify factors that contribute to Mr. Washington's incontinence by using an incontinence diary.	Identifying activities or other factors that cause loss of urine control can guide specific interventions. A diary facilitates monitoring over time and can identify patterns that could otherwise be missed (National Institute for Health and Clinical Excellence [NICE], 2006).
3. Teach pelvic floor muscle exercises (PFME).	PFME strengthen pelvic muscles and enhance sphincter control. They have been shown to increase urinary continence without side effects in men who have undergone prostatectomy (National Collaborating Centre for Women's and Children's Health, 2006; NICE, 2006; Sampselle, Wyman, Thomas, et al., 2006; van Kempen, De Weerdt, van Poppel, et al., 2000).

Nursing Care Plan (continued)

Nursing Activities	Rationale
4. Use biofeedback when needed in conjunction with PFME training to help Mr. Washington isolate pelvic floor muscles.	Biofeedback allows clients to receive auditory or visual (or both) cues when the proper muscles are contracted, so they learn what the proper muscle contraction feels like. Biofeedback also allows the nurse or therapist to objectively measure strength of contractions (Burgio, Goode, Urban, et al., 2007; Hunter, Moore, Cody, et al., 2007; UCGP, 1992).
5. Teach timed voiding. Have Mr. Washington void on a schedule of every 2 hours.	Voiding on a schedule of every 2 hours can reduce the amount of urine in the bladder, thus reducing the likelihood of leakage with activities of daily living (National Collaborating Centre for Women's and Children's Health, 2006; NICE, 2006; Sampselle, Wyman, & Thomas, 2006; UCGP, 1992).
6. Explain the need to drink adequate fluids and *not* limit fluids in an effort to prevent incontinence. Help Mr. Washington identify ways to drink a minimum of 1,500 mL/day.	Adequate fluid intake is important to maintain dilute urine, which is less irritating to the bladder; to maintain systemic hydration; and to reduce the risk for constipation, which can contribute to urinary incontinence (Dowling-Castronovo & Bradway, 2003, updated 2008; IOM, 2004; UCGP, 1992).
7. Assist the client in selecting appropriate absorbent products that collect urine strictly for temporary management while continence management is ongoing.	Proper absorbent garments and pads can collect and trap urine, keep skin clean and dry, reduce odor, and minimize the risk of soiling accidents (NICE, 2006; UCGP, 1992).
8. Help the client develop a personal hygiene routine that will maintain skin integrity.	Proper hygiene will reduce the risk of skin irritation and infection. Use warm (not hot) water, and pat (don't scrub) the perineal area. A barrier cream will repel fluid and protect the skin from urine.
9. Offer referral to a support group.	Support groups provide a sense of community and enhance members' problem-solving skills. Mr. Washington may feel less embarrassment when he discovers that others share his problems.
10. Explain that urinary incontinence is common after prostatectomy, but that it may be only temporary.	Urinary incontinence can be a troubling complication of prostatectomy for many men. Fortunately, it usually resolves with active management within 6 to 12 months of surgery (Burgio, Goode, Urban, et al., 2007).

There are many treatment recommendations that are not supported by research. Anecdotally, they may work for some clients. These include reducing caffeine consumption; eliminating bladder irritants, such as artificial sweeteners, spicy foods, and citrus from the diet; losing weight; and quitting smoking. In addition, it is important for nurses to understand that the pathophysiology of urinary incontinence differs between men and women and that interventions that are successful in women may or may not be equally successful in men.

Evaluation

At the end of the visit, Mr. Washington said, "I didn't know there were things I could do about the leaking urine. Before surgery, all I cared about was getting rid of the cancer. I don't need a support group for me but maybe I'll lead one!" Mr. Washington had been placing folded paper towels in his underwear to collect urine because he thought absorbent products were too expensive, but with guidance from his nurse, he identified products he could afford. He liked that they would not be visible through his clothing.

At Mr. Washington's next visit, the nurse will review the initial collaborative goals and stated outcomes and perform a client assessment to determine whether the goals were reached in the stated time frame.

(continued)

Nursing Care Plan (continued)

Mr. Washington currently has a positive attitude and is focused on "beating" his cancer first and on managing complications of surgery second. As time passes, incontinence may persist and may become more frustrating for him once he is fully recovered from surgery. Mr. Washington initially declined referral to a support group, but he may be more interested in joining one in the future for help dealing with long-term consequences of prostatectomy.

References

Burgio, Goode, Urban, et al., 2007; Dowling-Castronovo & Bradway, 2003, updated 2008; Hunter, Moore, Cody, et al., 2007; National Collaborating Centre for Women's and Children's Health, 2006; Nazarko, 2008; NICE, 2006; UCGP, 1992; VanKampen, DeWeerdt, VanPoppel, et al., 2000; Wilde & Getliffe, 2006.

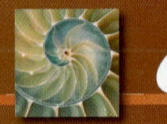

Care Map

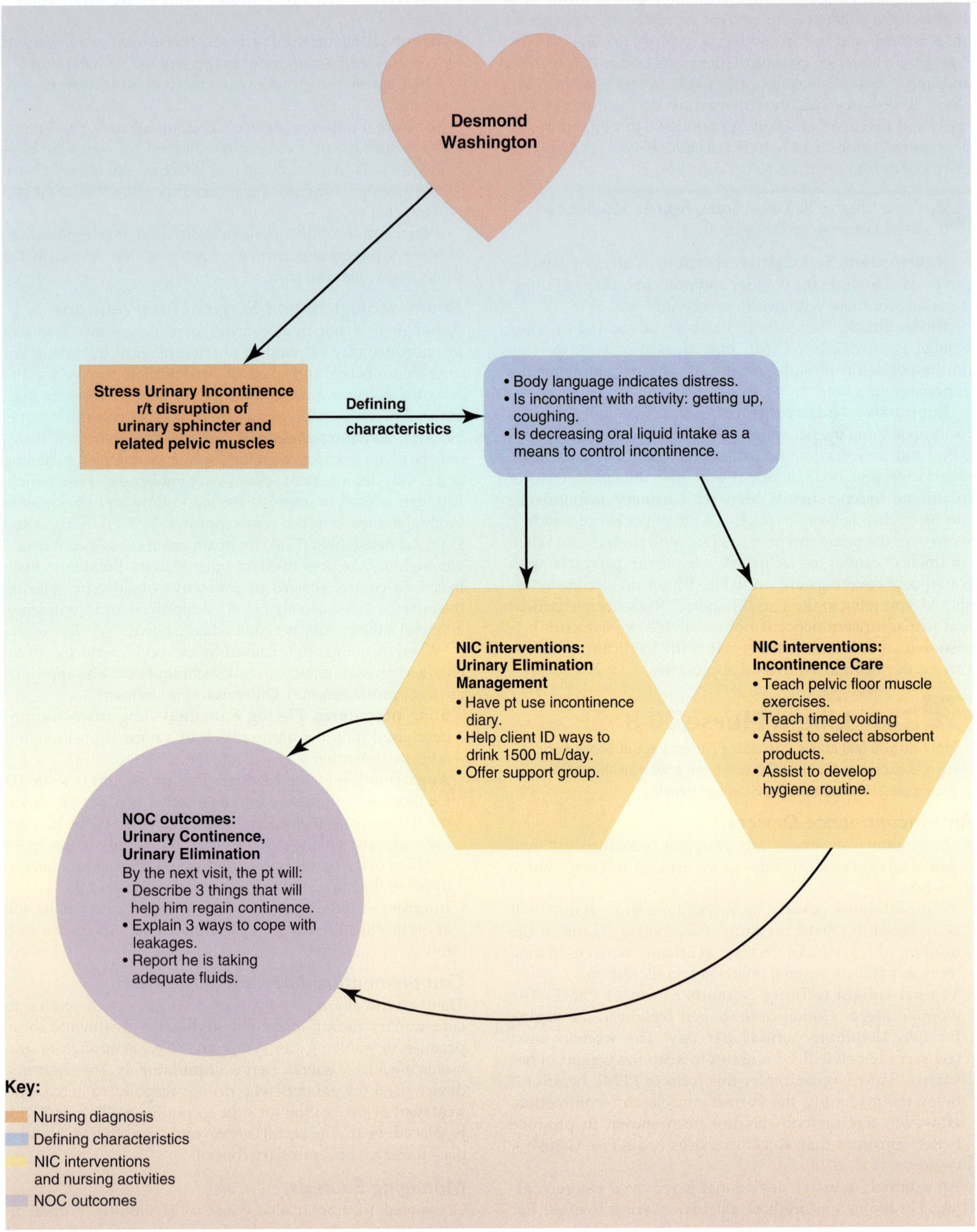

Desmond Washington

Stress Urinary Incontinence r/t disruption of urinary sphincter and related pelvic muscles

Defining characteristics

- Body language indicates distress.
- Is incontinent with activity: getting up, coughing.
- Is decreasing oral liquid intake as a means to control incontinence.

NIC interventions: Urinary Elimination Management
- Have pt use incontinence diary.
- Help client ID ways to drink 1500 mL/day.
- Offer support group.

NIC interventions: Incontinence Care
- Teach pelvic floor muscle exercises.
- Teach timed voiding
- Assist to select absorbent products.
- Assist to develop hygiene routine.

NOC outcomes: Urinary Continence, Urinary Elimination
By the next visit, the pt will:
- Describe 3 things that will help him regain continence.
- Explain 3 ways to cope with leakages.
- Report he is taking adequate fluids.

Key:

■ Nursing diagnosis

■ Defining characteristics

■ NIC interventions and nursing activities

■ NOC outcomes

Pelvic Floor Muscle Rehabilitation. Pelvic floor muscle exercises (PFME) are a mainstay of UI treatment for women. PFME strengthen perineal muscles and help to prevent and treat stress, urge, and mixed UI. **Kegel exercises** are the most commonly used method for preventing or reversing incontinence in women for the first year after giving birth. This approach may also prevent or reduce urinary incontinence in older women and in men undergoing prostate surgery. Cure rates of UI, based on patient diaries, range from 16% to 27%, and improvement rates vary from 48% to 80.7% with PFME alone. To be successful, the patient must do the exercises correctly and practice them daily. A period of 6 to 12 months may be required before treatment is effective. If you need specific instructions for how to do Kegel exercises,

 Go to Chapter 30, **Tables, Boxes, Figures: ESG Box 30-1: Kegel Exercises,** on Davis*Plus*.

Intermittent Self-Catheterization. A straight catheter can be used to drain the bladder and prevent leakage of urine, especially for those with overflow incontinence.

Biofeedback. Biofeedback has been advocated by some women as an adjunct to PFME. Electrodes attached to the skin on the perineum provide feedback to the patient about the perineal contraction.

Supportive Interventions. Supportive interventions focus on helping the patient reach the toilet, urinate independently, and perform toileting self-care. A bedside commode, raised toilet seat, bedpan, urinal, and other aids make it easier to urinate independently. Men with urinary incontinence can use a drip collector, which is a small pocket of padding worn over the penis and held in place with underwear. When continence cannot be achieved, absorbent products with waterproof coverings are available. Under no circumstances should you refer to these as "diapers." Reassure the patient that urinary incontinence is not inevitable or shameful. It is treatable, and, if not, manageable with medication and/or various devices and behavioral approaches.

 Think**Like a Nurse** 30-8

How do you feel about instructing patients about pelvic floor muscle exercises (PFME)? Do you think a woman should always provide this instruction? Explain your thinking.

Anti-Incontinence Devices

Anti-incontinence devices are designed to reduce the incidence of UI or provide a pathway for urine flow. They include the following:

- An **incontinence pessary,** or intravaginal support device. It is designed to relieve pressure of the pelvic organs on the urethra, which reduces the urge to urinate. When used long term, monitor for vaginal infection and ulceration.
- **Vaginal weight training** is another form of PFME. The woman inserts a small cone-shaped weight in the vagina for two 15-minute periods per day. The woman must contract the pelvic floor muscles to keep the weight in her vagina. Some women prefer this form of PFME because it helps them identify the correct muscles for contraction. However, this method has not been shown to produce better outcomes than Kegel exercises (Gamiero, Gamiero, Gamiero, et al, 2010).
- An **external occlusive device** that is removed before voiding. For women, a urethral meatus covering is used. For men, a penis clamp is a reusable, soft spongy rubber device

used to control stress incontinence or dribbling urine, common with enlarged prostate.

- An **internal urethral meatus plug,** which may be used by men and women. This is a disposable, single-use device, typically used for activities that cause stress incontinence.
- A **valved catheter** that allows urine to be drained on a schedule.
- An **indwelling urethral catheter.** This is used as a last resort to control the flow of urine and protect the perineal skin.
- A **bed alarm,** which will wake the patient if incontinence occurs.
- An **external collection device.** Condom catheters, also known as uro-sheaths, are most commonly used for men who have adequate bladder emptying and intact genital skin. To learn how to apply a condom catheter, see Procedure 30-5, at the end of this chapter.

When anti-incontinence devices are used, it is important to observe for vaginal or urinary tract infection, blood in the urine, and vaginal erosion.

Pharmacological and Surgical Interventions

Although it is not the treatment of choice, some forms of incontinence may respond to pharmacological treatment. For urge incontinence, anti-spasmotic medication may be used to relax the detrusor muscle and increase bladder capacity (e.g., anticholinergics, smooth-muscle relaxants, calcium-channel blockers, and antidepressants). For stress incontinence, drugs may be given to improve urethral sphincter muscle functioning (e.g., the decongestant phenylpropanolamine [Triaminic]). Estrogen is used to improve the blood flow and thickness to urethral tissues. Estrogen is not approved by the U.S. Food and Drug Administration (FDA) for treatment of stress incontinence, although may be prescribed for other reasons. Botulinum toxin injections control spasms of overactive bladder by relaxing the muscles. It is currently not FDA-approved for incontinence, although a therapeutic benefit has been shown.

When incontinence is caused by cystocele, rectocele, or an enlarged prostate gland, surgical techniques may be appropriate (e.g., prostatectomy). Other examples follow:

- **Sling procedures.** Placing a urethral sling treats incontinence by lifting the urethra back to a normal position and relieving pressure.
- **Augmentation of the bladder.** This procedure is reserved for those who do not benefit from other bladder therapies, medication, or self-catheterization. Segments of the bladder are surgically enlarged to improve the bladder capacity. A segment of the bowel is wrapped around the bladder neck to improve the muscle-squeezing action of the bladder.
- **Injection of bulking agents.** Collagen is injected alongside of the urethra. Effectiveness often lasts a period of years with few complications.

Complementary Alternative Methods

There are no alternative methods that have been proven to cure urinary incontinence, although some treatments show promise in reducing the symptoms (e.g., acupuncture and biofeedback). A **sacral nerve stimulator** is an electronic device used for patients who do not respond to behavioral treatment or medication for urge incontinence. The lead wire is placed near the sacral nerve and acts like a bladder pacemaker for better urinary control.

Managing Enuresis

Occasional wetting (called *enuresis*) is entirely normal in children even in the early school years. Parents should accept

such events calmly and not punish the child (see the Home Care box Managing Enuresis in Children)

Children, especially older ones, can be embarrassed by *nocturnal enuresis,* or bedwetting, not to mention the inconvenience it poses. Young children may feel anxious about using the bathroom in a clinic, hospital, or any unfamiliar environment. They may be especially anxious about using a bedpan. Also, be aware that the stress of an illness or hospitalization may cause a child to regress in his ability to toilet independently. You may need to schedule regular trips to the bathroom and to watch for nonverbal cues that the child needs to void.

Home Care

Managing Enuresis in Children

➤ Medication and moisture alarms can be effective for managing nocturnal enuresis for children younger than age 10. Medication is helpful when the child is not sleeping at home.

ThinkLike a Nurse 30-9

What treatment options for incontinence have you seen used in your clinical experience? What options do you believe should be used more frequently? Less frequently? Explain your thinking.

Caring for a Patient With a Urinary Diversion

A patient with a urinary diversion requires physical and psychological care. Initially you will care for the ostomy. However, the goals are for the patient to become comfortable with his changed body and to assume self-care.

What Are Urinary Diversions?

A **urinary diversion,** or **urostomy,** is a surgically created opening for elimination of urine. Urostomies are used to treat patients who have conditions such as birth defects, cancer, trauma, or disease of the urinary system. A patient with a urinary diversion does not eliminate urine via the urethra. Instead, urine bypasses the bladder and is expelled through the **stoma** or **ostomy.** The patient no longer has voluntary control of urination. Urine constantly flows through the stoma and is collected in a pouch the patient wears. Risks associated with urinary diversions are primarily infection and permanent kidney damage, which can occur from hydronephrosis (distention of the kidneys with urine, resulting from obstruction of the ureter). The following are three types of urinary diversions:

- A **cutaneous ureterostomy** reroutes the ureter(s) directly to the surface of the abdomen, forming a small stoma. It may be unilateral or bilateral. This procedure has limited use because it provides a pathway for pathogens on the skin to directly enter the kidney. The stomas are small and difficult to fit with a collection appliance.
- An **ileal conduit,** also known as a **Bricker's loop** or **ileal loop,** is the most common type of urinary diversion (Fig. 30-11). A small piece of ileum is removed with blood and nerve supply intact. The remainder of the ileum is reconnected to prevent disruption of flow through the bowel. The free segment of ileum is sutured closed at one end, and the other end is brought out to the abdominal wall to create a stoma. The result is a small pouch into which the ureters are implanted.

Urine, along with mucus from the ileum, drains continuously from the stoma. This procedure is preferable to a cutaneous ureterostomy because the mucous membrane lining the ileum protects the kidneys from ascending infection. In addition, the ileum creates a stoma that is easier to fit with an appliance.

- A **continent urostomy,** also known as an **ileal bladder conduit,** or **Kock pouch** (Fig. 30-12), is a variation of the ileal conduit. Urine drains from the ureters into a surgically created ileal pouch. The stoma created on the abdomen contains a nipple valve to keep urine from leaking. Rather than having urine flow constantly, the patient with an ileal bladder conduit inserts a catheter into the stoma to drain urine through the valve. A second valve prevents reflux of urine back into the kidneys.

INTERVENTIONS/IMPLEMENTATION FOR PATIENTS WITH URINARY DIVERSIONS

Patients experience a variety of reactions to the stoma. Patients with continent ostomies are usually more comfortable with their stoma because of the control it offers while avoiding the embarrassment, odor, and inconvenience of UI. Your attitude and willingness to discuss the body changes associated with an ostomy will help your patient begin his adjustment. In many communities, the local ostomy association has counselors available to visit patients, discuss the psychological changes

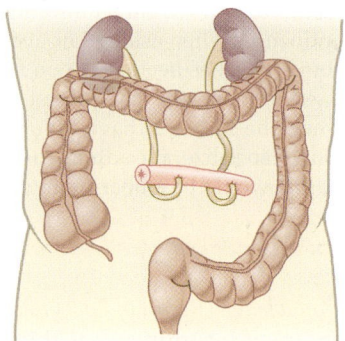

FIGURE 30-11 An ileal conduit is the most common urinary diversion.

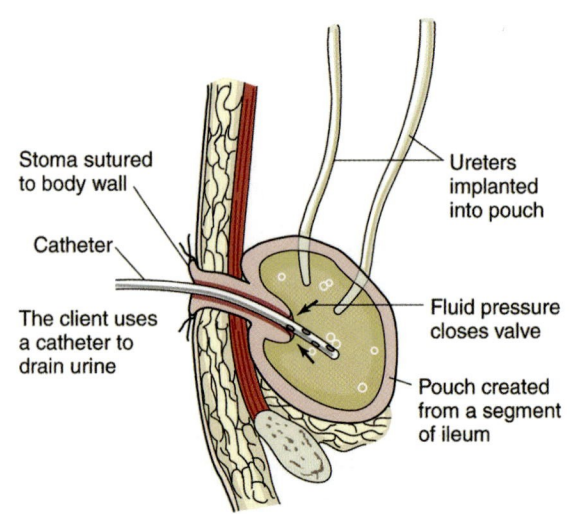

FIGURE 30-12 A continent urostomy allows the client to manage urine without the need to wear an ostomy appliance.

associated with a urinary diversion, and help them with physical care of the stoma. Most counselors are adept because they too have ostomies. They are able to share practical and personal information with patients based on their own experience with similar challenges.

Nursing care of a patient with a urinary diversion should begin with a thorough assessment. A healthy stoma ranges in color from deep pink to brick red, regardless of skin color, and is shiny and moist at all times. A pale, dusky, or black stoma often indicates inadequate blood supply. Immediately document and report such findings to the surgeon.

Assess the skin surrounding the stoma for signs of irritation, such as redness, tenderness, breakdown, and drainage.

Skin care is critical. When the normally acid urine remains in contact with the skin, it becomes alkaline. Encrustations collect on the skin and the skin becomes macerated and excoriated. Skin breakdown may lead to infection, pain, and leakage.

Empty the drainage device frequently during the day; connect it to a larger connection bag at night when the patient is sleeping. Monitor the amount and type of drainage.

A moisture-proof skin barrier is usually placed snugly around the stoma to protect surrounding skin. Barrier creams may also be prescribed. More extensive discussion about stoma care is covered in Chapter 29, Bowel Elimination, and in Procedure 29-7, Changing an Ostomy Appliance.

CLINICAL**REASONING:**
Applying the **Full-Spectrum Nursing Model**

Because the following critical thinking activities allow you to practice the kind of thinking you will use as a full-spectrum nurse, they usually have no single right answer. Discuss them with your peers—if you have difficulty with any of the questions, consult your instructor.

PATIENT SITUATION

You are providing care to an older-adult woman, Mrs. Patel, who has a number of health concerns, including diabetes and obesity. Mrs. Patel seeks healthcare because she is experiencing burning with urination, frequency, and urgency. You explain to her these are signs of a urinary tract infection. You discover while taking your nursing history that she also has difficulty with urinary continence. When asking her about toileting habits, she tells you she often doesn't "make it to the bathroom" even while at home. This has been going on for about 3 years now. She has trouble getting up and walking upstairs to the bathroom because of a foot ulcer that doesn't seem to be healing well. Mrs. Patel's affect is flat with little expression. During your time with her, she seems to have little interest in talking about her health concerns. When you ask her about what she does to get out or socialize, she admits to being hesitant to go far because she is afraid of wetting without knowing it and carrying an odor that would be embarrassing to her.

THINKING

1. *Theoretical Knowledge (Recall of Facts and Principles):*
   a. What kind(s) of incontinence is this patient likely to have?
   b. What are this patient's risk factors for incontinence?
2. *Critical Thinking (Contextual Awareness):*
   a. What aspects of this situation have you experienced or observed before in your role as a caregiver?
   b. How might those past experiences affect your perception in this situation?

DOING

3. *Practical Knowledge (Patient Teaching):*
   a. How could you encourage this woman to seek healthcare for managing her urinary incontinence?
   b. What might you ask your patient to do in order to get a better idea of her bladder history and toileting habits?
   c. By looking at Mrs. Patel's bladder diary, you see a pattern suggestive of urinary incontinence. What other behavioral strategies might you suggest to improve her ability to have control of her bladder?

CARING

4. *Self-Knowledge:*
   a. Have you ever personally experienced urinary urgency when you had trouble getting to the bathroom in time? Reflect on this experience and examine how you might feel if you were incontinent much of the time.
   b. In what way(s) can you show compassion for the patient who has urinary incontinence?

 Go To Chapter 30, **Clinical Reasoning: Applying the Full-Spectrum Nursing Model Response Sheet,** on Davis*Plus.*

Practical Knowledge
procedures

Procedure 30–1 ■ Measuring Urine

➤ For steps to follow in *all* procedures, refer to Universal Steps for All Procedures found on the page facing the inside back cover of this book.

- Bedpan or urinal
- Clean procedure gloves
- Graduated container
- Toilet paper, as indicated
- Washcloth or towel
- Mild soap and water for patient's hands

Delegation

The procedure may be delegated to nursing assistive personnel (NAPs), but you must be sure that that they know how to perform the procedure correctly, including proper cleansing of the bedpan/urinal and the graduated container according to the facility's policies. Complete the following assessments

and instruct the NAP to report any abnormalities seen in the urine (e.g., blood, foul odor, mucus) or any complaints of dysuria by the patient.

Pre-Procedure Assessments

- Cognitive status
  To determine whether the patient can follow directions and complete this procedure on her own.
- Mobility status
  To determine whether the patient can get out of the bed to use the toilet.
- Urinary status
  To determine the patient's ability to control bladder function.

Procedure 30-1A ■ Measuring Urine Output From a Bedpan or Urinal

➤ When performing the procedure, always identify your patient according to agency policy and be attentive to standard precautions, hand hygiene, patient safety and privacy, body mechanics, and documentation.

Procedure Steps

1. **Wash your hands and don clean** procedure gloves.
   Prevents transmission of bacteria.
2. **Place a bedpan or urinal** in the appropriate position (see Procedure 29-2).
3. **Remove the bedpan or urinal**, being careful not to spill the urine. Reposition the patient and transport the urine to the bathroom.
4. **While still wearing** procedure gloves, pour the urine into a graduated

cylinder or calibrated measuring container.
   a. Be sure that the measuring device is labeled with the correct patient information (in many institutions, labels are preprinted or bar coded).
   b. Do not use a measuring device for more than one patient.
5. **Place the measuring device** on a flat surface (e.g., shelf, table), and read the amount at eye level.
6. **Observe the urine for color**, clarity, and odor.

7. **Discard the urine** in the toilet. If a specimen is required, transfer at least 30 mL of urine to the designated container.
8. **Clean the measuring container** and store in the patient's bathroom.
9. **Remove gloves. Wash your hands**.
10. **Record the time and volume** on the I&O record.

Procedure 30-1B ■ Measuring Urine From an Indwelling Catheter

➤ When performing the procedure, always identify your patient according to agency policy and be attentive to standard precautions, hand hygiene, patient safety and privacy, body mechanics, and documentation.

Procedure Steps

1. **Wearing clean gloves**, place the drainage spout for the collection bag inside a calibrated measuring container. Avoid touching the spout to the inside of the container.
   Gloving prevents transmission of bacteria.

2. **Unclamp the drainage spout**, and direct the flow of urine into the measuring device, still keeping the spout away from the sides of the container.
   Prevents contaminating the drainage spout. ➤

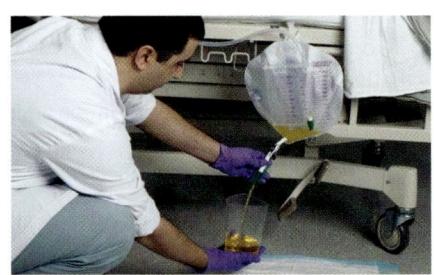

(continued on next page)

Procedure 30–1 ■ **Measuring Urine** (continued)

3. **Reclamp the spout** when the collection bag is empty.
4. **Wipe the drainage spout** with an alcohol pad, and replace the spout into the slot on the collection bag.
   A clean spout reduces transmission of bacteria.
5. **Measure urine output** from the indwelling catheter at the end of each shift unless otherwise ordered. Record the time and amount on the I&O record; record urine color, clarity, and odor. ➤

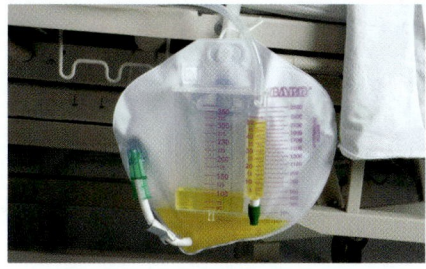

6. **Discard the urine in the toilet**.
7. **Remove gloves. Wash your hands**.

? What if . . .

■ **The physician orders hourly monitoring of the patient's urine output?**
You will need to obtain a special collection bag with a small measuring chamber; document urine output on the I&O record every hour.

Evaluation

- Note any unusual characteristics of the urine (e.g., color, odor, presence of sediment or mucus).
- Note any difficulties with urination (e.g., pain, dribbling, difficulty beginning urination).
- Continue to assess that drainage from the indwelling catheter is not obstructed and that the drainage bag is below the level of the bladder.
- Assess for bladder distention.
  Bladder distention indicates poor bladder emptying. Note: Some facilities have a bladder-scanning device that will allow you to determine whether there is residual urine.

Patient Teaching

Instruct the patient and/or primary caregiver to document the urine intake and output on the I&O worksheet at the bedside.

Home Care

Teach the patient and/or the primary caregiver how to collect and measure the urine

Documentation

- Document urine volume and record the time and date the specimen was collected, per agency policy. You may chart specimen collection in the patient's health record (nurse's notes) or a patient graphic flow sheet, depending on the agency.
- Document the characteristics of the urine: color, odor, particulate matter, blood, clarity, or other qualities.
- Document any difficulty with voiding, including pain or burning with urination, frequency, or difficulty starting the urine flow.

Practice Resources

Siegel, Rhinehart, Jackson, et al. & the Healthcare Infection Control Practices Advisory Committee of the Centers for Disease Control and Prevention, 2007.

Procedure 30–2 ■ **Obtaining a Urine Specimen for Testing**

➤ For steps to follow in *all* procedures, refer to the Universal Steps for All Procedures found on the page facing the inside back cover.

Equipment

Collecting a Clean-Catch Urine Specimen

- Prepackaged collection kit
- If no kit is available:
  - Sterile specimen container
  - Antiseptic solution
  - Sterile cotton balls or 2 in. × 2 in. gauze pads
- Washcloth or towel
- Mild soap and water
- Two pairs of clean procedure gloves
- Patient identification labels
- Bedpan or bedside commode for an immobile patient

Obtaining a Sterile Urine Specimen From a Catheter

- Clean gloves
- Antiseptic swab

- Sterile specimen container with a lid
- Patient identification label
- Sterile syringe with a sterile 21- to 25-gauge needleless access device (a 5- to 10-mL syringe is usually sufficient)

Collecting a 24-Hour Urine Specimen

NOTE: Some tests require using a double-storage container. Be sure to find out if you need a double-storage container, preservative, or if there are special instruction for collection of the sample.

- Basin and ice, possibly. Check with the laboratory to determine whether the specimen needs to be kept on ice.
- Large collection container.

Delegation

This procedure may be delegated to the NAP but you must be sure they know how to perform the procedure correctly, including proper cleansing and maintaining sterility of the container. You must complete the following assessments and instruct the NAP to report any abnormalities seen in the urine (e.g., blood, foul odor, mucus). In addition, the NAP should report any complaints of dysuria by the patient and she should bring the specimen to you for inspection.

Pre-Procedure Assessments

- Cognitive status
  Helps you to determine whether the patient can follow directions and complete this procedure on her own.
- Mobility status
  Helps you to determine where the specimen will be collected (e.g., bed, commode, bedpan)
- Urinary status
  Patients with impaired ability to control urinary flow may not be able to collect a specimen in this manner.

Procedure 30-2A ■ Collecting a Clean-Catch Urine Specimen

➤ When performing the procedure, always identify your patient according to agency policy and be attentive to standard precautions, hand hygiene, patient safety and privacy, body mechanics, and documentation.

Procedure Steps

1. **Don procedure gloves.**
2. **Open the prepackaged kit** (if available), and remove the contents.
3. **Cleanse, or instruct the patient** to cleanse, around the urinary meatus. Allow the area to dry.
   Cleansing prevents contamination of the specimen with surface bacteria.

For Women

a. Wash the perineal area with warm water and mild soap, if soiled.
   Cleansing the perineum will help healthcare providers to determine whether bacteria found in the specimen could be assumed to have come from the bladder and urethra rather than the perineal skin.

b. Open the antiseptic towelette provided in the prepackaged kit. If there is no kit, pour the antiseptic solution over the cotton balls.

c. To cleanse the perineum, wipe down one side of the meatus using one pad and discard it. Then wipe the other side with a second pad. Wipe down the center over the urinary meatus with the third pad; then discard it. Clean the perineal area at least twice. Use each towelette or cotton ball only once.
   Following the "clean-to-dirty" principle decreases the likelihood of contamination of the specimen with feces. Antiseptic helps reduce the number of bacteria. ➤

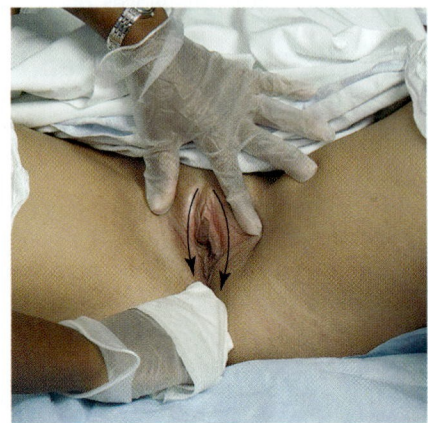

For Men

d. If the penis is uncircumcised, retract the foreskin from the end of the penis.
   Allows for better access when cleansing the area around the meatus.

e. Use the towelette provided in the prepackaged kit or pour antiseptic solution over cotton balls. You might also use 2 in. × 2 in. gauze pad soaked with povidone-iodine to cleanse the periurethral area.

➕ Before using an iodine-based solution, be sure to check the patient's health history for allergy to iodine.

f. With one hand, grasp the penis gently. With the other hand, cleanse the meatus in a circular motion from the meatus outward away from the urethral opening, and cleanse for a few inches down the shaft of the penis. Cleanse around the meatus at least twice,

using each towelette or cotton ball only once. Repeat the cleansing three times, each time with a fresh 2 in. × 2 in. gauze pad, towelette, or cotton ball.
   Cleansing the site in this manner helps prevent contaminating the specimen with bacteria.

4. **Remove gloves. Wash your hands,** and don the second pair of clean procedure gloves.
   Helps prevent transmission of bacteria when opening a sterile specimen container.

5. **Open the sterile specimen** container, being careful not to touch the inside of the lid or container.

6. **Holding the container** near the meatus, instruct the patient to begin voiding.

For Men

a. Keep the foreskin retracted during voiding, if uncircumcised. For a male patient who is unable to assist, it will be necessary to hold the penis.

For Women

b. Separate and hold the labia apart, or have the patient do so.
   To help keep bacteria from the foreskin (or labia) from contaminating the urine specimen.

7. **Allow a small stream of urine** to pass; and then without stopping the urine stream, place the specimen container into the stream, collecting approximately 30 to 60 mL.

(continued on next page)

Procedure 30–2 ■ Obtaining a Urine Specimen for Testing (continued)

8. **Remove the container** from the stream, and allow the patient to finish emptying the bladder. *Note:* For men, if the penis is uncircumcised, replace the foreskin over the glans when the procedure is finished.

9. **Carefully replace the container lid**, touching only the outside of the cap and container. Avoid touching the rim of the cup to the genital area. Do not get toilet paper, feces, pubic hair, menstrual blood, or anything else in the urine sample.

These measures maintain sterility of specimen and prevent cross-contamination of others with urine.

10. **Label the container** with the correct patient information (in many institutions, labels are preprinted or bar coded). Place the container in a facility-specific carrier (usually a plastic bag) for transport to the lab.

11. **Remove your gloves and wash** your hands. If the specimen has been obtained from a patient on a bedpan, leave your gloves on until

you have removed, emptied, and stored the bedpan properly.
Hand hygiene and gloving prevent transmission of bacteria.

12. **Assist the patient back to bed,** or remove the bedpan or urinal, if applicable. (See Procedure 29-2 for removing a bedpan.)

13. **Transport the specimen** to the lab in a timely manner.
Delayed testing can cause inaccurate results (e.g., casts in the urine will break up if urine is allowed to sit for an extended period of time).

Procedure 30–2B ■ Obtaining a Sterile Urine Specimen From a Catheter

➤ When performing the procedure, always identify your patient according to agency policy and be attentive to standard precautions, hand hygiene, patient safety and privacy, body mechanics, and documentation.

Procedure Steps

1. **Empty the drainage tube of urine.**

2. **Clamp the drainage tube** below the level of the specimen port for 15 to 30 minutes to allow a fresh sample to collect. If the client's urine is flowing briskly, you may not need to clamp the catheter.

3. **Don clean gloves**, and swab the specimen port with an antiseptic swab.

4. **Insert the needleless access device** with a 20- or 30-mL syringe into the specimen port, and aspirate

to withdraw the amount of urine you need.

5. **Once you have the sample**, transfer the specimen into a sterile specimen container.

6. **Discard the needleless access** device and syringe in a safe container.

7. **Tightly cap the specimen container.**

8. **Remove the clamp** from the catheter.

✚ Be sure to unclamp the tubing of the urinary collection bag after you obtain the sample.

Urine backflow can cause bladder distention and lead to stasis-induced UTI.

9. **Label and package the specimen** with the correct patient identification according to agency policy.

10. **Transport the specimen** to the lab. If immediate transport is not possible, refrigerate the sample.

✚ *Note:* Never disconnect the catheter from the drainage tube to obtain a sample. Interrupting the system creates a portal of entry for pathogens, thereby increasing the risk of contamination.

Procedure 30–2C ■ Collecting a 24-Hour Urine Specimen

➤ When performing the procedure, always identify your patient according to agency policy and be attentive to standard precautions, hand hygiene, patient safety and privacy, body mechanics, and documentation.

Procedure Steps

1. **Use a large collection container** (usually supplied by the lab), and collect all urine voided in the 24-hour period. If you need to use more than one container during the 24-hour period, use one container at a time. When it is full, collect your urine in the next container. Occasionally you will be asked to collect each voiding in a separate container.

2. **To begin collection,** have the client void, and record the time. Discard this first voiding.

3. **Collect all urine voided** during the next 24 hours (e.g., if the first voiding was at 9:00 a.m. on Monday,

collect all urine voided until 9:00 a.m. on Tuesday).

4. **Inform the client and all staff** about the collection.
Communication can help to prevent accidental discarding of urine.

5. **Post signs in prominent locations**, such as the client's bathroom or entry door, to remind staff of the ongoing collection.
It is essential to collect all urine voided during the 24-hour period in order for the test results to be accurate.

6. **Apply a label on the specimen**, with the patient's name, date, and time the test ended on your storage container.

? What if . . .

■ **A urine culture is ordered on the specimen?**

Be sure to list current antibiotic therapy on the laboratory request form.
This information is important to determine sensitivity of the microorganisms.

■ **A clean-catch urine sample is needed for an immobile patient?**

For the patient using a bedpan, raise the head of the bed to a semi-Fowler's position. Facilitates correct direction of urine flow down into the specimen container you are holding.
In addition, this is the anatomical position for voiding.

■ **The catheter drainage tube is made of rubber and has no sampling port?**

In that case, you can obtain the specimen directly from the rubber catheter. Be sure to properly cleanse the tubing with an antiseptic pad before inserting a needleless access device at a 45° angle. Withdraw the specimen. Put the sterile specimen into a sterile container; label it with the correct patient identification. Send it to the lab or put it on ice until it is transported.

✚ Never insert a needle into the shaft of the catheter because this can puncture the lumen and cause damage to the balloon holding the catheter in place.

Catheters made of materials other than rubber will leak after you take the needle out.

■ **You need to collect a urine sample from an infant?**

For infants and very young children, you will apply a special collection device over the genitals to collect the specimen.

1. Remove the paper covering adhesive patches on the back side of the specimen bag before applying it to the clean and dry perineal area. Start at the narrow area between the anus and vaginal or penile area. Press the adhesive sides firmly against the skin while avoiding wrinkles in the skin against the patch.
2. It is easier to apply the lower portion of the bag first. The area must also be dry in order for the adhesive to stick to the skin. Since infants urinate frequently, it is best to work quickly to catch the specimen.
3. After the specimen bag is adhering to skin, put a diaper on the infant/child. Remember to check the collection bag every 15 to 30 minutes to see if there is a specimen. If the infant has not urinated in 2 to 3 hours, discard the bag, re-cleanse the area, and apply a new bag.
   It is possible there was a leak in the seal between the skin and the adhesive sides of the specimen collection bag.
4. Once a specimen is obtained in the bag, remove it gently and pour the urine into a sterile specimen cup. Label it with the patient identifying information. ▼

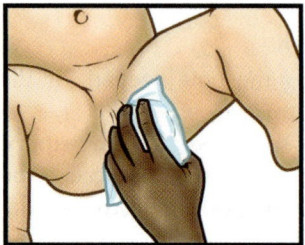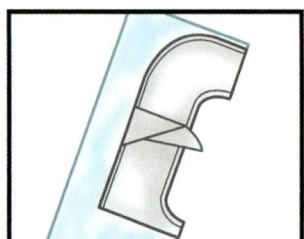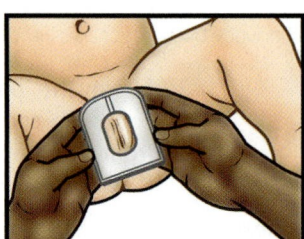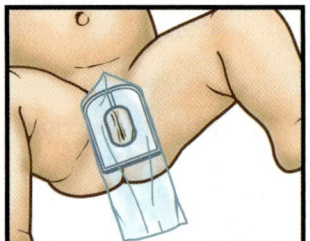

Evaluation

■ Note any unusual characteristics of the urine (e.g., color, odor, clarity, crystals, blood, mucus).
■ Note any difficulties with urination (e.g., pain, burning, dribbling, difficulty beginning).

Patient Teaching

■ Teach cognitively intact ambulatory patients to obtain a clean-catch specimen independently.
■ For clean-catch and 24-hour urine specimen collection, teach the patient the steps of the procedure, focusing on how to maintain sterility of the specimen.
■ Tell the patient to refrigerate a urine specimen for up to 24 hours until it can be transported to the lab. Instruct the patient to place the specimen in a plastic bag, separate it from food items, and label it appropriately.
■ Explain that prepackaged antiseptic wipes cannot be flushed down the toilet.
■ For clean-catch and 24-hour urine specimens, instruct a menstruating woman that perineal cleansing is especially important. The woman may use a tampon to prevent leakage during specimen collection. Instruct her to notify the lab that she is menstruating.

Documentation

■ Document urine volume and the time and date that the specimen was collected per agency protocol. Some facilities use a Kardex or flow sheet; others require documentation in nursing notes or electronic health records.
■ Document the characteristics of the urine: color, odor, particulate matter, blood, clarity, or other qualities.
■ Document any difficulty with voiding, including pain or burning with urination, frequency, or difficulty starting the urine flow.

Practice Resources

National Institutes of Health, Warren Grant Magnuson Clinical Center, 1999, last updated 2009; Saint Jude's Children's Research Hospital, 2004.

Procedure 30–3 ▪ Testing Urine at the Bedside

➤ For steps to follow in *all* procedures, refer to the Universal Steps for All Procedures found on the page facing the inside back cover.

Equipment

Dipstick Testing

- Procedure gloves
- Dipstick testing kit

Refractometer Testing

- Refractometer
- Procedure gloves
- Distilled water
- Dropper
- Small urine sample

Delegation

You may delegate bedside urine testing to the NAP if you know that he has the knowledge and skill to perform the procedure. Ask the NAP to report the test results to you and to save the urine sample in case you should need to repeat the test.

Pre-Procedure Assessments

- Mobility status

  Helps you determine where the specimen will be collected (e.g., toilet, bedside commode, bedpan).

- Urinary status

  Helps you to determine how the specimen will be collected (e.g., via catheter or commode).

Procedure 30–3A ▪ Dipstick Testing of Urine

➤ When performing the procedure, always identify your patient according to agency policy and be attentive to standard precautions, hand hygiene, patient safety and privacy, body mechanics, and documentation.

Procedure Steps

1. **Read the instructions** on the diagnostic kit and obtain the reagent and a test strip.
2. **Wash your hands** and don clean procedure gloves.
   Prevents the transmission of bacteria.
3. **Have the patient void** into the collection container or obtain urine from the indwelling urinary catheter. (See Procedures 30-1A and B for measuring urine.)
4. **Obtain a test strip from the kit**, dip it into the urine, and begin timing. Follow the manufacturer's directions regarding the time needed for the reagent to develop.
5. **At the specified time, compare** the results to the color chart. You will need good lighting to evaluate the results.
6. **Document the test results.**

Procedure 30–3B ▪ Measuring Specific Gravity of Urine

➤ When performing the procedure, always identify your patient according to agency policy and be attentive to standard precautions, hand hygiene, patient safety and privacy, body mechanics, and documentation.

Procedure Steps

1. **Clean the equipment lens** with distilled water and dry with dry lens paper or a soft, nonabrasive cloth.
2. **Before use, confirm** the refractometer calibration by testing with distilled water and commercial urinalysis controls (follow the manufacturer's instructions). When calibrated the refractometer should read 1.000.
3. **Wash your hands** and don clean procedure gloves.
   Prevents the transmission of bacteria.
4. **Use fresh urine**; if you cannot perform the test within 1 hour, refrigerate the specimen.
5. Wearing procedure gloves, use the dropper to place one or two drops of urine on the prism surface (at the notched bottom of the cover).
6. **Hold the refractometer horizontally**, and turn toward the light. Rotate the eyepiece until the scale is in focus.
7. **Read the scale at the point** where the dividing line between bright and dark fields crosses the scale. The scale reads from 1.000 to 1.035 in increments of 0.001.
8. **Record the results.**
9. **When you are finished**, dry the refractometer, and add a drop of distilled water to cleanse the prism. Dry the equipment with lens paper.

? What if . . .

- **The diagnostic kit is outdated?**

  Contact the pharmacy and/or work with the patient's caregiver to obtain a valid kit.

Evaluation

- Characteristics of urine output (e.g., volume of output, color, clots, mucus)
- Abnormally concentrated or dilute urine

Patient Teaching

- Explain test procedures to the patient and the patient's caregiver and family members as indicated.

Home Care

- Teach the patient or caregiver the steps of the procedure.
- Tell the patient or caregiver the urine must be tested within an hour or refrigerate the specimen to test later.
- Instruct the patient or caregiver that the specimen should be tested as ordered by the healthcare provider.
- Teach the patient or caregiver to record results on the flow sheet per agency protocol.

Documentation

- Document urine volume and the time and date that the specimen was collected per agency protocol (e.g., on a Kardex, checklist, or nursing notes).
- Document the urine specific gravity and pH and note the presence of hemoglobin, glucose, ketones, protein, white blood cells, bilirubin, casts, crystal, and nitrites.
- Chart other characteristics of the urine: color, odor, clarity, particulate matter, gross blood, mucous shreds, or other qualities.
- Document any difficulty with voiding, including pain or burning with urination, frequency, or difficulty starting the urine flow.

Practice Resources

Stuempfle & Drury, 2003.

Procedure 30–4 ■ Inserting a Urinary Catheter

➤ For steps to follow in *all* procedures, refer to the Universal Steps for All Procedures found on the page facing the inside back cover.

Equipment

Intermittent Urinary Catheter (Straight Catheter)

- Washcloth and towel
- Soap and water
- Procedure gloves, at least two pairs
- Catheter insertion kit containing:
  Sterile gloves
  Urinary catheter
  Antiseptic cleansing agent
  Forceps
  Cotton balls
  Sterile waterproof drapes
  Sterile lubricant
  Urine receptacle
  Specimen container
- Extra pair of sterile gloves and extra sterile catheter
  Obtaining extra supplies prevents the need to leave the bedside to obtain additional supplies should the gloves or catheter become contaminated.
- Bath blanket
- Procedure lamp or flashlight

- 2% lidocaine (Xylocaine) gel (according to agency policy and patient need) ▼

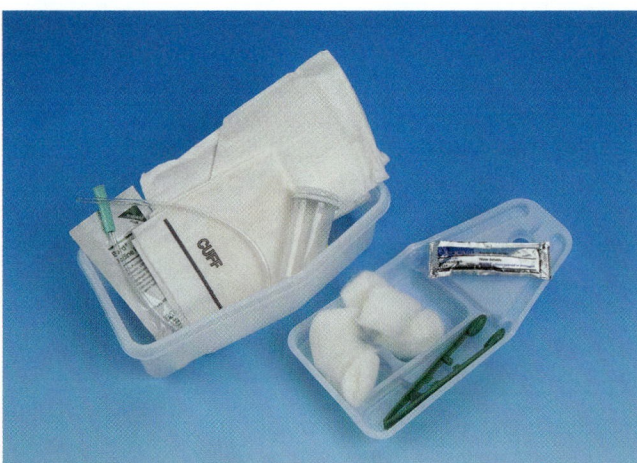

Indwelling Urinary Catheter

An indwelling catheter is designed to remain in the urinary bladder. Therefore, in addition to the supplies contained in a straight-catheter kit, an indwelling catheter kit will include the following:

- A double-lumen or triple-lumen catheter with a balloon tip for inflation instead of a single-lumen rubber catheter
- A syringe prefilled with sterile water (to inflate the catheter balloon)

(continued on next page)

Procedure 30–4 ■ Inserting a Urinary Catheter (continued)

- Urine collection bag with drainage tubing attached; often the tubing is also attached to the catheter
- Tube holder, tape, or leg strap (to secure the catheter)
- Safety pin and elastic band (if needed to secure the tubing to the bed; you can usually use the clamp on the drainage tubing) ▼

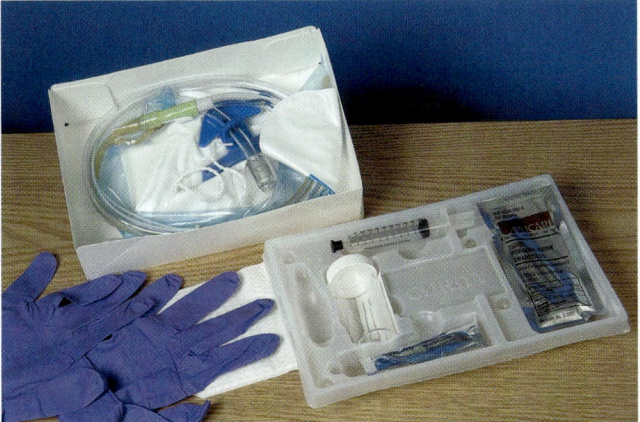

Delegation

In some institutions, NAPs undergo special training to learn this skill. In such instances, you may delegate this task to the NAP. However, you must complete the following assessments and instruct the NAP when to stop the procedure and what abnormal findings to report. Otherwise, you should not delegate catheter insertion to a NAP. If you do delegate to an NAP, you must from time to time supervise to ensure that the procedure is being performed correctly.

Pre-Procedure Assessments

- Assess the patient's cognitive level.
  To determine whether the patient will be able to follow instructions.
- Assess for conditions that may impair the patient's ability to assume the necessary position.
  To determine whether you will need assistance to help the patient maintain the correct position for catheter insertion.
- Assess the presence and degree of bladder distension.
  To establish a baseline against which to evaluate future data.
- Determine time of last voiding or last catheterization.
  To gain information you need to interpret the significance of the amount of urine obtained in this catheterization.
- Assess the general body size of the patient and size of the urinary meatus.
  To determine whether you need to choose a different size catheter.
- ✚ Determine whether the patient has an allergy to iodine (if that is the antiseptic solution in the kit). Use a different solution if the patient is allergic to Betadine.
- ✚ Determine whether the patient is allergic to latex.
  Many catheters are made of latex.
- Note signs and symptoms of bladder infection (e.g., elevated temperature, urinary frequency, dysuria).
- Note conditions (e.g., enlarged prostate in men) that may make it difficult to pass the catheter.
- Assess the need for extra lighting.
  It is sometimes difficult to visualize a woman's urinary meatus. Supplemental, direct lighting helps.

Procedure 30–4A ■ Inserting an Intermittent Urinary Catheter (Straight Catheter)

➤ When performing the procedure, always identify your patient according to agency policy and be attentive to standard precautions, hand hygiene, patient safety and privacy, body mechanics, and documentation.

➤ *Note:* The following steps are described for a female patient. For steps with an asterisk (*), if your patient is a male, refer to the Procedure Variations for Men list, immediately following the procedure steps.

Procedure Steps

*1. **Place the patient in a position** (usually supine) to allow you to see the urinary meatus:
  a. Flex the patient's knees, and place her feet flat on the bed (dorsal recumbent position).
  b. Instruct the patient to relax her thighs and allow them to rotate externally. If patient is confused, unable to follow directions, or unable to hold her legs in correct position, obtain help.
  The urinary meatus is sometimes difficult to visualize on women because it may resemble skinfolds or other anatomical landmarks in the area.

2. **If you are right-handed**, stand and work at the patient's right side;

if you are left-handed, stand and work on the patient's left side.

*3. **Drape the patient**. Fold the blanket in a diamond shape, wrapping the corners around the patient's legs and folding the upper corner down over the perineum. (To review draping, see Procedure 24-4: Providing Perineal Care, in Chapter 24.) ▼

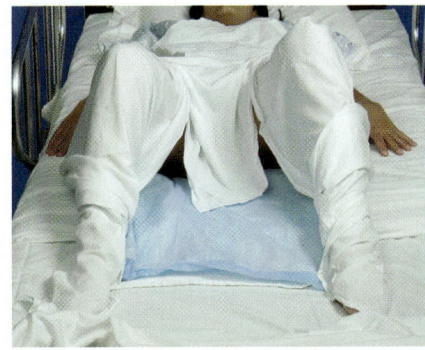

*4. **Don clean procedure gloves**. Lift the corner of the privacy drape to expose the perineum; wash the perineal area with soap and water; dry. At the same time, visualize and locate the urinary meatus.
  Cleansing the perineum before inserting the catheter will reduce the number of skin bacteria, thereby helping to prevent transmission of microorganisms into the bladder. Locating the meatus during this step, especially if the patient is a woman, will help prevent delays at subsequent steps when it is important to maintain sterile technique.

5. **Remove and discard gloves**. Wash your hands.
  Prevents transmission of microorganisms.

6. **Organize your work area.**
   a. Arrange the bedside table or overbed table within your reach.
   b. Open the sterile catheter kit according to directions, and place it on the bedside table.
   c. Position a biohazard bag or other trash receptacle so that you will not have to reach across the sterile field (between the patient's legs) to dispose of soiled cotton balls and so forth. For example, you may have a trash can on the floor beside the bed, or a trash bag on the bed near, but not between, the patient's feet. The outer wrapping of the catheter kit may be used for collecting discarded waste.
   Carrying contaminated objects above a sterile field can contaminate the field.
   d. Position the procedure light positioned to illuminate the perineum.
   To allow visualization of the site.

*7. **Apply sterile underpad** and drape. (*Note:* This step assumes the waterproof drape is packed as the top item in the kit. If your kit is different, see the What if . . . ? section.)
   These drapes provide sterile work surfaces and help prevent contaminating your gloves and sterile supplies.
   *a. Place the sterile underpad: Remove the underpad from the kit carefully, allowing it to fall open as you remove it. Do not touch other kit items. Place it flat on the bed, shiny side down, and tuck the top edge under the buttocks, taking care to touch only the corners of the drape.
   b. Lift the corner of the privacy drape to expose the perineum.
   c. Remove the sterile glove package, and don sterile gloves (see Procedure 22-7: Sterile Gloves, Open Method, in Chapter 22). *Note:* Once you have donned the sterile gloves, you may touch items inside the catheter kit, arranging the supplies as needed.

*d. Place the fenestrated drape: This has a hole in the center. Pick up the drape, allowing it to unfold as you remove it, without touching any other objects from the kit. For women, place the drape over the perineum with the hole over the labia (see photos in Steps 9 and 11).

*8. **Organize kit supplies** on the sterile field, and prepare the supplies in the kit.
   a. Pour antiseptic solution over the cotton balls.
   NOTE: Some kits contain a packet of sterile antiseptic swabs. Open the end of the packet where you feel the "stick," leaving the swab portions covered by the packet.
   b. Lay the forceps near the cotton balls.
   c. Open the specimen container if you are to collect a specimen.
   d. Remove any unneeded supplies, such as the urine specimen container, from the urine collection basin.
   e. Remove the plastic covering (if there is one) from the catheter.
   f. Open the packet or uncap the syringe filled with sterile lubricant.
   *g. Squeeze sterile lubricant into the kit tray; roll the catheter slowly in the lubricant. Lubricate the first 2.5 to 5 cm (1 to 2 in.) of the catheter. Leave the catheter tip in sterile lubricant or on the sterile field until ready to use.
   Lubrication allows for ease of insertion of the catheter. Prevents trauma to the mucosa.
   *h. Touching only the box or sterile side of the wrapping, place the sterile catheter kit down onto the sterile field between the woman's legs or bedside.
   This approach allows you to reach supplies during catheter insertion. It also extends the sterile field created by the sterile underpad.

*9. **Cleanse the urinary meatus.**
   *a. Place your nondominant hand above the labia, and with your thumb and forefinger spread the patient's labia, pulling up (or anteriorly) at the same time, to expose the urinary meatus. Hold this position throughout the procedure—firm pressure is necessary. If the labia slip back over the urinary meatus, it is considered contaminated, and you will need to repeat the cleansing procedure.
   When a woman is supine, gravity may cause tissues above the meatus to fall downward and obscure the meatus from sight. Once placed on the patient's perineal area, your hand is considered contaminated.
   *b. With your dominant hand, pick up a moistened cotton ball with the forceps and cleanse the perineal area, taking care not to contaminate your sterile glove.
   - Use one stroke and a new cotton ball for each area.
   - Wipe from front to back (clitoris to anus).
   - Wipe in this order: far labium majora, near labium majora, inside far labium, inside near labium, and directly down the center over the urinary meatus. If the kit has only three cotton balls, cleanse only the inside far labium minora, inside near labium minora, and down the center of the urethral meatus.
   - Discard the used cotton balls as you use them. Be careful not to move them across the open and sterile kit.
   Because the urethra is close to the anus in female patients, thorough cleansing of the perineum is essential to reduce contamination of the catheter and prevent bacteria from being introduced into the urethra. Following the "clean-to-dirty"

(continued on next page)

Procedure 30–4 ■ **Inserting a Urinary Catheter** (continued)

principle prevents recontamination of the cleansed area. ▼

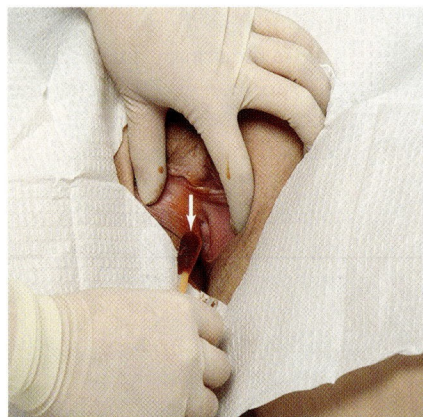

10. **Prepare the urine receptacle.** Place it 10 cm (4 in.) from the meatus (for women); between the patient's thighs (for men).
The end of the catheter will need to reach into the container to catch the draining urine.

*11. Insert the catheter. ▼

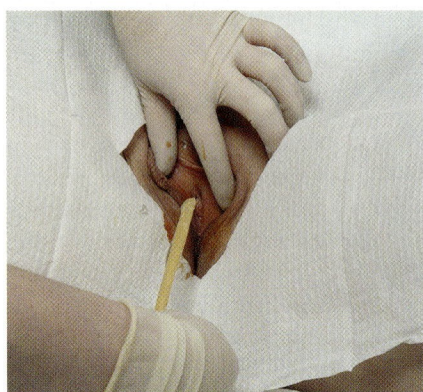

*a. Ask the woman to bear down as though she is trying to void. Grasp the catheter with your dominant hand, no more than 3 to 5 cm (1½ or 2 in.) from the distal end, holding it in a coil in your palm. Slowly insert the end of the catheter into the meatus. Ask the patient to take slow, deep breaths until the initial discomfort has passed.
Bearing down helps relax the external sphincter and makes

insertion easier and more comfortable. Holding the catheter close to the distal end will help to keep the tip stable and prevent it from being inserted into the vaginal opening.

*b. Continue inserting the catheter gently until urine flows, for a distance of 5 to 7.5 cm (2 to 3 in.). After you see urine, insert the catheter another 2.5 to 5 cm (1 to 2 in.).

✚ You may feel slight resistance as the catheter goes through the sphincters. Twist the catheter slightly or apply gentle pressure, but do not force the catheter while inserting it. You might need to remove it and cautiously attempt the insertion action again using a new catheter.

Deep breathing helps to relax the sphincters. Forcing may damage mucosa. Insert the catheter more deeply after urine flow to be sure the catheter is well into the bladder so that the bladder can empty completely. The catheter might not advance while inserted when it is misplaced in the vagina or if there is a stricture within the urethra or sphincter spasm.

c. If the catheter touches the labia or unsterile linens, or if you inadvertently place it in the vagina, it is contaminated; you must insert a new, sterile catheter. Leave the contaminated catheter in the vagina while you are inserting the new one into the meatus.
Leaving the catheter in the incorrect location helps to serve as a visual landmark and helps you to avoid making the same mistake again.

12. **Manage the catheter** and or/urine collection device.
a. Continue to hold the catheter securely with your nondominant hand while the urine drains from the bladder.

Prevents the catheter from being expelled by bladder or urethral contractions.

b. If you are to collect a urine specimen, use your dominant hand to take the specimen container and put it into the flow of urine until you obtain the correct amount of urine. Cap the container, maintaining sterile technique. See Procedure 30-2B.

c. When the flow of urine has ceased and the bladder has been emptied, pinch the catheter and slowly withdraw it from the meatus. Discard the catheter in an appropriate receptacle.
Withdrawing slowly promotes adequate urinary drainage, preventing urinary stasis. Pinching prevents urine from dribbling out of the end of the catheter.

d. Remove the urine-filled receptacle, and set it aside outside the patient care area to be emptied when the procedure is finished.
Moving the urine collection receptacle keeps it from spilling onto the bed.

13. **Cleanse the patient's perineal area** as needed; dry.
This removes residual antiseptic solution from the area, an especially important step if you used povidone-iodine (Betadine). Betadine left on intact healthy skin can cause irritation.

14. **Remove and discard** disposable supplies (e.g., drapes).

15. **Remove your gloves and wash your hands.**
Prevents transmission of bacteria.

16. **Return the patient to a position of comfort.**

Procedure Variations **for Men (Straight Catheter)**

Procedure Steps (above)	Nursing Action
1. Position the patient.	Position the patient supine, legs straight and slightly apart.
3. Drape the patient.	Cover the patient's upper body with a blanket; fold bed sheets down to expose the penis.
4. Wash the perineum.	Wash the penis and perineal area with soap and water; dry. If you are using 2% lidocaine (Xylocaine) gel, use a syringe (no needle) to insert it into the urethra now.
7a. Place the sterile underpad.	Drop the sterile underpad across the thighs.
7d. Place the fenestrated drape.	Place the fenestrated drape with the center hole over the penis. Lift the penis up and through the opening when cleansing the meatus.
8g. Lubricate the catheter.	Do not lubricate the catheter if you have already inserted a lubricant (lidocaine-based product) directly into the urethra.
8h. Place the kit on the sterile field.	Touching only the box or sterile side of the wrapping, place the sterile catheter kit down onto the sterile field at the bedside or on top of the thighs. You may, as an alternative, set up the sterile field between his legs.
9a(1) Expose the urinary meatus.	With your nondominant hand, reach through the opening in the fenestrated drape and grasp the penis, taking care not to contaminate the surrounding drape. If the penis is uncircumcised, retract the foreskin to fully expose the meatus. If the foreskin accidentally falls over meatus and does not remain retracted or if you drop the penis during cleansing, you must repeat the cleansing procedure.
9a(2) Cleanse the urinary meatus.	Continuing to hold the penis with your nondominant hand, hold the forceps in your dominant hand and pick up a cotton ball. Starting at the meatus, cleanse the glans in a series of circular motions and partially down the shaft of the penis. Repeat with at least one more cotton ball.
11a(1) Grasp the penis and the catheter.	Using your nondominant hand, hold the penis gently but firmly at a 90° angle to the body, exerting gentle traction. To gain firm control of the catheter, grasp the catheter 4–5 cm (1 1/2 to 2 in.) from the proximal end, with the remainder coiled in the palm of the hand. *Holding the penis at 90° and supporting the shaft with the fingers straightens the urethra, easing insertion of the catheter. Grasping the catheter close to the distal end of the catheter allows for control and helps to avoid inadvertent contamination.*
11a(2) Insert the lubricant.	If you have not inserted lidocaine gel into the urethra, make sure the kit contains a prefilled syringe of lubricant rather than a packet of lubricant. Gently insert the tip of the prefilled syringe into the urethra and instill the lubricant. *Lubricant in a Packet* If the kit contains only a single packet of lubricant and if no other kits are available, then lubricate 12.5 to 17.5 cm (5 to 7 in.) of the catheter. This is not the technique of choice, however.
11a&b Insert the catheter.	Ask patient to bear down as though trying to void; slowly insert the end of the catheter into the meatus. Have the patient take slow, deep breaths until the initial discomfort has passed. *Helps relax the external sphincter and makes insertion easier and more comfortable.* ✚ If you feel resistance, withdraw the catheter. Do not force against resistance. Continue inserting the catheter to about 17.5 to 22.5 cm (7 to 9 in.) or until urine flows. Continue to advance the catheter to the bifurcation (Y connector). Then lower the penis. When bladder is drained, replace the foreskin.

(continued on next page)

Procedure 30–4 ■ Inserting a Urinary Catheter (continued)

Procedure 30-4B ■ Inserting an Indwelling Urinary Catheter

➤ When performing the procedure, always identify your patient according to agency policy and be attentive to standard precautions, hand hygiene, patient safety and privacy, body mechanics, and documentation.

➤ *Note:* The following steps are described for a **male** patient. For steps with an asterisk (*), if your patient is a female, refer to the Procedure Variations for Women list, immediately following the procedure steps.

Procedure Steps

*1   **Place the patient supine** with legs straight and slightly apart. If the patient is confused, unable to follow directions, or unable to maintain correct position, obtain help with the procedure.
This position allows easy access.

2.   **If you are right-handed,** stand and work at the patient's right side; if you are left-handed, stand and work on the patient's left side.

*3.   **Drape the patient.** Cover the patient's upper body with a blanket; fold the bedsheets down to expose the penis.
Preserves modesty and enhances a feeling of security, while ensuring that you can expose the urinary meatus easily.

*4.   **Don clean procedure gloves.** Wash the penis and perineal area with soap and water; dry.
Cleansing the area reduces the risk of transmitting microbes into the bladder.

5.   **If you are using 2% Xylocaine** gel, use a syringe (no needle) to insert it into the urethra now.
This is frequently used for men to provide local anesthesia. You will need to wait at least 5 minutes for the gel to take effect before inserting the catheter.

6.   **Remove and discard gloves.** Wash your hands.
Helps prevent cross-contamination.

7.   **Organize your work area:**
   a. Arrange the bedside table or overbed table within your reach.
   b. Open the sterile catheter kit according to the directions, and place it on the bedside table.
   c. Position a plastic bag or other trash receptacle so that you will not have to reach across the sterile field to dispose of soiled cotton balls and so forth. For example, you may have a trash can on the floor beside the bed, or a trash bag on the bed near, but not between, the patient's feet, but not where you could trip on it. The outer wrapping of

the catheter kit may be used for collecting discarded waste.
Carrying contaminated objects above a sterile field can contaminate the field.

*8.   **Place the waterproof underpad** and sterile drape(s). (*Note:* This step assumes the waterproof drape is packed as the top item in the kit. If your kit is different, see the What if . . . ? section.)
These drapes provide sterile work surfaces and help prevent contaminating your gloves and sterile supplies.

   *a.   Remove the underpad from the kit carefully, allowing it to fall open as you remove it. Do not touch other kit items. Drop the underpad across the patient's thighs, touching only the corners.

   b.   Remove the sterile glove package and don sterile gloves (see Procedure 22-7, in Chapter 22).

   NOTE: Once you have donned the sterile gloves, you may touch any items inside the catheter kit, arranging the supplies as needed.

   *c.   Place the fenestrated drape: This has a hole in the center. Pick up the drape, allowing it to unfold as you remove it, without touching any other objects. Place the drape with the center hole over the penis.

*9.   **Organize the kit supplies** on the sterile field, and prepare the supplies in the kit.
   a. Pour antiseptic solution, such as Betadine, over the cotton balls. *Note:* Some kits contain a packet of sterile antiseptic swabs. Open the end of the packet where you can feel the "stick," leaving the swabs covered by the remainder of the packet.
   b. Lay the forceps near the cotton balls.
   c. Open the specimen container, if you are to collect a specimen.
   d. Remove any unneeded supplies, such as the specimen container,

from the kit. Remove the packaging from the catheter, if it is covered.

   *e.   Do not lubricate the catheter if you have already inserted a lubricant (Xylocaine gel) directly into the urethra. If you did not do that, be certain that the lubricant in the kit is packaged in a syringe rather than a packet.

   *f.   Touching only the box or sterile side of the wrapping, place the sterile catheter kit down onto the sterile field on top of the man's thighs. You may, as an alternative, set up the sterile field between his legs.
   Placement of supplies in this manner allows you to reach supplies during catheter insertion.

   g.   If the bedside bag is preconnected to the catheter itself, leave the bag on or near the sterile field until after the catheter is inserted.

*10.   **Cleanse the urinary meatus.** Discard the used cotton balls as you use them, taking care not to move them across the open and sterile kit.
Disposing of the used cotton balls reduces the risk for contaminating the sterile field. ▼

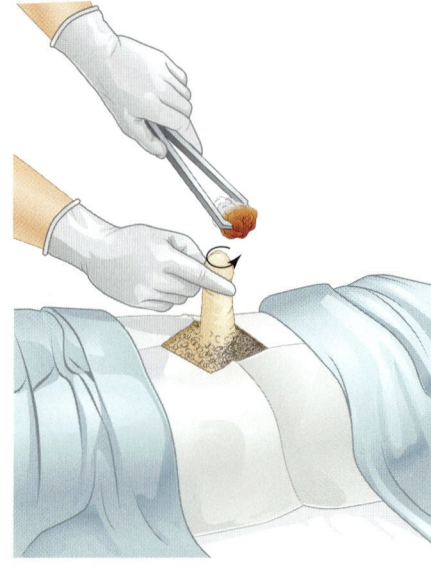

*a. With your nondominant hand, reach through the opening in the fenestrated drape and grasp the penis. Be careful not to contaminate the surrounding drape. If the penis is uncircumcised, retract the foreskin to fully expose the meatus. If the foreskin accidentally falls over the meatus or if you drop the penis during cleansing, you must repeat the cleansing procedure.
Retracting the foreskin allows for full cleansing of the area.

*b. Continuing to hold the penis with your nondominant hand, hold the forceps in your dominant hand and pick up a cotton ball. Starting at the meatus, cleanse the glans in a series of circular motions from the inside to the outside and partially down the shaft of the penis. Repeat with at least one more cotton ball. Discard cotton balls or swabs as they are used and do not move them across the open, sterile kit and field.
Following the "clean-to-dirty" principle prevents recontamination of the cleansed area.

c. Continue to grasp the penis with your nondominant hand. This glove is no longer sterile.

11. **Instill lubricant** (if not done previously).

Lubricant Packaged in a Syringe
Before beginning the procedure, you should have made sure that the catheter kit contains a prefilled syringe of lubricant rather than a packet. Gently insert the tip of the prefilled syringe into the urethra and instill the lubricant (unless you have already inserted Xylocaine gel).

Lubricant Packaged in a Packet
If the kit contains only a single packet of lubricant and if no other kits are available, then lubricate 12.5 to 17.7 cm (5 to 7 in.) of the catheter. This is not the technique of choice, however.

*12. **Insert the catheter.** ▼

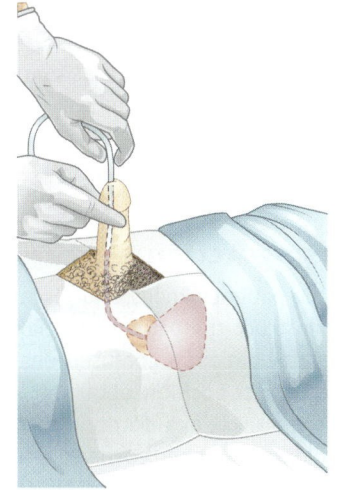

a. With your dominant hand, stabilize the catheter before inserting it by holding the catheter approximately 7.5 cm (3 in.) from the proximal end. Keep the rest of the catheter coiled in the palm of your hand or make sure the distal end of the catheter is connected to the drainage bag.
Coiling the catheter in your hand keeps you from contaminating the catheter. When you preconnect the drainage bag before you insert the catheter, you keep the urine from draining onto the bed. Frequently the catheter and drainage bag are connected by the manufacturer.

b. With your nondominant hand, hold the penis gently but firmly at a 90° angle to the body, exerting gentle traction.
Supporting the shaft with the fingers straightens the urethra, easing insertion of the catheter.

c. Ask the patient to bear down as though trying to void; slowly insert the end of the catheter into the meatus. Ask the patient to take slow deep breaths until the initial discomfort has passed.
These are strategies to help the patient to relax the external sphincter and make insertion easier and more comfortable.

d. Continue inserting the catheter to about 17 to 22.5 cm (7 to 9 in.) or until urine flows. You will feel slight resistance at the level of the external sphincter. Continue to advance to the bifurcation (Y connector).

➕ You will commonly feel resistance at the prostatic sphincter. Hold the catheter firmly against the sphincter until the sphincter relaxes. Then advance it, but do not force it.

e. Lower the penis and replace the foreskin.
This prevents compromised circulation and painful swelling.

13. **Manage the catheter.**

a. Continue to hold the catheter securely with your nondominant hand to stabilize the catheter's position in the urethra. Use your other hand to pick up the saline or sterile water-filled syringe and inflate the catheter balloon slowly.
Holding the catheter until the balloon is inflated reduces the chance of the catheter's being expelled by the bladder or urethral contractions. The inflated balloon prevents the catheter from slipping out of the bladder.

b. ➕ If the patient complains of pain on inflation of the balloon, withdraw the water from the balloon, and reposition the catheter by advancing it 1 inch (2.5 cm).

Pain usually indicates that the balloon was in the urethra instead of in the bladder.

14. **Connect the drainage bag** to the end of the catheter if it is not already preconnected. Hang the drainage bag on the side of the bed, below the level of the bladder.
Hanging the drainage bag below the bladder promotes adequate urinary drainage, preventing urinary stasis.

*15. **Using hypoallergenic** medical tape or a catheter strap, secure the catheter to the thigh or the abdomen.
Prevents urethral irritation related to tugging or pulling of the catheter.

(continued on next page)

Procedure 30–4 ■ Inserting a Urinary Catheter (continued)

16. Cleanse the patient's perineal area as needed; dry. Cover the patient with a gown.
Removes residual antiseptic solution from the area, an especially important step if you used povidone iodine (Betadine), which is not commonly used for this procedure. Betadine left on intact healthy skin can cause irritation.

17. Return the patient to a comfortable position.

18. Remove your gloves and discard them with supplies into biohazard receptacle. Wash your hands.

Procedure Variations for Women

Procedure Step (above)	Nursing Action
1. Position the patient.	Flex the patient's knees, and place her feet flat on the bed (dorsal recumbent position). Instruct the patient to relax her thighs and allow them to rotate externally. *Note:* If the patient is confused, unable to follow directions, or unable to hold her legs in the correct position, obtain help.
3. Drape the patient.	Fold the blanket in a diamond shape, wrapping the corners around the patient's legs and folding the upper corner down over the perineum (see Procedure 30-4A).
4. Wash the perineal area.	Don clean procedure gloves. Lift the corner of the privacy drape to expose the perineum; wash the perineal area with soap and water; dry. At the same time, visualize and locate the urinary meatus.
8a. Place the underpad and sterile drape.	(This step assumes the sterile underpad is packed as top item in the kit. If it is not, see the What If . . . ? section.) Remove the sterile underpad from the kit carefully before donning sterile gloves. Do not touch other kit items. Allow the underpad to fall open as you remove it from the kit. Place it flat on the bed shiny side down, and tuck the top edge under the buttocks, taking care to touch only the corners of the drape. Lift the corner of the privacy drape to expose the perineum.
8c. Place the fenestrated drape.	Pick up the drape, allowing it to unfold as you remove it, without touching any other objects. Place the drape over the perineum with the hole over the labia.
9e. Lubricate the catheter.	Squeeze sterile lubricant into the kit tray; roll the catheter slowly in the lubricant. Lubricate the first 2.5 to 5 cm (1 to 2 in.) of the catheter. Leave the catheter tip in sterile lubricant or on the sterile field until ready to use.
9f. Move the kit to the bed.	Touching only the box or sterile side of the wrapping, place the sterile catheter kit down onto the sterile field between the woman's legs.
10a. Spread the labia.	Place your nondominant hand above the labia, and with your thumb and forefinger spread the patient's labia, pulling up (or anteriorly) at the same time, to expose the urinary meatus. Hold this position throughout the procedure—firm pressure is necessary. If the labia slip back over the urinary meatus, it is considered contaminated, and you will need to repeat the cleansing procedure. *When a woman is supine, gravity may cause tissues above the meatus to fall downward and obscure the meatus from sight. Once placed on the patient's perineal area, your hand is considered contaminated.*
10b. Cleanse the perineal area.	With your dominant hand, pick up a wet cotton ball with the forceps and cleanse the perineal area, taking care not to contaminate your sterile glove. ■ Use one stroke and a new cotton ball for each area. Wipe from front to back (clitoris to anus). Wipe in this order: far labium majora, near labium majora, inside far labium, inside near labium, and directly down the center over the urinary meatus. ■ If the kit has only three cotton balls, cleanse only the inside far labium minora, inside near labium minora, and down the center of the urethral meatus. *Because the urethra is close to the anus in female patient, thorough cleaning of the perineum is essential to reduce contamination of the catheter and prevent it from it from being introduced into the urethra.*
12. Insert the catheter.	a. Ask the woman to bear down as though she is trying to void. Grasp the catheter no more than 11/2 or 2 in. (4 or 5 cm) from the distal end. Slowly insert the end of the catheter into the meatus. Ask the patient to take slow, deep breaths until the initial discomfort has passed. *Bearing down and deep breathing helps relax the external sphincter and makes insertion easier and more comfortable. Holding the catheter close to the distal end will help to keep the tip stable and prevent it from being inserted into the vaginal opening.*

b. Continue inserting the catheter gently until urine flows, for a distance of 5 to 7.5 cm (2 to 3 in.). After you see urine, insert the catheter another 2.5 to 5 cm (1 to 2 in.).

c. If the catheter touches the labia or unsterile linens, or if you inadvertently place it in the vagina, it is contaminated; you must insert a new, sterile catheter. Leave the contaminated catheter in the vagina while you are inserting the new one into the meatus.

Leaving the catheter in the incorrect location serves as a visual landmark and helps you to avoid making the same mistake again.

15. Secure the catheter.

Using a tape or catheter strap, secure the catheter to the thigh.

? What if . . .

- **The sterile gloves are packed as the top item in the catheter kit?**
  - Don sterile gloves: Remove the sterile glove package and don sterile gloves (see Procedure 22-7, in Chapter 22). *Note:* Once you have donned the sterile gloves, you may touch any item inside the catheter kit, arranging the supplies as needed.
  - Place the sterile underpad: Grasp the edges of the sterile drape. Fold the entire edge down 2.5 to 5 cm (1 to 2 in.) and toward you, making a "cuff" to protect your gloves. Take care not to touch unsterile objects with your gloves or the drape.
  For women: Carefully slide the drape under the patient's buttocks without contaminating your gloves. Ask the patient to raise her hips slightly if she can.

For men: Drop the sterile underpad across thighs.▾

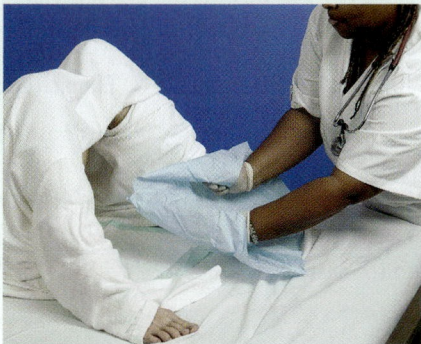

- Place the fenestrated drape: Pick up the drape, allowing it to unfold as you remove it, without touching any objects. Protect sterility as you did with the underpad (preceding step).
  For women: Place the fenestrated drape over the perineum so that the hole is over the labia.
  For men: Place the fenestrated drape so that the center hole is over the penis. You will pull the penis up and through the opening when cleansing the meatus.

- **A woman is unable to maintain a dorsal recumbent position?**
  Use Sims' position (side-lying with the upper leg flexed at the hip). Cover the rectal area.
  Prevents contamination from the rectal area to the urethra.

- **The patient is having a menstrual period?**
  Note on the lab form that the patient is having a menstrual period before sending a specimen for diagnostic testing.
  Blood in the urine from a menstrual period might lead to misinterpretation of the result.

Evaluation

- Note any difficulty with catheter insertion.
  This can indicate structural problems, especially in an older male patient with an enlarged prostate gland.
- Note the characteristics of the urine obtained (e.g., amount, color, odor, presence of sediment or mucus).
- Assess and palpate for absence of bladder distention. *Note:* Some facilities have a bladder-scanning device that will allow you to determine whether residual urine remains.
  Palpating the bladder helps you to determine if it has been emptied.
- For indwelling catheters, continue to assess that drainage is not obstructed and that the drainage bag is below the level of the bladder

Home Care

Indwelling Catheter

For inserting indwelling catheters in the home, teach clients:
- When to change the catheter
  Patients who are at higher risk for catheter blockage may need to change catheters more frequently than the usual 4-week period.
- How to prevent catheter blockage (e.g., increase fluid intake, use bladder irrigation)
  Fluids increase the urine volume, helping to reduce the deposit of sediment or other particles in the tubing.
- To empty the drainage bag frequently and to keep the bag below the level of the bladder
- How to prevent UTIs (e.g., use new silver/hydrogel-coated catheters, use clean technique when inserting catheter,

(continued on next page)

Procedure 30–4 ■ Inserting a Urinary Catheter (continued)

prevent blockage of urine outflow, avoid carbonated beverages)
- To take a shower rather than a bath to decrease the risk for UTIs
- How to prevent discomfort at the urethra
- Use of a leg bag
- To eat foods that help acidify the urine: meat, eggs, cheese, prunes, cranberries, and whole grains

Documentation

- Document the time and date of the procedure.
- Document the size of catheter used.
- Record the amount of urine obtained on the I&O portion of the graphics sheet. Record the color of urine, odor, presence of mucus, blood, and so on, in the nursing notes.
- Record the patient's subjective statements.
- Document if you collected a specimen, and note the time it was sent to the lab.
  For an indwelling catheter: In addition, some facilities require that you record the amount of saline used to inflate the balloon.

Practice Resources

Grabe, Bishop, Bjerklund-Johansen, et al., 2008; Gould, Umpshied, Agarwal, et al., and the Healthcare Infection Control Practices Advisory Committee (HICPAC), 2009; Joanna Briggs Institute, 2010; Lo, Nicolle, Classen, et al., 2008; Prevention of catheter-associated urinary tract infections, 2008; Ramakrishnan and Mold, 2005.

Thinking About the Procedure

 Go to the *Fundamentals of Nursing Skills Videos,* **Urinary Elimination: Catheterization: Male, Straight.**

1. When preparing equipment for inserting a straight catheter, what additional item might you bring with you? Why would this be a good idea?
2. What does the nurse do to help relax the patient before starting the procedure?

 Also go to the *Fundamentals of Nursing Skills Videos,* **Urinary Elimination: Catheterization: Female Indwelling, Inserting.**

1. How does the nurse position the patient when inserting a urinary catheter?
2. Is it necessary for the patient to be shaved before inserting the urinary catheter?
3. The nurse uses which hand to spread the urinary meatus?
4. What does the nurse do to make sure the catheter is secure?

 For suggested responses, go to Chapter 30, **Thinking About the Procedure Suggested Responses,** on Davis*Plus.*

Procedure 30–5 ■ Applying an External (Condom) Catheter

➤ For steps to follow in *all* procedures, refer to the Universal Steps for All Procedures found on the page facing the inside back cover.

Equipment

- Condom catheter
- Two pairs of clean procedure gloves
- Washcloth and towel
- Basin of soap and water
- Bath blanket
- Urine collection bag (e.g., bedside drainage bag or leg bag)
- Disposable tape measure
- Skin prep (per agency policy)
- Scissors
- Commercial leg strap

Delegation

You may delegate the application of a condom catheter to the NAP once you have assessed the NAP's skill level and completed the following assessments. Instruct the NAP to report any alterations in the skin integrity along the shaft of the penis.

Pre-Procedure Assessments

- Assess the patient's cognitive status.
  Knowing whether the patient can follow directions helps you to determine how to approach the procedure and also to know if the patient may be prone to pulling on the catheter.
- Assess pattern of voiding (e.g., degree, amount, and time of incontinence).
  Helps you to determine when the condom catheter should be applied.
- Assess the skin along the shaft of the penis, the glans, and the meatus (for swelling or excoriation).
  The condom catheter cannot be used on excoriated, irritated skin or over areas of impaired skin integrity.
- Note whether and how much the penis is retracted toward the body.
  There is an increased risk of nonadherence and leakage of urine in a patient with a retracted penis.
- Assess for neuropathy.
  Patients with neuropathies that affect sensation in the penis may not feel skin irritation from the condom catheter and will need to be assessed more frequently.

➤ When performing the procedure, always identify your patient according to agency policy, explain what you're going to do, and be attentive to standard precautions, hand hygiene, patient safety and privacy, body mechanics, and documentation.

Procedure Steps

1. **Don procedure gloves** and determine appropriate size of the external catheter by measuring the circumference of the penis using a disposable paper tape. Obtain a correctly sized catheter.

   A catheter that is too small impairs circulation. A catheter that is too large allows leakage of urine.

2. **Wash your hands** and don clean procedure gloves.

   Prevents the transmission of bacteria.

3. **Organize supplies** and prepare the leg bag or bedside drainage bag for attachment to the condom catheter by removing it from the packaging and placing the end of the connecting tubing near the perineal area.

4. **Place the patient supine.** If the patient has difficulty breathing, raise the head of the bed to 30°.

5. **Fold down the bedcovers** to expose the penis, and drape the patient using the bath blanket.

   Covering the patient reduces patient embarrassment.

6. **Gently cleanse the penis** with soap and water. Rinse and dry it thoroughly. If the patient is uncircumcised, retract the foreskin, cleanse the glans, and replace the foreskin. Excess hair along the shaft of the penis may be carefully clipped off with the scissors.

   Cleansing the penis helps to prevent infection and increases adherence of the condom catheter to the shaft.

7. **Wash your hands** and change procedure gloves.

8. **Apply skin prep** (if used by your agency), and allow it to dry. *Note:* Some external condom catheters require the placement of the special adhesive strip onto the penis before the application of the condom. Read the manufacturer's directions.

9. **Hold the penis** in your nondominant hand. With your dominant hand, place the condom catheter at the end of the penis, and slowly unroll it along the shaft toward the patient's body. Leave 2.5 to 5 cm (1 to 2 in.) between the end of the penis and the drainage tube on the catheter.

   Unrolling in this manner helps to prevent irritation of the glans due to rubbing and allows for expansion of the penis if an erection were to occur. ▼

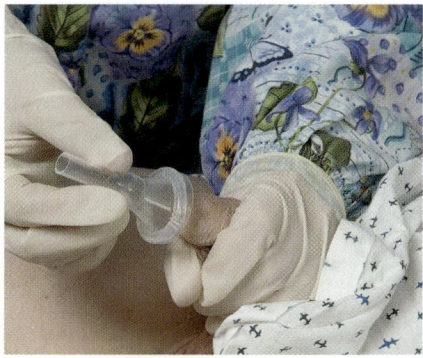

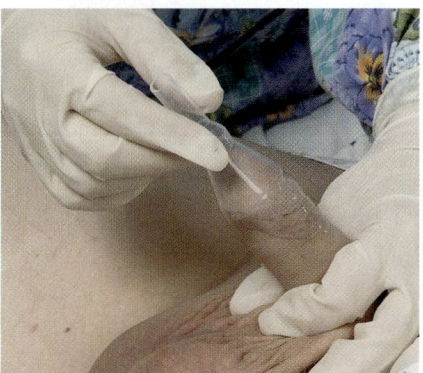

10. **Secure the condom** catheter in place on the penis.
    a. Ensure that the condom is not twisted.

       Twisting can obstruct urine flow.

    b. Do not use regular bandage or surgical dressing tape to hold an external condom catheter in place.

       Regular surgical dressing tape does not expand and could lead to decreased blood flow to the penis.

Catheter With Internal Adhesive

    c. Gently grasp the penis and compress so that the entire shaft comes in contact with the condom.

Catheter With External Adhesive Strip

    d. Wrap the strip around the outside of the condom in a spiral direction, taking care not to overlap the ends.

       Prevents constriction of blood flow to the penis.

11. **Assess the proximal end** of the condom catheter. If a large portion of the condom is still rolled above the adhesive strip, you may need to clip the roll.

    Clipping the roll helps prevent constriction of blood flow.

12. **Attach the tube end** of the condom catheter to a drainage system (e.g., a leg bag). Make sure there are no kinks in the tubing.

    Kinks impede the flow of urine. Urine that does not drain away from the meatus can cause irritation and skin breakdown and possibly cause the condom catheter to fall off.

13. **Secure the drainage tubing** to the patient's thigh using tape or a commercial leg strap (follow facility protocol).

    Controls movement of the tubing and accidental pulling on the condom catheter. ▼

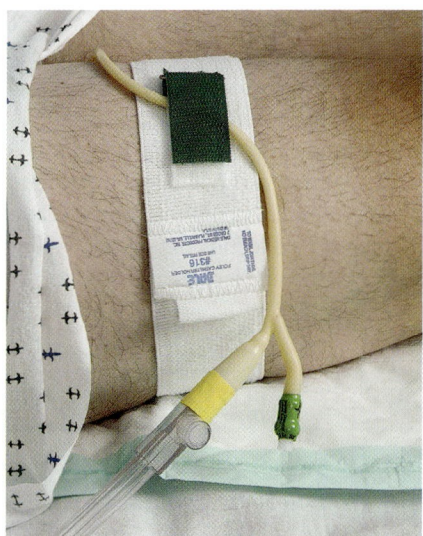

(continued on next page)

Procedure 30–5 ■ Applying an External (Condom) Catheter (continued)

14. **Cover the patient** and return him to a comfortable position. Raise the siderails and lower the bed.
15. **Remove your gloves and wash your hands.**
16. **Change the condom daily** or more often if needed.
    This helps to prevent UTI.

? What if . . .

- **The urine flow becomes obstructed?**

Check the catheter and collecting tube for kinking; readjust if needed. If that does not solve the problem, irrigate the tubing (see Procedure 30-7). Replace the catheter and tubing, if necessary.

Evaluation

Within 30 minutes of condom application, assess for:
- Urine flow (should not be obstructed)
- Swelling or discoloration of the penis
  Swelling or discoloration might indicate that the condom is too tight.

Monitor:
- The penis for circulatory changes
- Position and patency of the drainage tubing
- Characteristics of the urine (e.g., amount, color, odor, bleeding)
- Patient comfort
- Leakage of urine

Home Care

- Clients and caregivers should wash their hands before and after any manipulation of the penis or apparatus.
- Daily bag decontamination with a diluted (1:10) bleach solution has been found effective in reducing bacteria.
- Teach the client and caregiver to recognize the signs and symptoms of skin irritation and excoriation, as well as the symptoms of a UTI.
- Teach the client /caregiver to notify the care provider and discontinue use of the condom catheter if: skin irritation or swelling occurs; if the urine becomes thick and cloudy, pink or red; if the urine has mucus in it; if no urine has drained from the catheter in 6 to 8 hours.
- Change the external condom catheter every 24 hours. Use paper tape to secure the condom catheter to the inner thigh.
- Keep the collecting bag below the level of the bladder.
- Empty the urine collection device.

- Regularly empty the collection bag before it becomes completely full.
- Never allow the draining spigot to come in contact with the nonsterile collecting container.
- Disinfect the catheter–tubing junction before disconnecting them (if they must be disconnected).
- Avoid disconnecting the catheter and drainage tube unless the catheter must be irrigated.

Documentation

- Document the date and time of application of the external catheter in the nursing notes.
- Note any unusual findings in your assessment of the skin on the penis.
- Document characteristics of urine (e.g., color, odor, consistency, blood).

Practice Resources

Madigan & Neff, 2003; McConnell, 2001; Wong, 1981, updated 2005.

Thinking About the Procedure

 Go to the *Fundamentals of Nursing Skills Videos,* **Urinary Elimination: Catheter: External Condom.**

1. What does the nurse do prior to applying the condom catheter?
2. What type of adhesive for the condom catheter did the nurse use for the patient in the DVD?

 For suggested responses, go to Chapter 30, **Thinking About the Procedure Suggested Responses,** on DavisPlus.

Procedure 30–6 ■ Removing an Indwelling Catheter

➤ For steps to follow in *all* procedures, refer to the Universal Steps for All Procedures found on the page facing the inside back cover.

Equipment

- Syringe (5 to 30 mL, depending on balloon size)
- Towel or drape (and a towel as a receptacle for the catheter)
- Hygiene supplies (washcloth, warm water, towel)

Delegation

In some institutions, unlicensed NAPs undergo special training to learn this skill. In such instances, you may delegate this task to the NAP. However, you must complete the following assessments and instruct the NAP about what abnormal findings to report.

Pre-Procedure Assessments

- Assess the patient's cognitive level.
  Knowing whether the patient can follow directions helps you to determine how to approach the procedure and also to know if the patient may be prone to pulling on the catheter or your hands when you are removing the catheter.

■ Assess for conditions that may impair the patient's ability to assume the necessary position.
Knowing if there are physical limitations helps you to determine whether you will need assistance to help the patient maintain the correct position for catheter insertion

■ Assess the condition of bladder (e.g., distention), perineum, and meatus (e.g., color, swelling, crusting, drainage, lesion).
This information helps you to establish a baseline for later assessment.

➤ When performing the procedure, always identify your patient according to agency policy and be attentive to standard precautions, hand hygiene, patient safety and privacy, body mechanics, and documentation.

Procedure Steps

1. **Wash hands before and after** removing the catheter.
2. **Wear clean gloves** during the removal.
   Hand hygiene and gloving prevent transmission of bacteria.
3. **Explain that this procedure** is nearly always pain free.
4. **Instruct the patient** to assume a supine position (for males) or a dorsal recumbent position (for females).
5. **Place the catheter receptacle** near the patient (e.g., on the bed).
6. **For a woman, place a towel** or waterproof drape between the patient's legs and up by the urethral meatus. For a man, place the drape on his legs.
   These methods preserve modesty and a feeling of security and prevent soiling of the linens.
7. **Obtain a sterile specimen** (see Procedure 30-2B), if needed. Some agencies require a culture and sensitivity test of the urine when an indwelling catheter is removed.
8. **Remove the tape or device** securing the catheter to the patient.

9. **Deflate the balloon completely** by inserting a syringe into the balloon valve and allowing the balloon to self-deflate. Allow at least 30 seconds for the balloon to deflate. Verify that the total fluid volume has been removed by checking the balloon size written on the valve port.
10. **Ask the patient to relax** and take a few deep breaths as you slowly withdraw the catheter from the urethra.
    Deep breathing helps the patient to relax the sphincters.
11. **Wrap the catheter** in the towel or drape.
12. **Use warm water and a washcloth** to cleanse the perineal area. A mild soap may also be used. Be sure to rinse well if you use soap.
    Cleansing the perineum prevents transmission of bacteria. Soap is drying to the skin and mucosa.
13. **Measure the urine** and then empty it in the toilet; discard the catheter, drainage tube, and collection bag in the biohazard waste.
14. **Explain to the patient the need** to monitor the first few voidings

after catheter removal. If the patient toilets independently, place a receptacle in the toilet or bedside commode; ask him to notify the nurse when he voids and to save the urine.
15. **Remove and discard gloves;** wash hands.
16. **Record the date and time** of the procedure; the volume, color, and clarity of the urine; and your patient teaching.
17. **Return the patient to a position of comfort.**

? What if . . .

■ **You cannot aspirate all the fluid from the balloon?**

Do not pull on the catheter. Report to the charge nurse or the primary care provider before continuing the procedure.
Pulling on the catheter could cause injury to the urethra.

Evaluation

■ Observe for signs and symptoms of infection.
■ Observe the condition of the meatus.
■ After removing the catheter, monitor the next few voidings.
■ Assess the characteristics of the urine at the time the catheter is removed. Then note the time of the first voiding and the amount voided, and observe the urine for color, amount, odor, and presence of blood.
■ Compare voidings over the next 8 to 10 hours to the patient's intake.
■ Monitor for bladder distention.

Patient Teaching

■ Explain that you need to monitor the first few voidings after catheter removal to ensure that he does not have difficulty re-establishing bladder control.

■ Ask the patient to notify you when he voids and to save the urine (if the patient toilets independently)

Home Care

■ For patients who will have catheters at home, teach the family the steps for removing the catheter.
■ Teach the patient and caregiver to notify a healthcare provider if the client is unable to urinate within 8 hours after catheter removal, or if his abdomen becomes distended and painful.
■ Teach signs and symptoms of a UTI.
   Not everyone with a UTI develops recognizable signs and symptoms, but most people have some. Signs and symptoms of a UTI develop rapidly and can include a strong, persistent urge to urinate; a burning sensation when urinating; passing frequent, small amounts of urine; blood in the urine (hematuria); cloudy, strong-smelling urine; or bacteria in the urine.

(continued on next page)

Procedure 30–6 ■ Removing an Indwelling Catheter (continued)

- Increase fluid intake if not contraindicated by other health conditions.

- Caution the client never to remove a catheter unless trained by a healthcare provider. Remove the catheter only when prescribed by the provider.

Documentation

- Date and time the catheter was removed
- Amount of urine (on the I&O portion of the graphics sheet).
- Characteristics of urine (e.g., color, odor, cloudiness, turbidity, or blood).
- The time the specimen was sent to the lab
- The amount of fluid removed from balloon, client response to removal of the Foley catheter, urine in drainage bag, and notification of first void
- Any unusual findings in your assessment of the perineum
- How the patient tolerated the procedure
- Patient teaching

Practice Resources

Best practices: Evidence-based nursing procedures, 2008; Griffith & Fernandez, 2007, republished 2009; Madigan & Neff, 2003; Moore, Fader, & Getliffe, 2007; Wong & Hooton, 1981, updated 2005.

Thinking About the Procedure

 Go to the *Fundamentals of Nursing Skills Videos,* **Urinary Elimination: Catheterization: Female Indwelling, Removing.**

1. What does the nurse do that you would not do in real life with a patient?
2. Before removal, would the nurse tell the patient that removing the catheter is painful or pain-free?
3. Where would the nurse dispose of the catheter after removal?

For suggested responses, go to Chapter 30, **Thinking About the Procedure Suggested Responses,** on *DavisPlus.*

Procedure 30–7 ■ Irrigating the Bladder or Catheter

➤ For steps to follow in *all* procedures, refer to the Universal Steps for All Procedures found on the page facing the inside back cover.

Equipment

Intermittent Irrigation Through a Three-Way Catheter

- Bag of sterile irrigation solution
- Connecting tubing (to connect the bag to the irrigation port)
- IV pole
- Antiseptic swabs
- Bath blanket

Intermittent Irrigation via the Specimen Port Using a Syringe

- Sterile container
- Sterile 60-mL syringe with large-gauge needleless access device
- Two pairs of clean procedure gloves

Continuous Bladder Irrigation

- Three-way (or triple-lumen) indwelling catheter in place
- Sterile irrigation solution at room temperature
- Connecting tubing
- Antiseptic swabs
- IV pole
- Bath blanket
- Measuring container
- Pair of clean procedure gloves

Delegation

Irrigation of an indwelling catheter requires nursing assessment and clinical decision-making. Because of the high potential for UTI, you should not delegate this procedure to the NAP. Bladder/catheter irrigation may be delegated with supervision to qualified LPNs who are trained in the procedure.

Pre-Procedure Assessments

- Note the characteristics of the urine (e.g., amount, color, odor, presence of clots or mucus).
- Assess for the presence and degree of bladder distension.
  This information helps you to establish a baseline for assessment.
- Note patient complaints of discomfort.
- Assess the patient's cognitive status.
  Helps you determine whether the patient can follow directions and remain still during the procedure.
- Check the chart for the amount and type of sterile solution to use.
- Determine whether the irrigant is to remain in the bladder for any length of time.

Procedure 30-7A ■ Intermittent Bladder or Catheter Irrigation

➤ When performing the procedure, always identify your patient according to agency policy and be attentive to standard precautions, hand hygiene, patient safety and privacy, body mechanics, and documentation.

✚ *Note:* This is the procedure for the closed methods of irrigation. The "open" method is no longer recommended. Because of the risk for infection, you should never disconnect the drainage tubing from the catheter.

Procedure Steps

Procedure Variation Three-Way (Triple-Lumen) Indwelling Catheter

1. **Before starting bladder irrigation**, prepare the connection tubing and irrigation solution warmed to room temperature.
   a. Close the clamp on the connection tubing.
   b. Spike the tubing into the appropriate port on the irrigation solution bag, using aseptic technique.
   c. Invert the solution and hang it on an IV pole.
   d. Remove the protective cap from the distal end of the connection tubing. Hold the end of the tubing over the sink or trash receptacle. Open the roller clamp, and allow the solution to fill the tubing. Be sure to keep the end sterile.
   e. Reclamp the roller on the tubing to stop the flow of irrigation solution.
   f. Recap the tubing.
2. **Don procedure gloves.**
   Helps prevent transfer of microorganisms.
3. **Position the patient supine.**
4. **Drape the patient** so he is not exposed and only the connection port on the indwelling catheter is visible.
5. **Before beginning the flow** of irrigation solution, empty any urine that is in the drainage bag, and wash your hands. Then document the volume on the I&O record.
   Starting the procedure with an empty draining bag gives you a baseline for correct calculation of true urine output

during irrigation. I&O provides data for evaluating fluid balance and urinary system function.
6. **Cleanse the catheter port** with antiseptic solution.
   To remove microorganisms and help prevent UTI.
7. **Connect the irrigation tubing** to the catheter port.
8. **Slowly open the roller clamp** on the irrigation tubing to the desired flow rate.
   Slow instillation prevents patient discomfort.
9. **Instill or irrigate** with the prescribed amount of irrigant. If the irrigant is to remain in the bladder for a prescribed time period, clamp the drainage tubing for that time.
10. **When the correct amount** of irrigant has been used and/or the goals of the irrigation have been met, close the roller clamp on the irrigation tubing, leaving the tubing connected to the catheter for use during the next irrigation.
    You can assess whether the goals of irrigation have been met by inspecting the color of the urine and assessing for presence of clots, mucus, or blood. Clamping the drainage tubing prevents immediate outflow.
11. **Remove gloves, wash your hands**, and return the patient to a position of comfort.

Procedure Variation Two-Way Indwelling Catheter

12. **Don clean procedure gloves**. Empty any urine currently found in the bedside drainage bag.
    Emptying the bag will ensure accurate output results.
13. **Wash your hands** and then apply clean gloves.
    Handwashing and gloving prevent the transmission of microorganisms.
14. **Drape the patient** so that only the specimen removal port on the

drainage tubing is exposed. Place a sterile waterproof drape beneath the exposed port.
    Draping ensures patient privacy and prevents soiling of the bed linens.
15. **Open the sterile irrigation** supplies. Pour approximately 100 mL of the irrigating solution, warmed to room temperature, into the sterile container, using aseptic technique.
    Warm solution is more comfortable to the patient. Aseptic technique helps prevent UTI.
16. **Scrub all surfaces** of the specimen removal port with antiseptic swab.
    Cleaning the port reduces the risk of transmission of pathogens into the bladder.
17. **Draw up irrigation solution** into the syringe. Connect the syringe to the specimen port. For catheter irrigation, use a total of 30 to 40 mL; for bladder irrigation, the amount is usually 100 to 200 mL).
18. **Clamp or pinch the drainage** tubing distal to the specimen port.
    Clamping prevents irrigant from draining into the drainage bag instead of into the catheter and/or bladder.
19. **Inject the solution into the port**. Hold the specimen port slightly above the level of the bladder. If you meet resistance, have the patient turn slightly, and attempt a second time. If resistance continues, stop the procedure and notify the primary care provider.
    Holding the port above the level of the bladder enhances gravitational flow of irrigant into the bladder. Resistance might indicate trauma to the mucosa tissue or surgical site. ▼

(continued on next page)

Procedure 30–7 ■ **Irrigating the Bladder or Catheter** (continued)

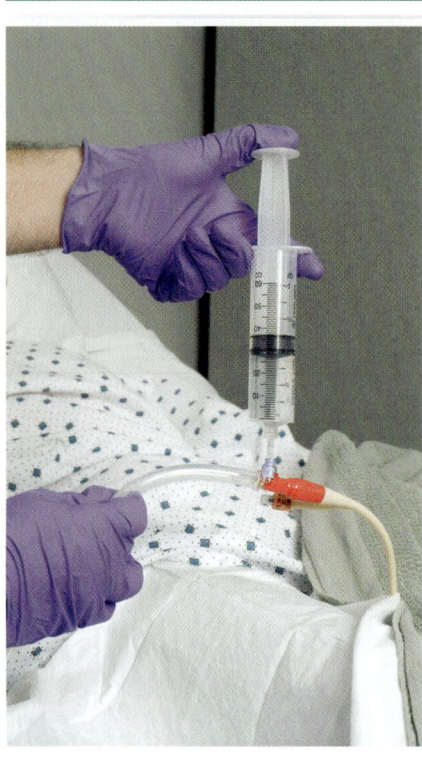

20. **When the irrigant has been** injected, remove syringe. Refill the syringe if necessary.

21. **Unclamp or release the drainage** tubing, and allow the irrigant and urine to flow into the bedside drainage bag by gravity. (If the solution is to remain in the bladder for a prescribed time, leave the tubing clamped for that time period.)

22. **Repeat the procedure** as necessary until the prescribed amount has been instilled or until the goal of the irrigation is met (e.g., removal of clots and mucus, free-flowing urine).

23. **Remove gloves, wash your hands,** and return the patient to a position of comfort.

Procedure 30-7B ■ **Continuous Bladder Irrigation**

> ➤ When performing the procedure, always identify your patient according to agency policy and be attentive to standard precautions, hand hygiene, patient safety and privacy, body mechanics, and documentation.

Procedure Steps

1. **If one is not already present,** insert a three-way (triple-lumen) indwelling catheter.

    A triple-lumen catheter provides an access for the irrigation solution without disrupting the sterile drainage unit.

2. **Prepare the irrigation fluid** and tubing:

    a. Roll the clamp on the connecting tubing to the "closed" position.

    Prevents air from filling the tubing.

    b. Spike the tubing into the portal on the irrigation solution container, using aseptic technique.

    Prevents introduction of microorganisms into the solution.

    c. Invert the container, and hang it on the IV pole.

    Elevating the bag allows the solution to flow by gravity.

    d. Remove the protective cap from the distal end of the connecting tubing. Hold the end of the tubing

over a sink or other receptacle. Open the roll clamp slowly, and allow the solution to fill the tubing completely. Recap the tubing.

    Priming the tubing flushes air from tubing, preventing bladder distension.

3. **Perform hand hygiene** and don clean procedure gloves.

    These two actions prevent the spread of microorganisms.

4. **Place the patient supine** and drape her so that only the connection port on the indwelling catheter is visible.

    Draping prevents exposure of the genital area and protects patient privacy.

5. **Place a waterproof barrier** drape under the irrigation port. If the irrigation kit comes with a sterile drape, use that. Pinching the tubing and using aseptic technique, connect the end of the irrigation infusion tubing to the side port of the catheter.

6. **Before beginning the flow** of irrigation solution, empty any urine that is in the bedside drainage bag, and document the volume on the I&O record.

    Starting the procedure with an empty bag gives you a baseline for correct calculation of true urine output during irrigation. I&O record provides data for evaluating urinary status.

7. **Remove your gloves** and wash your hands.

    Gloving prevents the transmission of microorganisms.

8. **Cover the patient,** and return him to a position of comfort.

9. **Open the roller clamp** on the tubing, and regulate the flow of the irrigation solution to meet the desired outcome for the irrigation.

    The goal of continuous bladder irrigation for patients who have had a transurethral resection of the prostate is to keep the urine light pink to clear. ➤

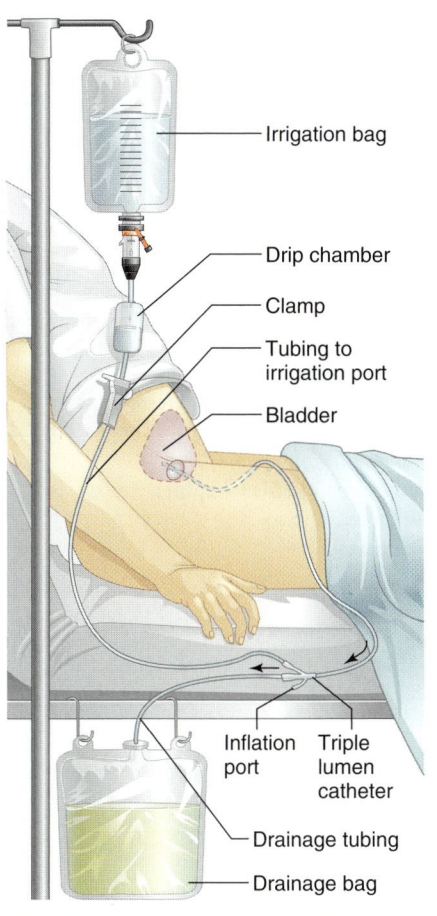

Irrigation bag

Drip chamber

Clamp

Tubing to irrigation port

Bladder

Inflation port

Triple lumen catheter

Drainage tubing

Drainage bag

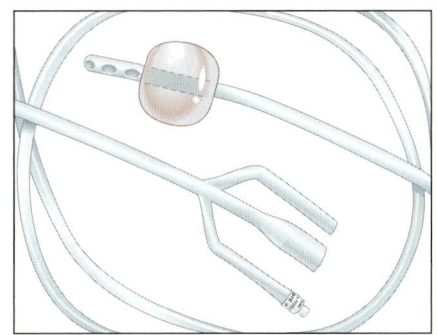

10. Monitor the flow rate for 1 to 2 minutes to ensure accuracy.

Infusing irrigation fluid for a minute or two prevents rapid introduction of solution into the bladder, which would cause patient discomfort.

? What if . . .

- **The draining irrigant solution and/or urine appears to have red blood cells in it?**

Stop the irrigation and report to the primary care provider.

Signs of increased red cells in urine may indicate bladder irritation and possible destruction of the inner mucosal lining of the bladder.

Evaluation

- Note the flow rate of irrigant and/or inability to instill irrigant into the catheter.
- Note the characteristics of urine output (e.g., presence of output, color, amount, clots, mucus).
- Note patient report of discomfort (e.g., pain, spasms).
- Assess for development of bladder distention accompanied by lack of urine outflow.

Home Care

For patients who will have continuous bladder irrigation at home, you will need to teach the family the necessary steps of the procedure. Also teach them to:

- Empty the urine collection device before beginning the procedure.
- Utilize strict aseptic technique when irrigating the bladder or catheter, and not disconnect the catheter and drainage tube.
- Irrigate the catheter using the closed method, which carries the least risk for introducing bacteria into the bladder.

- Identify signs and symptoms of urinary retention and UTI.
- Wash their hands before and after any manipulation of the catheter site or apparatus.
- Be certain to maintain unobstructed flow.
- For the syringe method, the patient will need access to syringes and needleless access devices and a process to dispose of them properly.

Documentation

- Date and time of procedure, the type of irrigant, and the total volume infused.
- Characteristics of the urine (e.g., color, odor, clarity, sediment, presence of clots or mucus).
- Evidence of catheter patency (e.g., flow of urine, absence of distension).

Practice Resources

Jahn, Preuss, Kernig, et al., 2007; Sinclair, Cross Hagen, et al., 2006, amended 2009; Wong & Hooton, 1981, last modified 2005.

(continued on next page)

Procedure 30–7 ■ Irrigating the Bladder or Catheter (continued)

Thinking About the Procedure

 Go to the *Fundamentals of Nursing Skills Videos,* **Urinary Elimination: Bladder Irrigation, Intermittent Two-Way.**

1. What does the nurse do after draining the urine out of the drainage collection bag?
2. What size syringe does the nurse use to draw up the irrigation solution?
3. What do you notice different about the urine before and after the bladder irrigation procedure?

 Go to the *Fundamentals of Nursing Skills Videos,* **Urinary Elimination: Bladder Irrigation, Intermittent Three-Way.**

1. What does the nurse do with the clamp if the irrigation solution is not to remain in the bladder?

 For suggested responses, go to Chapter 30, **Thinking About the Procedure Suggested Responses,** on Davis*Plus.*

 To explore learning resources for this chapter,

 Go to Davis*Plus* at http://www.Davisplus.fadavis.com, keyword Treas.

Chapter Resources for Chapter 30:
   Knowledge Check and Think Like a Nurse Response Sheets
   Knowledge Check Answers
   Resources for Caregivers and Health Professionals
   Reading More About Urinary Elimination (Suggested Readings)
   What Are the Main Points in This Chapter?
NCLEX-Style Review Questions
Chapter Overview Podcasts

Concept Map

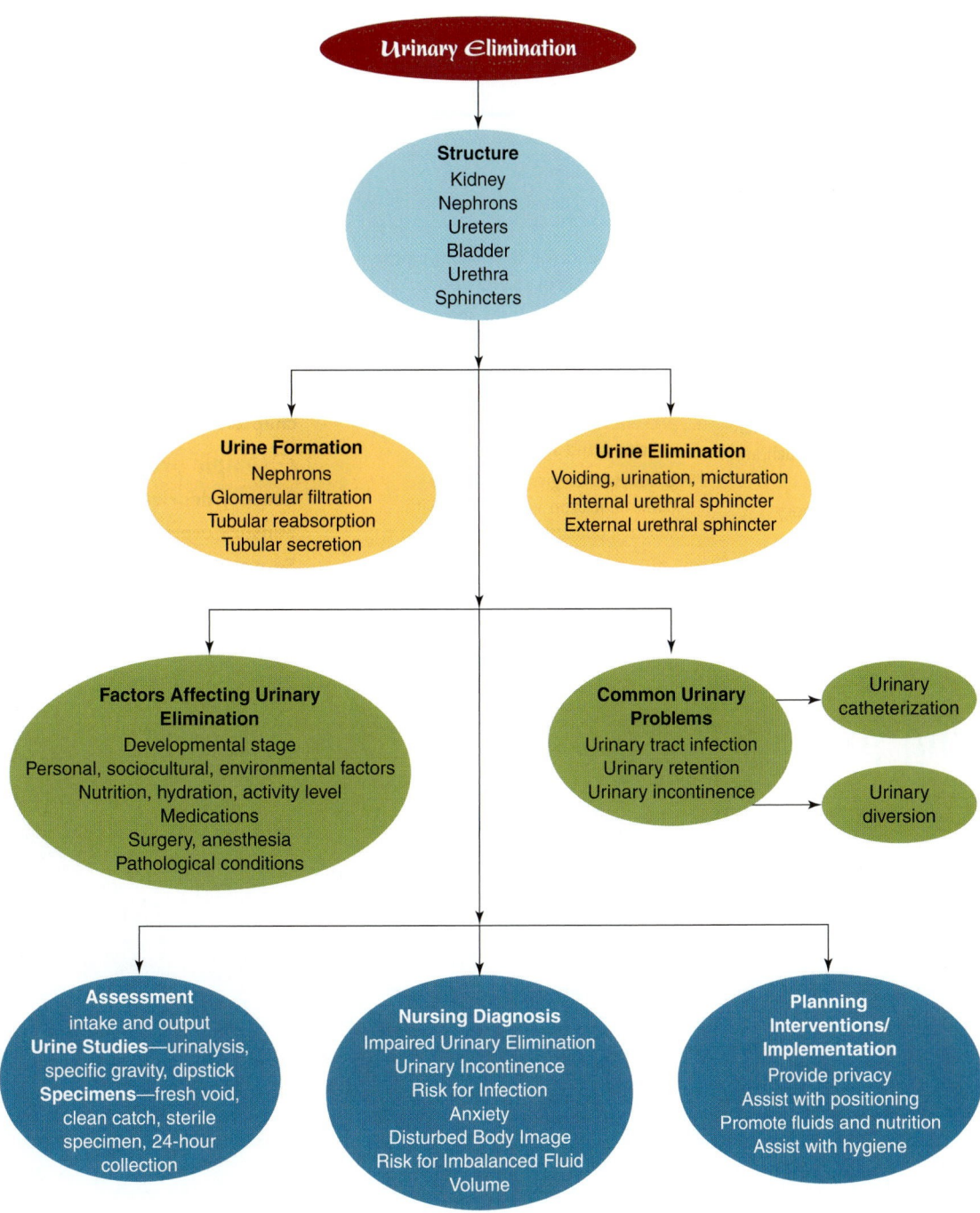

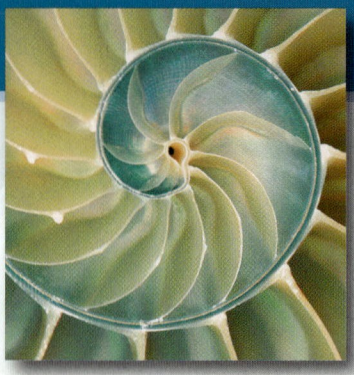

CHAPTER 31

Sensory Perception

Learning Outcomes

After completing this chapter, you should be able to:

➤ Identify the components of the sensory experience.

➤ Compare and contrast sensory deprivation and sensory overload.

➤ List factors placing clients at risk for altered sensory perception.

➤ Discuss the hazards of sensory deficits in vision, hearing, taste, smell, touch, and proprioception.

➤ Identify factors that affect sensory stimulation.

➤ Assess clients for signs and symptoms of altered sensory perception.

➤ State nursing diagnoses and outcomes appropriate for clients with problems of sensory perception.

➤ Describe nursing interventions to prevent sensory deprivation, sensory overload, and sensory deficits.

➤ Discuss strategies to enhance communication with clients with sensory deficits.

Key Concepts

Perception

Reception

Sensation

Related Concepts

See the Concept Map at the end of this chapter.

Example problems

Sensory deprivation

Sensory overload

Sensory deficits

Caring for the Nguyens

This feature allows you to practice the kind of thinking you will use as a full-spectrum nurse. There is usually more than one correct answer to a critical thinking question, so we do not provide answers for these features. It is more important to develop your nursing judgment than to "cover content." Discuss the questions with your peers. If you are still unsure, consult your instructor.

Mai Nguyen, Nam Nguyen's mother, has been experiencing blurred vision. At a recent ophthalmology appointment, she was told she has bilateral cataracts that will require surgical removal. She reports to the primary care clinic today, accompanied by Nam. Mai tells you, "I don't know what happened. I was pulling into a parking space at the grocery store, and the next thing you know, I hear this loud boom. I don't know how I did it, but I hit the car next to me. I just didn't see it."

Nam is very concerned and questions whether his mother should be allowed to drive. Mai is visibly upset. "I don't want to hurt anyone, but I don't want to lose all my freedom." Nam insisted on this appointment to discuss his concerns.

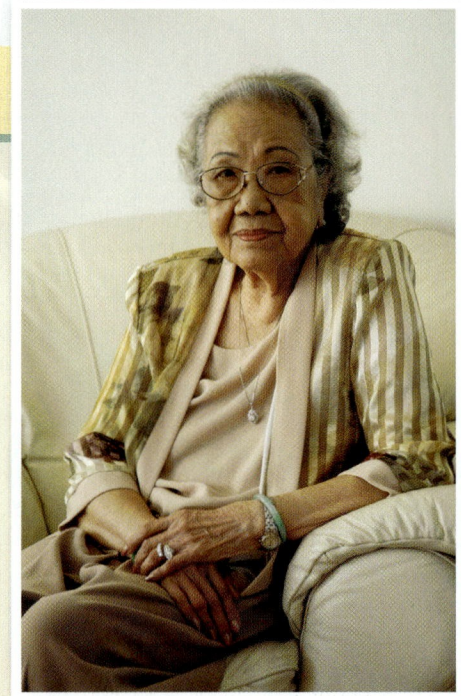

Caring for the Nguyens (continued)

A. What data will you need to gather from Mai and Nam?

B. What assessments will you need to perform?

C. How will cataract surgery most likely affect Mai? You will need to learn about the surgery and recovery to answer this question. Use a textbook, or, for a list of helpful Web sites you can access,

 Go to Chapter 31, **Resources for Caregivers and Healthcare Professionals**, on Davis*Plus*.

D. What information would you offer to Mai and Nam?

 Go to **Caring for the Nguyens Response Sheet** on Davis*Plus*.

Meet Your Patients

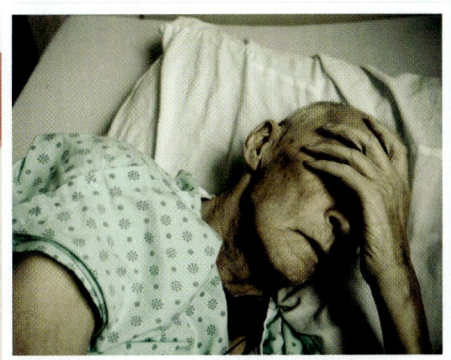

■ Joshua is a 28-year-old patient in the intensive care unit (ICU). He had a car accident 3 weeks ago and has had several surgeries to repair a fractured femur, ruptured spleen, and intracranial bleeding. He was ventilated mechanically for 10 days and has had numerous invasive procedures. The nurses report that he is very confused and has been hallucinating.

■ Richard is a 90-year-old man who has been a resident at a skilled nursing facility for 10 years. He has no visitors, never leaves his room, has no television or radio in the room, and no longer speaks. He does not respond to verbal or tactile stimulation. He lies in bed in a fetal position. When staff members try to move him, he moans and howls.

Consider how these patients are similar and how their care might overlap. It seems hard to imagine that these patients could have much in common. What similarities can you see? What differences? After you read this chapter, see if you answer these questions the same.

Theoretical Knowledge
knowing **why**

We experience the world through our senses. Vision, hearing, smell, taste, touch, and our sense of our body in space all help us to interpret and interact with our environment in a meaningful way. To grow, develop, and function, we must be able to sense and respond to sensory input.

Many patients who are being treated for one condition also have a preexisting sensory deficit (e.g., a diabetic client whom you are teaching self-injection may also be blind). Others develop alterations in sensory function as a result of their illness or of medications they are taking. The Joint Commission (2008) requires that you address the communication needs of patients with vision, speech, hearing, language, and cognitive impairments. This chapter will help you provide care for such patients.

ABOUT THE KEY CONCEPTS

Throughout your nursing career, you will care for patients with altered sensory function. To best meet their patient care needs, you will need to understand how the concepts of sensation, reception, and perception influence their sensory experience. In this section you will also learn about related concepts, including those needed to care for patients who experience sensory deprivation, overload, or deficits.

COMPONENTS OF THE SENSORY EXPERIENCE

The purpose of sensation is to allow the body to respond to changing situations and maintain homeostasis. A sensory experience involves four components in the nervous system: stimulus, reception, perception, and an arousal mechanism. A **stimulus** may be a sight, sound, taste, touch, pain, or anything that stimulates a nerve receptor. The brain must receive and process it to make it meaningful.

Reception

Reception is the process of receiving stimuli from nerve endings in the skin and inside the body. A receptor converts a stimulus to a nerve impulse and transmits the impulse along sensory neurons to the central nervous system (CNS). Some receptors remain activated for as long as the stimulus is applied. However, most receptors *adapt* to stimuli; that is, their response declines with time. Adaptation explains why, over time, you become unaware of an unpleasant smell or the persistent hum of an air conditioner.

Receptors usually respond to only one type of stimulus. For example, taste buds in the mouth detect sweet, sour, salty, or

bitter, whereas receptors in the retina detect light rays. The following are examples of the many types of sensory receptors in the body:

- *Mechanoreceptors* in the skin and hair follicles detect touch, pressure, and vibration.
- *Hair cells* are receptors for hearing. Located in the cochlea of the ear, they detect sound waves. In the vestibular apparatus of the ear, receptors for equilibrium and balance also detect acceleration of the body and position of the head.
- *Thermoreceptors* in the skin detect variations in temperature.
- *Proprioceptors* in the skin, muscles, tendons, ligaments, and joint capsules coordinate input to enable us to sense the position of our body in space (proprioception).
- *Photoreceptors* located in the retina of the eyes detect visible light.
- *Chemoreceptors* for taste are located in our taste buds. *Olfactory receptors* (chemoreceptors for smell) are located in the epithelium of the nasal cavity.

Perception

Perception is the ability to interpret the impulses transmitted from the receptors and give meaning to the stimuli. After the receptors generate nerve impulses, the impulses travel along neural pathways to the spinal cord and brain. They are then relayed to specialized locations in the brain where perception and awareness of the stimuli occurs (Fig. 31-1). For example, vision is perceived in the occipital lobes, hearing in the temporal lobes, and touch in the somatosensory area. Perception requires functioning of the sensory receptors, the reticular activating system, neural pathways, and brain.

It would not be possible to process all the stimuli that constantly bombard us. The brain discards about 99% of all sensory information as irrelevant and unimportant. For example, you are usually unaware of your clothing touching your body. However, if you focus on it, you can feel it. Perception of a stimulus is affected by past experiences, knowledge, and attitude, as well as the factors:

- *Location* of the receptors and pathway activated
- *Number* of receptors activated
- *Frequency* of action potentials generated (which varies according to the intensity of the stimulus)
- *Changes* in location, number, and frequency

Arousal Mechanism

For the central nervous system to perceive, interpret, and react to incoming stimuli, it must be active. The **reticular activating system (RAS),** located in the brainstem, controls consciousness and alertness. The neurons of the RAS make connections between the spinal cord, cerebellum, thalamus, and cerebral cortex. These connections relay visual, auditory, and other stimuli that help keep us awake, attentive, and observant. Without such stimuli, the CNS becomes lethargic, and the person may lose consciousness. Anesthesia, sedatives, opioids, and some other drugs depress the RAS, as does a darkened, quiet environment. Not surprisingly, as you will learn in Chapter 35, sleep is regulated by the RAS (see Fig. 35-4).

The level of stimuli needed to maintain arousal varies: Some people feel optimally alert in bright, noisy, fast-paced environments, whereas others prefer much lower levels of stimulation. As discussed earlier, the brain adapts to constant stimuli, such as a ticking clock. Thus, to maintain arousal, some variation in stimuli is required, such as different pieces of music or an ever-changing view.

Responding to Sensations

Once a stimulus is perceived, the brain either discards it, stores it in memory, or sends impulses along motor pathways to various parts of the body (e.g., the muscles, the heart), bringing about a response. Humans respond to sensations when they are alert and receptive to stimulation. For example, a fatigued new mother may wake up to the soft cry of her infant yet sleep through the persistent ringing of the doorbell. The response to a stimulus is based on the following factors:

Intensity. An intense stimulus excites more receptors, leading to a stronger response. For example, a bright, glaring light can cause you to respond by squinting and shielding your eyes, whereas a dim light may cause little reaction.

Contrast. Contrast is also stimulating. Imagine being outside in cold, windy weather. If you enter an unheated garage, you instantly feel warmer because the building blocks the wind. If you then go inside a room with a blazing fireplace, you will need to take off layers of clothing rapidly because the contrast in temperature will make you feel hot.

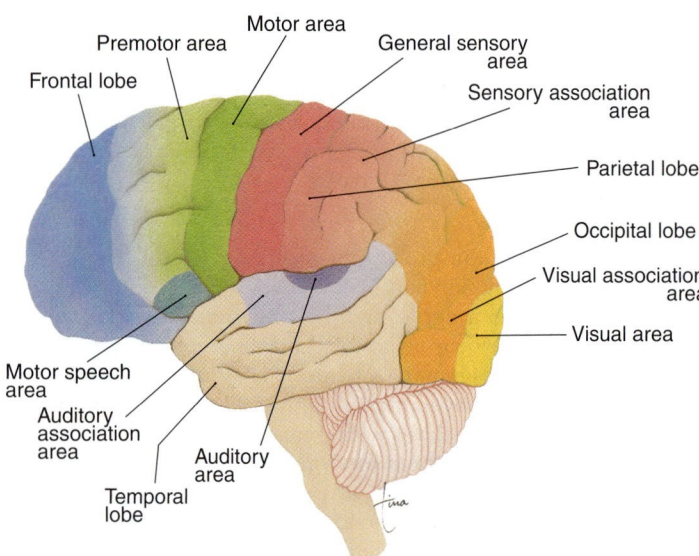

FIGURE 31-1 Special sensory areas of the brain receive and interpret stimuli from the sensory receptors. (*Source:* Scanlon, V., & Sanders, T. [2011]. *Essentials of anatomy and physiology* [6th ed.]. Philadelphia: F. A. Davis. Used with permission.)

Adaptation. Often we take stimuli for granted. Recall your first clinical experience. Did you notice the noise and activity on the unit? Nurses become accustomed to the noise, lights, activity, and even alarms and are able to "tune them out." Unfortunately, these stimuli are all new to patients, so they notice them and may have difficulty resting.

Previous Experience. Prior experience with a stimulus affects ongoing responses to the same stimulus. Have you ever seen a patient scrunch her eyes, grit her teeth, or turn away from an injection before you are even ready to give it? This may mean that she has memory of a prior negative experience with injections.

KnowledgeCheck 31-1

- What is the difference between reception and perception?
- What are the four components of a sensory experience?
- What is the role of the reticular activating system in the sensory experience?

FACTORS AFFECTING SENSORY FUNCTION

Among the many factors affecting sensory function are developmental stage, culture, health status, medications, stress level, personality, and lifestyle.

Developmental Variations

People have differing sensory perceptual abilities at different stages of life. In addition, the need and use for sensory stimulation differs throughout life.

Newborns. Newborns can track objects and respond to light, but their vision is far less acute than that of older children and adults. Their hearing is especially acute at low frequencies. Newborns can also discriminate between different tastes, and they prefer sweet over sour. They react to odors and

seem to be able to discriminate between the smell of their own mother's breast milk and that of another woman. The sense of touch is keenly present at birth; the face, hands, and soles of the feet are the most sensitive (Polan & Taylor, 2007).

Infants. Infants require sensory stimulation to grow and develop normally. Tactile stimulation through cuddling, feeding, and soothing creates a bond between infant and caregivers, provides comfort and pleasure, and teaches the infant about the external environment. Exposure to voices, music, and ambient noise develops the auditory nervous system. By age 1 year, the child can discriminate between different sounds and often recognizes the source. Lights, colors, and contrast allow the infant to observe the world in which she lives.

Children and Adolescents. In early childhood, visual acuity improves; full depth perception is achieved during the preschool period. Hearing is usually fully developed in young children; however, they may experience reversible hearing loss as a result of frequent ear infections and cerumen impaction. In contrast to toddlers, who often lose their balance when walking, older children are sure and steady on their feet. During the school-age years and adolescence, children are developmentally driven toward peers, and the increased social interaction provides a wealth of sensory stimulation.

Adults and Older Adults. By early adulthood, senses are at their peak, unless they are affected by illness or injury. As the adult ages, all of the senses are affected. Table 31-1 describes sensory changes associated with aging. Older adults experience a generalized decrease in the number of nerve conduction fibers, resulting in slower reflexes and delayed response to stimuli. Structural changes also occur in the aging eye and ear. Sensory decline with aging may cause withdrawal, depression, social isolation, and hallucinations. Keep in mind that aging is not the only cause of sensory deficits in older adults.

Table 31-1 ▶ Sensory Function Changes With Aging	
SENSE	**CHANGES ASSOCIATED WITH AGING**
Vision	Decreased peripheral vision
	Decreased tear production
	All structures of the eyes undergo changes:
	The vitreous humor becomes thinner, and "floaters" appear in the visual field.
	The lens becomes discolored and opaque; the pupil becomes smaller. Therefore, less light reaches the retina, limiting vision.
	The lens becomes less flexible and less able to focus on near objects.
	The ciliary body contracts and the lens thickens, bringing loss of visual acuity, decreased ability to accommodate to distance and sudden changes in illumination, and decreased night vision.
Hearing	Cerumen is drier and more solid, creating hearing loss.
	Scarring occurs (e.g., from previous inflammation over the life span).
	Hearing changes commonly include presbycusis (hearing loss of high-frequency tones) and decreased speech discrimination.
Taste	Taste buds atrophy and decrease in number, reducing the ability to perceive tastes, especially sweetness.
	Dry mouth may alter the sense of taste.

(Continued)

Table 31-1 ➤ Sensory Function Changes With Aging—cont'd

SENSE	CHANGES ASSOCIATED WITH AGING
Smell	Atrophy and loss of olfactory neurons decreases the ability to perceive smell (which may also alter the sense of taste).
Touch	Loss of sensory nerve fibers and changes in the cerebral cortex decrease the ability to perceive light touch, pain, and temperature variations.
Kinesthesia	Kinesthetic changes include a decrease in muscle fibers and diminished conduction speed of nerve fibers, resulting in slowed reaction time, decreased speed and power of muscle contractions, and impaired balance. These place older adults at increased risk for falling.

Culture

Culture affects the nature, type, and amount of interaction and stimulation that people feel comfortable with. People of different cultural backgrounds tend to prefer differing amounts of eye contact, personal space, and physical touch. Compare the day-to-day experience of an older adult living in a remote farming community with someone living in an extended family home in the center of a large city. The amount of stimulation perceived as normal would be very different for each of these people. For example, you may think your hospitalized patient needs quiet time alone to rest. However, if he is accustomed to being surrounded by a large family, he may actually rest better in the midst of what seems like chaos to you. Also, use touch advisedly. For some people, it is comforting; for others, it may be offensive.

Illness and Medications

Neurological disorders, such as multiple sclerosis, slow the transmission of nerve impulses. Diseases that affect circulation (e.g., atherosclerosis) may impair function of the sensory receptors and the brain, thereby altering perception and response. Some diseases affect specific sensory organs. For example, diabetic retinopathy is the leading case of blindness among adults ages 20 to 74. Hypertension, too, can damage the retina of the eyes.

Several medications affect sensory function. For example, aspirin and furosemide (Lasix) become ototoxic if taken for a long period of time and impair function of the auditory nerve. CNS depressants, such as opioid analgesics and sedatives, blunt reception and perception of stimuli.

Stress

Have you ever been under a great deal of stress? How did it feel? When you are under stress, do you find yourself looking for or avoiding stimuli? Obviously, stress provides added stimulation. As a result, a person who is bored may add stress. By setting a goal, such as running a marathon, the person undertakes a series of activities to reach that goal. In that regard, stress provides sensory stimulation at a time when the person may have been experiencing deprivation.

However, stress can cause too much stimulation. Physical illness, pain, hospitalization, tests, and surgery are all stressors that can lead to sensory overload—more stimuli than the person can handle. Jason (Meet Your Patients) has been under tremendous physical and emotional stress as a result of his injuries and surgeries. His situation is one in which you might want to limit unnecessary stimuli (e.g., noise, lights, too many visitors).

Personality and Lifestyle

Are you the kind of person who likes to have people around all the time? Do you thrive on noise and action? Or are you the kind of person who loves to curl up with a book and a cup of tea? Clients, too, vary in their personalities and lifestyles. Some people, by nature, like excitement, change, and stimulation; others prefer a more predictable and quiet life. Clients are at risk for sensory alterations if their previous level of stimuli does not match their current level. Health problems, a change of environment, or loss of a partner can each create changes in stimuli.

KnowledgeCheck 31-2

- List five major factors that affect sensory function.
- Compare and contrast the sensory changes in childhood with those in older adulthood.

SENSORY ALTERATIONS

Humans are constantly striving to achieve **sensoristasis,** a state of optimum arousal. Sensory alterations occur when the body experiences meaningless or limited stimulation (sensory deprivation), excessive stimulation (sensory overload), or sensory deficits.

Example Problem: Sensory Deprivation

Sensory deprivation is a state of RAS depression caused by a lack of meaningful stimuli. When environmental stimuli are deficient, the remaining stimuli, such as distant noises, minor pain, and cold extremities, can become overly noticeable or distorted, filling in the "sensory gap" and causing the patient a level of distress that is out of proportion to the intensity of the stimulus. Clinical manifestations include problems with perception, cognition, and emotion (Table 31-2).

The following situations increase the risk for sensory deprivation:

- Impaired sensory reception (e.g., neurological injury, dementia, depression, sleep deprivation, and CNS-depressant medications)
- Inability to transmit or process stimuli (e.g., nerve or brain injury)
- Restricted mobility
- Sensory deficits (e.g., vision, hearing)
- A nonstimulating, monotonous environment. Examples include children in orphanages; people in prison; homebound disabled and older people; patients in nursing homes and

Table 31-2 ➤ Signs of Sensory Deprivation and Sensory Overload

SENSORY DEPRIVATION	SENSORY OVERLOAD
Irritability	Irritability
Confusion	Confusion
Reduced attention span	Reduced attention span
Decreased problem-solving ability	Decreased problem-solving ability
Drowsiness	Drowsiness (due to insomnia)
Depression	Muscle tension
Preoccupation with somatic complaints (e.g., heart palpitations)	Anxiety
Delusions (misinterpretations of external stimuli)	Inability to concentrate
Hallucinations (seeing, hearing, feeling, tasting, or smelling something that is not there)	Decreased ability to perform tasks
	Restlessness
	Disorientation

other institutions; and hospitalized patients in isolation, seclusion, or private rooms.

- Being from a different culture and unable to interpret received cues

Example Problem: Sensory Overload

Sensory overload develops when either environmental or internal stimuli—or a combination of both—exceed a higher level than the patient's sensory system can effectively process. This sometimes occurs in patients who, because of neurological or psychiatric disorders, are unable to adapt to continuing, nonmeaningful stimuli. Or it might be that the environment provides more stimuli than is usual for a person. Some clinical manifestations of sensory overload are similar to those of sensory deprivation (see Table 31-2).

Hospitalized patients often experience sensory overload due to a combination of physical discomfort, anxiety, separation from loved ones, and the experience of being in the unfamiliar hospital environment. Medications that stimulate the CNS may also contribute to overload, as will substances, such as caffeine and over-the-counter weight-loss pills. In addition, physical conditions that activate the CNS (e.g., hyperthyroidism) contribute to sensory overload.

KnowledgeCheck 31-3

- How does sensory deprivation occur?
- Identify five signs of sensory deprivation.
- How does sensory overload occur?
- Identify five signs of sensory overload.

ThinkLike a Nurse 31-1

Review the stories of Joshua and Richard (Meet Your Patients). How are these patients similar? What factors may have contributed to each patient's current concerns?

Example Problem: Sensory Deficits

Sensory deficits may stem from impaired reception, perception, or both. Of the six basic sensory deficits discussed here, impaired vision and hearing are the two that you are most likely to encounter in nursing practice. How many people do you know personally who wear glasses or contact lenses or who wear a hearing aid? How many do you know whose vision or hearing is not completely corrected by such aids? You can see that sensory deficits are common.

A sudden onset of a deficit is unnerving and may lead to disorientation and anxiety. Gradual changes allow the person to adapt, often without even realizing the extent of it. The patient who has progressively lost hearing may, over time, keep turning up the sound on his radio and telephone and not realize that others find the sound blaring. When there is a deficit in one sense, the other senses may become sharper to compensate (e.g., a person who is blind may develop more acute hearing). Six sensory deficit example problems are discussed in the following sections.

Sensory Deficit: Impaired Vision

Vision occurs when light rays that focus on the retina trigger a nerve impulse that is transmitted to the visual area of the brain in the occipital region. Visual deficits may result from trauma or disease of the eye, microvascular problems, or CNS disorders. Common causes of visual deficits include age-related changes, refractive errors, orbital trauma, cataracts, glaucoma, diabetic or hypertensive retinopathy, macular degeneration, or loss of visual fields after a stroke (Box 31-1). Changes in vision affect all aspects of daily living and may severely limit mobility and interaction.

Sensory Deficit: Impaired Hearing

Hearing occurs when sound waves entering the ear canal are converted to vibrations and transferred from the middle ear to the inner ear. Vibrations cause the hair cells in the cochlea to bend, generating impulses that are carried by cranial nerve VIII to the brain. The auditory area in the brain is located in the temporal lobes. The auditory area interprets the sound and allows you to determine the direction from which the noise is coming. See Chapter 21, Figure 21-4, for an illustration of the structures of the ear.

Hearing deficits may result from injury or disease in structures of the ear, the nerves, or the brain (Box 31-2). Inability to hear decreases the ability to communicate and thus hampers

BOX 31-1 ■ Common Visual Deficits

- **Myopia,** or nearsightedness, means that the patient is able to see close objects well but not distant objects. For example, a person with 20/200 vision can see an object from 20 feet away that a person with normal sight could see from a distance of 200 feet.
- **Hyperopia,** or farsightedness, implies that the eye sees distant objects well. A person with hyperopia may have 20/10 vision—he can see an object from 20 feet that a normal eye can see from 10 feet; however, near vision is impaired.
- **Presbyopia** is a change in vision associated with aging. The lens becomes less elastic and less able to accommodate to near objects. If you're older than age 40 years, there's a good chance you may be experiencing this problem.
- **Astigmatism** is caused by an irregular curvature of the cornea or lens that scatters light rays and blurs the image

on the retina. The person has blurred vision with distortion.
- **Cataracts** are a clouding of the lens, resulting in blurred vision, sensitivity to glare, and image distortion.
- **Glaucoma** is a type of vision loss caused by increased pressure in the anterior cavity of the eyeball that distorts the shape of the cornea and shifts the position of the lens, resulting in loss of peripheral vision. It can eventually lead to blindness.
- **Macular degeneration** is the loss of central vision due to damage to the macula lutea, the central portion of the retina. The leading cause of visual impairment in U.S. residents older than age 50, it is characterized by slow, progressive loss of central and near vision. It is usually present in both eyes.
- **Strabismus** (crossed eyes), in which one eye deviates from a fixed image, can cause permanent vision loss.

---

social interaction. It may interfere with a patient's ability to understand instructions from healthcare professionals and create a safety hazard due to inability to hear warnings.

Sensory Deficit: Impaired Taste

Taste imparts flavor and interest to food. Taste deficits may decrease the pleasure associated with eating; weight loss and malnutrition may result. Taste depends on the functioning of the taste buds on the tongue and, to a lesser extent, on the soft palate. Four types of taste buds exist: sweet, sour, salty, and bitter. A proposed fifth taste bud, umami (produced by the amino acid glutamate), can detect savory flavors. The buds for sweet and salty tastes are primarily on the tip of the tongue; for sour taste, on the two lateral sides of the tongue; and for bitter taste, primarily on the posterior tongue and the soft palate (Fig. 31-2). When stimulated, taste buds generate nerve impulses that travel along the facial and glossopharyngeal nerves (cranial nerves VII and IX, respectively) to the taste area in the parietal–temporal cortex. Foods stimulate different combinations of taste buds. That stimulation, together with

the sense of smell, produces the vast number of tastes we can perceive.

Impaired taste most commonly results from **xerostomia** (excessively dry mouth), which may be caused by medications, decreased saliva production, inadequate fluid intake, poor nutrition, or poor oral hygiene. Other causes of taste deficits include the common cold; infections of the nose, sinuses, mouth, or salivary glands; smoking; vitamin B_{12} or zinc deficiency; and injury to the mouth, nose, or head (Box 31-3).

Sensory Deficit: Impaired Smell

The sense of smell is triggered when chemoreceptors in the upper nasal cavities detect vaporized chemicals. Chemoreceptors generate impulses carried by the olfactory nerve (cranial nerve I) into the olfactory area in the temporal lobes (see Fig. 31-2). Vaporized molecules can be detected from a distance, so the sense of smell can serve as an early warning system for detection of smoke and noxious chemicals.

The sense of smell is vital to the sense of taste. When the sense of smell is lost **(anosmia),** food does not taste the same.

BOX 31-2 ■ Common Hearing Deficits

- **Conduction deafness** results when one of the structures that transmits vibrations is affected. It may be a temporary or permanent condition caused by infection of the middle ear, a punctured tympanic membrane, or arthritis of the auditory bones. A hearing aid may be helpful for conduction deafness.
- **Nerve deafness** occurs when there is damage to cranial nerve VIII or the receptors in the cochlea. It may result from ototoxic medications (e.g., gentamicin) or viral infections. Chronic exposure to loud noise may also lead to nerve and receptor impairment.
- **Presbycusis** is a progressive sensorineural loss associated with aging. The person experiences diminished ability to hear high-pitched sounds and to distinguish sounds in a noisy environment. Presbycusis results from deterioration of the hair cells in the cochlea. Hearing aids may be of no value in sensorineural hearing loss.
- **Central deafness** results from damage to the auditory areas in the temporal lobes. Tumor, trauma, meningitis, or

CVA (cerebrovascular accident, i.e., stroke) in the temporal lobe may cause this.
- **Tinnitus** is a term used to describe ringing in the ears. Most tinnitus comes from damage to the microscopic endings of the nerve in the inner ear, for example, trauma, turbulent blood flow, hypertension, ear infection, medications, otosclerosis, or arthritic changes of the bones of the ear.
- **Impacted cerumen** is a condition in which earwax becomes tightly packed in the ear canal, blocking the canal. Patients with impacted cerumen may experience a feeling of fullness or pain, decreased hearing, or tinnitus.
- **Otosclerosis** is a hardening of the bones of the middle ear, especially the stapes. The stapes becomes fixed, leading to poor sound transmission to the inner ear. The cause of this disorder is unknown.
- **Otitis media** is a middle ear infection. It is a common childhood illness that may be caused by viruses or bacteria.

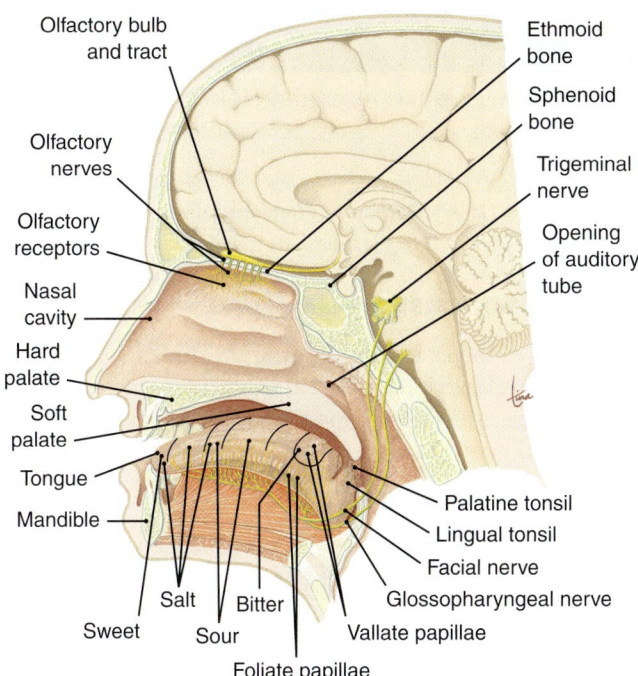

Olfactory bulb and tract

Olfactory nerves

Olfactory receptors

Nasal cavity

Hard palate

Soft palate

Tongue

Mandible

Sweet

Salt

Sour

Bitter

Foliate papillae

Ethmoid bone

Sphenoid bone

Trigeminal nerve

Opening of auditory tube

Palatine tonsil

Lingual tonsil

Facial nerve

Glossopharyngeal nerve

Vallate papillae

FIGURE 31-2 Structures concerned with the sense of smell and taste. (*Source:* Scanlon, V., & Sanders, T. [2011]. *Essentials of anatomy and physiology* [6th ed., p. 217]. Philadelphia: F. A. Davis. Used with permission.)

For patients who are unable to smell, food does not taste the same. They lose their appetite and nutritional deficits may result. Permanent anosmia may develop after cranial nerve damage, a tumor, or atherosclerosis. It may also be inherited and nonpathological. Zinc deficiency, heavy smoking, cocaine use, rhinitis, and sinusitis can cause reversible anosmia.

Nurses may make therapeutic use of a patient's sense of smell. **Aromatherapy,** the use of odors for therapeutic effect, has become one of the most widely practiced complementary therapies among nurses in the United States. See the Complementary & Alternative Modalities (CAM) box, Essential Oils box.

BOX 31-3 ■ Medications That Cause Taste Disturbance

Numerous medications affect the sense of taste. A study by Zervakis and Schiffman (2004) found that most prescription medications are foul tasting and may have a profound effect on the sense of taste. In a test of 62 prescription medications, "bitter, sour, and metallic" described all the medications. Medications with the highest incidence of taste disturbance include the following:

- Antibiotics
- Anticonvulsants, such as phenytoin (Dilantin) and carbamazepine (Tegretol)
- Antihistamines and decongestants
- Antihypertensive and cardiac medications
- Chemotherapy agents
- Lithium carbonate (Lithobid)
- Antipsychotics
- Antidepressants
- Statins
- Muscle relaxants

For more information about aromatherapy,

 Go to Chapter 46, **Holistic Healing,** on Davis*Plus.*

Olfaction has been shown to play a role in memory, mood, and safety. See the Toward Evidence-Based Practice box for a discussion of current research on smell, memory, and mood.

Complementary & Alternative Modalities (CAM)

Essential Oils

Aromatherapy is the use of naturally extracted aromatic essences from plants to balance, harmonize, and promote the health of body, mind, and spirit. It is a natural, noninvasive treatment system designed to affect the whole person, not just the symptom or disease. Essential oils are thought to work by promoting the body's natural ability to balance, regulate, heal, and maintain itself. Some oils may be used topically in certain situations (e.g., minor burns). Beginning research supports the following; however, the evidence base is not strong.

- **Eucalyptus,** *Eucalyptus globulus or Eucalyptus radiata.* Helpful in treating respiratory problems, such as coughs, colds, and asthma. Used to treat burns, wounds, and insect bites. Also helps to boost the immune system and relieve muscle tension.
- **Ylang Ylang,** *Cananga odorata.* Promotes relaxation and can reduce muscle tension. Good antidepressant. Used to counteract anxiety, hypertension, and stress.
- **Geranium,** *Pelargonium graveolens.* Helps to balance hormones in women. Can be both relaxing and uplifting, as well as antidepressant. Used to control acne and oily skin.
- **Peppermint,** *Mentha piperita.* Used in treating headaches, sinusitis, vertigo, muscle aches, asthma, slow digestion, indigestion, nausea, and flatulence.
- **Lavender,** *Lavandula angustifolia.* Relaxing; also useful in skin care and treating wounds and burns. Used to alleviate asthma, itching, labor pains, colic, and dysmenorrhea.
- **Lemon,** *Citrus limon.* Uplifting, yet relaxing. Helpful in treating wounds and infections, and for house cleaning and deodorizing. Sometimes used to treat athlete's foot, colds, and warts.
- **Clary sage,** *Salvia sclarea.* Natural pain killer, helpful in treating amenorrhea and muscular aches and pains. Relaxing, and can help with insomnia. Used to balance hormones and treat sore throat, stress, and exhaustion.
- **Tea tree,** *Melaleuca alternifolia.* A natural antifungal oil, good for treating fungal infections including vaginal yeast infections, "jock itch," athlete's foot, and ringworm. Used for insect bites, itching, and migraine. Also helps to boost the immune system.
- **Roman chamomile,** *Anthemus nobilis.* Relaxing, and can help with sleeplessness and anxiety. Also good for muscle aches, arthritis, and tension. Useful in treating wounds and infection, insomnia, nausea, premenstrual syndrome (PMS), and earache.
- **Rosemary,** *Rosmarinus officinalis.* Uplifting and promotes mental stimulation. Also stimulating to the immune, circulatory, and digestive systems. Good for muscle aches and tension.

Toward Evidence-Based Practice

Jirovetz, L., Buchbauer, G., Stoilova, I., et al. (2006). **Chemical composition and antioxidant properties of clove leaf essential oil.** *Journal of Agricultural and Food Chemistry, 54*(17), 6303–6307.

These researchers studied the chemical properties of clove leaf essential oil in laboratory experiments. They found it to have antioxidant properties.

Sonboli, A., Babakhani, B., & Mehrabian, A. (2006). **Antimicrobial activity of six constituents of essential oil from** *Salvia. Zeitschrift fur Naturforschung, 61*(3–4), 160–164.

Using bioassay research, this laboratory found that *Salvia* has some antimicrobial activity, the degree of which varies among different species of the herb.

Kyle, G. (2005). **Evaluating the effectiveness of aromatherapy in reducing levels of anxiety in palliative care patients: Results of a pilot study.** *Complementary Therapies in Clinical Practice, 12*(2), 148–155.

This pilot study evaluated the effectiveness of aromatherapy massage with a sweet almond carrier oil as compared to two different types of sandalwood in reducing anxiety in patients receiving palliative care. No firm conclusions could be drawn, but the results seemed to support the notion that sandalwood oil is effective in reducing anxiety.

McCaffrey, R., Thomas, D., & Kinzelman, A. (2009). **The effects of lavender and rosemary essential oils on test-taking anxiety among graduate nursing students.** *Holistic Nursing Practice, 23*(2), 88.

Researchers studied the use of rosemary and lavender essential oil sachets on test-taking stress in graduate nursing students. The intervention reduced stress as measured by scores on a test anxiety measure, personal statements, and pulse rates.

Jayasekara, R. (2009). **Dementia: Wandering.** *Evidence Summaries—Joanna Briggs Institute.* Retrieved May 12, 2012, from http://www.jbiconnect.org/agedcare/docs/cis/es_html_viewer.php?SID=6782&lang=en&region=AU

One finding of this systematic review of 11 studies suggested that there is no robust evidence to recommend aromatherapy as an intervention to reduce wandering in patients with dementia.

Several of these studies provide beginning support for the usefulness of a specific oil for a specific purpose. For each of the following questions, (a) state whether one of the studies can answer the question for you; (b) if it can, give the answer; and (c) if it cannot, say why.

1. Is there research to support that aromatherapy with clove leaf essential oil may help prevent aging because of its antioxidant properties?

2. What essential oil is thought to have antimicrobial properties?

3. What would be a good way to deliver rosemary and lavender essential oils for the purpose of reducing stress?

4. Is there research to support that sandalwood oils help to reduce stress?

 Go to Chapter 31, **Toward Evidence-Based Practice Suggested Responses,** on Davis*Plus*.

Sensory Deficit: Impaired Tactile Perception

Touch is crucial to growth and development. It provides pleasure, warns us of injury, and transmits information about the external environment. The dermis of the skin contains receptors for the cutaneous sensations of light touch, pressure, heat, cold, and pain. Information from these receptors is transmitted to the sensory areas in the parietal lobes. The number of cutaneous receptors determines the sensitivity of an area and the amount of space devoted to that region in the sensory cortex area. The hands and face have the most receptors and therefore the largest area in the sensory cortex.

A person's ability to perceive touch is often measured in terms of *two-point discrimination*, that is, the ability to perceive as distinct two close but separate points pressed against the skin. On the lips and fingertips, a person can normally distinguish between points less than 4 mm apart, whereas on the torso, normal two-point discrimination is greater than 2 cm.

Loss of tactile sensitivity can be caused by a cerebrovascular accident (stroke), brain or spinal tumor or injury, or peripheral nerve damage caused by diabetes, Guillain-Barré syndrome, or chronic alcoholism.

ThinkLike a Nurse 31-2

- Why do you think a person with impaired tactile perception is at risk for injury?
- Speculate as to the possible nature of injuries that might occur.

Sensory Deficit: Impaired Kinesthetic Sense

Kinesthesia, or muscle sense, is a complex process involving **proprioceptors** that detect stretch in muscles to create a mental picture of how the body is positioned. Conscious muscle sense is perceived in the parietal lobes. Unconscious muscle sense occurs in the cerebellum, which coordinates movement.

Problems of the inner ear commonly impair kinesthesia. The vestibular apparatus of the inner ear has hair cells that detect rotation or acceleration of the body. Because the vestibular cell nuclei also receive input from neurons involved in vision, a mismatch between the position or acceleration of the head and the visual field can result in motion sickness. This is why it is not advisable to read a book while riding in a car traveling on a winding road.

Parkinson's disease, other neurological disorders, tumors, cerebrovascular accident, and even certain medications can

impair kinesthesia. Kinesthetic deficits place the patient at risk for balance and coordination problems and falls.

Seizures

A **seizure** is the abrupt onset of disturbance in electrical activity in the brain—a group of neurons fires abnormally. This results in motor symptoms, such as rhythmic jerking of the limbs. Symptoms and the duration of the seizure vary, depending on the area of the brain affected. In addition to motor symptoms, the person may have a decreased level of consciousness or a loss of consciousness. This places the patient at high risk for injury from falls.

Seizures are not uncommon. Incidence is highest for those younger than age 10 or older than age 65, and higher among males than among females, especially in children. Most seizures last less than 3 or 4 minutes. In 7 out of 10 people with seizures, no identifiable cause can be found. Among adults, the most common cause is a tumor or head trauma. The most common reason for seizures in a person with epilepsy is failure to take prescribed antiseizure medication. Other common triggers are ingesting substances, sleep deprivation, stress, illness, and hormone fluctuations. Half of the people newly diagnosed with a seizure disorder will have generalized seizures. Three-quarters of children with seizures outgrow the events (Epilepsy Foundation of America, n.d.).

✚ You need to take measures to protect patients who are at risk for seizures. Pad the head, foot, and siderails of the bed and place oral suction at the bedside. If a seizure occurs, you may need to perform suctioning after the episode to prevent aspiration of oral secretions. Do not attempt to open the mouth and insert a padded tongue depressor. This can result in airway obstruction by pushing the tongue back into the pharynx. When anxious, the first responder also could break teeth trying to insert the depressor. For guidelines, see Clinical Insight 31-1.

Clinical Insight 31-1 ▸ Seizure Precautions

Institute seizure precautions for patients with a new diagnosis of a seizure disorder or any seizure activity within the past 12 months; frequent seizure activity; history of head trauma (including surgery) within the past 3 years; withdrawal of antiseizure medication or adjustment of the medication regimen.

The goal of seizure precautions is to protect the patient from injury and prevent serious complications.

Before a Seizure Event

- Explain to the patient the reasons for the precautions.
- If the patient has frequent or prolonged seizures, establish intravenous (IV) access. To provide a route to administer medications (e.g., diazepam [Valium]) in the event of a seizure. For intermittent episodes, you can use rectal diazepam (Diastat), lorazepam (Ativan), or midazolam (Versed).
- Obtain a bed with full-length siderails.
- Cover the headboard, footboard, and siderails with commercial pads or bath blankets. Tape the blankets in place. Padding protects the patient's limbs and head from injury if he has a seizure.
- Keep the rails raised and the bed in low position. To prevent falls and minimize injuries.
- Place oral or nasal suction equipment at the bedside. Test to be certain it is working.
- Place an airway at the bedside or tape to the wall, depending on your agency protocol.
- Make sure the family knows how to use a call device. To summon help in the event of a seizure.
- Assign the patient to a room close to the nurses' station. To allow closer monitoring.
- You may delegate to the nursing assistive personnel (NAP) the tasks of setting up seizure precautions.

When a Seizure Occurs

- If you are present when the patient reports having an aura, help him into bed, lower the head, and raise the siderails. Or if in another location, help him to the floor and put something soft under his head. To keep the head from being injured by hitting the floor.
- Provide privacy.
- Stay with the patient.
- You may insert an oral airway. To keep the tongue from blocking the airway.
- Don't put anything into the patient's mouth and don't force the airway in place. This might break the teeth or cause other injury.
- Don't try to hold the jaw open or put your hands in the mouth. You may be bitten.
- Turn the patient on his side. This allows secretions to drain and the tongue to fall forward, keeping the airway patent.
- Loosen restrictive clothing.
- Move hard or sharp objects out of the way.
- Do not try to restrain the patient or control his movements. This might cause muscle and joint injury to the patient.
- If the seizure is prolonged or hypoxemia is present, administer oxygen as prescribed. To avoid hypoxia during the event.
- Usually little nursing action is required beyond preventing physical injury and maintaining a patent airway. The exception is with status epilepticus, in which the patient has repeated seizures without regaining consciousness. In that event, notify a physician immediately.
- Observe the characteristics of the seizure: how it started, location and duration of motor activity type of movements (e.g., stiffening, jerking, twitching, loss of muscle

(Continued)

Clinical Insight 31-1 ➤ Seizure Precautions—cont'd

tone), crying out, visual and auditory symptoms, tachycardia, pupil dilation, change in level of consciousness). Note the first symptom and how the seizure progressed. To help identify the area of the brain involved.

- You cannot delegate care of a patient who is having a seizure. Nursing assessments and interventions are required. You can ask the NAP to obtain help.
- Administer diazepam (Valium) as prescribed if the seizure is prolonged, typically more than 6 minutes.

After the Seizure

- Turn the patient on his side and apply suction, if needed. To allow secretions to drain and maintain a patent airway.
- Reorient and reassure the patient, and make him comfortable. If the patient was incontinent, change bedding and clothing.
- Examine for injuries.
- Keep the room quiet and the lighting dim.
- Stay with the patient, as he may be sleepy or confused.
- Do not give any food or drink until the patient is fully conscious and alert.

- Monitor vital signs and mental status every 15 to 30 minutes for 2 hours. You can delegate this activity to a NAP.
- Observe post-seizure behavior: Evaluate muscle strength, ability to speak, memory, and orientation.
- Pad the siderails, if not already done.
- Ask the patient whether he experienced an aura and what activities preceded the seizure. The type of aura helps locate the area in the brain where the seizure originated.
- Document what happened and your post-procedure assessment.

Lifestyle Management

Sleep deprivation lowers the threshold for seizure activity. The patient should have sufficient rest and a healthy diet. Advise the patient to visit his primary care provider regularly and avoid excess alcohol and any drugs that may interact with seizure medications.

References

American Association of Neuroscience Nurses, 2007; Wiegand, 2005.

KnowledgeCheck 31-4

- Discuss the difference between myopia and hyperopia.
- What is the difference between conduction deafness and nerve deafness?
- Identify three factors that may impair the sense of taste.
- How is the sense of smell triggered?
- What areas of the body have the greatest number of tactile receptors?
- What type of health concerns may be generated by kinesthetic deficits?

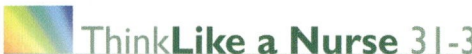 ThinkLike a Nurse 31-3

Imagine that you are experiencing sensory deficits. Which deficits would you find most challenging?

PracticalKnowledge
knowing how

As a nurse, you should always consider your client's sensory perceptual status. Sensory deficits, excess, and overload influence a person's safety and quality of life and may be especially troublesome for those in inpatient facilities.

ASSESSMENT

Assessment of sensory perception includes a history and physical exam to gather data about the following items (see Chapter 21):

- Factors affecting sensory perception (e.g., culture)
- Mental status
- Level of consciousness
- Recent changes in sensory stimulation

- Use of sensory aids (e.g., glasses, contact lenses, hearing aids, canes, and walkers)
- The client's environment
- The support network
- Focused examination of vision, hearing, taste, smell, touch, and balance

Nursing Interview. In your nursing interview, you will assess the client's usual and current state of sensory function, as well as gather a history of sensory problems and use of sensory aids. See the Focused Assessment box, Nursing History: Sensory Perceptual Status.

In addition to interviewing the client and family, assess the environment and client situation. This section provides a brief overview of each of those items.

Physical Assessment. Physical assessment of sensory function requires assessment of the six senses. For guidelines, refer to Procedures 21-6, 21-7, and 21-16, in Chapter 21. Also see the Focused Assessment box Bedside Assessment of Sensory Function.

Assess Risk Factors for Impaired Sensory Perception

You should perform a comprehensive assessment for any client at increased risk for sensory alterations: older adults, clients with limited mobility, clients who are bedbound or homebound, clients in intensive care units, and clients with known sensory deficits, especially if the change has been acute. Routinely assess developmental level, health status, medications, stress and coping mechanisms, personality, and lifestyle related to sensory alterations.

Assess Mental Status

Sensory alterations may trigger changes in mental status and, conversely, altered mental status can interfere with sensory perception. A check of mental status includes assessment of

Nursing History: Sensory Perceptual Status

Ask questions such as the following:

Usual Sensory Function

➤ How would you rate your vision?
➤ How would you evaluate your ability to see objects up close or at a distance?
➤ Do you have any difficulty hearing conversations or listening to the radio or television?
➤ Have you experienced any difficulty locating sounds?
➤ Do you experience ringing or buzzing in your ears?
➤ Do you enjoy the taste of food?
➤ Do you notice any difficulty with your ability to smell?
➤ Are you experiencing any pain or discomfort?
➤ Do you have any areas of numbness or tingling on your body?
➤ Do you have any difficulty with sensing hot or cold?
➤ Describe your level of coordination.
➤ What medications are you taking? Have they had any effect on your vision; hearing; or sense of taste, smell, touch, or balance?
➤ What is your current stress level?
➤ What is your usual activity level?
➤ What is your preferred activity level?

Risk Factors for Impaired Sensory Function

➤ Developmental level (e.g., older adults)
➤ Health status (usual and current state of health, current health concerns, e.g., Ménière's disease), history of hospitalizations and surgeries)
➤ Medications (i.e., look up side effects to determine what, if any, effect the medications have on sensory function)
➤ Stress (current and usual stress level, major sources of stressors, usual coping mechanisms)
➤ Lifestyle (normal activity, noise, interaction levels, hobbies, and usual lifestyle)

History of Sensory Problems

➤ Have you experienced any problems with blurred vision, double vision, sensitivity to light, blind spots, objects moving in front of your eyes, or eye pain?
➤ Have you ever felt unable to follow a conversation because of difficulty hearing?
➤ Have you ever had problems with your ability to taste or smell?
➤ Have you ever had areas of numbness or tingling?
➤ Has anyone in your family ever been diagnosed with a stroke or circulation problem?
➤ Have you ever had episodes of confusion or disorientation?

Use of Sensory Aids, Including Diet, Exercise, Medications, and Remedies

➤ Does the client wear glasses or contact lenses at any time? If so, determine the following:
  When was the client's last eye exam?
  Are the glasses clean and in good repair? Are the glasses within easy reach?
  Are contact lenses in good condition? Is the client able to care for them?

➤ Does the client wear a hearing aid? If so, determine the following:
  Can the client hear adequately with the hearing aid in place?
  Are the batteries working?
  Is the hearing aid clean?
  How much help does the client need to place the aid in his ear?
➤ Does the client use a cane or walker? If so:
  Has the cane or walker been properly fitted to the client?
  How often does the client use the device when walking?
➤ What factors determine when the device will be used?

Assess Mental Status

➤ Assess behavior, appearance, response to stimuli, speech, memory, and judgment. If you need more specific instructions, see Procedure 21-16 and Questions for Evaluating Cognitive Status at the end of the procedure.
➤ For older adults, a tool called the Mini-Cog is especially useful (Borson, Scanlan, Brush, et al., 2000). It consists of three memory questions and instructions to draw a clock face. To use this tool,

 Go to http://consultgerirn.org/uploads/File/trythis/try_this_3.pdf

➤ Assess level of orientation: Have the client tell you his name, the date, and his current location. If he can answer these questions correctly, describe him as "awake, alert, and oriented to person, place, and time" (AA&Ox3).
➤ Assess level of consciousness:

Alert	Is the patient awake and aware of the environment and himself, speaking clearly, making eye contact?
Confused	Are actions and speech inappropriate?
Lethargic	Is speech slow or sluggish? Are mental processes and movements sluggish?
Obtunded	This is a low level of awareness and response to environment. Document it if it occurs.
Stuporous	This occurs when the patient can be aroused by vigorous stimulation but seems confused during periods of arousal.
Comatose	In this state, there is no spontaneous movement, no verbalization, and only nonpurposeful movement with stimulation. (Huntley, 2008)

➤ Also see Chapter 21, Procedure 21-16, Assessing the Sensory-Neurological System, Glasgow Coma Scale and Full Outline of UnResponsiveness Scale.

Assess Support Network for Clients With Sensory Deficit

➤ Are there support persons to help the client by assuming chores he can no longer perform?
➤ Are there people who provide comfort to ease the client's distress about sensory losses?
➤ Who can provide sensory stimulation?
➤ Who can help reorient and calm the client?
➤ Does the client need help with transportation in order to maintain social contact?

Bedside Assessment of Sensory Function

SENSE	ASSESSMENT PROCESS
Vision	Use the Snellen chart, or have the client read a newspaper.
	Observe for squinting.
Hearing	Perform the whisper test.
	Inspect the ear canals for hardened cerumen.
	Observe client conversations. Are there frequent requests for repeating information or misunderstandings?
	How loud is the client's radio or television?
	To screen hearing in older adults, you will find a useful tool if you Go to http://consultgerirn.org/resources
Smell	Ask the client to close his eyes and identify common smells (e.g., coffee, vanilla, cloves, tobacco).
Taste	Ask the client to close his eyes and identify common tastes (e.g., salt, lemon, sugar). Give water between tastes.
Tactile	With his eyes closed, touch the client with a wisp of cotton. Have him identify when you have touched him. Repeat this process with a sharp object, such as a needle.
	With his eyes closed, ask the client to identify where you are touching his body.
Kinesthesia	Have the client perform the Romberg test. See Procedure 21–7.
	Have the client perform alternating rapid motions, such as tapping heels or clapping.
	Observe the client's gait and movement.

behavior, appearance, response to stimuli, speech, memory, and judgment. Normal findings include an ability to express and explain realistic thoughts with clear speech, follow directions, listen, answer questions, and recall significant past events.

You can assess many of those factors as you interact with the client. For example, if you have asked the client the questions covered in the previous section, you have already formed an impression about his appearance, speech, ability to express himself, and other facets of mental status. In addition, you must specifically assess the client's level of orientation. Chapter 21 presents additional discussion of mental status screening and orientation.

Assess Level of Consciousness

Level of consciousness (LOC) is one indicator of cerebral function. It includes arousal (from alert to deeply comatose) and orientation (to time, place, person, and situation). An alert client will respond to auditory stimuli. If the client does not respond, progress to tactile and then painful stimuli (refer to Chapter 21). Remember, however, that if your client does not speak your language he may not respond to questions or commands. The Glasgow Coma Scale is commonly used to assess LOC. It assesses eye, motor, and verbal responses. The FOUR (Full Outline of Un-Responsiveness) scale adds to that, brainstem reflexes and respirations. To use the Glasgow Coma Scale

or the FOUR Scale for assessing level of consciousness, see Procedure 21-16, in Chapter 21.

If you are not using a coma scale, document your findings specifically and objectively in your nursing notes. Be sure to assess whether the patient is alert, confused, lethargic, obtunded, stuporous, or comatose.

Assess the Environment

The environment is an important source of stimulation. Consider how different the environment is for Joshua and Richard (Meet Your Patients). Joshua is in a crowded space with lights and noise 24 hours a day. He has had a number of invasive procedures and is most likely receiving pain medication. In contrast, Richard is in a quiet room with little exposure to light, noise, or touch. As Joshua's and Richard's situations demonstrate, a healthcare environment can have too many or too few stimuli. As part of your assessment, assess how the client is responding to the conditions of the environment.

- **Compare your data about the patient's personality and lifestyle with the current environmental situation.** In healthcare facilities, patients are subjected to lights, noises, and odors that cause them anxiety. They may hear others who are crying out in pain. For most, this environment is very different from anything they are used to. A patient from a small family and a quiet environment may

become overwhelmed and develop sensory overload in a hospital setting. Even a client used to a rapid-paced lifestyle may experience overload if he also feels pain, nausea, dizziness, or other symptoms of illness. In contrast, a client used to an active life may find the hospital setting boring.

- **Assess the effect of the environment on sensory deficits.** For example, for a patient with age-related hearing changes, the background noise of the healthcare environment may make it difficult to hear voices. A patient with visual deficits or impaired balance will often modify his home environment to allow optimal function; however, when the patient is in an institution, these aids are no longer present. To assist the patient, you must determine which environmental factors make his deficits worse and which help to compensate.

Assess the Support Network

For a client with a sensory deficit, his support network may serve as a buffer or a hindrance. For example, an older adult with macular degeneration has progressive loss of vision. If he lives alone, the effect of the visual loss will be quite different than if he lived with an extended family. Support persons may help the client to adapt to deficits by assuming chores that the client can no longer perform or by providing comfort to the client so he is less distressed by the sensory losses.

A support network can also be influential when clients are experiencing sensory deprivation or overload. Recall that Richard (Meet Your Patients) has no visitors. What influence do you think frequent visits by family members would have on Richard? If you say that Richard would receive more stimulation and may have less sensory deprivation, you are correct. Family members can also help clients who are confused from sensory alterations by reorienting and calming them.

KnowledgeCheck 31-5

- Identify six areas you should assess for a client with known or suspected sensory alterations.
- What factors must be evaluated when it is known that a client uses a sensory aid?
- Identify at least two ways that you can assess vision and hearing deficits at the bedside.

 ThinkLike a Nurse 31-4

How would you assess Joshua and Richard (Meet Your Patients) for sensory alterations? You may need to review the scenario at the beginning of this chapter to answer this question.

ANALYSIS/NURSING DIAGNOSIS

NANDA International (NANDA-I) (2012) identifies the following diagnostic labels for use with sensory-perceptual problems.
Acute Confusion
Risk for Acute Confusion
Chronic Confusion
Impaired Environmental Interpretation Syndrome
Impaired Memory
Risk for Peripheral Neurovascular Dysfunction
Unilateral Neglect
For definitions of the preceding labels,

 Go to Chapter 31, **Standardized Language: Selected NOC Outcomes and NIC Interventions for Sensory Perceptual Nursing Diagnoses,** on DavisPlus.

Impaired sensory perception may be the etiology of other nursing diagnoses. Examples include the following:
Risk for Falls r/t visual impairment
Risk for Injury r/t reduced tactile sensation
Self-Care Deficit: Bathing and Dressing r/t kinesthetic impairment
Deficient Diversional Activity r/t reluctance to be in social situations because of hearing impairment
Imbalanced Nutrition: Less Than Body Requirements r/t loss of appetite secondary to impaired taste
Social isolation r/t embarrassment about Impaired Memory

PLANNING OUTCOMES/EVALUATION

For *NOC standardized outcomes* associated with sensory perception diagnoses,

 Go to Chapter 31, **Standardized Language: Selected NOC Outcomes and NIC Interventions for Sensory Perceptual Nursing Diagnoses,** on DavisPlus.

Individualized goals/outcomes statements you might write for a client with Disturbed Sensory Perception include the following:

- Compensates for visual impairment by maximizing the use of touch and hearing.
- Verbalizes the importance of eating nutritious foods, despite the fact they "taste funny."
- Demonstrates proper use of her hearing aid.
- Participates in at least one unit activity daily.

As always, use the goals and outcomes you write to evaluate the client's responses to nursing interventions. The outcomes focus your data collection; comparing the new data against the outcomes allows you to determine patient progress.

PLANNING INTERVENTIONS/IMPLEMENTATION

For *NIC standardized interventions* associated with sensory perception nursing diagnoses,

 Go to Chapter 31, **Standardized Language: Selected NOC Outcomes and NIC Interventions for Sensory Perceptual Nursing Diagnoses,** on DavisPlus.

Specific nursing activities to address sensory perception problems are based on the nursing diagnosis chosen, especially on its etiology. Common nursing activities are discussed in the following sections.

Promoting Optimal Sensory Function

Optimal sensory function requires periodic health screening along with early identification and treatment of health problems. Comprehensive healthcare is the ideal approach, because sensory problems are often related to other health disorders. For example, to protect his vision, a client with hypertension needs to have periodic eye examinations and to control his blood pressure. See the Self-Care box, Teaching Your Client About Sensory Perceptual Health for information to teach your clients about their vision and hearing. For additional information on health promotion and health screening, see Chapter 27.

Self-Care

Teaching Your Client About Sensory Perceptual Health

Vision

➤ Have regular eye examinations.

Infants and preschoolers—Screen at their routine office visits.

Young adults—Complete eye exam at least three times between the ages of 20 and 39.

At age 40—Have a baseline screening, and based on that information, the ophthalmologist will determine how frequently your eyes need to be re-examined.

Age 65 and older—Complete eye exam every 1 to 2 years to check for cataracts and other eye conditions (Foundation of the American Academy of Ophthalmology, 2007).

➤ If you are at risk for eye disease, have more frequent eye exams, regardless of your age—for example, if you (1) take steroids; (2) are of African ancestry; (3) have a family history of eye disease, diabetes, or high blood pressure; (4) or if you have any symptoms. Your ophthalmologist will recommend how often you should have an exam.

➤ Call your healthcare provider for prompt examination if you have eye pain, discharge, a change in vision, or bleeding.

➤ Have your prescriptions for glasses or contact lenses reviewed at each screening and updated if needed.

➤ Be sure that visual screening is done at your child's elementary school. If not, consult your pediatrician or other care provider.

➤ Work with your primary healthcare provider to control conditions such as hypertension and diabetes.

➤ If you are pregnant, obtain early and adequate prenatal care to prevent the danger of premature birth and exposure of the newborn to high-volume oxygen.

➤ Keep sharp or pointed tools (e.g., scissors) out of reach of infants, toddlers, and preschoolers.

➤ Teach children to walk carefully, tool point downward, when carrying pointed tools or other objects.

➤ Teach children to stay away from projectile activities, such as lawn mowing.

➤ Keep the child away from firearms and fireworks.

➤ Insist that your child use eye protection when playing sports such as tennis or baseball.

➤ Insist that children wear helmets when skating or riding bicycles and that teenagers wear helmets when riding motorcycles.

➤ For children who wear glasses, be sure the lenses are made of shatterproof safety glass.

Hearing

➤ Auditory screening is often performed in elementary school; however, most adults do not have their hearing screened regularly. If you work in an area with a high noise level, you should have your hearing checked regularly. Early detection may prevent hearing loss.

➤ If you are pregnant:

Obtain early prenatal care.

Avoid ototoxic drugs.

Be sure you are tested for syphilis and rubella (German measles).

Avoid anyone you suspect may have rubella.

➤ Children with frequent ear infections require evaluation to determine whether hearing loss has occurred.

➤ Middle and older adults may begin to experience difficulty distinguishing voices in a crowd or hearing the television or radio. These are indications of hearing loss and should be evaluated; you may need a hearing aid. Hearing loss is not a "natural part of aging."

Taste

Decayed teeth, gum disease, and other disorders of the mouth may affect the ability to taste. Have your teeth cleaned and examined at least yearly. You may need additional dental work to promote oral health.

Interventions for Example Problem: Sensory Deprivation

If your assessment indicates that the client is at risk for sensory deprivation, include that information in the nursing care plan, along with specific strategies for prevention. Be sure to communicate this information to nursing assistive personnel (NAPs) so they can participate in this aspect of care. To prevent and treat sensory deprivation, you will need to (1) provide stimulation and (2) support the patient's ability to perceive and interpret stimuli. Ideally you will use the following as preventive actions.

Visual Stimulation. For visual stimulation, help the patient with eyeglasses to apply them whenever she is not sleeping. Make sure glasses are clean and in good repair. This will allow the patient to receive available stimuli. Put artwork on the walls, furnish colorful pajamas and robes, and place pictures or flowers where the patient can see them. Unless the patient objects, open curtains during the daytime to allow sunlight to enter the room. Avoid keeping the patient in a dark room, except to promote sleep.

Auditory Stimulation. To stimulate hearing, help the patient with a hearing aid to apply it whenever she is not sleeping. Check that the hearing aid has working batteries and the sound is set at the appropriate level. When possible, move the patient to a quiet area to avoid background noise when communicating.

Olfactory Stimulation. Stimulate the sense of smell with fruits and flowers, or even aromatherapy. Pleasant smells may also stimulate appetite.

Tactile Stimulation. Use touch carefully in your patient care activities. You might hold a patient's hand while talking or provide a back rub with morning and bedtime care. Gentle hand massage is sometimes effective in calming agitated patients. However, people do respond differently to being touched, so adjust the amount of touch you provide according to the patient's reaction.

Media. A television, radio, or computer in the room may provide meaningful stimulation. Teach NAPs to choose appropriate music and programs for the patient. Inappropriate choices (e.g., cartoons with laugh tracks) offer meaningless stimulation and may lead to sensory deprivation.

Social Interaction. Social interaction is a type of stimulus. The following are some social interaction measures:

- Make regular contact with the patient. Introduce yourself, and address the patient by name.
- Provide continuity of care by assigning the same personnel whenever possible.
- Encourage patients to have some form of social interaction. For example, urge long-term care patients to take part in scheduled activities. Assist acute care patients out of bed for meals or visits from family and friends. Encourage patients to leave their rooms. Children may play video games with others online.
- Avoid isolating the patient when at all possible. Ensure that any patient in isolation receives adequate stimulation from nurses, family members, or assistive personnel.

Minimizing Anxiety and Confusion. Minimize anxiety and confusion so the patient can accurately perceive stimuli. For example:

- Explain all procedures and care. This will decrease anxiety and help orient confused clients.
- Place clock and a calendar in the room, along with a schedule of activities.
- Encourage family members to bring in familiar objects from home.
- If the patient is disoriented, provide information at each visit. For example, "Good morning, Mr. Booker. My name is Elsa. I am the nurse taking care of you this morning. It is a few minutes after eight in the morning. I'm going to take your blood pressure and get you ready for breakfast."

Facilitating Communication. Develop alternative methods of communication when interacting with clients with aphasia, or who speak another language, or who have difficulty hearing. Communication boards, a magic slate, pictures, or writing may be helpful. You might also hang a message board in the room and ask family members to post photos, cards, or notes. Computers are useful if the patient has one; and telephone texting might also be used.

Pet Therapy. Many facilities have resident pets or can arrange to have pets visit. A singing bird may delight a resident who cannot be out of bed. In long-term care facilities, resident cats often favor bedbound clients for their frequent naps. Pet therapy can increase socialization, lower blood pressure, and decrease loneliness and pain (Braun, Stangler, Narveson, et al., 2009; Hooker, Freeman, & Stewart, 2002).

Collaboration. Collaborate with other healthcare team members in caring for clients with sensory deprivation. Music therapy, activities, physical therapy, speech therapy, nutritional therapy, and occupational therapy may all be valuable in the care of the client. Carefully monitor the use of sedating medications that may contribute to sensory deprivation.

Self-Stimulation. Finally, teach patients, when they are able, to provide their own stimulation by counting, singing, reading, playing computer video games, or reciting poetry.

ThinkLike a Nurse 31-5

Which of the strategies to treat sensory deprivation would be most appropriate for Richard (Meet Your Patients)?

Intervention for Example Problem: Sensory Overload

Sensory overload is sometimes an unfortunate outcome of hospitalization. To prevent or treat sensory overload, consider the following strategies. Oddly, some of the interventions are the same as those for preventing sensory deprivation.

- **Control Visual Stimuli.** Minimize unnecessary light. Instruct NAPs to be aware of appropriate light levels, especially at night. Use a flashlight instead of turning on room lights, for example.
- **Control Auditory Stimuli.** Minimize unnecessary noise. Instruct NAPs to be aware of appropriate noise levels, especially at night. Speak in a moderate tone of voice, using a calm and confident manner. Do not speak about the client to others in his presence, even when he seems unresponsive. Consider the use of earplugs for the client.
- **Control Olfactory Stimuli.** Reduce noxious odors by promptly emptying commodes and bedpans, removing meal trays, using deodorant sprays, and keeping wounds covered.
- **Use Radio and TV Appropriately.** Choose programs to meet the client's interests. Do not leave the TV or radio on 24 hours a day.
- **Promote Adequate Sleep and Rest.** Establish a schedule for care that allows for uninterrupted periods of sleep and rest. Besides preventing interruptions during rest periods, a schedule will provide the client with advance notice of what to expect during the day. Instruct NAPs on the importance of allowing the client adequate rest and the need to avoid interruptions.
- **Minimize Stress.** Stressors create internal stimuli such as anxiety.
  Observe for the client's reaction to environmental stimuli. Remove annoying or bothersome stimuli if possible.
  Introduce yourself when meeting the client and address him by name. Provide a calm presence: do not hurry with care or speak rapidly.
  If possible, provide a private room and limit visitors.
  Minimize nonessential tasks by other health team members.
  Control pain and nausea with prescribed medications.
  Teach clients about stress reduction techniques.
  Provide relaxing music that facilitates both visualization and deep-breathing techniques.

ThinkLike a Nurse 31-6

Review the scenario of Joshua, the young ICU patient with sensory overload (Meet Your Patients).

- Which strategies to prevent sensory overload would be most appropriate for an ICU patient?
- Which would be least likely to be successful or not feasible based on the setting?

Provide rationale for your choices. You may need to visit an ICU or talk with classmates who have been to an ICU to answer this question.

Interventions for Example Problem: Sensory Deficits

Recall that in addition to sensory deprivation and sensory overload, many clients have sensory deficits. The Joint Commission (2008) requires that you address the communication needs of patients with vision, speech, hearing, language, and cognitive impairments. Regardless of the primary medical diagnosis, you may need to modify your approach to the client or alter the environment. The specific interventions depend on the type of deficit. Describe the sensory deficits on the nursing care plan, along with strategies to deal with them. For example, if the patient recovering from an abdominal surgery has no vision in his left eye, nursing orders should specify to approach the patient from the right.

Interventions for Visual Deficits

Visual deficits range from minor problems requiring corrective lenses to complete blindness. Surgical procedures of the eye may cause temporary visual problems. Problems that limit movement of the head may limit peripheral vision but have no effect on central vision. To provide care for the client with visual deficits, you will need to describe fully the scope of the deficit on the care plan. For the client with sight, your interventions focus on enhancing vision.

- Make sure eyeglasses are clean, in good repair, and of the proper prescription. Place them within easy reach or help the client put them on if necessary.
- Offer a magnifying lens or large-print books and magazines for clients with presbyopia.
- Provide enough light, but avoid glare: (1) use soft, diffuse lighting; (2) provide sunglasses, visors, or hats with brims when the client is outdoors.
- For information on caring for contact lenses, see Chapter 24 and Procedure 24-12.
  For clients with severely limited vision:
- Be sure that all staff are aware of the client's limited vision.
- Provide an uncluttered environment, and do not rearrange furniture.
- Place the call device, phone, and self-care items within easy reach.
- Consider books on tape or Braille for the client's enjoyment.
- Keep the bed in a low position.
- When helping the client walk, ask which side she prefers to have you on. Offer her your arm and allow her to grasp it.
- If the client refuses an offer of help, don't insist.
- For safety measures, see Home Care box, Sensory Deficits—Safety and Health Measures.
- If a visually impaired client uses a guide dog, do not distract the dog. A guide dog in a harness is working and should be approached only with the owner's permission.
- To learn about communicating with visually impaired clients, see Clinical Insight 31-2.

Interventions for Hearing Deficits

A hearing impairment can limit communication and place the client at risk for social isolation. In addition, clients with impaired hearing are unable to receive warnings. This places them at risk for injury (e.g., they may not hear a fire alarm). Your nursing interventions should focus on supporting auditory function, improving communication, and creating a safer environment.

Support Auditory Function. See that hearing aids are functioning properly. If the client has a hearing aid, check to make sure that it is working, the batteries are functional, and the sound is adjusted to a comfortable level. Encourage your client to wear her hearing aid as often as possible. A significant number of people with hearing impairment do not wear hearing aids. To review care of a hearing aid, refer to Procedure 24-16, in Chapter 24.

Inspect ear canals regularly to detect cerumen impaction, a common cause of conduction hearing loss. For key information about otic irrigation, see Procedure 31-1.

Other support measures include closed-caption television, which allows the client to read the dialogue and continue to enjoy his favorite shows or stay current with the news. For telephones, the client might want to consider sound amplification or conversion to text-telephone service. Finally, some clients may also be candidates for hearing aid dog service.

Adapt and Improve Communication. For a client with hearing impairment, provide written instructions to ensure that she understands the teaching and instructions. For additional suggestions for communicating with hearing-impaired persons, see Clinical Insight 31-3.

Promote Safety. ✚ Suggest that your client modify the home environment. For example, install blinking lights that alert the person to an incoming phone call or the ring of a doorbell. Blinking alarm clocks, burglar alarms, and smoke detectors are also available. Also refer to the accompanying Home Care box, Sensory Deficits—Safety and Health Measures. For institutionalized patients, keep background noise to a minimum, and keep a call bell within easy reach of the patient.

KnowledgeCheck 31-6

- Identify three safety measures that may be used with clients with visual impairment.
- Identify three safety measures that may be used with clients with hearing impairment.

Clinical Insight 31-2 ▶ Communicating With Visually Impaired Clients

The Joint Commission (2008) requires that institutions address the communication needs of patients with impaired vision.

- Introduce yourself when you enter the room.
- Call the client by her name so that she can be certain that you are addressing her.
- When you enter a room with a client who is visually impaired, describe the room, room layout, and activities that are occurring.
- Explain unfamiliar sounds, such as the paging system and monitor and pump alarms.
- If the client has limited vision, be sure to position yourself in the client's field of vision.

- Speak to the visually impaired person before you touch her so that she is prepared for your touch.
- Do not speak loudly unless the client has a hearing impairment.
- Let the client know when you are leaving the room.
- Use the words *see* and *look* as you would with a sighted person.
- Avoid expressions such as "over there" or "right here." Guide the client to the location or place her hand on the object.

Clinical Insight 31-3 ➤ Communicating With Hearing-Impaired Clients

Healthcare agencies should address the communication needs of those with vision, speech, hearing, language, and cognitive impairments (The Joint Commission, 2008, p. 156).

Assess the patient's method of receiving speech.

- If the patient wears a hearing aid, check to see that it is turned on.
- If not, does the patient read lips or use sign language? Remember that only about a third of spoken words can be understood by speech reading.
- If possible, arrange a hearing evaluation for the client and construction of any required hearing aids.

Position yourself and minimize noise.

- Don't chew gum or eat while talking. Many clients use lipreading to help them interpret your speech.
- Make sure you are clearly visible to the client before you start speaking. Use touch to get the client's attention.
- Face the client directly; keep your hands away from your mouth.
- If the hearing deficit is predominantly in one ear, move closer to the less affected ear.
- Minimize environmental noise (e.g., turn off the TV).

Send the message.

- Speak slowly and articulate clearly, in a natural way. Don't shout. Shouting distorts your words.

- Don't drop your voice at the end of a sentence.
- Use simple, plain language, but longer phrases (e.g., "Would you like for me to get you a drink of water?" instead of "Do you want a drink?")
- Use gestures to provide visual cues (e.g., act out what you want the patient to do).
- Use paper, pencil, or computer communication when necessary. Consider literacy skills.

Interpret the client's responses.

- Observe the client's verbal responses, facial expressions, and body language for clues to understanding. An inappropriate response indicates misunderstanding.
- Be aware the person may nod agreement or say yes even when she does not understand what is being said.
- Confirm that the client understood you by asking her to repeat what you said, especially if you are giving specific information, such as a time or place. Many numbers and words sound alike (e.g., "fifteen" and "fifty"; or "Prozac" and "Prograf").
- If the person does not understand what you've said, rephrase your statement. Don't repeat the same words.

For older adults: Use a low-pitched voice. The ability to hear high-pitched tones is lost first with aging.

Interventions for Olfactory Deficits

An impaired sense of smell diminishes taste and denies the client the pleasure of enjoying food. This often leads to weight loss. Home safety issues are also a concern for the client who cannot smell. Measures to protect the client with olfactory deficits are found in the Home Care box.

Interventions for Gustatory Deficits

Many people find great pleasure from the different tastes of food. Without the gustatory sense, a client may eat less and be at risk for nutritional deficits and weight loss. If the client has lost weight, be sure to check the fit of any dentures or dental appliances. Weight changes may affect their fit and make it even harder to eat.

For hospitalized clients, provide frequent oral hygiene. Assess for sores or open areas in the mouth. These require prompt treatment because they may become infected and further damage the sense of taste. Teach clients to eat foods separately or drink water between bites to distinguish the taste of the food more readily. Seasonings, salt substitutes, spices, or lemon may improve the taste of foods and encourage the client's appetite (see Home Care box).

Interventions for Tactile Deficits

Patients with peripheral vascular disease, spinal cord injury, diabetes, cerebrovascular accident, trauma, or fractures are at risk for diminished tactile sensation. They may not notice a cut or wound in an area with limited sensation. For institutionalized patients, inspect the affected area daily and teach the patient to continue this practice at home. Look for open areas,

cuts, abrasions, or areas of erythema. Any of these findings requires care. Also see the Home Care box.

If the patient consents, you can stimulate the sense of touch by brushing his hair, giving a back rub, or touching him when giving care. You may need to use firm pressure for him to feel the touch. Frequent turning and positioning may also help. In contrast to tactile deficit, some patients are overly sensitive to touch. In those instances, you must minimize irritating stimuli: Use a bed cradle, and keep bed linens loose to keep them off the skin as much as possible.

Although traditionally we have thought of touch as a caring and healing intervention, there is actually not a lot of empirical evidence that supports its use as a nursing intervention. Furthermore, there are wide differences in how touch is perceived among both patients and nurses. Although many patients are comforted by touch, others are not. Use touch carefully, observing the patient's reaction, until research evidence provides clear guidelines for practice (Gleeson & Higgins, 2009; Gleeson & Timmins, 2005).

Interventions for Kinesthetic Deficits

Kinesthesia, or muscle sense, is enhanced by activities that tone muscles and increase coordination. Examples of activities that are helpful for individuals of any age include the following:

- Rhythmic movement (e.g., tai chi, dance, yoga)
- Aerobic activities, such as walking, running, or bicycling
- Strength training, such as weight-bearing exercise or use of light weights
- Flexibility activities, such as stretching

Sensory Deficits—Safety and Health Measures

To promote safety and health, instruct clients on the following points:

Visual Deficits

➤ Do not use throw or area rugs on any floors.
➤ Keep spaces uncluttered.
➤ Orient the client to new surroundings, for example, "The couch is directly ahead 3 feet. There is a table next to it."
➤ Do not rearrange furniture.
➤ Keep the bed in a low position.
➤ Clients with significant visual impairment should be evaluated for the ability to drive. Many people resist giving up driving privileges, because this severely limits their lifestyle. However, poor vision places the driver, passengers, pedestrians, and other drivers at risk for harm.

Hearing Deficits

➤ Install blinking lights that alert the person to an incoming call or the ring of a doorbell.
➤ Install blinking alarm clocks, burglar alarms, and smoke detectors.

Olfactory Deficits

➤ Have gas appliances regularly inspected and maintained to prevent gas leaks.
➤ Check smoke detectors and replace batteries regularly.

➤ If you cannot detect food spoilage by smell or taste, date foods and inspect them for any evidence of spoilage. Spoilage usually causes changes in the color and consistency of canned, fresh, or leftover foods.

Gustatory Deficits

➤ Perform frequent oral hygiene to encourage appetite and enhance the sense of taste.
➤ Enhance the meal experience by concentrating on the visual appeal of the meal, the plates, and the dinner table.
➤ Avoid bland, overcooked food. Use spices liberally unless they are contraindicated.
➤ Vary food texture, color, and temperature to provide more interest.

Tactile Deficits

➤ Use a bath thermometer to monitor water temperature and prevent burns.
➤ Change position frequently to relieve pressure on bony prominences.
➤ Use properly fitting shoes and socks.
➤ Immediately report any signs of circulatory impairment (e.g., declining motor function, cool temperature, gray-blue coloration).
➤ Inspect daily for open areas, cuts, abrasions, or areas of redness.

■ Balance conditioning with eyes open and closed (e.g., standing on one foot)
■ Putting joints through full range of motion, especially rotational movements

Interventions for Confused Clients

Confusion interferes with the ability to interpret stimuli accurately. It can be temporary or permanent. Confusion is an aspect of both delirium and dementia. **Delirium** is an acute, reversible state of confusion caused by medications and a variety of physiological processes, such as hypoxia, metabolic disturbances, infection, or sensory alterations. It may be accompanied by changes in the level of consciousness. In contrast, **dementia** is a chronic and progressive deterioration in mental function caused by physical changes in the brain and is not associated with changing levels of consciousness.

Your nursing care should promote orientation, use simple communication, decrease anxiety, keep the patient safe, and provide continuity of care. Notice that some of the following interventions are the same as those for preventing sensory deficit.

Promote Orientation. Introduce yourself and state the client's name each time you meet with him. Wear a readable (large, plain type) name tag to reinforce your introduction. Also identify the day, date, and time as you interact. Provide visual clues to time, such as opening the drapes during the day and closing them at night, and placing calendars and clocks where they are easy to see. Also place personal objects, photos, and mementos in the immediate environment, and discuss them with the client. Encourage the patient to participate in familiar activities, such as bathing.

Simplify Your Communications. The patient cannot interpret stimuli accurately and may not understand what you

say. Take an unhurried approach, allowing adequate time for the client to answer any questions you raise. Face the client and speak calmly, simply, and directly. Provide simple explanations for all care and treatments. Use short sentences with few words: "It's bath time," rather than, "Let's go have a bath and get you all nice and clean for visitors." Do not offer too many choices because this confuses the confused patient.

Relieve Anxiety. People with dementia are often anxious, worried, and fearful. Find ways to make the person feel more secure and comfortable before you focus on the content of your conversations.

■ Gently hold or pat the patient's hand.
■ Realize that the person is probably distressed and is doing the best he can. Be affectionate, reassuring, and calm, even when things make no sense.
■ Try to respond to the person's feelings instead of the content of his words. This helps to reassure her. For example, if a woman is constantly searching for her husband, don't say, "Your husband is not here." Rather, say, "You must miss your husband," or "Tell me about your husband."
■ If the person has difficulty finding the right word, supply it for him unless it upsets him. This helps control his frustration.
■ If you do not understand what the patient is trying to say, ask him to point to it or describe it (e.g., "What does a zishmer look like?").
■ Consider using alternative therapy, such as music therapy.

Provide for Safety. ✚ Recognize that the client's decision making may be poor. Maintain a safe environment. For example, store medications away from the patient's reach, keep doors and windows closed securely, and use bed or chair monitors to prevent wandering.

Provide Continuity of Care When Possible. It helps to establish a routine for care and assign the same caregivers each day.

KnowledgeCheck 31-7

- What are the major concerns associated with loss of smell and taste?
- What safety measures should be taught to a client with tactile impairment?
- How can you best assist a client who is confused?

Interventions for Unconscious Clients

The unconscious client is unable to interact with you but requires reality orientation nevertheless. In addition to some of the preceding suggestions, you should include the patient's support persons in the care. Teach them the necessary strategies. You can usually incorporate more touch into the plan of care.

 Safety measures are a priority for unconscious patients. Keep the bed in low position when you are not at the bedside, and keep the siderails up. If the patient's blink reflex is absent or her eyes do not close totally, you may need to give frequent eye care to keep secretions from collecting along the lid margins. The eyes may be patched to prevent corneal drying, and lubricating eye drops may be ordered. Oral care is also important because the unconscious patient can have no oral fluids.

 Think**Like a Nurse** 31-7

What types of interventions would be most appropriate for Joshua and Richard (Meet Your Patients)—that is, interventions for sensory deficits, sensory deprivation, sensory overload, or confusion?

CLINICALREASONING:
Applying the **Full-Spectrum Nursing Model**

Because the following critical thinking activities allow you to practice the kind of thinking you will use as a full-spectrum nurse, they usually have no single right answer. Discuss them with your peers—if you have difficulty with any of the questions, consult your instructor.

PATIENT SITUATION

Clint Gossage is an 85-year-old man who lives at home alone. His wife moved to a nursing home a year ago. Although Mr. Gossage has many self-care deficits, he is still able to live at home with regular visits from a home health nurse and community services to help with some meals and bathing. When you visit him, you notice that he shouts when talking to you, looks at you intently when you speak, and constantly asks you to repeat what you say. You examine his external ear canal and note that there is some hardened cerumen in the canal. He is not wearing a hearing aid. The patient record reveals tympanic membrane scarring and a diagnosis of conductive hearing loss.

THINKING

1. *Theoretical Knowledge:* Describe the pathophysiology of conductive hearing loss.
2. *Critical Thinking (Considering Alternatives):* Based on your knowledge of conductive hearing loss and your assessment of Mr. Gossage, what is the first follow-up question you would ask him about his hearing?

DOING

3. *Practical Knowledge:* At a subsequent visit, you discover that Mr. Gossage has impacted cerumen in his left ear. After obtaining a medical order, you prepare to perform an otic irrigation.
   a. To what temperature will you warm the solution?
   b. What position would you use for Mr. Gossage?
   c. Describe how you would place the tip of the syringe (or ear wash system) for irrigating.
   d. After the ear is cleared of cerumen and you have finished irrigating, what should you do next? And what position will you have Mr. Gossage assume when you do it?
4. *Nursing Process (Diagnosis):*
   a. Write a nursing diagnosis that focuses on Mr. Gossage's safety and that relates to hearing.
   b. Based on your nursing diagnosis, what safety measures would you recommend for Mr. Gossage's home? (Do not address the hearing aid issue here.)

CARING

5. *Ethical Knowledge:* Now think back to the first visit with Mr. Gossage. What are some reasons that he might not have been wearing a hearing aid? Consider physical changes associated with aging.

 Go To Chapter 31, **Clinical Reasoning: Applying the Full-Spectrum Nursing Model Response Sheet,** on *DavisPlus.*

PracticalKnowledge
procedures

Procedure 31-1 ■ **Performing Otic Irrigation**

> ➤ For steps to follow in *all* procedures, refer to the Universal Steps for All Procedures found on the page facing the inside back cover.

Equipment

- An ear irrigation system, such as the Welch Allyn ear wash system or an electronic jet ear irrigator.
  Using a metal syringe is no longer recommended and is considered dangerous. An ear irrigation system is also preferred over an Asepto or bulb syringe because of the better ability to control pressure and remove cerumen (Burtin & Doree, 2009; Harkin, 2008).
- Asepto syringe, or rubber bulb syringe (if an ear irrigation system is not available)
- Irrigating solution (usually water, but may be an antiseptic solution), warmed to 98.6°F (37°C).
- Bath towel and moisture-resistant towel
- A headlight if one is available
- Emesis basin
- Otoscope
- Cotton balls
- Procedure gloves

Delegation

You must assess the client before performing this procedure and evaluate client responses during and after the procedure. The procedure requires knowledge of anatomy and physiology, use of an otoscope, and, sometimes, use of sterile technique. Therefore, you should not delegate otic irrigation to nursing assistive personnel (NAP).

Pre-Procedure Assessments

- Determine whether there are contraindications for ear irrigation.
  Contraindications include ruptured tympanic membrane, present or recent middle ear infection, prior surgery on the ear, cleft palate, or acute inflammation of the ear canal.

- ✚ Assess the external ear for drainage. Do not irrigate the ears if drainage is present.
  Drainage from the ear may be a sign of rupture of the tympanic membrane.

- Assess the external ear for cerumen.
  Impacted cerumen is the most common reason for performing an ear irrigation.

- ✚ Assess the external ear canal for redness, swelling, or foreign objects; visualize the tympanic membrane. If a foreign object is present, attempt to remove it before irrigation.
  Establishes the baseline. If you irrigate with a foreign object in the ear, it may cause the object to swell and become more difficult to remove. Also, if you cannot visualize the tympanic membrane, it may be perforated; if so, otic irrigation is contraindicated.

- Assess for pain or hearing loss.
  Establishes the baseline. Cerumen blockage in the ear canal may result in a conductive hearing loss.

> ➤ When performing the procedure, always identify your patient according to agency policy and be attentive to standard precautions, hand hygiene, patient safety and privacy, body mechanics, and documentation.

Procedure Steps

1. **Warm the irrigating solution** to body temperature (98.6°F [37°C]), and fill the reservoir of the irrigator.
   Placing cool solutions in the ear can cause dizziness.

2. **Assemble the irrigator** if necessary, and place a clean disposable tip on it.

3. **Assist the client into a sitting** or lying position, with the head tilted with the affected ear up. Explain what you are going to do.
   Positioning facilitates administering the solution and allows fluid to run along the roof of the ear canal. Knowing what to expect may decrease patient anxiety and improve his ability to cooperate during the procedure.

4. **Don gloves; put on the headlight.**
   The gloves are needed because of the risk of exposure to body fluids. The headlight facilitates direct vision.

5. **Drape the client** with a plastic drape, and place a towel on the client's shoulder on the side being irrigated. Ask the client to hold an emesis basin under his ear to collect the irrigating fluid that drains out of the ear.

   NOTE: An emesis basin is not necessary if a comprehensive ear wash system is used.

   Drape and towel protect the client's clothing.

6. **Set the irrigator pressure** to the minimum level. Let it run for 20 to 30 seconds to prime the tubing or nozzle before irrigation. (If you must use an Asepto or rubber bulb syringe, fill the syringe with about 50 mL of the irrigating solution, and expel any remaining air.)

7. **Straighten the ear canal.**
   a. For a child younger than age 3 years, pull the pinna down and back.
   b. For older children and adults, pull the pinna upward and outward.
      Straightens the ear canal so that the solution can flow through the length of the canal.

8. **Instruct the client to notify you** if he experiences any pain or dizziness during the irrigation. Explain to the client that he may feel warmth,

fullness, or pressure when the fluid reaches the tympanic membrane.
Pain or dizziness may indicate a contraindication to the procedure.

9. **Place the tip of the nozzle** (or syringe) about 1 cm (½ in.) above the entrance of the ear canal, and direct the stream of irrigating solution gently along the top of the ear canal toward the back of the client's head.

   a. Do not occlude the ear canal with the nozzle.

   b. Instill the solution slowly.

   c. Allow the solution to flow out as it is instilled.

   d. Repeat these steps for 5 minutes or until you can see cerumen in the return solution.

   ✚ Directing the flow directly onto the tympanic membrane could injure the membrane. Strong pressure can cause discomfort and may even damage the tympanic membrane. ➤

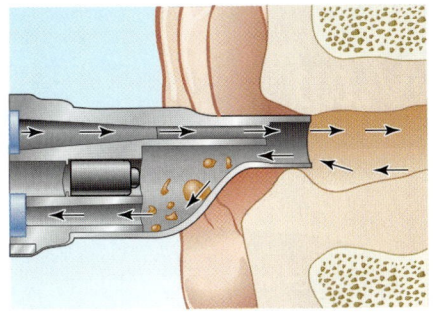

10. **Inspect the ear with an otoscope** to evaluate cerumen removal. See Procedure 21-7 if you need to review otoscopic examination.
    Allows visualization of the canal.

11. **Continue irrigating** until the examination indicates the canal is cleaned of cerumen and debris.
    The irrigating solution will soften the cerumen, easing removal. Blocking the canal prevents the outward flow of the solution.

12. **Place a cotton ball loosely** in the ear canal, and ask the client to lie on the side of the affected ear.
    The cotton ball will absorb excess fluid that drains by gravity.

13. **Clean and disinfect the irrigator,** according to the manufacturer's instructions or agency protocols. Dispose of the disposable tips.

 What if . . .

- **The cerumen is very hard or you have difficulty removing it?**

  The irrigating solution will help soften it, so you may attempt again after 15 minutes.

- **The patient is an infant or young child?**

  Ask another caregiver to immobilize the child during the irrigation.

Evaluation

- Observe the quantity and quality of ear cerumen you removed.
- Observe the appearance of the ear canal.
- Assess for complaints of pain or dizziness.
- Assess for improvement in hearing acuity.
- Reassess for drainage on the cotton ball.

Patient Teaching

- Avoid use of cotton-tipped swabs.
  They simply push cerumen deeper into the ear.
- Keep the ear dry for a few days. Use cotton balls coated with petroleum jelly when bathing.
  Exposure to a wet environment, such as a swimming pool, may increase the risk of bacterial or fungal infection. Petroleum jelly serves as a barrier to keep water from entering the ear.
- Clean ears daily with washcloth, soap, and water. If earwax is a problem, over-the-counter preparations (oils) can be used to prevent wax buildup.
- Notify the primary care provider if you experience ear pain, vertigo, or "ringing in the ears."
  Ear irrigation is an invasive procedure and may result in otitis media, trauma to the external meatus, vertigo, tinnitus, and perforation of the tympanic membrane, although this is not common.

Home Care

- Provide the caregiver with instructions on ear care as stated above.
- Teach parents that it is best to avoid irrigation in young children unless absolutely necessary. Oil- or water-based ear drops may be used to treat a wax problem in a child, applying the oil when the child is asleep.

Documentation

- Document the ear solution used, the quantity, character, and odor of cerumen or drainage.
- Chart the condition of the ear canal and tympanic membrane after the irrigation.

Practice Resources

Roland, P. S., Smith, T. L., Schwartz, S. R., et al. (2008).

 To explore learning resources for this chapter,

Go to Davis*Plus* at http://davisplus.fadavis.com, keyword **Treas**

Chapter Resources for Chapter 31:
Knowledge Check and Think Like a Nurse Response Sheets
Knowledge Check Answers
Resources for Caregivers and Health Professionals
Reading More About Sensory Perception (Suggested Readings)
What Are the Main Points in This Chapter?
Practice Documentation Exercises and Suggested Responses
Care Planning Exercises and Care Map Response
NCLEX-Style Review Questions
Chapter Overview Podcasts

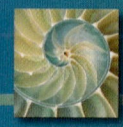

Concept Map

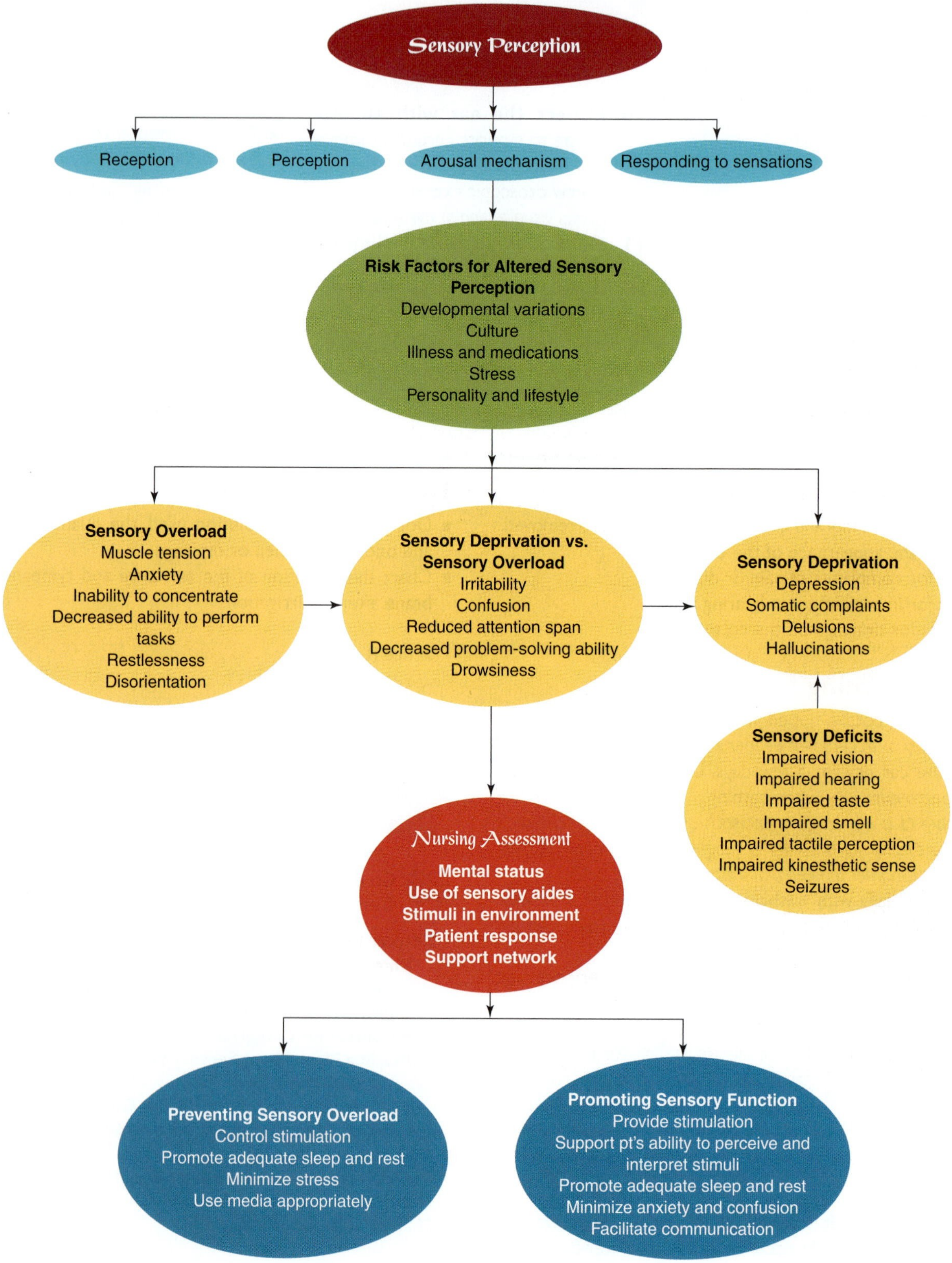

Sensory Perception

- Reception
- Perception
- Arousal mechanism
- Responding to sensations

Risk Factors for Altered Sensory Perception
Developmental variations
Culture
Illness and medications
Stress
Personality and lifestyle

Sensory Overload
Muscle tension
Anxiety
Inability to concentrate
Decreased ability to perform tasks
Restlessness
Disorientation

Sensory Deprivation vs. Sensory Overload
Irritability
Confusion
Reduced attention span
Decreased problem-solving ability
Drowsiness

Sensory Deprivation
Depression
Somatic complaints
Delusions
Hallucinations

Sensory Deficits
Impaired vision
Impaired hearing
Impaired taste
Impaired smell
Impaired tactile perception
Impaired kinesthetic sense
Seizures

Nursing Assessment
Mental status
Use of sensory aides
Stimuli in environment
Patient response
Support network

Preventing Sensory Overload
Control stimulation
Promote adequate sleep and rest
Minimize stress
Use media appropriately

Promoting Sensory Function
Provide stimulation
Support pt's ability to perceive and interpret stimuli
Promote adequate sleep and rest
Minimize anxiety and confusion
Facilitate communication

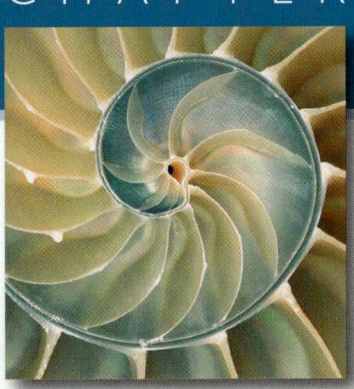

CHAPTER 32

Pain

Learning Outcomes

After completing this chapter, you should be able to:

➤ Define *pain*.

➤ Classify pain according to origin, cause, duration, and quality.

➤ Describe the physiological changes that occur with pain.

➤ Discuss two physiological mechanisms involved in pain modulation.

➤ Discuss factors that influence pain.

➤ Identify the effect of unrelieved pain on each of the body systems.

➤ Discuss nonpharmacological pain relief measures.

➤ Describe pharmacological measures, including nonopioid analgesics, opioid analgesics, and adjuvant analgesics.

➤ Describe chemical and surgical pain relief measures.

➤ Explain why pain should be considered the fifth vital sign.

➤ Identify the steps involved in creating a pain management program for a client.

➤ Write individualized goals and interventions for clients with a nursing diagnosis of Acute Pain.

➤ Write individualized goals and interventions for clients with a nursing diagnosis of Chronic Pain.

➤ Explain how to use a patient-controlled analgesia (PCA) system.

➤ Describe a method for evaluating a pain management program.

Key Concepts

Pain

Pain management

Related Concepts

See the Concept Map at the end of this chapter.

Caring for the Nguyens

This feature allows you to practice the kind of thinking you will use as a full-spectrum nurse. There is usually more than one correct answer to a critical thinking question, so we do not provide answers for these features. It is more important to develop your nursing judgment than to "cover content." Discuss the questions with your peers. If you are still unsure, consult your instructor.

Review the introduction to the Nguyens at the front of the textbook. Mr. Nguyen has bilateral knee pain secondary to osteoarthritis.

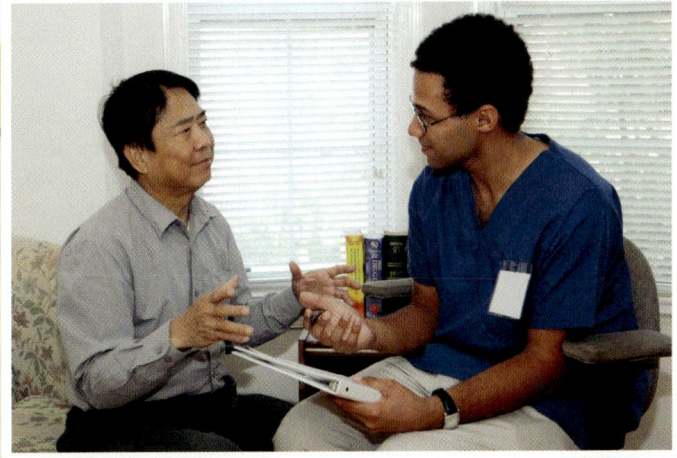

(Continued)

Caring for the Nguyens (continued)

A. To develop a pain-management plan, what patient data do you need?

B. How will you get the data you need? What sources should you use?

C. What types of nursing knowledge (theoretical, practical, ethical, or self-knowledge) are needed to develop a pain-management plan?

 Go to **Caring for the Nguyens Response Sheet** on Davis*Plus*.

Meet Your Patient

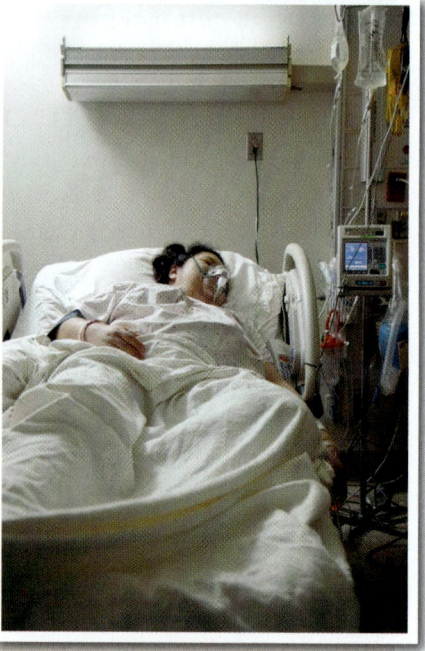

As a special experience, your instructor has arranged for you to spend a half day in the intensive care unit (ICU). As you enter the ICU, you are a little apprehensive. Your patient today is a 23-year-old Asian woman who was in an automobile accident yesterday and sustained chest and abdominal injuries. You walk into the room with your clinical instructor to meet your patient, Ms. Eunice Chu Ling. She was taken to surgery during the night to have her spleen removed. She is intubated (has an endotracheal tube in her airway that is connected to a ventilator), has an intravenous line infusing, and a chest tube on the left side that is draining bloody fluid. Her parents and siblings are in the room sitting rigidly in the chairs, smiling at you. Ms. Chu Ling is awake and grimacing. You want to ask her if is she is in pain, but she cannot speak.

Theoretical Knowledge
knowing **why**

Pain is one of the most distressing symptoms nurses deal with, and it is the most frequent reason people seek medical attention (American Academy of Pain Management, 2008). Most of the top 10 causes of death, such as heart disease, cancer, and chronic lower respiratory diseases, are associated with pain. As more people age and experience these chronic illnesses, you are likely to encounter more patients in pain. The following are some facts about the incidence of pain:

- More than 1 in 4 American adults experience pain lasting more than 24 hours.
- One in 6 American adults live in chronic pain (American Academy of Pain Management, 2008).
- About ¼ to ½ of all community-dwelling older adults report pain that interferes with normal functioning.
- An estimated 1 in 5 adults experiences pain or physical discomfort that disrupts sleep a few nights a week or more.
- In spite of measures to relieve pain, ½ to ¾ of all hospitalized patients die in moderate to severe pain.
- Non-Hispanic white adults reported pain more often than adults of other races. Women and men reported pain at about the same frequency.

- The most commonly reported types of pain are severe headaches and lower back, neck, and facial ache or pain. People with arthritis and joint issues account for a large proportion of pain sufferers (American Pain Society, 2008).

ABOUT THE KEY CONCEPTS

In this chapter, you will begin to understand the key concept of pain. Related concepts, such as transduction, transmission, perception, and modulation will help you to know what pain is and why it occurs; how to better assess it; and how to manage patients' experience acute and chronic pain (acute and chronic pain are also related concepts you will learn in the chapter).

WHAT IS PAIN?

The American Academy of Pain Medicine (2008) defines pain as "an unpleasant sensation and emotional response to that sensation." Pain is the most common reason people seek medical care in the United States. The pain experience can significantly interfere with a person's quality of life, affecting nearly every aspect of life. For instance, severe back pain can affect a patient's job performance, engagement in social activities, sexual intimacy, sleep and rest, ability to exercise, and ability to perform activities of daily living. These factors, in turn, can

affect the intensity of the patient's pain, as well as his response to pain.

Margo McCaffery, a nursing expert on pain, describes pain as "whatever the person says it is, and existing whenever the person says it does" (1968). In other words, pain is a subjective experience. Unlike a pulse or blood pressure, you cannot measure pain objectively. In addition, your expectations of your patients' pain will be influenced by your own values, ideals, and life experiences. As McCaffery's definition indicates, you will need to put aside your personal beliefs about pain and focus on the *patient's* experience.

Pain can cause sleep loss, irritability, cognitive impairment, functional impairment, and immobility, and thus it can be destructive to both the patient and her family. Although we usually think of pain in this negative context, pain is also protective, warning us of potential injury to the body. For example, if you touch a hot object with your bare hand, you will quickly pull your hand away when you feel discomfort. Without the ability to sense pain, you might be burned. Pain can also prompt us to change our actions. For example, after you have been working at the computer for a while, muscle pain may prompt you to get up and stretch; or the gastrointestinal discomfort you experience after overeating may remind you to eat more moderately in the future.

You will be able to manage pain more effectively if you can classify the type of pain the patient is experiencing. But remember that patients often experience more than one kind of pain (Institute for Clinical Systems Improvement [ICSI], 2008). Pain can be classified by the region of the body involved; cause, duration, and pattern of occurrence; and quality, intensity, and time since onset.

Origin of Pain

The origin of pain refers to the site where pain is felt, and not necessarily the source of pain.

Cutaneous or **superficial pain** arises in the skin or the subcutaneous tissue. If you have ever touched a hot object or received a paper cut, you have experienced superficial pain. Although the injury is superficial, it may cause significant short-term pain.

Visceral pain is caused by the stimulation of deep internal pain receptors, most often in the abdominal cavity, cranium, or thorax. Visceral pain may vary from local, achy discomfort to more widespread, intermittent, and crampy pain. Menstrual cramps, labor pain, gastrointestinal infections, bowel disorders, and organ cancers all produce visceral pain. The description of the quality and extent of the pain often serves as a strong clue to the cause.

Deep somatic pain originates in the ligaments, tendons, nerves, blood vessels, and bones. Deep somatic pain is more diffuse than cutaneous pain and tends to last longer. A fracture or sprain, arthritis, and bone cancer can cause deep somatic pain.

Radiating pain starts at the origin but extends to other locations. For instance, the pain of a severe sore throat may extend to the ears and head. Or the pain of gastroesophageal reflux ("heartburn") may radiate outward from the sternum to involve the entire upper thorax.

Referred pain occurs in an area that is distant from the original site. For example, the pain from a heart attack may be experienced down the left arm, through the back, or into the jaw. See Figure 32-1 for other examples of referred pain.

Phantom pain is pain that is perceived to originate from an area that has been surgically removed. Patients with

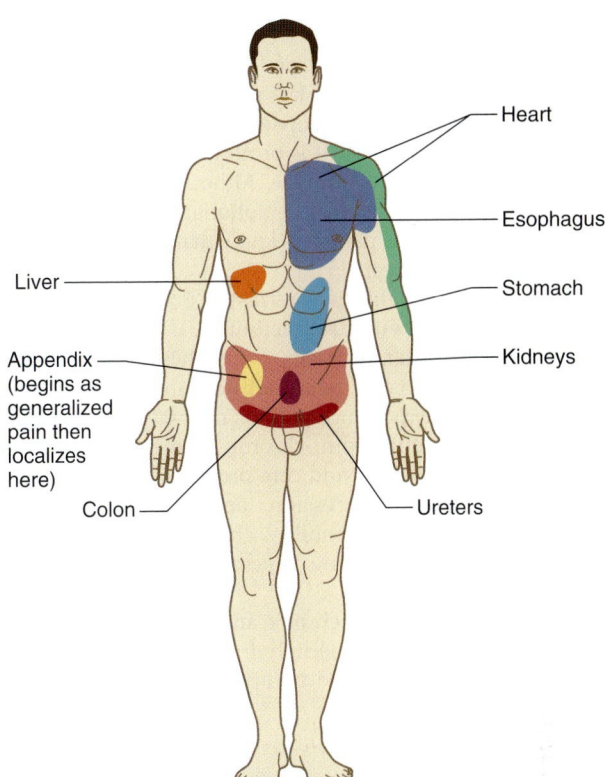

FIGURE 32-1 Most common areas of referred pain.

amputated limbs may still perceive that the limb exists and experience burning, itching, and deep pain in that area.

Psychogenic pain refers to pain that is believed to arise from the mind. The patient perceives the pain despite the fact that no physical cause can be identified. Psychogenic pain can be just as severe as pain from a physical cause. See the discussion of somatoform pain disorder in Chapter 12, if you would like more information.

Cause of Pain

Physical pain is either nociceptive or neuropathic. These two types of pain differ in the way that they affect the patient as well as in how they are treated.

Nociceptive pain is the most common type of pain. It occurs when pain receptors, which are called **nociceptors,** respond to stimuli that are potentially damaging, (e.g., noxious thermal, chemical, or mechanical stimuli). Nociceptive pain may occur as a result of trauma, surgery, or inflammation. It is most commonly described as aching. There are two types of nociceptive pain:

- Visceral pain (i.e., pain originating from internal organs)
- Somatic pain (i.e., pain originating from the skin, muscles, bones, or connective tissue).

Neuropathic pain is a complex and often chronic pain that arises when injury to one or more nerves results in repeated transmission of pain signals even in the absence of painful stimuli. The nerve injury may originate from any of a variety of conditions, such as poorly controlled diabetes, a stroke, a tumor, alcoholism, amputation, or a viral infection (e.g., shingles or HIV/AIDS). Some medications, such as chemotherapeutic agents, can trigger nerve injuries that may cause neuropathic pain even after the medication is discontinued. Neuropathic pain is described as burning, numbness, itching, and "pins and needles" prickling pain.

Duration of Pain

Acute pain has a short duration and is generally rapid in onset. It varies in intensity and may last up to 6 months (American Pain Society, 1994). This type of pain is most frequently associated with injury or surgery. It is protective in that it indicates potential or actual tissue damage. Although acute pain may absorb a patient's physical and emotional energy for a short time, it is helpful for the patient to know that it will usually disappear as the tissues heal.

Chronic pain is pain that has lasted 6 months or longer and often interferes with daily activities. It can be related to a progressive disorder, or it can occur when there is no current tissue injury, as in neuropathic pain. Patients with chronic pain may experience periods of remission and exacerbation. Unlike acute pain, chronic pain is often viewed as insignificant by family and care providers. It may lead to patient withdrawal, depression, anger, frustration, and dependence. Next to incurability, chronic pain is the most feared aspect of contracting cancer or other progressive diseases.

Intractable pain is both chronic and highly resistant to relief. This type of pain is especially frustrating for the patient and care provider. It should be approached with multiple methods of pain relief.

Quality of Pain

The words patients use to describe the quality of their pain help care providers to determine the probable cause and most effective treatment. Patients may describe their pain quality as *sharp* or *dull, aching, throbbing, stabbing, burning, ripping, searing,* or *tingling.* They may refer to its periodicity as *episodic, intermittent,* or *constant.* Patients also use a variety of terms to convey the intensity of their pain, such as *mild, distracting, moderate, severe,* or *intolerable.*

KnowledgeCheck 32-1

How would you classify the pain that the following patients are experiencing?

- A patient with metastatic cancer
- A patient with back pain that was the result of an automobile injury a year ago
- A patient who had bowel surgery yesterday
- A patient with a fractured leg
- A patient who just had his leg amputated but feels as though the leg is still there
- You just received a paper cut while turning the pages of a book.

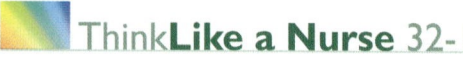 ThinkLike a Nurse 32-1

How would you expect a patient with neuropathic pain to appear?

WHAT HAPPENS WHEN SOMEONE HAS PAIN?

Review the story of Eunice Chu Ling in the Meet Your Patient scenario. Eunice was severely injured in an auto accident. She has had surgery and requires monitoring and invasive devices, such as a ventilator and IV line. Through the maze of equipment you can see that she is restless and grimacing. Consider these aspects of Eunice's experience as we explore the physiology of pain.

Transduction

Pain-sensitive nociceptors are found in the skin, subcutaneous tissue, joints, walls of the arteries, and most internal organs. The skin has the highest density of nociceptors, and the internal organs the least. In a process called **transduction,** nociceptors become activated by the perception of mechanical, thermal, and chemical stimuli. Tissue damage prompts the release of substances such as bradykinin, histamine, and prostaglandins, which activate nociceptors in the surrounding tissues. Bradykinin is also a powerful vasodilator that triggers a release of inflammatory chemicals that cause the injured area to become red, swollen, and tender. Inflammation is the most frequent cause of pain.

Mechanical stimuli are external forces that result in pressure or friction against the body. They involve stretching of body tissues related to bleeding and swelling, and compression of tissues caused by the force of the trauma. Other types of mechanical stimuli are surgical incisions, friction or skin shearing that occurs from sliding down in bed, or pressure from a mechanical device, such as a cast or brace.

Thermal stimuli result from exposure to extreme heat or cold. If you've ever touched a hot object or suffered an earache when outdoors on a cold day without a hat, you have experienced pain from thermal stimuli.

Chemical stimuli can be internal or external. Lemon juice or any acidic substance on an open area in the skin causes sharp, sudden pain. This is an example of pain from *external* chemical stimuli. In contrast, the chest pain experienced during a myocardial infarction (heart attack) is caused by *internal* chemical stimuli, specifically, the chemical changes that result from tissue ischemia.

Transmission

Peripheral nerves carry the pain message to the dorsal horn of the spinal cord in a process known as **transmission** (Fig. 32-2). Pain messages are conducted to the spinal cord along either of two types of fibers:

- **A-delta fibers** are large-diameter myelinated fibers that transmit impulses at 6 to 32 meters per second. These fibers transmit *fast pain impulses* from acute, focused mechanical and thermal stimuli (e.g., the initial sharp pain when you bump your knee).
- **C fibers** are smaller unmyelinated fibers that transmit *slow pain impulses,* that is, dull, diffuse pain impulses that travel at a slow rate. C fibers conduct pain from mechanical, thermal, and chemical stimuli. If you bump your knee, the lingering ache in the tissue will be carried by C fibers.

At the dorsal horn of the spinal cord, the impulses ascend through via spinothalamic tracts to the brainstem and the thalamus. This process requires chemicals called neurotransmitters (e.g., *substance P*). Most pain impulses are sent to the thalamus of the brain, which acts as an integrating center to direct the impulses to three regions of the brain: (1) the somatosensory cortex perceives and interprets physical sensations; (2) the limbic system is involved in emotional reactions to stimuli; and (3) the frontal cortex is involved in thought and reason. The person now perceives pain.

Pain Perception

Perception involves the recognition and definition of pain in the frontal cortex. The point at which the brain recognizes and defines a stimulus as pain is called the **pain threshold.** The number and intensity of stimuli necessary to produce pain, as well as the duration and characteristics of the pain produced,

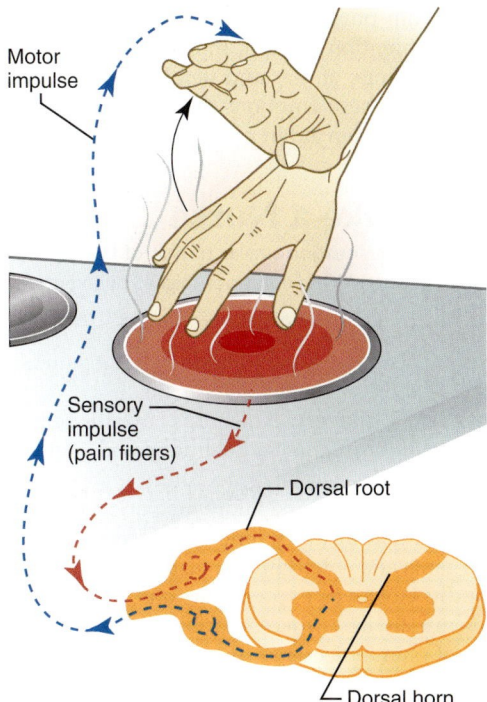

FIGURE 32-2 After nociceptors are activated, pain is transmitted along A-delta fibers or C fibers to the dorsal horn of the spinal cord. From there, the pain message is sent to the brain for perception.

vary from patient to patient. Although the pain threshold usually remains fairly constant for an individual over time, repeated experience with pain can reduce a patient's threshold.

Pain tolerance is the duration or intensity of pain that a person can endure. This varies not only from person to person but also for the same person in different situations. For example, a mother donating a kidney to her child may not report as much postoperative pain as if she had a kidney removed because it was cancerous. Extreme sensitivity to pain is called **hyperalgesia.**

Pain Modulation

A process called **modulation** changes the perception of pain by either facilitating or inhibiting pain signals through the endogenous analgesia system and the gate-control mechanism.

The Endogenous Analgesia System

In the **endogenous analgesia system,** neurons in the brainstem activate descending nerve fibers that conduct impulses back to the dorsal horn of the spinal cord. These impulses trigger the release of serotonin, norepinephrine, and endogenous opioids. *Endogenous opioids* are naturally occurring analgesic neurotransmitters that inhibit the transmission of pain impulses and the release of substance P. Endogenous opioids bind to opiate receptor sites in the central and peripheral nervous system at four receptor sites, designated as mu (μ), kappa (κ), delta (δ), and sigma (σ). Each of the receptor sites has a different affinity for various pain medications. Nonpharmacological measures can also stimulate the endogenous analgesia system.

The Gate-Control Theory

Pain impulses can also be modulated at the spinal level. The **gate-control theory of pain modulation** describes the mechanism of pain sensation, based on the idea that the perception of pain does not occur by direct stimulation of only nociceptors (pain-producing fiber). Instead, pain is perceived by the interplay between two different kinds of fibers—those that produce pain and those that inhibit pain.

As slow-pain impulses travel along C (small) fibers from the periphery to the brain, they encounter a "gate" that either allows or blocks the transmission of pain sensation to the brain. If the source of stimulation is non-painful, the gate would be blocked to feeling pain. Likewise, noxious stimulation keeps the gate open to pain. Imagine that you've just hit your arm against a hard surface. Almost without thinking, you reach down and rub the area. Your massage stimulates skin receptors. These send sensory impulses along fast A-delta (large) fibers, which quickly excite inhibitory neurons at the "gate." These neurons in turn block some of the pain signals being carried along the slower C fibers (Fig. 32-3). The gate control theory is the basis for development and use of transcutaneous electrical nerve stimulation (TENS) to relieve pain (Melzack and Wall, 1965).

Descending impulses from the brain, including impulses related to mood or emotion, are also thought to open or close the gate. For this reason, medications for depression are sometimes used for patients with chronic pain. Nonmedication therapies, such as meditation, exercise, relaxation techniques, and laughter, may also compete with C fiber impulses and block the gate. These strategies are discussed later in this chapter.

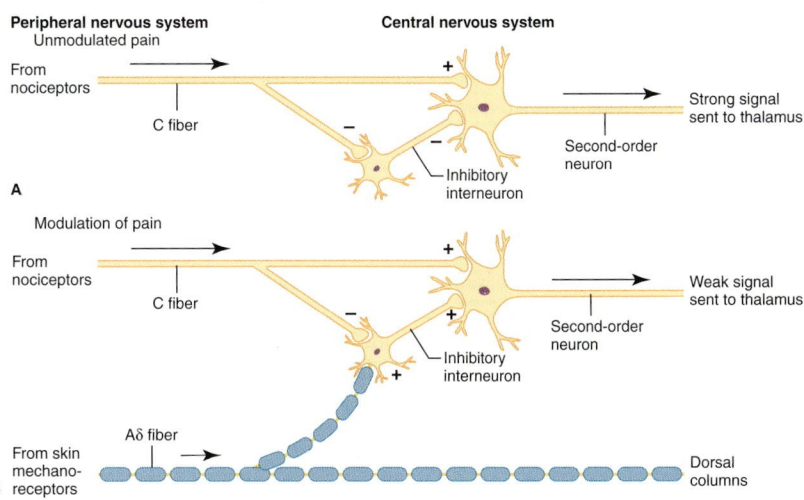

FIGURE 32-3 The gate-control theory of pain modulation. A, Normally, C fibers carrying slow-pain signals block inhibitory interneurons and transmit their signals across the synapse unimpeded. B, A-delta fibers carrying pleasurable signals (e.g., from touch) excite inhibitory interneurons, which then block the transmission of slow-pain signals (+ equals transmission, − equals no transmission).

In summary, on a purely physiological basis, pain is simply transduction, transmission, perception, and modulation. However, as we discuss next, our experience of pain involves far more than these four processes.

KnowledgeCheck 32-2

- What must occur to generate pain?
- What are the four physiological steps involved in the pain process?

ThinkLike a Nurse 32-2

Based on what you have learned about pain modulation, what nursing interventions might help Eunice (Meet Your Patient) be more comfortable?

WHAT FACTORS INFLUENCE PAIN?

Pain is universal, yet each person experiences and responds to pain differently. This demonstrates that pain is a complex phenomenon that influences and is influenced by emotions, age, sociocultural factors, and communication and cognitive impairments.

Emotions

The most common emotions associated with pain are fear, guilt, anger, helplessness, and loneliness. In Meet Your Patient, imagine how Eunice Chu Ling must be feeling. How might her feelings affect and be affected by her pain?

Fear. Some patients (e.g., Eunice) fear that their pain means their illness or injury is life threatening. Others fear their pain will eventually become intolerable. Many fear that if they ask for pain relief, they will be judged as weak or that they will become addicted to pain medications. Such fears can prolong or increase the patient's pain.

Confusion and Helplessness. In addition to fear, Eunice is also probably experiencing confusion and helplessness. Depending on her role in the accident, she may also feel some guilt. When Eunice is by herself, she may experience loneliness or even a sense of abandonment.

Anger and Depression. As you learned in Chapter 13, anxiety and depression are common in people who are ill or hospitalized. Anxiety is most often associated with acute pain, but the anticipation of pain may also trigger anxiety. Waiting for surgery or a procedure that you know will be painful offers plenty of time to think about the unpleasantness and to become anxious. In contrast, depression is most often linked with chronic pain, especially intractable pain.

Previous Pain Experience. Emotional responses to pain are affected by previous pain experiences. Often patients who have had numerous painful experiences are more anxious about the prospect of experiencing pain and are more sensitive to pain. This is especially troublesome for children and adults who require a series of surgeries or painful treatments for their medical conditions. Conversely, patients who have had effective pain relief in the past are usually less anxious and are more confident they will achieve satisfactory pain relief.

People in pain do not experience one single emotional response. Instead, a flood of feelings may overwhelm them, and these emotions may escalate their pain. Patients may get in a vicious cycle: Illness and pain trigger emotional reactions, and the emotional reactions exacerbate the pain.

Rarely is pain purely physical or emotional. Instead, it is usually a combination of both. Interventions to relieve pain may relieve feelings of fear and helplessness, and interventions addressing these emotions, such as reflective listening and gentle touch, often aid in pain relief.

ThinkLike a Nurse 32-3

Imagine being in a situation similar to that of Eunice Chu Ling (Meet Your Patient). What emotions might you experience?

Developmental Stage

The behavior people exhibit when they have pain is strongly influenced by their stage of development.

Infants and Children. Newborns have the same sensitivity to pain as older infants and children, and preterm infants may have a greater sensitivity (McCaffery & Pasero, 1999). The most common kind of pain children experience is acute pain, usually resulting from injury, illness, or necessary medical procedures. Infants and small children usually respond to pain by crying loudly. However, in premature and term newborns, the pain does not always evoke detectable behavioral response. Indicators of pain in neonates might be as subtle as skin mottling, grimacing, twitching, crying, poor feeding, increased or decreased activity, averting gaze, temperature fluctuation, elevated blood pressure, and decreased oxygen saturation. As a result, even though an infant has a low pain score based on behavioral assessment tools, he may not be pain free (Slater, Cantarella, Franck, et al., 2008).

Older Adults. Pain occurs in approximately ½ to ¾ of the geriatric population. Estimates are that as many as 45% to 80% of nursing home residents have significant undertreated pain (Takai, Yamamoto-Mitani, Okamoto, et al., 2010). Some older adults may be unable to report pain because of cognitive impairment. Often their discomfort is evident only in nonverbal cues, such as grimacing, rapid blinking, withdrawal, labored breathing, altered gait, or decreased activity. Some older patients respond to pain in atypical ways, such as mental confusion or collapse (American Geriatrics Society, Panel on Persistent Pain in Older Persons, 2002; Flaherty, 2007). Undertreated pain often leads to other problems that diminish the quality of life, such as social isolation, depression, sleep disturbances, and mobility-related problems.

Sociocultural Factors

We learn behaviors associated with pain through interactions with family (Shin & Kolanowski, 2010), and social support groups. Beliefs about the value of expressing pain or minimizing it are often tied to culture. As you care for clients of various backgrounds, you may notice patterns of behavior. For example, some patients may gain comfort from crying or moaning, whereas some may value silence and brave endurance of pain. Be careful, however, not to assume that patients will react according to responses you have seen in others of the same ethnic or cultural group. Each patient is unique. For example, do you respond to pain in exactly the same way as your parents and siblings?

The family and friends of patients in pain also have culturally influenced responses to the experience. From the Meet Your Patient scenario, recall how Eunice Chu Ling's family is responding. Although you may think it odd that they are smiling, they may be doing so because they want to make a favorable connection with you as the nurse responsible for providing care

to Eunice. As a nurse, you will be caring for many people in pain and will see a variety of responses.

Most nurses respond compassionately to those in pain. However, if you fail to recognize that pain is a unique, multi-dimensional experience, you may misjudge a patient's reaction to injury, surgery, or other discomforts. Disparities exist in the treatment of chronic pain among people of different racial backgrounds. Clinicians should strive to provide culturally competent care and adequate pain control to every patient.

Communication and Cognitive Impairments

One of your greatest challenges as a nurse will be caring for patients in pain who have impaired cognition or communication (e.g., from stroke or dementia, intubation, or limited command of language). Although people with dementia might not appear to be experiencing pain, there is no evidence they have less pain than others. Cognitively impaired adults are not less sensitive to pain but rather may (1) fail to interpret sensations as painful, (2) be unable to effectively communicate their pain, or (3) be unable to recall their pain. Nevertheless, they do experience it (American Geriatrics Society, Panel on Persistent Pain in Older Persons, 2002). These patients are at risk for underassessment of pain and inadequate pain relief (Baldridge & Andrasik, 2010; Horgas, 2007). You will need to consider their behavioral cues as a form of self-report.

Common nonverbal cues of pain include decreased activity, grimacing, frowning, crying, moaning, and irritability. Less obvious indicators you may see in cognitively impaired patients include the following:

- Facial expressions (e.g., a sad or frightened expression, rapid eye blinking)
- Vocalizations (e.g., noisy breathing, profanity, verbally abusive language)
- Changes in physical activity (e.g., fidgeting, increased pacing or rocking, disruptive behavior)
- Changes in routines (e.g., refusing food, difficulty sleeping)
- Mental status changes (e.g., increased confusion)
- Physiological cues include elevated blood pressure, respiration, and pulse.

Be aware, however, that the absence of these cues does not automatically mean that pain is absent (Bjoro, Bergen, & Herr, 2008; Herr, 2004; Herr, Coyne, Key, et al., 2006).

KnowledgeCheck 32-3

- What are the most common emotional responses to pain?
- What factors influence behavioral responses to pain?

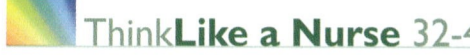

ThinkLike a Nurse 32-4

Eunice Chu Ling (Meet Your Patient) is unable to communicate verbally because of her intubation. She is grimacing in pain. After you medicate her for pain, how would you determine whether her pain has been relieved?

HOW DOES THE BODY REACT TO PAIN?

Our bodily reactions to pain are influenced by the stage of the pain experience and the intensity, duration, and quality of the pain. Pain triggers a variety of changes in the body. The onset of acute pain activates the sympathetic nervous system. As discussed in Chapter 12, this fight-or-flight (stress) response is protective. It minimizes blood loss, maintains perfusion to vital organs, prevents and fights infections, and promotes healing.

If the pain continues, the body adapts, and the parasympathetic nervous system takes over. However, the pain receptors continue to transmit the pain message so that the person remains aware of the tissue damage. Again, this is largely protective; for example, the pain you feel for several days after you sprain your ankle reminds you to stay off it until it is fully healed.

The severity and duration of the pain significantly affect how the person continues to respond to it. Often the person is able to ignore mild pain, but pain that is severe and unrelieved can consume thoughts and change daily living patterns. Box 32-1 identifies common pain responses.

Unrelieved Pain

Unrelieved pain can produce harmful effects in various body systems.

Endocrine System. Ongoing pain triggers excessive release of the hormones adrenocorticotropic hormone (ACTH), cortisol, antidiuretic hormone (ADH), growth hormone (GH), catecholamines, and glucagon. Insulin and testosterone levels decrease. These hormone shifts activate carbohydrate, protein, and fat catabolism (breakdown); hyperglycemia; and poor glucose use. The inflammatory process, combined with these

---

BOX 32-1 ■ Common Pain Responses

Physiological (Involuntary) Responses

Sympathetic Responses (Acute Pain)

Dilated blood vessels to the brain, increased alertness
Dilated pupils
Increased heart rate and force of contraction
Increased respiratory rate
Increased systolic blood pressure
Rapid speech
Pallor

Parasympathetic Responses (Deep or Prolonged Pain)

Changeable breathing patterns
Constricted pupils
Decreased pulse rate
Decreased systolic blood pressure, feeling faint, possible syncope
Slow, monotonous speech
Withdrawal

Behavioral Responses (Voluntary)

Agitation
Crying
Facial grimacing
Guarding the painful area
Moaning
Withdrawing from painful stimuli

Psychological (Affective) Responses

Anger
Anxiety
Depression
Exhaustion
Fear
Hopelessness
Irritability

endocrine and metabolic changes, can result in weight loss, tachycardia, fever, increased respiratory rate, and even death.

Cardiovascular System. Unrelieved pain leads to hypercoagulation and an increase in heart rate, blood pressure, cardiac workload, and oxygen demand. The combination of hypercoagulation and increased cardiac workload may lead to unstable angina (chest pain), intracoronary thrombosis (clot formation in the vessels that supply the heart), and myocardial ischemia and infarction (heart attack).

Musculoskeletal System. Unrelieved pain causes impaired muscle function, fatigue, and immobility. Poorly controlled pain can prevent the patient from performing activities of daily living and engaging in physical therapy.

Respiratory System. Patients in pain tend to breathe shallowly—to limit thoracic and abdominal movement—in an effort to reduce pain. This is called **splinting.** Splinting reduces tidal volume (air exchanged with each breath) and increases inspiratory and expiratory pressures. These changes can lead to pneumonia and atelectasis as well as underventilation (retained carbon dioxide, also called *hypercarbia*) and respiratory acidosis.

Genitourinary System. Unrelieved pain causes release of excessive amounts of catecholamines, aldosterone, ADH, cortisol, angiotensin II, and prostaglandins. These hormones lead to decreased urinary output, urinary retention, fluid overload, hypokalemia, hypertension, and increased cardiac output.

Gastrointestinal (GI) System. In response to pain, intestinal secretions and smooth muscle tone increase, and gastric emptying and motility decrease.

KnowledgeCheck 32-4

- What are the effects of untreated pain on each of the body systems?
- How might untreated pain affect the progress of a patient recovering from major illness?

PracticalKnowledge
knowing **how**

As discussed earlier, a person's *pain threshold* is the point at which that person perceives a stimulus as painful, whereas *pain tolerance* is the amount of pain a person is willing or able to endure. Both differ greatly from person to person. You should regularly assess for pain. Increases in pain may indicate change in condition or a need for more aggressive pain management.

■ ASSESSMENT

A comprehensive pain assessment includes pain location and quality, intensity, aggravating and alleviating factors, timing and duration, pain relief and goals for pain relief.

The patient self-report is the most reliable indicator of pain, including report from those with mild cognitive impairment (ICSI, 2008; National Institutes of Health [NIH], National Institute on Drug Abuse, 2005, revised; National Guideline Clearinghouse (NGC), 2003, updated 2005). Self-report is especially important for patients with chronic pain. When pain is ongoing, the autonomic nervous system eventually adapts, so physiological and behavioral signs become less evident (Schneider, 2006–2007).

To treat pain effectively, you must first understand the patient's perception of pain. Begin with a pain history. Each agency will have different assessment forms for this history. For a list of questions that are typically asked, and for nonverbal indicators of pain, see the Focused Assessment box, Pain Assessment.

Pain, the Fifth Vital Sign

The American Pain Society (1999) recommends assessing for pain as the fifth vital sign. This means that you should ask patients to rate their pain intensity whenever you take a full

---

Focused Assessment

Pain Assessment

Taking a Pain History

Taking a pain history is the most effective way to perform an assessment. Each agency has a different assessment form for this history, but the questions typically will include the following:

   Do you have pain now?
   When did the pain begin?
   Where is the pain located?
   How do you rate your pain? (Use a pain scale.)
   How would you describe your pain? Sharp? Dull? Achy? Burning?
   How often do you have pain? Is it constant or intermittent?
   Is there a rhythm or pattern to your pain?
   What makes the pain better?
   What makes it worse?
   How many days this past week has pain interfered in your ability to do what you would like to do?
   Does pain interfere with your ability to take care of yourself?

Does pain wake you up at night?
Does pain interrupt your concentration and reduce your ability to think clearly?
Have you experienced this type of pain in the past?
Do you have any other associated symptoms (such as nausea and vomiting) when you are experiencing pain?
Does pain prevent you from participating in pleasurable activities, hobbies, and socializing with friends?
Have you used any medications to treat the pain? If so, were they effective? How often do you need to take pain relievers?
What, if any, alternative treatments have you used for pain?
What past experiences or cultural factors, if any, influence the pain?

Observing for Nonverbal Indicators of Pain

Physiological (Involuntary) Responses

Sympathetic Responses (Acute Pain)
Increased systolic blood pressure
Increased heart rate and force of contraction

Focused Assessment

Pain Assessment—cont'd

Increased respiratory rate
Dilated blood vessels to the brain, increased
    alertness
Dilated pupils
Rapid speech
**Parasympathetic Responses (Deep or Prolonged
    Pain)**
Decreased systolic blood pressure, possible syncope
Decreased pulse rate
Changeable breathing patterns
Withdrawal
Constricted pupils
Slow, monotonous speech

Behavioral Responses (Voluntary)

Withdrawing from painful stimuli
Moaning
Facial grimacing
Crying
Agitation
Guarding the painful area

Psychological (Affective) Responses

Anxiety
Depression
Anger
Fear
Exhaustion
Hopelessness
Irritability

Using Pain Scales

The most commonly used pain scales are the visual analog scale (VAS), the numerical rating scale (NRS), the simple descriptor scale (SDS), and the Wong-Baker FACES rating scale.

The Visual Analog Scale

The visual analog scale (VAS) is a 10-cm horizontal line in which "No pain" is written on the left side and "Worst pain imaginable" is written on the right. Patients point to a location on the line that reflects their current pain. Although this rating system is simple and quick, some patients have problems with the abstract nature of the scale.

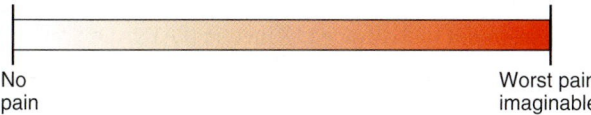

No   Worst pain
pain   imaginable

The Numerical Rating Scale

The numerical rating scale (NRS) is a line numbered from 0 to 10. Zero indicates no pain at all, whereas a 10 indicates the worst possible pain. Patients choose a number from 0 to

10 to denote their level of pain. To use this scale, the patient must be able to count to 10. A scale of 0 to 5 may be more helpful for cognitively impaired patients.

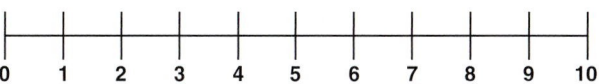

The Simple Descriptor Scale

The simple descriptor scale (SDS) is a list of adjectives that describe different levels of pain intensity. The simplest version of this scale uses the words *mild, moderate,* and *severe.* An SDS with many words is not recommended; it is time consuming to describe and may not be understood by many patients.

The Wong-Baker FACES Pain Rating Scale

The FACES scale uses simple illustrations of faces to depict various levels of pain. It requires no numerical or reading skill. Initially developed for use with children older than the age of 3, the scale also has proven to be extremely useful for adults with communication and cognitive impairments.

Wong-Baker FACES Pain Rating Scale

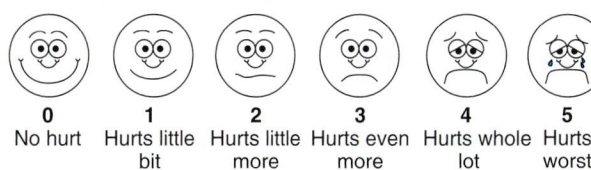

| 0 | 1 | 2 | 3 | 4 | 5 |
| No hurt | Hurts little bit | Hurts little more | Hurts even more | Hurts whole lot | Hurts worst |

Explain to the person that each face is for a person who feels happy because he has no pain (hurt) or sad because he has some or a lot of pain. Face 0 is very happy because he doesn't hurt at all. Face 2 hurts a little more. Face 3 hurts even more. Face 4 hurts a whole lot. Face 5 hurts as much as you can imagine, although you do not have to be crying to feel this bad. Ask the person to chose the face that best describes how he is feeling. Rating scale is recommended for persons age 3 and older.

Revised Faces Pain Scales

We commonly ask patients to rate their pain on a scale of 0 to 10. However, the Wong-Baker FACES scale uses a 0 to 5 scale. To see a revised faces scale adapted to a 10-point scoring system, see Spragud, L. J., Piira, T., & Baeyer, C. L. (2003). Children's self-report of pain intensity, *American Journal of Nursing, 103*(12), 62–64, or

 Go to the Pediatric Pain Sourcebook Web site at http://www.iasp-pain.org//AM/Template.cfm?Section=Home

To see FACES scales using photos of children of various ethnicities,

 Go to the OUCHER!™ Web site at http://www.oucher.org

set of vital signs (Berdine, 2002; Molony, Kobayashi, Holleran, et al., 2005; Pasero, 1997; Pasero & McCaffery, 2010). By simply raising the question with each vital signs check, you will prompt your clients to report pain more often. Also, teach nursing assistive personnel (NAPs) to ask patients about their pain when taking vital signs and to report their findings to you. Box 32-2 provides the clinical approach to pain assessment recommended by the Agency for Healthcare Policy and Research (AHCPR, 2004). Perform pain assessments routinely, but not limited to:

- On admission to a healthcare facility
- Before and after each potentially painful procedure or treatment
- When the patient is at rest, as well as when involved in a nursing activity
- Before you implement a pain management intervention, such as administering an analgesic drug, and 30 minutes after the intervention
- With each check of vital signs, if the pain is an actual or potential problem
- When the patient complains of pain

How Do I Use Pain Scales?

To help you assess the intensity of the pain as well as any changes in the pain, you can choose from among a variety of pain scales. Select a pain scale by considering the patient's age, level of education, language skills, eyesight, and developmental level. Keep in mind that when using a simple pain intensity scale, children can communicate the quality of pain before they are developmentally capable of indicating the intensity (O'Rourke, 2004). Once you choose a particular pain scale for a patient, use it consistently to prevent confusion and allow for comparison. To see some pain scales you might use, see the preceding Focused Assessment box, Using Pain Scales.

How Do I Assess for Nonverbal Signs of Pain?

In addition to the patient's verbal report of pain, you must recognize other responses that may signal pain. Pay attention to the patient's physical signs and symptoms (see Box 32-1).

BOX 32-2 ■ Recommended Clinical Approach to Pain Assessment—Agency for Healthcare Policy and Research

*A*sk about pain regularly. *A*ssess pain systematically.
*B*elieve the patient and family in their reports of pain and what relieves it.
*C*hoose pain control options appropriate for the patient, family, and setting.
*D*eliver interventions in a timely, logical, coordinated fashion.
*E*mpower patients and their families.
*E*nable patients to control their course to the greatest extent possible.

Source: Jacox, A. (1994). Management of cancer pain. [AHCPR Pub. No. 94-0592]. Rockville, MD:.Agency for Healthcare Policy and Research, Public Health Service, U.S. Department of Health and Human Services. (2004). AHCPR Publication no. 94-0592.

You will see sympathetic nervous system responses if the pain is acute. If the pain is unresolved or chronic, you may see signs of parasympathetic nervous system stimulation. For guidelines to help you assess for nonverbal signs of pain, see Clinical Insight 32-1, Guidelines for Assessing Nonverbal Signs of Pain.

Assessing Pain in Children

You can assess pain in children through self-report, behavioral observation, or physiological measures. Be sure to consult the parents about the child's stress signals and reaction to pain. With children, use art and play as a way to assess the child's understanding of pain and the pain management plan. Choose age-appropriate toys to engage the child in acting out feelings. Sometimes this indirect method is more effective than directly asking the child. Remember, most children are fearful about injections and may deny pain if they think that describing their pain will lead to an injection. You can also use a pain-rating scale consisting of simple illustrations of faces. For an example, see the Focused Assessment box, Pain Assessment (Using Pain Scales).

Culturally Competent Assessments

Three words—*pain, hurt,* and *ache*—seem to be used across many cultures to describe pain (American Geriatrics Society, Panel on Persistent Pain in Older Persons, 2002). You might also use descriptions of *burning, itching,* and *cramping* when asking patients about their pain experience. If you work in an area where there are many non-English-speaking patients, you may benefit from pain assessment tools that have been translated into the languages you are most likely to encounter. To see the word *pain* translated into common languages,

 Go to Chapter 32, **Tables, Boxes, Figures: ESG Box 32-1: Pain in a Sample of Languages,** on Davis*Plus.*

Difficult-to-Assess Patients

Patients who are under anesthesia or those receiving pancuronium bromide (Pavulon) are difficult to assess for pain. Those with brain injury may mimic pain-like behavior. Patients with Alzheimer's disease with severe cognitive and expressive deficits are also a challenge for assessing the extent of pain. It may not be possible to elicit a reliable self-report for pain, and their behavioral cues might not be reflective of the pain experience either.

When using a pain scale for cognitively impaired patients, you must allow sufficient time for the patient to respond. Although there are many pain assessment tools, the Pain Assessment in Advanced Dementia (PAINAD) Scale is a five-item, observational tool, specifically geared to older adults with dementia. To see this tool,

 Go to Chapter 32, **Tables, Boxes, Figures: ESG Table 32-1: Pain Assessment in Advanced Dementia (PAINAD) Scale,** on Davis*Plus.*

You will need to judge the intensity and quality of pain based on patient history and current environment. Does the patient have an underlying painful condition? What is the likely source of pain? Are there physical signs that indicate that the patient has increased pain with movement? Nonverbal signs of pain become important cues for such patients.

Clinical Insight 32-1 ▶ Guidelines for Assessing for Nonverbal Signs of Pain

When assessing for nonverbal signs of pain, keep the following guidelines in mind:

- **Facial expression, posture, and body position are reliable indicators of the intensity of pain.**

  Basic and common facial expressions that signal pain are lowering the brow, wincing, clenching jaws, and closing eyelids (ICSI, 2008). Guarding a painful site or maintaining a tense position is also a sign of pain.

- **Changes in vital signs generally last only a short time.**

  The body seeks equilibrium; thus, after an hour or so, the vital signs typically return to baseline even though the patient may still be in pain. Continuous, severe pain may elevate the vital signs again from time to time, but they rarely remain elevated. **Key Point:** *Normal vital signs do not mean that the patient is free of pain.*

- **Patients may be in pain even if they don't "act like" they are.**

  Unfortunately, it has been well documented that healthcare professionals fail to assess pain and tend to underrate the pain that the patient is experiencing (American Geriatric Society, Panel on Persistent Pain in Older Persons, 2002; McCaffery & Pasero, 1999). They expect to see frowning, crying, or scowling. Patients who use laughter, distraction, or even sleep to cope with their pain are often undertreated. **Key Point:** *To assess pain accurately, you must ask your patients and then believe them.*

- **Use an interpreter if the patient speaks a different language.**

  Ask the interpreter to explain to the patient that it is important to manage pain and that you will be using a pain scale regularly to assess his pain. Have the interpreter translate and write out the explanation and directions for the pain scale so that you can refer to these when you assess your patient. With written directions, patients can point to a face or numeric line to tell you about their pain when no one is present to translate.

- **Some patients feel that they are being "bad" or "weak" if they express pain.**

  Such patients may withdraw or become stoic. It is important that you establish a trusting relationship with them. Convey your concern, and acknowledge the person's pain. If the patient trusts you, she will feel free to verbalize thoughts and feelings.

- **Remember to assess for depression** (see Chapter 13 if you need to review).

  Depression is often overlooked in the patient in pain. If depression is not treated aggressively, efforts to manage the pain may not be successful. Avoid the misconception, however, that pain is the cause of the depression and that controlling the pain will eliminate the depression. This is rarely the case.

QSEN

Assessing and Treating Pain in Cognitively Impaired Patients

Competency: Patient-Centered Care (Knowledge, Skills, Attitudes)*

Scenario: Mr. Fagin, who has dementia, has been hospitalized for prostate cancer that has metastasized to his pelvis, femur, and ribs. Mr. Fagin seems confused and is loudly singing hymns and banging his hands against his table in rhythm. The RN goes to Mr. Fagin's room, observes him carefully, and speaks with him. When asked if his bones hurt, he nods his head yes. She also asks Mrs. Fagin about her husband's usual responses to pain. Mrs. Fagin states that her husband has always been very religious and often sings hymns when upset. She also says that he never complained about aches and pains in the past and that she believes he is now having "quite a bit of pain." She says, "I can't stand to see him suffer." The nurse checks the medication administration record (MAR). While Mrs. Fagin speaks gently to her husband, the nurse administers an opioid analgesic. She documents the medication in the MAR, noting Mr. Fagin's behaviors prior to being medicated. Thirty minutes later the nurse observes Mr. Fagin eating dinner with his wife. His body and facial expression are relaxed, and he has stopped singing. Before leaving, the nurse asks Mr. and Mrs. Fagin if they would like a visit from the hospital chaplain.

Think about it: A central nursing duty in the patient-centered care competency is alleviating pain and suffering.

(1) How is Mr. Fagan's situation different from that of a patient with normal cognitive function? (2) What knowledge, skills, and attitudes did the nurse apply that demonstrate competency in pain management (and, therefore, in patient-centered care), particularly for the patient with dementia? As you think about it, consider the following:

➤ Why was it important to ask Mrs. Fagin about her husband's usual behavior?

➤ Was it appropriate to ask the Fagins if they wanted a visit from the chaplain?

➤ How did the nurse show respect for Mr. and Mrs. Fagin's preferences, values, and needs?

➤ Singing loudly doesn't seem to be an obvious indication of pain; what other factors let the nurse know Mr. Fagin was in pain?

➤ How is pain assessment modified for cognitively impaired patients?

➤ Do you see how the nurse recognized Mr. Fagin and his wife as full partners in care?

*For specific Knowledge, Skills, and Attitudes,

 Go to the QSEN web site at **http:www.qsen.org.ksas_prelicensure.php**

KnowledgeCheck 32-5

- How often should you assess the patient for pain, if pain is a potential problem for the patient?
- What are some of the common pain scales used?
- Who should determine if the patient is in pain?

ThinkLike a Nurse 32-5

What pain rating scale would you use to assess Eunice (Meet Your Patient)? Why?

ANALYSIS/NURSING DIAGNOSIS

The following NANDA International (NANDA-I) labels are commonly used when pain is the focus of the problem:

- *Acute Pain.* Pain with an anticipated or actual duration of less than 6 months.
- *Chronic Pain.* Pain with an anticipated or actual duration of greater than 6 months.

Notice that NANDA-I uses only duration, not speed of onset or severity, to differentiate between Acute Pain and Chronic Pain.

When writing a pain nursing diagnosis, specify the location of the pain and any etiological or precipitating factors that you are aware of. Also identify any knowledge deficits, fear of addiction, or any other fears or beliefs that may interfere with effective pain management. Focusing on the specific nature of pain enables you to choose the most useful interventions. For example:

Acute Pain (headache) related to changes of position and secondary to increased intracranial pressure

Pain affects many areas of functioning. Therefore, it is often the etiology of other nursing diagnoses. For nursing diagnoses, NOC outcomes, and NIC interventions associated with Pain,

Go to Chapter 32, **Standardized Language: NANDA-I Diagnoses, NOC Outcomes, and NIC Interventions Associated With Pain,** on Davis*Plus.*

PLANNING OUTCOMES

The overall objective when working with a client in pain is to prevent pain or, if that is not possible, to reduce or eliminate pain.

Individualized goals/outcome statements you might write for a client with pain include the following:

- By day 2 post-op, will require only oral analgesics.
- Within 15 minutes of PCA injection, reports pain is < 3 on a 0–10 scale.
- Reports that chronic pain does not prevent her from performing activities of daily living.
- Pain Control: Uses pain diary (4: Often demonstrated) (NOC)

Use the goals set in the planning outcomes phase to evaluate the pain relief obtained from nursing and medical interventions.

PLANNING INTERVENTIONS/IMPLEMENTATION

When planning care, remember that each situation is unique. For example, one terminally ill patient may request complete relief of pain even if this leads to heavy sedation. Another patient with the same diagnosis and prognosis may prefer that the pain be kept at a just manageable level so he can interact with his family or complete unfinished business. Generally, the most effective and least invasive method

of pain control is preferable. Remember to include nonpharmacological interventions.

Although overall care of the patient depends on the cause of the pain, whether pain is acute or chronic, and on the patient's unique situation, there are nursing interventions and activities that address pain, regardless of its cause.

Specific nursing activities (including focused assessments) for clients with Acute Pain and Chronic Pain include the following:

- Actively listen to the patient's reports of pain.
- Support the patient and family in maintaining an active role in treatment by including them as part of the pain management team.
- Provide prescribed analgesics promptly.
- Assess responses to analgesics and nonpharmacological measures, including level of sedation. Make assessments approximately 30 to 60 minutes after the administration of an oral medicine. Injectable medications work more quickly, so adjust the assessment time accordingly.
- Provide interventions to manage the side effects of medications.
- Reduce anxiety and fear by offering explanations about care and medications, by allowing the patient to be in control of his pain management, and by providing positive encouragement.
- Consult with the healthcare team about complex pain management issues.
- Alter the treatment if the pain is not adequately relieved.
- Delegate appropriate pain management strategies to NAPs. See Box 32-3 for a list of strategies that may be delegated to NAPs.

Nonpharmacological Pain Relief Measures

Integrating complementary therapies into a pain management plan can help ease chronic pain and reduce the need for drug therapy (Bishop, Yardley, & Lewith, 2008; Ernst, 2008; Hart, 2008). According to a recent National Health Interview Survey, one-third of adults used some form of complementary alternative medicine (CAM) when confronted with pain or stress (Barnes, Bloom, & Nahin, 2008).

Nonpharmacological measures, such as exercise, meditation, visualization, and music therapy, can prompt the release of endogenous opioids. They offer an alternative for people with mild pain who do not wish to take potent drugs for pain relief. For many patients, they are satisfying and empowering.

BOX 32-3 ■ Pain Management Tasks That May Be Delegated to Nursing Assistive Personnel

Nursing assistive personnel (NAPs) may assist you in caring for patients with pain. However, you may never delegate the responsibility to assess the patient's pain, monitor the patient's response to pain management strategies, or evaluate the pain management plan. The following tasks may be delegated:

- Repositioning, using pillows for support
- Back rub or massage
- Providing darkness and quiet in the room for sleep
- Straightening sheets
- Mouth care
- Soft music of the patient's preference
- Using distraction (talking or setting up a favorite game for the patient)

However, they should be used as an adjunct to pharmacological therapies for patients with moderate to severe pain.

Cutaneous Stimulation

Cutaneous stimulation (stimulation of the skin) is a pain relief method based on the gate-control theory. As discussed earlier, skin stimulation sends impulses along the large sensory fibers, which in turn excite inhibitory interneurons in the spinal cord to "close the gate." This process diminishes the patient's perception of pain. Cutaneous stimulation works best on pain that is localized and not diffuse.

TENS Units. A **transcutaneous electrical nerve stimulator (TENS)** is a battery-powered device about the size of a pager that is worn externally. TENS units consist of electrode pads, connecting wire, and the stimulator. The pads are directly applied to the painful area. Once activated, the unit stimulates A-delta sensory fibers. A TENS unit can be worn intermittently or for long periods of time, depending on the patient's pain.

PENS Units. **Percutaneous electrical stimulation (PENS)** combines a TENS unit with percutaneously placed (through the skin) needle probes to stimulate peripheral sensory nerves. PENS is effective in short-term management of acute and chronic pain. PENS therapy in some patients promotes physical activity, increases the sense of well-being, reduces the use of nonopioid medication, and improves sleep.

Spinal Cord Stimulator. Chronic neurological pain may be treated by a surgically implanted **spinal cord stimulator (SCS).** The SCS produces a tingly sensation that interferes with the perception of pain (Mailis-Gagnon, Sandoval, & Taylor, 2004, reviewed 2009).

Acupuncture. Application of extremely fine needles to specific sites in the body to relieve pain is called **acupuncture.** It is believed to stimulate the endogenous analgesia system. Acupuncture is well documented to provide relief from dental pain and has been used extensively after surgery and chemotherapy to treat nausea. Of all the complementary therapeutic approaches, acupuncture enjoys the most credibility in the medical community (Hart, 2008). There have been some reports in which acupuncture has led to lightheadedness, which may be a concern for patients who are at risk for falls. Assess these patients carefully after the treatment.

Acupressure. Similar to the ancient art of acupuncture, from which it evolved, **acupressure** stimulates specific sites in the body. However, instead of needles, fingertips provide firm, gentle pressure over the various pressure points. This process may have a calming effect through the release of endorphins. Patients can be readily taught key points to stimulate so that they can self-administer acupressure at any time.

Massage. Massage has been shown to be effective in reducing pain (Cassileth, Trevissan, & Jyothirmai, 2007). By providing cutaneous stimulation and relaxing the muscles, **massage** helps to reduce pain. **Effleurage,** or the use of slow, long, guiding strokes, is used for obstetrical patients during labor and as back rubs for postsurgical patients. Massage requires little effort from the patient and may improve sleep. For most patients, superficial massage is soothing and relaxing, both mentally and physically. However, some patients do not like to be touched, and you should always obtain verbal permission for a massage.

Application of Heat and Cold. The application of cold causes vasoconstriction and can help prevent swelling and bleeding. Cold can be especially effective in reducing the amount of pain that occurs during procedures. Apply a cold pack to the site before and after a procedure to reduce pain. Heat promotes circulation, which speeds healing. Use caution

with these methods, however, because the skin may be injured by extremes of either hot or cold. Also, because the addition of moisture to heat or cold amplifies the intensity of the treatment, take extra precautions when applying moist heat or cold.

 To safely use heat and cold:
- Avoid direct contact with the heating or cooling device. Cover the hot or cold pack with a washcloth, towel, or fitted sleeve.
- Apply heat or cold intermittently, for no more than 15 minutes at a time, to avoid tissue injury.
- Check the skin frequently for extreme redness, blistering, cyanosis (blue color), or blanching (white color).
- If any of these occur, discontinue the treatment immediately and notify the provider.

Contralateral Stimulation. Why does a patient experiencing pain in the right arm experience some relief when lotion is applied and rubbed into the left arm? The principle involved is called **contralateral stimulation**—stimulating the skin in an area opposite to the painful site. Stimulation may be in the form of scratching, rubbing, or applying heat or cold. This intervention is especially helpful if the affected area is painful to touch, under bandages, or in a cast. It has provided some relief to patients who have phantom pain after an amputation.

Immobilization

Immobilizing a painful body part (e.g., with splints) may offer some relief. It is particularly helpful with arthritic joints. You must remember to remove the splints at regular intervals so that the patient can exercise the area to strengthen the site and prevent further injury. Patients in severe pain have the tendency to immobilize a painful area by limiting its use.

Cognitive–Behavioral Interventions

Cognitive–behavioral therapy attempts to alter patterns of negative thoughts and to encourage more adaptive thoughts, emotions, and actions. It is used to decrease depression and anxiety, both of which play a role in pain. Cognitive therapy helps patients to deal with their pain by fostering a sense of control over their illness and decreasing feelings of helplessness. Be sure to obtain the patient's permission before using these methods, because psychological or spiritual distress may occur if she considers them inconsistent with her belief system. Because they are complementary therapies, several of these interventions are discussed in more detail in Chapter 46. To read about holistic nursing, including complementary therapies,

 Go to Chapter 46, **Holistic Healing,** on DavisPlus.

Distraction. You can use **distraction** as a method of drawing the patient's attention away from the pain and focusing on something other than the pain. It is based on the belief that the brain can process only so much information at one time. When distraction works, the patient has only a peripheral awareness of pain. You may have responded to this strategy in the past. Have you ever had a headache or muscle pain go away when you became busy with other activities?

Distraction can be visual, tactile, intellectual, or auditory. The usefulness of the different methods varies among patients. For some patients, *visual* tactics, such as watching a football game on TV, serve as effective distraction. Others may respond better to *tactile* distraction such as massage, hugging a favorite toy, holding a loved one, or stroking a pet. Examples of *intellectual* distraction include becoming engrossed in a crossword puzzle or playing a challenging game. *Auditory* distraction in

the form of music therapy has been shown to reduce anxiety during childbirth and appears to improve mood and pain tolerance. Music should not be limited to adults; it can be used for infants and children as well (Evans, 2002). Distraction is useful with all ages, but it should not be used in place of analgesics.

Although distraction can be used for severe pain, it is most effective for mild to moderate pain and for brief periods of time (e.g., for a short procedure such as an injection or infusion). Some patients experience an increase in pain and may become fatigued and irritable when they are no longer distracted.

Relaxation Techniques. Relaxation techniques are especially useful for reducing chronic pain. In **sequential muscle relaxation (SMR),** or progressive relaxation, the person sits comfortably and tenses a group of muscles for 15 seconds and then relaxes the muscle while breathing out. After a brief rest, this sequence is repeated using another set of muscles. Patients often start at the facial muscles and work downward to the feet.

Guided Imagery. The use of auditory and imaginary processes to affect emotions and help calm and relax is called **guided imagery**. Acute and chronic pain, both physical and psychological, may respond to guided imagery; however, it is more effective for chronic pain. Audio media featuring guided imagery can help patients use their imagination to create images of temporary escape that will elicit a sense of well-being (Lewandowski, Good, & Draucker, 2005). For a script for a guided imagery session,

 Go to Chapter 12, **Tables, Boxes, Figures: ESG Box 12-2: Script for Visualization,** on *DavisPlus*.

Hypnosis. **Hypnosis** involves the induction of a deeply relaxed state. Once the person is in this state, the hypnotist offers therapeutic suggestions to provide relief of symptoms. For example, the hypnotist may suggest to a patient with arthritis

that the pain can be turned down, like the volume of a radio. Special training in hypnotherapy is required.

Therapeutic Touch. **Therapeutic touch (TT)** was developed by nurses and derived from the ancient practice of laying on of hands. Despite its name, TT does not require physical contact. It focuses on the use of the hands to direct energy fields surrounding the body. Although research studies on its effect are not consistent, some patients become relaxed and require less pain medication after a TT session.

Humor. For most people, laughter is positive and indicates mental well-being. **Humor** has positive effects on a patient's physical and emotional health. Humor may boost the immune system as well. It is especially helpful when used before a painful procedure because it lessens anxiety and serves as a form of distraction. Some institutions have humor carts and even humor rooms containing videos, books, and playful items, such as bubbles, finger paints, and puppets. Humor is helpful for both children and adults, but it must always be in good taste and age appropriate. Involve the patient in choosing the humor material, because what one person considers very funny another person may not.

Expressive Writing. **Expressive writing** can help reduce chronic pain. Some recommend structured writing sessions in which the patient describes stressful events for a specified period of time over consecutive days. This type of therapy is best when done in conjunction with a knowledgeable practitioner who provides direction and support (Hart, 2008). Others benefit from frequent journaling in an informal way, expressing feelings, fears, or what comes to mind.

 Think**Like a Nurse** 32-6

What has been your experience with using nonpharmacological pain relief measures to manage your own pain? How would you incorporate these methods into your nursing practice?

Toward Evidence-Based Practice

Lewandowski, C. S., Good, M., & Draucker, C. B. (2005). Changes in the meaning of pain with the use of guided imagery. *Pain Management Nursing,* 6(2), 58–67.

In a sample of 44 people experiencing chronic pain in the home setting, participants in the treatment group learned the guided imagery technique to reduce pain. Of the 210 verbal descriptions of pain reported by participants who used guided imagery and those who did not use the technique, six categories emerged from the data: pain is never-ending, pain is relative, pain is explainable, pain is torment, pain is restrictive, and pain is changeable. Before introducing the imagery technique, pain was described most often as never-ending in both groups. However, this phrase was not expressed by participants after using guided imagery.

Smith, C. A., Collins, C. T., Cyna, A. M., et al. (2006). Complementary and alternative therapies for pain management in labour. Cochrane Database of Systematic Reviews, Issue 4. Retrieved January 2, 2012, from http://www. cochrane.org/reviews/en/ab003521.html

Some women experience labor and childbirth without using drugs and turn to alternatives to manage pain. Alternative

methods include acupuncture, mind–body techniques, massage, reflexology, herbal medicines or homoeopathy, hypnosis, and music. Researchers found evidence that acupuncture and hypnosis may help relieve pain during labor. More research is needed on these and other complementary therapies.

1. For patients using alternative therapies, such as guided imagery, acupuncture, and hypnosis to manage pain in various situations, why do you think these techniques might be effective?

2. When teaching alternative therapies for managing pain, how might you best prepare the setting in order to maximize the effectiveness of the technique?

3. Can you think of reasons why patients might resist trying alternative methods for managing chronic pain? What would you do to encourage patients who seem to oppose the idea of practicing nonpharmacological pain management?

 Go to Chapter 32, **Toward Evidence-Based Practice Suggested Responses,** on *DavisPlus*.

Pharmacological Pain Relief Measures

Analgesics are classified into three groups: nonopioids, opioids, and adjuvants. Many health practitioners use the World Health Organization's (WHO) three-step ladder to assist in the selection and titration of an analgesic (Fig. 32-4). Each step in the ladder represents severity of pain, by which the analgesic selection is determined. Patients in severe pain should start at the third step. Titration is accomplished according to the patient's response. Monitoring should be regular and continuous. If the patient's pain is not controlled, adjust by moving up the pain ladder. To apply the ladder correctly, you need to know the interactions and side effects of all the drugs recommended on each step.

Around-the-Clock Dosing. Administer analgesics at regular times throughout the day if the patient has pain that lasts throughout the day. First, determine the dosage that relieves pain at the desired level; then observe how long the first dose lasts. Administer the next dose before the last dose wears off. Around-the-clock dosing prevents the patient from experiencing severe pain several times a day and is believed to be better than prn (as needed) dosing for pain. Explain to the patient that such dosing will keep pain at an acceptable level throughout the day and allow her to function at an optimal level.

Nonopioid Analgesics

Nonopioid analgesics include a variety of medications that relieve mild to moderate pain. Several of these medications, including acetaminophen (Tylenol), aspirin, ibuprofen (Advil, Motrin), and naproxen (Aleve), are available over the counter. All may be used for acute and chronic pain. Many also reduce inflammation and fever. Most have an onset of action within 1 hour. For more examples of commonly used nonopioid analgesics,

 Go to Chapter 32, **Tables, Boxes, Figures: ESG Box 32-2: Commonly Used Nonopioid Analgesics,** on Davis*Plus*.

The analgesic properties of nonopioid analgesics are often underestimated. Research indicates that 650 mg of aspirin or acetaminophen may relieve as much pain as does 50 mg of oral meperidine or 3 to 5 mg of oxycodone, both of which are narcotic analgesics. Nevertheless, nonopioid analgesics are often compounded with opioids. This allows for a lower dose of opioid to be administered and reduces the incidence of side effects.

Nonsteroidal Anti-Inflammatory Drugs

The largest group of nonopioid analgesics is made up of nonsteroidal anti-inflammatory drugs (NSAIDs). These include aspirin and ibuprofen, as well as several others. NSAIDs act primarily in the peripheral tissues by interfering with the production of prostaglandins. Prostaglandins sensitize pain receptors and are involved with inflammation.

One of the most common side effects of NSAIDs is gastric irritation. Taking the medication with food, lowering the dose, or using enteric-coated pills can reduce the incidence of this side effect. Some of the newer NSAIDs are less irritating to the GI tract, so they markedly decrease gastric irritation and bleeding. However, they are expensive and available only by prescription. NSAIDs should be used with caution in patients with impaired blood clotting, renal disease, and gastrointestinal bleeding or ulcers.

In addition to reducing inflammation, fever, and pain, aspirin can inhibit platelet aggregation (clumping), the first step in clot formation. Myocardial infarction (heart attack), stroke, and thrombophlebitis (a clot in the peripheral veins) are all associated with platelet aggregation. Because of this property, low-dose aspirin (usually 81 mg) is prescribed to decrease risk of these disorders. Regular use of aspirin prolongs clotting time, so teach patients who use aspirin that they will bruise easily and will bleed more if cut.

Combining two NSAIDs is not recommended because it increases the risks of side effects and may not be more effective. However, taking a small daily dose of aspirin to prevent myocardial infarction does not seem to increase the side effects for patients taking other NSAIDs.

Acetaminophen

Unlike most nonopioid analgesics, acetaminophen has very little anti-inflammatory effect. Instead it has analgesic and fever-reducing properties. It has fewer side effects and is probably the safest of the nonopioids. It does not affect platelet function, rarely causes gastrointestinal problems, and can be used in patients who are allergic to aspirin or other NSAIDs. However, even in recommended doses (up to a maximum of 4,000 mg daily), it can cause severe hepatotoxicity (liver toxicity) in patients who consume alcohol and in patients with liver disease.

KnowledgeCheck 32-6

- How do NSAIDs induce pain relief?
- What is the main side effect of NSAIDs?
- In which patients are NSAIDs contraindicated?

Adjuvant Analgesics

Adjuvant analgesics may be used as a primary therapy for mild pain or in conjunction with opioids for moderate to severe pain. Drugs in this category include anticonvulsants, antidepressants, local anesthetics, topical agents, psychostimulants, muscle relaxants, neuroleptics, corticosteroids, and others. **Adjuvant analgesics** reduce the amount of opioid the patient requires. They are especially useful if the patient experiences significant side effects from escalating doses of opioids. Adjuvant analgesics are frequently used in managing

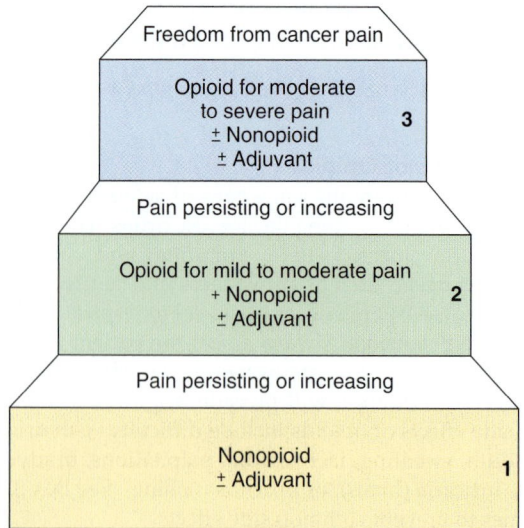

PAIN

FIGURE 32-4 The WHO three-step analgesic ladder. *(Source: World Health Organization [WHO, 1990]. Cancer pain relief and palliative care: Report of a WHO expert committee. WHO Technical Report series, No. 804. Geneva, Switzerland: Author. Used with permission.)*

neuropathic pain, in which they may be the primary treatment or may be used in conjunction with opioids.

Opioid Analgesics

Opioids are natural and synthetic compounds that relieve pain, although they vary in potency. Although analgesia is a complex process, in general opioids work by either stimulating pain receptors or binding with them to block pain impulse. Opiate receptors include mu, delta, kappa, and sigma receptors; however, mu receptors are most effective in relieving pain.

- **Mu (μ) agonist** opioids stimulate mu receptors and are used for acute, chronic, and cancer pain. They include codeine, morphine, hydromorphone (Dilaudid), fentanyl, methadone, and oxycodone. These are excellent medications for **breakthrough pain**—pain that "breaks through" relief provided by analgesics. *Breakthrough analgesia* refers to a rescue, or extra, dose. Drugs used for breakthrough pain should have a rapid onset and short duration. Whenever possible, use the same drug as that given for ongoing pain relief. There is no maximum daily dose limit and no "ceiling" to the level of analgesia from mu agonists. You can steadily increase the dose to relieve pain.
- **Agonist–antagonists** are another group of opioids. These medications stimulate some opioid receptors but block others. Commonly used medications include mixed agonist–antagonists, such as pentazocine (Talwin) and nalbuphine (Nubain), and partial agonists, such as buprenorphine (Buprenex). These medications are appropriate for moderate to severe acute pain. Agonist–antagonists should not be given to patients taking mu agonists (e.g., morphine) because they may act as antagonists at the mu receptor sites and reduce or reverse the analgesia from the mu agonist.

Opioid Effectiveness

The effectiveness of opioids for pain relief can vary depending on people's individual differences in metabolism. Some are classified as poor, intermediate, extensive, and ultrarapid metabolizers. Body size has little to do with appropriate opioid dosing (D'Arcy, 2008b). For instance, a person weighing almost 300 pounds may not receive the same therapeutic effect with the dosage that effectively treats a 90-pound frail, older adult.

Opioids are most effective for certain types of pain. For instance, visceral pain, which is more generalized, is most responsive to opioid treatment, whereas pain of neurological origin tends to be resistant to opioids, requiring that they be given as an adjunct to other therapies (ICSI, 2008).

Patient Misconceptions About Opioids

Some people may be concerned about using opioids because they fear respiratory depression, drug tolerance, drug dependence, and addiction. To help them, you should understand the following concepts:

- **Respiratory depression** can be treated with naloxone (Narcan), an opioid antagonist.
- **Tolerance** to opioids can occur, but increasing the dose or changing the route of administration can correct that problem. There is no ceiling on the analgesic effects of opioids. Because of the problem of cross-tolerance, opioid rotation and new opioid compounds are used to produce better pain relief (D'Arcy, 2008b).
- **Physical dependence** leads to withdrawal symptoms when the drug is removed abruptly; it can be prevented by decreasing the dose slowly over time.
- **Psychological dependence,** commonly called *addiction,* occurs in less than 1% of patients even after long-term

prescribed use of opioids for pain. Thus, fear of addiction should not prevent patients from receiving opioids for appropriate pain relief (Pasero, Manworren, & McCaffery, 2008; Patterson, 2008).

Screening for Abuse Potential

Patients with chronic pain *can* become addicted or abuse drugs. But the addiction is not necessarily *only* because they're taking opioids, but because of their tendencies toward abuse. Considering the prevalence of substance abuse in the general population, assessing the risk for abuse is particularly important for the patient with chronic, nonmalignant pain.

Healthcare professionals often fail to recognize substance abuse unless they actively screen for it. Although you may be uncomfortable asking questions about alcohol and illicit drug use, gathering a reliable substance use history is important to provide a foundation for good pain management, especially for those with chronic pain. This history should include information on the pattern and amount of alcohol intake because patients whose tolerance for alcohol is high may require a higher dose of opioids. You can't rely on the normalcy of behavior to indicate opioid abuse. Random drug screening will show opioid use even when aberrant behavior is not evident (Schneider, 2006–2007). To screen for abuse, use validated risk assessment tools, such as the following:

- The **Opioid Risk Tool (ORT).** This is a five-question, yes/no self-report designed to predict a patient's tendency for aberrant behaviors when prescribed opioid analgesia. To use the Opioid Risk Tool,

 Go to Chapter 32, **Tables, Boxes, Figures: ESG Table 32-2: Using the Opioid Risk Tool,** on Davis*Plus.*

- The **Screener and Opioid Assessment for Patients with Pain (SOAPP®).** This is longer than the ORT and is a highly reliable tool used for assessing patients experiencing chronic pain who might be helped with long-term opioid treatment.
- The **Current Opioid Misuse Measure (COMM™)** is used to identify opioid misuse among patients currently taking long-term opioid medication.

  For more information about the SOAPP® and the COMM™,

 Go to the PainEDU.org Web site at http://www.painedu.org/soapp.asp

Side Effects of Opioids

Most opioids share the same general side effects, but there are some differences among the specific drugs. The most common are drowsiness, nausea, vomiting, and constipation. Some side effects, such as drowsiness and nausea, improve after a few doses. Large doses may lead to respiratory depression and hypotension. Always assess the patient for level of alertness and respiratory status before you administer an opioid. Excessive sedation will precede respiratory depression. Other side effects of opioids include difficulty with urination, dry mouth, sweating, tachycardia, palpitations, bradycardia, rashes, urticaria (hives), or pruritus (itching). See Box 32-4 for strategies to prevent common side effects.

- *Paradoxical reactions.* For some individuals, opioids may lead to a paradoxical increase in pain despite receiving increasing doses of opioids (ICSI, 2008).
- *Sedation.* Most patients experience some degree of sedation at the beginning of opioid therapy or when the dose is increased. For postoperative patients who receive opioids,

BOX 32-4 ■ Preventing and Treating Side Effects From Opioids

Before deciding to add another medication to treat a side effect, consider changing the dose or frequency of the current opioid or changing to another opioid.

Side Effect: Constipation

- Add more fruits, vegetables, and fiber to the diet. Keep in mind, though, that this does not help relieve opioid-induced constipation unless the patient's current fiber intake is deficient. Excessive fiber might even put the patient at risk for bowel obstruction due to the opioid-induced decreased peristalsis (refer to Chapter 29, as needed).
- Increase exercise. Even walking short distances will help.
- Increase oral fluid intake to eight 8-oz. glasses of water per day.
- If needed, administer stool softeners.
- If the above are not effective, administer a mild laxative.
- If constipation continues, soften stool with glycerin suppository and follow up with a soapsuds enema.

Side Effect: Nausea and Vomiting

- Reduce opioid dose by combining nonopioid or adjuvant drugs.
- Teach patients that nausea will usually subside after several doses.
- Premedicate or medicate consecutively with an antiemetic. Be aware this may increase sedation, depending on the antiemetic chosen.
- Teach relaxation techniques.

Side Effect: Pruritus

- Reduce opioid dose by combining with nonopioid or adjuvant drugs.
- Use cool packs, lotion, or topical anesthetics.

- Administer antihistamines, such as diphenhydramine (Benadryl). Be aware that this may increase sedation.
- Teach the patient that he can generally expect to develop a tolerance to pruritus.
- Use distraction techniques, which frequently work well.

Side Effect: Respiratory Depression

- Assess the patient's respiratory status *before* administering the opioid and frequently afterward.
- Reduce the opioid dose by combining with nonopioid or adjuvant drugs.
- Reduce the opioid dose by 25% when you observe signs of oversedation.
- If the patient is not responsive or is only minimally responsive, stop the opioid and administer an antagonist, such as naloxone (Narcan). After dosing with a narcotic antidote, reassess the patient for respiratory depression. Naloxone is metabolized more quickly than opioids and therefore, repeat dosing might be needed.

Side Effect: Drowsiness

- Assess the patient to ensure that the drowsiness is due to opioid administration and not from another cause.
- Teach the patient that drowsiness will generally subside after a few days as she develops tolerance.
- If analgesia is adequate, reduce the opioid by 25%.
- Discontinue all other nonessential CNS depressant medications.
- During the daytime, offer simple stimulants, such as caffeine.
- Offer a lower dose more frequently to decrease peak concentration.
- Consider another opioid or route of administration.

---

use oxygen saturation and transcutaneous CO_2 monitoring to assess for sedation and respiratory depression every 1 to 2 hours during the first 12 to 24 hours after surgery (Jarzyna, Jungquist, Pasero, et al., 2011). For an example of a sedation scale, see the Focused Assessment box, Sedation Rating Scale.

KnowledgeCheck 32-7

- What are the most common side effects of opioids?
- Identify at least three things that you should monitor when administering opioids.
- What is the risk of addiction to opioids for patients with acute pain?

Equianalgesia

Equianalgesia refers to the approximately equal analgesia that a variety of opioids will provide. Equianalgesic dose calculations provide a starting point when changing from one opioid to another or from one route of administration to another. For example, a parenteral dose of 5 mg of morphine is equivalent to 60 mg of parenteral codeine or 100 mg of oral codeine in terms of the analgesic effect that it produces. As another example, 5 mg of parenteral morphine is the equivalent of 15 mg of oral morphine. These doses are approximate and vary according to the number of doses, the variety of opioids the patient has received, and the needs of the patient. To see a table of equianalgesic dosages among opioids,

 Go to Chapter 32, **Tables, Boxes, Figures: ESG Table 32-3: Equianalgesic Doses of Commonly Used Opioid Analgesics,** on Davis*Plus*.

Routes of Administration for Opioid Analgesics

Use the safest and least invasive route to administer opioids. See Box 32-5 for an overview of opioid administration routes.

Patient-Controlled Analgesia (PCA). PCA pumps are a safe way to deliver opioids by IV, epidural, or subcutaneous routes. They provide excellent pain relief and give the patient a sense of control over the pain. The system consists of a programmable infusion pump, a syringe, IV tubing, and a trigger that the patient presses to self-administer a dose. The pump must be programmed so that a dose that can be administered frequently enough to manage the patient's pain effectively. Some providers order a low continuous rate of infusion as a base that can be supplemented with patient-initiated doses. Most PCA pumps can be programmed with 1- or 4-hour maximum medication limits.

If the patient reaches the limit set, the pump will automatically trigger a "lockout" even if the patient keeps pressing the button. Teach patients about this lockout feature; some may not activate the pump enough because they fear overdosing. If you are educating the patient in the postoperative period, make sure she is alert enough to understand the directions and has been given a hearing aid or glasses, if needed.

Sedation Rating Scale

Richmond agitation–sedation scale

Score	Term	Description
+4	Combative	Overtly combative or violent; immediate danger to staff
+3	Very agitated	Pulls on or removes tube(s) or catheter(s) or has aggressive behavior toward staff
+2	Agitated	Frequent nonpurposeful movement or patient–ventilator dyssynchrony
+1	Restless	Anxious or apprehensive but movements not aggressive or vigorous
0	Alert and calm	
−1	Drowsy	Not fully alert, but has sustained (more than 10 seconds) awakening, with eye contact, to voice
−2	Light sedation	Briefly (less than 10 seconds) awakens with eye contact to voice
−3	Moderate sedation	Any movement (but no eye contact) to voice
−4	Deep sedation	No response to voice, but any movement to physical stimulation
−5	Unarousable	No response to voice or physical stimulation

Sessler, C. N., Gosnell, M.S., Grap, M. J., et al. (2002). The Richmond Agitation–Sedation Scale: Validity and reliability in adult intensive care unit patients. *American Journal of Respiratory Critical Care Medicine, 166,* 1338–1344, Retrieved on March 24, 2012, from http://ajrccm.atsjournals.org/content/166/10/1338.full.pdf+html

Focused Assessment

BOX 32-5 ■ Opioid Administration Routes

Oral

The oral route is convenient, safe, and generally produces steady analgesic levels. It is the preferred route of administration unless rapid onset of analgesia is desired. It includes medications that are swallowed but also includes sublingual, transmucosal, buccal, and gingival routes. Use the oral route to relieve mild to severe pain. Oral patient-controlled analgesia (oral PCA) is being used in some hospitals to eliminate the delay between the patient's request for medication and the nurse's administration of it.

Nasal

The intranasal route of administration of drugs has been used for centuries. A rich supply of blood in this area provides the drug easy access to systemic circulation. The mixed agonist–antagonist opioid and the mu agonist can be administered intranasally. One drawback to this route is that it may cause burning or stinging.

Transdermal

The transdermal route delivers a continuous release of drug for up to 72 hours. It is a convenient alternative for a patient who requires constant opioid treatment for pain. Fentanyl (Duragesic) is commonly given as a transdermal patch. Use this route with care on patients who are febrile, because their increased temperature will increase absorption of the drug. This route is effective for ongoing pain relief but does not provide immediate relief. Inform the patient and family about safe storage and proper disposal of transdermal patches. Proper dating and removing patches after the dose is complete can prevent confusion and dosing errors.

Rectal

Suppositories are an excellent alternative to the oral route, especially in infants and young children. This route is effective when the patient is vomiting, has a gastrointestinal obstruction, or is at risk for aspiration of oral medications. The rectal route may be contraindicated in patients with neutropenia or thrombopenia because of the potential to cause rectal bleeding while inserting the suppository.

Subcutaneous

The subcutaneous route may be used for intermittent injections and continuous administration of opioids. Continuous subcutaneous infusion (CSCI) of opioids is gaining popularity. CSCI is appropriate for people who cannot tolerate oral opioids or who have dose-limiting side effects from oral administration (e.g., nausea) and who also have limited venous access. Absorption and distribution vary based on the placement site chosen. Hydromorphone and morphine are the drugs most commonly used. Frequently, CSCI of opioids is used for chronic cancer pain and in palliative care. Continuous infusion is better absorbed, is safer, and provides more continuous relief than the intramuscular (IM) route.

Small portable medication pumps allow the patient to be mobile. However, some patients find this method painful and time consuming. You will need to teach patients and their families how to use the pumps, needles, syringes, and other equipment. Because of the small volume of drug (2 to 3 mL/hr) that can be absorbed, two sites may be needed if higher doses are required.

BOX 32-5 ■ Opioid Administration Routes—cont'd

Intramuscular (IM)

This is not the preferred route of administration of pain medication because IM injections are painful, the onset of action is slow, and absorption is unreliable. With repeated administration, sterile abscesses and fibrotic tissue can result. Nevertheless, the IM route is often used for short-term pain relief postoperatively. This route should be avoided in children because they often refuse pain medication to avoid having an injection.

Intravenous (IV)

The IV route produces immediate pain relief and is desirable for acute or escalating pain. It is most commonly used for short-term therapy and for hospitalized patients who can be monitored. It is also used in the home care setting for patients with cancer and other pain who are unable to tolerate oral opioids. Methods of IV delivery include continuous infusions, bolus, and patient-controlled analgesia (PCA). Patients using a continuous infusion can deliver a bolus for breakthrough pain or procedures such as wound care. Drawbacks to the IV route include the need for venous access and the need to maintain a patent line. Patients who previously used oral opioids may find the IV equipment cumbersome but they typically report less pain and fewer side effects than with the oral route.

Intra-articular

A pain pump is implanted into a joint during arthroscopic surgery to control postsurgical pain. A pain pump provides relief to patients by delivering continuous infusion of local anesthetic directly to the joint.

Intraspinal and Epidural Analgesics

Intraspinal analgesia requires placement of a catheter in the subarachnoid space (for intrathecal analgesia) or the epidural space by an anesthesiologist or a certified registered nurse anesthetist (CRNA). The epidural space (Fig. 32-5) is generally preferred because it poses less risk of complications although they can occur (e.g., dural puncture, infection, hematoma, and nerve damage). Placement of the catheter, as well as the type

and concentration of medication, determines the area affected by the medication. Higher doses are needed for epidural than for intrathecal administration.

The most commonly used opioids for epidural administration are morphine sulfate (Duramorph), fentanyl citrate (Sublimaze), and hydromorphone (Dilaudid, Palladone). Local anesthetics are frequently combined with the opioids to reduce the total amount of drug necessary to produce analgesia. For nursing care activities associated with caring for a client with an epidural catheter for pain management, see Clinical Insight 32-2.

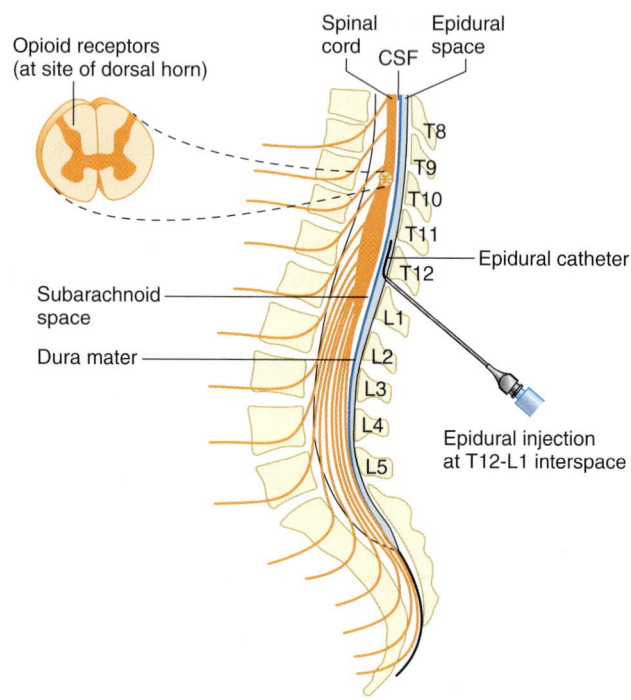

FIGURE 32-5 Placement of an epidural needle and catheter.

Because of the potential to overdose the patient, only nurses who are trained in PCAs should set up and program the pump. As a safeguard, another nurse should double-check the setup before patient use. Encourage patients to administer a dose before potentially painful activities, such as walking or physical therapy. PCA pumps are contraindicated in patients who have limited ability to understand directions. For detailed instruction on using a PCA pump, see Procedure 32-1.

ThinkLike a Nurse 32-7

- What routes of opioid administration have you seen in your clinical rotation?
- What types of pain relief and side effects have you observed?
- What routes of administration would you like to see? Why?

Chemical Pain Relief Measures

Nerve blocks and **epidural injection** are types of regional anesthesia. An anesthetic agent is injected into or around the nerve or network of nerves (*plexus*) that supplies sensation to a specific part of the body. Nerve blocks may be used for

short-term pain relief after surgical procedures or for long-term management of chronic pain. See Clinical Insight 32-2 to learn about caring for a patient with an epidural catheter.

Local anesthesia is the injection of local anesthetics into body tissues. Short-acting agents (e.g., lidocaine) and long-acting agents (e.g., marcaine) may be used. Local anesthetics are injected into subcutaneous tissue for minor surgical procedures. They may also be injected into joints and muscle for pain relief. Pumps are commonly used to administer local anesthetics at surgical sites for postoperative pain relief.

Topical anesthesia involves applying an agent that contains cocaine, lidocaine, or benzocaine directly to the skin, mucous membranes, wounds, or burns. Topical anesthesia is quickly absorbed and provides pain relief for mild to moderate pain. Many topical anesthetics are available over the counter. Sunburn relief agents, gel products for tooth and gum pain, and first aid sprays are forms of topical anesthetics.

Radiofrequency Ablation Therapy

Radiofrequency ablation therapy uses electromagnetic waves that travel at the speed of light to target nerves that carry pain impulses. This procedure is used to provide longer-term pain

Clinical Insight 32-2 ➤ Caring for the Patient With an Epidural Catheter

Intraspinal analgesia is contraindicated in patients who received anticoagulant therapy or who have spinal defects, local or systemic infections, or increased intracranial pressure.

Monitoring

- Monitor for respiratory depression (every hour for the first 24 hr, then every 4 hr if the patient is stable).
- Monitor the site for leaking or drainage.
- Check connections for leaks. This can be fixed by carefully retightening connections. If the filter is cracked, replace with a new one using sterile technique.
- Assess for urine retention. Keep careful intake and output (I&O) records. Urinary retention is one side effect of epidural opioids.
- Observe for signs of headache in the patient as a result of dural puncture. Treatment consists of bedrest, analgesics, and liberal hydration. Caffeine is also helpful and may be administered IV. If unresolved after 72 hours, patient might receive an epidural blood patch.
- Observe for signs of catheter migration: nausea, a decrease in blood pressure, and a loss of motor function without a recognizable cause.

Prevention

- Mark all epidural lines *clearly,* for patient safety. This line must not be confused with an arterial or venous catheter.

- Ensure that the tape on the tubing connected to the patient is secure. To prevent catheter migration.
- Use strict aseptic technique when changing tubing, including mask and sterile gloves for access and maintenance procedures.

Discontinuing the Catheter

- If you are specially trained to remove an epidural catheter, first loosen the tape securing the catheter. While wearing clean gloves, apply slow, steady pressure to withdraw the catheter. Inspect the catheter on removal. You must be able to see the tip of the catheter. If not, a portion of the catheter may still be lodged in the patient's epidural space. Notify the anesthesia team immediately of this finding.
- If the catheter cannot be withdrawn with minimal force, try repositioning the patient to the same position for removal as the patient was in during insertion of the catheter.
- Cleanse the insertion site, and cover with a dry sterile dressing.

---

relief than that provided by injections of steroids or pain relievers and nerve blocks.

Surgical Interruption of Pain Conduction Pathways

Surgical interruption of pain conduction pathways results in permanent destruction of nerve pathways. It is used as a last resort for intractable pain. The various options depend on the type and location of pain.

- **Cordotomy** interrupts pain and temperature sensation below the tract that is severed. This is most frequently done for leg and trunk pain.
- **Rhizotomy** interrupts the anterior or posterior nerve route that is located between the ganglion and the cord. Anterior interruption is generally used to stop spastic movements that accompany paraplegia, and posterior interruption eliminates pain in the area innervated. This procedure may be safely performed at any level along the spine but is most often used for head and neck pain produced by cancer.
- **Neurectomy** is used to eliminate intractable localized pain. The pathways of peripheral or cranial nerves are interrupted to block pain transmission.
- **Sympathectomy** severs the paths to the sympathetic division of the autonomic nervous system. This procedure is performed to improve vascular blood supply and eliminate vasospasm. It is used to treat the pain from vascular disorders, such as Raynaud's disease.

Surgical therapies disrupting pain pathways are not widely used due to advances in oral and transdermal opioid therapies.

Knowledge Check 32-8

- Identify three types of chemical pain relief measures.
- What type of patient might be suitable for surgical interruption of a pain pathway?

Misconceptions That Interfere With Pain Management

Pain is invisible to others but it exists when the patient says it does. It exists even when there are no sure signs of pain or an apparent cause.

Patients, caregivers, and clinicians sometimes have beliefs about pain or pain management strategies that interfere with the treatment plan. For instance, one older patient may fear that severe pain is a sign of weakness and try to endure it; another might perceive pain as a part of the normal physical declines that accompany aging instead of an acute situation that requires treatment. An athlete might believe "no pain, no gain," but actually pain can signal a problem. Or one family member may worry that pain medication may make the patient nonfunctional; whereas others might fear addiction to pain medication even though non-narcotic analgesics are not addictive.

The beliefs of healthcare providers can also interfere with pain management. For example, nurses and other caregivers

sometimes doubt the patient's report of pain because of the following:

- Most people don't have pain from that particular illness or procedure.
- There is no obvious, physical cause for the pain.
- They are concerned about drug-seeking behavior and patient addiction.

As you care for patients in pain, remain open to the patient's description of pain, and work with the patient and caregivers to provide pain control. Table 32-1 highlights some of the most common misconceptions about pain.

Managing Pain in Older Adults

Pain, particularly persistent pain, is common among older adults, especially those suffering from degenerative spine conditions, arthritis, nightly leg pain, or pain as a result of cancer. Pain management among older patients is especially difficult. Most older adults have at least one chronic condition and take multiple medications. Adding analgesics to an already complex medication regimen increases the likelihood of drug interactions. In addition, drug distribution is altered in older patients because of changes in blood flow to the organs, protein binding, and the difference in body composition. Older adults are at great risk for undertreatment of pain because they and their caregivers may be reluctant to administer analgesics for fear of producing confusion, excessive sedation, drug interactions, and respiratory depression (American Geriatrics Society, 2009).

Another problem for sufficiently treating pain in older adults is that healthcare providers often fail to recognize because of the patient's dementia, coexisting medical conditions, sensory impairment, or inability to verbally communicate the quality or intensity of pain. At the same time, there is a risk of overtreatment due to the higher peak effect and longer duration of pain relief that they experience as a result of changes associated with aging (American Geriatrics Society, Panel on Persistent Pain in Older Persons, 2002; Christo, 2009). Poor pain management can result in falls, poor sleep, delayed healing, reduced activity, prolonged hospitalization, anxiety, and poor quality of life (Horgas, 2007).

Persistent pain is not a normal part of aging and should not be ignored. There is a major change in the 2009 American Geriatrics Society guidelines for managing persistent pain in older adults. Original guidelines recommended seniors use over-the-counter or prescription NSAIDs, such as aspirin or ibuprofen, before being prescribed an opioid drug. However, in light of increased cardiovascular risk and gastrointestinal toxicity in this population, the American Geriatrics Society, Panel on Persistent Pain in Older Persons now recommends that all patients with moderate to severe pain or diminished quality of life due to pain should be considered for opioid therapy. Acetaminophen should be considered for treatment of persistent pain, particularly musculoskeletal pain, in light of its effectiveness and safety. The guidelines also provide recommendations about the use of adjuvant therapy for older persons with recurring pain.

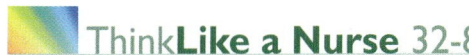

ThinkLike a Nurse 32-8

Which groups of patients are most at risk for inadequate pain management?

- What can you do to assist each group?
- How do past pain experiences affect present pain experience?

Managing Pain in Patients With Substance Abuse or Active Addiction

It is important to differentiate between physical dependence, which is expected and treatable, and addiction. **Addiction** is a state of psychological dependence in which a person uses a drug compulsively and will engage in self-destructive behavior to obtain the drug. Many studies have shown that the properly managed, short-term medical use of opioid analgesic drugs is safe and rarely causes addiction with the exception of those with a personal or family history of drug abuse or mental illness (NIH, National Institute on Drug Abuse, 2005).

Nevertheless, substance abuse is a common problem within our society and is a problem among individuals from all backgrounds. Behaviors that may indicate substance abuse or addiction include the following:

- Repeated requests for injections of an opioid or atypical high dosing when pain should normally be diminishing with recovery from an injury or surgery
- Refusal to try oral medication for pain relief

Table 32-1 ➤ Common Misconceptions Among Patients and Caregivers About Pain	
FALLACY	**TRUTH**
The caregiver is more objective than the patient about the amount of pain experienced.	The patient's report is the "gold standard," and the patient is the authority.
You should wait until the pain is severe before taking medication.	You should take pain medication early and on a regular basis if pain is severe.
There is a significant danger of addiction to pain medications.	Patients in pain rarely become addicted to their pain medications.
Pain is a normal component of aging.	Pain is a symptom that something is wrong and should be treated.
Complaining of pain will label the person as a "bad patient."	The patient should report pain so that it can be treated.
Patients should have severe pain only if they have major surgery.	Even minor surgery and injury can produce severe pain.
Patients will have visible physical or behavioral signs if they are really in pain.	Even when patients are in severe pain, they may not exhibit physical or behavioral signs.

- "Doctor shopping"—moving from provider to provider in an effort to obtain multiple prescriptions for the drug(s) the person abuses
- "Pharmacy shopping"—using multiple pharmacies to dispense controlled substances

If you observe these signs, assess the patient carefully because the signs may also indicate untreated withdrawal or increased pain due to complications. When dealing with clients with active addiction, try to assume a nonjudgmental approach.

Although it is important to recognize opioid addiction, you must be careful not to undertreat pain in patients whom you know or suspect to abuse substances. As a nurse, you will be in a position to help maintain the balance between providing adequate pain relief and protecting against inappropriate drug use.

 Think**Like a Nurse** 32-9

You are preparing to give your patient a bath. When you remove his bath equipment from under the bedside table, you find illicit drugs mixed in with the bath equipment. What would you do?

Pain Relief From Placebos

A **placebo** is defined as "any medication or procedure, including surgery, that produces an effect in a patient because of its implicit or explicit intent, not because of its specific physical or chemical properties" (McCaffery & Pasero, 1999, p. 36). Placebos contain inactive substances that do not chemically provide analgesia. Clearly, placebos can relieve pain for some patients, but how they do so is not well understood. Theories include operant conditioning, faith, anxiety reduction, and endorphin release. Although use of placebos may be appropriate in clinical trials, they are not suitable for pain management for the following reasons:

- If the patient responds to a placebo, it does not mean that the patient did not have pain. In classic studies done in the 1950s, 36% of patients demonstrated adequate pain relief from a placebo injection the day after abdominal surgery (Evans, 1974). However, there is no way to determine in advance which patients will experience pain relief; therefore, you risk inadequately treating the patient.
- Even in the same patient, placebos may relieve pain at one time and not at another.
- Ethically, the most important reason for not using placebos is that their use involves deceit. If discovered, and it frequently is, the patient's trust in healthcare professionals may be diminished, if not destroyed.

Teaching the Patient and Family About Pain

Patients and caregivers tend to cope more effectively when they are well informed. Because pain can interfere with a patient's learning, be sure to include the patient's family in your teaching. If the patient is discharged from the facility with a prescription for opioids, teach the family how to monitor for excessive sedation and to call the healthcare provider if pain relief is not adequate. You should discuss the following topics with the patient and family:

- The cause of the pain, if it is known
- The normal duration of the pain, if known (e.g., postoperative pain generally decreases every day as tissues heal)
- How to use the selected pain scale; ask for a demonstration of use

- The overall pain management plan
- Information about the analgesic prescribed—dose, interval, and route of administration
- If opioids are prescribed, explanation that the risk of addiction is extremely low
- Nonpharmacological ways to treat pain
- Side effects to assess
- The need to alter the treatment plan if relief is not achieved
- How to contact the healthcare team regarding side effects, missed doses, change in condition, or ineffective pain management

Documentation

Thoroughly document the pain management plan and the patient's responses. Documentation may be narrative, in either nursing or interdisciplinary notes, or recorded on a pain management flow sheet. Although documentation varies from facility to facility, it typically reflects the entire spectrum of the nursing process:

- The expected outcome for pain management
- The patient's present pain level
- The patient's responses to any intervention for pain
- Any adverse reactions that may have resulted from the analgesic
- Planned interventions to improve pain relief if needed

Typically, pain management flow sheets contain a column for time, pain ratings, and analgesic used, including dose and route, vital signs, and side effects. They are tailored to the patient population, the type of pain being monitored, and the clinical setting. For example, the pain flow sheet for a patient using an IV PCA pump is more complex than a pain flow sheet for a patient taking oral medications at home. Documentation is important because typically pain recall is poor and patients often underestimate their pain after the fact. If pain is not adequately documented, there is no way to prove that it was accurately assessed. For an example of a pain flow sheet,

 Go to Chapter 32, **Tables, Boxes, Figures: ESG Table 32-4: Pain Flow Sheet,** on Davis*Plus*.

 EVALUATION

Evaluation is critical to pain management. Compare your findings with the expected outcomes to determine whether the pain management strategy is effective. Questions to ask include the following:

- Are the patient's pain scores consistently at or better than the desired level? Are they improving?
- Is the patient's behavior, mobility, range of motion, mood, and affect consistent with pain relief?
- What is the quality of the patient's life, according to the patient's standards?

In addition to evaluating the extent of pain relief, you need to determine which interventions were or were not effective, as well as any adverse reactions to the interventions. Close examination of the patient's pain diary should provide most of the data you need for evaluation.

It is important to reassess the patient's pain regularly. An increase in pain may be a sign of inadequate pain management, but it may instead be a sign of developing complications. Before changing the treatment plan, you should determine whether the plan was carried out correctly. If the healthcare team decides to make a change, remember to again

evaluate the effect of the change. Do not assume the new intervention will provide adequate pain relief.

NURSING PROCESS IN ACTION

Mary Jean Thompson, 30 years old, was admitted to the hospital with severe abdominal pain and underwent an appendectomy yesterday. The physician has prescribed hydromorphone (Dilaudid) 2 mg tablet PO q 4–6 hr prn for pain. Ms. Thompson doesn't like the idea of taking pain medication and waits until she rates her pain a 9 or 10 on a scale of 0 to 10 before requesting an injection. Even after the medication, her pain never drops below a 7 on a scale of 0 to 10 and she is unwilling to turn or ambulate due to the pain.

When you perform your assessment, she tells you she does not want to be sedated. "I hate that groggy, drugged feeling. I'm willing to have some pain to avoid that." After you discuss the importance of pain management to aid in healing and ability to participate in activities and therapy, Ms. Thompson states that she would like to have a pain score of 3 to 4 today. See the accompanying care plan, Pain Management: Nursing Care, and Care Map for the nurse's application of nursing process for Ms. Thompson.

Nursing Diagnosis: Acute Pain (surgical incision) related to possible inadequate analgesia (drug and dosing) because of reluctance to have IM injection, as manifested by not requesting medication until her pain is at a score of 9.

EXPECTED OUTCOMES	NURSING INTERVENTIONS	RATIONALE
On a scale of 0–10, the patient will verbalize pain relief at a score of 3 or below while in bed and 4 or below while ambulating at all times.	Assess and document the patient's verbal and nonverbal expressions of pain relief with each check of vital signs, with every procedure and ambulation, and when the patient is at rest.	Assessment is necessary to determine the effectiveness of the prescribed medications. Assessment and documentation are legal responsibilities for the nurse as well.
	Discuss with the prescriber the need to modify prescriptions if pain relief measures are ineffective. Recommend PCA.	Ineffective pain management will cause the patient increased stress and can lead to further complications because the patient will be unwilling to move.
	When you obtain new pain orders for a PCA morphine pump, educate the patient about the pump.	A patient using PCA requires instruction about safe use of the pump.
	Provide nonpharmacological interventions, such as a back rub or other techniques described in this chapter, before rest or sleep, with any exacerbation of pain, and after painful procedures such as ambulation.	Nonpharmacological interventions are synergistic and enhance the relief the opioid gives.
The patient will demonstrate pain relief by participating in ambulation and turning within 24 hours.	Teach the patient to press the PCA pump before activities.	Peak blood levels enable the patient to ambulate, cough and deep-breathe, and perform activities of daily living.

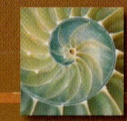

Care Map

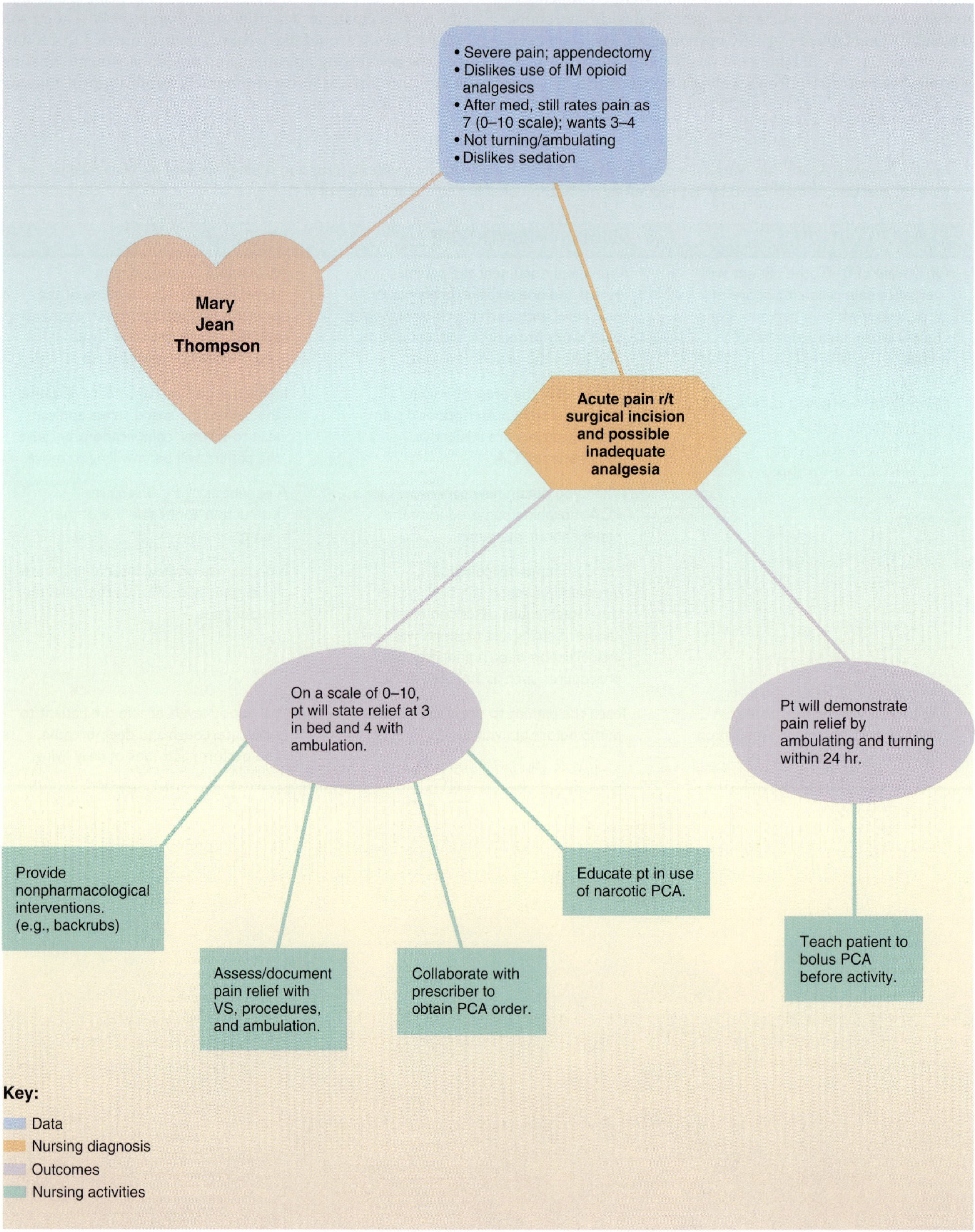

Data:
- Severe pain; appendectomy
- Dislikes use of IM opioid analgesics
- After med, still rates pain as 7 (0–10 scale); wants 3–4
- Not turning/ambulating
- Dislikes sedation

Mary Jean Thompson

Acute pain r/t surgical incision and possible inadequate analgesia

On a scale of 0–10, pt will state relief at 3 in bed and 4 with ambulation.

Pt will demonstrate pain relief by ambulating and turning within 24 hr.

Provide nonpharmacological interventions. (e.g., backrubs)

Assess/document pain relief with VS, procedures, and ambulation.

Collaborate with prescriber to obtain PCA order.

Educate pt in use of narcotic PCA.

Teach patient to bolus PCA before activity.

Key:
- Data
- Nursing diagnosis
- Outcomes
- Nursing activities

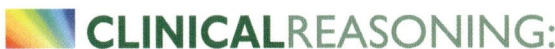 **CLINICAL**REASONING:
Applying the **Full-Spectrum Nursing Model**

Because the following critical thinking activities allow you to practice the kind of thinking you will use as a full-spectrum nurse, they usually have no single right answer. Discuss them with your peers—if you have difficulty with any of the questions, consult your instructor.

PATIENT SITUATION

Mr. Dieter Schmidt is a 48-year-old with a 2-year history of cervical spine injury that began after a motor vehicle accident (MVA). Three years prior to the accident, Mr. Schmidt fell through a roof to the cement basement when inspecting a building under construction. Presenting symptoms were neck pain when turning his head, biceps weakness, and pain down the arm with tingling into the fingertips. He is unable to sit for extended periods or walk distances. Initially he received treatment with medication, TENS to the site, physical therapy, and cervical fusion. Despite trying all treatments available to him, including surgery, Dieter continues to suffer chronic pain and fatigue. After prolonged suffering with no relief, he develops a cynical attitude toward healthcare. Dieter begins missing more and more scheduled appointments for physical therapy. He describes stress he feels with an economic downturn affecting his land development business and fears bankruptcy. As a result, he has given up previous hobbies and most social activities. His relationships with his family and friends are increasingly strained as the pain persists over time.

THINKING

1. *Theoretical Knowledge:* What is the mechanism that explains how pain is transmitted in the spine?
2. *Critical Thinking (Considering Alternatives, Deciding What to Do):*
   a. When planning care for Mr. Schmidt, what approach would you take in helping him to set goals for his rehabilitation?
   b. Why do you think Mr. Schmidt displays a negative attitude and reduced compliance toward rehabilitative therapies?

DOING

3. *Practical Knowledge:*
   a. *Nursing Process (Assessment):* What questions would you ask Mr. Schmidt to assess the impact of pain on his daily living and quality of life?
   b. *Nursing Process (Interventions):* In addition to drug therapy, what other measures might you teach your patient to perform for controlling pain and promoting comfort?

CARING

4. *Self-Knowledge:* Have you experienced chronic pain, such as back pain, fibromyalgia, arthritis, migraines, sports injuries, or other types? If so, how has it affected your daily life? Has your pain affected your relationships? Has it interfered with your job or recreational activities? What other ways would you say chronic pain has reduced the quality of your life?

 Go To Chapter 32, **Clinical Reasoning: Applying the Full-Spectrum Nursing Model Response Sheet,** on Davis*Plus.*

PracticalKnowledge
procedures

The following procedure provides the practical knowledge you will need to assist patients with reducing pain. More and more, medication is being administered by patient-controlled analgesia. Although pump operation differs among manufacturers, you should understand in general how pumps work. Be prepared to consult manufacturers' directions when you must use an unfamiliar pump in the clinical setting.

Procedure 32–1 ■ Setting Up and Managing Patient-Controlled Analgesia by Pump

➤ For steps to follow in *all* procedures, refer to the Universal Steps for All Procedures found on the page facing the inside back cover.

Equipment

- PCA pump (infuser and central unit)
- Manufacturer's instructions for the pump
- Cartridge, syringe, or other type of sealed unit containing the medication
- Connecting tubing (to connect the PCA device to the patient's IV line)
- Maintenance IV supplies, as needed
- IV pole
- Antiseptic swab
- Flow sheet
- One pair of clean procedure gloves (if venipuncture is necessary)

Delegation

Because a narcotic medication is delivered intravenously to the patient, this procedure is outside the scope of practice of nursing assistive personnel (NAP) and should never be delegated. Furthermore, the NAP should not administer a dose for the patient, even if he asks her to do so. You can inform the NAP of expected side effects and ask her to report her observations to you.

Pre-Procedure Assessment

- Assess physical conditions that can affect respirations.
  Respiratory diseases (e.g., chronic obstructive pulmonary disease [COPD] and asthma) and conditions such as head injury and sleep apnea increase the risk for respiratory depression with opioid use.
- Assess level of consciousness and cognitive level.
  Determines whether the patient will be able to follow directions for self-dosing.

- Review lab values reflecting liver and kidney function, such as blood urea nitrogen [BUN], creatinine, and liver enzymes.
  Narcotic analgesics are typically metabolized through the liver or kidneys.
- Assess the baseline respiratory rate, pulse, blood pressure, and oxygen saturation.
  A change in vital signs (e.g., hypotension, respiratory rate below 12) may indicate adverse responses to narcotic administration.
- Be aware of the patient's age and weight.
  Age is a factor when you are verifying the dose. Older patients and very young children are at increased risk for respiratory suppression, so require lower doses. Pediatric doses are based on the child's weight.
- Assess the patient's baseline pain level using a standardized pain assessment tool or numeric scale ranging from 0 to 10.
- Assess the patient's manual dexterity.
  Patients with impaired fine motor control or upper extremity injury may not be able to operate the self-dosing mechanism.
- Review medications currently in use.
  The risk of respiratory suppression increases when a PCA pump is used in conjunction with other central nervous system (CNS) depressants, such as diazepam (Valium).
- Assess the extent of family involvement. Identify any family anxiety over the patient's pain. Reinforce that only the patient should use the PCA button.
  Only the patient should administer the medication. "PCA by proxy" (someone other than the patient pushing the dosing button) is a major factor contributing to adverse patient outcomes (Hagle, Lehr, Brubakken, et al., 2004).

➤ When performing the procedure, always identify your patient according to agency policy and be attentive to standard precautions, hand hygiene, patient safety and privacy, body mechanics, and documentation.

Procedure Steps

1. **Don clean procedure gloves**, and initiate IV therapy if the patient does not currently have an IV solution infusing. Refer to Procedure 39-1 as needed.

2. **Obtain the medication and double-check** it with the original prescription. You may need to remove air from the vial by pushing the injector into the vial. Connect the PCA tubing to the vial (or cartridge).
   Some vials may not be completely filled with medication. Ejecting the air makes it faster to prime the connecting tubing.

3. **Double-check your dose calculation** with another nurse before starting the infusion or wasting medication.
   To prevent medication errors in dosing.
   a. One-time "bolus" (or loading) dose, which you administer after setting up the pump
   b. Basal rate (the amount of medication to be delivered automatically by the pump over 1 hour)
   c. "On-demand" dose (the amount of drug to be delivered with each push of the button)
   d. The "lockout" interval (the number of minutes allowed between each

administration of an on-demand dose [e.g., q10 min]). Even if the patient pushes the button more frequently, the PCA pump will not administer a dose until the preset time between doses has been met.
   e. The 1-hour or 4-hour lockout dosage limit (the maximum dose allowed in that time frame). For example, if the patient has a 4 mg on-demand dose with a 10-minute lockout interval, the patient can receive a maximum of six 4-mg doses per hour for a total of 24 mg/hr and a maximum dose of 96 mg in 4 hours.

NOTE: PCA prescriptions are usually written in milligrams; however, pump settings may be in milliliters. In such cases, you must verify the concentration (milligrams per milliliter) to set the pump correctly.

4. Prime the tubing; then clamp the tubing above the connector.

Priming prevents air from entering the pump and causing malfunction. Clamping prevents accidental bolus of medication to the patient.

5. Insert the cartridge or vial injector into the pump, and lock the pump. Follow the manufacturer's instruction manual (e.g., some pumps can be set only if the door is closed and locked).

Depending on the pump, it may be a syringe, a cartridge, or other sealed container that can be "locked" into the pump. Locking the pump prevents unauthorized access to the narcotic and dosing features.

6. Turn the pump on, and set the parameters according to the prescriptions and your calculations. The settings may include the following:
- One-time bolus dose
- Basal rate
- On-demand
- The lockout interval
- The 1-hour or 4-hour lockout dosage limit

7. Scrub the port on the IV tubing closest to the patient, using alcohol or chlorhexidine alcohol-based product; then connect the PCA pump tubing.

Removes gross contamination and discourages growth of pathogens.

8. Open the clamp and administer the bolus (loading) dose if prescribed. Remain with the patient as the dose is delivered. To administer a loading dose, set the pump lockout time to 0 minutes. Set the volume to be delivered as the bolus volume you calculated (e.g., if 10 mg = 0.2 mL, set the volume to 0.2 mL); press the button that controls the loading dose.

A loading dose is usually larger than the basal and on-demand doses because pain is likely to be more severe before the pump is initiated. Remaining with the patient allows you to observe for adverse effects.

9. Close the pump door, and lock the machine with the key.

10. Check for flashing lights or alarms that may indicate the need to correct settings.

11. If you clamped the tubing, be sure to release tubing clamps; press the start button to begin the basal infusion.

12. Ensure that the battery life is sufficient or, preferably, that the pump is plugged into an appropriate electrical outlet.

To avoid battery failure.

13. Put the control button for on-demand doses within the patient's reach. Be sure the PCA cord is placed away from the call bell.

To avoid error in self-dosing with PCA.

? What if . . .

- **The patient cannot verbally communicate pain status?**

  Use an alternate standardized pain tool such as the FACES pain scale or a behavioral measure to determine pain level.

  Pain assessment in patients who are uncommunicative may include behavioral or physiological indicators to assess and monitor the effectiveness of pain medication.

- **The infusion infiltrates?**

  Discontinue the IV and establish another IV site. Follow facility policy for application of cold or warm compresses to the infiltrated area. Assess pain level. You may need to contact the prescriber for a bolus dose if the IV has been interrupted for an extended period or the patient has insufficient pain relief.

Evaluation

- Monitor the patient's pain level, sedation level, and respiratory rate at least every hour for the first 24 hours or according to facility policy after initiating PCA.

  Promotes the early detection of respiratory depression, oversedation, or inadequate pain control.

- Perform routine assessment of number and frequency of doses and pump settings per facility protocol.
- Check the IV site for redness, infiltration, or phlebitis.
- Check the IV tubing for patency (e.g., for kinks) to be sure the medication is infusing.

Patient Teaching

Patients who are candidates for use of PCA should be trained before surgery rather than in the immediate postoperative period, when the effects of anesthesia impair learning. Reinforce or teach the patient and family the following:
- Safe and correct use of the PCA pump
- The benefits of PCA for controlling pain

- The pump will deliver only the amount of medication prescribed. Pushing the button too many times will not result in overdosing.
- The patient cannot accidentally roll over on the button and unintentionally give additional medication.
- If pain is not being relieved, the patient should tell the nurse so adjustments can be made to the PCA.
- The pump will alarm when nearly empty, alerting nurses to change the syringe.
- The PCA button is to relieve pain—not to help the patient sleep.
- Signs and symptoms of allergic reaction and which ones to report.
- How to rate pain using a standard pain scale
- ✚ The patient is the only one who may push the pain-dosing button. Explain why family members should not give "doses by proxy."

Procedure 32-1 ■ Setting Up and Managing Patient-Controlled Analgesia by Pump (continued)

Documentation

You will usually document PCA initiation on a specialized flow sheet. Items charted include the following:

- Time the infusion was begun, including the drug, the loading dose, the basal dose, and lockout and hourly limit
- Patient's baseline pain level and evaluation of subsequent pain level performed at intervals determined by facility policy
- Baseline respiratory rate, pulse, blood pressure, and oxygen saturation; routine evaluation of subsequent vital signs performed at intervals determined by facility policy
- Sedation level
- Continuous monitoring of vital signs, level of consciousness, and pain status as well as the number and frequency of doses
- Unusual occurrences (e.g., oversedation, IV infiltration) in the nursing notes

To explore learning resources for this chapter,

  Go to Davis*Plus* at http://davisplus.fadavis.com, keyword Treas:

Chapter Resources for Chapter 32:
   Knowledge Check and Think Like a Nurse Response Sheets
   Knowledge Check Answers
   Resources for Caregivers and Health Professionals
   Reading More About Pain (suggested readings)
   What Are the Main Points in This Chapter?
NCLEX-Style Review Questions
Chapter Overview Podcasts

Thinking About the Procedure

  Go to the *Fundamentals of Nursing Skills Videos,* **Pain Management: Patient-Controlled Analgesia.**

1. Why does the nurse close the door of the pump before priming the IV tubing?
2. What vital step does the nurse do before connecting IV tubing to the patient's IV line?

  For suggested responses, go to Chapter 32, **Thinking About the Procedure Suggested Responses,** on Davis*Plus.*

Practice Resources

Best practices, 2008; Cohen, Weber, & Moss, 2006; d'Arcy, 2008; National Guideline Clearinghouse, 2009.

Concept Map

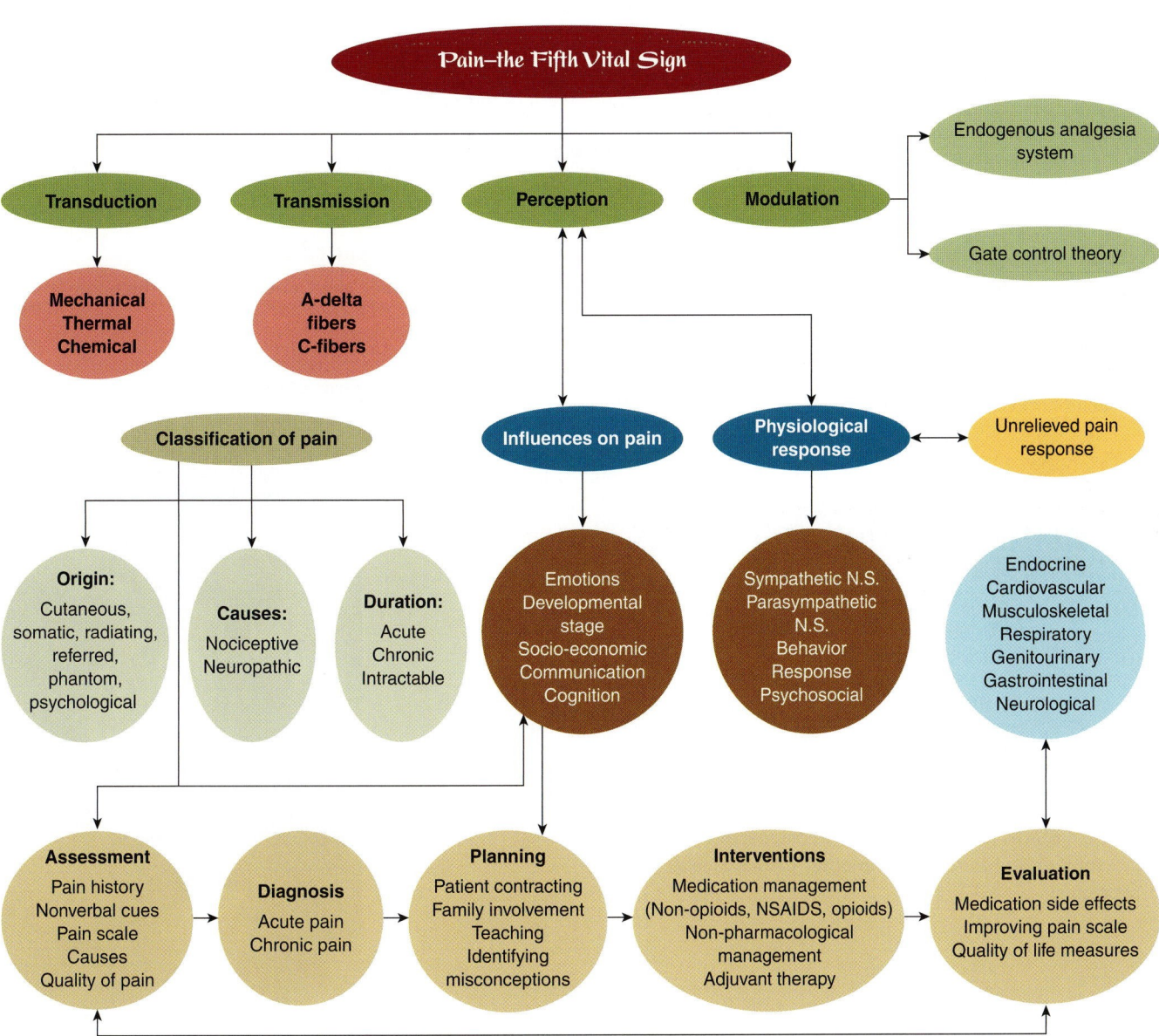

Pain–the Fifth Vital Sign

Transduction

Transmission

Perception

Modulation

Endogenous analgesia system

Gate control theory

Mechanical Thermal Chemical

A-delta fibers C-fibers

Classification of pain

Influences on pain

Physiological response

Unrelieved pain response

Origin: Cutaneous, somatic, radiating, referred, phantom, psychological

Causes: Nociceptive Neuropathic

Duration: Acute Chronic Intractable

Emotions Developmental stage Socio-economic Communication Cognition

Sympathetic N.S. Parasympathetic N.S. Behavior Response Psychosocial

Endocrine Cardiovascular Musculoskeletal Respiratory Genitourinary Gastrointestinal Neurological

Assessment Pain history Nonverbal cues Pain scale Causes Quality of pain

Diagnosis Acute pain Chronic pain

Planning Patient contracting Family involvement Teaching Identifying misconceptions

Interventions Medication management (Non-opioids, NSAIDS, opioids) Non-pharmacological management Adjuvant therapy

Evaluation Medication side effects Improving pain scale Quality of life measures

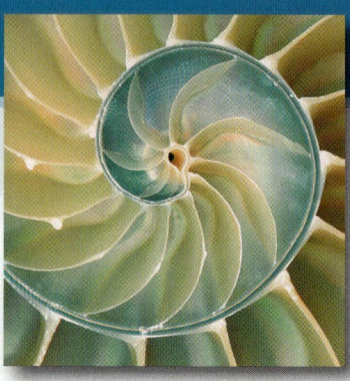

Activity & Exercise

Learning Outcomes

After completing this chapter, you should be able to:

- Discuss the physiology of movement
- Use proper body mechanics when providing patient care.
- Discuss the concept of fitness.
- Describe the five types of exercise discussed in this chapter.
- Compare the effects of exercise and immobility on the body.
- Describe the physical activity recommended for health promotion,

cardiovascular fitness, and maintenance of healthy weight.
- Discuss factors that affect body alignment and activity.
- Identify patients who are at risk for immobility or activity intolerance.
- Develop a plan of care for patients with decreased activity tolerance.
- Implement care related to a patient's mobility problems.

Key Concepts

Activity
Fitness
Mobility

Related Concepts

See the Concept Map at the end of this chapter.

Example Problem

Hazards of immobility

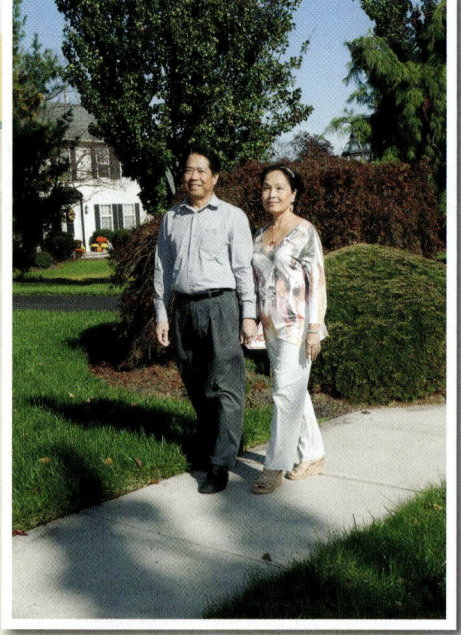

Caring for the Nguyens

This feature allows you to practice the kind of thinking you will use as a full-spectrum nurse. There is usually more than one correct answer to a critical thinking question, so we do not provide answers for these features. It is more important to develop your nursing judgment than to "cover content." Discuss the questions with your peers. If you are still unsure, consult your instructor.

As you may recall, Nam Nguyen has been advised to diet and exercise as part of the treatment plan for hypertension, type 2 diabetes mellitus, obesity, and osteoarthritis. Zach Jackson's exam has revealed no other cardiovascular problems.

A. Design a fitness program for Nam. Describe the program in detail. Recall that Nam has been relatively sedentary.

B. Compare the type of program you would recommend for Nam with the type of program appropriate for his grandson, Kim.

C. What type of fitness program would be most appropriate for Mai Nguyen, Nam's mother? What additional information do you need to know to answer this question?

 Go to **Caring for the Nguyens Response Sheet** on *DavisPlus*.

Meet Your Patients

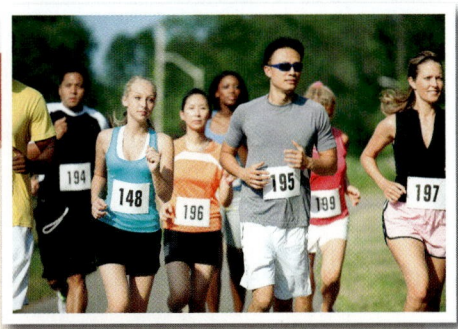

You are attending a health promotion series at the local hospital in order to fulfill your state's requirement for continuing nursing education. For the next 4 weeks, the topic is exercise. In the group, you meet the following people:

- Phillip Flanders is a 40-year-old accountant. He works long hours in an office setting doing work that is sedentary and requires concentration. Although he is not physically active, he often feels tired. He does not exercise regularly. Many of his friends have suggested that he begin some kind of exercise program to improve his energy and health. Phillip would like to learn how to get started with an overall fitness program that works with his job and family life. Before getting started, he makes an appointment with his primary care provider for a thorough health evaluation.
- Peter Phan is 28 years old and is a marathon runner and triathlete. On average, he runs 35 miles per week and cycles at least twice per week. Peter has had plantar fasciitis in the past that was painful and caused him to miss exercising. Peter would like to learn what he can do to prevent other injuries.

- Helen Jillian is 72 years old. She has hypertension and high cholesterol levels for which she takes four medications. She is 5 feet 1 inch tall and weighs 290 pounds. Recently she began having chest pain when starting a brisk walk. Her physician prescribed nitroglycerin for the chest pain, and after a thorough cardiac evaluation told her to enroll in the health promotion series and the CardioFit program at the hospital. She does not understand why she is being asked to do these things because activity seems to trigger her chest pain.

In this chapter, you will find answers to each of these patient questions about activity and exercise. In addition, you will learn more about assisting patients with mobility problems.

Theoretical Knowledge
knowing why

Primitive nomadic people were active just meeting their daily needs. Tribes commonly journeyed to hunt for game; women were on foot gathering roots, fruits, and other edible plants. Survival depended on physical activity, such as changing locations to find food or escape a dangerous situation. Later, the shift to an agricultural society reduced the need for most people to hunt and gather food. However, farming itself was hard work and people were physically active most of the year.

Today, with modern grocery distribution systems, we expend little to no energy to obtain food. In addition, there are many occupations at which people spend hours at a desk or in front of a computer screen. Many of today's leisure activities, (e.g., watching television, playing video games) are sedentary. Even though fitness equipment and health clubs are popular, the overall level of fitness in the United States is declining. Nearly half of adolescents do not engage in moderate to vigorous activity on a regular basis. And, more than two-thirds of adults do not achieve the recommended amount of physical activity needed for health and fitness. To get enough exercise, most people need to make a conscious effort to build exercise and activity into their lives. This chapter will help you to understand why that is important.

ABOUT THE KEY CONCEPTS

Two concepts are widely used to describe human movement: physical activity and exercise. **Physical activity** is bodily movement produced by the contraction of skeletal muscle that increases energy expenditure above a baseline level (U.S. Department of Health and Human Services [USDHHS], 2008,

updated 2011). **Mobility** refers to a person's ability to move within the environment. **Fitness** (or physical fitness) is the ability to carry out activities of daily living with vigor and alertness, without undue fatigue, and with enough energy for leisure pursuits and to respond to emergencies (USDHHS, 2008, updated 2011).

Exercise is a subconcept of physical activity. It is planned, structured, and repetitive and purposeful for improving or maintaining physical fitness, physical performance, or health (Caspersen, Powell, & Christenson, 1985). As you read this chapter, you will learn how the key concepts of activity, fitness, and mobility are related, and how they relate to subconcepts such as fitness, exercise, and body mechanics. Once you have a grasp of these concepts, you should be able to apply them to any patient, regardless of their particular health problem or medical diagnosis.

PHYSIOLOGY OF MOVEMENT

Physical activity and exercise depend on the coordination of skeleton, the muscles, and the nervous system.

Skeletal System

The skeletal system includes bones, cartilage, ligaments, and tendons. The skeleton forms the framework of the body, protects the internal organs, produces blood cells, and stores mineral salts (e.g., calcium) and fat.

Bones consist of a hard outer shell with a spongy interior (Fig. 33-1). There are 206 bones in the human body. Some bones are long (e.g., femur and humerus), some short (e.g., phalanges and metacarpals), some flat (e.g., sternum and cranial bones), and some are irregularly shaped (e.g., vertebrae and tarsal bones). The short, flat, and irregular bones contain red bone marrow that produces red blood cells.

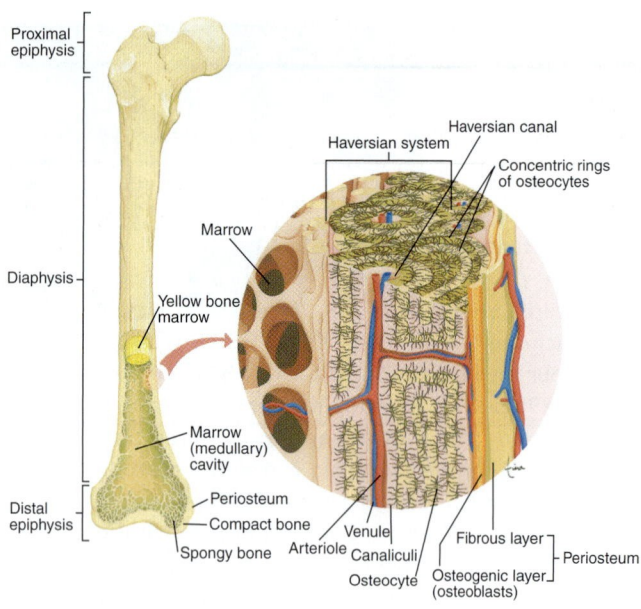

FIGURE 33-1 Bone is complex living tissue.

Bones feel strong and tough, so it is easy to forget that they are composed of living tissue that is constantly building and remodeling. **Osteoclasts** are specialized cells that function as housekeepers in the bone by breaking down old or damaged tissue. **Osteoblasts** repair damaged bone and build new bone to keep the skeleton strong. A delicate balance exists between the actions of the osteoblasts and the osteoclasts.

When two bones come close together **(articulate),** a joint is formed. Body movement occurs at the joints. Joints are classified based on the amount of movement they permit:

- **Synarthroses** are immovable joints (e.g., the sutures between the cranial bones). In youth, these joints have some flexibility to allow growth, but they gradually become rigid.
- **Amphiarthroses** allow for limited movement. Examples are the joints between the vertebrae and pubic bones.

- **Diarthroses,** or **synovial joints,** are freely movable because of the amount of space between the articulating bones. Synovial joints are filled with **synovial fluid,** and the joint surfaces of the articulating bones are covered with smooth **articular cartilage** (connective tissue found in the joints and skeleton). The synovial fluid and articular cartilage prevent friction as the bones move. Table 33-1 identifies the types of movable joints in the body.

Cartilage, ligaments, and tendons serve as the interface between the skeleton and the muscles. Ligaments are fibrous tissues that connect most movable joints. Ligaments are flexible to allow freedom of movement, but strong and tough so they do not yield under force of movement. Tendons are fibrous connective tissues that attach muscles to the bone. Muscles span a joint and attach by tendons to two different bones.

Muscles

Muscles make up 40% to 50% of body weight. When they contract, they cause movement. The type of movement depends on the type of muscle: skeletal, smooth, or cardiac.

- **Skeletal muscle** moves the skeleton.
- **Smooth muscle,** occurring in the digestive tract and other hollow structures, such as the bladder and blood vessels, produces movement of food through the digestive tract, urine through the urinary tract, and blood through the circulatory system.
- **Cardiac muscle** is a unique form of muscle that has the ability to contract spontaneously. It is responsible for the beating of the heart.

Muscles attach to bone at two points: (1) at the *point of origin,* to the more stationary bone, and (2) at the *point of insertion,* to the more movable bone. The "belly" (thickest part) of the muscle lies between these two points. When a skeletal muscle contracts, it shortens, thus causing one bone to move at the joint. Muscles work in pairs. For example, the biceps brachii contracts to flex the forearm (bend the elbow joint). When the biceps contracts, the opposing muscle, the triceps brachii, relaxes. Similarly, contraction of the triceps is associated with relaxation of the biceps (Fig. 33-2).

Table 33-1 ➤ **Types of Synovial Joints**		
TYPE	**DESCRIPTION**	**EXAMPLES**
Ball-and-socket	A rounded head (ball) fits into a cup-like structure (socket) to allow movement in all planes in addition to rotation.	Shoulder and hip joints
Condyloid	An oval-shaped bone fits into an elliptical cavity to allow movement in two planes at right angles to each other.	Wrist
Gliding	Two flat plane surfaces move past each other.	Intervertebral joints
Hinge	A convex surface fits into a cavity, allowing flexion and extension.	Knee and elbow
Pivot	The joint is formed by a ring-like object that turns on a pivot. Motion is limited to rotation.	The atlas and axis of the first vertebrae and base if the skull
Saddle	One bone surface is concave in one direction and convex in the other. The other surface has the opposite construction so that the bones fit together. Movement is possible in two planes at right angles to each other.	Carpal–metacarpal joint of the thumb

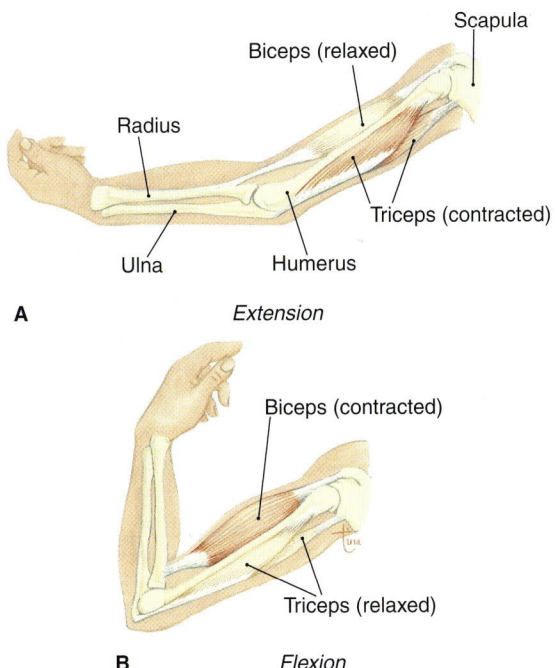

FIGURE 33-2 Antagonistic muscles. A. Extension of the forearm. B. Flexion of the forearm.

Nervous System

The nervous system controls the movement of the musculoskeletal system. Motor nerves are either autonomic or somatic. The **autonomic nervous system** consists of the sympathetic and parasympathetic nervous systems, which innervate involuntary muscles, such as the heart, blood vessels, and glands. The **somatic nervous system** innervates the voluntary skeletal muscles.

When you make a conscious decision to bend your elbow, the thought originates in the motor area of your cerebral cortex. The upper motor efferent nerves communicate with the lower motor neurons that conduct impulses to the muscles. When the muscle receives sufficient stimuli, it contracts the biceps as the triceps relaxes and moves the elbow. Movement also occurs through reflex mechanisms. Common reflexes include the knee-jerk reflex and corneal reflex. Reflexes are discussed at length in Chapter 21.

A muscle contraction, whether conscious or reflexive, stimulates afferent nerves that convey information to the cerebral cortex and the cerebellum. This information helps control and coordinate movements.

KnowledgeCheck 33-1

- Name three purposes of the skeletal system.
- Identify three types of muscle.
- How do the muscles and the nerves interact?

BODY MECHANICS

Body mechanics is a term used to describe the way we move our bodies. It includes four components: body alignment, balance, coordination, and joint mobility. You should always use good body mechanics and teach them to patients as part of your health promotion and disease prevention efforts. In addition to discussing those components, this chapter also presents some guidelines to use when teaching your patients about safe movement and lifting. The following are concepts used to describe problems with muscle mass, strength, or mobility.

Body Alignment

Body alignment, or posture, is an important aspect of body mechanics. Proper posture places the spine in a neutral (resting) position. There are four natural curves to the spine (Fig. 33-3). Proper posture maintains these natural curves because it allows movement to occur with less stress and fatigue; the bones are aligned, and the muscles, joints, and ligaments can work at peak efficiency. Good posture contributes to the normal functioning of the nervous system and improves feelings of well-being (see the Self-Care box, Tips to Maintain Proper Posture). Most posture problems result from a combination of the following:

Accidents, injuries, and falls
Careless sitting, standing, or sleeping habits
Excessive weight
Foot problems or improper shoes
Negative self-image
Occupational stress
Poor sleep support (mattress)
Poorly designed workspace
Visual difficulties
Weak muscles or muscle imbalance

Balance

The body achieves balance when it is in alignment. For your body to be balanced, your line of gravity must pass through your center of gravity, and your center of gravity must be close to your base of support. The **line of gravity** is an imaginary vertical line drawn from the top of the head through the center of gravity. The **center of gravity** is the point around which mass is distributed. In the human body, the center of gravity is below the umbilicus at the top of the pelvis. The **base of support** is what holds the body up. The feet provide the base of support.

To avoid injury when moving objects, place your center of gravity closest to your base of support and stand with your head erect, buttocks pulled in, abdominal muscles tight, chest

Lateral (side) spinal column

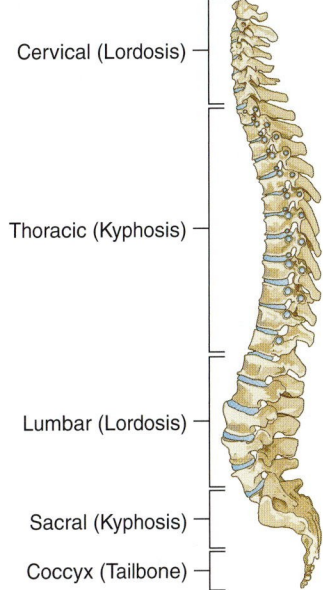

Cervical (Lordosis)

Thoracic (Kyphosis)

Lumbar (Lordosis)

Sacral (Kyphosis)

Coccyx (Tailbone)

FIGURE 33-3 There are four natural curves to the spine.

Tips to Maintain Proper Posture

➤ Avoid standing in one position for a lengthy period. If you cannot change positions, elevate one foot on a stool or box, and alternate foot placement frequently.
➤ Do not lock your knees when standing upright.
➤ Keep your stomach muscles tight to support your back.
➤ Do not bend forward at the waist or neck when you are working in a low position.
➤ When you are seated at your desk, work at a comfortable height.
➤ Do not wear high-heeled or platform shoes for long periods of time.
➤ Do not slump when you sit.
➤ Sit close to your work.
➤ Use a chair that supports your back in a slightly arched position.
➤ Sit with your feet flat on the floor and your knees below your hips.
➤ Sleep on a mattress that is firm but not extremely hard.

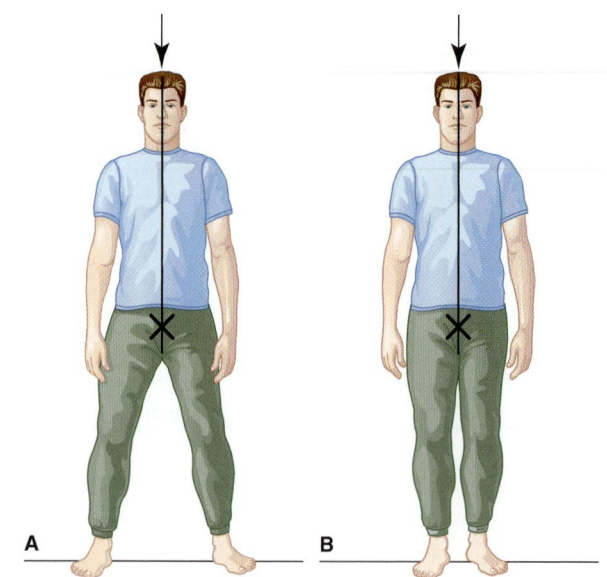

FIGURE 33-4 A. With a wide stance, the center of gravity (x) is closer to the base of support. B. With a narrow stance, the body is less stable.

high, shoulders pulled back, and feet wide (Fig. 33-4). Use a wide stance, with feet apart and one foot forward when standing for a long period of time. The broader the base of support, the lower the center of gravity, and the easier it is to maintain balance.

Coordination

Smooth movement requires coordination between the nervous system and the musculoskeletal system. Voluntary movement is initiated in the cerebral cortex. However, the cerebellum coordinates movements. As you may recall, *proprioception*—the awareness of posture, movement, and position sense—is largely controlled by the cerebellum. The basal ganglia, located deep in the cerebrum, assist with coordination of movement. Damage to the motor cortex, cerebellum, or basal ganglia affects coordination of movement. For example, a stroke affecting the motor cortex alters gait and changes posture.

Joint Mobility

The key concept **mobility** refers to a person's ability to move within the environment (*Taber's Cyclopedic Medical Dictionary*, last updated 2009). Joint movement allows us to sit, stand, bend, walk, and perform other activities. **Range of motion (ROM)** is the maximum movement possible at a joint. **Active range of motion** (AROM) is defined as the movement of the joint through the entire ROM by the individual. Full ROM is part of being physically fit; for that reason, stretching exercises are included in a comprehensive exercise program. **Passive ROM (PROM)** is a nursing activity that is discussed later in this chapter. It involves moving joints through their ROM when the patient is unable to do so for himself. Other terms describing body movement are listed in Table 33-2.

Table 33-2 ➤ Range of Motion at the Joints	
JOINT	**ILLUSTRATION**
Neck (Pivot Joint)	

Flexion—Move the head from upright midline position to the chin, resting the head on the chest.
  Normal Range: 45° from midline
Extension—Move the head from flexed to upright midline position.
  Normal Range: 45° from midline
Hyperextension—Move the head from upright midline position to as far back as possible.
  Normal Range: 10°
	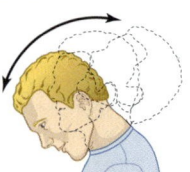

Lateral flexion—Tilt the head laterally from midline position toward the shoulder. *Normal Range:* 40° from midline	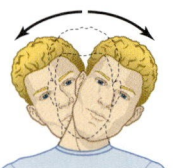

Table 33-2 ➤ Range of Motion at the Joints—cont'd

JOINT	ILLUSTRATION

Rotation—Rotate the head in a circular motion from upright midline position to as far right or left as possible.

Normal Range: 180°

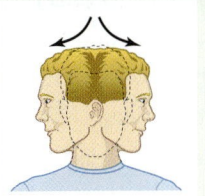

Shoulder (Ball-and-Socket Joint)

Flexion—Raise the arm from a neutral position at the side to alongside the head.

Normal Range: 180°

Extension—Move the arm from flexed to a neutral position at the side of the body.

Normal Range: 180°

Hyperextension—Move the arm, keeping the elbow straight, from a neutral position at the side of the bed to behind the body.

Normal Range: 45°–60°

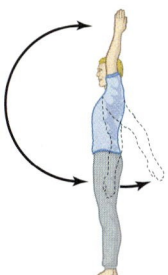

Abduction—Raise the arm laterally from a neutral position at the side of the body to a position at the side of the head, palm facing outward.

Normal Range: 180°

Adduction—Move the arm downward from a position beside the head to across the front of the body as far as possible.

Normal Range: 230°–320°

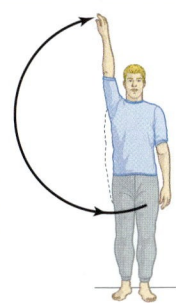

Circumduction—Circle the arm from the shoulder.

Normal Range: 360°

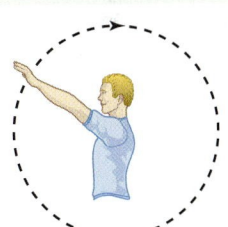

External rotation—Keeping arm held out to the side at shoulder level and bent to a right angle, fingers pointing down, move the arm upward so that the fingers point upward and are above the shoulder.

Normal Range: 90°

Internal rotation—Move the arm forward and down to return to the starting position, fingers pointing down.

Normal Range: 90°

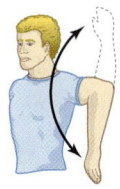

(Continued)

Table 33-2 ▶ Range of Motion at the Joints—cont'd

JOINT	ILLUSTRATION

Elbow (Hinge Joint)

Flexion—Bend at the elbow to move the forearm from a straightened position up toward the shoulder.

Normal Range: 150°

Extension—Straighten the arm by bringing the lower arm forward and down.

Normal Range: 150°

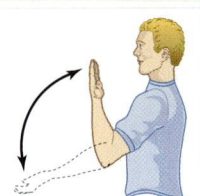

Rotation (for supination)—With the arm at the side, elbow bent, move the hand and forearm so that the palm is facing upward.

Normal Range: 70°–90°

Rotation (for pronation)—With the arm at the side, elbow bent, move the hand and forearm so that the palm is facing downward.

Normal Range: 70°–90°

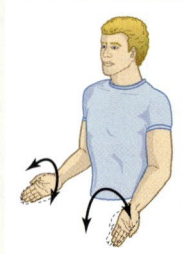

Wrist (Condyloid Joint)

Flexion—Bend the fingers of the hand toward the inner aspect of the forearm.

Normal Range: 80°–90°

Extension—Straighten the wrist so that it is on the same plane as the forearm.

Normal Range: 80°–90°

Hyperextension—Bend the wrist as far back as possible toward the outer aspect of the forearm.

Normal Range: 70°–90°

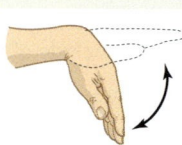

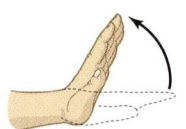

Abduction (radial flexion)—With the hand supinated, bend each wrist laterally toward the thumb side.

Normal Range: 0–20°

Adduction (ulnar flexion)—With the hand supinated, bend each wrist laterally toward the fifth finger side.

Normal Range: 30°–50°

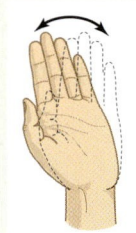

Flexion—Bend the fingers into a fist.

Normal Range: 90°

Extension—Straighten the fingers.

Normal Range: 90°

Hyperextension—Bend the fingers back.

Normal Range: 30°

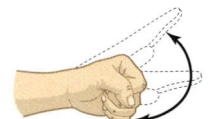

Table 33-2 ➤ Range of Motion at the Joints—cont'd

JOINT	ILLUSTRATION
Abduction—Spread the fingers apart. *Normal Range:* 20° *Adduction*—Bring the fingers together. *Normal Range:* 20°	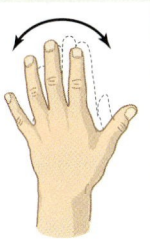

Thumb (Saddle Joint)

Flexion—Move the thumb across the palm of the hand toward the fifth finger. *Normal Range:* 90° *Extension*—Move the thumb laterally away from the fingers. *Normal Range:* 90°	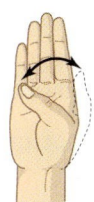
Opposition—Touch the thumb to the top of each finger of the same hand. *Normal Range:* NA	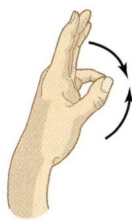

Hip (Ball-and-Socket Joint)

Flexion—Move the leg forward and up. *Normal Range:* Knee extended 90° *Extension*—Move the leg back down beside the other. *Normal Range:* Knee flexed 120° *Hyperextension*—Move the leg back behind the body. *Normal Range:* 30–50°	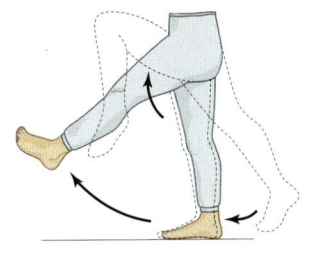 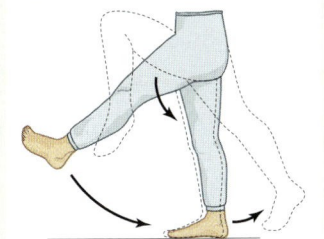
Abduction—Move the leg laterally. *Normal Range:* 45–50° *Adduction*—Sweep the leg inward across the midline. *Normal Range:* 20–30° beyond the other leg	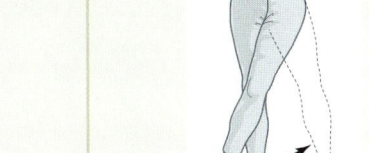

(Continued)

Table 33-2 ➤ Range of Motion at the Joints—cont'd

JOINT	ILLUSTRATION
Circumduction—Circle the leg, keeping the knee straight. *Normal Range:* 360°	

Internal rotation—Turn the foot and leg inward toward the other leg.
 	
  Normal Range: 90°
 	
External rotation—Turn the foot and leg outward, pointing the toes as far as possible away from the other leg.
 	
  Normal Range: 90°	

Knee (Hinge Joint)

Flexion—Bend at the knee, bringing the heel back toward the buttocks.
 	
  Normal Range: 120°–130°
 	
Extension—Straighten the knee, returning the leg to its original position.
 	
  Normal Range: 120°–130°	

Ankle (Hinge Joint)

Extension (plantar flexion)—Point the toes and foot downward.
 	
  Normal Range: 45°–50°
 	
Flexion (dorsiflexion)—Pull the toes and foot upward.
 	
  Normal Range: 20°	

Foot (Gliding Joint)

Eversion—Turn the sole of the foot laterally.
 	
  Normal Range: 5°
 	
Inversion—Turn the sole of the foot medially.
 	
  Normal Range: 5°
	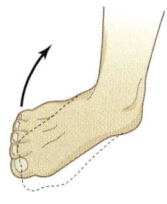

Table 33-2 ➤ Range of Motion at the Joints—cont'd

JOINT	ILLUSTRATION

Flexion—Curl the toes downward.
 	
   Normal Range: 35°–60°
 	
 Extension—Straighten the toes.
 	
   Normal Range: 35°–60°	

Abduction—Spread the toes apart.
 	
   Normal Range: 0–15°
 	
 Adduction—Bring the toes together.
 	
   Normal Range: 0–15°	

Trunk	

Flexion—At the waist, bend forward toward the toes.
 	
   Normal Range: 70°–90°
 	
 Extension—Straighten the trunk from the flexed position.
 	
   Normal Range: 70°–90°
 	
 Hyperextension—Bend the trunk backward.
 	
   Normal Range: 20°–30°	

Lateral flexion—Bend the trunk to the side. *Normal Range:* 20°–40°	
Rotation—Turn the upper body from side to side (twist at the waist). *Normal Range:* 30°–45°	

To see animations of joints and range of motion,

 Go to **Animations: Range of Motion Animations,** on *DavisPlus.*

Body Mechanics Guidelines

Principles of body mechanics are the rules that allow you to move your body while reducing your risk for injury. Historically, nurses have used body mechanics guidelines as the cornerstone of safe practice for moving and lifting patients. However, patient characteristics and condition (e.g., obesity), as well as the patient care environment, make it difficult to rely on body mechanics alone to prevent injury (Nelson, Fragala, & Menzel, 2003). There is no reason to "prove yourself" by transferring without the use of an assistive device (e.g., lift, transfer board, or other staff). The American Nurses Association launched the Handle With Care national campaign to

reduce the risk of back and musculoskeletal injuries among nurses. Handle With Care emphasizes the use of assistive devices to decrease the risk of injury and recommends virtually no manual lifting. Even though more assistive devices are becoming increasingly available in clinical facilities, to avoid injury it is essential to continue to use good body mechanics as you move and lift patients (American Nurses Association [ANA], 2006). For guidelines to help you assess patients' transfer abilities and use good body mechanics, see Clinical Insight 33-1.

KnowledgeCheck 33-2

- Identify the four components of body mechanics.
- Give at least five guidelines for good body mechanics.
- Define the following movements: abduction, adduction, flexion, extension, circumduction, internal rotation, supination, and pronation.

 ThinkLike a Nurse 33-1

While you are attending the health promotion class, Helen Jillian (Meet Your Patients) develops chest pain and must be assisted to a wheelchair for transport to the emergency department.

- Based on what you know about body mechanics, how would you be able to assist Ms. Jillian?
- What additional information do you need to know?

PHYSICAL ACTIVITY AND EXERCISE

Physical activity is bodily movement that can be grouped into two basic categories:

- **Baseline activity** refers to the light-intensity activities of daily living, such as standing, walking slowly, and lifting lightweight objects.
- **Exercise (health-enhancing physical activity)** is purposeful, bodily exertion to produce health-enhancing benefits **(fitness).** People who are physically fit are able to perform activities of daily living with vigor and alertness and with enough energy to enjoy work and leisure activities (USDHHS, 2008).

Types of Exercise

Exercise may be classified according to the type of muscle contraction it involves and according to whether it uses oxygen for energy.

Isometric exercises involve muscle contraction without motion. They are usually performed against an immovable surface or object, for example, pressing the hand against a wall. The muscles of the arm contract, but the wall does not move. Each position is held for 6 to 8 seconds and repeated 5 to 10 times. Isometric training is effective for developing total strength of a particular muscle or group of muscles. It is often used for rehabilitation because the exact area of muscle weakness can be isolated and strengthening can be administered at the proper joint angle. This kind of training requires no special equipment, and there is little chance of injury.

Clinical Insight 33-1 ▶ Applying Principles of Body Mechanics

Principles of body mechanics are the rules that enable you to move your body without causing injury. Use the following guidelines to decrease the risk of back and other injuries. Teach them to your patients as well. Remember that the ANA states you should use mechanical equipment for lifting and transferring whenever possible and not rely on body mechanics alone to prevent injury.

- **Assess patient dependency levels** and select equipment after determining the patient's ability to assist in the transfer (Table 33-4). You will also want to be aware of the patient's strength and ability to bear weight. The patient's height and weight factor into how you transfer the patient safely.
- **Use a wide base of support** (feet spread apart).
- **Minimize bending and twisting.** These movements increase the stress on the back. Instead, face the object or person, and bend at the hips or squat.
- **Squat to lift heavy objects from the floor.** (Squatting lowers your center of gravity.) Push against the strong hip and thigh muscles to raise yourself to a standing position. Avoid bending at the waist.
- **Use the muscles in your legs** as the power for lifting. Bend your knees, keep your back straight, and lift smoothly. Repeat the same movements for setting the object down.
- **Keep objects close to your body** when you lift, move, or carry them. The closer an object is to the center of gravity, the greater the stability and the less strain on the back.

- **Use both hands and arms** when you lift, move, or carry heavy objects.
- **Raise the height of the bed and over-the-bed table to waist level** when you are working with a patient.
- **When possible, keep your elbows bent** when you carry an object.
- **Do not stand on tiptoes to reach an object.** If you must use a ladder or stepstool to reach an object, make sure it is stable and adequate to position your body close to the object.
- **Push, slide, or pull heavy objects** whenever possible rather than lifting.
- **Maintain a good grip on the patient or object** you are moving before attempting to move it.
- **Work with smooth and even movements.** Avoid sudden or jerky motions.
- **Get help to move a heavy object or patient.** Assess the object or patient you are going to lift. If you have any doubt that you can do it by yourself, get help from a coworker.
- **Use assistive devices at all times** to limit the risk of back and musculoskeletal injury.
- **Maintain competency** in using all assistive and transfer devices.

Patients who are bedbound can use this form of exercise to maintain or regain muscle strength.

Isotonic exercise involves movement of the joint during the muscle contraction. A classic example of an isotonic exercise is weight training with free weights. As the weight is moved throughout the ROM, the muscle shortens and lengthens. Calisthenics, such as chin-ups, push-ups, and sit-ups, all of which use body weight as the resistance force, are also isotonic exercises.

Isokinetic exercise is performed with specialized apparatuses that provide variable resistance to movement. Isokinetic exercise combines the best features of both isometrics and weight training by providing resistance at a constant, preset speed while the muscle moves through the full ROM. Specialized machines available at health clubs and physical therapy departments are used for this form of exercise.

Aerobic exercise acquires energy from metabolic pathways that use oxygen—the amount of oxygen taken into the body meets or exceeds the amount of oxygen required to perform the activity. Aerobic exercise uses large muscle groups, can be maintained continuously, and is rhythmic in nature. It increases the heart and respiratory rates, thereby providing exercise for the cardiovascular system while simultaneously exercising the skeletal muscles. Jogging, brisk walking, and cycling are common forms of aerobic exercise.

Anaerobic exercise occurs when the amount of oxygen taken into the body does not meet the amount of oxygen required to perform the activity. Therefore, the muscles must obtain energy from metabolic pathways that do not use oxygen. Some examples of rapid, intense anaerobic exercise include lifting heavy objects or sprinting.

Fitness Program Guidelines

A well-rounded fitness program focuses on flexibility, resistance training, and aerobic conditioning. Factors when designing or evaluating a fitness program include the following:

Flexibility Training. Stretching before exercise helps warm up the muscles and prevents injury during exercise.

Stretching after exercise cools the muscles and limits post-exercise stiffness. As we get older, joints and muscles become stiffer. A regular flexibility program helps maintain mobility as aging progresses.

Resistance Training. Movement against resistance increases muscular strength and endurance. Perhaps the most common type of resistance training is weight lifting. When a person is exercising for strength, the goal is to increase the amount of resistance with each exercise (i.e., lift more weight). When a person is exercising for endurance, the goal is to increase the number of repetitions with each exercise (i.e., lift the weight more times).

Aerobic Conditioning. Fitness and body composition are improved by aerobic conditioning. Components of aerobic conditioning include intensity, duration, frequency, and mode. Intensity is how hard one is exercising. Box 33-1 describes three common tests used to evaluate exercise intensity.

Amount of Physical Activity. Duration is the amount of time one is exercising. To achieve and maintain a healthy level of fitness, the USDHHS recommends 2.5 hours/week (150 min/wk) or more of moderate-intensity physical activity (e.g., brisk walking) coupled with increasing the activity every day (USDHHS, 2008). The **frequency** of exercise should be 3 to 5 days/week, although the more often and the longer duration the better.

Mode of Exercise. The **mode** of exercise is the type of activity. Aerobic (endurance) and muscle-strengthening (resistance) physical activities both promote better health. See Box 33-2.

Many people become discouraged because they don't see immediate results from their efforts. However, subtle changes occur long before the person sees changes in weight or shape. Some tips to help develop an exercise program are included in the Self-Care box, Teaching Clients How to Set Up a Fitness Program.

BOX 33-1 ■ Tests for Determining Exercise Intensity

Target Heart Rate Method

In the target heart rate method, the target heart rate (THR) is calculated from an estimate of maximum heart rate. The estimated maximum heart rate is calculated using the following formula:

$$\text{Maximum heart rate} = 220 - \text{age}$$

The THR is calculated as a percentage of the maximum heart rate. Most persons can exercise at 60% to 80% of the maximum heart rate.

For example, consider a 50-year-old woman. Her maximum heart rate is 170 beats/min. To exercise at 75% intensity, her target heart rate is 128 beats/min.

$$\text{Maximum heart rate} = 220 - 50 = 170$$
$$\text{THR} = 0.75 - 170 = 128$$

The person's heart rate during exercise should be 128 beats per minute, excluding warm-up and cool-down.

Talk Test

The talk test evaluates exercise intensity based on the person's ability to talk while exercising. Short phrases interspersed with breaths or feeling like you can "just respond" is considered an appropriate level of exercise. If you are too short of breath to answer, the level of intensity is too high. An ability to carry on a conversation indicates that you are not exercising hard enough.

Borg Rate of Perceived Exertion Scale®

The rate of perceived exertion (RPE) scale is easy to use. The person who is exercising selects the rating based on how difficult the exercise feels at that time. The exerciser selects one of eight categories that best describes the intensity of activity. RPE ratings range from No Exertion at All to Extremely Hard. Extremely Hard is associated with exercise that corresponds to almost 100% of maximum heart rate. Somewhat Hard corresponds with 75% of maximum heart rate; this is the level you should encourage for most individuals.

Sources: Borg, G. (1998). *Borg's perceived exertion and pain scales.* Stockholm, Sweden: Human Kinetics; and Foster, C. (2004). "Talk test" measures exercise intensity. *Medicine & Science in Sports & Exercise, 36*(9), 1632–1636.

BOX 33-2 ■ U.S. Department of Health and Human Services. 2008 Physical Activity Guidelines for Americans

Children and Adolescents

- Engage in at least 1 hour of physical activity daily.
- Physical activity should be enjoyable. A variety of activities will improve adherence.
- Most activity should be aerobic, either moderate- or vigorous-intensity.
- At least 3 days/week, children and teens should participate in vigorous-intensity exercise as well as muscle- and bone-strengthening physical activity.

Adults and Older Adults

- To gain substantial health benefits, get at least 150 minutes per week of moderate-intensity or 75 minutes a week of vigorous-intensity aerobic physical activity, or an equivalent combination of moderate- and vigorous-intensity aerobic activity. More frequent exercise (i.e., 300 min/wk) is even more beneficial.
- Engage in aerobic activity throughout the week in episodes of at least 10 minutes. Longer periods of time provide additional benefits.
- For additional health benefits, perform moderate or high-intensity muscle and bone-strengthening activities on 2 or more days per week.

Specific to Older Adults

- Older adults unable to perform 150 minutes of moderate-intensity aerobic activity per week should be as physically active as abilities and conditions allow.
- Include exercises that maintain or improve balance and core strength.

Adults, Children, and Adolescents With Disabilities

- Be as physically active as abilities allow with guidance from their healthcare provider.

Healthy Pregnant and Postpartum Women

- Consult with the healthcare provider regarding activity level throughout pregnancy. If the pregnancy or postpartum recovery is uncomplicated, then those who regularly engage in vigorous-intensity aerobic activity or in high amounts of activity can continue with this regimen.
- If not already engaged in vigorous-intensity physical activity, get at least 150 minutes of moderate-intensity aerobic activity per week, preferably spread throughout the week after consulting with healthcare provider.

Source: Adapted from USDHSS. (2008). 2008 physical activity guidelines for Americans. Retrieved from http://www.health.gov/paguidelines

---

Self-Care

Teaching Clients How to Set Up a Fitness Program

If you are older than 40, smoke or drink, are sedentary, are overweight, or have a chronic health condition, then you should have a medical evaluation before starting an exercise program.

Getting Started

- Choose a variety of exercises that you enjoy and feel comfortable doing, such as walking, biking, dancing, or a team sport.
- Find allies. Exercising with someone else can make it more fun. If you choose to exercise by yourself, pick a friend with whom you can discuss your exercise progress.
- Vary your routine. You may be less likely to get bored or injured.
- Choose a comfortable time of day.
- Don't get discouraged. It can take weeks or months before you notice some of the changes from exercise.
- Forget "no pain, no gain." Although a little soreness is normal after you first start exercising, pain isn't. Stop if you hurt.
- Make exercise fun. Find fun things to do, such as taking a walk through the park or watching your favorite show while riding a stationary bike.
- Sign a contract committing yourself to exercise.
- Find an accountability partner. A fitness program is not only more enjoyable when shared with someone else but also is more successful with others for whom you are accountable.
- Keep a daily log of your activities.
- Think about joining a health club. The cost gives some people an incentive to exercise regularly.

Exercise Tips

- Warm up your muscles for 5 to 10 minutes before your main session of aerobic exercise.
- Maintain your exercise intensity for 30 to 45 minutes.
- Gradually decrease the intensity of your workout (cool down) and then stretch for 5 to 10 minutes at the end of your workout.
- Accumulate physical activity throughout the day. For example:
  - Take the stairs instead of the elevator.
  - Go for a walk during your coffee break or lunch.
  - Walk all or part of the way to work.
  - Park your car at the far end of the parking lot.
- Wear good, shock-absorbing footwear. Shoes that do not support your feet will cause stress on leg bones and the back and, over time, lead to injury.
- Alternate easy and hard exercise days, or alternate modes of exercise (e.g., alternate running, swimming, and biking).
- Take a day off periodically. The body needs a chance to rest and allow bones, joints, and muscles to rest and repair.
- To avoid becoming dehydrated, drink at least 8 ounces of fluid before the exercise, and then pause regularly during the exercise for more. If you are thirsty after the exercise session, drink until you feel satiated. Water is still the best liquid to drink during and after exercise. However, you can't rely on feeling thirsty as a reminder to replace fluid lost through sweating; one of nature's dirty tricks is that exercise suppresses thirst.

Source: Adapted from USDHHS. (2008). 2008 physical activity guidelines for Americans. Retrieved November 1, 2011, from http://www.health.gov/paguidelines

Benefits of Regular Physical Activity

Regular exercise or other physical activity each week, sustained for months and years, can produce long-term health benefits. Strong evidence links regular physical activity with a lower risk for early death, heart disease, stroke, type 2 diabetes, hypertension, hyperlipidemia, metabolic syndrome, colon and breast cancers, and depression. Regular physical activity also promotes weight loss and maintenance of normal weight when combined with diet, better heart and lung function, muscular fitness, fall prevention, and improved memory and mental clarity in older adults. People with disabilities also benefit from physical activity (USDHHS, 2008).

Weight-bearing exercise reduces loss of bone density in adults and older adults (Jitramontree, 2002, updated 2007; USDHHS, 2008). Resistance training does not lead to weight loss; instead, it may increase loss of fat mass and improve muscle tone and strength (American College of Sports Medicine [ACSM], 2009). Exercise is associated with an overall decrease in mortality in men and women of all ages and an overall improvement in quality of life for people in all ethnic groups and across the lifespan. People with disabilities also benefit from physical activity (USDHHS, 2008). Box 33-3 presents numerous other benefits of regular exercise.

Toward Evidence-Based Practice

Frimel, T. N., Sinacore, D. R., & Villareal, D. T. (2008, July). Exercise attenuates the weight-loss induced reduction in muscle mass in frail obese older adults. *Medicine & Science in Sport & Exercise, 40(7), 1213–1219.*

The goal of this study was to assess the effect of adding exercise to a low-calorie diet on changes in lean mass and strength in frail, obese older adults who were voluntarily losing weight. Researchers found when exercise is added to weight-reducing diet, less muscle mass is lost as compared to diet alone. In adults ages 65 years and older, regular exercise that incorporates resistance training, combined with a diet for weight loss for 6 months, reduces the amount of lean muscle mass lost and increased strength.

Simoes, E. J., Kobau, R., & Waterman, B., et al. (2006, December). Associations of physical activity and body mass index with activities of daily living in older adults. *Journal of Community Health, 31(6), 453–467.*

This study was done to find out more about physical activity and the effect on body mass index (BMI) and activities of daily living (ADLs) and instrumental ADLs. Physically active individuals were less likely than inactive people to be dependent with ADLs/IADLs. Researchers supported a strategy to improve the quality of life for older adults by improving physical activity.

Maddalozzo, G. F., & Snow, C. M. (2000). High intensity resistance training: Effects on bone in older men and women. *Calcified Tissue International, 66, 399–404.*

This classic study revealed that high-intensity resistance exercise improves bone mineral density, lean mass, and muscle strength. It is important to emphasize careful progression in order to prevent overtraining and possible injuries. Older adults should include resistance training within their lifestyles.

1. Based on these three studies, what benefits can you think of for older adults that support starting a community-based physical fitness program?

2. You are in charge of an outpatient healthy lifestyle program for adults 65 years and older. The program is geared for obese, sedentary older adults who want to lose weight and improve physical fitness. Based on the Maddalozzo and Snow study, how would you design the program?

 Go to Chapter 33, **Toward Evidence-Based Practice Suggested Responses,** on Davis*Plus.*

Risks Associated With Exercise

Armed with theoretical knowledge, you should be able to teach your clients realistically about the risks associated with exercise and thereby help them to exercise safely. Risks include cardiac injury, musculoskeletal injury, dehydration, hypoglycemia, and temperature regulation problems. Keep in mind that the benefits of exercise far outweigh the risks. Advise clients to follow the tips in the Self-Care box, Teaching Your Patient How to Prevent Back Injury to exercise safely and help prevent injury.

Cardiac Injury. Fear of triggering a cardiac event prevents some people from exercising. However, exercise itself is rarely life threatening, especially when compared with the alternative (*not* exercising). Before starting an exercise pro-

gram or significantly increasing the intensity of normal workouts, seasoned athletes as well as rank beginners should be screened for underlying health problems, such as high blood pressure, thickened heart muscle (cardiac hypertrophy), electrical abnormalities, and blood vessel abnormalities. In people without underlying heart disease, recreational drug use is an important cause of sudden cardiac arrest, whether during exercise or at rest.

Musculoskeletal Injury. High-impact exercises, such as running or aerobic dance, may pose a risk for injuries to bones, joints, and muscles. However, you can prevent most such injuries by gradually increasing the activity level or varying activities. Walking is an exercise that most people can do without injury. Injury can also occur from lifting weights. Free weights

Teaching Your Older Adult Patient About Increasing Physical Activity and Exercise

What Are the Benefits of Physical Activity for an Older Adult?

➤ Improves and maintains strength so you can stay as independent as possible.
➤ Maintains balance and prevents falls.
➤ Gives you more energy to do the things you want to do.
➤ Helps you to sleep better and feel more rested.
➤ Perks up your mood and helps reduce depression.
➤ Prevents or delays some diseases like diabetes, heart disease, and cancer.

What Kind of Physical Activity Should I Do?

➤ Get at least 30 minutes of *endurance* activity almost every day. Exercise that makes you breathe hard builds strength and staying power.
➤ Incorporate *resistance* into your exercise: Use some kind of weight or isometric activity to build strength. Remember that you can do more and are less likely to fall when your muscles are strong.
➤ Do things to work on your *balance* (e.g., standing on one foot). This can help to prevent falls.

➤ Daily stretching will help you be more *flexible* and prevent injury.

Who Should Exercise?

Almost anyone can do some type of physical activity, but before starting a new exercise program check with your healthcare provider if you experience any of the following:
➤ Any change in your health in the past 6 months
➤ Shortness of breath or dizziness
➤ Chest pain or pressure, or fluttering heart
➤ Joint pain or swelling
➤ Unexplained weight loss
➤ An infection with fever
➤ Eye problems
➤ Blood clot
➤ Hernia
➤ Recent hip surgery or joint injury

Source: Adapted from the National Institutes of Health, National Institute on Aging. (2006, October, updated 2009, February. Exercise and physical activity: Getting fit for life. Retrieved February 4, 2012, from http://www.nia.nih.gov/HealthInformation/Publications/exercise.htm

---

BOX 33-3 ■ Benefits of Regular Exercise

Cardiovascular System

- Improves pumping action of the heart.
- Decreases heart rate and blood pressure.
- Improves circulation by increasing the number of capillaries.
- Improves venous return to the heart.
- Increases high-density lipoprotein (HDL).
- Decreases low-density lipoprotein (LDL) and total cholesterol.
- Decreases risk of thrombophlebitis.

Respiratory System

- Improves pulmonary circulation.
- Improves gas exchange at the alveolar–capillary membrane.
- Dilates bronchioles to increase ventilation.

Musculoskeletal System

- Improves skeletal development in children.
- Increases muscle strength.
- Improves flexibility.
- Increases coordination.
- Helps maintain joint structure and function; reduces risk of osteoarthritis.
- Improves bone mineral density.
- Improves bone mass with aging; reduces risk of osteoporosis.
- Reduces risk of falls and helps older adults maintain an independent lifestyle.

Nervous System

- Speeds nerve impulse transmission.

Endocrine System

- Increases sensitivity to insulin at the receptor sites.
- Increases efficiency of metabolic processes.
- Improves temperature regulation.
- Facilitates weight management.

Gastrointestinal System

- Improves appetite.
- Improves abdominal muscle tone.
- Decreases risk of colon cancer.

Urinary System

- Increases efficiency of kidney function.

Integumentary System

- Improves skin tone as a result of improved circulation.

Immune System

- Reduces susceptibility to minor viral illnesses.

Mental Health

- Boosts energy level.
- Release endorphins, which assist with pain control and stress management.
- Improves self-esteem and body image.
- Provides a nonpharmacological way to relieve symptoms of anxiety and depression.
- Leads to positive outlook and sense of optimism.
- Promotes clearer thinking and improved memory in older adults.
- Enhances feelings of well being and diminishes depressive symptoms.
- Relieves some stress.
- Can be a source of social interaction.

Overall Health

- Burns calories to achieve and maintain healthy body weight.
- Leads to reduced abdominal obesity.
- Improves overall stamina.
- Reduces fatigue.
- Increases time spent in stage IV and REM sleep.

Self-Care

Teaching Your Patient How to Prevent Back Injury

➤ Poor posture is one of the main causes of back pain. Make a conscious effort to maintain good posture at all times.

➤ Use a firm mattress that provides adequate support.

➤ Sit with your knees slightly lower than your hips.

➤ If you must stand for a long period of time, flex your hip and raise one foot on a stool or object 6 to 8 inches off the ground. Periodically switch legs.

➤ Wear comfortable, low-heeled shoes. Avoid high heels as much as possible.

➤ Avoid restrictive clothing that inhibits your ability to use good body mechanics.

➤ Follow principles of body mechanics at all times (e.g., use wide base of support, and do not lift with your back).

➤ Exercise regularly to maintain your optimal weight and strengthen the muscles of your body.

➤ Include abdominal exercises in your routine. Strong abdominal muscles help support the back.

➤ Avoid lifting excessive weight.

➤ Avoid exercises or movements that cause spinal flexion (e.g., toe-touches, sit-ups with knees extended), excessive flexion of the neck (e.g., abdominal crunches with neck curved to chest), or spinal rotation (twisting).

can cause injury if the person lifts too much weight or uses poor body mechanics when lifting. Working with a fitness trainer to learn correct form and appropriate weights markedly decreases the risk of injury. In addition, exercise machines provide some degree of control and are less likely to cause injury.

Dehydration. It is possible to become dehydrated with prolonged exercise, with warm temperatures, or as a result of health problems or medications. During an intense exercise period, the body can lose 2 liters of fluid for every hour of exercise. It is important to drink water before, during, and after the exercise period. Water is still the best choice during and after exercise. Some sports drinks have glucose and electrolytes for replacement and quick energy and can be used for endurance activities or prolonged, intense activity.

Temperature Regulation Problems. **Hyperthermia** can occur when the person exercises in a hot climate. Hyperthermia is often accompanied by dehydration. **Heat exhaustion** is a potentially life-threatening event. Signs of heat exhaustion include lightheadedness, nausea, headache, fatigue, hyperventilation, loss of concentration, and abdominal cramps. Body temperature rises, but the skin is clammy and cold. In contrast, **hypothermia** can occur when the person does not wear proper clothing or is exposed to cool water for an extended period of time. Hypothermia is characterized by fatigue, confusion, and lack of coordination.

KnowledgeCheck 33-3

■ Identify and describe four types of exercise.
■ State the components of an exercise program.

ThinkLike a Nurse 33-2

■ How would you address Helen Jillian's (Meet Your Patients) concerns about the risks associated with engaging in an exercise program?

■ Peter Phan (Meet Your Patients) has experienced a number of injuries as a result of his exercise. Based on your knowledge of exercise, what questions would you like to ask Peter about his exercise program?

FACTORS AFFECTING MOBILITY AND ACTIVITY

Recall that physical activity is bodily movement produced by the contraction of skeletal muscles. **Mobility** refers to a person's capacity for bodily movement, or how well the person is able to move about in the environment. Factors influencing activity and mobility include developmental stage, nutrition, lifestyle, attitudes, external factors, diseases, and physical abnormalities. These factors are discussed in the next sections.

Developmental Stage

Neuromuscular development is related to age. A newborn can move his extremities and turn his head from side to side, but he is unable to get from place to place. As the child matures, motor skills and coordination develop. In spite of that, children in the United States are becoming more sedentary, contributing to the continuing rise of obesity among children. Using 2005–2006 data, the Centers for Disease Control and Prevention (CDC) reported the following:

■ Obesity rates for young adults tripled compared to the 1971–1974 data.

■ Only 36% of young adults get regular physical activity in their spare time.

■ Only 26% of young adults were doing strength training at least twice per week, which is a minimum recommendation for adults of all ages (CDC, 2008, updated 2011).

Healthy People 2020 goals recommend that older adults also need to increase physical activity (USDHHS, 2011). The expected physiological changes associated with growing older make it harder to start or maintain an exercise program. The result is increased risk for chronic health problems. For a discussion of neuromuscular development across the life span and associated nursing considerations as it affects activity and exercise,

 Go to Chapter 33, **Tables, Boxes, Figures: ESG Table 33-1: The Influence of Developmental Stage on Activity and Exercise,** on Davis*Plus*.

Nutrition

In the United States, obesity is a major health problem. For example, 24% of young adults are obese and 28% more are overweight. Obesity often leads to health problems, which indirectly reduce activity and can in turn contribute to further obesity. For example, joint injuries and osteoarthritis are more prevalent with obesity, which in turn reduces a person's physical activity. Unhealthy eating patterns, such as consuming large portions, eating mostly convenience foods, and having a diet high in saturated fat and simple carbohydrates, play a major role in the obesity problem. Although the obese person has plenty of calories available to expend on exercise, movement becomes more difficult as body size increases. For more information about nutrition, see Chapter 28.

In contrast, people with chronic disease may be in negative nitrogen balance—that is, they do not have adequate protein stores available to maintain or repair body tissue. They experience muscle wasting and fatigue, which lead to decreased activity levels.

Lifestyle

Over the past century, manual labor has declined and work environments have become increasingly sedentary. As a result, individuals need to look toward leisure time for exercise and fitness activities. This requires making time for exercise. Personal values about exercise and fitness determine when, or whether, exercise becomes part of a person's routine.

Some people enjoy exercise. Others see it as pure drudgery or as "something I have to do." A person's culture and support system define what exercise the person is likely to accept. For example, swimming requires wearing a bathing suit. People brought up in a culture that values modesty may not choose swimming as a form of exercise. Walking, which allows a person to dress in modest clothing, would be a preferred form of exercise.

Stress

How is your stress level? A high stress level can produce fatigue. Although you may view exercise as one more thing you don't have time for, exercise is energizing and can be used to relieve stress. For example, taking a brisk 20-minute walk during a study break may allow you to continue working for several more hours. You can also use this technique when caring for patients. Hospitalized patients and family members often experience a great deal of stress. Helping the patient take a walk to the courtyard, or instructing family members how to handle the wheelchair so they can take a walk around the block, often will help lessen some of the strain.

Environmental Factors

Environmental factors affecting exercise include weather, pollution, neighborhood conditions, finances, and support systems. Weather has a strong influence on activity level. When it is cold, damp or even hot and humid outside, people tend to avoid strenuous activity outside. Encourage patients to choose a variety of activities that they enjoy so they can be active, regardless of the weather. When air quality is poor, suggest indoor activities in order to reduce exposure to allergens and pollutants.

Neighborhood conditions, such as crime or lack of parks, influence attitudes about outside activities. Mall walking is an example of a successful way to incorporate exercise into daily patterns when neighborhood conditions do not encourage activity. Joining a gym or engaging in some sports (e.g., skiing, golfing) might not be practical for some budgets. However, many activities, such as walking or playing basketball or tennis in the community park, are inexpensive.

The support system is perhaps the most influential external factor. Family and friends who are active are likely to promote and support your efforts to exercise. Those who are themselves sedentary may not encourage you to be more active or lose weight.

Diseases and Abnormalities

Diseases and abnormalities in various body systems can negatively influence body alignment, balance, coordination, and joint mobility. In the next sections, we describe some disorders that affect activity and exercise.

Congenital Abnormalities of the Musculoskeletal System

The following are common congenital abnormalities that affect appearance, motor function, and mobility:

- **Syndactylism** is the fusion of two or more fingers or toes. Most cases involving the hands are treated surgically at an early age to limit the effect on fine motor development.

- **Developmental dysplasia of the hip (DDH)** is a congenital abnormality of the development of the femur, acetabulum, or both that shows as hip dislocation.
- **Foot deformities,** such as clubfoot (talipes equinovarus), occur in about 4% of all newborns. Serial casts or surgery may be used to correct the defect and preserve function.
- **Scoliosis** is a lateral curvature of the spine. Scoliosis can result from congenital bone disorders, neuromuscular impairment, or trauma, but approximately two-thirds of cases have no known cause and are termed idiopathic scoliosis. Idiopathic scoliosis is classified as infantile, juvenile, or adolescent depending on the age at onset.

Diseases Related to Bone Formation or Metabolism

Bone formation abnormalities may be congenital, related to dietary deficiencies, or the result of bone disease.

- **Osteogenesis imperfecta (OI)** is a congenital disorder of bone and connective tissue that is characterized by brittle bones that fracture easily. Infants with OI are often born with fractures and continue to fracture with minimal trauma or even spontaneously. Prompt recognition and treatment of fractures helps prevent deformities.
- **Achondroplasia,** or dwarfism, occurs when the bones ossify (harden) prematurely.
- **Paget's disease** is a metabolic bone disease in which increased bone loss results in pain, pathological fractures, and deformities. This disorder usually affects the skull, vertebrae, femur, and pelvis.
- **Vitamin D and calcium** are needed to form and maintain bone. Deficiencies lead to porous bones. In children, prolonged deficiencies can cause the long bones of the legs to become bowed, retard growth, and lead to frequent fractures.

Diseases Affecting Joint Mobility

Diseases of the joints may be degenerative or inflammatory. The most prevalent type of degenerative joint disease is **osteoarthritis (OA)**. OA involves a loss of articular cartilage in the joint, with pain and stiffness as the primary symptoms. Patients may also have decreased ROM and **crepitus,** a creaking or grating sound, with joint motion. Symptoms are aggravated by weight-bearing and joint use and are relieved by resting the affected joints. OA is more common in women, older adults, and people who are overweight.

Rheumatoid arthritis (RA) is a systemic autoimmune disease involving chronic inflammation of the joints and surrounding connective tissue. RA causes joint pain, deformity, and loss of function; patients may also experience fever, fatigue, weakness, and weight loss. RA occurs most frequently in the fingers, wrists, elbows, ankles, and knees. RA occurs in 1% to 2% of the population, with a greater incidence in women. The illness usually begins in mid-life, but persons in any age group can be affected. Swann (2007) identified the most frequently affected age group as those in the 30- to 50-year-old range. Unlike OA, RA does not improve with rest. Pain is most intense when the person arises from bed. Pain and joint deformities may so severely affect mobility that patients cannot care for themselves.

Ankylosing spondylitis is a chronic inflammatory joint disease characterized by stiffening and fusion of the spine and sacroiliac joints. The inflammation occurs where the ligaments, tendons, and joint capsule insert into the bone. The disease usually develops in young adults, equally in men and women. Signs and symptoms include low back pain and

stiffness and decreased ROM of the spine. The convex lumbar curve is lost, and the upper spine curve increases, causing kyphosis (see Chapter 21 for review).

Gout is an inflammatory response to high levels of uric acid. Crystals form in the synovial fluid, and small white nodules, or *tophi,* form in the subcutaneous tissues. Gout produces painful joints and severely limits activity during acute flare-ups.

Nursing activity for patients with joint mobility problems focuses on assisting with movement, providing comfort, and teaching about medications. If mobility is severely restricted, you will also assist patients with activities of daily living (ADLs).

Problems Affecting Bone Integrity

Osteoporosis is a decrease in total bone density, which occurs when osteoclast activity outpaces that of the osteoblasts. The internal structure of the bone diminishes, and the bone collapses in on itself. Normally bone mass continues to increase up to the third decade of life. After age 30, bone loss begins. Women experience a rapid decline in bone mass at menopause. In men, a gradual loss continues. As bones become porous, they become weak, leading to vertebral collapse or fractures of the long bones of the arms and legs. Fractures may occur spontaneously or with very slight trauma.

The best treatment for osteoporosis is prevention. Teach adolescents to eat a diet high in calcium, fluoride, and other minerals, and to start an exercise program they can continue throughout their lives. Advise older women that weight-bearing exercise can help decrease the rate of bone loss, and advise them to ask their provider about medications to reduce bone mineral loss.

The National Osteoporosis Foundation recommends calcium intake for adults age 50 and older to be 1,200 mg/day and vitamin D 800 to 1,000 IV/day to prevent bone loss. The foundation also urges people of all ages, but particularly postmenopausal women, to avoid smoking because tobacco reduces the absorption of calcium in the intestine. In addition, more than two drinks of alcohol per day decreases the matrix of the bone and reduces the body's ability to absorb calcium ("Management of Osteoporosis," 2010).

Osteomyelitis (infection of the bone) may develop after bone injury or surgery. It can be difficult and expensive to treat and can leave the patient with permanent disability. Bone contains microscopic channels that are impermeable to most of the natural defenses of the body. Once bacteria enter these channels, they multiply rapidly.

Bone tumors may also affect form and function. Tumors in the bone cause considerable pain and severely limit activity. Nursing responsibilities for patients with osteomyelitis or bone tumors include collaborative treatments, patient education about the treatment plan, and providing comfort.

Trauma

Trauma can affect the entire musculoskeletal system. One of the most significant forms of trauma is a **fracture,** or a break in the bone. Signs and symptoms of a fracture include tenderness at the site, loss of function, deformity of the area, and swelling of the surrounding tissues. However, x-ray is required for definitive diagnosis. Fractures are classified according to the extent of damage. The type and severity of fracture determine whether casting, traction, or surgical repair is necessary. To learn about caring for a cast in the home, refer to the accompanying Home Care box, Teaching Care of a Cast at Home. For a classification and description of several types of fractures,

 Go to Chapter 33, **Tables, Boxes, Figures: ESG Figure 33-1, Types of Fractures,** on *DavisPlus.*

Home Care

Teaching Care of a Cast at Home

➤ Always keep the cast clean and dry.
➤ Before bathing, cover the cast with a plastic bag and tape the opening shut or use a special cast cover with Velcro straps. Do not place the cast into water unless it is made of water-repellent material. Keep in mind that waterproof casts are not for all types of fractures. They can't be used for recently manipulated fractures or when skin pins are used.
➤ If the cast gets wet enough that the skin gets wet under the cast, it may break down and infection may occur. Dry it immediately with a blow dryer on the cool setting. Be careful—skin can be burned using the hot setting. If you have any trouble getting the cast dry, the cast may need to be replaced. Call the healthcare provider if the cast doesn't dry properly.
➤ Sweating under the cast enough to make it damp may cause mold or mildew to develop. Call the healthcare provider if you notice odor coming from the cast.
➤ Never put anything inside the cast. Do not try to scratch the skin under the cast with any sharp objects, such as a hanger or pencil. This may break the skin under the cast and cause it to become infected. Do not use powders, ointments, or lotions inside the cast.

➤ Sometimes when swelling goes down, the cast can become loose and rub on the skin. If this is the case, advise your patient to call the primary provider to look at the cast.
➤ Check the circulation by gently squeezing a finger or toe below the cast. It should blanch (turn lighter) and quickly return to a pink color. The fingers and toes should be warm to the touch, able to move freely, and not tingling or numb.
➤ Do not trim the cast or break off any rough edges. This may weaken or break the cast. If a fiberglass cast has a rough edge, use a metal file to smooth it or call the healthcare provider.
➤ A sling may be needed for support if the cast is on the hand, wrist, arm, or elbow. It is helpful to wrap soft sheepskin or padding behind the neck to protect the skin and make it feel more comfortable.
➤ If the cast is on the foot or leg, do not walk on or put any weight on the injured leg, unless the doctor allows it.
➤ If the primary provider allows walking on the cast, be sure to wear the cast boot. The boot is to reduce wear and tear on the bottom and has a tread to prevent slipping and falling.
➤ Crutches may be needed to walk if a cast is on the foot, ankle, or leg. Make sure the crutches are adjusted properly before leaving the hospital or the doctor's office.

Sprains and strains are more common than fractures. A **sprain** is a stretch injury of a ligament that causes the ligament to tear. A partial tear can usually heal with rest, but a complete tear often requires surgery to stabilize the joint. A **strain** is an injury to muscle caused by excessive stress on the muscle. Both strains and sprains cause pain at the site of injury, swelling, and loss of function. As you can see, the signs and symptoms are the same as those of a fracture. As a result, x-ray studies are used to distinguish these injuries. Initial treatment of fractures, sprains, and strains include rest, ice, compression, and elevation.

Stretching and tearing injuries to the meniscus (knee cap), lateral knee ligaments, and Achilles' tendon are also fairly common. Magnetic resonance imaging (MRI) studies are done to determine the extent of injury. Rest and ice are necessary, but often, surgical repair is needed to achieve full healing.

Disorders of the Central Nervous System

Any disorder that affects the motor centers of the brain or the transmission of nerve impulses will affect mobility. Cerebrovascular accident (stroke), head or spinal cord injury, multiple sclerosis (a disorder affecting nerve transmission), and myasthenia gravis (a disease caused by antibodies to the acetylcholine receptors at the neuromuscular junction) are examples. Progressive degenerative disorders of the neurological system also affect mobility and coordination. For example, Parkinson's disease is a progressive degeneration of the basal ganglia. It produces tremor, rigidity, and difficulty coordinating movement.

Diseases of Other Body Systems

Diseases affecting other body systems may affect mobility and activity tolerance, as in the following examples:

- *Respiratory disorders.* Any disorder that affects oxygenation limits exercise tolerance. Chronic obstructive pulmonary disease, asthma, and pneumonia are associated with shortness of breath, which becomes worse with increased activity. Consequently, patients limit their activity.
- *Circulatory disorders* affect mobility. Impaired arterial circulation limits oxygen delivery to the tissue. As activity increases, skeletal muscle pain develops. Impaired venous circulation causes leg swelling and discomfort, which are relieved by elevating the legs. As a result, patients may become relatively sedentary to relieve the pain and discomfort.
- *Fatigue* also affects activity level. Acute illnesses, such as influenza, produce fatigue during the acute illness and limit activity for short periods of time. Disorders that produce long-standing fatigue include anemia, anorexia nervosa, cancer, depression, and grief.
- *Bedrest* is part of the treatment for a variety of disorders. For example, a woman with a high-risk pregnancy may be placed on bedrest. You will learn more about bedrest and the effects of immobility in the following section.

KnowledgeCheck 33-4

- In which age groups are you more likely to see health concerns that affect mobility?
- What types of disorders limit activity or mobility?
- What are the signs and symptoms of a fracture?
- What is the difference between a strain and a sprain?

ThinkLike a Nurse 33-3

- Your teenage daughter complains when you ask her to take a calcium supplement and encourage her to exercise. What information should you provide so she understands why these measures are important?
- Phillip Flanders (Meet Your Patients) has never been involved in a regular exercise program. Phil works as an accountant, and most of his friends are work associates. Phil's siblings are overweight and do not exercise. Both of his parents died of heart disease. Many of Phil's friends have suggested that he begin exercising to improve his energy and health. What recommendations can you make to Phil to make it more likely that he will start and continue an exercise routine?

Example Problem: Hazards Of Immobility

Most people take their mobility for granted until illness, disease, or trauma affects their ability to move. Even short periods of immobility may be difficult. If you've ever had the flu or an illness that sent you to bed, you know that it can take several days to return to your pre-illness state, especially for older adults and people with underlying chronic illness. Severe illness associated with prolonged immobilization causes physiological changes in almost every body system, along with psychological changes. Some changes are reversible, but others are not. The effects of immobility on the following systems are discussed.

Effect of Immobility on Muscles and Bones. Even a couple of days in bed can leave you feeling tired and weak, because the musculoskeletal system is one of the first systems affected by immobility. Inactivity causes significant wasting of the gastrocnemius, soleus, and leg muscles that control flexion and extension of the hip, knee, and ankle. Confinement to bed leads to 7% to 10% loss of muscle strength (atrophy) per week. Immobility also causes the joints to become stiff. The strongest muscles, usually the flexors, pull the joints in their direction, leading to contractures, or joint ankylosis (fusion of the joints).

Immobility affects parathyroid function, calcium metabolism, and therefore bone formation. The result of these changes is osteoporosis, calcium depletion in the joints, and **renal calculi** (kidney stones) due to increased excretion of calcium. These changes place the patient at risk for pathological fractures with minimal trauma.

Effects of Immobility on the Lungs. Immobility decreases the strength of all muscles, including those involved in chest wall expansion, which also affects ventilation. When a patient is in bed, the depth of respirations decreases, and secretions pool in the airways. The ability to effectively cough and expectorate secretions diminishes as muscle tone of the abdomen and chest decrease. As a result, pooled secretions block air passages and alveoli, decrease oxygen and carbon dioxide exchange, and often lead to atelectasis, (collapse of air sacs), or pneumonia. Even a sedentary lifestyle affects the capacity to increase ventilation in response to exercise (see Chapter 37 if you want more information about ventilation).

Effect of Immobility on the Heart and Vessels. Immobility increases the workload of the heart and promotes venous stasis. When you are active, the skeletal muscles of the legs help pump blood back to the heart. Recall that the veins are thin-walled vessels with valves. Muscle activity propels blood toward the right side of the heart, and the valves prevent backflow of blood. To compensate for immobility, heart rate and stroke volume increase to maintain blood pressure. But with immobility, cardiac reserves are lessened, which means the

heart is less able to respond to demands above baseline. Without muscle activity, the force of gravity causes blood to pool in the periphery, which leads to edema. Fluid in the tissue (e.g., heels or sacrum) is more prone to pressure injury.

In addition to venous pooling, immobility leads to compression and injury of the small vessels in the legs and decreased clearance of coagulation factors, causing blood to clot faster. These three changes—stasis, activation of clotting, and vessel injury—make up what is known as **Virchow's triad,** a trilogy of symptoms associated with a greater chance of thrombus formation, such as deep vein thrombosis (DVT).

An immobile person is also more prone to **orthostatic hypotension**. Prolonged bedrest inactivates the baroreceptors involved with constriction and dilation of the blood vessels. As a result, when a person who has been immobilized changes position, he is less able to maintain his blood pressure. The patient complains of feeling dizzy and light-headed and may be unable to support his own weight.

Effects of Immobility on Metabolism. Inactivity increases the level of serum lactic acid and decreases adenosine triphosphate (ATP) concentrations. As ATP concentrations decrease, so do the body's energy reserves. In response, metabolic rate drops, protein and glycogen synthesis decrease, and fat stores increase. Together, these effects cause glucose intolerance and reduced muscle mass. Immobility also triggers the release of epinephrine, norepinephrine, thyroid hormones, adrenocorticotropic hormone (ACTH) from the pituitary gland, and aldosterone from the kidneys. These changes in hormones are the same as occur in the stress response; so, as you can see, immobility can be a stressor in itself.

Effects of Immobility on the Integumentary System. External pressure from lying in one position compresses capillaries in the skin, obstructing skin circulation. Lack of circulation causes tissue ischemia and possible necrosis (death). Nursing interventions include frequent turning and skin care to prevent wounds, known as pressure ulcers, from forming (see Chapter 36 as needed).

Effects of Immobility on the Gastrointestinal System. Immobility slows peristalsis, which leads to constipation, gas, and difficulty evacuating stool from the rectum. In extreme circumstances, a paralytic ileus (cessation of peristalsis) may occur. When peristalsis slows, appetite diminishes and food also is digested slowly. The net effect is usually decreased calorie intake and inability to meet the protein demands of the body. Body muscle is broken down as a fuel source, causing further wasting.

Effects of Immobility on the Genitourinary System. Being supine inhibits drainage of urine from the renal pelves and bladder. Urine becomes stagnant, which creates an ideal environment for infection and kidney stone formation. Immobility triggers a rise in calcium levels, which also contributes to stone formation. Diminished muscle tone leads to a decrease in bladder tone, and many patients have difficulty voiding in a bedpan or urinal.

Psychological Effects of Immobility. Prolonged immobility, whether in the hospital or at home, leads to isolation and mood changes. In the 1960s, the effects of immobility were studied among astronauts. Along with the many physical effects of immobility, these healthy men showed signs of depression, anxiety, hostility, sleep disturbances, and changes in their ability to perform self-care activities. Patients who are in bed for long periods can suffer all these problems, as well as disorientation, apathy, and altered body concept. Other notable psychological effects of immobility/bedrest include a diminished ability to concentrate, recall sequential events, problem solve, and perform self-care.

Interventions for Patients on Bedrest. Interventions for patients on bedrest focus on preventing additional problems caused by immobility, such as pressure injury, constipation, joint contracture, muscle weakness, balance problems, DVT, pooling of secretions, orthostatic hypotension, and various other hazards. The following tips will help you to minimize hazards of immobility for your patients:

- Position the patient to allow for lung expansion and prevent atelectasis and pneumonia.
- Provide a healthy diet to prevent loss of muscle mass.
- Prevent orthostatic hypotension by having the patient sit on edge of bed before the first time out of bed.
- Turn the patient every 2 hours to prevent pressure on the skin and minimize edema.

KnowledgeCheck 33-5

- Identify the effects of immobility on the cardiovascular, musculoskeletal and integumentary systems.
- Why might immobility be referred to as a stressor?
- What are three effects of immobility on the GI system?
- What changes in mood might be seen with immobility?

PracticalKnowledge
knowing **how**

As you have seen in the preceding sections, immobility can result in serious health consequences. In the remainder of the chapter, we discuss nursing actions to promote activity and exercise and eliminate the hazards of immobility.

ASSESSMENT

Perform an assessment focused on mobility and exercise for any patient who has musculoskeletal concerns, is obese, has limited mobility, or is confined to bed or home. As always, you will validate the nursing history data with physical examination. Box 33-4 defines a variety of terms used to describe problems with muscle mass, strength, or mobility. To help you with focused mobility assessments in the home, see the Home Care box Home Assessment for a Patient With Mobility Concerns.

Focused Nursing History

A nursing history focused on activity and exercise addresses usual activity, fitness goals, mobility problems, underlying health problems, lifestyle, and external factors. For questions to ask, see the accompanying Focused Assessment box, Activity and Exercise.

When caring for patients with very limited activity, assessing the ability to perform ADLs or instrumental activities of daily living (IADLs) may be more appropriate. Recall that ADLs focus on hygiene, feeding, toileting, and transfer out of bed. In contrast, IADLs focus on tasks that are instrumental in helping a patient maintain independent living status. Assessment tools for ADLs and IADLs were presented in Chapter 3.

Focused Physical Assessment

Important data to include in a physical assessment related to activity and exercise include vital signs, height, weight, body mass index, body alignment, joint function, gait, muscle

Home Assessment for a Patient With Mobility Concerns

Assess the Environment

➤ Are there stairs or other obstacles that the patient must negotiate?

➤ What aspects of the home environment assist with patient care?

➤ What aspects of the home environment hinder patient care?

➤ What is the patient's history of falls or other mobility concerns?

➤ Would the patient benefit from assistive equipment (e.g., hospital bed, walker)?

➤ Can the patient negotiate the distance between the bedroom, bathroom, and kitchen?

Assess the Family or Caregivers' Abilities and Needs

➤ Who is providing care?

➤ Is the available care sufficient to meet the patient's needs?

➤ Are additional support persons available to assist with care?

➤ Can the caregiver safely move the patient in bed or assist the patient out of bed?

➤ What are the health concerns or physical limitations of the caregivers?

➤ What is the backup plan if the family or caregiver can no longer meet the patient's needs?

Assess Resources

➤ What community resources are available to the patient or caregiver (e.g., Meals on Wheels, physical therapy, Visiting Nurses Association)?

➤ Are the patient and caregiver willing to use community resources?

➤ What services are provided by the patient's insurance?

➤ Can the patient or family afford private services? If so, what services are they interested in?

> **BOX 33-4 ■ Terms Used to Describe Problems With Muscle Mass, Strength, or Mobility**
>
> **Atrophy** is a decrease in the size of muscle tissue due to lack of use or loss of innervation.
> **Clonus** is spasmodic contraction of opposing muscles resulting in tremorous movement.
> **Flaccidity** is a decrease or absence of muscle tone.
> **Hemiplegia** is paralysis of one side of the body.
> **Hypertrophy** is an increase in the size or bulk of a muscle or organ.
> **Paraplegia** is paralysis of the lower portion of the trunk and both legs.
> **Paresis** is partial or incomplete paralysis.
> **Paresthesia** is numbness, tingling, or burning due to injury of the nerve(s) innervating the affected area.
> **Quadriplegia** is paralysis of all four extremities.
> **Spasticity** is a motor disorder characterized by increased muscle tone, exaggerated tendon jerks, and clonus.
> **Tremor** is involuntary quivering movement of a body part.

strength, and activity tolerance. This section summarizes a few of these components. For a description of all the components, see the accompanying Focused Assessment box.

Before beginning the exam, be fully aware of the patient's mobility status and any restrictions in movement, pain, injury, or otherwise. As you move through the exam, observe for pain, inflammation and mobility limitations in all areas. For a thorough discussion of physical assessment of the musculoskeletal system, see Chapter 21.

The Functional Independence Measure

Also known as the FIM Scale, the functional independence measure is used to measure multiple areas of a patient's care needs, such as ADLs, mobility, problem solving, memory, and others. On admission, patients are scored for baseline and then serially until discharge and later in the outpatient or home setting to monitor improvement.

Gait

The way a person moves communicates a great deal about his general state of health, mood, and risk for falls. You might want to assess abnormal gaits in patients with injury, neurological issues, or with the following characteristics:

- **Antalgic gait**—limp to avoid pain when bearing weight on the affected side
- **Propulsive gait**—a stooped, rigid posture, with the head and neck bent forward; movement forward is by small, shuffling steps with involuntary acceleration; also known as festinating gait; common in Parkinson's disease
- **Scissors gait**—legs flexed slightly at the hips and knees with the thighs crossing in a scissors-like movement; common with cerebral palsy, stroke, or spinal tumor
- **Spastic gait**—a stiff, foot-dragging walk caused by one-sided, long-term muscle contraction; seen with cerebral palsy, head trauma, or brain tumor
- **Steppage gait**—an exaggerated motion of lifting the leg to avoid scraping the toes of a foot with foot drop (foot appears floppy with the toes pointing down); seen with Guillain-Barré syndrome
- **Waddling gait**—a distinctive rolling motion in which the opposite hip drops; seen in patients with muscular dystrophy or developmental dysplasia of the hip; characteristic gait in late pregnancy.

To see illustrations of these gaits,

 Go to Chapter 21, **Tables, Boxes, Figures: ESG Table 21-3: Abnormal Atlas: Abnormal Gaits,** on DavisPlus.

Activity Tolerance

To promote the benefits of physical activity, people need to pace themselves during exercise, especially those who have been inactive. Health professionals can teach people to rate the perceived level of exertion and monitor target heart rate. Target heart rate requires a pulse check during exercises and staying within 50% to 85% of the maximum rate. To figure this out, take 220 and then subtract the person's age and then multiply times 0.5 to 0.85.

Focused Assessment

Activity and Exercise

Suggested History Questions for Assessing Activity and Exercise

Usual Activity

Describe your typical daily activity level.

If the patient has very restricted activity, ask the following questions:

➤ Are you able to care for yourself in regard to hygiene, dressing, toileting, and getting out of bed?

➤ If the patient has ADL limitations: Who helps you with these daily activities?

If the patient does not indicate restricted activity, ask the following questions:

➤ What is your usual form of exercise?

➤ How often do you exercise?

➤ How long are your exercise sessions?

➤ How long have you been engaged in this type of activity?

➤ What types of exercise or sports have you participated in the past?

➤ Describe your activity level over the past 10 years.

➤ Are you exercising more or less than in the past?

➤ What factors have changed your activity level?

Fitness Goals

What aspects of exercise do you enjoy? What aspects of exercise do you dislike?

What do you think are the benefits of exercise?

How do you schedule your exercise?

What motivates you to exercise?

What are your current fitness goals?

Mobility Concerns

Do you have any pain or discomfort with activity?

Do you avoid any activities because of pain, discomfort, shortness of breath, or chest pain?

If you answered yes to either question, describe the following:

➤ Type of problem

➤ Onset of concern

➤ Frequency of problem

➤ Activities that trigger and relieve

➤ Severity and type of symptoms

➤ Effect of problem on day-to-day activities

➤ Treatments used to alleviate and how they worked

Underlying Health Concerns

Do you have any healthcare problem that affects your ability to engage in activity or exercise?

If so, describe the problem and the effect.

What medications do you take?

Have you ever been told you have a bone problem? If so, what was the nature of the problem?

Have you ever experienced a fracture, strain, or sprain? If so, where was the problem? When did it occur? How did it occur?

Have you ever had weakness of the muscles or problems coordinating movement?

Do you have any cardiac or respiratory problems that affect your ability to perform activities?

Have you ever experienced anxiety or depression that affected your ability to participate in activities?

Lifestyle

What kind of work do you do?

Describe your typical work activities.

How many hours per week do you work?

What other commitments do you have (school, family, other obligations)?

External Factors

Are there any restrictions in your home that limit your ability to be active?

Do you feel you need an assistive device?

Are you comfortable exercising outside your home or in your neighborhood?

Focused Physical Assessments for Activity and Body Alignment

With the patient standing, observe from the anterior, posterior, and lateral views. Check for the following:

Shoulders and hips are level.

Toes are pointed forward.

The spine is straight, with no abnormal curvatures noted.

The posture is not slumped.

Ask the patient to sit down; observe as he does so.

Does he have difficulty lowering his torso?

Can he control the movement?

Is he able to get into this position with ease?

When he sits, does he slump?

If the patient cannot stand or sit, assess his alignment in bed. Look for ability to move in bed, as well as the posture the patient maintains.

Joint Function

Assessing joint function includes inspection and palpation of the joints and assessment of range of motion.

Begin your assessment at the neck and systematically work your way through each of the joints.

At each joint observe for swelling, erythema, asymmetry, or obvious deformity.

Compare the size of the muscles above and below the joint and on each side of the body.

Palpate the joint for temperature and crepitus. Warmth over a joint indicates inflammation or infection. Be sure to compare body temperature over several joints and right to left. **Crepitus** is a grating sensation when the joint is moved. It can often be heard as well as felt. Crepitus is associated with degenerative joint disease or arthritic changes in the joint.

As you palpate the joint, move it through its range of motion.

Muscle Strength

Assess muscle strength by having the patient push and then pull against your hands.

Start at the neck, and test the strength of all major joints' range of motion.

To see a nurse using a performing passive range-of-motion exercises,

 Go to the *Fundamentals of Nursing Skills Videos,* **Activity & Exercise: Passive Range-of-Motion Exercises.**

(Continued)

Focused Assessment

Activity and Exercise—cont'd

Gait

Gait is divided into two phases: stance and swing.

Stance—In the stance phase, the heel of one foot strikes the ground while the opposite foot pushes off and leaves the ground.

Swing—In the swing phase, the leg from behind moves in front of the body. When the right leg is in stance mode, the left leg is in swing mode.

You must observe the patient walking. Normal gait includes the following features:

➤ Head is erect, gaze forward.
➤ Heel strikes the ground before the toe.
➤ Opposite arm moves forward at the same time.
➤ Feet are dorsiflexed in the swing phase.
➤ Gait is coordinated and rhythmic.
➤ Weight is evenly distributed, with minimal swing from side to side.
➤ Movement starts and stops with ease.
➤ Movement is at a moderate pace.

If the patient uses an assistive device, such as a cane, crutch, or walker, pay attention to how he uses it. Ask the patient to ambulate a short distance with and without the device to determine if the device is actually providing stability.

Activity Tolerance

Assess and record vital signs before having the patient engage in 3 minutes of activity.

Select an activity appropriate for the patient. For example, if the patient uses a walker, ask the patient to walk down the

hallway. For a patient without obvious health limitations, consider asking her to run in place for 3 minutes.

Observe the patient throughout the exercise. If she shows any signs of distress, stop the exercise, immediately take a set of vital signs, and repeat the vital signs every minute until they have returned to baseline.

If the patient can exercise continuously for 3 minutes, assess the patient at the end of the 3-minute period and at 1-minute intervals. Note the change in heart rate, blood pressure, and respiratory rate.

✚ This type of approach is not appropriate for patients who easily become short of breath, develop chest pain, or are very unsteady on their feet. Instead, for example, limit your assessment to determining the amount of assistance the patient needs to turn in bed or get out of bed.

Muscle Mass and Strength

As you observe the patient, compare muscle mass on the right and left sides. If you notice an obvious discrepancy in size, measure the circumference of the limbs and compare.

To assess strength, ask the patient to push against your hand with the hands and feet. Once again, compare both sides.

For guidelines for assessing mobility in the home, see the Home Care box Home Assessment for a Patient With Mobility Concerns.

For more information about optimal target heart rates during exercise, see Box 33-1 or

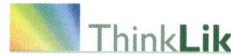 Go the American Heart Association Web site. **Target Heart Rates** are available at http://www.heart.org/HEARTORG/GettingHealthy/PhysicalActivity/Target-Heart-Rates_UCM_434341_Article.jsp#.TyqdCpjrS-8

KnowledgeCheck 33-6

- Describe a focused assessment for a patient experiencing mobility concerns.
- Identify the assessment methods (inspection, palpation, percussion, and auscultation) used when performing a physical examination focused on mobility concerns.

 ## ThinkLike a Nurse 33-4

Review the Meet Your Patients scenario. Which, if any, of the class participants requires a physical examination focused on mobility concerns? Explain your reasoning.

ANALYSIS/NURSING DIAGNOSIS

Nursing diagnoses that specifically describe activity and exercise problems include the following:

- *Activity Intolerance* is a state in which a patient has insufficient physical or psychological energy to carry out daily activities.

- *Impaired Physical Mobility* is limitation of independent purposeful movement of the body. Impaired Physical Mobility is a broad, general diagnosis. Use the following, more descriptive diagnoses when the patient has specific deficits: Impaired Bed Mobility, Impaired Walking, Impaired Wheelchair Mobility, and Impaired Transfer Ability.
- *Risk for Disuse Syndrome* exists when a patient's prescribed or unavoidable inactivity creates the risk for deterioration of other body systems.
- *Sedentary Lifestyle* is a habit of life that is characterized by a low physical activity level.

Mobility problems may also be the etiology of other diagnoses. The following are examples:

- Acute Pain r/t musculoskeletal injury.
- Risk for Injury r/t unsteady gait.

Keep in mind that Immobility, especially bedrest, can be the etiology of problems in all body systems, as well as psychosocially. For more examples and for further information about mobility diagnoses,

 Go to Chapter 33, **Standardized Language: NANDA-I Diagnoses for Activity and Exercise Problems,** on DavisPlus.

PLANNING OUTCOMES/EVALUATION

For *associated NOC standardized outcomes* for mobility diagnoses,

 Go to Chapter 33, **Standardized Language: Selected NOC Outcomes for Energy Maintenance and Mobility,** on DavisPlus.

Effects of Teamwork and Collaboration on Activity and Exercise Outcomes

Competency: Teamwork and Collaboration (Knowledge, Skills, Attitudes); Patient-Centered Care (Knowledge, Skills, Attitudes)*

Scenario: Mr. Lee underwent surgery to repair a ruptured quadriceps tendon in his left leg. His discharge instructions provided general guidelines about wound care, signs and symptoms to report, and when to follow up with the surgeon.

At his two week post-op visit, Mr. Lee was making good progress. The surgeon gave him a prescription to begin physical therapy, telling him that the referred therapists knew his protocols. He also told Mr. Lee that he could drive and return to work, but that he should "listen to his body" and rest when he was tired or in pain. Mrs. Lee mentioned that the drive to work was 1 hour each way and wondered if that was too much. After the surgeon left, the nurse removed the staples from the incision and talked to Mr. and Mrs. Lee about potential complications and how to perform wound care.

The next day, the physical therapist scheduled Mr. Lee for therapy on Mondays, Wednesdays, and Thursdays. During the first therapy session, Mr. Lee moaned with pain. On the second visit, Mrs. Lee remarked that his knee was very swollen but the therapist disagreed with her, noting that other patients had much more swelling than Mr. Lee. One week later Mr. Lee, fearing something was wrong, went to the surgeon's office. He had a fever of 101°F and was in severe pain. The surgeon said, "Your knee is not damaged or infected, but it is very inflamed. You should not have scheduled back-to-back therapy sessions. You've been overdoing it."

Outcome: It was two weeks before Mr. Lee's pain, swelling, and fever subsided.

Think about it: Patient-centered care, teamwork, and collaboration are considered integral to patient safety and quality care. Reflect on this scenario, considering the following questions and concepts:

➤ How would you describe this team's functioning?
➤ What barriers to team functioning do you think might exist in this scenario?
➤ What could the office nurse have done to improve collaboration?
➤ How did teamwork and communication affect Mr. Lee's activity outcomes?
➤ Did the teamwork and communication affect his safety? If so, in what way?
➤ What system changes would you make to improve communication?
➤ Think about patient-centeredness. Did the team value Mrs. Lee's input (give examples)? How might outcomes have been different if Mrs. Lee had been recognized as a full partner in planning or providing care? Do you think quality, safety, costs, and patient satisfaction were affected?

_____
*For specific Knowledge, Skills, and Attitudes,

 Go to the QSEN web site **at http:www.qsen.org. ksas_prelicensure.php**

Individualized goals/outcome statements depend on the nursing diagnosis used. Because activity and exercise abilities are individualized, goals must consider the patient's current condition, expected condition changes, lifestyle, and values. Examples:

Will independently transfer to the wheelchair by [date].

Will discuss his feelings about his activity restrictions by [date].

 ### PLANNING INTERVENTIONS/IMPLEMENTATION

Because attitudes about fitness and activity vary widely, mobility is often a difficult topic. Some people are devastated by activity limitations caused by disease or treatment. Others are able to accept these changes. For these reasons, it is important for you to convey an attitude of acceptance about the patient's current activity level and provide care that helps the patient achieve his optimal level of function.

For *NIC standardized interventions and activities* for patients with mobility problems,

Go to Chapter 33, **Standardized Language: Selected NIC Interventions for Activity and Exercise Management and Immobility Management,** on *DavisPlus.*

Specific nursing activities to promote exercise and mobility include caring for patients with diseases and abnormalities that affect mobility, promoting exercise, preventing injury from exercise, positioning patients, moving patients in bed, transferring patients out of bed, performing ROM exercises, and assisting with ambulation.

Promoting Exercise

Nurses are in an ideal role to encourage and educate people of all ages to be active for healthy living. Here are some common steps to help people attain and maintain fitness. Also see the Self-Care box, Teaching Clients How to Set Up a Fitness Program.

- *Personalize the benefits of regular physical activity.* In other words, find out what motivates your patient. For instance, your patient might want to lose weight and improve his physical appearance. Yet another patient might be interested in improving the quality of sleep or overcoming periods of low energy during the day.
- *Set personal goals for physical activity.* Simple, realistic goals tend to be best. Be sure to define them so they are specific and measurable.
- *Include a variety of activities to keep the patient from feeling bored.*
- *Remind your patient to recognize and appreciate success.*
- *Suggest strategies to achieve the patient's goals.* For instance, you might suggest a fitness program that is fun and entertaining. You can also inform your patient about ways to avoid joint injury or falls.
- *Provide encouragement.* Sometimes just the right approach is a positive, enthusiastic one. You might offer praise for taking steps toward health and fitness. Support from spouse, family members, friends, and coworkers can improve compliance and consistency.

■ *Promote physical exercise as an enjoyable activity.*
■ *Discuss barriers to regular activity and elicit ways to overcome those obstacles.*

People give various reasons for failing to develop a regular exercise program. See Box 33-5 for suggestions on dealing with such objections.

Preventing Injury From Exercise

As previously discussed, the benefits of exercise outweigh any associated risks. Advise clients to follow the tips in the Self-Care boxes, Teaching Clients How to Set Up a Fitness Program and Teaching Your Patients How to Prevent Back Injuries. Also re-read the theoretical knowledge in the section Risks Associated With Exercise if you need a review.

Positioning Patients

Healthy people regularly shift position to maintain comfort. However, many patients are unable to move without assistance. They require a change of position at least every 2 hours to prevent skin breakdown, muscle discomfort, damage to superficial nerves and blood vessels, and contractures. Immobile people are more prone to pressure injury as a result of reduced circulation, impaired oxygen exchange to the tissues, and edema.

A firm mattress provides support to the patient's body and makes it easier to turn the patient (because he does not sink down into the mattress). Most hospital mattresses are firm. However, when you provide home care, you will find mattresses of various types and conditions. To provide additional support, you can place a large piece of plywood under a sagging mattress.

A clean, dry bed also makes it easier to turn the patient and decreases the risk of skin maceration or pressure ulcer formation. Bedding should provide coverage and warmth but not be tucked in so tightly as to restrict movement.

✚ To protect yourself from back injury as you move patients, avoid manual lifting as much as possible. Use assistive equipment and devices, as recommended by the ANA (2006), and always make sure you have adequate help. The amount of help you need depends on the size of the patient, the level of assistance the patient can offer, your size and strength, and the equipment or lines attached to the patient.

Positioning Devices

Devices used to maintain body alignment, prevent contractures, and promote comfort are briefly discussed in the next sections. Positioning devices are commonly used to help minimize the risk for the example problem, Hazards of Immobility. For guidelines for using common positioning devices, including hip abduction pillows, see Clinical Insight 33-2.

BOX 33-5 ■ Suggestions for Overcoming Objections to Exercise

OBJECTION	SUGGESTION
"I hate to exercise."	Pick several activities that you enjoy.
"I burn out on exercise."	Plan ahead and build in rest days and varied activities.
"I am self-conscious about going to the gym and don't have the motivation to exercise by myself."	Find a friend to exercise with, or develop a reward system for yourself if you continue to exercise.
"I am too busy with work or family."	Develop a routine that you can do at lunchtime, or exercise *with* your family.
"I find exercise boring."	Change your routine frequently.
"Exercise hurts."	Make sure to exercise at your target heart rate, and plan a rest day after every weightlifting session.
"I don't have time."	Schedule your exercise time. If need be, schedule several short 10- to 15-min sessions throughout the day.
"I have pain about all the time."	Take pain medication an hour or so before starting physical activity. If fatigue is the problem, try to arrange schedule to keep a balance of rest and activity as well as avoid stimulants (e.g., caffeine or nicotine) that might interfere with the quality of sleep.
"I have difficulty getting around sometimes."	Stretch adequately before starting exercise, but not to overstretch joints. Walk on smooth, even surfaces.
"I am diabetic and have trouble with my feet. My vision is not very good, either."	Be sure shoes fit properly and the area is well lit.

Clinical Insight 33-2 ➤ **Using Common Positioning Devices**

Applying a Trochanter Roll

Trochanter rolls prevent external hip rotation when the patient is in a supine position.

- Fold a towel or bath blanket lengthwise.
- Roll the towel or bath blanket tightly.
- Invert the roll. Turning the patient to one side, place the bath blanket or towel under the patient's hip and thigh. Repeat on the other side if needed.
- Roll the sheet or towel under until it is snug against the patient's hip and thigh. The patient's weight should keep the roll from moving and help to prevent external (outward) rotation of the hips.

- Make sure the roll does not extend as far as the knee. To avoid nerve compression and palsy that can lead to foot drop.
- Alternately, you can place the patient on a sheet that has been folded so that the top edge is at the top of the hips, and the lower edge is about one-third of the way down the thighs. Then place the rolled towels under the sheet and roll the sheet under tightly.

To see a nurse using a trochanter roll,

 Go to the *Fundamentals of Nursing Skills Videos*, **Activity and Exercise: Trochanter Roll.**

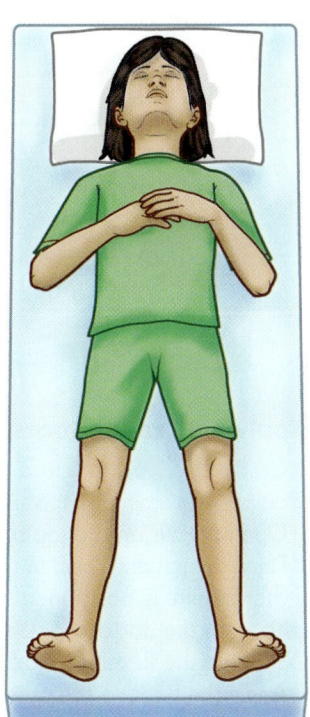 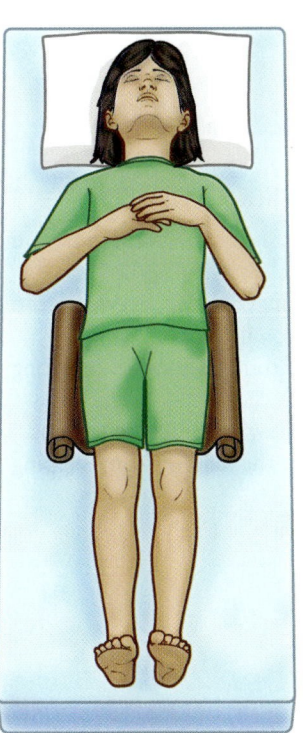

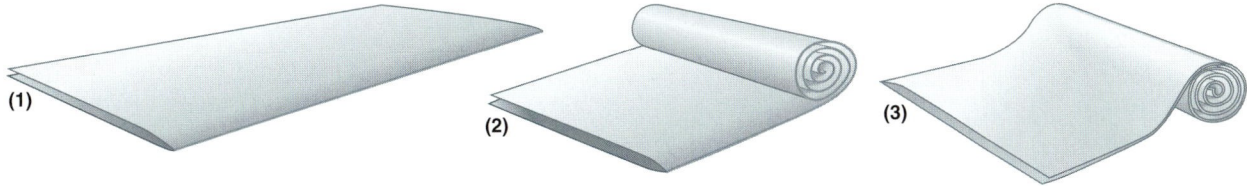

(1)   (2)   (3)

(Continued)

Clinical Insight 33-2 ➤ Using Common Positioning Devices—cont'd

Applying Hand Rolls

- Place a rolled up washcloth or commercial hand roll in the patient's palm. The roll maintains neutral position.
- Secure the strap, if present.
- Roll soft gauze around the hand and secure with nonallergenic, adhesive tape. Wrapping the roll in gauze keeps it from falling out of the patient's hand.
- Place another roll in the patient's other hand, if needed. Hand rolls help prevent hand contractures.

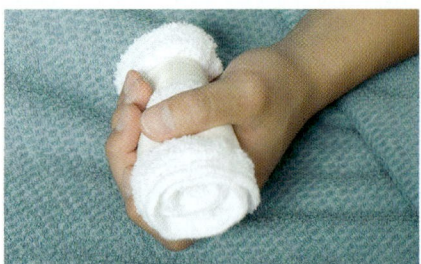

Applying Hip Abduction Pillow

Hip abduction pillows prevent internal hip rotation and hip adduction when the patient is in a supine position.

- Place the wedge-shaped, spongy pillow between the patient's legs when she is lying on her back.
- Slide it toward the groin so it touches the legs all along the inside of the thigh.
- Place both upper legs in the pillow's lateral indentations.
- Secure the straps to prevent the pillow from slipping down the mattress.

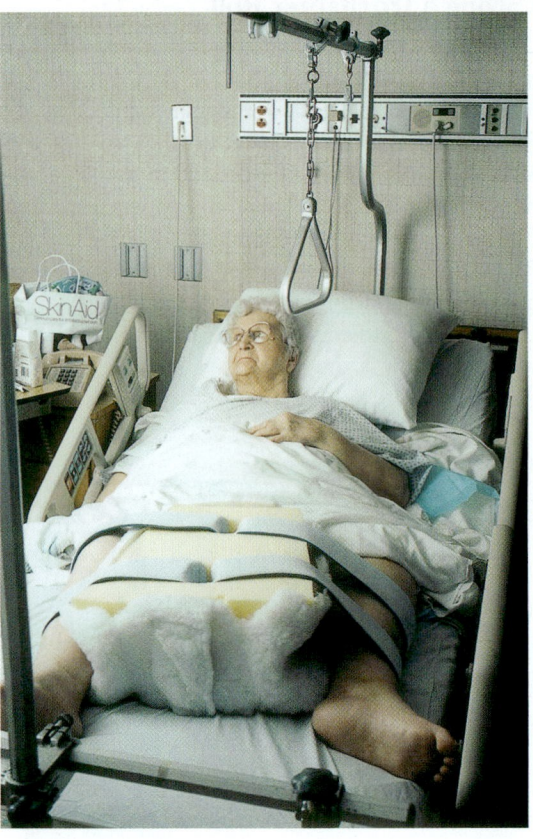

Applying Cradle Boots

Cradle boots prevent foot drop, hip rotation, and pressure on bony prominences, which lead to skin breakdown.

- Open the slit on the top surface of the boot.
- Place the patient's heel in the round cutout for the heel. If the patient is positioned on her side, you may put the boot on the bottom foot.
- Support the flexed top foot with a pillow.
- Apply the boot to the other foot, as needed.
- Position the patient's legs in neutral alignment with slight flexion. Neutral positioning prevents strain on hip ligaments.

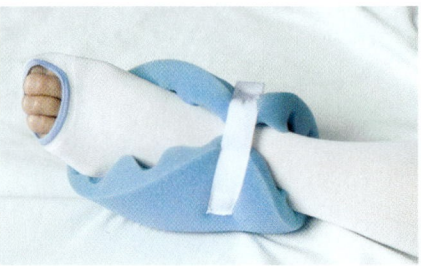

Adjustable Beds

An adjustable bed, often referred to as a *hospital bed*, assumes a variety of positions. You can elevate or lower the head of the bed, and elevate the foot of the bed. Often the bed breaks, or "gatches," at the knee to keep the patient from sliding down when the head is elevated. You can also adjust the height of the bed. You should raise the bed to waist height when providing care so that you can use proper body mechanics; place the bed in its lowest position before helping a patient get out of bed or if the patient is at risk for falling.

Several types of specialized beds are used in treating and preventing pressure ulcers. These include alternating, low air loss, immersion (air-fluidized), and oscillating beds. The mattresses may be composed of air, water, or gel A circular bed and Stryker frame are used in the care of patients with severe mobility restrictions. Both can rotate a patient from supine to prone. With the advent of low-pressure specialized beds, these latter two types of beds are now in limited use.

Pillows

Pillows are the most common devices used to assist with positioning, provide support, and elevate body parts. They help position a patient by molding to the body and expanding the weight-bearing area. You will need a variety of sizes to position patients who are unconscious, paralyzed, frail, or who have had surgery. To obtain the right size or type (e.g., abductor pillows), or if pillows are not available, you can use folded blankets or towels. Foam wedge pillows are useful for elevating the upper body when an adjustable bed is not available and for abducting the hips after hip surgery.

Siderails

Most hospital beds are equipped with siderails. The rails may run the full length of each side of the bed or consist of an upper or lower rail on each side.

✚ Siderails are designed to ensure patient safety. They serve as a reminder that the patient should call for assistance before getting out of bed and provide a grip for the patient who is able to reposition himself in bed. Although siderails are designed to protect patients, they can be a source of injury. Patients can get tangled in the railing or fall between the bed and rail, and confused patients may injure themselves trying to climb over the rails.

Siderails may also be considered a form of restraint, so follow your agency's policy for use and be sure to discuss their purpose with patients and family. See Chapter 23 if you need to review restraint use.

Trapeze Bar

A trapeze bar is a triangular-shaped device that is attached to an overhead bed frame (see Clinical Insight 33-2). The patient can use the base of the triangle as a grip bar to move up in bed, turn, and pull up in preparation for getting out of bed or getting on and off the bedpan. Patients can use the trapeze to move about in bed and to exercise their upper extremities. Frail patients may not be able to use a trapeze bar because of the amount of effort it requires.

Footboard

When a person is supine, the toes tend to point downward toward the bed **(footdrop)**, and the feet are in plantar flexion. Able-bodied persons usually shift position throughout the night, so the foot and leg muscles are periodically contracted and relaxed. In contrast, the patient who is unable to move independently will experience a shortening of the gastrocnemius muscle and may have difficulty walking again if prolonged

plantar flexion occurs. A footboard is a device placed at the end of the bed to prevent foot drop and outward hip rotation, but it does not relieve heel pressure (Fig. 33-5). For the footboard to be effective, the heels must be touching it. Each time you turn the patient, you may need to reposition the footboard to ensure proper position.

Other Positioning Devices

The following are other positioning devices used in the clinical setting.

- *Trochanter rolls* are made from tightly rolled towels, bath blankets, or foam pads. They are placed snugly adjacent to the hips and thighs to prevent external rotation of the hips. To learn how to make them, see Clinical Insight 33-2.
- *Hand and wrist splints* may be manufactured or fashioned from rolled washcloths. Often splints are custom made for patients. The purpose of splints is to hold the wrist and hand in natural position and prevent claw-hand deformities.
- *Hand rolls* prevent hand contractures. Some are commercially made. Otherwise, you can make a hand roll from a tightly rolled washcloth.
- *Hip abduction pillows* prevent internal hip rotation and hip adduction when the patient is in a supine position. These wedge-shaped pieces of spongy material are used after femoral fracture, hip fracture, or surgery. Lateral indentations and straps that wrap around the patient's thighs hold the patient in the correct position.
- *Boots* made of spongy rubber with heel cutouts and ankle cushioning prevent footdrop, skin breakdown, and external hip rotation.

✚ If any part of the boot is made of a latex product, be sure the patient does not have a latex allergy before applying.

- *Foot cradles* are metal or plastic devices that are secured at the foot of the bed to hold bedding up off the toes and feet, allowing for free movement.
- *High-top sneakers* may be used to prevent heel drop, but they do not reduce heel pressure. They do help in positioning hips and pelvis to prevent hip rotation.

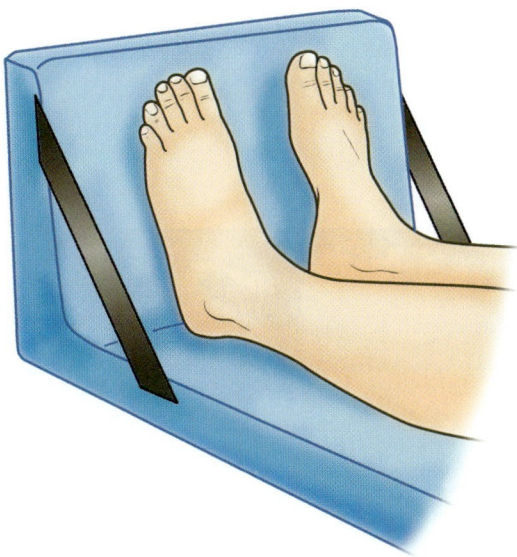

FIGURE 33-5 A footboard is placed at the end of the bed to prevent foot drop.

- *Sandbags* are small fabric bags filled with sand. They are used in the same manner as pillows and trochanter rolls; however, they provide firmer support.

Positioning Techniques

In the next section we briefly describe the various ways to position patients. Table 33-3 illustrates these positions; identifies potential problems associated with them; and offers solutions to prevent the problems. The positions are also described and illustrated in Chapter 21, Table 21-1.

Fowler's Positions

Fowler's position is a semisitting position, in which the head of the bed is elevated 45° to 60°. This position promotes respiratory function by lowering the diaphragm and allowing the greatest chest expansion. It is also an ideal position for some patients with cardiac dysfunction. Common variations include **semi-Fowler's position,** in which the head of the bed is elevated only 30° and **high-Fowler's position,** in which the head is elevated 90°.

In the **orthopneic position,** the head of the bed is elevated 90° and an overbed table with a pillow on top is positioned in front of the patient (Fig. 33-6). Have the patient lean forward, resting his arms and head on the pillow. This position is helpful for a patient with shortness of breath.

Lateral Positions

The **lateral position** is a side-lying position with the top hip and knee flexed and placed in front of the rest of the body. The lateral position creates pressure on the lower scapula, ilium, and

Table 33-3 ➤ Positioning a Bed-Bound Patient

POSITION	POTENTIAL PROBLEM	SOLUTION
Fowler's	Hyperextension of the neck	Use a small pillow under the head and neck.
	Posterior flexion of the lumbar curvature	Use a firm mattress. Position the patient so that the angle of elevation begins at the hip.
	Dislocation of the shoulders	Position a pillow under the forearms to prevent pull on the shoulders.
	Flexion contracture of the wrist and edema of the hands	Support the hands on pillows in alignment with the forearms.
	Flexion contracture of the fingers and abduction of the thumbs	Use hand splints if appropriate, or provide a large roll in the palm of the hand.
	External rotation of the legs	Place sandbags or rolls alongside the trochanters and upper thighs.
	Hyperextension of the knees	Place a small pillow under the lower legs from the ankles to below the knees. Do this for short periods only; avoid pressure on the popliteal area.
	Foot drop	Use a footboard or high-top sneakers to hold the feet in dorsiflexion.
Lateral	Lateral flexion of the neck	Place a pillow under the head and neck to provide alignment.
	Internal rotation and adduction of the upper shoulder and limited respirations	Place a pillow under the upper arm, and comfortably flex the lower arm.
	Internal rotation and adduction of the femur	Support the upper leg from groin to foot with pillows.
	Twisting of the spine	Align the shoulders with the hips.
	Twisting of the spine	Align the shoulders with the hips.
	Flexion of the cervical spine	Place a pillow under the head and neck to provide alignment, unless drainage from the mouth is desired.

Table 33-3 ➤ Positioning a Bed-Bound Patient—cont'd

POSITION	POTENTIAL PROBLEM	SOLUTION
Prone	Hyperextension of the lumbar curvature, pressure on the breasts in women or genitals in men, impaired respirations	Place a small pillow under the abdomen.
	Foot drop	Move the patient down in bed so the feet extend over the edge of the mattress, or place a small pillow under the shins so that the toes do not touch the bed.
	Lateral flexion of the neck	Place a pillow under the head and neck to provide alignment, unless drainage from the mouth is desired.
Sims'	Internal rotation and adduction of the upper shoulder and limited respirations	Place a pillow under the upper arm, and comfortably flex the arm at the elbow.
	Pressure on the shoulder and axilla of the inferior arm	Position the lower arm behind and away from the back.
	Internal rotation and adduction of the femur	Support the upper leg from groin to foot with pillows.
	Twisting of the spine	Align the shoulders with the hips.
	Foot drop	Support the feet in dorsiflexion with sandbags.
	Hyperextension of the neck	Place a pillow under the head and neck to provide alignment.
Supine	Internal rotation of the shoulders and extension of the elbows	Position the upper arms next to the body. Place pillows under the forearms, and position the wrists in slight pronation.
	Flexion of fingers and abduction of the thumbs	Use hand splints if appropriate, or provide a large roll in the palm of the hand.
	Flexion of the lumbar curvature and hips	Provide a firm mattress, or place a small pillow under the lumbar curvature.
	External rotation of the legs	Place sandbags or rolls alongside the trochanters and upper thighs.
	Hyperextension of the knees	Place a small pillow under the lower legs from the ankles to below the knees.
	Foot drop	Use a footboard or high-top sneakers to hold the feet in dorsiflexion.

trochanter but relieves pressure from the heels and sacrum. The **lateral recumbent position** is side-lying with legs in a straight line. The **oblique position** is an alternative to the lateral position that places less pressure on the trochanter. The patient turns on the side with the top hip and knee flexed; however, the top leg is placed behind the body (Fig. 33-7).

Prone Position

In the **prone position,** the patient lies on his abdomen with his head turned to one side. This is the only position that allows full extension of the hips and knees. It also allows secretions to drain freely from the mouth and thus is helpful for an unconscious patient. However, this is the most difficult position to

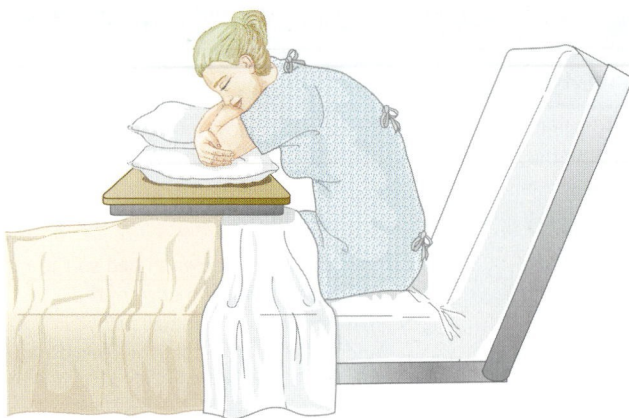

FIGURE 33-6 The orthopneic position is ideal for a patient with shortness of breath.

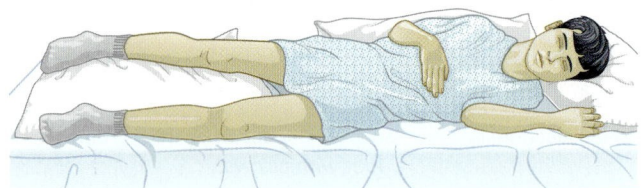

FIGURE 33-7 The oblique position is a modified lateral position that places less pressure on the trochanter.

move an unconscious or frail patient into, because it requires the greatest amount of manipulation to position the patient appropriately. The prone position creates a significant lordosis (inward curving of the spine in the lower back) and rotation of the neck. Therefore, it should not be used for patients with cervical or lumbar spine problems. You should not use the prone position for patients with cardiac or respiratory difficulty because it inhibits chest wall expansion and, therefore, oxygenation. As a rule, you can use this position only for short periods of time.

Sims' Position

Sims' position is a semiprone position. The lower arm is positioned behind the patient, and the upper arm is flexed. The upper leg is more flexed than the lower leg. Sims' position facilitates drainage from the mouth and limits pressure on the trochanter and sacrum. This is an ideal position for administering an enema or a perineal procedure.

Supine Position

In the **supine position,** also known as the **dorsal recumbent position,** the patient lies on his back with head and shoulders elevated on a small pillow. The spine is aligned and the arms and hands comfortably rest at the side.

KnowledgeCheck 33-7

- Describe the following positions: Fowler's, lateral, prone, Sims', and supine.
- What is the advantage of the oblique position versus the lateral position?
- Identify and describe six positioning devices.
- What are three uses for siderails?

ThinkLike a Nurse 33-5

You are providing care for a young man who is recovering from Guillain-Barré syndrome, which produces a reversible paralysis after viral illness. He has been healthy until this present illness. How would you position this patient? Explain your reasoning.

Moving Patients in Bed

To position patients, you must be adept at moving and lifting them in bed. This involves positioning the patient in the length of the bed, as well as turning with as little friction and shearing on the skin as possible. Moving positions in bed is a commonly used intervention to help minimize the risk for the Example Problem, Hazards of Immobility

Moving Up in Bed. Frail patients slide down in bed because of gravity and their inability to correct their position. Elevating the head of the bed accentuates the slide and places the patient in an awkward position. If the patient is light in weight or able to provide assistance, you will be able to move her independently. For complete instructions, refer to Procedure 33-1A.

Turning in Bed. Turn patients at least every 2 hours to protect their skin and prevent other complications of immobility. For efficient use of time, try to time turning to coincide with moving the patient up in bed. Use pillows and other positioning devices to help the patient maintain the new position. For a complete description, see Procedure 33-1B.

Logrolling. Logrolling is a special turning technique used when the patient's spine must be kept in straight alignment. You will need at least two nurses for this procedure, more if the patient is large. Logrolling moves the patient's body as a unit. One nurse is positioned at the level of the patient's head. The other staff members are distributed along the length of the patient. All must move the patient in unison. For a complete description, see Procedure 33-1C.

Friction-Reducing Devices. You can use one of a variety of friction-reducing devices when moving a patient in bed. **Transfer roller sheets** are thin, low-friction fabric sheets that may be placed beneath the drawsheet to facilitate moving the patient in bed (Fig. 33-8). A **scoot sheet** is also a thin, low-friction fabric sheet that is often positioned under the

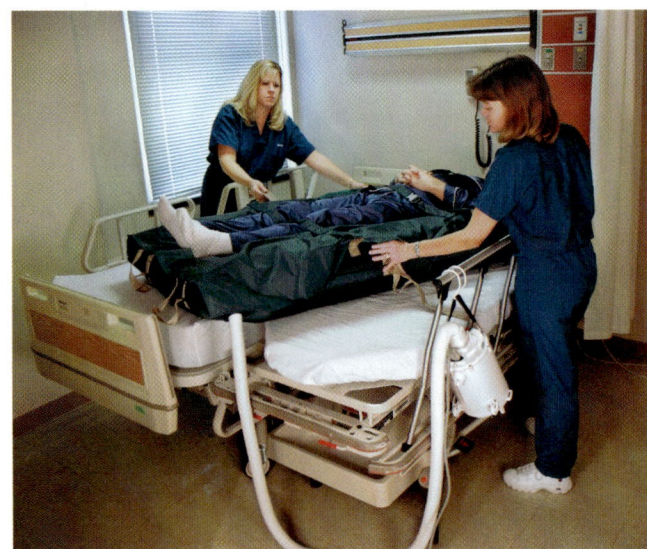

FIGURE 33-8 A transfer roller sheet reduces friction and facilitates movement.

drawsheet of the patient, but it is attached to a mechanical crank (Fig. 33-9). By turning the crank, a single person can move a patient up in bed. Transfer roller sheets are relatively inexpensive and are widely available on clinical units. If one is not available, you can improvise by placing a large, clean, unused plastic bag under the drawsheet to help you move the patient. The plastic bag reduces drag and facilitates movement. However, unlike the thin fabric of transfer sheets, plastic allows moisture to pool under the patient. Consequently, you should not leave a bag in place under the drawsheet.

Transferring Patients Out of Bed

Stretchers and wheelchairs are used to transport patients between units and to tests or procedures. A stretcher is usually reserved for the patient who is weak, sedated, or has a condition that does not permit transfer by wheelchair. A wheelchair may be used for transport or as part of an activity program. In addition, you may transfer patients to a stationary chair to increase their general activity level. For detailed information about transferring patients in or out of bed, see Procedure 33-2.

Transfer Board

A **transfer board** is a wood or plastic device designed to assist with moving patients. Using a transfer board reduces your risk of injury and promotes a smooth transfer. Place the board under the patient on the side to which he will be moved. It is best to use a drawsheet to slide the patient across the board (Fig. 33-10). Transfer boards are also used by patients with long-standing mobility problems to increase their independence.

Mechanical Lift

A **mechanical lift** is a hydraulic device used to transfer patients. Place a fabric sling under the patient, and attach chains or straps from the sling to the lifting device (Fig. 33-11). A mechanical lift is especially useful when providing care for obese and immobile patients. Lifts are often used in home care because they allow one person to transfer the patient safely. Most lifts position patients in a seated position and thus are ideal for assisting the patient into a chair. Others suspend the patient in a supine position; they may be used to transfer the patient from bed to stretcher or to suspend the patient while the bed is made. Many such lifts include scales that weigh the patient while he is suspended in the sling. Some

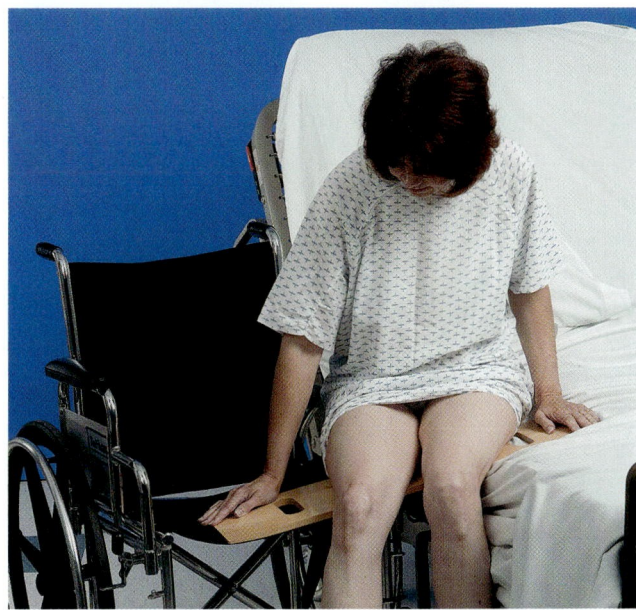

FIGURE 33-10 Transfer boards are used by patients with chronic mobility problems to increase their independence.

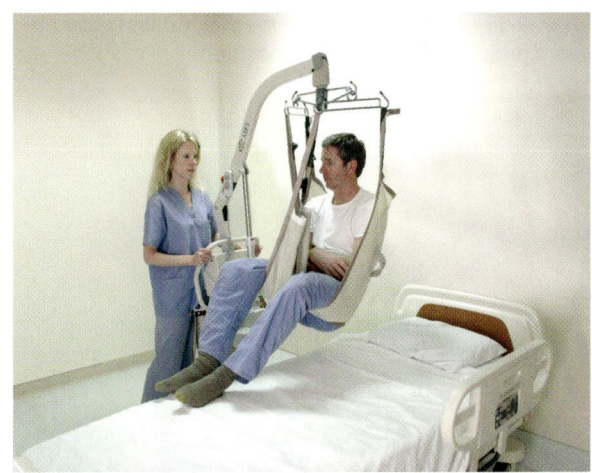

FIGURE 33-11 A mechanical lift is useful when providing care to patients with impaired mobility.

mechanical lifts are mounted on the ceiling to reduce caregiver back injuries and increase patient safety (see Fig. 33-12).

Standing assist devices are mechanical lifts that help the patient move from a sitting to a standing position or support a patient in the standing position. A sling is positioned around the back and under the arms of the patient (Fig. 33-13). Specialized chairs and wheelchairs are also available. Each has a mechanical lift in the seat that rises to assist the patient to a standing position. Mechanical lift devices reduce the risk of back and musculoskeletal injury.

Transfer Belt

A **transfer belt** is a heavy belt several inches wide that is used to facilitate transfer or provide a secure mechanism to hold the patient when ambulating. Apply the belt around the patient's abdomen, close to the patient's center of gravity. The belt may have external grip holds, or you may grip the entire belt with your hand (Fig. 33-14).

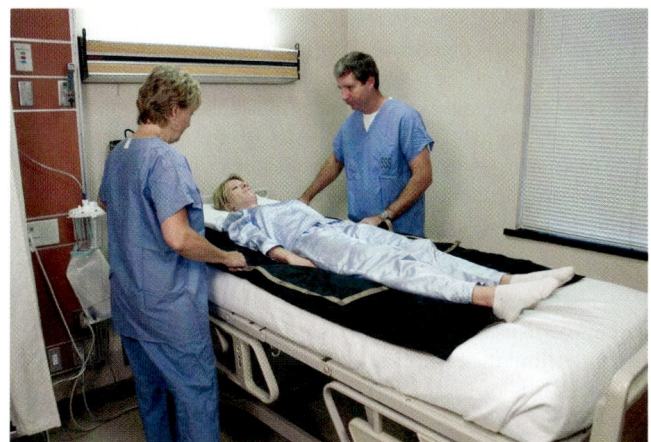

FIGURE 33-9 A scoot sheet allows a single person to move a patient up in bed.

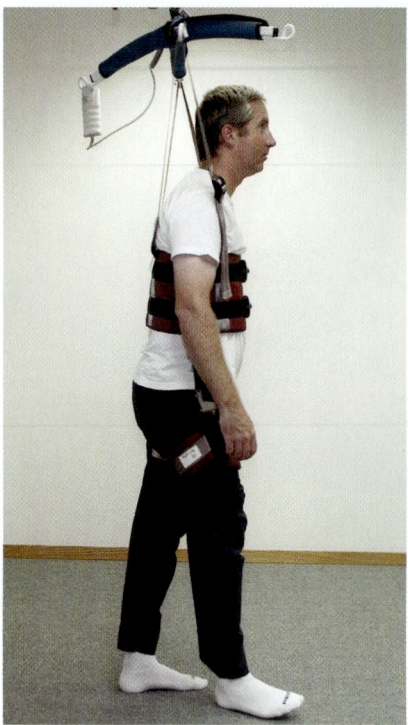

FIGURE 33-12 A ceiling mounted mechanical lift is used to support patients in the standing position.

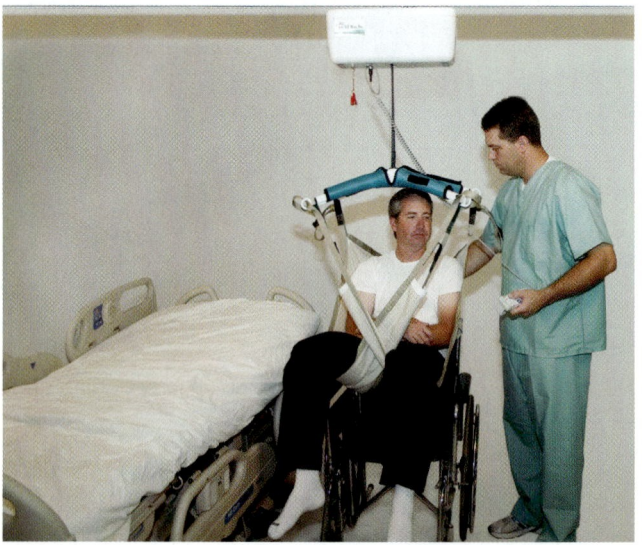

FIGURE 33-13 A mechanical lift with a sling chair is used to safely transfer an immobile patient into a wheelchair.

The fit should not be overly tight or cause the patient discomfort. You should be able to easily place your hand under the belt. Do not place it over the rib cage, as this could compromise breathing. Do not use a transfer belt around the patient's hip. This could cause unsteadiness and lead to a patient fall. You would not use a transfer belt after abdominal surgery or with other abdominal wound, colostomy, or internal organ contusion or other injury.

To know what type of assistive device is appropriate for patient safety and to prevent back injury to the nurse, see Table 33-4.

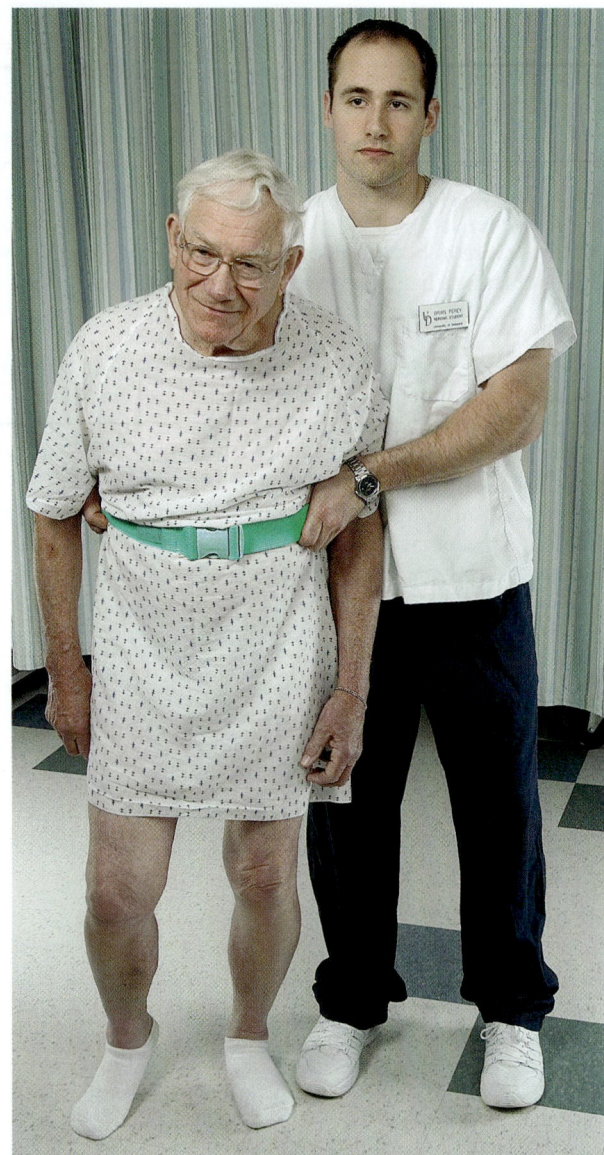

FIGURE 33-14 A transfer belt is placed close to the patient's center of gravity. It may have external grip holds to facilitate transfer or provide a secure mechanism to hold the patient when ambulating.

KnowledgeCheck 33-8

- What criteria determine whether your patient should be logrolled when he is repositioned?
- How often should you turn and reposition a patient?
- Identify the most appropriate device for the following activities:
  Transferring an obese patient from a bed to a stretcher
  Assisting an immobile patient to a recliner chair
  Helping a weak patient from bed to chair

Performing Range-of-Motion Exercises

Patients with limited mobility are at risk for developing complications of disuse, such as muscle atrophy and contractures. ROM exercises limit the complications of this chapter's Example Problem, Hazards of Immobility. **Active range of motion (AROM)** occurs when the patient independently moves his joints through flexion, extension, abduction, adduction, and circular rotation. Patients recovering from illness, injury, or surgery often perform this exercise as a rehabilitation procedure. Performing ADLs

Table 33-4 ➤ Transferring Patients According to Dependency Level

PATIENT LEVEL OF DEPENDENCE	ASSISTIVE DEVICE
Complete dependence (immobile; no assistance)	Mechanical lift with full sling
Extensive dependence (holds on to device but with minimal strength)	Mechanical lift with full sling or stand/assist lift
Moderate dependence (no patient assist for lifting from floor)	Mechanical lift with full sling, or if transfer is manual, more than one helper might be needed
Patient assists with limited mobility	Transfer belt or gait belt
Limited dependence	Stand/assist lift or friction-reducing device

Source: Adapted from ANA. (2006). Preventing back injuries: Safe patient handling and movement. Retrieved February 1, 2012, from http://www.nursingworld.org/MainMenuCategories/WorkplaceSafety/SafePatient/PreventingBackInjuries.pdf

exercises most joints. **Passive range of motion (PROM)** is movement of the joints through their range of motion by another person. Both AROM and PROM improve joint mobility, increase circulation to the area exercised, and help maintain function. However, AROM also improves muscle strength and tone, as well as respiratory and cardiac function. For an explanation of how to perform PROM, see Clinical Insight 33-3.

Continuous passive motion (CPM) is a device that is used to gently flex and extend the knee joint. The CPM machine is often used after knee replacement or other knee procedures to allow the joint to improve range of motion, eliminate the problem of stiffness, and prevent the development of adhesions, which can limit motion further.

Assisting With Ambulation

Prolonged bedrest is no longer the standard of care. However, as a nurse, you will provide care to patients whose illnesses and injuries curtail their ability to walk and be active. Assisting patients with ambulation includes physical conditioning to prepare the patient for ambulation, as well as assisting the patient to walk. These activities help to minimize the effects of the Example Problem, Hazards of Immobility.

Physical Conditioning

Patients who have been confined to bed for more than a week or who have sustained major injury require conditioning before they are able to resume walking. The following conditioning exercises are summarized here; they are explained in detail, see Clinical Insight 33-4.

Quadriceps and Gluteal Drills. The quadriceps muscle group and the gluteal muscles are the largest muscles of the body. Patients who are confined to bed can perform isometric exercises to prepare them for walking.

Arm Exercises. Patients use the biceps and triceps muscles when getting out of bed and for crutch walking. Exercises to help prepare the patient for ambulation include using a trapeze bar, and doing "push-ups" off the mattress or a chair.

➕ Be mindful of any cardiac or musculoskeletal precautions that restrict arm movement, weight-bearing on the hands and wrists, or other upper body injury. If lymphedema is present in the upper extremities, do not encourage arm exercises or use of the trapeze, unless directed by the primary care provider.

Dangling. Use this position to prepare the patient to get up in a chair, to stand, or to ambulate.

Clinical Insight 33-3 ➤ Performing Passive Range-of-Motion Exercises

- **Explain the purpose of PROM.** You may also wish to teach family members and caregivers about the importance of ROM exercises and enlist their help in exercising the patient when they visit.
- **Observe the patient as you perform PROM.** You may need to perform the exercises in several short segments if the patient tires easily or experiences discomfort.
- **Support the patient's limb** above and below the joint that is to be exercised.
- **Move the joint in a slow, smooth, rhythmic manner.** Avoid fast movements; they may cause muscle spasm.
- **Never force a joint.** Some patients may have limited ROM. Move each joint to the point of resistance. This should not be painful.

- **Perform PROM** at least twice daily. Move each joint through ROM three to five times with each session. Consider incorporating PROM into care activities, for example, while bathing or turning the patient.
- **Return the joint to a neutral position** when exercise is complete.
- **Encourage active exercise** whenever possible.

To see a nurse performing passive range-of-motion exercises,

 Go to the *Fundamentals of Nursing Skills Videos,* **Activity and Exercise: Passive Range-of-Motion Exercises.**

Clinical Insight 33-4 ➤ **Assisting With Physical Conditioning Exercises to Prepare for Ambulation**

Conditioning exercises include the following.

Quadriceps and Gluteal Drills

- Ask the patient to tighten her thigh muscles by pushing downward with her knees and flexing her feet. Each leg may be done separately if moving both is contraindicated.
- Ask the patient to hold the position for a count of 5 and then relax.
- Repeat this process two to three times per hour during the waking hours.
- To exercise the gluteal muscles, ask the patient to pinch her buttocks together.
- Do this exercise when the patient exercises her quadriceps muscles.
- Instruct the patient not to hold her breath as she exercises.

Arm Exercises

- Install a trapeze bar on the patient's bed. Ask the patient to do pull-ups on the bar from a lying position. This exercises the biceps muscles.
- To exercise the triceps muscles, ask the patient to lift his upper body off the mattress by firmly pressing down with the palms.
- The patient can also do push-ups from a seated position at the side of the bed or from a stationary chair or wheelchair.

Dangling

- Dangling is a seated position at the side of the bed, feet resting on the floor.
- Provide a footstool if the patient's feet do not reach the floor.
- Assess for light-headedness or postural hypotension.
- Do not progress to ambulation until the patient is comfortable and stable in the dangling position.

Daily Activities

- Encourage your patient to be active in bed by repositioning and turning herself.
- Encourage the patient to get out of bed and into a chair before attempting to walk.
- Encourage the patient to perform as much of her ADLs as possible.

   ADLs exercise many of the muscle groups used in ambulation.

   To see a nurse performing PROM exercises,

 Go to the *Fundamentals of Nursing Skills DVDs,* **Activity and Exercise: Physical Conditioning Exercises: Quadriceps, Gluteal, Arm, and Dangling.**

✚ Patients who have been confined to bed frequently become lightheaded or develop orthostatic hypotension when first getting up. Dangling allows the patient to experience being upright with limited risk of falling.

Some common approaches used for orthostatic problems include antiembolism stockings with compression wraps to prevent pooling of venous blood. Sometimes abdominal binders are used for this purpose as well. Medication is available to control orthostatic hypotension. Patients with spinal cord injury experiencing autonomic dysfunctions need a high-backed reclining wheelchair so the back of the chair can be lowered (and someone might even have to lift up their legs for a few minutes) until blood pressure stabilizes. Tilt-table therapies are also used.

Daily Activities. Moving around in bed and performing ADLs (e.g., brushing ones hair) exercise many of the muscle groups needed for ambulation. Getting up into a chair accustoms the patient to an upright posture and is an important predictor of success with ambulation.

Assisting the Patient to Walk

Before getting the patient out of bed, assess his readiness to walk. Also obtain the appropriate equipment and assistance. Move floor rugs and loose objects from the path of the patient and caregiver. Be sure the floor is not slippery. When possible, use a transfer belt. Have a chair or additional assistance available on the first few attempts at ambulation.

✚ If the patient becomes faint or begins to fall, do not attempt to hold him up by yourself. Instead, protect the patient as you guide him to a seated or lying position. Create a wide base of support, and project forward the hip closest to the patient. Help the patient slide down your leg as you call for help (Fig. 33-15). Protect the patient's head as his body descends.

To learn procedures for assisting with ambulation, see Procedures 33-3A and 33-3B, at the end of this chapter.

   Assisting Older Adults. When assisting older adults to ambulate, find out how much assistance, if any, the patient typically requires and modify support as needed. Consider the following nursing interventions.

- Observe constantly during ambulation for weakness and fatigue. Plan for periods of rest during ambulation, if needed. The older adult might become fatigued more quickly and recover more slowly from the physical demands of walking, especially if a heart or lung condition is present.

- ✚ Move the patient gradually to a sitting position and allow him to dangle at the bedside before coming to a standing position. Observe for dizziness or lightheadedness.

- Assess for falls risk factors. For example, some medications cause dizziness or lethargy; and patients with neurological or cognitive disorders, such as Parkinson's or Alzheimer's disease, have a greater potential for falls. For more information about assessing a patient's risk for a fall, see Chapter 23.

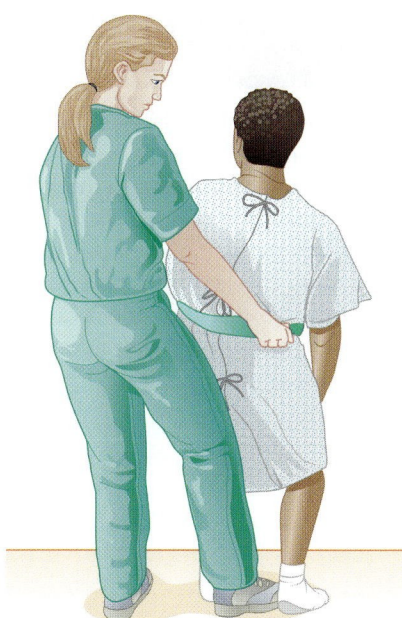

FIGURE 33-15 If the patient begins to fall, the nurse guides the patient gently to the floor or to a chair.

- To reduce the risk for falling in the home, recommend family place nonskid strips on stairs or other smooth flooring.
- Assistive devices, such as walkers, canes, and transfer belts, can be useful for older adults who require more support.

✚ Be cautious when using a transfer belt for the patient with osteoporosis or back pain. Too much pressure from the belt can cause injury or pain.

KnowledgeCheck 33-9

- Identify four principles to be followed when performing PROM.
- Describe activities that can promote a patient's readiness for ambulation.
- What action should you take if a patient begins to fall when ambulating?

Mechanical Aids for Walking

There are several aids available to promote stability and independence when walking. Some aids are intended for short-term use; others will be incorporated into the patient's lifestyle. Some patients consider the use of aids a sign of weakness or inconvenience. As a result, they avoid using the aid and increase their risk of falls. However, most people dread loss of independence, so you can promote the use of walking aids by stressing their importance in helping the person maintain independence. For instructions on sizing canes, walkers, and crutches, see Clinical Insight 33-5. For instructions on teaching patients to use these aids, refer to Clinical Insight 33-6.

Canes

The following are three basic types of canes used (Fig. 33-16):
- *Single-ended cane with a half-circle handle.* This is ideal for the patient who needs minimal support and is able to negotiate stairs.
- *Single-ended cane with a straight handle.* This is ideal for the patient with hand weakness who has good balance.
- *Multiprong canes.* A multiprong cane usually has three or four prongs, and all types have a straight handle. These

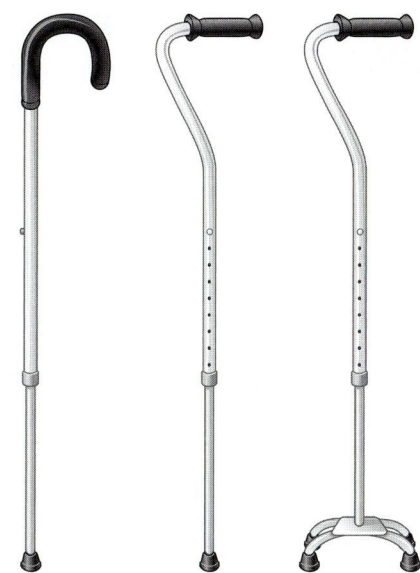

FIGURE 33-16 Three types of canes.

canes provide a wide base of support and are useful for patients with balance problems.

Walkers

A walker is a lightweight metal frame device with four legs that provides a wide base of support as a patient ambulates (Fig. 33-17A). Various forms of walkers are available. Some models have wheels that allow the walker to be rolled forward; others have a seat that allows the patient to rest periodically (Fig. 33-17B). These walkers are best for patients whose mobility problems are related to fatigue or shortness of breath rather than gait instability.

Braces

Braces support joints and muscles that cannot independently support the body's weight. They are most commonly used in the lower extremities. Physical medicine specialists usually fit the brace. Nursing responsibilities include assisting the patient into and out of the brace and monitoring the condition of the skin under the brace.

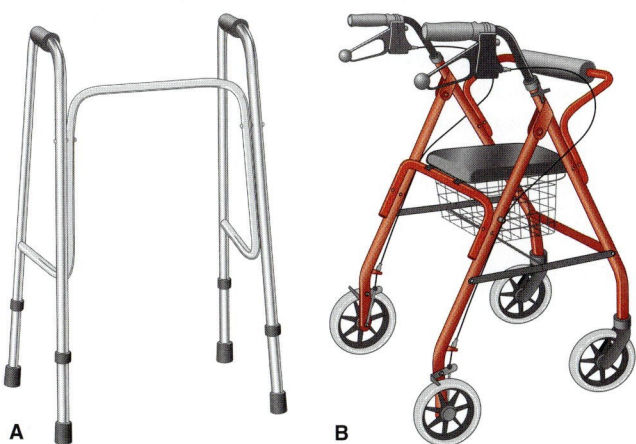

A   B

FIGURE 33-17 Walkers. A. The basic walker is picked up and advanced as the patient steps ahead. B. Some walkers have wheels and seats that allow the patient to rest periodically.

Clinical Insight 33-5 ➤ Sizing Walking Aids

Sizing Canes

- Ask the patient to stand erect, and place the cane tip 20 cm (4 in.) to the side of the foot.
- The top of the cane should reach the top of the hip joint so that the patient can hold the cane with her elbow flexed 30°.

Sizing Walkers

- Ask the patient to stand erect, holding onto the walker.
- The walker should extend from the floor to the hip joint so that the patient can comfortably hold the walker with 30° flexion of the elbow.

Sizing Crutches

To measure a patient for an axillary crutch, follow these guidelines:
- Ask the patient to lie down wearing the nonskid shoes that will he use when walking.

- Measure the distance between the heel and the anterior fold of the axilla, then add 2.5 cm (1 in.).
- Select a crutch that can be adjusted to this height.
- Have the patient stand, and position the crutch tip 10 to 15 cm (4 to 6 in.) to the side of the heel. Adjust the axillary crutch pad three fingerbreadths below the axilla.
- Adjust the handgrips so that the patient can comfortably grasp the bar while the elbow is slightly flexed. The patient's axilla should not rest on the crutchpad.

Clinical Insight 33-6 ➤ Teaching Patients to Use Canes, Walkers, and Crutches

Canes

After ensuring the cane is the proper size (refer to Clinical Insight 33-5), instruct the patient to do the following:
- Hold the cane on the stronger side.
- Distribute weight evenly between the feet and cane.
- Advance the cane and weaker leg simultaneously, then bring the stronger leg through.
- Avoid leaning over or on the cane.
- Maintain the integrity of the rubber tip for traction.

Walkers

After ensuring the walker is the proper size (refer to Clinical Insight 33-5), instruct the patient to do the following:
- Stand between the back legs of the walker. Do not stand too far behind the walker.
- Pick up the walker, and advance it as you step ahead. Do not advance it so far as to lose balance.
- If one leg is weaker, move it forward as the walker moves forward.
- Pick up, rather than slide, the walker (unless it has wheels).

Crutches

After ensuring the crutches are the proper size (refer to Clinical Insight 33-5), do the following:
- When first teaching crutch walking, instruct the patient to stand near a wall with a chair behind him. Help the patient

to stand and grip the crutches. Ask the patient to sway from side to side on the crutches to become accustomed to weight-bearing by the arms.
- *Tripod position* is the basic crutch gait standing position. Place crutches 15 cm (6 in.) in front of the feet, with the crutch point 15 cm from the patient's center. In this position, a triangle is formed by the crutches and the body.
- Five crutch gaits exist (see accompanying chart): 2-point gait, 3-point gait, 4-point gait, swing-to gait, and swing-through gait.
- To teach the patient how to go down stairs, instruct him to hold his injured leg in front and hop down each stair on his good leg, one step at a time. When going up stairs with no handrail, he should lead with his good leg by standing close to the first step with weight on the crutches, and lift the uninjured leg, landing it solidly on the step. Then bring the crutches up to that same step, and repeat. If there is a handrail, then patient holds the crutches in one hand and handrail with the other. He then brings the good leg up one step, while the injured leg bears no weight.

⊕ Navigating stairs with crutches can be dangerous. When possible, have the patient practice this technique before discharge. When having a patient practice, someone should always stand below the patient on the stairs to prevent falling. If this is too difficult, he should try sitting on the stairs and inch down each step slowly and carefully.

Clinical Insight 33-6 ▶ **Teaching Patients to Use Canes, Walkers, and Crutches—cont'd**

Read this table from bottom to top.

2-Point gait	3-Point gait	4-Point gait	Swing to	Swing through
• Partial weight bearing, both feet; faster, but less support than a 4-point gait	• Non-weight bearing; faster than a 4-point gait; can use with walker	• Partial weight bearing, both feet; patient must shift weight constantly	• Weight bearing, both feet; can use with walker	• Weight bearing; requires the most coordination and balance
4. Advance right foot and left crutch	**4.** Advance right foot	**4.** Advance right foot	**4.** Lift both feet; swing them forward, landing feet next to the crutches	**4.** Lift both feet; swing them forward, landing feet in front of the crutches
3. Advance left foot and right crutch	**3.** Advance left foot and both crutches	**3.** Advance left crutch	**3.** Advance both crutches	**3.** Advance both crutches
2. Advance right foot and left crutch	**2.** Advance right foot	**2.** Advance left foot	**2.** Lift both feet; swing them forward, landing feet next to the crutches	**2.** Lift both feet; swing them forward, landing feet in front of the crutches
1. Advance left foot and right crutch	**1.** Advance left foot and both crutches	**1.** Advance right crutch	**1.** Advance both crutches	**1.** Advance both crutches
Tripod position	Tripod position	Tripod position	Tripod position	Tripod position

Crutch gaits. The shaded area represents weight-bearing. The arrow shows movement.

Crutches

Crutches are commonly used for rehabilitation of an injured lower extremity. The purpose of using crutches is to limit or eliminate weight-bearing on the leg(s) by forcing the user to rely on strength in the arms and shoulders for support. Two forms of crutches are available.

The *forearm support crutch* is more likely to be used by a patient with permanent limitations. It is usually constructed of lightweight aluminum with a hand hold and a forearm support (Fig. 33-18A).

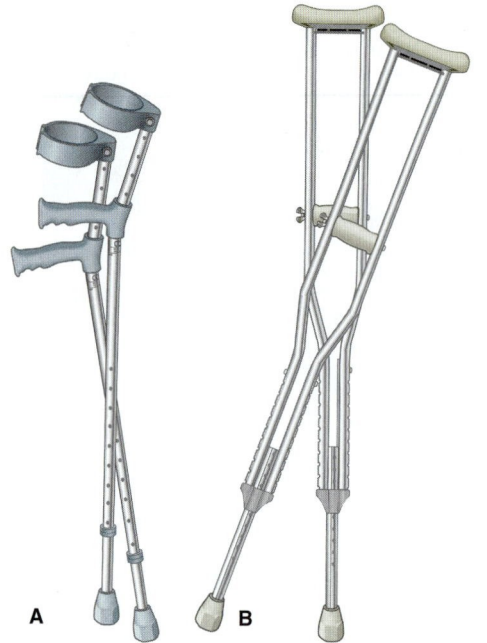

A   **B**

FIGURE 33-18 Crutches. A. Forearm support crutches. B. Axillary crutches.

Axillary crutches are for both short- and long-term use (Fig. 33-18B). Properly fitted axillary crutches support the body weight in the hands and arms, not the axilla. For guidelines on how to measure a patient for an axillary crutch, see Clinical Insight 33-5.

Crutch walking taxes the arms and hands and may cause discomfort to the axillae, arms, and palms where the patient is bearing weight. There are five crutch gaits: two-point gait, three-point gait, four-point gait, swing-to gait, and swing-through gait. Two-point and four-point gait are used for partial weight-bearing, whereas three-point gait is used when weight-bearing must be avoided. Swing-to and swing-through are used when weight-bearing is permitted. For basic gaits and guidelines for teaching patients to use crutches, refer to Clinical Insight 33-6.

To see animations of crutch gaits,

 Go to **Animations: 5 Types of Crutch Gaits,** on Davis*Plus*.

Navigating stairs with crutches can be quite dangerous. When possible, have the patient practice this technique before discharge.

KnowledgeCheck 33-10

- What type of cane should a patient with significant balance problems use?
- When are forearm support crutches used?
- Identify five crutch gaits.

 Think**Like a Nurse** 33-6

Discuss crutch walking with your peers and family. What instruction would facilitate the best understanding of proper crutch-walking technique?

 CLINICALREASONING
Applying the **Full-Spectrum Nursing Model**

Because the following critical-thinking activities allow you to practice the kind of thinking you will use as a full-spectrum nurse, they usually have no single right answer. Discuss them with your peers—if you have difficulty with any of the questions, consult your instructor.

PATIENT SITUATION

Mr. Ronald Ornduff is a 72-year-old retired man who lives with his wife in a one-story home. He has excellent general health with no significant health problems. Ronald typically walks with a moderate to fairly vigorous pace in his neighborhood or at the mall in the winter. He belongs to a health club and works out two or three times a week, walking on the treadmill or using the weight machines or taking a basic conditioning class. Mr. Ornduff considers himself fit and of an acceptable weight for his age. When going outdoors to pick up the morning paper, he slipped on a patch of ice and fell. You are now caring for him 2 days after hip surgery. He is experiencing pain and seems fearful his injury could be the beginning of a decline in his health.

THINKING

1. *Theoretical Knowledge:*
   a. Based on Mr. Ornduff's age, physical condition, and activity level, make a rough estimate of the number of minutes/week of physical activity he should have after he recovers from surgery and resumes full mobility. What are the benefits of this physical activity?
   b. As a nurse planning the care for a patient after hip surgery, what complications of immobility can occur?

2. *Critical Thinking (Considering Alternatives):* What are some possible barriers for an older adult's participating in physical activity? What might you teach your patient to do to overcome those barriers?

DOING

3. *Practical Knowledge:*
   a. How might you position your patient after hip surgery?
   b. What equipment would you need to position your patient after surgery? Is there anything you can set up that will help your patient move around in bed when he can tolerate it?
   c. What type of physical activity would you recommend Mr. Ornduff incorporate into his exercise plan after he experiences full recovery from his surgery? What benefit will these exercises provide?
   d. *Nursing Process (Diagnosis):* Write at least two nursing diagnoses for Mr. Ornduff. Use just the data provided in the situation. Assume he is 2 days post-op.

CARING

4. *Self-Knowledge:* What would you be feeling if you were in Mr. Ornduff's situation of being physically fit one day and suffering pain and immobility the next?
5. *Ethical Knowledge:* What are one or two things you would do to help Mr. Ornduff feel cared for and cared about?

 Go To Chapter 33, **Clinical Reasoning: Applying the Full-Spectrum Nursing Model Response Sheet,** on Davis*Plus*.

PracticalKnowledge
procedures

In this section you will learn about procedures and techniques for positioning, moving, turning, transferring, and ambulating patients safely. Although the ANA (2005) recommends that you use assistive equipment for all lifting and transferring, you may encounter situations in which equipment is not available or you do not have time to get it. In such situations, using good body mechanics may help you decrease the risk of injury to you and the patient.

Procedure 33-1 ■ Moving and Turning Patients in Bed

➤ For steps to follow in *all* procedures, refer to the Universal Steps for All Procedures found on the page facing the inside back cover.

Equipment
- Nonlatex gloves, if you may be exposed to body fluids
- Friction-reducing device, such as a transfer roller sheet or scoot sheet
- Pull or lift (draw) sheet
- Pillows, as needed

Delegation
You may ask nursing assistive personnel (NAP) to assist with moving a patient up in bed, turning a patient, or logrolling a patient after ensuring that the NAP has the necessary skills and that the patient's condition is stable. Complete the assessment, and inform the NAP of any special considerations when moving the patient.

Pre-Procedure Assessment
- Assess the patient's level of comfort.
  If the patient is uncomfortable, you may need to administer an analgesic before moving.

- Assess the patient's level of consciousness, ability to follow directions, and ability to assist with the move.
- Assess for restrictions in movement or position by asking the patient and checking the provider's orders.
- Assess the physical size of the patient and the assistive devices available.
- Review the patient's medical diagnoses. Identify problems that may affect positioning (e.g., respiratory or cardiac problems, pain).
- Observe for the presence of equipment such as IV setups, pumps, or casts and know what must be moved with the patient.
  The preceding assessments all help determine how many assistants and equipment you need, the patient's ability to assist in the procedure, and how to proceed with the move safely.

(continued on next page)

Procedure 33-1 ■ Moving and Turning Patients in Bed (continued)

Procedure 33-1A ■ Moving a Patient Up in Bed

➤ When performing the procedure, always identify your patient according to agency policy and be attentive to standard precautions, hand hygiene, patient safety and privacy, body mechanics, and documentation.

➤ *Note:* This procedure employs the use of a transfer roller sheet. This device is inexpensive and readily available. Scoot sheets further reduce the risk of back and musculoskeletal injury; however, their availability varies. However, having a second person to help move a patient up in bed is the safest approach for staff and patients. Follow the body mechanics guidelines in Clinical Insight 33-1.

Procedure Steps

Note: Medicate the patient for pain, if needed, before moving the patient in bed.

1. **Lock the bed wheels.** Lower the head of the bed, and place the patient in a supine position. Position one nurse on each side of the bed. Lower the siderails on the "working" side of the bed. Raise the height of the bed to waist level.
   Lowering the siderails and raising the bed allows you to move the patient while maintaining good body mechanics and working with gravity.

2. **Ensure that a friction-reducing** device, such as a transfer roller sheet, is in place under the drawsheet. If not, turn the patient from side to side to place the device under the drawsheet. You can improvise this device by placing a clean, unused plastic bag or plastic film under the drawsheet.
   A transfer roller sheet facilitates movement by reducing friction. This also helps to reduce back injury to the nurse.

3. **Remove the pillow** from under the patient's head. Place it at the head of the bed.
   A pillow prevents patient from hitting his head on the headboard.

4. **Instruct the patient** to fold his arms across his chest. If an overhead trapeze is in place (e.g., see Clinical Insight 33-2), ask the patient to hold the trapeze with both hands if able. Have the patient bend his knees with feet flat on the bed.
   This position facilitates patient's assistance with move.

5. **Instruct the patient to flex** his neck.
   Flexion protects the neck with movement.

6. **With a nurse positioned** on either side of the patient, grasp and roll the drawsheet close to the patient.

7. **Instruct the patient**, on the count of 3, to lift his trunk and push off with his heels toward the head of the bed.

8. **Position your feet with a wide base** of support. Point your feet toward the direction of the move. Flex your knees and hips.
   Allows you to maintain proper body mechanics and prevents injury while moving the patient. ▼

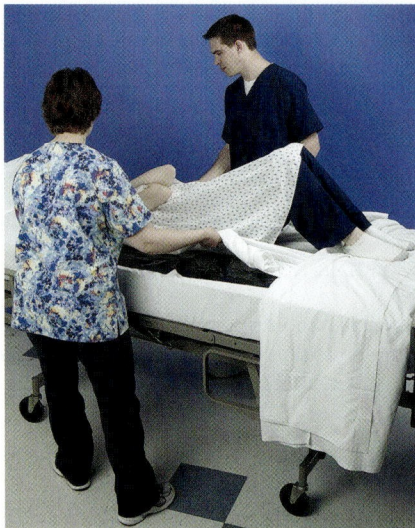

9. **Place your weight on your foot** nearest to the foot of the bed. Count to 3, and shift your weight forward toward the head of the bed.
   Shifting your weight allows you to use your momentum to move the patient, which helps protect your back from injury.

10. **Repeat until the patient** is positioned near the head of the bed. If you used a plastic bag or film to reduce friction, remove it now.
    Plastic is water impermeable, so it allows moisture to pool under the patient. This creates a risk for Impaired Skin Integrity.

11. **Straighten the drawsheet,** and tuck it in tightly at the sides of the bed.
    A wrinkle-free sheet prevents uneven pressure, discomfort, and skin irritation.

12. **Place a pillow under** the patient's head, and assist him to a comfortable position.

A pillow provides comfort and good body alignment.

13. **Place the bed in low position**, and raise the siderail.
    Helps prevent falls.

14. **Place the call light** in a position where the patient can easily reach it.
    Allows patient to call for help, if needed.

Procedure Variation Use of an Approved Mechanical Lifting Device

15. **Lock the bed wheels.** Lower the head of the bed, and place the patient in a supine position. Position at least one nurse on each side of the bed. Lower the siderails. Raise the height of the bed to waist level.

16. **Using the drawsheet**, turn the patient to one side of the bed. Position the midline of the full body sling at the patient's back. Tightly roll the remaining half of the sling, and tuck the fabric under the drawsheet. ▼

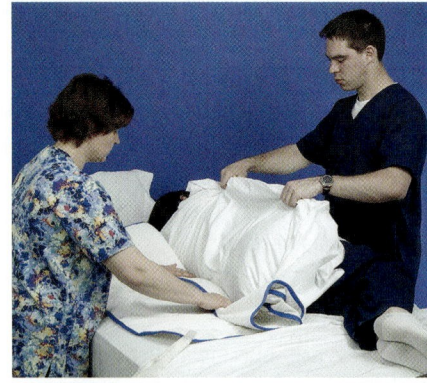

17. **With a second nurse positioned** on either side of the patient, use the drawsheet to turn the patient to the opposite side of the bed. Unroll the full body sling, and reposition the patient supine.

18. **Attach the sling** to the overbed lifting device or mechanical lift.

19. Engage the lift to raise the patient off the bed. Advance the lift toward the head of the bed until the patient is at the desired level. ➤

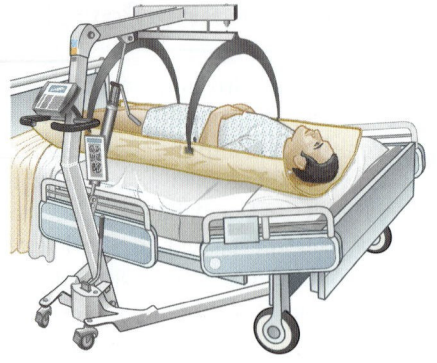

20. Lower the lift, and turn the patient to the desired position. You may leave the sling in place for future movement, or you may remove it by turning the patient from side to side.

NOTE: If a full body sling is not available, use a friction-reducing device, such as a transfer roller sheet, and at least three staff members.

Procedure 33-1B ■ Turning a Patient in Bed

➤ When performing the procedure, always identify your patient according to agency policy and be attentive to standard precautions, hand hygiene, patient safety and privacy, body mechanics, and documentation.

➤ *Note: This procedure describes the use of a transfer roller sheet. This device is inexpensive and readily available.*

Procedure Steps

1. Lock the bed wheels. Lower the head of the bed, and place the patient in a supine position. Position one nurse on each side of the bed. Lower the siderails. Raise the height of the bed to waist level.
Lowering the siderails and raising the bed allow you to move the patient while maintaining good body mechanics and working with gravity to prevent injury.

2. Remove the pillow from under the patient's head and place it at the head of the bed.
a. Roll the patient side to side and place a friction-reducing device under the drawsheet. You can improvise this device by placing a large, clean plastic bag or plastic film under the drawsheet.
b. Move the patient to the side of the bed you are turning him away from by rolling up the drawsheet close to the patient's body and pulling it.
c. Align the patient's legs and head with the trunk.
This allows you to position the patient in the center of the bed after turning. ➤

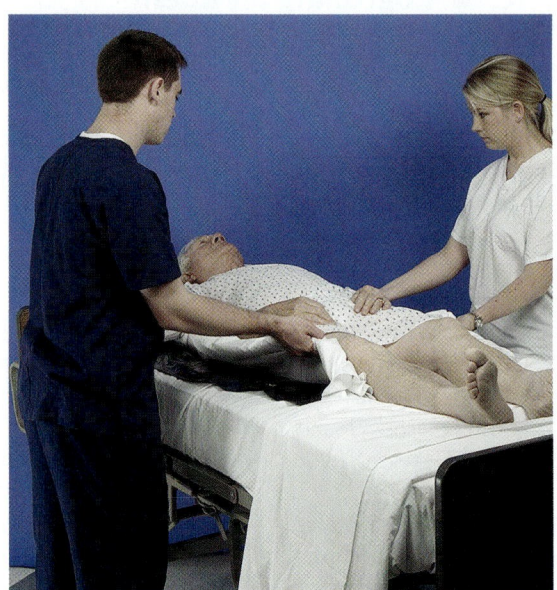

3. Place the patient's near leg and foot across the far leg (e.g., when turning the patient to his right, place his left leg over his right leg).

4. Place the patient's near arm (e.g., left when turning right) across his chest. Abduct and externally rotate the other arm and shoulder.
Positioning the patient's legs and his near arm facilitates turning. Abducting and rotating the other arm prevents it from being caught under the patient during the turn.

5. Each nurse positions her feet with a wide base of support with one foot forward of the other. Bend from the hips, and place one hand on the drawsheet at the level of the patient's hip and the other at the level of the shoulder.
A wide base of support allows you to maintain good body mechanics while performing the move.

6. Instruct the patient that the turn will occur on the count of 3.
Counting coordinates and facilitates patient cooperation with the move.

7. On the count of 3, flex your knees and hips and shift your weight. The nurse positioned on the side toward which the patient will turn shifts his weight to the back foot. The nurse on the opposite side shifts her weight forward.
Provides the best leverage to turn the patient. ➤

(continued on next page)

Procedure 33-1 ■ **Moving and Turning Patients in Bed** (continued)

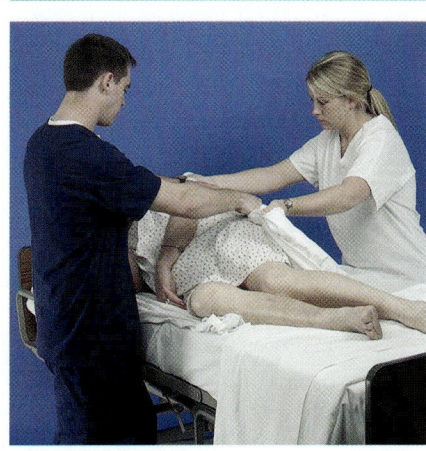

8. **If a plastic film is used**, remove it after you turn the patient.

9. **Position the dependent shoulder** forward. Place pillows behind the patients back and between legs to maintain the patient in the lateral position. Replace the pillow under the patient's head. See Table 33-3 if you need to review positioning.

Positioning ensures that patient is not putting excess pressure on the inferior shoulder. Pillows help maintain good body alignment.

10. **Place the bed in low position**, and raise the siderail.
    Helps ensure patient safety.

11. **Place the call light** in a position where the patient can easily reach it.
    Allows patient to call for help, if needed.

Procedure 33-1C ■ **Logrolling a Patient**

➤ When performing the procedure, always identify your patient according to agency policy and be attentive to standard precautions, hand hygiene, patient safety and privacy, body mechanics, and documentation.

Procedure Steps

1. **Lock the bed wheels.** Lower the head of the bed with the patient supine. Lower the siderail on the side where you are standing, but keep the opposite rail in the up position. Raise the height of the bed to waist level.
   Lowering the siderail and raising the bed allows you to move the patient while maintaining good body mechanics and working with gravity to prevent back injury.

2. **You should already have** a drawsheet with an underlying friction-reducing device, such as a transfer roller sheet, to move the patient to the side of the bed on which you are standing. (You can improvise this device by placing a clean, unused plastic bag or plastic film under the drawsheet.)

3. **Position one staff member** at the patient's head and shoulders; she is responsible for moving the head and neck as a unit. Position the other person at the patient's hips. If you need three staff members, position one at the shoulders, one at the waist, and the third at thigh level. One staff member must maintain the patient's head and neck in alignment. The other members assist with moving the rest of the body in alignment.

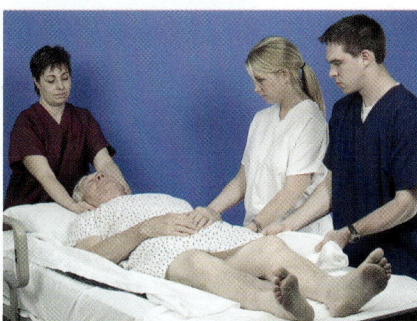

4. **Each nurse should position her feet** with a wide base of support with one foot slightly more forward than the other.
   Facilitates proper body mechanics and minimizes risk of injury to staff members.

5. **Use the drawsheet** or transfer sheet to move the patient to the side of the bed on which the nurses are standing. The move must be smooth so that the patient's head and hips are kept in alignment. Position the patient's head with a pillow.
   A transfer sheet maintains straight alignment of the spine.

6. **Instruct the patient to fold** his arms across his chest.

7. **Place a pillow between** the patient's knees.
   A pillow prevents internal rotation of the hip and spine with movement. Maintains straight alignment of the spine.

8. **Raise the siderail, and move** to opposite side of the bed.
   Siderails keep the patient from falling out of bed.

9. **Lower the siderail** on the "new" side of the bed, and face the patient. All nurses should position their feet with a wide base of support, with one foot forward of the other. Place your weight on the forward foot. Bend from the hips, and position your hands evenly along the length of the drawsheet.
   Provides the best leverage to turn the patient while maintaining spine alignment. ▼

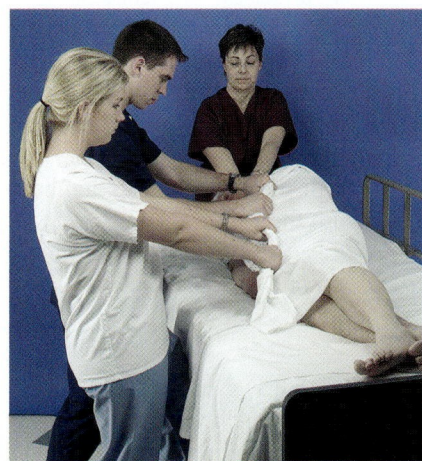

10. **All nurses flex their knees and hips** and shift their weight to the back foot on the count of 3. Be sure to support the head as the patient is rolled to his side.

    Allows you to maintain straight alignment and body mechanics while performing the move.

11. **Place pillows to maintain** the patient in the lateral position (see Table 33-3 as needed).

    A pillow provides support and maintains proper alignment.

12. **Place the bed in low position**, and raise the siderail.

13. **Place the call light** in a position where the patient can easily reach it.

    Allows patient to call for help, if needed.

? What if . . .

- **Your facility has instituted a no-lift policy and you have to pull the patient up in bed?**

Use assistive equipment, such as friction-reducing devices, mechanical lifts, air-powered mattresses, and/or lateral transfer devices to help prevent work-related injuries.

- **Your patient is obese or unable to assist (totally dependent) and you need to lift him?**

Minimize manual lifting in all cases and eliminate it where feasible. Therefore, follow facility recommendations/protocols and use approved devices. You should be familiar with the lift devices in your facility.

- **The patient has had a total hip replacement and you have to turn or log roll your patient?**

Maintain the affected leg in abduction, by using a pillow or abduction wedge between the legs.

To ensure the hip will not become dislocated during turning.

- **The patient has a cast or is in traction and you have to turn or log roll your patient?**

Designate a third person to assist in the turning by guiding the affected extremity.

- **The patient has an external fixation device and you have to turn or log roll your patient?**

Secure the device in place to keep it from moving when lifting or moving the limb as needed.

By holding onto the device to secure it and keep it from moving, there is less movement of the healing bone, and therefore less trauma and pain.

Evaluation

- Assess the patient's comfort level after the position change.
- Assess body position and alignment after position change.
- Assess skin for pressure areas.

Patient Teaching

- Explain to the patient the importance of maintaining spine alignment.
- Explain to the patient the importance of frequent position changes.
- Instruct the patient to ask the nurse when she needs to be turned sooner than scheduled.
- Teach the patient how she can assist with moving and turning.

Home Care

- Instruct the family member or caregiver in the techniques for moving, turning, or logrolling the client.
- Discuss the shearing effects on the skin from sliding down in bed (see Chapter 36).
- Provide instruction on importance of changing position and maintaining proper body alignment.

Documentation

Repositioning and turning patients are considered routine aspects of care and are not usually charted every time they are done. However, document in the nursing notes any problems with positioning the patient or any areas of skin breakdown. You might also chart turning as an intervention when charting

to a specific problem. For example, if the patient has Impaired Skin Integrity, you might describe the skin and chart, "Position changed hourly." Some facilities have flow sheets on which you indicate by a checkmark each time a patient is repositioned.

Practice Resources

Collins, Nelson, & Sublet, 2006; Nelson & Baptiste, 2004.

Thinking About the Procedure

 Go to the *Fundamentals of Nursing Skills Videos*, **Activity and Exercise: Moving a Patient Up in Bed and Moving a Patient Up in Bed: Mechanical Lift; Logrolling.**

Moving a Patient Up in Bed: Mechanical Lift

1. When does the nurse first lower the siderails when moving a patient up in bed?
2. In what instance is the mechanical assist used to move a patient up in bed?

Turning a Patient in Bed

1. When the nurse positions the patient to prepare for turning in bed, where does she place the arms when turning to the left? How does she position the legs?

Logrolling

1. What might the nurses do to improve the positioning of the patient during and after logrolling?

 For suggested responses, go to Chapter 33, **Thinking About the Procedure Suggested Responses,** on *DavisPlus.*

Procedure 33-2 ■ Transferring Patients

➤ For steps to follow in *all* procedures, refer to the Universal Steps for All Procedures found on the page facing the inside back cover.

Equipment

- Nonlatex gloves, if you may be exposed to body fluids
- Transfer board (for transferring from bed to stretcher, and sometimes bed to chair)
- Pull or lift (draw) sheet (for transfers)
- Gait transfer belt (for dangling and transferring from bed to chair)

Delegation

You may ask nursing assistive personnel (NAP) to dangle, transfer a patient from bed to stretcher, or transfer a patient from bed to chair. Ensure that the NAP has the necessary skills and that the patient's condition is stable. Inform the NAP of any special considerations when dangling or transferring the patient and evaluate the patient after transfer.

Pre-Procedure Assessment

- Assess for any restrictions in movement or position by asking the patient and checking the physician's orders.

- Observe for the presence of equipment such as IV lines, drains, or catheters.
- Assess possible side effects of medications (e.g., dizziness and sedation). Assess the patient's level of consciousness, ability to follow directions, and ability to assist with the move.
- Assess the physical size of the patient and your own strength and ability to move the patient.
- Before transferring a patient to a chair, assess the patient's tolerance of dangling.
  The preceding assessments inform you about activity tolerance, readiness to get out of bed, and ability to participate in the transfer. They help you determine how many assistants you need, the appropriate transfer device, and how to proceed with the move while preventing injury and dislodging of equipment.
- Assess vital signs, and monitor for postural hypotension.
  If the patient is at risk for postural hypotension, you may need to allow additional time for the patient to change position.
- Assess the patient's level of comfort using a standardized pain scale.
  If the patient is experiencing pain, you may need to administer an analgesic before moving.

Procedure 33-2A ■ Transferring a Patient From Bed to Stretcher

➤ When performing the procedure, always identify your patient according to agency policy and be attentive to standard precautions, hand hygiene, patient safety and privacy, body mechanics, and documentation.

Procedure Steps

1. Lock the wheels on the bed. Position the bed so that it is flat (if the patient can tolerate being supine) and at the height of the stretcher.
   Locking the wheels ensures client safety during the transfer. Having the bed flat helps prevent injury to staff, because the patient is easier to move.

2. **Lower the siderails**, and position at least one nurse on each side of the bed. Move the patient to the side of the bed where the stretcher will be placed by rolling up the drawsheet close to the patient's body and pulling it toward the designated side. Align the patient's legs and head with her trunk.
   Positions patient to enable nurses to move her to the stretcher efficiently.

3. **Position the stretcher** next to the bed. Lock the stretcher wheels.
   Keeps the stretcher from moving during the transfer; prevents falls.

4. **Place the transfer board** against the patient's back.

   a. Place a friction-reducing device, such as a transfer roller sheet, over the transfer board. (You can improvise this device by placing a clean, unused plastic bag or plastic film under the drawsheet.)

   b. The nurse on the side opposite the stretcher uses the drawsheet to turn the patient away from the

stretcher, while the other nurse places the transfer board against the patient's back halfway between bed and stretcher. Turn the patient to her back and onto the transfer board.
   Safely positions the transfer board under the patient without friction. ▼

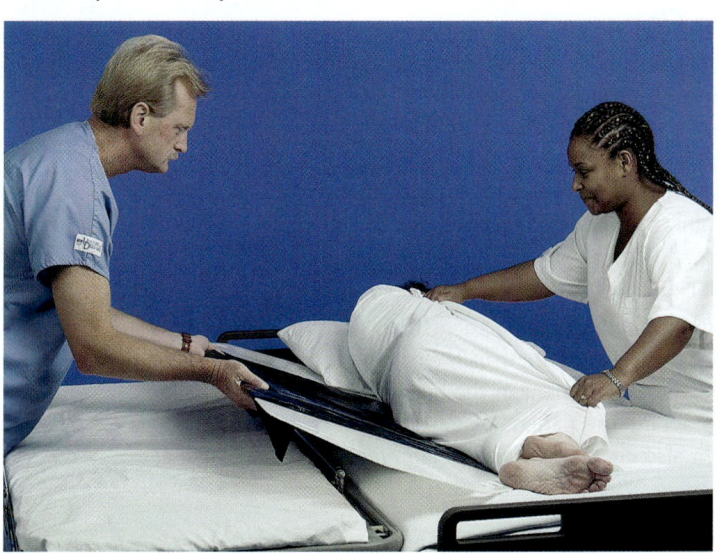

5. **Ensure the patient's feet** and shoulder are over the edge of the transfer board.
   To prevent injury to the patient from the edge of the board.

6. **Have the patient raise her head** if able. Use the drawsheet to slide her across the transfer board onto the stretcher.
   These devices facilitate the move to stretcher and prevent friction on patient's skin. ▼

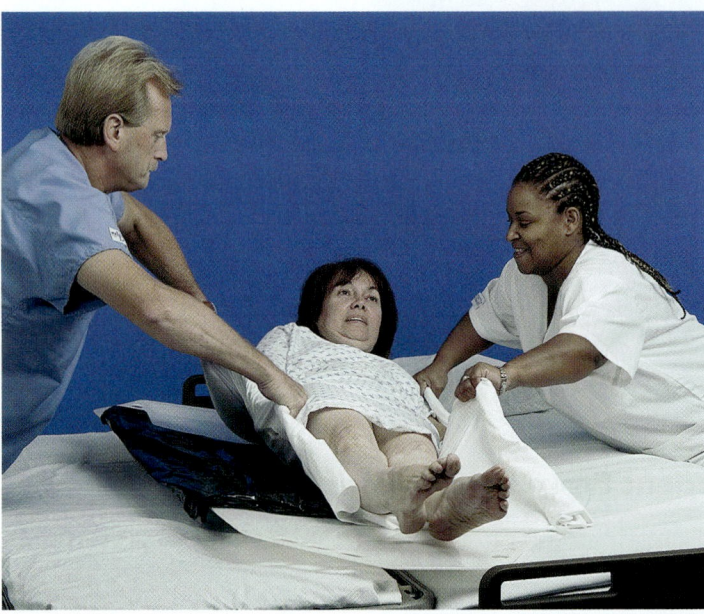

Procedure Variation Transferring a Patient From Bed to Stretcher With a Slipsheet

NOTE: A slipsheet may be used instead of a transfer board. A slipsheet is a large, low-friction fabric that facilitates transfer.

7. **Use the drawsheet to turn** the patient away from the bed; remove the board and roller sheet.

8. **Reposition the patient** on the stretcher for comfort and alignment.
   Provides support and maintains proper alignment.

9. **Provide a blanket**, if needed for warmth or privacy.

10. **Fasten safety belts**, and raise the siderails on the stretcher.
    Prevents falls.

11. **Lock the bed.** Position the bed so that it is flat (if the patient can tolerate being supine) and at the height of the stretcher.

Ensures patient safety during the transfer. Helps prevent injury to staff because the patient is easier to move if the bed is flat.

12. **With the drawsheet, turn** the patient to the side opposite where the stretcher will be placed. Position the midline of the slipsheet under the patient. Roll the remaining half tightly, and tuck it under the patient.

13. **Turn the patient to the opposite** side, and pull the slipsheet through from under the patient.

14. **Place the patient supine**, and lower the siderail on the side where the stretcher will be placed.

15. **Move the stretcher** next to the bed and lock the wheels on the stretcher.

16. **Position at least two nurses** on the far side of the stretcher. Using the slipsheet, pull the patient onto the stretcher. ▼

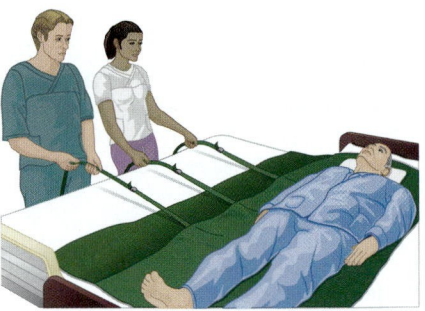

Procedure 33-2B ■ Dangling a Patient at the Side of the Bed

➤ When performing the procedure, always identify your patient according to agency policy and be attentive to standard precautions, hand hygiene, patient safety and privacy, body mechanics, and documentation.

Procedure Steps

1. Lock the bed wheels. Place the patient in a supine position, and raise the head of the bed to 90°. Keep the siderail elevated on the side opposite where you are standing.
   Locking the wheels prevents the bed from moving as you move the patient. Raising the head of the bed prepares the patient to be dangled and requires less effort from you to help the patient sit erect.

2. **Apply a gait transfer belt** to the patient at waist level. Place the bed in the low position.
   Ensures patient safety and proper body mechanics.

3. **Instruct the patient to bend** his knees and turn the patient onto his side, if possible, keeping knees flexed.
   Prepares the patient to be able to dangle his legs over side of bed.

4. **Stand on the side of the bed**, facing the patient and using a wide base of support. Place your foot closest to the head of the bed forward of the other foot. Lean forward, bending at the hips, with your knees flexed. Instruct the patient to use his arm to push off the bed.
   Allows you to maintain proper body mechanics and prevents injury. ➤

(continued on next page)

Procedure 33-2 ■ **Transferring Patients** (continued)

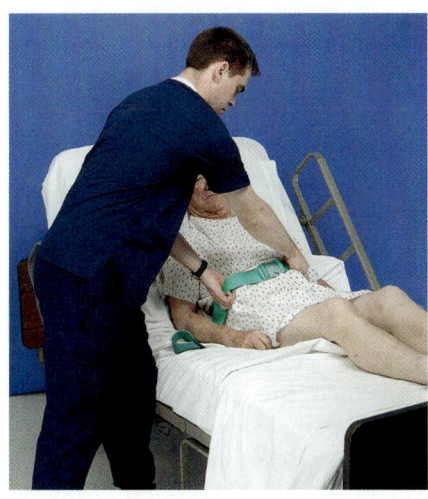

5. Position your hands on each side of the gait transfer belt.

6. Rock onto your back foot as you assist the patient toward you with the gait transfer belt, thereby moving the patient into a sitting position at the side of the bed.

Uses your body weight as leverage to reposition the patient, preventing injury to your back. ▼

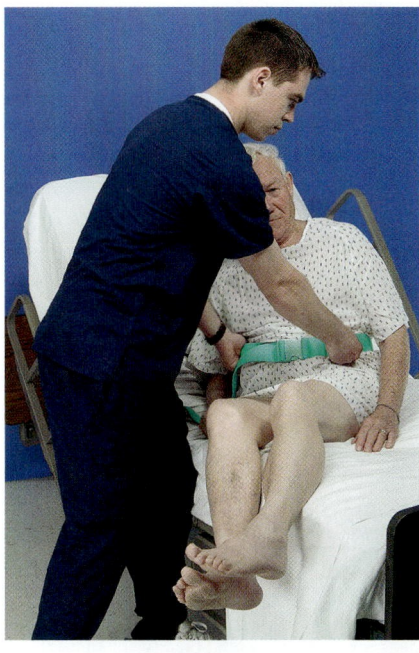

7. Stay with the patient as he dangles. Reassess comfort level and for dizziness.
Helps prevent falls.

Procedure 33-2C ■ **Transferring a Patient From Bed to Chair**

➤ When performing the procedure, always identify your patient according to agency policy and be attentive to standard precautions, hand hygiene, patient safety and privacy, body mechanics, and documentation.

Procedure Steps

1. Position the chair next to the bed. If possible, lock the chair.
   Prevents the chair from moving during transfer. Ensures patient safety.

2. **Put nonskid footwear** on the patient.
   Prevents the patient from slipping during transfer.

3. **Place the bed in a low position**, and lock the bed wheels.
   Prevents the bed from moving during the transfer. Low position allows patient to place feet firmly on the floor.

4. **Assist the patient to dangle** at the side of the bed (see Procedure 33-2B). Be sure the patient doesn't need support before releasing him.

5. **Apply a transfer belt.**
   Facilitates transfer of the patient to the chair and helps prevent back injury to the nurse. ➤

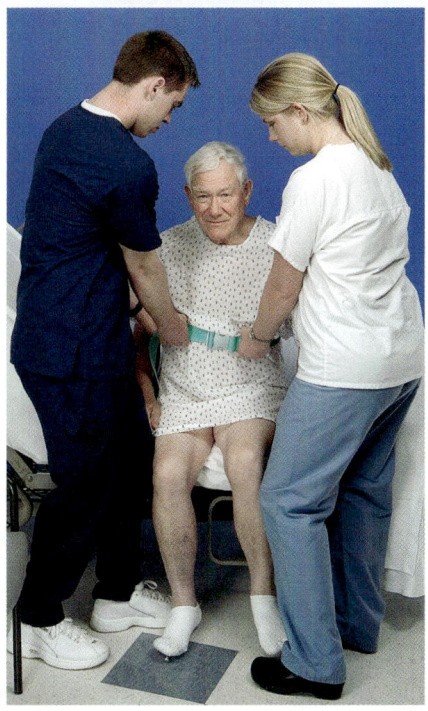

6. **Stand toward the bed**, facing the patient. Brace your feet and knees against the patient. Pay particular attention to any known weakness. Bend your hips and knees, and, keeping your back straight, hold onto the transfer belt on both sides. If two nurses are available to assist with the transfer, one nurse should be on each side of the patient.
   Bracing provides stability. Bending the hips and knees allows you to use the major muscle groups and limit the risk of injury. Lifting the patient at waist level prevents injury to the arm or shoulder.

7. **Instruct the patient** to place his arms around you between the shoulders and waist (the location depends on your height and the height of the patient).
   Prevents injury to your neck.

8. **Ask the patient to stand** as you move to an upright position by straightening your legs and hips.
Straightening your thighs and hips uses your large muscle groups and prevents injury to your back.

9. **Allow the patient to steady himself** for a moment.
Provides the patient an opportunity to rest before further movement. Allows you to evaluate his tolerance to activity and ability to maintain an upright posture before continuing.

10. **Instruct the patient to pivot** and turn with you toward the chair.
Pivoting helps prevent twisting and straining the patient's back muscles.

11. **Assist the patient to position** himself in front of the chair. Have the patient flex his hips and knees, and as he lowers himself to the chair, reach for arms of the chair. Guide his motion while maintaining a firm hold on him and keeping your back straight.
Maintains good body mechanics and balance and ensures patient safety. ➤

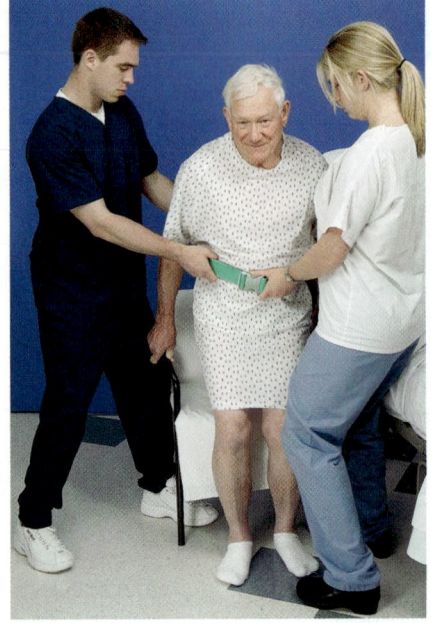

12. **Assist the patient** to a comfortable position in the chair.

13. **Provide a blanket if needed** for warmth or privacy.

14. **Place the call light in reach** of the patient or position the patient where staff members can see him at all times.

? What if . . .

- **The patient is obese?**

  If the patient is obese or unable to assist, use a full body sling that allows the patient to assume a seated position. You may also use a powered standing assist lift, if one is available.

- **The patient has had hip surgery (replacement or fracture repair).**

  When assisting the patient out of bed, raise the bed to a higher position, allowing the patient to exit the bed without acute hip flexion.
  To avoid hip dislocation

- **The patient becomes dizzy during the transfer?**

  Return the patient to recumbent position and assess his vital signs.

- **The patient has a weaker side, for example, from a CVA or surgical procedure?**

  Instruct the patient to exit the bed from his unaffected side. Stand on the patient's weaker side.
  The stronger side should lead a transfer.

Evaluation

- Assess the level of patient participation in the transfer.
- Assess the patient's comfort level during the transfer and in the new position.
- Assess proper body position and alignment after his position change.
- Assess the patient's vital signs for postural hypotension after dangling or transferring to a chair.

Patient Teaching

- Explain the importance of frequent position changes and getting out of bed to avoid complications of immobility.

Home Care

- Instruct the family member or caregiver in the proper technique for assisting the client to dangle at the bedside or transfer to a chair.
- Provide instruction in the importance of changing position and maintaining proper body alignment.

Documentation

Patients are usually moved to a stretcher for transport to a test or procedure. Moving patients is a routine aspect of care and is not documented. When dangling or transferring a patient to a chair, document in the nursing notes how much assistance was required, the use of assistive devices, any problems with positioning the patient, how long the patient was out of bed, and how the patient tolerated the activity.

Practice Resources

Collins, Nelson, & Sublet, 2006; Occupational Safety and Health Administration, U.S. Department of Labor, 2009.

Thinking About the Procedure

 Go to the *Fundamentals of Nursing Skills Videos*, **Activity and Exercise: Transferring From Bed to Stretcher and Transferring From Bed to Chair.**

Transferring Patients Bed to Stretcher

1. What kind of friction-reducing device do the nurses use to transfer the patient from the bed to the stretcher?

Transferring Patients: Bed to Chair

1. For those who can assist in transferring from the bed to the chair, how should the patient hold on to the nurse?

 For suggested responses, go to Chapter 33, **Thinking About the Procedure Suggested Responses,** on *DavisPlus.*

Procedure 33-3 ■ Assisting With Ambulation

➤ For steps to follow in *all* procedures, refer to the Universal Steps for All Procedures found on the page facing the inside back cover.

Equipment
- Nonlatex gloves, if you may be exposed to body fluids
- Transfer belt
- Nonskid footwear

Delegation
You may ask nursing assistive personnel (NAP) to assist with ambulation. Ensure that the NAP has the necessary skills and that the patient's condition is stable. Inform the NAP of any special considerations when assisting a patient with ambulation and evaluate the patient after the activity.

Pre-Procedure Assessment
- Assess for any restrictions in movement or position by asking the patient and checking the physician's orders.
- Observe for the presence of equipment such as IV lines, drains, or catheters.
- Assess possible side effects of medications (e.g., dizziness and sedation).
- Assess the patient's level of consciousness, ability to follow directions, and ability to assist with the move

- Assess the physical size of the patient and your own strength and ability to move the patient.
- Assess the patient's tolerance when dangling before beginning to ambulate.
  The preceding assessments inform you about activity tolerance, readiness to get out of bed, and ability to participate in the transfer. They help you determine how many assistants you need, the appropriate transfer device, and how to proceed with the move while preventing injury and dislodging of equipment.
- Assess vital signs, and monitor for postural hypotension.
  If the patient is at risk for postural hypotension, you may need to allow additional time for the patient to change position and plan for adequate help.
- Assess the patient's level of comfort using a standardized pain scale.
  If the patient is uncomfortable, you may need to administer an analgesic before moving.
- Assess for factors that may increase the risk of falls (elderly, muscle weakness, chronic disease, gait disturbance).
  Identifies patients at risk.

Procedure 33-3A ■ Assisting With Ambulation (One Nurse)

➤ When performing the procedure, always identify your patient according to agency policy and be attentive to standard precautions, hand hygiene, patient safety and privacy, body mechanics, and documentation.

Procedure Steps

1. Put nonskid footwear on the patient.
   Prevents the patient from slipping while transferring and ambulating.
2. **Place the bed in a low position**, and lock the bed.
   Prevents the bed from moving during transfer. Makes it easier for the patient's feet to reach the floor.
3. **Apply the transfer belt.**
   Allows you to safely support the patient during the transfer and ambulation.
4. **Assist the patient to dangle** at the side of the bed (see Procedure 33-2B, if you need to review).
5. **Face the patient**. Brace your feet and knees against the patient's feet and knees. Pay particular attention to any known weakness. Bend your

hips and knees, and hold onto the transfer belt.
Bracing provides stability of the patient's legs. Bending the hips and knees allows you to use the major muscle groups and limit injury. Lifting at the patient's waist level prevents injury to his arm or shoulder.

6. **Instruct the patient to place** his arms around you between the shoulders and waist (the location depends on your height and the height of patient). Ask the patient to stand as you move to an upright position by straightening your legs and hips.
   Having the patient hold you on your trunk prevents injury to your neck. Straightening your thighs and hips uses your large muscle groups and promotes good body mechanics.

7. **Allow the patient to steady himself** for a moment.
   Allows the patient an opportunity to rest before further movement and to regain equilibrium before walking.

8. **Stand at the patient's side**, placing both hands on the transfer belt. If the patient is weak on one side, position yourself on the weaker side.
   By standing on the weaker side, the patient is freer to reach with the stronger arm and grip wall or bed rails with his strong-side hand, and use the stronger side for strength and balance. This position also keeps you clear of a cane or other assistive device, which would be used on the strong side, and allows you to support the weaker side to prevent the patient from falling. ➤

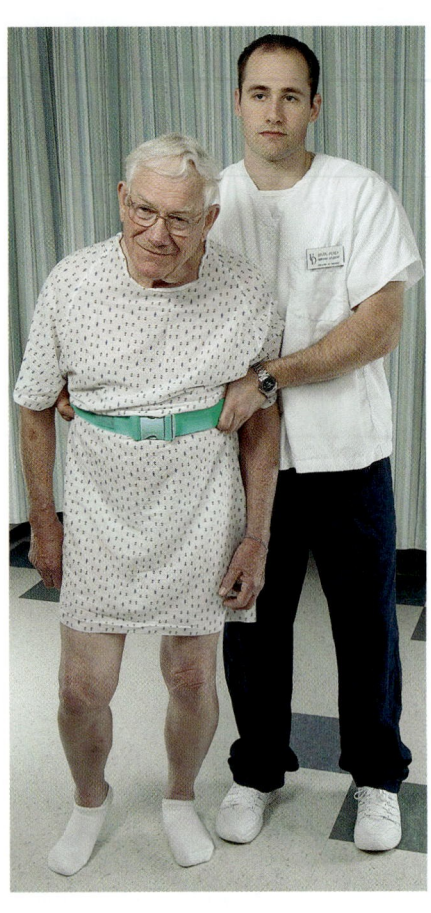

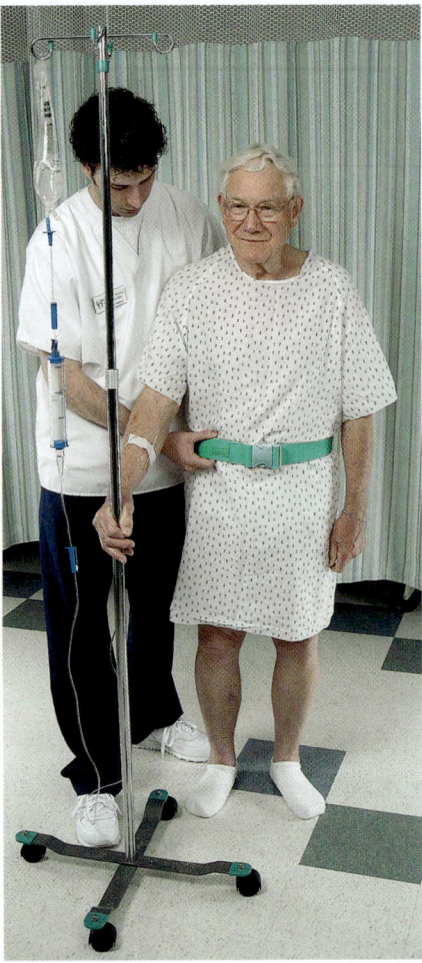

9. **Slowly guide the patient for-ward.** Observe for signs of fatigue or dizziness.
   Helps prevent falls.
10. **If the patient has an IV pole,** ask him to hold on to the pole on the side where you are standing. Assist the patient to advance the pole as you ambulate. Be sure the patient does not rely on the pole for support. ➤
    Using an IV pole on wheels for balance could lead to a fall.

Procedure 33-3B ■ Assisting With Ambulation (Two Nurses)

➤ When performing the procedure, always identify your patient according to agency policy and be attentive to standard precautions, hand hygiene, patient safety and privacy, body mechanics, and documentation.

Procedure Steps

1. Put nonskid footwear on the patient.
   Prevents the patient from slipping during the transfer and ambulation.
2. **Place the bed in low position,** and lock the bed.
   Prevents the bed from moving during transfer and prevents the patient from falling.
3. **Apply the transfer belt.**
   Allows you to support client during transfer and ambulation.
4. **Assist the patient to dangle** at the side of the bed (see Procedure 33-2B, as needed).
5. **Each nurse should stand facing** the patient on opposite sides of the

patient. Brace your feet and knees against the patient, paying particular attention to any known weakness. Bend from the hips and knees and hold onto the transfer belt.
Bracing provides stability. Bending the hips and knees allows you to use the major muscle groups and limit injury. Lifting at the patient's waist level prevents injury to his arm or shoulder.

6. **Instruct the patient to place** his arms around each of you between the shoulders and waist (the location depends on your height and the height of the patient). Ask the patient to stand as each of you move to an upright position by straightening your legs and hips.

7. **Allow the patient to steady him-self** for a moment.
   Provides an opportunity for the patient to rest before further movement and to regain equilibrium. Allows you to evaluate the patient's tolerance to activity and ability to maintain an upright posture before ambulating.
8. **Each nurse stands** at the patient's sides, grasping hold of the transfer belt. If no belt is available, the nurses grasp each other's arms at the patient's waist.
   Helps patient maintain an erect posture. ➤

(continued on next page)

Procedure 33-3 ■ Assisting With Ambulation (continued)

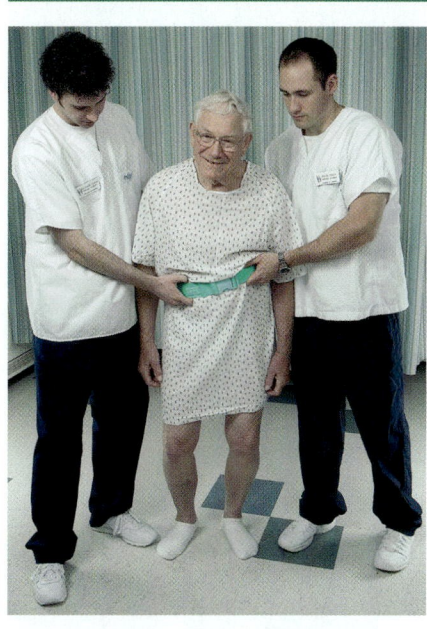

9. **Slowly guide the patient forward.** Observe for signs of fatigue or dizziness.
   Ensures client safety.

10. **If the patient has an IV pole,** one nurse advances the IV pole along the side of the patient by holding the pole with the outside hand. Remind the patient not to use the IV pole for support.
    Positions the IV pole out of the path of the patient. Because the IV pole is on rollers, it will not support the patient if he starts to fall.

 What if . . .

■ **The patient has a weaker side (i.e., stroke)?**

If the patient has weakness on one side, provide additional support but allow him to use that side as he is able.
This will force him to use his weaker side.

Evaluation

■ Assess the level of patient participation in the transfer.
■ Assess patient comfort with ambulation.
■ Assess posture and base of support.
■ Assess vital signs for postural hypotension.

Patient Teaching

■ Instruct the patient to inform you if he feels dizzy or weak.
■ Explain the importance of ambulation to prevent complications of immobility.

Home Care

■ Teach family members or caregivers how to assist the client with ambulation.
■ Provide instruction on importance of ambulation.

Documentation

Document in the nursing notes how much assistance was required, any problems with ambulation, and the distance walked.

Sample Documentation:

11/11/14   0630   Pt. assisted to ambulate to doorway. Required minimal assistance from one nurse. Placed in chair for 30 minutes, then assisted back to bed. Required maximum assist from two nurses to return to bed.   — B. Bowen, RN

Practice Resources
Occupational Safety and Health Administration, U.S. Department of Labor, 2009.

Thinking About the Procedure

 Go to the *Fundamentals of Nursing Skills Videos,* **Activity and Exercise, Dangling and Ambulation: One Nurse Assist.**

1. How does the patient steady herself before dangling?

 Go to the *Fundamentals of Nursing Skills Videos,* **Activity and Exercise, Dangling and Ambulation: Two Nurse Assist.**

1. What does the nurse do with the transfer belt to keep it from becoming looser?

2. What could nurses do to assist the patient who requires assistance with ambulation if no transfer belt is available?

 For suggested responses, go to Chapter 33, **Thinking About the Procedure Suggested Responses,** on DavisPlus.

To explore learning resources for this chapter,

Go to DavisPlus at http://davisplus.fadavis.com/, **keyword Treas.**

Chapter Resources for Chapter 33:
   Knowledge Check and Think Like a Nurse Response Sheets
   Knowledge Check Answers
   Resources for Caregivers and Health Professionals
   Reading More About Activity and Exercise (Suggested Readings)
   What Are the Main Points in This Chapter?
   Nursing Care Plan, Impaired Physical Mobility
   Care Planning & Mapping Practice
NCLEX-Style Review Questions
Chapter Overview Podcasts

Concept Map

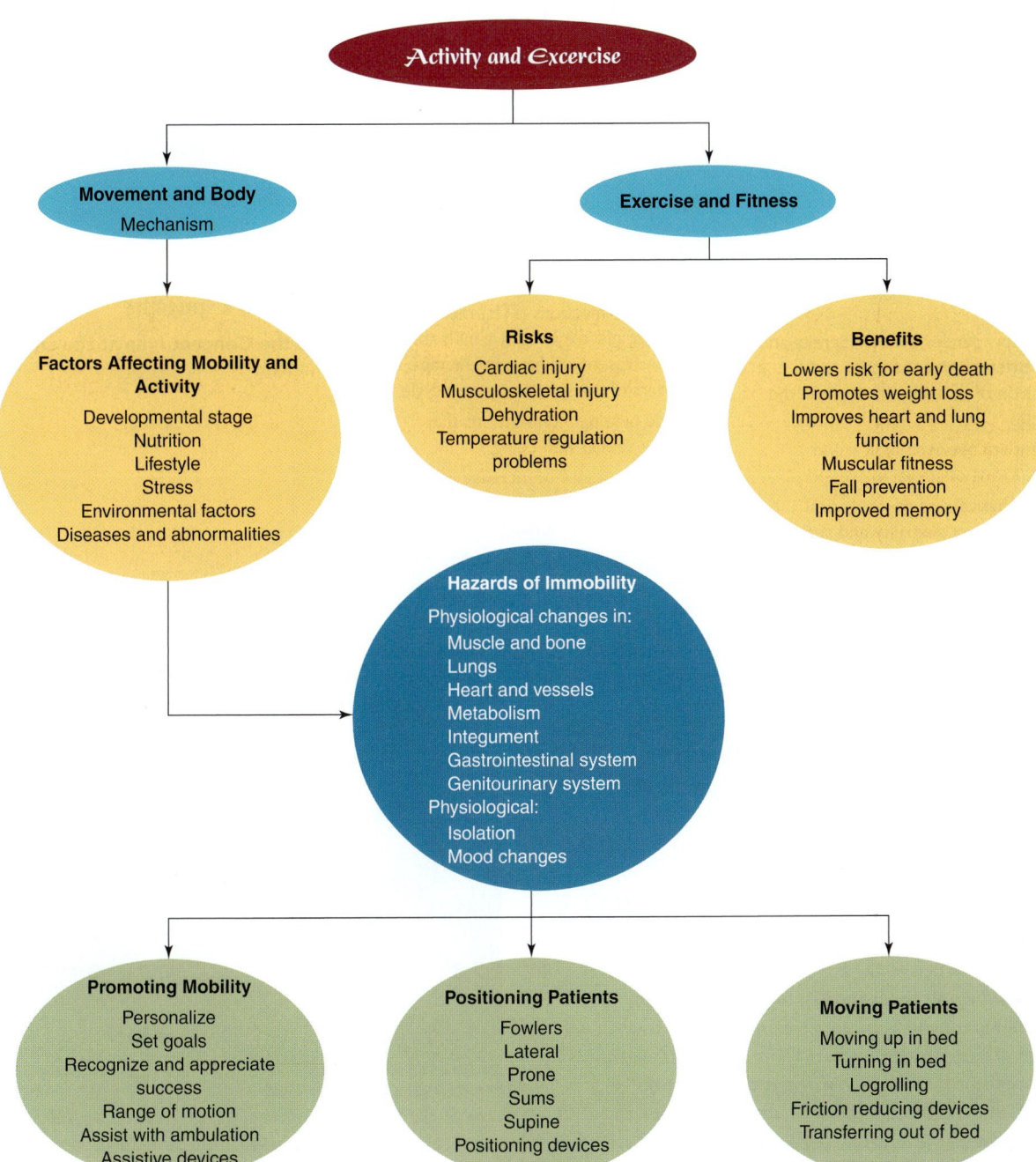

Activity and Exercise

Movement and Body Mechanism

Exercise and Fitness

Factors Affecting Mobility and Activity

Developmental stage
Nutrition
Lifestyle
Stress
Environmental factors
Diseases and abnormalities

Risks

Cardiac injury
Musculoskeletal injury
Dehydration
Temperature regulation problems

Benefits

Lowers risk for early death
Promotes weight loss
Improves heart and lung function
Muscular fitness
Fall prevention
Improved memory

Hazards of Immobility

Physiological changes in:
  Muscle and bone
  Lungs
  Heart and vessels
  Metabolism
  Integument
  Gastrointestinal system
  Genitourinary system
Physiological:
  Isolation
  Mood changes

Promoting Mobility

Personalize
Set goals
Recognize and appreciate success
Range of motion
Assist with ambulation
Assistive devices

Positioning Patients

Fowlers
Lateral
Prone
Sums
Supine
Positioning devices

Moving Patients

Moving up in bed
Turning in bed
Logrolling
Friction reducing devices
Transferring out of bed

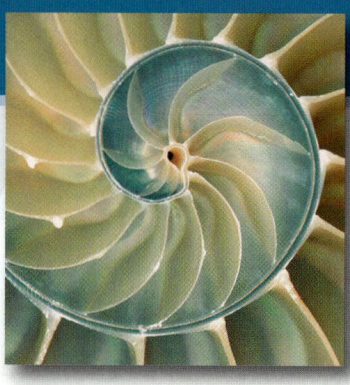

CHAPTER 34

Sexual Health

Learning Outcomes

After completing this chapter, you should be able to:

➤ Identify the female and male reproductive organs.

➤ Describe the physical, emotional, social, and spiritual aspects of human sexuality.

➤ Explain how gender, gender identity, and sexual orientation contribute to expression of sexuality throughout the life cycle.

➤ Differentiate between typical and atypical forms of sexual expression.

➤ Explore physical and psychological issues that affect sexuality and sexual functioning.

➤ Complete a sexual history as part of a comprehensive nursing assessment.

➤ State nursing diagnoses to describe sexuality problems.

➤ Explain how sexual health is challenged by high-risk sexual behaviors, sexually transmitted infections (STIs), menstrual problems, infertility, negative intimate relationships, sexual harassment, rape, and disorders of the sexual response cycle.

➤ Provide nursing interventions that enhance sexual well-being.

➤ Discuss strategies to increase your personal comfort and confidence in providing holistic nursing care.

➤ Describe approaches for dealing with inappropriate sexual behavior from patients or in the work environment.

Key Concepts

Sexual dysfunction

Sexual health

Sexuality

Related Concepts

See the Concept Map at the end of this chapter.

Caring for the Nguyens

This feature allows you to practice the kind of thinking you will use as a full-spectrum nurse. There is usually more than one correct answer to a critical thinking question, so we do not provide answers for these features. It is more important to develop your nursing judgment than to "cover content." Discuss the questions with your peers. If you are still unsure, consult your instructor.

As you may recall, Nam and Yen Nguyen are raising their 3-year-old grandson, Kim. Kim has made friends with Dinh, another little boy at preschool. Kim has asked whether they can play together. Yen works at the preschool and knows Dinh and his family. She is unsure whether she should allow her grandson to play with Dinh because Yen is uncomfortable with the boy's family. Dinh was conceived

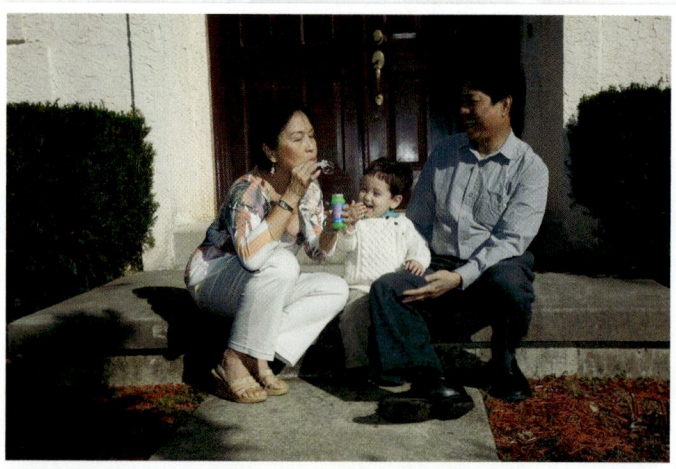

via artificial insemination and is being raised by a lesbian couple. Her parents are open about the relationship and shared the conception information with Yen voluntarily.

Caring for the Nguyens (continued)

A. Yen calls the clinic to speak with you. She explains the situation and asks you whether you think it would be a problem to allow the children to play together. She is concerned that being around this family may be a bad influence on Kim. How would you respond?

B. Yen remains concerned and presses you for more information. She is concerned that Kim's interest in

Dinh may indicate that Kim has homosexual tendencies. How would you address her concerns?

C. Yen admits that Nam does not agree with her. "He told me that sexual orientation is genetic." How would you react to this statement?

 Go to **Caring for the Nguyens Response Sheet** on *DavisPlus.*

Meet Your Patients

Jocelyn Carter. Two days after undergoing a fine-needle aspiration to evaluate a small breast mass, Jocelyn Carter's surgeon informed her that the mass was malignant. He recommended a mastectomy (removal of the breast). Today, she arrives alone at the surgery registration area. You ask how she is feeling, and she tells you that the last week has been a whirlwind of activity. "I had to arrange child care, cancel a business trip, and organize the house so that I could take a few days off to have the surgery. My husband is working overseas this fall, so he couldn't be here to help me. Honestly, I don't know how I'm feeling. I haven't had time to think about it." A few minutes later, as she waits in the surgery holding area, she begins to cry. You hold her hand and ask whether she would like to talk. She asks you, "Do you think my husband will still want me? I'm afraid he will be turned off when he looks at me."

   Gabriel Thomas comes to the outpatient clinic complaining of a throbbing headache over the past 3 days. He explains that he has tried several over-the-counter medicines and has had no relief. You check his blood pressure, and measure the reading at 240/130 mm Hg. When you ask whether he has ever been treated for high blood pressure, he replies, "Are you another one of these people trying to get me to take drugs that will ruin my sex life?"

   Frank Thanee, who has heart disease, had a mitral valve replacement 3 days ago. He has been transferred to the

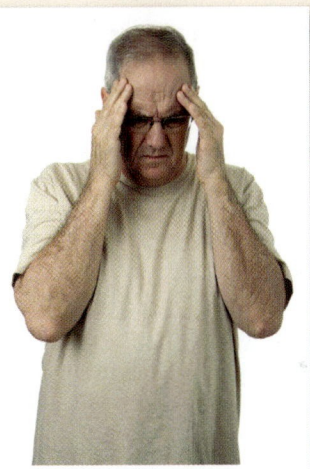
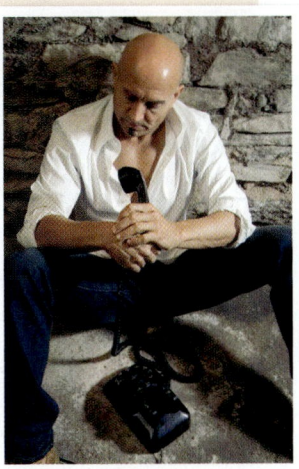

cardiology floor for an additional day of hospitalization. His partner, Greg, has spent the last 3 days at the hospital and has just left to check on the apartment and feed their cat. Frank confides that he is worried about his parents' expected visit. "I've never been able to tell them about Greg. They wouldn't be able to understand it, never mind approve. I don't know how to handle this. What do you think I should do?"

   Although each of these clients has a different medical diagnosis, all are experiencing a concern related to sexuality. In this chapter, we explore the relationship between health and sexuality, as well as the nurse's role in promoting sexual health.

Theoretical Knowledge
knowing **why**

When a baby is born, the first question the parents ask is, "Is it a boy or a girl?" In fact, many parents want to know the gender of their baby at the first sonogram, early in the pregnancy. Hopes and dreams of future gender-specific parent–child relationships often begin to form even during the first months of pregnancy. As you will learn, sexuality encompasses much more than gender. It includes how we perceive ourselves, how we relate to others, and how we express ourselves as sexual beings.

ABOUT THE KEY CONCEPTS

Like many people, you may have been socialized to avoid talking openly about sexuality. As a nurse, though, you will find that you must discuss a variety of issues pertaining to sexuality that are vital for clients' optimal wellness. Some of these discussions may include sexual dysfunctions or behaviors. As you learn about concepts relating sexuality and sexual function, you will be challenged to confront your own biases and to set those aside in order to address your clients' sexual health needs comfortably and competently.

SEXUAL AND REPRODUCTIVE ANATOMY AND PHYSIOLOGY

The role of the reproductive system in human life extends far beyond its basic function of producing children. It influences body image, sexual desire, and sense of sexual identity. The first step in exploring human sexuality is to understand the basics of reproductive anatomy and physiology.

Female Reproductive Organs

The female reproductive system consists of a pair of ovaries and fallopian tubes, the uterus, vagina, and external genital tissues (Fig. 34-1). **Ova** (eggs) are produced in the ovaries and travel through the fallopian tubes to the uterus. If fertilization occurs, the embryo embeds in the wall of the uterus for further development.

The **vagina** is a muscular tube that receives sperm during sexual intercourse, allows the exit of menstrual flow if fertilization does not occur, and serves as a birth canal at the end of pregnancy.

The external genitalia and the mons pubis are a source of pleasurable sensations. The **mons pubis** is a pad of fatty tissue over the symphysis pubis. The external genitalia, or **vulva,** consist of the clitoris, labia majora, labia minora, Bartholin's glands, urinary meatus, and vaginal introitus. The **clitoris** contains erectile tissue, blood vessels, and nerves. It is extremely sensitive and reacts to pleasurable stimuli. The **labia minora** also engorge and become sensitive during sexual stimulation. The **labia majora** protect external genitalia, such as the clitoris.

The breasts are important to female sexual arousal. The mammary glands, enclosed within the breasts, are also part of the reproductive system. Their function is to produce milk after the birth of an infant.

The Menstrual Cycle

Menstruation begins with puberty and involves hormone changes that prepare the body for pregnancy. The phases of the menstrual cycle are triggered by hormonal changes (Fig. 34-2).

Menstrual Phase. Menstruation usually lasts 3 to 7 days, averaging 5 days. During this phase, the uterus sheds the endometrial lining and several ovarian follicles develop. Follicle-stimulating hormone (FSH) from the anterior pituitary begins to increase during this phase, leading to a rise in estrogen levels.

Follicular Phase. This phase begins on the first day of menstrual bleeding and is associated with growth of ovarian follicles and regrowth of the endometrium of the uterus. This phase ends with **ovulation,** or release of the ovum from the mature follicle, around day 13 or 14 of the menstrual cycle. Luteinizing hormone (LH) levels from the anterior pituitary rise, as does the estrogen level.

Ovulatory Phase Lasting about 16 to 36 hours, a surge in LH and FSH occurs. The follicle then ruptures and the egg is released for fertilization. Estrogen peaks and progesterone rises, stimulating growth of the endometrium.

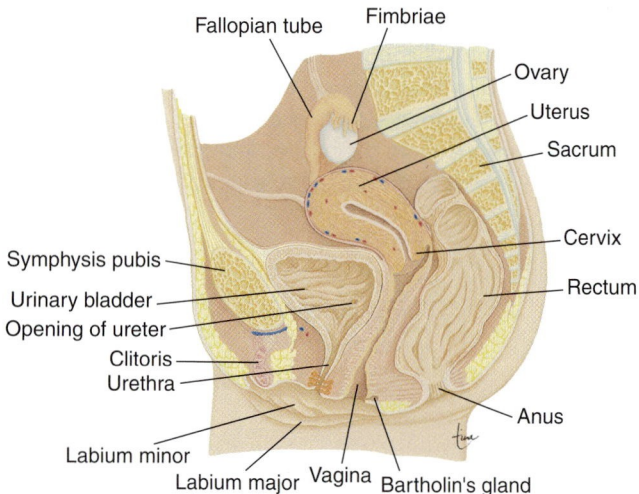

FIGURE 34-1 The female reproductive system.

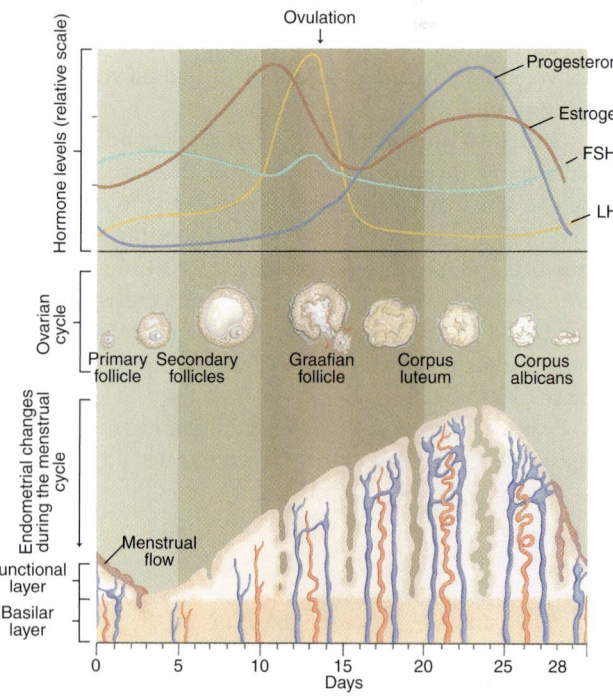

FIGURE 34-2 The menstrual cycle. Hormone levels and endometrial thickness throughout the cycle are shown.

Luteal Phase. If fertilization occurs, the endometrium thickens to support an embryo. The pregnancy hormone, called chorionic gonadotropin, is produced. Pregnancy tests are based on detecting levels of this hormone. If fertilization does not occur, progesterone levels drop, and menses begins.

Male Reproductive Organs

The male reproductive system consists of the testes and a series of ducts and glands that transport sperm. Sperm are produced in the testes and transported through the epididymis, ductus deferens, ejaculatory duct, and urethra (Fig. 34-3). Along the path, the reproductive glands (seminal vesicles, prostate, and bulbourethral glands) add secretions that mix with the sperm to produce semen.

The penis functions in the urinary system to transport urine from the bladder to the outside of the body. It has important functions in the reproductive system as well. Within the penis are three sections of erectile tissue: the corpus cavernosum and sections of corpus spongiosum above and below the urethra. During sexual arousal these erectile tissues fill with blood, making the penis erect. **Ejaculation** (the expulsion of semen) is brought about by peristalsis of the reproductive ducts and contraction of the prostate and muscles of the pelvic floor. With each ejaculation, approximately 100 million sperm cells are expelled in 2 to 4 mL of semen.

KnowledgeCheck 34-1

- Identify the major structures of the female reproductive system.
- Summarize the phases of the menstrual cycle.
- Identify the major structures of the male reproductive system.

SEXUALITY

The World Health Organization (WHO) describes the concept of **sexuality** as a "central aspect of being human throughout life and encompasses sex, gender identities and roles, sexual orientation, eroticism, pleasure, intimacy and reproduction" (WHO, 2002). **Sexual identity** is a person's perception of his or her gender, gender identity, gender role, and sexual orientation. All of these are also a part of the person's overall self-concept (see Chapter 13 to review self-concept).

What Is Gender?

People often think of *sexuality* as a synonym for *sex*. This is inaccurate. In fact, even the word *sex* has multiple meanings. For example, *sex* is commonly used to describe intimate pleasurable activity or to indicate whether an individual is male or female (e.g., "What sex is your baby?"). In this chapter, we use the term **gender** to indicate biological sex status (male or female) and follow WHO's definition of sexuality.

Gender is determined at the moment of conception, when an ovum is fertilized by a sperm. The ovum always provides an X chromosome, whereas the sperm may contribute either a second X chromosome, which results in a female offspring, or a Y chromosome, resulting in a male offspring (Fig. 34-4).

Gender Roles

Gender roles are the societal norms for gender-appropriate behavior. During the 1950s, the media portrayed the father-in-a-suit who went off to work to support his family. Mother, in her apron, spent the day cooking, cleaning, and caring for her perfect children and devoted husband. Even then, many Americans did not identify with this stereotype, and today it may seem absurd. But many of these values remain embedded at some level within our contemporary culture.

Historically in Western culture, people expected men to be strong and to control their feelings, and women to be gentle and to express their feelings. Boys received positive reinforcement for "masculine" behaviors, such as competitiveness, and may have endured teasing if they showed passivity. In girls, "feminine" behaviors, such as cooperation, were reinforced, whereas assertiveness was often labeled aggression. In the past 50 years, expectations regarding gender roles have changed and expanded. Now women commonly perform jobs formerly thought to be "for men only" (e.g., physician, police officer); and men are entering predominately female professions (e.g., nursing).

Today, many parents encourage some **androgyny** in their children. The word *androgyny* is a combination of the Greek words for "male," *andro*, and "female," *gyn*. By one definition, *androgyny* refers to a blending of traditional masculine and feminine roles. It means that everyone has some skills, traits, and behaviors that may be classified as masculine and some that may be feminine. Androgyny is a positive trait in that it gives an individual greater adaptability in life situations.

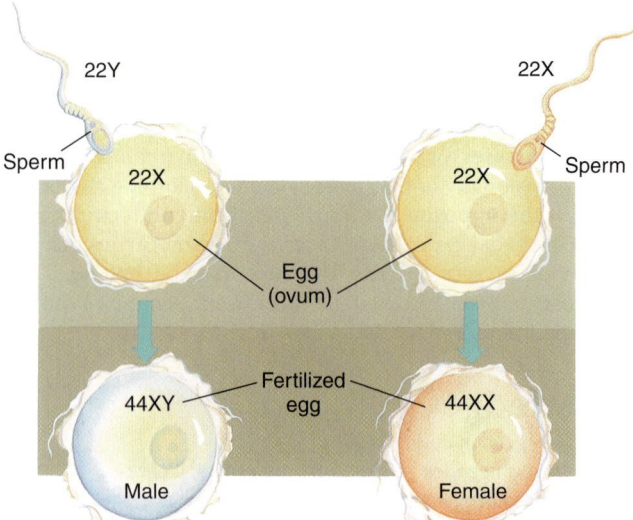

FIGURE 34-4 The woman provides the X chromosome, and the man may contribute either a second X chromosome, which results in a female offspring, or a Y chromosome, resulting in a male offspring.

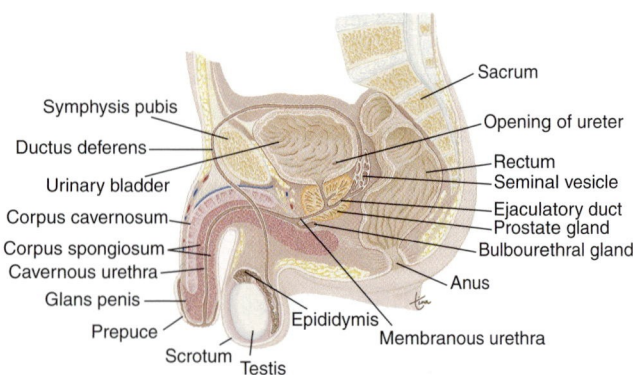

FIGURE 34-3 The male reproductive system.

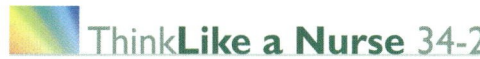

ThinkLike a Nurse 34-1

- Provide at least three examples of nonconformity to traditional gender role expectations.
- As a parent, how might you encourage androgyny in your children, if you wished to do so?

Gender Identity

Gender identity, one component of sexual identity, is the image we have about ourselves as a man or woman. It is an internal experience: whether we "feel like" a woman or a man. However, when a person forms a gender identity that is not the same as his biological gender, she is considered **transgendered** (or "differently gendered"). For example, a woman might think of herself as female even though she has male genitalia. Longitudinal studies have shown that transgendered persons may be transsexual, intersexed, or cross-dressing; and heterosexual, homosexual, or bisexual (Zucker, 2000).

- **Transsexuals** are people who identify with the opposite gender from their biology—for example, a person with the physical appearance and reproductive organs of a woman who "feels" and perceives herself to be a man. It is common for transsexuals to express dissatisfaction with their gender at an early age. Their preference for dress and play is more typical of those of the other gender.
- **Preoperative transsexuals** are adults who alter their physical appearance through dress, make-up, and/or the use of hormones so that their external appearance corresponds to their gender identity. After extensive counseling and successfully living in the opposite gender role for period of time, they may decide to undergo surgery to reconstruct their external genitalia and remove the reproductive organs of the biological birth gender. After sex reassignment surgery, the **postoperative transsexual individual** legally changes gender. For the transsexual or transgender person in an inpatient facility, single rooms are best.
- **Intersexed** people are born with ambiguous sexual organs. For example, the person may have female internal organs (ovaries, a uterus), but enlarged clitoral tissue resembling a penis. You may have heard an old-fashioned term, **hermaphrodites,** used to describe this condition. Initially, a developing embryo is in an **undifferentiated sexual state—** neither male nor female—until about the seventh week of pregnancy when the gonads form into either testes or ovaries. A mutation of any of the genes during this process may result in altered genitalia.
- A **cross-dresser** (or **transvestite**) is a person (man or woman) who occasionally or frequently wears the clothing characteristic of the opposite sex, particularly the underwear, as a form of sexual expression. Often the person carries out this behavior in secret. Cross-dressers may be heterosexual, homosexual, or bisexual (see the next section, What Is Sexual Orientation?).

KnowledgeCheck 34-2

- How is gender determined?
- Distinguish gender, gender role, and gender identity.
- What is androgyny?

ThinkLike a Nurse 34-2

Do you believe that androgyny is a positive attribute? Explain your thinking.

What Is Sexual Orientation?

Sexual orientation refers to the general tendency of a person to feel sexually attracted to people of a certain gender. Because most people in Western culture are thought to be **heterosexual** (sexually attracted to members of the opposite sex), heterosexuality is the predominant cultural expectation. However, in the mid-20th century, the research of Alfred C. Kinsey indicated that a population's sexual orientation falls on a bell curve, with the majority of people experiencing at least some attraction to people of the same gender.

Klein, Sepekoff, and Wolf (1985) described sexual orientation as an ongoing dynamic process, with people's gender-based inclinations changing over time. In truth, we do not fully understand what makes up sexual orientation or how it develops. With increasing research on the biological aspects of sexual orientation, more professionals are concluding that people come to "recognize" the object of their sexual desire rather than "choose" or "prefer" it. Therefore, *sexual orientation* is probably a more accurate term than *sexual preference*.

Heterosexuality

As just mentioned, **heterosexuals** are people who are sexually and emotionally attracted to members of the opposite sex. In informal discourse, this segment of the population is commonly referred to as *straight*. Many major religious traditions reinforce heterosexual behaviors and gender roles. Although some heterosexuals have had same-gender sexual thoughts or limited experiences during childhood, adolescence, or adulthood, they still consider themselves heterosexual and have relationships with people of the opposite gender.

Homosexuality

The focus of sexual attraction for **homosexuals** is a person of the same gender. Homosexuals are also referred to as *gay* men and *lesbian* women. Accurate prevalence statistics are difficult to obtain because most studies rely on self-report data. Because homosexuality is not an aspect of the dominant culture and is prohibited by some religions, it can be difficult for gays and lesbians to share this aspect of their lives with employers, colleagues, family, and friends, much less with researchers and pollsters. Some homosexuals openly acknowledge that they are gay; others hide their sexual preference from family, friends, employers, and others. Of note, the *Diagnostic and Statistical Manual of Mental Disorders* (4th ed.) (*DSM-IV-TR*) of the American Psychiatric Association (2000) does not classify homosexuality as a psychiatric disorder.

Bisexuality

A person who is **bisexual** is sexually and emotionally attracted to both males and females. This group is perhaps least understood and least accepted by both the heterosexual and homosexual communities. They are less likely to be found in long-term monogamous relationships and often experience feelings of isolation. However, some bisexuals maintain stable and satisfying marriages because of their sustained sexual attraction to and amiable relationship with their spouse and the importance they place on parenting.

KnowledgeCheck 34-3

- What are the majority and minority sexual orientations in our culture?
- What is meant by transgender?

ThinkLike a Nurse 34-3

- What sexual orientations are you comfortable working with?
- Would you have difficulty working with a transsexual or other transgendered client?

How Does Sexuality Develop?

We are sexual beings from birth to death. Expression of our sexuality evolves through the life span. If you require additional discussion on sexuality and developmental stages, refer to Chapters 9 and 10.

Birth Through Preschool

Beginning at birth, parents, caregivers, and others respond to the infant with preconceived thoughts of what that gender role entails. The first 2 years of life can be highly sensual; as infants are nursed, stroked, bathed, and massaged, they develop their first attachment experience through bonding with the parent or other caregiver (Fig. 34-5). It is not unusual for children in this age group to touch their genitals and enjoy being nude. This behavior is part of their exploration of their bodies and is a normal part of child development. By age 3, most children recognize gender differences and know the names of body parts. Toddlers are interested in their bodies and curious to see the genitals of others. By age 5, children mimic adults by holding hands or hugging. It is not unusual for preschool children to masturbate and ask questions about "where babies come from." Parents should give factual information without offering explanations beyond what the child asks.

School Age Through Puberty

The school-age child strongly identifies with the same-sex parent and has mostly same-sex friends. Through interaction at home, school, and other activities, children gain awareness of gender roles and emerging gender identity.

From age 8 to 12 years, the child is in transition between childhood and puberty. Secondary sex characteristics become apparent. In females, breast buds form, and pubic hair appears. For a significant number of girls, **menarche** (beginning of menstruation) occurs. Boys become more muscular, the voice deepens, hair in facial and axillae develop, and the genitals begin to increase in size. The first attraction, either heterosexual or homosexual, may occur during this stage, and the

child may begin to masturbate more frequently, but privately. For information on the Tanner stages of sexual development in boys and girls, see the tables in Procedures 21-17 and 21-18.

Many school-age children are curious about sexual activity, reproduction, and sex roles, and they may ask explicit questions. By the time children reach the age range of 10 to 12, parents should begin teaching them basic information about approaching body changes, menstruation, sexual intercourse, and reproduction.

Adolescents

Adolescence is a time of heightened sexual interest and activity. There are two reasons for this: (1) the hormonal changes accompanying puberty and (2) cultural emphasis on sex. Masturbation is common. It is a safe and comforting sexual activity that has neither interpersonal nor disease risks. However, some adolescents may encounter parental, cultural, or religious disapproval of masturbation.

Sexual exploration usually begins with kissing, moves on to fondling, and can lead to genital contact. This progression may occur over a period of years, or there may be an early initiation of oral, vaginal, or anal intercourse. Although about 75% of adolescents are sexually active by their late teen years, the teen pregnancy rate is slowly dropping (Alan Guttmacher Institute, 2002, updated December 2006; U.S. Department of Health and Human Services [USDHHS], 2006, updated 2010).

Sexuality education in the home and school dispels myths and prepares teens for adult roles. To make informed choices as they move toward adulthood, adolescents need information about body changes, interpersonal relationships, **contraception** (birth control), and preventing sexually transmitted infections (STIs). To review physical changes of adolescence, see Chapters 9 and 21.

Young Adults

Not so many years ago it was generally assumed that young adults would abstain from sexual intercourse until marriage, when the husband and wife could become sexually active and start a family. Today, the age of first marriage is higher than in previous decades, and young adults engage more openly in sexual activity outside of marriage. Many young adults practice **serial monogamy,** in which the partners are mutually faithful but make no lifelong commitment. When the relationship ends, each partner usually enters another monogamous relationship.

During early adulthood, people define their sexual identity and resolve issues related to their sexual orientation and self-concept. As a part of sexual maturity, they develop an intimate relationship in which there is both communication and respect. Many people find a life partner during this period and make long-term plans, which often include parenting. However, some adults continue to struggle with their sexual identity, sexual orientation, or ability to form or commit to intimate relationships.

Young adults often wonder whether their sexual behaviors and responses are normal (e.g., "How often do most people have intercourse?" "Do other women have an orgasm every time they have sex?"). Many still need information about birth control, prevention of STIs, and sexual expression, and communication issues.

Middle Adults

Many adults in the middle years experience life changes that may enhance physical and emotional intimacy. For many, their children are now young adults who no longer rely on parental

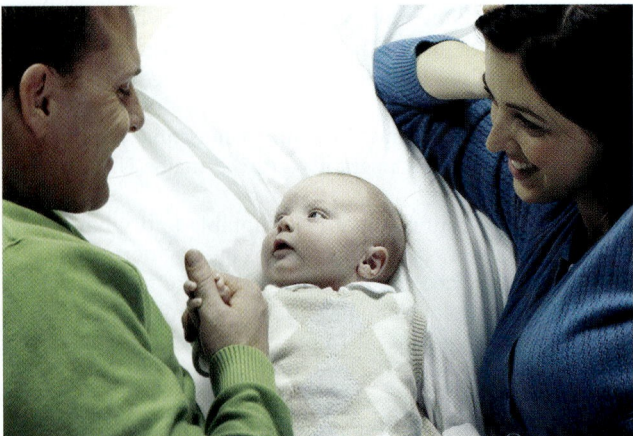

FIGURE 34-5 Parent infant attachment occurs through daily contact and care through activities such as feeding, bathing, and holding.

support, and the parents may have more privacy and time to spend together. However, it should be noted that new stressors might arise. In times of economic downturn, for example, middle adults are also one of the groups most seriously affected. In addition, this may also be a time when physical changes and chronic diseases emerge to affect sexual patterns.

Female Transitions. Women transition through **menopause** (cessation of menstruation). Some are relieved that the prospect of childbearing has ended; others may mourn the loss of the ability to give birth. Normal physiological changes include decreased vaginal secretions and vaginal wall thinning, which result from decreased levels of estrogen and progesterone. These changes may result in painful intercourse and diminish a woman's desire for sexual activity. Some women also experience hot flashes, sleep disturbances, and mood changes.

Male Transitions. As a result of the aging process or health conditions (e.g., type 2 diabetes or hypertension), men may experience erectile difficulty. They may perceive this problem as a threat to their masculinity and sexual attractiveness, and their self-image may suffer. Men also experience a decrease in the sex hormone testosterone. Sexual desire and the ability to achieve and maintain erection may decrease gradually, but many men remain fertile into old age.

Aging Adults

Most older adults are sexually active and regard sexuality as an important part of life, according to national data from the National Social Life, Health, and Aging Project (NSHAP). Sexual activity does decline with age, yet a substantial number of men and women engage in vaginal intercourse, oral sex, and masturbation even in their 80s and 90s (Lindau, Schumm, Laumann, et al., 2007). Sexual problems are more likely to result from failing physical health and medication side effects than from age alone. For example, as noted earlier, men with diabetes are more likely to have difficulty achieving and maintaining an erection. Other obstacles for sexual expression are lack of a partner (especially for women) and lack of privacy (e.g., for those who live with family members or in a long-term care facility).

As a result of age-related changes, postmenopausal women report less sexual stimulation and reduced desire, so they tend to need more foreplay and direct clitoral stimulation for sexual enjoyment. They may have fewer orgasms or orgasms that are weaker in intensity. Nevertheless, some women rediscover sexual desire after menopause.

Older women with poorer health are less likely to engage in masturbation (Laumann, Paik, Glasser, et al., 2006). Many older women complain of loss of vaginal lubrication. Some have pain during intercourse, usually caused by vaginal thinning and dryness. You can help your patients by suggesting water-soluble lubricants to counteract vaginal dryness and enhance pleasurable sensations during sexual activity.

Some men report erectile difficulty and need more time and more direct genital stimulation to achieve erection. It may take longer to ejaculate, and the orgasmic contractions may be less intense. When penetration is not possible (e.g., because of male erectile dysfunction), many couples find satisfaction with alternate forms of sexual stimulation and expression.

Older adults frequently experience sexual problems, but may hesitate to discuss them unless encouraged to do so. But if you bring up the subject and people feel comfortable, then they are eager for advice. In the past, many healthcare providers have hesitated to offer sexual counseling, fearing that such intimate discussion might offend their patients. But

if you bring up the subject and people feel comfortable, they are eager for advice (American Geriatrics Society Foundation for Health in Aging, n.d.). Even terminally ill people have sexual needs (e.g., reassurance from sexual partner or sexual stimulation) or sexual problems (e.g., lack of closeness).

KnowledgeCheck 34-4

- Why is it important to consider sexuality throughout the life cycle?
- What are the two major contributing factors to adolescents' heightened sexual interest and activity?
- What aspects of human sexuality are associated with young and middle adulthood?
- What challenges to sexuality may be found in the aging adult?

What Factors Affect Sexuality?

Culture, religion, lifestyle, sexual knowledge, and physical health all influence our attitudes toward sexuality, sexual behaviors, and intimate relationships. This knowledge can help you to provide nonjudgmental, holistic care to people who have a wide range of values, lifestyles, and states of well-being.

Culture

Culture influences our ideas about gender role, gender identity, marriage, sexual expression, and social responsibilities. However, it is not unusual for people to be **ethnocentric**— that is, to see their own culture and sexual behaviors as the norm for all. Because the United States is a multicultural country, beliefs and practices related to human sexuality vary widely. Consider the following examples of cultural influences.

- Victorian-era and later puritanical legacies have influenced many European Americans, some of whom consider sex to be "not nice," particularly if engaging in certain sexual activities or positions.
- African Americans are influenced by the dominant Anglo-Saxon culture as well as by their African heritage, history in America, and current economic and social situation. Marriage rates for African Americans are lower than for other ethnic groups, in part because of an unequal gender ratio (84 males per 100 females), as well as cultural acceptance of single parenting (Hyde & DeLamater, 2008).
- Many Latinos have strong ties to the Roman Catholic Church and a tradition of rigidly defined gender roles. The norm in Hispanic culture is for the male to be given more freedom as a child, but he is expected to be a virile, responsible provider for his family as an adult. In contrast, the female is typically raised to be more passive and obedient throughout her life.
- Asian Americans and Muslim Americans tend to be the most sexually conservative of the major U.S. cultural groups.

Culture determines what is acceptable and what is not. In some societies, **polygamy** (marriage to more than one partner) may be acceptable. Another culture may permit or prohibit sexual play among children. Many cultures have special rites of passage at puberty, such as the Jewish bar mitzvah for boys and bat mitzvah for girls, or the Native American vision quest.

Generally, you should honor cultural practices unless they are harmful. An example of a harmful practice is female genital mutilation (formerly known as **female circumcision),** which is illegal in most countries but is still performed among

certain tribes. In this procedure, the labia majora, labia minora, and clitoris are excised, and/or the vagina is sutured closed (**infibulation**). Infibulation may be done to ensure that the girl remains a virgin, whereas clitoral excision is meant to reduce sexual desire and ensure that the woman remains faithful to her husband. In addition to its psychosocial consequences, the procedure carries a high risk of infection and can cause the development of scar tissue that makes vaginal birth impossible. The U.S. Congress passed a law in 1996 making female genital mutilation of girls younger than 18 a federal offense. In 1997 and again in 2010, the World Health Organization issued a statement, with United Nations support, to abolish the practice of female genital mutilation (WHO, 2010).

Religion

Religion also has a powerful influence on sexuality. Religious practices restricting premarital sex, birth control, homosexuality, abortion, extramarital relationships, and masturbation are common. Some religions have rules about body coverings, modesty, and restricting opposite gender healthcare providers. Even education about the structure and function of the human body is governed by some religions. The "sexual revolution" that began in the 1960s has led to permissive sexual values in the broader Western culture. When these values conflict with a person's traditional religious values, anxiety and sexual dysfunction may result. To review the influence of religion on health, see Chapter 16.

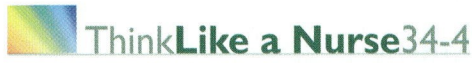 ThinkLike a Nurse34-4

How have religion and culture influenced your views on sexuality?

Lifestyle

Life experiences encompass our interactions with others and the environment. Family, socioeconomic status, employment factors, and interpersonal relationships shape our lifestyle, although they do not fully determine it. Consider the following examples:

- Having a beloved brother reveal to you that he is gay might alter your perception of homosexuality. Similarly, being raised by a lesbian couple might affect your view of gender roles.
- Growing up in a low-income neighborhood in which prostitution is a visible and accepted part of the environment might influence your views on what is acceptable sexual behavior.
- Dedication to a high-stress job or the demands of raising young children might leave you too exhausted to desire sex with your spouse.
- Being in an abusive relationship would affect your self-concept and might cause you to avoid intimacy in the future.

Lessons learned through day-to-day experience create powerful impressions on our views and often modify cultural and religious influences.

Sexual Knowledge

Although sexuality and family life are part of the curriculum in many public schools, you cannot assume that young adults have adequate sexual knowledge. Community values play a large role in determining how sexuality is viewed and taught. Thus, even if a state mandates sex education, a particular school may limit discussion on reproduction, STIs, birth control, intimacy, exploitive relationships, domestic abuse, or rape, believing that these topics are best addressed by the

family or religious institution. In addition, many children are home-schooled or taught in private or church-affiliated schools that do not allocate any class time to sex education. Even in schools with a comprehensive curriculum, parents have the right to exclude their child from sex education classes. Do not let your clients' age, level of education, or life experiences lead you to make assumptions about their knowledge of sexuality. For example, consider the following:

- A married person may not be sexually active.
- A woman with several children may not know what is involved in a pelvic exam or how conception occurs.
- A highly educated person may be uninformed regarding his body's structure and function.

It is difficult for most people to admit to a professional that they lack knowledge. Therefore, you must assess each client's knowledge and understanding of sexual terms. At times you may need to use the vernacular or "street" terminology to be understood. You can then introduce medically specific terminology.

KnowledgeCheck 34-5

- What sexual knowledge would you expect an adult male with children to have?
- What sexual knowledge would you expect a nursing student to have?

Health and Illness

Sexuality involves body, mind, and spirit; so it is not surprising that health status affects sexuality. For example, healthful nutrition and physical exercise are commonly reported to increase satisfaction in sexual relationships, whereas obesity and inactivity can undermine one's own feelings of attractiveness or one's attraction for one's partner. The importance of sexuality is readily apparent in the clinical setting. For example, the clients in the Meet Your Patients scenarios all expressed concerns related to their sexuality.

Physical Illness

Diseases, injuries, and medical treatments may demand lifestyle changes in multiple areas, including sexual functioning. To see examples of physical illnesses and how they affect sexual health,

 Go to Chapter 34, **Tables, Figures, and Boxes: ESG Box 34-1: Physical Illnesses Affecting Sexual Health,** on Davis*Plus*.

If a person becomes disabled while in a marriage or other committed relationship, the strain can threaten the partnership. In contrast, a person who is single or has a life-long disability may experience difficulty establishing an intimate relationship because of physical limitations, social isolation, poor self-image, or discrimination. Even when people lose interest in sexual intercourse, a need for intimacy still exists. Communication about sexual needs and desires may be difficult for couples, but as a nurse, you can support and facilitate it. Rehabilitation programs ideally offer holistic services and facilitate discussion regarding sexuality and relationship issues.

Mental Health Disorders

Mental health disorders can lead to interpersonal disruptions and difficulty with sexual expression.

- A depressed person experiences significant loss of interest in activities that previously brought pleasure. Thus it is

common for people with depression to avoid engaging in interpersonal activities, including sex.

- Conversely, a person with hypomania or mania may be preoccupied with pleasurable activities and increased sexual activity, as well as verbalization and acting out. Both extremes are disruptive to a relationship.
- For a person with psychosis, interpersonal relationships and sexual patterns are disrupted by lack of contact with reality or frank delusions.

Counseling for the couple is important when symptoms are controlled. During times of acute illness, support for the partner is vital.

Medication

Many medications used to treat health problems have unwelcome sexual side effects. Gabriel Thomas (Meet Your Patients) clearly illustrates the concern some clients have about commonly prescribed medications. Table 34-1 lists a number of medications and their effects on sexual function.

Medications may be prescribed to enhance sexual function, particularly for men experiencing erectile dysfunction (ED), for example, those with diabetes mellitus, or who are

Table 34-1 ▶ Effects of Drugs on Sexual Function	
MEDICATION	**POSSIBLE EFFECT**
Alcohol	In limited quantities, alcohol may enhance desire and function. However, heavy or chronic use may lead to decreased libido, orgasmic dysfunction, and erectile dysfunction.
Anti-anxiety agents	Decreased libido, delayed ejaculation
Anticonvulsants	Decreased libido, prolonged painful erections, difficulty achieving orgasm
Antidepressants	Decreased libido, difficulty achieving orgasm
	Bupropion (Wellbutrin) and trazodone (Desyrel) are least likely to cause sexual side effects.
Antihistamines	Decreased libido, decreased vaginal lubrication
Antihypertensives	Decreased libido, erectile dysfunction, delayed ejaculation
	Calcium channel blockers are least likely to cause sexual difficulties.
Chemotherapy	Fatigue, decreased libido
Opioids	Decreased libido, erectile dysfunction
Stimulants (cocaine, methamphetamines)	Initially stimulants cause increased intensity of the sexual encounter; however, with continued use, sexual dysfunction develops.

taking beta-adrenergic blocking agents to treat high blood pressure. Oral drugs are available for impotence (e.g., sildenafil, vardenafil, or tadalafil). These drugs generally work within 1 hour of administration, but have no effect without sexual stimulation. They increase blood flow to the corpus cavernosum of the penis.

KnowledgeCheck 34-6

- Identify four factors associated with physical illness that may affect sexuality or sexual functioning.
- What determines our sexual attitudes?

SEXUAL HEALTH

WHO defines **sexual health** (a key concept in this chapter) as a state of physical, emotional, mental, and social well-being related to sexuality; it is not merely the absence of disease, dysfunction, or infirmity. Sexual health requires a positive and respectful approach to sexuality and sexual relationships, as well as the openness and opportunity to have pleasurable and safe sexual experiences, free of coercion, discrimination, and violence. For sexual health to be attained and maintained, the sexual rights of all persons must be respected, protected, and fulfilled (WHO, 2002). To promote sexual health effectively, you will need theoretical knowledge about sexual responses, modes of sexual expression, and problems affecting sexuality.

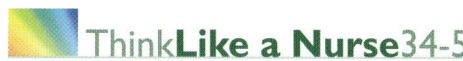

ThinkLike a Nurse 34-5

Examine your own beliefs about sexuality. Identify areas of concern you have regarding sexuality. How do you think this will affect your ability to assist patients with sexual health concerns?

What Is the Sexual Response Cycle?

The **sexual response cycle** is the sequence of physiological events that occur when a person becomes sexually aroused. Based on research conducted in the 1950s, Masters and Johnson (1966) identified a four-stage sexual response: excitement, plateau, orgasm, and resolution (Fig. 34-6). A growing body of research has called into question this four-stage model. One suggested alteration of the original Masters

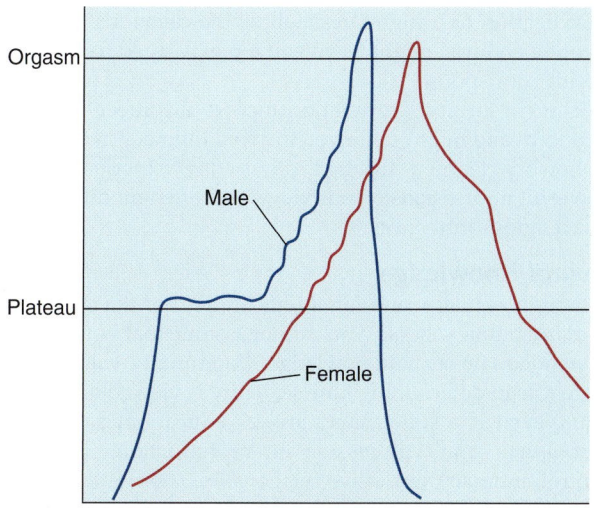

FIGURE 34-6 The sexual response cycle.

and Johnson model is to add a stage of desire, which in some people precedes and in some people follows excitement (Basson, 2001).

Although it is most intense in the genitals, sexual response is a total body response, involving many physiological changes (e.g., increased heart rate, flushing). The emotional and mental aspects of sexual activity are equally important to the person's satisfaction. The body has many **erogenous zones** (areas that cause sexual arousal when stimulated): the genitals, the skin, lips, ears, breasts, buttocks, and thighs. Box 34-1 shows normal physiological changes in sexual response that occur with aging.

Desire

Desire is a stage of varying length characterized by an interest in sexual intimacy. Desire occurs in the mind and is communicated verbally or through body language. This communication may be subtle and easily misread. **Libido** is an individual's typical level of desire. Desire increases in proportion to the level of the sex hormones (e.g., a man with low testosterone is not as interested in sex). For women, desire reaches a peak each month near the time of ovulation, when estrogen levels are high.

In many people, desire is readily aroused by erotic stimuli, such as sights, sounds, and fantasies. However, recent research indicates that a majority of women and a minority of men do not experience desire until after they have become aroused; in these people, physical excitement prompts the desire for sex (Basson, 2001).

What is considered sexual or attractive can vary greatly, because societal, cultural, and personal values influence the range of stimuli that provoke sexual desire. Desire may last only moments or be ongoing for years. Transient sexual thoughts are fleeting moments of desire that might be triggered by exposure to sexually explicit media or erotic thoughts, words, or actions.

Excitement

Excitement is the body's physical response to desire. During excitement the following bodily changes occur: heart rate, blood pressure, and respiratory rate increase; muscles tense **(myotonia);** nipples become erect; and genital and pelvic blood supply increases **(vasocongestion).** In women, vasocongestion leads to vaginal lubrication, swelling of the breasts, rise of the uterus, and swelling of the labia and clitoris. In men, erection begins as the penis increases in length and diameter. The testes rise closer to the body, and the scrotum thickens.

Excitement may lead to further sexual activity, but this is not inevitable. For both sexes, the person may lose and regain initial physical excitement many times without advancing to the next stage. Excitement may be communicated verbally or through body language.

Plateau

If stimulation continues, the person reaches the **plateau** phase. Plateau is associated with continued increases in pulse, respiratory rate, blood pressure, and muscle tension. Some people flush around the face, neck, and chest in this phase. In women, the areolae become firmer, the clitoris retracts into the clitoral hood, Bartholin's glands lubricate, and the lower vagina swells and narrows. With a male partner, the vagina tightens around

---

BOX 34-1 ■ Normal Physiological Changes in Sexual Response That Occur With Aging

Sexual Response Stage	Changes in Women	Changes in Men
Desire	Decreased libido	Decreased libido
Excitement and plateau	Delayed nipple erection	Delayed nipple erection
	Reduced labial separation and swelling	Delayed and less-firm erection
	Reduced vaginal expansion	Longer excitement stage
	Reduced lubrication	Decreased pre-ejaculatory emissions
	Decreased elevation of the uterus	Reduced muscle tension
	Reduced muscle tension	Reduced lifting of the scrotum and testes
	Reduced vaginal tone (in those who have had multiple vaginal deliveries); results in less stimulation during intercourse	Shorter phase of impending orgasm
		May require more direct stimulation to achieve and maintain an erection
Orgasm	Reduced spread of sexual flush	Shorter ejaculation time
		Fewer ejaculatory contractions
		Reduced volume of ejaculate
Resolution	No cervical dilation	More rapid loss of erection
		Longer refractory period
		Nipple erection lasts longer after orgasm

Sources: EngenderHealth. (2007). Sexual response and sexual practices: Normal changes in response with aging. *Sexuality and Sexual Health: An Online MiniCourse.* Retrieved September 12, 2011, from http://www.engenderhealth.org/res/onc/sexuality/response/miw/pg5.html; Kennedy-Malone, L., Fletcher, K., & Plank, L. (2004). *Management guidelines for nurse practitioners working with older adults.* Philadelphia: F. A. Davis; Running, A., & Berndt, A. (2003). *Management guidelines for nurse practitioners working in family practice.* Philadelphia: F. A. Davis; and Stanley, M., Blaire, K. A., & Beare, P. G. (2005). *Gerontological nursing: Promoting successful aging with older adults* (3rd ed.). Philadelphia: F. A. Davis.

Toward Evidence-Based Practice

Relatively little is known about the sexual behaviors of older people, and the relationship between quality of life and sexuality in older adults has not been fully explored.

> **Lindau, S. T., Schumm, P., Laumann, E. O., et al. (2007). A study of sexuality and health among older adults in the United States.** *New England Journal of Medicine, 357*(8), 762–774.

This study was conducted to explore the sexual behaviors and sexual function of older people. In a sample of 3,005 U.S. adults 57 to 85 years of age, researchers found that sexual activity declined with age. Women were significantly less likely than men at all ages to report sexual activity. Of those who were sexually active, about half of both men and women reported at least one sexual problem. The most common complaints among women were low desire, difficulty reaching climax, and difficulty with vaginal lubrication. Men reported erectile difficulty. Men and women who rated their health as poor were less likely to be sexually active. Sexual problems are frequent among older adults, but these problems are infrequently discussed with healthcare providers.

> **Kleinplatz, P. J. (2008). Sexuality and older people.** *BMJ, 337,* a239.

Much of the literature on sexuality in older adults focuses on sexual problems, leaving healthcare providers with the impression that older adults have either dismal or nonexistent sex lives. Little research is available as it pertains to normal sexuality in older adults. This study reports sexual satisfaction is increasing among older adults, especially in women, even if sexual dysfunctions are present. Some dysfunctions, such as erectile dysfunction and female lack of orgasm, are decreasing, whereas sexual problems, such as ejaculatory dysfunction in men, have increased over the past 30 years.

> **Beckman, N., Waern, M., & Gustafson, D. (2008). Secular trends in self reported sexual activity and satisfaction in Swedish 70 year olds: Cross sectional survey of four populations, 1971–2001.** *BMJ, 337,* a279.

Researchers studied trends in sexual behavior among 70-year-olds. They interviewed four samples of Swedish

people over a 30-year period and found the 70-year-olds born more recently reported higher satisfaction with sexuality, fewer sexual dysfunctions, and more positive attitudes in sexuality in later life than those who were interviewed earlier in the century. Overall, self-reported quantity and quality of sexual experiences among 70-year-olds improved over time. At the same time, a relatively large proportion of participants had stopped having intercourse. However, most elderly people consider sexual activity and associated feelings a natural part of later life.

> **Penhollow, T. M., Young, M., & Denny, G. (2009, January/February). Predictors of quality of life, sexual intercourse, and sexual satisfaction in older adults.** *American Journal of Health Education, 40*(1), 13–22.

This study attempted to find out what aspects of sexuality have the greatest influence on sexual intercourse, sexual satisfaction, and overall quality of life in residents of a large active retirement community. Sexual self-confidence was found to be the single most important predictor of sexual intercourse and sexual satisfaction and (for women) quality of life. Cultural (sexual acceptance, sexual priority), psychological (sexual desire, sexual self-confidence, and control), and social factors (satisfaction in relationship and social life) help to explain sexual satisfaction beyond the physical health.

---

1. What trend in the research about sexuality in older adults do you see?

2. In the Penhollow et al. study, what was the single most important factor influencing sexual satisfaction and quality of life, other than physical health? What do you think nurses can do to promote it?

3. Based on these studies, how do you think nurses can affect the quality of sexuality in older adults?

 Go to Chapter 34, **Toward Evidence-Based Practice Suggested Responses,** on Davis*Plus.*

---

the man's penis, increasing his sexual stimulation. In men, the ridge of the glans penis becomes more prominent, pre-ejaculate (two or three drops of fluid) is emitted, and the testes rise closer to the body. The person may achieve, lose, and regain the plateau phase several times without experiencing orgasm.

Orgasm

Orgasm occurs at the peak of the plateau phase. At the moment of orgasm, the sexual tension that has been building is released. The heart rate, respiratory rate, and blood pressure reach their peak, and there is loss of voluntary muscle tone.

- *In women,* spinal cord reflexes cause powerful rhythmic contractions of the vagina, uterus, anus, and pelvic floor

muscles; feelings of warmth spread through the pelvic area. The cervical canal dilates, allowing easy transport of the sperm to the uterus. Orgasm may last for a few seconds or up to nearly a minute.

- *In men,* spinal cord reflexes cause the urethra, anus, and pelvic floor muscles to contract, followed by **ejaculation** (the expelling of semen through the urethra). For men, orgasm usually lasts no more than 30 seconds.

The intensity of orgasm varies among individuals and in each individual from one sexual experience to another. Orgasm may involve intense spasm associated with intense focus on the sexual pleasure, or it may be signaled by as little as a sigh or subtle relaxation.

Resolution

Resolution is the period of time following orgasm. The muscles relax, and the body returns to its pre-excitement state. Immediately after orgasm, men experience a **refractory period,** during which they cannot achieve an erection. The duration of this period varies among individuals and increases with age. Women experience no refractory period—they can either enter the resolution stage or return to the excitement or plateau stage immediately following orgasm.

KnowledgeCheck 34-7

Identify the phase of the sexual response cycle described.

- This phase is reached if there is ongoing stimulation. This stage may be achieved, lost, and regained several times without the occurrence of orgasm.
- This stage occurs in the mind and may be communicated between potential sexual partners either verbally or through body language.
- This phase is associated with the release of sexual tension.

 ThinkLike a Nurse 34-6

Critique the theory of Masters and Johnson, as represented in the preceding discussion of the sexual response cycle. How would you respond to the statement that the theory does not adequately address variation among individuals and even within an individual's sexual response?

What Are Some Forms of Sexual Expression?

People express their sexuality and gain sexual satisfaction in many different ways. Although opinions vary, there is a range of behaviors that are socially acceptable and therefore considered "normal" by most people in our society. These are discussed in the next few sections.

Developing Intimate Relationships. Developing intimate relationships involves a willingness to take risks and offer trust. Intimacy involves openness, mutual respect, caring, commitment, protection, honesty, and devotion. Although we often think of intimate relationships as sexual, they are not necessarily so. Furthermore, in our society, many sexual relationships occur without intimacy.

Fantasies and Erotic Dreams. Most men and women have sexual fantasies. They may be related to past experiences, dreams, desire; or stories heard, seen, or read. Sexual fantasies serve to increase self-esteem and sexual arousal and as an outlet to explore sexual desires. People in long-term monogamous relationships may fantasize to bring variety and excitement into a routine sexual encounter. Erotic dreams are also common among both men and women. Nocturnal orgasm may or may not occur with the dream.

Masturbation. Masturbation is self-stimulation of the genitals. Although there are many techniques, men typically stroke the shaft of the penis, and women typically stimulate the clitoris manually. Young children touch their genitals as a part of body exploration, but they quickly learn either that touching certain areas is not acceptable or that it should be done in private. Adolescents, particularly males, may masturbate frequently. Adults may masturbate for sexual release when a partner is not available or for variety in a partnered

relationship. Sex therapists often recommend masturbation as a means to resolve orgasm difficulties in women and ejaculatory problems in men.

Religious and social taboos discouraging masturbation are common. Some people mistakenly believe that masturbation is harmful, causing acne, warts, blindness, or insanity. More commonly masturbation is considered a "dirty," shameful, or perverted act. Although most people masturbate at some point in life, most do not talk about it openly in our society.

Shared Touching. Mutual masturbation, or shared touching, may be an alternative to sexual intercourse. This is particularly appealing to individuals who seek to maintain virginity, wish to decrease the risk of STIs, or have mobility or other physical problems that make intercourse difficult. Mutual masturbation is recognized as a form of safer sex because body fluids are not likely to be exchanged. This behavior can be satisfying because it allows for a significant level of sexual intimacy and allows participants to experience orgasm.

Sexual Intercourse. *Sexual intercourse* and *coitus* are terms used to describe penile penetration of the vagina. People use a variety of positions for intercourse, depending on preference, mobility, cultural and religious influences, the relationship, and other personal beliefs. For some women, manual stimulation of the clitoris is also necessary to achieve orgasm. Partners typically do not reach orgasm at the same time, despite the romantic preoccupation with this phenomenon.

Unprotected intercourse may lead to conception, so the couple should use some method of contraception if they want to avoid pregnancy. Because it involves exchange of body fluids, sexual intercourse may also lead to the transmission of infections. Using a lubricated latex condom decreases this risk but is not a foolproof measure to prevent STIs.

Oral–Genital Stimulation. Both heterosexual and homosexual couples practice oral–genital stimulation (oral sex). Couples in committed relationships may engage in it for sexual variety or as foreplay. Others may engage in oral sex because it provides intimacy yet cannot result in pregnancy; many believe that it does not affect their virginity status. For the latter reasons, oral sex has become more prevalent among adolescents. Oral–genital contact may, however, lead to STIs. **Cunnilingus** is the oral stimulation of a woman's genitals. **Fellatio** is stimulation of the male genitals by a partner's mouth. Although swallowing semen is not a health issue, it may be a matter of personal preference whether the recipient ejaculates in his partner's mouth. If the couple is not in a long-term monogamous relationship, dental dams, plastic wrap, or latex condoms should be used to prevent the transmission of STIs.

Anal Stimulation and Anal Intercourse. Both homosexual and heterosexual couples engage in oral–anal stimulation (called **anilingus**). Objects for sexual stimulation, or the partner's, finger, tongue, and mouth, may be used to stimulate the anus. **Anal intercourse** (also termed *sodomy*) is the insertion of the penis into the partner's rectum. When engaging in anal intercourse, lubrication is essential to lessen the chance of tiny tears to the rectal mucosa or damage to the anal sphincter. Unless the couple is in a long-term monogamous relationship, they should use a lubricated latex condom to lessen the chance of STIs. The condom must be changed before vaginal penetration to

avoid the transfer of *Escherichia coli* bacteria from the rectum to the vagina. Couples should follow the same precaution when using objects for sexual pleasure.

Celibacy. Celibacy, or *abstinence*, is a state in which a person refrains from sexual activity. Traditionally, a celibate is one who remains unmarried, often for religious reasons, and sublimates sexual desire through prayer, meditation, and service. However, the following are other reasons some people choose to remain celibate:

- Fear of or lack of desire for intimate relationships
- Childhood sexual trauma
- A developmental or physical disability that limits opportunities for meeting prospective partners, limits privacy, or interferes with the ability to communicate or act on desires.
- Focusing energies elsewhere secondary to a low libido

Married couples may be happily celibate. Others might be celibate after the loss of a relationship, whether through separation, divorce, or death, often feeling a considerable void.

Alternative Forms of Sexual Expression. The *DSM-IV-TR* (American Psychiatric Association, 2000) describes eight categories of sexual deviation, or paraphilias: exhibitionism, fetishism, frotteurism, pedophilia, sexual masochism, sexual sadism, transvestic fetishism, and voyeurism. Whereas some people experience guilt, shame, and depression about their paraphilia, others are distressed only by the societal disapproval, restrictions, and possible criminal charges associated with their mode of expression. If you need more detailed information about paraphilias,

 Go to Chapter 34, **Supplemental Materials: Alternative Forms of Sexual Expression,** on Davis*Plus*.

There are some important things you can teach parents and other caregivers to do to reduce children's risk of sexual violence, predators, or other unhealthy exposure (see the Self-Care box Teaching Children About Predators).

KnowledgeCheck 34-8
- What are aspects of an intimate relationship?
- Identify solitary types of sexual expression and those that may be conducted with a partner.

What Problems Affect Sexuality?

Sexual well-being is a complex mesh of physical, emotional, cognitive, social, and spiritual components. Therefore, it is not surprising that many people experience challenges to their sexual health. Difficulties can arise in loving, healthy relationships as well as in dysfunctional couplings. Sexual dysfunction may be temporary and situational, or it may be long standing.

Sexually Transmitted Infections

An STI may be caused by bacteria, viruses, fungi, or parasites. They are spread through direct sexual contact with an open wound or with body fluids, such as semen, vaginal secretions, or blood that contains pathogens. STIs are not transmitted by casual touching, sitting on toilet seats, shaking hands, or sharing a glass with someone.

STIs are among the most common infectious diseases in the United States today. More than 20 different STIs have been identified, and they affect millions of men and women each year. **Reportable** (or **notifiable) diseases** are diseases that have a significant effect on public health. When healthcare providers diagnose a reportable disease, laws require it be reported to the Centers for Disease Control and Prevention (CDC). Examples include the following:

- *Chlamydia trachomatis.* In 2007, over 1.1 million cases of sexually transmitted *C. trachomatis* infection were reported to CDC. This is the largest number of cases ever reported to CDC for any condition (CDC, 2007b).
- *Gonorrhea.* The incidence of gonorrhea has been declining for the past 20 years, and has now reached a plateau at about 350,000 new cases per year.

Self-Care

Teaching Children About Predators

Set the Stage for Open Discussion

➤ Talk openly and directly with your child about her own development and sexuality. This establishes trust and makes it easier for the child to come to you when she has questions.

➤ Be open to your child's questions. Acting embarrassed discourages further conversation.

➤ Assure your child that she won't get in trouble for "tattling" on someone who asks her to keep a secret about sexual encounters.

➤ Make discussion a natural part of growing up—don't save it "for later."

Know What's Going On

➤ Be involved in your child's everyday life and ask questions—that is, where he is, who he's with, what he's doing.

➤ Go to your child's activities and get to know the other adults your child is around.

➤ Know what the child watches on television or media games.

➤ Locate computers in a central area in the home where you can monitor Internet use.

➤ Install a parental control to limit access to and monitor Web sites where your child could be exposed to sexual content or predators.

➤ Know if sexual predators live near you. Check out the sexual predators registry in your area.

Just Say No

➤ Teach your child about body parts that are private and should not be touched or looked at by others—except for medical reasons.

➤ Teach your child to firmly say no and get away if someone tries to touch or look at her in a way that makes her feel uncomfortable.

➤ Urge your child to tell you or another trusted adult if someone tries to touch or look at private areas or if the person tries to show the child his or her own private body parts.

➤ Place limits on Internet use.

➤ Teach children not to disclose personal information in public settings or on the Internet, even social networking sites.

- *Syphilis.* Although less common, syphilis is important because of the serious neurological complications it can lead to.

Nearly two-thirds of all STIs occur in people younger than 25 years. However, at least one in ten newly diagnosed cases of HIV occurs in a person older than 50 years.

Many STIs have few or no initial symptoms, allowing an infected person to transmit the infection without knowing it. For example, up to 90% of women infected with gonorrhea or chlamydia have no symptoms. To find out whether a patient has an STI, you must obtain a culture, that is, a swab of secretions from the genitals. In a man, the swab is put into the urethral opening. In a woman, the swab is obtained from secretions near the cervix. A culture of the throat or rectum is obtained if the person has had oral or anal sex.

Many STIs can be treated fairly easily with antibiotics; however, if left untreated, they may cause serious problems. For example, in women, the pathogens can travel up through the uterus into the fallopian tubes and cause pelvic inflammatory disease (PID). Untreated PID may cause infertility. One STI, human papillomavirus infection (HPV), causes genital warts and cervical and other genital cancers.

The best way to prevent STIs is to be abstinent or to participate only in a mutually monogamous sexual relationship with someone who has never had an STI and has never shared needles. Risk for an STI increases if a person has unprotected sex or has more than one sex partner. The more sex partners, the greater the risk (CDC, 2010). Other risk factors include alcohol and drug use, sexual activity at an early age, intercourse with a new partner, prior history of an STI, failure to utilize latex barriers with sexual contact, genital piercings, intercourse between men, intercourse with someone who has recently been in prison, sexual assault, sexual abuse, and failure to comply with prescribed treatment for an STI (Davidson, 2004).

To read about various STIs, their symptoms; treatment; and effect on sexual functioning, fertility, and childbearing,

 Go to Chapter 34, **Tables, Boxes, Figures: ESG Table 34-1: Common Sexually Transmitted Infections (STIs),** on DavisPlus.

Dysmenorrhea

Dysmenorrhea is painful menstruation caused by strong uterine contractions that lead to ischemia of the uterus. The patient may experience cramping, lower abdominal pain, back and upper thigh pain, headache, vomiting, and diarrhea. Interventions are discussed later in the chapter.

Premenstrual Syndrome

Premenstrual syndrome (PMS) is characterized by physical and emotional changes occurring 3 to 14 days before the onset of the woman's menstrual period. Physical symptoms include headaches, constipation, breast tenderness, and weight gain associated with bloating, abdominal swelling, or swelling of the hands and feet. Some women feel as though they are on an emotional roller coaster, with periods of depression, anxiety, irritability, tension, and an inability to concentrate. Some have difficulty maintaining social interactions because of severe emotional symptoms. Client teaching for PMS is discussed later in this chapter.

Women experiencing a more severe form of menstrual cycle dysfunction **(premenstrual dysphoric disorder [PMDD])** become seriously depressed for a week or more before their periods. In contrast, PMS is shorter, usually milder, and involves more physical symptoms. A woman can suffer from both PMS and PMDD at the same time, or may have one and not the other.

KnowledgeCheck 34-9

- Identify three methods to decrease the transmission of STIs.
- What are physical and emotional symptoms of premenstrual syndrome (PMS)?

Negative Intimate Relationships

Some intimate relationships are not mutually satisfying, even when they do not involve neglect, or physical or emotional abuse. Couples may be involved in a celibate or loveless union for financial security, social status, for "the sake of the children," or because of cultural or religious restrictions regarding divorce. In reality, many relationships fall somewhere in between—sometimes satisfying and other times less so—depending on a wide variety of factors, including stress, physical and mental illness, hormones, fatigue, distractions, low self-esteem, financial pressure. The most negative relationships involve *domestic violence* (also called *intimate partner violence*), which may include physical and/or emotional intimidation, assault, and rape.

Although either gender partner may be a victim of domestic violence, most often the woman is the victim. The anger, domination, and physical violence of the partner lead to fear, intimidation, and submission in the victim. Often victims come to believe that they deserve the abuse and thus may hesitate to admit the cause of their injuries, even in the hospital setting. Many abused women are either emotionally or financially dependent on their partner and believe that they have no options except to stay in the relationship.

Sexual Harassment

Sexual harassment occurs when a person in power makes unwanted sexual advances that implicitly or explicitly relate to the victim's employment, academic status, or success. "Advances" can take the form of sexual comments or behaviors (such as touching). Because of the power imbalance, the victim may keep silent. **Sexual assault** includes contact with or without penetration; touching sexual or intimate parts; and any unwanted sexual activity in situations of intoxication, coercion, or misconception.

Sexual harassment may take two forms: (1) In *quid pro quo* cases, the employer makes the employee feel that she must engage in unwelcome sexual advances to maintain employment; (2) in *hostile environment* cases, the sexual advances are more subtle, but persistent, and create an intimidating environment.

Rape

Although rape is actually a crime of violence rather than of sex, we discuss it here because it involves the sexual organs and usually has negative effects on the victim's sexuality. **Rape** is nonconsensual vaginal, anal, or oral penetration. It occurs through force, by the threat of bodily harm, or when the victim is incapable of giving consent. In all 50 states, laws consider rape, even within a marriage, to be a crime.

Victims of rape range from infants to older adults and may be either gender, although girls and young women are more than 13 times more likely than males to be victims (American Academy of Pediatrics [AAP], Committee on Adolescents, 2001). In two-thirds of cases, the victim knows or is related to

the assailant, especially when the victim is a young child (Homor, 2010; Rennison & Rand, 2008). People with developmental disabilities, especially mental retardation, are at twice the risk for sexual assault than the general population.

Group rape (also called gang rape) occurs when more than one person sexually assaults a victim. Group rape usually occurs when drugs and alcohol are involved. **Statutory rape** is sexual activity between an adult and a person under the "age of consent" (this ranges from 14 to 18 years of age, depending on state regulations). This charge may be filed even when the sex is consensual. **Date rape** is rape by an acquaintance when the assault occurs during an agreed-on social encounter. Although date rape is not a lesser violation, our society tends to blame the woman when date rape occurs.

Many rapes go unreported. An assault that involves significant physical injury is most likely to become known to the authorities because the victim requires medical attention. After a rape or other forms of sexual assault, care is more likely to be delayed, particularly for teens, if alcohol or drugs are involved. Other reasons for not reporting rape include fear of the assailant, fear of consequences to the assailant, knowledge of the low conviction rate for rapists, the desire to avoid a trial, shame and embarrassment, past sexual history, self-blame, wanting to "move on," and the wish to deny the event and its possible consequences.

In addition to psychological and physiological trauma, the rape victim is at risk for STIs and pregnancy. Three-quarters or more of sexually assaulted teens experience post-traumatic stress disorder. Referral to a local sexual assault support group is critical. A *sexual assault nurse examiner (SANE)* is a registered nurse who has received special training in the immediate care of sexual assault victims. To learn about providing care for sexual assault victims, refer to Clinical Insight 34-1.

Sexual Response Cycle Disorders

Disorders in various stages of the sexual response cycle may affect desire, arousal, excitement, and orgasm.

Low Libido

Low libido (hypoactive sexual desire) manifests as a significant decrease in or absence of sexual fantasies and sexual activity. Low libido may affect both men and women. It can be transient or long term. The person may experience low libido only with one particular partner, or the lack of desire can extend to all sexual activity. Persons with low libido may reluctantly engage in sexual encounters or avoid all sexual contact. However, once sexual activity has been initiated, the person is usually able to achieve orgasm.

Factors contributing to hypoactive sexual desire include sexual trauma, a negative attitude toward sex, negative relationships, and biological factors, including hormone deficiencies, perimenopause, and side effects of various medications. Low sexual desire, in both men and women, sometimes responds positively to testosterone administration.

Arousal Disorders

In women, arousal disorders manifest as minimal or absent pelvic congestion and vaginal lubrication even though desire may be present. Hormonal changes, the aging process, tampons, and medications (including antihistamines) also cause vaginal dryness. Vaginal dryness may result in **dyspareunia**, or painful intercourse, which further reduces sexual desire. A water-based lubricant or saliva helps to resolve vaginal dryness. Other causes of female dyspareunia include vaginal or urinary tract infections, pelvic inflammatory disease, and endometriosis.

Clinical Insight 34-1 ▶ Providing Care After Sexual Assault

- **Carefully collect information about the incident** and document findings in a fact-based manner, following your institution's protocol.
- **Be sensitive to the victim's fear, anxiety, and guilt** related to the event.
  Open discussion without communicating judgment or disapproval helps with fact finding for better care.
- **Assess the victim's emotional status,** including sexual identity, stress disorder, and risks for suicide and self-harm. Also discuss the potential for sexual and physical violence, including violence within relationships.
- **When collecting a nursing history for people with disabilities, be sure to screen for sexual violence**.
- **Administer prophylactic treatment** for STIs, such as chlamydia and gonorrhea, to patients who have been assaulted (vaginally, anally, or orally). If there is a significant risk for HIV, prophylaxis may be prescribed within 72 hours of exposure.
- **Administer vaccines to prevent hepatitis B and HPV,** as prescribed and according to your agency's policy.
- **Administer emergency pregnancy prevention** (e.g., the "morning-after" pill) to patients who have been

vaginally assaulted even if penetration is uncertain, according to your agency's policy.
- **Document pregnancy status** with a urine or blood sample.
- **Advise the female victim who has had vaginal penetration to obtain pregnancy testing** again 2 weeks after the event. The victim should receive follow-up care within 1 week after the event to assess for healing of injuries and presence of STIs.
- **Know the current reporting requirements** for sexual assault in your state. Some states require reporting assault of children and adolescents, even if they do not consent to the reporting.
- **Be familiar with support services** available in your community for victims of abuse. Consider referring the victim to a sexual assault center for support, counseling, and additional information.
  Because of the long-term psychological and emotional consequences of sexual assault, most victims benefit from counseling.

Dyspareunia in men most commonly results from urinary tract infection or **phimosis,** a condition in which the foreskin of the penis is too tight. **Balanitis,** inflammation of the penis, is another cause of dyspareunia in men.

Vaginismus is a rare female disorder affecting desire and arousal. It is characterized by intense involuntary contractions of the perineal muscles, which close the vaginal opening and prevent penile penetration. Vaginismus may be associated with negative attitudes toward sex or a history of sexual abuse or trauma. Physiological disorders may also be the cause.

Sexual arousal disorders in men manifest as **erectile dysfunction (ED),** formerly known as *impotence.* Men with ED have persistent or recurring inability to achieve or to maintain an erection sufficient for satisfactory sexual performance. The most common cause of ED is diseases of the blood vessels (e.g., hypertension, high cholesterol, or diabetes). ED may also result from underlying neurological problems (e.g., spinal cord injury, Parkinson's disease, stroke) or endocrine problems (diabetes). Testosterone plays a minor role in erectile function and a major role in libido (desire). Common psychological causes include performance anxiety, childhood sexual abuse, relationship issues, or mental illness. Some medications can also cause ED (e.g., antihistamines, antidepressants, antipsychotics, and antihypertensives).

Orgasmic Disorders

Orgasmic disorder is a delay in or absence of orgasm after a normal sexual excitement phase. Once a woman has had orgasms, it is uncommon for her to lose that ability unless there has been a sexual trauma, poor sexual communication, a conflicted sexual relationship, a mood disorder, a medical condition, or direct physiological effects from a drug. Orgasmic disorder is more prevalent in younger women who have not had adequate sexual experience to learn how to reach orgasm. It is not unusual for a woman to require manual clitoral stimulation to reach orgasm; not all women can achieve orgasm through intercourse alone.

Men, too, can experience orgasmic disorders. Some cannot achieve orgasm during intercourse but are able to reach orgasm through masturbation or manual or oral stimulation by their partner.

In **premature ejaculation,** the male reaches orgasm and ejaculates before, at the time of, or shortly after penetration. The disappointment of both partners may lead to issues with self-esteem, sexual avoidance, and ED. There are sexual techniques as well as medications that help to delay ejaculation.

Retrograde ejaculation occurs when the semen empties into the bladder instead of being ejaculated through the urethra. Normally this cannot occur because the internal bladder sphincter closes in the orgasmic phase. However, some medications, prostate surgery, and spinal cord injuries may lead to retrograde ejaculation, resulting in sterility.

KnowledgeCheck 34-10

- Identify three forms of sexual victimization.
- In which phases of the sexual response cycle can sexual dysfunction occur?

PracticalKnowledge
knowing **how**

Although you understand the importance of comprehensive client assessment, you may find it difficult to gather information related to sexuality. Some students and nurses may be shy, or may be concerned that the client will be embarrassed to talk openly about sexual topics. These matters are personal and private, and they can threaten a person's self-esteem. But including sexuality as a routine part of your nursing assessment reinforces the concept that sexuality is an integral part of life, and provides an opportunity for much-needed patient teaching. Many patients will not raise the topic of sexuality, so if you do not mention it, you may not meet patient needs.

ASSESSMENT

The extent to which you will assess a client's sexual health status varies. For example, if a patient has a suspected STI, you would perform a comprehensive health assessment in addition to a focused sexual health assessment. Similarly, clients with illnesses that affect their sexual functioning should receive a full assessment. Jocelyn Carter (Meet Your Patients) is an example. Recall that chronic health problems have a profound effect on sexual functioning (e.g., recall Frank Thanee and Gabriel Thomas, in the Meet Your Patients scenario). A focused sexual health assessment is needed in the following situations:

Pregnancy, infertility workup, request for birth control
Menstrual cycle irregularities or problems
Annual health visit
Unusual discharge from or change in genital organs
Urination problems
As part of a comprehensive physical examination
A known sexual problem (e.g., dyspareunia)
Illness that may affect sexual function (e.g., arthritis)
Victim of unwanted sexual activity (e.g., rape)
Medications

Tailor your assessment to meet the client's needs. For example, Frank Thanee (Meet Your Patients) is concerned about his family's reaction to his lifestyle and sexual orientation. In his situation, you would focus your assessment on his sexual self-concept, family relationships, present sexual functioning, and specific concerns about his heart and the impending family visit.

Sexual History

Most healthcare facilities use a standard nursing assessment form. Some address sexuality in a comprehensive manner, but most have only a few superficial questions or nothing at all. You will need to be sensitive to your client's verbal and nonverbal cues to identify and explore relevant issues that are not on the form. For topics to include in a sexual history and for suggestions for questions to ask, see the accompanying Focused Assessment box, Guidelines and Questions for Taking a Sexual Health History.

When you are asking personal questions, be sure to provide privacy. It is one thing to discuss blood pressure in the presence of family, but quite another to discuss sexual health issues, which may threaten the very core of a relationship. For example, an 18-year-old man may not admit to having sex with another man when his father is present; and an adolescent daughter may not want to discuss her STI in front of her mother. For guidelines about your approach when taking a sexual history, see Clinical Insight 34-2.

Focused Physical Examination

Sexual health assessment includes a physical examination focused on the reproductive system. For detailed instructions about performing these examinations, see Procedure 21-17 and Procedure 21-18.

KnowledgeCheck 34-11

What techniques can you use to increase comfort and communication during a sexual history assessment?

Guidelines and Questions for Taking a Sexual Health History

Topics to Include in a Sexual Health History

Topics to include in the sexual history depend on the nature of the patient's concern. The following topics are most commonly included:

➤ Reproductive history
➤ Sexual self-concept
➤ History of STIs
➤ History of sexual dysfunction
➤ Present sexual functioning
➤ Other factors that affect sexuality, such as medications and diseases
➤ Signs or symptoms of sexual abuse (see Procedure 9-1)
➤ Knowledge level about sex, reproduction, and contraception

Sexual Health History: Questions to Ask Women

Menstrual Cycle

➤ How old were you when you started your menstrual periods?
➤ When was your last menstrual period?
➤ How often are your periods? How would you describe the flow? How long does your period last?
➤ Do you have any problems with your periods, such as cramping, breast pain, or heavy flow?
➤ Does your menstrual period ever prevent you from going to work or school or doing the activities you enjoy?
➤ What products do you use during your period, such as tampons and pads? Do you ever use douches, either during your period or at other times?

Cancer Screening

➤ When was your last Pap smear?
➤ Have you ever had an abnormal Pap smear? If so, how was it treated?
➤ Have you received a vaccine for HPV?
➤ Do you examine your breasts? If so, how often?
➤ Have you noticed asymmetry, lumps, or masses in your breasts? If so, describe them and show me where they are.
➤ When was your last mammogram? What were the results?
➤ Is there any history of breast cancer in your family?

Childbearing History

➤ How many living children do you have?
➤ How many times have you been pregnant?
➤ Have you ever had a miscarriage? An abortion?
➤ How many of your births were preterm (prior to 38 weeks)? Term?

Sexual Activity

➤ How often do you typically have sexual intercourse per month?
➤ Are you satisfied with the frequency or quality of sexual activity?
➤ Is there anything in your life that prevents you from sexual activity?
➤ Do you have any difficulty achieving orgasm?
➤ Is sexual intercourse ever painful for you?
➤ Are you sexually attracted to women? Have you had oral or genital sexual intercourse with women?

Sexual Health History: Questions to Ask Men

Sexual Activity

➤ How many times a month do you typically have sexual intercourse?
➤ Do you have any difficulty achieving or maintaining an erection or orgasm?
➤ Are you satisfied with the firmness of your erection?
➤ Do you experience either premature ejaculation or have difficulty achieving sexual orgasm?
➤ Are you sexually attracted to men? Have you had oral or anal intercourse with men?

Cancer Screening

➤ Have you been taught to examine your testicles? Do you practice testicular self-exam?
➤ Is there a history of testicular cancer in your family?

Sexual Health History: Questions to Ask Both Men and Women

Illnesses and Medications

➤ What types of illnesses have you been treated for in the past?
➤ Have you ever been hospitalized? Have you ever had surgery?
➤ What medications, herbal remedies, or over-the-counter medicines do you take?

Family Responsibilities

➤ Do you have children? If so, how many? How many are still at home? Dependent on you?
➤ Are you responsible for other children or adults? [This question may reveal whether the person continues to care for an adult disabled child or for grandchildren.]

Genitalia

➤ Have you noticed any redness, swelling, discharge, itching, or odor in your genital area?
➤ Have you noticed asymmetry, lumps, or masses in the genitals? If so, describe them and show me where they are.
➤ Have you ever been told you have a hernia?
➤ Have you ever had trauma to your genitals?
➤ Are you having any problems urinating?

Sexual Patterns

➤ Are you sexually active? If not, have you ever been?
➤ Do you have sex with men, women, or both?
➤ What types of sexual activity do you engage in? Oral, anal, or genital?
➤ How many partners do you currently have? How many partners have you had in the past 6 months?
➤ How would you describe your satisfaction with your current sexual relationship?
➤ What are your thoughts about how this procedure/illness may affect your sexual relationship?
➤ Have you experienced any recent changes in your sexual function—in your level of desire, your sexual activity, participation, or satisfaction?
➤ Do you have any concerns about your sexual function, including your level of desire, activity, participation, or satisfaction?

Guidelines and Questions for Taking a Sexual Health History—cont'd

Contraception (as appropriate)

➤ Do you use birth control? If so, what type and how often?
➤ How satisfied are you with your method of contraception?

Sexually Transmitted Infections

➤ Have you ever been treated for an STI? If so, what type?
➤ Are you concerned about STIs or HIV?
➤ Do you take any precautions to avoid infections?

➤ If there is reason to suspect that a client has a STI, you should obtain cultures of any discharge or lesions. Other laboratory tests may be ordered as well.

Abuse

➤ Have you ever been forced to have sex against your will?
➤ Have you ever been threatened or abused by a partner?
➤ Do you ever feel threatened by your partner?

Clinical Insight 34-2 ➤ Tips for Taking a Sexual History

1. **Provide privacy.**
   - Usually it is not enough merely to pull the curtains around the bed. If others could overhear private conversation behind the curtain, ask them to leave the room.
   - Talk to the client alone.
   - In some situations it is good to also talk to the partners as a unit, with the consent of both of course.
2. **Protect confidentiality.** Assure your client that information will not be shared with others unless directly related to planning or delivering healthcare.
3. **Be relaxed in your approach,** and allow the client time to answer your questions fully. Your manner and attitude are critical.
4. **Make eye contact.** Do not act embarrassed or allow your body language to show your discomfort.
5. **Avoid communication stoppers,** such as:
   - "I'm only asking you these questions because I have to."
   - "I know that you probably won't want to tell me but . . ."
   - "You're not having any sexual problems, are you?"
6. **Consider a more inviting opening,** such as:
   - "Many people are embarrassed when asked questions about their sexuality, but whatever you tell me will remain confidential."
   - "Many people hesitate to talk about sexual problems. However, your sexual health is important to your overall health, and I would like to ask you a few questions about that."

7. **Be aware of verbal and nonverbal cues** that indicate concerns. Many people will cloak their concerns in comments such as, "I suppose that I won't need to worry about sexy lingerie any longer," or "Sex is for the young. I just have to accept that I'm sick and older now." Be careful your response does not either negate or validate your patient's identity as a sexual being. Follow up with comments that encourage the client to provide more details (see Chapter 20 if you would like to review communication techniques).
8. **Realize the client may be embarrassed.** If the client is uncomfortable discussing topics about his own sexual health, reassure him by letting him know that some information, because of its private nature, may be difficult to discuss but important.
9. **Encourage your client to use terminology that he is comfortable with.**
10. **Help the client feel comfortable.** Consider statements such as the following:
    - "Most people wonder how this surgery (or illness) may affect their sexual functioning."
    - "Whenever these medications are suggested, there are questions about sexual side effects."
    - "Have you thought about the kinds of adaptations you may have to make in your sex life after this surgery/treatment/illness?"
11. **Begin with a less sensitive topic,** such as "How is your relationship with your partner (spouse)?" Then you can move into more sensitive areas: "Many older women have some vaginal dryness that creates discomfort during intercourse. Do you have any concerns about this?"

ThinkLike a Nurse 34-7

Review the three case scenarios in the Meet Your Patients discussion. Consider the following questions for each patient:

- Would you be comfortable caring for and responding to each of these clients?
- What topics, if any, have been raised by these clients that would be difficult for you to handle?
- How would you answer each of the client's questions?

ANALYSIS/NURSING DIAGNOSIS

NANDA International (NANDA-I) has two nursing diagnoses for describing sexual problems. Although there is much overlap between these two diagnoses, the following should help you differentiate between them:

Sexual Dysfunction. Use this label when there is an actual change in sexual function that the patient views as unsatisfying, unrewarding, or inadequate. This includes sexual response cycle disorders, such as low libido, arousal disorders,

orgasmic disorders, vaginismus, premature ejaculation, and erectile dysfunction. Sexual Dysfunction is a more specific diagnosis than Ineffective Sexuality Patterns, and is a better fit for physiological problems and for concerns about sexual performance. Thus, it is best to diagnose Sexual Dysfunction when the patient has one or more of the following defining characteristics:

> Changes in achieving sexual satisfaction
> Change of interest in self or others
> Inability to achieve sexual satisfaction
> Verbalization of a sexual problem
> Actual or perceived limitations imposed by disease or therapy
> Changes in ability to achieve perceived sex role
> Seeking confirmation of desirability

You could diagnose Sexual Dysfunction for Frank Thanee (Meet Your Patients) because he is experiencing a values conflict. He is expressing concerns, not about his sexual identity, performance, or satisfaction, but about how his homosexuality will affect his parents.

Ineffective Sexuality Patterns. Use this diagnosis when the patient expresses concerns about his own sexuality. Examples of such concerns might include conflict about sexual orientation, values conflicts, fear of acquiring an STI, lack of knowledge about how to adapt sexual techniques to altered body function, lack of privacy, not having a partner, or impaired relationship with the partner. If these defining characteristics for Sexual Dysfunction do not seem to "fit" the patient, then use this more general diagnosis (Ineffective Sexuality Patterns). The only defining characteristic needed to make this diagnosis is that the patient reports difficulties, limitations, or changes in sexual behaviors or activities. Jocelyn Carter (Meet Your Patients), for example, is not actually experiencing problems with sexual satisfaction or performance. She is expressing a broader concern about her sexuality—about her future desirability as a sex partner. Therefore, the better diagnosis for her is Ineffective Sexuality Patterns. The same is true for Gabriel Thomas, who is expressing fear that he may have sexual problems in the future.

Etiologies of Sexuality Diagnoses

Several nursing diagnoses may be the cause of sexuality problems. The following are the more common:

- *Activity Intolerance* and *Fatigue* (e.g., from cardiac or respiratory disease) may cause the person to alter his lifestyle, including sexual activity, to conserve energy. Lack of energy may decrease the person's interest in sex, or it may require a change in the mode of sexual expression.
- *Impaired Physical Mobility* (e.g., as occurs with arthritis or spinal cord injuries) may affect a person's ability to interact, meet potential partners, and perform sexually (e.g., assume certain positions, make certain movements).
- *Fear* that sexual activity may be dangerous can inhibit desire and the ability to perform (e.g., after heart surgery). This diagnosis may also apply to the client's partner, who may be afraid that sexual activity will hurt the client after surgery, or hurt a pregnant partner or the baby.
- *Chronic Pain* may directly affect interpersonal relationships, interest in sex, or comfort during sexual intimacy. It may cause fatigue, indirectly affecting sexuality.
- *Chronic Low Self-Esteem* may result from chronic health problems and their consequences (e.g., loss of employment, inability to perform parenting roles). Sexual expression may also become a challenge, yet the intimacy and reassurance

that accompanies sexual encounters can be vital to self-esteem and a sense of wholeness.

- *Self-Care Deficits.* For clients who need assistance with activities of daily living (ADLs), for example with toileting, family or caretakers often find it difficult to accept and facilitate sexual relationships. When a person with a physical disability lives in a residential facility, lack of opportunity and privacy may interfere with sexual expression (Fig. 34-7).
- *Risk for Delayed Development.* Relationship challenges also exist for people who are developmentally disabled. Those with very low cognitive functioning are unable to seek out or understand sexual relationships. Unfortunately, this makes them vulnerable to sexual abuse. Sex education is vital for these individuals to help them understand body structure and function, relationship issues, and ways to avoid exploitation and abuse.

Sexuality Problems as Etiologies of Other Diagnoses

Sexuality problems can be the etiology of other nursing diagnoses, for example:

- *Disturbed Body Image* related to change in appearance secondary to orchiectomy (removal of a testicle)
- *Pain (during coitus)* related to inadequate vaginal lubrication secondary to aging
- *Fear* related to sexual abuse by father
- *Rape-Trauma Syndrome* (Note that you do not need an etiology for this nursing diagnosis. It is self-explanatory, as are most syndrome diagnoses.)

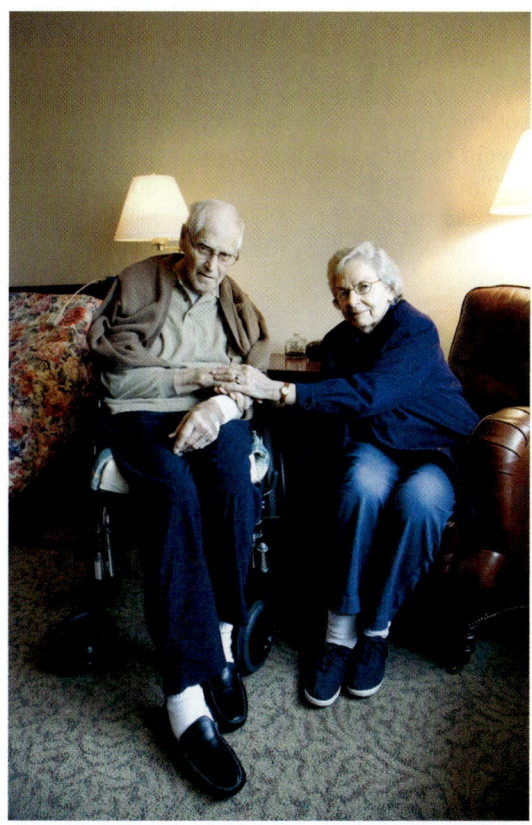

FIGURE 34-7 Sexual expression may be a challenge, yet the intimacy and reassurance that accompanies sexual encounters can be vital to self-esteem and a sense of wholeness.

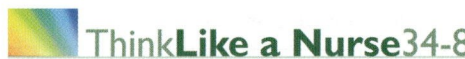 ThinkLike a Nurse34-8

Give a specific example (patient situation) for each of the defining characteristics of Sexual Dysfunction given in the preceding section.

PLANNING OUTCOMES/EVALUATION

For *NOC standardized outcomes* associated with Ineffective Sexuality Patterns and Sexual Dysfunction,

 Go to Chapter 34, **Standardized Language: Examples of NOC Outcomes for Sexuality Problems** on Davis*Plus.*

Individualized client outcomes and goals depend on the nursing diagnosis you identify. For Sexual Dysfunction and Ineffective Sexuality Patterns, you might write the following desired outcomes:

- Expresses comfort with sexual orientation.
- Describes plans for resolving values conflicts about extramarital sex (e.g., will talk to his minister).
- Describes techniques for preventing STIs.
- Reports using a condom for all sexual activities involving exchange of body fluids.

The following are examples of outcomes that apply specifically to Sexual Dysfunction:

- Communicates sexual needs and preferences to partner.
- Maintains penile erection through orgasm.
- Describes ways to adapt positions for intercourse to accommodate painful knee joints.

PLANNING INTERVENTIONS/IMPLEMENTATION

For *NIC standardized interventions* and selected nursing activities for sexuality,

 Go to Chapter 34, **Standardized Language: Examples of NIC Interventions and Nursing Activities for Sexuality Problems,** on Davis*Plus.*

Specific nursing activities for sexuality problems depend on the etiology of the problem and on the goals selected. Broadly speaking, nursing interventions involve teaching about sexual health and self-care, counseling for altered sexual functioning, and dealing with inappropriate sexual behavior. Those interventions are discussed in the following sections.

You will also find a nursing care plan and care map for Ineffective Sexuality Problems on the following pages.

Nursing Care Plan

Client Data

Emilio Juarez is a 50-year-old man hospitalized for cardiac monitoring after an acute myocardial infarction (MI; heart attack). He has no history of diabetes or hypertension. Mr. Juarez owns a computer software company and is active in the community as president of the chamber of commerce.

After dinner, Mr. Juarez's nurse sits down to teach Emilio and his wife, Luz, about the medications that he will be taking. She also begins to talk to them about a cardiac rehabilitation program. Mr. Juarez asks, "What do you mean by 'activity restriction'? Do I have to stop doing all the things I did before?" The nurse asks, "What things are you thinking about?" Mr. Juarez hesitates, then says, "Oh, like working in the yard, going up the stairs, and, you know, personal things." Mrs. Juarez immediately says, "There is no need to talk about that now. The most important thing is for my Emilio to feel better and get home—there is plenty of time for other things later." The nurse tells the two that many couples are anxious about resuming sexual activity after a heart attack and says, "I'd like to give you some information about that and answer any questions you might have."

Nursing Diagnosis

Ineffective Sexuality Patterns related to lack of knowledge about post-MI sexual activity and reluctance to ask questions, as evidenced by Mrs. Juarez's comment, "There is no need to talk about that now."

NOC Outcomes	Individualized Goals / Expected Outcomes
Sexual Identity (1207) Sexual Functioning (0119) Body Image (1200)	*By discharge, Mr. Juarez will:* 1. Be able to identify two resources he can use to learn more about sexual activity after myocardial infarction. 2. Commit to attending the cardiac rehabilitation classes offered at the hospital. *During and by the end of the cardiac rehabilitation program, Mr. Juarez will:* 1. Identify stressors in his life related to sexual activity. 2. Report a desire to resume sexual activity to pre-MI levels. 3. Resume previous sexual activity.

NIC Interventions / Activities

NIC Interventions
Sexual counseling (5248)
Body image enhancement (5220)
Anxiety reduction (5820)

Nursing Activities	Rationale
1. Initiate discussions about sexual activity after MI, beginning with general, nonthreatening statements.	Clients and significant others are often too embarrassed to ask about sexual matters. The client's perception of his sexuality impacts personal and social behavior outside the bedroom (Steinke, 2002; Steinke & Patterson-Midgley, 1996). Patients should be reassured that after recovery from an MI, sexual activity presents no great risk of another MI (Cooper, Skinner, Nherera, et al., 2007).

Nursing Care Plan (continued)

Nursing Activities	Rationale
2. Allow Mr. Juarez to control the discussion of sexual matters.	The subject of sexual activity should be raised with patients within the context of cardiac rehabilitation (Cooper et al., 2007; Miner, 2006). This shows respect for the client's privacy and his sexual being. Controlling what issues are discussed and when enhances self-esteem (Steinke, 2000).
3. Listen carefully to Mr. Juarez's verbal and nonverbal expression of concerns.	Anxiety interferes with patients' return to sexual activity after an acute cardiovascular event (Moser, 2007). Some men may overtly express disinterest in discussing sexual matters; others avoid the topic by joking, avoiding eye contact, or brushing off concerns as not pressing. Commonly, men avoid verbalizing feelings in this area because of the personal nature and threats to masculine identity. Although depressive symptoms are more common in women after an MI and contribute to higher rates of rehospitalization, men also show depression (Moser, 2007; Parashar, Rumsfeld, Reid, et al., 2008).
4. Seek consultation from other members of the healthcare team as needed.	When nurses are uncomfortable talking about sexual matters and do not initiate the conversation, the client may think sexual activity is prohibited after MI. If the nurse is personally uncomfortable discussing these matters, it is imperative to consult with other members of the team who can meet the client's needs (Steinke, 2000; Steinke & Patterson-Midgley, 1996).
5. Include Mrs. Juarez in counseling as much as possible, with Mr. Juarez's consent.	Marriage and close interpersonal relationships allow each member to support the other and alleviate negative effects of stress. The client's ability to adapt physically and emotionally after MI depends on the spouse's ability to cope with situational stressors (Beach, Maloney, Plocica, et al., 1992).
6. Be clear about exploring Mr. and Mrs. Juarez's specific concerns, and correct any misinformation.	Anxiety about sexual activity after MI often arises from misconceptions. Less than 1% of MIs and 5% of angina attacks occur during sexual activity (Miner, 2006; Salamon, 2008). There is no evidence suggesting that sexual activity poses a risk for sudden death (Cooper, Skinner, Nherera, et al., 2007). Regular exercise, such as in a cardiac rehab program, reduces the risk of MI from sexual activity (DeBusk, Drory, Goldstein, et al., 2000; Muller, 2000). For some cardiac patients, sexual problems begin before a heart attack. Erectile dysfunction, the consistent inability to sustain an erection, affects more than 50% of men older than 60 and is a recognized symptom of cardiovascular disease. The typical period of maximum risk (which is still very low) is within 4 weeks of the MI (DeBusk, Drory, Goldstein, et al., 2000). Exercise training after acute MI improves cardiovascular efficiency and reduces myocardial oxygen demand during customary activities, including sexual activity (Miner, 2006). Erectogenic drugs, when used correctly, do not increase overall cardiovascular risk in patients after an MI (Cooper, Skinner, Nherera, et al., 2007).

(continued)

Nursing Care Plan (continued)

Nursing Activities	Rationale
7. Discuss the risks of using drugs for erectile dysfunction together with nitrates.	An unsafe drop in blood pressure can occur when erectile dysfunction medication is taken with nitrates (Cooper, Skinner, Nherera, et al., 2007; Miner, 2004). Men should be taught to contact their prescribers if they experience an erection lasting more than 4 hours or if a change in vision occurs.

Evaluation

After Mrs. Juarez left for the evening, the nurse returned to bring Mr. Juarez a medication. He said, "Thanks for bringing that up and for leaving the booklet. I love my wife, and I was worried. I sure didn't want to have another heart attack. She was embarrassed to let on that it is important to her, but we will be sure to make use of the rehab program." The nurse followed up later by giving the Juarezes a DVD that discusses sexual issues, which they can take home and watch in privacy and comfort when they are ready to do so.

References

Beach, Maloney, Plocica, et al., 1992; Cooper, Skinner, Nherera, et al., 2007; DeBusk, Drory, Goldstein, et al., 2000; Friedman, 2000; Miner, 2006; Moser, 2007; Muller, 2000; Parashar, Rumsfeld, Reid, et al., 2008; Salaman, 2008; Steinke, 2000; Steinke, 2002; Steinke & Patterson-Midgley, 1996.

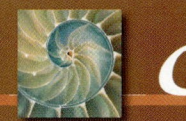

Care Map

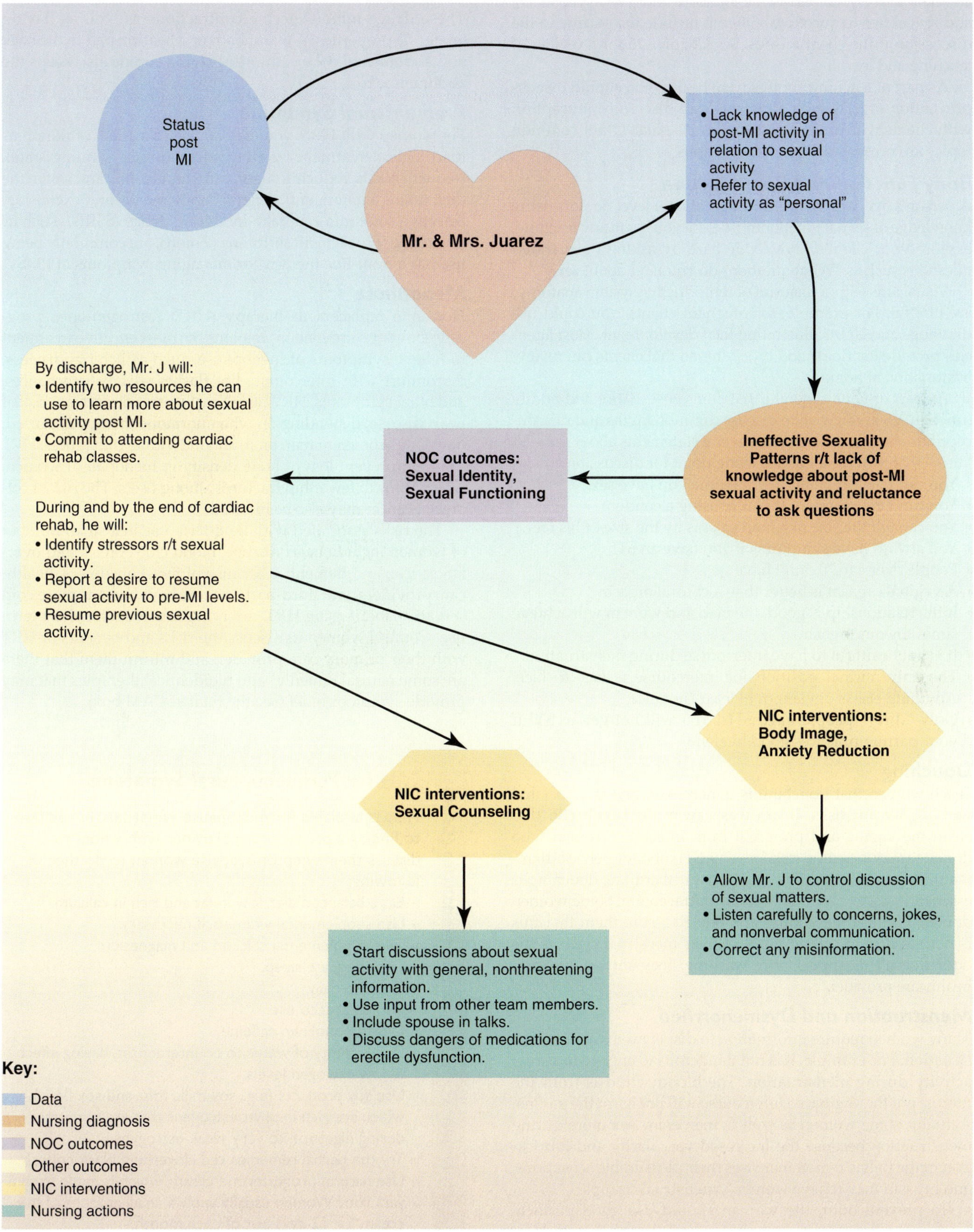

Status post MI

Mr. & Mrs. Juarez

- Lack knowledge of post-MI activity in relation to sexual activity
- Refer to sexual activity as "personal"

Ineffective Sexuality Patterns r/t lack of knowledge about post-MI sexual activity and reluctance to ask questions

NOC outcomes: Sexual Identity, Sexual Functioning

By discharge, Mr. J will:
- Identify two resources he can use to learn more about sexual activity post MI.
- Commit to attending cardiac rehab classes.

During and by the end of cardiac rehab, he will:
- Identify stressors r/t sexual activity.
- Report a desire to resume sexual activity to pre-MI levels.
- Resume previous sexual activity.

NIC interventions: Sexual Counseling

NIC interventions: Body Image, Anxiety Reduction

- Start discussions about sexual activity with general, nonthreatening information.
- Use input from other team members.
- Include spouse in talks.
- Discuss dangers of medications for erectile dysfunction.

- Allow Mr. J to control discussion of sexual matters.
- Listen carefully to concerns, jokes, and nonverbal communication.
- Correct any misinformation.

Key:

- Data
- Nursing diagnosis
- NOC outcomes
- Other outcomes
- NIC interventions
- Nursing actions

Teaching About Sexual Health

Before you begin teaching, take the time to get to know your client and find out what she already knows about sexuality. Take time to put the client at ease. When you develop rapport and trust, the client is more likely to speak openly with you about sensitive or embarrassing topics, to retain what you teach, and to feel free to questions. Offer to include the partner in the discussion if the client wishes. See Chapter 26 for a review of teaching and learning.

As part of teaching about sexual health, you should discuss prevention of STIs with all clients and discuss contraception with clients who are heterosexual or bisexual. Other common topics are presented in the next sections.

Body Function and Reproduction

A person's age, experience, and educational level do not ensure knowledge of sexual functioning. Before you begin any teaching, explore your client's knowledge base by asking open-ended questions such as "What questions do you have about sex?"

Visual aids (e.g., a diagram of reproductive system anatomy) are helpful. For example, for pregnant clients, you could use drawings and charts illustrating fetal development. Most agencies provide handouts and brochures so that clients can review information at home.

As part of your general discussion on sexuality and bodily function, you may wish to discuss common myths and misconceptions about sex. Below are several statements about sex—all false—that provide a good starting point for discussion.

- You can't get pregnant the first time you have sex.
- You can't get pregnant if you're using a condom.
- You can tell the size of a man's penis by the size of his feet.
- You always have symptoms if you have an STI.
- People over age 70 don't have sex.
- A vaginal orgasm is better than a clitoral orgasm.
- If the relationship is good, the man and woman will achieve simultaneous orgasm.
- It is not healthful to have intercourse during menstruation.
- The only normal position for intercourse is face to face. Anything else is deviant or at least "not nice."
- Only "dirty" people have STIs. You will not get an STI if your partner practices good hygiene.

Douching

Teach women that douching is unnecessary and is associated with significant risks. It can wash away the lactobacilli that clean the vagina and protect it from infection. Women who douche are at increased risk for some STIs and for pelvic inflammatory disease (Iannacchione, 2004). Furthermore, douching is essentially useless as a method of contraception. Some women douche because they notice an odor. Reassure them that this is normal during certain times of their menstrual cycle. If the odor doesn't disappear after washing, they should see their healthcare provider.

Menstruation and Dysmenorrhea

Many women require information to dispel myths about menstruation. For example, it is not dangerous to engage in sexual activity during menstruation. The bloody fluid is from the uterus, not the vagina, so intercourse will not harm the vagina. Actually, some women as well as men enjoy sex more during menstruation because the increased vascularity and lubrication in the pelvic region increases their pleasurable sensations, and orgasm may relieve women's menstrual cramps.

To prevent odor, the woman should use good perineal hygiene, bathe or shower every day, and change pads or tampons frequently. Advise women to follow the manufacturer's directions for reducing the risk for toxic shock syndrome. Deodorized pads and tampons are not very effective and can cause irritation to the vulva and vagina.

For mild cramping occurring before or during menses, aspirin and NSAIDs, such as ibuprofen or naproxen, are effective and can be taken unless contraindicated for other reasons. These drugs inhibit uterine contractions as well as having analgesic properties. A warm bath or a heating pad to the back and abdomen may be comforting; lying supine also keeps the abdomen warm.

Premenstrual Syndrome

For women with PMS, you may suggest a variety of nonpharmacological treatments: getting adequate sleep; eating small, frequent meals; reducing sugar, caffeine, alcohol, and salt in the diet; taking vitamin and mineral supplements; and exercising. Selective serotonin reuptake-inhibiting drugs (SSRIs), such as fluoxetine (Prozac) and sertraline (Zoloft), are commonly being used as a front-line therapy for managing symptoms of PMS.

Menopause

Hormone replacement therapy (HRT) (estrogen-only, progestin-only, or combination) remains the most effective treatment to relieve symptoms of menopause, such as itching, dryness, discomfort with intercourse, hot flashes, sleep disturbances, and other symptoms. HRT can either increase or decrease risk of heart disease, depending on when hormone therapy is started; how long women remain on it; and individual differences. HRT can help prevent loss of bone density in menopausal women, which leads to fewer hip fractures among users. The risk of colorectal cancer may also be reduced.

The risks associated with long-term use in a small number of women include heart disease, blood clots, breast and ovarian cancer, and dementia. Because of this, consumers, healthcare providers, and third-party payors have become more conservative about using HRT, reserving treatment for short-term use. Counsel women to discuss the risks and benefits of HRT with their primary care provider, and inform them that there are some natural remedies and bioidentical therapies that may provide symptom relief (see the related CAM box).

Complementary & Alternative Modalities (CAM)

CAM for Perimenopausal Symptoms

Help is available for menopause symptoms. In addition to finding a primary care provider with whom to discuss their symptoms, advise women to do the following:

➤ Eat a balanced diet, low in fat and rich in calcium.
➤ Use supplemental vitamins, if necessary.
➤ Take supplemental calcium and magnesium.
➤ Get adequate sleep.
➤ Exercise daily.
➤ Avoid tobacco use.
➤ Limit alcohol and caffeine.
➤ Drink plenty of water to counteract the drying effect of low estrogen levels.
➤ Use soy products (e.g., soy milk, tofu, and soy flour), which are rich in phytoestrogens that are converted during digestion to very weak estrogens.
➤ Try the herbal remedies red clover and black cohosh.
➤ Use natural progesterone cream, which is made from a yam root. Women usually apply a small amount of the cream for 12 days out of each month.

Self-Examination

Breast self-examination is a vital aspect of sexual health. Any change in how the breasts normally look and feel should be immediately provided to the healthcare provider. Although there is controversy about whether to advise routine breast self-examination, the American Cancer Society (ACS, 2010) recommends it as an option for women in their 20s. Women should have yearly mammograms to screen for breast cancer after age 40. These guidelines represent an extensive review of the health literature and input from an expert advisory group. However, some researchers have concluded there is no clear benefit for performing breast self-exam in detecting cancer.

The ACS advises men to be aware that a lump in the testicle could be a sign of testicular cancer. However, because the benefit of testicular self-exams has not been studied enough to show they reduce the death rate from this cancer, the ACS does not make a recommendation about monthly self-exams. However after puberty, checking for lumps is a good idea, especially if the man had undescended testicle or family history of testicular cancer.

For more information and for details about the assessments, see Chapters 9, 21, and 27.

Preventing Sexually Transmitted Infections

STIs are a worldwide health concern, and education is a key component of prevention. The only absolutely safe sex is total avoidance of sexual activity with a partner. However, most adults do not choose abstinence. The next safest sex occurs within a long-term, mutually monogamous relationship. Other safer sex practices involve the consistent, correct use of a condom and limiting the number of sexual partners. See Clinical Insight 34-3 for information about the use of male and female condoms.

Teach your clients the proper use of condoms and encourage them to discuss sexual feelings, activity, and safety with their partners. If people are not comfortable talking about birth control, STIs, and safer sex with a potential partner, they need to consider whether it is wise to begin a sexual relationship. Planned Parenthood advocates the following behaviors for safer sex:

- Be honest about current sexual practices and sexual history, as well as sexual health concerns.
- Avoid the exchange of body fluids, including semen, blood, and vaginal secretions, by correctly and consistently using latex barriers.
- Avoid contact with genital sores or growths.
- Have routine checkups for infection.
- Consult a healthcare provider for diagnosis and treatment of symptoms such as abnormal discharge from the vagina, penis, or rectum; a burning sensation with urination; sores in the genital area; or painful intercourse.
- Accept responsibility for your actions.

Also advise clients to choose a healthcare provider with whom they can comfortably discuss these issues. Freedom to speak frankly and openly about their sexual health concerns is important to their health. Assure them that testing, examination, and treatment for STIs are always confidential.

Clinical Insight 34-3 ▶ Teaching Your Patient to Use a Condom

Using Male Condoms

The male condom is a sheath that covers the penis during sexual activity.

- Put the condom on before the penis touches the vagina, mouth, or anus.
- Inspect the package to ensure that the condom has not been damaged.
- Open the package without tearing the condom.
- Squeeze out the air at the tip of the condom, and unroll it over the erect penis, leaving some space at the tip to collect the ejaculate.
- After sex, to avoid breaking the condom, hold the condom at the rim as the penis is withdrawn. Wash your hands.
- Use a new condom if you want to have sex again.

Using Female Condoms

The female condom is a plastic pouch that fits inside the vagina so that all vaginal tissue is protected from contact with the penis. The condom is inserted with the inner ring placed high in the vagina near the cervix and the outer ring on the labia.

- Insert the condom before the penis touches the vagina.
- Inspect the package to ensure that the condom has not been damaged.
- Open the package without tearing the condom.
- Put the inner ring and pouch inside the vagina.
- Push the inner ring as far into the vagina as it will go.
- Ensure that the outer ring stays outside the vagina.
- If needed, add lubricant to the inside of the condom.
- After sex, gently pull out the condom and discard.

Do

- Use latex condoms unless you or your partner are allergic to latex, or use polyurethane condoms.
- Treat condoms gently, and keep them out of the sun.
- Use only water-based lubricants to reduce friction and prevent tearing.
- Check the expiration date of the condom and packaging. Old condoms may be brittle and more likely to break.

Don't

- Don't store condoms in your wallet or other place where body heat can break down the latex.
- Don't use fingernails or teeth to open the condom wrapper; doing so can tear the condom.
- Don't reuse a condom.
- Don't use lotions or oils with condoms; these may cause breakage.

Contraception

For clients who are heterosexual or bisexual, your sexual health teaching may include methods for preventing unwanted pregnancies. We discussed condom use in the preceding section. The only 100% effective method is abstinence, or refraining from sexual intercourse. Several other fertility control and family planning strategies are available, including the following:

- Fertility awareness (natural family planning, rhythm method)—Having intercourse only when a woman is thought to be in the infertile phase of her menstrual cycle
- Withdrawal (coitus interruptus)—Removal of the penis from the vagina before ejaculation
- Spermicides—Jelly, creams, or foams placed in the vagina
- Oral contraceptives (birth control pills)
- Depo-Provera injections
- Intrauterine device (IUD)—A small piece of plastic placed through the cervix into the uterus by a healthcare provider
- Diaphragm—Latex dome-shaped cup with a flexible rim, inserted into the vagina; fits over the cervix
- Hormonal implant—Small rod(s) containing hormones, inserted under the skin in the back of the upper arm
- Sterilization—Tubal ligation for females; Vasectomy for males
    To read about the advantages and disadvantages of each method,

 Go to Chapter 34, **Tables, Boxes, Figures: ESG Table 34-2: Fertility Control Methods,** on Davis*Plus.*

Promoting Sexual Health in Older Adults

You can help aging clients to understand that sexual feelings do not necessarily disappear with age, and sexual expression need not stop (Fig. 34-8). Suggest alternatives to intercourse when illness or disability interferes. For example, sexual expression may include hugging, caressing, oral sex, and mutual manual stimulation. In addition, you may suggest ways to adapt coital positions to accommodate bodily changes, for example, when a partner is obese or has joint immobility.

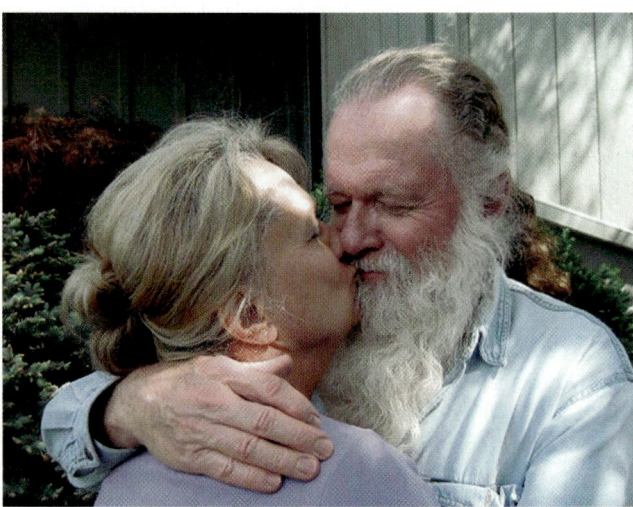

FIGURE 34-8 Healthy older adults maintain sexual intimacy.

Counseling for Sexual Problems

The PLISSIT model was developed as a guideline for counseling for sexual problems (Annon, 1974). Basic nursing education does not prepare you to provide sex therapy. However, the first three PLISSIT steps have been successfully adapted to address sexual knowledge deficits, which you are qualified to treat. The acronym PLISSIT represents the following:

*P*ermission. Permission means that you communicate an open, accepting attitude so that the client feels free to ask open-ended questions and express concerns and feelings and to engage in sexual behaviors with a consenting partner. For example, you might state, "Many women experience decreased vaginal lubrication after menopause. Tell me how well you have been lubricating."

*L*imited *I*nformation. Supplying limited information may include teaching about normal sexual functioning, expected changes in sexual functioning, medication side effects, and medical and surgical impacts on sexuality. For example, you might say, "Some women experience decreased vaginal lubrication because of decreased levels of certain hormones."

*S*pecific *S*uggestions. You might make specific suggestions for self-care, as presented in this chapter. For example: "You might consider using a water-soluble lubricant."

*I*ntensive *T*herapy. If these interventions do not relieve the client's concerns, you should refer the client to someone with specialized knowledge of sexual health. For example: "You might consider discussing this with your gynecologist."

Dealing with Inappropriate Sexual Behavior

Nursing involves intimate contact. We see people disrobe, literally touch bodies, and discuss private topics. In most cases, patients recognize this as professional behavior associated with providing health care. Occasionally they may respond inappropriately. For example, a client may make sexually suggestive comments, request sexually related care that is not required (e.g., ask you to bathe his genitalia when he can do it adequately himself), disrobe or expose body parts that are not involved in the care delivered, or touch or grab you as you provide care. The following are the most common reasons for sexually inappropriate behaviors:

- Confusion
- Neurological disorders, especially those involving the frontal lobe
- Poor impulse control
- Misinterpretation of nursing care
- Need to have power or control over others, especially when the client feels powerless in other aspects of his life
- Worries about sexual functioning
- Unrealistic view of nursing based on sexual stereotypes

    If you believe a client is demonstrating inappropriate sexual behaviors, immediately tell the client that the behavior is inappropriate. Do not express anger, but use clear statements, such as, "I don't like your comments. They are inappropriate. Please stop." Next, let the client know what behavior you expect. Be direct with your comments. If the client is exposing himself, let him know what you expect him to wear ("I expect you to keep your pajama pants on"). If the client is attempting to touch you, tell him, "Don't touch me." Refocus the client's attention to the care you are delivering ("Hold still now, while I tape your IV"). If you are extremely uncomfortable or the

client persists in the comments or actions, leave the room and report the incident to the charge nurse. You may also wish to consider discussing the situation with the client while another person is in the room.

Sexual harassment is a unique form of inappropriate sexual behavior (refer to Sexual Harassment in the Theoretical Knowledge section). If you believe you are being sexually harassed, you should confront your harasser and clearly state your concerns. If you feel unable to confront your harasser (e.g., if the harasser is a teacher or supervisor), keep a written record of the events, and report your concerns to the worksite or school official in charge of personnel. By law, all worksites and educational environments must have a written procedure for handling cases of sexual harassment. It will tell you how to file a grievance, what forms you need to use, to whom the incident is reported, and details of the procedure for a hearing and resolution.

PUTTING IT ALL TOGETHER

Consider the three patients discussed in the Meet Your Patients scenario. Each situation illustrates how important sexual identity is to the sense of self. Each of the patients is concerned about how their medical problem would affect their sexuality: Jocelyn Carter is worried about her relationship with her husband; Gabriel Thomas is concerned that blood pressure medications would impair his sexual abilities; Frank Thanee, though recovering from open heart surgery, is focused on explaining his long-term relationship to his family.

A sound knowledge base enables you to teach and respond sensitively to all your clients. Many myths and taboos surround the subject of sexuality; so it is important that you remain objective and current regarding these topics. You also need to focus on what patients are experiencing and critically examine their concerns in light of their medical conditions and treatments. Try to help your patients balance their sexual needs with the need to control and treat their medical conditions. Help them consider the consequences of various approaches, for example, by discussing alternative forms of sexual expression.

When dealing with sexuality, communication skills are essential practical knowledge. Your verbal and nonverbal skills demonstrate to patients your comfort with sensitive topics. When working with patients with sexual health concerns, tailor your approach and interventions to each individual's needs, just as you do in all areas of health.

To help patients identify and resolve sexual health concerns, you will need to examine your own beliefs and values. The self-knowledge gained from examining your own views on sexuality will help you to be open to your patients' sexual concerns.

▰▰CLINICALREASONING:
Applying the Full-Spectrum Nursing Model

Because the following critical thinking activities allow you to practice the kind of thinking you will use as a full-spectrum nurse, they usually have no single right answer. Discuss them with your peers—if you have difficulty with any of the questions, consult your instructor.

PATIENT SITUATION

Debra is perimenopausal at age 52, and her husband, Roberto, is 59. She has been feeling tired in the afternoon and moody at times. At her annual women's health visit, Debra tells you that she feels a lower level of sexual desire than she used to. Debra says, "I chalk it up to being very busy at work and yet still having so many demands on my time and energy with care of our three kids and housework." Debra is physically active, exercising four times a week, and is in good general health. She takes no medication and is within 15 pounds of her normal weight. Debra still has her period, but the flow is very heavy and cramping is more uncomfortable than it had been.

Recently, Debra has noticed that Roberto has been taking longer to achieve an erection, and his erection is not as firm as it used to be. His health is generally healthy except for high blood pressure and high blood cholesterol levels. He takes medication for both conditions.

THINKING

1. *Theoretical Knowledge (Factual Information):*
   a. What are the common physical and emotional manifestations occurring with perimenopause?
2. *Critical Thinking (Analyzing Alternatives, Deciding What to Do):*
   a. How would you respond to Debra when she asks for information and support regarding her husband's erectile dysfunction?
   b. Debra asks you if her desire for sexual intimacy will continue to decline after she goes through "the change of life." Describe in detail what you would tell her.

DOING

3. *Practical Knowledge:*
   a. What general topics would you explore with Debra to assess her sexual history?
   b. What questions would you ask Roberto to assess his sexual history?

(continued on next page)

CARING

4. *Self-Knowledge:* What might you be feeling if you were in Debra's situation?
5. *Ethical Knowledge:* What are one or two things you would do to help Debra and Roberto feel cared for and cared about?

 Go To Chapter 34, **Clinical Reasoning: Applying the Full-Spectrum Nursing Model Response Sheet,** on Davis*Plus.*

 To explore learning resources for this chapter,

 Go to Davis*Plus* at http://davisplus.fadavis.com/, **keyword Treas**

Chapter Resources for Chapter 34:
 Knowledge Check and Think Like a Nurse Response Sheets
 Knowledge Check Answers
 Resources for Caregivers and Health Professionals
 Reading More About Sexual Health (suggested readings)
 What Are the Main Points in This Chapter?
NCLEX-Style Review Questions
Chapter Overview Podcasts

Concept Map

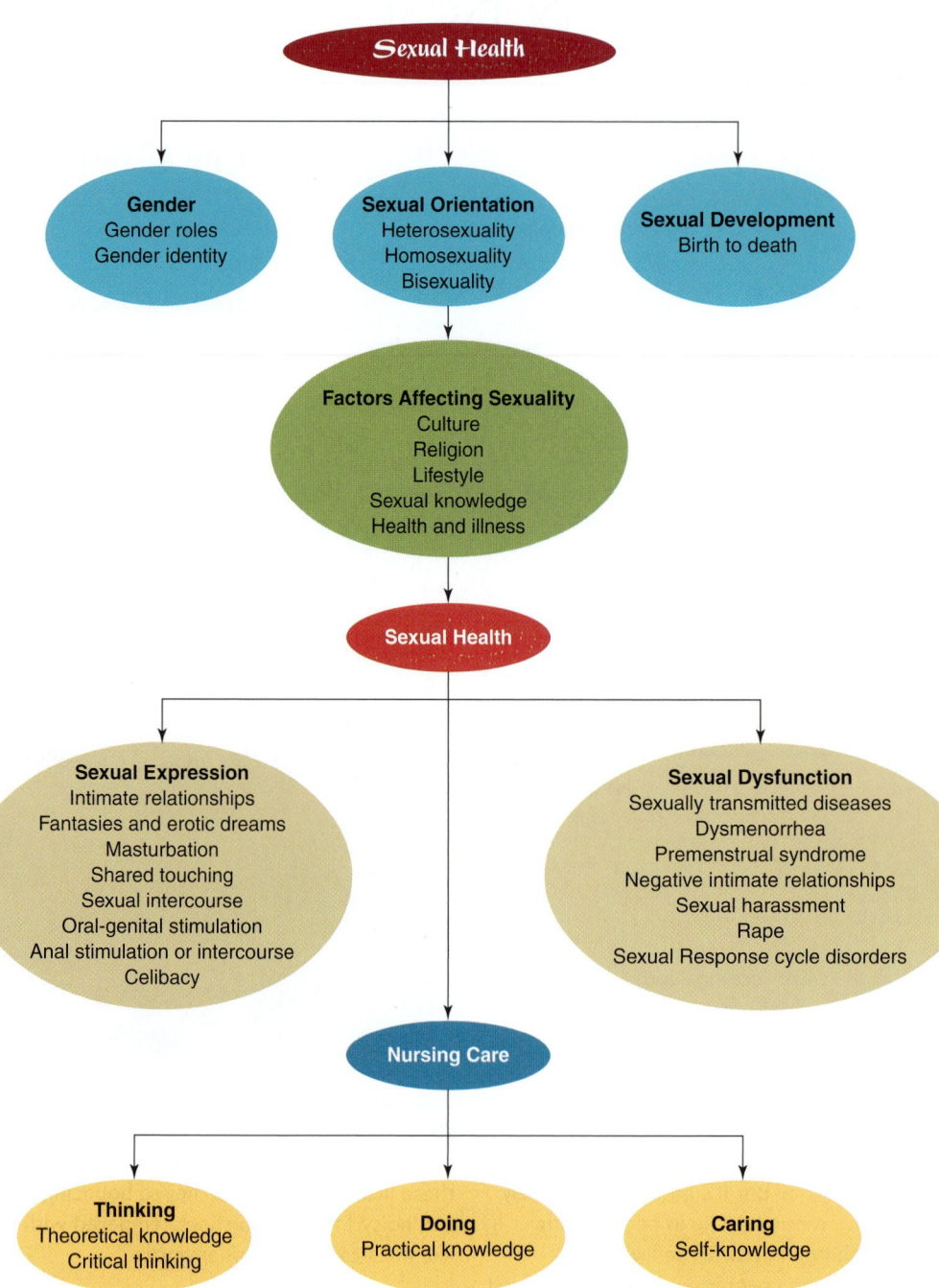

Sexual Health

Gender
Gender roles
Gender identity

Sexual Orientation
Heterosexuality
Homosexuality
Bisexuality

Sexual Development
Birth to death

Factors Affecting Sexuality
Culture
Religion
Lifestyle
Sexual knowledge
Health and illness

Sexual Health

Sexual Expression
Intimate relationships
Fantasies and erotic dreams
Masturbation
Shared touching
Sexual intercourse
Oral-genital stimulation
Anal stimulation or intercourse
Celibacy

Sexual Dysfunction
Sexually transmitted diseases
Dysmenorrhea
Premenstrual syndrome
Negative intimate relationships
Sexual harassment
Rape
Sexual Response cycle disorders

Nursing Care

Thinking
Theoretical knowledge
Critical thinking

Doing
Practical knowledge

Caring
Self-knowledge

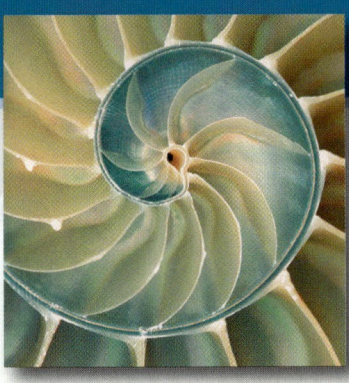

Sleep & Rest

Learning Outcomes

After completing this chapter, you should be able to:

➤ Explain why rest and sleep are important.

➤ Describe the functions and physiology of sleep.

➤ Explain circadian rhythms and how they relate to sleep.

➤ Identify factors that influence rest and sleep.

➤ Describe nursing implications for age-related differences in the sleep cycle.

➤ Identify at least five common sleep disorders.

➤ Perform a comprehensive sleep assessment using appropriate interview questions, a sleep diary, and a sleep history.

➤ Formulate nursing diagnoses that identify sleep problems that may be treated through specific nursing interventions.

➤ Plan, implement, and evaluate nursing care related to specific nursing diagnoses addressing sleep problems.

Key Concepts

Sleep

Rest

Related Concepts

See the Concept Map at the end of this chapter.

Caring for the Nguyens

This feature allows you to practice the kind of thinking you will use as a full-spectrum nurse. There is usually more than one correct answer to a critical thinking question, so we do not provide answers for these features. It is more important to develop your nursing judgment than to "cover content." Discuss the questions with your peers. If you are still unsure, consult your instructor.

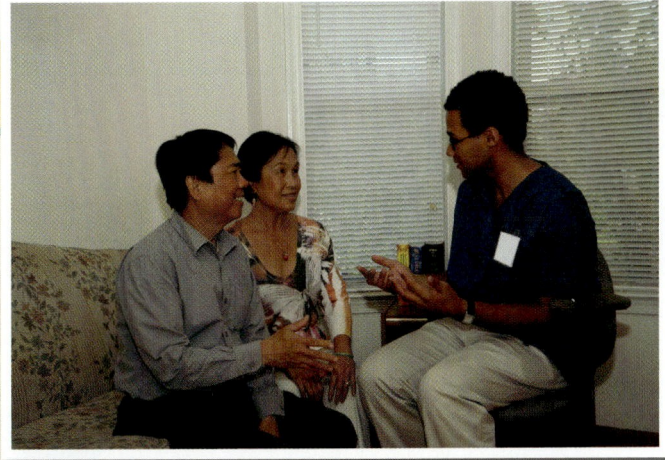

Yen Nguyen arrives at the clinic accompanied by her husband, Nam. She appears very tired. Nam tells you that she has been sleeping poorly. "She worries so much. She worries about Kim, our grandchild. She worries about our kids. Now she's worried about my mother. When we were going through that mammogram scare, she was even worse!"

Mrs. Nguyen shrugs her shoulders. "I can't help it. I'm like that. I've always been a worrier. But it's gotten worse lately. Now I worry and get so emotional. I lie in bed thinking about all this stuff and end up in tears. Then, when I finally get to sleep, I wake up covered with sweat. I've tried

extra soy for hot flashes, melatonin from the health food store, herbal tea, and even Benadryl—but nothing seems to work. I'm so tired. But when I get up, I have to deal with all these little kids at work. They're bouncing all over the place and noisy. I just get so short-tempered with them. That's not like me. I can't take this anymore."

Caring for the Nguyens (continued)

A. *Patient data:* Clearly Mrs. Nguyen has a sleep problem. Underline the data that are defining characteristics (symptoms) of a sleep problem.

B. *Patient data:* Which data suggest ideas about the etiologies (causes) of Mrs. Nguyen's sleep problem?

C. *Nursing diagnosis:* Two NANDA-I sleep-related nursing diagnoses are Sleep Deprivation and Disturbed Sleep Pattern. You have already identified the patient's defining characteristics. Now, what *knowledge* do you need to decide which of these NANDA-I labels to use?

D. How could you obtain this knowledge?

E. Sleep Deprivation is defined as "prolonged periods of time without sleep" and Disturbed Sleep Pattern is defined as "time-limited disruption of sleep." Can you make the diagnoses on the basis of this knowledge? Why or why not?

F. Following are some of the defining characteristics for these two nursing diagnoses. Certainly there is some overlap between the two sets of symptoms. Nevertheless, which set seems to be a better fit for Mrs. Nguyen? Why?

G. Write a nursing diagnosis for Mrs. Nguyen.

Disturbed Sleep Pattern	**Sleep Deprivation**
Verbal complaints of not feeling well rested	Daytime drowsiness
Dissatisfaction with sleep	Decreased ability to function
Change in normal sleep pattern	Agitation
Decreased ability to function	Irritability
Reports being awakened	Hallucinations
Reports no difficulty falling asleep	Anxiety
	Inability to concentrate
	Apathy
	Slowed reactions
	Combativeness
	Fatigue
	Fleeting nystagmus
	Hand tremors
	Heightened sensitivity to pain
	Lethargy, listlessness, malaise
	Perceptual disorders (e.g., disturbed body sensation, delusions, feeling afloat)
	Restlessness
	Transient paranoia

 Go to **Caring for the Nguyens Response Sheet** on Davis*Plus*.

Meet Your Patient

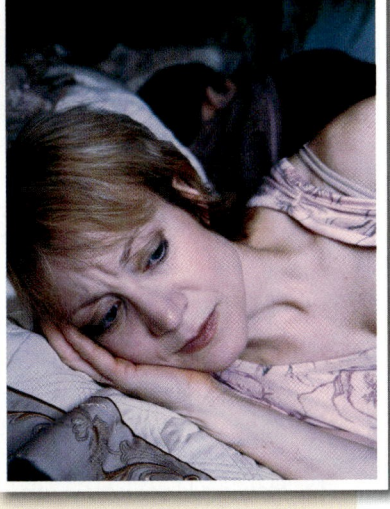

You are a nurse working on a surgical unit. Today you are meeting with Anne for preoperative teaching. She is scheduled for a complete hysterectomy next Monday. She has a secondary diagnosis of fibromyalgia, a chronic disorder characterized by widespread muscle pain and nonrestorative sleep.

Anne is a 49-year-old married woman with three children. She works full time and manages the family with her husband. She says, "I'm a little nervous about the surgery, but I know I need it. But I haven't been sleeping well because of thinking about it." Anne tells you that she has actually had trouble sleeping for the past 20 years. "I take an Ambien pill, 10 mg, every night to help me sleep. Will I be able to get that in the hospital? I really can't sleep at all without it," explains Anne.

As you continue the interview, Anne explains that she suffered from physical and emotional abuse as a young woman and has had sleep problems ever since. She has been to counseling, but that did not improve her sleep. Recently her sleep has been even more troublesome. Aside from her upcoming surgery, she has been coping with the recent death of her father. After meeting with Anne, you realize that sleep-promoting measures will be an important part of her nursing care while she is in the hospital.

What clues in Anne's situation would cause you to suspect that she will have difficulty sleeping while in the hospital? What characteristics of the hospital environment might interfere with Anne's sleep? You may not have enough theoretical knowledge and experience to feel confident about your answers to these questions, but use your present knowledge base and your life experiences to think about them.

Theoretical Knowledge
knowing **why**

Have you felt tired after waking up from a night's sleep? Have you ever been tired, but not sleepy, and, after relaxing a while, felt your normal energy return? How do you think sleep and rest are different? How are they alike? This chapter will help you to make those distinctions.

ABOUT THE KEY CONCEPTS

In this chapter we will examine the concepts of rest and sleep, along with related concepts (e.g., stages of sleep, sleep disorders).

Rest is a condition in which the body is inactive or engaging in mild activity, after which the person feels refreshed. A person at rest is calm, at ease, relaxed, and free of anxiety and stress (Fig. 35-1). People rest by doing things that they find calming and relaxing (e.g., reading, listening to music, surfing the Internet, doing needlework, praying or meditating, gardening, playing golf).

Sleep is a cyclically occurring state of decreased motor activity and perception (Germann & Stanfield, 2008) (Fig. 35-2). Body functions slow, and metabolism falls by 20% to 30%, so the body conserves energy. Sleep is characterized by altered consciousness: A sleeping person is unaware of the environment and responds selectively to external stimuli. For example, an alarm clock, bright light, or other meaningful stimuli usually awaken a sleeper, but everyday background noises and soft light do not.

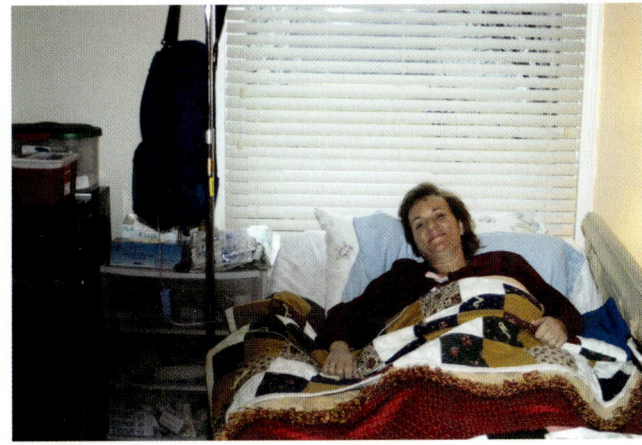

FIGURE 35-1 Woman receiving hospice care resting comfortably.

Although necessary and beneficial, rest without sleep is inadequate. At rest, the body is disturbed by all exterior stimuli, whereas in sleep it is screened from them by altered consciousness. Thus, sleep restores the body; rest alone cannot do this.

WHY DO WE NEED TO SLEEP?

We spend more time sleeping than in any other single activity: about 8 hours a day, or 2,688 hours a year—nearly one-third of our lives! So why is sleep so important? Before you try to answer, think back to the last time you slept poorly. Remember

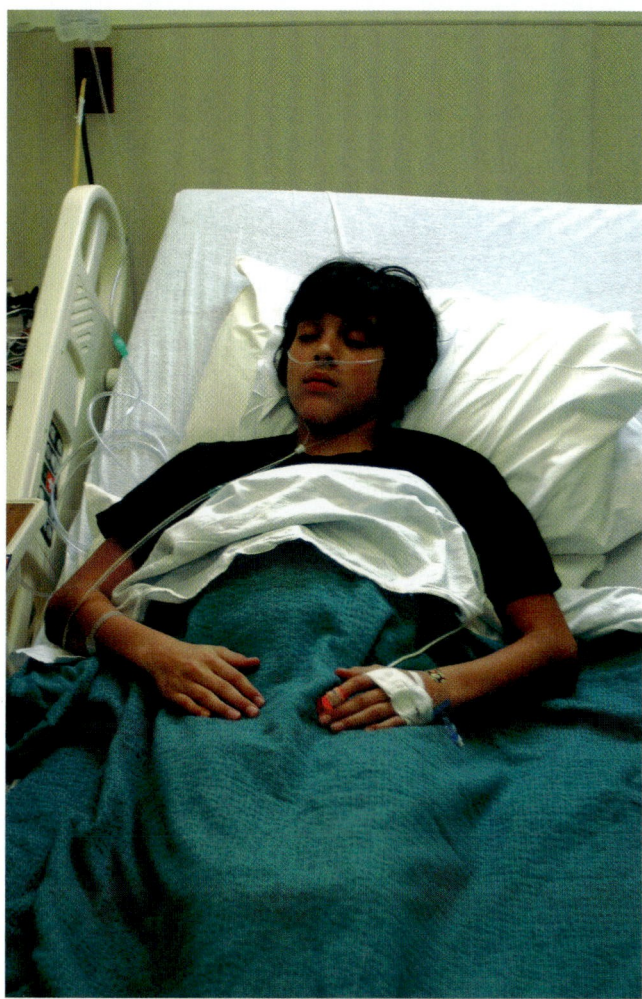

FIGURE 35-2 Boy sleeping in hospital setting.

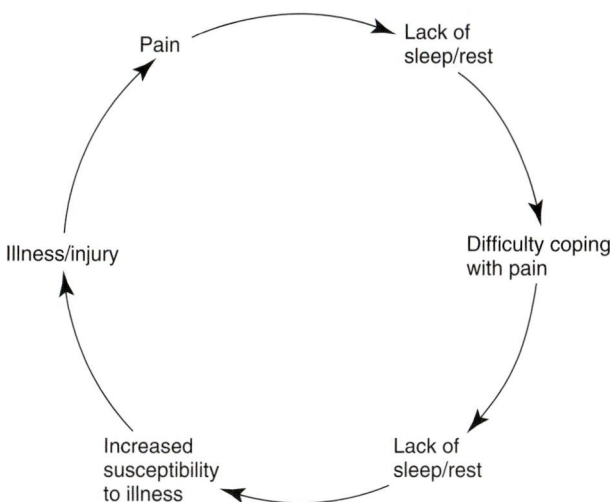

FIGURE 35-3 Relationship between sleep/rest and illness. Lack of sleep and rest increases susceptibility to illness. Likewise, the pain and stress of illness disturb sleep.

People who are ill or injured need more sleep than usual to restore energy needed for tissue repair and healing. However, they often have difficulty resting because of pain and other symptoms of their illness.

For further discussion of sleep theories,

 Go to Chapter 35, **Supplemental Materials: Theories of Sleep,** on Davis*Plus*.

KnowledgeCheck 35-1

- Compare and contrast sleep and rest. How are they different? Alike?
- Why is promoting sleep an important nursing intervention?

ThinkLike a Nurse 35-1

What effect do you think surgery will have on your patient's sleep? Why?

HOW MUCH SLEEP DO WE NEED?

Sleep needs vary widely among individuals. Even though the accepted standard has been 8 hours per night for adults, there is really no universal amount or pattern of sleep that is best suited for all people. Nevertheless, different sleep patterns are characteristic of different age groups.

Infants and Children. Infants have an overall greater total sleep time than any other age group. Newborns sleep as much as 16 to 20 hours a day, in periods ranging from one to several hours. Sleep time gradually decreases over the next few months, but throughout the first year of life, a minimum of 14 hours of sleep per day is recommended (Tuller, 2004). Most infants sleep several hours during one overnight period, with a morning and afternoon nap each day.

Adults. After the first year of life, sleep duration gradually lessens (Table 35-1). In most adults, sleep of 7 to 8 hours is fully restorative; however, there are wide individual variations. In some cultures, total sleep time is divided into an overnight sleep period and a mid afternoon nap.

Older Adults. Older adults spend significantly less time sleeping but need more rest than younger adults. Usually older

the mental fogginess, the physical fatigue, the feeling of slight nausea? Poor quality or insufficient length of sleep for even one night can reduce mental performance, and long periods of sleep deprivation can result in stress-related illnesses and injuries (e.g., from an automobile accident). Sleep and rest are essential for physical, mental, and spiritual well-being.

Theorists do not agree on all of the functions of sleep, but studies have shown that adequate sleep restores energy. Despite the fact that some regions of the brain are more active during sleep than when we are awake, total energy output is reduced during sleep, giving the body time for restoration and repair. Research also indicates that sleep strengthens the immune system (Cohen, Doyle, Alper, et al., 2009; Ranjbaran, Keefer, Stepanski, et al., 2007) and helps the body to fight infection. Sleep may also improve learning and adaptation, giving the person a chance to mentally repeat and rehearse facts and situations before they are encountered in wakeful life. Some evidence suggests that sleep and dreaming may facilitate long-term memory (Germann & Stanfield, 2008), perhaps by assisting the brain in reorganizing and storing information. Sleep also appears to reduce stress and anxiety, improving our ability to cope and concentrate on activities of daily living.

Sleep/rest and illness are interrelated (Fig. 35-3). Illness and injury increase the need to sleep and at the same time make it difficult to sleep. In turn, lack of sleep increases the susceptibility to illness by compromising the immune system.

Table 35-1 ➤ Average Sleep Requirements

AGE GROUP	HOURS PER DAY
Newborns (birth–4 wk)	16–20
Infants (4 wk–1 yr)	14–16
Toddlers (1–3 yr)	12–14
Preschoolers (3–6 yr)	11–13
Middle and late childhood (6–12 yr)	10–11
Adolescents (12–18 yr)	8–9
Young adults (18–40 yr)	7–8
Middle-aged adults (40–65 yr)	7
Older adults (65 years and older)	5–7

adults rest or nap during the day, go to bed early, and get up early. They take longer to fall asleep, and their arousal periods during sleep are longer and more frequent. Frequent waking is commonly due to physical discomfort, anxiety, and nocturia (Polan & Taylor, 2007). If sleep is interrupted, the person needs to sleep longer to feel restored. If the older adult does not increase the total time in bed, she may experience fatigue, irritability, and impaired cognition.

ThinkLike a Nurse 35-2

- How much sleep might you expect your patient, Anne (Meet Your Patient), to need in a normal night?
- How will a good night of sleep benefit Anne while she is in the hospital?
- If you were preparing for an important test, would it be better to stay up all night studying, or should you try to get a good night of sleep?
- How many hours of sleep do *you* need to feel rested and function well the next day? Compare notes with family members, friends, and classmates. Do they all need the same amount of sleep as you?

PHYSIOLOGY OF SLEEP

The environment plays a role in the physiology of sleep, so we begin with an exploration of circadian rhythms, by which the body maintains synchrony with nature. **Synchrony** occurs when things happen at the same time, or work or develop on the same time scale as something else.

How Do Circadian Rhythms Influence Sleep?

Biorhythms are "biological clocks" that are controlled within the body and synchronized with environmental factors (e.g., gravity, electromagnetic forces, light, darkness). Biorhythms influence many physical and mental functions. For example, body temperature is typically lowest when the person wakes up in the morning. As another example, female menstruation follows an approximately 28-day cycle, like the lunar cycle on which our calendar months are based.

A **circadian rhythm** is a biorhythm based on the day–night pattern in a 24-hour cycle. The term comes from the Latin words *circa,* meaning "about" and *dies,* meaning "day"—once

a day. Circadian rhythm is regulated by a cluster of cells in the hypothalamus of the brainstem that respond to changing levels of light. Circadian rhythm affects our overall level of functioning; most people have a higher energy level in the daytime and less energy at night. However, some people are more alert and active in the morning, whereas others function at a higher level in the afternoon or evening.

Do you feel sleepy at about the same time each night? Do you often awaken before the alarm clock goes off? If so, that's because the timing of sleep and waking is also influenced by your circadian biorhythm. Sleep quality is best when the time at which you go to sleep and wake up is in synchrony with your circadian rhythm. For this reason, people who work evening and night shifts (e.g., healthcare workers, police officers) can suffer significant sleep deprivation until their bodies adjust to the new pattern. Changing time zones can also disrupt sleep–wake cycles and can thus be troublesome for people who travel frequently. Hospitalization can also interfere with a patient's circadian rhythm. Noises, lights, waking the patient for vital signs or medications, altered normal bedtime rituals, absence or presence of family members, recent losses, or fear of the unknown may compromise the patient's quality of sleep and the ability to fall and stay asleep.

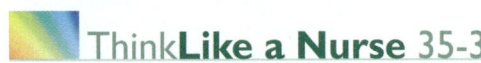
ThinkLike a Nurse 35-3

What may upset your patient, Anne's (Meet Your Patient), circadian rhythm?

How Is Sleep Regulated?

The mechanisms of sleep are complex and poorly understood, but we know that sleep is controlled by centers in the lower part of the brain, which produce sleep by actively inhibiting wakefulness. As just noted, a major factor in regulating sleep is the amount of light received through the eyes. The increasing light of a dawning sky signals the hypothalamus (Fig. 35-4) to

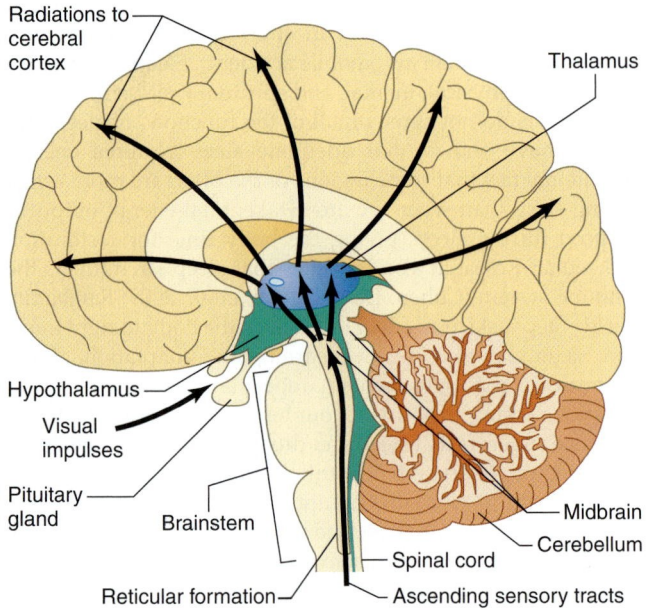

FIGURE 35-4 The reticular activating system works to regulate sleep and wakefulness.

induce gradual arousal from sleep. Another collection of nerve cell bodies within the brainstem, called the **reticular formation,** is responsible for maintaining wakefulness. The reticular formation is activated by stimuli from the cerebral cortex. Together, these reticular and cortical neurons are called the **reticular activating system (RAS).** Neurotransmitters associated with excitatory and inhibitory sleep mechanisms include catecholamines, acetylcholine, serotonin, histamine, and prostaglandins. L-Tryptophan and adenosine promote feelings of sleepiness.

An **electroencephalogram (EEG)** is used to record the electrical activity of the neurons in the brain. Electrical impulses are transmitted from the brain through electrodes attached to the scalp. These impulses create five different wave patterns, or *brain waves*. Figure 35-5 shows examples of different types of brain waves during sleep:

- *Alpha waves* are high-frequency, medium-amplitude, irregular waves. These occur in the drowsy stage.
- *Beta waves* are high-frequency, low-amplitude irregular waves. These occur during periods of wakefulness.
- *Spindles* or *K-complexes* are peaked, irregular waveforms that occur in the earlier phases of NREM sleep.
- *Theta waves* are high-amplitude waves that are common in children but rare in adults. These occur with delta waves when transitioning to a deeper sleep stage.
- *Delta waves* are low-frequency, high-amplitude regular waves common in deep sleep.

The EEG of a waking person differs greatly from that of a sleeping person. In general, the greater the brain activity, the more rapid the brain waves will be on the EEG. While the person is awake, brain waves are very rapid, irregular, and low in amplitude, mostly alpha and beta waves. Many neurons are firing at different intervals, at different times, and with different strengths. When a person is relaxed without intense stimulation of the senses, the EEG records mostly alpha activity. During sleep, alpha waves disappear. They are replaced by slower, higher amplitude delta waves.

What Are the Stages of Sleep?

There are two distinct types of sleep:

- **NREM** (non–rapid eye movement) sleep is generally the restful phase of sleep where physiological function slow.
- In **REM** (rapid eye movement) sleep, the brain is highly active, with brain waves similar to those that occur when a person is awake and alert.

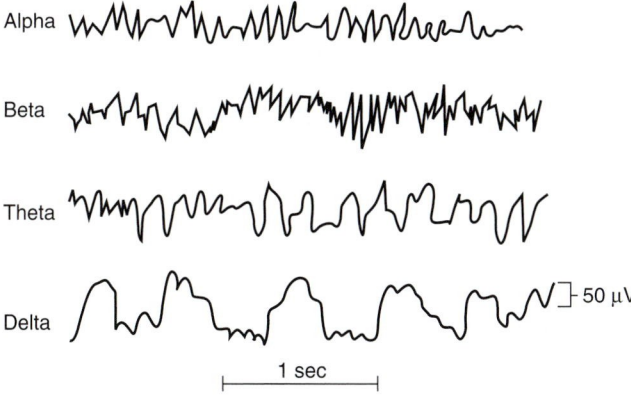

FIGURE 35-5 Four different types of brain waves.

The sleep cycle is typically 90 to 120 minutes. Cycling between REM and NREM sleep produces restorative rest. The American Association of Sleep Medicine (2007) identifies four stages of sleep (three NREM stages and the REM stage), based on brain activity and other physiological characteristics (Table 35-2).

NREM Sleep

NREM sleep is also called *slow-wave sleep (SWS)* because it is characterized by the presence of delta waves. NREM is divided into three stages, each deeper than the one preceding it. The parasympathetic branch of the autonomic nervous system becomes progressively more dominant during each stage of NREM sleep. During this phase, muscles relax, body temperature lowers, and heart rate, respirations, and blood pressure decrease.

REM Sleep

About 90 minutes after the onset of sleep and after the deep sleep of stage III, the brain becomes highly active; the brain waves resemble those of a person who is fully awake. This stage is called REM sleep because of the characteristic rapid eye movements, which can often be detected even though the sleeper's eyelids are closed. More spontaneous awakenings occur during this stage than any other.

REM sleep is essential for mental and emotional restoration. Loss of REM sleep impairs memory and learning. A person deprived of REM sleep for several nights will usually experience REM rebound. That is, the person will spend a greater amount of time in REM sleep on successive nights, keeping the total amount of REM sleep constant over time.

Sleep Cycles

Sleep is cyclic. The NREM/REM sleep cycle repeats four to six times throughout the night, depending on the total amount of time spent sleeping (Fig. 35-6). Each cycle lasts approximately 100 minutes. The first REM period may last only about 20 minutes, but with each cycle, the REM period lengthens until, in the last cycle of a typical 8-hour sleep period, REM may last as long as 60 minutes. The amount of time spent in each sleep stage varies over the life span.

KnowledgeCheck 35-2

- List the stages of sleep.
- Describe the progression of a typical sleep cycle for a young adult.
- Describe the physiological activity characteristic of each stage of sleep.
- What is the stage that must be "made up" if not enough time is spent in it?

ThinkLike a Nurse 35-4

- A physician has prescribed zolpidem (Ambien) for your patient, Anne (Meet Your Patient). This sedative/hypnotic (nonbarbiturate) is used as a short-term treatment for insomnia. Why do you think the doctor prescribed a sleeping medication even though she is physiologically and psychologically dependent on the medication?
- Anne will likely receive narcotic analgesics after surgery. How do you think they will affect her sleep?

Table 35-2 ➤ Characteristics of Stages of Sleep

STAGE	TYPICAL BRAIN WAVE TYPE	CHARACTERISTICS
W (Wakefulness)	Beta waves with some alpha waves	Ranges from full alertness to the early stages of drowsiness. Reading eye movements Eye blinks with eyes open or closed
NI (NREM)	Alpha waves with occasional low frequency theta waves	Transition between wakefulness and sleep Slow eye movements Light sleep; can be awakened easily Relaxed but aware of surroundings Groggy, heavy lidded Regular, deep breathing; eyelids open and close slowly. Accounts for about 5% of total sleep. Dreams are usually not remembered.
NII (NREM)	Theta waves, K-complexes and sleep spindles	Light sleep Easily roused Temperature, heart rate, and blood pressure decrease slightly. Accounts for about 50% of total sleep
NIII (NREM)	Delta waves; sawtooth waves	Deep sleep Difficult to rouse; if awakened in this stage, may be confused. Parasympathetic nervous system predominates: temperature, pulse, respirations, and blood pressure slow even more Skeletal muscles are very relaxed. Snoring may occur. Some dreaming may occur, but dreams are less vivid than those that occur in REM sleep. This sleep stage is especially important for restorative processes such as healing, growth, and tissue renewal. Makes up 20–25% of total sleep time.
REM	5–30 min (usually at least 20–30)	Highly active sleep with spontaneous awakenings Less restful than NREM sleep Eyes move rapidly and small muscles twitch. Essential for mental and emotional restoration Metabolism, temperature, pulse, and blood pressure increase. Pulse may be rapid and irregular. Apnea may occur. Gastric secretions increase. Deep-tendon reflexes are depressed. Dreaming occurs. If awakened, person will react normally. Accounts for about 25% of total sleep.

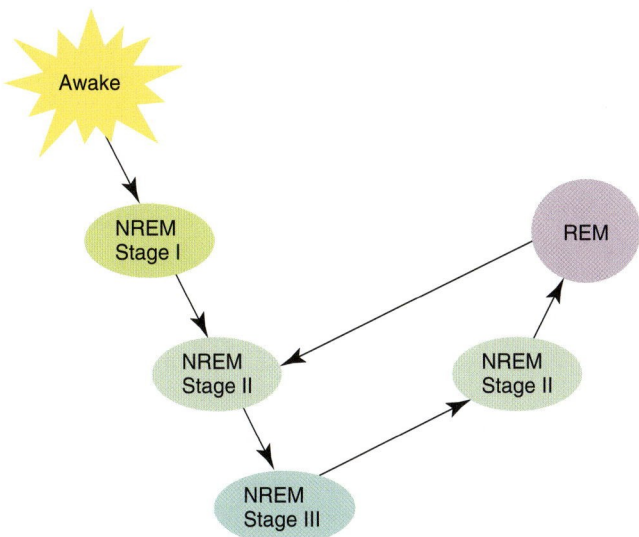

FIGURE 35-6 The normal adult sleep cycle. All but NREM stage I are repeated four or more times a night.

WHAT FACTORS AFFECT SLEEP?

People vary not only in the amount of sleep they need, but also in their sleep patterns. Some people are refreshed after napping for 15 or 20 minutes; others feel groggy after napping; others cannot nap at all. Many people routinely waken several times a night and do not report being tired, whereas others report fatigue and loss of mental clarity if their sleep is even minimally interrupted. In short, **sleep quality** has both subjective and objective components. It is related to (1) the total amount of sleep, (2) how well the person slept, and (3) whether the person obtained the needed amounts of NREM and REM. Several factors affect the amount and quality of sleep.

Age

Age is an important factor affecting the duration of sleep (see Table 35-1). But sleep *patterns* are also affected by age. For example, newborns and young children experience prolonged REM sleep periods; young adults spend about 25% of their sleep in REM sleep; and older adults typically enter REM sleep quicker and spend more time in this active phase of sleep.

Children and Adolescents

A survey by the National Sleep Foundation found that two out of three young children experience sleep-related problems a few times a week. The problems included trouble falling asleep, frequent awakenings, nightmares, and heavy snoring (Tuller, 2004). Environmental stimuli, such as the sounds and lights of older family members' activities, may make it difficult for a young child to sleep, or the child may have difficulty "winding down" after hectic activities in the late afternoon and early evening hours. Toddlers and preschoolers may be frightened to go to bed because of imaginary figures or intruders, or they may waken frequently at night because of bad dreams, the need to use the bathroom, illness, heavy snoring, tossing off the bedclothes, or falling out of bed. Some have difficulty self-calming

enough to achieve a restful state before falling asleep. Some school-age children may suffer significant sleep disturbances because of anxiety or depression. Others might have more temporary sleep difficulty related to isolated situations, stress, excitement, or social concerns, such as anticipating a school event or sports competition.

The growth spurt that occurs during adolescence increases the need for sleep (Polan & Taylor, 2007). At the same time, teenagers may not sleep well because of increased demands at school; staying up late to watch television, texting or other social networking, or study; dating or staying out late with friends; or the effect of alcohol or drugs. Some teens consume large amounts of caffeinated colas and other beverages that can delay or disturb sleep.

Young Adults

College students may pull "all-nighters" to cram for exams or experience insomnia because of worries about grades or future career choices. Young adults may drive themselves too hard to succeed, prompting late nights at work or sleep loss due to hectic travel schedules or work-related stress. Others might not obtain enough sleep because of social choices and personal entertainment choices during the night. Others might work the evening or night shift.

Parents of young children often sleep poorly. Breastfeeding mothers typically need to feed their infants one or more times each night until the infant begins solid foods. Parents of toddlers often wake to care for a child who is having a nightmare, is ill, or needs to use the bathroom. The National Sleep Foundation survey found that some parents lose as many as 200 hours of sleep a year because of their children's poor sleeping patterns (Tuller, 2004).

Middle-Aged and Older Adults

Middle-aged adults may experience insomnia for any number of transient reasons with stress or reaction to change being the most common. It might also occur because of the depression, anxiety, and tension that result from the stress of career demands, the need to care for a parent, loss of a loved one, marital discord, worry about teenaged children, or financial problems. The lack of sleep compounds the problem, leading to reduced ability to cope, and again to lack of sleep. Female hormonal fluctuations, particularly progesterone, can disrupt normal sleep patterns and play a role in insomnia during menstruation, pregnancy, or menopause.

Older adults are particularly at risk for insomnia. Many suffer sleep disturbances because of nocturia, the side effects of medications, discomfort or pain, or even a partner's sleep habits that includes snoring or restlessness. In addition, the levels of melatonin, the natural hormone that controls sleep, decline in the latter decades of life.

Lifestyle Factors

Lifestyle factors influencing sleep include work, exercise, nutrition, and use of alcohol, nicotine, caffeine, medications and drugs. As noted earlier, a person who changes work shifts frequently may find it difficult to sleep at the right time. Moreover, people who cross time zones frequently because of travel may experience difficulty falling asleep, early wakening, or daytime fatigue.

Exercise. If it occurs at least 2 hours before bedtime, exercise promotes sleep for most people. Fatigue from a normal physically active day is thought to promote a restful night's sleep. However, the more tired a person is, the shorter the first period of REM sleep.

Diet. Foods can either promote or interfere with sleep. A meal high in saturated fat near bedtime may interfere with sleep. Dietary L-tryptophan, an amino acid found in milk and cheese, may help to induce sleep, although some studies indicate that the protein in these foods actually increases alertness and concentration. Carbohydrates seem to promote relaxation through their effects on brain serotonin levels. In general, satiation induces sleep, whereas many people, especially infants and children, have difficulty falling asleep when they are hungry.

Nicotine and caffeine. Central nervous system stimulants, such as nicotine and caffeine, interfere with sleep. Smokers tend to have more difficulty falling asleep and are more easily roused than nonsmokers. People who stop smoking often experience temporary sleep disturbances during the withdrawal period. Caffeine blocks adenosine and thereby inhibits sleep. However, individuals vary greatly in their sensitivity to caffeine. Some people can consume caffeine throughout the day and evening and suffer no loss of sleep, whereas others cannot consume even small amounts early in the day without suffering insomnia later.

Alcohol. Consumption of alcohol, especially if heavy, may hasten the onset of sleep; however, it disrupts REM and slow wave sleep and may cause spontaneous awakenings with difficulty returning to sleep. In addition, heavy alcohol ingestion can prompt vivid dreams during REM sleep. Because alcohol is a diuretic, it can also interrupt sleep by inducing nocturia.

Medications. Medications can either promote or interfere with sleep. For those with insomnia, there are various types of drugs that may be used to help people fall asleep or stay asleep. Over-the-counter sleep aids are commonly used to induce drowsiness. Prescription medications to improve sleep are sedative hypnotics—either benzodiazepines or nonbenzodiazepines. These carry risk for dependency, tolerance, rebound insomnia, and withdrawal.

Amphetamines, tranquilizers, and antidepressants reduce the amount of REM sleep; barbiturates, in addition, interfere with NREM sleep. Opioids, such as morphine, suppress REM sleep and cause frequent awakening. Beta-blockers are reported to cause insomnia and nightmares.

Illness

Illness increases the need for sleep and rest. At the same time, its associated mental and physical distress can cause sleep problems. Fear of the unknown outcome of an illness and role changes associated with hospitalization can cause anxiety. Disease symptoms, such as fever, pain, nausea, and respiratory conditions (e.g., shortness of breath, dyspnea, sinus congestion), can also interfere with sleep. Specific disease conditions altering the quality of sleep are allergies, hyperthyroidism, and Parkinson's disease.

Anxiety increases gastric secretions, intestinal motility, heart rate, and respirations, all of which contribute to a restless night. Anxiety also stimulates the sympathetic nervous system, increasing the level of norepinephrine. This decreases stage III and REM sleep and leads to more awakenings. Depression may be associated either with almost constant sleeping or with insomnia.

Environmental Factors

Environmental factors can promote or inhibit sleep. Some people need a cool room, whereas others need warmth. Some prefer heavy blankets, and others like to sleep with just a light sheet. Noise can also inhibit sleep, but a person can become habituated to noise over time and be less affected by it. Some people routinely fall asleep to music or while listening to a radio or television. Often loud noises are needed to awaken a person in NREM stage III and REM sleep.

Any change in the usual environmental stimuli can affect sleep. For example, a patient used to falling asleep next to his wife may have trouble sleeping alone in a hospital bed. Equipment noise, the muffled sounds of a busy medical–surgical unit, or the labored breathing or snoring of a roommate also can interfere with the patient's ability to sleep.

When people who are accustomed to sleeping in a dark room are hospitalized, they may have trouble falling asleep because of light outside their window or filtering into the room from the hallway. However, light can be therapeutic for some patients suffering from sleep problems. Exposure to bright light can alter circadian rhythms in some adults. However, light therapy has not been shown to be effective in older adults with dementia living in skilled nursing facilities (Haesler, 2004).

KnowledgeCheck 35-3

- For each of the following patients, propose at least two factors that might affect sleep:
  A newborn in the neonatal intensive care unit (NICU)
  A preschooler being treated for pneumonia
  An adolescent with cancer
  A breastfeeding mother of a newborn
  An elderly man who has fractured his hip
- Identify at least three types of environmental stimuli that can disturb sleep.

WHAT ARE SOME COMMON SLEEP DISORDERS?

Sleep disorders are classified by their signs and symptoms. The more common disorders fall into two groups:

- **Dyssomnias**—Sleep disorders characterized by difficulty falling or staying asleep, early awakening, or excessive sleepiness. They include insomnia, sleep–wake schedule (circadian) disorders, sleep apnea, restless leg syndrome, hypersomnia, and narcolepsy.
- **Parasomnias**—Patterns of waking behavior that appear during sleep (e.g., sleepwalking)

Insomnia

Insomnia is the inability to fall asleep, remain asleep, or go back to sleep. Insomnia may be *transient/short term* (less than a month) or *chronic* (longer than a month). People with insomnia usually report an insufficient quantity and quality of sleep and wake without feeling refreshed, even though they are often observed to sleep more than they perceive that they do. Most people are distressed by the daytime consequences of insomnia, which include symptoms of excessive daytime sleepiness, poor concentration, fatigue, lethargy, and irritability.

Insomnia is the most common sleep disorder. Two out of three people say they have insomnia at least once a week (National Sleep Foundation [NSF], 2008). It is more prevalent in women and in adults older than 60 years. Recent evidence suggests a link between neuroendocrine activity insomnia and depression, linking abnormal hypothalamic–pituitary–adrenal gland activity with insomnia and mood disorders (Roth, Roehrs, & Pies, 2007). Insomnia may occur as a result of illness,

depression, anxiety disorders, acute stress, substance abuse, side effects of medications (e.g., steroids, central adrenergic blockers, bronchodilating agents), or inadequate sleep hygiene (e.g., watching television in bed, drinking caffeine-containing beverages before bedtime). It may also be the presenting symptom of other primary sleep disorders, such as restless leg syndrome.

Primary care providers can diagnose and manage most cases of insomnia. Once underlying medical or psychiatric conditions have been identified and treated, a combination of behavioral and pharmacological therapy may be effective. The use of medication to induce sleep is considered the last alternative because some types can become habit-forming, become less effective when taken continuously, and can have serious side effects. However, sedative–hypnotic treatment is justified in short-term insomnia to avoid the negative effects of insomnia on mood and performance. Short-term aggressive treatment may prevent the development of chronic insomnia.

Sleep–Wake Schedule (Circadian) Disorders

Abnormalities in sleep–wake schedules may be caused by rapid time-zone changes (jet lag), shift work, or a change in total sleep time from day to day. Symptoms include decreased vigilance, decreased ability to perform psychomotor tasks, and short sleep episodes *(microsleeps)* that the person is not aware of. People suffering jet lag need several days to adjust their sleep–wake schedule.

Restless Leg Syndrome (RLS)

Restless leg syndrome (RLS) is a disorder of the central nervous system characterized by an overwhelming urge to move the legs while resting or before sleep onset (National Sleep Foundation, n. d.; U.S. Department of Health and Human Services [USDHHS], National Institutes of Health [NIH], 2010). It tends to run in families. Children and young adults experience this condition, but it is especially common in older adults, and is sometimes associated with low levels of iron (Ball & Caivano, 2008; Hening, 2007; NSF, n.d.) and use of some antidepressants. Symptoms include unpleasant creeping, crawling, itching, or tingling sensations in the legs. Symptoms are relieved only by moving the legs, which prevents the person from relaxing and falling asleep. If RLS is severe, treatment may include neuroleptic agents and medication used to treat Parkinson's disease (Birath & Martin, 2008; NSF, n.d.). People with RLS should avoid stimulants (e.g., caffeine). Other self-care measures include walking, massaging, stretching, heat or cold compresses, medication, vibration, and acupressure.

Sleep Deprivation

Sleep Deprivation is a NANDA International (NANDA-I) nursing diagnosis. It is not actually a sleep disorder, but rather a result of prolonged sleep disturbances (e.g., insomnia and parasomnias). It can result from NREM or REM deprivation, or both. Signs and symptoms of sleep deprivation include daytime drowsiness, impaired cognitive functioning, restlessness, perceptual disorders, slowed reaction time, irritability, somatic (body) complaints (e.g., hand tremors), and a general feeling of malaise. Functional imaging studies contrasting sleep-deprived and well-rested brains reveals the importance of adequate sleep for memory and learning (Chee & Chuah, 2008). If sleep deprivation is severe and prolonged, delusions, paranoia, and other psychotic behavior may occur. Studies of sleep-deprived adults revealed changes in the levels of certain immunoglobulins and other markers of the immune system (Hui, Hua, Diandong, et al., 2007; Ranjbaran, Keefer, Stepanski, et al., 2007), which means going without sleep can weaken the body's protection against infection,

Illness and hospital care are common causes of sleep deprivation, especially for patients in critical care units (CCUs). In this environment, lights are on most of the time, and equipment noise, frequent treatments, and assessments all combine with the client's fragile physical condition to create

Toward Evidence-Based Practice

Kazuo. E., Pickering, T. J., Phil, D., et al. (2008). Short sleep duration as an independent predictor of cardiovascular events in Japanese patients with hypertension. *Archives of Internal Medicine.* **168,** 2225–2231.

Researchers found that short duration of sleep is a predictor of future cardiovascular events in patients with hypertension. Healthcare providers should ask patients with high blood pressure about how many uninterrupted hours of sleep they get.

Ong, J. C., Stepanski, E. J., & Gramling, S. E. (2009, February 15). Pain coping strategies for tension-type headache: Possible implications for insomnia. *Journal of Clinical Sleep Medicine,* **5(1),** 52–56.

Study participants reported sleep problems as a trigger of headaches, stress as a trigger of headache, and going to sleep as a strategy for dealing with pain. Study findings suggest too much or too little sleep can lead to headaches; and people with headaches often take naps to deal with

headache pain. Chronic insomnia can occur from napping during the day.

1. Sleep deprivation produces detrimental effects for many people, especially for those with high blood pressure and those experiencing stress. In what other ways do you think sleep deprivation creates problems for the physical body?

2. Considering the findings of the Kazuo, Pickering, Phil, et al., study, what else would you want to know about your patient with high blood pressure?

3. On one hand, sleep can be a way for people with headaches to deal with the pain. On the other hand, too much sleep, such as daytime naps, can wreak havoc on getting a good, restful sleep at night. How would you use the Ong, Stepanski, and Gramling study to guide patients who are dealing with the pain of a migraine?

 Go to Chapter 35, **Toward Evidence-Based Practice Suggested Responses,** on DavisPlus.

sleep deprivation. Likewise, healthcare providers who work long and late hours or rotating day–night shifts experience serious fatigue that can lead to medical error and patient injury or death (Lockley, Barger, Ayas, et al., 2007).

Hypersomnia

Hypersomnia is excessive sleeping, especially in the daytime. People with excessive daytime sleepiness doze, nap, or fall asleep at times and in situations when they need or wish to be awake and alert. The sleep disorders that commonly cause hypersomnia are obstructive sleep apnea and narcolepsy. Hypersomnia may also be caused by disorders of the central nervous system, kidney, or liver or by metabolic disorders (e.g., diabetic acidosis and hypothyroidism). It can also be a symptom of depression where the person is only interested in sleeping.

Sleep Apnea

Sleep apnea is a periodic interruption in breathing during sleep—an absence of air flow through the nose or mouth during sleep. Typically the soft tissue of the pharynx and soft palate collapse and obstruct the airway. Episodes may occur several or a hundred times a night and may last for as long as 1 minute or longer (American Sleep Apnea Association, 2008). During periods of apnea, the oxygen level in the blood drops, and the carbon dioxide level rises, causing the person to wake up. This may result in cardiac dysrhythmias (irregularities) and increases in pulse and blood pressure. Many people with sleep apnea complain of fatigue and morning headache; however, some may experience mild sleep apnea without any symptoms.

To diagnose sleep apnea, a sleep study consisting of an EEG, monitoring of arterial oxygen saturation, and an electrocardiogram (ECG) is recommended. Treatment depends on the type of apnea involved. Untreated sleep apnea is associated with polycythemia, hypertension, angina, coronary artery disease, right-sided heart failure, stroke, impotence, depression, personality changes, and mood swings.

The two main types of sleep apnea have different etiologies. **Mixed apnea** is a combination of the two main types. **Obstructive sleep apnea (OSA)** is caused by airway occlusion when the muscles of the upper airway and tongue relax and block the airway, stopping breathing. Sometimes rescue breathing is required to wake the sleeper. More often, people with OSA experience partial awakenings from sleep and resume breathing without realizing it. They typically snore, snort, grunt, or thrash about during sleep. Those with untreated OSA may feel sleepy or experience irritability during the day. They often have morning headaches or wake up with dry mouth or sore throat. Although most often males over age 40, particularly if overweight, are affected by sleep apnea, the condition occurs in females of any age and weight. Treatment of OSA might involve surgery to remove any obstruction within the airway or applying continuous positive airway pressure (CPAP) treatment. This is a device that delivers oxygen using forced air pressure and keeps the airways open when apnea occurs. Patients with OSA should avoid alcohol and smoking, lose excess weight, and maintain normal blood pressure (American Sleep Apnea Association, 2008; Marshall, Glazier, & Grunstein, 2008).

Central sleep apnea (CSA) is a complete suspension of breathing resulting from a dysfunction in central respiratory control. Only about 10% of sleep apnea is central in origin. People with CSA tend to awaken during sleep and, therefore, experience daytime sleepiness.

Snoring. Snoring is a hallmark sign of obstructive sleep apnea, but it does not necessarily indicate OSA. Even so, snoring can significantly reduce the quality of sleep for the bed partner. Snoring results when the muscles at the back of the mouth relax during sleep, obstruct the airway, and vibrate with each breath. Obstruction is usually more pronounced when the person sleeps on his back. Many treatments have been invented to open the air passages, such as nose tapes or even surgery. Saline sprays, nose drops, and cortisone sprays are also used—all with mixed success.

Narcolepsy

Narcolepsy is a chronic disorder caused by the brain's inability to regulate sleep–wake cycles normally. At various times the person with narcolepsy experiences a sudden, uncontrollable urge to sleep lasting from seconds to minutes, even though the person sleeps well at night. The person cannot avoid the sleep episodes but awakens easily. Narcolepsy is characterized by sleepiness, slurred speech, slackening of the facial muscles, a feeling of impending weakness of the knees, paralysis, and hallucinations. Performance is impaired during these micro-sleep episodes. Sleep episodes can come on suddenly, even while the person is having a conversation. If they occur while the person is driving, working, or even operating machinery, they can be dangerous. People with narcolepsy will awaken from episodes of unavoidable sleep feeling refreshed (National Institute of Neurological Disorders and Stroke [NINDS], 2009). Some have other symptoms, such as **cataplexy,** a sudden loss of muscle tone usually triggered by an emotional event (e.g., laughter, surprise, anger), but most only have hypersomnia.

Narcolepsy affects up to 1 in every 2,000 Americans, males about as often as females (NINDS, 2009). It is thought to be caused by a genetic defect of the central nervous system in which REM sleep cannot be controlled. Each micro-sleep episode begins in the REM stage instead of progressing through the NREM stages first. People with narcolepsy do not tolerate irregular sleep–wake patterns, such as shift work, and have difficulty staying awake with passive activity, such as watching television. The condition is controlled by central nervous system stimulants, such as methylphenidate (Ritalin), with little evidence of tolerance, dependence, or abuse.

Other individuals might suffer pseudo-narcolepsy, which is characterized by involuntary episodes of sleep but are related by acute or chronic sleep deprivation. In this case, when the person is well rested, the episodes resolve.

KnowledgeCheck 35-4

- What is the most common dyssomnia?
- What factors in the hospital may contribute to sleep deprivation in patients?
- What are the clinical signs of sleep deprivation?
- Why are sleeping pills not recommended for chronic insomnia?
- Why is snoring significant?

ThinkLike a Nurse 35-5

Compare and contrast insomnia and hypersomnia. How are they different? How are they alike?

Parasomnias

The parasomnias include sleepwalking, sleeptalking, bruxism, night terrors, REM sleep behavior disorders, and nocturnal enuresis.

Sleepwalking (somnambulism) occurs during stage III of NREM sleep, usually 1 to 2 hours after the person falls asleep. The sleeper leaves the bed and walks about, with little awareness of surroundings. He may perform what appear to be conscious motor activities (e.g., brush his teeth, make coffee), but he does not wake up. The person is not aware of sleepwalking and has no memory of the event on awakening. The event may last 3 to 4 minutes or longer. Children sleepwalk more than adults do. If the child does not outgrow the condition or serious safety risks exist, medication may be given to suppress the deepest stage III sleep. Stress, fatigue, and some drugs can trigger sleepwalking.

Sleeptalking occurs during NREM sleep, just before the REM stage. It does not usually interfere with the person's rest but may be disturbing to a bed partner.

Bruxism, grinding and clenching of the teeth, usually occurs during stage II NREM sleep. It can eventually erode tooth enamel and loosen the teeth. The noise can also disturb the bed partner's sleep.

Night terrors are sudden arousals in which the person (often a child) is physically active, often hallucinatory, and expresses a strong emotion such as terror. Children experiencing night terrors typically cry or scream in fear, thrash about, and resist all attempts by their parents or other caregivers to hold or console them. The child appears to be fully awake, but she is not; in fact, children in the midst of night terrors are extremely difficult to awaken. Episodes may last from 10 to 30 minutes. However, the child typically returns to sleep without awakening, and in the morning has no memory of the event (Cohen, 2004). Unlike *nightmares* (unpleasant, frightening dreams), which occur during REM sleep, night terrors occur during stage III (deep NREM) sleep.

REM sleep behavior disorders are associated with REM (or dreaming period) sleep, in which the sleeper violently acts out the dream. People have actually injured themselves or others without waking.

Nocturnal enuresis (bedwetting) is nighttime incontinence past the stage at which toilet training has been well established (Polan & Taylor, 2007). It has incorrectly been associated with dreaming; however, most incidents occur during NREM sleep, during the first third of the night when the child is difficult to rouse. It may be distressing to the child and family because of the importance society places on continence, the inconvenience of keeping bed linens clean, and the misconception that the child is bedwetting to act out against parents. Because the great majority of children outgrow enuresis, the best strategy is patience (McCance & Huether, 2005). If the problem persists, the child should have a full medical evaluation.

Secondary Sleep Disorders

Secondary sleep disorders occur when a disease causes alterations in sleep stages or in quantity and quality of sleep. The following are the most common causes:

- *Depression.* Depressed people may spend a great deal of time in bed. However, in general, they have difficulty falling asleep, experience less slow-wave (deep) sleep, spend less time in REM sleep, awaken early, and have less total sleep time.
- *Hyperthyroidism or hypothyroidism.* An increase in thyroid secretion causes an increase in stage III sleep; hypothyroidism causes a decrease in that stage. Hyperthyroidism increases metabolic rate, making it difficult for the person to fall asleep.

- *Pain.* Both acute and chronic pain interfere with sleep. Chronic pain affects both the quality and quantity of sleep. It inhibits sleep, increases arousals during sleep, and causes longer waking intervals during the night.
- *Airway passage obstruction or central nervous system (CNS) dysfunction, which cause sleep apnea.* These conditions were discussed under "Sleep Apnea."

Disorders That Are Provoked by Sleep

Sleep-provoked disorders are those that occur when signs and symptoms of the disease appear or become worse during sleep. Diseases affected by sleep include the following (McCance & Huether, 2005):

- *Coronary artery disease.* During REM sleep, dreams may increase heart rate and provoke angina and ECG changes.
- *Asthma.* People with asthma may experience bronchospasm during REM sleep. In adults, asthma attacks frequently occur during the night as the esophageal sphincter relaxes and reflux results. In children, they occur mostly during the final two-thirds of the night, when there is less stage III sleep.
- *Chronic obstructive pulmonary disease (COPD).* Persons with COPD experience lowered oxygen tension and increased carbon dioxide retention during sleep, especially during REM sleep, when neuromuscular control is normally depressed. This can result in pulmonary spasm and transient pulmonary hypertension.
- *Diabetes.* Blood glucose levels vary during sleep. When diabetes is uncontrolled, it may profoundly affect the blood sugar level during sleep, when the person is not alert enough to deal with it. Therefore, patients with uncontrolled diabetes may need to have blood glucose levels monitored during sleep.
- *Gastric and intestinal ulcers.* During REM sleep, people with duodenal ulcers secrete up to 20 times more gastric acid than do people who do not have duodenal ulcers. Peptic ulcers also contribute to increased acid, often producing nocturnal epigastric pain and sleep loss.

KnowledgeCheck 35-5

- List and define at least three parasomnias.
- Describe ways in which depression can affect sleep.
- List two sleep-provoked disorders, and explain how the sleep stage affects the disease.

PracticalKnowledge
knowing **how**

Because sleep enhances wellness and speeds recovery from illness, promoting sleep is an important independent nursing intervention. In this chapter, you will learn how to recognize signs of sleep disturbance, and factors that interfere with patients' sleep, as well as specific measures to facilitate sleep for each client.

▓ ASSESSMENT

It is important to assess usual sleep patterns and rituals for all patients who are being admitted to the hospital or seeking help for a sleep problem. A brief assessment for all patients should include questions about the following:

- Usual sleeping pattern
- Sleeping environment

- Bedtime routines/rituals
- Sleep aids
- Sleep changes or problems

If the person reports experiencing satisfactory sleep, that is an adequate assessment, and you merely need to support her usual sleep patterns and rituals. When you suspect a sleep problem, you will perform a more in-depth assessment, such as a detailed sleep history or sleep diary.

A **sleep history** includes in-depth questions about the person's usual times for sleep, any preparation, preferences and routines, quality of sleep, napping habits (if any), and whether she wakes early and cannot return to sleep. See the accompanying Focused Assessment box, Questions for a Sleep History.

A **sleep diary,** such as the one in the Focused Assessment box Sleep Diary, provides very specific information on your patient's patterns of sleep. This allows you to identify trends in sleep/wakefulness and associate behaviors interfering with sleep. You will usually tell the patient to keep the diary for 14 days; remind him that it is important to be diligent in maintaining it.

A **sleep study** is most useful in detecting sleep apnea and other sleep disorders, such as narcolepsy, night terrors, and periodic limb movement disorder. One of the most common sleep studies performed in a sleep lab is polysomnography, which records brain activity, eye movement, oxygen and carbon dioxide levels, vital signs, and body movements during the sleep phases.

Focused Assessment

Questions for a Sleep History

A brief assessment for all patients should include questions about the following:

Usual Sleeping Pattern

When do you go to sleep and wake up?
How many hours do you sleep?
Do you have a regular sleep schedule?
How would you rate the quality of your sleep on a scale of 1 to 10, with 10 meaning "great"?
Do you take a nap? If you do, for how long?
How often do you waken during sleep, for example, to go to the bathroom?
Do you feel adequately rested when you wake up?

Sleeping Environment

Would you like a night-light?
What room temperature do you prefer?
What noise level do you prefer (for example, radio, television, absolute quiet)?

Bedtime Routines/Rituals

What do you typically do in the hour before bedtime?
What do you do to help you fall asleep?

Sleep Aids

Do you need a special pillow or positioning aid?
Do you take any sleep medications or other drugs, natural sleep aids, or homeopathic remedies that may affect sleep?

Sleep Changes or Problems

Have your sleep patterns changed? If so, how?
How often do you experience difficulty falling asleep? Staying asleep?
Do you currently, or have you in the past, ever experienced a sleep disorder (e.g., narcolepsy, insomnia)?
Do you remember your dreams after you wake? Do you ever have night terrors? Do you sleepwalk?
Do you ever experience an unpleasant creeping feeling, crawling, or tingling, relieved only by moving the legs at night?
Do you snore? Does your own snoring or grunting ever wake you or anyone in the room?
Do you wear a cap at night? Do you require oxygen at night or any other medical aid or therapy while you sleep?
Do you grind your teeth while you sleep? Do you wear a dental appliance to prevent grinding?
Do you experience any kind of pain that makes it difficult for you to fall asleep or stay asleep?
Is there anything that I have not asked that might help you sleep while you are in the hospital (having surgery, receiving home care)?

If the client reports experiencing satisfactory sleep, that is an adequate assessment, and you merely need to support her usual sleep patterns and rituals. When you suspect a sleep problem, you will perform a more in-depth assessment, such as a detailed sleep history or sleep diary.

Focused Assessment

Sleep Diary

A sleep diary provides specific information on the patient's sleep–wakefulness patterns over a long period. The diary is usually kept for 14 days and may include the following:

1. Time you went to bed:_____
2. What did you eat or drink just before bedtime?

_____

3. What mental and physical activities did you engage in the 2 to 3 hours before bedtime? _____
4. Were you worried or anxious about anything when you went to bed? _____

5. Approximate time you fell asleep: _____
6. Times you woke during the night: _____
7. Times you fell back to sleep: _____
8. Time you woke up: _____
9. Sleep medications you have taken: _____
10. Any repeated doses? _____ Times: _____
11. Episodes of "disorientation": _____
12. Frequency of pain medication taken and times: _____
13. Did you feel refreshed in the morning? _____

ANALYSIS/NURSING DIAGNOSIS

It is important to determine whether lack of sleep is a problem, is a symptom of a problem, or is contributing to (etiology of) a different problem. For health promotion applications, use the NANDA-I diagnosis Readiness for Enhanced Sleep when a client has no particular sleep problem but wishes his sleep to improve in quality.

Sleep as the Problem

When you wish to focus on interventions to promote sleep, use the diagnoses Insomnia, Sleep Deprivation, or Disturbed Sleep Pattern on the problem side of the nursing diagnosis.

Use *Insomnia* for patients who have a disruption in the amount of quality of sleep to the extent that it impairs functioning.

Use *Sleep Deprivation* as the nursing diagnosis when the patient's amount, consistency, or quality of sleep is decreased over prolonged periods of time. Defining characteristics of Sleep Deprivation are more severe than those for Disturbed Sleep Pattern, so nursing activities may focus as much on relieving symptoms (e.g., confusion, paranoia) as on sleep promotion.

Use *Disturbed Sleep Pattern* as the diagnosis when assessment data points to a time-limited sleep problem due to external factors (e.g., inability to sleep in the unfamiliar hospital environment). The problem should be one that can be treated by nursing therapy. Add modifying words to specify the type of sleep problem, as in the examples. This will help you to focus goals appropriately.

- Disturbed Sleep Pattern (difficulty falling asleep) related to worries about family
- Disturbed Sleep Pattern (difficulty falling and remaining asleep) related to noise of hospital environment and need for scheduled treatments
- Disturbed Sleep Pattern (premature awakening) related to sleeping aid dependence and lack of knowledge of nonpharmacological aids for insomnia
- Disturbed Sleep Pattern (excessive daytime sleeping) related to effects of biological aging and depression
- Disturbed Sleep Pattern (altered sleep–wake patterns) related to frequent rotations of shift and overtime

Carefully describe the etiologies for sleep problems, because they determine your interventions.

ThinkLike a Nurse 35-6

In the following nursing diagnoses, how do you think your interventions would be different for each diagnosis?
  Disturbed Sleep Pattern related to:
- Changes in bedtime routines
- Exercising within 2 hours before sleep
- Drinking caffeinated beverages, eating chocolate, and drinking alcohol
- Emotional or physical pain
- Drug dependence or withdrawal
- Physical illness

Sleep Pattern as an Etiology

Disturbed Sleep Pattern and Sleep Deprivation affect many areas of functioning, so they often are the etiology of other nursing diagnoses, as in these examples:

- Risk for Injury or Falls r/t sleepwalking (or REM sleep behavior disorder or narcolepsy)
- Fatigue (or Activity Intolerance) r/t chronic insufficient quality or quantity of sleep (e.g., secondary to insomnia)

- Ineffective Coping r/t decreased cognitive functioning and awareness, secondary to lack of sleep
- Disturbed Thought Processes r/t decreased cognitive functioning, secondary to lack of sleep
- Anxiety (or Fear) r/t fear of death from sleep apnea

Sleep Pattern as a Symptom

Difficulty sleeping may be one of the symptoms of another problem. For example, a client may have Spiritual Distress related to challenges to belief system *as manifested by nightmares, sleep disturbances, and verbalization of inner conflict about beliefs.* In this instance, you would focus on interventions for Spiritual Distress, assuming that the sleep pattern would improve as the Spiritual Distress is resolved. Other nursing diagnoses that may cause sleep loss include Anxiety, Chronic Sorrow, Death Anxiety, Complicated Grieving, Diarrhea, Impaired Gas Exchange, Nausea, Pain, and Relocation Stress Syndrome.

KnowledgeCheck 35-6

- For a chronic, long-term sleep problem, would you use a diagnosis of Sleep Pattern Disturbance, Sleep Deprivation, or Readiness for Enhanced Sleep?
- Name at least two nursing diagnoses that might have a sleep problem as the etiology.
- Name at least one nursing diagnosis that might have a sleep problem as the defining characteristic.

PLANNING OUTCOMES/EVALUATION

NOC standardized outcomes linked to the NANDA sleep labels are as follows:
- For Disturbed Sleep Pattern: Rest, Sleep, and Personal Well-Being
- For Sleep Deprivation: Rest, Sleep, and Symptom Severity
- For Insomnia: Concentration, Endurance, Fatigue Level, Mood Equilibrium, Personal Health Status, Personal Well-Being, Quality of Life, Rest, and Sleep

When sleep disturbances are the etiology of another nursing diagnosis, you will need to use the NOC outcomes associated with that diagnosis. For example:

Nursing diagnosis: Anxiety related to Sleep Deprivation
NOC outcomes for Anxiety: Anxiety Control, Coping

Individualized goals/outcome statements you might use to evaluate the success of interventions to promote sleep include the following:
- Verbalizes feeling rested or feeling less fatigue.
- Falls asleep within 30 minutes; sleeps 6 hours without awakening.
- Maintains a sleep–wake pattern that provides sufficient energy for the day's tasks.
- Demonstrates self-care behaviors that provide a healthy balance between rest and activity.
- Identifies stress-relieving rituals that enable falling asleep more easily.
- Demonstrates decreased signs of sleep deprivation.
- Verbalizes feeling less fatigued and more in control of life activities.

For examples of Selected NOC Outcomes and NIC Interventions for Sleep Diagnoses,

 Go to Chapter 35, **Standardized Language: Selected NOC Outcomes and NIC Interventions for Sleep Diagnoses,** on Davis*Plus.*

PLANNING INTERVENTIONS/IMPLEMENTATION

NIC standardized interventions for Sleep Deprivation and Sleep Pattern Disturbance include the following: Coping Enhancement, Energy Management, Environmental Management: Comfort, Simple Relaxation Therapy, and Sleep Enhancement. Linkages have not yet been established for Insomnia.

Specific nursing activities for clients with sleep problems are described in the next sections. For a care plan for Sleep Pattern Disturbance,

 Go to Chapter 35, **Nursing Care Plan,** on Davis*Plus.*

Schedule Nursing Care to Avoid Interrupting Sleep

Use nursing judgment to decide when a procedure must be done and when it is more important for your patient to sleep. Healthcare routines usually allow time for rest periods. In addition, you may consider the following:

- Some patients need to rest after a procedure or after meals.
- If the person looks sleepy, give a prescribed sleeping pill early to avoid waking him later in the evening.
- You can often alter routines; for example, you can allow the patient to sleep as long as he can in the morning and bring his breakfast later.
- Cluster care to avoid unnecessary interruptions in sleep. Unless the patient is critically ill, do not wake him for morning vital signs if he is sleeping.
- Keep the noise level to a minimum. Be aware that activities, conversation, and equipment, even outside the patient's room, can disrupt sleep.

Create a Restful Environment

Many people find it difficult to sleep in a strange bed, even a comfortable one. Hospital beds are not noted for their luxury, but you can help make them more comfortable.

- Be sure the bed linens are tight on the bottom and loose on top to allow movement.
- Keep linens clean, dry, and free of irritants. Perspiration on the hospital gown or linens can lead to chill.
- Good body alignment also facilitates relaxation. Use extra pillows, a blanket from home, or any other item that may help the patient rest.
- Keep the room dark and quiet, unless the patient prefers a light.
- As much as possible, control the temperature of the room and provide good ventilation.

Promote Comfort

Pain, itching, and nausea may all be deterrents to rest and sleep in an ill person. Be sure to offer pain medications at their scheduled times, and before the patient's sleep time. Other comfort measures include providing a restful environment (see the preceding intervention) and offering fluids, cool cloths, or a massage or back rub. For detailed instructions for back massage, see Procedure 35-1 at the end of this chapter.

Support Bedtime Rituals and Routines

Most people have some kind of a routine before bed, be it reading, watching television, drinking warm milk, or praying or meditating, to allow them to prepare for sleep. For children, a favorite doll, blanket, bedtime story, as well as brushing their teeth and hair, may enhance sleepiness. Be sure to include any routines or rituals in the nursing plan of care to ensure continuity. Advise patients who smoke not to smoke after the evening meal.

Offer Appropriate Bedtime Snacks or Beverages

Complex carbohydrates (e.g., bread, cereal) seem to help most people sleep. A small amount of protein (e.g., milk, cheese) with the snack reduces the sugar boost and keeps blood glucose more stable. The dietary amino acid L-tryptophan promotes sleep. Advise the client to avoid alcohol, especially in the evening. Although it may induce sleepiness at first, alcohol interferes with the deep sleep cycle. The client should also avoid taking caffeine-containing foods and beverages (e.g., tea, coffee, chocolate, colas) after the evening meal. Advise the client to drink plenty of fluids during the day but to restrict fluids close to bedtime. Nicotine is a stimulant and should be avoided.

Promote Relaxation

You will base your choice of relaxation strategies on your repertoire of techniques and on patient preference. Relaxation strategies may include a massage, a warm bath, or one of the following:

- *Guided imagery* can be used to help your patient move in his mind to a safe place, where relaxation is possible. You may ask the patient what type of place will soothe him and "guide" him there through visualization. See Chapter 12 and

 Go to Chapter 12, **Tables, Boxes, Figures: ESG Box 12-2, Script for Visualization,** on Davis*Plus.*

- *Progressive muscle relaxation,* relaxing each muscle independently and progressing from head to toe, may help to promote sleep.
- *Music therapy* has been shown to be effective in promoting relaxation. Some patients respond well and can put away their troubles while listening to music, whereas others may find music irritating. Slow, quiet music or a recording of forest or ocean sounds may be soothing.

If you want more details about relaxation strategies,

 Go to Chapter 46, **Holistic Healing,** on Davis*Plus.*

Maintain Patient Safety

A person who sleepwalks needs protection from injury, because the risk of falling is great (e.g., stairs). Intravenous infusions, catheters, and nasogastric tubes can produce injury if they are pulled out of the body when the person gets out of bed. Guide sleepwalkers back to bed, and remember that they startle easily, so be gentle and quiet.

Teach About Sleep Hygiene

Most people with sleep problems manage them at home by creating a restful environment, relaxing, avoiding distractions, and trying various sleep strategies without using sleep-inducing medication. Refer to the Self-Care box Teaching Your Client About Sleep Hygiene.

Administer and Teach About Sleep Medications

When considering sleep medications, it is important for the patient to understand the options, be aware of potential side effects, and know what questions to ask. Some medications are

Teaching Your Client About Sleep Hygiene

➤ Follow a regular routine for bedtime and morning awakenings.

➤ Go to bed each night at the same time, even on days you are off work.

➤ If you cannot fall asleep in 30 minutes, get up and do something nonstimulating. When you feel sleepy, go back to bed.

➤ Use relaxation methods to promote sleep; read a book, pray, or meditate.

➤ Avoid going to bed angry.

➤ Don't depend on sleeping aids; be aware of the potential dangers of sleeping medications.

➤ Use your bedroom only for sleep; do not turn your bedroom into the family room.

➤ Avoid caffeine, alcohol, smoking, and heavy meals before going to sleep. Remember that beverages and foods, such as black tea, chocolate, and cola, contain caffeine. Alcohol interferes with the transition to deeper phases of sleep.

➤ Eat a small amount of carbohydrates (e.g., crackers, cereal, or bread) before bed; they aid in sleeping.

➤ Use aromatherapy to relax.

➤ If you take prescription drugs, ask your prescriber or pharmacist about the side effects.

➤ Use earplugs to block out noise.

➤ Walk or exercise in the early evening at least one hour before going to sleep; doing so will raise your body temperature and tire your muscles. Even 15 minutes a day of exercise will give your body the activity and oxygen it needs to help you relax more and sleep better.

➤ Take a warm bath just before going to sleep. This will raise your body temperature and relax you to help you fall asleep more easily.

➤ Avoid naps during the day, unless you are an older adult who takes short "power naps." Daytime napping can lead to nighttime insomnia.

➤ Don't try to "catch up" on sleep. Rise at your regular time, even if you went to bed later than usual.

➤ Try to keep your bedroom as dark as possible. An illuminated bedroom clock is a source of light that can be distracting when trying to fall asleep. Either replace the clock or block the light with something.

➤ Close your eyes and visualize something peaceful when trying to fall asleep. Imaging your favorite, relaxing place where you find comfort or familiarity can relax you and help you get to sleep.

➤ Try progressive relaxation to fall asleep. Follow recorded instructions directing you in a sequence of relaxing certain muscle groups.

habit forming; others may have unpleasant side effects. As a general rule, they are not recommended for long-term use. Others are considered safe and indicated for longer-term use. Some natural or homeopathic aids can lead to rest and sleep. The most common side effects of sleep medicines include dizziness, lightheadedness, daytime drowsiness, diarrhea, and difficulty with coordination.

Prescription Sleep Medications

You should be familiar with the various prescription and nonprescription sleep medications your patients may be taking.

Nonbenzodiazepines. This class of sedative/hypnotics have a short half-life, which means that they are eliminated from the body quickly and do not cause "hangover" (daytime sleepiness). They are also selective, which means they target specific receptors that are thought to be associated with sleep rather than depressing the entire central nervous system. Examples are zolpidem tartrate (Ambien), zaleplon (Sonata), and eszopicione (Lunesta). The newest type of sedative hypnotic, although not technically a nonbenzodiazepine, is ramelteon (Rozerem), is the first sleep drug not designated as a controlled-substance. It works by targeting melatonin receptors. General side effects of nonbenzodiazepine drugs include drowsiness, dizziness, fatigue, headache, and unpleasant taste. When patients first start taking prescription sleep aids, they should use caution during morning activities until they are sure how the drug affects them. Long-term effects of these medications are not yet known.

Benzodiazepines. This class of sedative/hypnotics includes both long-acting and short-acting drugs. Long-acting medications linger in the body and potentially cause daytime drowsiness. The risk for rebound insomnia and dependency and tolerance, especially in older adults, is greater with this class of sleep inducing drugs. They are potentially dangerous when combined with alcohol and some medications. Examples are diazepam (Valium), alprazolam (Xanax), flurazepam (Dalmane), lorazepam (Ativan), temazepam (Resoril), and triazolam (Halcion).

Barbiturates. These sedative/hypnotics and anticonvulsants are rarely prescribed for insomnia because of the risk of addiction, abuse, and overdose. Examples are amobarbital (Amytal), pentobarbital (Nembutal), and secobarbital (Seconal).

Tricyclic antidepressants. At times, primary care providers prescribe antidepressants to promote sleep. Although none of these medicines is specifically approved by the U.S. Food and Drug Administration (FDA) for this purpose they have shown clinical benefit for some people with insomnia. Examples are amitriptyline (Elavil), doxepin (Sinequan), imipramine (Tofranil), and nortriptyline (Aventyl, Pamelor). Elderly patients can be particularly at risk for daytime sleepiness and dizziness.

Nonprescription Sleep Medications

Nonprescription sleep medications usually contain an antihistamine, which may induce drowsiness that lasts into the next day. It is important to check the ingredient label of any over-the-counter (OTC) medication to see whether it contains an antihistamine, commonly diphenhydramine (Benadryl), to induce sleepiness. Advise clients that OTC sleep medications can interact with other medicines they may be taking, so they should consult their prescriber or pharmacist before using them. Other nonprescription sleep aids include the following:

- *Melatonin.* This is widely sold as a sleep aid but remains controversial in medical circles. Melatonin is a natural hormone produced by the pineal gland.
- *Herbal sleep aids.* Herbal remedies for sleep problems include chamomile tea, valerian root, hops, lavender, and

passionflower. The American Academy of Sleep Medicine states there is only limited scientific evidence to show herbal products are effective sleep aids. Patients should consult with their healthcare providers before using them as some of these products can interact with prescription medication.

KnowledgeCheck 35-7

- What is the classification of zolpidem (Ambien)? Why is it an especially desirable medication for sleep?
- What are two other classes of medications that are sometimes prescribed for sleep?
- Describe three independent nursing interventions to promote sleep.
- Why should people contact their prescriber before taking nonprescription sleep aids?

PUTTING IT ALL TOGETHER

Anne (Meet Your Patient) has arrived back on the surgical unit after her surgery. She has a urinary catheter, oxygen mask, IV line, and morphine by patient-controlled analgesia (PCA) for pain control. She is nauseated from the anesthesia and moaning in pain. Her husband, Eric, and their three children are there to greet her, and they are worried. Anne looks dreadful! "With all this equipment, and her moaning, is she going to be OK?" Eric asks. He tells you that Anne didn't sleep at all the night before surgery. "She was nervous and didn't want to take a sleeping pill because we were supposed to be at the hospital by 5:30 a.m.," he explains.

You perform an initial assessment. Anne's vital signs are as follows: BP, 118/74 mm Hg; pulse, 88 beats/min and regular; respirations, 26 breaths/min; and temperature, 99.48°F. Her lungs are clear, the dressing is dry and intact, and the urinary catheter shows a small amount of light yellow urine draining from the bladder. The oxygen mask is partially off. You check Anne's oxygen saturation. It is 99%. The notes from the operating and recovery rooms indicate that Anne has not received anything for pain in more than 90 minutes. The PCA is connected, but the pump supplies analgesia only when the patient triggers the device. Anne has been groggy and does not understand or remember that she must push the button to obtain pain medication. You trigger a bolus of morphine and show Anne and the family how the PCA works. You realize that she is sedated and may not remember what you have taught her, but Eric assures you that they will be staying for the day and will reinforce your instruction.

Several minutes later Anne is calm. Her respirations have slowed to 20 breaths/min, and she is lightly snoring. Eric sighs in relief. "I guess she'll sleep for a while now," he says. You explain that she will sleep with the pain medication, but it will not be as restful as good-quality sleep. "With the morphine she will wake frequently and not get much REM sleep—that's a type of sleep we all require for health," you explain.

You were able to gather data preoperatively from Anne about her sleep habits and routines. You are also aware that Anne has had chronic sleep problems. In the nursing care plan, you have written the diagnosis Disturbed Sleep Pattern related to pain, dependence on Ambien, anxiety and other stresses of surgery and the recent loss of father, and unfamiliar environment; and secondary to fibromyalgia. You tell Eric that you would like him to bring from home Anne's pillow, toothbrush, and face cream because she has indicated that these are all part of her usual bedtime ritual. When Eric volunteers that Anne sometimes listens to music before bedtime, you suggest that he also bring her favorite music.

At dinnertime, Eric and the kids go home and gather Anne's belongings. When they return, she is more alert and comfortable. She tells them she feels exhausted, but not in pain. When you make your rounds, you explain that you would like to keep her usual bedtime routine and that she will be getting Ambien this evening. She is visibly relieved by your comments.

This scenario demonstrates full-spectrum nursing and shows how a nurse can make a difference for patients and their families by recognizing the need for sleep and providing appropriate interventions.

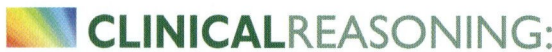

CLINICALREASONING:
Applying the **Full-Spectrum Nursing Model**

Because the following critical thinking activities allow you to practice the kind of thinking you will use as a full-spectrum nurse, they usually have no single right answer. Discuss them with your peers—if you have difficulty with any of the questions, consult your instructor.

PATIENT SITUATION

A 43-year-old healthy woman, Maria Lupe, is being seen for her annual women's health visit. She tells you she lies awake in bed for hours before falling asleep at night. Sometimes she falls asleep OK but will wake up and then have trouble going back to sleep. After feeling like she was awake nearly all night, Maria wakes in the morning feeling exhausted. She tells you she feels tired all the time and can't seem to get things done during her time off because of her fatigue. Maria admits to feeling irritable with her co-workers and children. Because of her lack of rest, she doesn't have the desire to do things socially anymore.

THINKING

1. *Theoretical Knowledge:* The NANDA-I definition and defining characteristics of Insomnia differ slightly from the medical diagnosis of insomnia.
   a. What is insomnia, as defined medically (e.g., by the National Sleep Foundation)?
   b. What other health conditions might a medical diagnosis of insomnia be confused with?
   c. What factors either lead to or aggravate insomnia, as described medically?

2. *Critical Thinking (Contextual Awareness):*
   a. Obviously Maria has trouble sleeping. Based on the data you have, do you consider her difficulty sleeping significant enough to require consultation with her primary healthcare provider? Explain your thinking.

DOING

3. *Nursing Process (Assessments):*
   a. When conducting a sleep history for Maria, what questions would you ask her in order to (1) describe more fully her sleeping problem and (2) identify the cause of her sleeping problem?
   b. What would you suggest Maria do to help you gain more information about her sleeping problem?
4. *Nursing Process (Nursing Diagnosis):* Based on the data in the Patient Situation, would you use a nursing diagnosis of Sleep Deprivation or Insomnia for Maria? Explain your thinking. Use a nursing diagnosis handbook, as needed, to compare the defining characteristics of the two diagnoses.
5. *Nursing Process (Interventions):* How might you help your patient manage her Insomnia other than using prescription medication? What might you suggest?

CARING

6. *Self-Knowledge:*
   a. Have you ever had trouble falling or staying asleep? How did you feel at the time and in the morning? Describe your experience.
   b. How might you provide better emotional care and support to your patient after recalling your own episodes of sleeping difficulty?

 Go To Chapter 35, **Clinical Reasoning: Applying the Full-Spectrum Nursing Model Response Sheet,** on Davis*Plus.*

 To explore learning resources for this chapter,

 Go to Davis*Plus* at http://davisplus.fadavis.com/, keyword Treas:

Chapter Resources for Chapter 35:
   Knowledge Check and Think Like a Nurse Response Sheets
   Knowledge Check Answers
   Resources for Caregivers and Health Professionals
   Reading More About Sleep and Rest (Suggested Readings)
   What Are the Main Points in This Chapter?
   NCLEX-Style Review Questions
Chapter Overview Podcasts

PracticalKnowledge
procedures

In the not-so-distant past, a relaxing back massage was a part of the evening care routine for every hospitalized patient. In this era of cost containment, this sleep enhancer has become a "nice but not essential" procedure in most agencies. Massage has therapeutic benefits, however. It promotes circulation, physical and emotional comfort, and sleep. Furthermore, it is an independent nursing activity for which you do not need a medical prescription (except in very rare circumstances). Try to offer a back rub whenever you can, and teach and encourage nursing assistive personnel (NAP) to do so as well. Refer to the following procedure.

Procedure 35–1 ■ Giving a Back Massage

➤ For steps to follow in *all* procedures, refer to the Universal Steps for All Procedures found on the page facing the inside back cover.

Equipment
Skin care lotion

Delegation
You can delegate back massage to the NAP if the patient's condition and the NAP's skills allow. However, giving the back

rub yourself provides an excellent opportunity to assess the patient, develop rapport, and provide emotional support.

Pre-Procedure Assessment
Check the skin for reddened areas or skin breakdown.

➤ When performing the procedure, always identify your patient according to agency policy and be attentive to standard precautions, hand hygiene, patient safety and privacy, body mechanics, and documentation.

Procedure Steps

1. **Warm the lotion** by placing the bottle in warm water.
   Cold lotion can cause muscle contraction; warming the lotion helps relax the muscles.
2. **Raise the bed to working height.**
   Prevents back strain of the nurse.
3. **Position the patient comfortably** on her side or prone.
   a. Untie the patient's gown, and expose her back.
   b. Raise the siderail on the opposite side of the bed.
      Siderails prevent the patient from falling off the bed when you turn her toward the side of the bed away from you.
   c. Wash the patient's back with warm water, if needed.
      Warm water will help relax the muscles while removing any sweat and soiling.
4. **Place lotion on your hands.**
   Placing the lotion directly on the back may cause the patient's muscles to tighten.
5. **Place your hands on either side** of the spine at the base of the neck.

Using gentle, continuous pressure, rub down the length and then up the sides of the back.
   a. Repeat this motion several times.
   b. Never rub directly over the spine.
      The spine is a vulnerable area. ▼

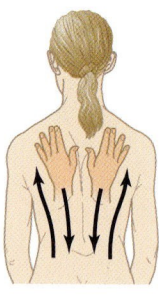

6. **Apply gentle thumb pressure** (using the fleshy part of your thumbs) on either side of the spine at the mid back, pushing outward for about 2.5 cm (1 in.).
   a. Repeat from the mid back to the base of the neck in a series of small, outward strokes.
      Strokes should be along the muscle length and not across the muscle to help stretch and relax it.

b. Ask the patient whether the amount of pressure is comfortable. Be careful not to cause the patient discomfort, which might cause further muscle tightness.
c. Always apply pressure away from the spine, not toward it.
   This gently stretches the muscles and helps prevent placing pressure on the spine.
d. If you are unable to massage both sides at the same time, work on one side and then the other.
   Work as symmetrically as possible to increase muscle relaxation. ▼

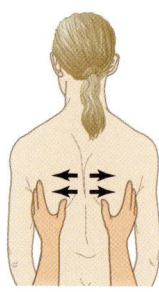

7. **Now go to the spots that felt** the tightest or that the patient states are

tight. Work in small circles, using gentle thumb pressure.

Small circular movements can help release muscle "knots" and relax tightened muscles. ▼

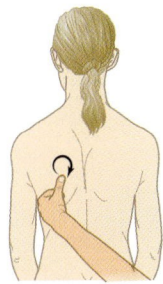

8. **Gently shake the scapulae.** Place your palm on one scapula, and gently shake it by quickly moving your palm back and forth. Repeat on the other side.

Movement of the scapula decreases when muscles tighten; gently vibrating the scapula helps loosen the muscles. ▼

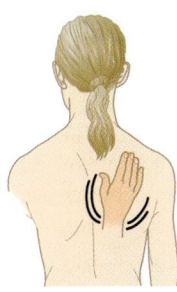

9. **Apply horizontal strokes** across the scapula, using your thumb.

Using horizontal strokes from near the spine across the bottom of the scapula, push out all the way across the scapula from the spine. Move up and repeat until you have covered the entire scapula and top of the shoulder. Repeat on the other side.

This movement helps loosen the trapezius muscle. ▼

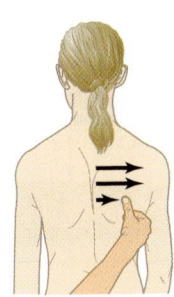

10. **If you find tender spots**, use the fleshy parts of your fingers in a small circular motion.

11. **Apply pressure in circles** using the heels of your hands down both sides of the spine. Beginning at the upper shoulder and working down to the lower back, apply pressure in medium-sized circles down the sides of the spine with the heels of your hands. Be cautious not to apply too much pressure. Assess patient for comfort.

The circular motion helps relax tightened areas in the paraspinal muscles. ▶

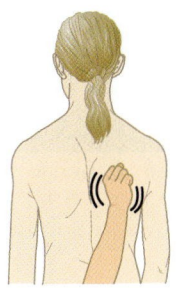

12. **Apply horizontal strokes** using the heels of your hands across the latissimus dorsi muscle. Using horizontal strokes from near the spine below the scapula, push out from the spine across to the ribs, and work down across the lower back with the heels of your hands.

This movement helps relax the latissimus dorsi muscle.

13. **Gently rub your hands up** either side of the spine from the base of the back to the base of the neck and then down the sides of the back. Repeat several times.

Long strokes help increase circulation and promote relaxation of the back muscles.

NOTE: If you are unable to do a complete back massage, ask the patient where she is most uncomfortable, and massage those areas. If the patient has general tightness, use the long strokes down each side of the spine and back up the sides.

Evaluation

Assess the patient's report of comfort, relaxation, and how soon she falls asleep.

Documentation

This is a routine aspect of care and is usually documented on a flow sheet.

Thinking About the Procedure

 Go to the *Fundamentals of Nursing Skills Videos,* **Hygiene: Back Massage.**

1. What does the nurse do between the bed bath and back massage?
2. What does the narrator say the benefit of the back rub is to this patient in bed?

 For suggested responses, go to Chapter 35, **Thinking About the Procedure Suggested Responses,** on DavisPlus.

Concept Map

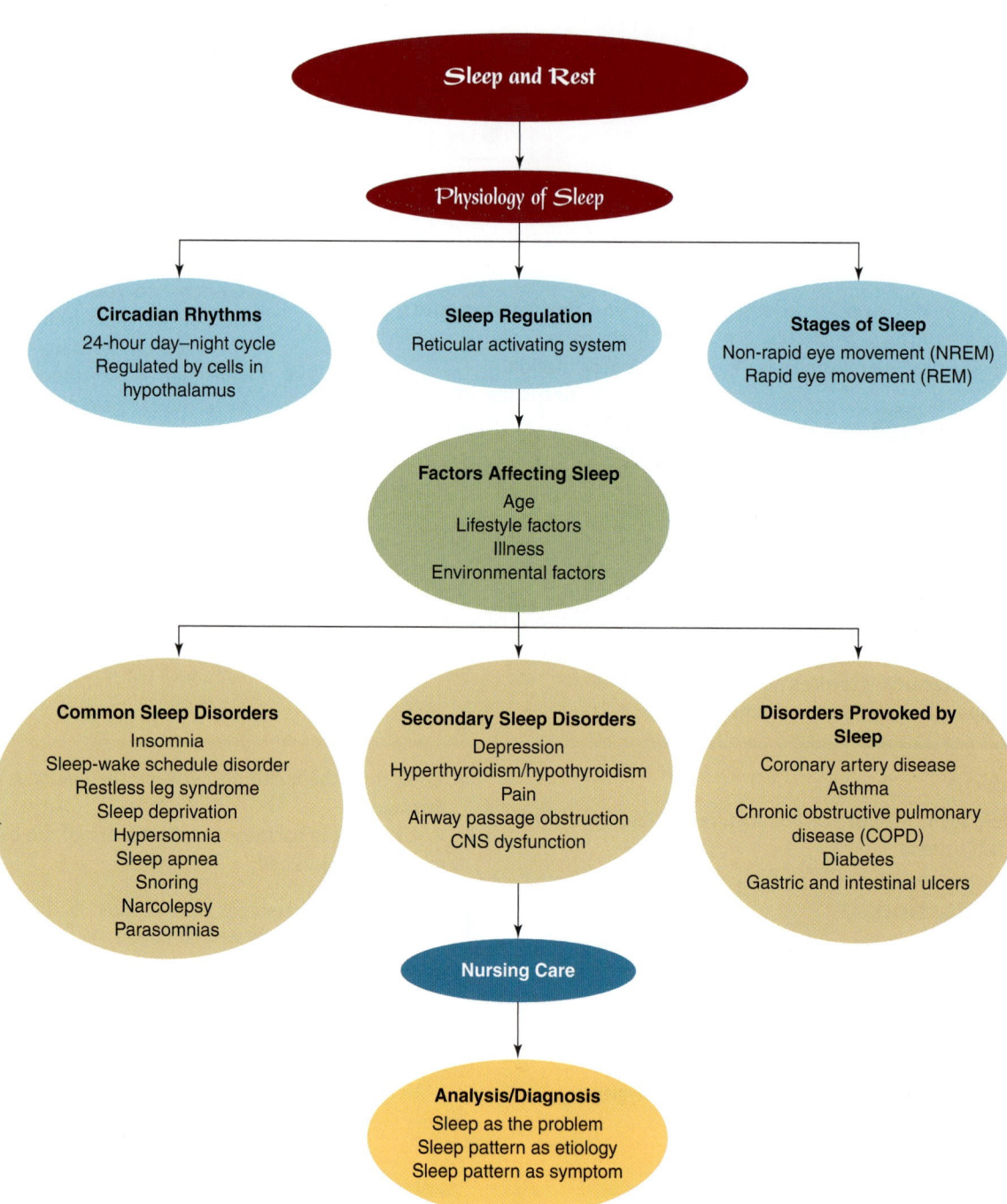

Sleep and Rest

Physiology of Sleep

Circadian Rhythms
24-hour day–night cycle
Regulated by cells in
hypothalamus

Sleep Regulation
Reticular activating system

Stages of Sleep
Non-rapid eye movement (NREM)
Rapid eye movement (REM)

Factors Affecting Sleep
Age
Lifestyle factors
Illness
Environmental factors

Common Sleep Disorders
Insomnia
Sleep-wake schedule disorder
Restless leg syndrome
Sleep deprivation
Hypersomnia
Sleep apnea
Snoring
Narcolepsy
Parasomnias

Secondary Sleep Disorders
Depression
Hyperthyroidism/hypothyroidism
Pain
Airway passage obstruction
CNS dysfunction

Disorders Provoked by Sleep
Coronary artery disease
Asthma
Chronic obstructive pulmonary
disease (COPD)
Diabetes
Gastric and intestinal ulcers

Nursing Care

Analysis/Diagnosis
Sleep as the problem
Sleep pattern as etiology
Sleep pattern as symptom

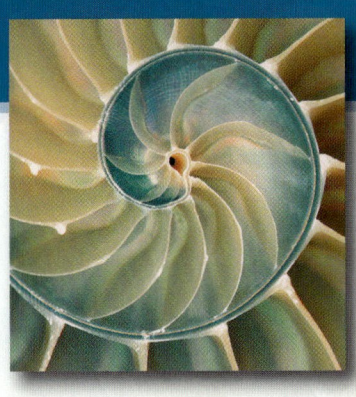

CHAPTER 36

Skin Integrity & Wound Healing

Learning Outcomes

After completing this chapter, you should be able to:

- ➤ Discuss the factors that affect skin integrity.
- ➤ Identify wound type based on accepted classification schemes.
- ➤ Describe the three phases of wound healing.
- ➤ Distinguish primary intention healing, secondary intention healing, and tertiary intention healing.
- ➤ Describe three types of wound drainage.
- ➤ Review the major complications of wound healing.
- ➤ Explain the factors involved in the development of pressure ulcers.
- ➤ Use the Braden scale to assess risk for pressure ulcers.
- ➤ Assess and categorize pressure ulcers based on the pressure ulcer staging system.
- ➤ Provide nursing care that limits the risk of pressure ulcer development.
- ➤ Differentiate the kinds of chronic wounds.
- ➤ Accurately document assessment of a wound.
- ➤ Demonstrate appropriate technique for irrigating a wound.
- ➤ Describe care of a wound with a drain.
- ➤ Differentiate the five forms of wound débridement.
- ➤ Discuss the different kinds of tissue found in wounds.
- ➤ Discuss when and how to use absorbent, alginate, collagen, gauze dressings, transparent films, hydrocolloids, hydrogels, and foam and antimicrobial dressings.
- ➤ Describe guidelines to follow when applying heat or cold therapy.
- ➤ Demonstrate bandage and binder application.

Key Concepts

Skin integrity
Wound
Wound healing

Related Concepts

See the Concept Map at the end of this chapter.

Example Problem

Pressure ulcers

Caring for the Nguyens

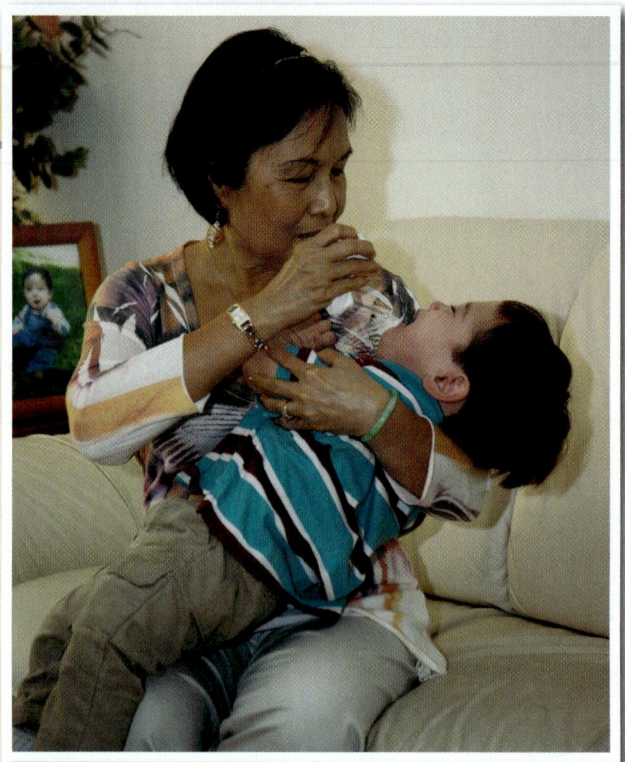

This feature allows you to practice the kind of thinking you will use as a full-spectrum nurse. There is usually more than one correct answer to a critical thinking question, so we do not provide answers for these features. It is more important to develop your nursing judgment than to "cover content." Discuss the questions with your peers. If you are still unsure, consult your instructor.

Kim Phan, Nam and Yen Nguyen's 3-year-old grandchild, fell at the neighborhood playground. He has abrasions on his knees, a deep puncture wound on his left hand, and a laceration on his scalp. Mr. and Mrs. Nguyen bring him to the clinic for assessment. He is crying loudly and moving all extremities. No treatment has been given.

A. What should be your first course of action?

B. What kind of care will Kim need at the clinic?

C. You determine that the scalp laceration will need to be sutured. What actions should you take to prepare Kim for the suturing?

D. One week later Kim arrives at the clinic with his grandmother to have the sutures removed. The scalp laceration is dried and healed. When you inspect his other wounds, you notice that his left knee is erythematous, warm and painful to touch, and draining a moderate amount of purulent drainage. What assessment questions should you ask?

E. Yen Nguyen tells you that Kim would not allow her to clean or dress the abraded knees. You cleanse the knee and remove several small pieces of gravel from the wound bed. The wound is yellow and malodorous. What kind of care will Yen need to provide to Kim to heal the left knee?

 Go to **Caring for the Nguyens Response Sheet** on Davis*Plus.*

Meet Your Patient

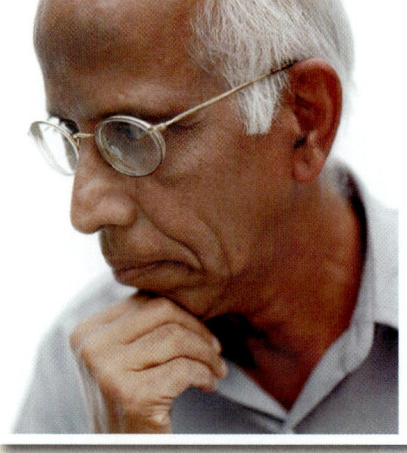

William Harmon is a 78-year-old man who fell 3 days ago. His fall resulted in a fractured left hip. He was admitted to the hospital and underwent an open reduction and internal fixation (ORIF) of the left hip. Today is his second postoperative day. He is still bed bound and is unable to roll or pull himself up in bed.

Mr. Harmon weighs 140 lb (63.64 kg) and is 73 inches tall. His family reports that he has been steadily losing weight. He expresses little interest in eating and says he has been depressed since his wife died last year.

While performing your assessment, you notice that a large dressing covers Mr. Harmon's hip incision. You loosen the dressing and see the staples are intact at the incision site and there is a minimal amount of serosanguineous drainage on the bandage. As you turn him in bed, you see a 10 cm by 6 cm reddened area on his coccyx and a 2 cm by 3 cm purple bruise-like area on his left heel. William now has three wounds, an intentional surgical wound and two pressure ulcers that have resulted from his impaired mobility. How will you care for each of these wounds? What factors contributed to each of the wounds, and how will you promote healing?

Theoretical Knowledge
knowing **why**

The integumentary system consists of the skin, hair, nails, sweat glands, and the subcutaneous tissue below the skin. The skin is the largest organ of the body. The major functions of the skin include protection of the internal organs, unique identification of an individual, thermoregulation, metabolism of nutrients and metabolic waste products, and sensation.

ABOUT THE KEY CONCEPTS

From the preceding paragraph, you can see how important the skin is to a person's health. For optimal function, *skin integrity* must be preserved—that is, all layers of the skin must be intact. A *wound* is a disruption in the normal skin integrity. It is easy to see how the concepts of skin integrity and wound are related; they are opposites. You will use your knowledge of both these concepts as you protect your patients' skin and promote the physiological process of *wound healing*.

WHAT FACTORS AFFECT SKIN INTEGRITY?

To understand skin integrity you need to know about the structure of the skin—the dermis, the epidermis, and the subcutaneous tissue (Fig. 36-1).

Epidermis. The **epidermis** is the outer portion of the skin. The epidermis is made up of four or five layers, of which the most important are the inner and outer layers.

- The **stratum corneum,** the outermost layer, is composed of numerous thicknesses of dead cells. Functioning as a barrier, it restricts water loss and prevents fluids, pathogens, and chemicals from entering the body.
- The **sratum germinativum,** the innermost layer, continually produces new cells, pushing the older cells toward the skin surface. **Keratinocytes** are protein-containing cells that give the skin strength and elasticity. Deeper in the epidermis are **melanocytes,** which produce **melanin,** a pigment that gives skin its color and provides protection from ultraviolet light. **Langerhans cells** are mobile. Their function is to phagocytize (engulf) foreign material and trigger an immune response.

Dermis. The **dermis** lies below the epidermis and above the subcutaneous tissue. It is made of irregular fibrous connective tissue that provides strength and elasticity to the skin and is generously supplied with blood vessels. Within the dermis are sweat glands, sebaceous (oil) glands, ceruminous (wax) glands, hair and nail follicles, sensory receptors, elastin, and collagen.

Subcutaneous Tissue. The **subcutaneous layer** is composed primarily of connective and adipose tissue. It provides insulation, protection, and a reserve of calories in the event of severe malnutrition. This layer varies in thickness in different body sites. Sex hormones, genetics, age, and nutrition also influence the distribution of subcutaneous tissue.

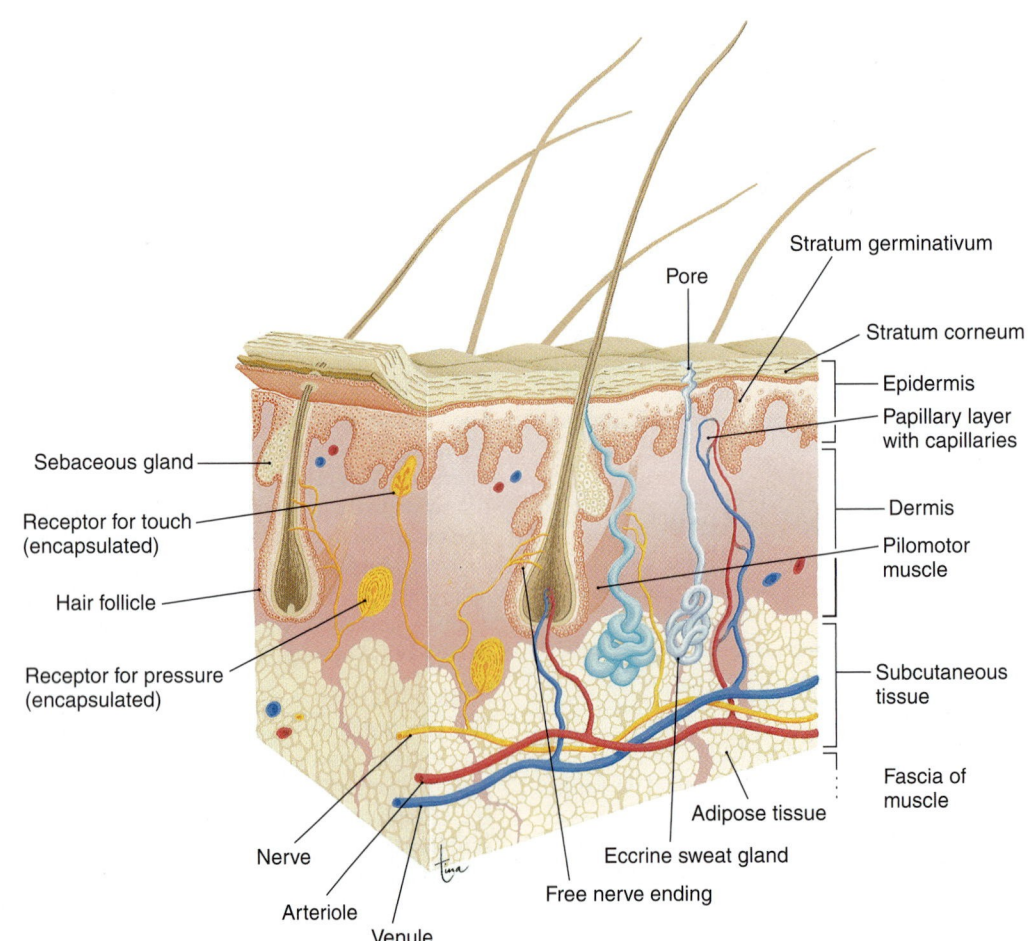

FIGURE 36-1 The structure of the skin.

All layers of healthy skin are intact. Breaks in the skin (as with surgery or injury) increase the risk of infection. In the following sections you will learn about factors that influence skin integrity and wound healing.

Age-Related Variations

Age affects the condition and structure of the skin. Infants, for example, are born with varying amounts of *vernix caseosa*, a creamy substance that protects their skin. Their skin is thinner and more permeable than that of adults, which predisposes infants to skin breakdown (e.g., diaper rash). The subcutaneous layer (brown fat) and sweat glands are not fully developed, especially for preterm infants. As a result, in the first few weeks of life infants' temperature-regulating systems are immature, which is why they need be swaddled to maintain body heat.

As children are exposed to sun and other elements, skin texture becomes coarser. Sex hormones released during puberty increase sebaceous and sweat gland activity, which leads to perspiration odor and sometimes acne. In women, high estrogen levels may contribute to the softening of connective tissue and cause striae and darkening of the skin, particularly on the face, areolae, nipples, vulva, and umbilicus, especially in people with dark skin.

Older Adults. The activity of the sebaceous and sweat glands diminishes with aging, resulting in drier skin. **Xerosis** (itchy, red, dry, scaly, cracked, or fissured skin) is a problem for up to 85% of older adults and can be a threat to the integrity of their skin. Along with loss of lean body mass, the subcutaneous tissue layer thins, giving the normal-weight individual a sharp, angular appearance. Changes in collagen fibers decrease the elasticity of the dermal layer, thus weakening the strong bond between the epidermis and dermis. These changes make the skin prone to breakdown and prolong wound-healing time. Regeneration of healthy skin takes at least twice as long in an 80-year-old as in a 30-year-old. In addition, many older adults have chronic diseases that interfere with healing. Diabetes, for instance, predisposes to infection; and liver dysfunction interferes with synthesis of blood-clotting factors.

Impaired Mobility

A healthy person moves and shifts position unconsciously when he senses pressure or discomfort. However, for people who cannot move independently, the weight of the body on the bed or chair causes an increase in pressure and may lead to skin breakdown. Impaired mobility is caused by conditions that require complete bedrest or that severely limit activity (e.g., paralysis, high-risk pregnancy, sedation, casts, and altered sensory perception).

KnowledgeCheck 36-1

- Identify the major functions of the skin.
- What is the function of the stratum corneum, the outermost layer of the skin?
- What is the function of the subcutaneous layer?
- What effect does aging have on skin?
- What effect does immobility have on skin?

Nutrition and Hydration

Skin condition reflects overall nutritional status, and at the same time, nutritional intake affects the skin. Adequate intake of nutrients and fluid are essential to maintaining skin integrity.

Protein. Healthy skin requires protein to maintain integrity, repair minor defects, and preserve intravascular volume. If protein levels decline from excess loss or inadequate intake, minor defects cannot be repaired, fluid leaks from the vascular compartment of dependent areas, and *edema* (excess fluid in the tissues) develops. Edema decreases skin elasticity and interferes with the diffusion of oxygen to the cells. Therefore, the skin becomes prone to breakdown.

Cholesterol. Abnormally low cholesterol levels predispose patients to skin breakdown and inhibit wound healing. Patients on low-fat tube feedings may experience deficiencies in fatty acids and linoleic acid, as well as cholesterol. Together, these fats aid in providing calories for wound healing and maintain a waterproof barrier in the stratum corneum.

Calorie Intake. If calorie intake is inadequate, the body uses proteins for energy (catabolism). Proteins are then unavailable for building and maintenance functions (anabolism) (see Chapter 28 as needed). When undernutrition is prolonged, the person experiences loss of subcutaneous tissue, and muscle atrophy. As a result, there is less padding between the skin and the bones, predisposing the skin to pressure ulcers.

Ascorbic Acid, Zinc, and Copper. Vitamin C, or ascorbic acid, is involved in the formation and maintenance of collagen, so a deficiency can delay wound healing. Zinc and copper are also involved in collagen formation, and deficiencies of either may impair healing.

Hydration. Poor skin turgor may occur as a result of dehydration, whereas edema may result from overhydration. For further discussion on fluid requirements, see Chapter 39.

Diminished Sensation or Cognition

Clients with peripheral vascular disease, spinal cord injury, diabetes, cerebrovascular accident, trauma, or fractures often have diminished tactile sense. They are therefore more prone to skin breakdown. If you've ever touched a hot surface and quickly pulled back your hand, you know the importance of tactile sensation.

A *client with diminished sensation* is less able to sense a hot surface and would likely suffer a burn. A cut or wound in an area with limited sensation may go unnoticed and therefore untreated. The client with diminished sensation is also unable to feel pressure in an affected area. As a result, he may not shift position to relieve pressure over bony prominences or be aware that shoes or clothing are constricting.

Clients with impaired cognition (i.e., Alzheimer's disease, dementia, altered level of consciousness) are at higher risk for skin breakdown because they are not aware of the need to reposition.

Impaired Circulation

The vascular system brings oxygen-rich blood to the tissues and removes metabolic waste products. Circulatory impairment interferes with tissue metabolism. *Impaired arterial circulation* restricts activity, produces pain, and leads to muscle atrophy and thin tissue that is prone to ischemia and necrosis. *Impaired venous circulation* results in engorged tissues with high levels of metabolic waste products, thereby increasing the risk for edema, ulceration, and breakdown. Both forms of circulatory impairment delay wound healing, and may lead to chronic wounds.

Medication

Side effects and idiosyncratic reactions to medications can affect skin integrity and wound healing. Any medication that causes pruritus (itching), dermatoses (rashes), photosensitivity, alopecia, or pigmentation changes can result in changes that impair skin integrity or delay healing. The following are examples:

- *Blood pressure medications* decrease the amount of pressure required to occlude blood flow to an area, creating a risk for ischemia.

- *Anti-inflammatory medications*, such as over-the-counter (OTC) nonsteroidal anti-inflammatory drugs (NSAIDs) and steroids, inhibit wound healing.
- *Anticoagulants* (e.g., heparin, warfarin) can lead to extravasation of blood into subcutaneous tissue. As a result, even minimal pressure or injury can cause a hematoma.
- *Chemotherapeutic agents* delay wound healing because of their cellular toxicity.
- *Certain antibiotics, psychotherapeutic drugs,* and *chemotherapy agents* for cancer increase sensitivity to sunlight, increasing the risk for sunburn.
- *Several herbal products*, such as those containing lavender and tea tree oil, have a drying effect on the skin.

Moisture on the Skin

Moisture leads to **maceration** (softening of the skin) and increases the likelihood of skin breakdown. Incontinence and fever are the most common sources of moisture. Bowel incontinence is particularly troublesome because feces contain digestive enzymes and microorganisms that readily lead to **excoriation** (denuding) of superficial skin layers, placing such a patient at risk for **moisture-associated skin damage (MASD)**, **dermatitis** (inflammation of the skin), pressure ulcers, and infection.

Fever

Fever leads to sweating, which can cause maceration. In addition, it increases the metabolic rate, thereby raising the tissue demand for oxygen. An increased demand for oxygen is difficult to meet if there is any circulatory impairment or tissue compression from immobility.

Contamination or Infection

Contamination of a wound refers to the presence of microorganisms in the wound. All chronic wounds are contaminated.

As bacteria begin to increase in number, a wound is said to be **colonized,** though the microorganisms are causing no harm. Wounds are colonized from the surrounding skin and local skin organisms, the external environment, and internal sources, usually from the mucous membranes of the gastrointestinal system. A wound becomes **critically colonized** when the bacteria begin to overwhelm the body's defenses. Critical colonization may be detected by subtle signs, such as an increase in drainage, or by more pronounced signs such as a new foul odor, a change in color of the wound bed, new tunneling of the wound, or absent or friable granulation tissue.

An **infection** implies the microorganisms are causing harm by releasing toxins, invading body tissues, and increasing the metabolic demand of the tissue. Infection of the skin makes it more vulnerable to breakdown and impedes healing of open wounds. If not stopped, bacteria can then gain access to the systemic circulation.

Lifestyle

The following are some lifestyle habits that affect skin integrity:
- *Tanning* exposes the skin to ultraviolet radiation, thereby increasing the risk for skin cancer.
- *Hygiene habits* involving either excessive or insufficient skin hygiene are not healthy for skin integrity. Frequent bathing and use of soap remove skin oils and may lead to drying, which jeopardizes the skin's barrier function. Infrequent cleansing of the skin contributes to excessive oiliness, clogged sebaceous glands, and inadequate removal of microbes on the skin, which can infect a wound or lesion.
- *Regular exercise* improves circulation.

- *A nutritious diet* provides the nutrients needed to maintain skin integrity.
- *Smoking* compromises the oxygen supply to the tissues, making skin more prone to breakdown and delaying wound healing. It also interferes with vitamin C absorption, which is needed for collagen formation.
- *Body piercings and tattoos* present a risk for infection and scarring. Complications, which occur in about 20% of piercings, include local infections, sepsis, endocarditis, hepatitis, and toxic shock syndrome. Intraoral and perioral piercings can result in gingivitis, damage to teeth and gums, and choking. Advise patients to become informed about the procedure and about aftercare and to find reputable piercers.

KnowledgeCheck 36-2

- Identify the factors that affect skin integrity.
- What nutritional components are essential to maintain skin?

ThinkLike a Nurse 36-1

- Review the case of William Harmon (Meet Your Patient). What risks, if any, does William have for skin breakdown or delayed healing?
- What additional information do you need to know to fully evaluate his risk?
- What risks do you have for impaired skin integrity? What actions can you take to protect your skin?

WOUNDS

Wounds are a disruption in the normal integrity of the skin. Wounds may be intentional, such as a surgical incision, or unintentional, such as a cut or a pressure ulcer.

Types of Wounds

Wounds are classified according to the degree of skin integrity, length of time the wound has existed, level of contamination, and depth or severity of the wound.

Skin Integrity. This is the simplest wound classification system. If there are no breaks in the skin, the wound is described as **closed.** *Contusions* (bruises) or tissue swelling from fractures are common closed wounds. A wound is considered **open** if there is a break in the skin or mucous membranes. Open wounds include abrasions, lacerations, puncture wounds, compound fractures (projection of bone through the skin), and surgical incisions. Several open and closed wounds are described in Table 36-1.

Length of Time for Healing. The length of time for wound healing varies according to the skin integrity and the factors affecting it, discussed in the previous section. **Acute wounds** are expected to be of short duration. In a healthy person, these wounds heal spontaneously without complications through the three phases of wound healing (inflammation, proliferation, and maturation). Wounds that exceed the expected length of recovery are classified as **chronic wounds.** The natural healing progression has been interrupted or stalled because of infection, continued trauma, ischemia, or edema. Chronic wounds include pressure, arterial, venous, and diabetic ulcers. These wounds are frequently colonized with several types of bacteria, and healing is slow because of the underlying disease process. Unless the wound is properly diagnosed and the underlying disease treated, a chronic wound may linger for months or years (Table 36-2).

Table 36-1 ➤ Types of Wounds	
TYPE	**DESCRIPTION**
Abrasion	A scrape of the superficial layers of the skin; usually unintentional but may be performed intentionally for cosmetic purposes to smooth skin surfaces
Abscess	A localized collection of pus due to invasion from a pyogenic bacterium or other pathogen; must be opened and drained to heal
Contusion	A closed wound caused by blunt trauma. May be referred to as a bruise or ecchymotic area.
Crushing	A wound caused by force leading to compression or disruption of tissues. Often associated with fracture. Usually there is minimal or no break in the skin.
Incision	An open, intentional wound caused by a sharp instrument
Laceration	The skin or mucous membranes are torn open, resulting in a wound with jagged margins.
Penetrating	An open wound in which the agent causing the wound lodges in body tissue.
Puncture	An open wound caused by a sharp object. Often there is collapse of tissue around the entry point, making this wound prone to infection.
Tunnel	A wound with an entrance and exit site

Table 36-2 ➤ Chronic Wounds		
TYPE	**ETIOLOGY**	**CHARACTERISTICS**
Pressure Ulcers	Caused by pressure, resulting in tissue ischemia and injury	Appearance depends on the stage or tissue layers involved. Pressure ulcers tend to be located over bony prominences. Can cause serious tissue damage.
Arterial Ulcers	Caused by inadequate circulation of oxygenated blood to the tissue, which leads to tissue ischemia and damage	Ulcer appears "punched out," small and round with smooth borders. The wound base is usually pale with or without necrotic tissue. Ulcers tend to occur over the distal part of the leg, especially the ankles, toes, side of the foot, and shin. The surrounding skin appears shiny, thin, and dry and is cool to touch. Often there is loss of hair in the surrounding area. The area has delayed capillary refill time, and patients may complain of pain that worsens with increased activity. Arterial ulcers are most common in lower extremities but can occur anywhere. This type of ulcer can lead to serious injury and even death
Venous Stasis Ulcers	Caused by incompetent venous valves, deep vein obstruction, or inadequate calf muscle function, resulting in venous pooling, edema, and impaired microcirculation of the skin	Located usually around the inner ankle, or in the lower part of the calf. Surrounding skin is reddened or brown and edematous. Wounds are usually shallow, with irregular wound margins. The wound bed appears "ruddy" or "beefy" red and granular. Drainage may be moderate to heavy depending on amount of edema. Pain usually occurs with leg dependence and dressing changes.

Level of Contamination. **Clean wounds** are uninfected wounds with minimal inflammation. They may be open or closed and do not involve the gastrointestinal, respiratory, or genitourinary tracts (these systems frequently harbor bacteria). There is little risk of infection for a clean wound. **Clean-contaminated wounds** are surgical incisions that enter the gastrointestinal, respiratory, or genitourinary tracts. There is an increased risk of infection for these wounds, but there is no obvious infection.

Contaminated wounds include open, traumatic wounds or surgical incisions in which a major break in asepsis occurred.

The risk of infection is high for these wounds. Wounds are considered **infected** when bacteria counts in the wound tissues are above 100,000 organisms per gram of tissue. However, the presence of *beta-hemolytic streptococci,* in any number, is considered an infection. Signs of wound infection include erythema and swelling around the wound, fever, foul odor, severe or increasing pain, a large amount of drainage, or warmth of the surrounding soft tissue.

Depth of the Wound. **Superficial wounds** involve only the epidermal layer of the skin. The injury is usually the result of friction, shearing, or burning. **Partial-thickness wounds**

extend through the epidermis but not through the dermis. **Full-thickness wounds** extend into the subcutaneous tissue and beyond (National Pressure Ulcer Advisory Panel [NPUAP], 2007c). The descriptor **penetrating** is sometimes added to indicate that the wound involves internal organs. Wound depth is a major determinant of healing time: The deeper the wound, the longer the healing time.

KnowledgeCheck 36-3

- Explain the difference between an acute and a chronic wound.
- Describe the wound categorization system based on the level of contamination.
- How does wound depth affect healing?

Wound-Healing Process

All wounds heal through a physiological process in which epithelial, endothelial, and inflammatory cells, platelets, and fibroblasts migrate into the wound to bring about tissue repair and regeneration. The process is essentially the same regardless of the type of injury or the type of tissues involved. Wounds may heal by regeneration or by primary, secondary, or tertiary intention.

Regenerative/Epithelial Healing. When a wound affects only the epidermis and dermis, **regenerative/epithelial healing** takes place. No scar forms, and the new (regenerated) epithelial and dermal cells form new skin that cannot be distinguished from the intact skin. Partial-thickness wounds heal by regeneration.

Primary Intention Healing. When a wound involves minimal or no tissue loss and has edges that are well approximated (closed), **primary** (first) intention healing takes place (Fig. 36-2A). Little scarring is expected. A clean surgical incision heals by this method.

Secondary Intention Healing. Healing by **secondary (second) intention** occurs when a wound (1) involves extensive tissue loss, which prevents wound edges from approximating, or (2) should not be closed (e.g., because it is infected). Because the wound is left open, it heals from the inner layer to the surface by filling in with beefy red **granulation tissue** (a form of connective tissue with an abundant blood supply) (Fig. 36-2B). Epithelial tissue may appear in the wound as small pink or pearl-like areas. Do not mistake this as a sign of infection. Wounds that heal by secondary intention heal more slowly, are more prone to infection, and develop more scar tissue. Pressure ulcers (discussed later) and infected wounds are examples.

Tertiary Intention Healing. A wound heals by **tertiary (third) intention,** also called *delayed primary closure,* when two surfaces of granulation tissue are brought together (Fig. 36-2C). This technique may be used when the wound is clean-contaminated or contaminated. Initially the wound is allowed to heal by secondary intention. When there is no evidence of edema, infection, or foreign matter, the wound edges are closed by bringing together the granulating tissue and suturing the surface. Such wounds require strict aseptic technique during all dressing changes because they are prone to infection. Tertiary

Primary intention

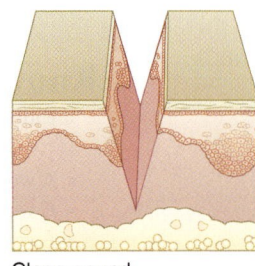
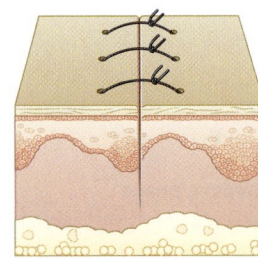
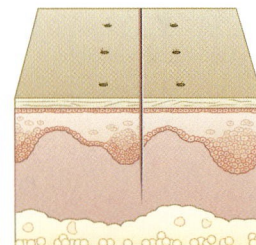

A Clean wound Sutured early Results in hairline scar

Secondary intention

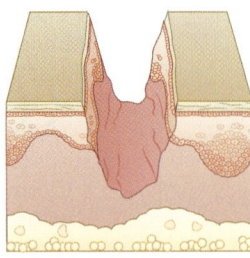
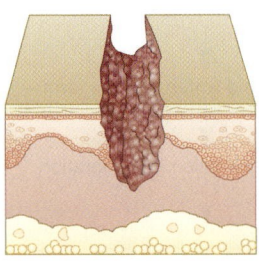

B Wound gaping and irregular Granulation occurring Epithelium fills in scar

Tertiary intention

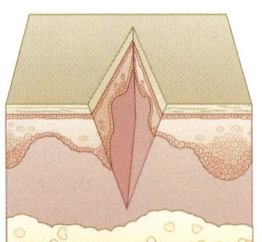
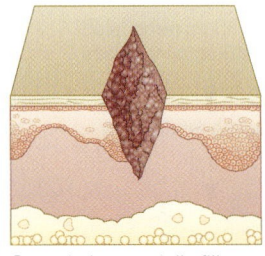
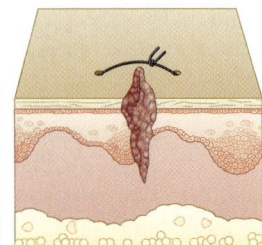

C Wound not sutured Granulation partially fills in wound Granulating tissue sutured together

FIGURE 36-2 A. In a wound with minimal tissue loss, the edges may be sutured together, resulting in rapid healing and minimal scarring. B. A wound that heals by secondary intention heals from the inner layer to the surface. Healing takes longer, and there is scarring. C. A wound that heals by tertiary intention is initially healed by secondary intention and later sutured.

intention healing creates less scarring than does secondary, but more than primary intention healing.

Phases of Healing

Wound healing occurs in three stages: inflammatory, proliferative, and maturation (Fig. 36-3).

The inflammatory phase—cleansing—lasts from 1 to 5 days and consists of two major processes: hemostasis and inflammation.

- *Hemostasis.* At the time of injury, tissue and capillaries are destroyed, causing blood and plasma to leak into the wound.

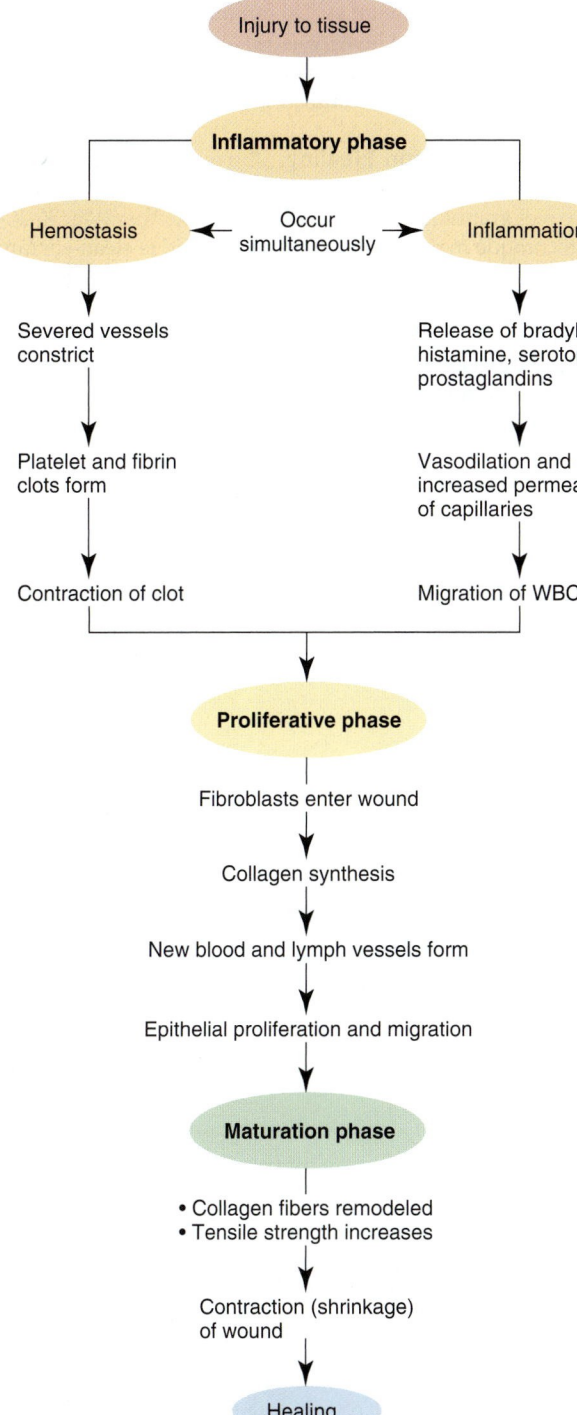

FIGURE 36-3 Stages in the wound-healing process.

Area vessels constrict to limit blood loss. Platelets are activated and aggregate (clump together) to slow bleeding. At the same time, the clotting mechanism is activated to form a blood clot.

- *Inflammation.* The inflammatory reaction is characterized by edema, erythema, pain, temperature elevation, and migration of white blood cells into the wound tissues. Within 24 hours, macrophages begin engulfing bacteria **(phagocytosis)** and clearing debris. In conjunction with plasma proteins and fibrin, they form a scab at the surface of the wound, which seals the wound and helps prevent microbial invasion.

The proliferative phase—granulation—is also called the regeneration phase. It occurs from days 5 to 21. Cells develop to fill the wound defect and resurface the skin. **Fibroblasts** (connective tissue cells) migrate to the wound where they form **collagen,** a protein substance that adds strength to the healing wound. New blood and lymph vessels sprout from the existing capillaries at the edge of the wound. The result is the formation of granulation tissue, a beefy red tissue that bleeds readily and is easily damaged. As the clot or scab is dissolved, epithelial cells begin to grow into the wound from surrounding healthy tissue and seal over the wound **(epithelialization).**

The maturation phase—epithelialization (or remodeling)—is the final phase of the healing process. It begins in the second or third week and continues even after the wound has closed. Over the next 3 to 6 months, the initial collagen fibers that were laid in the wound bed during the proliferative phase are broken down and remodeled into an organized structure (e.g., scar tissue), increasing the tensile strength of the wound. A wound that has healed by primary intention leaves little scarring. Even so, a scar is only 80% as strong as the original tissue.

KnowledgeCheck 36-4

Identify the type of wound healing (primary, secondary, or tertiary intention):

- A wound that heals from inner layer to the surface
- A wound with approximated edges
- A wound that heals by approximating two surfaces of granulation tissue
- A wound that is sutured and has minimal or no tissue loss

Wound Closures

Wounds that heal by primary and tertiary intention may be closed in a number of ways. The following are the current choices.

Adhesive Strips. In the following situations, adhesive strips (e.g., Steri-Strips™) are used:

- Closing superficial low-tension wounds, such as skin tears or lacerations
- Closing the skin on a wound that has been closed subcutaneously
- Giving additional support to a wound after sutures or staples have been removed.

Adhesive strips are often kept in place until they begin to separate from the skin on their own. For instructions on applying adhesive strip closures (Steri-Strips™), see Procedure 36-10.

Sutures. The traditional wound closures are sutures ("stitches"). Suturing leads to small puncture wounds along the track of the laceration or incision. Several types of suture materials are available.

- *Absorbent sutures* are used deep in the tissues, for example, to close an organ or **anastomose** (connect) tissue. Because they

are made of material that will gradually dissolve, there is no need to remove absorbent sutures.

- *Nonabsorbent sutures* are placed in superficial tissues and require removal, often by a nurse. For instructions on removing sutures and staples, see Procedure 36-13.

Surgical Staples. Made of lightweight titanium, surgical staples provide a fast, easy way to close an incision. They are also associated with a lower risk of infection and tissue reaction than sutures. The downside of staples is that some wound edges are more difficult to align. The most common sites for wound stapling are arms, legs, abdomen, back, scalp, or bowel. Wounds on the hands, feet, neck, or face should not be stapled.

Surgical Glue. This is a relatively new method for wound closure. It is safe for use in clean, low-tension wounds. It is an ideal closure method for skin tears.

Negative Pressure Wound Therapy. Negative pressure wound therapy promotes healing by secondary and tertiary intention. Using a specialized pump, negative pressure is placed on a wound packed with foam or gauze dressings to create a vacuum. The subatmospheric pressure improves wound healing by reducing edema from swollen tissues; promoting granulation tissue formation; and removing exudate and infectious material. Negative pressure promotes granulation tissue formation by "stretching" cells and stimulating blood vessel growth and wound perfusion. See Procedure 36-7 for further information.

Advanced Wound Treatments

Collaborative treatments are necessary for wounds that will not heal despite aggressive care. Such treatments include the following:

- **Surgical options**, such as extensive débridement, skin grafts, secondary closure of the wound, and **flap techniques** (partially detached tissue placed over a wound) are used for complicated wounds.
- **Hyperbaric oxygen therapy (HBOT)** is the administration of 100% oxygen under pressure to a wound site. HBOT increases oxygen concentration in the tissue, stimulates the growth of new blood vessels, and enhances white blood cell (WBC) action.
- **Platelet-derived growth factor** augments the inflammatory phase of wound healing and accelerates collagen formation in the wound.

Types of Wound Drainage

Drainage is the flow of fluids from a wound or cavity. It is often referred to as exudate—fluid that oozes as a result of inflammation. Exudate may take several forms.

- **Serous Exudate.** Clean wounds typically drain serous exudate. It is watery in consistency and contains very little cellular matter. Serous exudate consists of *serum,* the straw-colored fluid that separates out of blood when a clot is formed.
- **Sanguineous Exudate.** You will often see sanguineous exudate (bloody drainage) with deep wounds or wounds in highly vascular areas. It indicates damage to capillaries. Fresh bleeding produces bright red drainage, whereas older, dried blood is a dark, red-brown color.
- **Serosanguineous Drainage.** In new wounds, you will most commonly see serosanguineous drainage, a combination of bloody and serous drainage.
- **Purulent Exudate.** The thick, often malodorous, drainage that is seen in infected wounds is called purulent exudate. It contains pus, a protein-rich fluid filled with WBCs, bacteria, and cellular debris. It is commonly caused by infection from **pyogenic** (pus-forming) bacteria, such as streptococci or staphylococci. Normally, pus is yellow in color, although it may take on a blue-green color if the bacterium *Pseudomonas aeruginosa* is present.
- **Purosanguineous Exudate.** Red-tinged pus is called purosanguineous exudate. It indicates that small vessels in the wound area have ruptured.

Complications of Wound Healing

Recall that wounds heal by moving through the phases of inflammation, proliferation, and maturation. At times, this process is interrupted by complications. The most common complications are hemorrhage, infection, dehiscence, evisceration, and fistulas.

Hemorrhage

Whenever a capillary network is interrupted or a blood vessel is cut, bleeding occurs. **Hemostasis** (cessation of bleeding) usually occurs within minutes of the injury. Hemostasis is delayed, however, when large vessels are injured, a clotting disorder exists, or the client is on anticoagulant therapy. If bleeding begins again after initial hemostasis, something is probably wrong. Possible causes include a slipped suture, erosion of a blood vessel, a dislodged clot, or infection. The risk of hemorrhage is greatest in the first 24 to 48 hours following surgery or injury. Bleeding may be internal or external.

Internal Bleeding. Swelling of the affected body part, pain, and changes in vital signs (i.e., decreased blood pressure, elevated pulse) may indicate internal bleeding. *Internal bleeding,* in this chapter, includes **hematoma,** a red-blue collection of blood under the skin, which forms as a result of bleeding that cannot escape to the surface. The amount of blood in a hematoma varies. A large hematoma causes pressure on surrounding tissues. If it is located near a major artery or vein, it may impede blood flow.

External Hemorrhage. Compared to internal bleeding, external hemorrhage is easier to recognize. You will see bloody drainage on the dressings and in the wound drainage devices. When there is a brisk hemorrhage, blood often pools underneath the client as the dressings become saturated. To be sure that you recognize the full extent of the bleeding, remember to look underneath the patient.

Infection

Microorganisms can be introduced to a wound during an injury, during surgery, or after surgery. Suspect infection if a wound fails to heal. Localized swelling, redness, heat, pain, fever (temperatures higher than 38°C [100.4°F]), foul-smelling or purulent drainage, or a change in the color of the drainage may also indicate infection. The symptoms are likely to occur in a contaminated or traumatic wound within 2 to 3 days. In a clean surgical wound, you will usually not see signs and symptoms of an infection until the fourth or fifth postoperative day. Incisions that begin draining within 5 to 7 days of surgery are at risk for dehiscing.

Dehiscence

Rupture (separation) of one or more layers of a wound is called **dehiscence** (Fig. 36-4). Wound dehiscence is most likely to occur in the inflammatory phase of healing, before large amounts of collagen have been deposited in the wound to strengthen it. The most common causes of dehiscence are poor nutritional status, inadequate closure of the muscles, or wound infection. Obese clients are also more likely to experience dehiscence because fatty tissue does not heal readily and the patient's mass increases the strain on the suture line.

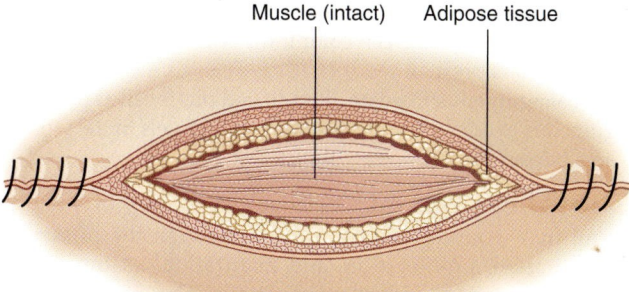

FIGURE 36-4 Dehiscence is separation of one or more layers of a wound. It is most common in the inflammatory phase of healing.

Dehiscence is usually associated with abdominal wounds. Patients often report feeling a pop or tear, especially with sudden straining from coughing, vomiting, or changing positions in bed. Usually there is an immediate increase in serosanguineous drainage. Nursing interventions include maintaining bedrest with head of bed elevated at 20° and the knees flexed. To prevent evisceration, a binder may be applied and activity modified. The surgeon should be notified of the dehiscence and may visit the patient to examine the wound.

Evisceration

Evisceration is total separation of the layers of a wound in which internal viscera protrude through the incision (Fig. 36-5).

Evisceration is a rare complication and is a surgical emergency. Immediately cover the wound with sterile towels or dressings soaked in sterile saline solution to prevent the organs from drying out and becoming contaminated with environmental bacteria. Have the patient stay in bed with knees bent to minimize strain on the incision. Notify the surgeon and ready the patient for a surgical procedure (see Chapter 40 for perioperative care).

Fistulas

A **fistula** is an abnormal passage connecting two body cavities or a cavity and the skin. Fistulas often result from infection. An abscess forms, which breaks down surrounding tissue and creates the abnormal passageway. Chronic drainage from the fistula may lead to skin breakdown and delayed wound healing. The most common sites where fistulas form are the gastrointestinal and genitourinary tracts. Figure 36-6 illustrates a fistula between the rectum and vagina.

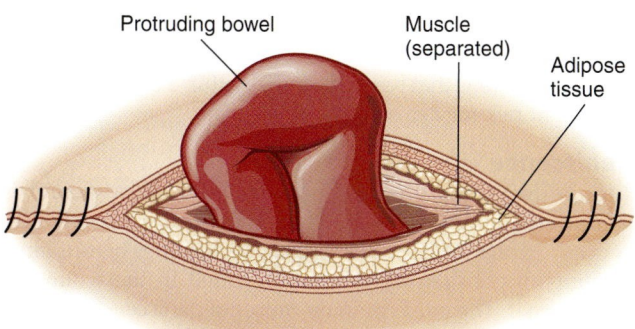

FIGURE 36-5 Evisceration is total separation of the layers of a wound with internal viscera protruding through the incision.

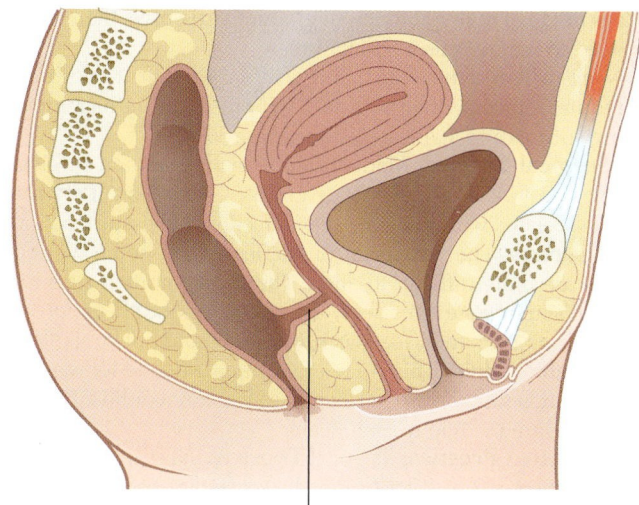

Fistula between rectum and vagina (enterovaginal)

FIGURE 36-6 A fistula is an abnormal passage connecting two body cavities or a cavity and the skin. Fistulas are most common in the gastrointestinal and genitourinary tracts.

KnowledgeCheck 36-5
- Describe four types of wound closures.
- Identify five types of wound complications.
- Describe three signs of internal hemorrhage.
- Differentiate between dehiscence and evisceration.

ThinkLike a Nurse 36-2

Recall the case of Mr. Harmon (Meet Your Patient). What form of wound healing (primary, secondary, or tertiary) is he undergoing? How long would you expect it to take before his wounds heal?

CHRONIC WOUNDS

A chronic wound is one that has not healed within the proper time frame. It has not moved through the repair process in an orderly fashion (inflammation, proliferation, maturation). Wounds that do not heal within 2 to 4 weeks may be considered chronic.

Example Problem: Pressure Ulcers

A pressure ulcer is a type of chronic wound. We discuss it separately because vigilant nursing care can prevent pressure ulcers. In the event pressure ulcers do form, nurses play a major role in their treatment. About 15% of hospital patients, 10% of home care patients, and 20% of long-term care patients have pressure ulcers (Ayello & Lyder, 2008; Black, Baharestani, Cuddigan, et al., 2007a). Unless the pressure injury is present on admission (POA), in most circumstances Medicare will decline payment for treatment for that ulcer. Costs in lives can be high as well, with reported mortality rates of 70% for older adults within 6 months of developing a pressure ulcer (Brown, 2003).

How Do Pressure Ulcers Develop?

Pressure ulcers (formerly called *decubitus ulcers*, *pressure sores*, and *bedsores*) are localized areas of injury to the skin, and possibly the underlying tissue, usually over a bony prominence. They are caused by unrelieved pressure, or pressure in combination with shearing forces, which compromises blood flow to an area, resulting in *ischemia* (inadequate blood supply) in the underlying

tissue (NPUAP, 2007e). Tissue ischemia leads to tissue anoxia (lack of oxygen) and cell death.

The key variables in ischemia are time and pressure. Small amounts of pressure over an extended period of time or a large amount of pressure for a short period of time results in tissue ischemia. Pressure ulcers can occur in as little time as 2 hours, though it may take as long as 5 days for the full extent of tissue damage to be known.

When ischemia first occurs, the skin over the area is pale and cool. When you relieve the pressure (e.g., by turning the patient), vasodilation occurs, and extra blood rushes to the area to compensate for the ischemic period. The area flushes bright red **(reactive hyperemia).** If the redness does not disappear quickly, tissue damage has occurred. The redness should last about half as long as the duration of the ischemia. For example, if the tissue was compressed for an hour, reactive hyperemia should not last more than about 30 minutes.

Although time and pressure are the key variables, several other factors predict the likelihood of pressure ulcer formation (Fig. 36-7). Some factors are intrinsic and some are extrinsic.

Intrinsic Factors. Certain intrinsic (internal) factors alter skin and tissue integrity or oxygen delivery capabilities, decreasing the amount of force required to create a pressure ulcer. Examples include immobility and impaired sensation, as occur with spinal cord injuries, stroke, or coma; poor nutrition; edema; aging; low arteriolar pressure; and fever. Septicemia is one of the most common principal reasons for hospitalization among patients with secondary pressure ulcers (Russo, Steiner, & Spector, 2008).

Poor nutrition or dehydration can weaken the skin and lead to pressure ulcers. Adequate intake of calories, protein, vitamin C, and zinc is necessary to prevent pressure ulcers and promote healing of injured tissue (Institute for Clinical Systems Improvement (ICSI), 2007, updated 2010).

Extrinsic Factors. The following extrinsic (external) factors contribute to the development of pressure ulcers.

- *Friction* damages the outer protective epidermal layer, decreasing the amount of pressure needed to develop skin lesions (Black, Baharestani, Cuddigan, et al., 2007a).

- *Shearing* occurs when the epidermal layer slides over the dermis, causing damage to the vascular bed. It most commonly occurs when the head of the bed is elevated and the patient slides downward, causing shear to develop in the sacral area. When shearing occurs, the amount of pressure needed to occlude circulation is cut in half.

- *Moisture,* especially in the form of urine or feces, macerates the skin and also decreases the amount of pressure required to produce ulceration.

Pressure ulcers most commonly develop over **bony prominences,** but can occur under casts, splints, or other assistive devices. Skin is compressed between the bone and the hard surface of the bed or chair, reducing blood flow to the area. Figure 36-8A–D illustrates the pressure points in the supine, lateral, prone, and sitting positions.

- Wounds caused by **trauma** have a greater risk of infections and slower healing (ICSI, 2007, updated 2010).

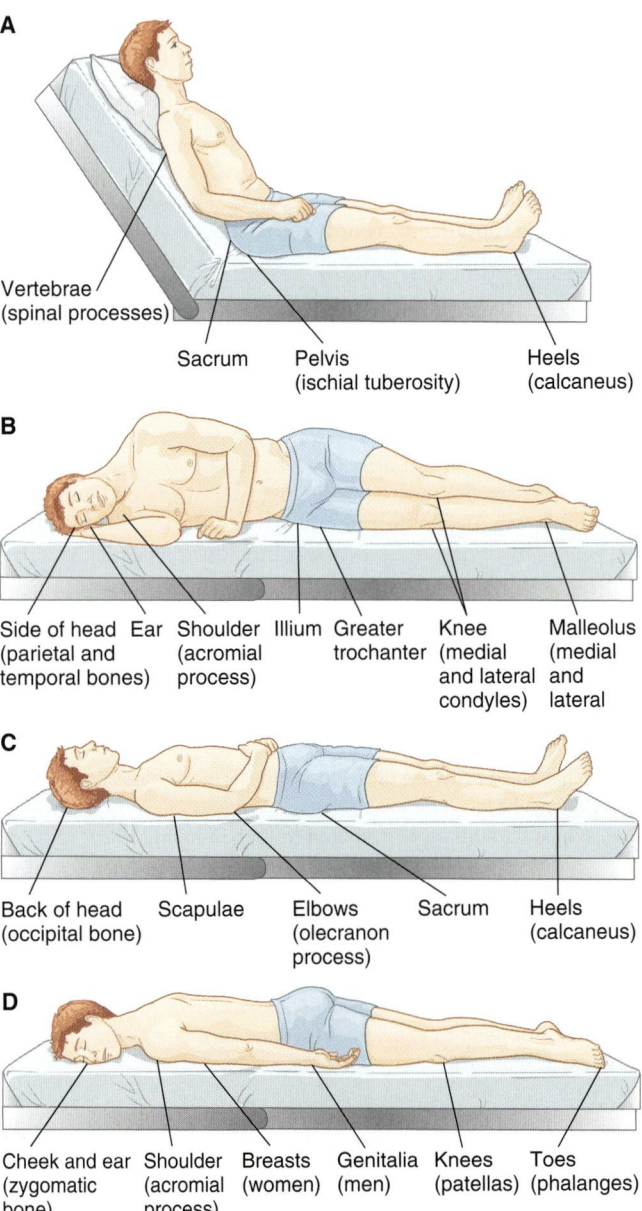

FIGURE 36-8 Most commonly, pressure ulcers develop over the bony prominences. A, Sitting. B, Lateral. C, Supine. D, Prone. (*Source:* Adapted from AHRQ Clinical Practice Guidelines.)

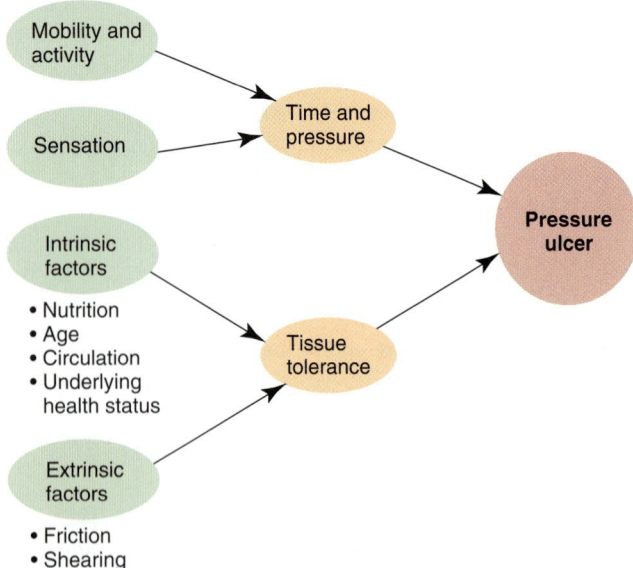

FIGURE 36-7 Several factors contribute to the development of pressure ulcers.

How Are Pressure Ulcers Staged?

Pressure ulcers are classified by the degree of tissue involvement (Table 36-3). The National Pressure Ulcer Advisory Panel developed a standardized staging system (European Pressure Ulcer Advisory Panel [EPUAP] and NPUAP, 2009a). Only wounds that are caused by pressure should be "staged" (NPUAP, 2007e). Other classification systems exist to describe other chronic wounds, such as diabetic foot ulcers and venous stasis ulcers.

Key Point: *Reverse staging does not occur as an ulcer heals. The healing process cannot cause a stage IV pressure ulcer to become a stage III ulcer. Pressure ulcers become progressively more shallow by filling with granulation tissue, but lost muscle, subcutaneous fat, and dermis are not replaced. Therefore, reverse staging does not accurately characterize what is physiologically occurring in the ulcer. Instead, pressure ulcers maintain their original staging classification throughout the healing process, but they are described as healing (e.g., "stage IV ulcer: healing" or "stage I ulcer: healing").*

Other Types of Ulcers

This chapter focuses primarily on pressure ulcers. However, not all lower extremity ulcers are related to pressure.

Venous stasis ulcers are open lesions caused by venous stasis that results from damage to valves in the veins (e.g., from deep vein thrombosis). They occur usually between the inside ankle and the knee, not necessarily over a bony prominence.

Diabetic foot ulcers occur when diabetes causes narrowing of arteries, decreasing oxygenation to the feet and resulting in delayed healing and tissue necrosis. Because people with diabetes lose protective sensation, they may walk on sores, continuously damaging the tissues. Diabetic foot ulcers, often painless, occur mainly on the plantar surface of the foot, the ball of the foot, or top and bottom of the toes.

Arterial ulcers occur when a nonpressure-related blockage of arterial blood to an area (e.g., by a clot or stenosis of the arterioles) causes tissue necrosis, Arterial ulcers usually occur over the lower leg, ankle, or bony areas of the foot. The wound bed tends to be dry and pale, with little drainage.

For more detailed information about these three types of ulcers,

 Go to Chapter 36, **Supplemental Materials,** on Davis*Plus*

KnowledgeCheck 36-6

- What stage pressure ulcer does Mr. Harmon (Meet Your Patient) have?
- What factors have contributed to its development?

 ## ThinkLike a Nurse 36-3

Based on your knowledge of the factors that have contributed to Mr. Harmon's pressure ulcer development, what actions may lead to healing of the pressure ulcer? *Note:* To answer this question, you do not need to know about wound care (e.g., irrigation) for a pressure ulcer.

PracticalKnowledge
knowing **how**

As a nurse, you will care for many patients who have wounds or who are at risk for skin breakdown. In the remainder of the chapter, we will discuss how to maintain skin integrity, prevent pressure ulcers, and treat wounds.

ASSESSMENT

A thorough skin assessment includes a nursing history, physical examination, and diagnostic testing. The NPUAP recommends that nurses perform a comprehensive wound assessment while identifying other health problems and their impact on wound healing. Existing wounds require additional assessment. For a list of competencies for nurses preventing pressure ulcers (NPUAP, 2010),

 Go to Chapter 36, **Tables, Boxes, Figures: ESG Box 36-1: Competencies for Registered Nurses Preventing Pressure Ulcers,** on Davis*Plus*

Focused Nursing History

To assess wound healing ability and the risk for skin breakdown, you will need data on factors that affect skin integrity (discussed previously): age, mobility, nutrition, hydration, sensation, circulation, medications, moisture, lifestyle, underlying health and disease status, and the presence of microorganisms. Also consider the psychosocial issues related to coping with chronic wounds. For instance, with care and compassion you will assess how patients cope with the pain of a chronic wound, handle the loss of control and independence, adapt to changes in body image, deal with the financial burden of caring for complex wounds, and adjust to the social isolation that comes with impaired mobility and chronic illness. For history questions to help you assess these factors, see the Focused Assessment box, History Questions for Skin and Wound Assessment.

Assessment

History Questions for Skin and Wound Assessment

- ➤ What is your typical activity level?
- ➤ Do you ever use a wheelchair or mobile device to get around? Do you require assistance to get out of bed or a chair?
- ➤ Tell me about your usual diet.
- ➤ How much liquid do you drink each day?
- ➤ Do you have any areas of numbness and tingling?
- ➤ Have you had any recent changes in your skin?
- ➤ Do you have any sores or open areas? If so, how long have you had the wound?
- ➤ Have you ever had difficulty with wound healing?
- ➤ What kinds of healthcare problems have you been experiencing?
- ➤ What medications—prescribed, herbal, or OTC—are you taking?
- ➤ What is your typical hygiene routine?
- ➤ Do you ever lose control of your bladder or bowels?
- ➤ Do you smoke?
- ➤ How much time do you spend outdoors?
- ➤ Do you have diabetes? If so, how often do you check your feet? How often do you see a podiatrist? What is your average blood sugar?

Table 36-3 ➤ Staging Pressure Ulcers

STAGE	CLINICAL FINDINGS	DISCUSSION
Suspected Deep Tissue Injury (DTI) 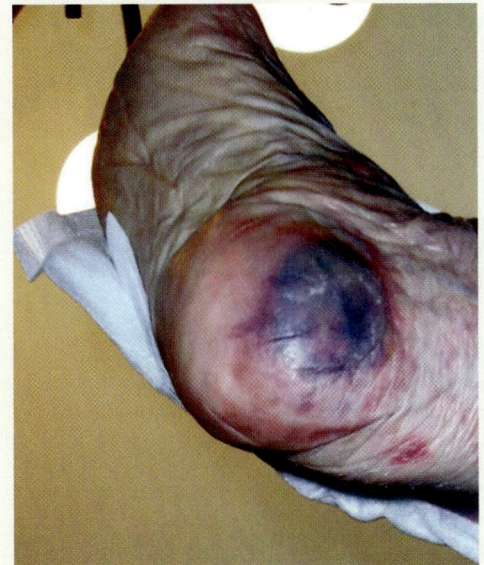	An area of skin that is intact but discolored. It might be purplish or deep red, painful, boggy, or have a blister.	Occurs due to damage of underlying soft tissue from pressure or shear. Findings can be subtle enough that often DTI is not recognized until after severe tissue damage has occurred. May heal or evolve further and become covered by thin eschar, rapidly exposing additional layers of tissue even with optimal treatment. In darker pigmented individuals, discoloration might go undetected.
Stage I Pressure Ulcer 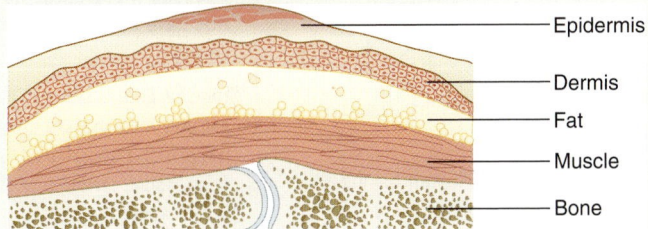 Epidermis Dermis Fat Muscle Bone **Stage I**	Localized area of intact skin with nonblanchable redness, usually over a bony prominence. The area may be painful, firm, soft, or warmer or cooler as compared to adjacent tissue. Discoloration will remain for > 30 min after pressure is relieved.	Dark skin may not have visible blanching; its color may differ from that of the surrounding area. Therefore, stage I may be difficult to detect.
Stage II Pressure Ulcer 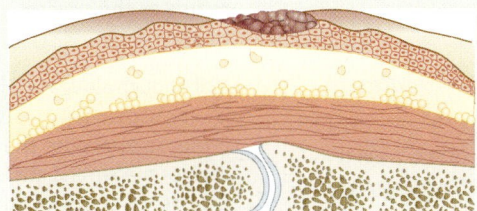 **Stage II**	Involves partial-thickness loss of dermis. Stage II pressure ulcers are open but shallow and with a red pink wound bed. There is no slough. May also be an intact or open/ruptured serum-filled blister, or a shiny or dry shallow ulcer without slough or bruising.	Do not use this stage to describe skin tears, tape burns, perineal dermatitis, maceration, or excoriation. Do not mistake moisture-associated skin damage or fungal infections for stage II pressure ulcer. Stage II ulcers do not involve sloughing or bruising.

(Continued)

Table 36-3 ➤ Staging Pressure Ulcers—cont'd

STAGE	CLINICAL FINDINGS	DISCUSSION
Stage III Pressure Ulcer **Stage III**	A deep crater characterized by full-thickness skin loss with damage or necrosis of subcutaneous tissue. May extend down to, but not through, underlying fascia. Undermining (deeper-level damage under boggy superficial layers) of adjacent tissue may be present. Bone/tendon is not visible or directly palpable.	Some stage III pressure ulcers can be extremely deep when located in an area with significant adipose layers.
Stage IV Pressure Ulcer **Stage IV**	Involves full-thickness skin loss with extensive destruction, tissue necrosis, or damage to muscle, bone, or support structures. Exposed bone/tendon is visible or directly palpable. Slough or eschar may be present. Undermining and sinus tracts (blind tracts underneath the epidermis) are common.	The depth of a stage IV pressure ulcer varies by location. They can be shallow on the bridge of the nose, ear, occiput, and malleolus because these areas do not have subcutaneous tissue. Stage IV ulcers can extend into muscle and supporting structures (e.g., fascia, tendon, or joint capsule). Often require a full year to heal. Even once healed, the site remains at risk for future injury because the scar is not as strong as the original tissue.
Unstageable Pressure Ulcer 	Involves full-thickness skin loss. The base of the wound is obscured by *slough* (tan, yellow, gray, green, or brown necrotic tissue) or *eschar* (tan, black, or brown leathery necrotic tissue).	Until enough slough and/or eschar is removed to expose the base of the wound, the true depth, and therefore stage, cannot be determined. *Stable eschar* is dry, adherent, and intact without erythema or fluctuance. Do not remove stable eschar, as it serves as "the body's natural cover."

Source: NPUAP. (2007). Pressure ulcer stages revised by NPUAP. Retrieved October 26, 2011, from http://npuap.org/pr2.htm.

Reprinted with permission. Photo of suspected deep tissue injury from WOCNS. (2007). Position statement: Pressure ulcer staging. Mount Laurel, NJ: Author, 52.

For example, patients with poor circulation are at risk for tissue injury (e.g., those with diabetes, atherosclerosis, or low blood pressure). Patients who use tobacco or are anemic have reduced oxygen supply in the blood, predisposing them to pressure ulcers. Those who have limited mobility or reduced sensation because of nerve damage, head injury or stroke, spinal cord injury, or diabetes, experience a loss of protective sensations to reposition themselves (ICSI, 2007, updated 2010).

Example Problem Assessment: Pressure Ulcer Risk Assessment Measures

Patients may have multiple risk factors for skin problems. A comprehensive risk assessment tool enables you to evaluate the cumulative risk. Among the most commonly used tools are the Braden and Norton scales.

The Braden scale is used to identify persons at risk for developing pressure ulcers. The Braden scale evaluates six major risk factors: sensory perception, moisture, activity, mobility, nutrition, and friction and sheer (see the Focused Assessment box, The Braden Scale for Predicting Pressure Sore Risk). The final score reflects the patient's risk; the lower the score, the more likely the patient will develop a pressure ulcer. A score of 18 or less for hospitalized patients indicates risk. Interventions should be based on the individual risk factors, as well as the total score. You should use this scale to assess the patient on admission to the facility and again in 48 to 72 hours. Studies have shown the second score to be more predictive, probably related to increased awareness of the patient's status. The Braden Q is a modified scale used in children.

The Norton scale assesses risk based on the patient's physical condition, mental state, activity, mobility, and incontinence. A low score indicates a high risk. Some have suggested that the Norton scale should be modified by adding categories for skin appearance, medication, and nutrition. For a printable version of the Norton scale,

 Go to Chapter 36, **Tables, Boxes, Figures: ESG Figure 36-1, Norton Scale for Assessing the Risk of Pressure Sores,** on Davis*Plus*.

ThinkLike a Nurse 36-4

Review the Braden scale. Apply this risk assessment scale to Mr. Harmon (Meet Your Patient).

- What additional information, if any, do you need to complete these assessments?
- Calculate a Braden score based on Mr. Harmon's risk factors, if he had also been incontinent of urine twice that day.

Focused Physical Examination

Physical assessment of skin integrity focuses on the two following areas.

Inspecting the Skin. Inspect all areas of the body routinely. Evaluate the skin for color, integrity, temperature, texture, turgor, mobility, moisture, lesions, and hair distribution. Check pressure points for erythema, tenderness, or edema. Assess all bony prominences of individuals "at risk" for skin breakdown routinely. Include skin under special garments, such as shoes, heel elevators, and antiembolism stockings. Also assess vulnerable pressure points for bed- or chair-bound patients. See Chapter 21 if you need more details on skin assessment.

Assessing Mobility and Activity Level. As you know, activity level and mobility affect skin integrity, so they will be a part of your focused assessment. See Chapter 21 if you need to review assessment of the musculoskeletal system. See Chapter 33 if you need additional information on activity and mobility.

Assessing Treated Wounds

All wounds require a focused assessment. Assessment frequency depends on the condition of the wound, the work setting, the patient's overall condition and underlying disease process, the type of wound, and the type of treatment used for the wound. If you are providing wound care, you will assess the wound with every treatment. Assessment parameters include the following. Also refer to the Focused Assessment box, Physical Examination: Wound Assessment.

Location. Describe the wound location in anatomical terms. For example, describe an incision from cardiac surgery as a midsternal incision extending from the manubrium to the xiphoid process. An accurate description of the location is important because:

- *Location influences the rate of healing.* Wounds in highly vascular regions, such as the scalp or hands, heal more rapidly than wounds in less vascular regions, such as the abdomen or a heel.
- *Location affects movement.* Wounds that can be readily stabilized heal more rapidly than those in areas that are affected by the constant stress of movement.
- *Location can give you clues to the wound etiology.* A wound over a bony prominence could be related to pressure, whereas one on the bottom of the foot could be a diabetic foot ulcer.

Type of Wound. Is it an acute wound? If the wound is sutured, examine the closure. Are the wound edges approximated (together)? Is there tension on any aspect of the wound? Are the stitches intact? Or is this a chronic wound?

Size. Measure the length and width of the wound in centimeters. It is important that nurses using a ruler measure a wound the same way. The NPUAP recommends using a head-to-toe orientation, the longest length head to toe, and the widest width side-to-side, perpendicular (90° angle) to length, encompassing the entire wound (NPUAP, 2007a). Use serial photographs showing the wound's dimensions to document the baseline and wound healing, especially if the wound has an irregular border (EPUAP and NPUAP, 2009a). To measure wound depth, gently insert a sterile cotton-tip applicator into the deepest part of the wound. Measure the applicator from skin level to the tip (NPUAP, 2007a).

Undermining or Tunneling. Assess the wound edges for any undermining or tunneling. Pay close attention to any tissue that appears to have a separation either in tissue type or plane, as frequently tunnels may be found in that area. Measure the depth and location of any undermining or tunneling using the face of a clock as a guide. If the top of the wound is 12:00 and the bottom of the wound is 6:00, for example, record "2 cm of undermining is present from 1:00 to 4:00" or "6 cm tunnel exists at the center of the wound tracking in the 3:00 direction."

Periwound. Examine the skin surrounding the wound. Skin discoloration may indicate a hematoma or additional

The Braden Scale for Predicting Pressure Sore Risk

Patient's Name _____   **Evaluator's Name** _____   **Date of Assessment**

Category	1	2	3	4												
Sensory perception Ability to respond meaningfully to pressure-related discomfort	**1. Completely limited:** Unresponsive (does not moan, flinch, or grasp) to painful stimuli, due to diminished level of consciousness or sedation, OR limited ability to feel pain over most of body surface.	**2. Very limited:** Responds only to painful stimuli. Cannot communicate discomfort except by moaning or restlessness, OR has a sensory impairment which limits the ability to feel pain or discomfort over ½ of body.	**3. Slightly limited:** Responds to verbal commands but cannot always communicate discomfort or need to be turned, OR has some sensory impairment which limits ability to feel pain or discomfort in 1 or 2 extremities.	**4. No impairment:** Responds to verbal commands. Has no sensory deficit, which would limit ability to feel or voice pain or discomfort.												
Moisture Degree to which skin is exposed to moisture	**1. Constantly moist:** Skin is kept moist almost constantly by perspiration, urine, etc. Dampness is detected every time patient is moved or turned.	**2. Moist:** Skin is often but not always moist. Linen must be changed at least once a shift.	**3. Occasionally moist:** Skin is occasionally moist, requiring an extra linen change approximately once a day.	**4. Rarely moist:** Skin is usually dry; linen requires changing only at routine intervals.												
Activity Degree of physical activity	**1. Bedfast:** Confined to bed.	**2. Chairfast:** Ability to walk severely limited or nonexistent. Cannot bear own weight and/or must be assisted into chair or wheel chair.	**3. Walks occasionally:** Walks occasionally during day but for very short distances, with or without assistance. Spends majority of each shift in bed or chair.	**4. Walks frequently:** Walks outside the room at least twice a day and inside room at least once every 2 hours during waking hours.												
Mobility Ability to change and control body position	**1. Completely immobile:** Does not make even slight changes in body or extremity position without assistance.	**2. Very limited:** Makes occasional slight changes in body or extremity position but unable to make frequent or significant changes independently.	**3. Slightly limited:** Makes frequent though slight changes in body or extremity position independently.	**4. No limitations:** Makes major and frequent changes in position without assistance.												

Focused Assessment

Focused Assessment

	1. Very poor:	2. Probably inadequate:	3. Adequate:	4. Excellent:				
Nutrition Usual food intake pattern	**1. Very poor:** Never eats a complete meal. Rarely eats more than 1/3 of any food offered. Eats 2 servings or less of protein (meat or dairy products) per day. Takes fluids poorly. Does not take a liquid dietary supplement, OR is NPO[1] and/or maintained on clear liquids or IV[2] for more than 5 days.	**2. Probably inadequate:** Rarely eats a complete meal and generally eats only about 1/2 of any food offered. Protein intake includes only 3 servings of meat or dairy products per day. Occasionally will take a dietary supplement, OR receives less than optimum amount of liquid diet or tube feeding.	**3. Adequate:** Eats over half of most meals. Eats a total of 4 servings of protein (meat, dairy products) each day. Occasionally will refuse a meal, but will usually take a supplement if offered, OR is on a tube feeding or TPN[3] regimen, which probably meets most of nutritional needs.	**4. Excellent:** Eats most of every meal. Never refuses a meal. Usually eats a total of 4 or more servings of meat and dairy products. Occasionally eats between meals. Does not require supplementation.								
Friction and shear	**1. Problem:** Requires moderate to maximum assistance in moving. Complete lifting without sliding against sheets is impossible. Frequently slides down in bed or chair, requiring frequent repositioning with maximum assistance. Spasticity, contractures, or agitation leads to almost constant friction.	**2. Potential problem:** Moves feebly or requires minimum assistance. During a move skin probably slides to some extent against sheets, chair, restraints, or other devices. Maintains relatively good position in chair or bed most of the time but occasionally slides down.	**3. No apparent problem:** Moves in bed and in chair independently and has sufficient muscle strength to lift up completely during move. Maintains good position in bed or chair at all times.								
Total Score:								

Physical Examination: Wound Assessment

All Wounds

Assess all wounds for the following:

Location

Describe the location of the wound in anatomical terms. For example, you would describe an incision from cardiac surgery as a midsternal incision extending from the manubrium to the xiphoid process.

Size

➤ Measure the length and width of the wound in centimeters.
➤ To measure wound depth, gently insert a sterile cotton tip applicator into the deepest part of the wound. Measure the applicator from the skin level to the tip.
➤ If possible, use photo documentation, indicating the dimensions on the photo. This is especially useful in the case of a wound with an irregular border.

Appearance

Your description of the appearance of the wound should be very detailed. You must describe:

➤ **Type of wound** (open or closed)
➤ **If the wound is sutured**, examine the closure. Are the wound edges approximated? Is there tension on any aspect of the wound? Are the stitches intact?
➤ **The color of the wound**. Redness and inflammation for the first 2 to 3 days are normal, but erythema or swelling beyond that time may indicate infection.
➤ **Condition of the wound bed (in an open wound).** A beefy red, moist appearance is evidence of healing. A pale color or dry texture indicates a delay in healing.
➤ **Examine for necrosis, slough, and eschar.** Examine for a tunnel or sinus tract in the wound bed; if there is one, inspect and probe it for depth and characteristics.
➤ **The skin surrounding the wound.** Observe for skin discoloration, hematoma, or additional injury to the surrounding tissue. Observe for maceration, tunneling, crepitus, blistering, or erythema. Examine the edges of the wound for epithelial tissue and contraction. Look for undermining beneath the wound margins.

Drainage

➤ **Presence of drainage or exudate.** Describe the color, consistency, amount, and odor.

➤ **Assess the quantity of wound drainage** by weighing dressings before they are applied and again when they have been removed. The change in weight reflects the amount of drainage that they have absorbed.
➤ **If a drain is present**, measure the amount of fluid in the collection container.
➤ **Odor may indicate** fistula formation or contamination with bacteria. If a new odor develops, assess carefully for presence of a fistula.

Patient Responses

Ask your patients about pain, discomfort, or itching related to the wound or wound care.

Assessing an Untreated Wound

Your assessment should determine what, if any, additional professional support is necessary. Assess the following same aspects as for treated wounds above: location, size, appearance, description of drainage, condition of wound margins, condition of surrounding skin, and effect of the wound on the patient. In addition, assess the following:

➤ **Bleeding.** If bleeding is profuse, apply direct pressure to the site. If bleeding continues after you apply pressure for 5 minutes or if blood is spurting from the wound, call the physician immediately.
➤ **Severity of the wound.** A gaping wound, or a deep wound with fat, fascia, or muscle exposed, will need additional care.
➤ **Last tetanus immunization.** Immunization should be given if (1) the last immunization was 10 years ago or longer, (2) the wound is contaminated with dirt or debris and the tetanus injection was given more than 5 years ago, or (3) it is uncertain when the patient last received an immunization.
➤ **Whether the wound was caused by a bite.** Determine whether the wound was caused by any type of bite, animal or human. A deep bite wound usually requires additional observation and/or antibiotics.
➤ **Pain.** Assess for pain. Any wound causing severe pain requires a comprehensive evaluation.
➤ Numbness or loss of movement. If any deficit is detected, the patient will need immediate evaluation.
➤ **Presence of chronic medical conditions.** Examples include diabetes, malnutrition, immunocompromise, or a bleeding disorder. Patients with conditions that affect wound healing will need ongoing evaluation.

injury to the surrounding tissue. Look for maceration; undermining; crepitus; blistering; erythema; and epiboly, slough, and eschar.

Maceration is caused by excessive moisture on intact skin for extended periods of time—as can result when there is pooled drainage or when a moist dressing is inappropriately applied, left on too long, or overlaps onto healthy skin. The skin may appear as pale and wrinkled or "pruned," and may flake and peel.

Undermining will produce a boggy feel around the wound.

Blister is injured epidermis containing clear, watery fluid, usually caused by irritation or burn. It looks like bubbled skin and is usually tender.

Crepitus is gas trapped under the skin. If you palpate the surrounding skin and feel a crackling sensation, this is crepitus. Crepitus may be due to air leaking from the lung in a chest wound or may indicate the presence of gas-producing bacteria.

Erythema, swelling, or other signs of irritation indicate that the surrounding tissue is in jeopardy.

Epiboly is a closed or rolled wound edge. Examine wound edges for epithelial tissue and contraction. Epibolies

may indicate that epithelial cells have moved down and rolled under the wound edges. Once the cells reach the wound bed, they will stall wound healing.

Slough is usually soft, stringy, and pale yellow or gray.

Eschar is thick, hard, and black or brown, also known as an unstageable pressure ulcer.

Extent and Type of Tissue in Wound Base. Assessment of the types of tissue and their amounts can give you an idea of the severity of the wound, needed treatment options, and/or healing of the wound. Table 36-4 outlines different types of tissue you might see in a wound bed. Viable (living) tissue must be distinguished from nonviable tissue. Many wounds may have different types of tissue at the same time. Describe each type with percentages. For example, "80% of the wound bed contains granulation tissue, and 20% remains necrotic." Granulation tissue is evidence of healing. A pale color or dry texture may indicate a delay in healing. Necrotic tissue of any type will delay wound healing and should be removed. The exception is stable eschar on a heel that is firmly attached to the healthy wound edges without signs of infection.

Drainage. Determine whether exudate is present. If so, describe the amount, color, consistency, and odor. Compare changes in the exudate to the patient's previous status.

- *Amount.* Describe the amount as none, light, moderate, or heavy. Drainage amounts vary according to the type of wound (i.e., venous stasis ulcers usually produce more drainage than do arterial ulcers).
- *Drains.* If a drain is present, measure the amount of fluid in the collection container.
- *Color.* Describe the color or consistency as serous or clear, serosanguineous, sanguineous, purulent, or seropurulent.
- *Odor.* Describe odor as absent, faint, moderate, or strong. Clean the wound of all exudate or foreign material before assessing for odor because odor characteristics vary depending on the wound moisture, organisms, amount of nonviable tissue or types of dressings used. Odor may indicate fistula formation or bacterial contamination. For example, if a patient has an abdominal wound that was odorless but begins to smell of bile or feces, you should carefully assess for presence of a fistula.

Wound and Tissue Pain. Routinely ask your patients about pain or discomfort related to the wound or wound care. You will need to develop a pain management plan if the patient is uncomfortable. Always take seriously the patient's complaint of pain, especially if there is a sudden increase. Pain is often an early symptom of infection. In the immunocompromised patient, pain may be the only symptom of infection (Branom, 2002).

Nutritional Status. Screen and assess nutritional status for each patient with a pressure ulcer at admission. If nutritional problems are present, a referral to the dietitian for early assessment of and intervention may be necessary. Sufficient calories are needed for wound healing. This may involve adding oral supplemental meals, or even enteral or parenteral nutrition (EPUAP and NPUAP, 2009a).

Assessing Untreated Wounds

For an untreated wound, make the same assessments as for a treated wound (see the Focused Assessment box, Physical Examination: Wound Assessment). Also, make additional assessments that allow you to determine the immediate treatment needed. For example, assess for bleeding. If bleeding is profuse, apply direct pressure to the site. If bleeding continues after you apply pressure for 5 minutes or if blood is spurting from the wound, call the provider immediately. Severe pain, numbness, or loss of movement below the wound also requires immediate, comprehensive evaluation.

Also determine whether the patient needs a tetanus immunization. Tetanus-prone wounds include compound fractures, gunshot wounds, crush injuries, burns, punctures, foreign object injuries, wounds contaminated with soil, and wounds neglected for more than 24 hours. An immunization should be given if:

- The last immunization was 10 years ago or longer (Immunization Action Coalition, 2007 [reviewed by the Centers for Disease Control and Prevention (CDC), 2009]).
- The wound is contaminated with dirt or debris, and the most recent tetanus immunization was given more than 5 years ago.
- It is uncertain when the patient last received an immunization.

Evaluating Pressure Ulcer Healing

In addition to the Braden and Norton risk assessments previously described, the Agency for Healthcare Research and Quality (AHRQ) and NPUAP recommend use of the *PUSH Tool* to evaluate existing pressure ulcers (NPUAP, 2003). The tool provides a comprehensive means of reporting the progression of a pressure ulcer. Surface area, exudate, and type of wound tissue are scored and totaled. As the ulcer heals, the total score falls. See the Focused Assessment box, The PUSH Tool for Evaluation of Pressure Ulcers.

Table 36-4 ➤ Types of Tissue in the Wound Bed		
TYPE OF TISSUE	**DESCRIPTION**	**NURSING GOAL**
Slough (moist, devitalized tissue)	Soft, moist, devitalized (necrotic) tissue; may be white, yellow, tan; may be stringy, loose, or adherent to bed.	Débride the wound.
Eschar	Necrotic tissue; dry, thick, leathery; may be black, brown, or gray depending on moisture level.	Débride the wound.
Granulation Tissue	Pink to red moist tissue; made of new blood vessels, connective tissue, and fibroblasts; surface is granular or pebble-like.	Cleanse, protect.
Clean, Nongranulating	Absence of granulation tissue, but bed is pink, shiny, and smooth	Cleanse, protect.
Epithelial	Regenerating epidermis; may appear pink or pearly white as it crosses the wound bed; may begin as a ring around the wound or from epithelial cells lining hair follicles.	Cleanse, protect.

The PUSH Tool for Evaluation of Pressure Ulcers

PUSH Tool - Version 3.0

Patient Name:_____   Patient ID#:_____

Ulcer Location: _____   Date:_____

DIRECTIONS:
Observe and measure the pressure ulcer. Categorize the ulcer with respect to surface area, exudate, and type of wound tissue. Record a sub-score for each of these ulcer characteristics. Add the sub-scores to obtain the total score. A comparison of total scores measured over time provides an indication of the improvement or deterioration in pressure ulcer healing.

	0	1	2	3	4	5	Subscore
Length x Width	0 cm^2	<0.3 cm^2	0.3 - 0.6 cm^2	0.7 - 1.0 cm^2	1.1 - 2.0 cm^2	2.1 - 3.0 cm^2	
	6	**7**	**8**	**9**	**10**		
	3.1 - 4.0 cm^2	4.1 - 8.0 cm^2	8.1 - 12.0 cm^2	12.1 - 24.0 cm^2	> 24 cm^2		
	0	**1**	**2**	**3**			Subscore
Exudate Amount	None	Light	Moderate	Heavy			
	0	**1**	**2**	**3**	**4**		Subscore
Tissue Type	Closed	Epithelial Tissue	Granulation Tissue	Slough	Necrotic Tissue		
							Total Score

Length x Width: Measure the greatest length (head to toe) and the greatest width (side to side) using a centimeter ruler. Multiply these two measurements (length • width) to obtain an estimate of surface area in square centimeters (cm^2). **Caveat:** Do not guess! Always use a centimeter ruler and always use the same method each time the ulcer is measured.

Exudate Amount: Estimate the amount of exudate (drainage) present after removal of the dressing and before applying any topical agent to the ulcer. Estimate the exudate (drainage) as none, light, moderate, or heavy.

Tissue Type: This refers to the types of tissue that are present in the wound (ulcer) bed. Score as a "4" if there is any necrotic tissue present. Score as a "3" if there is any amount of slough present and necrotic tissue is absent. Score as a "2" if the wound is clean and contains granulation tissue. A superficial wound that is reepithelializing is scored as a "1". When the wound is closed, score as a "0".

  4 - Necrotic Tissue (Eschar): black, brown, or tan tissue that adheres firmly to the wound bed or ulcer edges and may be either firmer or softer than surrounding skin.

  3 - Slough: yellow or white tissue that adheres to the ulcer bed in strings or thick clumps, or is mucinous.

  2 - Granulation Tissue: pink or beefy red tissue with a shiny, moist, granular appearance.

  1 - Epithelial Tissue: for superficial ulcers, new pink or shiny tissue (skin) that grows in from the edges or as islands on the ulcer surface.

  0 - Closed/Resurfaced: the wound is completely covered with epithelium (new skin).

Note: Refer to the NPUAP Website (www.npuap.org) for further information regarding development and use of the PUSH Tool.

Focused Assessment

PRESSURE ULCER HEALING CHART
(use a separate page for each pressure ulcer)

Patient Name:_____   Patient ID#:_____

Ulcer Location: _____   Date:_____

Directions: Observe and measure pressure ulcers at regular intervals using the PUSH Tool. Date and record PUSH Sub-scale and Total Scores on the Pressure Ulcer Healing Record below.

PRESSURE ULCER HEALING RECORD

DATE												
Length × Width												
Exudate Amount												
Tissue Type												
Total Score												

Graph the PUSH Total Score on the Pressure Ulcer Healing Graph below.

PUSH Total Score	PRESSURE ULCER HEALING GRAPH											
17												
16												
15												
14												
13												
12												
11												
10												
9												
8												
7												
6												
5												
4												
3												
2												
1												
Healed 0												
DATE:												

Version 3.0: 9/15/98
© National Pressure Ulcer Advisory Panel

Laboratory Data

The most common laboratory assessments performed on clients with wounds or risk for impaired skin integrity are protein levels, complete blood count, erythrocyte sedimentation rate, glucose, thyroid and iron levels, coagulation studies, and wound cultures. See the accompanying Diagnostic Testing box.

Wound cultures may be ordered to determine the types of bacteria present in the wound. Local or systemic signs of infection, suddenly elevated glucose levels, pain in a neuropathic extremity, or lack of healing after 2 weeks in a clean wound may indicate the need for a wound culture. Cultures may be obtained by swab, aspiration, or tissue biopsy.

Swabbing. The most common and most noninvasive method to obtain a culture is with a swab. Swab specimens are acceptably accurate in representing bacteria counts biopsied from wound tissue (Bill, Ratliff, Donovan, et al., 2001; Gardner, Frantz, Saltzman, et al., 2006). The Wound, Ostomy and Continence Nurses Society (WOCNS, 2007) recommends using swab cultures as a reasonable alternative to biopsy in the clinical setting. See Procedure 36-1.

Needle Aspiration. Specially trained providers may perform needle aspiration of a wound. This involves insertion of a needle in the tissue to aspirate tissue fluid. Organisms present in the tissue fluid can then be detected. Needle aspiration is an invasive procedure, with the risk of inadvertent needle damage to tissue and underlying structures (Procedure 36-2).

Tissue Biopsy. The most accurate method for culturing a chronic wound is *tissue biopsy*. It has long been considered

Diagnostic Testing

Tests for Assessing Wounds

Test	Normal Range	Comments
Leukocyte (WBC) count	4,500–11,000/mm^3	Usually done as a part of a complete blood count (CBC) but may be ordered as an independent test. WBCs may increase when a wound develops; continued elevation may signal infection. A low WBC count may delay wound healing. Leukocytes are responsible for an inflammatory reaction at the wound site, phagocytosis of bacteria and cellular debris, and the creation of antibodies.
Serum protein Serum albumin Serum prealbumin	6.0–8.0 g/dL 3.4–4.8 g/dL 12–42 mg/dL	Low serum levels indicate limited nutritional stores that delay wound healing or place the patient at high risk for pressure ulcers. Serum protein may be monitored as an indicator of the ability to heal a wound or prevent a pressure ulcer. Serum protein and albumin levels are closely related. However, both fluctuate slowly. A more accurate measure of a patient's immediate protein stores is reflected in prealbumin level.
Erythrocyte sedimentation rate (ESR)	Younger than 50 yr: 0–15 mm/hr; older than 50 yr: 0–20 mm/hr	In the presence of an inflammatory and necrotic process, blood proteins are altered. This test indicates whether the RBCs stick together, become heavier, and settle at the bottom of a lab tube when held vertically.
Coagulation studies: Partial thromboplastin time, activated (aPTT)	Varies with respect to equipment and reagents used. Critical values: >70 sec or <53 sec	Prolonged coagulation times may result in excessive blood loss or ongoing bleeding in the wound bed. Shortened coagulation times increase the risk for blood clot formation problems, such as deep vein thrombosis, pulmonary embolus, or stroke.
Prothrombin time (clotting time)	Critical values: >20 sec (uncoagulated) or 3 times normal control (anticoagulated)	Altered coagulation may result from anticoagulant medications, a concurrent illness, trauma, or reaction to transfusions.
International normalized ratio (INR)	< 2.0 for patients not receiving anticoagulation therapy; 2.0–3.0 for those receiving coagulation therapy	A standardized test to evaluate clotting times, considered the gold standard.
Wound cultures	Negative; no growth of pathogens	Wound cultures may be prescribed to determine the types of bacteria present in the wound. Cultures may be obtained by swab, aspiration, or tissue biopsy. A positive culture may not indicate an infection as chronic wounds are colonized with bacteria.
Tissue biopsy	Negative; no growth of pathogens	Wounds are not considered infected unless the bacteria count exceeds 100,000 organisms per gram of tissue. Exception: The presence of beta-hemolytic streptococci in any number indicates infection.

the gold standard. Tissue is removed from the wound edge by a specially trained provider. However, many facilities do not have the equipment needed to process tissue samples. This is an invasive procedure, causes pain, and disrupts the wound bed, sometimes delaying healing. Biopsy also creates a risk of sepsis.

KnowledgeCheck 36-7

- What should be included in a wound assessment?
- What is the preferred method of wound culture that may be performed by a registered nurse?
- Identify three types of laboratory data that may be associated with a delay in wound healing.

What Assessments Can I Delegate?

Initial assessment of a wound, as well as ongoing evaluation of a wound that requires treatment, must be done by the registered nurse. You may delegate to nursing assistive personnel (NAP) inspection of the skin for evidence of skin breakdown. Instruct the NAP to notify you of redness, tissue warmth, or drainage. You may also delegate turning and position changes to the NAP. Turning and movement prevent tissue damage from ischemia, thereby preventing pressure ulcers.

ANALYSIS/NURSING DIAGNOSIS

The following nursing diagnoses are appropriate for patients who are at risk for skin breakdown or for patients who have wounds.

- *Risk for Impaired Skin Integrity* is appropriate for patients who have one or more risk factors for skin breakdown (e.g., immobility, incontinence, extremes of age, impaired circulation, emaciation). NANDA International (NANDA-I, 2012) recommends that you use a risk assessment tool (e.g., Norton or Braden scale) to identify these patients.
- *Impaired Skin Integrity* is appropriate for patients who have experienced damage to the epidermis or dermis, for example, patients who have superficial wounds or stage I or II pressure ulcers.
- *Impaired Tissue Integrity* is appropriate for patients with wounds that extend into the subcutaneous tissue, muscle, or bone. Use this diagnosis for patients with deep wounds or stage III or IV pressure ulcers.
- *Risk for Impaired Tissue Integrity* is appropriate for clients with Impaired Skin Integrity who are at risk for delayed healing. For example, Mr. Harmon (Meet Your Patient) has a stage I pressure ulcer but is at risk for further progression of the ulcer because of his age, nutritional state, and the presence of another wound. Note that this is not a NANDA-I diagnosis; however, it is useful in the situation described.

 Skin problems and wounds can be the etiology for other nursing diagnoses, for example:

- *Risk for Infection* is an appropriate diagnosis if the patient has a traumatic wound or is immunosuppressed, undernourished, or immobile.
- *Pain* is a diagnosis that may be used for patients who are experiencing discomfort from the wound or from the treatments for it.
- *Disturbed Body Image* should be used if the patient is experiencing distress about the wound. Consider this diagnosis even if the patient is expected to make a complete recovery.

Some patients experience extreme distress about wounds. You will certainly want to consider this diagnosis if the patient experiences an injury that is expected to result in disfigurement.

PLANNING OUTCOMES/EVALUATION

For associated NOC standardized outcomes for skin and tissue integrity diagnoses,

 Go to Chapter 36, **Standardized Language: Selected Standardized Outcomes and Interventions for Skin and Wound Diagnoses,** on Davis*Plus*.

Individualized goals/outcome statements should address the need to maintain intact skin or heal the wound. For patients who have a diagnosis of Risk for Impaired Skin Integrity, you might write a goal such as the following:

 Maintains intact skin throughout treatment, as evidenced by good skin turgor with no erythema, edema, or breaks in the skin.

For patients who have a wound (actual Impaired Skin Integrity or Impaired Tissue Integrity), you might write a goal such as the following:

 Wound will heal by May 1, as evidenced by a progressive decrease in the size of the wound, a decrease in drainage from the wound, improvement in the condition of the surrounding skin, and no evidence of infection (erythema, purulent drainage, or odor).

PLANNING INTERVENTIONS/IMPLEMENTATION

For NIC standardized interventions for skin and tissue integrity problems,

Go to Chapter 36, **Standardized Language: Selected Standardized Outcomes and Interventions for Skin and Wound Diagnoses,** on Davis*Plus*.

Specific nursing activities directed at maintaining skin integrity or healing wounds focus on preventing and treating pressure ulcers and other chronic wounds, providing wound care, and applying heat and cold therapies. In the next section, we discuss these nursing therapeutic measures.

Interventions for Example Problem: Pressure Ulcers

Pressure ulcers are extremely difficult and time-consuming to treat. As a result, prevention is the most important nursing intervention. *Healthy People 2020* proposed two public health objectives focused on pressure-related skin injury: (1) to reduce the proportion of nursing home residents with a current diagnosis of pressure ulcers, and (2) to reduce the rate of pressure ulcer-related hospitalizations among older adults by the year 2020 (USDHHS, 2010). The Institute for Healthcare Improvement (IHI, 2011) has made preventing pressure ulcers one of twelve goals in its 5 Million Lives Campaign. IHI recommended the six crucial elements in preventing pressure ulcers discussed following.

Conduct a Pressure Ulcer Admission Assessment for All Patients

Most agencies use a standardized risk assessment, such as the Braden and Norton scales, to assess the risk of pressure ulcers (see Pressure Ulcer Risk Assessment Measures in the Assessment

section). You should use these scales to assess the patient on admission to any type of facility (hospital, nursing home or with home healthcare). Risk factors not found on those scales will place your patient at even higher risk. Examples include age, fever, hypotension, and poor dietary intake.

Reassess Risk for All Patients Daily

✚ Reassess your hospitalized patient for risk daily because his condition can change frequently and rapidly. Any time your patient's condition changes or he is transferred to another unit, reassess his risk. Monitor a nursing home resident weekly for the first 4 weeks, then quarterly or whenever the patient's condition changes or deteriorates. Reassess home patients with every visit (WOCNS, 2007).

Once a patient is identified as being at risk for developing pressure ulcers, strategies can be implemented. Inform all members of the healthcare team (i.e., physical therapists, transporters, physicians, dietitians). Using visual cues, such as stickers on charts or dots on ID bands, can help remind staff.

Inspect Skin Daily

Skin care begins with regular inspection of the skin—at least daily for patients at risk—and usually every 8 to 12 hours for institutionalized patients. You must have adequate light to detect subtle, early skin changes. Use a penlight to inspect bony prominences if direct sunlight is not available. Be sure to check pressure points for erythema, tenderness, or edema. Instruct family members and caregivers about the importance of early detection of skin problems. In obese patients, skin damage can occur under breasts, abdominal folds, or anywhere skin contacts skin.

Manage Moisture

Excess moisture creates a risk for skin breakdown. Use the following nursing actions to help you manage moisture:

Incontinence Care. Provide skin care regularly soon after each incontinence episode. Apply incontinence or moisture barrier cream to protect perineal skin from urine and stool. Keep these products readily available for use by all staff members and family. Use undergarments or products that will wick moisture away from the skin.

Bathing. Soaps and bathing techniques can contribute to skin breakdown, so be careful to keep the skin clean and intact. Diaphoretic (sweaty) patients may need frequent bathing as sweat can be irritating to sensitive or injury-prone skin. Older adults most likely will not need daily bathing due to decreased oil and sweat production. Use warm water; hot water dries the skin. Gently bathe fragile skin, using a minimum of force and friction, as washcloths can be abrasive. Use a mild, emollient cleansing soap only as needed and not routinely; and be sure to rinse thoroughly and gently pat the skin dry (Joanna Briggs Institute, 2007). Soaps are drying to the skin because they remove oils from the skin and may interfere with the ability of the skin to hold water.

Lotion and Massage. If the patient's skin is dry, apply a moisturizing lotion using a gentle massaging motion to promote circulation and wound healing. ✚ Do not massage over bony prominences, which can irritate the area and lead to tissue injury (EPUAP and NPUAP, 2009b).

Linens. Keep the linen soft, clean, dry, and free from wrinkles by changing it frequently. Moisture and wrinkles in the sheets can damage to skin integrity.

Optimize Nutrition and Hydration

Nutrition is vital to skin integrity. Patients with rapid weight loss, high metabolic demands, limited intake, or decreased serum albumin are particularly at risk for developing pressure ulcers. Monitor hydration status and offer water (if appropriate) whenever you reposition the patient.

Carefully review the diet ordered for at-risk patients, and assess what the patient is eating. The diet may need to be modified to achieve adequate calorie and protein intake. Protein requirements may be as high as 2 grams per kilogram of body weight in a malnourished individual with a wound, so high-protein supplements may be necessary.

Consider the consistency of the diet as well. A soft diet may be helpful for a patient who is frail or is missing teeth. Tube feeding or parenteral nutrition may be prescribed to supplement oral intake if the patient is unable to consume adequate quantities of calories and protein. You may need to make a dietary referral.

Minimize Pressure

Most patients who are at risk for pressure ulcers have mobility problems. As a result, you must provide frequent position changes. This is one of the most important interventions for preventing pressure ulcers. You may delegate turning and position changes to the NAP. Turning and movement prevent tissue damage from ischemia, thereby preventing pressure ulcers (Joanna Briggs Institute, 2008a, 2008b).

Turning and Repositioning. Reposition the patient at least every 2 hours (Armstrong, Ayello, Capitulo, et al., 2008; Bergstrom, Bennett, Carlson, et al., 1994; Buss, Halfens, & Abu-Saad, 2002). However, patients with very fragile skin or little subcutaneous tissue might need to be repositioned more frequently. At-risk individuals who are chair bound should be repositioned every hour or taught to shift their weight every 15 minutes. Place a turning schedule at the bedside so that all caregivers can participate in the prevention strategy. For an example of a patient turning schedule,

 Go to Chapter 36, **Tables, Boxes, Figures: ESG Box 36-2: Scheduled Position Changes,** on Davis*Plus.*

Use the "rule of 30" to guide your positioning:

✚ Elevate the head of the bed 30° or less, and when the patient is on her side, position the patient at a 30° angle to avoid direct pressure on the trochanter. If the head of the bed is elevated more than 30°, limit the time in this position to minimize pressure and shear.

✚ To protect skin during turning or repositioning, use lift devices or drawsheets, heel and elbow protectors, or sleeves and stockings. Never drag a patient when pulling her up in bed.

Support Surfaces. Numerous support surfaces are available for preventing and treating pressure ulcers. They do so by redistributing pressure and controlling moisture to prevent bacterial growth on the skin (microclimate between the skin and the surface of the bed). Support surfaces include specialty mattresses, integrated bed systems, mattress replacements, and overlays. These products may consist of air, gel, foam, or water, and are available in various sizes and shapes for beds, chairs, exam tables, and operating room tables (Fig. 36-9).

✚ Any patient at risk should be placed on a pressure-redistributing device. Of course, use of support surfaces should not be the only prevention measure, but should be coupled with effective turning and positioning schedules (NPUAP and EPUAP, 2009b).

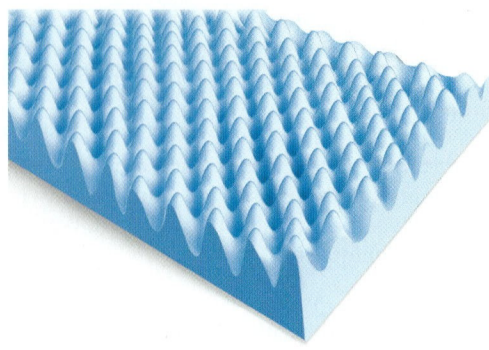

FIGURE 36-9 An egg crate mattress is a nonpowered foam mattress overlay used to redistribute pressure.

 Protect heels by using products that completely raise the heels off the bed. Pillows may not be enough to redistribute the weight of your patient's foot, and donut-type devices should not be used. Pressure redistributing devices are made for chairs and wheelchairs too.

To see a decision-making tree developed by the AHRQ to guide the selection of appropriate support surfaces,

 Go to Chapter 36, **Tables, Boxes, Figures: ESG Figure 36-2: Decision Tree Guiding Selection of Appropriate Support Surfaces,** on Davis*Plus*.

What Are Adjunctive Wound Care Therapies?

The use of adjunctive therapies is the fastest growing area in pressure-related wound management. Nurses apply adjunctive therapies that include negative pressure wound therapy, electrical stimulation, hyperbaric oxygen, radiant heat, tissue growth factors, ultrasound, bioengineered skin equivalents, and surgical options. Hyperbaric oxygen therapy and surgical options were discussed under Advanced Wound Treatments, in the Theoretical Knowledge section; they are listed but not discussed here.

- **Negative Pressure Wound Therapy.** Using a specialized pump, negative pressure is placed on a wound packed with foam or gauze dressings to create a vacuum. The subatmospheric pressure reduces edema from swollen tissues, promotes granulation tissue formation, and removes exudate and infectious material (Procedure 36-7).
- **Silver Dressing.** Silver-coated dressings or silver-based cream may act as a barrier to bacterial penetration in the wound bed. Silver may eradicate biofilms of colonized bacteria.

 Go to Chapter 36, **Tables, Boxes, Figures: ESG Table 36-1: Silver Dressings Used in Chronic Wound Management,** on Davis*Plus*.

- **Electrical Stimulation.** Electrical currents are transferred across tissues to aid in chronic wound healing. Electrodes are placed around the wound bed and connected to a machine that produces an electrical impulse. This therapy stimulates cellular growth through development of fibroblasts, new collagen, and increased blood flow and tissue oxygenation.
- **Hyperbaric Oxygen Therapy.** High oxygen therapy can be used to accelerate healing.

- **Tissue Growth Factors.** Tissue growth factors are proteins that occur naturally in the body and cause specific cells to grow and replicate. Platelet-derived growth factor has been used in chronic wound healing. It is indicated for diabetic and other nonhealing wounds that are clean of necrotic tissue and have good vascularity.
- **Ultrasound.** Another adjunctive therapy used in chronic wound healing, is ultrasound. Sound waves are emitted by a control unit and handheld sound head or transducer. Vibrations from the transducer create sound waves that pass into the tissue, causing it to vibrate and heat up. This stimulates movement of fluid within and between cells and aids in débridement and increased cell metabolism.
- **Bioengineered Skin Substitutes.** This is a group of substances that aid in the temporary or permanent closure of wounds. Substitutes may be actual human epidermis or dermis, animal cells, or synthetic material. They can be used to treat partial- and full-thickness wounds.
- **Surgical Options.** Surgical excision and débridement, skin graft, drain, flaps and other methods may be used to treat wounds and promote healing.

What Patient and Family Teaching Do I Need to Do?

Teaching the at-risk patient and family about pressure ulcer prevention is a key prevention strategy. Include the following topics in your teaching:
- Characteristics of healthy skin
- Appearance of skin that has experienced unrelieved pressure
- Skin care and hygiene
- Protection of the skin and prevention of pressure ulcers
- Importance of adequate nutrition
- Techniques for turning and positioning
- Importance of frequent position changes
- Use of pressure-redistributing devices
- Skin changes that should be reported to healthcare professionals

The following are some simple tips for taking care of wounds at home that you can teach families (ICSI, 2008). If the wound is:

Wet → dry it
Open → cover it
Unclean → clean it
Necrotic → don't scrub it
Dry → moisten it

KnowledgeCheck 36-8

- Identify the major interventions for preventing pressure ulcers.
- What nursing diagnosis is most appropriate for a patient at risk for pressure ulcer development?

What Wound Care Competencies Do I Need?

Care planning to meet the complex, individualized needs of a patient with a chronic wound involves the entire multidisciplinary team (e.g., physical therapists, dietitians, infection control specialist, wound specialist). Your wound assessment will guide your choice of interventions, which depend on the nature of the wound. Consider these two examples:
- A patient with a diabetic foot ulcer must have all the pressure taken off that area because every step traumatizes healing tissues. This patient will also need to wear a special shoe that is especially made for patients with neuropathy.

■ A patient with a venous stasis ulcer will need to wear a compression garment (hose, stocking or multilayer compression wrap). These apply continuous pressure to the veins, which helps venous return and allows the ulcer to heal. See Chapter 40 if you need more information about compression (antiembolism) stockings.

Wound care is more than placing a dressing into a wound. It incorporates all of the strategies for preventing that wound, as well as treating it. These interventions can also be used in treating other types of acute and chronic wounds. For an example of how wound management software can help you to more efficiently care for your patients' wounds, see the QSEN box, Improving Wound Care With Information Technology.

Cleansing Wounds

Wounds are cleansed to remove exudate, slough, foreign materials, and microorganisms. Cleansing also helps to promote healthy tissue healing. Historically, antiseptic solutions, such as Dakin's, acetic acid, hydrogen peroxide, povidone-iodine, and alcohol, were used to cleanse all types of wounds. However, research shows that these antiseptic solutions can damage granulating tissue and should not be used on healing tissue. Antiseptic solutions should be reserved for wounds that won't heal or those in which the bacterial burden is more harmful than the solution itself.

Because normal saline is physiological, it is safe and it will not harm injured or healing tissue. It will adequately cleanse most wounds if a sufficient amount is used to thoroughly flush the wound. Drinkable tap water is as effective as saline to cleanse a wound (Fernandez & Griffiths, 2010). Liquid or foam skin cleansers that are pH balanced may be used to cleanse

periwound skin or incontinence effluent. They are not for use in wounds. **Key Point:** *Regardless of the type of solution used, be sure to use universal precautions to minimize the risk of cross-contamination.*

Always clean a wound initially and with each dressing change. To cleanse a wound, gently pat the surface with gauze soaked with saline or other prescribed wound cleanser. If there is granulation tissue, be careful not to disrupt it. Wound irrigation is a gentle technique.

Irrigating Wounds

Nurses commonly use irrigation **(lavage)** to cleanse wounds gently by flushing. To remove debris from a wound, you must introduce the irrigation solution with a mild amount of force. Ideal irrigation pressures range from 4 pounds per square inch (psi) to 15 psi. To remove material adhering to the wound bed, use a 35-mL syringe attached to a 19-gauge angiocatheter to deliver the solution at approximately 8 psi (Branom, 2002; Campton-Johnston & Wilson, 2001; ICSI, 2007, updated 2010). Pressures above 15 psi increase the risk of driving bacteria into the tissues, as well as causing mechanical damage.

Some agencies use a piston syringe for irrigation. Do not use a bulb syringe; it increases the risk of aspirating the drainage. Commercial irrigation systems are also available. Closely evaluate the amount of pressure they deliver before you use these devices.

There is a risk of splattering with this technique, so you must use gowns, masks, and goggles. Sterile technique is used for acute surgical wounds, wounds that have recently undergone sharp débridement, or when prescribed by the physician (Procedure 36-3). The majority of wound irrigation uses clean technique.

Improving Wound Care With Information Technology

Competency: Informatics (Knowledge); Quality Improvement (Knowledge); Evidenced-Based Practice (Attitudes)*

Information technology (IT) can have a significant impact on wound care management—from reducing documentation time to tracking outcomes:

➤ Extensive documentation of wound care is required for both clinical and reimbursement.

➤ Electronic documentation systems save time by using data entered once and adding it in all the other fields where it is required. Eliminating duplication allows for more time to spend in patient care.

➤ Wound management software incorporates best practices into care management algorithms, decision supports, and alerts based on the type and stage of each wound. Changes in wound characteristics or new patient information initiate computer prompts that request more information or suggest treatment changes. For example, if the patient begins a new medication that can delay wound healing, a prompt may ask if another medication can be used instead; or the prompt might suggest more frequent monitoring of wound characteristics.

➤ When you upload photographs and multiple measurements of the patient's wound(s), they become part of the

electronic care plan and pop up in chronological order so that you can visualize how the wound is healing.

➤ Clinicians can also set reminders for initiating future steps or referrals, eliminating the need to rely on memory and reducing errors.

Think about it: Informatics is the use of information and technology to communicate, manage knowledge, mitigate error, and support decision making. Can you think how other patient conditions can benefit from specific management software? What might the information technology software look like for patients with high blood pressure or obesity?

➤ What data would be collected?

➤ What information might be generated from the data?

➤ What errors might be prevented?

---

*For specific Knowledge, Skills, and Attitudes,

 Go to the QSEN web site at http:www.qsen.org.ksas_ prelicensure.php

Sources: Health Leaders Media. (2007, January). New-age wound care solutions drive improved efficiency, outcomes, and patient satisfaction. Retrieved January 8, 2012, from http://www.healthleadersmedia. com/HOM-67349-4625/Newage-wound-care-solutions-drive-improved-efficiency-outcomes

Toward Evidence-Based Practice

Fernandez, R., & Griffiths, R. (2010, March 14). Water for wound cleansing. *Cochrane Database of Systematic Reviews*, Issue 1. Art. No.: CD003861. DOI: 10.1002/14651858. CD003861.pub2. Retrieved November 11, 2011, from http://onlinelibrary.wiley.com/doi/10.1002/14651858.CD003861.pub3/abstract;jsessionid=94E5F79C171A975B6C84A39DA9082.

Use of saline versus tap water for cleansing wounds is debated. Normal saline is traditionally preferred because it cleanses without interfering with the normal healing process. Yet, tap water is used commonly in the community for cleaning wounds and for care of chronic wounds because it is generally free of pathogens, yet easily accessible and inexpensive. Researchers wanted to know if rates of infection and healing differ depending on whether tap water or normal sterile saline is used to clean acute and chronic wounds. They analyzed findings from 24 clinical studies. Results showed no differences in the rates of infections among acute and chronic wounds in adults and children cleansed with tap water as compared to those washed with saline.

1. What trend in the research about cleansing wounds do you see as compared to previous times?

2. If study findings indicate little difference in wound infection when tap water is used for cleansing, then what would you recommend to those using tap water in the community?

3. What implications does using tap water for cleaning wounds have when sending patients home after surgery?

 Go to Chapter 36, **Toward Evidence-Based Practice Suggested Responses,** on *DavisPlus*.

Caring for Wounds With Drainage Devices

By allowing fluid and exudate to exit, drains prevent excessive pressure from building up in the tissues. Drains are usually placed during a surgical procedure. Some are sutured into place, whereas others are simply placed into the cavity.

Types of Drains

A *Penrose drain* is a flexible latex tube that is placed in the wound bed but usually not sutured into place. A clip or pin may be attached to keep it from slipping further into the wound. You may be asked to advance the drain by gradually removing it from the wound bed. For example, the surgeon may prescribe: "Advance the Penrose drain 6 mm (¼ in.) per day." Each day you pull the drain out of the wound 6 mm (¼ in.) until the drain is finally removed Procedure 36-14 explains how to shorten a drain.

Some drains are attached to a collection device. Examples include Hemovac, Jackson-Pratt, and Davol drains (Fig. 36-10). The surgeon may order a device to be "placed to suction." This means that you will compress the device to create suction and facilitate removal of drainage (Fig. 36-11). To learn to empty closed drains, see Procedure 36-15.

If a specific pressure is to be applied, some drains can be connected to wall suction. The provider will prescribe the amount of suction. For example, a surgeon may prescribe: "Place Hemovac to 20 mm Hg suction at all times."

Nursing Activities for Maintaining Drains

You are responsible for monitoring wound drains. The surgeon will describe the number and type of drains present. Describe drain placement according to the position on the clock face. Consider the patient's head to be at the 12 o'clock position. Some patients have more than one drainage device in a wound. Label the drains numerically with a marker or by placing tape on the collection apparatus so that each caregiver provides consistent care.

When removing dressings or irrigating wounds, take care to avoid dislodging any drains. Remember, many drains are not sutured in place. Monitor the amount and character of the drainage and the condition of the collection apparatus. Record

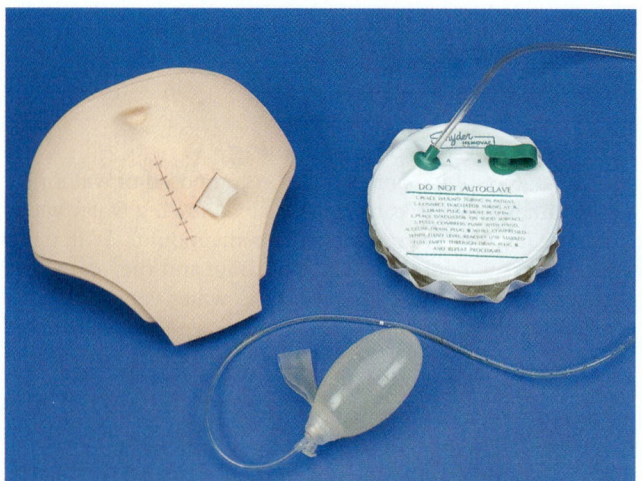

FIGURE 36-10 *Left,* Penrose drain. *Center,* Jackson-Pratt device. *Right,* Hemovac drainage system.

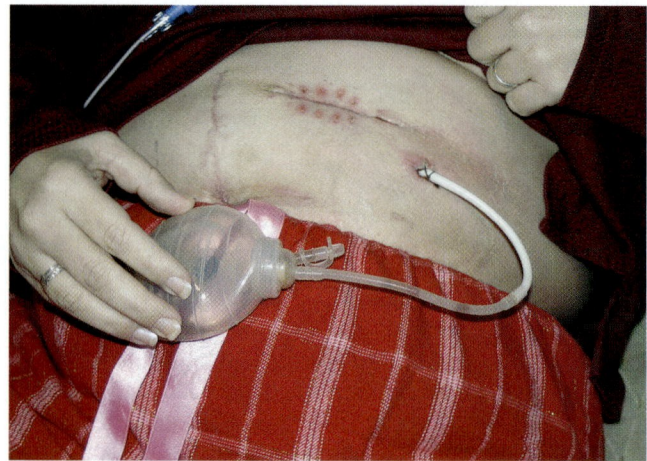

FIGURE 36-11 Compress the bulb of the Jackson–Pratt drain to create suction and remove wound drainage.

this information in your nursing notes as well as on the intake and output (I&O) record. Report to the surgeon any change in the amount or character of the drainage.

You need to empty the collection apparatus at a designated volume to maintain suction. As the device fills, suction pressure decreases. If there is significant drainage, you may need to empty the device several times during your shift. If you suspect a drain is occluded, check the drain line from the insertion site to the collection device. Remove any kinks in the tubing. If this does not correct the problem, notify the provider of the blockage.

KnowledgeCheck 36-9

- Identify goals for wound care before applying a dressing to a wound.
- What solutions are used to cleanse a wound?
- How can you control the amount of force applied for wound irrigation?
- Identify three nursing responsibilities when caring for a client with a wound drain.

 ## ThinkLike a Nurse 36-5

- Describe the percentage and type of tissue found in Mr. Harmon's wounds.
- What are the goals of treatment with both of Mr. Harmon's wounds?

Débriding a Wound

Débridement is the removal of devitalized tissue or foreign material from a wound. It also helps remove cells that are alive but not functioning **(senescent)** from the wound bed and edges. Removal of necrotic tissue, exudate, and infective material helps stimulate wound healing and prepare the wound bed for advanced therapies or biological agents. There are five types of débridement: sharp or surgical, mechanical, enzymatic, autolytic, and biotherapy or maggot therapy.

Sharp Débridement

Sharp débridement is the use of a sharp instrument, such as scalpel or scissors, to remove devitalized tissue. This method provides an immediate improvement of the wound bed and preserves granulation tissue. However, it requires specialized training. A physician, nurse, or physical therapist may perform this procedure at the bedside. If a wound requires extensive débridement, it may be performed in the operating room. Many stage IV ulcers extend into the bone, so a bone biopsy is often performed at the same time. A biopsy will detect **osteomyelitis**, extension of the infection into the bone.

Mechanical Débridement

Mechanical débridement may be performed via lavage (discussed in a preceding section), the use of wet-to-dry dressings, or hydrotherapy (whirlpool).

- **Wet-to-Dry Dressings.** Coarse gauze moistened with normal saline is packed into the wound, allowed to dry, and then removed, perhaps several times a day. This form of débridement was common once, but has declined in use because it provides only **nonselective débridement.** That is, it removes not only debris, but also granulation tissue, and it causes pain. If you must use this method, medicate the patient beforehand with opioid analgesics. Rewetting the gauze aids in its removal and decreases the pain, but it may eliminate the débriding action of the dressing change.

- **Hydrotherapy or Whirlpool Treatments.** Hydrotherapy or whirlpool treatments also provide nonselective débridement. This is a vigorous form of débridement reserved for wounds with a large amount of nonviable tissue, such as burns. Usually this treatment is performed in the physical therapy department once or twice per day. The wound is placed in a whirlpool containing tepid water for a prescribed amount of time (usually 5 to 15 minutes). Do not expose the wound directly to the water jets.

Whirlpool treatments increase the risk for periwound maceration, contamination by waterborne infections, and cross-contamination. Therefore, strict adherence to infection control measures is essential. Use hydrotherapy with caution in patients with venous stasis ulcers because it leads to vasodilation, which may increase edema and congestion. Persons with diabetic neuropathies are at increased risk for burns because of a decrease in sensory abilities.

Enzymatic Débridement

Enzymatic débridement uses proteolytic agents to break down necrotic tissue without affecting viable tissue in the wound. To use an enzymatic product, clean the wound with normal saline, apply a thin layer of the cream, and cover with a moisture-retaining dressing. This may be done once or twice daily, depending on the product. Apply the product only to devitalized tissue because it might cause some local irritation.

Autolysis

Autolysis is the use of an occlusive, moisture-retaining dressing and the body's own enzymes and defense mechanisms to break down necrotic tissue. This process takes more time than the other techniques, but it is tolerated better. The procedure involves applying the dressing and observing the fluid that collects under it (wound fluid may be tan in color). The dressing is normally changed every 72 hours. At that time, the wound is cleansed before a new dressing is applied. Observe the wound closely and regularly for signs of infection, such as an increase in pain or a foul odor. Autolysis is contraindicated in the presence of infection or immunosuppression.

Biotherapy or Maggot Débridement Therapy

Maggot débridement therapy is the use of medical-grade larvae of the green bottle fly to dissolve dead and infected tissue from wounds. The larvae secrete enzymes that liquefy dead tissue and create an alkaline environment. The enzymes are neutralized when they come in contact with normal tissue, so healthy tissue is unharmed. The larvae also digest bacteria from the wound. This therapy is effective and simple to use, although containing the larvae within the dressing can be problematic. Larvae are usually changed every 48 to 72 hours and disposed of as biohazardous medical waste.

Providing Moist Wound Healing

More than 65% of the human body is composed of water. The skin maintains this level of moisture by allowing water vapor to escape into the air around us in small amounts. With damage to the skin, body cells can dehydrate and die, so wound dressings must function as a barrier to water vapor loss. The type of dressing used on a wound depends on the characteristics of the wound and the goals of treatment. The dressing of choice should do the following:

- Prevent drying of the wound bed.
- Absorb drainage.
- Keep the surrounding tissue dry and intact.
- Protect from contamination and infection.
- Aid in hemostasis.

- Débride the wound.
- Eliminate dead space.
- Prevent heat loss.
- Splint the wound site.
- Provide comfort to the patient.
- Control odor.

Each wound must be treated individually based on the patient history and assessment. When choosing a dressing, ask yourself if it will achieve the purposes listed above (e.g., Can it be removed without damaging fragile skin or the wound itself?). Also consider how long it should stay in place and how often it needs to be changed.

New products are continually introduced, but the "newest" dressing is not necessarily the best for the wound. Perform ongoing reassessment of your dressing choice every time you assess the wound. Modify dressings and wound treatments as the wound evolves.

The goal of all wound care is to heal the wound in the most rapid and comfortable manner, protect it from further injury and infection, and minimize scarring when possible.

KnowledgeCheck 36-10

- What should you consider when choosing a dressing?
- Describe the five types of wound débridement.
- Identify the purposes of a wound dressing.

Primary dressings are ones that are placed in the wound bed and actually touch the wound. A **secondary dressing** is one that covers or holds a primary dressing in place. Many dressings can act as both, touching the wound bed and securing themselves to the wound with some type of adhesive (Table 36-5).

KnowledgeCheck 36-11

- Differentiate among the different categories of dressings.
- What types of dressings may be used for wounds with a large amount of exudate?
- What form of dressing is appropriate for a wound with an eschar that needs to be eliminated?

Securing Dressings

What you will use to secure a dressing depends on wound size, location, amount of drainage, frequency of dressing changes, patient's activity level, and type of dressings used. Tape, ties, bandages, secondary dressings, and binders are among the choices. Tape is most commonly used. Tape is available in several forms:

- **Adhesive tape** provides stability to a dressing. It is tough and durable and can be used if you need to apply pressure to a wound. It leaves a residue on the skin and can cause trauma to surrounding intact skin when it is removed. However, commercial adhesive removers are available to remove the residue.
- **Foam tape** readily molds to the contours of the body and is ideal for dressings over joints.
- **Nonallergenic tape and paper tape** are best for sensitive skin. Ask patients whether they have any history of tape allergies or irritation, and use a tape that the patient has tolerated well in the past.

To tape a dressing, place strips of tape at the ends of the dressing, and space them evenly over the remainder of the dressing (Fig. 36-13A–C). Also see Procedure 36-4.

If a dressing requires frequent changes, you can use **Montgomery straps** with ties to secure the dressing (Fig. 36-14). Montgomery straps decrease the amount of pulling and irritation of skin around a wound. Apply the adhesive part of the straps to the skin at the ends of the dressing and at evenly spaced intervals. Lace the cloth ties between the straps to secure the dressing. Change the ties whenever they become soiled. Keep the straps in place until they begin to loosen from the skin.

Consider using thin hydrocolloids, low-adhesion foam dressings, or skin sealants under tape to help prevent skin tears. For the fragile skin of older adults or infants, use porous tapes and avoid unnecessary tape use.

Controlling Infection

A wound provides a portal of entry or exit for microorganisms. When caring for patients with closed wounds, follow CDC Standard Precautions. For patients with open or draining wounds, follow CDC Tier 2: Contact Level Precautions in addition to Standard Precautions. To review, see Chapter 22, and also, see Clinical Insights 22-3 and 22-4. Also observe the following guidelines:

Asepsis Measures. If the patient has an infection, place her in a private room or in a room with a patient who has an active infection caused by the same organism and no other infections. Follow any additional specific precautions for the microorganism identified. Most important, wash your hands frequently.

Use clean gloves when caring for the patient with a wound. Remove gloves, and wash your hands before coming in contact with another patient. Change your gloves after removing a soiled dressing, before applying a clean dressing.

If a patient has multiple wounds, treat the least contaminated wound first, then progress to the most contaminated. Wash your hands and change gloves between each wound.

Sharp Débridement. Use sterile instruments for sharp débridement. Monitor the patient for signs and symptoms of sepsis (fever, tachycardia, hypotension, altered level of consciousness) after sharp débridement.

Dressings and Supplies. Use clean dressings when treating a chronic wound. Acute wounds may require sterile dressings. An immunocompromised patient may require sterile dressings even if the wound is chronic. Carefully dispose of contaminated dressings in biohazard waste receptacles.

Store patient dressing supplies in a clean and dry area. Do not share supplies among more than one patient. Access only the number of supplies you need for the dressing change. Do not touch the supply of dressings with gloves that have come in contact with the wound. Discard unused dressings if they become contaminated.

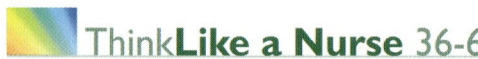

ThinkLike a Nurse 36-6

What would be the best method to secure dressings for Mr. Harmon (Meet Your Patient)?

How Are Wounds Supported and Immobilized?

Binders and bandages are used to hold a dressing in place, apply pressure to a wound to impede hemorrhage, and support and immobilize an injured area, thereby promoting healing and comfort. Before applying a bandage or binder,

Table 36-5 ▶ Types of Wound Dressings

DRESSING TYPES	DESCRIPTION	USES	CAUTION
Absorbent dressings (See Procedures 36-5 and 36-6 to learn how to remove and apply dry and wet-to-damp dressings.)	▪ Made from highly absorptive layers of fibers such as cellulose, cotton, or rayon ▪ May or may not have an adhesive border.	▪ For moderate to large wounds ▪ Can be used as a primary or secondary dressing to manage drainage from partial- or full-thickness wounds.	▪ Do not use to pack undermining wounds. ▪ Do not use if the wound is not draining.
Alginates	▪ Fibers derived from brown seaweed and kelp. ▪ Available in pad or rope form. ▪ Highly absorbent (20 to 40 times their weight).	▪ For large wounds ▪ Very high absorbency ▪ Promote a moist environment. ▪ Facilitate autolytic débridement. ▪ Ideal for wounds that have depth, tracts, tunneling, or undermining.	▪ Extremely absorptive and will adhere to the wound bed if there is no drainage. ▪ When the alginate comes in contact with exudate, a nonadhesive gel is created. ▪ Must irrigate this gel from the wound before placing the next dressing.
Antimicrobials	▪ Available as ointments, impregnated gauzes, pads, gels, foams, hydrocolloids, and alginates. ▪ Commonly contain silver and cadexomer iodine.	▪ For large wounds ▪ Reduce and prevent infection. ▪ Promote collagen deposition. ▪ Can be used on partial- or full-thickness wounds, malodorous wounds with little to large amounts of drainage, or highly contaminated or infected wounds.	▪ Allergy to antibiotic ingredient
Collagens	▪ Made from bovine (cow) or porcine (pig) sources and made into sheets, pads, powders and gels.	▪ For minimal to large wounds. ▪ Absorb exudate. ▪ Promote a moist wound bed for healing. ▪ Stimulate wounds to produce collagen fibers and granulation tissue in the wound bed. ▪ Do not stick to the wound bed and are easy to apply and remove.	
Foams	▪ Made from semipermeable hydrophilic foam that forms an impermeable barrier over the wound. ▪ Made into wafers, rolls, and pillows; have film coverings; and are adhesive or nonadhesive. ▪ Used to provide compression.	▪ For minimal to large wounds ▪ Absorbency ▪ Insulation ▪ Provide comfort. ▪ Promote a moist environment. ▪ Protects friable periwound skin. ▪ Can be shaped around body contours. ▪ May be used in combination with alginates or films.	▪ Do not use with wounds that have tunneling or tracts. ▪ Not recommended for dry, desiccated wounds. ▪ May macerate periwound skin if dressing becomes oversaturated.

| Gauze | ■ Simplest and most widely used dressings
■ Made of woven and nonwoven fibers of cotton, rayon, polyester, or a combination of these.
■ Impregnated with antimicrobial agents, medications, or moisture, and others contain petrolatum to keep the wound moist.
■ May be packed as sterile or nonsterile, in bulk or in smaller packages. | ■ For large wounds
■ Cleansing
■ Protection
■ For packing large wounds, cavities, or tracts, deep or dirty wounds, or heavily draining wounds.
■ Used in combination with **amorphous hydrogels**, saline, or medications. | ■ Labor intensive
■ Can stick to wound tissue and damage new, regenerated cells with the gauze removal.
■ Does not ensure a moist wound environment, as they allow for fluid evaporation.
■ May be applied incorrectly—must be fluffed to avoid pressure or overpacking of a wound.
■ Dressing change interval is dependent on the amount of fluid saturation of the gauze. Frequent dressing changes disrupt the wound bed and cause the wound to become hypothermic (cold), which physiologically impairs cell growth for healing. |
| **Hydrocolloids**
(See Procedure 36-9 to learn how to apply hydrocolloid dressings) | ■ Are wafers, pastes, or powders that contain hydrophilic (water-loving) particles.
■ Used under compression. | ■ For light to moderate drainage
■ Promote a moist environment.
■ Provide a protective layer against friction/caustic agents.
■ Promote autolysis.
■ Mold to the shape of the body, making them useful for difficult areas, such as heels or between buttocks. | ■ Not the dressing of choice for wounds that require frequent dressing changes.
■ Do not allow the wound to be visualized.
■ Not recommended for wounds surrounded by friable or sensitive skin (difficult to remove).
■ Should not be used on infected wounds because they are impermeable to oxygen, moisture, and bacteria.
■ May facilitate the growth of anaerobic bacteria.
■ Should not be used on wounds with tunneling or tracts because these wounds must be packed and allowed to drain. Wound should be shallow enough that the hydrocolloid touches the wound bed. |

(Continued)

Table 36-5 ▶ Types of Wound Dressings—cont'd

DRESSING TYPES	DESCRIPTION	USES	CAUTION
Hydrogels (See Procedure 36-9)	▪ Are sheets, granules, or gels, with a high water content, creating a jelly-like consistency that does not adhere to the wound bed.	▪ For minimal drainage ▪ Promote a moist environment. ▪ Rehydrate the wound bed. ▪ Promote autolysis. ▪ Promote comfort. ▪ Soften slough or eschar in necrotic wounds.	▪ Have limited absorptive capabilities (not practical for wounds with significant exudate). ▪ Easily macerate periwound skin due to high moisture content.
Skin sealants and moisture barriers	▪ Skin sealants — made from liquid transparent copolymer. ▪ Moisture-barrier ointments— petrolatum, dimethicone, or zinc-based products that can be applied to skin to protect it from exudate, moisture, urine, and feces.	▪ For all wound types ▪ Simple and fast to use, and if needed, should be used with each dressing change. ▪ Can be wiped or sprayed on skin to protect it from wound exudate and moisture, friction, and skin stripping from adhesives ▪ Provide a barrier of protection over vulnerable skin from the effects of moisture and mechanical and chemical skin injury.	▪ Ointments impair the adhesion of wound dressings or tapes.
Transparent Films (Fig. 36-12) (To learn how to apply transparent film dressings, see Procedure 36-8.)	▪ Clear and semipermeable.	▪ For minimal drainage to none ▪ Promote a moist environment. ▪ Occlusive with oxygen permeability. ▪ Promote autolysis. ▪ Often used to dress IV sites. ▪ Prevent external bacterial contamination. ▪ Allow wound assessment without removing or disturbing the dressing. ▪ Can be placed over joints without inhibiting movement.	▪ If used over wounds that are draining, the tissues will become macerated. ▪ Adhere to the skin, so do not use them on friable skin.

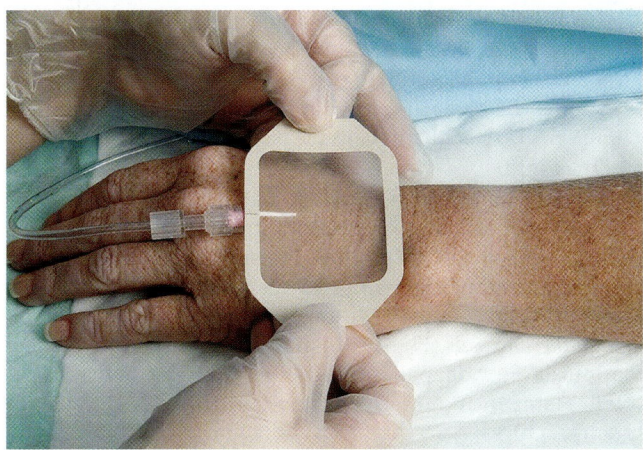

FIGURE 36-12 IV sites are commonly dressed with transparent film dressings.

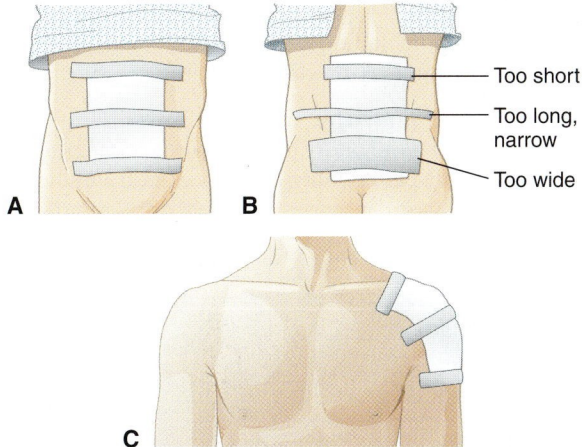

FIGURE 36-13 A, Place strips of tape at the ends of the dressing and space them evenly over the remainder of the dressing. B, Choose a tape width appropriate for the size of the dressing. Use strips that are sufficiently long to secure the dressing in place. C, When taping over a joint, place the tape at a right angle to the direction in which the joint moves.

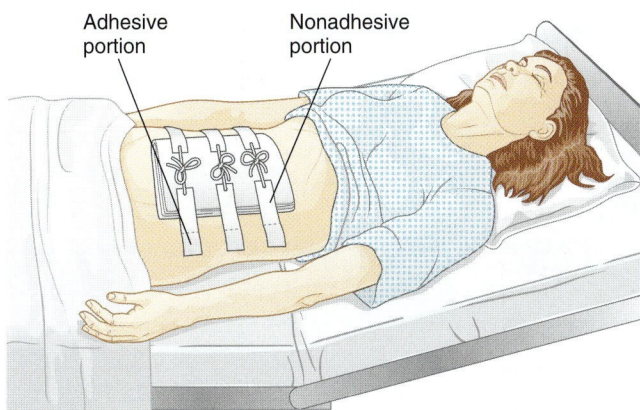

FIGURE 36-14 Montgomery straps with ties may be used to secure a dressing that requires frequent changing.

determine the intended purpose of the application and assess the part being bandaged. When a bandage is not needed, adhesive skin closures can provide support to wound margins (see Procedure 36-10).

Binders

Binders may be used to keep a wound closed when there is danger of dehiscence, or to immobilize a body part to aid in the healing process. They are typically used on large areas of the body and are designed for a specific body part. They may be made of cloth or elasticized material and fasten with straps, pins, or Velcro. The most common binders are the following:

- A *triangular arm binder or sling* is used to support the upper extremities. Because commercial slings are readily available, you will use the triangular sling infrequently.
- A *T-binder* is used to secure dressings or pads in the perineal area.
- An *abdominal binder* is used to provide support to the abdomen. It is often ordered when there is an open abdominal wound that is healing by secondary intention. The binder decreases the risk of dehiscence. Abdominal binders may be straight or multitailed.

To learn how to apply binders, see Procedure 36-11.

Bandages

A bandage is a cloth, gauze, or elastic covering that is wrapped in place. With the exception of a sling, most bandages come in rolls and in various widths, commonly 1.5 to 7.5 cm (0.5 to 3 in.). Use a narrow width on small body parts, such as a finger, and wider bandages on arms and legs.

- **Cloth bandages** are most commonly used as slings to immobilize an upper extremity or to hold large abdominal dressings in place.
- **Gauze** is the most frequently used type of bandage. It is available in many sizes and forms and readily conforms to the shape of the body. It may also be impregnated with medications for application to the skin or with plaster of Paris, which, when dried, hardens to form a cast.
- **Elastic bandages** are used to apply pressure and give support (e.g., to improve venous circulation in the legs). Ace bandages are the most common form of elasticized bandage.
- **A rolled bandage** is a continuous strip of material (gauze, stretchable gauze, or elastic webbing) that you unroll as you apply it to a body part. To apply a rolled bandage, hold the free end in place with one hand, and use the other hand to pass the roll around the body part. Exert equal tension on each pass (or turn). Each turn should overlap the last one-half to two-thirds the width of the bandage, except for the circular turn. There are five basic turns for rolled bandaging (see Procedure 36-12).

How Should I Use Heat and Cold Therapy?

Local application of heat or cold has been used for therapeutic purposes for centuries. Temperature-sensitive nerve endings respond readily to temperatures between 59°F and 113°F (15°C and 45°C). Response to heat or cold depends on the area being treated, the nature of the injury, duration of the treatment, age, physical condition, and the condition of the skin.

➕Monitor the patient especially carefully in the following situations:

- **Extremes of Age.** The very young and the very old are the least tolerant of heat and cold therapies.
- **Sensory Impairment.** May be at increased risk for injury because they may not perceive temperature changes, burns, or ischemia.
- **Highly Vascular Areas.** Fingers, hand, face, and perineum are very sensitive to temperature changes and thus are at high risk for injury from heat and cold.
- **Application to a Large Area.** Decreases the patient's tolerance of the treatment. Application to a small area is best tolerated.
- **Injured Skin or Wounds.** Intact skin tolerates heat and cold therapy better than skin that has been injured or has open wounds.

Safety Measures

➕For patient safety, observe the following precautions when applying either heat or cold:

- Avoid direct contact with the heating or cooling device. Cover the hot or cold pack with a washcloth, towel, or fitted sleeve.
- Apply hot or cold intermittently, leaving it on for no more than 15 minutes at a time in an area. This precaution helps prevent tissue injury (e.g., burns, impaired circulation). It also makes the therapy more effective by preventing **rebound phenomenon:** At the time the heat or cold reaches maximum therapeutic effect, the opposite effect begins.
- Check the skin frequently for extreme redness, blistering, cyanosis (blueness), or blanching. When heat or cold is first applied, the thermal receptors react strongly, and the person feels the temperature intensely. Over about a 15-minute period, the receptors adapt to the new temperature, and the person notices it less. Caution clients not to change the temperature when this occurs because doing so can cause tissue injury.

Applying Heat Therapy

Local application of heat is used to relieve stiffness and discomfort associated with musculoskeletal problems. It may also be used for patients with wounds. Heat increases blood flow to an area through vasodilatation, increased capillary permeability, and reduced blood viscosity. Increased blood flow brings oxygen and white blood cells to the wound and aids in the healing process. Heat promotes the delivery of nutrients and removal of waste products from the tissue, promotes relaxation, and decreases stiffness and muscle tension.

➕When heat is applied to a large area of the body, vasodilatation may cause a drop in blood pressure and a feeling of faintness. Warn patients to be alert for this effect if they will be administering heat at home.

Moist Heat

The addition of moisture to heat amplifies the intensity of the treatment. Moist heat can be applied in several forms. The form used depends on the skin condition.

- *Washcloth or towel.* If heat is being applied for relaxation and the skin is intact, you can soak a washcloth or towel in warm water and wring out the excess moisture before applying to the skin.
- *Gauze compress.* If there are any open areas, you will need to use a gauze compress (usually sterile).

- *Soaks and baths.* A **soak** involves immersion of the affected area. Soaking helps cleanse a wound and remove encrusted material. A **bath** is a modification of a soak in which a special tub or chair may be used. The most commonly used bath is a sitz bath (Fig. 36-15). A **sitz bath** soaks the patient's perineal area.

Dry Heat

Dry heat may be applied by several methods: electric heating pads, disposable hot packs, or hot water bags.

- *Electric heating pads* have the advantage of providing a constant temperature, but the risk of burns is high. Caution patients to place the pad over the body area and never to lie on the pad.
- *Aquathermia pads* (Fig. 36-16) may also be used for dry heat application. Aquapads are plastic or vinyl pads that circulate water in the interior of the pad to create a constant temperature.

- *Disposable hot packs and hot water bags or bottles* are also available.
➕Hot water bags are common in home use, but not in healthcare agencies because of the danger of burns from improper use.

For guidelines (including water temperatures) for applying moist and dry heat, see Clinical Insight 36-1.

Applying Cold Therapy

The application of moist or dry cold causes vasoconstriction and decreases capillary permeability. It produces local anesthesia, reduces cell metabolism, increases blood viscosity, and decreases

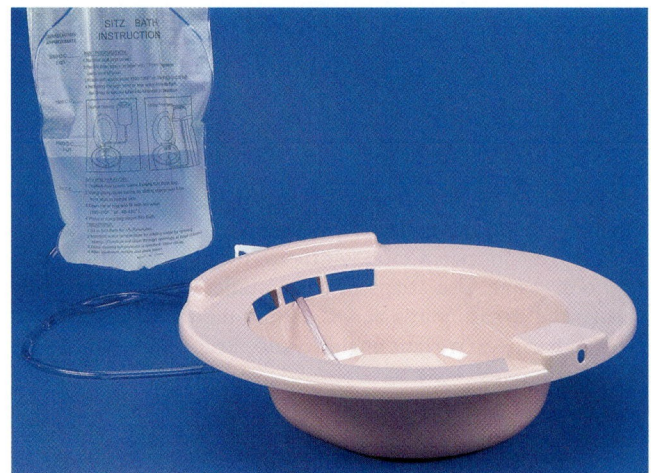

FIGURE 36-15 A sitz bath soaks the patient's perineal area.

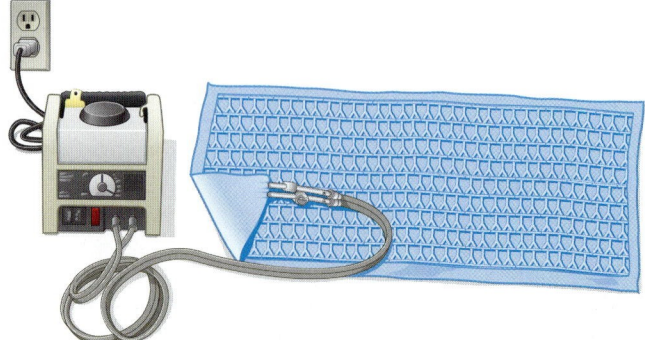

FIGURE 36-16 Aquapads circulate water in the interior of the pad to create a constant temperature.

Clinical Insight 36-1 ➤ **Applying Local Heat Therapy**

Preparation

- Determine whether there are any contraindications to the treatment, such as impaired circulation, bleeding, wound complications, or inability to tolerate the treatment.
- Explain the application and rationale to the client.

Moist Heat (Irrigations, Compresses, Hot Soaks)

If skin is intact:

- Soak a washcloth or towel in warm water (105°F to 115°F [40°C to 46°C]), and wring out the excess before applying to the skin. Reapply and change water frequently to maintain a constant temperature.

For open areas, use a compress, a soak, or a bath:

- To make a compress, soak gauze in the heated solution (105°F to 115°F [40° to 46°C]), and then apply it to the wound. Usually, you will use sterile gloves, gauze, and solution.
- Reapply compresses or towels, and change the water frequently to maintain a constant temperature. Heat disperses quickly.
- **For a soak** you will need to immerse the affected area. Sterilized tubs are often used for this procedure.
- **A sitz bath** soaks the client's perineal area. A special tub or chair may be used. Because of infection control concerns, disposable sitz baths are preferred. Check that the water temperature is from 105°F to 110°F (40°C to 43°C). Instruct the client to soak for 15 minutes.

Dry Heat (Electric Heating Pads, Disposable Hot Packs, Hot Water Bags)

Aquathermia pads (also called K-pads) are plastic or vinyl pads that circulate water in the interior.

- Connect the pad via tubing to the electric heating unit, which constantly exchanges water that has been heated to the specified temperature.
- Fill the reservoir about two-thirds full of distilled water.
- Set the temperature control to 98°F to 105°F (37°C to 40.5°C).
- Cover the pad, and apply it to the body part.

Disposable hot packs and hot water bags or bottles:

- Use water that is 115°F to 125°F (46°C to 52°C).
- Fill the bag about two-thirds full of warm tap water, expel the air from the bag, and close the top.
- Tip the bag upside down to test for leaking.
- Wrap the bag in a towel, and place it on the client.
- Never place a heat source directly on the client's skin. Burns can occur.

Electric heating pads:

- Be sure that the body part is dry or that the pad has a waterproof cover.

✚ Safety Precautions for Electric Heating Pads

- Do not use pins (e.g., to hold a cover in place) or other sharp objects on the pad. The pin could go through a wire and cause an electric shock.
- Tell the client to report any discomfort during the treatment.
- Measure water temperature with a bath thermometer.
- For home use, warn the client about the danger of burns from high settings. Use pads with a switch that the client cannot turn up.
- Avoid direct contact with the heating device. Cover the heat source with a washcloth, towel, or fitted sleeve.
- Do not place the heating device (pad, bag) under the client; place it over the body part. This helps prevent burns.
- Apply heat intermittently, leaving it on for no more than 15 minutes at a time in an area. This helps prevent tissue injury (e.g., burns, impaired circulation). It also makes the therapy more effective by preventing rebound phenomenon.
- Check the skin frequently for extreme redness or blistering.
- Assess for hypotension and faintness. If they occur, discontinue the treatment. Have the client lie down for several minutes. When the faint feeling passes, assist the client to sit up slowly. Recheck the blood pressure (BP) when the client is in the sitting position. If the BP remains low, encourage the client to remain seated. If the client is ambulatory, have her dangle her feet for several minutes before she gets up.

---

muscle tension. It also slows bacterial growth. Applications of cold are used to prevent or limit edema and reduce inflammation, pain, oxygen requirements, and bleeding. Cold therapy is often used to treat fevers and sports injuries (e.g., sprains, strains, fractures, and contusions), and to prevent swelling after surgery (e.g., an ice bag may be applied to the perineum after childbirth; an ice collar may be applied to the throat after a tonsillectomy). Cold applications have the following side effects:

- *Elevated blood pressure.* Because cold causes vasoconstriction, it may increase the patient's blood pressure.
- *Shivering.* Prolonged cold may cause shivering, a normal response as the body attempts to produce heat.

- *Tissue damage.* Prolonged exposure to cold may cause tissue damage due to impaired circulation.

For guidelines in applying cold therapy, see Clinical Insight 36-2.

KnowledgeCheck 36-12

- What is the effect of adding moisture to heat or cold treatments?
- For how long should heat or cold be applied to an area?
- What precautions should you take before using heat or cold therapy?

Clinical Insight 36-2 ➤ Applying Local Cold Therapy

Preparation

- Determine whether there are any contraindications to the treatment, such as impaired circulation, bleeding, wound complications, or inability to tolerate the treatment.
- Explain the application and rationale to the client.
- Assess for indications for cold application (e.g., fever above 104°F [40°C]). Measure the client's temperature.

Cooling Baths

A cooling bath is often used to treat a high fever (above 104°F [40°C]). It promotes heat loss through conduction and vaporization.

- Prepare a pan of water with a temperature from 65°F to 90°F (18°C to 32°C).
- You may add a fan to increase heat loss if the temperature is markedly elevated.
- Slowly sponge the face, arms, legs, back, and buttocks with the cool water. Do not dry the areas; cover with a damp towel.
- Take about 30 minutes to complete the bath.
- Cooling the body too rapidly will cause shivering, which will increase heat production.
- You may also place ice bags or cold packs on the forehead and in the axillae and the groin.
- Assess the client constantly during a cooling bath. If the client begins to shiver, his temperature may actually rise.

Cold Compresses

- Apply a cool, damp cloth or towel to the body part.
- Renew the compress or cloth frequently.

- The temperature of the compress or cloth will rapidly rise toward body temperature.

Ice Collars, Ice Bags, Commercially Prepared Cold Packs, Aquapads

- You can make an ice bag out of a procedure glove or small plastic bag by filling it with ice chips and tying a knot in the top.
- Fill the ice bag with ice chips or an alcohol-based solution.
- Cover ice bags or packs with a towel or soft cover.
- Apply to the skin for a maximum of 15 minutes, then remove. You may reapply the cold pack in 1 hour.

✚ Safety Precautions for Cooling Devices

- Measure water temperature with a bath thermometer.
- Tell the client to report any discomfort during the treatment.
- Avoid direct contact with the cooling device. Cover the cold pack with a washcloth, towel, or fitted sleeve.
- Apply cold intermittently, leaving it on for no more than 15 minutes at a time in an area. This helps prevent tissue injury (e.g., impaired circulation). It also makes the therapy more effective by preventing rebound phenomenon.
- Observe for tissue damage: bluish purple mottled appearance of the skin, numbness, and sometimes blisters and pain.
- Monitor for elevated blood pressure.

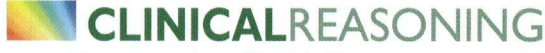

CLINICAL REASONING:
Applying the **Full-Spectrum Nursing Model**

Because the following critical thinking activities allow you to practice the kind of thinking you will use as a full-spectrum nurse, they usually have no single right answer. Discuss them with your peers—if you have difficulty with any of the questions, consult your instructor.

PATIENT SITUATION

A 66-year-old obese man with diabetes and hypertension, Tio Santos, is being seen for a wound on his right foot that does not seem to be healing. He injured his foot when repairing drywall at home. He is otherwise relatively sedentary at home. The wound is oozing, swollen, tender, and warm to the touch. Mr. Santos is now running a low-grade fever of 100.4°F at home. He tells you his foot is very painful, especially with any weight bearing, and throbs when sitting or lying still. You measure the wound bed to be 6 cm × 4 cm and note purulent exudate at the distal edge. He is referred to an outpatient wound care center for treatment.

THINKING

1. *Theoretical Knowledge:*
   a. What is the Braden Scale and why might it be used for Mr. Santos?
   b. What risk factors for delayed wound healing does Mr. Santos have?

2. *Critical Thinking (Considering Alternatives, Deciding What to Do):*
   a. To care for Mr. Santos' wound, should you use sterile gloves, clean nonsterile gloves, or no gloves? Explain your thinking.

DOING

3. *Practical Knowledge (Assessment):*
   a. What symptoms of infection does Mr. Santos have?
   b. To be certain the wound is infected, what would you need to know or do?

CARING

4. *Self-Knowledge:* Imagine you have had a wound on your foot for 6 weeks. It has not healed and you have all Mr. Santos' symptoms and, in fact, are in his situation. What would be the most troublesome symptom in your daily life? What would worry you the most?

 Go To Chapter 36, **Clinical Reasoning: Applying the Full-Spectrum Nursing Model Response Sheet,** on Davis*Plus*.

PracticalKnowledge
procedures

As a nurse, you will care for many patients who have wounds or who are at risk for impaired skin integrity. You will need practical knowledge of wound assessment and wound care. Specific nursing interventions focus on providing wound care and applying heat and cold therapies. In this section, you will find procedures for obtaining wound cultures, cleansing wounds, and dressing wounds, for placing and removing wound closures, caring for wound drains, and applying binders and bandages.

Procedure 36-1 ■ Obtaining a Wound Culture by Swab

➤ For steps to follow in *all* procedures, refer to the Universal Steps for All Procedures found on the page facing the inside back cover.

➤ *Note:* This procedure uses modified sterile technique because wound care is now usually performed using clean rather than sterile technique.

Equipment

- Three pairs of clean procedure gloves
- Culturette tube
- Sterile 4 in. × 4 in. gauze in an impermeable tray or separate 4 × 4 packs and an impermeable barrier
- Sterile 0.9% (normal) saline solution for irrigation, warmed to body temperature when possible
- Cold solution lowers the temperature of the wound bed and slows the healing process.
- 35-mL syringe
- 19-gauge angiocatheter
- Gown and face shield
- Emesis basin
- Water-resistant disposable drapes

Delegation

This is an invasive procedure that requires knowledge of wound healing. It should be performed by a licensed nurse. Do not delegate this skill to nursing assistive personnel (NAP).

Pre-Procedure Assessments

NOTE: If the wound is covered when you begin, you will make these assessments when you remove the soiled dressing and after cleansing the wound.

- Assess for pain.

  Wounds may be very painful, and wound irrigation may increase pain. Provide prescribed pain medication 30 minutes before performing the procedure, if indicated.

- Determine whether the wound requires sterile, modified sterile, or clean technique.

  Sterile technique is used for acute surgical wounds and for wounds that have undergone recent sharp débridement, or when the physician prescribes it. Chronic wounds are colonized with bacteria and may be cared for using clean technique, as in this procedure. To perform sterile wound irrigation, see Procedure 36-3.

- Assess the amount and type of tissue present in the wound bed.

  Granulating tissue is beefy red with a velvety appearance. It appears with the growth of new blood vessels and connective tissue. Pale pink tissue may indicate compromised blood supply to the

(continued on next page)

Procedure 36–1 ■ **Obtaining a Wound Culture by Swab** (continued)

wound bed. Necrotic tissue, which is black, brown, or yellow in appearance, is nonviable, and inhibits healing. Only red granulating tissue should be swabbed for a culture.

- **Assess the type and amount of exudate.**
  Exudate may be a sign of infection.
- **Assess the wound for odor.**

A foul odor may indicate infection. Cleanse wounds before you assess for odor, because some dressings interact with wound drainage to produce an odor.

- **Assess the tissue surrounding the wound edge.**
  Surrounding tissue that is red, warm, and/or edematous may indicate infection

➤ When performing the procedure, always identify your patient according to agency policy and be attentive to standard precautions, hand hygiene, patient safety and privacy, body mechanics, and documentation.

Procedure Steps

1. **Place the patient in a comfortable position** that provides easy access to the wound and will allow the irrigation solution to flow freely from the wound with the assistance of gravity. Position a water-resistant disposable drape to protect the bedding.

2. **After washing and drying hands**, apply a gown, face shield, and clean gloves.
   Protects against splattering that may occur during irrigation.

3. **Remove the soiled dressing.** Dispose of gloves and soiled dressing in a biohazard bag.
   Soiled dressings contain contaminants and should be treated as biohazardous waste.

4. **Don clean procedure gloves**.

5. **Place an emesis basin** at the dependent edge of the wound to collect irrigation runoff. Avoid touching the wound with the basin.
   Prevents contamination of wound from the emesis basin; protects linens from runoff.

6. **Using a 19-gauge angiocatheter**, remove the metal stylet needle and dispose into a sharps container. Attach the angiocatheter to a 35-mL syringe and fill with normal saline irrigation solution.
   Prevents contamination and needlestick injury. A 19-gauge angiocatheter with a 35-mL syringe provides 8 psi (pounds per square inch) of pressure and is effective for removing bacteria, necrotic tissue, exudate, and/or metabolic wastes.

   NOTE: This procedure follows guidelines established by the Agency for Healthcare Research and Quality (AHRQ). Commercial irrigation kits containing a piston tip syringe

may also be used. Their use is discussed in Procedure 36-3.

7. **Holding the angiocatheter** tip 2 cm from the wound bed; gently irrigate the wound with a back-and-forth motion, moving from the upper aspect to the lower, dependent aspect.
   Irrigating from top to bottom prevents flow of contaminated solution over the cleansed area. ▼

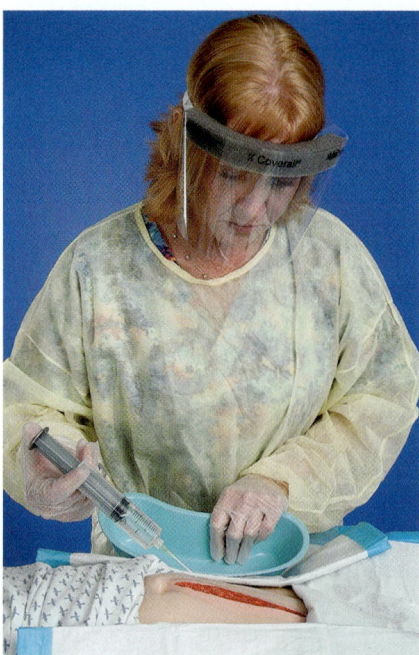

8. **Dispose of the syringe** and angiocatheter in the sharps container, and gloves in the biohazardous waste receptacle.
   Prevents contamination and needlestick injury.

9. **Obtain a culturette tube**, and twist the top of the tube to loosen the swab.

10. **Don clean procedure gloves**, and locate an area of red, granulating tissue in the wound bed.

11. **Withdraw the swab** from the culturette tube. Press the swab against the granulating area with sufficient pressure to express fluid from the wound tissue, and rotate the swab.
    a. Do not allow the swab to touch anything other than the granulating area of the wound.
    b. Do not swab culture areas where slough or eschar is present.
       These are areas of avascular or necrotic tissue and are contaminated with bacteria. Swab cultures detect only surface bacteria and are not a reliable means for diagnosing wound infection.
    c. Do not roll the swab around in a pool of exudate.
       Pus is a collection of white blood cells that have already done their work, and includes the microorganisms that have already died. Obtaining a culture from this material would not produce reliable culture result. The culture specimen must be of tissue or tissue fluid, not surface fluid or exudate. ▼

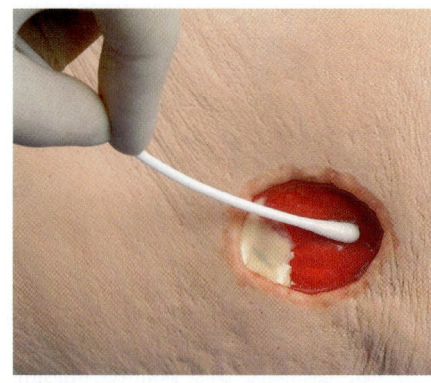

12. **Carefully insert the swab** back into the culturette tube, making sure it does not make contact with

the opening of the tube upon reinsertion. Twist the cap to secure the tube.

Decreases risk of contamination; ensures that any microorganisms that grow in the culture are from the wound and were not introduced from the environment.

13. **Crush the ampule** of culture medium at the bottom of the tube. (*Note:* Inspect the culture tube to determine whether this step is required.)

The ampule contains medium for growth of microorganisms.

14. **Label the culturette tube** with the patient's name, patient identification number, birth date, source of specimen, and date and time of collection.

Labeling ensures obtaining the results for the correct patient.

15. **Transport the specimen** for culture to the lab.

16. **Apply a clean dressing** to the wound as ordered.

? What if . . .

- **You determined this wound requires sterile technique?**

  After removal of soiled dressing, apply sterile gloves for irrigating, obtaining culture, and applying new sterile dressing.

  Sterile technique is used for acute surgical wounds and for wounds that have undergone recent, sharp débridement, or when the provider prescribes it.

- **The culture tube is not sent to the lab within 72 hours?**

  If the culture swab is not sent to the lab within 48 to 72 hours, it must be discarded. Be sure to check the policy within your institution.

  The swab culture needs to be exposed to ideal laboratory conditions to allow microbial growth. If the culture sits on the unit too long, the culture medium might not produce reliable results. Most swab transport systems are validated for 48 to 72 hours after collection. However, if bacteria are suspected, the quicker the specimen is sent to the lab, the better.

- **The wound care and culture supplies are kept on a common treatment cart?**

  Common treatment carts should be left in the hall and not taken into individual rooms.

  When a mobile cart is rolled into a room, it is a source for possible cross-contamination.

Evaluation

- Assess patient's pain level. Medicate according to prescriptions.
- Monitor lab reports for results of the swab culture.

Documentation

Document the following information (some agencies use a wound/skin flow sheet):

- Appearance and location of the wound and surrounding tissue. Note type, consistency and amount of exudate, and odor, if present, after irrigation.
- Patient's pain level before you obtained the culture

- If the patient was medicated for pain, document the drug and dose used, time given, and patient response.
- Method by which the wound was cleansed before you obtained the swab culture
- Description of the area where the culture was obtained
- Dressing reapplied to wound, if applicable
- Education provided to the patient

Practice Resources

ICSI, 2010; National Guideline Clearinghouse (NCG), 2006, revised 2008; Moore & Cowman, 2007; NPUAP, 2007d.

Procedure 36-2 ■ Obtaining a Needle Aspiration Culture From a Wound

➤ For steps to follow in *all* procedures, refer to the Universal Steps for All Procedures found on the page facing the inside back cover.

➤ *Note:* This procedure uses modified sterile technique because wound care is now usually performed using a clean approach rather than sterile technique. Recall that the basic differences in sterile and modified sterile technique are that modified sterile technique uses nonsterile procedure gloves and tap water.

Equipment

- One pair of clean procedure gloves and one pair of sterile gloves
- Gown and face shield
- 0.9% (normal) saline solution for irrigation, warmed to body temperature when possible
- Cold solution lowers temperature of wound bed and slows the healing process.
- Sterile 4 in. × 4 in. gauze pads in an impermeable tray
- Vial of 0.9% (normal) saline for injection

- 22-gauge needle
- 3-mL syringe
- Lab tube with culture medium

Delegation

This is an invasive procedure that requires knowledge of wound healing. It should be performed by a registered nurse or an LPN trained in the correct procedure. Do not delegate this skill to nursing assistive personnel (NAP).

(continued on next page)

Procedure 36–2 ■ Obtaining a Needle Aspiration Culture From a Wound (continued)

Pre-Procedure Assessments

NOTE: If the wound is covered when you begin, you will make these assessments when you remove the soiled dressing and after cleansing the wound.

■ **Assess for pain.**
Wounds may be painful, and wound irrigation may increase pain. Provide prescribed pain medication 30 minutes before performing the procedure, as indicated.

■ **Assess the amount and type of tissue present in the wound bed.**
Granulating tissue is beefy red with a velvety appearance. It appears with the growth of new blood vessels and connective tissue. Pale pink tissue may indicate compromised blood supply to the wound bed. Necrotic tissue, which is black, brown, or yellow in appearance, is nonviable and inhibits healing.

■ **Assess the type and amount of exudate.**
Exudate may be a sign of infection.

■ **Assess the wound for odor.**
A foul odor may indicate infection. Cleanse wounds before you assess for odor, because some dressings interact with wound drainage to produce an odor.

■ **Assess the tissue surrounding the wound edge.**
Surrounding tissue that is red, warm, and/or edematous may indicate infection.

➤ When performing the procedure, always identify your patient according to agency policy and be attentive to standard precautions, hand hygiene, patient safety and privacy, body mechanics, and documentation.

Procedure Steps

1. **Position the patient** so the wound is easily accessible. Position a water-resistant disposable drape under the patient to collect fluid runoff.
   A drape protects the linens.

2. **After washing and drying your hands**, apply a gown, face shield, and clean gloves.
   Protects you from splattering of contaminated bodily fluid or drainage.

3. **Remove the soiled dressing.** Dispose of gloves and soiled dressing in a biohazardous waste bag.
   Soiled dressings contain wound exudate, blood, or debris and should be treated as biohazardous waste.

4. **Open a tray of sterile 4 in. × 4 in. gauze.** Moisten the gauze with normal saline solution for irrigation.
   The sterile container tray is impermeable.

5. **Attach a 22-gauge needle** to a 3-mL syringe, and aspirate 1 mL of sterile normal saline from the vial. Cap the needle, using a one-handed technique (see Procedure 25–10), and place the syringe on the bedside table.
   Maintains sterility and prevents needle-stick injury.

6. **Don sterile gloves.**
   Reduces the incidence of introducing microorganisms into the wound to be cultured.

7. **Gently cleanse the wound** with the saline-moistened gauze by lightly wiping a section of the wound from the center toward the wound edge. Discard the gauze in a biohazard receptacle, and repeat in the next section using a new piece of gauze with each wiping pass.
   Removes surface bacteria and exudate. ▼

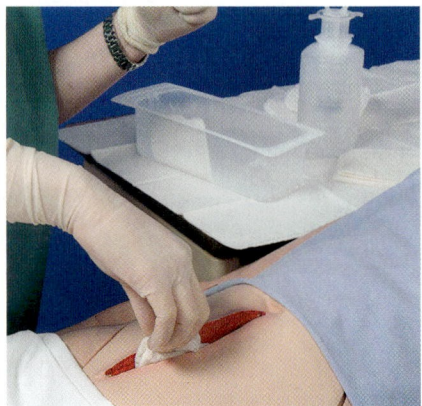

8. **Uncap the syringe** from the bedside table, and insert the needle 1 to 2 mm into the wound bed. Inject 1 mL of normal saline into the wound tissue.
   Allows for an adequate amount of culture fluid to be aspirated. ▼

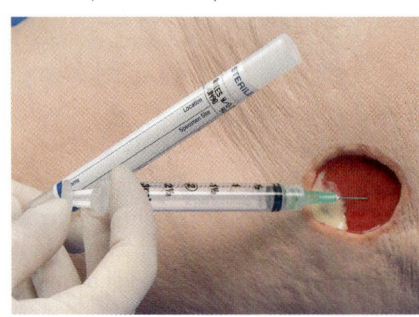

9. **Pull back on the syringe plunger** to aspirate approximately 0.5 to 1.0 mL of fluid into the barrel of the syringe. Remove the needle from the wound bed after you have collected the aspirate.
   This method assesses for bacteria within the tissue, rather than surface colonization.

10. **Without contaminating** the end of the needle, place the collected fluid into a culture tube containing culture medium.
    Culture medium supports the growth of microorganisms. ▼

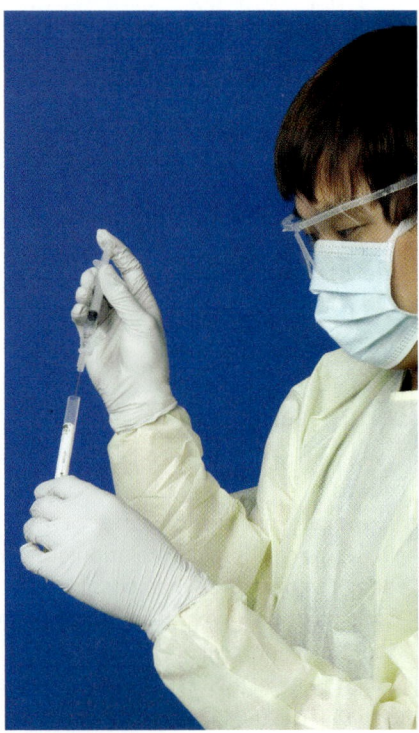

11. **Label the culture tube** with the patient's name, birth date, source of specimen, and date and time of collection. (A label may be supplied with the culture kit.)

Labeling ensures obtaining culture results for the correct patient.

12. **Arrange for transport** of the specimen for culture to the lab.

13. **Apply a clean dressing** to the wound as ordered.

? What if . . .

■ **The wound is covered in eschar or slough?**

Since only red granulating tissue is appropriate for culture, you would need to consult the primary care provider.

■ **The wound has deep tunneling or sinus tracts?**

These types of wounds may provide an oxygen-depleted environment that could allow proliferation of anaerobic microbes. You may need to culture this type of wound for both aerobic and anaerobic microorganisms.

■ **The wound covers a large surface area?**

Large wounds should have separate cultures taken from different areas of the wound bed.

Evaluation

■ Determine whether the patient remains comfortable. If not, medicate as prescribed.

■ Monitor the wound bed at the puncture site for evidence of bleeding.

■ Monitor lab reports for results of the aspirate culture.

Documentation

Document the following information (many agencies use a wound/skin flow sheet):

■ Appearance and location of the wound and surrounding tissue. Note type, consistency and amount of exudate, and odor, if present, after irrigation.

■ Length, width, and depth of wound when the patient's condition changes or at regular intervals

■ The patient's pain level before and after you obtained the culture

■ If the patient was medicated for pain, document the drug and dose used, time given, and patient response.

■ Method by which the wound was cleansed before you obtained the aspiration culture

■ Description of the area where the culture was obtained

■ Dressing reapplied to wound, if applicable

■ Education provided to patient

Practice Resources

Myers, 2008; NCG, 2006, revised 2008; NPUAP, 2007d; Sussman & Bates-Jensen, 2007. WOCN, 2001, revised 2011).

Procedure 36-3 ■ Performing a Sterile Wound Irrigation

➤ For steps to follow in *all* procedures, refer to the Universal Steps for All Procedures found on the page facing the inside back cover.

Equipment

■ Clean gloves
■ Sterile gloves
■ Gown and face shield
■ Water-resistant, disposable drapes
■ Tepid (body temperature) irrigation solution
■ Cold solution lowers temperature of wound bed and slows the healing process.
■ Sterile gauze
■ Dressing supplies
■ Biohazardous waste container
■ Sterile impermeable barrier
■ Sterile bowl

For Step Variation: Using an Angiocatheter

■ Sterile emesis basin
■ 35-mL syringe
■ 19-gauge angiocatheter (needle removed)

For Step Variation: Using a Piston-Tip Syringe

■ Sterile commercial irrigation kit containing a sterile basin and piston-tip syringe

Delegation

This is an invasive, sterile procedure that requires nursing assessment, judgment, evaluation, and teaching during the procedure. It requires knowledge of wound healing and should be performed by a registered nurse. Do not delegate this skill to nursing assistive personnel (NAP).

Pre-Procedure Assessments

NOTE: If the wound is covered when you begin, you will make these assessments when you remove the soiled dressing and after cleansing the wound.

(continued on next page)

Procedure 36-3 ■ Performing a Sterile Wound Irrigation (continued)

- Assess the amount and type of tissue present in the wound bed.

  Granulating tissue is beefy red with a velvety appearance. It appears with the growth of new blood vessels and connective tissue. Pale pink tissue may indicate a delay in wound healing due to compromised blood supply to the wound bed or lack of proper nutrition. Necrotic tissue, which is black, brown, or yellow in appearance, is nonviable, inhibits healing, and is a source of bacterial growth.

- Determine whether the wound requires sterile, modified sterile, or clean technique for irrigation.

  Irrigation helps wounds to heal because it removes bacteria, old drainage, and necrotic tissue from the wound bed. Sterile technique is used for acute surgical wounds, for wounds that have undergone recent sharp débridement, or when the primary care provider has ordered it. Chronic wounds are colonized with bacteria and may be irrigated with clean technique.

Irrigation using clean technique is presented in steps 1 through 7 of Procedure 36-1.

- Assess the wound for signs of infection (erythema, induration, amount and type of drainage).

  Infected wounds require higher flow pressures for irrigation.

- Assess the wound for odor.

  A foul odor may indicate infection. Cleanse wounds before you assess for odor, because some dressings interact with wound drainage to produce an odor.

- Assess the tissue surrounding the wound edge.

  Surrounding tissue that is red, warm, and/or edematous may indicate infection. Tissue that is macerated (white and moist) indicates too much fluid is being held against the skin, usually from saturated dressings.

- Assess for pain.

  Wound irrigation may be very painful.

➤ When performing the procedure, always identify your patient according to agency policy and be attentive to standard precautions, hand hygiene, patient safety and privacy, body mechanics, and documentation.

Procedure Steps

1. **Administer pain medication** 30 minutes before the treatment, if necessary.

2. **Place the patient in a comfortable position** that provides easy access to the wound and will allow the irrigation solution to flow freely from the wound with the assistance of gravity. Position a water-resistant disposable drape to protect the bedding from any possible runoff.

3. **After washing and drying** your hands, apply a gown, face shield, and clean gloves.

   Personal protective equipment (PPE) provides a barrier against splattering that commonly occurs during wound irrigation.

4. **Remove the soiled dressing.** Dispose of gloves and soiled dressing in a biohazard bag.

   Soiled dressings contain body fluids and other contaminants and should be treated as biohazardous waste.

5. **Set up a sterile field** on a clean, dry surface. Add the following supplies to the field based on the type of irrigation to be performed:
   Sterile gauze
   Sterile bowl
   Dressing supplies
   A sterile commercial irrigation kit *or* a 19-gauge angiocatheter,

35-mL syringe, and sterile emesis basin.

Setting up a sterile field at bedside provides easy access to equipment for irrigation and reduces the risk for contamination when retrieving supplies after getting started. ▼

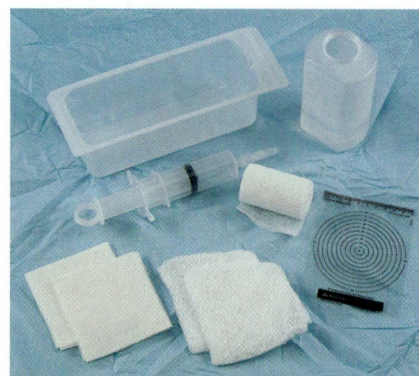

6. **Select irrigation solution** based on the wound assessment, goals of therapy and primary care provider's orders. Potable water is the solution of choice unless the patient is immunocompromised. Consider solutions with surfactants and/or antimicrobials for pressure ulcers with debris, infection or suspected high levels of bacterial colonization.

   ✚ Do not use povidone-iodine (Betadine) if the patient has an iodine allergy.

Some common commercial wound-cleansing solutions might contain antimicrobial ingredients that can damage wound cells.

7. **Pour the tepid** (room-temperature) irrigation solution into the sterile bowl.

   Local cooling of wound tissues impairs healing. This can occur if you irrigate with refrigerated solutions and change dressings frequently.

8. **Don sterile gloves.**

   Maintains sterile technique.

9. **Place the sterile basin** at the bottom of the wound to collect irrigation runoff.

10. **Fill the irrigation syringe.**

Using an Angiocatheter

a. Attach the 19-gauge angiocatheter (with needle removed) to the 35-mL syringe, and fill with the irrigation solution.

   A 19-gauge angiocatheter (with needle removed) and 35-mL syringe provides 8 psi of pressure and is effective for removing bacteria, necrotic tissue, exudate, and/or metabolic wastes.

Using a Piston-Tip Syringe

b. Fill a piston-tip syringe with irrigation solution.

11. **Holding the angiocatheter** tip or syringe tip 2 cm from the wound bed, gently irrigate the wound with a back-and-forth motion, moving from the superior aspect to the inferior aspect.

Irrigating from superior to inferior prevents flow of contaminated solution over cleansed area. Irrigating a clean, noninfected wound with gentle low-pressure (8 psi) reduces disruption of the healthy, healing tissue. Irrigating an infected wound with higher flow (but < 15 psi) selectively débrides necrotic tissue while protecting healthy tissue. ▼

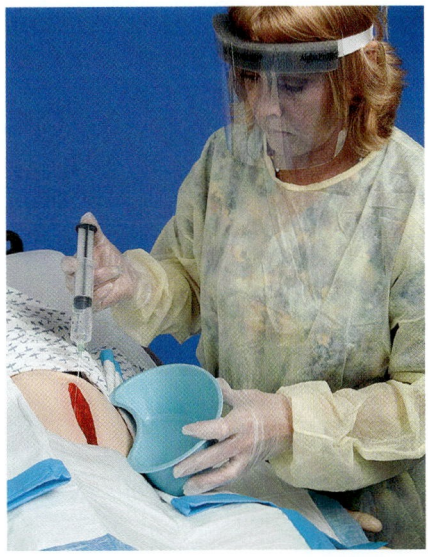

   a. Ensure any undermining or tunneling is irrigated as well.

b. Repeat the irrigation until the solution returns clear.

Flushing removes exudate, debris, and some surface bacteria.

12. **Remove the basin** or sterile container from the base of the wound.

13. **Pat the skin surrounding** the wound dry with sterile gauze, beginning at the top of the wound and working downward.

Moisture on the surrounding tissue may lead to maceration and further breakdown of the wound margins.

14. **Dress the wound as prescribed.**

15. **Consider applying a waterproof** skin protectant around the wound if drainage is heavy.

Wound drainage contains irritating chemicals that can damage healthy tissues, especially at the wound edge and surrounding skin. Solutions used to keep the wound bed moist can also macerate or damage healthy skin if allowed to remain on intact skin.

16. **Dispose of the contaminated** irrigation fluid in a biohazardous receptacle.

To prevent cross-contamination.

17. **Remove soiled drapes** from the patient area.

18. **Remove your gloves, face shield**, and gown. Dispose of these items appropriately.

Contaminants from the irrigation may be present on these items, and they should also be considered biohazardous.

19. **Reposition the patient** to a comfortable position.

20. **Wash your hands.**

Hand hygiene is one of the most important interventions for preventing cross-contamination.

? What if . . .

- **The client has a wound covering a large area of the body?**

A general rule is that the larger the wound, the more solution needed to clean it.

Remember that the purpose of cleansing a wound is to remove bacteria and debris by flushing the wound.

- **Peroxide or another antiseptic solution is prescribed?**

First, identify the reason that the solution was ordered for the wound type. Then identify the length of time it is to be used. Weigh the benefit of using the solution with the potential risks to healing tissues. Finally, discuss any concerns with the primary care provider.

Peroxide is indicated more for acute, traumatic wounds to remove dirt and other debris. Peroxide and other commercial antiseptics can damage fibroblasts, and cause air embolism if used to forcefully irrigate or pack a tunneling wound. Fibroblasts produce collagen, the major structural protein of skin and healing tissues.

Evaluation

- Determine whether the patient remains comfortable. If not, medicate according to prescriptions.
- Reassess the wound at regular intervals.

Patient Teaching

- Answer any questions the patient may have.
- Teach the patient about the expected healing process.
- Inform the patient and caregiver about signs and symptoms of infection and the need to report these findings.

Home Care

- Wound irrigation is commonly done in the home. In most cases, clean technique is used in the home setting.
- Irrigation solutions, such as saline, can be made and stored up to 7 days if refrigerated.
- Review with the family proper disposal of contaminated supplies.

Documentation

Document the following information (many agencies use a wound/skin flow sheet):

- Appearance and location of the wound, size, tissue in wound base, periwound tissue, type and amount of exudate, and odor, if present, after irrigation
- The patient's pain level. If the patient was medicated for pain, document the drug and dose used, time given, and patient response.
- Method by which the wound was cleansed
- Dressing reapplied to the wound, if applicable
- Education provided to the patient

Practice Resources

Bergstrom, Bennett, Carlson, et al., 1994; Hess, 2007; Myers, 2008; Rolstad & Ovington, 2007; Stotts & Gunningberg, 2007.

Procedure 36-4 ■ Taping a Dressing

➤ For steps to follow in *all* procedures, refer to the Universal Steps for All Procedures found on the page facing the inside back cover.

➤ *Note:* This procedure uses clean technique because wound care is now usually performed using a clean, rather than sterile, technique.

Equipment
- Procedure gloves
- Tape (cloth, plastic, foam, silk-like, etc.)

Delegation
As a nurse, you are responsible for assessing the wound and evaluating interventions. However, this procedure may be delegated to nursing assistive personnel (NAP).

Pre-Procedure Assessments
- Assess the degree of importance of the dressing.
  The more critical the dressing is, the more adhesion will be required.
- Assess the characteristics the dressing material, weight and conformability, and the device or tubing to be held.

Heavier dressings require higher adhesion. Bulky dressings may need high conformability or greater adhesion.
- Assess the skin surface (i.e., dry, damp, diaphoretic, oily, hairy, edematous, fragile, or impaired skin integrity).
  Fragile skin may require less adhesion while damp or oily skin may require higher adhesion.
- Assess the anticipated wear time.
  Tape adhesion gets stronger over time. Breathable tapes can be used longer. Occlusive plastic tapes build up moisture and are used when adhesion is intended for a shorter period of time.
- Assess the patient's history and current medical conditions.
  Review allergies or sensitivities to tapes. Review medical conditions that may be affected by adhesives.
- Assess activity level and the anticipated length of time the dressing will be needed.
  The more active the patient, the more adhesion required.

➤ When performing the procedure, always identify your patient according to agency policy and be attentive to standard precautions, hand hygiene, patient safety and privacy, body mechanics, and documentation.

Procedure Steps

1. **Wash your hands. Don gloves**.
2. **Choose the type of tape** based on wound size, location, amount of drainage or edema, frequency of dressing changes, patient's activity level, and type of dressings used.
   Tapes come in many different adhesive types and backings. Select the tape based on individual characteristics.
   a. Choose tape of the width that is appropriate for the size of the dressing. The larger the dressing, the wider the tape needed for securing.
      For example, a large abdominal dressing may require 3-inch tape, whereas a small incision on an extremity may need only ½-inch tape.
   b. Choose a tape that stretches if the area is at risk for distention, edema, hematoma formation, or movement.
      Skin distention under tape may cause blistering or skin tears.
3. **Tear strips that extend ½-inch** beyond the dressing.
   To anchor the dressing to the skin.

4. **Place the tape perpendicular** to the incision.
   Fewer skin tension injuries occur with taping perpendicular to the incision.
   a. When taping over joints, apply the tape at a right angle to the direction of joint movement, or at a right angle to a body crease. For example, tape a shoulder or knee horizontally, not lengthwise.
   b. Apply tape with an even amount tension on both sides, being careful not to pull at the edges.
      This reduces the risk of skin damage.
5. **Smooth tape in place** by gently stroking the surface to maximize adhesion.
6. **Replace tape if site** becomes edematous, or the skin is not intact.

? What if . . .

- **The tape will not adhere to the patient's skin due to excess hair?**

  Remove the hair with clippers or scissors. Do not shave the site with a razor.

Shaving can cause nicks or abrasions to the skin that could become a portal of entry for bacteria.

- **The patient's skin is diaphoretic or excessively oily?**

  Cleanse the skin with soap and water before the dressing change. You may use polymer skin barriers to place a seal over the skin and allow the tape adhesive to adhere.

- **The patient has fragile skin (e.g., older adult)?**

  Use skin sealant preparations under adhesives. Use the least adhesive product possible for the need.
  The junction between the epidermis and dermis on the older adult is not as strong as in a younger person.

- **The patient is allergic to tape adhesives?**

  Use hypoallergenic products.
  Circular wraps, ace bandages, or other such products may be used to secure dressings.

Evaluation

- Verify type of tape that is appropriate for the patient and dressing.
- Note whether the tape adheres comfortably to the skin.
- Ensure that the patient verbalized understanding of the treatment.
- Inspect the dressing daily for intactness, edema, or hematoma.

Patient Teaching

- Teach the patient about the expected healing process.
- Educate the patient about the purpose of the procedure.
- Instruct the patient to keep the dressing dry.

Documentation

Document the following information (many agencies use a wound/skin flow sheet):
- Type of dressing and tape applied
- Location and characteristics of wound
- Education given to patient

Practice Resources

Association of periOperative Registered Nurses (AORN), 2008; Fletcher, 1999; 3M, 2004.

Procedure 36-5 ■ Removing and Applying Dry Dressings

➤ For steps to follow in *all* procedures, refer to the Universal Steps for All Procedures found on the page facing the inside back cover.

➤ *Note:* This procedure uses clean technique because wound care is now usually performed using clean rather than sterile technique.

Equipment

- Three pairs of clean nonsterile gloves
- Sterile normal saline solution for irrigation, warmed to body temperature when possible
  Cold solution lowers the temperature of wound bed and slows the healing process.
- Tray of sterile 4 in. × 4 in. gauze
- Sterile gauze for dressings
- Tape

Delegation

This procedure requires knowledge of wound healing. It should be performed by a registered nurse. Do not delegate this skill.

Pre-Procedure Assessments

NOTE: *When you begin, the wound will likely be covered with a dressing. You will make these assessments when you remove the soiled dressing and after cleansing the wound.*

- Assess for pain at least 30 minutes before performing the procedure.
  Wounds may be very painful. Provide pain medication 30 minutes before performing the procedure if needed, to allow the medication time to be distributed in target tissues. Changes in the quality or severity of pain are some symptoms linked with infection.
- Assess the type and amount of exudate.
  Exudate may be a sign of infection.
- Assess the wound for odor.
  A foul odor may indicate infection. Clean wounds before you assess for odor, because some dressings interact with wound drainage to produce an odor.
- Assess the tissue surrounding the wound edge.
  Surrounding tissue that is red, warm, and/or edematous may indicate infection.
- Determine the type of dressing needed.
  The type of dressing depends on the characteristics of the wound and the goal of treatment. Dry dressings are appropriate when there is no need to keep the wound bed moist, such as a wound healing by primary intention or a wound covered by eschar.

➤ When performing the procedure, always identify your patient according to agency policy and be attentive to standard precautions, hand hygiene, patient safety and privacy, body mechanics, and documentation.

Procedure Steps for Removing the Dressing

1. **Place the patient in a comfortable position** that provides easy access to the wound.
   Provides for patient comfort and proper nurse body mechanics during dressing change.

2. Wash your hands, and **don clean, nonsterile gloves**.

Handwashing is one of the most important measures for preventing infection transmission.

3. **Gently loosen the edges of the tape** of the old dressing at an angle parallel to the skin.
   - Hold that edge with one hand and gently raise the edge until it is taut, but not pulling on the skin.
   - Using your other hand, push down on the exposed skin at the point

where the tape and skin meet. Push the skin off of the tape.
   The pull–push method helps prevent skin stripping from the adhesive and reduces discomfort and skin trauma as you remove the tape.

4. Beginning at the edges of the dressing, **lift the dressing** toward the center of the wound. If the dressing sticks, moisten it with normal saline before removing it completely.

(continued on next page)

Procedure 36–5 ■ Removing and Applying Dry Dressings (continued)

Moistening the dressing decreases the risk of bleeding and/or removal of granulating tissue.

5. **Assess the type and amount** of drainage on the soiled dressing.
   Allows for evaluation of wound healing. Purulent drainage is an indication of infection.

6. **Dispose of the soiled dressing** and gloves in a biohazard receptacle.
   Soiled dressings contain bodily fluids and other contaminants.

7. **Remove the cover of a tray** of sterile 4 in. × 4 in. gauze. Moisten the gauze with sterile saline.
   The sterile container tray is impermeable and allows you to moisten the gauze while maintaining sterility. Gauze will not shed fibers into the wound (as do cotton balls). Fibers and any other foreign bodies in a wound promote inflammation and delay healing.

8. **Don clean nonsterile gloves.**

9. **Gather a gauze pad by pulling** the four corners up toward the middle. Use the center ball of the gauze to cleanse the wound.
   Forming a ball with the gauze pads prevents contamination of gloved hands during cleansing.

10. **Gently cleanse the wound** with the saline-moistened gauze by lightly wiping a section of the wound.
    - Wipe from the center toward the wound edge or from top to bottom or dirty to clean, depending on the wound.
    - Repeat as needed, discarding the gauze in a biohazard receptacle, using a new piece of gauze with each wiping pass.
    Removes surface bacteria and exudate. Prevents transfer of microorganisms

from the surrounding skin into the wound.

11. **Discard the gloves** and soiled gauze into a biohazard bag.

12. **Reassess wound** for size, color of tissue, amount and type of exudate, and odor.

Procedure Steps for Applying Dry Dressing

13. **Wash your hands**, or use an antiseptic handrub at the bedside.

14. **Open sterile gauze packages** on a clean, dry surface.
    Maintains sterility of gauze. ▼

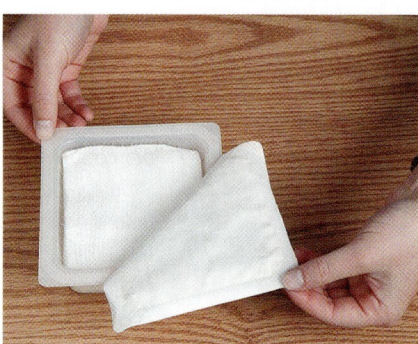

15. **Don clean nonsterile gloves.**

16. **Apply a layer of dry dressings** over the wound. If drainage is expected, use an additional layer of dressings.
    The first layer serves as a wick for drainage. A second layer is needed if increased absorption is required.

17. **Place strips of tape at the ends** of the dressing and evenly spaced over the remainder of the dressing. Use strips that are sufficiently long to secure the dressing in place. Tape the dressing around all edges, "windowpaning," if appropriate.
    Edges remain taped down and dressing stays intact. ➤

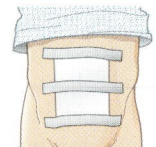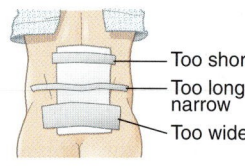

| Too short |
| Too long, narrow |
| Too wide |

Correct   Incorrect

18. **Remove gloves**, turning them inside out, and discard them in a biohazard receptacle.

19. **Assist the patient to a comfortable position.**

? What if . . .

- **Signs of infection are noted with wound assessment?**

  Notify the primary care provider. Cultures, wound care interventions, and perhaps antibiotics may be required.

- **The wound is not approximated?**

  Place the patient in a supine position, apply Steri-Strips™, and cover with sterile saline dressings. Notify primary care provider.
  This could indicate wound dehiscence.

- **The skin surrounding the incision is not intact?**

  Clean the area with sterile saline, dry thoroughly, and apply protective moisture barrier dressing. Consider using Montgomery straps.
  Montgomery straps are useful when dressings must be changed frequently because they do not cause trauma to the skin.

- **A drain or drainage tube is present?**

  Always clean the drain site after cleaning the primary incision site.
  Reduces the risk of cross-contamination.

Evaluation

- Determine whether the dressing is clean, dry, and intact.
- Verify that the patient experienced minimal discomfort during the procedure.

Patient Teaching

- Teach the patient about the expected healing process.
- Relate the signs and symptoms of infection and the need to report these findings.

Home Care

- Help the client to store dressings appropriately to keep them clean, for example, in a plastic container with a lid.
- Teach the client or caregivers to dispose of contaminated dressings and gloves by double-bagging them in moisture-proof bags (e.g., plastic grocery bags).
- Advise the client and family whether they can get the wound wet (e.g., during bathing). If it must be kept dry, demonstrate how to cover it with a waterproof barrier (e.g., a plastic bag).

Documentation

Document the following information (many agencies use a wound/skin flow sheet):

- Appearance and location of the wound, type and amount of exudate, and odor, if present, after cleansing
- The patient's pain level before the procedure. If the patient was medicated for pain, document the drug and dose used, time given, and patient response.
- Method of cleansing the wound
- Type of dressing applied to the wound
- Education provided to the patient

Practice Resources

Atiyeh & Hayek, 2004; Dunaway & Goldrick, 2007; Joanna Briggs Institute, 2008a; NPUAP, 2007d; NPUAP and EPUAP, 2009.

Thinking About the Procedure

 Go to the *Fundamentals of Nursing Skills Videos,* **Wound Care: Dressings: Dry.**

1. What kind of personal protective equipment did the nurse don to protect herself from infection when changing the patient's bandage?
2. What should the nurse do to remove the dressing if it sticks to the wound?

 For suggested responses, go to Chapter 36, **Thinking About the Procedure Suggested Responses,** on Davis*Plus.*

Procedure 36-6 ■ Removing and Applying Wet-to-Damp Dressings

➤ For steps to follow in *all* procedures, refer to the Universal Steps for All Procedures found on the page facing the inside back cover.

➤ *Note:* This procedure uses clean technique because wound care is now usually done using a clean or modified sterile approach rather than sterile technique. However, sterile technique is recommended for wounds that have recently had sharp débridement, have a drain, or are fresh surgical wounds.

Equipment

- Three pairs of clean nonsterile gloves
- Sterile solution for irrigation, warmed to body temperature when possible

  Cold solution reduces the temperature of wound bed and slows the healing process.
- Water-resistant disposable drapes
- Sterile fine-mesh gauze in a tray
- Surgipad
- Tape or Montgomery straps

Delegation

This is an invasive procedure that requires knowledge of wound healing. It should be performed by a registered nurse. Do not delegate this skill to nursing assistive personnel (NAP).

Pre-Procedure Assessment

NOTE: When you begin, the wound will likely be covered with a dressing. You will make these assessments when you remove the soiled dressing and after cleansing the wound.

- Assess the amount and type of tissue present in the wound bed.

  Granulating tissue is beefy red with a velvety appearance. It appears with the growth of new blood vessels and connective tissue. Pale pink tissue may indicate compromised blood supply to the wound bed. Necrotic tissue, which is black, brown, or yellow in appearance, is nonviable and inhibits healing.
- Assess the type and amount of exudate.

  Exudate may be a sign of infection.
- Assess the wound for odor.

  A foul odor may indicate infection. Clean wounds before you assess for odor, because some dressings interact with wound drainage to produce an odor.
- Assess the tissue surrounding the wound edge.

  Surrounding tissue that is red, warm, and/or edematous may indicate infection.
- Assess for pain.

  Wounds may be very painful. Assess for pain and provide prescribed pain medication 30 minutes before performing procedure, if needed. A change in the quality or intensity of pain may be a sign of infection.

➤ When performing the procedure, always identify your patient according to agency policy and be attentive to standard precautions, hand hygiene, patient safety and privacy, body mechanics, and documentation.

Procedure Steps for Removing the Wet-to-Damp Dressing

1. **Place the patient in a comfortable position** that provides easy access to the wound.

2. Wash your hands, and **don clean gloves.**

   Handwashing complies with standard precautions, helping to prevent transfer of pathogens.

3. **Gently loosen the edges** of the tape of the old dressing.
   - Hold that edge with one hand and gently raise the edge until it is taut, but not pulling on the skin.

(continued on next page)

Procedure 36–6 ▪ **Removing and Applying Wet-to-Damp Dressings** (continued)

- Using your other hand, push down on the exposed skin at the point where the tape and skin meet.
- Push the skin off of the tape.

The pull–push method will help prevent skin stripping from the adhesive and reduce discomfort and skin trauma as you remove the tape.

4. **Beginning with the top layer,** lift the dressing from the corner toward the center of the wound. If the dressing sticks, moisten it with normal saline or tap water before completely removing it.
   - Remove first from one side of the wound, first toward the wound, and then from the other side.
   - Continue to remove layers until you have removed the entire dressing.

Moistening the dressing decreases the risk of bleeding and/or removal of granulating tissue. ▼

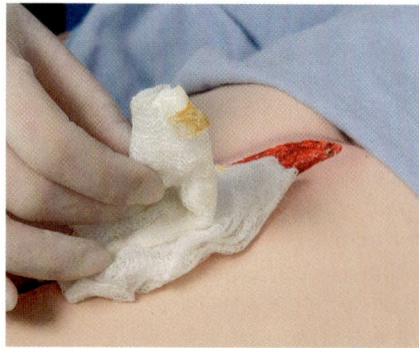

5. **Assess the type and amount** of drainage present on the soiled dressing.

Type of drainage is an indication of the stage of healing. Purulent drainage is an indication of infection.

6. **Dispose of the soiled dressing** and gloves in a biohazard container. Wash your hands.

Soiled dressings contain body fluids contaminants and should be disposed of as biohazardous waste.

7. **Remove the cover of a tray** of sterile 4 in. × 4 in. gauze. Moisten the gauze with sterile saline or water.

The sterile container tray is impermeable and allows you to moisten the gauze while maintaining sterility.

8. **Don clean procedure gloves**.
   Avoids introducing microorganisms into the wound.

9. **Gather a gauze pad by pulling** the four corners up toward the middle. Use the center of the gauze to cleanse the wound.
   Prevents contamination of your gloves during wound cleansing.

10. **Gently cleanse the wound** with the saline- or water-moistened gauze by lightly wiping a section of the wound from the center toward the wound edge. Discard the gauze in a biohazard receptacle, and repeat in the next section using a new piece of gauze with each wiping pass.
    Removes surface bacteria and exudate. Prevents transfer of microorganisms from the skin to the wound.

11. **Assess the wound for location**, amount of tissue present, exudate, and odor.
    Allows for determination of most effective treatment and type of dressing.

12. **Discard the gloves** and soiled gauze into a biohazard bag.
    Soiled gauze contains contaminants.

Procedure Steps for Applying a Wet-to-Damp Dressing

13. **Open a sterile gauze pack tray** and a surgipad. The amount of gauze you use depends on the size of the wound.
    Maintains sterile field and supplies.

14. **Moisten sterile gauze with saline** solution or water for irrigation.

15. **Don clean gloves.**

16. **Squeeze out excess moisture** from the gauze. Apply a single layer of moist, fine-mesh gauze to the wound.
    Be sure to place gauze in all depressions or crevices of the wound.

You may need to use forceps or a cotton applicator to ensure that you fill deep depressions or sinus tracts with gauze.

Maintains a moist environment for the wound bed. ▼

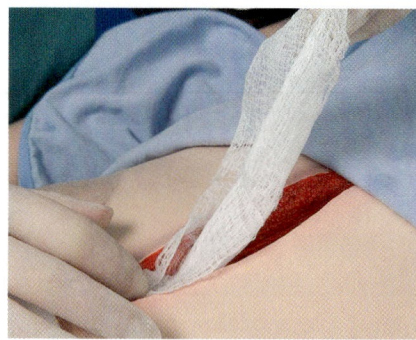

17. **Apply a secondary moist layer** over the first layer. Repeat this process until the wound is completely filled with moistened sterile gauze—but do not tightly *pack* the gauze into the wound. Do not extend the moist dressing onto the surrounding skin.
    Packing the gauze can restrict blood flow to the area. Moist dressing on the surrounding skin can cause maceration.

18. **Cover the moistened gauze** with a surgipad.
    Protects the wound from external contaminants. ▼

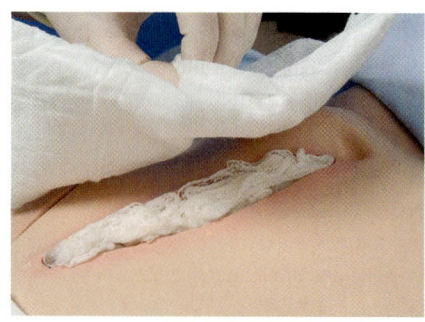

19. **Secure the dressing** with tape or Montgomery straps.
    Montgomery straps are useful when dressings must be frequently changed because they do not cause trauma to the skin. ➤

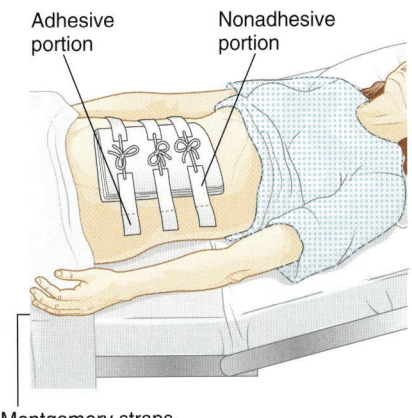

Adhesive portion   Nonadhesive portion

Montgomery straps

21. Assist the patient to a comfortable position.

? What if . . .

- **Gauze becomes dry between dressing changes?**

  Moisten with sterile saline before removing dressings, change dressing more frequently, and consider using a semi-occlusive dressing.
  A moistened dressing prevents débridement of granulating tissue, maintains a moist environment, and prevents tissue injury. Dressings that become too dry will injure healthy tissue and impair healing.

- **The patient has multiple wounds?**

  The most infected wound should be treated last, and change your gloves in between wound dressing changes.
  The risk of cross-contamination is reduced when moving from clean to dirty and with fresh gloves.

20. Dispose of gloves and materials in the biohazard waste receptacle.

Evaluation

- Verify that the patient experiences minimal discomfort with the procedure.
- Note whether the patient verbalizes understanding of the procedure.

Patient Teaching

- Teach the patient about the expected healing process.
- Inform the patient and caregiver about signs and symptoms of infection and the need to report these findings.

Home Care

- Help the client store dressings appropriately to keep them clean, for example, in a plastic container with a lid.
- Teach the client or caregivers to dispose of contaminated dressings and gloves by double-bagging them in moisture-proof bags (e.g., plastic grocery bags).
- Advise the client and family whether they can get the wound wet (e.g., during bathing). If it must be kept dry, demonstrate how to cover it with a waterproof barrier (e.g., a plastic bag).

Documentation

Document the following information (many agencies use a wound/skin flow sheet):
- Appearance and location of the wound, type and amount of exudate, and odor, if present, after cleansing

- Pain level before and after the procedure
- Pain medication given including the dose, time, your name, and the patient's response.
- Method of cleansing the wound
- Type of dressing applied to the wound
- Education provided to the patient

Practice Resources

Atiyeh & Hayek, 2004; Dunaway & Goldrick, 2007; NPUAP, 2007d; NPUAP and EPUAP, 2009.

Thinking About the Procedure

 Go to the *Fundamentals of Nursing Skills Videos,* **Wound Care: Dressings: Wet-to-Damp Dressing.**

1. Did the nurse use clean or sterile technique for the dressing change?
2. Where is the patient's wound located? And how did the nurse protect his privacy when changing a wound dressing?

 For suggested responses, go to Chapter 36, **Thinking About the Procedure Suggested Responses,** on *DavisPlus.*

Procedure 36-7 ■ Applying a Negative Pressure Wound Therapy (NPWT) Device

▶ For steps to follow in *all* procedures, refer to the Universal Steps for All Procedures found on the page facing the inside back cover.

Equipment

- Suction unit (pump)
- Collection canister with connecting tubing
- Appropriate dressing per manufacturer
- Semipermeable transparent adhesive dressing
- Skin preparation product or sealant (skin prep)
- Sterile 4 in. × 4 in. gauze
- Clean procedure gloves

(continued on next page)

Procedure 36–7 ■ **Applying a Negative Pressure Wound Therapy (NPWT) Device** (continued)

- Two pairs of sterile gloves (if using sterile technique)
- Sterile scissors (if using sterile technique)
- Waterproof pad
- Bath blanket
- Goggles or safety glasses, mask, and protective gown
- 10- to 20-mL irrigation syringe
- Normal saline for irrigation
- Emesis basis
- Biohazard bag for contaminated materials

For Procedure 36-7A: Vacuum-Assisted Closure (V.A.C.) Therapy

GranuFoam (black), white or silver foam dressing
Therapeutic regulated accurate care (TRAC) pad

For Procedure 36-7B: Chariker–Jeter Dressing Application

Fenestrated drain
Ostomy paste

Delegation

As a nurse, you are responsible for assessing the wound and evaluating interventions. You should not delegate application of a negative pressure wound therapy device to a NAP. However, you may ask the NAP to report to you any changes in the wound dressing, pressure in the unit, or alarms.

Pre-Procedure Assessments

- **Assess the type of wound to be treated with negative pressure.**
  Negative pressure wound therapy is used to promote wound healing by secondary or tertiary intention in acute, chronic, traumatic, and dehisced wounds; partial-thickness burns; or flaps and grafts. NPWT will prepare the wound bed for closure, reduce edema, promote granulation formation, and remove exudate and infective material.

- **Determine if there is any contraindication to use of a NPWT:** nonenteric or unexplored fistulas; necrotic tissue with eschar; untreated osteomyelitis; malignancy in the wound or in exposed blood vessels, anastomotic sites, organs, or nerves.

- **Assess patients for active or prolonged bleeding; patients** who are on anticoagulant therapy or platelet aggregation inhibitors; or patients with infected, damaged, irradiated, or sutured blood vessels.
  Patients who are at increased risk for bleeding should be closely monitored. These conditions could be fatal if negative pressure is applied and bleeding is uncontrolled (exsanguination could occur). Notify the primary care provider of these conditions.

- **Assess the wound for bone fragments or sharp edges.**
  When NPWT is activated, mechanical stress is placed upon the wound. Sharp edges or bone may puncture protective barriers, vessels, or organs, causing injury, and bleeding, if uncontrolled, could be fatal.

- **Assess the wound for infection.**
  Monitor infected wounds closely, as they may require more frequent dressing changes than noninfected wounds.

- **Assess the wound for size (length, width, and depth in cen-** timeters); location and depth of undermining or tunneling; amount, character, and odor of drainage; type and percentage of tissue present in wound bed (granulation, slough, fibrin, necrotic); and periwound condition (i.e., intact, denuded, erythema, induration, or maceration).
  If no response or improvement in the wound condition occurs in 2 weeks, use of NPWT should be reevaluated.

- **Assess the patient's nutritional status.**
  Adequate protein stores are needed for wounds to heal. Evaluate the patient's albumin or prealbumin level before initiating therapy, as NPWT may deplete these levels and prevent healing.

- **Assess for pain.**
  Wound care is very painful. Wound pain that is inadequately treated can lead to wound bed hypoxia that impairs wound healing and increases infection rates. Wound pain also negatively affects the patient's quality of life.

➤ When performing the procedure, always identify your patient according to agency policy and be attentive to standard precautions, hand hygiene, patient safety and privacy, body mechanics, and documentation.

➤ *NOTE:* The success of NPWT can depend on the training and expertise of the clinician. Allow adequate time for this procedure. Experienced nurses need at least 15 to 30 minutes. You will need more time if problems arise, and even more if you are a novice.

➤ *NOTE:* This procedure assumes you are performing the initial application of V.A.C. therapy. If you are changing the dressing, first read the What If . . . ? section near the end of this procedure.

Procedure Steps

1. **Consider administering pain medication** before initiating negative pressure wound therapy. Allow sufficient time for the medication to take effect.

2. **Select the appropriate dressing** (per NPWT system used) to fill the entire wound cavity.

Dressings should be placed directly against the wound surface to allow for equal suction/pressure throughout the wound bed.

3. **Obtain suction pump unit** as prescribed.
Negative pressure wound therapy is provided by several different manufacturers.

Use the unit and dressing method that is approved by your facility.

a. Place the suction unit upright on a level surface.
b. Remove the canister from the sterile package and insert it into the pump.
c. Connect the tubing to the canister.

d. Ensure the opposite end of the tubing remains clean before connecting with the tubing from the dressing.

e. Place the suction unit at the end of the bed or hang on an IV pole.

f. Do not place the unit on the floor. Ensure it is not knocked over, as drainage from the canister can back up and contaminate the pump's filter, blocking suction.

4. **Place the trash receptacle** so you can reach it easily during the procedure.

Convenient placement facilitates access to safe disposal of the dressing into a trash receptacle for biohazardous waste.

5. **Assist the patient to a comfortable position** that allows for easy access to the wound.

Facilitates access to the wound site with less contamination and promotes good body mechanics.

6. **Expose the wound area and drape** the patient (use a bath blanket if needed) to expose only the wound area.

Provides privacy and comfort.

7. **Place a waterproof pad as needed**.

An underpad protects the linens from moisture and drainage.

8. **Prepare a sterile or clean field** and add all supplies: gloves, scissors, irrigation supplies, gauze pad, selected wound dressings, tubing, and/or connectors.

9. **Don sterile or clean procedure gloves**. Use gown and protective eyewear.

Using sterile/aseptic versus clean technique is based on the wound type, physician preference, or facility protocol. A safe rule to follow is to use sterile gloves for a fresh noninfected wound; clean gloves for other wounds.

10. **Irrigate the wound** with 10 to 30 mL of normal saline or other prescribed solution before all dressing changes. Use a 35-mL syringe and a 19-gauge angiocatheter (needle removed) to direct the flow of the irrigant from the clean end toward the dirty end of the wound.

Loosens adherent tissue and removes debris and exudate. Observes infection control principles of clean-to-dirty.

11. **Remove the excess solution** from the wound. Clean and dry periwound skin with sterile gauze sponge, as needed. Consider a skin protectant around the wound edges.

Excess moisture predisposes skin to maceration. Skin protectant assists the drape to stick to the skin, and protects the skin when the drape is removed (i.e., from stripping of skin by the adhesive).

12. **Remove soiled gloves** and don new, nonsterile ones.

Change gloves during patient care if the hands will move from a contaminated body site (e.g., perineal area or wound) to a clean body site.

13. **To apply appropriate dressing** per preferred negative pressure wound therapy unit, follow Procedure 36-7A or 36-7B.

Procedure 36-7A ■ Open-Pore Reticulated Polyurethane Foam Therapy (i.e., Vacuum-Assisted Closure [V.A.C.])

➤ When performing the procedure, always identify your patient according to agency policy and be attentive to standard precautions, hand hygiene, patient safety and privacy, body mechanics, and documentation.

➤ Begin with Procedure steps 1 through 13, at the beginning of Procedure 36-7. Then proceed as follows.

1. **Select the appropriate foam** dressing: black, white, or silver.

Black foam is sufficient for most wounds unless individual patient circumstances require white or silver. White foam is denser and will limit granulation formation. It may be used for painful or superficial wounds, tunneling/sinus tracts/undermining, or where granulation tissue growth needs to be limited. Silver dressings may act as a barrier to bacterial penetration in the wound bed. Silver may eradicate biofilms of colonized bacteria.

2. **Cut the foam dressing** to the appropriate size to fill the wound cavity. Do not cut the foam dressing over the wound. Rub the cut edges to remove any loose pieces.

If you cut the foam over the wound, particles may fall into the wound and create irritation. ▼

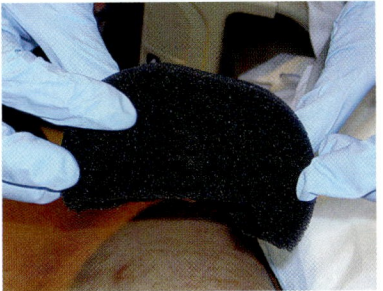

3. **Gently place the foam dressing** into the cavity without overlapping onto intact skin. Do not overfill the cavity or pack into deep crevices.

a. Do not place foam into blind/unexplored tunnels.

Forcing foam dressings into any area may damage tissue, alter the delivery of negative pressure, or hinder exudates or foam removal.

b. Do not allow foam dressing to overlap onto healthy skin.

Foam dressing becomes very wet during therapy and will macerate and damage intact skin.

c. If you use more than one piece, note the total number of pieces that were placed into the wound so you can document them on the transparent dressing and in the patient record.

An accurate record of the number of foam pieces is necessary to prevent retained material within the wound.

(continued on next page)

Procedure 36-7 ■ Applying a Negative Pressure Wound Therapy (NPWT) Device (continued)

4. **Apply a liquid skin preparation** product to periwound, if needed.

   Skin preps can protect the periwound skin from excess fluid, adhesive stripping, or other damage.

5. **Apply transparent film/drape** 3 to 5 cm (1 to 2 in.) from wound margins without pulling, stretching, or wrinkling the drape. Do not push down or compress foam while placing drape.

   The occlusive dressing creates a seal to help create negative pressure within the wound. Tension from pulling, stretching, or wrinkling the dressing may lead to tissue injury. More pressure will be placed on the wound bed than necessary if you have flattened the foam before turning on the suction unit.

6. **Avoid placing dressings that wrap** all the way around an extremity. If necessary, place several smaller pieces of drape rather than one continuous piece.

   When pressure is applied, a circumferential dressing may interfere with circulation, if wrapped too tightly.

7. **Identify a site over the dressing** for the suction track tubing apparatus.

8. **Pinch up a piece of drape** and cut at least a 2-cm round hole. Do not make a slit or X, as this may close off under pressure. ▼

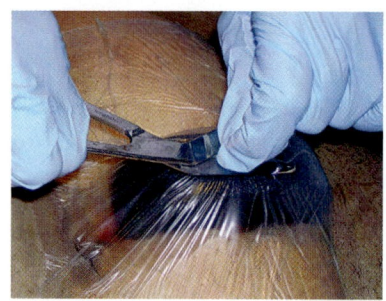

9. **Place the track adhesive** and suction device directly over the hole in the drape and apply gentle pressure to secure.

   Negative pressure removes excess wound exudate from the wound bed. ▼

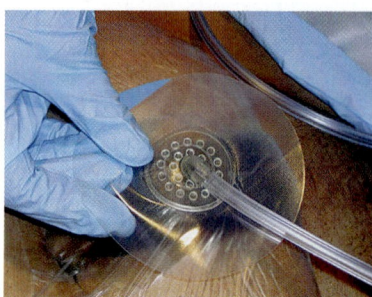

10. **Connect suction track tubing to the canister tubing and open clamps.** The canister is attached to a vacuum pump that provides either continuous or intermittent negative pressure, adjusted for the type of wound. Pressure is applied in the range of −5 to −125 mm Hg (adjustable pressures, depending on the particular device used).

    Suction draws excess exudate away from the wound and into an evacuation container.

11. **Connect tubing from the dressing to the suction** track tubing going to the collection canister.

    Allows for collection and measurement of drainage.

12. **Position the tubing and connector** away from bony prominences and skin creases.

    Prevents pressure injury to the skin.

13. **Ensure clamps are open** on all tubing.

14. **Turn on power to the pump** and set to the prescribed therapy settings to initiate therapy.

    Therapy should be maintained for at least 22 out of 24 hours daily. Alternate wound care should be considered if vacuum couldn't be tolerated for this length of time.

15. **Listen for audible leaks** and observe dressing collapse or wrinkling as pressure is applied to the wound bed.

    With an adequate seal, the dressing will collapse almost immediately. Any leak (i.e., between the dressing and drape, around tubing, at skin crevices, or at tubing connection sites) will prevent collapse. ▼

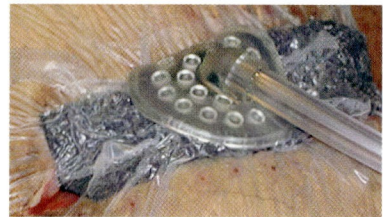

16. **Change the canister at least once a week** or when it is filled. Write the date on the canister.

    This will help to know when it was changed last as well as how often it is being changed for fluid loss.

Procedure 36-7B ■ Gauze Dressing Application (i.e., Chariker–Jeter Method)

➤ When performing the procedure, always identify your patient according to agency policy and be attentive to standard precautions, hand hygiene, patient safety and privacy, body mechanics, and documentation.

Begin with Procedure steps 1 through 13, at the beginning of Procedure 36-7. Then proceed as follows.

1. **Measure the length of drain** from wound margin, starting with the first hole perforation and pull back 1 cm.
2. **Moisten gauze with normal saline.**
3. **Wrap or "sandwich" the drain** in the moistened gauze and place in the wound base. Tuck gauze into any undermining areas to ensure contact with the wound bed.
4. **Apply a strip or small amount** of ostomy paste 1 cm from the wound edge and secure the drain as needed.

   Paste is occlusive and will help maintain a seal between the drain and the transparent film dressing. If placed too close to the wound edge, paste can get sucked into the drain, and occlude pressure.

5. **Apply liquid skin preparation** product to periwound, if needed. Extra drape, hydrocolloid, or transparent dressing may be used to protect fragile skin.

   Skin preps help protect the periwound skin from excess fluid, adhesive stripping, or other damage.

6. **Apply transparent film** approximately 1.0 to 2.5 cm (½ to 1 in.) beyond the wound margin to intact skin. Pinch the film around the drain tubing to ensure a tight seal.
7. **Avoid wrapping dressings around** an extremity. If necessary, place several smaller pieces of drape rather than one continuous piece.

   When pressure is applied, a circumferential dressing may interfere with circulation.

8. **Attach filter tubing to the canister spout.**
9. **Connect tubing from the dressing** to the evacuation tubing going to the collection canister.

   Allows for collection and measurement of drainage.

10. **Position the tubing and connector** away from bony prominences and skin creases. ▾

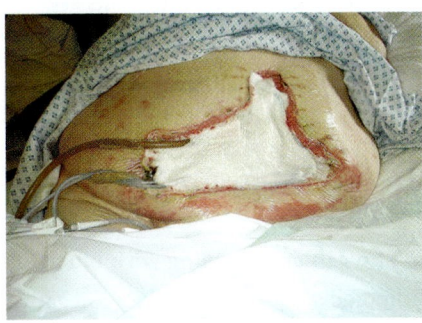

Prevents pressure injury to the skin.

11. **Ensure clamps are open** on all tubing.
12. **Turn on power to pump** and set to the prescribed therapy settings to initiate therapy.

    Therapy should be maintained for at least 22 out of 24 hours daily. Alternate wound care should be considered suction couldn't be tolerated for this length of time.

13. **Listen for audible leaks** and observe dressing collapse as pressure is applied to the wound bed.

    With an adequate seal, the dressing will collapse almost immediately. Any leak (i.e., between the dressing and drape, around tubing, at skin crevices, or at tubing connection sites) will prevent collapse.

14. **Change the canister at least once a week** or when it is filled. Write the date on the canister.

    This will help to know when it was changed last as well as how often it is being changed for fluid loss.

? What if . . .

■ **You are changing the dressing instead of applying it for the first time.**

Follow the procedure steps below. *Note:* Dressings should be changed every 48 to 72 hours.

Dressings left in the wound longer than the recommended time frame can be difficult to remove if tissue grows into the foam, or can lead to infection.

a. Evaluate the need for analgesia.
b. Turn the suction pump unit off during the procedure.
c. Place a waterproof, biohazard pad under the body part requiring the dressing change.
d. Perform hand hygiene and don sterile or clean gloves as appropriate.
e. Remove the transparent dressing, using a push–pull method to gently pull up drape while pushing it slowly from the skin. Separating the drape from the skin in this manner will decrease the risk of tape stripping.
f. Gently remove gauze or foam dressing. If dressing is difficult to remove, instill normal saline onto the dressing for 15 to 30 minutes.

   Dressing removal can damage new granulation tissue if tissue has grown into the dressing.

g. Count all pieces of gauze or foam dressing that were removed to ensure none remain in the wound bed. Ensure no dressing is left in tunneled or undermined areas.

   Dressings are not bioabsorbable and can abscess if left in the wound.

h. Discard soiled dressings in a biohazardous waste receptacle.
i. Start at the beginning of Procedure 36-7 and perform steps 1 through 13. Then, as instructed in step 13, follow either Procedure 36-7A or 36-7B.

(continued on next page)

Procedure 36–7 ■ Applying a Negative Pressure Wound Therapy (NPWT) Device (continued)

■ **After 2 weeks, you see that the wound is not improving?**

Consult with the primary provider or a wound care specialist. Average length of therapy is usually 4 to 6 weeks. Therapy should be discontinued if the wound shows no improvement in 1 to 2 consecutive weeks, the patient is unwilling or unable to follow the medical plan, or the goal of therapy has been met.

The longer a wound is open, the longer it takes to heal, and places the patient at risk for complications. A steady decrease in wound size should be seen every week. If NPWT is not effective, alternate wound care should be evaluated.

■ **You cannot find or remove a piece of foam?**

Notify the provider, as this may necessitate surgery.

The material could be retained in the patient and create an inflammatory response.

■ **There is a foul odor when the dressing is removed?**

Clean the wound with normal saline to ensure odor is not emanating from the soiled dressing. If other signs of infection are present (i.e., fever, tenderness, redness, swelling, purulent drainage), notify the provider.

■ **Suction cannot be maintained?**

Identify why the seal cannot be maintained. If the wound is very near the coccyx and gluteal fold, use a small amount of paste to help fill in the crack and maintain a seal. If the skin around the wound is moist, adhesive drape will not adhere to skin. Use a skin prep product or drape to protect the skin. If the tube is pulling away from the dressing or tension is being placed on the tube, anchor it with additional drape or tape several centimeters from the dressing or wound.

■ **The canister is filling with blood?**

Immediately discontinue negative pressure therapy. The gauze or foam dressing will not stop the bleeding, so take measures to control bleeding (i.e., hold pressure on wound). Do not remove dressing until the treating primary care provider is consulted.

■ **Dressing does not collapse or the alarm sounds?**

a. Press firmly around the transparent dressing to seal.

b. Verify the machine is turned on, and all clamps are open and tubing is not kinked.

c. Check tubing and drape for leaks. Listen for leaks with a stethoscope or by moving your hand around the wound margins while applying slight pressure.

d. Additional small pieces of transparent dressing may be used to seal around hardware, skin fold, or creases.

e. Do not place multiple layers of drape or adhesive dressing.
Several layers may decrease the dressing's moisture vapor transmission rate, increasing the risk of maceration.

f. Never leave foam in place without an adequate seal for more than 2 hours. If an adequate seal cannot be achieved in that time, remove the foam and apply a saline moistened gauze dressing.

Evaluation

- Note the patient's response to the procedure.
- Continue to monitor wound healing and changes in periwound tissues.
- Monitor dressing every 2 hours to ensure it is firm and collapsed in the wound bed while therapy is on.
- Monitor the seal of the dressing, and pressure settings.
- Monitor for brisk or bright bleeding, evisceration or dehiscence, and symptoms of infection.
  You must report these to the provider.

Home Care

- Refer the client to a home health agency for wound care.
- In limited circumstances, some clients or caregivers may be able to perform dressing changes. Determine their ability to perform dressing changes teach and demonstrate as needed.
- Instruct the client or family to visually check the dressing every 2 hours to ensure it is firm and collapsed in the wound bed.
- Review safety labeling, alarms, and pump instructions.
- Review conditions in which to seek medical care: bleeding, infection, unresolved alarms, or loss of suction.
- Review proper disposal of contaminated supplies.

Documentation

Document the following information:

- Date and time of dressing change
- Wound assessment: location of the wound, size (length, width, diameter), undermining or tunneling, amount and character of drainage, odor, wound bed including type and percentage of tissue seen, and periwound appearance
- Evaluation of therapy with evidence of healing
- Treatment selected: type of NPWT, type of gauze or foam, number of pieces placed in the wound
- Treatment settings: pressures, intermittent vs. continuous, or variable pressures
- Patient response to dressing change

Practice Resources

Armstrong, Attinger, Boulton, et al., 2004; Chariker, 2009; Kinetic Concepts Inc., 2007, 2008; Krasner, Shapshak, & Hopf, 2007; Medica-Rents Co. 2008); NGC, 2006, revised 2008; Samson, Lefevre, & Aronson, 2004; Siegel, Rhinehart, Jackson, et al., 2007; Sullivan, Snyder, Tipton, et al., 2009.

Procedure 36-8 ■ Applying and Removing a Transparent Film Dressing

➤ For steps to follow in *all* procedures, refer to the Universal Steps for All Procedures found on the page facing the inside back cover.

Equipment

- Clean nonsterile gloves
- Sterile gauze
- Normal saline solution or specified cleansing agent, warmed to body temperature when possible
  Cold solution lowers the temperature of the wound bed and slows the healing process.
- Scissors (if needed)
- Liquid skin preparation (if needed)
- Transparent film dressing (e.g., Op-Site, Tegaderm, Bio-Occlusive)

Delegation

Because assessment of the wound and knowledge of clean technique are important, you should not delegate this procedure to a NAP.

Pre-Procedure Assessment

- Assess the area to determine whether a transparent film dressing is appropriate.

Transparent film dressings are indicated as primary dressings (dressings that touch the wound or area to be treated) to protect high-risk intact skin; for superficial or partial-thickness wounds that have little to no drainage (i.e., stage I or II pressure ulcers); and to assist in débriding eschar by autolysis. Films may be used as a secondary dressing to protect other types of dressings from bodily fluids (i.e., wounds near the perineum).

- Assess the wound to determine if use of a transparent film is contraindicated.
  Films are contraindicated in third-degree burns, arterial ulcers, and infected wounds. Films should not be used to fill dead space.
- Determine the size of the wound.
  Film dressings are available in many sizes. Select the appropriate size based on wound measurements, allowing for a 2.5 cm (1 in.) perimeter of intact skin around the wound for the adhesive to stick.
- Assess the periwound area.
  Film dressings should be attached to intact skin. The adhesive is not waterproof and will not adhere to wet or moist skin.

➤ When performing the procedure, always identify your patient according to agency policy and be attentive to standard precautions, hand hygiene, patient safety and privacy, body mechanics, and documentation.

Procedure Steps

1. **Place the patient in a comfortable position** that provides easy access to the wound.

Procedure Steps for Applying the Dressing

2. **If a dressing is present**, wash your hands, don clean nonsterile gloves, and remove the old dressing.
3. **Dispose of the soiled dressing** and gloves in the biohazard waste receptacle.
   Observe universal precautions, preventing transfer of pathogens.
4. **Don clean gloves** and cleanse the skin surrounding the wound with normal saline or a mild cleansing agent. Be sure to rinse the skin well if you use a cleanser. Allow the skin to dry.
   Cleansing prepares the skin for application of the dressing. Skin must be dry for the dressing to adhere.
5. **Cleanse the wound** as prescribed or according to agency procedure.

Cleansing of wounds removes bacteria and necrotic debris from wound beds.

6. **Consider placing a skin barrier** around the wound before transparent film dressing application.
   Skin sealants may be applied to skin before tape to protect fragile skin from tears or epidermal stripping.
7. **Remove the center backing liner** from the transparent film dressing. ▼

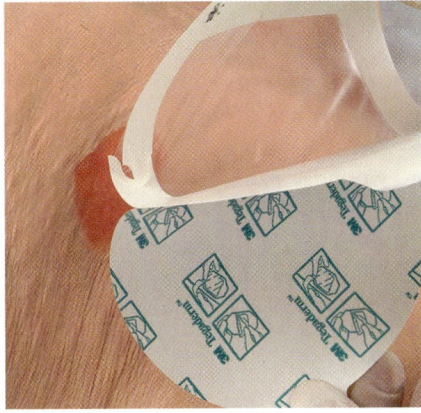

8. Holding the dressing by the edges, **apply the transparent film** to the wound without stretching or pulling the dressing or the skin.
   This reduces the risk of skin damage to skin.
9. **Remove the edging liner** from the dressing.
10. **Gently smooth and secure** the dressing to skin.
    Allows the dressing to adhere fully to the patient's skin.
11. **Dispose of soiled equipment**, and remove your gloves.

Procedure Steps for Removing the Dressing

Transparent film dressings are typically changed every 3 days. Change dressing sooner if drainage extends beyond the edges of the wound onto periwound skin. To remove the dressing, do the following:

12. **Grasp one edge of the film dressing.**

(continued on next page)

Procedure 36–8 ■ Applying and Removing a Transparent Film Dressing (continued)

13. **Gently lift the edge.**
14. **Stabilize the skin underneath** the elevated edge with your finger.
    Stabilizing the skin as the adhesive is taken off will prevent epidermal stripping.
15. With your other hand, **slowly peel the dressing back over itself**, "low and slow," in the direction of hair growth.
    Removing the dressing at an angle will increase the risk of pulling on the epidermis and causing mechanical trauma.
16. As dressing is removed, **keep moving your finger** as necessary to avoid newly exposed skin.

? What if . . .

■ **The adhesive will not adhere to the patient's skin due to excess hair?**

Hair may be removed with clippers/scissors. Do not shave the site with a razor.

Shaving can cause nicks or abrasions to the skin that could become a portal of entry for bacteria.

■ **The patient's skin is diaphoretic or excessively oily?**

Cleanse the skin with soap and water before the dressing change. Also, polymer skin barriers may be used to place a seal over the skin and allow the tape adhesive to adhere.

■ **The patient has fragile skin (i.e., elderly patient)?**

Skin sealant preparations may be used under adhesives.
The junction between the epidermis and dermis on the older adult is not as strong as with a younger person. Less pressure or tension is needed to break those bonds and cause skin damage.

■ **The dressing sticks to itself before it can be applied?**

If a small portion of the dressing is stuck to itself, gently stretch or pull the edges in opposite directions. If a large portion is involved, throw the dressing away and start over.
Transparent dressings can be difficult to apply because they are polyurethane sheets coated on one side with an acrylic, hypoallergenic adhesive and are flimsy in nature, making them clumsy to work with at times.

■ **Purulent-appearing fluid has collected underneath the film dressing?**

This does not necessarily mean the wound is infected. Remove the dressing and clean the wound per policy. Select an alternate dressing that will be more absorptive.
Because films do not have absorptive capabilities, any drainage produced by the wound will pool underneath.

Evaluation

■ Verify the transparent film dressing is appropriate for the wound.
■ Determine whether the dressing adheres comfortably to skin.
■ Ensure that patient verbalizes understanding of treatment.

Patient Teaching

■ Teach the patient about the expected healing process.
■ Teach the patient about the use of transparent film dressings.
■ Inform the patient and caregiver about signs and symptoms of infection and the need to report these findings.

Documentation

Document the following information (many agencies use a wound/skin flow sheet):
■ Wound assessment: location of the wound, size (length × width × diameter) undermining or tunneling, amount and character of drainage, odor, wound bed including type and percentage of tissue seen, and peri-wound appearance
■ Appearance and location of the wound, type and amount of exudate, and odor, if present, after cleansing
■ The patient's pain level before the procedure. If the patient was medicated for pain, document the drug and dose used, time given, and the patient's response to analgesia.
■ Method of cleansing the wound and surrounding skin
■ Type of dressing applied to the wound
■ Education provided to the patient

Practice Resources

AORN, 2008; Bryant & Nix, 2006; 3M, 2004.

Procedure 36-9 ■ Applying a Hydrating Dressing (Hydrocolloid or Hydrogel)

➤ For steps to follow in *all* procedures, refer to the Universal Steps for All Procedures found on the page facing the inside back cover.

Equipment

- Clean nonsterile gloves
- Hydrating dressing 3 to 4 cm (1.5 in.) larger than the wound
- Moisture-proof bag
- Obtain the following items, only if needed:
- Sterile normal saline solution or tap water according to agency policy or as prescribed for irrigation, warmed to body temperature when possible
  Cold solution lowers the temperature of wound bed and slows the healing process.
- Emesis basin
- Sterile gauze for cleansing
- Disposable clippers or scissors (to trim hair or dressing)
- Skin prep
- Measuring device
- Tape

Delegation

This procedure requires knowledge of wound healing, dressings, and infection control and prevention. You should not delegate this procedure to a NAP.

Pre-Procedure Assessments

- Assess the area to determine whether a hydrating dressing is appropriate.
  Hydrating dressings are appropriate for wounds with minimal drainage. These dressings autolytically débride necrotic tissue from the wound bed. They may also be used to protect skin at risk for breakdown.
- Determine the size of the wound.
  Allows you to select a dressing of the appropriate size. Choosing a dressing size that extends beyond the ulcer ensures complete coverage.

➤ When performing the procedure, always identify your patient according to agency policy and be attentive to standard precautions, hand hygiene, patient safety and privacy, body mechanics, and documentation.

Procedure Steps

1. **Place the patient in a comfortable position** that provides easy access to the wound.
   Provides for patient comfort and proper nurse body mechanics during dressing change.

2. If a dressing is present, wash your hands, **don clean nonsterile gloves, and remove the old dressing**.
   Prevents transfer of pathogens.

3. **Dispose of the soiled dressing** and gloves in the biohazard waste receptacle.
   Dressings may contain body fluids and other contaminants, so they must be disposed of moisture-proof containers.

4. **Wash your hands**. Don clean gloves, and cleanse the skin surrounding the wound with normal saline or a mild cleansing agent. Be sure to rinse the skin well if you use a cleanser. (You might need a linen saver pad under the patient.) Allow the skin to dry. Do not attempt to remove residue that is left on the skin from the old dressing.

Cleansing and drying prepare the skin for application of the dressing. Removing residue irritates the surrounding skin.

5. **Cleanse the wound as directed**. Wound cleansing may be performed with clean or sterile technique, depending on the type of wound.
   Cleansing the wound removes microbes and necrotic debris from wound bed. Studies show that both saline and tap water are similarly effective for cleansing.

6. **Apply skin prep** to the area covered by tape.
   Skin prep protects intact skin from breakdown from tape removal.

7. **Remove soiled gloves**, and assess the condition of the wound. Note the size, location, type of tissue present, amount of exudate, and odor.
   Granulating tissue is beefy red with a velvety appearance. It appears with the growth of new blood vessels and connective tissue. Pale pink tissue may indicate compromised blood supply to the wound bed. Necrotic tissue, which is black, brown, or yellow in appearance, is nonviable and inhibits healing. A hydrocolloid dressing will interact with wound drainage to produce a thick, yellow gel that may have a foul

odor. Clean the wound before assessing for exudate and odor.

8. With the backing still intact, **cut the hydrating dressing**, if necessary, to the desired shape and size. Size the hydrocolloid dressing so it will extend 3 to 4 cm (1.5 in.) beyond the wound margin on all sides and cover all areas of nonintact skin.
   Provides complete coverage of the wound.

9. Don clean gloves, and remove the backing of the hydrocolloid dressing, starting at one edge. **Place the exposed adhesive portion on the patient's skin**. Position the dressing to cover the wound. ▼

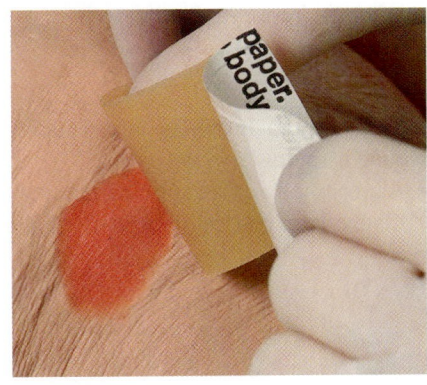

(continued on next page)

Procedure 36–9 ■ Applying a Hydrating Dressing (Hydrocolloid or Hydrogel) (continued)

10. Gradually peel away the remaining liner, and smooth the hydrocolloid dressing onto the skin by placing your hand on top of dressing and holding in place for 1 minute. *Warmth helps the dressing adhere to the skin.* ▼

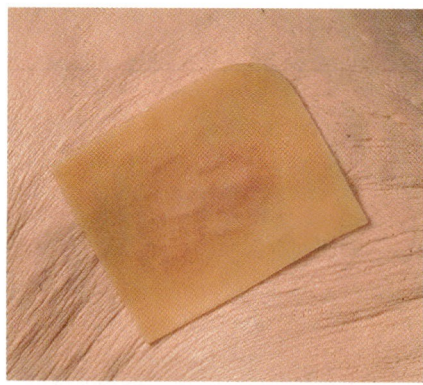

11. Assist the patient to a comfortable position, and remove your gloves. Wash your hands.

? What if . . .

- **Signs of infection are noted?**

  Notify primary care provider. Cultures may be prescribed. A different type of dressing may be prescribed, as well.

- **The surrounding skin is not intact?**

  Choose a larger size hydrocolloid dressing to cover the nonintact area. Document your observations and report new findings to the primary care provider.

Evaluation

- Verify that a hydrocolloid dressing is still appropriate for the wound.
- Note whether the dressing adheres comfortably to the skin.
- Ensure the patient verbalizes understanding of treatment.
- Inspect the dressing daily. Change it if it becomes dislodged, leaks, or wrinkles or if it develops an odor.

Patient Teaching

- Teach the patient about the expected healing process.
- Inform the patient and caregiver about signs and symptoms of infection and the need to report these findings.

Home Care

- Hydrating dressings may be required in the home setting. Teach caregivers to use the appropriate size and change the dressing if it begins to leak, develops an odor, or begins to separate from the skin.

Documentation

Document the following information. (Many agencies use wound care flow sheets.)
- Appearance and location of the wound, type and amount of exudate, and odor, if present, after cleansing. Include

wound measurements, if taken, and condition of surrounding skin.
- The patient's pain level before the procedure. If the patient was medicated for pain, document the drug and dose used, time given, and patient response.
- Method of cleansing the wound and surrounding skin
- Type of dressing applied to the wound
- Use of skin prep
- Education provided to the patient

Practice Resources

Atiyeh & Hayek, 2004; Dunaway & Goldrick, 2007; Joanna Briggs Institute, 2008a.

Thinking About the Procedure

 Go to the *Fundamentals of Nursing Skills Videos*, **Wound Care: Dressings: Hydrocolloid.**

1. Did the nurse place a pad under the patient when changing the dressing? Why or why not?
2. What kind of wound is the nurse dressing with the hydrocolloid dressing in this demonstration?

 For suggested responses, go to Chapter 36, **Thinking About the Procedure Suggested Responses,** on *DavisPlus*.

Procedure 36-10 ■ Placing Skin Closures

➤ For steps to follow in *all* procedures, refer to the Universal Steps for All Procedures found on the page facing the inside back cover.

Equipment
- Adhesive skin closures
- Skin preparation product
- Forceps
- Normal saline
- Gauze
- Gloves (sterile if indicated)

Delegation
This procedure itself may be delegated to a NAP unless it is a new wound requiring sterile technique. Assessment of the incision line or wound is a licensed professional's responsibility and should not be delegated.

Pre-Procedure Assessment
- Assess the type of wound to be closed.
  Adhesive closures are frequently used to keep surgical incisions well approximated. They may be used in conjunction with staples or sutures or following early staple/suture removal. Closures may be used to approximate the edges of lacerations or skin tears.

- Assess the wound for skin edge approximation.
  Wounds that are gaping or appear to have undermining should not be closed using adhesive closures.
- Assess the wound for drainage, amount, type, and odor.
  Wounds that are draining heavily might not be suitable for Steri-Strips™ because the adhesive would not stick to the skin.
- Assess the periwound area or surrounding skin. Assessment should include skin color, texture, temperature, and integrity of the surrounding skin. Look for maceration (caused by heavy drainage), excoriation (from caustic effluent), stripping (from inappropriate adhesive removal), pustules, papules, or lesions.
  Adhesive closures should be placed only on intact skin.
- Assess the length of the wound, the location (over a joint), or if edema may occur, to determine the size of the skin closure used. Consider elastic skin closures if distention or movement is anticipated.
  Closures come in several different lengths, widths, and flexibility capabilities to meet elasticity and conformability needs.

➤ When performing the procedure, always identify your patient according to agency policy and be attentive to standard precautions, hand hygiene, patient safety and privacy, body mechanics, and documentation.

Procedure Steps

1. **Don clean nonsterile gloves.**
   Gloving prevents cross-contamination.
2. **Cleanse the skin** at least 5 cm (2 in.) around the wound with a saline-moistened gauze. Pat the skin dry, allowing it to dry thoroughly.
   The skin surrounding the wound must be clean and dry in order for the strips to adhere.
3. **Apply skin preparation product**, and allow it to dry (or follow agency procedures). Avoid benzoin on fragile skin.
   Skin preparation product enhances adhesion of the strips.
4. **Do not allow skin preparation** product to contact the wound.
   It may impair healing.
5. **Peel back package tabs** to access the adhesive closures.
6. **Remove the card from the package** using modified sterile technique as necessary.
   Careful technique should be followed when applying to a surgical wound to
minimize contamination and promote healing.
7. **Grasp end of skin closure** with forceps or gloved hand and peel strip from the card at a 90° angle.
   Closures lifted at a lesser angle or directly back on themselves may "curl," complicating handling.
8. Starting at the middle of the wound, **apply strips across the wound**, drawing the wound edges together. Apply closures without tension; do not stretch or strap closures.
   a. Apply half of the closure to the wound margin and press firmly in place.
   b. Using fingers or forceps, ensure skin edges are approximated.
   c. Press free half firmly on the other side of the wound.
   d. Place the strips so that they extend at least 2 to 3 cm (¾ to 1 in.) on either side of the wound to ensure closure.

   e. Place the wound closure strips 3 mm (⅛ in.) apart along the wound. ▼

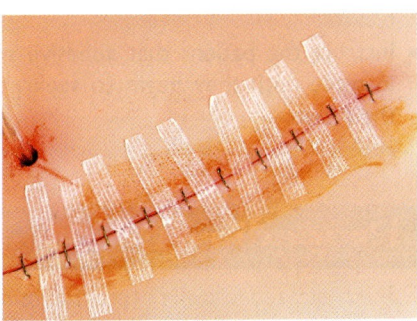

? What if . . .
- **A flap of skin rolls up on the edges?**
  Cleanse the wound with normal saline and reapproximate the edges of the skin flap with the intact epidermis. Apply skin closures across the flap.
  Elderly or immature skin can experience delayed wound healing.

(continued on next page)

Procedure 36–10 ■ Placing Skin Closures (continued)

■ **The skin around the wound is swollen?**

Apply skin closures without tension, and reapply as swelling increases.
This prevents pulling on the skin that can delay healing or disrupt the approximated borders of the wound, which is more likely to lead to scarring.

■ **Edges are not accurately approximated or tension has been placed on the skin?**

Remove the closure over the affected area, peeling each side toward the wound, and reapply.

Use of adhesive products can cause superficial skin damage if the skin is stretched during application or with edema formation. Tension blisters are the most common problem associated with taping.

Patient Evaluation

- Verify that skin closures are appropriate for the wound.
- Note whether the closures adhere comfortably to the skin.
- Ensure the patient verbalized understanding of the treatment.
- Inspect the wound daily. Lifted closure edges may be trimmed or closures replaced if less than half of the strip remains.

Patient Teaching

- Teach the patient about the expected healing process.
- Inform the patient or caregiver about signs and symptoms of infection and the need to report these findings.
- Instruct patients not to pull or tug on the strips.
  Improper removal may damage the underlying skin or the wound itself.
- Instruct patients that they do not need to keep the strips dry.
  They can bathe and shower as directed by the healthcare provider.
- Instruct the patient that adhesive strips are often kept in place until they begin to separate from the skin on their own.

Documentation

Document the following information. (Many agencies use specialized wound care flow sheets.)
- Appearance and location of the wound, type and amount of exudates, and odor, if present, after cleansing
- The patient's level of pain before the procedure. If the patient was medicated for pain, document the drug and dose used, time given, and the patient response to analgesia.
- Method of cleansing the wound and surrounding skin
- Type of skin closures applied
- Education provided to the patient

Practice Resources
Bryant & Nix, 2006; 3M, 2004.

Thinking About the Procedure

 Go to the *Fundamentals of Nursing Skills Videos*, **Wound Care: Steri–Strips.**

1. How are the skin closure strips positioned on the patient's wound?

 For suggested responses, go to Chapter 36, **Thinking About the Procedure Suggested Responses,** on *DavisPlus.*

Procedure 36–11 ■ Applying Binders

➤ For steps to follow in *all* procedures, refer to the Universal Steps for All Procedures found on the page facing the inside back cover.

Equipment

- Abdominal binder, triangular arm binder, or T-binder
- Clean nonsterile gloves
- Measuring tape

Delegation

This procedure itself may be delegated to a NAP. Assessment of the incision line or wound is a licensed professional's responsibility and should not be delegated.

Pre-Procedure Assessments

- Assess the condition of the wound (if one is present). Note the amount and type of drainage. A wound must be dressed before it is bandaged; if there is a significant amount of exudate, you will need to apply a secondary dressing.
- Assess for pain, and check the circulation of the underlying body parts before and after applying the binder. Look for cool, pale, or cyanotic skin, tingling, and numbness.
- Determine whether the client or family has the skills to reapply the binder when necessary.

➤ When performing the procedure, always identify your patient according to agency policy and be attentive to standard precautions, hand hygiene, patient safety and privacy, body mechanics, and documentation.

➤ Observe steps 1 through 6, regardless of the type of binder you use:

Procedure Steps

1. **Choose a binder of the proper size.**
2. **Wash hands. Don gloves.**
3. **Thoroughly clean and dry the part** to be covered.
   Moisture contributes to skin breakdown.
4. **Place the body part** in its natural, comfortable position (e.g., with the joint slightly flexed), whenever possible.
   Prevents strain on ligaments and muscles.
5. **Pad between skin surfaces** (e.g., under the axilla) and over bony prominences.
   Prevents pressure and abrasion of the skin.
6. **Fasten from the bottom up**, especially for abdominal binders.

   ✚ Make sure the binder is secured with enough pressure to provide the needed support and control bleeding, but not so tightly as to compromise circulation or impair breathing.

   Provides upward support.
7. **Change binders** whenever they become soiled or wet.
   Proceed to step 8, 14, or 20, depending on the type of binder you are using.

Procedure Variation **Applying an Abdominal Binder**

8. **Measure the patient** for the abdominal binder.
   a. Place the patient in supine position.
   b. With a measuring tape, encircle the abdomen at the level of the umbilicus. Note the measurement. This is the length of the binder. ▼

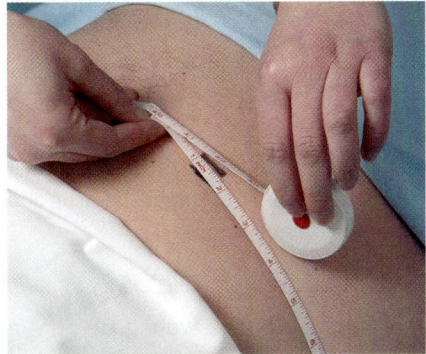

   c. Measure the distance from the costal margin to the top of the iliac crests. This is the width of the binder.
   d. Dispose of gloves and measuring tape, and wash your hands.
   e. Based on the measurements, obtain an abdominal binder.
9. **Assist the patient to roll** to one side. Roll one end of the binder to the center mark. Place the rolled section of the abdominal binder underneath the patient. Position the binder appropriately between the costal margin and iliac crest.
10. **Make sure the binder** does not slip upward or downward.
    If the binder is positioned too high, it could impair lung expansion and gas exchange. If it is positioned too low, the binder will not provide adequate support.
11. **Assist the patient to turn** to the other side as you unroll the binder from underneath him.

    ✚ Pad any pressure areas or skin abrasions to avoid pressure injury.
12. **With your dominant hand**, grasp the end of the binder on the side furthest from you, and steadily pull toward the center of the patient's abdomen. With your nondominant hand, grasp the end of binder side closest to you, and pull toward the center. Overlap the ends of the binder so that the hook and loop fasteners (e.g., Velcro) meet. ▼

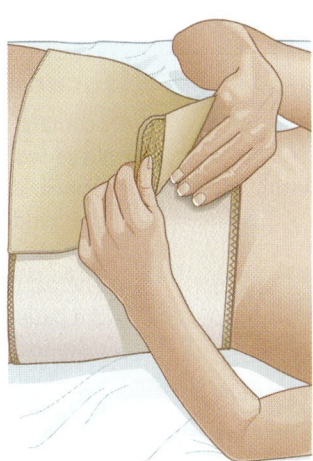

13. **Remove the abdominal binder every 2 hours,** and assess the underlying skin and dressings. Change wound dressings if they are soiled, or as prescribed.

Procedure Variation **Applying a Triangular Arm Binder**

A triangular arm binder or sling is used to support the upper extremities. Obtain a commercial sling (consisting of a sleeve for the arm and a strap to go around the neck) or a triangular piece of fabric. To form a splint from a triangular cloth, follow these steps:

14. **Ask the patient to place** the affected arm in a natural position across the chest, elbow flexed slightly.
    Slight flexion prevents swelling of the hand and relieves pressure on the shoulder.
15. **Place one end of the triangle** over the shoulder of the uninjured arm, and allow the triangle to fall open so that the elbow of the injured arm is at the apex of the triangle.
16. **Move the sling behind the injured arm.**
17. **Pull up the lower corner** of the triangle over the injured arm to the shoulder of the injured arm.
18. **Tie the sling with a square knot** at the neck on the side of the arm requiring support.
    A square not will not slip and is easy to untie.
19. **Adjust the injured arm** within the sling.
    To ensure patient comfort. ▼

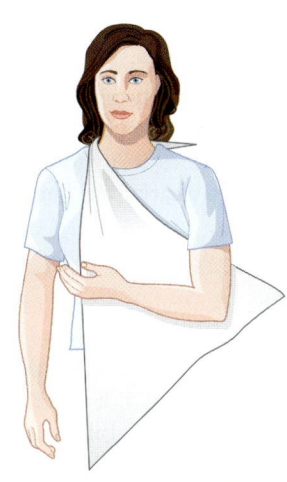

(continued on next page)

Procedure 36-11 ■ **Applying Binders** (continued)

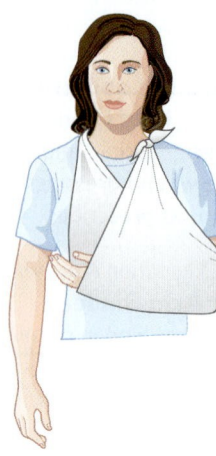

Procedure Variation Applying a T-Binder

A T-binder is used to secure dressings or pads in the perineal area. A single T-binder is often used for women. A double T-binder is most commonly used for men. To apply a T-binder, follow these steps:

20. **Position the waist tails** under the patient at the natural waistline. Bring the right and left tails together, and secure them at the waist with pins or clips.

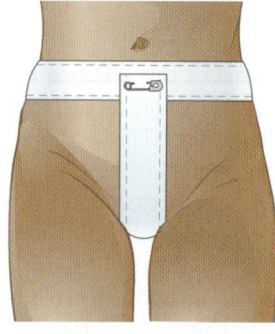

21. **For a single T-binder**, bring the center tail up between the legs of the patient. Secure the tail at the waist with pins or clips.
22. **For a double T-binder**, bring the tails up on either side of the penis. Secure the tail at the waist with pins or clips. ▼

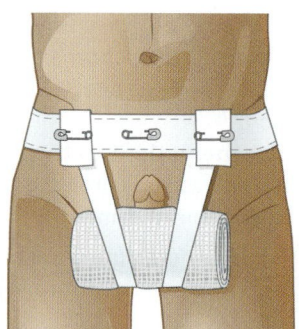

23. **Fasten the ties at the waist** using pins or clips.

? What if . . .

■ **The patient is obese?**

Obtain a binder of the appropriate size before applying. Do not try to position a binder that is too small for the patient.

A poorly fitting binder can constrict circulation, cause pressure points that can injure the skin, and can restrict movement of the chest for adequate breathing. A binder that is too tight is uncomfortable and it will not provide the proper support of an incision or wound needed for healing.

Evaluation

■ Evaluate whether the patient's physical condition has changed since using the binder.
■ Assess circulation to be sure the binder is not securely too tightly. Check color, warmth, tingling, sensation, and capillary refill.
■ Assess the depth of breathing to be sure the binder is not restricting ventilation.
■ Check the skin under the binder to be sure there are no areas of irritation, pressure, or skin abrasion.
■ Assess incisions or wounds under the binder to be sure they are not bleeding and are healing properly.
■ Monitor comfort regularly.
■ Assess the client's ability to perform activities of daily living (ADLs) while wearing the binder.

Home Care

■ Teach the client and/or caregiver how to apply the binder in the proper position, snugly but not too tightly.
■ Teach the family to inspect the site under the binder to be sure the skin is not pinched or with other points of pressure. This is especially crucial for older adults.
■ Clean binders in warm, soapy water when soiled. Use a mesh laundry bag to keep the Velcro straps from catching other clothing in the washer. Air dry thoroughly. Clients should have two binders at home—a clean one to wear while the other is laundered.
■ Apply and remove binder to promote comfort and ensure good circulation. This also allows the patient and caregiver to inspect any incision or wound underneath.
■ Binders for children at home could be decorated with permanent marking pens.
■ Allow children to help with applying and removing the binder.

Documentation

Document the following information. (Many agencies use specialized wound care flow sheets.)

■ Appearance and location of the wound or incision under the binder, type and amount of exudates, and odor, if present, after cleansing
■ The patient's level of pain before and after the procedure. If the patient was medicated for pain, document the drug and dose used, time given, and patient response.
■ Type of binder applied
■ Date and time the binder was applied and removed
■ Any change in the appearance of the wound or skin in contact with the binder
■ Education provided to the patient

Procedure 36-12 ■ **Applying Bandages**

➤ For steps to follow in *all* procedures, refer to the Universal Steps for All Procedures found on the page facing the inside back cover.

Equipment

- Appropriate bandage dressing
- Clean procedure gloves (2 pairs)
- Gauze sponges
- Normal saline
- Primary dressing (as prescribed)
- Scissors
- Tape or metal closures

Delegation

This procedure itself may be delegated to a NAP who has the appropriate training. Assessment of the incision line or wound is a licensed professional's responsibility and should not be delegated.

Pre-Procedure Assessment

- Determine the body part or area to be bandaged.
  This allows you to choose the correct width of gauze or elastic bandage to use.

- Assess the condition of the wound (if one is present).
- Assess the wound for size (length, width, and depth in centimeters); location and depth of undermining or tunneling; amount, character and odor of drainage; type and percentage of tissue present in wound bed (granulation, slough, fibrin, necrotic); and periwound condition (intact, denuded, erythema, induration, or maceration)
  Wound dressings should be chosen based on the characteristics of the wound.
- Assess for pain, and check the circulation of the underlying body parts before and after applying the bandage. Look for cool, pale, or cyanotic skin, tingling, and numbness.
  Circulation to an extremity can be compromised if the bandage is too tight or the extremity swells after application.
- Determine whether the client or family has the skills to reapply the bandage when necessary.
  Teaching might be needed for home care.

➤ When performing the procedure, always identify your patient according to agency policy and be attentive to standard precautions, hand hygiene, patient safety and privacy, body mechanics, and documentation.

Procedure Steps

Observe the following guidelines, regardless of the type of bandage you use:

1. **Choose a bandage** of the proper width. For example, use a 2.5-cm (1-in.) wide bandage for a finger, a 5-cm (2-in.) wide bandage for an arm, and a wider bandage for a leg.
   This prevents pressure and abrasion of the skin.

2. **Thoroughly clean and dry** the part to be covered. Use a nontoxic cleansing solution, such as normal saline.
   Cleaning the wound removes debris, exudates, and bacteria. Drainage and moisture on the skin contribute to irritation.

3. **Remove excess fluid** by gently patting the wound and surrounding skin with gauze sponge.
   Drainage and moisture contribute to skin breakdown.

4. **Stand facing the patient.**
   In this position you can wrap the bandage evenly in the proper direction.

5. **Bandage the body part** in a comfortable position (e.g., with the

joint slightly flexed), whenever possible.
This prevents strain on ligaments and muscles. Movement of the extremity (extension) may cause skin damage if the bandage is too tight or the extremity is not properly positioned.

6. **Always work from distal** to proximal (or peripheral to central).
   This improves venous return and helps to prevent edema.

7. **If a wound is present,** apply a primary dressing, as prescribed, over the wound.
   A primary dressing is any dressing that is placed first in the wound bed. It provides exudates absorption, holds medications in place, provides antimicrobial coverage, or maintains a moist wound bed.

8. **Apply the bandage with enough** pressure to provide the needed support, but do not bandage too tightly. Make sure circulation to the area is not interrupted.

9. **If possible, leave the fingers** (if you are bandaging an arm) or toes (if you are bandaging a leg or foot) ex-

posed so you can assess the circulation to the extremity. Begin the wrap along the pad of the foot or hand, just under the first bend of the toes or fingers (metatarsal or metacarpal joints).

10. **Begin the wrap** with the bandage against the skin. Unwind the bandage as if rolling it over the extremity.
    This helps to keep the bandage snug against the skin.

11. **Pad bony prominences** before bandaging if there are pressure concerns.

12. **Change bandages** whenever they become soiled or wet from external sources (stool, urine, etc.) and internal sources (drainage that has wicked on the outer surface of the bandage).
    Wound drainage contains chemicals, enzymes, and bacteria that can damage fragile healing tissues.

13. **After bandaging, assess circulation** and comfort regularly.

Proceed to step 14, 16, 19, 25, or 28, depending on the type of bandaging you are using.

(continued on next page)

Procedure 36–12 ■ **Applying Bandages** (continued)

Procedure Variation **Circular Turns**

Use this technique to wrap a finger or toe, or as an anchor at the beginning and end of another wrapping technique.

14. With one hand, **hold one end of the bandage in place**. With the other hand, encircle the body part two times with the bandage—the second wrap should partially cover the first wrap. Continue to wrap the body part by overlapping two-thirds of the width of the bandage. ▼

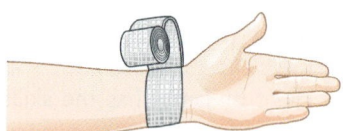

15. If circular turns are not being combined with another technique, **secure the bandage** with tape or metal clips when you are finished.

Procedure Variation **Spiral Turns**

Spiral turns are a variation of the circular turn technique. Spiral turns are most commonly used to wrap an extremity.

16. **Anchor the bandage** by making two circular turns—the second wrap completely covering the first one.

17. **Continue to wrap the extremity** by encircling the body part with each turn angled at approximately 30° so that you are overlapping the preceding wrap by two-thirds the width of the bandage. ▼

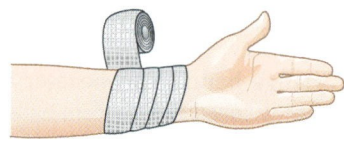

18. **Complete the wrap** by making two circular turns and securing the bandage with tape or metal clips.

Procedure Variation **Spiral Reverse Turns**

Spiral reverse turns are used to bandage cylindrical body parts that are not uniform in size.

19. **Anchor the bandage** by making two circular turns.
20. **Bring the next wrap up at a 30° angle.**
21. **Place the thumb** of your nondominant hand on the wrap to hold the bandage. ▼

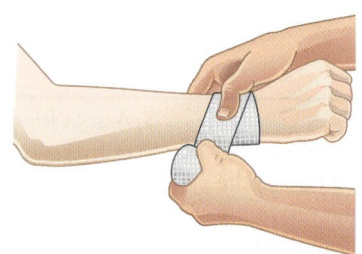

22. **Fold the bandage back on itself**, and continue to wrap at a 30° angle in the opposite direction. ▼

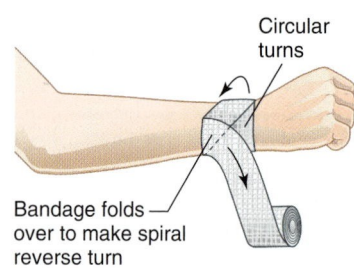

Circular turns

Bandage folds over to make spiral reverse turn

23. **Continue to wrap the bandage**, overlapping each turn by two-thirds. Align each bandage turn at the same position on the extremity. ▼

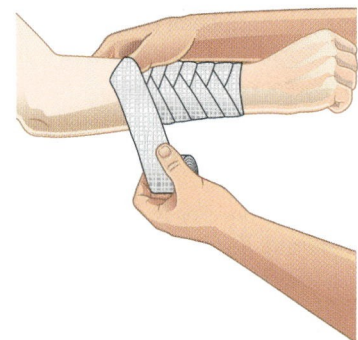

24. **Complete the wrap** by making two circular turns and securing the bandage with tape or metal clips.

Procedure Variation **Figure-8 Turns**

The figure-8 wrap is used on joints (e.g., ankle, elbow).

25. **Anchor the bandage** by making two circular turns.
26. **Wrap the bandage** by ascending above the joint and descending below the joint to form a figure 8. Continue to wrap the bandage, overlapping each turn by two-thirds. Align each bandage turn at the same position on the extremity. ▼

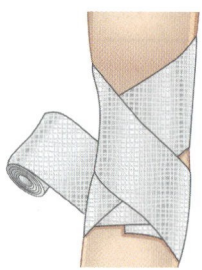

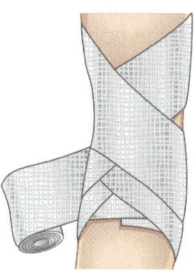

27. **Complete the wrap** by making two circular turns and securing the bandage with tape or metal clips.

Procedure Variation **Recurrent Turns**

28. **Anchor the bandage** by making two circular turns.
29. **Fold the bandage back on itself**; hold it against the body part with one hand. With the other hand, make a half turn perpendicular to the circle turns and central to the distal end being bandaged. ▼

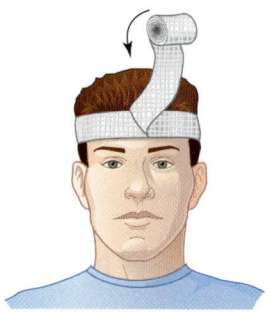

30. **Hold the central turn** with one hand, and fold the bandage back on itself; bring it over the distal end of the body part to the right of the center, overlapping the center turn by two-thirds the width of the bandage. ▼

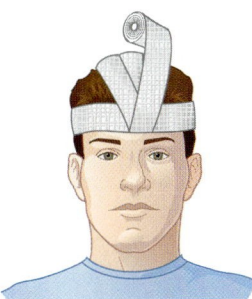

31. **Next, hold the bandage** at the center with one hand as you bring the bandage back over the end to the left of center. Continue holding

and folding the bandage back on itself, alternating right and left until the body part is covered. Overlap by two-thirds the bandage width with each turn. ▼

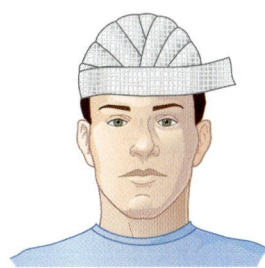

32. **Start and return each turn** to the midline or center of the body part, and angle it slightly more each time to continue covering the body part.
33. **Complete the bandage** by making two circular turns and securing the bandage with tape or metal clips.

> **? What if . . .**
>
> ■ **Drainage breaks through the outer bandage more frequently than expected?**
>
> Determine the cause of the drainage if possible (i.e., Is it blood or serum?). Increased drainage may be a sign of infection and should be evaluated. The dressing change frequency may need to be increased or an alternate dressing with a higher degree of exudate absorption may be needed.
>
> *Wound exudates can harm healing tissues. Dressings that are saturated should be changed as soon as possible to prevent prolonged moisture exposure or maceration.*

Evaluation

■ Be sure the bandage is firmly wrapped without being too tight.
■ Check the circulation is not compromised to the area distal of the bandage.
■ Evaluate for numbness or pain around or distal to the bandaged area.

Patient Teaching

■ Teach the patient about the expected healing process.
■ Inform the patient and caregiver about signs and symptoms of infection and the need to report these findings.
■ Instruct the patient and family about signs of circulation problems and how to remove bandage if needed.

Home Care

■ Refer the client to a home health agency for wound care.
■ Some clients or caregivers may be able to perform dressing changes. Determine the client and/or caregiver's ability to perform dressing changes; teach and demonstrate as needed.

Documentation

Many agencies use wound care flow sheets, which assess for the following:
■ Appearance and location of the wound, type and amount of exudates, and odor, if present, after cleansing.

■ Level of pain before the procedure. If the patient was medicated for pain, document the drug and dose used, time given, and patient response.
■ Method of cleansing the wound and surrounding skin, if performed
■ Application of primary and secondary dressings
■ Education provided to the patient

Practice Resources

Bergeron, Bizjak, Le Badour, et al., 2009; Rolstad & Ovington, 2007.

Thinking About the Procedure

Go to the *Fundamentals of Nursing Skills Videos,* **Wound Care: Bandaging With Circular and Spiral Turns.**

1. Name three tips the nurse suggested for bandaging using circular and spiral turns?

For suggested responses, go to Chapter 36, **Thinking About the Procedure Suggested Responses,** on *DavisPlus.*

Procedure 36-13 ■ Removing Sutures and Staples

➤ For steps to follow in *all* procedures, refer to the Universal Steps for All Procedures found on the page facing the inside back cover.

Equipment
- Nonsterile procedure gloves
- Suture removal kit or sterile scissors and forceps (Procedure 36-13A)
- Staple remover (Procedure 36-13B)
- Gauze

Delegation
This procedure itself may be delegated to a NAP who has been trained in the skill. Assessment of the incision line or wound is a licensed professional's responsibility and should not be delegated.

Pre-Procedure Assessment
- Assess staples to ensure none have rotated or turned instead of lying flat along the incision.

Procedure 36-13A ■ Removing Sutures

➤ When performing the procedure, always identify your patient according to agency policy and be attentive to standard precautions, hand hygiene, patient safety and privacy, body mechanics, and documentation.

Procedure Steps
1. **Obtain a suture removal kit.**
2. **Use the forceps to pick up** one end of the suture. ▼

3. **Slide the small scissors** around the suture, and cut near the skin. *This helps you avoid pulling the exposed portion of the suture through the underlying tissue.*

4. **With the forceps, gently pull** the suture in the direction of the knotted side to remove it. ▼

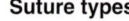
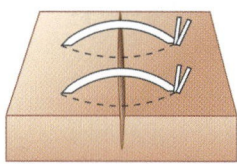

Suture types

Plain interrupted

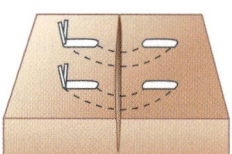

Suture types

Mattress interrupted

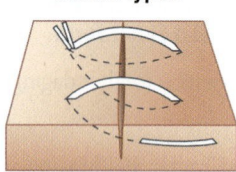

Suture types

Plain continuous

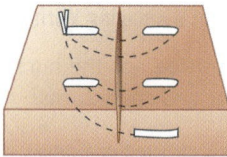

Suture types

Mattress continuous

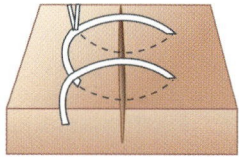

Suture types

Blanket continuous

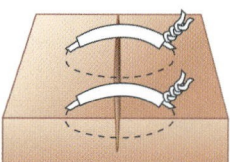

Suture types

Retention

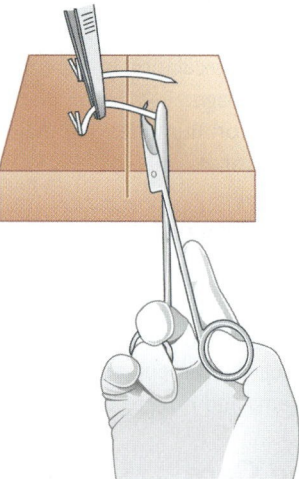

Removing interrupted sutures

5. **Apply dressing if needed.**
6. **Remove gloves and perform hand hygiene.**

Procedure 36-13B ■ Removing Staples

➤ When performing the procedure, always identify your patient according to agency policy and be attentive to standard precautions, hand hygiene, patient safety and privacy, body mechanics, and documentation.

Procedure Steps

1. **Wash hands. Don gloves.**
2. After cleansing the wound or incision, **position the staple remover** so that the lower jaw is on the bottom.
3. **Place both tips of the lower jaw** of the remover under the staple. ▼

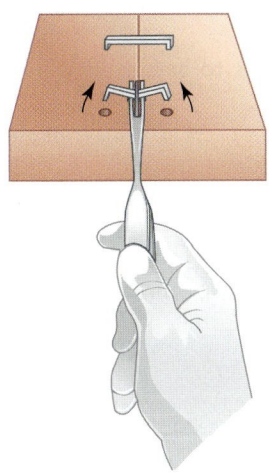

Removing staples

4. **Ensure the staple is perpendicular** to the plane of the skin. If not, reposition the staple with the tips of the lower jaw and apply gentle pressure, causing it to straighten the ends for easier removal.
5. **Lift slightly on the staple** ensuring that it stays perpendicular to the skin.
6. **Continue to lift slightly** as you gently squeeze the handles together to close.

   This spreads the ends of the staples apart, freeing them from the skin.
7. **Lift the reshaped staple** straight up from the skin.
8. **Remove every other staple**, and check the tension on the wound.
9. If there is no significant pull on the wound, **remove the remaining staples**.
10. **Place the removed staples** on a piece of gauze.

    Staples are small and can be easily lost. Keeping them in one place prevents this.
11. **Apply dressing if needed.**
12. **Dispose of the removed staples** in the sharps container.

    Ends of the staples are sharp and should be handled with care.
13. **Remove gloves and wash hands.**

? What if . . .

■ **A staple gets stuck?**

Gently manipulate the staple with the remover until it is perpendicular to the skin.

When the skin is stapled, the edges of the staple are crimped to hold the incision together. To be removed, those edges must be reshaped and straightened. If one edge of the staple is reshaped and the other is not, it can be painful to remove if not further manipulated.

■ **The incision needs a dressing once the staples or sutures have been removed?**

New surgical incisions should be covered with a sterile dressing the first 24 to 48 hours, but not necessarily after that time. Apply a dressing if you are concerned about soiling or per your institution's policy.

In a healing incision, epithelial resurfacing is complete in 24 to 48 hours. Although only a few cells thick, this epithelium is enough to keep the wound closed and provide a bacterial barrier.

Evaluation

- Note whether the incision is well approximated after the procedure.
- Ensure that the patient verbalized understanding of the treatment.
- Inspect the wound daily.

Patient Teaching

- Instruct the client of signs and symptoms of wound infections (i.e., redness, drainage) and the need to report these findings.
- Instruct the client that he may be able to shower once sutures or staples are removed, if approved by the provider.

Documentation

Document the following information. (Many agencies use wound care flow sheets.)

- Appearance and location of the wound, type and amount of exudates, and odor, if present, after cleansing
- The patient's level of pain before and after the procedure. If the patient was medicated for pain, document the drug and dose used, time given, and patient response.
- Method of cleansing the wound and surrounding skin, if performed
- Removal of staples or sutures
- Education provided to the patient

Practice Resources

Autio & Olsen, 2002.

Procedure 36–14 ■ Shortening a Wound Drain

> For steps to follow in *all* procedures, refer to the Universal Steps for All Procedures found on the page facing the inside back cover.

Equipment
- Nonsterile procedure gloves
- Sterile gloves
- Sterile scissors
- Two safety pins or other clips (sterile)
- Sterile gauze

Delegation
This procedure may be delegated to a NAP who has been appropriately trained in the skill. Assessment of the incision line or wound is a licensed professional's responsibility and should not be delegated.

Pre-Procedure Assessment
- Inspect the site around the drain, noting skin excoriation, tenderness, erythema, warmth to the touch, and drainage seeping from the wound.
  These symptoms could indicate a wound infection or irritation at the skin site. Excoriation can be the result of seeping drainage
  around the tube (e.g., if the tube diameter is not sufficient size to handle drainage output) or more likely, an obstruction within the tubing.
- Assess the characteristics of the drainage, including color, volume drainage, presence of blood, odor, pus, and any change in the type or amount of drainage through the tubing.
  A sudden decrease in drainage might indicate a blocked drain. Presence of fresh blood might be a sign of irritation within the wound. Pus and odor in the drainage could indicate wound infection.
- Check the suction apparatus to be sure it is functioning properly.
  A self-suction apparatus might need to be recompressed from time to time to maintain effective vacuum. Electric suction units can fail, delivering too much suction, which can lead to injury. Too little suction can contribute to insufficient drainage, which can lead to pressure on sutures if present, or cause the wound to become infected or heal more slowly.

> When performing the procedure, always identify your patient according to agency policy and be attentive to standard precautions, hand hygiene, patient safety and privacy, body mechanics, and documentation.

Procedure Steps
1. After donning procedure gloves, **remove wound dressings**.
2. **Remove soiled gloves** and discard in a moisture-proof biohazard collection container.
3. **Open sterile supplies** (scissors, etc.).
4. Don sterile gloves; use sterile scissors **to cut halfway through a sterile gauze dressing** (for later use), or use a sterile precut drain dressing.
5. If the drain is sutured in place, **use sterile scissors to cut the suture.**
6. Firmly grasp the full width of the drain at the level of the skin and **pull it out by the prescribed amount** (e.g., 6 mm [¼ in.]).
7. **Insert a sterile safety pin** through the drain at the level of the skin. Hold the drain tightly, and insert the pin above your fingers.
   This will keep from sticking the client or your fingers. The pin keeps the drain from disappearing into the wound.

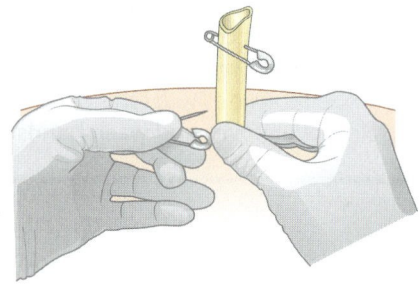

8. **Using sterile scissors**, cut off the drain at about 2.5 cm (1 in.) above the skin. ▼

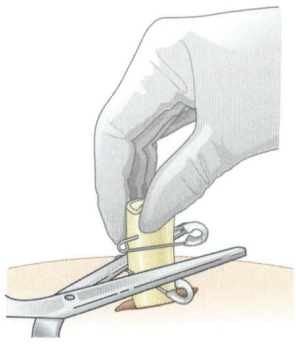

9. **Cleanse the wound**, using sterile gauze swabs and the prescribed cleaning solution. In some situations,
   you may use sterile forceps to manipulate the swabs.
10. **Apply precut sterile gauze** around the drain; then redress the wound. ▼

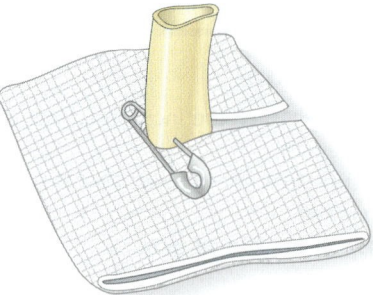

11. **Remove gloves and discard** in a biohazard container. Wash your hands.
12. **Leave the patient in a safe and comfortable position.**

? What if . . .

- **You shorten the drain too much?**
  Immediately notify the surgeon who placed the drain.
  Drainage tubing is secured under the skin surface and will probably not be dislodged with shortening.

Patient Evaluation

- Assess the local area of skin around the drain after manipulating it.
- Note the patency of the drain after shortening it.
- Be sure the drain is secure after shortening.
- Evaluate for complications occurring related to shortening procedure.
- Patient Teaching
- Patients should not shorten their own drains. Consult a healthcare provider if concerned about the length of tubing or drains.

Documentation

- Record the intervention.
- Note the amount and characteristics of the drainage.
- Document the appearance of the wound.

- Note any complications that occur with shortening a drain (e.g., manipulation of tubing causes bleeding or drainage at the site).

Thinking About the Procedure

 Go to the *Fundamentals of Nursing Skills Videos,* **Wound Care: Wound Drainage Systems: Penrose.**

1. In what manner does the nurse clean around the penrose drainage tubing?
2. Where is the drain positioned when redressing the wound?

 For suggested responses, go to Chapter 36, **Thinking About the Procedure Suggested Responses,** on Davis*Plus.*

Procedure 36-15 ▪ Emptying a Closed-Wound Drainage System

➤ For steps to follow in procedures, refer to the Universal Steps for All Procedures found on the page facing the inside back cover.

Equipment

- Drainage container with graduated markings
- Nonsterile procedure gloves
- Disposal sink for biomaterial
- Biohazard disposal receptacle

Delegation

This procedure itself may be delegated to a NAP who is trained in the skill. Assessment of the incision line or wound is a licensed professional's responsibility and should not be delegated.

Pre-Procedure Assessment

- Assess the appearance of the drainage tube site and sutures, if in place.
- Inspect for warmth, edema, redness, or pus where tubing penetrates the skin.
- Check to be sure the closed-wound drainage system is securely fastened at the connections and within the wound.
- Determine whether suction (electric, portable, or manual) is working properly.

➤ When performing the procedure, always identify your patient according to agency policy and be attentive to standard precautions, hand hygiene, patient safety and privacy, body mechanics, and documentation.

Procedure Steps

1. **Read the instructions** about the drainage device.
   Procedures vary among manufacturers and different systems.
2. **Don procedure gloves and goggles** or mask.
3. **Unpin the drainage device** from the patient's gown.
   The drainage device is often pinned to the patient's gown to prevent it from dislodging.
4. **Open the drainage port**, and empty the drainage into a small graduated container. ➤

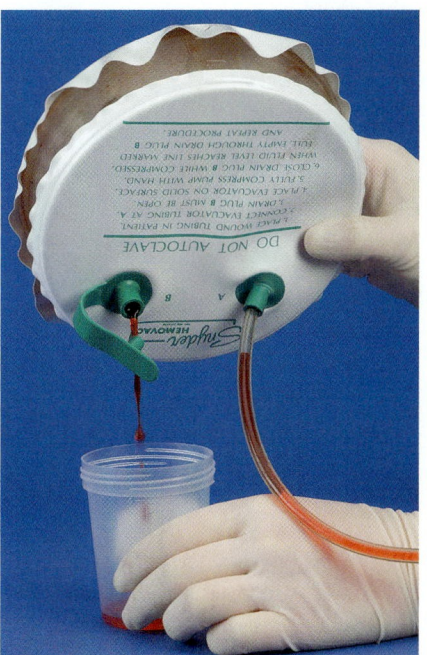

5. With the port still open, **place the collection device on a firm, flat surface** (e.g., the overbed table).
6. Use the palm of one hand to **press down on the device and eject air from it.** Do not stand directly over the air vent. Do not touch the drainage port.
   It can splash or bubble.
7. **Use the other hand to scrub** the port and plug with an alcohol-based antiseptic or povidone iodine swab (Betadine), if the patient is not allergic to iodine. ➤

(continued on next page)

Procedure 36–15 ■ Emptying a Closed-Wound Drainage System (continued)

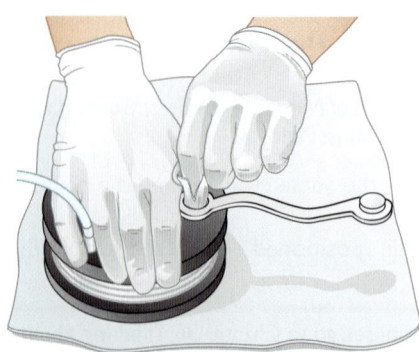

This will create a constant, negative pressure vacuum to facilitate suction.

9. Repin the drainage device to the patient's gown.
Pinning keeps it secure and prevents it from accidentally dislodging.

10. Measure the drainage in the graduated container; discard drainage in the disposable container for biohazardous material. Wash the graduated container. Do not stand in front of an air vent while doing so.
Forced air in the room can cause the drainage to splash or bubble, introducing biohazard into the environmental air.

8. Continuing to press down on the device, **replace the plug in the port.** Do not touch the open port or the part of the plug that goes into the port.

11. Remove your gloves. Perform hand hygiene.

12. Document in the patient's record.

? What if . . .

■ **The wound drainage spills?**

Don procedure gloves. Wipe up the spilled biomaterial (patient body fluid). Dispose of contaminated materials in a biohazard waste receptacle.
Proper handling of contaminated biomaterials is important to prevent transmission of infectious organisms.

Home Care

■ Teach family members who are emptying drainage systems at home to wear gloves and avoid touching the drainage port.

Documentation

■ Note the date and time the drainage system is emptied.
■ Record the volume lost. Report excess fluid loss to the primary care provider.
■ Describe the appearance of drainage, including presence of blood or purulent material.

Thinking About the Procedure

 Go to the *Fundamentals of Nursing Skills Videos*, **Wound Care: Wound Drainage Systems: Negative Pressure.**

1. What does the nurse empty the wound drainage into? Where is the drainage discarded?

 For suggested responses, go to Chapter 36, **Thinking About the Procedure Suggested Responses,** on *DavisPlus*.

 To explore learning resources for this chapter,

 Go to DavisPlus at http://davisplus.fadavis.com, keyword Treas

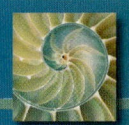

Concept Map

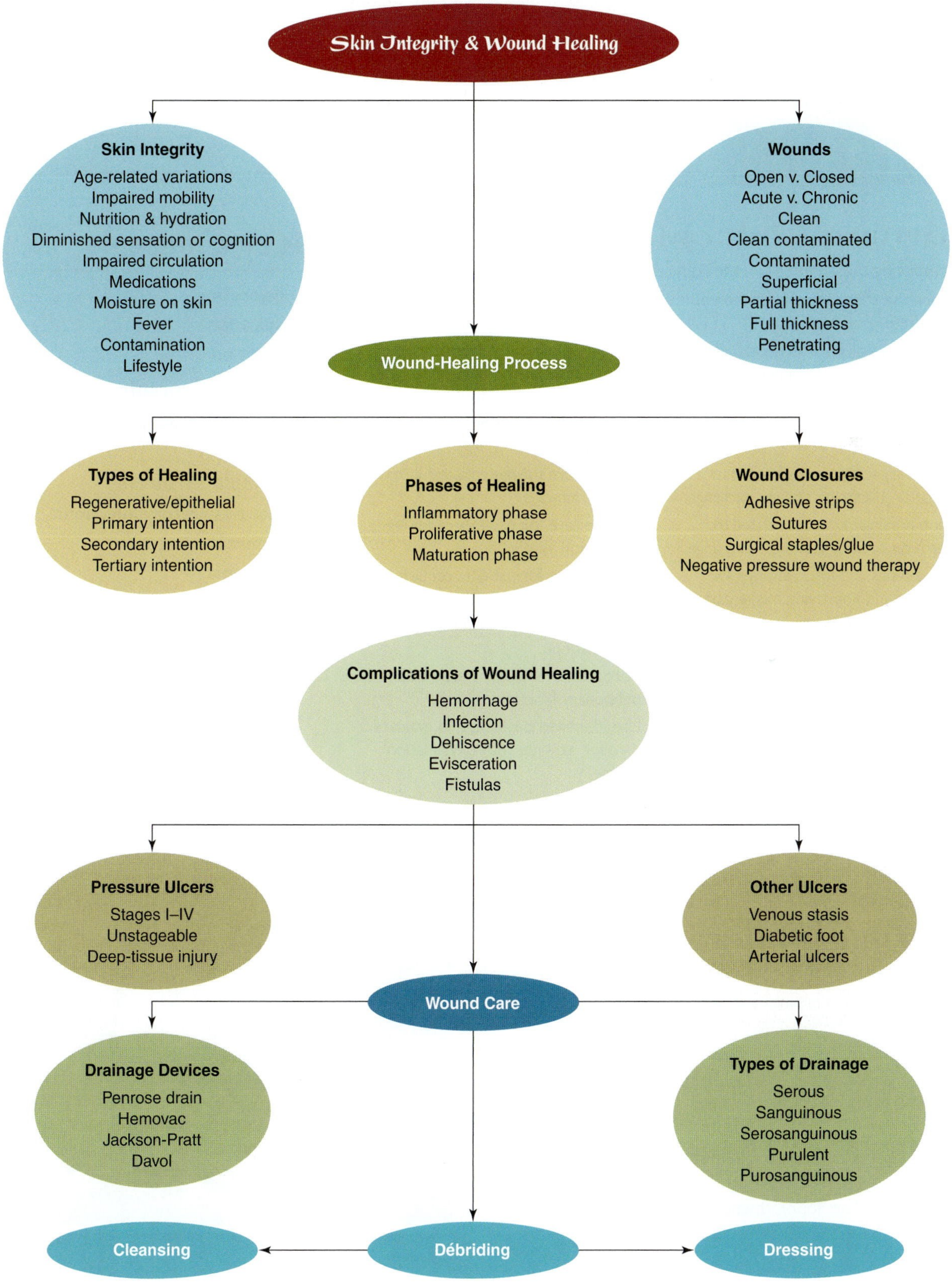

Skin Integrity & Wound Healing

Skin Integrity
Age-related variations
Impaired mobility
Nutrition & hydration
Diminished sensation or cognition
Impaired circulation
Medications
Moisture on skin
Fever
Contamination
Lifestyle

Wounds
Open v. Closed
Acute v. Chronic
Clean
Clean contaminated
Contaminated
Superficial
Partial thickness
Full thickness
Penetrating

Wound-Healing Process

Types of Healing
Regenerative/epithelial
Primary intention
Secondary intention
Tertiary intention

Phases of Healing
Inflammatory phase
Proliferative phase
Maturation phase

Wound Closures
Adhesive strips
Sutures
Surgical staples/glue
Negative pressure wound therapy

Complications of Wound Healing
Hemorrhage
Infection
Dehiscence
Evisceration
Fistulas

Pressure Ulcers
Stages I–IV
Unstageable
Deep-tissue injury

Other Ulcers
Venous stasis
Diabetic foot
Arterial ulcers

Wound Care

Drainage Devices
Penrose drain
Hemovac
Jackson-Pratt
Davol

Types of Drainage
Serous
Sanguinous
Serosanguinous
Purulent
Purosanguinous

Cleansing   **Débriding**   **Dressing**

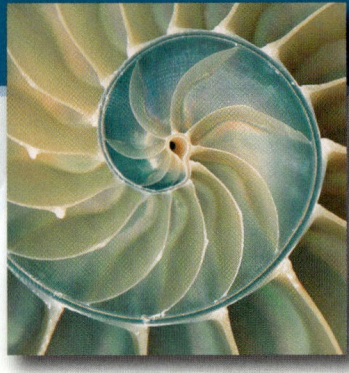

CHAPTER 37

Oxygenation

Learning Outcomes

After completing this chapter, you should be able to:

➤ Describe the structure and function of the respiratory system.

➤ Identify individual, environmental, and pathological factors that influence oxygenation.

➤ Assess oxygenation, breathing, and gas exchange.

➤ Interpret diagnostic testing related to oxygenation, breathing, and gas exchange.

➤ Develop nursing diagnoses related to oxygenation, breathing, and gas exchange.

➤ Plan outcomes and interventions for maintaining and improving oxygenation.

➤ Safely and correctly perform common nursing procedures related to oxygenation, breathing, and gas exchange.

➤ Evaluate adequacy of oxygenation, breathing, and gas exchange, and modify nursing activities appropriately based on outcomes.

➤ Describe a procedure for safe oxygen administration.

➤ Describe measures for mobilizing airway secretions.

➤ Implement measures for promoting optimal respiratory function (e.g., positioning).

➤ Explain how to suction the upper and lower airways.

➤ Provide care for patients requiring artificial airways.

➤ Provide care for patients requiring mechanical ventilation.

➤ Provide care for patients requiring chest tubes.

➤ Provide measures to promote oxygenation.

➤ Recognize medications used to enhance pulmonary function.

➤ Use identified outcomes to evaluate care for patients with oxygenation problems.

Key Concepts

Oxygenation
Respiration
Ventilation

Related Concepts

See the Concept Map at the end of this chapter.

Example Problems

Upper Respiratory Infections
Influenza
Pneumonia

Caring for the Nguyens

This feature allows you to practice the kind of thinking you will use as a full-spectrum nurse. There is usually more than one correct answer to a critical thinking question, so we do not provide answers for these features. It is more important to develop your nursing judgment than to "cover content." Discuss the questions with your peers. If you are still unsure, consult your instructor.

Mai Nguyen, Nam's 76-year-old mother, has been complaining of fatigue and a persistent cough for approximately 2 weeks. Nam scheduled an appointment for his mother at the family clinic. You are the nurse at the clinic. Mrs. Nguyen appears

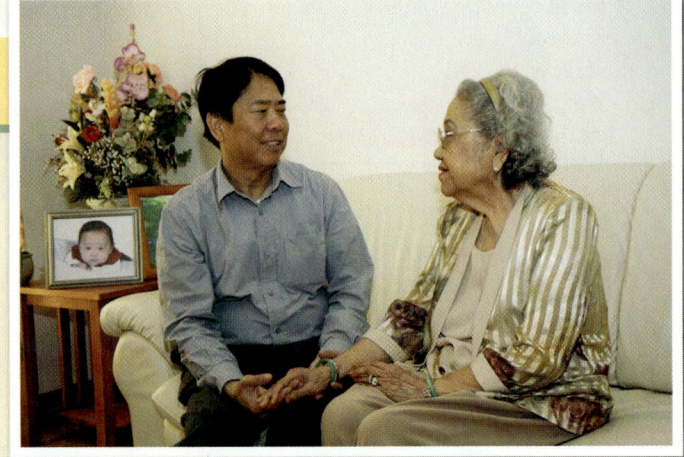

Caring for the Nyugens (continued)

disheveled. Her clothes are mismatched and rumpled, and her hair is tousled. Normally she appears at the clinic dressed neatly and wearing makeup. She has a hard time signing in at the desk and tells the receptionist she has a 1:00 p.m.

appointment, but it is 9:00 a.m. Mrs. Nguyen's vital signs are as follows: BP, 142/90 mm Hg; pulse, 94 beats/min and regular; respirations, 24 breaths/min and labored; temperature, 99.6°F (37.5°C) oral.

A. What additional assessment data would be useful to gather at this time?

B. During her visit at the clinic, you notice that Mrs. Nguyen is very confused. Her weight has dropped 7 pounds since her visit last month, her mucous membranes are dry, and she is dyspneic with any activity. She is diagnosed with pneumonia. Because of her rapid decline, Mrs. Nguyen is admitted to the hospital to receive antibiotics administered intravenously. At the hospital, her initial pulse oximetry reading is 90%, and she is unable to cough up secretions. Write the most appropriate nursing diagnosis to focus interventions for Mrs. Nguyen.

C. What actions should you anticipate taking?

D. The hospitalist (hospital-based physician) writes prescriptions for IV fluids, antibiotics, suction prn, and

continuous pulse oximetry. What additional prescriptions will you need to provide care for Mrs. Nguyen? What therapy would you suggest?

E. Mrs. Nguyen requires suctioning to help remove secretions. She has a weak cough and crackles and rhonchi throughout all lung fields. There are few secretions in her oropharynx, and she bites down on the catheter. What technique would you use to suction her? Explain your choice.

F. After 4 days in the hospital, Mrs. Nguyen is discharged to home. She asks the hospital nurse, "What can I do to make sure I never get that sick again?" How would you answer this question?

 Go to **Caring for the Nguyens Response Sheet** on DavisPlus.

Meet Your Patients

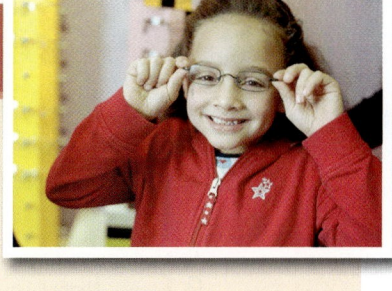

In a pulmonary clinic, your student assignment is to (1) perform a focused assessment related to breathing and oxygenation, (2) perform common therapeutic interventions related to breathing and oxygenation, (3) identify desired outcomes and evaluate achievement of those outcomes, and (4) plan for follow-up and home care needs. In the course of your clinical day, you care for the following clients:

- Mary is a 4-year-old girl with a history of asthma. Her mother, Ms. Green, has brought her in because of an "asthma attack." Mary is sitting in her mother's lap and breathing rapidly through an open mouth. Her cough sounds congested and wheezy. The nurse practitioner has prescribed a nebulized treatment containing albuterol (Proventil) and ipratropium bromide (Atrovent).
- Mr. Chu is a 78-year-old man complaining of cough, sore throat, fatigue, and weakness. His temperature is

100.4°F (38°C), pulse is 90 beats/min, respirations are 26 breaths/min, and blood pressure (BP) is 166/82 mm Hg.

- William is a 19-year-old male who has had a sudden onset of right-sided chest pain and shortness of breath. His chest x-ray revealed a right pneumothorax, and he is currently receiving 35% oxygen by face mask while waiting for an ambulance to transport him to the hospital for further evaluation.

Each of these patients is experiencing an oxygenation problem. In this chapter you will learn a variety of assessment techniques and interventions to support breathing, oxygenation, and gas exchange for patients such as these.

Theoretical Knowledge
knowing **why**

The pulmonary, cardiovascular, musculoskeletal, and neurological systems work together to achieve oxygenation. The musculoskeletal and neurological systems regulate the movement of air into and out of the lungs. The lungs oxygenate the blood, and the heart circulates the blood throughout the body and back to the lungs. In this chapter, we focus on the pulmonary system; Chapter 38 presents the cardiovascular system. Remember, however, that the two systems work together. Changes in one system create changes in the other.

ABOUT THE KEY CONCEPTS

The concept **oxygenation** refers to how well the cells, tissues, and organs of the body are supplied with oxygen. The concepts of *respiration* and *ventilation* are the two major processes that occur in the pulmonary system to oxygenate the blood. All of the problems and interventions in this chapter relate in some way to oxygenation, respiration, or ventilation. Knowledge of these concepts will help you to understand the rationale for interventions such as airway suctioning, oxygen, mechanical ventilation, and chest tubes.

THE PULMONARY SYSTEM

The pulmonary system has two major components: the *airway* and the *lungs*. The following presents a brief review of the anatomy and physiology of the pulmonary system and explains how breathing is controlled. For more in-depth information, consult anatomy and physiology texts, or

 Go to Chapter 37, **Supplemental Materials: Structures of the Pulmonary System,** on Davis*Plus.*

The Airway

The airway consists of the nasal passages, mouth, pharynx, larynx, trachea, bronchi, and bronchioles (Fig. 37-1). Air flows through these structures into and out of the lungs. In addition, the airway structures do the following:

- *Moisten the air*—A moist mucous membrane lining adds water to inhaled air.
- *Warm the air*—Blood flowing through the vascular airway walls transfers body heat to the inhaled air.
- *Filter the air*—(1) Specialized cells in the lining of the airways secrete sticky mucus to trap foreign particles. (2) **Cilia,** tiny hair-like projections from the walls of the airways, move rhythmically to sweep trapped debris up and out of the airway.

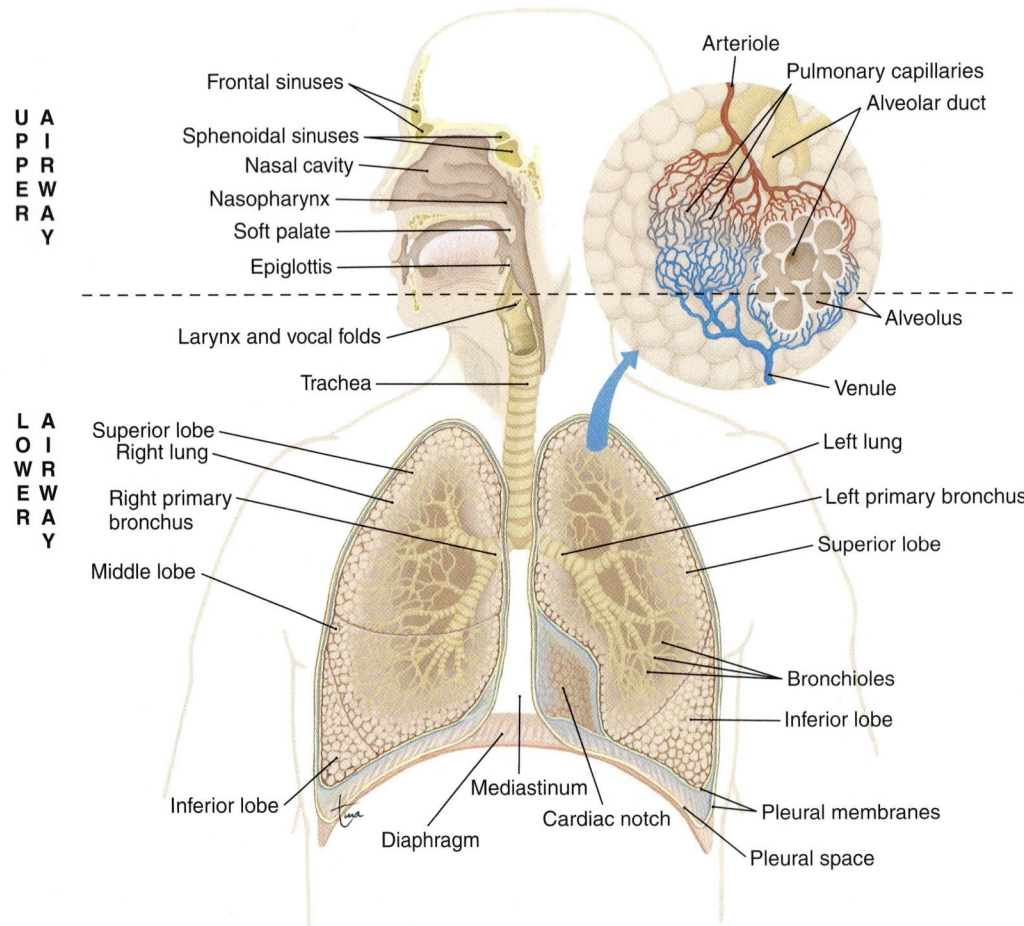

FIGURE 37-1 An anterior view of the respiratory system. The upper airway lies above the larynx. The lower airway, located below the larynx, is considered sterile.

The **upper airway,** located above the larynx, includes the nasal passages, mouth, and pharynx. The *pharynx* (throat) contains the openings to the esophagus and trachea. The *trachea* lies just in front of the esophagus. The *epiglottis,* a small flap of tissue superior to the larynx, closes off the trachea during swallowing so that food and fluids do not enter the lower airway. The epiglottis opens during breathing to allow air to move through the airway.

The **lower airway,** located below the larynx, includes the trachea, bronchi, and bronchioles. The lower airway is considered sterile. The **trachea** extends from the larynx to where it divides to form the right and left mainstem bronchi. As the airways branch and become smaller, they have progressively thinner and less cartilage, until it disappears completely in the smaller bronchioles. Spasm of the layers of smooth muscle in the bronchi and bronchioles **(bronchospasm)** narrows the airway and obstructs airflow.

The Lungs

The *lungs* are soft, spongy, cone-shaped organs. They are separated by the **mediastinum,** which contains the heart and great vessels. The right lung has three lobes; the left lung has two lobes. The upper portion of each lung, the *apex,* extends upward above the clavicle. The lower portion of each lung, the *base,* rests on the diaphragm. Knowing the location of lung tissue beneath the chest wall helps you to perform a complete and accurate assessment of the lungs.

The lungs are composed of millions of **alveoli**—tiny air sacs with thin walls surrounded by a fine network of capillaries. Gases (oxygen and carbon dioxide) easily pass back and forth between the alveoli and capillaries. Alveoli are composed of two types of cells:

- *Type I alveolar cells* are the gas exchange cells.
- *Type II alveolar cells* produce **surfactant,** a lipoprotein that lowers the surface tension within alveoli to allow them to inflate during breathing.

To see an illustration of the alveolar structure,

 Go to Chapter 37, **Tables, Boxes, and Figures: ESG Figure 37-1,** on Davis*Plus.*

Knowledge Check 37-1

- What happens to inhaled air in the airways? How does this occur?
- In which structures of the lung does gas exchange take place?
- What does surfactant do for alveoli?

 Think**Like a Nurse** 37-1

You are assigned to care for an adult patient who has a medical condition with which you are not familiar. You look it up and find that the condition causes a dramatic loss of surfactant. Based on your knowledge of the function of surfactant, what problems is this patient at high risk for developing?

WHAT ARE THE FUNCTIONS OF THE PULMONARY SYSTEM?

Two of the key concepts in this chapter are major processes that occur in the pulmonary system: ventilation and respiration. **Ventilation** is the movement of air into and out of the lungs through the act of breathing. **Respiration** is the exchange of the gases oxygen and carbon dioxide in the lungs.

Pulmonary Ventilation

Oxygenation of the blood, and ultimately of organs and tissues, depends on adequate ventilation. Ventilation must move enough air through the lungs to make adequate oxygen available to the alveoli. Ventilation is accomplished through cycles of inhalation and exhalation. To see an animated demonstration of the physiology of ventilation,

 Go to **Cardiovascular/Pulmonary Animations: Pulmonary Ventilation,** on Davis*Plus.*

Inhalation. Expansion of the chest cavity and lungs creates negative pressure inside the lungs, causing air to be drawn in through the nose or mouth and airways. This is **inhalation.** The *diaphragm* is the major muscle of breathing. When it contracts with each inhalation, the chest cavity is pulled downward, pulling the lung bases downward with it. *Intercostal muscles,* the small muscles around the ribs, also contract on inhalation and pull the ribs outward, slightly expanding the chest cavity and lungs. The pleural membrane covering the lungs adheres ("sticks") to the pleural membrane lining the chest cavity, so the lungs expand. Lung expansion creates negative pressure and draws air in through the only opening to the outside, the trachea. See Figure 37-2A.

Exhalation. Exhalation occurs when the diaphragm and intercostal muscles relax, allowing the chest and lungs to return to their normal resting size. See Figure 37-2B. The reduction in size causes the pressure inside the chest and lungs to rise above atmospheric pressure, so air flows out of the lungs. Exhalation requires no energy or effort.

What Factors Affect Ventilation?

The adequacy of ventilation is affected by the rate and depth of respirations, lung compliance and elasticity, and airway resistance.

- **Respiratory rate and depth** are almost self-explanatory: **Rate** is how fast you breathe and **depth** is how much your lungs expand to take in air. These processes affect oxygen and carbon dioxide levels in the blood.
- **Hyperventilation** occurs when a person breathes fast and deeply to move a large amount of air through the lungs,

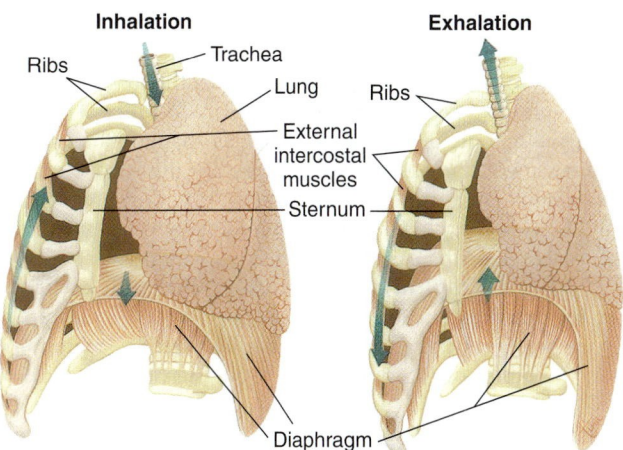

FIGURE 37-2 A, During inhalation, the diaphragm contracts, pulling the chest cavity and lung bases downward; the intercostal muscles pull the rib cage up and outward. B, In exhalation, the diaphragm relaxes, the lung bases move upward, and the ribs and intercostal muscles move down and in, resulting in lung compression.

causing too much carbon dioxide to be removed by the alveoli. Mild hyperventilation can occur in response to **hypoxemia** (a low level of oxygen in the blood). When blood oxygen is low, ventilation increases to draw additional air (and oxygen) into the lungs. However, as ventilation increases, carbon dioxide levels fall. Severe hyperventilation is usually triggered by medication, central nervous system abnormalities, high altitude, heat, exercise, panic, fear, or anxiety.

- **Hypoventilation** occurs when a decreased rate or shallow breathing moves only a small amount of air into and out of the lungs. Hypoventilation can lead to hypoxemia because less air (carrying oxygen) reaches the alveoli. The concern is that hypoxemia will lead to **hypoxia** (an oxygen deficiency in the body tissues).

- **Lung compliance** refers to the ease of lung inflation. Normally the lungs inflate easily. Lung compliance is reduced by increased lung water (edema), loss of surfactant, or conditions that cause elastin fibers in the lungs to be replaced with scar tissue (collagen).

- **Lung elasticity** (or elastic recoil) refers to the tendency of the elastin fibers to return to their original position away from the chest wall after being stretched (think of stretching a rubber band, then letting go of it). Alveoli that have been overstretched, as with emphysema, lose their elastic recoil over time. This loss of elasticity allows the lungs to inflate easily but inhibits deflation, leaving stale air trapped in the alveoli.

- **Airway resistance** is the resistance to airflow within the airways. The larger the diameter of the airway, the more easily air moves through it. Normally, airway resistance is very low, so it takes little effort to move large volumes of air into and out of the lungs. However, even small decreases in airway diameter (as might occur with secretions in the airway or mild bronchospasm) markedly increase airway resistance. Mary, the little girl with asthma (Meet Your Patients), is undoubtedly experiencing airway resistance.

KnowledgeCheck 37-2

- What is the difference between ventilation and respiration?
- Describe how the diaphragm, accessory muscles, and pressure changes within the lungs create inhalation and exhalation.
- How does hypoventilation affect risk for hypoxemia and hypoxia?

Respiration (Gas Exchange)

Respiration refers to gas exchange, that is, the oxygenation of blood and elimination of carbon dioxide in the lungs. Although nurses commonly use the term *respirations* to mean "breaths" in an assessment of vital signs, strictly speaking this is not accurate: You cannot measure gas exchange by counting breaths per minute. Gas exchange occurs at two equally essential levels: external (in the lungs) or internal (in other body tissues).

External Respiration. **Alveolar–capillary gas exchange** (or **external respiration**) occurs in the alveoli of the lungs. Oxygen (O_2) diffuses across the alveolar–capillary membrane into the blood of the pulmonary capillaries; carbon dioxide (CO_2) diffuses out of the blood and into the alveoli to be exhaled (Fig. 37-3). The rate of diffusion depends on the thickness of the membrane and the total surface of lung tissue available for gas exchange. Examples of conditions that slow diffusion are pleural effusion (fluid in the lungs), pneumothorax (lung collapse), and asthma (bronchospasms). If blood is not adequately oxygenated in the alveoli, **hypoxemia** (low blood-oxygen levels) occurs. Getting oxygen into the blood as it flows through the lungs is only the first step in oxygenation.

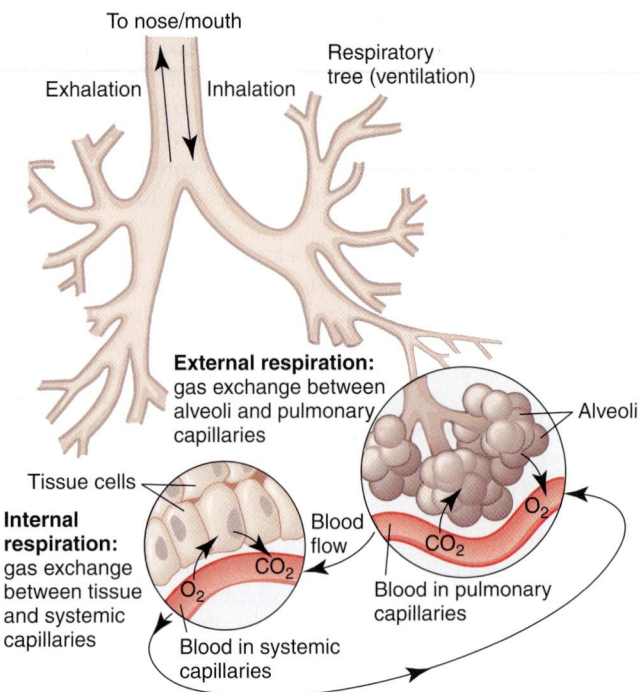

FIGURE 37-3 External respiration occurs at the alveolar–capillary membrane. Internal respiration occurs at the tissue–capillary membrane.

Internal Respiration. **Capillary–tissue gas exchange** (or **internal respiration**) occurs in body organs and tissues. Oxygen diffuses from the blood through the capillary–cellular membrane into the tissue cells, where it is used for metabolism. From the cells, CO_2, a waste product of cellular metabolism, diffuses through the capillary–cellular membrane into the blood, from where it is transported to the lungs and exhaled. Tissue oxygenation requires both adequate external respiration and adequate peripheral circulation. Limitations in either function may lead to **hypoxia** (oxygen deficiency in body tissues). In addition, if tissue cells are using more oxygen for metabolism than normal (e.g., during a high fever), hypoxia will occur unless more oxygen is made available to the tissues.

ThinkLike a Nurse 37-2

William (Meet Your Patients) has a right pneumothorax. Which of the two factors affecting the rate of gas diffusion is causing William to be hypoxemic? If you do not know what a pneumothorax is, look it up.

How Is Breathing Controlled?

The respiratory centers in the brainstem control breathing using feedback from chemoreceptors and lung receptors. Voluntary control from the **motor cortex** can override the involuntary respiratory centers, but only temporarily. This allows a person to continue breathing while doing activities such as talking, singing, swallowing, whistling, and blowing.

- **Chemoreceptors,** located in the medulla of the brainstem, the carotid arteries, and the aorta, detect changes in blood pH, O_2, and CO_2 levels and send messages back to the central respiratory center in the brainstem. In response, the respiratory center increases or decreases ventilation to maintain normal blood levels of pH, O_2 (PO_2), and CO_2 (PCO_2). Normally the blood CO_2 level provides the primary stimulus to breathe.

High CO_2 levels stimulate breathing to eliminate the excess CO_2. A secondary, though important, drive to breathe is hypoxemia. Low blood O_2 levels stimulate breathing to get more oxygen into the lungs.

- **Lung receptors,** located in the lung and chest wall, are sensitive to breathing patterns, lung expansion, lung compliance, airway resistance, and respiratory irritants. The respiratory center uses feedback from the lung receptors to adjust ventilation. For example, if the lung receptors sense respiratory irritants such as dust, cold air, or tobacco smoke, the respiratory center triggers airway constriction and a more rapid, shallow pattern of breathing.

For a brief overview of the nervous system,

 Go to Chapter 37, **Supplemental Materials: The Nervous System,** on DavisPlus.

KnowledgeCheck 37-3

- Describe two ways in which breathing is controlled.
- The level of which gas (oxygen or carbon dioxide) is the primary stimulant for breathing?

 ThinkLike a Nurse 37-3

A patient has adequate blood oxygen levels, based on a pulse oximeter reading of 98%. Can you conclude that organ and tissue oxygenation are adequate? Explain your thinking.

WHAT FACTORS INFLUENCE PULMONARY FUNCTION?

Factors that influence pulmonary function include developmental stage, the environment, individual and lifestyle factors, medications, and pathophysiological states.

Developmental Stage

Normal development influences lung, heart, and circulatory function, all of which affect oxygenation. Developmental factors have less effect on function in young and middle adults than in older adults.

Infants

Premature infants (less than 35 weeks' gestation) do not have a fully developed alveolar surfactant system. Surfactant is the substance that keeps air sacs inflated for effective respiration. Therefore, premature infants are at high risk for **respiratory distress syndrome (RDS).** RDS is characterized by widespread **atelectasis** (collapse of alveoli). The premature infant also has immature pulmonary circulation. Together with hypoventilation, this leads to hypercarbia (high CO_2 blood levels) and hypoxemia.

Infants born at term are also at risk for oxygenation problems (e.g., infection and airway obstruction) for the following reasons:

- Because the newborn's lower airway structures are immature and small, an infectious agent can spread rapidly.
- The infant's airways are quite narrow in diameter and, therefore, easily obstructed by edema, mucus, or a foreign body, such as meconium passed at birth.
- The central nervous system for preterm, and even some term, infants is immature, leading to periodic breathing patterns and apnea.
- In the first few months of life, the immune system of infants is immature. Although at birth, infants enjoy the benefit of some maternal immunoglobulin circulating in their system; this

protection is limited and not sufficient for fighting certain infections.

- By age 6 months, infants can grasp small objects and put them in their mouths. This new skill, combined with small airway diameter, puts them at risk for choking on small objects.

Toddlers

Although the toddler's risk for frequent and serious infections diminishes, *upper respiratory infections* (URIs) remain common because (1) the tonsils and adenoids are relatively large, predisposing to tonsillitis, and (2) many children are exposed to new infectious agents in preschool and day care. Most children recover from URIs without difficulty.

Toddlers actively explore the environment and often put objects in their mouths, which puts them at risk for other respiratory problems, for example:

- *Acquiring and transmitting infections* through toys and other objects
- *Airway obstruction* from aspiration of small objects (e.g., candy, buttons, coins, peanuts, grapes). The toddler's airway is still relatively short and small and may be easily obstructed.
- *Drowning* in very small amounts of water around the home (e.g., in a bucket of water or toilet bowl).

Preschool and School-Age Children

Preschool and school-age children have developed mature lungs, heart, and circulatory systems that can adapt to moderate stress and change. Healthy children typically have bouts of tonsillitis or URIs, which usually resolve without difficulty. Viral infections, such as croup and pneumonia, are common, especially in preschoolers and younger school-age children. Exercise-induced (and other) asthma is also a problem. A few children as young as middle-school-age begin social habits, such as tobacco use, that can have long-term adverse effects on oxygenation in both the pulmonary and cardiovascular systems.

Adolescents

In adolescence, the lungs develop adult characteristics. The average adolescent is developmentally at little risk for lung diseases. Some may, however, be developing behaviors and habits that can create risk throughout life. As do adults, young people often begin smoking for social reasons (e.g., peer pressure, advertising, desire to feel cool), but nicotine addiction perpetuates the habit. In addition, many adolescents do not receive the recommended influenza vaccines. And finally, exercise-induced asthma is still a problem in this age group.

Young, Middle, and Older Adults

Unhealthful practices (e.g., smoking and a lack of aerobic exercise) often continue into, or may begin in, adulthood. About one in five U.S. adults is a cigarette smoker ("Vital Signs," 2011). More than half the adults who smoke were regular smokers by their 18th birthday (American Lung Association [ALA], 2011; Centers for Disease Control and Prevention [CDC]/National Center for Health Statistics [NCHS], 2008).

Changes in the respiratory system that begin in middle age may become significant when the person experiences stressors such as infection, surgery, anesthesia, and emotional problems. The number of cells and the efficiency of the organs decline in a subtle and progressive way as a person ages. Keep in mind, though, that endurance training and regular exercise minimize the rate of these changes. In fact, an older person who is physically conditioned by regular exercise may have better lung function than a younger adult who is not well conditioned.

Older adults tend to experience the following changes:

- *Reduced lung expansion and less alveolar inflation.* This is because (1) costal cartilage begins to calcify, reducing chest wall movement during breathing; (2) the lungs have less recoil ability; and (3) the alveoli lose elasticity.
- *Difficulty expelling mucus or foreign material* due to a less effective cough reflex, drier mucus, and fewer cilia in the airways.
- *Diminished ability to increase ventilation* when oxygenation demands increase (e.g., with exercise). As diaphragm strength decreases, vital capacity is reduced; so exhalation becomes less efficient, causing progressive air trapping.
- *Declining immune response,* especially cell-mediated immunity, T-cell activity, and the inflammatory response
- *Gastroesophageal reflux disease* is more common in older adults, creating a risk for aspirating stomach contents into the lungs. This may result in an inflammatory response.
- *Chemoreceptors* that control breathing respond more slowly to increased O_2 demand or rising levels of CO_2, making hypoxemia more likely when respiratory problems occur.

All of these changes put older adults at risk for respiratory infections. URIs that would be mild and short lived in a younger person may quickly lead to pneumonia in an older adult.

Environment

Environmental factors, such as stress, allergic reactions, altitude, and temperature, affect oxygenation.

Stress

The stress response stimulates the release of catecholamines from the sympathetic nervous system, resulting in (1) increased tendency of blood to clot (e.g., as in pulmonary embolus), and (2) suppression of the immune system and inflammatory response. A chronically suppressed immune and inflammatory response increases the risk for all infections, including respiratory.

For additional information on the effects of stress, see Chapter 12.

Allergic Reactions

An **allergy** is a hypersensitivity, or over-response, to an antigen. Pulmonary allergens include such things as dust, dust mites, cockroach particles, pollen, molds, newsprint, tobacco smoke, animal dander, and sometimes foods.

- **Hay fever** is an allergic reaction affecting the eyes, nose, and/or sinuses. It causes the release of *histamine,* which is largely responsible for accumulation of nasal fluid; swollen nasal membranes; nasal congestion; and itchy, swollen, watery eyes. Antihistamines are effective in combating hay fever.
- **Asthma** is an allergic reaction occurring in the bronchioles of the lungs. *Slow reacting substance of anaphylaxis* is released, which causes bronchoconstriction and lower airway edema and spasms, making breathing difficult and ineffective. Because histamine is not a major factor in causing the asthmatic reaction, antihistamines have little effect in the treatment of asthma. Asthma is the most common serious chronic disease of childhood, and it can be life threatening. In adults, a significant amount of asthma is caused or made worse by their workplace environment, especially among adults ages 45 to 64 years, blacks, and other minorities (CDC, 2012).

Air Quality

Air pollution triggers respiratory problems (e.g., lung cancer, carbon monoxide poisoning) that interfere with oxygenation. Even healthy people may experience headache, coughing, and other symptoms when exposed to air pollution. People with existing respiratory disease may become unable to function.

Some sources of air pollution are natural (e.g., forest fires), but the most common and damaging sources result from human activities (e.g., automobile exhaust emissions). Indoor air pollutants include carbon monoxide, nitrogen oxides, radon, and suspended particles (e.g., dust, mold spores, aerosols, and tobacco smoke). Pollutants are most harmful to infants, toddlers, older adults, and people with heart or lung disease. For more information about air quality,

 Go to Chapter 37, **Supplemental Materials: Air Quality Affects Oxygenation,** on Davis*Plus.*

Altitude

Atmospheric pressure falls from 760 mm Hg at sea level to 523 mm Hg at 10,000 feet. Oxygen pressure falls proportionally, leading to decreased oxygen diffusion from alveoli into capillaries (impaired gas exchange). Low oxygen levels at high altitudes can cause hypoxemia and hypoxia. If a person is suddenly exposed to low oxygen levels, arterial chemoreceptors stimulate ventilation, making more oxygen available in the alveoli and at the tissue level. People who live at high altitudes gradually undergo physiological changes that facilitate oxygenation, including an increase in the following:

- Ventilation, which brings more oxygen into the lungs
- Production of red blood cells (RBCs), which aids in the transport of oxygen to organs and tissues
- Lung volume and pulmonary vasculature, which results in increased surface area for alveolar–capillary gas exchange
- Vascularity of body tissues, which allows for improved oxygen delivery to the tissues
- Production of hemoglobin, which readily binds with oxygen so that the tissue cells can use oxygen even when oxygen pressure is low in the environment.

Lifestyle

Lifestyle factors that affect oxygenation include pregnancy, occupational exposure to hazards, nutrition, obesity, exercise, smoking, and substance abuse.

Pregnancy. During pregnancy, oxygen demand increases dramatically. Maternal metabolism increases by approximately 15% during the last half of pregnancy, increasing the demand for O_2. At the same time, the enlarging uterus pushes upward against the diaphragm, limiting its downward movement. In response, the maternal respiratory rate increases in order to increase minute ventilation (amount of air moved into and out of the lungs in 1 minute) (Hall, 2011).

Occupational Hazards. Occupational hazards may affect pulmonary function by irritating airways or causing cancer. Toxic agents may be categorized as follows:

- *Chemicals and their fumes* irritate the sensitive membranous lining of the lungs and airways and may lead to lung cancer or leukemia. Even common household cleaners can emit toxic fumes.
- *Products of combustion* (e.g., carbon monoxide) are known causes of lung cancer and chronic lung disease.
- *Microorganisms,* such as viruses, fungi, and mold, may lead to infections and precipitate asthma.
- *Fine particles* (e.g., coal dust and asbestos) suspended in the air can be inhaled into the smallest airways, causing irritation and toxic reactions, including cancer.

Nutrition. The body needs an appropriate balance of proteins, carbohydrates, fats, and other nutrients for proper immune function. A healthy diet builds resistance to disease and infection, promotes normal cellular function and tissue repair,

and maintains a healthy weight. Poor nutrition, especially in those with pulmonary disorders, can lead to loss of ventilatory muscle strength, making breathing more difficult.

Obesity. Obesity is defined as a body mass index (BMI) above 30. Obesity causes certain health problems that affect pulmonary function. The following are two examples:

- *Respiratory infections.* Excess abdominal fat presses upward on the diaphragm, preventing full chest expansion, leading to hypoventilation and dyspnea on exertion. The risk for respiratory infection then increases because lower lung lobes are poorly ventilated and secretions not removed effectively.
- *Sleep apnea.* When the person lies down, chest expansion is limited even more. Excess neck girth and fat deposits in the upper airway often lead to obstructive sleep apnea, a condition characterized by daytime sleepiness, snoring, and periods of apnea lasting 10 to 120 seconds (Porth & Matfin, 2010).

Exercise. Exercise increases metabolic demands. The body responds by increasing the heart rate and the rate and depth of breathing. Lack of exercise has the opposite effect. A sedentary lifestyle reduces the capacity to increase ventilation in response to exercise.

Substance Abuse. People abuse various kinds of substances, including prescription medications. Excess use or overdose of respiratory depressants, such as opioids, sedatives, anti-anxiety agents, and hypnotics, can cause death due to hypoventilation, apnea, and respiratory failure. Over-the-counter (OTC) medications and other legally available products, such as alcohol, tobacco, caffeine, glue, aerosols, "bath salts" (a stimulant and hallucinogenic), and other inhalants, also have abuse potential and can be lethal. Large amounts of alcohol, for example, depress respiratory and vasomotor centers of the brain. Illicit drugs, including stimulants (e.g., amphetamines, cocaine), hallucinogens (e.g., LSD, PCP), marijuana, and in some states "bath salts," also have adverse effects on the respiratory system. And of course, an overdose of these substances can depress respirations and increase the risk for aspiration.

Smoking

Tobacco smoke contains tiny particles of tar and approximately 200 known toxic chemicals, more than 60 of which are known to cause cancer. There are two types of *second-hand smoke:*

- *Mainstream smoke* (inhaled directly from the cigarette and then exhaled)
- *Sidestream smoke* (released from the burning tip of a cigarette into the air)

Sidestream smoke has been found to have higher concentrations of harmful compounds than mainstream smoke, thus posing a significant health risk to nonsmokers (Schick & Glantz, 2005). However, both are harmful to everyone in the environment, especially children, older adults, and people with allergies or lung disorders.

Tobacco smoke constricts bronchioles, increases fluid secretion into the airways, causes inflammation and swelling of the bronchial lining, and paralyzes cilia. These effects lead to reduced airflow and increased production of secretions that are not easily removed from the airways. Lung inflammation stimulates the release of enzymes that break down elastin and other alveolar wall components. Continued smoking leads to chronic bronchitis, obstruction of bronchioles and alveolar walls, and emphysema. Cigarette smoking is estimated to be the cause of more than 80% of cases of lung cancer. The longer a person smokes and the more cigarettes he smokes, the greater the risk for cancer and other chronic lung diseases (ALA, 2010; MedlinePlus, n.d.).

Roughly one in every five American adults smokes. However, once a person stops smoking, the body begins to repair the damage. In the first few days, the person will cough more as the cilia begin to clear the airways. Then the coughing subsides, and breathing becomes easier. Even long-time smokers can benefit from smoking cessation (Box 37-1).

KnowledgeCheck 37-4

- What are the major risks to oxygenation related to developmental factors?
- What environmental and lifestyle factors that influence ventilation can be avoided or minimized?

ThinkLike a Nurse 37-4

Review the Meet Your Patients scenario at the beginning of this chapter.

- Which patient(s) may be experiencing developmental, environmental, or lifestyle-related problems with oxygenation?
- Identify any additional information you need to know to answer this question.

Medications

Many drugs can interfere with pulmonary function by depressing respirations. Respiratory depressants generally act by depressing central nervous system (CNS) control of breathing or by weakening the muscles of breathing. They include general anesthetics, opioids (e.g., morphine), anti-anxiety drugs (e.g., diazepam [Valium]), sedative-hypnotics (e.g., barbiturates), neuromuscular blocking agents, and magnesium sulfate. Drugs that block beta-2 adrenergic receptors (e.g., used to lower the blood pressure) have little effect on healthy lungs but can lead to serious bronchiole constriction in people with asthma.

Medications are also used to improve respiratory function. A few examples are bronchodilators, anti-inflammatory agents such as corticosteroids, cough suppressants, expectorants, and decongestants.

For a more extensive discussion of individual medications that either interfere with or improve respiratory function,

> Go to Chapter 37, **Supplemental Materials: Medications That Can Interfere With Oxygenation** and **Medications Used to Improve Oxygenation,** on Davis*Plus.*

BOX 37-1 ■ Health Effects of Smoking Cessation

- Life expectancy increases.
- Blood pressure and heart rate decrease.
- Circulation to the extremities improves within 2 hours.
- Carbon dioxide levels in the blood begin to drop within 4 hours.
- Oxygen levels in the blood begin to improve within 8 hours.
- Digestion improves.
- Coughing, congestion, and shortness of breath decrease.
- Overall energy increases.
- Lungs increase ability to clean themselves, thereby reducing the risk of infection.
- Risk of heart attack decreases and returns to that of a nonsmoker in 1 year.
- Risk of lung and other cancers, stroke, and chronic obstructive lung disease decreases.

Alterations in Gas Exchange

Poor exchange of oxygen and carbon dioxide at the alveolar–capillary membrane changes the levels of O_2 and CO_2 in the blood. Unchecked, it affects oxygenation in tissues and organs and can be life threatening. Box 37-2 describes some alterations in gas exchange.

Alterations in gas exchange are caused by a number of disorders that affect the structure, function, and regulation of the pulmonary and cardiovascular systems. Because it is difficult to separate pulmonary and cardiovascular causes and effects, both are included in the discussion of pulmonary disorders that follows. For a thorough description of these diseases and pathological conditions, consult a medical–surgical nursing text, or

 Go to Chapter 37, **Supplemental Materials: Pathophysiological Conditions That Influence Gas Exchange**, on Davis*Plus*.

KnowledgeCheck 37-5

- What are some indirect indicators of tissue oxygenation?
- How are hyperventilation and hypoventilation related to carbon dioxide levels?
- What are the effects of carbon dioxide levels on the nervous system?

 ThinkLike a Nurse 37-5

You are assessing a very anxious young man who looks frightened and is complaining of trouble breathing. His respiratory rate is 32 breaths/min and deep. He states his fingers and hands are numb.

- What is the most likely cause?
- What blood levels would help you clarify what is going on?

Example Problem: Respiratory Infections (URJs, Influenza, and Pneumonia)

Respiratory infections interfere with gas exchange. They are among the most common causes of short-term disability in the United States. URIs, influenza, and pneumonia (example problems in this chapter) are caused by viruses.

URIs and Influenza. URIs and influenza begin with similar symptoms. It is important to distinguish between them because antiviral medications are available for the flu. Diagnosis can be difficult because there are other conditions that start with cold-like symptoms (e.g., whooping cough, croup, allergies, measles, and pneumonia).

- **URI** symptoms include stuffy nose, sore throat, cough, sneezing, tearing, and a mild fever. Colds are more common in children, and tend to decline with age. They are rarely dangerous to healthy adults and children.
- **Influenza** is highly infectious viral disease and usually more severe than the common cold and may involve the lower airways. Most flu fatalities occur in children younger than age 2 and in older adults, especially the frail elderly. Symptoms include fever, headache, myalgia (muscle pain or tenderness), exhaustion, nasal inflammation and discharge, sore throat, and cough. In addition to cold-like symptoms, the person may experience headache, fatigue, weakness, exhaustion, and high fever. The flu virus is highly contagious. New strains of the virus continually emerge, so it is difficult to develop immunity to the disease. Influenza immunizations are manufactured for each season in an attempt to keep pace with the changing virus.

Lower respiratory tract infections. Pneumonia, acute bronchitis, respiratory syncytial virus [RSV], and tuberculosis are examples of lower respiratory tract infections. They occur more often, and are more severe, in children, older adults, and people with impaired immunity or lung function.

Pneumonia is an infection of the lungs caused by bacteria, fungi, or viruses. It occurs more often during winter months and often follows a recent URI or influenza. Pneumonia-causing organisms gain entry into the lungs from being released into the air with coughing, sneezing, or talking; from contaminated respiratory therapy equipment; from the blood spreading to the lung; or from the nose and throat. The invading pathogen releases toxins that damage bronchial and alveolar–capillary membranes. A full-scale

---

BOX 37-2 ■ Alterations in Gas Exchange

Hypoxemia—Low arterial blood oxygen levels.

Etiology: Poor oxygen diffusion across the alveolar–capillary membrane into the blood (ineffective external respiration) due to lung or pulmonary circulation disorders. Hypoventilation predisposes to the development of hypoxemia and may lead to hypoxia.

Comments: Even if the blood is adequately oxygenated, hypoxia may still occur in the organs and tissues because of poor circulation.

Hypoxia—Inadequate oxygenation of organs and tissues.

Etiology: Either hypoxemia or circulatory disorders

Comments: The effects of hypoxia depend on the organs affected. For example, hypoxic central nervous system tissue causes abnormal brain functioning (e.g., altered level of consciousness), whereas hypoxic renal tissue causes abnormal kidney functioning (e.g., poor urine output), and hypoxic limb tissue results in abnormal muscle functioning (e.g., muscle weakness and pain with exercise).

Hypercarbia (hypercapnia)—An excess of dissolved CO_2 in the blood.

Etiology: Hypoventilation is caused by abnormalities affecting the lungs or chest cavity or by neuromuscular abnormalities that interfere with normal breathing. Hypercarbia can occur suddenly, as in acute airway obstruction or drug overdose, or chronically, as in chronic lung disease.

Comments: Very high blood levels of CO_2 have an anesthetic effect on the nervous system and can lead to somnolence progressing to coma and death, a syndrome known as carbon dioxide narcosis.

Hypocarbia (hypocapnia)—A low level of dissolved CO_2 in the blood. In most cases (except high altitude), blood O_2 levels remain normal.

Etiology: Hyperventilation

Comments: Severe hypocarbia stimulates the nervous system, leading to muscle twitching or spasm (especially in the hands and feet) and numbness and tingling in the face and lips.

inflammatory response triggers edema in the small airways and deposits debris and exudate in the alveoli. Some toxins even cause lung tissue necrosis. The area of the lung affected becomes *consolidated* (solid rather than air filled).

Symptoms of pneumonia include cough, malaise, pleural pain from coughing, discolored sputum, fever, chills, dyspnea, and elevated WBC counts. Treatment includes antipyretics for fever, expectorants to enhance mobilization of secretions, humidity to moisten inhaled air, hydration to thin secretions, *pulmonary hygiene* (deep breathing, coughing, and chest percussion and vibration) to move secretions out of the airways, rest to conserve body energy stores, and, if needed, oxygen therapy. Curative therapy includes appropriate anti-infective agents to kill the causative organisms. Immunizations are available and are discussed in your textbook.

Pulmonary System Abnormalities

The following is a brief discussion of various pulmonary abnormalities that can lead to alterations in gas exchange.

Structural Abnormalities. Structural abnormalities include anything that restricts or limits the free movement of the chest wall (e.g., fractured ribs, kyphosis), interruptions in the chest cavity that inhibit inflation of the lungs (e.g., pneumothorax), or a collection of fluid (blood, lymph, pus) in the pleural space that inhibits lung expansion.

Airway Inflammation and Obstruction. Allergic reactions (e.g., asthma) or irritation from smoke or other irritants may cause airway inflammation. Obstruction may be mechanical, as with a foreign object or bolus of food, or due to spasm (e.g., laryngospasm). Swollen tonsils and a swollen epiglottis may also cause obstruction.

Alveolar–Capillary Membrane Disorders. These disorders are characterized by a change in the consistency of the lung tissue, especially at the alveolar level. The alveoli become stiff and difficult to ventilate, and gas exchange is impaired. Pulmonary edema, acute respiratory distress syndrome (ARDS), and pulmonary fibrosis are examples.

Atelectasis. Anything that reduces ventilation (e.g., tumor, obstructed airway) can cause **atelectasis,** or alveolar collapse.

Pulmonary Circulation Abnormalities

For gas exchange to occur in the alveoli, there must be adequate blood flow through the pulmonary circulation. The most common causes of impaired pulmonary circulation are pulmonary embolus and pulmonary hypertension. A **pulmonary embolus** is obstruction of pulmonary arterial circulation by a foreign substance (e.g., a blood clot, air, or fat).

Pulmonary hypertension is elevated pressure within the pulmonary arterial system. High pressure in the pulmonary circulation increases the workload of the heart. Over time, this causes right-sided heart failure, with a reduced amount of blood pumped into the pulmonary circulation. You will learn about the difference between right-sided and left-sided heart failure in a medical-surgical nursing course. However, if you need some information about it now,

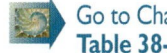 Go to Chapter 38, **Tables, Boxes, Figures: ESG Table 38-1,** on DavisPlus.

If you would like to see an animation demonstrating how blood is oxygenated in the heart and lungs,

 Go to **Cardiovascular/Pulmonary Animations: Blood Flow** and **Carbon Dioxide/Oxygen Transport** on DavisPlus.

Central Nervous System Abnormalities

Any condition that injures or alters the function of the CNS can interfere with the regulation of breathing and, therefore, gas exchange. Trauma and stroke (cerebrovascular accident) are the most commonly seen CNS problems in adults. Spinal cord injuries interfere with nerve transmission between the brain and the area below the level of the injury and may, for example, limit diaphragm function. Immature breathing patterns, such as apnea or periodic breathing, are common in preterm and term infants.

Neuromuscular Abnormalities

Neuromuscular abnormalities can affect gas exchange by interfering with the regulation of breathing or by limiting movement of the muscles involved with breathing. Trauma, stroke, and medications are the most common causes. Neuromuscular disorders that affect the nerves involved in breathing can also depress respiratory function (e.g., Guillain-Barré syndrome, amyotrophic lateral sclerosis, and myasthenia gravis).

KnowledgeCheck 37-6

- Identify four pathophysiological conditions that affect pulmonary function. How are they similar? How are they different?
- What types of injuries are most likely to cause oxygenation problems?

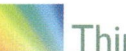 ## ThinkLike a Nurse 37-6

You are the nursing supervisor on the night shift in a small community hospital. At the beginning of the shift, you have only one critical care bed available. During your shift, you receive calls for assistance on the following patients:

- Patient A has burns on her face, scalp, and chest and is coughing up sputum with black streaks.
- Patient B has pneumonia and has suddenly become confused.
- Patient C is short of breath and complaining that he can't breathe. His skin is cool and moist, and he is coughing up clear sputum with small bubbles in it.

Which patient would you admit to the critical care bed? Why?

PracticalKnowledge
knowing how

Nursing care to support pulmonary functioning is directed at assessing for and maximizing the effectiveness of ventilation and gas exchange. In this part of the chapter, we discuss these nursing activities. In Chapter 19, the section entitled "Respirations" provides information about assessing respirations. Also see Procedure 19-5, Assessing Respirations.

 ### ASSESSMENT

Although this section focuses on respiratory assessments, recall that the pulmonary system is only a part of the concept of oxygenation. An evaluation of oxygenation includes a history and physical examination to assess lung, heart, and circulatory function. The order of data collection and the priorities of assessment vary with the patient's condition and the purpose of the assessment. For example, for someone in obvious respiratory distress, the immediate assessment focus is to ask simple questions about current symptoms while

performing a quick examination to determine adequacy of breathing, circulation, and oxygenation. In contrast, assessment for risk of respiratory disease in a healthy person might include more extensive questions about occupation, smoking habits, and living environment; a medical history; and an extensive physical examination. For a complete focused respiratory assessment, you will need to identify risk factors, perform a physical examination, and be familiar with certain diagnostic tests.

Assessing for Risk Factors

A health history related to pulmonary function includes questions about the presence of risk factors that affect lung and airway function. Topics to assess include demographic data, health history, respiratory history, cardiovascular history, environmental history, and lifestyle. For a detailed list of interview questions for each of these topics, see the Focused Assessment box, Oxygenation.

Key Point: *Ask every patient, not just those with oxygenation problems, if they use tobacco; and document their tobacco-use status regularly.*

Physical Examination

You will use all four examination techniques to assess respiratory function:

- *Inspect* to observe respiratory patterns, signs of respiratory distress, chest structures and movement, skin and mucous membrane color, presence or absence of edema, sputum

---

Focused Assessment

Oxygenation

Part I. Questions to Assess Risk for Impaired Oxygenation

Demographic Data

➤ What is your age?
➤ Where do you live?
➤ What is your occupation?

Health History

➤ What healthcare problems are you currently being treated for?
➤ Have you ever been hospitalized or had surgery? If so, when and for what reason?
➤ Do you have a history of allergies or asthma?
➤ What medications do you currently take?
➤ What over-the-counter medications or alternative treatments do you use? What do you use them for?

Respiratory History

➤ Have you ever been diagnosed with a respiratory problem? If so, what was the diagnosis? When was the diagnosis made?
➤ Have you noticed any changes in your breathing?
➤ How often do you cough?
➤ When you do cough, is it productive?
➤ What do the secretions you cough up look like and smell like?
➤ How much sputum do you produce?
➤ How do you treat your cough? What effect did it have?
➤ Do you ever wheeze or feel short of breath?
➤ What causes you to wheeze or feel short of breath?
➤ Do body positions affect your breathing pattern?
➤ What position do you lie in when you sleep? Do you use more than one pillow?
➤ Do you ever wake up short of breath?

Environmental History

➤ Are there pets in the house?
➤ What response, if any, do you have to pets, dust, pollen, or plants?
➤ Are you exposed to smoke or fumes in the home and workplace?
➤ Are you exposed to respiratory irritants such as asbestos, chemicals, coal dust, fungus, molds, or soot in the home or workplace?

➤ What type of heating, air conditioning, or air filtering system do you have in the home or workplace?

Lifestyle

➤ What is your current stress level? What are your major sources of stress?
➤ What is your usual diet? Is your current diet typical, or have you recently changed your eating habits?
➤ What is your usual activity level?
➤ What level of activity makes you feel short of breath?
➤ Do you smoke now, or have you ever smoked?
➤ If you smoke, how many packs per day and for how many years have you smoked?
➤ Do you smoke marijuana or use other substances?

Part II. Focused Physical Examination

Pulmonary System

➤ *Inspect* to observe respiratory patterns, signs of respiratory distress, chest structures and movement, skin and mucous membrane color, presence or absence of edema, sputum characteristics, and overall general appearance.
➤ *Palpate* skin temperature and areas of tenderness.
➤ *Percuss* over the lung fields (for consolidation or excess air pockets).
➤ *Auscultate* breath sounds and vascular sounds.
➤ *Assess breathing patterns:* eupnea, tachypnea, bradypnea, apnea, Kussmaul's breathing, Biot's breathing, and Cheyne–Stokes respirations.
➤ *Assess cough and related symptoms:*
   Nasal congestion, sneezing, water eyes, and nasal discharge suggest allergies.
   Fever, chest congestion, noisy breath sounds, sputum production suggest a URI.
   Dyspnea, chest tightness, and wheezing suggest airway obstruction (e.g., asthma).
➤ *Assess sputum:* appearance, color, odor, amount, and timing.
➤ *Obtain sputum samples* as needed.
➤ *Assess respiratory effort.* Breathing should be effortless. Observe for shortness of breath, dyspnea, nasal flaring, head bobbing, retractions, use of accessory muscles during inspiration, grunting, needing to sit upright to breathe, paroxysmal nocturnal dyspnea, conversational dyspnea, stridor, and wheezing.

characteristics, and overall general appearance. Refer to Chapter 21 to review the details of inspecting the skin and mucous membranes. Also see Procedure 21-2, Assessing the Skin.

- *Palpate* pulses, skin temperature, heart pulsations through the chest wall, and areas of tenderness.
- *Percuss* over the lung fields to screen for areas of consolidation or excess air pockets in the lungs.
- *Auscultate* breath sounds and vascular sounds. For a step-by-step discussion of how to assess the chest and lungs, refer to Procedure 21-12, Assessing the Chest and Lungs.

Assess breathing patterns, cough and associated symptoms, and respiratory effort, as follows. You may also need to monitor oxygenation and ventilation with pulse oximetry and capnography.

Poor peripheral circulation is characterized by weak or absent pulses; mottling (skin marbling); pale, ashen, or cyanotic skin and mucous membranes; and cool skin temperature. You can assess tissue oxygenation indirectly by determining whether organs are functioning normally. You will learn more about this in Chapter 38.

Assessing Breathing Patterns

Assess for normal and altered breathing patterns. They include the following: eupnea, tachypnea, bradypnea, apnea or periodic breathing, Kussmaul's breathing, Biot's breathing, and Cheyne–Stokes respirations. These patterns are shown and defined in Table 19-4. The significance of each pattern is described in Box 37-3.

Recall that pain alters the rate and depth of respirations. Often patients in pain breathe shallowly and are at risk for atelectasis. Regularly assess all patients for pain. Once you have medicated the patient, reassess breath sounds, and encourage the patient to breathe deeply and cough.

Assessing Respiratory Effort/Dyspnea

A healthy person breathes effortlessly. A patient experiencing shortness of breath or dyspnea requires a thorough assessment. However, you must take care not to increase his respiratory effort. Use closed questions that the patient can answer with yes, no, or only a few words. Ask whether the shortness of breath began suddenly or gradually, how severe it is right now,

and whether it is getting better or worse. At the same time, observe for or ask about the signs of increased respiratory effort discussed below. Note that these signs are most easy visible in infants and small children.

- **Nasal flaring**—The visible enlargement of the nostrils with inhalation. It helps reduce resistance to airflow in the nose and keep the nasal passages open to take in more air.
- **Retractions**—The visible "pulling in" of intercostal, supra-clavicular, and subcostal tissue, caused by excessive negative pressures generated in the chest to try to increase the depth of inhalation
- **Use of accessory muscles** during inspiration—The patient may use the intercostals, abdominal muscles, and muscles of the neck and shoulders when there is an increased demand for oxygen or problems with ventilation.
- **Grunting**—Noisy, difficult breathing. It is caused by forced expiration against a closed glottis, and by involuntary muscle contraction during expiration to help keep alveoli open and enhance gas exchange
- **Body positioning** to facilitate respirations—The patient usually finds an upright posture the most comfortable. In the upright position, gravity pulls the abdominal organs down and allows the diaphragm more room to contract. Most patients with dyspnea cannot tolerate lying down. **Orthopnea** is the term used to describe difficulty breathing when lying down. Ask how the patient usually sleeps. Some patients may report sleeping in a recliner or chair.
- **Paroxysmal nocturnal dyspnea**—Sudden awakening due to shortness of breath that begins during sleep. The patient feels panic and extreme dyspnea and must sit upright to ease breathing.
- **Conversational dyspnea**—The inability to speak complete sentences without stopping to breathe. The more frequently the patient pauses when speaking, the more severe the dyspnea.
- **Stridor**—A high-pitched, harsh, crowing, inspiratory sound caused by partial obstruction of the larynx or trachea. You can hear it without a stethoscope.

✚ Partial airway obstruction can easily become complete airway obstruction. Therefore, the patient with stridor needs immediate care.

BOX 37-3 ■ Breathing Patterns

Description	Significance
Eupnea—Rate is about 12 to 20 breaths/min	Normal respirations.
Bradypnea—Slow, < 10 breaths/min	May cause poor gas exchange. Causes include sedative and opioid medications and neuromuscular dysfunction.
Tachypnea—Faster than 24 breaths/min, usually shallow	Generally caused by hypoxemia or increased oxygen demand (e.g., exercise). Shallow respirations draw limited air into the alveoli and may result in hypoventilation.
Kussmaul's respirations—Regular, but abnormally deep and increased in rate	Can be a compensatory mechanism for metabolic disorders that lower blood pH, or a form of hyperventilation caused by fear, anxiety, or panic.
Biot's respirations—Irregular, of variable depth (usually shallow), alternating with periods of apnea	Often associated with damage to the medullary respiratory center or high intracranial pressure due to brain injury.
Cheyne-Stokes respirations—Gradual increase in depth of respirations followed by gradual decrease, and then a period of apnea	Often associated with damage to the medullary respiratory center or high intracranial pressure due to brain injury.
Apnea—Absence of breathing	Respiratory arrest requires immediate cardiopulmonary resuscitation.

- **Wheezing**—A musical sound produced by air passing through partially obstructed small airways. It is often heard in patients with asthma and lung congestion.

✚ **Diminished or absent breath sounds**—In a patient experiencing dyspnea these are signs of worsening ventilation and oxygenation. Oxygen therapy and measures to restore adequate ventilation may be required.

Assessing Cough

Everyone coughs from time to time to remove small amounts of mucus and debris from the airways. Coughing is a normal protective response to known respiratory irritants (e.g., cigarette smoke, irritating fumes, dust particles) or when food or fluid accidentally gets into the airways. A cough becomes significant if it persists, is recurring, or is productive. A persistent or recurring cough may indicate ongoing or recurring airway irritation. Advise patients to obtain medical evaluation for a cough that lasts more than 3 weeks and cannot be explained.

Assess the Cough. Is it dry, productive, or hacking? When does the cough occur and how long has the patient been coughing? What makes it worse? What seems to help it? What has been used to treat the cough, and what were the effects?

Assess for Other Clinical Findings Associated With a Cough. A cough associated with nasal congestion, sneezing, or watery eyes or nose discharge is most likely due to allergies and may be successfully treated with OTC remedies. A cough occurring with fever, chest congestion, noisy breath sounds, and sputum production is more likely to be due to a URI, which may require antibiotics. A cough associated with dyspnea, chest tightness, and wheezing may be due to an airway obstruction disorder such as asthma, which requires corticosteroids and bronchodilating medications.

Assess Sputum Appearance, Color, and Odor. A cough is described as **productive** if it raises sputum (mucus and debris) up from the airways. Sputum appearance and odor provide valuable clues about the cause and significance of a cough (see Box 37-4).

Assess Sputum Amount. The amount of sputum can vary from a teaspoon to pints. In general, sputum production increases with the severity of the underlying condition. However, limited sputum production does not always indicate that the problem is minor, because excess mucus and debris may be trapped in the airways and the patient is unable to cough it up and out of the body.

Assess Sputum Timing. Sputum production ranges from constant to once per day. Tobacco smokers often have a "morning cough," which helps clear their airways of mucus and debris accumulated overnight. In contrast, someone with a URI is more likely to produce sputum throughout the day.

KnowledgeCheck 37-7

- What areas should you include in a nursing history for a patient with oxygenation concerns who is undergoing a comprehensive assessment?
- When is a cough significant? What aspects of a cough should be assessed?
- Identify at least five signs that you may observe in a patient experiencing dyspnea.
- A patient has a respiratory rate of 30 breaths/min that is rhythmic and moderate in depth. What term would you use to describe this breathing pattern?

 ThinkLike a Nurse 37-7

Review the patients presented in the Meet Your Patients scenario.

- Which patients are experiencing respiratory distress? Identify the signs of distress in these patients.
- Which patients require a comprehensive assessment, and which patients will need a rapid assessment and immediate treatment because of the severity of their symptoms?

Diagnostic Testing

Diagnostic testing helps clinicians identify the causes of impaired oxygenation and monitor patient responses to treatment. You will need to assist with and be familiar with the results of the tests of respiratory function. We discuss several of these tests in the next sections. For others,

 Go to Chapter 37, **Diagnostic Testing: Tests Related to Oxygenation,** on DavisPlus.

Obtaining Sputum Samples

You may need to collect sputum samples. Sputum is examined microscopically and cultured in the lab to identify organisms and test for sensitivity to different anti-infective agents. To learn a procedure for collecting sputum specimens, refer to Procedure 37-1.

Skin Testing

Tuberculin skin testing is widely used to detect exposure and antibody formation to the tubercle bacillus. Annual screening is recommended for low-income populations, residents in congregate living conditions (e.g., dormitories, correctional facilities), immigrants from countries with a high prevalence of

---

BOX 37-4 ■ Significance of Sputum Appearance and Odor

Color/Appearance	Significance
White or clear	Usually present in viral infections (e.g., common cold, viral bronchitis), often requiring only supportive care
Yellow or green	A sign of infection
Black	Caused by coal dust, smoke, or soot inhalation
Rust colored	Associated with pneumococcal pneumonia, tuberculosis, and possibly the presence of blood
Hemoptysis	The coughing up of blood or bloody sputum. It may range from small streaks of blood to large amounts of frank blood.
Pink and frothy	Associated with pulmonary edema
Foul-smelling sputum	Bacterial infection (e.g., pneumonia, lung abscess).

tuberculosis (TB), and healthcare workers. For the skin test to be effective, you must administer the antigen intradermally, not subcutaneously. Read the test site 48 to 72 hours after administration. To review intradermal injection technique, see Procedure 25-11.

A positive skin test is defined as an area of induration (hardness) at the test site. The size of the induration that indicates a positive result depends on risk factors. Patients with positive TB skin tests must undergo further testing (chest x-ray study and sputum cultures) to determine whether they have merely been exposed to disease or whether they have active disease. For guidelines for interpreting test results, see the Diagnostic Testing box Reading a Tuberculin Skin Test Result.

Allergy testing uses skin testing to identify antigens that may cause hypersensitivity reactions in susceptible individuals. Testing is performed by scratching antigen samples onto the skin. The area is then observed for allergic skin reactions. Skin testing is performed in facilities with resuscitation equipment and personnel trained in its use, because life-threatening airway obstruction sometimes occurs in response to the allergens.

Pulse Oximetry

Pulse oximetry is a noninvasive estimate of arterial blood oxygen saturation (SaO_2). **SaO_2** reflects the percentage of hemoglobin molecules carrying oxygen. The normal value is 95% to 100%. Values below 94% are considered abnormal in healthy people and should be investigated to determine the cause. Well-oxygenated hemoglobin and deoxygenated hemoglobin in the circulating red blood cells absorb light differently. Using a light-emitting diode (LED), the oximeter is able to detect this difference and calculate the percentage of oxygenated hemoglobin.

Pulse oximetry is simple to perform, provides a rapid reading, and can be used intermittently or continuously. Frequency of measurement depends on the clinical condition of the patient. Recent recommendations are that pulse oximetry can be used to screen newborns for critical congenital heart disease (American Academy of Pediatrics, 2011).

Such factors as movement, acrylic fingernails, nail polish, or cold extremities can interfere with the accuracy of the readings. For tips to assure accuracy, refer to Clinical Insight 37-1. For the complete procedure, see Procedure 37-2.

Capnography

Capnography measures the carbon dioxide (CO_2) in inhaled and exhaled air. As a beam of infrared light passes through a sample of respiratory gases, more or less of it is absorbed depending on the amount of CO_2 present. The device displays the results digitally and prints out a graph showing CO_2 at various times in the breathing cycle. Capnography directly measures ventilation, and indirectly measures the partial pressure of CO_2 in the arterial blood. Normally the difference between arterial blood and expired CO_2 is very small.

Capnography is often used with pulse oximetry because (1) it provides information about ventilation because it shows accumulation or depletion of CO_2, whereas pulse oximetry reflects only oxygenation of the blood; and (2) capnography is a more reliable indicator of respiratory depression than is pulse oximetry. A few of the many situations in which capnography is used include the following: when a patient is receiving opioids, during general anesthesia, and for adjusting parameter settings in mechanically ventilated patients.

Although they do measure carbon dioxide, **CO_2 detectors** are different from capnography. They use chemically treated paper that changes color when exposed to CO_2. They do not give exact readings, but can measure only a range of values.

Spirometry

Spirometry is a measure of air that moves into and out of the lungs. To describe the events of pulmonary ventilation, the air in the lungs is divided into four volumes and four capacities. Normal lung volumes and capacities vary with body size, age, and exercise. Men, large people, and athletes have greater lung volume and capacity for ventilation. For a summary of this information, see the Diagnostic Testing box Lung Volumes and Capacities.

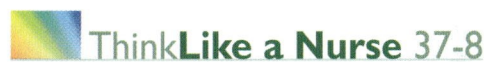

ThinkLike a Nurse 37-8

You hear a pulse oximeter alarm sound in a nearby patient room and find it reading 75%.

- What observations should you make?
- What actions should you take?

Reading a Tuberculin Skin Test Result

Size of Induration	Considered Positive For
5 mm	➤ People who have had recent close contact with someone with active TB ➤ People who have HIV or risk factors for HIV ➤ People with previous history of TB
> 10 mm	➤ IV drug users known to be HIV negative ➤ People with medical conditions that increase the risk of progressing from latent TB to active TB (e.g., diabetes mellitus, use of steroids, chronic renal failure, some malignancies) ➤ Residents and employees of high-risk congregate settings: prisons, skilled nursing facilities (SNFs) and other long-term facilities, healthcare facilities, and homeless shelters ➤ Foreign-born persons recently arrived (i.e., within the last 5 yr) from countries having a high incidence of TB ➤ Low-income groups ➤ Children younger than 4 years of age or exposed to adults in high-risk categories
> 15 mm	➤ People who do not meet any of the above criteria

Diagnostic Testing

Clinical Insight 37-1 ► Tips for Obtaining Accurate Pulse Oximetry Readings

Patient Movement. A nailbed is the most common site to place the probe. However, a tremor, twitch, shivering, or movement in bed can make pulse oximetry readings inaccurate. If the patient is unable to cooperate or control his movement, try using an ear probe or nasal sensor.

Acrylic Fingernails and Nail Polish. If the patient has acrylic nails, place the probe on a toe or earlobe. Many facilities stock individually packaged nail polish remover pads to remove nail polish before placing the probe.

Nail polish or acrylic nails may interfere with signal transmission, causing inaccurate SaO_2 measurement. However, a recent study found that nail polish did not cause a clinically significant change in readings in *healthy* people (Rodden, Spicer, Diaz, et al., 2007).

Dirt and Skin Oils. Dirt and oils on the site can interfere with passage of light waves.

Poor Perfusion. A low reading may result from poor perfusion of the area where the probe is placed.

A bent elbow, for example, may cause a slight decrease in circulation to the nailbed. If SaO_2 results are crucial to the patient's plan of care, use the earlobe to minimize the effect of movement on the reading.

Vasoconstriction due to cool extremities may also limit circulation. Keep the extremities warm to obtain a more accurate reading.

If poor perfusion is related to a disease process, use the earlobe or nose as the monitoring site.

Lighting. Bright fluorescent lighting may influence the accuracy of the reading. Dim the lights or cover the probe with bed covers or a towel to reduce error.

Anemia, Carbon Monoxide, Intravascular Dyes, and Dark Skin Color. These must be considered when interpreting oximetry readings. Because these factors cannot be controlled, watch for trend changes in the readings.

Equipment Function. Look for a displayed waveform; a reading is meaningless without the waveform. If there is a weak signal or no signal, check the patient's vital signs. If vital signs are satisfactory, check the circulation to the site. If that is satisfactory, check equipment connections.

Accuracy of the Reading. If there is an instantaneous change in saturation (e.g., from 99% to 82%), suspect an error. This is not physiologically possible. For any suspected inaccuracy, check the reading using the equipment on a healthy person. If it seems accurate, check the patient's medications and check for history of circulatory disorders; also check items listed above. When in doubt, rely on your clinical judgment more than the reading from the machine.

Arterial Blood Gases

Arterial blood gas (ABG) analysis measures the levels of oxygen and carbon dioxide in arterial blood. A blood sample is obtained from an artery (usually the brachial, radial, or femoral), either by arterial puncture or by withdrawal from an existing arterial line. Arteries are located deep under the skin and alongside nerves, making needle insertion painful. Nurses in critical care units routinely draw ABGs and monitor patients with invasive arterial monitoring; however, you may care for patients on medical–surgical units, or even outpatients, who will undergo periodic ABG evaluation. ABG analysis measures pH, partial pressure of oxygen (PO_2), partial pressure of carbon dioxide (PCO_2), saturation of oxygen (SaO_2), and bicarbonate (HCO_3) level. Here, we discuss only PO_2 and PCO_2. For a more thorough discussion of arterial blood gas values, see Chapter 39.

Measuring Arterial Blood Oxygen

Three values are important when assessing the degree to which the tissues are receiving oxygen:

- **Hemoglobin** is the iron-containing pigment of red blood cells that, as *oxyhemoglobin*, carries oxygen in the blood.

Lung Volumes and Capacities

The norms presented in this table are based on averages for a young adult man. The following are measured by spirometry.

Title	Definition	Significance
Tidal volume (V_T)	The amount of air moved into and out of the lungs with each normal breath. Normally around 500 mL.	In a healthy state, V_T increases when oxygen demand increases. Diseases that restrict lung inflation, create muscular weakness, or paralyze the diaphragm limit the ability of the body to increase tidal volume. When such disorders become severe, V_T will fall too low to support even resting oxygen demands.
Inspiratory reserve volume (IRV)	The maximum amount of air that can be inhaled above and beyond the normal tidal volume. Ranges from 2,000 to 3,000 mL.	IRV determines how much the tidal volume can increase when oxygen demands increase.

Diagnostic Testing

Lung Volumes and Capacities—cont'd

Diagnostic Testing

Title	Definition	Significance
Expiratory reserve volume (ERV)	The maximum extra amount of air that can be forcefully exhaled after the end of a normal tidal expiration. Ranges from 1,000 to 1,500 mL.	Some diseases (e.g., emphysema) cause collapse of alveoli and airways, which traps extra air in the lungs. This "trapped" air cannot be exhaled and lowers ERV.
Residual volume (RV)	The amount of air remaining in the lungs after the most forceful exhalation. Ranges from 1,000 to 1,500 mL.	Diseases that reduce ERV lead to an increase in RV. As more air is trapped in the lungs and cannot be exhaled even with forceful attempts (ERV), it becomes part of the residual volume that is never completely exhaled.
Inspiratory capacity (IC)	The combination of the tidal volume and inspiratory reserve volume (V_T + IRV). Ranges from 2,500 to 3,500 mL.	This is the amount of air that can be inhaled with maximum effort. It reflects the capacity one has to inhale deeply.
Functional residual capacity (FRC)	The combination of expiratory reserve volume and residual volume (ERV + RV). Ranges from 2,000 to 3,000 mL. Exhalation of additional air requires effort to force more air out.	This is the amount of air that stays in the lungs at the end of a normal passive, quiet exhalation. Disorders that cause air trapping increase the FRC.
Vital capacity (VC)	The combination of inspiratory reserve volume and expiratory reserve volume (IRV + ERV). Ranges from 3,000 to 4,500 mL.	This is the maximum amount of air that can be forcefully exhaled after filling the lungs to their maximum level with the deepest possible inspiratory effort.

- **PO₂ (partial pressure of oxygen)** is the amount of oxygen available to combine with hemoglobin to make oxyhemoglobin.
- **SaO₂ (saturation of oxygen)** reflects oxygen that is actually bound to hemoglobin.

At sea level, the normal PO₂ range in arterial blood is 80 to 100 mm Hg. After tissues have extracted oxygen from arterial blood and the blood enters the veins to return to the heart, the venous blood PO₂ has fallen to around 40 mm Hg. The SaO₂, along with the PO₂ and hemoglobin level, indicates the degree to which the tissues are receiving oxygen. Small changes in SaO₂ are associated with large changes in PO₂. For blood gas values, refer to the Diagnostic Testing box Arterial Blood Gas Values: Evaluating Adequacy of Oxygenation.

To fully interpret PO₂ and SaO₂ values, you need to know the percentage of oxygen in the air the patient is inhaling. This is known as the **fraction of inspired oxygen,** or **FIO₂.** At sea level, atmospheric air (commonly known as *room air*) is 21% oxygen (FIO₂ = 21%). The norms quoted for PO₂ and SaO₂ are based on an FIO₂ of 21%. If a healthy patient receives 100% oxygen for a few minutes, the arterial PO₂ would rise to 500 to 600 mm Hg, and the SaO₂ would remain at 100%. The reason is that the SaO₂ measures the oxygen *bound to hemoglobin*—and of course the hemoglobin cannot be "filled" with oxygen to more than 100% capacity. When gas exchange is impaired as a result of disease or injury, PO₂ and SaO₂ levels fall. However, they can be kept at normal levels if supplemental oxygen is given.

Measuring Arterial Blood Carbon Dioxide

The **partial pressure of carbon dioxide (PCO₂)** is a measure of the CO_2 dissolved in the blood. Normal arterial PCO₂ is 35 to 45 mm Hg. Carbon dioxide readily diffuses across the alveolar–capillary membrane in the lungs even when there are obstacles such as alveolar fluid or thickened membranes. As a result, PCO₂ levels remain normal until a severe disorder interferes with all gas exchange. Once in the alveoli, the amount of carbon dioxide exhaled from the lungs is directly influenced by how well air is moving into and out of the lungs (ventilation).

- **Hypocarbia.** When a person hyperventilates, he exhales large amounts of CO_2, causing arterial Pco₂ values to fall. Hyperventilation brings more oxygen into the lungs, so unless it is triggered by hypoxemia, oxygen levels (Po₂) usually remain normal.
- **Hypercarbia.** Conversely, in hypoventilation less CO_2 moves into the alveoli for exhalation, leaving more CO_2 in the arterial blood. This causes PCO₂ values to rise. High PCO₂ levels (hypercarbia) suppress the respiratory drive, have an anesthetic effect on the nervous system, and can be toxic. Hypoventilation severe enough to cause hypercarbia

Arterial Blood Gas Values: Evaluating Adequacy of Oxygenation

Diagnostic Testing

SAO₂	Arterial PO₂	Comment
95%–100%	80–100 mm Hg	Normal arterial values in healthy people.
90%	60 mm Hg	PO₂ > 60 mm Hg is required to sustain life and activity. This level is **not** normal in healthy people.
75%	40 mm Hg	Normal venous values; a **life-threatening arterial value** in anyone.

is usually associated with hypoxemia because not enough oxygen is inhaled.

For additional information on interpreting arterial blood gases, see Chapter 39, Interpreting ABGs, and Table 39-5.

KnowledgeCheck 37-8

- What does a pulse oximetry reading tell you?
- What is the relationship between arterial PO_2 and SaO_2 levels?
- Identify normal PO_2, SaO_2, and PCO_2 levels.
- What effect does ventilation have on arterial PCO_2?
- How is PCO_2 related to oxygenation?

 ## ThinkLike a Nurse 37-9

You are caring for two patients, both of whom have a PO_2 of 95 mm Hg and SaO_2 of 99%. Do they have similar lung function? Explain your answer.

Peak Flow Monitoring

Peak expiratory flow rate (PEFR) measures the amount of air that can be exhaled with forcible effort. Patients with asthma use PEFR monitoring to detect subtle changes in their condition, often before symptoms occur. A peak flow meter is used to monitor these changes (Fig. 37-4). Peak flow is expressed in liters per minute. Treatment protocols describe the use and frequency of medications based on individualized peak flow rates. The Home Care box Home Use of a Peak Flow Meter describes self-monitoring.

ANALYSIS/NURSING DIAGNOSIS

Alterations in pulmonary function may be nursing diagnoses, etiologies of other problems, or merely symptoms of other problems. In analyzing the assessment data, you must determine which. For example, suppose a patient is breathing shallowly and slowly. The pulmonary problem might be one of the following:

- **A nursing diagnosis:** *Ineffective Breathing Pattern (hypoventilation)* r/t pain secondary to rib fractures. In this case, you would provide pain relief; the desired outcome is that the patient will have effective (normal) ventilation. To sees a nursing care plan and care map for Ineffective Breathing Pattern,

 Go to Chapter 37, **Care Plan** and **Care Map,** on Davis*Plus.*

- **An etiology:** Risk for Ineffective Cerebral Tissue Perfusion r/t *Ineffective Breathing Pattern (hypoventilation).* In this case, you might address the etiology by administering oxygen; the desired outcome would be effective cerebral perfusion, evidenced by normal speech and alertness.
- **A symptom:** Decreased Intracranial Adaptive capacity r/t brain injury, *as manifested by Ineffective Breathing Pattern (hypoventilation),* and baseline ICP ≤ 10 mmHg. In this situation, you would, of course, support ventilation (the symptom) until the problem subsides. However, the primary interventions would be directed toward the head trauma and increased intracranial pressure (ICP). Once these etiologies were corrected, the hypoventilation would disappear. The goal would be normal intracranial pressure, evidenced in part by a normal breathing pattern.

Problems of Ventilation and Gas Exchange

Five NANDA International (NANDA-I) diagnoses directly describe problems with ventilation and gas exchange. Use these diagnoses when they are the central problem and you

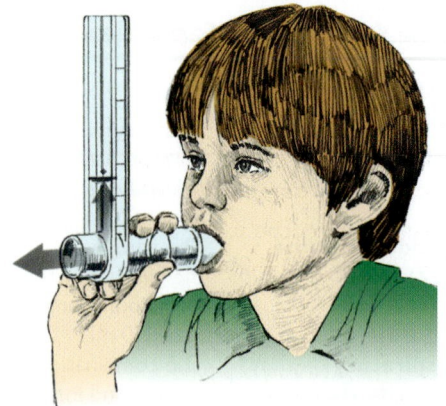

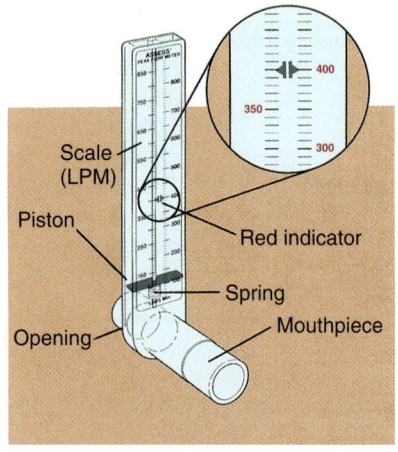

FIGURE 37-4 A patient with asthma using a peak flow meter to monitor peak expiratory flow rate (PEFR).

Home Care

Home Use of a Peak Flow Meter

People with asthma are often asked to monitor their peak flow readings at home and to compare their current readings to their baseline "personal best."

➤ Teach patients that to get an accurate reading, they need to take a deep breath and forcefully exhale.
➤ Teach patients to take a series of three readings and record the highest reading.
➤ Teach patients to maintain or adjust their medication according to their highest reading. They should follow the color-coded treatment protocols prescribed by their physician. These are individualized for each patient. Notice that these correspond to the color-coded markers on their peak flow meter.

Green = All clear: Baseline peak flow—Peak flow is within 80% to 100% of personal best baseline.

Treatment protocol calls for routine medication use.

Yellow = Caution: Peak flow is 50% to 80% of usual or "normal" rate. Said another way, there is a 20% to 50% reduction in peak flow—This reading signals the onset of airway changes.

Treatment protocols usually specify an increase in the dosage of maintenance medications, use of rescue therapies (e.g., fast-acting bronchodilators), or a call to

Home Use of a Peak Flow Meter—cont'd

the healthcare provider. These measures are designed to reverse acute exacerbations before they become severe.

Red = *Medical alert: Peak flow is less than 50% of personal best baseline.* *Severe reduction in peak flow.*

Treatment protocols usually specify immediate treatment with rescue medications and to seek emergency treatment if symptoms do not improve.

Source: Adapted from ALA. (2008b). Asthma & allergy: Peak flow meters. Retrieved from http://www.lungusa.org/lung-disease/asthma/living-with-asthma/take-control-of-your-asthma/AsthmaActionPlan-JUL2008-high-res.pdf

intend to use interventions to eliminate the cause of the problem.
- *Ineffective Airway Clearance* is the inability to maintain a clear airway.
- *Ineffective Breathing Pattern* is used to describe inadequate ventilation, such as hypoventilation, hyperventilation, tachypnea, or bradypnea.
- *Impaired Gas Exchange* is the appropriate diagnosis if the patient is ventilating adequately but diffusion of gases across the alveolar–capillary membrane is impaired.
- *Impaired Spontaneous Ventilation* describes a condition in which a patient, as a result of decreased energy reserves, is unable to maintain breathing adequate to support life.
- *Dysfunctional Ventilatory Weaning Response* represents a specific situation in which a patient who is being mechanically ventilated cannot adjust to lower levels of ventilator support, prolonging the ventilatory weaning process.
- *Risk for Aspiration* should be used when there is a risk for secretions, solids, or fluids entering into tracheobronchial passages (e.g., for patients who have had head or neck surgery or who have a reduced level of consciousness).

For further discussion of these diagnoses,

Go to Chapter 37, **Standardized Language: Nursing Diagnoses Associated With Impaired Ventilation and Gas Exchange,** on Davis*Plus.*

PLANNING OUTCOMES/EVALUATION

NOC standardized outcomes appropriate for patients with pulmonary function problems include the following:

Mechanical Ventilation Weaning Response: Adult
Respiratory Status: Airway Patency
Respiratory Status: Gas Exchange
Respiratory Status: Ventilation
Vital Signs.

For examples of NOC outcomes and NIC interventions for selected oxygenation nursing diagnoses,

Go to Chapter 37, **Standardized Language: Examples of NOC Outcomes and NIC Interventions Linked to Oxygenation Diagnoses,** on Davis*Plus.*

These provide a general care planning guide. Depending on individual patient needs, other NOC outcomes or NIC interventions may also be appropriate.

Individualized goals/outcome statements depend on the nursing diagnosis you identify. For diagnoses related to gas exchange, the following are examples of goals you might write:

Expectorates secretions effectively
No dyspnea or shortness of breath
Lungs clear; no adventitious sounds present

PLANNING INTERVENTIONS/IMPLEMENTATION

NIC standardized interventions related to oxygenation are found in the Respiratory Management category. They focus on maintaining a patent airway and promoting gas exchange, and include Airway Management, Airway Suction, Cough Enhancement, Oxygen Therapy, and Respiratory Monitoring.

Specific nursing interventions for patients with oxygenation problems include health promotion, prevention, and treatment activities. They are discussed in the sections that follow.

Administering Respiratory Medications

Respiratory medications promote ventilation and oxygenation by their effects on the respiratory system itself. Some need a prescription; others do not. The major types of respiratory medicines are shown in Table 37-1. See the accompanying Self-Care box, Cough and Cold Medicines: Tips for Parents for assistance in administering such medications to children. Refer to the accompanying CAM box for some common alternative cold remedies.

Promoting Optimal Respiratory Function

Deep, regular breathing promotes ventilation and optimizes gas exchange. Other interventions to promote optimal respiratory function include preventing URIs, performing immunizations, supporting smoking cessation, preventing and treating pneumonia, positioning, providing incentive spirometry, and preventing aspiration.

Example Problem: Upper Respiratory Infections (Prevention Interventions)

URIs may be viral or bacterial. Viral infections usually last about 10 to 21 days and are self-limiting. URIs may, however, lead to other respiratory diseases and seriously compromised oxygenation in children, older adults, and people who have other illnesses. Therefore, it is important to teach clients measures the importance of handwashing and other measures for preventing URIs (see the Self-Care box, Teaching Clients How to Prevent Upper Respiratory Infections in Chapter 27).

Overuse of antibiotics to treat URIs has contributed to the current crisis of antimicrobial resistance. Teach clients that antibiotics should be used only as prescribed for diagnosed bacterial infections. This includes taking the full course of prescribed antibiotics, even if symptoms are no longer present. Antibiotics are not without risks, and they are not effective for treating the common cold. Advise clients not to pressure clinicians for a prescription, nor to take any antibiotics left over from previous prescriptions or from others who might offer to share antibiotics.

Example Problem: Influenza (Prevention Interventions)

The most effective strategy for preventing influenza is annual vaccination. Vaccines are developed annually to closely match the major known strains of the virus that have evolved. Immunizations given to healthy young adults are 70% to 90% effective. Though less effective in preventing the disease in older

Table 37-1 ➤ Respiratory Medications that Promote Ventilation and Oxygenation

CLASS	ACTION	EXAMPLES AND COMMENTS
Bronchodilators	■ Relax the smooth muscles lining the airways. ■ Can be administered as oral or inhaled medicines.	Beta-2 adrenergic agonists Anticholinergics Methylxanthine
Respiratory Anti-inflammatory Agents	■ Combat inflammation in the airways. ■ Important in treating and controlling respiratory conditions characterized by hypersensitive airways and airway inflammation (e.g., asthma).	Corticosteroids Cromolyn Leukotriene modifiers
Nasal Decongestants	■ Relieve stuffy, blocked nasal passages by constricting local blood vessels through stimulation of alpha-1 adrenergic nerve receptors in the vessels. ■ Although the desired effect is on the nasal mucosa, these medications can have systemic adrenergic effects causing elevated blood pressure, tachycardia, and palpitations, especially in those with a history of cardiovascular conditions.	Ephedrine Pseudoephedrine Phenylephrine
Antihistamines	■ Prevent the effects of histamine release. ■ Used to treat upper respiratory and nasal allergy symptoms.	Diphenhydramine (Benadryl) Chlorpheniramine (Chlor-Trimeton) Brompheniramine (Dimetane) Loratadine (Claritin) Fexofenadine (Allegra) Cetirizine (Zyrtec)
Cough Preparations	■ *Antitussives* (cough suppressants) reduce the frequency of an involuntary, hacking, nonproductive cough. ■ *Expectorants* help make coughing more productive. ■ The goal is to reduce the frequency of dry, unproductive coughing while making voluntary coughing more productive.	These agents are often found mixed together in one preparation to achieve both desirable effects with one medication.

Self-Care

Cough and Cold Medicines: Tips for Parents

➤ Do not give children medicines labeled for adults only.

➤ ✚ Do not give OTC cough and cold remedies to children younger than age 4 years. There is a risk of serious and even life-threatening side effects.

➤ The safety and effectiveness of OTC cough and cold remedies for children ages 2 through 11 years is still in question. It is not certain they are safe, and they may not be effective.

➤ Read labels! Some labels are marked "Do not use for children under age 4."

➤ Choose medications with safety caps. Close caps tightly and store out of sight and reach of children.

➤ Do not give more than one medicine with the same active ingredient. Check the "active ingredients" on the label. Your child could be harmed by getting too much of the ingredient.

➤ Carefully follow the directions on the label for how to use the medicine. Overuse or misuse can cause serious side effects (e.g., drowsiness, breathing problems, and seizures).

➤ Measure carefully. Do not use household spoons because they come in different sizes.

➤ Understand that OTC medicines do not cure the cold or cough. They only treat symptoms such as runny nose, congestion, fever, and aches. They do not shorten the length of time your child is sick.

Source: U.S. Food and Drug Administration/Consumer Health Information. (2008). Using over-the-counter cough and cold products in children. Retrieved June 23, 2011, from http://www.fda.gov/ForConsumers/ConsumerUpdates/ucm048515.htm#TipsforParentsandCaregivers

Complementary & Alternative Modalities (CAM)

Common Cold Remedies

➤ Cold care products containing *Pelargonium sidoides*, an extract of the South African geranium, may reduce the intensity of the common cold. However, more evidence is needed ("Herbal Solution Hastens," 2008). In the United States, Zucol products are one example.

✚ Honey is more effective than dextromethorphan in children with nocturnal cough (Paul, Beiler, McMonagle, et al., 2007). However, avoid giving honey to children younger than the age of 1 year because it is a reservoir of *Clostridium botulinum* spores, and may cause botulism in infants.

➤ Vitamin C in daily doses of 200 mg or more has not been found to prevent colds, but it did reduce the length and severity of symptoms. Be aware that in amounts of 2,000 mg, it may cause diarrhea and gas (Hemilä, Chalker, Treacy, et al., 2007).

➤ A Cochrane Review found there is no evidence that Echinacea preparations are effective for preventing and treating the common cold (Linde, Barrett, Bauer, et al., 2006).

➤ Although lab studies are preliminary, elderberry (*Sambucus nigra*), an herb, has been found to help combat viruses, specifically influenza. It is thought to strengthen the immune system and keep the flu virus from adhering to cells.

adults, immunization decreases the severity of the disease, the development of secondary complications, and the incidence of death (Fiore, Shay, Broder, et al., 2008).

Another prevention measure is to avoid exposure to the virus. That is, avoid being around people who are sick, if possible; and use recommended hand hygiene measures.

Infection rates are highest among children. Rates of serious illness and death are highest among older adults, children younger than age 2 years, and people with certain medical conditions. However, the CDC has recently recommended universal vaccination—that is, that all people age 6 months and older receive annual influenza vaccination (CDC, 2010).

Example Problem: Pneumonia (Prevention Interventions)

Pneumonia is a leading cause of infectious death in the United States, with a mortality rate of approximately 50% in people older than age 65. Therefore, people who are most susceptible should be immunized against pneumonia. Historically this vaccine was thought to convey lifetime immunity, but recent data illustrate that this may not be so. As a result, the vaccine is recommended annually for high-risk groups, including the following (CDC, n.d., revised 2011):

- Adults age 65 years or older
- Children younger than age 5 years
- Children age 6 through 18 years who have certain medical conditions
- People age 2 through 64 years who have chronic illnesses (e.g., those with heart disease, diabetes, pulmonary disease, alcoholism, HIV infection) or lowered resistance to infection
- Adults age 19 through 64 years who have asthma or are smokers

CDC recommended immunization schedules change periodically. To be certain you have the most current information, always check the CDC Web site at

 http://www.cdc.gov/vaccines/recs/schedules/

Healthcare-Associated Pneumonia

Healthcare-associated pneumonia tends to be more complicated and to have a higher mortality rate than community-acquired pneumonia. Guidelines for preventing healthcare-associated pneumonia include following standard precautions for hand hygiene and gloving.

- ✚ Wear gloves for handling respiratory secretions or objects contaminated with respiratory secretions of all patients.
- Change gloves and decontaminate hands:
  - Between contacts with different patients
  - After handling respiratory secretions or contaminated objects and before contact with another patient, object, or environmental surface
  - Between contacts with a contaminated body site and the respiratory tract or respiratory device on the same patient (Tablan, Anderson, Besser, et al., 2004)

Support Smoking Cessation

Smoking cessation is important in preventing and treating all respiratory problems, including the example problems URIs, influenza, and pneumonia. Nurses can provide effective support to patients who want to quit smoking (Rice & Stead, 2008). *All* patients should be asked if they use tobacco. Furthermore, a systematic review of evidence indicates that their tobacco-use status should be documented regularly (e.g., by chart stickers or computer prompts) (National Guideline Clearinghouse [NGC], 2008). The U.S. Public Health Service guidelines suggest the 5A's model for treating tobacco dependence (Box 37-5) (Fiore, Jaén, Baker, et al., 2008).

Motivational counseling includes discussion about the connection between tobacco use and current health status, the risks of continued tobacco use, the rewards of quitting, anticipated barriers to quitting, and strategies for addressing barriers. It may also be important to refer the person to a tobacco cessation program. Most smokers are not able to quit "cold turkey."

Combining medication and counseling is more effective than either used alone. Encourage patients to contact their primary care provider for nicotine replacement therapy or other medications (e.g., antidepressants, clonidine) to treat tobacco dependence. For pregnant women, smokeless tobacco users, light smokers, and adolescents, medications may be contraindicated or may lack evidence of effectiveness (NGC, 2008).

Box 37-1 highlights some of the benefits of smoking cessation. Teach these to your patients. If you would like some smoking cessation tips to share with patients,

 Go to Chapter 37, **Tables, Boxes, Figures, ESG Self-Care: Smoking Cessation Tips,** on Davis*Plus.*

Position for Maximum Ventilation

An upright or elevated position pulls abdominal organs down, allowing maximum diaphragm excursion and lung expansion. Therefore, this intervention is applicable to almost all respiratory problems, including the example problems, UTI, influenza, and pneumonia.

- If the patient is short of breath, provide an overbed table to lean forward on. Patients with impaired respiratory function

BOX 37-5 ■ The 5A's for Treating Tobacco Dependence

Ask about tobacco use and document tobacco use status for every patient at every visit.
Advise to quit. Use a clear, strong, personalized approach to urge the patient to quit.
Assess willingness to make a quit attempt at this time.
Assist in a quit attempt. If the patient is willing, refer for counseling and medication. If the patient is not willing to quit at this time, provide interventions designed to increase future quit attempts.
Arrange follow-up. If the patient is willing to quit, make follow-up contacts beginning the first week after the quit date. If the patient is not willing to quit at this time, address tobacco dependence and willingness to quit at the next clinic (or other) visit.

Source: Adapted from Fiore, M., Jaén, C., Baker, T., et al. (2008). Treating tobacco use and dependence: 2008 update. Clinical Practice Guideline. Rockville, MD: U.S. Department of Health and Human Services. Public Health Service.

adopt a tripod position to allow maximum expansion. They may need to rest their arms on an overbed table.

- When the patient is lying on her side, provide pillows to support the upper arm.
- Assist with frequent position changes to keep all areas of the lungs well ventilated, and ambulate as often as possible without creating fatigue.

Assist With Incentive Spirometry

Incentive spirometers are designed to encourage patients to take deep breaths by reaching a goal-directed volume of air. Incentive spirometry is usually reserved for patients at risk for developing atelectasis or pneumonia, for example, patients who have had abdominal, chest, or pelvic surgery, patients on prolonged bedrest, or patients with a history of respiratory problems. Incentive spirometers offer various visual cues (such as elevation of a ball or piston) to show patients whether they are inhaling deeply enough. As a registered nurse (RN), you can delegate incentive spirometry coaching to licensed practical nurses (LPNs) and qualified nursing assistive personnel (NAPs). However, you are responsible for ensuring that incentive spirometry is carried out correctly and at required frequencies. You must also evaluate patient responses, airway clearance, and ventilation. See Figure 40-8 and the Self-Care box Teaching Your Patient About Incentive Spirometry in Chapter 40.

Take Aspiration Precautions

Aspiration is a risk for patients with a decreased level of consciousness, diminished gag or cough reflex, or difficulty with swallowing. Preventing aspiration requires you to have practical knowledge about positioning, enteral and oral feedings, and administering medications. For guidelines to use with at-risk patients, see Clinical Insight 37-2, Guidelines for Preventing Aspiration. Many of the guidelines involve basic care and can be delegated to qualified LPNs and NAPs. The RN is responsible for monitoring for aspiration. Record in the nursing notes any preventive measures taken.

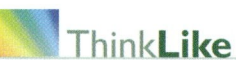 KnowledgeCheck 37-9

Identify at least three nursing interventions to promote optimal respiratory function in a hospitalized patient with chronic lung disease.

ThinkLike a Nurse 37-10

- Review the Meet Your Patients scenario. For which of these patients should you recommend annual flu or pneumonia immunizations? Why?
- A 24-year-old nursing student has no previous hospitalizations or known chronic health problems, takes no medications, and has no current respiratory symptoms. On routine purified protein derivative, or PPD, testing (tuberculin skin testing), the student has an area of induration measuring 5 mm. How would you interpret these results?

Clinical Insight 37-2 ▶ **Guidelines for Preventing Aspiration**

 To prevent aspiration, use the following guidelines.

For At-Risk Patients

Position the unconscious patient on his side to protect the airway.
Request medications in elixir or liquid form.
Break or crush pills, when appropriate.
Keep a suction setup available for routine and emergency use.
If the patient is intubated, keep the endotracheal or tracheostomy cuff inflated, and suction above the cuff before deflating the cuff.
Do not offer food or fluids if the patient is heavily sedated or in the initial recovery phase of anesthesia.

Enteral Feedings

Check the placement of the nasogastric tube before you administer enteral feedings.
Check gastric residual volume before administering the next enteral feeding. Hold the feeding if the residual volume is high.

(_Note:_ The amount of acceptable residual volume depends on the amount and frequency of feedings.)
If the patient is receiving continuous tube feedings, the head of the bed must remain elevated.
Also see Procedure 28-3 for step-by-step instructions for administering feedings through gastric and enteric tubes.

Oral Feedings

Position the patient upright or with the head of the bed elevated for feedings or meal.
Be sure the head of bed remains elevated for at least 30 minutes after each feeding or meal.
Offer small, frequent meals.
Avoid thin liquids, or use thickening agents.
Offer foods or liquids that can be formed into a bolus before they are swallowed.
Cut food into small pieces.

Mobilizing Secretions

Coughing promotes deep inhalation and forceful expulsion of secretions. Interventions that help enhance coughing and mobilize secretions include deep breathing, coughing exercises, and hydration. Mobilizing secretions is useful for many respiratory conditions, including the example problems, UTI, influenza, and pneumonia.

Teach Deep Breathing and Coughing

Deep breathing promotes ventilation and gas exchange. Coughing after deep breathing mobilizes secretions, which keeps airways and alveoli open and provides greater surface area for gas exchange. This intervention is important, for example, in treating pneumonia and preventing stasis pneumonia postoperatively. For information about teaching patients to deep-breathe and cough, see Procedure 40-1.

Alter this procedure for patients with chronic lung disease. Have the patient exhale through pursed lips and cough throughout expiration in several short bursts to avoid high expiratory pressures, which collapse diseased airways.

Maintain Hydration

The following activities are important to keep pulmonary secretions thin and mobile (e.g., in infections such as influenza and pneumonia):

- *Maintain systemic hydration.* Encourage oral fluid intake as much as possible. Supplement oral intake by intravenous fluid administration if the patient cannot ingest adequate amounts of fluid. For guidelines to use in teaching patients to maintain hydration, refer to the Self-Care box, Teaching Patients to Prevent Fluid and Electrolyte Imbalances in Chapter 39.
- *Humidify inhaled air.* You can accomplish this with humidification devices or nebulizers. A **humidifier** is a device that delivers small water droplets from a reservoir. Small humidifiers filled with sterile distilled water are attached to oxygen delivery systems to moisten the dry oxygen and keep secretions thin and mobile. A **nebulizer** is a device that turns liquids into an aerosol mist that can be inhaled directly into the lungs. Nebulizers are often used to deliver medications to the lungs, but they can also be used to deliver moisture to the airways and lungs. See Administering Respiratory Inhalations in Chapter 25, and Figure 25–8.

Perform Chest Physiotherapy

Chest physiotherapy moves secretions to the large, central airways for expectoration or suctioning (Fig. 37-5). It involves postural drainage, chest percussion, and chest vibration. In many institutions, respiratory therapists routinely perform chest physiotherapy. For a detailed description of chest physiotherapy, see Procedure 37-3.

- *Postural drainage* is the use of positioning to promote drainage from the lungs. Check chest x-ray results to see what segments of the lungs are affected. With this information, you can plan how to position your patient. Postural drainage uses gravity to drain the lungs, so you will place the affected area in an uppermost position so that secretions will drain down toward the large, central airways. Procedure 37-3 describes the various positions.
- *Chest percussion and chest vibration* are used in conjunction with postural drainage to loosen and mobilize secretions. Have the patient assume the desired drainage position for 10 to 15 minutes before percussing and vibrating. **Chest percussion** is the rhythmic clapping of the chest wall using cupped hands. **Chest vibration** is the vibration of the chest wall with the

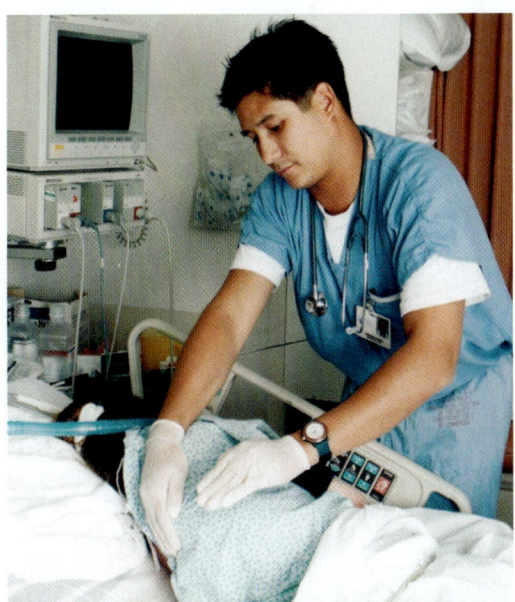

FIGURE 37-5 Patient receiving chest physiotherapy.

palms of the hands. Vibration is a gentle procedure, so you can use it in frail patients who cannot tolerate percussion. If one is available, you can use a vibrating machine instead of the palms of your hands.

ThinkLike a Nurse 37-11

Your patient has pneumonia in the right lower lobe. She is mildly dyspneic with any activity. Strategize how you would perform chest physiotherapy on this patient. What activities would you consider to make this procedure more tolerable for the patient?

Providing Oxygen Therapy

Oxygen therapy provides oxygen at concentrations greater than the level found in room air. Room air contains only about 21% oxygen. Because oxygen is a medication, it requires a medical prescription for dosage (concentration) and route. Many agencies have protocols with standing orders for oxygen administration in an emergency. (Note that oxygen therapy may be needed for the example problem, pneumonia.) Oxygen is supplied in several different ways:

- *Wall outlets* connected to a large central tank of oxygen are usually provided in healthcare facilities.
- *Compressed O_2 in portable tanks* may also be available.
- *Liquid oxygen units* are often used for home oxygen therapy (Fig. 37-6).
- An *oxygen concentrator* removes nitrogen from room air and concentrates O_2. It requires a battery pack or electrical outlet for power. Oxygen concentrators can deliver flow up to 4 liters per minute (L/min) to create an FIO_2 of approximately 36%. Concentrations are higher at lower flow rates (e.g., an FIO_2 of 95% at 1 L/min). These devices eliminate the need for buying oxygen cylinders, relieving clients' anxiety about running out of oxygen. However, they are expensive, noisy, and not portable; moreover, the client must still have backup oxygen in case of a power failure.

An oxygen flow meter must be connected to the oxygen source to control the flow rate of oxygen from its source to the patient. Flow meters are set in liters per minute.

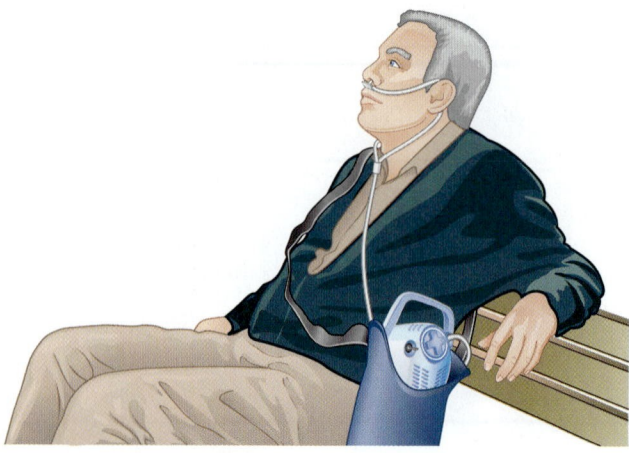

FIGURE 37-6 Liquid oxygen units are small and portable. They are ideal for home use.

Various devices (e.g., mask, cannula) are used to deliver oxygen to a patient. They differ in the amount of oxygen they can deliver and the degree to which they enclose the patient. Low-flow devices are the nasal cannula, simple face masks, and rebreather masks. High-flow devices include Venturi masks, aerosol face masks, face tents, and tracheostomy collars—all capable of reaching up to 100% oxygen concentration (Stich & Cassella, 2009). To see the various types of masks and learn how to set up apply or delegate oxygen therapy, refer to Procedure 37-4.

✚ **Oxygen Hazards.** The following risks are associated with oxygen therapy. Refer to Procedure 37-4 for guidelines to minimize these risks.

- *Oxygen toxicity can develop* in adults when O_2 concentrations of more than 50% are administered for longer than 48 to 72 hours. Prolonged use of high O_2 concentrations reduces surfactant production, which leads to alveolar collapse and reduced lung elasticity.
- *Oxygen supports combustion,* although it does not burn. High concentrations of oxygen will turn a small spark or fire into a large fire. Fire prevention precautions must be used near oxygen delivery systems.
- *Oxygen tanks contain oxygen under pressure.* If the tank ruptures or falls, compressed oxygen shoots forcefully from the tank, turning it into an unguided missile. Oxygen tanks have been known to hurtle through walls when ruptured.

Transtracheal Oxygen Delivery. A tracheostomy is a surgical opening into the trachea through the neck. It may be permanent or temporary. When a patient has a tracheostomy, inhaled air bypasses the upper airway, which normally warms and moistens air before it reaches the lower airway. Oxygen may be delivered through the tracheostomy via a collar or an adapter. A transtracheal catheter is a catheter placed into the tracheostomy to deliver O2 directly into the trachea. Because oxygen cannot be humidified through this device, it is rarely used.

KnowledgeCheck 37-10

- Why is oxygen humidified?
- Which oxygen delivery method is appropriate for the following patients?
  A patient prescribed to receive 2 L/min of oxygen
  A patient who complains of being claustrophobic and requires low-flow humidified oxygen
  A patient with chronic obstructive pulmonary disease (COPD) with an order for oxygen at an FIO_2 of 24%
  A patient who wants to avoid intubation but requires an FIO_2 of 100%

Using Artificial Airways

Artificial airways provide an open airway for patients who have or who are at risk for airway obstruction. Airways may be placed into the pharynx or deeper, into the trachea.

Pharyngeal Airways

Pharyngeal airways provide an open air passage by holding the tongue away from the back of the pharynx. When artificial airways are properly placed, air can flow around and through them, and suction catheters can be passed through them. Pharyngeal airways may be placed through the mouth or the nose.

Oropharyngeal Airways. Oropharyngeal airways are C-shaped, hard plastic devices inserted through the mouth into the pharynx. They should be used only in unconscious patients because they are likely to trigger gagging, vomiting, or laryngospasm in responsive patients with intact airway reflexes. It is important to select the proper size airway. If it is *too short,* it will not keep the tongue pulled forward; if it is *too long,* it may push the epiglottis against the laryngeal opening and completely obstruct the airway. To learn how to size, insert, and care for an oropharyngeal airway, see Clinical Insight 37-3.

Nasopharyngeal Airways. Nasopharyngeal airways are flexible rubber tubes that are inserted through a nostril into the pharynx. Patients who are semiconscious can tolerate nasal airways because they do not stimulate the gag reflex.

Clinical Insight 37-3 ➤ **Inserting an Oropharyngeal Airway**

✚ The American Heart Association (AHA) guidelines (2005) direct that you should insert an oropharyngeal airway only if you are trained in its use.

- You should not delegate this procedure because it requires specialized knowledge, training, and assessment skills.
- You will need a variety of sizes of airways, procedure gloves, tongue blade, suction equipment, and possibly a handheld resuscitation bag and oxygen source.

- Explain the procedure to the patient, even if he seems unresponsive. He may be able to hear you, so this will help relieve his anxiety.
- Select the correct size airway. Measured on the outside of the cheek, the airway should extend from the front teeth to the end of the jaw line.
- Position patient in supine or semi-Fowler's position, neck hyperextended (unless contraindicated).

Clinical Insight 37-3 ▶ Inserting an Oropharyngeal Airway—cont'd

- Clear the mouth of debris and secretions. Suction if needed.
- Lubricate the airway with water-soluble gel.
- Gently open the mouth with a tongue blade, or with thumb and index finger push the teeth apart.
- Hold the tongue down with a tongue blade, as needed, and insert the airway along the top of the tongue, in the upside-down position (the "C" faces upward toward the nose).

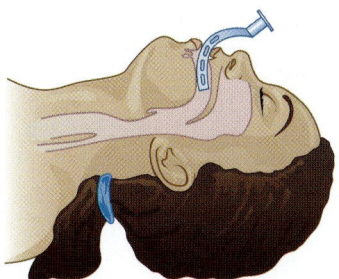

- When the distal end of the airway reaches the soft palate, rotate the airway 180° and continue inserting until the front flange is flush with the lips.

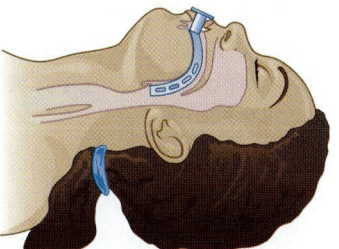

- Check to be sure the patient's lips and tongue are not caught between the teeth and the airway.
- Keep the patient's head slightly tilted and chin elevated for optimal airway function.
- Auscultate breath sounds to verify airway patency.
- Do not tape the airway in place. Remove it when the patient begins to cough or gag.
- Position the patient on his side or with his head turned to the side to allow secretions to drain from the mouth.
- Keep suction available at the bedside; suction the oropharynx as needed.
- Provide oral hygiene every 2 to 4 hours and assess the mucous membranes. Remove and cleanse the airway at that time (use hydrogen peroxide and then rinse well with water).
  Document the following:
- Date and time of airway insertion
- Type and size of airway (oropharyngeal or nasopharyngeal)
- Assessments before and after the procedure, including breath sounds and focused respiratory assessment
- Any suctioning performed
- Patient's tolerance of the procedure, adverse reactions and interventions taken

Sources: American Association for Respiratory Care (2004b); American Heart Association (2005).

Nasopharyngeal airways are available in a variety of pediatric and adult sizes. Generally, the larger the internal diameter, the longer the tube. To learn about sizing and inserting a nasopharyngeal airway, refer to Clinical Insight 37-4.

Endotracheal Airways

Patients who cannot breathe effectively because of airway obstruction or respiratory or cardiac failure need an airway inserted directly into the trachea. **Endotracheal airways** are pliable tubes inserted into the trachea through the following routes:

Orotracheal tube—the mouth
Nasotracheal tube—the nose
Tracheostomy tube—an opening directly into the trachea

There are several types of tracheostomy tubes, made of various materials. They may be cuffed or uncuffed and may have a single or double lumen. A cuffed tube is used for patients who are being ventilated or who have difficulty swallowing. For self-care at home, a tube with an inner cannula is preferred because the inner tube can be removed and cleaned to avoid tube occlusion, primarily due to accumulation of secretions in the airway.

Because tracheostomy tubes bypass the upper airway, the patient inhales air directly into the lower airway without humidification, filtering, or warming. For this reason, devices that warm and humidify inhaled air are used with endotracheal

airways. Figure 37-7A illustrates the parts of an endotracheal tube. Figure 37-7B shows the placement of an orotracheal tube. Nursing responsibilities related to endotracheal airways are to assist in their insertion, maintain stabilization, and provide routine suctioning and management.

Assisting With Endotracheal Airway Insertion

Insertion of endotracheal airways is within the scope of practice of certain specially trained nurses (e.g., nurse anesthetist). As a nurse in general practice, you will assist with insertion by gathering equipment and preparing the patient. On most units, you will find intubation equipment in the resuscitation cart. Intubation must often be done quickly, in response to a temporary decline in the patient's respiratory function during a procedure. See Clinical Insight 37-5 for guidelines for assisting with and managing endotracheal airways.

Managing Endotracheal and Tracheostomy Tubes.

Managing endotracheal and tracheostomy tubes generally requires the expertise of a respiratory therapist or an RN, but you can delegate this activity to specially trained and skilled LPNs, especially in critical care areas. Once the ostomy is well healed, the airway will not collapse if the tracheostomy tube is dislodged; so a NAP, or even the patient, can reinsert it if necessary. Many patients with permanent tracheostomies perform self-care at home.

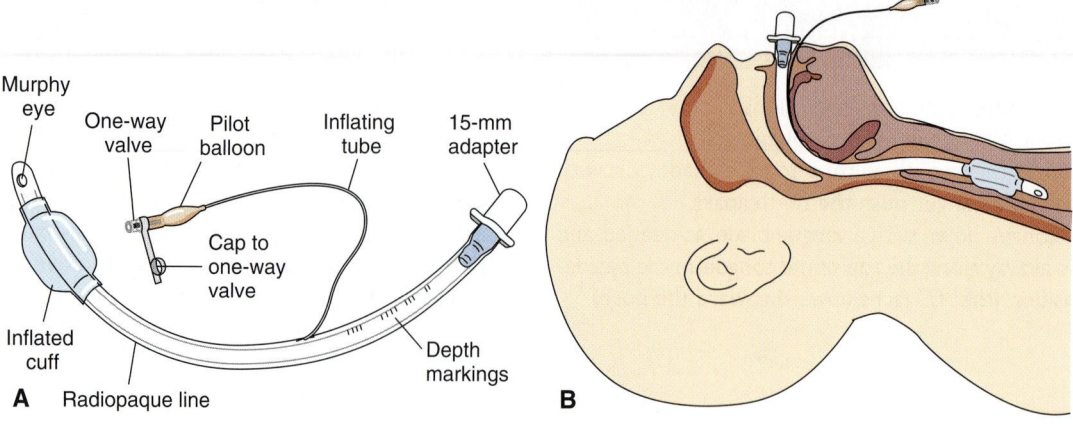

Murphy
eye
One-way   Pilot   Inflating   15-mm
valve   balloon   tube   adapter

Cap to
one-way
valve

Inflated
cuff   Depth
                                                    markings
A   Radiopaque line   **B**

FIGURE 37-7 A, An endotracheal tube. B, Placement of an orotracheal tube.

Clinical Insight 37-4 ➤ Inserting a Nasopharyngeal Airway

✚ The AHA guidelines (2005) direct that you should insert an oropharyngeal airway only if you are trained in its use.

■ You should not delegate this procedure because it requires specialized knowledge, training, and assessment skills.
■ Assess for contraindications to a nasopharyngeal airway (e.g., anticoagulant therapy, hemorrhagic disorder, nasopharyngeal deformity, sepsis). *Up to 30% of patients experience airway bleeding after insertion of a nasopharyngeal airway.*
■ You will need a correctly sized nasopharyngeal airway, procedure gloves, tongue blade, water-soluble lubricant, suction equipment, and possibly a handheld resuscitation bag and oxygen source.
■ Explain the procedure to the patient, even if he seems unresponsive. He may be able to hear you, so this will help relieve his anxiety.
■ Perform hand hygiene and don procedure gloves.
■ Select the appropriate airway size: (1) Measure the diameter of the patient's nostril and use an airway that is slightly smaller than that; and (2) Measure on the outside of the cheek, the distance from the tip of the patient's nose to the earlobe, and use an airway about 2.5 cm (1 in.) longer than that measurement. Airways are sized by their internal diameter. Generally, the larger the internal diameter, the longer the tube. Airways are available in a variety of pediatric and adult sizes. It should be slightly smaller than the nares.
■ Position the patient in supine or semi-Fowler's position.
■ Lubricate the airway with water-soluble lubricant.
■ Tilt the patient's head backward to hyperextend the neck, unless contraindicated.
■ Push up the tip of the nose and gently insert the airway through the naris along the floor of the nostril until the

outer flange rests on the nostril. If you meet resistance, rotate the tube slightly. Do not force.
■ Depress the tongue with a tongue blade and inspect the pharynx for proper placement of the tube tip. Use a penlight for better visualization

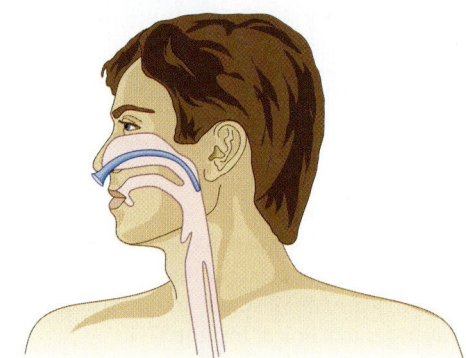

■ Close the patient's mouth and place your finger near the tube opening to feel for air exchange at the naris.
■ Auscultate the lungs bilaterally.
■ If the patient coughs, gags, vomits, or has laryngospasm after insertion of the airway, the tube may be too long. If the tip extends beyond the top of the posterior pharynx, remove it and insert a shorter one.
■ Keep suction available at the bedside. Suction as needed.
■ Remove the airway at least every 8 hours to check the nasal mucosa for ulceration or irritation. Clean the airway at this time by placing it in a basin, cleansing with hydrogen peroxide, then rinsing with water. Use a pipe cleaner to remove secretions, if needed.

Clinical Insight 37-4 ▶ Inserting a Nasopharyngeal Airway—cont'd

- Alternate nostrils each time the airway is removed and replaced, to avoid skin and mucous membrane breakdown. Document the following:
- Date and time of airway insertion
- Type and size of airway (oropharyngeal or nasopharyngeal)
- Assessments before and after the procedure, including breath sounds, focused respiratory assessment, and condition of the mucous membranes

- Any suctioning performed
- Patient's tolerance of the procedure
- Adverse reactions and interventions taken
- Removal of the airway, cleaning, and replacement in the other nostril

Sources: American Association for Respiratory Care, 2004b; American Heart Association, 2005; Roberts, Whalley, & Bleetman, 2005.

Clinical Insight 37-5 ▶ Caring for Patients With Endotracheal Airways

Assisting With Endotracheal Airway Insertion

- **Gather equipment.** You will need an oxygen source and a bag (e.g., Ambu or nonrebreather bag) to inflate the lungs, a laryngoscope, endotracheal tubes of various sizes, water-soluble lubricant, a syringe to inflate the cuff, and tape to secure the tube in place.
- **Keep suction at the bedside** to clear the mouth and airway if secretions are obstructing your view of the cords.
- **You will need a surgical tray** if a tracheostomy is performed to create the direct opening into the trachea.
- **Remain calm, and explain** to the patient that the airway will enable him to breathe effectively.
- **Once the airway is in place, listen to breath sounds** to establish that both lungs are ventilated.
- **Reassess breath sounds periodically.** After the airway is inserted, record the type and size, as well as the patient's response to the procedure.
- **Expect that a portable chest x-ray will be prescribed** to confirm correct placement.

Managing and Monitoring Endotracheal Airways

The following are activities associated with the care of all types of endotracheal airways.

- ✚ **Have emergency equipment,** including a duplicate tracheostomy kit, extra cannula, and suction setup, immediately available for reintubation if the tube should become dislodged.
  - **Keep an extra cannula at the bedside,** as patients may accidentally decannulate.
  - **Secure the endotracheal tube** with ties, Velcro tapes, or a commercial holder to prevent accidental displacement.

- **Provide tracheostomy care every 4 to 8 hours** (Dennis-Rouse & Davidson, 2008).
- **Change the endotracheal or tracheostomy ties every 24 hours.**
- **Secure the orotracheal tube** to the opposite side of the mouth with each change of tape or ties to prevent skin erosion and breakdown.

- **Inspect skin around the tube** or tracheal stoma for redness, swelling, drainage, or irritation at least every 8 hours.
- **Provide skin care** around the tube and tape or holder at least daily.
- **Perform regular oral care.**
- **Inflate the cuff of the tube with a minimal occlusive volume and monitor cuff pressures** to prevent pressure necrosis inside the trachea. (This is a joint responsibility with the respiratory therapist.) Maximum acceptable tube cuff pressure is 25 mm Hg. The following is a method for checking for minimal occluding volume:
  1. Place stethoscope on patient's neck over the carotid pulse.
  2. Attach a 10-mL syringe to the pilot balloon of the inflated cuff.
  3. Remove air from the cuff—(1 mL at a time) until you hear a slight leak at the peak of inspiration.
  4. When you hear the leak, inject 1 mL of air back into the cuff.
- **Monitor and document cuff pressure** once per shift and when the tube is changed or repositioned.
- **Note the centimeter reference marking** on the endotracheal tube to monitor for possible displacement.
- **Minimize pulling and traction** on the artificial airway by supporting all tubing connected to the airway and using flexible catheter mounts and swivels.
- If the patient is conscious, **remind him not to pull on the airway.**
- **Use a bite block** between the teeth to prevent the patient from occluding an orotracheal tube.
- **Provide 100% humidification** of inspired air. Check the oxygen setup regularly.
- **Routine saline instillation** to thin secretions is no longer recommended.
- **Ensure adequate hydration** with oral or IV fluids to keep the mucosa moist and thin secretions.
- **Suction the airway** when secretions collect. Remember, the patient probably can't cough effectively to clear secretions.

Evidence is still mixed about whether to use sterile or clean gloves when performing endotracheal care. The following are the different levels of asepsis currently in use for tracheostomy care:

- **Sterile technique** is the use of a sterile suction catheter and other supplies with sterile gloves. For new tracheostomies, most facilities use sterile technique. However, some use sterile technique only for patients who have increased susceptibility to infection.
- **Modified sterile technique** is use of a sterile suction catheter and supplies, but with nonsterile procedure gloves. For healed tracheostomies, and in many institutions for all tracheostomies, the trend is toward a modified sterile technique.
- **Clean technique** is use of a clean catheter and clean hands or nonsterile gloves. The portion of the catheter that will be inserted in the tracheostomy tube is protected to avoid contact with unclean surfaces. Clean technique is the usual method in the home setting. Anyone who is not a family member and anyone concerned about acquiring an infection should wear nonsterile procedure gloves, even in the home setting.

You should follow the procedure used in your healthcare facility or school. To learn a procedure and guidelines for tracheostomy care, respectively, see Procedure 37-6 and Clinical Insight 37-5.

KnowledgeCheck 37-11

- In what circumstances would you use an oropharyngeal airway? A nasopharyngeal airway?
- What facts should you record if a patient is intubated?
- Describe seven interventions associated with caring for a patient with an endotracheal tube.

Suctioning Airways

Airways are suctioned to remove secretions and maintain patency. Signs that indicate the need for suctioning include agitation, gurgling sounds during respiration, restlessness, labored respirations, decreased oxygen saturation (SaO_2), increased heart and respiratory rates, and adventitious breath sounds on auscultation. Although suctioning helps remove secretions, it also removes air from the airways and causes the patient's O_2 levels to fall. As a result, suctioning must be done quickly and is often accompanied by supplemental oxygen. Suctioning can also irritate mucous membranes if done too frequently.

Suction catheters may be open tipped or "whistle tipped" (Fig. 37-8A and B). Most suction catheters have a port on the side, over which you place your thumb to control the suction. A Yankauer tube (Fig. 37-8C) is a rigid device for suctioning the oral cavity.

You will need to collaborate with respiratory therapists in managing a patient's airway. Both respiratory therapists and nurses are responsible for suctioning and tracheostomy care. The respiratory therapist and the nurse should keep each other informed of changes in the patient's condition. Airway suctioning is usually performed by RNs and LPNs, but not by NAPs. NAPs may use a Yankauer tube to suction the oral cavity as part of maintaining hygiene and preventing aspiration of oral secretions.

Suctioning the Upper Airway

Pharyngeal suctioning is performed to prevent oral and nasal secretions from entering the lower airway when the patient is too weak to cough up secretions. Suctioning the pharynx triggers a cough, which helps loosen and mobilize secretions. The patient's condition determines whether you suction the pharynx through the mouth or nose. Most patients find oropharyngeal suctioning more comfortable than the nasal approach. However, if the patient is unable to cooperate and automatically bites down when anything is placed in his mouth or if the jaw is wired, use a nasal approach. To learn how to suction the pharynx, refer to Procedure 37-9.

QSEN

Removing Barriers to Patient and Family Involvement in Care

Competency: Patient-Centered Care (Knowledge, Skills, Attitudes); Teamwork (Knowledge)*

Scenario: Mrs. Yablonski, a 66-year-old former smoker, has recently had a permanent tracheostomy but can speak using an electromechanical device. She needs to learn how to suction herself and change the tracheotomy dressing. For three days in a row, different nurses have tried to explain how to perform the care. Each time she became tearful and frustrated. The nurse manager speaks with her to identify problems that may be occurring. Mrs. Yablonski cites several issues:

> *"Sometimes it's me. I may just feel too overwhelmed or I may just not have any energy. But the nurses don't always ask me if I feel well enough to learn. None of them really know me, and they don't take enough time with me. And sometimes my nurse would rather just do it herself and get it over with.*
>
> *There are too many nurses trying to teach me. They tell me different ways to do it or make me go over what I already know, so I get confused. I try to tell them what I already know or what another nurse told me to do, but they want to do it their way. They should have this all written down somewhere.*
>
> *I want my husband to learn, but he can't be here during the day, and that's the only time anyone tries to show me how to do it. I asked the doctor about learning about it later on in his office but he didn't want to talk about it. He said the nurses here would teach me."*

Think about it: Including patients or their significant others as equal partners in care is the foundation of patient-centered care. Think about the following questions:

➤ What barriers to participating in her own care does Mrs. Yablonski identify? Would they be applicable to other patients?

➤ How is team communication affecting this situation?

➤ Does Mrs. Yablonski see herself as a valuable partner in her care?

➤ What might the effects be if Mrs. Yablonski felt more empowered?

➤ Does she seem to have a conflict regarding how much care she wants to take over? If so, how should her nurse manage the conflict?

➤ What are the potential negative outcomes if Mrs. Yablonski goes home before she masters her tracheostomy care?

➤ What can the nurse manager do to make Mrs. Yablonski's care more patient-centered?

*For specific Knowledge, Skills, and Attitudes,

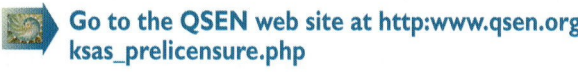

Go to the QSEN web site at http:www.qsen.org. ksas_prelicensure.php

Source: Larsson, Sahlsten, Segesten, & Plos, 2011.

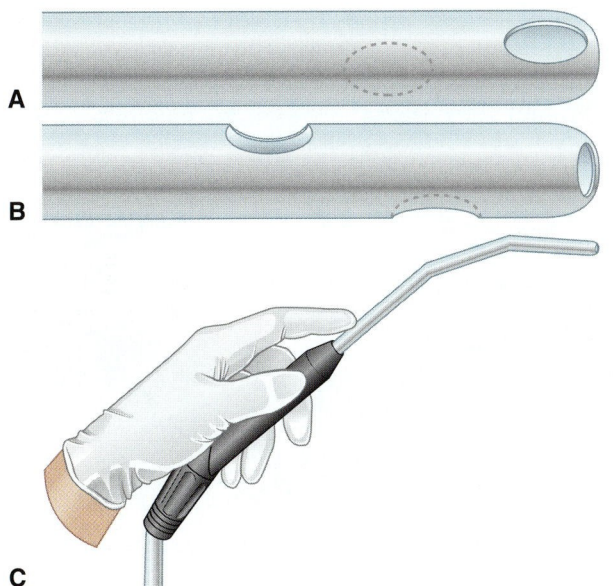

FIGURE 37-8 A, Whistle-tipped suction catheter. B, Open-tipped suction catheter. C, Yankauer (oral) suction tube.

Suctioning the Lower Airway

In tracheal suctioning, a catheter is passed beyond the pharynx into the trachea to remove secretions from the lower airways. The catheter may be inserted through the mouth, nose, or an endotracheal airway. In the healthcare setting, deep tracheal suctioning is a sterile procedure.

Orotracheal or Nasotracheal (NT) Approach. When suctioning through the nose or mouth, insert the catheter into the pharynx, and advance it into the trachea during inspiration. This prevents the catheter from entering the esophagus

and causing the patient to gag or vomit. When the suction catheter enters the trachea, it will stimulate coughing. Except in an emergency, NT suctioning should be done through a nasopharyngeal airway. For complete procedure steps, see Procedure 37-8.

Endotracheal or Tracheostomy Approach. An endotracheal or tracheostomy tube provides a direct path into the trachea. To suction, insert the catheter through the artificial airway into the trachea. You do not need to insert the catheter as far into a tracheostomy tube, because you are bypassing the long upper airway. Before suctioning, make sure the airway is secured so it is not dislodged by coughing or suctioning. You will find instructions for this skill in Procedure 37-7.

KnowledgeCheck 37-12

- Describe the difference between pharyngeal and tracheal suctioning.
- How can you ensure that the suction catheter enters the trachea and not the esophagus?

Caring for a Patient Requiring Mechanical Ventilation

A **mechanical ventilator** is a machine that assists a patient to breathe. Usually the patient is intubated before he is connected to the ventilator. An endotracheal tube or a tracheostomy tube is connected by oxygen tubing to the ventilator. Before initiating ventilation, be certain that the healthcare team is aware of advance directives and consults with family members. Many patients do not wish to be mechanically ventilated if it might be a permanent intervention. Mechanical ventilation is indicated for acute or chronic respiratory failure, and may be a short- or long-term therapy.

Toward Evidence-Based Practice

Fields, L. (2008). Oral care intervention to reduce incidence of ventilator-associated pneumonia in the neurologic intensive care unit. *Journal of Neuroscience Nursing, 40*(5), 291–298.

This was a study of patients in a neurological intensive care unit who were intubated and mechanically ventilated. Nurses were already implementing the Institute of Healthcare Improvement's ventilator-associated pneumonia (VAP) bundle (which includes elevating the head of the bed to 30°, practicing good hand hygiene, and other interventions). A control group received the VAP bundle and the usual oral care. The intervention group used the VAP bundle and increased tooth brushing to every 8 hours. In the intervention group, the VAP rate dropped to zero within a week.

Hugonnet, S., Uckay, I., & Pittet, D. (2007). Staffing level: A determinant of late-onset ventilator-associated pneumonia. *Critical Care, 11*(4), R80.

In this observational study of 936 patients who underwent mechanical ventilation during their stay in ICU, 262 VAP cases were diagnosed. Using statistical methods, researchers concluded that lower nurse-to-patient ratio is associated with increased risk for late-onset VAP.

Mateoso, J., Gonzalez, N., Sadaba, M., et al. (2011). Nursing care in the prevention of ventilator-associated pneumonia. *Enferm Intensive, 22*(1), 22–30.

Researchers observed and described the care of 26 patients with more than 24 hours of invasive mechanical ventilation. They reported good nursing compliance with established protocols for oral hygiene, oropharyngeal suction, turning of patients, and patient tolerance of enteral nutrition. Incidence of VAP was low and well within internationally established ranges. They concluded, nevertheless, that incidence of VAP could be further reduced with better control of endotracheal tube cuff pressures and by elevating the head of the bed to between 30° and 45°.

1. Based on these study findings, list two interventions a staff nurse could do to help prevent VAP.

2. Which study might you use to convince a hospital administrator to hire more nurses?

 Go to Chapter 37, **Toward Evidence-Based Practice Suggested Responses,** on DavisPlus.

Negative pressure ventilators consist of shells that fit externally around the chest. Negative pressure generated inside the shell pulls the chest outward and forces the patient to inhale air, similar to normal breathing. These ventilators are rarely used for acutely ill patients, but they are occasionally used for chronic conditions, for example, in patients with muscle weakness from neuromuscular disease.

Positive pressure ventilators, the most widely used type, require the patient to have an artificial airway (Fig. 37-9). Positive pressure ventilation carries risks, including *barotrauma* (injury to the airways due to pressure changes) and drop in cardiac output as the positive pressure in the chest decreases venous return to the heart.

To care for a patient receiving mechanical ventilation (also called *positive pressure ventilation*), you need a thorough understanding of the ventilator, its settings, and how to troubleshoot problems. You will need to be familiar with the types of ventilators in use. In the event of a malfunction, if the repair is not readily obvious, manually ventilate the patient with an Ambu bag (resuscitation bag) connected to supplemental oxygen while a colleague troubleshoots the problem. Procedure 37-10 describes care of the patient on a mechanical ventilator, including ventilator terminology and delegation of care.

Patients being mechanically ventilated, even for a short period, are at high risk for developing *ventilator-associated pneumonia (VAP)*. VAP is associated with high mortality rates (Maselli & Restrepo, 2011). Procedure 37-10 includes guidelines for nursing interventions to help prevent VAP. For ventilator terminology, refer to Table 37-2.

Caring for a Patient Requiring Chest Tubes

Normally there is negative pressure in the pleural space and only a thin layer of fluid between the lung and chest wall membranes. Accumulation of fluid and blood in the pleural space

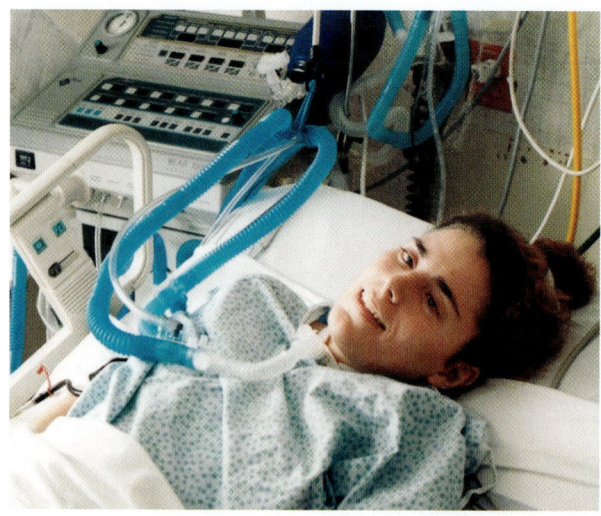

FIGURE 37-9 A patient on a ventilator via tracheosotomy.

(hemothorax) interferes with lung expansion, ventilation, and gas exchange. Air in the pleural space **(pneumothorax)** creates positive pressure, causing lung tissue to collapse. To see diagrams of different types of pneumothorax,

 Go to Chapter 37, **Tables, Boxes, Figures: ESG Figures 37-2, 37-3,** and **37-4,** on *DavisPlus*.

The purpose of a chest-drainage system is to make room for the lungs to fully expand. This is done by removing air and fluid from the pleural space. A valve in the line or a water-sealed compartment prevents reentry of air and fluid. A chest-drainage system is composed of a chest tube inserted into the pleural space and a drainage collection system. The system usually is attached to some form of suction.

Table 37-2 ▶ Ventilator Terminology	
TERM	**EXPLANATION**
FIO₂	Fraction of inspired oxygen
Modes of ventilation	Describes the setting on the ventilator that assists the patient to breathe. Can be controlled (CMV), intermittent mandatory (IMV), or synchronized intermittent mandatory (SIMV).
Tidal volume	Amount of air delivered from the ventilator with each breath
Assist-control mode—also known as continuous mechanical ventilation (CMV)	The preset number of breaths per minute delivered by the machine. If the patient is able to initiate breaths, the machine will deliver a breath when the patient begins to inspire. If the patient is unable to breathe on his own, the machine will deliver the preset number of breaths in a rhythmic fashion.
Intermittent mandatory ventilation	A ventilator setting that delivers a minimum number of breaths per minute if the patient does not ventilate independently.
Synchronized intermittent mandatory ventilation (SIMV)	A ventilator setting that delivers a minimum number of ventilations per minute if the patient does not ventilate independently. The ventilator breaths are synchronized with the patient's breaths. This mode is used for weaning patients from the ventilator.
Pressure support	Provides positive pressure on inspiration to decrease the workload of breathing.
Continuous positive airway pressure (CPAP)	Provides positive pressure during inspiration and expiration to keep alveoli open in a spontaneously breathing patient.
Positive end expiratory pressure (PEEP)	Provides positive pressure on expiration to keep airways open for patients on CMV or SIMV mode ventilation.

Flow of air and fluid must be in one direction: from the patient to the collection system. Think of the chest tube as an extension of the pleural space. To provide negative pressure within the chest tube, the open end of the tube is placed under water. With each exhalation, air is expelled through the chest tube into the water, but no air is drawn in during inhalation (Fig. 37-10). Once all air is expelled from the pleural space, negative pressure is reestablished and the lung can fully expand. When the lung tissue is re-expanded, the chest tube can be safely removed.

Types of Drainage Systems

Various chest drainage systems are available, including the older, reusable glass, three-bottle, water-seal system. However, you will most often use a disposable system. These are more compact and lightweight. Disposable systems may be water-seal or dry-seal, and may or may not use suction. To learn how to set up disposable chest drainage systems, see Procedure 37-11.

Water-Seal Systems

Water-seal systems can consist of one, two, or three chambers (or bottles, in the traditional glass bottle system).

- **A one-chamber device** is the simplest chest drainage system. The chest tube connects to one drainage chamber, which serves as both a collector and a water seal. This system can handle only small volumes of fluid or air. As fluid drains through the chest tube, it raises the fluid level in the chamber, making it harder for the patient to exhale. It is important that the device not be tipped over because the vent tube would no longer be below water and air would enter the pleural space.

- **A two-chamber system** has one chamber that connects directly with the chest tube and serves as a collection bottle. The second chamber serves as the water seal; it maintains negative pressure as air flows through it. Because the chest drainage never enters the water-seal chamber, you can measure the amount of drainage more accurately. The two-chamber system can handle large amounts of fluid drainage, but its design can still contribute to labored breathing.

- **A three-chamber system** adds a third chamber, which connects to the water-seal chamber and placed to suction (see Fig. 37-10). This creates controlled negative pressure within the system. The suction control chamber has three vent tubes: one connected to suction, one connected to the water seal chamber, and a long middle tube with one end open to air at the top. The amount of sterile water in the suction chamber determines the maximum suction possible within the system. Suction pressure is expressed in centimeters of water.

- Adjusting the suction regulator does not increase the amount of suction. Instead, it simply draws more air in from the atmosphere and causes more bubbling within the bottle. This is a safety feature that prevents excessive negative pressure from being created in the system. For proper functioning, adjust the suction regulator to create gentle bubbling in the suction control bottle.

Dry-Seal Systems

Dry-seal systems are a one-piece device with three chambers: fluid collection, dry seal, and dry suction control. They do not use water in the suction chamber, relying instead on a mechanical automatic control valve (ACV) and an air leak monitor. The valve allows air to pass out of the patient and prevents it from returning to the patient—even if the system is knocked over. Pressure is set by adjusting the rotary suction dial. The ACV keeps the pressure constant by adjusting to changes in air leaks and fluctuations in the suction source.

Portable Systems

Portable or mobile systems consist of a single, dry-seal chamber attached to the patient's chest tube (Fig. 37-11). It drains by gravity, but can be connected to wall suction. Portable systems improve ambulation and reduce the risk of

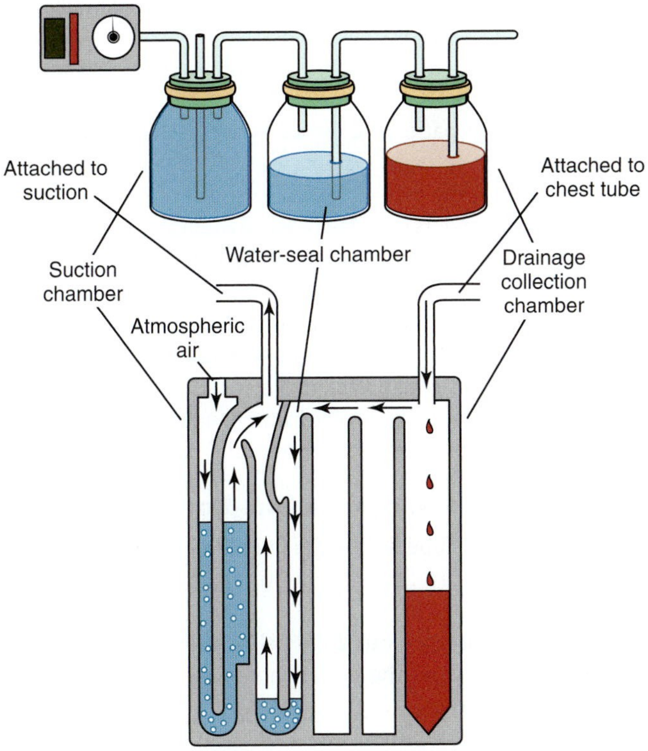

Attached to suction
Suction chamber
Water-seal chamber
Atmospheric air
Drainage collection chamber
Attached to chest tube

FIGURE 37-10 A disposable chest drainage system.

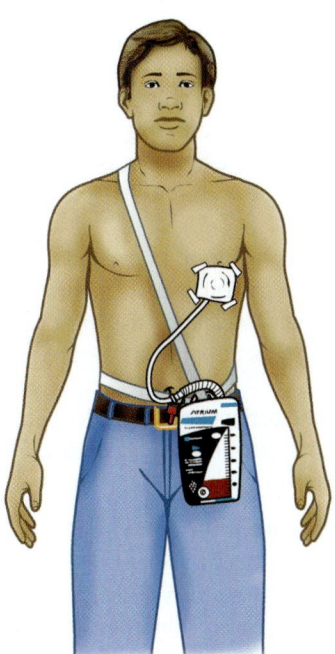

FIGURE 37-11 A one-chamber, dry-seal, portable chest drainage system.

deep vein thrombosis and pulmonary embolism. They are thought to decrease the length of time a patient must stay in the hospital. The collection chamber holds a maximum of 500 mL, so portable systems are not practical for patients whose drainage is more than 500 mL daily.

Preventing Complications of Chest Drainage

Drainage is usually greatest when the chest tube is initially inserted and decreases as the lung reexpands. Care of a patient with a chest drainage system involves four broad nursing interventions: monitoring, maintaining a properly functioning drainage system, promoting lung reexpansion, and recognizing

and intervening promptly should complications develop. For guidelines to help you manage care for patients with chest tubes, see Clinical Insight 37-6.

KnowledgeCheck 37-13

- What is the purpose of mechanical ventilation?
- Why is a chest tube inserted?
- What is the advantage of a three-chamber system (compared to a one-chamber or two-chamber system)?
- How does a portable chest drainage system compare to a water-seal drainage system?

Clinical Insight 37-6 ➤ Managing Chest Tubes

Monitor breathing, gas exchange, and drainage.

- Frequently assess breathing patterns, breathing effort, and breath sounds.
- Assess mental status, heart rate and rhythm, and pulse oximetry readings. These reflect adequacy of oxygenation.
- Monitor character, color, and amount of chest drainage. Immediately report sudden or large increases in drainage or new onset of bright red blood, along with an assessment of the patient's condition at that time. Drainage is usually greatest when the chest tube is initially inserted and decreases as the lung reexpands. The chest drainage unit (CDU) must be replaced when the drainage compartment is almost full.

Prevent complications or intervene if they occur.

- Observe the dressing at least every 4 hours. Make sure that the chest dressing around the tube insertion site is occlusive (e.g., not wet or loose). Usually, petroleum gauze is wrapped around the insertion site to ensure occlusion.
- Inspect for excessive, abnormal, or foul-smelling drainage. This may indicate hemorrhage or infection.
- Palpate around the dressing for **subcutaneous emphysema** (air in the subcutaneous tissues). This may be caused by an incomplete seal at the chest tube insertion site.
- Assess for pain; medicate as needed.
- Reposition the patient every 2 hours and use pillows to keep the patient's weight off the chest tube. To prevent occlusion of the tube, to promote drainage, and to preserve skin integrity.
- Encourage the patient to use the arm on the affected side. Assist with range-of-motion exercises, if necessary. To maintain joint mobility.

- A **tension pneumothorax** is a life-threatening complication of chest drainage. It occurs when positive pressure builds up in the pleural space and pushes the lungs, great vessels, and heart toward the other side of the chest. If a patient with a chest drainage system becomes acutely short of breath, immediately

check for occlusion of the system. Relieve the occlusion to prevent pressure buildup.

- ✚ **Recollapse of the lung** can occur because of loss of negative pressure within the system. This is commonly caused by air leaks, disconnections, or breaks or cracks of the bottles or chambers. If any of these occur, immediately place the disconnected end nearest the patient into a bottle of sterile water or saline.
- ✚ Do not clamp the chest tube. Clamp chest tubes only for changing the drainage system. Limit the clamp time and monitor respiratory status constantly until the clamp is removed. Clamping can rapidly lead to a tension pneumothorax.
- ✚ If the tube is accidentally pulled out, immediately cover the wound with a dry, sterile dressing. Listen for air leaking out of the site. If you can hear air, tape the dressing loosely so that you do not occlude the site. If air cannot escape from the chest, a tension pneumothorax will occur, eventually compromising cardiovascular function.

Promote Lung Reexpansion.

- Encourage the patient to be as active as his condition permits. Chest drainage systems are bulky, but with disposable systems, some patients can still get out of bed and ambulate. Most patients will need assistance from one or two staff members to protect and monitor the system and the patient.
- Instruct the patient to perform deep-breathing and coughing every 2 hours, unless contraindicated. Assist the patient to sit upright and splint the chest with a pillow or the hands, and provide analgesia as needed. These interventions help to minimize discomfort.

Key Points for Managing a One-Bottle System

- Keep the intake tube below the fluid level in the drainage bottle to prevent drawing air into the pleural space with inhalation.
- Maintain the tubing about 2 cm below the water level. As tubing length below the water increases, more effort is required to exhale.

Clinical Insight 37-6 ➤ Managing Chest Tubes—cont'd

■ Take precautions to see that the bottle is not accidentally tipped over, uncovering the long vent tube and allowing air to enter the pleural space.

Maintain the drainage system.

For All Types of CDUs:

■ Make sure the drainage system is located below the insertion site. If the drainage system is higher than the insertion site, fluid may flow back into the pleural cavity, compromising the patient's respiratory status.

■ Regularly inspect tubing to ensure that connections are airtight and tubing is not kinked or occluded. Kinks in the drainage tubing increase pressure in the pleural cavity and prevent fluid drainage.

■ Monitor drainage. Blood or purulent matter can occlude the tubing.

■ Inspect the air vent in the drainage system to make sure it is patent. If air builds up in the pleural cavity, pneumothorax may occur.

■ Monitor to ensure the system is maintaining consistent negative pressure levels.

■ ✚ Do not "milk" or strip the tubing. Doing so can create excess negative pressure and damage lung tissue.

■ Most systems will have some type of check system to ensure that the system is operating correctly. Always be sure to verify operation through the users' manual or with the product's vendor.

■ To transport or ambulate a patient: (1) keep the CDU upright below chest level; (2) disconnect the CDU from suction source and make sure the air vent is open.

Water-Seal Drainage Systems:

■ Take precautions that the CDU is not tipped over (e.g., tape it to the floor).

■ Observe for **tidaling** (fluctuations in the water-seal chamber's fluid level that correspond with respiration).

The level will increase on inspiration and decrease on exhalation. This will be opposite for a patient on a mechanical ventilator.

■ Bubbling in the bottom of the water-seal chamber indicates an air leak. When this occurs, check for poor tubing connections. A small amount of bubbling right after insertion or with exhalation or cough is normal.

■ Check the water in the suction control chamber; replace as needed. The water can evaporate.

■ ✚ If the chest tube disconnects from the drainage unit, establish a temporary water seal by immersing the open end of the chest tube in a bottle of sterile water to a depth of 2 cm until a new system can be connected. Cleanse the end of the patient connector on the drain system with alcohol and reconnect it if it has not been contaminated. If the patient connector on the drain system is contaminated, you must initiate a new CDU.

Dry-Seal Drainage Systems:

■ Inspect the air vent in the drainage system to make sure it is patent. The air vent must remain patent to allow air to escape. If air builds up in the pleural cavity, pneumothorax may occur.

■ Check the indicators on the CDU to be certain that suction is operating properly. A dry chest drainage system doesn't use water in the suction chamber. A valve inside the regulator continuously balances the forces of suction and the atmosphere. The valve automatically responds and adjusts to changes in patient air leaks and fluctuations in suction source vacuum to deliver accurate suction to the patient. Pressure can be set from -10 cm H_2O to -40 cm H_2O by adjusting the rotary dry suction dial.

■ Observe for bubbling. If the water in a dry-seal CDU is bubbling, it means there is an air leak.

CLINICALREASONING:
Applying the **Full-Spectrum Nursing Model**

Because the following critical thinking activities allow you to practice the kind of thinking you will use as a full-spectrum nurse, they usually have no single right answer. Discuss them with your peers—if you have difficulty with any of the questions, consult your instructor.

PATIENT SITUATION

Haley, a 15-year-old female high-school student, was admitted to the hospital with shortness of breath and right-sided chest pain when breathing. She states that she has had "the flu" for 3 days. She has a history of asthma since age 6, and smokes a half pack of cigarettes a day. Both her parents are heavy smokers, as well. An IV was initiated, and she is receiving 800 mg of vancomycin (an antibiotic) intravenously every 12 hours. She is not on oxygen therapy, but receives 10 incentive spirometer

treatments per hour while awake. Her heart rate is 80 beats/min, respiratory rate 24 breaths/min, and blood pressure 110/70 mm Hg. Her skin is pale but warm, and capillary refill time is 2 seconds. She has no clubbing of the fingers. She is urinating approximately 400 mL of clear yellow urine every 8 hours and maintaining a normal bowel elimination pattern. Laboratory results are:

Red blood cell count (RBCs): 3.56×10^6 (3.56 million/mm³)
White blood cell count (WBCs): 11,800/mm³
Hemoglobin: 11.2 g/dL
Hematocrit: 32.7%

Haley says, "I feel really tired, and too weak to even pick up a glass of water." Her cough produces white, thick sputum. Sputum culture on admission confirms a diagnosis of streptococcal pneumonia. (Case adapted from C. Green, 2000, pp. 233–234.)

THINKING

1. *Theoretical Knowledge:*
   a. According to the Centers for Disease Control and Prevention, should Haley have received a pneumonia immunization? Why or why not?
   b. What is clubbing of the fingers? You may wish to refer to Chapter 21 for review, or to a medical–surgical nursing text.
2. *Critical Thinking (Analyzing Assumptions):*
   Why is it a positive finding for Haley that she does not have clubbed fingers?

DOING

3. *Practical Knowledge:*
   Twenty-four hours after the antibiotics were started, Haley's respiratory status becomes worse. She says, "It's so hard to breathe." It is decided to begin administering oxygen. Another sputum culture is prescribed. You are to collect a sputum specimen from the patient.
   a. What position should Haley assume for this procedure?
   b. What kind of protective clothing do you need for this procedure?
   c. You remove the lid from the specimen container. When you hand it to Haley, she touches the inside of the container with her fingers. What should you do?
   d. What would you tell Haley to do in order to expectorate the sputum specimen?
4. *Nursing Process (Assessment):*
   In the admission data, what important information is missing with regard to her respiratory status?

CARING

5. *Self-Knowledge:*
   Describe one or two patient care experiences you might draw upon to help you in caring for Haley. In what ways were those patients similar to Haley, and how might that help you?
6. *Ethical Knowledge:*
   After you finish collecting the sputum specimen, what do you think Haley's biggest concern is right now?

 Go To Chapter 37, **Clinical Reasoning: Applying the Full-Spectrum Nursing Model Response Sheet,** on *DavisPlus.*

Practical Knowledge procedures

In this section you will find the procedures necessary for supporting oxygenation. As you perform the procedures, apply your theoretical knowledge you obtained. The registered nurse is responsible for assessing patients' oxygenation and their responses to procedures.

Procedure 37-1 ■ Collecting a Sputum Specimen

➤ For steps to follow in *all* procedures, refer to the Universal Steps for All Procedures found on the page facing the inside back cover.

Equipment

For all sputum specimens, you will need a patient identification label, a completed laboratory requisition form, and a small plastic bag with a biohazard label (or container designated by the agency) for delivering the specimen to the laboratory. Depending on how you obtain the specimen, you also need the following:

Procedure 37-1A: Obtaining an Expectorated Specimen

- Sterile specimen container with lid
- Procedure gloves
- Glass of water
- Emesis basin
- Tissues
- Pillow (if abdominal or chest incision is present)

Procedure 37-1B: Obtaining a Specimen by Suction

- Sterile suction catheter or sterile suction kit
- Suction device (portable or wall)
- Sterile gloves
- Protective eyewear
- Inline sputum specimen container or trap
- Sterile saline solution
- Oxygen therapy equipment, if indicated
- Linen-saver pad or towel

Delegation

You can delegate collection of an expectorated sputum specimen to a NAP who has been adequately trained in performing the skill. Assess the patient's respiratory status first; if the patient's condition is unstable, do not delegate the procedure. Do not delegate obtaining a specimen by tracheal suctioning.

Pre-Procedure Assessment

- Assess the patient's comprehension of the procedure.
  Understanding allays anxiety and promotes cooperation.
- Assess breath sounds; respiratory rate, depth, and pattern; skin and nailbed color; and tissue perfusion.
  You may need to delay sputum collection if the patient is in respiratory distress.
- Assess ability to deep-breathe, cough, and expectorate.
  If the patient is unable to deep-breathe, cough, and expectorate, suctioning may be necessary to obtain an adequate sputum specimen.
- Determine when the patient last ate or had a tube feeding, especially for a specimen obtained by suction.
  Specimen collection should be delayed for 1 to 2 hours after eating because the procedure may cause vomiting, which creates a risk for aspiration of stomach contents.
- If suctioning is required to obtain the specimen, check for factors such as anticoagulant therapy, bleeding disorders, or low platelet count.
  These factors place the patient at risk for bleeding when the suction catheter is introduced.

➤ When performing the procedure, always identify your patient according to agency policy and be attentive to standard precautions, hand hygiene, patient safety and privacy, body mechanics, and documentation.

Procedure Steps

1. **Verify the medical prescription** for type of sputum analysis.
   The type of sputum specimen determines the number of specimens required and the time of day the specimen should be collected. For example, specimens to confirm tuberculosis typically require three consecutive morning samples.

2. **Position the patient** according to the required specimen collection technique.
   a. *For an expectorated specimen,* assist the patient to high or semi-Fowler's position or to a sitting position at the edge of the bed.
   b. *For a suctioned specimen,* position the patient in high or semi-Fowler's position.
   These positions facilitate insertion of the suction catheter and the ability to cough. They also promote lung expansion and prevent aspiration should the patient vomit during the procedure.

3. **Drape a towel or linen-saver pad** over the patient's chest. Ask the patient to rinse his mouth and gargle with water.
   A towel or pad protects the patient's gown from soiling during specimen collection. Rinsing the mouth removes flora that may contaminate the specimen; however, evidence is not conclusive on this point.

4. **If the patient has an abdominal or chest incision,** have the patient splint the incision with a pillow.
   Splinting the incision decreases discomfort when the patient coughs.

(continued on next page)

Procedure 37-1 ■ Collecting a Sputum Specimen (continued)

Procedure 37-1A ■ Collecting an Expectorated Specimen

Procedure Steps

Follow steps 1 through 4, above.

5. **Provide the patient with the specimen container.** Advise the patient to avoid touching the inside of the container. If you must hold the container for the patient, first don procedure gloves.

   The inside of the container must remain sterile. Wear gloves because you may come in contact with secretions or airborne bacteria when the patient coughs and expectorates.

6. **Ask the patient to breathe deeply** for three or four breaths, and then ask him after a full inhalation to hold his breath and then cough.

   Deep breathing opens airways and stimulates the cough reflex. Coughing after a full inhalation creates enough force to mobilize secretions through the airways and into the pharynx.

7. **Instruct the patient to expectorate** the secretions directly into the specimen container.

   Prevents specimen contamination from outside organisms.

8. **Tell the patient to repeat deep breathing** and coughing until an adequate sample is obtained. Typically 5 to 10 mL of sputum is required to ensure adequate sputum analysis.

9. **Don procedure gloves**, if you are not already wearing them; cover the specimen container with the lid immediately after the specimen is collected.

   Gloves protect you in the event the patient's coughing has contaminated the outside of the container. Covering the container immediately prevents spread of microorganisms.

10. **Label the specimen container** with a patient identification label that contains the name of the test and collection date and time.

    Correctly identifying the specimen ensures accurate diagnosis and treatment.

11. **Place the specimen in a plastic bag** labeled with a biohazard label. Attach a completed laboratory requisition form.

    The plastic bag protects healthcare workers from exposure to microorganisms. Completing the laboratory requisition form ensures proper processing of the specimen.

12. **Send the specimen to the laboratory** immediately, or refrigerate it if transport might be delayed.

    If bacterial cultures are delayed, contaminating organisms may grow, producing false culture results and possibly inappropriate treatment.

Procedure 37-1B ■ Collecting a Suctioned Specimen

Procedure Steps

Follow steps 1 through 4, on the preceding page.

5. **Administer oxygen** to the patient, if indicated.

   Suctioning may cause hypoxemia.

6. **Prepare the suction device**, and make sure it is functioning properly.

7. **Don protective eyewear** (and other personal protective equipment if needed)

   Protects your eyes from splattering of secretions during suctioning.

8. **Attach the suction tubing** to the male adapter of the inline sputum specimen container. ▼

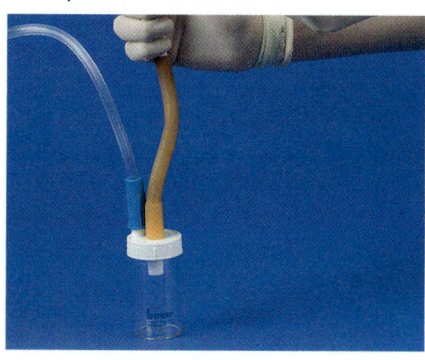

9. **Don sterile gloves**.

   Protects the patient's sterile airways from contamination by outside organisms.

10. **Attach the sterile suction** to the flexible tubing on the sputum specimen container. The hand that touches the specimen container is no longer sterile.

    Ensures that the sputum specimen goes directly into the specimen container instead of the suction tubing. ▼

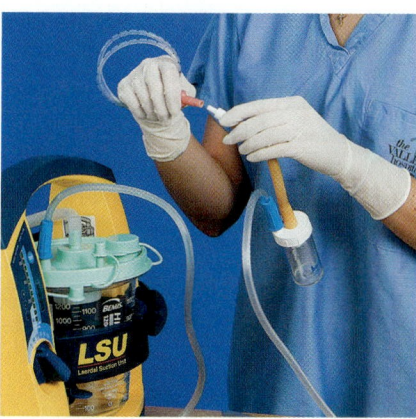

11. **Lubricate the suction catheter** with sterile saline solution.

    Lubrication eases insertion and prevents trauma to mucosa.

12. **Insert the tip of the suction catheter** gently through the nasopharynx, endotracheal tube, or tracheostomy tube. Advance the tip into the trachea (see Procedure 37-6 or Procedure 37-8).

    Gentle insertion prevents airway trauma.

13. **When the patient begins coughing**, apply suction by placing your finger over the suction control port for 5 to 10 seconds to collect the specimen.

    Applying suction for longer than 10 seconds can cause hypoxia.

14. **If an adequate specimen (5 to 10 mL)** is not obtained, allow the patient to rest for 1 or 2 minutes, and then repeat the procedure. Administer oxygen to the patient at this time, if indicated.

    Allowing the patient to rest and administering oxygen prevent hypoxia. You must assess your patient continually during this procedure to ensure patient safety and respiratory status.

15. **When you have collected** an adequate specimen, discontinue suction, then gently remove the suction catheter.
Applying suction during catheter removal can damage the airway mucosa.

16. **Remove the suction catheter** from the specimen container, and dispose of the catheter in the appropriate container.
Disposal of contaminated supplies prevents the spread of infection.

17. **Remove the suction tubing** from the specimen container, and connect the rubber tubing on the specimen container to the plastic adapter. ▼

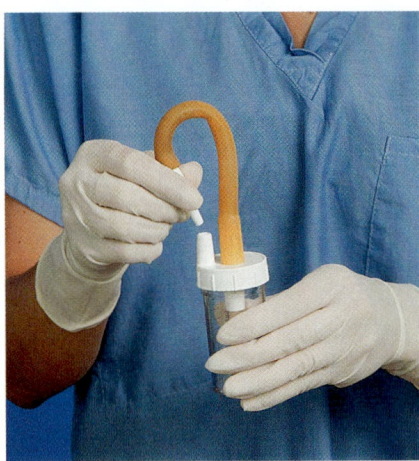

18. **If sputum comes in contact** with the outside of the specimen container, clean the outside with a disinfectant, according to agency policy.
Prevents spread of infection to staff members who must handle the specimen.

19. **After the patient expectorates**, offer tissues and provide mouth care.
Promotes patient comfort.

20. **Label the specimen container** with a patient identification label that contains the name of the test and collection date and time.
Correctly identifying the specimen ensures accurate diagnosis and treatment.

21. **Place the specimen in a plastic bag** affixed with a biohazard label.

Attach a completed laboratory requisition form.
Placing the specimen in a plastic bag protects healthcare workers from exposure to microorganisms. Completing the laboratory requisition form ensures proper processing of the specimen.

22. **Send the specimen to the laboratory** immediately, or refrigerate it if transport might be delayed.
If bacterial cultures are delayed, contaminating organisms may grow, producing false culture results and possibly inappropriate treatment.

Evaluation

- Evaluate the patient's respiratory status during and after the procedure, especially if suctioning was necessary.
- Examine the color, consistency, and odor of the sputum specimen.
- Promptly report laboratory results to the primary care provider.
- Evaluate the patient's understanding of the procedure and test results.

Patient Teaching

- Explain proper collection techniques to avoid specimen contamination.
- Show the patient proper coughing techniques to ensure an adequate specimen.
- Explain the importance of avoiding mouthwash before the procedure, as it may alter laboratory results.
- If the patient has an incision, show him how to splint his incision to avoid discomfort during coughing and expectoration.

Home Care

Explain how to collect an expectorated sputum specimen and the importance of sending the specimen to the laboratory immediately after collection.

Documentation

- Record the date and time the specimen was collected, the method of collection, and the type of specimen ordered.
- Note the amount, color, consistency, and odor of the specimen.
- Document the patient's tolerance of the procedure.

Sample documentation:

06/05/14   0700   Patient suctioned via tracheostomy. Sputum specimen obtained and sent for acid-fast bacillus (AFB) analysis. Specimen contained 15 mL of yellow, tenacious, odorless sputum. Patient became short of breath with suctioning. 100% O_2 administered via tracheostomy hood for 10 minutes after suctioning. Shortness of breath abated with treatment. O_2 returned to 40% ————— S. Ryan, RN

Practice Resources

California Department of Public Health, 2007; Texas Department of State Health Services, Laboratory Services Section Home, 2009.

Procedure 37-2 ■ Monitoring Pulse Oximetry (Arterial Oxygen Saturation)

➤ For steps to follow in *all* procedures, refer to the Universal Steps for All Procedures found on the page facing the inside back cover

Equipment

- Nail polish remover, if necessary
- Oximeter and probe sensor appropriate for patient age, size, and weight, and for the desired location

Delegation

Because it is noninvasive and simple to perform, the RN can delegate application of the pulse oximeter probe and measurement of arterial oxygen saturation (SaO_2) to a NAP or LPN who is adequately trained to perform the skill. Inform the NAP or LPN how often to take measurements, and instruct them to notify you immediately if SaO_2 falls below 95%. Although this procedure can be delegated, it is the responsibility of the RN to interpret the results, assess the patient, and notify the primary care provider.

Pre-Procedure Assessment

- Assess the patient's need for SaO_2 monitoring: risk factors, such as heart or pulmonary disease; low hemoglobin level; confusion, decreased level of consciousness, or respiratory distress.

  SaO_2 monitoring helps detect oxygenation problems early. Monitoring is especially important in patients at risk, such as those with heart and pulmonary disease, those recovering from anesthesia, and those who are ventilator dependent. Patients with underlying pulmonary disease may be accustomed to low

oxygen saturation levels, so you may need to adjust the lower limit alarm and, if you have delegated the procedure, the level for notification for these patients.

- Assess the patient's respiratory status, including breath sounds; respiratory rate, depth, and pattern; tissue perfusion; SaO_2; and skin and nailbed color.

  Assessment findings may suggest a decrease in oxygen saturation and validate oximetry readings.

- Determine the optimal location for the oximeter probe sensor, for example, the fingertip, earlobe, forehead, or bridge of the nose. Check the capillary refill and pulse at the pulse closest to the site.

  To ensure accurate monitoring, choose a site that has adequate circulation, is free of artificial nails, and contains no moisture. Clinical Insight 37-1 offers suggestions on site placement based on patient factors.

- Assess for factors that may interfere with pulse oximetry measurement, such as hypotension, hypothermia, and tremors.

  The sensor requires adequate circulation to recognize hemoglobin molecules that absorb the emitted light. Tremors may produce artifact that may be misinterpreted by the oximeter, causing false readings.

- Check patient history for allergy to adhesive.

  An allergic reaction may occur if an adhesive-backed disposable probe sensor is used in a patient with a history of allergy to adhesives.

➤ When performing the procedure, always identify your patient according to agency policy and be attentive to standard precautions, hand hygiene, patient safety and privacy, body mechanics, and documentation.

NOTE: This procedure explains how to apply a pulse oximeter. Refer to Clinical Insight 37-1 for tips for obtaining accurate pulse oximetry readings.

Procedure Steps

1. **Choose a sensor appropriate** for the patient's age, size, and weight and for the desired location. If the patient is allergic to adhesive, use a clip-on probe sensor. If the patient's peripheral circulation is compromised, use a nasal sensor.

   An appropriate type of sensor is more comfortable for the patient and ensures accurate readings.

2. **Prepare the site** by cleansing and drying it. If the finger is the desired location, remove nail polish or an acrylic nail, if present.

Dirt and skin oils on the site can interfere with passage of light waves. Nail polish or acrylic nails may interfere with signal transmission, causing inaccurate SaO_2 measurement. However, a recent study found that nail polish did not cause a clinically significant change in readings in healthy people (Rodden, Spicer, Spicer, et al., 2007).

3. **Remove the protective backing** if you are using a disposable probe sensor that contains adhesive.

4. **Attach the probe sensor** to the chosen site. Make sure the photodetector and LEDs on the probe sensor face each other. Most probe sensors contain markings to facilitate correct placement.

Clip-On Probe Sensor

If you are using a clip-on probe sensor, warn the patient that he may feel a pinching sensation. Choose the site based on the status of circulation to the extremity and patient movement.

Inadequate circulation to the site and artifact caused by motion may alter SaO_2 results. The photodetector diodes and LEDs must be properly placed to ensure accurate readings.

5. **Connect the sensor probe** to the oximeter and turn it on. Check the pulse rate displayed on the oximeter to see whether it correlates with the patient's radial pulse. (Be sure the pulse oximeter is plugged in to an electrical socket.)

   Correlation between the oximeter pulse display and the patient's radial pulse confirms accurate readings.

6. Read the SaO₂ measurement on the digital display when it reaches a constant value, usually in 10 to 30 seconds, but may take up to 2 minutes.

The oximeter requires time to detect the pulse, calculate oxygen saturation, and register an accurate reading. ▼

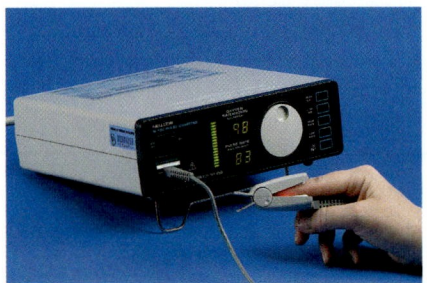

7. Set and turn on the alarm limits for SaO₂ and pulse rate, according to the manufacturer's instructions, patient condition, and agency policy if continuous monitoring is necessary.

Alarms must be set at appropriate levels to signify when SaO₂ or pulse rate falls below predetermined levels. Alarms help ensure prompt recognition and treatment of hypoxia.

8. Obtain readings as prescribed or indicated by the patient's respiratory status.

Some agencies require a prescription for pulse oximetry to ensure reimbursement.

9. Rotate the site if continuous monitoring is indicated.

Adhesive Probe Sensor
Rotate the site every 4 hours.

Clip-on Probe Sensor
Rotate the site every 2 hours.
Probe sensors and prolonged pressure may irritate the skin; rotating the site prevents skin breakdown.

10. Remove the probe sensor, and turn off the oximeter when monitoring is no longer necessary.
Some oximeters are battery powered; leaving them on after use depletes the battery.

Evaluation

- Evaluate the patient's understanding of the procedure and the obtained values.
- Compare pulse oximetry results with the patient's clinical presentation.
- Evaluate the effectiveness of therapy by comparing SaO₂ results before, during, and after treatment.
- Assess the site every 4 hours if you are using an adhesive probe sensor or every 2 hours if you are using a clip-on probe sensor.

Patient Teaching

- Demonstrate the procedure to the patient and caregiver, especially if the patient will be continuing pulse oximetry at home.
- Explain to the patient and caregiver the significance of SaO₂ results.
- Discuss the signs and symptoms of hypoxia (confusion, restlessness, shortness of breath, dyspnea, cyanosis, and somnolence) with the patient and caregiver.

Home Care

- Explain where to obtain a pulse oximeter.
- Tell the client and caregiver them when to notify the primary provider of abnormal results or signs and symptoms of hypoxia.
- Help the client identify risk factors that decrease SaO₂ levels.

Documentation

- Record the date and time of each pulse oximetry reading obtained. Most agencies use a flow sheet if frequent monitoring is necessary.
- Document whether readings are intermittent or continuous.
- If readings are continuous, record alarm parameters.
- Chart the patient's vital signs and SaO₂ results, and indicate whether the patient is breathing room air or receiving oxygen therapy. For oxygen therapy, note the oxygen concentration and the mode of delivery.
- Document acute decreases in SaO₂, any precipitating factors, treatment interventions, and the patient's response.

Practice Resources

American Association of Critical-Care Nurses (AACN), 2005; Hill & Stoneham, 2000; Rajkumar, Karmarkar, & Knott, 2006; Rodden, Spicer, Diaz, et al., 2007.

Thinking About the Procedure

 Go to the *Fundamentals of Nursing Skills Videos,* **Oxygenation: Pulse Oximetry.**

1. Based on the type of sensor used, would you infer that the patient's peripheral circulation was adequate or inadequate?
2. Which kind of sensor did the nurse use: clip-on or adhesive?
3. What did the nurse do after reading the SaO₂ measurement on the pulse oximeter?

 For suggested responses, go to Chapter 37, **Thinking About the Procedure Suggested Responses,** on Davis*Plus.*

Procedure 37-3 ■ Performing Percussion, Vibration, and Postural Drainage

➤ For steps to follow in *all* procedures, refer to the Universal Steps for All Procedures found on the page facing the inside back cover.

Equipment

- Bed capable of being placed in the Trendelenburg position
- Pillows
- Patient gown
- Facial tissues
- Emesis basin
- Sputum specimen container, if needed
- Suction equipment, if needed
- Stethoscope

Delegation

You should assess the patient to determine the need for the procedure and to evaluate whether the patient can tolerate the procedure. You must perform the initial procedure, but you can delegate subsequent treatments to a respiratory therapist or NAP who is adequately trained. Instruct the respiratory therapist or NAP to report any changes in the patient's condition immediately. The RN is responsible for ongoing assessment and monitoring of airway clearance and respiratory status.

Pre-Procedure Assessment

- Check the patient's chest x-ray results.
  Identifies which lung fields require treatment.
- Assess the patient's respiratory status, including respiratory rate, depth, and rhythm; breath sounds; color; and pulse oximetry results.
  Determines the need for and effectiveness of percussion, vibration, and postural drainage.
- Determine when the patient has last eaten.
  Postural drainage should not be performed for at least 2 hours after meals to prevent nausea, vomiting, and aspiration.
- Assess for dysrhythmias, coagulopathy (a defect in blood clotting), hypertension, and pain or tenderness in the chest area being treated.
  If any of these are present, the procedure should be avoided because it might worsen these conditions.

➤ When performing the procedure, always identify your patient according to agency policy and be attentive to standard precautions, hand hygiene, patient safety and privacy, body mechanics, and documentation.

Procedure Steps

1. **Help the patient assume** the appropriate position, based on the lung field that requires drainage.
   Helps mobilize secretions in the affected lung field by gravity.
   a. *Apical areas of the upper lobes.* Ask the patient to sit at the edge of the bed. If needed, place a pillow at the base of the spine for support. If the patient is not able to sit at the edge of the bed, use high-Fowler's position. ▼

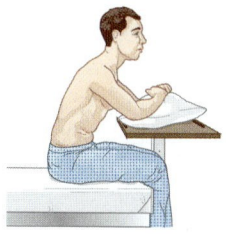

   b. *Posterior section of the upper lobes.* Position supine with a pillow under the hips and knees flexed. Have the patient rotate slightly away from the side that requires drainage.

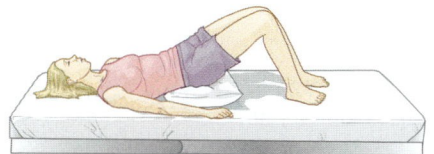

   c. *Middle or lower lobes.* With the bed in he Trendelenburg position, position the patient in Sims' position. To drain the left lung, position the patient on his right side. For the right lung, position the patient on his left side. ▼

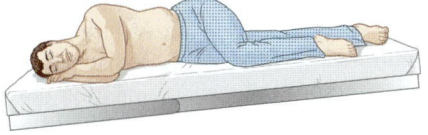

   d. *Posterior lower lobes.* Keeping the bed flat, position the patient prone with a pillow under her stomach. ▼

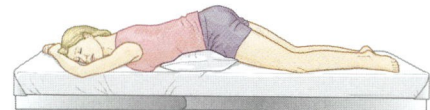

2. **Have the patient remain** in the desired position for 10 to 15 minutes, if tolerated.

Allows adequate drainage of secretions by gravity from the desired lung field.

3. **Perform percussion** over the affected lung area while the patient is in the desired drainage position.
   Loosens and mobilizes secretions.
   a. Instruct the patient to breathe deeply and slowly.
   Relaxation helps the patient tolerate the procedure.
   b. Place a towel over the patient's skin or cover with the patient's gown the area to be percussed.
   Protects the skin and promotes patient privacy and comfort.
   c. ✚ Avoid clapping over bony prominences, female breasts, or tender areas of the chest.
   Percussing over these areas may cause discomfort and compromise tissue integrity.
   d. Cup your hands, keeping your fingers flexed and your thumbs pressed against your index fingers.
   Cupping your hands promotes patient comfort during percussion.

e. Place your cupped hands over the lung area that requires drainage.

f. Percuss the lung area for 1 to 3 minutes by alternately striking your cupped hands rhythmically against the patient. ▼

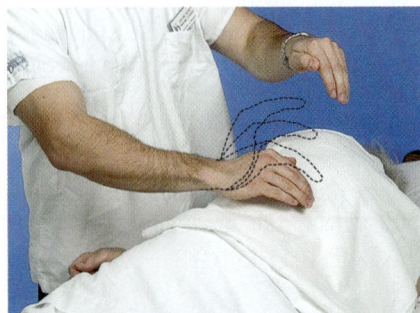

4. **Perform vibrations** while the patient remains in the desired drainage position. ▼

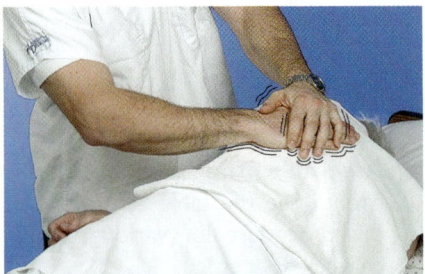

a. Place the flat surface of one hand over the lung area that requires vibration. Place your other hand on top of that hand at a right angle.
Using the flat surfaces of the hands provides a large surface area to transmit vibrations through the chest. Placing one hand on top of the other provides better leverage for vibrating.

b. Instruct the patient to inhale slowly and deeply.
Promotes relaxation and lung expansion.

c. Instruct the patient to make an "fff" or "sss" sound as she exhales.

d. As the patient exhales, press your fingers and palms firmly against her chest wall.
Vibrating during exhalation enhances the downward movement of the rib cage that occurs during exhalation.

e. Push down, and gently vibrate with your hands over the lung area.
Vibration helps mobilize secretions.

f. Continue performing vibrations for three exhalations.

5. **After performing postural drainage**, percussion, and vibration, allow the patient to sit up. Ask her to cough at the end of a deep inspiration. Suction the patient if she is unable to expectorate secretions. If a sputum specimen is needed, collect it in a specimen container.
Coughing helps clear the airway of secretions.

6. **Repeat steps 1 through 5** for each lung field that requires treatment. The entire treatment should not exceed 60 minutes.
Treating for longer than 60 minutes fatigues the patient.

7. **Provide mouth care.**
Cleanses the mouth of secretions and promotes patient comfort.

Evaluation

- Evaluate the effectiveness of percussion, vibration, and postural drainage.
- Auscultate breath sounds every 2 to 4 hours, as indicated.
- Monitor pulse oximetry and arterial blood gas (ABG) results.
- Evaluate the need for further treatments.

Patient Teaching

- Demonstrate percussion, vibration, and postural drainage if the patient will be continuing it at home.
- Reinforce the importance of immediately reporting shortness of breath or any difficulty breathing.
- Explain the importance of drinking fluids to help thin and mobilize secretions.
- Teach coughing and deep-breathing exercises.

Home Care

- Be sure the client family/caregiver knows how to perform percussion, vibration, and postural drainage, how often the procedure should be done, and why the treatments are important. There should be a prescription from the primary care provider.
- Most homes will not have a bed that can be placed in the Trendelenburg position.

- Demonstrate how to position the client with hips elevated on pillows, higher than the chest, or, if the client is able, to assume a knee–chest position.
- Provide contact information of healthcare personnel who can be reached for advice or emergencies.

Documentation

- Document the date and time you performed percussion, vibration, and postural drainage.
- Note the positions used for postural drainage and the length of time the patient maintained each position.
- Note the locations in which you performed percussion and vibration.
- Document the patient's tolerance of the procedure, as well as any complications and the nursing interventions you used to treat the complication.
- Document the amount, color, odor, and consistency of sputum you obtained during the procedure and whether you sent a sputum specimen to the lab.

Practice Resources

Best Practices, 2007.

Procedure 37-4 ■ Administering Oxygen

> For steps to follow in *all* procedures, refer to the Universal Steps for All Procedures found on the page facing the inside back cover.

Equipment

- Oxygen source
- Flow meter
- Oxygen tubing
- Nasal cannula, oxygen mask, or face tent
- Prefilled humidification device

Delegation

The RN is responsible for assessing respiratory function and initiating and monitoring response to oxygen therapy. However, you may delegate reapplication and maintenance of oxygen therapy (e.g., adjusting the face mask) to appropriately trained assistive personnel when necessary.

Pre-Procedure Assessment

- Assess the patient's understanding of oxygen therapy.
- Assessment of the patient's respiratory status; includes respiratory rate, depth, and rhythm; breath sounds; color; capillary refill and pulse oximetry results.
  Determines the need for further treatment and effectiveness of oxygen therapy.
- Assess nares for patency (if a nasal cannula is being used) and behind the ears for signs of skin breakdown.

> When performing the procedure, always identify your patient according to agency policy and be attentive to standard precautions, hand hygiene, patient safety and privacy, body mechanics, and documentation.

> *NOTE:* Oxygen requires a medical prescription. In an emergency, administer oxygen to prevent respiratory distress, then notify the primary care provider for a prescription.

Procedure Steps

✚ Also refer to the box Oxygen Therapy Safety Precautions following the Documentation section at the end of this procedure.

1. **Attach the flow meter** to the wall oxygen source. ▼

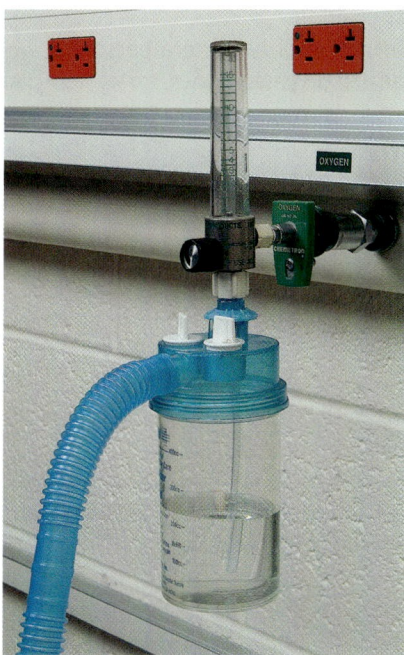

Portable Oxygen Tank
Attach the flow meter to the tank if it is not already connected. Once tubing is attached to the portable tank, check the amount of oxygen in the tank by looking at the meter.
The flow meter regulates the amount of oxygen delivered per minute. ▼

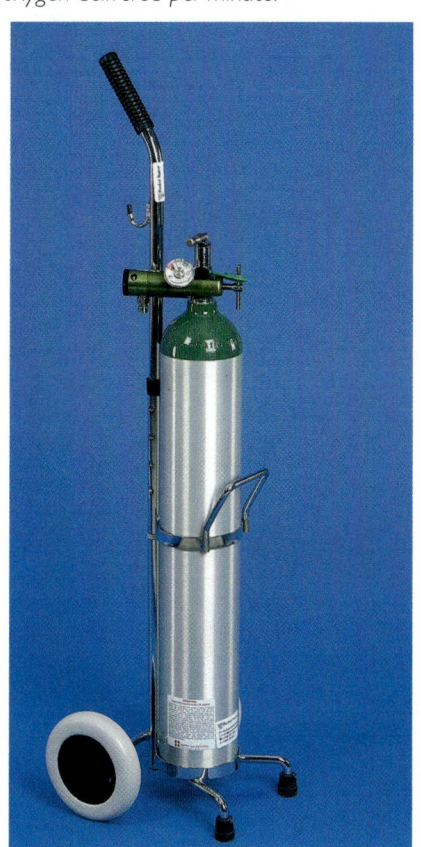

2. **Assemble the oxygen equipment.** (See the table at the end of this procedure for various oxygen delivery devices.)

3. **Attach the humidifier** to the flow meter. The humidifier is simply a small plastic container containing normal saline. If you are not using a humidifier, attach the adapter to the flow meter.
   The humidifier adds moisture in with the oxygen, which can dry the nasal or oral cavity.

Procedure Variation Nasal Cannula

Follow steps 1 through 3.

4. **Attach the nasal cannula tubing** to the humidifier or the adapter.

5. **Place the nasal prongs** in the patient's nares—prongs curved downward—and then place the tubing around each ear.
   Properly positions the device for optimal oxygen delivery.

6. **Use the slide adjustment device** to tighten the cannula in place under the patient's chin. Then go to Step 11.
   The nasal cannula must fit securely to maximize the amount of oxygen inhaled by the patient. A good fit minimizes the amount of oxygen lost around the prongs.

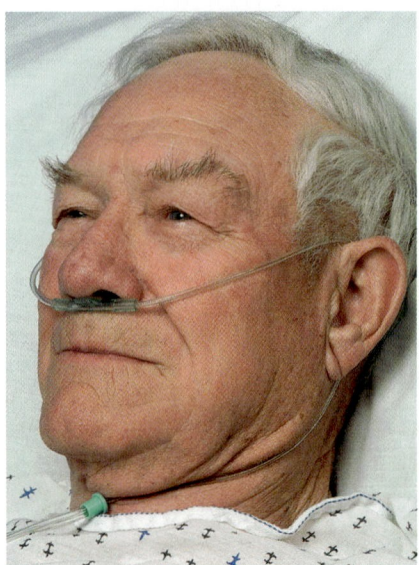

Nasal Cannula

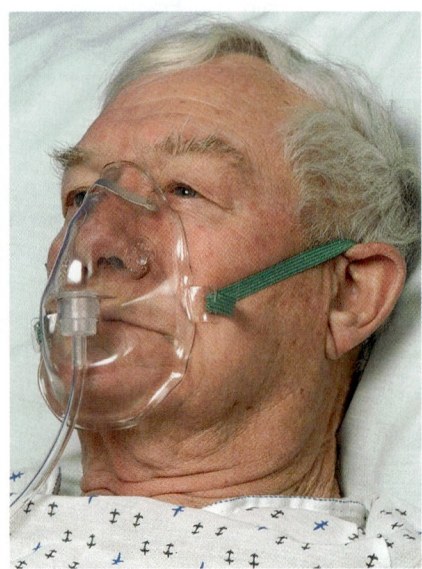

Face Mask

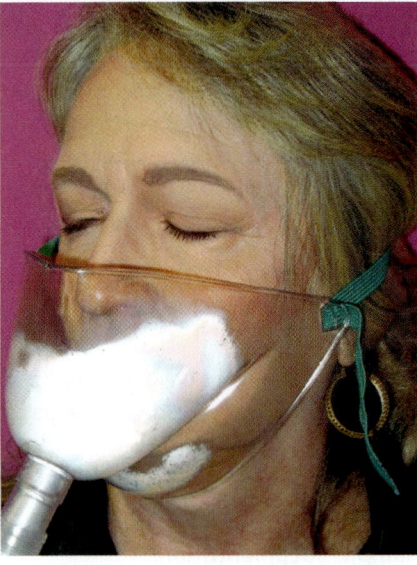

Face Tent

mask. If the mask is too tight, it may cause skin breakdown. ▼

Procedure Variation **Face Mask**

Follow steps 1 through 3.

7. **Gently place the face mask** on the patient's face, applying it from the bridge of the nose to under the chin.

8. **Secure the elastic band** around the back of the patient's head. Make sure the mask fits snugly but comfortably. Go to step 11.
   The mask must fit snugly so that oxygen cannot escape around the edges of the

Procedure Variation **Face Tent**

Follow steps 1 through 3.

9. **Gently place the face tent** in front of the patient's face, making sure that it fits under the chin.

10. **Secure the elastic band** around the back of the patient's head. Go to step 11.

11. **Turn on the oxygen** at the flow meter, and adjust to the prescribed flow rate.

12. **Double check that the oxygen** equipment is set up correctly and functioning properly.
    Ensures that the oxygen is delivered at the prescribed rate. Oxygen delivered at an incorrect rate can cause patient injury.

13. **Assess the patient's respiratory status** before leaving the bedside.
    To be certain it is safe to leave the patient.

Evaluation

- Assess respiratory rate, depth, and effort.
- Auscultate breath sounds before leaving the bedside, then monitor every 2 to 4 hours, and as indicated.
- Monitor pulse oximetry until respiratory status improves.
- Monitor ABG results if prescribed.
- Evaluate for skin breakdown, paying close attention to areas behind the ears, cheekbones, and under the chin—areas that are in contact with the oxygen delivery system.
- Notify the primary provider of respiratory status, oxygen, and response and any additional prescriptions needed.

Patient Teaching

- Demonstrate oxygen administration to the patient and caregiver if the patient will be continuing oxygen therapy at home. Allow for time to answer questions, and return demonstration of attaching and turning on the oxygen.
- Explain the importance of immediately reporting shortness of breath or any difficulty breathing to the nursing staff before discharge. If the patient is at home, he will need to report the difficulty to the home health and/or primary care provider, and, if needed, to call 911.

Home Care

- Explain to the family and caregiver where to obtain oxygen equipment and what services are available. Make sure they choose a supplier who has 24-hour emergency services.
- Instruct the client and caregiver about oxygen therapy and its use, as well as safety measures that they must institute. Safety measures include keeping oxygen away from items that may cause ignition such as lighters, cigarettes, fireplaces, heaters, etc.
- To demonstrate the oxygen is on, client can hold nasal prongs on the side of the cheek to feel air flow or over a glass of water to see air moving water.
- Teach the client and caregiver to clean the nasal cannula or face mask with soap and warm water when it becomes soiled. The mask needs to air dry.
- Provide the client and caregiver with contact information of healthcare personnel who can be reached for advice or emergencies.
- Explain the importance of immediately reporting shortness of breath or any difficulty breathing to the home health and/or primary care provider; and if needed, to call 911.
- In the home, liquid oxygen and oxygen concentrators are more commonly used than portable oxygen tanks. Liquid

(continued on next page)

Procedure 37-4 ■ Administering Oxygen (continued)

oxygen may be kept in small, portable containers; an oxygen concentrator removes nitrogen from room air and concentrates O_2. It requires a battery pack or electrical outlet for power. Oxygen concentrators can deliver a flow of 6 to 8 L/min.

Documentation

- Document the date, time, and reason oxygen therapy was initiated.
- Note the type of oxygen delivery system used, the amount of oxygen administered, and the patient's response to oxygen therapy.
- Document vital signs, pulse oximetry values, breath sounds, skin color, and respiratory effort.

Sample documentation:

12/14/14   2014   Patient developed acute shortness of breath. RR 36/min & labored, P = 126 beats/min, and BP 212/110 mm Hg. Pulse ox 80% on room air. Crackles and expiratory wheezes auscultated throughout both lungs. Dr. Chow notified of patient's condition. Partial rebreather mask @ 10 L/min and Lasix 40 mg IV prescribed and administered. Pulse ox on partial rebreather = 90%. ——————
———————————————————————— S. Peters, RN

Practice Resources

Best Practices, 2007.

> ### Oxygen Therapy Safety Precautions
>
> - ✚ Post signs indicating that oxygen is in use.
> - Do not permit smoking near oxygen
> - Ensure that three-pronged plugs are used for electrical devices (to prevent sparks).
> - Allow no open flames (e.g., candles) near oxygen.
> - Avoid electrical equipment with frayed wires or loose connections.
> - Avoid using petroleum products, aerosol products, and products containing acetone where oxygen is in use. (These are flammable substances that are easily ignited.)
> - Secure oxygen tanks to rigid stands.
> - Secure portable oxygen cylinders in holders or carriers provided.

Oxygen Delivery Systems

DELIVERY METHOD	FIO₂	DISCUSSION	NURSING RESPONSIBILITIES
Nasal cannula	1 L/min = 24% 2 L/min = 28% 3 L/min = 32% 4 L/min = 36% 5 L/min = 40% 6 L/min = 44%	■ Relatively comfortable. ■ Patients can eat, talk, and cough with a nasal cannula in place. ■ Works best if the patient breathes through his nose.	■ Check frequently that the prongs are in the patient's nose. ■ Assess for dryness of the nasal mucosa. ■ Humidify flow at rates above 3 L/min (flow rates > 3 L/min are drying). ■ Encourage the patient to take slow, deep breaths, so he will inhale more oxygen and less room air.
Simple face mask: A clear, flexible mask that covers the nose and mouth and delivers oxygen flow into the mask.	5–10 L/min = 40%–60% FIO₂	■ Requires flow rates greater than 5 L/min to prevent accumulation and rebreathing of exhaled CO_2 from within the mask. ■ Masks are not easily tolerated because they fit tightly and keep heat from radiating from the face, making patients feel hot. ■ Talking is muffled by the mask, and it must be removed for the patient to eat or drink. ■ Condensation within the mask might be irritating to the patient's skin.	■ Place face mask securely over the mouth and nose. ■ Elastic straps fit around the head to hold the mask in place. Place the straps well above the ears to prevent skin irritation and breakdown. ■ Place gauze or other soft material beneath the straps to prevent irritation. ■ Check the skin around the mask frequently. ■ Check the skin over the ears where the mask strap rubs. ■ Encourage the patient to take slow, deep breaths, so he will inhale more oxygen and less room air. ■ Wipe the moisture out of the mask occasionally.

Oxygen Delivery Systems—cont'd

DELIVERY METHOD	FIO$_2$	DISCUSSION	NURSING RESPONSIBILITIES
Partial rebreather mask: Uses the reservoir bag to capture some exhaled gas for rebreathing	6–15 L/min = 50%–90% FIO$_2$	▪ Allows higher FIO$_2$ levels to be delivered because O$_2$ is collected in the reservoir bag for inhalation. ▪ Exhalation ports allow most exhaled air to escape. ▪ Several types are available. ▪ Can deliver an FIO$_2$ above 50% at flow rates of 6–15 L/min. ▪ Patient rebreathes some exhaled air along with O$_2$.	▪ Maintain the flow at a high enough rate to prevent the reservoir bag from collapsing during inhalation. ▪ Encourage the patient to take slow, deep breaths, so he will inhale more oxygen and less room air.
Nonrebreather mask: A type of reservoir bag mask; a valve keeps exhaled air from entering the reservoir bag.	6–15 L/min = 70%–100% FIO$_2$	▪ Contains only O$_2$, which allows higher FIO$_2$ delivery. An FIO$_2$ of 60–100% can be delivered at flow rates of 6–15 L/min. ▪ This mask is the only external device capable of delivering an FIO$_2$ of 100% (in practice, it is rare to achieve a concentration over 75% because the mask does not seal perfectly with the face).	▪ Maintain the flow at a rate high enough to keep the reservoir at least one-third to one-half full during inhalation. ▪ Be sure the mask fits snugly so the patient will breathe in less room air.
Venturi mask: A cone-shaped adapter that serves as a mixing valve to control the amount of O$_2$ and room air that flows through the mask.	24%–50% FIO$_2$	▪ The cone-shaped adapter at the base of the mask allows a precise FIO$_2$ to be delivered. This is very useful for patients with chronic lung disease. ▪ Exhalation ports keep CO$_2$ buildup to a minimum.	▪ The adapter indicates the required oxygen flow rate needed to deliver the desired FIO$_2$. Ensure that flow is set at the rate specified to deliver the FIO$_2$ desired.

(continued on next page)

Procedure 37-4 ■ **Administering Oxygen** (continued)

Oxygen Delivery Systems—cont'd

DELIVERY METHOD	FIO₂	DISCUSSION	NURSING RESPONSIBILITIES
Face tent: A large, open plastic mask that fits under the chin. It is open at the top and is held in place with an elastic band around the head.	8–12 L/min = 30%–55% FIO_2	■ Less reliable than a face mask for delivering precise FIO_2 levels. ■ Allows moderate- to high-density aerosol delivery for humidification. ■ Patients who feel claustrophobic in a face mask often tolerate a face tent.	■ Check the skin over the ears where the mask strap rubs.
Tracheostomy collar: A small, cup-shaped device that fits over the tracheostomy opening and is held in place with elastic straps around the neck.	4–10 L/min = 24%–100%	■ It is possible to deliver both high FIO_2 and high humidity with a tracheostomy collar. ■ Large-bore tubing is used to deliver humidification to the trachea; however, water frequently condenses inside the tubing and can be accidentally drained into the tracheostomy. Usually, a water trap of some sort is placed in the tubing to prevent this problem.	■ Watch for water accumulation in the tubing.
T-piece: A T-shaped plastic piece; the bottom of the T fits directly and tightly onto the tracheostomy tube.	4–10 L/min = 24%–100% FIO_2	■ Oxygen and humidity are delivered into one side of the T and exhaled through the other side.	■ Take care that the oxygen delivery tubing does not pull on the T-piece, which can dislodge the tracheostomy tube and create an airway emergency.

Thinking About the Procedure

 Go to the *Fundamentals of Nursing Skills Videos,* **Oxygenation: Administration, Cannula.**

1. Does the nurse wear gloves for this procedure? What do you think is the reason for that

 Go to the *Fundamentals of Nursing Skills Videos,* **Oxygenation: Administration, Face Mask.**

2. Why does the nurse not attach a humidifier to the oxygen delivery system?

 Go to the *Fundamentals of Nursing Skills Videos,* **Oxygenation: Administration, Face Tent.**

3. Compare this procedure to **Oxygenation: Administration, Cannula.** Both procedures attach a humidifier to the flow meter. But what is different in the tubing that delivers the oxygen to the patient?

 For suggested responses, go to Chapter 37, **Thinking About the Procedure Suggested Responses,** on *DavisPlus.*

Procedure 37-5 ■ Performing Tracheostomy Care Using Sterile Technique

➤ For steps to follow in *all* procedures, refer to the Universal Steps for All Procedures found on the page facing the inside back cover.

➤ Also refer to Clinical Insight 37-5.

➤ Recall that the basic differences in sterile and modified sterile technique are that modified sterile technique uses nonsterile procedure gloves and tap water.

Equipment

- Tracheostomy suction equipment (see Procedure 37-6)
- Tracheostomy care kit or the following sterile supplies: several cotton-tipped applicators, two basins, a brush, sterile 4 in. × 4 in. gauze pads, sterile precut tracheostomy dressing
- Two pairs of sterile gloves (for modified sterile technique, use procedure gloves)
- Disposable inner cannula that is the same size as the tracheostomy, if available. Most tracheostomy tubes have disposable inner cannulas.
- Sterile normal saline solution (for modified sterile technique, you can use tap water if agency policy allows)
- Hydrogen peroxide for cleaning of reusable inner cannula only
- Roll of twill tape or hook and loop fastener (Velcro) tracheostomy holder
- Bandage scissors
- Towel or linen-saver pad
- Overbed table
- Face shield and protective gown
- For modified sterile technique: mild soap and two clean washcloths

✚ Use only the sterile precut dressing, or open and refold a 4 in. × 4 in. gauze pad into a V-shape. Do not cut 4 in. × 4 in. gauze, and do not use cotton-filled gauze squares.
The patient may aspirate the cotton or gauze fibers.

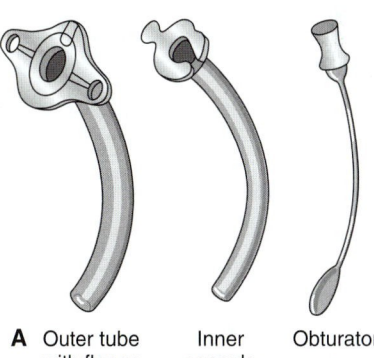

A Outer tube   Inner   Obturator
with flange   cannula

A, Nondisposable tracheostomy equipment

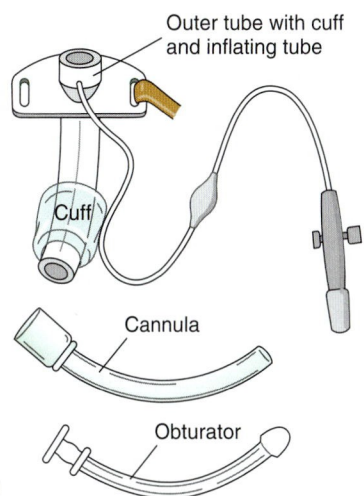

Outer tube with cuff and inflating tube

Cuff

Cannula

Obturator

B

B, Disposable tracheostomy equipment

(continued on next page)

Procedure 37-5 ■ Performing Tracheostomy Care Using Sterile Technique (continued)

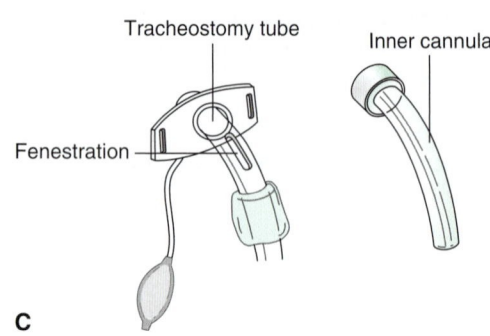

C, Fenestrated tracheostomy equipment

Delegation

In acute care settings and with new tracheostomies, you should not delegate this procedure to the NAP. For long-standing and well-healed tracheostomies, you can safely delegate care to a NAP or LPN who is adequately trained to perform the skill.

This varies by state. In some states only RNs can perform tracheostomy care. If you are not familiar with your state's nurse practice act, contact your state board of nursing.

Pre-Procedure Assessment

- Assess the patient's respiratory status, including respiratory rate, depth, and rhythm; breath sounds; color; and pulse oximetry results.
  Helps determine whether the patient can tolerate tracheostomy care.
- Assess the tracheostomy site for drainage, redness, or swelling.
  Drainage, redness, or swelling may indicate infection.
- Determine when the patient last ate.
  It is best to schedule this procedure at least 3 hours after a meal to decrease the risk of the patient vomiting and aspirating stomach contents.

➤ *NOTE: Asterisks indicate steps that differ when using modified sterile technique.*

➤ When performing the procedure, always identify your patient according to agency policy and be attentive to standard precautions, hand hygiene, patient safety and privacy, body mechanics, and documentation.

Procedure Steps

1. **Position the patient** in semi-Fowler's position, and place a towel or linen-saver pad over the patient's chest.
   A semi-Fowler's position promotes lung expansion and prevents back strain for the nurse. A towel or linen-saver pad prevents soiling of the patient's gown.

*2. **Don sterile gloves, gown, and face shield or mask.** (For modified sterile technique, don clean procedure gloves.)

One Sterile Glove

Put a sterile glove on your dominant hand and a clean glove on your other hand.

3. **Suction the tracheostomy** (see Procedure 37-6 or 37-7).
   Suctioning clears the tracheostomy of secretions that could occlude the outer cannula after the inner cannula is removed for care.

Passy–Muir Valve

Remove the Passy–Muir valve (PMV) before suctioning the patient to prepare for tracheostomy care. (A PMV is a device that is used to enable the patient with a tracheostomy to speak. It is attached to the end of the inner cannula at the tracheostomy site.)

4. **Remove and discard** the soiled tracheostomy dressing in the appropriate receptacle, and then remove and discard your gloves. Wash your hands.

*5. **Place the tracheostomy care equipment** on the overbed table, and prepare the equipment, using sterile technique.
   Ensures efficiency and helps maintain sterility during tracheostomy care.

   *a. *Disposable inner cannula*—Pour sterile normal saline solution into the two sterile containers. (For modified sterile technique, use tap water or sterile normal saline [per agency policy]).

   b. *Reusable inner cannula*—Pour hydrogen peroxide into one of the sterile solution containers, and pour normal saline solution into the other one. If the inner cannula is not disposable, use hydrogen peroxide to clean only the inner cannula. Use the normal saline (or tap water) to rinse the inner cannula and clean the faceplate and tracheostomy site.

   *c. *Steps c through g apply to both types of cannula.* Open two 4 in. × 4 in. gauze packages. Wet the gauze in one package with normal saline solution, and keep the second package dry. (For modified sterile technique, instead of sterile gauze, wet one washcloth with tap water or saline and keep the second washcloth dry.)
   You will use the second package of gauze to dry the skin around the tracheostomy site after cleaning.

   *d. Open one cotton-tipped applicator package. Wet the applicators with normal saline solution. (For modified sterile technique, wet the applicators with tap water or normal saline solution.)
   Prepares the applicators for cleaning the exposed surface of the outer cannula and the stoma site located under the faceplate of the tracheostomy tube, respectively.

   e. Open the package containing a new disposable inner cannula, if available.
   Allows for quick replacement of the inner cannula.

   f. Open the package of Velcro tracheostomy ties, or cut a length of twill tape long enough to go around the patient's neck two times. Make sure to cut end of the tape on an angle.

Allows for quick stabilization of the tracheostomy tube, preventing dislodgement. Cutting the twill tape on an angle allows for easy insertion through the faceplate eyelets.

g. Position a biohazard bag within reach.

Allows you to dispose of contaminated supplies safely as you use them without leaving the patient or interrupting the procedure.

*6. Don sterile gloves (or a sterile glove on your dominant hand and a clean glove on your nondominant hand); keep the glove on your dominant hand sterile. Handle the sterile supplies with the dominant hand only. (For modified sterile technique, don clean procedure gloves. Consider your dominant hand to be clean and handle supplies with that hand only.)

7. For patients receiving oxygen: With your nondominant (nonsterile) hand, remove the oxygen or humidification source. Attach the oxygen source to the outer cannula, if possible. If not possible, have the respiratory therapist set up oxygen blow-by to use while you are cleaning the reusable inner cannula.

Prevents oxygen desaturation in the patient during the procedure.

8. Unlock and remove the inner cannula with your nondominant hand, and care for it accordingly.

Disposable Inner Cannula

a. Dispose of the inner cannula in the biohazard receptacle according to agency policy. You should never clean and reuse a disposable inner cannula.

Prevents contamination by bacteria contained in the inner cannula.

b. With your dominant hand, insert the new inner cannula into the patient's tracheostomy in the direction of the curvature. Following the manufacturer's instructions, lock the inner cannula in place securely to prevent it from dislodging. Remember to keep your dominant hand sterile (or clean, for modified sterile technique).

Reusable Inner Cannula

c. If a reusable inner cannula was used, place the inner cannula into the basin filled with hydrogen peroxide.

Hydrogen peroxide helps loosen tenacious (sticky) secretions.

d. Pick up the reusable inner cannula from the container of hydrogen peroxide with your nonsterile hand, and scrub it with the sterile nylon brush, using your sterile dominant hand.

*e. Immerse the inner cannula in the container of sterile normal saline solution, and agitate it until it is rinsed thoroughly. (If using modified sterile technique, you may hold the inner cannula under running tap water briefly and agitate it.)

Immersing the inner cannula in normal saline solution (or tap water) and agitating it removes the hydrogen peroxide and debris from the inner cannula, minimizing tissue irritation.

*f. Tap the inner cannula against the side of the container if using sterile saline. (If using tap water, shake the cannula to remove water.)

Removes excess fluid so the patient does not aspirate it when you reinsert the cannula.

g. With your dominant hand, reinsert the inner cannula into the patient's tracheostomy in the direction of the curvature. Following the manufacturer's instructions, lock the inner cannula in place securely to prevent it from dislodging. Remember to keep your dominant hand sterile.

Passy–Muir Valve

h. Swish the PMV in warm tap water with mild soap.

i. Rinse the PMV thoroughly in warm tap water.

j. DO NOT use hot water, peroxide, bleach, vinegar, alcohol, brushes, or cotton-tipped applicators to clean PMV.

These could damage the valve.

k. Shake the PMV to remove excess fluid. If you are going to store the valve, be sure to air-dry the valve before placing it in a storage container.

Removes moisture, which can promote bacterial growth.

l. Set the PMV aside on clean surface to be replaced when the inner cannula is replaced.

For Patients Receiving Oxygen

m. Remove the humidification or oxygen source from the outer cannula, if indicated, using your nondominant hand.

n. Reinsert the inner cannula into the patient's tracheostomy in the direction of the curvature.

o. Following the manufacturer's instructions, lock the inner cannula in place securely. Remember to keep dominant hand sterile.

p. Lock the inner cannula in place securely to prevent it from dislodging.

q. Reattach the humidification or oxygen source, if indicated.

Provides the patient with needed humidity or oxygen and prevents oxygen desaturation.

*9. Clean the stoma under the faceplate with cotton-tipped applicators saturated with normal saline solution, using a circular motion from the stoma site outward. Use each applicator only once, and then discard it. (If using modified sterile technique, applicators may be saturated with tap water.)

Prevents contamination of the cleaned area. ▼

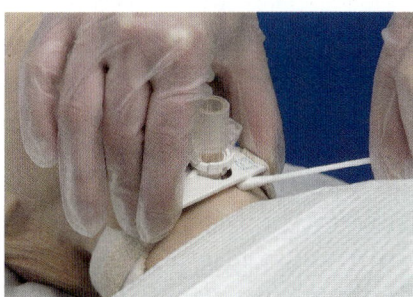

*10. Clean the top surface of the faceplate and the skin around it with the gauze pads saturated with normal saline solution. Use each

(continued on next page)

Procedure 37-5 ■ Performing Tracheostomy Care Using Sterile Technique (continued)

gauze pad only once, and then discard it. (For modified sterile technique, use a washcloth saturated with tap water. Or you can use the gauze pads if they are contained in the tracheostomy kit.)

Removes secretions that provide a medium for microbial growth; prevents contamination of cleaned areas.

*11. **Dry the skin and outer cannula** surfaces by patting them lightly with the remaining dry gauze pad.

Clean, dry skin is needed to avoid skin breakdown and removes moisture, which can promote bacterial growth around the stoma site.

12. ✚ **Seek assistance from another** staff member to help with changing the tracheostomy stabilizers.

Prevents accidental dislodging should the patient begin coughing during the procedure.

13. **Remove soiled tracheostomy stabilizers.**

Removing a Soiled Velcro® Tracheostomy Holder

a. With an assistant stabilizing the tracheostomy tube, disengage the Velcro on both sides of the soiled holder, and remove it gently from the eyes of the faceplate. Discard the Velcro holder in the nearest biohazard receptacle.

Removing the soiled holder promotes hygiene and prevents the spread of infection.

Removing Soiled Twill Tape Tracheostomy Ties

b. With an assistant stabilizing the tracheostomy tube, cut the soiled tracheostomy ties using bandage scissors. *Do not* cut the tube of the tracheostomy balloon (if you do, the tracheostomy tube must be replaced). Remove the ties gently from the eyes of the faceplate, and discard them in the nearest biohazard receptacle.

The tracheostomy balloon helps stabilize the tracheostomy in the trachea and prevents an air leak. *Cutting the tube to the balloon prevents the balloon from holding air. Removing the soiled holder promotes hygiene and prevents the spread of infection.*

14. **Ask the patient to flex his neck**, or, if he is unable, ask the assistant to hold the patient's head forward, and apply new tracheostomy ties.

Flexing the neck provides the same neck circumference as when the patient coughs and thus ensures you do not place and secure the tracheostomy stabilizers too tightly.

Using a Velcro Tracheostomy Holder

a. Unfasten the Velcro. Thread one end of the tracheostomy holder through the eyelet of the faceplate, and fasten the Velcro.

b. Bring the holder around the back of the patient's neck.

The holder must be placed around the patient's neck to adequately secure the tracheostomy.

c. Thread the remaining end of the tracheostomy holder through the empty eyelet of the faceplate and fasten the Velcro®, making sure that the holder fits securely.▼

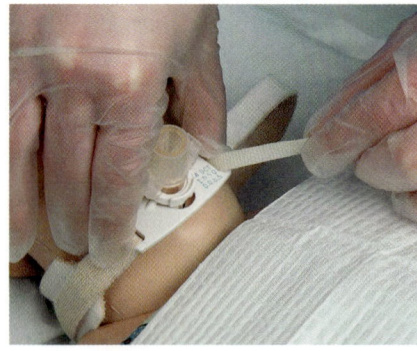

d. ✚ Place one finger under the holder to make sure that the holder is securing the tracheostomy effectively but isn't too tight.

Securing the tracheostomy too tightly might place pressure on the jugular veins, interfere with coughing, or cause necrosis at the tracheostomy insertion site.

Using Twill Tape

e. Thread one end of the twill tape into one of the eyelets on the tracheostomy faceplate.

f. Continue to thread the twill tape through the eyelet, bringing both ends of the tape together.

g. Bring both ends of the twill tape around the back of the patient's neck.

To adequately secure the tracheostomy.

h. Thread the end of the twill tape that is closest to the patient's neck through the back of the eyelet on the faceplate.

i. Have your assistant place one finger under the twill tape while you tie the two ends together in a square knot.

Ensures you do not secure the tracheostomy too tightly.

j. Place one finger under the holder to make sure that the holder is securing the tracheostomy effectively but isn't too tight.

See Step 14 d.

15. **Insert a precut, sterile** tracheostomy dressing under the faceplate and new tracheostomy stabilizers or fold a 4 in. × 4 in. gauze pad into a V shape (below).▼

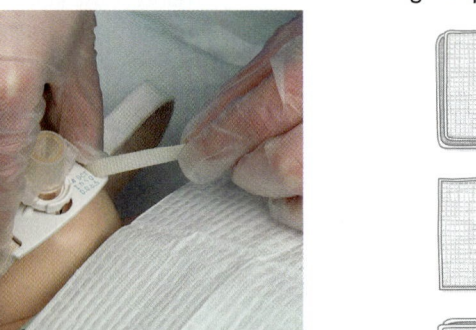

The new dressing absorbs secretions and prevents skin breakdown under the faceplate. Never cut the gauze to make a dressing because lint and fibers from the cut edge could enter

the trachea and cause respiratory distress. ▼

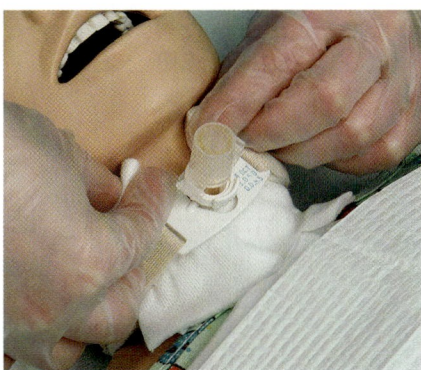

16. **Dispose of the used equipment** in the appropriate biohazard receptacle according to agency policy.
Helps prevent cross-contamination.

? What if . . .

- **Your patient begins coughing?**
  1. If the tracheostomy is still secured with ties or Velcro holder, wait to continue tracheostomy care until coughing has ended.
  2. If tracheostomy is unsecured, stabilize the tube so that it does not become dislodged being careful not to press too hard on the site. Continue with tracheostomy care when the patient finishes coughing.
  Pressing too hard at the tracheostomy site will stimulate the coughing reflex.
  3. If coughing continues, suspend tracheostomy care and suction the patient to remove any retained secretions.
  Retained secretions may cause increased airway irritation and coughing. Removing secretions will reduce this irritation.

- **You do not have an assistant to hold the cannula in place while you replace the soiled tracheostomy ties?**

  ✚ Never cut the soiled tape before applying the clean tape. Always place the new tape/holders, be certain the tracheostomy is secured, and then cut off the soiled tape or holder.

- **The tracheostomy tube becomes dislodged?**
  1. To prevent this, plan ahead and always have another staff member with you to secure the tracheostomy tube while you change the tracheostomy ties or Velcro® holder.
  2. If the tracheostomy tube slips out slightly but is still in the trachea site, gently push it back into the stoma and secure it.
  The pilot balloon will help to keep the tracheostomy tube from completely dislodging.
  3. If the tracheostomy tube becomes completely dislodged, stay with the patient and ask your assistant to call for the respiratory therapist or trained person in your facility to insert a new tracheostomy tube.

- **At step 9, there are crusts around the stoma when you are cleaning the stoma?**

  Remove the crusts with a cotton-tipped swab soaked in hydrogen peroxide; then rinse with a swab soaked in normal saline (or tap water in modified sterile technique). Have the patient hold his breath while you remove crusts so he does not inhale them.

Evaluation

- Assess the area around the stoma site for signs of skin breakdown.
- Evaluate the patient's tolerance of the procedure. Note whether there were any signs of respiratory distress.

Patient Teaching

- Explain to the patient and his family that bloody secretions are normal for 2 to 3 days after tracheostomy tube insertion or for 24 hours after a tracheostomy tube change.
- Tell the patient and/or family to inform the nurse immediately if the tracheostomy tube becomes dislodged.
- Teach tracheostomy care to the patient and caregiver if the tracheostomy is expected to remain long term.

Home Care

- Clean, rather than sterile, technique can be used for tracheostomy care if the tracheostomy is more than 1 month old.
- Instruct the client and caregiver about home oxygen therapy and suctioning, if necessary.
- Demonstrate tracheostomy care to the caregiver, and ask for a return demonstration.
- Provide the client and caregiver with information about where to obtain tracheostomy care supplies.
- Supply the client and caregiver with contact information of healthcare personnel who can be reached for advice or emergencies.

- Recommend ways of adding moisture to the air, with a goal of maintaining a relative humidity of 50% (e.g., a large humidifier, house plants, wearing damp gauze over the stoma, closing the bathroom door and turning on the hot water to fill the room with steam).
- The stoma should be cleaned using clean technique, at least twice daily (or more often, depending on the amount of secretions).
- Stress good handwashing before and after doing any part of tracheostomy care.
- Remind client and caregiver not to use cotton or gauze.
  These can leave fibers that may get into the airway and increase the incidence of infection.

Documentation

- Document the date and time you performed tracheostomy care.
- Record the color, amount, consistency, and odor of secretions.
- Record the condition of the stoma and skin around the stoma site; note the presence of drainage, redness, or swelling.
- Document respiratory status, including respiratory rate, depth, and pattern; skin color; and breath sounds.
- Document the patient's tolerance of the procedure.
- If problems arose, document any interventions that were necessary.

(continued on next page)

Procedure 37-5 ■ **Performing Tracheostomy Care Using Sterile Technique** (continued)

Practice Resources

American Thoracic Society and the Infectious Diseases Society of America, 2005; Barnett, 2005; Johnston, Davis, & Sherman, n.d.; Lewarski, 2005; Pierson, Epstein, Durbin, et al., 2005; Siegel, Rhinehart, Jackson, et al., 2007; Tablan, Anderson, Besser, et al., 2004.

Thinking About the Procedure

 Go to the *Fundamentals of Nursing Skills Videos,* **Oxygenation: Tracheostomy Care (Passy–Muir Valve), Disposable Inner Cannula Change, Dressing Change, and Stabilizer Change.**

1. Where does the nurse place the biohazard container?
2. What kind of gloves does the nurse wear to remove the soiled dressing and the Passy–Muir valve?
3. When is the first time the nurse changes her gloves?

 For suggested responses, go to Chapter 37, **Thinking About the Procedure Suggested Responses,** on Davis*Plus.*

Procedure 37-6 ■ **Performing Tracheostomy or Endotracheal Suctioning (Open System)**

➤ For steps to follow in *all* procedures, refer to the Universal Steps for All Procedures found on the page facing the inside back cover.

Equipment

- Portable or wall suction device with tubing and a collection canister
- Linen-saver pad or towel
- Resuscitation bag connected to oxygen source
- Sterile suction catheter kit: adults: 12 to 18 Fr, children: 8 to 10 Fr, infants: 5 to 8 Fr
- If a kit isn't available, collect the following: sterile gloves, sterile suction catheter of the appropriate size, and a sterile container.
- Pour-bottle of sterile, normal saline solution
- Sterile basin or container for fluids
- Prefilled 10-mL containers of normal saline solution
- Face shield or goggles
- Sterile gloves (or procedure gloves; follow agency policy)
- Protective gown

Delegation

As a rule you should not delegate tracheostomy or endotracheal suctioning to an LPN or NAP, because both procedures require professional-level theoretical knowledge, assessment skills, and problem-solving ability. However, if the patient has a permanent tracheostomy tube in place and will require long-term care, you can delegate care to trained personnel. Refer to individual state board of nursing for rules on delegating this procedure.

Pre-Procedure Assessment

- Assess the patient's respiratory status, including rate, depth, and rhythm; breath sounds; color; and pulse oximetry results.
- Assess for signs that indicate the need for suctioning: restlessness, cyanosis, labored respirations, decreased oxygen saturation, increased heart and respiratory rates, visible secretions in the airway, increased peak airway pressures on the ventilator, decreasing SaO_2 or PaO_2, and presence of adventitious breath sounds during auscultation.

Suctioning should be performed only when necessary to prevent unnecessary oxygen desaturation and tissue trauma.

➤ When performing the procedure, always identify your patient according to agency policy and be attentive to standard precautions, hand hygiene, patient safety and privacy, body mechanics, and documentation.

Procedure Steps

1. **Position the patient** in semi-Fowler's position, unless contraindicated.
   Promotes lung expansion and oxygenation.
2. **Place the linen-saver pad** or towel on the patient's chest.
   Prevents soiling of the patient's gown during suctioning.
3. **Put on a face shield or goggles and a gown.**

Protects you from contamination with secretions that may splash during suctioning.

4. **Turn on the wall suction** or portable suction machine, and adjust the pressure regulator according to agency policy, using the lowest possible suction pressure. Typically, this is:
   Adults: 100 to 150 mm Hg
   Children: 100 to 120 mm Hg
   Infants: 50 to 95 mm Hg

Using the appropriate pressure prevents tissue trauma and ensures successful suctioning. Higher pressures are associated with hypoxemia, tissue trauma, and atelectasis, yet do not improve removal of secretions

5. **Don a nonsterile glove** and face shield or goggles. Test the suction equipment by occluding the

connection tubing. Remove and discard the glove. Perform hand hygiene.

Ensures proper functioning before you insert suction catheter.

6. **Open the suction catheter kit** or (if a kit isn't available) the gathered equipment.

Sterile technique is used to avoid contaminating the upper airway when you introduce the suction catheter.

7. **Pour sterile saline** into the sterile container.

Sterile saline is used to clear the suction catheter of secretions after suctioning.

8. **Don sterile gloves**; consider your dominant hand sterile and your nondominant hand nonsterile.

Keeping your dominant hand sterile prevents contamination of the suction catheter.

Modified Sterile Procedure

Some guidelines allow for clean procedure gloves; follow agency policy. Consider your dominant hand clean and your nondominant hand contaminated.

9. **Pick up the suction catheter** with your dominant hand, and attach it to the connection tubing. Do not touch the connection tubing with your sterile glove.

10. **Put the tip of the suction catheter** into the sterile container of normal saline solution, and suction a small amount of normal saline solution through the suction catheter. Apply suction by placing a finger over the suction control port of the suction catheter.

Lubricates the catheter and helps ensure that the suction equipment is functioning properly.

11. **If the patient is receiving oxygen**, hyperoxygenate the patient according to agency policy. If the patient does not require oxygen, you do not need to hyperoxygenate.

Helps prevent hypoxia and related complications (cardiac arrhythmias, seizures, arrest) during suctioning. Suctioning clears secretions, but it also removes oxygen from airways.

Patient Requiring Mechanical Ventilation

a. Press the 100% O_2 button on the ventilator. Some agencies require the nurse to manually hyperoxygenate the patient; follow agency policy.

Ventilators typically have a button that allows you to hyperoxygenate the patient for a total of 2 minutes. Once this time period elapses, the ventilator automatically resumes its previous settings.

Patient Not Requiring Mechanical Ventilation

b. Obtain the assistance of a second provider.

c. Have your partner attach the resuscitation bag to the tracheostomy or endotracheal tube, and hyperoxygenate the patient by compressing the resuscitation bag three to five times as the patient inhales. Remove the resuscitation bag, and place it next to the patient when you are finished.

You must perform hyperoxygenation manually if the patient does not require mechanical ventilation. You will need assistance from a second provider in order to maintain sterile technique while suctioning.

12. **Perform suctioning.**

a. Lubricate the suction catheter tip with the normal saline solution.

Lubrication eases passage of the suction catheter through the endotracheal tube or tracheostomy tube.

b. Using your dominant hand, gently but quickly insert the suction catheter into the endotracheal tube or tracheostomy tube. ▼

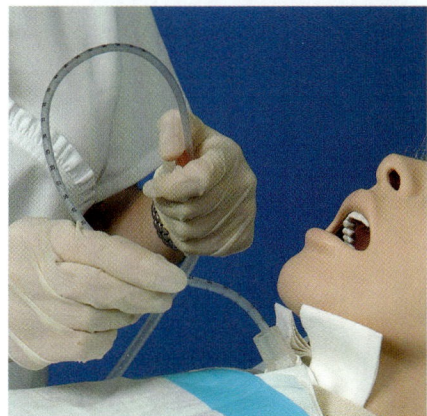

c. ✚ Advance the suction catheter, with suction off, gently aiming downward, and being careful not to force the catheter. Insert to the premeasured length: no farther than the **carina tracheae** (the ridge at the lower end of the trachea that separates the openings of the two mainstem bronchi); do not insert more than 6 inches (15 cm).

Premeasure the catheter insertion distance for 0.5 to 1 cm (1/4 to 1/2 in.) past the distal end of the endotracheal tube (ETT); the ETT normally sits between 3 and 7 cm (1 to 23/4 in.) above the carina. Forcing the catheter during insertion may cause tissue trauma.

d. Apply suction while you withdraw the catheter; rotate the catheter (roll it between your thumb and forefinger) as you remove it. Make sure to apply suction for no longer than 15 seconds.

Applying suction for longer than 15 seconds causes hypoxia and may cause tissue trauma.

13. **Repeat suctioning** as needed. Several passes with the suction catheter may be needed to clear the airway of secretions.

a. Allow at least 30-second intervals between suctioning.

b. Make sure to hyperoxygenate the patient between each pass.

c. Limit total suctioning time to 5 minutes.

14. **Replace the oxygen source**, if it was removed during suctioning.

To prevent hypoxia.

15. **Coil the suction catheter** in your dominant hand (alternatively, wrap it around your dominant hand). Pull the sterile glove off over the coiled catheter. Discard the glove containing the catheter in a fluid-resistant receptacle designated by your agency.

Prevents contaminating the environment with secretions.

16. **Don clean procedure gloves** and provide mouth care.

Clears the mouth of secretions and bacteria, which place the patient at risk for hospital-acquired pneumonia.

(continued on next page)

Procedure 37-6 ■ Performing Tracheostomy or Endotracheal Suctioning (Open System) (continued)

17. Using your nondominant hand, clear the connecting tubing of secretions by placing the tip into the container of sterile saline.
Prepares the tubing for later reuse.

18. Turn off the oxygen and suction units.

19. Reposition the patient.
Promotes comfort and prevents skin breakdown.

? What if . . .

■ **The patient has a cuffed tracheostomy tube?**

Check to see that it is properly inflated before suctioning. Usually this is 20 to 25 mm Hg or less, but follow the manufacturer's instructions and use a cuff manometer. See Clinical Insight 37-5 to learn how to check cuff inflation.

Evaluation

■ Assess the color, amount, and consistency of secretions.
■ Evaluate the patient's tolerance of the procedure (e.g., were there signs of respiratory distress during the procedure)?
■ Evaluate the effectiveness of the procedure by comparing breath sounds, vital signs, and pulse oximetry before and after suctioning.

Patient Teaching

■ Teach the patient and caregiver how to perform suctioning if the patient will be discharged with an artificial airway. Have them provide a satisfactory return demonstration.
■ Teach the caregiver strategies for managing the patient's airway at home.

Home Care

■ Provide the family and caregiver information about where to obtain suction equipment, contact information for healthcare personnel who can be reached for advice or emergencies, and information about home oxygen therapy.
■ Guidelines recommend clean technique for home care, and for repeated catheter use as long as the catheter is still clear.
■ Teach the family and caregiver how to clean catheters for reuse (soak in hot, soapy water; rinse inside and out with clean water; air dry; store in a dry container).

Documentation

■ Document the date, time, and reason you performed suctioning.
■ Note the size of the suction catheter you used.
■ Note the amount, color, consistency, and odor of secretions.
■ Document the patient's respiratory status before and after the procedure.
■ Document the patient's tolerance of the procedure.
■ Document any complications that occurred as a result of the procedure, and interventions you made in response.

Practice Resources

Johnston, Davis, & Sherman, n.d.; Kuriakose, 2008; Morrow & Argent, 2008; Rauen, Chulay, Bridges, et al., 2008; Tablan, Anderson, Besser, et al., 2004; Thompson, 2000.

Thinking About the Procedure

 Go to the *Fundamentals of Nursing Skills Videos,* **Oxygenation: Suctioning: Tracheostomy, Portable Open System.**

1. What personal protective equipment did this nurse use?
2. What did the nurse do right after she donned the one clean procedure glove?
3. Did the nurse wear gloves to pour the sterile saline into the sterile container? Why (or why not?)

 For suggested responses, go to Chapter 37, **Thinking About the Procedure Suggested Responses,** on Davis*Plus.*

Procedure 37-7 ■ Performing Tracheostomy or Endotracheal Suctioning (Inline Closed System)

➤ For steps to follow in *all* procedures, refer to the Universal Steps for All Procedures found on the page facing the inside back cover.

Equipment

For the once-a-day steps: Procedure gloves and inline suction catheter
When suctioning: Sterile normal saline

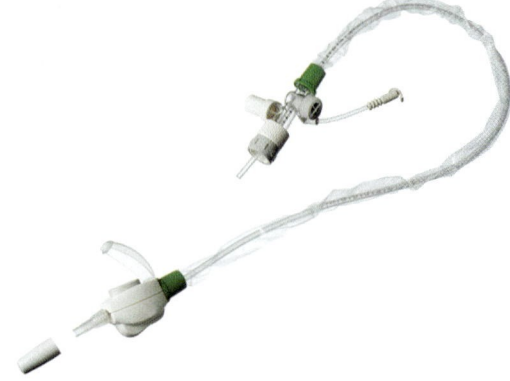

Inline suction catheter © Unomedical a/s, used with permission.

Delegation

As a rule, you should not delegate tracheostomy or endotracheal suctioning to an LPN or NAP, because both procedures require professional-level theoretical knowledge, assessment skills, and problem-solving ability. Refer to the individual state board of nursing for rules on delegating this procedure.

Pre-Procedure Assessment

■ Assess respiratory status, including respiratory rate, depth, and rhythm; breath sounds; color; and pulse oximetry results.

■ Assess for restlessness, cyanosis, labored respirations, decreased oxygen saturation, increased heart and respiratory rates, visible secretions in the airway, and the presence of adventitious breath sounds during auscultation.

These assessments help determine whether the patient requires suctioning. Suctioning should be performed only when necessary to prevent unnecessary oxygen desaturation and tissue trauma.

➤ When performing the procedure, always identify your patient according to agency policy and be attentive to standard precautions, hand hygiene, patient safety and privacy, body mechanics, and documentation

---

Daily Procedure Steps

You need to perform these steps only once per day:

1. Prepare the equipment. An inline suction unit is available only for patients using a mechanical ventilator.
2. Open the inline suction catheter package, using sterile technique.
3. Remove the adapter on the ventilator tubing.
4. Attach the inline suction catheter equipment to the ventilator tubing.
5. Reconnect the adapter on the ventilator tubing.
6. Attach the other end of the inline suction catheter to the connection tubing placed to suction.

Suctioning Procedure Steps

1. **Place the patient in semi-Fowler's** position, unless contraindicated, and don clean procedure gloves. Place a linen-saver pad or towel on the patient's chest.
   The suction catheter is contained within a sterile unit, so you do not need to wear sterile gloves.
2. **If a lock is present** on the suction control port, unlock it.
3. **Turn on the wall suction** or portable suction machine, and adjust the pressure regulator according to agency policy or provider's prescription.
   Using the appropriate pressure prevents tissue trauma and ensures successful suctioning.

4. **Pick up the catheter** with your dominant hand and use your non-dominant hand for the suction port.
   Using the dominant hand improves dexterity.
5. **Unlock the inline catheter** and gently insert the suction catheter into the airway by maneuvering the catheter within the sterile sleeve.▼

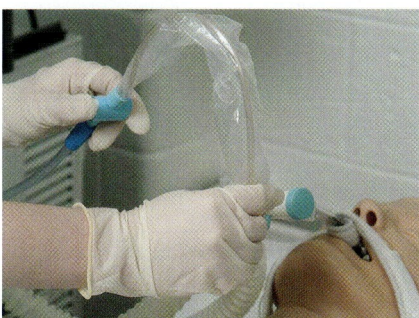

6. ✚ **Advance the suction catheter** into the airway, being careful not to force the catheter. Ask the patient to take slow, deep breaths if she can cooperate. Advance the catheter to the predetermined and premarked distance. Do not apply suction while advancing.
   Forcing the catheter during insertion may cause airway trauma.
7. **Apply suction** by depressing the button over the suction control port as you withdraw the catheter. Apply suction for no longer than 15 seconds.
   Applying suction for longer than 15 seconds causes hypoxia and may cause tissue trauma.

8. ✚ **Withdraw the inline suction catheter** completely into the sleeve. The indicator line on the catheter should appear through the sleeve.
   The indicator line is a safety mechanism designed to make sure the suction catheter is withdrawn completely to prevent airway obstruction.
9. **Attach the prefilled, 10-mL container** of normal saline solution to the saline port located on the inline equipment.
10. **Squeeze the 10-mL container** while applying suction.
    Clears the catheter of secretions, preparing the catheter for repeat use. If allowed to remain in the catheter or suction line, secretions may dry and harden, reducing line suction efficiency.
11. **Lock the suction regulator port.**
    Prevents you from inadvertently applying suction.

? What if . . .

■ **The patient experiences a dysrhythmia?**

Stop suctioning and hyperoxygenate the patient. If a further attempt at suctioning promotes a dysrhythmia, notify the medical care provider.

For Evaluation, Patient Teaching, and Documentation, see Procedure 37-6. Typically, you would not be doing inline suctioning in the home.

Practice Resources

Cleveland Clinic, 2009; Kuriakose, 2008; Morrow & Argent, 2008; National Institutes of Health (NIH), 2000.

Procedure 37–8 ■ Performing Orotracheal and Nasotracheal Suctioning (Open System)

➤ For steps to follow in *all* procedures, refer to the Universal Steps for All Procedures found on the page facing the inside back cover.

Equipment

- Portable or wall suction device with connection tubing and a collection canister
- Linen-saver pad or towel
- Sterile, flexible, multiple-eyed suction catheter kit (12 to 18 Fr for adults, 8 to 10 Fr for children, and 5 to 8 Fr for infants). If a kit isn't available, collect the following: sterile gloves, sterile suction catheter of the appropriate size, and a sterile container
- Sterile gloves
- Pour-bottle of sterile water or normal saline solution
- Sterile basin or other container for fluids
- Face shield or goggles and gown
- Water-soluble lubricant for NT suctioning
- Sputum trap, if a specimen is needed
- Nasopharyngeal airway when frequent NT suctioning is required
- Resuscitation bag with mask

Delegation

You should not delegate orotracheal and nasotracheal suctioning to an LPN or NAP, because these procedures require professional-level theoretical knowledge, assessment skills, and problem-solving ability.

Pre-Procedure Assessment

- Assess respiratory status, including respiratory rate, depth, and rhythm; breath sounds; skin color; and pulse oximetry results.
- Assess for gurgling sounds during respiration, restlessness, labored respirations, decreased oxygen saturation, increased heart and respiratory rates, and the presence of adventitious breath sounds during auscultation.

  The preceding assessments help determine whether the patient requires suctioning. Suctioning removes oxygen from airways and can cause tissue trauma, so it should be done only when essential (i.e., only when less invasive techniques have proved unsuccessful and when the secretions are causing physiological deterioration and/or distress).

- Assess the effectiveness of the cough.

➤ When performing the procedure, always identify your patient according to agency policy and be attentive to standard precautions, hand hygiene, patient safety and privacy, body mechanics, and documentation.

Procedure Steps

1. Position the patient.

Orotracheal Suctioning

a. Position the patient in semi-Fowler's position, with the head turned to face you.

Nasotracheal Suctioning

b. Position the patient in semi-Fowler's position, with his neck hyperextended, unless contraindicated.

Hyperextending the neck makes it easier to insert the suction catheter. Upright position helps to prevent back strain.

2. Place the linen-saver pad or towel on the patient's chest.

Prevents soiling of the patient's gown during suctioning.

3. Put on a face shield or goggles and gown.

Protects you from contamination with secretions that may splash during suctioning.

4. Turn on the wall suction or portable suction machine, and adjust the pressure regulator according to agency policy. Guidelines from American Association for Respiratory Care (AARC) specify:
Adults: 100 to 150 mm Hg
Children: 100 to 120 mm Hg
Infants: 80 to 100 mm Hg
Neonates: 60 to 80 mm Hg
The suction regulator must be set appropriately to prevent tissue trauma and hypoxia and yet remove secretions effectively.

5. Don a procedure glove and test the suction equipment by occluding the connection tubing. Discard the glove and perform hand hygiene.
Testing the equipment ensures proper functioning before you insert the catheter in the patient's airway.

6. Open the suction catheter kit or, if a kit isn't available, the gathered equipment.

Nasal approach: If you are using the nasal approach, open the

water-soluble lubricant and, preferably, a nasopharyngeal airway.

7. Don sterile gloves. Alternatively, put a sterile glove on your dominant hand and a clean procedure glove on your nondominant hand. Consider your dominant hand sterile and your nondominant hand nonsterile.

Keeping the dominant hand sterile prevents contaminating the upper airways with a nonsterile suction catheter. This is actually a modified sterile suction technique because the catheter enters the trachea via nose or the mouth—which are not sterile. However, take care to keep the catheter free from other contaminants.

8. Pour sterile saline into the sterile container, using your nondominant hand.
Sterile saline will be used to clear the suction catheter of secretions after suctioning.

9. Pick up the suction catheter with your dominant hand, and attach it to the connection tubing, maintaining sterility of your hand and the catheter.

10. **Put the tip of the suction catheter** into the sterile container of normal saline solution, and suction a small amount of normal saline solution through the suction catheter. Apply suction by placing a finger over the suction control port of the suction catheter.

    Lubricates the catheter and helps ensure that the suction equipment is functioning properly.

11. **Ask the patient to take several slow, deep breaths.**

    Taking several slow deep breaths promotes relaxation and helps hyperoxygenate the patient before suctioning.

12. Using your nondominant hand, **remove the oxygen delivery device**, if present.

Oral Approach, Patient Receiving Nasal Oxygen

    a. If the patient is receiving nasal oxygen and you are doing orotracheal suctioning, you do not need to remove the oxygen source.

Nasal Approach, Patient Receiving Nasal Oxygen

    b. Remove the nasal oxygen and place the nasal cannula in the patient's mouth. See Procedure 37-4.

    Placing the cannula in the patient's mouth makes it easier to access the nares for suctioning while still delivery oxygen to the patient (orally).

13. **Premeasure to approximate** the depth you should insert the suction catheter. For adults, insert the catheter about 15 cm (6 in.) for an oral approach and 20 cm (8 in.) for a nasal approach. Be careful not to contaminate the catheter while you measure.

    Prevents trauma at the carina and ensures suctioning of the full length of the trachea.

Oral Approach

    b. Measure the distance between the edge of the patient's mouth to the tip of the ear lobe and down to the bottom of the neck.

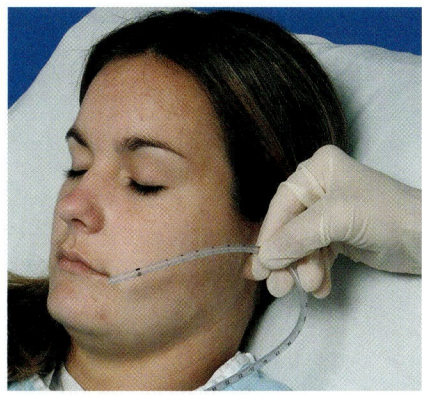

Nasal Approach

    c. Measure the distance from the tip of the nose to the tip of the ear lobe and down to the bottom of the neck.

14. **Lubricate and insert** the suction catheter.

    Lubrication helps prevent irritation of the nares.

Orotracheal Suctioning

    a. Lubricate the suction catheter tip with normal saline solution.

    b. Using your dominant hand, gently but quickly insert the suction catheter along the side of the patient's mouth into the oropharynx.

    Quick insertion along the side of the mouth prevents gagging.

    c. When the patient inhales, advance the suction catheter to the predetermined distance, being careful not to force the catheter.

    Advancing the suction catheter when the patient inhales ensures that the catheter enters the trachea rather than the esophagus. Forcing the catheter during insertion may cause tissue trauma.

Nasotracheal Suctioning

    d. Lubricate the catheter tip with the water-soluble lubricant.

    Water-soluble lubricant will dissolve if it accidentally enters the lungs, whereas an oil-based lubricant (e.g., petroleum jelly) won't dissolve in the respiratory tract and causes complications if it enters the lungs.

    e. Using your dominant hand, gently but quickly insert the suction catheter into the naris and down to the pharynx. When the patient

inhales, advance the suction catheter, gently aiming downward to the predetermined distance, being careful not to force the catheter.

Ensures that the catheter enters the trachea. Forcing the catheter during insertion may cause tissue trauma.

15. **Place a finger or thumb over** the suction control port of the catheter.

    ✚ Apply suction while you withdraw the catheter, using a continuous rotating motion. Apply suction for no longer than 15 seconds.

    Using a continuous rotating motion and suctioning while withdrawing the catheter prevents trauma to any one area of the airway. Limiting suctioning to less than 15 seconds prevents hypoxia. ▼

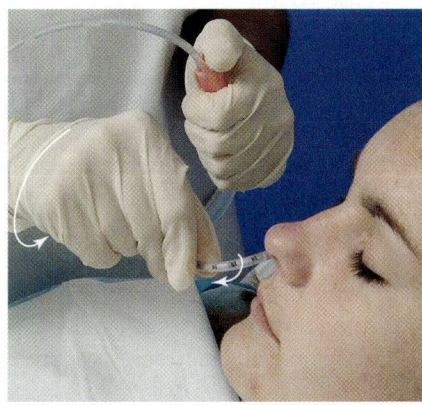

16. **After you withdraw the catheter,** clear it by placing the tip of the catheter into the container of sterile saline and applying suction. ▼

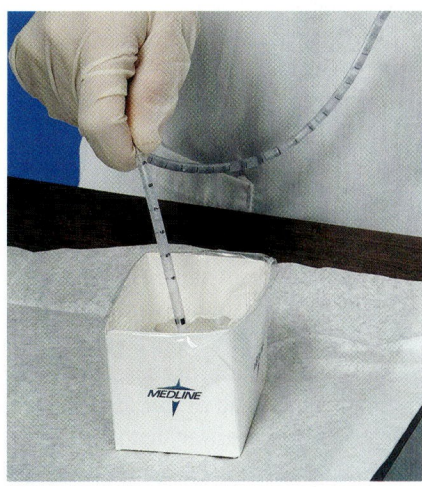

(continued on next page)

Procedure 37-8 ■ Performing Orotracheal and Nasotracheal Suctioning (Open System) (continued)

17. Lubricate the catheter, and repeat suctioning as needed, allowing intervals of at least 30 seconds between suctioning. Reapply oxygen between suctioning efforts, if required.

Several passes with the suction catheter may be needed to clear the airway of secretions. Total suctioning time should be limited to 5 minutes, however, to prevent trauma and hypoxia.

18. Replace the oxygen source.

Prevents hypoxia.

19. Coil the suction catheter in your dominant hand (alternatively, wrap it around your dominant hand). Hold the catheter while you pull the sterile glove off over it. Discard the glove containing the catheter in a biohazard receptacle

(e.g., bag) designated by your agency.

Coiling the catheter inside the glove and using a biohazard receptacle prevent contaminating the environment with secretions.

20. Using your nondominant hand, clear the connecting tubing of secretions by placing the tip into the container of sterile saline.

21. Dispose of equipment, and make sure new suction supplies are readily available for future suctioning.

The patient may require suctioning at any time, so equipment must be readily available.

22. Provide mouth care.

Promotes patient comfort and clears the mouth of any secretions the patient may have expectorated.

23. Position the patient in a comfortable position, and allow him to rest.

Comfort and rest help the patient recover from the stress of suctioning.

? What if . . .

■ **The patient's oxygen saturation is less than 94%, or if he is in any distress?**

Administer supplemental oxygen before, during, and after suctioning. Notify the patient's primary provider if the patient does not respond to additional oxygen.

Evaluation

- Assess the color, consistency, and amount of secretions.
- Evaluate the patient's tolerance of the procedure. Note whether there were signs of respiratory distress during the procedure.
- Evaluate the effectiveness of the procedure by comparing breath sounds, vital signs, and pulse oximetry or blood gas data before and after the procedure.

Patient Teaching

- Explain the importance of administering supplemental oxygen or of taking several deep breaths before suctioning.
- Inform the patient that coughing typically increases with suctioning.
- Demonstrate orotracheal or nasotracheal suctioning to the caregiver, and ask for a return demonstration if suctioning will be required at home.

Home Care

- Instruct the family and caregiver about where to obtain suction equipment.
- Provide the client and caregiver with contact information of healthcare personnel who can be reached for advice or emergencies.
- Explain that the procedure can be performed using clean technique instead of sterile technique in the home.
- Instruct the caregiver that suction catheters can be cleaned for reuse by washing them with soapy water and then boiling them for 10 minutes. After they are cleaned, rinse the catheters with normal saline solution or tap water.

- Teach to change the secretion collection container every 24 hours, or clean it according to home care agency guidelines every 24 hours.

Documentation

- Document the date, time, and reason you performed suctioning.
- Note the suction technique you used and the catheter size.
- Note the color, consistency, and odor of secretions.
- Document the patient's respiratory status before and after the procedure.
- Document the patient's tolerance of the procedure and any complications that occurred as a result of the procedure.
- Document any interventions you performed to address complications that occurred.

Practice Resources

AARC, 2004a; American Thoracic Society and the Infectious Diseases Society of America, 2005; CDC, 2004.

Thinking About the Procedure

 Go to the *Fundamentals of Nursing Skills Videos,* **Oxygenation: Suctioning: Orotracheal, Inline Closed System.**

1. This procedure in your text describes oro- and nasotracheal suctioning by the open method. The video shows orotracheal suctioning using the closed method. Why do you think the closed method was used for this patient?

 For suggested responses, go to Chapter 37, **Thinking About the Procedure Suggested Responses,** on *DavisPlus.*

Procedure 37-9 ■ Performing Upper Airway Suctioning

➤ For steps to follow in *all* procedures, refer to the Universal Steps for All Procedures found on the page facing the inside back cover.

Equipment

- Portable or wall suction device with connection tubing and a collection canister
- Linen-saver pad or towel
- Sterile suction catheter kit (12 to 18 Fr for adults, 8 to 10 Fr for children, and 5 to 8 Fr for infants). If a kit isn't available, collect the following: sterile suction catheter of the appropriate size, and a sterile container. If you plan to suction both the oropharynx and the nasopharynx, you need a separate sterile catheter for each.
- Yankauer device can be used for oropharyngeal suction.
- Pour-bottle of sterile normal saline solution
- Sterile basin or other container for fluids
- Face shield or goggles and gown
- Procedure gloves
- Water-soluble lubricant for nasopharyngeal suctioning
- Sputum trap, if a specimen is needed
- Biohazard bag

Delegation

Do not delegate oropharyngeal and nasopharyngeal suctioning to an LPN or NAP, because these procedures require professional-level theoretical knowledge, assessment skills, and problem-solving ability. However, the NAP (and the client or family) can use a Yankauer tube to suction the oral cavity because there is less risk for trauma to mucosa than with oro- or nasopharyngeal suctioning.

Pre-Procedure Assessment

- Assess respiratory status, including rate, depth, and rhythm; breath sounds; color; and pulse oximetry results. Note signs that indicate the need for suctioning: restlessness, cyanosis, labored respirations, decreased oxygen saturation, increased heart and respiratory rates, visible secretions in the airway, and the presence of adventitious breath sounds during auscultation.

You must be certain the patient requires suctioning. Suctioning should be performed only when necessary to prevent unnecessary oxygen desaturation and tissue trauma.

➤ When performing the procedure, always identify your patient according to agency policy and be attentive to standard precautions, hand hygiene, patient safety and privacy, body mechanics, and documentation.

➤ NOTE: This procedure describes modified sterile technique: sterile supplies with clean procedure gloves. Although the oropharynx and nasopharynx are not sterile, you should keep the suction catheter free from other contaminants as much as possible. Some facilities do use sterile gloves for this procedure.

Procedure Steps

1. **Position the patient**. Explain that suctioning may stimulate coughing or gagging, but that coughing helps mobilize secretions.

Oropharyngeal Suctioning
Position the patient in a semi-Fowler's or high Fowler's position, with his head turned toward you.
This position facilitates insertion of the suction catheter and prevents straining your back. It also promotes lung expansion and effective coughing.

Nasopharyngeal Suctioning
Position the patient in semi-Fowler's or high Fowler's position with his neck hyperextended, unless contraindicated.

2. **Place the linen-saver pad** or towel on the patient's chest.
Prevents soiling of the patient's gown during suctioning.

3. **Put on a face shield or goggles and gown.**
Protects you from contamination with secretions that may splash during suctioning. Not all guidelines specify wearing a gown for this procedure.

4. **Turn on the wall suction** or portable suction machine, and adjust the pressure regulator according to agency policy, typically:
Adults: 100 to 150 mm Hg
Children: 100 to 120 mm Hg
Infants: 50 to 95 mm Hg
The suction regulator must be set appropriately to prevent tissue trauma and hypoxia and to function effectively to remove secretions. Higher pressures are associated with hypoxemia, tissue trauma, and atelectasis, yet do not improve removal of secretions.

5. **Test the suction equipment** by occluding the connection tubing.
Testing the equipment ensures proper functioning before use.

6. **Open the suction catheter kit** or the gathered equipment. If you are using the nasal approach, open the water-soluble lubricant.

7. **Don procedure gloves**; consider (and keep) your dominant hand clean; consider your nondominant hand to be contaminated.
This is not a sterile suction procedure but care should be taken to keep the suction catheter free from other contaminants. Keeping the dominant hand clean prevents contaminating the upper airways with an unclean suction catheter.

8. **Pour sterile saline** into the sterile container, using your nondominant hand.
Sterile saline is necessary to clear the suction catheter of secretions after suctioning. The outside of the saline container is not sterile; it would contaminate your dominant hand.

(continued on next page)

Procedure 37–9 ■ **Performing Upper Airway Suctioning** (continued)

9. **Pick up the suction catheter** with your dominant hand, and use your other hand to hold the connection tubing (to suction) while you attach it.

10. **Put the tip of the suction catheter** into the sterile container of normal saline solution, and suction a small amount of normal saline solution through the suction catheter. Apply suction by placing a finger over the suction control port. When using a Yankauer-type device, the suction is continuous and there is no port to occlude.
Ensures that the suction equipment is functioning properly. If you need to see a Yankauer device, see Figure 37-8.

11. **Approximate the depth** to which you will insert the suction catheter.

Oropharyngeal Suctioning
Measure the distance between the edge of the patient's mouth and the tip of the patient's ear lobe.
Determines the proper distance you should insert the suction catheter for oropharyngeal suctioning.

Nasopharyngeal Suctioning
Measure the distance between the tip of the patient's nose and the tip of the patient's ear lobe.
Helps determine the correct distance you should insert the suction catheter for nasopharyngeal suctioning.

12. **Using your nondominant hand,** remove the oxygen delivery device, if present (for nasopharyngeal suctioning only). Have the patient take several slow, deep breaths.
Deep breathing helps to hyperoxygenate the patient and helps prevent hypoxia during suctioning.

13. **Lubricate and insert the suction catheter**.

Oropharyngeal Suctioning
a. Lubricate the catheter tip with the normal saline solution.
b. Using your dominant hand, gently but quickly insert the suction catheter along the side of the patient's mouth into the oropharynx.
Inserting the suction catheter along the side of the mouth prevents gagging.

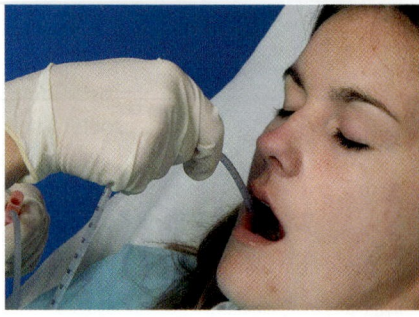

c. Advance the suction catheter quickly to the premeasured distance—usually 7.5 to 10 cm (3 to 4 in.) in the adult—being careful not to force the catheter.
Ensures that the suction catheter will reach the pharynx. Forcing the catheter during insertion may cause tissue trauma.

Nasopharyngeal Suctioning
d. Lubricate the catheter tip with the water-soluble lubricant.
Eases passage of the suction catheter through the naris. Water-soluble lubricant is preferred because it will dissolve if it accidentally enters the lungs, whereas an oil-based lubricant (e.g., petroleum jelly or lotion) will not dissolve in the respiratory tract and causes complications if it enters the lungs.

e. Using your dominant hand, gently but quickly insert the suction catheter into the naris.
Prevents trauma to the naris. ▼

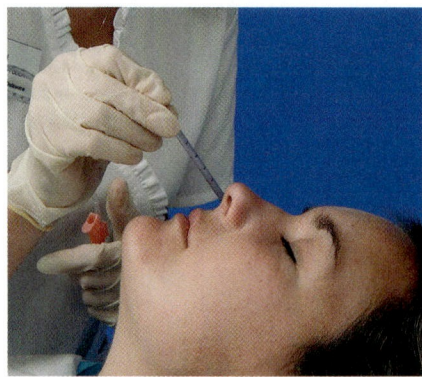

f. Advance the suction catheter, aiming downward to the premeasured distance—usually 13 to 15 cm (5 to 6 in.) in the adult—and being careful not to force the catheter. If you meet resistance, you may need to try the other naris.
Advancing the suction catheter the premeasured distance ensures that

the suction catheter will reach the pharynx. Forcing the catheter during insertion may cause tissue trauma.

14. **Place a finger or thumb over** the suction control port of the suction catheter, and start suctioning the patient. Apply suction while you withdraw the catheter, using a continuous rotating motion.

✚ Limit suctioning to 10 to 15 sec. *Using a continuous rotating motion while withdrawing the catheter prevents trauma to any one area of the airway. Limiting suctioning to less than 10 to 15 seconds prevents hypoxia.*

15. **After you withdraw the catheter,** clear it by placing the tip of the catheter into the container of sterile saline and applying suction.
Ensures patency of the catheter for repeat suctioning.

16. **Lubricate the catheter, and repeat** suctioning as needed, allowing at least 20-second intervals between suctioning. Limit total suctioning time to 5 minutes.
Several passes with the suction catheter may be needed to clear the airway of secretions. The total suctioning time should be limited, however, to prevent hypoxia and trauma to the mucosal membranes.

Nasopharyngeal Suctioning
Each time you repeat suction, alternate nares.
Prevents trauma that would occur if you used only one naris.

17. **Coil the suction catheter** in your dominant hand. Pull the sterile glove off over the coiled catheter. (Alternatively, wrap the catheter around your dominant, gloved hand, and hold the catheter as you remove the glove over it.) Discard the glove containing the catheter in a biohazard receptacle designated by your agency.
Prevents contamination with secretions.

18. **Using your nondominant hand,** clear the connecting tubing of secretions by placing the tip into the container of sterile saline.
Ensures patency and prepares the equipment for future use.

19. Dispose of equipment in biohazard waste container/bag, and make sure new suction supplies are readily available for future suctioning needs. *The patient may require suctioning at any time, so equipment must be readily available.*

20. Provide mouth care. *Promotes patient comfort and clears the mouth of any secretions the patient may have expectorated.*

21. Discard your other glove and remaining supplies.

22. Position the patient in a comfortable position, and allow him to rest. *Promoting comfort and allowing for a period of rest helps the patient recover from suctioning, which may be very tiring.*

? What if . . .

■ **The patient's oxygen saturation is less than 94%, or if he is in any distress?**

You may need to administer supplemental oxygen before, during, and after suctioning. See Procedure 37-4.

Evaluation

■ Assess the color, consistency, and amount of secretions.
■ Evaluate the patient's tolerance of the procedure. Note whether there were signs of respiratory distress during the procedure.
■ Evaluate the effectiveness of the procedure by comparing breath sounds, vital signs, and pulse oximetry before and after the procedure.

Patient Teaching

■ Explain the importance of administering supplemental oxygen to the patient before suctioning.
■ Inform the patient that coughing typically increases with suctioning.
■ Demonstrate oropharyngeal or nasopharyngeal suctioning to the caregiver, and ask for a return demonstration if suctioning will be required at home.

Home Care

■ Instruct the family and caregiver where to obtain suction equipment.
■ Provide the client and caregiver with contact information for healthcare personnel who can be reached for advice or emergencies.
■ Explain that the procedure can be performed using clean technique instead of sterile technique in the home setting.
■ Instruct the caregiver that suction catheters can be cleaned for reuse by washing them with soapy water and then boiling them for 10 minutes. After they are cleaned, rinse the catheters with normal saline solution or tap water.
■ Teach to change the secretion collection container every 24 hours, or clean it according to home care agency guidelines every 24 hours.

Documentation

■ Document the date, time, and reason you performed suctioning.

■ Note the suction technique you used and the catheter size.
■ Note color, consistency, and odor of secretions.
■ Document the patient's respiratory status before and after the procedure.
■ Document the patient's tolerance of the procedure and any complications that occurred as a result of the procedure, with resulting interventions.

Sample documentation:

3/15/14   2200   Resp. labored, rate 28 breaths/min. Pulse oximetry on room air 92%. Breath sounds with rhonchi scattered throughout. Gurgling audible in upper airways. Patient unable to mobilize secretions with coughing. Suctioned by nasopharyngeal route using a 14 Fr. Catheter. Approximately 30 mL thin, tan, odorless secretions obtained. After suctioning, resp. nonlabored, rate 20 breaths/min, and lungs clear on auscultation, with no gurgling audible. Pulse oximetry 96%. Patient tolerated procedure with no difficulty. — C.F. Hiam, RN

Practice Resources

Birmingham East and North Primary Care Trust, 2006); CDC, 2004); Roberts, 2004; Siegel, Rhinehart, Jackson, et al., 2007; Tablan, Anderson, Besser, et al., 2004; Vandenberg, Lutz, Vinson, 1999; Vandenberg & Vinson, 1999.

Thinking About the Procedure

 Go to the *Fundamentals of Nursing Skills Videos*, **Oxygenation: Suctioning, Nasopharyngeal, Open System.**

1. In what position did the nurse place this patient?
2. What did the nurse use to lubricate the suction catheter?

 For suggested responses, go to Chapter 37, **Thinking About the Procedure Suggested Responses,** on *DavisPlus*.

Procedure 37-10 ■ Caring for Patients Requiring Mechanical Ventilation

➤ For steps to follow in *all* procedures, refer to the Universal Steps for All Procedures found on the page facing the inside back cover.

Equipment

- Two oxygen sources
- Air source that provides 50 psi
- Mechanical ventilator
- Humidification device
- Ventilator tubing, connectors, and adaptors
- Condensation collection device
- Inline thermometer
- Resuscitation bag with oxygen connection tubing
- Pulse oximetry device
- Procedure gloves, protective gown, and eye covering
- Sterile gloves and suction equipment, if you will perform suctioning
- Sterile water for the humidifier

Delegation

Care of a mechanically ventilated patient requires advanced knowledge of pulmonary anatomy and physiology and should not be delegated to assistive personnel. In critical care settings, specially trained LPNs may provide care, but the RN is responsible for ensuring that procedures are implemented safely and effectively. RNs also provide ongoing assessment of the patient's ventilatory and oxygenation status. Patients requiring long-term ventilation are often cared for at home or in specialized long-term care units, where LPNs and family members may provide care.

Pre-Procedure Assessment

- Review the health record to make sure that mechanical ventilation is included in the options outlined in the patient's advance directive.
  The patient may not wish to pursue mechanical ventilation as a care option. If a patient who does not wish to be ventilated mechanically is currently on a ventilator, consult your hospital ethics committee.
- If the patient's condition allows, assess his understanding of mechanical ventilation therapy.
  Understanding helps allay the patient's anxiety and promotes cooperation.
- Assess respiratory status, including rate, depth, and rhythm; breath sounds; color; and pulse oximetry results.
  Confirms the need for mechanical ventilation.
- Blood will probably be drawn for an ABG analysis
  To establish a baseline and, after that, to monitor response to therapy.

➤ When performing the procedure, always identify your patient according to agency policy and be attentive to standard precautions, hand hygiene, patient safety and privacy, body mechanics, and documentation.

➤ Refer to Table 37-2 if you need to review ventilator terminology.

Procedure Steps

Initial Ventilator Setup

1. **Prepare the resuscitation bag**.
   The resuscitation bag should be readily available to provide ventilation in the event of an emergency. ▼

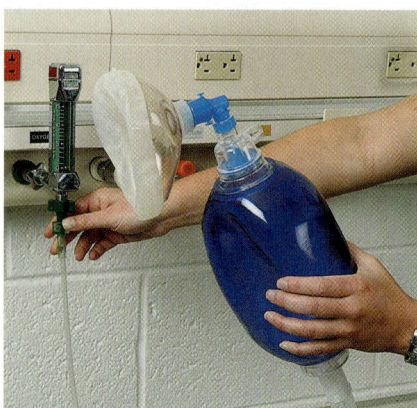

   a. Attach a flow meter to one of the oxygen sources.

   To help regulate and adjust oxygen flow.

   b. Attach an adapter to the flow meter, and connect the oxygen tubing to the adapter.

   c. Turn on the oxygen, and adjust the flow rate

2. **Respiratory therapists** are responsible for setting up mechanical ventilation in most agencies because they are specially trained. If you must assume the responsibility, refer to the manufacturer's instructions.

3. **Plug the ventilator** into a grounded electrical outlet and turn it on.

4. **Verify ventilator settings** and adjust as medically prescribed.
   Ventilator settings must be individualized according to the patient's need for respiratory support. Incorrect settings may cause harm (e.g., hypoxia or barotrauma) to the patient. ➤

5. **Make sure that ventilator alarm** limits are set appropriately.
   Inappropriately set alarm limits can result in harm to the patient.

6. **Make sure the humidifier** is filled with sterile distilled water.

7. **Don gloves, gown, and eye** protection if you have not already done so.

8. **Attach the ventilator tubing** to the endotracheal tube or tracheostomy tube.

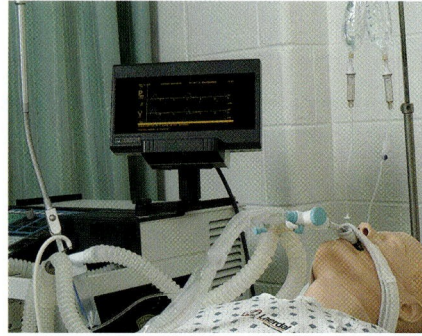

9. **Place the ventilator tubing** in the securing device.

Prevents dislodging the endotracheal tube or tracheostomy when the patient moves.

10. **Attach a capnographic device**, if available.

To measure levels of carbon dioxide. These data are used to confirm placement of the endotracheal tube and disconnection from or malfunction of the ventilator. Oxygen levels alone are not sufficient for the ventilated patient.

11. **Prepare the inline (closed) suction** equipment (see Procedure 37-7).

Suctioning equipment should be readily available when the patient requires suctioning. Closed catheters are recommended to prevent ventilator-associated pneumonia.

After Initial Ventilator Setup

12. **Check respiratory status** and ABGs about 30 minutes after setup. Also check whenever there are changes in the ventilator settings and as the patient's condition indicates.

To be certain the patient is being adequately ventilated and not experiencing oxygen toxicity

13. **Check the ventilator tubing** frequently for condensation. Drain the fluid into a collection device, or briefly disconnect the patient from the ventilator and empty the tubing into a waste receptacle, according to agency policy. ✚ Never drain the fluid into the humidifier.

Condensation in the ventilator tubing can cause resistance to airflow. Moreover, the patient can aspirate it. The fluid should not be drained into the humidifier because the patient's secretions may have contaminated it.

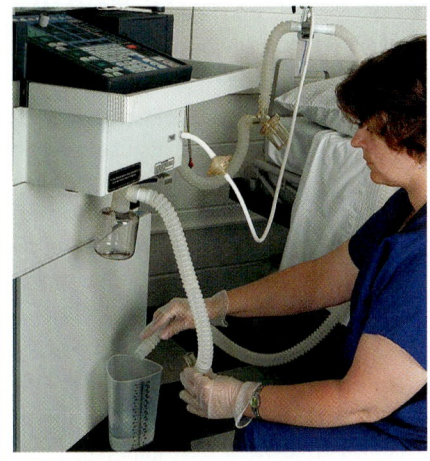

14. ✚ **Maintain the patient in** a semirecumbent position (head of bed elevated 30° to 45°). This is extremely important.

To promote lung expansion, reduce gastric reflux, and prevent ventilator-associated pneumonia.

15. **Check ventilator and humidifier** settings regularly.

16. **Check the inline thermometer**.

To ensure that the air being delivered to the patient is close to the body temperature to prevent scalding of the mucosal tissue or cooling the patient (core temperature).

17. **Provide the patient with** an alternative form of communication, such as a letter board or white board.

A patient being mechanically ventilated is unable to speak, which can produce extreme anxiety. The patient must have a way to express her needs and concerns.

18. **Reposition the patient regularly** (every 1 to 2 hours), being careful not to pull on the ventilator tubing.

Repositioning protects skin integrity. However, pulling on the tubing creates pain. Patient comfort promotes relaxation, which improves the effectiveness of the ventilator.

19. **Keep the patient's lips moistened** with a cool, damp cloth

and water-based lubricant; and provide regular antiseptic oral care. A recommended regimen includes the following:

- Brush the teeth twice a day.
- Use a soft toothbrush.
- Moisturize oral mucosa and lips every 2 to 4 hours.
- Use a chlorhexidine gluconate (0.12%) rinse twice a day during the perioperative period for patients who undergo cardiac surgery (adult patients).
- Use mouthwash twice a day for adult patients. (AACN, 2007)

Mouth care provides comfort and preserves integrity of the mucous membranes. Patients being mechanically ventilated, even for a short period, are at high risk for developing ventilator-associated pneumonia (VAP). VAP is not uncommon, and it is associated with high mortality rates. This regimen is thought to help prevent VAP.

20. **Make sure the call light is always** within reach, and answer call light and ventilator alarms promptly.

Provides the patient with immediate access to help if a breathing problem occurs; reassures the patient and thus relieves anxiety.

21. **Monitor the tracheostomy tube** for proper cuff inflation (usually 20 to 25 mm Hg); see Clinical Insight 37-5.

22. **Check for gastric distention** and take measures to prevent aspiration.

Aspiration creates high risk for pneumonia.

23. **Clean, disinfect, or change** ventilator tubing and equipment according to agency policy.

There is no good evidence to indicate how often this should be done. Research so far indicates that tubing and equipment should not be "routinely" changed for infection control purposes.

24. **Give sedatives or anti-anxiety drugs as prescribed**.

(continued on next page)

Procedure 37–10 ■ Caring for Patients Requiring Mechanical Ventilation (continued)

Evaluation

- After mechanical ventilation is instituted, assess for chest expansion and auscultate for bilateral breath sounds.
- Evaluate the patient's tolerance of mechanical ventilation. Verify that the patient is being adequately ventilated and that she is breathing in synchrony with the ventilator.
- Auscultate breath sounds every 2 to 4 hours, according to agency policy.
- When monitoring vital signs, count spontaneous breaths as well as those delivered by the ventilator.
- Monitor continuous pulse oximetry, capnography, and ABGs.

Patient Teaching

- Explain mechanical ventilation to the patient and her family. Include information about the alarms they will hear.
- Demonstrate an alternative form of communication to the patient and family.
- When appropriate, explain the weaning process to the patient and family.
- If the patient requires mechanical ventilation after discharge, make arrangements for a home ventilator, and teach the patient and caregiver how to use it.

Home Care

- Consult with your facility discharge planning program and/or case management for discharge plans.
- Explain to the family and caregiver where to obtain a home ventilator, resuscitation bag, and oxygen equipment and what services are available. Make sure they choose a supplier who has 24-hour emergency services available.
- Help the client and caregiver devise a backup plan for ventilating the client in the event of a power failure.
- Tell the caregiver to notify the utility company and area emergency personnel that the client is being maintained on a ventilator at home.

- Instruct the client and caregiver about oxygen therapy and its use, as well as safety measures that they must institute.
- Teach the client and caregiver to clean the ventilator tubing with soap and warm water when it becomes soiled.
- Provide the client and caregiver with contact information of healthcare personnel who can be reached for advice or emergencies.

Documentation

- Document the date and time mechanical ventilation was initiated.
- Note the type of ventilator used and the prescribed settings used.
- Document the client's response to mechanical ventilation, including vital signs, breath sounds, ease of breathing, pulse oximetry, intake and output, skin color, and ABG and chest x-ray results.

Sample documentation:

02/26/14   0800   Patient found difficult to arouse. Dr. Henry made aware. ABG obtained; results included: pH 7.28; PCO_2 78 mm Hg; PO_2 48 mm Hg. Dr. Henry in to evaluate patient. Anesthesia called to intubate patient. Medicated with Versed 5 mg IV and intubated orally with a 7.5 Fr. ET tube. Placed on mechanical ventilator: TV 700 mL; FiO_2 80%, respiratory rate 14 breaths/min. Portable chest x-ray confirms ideal placement of ET tube as well as white-out of both lung fields. ABGs to be obtained in 30 min. Pulse oximetry 90% since being placed on ventilator. —————
———————————————— L. Biello, RN

Practice Resources

AACN, 2007, 2008; Bozyk & Hyzy, 2008; Coffin, Klompas, Classen, et al., 2008; Maselli & Restrepo, 2011; Munro, Grap, Jones, et al., 2009; Tablan, Anderson, Besser, et al., 2004; Thille, Rodriguez, Cabello, et al., 2006.

Procedure 37–11 ■ Setting Up Disposable Chest Drainage Systems

➤ For steps to follow in *all* procedures, refer to the Universal Steps for All Procedures found on the page facing the inside back cover.

Equipment

- Two disposable drainage systems
- Chest tube insertion kit (common tube size for adults is 36 Fr). Should contain povidone-iodine, local anesthetic, syringe, needles, drapes, scalpel, suture.
- 5-in-1 or Y-connector for two chest tubes, if not contained in insertion kit
- Sterile water (for water-seal system)
- Two rubber-tipped hemostats
- Sterile gloves, masks, and sterile gowns
- Dressings: sterile 4 in. × 4 in. gauze dressings, precut drain dressings, petroleum gauze dressings, and large drainage dressings
- Tape: 2-in. silk tape, 1-in. silk tape (or nylon banding system)

For disposable dry-seal systems:

- 50-mL syringe and 45 mL of sterile water or saline. Some dry-seal CDUs include these.

Delegation

Some agencies permit only registered nurses in the critical care units to perform dressing changes. The physician must perform dressing changes on other units. You should not delegate this procedure, because it requires advanced knowledge of pulmonary anatomy and physiology. As needed, teach the LPN and NAP how to safely provide care for the patient with chest tubes. Instruct them to notify a registered nurse immediately if the chest drainage system becomes disconnected,

the chest tube becomes dislodged, sudden bleeding occurs, or the patient develops respiratory distress.

Pre-Procedure Assessment

- Ensure that the patient has venous access.
- Assess vital signs.
- Assess indicators of hypoxemia: level of consciousness, orientation, responsiveness, anxiety, and restlessness.

- Assess the patient's knowledge of chest tube therapy. *Understanding helps allay fears and anxiety.*
- Assess cardiac and respiratory status, including respiratory rate, depth, and rhythm; breath sounds; skin color; pulse oximetry and ABG results. *Provides a baseline for comparison after chest tube insertion. Evaluates chest tube functioning afterward.*

> ➤ When performing the procedure, always identify your patient according to agency policy and be attentive to standard precautions, hand hygiene, patient safety and privacy, body mechanics, and documentation.

Procedure Steps

Preparing the CDU

1. **Obtain and prepare the prescribed** chest drainage unit (CDU). ▼

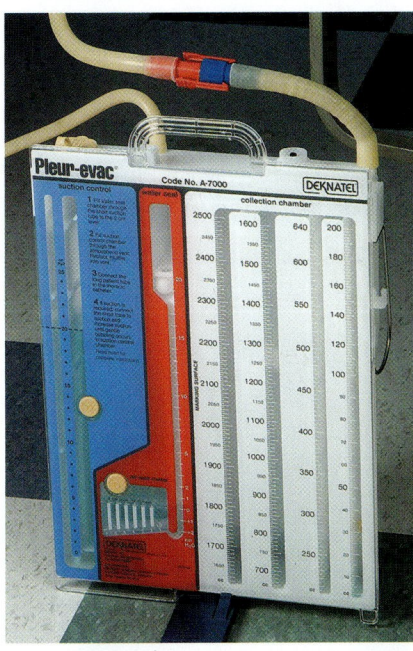

Disposable water-seal system

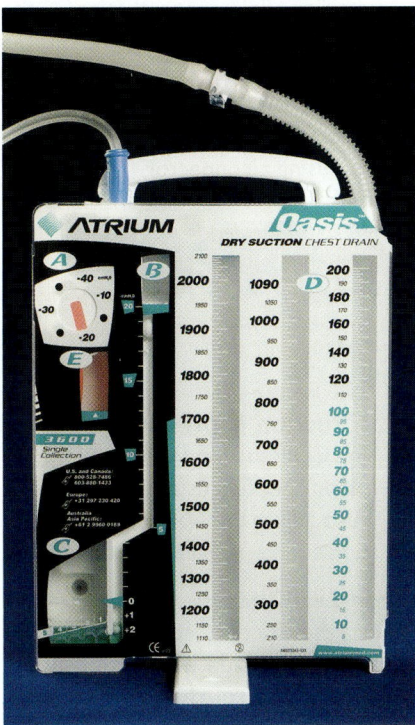

Disposable dry-seal system

Procedure Variation **Disposable Water-Seal CDU Without Suction**

2. **Remove the cover** on the water-seal chamber, and, using the funnel provided, fill the second (water-seal) chamber with sterile water or normal saline. Fill the chamber to the 2-cm mark, or as indicated. (Note that some systems come prefilled.)
   The water-seal chamber allows air to exit from the pleural space during exhalation and prevents air from entering the pleural space during inspiration.

3. **Place the chest drainage unit (CDU) upright,** usually on the floor, and at least 30 cm (1 ft) below the patient's chest level.

4. **Replace the cover** on the water-seal chamber.
   Protects the chamber from contamination.
   Go to step 13.

Procedure Variation **Disposable Water-Seal CDU With Suction**

5. **Remove the cover on the** water-seal chamber, and, using the funnel provided, fill the water-seal chamber (second chamber) with sterile water or normal saline to the 2-cm mark. (Note that some systems come prefilled.)
   The water-seal chamber allows air to exit from the pleural space during exhalation and prevents air from entering the pleural space during inspiration.

6. **Add sterile water or normal saline** solution to the suction control chamber in the amount prescribed, typically 20 cm (7 in.). Place the CDU upright, usually on the floor, and at least 30 cm (1 ft) below the patient's chest level.
   Suction is regulated by the height of fluid in the suction control chamber.

7. **Attach the tubing** from the suction control chamber to the suction source tubing. Turn on the wall (or other) suction source. A wall suction of −80 cm H_2O is common.
   Go to step 13.

Procedure Variation **Disposable Dry-Seal CDU With Suction**

8. **Remove the nonsterile outer** protective bag and the sterile inner wrapper following agency policy.

9. **Place the CDU upright,** usually on the floor, and at least 30 cm (1 ft) below the patient's chest level. Some CDUs have hangers for hanging at the bedside.

(continued on next page)

Procedure 37–11 ■ **Setting Up Disposable Chest Drainage Systems** (continued)

10. **If suction will be required,** attach the tubing from the suction control chamber to the connecting tubing attached to the suction source.

11. **Fill a syringe with 45 mL** of sterile water or saline (follow agency policy and the manufacturer's recommendation for type of fluid), or use the small bottle of sterile fluid in the CDU package. Fill the air leak monitor on the CDU by injecting the fluid via the needleless injection port on the back until it reaches the fill line.

   Once filled, the water may become colored for improved visibility of air leaks. Bubbles in this section of the CDU indicate an air leak.

   Go to step 13.

Procedure Variation **Heimlich Valve**

12. **When a patient has little or no** drainage and does not require suction, the chest tube may be connected to a Heimlich valve instead of a CDU. These valves are attached to the end of the chest tube and allow one-way flow of air out of the chest tube. They contain "flutter" leaflets that allow air to exit but not reenter the pleural space. These valves can also be used for emergency transport until a chest drainage system is available.

   Go to step 13.

Inserting and connecting the chest tube

NOTE: The remaining steps apply to all the preceding variations.

13. **Position the patient** according to the indicated insertion site.
   - For removing air: second intercostal space at the midclavicular line
   - For fluid drainage: on the midaxillary line in the fifth or sixth intercostal space.

14. **Open the chest tube insertion** tray and set up the sterile field. Using sterile technique, drop any necessary supplies on the field (e.g., 4 in. × 4 in. gauze pads, petroleum gauze, syringes).

15. **Don a mask, gown, and sterile gloves,** and organize the supplies you will need for dressing the chest tube insertion site.

   Protective clothing prevents contamination of the surgical site and protects you from splashing.

16. **Provide support to the patient** while the physician prepares the sterile field, anesthetizes the patient, and inserts and sutures the chest tube.

17. **As soon as the chest tube** is inserted, attach it to the CDU tubing, using a connector.

   Usually the nurse holds the nonsterile tubing that leads to the collection chamber and the physician attaches the sterile chest tube to it. Immediately attaching the chest tube to the drainage system prevents air from entering the pleural cavity.

18. **If suction is prescribed,** adjust the CDU suction to the level the clinician specifies, usually –20 cm H_2O. Also adjust the wall (or other) suction source, usually to –80 cm H_2O.

Water-Seal Drainage Unit

Adjust the suction source (e.g., wall suction) until gentle bubbling occurs in the suction control chamber. When the tube is functioning properly, the height of the fluid level in the drainage tube fluctuates with the respiratory cycle.

NOTE: Increasing suction at the suction source increases airflow through the system and creates more bubbling, but it does not increase the amount of suction placed on the chest cavity.

Dry-Seal Drainage Unit

Adjust the CDU suction (e.g., to –20 cm H_2O) by turning the suction control dial on the CDU. Adjust the wall (or portable) suction pressure to –80 mm Hg or greater until the display on the suction-control chamber confirms adequate suction.

Suction Is Not Prescribed.

Leave the suction tubing on the drainage system open to maintain negative pressure. Follow the manufacturer's directions on the CDU, as models will differ.

Dressing the Chest Tube.

19. **When the chest tube** is functioning properly, the clinician will suture it in place. Then don a new pair of sterile gloves. Using sterile technique, wrap petroleum gauze around the chest tube at the insertion site. (Note: Sometimes the physician dresses the site.)

   Petroleum gauze creates a seal that prevents air from leaking around the site. However, continued use of petroleum gauze or ointments can macerate the skin, so they should be used with caution.

20. **Place a precut, sterile split-drain dressing** over the petroleum gauze.

   Absorbs drainage from the insertion site, thereby reducing skin irritation and possible breakdown. ▼

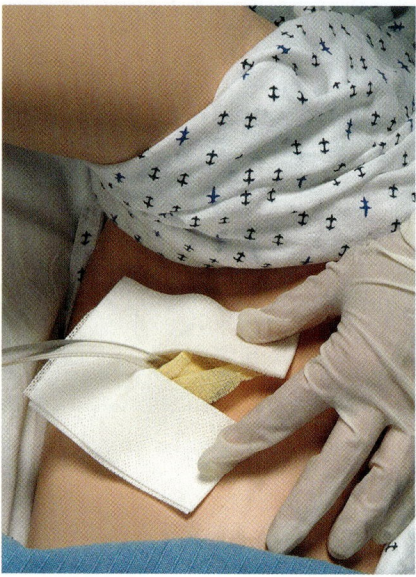

21. **Place a second sterile, precut** drain dressing over the first drain dressing with the opening facing in the opposite direction from the first.

   The second drain dressing helps secure the first drain dressing and provides reinforcement against drainage.

22. **Place a large drainage dressing** (e.g., ABD) over the two precut drain dressings.

   The large dressing covers the insertion site, protecting it from outside sources of infection.

23. **Secure the dressing in place** (e.g., with 2-in. silk tape), making

sure to cover the dressing completely.

Creates an occlusive dressing that protects the chest tube from becoming dislodged and provides a seal over the insertion site, protecting it from outside sources of infection.

24. **Date, time, and initial the dressing.**

Informs other staff members when the dressing change was completed and by whom.

25. ✚ Using the spiral taping technique, wrap 1-in. silk tape around the chest tube, starting above the connector and continuing below the connector. Reverse your wrapping by taping back up the tubing (using the spiral technique) until the wrapping is above the connector. The CDU may come with locking connections or bands; if so, use those.

Ensures a tight connection between the two tubings, thereby preventing an air leak at the connection site. ▼

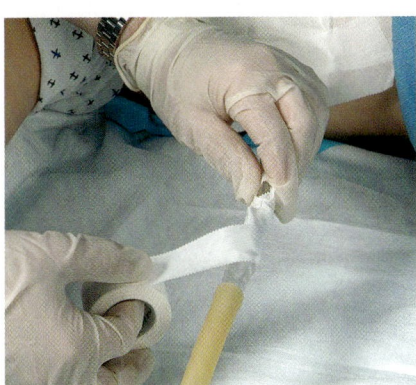

26. **Cut an 8-in.-long piece of 2-in. tape.** Loop one end around the top portion of the drainage tube, and secure the remaining end of the tape to the chest tube dressing.

Prevents pulling at the chest tube site when the patient moves.

27. **Make sure the drainage tubing** lies with no kinks from the chest tube to the drainage chamber.

Facilitates drainage and prevents fluid from accumulating in the pleural cavity. ➤

28. **Prepare the patient for a portable chest x-ray.**

A chest x-ray should be performed after the chest tube is inserted to ensure proper placement.

29. ✚ **Institute safety measures.**

a. Place two rubber-tipped clamps at the patient's bedside for special situations.

Rubber-tip clamps are used to clamp the chest tube to check for an air leak, to change the drainage system, and to assess whether the chest tube can be safely removed.

b. Place a petroleum gauze dressing at the bedside in case the chest tube becomes dislodged.

If the tube becomes dislodged, place a petroleum gauze dressing over the insertion site to prevent air from entering the pleural cavity.

c. Keep a spare disposable drainage system at the patient's bedside.

To use in case the drainage system in use is accidentally upended or the drainage collection chamber becomes filled.

30. **Position the patient** for comfort, as indicated, but with the head of the bed elevated to at least 30°.

- If the patient received a chest tube to relieve a pneumothorax, the preferred position is semi-Fowler's position.
- If the chest tube was inserted to promote fluid drainage, high-Fowler's position is recommended.

31. **Maintain patency** of the chest tube and drainage system. See Clinical Insight 37-6.

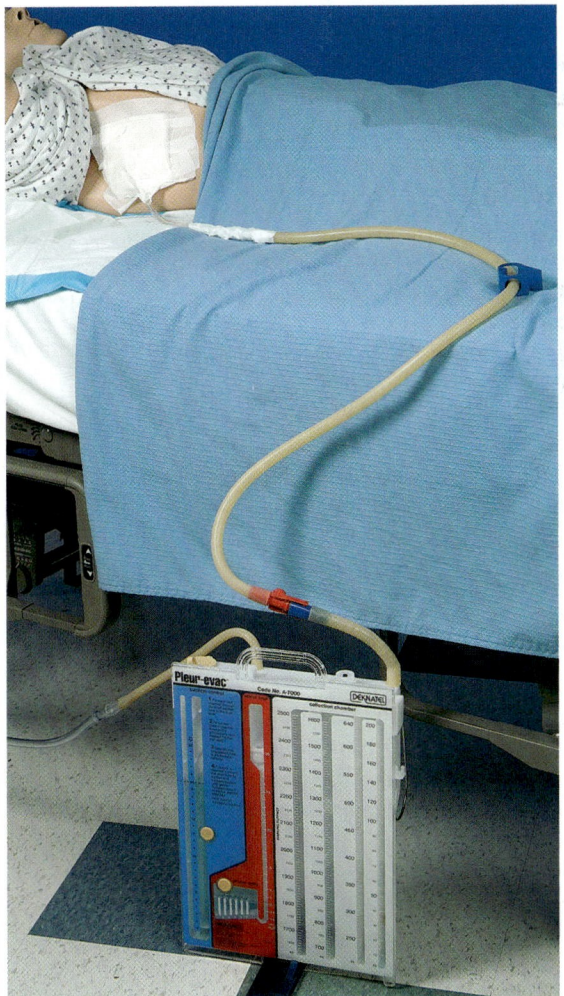

(continued on next page)

Procedure 37-11 ■ Setting Up Disposable Chest Drainage Systems (continued)

Evaluation

- For monitoring and managing chest tubes, refer to Clinical Insight 37-6.
- Evaluate tolerance to the chest tube insertion. Determine whether the respiratory status has changed.
- Auscultate breath sounds every 2 hours.
- Check chest drainage every 15 minutes for the first 2 hours, and then check as prescribed. Observe type, color, and amount.
- Monitor the chest tube insertion site for drainage and subcutaneous emphysema at least every 4 hours.
  Crepitus is a sign that air is leaking into the subcutaneous tissues. Drainage is a sign that fluid is leaking around the insertion site. Both may indicate a compromise in tube patency.
- Confirm chest tube patency and determine whether bleeding is present.
- Monitor intake and output (I&O) every 8 hours.
- Check laboratory values to evaluate blood loss and oxygenation.
- Check the disposable chest drainage system for the presence of an air leak
  An air leak indicates that air is leaking from the chest and a tight seal has not yet formed over the site of injury.

Patient Teaching

- Teach the patient and family about chest tube insertion.
- Explain the importance of immediately reporting chest pain, shortness of breath, or tube dislodgement.

Home Care

- Explain to the client and caregiver how to care for the chest tube at home.
- Provide the client and caregiver with contact information should problems with the chest tube arise.

Documentation

- Assessment findings before, during, and after chest tube insertion (e.g., vital signs, breath sounds, cardiac status, pulse oximetry)
- Date and time of the chest tube insertion
- Name of the clinician who performed the procedure
- The location of the insertion site, the size of the chest tube, the type of drainage system, and the amount of suction applied, if any
- Any medications the patient received during the procedure
- Color and amount of drainage
- Chest tube output on the intake and output portion of the flow sheet (in most agencies)
- Patient's tolerance of the procedure
- Presence of subcutaneous emphysema or air leak, if any
- Complications and any interventions preformed as a result of the complications
- Chest x-ray findings

Practice Resources

Lazzara, 2002; Roman & Mercado, 2006; Siegel, Rhinehart, Jackson, et al., 2007; Tablan, Anderson, Besser, et al., 2004.

Thinking About the Procedure

 Go to the *Fundamentals of Nursing Skills Videos,* **Oxygenation: Chest Tube Care.**

1. What kind of a chest drainage unit was used in this video?
2. What is the first type of dressing the nurse used at the chest tube site?
3. How many sterile precut drain dressings did the nurse use?

 For suggested responses, go to Chapter 37, **Thinking About the Procedure Suggested Responses,** on Davis*Plus.*

 To explore learning resources for this chapter,

 Go to DavisPlus at http://davisplus.fadavis.com/, keyword Treas:

Chapter Resources for Chapter 37:
Knowledge Check and Think Like a Nurse Response Sheets
Knowledge Check Answers
Resources for Caregivers and Health Professionals
Reading More About Oxygenation (Suggested Readings)
What Are the Main Points in This Chapter?
NCLEX-Style Review Questions
Chapter Overview Podcasts

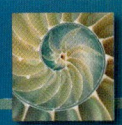

Concept Map

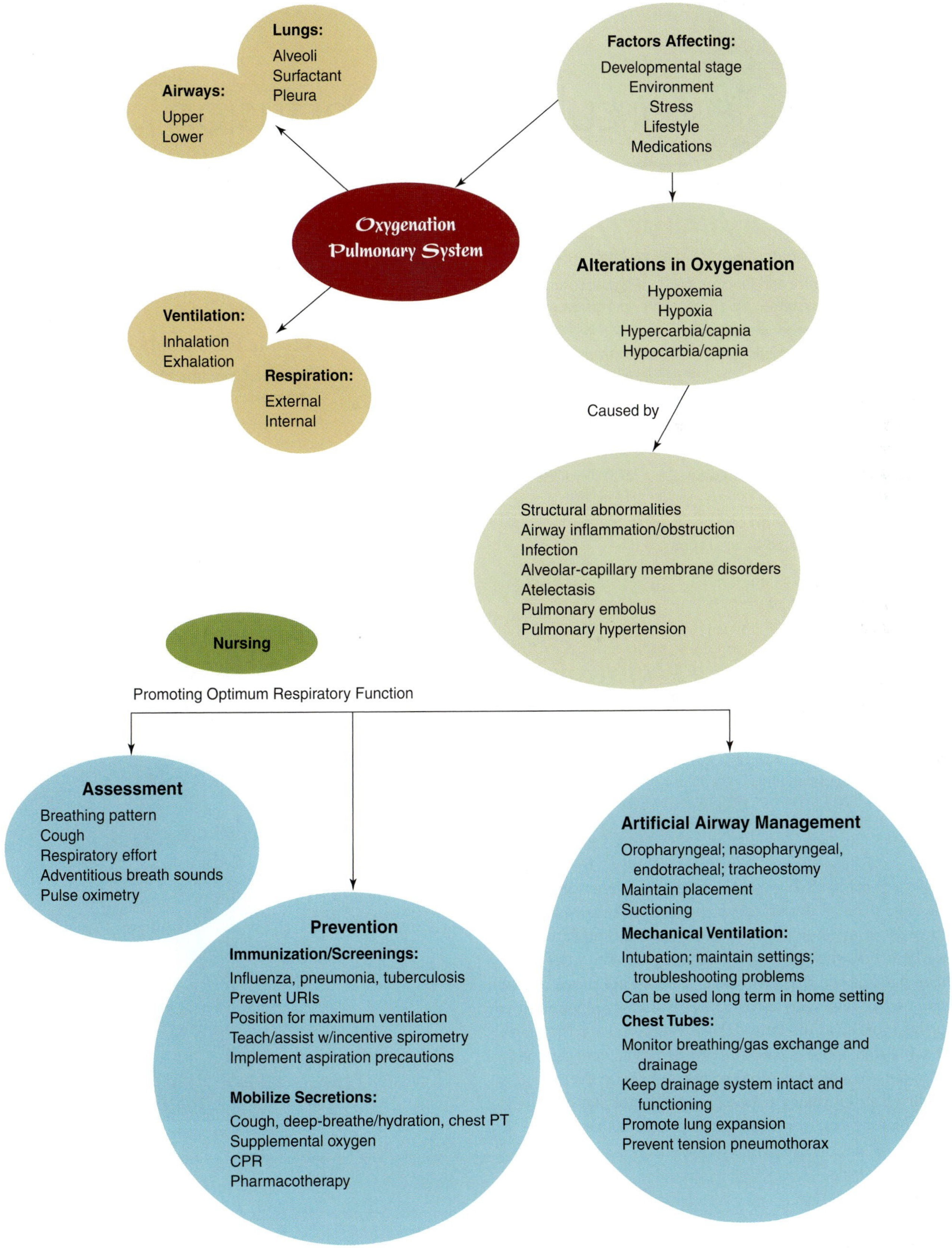

Lungs:
Alveoli
Surfactant
Pleura

Airways:
Upper
Lower

Factors Affecting:
Developmental stage
Environment
Stress
Lifestyle
Medications

Oxygenation Pulmonary System

Ventilation:
Inhalation
Exhalation

Respiration:
External
Internal

Alterations in Oxygenation
Hypoxemia
Hypoxia
Hypercarbia/capnia
Hypocarbia/capnia

Caused by

Structural abnormalities
Airway inflammation/obstruction
Infection
Alveolar-capillary membrane disorders
Atelectasis
Pulmonary embolus
Pulmonary hypertension

Nursing

Promoting Optimum Respiratory Function

Assessment
Breathing pattern
Cough
Respiratory effort
Adventitious breath sounds
Pulse oximetry

Prevention

Immunization/Screenings:
Influenza, pneumonia, tuberculosis
Prevent URIs
Position for maximum ventilation
Teach/assist w/incentive spirometry
Implement aspiration precautions

Mobilize Secretions:
Cough, deep-breathe/hydration, chest PT
Supplemental oxygen
CPR
Pharmacotherapy

Artificial Airway Management

Oropharyngeal; nasopharyngeal,
   endotracheal; tracheostomy
Maintain placement
Suctioning

Mechanical Ventilation:

Intubation; maintain settings;
   troubleshooting problems
Can be used long term in home setting

Chest Tubes:

Monitor breathing/gas exchange and
   drainage
Keep drainage system intact and
   functioning
Promote lung expansion
Prevent tension pneumothorax

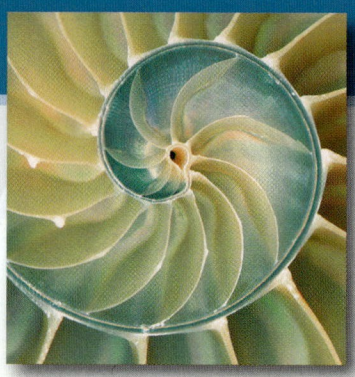

Circulation & Perfusion

Learning Outcome

After completing this chapter, you should be able to:

➤ Describe the structure and function of the cardiovascular system.

➤ Identify individual, environmental, and pathological factors that influence circulation and perfusion.

➤ Assess circulation and perfusion.

➤ Interpret diagnostic testing related to circulation and perfusion.

➤ Develop nursing diagnoses related to circulation and perfusion.

➤ Safely and correctly perform common nursing procedures related to circulation and perfusion.

➤ Evaluate adequacy of circulation and perfusion, and modify nursing activities appropriately based on outcomes.

➤ Provide measures to promote peripheral circulation.

➤ Recognize medications used to enhance cardiovascular function.

➤ Use identified outcomes to evaluate care for patients with circulation problems.

Key Concepts

Circulation

Perfusion

Related Concepts

See the Concept Map at the end of this chapter.

Caring for the Nguyens

This feature allows you to practice the kind of thinking you will use as a full-spectrum nurse. There is usually more than one correct answer to a critical thinking question, so we do not provide answers for these features. It is more important to develop your nursing judgment than to "cover content." Discuss the questions with your peers. If you are still unsure, consult your instructor.

Mai Nguyen, Nam's 76-year-old mother, has been complaining she feels tired all the time, like she just can't do what she normally does. She describes having a hard time catching her breath as she walks up stairs and goes about her day. Nam has noticed that his mother's ankles are more swollen than he has ever seen them. So he schedules an appointment for his mother at the family clinic where you are the nurse. Mrs. Nguyen appears pale and not her usual energetic self. Nam tells you that his mom is "not right" and seems to be confused about things at home, which is not like her. She has a history of chronic congestive heart failure.

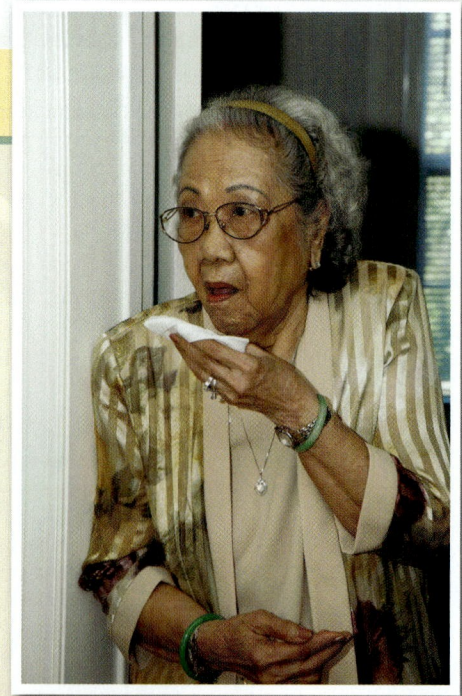

Caring for the Nguyens (continued)

A. What additional health history data would be useful to gather at this time?

B. During her visit at the clinic, you observe that Mai has a cough. She spits a small amount of pink, frothy mucous into a tissue. Mrs. Nguyen's vital signs are as follows: BP, 142/90 mm Hg; pulse, 96 beats/min and with some irregular beats; respirations, 38 breaths/min and shallow; temperature, 97.8°F (36.5°C) oral.
- Which of these symptoms and vital signs is/are not within normal limits?
- For each abnormal finding, explain why you think it is occurring.

C. You decide to include a nursing diagnosis of Acute Confusion in Mrs. Nguyen's plan of care.
- What symptoms does she have that support this nursing diagnosis?

- What physiological changes are causing these symptoms?

D. In addition to angiotensin-converting enzyme (ACE) inhibitor, beta-blocker, diuretic, and digoxin, what additional therapies do you anticipate the physician will prescribe?

E. Mrs. Nguyen asks you, "What can I do to make sure I never get this sick again?" How would you answer this question?

 Go to **Caring for the Nguyens Response Sheet** on Davis*Plus.*

Meet Your Patient

You are scheduled for a clinical placement in urgent care clinic. Your assignment is to (1) perform a focused assessment related to circulation, (2) perform common therapeutic interventions related to circulation, (3) identify desired outcomes and evaluate achievement of those outcomes, and (4) plan for follow-up and home care needs. One of your clients is Ms. Saunders, a 55-year-old accountant. She says she has been extremely tired, easily becomes short of breath, and is unable to complete her chores without frequent rest breaks. She is pale and moves slowly. Her vital signs are as follows: temperature 98.4°F (36.7°C); pulse, 86 beats/min; respirations 24 breaths/min and unlabored; BP 136/78 mm Hg; and pulse oximetry 98% on room air. She is now waiting for her lab results, which include a complete blood count (CBC).

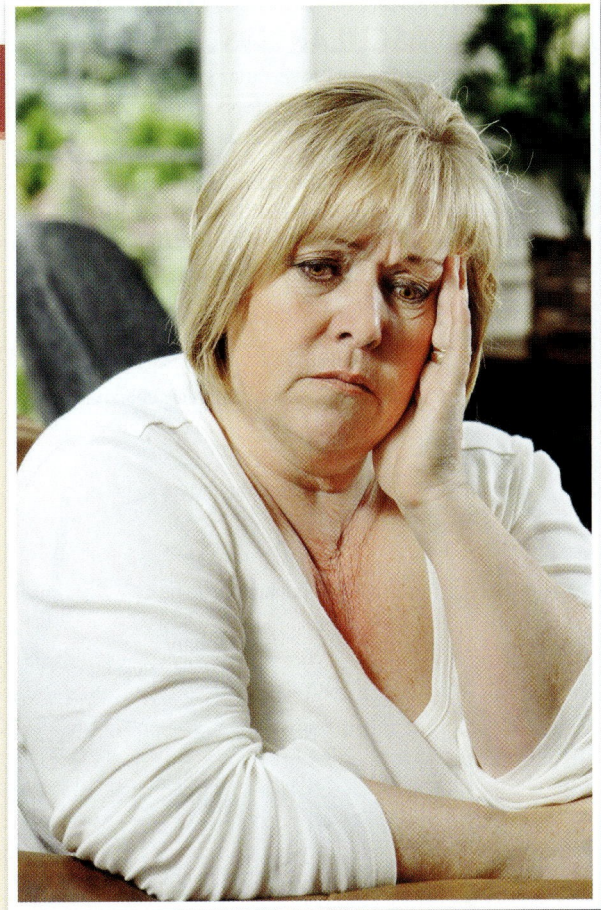

Theoretical Knowledge
knowing why

As you have you have already learned in Chapter 37, the pulmonary, cardiovascular, musculoskeletal, and neurological systems work together to achieve oxygenation. The lungs oxygenate the blood, and the heart circulates the blood throughout the body and back to the lungs. The circulatory system transports oxygenated blood throughout the body to meet physiological needs. We present the pulmonary and cardiovascular systems separately to make learning easier, but remember: the two systems work together. Changes in one system create changes in the other.

Theoretical knowledge in this chapter consists of the structures, functions, regulation, and factors affecting the cardiovascular system its functioning.

ABOUT THE KEY CONCEPTS

The concept of **circulation** refers to flow of blood throughout the heart and blood vessels. **Perfusion** describes blood flow to a capillary bed to provide nutrients and oxygen to tissues and organs. Although the distinction between these two concepts is subtle, they go hand in hand in explaining how a healthy circulatory system contributes to healthy functioning of every organ in the body.

WHAT ARE THE STRUCTURES OF THE CARDIOVASCULAR SYSTEM?

The structures of the cardiovascular system are the heart, the systemic and pulmonary blood vessels, and the coronary arteries.

Heart

The heart is a four-chambered muscular organ encased in the **pericardium** (a sac of connective tissue) located inside the chest cavity. The two thin-walled **atria** receive blood into the heart, and the two thick-walled **ventricles** pump blood out of the heart. Valves between the heart chambers open widely to allow blood to flow easily and without turbulence from one chamber to another, and the valves close tightly to prevent backflow of blood. The **base,** or broadest side of the heart, which houses the atria, faces upward. The **apex,** or tip of the heart, which houses the ventricles, faces downward (Fig. 38-1).

A strong, efficient heartbeat keeps blood flowing through the vascular system. Deoxygenated blood from organs and tissues flows through the venous system into the right side of the heart and then into the pulmonary circulation. At the alveolar–capillary membrane, external gas exchange occurs. The newly oxygenated blood then flows from the lungs into the left side of the heart and out into the arterial circulation.

The Cardiac Cycle

The **cardiac cycle** is the sequence of mechanical events that occurs during a single heartbeat. Very simply, it is the simultaneous contraction of the two atria, followed a fraction of a second later by the simultaneous contraction of the ventricles. The electrical activity of the myocardium regulates the cardiac cycle (Fig. 38-2).

Electrical Conduction

The heart contains specialized areas of nerve tissue that initiate electrical impulses.

- The **sinoatrial (SA) node** acts as the pacemaker. Located in the right atrium, it initiates an impulse that triggers each heartbeat. The impulse travels rapidly down the atrial conduction system so that both atria contract as a unit.
- At the **atrioventricular (AV) node,** there is a slight delay. From the AV node, impulses pass into the left and right *bundles of His* and into the *Purkinje fibers* to the ventricles.

In this way, myocardial fibers are electrically stimulated almost simultaneously to create a unified cardiac muscle contraction strong enough to pump blood out of a heart chamber.

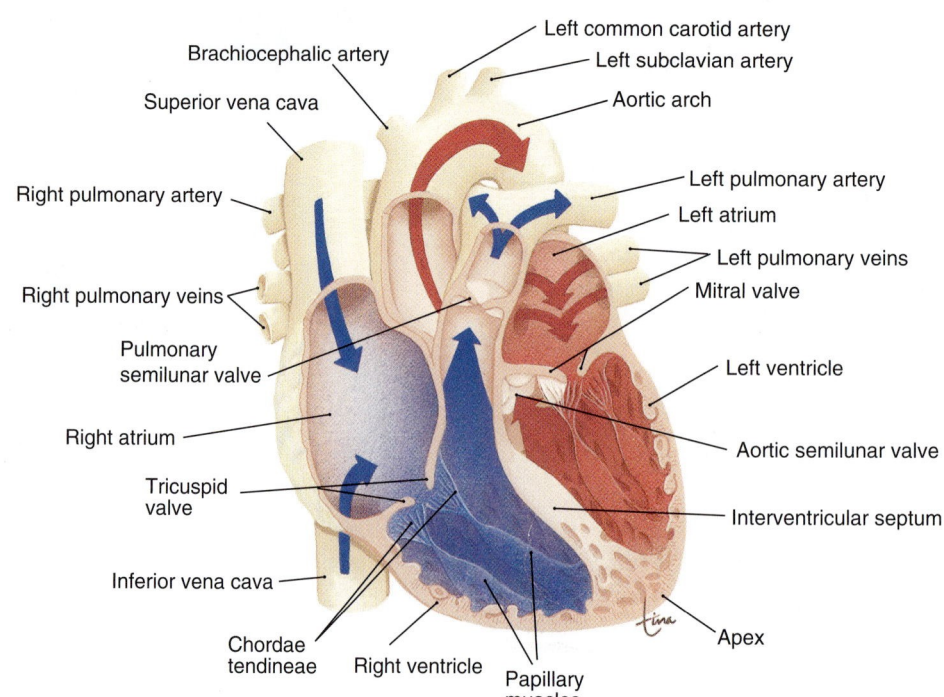

FIGURE 38-1 The atria receive blood into the heart; the ventricles pump blood out of the heart. Valves between the chambers allow blood to flow in one direction from one chamber to another without backflow.

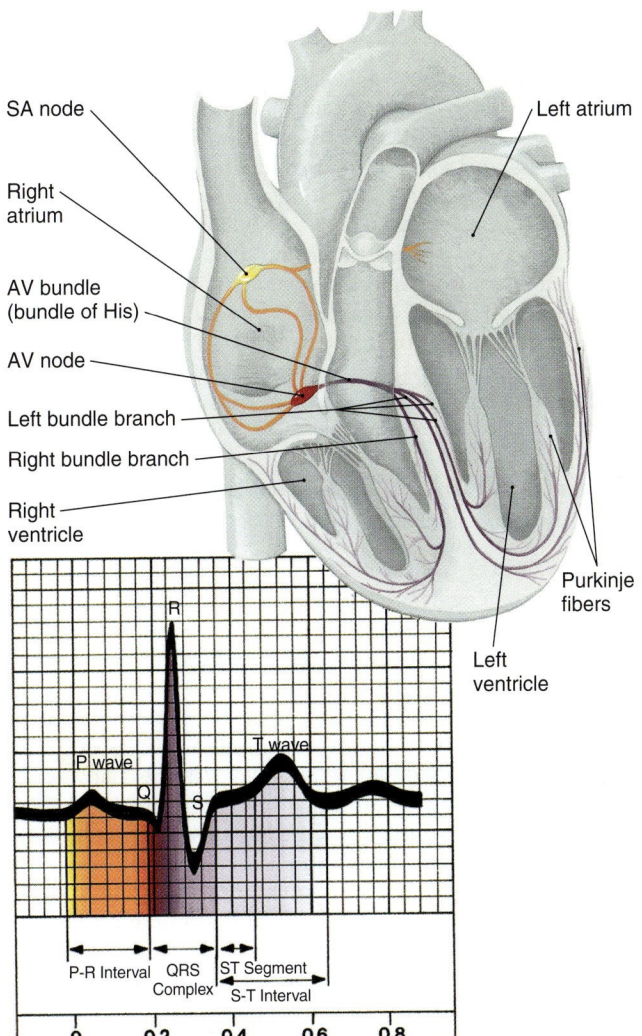

FIGURE 38-2 Conduction pathway of the heart. Anterior view of the interior of the heart. The electrocardiogram tracing is one of a normal heartbeat. See text for description.

This spontaneous rhythm of the heart is called **automaticity.** If there are defects in this electrical system, impulses travel more slowly through the heart and some areas contract before others. This can lead to ineffective heart pumping and decreased cardiac output.

Normally, the SA node initiates a rate of 60 to 100 beats/min, depending on the body's oxygen needs. If the SA node fails, the AV node can take over as the pacemaker, but it generally triggers a slower heart rate. If both the SA and AV nodes fail, the conduction fibers can initiate impulses. Ventricular conduction generates a very slow rate, usually less than 40 beats/min; however, this can be life saving if no other node or fiber is initiating an impulse.

Systemic and Pulmonary Blood Vessels

The vascular system is composed of three types of vessels: arteries and arterioles, veins, and capillaries. All vessels are lined with a smooth endothelial layer that promotes nonturbulent blood flow and prevents platelets from sticking to the sides of the walls and beginning a clot.

- **Arteries** have thick, elastic walls that allow them to stretch during cardiac contraction **(systole)** and to recoil when the heart relaxes **(diastole).**

- **Arterioles** are smaller branches of arteries. They are primarily smooth muscle and thinner than arteries. Under control by the sympathetic nervous system, the arterioles constrict or dilate to vary the amount of blood flowing into capillaries and help maintain blood pressure.

- **Capillaries** are microscopic vessels, created as arterioles branch into smaller and smaller vessels. Because they are only one cell thick, capillaries facilitate the exchange of gases, nutrients, and wastes between the tissue cells and the blood. Billions of capillaries provide blood flow to every cell in the body. Capillaries connect the arterial and venous systems and carry blood from arterioles to venules.

- The **venous system** returns the deoxygenated blood to the heart. **Veins** and **venules** have thin, muscular, but inelastic walls that collapse easily. These walls contract or relax in response to feedback from the sympathetic nervous system: When blood volume is low, the veins contract to provide a smaller space for smaller volume of blood; when blood volume is high, veins relax and enlarge to accommodate increased volume of blood. Think of the venous system as a holding tank for fluctuations in blood volume.

For illustrations of the systemic arteries and veins,

 Go to Chapter 38, **Tables, Boxes, Figures: ESG Figure 38-1** and **Figure 38-2,** on Davis*Plus.*

To see an animated illustration of the circulatory system,

 Go to **Animations, Cardiovascular/Pulmonary Animations: Blood Flow,** on Davis*Plus.*

The Coronary Arteries

The heart has its own blood supply through the coronary arteries (Fig. 38-3). The coronary sinus (not shown), located just above the aortic valve, fills with blood during diastole. From the coronary sinus, blood flows into the two main coronary arteries, which branch into several sections to supply the heart muscle with blood. The coronary arteries are the only arteries in the body that fill during diastole. To see an animated illustration of the coronary circulation,

 Go to **Animations, Cardiovascular/Pulmonary Animations: Blood Flow Through the Heart,** on Davis*Plus.*

KnowledgeCheck 38-1

- Describe oxygenation and perfusion.
- Trace the path of normal electrical impulses in the heart.
- How do the walls of arteries, veins, and capillaries differ?
- What is the importance of diastole to perfusion of the heart?

 ### ThinkLike a Nurse 38-1

Your patient has a condition that has caused the mitral valve to become stiff with only a narrow opening for blood flow. What type of problems related to circulation would you anticipate in this patient?

HOW ARE OXYGEN AND CARBON DIOXIDE TRANSPORTED?

The cardiovascular system circulates oxygenated blood to organs and tissues and returns deoxygenated blood to the heart. Maintaining this blood flow requires adequate circulation and effective regulation of cardiovascular function.

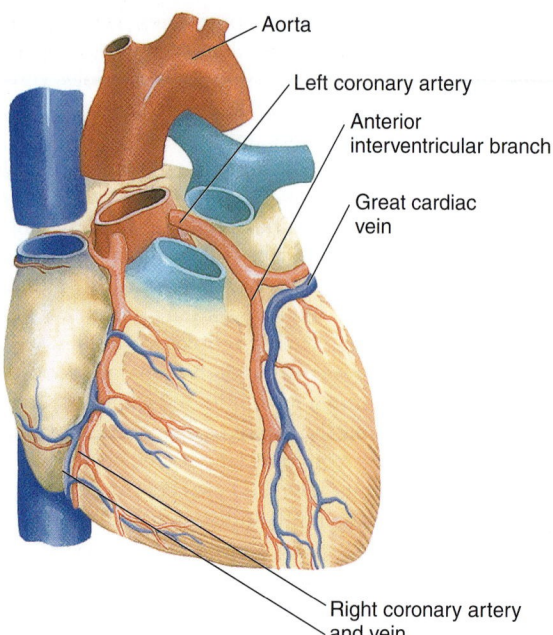

Aorta

Left coronary artery

Anterior
interventricular branch

Great cardiac
vein

Right coronary artery
and vein

FIGURE 38-3 Coronary vessels in anterior view. The pulmonary artery has been cut to show the left coronary artery emerging from the ascending aorta.

A full 97% of blood oxygen is bound to hemoglobin, the iron-containing protein in red blood cells; only 3% is in a dissolved state. At the tissue level, O_2 leaves the hemoglobin, becomes dissolved in the blood, and passes through the capillary membrane into the tissues. Only the dissolved form of O_2 can pass through capillary membranes. Hemoglobin thereby serves as a reservoir for oxygen until it is needed in the dissolved state.

Carbon dioxide is a waste product of normal aerobic tissue metabolism. Carbon dioxide can be carried in the blood in three ways: about 7% of CO_2 is dissolved in plasma, 23% attaches to hemoglobin, and 70% is converted into bicarbonate ions. However, CO_2 diffuses through cellular and alveolar–capillary membranes only in its dissolved state. The CO_2 bound to hemoglobin eventually detaches and becomes dissolved in the plasma for diffusion into the alveoli of the lungs. The bicarbonate ions in the plasma are converted back to CO_2, which becomes dissolved, diffuses into the alveoli, and is exhaled.

To see an animated explanation of CO_2 and O_2 transport,

 Go to **Animations, Cardiovascular/Pulmonary Animations: Carbon Dioxide/Oxygen Transport**, on DavisPlus.

HOW IS CARDIOVASCULAR FUNCTION REGULATED?

Cardiovascular function is regulated by the autonomic nervous system (ANS) and by control centers in the brainstem.

Autonomic Nervous System

The autonomic nervous system regulates cardiovascular function through its influence on cardiac rate and muscle contractility, as well as vascular tone.

Heart. Through branches at the thoracic level of the spinal cord, *sympathetic fibers* stimulate the heart to beat faster and contract more strongly. *Parasympathetic fibers* innervate the heart through the vagus nerve. Parasympathetic stimulation

results in a slowed heart rate, but it does not influence myocardial contractility.

Vascular System. All blood vessels are innervated by *sympathetic fibers* that maintain them in a constant baseline state of partial contraction (**tone**). Vascular tone maintains blood pressure and blood flow even when a person is resting or asleep. Sympathetic stimulation above and beyond baseline tone varies in response to body needs. Increased sympathetic stimulation causes constriction of some vessels (e.g., skin, gastrointestinal tract, and kidneys) and dilation of other vessels (skeletal muscle). This shunts blood flow to the skeletal muscles for a fight-or-flight response. The *parasympathetic nervous system* has no significant control over blood vessels.

For more complete information, consult an anatomy and physiology text. For a brief overview of the nervous system,

 Go to Chapter 37, **Supplemental Materials: The Nervous System,** on DavisPlus.

Brainstem Centers

The brainstem centers integrate feedback from baroreceptors and chemoreceptors in the body to regulate cardiac function and blood pressure. The *vasomotor center* controls sympathetic stimulation of the heart and vascular system. The *cardioinhibitory center* controls parasympathetic slowing of the heart rate.

Baroreceptors. Baroreceptors located in the walls of the heart and blood vessels are sensitive to pressure changes. The aortic arch and carotid artery baroreceptors are particularly important in the regulation of heart rate and vascular tone. When baroreceptors sense even a small drop in pressure, they send messages to the brainstem centers to stimulate the sympathetic nervous system to increase heart rate and induce vasoconstriction. This mechanism allows us to change positions and maintain blood pressure.

Chemoreceptors. Chemoreceptors located in the aortic arch and the carotid arteries are sensitive to changes in blood pH, oxygen levels, and carbon dioxide levels. Their main function is to regulate ventilation, but they also send information to the vasomotor center in response to lack of oxygen. The vasomotor center responds by activating sympathetic stimulation.

If you would like further review of nervous regulation of the heart,

 Go to Chapter 38, **Tables, Boxes, Figures: ESG Figure 38-3,** on DavisPlus.

KnowledgeCheck 38-2

- How are oxygen and carbon dioxide transported in the blood?
- How is the cardiovascular system regulated?
- Does poor peripheral perfusion increase the risk for hypoxemia?

 ThinkLike a Nurse 38-2

You are assigned the care of a 4-year-old girl, Mary, with a history of asthma (Meet Your Patient in Chapter 37). She is receiving a nebulized treatment containing Proventil (albuterol) and Atrovent (ipratropium bromide). These medications stimulate the sympathetic nervous system.

- What cardiovascular side effects can you anticipate?
- How might these side effects affect oxygenation?
- What do you need to know about the patient's history to safely administer the drugs?

WHAT FACTORS INFLUENCE CARDIOVASCULAR FUNCTION?

Similar to respiratory function, cardiovascular function is influenced by developmental stage, environment, lifestyle, substance abuse, medications, and pathophysiological conditions.

Developmental Stage

Normal development influences heart and circulatory function. Developmental factors exert more of an influence on infants and older adults than on young and middle adults.

Infants. Successful transition from life inside the uterus to the extrauterine environment depends on critical physiologic changes that occur at birth. Prior to delivery, the fetus uses the placenta for gas and nutrient exchange. Fetal circulation bypasses the lungs. When the umbilical cord is clamped and the newborn takes the first breath, the resistance in the pulmonary vessels then markedly decreases. The lungs inflate, and blood circulates without shunting as it did during fetal life.

Preschool and School-Age Children. Preschool and school-age children have body systems mature enough to adapt to moderate stress and change, including the heart and circulatory systems. However, children as young as school age sometimes begin social habits, such as tobacco use, that can have long-term adverse effects on the cardiovascular system. A diet with high in fats and sugars contribute to hyperlipidemia and the beginning of plaque lining the walls of blood vessels. Processed foods contain a great deal of salt and fat, which can contribute to high blood pressure and high cholesterol, even in children.

Adolescents. In adolescence, the heart and blood components develop adult characteristics. The average adolescent is developmentally at little risk for heart or circulatory disorders, although some athletes can be at risk for collapse and sudden cardiac dysrhythmia that is familial. New guidelines for health professionals performing sports assessments call for thorough investigation of the family history for fainting, collapse, or sudden death.

Some adolescents adopt behaviors and habits that can create risk throughout life. For instance, about half the adults who use tobacco were regular smokers by their 18th birthday, and 20% of high school students report they had smoked cigarettes on one or more of the 30 days preceding the survey (American Lung Association [ALA], 2011; Centers for Disease Control and Prevention [CDC], 2008). Childhood obesity is also rising to epidemic levels in the United States. As a result, some adolescents exhibit signs of cardiovascular disease (e.g., high blood levels of lipids and cholesterol, a known factor in the development of high blood pressure, heart disease, and blockages in the arteries of the heart).

Young and Middle Adults. Lifestyle in young and middle adulthood can create cardiac risk factors. Some adults become "too busy" to prepare and eat nourishing foods, or more often simply prefer the taste of high-fat, high-sugar foods. A sedentary lifestyle, lack of aerobic exercise, and tobacco use also contribute to cardiovascular disorders in this group. Crack cocaine and methamphetamine abuse can lead to sudden cardiac failure. Family history of cardiovascular disease is yet another risk factor for this age group.

Older Adults. Cardiac efficiency gradually declines as the heart muscle loses contractile strength and heart valves become thicker and more rigid. The peripheral vessels become less elastic, which creates more resistance to ejection of blood from the heart. As a result of these changes, the heart becomes less able to respond to increased oxygen demands, and it needs longer recovery times after responding. For example, in response to exercise, an older adult's heart rate does not increase as much as a younger person's, but it does remain elevated longer. Thus, older adults have lower exercise tolerance, need more rest after exercise, and are more prone to orthostatic hypotension. Keep in mind, though, that endurance training and regular exercise slow the rate of these changes. In fact, an older person who is physically conditioned by regular exercise may have better heart and circulatory function than a younger adult who is not well conditioned.

Environment

Environmental factors, such as stress, allergic reactions, altitude, and temperature, affect cardiovascular function.

Stress. The stress response stimulates *release of catecholamines* from the sympathetic nervous system. This results in increased heart rate and contractility, vasoconstriction, and increased tendency of blood to clot. Sustained stimulation of the sympathetic nervous system can lead to cardiovascular disease. In addition, a chronically suppressed immune and inflammatory response increases the risk for all infections. For additional information on the effects of stress, see Chapter 12.

Allergic Reactions. An **allergy** is a hypersensitivity, or over-response, to an antigen. Inflammatory substances released during an allergic response (e.g., histamine, protease) cause the following cardiovascular events:

- Blood vessels dilate in areas affected (which increases blood flow to the areas).
- Eosinophils and neutrophils are attracted to the reaction site.
- Local tissues are damaged by protease.
- Capillaries become more permeable, resulting in fluid leak into tissues.
- Local (e.g., vascular) smooth muscle cells contract.

Altitude. Oxygen pressure falls proportionally with increased altitude (to review, refer to Chapter 37), making more oxygen available in the alveoli and at the tissue level. Over the long term, people who live at high altitudes undergo physiological changes that facilitate oxygenation. Among the cardiopulmonary changes are the following:

- Increased production of red blood cells (RBCs)
- Increased vascularity of body tissues
- Increased ability of tissue cells to use oxygen even when atmospheric oxygen pressure is low

Heat and Cold. Heat generally causes vasodilation, which increases cardiac output and oxygenation. However, heat also increases metabolism. As a result, people are naturally more sedentary in hot weather.

Cold slows cell metabolism, reducing O_2 demand. It also causes vasoconstriction, and slows the heart rate. Induced hypothermia is used in some surgical procedures. As another example, victims of cold-water near drowning have been revived after long periods of time, in part because of the reduced O_2 demands associated with hypothermia. Prolonged exposure to cold causes frostbite, loss of hypothalamic temperature regulation, and death.

Lifestyle

Lifestyle factors that affect cardiovascular function include pregnancy, nutrition, obesity, exercise, tobacco use, and substance abuse.

Pregnancy. During pregnancy, oxygen demand increases dramatically, due to the needs of the fetus and an approximate 15% increase in maternal metabolism during the last half of

pregnancy. To compensate, the mother's blood volume increases by 30%. The woman requires additional iron to produce this blood as well as to meet fetal requirements. Failure to meet these iron demands can result in maternal anemia, reducing tissue oxygenation to the mother and fetus.

Nutrition. The body needs an appropriate balance of proteins, carbohydrates, fats, and other nutrients for proper immune function, resistance to disease and infection, normal cellular function and tissue repair, and maintenance of a healthy weight. A diet high in saturated fat predisposes to the development of atherosclerosis, coronary artery disease, and hypertension, all of which can compromise circulation and oxygenation. A low-fat, low-cholesterol, low-sodium diet is considered "heart healthy." Vitamins, minerals (especially iron), and protein are important to prevent anemia, which reduces blood-oxygen–carrying capacity. Green tea consumption has been associated with reduced mortality due to cardiovascular disease (Kuriyama, Shimazu, Ohmori, et al., 2007).

Obesity. Obesity is a body mass index (BMI) above 30 (see Chapter 28). Obesity causes multiple health problems, many of which affect the heart and circulation. Obesity increases the risk of developing atherosclerosis and hypertension. Excess fat stores in and around the heart itself reduce its effectiveness as a pump. At the same time, the workload of the heart is increased by the need to perfuse the excess body tissues.

Exercise. Exercise improves blood circulation and delivery of oxygen to tissues and cells. It also increases metabolic demands. The body responds by increasing the heart rate and the rate and depth of breathing. Like skeletal muscles, the heart muscle is strengthened with regular aerobic exercise. As the heart becomes stronger, it becomes a more efficient pump. As a result, resting heart rate is slower because a higher heart rate is not required to maintain cardiac output. Lack of exercise has the opposite effect. A sedentary lifestyle reduces the efficiency of the heart and the capacity to increase ventilation in response to exercise.

Tobacco Use. Tobacco use is a major risk factor in several chronic cardiovascular conditions: stroke, peripheral arterial disease, aortic aneurysm, and heart disease. Smoking has been shown to cause atherosclerosis (fatty buildups in the arteries), hypertension, and decreased high-density lipoprotein (HDL) (good) cholesterol—all of which lead to coronary heart disease and heart attack. The risk of coronary artery disease is four times higher in cigarette smokers than non-smokers. Cigarette smoking doubles a person's risk for stroke. Older adults who smoke have a 73% higher chance of developing heart failure than non-smokers. Former smokers' risks are related to how long they have smoked. Even light smoking increases the risk of sudden cardiac death. Cigar and pipe smoking are also implicated, but not to the extent of cigarettes (American Heart Association [AHA], 2011a).

Substance Abuse. People can abuse many substances, include over-the-counter (OTC) and prescription medications, commonly available commercial products, and illegal substances. Large amounts of alcohol depress respiratory, cardiac, and vasomotor centers of the brain. Chronic alcohol abuse causes fatty infiltration of the heart muscle, thrombi in the coronary arteries, heart enlargement, and dysrhythmias, all of which can ultimately lead to heart failure. Illicit drugs, including stimulants (e.g., methamphetamine, cocaine), hallucinogens [e.g., LSD (acid), mescaline (buttons)], and cannabinoids (e.g., marijuana) also have adverse effects on the cardiovascular system. For example, cocaine has been linked to myocardial dysfunction, dysrhythmias, endocarditis, and aortic dissection.

Medications

Various types of medication are used therapeutically to improve cardiac output and tissue oxygenation. They act to slow the heart rate or reduce the force of myocardial contraction; ease the workload of the heart; dilate blood vessels and reduce blood pressure in the pulmonary circulation and systemically; rid the body of excess fluid accumulation; and block abnormal heart rhythms (AHA, 2011c). See Table 38-1.

For a more complete discussion of medications,

 Go to Chapter 38, **Supplemental Materials: Cardiovascular Medications,** on Davis*Plus.*

KnowledgeCheck 38-3

- What changes occur in the cardiovascular system with aging?
- How does smoking affect the cardiovascular system?

Pathophysiological Conditions

Alterations in circulation and perfusion at the tissue or cellular level may be life threatening, particularly when hypoxemia and acidosis occur. Refer to Chapter 37 to review the effect of poor oxygenation on body systems.

Cardiovascular Abnormalities

Alterations in gas exchange are caused by a number of disorders that affect the structure, function, and regulation of the cardiovascular system. Cardiovascular abnormalities interfere with the flow of oxygenated blood to organs and tissues. Major abnormalities are as follows:

- **Heart failure** occurs when the heart becomes an inefficient pump and is unable to meet the body's demands. Blood is oxygenated when it passes through the lungs, but it is not well circulated to the organs and tissues. Impaired circulation leads to systemic and pulmonary edema, which further impairs gas exchange.
- **Cardiomyopathy** is a heart muscle disorder that results in heart enlargement and impaired cardiac contractility.
- **Cardiac ischemia** occurs when oxygen requirements of the heart are unmet. Prolonged ischemia leads to myocardial infarction (MI) as parts of the heart *necrose* (die) from inadequate oxygen. **Angina pectoris** is transient chest pain due to myocardial ischemia. The tissue becomes injured but does not necrose.
- **Coronary artery disease,** a leading cause of cardiac ischemia, is a condition in which plaque builds up inside the coronary arteries. Plaque narrows the arteries, reducing blood flow to the heart muscle and making it more likely that clots will form and block the arteries. If you are interested in seeing animated explanations of plaque buildup and coronary artery disease, respectively,

 Go to **Animations: Atherosclerosis,** and **Coronary Artery Disease,** on Davis*Plus.*

- **Dysrhythmias** (alterations in heart rate or rhythm) can lower cardiac output and decrease tissue oxygenation.
- **Heart valve abnormalities** create turbulent flow, leading to a decrease in cardiac output and compromised tissue oxygenation. Often there is an audible murmur. The valves most commonly affected are the mitral and aortic valves.

If you are interested in a more extensive discussion of cardiovascular abnormalities,

 Go to Chapter 38, **Supplemental Materials: Cardiovascular Abnormalities,** on Davis*Plus.*

Table 38-1 ➤ Medications That Promote Circulation

CLASS	ACTION	EXAMPLES AND COMMENTS
Vasodilators	▪ Enhance cardiac output, providing increased blood flow and oxygenation to organs and tissues. ▪ Cause vessel dilation, which eases workload of the heart. ▪ Control blood pressure. ▪ Treat heart failure.	Angiotensin-converting enzyme (ACE) inhibitors Angiotensin II receptor blockers Nitrates
Beta-Adrenergic Blockers	▪ Block norepinephrine and epinephrine (adrenaline) ▪ Reduce the workload of the heart and oxygen consumption. ▪ Control abnormal heart rhythms (dysrhythmias) by slowing conduction through the AV node. ▪ Control blood pressure.	Beta$_1$-selective: atenolol, metoprolol Nonselective: carvedilol, metoprolol, propranolol
Calcium-Channel Blockers	▪ Block the flow of calcium into the cells of the heart and blood vessels. ▪ Decrease blood pressure. ▪ Reduce the strength of myocardial contraction; slow heart rate. ▪ Dilate the arteries and arterioles.	Nifedipine
Positive Inotropic Agents	▪ Improve the effectiveness of the heart's pumping action without creating excess cardiac workload and oxygen demand. ▪ Reduce the heart muscle cells ability to trigger its own contraction (automaticity) ▪ Dilate blood vessels	Cardiac glycosides: digoxin Phosphodiesterase (PSE) inhibitors: PDE3 inhibitors (congestive heart failure) PDE5 inhibitors (erectile dysfunction)
Diuretics	▪ Remove sodium and water from the body through urine. ▪ Reduce the volume of circulating blood. ▪ Prevent accumulation of fluid in the pulmonary circulation and body tissues.	Thiazide diuretics: hydrochlorothiazide (HCTZ), metolazone Loop diuretics: furosemide Potassium-sparing diuretics: spironolactone Bumetanide Metolazone Triamterene

Peripheral Vascular Abnormalities

Disorders of peripheral blood vessels impair blood flow to and from organs and tissues.

Arterial abnormalities disrupt flow of oxygenated blood to tissues. Narrowing and hardening of the arteries to the legs and feet, called peripheral artery disease (PAD), occurs when fatty deposits build up on the blood vessels, causing them to be stiffer and less able to dilate when more blood and oxygen is needed. Poor circulation with PAD shows up as pain, aching, burning, and fatigue in the lower legs and feet. In the early phase, these symptoms appear when walking uphill, fast walking, and longer periods of exercise. Gradually, the pain comes on more quickly and with less exertion. When arterial blood flow is compromised, signs and symptoms include

pallor, pain, weak or absent pulses, poor capillary refill, cool skin, and tissue dysfunction. The symptoms may appear only when the person is walking uphill, walking faster, or walking for long distances. Gradually the symptoms will appear more quickly and with less exercise.

Venous abnormalities disrupt blood return to the heart. For example, peripheral venous disease (PVD) is a condition where damage or blockage occurs in the veins of the extremities, most commonly caused by a blood clot. A blood clot is deep within the body, it is called deep vein thrombosis (DVT); when it is closer to the skin, it is considered superficial thrombophlebitis. Clinical signs of compromised venous blood flow include edema, brown skin discoloration, and tissue dysfunction (e.g., stasis ulcers), or pain in the calf,

warmth, and redness (deep vein thrombosis [DVT]). If you are interested in a more extensive discussion of peripheral vascular abnormalities,

 Go to Chapter 38, **Supplemental Materials: Peripheral Vascular Abnormalities,** on Davis*Plus.*

Oxygen Transport Abnormalities

Even if the heart is functioning well and arterial blood flow is intact, tissues can become hypoxic if the blood is unable to carry adequate amounts of oxygen. The most common causes are anemia and carbon monoxide poisoning. **Anemia** is an abnormally low level of red blood cells, hemoglobin, or both. **Carbon monoxide** is a colorless, odorless gas produced by the combustion of flammable materials and fuels. When inhaled, carbon monoxide binds tightly to hemoglobin at the oxygen receptor sites, making it impossible for hemoglobin to carry oxygen. If you are interested in a more extensive discussion of oxygen transport abnormalities,

 Go to Chapter 38, **Supplemental Materials: Oxygen Transport Abnormalities,** on Davis*Plus.*

PracticalKnowledge
knowing **how**

Nursing care for patients with cardiovascular problems is directed at assessing for and maximizing the effectiveness of the heart and circulatory system.

▮ ASSESSMENT

Although this section focuses on cardiovascular assessments, evaluation of overall circulation and perfusion status includes a history and examination that gathers information about lung, heart, and circulatory function. The patient's condition and the purpose of the assessment determine your priorities for assessment and the order in which you gather information. For example, for someone with a cardiac emergency, the immediate assessment focus would be to ask simple questions about current symptoms while performing a quick examination to determine adequacy of circulation, perfusion, and oxygenation. In contrast, the assessment for risk of coronary artery disease in a healthy individual might include more extensive questions about occupation and smoking habits, a medical history, and an extensive physical examination.

You will need information about the patient's past and present cardiovascular signs and symptoms, risk factors, medications, activity level, tolerance of activity, and lifestyle factors that affect cardiovascular functioning.

Assessing for Risk Factors

A health history related to cardiovascular functioning includes questions about the presence of risk factors that affect the heart, and peripheral vascular function. Topics to assess include the following:

- Demographic data
- Health history
- Family history
- Respiratory history
- Cardiovascular history
- Environmental history
- Lifestyle

You should also assess the patient's level of anxiety. Patients with cardiac or respiratory problems are almost certain to be anxious, and anxiety interferes with achieving good outcomes for these patients. Pay close attention to verbal cues because heart rate and blood pressure changes may not be useful in assessing acutely ill patients for anxiety (Moser, 2007). For a detailed list of interview questions for each of these topics, see the Focused Assessment box, Circulation.

Focused Assessment

Circulation

Part I. Questions to Assess Risk for Impaired Circulation

Demographic Data

➤ What is your age?
➤ Where do you live?
➤ What is your occupation?

Health History

➤ Do you have current health problems? Describe.
➤ Do you have past health problems? Describe.
➤ Have you ever been hospitalized or had surgery? If so, when and for what reason?
➤ Do you take medication for your heart, blood pressure, cholesterol, or erectile dysfunction, diabetes, breathing difficulty, or other conditions?
➤ Do you have chronic fatigue, heartburn, anxiety, swelling of the ankles, difficulty breathing, chest discomfort, palpitations, dizziness or fainting spells, dental problems, pain in the calf when walking that stops with rest, chronic cough or wheezing, shortness of breath, or unexplained weight loss?
➤ Do you take over-the-counter products, such as vitamins, supplements, aspirin?
➤ What else do you want to tell me about your physical or mental health history?

Family History

➤ Did your father or a brother develop coronary artery disease or have a heart attack before the age of 55?
➤ Did you mother or sister develop coronary artery disease or have a heart attack before the age of 65?

Cardiovascular History

➤ Have you ever had or been diagnosed with a heart attack, angina, coronary artery disease, peripheral artery disease, stroke, aortic aneurysm?
➤ Do you have high or low blood pressure? Do you feel dizzy if you stand up quickly?
➤ Have you ever had chest pain? If so, describe the circumstances? What was done to relieve the symptoms? What measures do you take to prevent the pain?
➤ Do you become easily fatigued or feel your heart rate is rapid? Do you ever feel heart palpitations?
➤ Do you have pain in your legs when you are walking uphill or walking for a long time?
➤ Do you experience cold hands and feet? If so, how often?
➤ Do you have pain or tingling in your feet or toes with exercise? Do they feel numb when you are at rest? Does

Focused Assessment

Circulation—cont'd

the pain worsen when your leg is elevated and/or improve when you dangle your legs over the side of the bed?
➤ Do you have pain in your leg, foot, or toes that is so severe that shoes or the weight of a sheet at night is painful?
➤ If you are male, do you experience impotence?
➤ Do you have ulcers that do not heal?

Nutrition History

➤ In a typical day, how many servings of whole grains, fruits, vegetables, dairy products, eggs, nuts, and red meat or fish do you eat or drink per day?
➤ How many meals per week do you east fast food or other high-fat food?
➤ How many meals per week do you eat out? Where?
➤ How many times per day do you add salt or eat salty foods?
➤ How many times per week do you skip a meal?
➤ Do you have diabetes or prediabetes? Are you a normal weight?

Lifestyle and health promotion activities

➤ What is your current stress level? What are your major sources of stress? How do you relieve stress?
➤ What is you usual diet? Is your current diet typical, or have you recently changed your eating habits?
➤ What is your usual activity level? Do you exercise regularly? If so, how many minutes per week of moderate to vigorous physical activity do you get?
➤ Do you check your lipid profile (cholesterol and triglycerides) and blood sugar (fasting blood sugar and hemoglobin A_{1c}) on a regular basis?
➤ Do you smoke now, or have you ever smoked? If you smoke, how many packs per day and for how many years have you smoked?
➤ Do you use crack cocaine or other illicit substances?

Part II. Focused Physical Examination

Cardiovascular System

➤ **Inspect the neck** for carotid and jugular pulsations. Palpate each carotid separately. Auscultate the carotid arteries and jugular veins for bruits and hums.
➤ **Inspect the precordium** for pulsations. Palpate for pulsations, lifts, heaves, and thrills. Auscultate for heart sounds.

➤ Also review Procedure 21-13, Assessing the Heart and Vascular System.
➤ **Assess peripheral circulation.** Palpate peripheral pulses, assess skin color and temperature, note hair distribution on extremities. Inspect for skin ulcers and edema of the feet and ankles.
➤ **Inspect** for venous valve competence.
➤ **Perform the capillary refill test** anywhere you note signs of diminished blood flow.

Physical Examination

Start the physical exam by obtaining the patient's height and weight. Body mass index and waist circumference indicate obesity, which is a major risk factor for cardiovascular disease. Assessment of heart and peripheral vessels includes inspection, palpation, and auscultation (and occasionally percussion). Use inspection to observe for signs of distress (e.g., chest pain), skin and mucous membrane color, presence or absence of edema, and overall general appearance. Palpate pulses, skin temperature, edema, heart pulsations through the chest wall, and areas of tenderness. Auscultate heart sounds, vascular sounds, and blood pressure. Auscultate the lungs because adventitious sounds, such as rales, may signal decreased cardiac output. For a step-by-step discussion of how to assess the heart and vascular system, see Procedure 21-13, Assessing the Heart and Vascular System.

Assess Pain

If a patient has chest pain, evaluate it immediately because chest pain is the most common heart attack symptom. Ask the patient to describe the pain, its location, duration, frequency, and radiation. Chest pain may also be caused by musculoskeletal or respiratory conditions, for example, a fractured rib or pleuritis (inflammation in the pleural space). You can differentiate cardiac pain because it usually occurs in the center or on the left side of the chest and radiates to the left arm (most often in men). The pain typically lasts several minutes; it may subside and then return. Some women have milder chest pain, sometimes none at all. They are more likely than men are

to experience other symptoms, such as jaw or back pain, nausea, fatigue, and shortness of breath. Cardiac pain typically does not change with inhalation or exhalation. Ask the client to rate the pain on a scale of 0 to 10, with 0 representing no pain and 10 representing the worst possible pain. See Chapter 32 for pain assessment, as needed

Patients experiencing chest pain are likely to be fearful—most people are aware that chest pain may signal a heart attack. You need to work quickly but calmly to instill confidence in the patient. If the person is experiencing a cardiac event, anxiety and stress can make it worse by increasing oxygen consumption, thereby extending hypoxic damage to the heart.

Patients with impaired peripheral venous or arterial circulation often experience pain, cramping, tingling or numbness, burning in the affected limb (see Assess Peripheral Circulation). They might also be cool to the touch. Ulcers in the lower extremities are also slow to heal.

Assess Fatigue

Fatigue is a subjective experience. The patient feels tired and lacks endurance. Fatigue is a common symptom of various oxygenation problems, including anemia and heart failure. Ask your patient to rate his fatigue on a 0 to 10 scale, as you do for pain.

Assess Dyspnea

Dyspnea (shortness of breath) was discussed in chapter 37 in relation to respiratory conditions. Recall that dyspnea is a sign of hypoxia, which can be associated with cardiovascular

diseases and anemia, as well as with respiratory problems. As with pain, dyspnea provokes anxiety.

Assess Peripheral Circulation

Even if the lungs and heart are functioning well, pathology in the arteries and veins can interfere with tissue perfusion.

Peripheral Venous Circulation

When assessing for a clot in the veins (DVT), deep under the muscles of the leg, you will assess for pain, warmth, redness, and swelling of the leg. **Homan's sign** (pulling toes forward) and **Pratt's sign** (squeezing calf to trigger pain) have not been found to be reliable in diagnosing DVT. However, these signs may help confirm DVT when also considering the clinical signs of DVT, as well as the results of more accurate and specific diagnostic tests, such as ultrasound or venography (Rasavong, 2009).

Peripheral Arterial Circulation

During an exam for PAD, you will observe shiny, tight skin and hair will be absent. The skin may appear pale or even purple in the later stages. Calf muscles tend to shrink and toenails thicken. There might be painful ulcers (often black) on the feet or toes that don't seem to heal. Pulses in the feet or lower limb

are diminished or absent with palpation. Legs and feet will feel cool to the touch. In the later stages, pain can be so severe that even light touch can be intolerable. You may auscultate a whooshing sound with a stethoscope (arterial bruit) might be present.

KnowledgeCheck 38-4

Why would you auscultate the lungs as a part of your assessment of cardiac function?

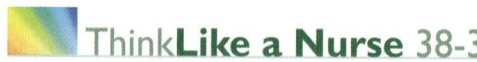

ThinkLike a Nurse 38-3

Why might it be more difficult to recognize a heart attack in a woman than in a man?

Diagnostic Testing

Diagnostic testing helps clinicians identify the causes of cardiovascular symptoms and monitor patient responses to treatment. We discuss several of these tests in the next sections. For others, see the Diagnostic Testing box, Tests Related to Circulation.

Diagnostic Testing

Tests Related to Circulation

TEST	PURPOSE
Angiogram	A contrast dye is injected into a vein, and serial films are taken to assess patency of the vessels.
Arterial blood gases (ABGs)	An analysis of arterial blood that evaluates the effectiveness of gas exchange and perfusion
Cardiac catheterization	A catheter is passed into the heart to assess pressures, blood flow, and the size and patency of chambers.
Chest x-ray study (CXR)	Provides an anterior–posterior or lateral view of the heart and lungs, shows tissue density (e.g., to evaluate size, masses, fluid).
Cholesterol, lipid profile	Indicates risk for cardiovascular disease long-term.
Creatine kinase-MB (CK-MB)	The MB isoenzyme is present only in the heart muscle. A serum measurement of the MB band is used to detect a myocardial infarction (MI). Levels rise with an acute MI.
Echocardiogram	An ultrasound evaluation of the heart that examines heart function and blood flow
Electrocardiogram (ECG)	Electrodes placed on the extremities and chest wall conduct electrical activity from the heart. ECG illustrates heart rate, rhythm, and size and helps evaluate heart damage.
Hemoglobin (Hgb)	A serum measurement that affects the oxygen-carrying capacity of the blood. May be measured separately or as part of a complete blood count.
Holter monitor	A continuous ECG tracing used to correlate symptoms and cardiac activity. Typically the tracing lasts 48 hours to 7 days.
Magnetic resonance angiography (MRA)	This is an MRI exam of the blood vessels. Unlike a traditional angiography, there is no tube (catheter) placed into the body. MRA is noninvasive.
Technetium scan	Technetium-99m sestamibi is injected intravenously. Approximately 90 to 120 minutes later, the heart is scanned. Areas of myocardial damage appear as "hot spots" on the scan.
Treadmill test	Evaluates the effect of exercise on the heart and circulation via continuous ECG and vital sign monitoring during exercise.
Troponin	A serum evaluation of a complex of proteins is used to detect myocardial infarction (MI). Levels of these contractile proteins remain elevated for up to 7 days after MI.

Diagnostic Testing

Tests Related to Circulation—cont'd

TEST	PURPOSE
Ultrasound (Doppler)	A transducer, which directs high-frequency sound waves to the artery or vein, is used to examine blood flow. A normal result shows no areas of narrowing or closure in the blood vessels.
Venography	Using dye and x-ray technology, a narrow tube (catheter) is inserted into a large vein to identify any blood clots or unusual narrowing or blockage of venous blood flow.
VQ scan	This test is used to detect a blood clot in the lungs.

Tests of Blood Oxygenation

Pulse oximetry, capnography, and arterial blood gases were discussed in the Diagnostic Testing box in Chapter 37. You should understand, though, that results from all of those tests are pertinent to cardiac conditions. Remember: The heart and lungs work together to provide oxygenation; a problem in one creates a problem in the other. See Chapter 37, Procedure 37-2, Monitoring Pulse Oximetry (Arterial Oxygen Saturation), and Clinical Insight 37-1, Tips for Obtaining Accurate Pulse Oximetry Readings.

To review (and use in clinical assignments) arterial blood gas values and other tests of blood oxygenation, respectively, see the Diagnostic Testing box in Chapter 37, Arterial Blood Gas Values: Evaluating Adequacy of Oxygenation. Also,

 Go to Chapter 37, **Diagnostic Testing Box, Tests Related to Oxygenation,** on Davis*Plus.*

Laboratory Testing

Cholesterol, lipid panel, C-reactive protein (CRP), and glucose testing are a valuable part of cardiovascular risk assessment. The National Heart, Lung, and Blood Institute (NHLBI) (2002, updated 2012) recommend testing total cholesterol, HDL and low-density lipoprotein (LDL), triglyceride levels every five years for adults over age 20. For adults with total cholesterol greater than 200 mg/dL, a fasting measurement is recommended. The maximum LDL cholesterol would be 176 mg/dL. Glucose testing is indicated, particularly those at risk for metabolic syndrome, which includes heart disease. The CRP appears to be the most reliable marker for arterial inflammation currently available.

An Expert Panel appointed by the NHLBI (2011) is recommending aggressive cholesterol screening for all children, regardless of family history. The panel recommends that children undergo select lipid screening between the ages of 9 and 11 years followed by another full lipid screening test between 18 and 21 years of age. The panel also recommends measuring fasting glucose levels to test for diabetes in children 10 years of age (or at the onset of puberty) who are overweight with other risk factors, including a family history, for type 2 diabetes mellitus.

Cardiac Monitoring

Cardiac monitoring is the continuous monitoring of the electrocardiogram (ECG), a rendering of the electrical activity of the heart. Three to five electrodes placed on the skin of the chest display a waveform on a monitor screen or printout (Fig. 38-4). The ECG illustrates electrical activity, but not mechanical activity. In other words, the ECG reflects what the nerves are telling the heart muscle to do, but not what the heart muscle is actually doing in response.

The purposes of cardiac monitoring are to:
- Identify the patient's baseline rhythm and rate.
- Recognize significant changes in the baseline rhythm and rate.
- Recognize lethal dysrhythmias that require immediate intervention.

The ECG reading illustrates the complete cardiac cycle. Each part of the ECG complex has been given a letter to identify it: **P, Q, R, S,** and **T** (see Fig. 38-2).
- The **P wave** represents the firing of the SA node and conduction of the impulse through the atria. In the healthy heart, this leads to atrial contraction.
- The **QRS complex** represents *ventricular depolarization* and leads to ventricular contraction.
- The **T wave** represents the return of the ventricles to an electrical resting state so they can be stimulated again (*ventricular repolarization*). The atria also repolarize, but they do so during the time of ventricular depolarization; thus, they are

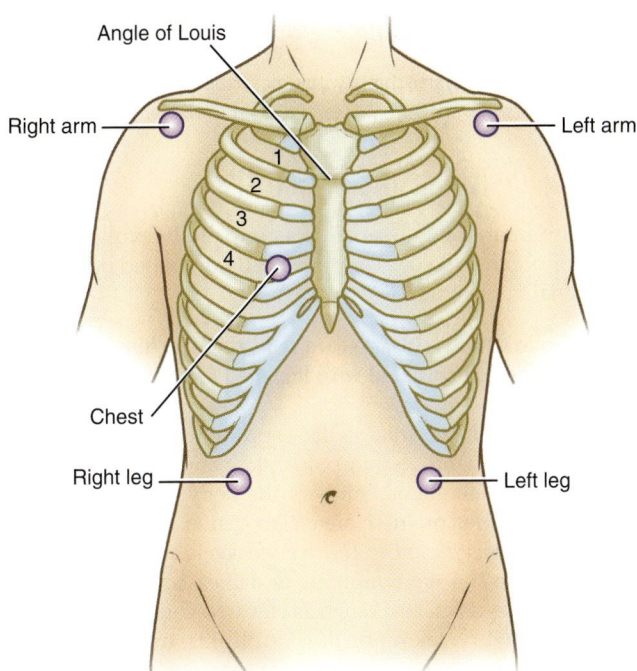

FIGURE 38-4 Electrodes placed for continuous cardiac monitoring.

obscured by the QRS complex and cannot be seen on the ECG complex.

- The **U wave** is not always seen on the ECG, but may be detected with electrolyte imbalance, such as hypokalemia or hypercalcemia. U waves sometimes occur in response to certain medication (e.g., digitalis, epinephrine). Inverted U wave may occur with ischemia to the cardiac muscle.

Dysrhythmias are abnormal heart rhythms. Dysrhythmias can be broadly categorized according to rhythm as follows:

Tachydysrhythmias—Rates >100 beats/min

Bradydysrhythmias—Rates <60 beats/min

Ectopy—extra beats

Within each or those categories, dysrhythmias can be further classified by their site of origin:

Supraventricular—Above the ventricles

Junctional—Within the AV node

Ventricular—In the ventricles

Note that a tachy- or bradydysrhythmia depends on the patient's baseline heart rate. Some people have a low resting heart rate (less than 60 beats/min) without distress. Keep this in mind before assuming that the heart rate is abnormal.

All dysrhythmias have the potential to decrease cardiac output, resulting in hypotension and tissue hypoxia. Skill in identifying cardiac rhythms (both normal and abnormal) requires study and experience and is beyond the scope of this chapter. For the complete procedure, see Procedure 38-1.

In contrast to cardiac monitoring, *electrocardiography* uses 12 "leads" (views of the heart). These are done by specially trained nurses or technicians. If you are interested in reading more about 12-lead ECGs,

 Go to Chapter 38, **Supplemental Materials: 12-Lead Electrocardiography, and Tables, Boxes, Figures: ESG Figures 38-4 and 38-5,** on Davis*Plus*.

KnowledgeCheck 38-5

- What do the P wave, QRS complex, T, and U wave of an ECG complex represent?
- What kind of dysrhythmia would describe a heart rate of 140 beats/min that originates in the ventricles?

ANALYSIS/NURSING DIAGNOSIS

Several nursing diagnoses address impaired circulation and tissue or organ hypoxia. They are briefly discussed below. For additional information,

 Go to Chapter 38, **Standardized Language: Nursing Diagnoses Associated with Impaired Circulation,** on Davis*Plus*.

- *Decreased Cardiac Output* is the appropriate diagnosis when the heart is unable to pump adequate amounts of blood to meet the metabolic demands of the body. Definitive interventions for this problem are collaborative.
- *Risk for Decreased Cardiac Tissue Perfusion* is appropriate for a patient who has no symptoms of decreased cardiac perfusion, but has risk factors such as elevated C-reactive protein, cardiac surgery, taking birth control pills, hyperlipidemia, and substance abuse.
- *Ineffective Peripheral Tissue Perfusion* is appropriate for a patient experiencing poor perfusion to the arms and/or legs (e.g., PAD or DVT).

- *Risk for Ineffective Cerebral, Gastrointestinal, or Renal, Tissue Perfusion* are appropriate for a patient who is at risk for experiencing poor perfusion to the brain, GI system, or kidneys (e.g., a patient with a brain tumor, certain heart problems, embolism, substance abuse).
- *Risk for Shock* should be used for patients who have inadequate blood flow to body tissues that may lead to life-threatening cellular dysfunction (e.g., patients with sepsis and hypovolemia).

Cardiovascular functioning can also be the etiology of other nursing diagnoses, such as the following examples:

- Risk for Activity Intolerance related to decreased oxygen-carrying capacity of the blood secondary to anemia
- Acute Pain secondary to myocardial ischemia
- Anxiety related to shortness of breath
- Death Anxiety related to diagnosis of myocardial infarction (heart attack)
- Ineffective Coping related to hospitalization for oxygenation impairment

PLANNING OUTCOMES/EVALUATION

NOC standardized outcomes and evaluation criteria related to cardiovascular status are included in the Cardiopulmonary class of NOC Domain II: Physiologic Health. They include the following: Blood Loss Severity, Cardiac Pump Effectiveness, Circulation Status, Tissue Perfusion (Abdominal Organs, Cardiac, Peripheral, Pulmonary), and Vital Signs.

Individualized goals/outcome statements depend on the nursing diagnosis you identify. For diagnoses related to cardiac function or circulation, the following are examples of goals you might write the following:

- No dyspnea or shortness of breath
- Heart rate in expected range
- Peripheral pulses strong and equal bilaterally
- Brisk capillary refill
- Normal skin color (no pallor or cyanosis)

For examples of NOC outcomes and NIC interventions for selected oxygenation nursing diagnoses,

 Go to Chapter 38 **Standardized Language: Examples of NOC Outcomes and NIC Interventions Linked to Circulation Diagnoses,** on Davis*Plus*.

PLANNING INTERVENTIONS/IMPLEMENTATION

NIC standardized interventions related to the cardiovascular system are found in NIC Domain 2: Physiological Interventions: Complex, in the subcategory of Tissue Perfusion Management. Tissue Perfusion Management focuses on optimizing circulation. These provide a general care planning guide. Depending on individual patient needs, other NOC outcomes or NIC interventions may also be appropriate.

Specific nursing interventions for patients with cardiovascular problems focus on relieving anxiety, promoting circulation, administering medications, and performing cardiopulmonary resuscitation (CPR).

Manage Anxiety

Almost everyone who experiences dyspnea or chest pain becomes anxious—some, extremely so. It is important to reduce anxiety because anxiety activates the sympathetic nervous system and triggers the stress response. Hormone changes occur, including the release of aldosterone, which promotes

fluid retention and increases blood pressure. The heart rate and contraction force increase; peripheral and visceral vessels constrict, and the blood clots more readily. All of these make a cardiac or vascular condition more serious.

Prioritize your interventions. You will, of course, need to intervene first to prevent life-threatening situations. But try not to appear rushed, and speak calmly and quietly to the patient and to those around you. Do not leave the patient alone. Provide clear factual information and keep the patient and family informed about treatments being given. Many patients are reassured by the presence of a family member. If you need a review of detailed information about assessments and interventions for anxious patients, see Chapter 13.

Promote Circulation

Adequate circulation ensures that oxygenated blood reaches tissues and organs and that venous blood returns to the heart. Three important nursing interventions are to promote venous return and prevent clot formation.

Promote Venous Return

Measures that promote venous return increase the flow of blood back to the vena cava and the right side of the heart.

- Elevate the patient's legs above the level of the heart. Gravity promotes venous return from the feet and legs.
- Flexion of the hips, legs, and knees constricts the veins and slows venous blood flow. If a recliner is available, have the patient sit in one that elevates the legs rather than sitting upright in a chair with legs elevated on a stool.
- Teach patients to avoid sitting with the legs crossed; doing so interferes with blood flow.
- Encourage and support early and frequent ambulation (e.g., after surgery). Contraction of the muscles in the legs moves blood upward against gravity.
- Encourage or provide range-of-motion (ROM) exercises, which increase venous blood flow through rhythmic massaging of the veins by the active muscles (see Chapter 33 to review ROM).
- Apply compression devices. *Antiembolism stockings (TED hose)* are elastic stockings that compress superficial leg veins and promote venous return. *Sequential compression devices (SCDs)*, also called *pneumatic compression devices*, are cuffs that surround the legs and alternately inflate and deflate to promote venous return to the heart. Antiembolism stockings and SCDs are frequently used in perioperative patients to promote venous return and prevent clot formation. See Chapter 40 for further discussion and instructions on how to apply these stockings and appropriate follow-up care. See Procedure 40-2, Applying Antiembolism Stockings.

Promote Peripheral Arterial Circulation

Peripheral arterial disease, usually found in the legs and feet, occurs when tissues don't receive enough blood flow to keep up with the demand for oxygen. It is caused by the buildup of fatty deposits and plaque within the arteries (atherosclerosis). When arteries that supply blood to the legs are narrowed, leg pain occurs, especially with walking. This is called **intermittent claudication**. As the blood flow becomes more restricted, pain occurs at rest, as well as numbness or a cold feeling to the leg or foot, especially on one side, weak pulse, change in color, hair loss or shiny skin on the legs, sores that won't heal, and erectile dysfunction in men. Teach the patient and family the following:

- Patients with poor peripheral circulation need to quit using tobacco because smoking restricts blood flow.

- When circulation is poor, it is especially important to take good care of the feet and prevent injury to the feet. Even dry, cracked skin can result in a sore and become infected. Patients need to wear well-fitting shoes with smooth, dry socks.
- Regular exercise improves circulation and oxygen delivery to body tissue.
- Medication might be needed to control blood pressure, control pain, lower cholesterol, prevent clots, and control blood sugar if the patient has diabetes.
- Angioplasty using a mesh stent or graft bypass surgery might be necessary to create a new path for blood flow to go around the damaged area of the blood vessel.

When treated properly, new, collateral blood vessels can form, allowing blood to circulate around the damaged area.

Prevent Clot Formation

A **thrombus** is a stationary clot adhering to the wall of a vessel. An **embolus** is a clot that travels in the bloodstream. Clots can form after injury to vessels, or in response to hypercoagulability. Of course, all the strategies to promote venous return also help prevent clot formation.

- Turn patients frequently; teach patients to change positions frequently. This prevents vessel injury from prolonged pressure in one position.
- Use scrupulous sterile technique when inserting or handling intravenous lines. This prevents infection that can damage the vessel lumens.
- Be sure intravenous medications are adequately diluted. This prevents chemical irritation of veins during IV medication therapy.
- Promote adequate hydration (i.e., monitor intake and output [I&O], assess hydration, manage fluid intake, teach patients to drink plenty of fluids). Unless contraindicated, adult fluid intake should be approximately 2,000 mL per day to keep urine output around 1,500 mL per day. Adequate hydration keeps respiratory secretions thin but also keeps the blood from becoming viscous ("thick"). Viscous blood clots more readily.
- Promote smoking cessation. Nicotine increases the risk for thrombus formation because of its constricting effects on vessel walls.
- Patients at particularly high risk for thrombus formation may receive anticoagulant therapy to help prevent abnormal clot formation.

Administer Medications

Cardiovascular medications are used to enhance cardiac output, thus providing increased blood flow and oxygenation to organs and tissues. They include vasodilators, beta-adrenergic blocking agents, diuretics, and positive inotropes.

- *Vasodilators* cause vessel dilation, which eases the work of the heart. Drugs that dilate arterioles decrease the resistance against which the heart pumps (afterload). Drugs that dilate veins decrease venous return to the heart (preload). Vasodilators can cause hypotension, especially when the person rises from a sitting or lying position. Patients should be warned of this effect. You will need to monitor the patient's blood pressure and observe for symptoms of hypotension. Vasodilating agents include angiotensin-converting enzyme (ACE) inhibitors, angiotensin II receptor blockers, and nitrates.
- *Beta-adrenergic agents* block stimulation of beta receptors, which are located primarily in the heart, lungs, and blood vessels. Beta-1 selective agents are used to treat angina, acute myocardial infarction, and congestive heart failure (CHF).

Toward Evidence-Based Practice

> **Wood, S., & Nghiem, H. (2007). Raw garlic and garlic supplements offer no effect on lipids. *Archives of Internal Medicine, 167*, 125–126, 346–353.**

Researchers randomly divided 192 adults with low-density lipoprotein (LDL) cholesterol concentrations of 130 to 190 mg/dL into four groups. One group received treatment with raw garlic, another with powdered garlic supplement, another with garlic extract, and another with placebo. None of the forms of garlic used had statistically or clinically significant effects on LDL cholesterol or other plasma lipids.

> **Jenkins, D., Kendall, C., Faulkner, D., et al. (2008). Long-term effects of a plant-based dietary portfolio of cholesterol-lowering foods on blood pressure. *European Journal of Clinical Nutrition, 62*, 781–788.**

The intent of this study was to determine the effect of a cholesterol-lowering diet on blood pressure. Sixty-six subjects who had high blood lipid levels and hypertension were followed for 1 year. They consumed a diet of plant-based, cholesterol-lowering foods. Those who complied with almond intake advice experienced significant reduction in blood pressure; the rest did not.

> **Sesso, H., Buring, J., Christen, W., et al. (2008). Vitamins E and C in the prevention of cardiovascular disease in men. *JAMA, 300*(18). Retrieved from http://jama.ama-assn.org/cgi/content/full/300/18/2123.**

This 10-year longitudinal research evaluated 14,641 men at low risk of cardiovascular disease to determine whether long-term vitamin E or vitamin C supplementation decreases the risk of major cardiovascular events among men. They concluded that there was no support for the use of these supplements for prevention of cardiovascular disease in middle-aged and older men.

> **Spangler, L., Newton, K., Grothaus, L., et al. (2007). The effects of black cohosh therapies on lipids, fibrinogen, glucose and insulin. *Maturitas, 57*(2), 195–204.**

Black cohosh is an herb commonly used to treat menopausal symptoms. The researchers randomly assigned 351 peri- or postmenopausal women, 45 to 55 years old, either black cohosh, a multibotanical including black cohosh, a multibotanical plus soy diet counseling, estrogen, or placebo. Baseline blood lipids levels were established at the beginning of the study. At the end of 3 months, there were no differences among the herbal groups and placebo in total cholesterol, LDL, HDL, or triglycerides.

Use the information provided above as you answer the following questions:

1. If you had several risk factors for cardiovascular disease, specifically coronary artery disease, which of the following might help lower your risk? Explain your thinking.
   a. Taking a garlic supplement and cooking with garlic
   b. Eating a handful of almonds every day
   c. Taking vitamin E and vitamin C supplements daily
   d. Taking black cohosh every day
2. A male client says, "I've heard that black cohosh will help lower my cholesterol. Is that true?" Based on the Spangler study, how would you answer: Yes, no, I don't know? Explain your thinking.

Go to Chapter 38, **Toward Evidence-Based Practice Suggested Responses,** on Davis*Plus*

They decrease heart rate, slow conduction through the AV node, and decrease myocardial oxygen demand by reducing myocardial contractility.

- *Diuretics* increase removal of sodium and water from the body by increasing urine output. In patients with CHF, diuretics are used to reduce the volume of circulating blood and prevent accumulation of fluid in the pulmonary circulation.
- *Positive inotropes* increase cardiac contractility. They are used therapeutically to make the heart a more effective pump. The goal is to improve pumping effectiveness without creating excess heart work and oxygen demand. The two main classes of positive inotropes are cardiac glycosides and phosphodiesterase inhibitors.

Performing Cardiopulmonary Resuscitation

All of the previously discussed interventions are designed to promote circulation and perfusion. However, the patient's condition can rapidly deteriorate. You must be prepared to perform *cardiopulmonary resuscitation (CPR)* in the event your patient experiences a respiratory, cardiac, or cardiopulmonary arrest. **Cardiac arrest** is the cessation of heart function. Signs of cardiac arrest are pale, cool, grayish skin; absence of femoral or carotid pulses; apnea; and pupil dilation. In the event of cardiac arrest, you have only 4 to 6 minutes before the brain is damaged by lack of oxygen. **Respiratory (pulmonary) arrest** is cessation of breathing. It can be caused by a blocked airway or occur after a cardiac arrest; it may be sudden or preceded by increasingly labored breathing.

CPR procedures are regularly updated as new knowledge is gained. The American Heart Association provides training sessions for healthcare professionals to become certified in CPR. This is a prerequisite for employment and clinical practice. We recommend you obtain CPR training from certified professionals. However, if you are already trained and just want to review the procedure,

Go to Chapter 38, **ESG Procedure 38-1: Performing Cardiopulmonary Resuscitation, One- and Two-Person Rescue,** on Davis*Plus*.

Key points of the most recent guidelines *for trained professionals* include the following:

- Focus on effective, uninterrupted chest compressions.
- Push hard, push fast in the center of the chest.

- Administer about 100 compressions per minute.
- Perform 30 compressions to 2 breaths—for all victims except newborns
- Give breath over 1 second and make the chest rise visibly (Sayre, Berg, Cave, et al., 2008).

In-Hospital Arrests

All agencies have procedures (called a Code Blue in many agencies) for announcing cardiac or respiratory arrest, and there is usually an emergency alert system in the patient rooms in acute care facilities. Activating the alert system (e.g., by pulling down a handle) summons a code team, trained in CPR. However, you will probably need to begin CPR before they arrive. Begin CPR immediately after activating the alert, and following the instructions given by an automatic external defibrillator (AED) or manual defibrillator as soon as one is available. For a manual defibrillator, use a dose of 2 joules/kg for the first shock and a dose of 4 J/kg for the second and subsequent shocks. Before beginning CPR, you are responsible for knowing whether your patient has an advance directive stating whether or not he would want CPR.

Hands-Only™ CPR

The American Heart Association (2011b) recommends different responses for laypersons, first responders, and CPR-trained professionals. The goal of these changes is to make it easier to learn, remember, and perform CPR. Referred to as Hands-Only™ CPR, the method is recommended for people who see an adult collapse suddenly in the community.

See the Self-Care box, Teaching Your Client Hands-Only™ CPR for a detailed description of CPR that you can teach to lay persons.

Rescuers should use Hands-Only™ CPR only for adults they observe to suddenly collapse. They should use CPR that combines breaths and compressions for:

Adults found already unconscious and not breathing normally

Victims of drowning or collapse due to breathing problems

All infants and children

KnowledgeCheck 38-6

- Identify three strategies that prevent clot formation.
- How do diuretics affect oxygenation?

Self-Care

Teaching Your Client Hands-Only™ CPR for a Single Rescuer, Adult Victim

Collapse

If you see an adult suddenly collapse in an "out-of-hospital" setting:

1. Call 911 (or send someone to do that).
2. Push hard and fast in the center of the chest (100 pumps per minute)
3. Continue until help arrives.

For an unwitnessed collapse of an adult victim:

1. Establish unresponsiveness (ask, "Are you OK?")
2. Call 911 (or send someone to do it).
3. Obtain an AED, if possible.
4. Start traditional CPR, if you know how, while waiting for the AED.

Traditional CPR

1. When the AED arrives, turn it on for rhythm analysis.
2. After turning on the AED, open the airway (tilt the head, lift the chin).
3. Check for breathing.
4. Give two rescue breaths (each 1 second long). Look for chest movement, listen for breathing, and feel for air coming from the mouth or nose.
5. Administer one shock and wait for the AED to tell you what to do next.
6. When the AED says to continue CPR, start alternating 30 compressions with 2 breaths. Continue until help arrives. Stop only to check the AED for rhythm.

   Key POINT: *The most important action is to deliver uninterrupted, hard and fast chest compressions.*

Source: American Heart Association (AHA). (2011b, February 24). Hands Only™ CPR. Retrieved November 22, 2011, from http:// handsonlycpr.eisenberginc.com/

CLINICALREASONING:
Applying the **Full-Spectrum Nursing Model**

Because the following critical thinking activities allow you to practice the kind of thinking you will use as a full-spectrum nurse, they usually have no single right answer. Discuss them with your peers—if you have difficulty with any of the questions, consult your instructor.

PATIENT SITUATION

Margarita, a 62-year-old Director of Management Technology for a large company, was admitted to the hospital with shortness of breath, sudden and intense fatigue, and intense chest pressure that she describes as feeling like a steel band tightening around her rib cage. She reports the pain moved up to her jaw. The pain began suddenly but lasted approximately 5 to 7 minutes. During the episode, her husband tells you that Margarita acted as though she had a feeling of doom.

Margarita also has a history of sudden onset neck pain that seems to be triggered by heightened stress at work. Margarita is pale and clammy. She states she feels nauseated and has burning in her epigastric area. Her heart rate is 80 beats/min, respiratory rate 12 breaths/min, and BP 168/92 mm Hg. Skin is pale but warm, and capillary refill time is 4 seconds. Height is 5 ft 4 in. Weight is 156 lb. Body mass index (BMI) is 29.2. Waist circumference is 36 in.

(continued on next page)

The health history includes type 2 diabetes mellitus, high blood pressure, and tobacco use (half pack of cigarettes a day). Margarita's mother had a heart attack in her 50s.

Lab work prior to admission:
Fasting lipids: Total cholesterol 288 mg/dL, LDL 148 mg/dL, HDH 44 mg/dL, triglycerides 222 mg/dL
Serum glucose: 244 mg/dL
Hs-CRP: 3.1 mg/dL

THINKING

1. *Theoretical Knowledge:*
   a. What predisposing factors increase Margarita's risk for myocardial infarction?
   b. What does it mean to have infarcted myocardial tissue?
2. *Critical Thinking (Analyzing Assumptions):*
   Based on your knowledge of vascular causes of myocardial infarction, what are the most likely causes in this patient?

DOING

3. *Practical Knowledge:*
   After your patient's vital signs are stable and her pain is controlled, the emergency physician prescribes further diagnostic testing to determine the extent of damage to her heart.
   a. What tests would you expect your patient to have?
   b. You attempt to adhere electrodes for cardiac monitoring to Margarita's chest. The ECG tracing shows a great deal of artifact rather than a clear ECG tracing. What should you do to obtain an accurate tracing?
   c. You notice your patient is experiencing multiple "runs" of aberrant heartbeats. What should you do in response to the abnormal ECG tracing?
4. *Nursing Process (Assessment):*
   In the admission data, what important information is missing with regard to her cardiac status?

CARING

5. *Self-Knowledge:*
   Describe a personal experience involving someone in your own family or a friend who experienced a life-threatening event. How did you feel when your loved one was faced with a potentially life-altering heart condition? How might you draw upon this experience to help you in caring for Margarita?
6. *Ethical Knowledge:*
   a. After Margarita is finished with the last diagnostic test, what do you think her biggest concern is likely to be?
   b. Margarita tells you that she does not want anyone to know she has a heart problem. Yet, her husband wants to tell other family members. How do you best respond to her concerns for privacy?

 Go To Chapter 38, **Clinical Reasoning: Applying the Full-Spectrum Nursing Model Response Sheet,** on DavisPlus.

PracticalKnowledge
procedures

In this section you will find the procedures necessary for supporting circulation and perfusion. As you perform the procedures, apply the theoretical knowledge you obtained in the preceding material. The registered nurse is responsible for assessing patients' circulation and perfusion and their responses to procedures. Some, but not all, of the procedures in this section can be delegated to qualified nursing assistive personnel (NAPs). Refer to the delegation notes in the procedures and to agency policies.

Procedure 38–1 ■ Performing Cardiac Monitoring

➤ For steps to follow in *all* procedures, refer to the Universal Steps for All Procedures found on the page facing the inside back cover.

Equipment

- Alcohol pads
- Gauze dressing
- Washcloth
- Shaving supplies or scissors, if necessary
- Disposable electrodes

For Hardwire Monitoring, Add:

- Cardiac monitor
- Cable with lead wires
- Safety pin
- 1-in. tape

For Telemetry, Add:

- Transmitter with lead wires (with a new battery inserted before each use)
- Pouch to carry transmitter

Delegation

You should not delegate this procedure to the LPN or NAP because it requires knowledge of anatomy, physiology, and advanced assessment techniques.

Pre-Procedure Assessment

- Assess cardiovascular status, including heart sounds, pulse rate, and blood pressure, and check for the presence of pain.
- Assess skin integrity of the chest before applying electrodes. *Skin lesions contraindicate the application of leads to the affected area.*
- Assess for history of dysrhythmias. *Early recognition of dysrhythmias allows for prompt treatment, which improves patient outcomes.*

➤ When performing the procedure, always identify your patient according to agency policy and be attentive to standard precautions, hand hygiene, patient safety and privacy, body mechanics, and documentation.

Procedure Steps

1. Prepare the monitoring equipment.

Hardwire Monitoring

a. Plug the cardiac monitor into an electrical outlet, and turn it on. *Allows the monitor to warm up while you prepare the patient for monitoring.*

b. Connect the cable with lead wires into the monitor. *The cable and lead wires must be properly connected to the monitor to obtain an accurate ECG tracing. Most are color coded.*

Telemetry Monitoring

c. Insert a new battery into the transmitter. *A new battery should be inserted with each use to ensure transmitter function.*

d. Turn on the transmitter. *Tests the unit to make sure that the battery is functional.*

e. Connect the lead wires to the transmitter, if they are not permanently attached. Be sure to attach each one to its correct outlet. *The lead wires must be properly connected to the transmitter to obtain an accurate ECG tracing.*

2. Expose the patient's chest, and identify electrode sites based on the monitoring system being used and the patient's anatomy. Gently rub the placement sites with a washcloth or gauze pad until the skin reddens slightly. *The monitoring system will dictate lead placement. Sites over soft tissues or close to bone provide accurate waveforms; sites over bony prominences, thick muscles, and skinfolds can produce artifact.*▼

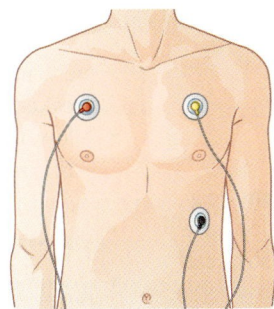

3. If the patient's chest has dense hair, shave or clip the hair with scissors at each electrode site. *Hair may interfere with electrical contact, preventing accurate ECG waveform transmission.*

4. With an alcohol pad, clean the areas chosen for electrode placement, and allow them to dry. *Alcohol removes oil on the skin that may prevent the electrodes from adhering.*

5. Remove the electrode backing, and make sure the gel is moist. Discard the electrode if the gel is dry. The number of electrodes needed depends on the monitoring system being used. It will be three to five electrodes. *A dry electrode will not conduct electrical activity.*

6. Attach the lead wires to the electrodes by snapping or clipping them in place.

7. Apply the electrode to the site by pressing it firmly. Repeat with the remaining electrodes. *Pressing the electrode firmly creates a tight seal, which ensures electrical contact.*

8. Secure the monitoring equipment.

Hardwire Monitoring

a. Wrap a piece of 1-in. tape around the cable, and secure it to the patient's gown with a safety pin. *Secures the cable so leads are not disconnected with patient movement.*

(continued on next page)

Procedure 38–1 ■ Performing Cardiac Monitoring (continued)

Telemetry Monitoring

    b. Place the transmitter in the pouch, and tie the pouch strings around the patient's neck. Place the transmitter into the patient's robe or gown pocket if a pouch is not available.

    Allows the patient independence with ambulation.

9. **Check the patient's ECG tracing** on the monitor. If necessary, adjust the gain on the monitor to increase the waveform size.

    The ECG tracing should be of adequate size to accurately assess all of the waveform components.

Telemetry Monitoring

    You may need to call a monitoring room to verify ECG tracing and rhythm.

10. **Set the upper and lower** heart rate alarm limits according to agency policy or patient condition, and turn them on.

11. **Obtain a rhythm strip** by pressing the "record" button.

    You must obtain a rhythm strip to document the patient's cardiac rhythm.

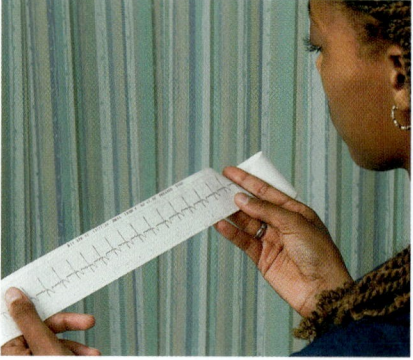

Hardwire Monitoring

    a. Press the "record" button on the bedside monitor.

    The "record" button, located on the monitor at the bedside, allows you to print a rhythm strip immediately when cardiac symptoms occur.

Telemetry Monitoring

    b. Press the "record" button on the transmitter of the telemetry unit, or call the monitoring room to have the ECG trip printed.

    The "record" button on the telemetry transmitter allows you or the patient to print a rhythm strip immediately when cardiac symptoms occur.

12. **Interpret the rhythm strip**, and mount it appropriately (e.g., with transparent tape) in the patient's chart.

    Provides a permanent record of the patient's heart activity; identifies abnormalities in the patient's rhythm.

? What if . . .

■ **The patient is diaphoretic?**

Remove electrodes, clean the area with alcohol, allow the area to dry, and then reapply electrodes.

Clean, dry skin is necessary for an accurate ECG tracing.

■ **The patient is receiving a cardiac medication?**

Print a strip before giving medication and after giving medication. You may also need to call the telemetry station to have the ECG monitored.

To assess and monitor effects of medication.

■ **You are not getting a good reading on the monitor?**

Recheck the leads; replace leads or move leads if necessary.

New leads might be needed for accurate ECG tracing.

Evaluation

■ Evaluate changes in the patient's cardiac rhythm.

■ Check skin integrity, and replace the electrodes at least every 24 hours.

Avoids skin irritation at the electrode sites. In addition, the gel begins to dry, so replacement ensures an adequate waveform.

Patient Teaching

■ Explain the rationale for cardiac monitoring.

■ Teach the patient that if he experiences symptoms (e.g., shortness of breath, chest pain, dizziness, palpitations) he should notify the nurse immediately so a rhythm strip can be recorded.

■ Tell the patient being monitored by telemetry to remove the transmitter before showering. Ask the patient to inform you before removing it.

■ Discuss home telemetry monitoring with the patient and caregiver if the patient requires telemetry monitoring after discharge.

Home Care

■ Evaluate the client's and caregiver's ability to continue telemetry monitoring at home with help from an outside agency.

■ Help the client and caregiver arrange for home telemetry monitoring by contacting the monitoring agency.

■ Explain to the caregiver and patient that the emergency medical service will be notified by the monitoring agency if a dysrhythmia develops.

■ Instruct the caregiver and patient about proper lead placement and the need to rotate electrode sites to prevent skin breakdown.

■ Allow the caregiver and client time for questions and to verbalize concerns.

Documentation

■ Document the date and time that monitoring was instituted.

■ Note the monitoring lead selected.

■ Document a rhythm strip every 8 hours and with changes in the patient's condition according to agency policy. Label the rhythm strip (if the monitor does not label it for you) with the date, time, patient's name, and room number. Indicate on the strip when symptoms and treatment interventions occurred.

■ Document the patient's response to treatment.

To explore learning resources for this chapter,

Go to Davis*Plus* at http://davisplus.fadavis.com/, keyword Treas

Chapter Resources for Chapter 38:
   Knowledge Check and Think Like a Nurse Response Sheets
   Knowledge Check Answers
   Resources for Caregivers and Health Professionals
   Reading More About Circulation (Suggested Readings)
   What Are the Main Points in This Chapter?
NCLEX-Style Review Questions
Chapter Overview Podcasts

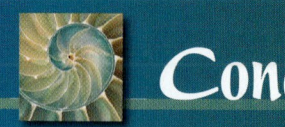

Concept Map

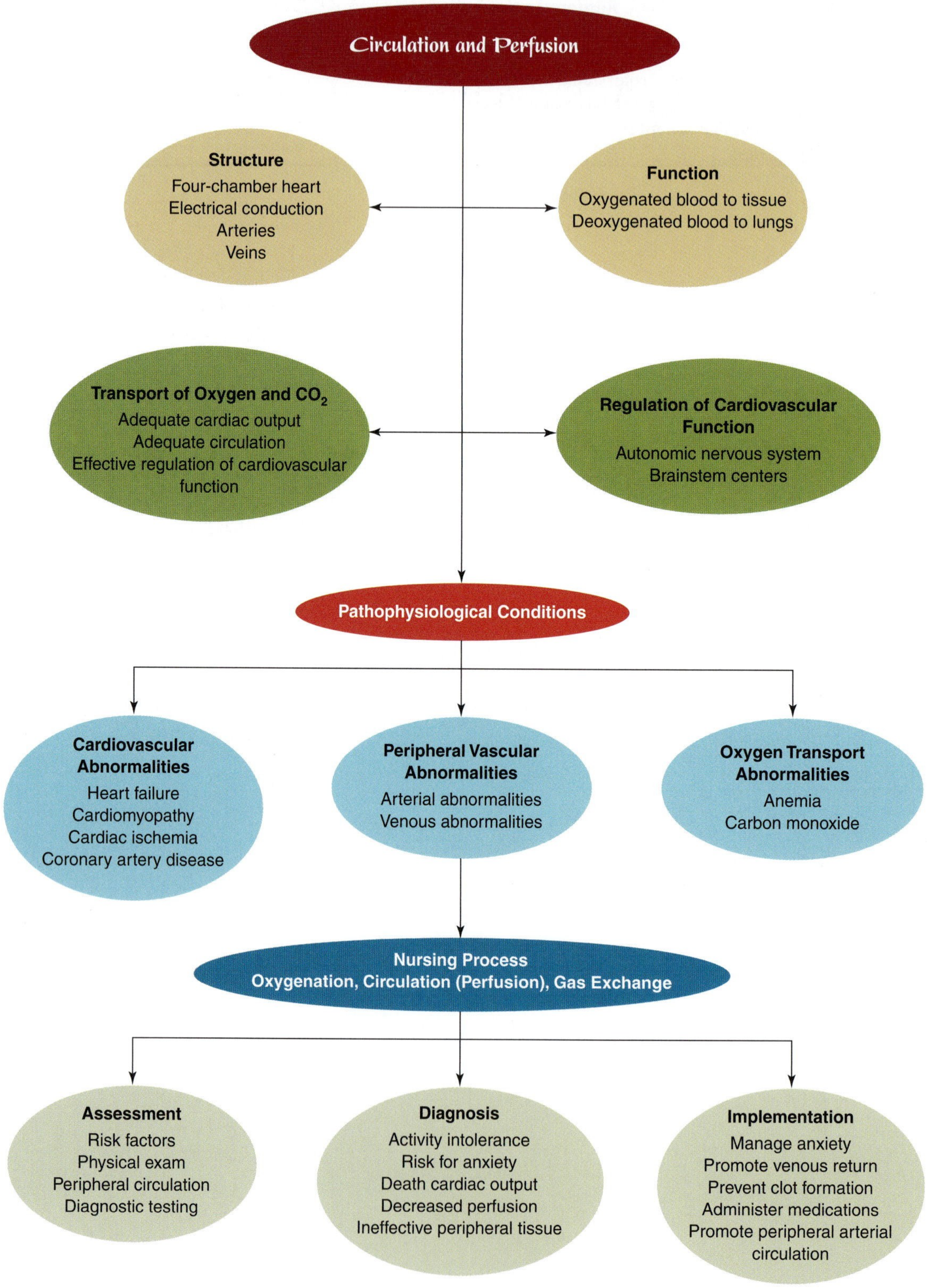

Circulation and Perfusion

Structure

Four-chamber heart
Electrical conduction
Arteries
Veins

Function

Oxygenated blood to tissue
Deoxygenated blood to lungs

Transport of Oxygen and CO$_2$

Adequate cardiac output
Adequate circulation
Effective regulation of cardiovascular
function

**Regulation of Cardiovascular
Function**

Autonomic nervous system
Brainstem centers

Pathophysiological Conditions

**Cardiovascular
Abnormalities**

Heart failure
Cardiomyopathy
Cardiac ischemia
Coronary artery disease

**Peripheral Vascular
Abnormalities**

Arterial abnormalities
Venous abnormalities

**Oxygen Transport
Abnormalities**

Anemia
Carbon monoxide

**Nursing Process
Oxygenation, Circulation (Perfusion), Gas Exchange**

Assessment

Risk factors
Physical exam
Peripheral circulation
Diagnostic testing

Diagnosis

Activity intolerance
Risk for anxiety
Death cardiac output
Decreased perfusion
Ineffective peripheral tissue

Implementation

Manage anxiety
Promote venous return
Prevent clot formation
Administer medications
Promote peripheral arterial
circulation

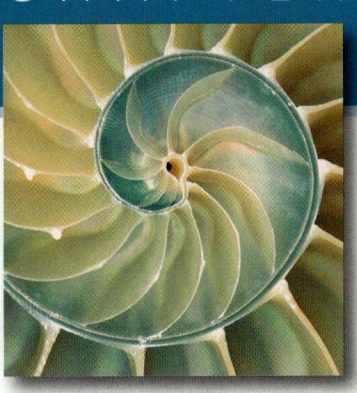

CHAPTER 39

Fluids, Electrolytes, & Acid–Base Balance

Learning Outcomes

After completing this chapter, you should be able to:

➤ Identify the fluid compartments within the body.

➤ Describe the location and function of the major electrolytes of the body.

➤ Differentiate among active and passive transport, osmosis, diffusion, and filtration.

➤ Describe the body mechanisms for maintaining fluid and electrolyte balance.

➤ Summarize the major fluid and electrolyte balance disorders.

➤ Compare and contrast respiratory and metabolic acidosis and alkalosis.

➤ Describe compensatory mechanisms for acid–base imbalances.

➤ Provide nursing interventions for clients with fluid, electrolyte, and acid–base imbalances.

Key Concepts

Acid–base balance

Electrolyte balance

Fluid balance

Related Concepts

See the Concept Map at the end of this chapter.

Example Problem

Fluid, electrolyte, and acid–base imbalances

Caring for the Nguyens

This feature allows you to practice the kind of thinking you will use as a full-spectrum nurse. There is usually more than one correct answer to a critical thinking question, so we do not provide answers for these features. It is more important to develop your nursing judgment than to "cover content." Discuss the questions with your peers. If you are still unsure, consult your instructor.

Nam Nguyen has been prescribed the following medicines:
    lisinopril (Prinivil) 20 mg PO daily
    hydrochlorothiazide (Diuril) 25 mg PO daily in the a.m.
    metformin (Glucophage) 500 mg PO before breakfast
        and lunch
Today he had blood drawn for analysis. Following are the electrolyte panel results.

Sodium	136 mEq/L
Potassium	3.0 mEq/L
Chloride	96 mEq/L
Bicarbonate	24 mEq/L
BUN	18 mg/dL
Creatinine	0.8 mg/dL

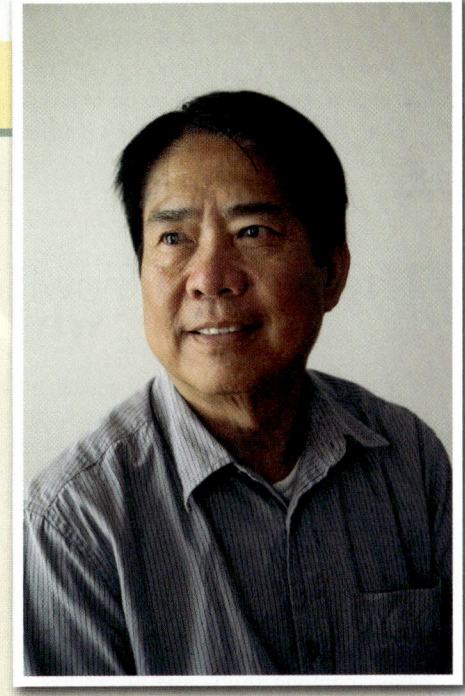

(Continued)

Caring for the Nguyens (continued)

A. Review the lab results. Compare Nam's lab work with the established norms for these values. Based on the lab results, what kind of assessment questions would be appropriate to ask Nam?

B. Use your pharmacology text to review Nam's medications. Which, if any, of these medicines might be contributing to Nam's lab results?

C. What teaching would be appropriate for Nam?

 Go to **Caring for the Nguyens Response Sheet** on *DavisPlus.*

Meet Your Patients

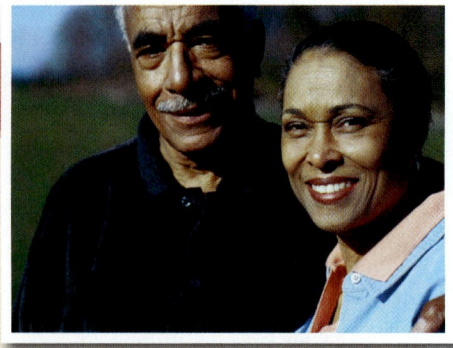

Your instructor has assigned you to care for Jackson LaGuardia, a 60-year-old man with end-stage renal disease. You have arrived at the hospital to review his chart so you can provide care the following day. When you arrive on the unit, the charge nurse informs you that Mr. LaGuardia is still in the emergency department (ED) while waiting to be admitted to the medical-surgical unit. You go to the ED to review his chart and gather data.

In the ED, you introduce yourself and explain your purpose. The charge nurse tells you that five members of the LaGuardia family have all come to the ED complaining of nausea, vomiting, and diarrhea related to severe gastroenteritis, a viral intestinal disorder. The family members include the following:
8-month-old Jason, grandson of Jackson
26-year-old Susanna, Jackson's daughter and Jason's mother

60-year-old Jackson
58-year-old Gemma, Jackson's wife
82-year-old Martha, Jackson's mother

Jason, Jackson, and Martha are being admitted to the hospital. However, Susanna and Gemma have been asked to follow up tomorrow in the urgent care clinic. As you prepare for your clinical day, you think, "If they all have the same disorder, why are only three family members being admitted? What makes these patients different?" In this chapter, we follow the LaGuardias and answer those questions.

Theoretical Knowledge
knowing **why**

When we are healthy, the fluid and chemical state of our bodies is in balance. However, illness can disturb this balance. In this chapter, we examine how fluid, electrolyte, and acid–base balances are maintained, as well as what happens when there are disturbances in each of these areas.

ABOUT THE KEY CONCEPTS

The concepts of *fluid balance* and *electrolyte balance* are intricately related. When one electrolyte changes, usually another does as well, and often fluids shift with it. Tipping the delicate balance among fluids and electrolytes leads to dysfunction and disease.

Likewise, the status of acid–base balance is a reflection of the overall body functioning. Disruption of the balance in pH (acidity and alkalinity) and other body chemicals has a profound effect on overall health. By the end of this chapter, you will become familiar with the various balances and imbalances among fluids, electrolytes, acids, and bases.

BODY FLUIDS

Body fluid is primarily water, with various dissolved substances. Gases, such as carbon dioxide and oxygen, readily dissolve in body fluids. In fact, body fluids transport gases throughout the body. Solid substances, called **solutes,** also dissolve in body fluids. Many solutes are **electrolytes**—substances (e.g., sodium, potassium) that develop an electrical charge when dissolved in water. Other solutes are nonelectrolytes. **Nonelectrolytes** (e.g., glucose, urea) do not conduct electricity. Body fluids perform several important functions:

- Maintain blood volume.
- Regulate body temperature.
- Transport material to and from cells.
- Serve as a medium for cellular metabolism.
- Assist with digestion of food.
- Serve as a medium for excreting waste.

Fluid makes up approximately 60% of an average adult's body weight. However, total body water content varies with the number of fat cells, age, and sex. Infants have very high body water content (70%–80%), and the percentage progressively decreases with age. Women have less body fluid than do men because they have proportionately more

body fat. An obese person has less fluid than does a person of lean build.

What Are the Body Fluids Compartments?

Most body fluid is contained within two compartments. **Intracellular fluid (ICF)** is contained within the cells. Essential for cell function and metabolism, it accounts for approximately 40% of body weight. **Extracellular fluid (ECF)** is outside the cells. ECF carries water, electrolytes, nutrients, and oxygen to the cells and removes the waste products of cellular metabolism. ECF accounts for 20% of body weight. ECF exists in three main locations in the body:

- *Interstitial fluid* lies in the spaces between the body cells. Excess fluid within the interstitial space is called *edema*.
- *Intravascular fluid* is the plasma within the blood. Its main function is to transport blood cells.
- *Transcellular fluid* includes specialized fluids, such as cerebrospinal, pleural, peritoneal, and synovial fluid; and digestive juices.

Figure 39-1 illustrates the distribution of body fluids. In times of illness, fluid may move into an area that makes it physiologically unavailable, such as the peritoneal space (a condition called *ascites*), the pericardial space (a condition called *pericardial effusion*), or the *vesicles* (blisters) produced by a burn wound. This type of fluid movement is known as **third spacing** because fluid is literally trapped in a third compartment—not within interstitial (cells) and not within intravascular spaces (blood vessels).

What Electrolytes Are Present in Body Fluids?

In addition to water, body fluid is composed of oxygen, carbon dioxide, dissolved nutrients, metabolic waste products, and electrolytes. Electrolytes that carry a positive charge are called **cations.** Electrolytes that carry a negative charge are called **anions.** See Table 39-2 for examples of cations and anions. Electrolytes are measured in milliequivalents per liter (mEq/L)

of water or milligrams per 100 mL (mg/100 mL or mg/dL). Note that 1 dL, or deciliter, equals 100 mL. *Milliequivalent* is a measure of chemical combining power, whereas *milligram* is a weight measure.

The composition of body fluids varies between compartments:

- **In the ICF**, the major cations are potassium and magnesium. The major anion is phosphate. Other electrolytes are present, but to a lesser degree.
- **In the ECF**, the major electrolytes are sodium, chloride, and bicarbonate. Albumin is also present in the ECF, mostly in the intravascular fluid. Gastric and intestinal secretions (transcellular fluids) also contain electrolytes.

Severe electrolyte imbalances can occur if electrolytes move into a compartment they do not normally occupy or if they are lost in excess amounts from the body through perspiration, wounds, injury, or illness.

KnowledgeCheck 39-1

- Define *solute, electrolyte, intracellular fluid, extracellular fluid, cation,* and *anion.*
- Identify the major electrolytes in the ICF and ECF.

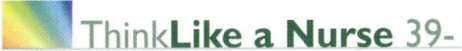

ThinkLike a Nurse 39-1

- Based on the information presented in the Meet Your Patients scenario, rank the members of the LaGuardia family based on total body water content.
- Does this information help you understand which family members were admitted to the hospital?

How Do Fluids and Electrolytes Move in the Body?

The selectively permeable membranes of cells and capillaries separate ICF and ECF (see Fig. 39-1). Fluid and electrolytes move across these membranes by passive and active mechanisms. In **active transport,** movement of fluid and solutes requires

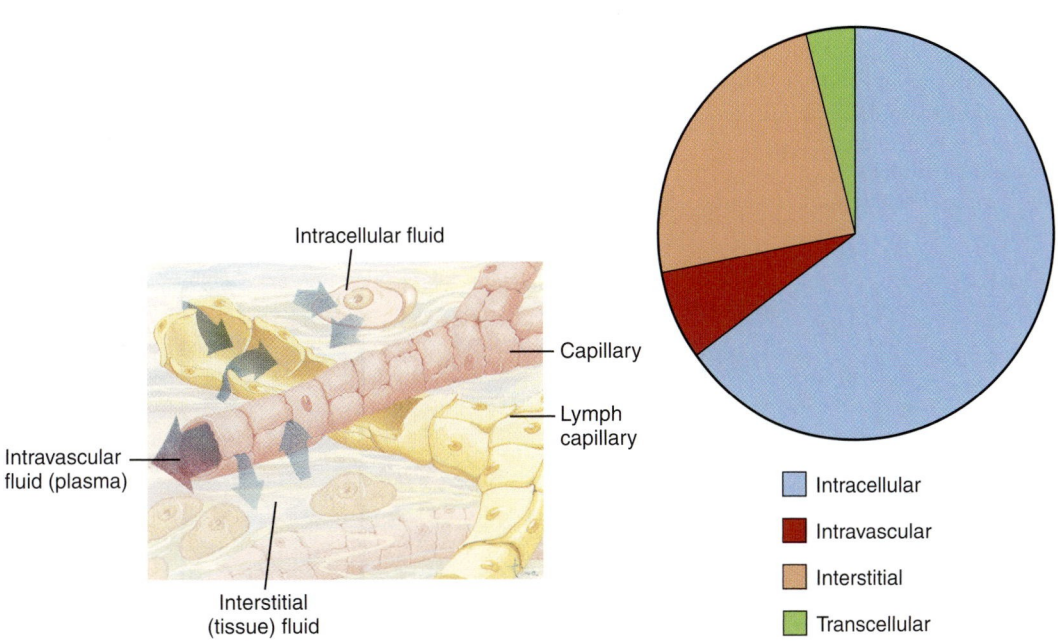

FIGURE 39-1 Normal distribution of body fluids. Transcellular fluid includes specialized fluids such as cerebrospinal and peritoneal fluid and digestive juices.

energy. **Passive transport** requires no energy. The three passive transport systems are osmosis, diffusion, and filtration. To see an animated illustration of these three systems,

 Go to **Animations: Osmosis, Diffusion, Filtration, and Active Transport,** on Davis*Plus*.

Osmosis

Osmosis involves movement of water (or other pure solute) across a membrane from an area of a less concentrated solution to an area of more concentrated solution. Water moves across the membrane to dilute the higher concentration of solutes (Fig. 39-2). Recall that a solute is a substance dissolved in body fluid. Solutes may be crystalloids or colloids. **Crystalloids** are solutes that readily dissolve (e.g., electrolytes). **Colloids** are larger molecules that do not dissolve readily (e.g., proteins).

The concentration of solutes providing pressure in body fluid is called **osmolality. Osmols** refers to the number of particles of solute per kilogram of water and is expressed as milliosmoles per kilogram (mOsm/kg). Sodium is the greatest determinant of serum osmolality, and potassium is the greatest determinant of intracellular osmolality. Glucose and urea also contribute to osmolality in the ICF and ECF.

Another term for osmolality is **tonicity.** A fluid that is of the same osmolality as blood is called **isotonic.** An isotonic solution is often given by intravenous (IV) infusion if blood volume is low. Because the solution is the same concentration as blood, the fluid will remain in the vascular space, and no osmosis will occur. A **hypotonic solution** is of lower osmolality than blood. When a hypotonic solution is infused, water moves by osmosis from the vascular system into the cells. A **hypertonic solution** contains a higher concentration of solutes than does blood. When a hypertonic solution is given to a patient, water moves by osmosis from the cells into the ECF.

Diffusion

Diffusion is a passive process by which molecules of a solute move through a cell membrane from an area of higher concentration to an area of lower concentration. Movement occurs (Fig. 39-3) until the concentrations are equivalent on both sides of the membrane. For an example of diffusion, pour yourself a cup of coffee. Now add cream to the coffee. Initially, the cream is concentrated in the area where you have poured it. However, within a short time the cream is evenly dispersed throughout the coffee. If you stir the coffee, the cream disperses even more quickly. Fluids within the human body work on a similar principle; body movement speeds the diffusion of molecules.

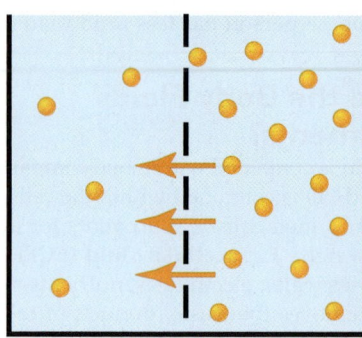

FIGURE 39-3 Diffusion is the movement of molecules of a solute through a cell membrane from an area of higher concentration to an area of lower concentration.

The rate of diffusion varies according to size of the molecules, concentration of the solution, and temperature of the solution. Small molecules move more rapidly than larger molecules. Large differences in concentration require a longer period of time to reach equilibration. Higher temperatures cause molecules to move faster, so that diffusion occurs more rapidly.

Filtration

Filtration is the movement of both water and smaller particles from an area of high pressure to one of low pressure (Fig. 39-4). **Hydrostatic pressure** is the force created by fluid within a closed system; it is responsible for normal circulation of blood. In other words, blood flows from the high-pressure arterial system to the lower pressure capillaries and veins. As fluid (plasma) moves through the capillary membrane, only solutes of a certain size can flow with it. For example, the membrane pores of Bowman's capsule in the kidneys are very small, and only albumin, the smallest of the proteins, can be filtered through the membrane. By contrast, the membrane pores of liver cells are extremely large, so a variety of solutes can pass through and be metabolized.

Osmotic pressure is the power of a solution to draw water. A highly concentrated solution (with many molecules in solution) draws water and has a high osmotic pressure. The plasma proteins in the blood exert osmotic, or colloidal, pressure to help maintain fluid in the vascular space. However, when hydrostatic pressure exceeds osmotic pressure, fluid leaves the vessels. This difference, known as the **filtration pressure,** represents the net pressures that move fluid and solutes.

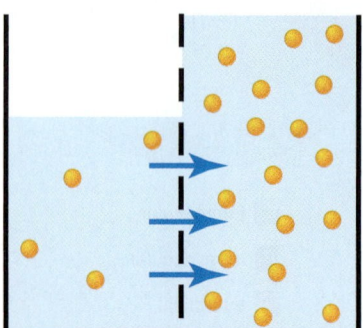

FIGURE 39-2 Osmosis is the movement of water across a membrane from a less concentrated solution to a more concentrated solution.

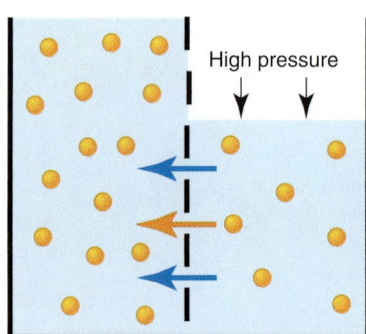

FIGURE 39-4 Filtration is the movement of water and smaller particles from an area of high pressure to an area of low pressure.

Active Transport

Active transport occurs when molecules (e.g., electrolytes) move across cell membranes from an area of low concentration to an area of high concentration. Active transport requires energy expenditure for the movement to occur against a concentration gradient (Fig. 39-5). Adenosine triphosphate (ATP) is released from the cell to enable certain substances to acquire the energy needed to pass through the cell membrane. For example, sodium concentration is greater in ECF; therefore, sodium tends to enter by diffusion into the intracellular compartment. This tendency is offset by the sodium-potassium pump, which is located on the cell membrane. In the presence of ATP, the sodium-potassium pump actively moves sodium from the cell into the ECF. Active transport is vital for maintaining the unique composition of both the extracellular and intracellular compartments.

Table 39-1 summarizes the processes of fluid and electrolyte movement.

If you would like to see some animations and further self-paced learning about fluids and electrolytes,

 Go to the Web sites listed in Chapter 39, **Resources for Caregivers & Health Professionals,** on *DavisPlus.*

KnowledgeCheck 39-2

Identify the appropriate mechanism: osmosis, diffusion, filtration, or active transport:
- Molecules move across a membrane to equalize concentration.
- Fluid moves across a membrane to equalize concentration.
- Molecules move against a concentration gradient.
- Molecules move to equalize pressure.

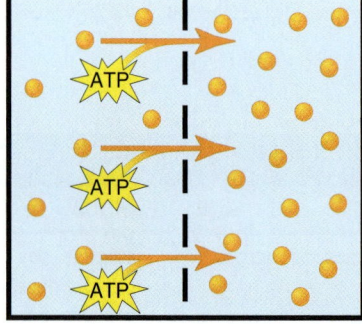

FIGURE 39-5 Active transport is the movement of electrolytes against a concentration gradient. For the movement to occur, active transport requires energy expenditure.

How Does the Body Regulate Fluids?

A balance between fluid intake and output is essential to maintain homeostasis. Excesses or deficits of intake or output can lead to severe disorders.

Fluid Intake

You have undoubtedly been told to drink eight to ten glasses of water per day. Did you ever wonder where that recommendation came from or why that volume is important? Eight to twelve 8-ounce cups of water provide 1,920 to 2,400 mL of fluid. The Institute of Medicine (IOM) (2004), however, recommends a total fluid intake of 2,700 mL per day for women and 3,700 mL per day for men. This is higher than the previous recommendation of 2,500 mL per day for the average adult engaged in moderate activity in moderate temperature, which you may have learned in a biology class. The IOM states we should obtain 80% of our intake from drinking fluids and the remaining 20% from food and cellular metabolism of foods. Prolonged exercise and heat exposure increase the requirements. The IOM did not set an upper limit on fluid intake for healthy adults.

Thirst is the major regulator of fluid intake. Changes in plasma osmolality signal the thirst center in the hypothalamus, which leads to the urge to drink. Situations that increase plasma osmolality (and promote thirst) include excessive fluid loss, excessive sodium intake, and decreased fluid intake. Situations that inhibit the thirst mechanism include a high intake of fluids, fluid retention, excessive IV infusion of hypotonic solutions, and low sodium intake.

Fluid Output

Fluid loss occurs throughout the day, creating a constant need to replenish fluid. In a healthy state, fluid losses are equivalent to fluid intake. **Sensible fluid loss** is measurable and perceived (e.g., urine, diarrhea, ostomy, and gastric drainage). **Insensible fluid loss** is loss that a person does not perceive and that is not easily measured. It occurs primarily by diffusion and evaporation through the skin, but also from the lungs, and accounts for about 900 mL per day. Insensible loss increases with open wounds, burns, or other breaks in the protective layer of the skin.

The following are common sources of fluid loss:
- *Urine* (1,500 mL/day). Urine accounts for the greatest amount of fluid loss. Urine output varies according to intake and activity, but should remain at least 30 to 50 mL/hour. The volume of urine increases as intake increases, and it decreases to compensate for other fluid losses (e.g., vomiting and excessive perspiration).
- *Feces* (100 to 200 mL/day). Soft stools contain more water than hard stools. As stool frequency increases, water loss also increases.
- *Skin* (about 600 mL/day). **Sensible (perceived) fluid loss** through the skin occurs through perspiration, at 300 to

Table 39-1 ➤ Processes of Fluid and Electrolyte Movement			
PROCESS	**WHAT MOVES**	**FROM AREA OF**	**TO AREA OF**
Diffusion	Molecules (solute)	High concentration	Low concentration
Active transport	Molecules (solute)	Low concentration	High concentration
Osmosis	Water	Low concentration	High concentration
Filtration	Water and small particles	High pressure	Low pressure

600 mL/day. Perspiration varies based on temperature, skeletal muscle activity, and metabolic activity. Fever, exercise, and some disease processes increase metabolic activity and heat production, leading to increased fluid loss.

- *Lungs* (about 300 mL/day). Insensible loss occurs through the lungs as water is exhaled with the breath. An increase in respiratory rate increases the amount of fluid lost.

Hormonal Regulation

The kidneys are the principal regulator of fluid and electrolyte balance. The following hormones are involved:

Antidiuretic Hormone. Pressure sensors in the vascular system stimulate or inhibit the release of **antidiuretic hormone (ADH)** from the pituitary gland. ADH causes the kidneys to retain fluid. If fluid volume within the vascular system is low, fluid pressures within the system decrease, and more ADH is released. If fluid volume (and therefore pressure) increases, less ADH is released, and the kidneys eliminate more fluid. ADH is also produced in response to a rise in serum osmolality, fever, pain, stress, and some opioids.

Renin–Angiotensin System. When extracellular (i.e., intravascular) fluid volume is decreased, receptors in the glomeruli respond to the decreased perfusion of the kidneys by releasing renin. **Renin** is an enzyme responsible for the chain of reactions that converts angiotensinogen to angiotensin II. **Angiotensin II** acts on the nephrons to retain sodium and water and directs the adrenal cortex to release aldosterone.

Aldosterone. When aldosterone is released, it stimulates the distal tubules of the kidneys to reabsorb sodium and excrete potassium. Sodium reabsorption results in passive reabsorption of water, thereby increasing plasma volume and improving kidney perfusion. When fluid excess is present, renin is not released, and this process stops.

Other Hormones. (1) *Thyroid hormone* affects fluid volume by influencing cardiac output. An increase in thyroid hormone causes an increase in cardiac output, thereby increasing glomerular filtration rate and urine output. A decrease has the opposite effect. (2) *Atrial natriuretic peptide (ANP), brain natriuretic peptide (BNP),* and *C-type natriuretic peptide (CNP)* are important in renal and cardiovascular regulation of fluid maintenance. **Natriuresis (natriuretic)** is the discharge of sodium through urine. BNP is actually released from both the brain and the right atrium. In clinical practice, BNP can be measured in the serum to help determine presence of heart failure with fluid excess and to distinguish heart failure from pulmonary edema. The test can be performed at the bedside.

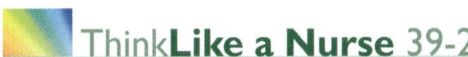

ThinkLike a Nurse 39-2

Apply the information on fluid balance to the LaGuardia family (Meet Your Patients). What have you learned that helps you explain why some family members require hospitalization? What additional information do you need to be able to predict each person's fluid balance?

How Does the Body Regulate Electrolytes?

To maintain health, the body must balance electrolyte losses and intake. For example, potassium lost through diarrhea and vomiting must be replaced by dietary potassium or potassium supplements. Table 39-2 provides information about the function, regulation, and food sources of major electrolytes in the body. Maintenance of normal serum electrolyte levels also depends on dietary intake, as well as various body regulatory mechanisms, discussed in the remainder of this section.

Sodium (Na⁺)

Sodium is the major cation in the ECF. Its primary function is to regulate fluid volume. When sodium is reabsorbed in the kidney, water and potassium are also reabsorbed, thereby maintaining ECF volume.

Table 39-2 ➤ Major Electrolytes

ELECTROLYTE	FUNCTION	REGULATION	SOURCES
Sodium (NA⁺) Major cation in the ECF Normal serum level is 135–145 mEq/L.	Regulates fluid volume. Helps maintain blood volume. Interacts with calcium to maintain muscle contraction. Stimulates conduction of nerve impulses.	Moves by active transport across cell membranes. Regulated by aldosterone and ADH levels Reabsorbed and excreted through the kidneys Minimal loss through perspiration and feces Low sodium may be caused by excess water intake.	Table salt, soy sauce, cured pork, cheese, milk, processed foods, canned products, and foods preserved with salt
Potassium (K⁺) Major cation in the ICF Normal serum level is 3.5–5 mEq/L.	Maintains ICF osmolality. Regulates conduction of cardiac rhythm. Transmits electrical impulses in multiple body systems. Assists with acid–base balance.	Regulated by aldosterone Excreted and conserved through the kidneys Lost through vomiting and diarrhea Loss triggered by many diuretics	Common food sources include bananas, oranges, apricots, figs, dates, carrots, potatoes, tomatoes, spinach, dairy products, and meats.

Table 39-2 ➤ Major Electrolytes—cont'd

ELECTROLYTE	FUNCTION	REGULATION	SOURCES
Calcium (Ca²⁺) Most abundant electrolyte in the body Normal serum level is 8.5–10.5 mg/dL.	Promotes transmission of nerve impulses. Major component of bone and teeth Regulates muscle contractions. Maintains cardiac automaticity. Essential factor in the formation of blood clots Catalyst for many cellular activities	Combines with phosphorus to form the mineral salts of the teeth and bones. Calcium and phosphorus levels inversely proportional Parathyroid hormone (PTH) stimulates release of calcium from bones and reabsorption from kidneys and intestines. Calcitonin (from the thyroid) blocks bone breakdown and lowers calcium levels. Absorption stimulated by vitamin D	See Table 39-3 for average daily requirements. Common food sources include milk, milk products, dark green leafy vegetables, and salmon, as well as calcium-fortified foods such as breads and cereals.
Magnesium (Mg²⁺) Present in skeleton and ICF; second most abundant cation in ICF Normal serum level is 1.6–2.6 mEq/L.	Involved in protein and carbohydrate metabolism Necessary for protein and DNA synthesis within the cell Maintains normal intracellular levels of potassium Involved in electrical activity in nerve and muscle membranes, including the heart May have a role in regulating blood pressure and may influence the release and activity of insulin (IOM, 2004).	Ingested in the diet and absorbed through the small intestine Excreted by kidneys Loss may be triggered by diuretics, poorly controlled diabetes mellitus, and excess alcohol intake.	Average daily requirement is 18–30 mEq. Found in most foods, but high levels are present in green vegetables, cereal grains, and nuts.
Chloride (Cl⁻) Major anion in the ECF Normal serum level is 95–105 mEq/L.	Works with Na⁺ to maintain osmotic pressure between fluid compartments. Essential for production of HCl for gastric secretions Functions as buffer in oxygen–carbon dioxide exchange in RBCs. Assists with acid–base balance.	Reabsorbed and excreted through the kidneys along with sodium Regulated by aldosterone and ADH levels Deficits lead to potassium deficits; potassium deficits lead to chloride deficits.	Found in foods high in sodium
Phosphate (PO₄⁻) Major anion in the ICF Normal serum level is 1.7–2.6 mEq/L.	Serves as a catalyst for many intracellular activities Promotes muscle and nerve action Assists with acid–base balance Important for cell division and transmission of hereditary traits	Combines with calcium to form the mineral salts of the teeth and bones Calcium and phosphorus levels inversely proportional Regulated by PTH; has inverse response to calcium Excreted and reabsorbed by the kidneys	Foods high in phosphorus are meat, fish, poultry, milk products, carbonated beverages, and legumes. Readily available in body as a result of metabolism
Bicarbonate (HCO₃⁻) Major buffer in the body In ECF and ICF Normal serum level is 22–26 mEq/L.	Maintains acid–base balance by functioning as the primary buffer in the body	Lost through diarrhea, diuretics, renal insufficiency Excess possible if person ingests quantities of acid neutralizers	Present in acid neutralizers (e.g., sodium bicarbonate)

According to the *Dietary Guidelines for Americans, 2010,* adults should limit intake of salt to 2,300 mg/day. Older adults; African Americans; people with chronic diseases including hypertension, diabetes, and chronic kidney disease (including children); and persons who are 51 and older are especially sensitive to the blood pressure–raising effects of salt. As a result, they are advised to limit salt to 1,500 mg/day. This applies to nearly half the U.S. population (U.S. Department of Agriculture (USDA), Center for Nutrition Policy and Promotion, 2011).

Potassium (K⁺)

Potassium is the major cation of the ICF; only 2% of body potassium is found in the extracellular fluid. Potassium is a key electrolyte in cellular metabolism. The *Dietary Guidelines for Americans, 2010* recommends that adults consume at least 4,700 mg/day. However, most American women age 31 to 50 years consume less than half of the recommended amount of potassium, and intake is only moderately higher for men. In short, most people do not consume enough potassium. Moderate potassium deficiency is associated with increases in blood pressure, salt sensitivity, risk of kidney stones, and risk of bone turnover (U.S. Department of Agriculture (USDA), 2004, updated 2010). Because of its effect on blood pressure, low intake of dietary potassium is associated with increased risk of stroke.

The Dietary Reference Intakes (DRIs) do not specify an upper limit of potassium intake because there is no evidence of problems associated with higher potassium intake (IOM, 2004). In a healthy person, a high potassium intake does not result in a high serum potassium level (hyperkalemia) because the kidneys efficiently eliminate excess dietary potassium.

Calcium (Ca²⁺)

Calcium is responsible for bone health and neuromuscular and cardiac function. It is also an essential factor in blood clotting. About 99% of body calcium is located in the bones and teeth. The remaining 1% circulates in the blood and affects system functions. Because calcium is so vital for cardiac and muscle function, serum levels are tightly regulated. As serum levels drop, calcium leaches from the bones into the blood to compensate. If dietary intake is not sufficient to replace it, bone loss occurs; prolonged deficiencies lead to osteoporosis.

Half the women older than age 50 and 90% of women older than age 75 have osteoporosis; about 30% of men older than age 50 are affected. About half of all Caucasian women will suffer an osteoporosis-related fracture at some point in life, as will approximately one in five men. Because most Americans do not include the recommended amount of calcium in their diets, the chances of bone loss increase with age. Most calcium should be obtained from naturally calcium-rich foods, such as dairy products. Calcium-fortified foods and calcium supplements can be used as a secondary source.

Calcium requirements are highest during childhood, adolescence, pregnancy, and breastfeeding. People who are immobile are at increased risk for reduced bone density. Older adults are at risk for calcium deficiencies because of reduced absorption that occurs with aging and chronic medical conditions (National Osteoporosis Foundation, 2008, revised 2010; U.S. Department of Health and Human Services, 2004-updated 2009). For recommended calcium intake by age group, see Table 39-3.

Table 39-3 ➤ Recommended Daily Calcium Intake

AGE	DIETARY REFERENCE INTAKE (DRI) FOR CALCIUM (MILLIGRAMS)	VITAMIN D* (INTERNATIONAL UNITS)
Birth to 6 mo	210	200
6–12 mo	270	200
1–3 yr	500	200
4–8 yr	800	200
9–18 yr	1,300	200
19–50 yr	1,000	200
51–70 yr	1,200	800–1,000
Older than 70 yr	1,200	800–1,000
Pregnant or Lactating Women		
18 yr or younger	1,300	200
19–50 yr	1,000	200

*Adequate intake of vitamin D is necessary for absorption of calcium.

Sources: Lim, L. S., Hoeksema, L. J., Sherin, K., and ACPM Prevention Practice Committee. (2009, April). Guideline summary: Screening for osteoporosis in the adult U.S. population: ACPM Position statement on preventive practice. In: National Guideline Clearinghouse (NGC) [Web site]. Rockville, MD. Retrieved November 28, 2011, from http://www.guideline.gov/summary/summary.aspx?view_id=1&doc_id=15270; and U.S. Department of Agriculture (USDA). (2004, updated 2010). Dietary Reference Intakes: Recommended intakes for individuals. National Academies of Sciences. Retrieved November 29, 2011, from http://www.iom.edu/Activities/Nutrition/SummaryDRIs/~/media/Files/Activity%20Files/Nutrition/DRIs/5_Summary%20Table%20Tables%201-4.pdf

Magnesium (Mg²⁺)

Magnesium is a mineral used in more than 300 biochemical reactions in the body. Like calcium, only about 1% of magnesium is found in the blood. The remaining 99% is divided between the ICF and bone (in combination with calcium and phosphorus). Although magnesium deficiency is rare, you may find low levels in individuals who have a high alcohol intake. Some malabsorption disorders may also cause magnesium depletion.

Chloride (Cl⁻)

Chloride is the most abundant anion in the extracellular fluid. It is usually bound with other ions, especially sodium or potassium (e.g., as sodium chloride, or salt). A healthy adult between the ages of 19 and 50 should consume 2.3 grams of chloride each day along with 1.5 grams of sodium to replace daily losses and maintain serum blood levels (IOM, 2004).

Phosphorus (Phosphate [PO₄⁻])

Most phosphorus in the body is combined with oxygen, forming phosphate—mostly bound with calcium in teeth and bones as calcium phosphate. Phosphate is the most abundant intracellular anion. Phosphate and calcium exist in an inverse relationship; as one increases, the other one decreases. As a result, high blood phosphate levels decrease the movement of calcium from the bones. Phosphate in the ECF is known as **phosphorus.**

Bicarbonate (HCO₃⁻)

Bicarbonate is present in both ICF and ECF. The kidneys regulate extracellular bicarbonate to maintain acid–base balance. When serum levels rise, the kidneys excrete excess bicarbonate. If serum levels are low, the kidneys conserve bicarbonate. Bicarbonate is not consumed in the diet but is produced by the body to meet current needs.

KnowledgeCheck 39-3

- Identify the major functions of sodium, potassium, calcium, magnesium, chloride, phosphate, and bicarbonate.
- What are the major concerns associated with sodium and potassium intake?
- Identify at least five potassium-rich foods.
- Identify the ideal calcium intakes for each member of the LaGuardia family (Meet Your Patients).

ThinkLike a Nurse 39-3

Based on the information you have learned about the major electrolytes of the body, which electrolytes are most likely to be out of balance in members of the LaGuardia family (Meet Your Patients)? Explain your answer.

How Is Acid–Base Balance Regulated?

Acids and bases are formed in the body as part of normal metabolic processes. An **acid** is any compound that contains hydrogen ions (H⁺) that can be released. For this reason, acids are referred to as cation donors. A common strong acid is hydrochloric acid (HCl), which is present in gastric secretions. A **base** or **alkali** is a compound that combines with (accepts) hydrogen ions in solution. Therefore, bases are referred to as cation (a positively charged particle) acceptors. A strong base has a tendency to bind hydrogen ions, whereas a weak base binds only a small portion of the available hydrogen ions.

The amount of acid or base present in a solution is measured as **pH.** The pH is reported on a scale of 1 to 14: 1 to 6.9 is acidic, 7 is neutral, and 7.1 to 14 is basic, or alkaline. The stronger an acid is, the lower the pH will be. In contrast, a strong base has a high pH. The pH is a *logarithmic* scale. For example, a pH of 4 is 10 times more acidic than a pH of 5. The body functions normally within a narrow range of pH values. Arterial blood and tissue fluid normally have a pH of 7.35 to 7.45; therefore, they are slightly alkaline. A serum pH below 7.30 or above 7.52 alters enzymatic activity and creates myocardial irritability. A serum pH below 6.9 or above 7.8 is usually fatal. Three complex mechanisms maintain acid–base balance: (1) buffers, (2) respiratory control of carbon dioxide, and (3) renal regulation of bicarbonate (HCO₃⁻).

Buffers

Buffer systems prevent wide swings in pH. A buffer system consists of a weak acid and a weak base. Buffer molecules keep strong acids or bases from altering the pH either by absorbing or releasing free hydrogen ions.

Carbonic Acid–Sodium Bicarbonate System. Carbonic acid (H₂CO₃) and sodium bicarbonate (NaHCO₃) buffer almost 90% of metabolic processes in the ECF. Blood and tissue fluid depend on this buffer system to maintain a relatively constant pH. During normal metabolism, blood and tissue fluids tend to become acidic; therefore, more sodium bicarbonate is required than carbonic acid. The usual ratio of NaHCO₃ to H₂CO₃ is 20:1. As long as this ratio is maintained, the pH remains within its normal range. If bicarbonate is depleted while neutralizing a strong acid, the pH may drop below 7.35, resulting in a condition called **acidosis.** If a strong base is added to extracellular fluid and depletes carbonic acid, the pH may rise above 7.45, resulting in a condition called **alkalosis.**

Phosphate System. The phosphate system helps regulate acid–base balance in intracellular fluids. The phosphate system works in the same way as the bicarbonate system but converts alkaline sodium phosphate (Na₂HPO₄) to acid sodium phosphate (NaH₂PO₄).

Protein System. Plasma proteins and the globin portion of hemoglobin (in red blood cells) contain chemical groups that can either combine with or free up hydrogen ions. This system helps buffer intracellular fluid and plasma to maintain pH balance.

Respiratory Mechanisms

The lungs are the second line of defense to restore normal pH. They control the body's carbonic acid supply via carbon dioxide retention or removal. When the serum pH is too acidic (pH is low), the lungs remove carbon dioxide through rapid, deep breathing. This reduces the amount of carbon dioxide available to make carbonic acid. If the serum pH is too alkaline (pH is high), the lungs try to conserve carbon dioxide through shallow respirations.

Renal Mechanisms

The last line of defense is the kidneys, which regulate the concentration of plasma bicarbonate. They can neutralize more acid or base than either the respiratory system or the chemical buffers. If the serum pH is too acidic, the kidneys conserve additional bicarbonate to neutralize the acid. If the serum pH is too alkaline, the kidneys excrete additional bicarbonate to lower the amount of base and thereby decrease the pH. The kidneys also buffer pH by forming acids and ammonium (a base).

Although the renal system is very effective at altering pH, it is slow. It may take up to 3 days to return the pH to normal limits. This process is known as *compensation*. The pH returns to normal, but the carbon dioxide or bicarbonate level is abnormal. Over time, or when the original problem is corrected, these levels also return to normal.

KnowledgeCheck 39-4

- Briefly describe the three mechanisms used to maintain pH.
- Rank in order the acid–base balance mechanisms from the most rapidly acting to the slowest acting.

Example Problem: Fluid, Electrolyte, and Acid–Base Imbalances

Illness or disease may lead to imbalances of fluid, electrolytes, or pH. These are discussed in the next sections. The Practical Knowledge section, later in the chapter, presents some interventions to correct these imbalances.

Fluid Imbalances

Fluid imbalances involve a deficit or excess in fluid volume or an alteration in distribution among the fluid compartments. Fluid deficit, regardless of the cause, is referred to as *hypovolemia*, whereas fluid excess, usually not blood, is referred to as *hypervolemia*.

Deficient Fluid Volume

Deficient fluid volume (hypovolemia) occurs when there is a proportional loss of fluid and electrolytes from the ECF. Loss of blood volume is called hypovolemia (*hypo* = low, *vol* = volume, *emia* pertains to blood). Hypovolemia may occur with surgery, trauma, or uterine rupture.

Categories of Dehydration

Dehydration describes a state of negative fluid balance in which there is a loss of water (*hydra* = water) from the intracellular, extracellular, or intravascular spaces. Dehydration can be categorized by three causes:

- Insufficient intake of fluids (e.g., as may occur in depression, sedation, or alcohol abuse)
- Excessive fluid loss (e.g., bleeding, vomiting, diarrhea, nasogastric [NG] suction)
- Fluid shifts (e.g., intravascular fluids leaking into body tissues, burns).

When dehydration occurs from the loss of body fluids, electrolytes may also be lost. Fluid loss can also lead to an increase in serum osmolarity.

Early Symptoms of Dehydration

The first symptom of volume loss is thirst. If the patient is able to recognize thirst and respond by drinking liquid, no further treatment may be required. If fluid is not available or the patient is unable to drink, or if blood loss continues faster than fluid is replaced (e.g., hemorrhage), fluid becomes deficient. Initially as fluid volume decreases, the heart rate increases and the blood vessels constrict. This increases the blood pressure, in order to continue to circulate the remaining fluid to meet the body's fluid demands.

Symptoms of Continuing Fluid Loss

If volume continues to be lost, the heart pumps faster but not as powerfully, resulting in a rapid, weak pulse, and orthostatic hypotension. This is known as **hypovolemic shock.** Orthostatic blood pressure is measured when the patient is lying, sitting, and standing. A drop in the systolic blood pressure (from lying or sitting to standing) greater or equal to 20 mm Hg is called **orthostatic hypotension.** Low fluid volume is just one of its causes.

As fluid loss continues, water is pulled from the interstitial spaces and the ICF into the vascular system, resulting in dry skin and mucous membranes, decreased skin and tongue turgor, decreased urine output, and flat neck veins. Patients complain of muscle weakness, fatigue, and feeling warm. Temperature increases because the body is less able to cool itself through perspiration. In an older adult, temperature will rise but may not be elevated above normal body temperature.

Weight is a sensitive measure of fluid loss. A sudden 5% loss of body weight is considered clinically significant. When weight loss approaches 8%, fluid loss is severe. A sudden loss of 15% of body weight due to fluid loss is usually fatal. The patient with fluid volume deficit usually has elevated blood urea nitrogen (BUN)-to-creatinine ratio and elevated hematocrit. Both values increase because there is less water in proportion to the solid substances being measured. Specific gravity of the urine increases as the kidneys attempt to conserve water, resulting in more concentrated urine.

Preventing Deficient Fluid Volume

You can help prevent fluid volume deficit by identifying patients who have the highest risk for developing this condition. High-risk patients include older adults, infants, children, and any patients with conditions associated with fluid loss (e.g., diabetes insipidus, vomiting, diarrhea, fever). You will learn how to facilitate fluid intake and provide parenteral fluid replacement in the Planning Interventions/Implementation section.

Excess Fluid Volume

Excess fluid volume (hypervolemia) involves excessive retention of sodium and water in the ECF. Fluid volume excess can result from excessive salt intake, disease affecting kidney or liver function, or poor pumping action of the heart. The retained sodium increases osmotic pressure in the ECF. This pressure pulls fluid from the cells into the ECF.

Signs of Fluid Overload. The vital sign changes in a patient with hypervolemia are the opposite of those in a patient with hypovolemia. The blood pressure is elevated, pulse is bounding, and respirations are increased and shallow. The neck veins may become distended. Along with increased intravascular volume, excess ECF may accumulate in the tissues, especially in dependent areas, as *edema.* The skin is pale and cool. Urine output becomes dilute, and volume increases. The patient rapidly gains weight. In severe fluid overload, the patient develops moist crackles in the lungs, dyspnea, and ascites (excess peritoneal fluid). Hemodilution causes BUN, hematocrit, and the specific gravity of the urine to decrease.

Preventing Fluid Overload. You can help prevent fluid overload by monitoring intake and output and observing patients for signs and symptoms of fluid overload. Electronic infusion pumps control the rate of infusion of intravenous fluid, thereby limiting the risk for patients receiving IV therapy (see the Planning Interventions/Implementation section).

KnowledgeCheck 39-5

- Define *deficient fluid volume* and *excess fluid volume.*
- Identify the signs and symptoms of deficient fluid volume and excess fluid volume.
- Describe dehydration and hypervolemia.

Table 39-4 ➤ Electrolyte Imbalances

DISORDER	COMMON CAUSES	SIGNS AND SYMPTOMS	TREATMENT
Hyponatremia $Na^+ < 135$ mEq/L	Diuretics GI fluid loss Adrenal insufficiency Excessive intake of hypotonic solutions, such as water or D_5W IV fluids Syndrome of inappropriate ADH	Anorexia, nausea, and vomiting Weakness Lethargy Confusion Muscle cramps or twitching Seizures	Monitor I&O. Monitor sodium level. Increase oral sodium intake. Administer IV saline infusion and take seizure precautions, if severe.

Hypernatremia $Na^+ > 145$ mEq/L	Excessive sodium intake
	
	Water deprivation
	
	Increased water loss through profuse sweating, heat stroke, or diabetes insipidus
	
	Administration of hypertonic tube feeding
		Thirst
		
		Elevated temperature
		
		Dry mouth and sticky mucous membranes
		
		If severe:
		  Hallucinations
		  Irritability
		  Lethargy
		  Seizures
			Monitor I&O.
			
			Monitor sodium level.
			
			Monitor vital signs and level of consciousness.
			
			Restrict sodium in the diet.
			
			Beware of hidden sodium in foods and medications.
			
			Increase water intake.
			
			Administer IV solutions that do not contain sodium.

Hypokalemia $K^+ < 3.5$ mEq/L	Diuretics GI fluid loss through vomiting, gastric suction, or diarrhea Steroid administration Hyperaldosteronism Anorexia or bulimia	Fatigue Anorexia, nausea, and vomiting Muscle weakness Decreased GI motility Dysrhythmias Paresthesia Flat T wave on ECG Increased sensitivity to digitalis	Monitor I&O. Monitor potassium level. If the client is taking digoxin, monitor pulse and observe for toxicity. Encourage intake of foods rich in potassium. Administer potassium supplements (*Note:* IV supplements must be well diluted and administered into a central vein slowly.)
Hyperkalemia $K^+ > 5.0$ mEq/L	Renal failure Potassium-sparing diuretics Hypoaldosteronism High potassium intake coupled with renal insufficiency Acidosis Major trauma Hemolyzed serum sample produces pseudohyperkalemia	Muscle weakness Dysrhythmias Flaccid paralysis Intestinal colic Tall T waves on ECG	Monitor I&O. Monitor potassium level. Caution about potassium-rich food intake in patients with elevated creatinine levels.

(Continued)

Table 39-4 ▶ Electrolyte Imbalances—cont'd

DISORDER	COMMON CAUSES	SIGNS AND SYMPTOMS	TREATMENT
Hypocalcemia $Ca^{2+} < 8.5$ mq/dL	Hypoparathyroidism Malabsorption Pancreatitis Alkalosis Vitamin D deficiency	Diarrhea Numbness and tingling of extremities Muscle cramps Tetany Convulsions Laryngeal spasms Cardiac irritability *Positive Trousseau's and Chvostek's signs	Monitor I&O. Monitor serum calcium. Encourage increased calcium intake. Administer calcium supplements. If severe, monitor patency of airway, institute seizure and safety precautions, and administer parenteral calcium.
Hypercalcemia $Ca^{2+} > 10.5$ mq/dL	Hyperparathyroidism Malignant bone disease Prolonged immobilization Excess calcium supplementation Thiazide diuretics	Muscle weakness Constipation Anorexia, nausea, and vomiting Polyuria and polydipsia Kidney stones Bizarre behavior Bradycardia	Monitor I&O. Encourage fluid intake to prevent stone formation. Encourage fiber to prevent constipation. Eliminate calcium supplements and limit calcium-rich foods. Avoid calcium-based antacids. Renal dialysis may be required.
Hypomagnesemia $Mg^{2+} < 1.3$ mEq/L	Chronic alcoholism Malabsorption Diabetic ketoacidosis Prolonged gastric suction	Neuromuscular irritability Disorientation Mood changes Dysrhythmias Increased sensitivity to digitalis	Monitor I&O. Encourage foods high in magnesium. Avoid alcohol intake. If the client is taking digoxin, monitor pulse and observe for toxicity.
Hypermagnesemia $Mg^{2+} > 2.1$ mEq/L	Renal failure Adrenal insufficiency Excess replacement	Flushing and warmth of skin Hypotension Drowsiness, lethargy Hypoactive reflexes Depressed respirations Bradycardia	Monitor vital signs and airway. Monitor reflexes. Avoid magnesium-based antacids and laxatives. Restrict dietary intake of foods high in magnesium.
Hypophosphatemia $PO_4^- < .7$ mEq/L	Refeeding after starvation Alcohol withdrawal Diabetic ketoacidosis Respiratory acidosis	Paresthesia Joint stiffness Seizures Cardiomyopathy Impaired tissue oxygenation	Monitor serum phosphorus level. Monitor calcium levels as phosphate is replaced. Start TPN slowly to avoid drops in phosphate.
Hyperphosphatemia $PO_4^- > 2.6$ mEq/L	Renal failure Hyperthyroidism Chemotherapy Excess use of phosphate-based laxative	Short term: tetany symptoms—tingling of extremities and cramping Long term: Calcification in soft tissue	Monitor serum phosphorus level. Monitor for tetany. If severe, administer aluminum hydroxide with meals to bind phosphorus.

*See Clinical Insight 39-2, Assessing for Trousseau's and Chvostek's Signs.

Electrolyte Imbalances

Any electrolyte may become imbalanced. Table 39-4 discusses the common causes; signs and symptoms; and treatment of sodium, potassium, calcium, magnesium, and phosphate imbalances. Disorders affecting chloride ions occur along with sodium disorders. As sodium levels rise, chloride levels also rise. Decreases also occur simultaneously. Clinical signs and treatments are identical to the treatments used for sodium imbalances. Because of the role of bicarbonate as a buffer, bicarbonate levels rise and fall to maintain pH. You will find further discussion of abnormal bicarbonate levels in the Acid–Base Imbalances section, which follows.

We can apply the information in Table 39-4 to the LaGuardia family (Meet Your Patients). Jackson LaGuardia has end-stage renal disease (ESRD), or renal failure. As a result, he is at risk for imbalances in all of his electrolytes. Now he is experiencing nausea, vomiting, and diarrhea. This will further aggravate the imbalance of potassium and sodium. Due to his complex imbalances, he is a candidate for admission to the hospital. He will need careful rehydration and monitoring of his electrolytes. The remaining family members are likely to be experiencing sodium, potassium, and fluid deficits.

ThinkLike a Nurse 39-4

Martha LaGuardia (Meet Your Patients) is taking the following medications: atenolol (Tenormin) 50 mg daily at bedtime, alendronate sodium (Fosamax) 10 mg daily, furosemide (Lasix) 20 mg every morning, and calcium carbonate 500 mg three times per day. She takes her medications regularly and sees her primary care provider monthly. Using your reference books, look up her prescribed medications. Given that Ms. LaGuardia is now experiencing nausea and vomiting, she may be at risk for developing problems and side effects related to her medications. Which medications may cause problems and what problems might they cause? Explain your rationale.

Acid–Base Imbalances

The two broad types of acid–base imbalance are acidosis and alkalosis. **Acidosis** occurs when the serum pH falls below 7.35. **Alkalosis** occurs when the serum pH increases above 7.45 (Fig. 39-6). Arterial blood gases (ABGs) are used to monitor acid–base balance. **ABG analysis** measures pH, partial pressure of oxygen (PO_2), partial pressure of carbon dioxide (PCO_2), saturation of oxygen (SaO_2), and bicarbonate (HCO_3^-) level. Acid–base balance is reflected by the pH, PCO_2, and HCO_3 values.

A respiratory disturbance alters the carbonic acid portion of the buffering system, and the resulting imbalance is labeled **respiratory acidosis** or **respiratory alkalosis.** A metabolic disturbance alters the bicarbonate portion of the buffering system, so the resulting imbalance would be labeled as **metabolic acidosis** or **metabolic alkalosis.** Metabolic and respiratory problems can coexist, resulting in disturbances of both sides of the buffering system. Compensatory mechanisms may also produce both bicarbonate and carbon dioxide abnormalities.

Interpreting ABGs

To determine acid–base balance, you must examine the ABG results. The pH, PCO_2, and HCO_3^- values are of primary importance (Table 39-5). The partial pressure of oxygen (PO_2) and saturation of oxygen (SaO_2) are also part of the ABG result, but they do not affect acid–base balance. Instead, they affect tissue oxygenation. For further discussion on those two measures, see Chapter 37. Table 39-6 describes the causes, manifestations, ABG results, and treatments of acid–base imbalances. Use the following steps to interpret acid–base balance of blood.

> **Step 1: Examine the blood pH. Is it too low or too high? Or normal?**

- If the pH is low (< 7.35), then the blood is *acidic*.
- If the pH is high (> 7.45), then it is *alkalotic*.
- If the pH is between 7.35 and 7.45, then it is *normal*

> **Step 2: Check the amount of carbon dioxide in the blood (PCO_2). Is there too little or too much?**

- If PCO_2 is < 35 mm Hg, then there is too little acid in the blood (respiratory alkalosis).
- If PCO_2 is > 45 mm Hg, then there too much acid in the blood (respiratory acidosis).
- If PCO_2 is 35 to 45 mm Hg, then the cause for the abnormal pH is not respiratory.

> **Step 3: Think about the bicarbonate level (HCO_3^-). Is there too little or too much?**

- If HCO_3^- is < 22 mEq/L, then there is too little base in the blood (metabolic acidosis).
- If HCO_3^- is > 26 mEq/L, then there too much base in the blood (metabolic alkalosis).
- If HCO_3^- is 22 to 26 mEq/L, then the cause for the abnormal pH is not metabolic.

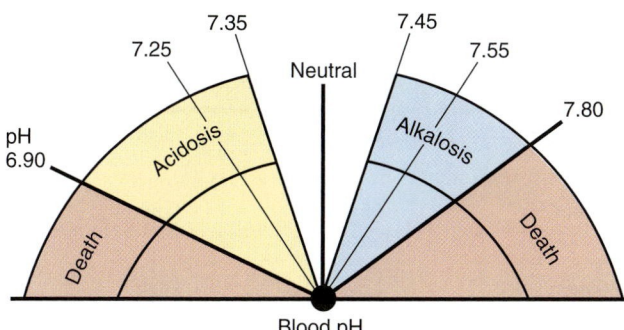

FIGURE 39-6 The pH scale ranges from 1 to 14. Normal blood pH is 7.35 to 7.45.

Uncompensated ABG	pH	$PaCO_2$	HCO_3^-
Respiratory acidosis	↓	↑	Normal
Respiratory alkalosis	↑	↓	Normal
Metabolic acidosis	↓	Normal	↓
Metabolic alkalosis	↑	Normal	↑

> **Step 4: Is there compensation? If so, is it partially or fully?**

Now let's look at what happens when the acid–base imbalance continues over a period of time. The body will naturally try to correct the unhealthy situation by using the lungs and kidneys to buffer the abnormality and return the pH into a normal range. If breathing is the reason for the abnormal pH, then the kidneys will pick up the slack and try to improve the situation. But if the problem is metabolic, then breathing (either faster and deeper or slower and more shallow) is the answer.

- **No compensation.** If the *pH is abnormal,* there is no compensation. The following example shows low pH and high carbon dioxide. This is *respiratory acidosis with no compensation.*

  pH = 7.30, PCO$_2$ = 50 mm Hg, HCO$_3^-$ = 24 mEq/L

- **Partial compensation.** Again, the *pH will be abnormal* unless it is fully compensated. If the pH and one ABG component are abnormal, with the second ABG value starting to change and the pH beginning to move toward normal, partial compensation is taking place. Compared to the uncompensated blood gas (above), this example shows the pH increasing but still acidotic. The PCO$_2$ remains high. This time the HCO$_3^-$ is going up to bring the pH closer to normal. This is *partially compensated respiratory acidosis.*

  pH = 7.32, PCO$_2$ = 50 mm Hg, HCO$_3^-$ = 28 mEq/L

Partial Compensation	pH	PaCO$_2$	HCO$_3^-$
Respiratory acidosis	↓	↑	↑
Respiratory alkalosis	↑	↓	↓
Metabolic acidosis	↓	↓	↓
Metabolic alkalosis	↑	↑	↑

- **Full compensation.** Full compensation occurs when the *pH returns to normal* range and both other ABG components are abnormal. The initial causal component is still abnormal, and the second ABG component (that had the normal values) has changed enough to return the pH to normal. Using the same respiratory acidosis example, below, the pH is now in the normal range and the PCO$_2$ is still high. But the HCO$_3^-$ is now also high; it has moved enough to raise the pH into

the normal range. The problem is now *fully compensated respiratory acidosis.*

pH = 7.35, PCO$_2$ = 50 mm Hg, HCO$_3^-$ = 30 mEq/L

Full Compensation	pH	PaCO$_2$	HCO$_3^-$
Respiratory acidosis	Normal, but < 7.35	↑	↑
Respiratory alkalosis	Normal, but > 7.35	↓	↓
Metabolic acidosis	Normal, but < 7.35	↓	↓
Metabolic alkalosis	Normal, but > 7.35	↑	↑

KnowledgeCheck 39-6

Interpret the following ABG results:

pH = 7.53	PCO$_2$ = 26 mm Hg	HCO$_3^-$ = 22 mEq/L
pH = 7.40	PCO$_2$ = 39 mm Hg	HCO$_3^-$ = 25 mEq/L
pH = 7.30	PCO$_2$ = 70 mm Hg	HCO$_3^-$ = 30 mEq/L
pH = 7.48	PCO$_2$ = 46 mm Hg	HCO$_3^-$ = 30 mEq/L

PracticalKnowledge
knowing **how**

In the remainder of this chapter, you will learn to apply theoretical knowledge of fluids, electrolytes, and acid–base balance to patient care.

ASSESSMENT

The purposes of a focused assessment of fluids, electrolytes, and acid–base status are to identify clients at risk for or already experiencing imbalances, to identify the nature of the disorder, and to evaluate responses to treatments.

Assessing for Example Problem: Fluid, Electrolytes, and Acid–Base Imbalances

Assessment for fluid, electrolyte, and acid–base imbalances includes collecting a focused nursing history, performing a physical assessment, and reviewing pertinent laboratory tests. For complete guidelines to use in obtaining a focused nursing history and physical assessment, see the Focused Assessment box, Focused Assessment for Fluid, Electrolyte, and Acid–Base Balance.

Focused Nursing History

A focused nursing history for fluids, electrolytes, and acid–base balance includes questions about demographic data, past medical history, current health concerns, food and fluid intake, fluid elimination, medications, and lifestyle.

Table 39-5 ➤ Using ABGs to Assess Acid–Base Balance

EXPLANATION OF CHANGES	ABG COMPONENT	NORMAL RANGE	ACIDOSIS	ALKALOSIS
Indicates acidosis, alkalosis, or normal acid–base balance	pH	7.35–7.45	Low	High
Carbon dioxide ("acid"). Signals respiratory cause	PCO$_2$	35–45 mm Hg	High	Low
Sodium bicarbonate ("base"). Signals metabolic cause	HCO$_3^-$	22–26 mEq/L	Low	High

Table 39-6 ➤ Acid–Base Imbalances

DISORDER	CLINICAL MANIFESTATIONS	INTERVENTIONS
Respiratory Acidosis May be caused by conditions or medications that impair gas exchange at the alveolar–capillary membrane, depressed respiratory rate and depth, or injury to the respiratory center in the brain.	*Acute:* Increased pulse and respiratory rate Headache, dizziness Confusion, decreased level of consciousness (LOC) Muscle twitching *Chronic:* Weakness Headache	Provide pulmonary hygiene. Institute measures to improve gas exchange, such as chest physiotherapy, bronchodilators, antibiotics possible. Provide supplemental oxygen. Maintain hydration.
Respiratory Alkalosis May be caused by hyperventilation due to anxiety, fever, sepsis, thyrotoxicosis, lesion in the respiratory center in the brain, or excessive ventilation with a mechanical ventilator.	Confusion, difficulty focusing Headache Tingling Palpitations Tremors	If caused by anxiety, encourage the patient to relax and breathe slowly. For other causes: Identify and treat the underlying disorder.
Metabolic Acidosis May be caused by retained acids in the blood due to renal impairment, poorly controlled diabetes mellitus, or starvation. Conditions that decrease bicarbonate, such as excessive GI loss, will also trigger metabolic acidosis. May be caused by excessive intake of acids, which may occur with aspirin poisoning, or by prolonged infusion of chloride-containing IV fluids.	Headache Confusion, drowsiness Weakness Peripheral vasodilatation Nausea and vomiting Kussmaul breathing (rapid and deep) Frequently associated with hyperkalemia	Treatment is directed at correcting the underlying problem. Bicarbonate may be ordered.
Metabolic Alkalosis May be caused by excessive acid loss due to vomiting or gastric suction, use of potassium-wasting diuretics, hypokalemia, excess bicarbonate intake, or hyperaldosteronism.	Dizziness Tingling of extremities Hypertonic muscles Decreased respiratory rate and depth	Treatment is directed at correcting the underlying problem. Treatment often includes administration of NaCl-rich fluids.

Focused Assessment

Focused Assessment for Fluids, Electrolytes, and Acid–Base Balance

Nursing History

Demographic Data

Age, gender, height, weight, body mass index (BMI)

Past Medical History

➤ Have you ever been hospitalized or had surgery? If so, when and for what reason?
➤ What healthcare problems are you currently being treated for?
➤ Have you ever been diagnosed with kidney disease, high blood pressure, diabetes, or thyroid or parathyroid problems?

Current Health Concerns

➤ What symptoms are you currently experiencing?
➤ Have you recently experienced any of the following symptoms?

Excessive thirst	Difficulty breathing
Fever	Swelling of your hands, feet, or ankles
Excessive perspiration	Dizziness or feeling faint
Nausea, vomiting, or diarrhea	Muscle weakness
Dry skin or mucous membranes	Excessive fatigue
Dark, concentrated urine	Numbness, tingling, or cramping sensations
Limited amounts of urine	

➤ Is your weight stable? Have you had any recent changes in your weight?
➤ Do you believe you have any problems with fluid loss?

Food and Fluid Intake

➤ How much fluid do you usually drink in a 24-hour period?
➤ Do you believe you drink adequate amounts of fluid?
➤ Describe your usual diet.
➤ Have you recently changed your diet or fluid intake?
➤ Are you following a special diet?
➤ Have you ever been placed on a restricted diet?
➤ Have you experienced any recent changes in your appetite or thirst?
➤ Do you salt your food?
➤ Do you ever use salt substitute?

Fluid Elimination

➤ How often do you urinate in a 24-hour period? Has that changed recently?
➤ How often do you get up during the night to urinate?
➤ Have you noticed any recent changes in the amount or appearance of your urine?
➤ How often do you experience vomiting, diarrhea, or constipation? Describe your experience.
➤ Do you have any wounds? If so, where are they, and how did they happen? What is the color of drainage and how much drainage are you experiencing?
➤ Do you have any breaks in your skin? If so, describe the problem, and show me the area.

Medications

➤ What prescribed medications do you currently take?
➤ What over-the-counter medications or alternative treatments do you use? What do you use them for?

➤ How often do you take laxatives or antacids?
➤ What vitamins, herbals, or supplements do you take?

Lifestyle

➤ What is your usual activity level?
➤ What type of exercise do you engage in? How often?
➤ How much fluid do you consume before, during, and after exercise?
➤ Do you drink alcohol? If so, how much do you consume in a day, week?
➤ Do you smoke? If so, how much? For how long?
➤ Do you use any illegal medications or drugs?

Physical Assessments

Skin

Assess the skin for color, temperature, moisture content, continuity, turgor, and edema.

➤ **Color and temperature** may be cues to the presence of fever and circulation status.
➤ **Moisture content** offers some indication of fluid status. A diaphoretic client is losing fluid at a faster rate than a client with dry skin. Dry, scaling skin may indicate a fluid deficit. Any breaks in the skin are potential areas for fluid loss.
➤ **Turgor** varies with age, weight, and skin condition but does offer information on fluid status. Pinch the skin over the sternum. Normally skin immediately returns to its usual position. In fluid volume deficit or malnutrition the skin may remain "tented" for a period of time before returning to its original position. You must, however, correlate skin turgor with context and other clinical signs. For example, the skin loses elasticity with aging, so clients older than age 65 often have decreased turgor, which is normal for them.
➤ **Edema** in dependent areas is a cue for fluid volume excess. In an ambulatory client, assess the lower extremities and hands. In a bedridden client, edema will shift as the client is turned.
➤ **To grade edema** (on a scale +1 to +4, +1 represents minimal edema and +4 represents the most severe edema), go to Chapter 21, Procedure 21-2.

Mucous Membranes

➤ Inspect the tongue and buccal mucosa. Mouth breathing alone usually does not change these areas.
➤ Dry, cracked, or dull mucous membranes are signs of fluid volume deficit.

Cardiovascular System

➤ Assess vital signs (see later section).
➤ If you suspect fluid volume deficit, assess for orthostatic hypotension:
  ➤ Assess blood pressure while client is lying or sitting.
  ➤ Have the client rise to a seated or standing position, and reassess the blood pressure (BP).
  ➤ A drop in systolic BP of more than 15 mm Hg is a sign of orthostatic hypotension.
➤ Check capillary refill. Delayed capillary refill is a sign of fluid volume deficit; rapid capillary refill indicates adequate circulation and volume. If capillary refill is delayed, evaluate feet and hands bilaterally. Delays in just one area indicate impaired circulation to the extremity rather than volume changes.

Focused Assessment for Fluids, Electrolytes, and Acid–Base Balance—cont'd

➤ Assess venous filling by observing the jugular and hand veins. Flat jugular or hand veins indicate low fluid volume. Distended vessels are a sign of overload.

Respiratory System

➤ Assess respiratory rate, depth, and pattern. The respiratory system rapidly responds to changes in pH. Similarly, alterations in gas exchange at the alveolar–capillary membrane may trigger pH changes.

➤ Assess breath sounds. Crackles or moist rales may indicate fluid overload. Areas of consolidation indicate impaired gas exchange.

Neurological System

➤ Assess level of consciousness and orientation.
➤ Assess neuromuscular irritability.
➤ Assess energy level and fatigue.
➤ Assess reflexes.

For specific neurological cues to alterations in fluid, electrolyte, or acid–base balance, see Table 39-4 and Table 39-6.

Vital Signs

➤ **Temperature.** An elevated body temperature increases the loss of body fluids.

In hypernatremia, body temperature elevates because less fluid is available for sweating.

In uncomplicated fluid volume deficit, body temperature decreases.

➤ **Pulse:**

1. Tachycardia is an early sign of fluid volume deficit.

2. Pulse rate is affected by fluid status and some electrolytes (primarily sodium, potassium, calcium, and magnesium).

3. Dysrhythmias are seen with potassium and magnesium imbalances.

4. The pulse volume is directly affected by fluid status. As fluid volume increases, the pulse volume also increases. Similarly, a drop in fluid volume leads to a drop in pulse volume.

➤ **Respiratory rate.** Alterations in respiratory rate may cause acid–base imbalances or be associated with compensation for a metabolic disorder.

➤ **Blood pressure:**

Blood pressure rises and falls with fluid volume.

Blood pressure is elevated by hypernatremia and fluid volume excess.

Respiratory acidosis causes increased heart rate, resulting in BP elevation.

High potassium intake may lower blood pressure.

Daily Weights

➤ Use the same balanced scale each day to monitor fluid status accurately.

➤ Weigh the client at the same time of day, making sure that the client is wearing the same amount of clothing.

➤ For clients undergoing hemodialysis, weigh the client before and after dialysis treatments.

➤ You may institute weight monitoring as an independent nursing order.

Fluid Intake and Output

See table in Clinical Insight 39-1.

Focused Physical Assessment

Correlate physical assessment data with the nursing history and laboratory studies. You will need to assess the following:

- *Skin.* Assess for color, temperature, moisture content, continuity, turgor, and edema. To describe edema, see Chapter 21, Procedure 21-2, Assessing the Skin.
- *Mucous membranes.* Inspect the tongue and buccal mucosa; assess the color, moisture, and continuity of the mucous membranes, as well as tongue turgor. Tongue turgor is not affected by age, so it is useful for all age groups.
- *Cardiovascular system.* Pulse and blood pressure are affected by fluid and electrolyte status. Also assess for orthostatic hypotension, capillary refill, jugular venous distension, and peripheral edema.
- *Respiratory system.* Assess respiratory rate, depth, and pattern, as well as breath sounds.
- *Neurological system.* As described in Tables 39-4 and 39-6, neurological status (e.g., level of consciousness) provides cues to fluid, electrolyte, and acid–base imbalance.

In addition to the above assessments, you will track vital sign changes, monitor daily weights, and record intake and output. These are independent nursing assessments. They do not require a medical prescription. You may delegate these tasks to assistive personnel, but you remain responsible for evaluating the data.

Vital Signs

All of the vital signs reflect information about fluid, electrolyte, and acid–base balance. These effects are briefly summarized below.

- *Temperature.* An elevated body temperature increases the loss of body fluids and also may indicate dehydration. In hypernatremia, body temperature rises because the fluid available for sweating decreases. In uncomplicated fluid volume deficit, body temperature decreases.
- *Pulse.* Tachycardia is an early sign of fluid volume deficit. Dysrhythmias can result from potassium, calcium, and magnesium imbalances. Fluid status directly affects the pulse volume: As fluid volume increases, the pulse volume also increases; similarly, a drop in fluid volume leads to a drop in pulse volume.
- *Respiratory rate.* Alterations in respiratory rate may cause acid–base imbalances or be associated with compensation for a metabolic disorder.
- *Blood pressure.* Blood pressure rises and falls with fluid volume. Postural hypotension occurs with dehydration. Blood pressure is also affected by electrolytes. High sodium intake is a factor in hypertension, whereas high potassium and magnesium intake may lower blood pressure.

Daily Weights

Monitoring daily weight is an accurate method of assessing fluid status. Weight changes over time are usually related

to diet and exercise. In contrast, short-term changes usually indicate changes in fluid status. Each kilogram (2.2 lb) of weight is equivalent to 1 liter (1,000 mL) of fluid. Thus, in a client with diarrhea, a sudden drop in weight of 5 pounds is equivalent to a fluid loss of almost 2,300 mL.

For weight to accurately reflect fluid status, you must use the same balanced scale each time. Weigh the client at the same time each day after emptying the bladder, making sure that he is wearing the same amount of clothing. Clients undergoing hemodialysis (blood cleansing through an artificial kidney) are usually weighed before and after dialysis treatments. Many lose 3 to 4 kg (6.6 to 8.8 lb) over the course of several hours of dialysis.

Weight monitoring is especially valuable data when it is impractical or impossible to measure intake and output. For example, it is not easy to know for sure how much fluid a breastfed infant receives with each feeding, nor how much fluid is lost in urine and stools. Incontinence, draining wounds, and limited resources may also make it difficult to monitor intake and output. Weight monitoring can be initiated as a nursing order.

Fluid Intake and Output

Intake and output (I&O) are monitored to assess fluid status. I&O are usually tallied at the end of each shift, as well as for each 24-hour period. In intensive care units, I&O are measured at least hourly. To monitor I&O, measure all fluids the client consumes or excretes. You must correlate I&O with daily weights to accurately determine overall fluid status (Pflaum, 1979, 2000, 2006).

- **Output.** Fluid output includes urine, liquid stools, emesis, gastrointestinal fluids (e.g., from suction devices), and drainage (e.g., from wounds and pressure ulcers). Output also includes insensible losses through perspiration and respiration, but these are not usually measured. For more information about I&O, refer to Chapter 30, Measuring Intake and Output. For procedure steps, see Procedure 30-1.
- **Intake.** Measuring fluid intake means including all oral fluids, semiliquid foods, ice chips, parenteral fluids, enteral feedings, and irrigations instilled and not withdrawn immediately. For more information about measuring intake, refer to Clinical Insight 39-1.

Clinical Insight 39-1 ▶ Guidelines for Measuring Intake and Output (I&O)

General Guidelines

Assessing

- Identify factors that can affect the patient's fluid intake or output (e.g., surgery, medical condition, or medications such as diuretics).
- Enlist the patient's help in keeping track of I&O if she is able.
- If you delegate the task of recording intake and output:
  - Be sure the assistive person understands its importance and knows how to perform the procedure correctly.
  - Be certain to evaluate the totals and the fluid sources. A patient or nursing assistive personnel (NAP) can collect the data, but a registered nurse (RN) must make the assessments.
  - For accuracy, use a graduated container and hold it at eye level when measuring fluids.

Recording

- You will usually record measurements on a bedside I&O form and transfer the 8-hr total to a graphic sheet or the 24-hour I&O on the patient's record. You may sometimes need hourly measurements.
- Document your findings in milliliters (mL). Describe any fluid restrictions and the patient's compliance with them.

Measuring Intake

It is most accurate to premeasure fluids before they are consumed. However, if that is not possible, you can use the following estimates:

Equivalents
- 1 oz = 30 mL
- 1 teaspoon = 5 mL
- 1 tablespoon = 15 mL
- 1 home measuring cup of fluid = 8 oz (240 mL)
- 1 pint of fluid = 16 oz (480 mL)
- 1 quart of fluid = 32 oz (960 mL)

Various containers
- Record ice chips as fluid at half their volume (1 cup ice = ½ cup fluid)
- Bowl (soup) = 180 mL
- Creamer (small) = 30 mL
- Custard cup = 100 mL
- Drinking cup = 180 mL
- Coffee mug = 240 mL
- Gelatin cup = 100 mL
- Ice cream serving = 120 mL
- Juice glass = 120 mL
- Paper cup, large = 200 mL
- Paper cup, small = 120 mL
- Water glass = 200 mL
- Water pitcher = 1,000 mL

Examples of fast food drinks
- Child-size drink = 12 oz
- Small drink = 16 oz
- Medium drink = 21 oz
- Large drink = 32 oz

Assessing

- Fluid intake includes the following:
  Oral fluids, including the liquid in prepared foods
  Soups
  Everything that melts into liquid at room temperature (e.g., gelatin, custard, ice cream, and ice)
  Liquid medications and fluids used to take pills or capsules
  IV fluids
  Enteral or parenteral nutrition fluids
  Instillations into the gastrointestinal (GI) tract
  Bladder irrigations
- Measure oral fluids according to agency policy.

Clinical Insight 39-1 ▶ Guidelines for Measuring Intake and Output (I&O)—cont'd

- For increased accuracy, use a graduated cup to measure and record fluid amounts before the patient consumes them. Subtract from the total any fluid that the patient throws away or saves for future consumption.
- Wash the measuring cup after each use, except after measuring water.
- Measure and teach the patient to measure and record the amount of fluid he drinks with each meal, with medicine, and between meals.
- In the home, cups come in many different sizes, as do the following:
  Use a measuring cup to measure how much the drinking cups and glasses hold.
  Always use the same drinking cup or glass.
  Explain that the labels on cans and bottles will help to determine precise fluid amounts.

Recording

- At least every 8 hours record the type and amount of all fluids the patient has received and indicate the route (oral, parenteral, rectal, or enteric tube).
- Record all forms of intake except blood and blood products

Measuring Output

Assessing

- Refer to Procedure 30-1 to review how to measure urine. Fluid output includes everything that leaves the body in fluid form: urine; watery stool; vomitus; wound drainage; output from surgical drains, NG tubes, and chest tubes; and any fluid aspirated from a body cavity.
- Use a calibrated container to measure fluids. Observe it at eye level and take the reading at the bottom of the fluid meniscus.
- Use a different graduated container for each patient; clean after use.
- Teach the patient to keep toilet paper out of the urine for accurate measurement.

- If irrigating an NG tube or the bladder, measure the amount instilled and subtract it from total output.
- You will need to empty wound drains or other devices to measure this volume.
- If a wound is draining but the fluid is not collected in a drainage device, you may measure the amount of fluid lost by weighing dressings before and after they are applied. If measuring the exact volume is not crucial, you may evaluate the degree of saturation of the dressing.

Recording

- Record the type, route, and amount of all fluids the patient loses.
- Insensible fluid losses can't be easily quantified. However, unusual losses (e.g., saturated dressing, excessive perspiration, rapid breathing patterns, and large burn areas) should be objectively described in narrative charting.

Tips for Analyzing I&O

- Measure and record all intake and output.
- Determine if output is more or less than intake.
- Evaluate trends over 24 to 48 hours.
- To identify problems, when evaluating total urine output, ask how many times the patient voided. For example, was the total of 300 obtained from 2 voids, or from 10 voids of 30 mL each?
- Evaluate patterns and values outside the normal range (e.g., frequent voiding, infrequent voiding), keeping in mind the normal range for 24-hour intake and output.
- The amount of output is important, but consider color, color changes, and odor too.
- Analyze intake and output holistically. Take into account the patient's usual pattern and amounts, age, medical problem, and type of surgical procedure.
- You must correlate I&O with daily weights to accurately determine overall fluid status (Pflaum, 1979, 2000, 2006).

Most healthcare facilities have standardized I&O forms for recording at the bedside and as a permanent part of the patient record (either paper or electronic). To see an electronic I&O record, see Figure 18-2 in Chapter 18. For an example of a paper I&O flow sheet, see Figure 18-7.

KnowledgeCheck 39-7

- Identify ten physical assessment components that can be used to monitor fluid, electrolyte, and acid–base balance.
- What aspects should be evaluated in a nursing history focused on fluid, electrolyte, and acid–base balance?

ThinkLike a Nurse 39-5

What vital sign changes would you expect to find when assessing Jackson LaGuardia (Meet Your Patients)?

Laboratory Studies

Several laboratory tests are performed to evaluate fluid, electrolyte, and acid–base status.

Complete Blood Count. Fluid status is reflected in a **complete blood count (CBC)**, which is a measure of red blood cells (RBCs), white blood cells (WBCs), and platelets. Included in the CBC is the hematocrit, a measure of the percentage of RBCs in whole blood. As fluid levels decrease, the percentage of blood made up by cells increases, and the hematocrit rises. As fluid levels increase, the hematocrit falls.

Serum Electrolytes. Venous blood samples are taken to measure sodium, potassium, chloride, and BUN/creatinine ratio and glucose. BUN and creatinine are sensitive measures of fluid status and kidney function. Physical assessment can also reveal hypocalcemia. See Clinical Insight 39-2.

Clinical Insight 39-2 ➤ Assessing for Trousseau's and Chvostek's Signs

Positive Trousseau's and Chvostek's signs are signs of hypocalcemia. To check for these signs, follow these instructions.

Trousseau's Sign

Inflate a blood pressure cuff above systolic pressure. Flexion of the wrist and hand constitutes a positive sign.

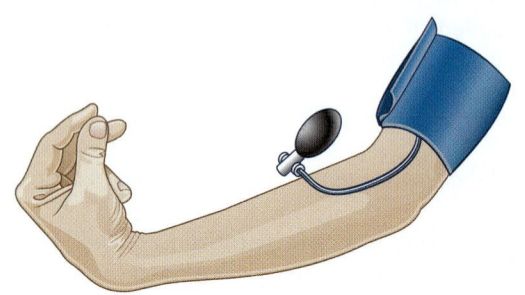

Chvostek's Sign

Tap the face in front of the ear and below the zygomatic bone (cheek bone). Facial twitching constitutes a positive sign.

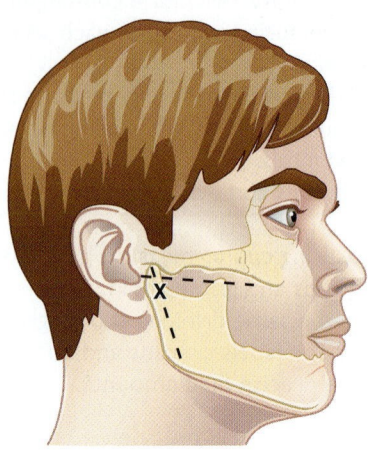

Serum Osmolality. A measure of the solute concentration of the blood is **serum osmolality.** It is expressed as milliosmoles per kilogram (mOsm/kg). Serum osmolality may be directly measured with venous blood or estimated by doubling the serum sodium level. A rise in serum osmolality indicates fluid volume deficit; a decrease indicates fluid volume excess. Changes in serum osmolality usually indicate alterations in sodium levels.

Urine Osmolality. The solute concentration of urine is measured by **urine osmolality**. The body excretes nitrogenous wastes as well as electrolytes. As a result, urine osmolality is substantially higher than serum levels. Fluid volume deficit increases urine osmolality; fluid volume excess decreases urine osmolality. This test may call for a 24-hour urine specimen, or for discarding the first morning specimen and collecting a clean-catch specimen 2 hours later.

Urinalysis. The routine screening test, **urinalysis,** includes a measure of urine pH and specific gravity. Urine pH normally ranges from 5.0 to 9.0, with an average of 6.0.

- *pH.* Urine becomes more acidic in respiratory or metabolic acidosis, starvation, or fluid volume deficit. Alkaline urine is associated with an alkaline state in the blood.
- *Specific gravity.* Specific gravity rises and falls in opposition to fluid status. A normal range is 1.001 to 1.029. A low specific gravity occurs when fluid is plentiful. When fluid levels decrease, urine becomes more concentrated, and specific gravity increases. For a procedure for testing specific gravity of urine, see Procedure 30-3B, in Chapter 30.
- *ABGs.* Interpretation of ABGs was discussed earlier in this chapter. For a list of these values, along with other lab studies discussed earlier, refer to Diagnostic Testing box Assessing Fluid, Electrolyte, and Acid–Base Balance.

ANALYSIS/NURSING DIAGNOSIS

Nursing diagnoses directly related to fluid, electrolyte, and acid–base balance include the following: Deficient Fluid

Diagnostic Testing

Assessing Fluid, Electrolyte, and Acid–Base Balance

Venous Blood Sample	Normal Ranges
Sodium	135–145 mEq/L
Potassium	3.5–5 mEq/L
Chloride	97–107 mEq/L
Bicarbonate	22–26 mEq/L
BUN	10–31 mg/dL
Creatinine	0.5–1.2 mg/dL
Serum osmolality	275–295 mOsm/kg
Urine osmolality	250–900 mOsm/kg
Hematocrit	43%–49% in men
	38%–44% in menstruating women

Freshly Voided Urine Sample

pH	5.0–9.0
Specific gravity	1.001–1.029

Arterial Blood Sample

pH	7.35–7.45
PCO_2	35–45 mm Hg
HCO_3^-	22–26 mEq/L

Volume, Excess Fluid Volume, Readiness for Enhanced Fluid Volume, Risk for Deficient Fluid Volume, Risk for Electrolyte Imbalance, Risk for Imbalanced Fluid Volume, Impaired Gas Exchange, and Risk for Vascular Trauma. For other defining characteristics and etiologies of these NANDA International (NANDA-I) diagnoses,

 Go to Chapter 39, **Standardized Language: NANDA-I Diagnoses Related to Fluid, Electrolytes, and Acid–Base Balance,** on Davis*Plus.*

Diagnoses for Example Problem: Fluid, Electrolytes, and Acid–Base Imbalances

Impaired Gas Exchange is appropriate for a client with a disorder affecting gas exchange at the alveolar–capillary membrane in the lungs (see Chapter 37). This condition limits the effectiveness of the carbonic acid–bicarbonate buffer system and alters serum pH, predisposing the patient to acid–base imbalances.

Fluid, electrolyte, and acid–base imbalances (e.g., dehydration, metabolic acidosis, respiratory alkalosis), as well as treatments imbalances, may be etiologies of other nursing diagnoses. Below are a few examples:

- Activity Intolerance r/t excess fluid and electrolyte loss through Diarrhea
- Impaired Oral Mucous Membrane r/t Deficient Fluid Volume
- Decreased Cardiac Output r/t hypovolemia
- Risk for Vascular Trauma (from insertion of an IV catheter)

▨ PLANNING OUTCOMES/EVALUATION

The overall goal for a client experiencing fluid, electrolytes, or acid–base imbalance is to restore balance.

Outcomes for Example Problem: Fluids, Electrolytes, and Acid–Base Imbalances

NOC standardized outcomes for describing fluid and electrolyte status include the following: Electrolyte & Acid/Base Balance, Fluid Balance, Fluid Overload Severity, and Hydration. For selected indicators for these outcomes,

Go to Chapter 39, **Standardized Language: Selected NOC Outcomes and NIC Interventions for Fluid and Electrolyte Problems,** on Davis*Plus*.

Individualized goals/outcome statements you might write for a client include the following examples:

- Maintains fluid balance, as evidenced by balanced 24-hour intake and output; good skin and tongue turgor; blood pressure and heart rate within normal limits; and no adventitious breath sounds.
- Electrolyte balance restored, as evidenced by alertness and cognitive orientation and no muscle cramping, seizures, or electrocardiogram changes.
- Drinks at least 2,500 mL in 24 hours.
- Urine specific gravity within normal limits.

▨ PLANNING INTERVENTIONS/IMPLEMENTATION

The following sections describe nursing interventions and activities for preventing and treating fluid, electrolyte, and acid-base problems.

Interventions for Example Problem: Fluid, Electrolyte, and Acid–Base Imbalances

NIC standardized interventions related to fluid, electrolyte, and acid–base imbalance include Acid–Base Management, Electrolyte Management, and Fluid Management. For a listing of other interventions,

Go to Chapter 39, **Standardized Language: Selected NOC Outcomes and NIC Interventions for Fluid and Electrolyte Problems,** on Davis*Plus*.

Individualized interventions are aimed at correcting the underlying disorder that led to imbalance. Nursing care focuses on preventing imbalances, modifying oral intake, providing parenteral fluids, and transfusing blood products, all of which are discussed in the rest of this chapter.

Preventing Fluid and Electrolyte Imbalances

It is better to prevent imbalances than to treat them. Use the data obtained from your assessment to plan how to help your client avoid imbalances. Common strategies are listed in the accompanying Self-Care box, Teaching Patients to Prevent Fluid and Electrolyte Imbalances.

Self-Care

Teaching Patients to Prevent Fluid and Electrolyte Imbalances

➤ Teach the client about usual fluid needs and circumstances that increase fluid needs, such as high environmental temperature, fever, GI fluid loss, or draining wounds. Base your teaching on the client's current intake and the changes required to meet fluid goals.

➤ Identify medications or conditions that place the client at risk for imbalances. For example, if the client is receiving a potassium-wasting diuretic, she will need to increase potassium intake, either by taking a supplement or by altering the diet.

Also teach clients to do the following:

➤ Drink at least eight to twelve 8-oz glasses of water per day unless your healthcare provider has told you to limit fluids.

➤ Healthy adults: Use thirst as a guide to fluid intake. However, adults over age 50 have diminished thirst sensation and cannot depend solely on thirst for fluid replacement.

➤ Vigorous exercise may delay the thirst mechanism. Athletes should become accustomed to consuming fluid at regular intervals (with or without thirst) during training sessions and competition so that they do not experience dehydration.

➤ Limit consumption of fluids high in salt, sugar, caffeine, or alcohol.

➤ Teach able individuals to use a urine color chart to monitor hydration status (Mentes, 2008).

➤ Drink water before, during, and after strenuous exercise.

➤ Avoid routine use of laxatives, antacids, weight-loss products, or enemas. All of these products may cause imbalances of fluids and electrolytes such as sodium and potassium.

➤ Weigh yourself daily if fluid balance is critical or if you are experiencing excessive loss or gain.

➤ Contact a health professional if there is a sudden change of weight, decreased urine output, swelling in dependent areas (e.g., hands and feet), shortness of breath, or dizziness.

➤ Contact a healthcare provider if you experience prolonged vomiting, diarrhea, or inability to tolerate liquids or food.

➤ Eat a well-balanced diet, including dairy products rich in calcium.

Dietary Changes

To promote fluid and electrolyte balance, most people need to limit their sodium intake and increase their dietary potassium and calcium. Some may need oral electrolyte supplements, as well (see the Self-Care box, Taking Oral Electrolyte Supplements). As previously discussed, most North Americans consume more sodium than they should and not enough potassium and calcium. Teach clients to eat foods rich in potassium and calcium every day and to avoid sodium-rich foods (see Chapter 28 to review foods, as needed). For example, instruct clients to read food labels, particularly when trying to limit sodium intake.

Oral Electrolyte Supplements

Many clients are unable to correct electrolyte disturbances with dietary changes alone. This is especially true for clients who have food intolerances, who rely on prepared meals, or who live in group settings. Such clients may need oral supplements to meet their dietary requirements. Potassium and calcium are among the most common supplements. Most adults, especially older adults, consume less dietary calcium per day than the recommended amount. Calcium supplements come in many forms, including tablet, liquid, and chewable form. Potassium supplements are available in pill and liquid form. Many have an unpleasant taste. See the Self-Care box, Taking Oral Electrolyte Supplements for suggested nursing activities to help improve your patients' compliance.

KnowledgeCheck 39-8

- Identify laboratory tests that monitor fluid, electrolyte, and acid–base balance.
- Give at least five strategies to prevent fluid and electrolyte imbalance.

Modifying Oral Fluid Intake

Clients experiencing fluid imbalances may need to restrict or increase their daily oral intake to correct the underlying disorder.

Facilitating Fluid Intake

Clients with actual or potential fluid volume deficit may need to increase their fluid intake. Whenever possible, clients should take fluids by mouth. You may provide replacement through a nasogastric or feeding tube if the client is unable to meet his needs independently but can tolerate fluids in the gastrointestinal tract. Parenteral fluid replacement is used only when enteral replacement cannot meet the client's fluid needs (for review, see Chapter 28).

You must first establish the desired amount of fluids for the client. The daily fluid goal reflects the client's current fluid balance and underlying condition. For example, if a client is dehydrated, an order might read: "Force fluids: 2,500 mL oral fluids per 24 hours." From this order you can develop a fluid schedule. Typically people drink more fluid during the day and early evening, when they are more likely to be active. A large volume of fluid late in the evening may interrupt sleep by prompting the need to urinate. Therefore, you should distribute fluids to reflect the time of day, for example:

    0700 to 1500—1,300 mL
    1500 to 2300—1,000 mL
    2300 to 0700—200 mL

Strategies to increase fluid intake include the following:

- Offer a variety of fluids throughout the day on a regular schedule. Vary hot and cold liquids, and offer a choice of juices and other drinks.
- Instruct nursing assistive personnel to make "fluids rounds" to offer and help with oral fluids.
- Each time you are at the bedside, remind the patient to drink.
- Break daily goals into hourly amounts. For example, in the preceding example, in the 8 hours between 0700 and 1500 have the patient drink 150 mL of fluid every hour. Give him a written schedule.
- Provide a glass or cup with milliliter markings on it so that the patient will know how much he is drinking.
- Always have fluid readily available to the patient. For example, keep a pitcher of water at the bedside.
- When possible, have the patient and family members participate in offering fluids and tracking fluid intake.
- Schedule diagnostic and surgical procedures to minimize the length of time the patient must fast.
- For ambulatory patients (e.g., residents in long-term care facilities) schedule "tea time" or "happy hour" to promote increased intake.

Facilitating Fluid Restriction

Patients may need to limit fluids for a variety of reasons (e.g., impaired cardiovascular, liver, or renal function). Inform patients and caregivers of the reason for the restriction, as well as the amount of fluid allowed.

Typically, fluid volume is divided into amounts allotted per shift. However, fluid restrictions usually include *all* forms of intake, not just oral. For example, an order might read: "Limit total fluid intake to 1,500 mL per 24 hours." If the patient is receiving IV antibiotics four times per day, you must include that volume as a part of the total fluids. If 75 mL is infused with each administration, total IV fluids equal 300 mL. So, the oral intake must be limited to 1,200 mL per day. This amount may be distributed as 700 mL on the day shift, 400 mL on the evening shift, and 100 mL at night. Strategies to restrict fluid intake include the following:

- Do not offer liquids with meals. Reserve liquids for between meals.
- Limit intake of dry, salty, or spicy foods; these foods increase thirst.
- Offer ice chips to help quench thirst.
- Provide frequent oral hygiene.

Self-Care

Taking Oral Electrolyte Supplements

➤ Encourage clients to take potassium supplements with juice to mask the taste.

➤ Teach clients to take supplements as prescribed to maintain electrolyte balance.

➤ Remind clients that supplements are medications and should be viewed as part of the treatment plan.

➤ If the client's medications are altered, review the continued need for supplements.

➤ Caution clients that salt substitutes contain potassium. If the client has been advised to use salt substitutes, review the need for potassium supplements.

➤ Encourage clients who take calcium supplements to consume at least 2,500 mL of fluid per day to avoid constipation and reduce the risk of kidney stone formation.

- Keep liquids away from the bedside.
- Provide diversional activities for the patient.

Parenteral Replacement of Fluids and Electrolytes

The word **parenteral** refers to any route other than through the alimentary canal (passage from the mouth to the anus). **Intravenous therapy** is the administration of fluids, electrolytes, medications, or nutrients by the venous route. Intravenous fluids are used to:

- Expand intravascular volume.
- Correct an underlying imbalance in fluids or electrolytes.
- Compensate for an ongoing problem that is affecting either fluid or electrolytes.

For instance, Martha LaGuardia (Meet Your Patients) is being treated in the ED for gastroenteritis. She is experiencing fluid loss from vomiting and diarrhea, complicated by her use of a diuretic. IV therapy will allow her to receive fluid to expand her intravascular volume and to maintain her hydration until the vomiting and diarrhea subside. It will also provide electrolyte replacement based on her laboratory studies. Mrs. LaGuardia will remain on IV fluids until she can meet her fluid and electrolyte needs orally. All of the members of the LaGuardia family are experiencing fluid losses and would benefit from increasing their fluid intake, but may not need IV fluid replacement. When fluid balance is fragile, or when the client cannot tolerate oral fluids, replacement may be supervised in an inpatient setting.

 When initiating and maintaining intravenous infusions, always use careful aseptic technique. Remember that the IV catheter provides a portal of entry for pathogens directly into the bloodstream. You should know that Medicare will not reimburse a hospital for the expenses (e.g., antibiotics, extra hospital days) caused by catheter-related infections that occur during hospitalization.

Types of Intravenous Solutions

As we explained earlier, solutions are classified according to how they compare to the osmolality of blood serum. Intravenous fluids are these classified as isotonic, hypotonic, and hypertonic solutions.

To help you remember, here is a somewhat oversimplified summary. When infused:

- *Isotonic* fluids remain in the blood vessels. Examples are lactated Ringer's solution and 0.9% saline (normal saline [NS]).
- *Hypotonic* fluids pull body water *out* of the blood vessels. Examples include 5% dextrose (D_5W) and 0.45% saline (1/2 NS).
- *Hypertonic* fluids pull body water *into* the blood vessels. Examples include D_5 0.9% NaCl (D_5 NS), D_5 0.45% NaCl (D_5 1/2 NS), and $D_{50\%}$ (50% dextrose in water) and volume expanders (albumin).

For more information about these types of IV solutions,

 Go to Chapter 39, **Supplemental Materials: Types of IV Fluids,** on Davis*Plus.*

Peripheral Vascular Access Devices

Intravenous therapy requires placement of a vascular access device. You will choose the type of device based on the client's condition, type of fluid that will be infused, and the anticipated length of treatment. IV catheters (and needles) are sized by their diameter, which is called the **gauge**. The smaller that the diameter is, the larger the gauge will be (e.g., a 16-gauge catheter is larger than a 21-gauge catheter). Therefore, the smaller the gauge, the more rapidly fluid can be delivered. Various types of catheters are used to access peripheral veins, including the following:

Over-the-Needle Catheters. These are also called **angiocaths,** short for angiocatheter (Fig. 39-7A). A polyurethane or Teflon catheter is threaded over a metal stylet (needle). You pierce the skin and vein with the needle, advance the catheter into the vein, and remove (or retract) the metal needle. In most cases, the plastic catheter is less than 7.5 cm (3 in.) in length. This type of access device is ideal for brief therapy. However, you cannot give highly irritating or hyperosmolar solutions through this type of catheter because it may cause severe damage to the vein. For an animated illustration of an over-the-needle IV catheter,

Go to **Animations: Insertion of an Over-the-Needle IV Catheter** on Davis*Plus.*

Inside-the-Needle Catheters. This type of catheter is similar to the over-the-needle catheter; however, the polyurethane or Teflon catheter lies inside the metal needle (Fig. 39-7B). After you advance the catheter into the vein, you withdraw the needle.

Butterfly Needle. Also called a *scalp vein needle* or *wing-tipped cathete*r, a **butterfly needle** is a short, beveled metal needle with flexible plastic flaps attached to the shaft (Fig. 39-8). You can pinch the flaps and hold them tightly together to facilitate insertion. After insertion, flatten them out and tape them against the skin to prevent dislodgement during the infusion process. These needles are commonly used for intermittent or short-term therapy for children and infants or for single-dose medications and drawing blood. Because the inflexible metal needle remains in the vein, a butterfly needle is more likely to **infiltrate** (damage the vein and allow fluid to leak into the interstitial spaces) than a plastic catheter.

Midline Peripheral Catheter. A **midline peripheral catheter** is a flexible IV catheter, typically inserted into the antecubital fossa and then advanced into the larger vessels of the upper arm for greater hemodilution. It is 15 cm (6 in.) long,

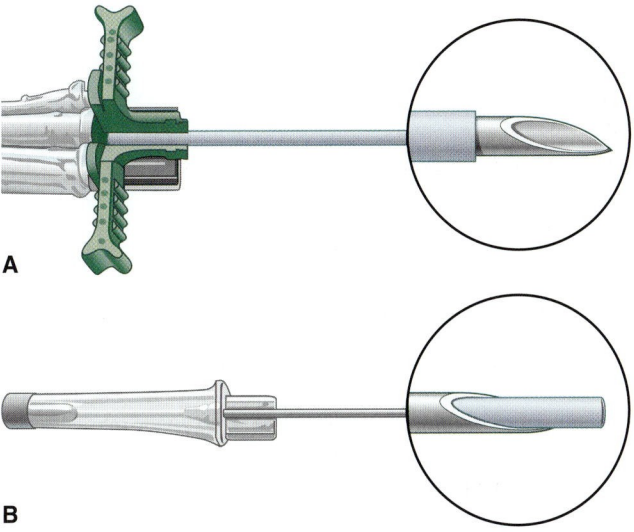

FIGURE 39-7 Typical IV access devices. A. An over-the-needle catheter. B. An inside-the-needle catheter.

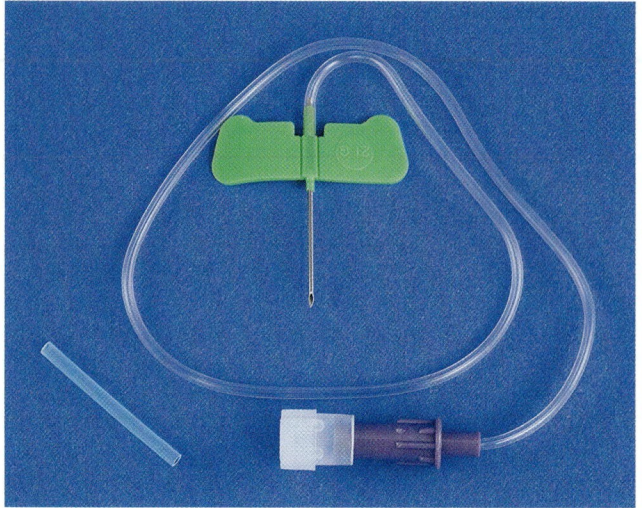

FIGURE 39-8 The butterfly needle is commonly used for intermittent or short-term therapy for children and infants.

so it can be used for a longer period of time than a shorter, over-the-needle catheter. A midline peripheral catheter may remain in place for as long as 49 days, although the median length of use is 7 days (Centers for Disease Control and Prevention [CDC], 2002). A midline catheter is still considered a peripheral line, so you cannot administer highly osmolar and irritating solutions through it.

✚ In response to the Needlestick Safety and Prevention Act passed by Congress in 2000, the CDC and the Occupational Safety and Health Administration (OSHA) require the use of "needleless" systems. Therefore, you will usually have available access devices with safety features to prevent accidental "sticks." But if you find you must use an older, nonsafety device, do not attempt to recap the needle after removing it from the vein.

Peripheral Intravenous Lock

A **peripheral intravenous lock** (also called a saline lock, a prn adapter, and sometimes a heparin lock) establishes a venous route as a precautionary measure for clients whose condition may change rapidly or who may require intermittent infusion therapy. A peripheral IV catheter or butterfly wing-tipped catheter is inserted into a vein, and the hub is capped with a lock port (Fig. 39-9). Patency of the lock is maintained by injecting normal saline or a dilute heparin solution, depending on agency policy. See Procedure 39-6.

Central Venous Access Devices

A **central venous access device (CVAD)** is an intravenous line inserted into a major vein. Typically, the subclavian or internal jugular vein is used. Using surgical asepsis, a catheter is advanced from the insertion site into the superior vena cava. CVADs are used to administer large volumes of fluid or highly irritating medications, when peripheral sites are unavailable, for monitoring central venous pressure, and for frequent blood draws. You will likely care for patients with central lines and perhaps assist with inserting them. To learn how to care for patients with central lines, see Clinical Insight 39-3, Procedure 39-5B, and Procedure 39-9.

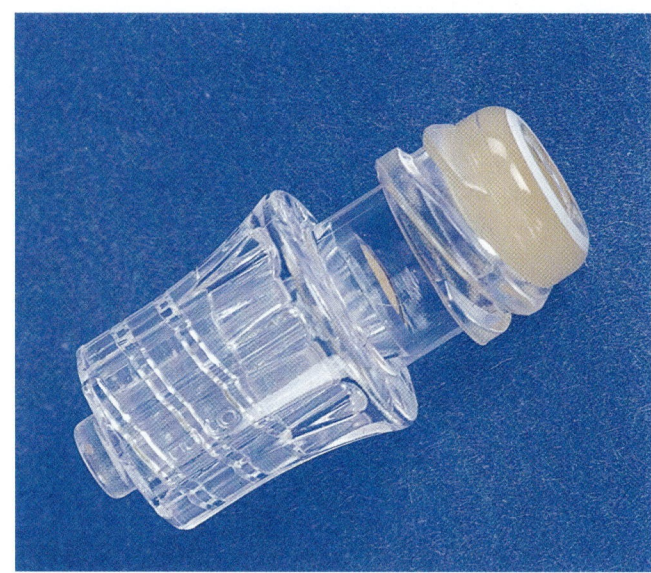

FIGURE 39-9 A peripheral intravenous lock establishes a venous route as a precautionary measure for clients whose condition may change rapidly or who may require intermittent infusion therapy.

Clinical Insight 39-3 ➤ **Caring for Patients With a Central Venous Access Device (CVAD)**

Asepsis

- ✚ Use good hand hygiene and follow agency protocols for site care. To protect yourself and the patient.
- Use strict aseptic technique when manipulating injection ports, catheter hub and extension legs, needleless connectors, insertion site, and dressing. This includes sterile gloves and supplies, mask, and in some agencies a mask for the patient. To minimize line contamination and infection.
- Scrub injection ports, extension legs, and catheter hubs vigorously for at least 15 seconds, preferably with 70%

alcohol, or 2% chlorhexidine preparation before accessing them.
- Appropriate antiseptics include alcohol and chlorhexidine gluconate. Do not use povidone-iodine and tincture of iodine to scrub ports unless there is some reason alcohol or CHG-alcohol combination products can't be used.
- Do not apply acetone or acetone-based products to the skin before insertion of a catheter or during dressing changes. These are organic solvents.

Clinical Insight 39-3 ➤ **Caring for Patients With a Central Venous Access Device (CVAD)—cont'd**

Assessments

- Check the patient record for radiographic confirmation of correct tip location before beginning prescribed therapies.
- Inspect catheter–skin junction sites through the transparent dressing and palpate for tenderness daily. Do not remove transparent dressing except when dressing change is required. If site is dressed with gauze, remove it to inspect the site. A high-risk route of infection is via migration of skin organisms at the insertion site into the cutaneous catheter tract, with colonization of the catheter tip.
- Observe for excessive bleeding at the insertion site. You may need to obtain a prescription for a topical hemostatic agent and use with a pressure dressing.
- If symptoms of infection occur (e.g., fever without obvious cause; redness, edema, induration, exudates, or tenderness at the site), remove the dressing and inspect the site directly. Anticipate that blood cultures will be needed from both the peripheral site and the central catheter.
- Be aware that risk of infection is higher with femoral catheters and with multilumen catheters. Multilumen catheters require more manipulation, which encourages more colonization and bacterial growth within the catheter lumen.
- Assess for compromised catheter integrity (wet dressing; kinked, cracked, or leaking external catheter).
- Inspect catheter connections and pump function, including flow rate.
- Observe for symptoms of catheter migration to the right atrium or ventricle (i.e., mid- to lower sternal pain, dysrhythmias).
- If there are signs of complications, notify the medical provider.
- Assess the patient daily for indications that the CVC is still needed. CVCs should be removed as soon as possible because the infection rate is closely related to the length of time that the CVC is in place.

Interventions

- The site should be covered with a semipermeable transparent dressing, the catheter secured with a sterile commercially manufactured stabilizer (instead of tape), and the lumens anchored near the ports with clear tape.
- Keep dressings dry, intact, and air occlusive. Protocols generally require a dressing change every 5 to 7 days unless the integrity of the dressing is compromised (e.g., it is damp, loosened, or soiled) or if the site must be examined (e.g., because of pain or odor).
- Perform site care with each dressing change. Cleanse the catheter–skin junction with an appropriate antiseptic

solution, apply a sterile stabilizer, and a new sterile dressing.

- Manipulate the catheter hub as little as possible. To minimize catheter movement, phlebitis, and contamination of the line. Less catheter manipulation is associated with fewer bloodstream infections.
- Flush catheters before and after any infusions or per agency protocol. This may be every 12 to 24 hours when not in use.
  - Flush volume should be twice the volume of the catheter and add-on devices (consult package label).
  - Use a syringe size recommended by the catheter manufacturer (10 mL is the smallest size recommended due to the pressure generated).
  - Type of flush solution depends on agency policy (saline versus heparin).
  - Use single-use, labeled syringes of flush solution. To prevent cross-contamination.
- If you have trouble flushing, the catheter may be kinked or malpositioned, the inline filter may be clogged, or a clamp may need to be released. You can correct these problems.

- ✚ Never flush against resistance. The catheter might be clogged and you would risk dislodging a small clot. This could also rupture the catheter.

- ✚ If the patient has a peripherally inserted central catheter (PICC) line, take blood pressures on the alternate arm. Using the arm with the PICC can cause bleeding at the site, thrombus formation, retrograde blood flow, and increased risk of catheter occlusion.

- If the patient is receiving parenteral nutrition, reserve and label one lumen just for that purpose.

Documentation

- Document routine assessments and the condition of the catheter–skin junction site. When site care is given, also document the patient's response and any actions taken to correct or prevent adverse reactions.

Related Information

For information about dressing changes, refer to Procedure 39-5B: Central Line Dressings.

For information about administering medications through a CVAD, refer to Chapter 25, Procedure 25-18: Administering Medication Through a Central Venous Access Device.

References

Betsy Lehman Center for Patient Safety and Medical Error Reduction, JSI Research and Training Institute, Inc., 2008; Infusion Nurses Society [INS], 2006b; Institute for Healthcare Improvement, n.d; Joanna Briggs Institute, 2008; Marschall, Mermel, Classen, et al., 2008; Rhoads & Meeker, 2008.

Advantages of Central Lines. A central line offers several advantages:

- A central vein can accommodate highly irritating and hyperosmolar solutions because the blood and solution mix rapidly at the infusion site.
- Central veins are accessible even if the patient is experiencing severe fluid depletion.
- Some types of central lines may also be used to monitor central venous pressure.
- Central lines can be left in longer than peripheral IVs, ranging from a week to long term, depending on the type of central line used.
- Nutrition can be given parenterally.
- Phlebitis, extravasation, and infiltration are less likely to occur with central lines.
- Central lines with extra ports allow you to withdraw blood to use for laboratory tests.

Disadvantages of Central Lines. There are some drawbacks to central lines:

- Practitioners must have specialized training in order to insert the catheter.
- You must obtain patient consent.
- Placement must be confirmed by radiography.
- Placement is treated as a minor surgical procedure, requiring strict sterility.
- Dressing changes require strict sterile technique.
- When placed via the neck, especially though the subclavian vein, there is a risk of pneumothorax.
- There is a risk that the catheter will float into the right side of the heart, where it may cause ventricular dysrhythmias.
- There is a greater risk of air embolus and infection when compared to peripheral IVs.
- Associated costs are greater than with peripheral lines.
- The risk for sepsis is much higher than for peripheral sites. CVCs account for about 90% of catheter-related bloodstream infections.

Preventing Bloodstream Infections From Central Lines. This is one of The Joint Commission's national patient safety goals for 2011. To help prevent CVC catheter-related infections:

Education and training—regarding proper infection control measures to prevent intravascular catheter-related infections. Encourage patients to report any changes or new discomfort in their catheter site.

Hand hygiene—Wearing gloves does not make handwashing or hand hygiene unnecessary.

Maximal barrier precautions for insertion—Includes sterile drape for patient, hat, mask, and sterile gown and gloves.

Chlorhexidine skin antisepsis—For patients older than 2 months, use 2% chlorhexidine gluconate in 70% isopropyl alcohol to prep the insertion site.

Optimal catheter site selection—The subclavian vein has the lowest rate of infection. The femoral vein should be avoided if possible.

Type of catheter—To reduce the risk of catheter-related infection, the catheter with the fewest number of ports or lumens needed to manage the patient is best.

Daily review of lines—The CVC should be removed as soon as it is no longer necessary. Risk of infection is closely related to the length of time the CVC is in place. (O'Grady, Alexander, Burns, et al., Healthcare Infection Control Practices Advisory Committee [HICPAC], 2011).

Types of Central Venous Catheters

There are four types of CVADs: peripherally inserted central catheters, nontunneled CVCs, tunneled CVCs, and implanted ports.

Peripherally Inserted Central Catheters (PICC Lines)

PICCs are long, soft, flexible catheters inserted at the antecubital fossa through the basilic or cephalic vein of the arm. The catheter is then advanced into the superior vena cava (Fig. 39-10). A physician or specially trained registered nurse performs the insertion. PICC lines are most commonly used for prolonged IV antibiotic therapy, parenteral nutrition, and chemotherapy. A PICC line is intended for intermediate to long-term use and does not need to be replaced unless the site appears infected or the catheter is no longer patent.

Nontunneled Central Venous Catheters

Nontunneled CVCs are inserted by a physician, specially trained nurse practitioner, or physician assistant through the skin into the jugular, subclavian, and occasionally, femoral veins. They are sutured in place. Often these are referred to as single, double, triple or quadruple-lumen catheters, depending on the number of ports in the line (Fig. 39-11). These CVADs are intended for shorter use than a PICC line (less than 6 weeks); however, guidelines advise that nontunneled CVADs not be routinely replaced (CDC, 2002; National Guideline Clearinghouse [NGC], 2008). Blood can be drawn from a nontunneled CVAD for diagnostic studies. However, if parenteral nutrition or blood is running in a port, you cannot use that same port for blood draws.

Example:

Imagine that you have a frail elderly patient who needs two different kinds of IV fluid, parenteral nutrition, and frequent blood draws for lab tests. This patient has fragile peripheral veins and is also at high risk for infection and other complications. With a multiple-lumen central catheter, the patient needs only one insertion site. You can run both fluids and the parenteral nutrition fluids, and still reserve one port for drawing blood. The patient has less risk for the catheter to become dislodged or infiltrate, or for phlebitis to develop.

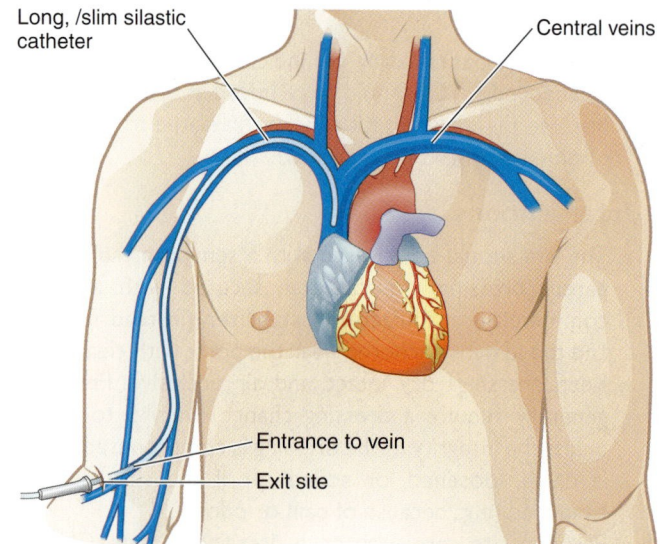

Long, /slim silastic catheter

Central veins

Entrance to vein

Exit site

FIGURE 39-10 A PICC line is a long, soft, flexible catheter inserted through a vein in the arm and threaded into a central vessel.

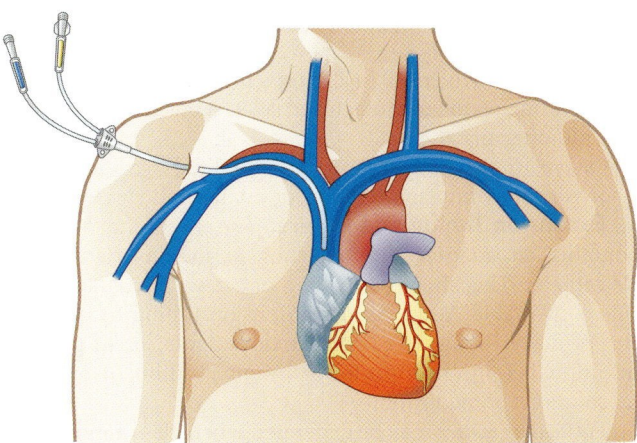

FIGURE 39-11 Nontunneled central venous catheters are inserted into the jugular, subclavian, and, occasionally, femoral veins.

Nontunneled central catheters can also be used to measure central venous pressure (CVP). CVP measurements offer information on volume status, with a low reading indicating hypovolemia and a high reading, hypervolemia.

Tunneled Central Venous Catheters

Tunneled CVCs are intended for long-term use. The catheter is inserted by a surgeon through a 7.5- to 15-cm (3- to 6-in.) subcutaneous tunnel in the chest wall and then into the jugular or subclavian vein (Fig. 39-12). The catheter can be sutured in place, with the sutures removed when fibrosis has developed around the catheter, or secured with an IV securing device. Because they are tunneled through the skin rather than through a vein, the risk of infection is lower than with PICCs or nontunneled central lines.

Implanted Ports

Implanted ports are devices made of a radiopaque silicone catheter and a plastic or stainless steel injection port with a self-sealing silicone-rubber septum. The catheter enters the internal jugular vein in the neck, and it may be tunneled or untunneled to a completely implanted subcutaneous reservoir (port) in the upper chest (Fig. 39-13). Implanted ports are placed by surgeons and only specially trained nurses are allowed to access an implanted port because of the risk of infiltration into the tissue if the needle placement is not correct. Implanted ports are also intended for long-term use.

✚ Blood pressures and blood draws should be avoided in the extremity of the side of the chest where the implanted port has been placed.

For a procedure for assisting with placement of a central venous catheter, refer to Procedure 39-9.

Intraosseous Devices

Designed for immediate access (within seconds) and short-term use (less than 24 hours), intraosseous (IO) access devices are used to administer fluids when a peripheral catheter cannot be inserted or when a central line insertion is not advisable, but especially in emergency situations. IOs are placed into the matrix of a bone. The venous sinusoids in the matrix can quickly absorb fluids to send to the central circulation. The most common access site is the proximal tibia in both children and adults. The sternum and the head of the humerus can also be used in adults. Osteomyelitis is a rare complication, occurring in fewer than 1% of cases. Contraindications for IO use include obesity, fracture, recent surgery, infection, or evidence of poor circulation at the proposed insertion site.

KnowledgeCheck 39-9

- What is the purpose of intravenous fluids?
- Describe the types and functions of three types of IV solutions: isotonic, hypotonic, and hypertonic.
- Under what conditions would a central venous access device be preferable to a peripheral device?

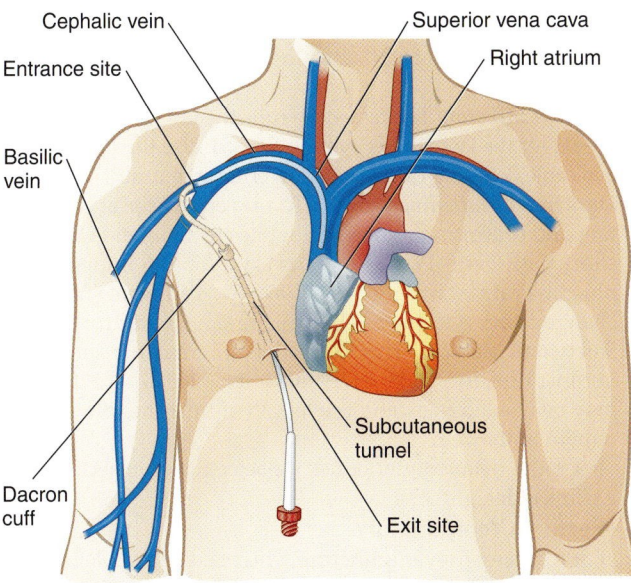

FIGURE 39-12 A tunneled central venous catheter is inserted through subcutaneous tissue in the chest wall into the jugular or subclavian vein.

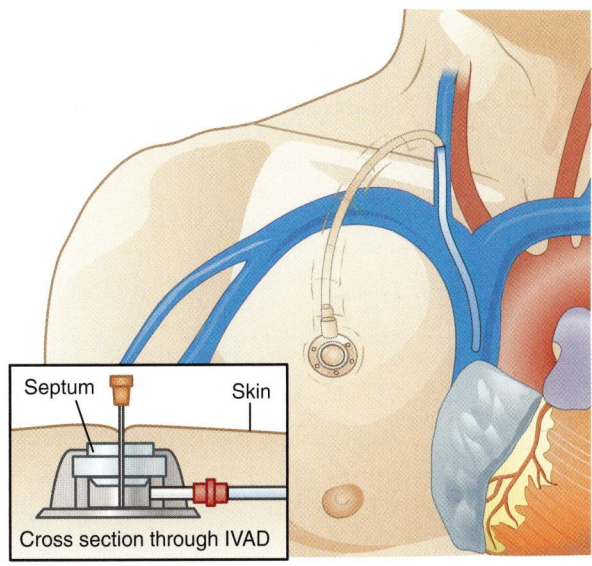

FIGURE 39-13 An implanted venous access port (IVAD) is a CVAD that enters the internal jugular vein in the neck but is tunneled to a completely implanted subcutaneous reservoir (port) in the upper chest.

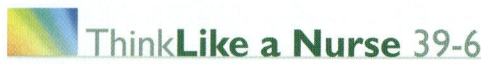

ThinkLike a Nurse 39-6

What type of venous access device would you expect Martha LaGuardia (Meet Your Patients) to receive in the hospital? Why?

Starting an Intravenous Infusion

To start an IV infusion, you will need to gather equipment and supplies, set up the solution and administration set, select a venipuncture site, and perform venipuncture.

Obtain Equipment and Supplies

Venipuncture supplies and IV infusion equipment are sterile, prepackaged, and disposable. They vary among manufacturers, so familiarize yourself with what is available in your facility. Set up the solution and administration set before performing the venipuncture.

IV Catheter. Select the smallest diameter and the shortest length catheter that will accommodate the prescribed therapy (Infusion Nursing Society, 2006b). Catheter sizes range from 16- to 24-gauge, depending on patient, type of fluid, and infusion rate. For most peripheral infusions, running at 50 to 175 mL per hour, a 24-gauge thin-walled catheter or a 22-gauge non–thin-walled catheter will deliver more than 1400 mL/hr if needed (Macklin, 2003). You will need a larger size for rapid infusions, viscous (thick) fluids, or surgical or trauma patients.

Administration Set (Infusion Kit). The administration set connects the fluid container to the catheter inserted in the patient. The set consists of tubing with a plastic insertion spike, a drip chamber, a roller clamp to regulate the flow, an injection port, and a catheter adapter (hub) (Fig. 39-14). Both ends of the infusion set (the spike and the hub) are sterile and must remain sterile.

The drip chamber is calibrated to allow a predictable amount of fluid to be delivered in each drop. The drop factor

is indicated on the package. A roller clamp on the tubing controls the rate of flow.

- A *macrodrip* delivers 10 to 20 drops per milliliter of solution, depending on the manufacturer; select a macrodrip for most adult infusions.
- A *microdrip* delivers 60 drops per milliliter; use a microdrip for very slow infusion rates or for infants and children.

Extension Tubing and Filters. The end of the IV tubing contains an adapter that attaches to the inserted sterile IV catheter. This should a locking or screw-on connection, if one is available. You may use extension tubing to lengthen the primary tubing (e.g., for active patients) or to provide additional Y-injection ports for administration of multiple IV solutions or medications.

Particulate matter may be generated when glass ampules are opened, or from additives or medications that have a tendency to clump. Occasionally, a filter will be used to remove particulate matter from the solution or to filter microorganisms. Some administration sets have built-in filters, or you may attach one to the end of the tubing. Some studies have shown that IV filters reduce the rate of phlebitis and bacteremia by as much as 40%; however, at present, guidelines do not recommend using filters routinely for infection-control purposes (Betsy Lehman Center for Patient Safety and Medical Error Reduction, JSI Research and Training Institute, Inc., 2008; CDC, 2002; Foster, Richards, and Showell, 2006, updated 2009; INS, 2006a).

Injection Port. Use the injection port to administer a secondary IV fluid or medication (see Chapter 25).

Solutions. Inspect the solution container to be certain that it contains the desired fluid, the fluid is clear, the bag is intact, and the solution has not expired. Most IV fluid containers are plastic, but a few are glass. Fluids for continuous infusions are packed in 1-L or 500-mL bags. Smaller bags (50 mL, 100 mL, and 250 mL) are used for intermittent infusions, such as antibiotics or other medications. Plastic containers collapse as fluid infuses, so you can use a nonvented administration set. Glass bottles do not collapse and therefore require a vented administration set.

Select a Peripheral Intravenous Site

To select a venipuncture site, consider age of the patient and type of solution (Clinical Insight 39-4), as well as the following:

- *Speed of infusion.* The faster the rate, the larger the vein (and the larger the IV catheter) you will need. Use the largest vein available, keeping other selection criteria in mind.
- *Duration of infusion therapy.* To prevent bacterial colonization and phlebitis, national guidelines recommend changing short peripheral IV catheters every 72 to 96 hours. If the phlebitis rate in an agency is above 5%, catheters should be changed every 48 hours (Betsy Lehman Center for Patient Safety and Medical Error Reduction, JSI Research and Training Institute, Inc. 2008; CDC, 2002; INS, 2006a). A PICC line may be needed to extend the length of time the catheter can remain in the vein.

For more detailed guidelines for selecting an insertion site, see Clinical Insight 39-4.

Perform Venipuncture

For a successful venipuncture, you need to be able to visualize or palpate the vein before attempting to insert the catheter. Use a vein viewer, if available, to aid in locating the vein. These instruments use infrared light and camera technology to project the patient's superficial veins onto the skin

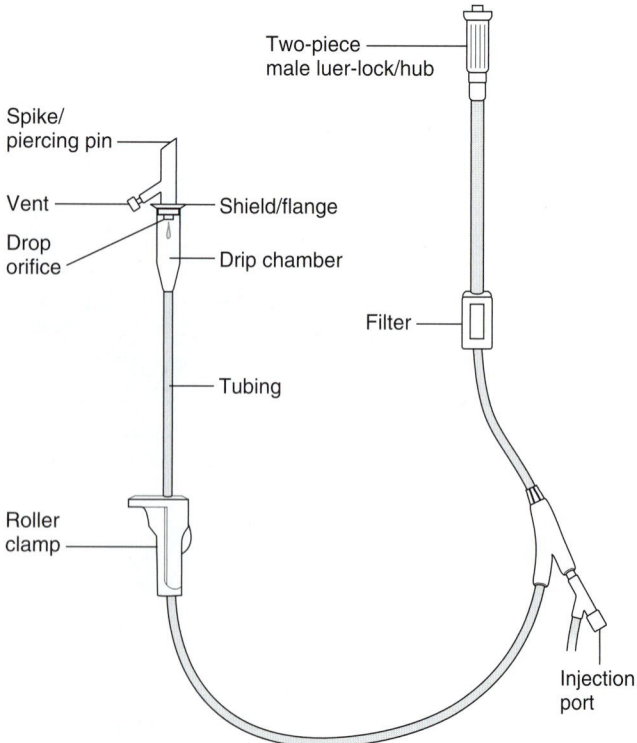

FIGURE 39-14 A basic administration set, or infusion kit.

Clinical Insight 39-4 ➤ Guidelines for Selecting a Peripheral Venipuncture Site

- As a general rule, select the most distal vein on an upper extremity.
- If available, use visualization technologies, such as portable ultrasound or imaging devices. This minimizes the number of needlesticks the patient must undergo.
- For adults, you will usually use veins in the hand or arm; for infants, veins in the scalp or dorsum of the foot can also be used.
- If possible, select a vein on the patient's nondominant hand or arm. Helps to preserve functional ability.

- Look for a vein that has a firm, round appearance with a relatively straight pathway. Do not use a red, hot, or hard vein.
- Avoid veins that are highly visible; they tend to roll.
- The cephalic vein of the arm is one of the best veins to use because it is relatively large, and the forearm provides a natural splint
- The dorsal veins of the hand are easy to access and are splinted by the metacarpals, but these veins are often quite small and fragile.
- Avoid the antecubital veins if possible. If the patient flexes her arm, the IV catheter may become displaced; so you

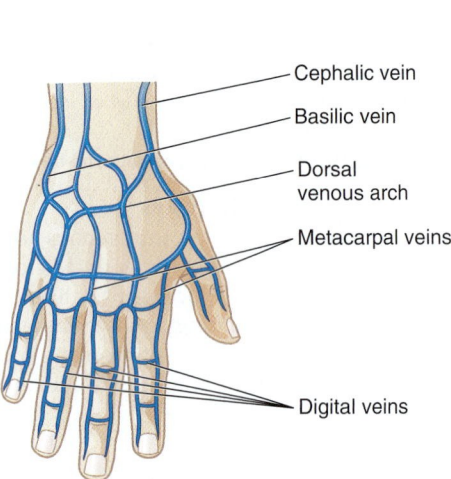

A Superficial veins of the hand

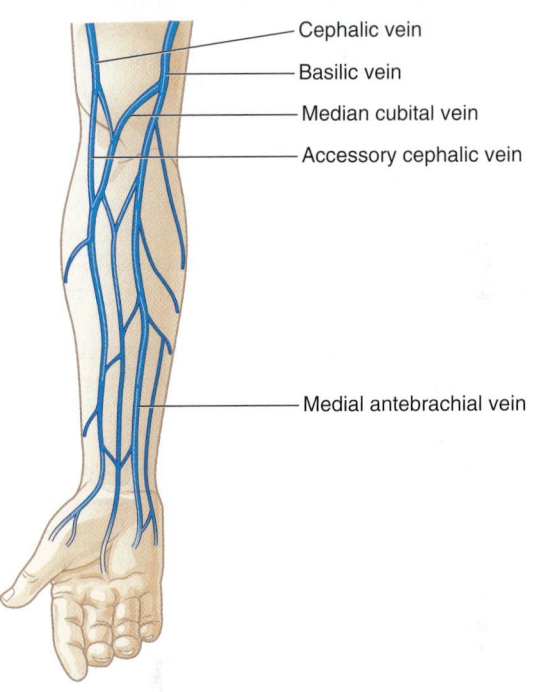

B Superficial veins of the forearm

would probably need to splint her elbow to prevent that. Furthermore, if a PICC line is needed at a later time, you will still have the antecubital veins available for it.
- For these situations, you need to use the largest vein available, keeping other selection criteria in mind:
  - Hypertonic solutions, viscous solutions, or irritating medications
  - Rapid rates (also require a larger IV catheter)
- Especially if the infusion is to be ongoing, begin the infusion with the best lowest vein and move proximal to the previous site (toward the heart) for subsequent insertions. Peripheral IV catheters are routinely changed every 72 to 96 hours. If you start the next IV below an already used site (i.e., to change the site or after a failed attempt at insertion), fluid may leak from the old site.
- Avoid areas where the vein crosses over joints. If you must use such an area, splint the joint to limit movement.

Splinting the joint helps preserve the vein for use, but it limits functional ability.
- Avoid areas with scarring, or with impaired circulation or neurological status. Examples are: the affected arm following a mastectomy; an area with signs of infection, previous infiltration or thrombosis; an arm with an arteriovenous fistula (shunt for dialysis); or the affected side after cerebrovascular accident (stroke). If you must use such an area, first obtain a medical prescription.
- Do not use veins in the legs and feet unless there is no other option. Peripheral circulation may not be adequate in the lower limbs, so there is increased danger of thrombus formation. In adults this location also interferes with mobility. Foot veins may be used for infants if the IV is taped securely.

surface. For other suggestions for locating a vein, refer to Procedure 39-1. This procedure also provides the "fine points" of venipuncture, such as how to stabilize the vein, the angle of insertion, and other related techniques.

If you are not successful with the venipuncture, you can make a second attempt above the initial site or in the opposite extremity. But do not make more than two attempts to start an IV on a patient. Get help from a more experienced colleague.

Regulating and Maintaining an Intravenous Infusion

Intravenous fluids can flow by gravity or be regulated by an electronic infusion control device (pump). You are responsible for maintaining the correct rate of flow and for monitoring the client's response to the infusion. Many factors can influence the flow rate of an IV solution, especially when using gravity flow.

- *Height of the solution container.* The greater that the distance is between the height of the container and the patient's heart, the faster the flow will be. Check the flow rate each time the client or IV solution is repositioned to ensure that it is correct.
- *Client position.* Pressure on the IV site decreases flow. If an IV is infusing in the right arm and the patient is positioned on his right side, the pressure on the right arm will be greater than if the client were positioned supine or on the left.
- *Blood pressure.* As blood pressure rises, more force is required to infuse into the vein.
- *Internal diameter of the IV catheter.* The smaller the diameter (the higher the gauge), the more you must open the roller clamp to achieve the flow rate desired.
- *Condition of the catheter and tubing.* If the catheter is dislodged from the vein, flow may stop entirely or continue at a slowed rate. A knot or kink at any point in the tubing will slow flow.

Gravity Flow

Most IV fluids are administered by a volume control pump. However, you may still encounter instances when you will need to regulate the rate with the roller clamp on the tubing. You should check gravity infusion rates hourly, and adjust the flow as needed. If the fluid is running too slowly, do not attempt to catch up by administering extra fluid rapidly. If the fluid is running too fast, slow the rate, and assess the client for signs of fluid volume excess.

If the client is ambulatory, attach the fluid container to a pole with wheels. Instruct the client to keep the solution container above the infusion site and to avoid pulling on the tubing or the infusion site. Procedure 39-2 describes how to regulate a gravity-flow IV.

Volume-Control Set

A volume-control set (e.g., Buretrol, Soluset, Volutrol) is another method for regulating an IV infusion (see Fig. 25-25). You will drain a small amount of fluid from the larger IV solution container into the volume-control container. Typically, the volume placed in the volume-control container is equal to the prescribed hourly infusion rate. The rate is regulated in the same way as other administration sets (the drip factor is usually 60 gtts/mL [gtts = drops]); however, the maximum amount of fluid that can enter a patient is limited to the volume in the volume-control set. You may use this type of equipment when the client is at risk for fluid volume excess and for infants and children, who require close supervision of fluid intake. However, more often, the policy will be to use

an infusion pump for continuous infusions for such patients. An advantage of this system is that medications can be added to the volume-control set and diluted with IV fluid for intermittent administration. To learn or review how to use a volume-control set, see Procedure 25-17A in Chapter 25.

Infusion Pump

If you are using an electronic volume-control device (pump), the machine will maintain the infusion rate after you program it. Most infusion pumps sound an alarm when the fluid bag is almost empty, when air is in the line, or when there is resistance to flow. Infusion control devices save time and prevent accidental delivery of large amounts of fluid. They do not, however, excuse you from regularly monitoring the flow rate and assessing the needle insertion site. ✚ You should know that absence of an alarm does not mean there is no problem. For example, if the IV is infiltrated, the pump may keep infusing fluid into the tissues.

To find out more about how to regulate an IV using an infusion pump, see Procedure 39-3.

KnowledgeCheck 39-10

- What factors should you consider when selecting an insertion site for a peripheral IV line?
- What are the preferred locations for peripheral IV lines?
- What equipment is needed when inserting an IV and starting an IV infusion?
- Identify three ways to regulate the flow rate of IV fluid.

Calculating Flow Rates

As you already know, intravenous administration sets are sized as microdrips or macrodrips. Microdrips deliver fluid at a rate of 60 gtts/mL. Macrodrips deliver fluid at a rate of 10 to 20 drops/mL (depending on the manufacturer). To begin, you need to know the ordered infusion rate and the flow rate of the administration set in drops per minute. See Box 39-1 to learn how to calculate flow rates.

BOX 39-1 ■ Calculating IV Flow Rates

Microdrips = 60 drops/mL
Macrodrips = 10 to 20 drops/mL

You need to know drops per minute: the prescribed infusion rate and the flow rate of the administration set.
1. Multiply the hourly rate (number of mL to be infused in 60 min) by the drop factor (in drops per mL) to obtain the total drops per hour.
2. Then divide by 60 to get the drip rate in drops per minute. For example, an hourly rate of 100 mL multiplied by 15 drops per mL and divided by 60 equals the drip rate. Therefore, the drip rate equals 25 drops per minute.

Use this formula to calculate flow:

$$\frac{\text{Hourly rate in mL} \times \text{drop factor (drops/mL)}}{60 \text{ min}} = \text{drip rate}$$

Example:

$$\frac{100 \text{ (mL per hour)} \times 15 \text{ (gtts/mL)}}{60 \text{ minutes}} = 25 \text{ gtts/min}$$

Managing Multiple Lines

When a patient has multiple IV solutions and multiple lines, you must label each line to identify what is infusing in it. Label the IV tubing close to the catheter so that it is easy to see which fluid is infusing the line. This is especially true when using double- and triple-lumen catheters. Multiple lines are often used because solutions are not compatible with each other such (e.g., you can never infuse blood, parenteral nutrition, or lipids through a line with anything else; and you can never draw blood samples from these lines).

The name of each line should also be reflected in your nursing notes and the intake form. For peripheral IVs, use RA for right arm, LA for left arm, and so on; and designate a number for each site because there may be more than one line or site in each arm (e.g., RA-1, RA-2, LA-1). If the lines are in separate arms, it may seem unnecessary to give each one a number; however, over the course of therapy, some lines may need to be discontinued and new ones started.

For multiport central lines, label each port. For example, with a triple-lumen central catheter, you might have named each lumen as proximal, mid, and distal, or CVAD-1, CVAD-2, CVAD-3. The finished labeling and nursing record may indicate "CVAD-1 – TPN, CVAD-2 – D_5-1/2 NS, CVAD-3 – insulin."

➕ Also be sure to always keep the lines untangled and know where your main IV fluid is (e.g., the D_5-1/2 NS), so that if a crisis occurs or intermittent infusions are needed, you can quickly identify the correct solution and tubing for use.

Complications of Intravenous Therapy

Complications at the IV site include infiltration, extravasation, infection, thrombus, and thrombophlebitis. Inserting an IV catheter breaks the body's first line of defense (the skin) and provides a portal of entry for microorganisms. In addition, trauma roughens the vein wall and predisposes the person to platelet clumping and thrombus formation. Minimize this effect by swiftly piercing the skin and anchoring the catheter and tubing to reduce tissue trauma. Systemic complications occur less frequently than local complications but may be life-threatening. They include fluid volume excess, sepsis, and embolus. Table 39-7 describes potential complications of IV therapy; and Clinical Insight 39-5 discusses managing infiltration and extravasation.

Table 39-7 ➤ Complications of Intravenous Therapy

COMPLICATION	CAUSES	SIGNS AND SYMPTOMS	NURSING RESPONSE
Local Complications			
Hematoma—a localized mass of blood outside the blood vessel	Nicking the vein during an unsuccessful insertion, discontinuing an IV line without holding pressure over the site, or applying a tourniquet too tightly above a previously attempted venipuncture site	Ecchymosis, localized mass, discomfort	Be gentle with venipuncture technique. Apply pressure when discontinuing an IV.
***Infiltration**—the seepage of nonvesicant solution or medication into surrounding tissues	IV catheter dislodges or the tip penetrates the vessel wall.	Slowed or stopped flow Swelling, tenderness, pallor, hardness and coolness at the site The patient may report a burning sensation in the area.	Stop the infusion immediately. Restart the IV infusion in a different vein, higher in the extremity or in another extremity. Elevate the affected arm on a pillow to promote absorption of excess fluid.
***Extravasation**—seepage of a vesicant substance into the tissues. (A *vesicant* is a solution that causes the formation of blisters and subsequent tissue sloughing and necrosis.)	IV catheter dislodges, or the tip penetrates the vessel wall.	Slowed or stopped flow Pain, burning, and swelling at IV site, blanching and coolness of the surrounding skin Blistering is a late sign. If extravasation was due to vasoconstricting medication may see necrosis (death) of dermis.	Treatment depends on the severity of the infiltration. Stop the IV infusion immediately. Administer an antidote, if one is available. (Antidotes alter the pH, alter DNA binding, neutralize the drug, or dilute the extravasated drug.) Apply cold compresses, and elevate the extremity.

(Continued)

Table 39-7 ➤ Complications of Intravenous Therapy—cont'd

COMPLICATION	CAUSES	SIGNS AND SYMPTOMS	NURSING RESPONSE
Phlebitis—inflammation of the vein	May be due to mechanical irritation, infusion of solutions that are irritating to the vessel, or sepsis. Dextrose solutions, potassium chloride, antibiotics, and vitamin C are associated with a higher risk of phlebitis. Trauma to the vessel, compression of the line by client movement, or a low flow rate	Redness, pain, and warmth at the site, local swelling, palpable cord along the vein, sluggish infusion rate, and elevated temperature Slowed or stopped infusion, localized warmth at the site, inability to restart flow of IV	Discontinue the IV infusion. Initially, apply cold compresses to the site. Thereafter, use warm compresses. Consult the primary care provider if there is streaking or erythema along the vein or a palpable cord. *Prevention measures:* Use the smallest catheter practical (usually 22-gauge or 24-gauge thin-walled catheter). Use polyurethane catheters instead of Teflon. Stabilize and secure the catheter to minimize movement in the vein. Rotate the site at least every 96 hr. Discontinue the IV infusion, and restart in a new location. Apply cold compresses to the site if the site is warm and tender. Assess for circulatory impairment.
Thrombophlebitis—thrombosis and inflammation	Use of veins in the legs for infusion, use of a hypertonic or highly acidic solution; can be a result of untreated phlebitis	Sluggish flow rate, edema, tender and cordlike veins, warmth and erythema at site	Discontinue the IV infusion, and restart in the opposite extremity, using all new equipment. Apply warm, moist compresses. Consult the primary care provider.
Local infection—microbial contamination of the cannula or IV site	Using poor technique when inserting the catheter, leaving the catheter in place for longer than 72 hours, or direct contamination	Redness, swelling, exudate, elevated temperature	Remove the IV line. Apply a sterile dressing over the site. Administer antibiotics, if necessary.
Nerve injury—A nerve is inadvertently injured during venipuncture (direct) or is compressed	Using veins on inner surface of the wrist and forearm; not anchoring the vein for puncture; using a large needle; advancing the needle across instead of with the vein; "probing" (excessive redirection of the needle at	*Direct injury:* Sharp, acute pain at the site or up and down the arm; pins and needles or electric shock sensation; pain, numbness, or tingling in fingers; pain that persists after the needle is removed	Do not make more than 2 venipuncture attempts. *If patient complains of symptoms:* Stop the procedure and withdraw the catheter. Apply pressure to prevent hematoma.

Table 39-7 ➤ Complications of Intravenous Therapy—cont'd

COMPLICATION	CAUSES	SIGNS AND SYMPTOMS	NURSING RESPONSE
	insertion); inserting too deeply and through the back wall of the vein; too many venipuncture attempts; infiltration, extravasation, tourniquet too tight or left on too long	*Compression injury:* Pain and tingling typically appear 24 to 96 hr after venipuncture.	Report to supervisor and physician. Do not start a new IV in the affected arm. Treat infiltration if it occurs. **Fasciotomy** (incisions around the area to let blood or fluid seep out) is the usual treatment; or fluid may be expressed.

Systemic Complications

COMPLICATION	CAUSES	SIGNS AND SYMPTOMS	NURSING RESPONSE
Septicemia—the presence of microorganisms or their toxic products in the circulatory system	A break in aseptic technique, or contaminated IV solution	Fluctuating fever, chills, tachycardia, confusion, hypotension, altered mental status, elevated WBC count	Discontinue the IV infusion immediately. Consult the primary care provider. Treatment often involves antibiotics, fluids, and medications to support vital signs.
Fluid overload	Infusing excessive amounts of IV fluids or administering fluid too rapidly.	Weight gain, edema, hypertension, shortness of breath, crackles, distended neck veins	Slow the IV flow rate. Place the client in high-Fowler's position. Monitor vital signs. Administer oxygen, if needed. If severe, diuretics may be ordered.
Air embolus—a rare complication involving the introduction of air into the vascular system	Loose connections, adding a new IV bag to a line that has run dry without clearing the line of air; air in tubing cassette of infusion pump	Palpitations, chest pain, lightheadedness, dyspnea, cough, hypotension, tachycardia, sudden change in mental status	Call for help. Place client in Trendelenburg's position on the left side. Administer oxygen. Have emergency equipment available.
Catheter embolus—a piece of catheter breaks off and travels through the vascular system	Reinserting a catheter used in an unsuccessful insertion; removing and reinserting a stylet, causing shearing of the catheter; placing the catheter in a joint flexion	Sharp, sudden pain at IV site, jagged catheter end on removal, dyspnea, chest pain, tachycardia, hypotension	Apply a tourniquet above the site. Notify the physician and radiologist. Start a new IV line. Prepare the patient for radiographic examination.

*For more information about interventions for infiltration and extravasation, see Clinical Insight 39-5.

Source: Phillips, L. D. (2010). *Manual of IV therapeutics* (5th ed.). Philadelphia: F.A. Davis.

Clinical Insight 39-5 ➤ Managing Infiltration and Extravasation

- At the first sign or symptom of infiltration or extravasation, stop the IV. Symptoms include slowed or stopped flow, swelling, tenderness, pallor, hardness, and coolness at the site.
- The patient may report a burning sensation in the area.

For a Central Venous Catheter:

- Clamp and cap the catheter hub.
- Do not remove the catheter.
- Follow agency policy for flushing when you suspect infiltration or extravasation.
- If the patient has an implanted port, aspirate, remove the port access needle, and apply a dressing.
- Notify the provider who inserted the catheter, who may order an x-ray to help determine the cause of the problem.

For a Short Peripheral Catheter:

- Disconnect the tubing from the catheter hub; attach a 3- to 5-mL syringe and try to aspirate fluid from the catheter lumen. Use aseptic technique.
- Photograph the site to create a record of its condition, if agency policy allows.
- Wearing gloves, remove the catheter and hold a dry gauze pad over the site to stop the bleeding. Apply a dry dressing. Do not apply excessive pressure to the site.
- If you are to start a new IV, start it on the other arm, if possible. If it is not possible, start it in a more proximal location on the same arm.
- Measure the circumference of the arm and compare it with the opposite arm.
- Assess capillary refill, sensation, and motion distal to the infiltrated site.

- Apply cold or warm compresses depending on which fluid has escaped into the tissues.
  - For alkaloids (e.g., vincristine) and epipodophyllotoxins (e.g., etoposide), use heat.
  - For hypertonic fluids or medications, use cold.
  - For isotonic or hypotonic fluids or medications, choose either heat or cold, or alternate them, based on patient comfort.
- Apply compresses for 15 to 30 minutes every 4 to 6 hours; continue for 24 to 48 hours.
- Estimate the volume of fluid that escaped into the tissues; notify the prescriber.
- Some medications leaked into the surrounding tissue can cause damage and even necrosis. For instance, when dopamine extravasates, you might need to give a prescribed amount of antidote (e.g., regitine injected subcutaneously) as well as hydrocortisone and an anti-inflammatory to minimize tissue damage. Be sure to check the protocol at your facility.
- Elevate the extremity and advise the patient to rest.
- Document all fluids and medications involved, equipment being used (e.g., pump), size and type of the catheter, description of the site (including location, size, and color), methods used to assess the site before administering the fluids (e.g., aspiration), patient's signs and symptoms, interventions, notifications, and patient teaching.
- Complete an occurrence (or incident) report, as required by your facility.

References

Hadaway, 2007; Polovich, White, & Kelleher, 2006.

Changing Intravenous Solutions, Tubing, and Dressings

Follow practice guidelines and agency policies for changing IV solutions, tubing, and dressings. As with IV insertion, use meticulous aseptic technique.

Changing IV Solutions. Hang a new container of fluid when the present container is nearly empty but fluid still remains at the appropriate level in the drip chamber. The infusion rate dictates how often you need to change the IV solution. For example, a liter of IV fluid infusing at 125 mL/hr must be changed every 8 hours; a liter infusing at 50 mL/hr will hang for 20 hours. Regardless of rate, the Infusion Nurses Society (2006a) recommends you not leave an IV solution hanging for more than 24 hours because the likelihood of contamination increases with time. There is not complete agreement about the allowable hang time for a container, though. The National Guideline Clearinghouse (2008) states that there is not enough evidence to make a recommendation about hanging time of parenteral fluids other than blood and parenteral nutrition. In any event, you will need to follow institutional policies. For more instructions for

changing solutions, tubing, and dressings, see Procedures 39-4A, 39-4B, and 39-5.

Changing Administration Sets. Administration sets for continuous peripheral and central infusions are usually changed every 72 hours (every 24 hours for total parenteral nutrition). Because most peripheral catheters are changed at least every 72 to 96 hours (CDC, 2002), changing the administration set often coincides with inserting a new intravenous catheter. As a rule, if you start an IV at a new site, use a new administration set. Reusing a set from a previous site increases the risk of contamination.

Changing IV Dressings. Change peripheral IV dressings routinely when the catheter is replaced, or at least weekly (CDC, 2002). CVCs usually remain in place for lengthy periods, but the dressing at the site must be changed periodically, usually every 72 hours in acute care settings. In home care, the dressing may be left in place for 1 week. Change any dressing, regardless of site, when it becomes soiled, damp, or loosened. It is best to dress both central and peripheral lines with transparent, semipermeable dressings. These dressings allow direct visualization of the site between

dressing changes, permit evaporation of moisture, and provide a secure anchor for the catheter. Use a catheter stabilization device, if one is available, although you may still sometimes see tape securing a catheter at the insertion site. This trend has diminished, though, because of the risk of contamination of the site (INS, 2006a).

Converting to a Peripheral Intravenous Lock

Recall that you may need a peripheral IV lock for intermittent infusions or for venous access for emergencies. Some clients do not need the additional fluids provided by a constant infusion of solution. A peripheral infusion can be easily converted to a peripheral lock when continuous infusion is no longer required. You simply remove the tubing from the IV catheter and replace it with a sterile injection cap (see Fig. 39-9). Some IV locks also contain a short segment of tubing. Procedure 39-6 describes how to convert an IV line to an IV lock.

Each time you give a medication through the lock, you will need to disinfect and flush the lock before and after you administer the medication. Consult your agency policy regarding the type of solution to use (saline or a dilute heparin solution). Research has shown that saline is as effective as heparin in maintaining IV lock patency and that there is no difference in the incidence of phlebitis (LeDuc, 1997; Niesen, Harris, Parkin, et al., 2003). To review how to administer IV push medications through an IV lock (with and without extension tubing) see Chapter 25, Procedures 25-16B, and 25-16C, respectively.

Discontinuing an Intravenous Line

Discontinue the IV line and IV catheter when IV fluids and medications are no longer needed or if the integrity of the line is compromised. Inspect the catheter to ensure that it is intact when you remove it. For complete steps to remove an IV catheter see Procedure 39-7.

KnowledgeCheck 39-11

- The order reads, "5% dextrose in water/ 0.45% saline solution (D_5-1/2 NS) with 20 mEq KCl; infuse 1 liter in 5 hours." Calculate the hourly rate and the drip rate using (1) a macrodrip administration set with 15 gtts/mL and (2) a microdrip set.
- Describe the difference between infiltration and extravasation as a complication of IV therapy.
- In general, how often are administration sets changed on peripheral IV lines? When TPN is infused?

Replacement of Blood and Blood Products

Intravenous fluids can replace fluid volume, but they do not restore oxygen-carrying capacity or replace clotting factors. Blood products are infused when the patient has experienced significant blood loss, diminished oxygen-carrying capacity, or a deficiency in one of the blood components. The AABB (an organization involved in the field of transfusion medicine) estimates that 10.8 million volunteers donate blood each year, for a total of 23 million units of whole blood and red blood cells (AABB, n.d.).

Each unit of donated blood is separated into multiple components, such as red blood cells, plasma, platelets, and clotting factors. Thus, one unit of donated blood may be used in the care of four clients. Unfortunately, fewer than 5% of eligible persons donate blood each year. To be eligible to donate blood, a person must be in good health (no cold or flu, uncontrolled hypertension, or diabetes), at least age 16 years (although some states permit younger people, with parental consent, to donate), have a hemoglobin at least 12.5 g/dL, and weigh at least 110 pounds. In addition, each potential donor is screened for travel to certain countries and for a variety of disorders, such as hepatitis, HIV, and Creutzfeldt-Jakob disease (the human form of "mad cow" disease).

Blood Groups

Human blood is classified into four main groups (A, B, AB, and O) based on the presence or absence of certain antigens and antibodies. You inherit the blood group you belong to from your parents.

If you belong to blood group A, you have A antigens on the surface of your RBCs, and B antibodies in your plasma. The opposite is true for persons with blood group B. Blood group AB has both antigens on the surface of the red blood cells and no antibodies at all in the plasma. In contrast, blood group O has neither A or B antigens on the surface of the red blood cells but both A and B antibodies in the blood plasma (Table 39-8). Patients must receive only blood that is compatible with their own blood group.

An additional antigen, known as Rh factor, is also important with blood typing. If the antigen is present, you are referred to as Rh positive (RH+). If it is absent, you are Rh negative (Rh−). Thus, you can belong to one of the following eight groups:

A Rh+	B Rh+	AB Rh+	O Rh+
A Rh−	B Rh−	AB Rh−	O Rh−

Blood Typing and Crossmatching

Once blood is donated, several tests are performed on the sample. First, the sample is tested for ABO group (blood type) and Rh type (positive or negative), as well as for any unexpected red blood cell antibodies that may cause problems in a recipient. Screening tests assess for evidence of donor infection with hepatitis B and C viruses, HIV, human T-lymphotropic viruses, West Nile Virus, and syphilis. If all disease screens are negative, the blood is acceptable for transfusion and is placed in the pool of available products.

When a potential donor is identified, crossmatching is performed. **Crossmatching** identifies possible minor antigens that will affect the compatibility of the donor blood in the recipient. RBCs from the donor blood are mixed with plasma from the potential recipient. A reagent is added, and the sample is observed for clumping or agglutination. If no clumping is observed, the risk of transfusion reaction is low, and it is considered safe to transfuse the sample of blood. Table 39-8 summarizes blood group matching. As you can see, people with blood group O are considered universal donors, whereas people with blood group AB are considered universal recipients. In regard to Rh factor, people who are Rh+ may receive blood with or without Rh factor. However, people who are Rh− may receive only Rh− blood.

When possible, **autologous** (self-donated) units of blood are given instead of blood from a donor. This negates the risk of a mismatch or exposure to undetected disease. The patient's blood is usually collected in the preoperative weeks for possible transfusion during elective surgery. Autologous donation is most often done with orthopedic, cardiac, and vascular surgery. The process of donating autologous blood stimulates

Table 39-8 ▶ Blood Transfusions

BLOOD GROUP	ANTIGENS	ANTIBODIES	CAN GIVE BLOOD TO	CAN RECEIVE BLOOD FROM
AB	A and B	None	AB	AB, A, B, and O
A	A	B	A and AB	A and O
B	B	A	B and AB	B and O
O	None	A and B	AB, A, B, and O	O

the bone marrow to produce new blood cells. Given adequate time for recovery, the collected cells may be wholly or partially replaced prior to surgery.

Blood Products

Several blood products are available for transfusion:

- *Whole blood* contains red blood cells, white blood cells, and platelets suspended in plasma.
- *Red blood cells* are prepared from whole blood by removing the plasma. RBCs can raise the client's hematocrit and hemoglobin levels while minimizing an increase in volume. RBCs are available for transfusion as packed RBCs (PRBCs).
- *Plasma* is the liquid portion of the blood. It is 90% water and makes up about 55% of blood volume. Plasma may be transfused whole or may be separated into specific products, such as albumin, clotting factor concentrates, and immune globulins.
- *Platelets* help the clotting process by sticking to the lining of blood vessels. Units of platelets are prepared by using a centrifuge to separate the platelet-rich plasma from the donated unit of whole blood. The platelet-rich plasma is then centrifuged again to concentrate the platelets further. Platelets are used to treat clients who have a shortage of platelets or have abnormal platelet function.

- *White blood cells (WBCs)*, specifically granulocytes, can be collected by centrifugation of whole blood. They are transfused within 24 hours after collection and are used for infections that are unresponsive to antibiotic therapy. The effectiveness of WBC transfusion is still being investigated.
- *Plasma derivatives* are concentrates of specific plasma proteins prepared from many units of plasma. Plasma derivatives include a variety of clotting factors, immune globulins, and albumin.

Initiating a Transfusion

It is critical to identify the patient and the blood product when transfusing blood. Before beginning a transfusion, obtain a set of vital signs. If the patient's temperature is elevated, inform the primary care provider before hanging the transfusion. Most patients experience a minor elevation in temperature after a transfusion is given. A preexisting elevated temperature may exacerbate this response. As a result, premedication may be prescribed.

Some patients will refuse a blood transfusion because of cultural, religious, or other beliefs. Be ready to discuss with them any available alternatives to whole blood administration.

Also inspect the IV site to be sure it is patent before hanging the blood product. Nurses commonly use a 20-gauge catheter to infuse blood—and a larger size for rapid flow rates. There is

Toward Evidence-Based Practice

Houck, D., & Whiteford, J. (2007). Transfusion with infusion pump for peripherally inserted central catheters and other vascular access devices. *Journal of Infusion Nursing, 30*(6), 341–344.

In a 500-bed community hospital, policy required that blood transfusions be infused by gravity flow. This policy necessitated that a peripheral IV be initiated if the patient had a peripherally inserted central catheter (PICC). Nurses sought to show that using a PICC line with an infusion pump was safe and efficient for transfusing blood. A literature search indicated that one of the main concerns was exceeding the psi (pressure per square inch) tolerance of the catheter. Further literature review showed no increased risk of hemolysis of red blood cells when given via pump as compared to gravity. In the study, a total of 169 units of blood products were infused via various types of PICCs and infusion ports, some using a pump and some using gravity flow. All

PICC lines remained patent during transfusion and no problems with using a pump were identified. The study also revealed that nursing time decreased by 30 minutes when using a pump—the time needed to start and maintain another IV site. Cost was decreased when using a pump because of the savings in nursing time and equipment needed for a new IV start. Based on the study, the policy for blood administration via PICC lines was changed.

1. Based on this study, how do you see nurses can affect institution policy and procedure?

2. Are there any other concerns related to infusing blood via an infusion pump that you might have, and why?

 Go to Chapter 39, **Toward Evidence-Based Practice Suggested Responses,** on DavisPlus.

evidence that a 22-gauge catheter can be used in adults without damage to the red blood cells (INS, 2006a; Macklin, 2003). Certainly, for children and the frail elderly, you will need a smaller, 22- or 24-gauge catheter. For the complete procedure for initiating and monitoring a blood transfusion and managing a transfusion reaction, see Procedure 39-8A and B.

Transfusion Reactions

Even though you use perfect technique, transfusion reactions can and do occur. Five types of reaction are possible: allergic, bacterial, febrile, or hemolytic reactions; and circulatory overload. Table 39-9 describes each of these reactions.

To help prevent transfusion reactions, be extremely careful in identifying the patient and the blood, start the transfusion slowly, remain with the patient for the first 5 minutes of the transfusion, and assess again at 15 minutes (see Procedure 39-8).

KnowledgeCheck 39-12

- Identify eight potential blood types.
- Describe the types of blood products that are available for transfusion.
- Identify and describe types of transfusion reactions.

Table 39-9 ➤ Transfusion Reactions

TYPE OF REACTION	SIGNS AND SYMPTOMS	NURSING RESPONSIBILITIES
Allergic—allergy to blood being transfused	Flushing, itching, wheezing, urticaria (hives); anaphylaxis, if severe	Stop the transfusion. Replace with a saline infusion. Notify the physician immediately. Administer prescribed antihistamine.
Bacterial—contamination of the blood	Fever, chills, vomiting, diarrhea, hypertension	Stop the transfusion. Replace with a saline infusion. Notify the physician. Administer antibiotics as ordered. Treat symptoms.
Febrile—temperature elevation due to sensitivity to WBCs, plasma proteins, or platelets	Fever, chills, warm, flushed skin, aches	Stop the transfusion. Replace with a saline infusion. Notify the physician. Treat symptoms.
Hemolytic reactions—destruction of RBCs as a result of infusing incompatible blood; occurs in 1 in 600,000 transfusions	Fever, chills, dyspnea, chest pain, tachycardia, hypotension; can be fatal	Stop the transfusion immediately. Replace with a saline infusion. Notify the physician immediately. Send the remaining blood, including tubing and filter; a sample of venous blood; and the first voided urine to the lab for analysis. Treat shock.
Circulatory overload—administering too great a volume or too rapidly	Persistent cough, crackles, hypertension, distended neck veins	Slow or stop the transfusion. Monitor vital signs. Place the client upright. Notify the physician.

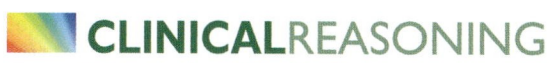

CLINICALREASONING
Applying the Full-Spectrum Nursing Model

Because the following critical thinking activities allow you to practice the kind of thinking you will use as a full-spectrum nurse, they usually have no single right answer. Discuss them with your peers—if you have difficulty with any of the questions, consult your instructor.

PATIENT SITUATION

Darlene Malone, age 42, has been admitted to the emergency department with complaints of fatigue, extreme weakness, and heart palpitations. She says she has not seen a healthcare provider in nearly 10 years. Suddenly, she slumps and falls over. She is not breathing, has no pulse, and does not respond to verbal stimuli. She is resuscitated with CPR and IV epinephrine, and an endotracheal tube is placed. Stat lab results show a potassium level of 7.7 mEq/L, BUN of 102 mg/dL, and creatinine of 5 mg/dL. A physician diagnoses acute renal failure. Among other interventions, an IV is started to administer 10% calcium chloride solution, 1,000 mg, by slow IV push to counteract the toxic effects of hyperkalemia on the cell membranes. The nurse used a 20-gauge over-the-needle catheter in Ms. Malone's right cephalic vein, about 5 cm (2 in.) above her wrist.

THINKING

1. *Theoretical Knowledge:*
   a. Which lab results are abnormal? Are they high or low?
   b. Which lab results directly reflect her renal failure?
   c. What term correctly describes serum potassium of 7.7 mEq/L?
2. *Critical Thinking (Considering Alternatives):*
   a. What do you think is causing Ms. Malone to have hyperkalemia? You should be able to think this through and make a reasonable guess even if you have not studied pathophysiology.
   b. Ms. Malone is to be given 50 mEq of sodium bicarbonate by slow IV push for an acid–base imbalance that is often associated with hyperkalemia. Which imbalance do you think would be treated with sodium bicarbonate: metabolic acidosis or metabolic alkalosis?

DOING

3. *Practical Knowledge:*
   a. When you prepare to administer the sodium bicarbonate (in question 2b), you notice that the IV infusion is barely flowing and that the insertion site is swollen and pale. What is the first thing you should do?
   b. You aspirate the catheter and do not obtain a blood return. Ms. Malone absolutely must have this medication. Describe what you would do in the order you would do it.
4. *Nursing Process (Planning Goals):* Choose the NOC outcome best suited to evaluating Ms. Malone's hyperkalemia. Also choose three outcome indicators you could use to evaluate her goal achievement for that problem.

CARING

5. *Self-Knowledge:* Ms. Malone will need dialysis to replace her inadequate renal function and control her serum potassium level. It is likely that her renal failure was brought on by years of illegal drug abuse. She has never held a full-time job and has not worked at all for the last 7 years. Her dialysis treatments will need to be paid for by Medicaid, which is funded by tax dollars. How do you feel about this—specifically, how do you feel about the issues of (a) a person's responsibility for her own health and (b) compassion for people who cannot afford to pay for healthcare? Focus on your own feelings, not on issues of what "should" be done.

 Go To Chapter 39, **Clinical Reasoning: Applying the Full-Spectrum Nursing Model Response Sheet,** on Davis*Plus*.

Practical Knowledge
procedures

To prevent, identify, and treat fluid, electrolyte, and acid–base problems, you will need to be skilled at initiating and managing intravenous infusions of fluids and blood, performing focused history and physical assessments, and interpreting arterial blood gas (ABG) values. When performing the procedures, apply the concepts and other theoretical knowledge you have learned.

Procedure 39–1 ■ Initiating a Peripheral Intravenous Infusion

➤ For steps to follow in *all* procedures, refer to the Universal Steps for All Procedures found on the page facing the inside back cover.

Equipment

- IV solution
- Administration set or IV lock and injection caps. (For a glass solution container, use vented tubing; for a plastic container you may use either vented or nonvented tubing.)
- Extension tubing with or without saline lock, possibly
- Prefilled syringe to prime extension tubing.
- Appropriately sized IV catheter
- Clean, unsterile gloves
- Scissors
- Antiseptic swabs that contain solutions such as chlorhexidine (preferred by the CDC, 2002) or 70% alcohol wipes.
- Tourniquet (nonlatex, if available)
- Sterile manufactured catheter stabilization device or ½-inch tape.
- 2-in. × 2-in. sterile gauze, and/or transparent semipermeable occlusive dressing
- 1-inch nonallergenic tape, preferably clear
- Labels, time tape
- Linen-saver pad
- Arm board, if necessary

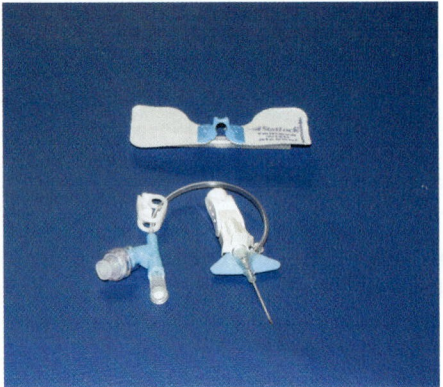

Catheter stabilization device.

Delegation

In some states and agencies you can delegate peripheral IV catheter insertion to a licensed practical nurse (LPN) who is adequately trained in the skill.

Pre-Procedure Assessment

- Assess the patient's need for IV therapy by checking vital signs, laboratory values, urine output, skin turgor, breath sounds, and the condition of mucous membranes.
- Check for any situations that may contraindicate administering the prescribed fluids to the patient.
- Assess for allergy to tape.
- Assess the veins on the arms and hands for a potential insertion site.
  Preferred sites are the upper extremities because of better blood flow, easier access, and less risk for complications than in other locations. Consider the best most distal sites first.
- Check the medical record for factors such as anticoagulant therapy, bleeding disorders, or low platelet count.
  These factors place the patient at risk for bleeding during IV catheter insertion.

➤ When performing the procedure, always identify your patient according to agency policy and be attentive to standard precautions, hand hygiene, patient safety and privacy, body mechanics, and documentation.

Procedure Steps

✚ *NOTE: Maintain scrupulous aseptic technique throughout this procedure.*
Any microorganisms introduced can cause infection at the site, which could quickly migrate into the bloodstream and cause sepsis.

1. **Place the patient in a comfortable position**, the bed at a comfortable working height, and supplies within reach. Explain the procedure to the patient.

Makes the procedure safer and easier, and decreases the risk for the nurse to develop back problems from improper body mechanics.

2. **Prepare the IV solution** and administration set or IV lock.
   a. Following the "rights" of medication administration, check the IV solution to make sure that you have the proper solution with the prescribed additives.
   IV solution is considered medication. Check it carefully to avoid

administration and compatibility errors.

   b. Check the expiration date on the IV solution. Do not use IV solution after that date.
   c. Check the IV solution for discoloration or particulate matter.
   Such solutions may be contaminated and should not be used.
   d. Label the IV solution container with the patient's name, date, and your initials. Place a time tape on the solution container with the

(continued on next page)

Procedure 39–1 ■ **Initiating a Peripheral Intravenous Infusion** (continued)

prescribed infusion rate, time the infusion begins, and the time it is to be completed.

Policies govern when solution containers, administration sets, dressings, and IV catheters need to be changed to avoid complications such as infection. Although not all agencies require a time tape, labeling infusion rates on the solution containers in this manner will alert others and makes it easy to see at a glance whether the solution is infusing on time. ▼

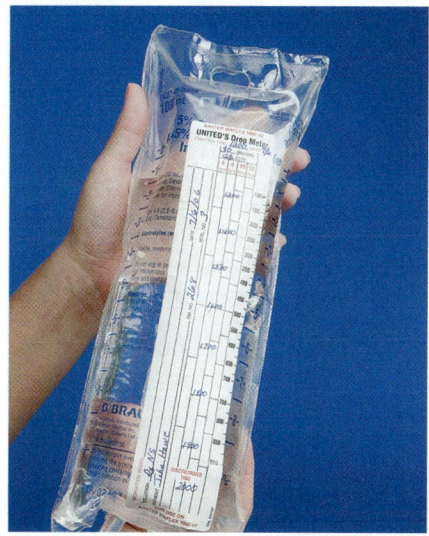

e. Take the administration set from the package and close the roller clamp by rolling it downward. Label the tubing with the date and time.
   Keeps the fluid does from flow through the line after the bag is spiked.

f. Remove the protective cover from the solution container port.

g. Remove the protective cover from the spike on the IV administration set, keeping the spike sterile. Place the spike into the port of the solution container. ▼

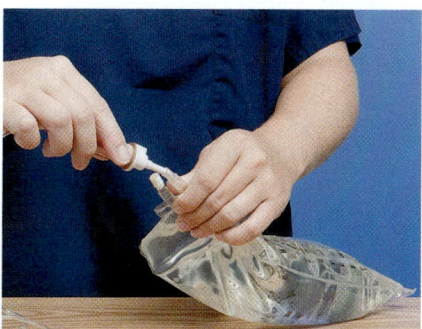

h. Lightly compress the drip chamber and allow it to fill up halfway. ▼

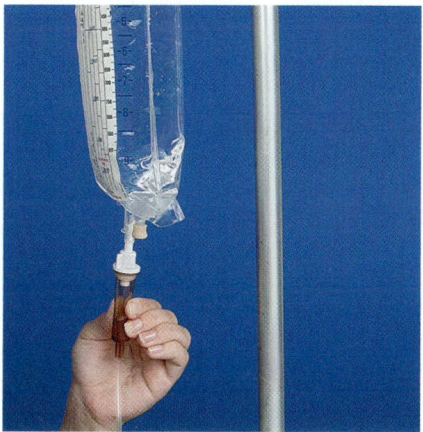

Glass Bottle

If using a glass bottle, clean the rubber stopper on the top of the bottle with an alcohol pad. Then insert the spike of the administration set through the stopper.

   i. Be certain the tubing is clamped. Hang the IV solution container on an IV pole.
      Clamping prevents loss of fluid.

   j. Lightly compress the drip chamber, and allow it to fill up halfway.
      Overfilling the drip chamber will impair your ability to see the drips and adequately regulate the flow rate.

No Extension Tubing

Prime the tubing by opening the roller clamp and allowing the fluid to slowly fill the tubing. When tubing is filled, close the clamp.

Using Extension Tubing

   k. If using extension tubing, either attach it to the end of the administration set now and prime it with the rest of the IV line, or prime it separately, as follows:

   (1) Scrub the injection port of the extension tubing, if there is one, with an alcohol pad and let it dry.

   (2) Attach a flush syringe filled with normal saline to the injection port or to the non-luer-lock end and slowly push the fluid through the tubing until completely primed. Consult packaging instructions for the amount of saline needed to flush the tubing.

   (3) Leave flush syringe attached to the extension tubing.
      IV extension tubing makes it easier to later convert an IV to a saline lock without disturbing the IV dressing and catheter. Manipulation of the IV catheter increases the risk of complications such as phlebitis, inflammation, infection, and infiltration.

   l. Inspect the tubing for air. If air bubbles remain in the tubing, flick the tubing with a fingertip to mobilize them into the drip chamber. Recap end of tubing firmly.
      Air in the tubing creates the potential for air embolism.

3. **Place a linen-saver pad under the patient's arm**.
   Protects the bed from soiling during venipuncture.

4. **Place the patient's arm** in a dependent position.
   Gravity helps fill and dilate the vein, making venipuncture easier.

5. **Apply a tourniquet** 10 to 20 cm (4 to 8 in.) above the selected site. Palpate the radial pulse. If no pulse is present, loosen the tourniquet, and reapply it with less tension.
   Occluding the arterial flow diminishes venous filling, making venipuncture difficult.

6. **Locate a vein for inserting the IV** catheter. Select the best most distal vein on the hand or arm. Check with the medical provider before using an arm or hand that contains a dialysis graft or fistula, or the affected arm of a patient who has undergone a mastectomy. See Clinical Insight 39-4 for more guidelines.
   Choose the most distal veins on the hand or arm so that you can perform subsequent venipuncture proximal to the previous site. This preserves veins for long-term therapy and prevents extravasation of fluid and medicines.

7. **Palpate the vein** and press it downward, making sure that it rebounds quickly. If the vein is not adequately dilated, ask the patient to open and close his fist; apply heat (e.g., a warm towel, a warming mitt); lightly tap the vein site; or stroke the extremity from distal to proximal, beginning

below the selected venipuncture site. If available in your agency, use an infrared or other visualization device to assist in locating a vein.

These maneuvers help bring blood to the local area to dilate the vein, making it easier to locate and making venipuncture easier.

8. **Loosen the tourniquet.** If excessive hair is present at the venipuncture site, clip it with scissors.

Loosening the tourniquet restores blood flow and allow for patient comfort while preparing for venipuncture. Clipping the hair helps the dressings to adhere after catheter insertion. Shaving is not recommended because it may abrade the skin, providing a portal of entry for pathogens.

9. **Don clean nonsterile gloves.**

Provides protection from inadvertent exposure to blood. Note that some nurses don gloves routinely, even when preparing supplies and equipment. However, there is no risk for coming in contact with body fluids before this step, so strictly speaking, CDC standard precautions require gloves only from this step forward.

10. **Select an appropriate IV catheter** based on the size of the vein, the solution to be infused, and the expected duration of therapy. Using aseptic technique, open the package.

Reduces the risk of extravasation and phlebitis. Always use the smallest diameter and shortest catheter that will deliver the desired solution flow. For most adults this will be a 20 to 24 gauge to minimize venous irritation and promote blood flow around the catheter. Aseptic handling reduces the risk of infection.

11. **Gently reapply the tourniquet** and scrub the site, using an antiseptic swab that contains chlorhexidine gluconate (preferred, [CDC, 2002]); if this is not available, use 70% alcohol wipes. Cleanse for 30 seconds, using friction.

Removes microorganisms from the skin so that they do not enter the venous system during venipuncture. Working "clean to dirty," or from the venipuncture site outward, avoids moving microorganisms toward the puncture site.

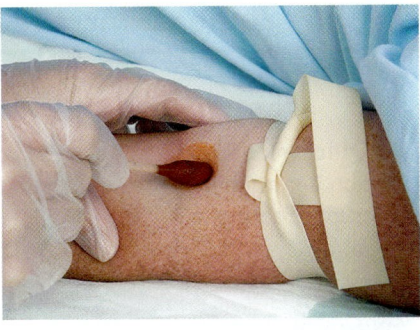

12. **Allow the antiseptic to air-dry.** Do not fan.

The antiseptic promotes adherence to the dressing. Fanning can cause contamination of the site.

13. **Pick up the catheter and inspect the tip.**

There should be no burrs (rough spots, ridges) on the needle or peeling of the catheter material.

14. **Inform the patient** that you are about to insert the catheter and that it may be uncomfortable.

Keeping the patient informed promotes cooperation and lessens anxiety.

Wing-Tipped Catheter (Butterfly)

Grasp the catheter by the wings, using the thumb and forefinger of your dominant hand and making sure that the bevel is up. Remove the protective cap from the needle.

Stabilizes the catheter for insertion. Inserting the needle bevel up makes it less likely that you will pierce both vein walls (go "through" the vein) as well as making piercing the skin less painful for the patient. ▼

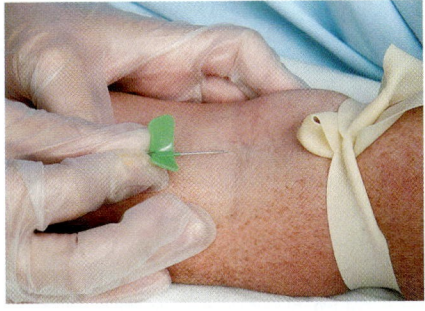

Over-the-Needle Catheter

Grasp the catheter by the hub, using the thumb and forefinger of your dominant hand and making sure that the bevel is up.

For both variations, inserting the needle with the bevel up makes it less likely that you will pierce both vein walls (go "through" the

vein) as well as making piercing the skin less painful for the patient. ▼

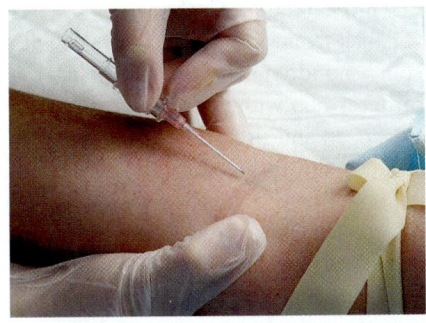

15. **Using your nondominant hand,** stabilize the vein by continuously pulling the skin taut below the puncture area (pull downward toward the hand or fingers). Do not press too hard, and make sure not to contaminate the insertion site.

Stabilizing the vein eases insertion and prevents damage to the underside of the vein as well as preventing the vein from rolling. Pressing too hard compresses blood flow in the vein and causes it to collapse. ▼

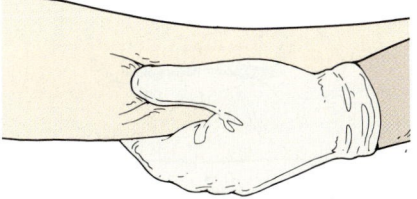

16. **Holding the catheter at** a 30° to 45° angle, pierce the skin directly over the vein. Penetrate all layers of the vein with one quick, smooth motion.

A 30° to 45° angle allows you to pierce the skin without inadvertently passing through the vein, and allows backflow of blood into the catheter.

17. **Watch closely for a flashback** of blood into the chamber of the catheter or the tubing of the winged catheter.

The flashback of blood indicates that the vein has been entered, but only by the needle when using an over-the-needle catheter.

18. **Lower the angle of the catheter** and needle to skin level and advance them into the vein.

Wing-Tipped Catheter

Fully advance the catheter.

(continued on next page)

Procedure 39–1 ■ Initiating a Peripheral Intravenous Infusion (continued)

Over-the-Needle Catheter

Still maintaining traction on the skin with your nondominant hand, hold the catheter hub with your thumb and middle finger, and use your index finger to advance the catheter to at least half of its length before you begin withdrawing the needle. When a steady backflow of blood occurs, partially withdraw the needle while advancing the catheter fully into the vein. For an animated illustration of an over-the-needle IV catheter,

 Go to **Animations: Insertion of an Over-the-Needle IV Catheter,** on Davis*Plus*.

Withdrawing the needle too early will result in the catheter not fully entering the vein, only the needle. There will be no bleeding from the catheter and infiltration will occur when starting the IV solution. The patient will also complain of pain. ▼

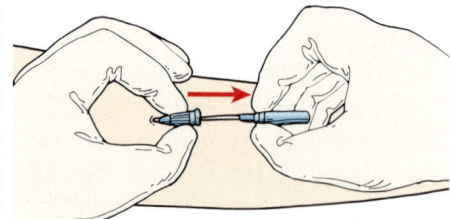

19. While holding the catheter in place with one hand, release the tourniquet and remove or retract the needle.

  a. For an over-the-needle catheter, hold the catheter in place by placing light pressure on the catheter, away from the hub and venipuncture site.

  b. For a winged needle, place a finger lightly on the same area plus a finger further along the vein away from the needle so the needle does not go through the vein.

> ✚ Never attempt to reinsert the needle after it is withdrawn. This can damage the catheter and even cause bits of it to break off within the vein.

Releasing the tourniquet restores full circulation to the patient's extremity and prevents injury. Placing light pressure on the catheter or vein minimizes bleeding from the

catheter or needle while you complete the procedure.

20. Quickly connect the administration set to the IV catheter, using aseptic technique.

To minimize bleeding and prevent infection. ▼

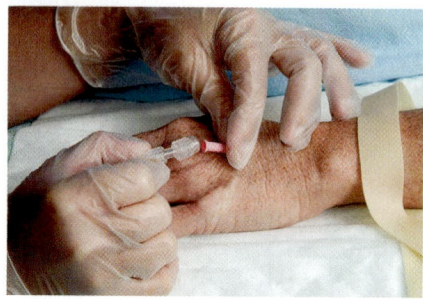

Saline Lock

If using extension tubing with a saline lock, once connected, flush with normal saline and then disconnect the flush. A common amount is 1 to 2 mL, but tubing varies, so check package instructions for the exact amount needed.

Flushing the catheter both clears it and keeps it sterile.

21. While still stabilizing the catheter, slowly open the roller clamp. Observe that flow is achieved. Adjust the drip to the prescribed flow rate.

22. Secure the connection between the tubing and the catheter. Many sets have luer-lock connections, so no further securing is needed. If not using luer-lock tubing, clasping devices and threaded devices can be used. Do not use tape.

Secure the connection to prevent separation of tubing from the hub.

> ✚ Taping is not recommended because the junction is not visible under tape; therefore, the tubing could separate from the catheter without being discovered, possibly leading to air embolism, bleeding, or infection.

23. Stabilize the catheter. Use an agency-approved device. Catheter stabilization devices include manufactured devices (such as StatLok®), or tape.

Stabilizing With Tape

If using tape, place a narrow (1/4-in.) strip of tape under the catheter hub and

crisscross the ends over the hub to form a chevron. Apply tape only to the catheter hub, not to the catheter itself, and do not apply tape directly to the site where the catheter enters the skin.

Luer locks are designed to prevent accidental disengagement of tubing and catheter; they do not stabilize the catheter. Catheter stabilization is important to minimize catheter movement and help prevent complications such as phlebitis, inflammation, infiltration, and infection.

24. Dress the site, following agency policy. If needed, clean the site with an antiseptic swab and allow it to dry before applying the dressing.

Transparent Dressing

  a. Open the package containing the dressing. Remove the protective backing from the dressing, making sure not to touch the sterile surface.

  b. Cover the insertion site and the hub or winged portion of the catheter with the dressing. Do not cover the junction with the administration tubing. ▼

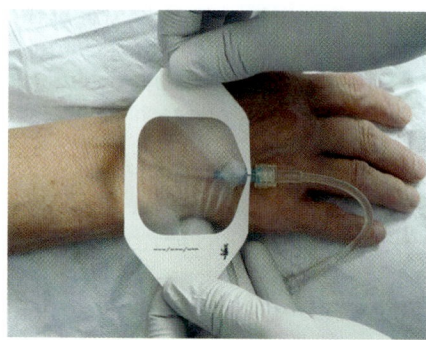

  c. Gently pinch the transparent dressing around the catheter hub to secure the hub further. Smooth the remainder of the dressing so that it adheres to the skin. ▼

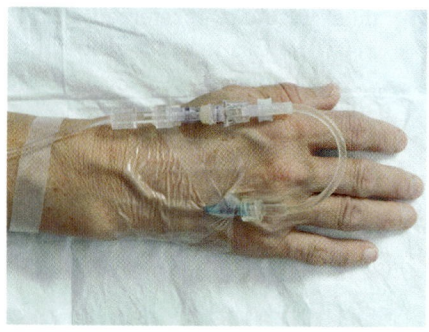

Gauze Dressing

d. Fold a 2 in. × 2 in. sterile gauze dressing in half, cover it with 1-inch tape (about 3 in. long).

e. Place under the tubing/hub junction and press down on the tape.
   Raises hub off the skin and prevents pressure on the skin.

f. Place a sterile gauze pad over the insertion site and catheter hub—but not over the catheter–hub junction.

g. Secure all edges with tape.

25. **Label the dressing** with the date and time of insertion, catheter size, and your initials.
   A label lets nurses see at a glance how long the dressing has been in place.

26. **Secure the IV administration tubing** by looping and taping the tubing to the skin.
   Helps prevent the IV catheter from becoming dislodged and decreases movement of the catheter, thereby decreasing the risk of phlebitis, inflammation and infiltration.

27. **If the insertion site** is located near a joint, place an arm board under the joint, and secure it with tape.
   An arm board stabilizes the joint and helps prevent the catheter from becoming dislodged. However, avoid inserting an IV near a joint when possible, as there is increased potential for movement of the IV catheter, leading to an increased risk of complications. IVs placed in the antecubital fossa are difficult to assess for infiltration. Arm boards are not widely used because of the high acuity of inpatients, many of whom have central lines instead of peripheral IVs.

28. **Dispose of all supplies**, including sharps, into appropriate receptacles; raise the siderail; lower the bed; and be sure the patient call system is within reach. Wash your hands.
   Prevents infection and ensures patient and staff safety.

? What if . . .

- **The patient is an older adult?**

  Do not scrub skin too vigorously.
  This can damage fragile surface tissue, creating a portal for pathogens.
  Use a softer tourniquet and do not apply tightly; for well-dilated veins do not use one at all.
  This increases the risk of rupture of fragile veins.
  Use the smallest catheter possible to meet the infusion needs.
  Insert the needle at an almost flat angle (10° to 20°).
  In most older adults, veins are close to the skin surface.
  Before penetrating the skin, apply traction to the vein below the insertion site.
  Insert the catheter on top of the vein; do not use the side access technique.
  If bleeding occurs, hold gentle pressure longer than for younger patients.
  A clot may take longer to form.

- **Patient is an infant younger than 2 months old?**

  Allow the antiseptic to air-dry on the skin. Do not fan.
  Increases the antiseptic's effectiveness; promotes patient comfort on puncture of the skin; promotes adherence of dressing. Fanning increases exposure to airborne microbes.

- ✚ **The patient is allergic to iodine or shellfish?**

  Use 70% alcohol or chlorhexidine for 30 seconds to cleanse the site, not povidone-iodine or iodine.

- **You are not successful with the first venipuncture attempt?**

  Use a new cannula and make a second attempt on the other arm or, if that is not possible, higher up on the same arm. Do not make more than two attempts to start an IV without seeking assistance.

- ✚ **When you insert the needle and catheter and connect the tubing, you see bright red blood quickly appear and start to advance up the tubing?**

  You may have inadvertently entered an artery. If this occurs, remove the catheter and apply direct pressure for at least 5 minutes. Notify the primary care provider. Monitor the extremity distal to the insertion site for pulses, color, and temperature.

Evaluation

- Monitor the IV site and flow rate regularly (many agency standards require hourly) while IV fluid is infusing. Check for signs of infiltration, inflammation, and phlebitis.
- Monitor the patient's tolerance of IV therapy by auscultating breath sounds and monitoring vital signs, urine output, laboratory values, and neck vein distention. Report to the primary provider any signs of fluid overload, such as crackles, edema, shortness of breath, diminished urine output, increased blood pressure, increased heart rate with bounding pulse, and distended neck veins. Fluid overload can lead to pulmonary edema and heart failure.

Patient Teaching

- Instruct the patient about IV therapy.

- ✚ Teach the patient the importance of notifying staff immediately if the catheter or administration set becomes dislodged; the insertion site becomes tender, red, or swollen; or if the patient notices moisture or fluid leakage.
- ✚ Explain the desired and adverse effects of IV therapy, and tell the patient to notify staff if he develops discomfort or breathing difficulty.
- Teach the patient measures to avoid dislodging the catheter.

Home Care

- Explain home IV therapy to the client and caregiver, and teach them how to identify complications.
- Provide the client with the name and phone numbers of people to contact in case problems arise with the catheter site or if there is a change in level of comfort.

(continued on next page)

Procedure 39-1 ■ **Initiating a Peripheral Intravenous Infusion** (continued)

Documentation

- Date and time of insertion, gauge and type of catheter, number of attempts, and location of the insertion site
- Tourniquet use (or nonuse)
- Blood return in catheter; whether the IV flushes, type and amount of flush solution used
- Dressing and tape type used
- Method of securing or stabilizing the IV line
- Type and rate of the IV fluid infusing
- Patient's tolerance of the procedure, any adverse reactions to the insertion or IV therapy, and the interventions required
- Patient teaching
- Often, IV care is documented on a flow sheet. Fluids infused are documented on the I&O record as well.

Sample Documentation:

06/07/14   0200   20-gauge, winged catheter inserted in cephalic vein, with tourniquet, without difficulty on first attempt. Obtained blood return. Catheter flushed easily. Dressed site with a transparent, semipermeable dressing and clear tape. Catheter stabilized with fixation device. 1 L of D5/0.9% NSS hung at 125 mL/hr. Patient tolerated venipuncture with no difficulty. Instructed to notify nursing staff immediately if pain or swelling occurs at the site. Also instructed about precautions to take to avoid dislodging IV catheter and importance of notifying staff immediately should it become dislodged. ——————S. Jiminez, RN

Practice Resources

AORN, 2009; Betsy Lehman Centre for Patient Safety and Medical Error Reduction, JSI Research and Training Institute, Inc., 2008; Camp-Sorrell, 2010; CDC, 2002; Gorski, 2007; INS, 2006a; Joanna Briggs Institute, 2008; Smith & Royer, 2007; Uslusoy & Mete, 2008.

Thinking About the Procedure

 Go to the *Fundamentals of Nursing Skills Videos,* **Medications, Intravenous: Peripheral IV: Initiating and Regulating.**

1. Describe how the nurse secures the connection between the IV tubing and the catheter.
2. When does the nurse put on her clean nonsterile gloves? In what step of Procedure 39-1 are you instructed to don your gloves? Either way is acceptable. Which way would you prefer to do it? Explain why.

 For suggested responses, go to Chapter 39, **Thinking About the Procedure Suggested Responses,** on Davis*Plus.*

Procedure 39-2 ■ **Regulating the IV Flow Rate**

> ➤ For steps to follow in *all* procedures, refer to the Universal Steps for All Procedures found on the page facing the inside back cover.

Equipment

- IV solution hanging on an IV pole and attached to an administration set
- Watch with a second hand or digital seconds
- Time tape

Delegation

Refer to your state nurse practice act and agency policy regarding delegation of this task to an LPN.

Pre-Procedure Assessment

- Assess the IV catheter for patency and date of insertion before starting the infusion and then regularly (many agencies specify hourly) while the IV fluid infuses.

Decreases risk of complications related to incorrect infusion rate, expired infusion solution, tubing, or catheter dwell time.

- Assess the IV site for signs of phlebitis, infiltration, infection, or inflammation.
  You must change the IV site before regulating the flow rate if any of these complications occur.
- Confirm the patient's need for IV therapy by verifying the order and checking laboratory values, urine output, vital signs, and breath sounds.
  Ensures that the patient still needs IV fluids and that the solution is correct. Laboratory values and assessment findings monitor the IV treatment plan. IV therapy creates a risk for fluid overload.

> ➤ When performing the procedure, always identify your patient according to agency policy and be attentive to standard precautions, hand hygiene, patient safety and privacy, body mechanics, and documentation.

Procedure Steps

1. **Follow all the "checks" and "rights"** of medication administration, including verifying the prescription. Check the solution to make sure that you have the proper IV fluid hanging with the prescribed additives, and that there is no discoloration of or particles or crystallization in the fluid. Also verify the infusion rate.

IV solution is considered medication, and you should check it carefully to avoid administration and compatibility errors. Do not simply pull a bag of fluid from a shelf assuming that the

shelf is labeled properly, as bags are often misplaced and this is a potential source of error.

NOTE: If you are using a volume-control pump, you can omit steps 2, 3, and 4.

2. **Calculate the hourly rate** if it is not specified in the order. Divide the volume to be infused by the number of hours it is to be infused. For example, if the physician prescribes 1,000 mL to run over 4 hours, the infusion rate is 250 mL/hr.
   You must carefully calculate the infusion rate to ensure that the patient receives the correct volume of fluid.

3. **Calculate the drip rate** by multiplying the number of milliliters to be infused in 60 minutes by the drop factor in drops/milliliter; then divide by 60 minutes:

$$\frac{\text{Hourly rate in mL} \times (\text{gtts/mL})}{60 \text{ min}} = \text{drip rate}$$

   For example, an hourly rate of 100 mL multiplied by 15 drops/mL and divided by 60 minutes equals 25. Therefore, the drip rate equals 25 drops per minute. Each administration set has a drip factor that is determined by the manufacturer.

4. **Verify your calculations.**
   To prevent dosage errors, either have a second person verify your calculations or check them a second time yourself.

5. **When hanging a new bag,** apply a time tape to the IV solution container next to the volume markings. Mark the time tape with the time that the infusion was started. Continue to mark 1-hour intervals on the time tape until you reach the bottom of the container.
   The time tape allows all nurses to accurately monitor the rate of administration.

6. **Open the roller clamp** so that IV fluid begins to flow (when hanging a new bag).
   The roller clamp must be opened to allow the flow of fluid.

7. **Set the rate.**

Gravity Drip
Using a watch placed next to the drip chamber, count the number of drops entering the drip chamber in 1 minute. Adjust the roller clamp by increasing or decreasing the flow until you achieve the prescribed drip rate.
Timing the drip rate for 1 minute helps to accurately achieve the correct drip rate and having the watch next to what you are counting will ensure that you do not miss seeing any drops. ▼

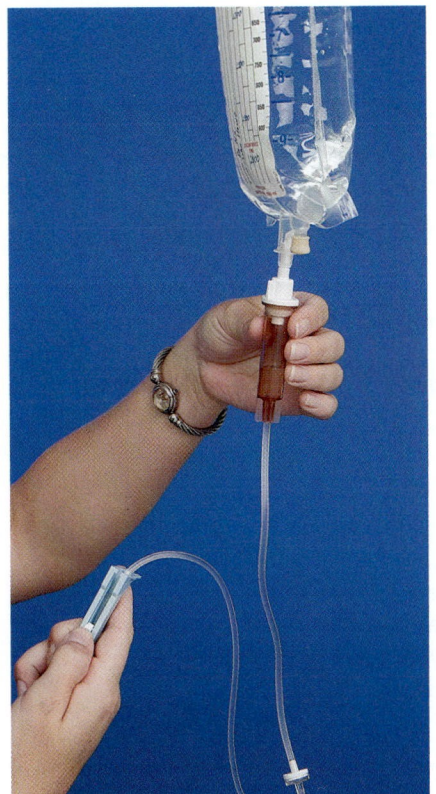

Volume-Control Pump
Program the ordered rate into the pump.
IV solution is considered a medication and must infuse at the prescribed rate.

8. **Monitor manually regulated** infusion rates closely for the 15 minutes after you begin an infusion; then monitor it regularly by counting drops per minute or reading the numbers on the pump.
   Changes in the patient's position may speed up or slow down the infusion rate; frequent monitoring of the infusion rate ensures that the correct volume of fluid infuses over the correct length of time.

? What if . . .

- **The prescription for the IV flow rate changes?**

  Recalculate the new flow rate and adjust the drops/minute to obtain the desired new flow rate. Also, remove the old time tape and place a new time tape with the new rate of infusion.

- **When you check the rate, you discover that the IV has been running too slowly for the past hour?**

  Adjust to the correct rate, but do not attempt to catch up by adjusting the flow to a rate higher than prescribed.
  Too rapid IV infusion can lead to fluid overload for patients with congestive heart failure or other cardiopulmonary problems.

- **When you check the rate, you discover that the IV has been running too fast for the past hour?**

  Slow the rate and assess the patient for signs of fluid volume excess.

Evaluation
- Evaluate the patient's response to IV therapy by checking for signs of excessive or deficient fluid volume.
- Evaluate the IV site for signs of infiltration, inflammation, infection, and phlebitis.
- Check laboratory studies to help evaluate the effectiveness of IV therapy.
- Monitor for correct IV rate at least hourly.
- Evaluate the tubing for kinks, patient lying on the tubing.
  Kinked tubing will interfere with the flow rate.

Patient Teaching
- Explain the desired and adverse effects of IV therapy.
- Discuss the importance of notifying staff immediately if the catheter or administration set becomes dislodged; if the insertion site becomes tender, red, or swollen; if the patient notices moisture or fluid leakage; or if he has difficulty breathing.
- Teach safety measures if the patient is permitted to ambulate while the IV is infusing.

(continued on next page)

Procedure 39–2 ■ Regulating the IV Flow Rate (continued)

Home Care

- Explain home IV therapy to the client and caregiver, and teach them how to identify complications.
- Provide the client and caregiver with the name and phone numbers of people to contact in case problems arise with the catheter, insertion site, or level of comfort.

Documentation

- Date and time the infusion was started
- Type of IV fluid, rate of infusion, and IV catheter site
- Whether rate is manual or pump controlled
- Patient's tolerance of IV therapy, any complications, and the interventions taken
- Document the volume infused on the I&O record. Often IV care is documented on a flow sheet.

Practice Resources

INS, 2006a, 2006b; Oncology Nursing Society (ONS), 2004; Phillips, 2010.

Thinking About the Procedure

 Go to the *Fundamentals of Nursing Skills Videos*, **Medications, Intravenous: Peripheral IV: Initiating and Regulating.**

1. Near the very end of the procedure, the nurse times the IV drip rate. Is the IV running by pump or by gravity?
2. What kind of administration set is hanging, macrodrip or microdrip?
3. Aside from the fact that the drops are difficult to see, why can you not count the drip rate accurately from the video?

 For suggested responses, go to Chapter 39, **Thinking About the Procedure Suggested Responses,** on DavisPlus.

Procedure 39–3 ■ Setting Up and Using Volume-Control Pumps

➤ For steps to follow in *all* procedures, refer to the Universal Steps for All Procedures found on the page facing the inside back cover.

Equipment

- Nonsterile gloves
- Alcohol wipes or chlorhexidine/alcohol antiseptic product
- Volume-control pump and IV pole
- Administration set appropriate for the pump
- IV fluid or medicated solution
- Tape for IV fluid solution time tape

Delegation

You can delegate the task of setting up a volume-control pump to an LPN who is specially trained in IV therapy, if covered by the agency's policy and procedure. Do not delegate this task to a nursing assistive personnel (NAP). Do, however, instruct the NAP to notify you of any pump alarms that sound.

Pre-Procedure Assessment

- Confirm the patient's need for IV therapy by checking vital signs, laboratory values, urine output, skin turgor, breath sounds, and the moisture of mucous membranes.
  IV therapy creates a risk for fluid overload and electrolyte imbalance, which may be revealed by assessment data.
- Assess the existing IV catheter for patency.
  Occlusion of the IV catheter prevents the infusion of IV fluid. If not patent, you will need to change the IV.
- Assess the IV site for signs of phlebitis, infiltration, infection, and inflammation.
  Complications of IV therapy retard the therapeutic benefit of the fluids as well as increase medical concerns, and treatment cost for the patient. You must change the IV catheter and site if any of these complications occur.

Procedure Steps

1. **Calculate the infusion rate** by dividing the volume to be infused by the number of hours it is to be infused. For example, if the order states 1,000 mL to run over 8 hours, divide 1,000 mL by 8 hours to determine the infusion rate of 125 mL/hr.
   This is to ensure that the patient receives the correct dose. Pumps are usually programmed in milliliters per hour instead of drops per minute.

2. **Verify your calculations.**
   To prevent dosage errors, either ask a second person verify your calculations or check them a second time yourself.

3. **Attach the pump to the IV pole**, and plug it into the nearest electrical outlet.

   ✚ Check to be sure the infusion pump has a safety sticker on it and that the cord and plug are intact.

   Volume-control pumps need regular maintenance checks. Using an electrical

   outlet saves battery power if needed for transport or electrical outage. As with gravity flow, the IV solution container needs to remain above the pump to prevent occlusion and for proper drainage of the container.

4. **Take the administration set** from the package, and close the clamp on the administration set.
   To prevent inadvertent loss of fluid.

5. **If a filter is required, attach** it to the end of the administration set.
   Filters are sometimes used to filter minute particles from the solution.

6. **Remove the protective covers** and spike the port of the solution container with the administration set, maintaining sterility. Label the IV tubing and solution container with the date and time, and place a time tape on the solution container. Hang the container on the IV pole.

   Labeling the administration set with the date and time informs the nursing staff when the administration set should be changed. The time tape allows you, and other nurses, to see at a glance whether the correct volume is infusing.

7. **Compress the drip chamber** of the administration set, and allow it to fill halfway. Consult the manufacturer's instructions for setup, as pumps differ. (On older-style gravity pumps, place the electronic sensor on the drip chamber between the fluid level and the origin of the drop.)

   Prepares the administration set for priming and prevents air from entering the tubing with the solution. Infusion pumps compress the tubing to move fluid; they measure the amount internally. On older gravity-type pumps, an electronic sensor counts the number of drops to ensure the proper rate.

8. **Prime the administration set** with fluid by opening the roller clamp and allowing the fluid to flow slowly through the tubing. Close the clamp.

   Priming removes air from the tubing to prevent air embolus.

9. **Inspect the tubing for** the presence of air. If air bubbles remain in the tubing, flick the tubing with a fingertip to mobilize the bubbles into the drip chamber.

   Air bubbles in the administration tubing interrupt flow and they can cause air emboli, which can be dangerous to the patient if they accumulate in the circulation.

10. **Turn on the pump, and load** the administration tubing into the pump according to the manufacturer's instructions.

    This process differs among manufacturers.

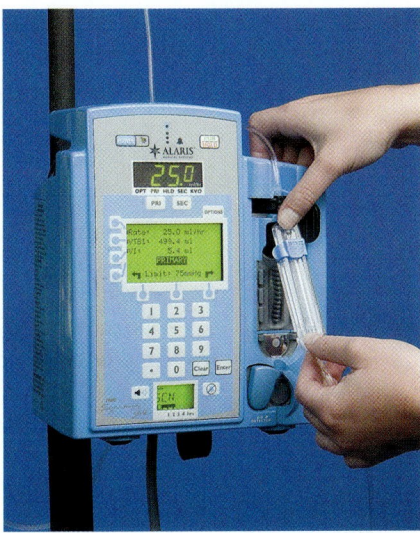

11. **Program the pump** with the prescribed information: total hours, infusion rate (hourly rate) and the volume to be infused (usually the total amount in the IV bag). *Note:* Some pumps have only total hours and volume to infuse and do not have a calculation-of-rate feature. ▼

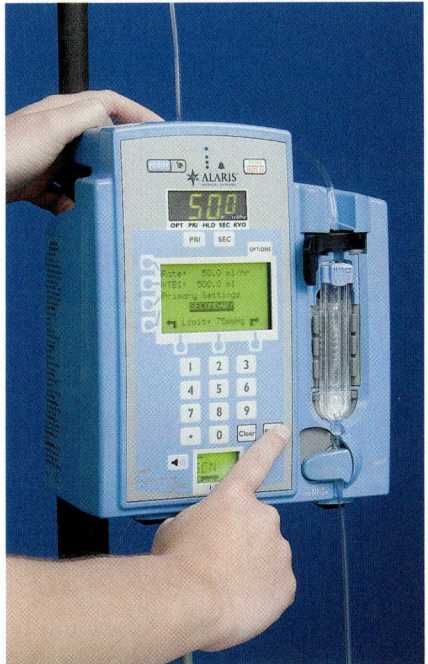

12. Don clean nonsterile gloves, check the IV site for patency, and scrub all surfaces of the injection port or needleless connector, including the threads, with an antiseptic pad for at least 15 seconds. Allow it to dry.

    Clean nonsterile gloves protect from exposure to body fluids when you connect the tubing to the IV catheter or port. Scrubbing the port helps prevent infection.

13. **Connect the administration set** adapter to the injection port, keeping the connecting ends sterile.

    Aseptic technique decreases the risk for contamination.

14. **Unclamp the administration set** tubing (open the roller clamp all the way), and press *Allows the IV fluid to flow through the administration set.*

15. **Make sure that the alarms are** turned on and audible.

    The alarms must be functioning so that the pump can alert you of problems, such as kinks, air in the tubing, or catheter occlusion. Do not depend on the pump alarms to indicate IV patency. Pumps can infuse fluid, even if the line is clogged or infiltrated into the surrounding tissue.

16. **Check the pump regularly** (often this is hourly) to make sure the correct volume is infusing.

    Infusion pumps sometimes malfunction, so frequent monitoring is essential.

17. **At the end of your shift** (or at the time specified by your healthcare facility), clear the pump of the volume infused and record the volume on the patient's I&O form.

    This helps the oncoming shift accurately monitor the fluid infused during their shift.

? What if . . .

- **In later evaluation you find the IV free flowing and not running via the pump setting?**

  Immediately slow the IV fluid down. At the same time, begin assessing the patient: vital signs, mental awareness, lung sounds, pulse oximetry. Depending on the type of fluid running, you may need to make other assessments as well. Calculate the amount of IV fluid actually infused compared to the prescribed amount. Notify the provider and write out an occurrence report. If the pump is malfunctioning, set it aside and notify biomedical engineering so they can repair it.

  Manufacturers sometimes recall certain pump models due to malfunctioning.

(continued on next page)

Procedure 39–3 ■ **Setting Up and Using Volume-Control Pumps** (continued)

Evaluation

- Monitor the correct functioning of the pump regularly, perhaps hourly.
- Assess the IV site hourly for signs of phlebitis, infiltration, infection, and inflammation.
  Complications of IV therapy retard the therapeutic benefit of the fluids as well as increase medical concerns, and treatment cost for the patient. You must change the IV catheter and site if any of these complications occur.

Patient Teaching

- Explain use of the IV infusion pump to the patient.
- Teach the patient the importance of notifying staff immediately if the infusion pump alarm sounds, the catheter or administration set becomes dislodged, the insertion site becomes tender, red, or swollen, or the dressing becomes wet.
- Teach the patient safety measures if he is able to ambulate while the infusion pump is in use.

Home Care

- Explain home IV infusion pump use to the client and caregiver, and teach them how to identify complications. Most home infusion pumps are smaller than institutional pumps.
- Provide the client with the name and phone numbers of people to contact in case problems arise with the catheter, insertion site, IV infusion pump, or other equipment.

Documentation

- Type and volume of IV fluid infusing, along with the infusion rate
- Use of the infusion pump, and patient's tolerance of IV therapy
- Any complications of IV therapy and the interventions taken
- Document volume infused on the patient's I&O record and/or an IV flow sheet.

Practice Resources
Phillips, 2010.

Thinking About the Procedure

 Go to the *Fundamentals of Nursing Skills Videos*, **Medications, Intravenous: Infusion Pump.**

1. When did the nurse spike the IV bag with the administration set: before or after hanging the bag on the IV pole?
2. When does the procedure in this book tell you to spike the bag?
3. Do you think it makes any difference which is done first? Explain your thinking.

 For suggested responses, go to Chapter 39, **Thinking About the Procedure Suggested Responses,** on *DavisPlus.*

Procedure 39–4 ■ **Changing IV Solutions and Tubing**

➤ For steps to follow in *all* procedures, refer to the Universal Steps for All Procedures found on the page facing the inside back cover.

Equipment

- Nonsterile gloves
- Administration set
- IV solution
- IV pole
- Antiseptic swabs that contain solutions such as 70% alcohol or 2% chlorhexidine (chlorhexidine is not recommended in infants younger than age 2 months). You may use iodine-based products if alcohol or chlorhexidine are contraindicated and the patient is not allergic to iodine.
- 1-in. nonallergenic tape
- Time tape
- Watch with a second hand or digital seconds

Delegation

You can delegate the tasks of changing IV solutions and tubing to an LPN who is specially trained in IV therapy. The task should not be delegated to a NAP. Do, however, instruct the NAP to notify you of any problems that occur with IV therapy, such as the disconnecting of the administration set; catheter dislodging; or complaints of pain, swelling, or redness at the insertion site.

Pre-Procedure Assessments

- Assess the IV catheter for patency before changing the solution container or administration set.
- Assess the IV site for signs of phlebitis, infiltration, infection, or inflammation.
  If any of these complications occur, this IV needs to be discontinued and a new IV started.
- Check IV catheter insertion date.
  IV catheters are replaced per agency guidelines, which are based on the Centers for Disease Control (CDC) recommendations of changing a peripheral IV site every 72 to 96 hours.

Procedure 39-4A ■ Changing the IV Solution

➤ When performing the procedure, always identify your patient according to agency policy and be attentive to standard precautions, hand hygiene, patient safety and privacy, body mechanics, and documentation.

Procedure Steps

1. **Following the "rights" of medication** administration, prepare and label your next container of IV solution at least 1 hour before the present infusion is scheduled to finish.

   Preparing the next IV solution container reduces the risk of the present container running dry and thereby causing clots to form that would occlude the catheter.

2. **Close the roller clamp** on the administration set.

   Prevents air from entering the tubing while changing the IV solution container.

3. **Wearing clean nonsterile gloves**, remove the old IV solution container from the IV pole. Remove the spike from the bag, keeping the spike sterile.

   The spike must remain sterile to prevent contamination of the new IV fluid. Clean nonsterile gloves protect you from exposure to body fluids.

4. **Remove the protective cover** from the new IV solution container port.

5. Place the spike into the port of the new solution container.

   Glass Bottle

   If the solution is contained in a glass IV bottle, first scrub the rubber stopper on the top of the bottle with an antiseptic pad; then, insert the spike of the administration set through the black rubber stopper.

   Cleansing the stopper removes particulate matter and microbes.

6. **Hang the IV solution** container on the IV pole.

   Allows the fluid to infuse by gravity.

7. **Inspect the tubing** to be sure that it is free of air bubbles and the drip chamber remains half-filled. Flick the tubing with a finger to mobilize the bubbles into the drip chamber.

   Prevents air from entering the system as the new solution is hung. If the drip chamber becomes too full, it will be difficult to impossible to count the drip rate properly and regulate the IV.

8. **Open the roller clamp** and adjust the drip rate, as prescribed.

   IV solution is considered a medication and must infuse at the prescribed rate for therapeutic effect and to prevent fluid overload.

9. **If practiced within your agency**, affix the time tape to the new IV solution container. Mark the tape with the time the infusion was started, and continue to mark 1-hour intervals on the time tape until you reach the bottom of the container.

   The time tape allows you and other nurses to monitor the rate of administration easily.

10. **Dispose of used supplies** into appropriate receptacles, according to agency policy in line with CDC guidelines.

Procedure 39-4B ■ Changing the IV Administration Tubing and Solution

➤ When performing the procedure, always identify your patient according to agency policy and be attentive to standard precautions, hand hygiene, patient safety and privacy, body mechanics, and documentation.

Procedure Steps

1. **Prepare the IV solution** and tubing as you would when initiating a new IV. (See Procedure 39-1, step 2.)

2. **Hang the new administration set** on the IV pole.

3. **Close the roller clamp** on the old administration set.

   Stops the flow of fluid from the old container.

4. **Disconnect the old tubing.**

   a. Wearing clean nonsterile gloves, place a sterile swab under the catheter hub.

   The swab absorbs any leakage from the catheter hub when you disconnect the tubing.

   b. Apply pressure to the vein about 3 inches above the insertion site, using the fourth or fifth finger of your nondominant hand. Hold the catheter hub firmly with the thumb and index finger of that hand, but do not apply downward pressure.

   Prevents blood from leaking out of the catheter during the tubing change. Holding the hub firmly keeps the catheter from moving about and traumatizing the vein.

   c. Then carefully remove the device securing the connection between the catheter and tubing. This may be as simple as unscrewing a luer-lock. The connection should not be covered by tape, but if it is, remove it so you can access the connection.

5. **Remove the protective cover** from the distal end of the new administration set.

   Cover keeps the distal end sterile until you are ready to connect it to the IV catheter.

6. **Continue to stabilize the IV** catheter with your nondominant hand while applying pressure over the vein.▼

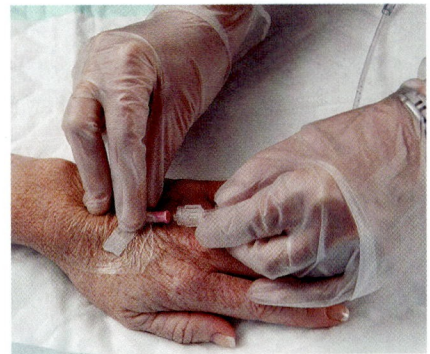

(continued on next page)

Procedure 39–4 ■ Changing IV Solutions and Tubing (continued)

7. **Gently disengage the used tubing** from the IV catheter, and place it in a basin or other receptacle. Quickly insert the new tubing into the catheter hub.

    IV tubing should be changed every 72 to 96 hours, depending on agency policy and solution. Certain solutions require more frequent, every 24 to 48 hours, tubing changes. Change it quickly to prevent microorganisms from entering the IV catheter.

8. **Open the roller clamp** on the new administration set, and allow the IV solution to infuse.

    This clears the IV catheter of blood, preventing catheter occlusion.

9. **Program and turn on** the volume-control pump. Or, for a gravity drip, use the roller clamp to adjust the flow to the prescribed rate.

IV solution is considered a medication and must infuse at the prescribed rate.

10. **Cleanse the IV site** and secure the IV catheter and tubing connection.

    Removes microorganisms and media for growth; helps preserve the integrity of the intact line; and prevents air and microorganisms from entering the line.

11. **Loop and tape tubing** to patient's skin.

    Helps minimize catheter movement, which contributes to phlebitis.

12. **Label tubing and solution** with date, initials, rate, and time tape.

    Alerts staff to when tubing and solution was changed and when they will need to be changed again to decrease the incidence of infection.

13. **Dispose of used supplies** into appropriate receptacles according to agency policy in line with CDC guidelines.

? What if . . .

- **The drip chamber becomes too full (over half) so that drops cannot be adequately counted?**

    Close the roller clamp, invert the bag or bottle, and squeeze the excess fluid back into the bag/bottle.

- **The tubing will not separate from the catheter connection when you attempt to disconnect it?**

    If the lock does not twist off, try using a hemostat ("mosquito" clamp) to gently twist the lock. Do not lock the hemostat; merely use it lightly as a grip. After the lock is off, if the tubing will not separate, use the hemostat to gently twist the tubing back and forth. If the catheter needs to be stabilized, wear a sterile glove or use a sterile hemostat.

Evaluation

- Evaluate the IV insertion site for signs of infiltration, inflammation, infection, and phlebitis.
- Evaluate the effectiveness of IV therapy by assessing the patient's hydration status or expected effect of the intravenous medication/solution.
- Evaluate proper IV rate regularly (usually hourly).

Patient Teaching

Discuss the importance of notifying staff immediately if the catheter or administration set becomes dislodged; if the insertion site becomes tender; red, or swollen; or if the IV dressing becomes wet.

Home Care

- Explain home IV therapy to the client and caregiver; teach them how to identify complications.

- Obtain a return demonstration to ensure the caregiver is able to perform fluid and tubing, changes when necessary.

Documentation

- Fluid and tubing changes are usually documented on a flow sheet.
- Document the date and time the IV fluid and tubing were changed; type of IV fluid and rate of infusion; and the location and condition of the IV catheter insertion site.
- Document any complications of IV therapy and the interventions taken.

Practice Resources

CDC, 2002; Gillies, Wallen, Morrison, et al., 2005; INS, 2006a, 2006b; ONS, 2004.

Procedure 39–5 ■ Changing IV Dressings

➤ For steps to follow in *all* procedures, refer to the Universal Steps for All Procedures found on the page facing the inside back cover. For this procedure, also refer to procedures and Clinical Insights in Chapter 22, if you need to review information about medical and surgical asepsis.

Equipment

Peripheral IV Dressings

- Clean nonsterile gloves
- Sterile transparent semipermeable dressing or dressing specified by institution

- Antiseptic swabs: alcohol or chlorhexidine (*Note:* Use iodine-based products only if the preferred antiseptics cannot be used. Chlorhexidine is not recommended in infants younger than age 2 months.)
- 1-in. nonallergenic tape or manufactured stabilization device

Central Line Dressings

- Clean nonsterile gloves
- Central line dressing kit. It should include sterile gloves, a mask, a sterile transparent semipermeable dressing, sterile tape, an antimicrobial agent, and a sterile catheter stabilization device. If it does not, obtain them. *Note:* It is acceptable to povidone-iodine followed by alcohol as the antimicrobial if the preferred chlorhexidine is contraindicated.
- A sponge containing the antimicrobial agent chlorhexidine gluconate may be used as a part of the dressing, as well.
  To reduce the risk for catheter-related infection.
- Mask for patient (possibly)

  NOTE: *Some institutions do not include this in their procedure and a few patients cannot tolerate wearing a mask.*

Delegation

You can delegate the tasks of changing dressings to an LPN who is specially trained in IV therapy. The task should not be delegated to a NAP. Do, however, instruct the NAP to notify you of any problems that occur with dressing such as soiling, blood, leakage, or loosening.

Pre-Procedure Assessments

For Peripheral Catheters

- Assess the IV catheter for patency before changing the dressing.
  Ensure that the IV is still working properly.
- Assess the IV site for signs of phlebitis, infiltration, infection, or inflammation.
  If any of these complications exist, the current IV will need to be discontinued and a new IV started.
- Assess for allergy to tape.
- Assess IV catheter start date.
  IV catheters are replaced per agency guidelines which are based on the CDC recommendations of changing a peripheral IV site every 72 to 96 hours. Changing more often than recommended actually increases the risk of infection.

Procedure 39-5A ■ Peripheral IV Dressings

➤ When performing the procedure, always identify your patient according to agency policy and be attentive to standard precautions, hand hygiene, patient safety and privacy, body mechanics, and documentation.

➤ *Note:* This procedure is usually performed at the same time the IV tubing is changed because the old dressing may need to be removed to do that. Most dressings may remain in place for 72 to 96 hours and are changed when the insertion site is rotated. However, dressings should be changed at other times if they become soiled, wet, or dislodged. Gauze dressings must be changed every 48 hours.

Procedure Steps

1. **Wearing clean nonsterile gloves,** stabilize the catheter with your nondominant hand, avoiding direct pressure on the catheter/hub junction, and carefully remove and discard the dressing and the catheter stabilization device. *Note:* If the catheter has an extended dwell time, sterile gloves are required for this step.
   Remove the dressing gently to avoid dislodging the catheter.
2. **Inspect the insertion site.** Look for erythema and drainage, and note any tenderness.
   If signs of infection, phlebitis, or infiltration are present, you must remove the IV catheter.
3. **Don a clean pair of nonsterile gloves.**
4. **Cleanse the insertion site,** and then allow the antiseptic to dry on the skin. Do not fan.

Using Chlorhexidine

Apply using a back-and-forth motion and friction for at least 30 seconds. (Avoid using chlorhexidine in infants younger than age 2 months).

Using Alcohol or 2% Tincture of Iodine

Using a circular motion, start at the insertion site and work outward 2 to 3 inches. Do not "go back over" any cleansed area.
Removes microorganisms from the skin to minimize the risk of their entering the venipuncture site. Allowing the antiseptic to dry increases the effectiveness of the antiseptic.

5. **Change procedure gloves** and apply a new sterile catheter stabilization device and dressing. For illustrations, see Procedure 39-1.

Transparent Dressing

a. Open the package containing the sterile, semipermeable, transparent dressing. Remove the protective backing from the dressing, making sure not to touch the sterile surface.

b. Cover the insertion site and the hub or winged portion of the catheter with the dressing. Do not cover the junction with the tubing of the administration set.

c. Gently pinch the transparent dressing around the catheter hub to secure the hub. Smooth the remainder of the dressing so that it adheres to the skin.
   Pinching the dressing around the hub prevents pressure of the hub on the underlying skin.

Gauze Dressing

d. Fold a 2 in. × 2 in. sterile gauze dressing in half, cover it with 1-in. tape (about 3 in. long).

e. Place under the tubing/hub junction and press down on the tape.
   Raises hub off the skin and prevents pressure on the skin.

f. Place a sterile gauze pad over the insertion site and catheter hub— but not over the catheter/hub junction

g. Secure all edges with tape.

6. **Secure the connection** between the catheter and the tubing, but do

(continued on next page)

Procedure 39–5 ■ Changing IV Dressings (continued)

not cover the catheter-tubing junction with tape.

Securing the connection helps maintain a closed system and prevent entry of microorganisms. You should not cover the junction with tape because removing the tape may interfere your ability to disconnect the tubing from the hub quickly, should you need to do so. Removing tape requires much manipulation; the more the catheter is manipulated, the higher the risk for infection.

7. **Secure the IV administration tubing** by looping and taping the tubing to the skin.

Looping the tubing supplies slack to prevent the IV catheter from becoming dislodged.

8. **Label the dressing** with the date and time of insertion, catheter size, and the date the dressing was changed and your initials.

Peripheral IV catheters should be replaced every 72 to 96 hours to prevent phlebitis. Labeling the dressing with the date and time of insertion helps communicate to other nurses when to change catheters. Gauze dressings covering the insertion site should be changed every 48 hours to inspect for signs of complications.

9. **Discard all supplies** in the appropriate containers according to agency policy in line with CDC guidelines.

? What if . . .

- **The patient is immunocompromised? Or the peripheral midline catheter must be in the same site for an extended time?**

  Use sterile gloves and a mask when changing the dressing and giving site care.

Thinking About the Procedure

 Go to the *Fundamentals of Nursing Skills Videos*, **Medications, Intravenous: Peripheral IV: Dressing Change.**

1. At what point in the procedure did the nurse don clean nonsterile gloves? That is, what does she do before donning the gloves, and what does she do immediately after?

2. Would it be acceptable for the nurse to do the steps in this order? Place the linen-saver pad and rolled towel under the patient's arm, open the dressing and antiseptic packages, don procedure gloves, and remove tape from the looped tubing.

 For suggested responses, go to Chapter 39, **Thinking About the Procedure Suggested Responses,** on *DavisPlus.*

Procedure 39–5B ■ Central Line Dressings

➤ When performing the procedure, always identify your patient according to agency policy and be attentive to standard precautions, hand hygiene, patient safety and privacy, body mechanics, and documentation.

➤ *Note:* This procedure focuses on dressing change. Refer to Clinical Insight 39-3 for assessments and maintenance of CVCs.

Procedure Steps

1. **Obtain sterile central line dressing** kit (or equivalent supplies if there is no kit) and mask for the patient, if one is needed.

   Because central lines have direct access to the central circulation, the risk of systemic infection is greater. Therefore, the procedure uses aseptic technique. All supplies must be sterile.

2. **Place the patient** in a semi-Fowler's position, if tolerated. Lower the siderail and adjust the bed to working height.

   Semi-Fowler's position and bed adjustments facilitate site cleansing and dressing application and reduce strain on the nurse's back.

3. **Explain the procedure** and ask the patient to turn his head to the opposite side from the insertion site. If he cannot cooperate, place a mask on the patient.

Explanation may reduce anxiety and enhance cooperation; turning helps prevent contamination of the insertion site.

4. **Don mask and clean nonsterile** gloves and carefully remove the old dressing and catheter stabilization device if present.

5. **Inspect the site** for signs and symptoms of infection and other complications.

   If a complication is suspected, notify the person who placed the central line.

6. **Remove and discard your gloves**, along with the soiled dressing. Wash your hands.

7. **Set up a sterile field** and arrange and open the dressing kit and supplies.

8. **Don sterile gloves** contained in the kit.

   To prevent contamination of the insertion site and the sterile supplies.

9. **Scrub the insertion site** and surrounding skin with an antiseptic swab.

Using Chlorhexidine

Use a back-and-forth motion with friction and scrub for at least 30 seconds.

Using Povidone-Iodine and Alcohol

The kit should contain three swabs of each. Beginning with a povidone-iodine swabs, start at the insertion site and work outward several inches ("dirty to clean"). Repeat with the other two povidone-iodine swabs. Then, using the same method, cleans with the three alcohol swabs. With each swab, do not "go back over" an area you have just cleaned with that swab.

To rid the site of any potential infectious microorganisms, working "from clean to contaminated."

10. **Scrub the sutures (if any),** and the catheter from insertion site to the hub or bifurcation, for at least 15 seconds with an alcohol swab or chlorhexidine/alcohol antiseptic product.

11. **Allow the site to dry**—do not fan. *Allows the antiseptic time to work completely and allows the dressing to stick properly. Povidone-iodine requires 1 minute to air-dry completely; chlorhexidine requires 30 seconds.*

12. **Apply the transparent dressing** that comes in the kit.

Gauze Under the Catheter Hub

You may first place a small piece of folded sterile gauze under the catheter hub.

To reduce pressure on the skin under the hub.

Chlorhexidine Gluconate Sponge as Part of the Dressing

Apply the sponge directly over the catheter insertion site, ensuring that the sponge is in full contact with the skin. Then apply the transparent dressing over the sponge.

Reduces the risk for catheter-related infection, especially in units with high infection rates or in high-risk patients (Timsit, Schwebel, Boudma, et al., 2009).

13. **Apply the new catheter** stabilization device, if one is used.

14. **Remove drape, if you used one.**

15. **Loop the catheter gently** and secure it with tape to the skin. Avoid securing it to the dressing. Or, depending on type of CVC, place a piece of clear tape across the ends of the catheter lumens, near but not on the hubs.

Ensures that accidental tugging on the catheter does not accidentally dislodge the catheter. Do not cover the hubs, as you may need to access them.

16. **Label the dressing** with the date changed, time, and your initials.

Alerts staff to when the next dressing change will be due.

17. **Place the patient** in a comfortable position, put siderail back up and be sure call light is accessible.

18. **Dispose of supplies** into the appropriate receptacles according to agency policy in line with CDC guidelines.

Evaluation

- Evaluate the IV insertion site and surrounding tissue for signs of infiltration, inflammation, infection, and phlebitis.
- Monitor the dressing for dampness, blood, soiling, or loosening.

  If these occur, the dressing must be changed.

Patient Teaching

- Explain the importance of notifying staff if the IV dressing becomes soiled, dampened, or loosened.
- Remind the patient to notify staff immediately for bleeding, pain, or swelling around the catheter or dressing area or discomfort in the hand, arm, or shoulder on the same side as the catheter.

Home Care

- Explain home IV therapy to the client and caregiver; teach them how to identify complications.
- Obtain a return demonstration by the client or caregiver to ensure competent performance of fluid, tubing, and dressing changes when necessary.

Documentation

- Chart the date and time the dressing was changed. Document the location and condition of the IV catheter insertion site.

- Document any complications of IV therapy and the interventions taken.
- Document the dressing change on your IV record. Often, IV care is documented on a flow sheet.

Practice Resources

CDC, 2002; Hadaway, 2010; INS, 2006a, 2006b; The Joint Commission, 2011; ONS, 2004; Pronovost, Needham, Berenholz, et al., 2006; Pronovost, Goeschel, Colantuoi, et al., 2010; Society for Healthcare Epidemiology of America, 2008; Timsit, Schwebel, Boudma, et al., 2009; Wenzel & Edmond, 2006.

Thinking About the Procedure

 Go to the *Fundamentals of Nursing Skills Videos,* **Medications, Intravenous: Central Venous Access Device: Dressing Change.**

1. What is the first piece of personal protective equipment the nurse puts on?
2. During the central line dressing change procedure, does the patient wear a mask or turn her head to help prevent contamination of the insertion site?
3. What does the nurse do immediately after donning the sterile gloves?

 For suggested responses, go to Chapter 39, **Thinking About the Procedure Suggested Responses,** on *DavisPlus.*

Procedure 39–6 ■ Converting a Primary Line to a Heparin or Saline Lock

➤ For steps to follow in *all* procedures, refer to the Universal Steps for All Procedures found on the page facing the inside back cover.

Equipment
- Clean nonsterile gloves
- Peripheral intermittent IV lock adapter
- Two syringes containing saline or dilute heparin solution
- Linen-saver pad
- Transparent semipermeable dressing
- Alcohol or chlorhexidine/alcohol or other antiseptic swab

Delegation
You can delegate the task of converting a primary IV line to an intermittent lock to an LPN who is specially trained in IV therapy. The task should not be delegated to a NAP. However, you should instruct the NAP to notify you of any problems with the intermittent lock device, such as dislodging of the catheter or client complaints of pain, swelling, or redness at the insertion site.

Pre-Procedure Assessment
- Assess the patient's readiness to have the IV fluid discontinued (e.g., tolerating oral fluids, adequate urine output, and laboratory values within normal limits).
  If the patient's condition indicates that he still requires IV fluids, notify the primary care provider and do not discontinue the IV line.
- Assess for allergy to tape.
- Assess the IV site for signs of phlebitis, infiltration, extravasation, or infection.
  If complications are present or the IV has been in place longer than 72 to 96 hours, remove the IV catheter instead of converting it to an intermittent lock.

➤ When performing the procedure, always identify your patient according to agency policy and be attentive to standard precautions, hand hygiene, patient safety and privacy, body mechanics, and documentation.
➤ Maintain sterility of supplies and equipment (e.g., do not touch catheter opening or ends of the IV lock; keep flush syringe connector sterile).

Procedure Steps

1. **Help the client assume** a comfortable position that provides access to the IV site.
   Promotes cooperation with the procedure and facilitates your ability to perform the procedure.

2. **Lower siderails, raise bed** to working height, and place linen-saver pad under extremity with the IV.
   Protects linens from blood and fluid that might leak from the vessel during catheter removal and ensures good body mechanics.

3. **Don clean nonsterile gloves.** Remove the IV lock from the package and flush the adapter with the first syringe of saline or dilute heparin, according to agency policy. Place the lock back loosely inside the sterile package, keeping it sterile. **Continue with step 5.**
   Removes air from the lock.

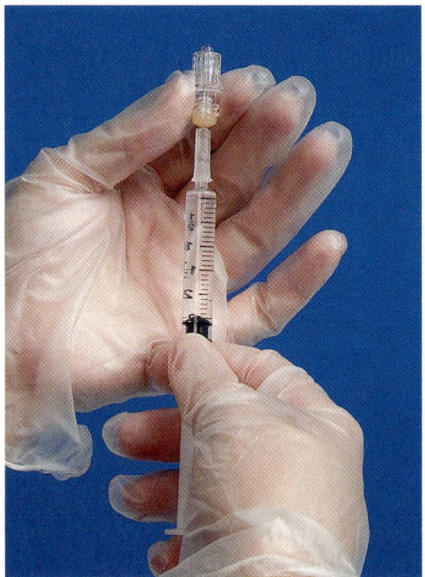

Procedure Variation for Primary Tubing Set Up With Extension Tubing With a Lock

4. **Merely discontinue the IV solution** and disconnect the primary tubing from the extension tubing with lock. Then, flush extension tubing per agency policy and **skip to step 14.**

5. **Carefully remove the IV dressing** and the tape that is securing the tubing.
   Provides access to the IV catheter.

6. **Close the roller clamp** on the administration set.
   Prevents loss of IV fluid during the procedure.

7. **With the side of your nondominant** hand, apply pressure over the vein just above the insertion site but not directly on the catheter–hub junction. At the same time, stabilize the catheter hub with your thumb and forefinger.
   Applying pressure over the vein stops blood from flowing from the catheter as you change the administration tubing.

8. **Gently disengage the used tubing** from the IV catheter. If the tubing does not separate from the catheter, see the What if . . . ? section at the end of step 14.

9. **Quickly insert the lock adapter** into the IV catheter and turn it to lock it in place.
   Insert the adapter quickly to prevent bleeding from the IV catheter. ▼

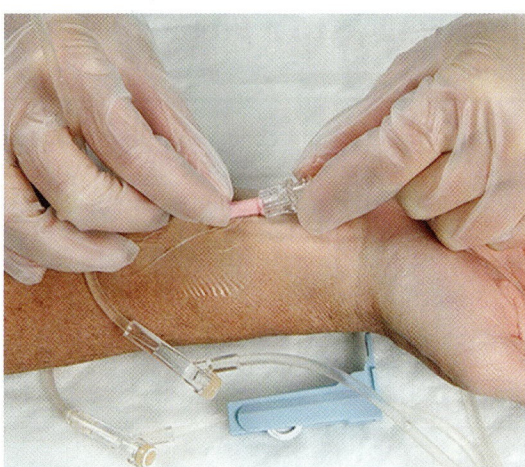

10. **Scrub the injection port** of the adapter with an antiseptic pad.

    Cleaning the port with antiseptic helps prevent contamination by microorganisms when the adapter is flushed.

11. **Insert the second syringe** containing saline or dilute heparin into the injection port of the adapter. Flush the catheter using the method recommended in your agency.

    Some experts recommend a turbulence (push-stop-push method) on the theory that turbulence ensures patency of the IV catheter by clearing the catheter and helping prevent reflux of blood back into the catheter. Others believe this method has undesired effects and recommend, instead, a steady, slow push. More evidence is needed to settle this question. In the meantime, follow agency policy regarding the flushing technique.

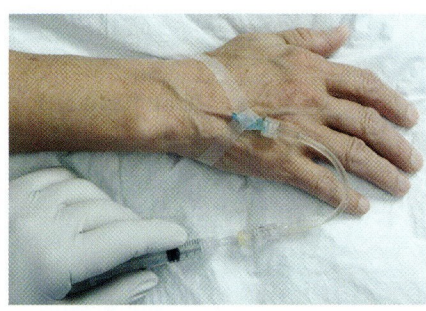

12. **Using aseptic technique**, cover the insertion site and catheter hub with a sterile transparent semipermeable dressing. Do not cover the junction of the catheter hub and the IV lock. See Procedure 39-5A for review of dressings.

    Secures the IV catheter and prevents contamination of the site.

13. **Label the dressing** with the date changed and your initials.

14. **Discard used supplies** into appropriate receptacles according to agency policy in line with CDC guidelines.

Discarding used equipment properly keeps the healthcare environment safe.

? What if . . .

■ **At step 8, the tubing will not separate from the catheter?**

First, if it is a luer-lock connection, be sure you have twisted the luer-lock "open." If so, place a hemostat ("mosquito" clamp) on the IV tubing and gently twist back and forth to loosen the connection. Then if the IV tubing still does not come loose, use the hemostat to gently twist the lock back and forth to loosen the connection. Do not lock the hemostat; merely use it lightly as a grip.

Use of hemostat may help loosen tubing from the catheter, but placement is critical so that the IV catheter and connector are not damaged.

■ **At step 8, the IV catheter becomes dislodged while trying to disconnect the tubing?**

If you can see as much as three-fourths of the catheter emerging from the site, you must remove it and start a new IV at a different site.

Trying to re-advance the catheter might cause it to pierce through the vein as well as increase the risk of infection from reinserting a catheter that is no longer sterile. It also causes tissue trauma and increases the risk of phlebitis from catheter manipulation.

Evaluation

■ Evaluate the patency of the catheter before each use according to institutional policy. Patency check and flushing are usually done every 8 to 24 hours.

■ Evaluate the patient's tolerance to intermittent IV therapy.

■ Evaluate the insertion site for signs of complications.

Patient Teaching

Explain the importance of notifying staff if the IV site becomes red, painful, or swollen; or if the dressing becomes soiled, damp, or loosened (indicating that the catheter has become dislodged or the connection is loose). Include the family in the teaching, as the patient may not be able to assess his own IV therapy.

Home Care

■ Explain home use of the intermittent lock to the patient and caregiver. Teach them how to flush the catheter before and after administering prescribed medications.

■ Provide the patient and caregiver with the name and phone numbers of people to contact in case problems arise with the catheter or insertion site.

(continued on next page)

Procedure 39–6 ■ Converting a Primary Line to a Heparin or Saline Lock (continued)

Documentation

- Chart the date and time the IV line was converted to an intermittent lock device.
- Note the size and location of the catheter, as well as the type and amount of flush solution used.
- Record on the I&O record the amount of IV fluid infused.

- Document the condition of the IV site and any complications noted.
- Often, IV care is documented on a flow sheet or the electronic patient record.

Practice Resources

CDC, 2002; Hadaway, 2006, 2010; INS, 2006a; ONS, 2004.

Procedure 39–7 ■ Discontinuing a Peripheral IV

➤ For steps to follow in *all* procedures, refer to the Universal Steps for All Procedures found on the page facing the inside back cover.

Equipment

- Clean nonsterile gloves
- Sterile 2 in. × 2 in. gauze dressings
- 1-in. tape or transparent semipermeable dressing
- Linen-saver pad

Delegation

You can delegate the task of discontinuing an IV to an LPN who is specially trained in IV therapy. The task should not be delegated to a NAP. However, you should instruct the NAP to notify you of any bleeding from the insertion site.

Pre-Procedure Assessment

- Assess the patient's readiness to have the IV fluid discontinued and verify the order. For example, determine whether he is tolerating oral fluids and has adequate urine output and whether laboratory values are within normal limits.
  If the patient's condition indicates that he still requires IV fluids, notify the physician and do not discontinue the IV line.

➤ When performing the procedure, always identify your patient according to agency policy and be attentive to standard precautions, hand hygiene, patient safety and privacy, body mechanics, and documentation.

Procedure Steps

1. **Assist the client to a comfortable position** and raise the bed to working height.
   Helps ensure patient cooperation with the procedure; supports good body mechanics for the nurse.

2. **Place a linen-saver pad** under the extremity with the IV.
   Protects linens from blood and fluid that might leak from the vein during catheter removal and ensures good body mechanics.

3. **Don clean nonsterile gloves**, and close the roller clamp on the administration set.
   Closing the roller prevents IV fluid from spilling onto the bed or client during catheter removal. Procedure gloves protect you from body fluid exposure.

4. **Carefully remove the IV dressing**, catheter stabilization device, and the tape that is securing the tubing.

Removing tape and dressings can be painful especially if over hair or sensitive or thin skin.

IV is running through an extension tubing or a saline lock.
Disconnect the administration set tubing and close the slide clamp on the extension tubing.

5. **Scrub the catheter–skin junction** with an alcohol prep pad or chlorhexidine/alcohol antiseptic product for at least 15 seconds.
   Removes microorganisms from the skin entry site.

6. **Apply a sterile 2 in. × 2 in. gauze** pad above the IV insertion site and gently remove the catheter, directing it straight along the vein. Do not press down on the gauze pad while removing the catheter.
   Directing the catheter along the vein prevents vein injury while you are removing the catheter.

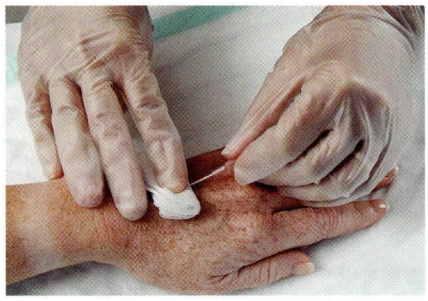

7. **Immediately apply firm pressure** with the gauze pad over the insertion site. Hold pressure for 1 to 3 minutes; hold longer if bleeding persists.
   This typically stops bleeding by hastening clot formation.

8. **Remove the soiled 2 in. × 2 in.** gauze pad, and replace it with a sterile 2 × 2 gauze pad folded over to form a pressure dressing. Secure it with 1-in. tape or a transparent semipermeable dressing.
   Protects the site from contamination.

9. **Return the bed to a low position.** Discard all supplies in the appropriate containers according to agency policy in line with CDC guidelines.

Evaluation

- Assess the integrity of the removed catheter; compare the length to the original insertion length to ensure the entire catheter is removed. If a catheter defect is noted, report to the manufacturer and regulatory agencies and complete an incident report according to agency policy.
- Evaluate the patient's response to oral fluids after IV therapy is discontinued.
- Monitor for changes in the patient's condition to assess whether IV therapy should be re-established.

Patient Teaching

- Instruct the client and family to notify staff if bleeding or discomfort occurs at the insertion site.
- Teach the importance of drinking adequate amounts fluid, within the prescribed plan of treatment, to prevent dehydration. (Some patients have fluid restrictions.)

Documentation

- Chart the date and time that IV therapy was discontinued.
- Note the condition of the site, including any complications. If complications are present, document your interventions, including physician notification.
- Often you will record this procedure on a flow sheet or in the electronic patient record.

Sample Documentation:

RA #2, 22-gauge catheter discontinued. Site without redness, swelling, tenderness, or exudate. Pressure applied to the site for 2 minutes. Bleeding stopped and sterile 2 × 2 gauze dressing applied. Informed patient to notify staff if bleeding or discomfort occurs. ————————S. Horowitz, RN

Practice Resources

Betsy Lehman Center for Patient Safety and Medical Error Reduction, JSI Research and Training Institute, Inc., 2008; CDC, 2002; INS, 2006a, 2006b; ONS, 2004.

Thinking About the Procedure

 Go to the *Fundamentals of Nursing Skills Videos*, **Medications, Intravenous: Peripheral IV: Discontinuing.**

1. Was this patient's IV being regulated by pump or by gravity?
2. Was the 2 in. × 2 in. gauze pad needed to absorb blood in this situation?

 For suggested responses, go to Chapter 39, **Thinking About the Procedure Suggested Responses,** on Davis*Plus.*

Procedure 39–8 ■ Administering a Blood Transfusion

➤ For steps to follow in *all* procedures, refer to the Universal Steps for All Procedures found on the page facing the inside back cover.

Equipment

- Clean nonsterile gloves
- Blood product
- Normal saline IV solution, 250 mL
  Normal saline is the only solution that is compatible with blood products; other IV solutions cause hemolysis of blood cells.
- Blood administration set (with a 200-micrometer filter and luer-lock connection). If there is no filter on the tubing, you must attach one.
- IV pole
- Watch with a second hand or digital seconds
- Thermometer
- Blood pressure cuff with sphygmomanometer
- Stethoscope

Delegation

Do not delegate this procedure to the LPN or NAP, because blood product administration requires advanced assessment and critical-thinking skills. The LPN and NAP can assist by monitoring vital signs. Instruct both about the complications associated with blood product administration, and instruct them to inform you if any occur.

Pre-Procedure Assessment

- Confirm the patient's need for blood products by assessing vital signs, urine output, and laboratory studies.
  Blood products may cause life-threatening complications; therefore, they should be administered only when needed.
- Check the patient's history for previous blood transfusions and reactions and verify her blood type.
  If the patient has a history of a blood transfusion reaction, precautions must be taken before she receives additional transfusions. For example, she may need premedication with acetaminophen, a corticosteroid, and diphenhydramine; specially treated blood products; and the use of a specialized administration set with greater filtering capabilities.
- Assess patency of the existing IV catheter, and make sure that it is the proper size for blood product administration.
  Nurses often use a 20-gauge catheter for blood administration. However, for routine transfusion, a 22-gauge or even a 24-gauge catheter can be used. You will need an 18- or 20-gauge catheter when large amounts of blood must be transfused rapidly. The primary consideration should be the size of the patient's veins and not an arbitrary catheter size.
- Assess for allergy to tape.

(continued on next page)

Procedure 39–8 ■ Administering a Blood Transfusion (continued)

Procedure 39-8A ■ Administering Blood and Blood Products

➤ When performing the procedure, always identify your patient according to agency policy and be attentive to standard precautions, hand hygiene, patient safety and privacy, body mechanics, and documentation.

Procedure Steps

1. **Verify that informed consent** has been obtained.

   Informed consent is required for blood product administration, as for any invasive or risk-bearing procedure.

2. **Verify the medical order**, noting the indication, rate of infusion, and any premedication prescriptions. Administer any pretransfusion medications as prescribed.

   Helps prevent administration errors.

3. **Obtain the blood product** from the blood bank, according to your institution's policy. Wear clean non-sterile gloves whenever handling blood products.

   Some blood banks require a pickup slip that verifies the presence of a functioning IV catheter, signed informed consent, and an order, because blood must be discarded after it has been out of refrigeration for 30 minutes.

4. **Verify that the blood product** matches the order. Inspect the blood. If you note any abnormality, return it to the blood bank and obtain a new bag.

   a. The plasma should not be pink. Pink indicates hemolysis.

   b. The red cells red should be red, not purple or black.

   c. There should be no clots visible.

   d. There should be no leakage.

5. **With another qualified staff** member (as deemed by your institution), verify the patient and blood product identification.

   Only one of the staff members is required by The Joint Commission to be qualified to administer blood products; however, agency policies may specify what those requirements are.

   a. Use two patient identifiers (e.g., ask the patient to tell you her full name and date of birth) and compare it to the name and date of birth located on the blood bank form and patient ID band.

   Allowing the patient to confirm her identity and comparing the information

against the blood bank form is a safety measure to ensure that the correct patient is receiving the blood product that is compatible with the patient's blood type.

   b. Compare the patient name and hospital identification number on the patient's identification bracelet with the patient's name and hospital identification number on the blood bank form attached to the blood product.

   Verifies that the correct patient is receiving the correct blood product.

   c. Compare the unit identification number located on the blood bank form with the identification number printed on the blood product container.

   Verifies that the blood bank has dispensed the correct blood product. ▼

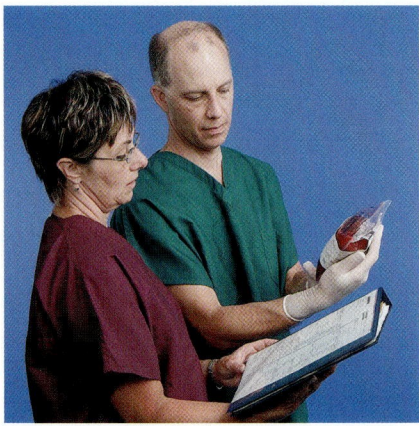

   d. Compare the patient's blood type listed on the blood bank form with the blood type listed on the blood product container.

   Verifies that the blood type of the product matches the patient's blood type.

   e. If all verifications are in agreement, both staff members should sign the blood bank form attached to the blood product container.

   ✚ Contact the blood bank immediately if any discrepancies occur during the identification process. If there are any discrepancies, do not administer the blood product.

Signing the blood bank form confirms that the blood product was identified and verified by two qualified staff members.

   f. Document on the blood bank form the date and time that the transfusion was begun.

   Blood cannot be infused past the expiration time; documenting the start time alerts the nurse of the expiration time.

   g. Make sure that the blood bank form remains attached to the blood product container until administration is complete.

   Ensures product identity should a transfusion reaction occur.

6. **Remove the blood administration** set from the package, and label the tubing with the date and time. Then close all clamps on the administration set.

   Labeling the administration set with the date and time informs the nursing staff when the administration set should be changed.

7. **Remove the protective covers** from the normal saline solution container port and from one of the spikes located on the "Y" of the blood product administration set. Place the spike into the port of the solution container.

8. **Hang the normal saline solution** container on the IV pole. Refer to the photo in step 13.

9. **Compress the drip chamber** of the administration set, and allow it to fill halfway.

   Prevents air from entering the tubing with the solution.

10. **Open the roller clamp** and prime the administration set tubing with normal saline.

   Removes air from the tubing.

11. **Close the roller clamp.** Inspect the tubing for the presence of air. If air bubbles remain in the tubing, flick the tubing with a fingertip to mobilize the bubbles up into the drip chamber.

   Air bubbles in the administration tubing can cause an air embolus.

12. **Gently invert the blood product** container several times but do not shake the bag.

Mixes the blood product with the preservatives that are added to the container without causing trauma (lysis) to the cells.

13. **Remove the protective covers** from the blood spike on the blood tubing and the blood product port. Carefully spike the blood product container through the port.

Careful spiking prevents inadvertent puncturing of the container. ▼

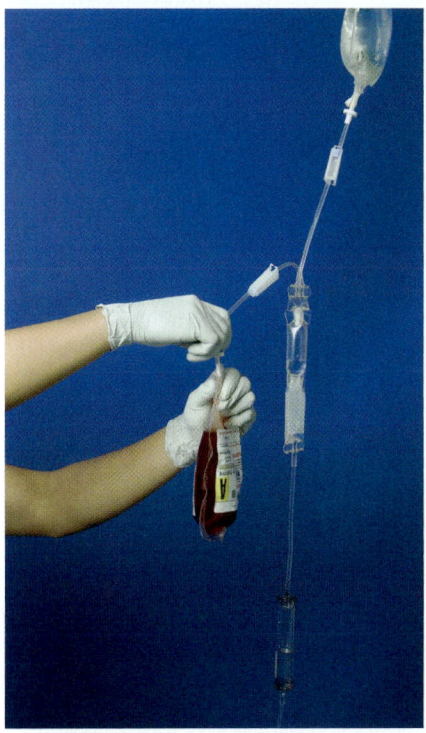

14. **Hang the blood product** container on the IV pole.

Enables the blood to flow by gravity.

15. **Obtain and record** the patient's vital signs, including temperature, pulse, and blood pressure, before beginning the transfusion.

Establishes a baseline to help monitor for transfusion reactions.

16. **Using aseptic technique**, attach the distal end of the administration set to the IV catheter.

Prevents contamination of the IV catheter and administration set.

17. **Slowly open the roller clamp** closest to the blood product.

Allows the blood product to slowly fill that side of the "Y" of the administration set tubing.

18. **Set the drip rate.** Start the rate slowly until 50 mL have infused; if there is no reaction, set to prescribed rate.

A unit of blood cannot hang for more than 4 hours; otherwise, bacterial growth may occur.

Volume-Control Infusion Pump
Program in the rate. Push "Start."

Gravity Flow
Using the roller clamp, adjust the drip rate. Keep in mind that blood administration sets have a drip factor of 10 drops/mL. Note: When using a 24-gauge needle, you will usually (but not always) use gravity infusion instead of a pump.

Forcing red blood cells through a smaller size catheter could result in some cell damage. Allowing the blood to flow by gravity allows time for the cells to change shape as they naturally do when flowing through small capillaries. However, certain models of infusion pumps have been approved that maintain a constant delivery of blood without significant hemolysis, even with small needle sizes (AABB, 2008).

19. **Remain with the patient** during the first 5 minutes, and then obtain vital signs.

Most severe blood transfusion reactions occur during the transfusion of the initial 50 mL of blood.

20. **Make sure that the patient's call** bell or light is readily available. Warn the patient to alert you immediately of any signs or symptoms of a transfusion reaction, such as back pain, chills, itching, or shortness of breath.

If the patient alerts you immediately, you should be able to stop the transfusion in time to prevent serious complications.

21. **Obtain vital signs again** in 15 minutes (follow agency procedures), then again in 30 minutes, and then hourly while the transfusion infuses. Blood and blood product infusions must complete within 4 hours.

Frequent monitoring alerts you to detect early signs of transfusion reaction or fluid overload.

22. **After the unit has infused**, close the roller clamp to the blood product container, and open the roller clamp to the normal saline solution to flush the administration set with normal saline solution.

Flushing the tubing with normal saline solution clears the tubing and avoids wasting any of the blood product.

23. **Close the roller clamp** to the normal saline, and then disconnect the blood administration set from the IV catheter, if an additional unit of blood has not been prescribed.

24. **If another unit of blood** is required, you may hang the second unit with the same administration set. However, administration sets and add-on filters need to be changed every 4 hours.

The same administration set can be used for two units of blood or per agency policy.

25. **Discard the empty** blood container and administration set in the proper receptacle, according to your institution's policy.

Promotes a safer healthcare environment.

? What if . . .

■ **Two individuals are not available to verify that the blood and the patient are a match, and the blood must be hung now?**

In this instance, if it is available, an automated identification technology (e.g., bar coding) may be used.

(continued on next page)

Procedure 39–8 ■ Administering a Blood Transfusion (continued)

Procedure 39-8B ■ Managing a Transfusion Reaction

➤ When performing the procedure, always identify your patient according to agency policy and be attentive to standard precautions, hand hygiene, patient safety and privacy, body mechanics, and documentation.

Procedure Steps

1. **If symptoms of a transfusion** reaction occur, stop the transfusion immediately. Do not flush the tubing.
   Flushing the tubing causes the patient to receive the blood that remains in the tubing.

2. **Disconnect the administration set** from the IV catheter. Call for help. Obtain vital signs, and auscultate heart and breath sounds.
   Severe transfusion reactions may cause respiratory distress and shock; early recognition and treatment improve patient outcomes.

3. **Maintain patency of the IV** catheter by hanging a new infusion of normal saline solution, using new tubing.
   Maintaining a patent IV catheter with normal saline solution provides IV access in which emergency medication can be administered if necessary.

4. **Notify the primary provider** as soon as you have stopped the blood, assessed the patient, and hung the new normal saline solution.

5. **Place the administration set** and blood product container, with the blood bank form attached, inside a biohazard bag. Send the bag to the blood bank immediately.
   The remainder of the blood must be sent to the blood bank, where it can be analyzed to help determine the cause of the reaction.

6. **Obtain blood** (in the extremity opposite the transfusion site) and urine specimens according to your institution's policy.
   Blood banks typically require (1) a specimen for a type and crossmatch to compare with the pretransfusion type and crossmatch, (2) a specimen for free hemoglobin, and (3) a specimen for serum bilirubin level. A urine sample

should also be sent to check for hemoglobinuria, a sign of acute hemolytic reactions.

7. **Continue to monitor vital signs** frequently, at least every 15 minutes.
   To quickly detect worsening of the patient's condition

8. **Administer medications, as prescribed.**
   Medications will vary depending on the type of transfusion reaction.

? What if . . .

■ **At step 2, you do not have a new bag of normal saline to hang?**

Clamp the normal saline line until you can obtain a new bag of normal saline, then disconnect the old normal saline. Do this as quickly as possible.
Preserves the patency of the IV catheter.

Evaluation

■ Evaluate the patient's response to the blood transfusion by checking for changes in blood pressure and oxygenation, improvement in color, or for signs of fluid overload.
■ Monitor for signs and symptoms of transfusion reaction.
■ Evaluate the IV insertion site for signs of infiltration, phlebitis, infection, or inflammation.
■ Check laboratory studies, such as complete blood count, to help evaluate the effectiveness of therapy and/or transfusion reaction.

Patient Teaching

■ Explain the signs and symptoms of transfusion reactions, and tell the client and family to notify staff immediately should they occur.
■ Warn the client or family to notify staff immediately if tenderness, redness, or swelling occurs at the IV catheter insertion site.
■ Explain the importance of notifying staff immediately if the administration set becomes disconnected from the IV catheter or the IV catheter becomes dislodged.

Documentation

■ Chart the date, time, and reason the transfusion was started.
■ Document transfusion vital signs according to institution policy (many institutions have a special form for transfusion vital signs).

■ Record the amount of blood transfused on the I&O record.
■ Chart any complications and the interventions taken.

Practice Resources

AABB, 2008; Blest, Roberts, Murdock, et al., 2008; Finnish Medical Society Duodecim (2008, updated 2008, update pending; INS, 2006a, 2006b; The Joint Commission, 2009; ONS, 2004.

Thinking About the Procedure

 Go to the *Fundamentals of Nursing Skills Videos,* **Oxygenation: Blood Transfusion.**

1. Where was the nurse when verifying the informed consent and the primary provider's prescription?
2. What size bag of normal saline did the nurse take into the room with her? What is the size usually used?
3. Why is it acceptable for the nurse, early in the video, to remove the blood product from the pneumatic tube system without wearing gloves?
4. What symptoms of transfusion reaction did the patient demonstrate (near the end of the video)?

 For suggested responses, go to Chapter 39, **Thinking About the Procedure Suggested Responses,** on *DavisPlus.*

Procedure 39–9 ■ **Assisting With Percutaneous Central Venous Catheter Placement**

➤ For steps to follow in *all* procedures, refer to the Universal Steps for All Procedures found on the page facing the inside back cover.

Equipment

- Sterile gloves (two or three pairs)
- Masks, hats, barrier gowns
- 10-mL vials of normal saline (three or four)
- Syringes with 1-inch needle (two or three)
- 25-gauge ⅝-inch, and 18-gauge 11/2-inch needles (two or three of each)
- Central venous catheter (CVC) kit containing: an introducer, antiseptic solution/swabs, sterile drapes, 10-mL syringe, 1% or 2% Xylocaine without epinephrine, suture, sterile scissors and needle holder, CVC kit (single- or multilumen)
- Injection caps
- Alcohol wipes

Delegation

Do not delegate this procedure because complex assessment and support skills are needed. The nurse must be alert to changes in the patient's condition and signs of developing complications. CVC placement at the bedside is associated with pneumothorax, hemothorax, cardiac tamponade, and air emboli.

Pre-Procedure Assessments

- Obtain baseline vital signs.
- Verify that informed consent has been given.
- Assess for allergy to tape.

➤ When performing the procedure, always identify your patient according to agency policy and be attentive to standard precautions, hand hygiene, patient safety and privacy, body mechanics, and documentation.

Procedure Steps

1. **Explain the procedure** to the patient.
   To relieve anxiety and increase the patient's ability to cooperate with the procedure.
2. **Gather supplies and perform hand hygiene**.
   Promotes efficiency; removes contaminants to help prevent infection.
3. **Set up the sterile field** and add supplies. Position the table so it is easily accessible by the physician or advanced practice nurse (APN) during the procedure.
   Promotes efficiency and makes the procedure faster, and therefore less burdensome for the patient.
4. **Position the patient** to facilitate the procedure, usually in the Trendelenburg position with a rolled towel between the shoulders.
   To prevent air embolism and dilate neck veins.
5. **After the physician or APN** performs hand hygiene, offer mask, gown, and sterile gloves (and possibly hat, depending on agency policy).

Maximum barrier precautions are required for central line placement.

6. **Don mask and then sterile gloves**.
   To prevent contamination of sterile areas and of the insertion site as you cleanse it. Don mask first to keep gloves sterile.
7. **Prep the marked site** with 2% chlorhexidine gluconate in 70% alcohol applicators, using a friction scrub.
   a. Use a back-and-forth motion to scrub an area at least 20 to 25 cm (8 to 10 in.) in diameter. Do not go back over an area with the same applicator.
   b. Repeat with three applicators. Total scrub should take at least 30 seconds (2 minutes for a moist site such as the femoral vein).
   c. Allow site to air dry completely (about 2 minutes). Never wipe or blot dry.
   Insertion kits and agency policies may vary. Follow agency policy. If it does not conform to evidence-based guidelines, work for policy change.
8. **Drape the insertion site** with a large sterile drape, exposing only the prepared skin area. Use other

large drapes to cover the patient from head to toe. If your agency does not have a policy that the patient wears a mask, have him turn his head in the opposite direction of insertion site.
   Creates a sterile field and decreases the chance of contamination by the patient's exhalations. Turning the head to the opposite side also helps to make it easier to advance the catheter when it passes through the subclavian site.

9. **Observe while the physician or APN performs the following steps:**
   a. Anesthetizes the area with lidocaine.
   b. Primes the central venous catheter with saline.
   c. Performs venipuncture with the insertion needle (in the internal jugular or subclavian site). The femoral site may be used in emergencies, but it is associated with a higher rate of complications than other sites.
   d. Attaches a syringe to the needle and aspirates for blood.
   To ensure the needle is in the vein.

(continued on next page)

e. After obtaining blood return, removes syringe from the needle and inserts a guidewire through the needle.

The guidewire guides the flexible catheter into the vein.

f. Aspirates all air out of the catheter lumens and then flushes them with normal saline.

To reduce the risk of air embolism.

g. Places injection caps on each lumen.

To prevent blood loss and maintain sterility of the lumens

h. Sutures the catheter in place.

To minimize movement and prevent catheter migration (in or out).

10. **After the physician or APN is finished, apply sterile transparent dressing over the site.**

Minimizes contamination of the site. The most common route of infection is via migration of skin organisms at the insertion site into the cutaneous catheter tract with colonization of the catheter tip. Transparent dressing allows for observation of the site without removing the dressing and manipulating the catheter.

11. **If there are clamps on the lumens,** close them.

12. **Place tape over the lumens** near the ends, but not on the injection caps.

To minimize movement of the catheter that increases the risk of dislodgement.

13. **Remove sterile drape** and assist the patient to a comfortable position.

14. **Dispose of used supplies** and equipment in the appropriate containers according to agency policy in line with CDC guidelines.

15. **Remove and dispose of mask** and gloves. Perform hand hygiene.

Observes standard precaution guidelines.

Guidelines

- The patient and all staff in the room should wear a mask.
- A health professional who has received appropriate education (e.g., a nurse) should observe the CVC insertion to ensure that aseptic technique is maintained.
- This person should stop the procedure if aseptic technique errors are made.
- A central line checklist should be used during the procedure. You may be responsible for auditing the procedure and completing the checklist.

? What if . . .

- **In step 8, a large sterile drape is not available?**

Use two small drapes to cover the patient from head to toe.

Evaluation

- Obtain vital signs.

To assess for complications.

- Auscultate the lungs and assess for respiratory distress, sharp chest pain, and coughing. Monitor for 24 hours for these signs.

To detect pneumothorax or cardiac tamponade.

- Obtain a chest x-ray.

To verify correct location of catheter tip in the distal third of the superior vena cava, as well as absence of thorax and cardiac puncture.

- Assess the patient daily to determine continuing need for the CVC.

Risk of infection is closely related to the length of time the CVC is in place.

- For further evaluation, refer to Clinical Insight 39-3 and Procedure 39-5B.

Documentation

- Date and time of catheter insertion
- Catheter type and size
- Site location
- Assessments and interventions performed at insertion and immediately after
- Patient's tolerance of procedure (subjective and objective data)
- X-ray verification of catheter placement

Practice Resources

Betsy Lehman Center for Patient Safety and Medical Error Reduction, JSI Research and Training Institute, Inc., 2008; INS, 2006a, 2006b; Institute for Healthcare Improvement, (IHI), n.d.; The Joanna Briggs Institute, 2008; Pronovost, Goeschel, Colantuoni, E., et al., 2010); Pronovost, Needham, Berenholtz, et al., 2006; Rhoads & Meeker, 2008; Riley, n.d.; Society for Healthcare Epidemiology of America, 2008; Wentzel & Edmond, 2006.

To explore learning resources for this chapter,

Go to DavisPlus at http://davisplus.fadavis.com/, keyword Treas:

Chapter Resources for Chapter 39:

Knowledge Check and Think Like a Nurse Response Sheets

Knowledge Check Answers

Resources for Caregivers and Health Professionals

Reading More About Fluids, Electrolytes, & Acid–Base Balance (suggested readings)

What Are the Main Points in This Chapter?

NCLEX-Style Review Questions

Chapter Overview Podcasts

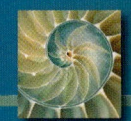

Concept Map

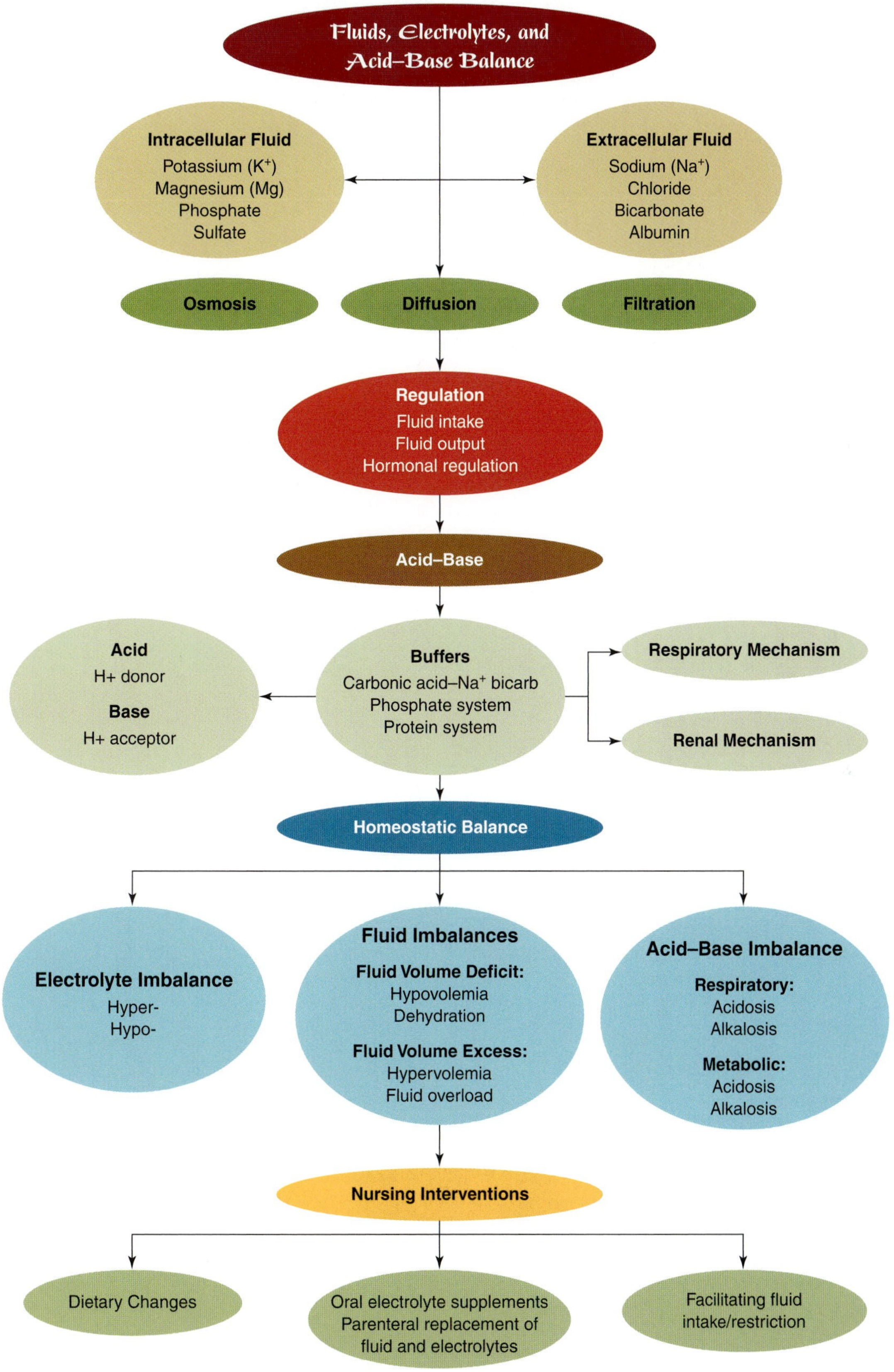

Fluids, Electrolytes, and Acid–Base Balance

Intracellular Fluid
Potassium (K⁺)
Magnesium (Mg)
Phosphate
Sulfate

Extracellular Fluid
Sodium (Na⁺)
Chloride
Bicarbonate
Albumin

Osmosis

Diffusion

Filtration

Regulation
Fluid intake
Fluid output
Hormonal regulation

Acid–Base

Acid
H+ donor

Base
H+ acceptor

Buffers
Carbonic acid–Na⁺ bicarb
Phosphate system
Protein system

Respiratory Mechanism

Renal Mechanism

Homeostatic Balance

Electrolyte Imbalance
Hyper-
Hypo-

Fluid Imbalances
Fluid Volume Deficit:
Hypovolemia
Dehydration
Fluid Volume Excess:
Hypervolemia
Fluid overload

Acid–Base Imbalance
Respiratory:
Acidosis
Alkalosis
Metabolic:
Acidosis
Alkalosis

Nursing Interventions

Dietary Changes

Oral electrolyte supplements
Parenteral replacement of
fluid and electrolytes

Facilitating fluid
intake/restriction

The Context for Nurses' Work

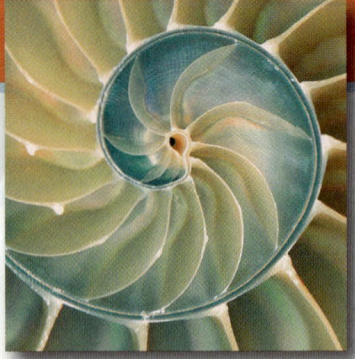

CHAPTER 40

Perioperative Nursing

Learning Outcomes

After completing this chapter, you should be able to:

> Discuss the importance of perioperative safety.

> Name and differentiate the three phases of the perioperative period.

> Describe the ways in which surgeries can be classified.

> Discuss factors that affect the degree of risk of surgery.

> Describe nursing actions associated with the preoperative phase, including physical preparations for surgery, preoperative teaching, and surgical consent forms.

> Compare and contrast the roles of the circulating and scrub nurse.

> Compare and contrast general anesthesia, local anesthesia, regional anesthesia, and conscious sedation.

> Discuss common nursing interventions during the intraoperative phase, including skin preparation, positioning for surgery, and intraoperative safety measures.

> Describe nursing assessments appropriate for surgical clients on admission to the nursing unit.

> Provide nursing care to prevent postoperative complications, including application of sequential compression devices, use of incentive spirometry, and management of gastric suction.

> Use nursing diagnoses appropriately to describe a patient's unique needs during the preoperative, intraoperative, and postoperative periods.

Key Concepts

Perioperative nursing
Preoperative care
Intraoperative care
Postoperative care

Related Concepts

See the Concept Map at the end of this chapter.

Caring for the Nguyens

This feature allows you to practice the kind of thinking you will use as a full-spectrum nurse. There is usually more than one correct answer to a critical thinking question, so we do not provide answers for these features. It is more important to develop your nursing judgment than to "cover content." Discuss the questions with your peers. If you are still unsure, consult your instructor.

Mai Nguyen, the 76-year-old mother of Nam Nguyen, has been experiencing blurred vision and decreased visual acuity. A local ophthalmologist diagnosed bilateral cataracts. The ophthalmologist has recommended cataract removal in the left eye, with insertion of an intraocular lens. He told Mai Nguyen to schedule the surgery "at your convenience" and explained that the surgery would be performed on an outpatient basis. The ophthalmologist gave Mai Nguyen a list

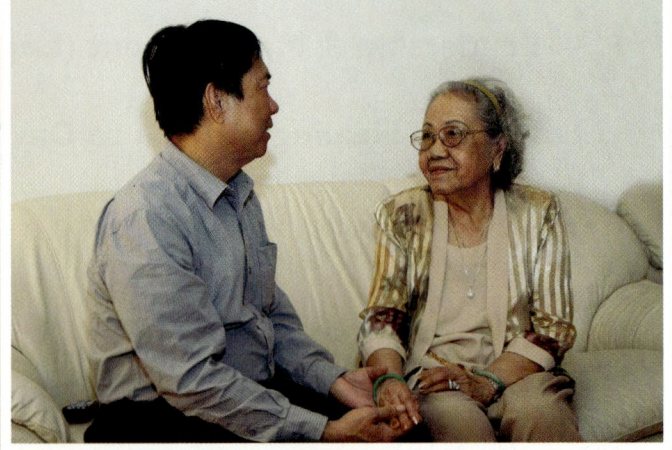

of activities to prepare for the surgery, containing the following information:

■ Schedule a date for your surgery. My receptionist will set up a time for your surgery. All surgeries are

(Continued)

Caring for the Nguyens (continued)

performed at Western Medical Center Same-Day Surgery Department.
- Please arrange to be seen by your primary care provider 1 to 2 weeks prior to the surgery to receive clearance for surgery.

- Make an appointment with the Preoperative Center at Western Medical Center Same-Day Surgery Department 1 to 2 days before surgery.
- Arrange to have a ride to and from the surgery.

A. What preoperative testing is Mrs. Nguyen likely to undergo? Explain your rationale.

B. The preoperative list states that the client must be seen by the primary care provider to receive clearance for surgery. Why is this an essential part of the preoperative period?

C. What theoretical knowledge do you need to perform preoperative teaching for Mai Nguyen? How could you obtain that information? Be specific about your sources.

D. What content would you include in Mrs. Nguyen's preoperative teaching?

E. The ophthalmologist has planned anesthesia via conscious sedation. What factors, if any, might keep Mrs. Nguyen from receiving this form of anesthesia? What additional information do you need to answer this question?

 Go to **Caring for the Nguyens Response Sheet** on *DavisPlus*.

Meet Your Patient

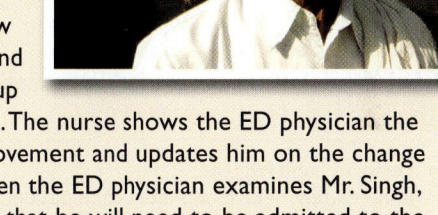

Nishad Singh is a 68-year-old man who came to the emergency department (ED) with sudden onset of rectal bleeding. He tells the ED nurse, "I've been real tired and dragging for several months. This morning I felt a little worse than usual. When I went to the bathroom, there was a lot of blood. I've never had that before, and it scared me. I've had to go to the bathroom a couple times this morning, and it's all blood." The ED nurse collects the following data:

BP: 138/88 mm Hg
Pulse: 104 beats/min and regular
Respiratory rate: 20 breaths/min
Temperature: 36.7°C (98.0°F)
Oxygen saturation: 98%

The ED nurse assesses that Mr. Singh is mildly anxious. His breath sounds are clear, but his abdomen is tender in the left lower quadrant (LLQ). The nurse draws blood to be sent to the lab. While they are waiting for the lab results, Mr. Singh tells the nurse, "My stomach is cramping down low, and I need to go to the bathroom." She provides him with a bedpan. He passes approximately 200 mL of bright red blood with a small amount of fecal material. He becomes sweaty and lightheaded after the

BM. The nurse rechecks his vital signs and notes that his BP is now 120/76 mm Hg and that his pulse is up to 120 beats/min. The nurse shows the ED physician the bloody bowel movement and updates him on the change in vital signs. When the ED physician examines Mr. Singh, he tells Mr. Singh that he will need to be admitted to the hospital for further evaluation of the bleeding.

You are the nurse assigned to care for Mr. Singh on the medical–surgical unit. Mr. Singh has been sent from the ED directly to radiology for a computed tomography (CT) scan of his abdomen. The scan reveals a tumor in the sigmoid colon. Since leaving the ED, Mr. Singh has had three more bloody bowel movements. His blood pressure is 100/72 mm Hg, and his pulse rate is now 134 beats/min. The physician prescribes a bolus of 1,000 mL of lactated Ringer's solution and a unit of packed red blood cells as soon as it is available. Mr. Singh is scheduled for colon resection surgery, which will occur as soon as the surgical team can be assembled and the room prepared.

ABOUT THE KEY CONCEPTS

The overarching concept for this chapter is *perioperative nursing,* which includes the key concepts of *preoperative, intraoperative,* and *postoperative care.* To help you understand and remember those concepts, we discuss in this chapter how to prepare a client for surgery and the activities that occur before, during, and after surgery, as we follow Mr. Singh (Meet Your Patient) through his perioperative experience. We will present definitions and examples of the key concepts, as well as numerous subconcepts that relate to each other in various ways. We begin with perioperative nursing.

PERIOPERATIVE NURSING

Perioperative nursing involves the care of clients before, during, and after surgery and some other invasive procedures. Historically, perioperative nursing practice was called *operating room nursing* and was limited to transferring patients into and out of operating rooms and handing instruments to surgeons during surgical procedures. Now nurses in all phases of the operative experience actively provide and manage care, teach, and study the care of perioperative patients.

The Association of periOperative Registered Nurses (AORN) is a specialty organization. Its *Standards and Recommended Practices* (2009) keep perioperative nurses up to date on current practice. For additional information about AORN,

 Go to the **AORN Web site** at http://www.aorn.org

Perioperative Safety

An important aspect of perioperative nursing is to help prevent complications of surgery. Hand hygiene is an important component of perioperative prevention (Box 40-1).

BOX 40-1 ■ Recommended Practices for Hand Hygiene

- Perform hand hygiene:
  Immediately before and after each patient contact
  After removing gloves. Wearing gloves does not
    substitute for hand hygiene.
  Any time you may have come in contact with blood or
    potentially infectious substances
  Before and after eating
  After using the restroom
- Remove rings, watches, and bracelets before performing hand hygiene.
- It is preferable that you do not wear rings. They have been associated with a significant increase in skin microorganism count.
- Keep fingernails short and clean. They should not extend beyond the fingertips.
- Replace nail polish when it is chipped or at least every 4 days.
- Do not wear artificial nails. Fungal growth often occurs under them.
- Be certain there are no lesions or breaks in skin integrity on your hands.
- For handwashing and handrub procedures, see Procedure 22-1, Hand Hygiene, in Chapter 22.

Sources: Adapted from AORN, 2009; Boyce & Pittet, 2002; Siegel, Rhinehart, Jackson, et al., 2007.

Preventable perioperative errors cause 10% of surgery-related deaths, have an unfavorable financial impact on health-care institutions, and result in physical and emotional harm to patients (Agency for Healthcare Research and Quality [AHRQ], 2008). Various government and private organizations, including the following, stress the importance of patient safety:

- ***The Association of periOperative Registered Nurses (AORN, 2009).*** Perioperative Safety is one of the three domains under which AORN organizes its perioperative patient outcomes. Specific safety outcomes include prevention of injury and freedom from infection.
- **The Joint Commission.** The Joint Commission's 2011 *National Patient Safety Goals* that are applicable to surgery include preventing infection, improving the accuracy of patient identification, improving staff communication, making sure the correct surgery is done on the correct patient and on the correct part of the patient's body, and performing a time-out immediately before starting procedures (The Joint Commission, 2011).
- ***The Institute for Healthcare Improvement (IHI).*** The IHI is an independent, not-for-profit organization that works to reduce morbidity and death in American healthcare. One goal of their 100,000 Lives Campaign and their 5 Million Lives Campaign was to reduce surgical complications and specifically, surgical infections. To see the entire list of IHI recommendations (IHI, 2011),

 Go to Chapter 23, **Tables, Boxes, Figures: ESG Box 23-1, The 100,000 Lives Campaign,** on *DavisPlus.*

"Never Events"

"Never events" are serious and costly errors resulting in severe consequences for the patient, and that are mostly preventable. Believing these events are reasonably preventable and should never happen in a hospital, Medicare no longer reimburses institutions for care related to such complications (Centers for Medicare & Medicaid Services, 2006, 2008). Several of the "never events" (also called *serious reportable events*) are also targeted by the national organizations listed earlier. Among the never events important to perioperative care are:

- Surgery on the wrong body part
- Surgery on the wrong patient
- Wrong surgery on a patient
- Deep vein thrombosis or pulmonary embolism after total knee or hip replacement
- Foreign body left in a patient after surgery (e.g., sponge, clip for draping)
- Surgical site infections after certain elective procedures (e.g., after bariatric surgery for obesity). AORN, The Joint Commission, National Priorities Partnership, and IHI extend that to include all infections. The Centers for Disease Control and Prevention (CDC) targeted certain antimicrobial-resistant bacterial infections.

PREOPERATIVE CARE

The **preoperative phase** begins with the client's decision to have surgery and ends when he enters the operating room.

TheoreticalKnowledge
knowing **why**

Nursing care during the preoperative phase focuses on identifying existing health concerns, planning for intraoperative and postoperative needs, and providing preoperative teaching.

Preoperative nursing care is delivered in a variety of settings. More than two-thirds of surgeries in the United States are performed in outpatient settings, such as endoscopy suites, physicians' offices, and ambulatory surgery centers (Centers for Disease Control [CDC] National Center for Health Statistics, 2009). The length of the preoperative period and the extent of the patient teaching depend on the type of surgery to be done and the patient's overall health status.

How Are Surgeries Classified?

Knowing the type of surgery helps you to identify the patient's perioperative needs and plan patient care. Surgeries can be classified by body system, purpose, level of urgency, and acuity. The classifications often overlap.

By Body System

The body system classification is useful for determining the postoperative risk of infection. For example, surgical incisions that enter the gastrointestinal, respiratory, or genitourinary tracts have a higher risk for infection than does surgery of other body systems. However, if an organ ruptures or surgery is required to repair a penetrating injury, the risk of infection is very high regardless of the body system involved. Mr. Singh (Meet Your Patient) will have surgery of the gastrointestinal system.

By Purpose

See whether you can identify which of the following purposes describes Mr. Singh's (Meet Your Patient) surgery.

- **Ablative surgery** involves removal of a diseased body part (e.g., a cholecystectomy removes the gallbladder.
- **Diagnostic (exploratory) surgery** is done to confirm or rule out a diagnosis. Examples include biopsy, fine-needle aspiration, and invasive tests, such as a cardiac catheterization.
- **Palliative surgery** is performed to relieve discomfort or other disease symptoms without producing a cure. Examples include nerve root destruction for chronic pain.
- **Reconstructive surgery** is performed to restore function (e.g., rotator cuff and torn ligament repair).
- **Cosmetic surgery** is done to improve appearance (e.g., face-lift).
- **Transplant surgery** replaces a malfunctioning body part, tissue, or organ. Joint replacements and organ replacement procedures are included in this category.
- **Procurement surgery** is related to transplant surgery. An organ or tissue is harvested from someone pronounced brain dead for transplantation into another person.

By Degree of Urgency

Based on the following definitions, how would you describe the degree of urgency for Mr. Singh's surgery?

- **Emergency surgery** requires transport to the operating suite as soon as possible to preserve the patient's life or function. The surgical team is summoned and preparations are made rapidly. Internal hemorrhage, rupture of an organ, and trauma are common causes of emergency surgery.
- **Urgent surgery** is scheduled within 24 to 48 hours to alleviate symptoms, repair a body part, or restore function. Removal of a cancerous breast and internal fixation of a fracture are examples.
- **Elective surgery** is performed when surgery is the recommended course of action, but the condition is not time sensitive. The client may delay surgery to gather information, consider options, or organize care for the family. Examples include repair of a torn ligament, removal of rectal polyps, or a rhinoplasty (repair of the nose).

By Degree of Risk

There is an old adage that "the only minor surgery is someone else's surgery." This statement reflects the anxiety that often accompanies surgery. Nevertheless, surgery is defined as major or minor based on the degree of seriousness or risk associated with the procedure. The degree of risk varies with the condition of the client, as well as with the type of surgery and anesthesia.

Major surgery is associated with a high degree of risk. For example, it may be associated with the potential for significant blood loss, involve vital organs, be a prolonged or complicated procedure, or have significant potential for postoperative complications. Some examples of major procedures are coronary artery bypass graft (CABG), nephrectomy (removal of a kidney), and colon resection. **Minor surgery,** often performed on an outpatient basis, involves little risk and usually has few complications. Examples include breast biopsy and inguinal hernia repair.

What Factors Affect Surgical Risk?

The following factors can contribute to increased surgical risk.

Age. The very young and very old are at greatest risk during surgical procedures.

Infants have limited ability to regulate temperature and have immature immune, cardiovascular, liver, and renal systems. They are at greater risk for infection, excess fluid volume, and deficient volume. Even minor blood loss may represent a substantial portion of an infant's total blood volume. In addition, infants may have difficulty calming. They are unable to understand what is happening, so you cannot use verbal reassurance and explanations to comfort them.

Toddlers understand simple explanations but may be anxious about separation from parents or caregivers. Many fear the dark. *Preschoolers* fear damage to body parts. Fear of pain or of needles is common for children of any age. *Teens* might fear disfigurement resulting from scars. *Young adults* commonly are anxious about the cost associated with hospitalization or surgery.

Older adults are at increased risk because they have less physiological reserve and often have comorbid conditions (other illness not related to the surgery). Many of the physiological changes of aging predispose older adults to increased risk. Among these changes are decreased kidney function, diminished immune function, decreased bone and lean body mass, increased peripheral vascular resistance, decreased cardiac output, decreased cough reflex, and increased time required for wound healing.

Type of Wound. Both preexisting wounds (e.g., from trauma) and the wounds (incisions) created by the surgical procedure can pose a risk for infection (Table 40-1). Risk to the patient increases along with the risk for or presence of infection. Which type of wound will Mr. Singh (Meet Your Patient) have immediately after surgery?

Preexisting Conditions. The ideal surgical candidate is a healthy young adult who takes no medications. Unfortunately, many surgical clients have underlying acute or chronic disorders that increase surgical risk (Box 40-2).

Mental Status. Patients with altered cognition, from either physical or mental illness, may be unable to understand preoperative instructions or give informed consent for surgical procedures. They may also require medications (e.g., antipsychotic agents) that interact with anesthetics and analgesics. Surgery and anesthesia may aggravate preexisting dementia, confusion, and disorientation.

Table 40-1 ➤ Wound Type and Potential for Infection

WOUND TYPE	WOUND CHARACTERISTICS	EXAMPLES OF SURGERY ASSOCIATED WITH THE WOUND
Clean Wounds	Uninfected; minimal inflammation; little risk of infection AND Surgery does not involve the gastrointestinal, respiratory, or genitourinary tract.	Face-lift, cataract surgery, joint replacement, breast biopsy, tonsillectomy
Clean-Contaminated Wounds	Not infected, but carry increased risk for infection	Surgical incisions that enter the gastrointestinal, respiratory, or genitourinary tract.
Contaminated Wounds	Not infected, but carry high risk for infection	Surgery to repair trauma to open wounds, such as compound fractures; surgery in which a major break in surgical asepsis occurred
Infected Wounds	Evidence of infection, such as purulent drainage, necrotic tissue, or bacterial counts above 100,000 organisms per gram of tissue	A postoperative surgical incision of any type that has evidence of infection

BOX 40-2 ■ Preexisting Conditions That Increase Surgical Risk

Chronic Conditions

Cardiovascular diseases (such as hypertension, congestive heart failure, and myocardial infarction) affect the ability of the heart to work as an efficient pump. If these disorders are well controlled (e.g., with blood pressure medications or cardiotonic medications), risk is limited.

Chronic respiratory disorders (such as emphysema, asthma, or bronchitis) decrease pulmonary function, increase the risk of respiratory infection, and may be exacerbated (made worse) by general anesthesia.

Coagulation disorders delay clotting and increase blood loss, placing the patient at risk for hemorrhage and hypovolemic shock. In contrast, a hypercoagulation state increases the risk of stroke, embolism, or intravascular clotting.

Diabetes mellitus delays wound healing and increases the risk of infection and cardiovascular disorders associated with diabetes.

Liver disease affects the body's ability to metabolize amino acids, carbohydrates, and fat; to manufacture prothrombin for clotting; and to detoxify medications. Therefore, the patient is at increased risk for poor wound healing, hemorrhage, and toxic reactions to anesthetics and medications.

Neurological disorders (such as paralysis or spinal cord injury) increase the risk for vasomotor instability and thus create the potential for wide swings in blood pressure. In addition, patients with seizure disorders are more likely to have a seizure in the perioperative period.

Nutritional disorders can affect surgical outcomes. Patients who are malnourished or obese are at risk for delayed wound healing, infection, and fatigue. Obese clients are also more prone to cardiovascular disorders and impaired pulmonary function.

Renal disease affects the patient's ability to excrete many medications, including anesthetic agents. It also affects the body's ability to regulate fluid and electrolytes.

Acute Conditions

Acute infections tax the patient's energy and physiological reserves, increasing the risk for various postoperative complications.

Upper respiratory tract infections are associated with increased risk of postoperative pneumonia, especially if the patient receives a general anesthetic.

Medications. Both prescribed and over-the-counter (OTC) medications may increase surgical risk (Box 40-3). For example, (1) patients who self-prescribe high doses of vitamin E may be at increased risk for bleeding and (2) certain herbal and alternative medications can have the following effects:

- Increase the risk for cardiac dysrhythmias secondary to potassium loss.
- Interfere with metabolism of anesthetics because of their effects on the liver.
- Increase the potential for excessive bleeding.
- Decrease cerebral blood flow.
- Cause hypertension.

- Increase the effects of opioids and sympathetic nervous system stimulants.

For a list of herbal products and associated surgical risks,

 Go to Chapter 40, **Tables, Boxes, Figures: ESG Box 40-1,** on *DavisPlus.*

Personal Habits. Substance abuse can increase surgical risk. Smoking affects pulmonary function; long-term alcohol use contributes to liver disease, predisposing the patient to bleeding. Alcohol and other drugs interact with anesthetic agents and medications to create adverse effects. Also, habitual substance abusers may have a cross-tolerance to anesthetic

BOX 40-3 ▪ Medications That Increase Surgical Risk

Antibiotics	May potentiate the action of anesthetic agents.
Anticoagulants	Increase risk for bleeding.
Antidysrhythmics	May impair cardiac function during anesthesia.
Antihypertensives	Increase the risk for hypotension during surgery; may interact with anesthetic agents to cause bradycardia and impaired circulation.
Aspirin	Increases risk for bleeding.
Corticosteroids	Delay wound healing and increase risk for infection.
Diuretics	Alter fluid and electrolyte balance (especially potassium balance).
Opioids	Increase the risk of respiratory depression.
NSAIDs	Inhibit platelet aggregation, increasing the risk for bleeding.
Tranquilizers	Increase the risk of respiratory depression.

and analgesic agents, causing them to need higher than normal doses.

Allergies. Patients may be allergic to medications (e.g., antibiotics, such as penicillins or cephalosporins), analgesics (e.g., codeine), tape, latex, and solutions used in surgery. Reactions range from unpleasant to life threatening.

KnowledgeCheck 40-1

- Define *preoperative phase*.
- What are four ways surgeries can be classified?
- What factors affect surgical risk?

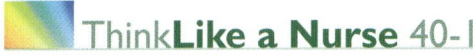 **ThinkLike a Nurse 40-1**

How would you evaluate Mr. Singh's (Meet Your Patient) surgical risk? What additional information do you need to answer this question?

PracticalKnowledge
knowing **how**

The nursing focus in the preoperative phase is to prepare the patient for surgery. You will use the nursing process to identify any unique nursing diagnoses a patient might have. However, many preoperative nursing interventions are routine preventive measures that you will use for *all* surgical patients.

Perioperative Nursing Data Set

The Perioperative Nursing Data Set (PNDS) is a standardized vocabulary specifically designed to describe the care of perioperative patients. It includes terminology for nursing diagnoses, nursing interventions, and nurse-sensitive patient outcomes appropriate for use in any surgical setting. It is the first nursing language developed by a specialty organization that has been recognized by the American Nurses Association.

Perioperative Patient-Focused Model. The PNDS is derived from the AORN's Perioperative Patient-Focused

model. The patient is at the center of the model and is the focus of care. The perioperative nurse assists the patient throughout the perioperative experience to achieve outcomes in the Health System domain and the Patient-Centered domains (which include Safety, Physiological Responses to Surgery, and Behavioral Responses to Surgery).

The Health System domain refers to the system in which perioperative care is given. It involves administrative and structural elements necessary for successful surgical outcomes—for example, equipment, supplies, staff, and policies (AORN, 2009).

In this chapter, we continue to use the NANDA-I, NOC, and NIC standardized languages, to which you have already been introduced in previous chapters.

◼ ASSESSMENT

For patient safety, data must be correct and complete. To prevent omission of important information, most organizations have developed a preoperative checklist. Although the forms may vary at each institution, the areas for assessment are the same and are discussed in the sections that follow.

Focused Nursing History. It is essential to determine whether the client is physiologically, cognitively, and psychologically prepared for the intraoperative and postoperative phases of surgery. For a complete and accurate nursing history, collect assessment data from the client, significant others, medical records, and other members of the healthcare team. Include the following topics in your preoperative assessment: health history, physical status, allergies, medications (including herbal products and over-the-counter medications), mental status, knowledge and understanding of the surgery and anesthesia, cultural and spiritual factors, access to social resources, coping strategies, and use of alcohol and drugs. For an example of a preoperative assessment form developed by the AORN, see the Focused Assessment box, Example of a Perioperative Checklist (AORN).

Additional assessments may be needed if the client is undergoing outpatient surgery or has a planned short stay after surgery (see the Home Care box Preoperative Assessment for the Surgical Client Who Will Be Discharged to Home).

Focused Physical Assessment. If you identify risk factors from the nursing history, focus on these aspects during your brief head-to-toe physical assessment. For example, if the patient states she had a cough last week, perform a focused assessment of the ear, nose, throat, and lungs to determine how the cough may affect the patient's risk. If the patient has lower airway congestion, as evidenced by rhonchi and productive cough, communicate these findings to the surgeon and the anesthesia team; if a general anesthetic is planned, it may be necessary to delay the surgery. For all patients, assess risk factors for thrombophlebitis, as venous thrombus is one of the never events that are important to prevent. For additional details on a brief bedside physical assessment, see Procedure 21-20 in Chapter 21.

Diagnostic Testing. Preoperative screening tests are usually prescribed before surgical procedures. The type of testing depends on the patient's age, health history, and facility policies. For example, most institutions require a complete blood count and urinalysis before surgery, as well as an electrocardiogram for patients older than age 50. Patients with chronic health problems may require additional testing. See the accompanying Diagnostic Testing box Common Preoperative Screening Tests.

Example of a Perioperative Checklist (AORN)

AORN *SAMPLE* Preoperative Assessment Form
(Facility Name and Address)

NOTE: *This record is a sample only. Clinical records should be customized to incorporate data fields that represent the setting, facility, procedure, and patient. Reproductions and variations are encouraged, provided credit is given to AORN.*

Date:_____

Addressograph

(Patient Information: name, age, gender, medical record number, date)

Structural Data:

Admitted via:
☐ Ambulatory ☐ Wheelchair ☐ Stretcher
☐ Other assistive devices:_____

Admitted from:
☐ Home   ☐ Transferring hospital
☐ Acute rehab facility ☐ Extended/skilled care facility

Date of preoperative assessment:_____

Planned procedure:_____

Language(s) spoken: ☐ English ☐ Spanish ☐ Other:_____

☐ Patient's records, belongings, valuables secured (I115)
    Belonging inventory: ☐ Watch   ☐ Jewelry
        ☐ Contacts/glasses ☐ Dentures/partial(s) ☐ Hearing aid

Identity confirmed (I26):   ☐ Yes   ☐ No
Advance directive signed: ☐ Yes   ☐ No
    Location:_____

Operative procedure, surgical site, and laterality verified (I143):   ☐ Yes   ☐ No

Consent for planned procedures verified (I124):
                                ☐ Yes   ☐ No

NPO status verified (I138):   ☐ Yes   ☐ No
    Since: (date/time)_____

Preadmission testing
☐ CBC_____   ☐ Urinalysis_____
☐ Potassium level_____ ☐ EKG_____
☐ CXR_____   ☐ Pregnancy test:_____
☐ Type and cross   # of units:_____

Nursing Data Elements:

General health status: (check when present)
☐ Diabetes   ☐ Cancer   ☐ Obesity   ☐ Pregnancy
☐ Hematologic disorders (anemia, sickle cell disease or conditions)

☐ Vital signs:
    Temperature:_____   Pulse:_____   BP:_____
    Respirations:_____   Height:_____   Weight:_____

☐ Allergies verified (note type of reaction) (I123)
    Latex allergy: ☐ Yes   ☐ No
    Medications: ☐ Yes:_____   ☐ No
                    _____

    Food: ☐ Yes:_____   ☐ No
                _____

☐ Daily medications (prescription, OTC, vitamins, alternative medication, herbal remedies, chemotherapy):
    _____
    _____
    _____
    Medications taken day of surgery:_____

☐ Alcohol/Drug social use:_____

☐ **Neurologic assessment:** ☐ Alert and oriented
    ☐ Speech intact   ☐ Follows simple commands
    ☐ Risk of falls   ☐ History of seizures
    LOC: ☐ Alert/oriented ☐ Drowsy   ☐ Sedated
        ☐ Asleep   ☐ Unresponsive ☐ Disoriented
        ☐ Other:_____

☐ **Sensory assessment:**
    ☐ No limitations   ☐ Hearing impairment   ☐ Visual impairment

☐ **Cardiovascular assessment:**
    ☐ Pacemaker   ☐ Implanted defibrillator
    ☐ Chest pain
    ☐ Peripheral edema: Location:_____
    ☐ DVT/PE risk:
        ☐ None ☐ Low ☐ Med ☐ High
        _____
        _____

☐ **Respiratory assessment:**
    ☐ Tracheotomy
    ☐ Intubated
    ☐ Chest tube
    Respirations: ☐ Regular   ☐ Labored
    Smoking history ☐ Yes   ☐ No
        Packs/day:____ Years smoked:_____
        Quit date:_____
    ☐ Cough   ☐ Cold symptoms
    ☐ Current or recent respiratory infection
    ☐ Preexisting respiratory problems (specify):
        _____
        _____

☐ **Musculoskeletal assessment:**
    ☐ No limitations
    ☐ Paralysis
    ☐ Traction
    ☐ Limited ROM
    ☐ Amputation:_____
    ☐ Prosthesis:_____

Focused Assessment

Example of a Perioperative Checklist (AORN)—cont'd

Nursing Data Elements (continued):

☐ **Skin assessment:**
  ☐ Cool   ☐ Warm   ☐ Intact
  ☐ Dry   ☐ Moist
  ☐ Body jewelry removed
  ☐ Makeup removed
  ☐ Tattoos: _____
  ☐ Rash: _____
  ☐ Bruises: _____
  ☐ Wounds: _____
  ☐ Ostomy: _____
  ☐ Catheter/Drain: _____
  ☐ Venous access device: _____

☐ **Gastrointestinal assessment:**
  Last bowel movement (date/time): _____
  Usual diet: _____
  _____

  Recent unexplained weight loss
  ☐ Yes: Amount: _____ Time frame: _____
  ☐ No
  Problems chewing or swallowing
  ☐ Yes   ☐ No
  Special needs:
  ☐ Chewing   ☐ Swallowing
  ☐ Appetite   ☐ Diet preferences

☐ **Genitourinary/Gynecology assessment:**
  ☐ Voided on call to OR
    Time: _____ Amount: _____
  ☐ Urinary catheter: Amount in bag: _____
  ☐ Urinary incontinence

☐ **Psychosocial assessment:**
  ☐ Calm/relaxed   ☐ Anxious   ☐ Talkative
  ☐ Crying   ☐ Restless   ☐ Withdrawn
  ☐ Other: _____
  ☐ Concerns regarding surgery or hospitalization:
  _____

  ☐ Religious/cultural concerns/requests:
  _____

  ☐ Receives help from:
    ☐ Children   ☐ Support person
    ☐ Other (specify):

  ☐ Patient cares for:
    ☐ Children: Ages: _____
    ☐ Self   ☐ Spouse
    ☐ Other (specify): _____
  _____

☐ Determine level of knowledge (I135):
  ☐ Barriers to learning: _____
  ☐ Motivation to learn
    ☐ excellent   ☐ average   ☐ limited

☐ Abuse screening
  Have you ever felt threatened verbally,
  emotionally, or physically in any of your
  relationships?
  ☐ Yes   ☐ No
  Have you been hit, slapped, kicked, or other-
  wise physically hurt by an intimate partner?
  ☐ Yes   ☐ No
  Are you afraid of your partner or anyone you
  live with?
  ☐ Yes   ☐ No
  If yes, describe and make appropriate referral

☐ **Pain assessment**
  ☐ Instructed on use of pain scale
  ☐ Pain assessment (0-10): _____
    Location: _____

☐ **Discharge planning**
  Will require assistance after discharge
  ☐ Yes   ☐ No
  Discharge plan:
  ☐ Home
  ☐ Home nursing service
  ☐ Short-term care facility
  ☐ Extended care facility
  ☐ Other: _____

  Individual who will escort patient home:
  Name: _____
  Phone number: _____
  Relationship: _____

Comments:
  _____
  _____
  _____
  _____
  _____

Preoperative nursing diagnoses
  ☐ Anxiety/fear (X4)
  ☐ Therapeutic regimen management ineffective (X33)
  ☐ Deficient knowledge (X30)
  ☐ Risk for injury (X29)
  ☐ Pain (X38)
  ☐ Other: _____

RN Signature:
X

Comments:

Example of a Perioperative Checklist (AORN). (*Source:* Reprinted with permission from AORN Perioperative Patient-Focused Model. Copyright AORN, Inc., 2170 Pakert Rd., Suite 300, Denver, CO 80231)

Preoperative Assessment for the Surgical Client Who Will Be Discharged to Home

The type of surgery, the client's condition, and the support system determine whether it is safe to discharge a client to home after surgery. Your assessment should focus on the following questions:

➤ What kind of care will be needed?

➤ Is the client able to take care of himself? If not, who is available to assist with care?

➤ Does the caregiver have the necessary skills to provide care?

➤ If not, can these skills be taught before the client is discharged?

➤ What features in the home environment will facilitate the client's progress? What features will inhibit progress? For example, can the client get to the bathroom? Can the client negotiate the stairs in the house?

➤ How will the client be followed after discharge? That is, how soon should he visit his physician? Will he receive home nursing care?

KnowledgeCheck 40-2

- List the information you should gather in the preoperative nursing history.
- What type of physical assessment is performed as part of the preoperative assessment?
- What laboratory tests are most commonly prescribed before surgery?

ThinkLike a Nurse 40-2

- What factors will affect your preoperative assessment of Mr. Singh (Meet Your Patient)?
- Describe how you might perform the assessment as well as provide physical care. What modifications, if any, should you make in his assessment?

ANALYSIS/NURSING DIAGNOSIS

As you learned in Chapter 4, nursing diagnoses describe the individualized needs of patients. However, preoperative patients share a common set of needs, regardless of their individual differences and the type of surgery they are to have. Consider the following examples:

- All preoperative patients need preoperative teaching, so it's not necessary to write a nursing diagnosis of Deficient Knowledge for every patient. Agency protocols or critical pathways will almost certainly mandate teaching.
- Almost all surgical patients have at least mild anxiety, and many of your routine actions will help to relieve anxiety, so there is no need to always include a diagnosis of Anxiety.

Key Point: *Do not put any nursing diagnosis on the care plan unless you plan to address it with something other than the routine preoperative interventions.*

Special Risks for Older Adults. Older adults, especially those older than age 70 and the frail elderly, are likely to need some individualized nursing diagnoses and collaborative problems (Table 40-2). They present unique risks because they often have other illnesses, but also because of certain physiological changes of aging. For example, older adults metabolize anesthetic agents differently from younger adults.

Individualized Nursing Diagnoses

Individualized nursing diagnoses for the preoperative patient evolve from your assessment. You should identify an actual nursing diagnosis only if the patient has the defining characteristics for it. Identify risk (potential) diagnoses only if the patient has an underlying condition that places him at higher risk than the average surgical patient. The following NANDA-I nursing diagnoses may be useful for certain preoperative patients.

- *Ineffective airway clearance* may be used for patients who have a preexisting health problem, such as bronchitis or emphysema.
- *Ineffective Coping* may be appropriate for a patient with extreme anxiety and concerns about the outcomes of the surgery.

Common Preoperative Screening Tests

Test	Uses
Urinalysis	To detect urinary tract infections (UTIs) and the presence of glucose or protein in the urine, which may indicate poorly controlled diabetes or renal disease
Complete blood count (CBC)	To detect irregularities in hemoglobin (Hgb) and hematocrit (Hct). A low Hg level is an indication of anemia, which may place the client at risk if significant blood loss occurs. Measures white blood cell (WBC) count as an indicator of immune function. Measures platelet count, which affects clotting ability
Electrocardiogram (ECG)	To detect cardiac dysrhythmias and other cardiac pathology
Chest x-ray examination	To detect underlying pulmonary disease; also to reveal heart size, as an indicator of heart function
Blood type and crossmatch	To identify blood type in the event that blood transfusion becomes necessary
Serum electrolytes	To detect sodium, potassium, chloride, magnesium, calcium, and pH imbalances, which affect cardiac and other organ function and fluid balance
Fasting blood sugar	To detect diabetes or poorly controlled diabetes
Comprehensive metabolic panel	Includes electrolytes, blood glucose, liver function tests (alanine aminotransferase [ALT], aspartate aminotransferase [AST]), serum albumin and protein, and renal function tests (blood urea nitrogen [BUN] and creatinine); used to detect underlying health problems that may affect surgical risk or outcome

Table 40-2 ➤ Special Risks for Older Adults

RISK FACTORS	POTENTIAL COMPLICATIONS (PC) AND NURSING DIAGNOSES
Most older adults have at least some degree of coronary artery disease.	▪ PC: Hypotension ▪ Risk for Falls secondary to postural hypotension
Age-related respiratory changes, such as decreased chest wall compliance, forced vital capacity, and diaphragmatic strength	▪ PC: Pneumonia ▪ PC: Atelectasis
Age-related skin changes: Dry, fragile skin; decreased turgor and elasticity	▪ Risk for Impaired Skin Integrity ▪ Risk for Impaired Tissue Integrity
Age-related musculoskeletal changes: Decreased bone mass and muscle fiber mass	▪ Risk for Impaired Mobility ▪ Risk for Falls
Comorbidities of the central nervous system are more common in older adults. Some conditions may be aggravated by surgery and anesthesia.	▪ PC: Dementia ▪ Risk for Acute Confusion
Age-related decrease in gastrointestinal motility	▪ PC: Ileus ▪ Risk for Aspiration secondary to vomiting
Age-related decreases in genitourinary function: decreased bladder tone, elasticity, and tone; decreased renal function	▪ PC: Side effects of medications ▪ PC: Renal complications ▪ PC: Urinary tract infection ▪ Risk for Impaired Skin Integrity r/t urinary incontinence

▪ *Latex Allergy Response* is appropriate for patients who have a known allergy to latex.
▪ *Risk for Latex Allergy Response* is appropriate for patients who have had multiple surgeries or urinary catheterizations; are in professions with daily exposure to latex; have a history of asthma; or are allergic to bananas, avocados, kiwi, chestnuts, or poinsettia plants. Do not use it routinely for all patients.

The following diagnoses are discussed in Table 40-3
▪ Anxiety
▪ Fear
▪ Disturbed Sleep Pattern
▪ Deficient Knowledge

ThinkLike a Nurse 40-3

Which, if any, of the preceding nursing diagnoses would be most appropriate for Mr. Singh (Meet Your Patient)? Do not use the potential complications in Table 40-2. Explain your reasoning.

PLANNING OUTCOMES/EVALUATION

The overall nursing goal in the preoperative phase is to prepare the patient adequately for surgery and to deliver him to the operating suite in the best condition possible. Outcomes that provide evidence of achieving this goal, and that are appropriate for nearly all preoperative patients, are that the patient:
▪ Is able to describe his surgical procedure in a basic manner.
▪ Provides informed consent.
▪ When asked, states what he can expect in the postoperative period.
▪ States he has very little anxiety.

Associated NOC outcomes for the preoperative nursing client depend, of course, on the nursing diagnoses you identify. For outcomes and goals using NOC terminology for the diagnoses Anxiety, Fear, Deficient Knowledge, and Disturbed Sleep Pattern, and for *individualized goals/outcome statements* you might write for those diagnoses, refer to Table 40-3.

PLANNING INTERVENTIONS/IMPLEMENTATION

For *NIC standardized interventions* and nursing activities designed to achieve the expected outcomes for the nursing diagnoses of Anxiety, Fear, Deficient Knowledge, and Disturbed Sleep Pattern, refer to Table 40-3.

Many preoperative nursing activities are routine interventions to be used for *all* preoperative patients, regardless of their nursing diagnoses. NIC has a special Perioperative Care domain (category) for such interventions. The following are the preoperative NIC interventions in that domain: Preoperative Coordination, Surgical Preparation, and Preoperative Teaching.

The following sections explain in more detail how to carry out routine interventions such as obtaining informed consent for the surgery, providing preoperative teaching, communicating with the surgical team, preparing the client physically, and transferring to the operating suite. Be sure to include parents and caregivers in your plan of care.

Confirm That Surgical Consent Has Been Obtained

Before a surgical procedure is performed, professional standards and the law require the surgeon to obtain the patient's informed consent. The signed consent form verifies that the

Table 40-3 ➤ Preoperative Patients: Selected Standardized Nursing Diagnoses, Outcomes, and Interventions

NURSING DIAGNOSES	SELECTED NOC OUTCOMES AND GOALS USING NOC INDICATORS	SELECTED NIC INTERVENTIONS AND NURSING ACTIVITIES (HIGHLIGHTED ACTIVITIES ARE ROUTINE NURSING MEASURES FOR ALL PREOPERATIVE PATIENTS)
Anxiety related to change in health 14 status **Comments:** *Anxiety may be mild, moderate, severe, or panic level. It may be related to the current change in health status or to concerns about being unable to provide care for loved ones. Make this diagnosis only if the client has symptoms such as restlessness, trembling, increased pulse, and so on that do not respond to routine preoperative interventions.*	**NOC outcomes:** Anxiety Level Anxiety Self-Control **NOC goals:** Patient will exhibit: ■ (5) No restlessness ■ (4) Only mild muscle and facial tension ■ (4) Only mild difficulty concentrating ■ (5) No increased blood pressure, pulse rate, or respiratory rate ■ (5) No physical signs of anxiety such as: dilated pupils, sweating, and dizziness ■ (3) Moderate verbalized anxiety **Individualized goals:** ■ Identifies symptoms that are indicators of her anxiety. ■ Communicates need for assistance.	**Anxiety Reduction** ■ Use a calm, reassuring approach. ■ Explain all procedures, including sensations likely to be experienced during the surgical procedure. ■ Seek to understand the patient's perspective of the situation. ■ Provide accurate factual information about the surgery. ■ Discuss common feelings and concerns that patients have about surgery. This helps the patient feel supported and less anxious. **Calming Technique** ■ Maintain eye contact with patient. ■ Encourage slow, purposeful deep breathing. **Presence** ■ Stay with the patient and provide assurance of safety and security during periods of anxiety. ■ Listen to the patient's concerns. ■ Administer medications as appropriate to reduce anxiety.
Fear related to unknown outcome of surgery and fear of pain that may result **Comments:** *Fear is a common reaction to surgery. Fear may be related to the unknown outcome of the surgery, to learning the diagnosis after a diagnostic procedure, and to the prospect of pain. Fear and Anxiety share several defining characteristics.*	**NOC outcomes:** Fear Level Fear Self-Control **NOC goals:** ■ (5) Exhibits no restlessness or irritability. ■ (5) Reports no difficulty concentrating. ■ (5) No physical signs of fear: increased BP, radial pulse rate, respiratory rate, sweating, dilated pupils, pale skin ■ (5) No verbalized fear ■ (5) No crying **Individualized goals:** ■ Does not exhibit physical signs of fear (e.g., pupil dilation; dry mouth; increased BP, pulse and respiratory rate). ■ Reports understanding of pain control measures to be used during and after surgery.	**Anxiety Reduction** ■ (See Anxiety diagnosis) **Coping Enhancement** ■ Assist the patient in developing an objective appraisal of the event ■ Evaluate the patient's decision-making ability. ■ Encourage the use of spiritual resources, if desired. **Preparatory Sensory Information** ■ Identify the typical sensations (what will be seen, felt, smelled, tasted, heard) the majority of patients describe as associated with each aspect of the procedure/treatment. ■ Personalize the information by using personal pronouns. **Security Enhancement** ■ Explain all tests and procedures to the patient/family. ■ Assist the patient to use coping responses that have been successful in the past.

Table 40-3 ➤ Preoperative Patients: Selected Standardized Nursing Diagnoses, Outcomes, and Interventions—cont'd

NURSING DIAGNOSES	SELECTED NOC OUTCOMES AND GOALS USING NOC INDICATORS	SELECTED NIC INTERVENTIONS AND NURSING ACTIVITIES (HIGHLIGHTED ACTIVITIES ARE ROUTINE NURSING MEASURES FOR ALL PREOPERATIVE PATIENTS)
Deficient Knowledge of preoperative procedures and postoperative expectations **Comments:** All patients need preoperative teaching, a routine intervention; so you do not usually need a Deficient Knowledge diagnosis. If you believe the patient may not learn, or that the information is too complex to remember, then identify the problem likely to result from the Deficient Knowledge (e.g., Ineffective Management of Therapeutic Regimen, or Risk for Infection)	**NOC outcomes:** Knowledge: Disease Process Knowledge: Treatment Procedure(s) **NOC goals:** Provides: ■ (3) Moderate description of specific disease process ■ (4) Substantial description of strategies to minimize disease progression ■ (4) Substantial description of signs and symptoms of disease complications **Individualized goals:** ■ Verbalizes rationale for pre- and postoperative interventions. ■ Describes or demonstrates. postoperative expectations (i.e., deep breathing, turning/position changes).	**Teaching: Preoperative** ■ Inform the patient/significant others how long surgery is expected to last. ■ Determine the patient's previous surgical experiences and level of knowledge related to surgery. ■ Provide time for the patient to ask questions and discuss concerns. ■ Instructing the patient or caregiver how to participate in the care ■ Describe preoperative routines (e.g., anesthesia, diet, bowel preparation, tests/labs, voiding, skin preparation, IV therapy, clothing, family waiting area, transportation to operating room). ■ Describe any preoperative medications, the effects these will have on the patient, and the rationale for using them. ■ Inform significant others of the place to wait for the results of the surgery. ■ Introduce the patient to perioperative staff as appropriate. ■ Discuss possible pain control measures. ■ Describe postoperative routines/equipment (e.g., medications, respiratory treatments, tubes, machines, support hose, surgical dressings, ambulation, diet, family visitation) and explain their purpose. ■ Instruct the patient in postoperative deep breathing exercises, splinting incision, coughing. ■ Reinforce information provided by other healthcare team members, as appropriate. ■ Include the family/significant others [in the teaching-learning process] as appropriate.
Disturbed Sleep Pattern related to anxiety about the upcoming surgery	**NOC outcome:** Sleep **NOC goals:** ■ (4) Mild interrupted sleep ■ (5) Hours of sleep (at least 5 hr/24 hr), not compromised ■ (4) Sleeps through the night consistently, mildly compromised. **Individualized goals:** ■ Reports minimal compromise in hours of sleep and sleep pattern. ■ No difficulty falling and staying asleep reported or observed	**Sleep Enhancement** ■ Determine the patient's usual sleep-activity pattern. ■ Determine effects of patient's current medications on sleep pattern. ■ Adjust environment (lighting, noise, temperature, etc.) to promote sleep. ■ Demonstrate and explain the procedure for progressive muscle relaxation. ■ Administer medication to promote sleep, as appropriate.

Sources: Bulechek, G. M., Butcher, H. K., & Dochterman, J. M. (Eds.). (2008). *Nursing interventions classification (NIC)* (5th ed.). St. Louis, MO: C.V. Mosby; Moorhead, S., Johnson, M., Maas, M., et al. (Eds.). (2008). *Nursing outcomes classification (NOC)* (4th ed.). St. Louis, MO: C.V. Mosby; and NANDA-I. (2012). *Nursing diagnoses: Definitions and classification 2012–2014.* Ames, IA: Wiley-Blackwell. Used with permission.

surgeon and patient have communicated adequately about the surgery (Dale, Rothrock, & McEwen, 2003). **Informed consent** requires that the patient understood the communication and was not coerced (pressured) to consent. The patient must be alert, rational, mentally competent, and not sedated when he signs; and the information must be given to him in a language and vocabulary that he can understand. If a patient is not capable of giving informed consent (e.g., is unconscious or has dementia) or if the patient is a minor child, in most states a family member, conservator, or legal guardian may give consent for the procedure.

Key Point: *The surgeon is responsible for (1) giving the patient the necessary information and (2) determining the patient's competence to make an informed decision about the surgery. You are responsible for verifying that the surgical consent form is signed and witnessed.*

Often you will obtain the patient's signature and document on the preoperative checklist that you have done so. As a patient advocate, you should first verify with the patient that the physician has explained the procedure and answered all his questions: Ask the patient to state what he was told during the consent process. If the patient has questions or if you have any questions about the patient's competence, notify the surgeon, and delay sending the patient to surgery. Be sure to document these conversations, and document in the nursing notes that the surgeon was notified of any additional questions or concerns.

Informed consent helps protect patients from having a surgery they do not understand or want, and the signed document protects the healthcare agency and workers from later claims that the patient did not consent to have the procedure. Also see Chapters 42 and 43 regarding informed consent, if you would like more information.

KnowledgeCheck 40-3

- Who is responsible for obtaining informed consent for the surgical procedure?
- What are the nursing responsibilities related to informed consent?

Provide Preoperative Teaching

Preoperative teaching prepares the patient for the surgical experience, allays fears, and decreases the risks of postoperative complications.

What to Teach

The type of surgery influences the content of your teaching. For example, if the patient is scheduled for an outpatient knee arthroscopy (visualization of the joint) under spinal anesthesia, the teaching plan needs to describe the procedure and the anticipated discharge of the patient within hours after surgery. This is different from the teaching for a patient who will have cardiac surgery and spend a number of days in the hospital. In general, preoperative teaching should focus on explaining what will happen before, during, and after surgery. You will find specific teaching content in the Preoperative Teaching interventions for Deficient Knowledge in Table 40-3. Also refer to Clinical Insight 40-1.

You will also need to explain what patients and families can do to help safeguard against surgical site infection (see the Self-Care box, Teaching Patients How to Help Prevent Surgical Site Infections).

Self-Care

Teaching Patients How to Help Prevent Surgical Site Infections

Before Surgery

- If you smoke, stop. Those who smoke are more likely to get infections.
- Discuss your health problems with your surgeon (e.g., diabetes, allergies). These can affect incision healing.
- Ask your surgeon if you should have antibiotics before surgery.
- Don't shave near where you will have surgery. Not all procedures require hair removal, but if they do, it should be done with electric clippers. If someone starts to use a razor to shave you, speak up.

After Surgery

- Be sure family and friends wash their hands or use alcohol-based hand rub before and after they visit you.
- When anyone examines you or checks your incision, ask them if they have washed their hands (or used alcohol-based hand rub).
- Wash your hands before and after caring for your own incision.
- Do not allow family and friends to touch your incision or the surgical dressing.
- Be sure you know how to care for your incision before you go home.
- If you have fever or redness, pain or drainage at the surgery site, call your physician right away.

Source: Adapted from CDC (n.d.) (updated 2010). Having surgery? What you should know before you go. Retrieved August 6, 2011, from http://www.cdc.gov/features/SafeSurgery/

How to Teach

You can use written instructions, video presentations, phone contact, or face-to-face discussion to provide preoperative teaching. Teach in a language that the patient understands and at a level that is easily understood. Use terms the patient understands clearly, that is, avoid medical jargon that the patient could misunderstand. Include family members in the teaching as much as possible and as much as desired by the patient; provide written materials to reinforce your instruction. See Chapter 26 if you need to review patient teaching techniques and information about health literacy.

Obtain an interpreter for translation if the patient speaks a language that you do not speak. When possible, avoid using family members as translators in order to protect the patient's privacy or avoid a bias in translation (see Chapter 15 if you need more information about using a translator).

If the patient is a child or dependent adult, be sure to include the parents or caregivers in the teaching and assessments. So that the child better understands what will happen before, during, and after surgery, you might teach using dolls or age-appropriate toys. Play can be one of the most effective ways for kids to learn. For instance, have the child

Clinical Insight 40-1 ➤ Preoperative Teaching

Explain what to expect before surgery.

- Explain the planned preoperative testing—lab tests, x-ray studies, ECG, and so on.
- Discuss skin preparation, including preoperative wash with an antibacterial product if this is included in the treatment plan.
- Discuss prescribed preoperative medications.
- Outline activities that will occur before surgery, such as insertion of an IV, placement of a urinary catheter, or cardiac monitoring.
- Review the preoperative restriction of fluid and food. Often the patient is to be NPO for at least 8 hours before the planned start of surgery. Some guidelines indicate that most children, and healthy adults, can drink clear liquids until 2 hours before surgery (The Joanna Briggs Institute, 2008b; "Practice Guidelines for Preoperative Fasting," 2011).
- If the patient is having surgery on the gastrointestinal (GI) tract, explain that an additional bowel prep may be ordered (e.g., a low-residue diet beginning 1 week before surgery, and a liquid diet for the 48 hours preceding surgery). Patients having GI surgery also may have enemas before surgery.
- Explain the need to remove jewelry, makeup, hearing aids, glasses, contact lenses, and any removable dental prostheses before being transported to the operating suite. It is best to have a family member take valuable belongings home for safekeeping.
- Tell the patient that a member of the anesthesia team will speak with him about the proposed anesthesia before surgery.
- Give the patient and family a tentative schedule for the operative day, including the time to arrive at the hospital or surgery center.

Explain what to expect in the operative suite.

- Inform the patient and family where relatives may wait during surgery.
- Describe the activities that may occur in the preoperative holding area.
- Describe the operating room and the activities that the patient may anticipate there.

- Explain that the anesthesiologist or nurse anesthetist will monitor the patient and is responsible for keeping him comfortable with medications throughout the entire procedure.
- Describe the types of people who may be present in the operative suite. This is particularly important if the patient is not receiving a general anesthetic.

Explain what to expect after surgery.

- Explain that the patient will initially be cared for in the postanesthesia care unit. After a period of observation, he will be transferred to the surgical unit. Note that some patients may be transferred directly to a critical care unit after surgery. If this is expected, inform the patient and family preoperatively.
- Family may visit after the patient has been admitted and assessed on the surgical unit.
- Tell the patient what to expect in terms of dressings, equipment, and monitoring devices.
- Describe the types of assessments that will be performed.
- Explain that pain medication will be given to keep the patient comfortable. If he experiences pain, he should tell the nursing staff.
- Discuss the usual progression of recovery, including activity level, deep breathing, coughing, leg exercises, and dietary intake.
- Discuss the anticipated length of stay.
- Teach the patient how to move into and out of bed after surgery.
- Teach the importance of deep breathing and coughing, especially after general anesthesia. Demonstrate how to splint the incision to facilitate deep breathing and coughing. Refer to Procedure 40-1.
- Teach and emphasize the importance of leg exercises to minimize the risk of thrombus formation. Refer to Procedure 40-1.
- If decreased activity or prolonged bedrest is anticipated, explain the use of anitembolism stockings or sequential compression devices. Refer to Procedure 40-2.

Note: If the patient is to be discharged the day of surgery, inform him in advance about what to wear to the facility, and explain that he must arrange for a responsible adult to drive him home.

give medicine to her doll with an empty syringe or listen to its "heart" with your stethoscope. Simple language is a must! For example, you'd say to a young child, "Lie on your tummy, please."

When to Teach

For elective surgery, many patients have a scheduled preoperative assessment about a week before the surgery. The session

may include preoperative testing, an appointment with the anesthesia staff, signing the consent form, and planned preoperative teaching.

Patients undergoing emergency surgery usually require extensive physical care preoperatively. You may need to give IV fluids, transfuse blood, treat for pain, and administer many medications, as in the case of Mr. Singh (Meet Your Patient). The urgency of such surgeries may limit the time you

have for teaching. However, you should always teach the patient as much as possible to prepare him for the surgical experience.

Prepare the Patient Physically for Surgery

Physical preparation of the patient for surgery involves several nursing concerns.

Maintaining Normothermia. Recent evidence-based guidelines stress that maintaining a normal body temperature helps produce good surgical outcomes (Hooper, Chard, Clifford, et al., 2009). In addition to monitoring temperature, you can provide passive thermal care measures, such as providing blankets, socks, and head coverings; and keeping the room temperature at or above 75°F (24°C). Some agencies use forced-air warming gowns or mattresses to pre-warm patients before surgery, as well as in the intraoperative and postoperative periods.

Nutritional Status. Anxiety and anesthesia reduce gastrointestinal motility. To decrease the risk of nausea and vomiting, patients usually fast, taking no food or liquids (NPO) for 8 hours before surgery. Stress to patients and family the importance of fasting (for the prescribed length of time) to avoid the danger of aspiration. You should know, though, that years of evidence support shorter fasting times than you will see used in most institutions. The American Society of Anesthesiologists (ASA) preoperative fasting guidelines for healthy patients, recommends ingesting clear liquids up to 2 hours before surgery – and even a light meal up to 6 hours before surgery (Crenshaw, 2011; "Practice Guidelines for Preoperative Fasting," 2011).

Skin Preparation. Depending on the surgery and facility, patients may be asked to shower or scrub the surgical site with soap or an antibacterial solution (e.g., 4% chlorhexadine gluconate, Betadine) the evening before surgery and the morning of the surgery. Studies demonstrate that this reduces bacterial colonization on the skin, but do not clearly prove that it reduces surgical infection (National Guideline Clearinghouse [NGC], 2009; National Institute for Health and Clinical Excellence [NICE], 2008). Final skin preparation and hair removal, if done, should be completed before taking the patient into the surgical suite.

Bowel Preparation. Enemas are now used primarily for surgical procedures of the colon, not for all surgeries. To empty the colon of feces, patients are asked to consume a low-residue diet for several days before surgery and are given a regimen of medications and/or enemas to clear the bowel. Stress the importance of adhering to the regimen to limit the risk of contaminating the operative site with feces.

Urinary Elimination. Indwelling catheters are not routinely inserted for surgery. Catheterization may be prescribed if it is important to keep the bladder empty during surgery or if fluid status is being carefully monitored. ✚ If a catheter is not prescribed, have the patient void before receiving preoperative medications. The patient could fall if he gets out of bed after being sedated or given opioids for pain.

Preoperative Medications. The anesthesiologist may prescribe preoperative medications to relax the patient, reduce respiratory secretions, or reduce the risk of vomiting and aspiration (Table 40-4). The medication is prescribed at a prearranged time (e.g., at 0615) or it may be prescribed to give "on call." You will give an on-call medication when the surgical suite staff notifies you it is time to do so.

Table 40-4 ➤ Preoperative Medications		
TYPE OF MEDICATION	**USE**	**EXAMPLES**
Antibiotics	Reduce the microbial burden of intraoperative contamination to a level that cannot overwhelm host defenses	Cephalosporins (e.g., cefazolin, cefoxitin), clindamycin, vancomycin
Anticholinergics (e.g., phenothiazines)	Reduce oral and pulmonary secretions, prevent laryngospasms, prevent bradycardia	Atropine (Atropisol), chlorpromazine (Thorazine), scopolamine (Maldemar), glycopyrrolate (Robinul)
Anxiolytics (e.g., benzodiazepines)	Control anxiety, calming	Alprazolam (Xanax), clonazepam (Klonopin), diazepam (Valium), lorazepam (Ativan), midazolam (Versed)
Antihistamines	Provide sedation and antiemetic effects	Hydroxyzine (Vistaril), diphenhydramine (Benadryl)
Barbiturates	Provide sedation without significant cardiopulmonary depression	Secobarbital (Seconal), pentobarbital (Nembutal)
H_2 receptor antagonists	Reduce gastric acidity	Cimetidine (Tagamet), ranitidine (Zantac)
Hypnotics	Provide sedation and increase the duration of sleep	Temazepam (Restoril)
Neuroleptics	Provide sedative, antiemetic, and anticonvulsant effects	Droperidol (Inapsine), Innovar (fentanyl and droperidol)
Opioid analgesics	Provide pain relief and sedation; induce anesthesia	Fentanyl (Sublimaze), meperidine (Demerol), morphine (Duramorph)

Antibiotics are often administered prophylactically to help prevent postoperative infections. You will usually administer the antibiotic intravenously, timed so that a bactericidal concentration of the drug will be present in serum and tissues by the time the incision is made (usually within the hour preceding incision, just as the patient is going to the surgical suite) (Mangram, Horan, Pearson, et al., 1999; NGC, 2009; NICE, 2008).

Routine Medications. Many routine medications are held (not administered) on the day of surgery. For example, an insulin-dependent diabetic patient may be instructed to hold her morning injection or administer half of the normal dose. The patient needs less insulin because her NPO status will keep her blood sugar lower than usual. The anesthesiologist will monitor the blood sugar in the operating room and give additional insulin if needed. Some patients may be instructed to stop routine medications several days before surgery. For example, a client receiving warfarin for anticoagulation may need to stop the medication 7 days before surgery.

Prostheses. Before being transported to the operating suite, the patient must remove all artificial body parts, such as dentures, artificial limbs, or contact lenses. Wigs, eyeglasses, makeup, and jewelry must also be removed.

Antiembolism Stockings. Also referred to as "TED hose," **antiembolism stockings** are elastic stockings that compress the veins of the legs and increase venous return to the heart (Fig. 40-1). They may be applied preoperatively to prevent venous pooling during surgery and decrease the risk of thrombus formation. Older adults and those with risk factors for venous thromboembolism are most in need of antiembolism stockings (Bartley, 2006). Risk factors include the following conditions:

- Venous stasis (such as occurs with bedrest, lengthy surgery, varicose veins, and heart failure)
- Vascular wall injury, which initiates clotting (e.g., surgery, IV catheter, irritating IV drugs, prior deep vein thrombus)
- Hypercoagulability (e.g., estrogen therapy, oral contraceptive use, cancer, dehydration, pregnancy)
- Older age, especially adults with other risk factors

Stockings may extend from foot to knee, or foot to thigh. Some have an opening at the toes that allows you to assess circulation in the feet. Antiembolism stockings must be sized and applied correctly in order to be effective (see Procedure 40-2). Stockings are contraindicated for some patients (e.g., those with peripheral arterial disease) (Joanna Briggs Institute, 2008a; Winslow & Brosz, 2008).

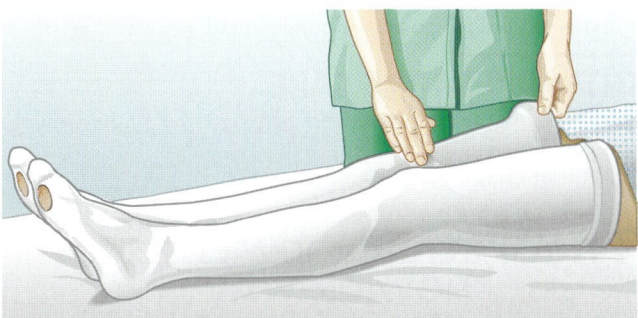

FIGURE 40-1 Antiembolism stockings compress the veins of the legs and increase venous return to the heart.

Take Measures to Prevent Wrong Patient, Wrong Site, Wrong Surgery

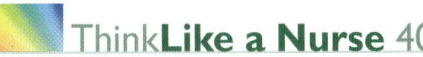 To help prevent patient misidentification and wrong-site surgery (The Joint Commission, 2011; Ridge, 2008):

- Use a preoperative checklist to confirm that appropriate documents are available and the appropriate activities have been performed.
- Verify the patient's identity before the patient leaves the preoperative area.
- Mark the surgical site before surgery. Use a permanent marker that will not be removed by the surgical skin prep, and involve the patient in the marking process.
- Take a time-out with all team members before starting the procedure.

Communicate With the Surgical Team

The most common root cause of medical errors is communication failure (AHRQ, 2003). For this reason, good communication is essential for patient safety in perioperative care. The following are elements of successful communication. Surgical team members:

- Receive a summary of the plan of care (e.g., a short briefing by the surgeon) and develop a shared understanding of the plan.
- Speak up and are assertive with concerns about the procedure or decisions.
- Ask questions to clarify confusion.
- Acknowledge that they have heard and understood.
- Ask for and provide feedback (e.g., read back) on critical information.
- Use standard terminology (e.g., checklists). In one large, long-term study, use of surgical checklists was found to reduce the number of deaths from surgery by more than 40% (Haynes, Weiser, Berry, et al., 2009).

Two-minute briefings just before surgery, led by the attending surgeon using a standardized format, have been found to improve communication and reduce delays and wrong-site surgery (Makary, Mukherjee, Sexton, et al., 2007). Surgical briefings encourage team members to talk when there is no problem, so they are more likely to speak up when they have misgivings or when problems occur (Hendrickson, Wadhera, & El Bardissi, 2008).

KnowledgeCheck 40-4

- Identify topics that should be discussed in preoperative teaching.
- Describe the typical physical preparation of a client undergoing surgery.

ThinkLike a Nurse 40-4

- What aspects of preoperative teaching should you stress when caring for Mr. Singh (Meet Your Patient)?
- A bowel preparation is typically part of preoperative preparation for a client having colon surgery. Do you think this will be part of Mr. Singh's physical preparation? Why or why not?

Transfer to the Operative Suite

Once you have completed your preoperative care, the patient is ready for transport by stretcher to the operative area, usually to the surgical holding area (Fig. 40-2). The completed

Toward Evidence-Based Practice

Makary, M., Mukherjee, A., Sexton, J., et al. (2007). Operating room briefings and wrong-site surgery. *Journal of the American College of Surgeons*, 204, 236–243.

These researchers evaluated the impact of operating room briefings on coordination of care and the perceived risk for wrong-site surgery. A questionnaire was administered to 154 surgeons, anesthesiologists, and nurses before and after beginning an OR briefing program. The authors compared care provider perceptions before and after implementation of the briefings. The OR briefings were found to significantly (1) reduce perceived risk for wrong-site surgery and (2) improve perceived collaboration among the OR team.

Haynes, A., Weiser, T., Berry, W., et al. (2009). A surgical safety checklist to reduce morbidity and mortality in a global population. *New England Journal of Medicine*, 360(5), 491–499.

These researchers investigated whether using a surgical safety checklist designed to improve team communication and consistency of care would reduce complications and deaths associated with surgery. Using eight hospitals in eight cities globally, they collected data from 3,733 patients 16 years of age and older before introduction of the checklist. They later collected data from similar patients after the introduction of the checklist. The death rate was 1.5% before the use of checklist and 0.8% afterward. Inpatient complications fell from 11.0% before to 7.0% after.

Imagine that you are the OR nurse manager and that the incidence of wrong-site surgery in your hospital is higher than the national average. You want to introduce some changes in the OR, and need to "start small," by introducing changes gradually, one at a time. You are trying to decide whether to use an OR briefing program or a surgical safety checklist. In practice, you would have more studies to rely on, but pretend you must base your decision on just the two studies described here.

1. Before introducing an OR briefing program, what would you like to know about briefings that the first study does not tell you?

2. What information is missing from the summary of the second study that you will need in order to know if a surgical safety checklist would be helpful in your situation?

 Go to Chapter 40, **Toward Evidence-Based Practice Suggested Responses,** on Davis*Plus*.

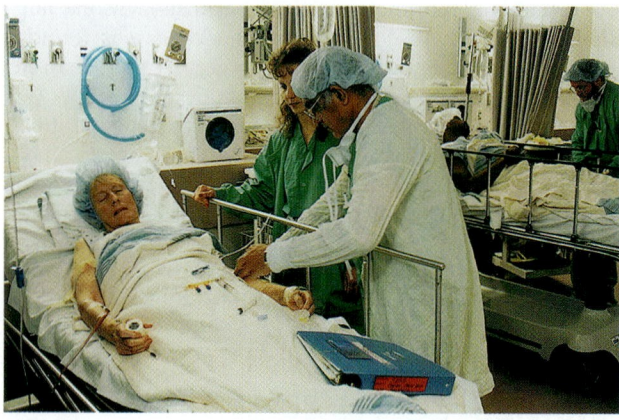

FIGURE 40-2 Surgical holding area.

preoperative checklist and the patient's chart must accompany the patient. Lock up valuables according to agency policy, or have the patient's family keep them. Occasionally, especially if the patient has a significant sensory deficit, the patient can wear his hearing aid or glasses to the surgical suite. You will need to arrange this in advance with the surgical staff or anesthesia team.

Often children are permitted to bring a favorite toy with them to the OR to provide comfort. Children may fear being separated from their parents, so arrange for parents to spend time with the child immediately before the surgery and as soon as possible after the surgery. Keep the parents informed, and let them know what to expect.

Prepare the Postoperative Room

If you transfer the patient to the surgical suite from a nursing unit in the hospital, you should prepare the room for the patient's return after surgery (see Figure 40-3). In many institutions, the patient is transported to surgery using the bed that is in his hospital room, so the following steps may vary:

- Put clean linens on the bed, including pads to protect the linen from drainage. Fold the linens back to the end of the bed.
- Raise the bed to stretcher height, and lock the wheels.
- Move furniture and equipment so that the stretcher can be placed directly against the bed.
- If needed, set up suction, oxygen, or other special equipment.
- Place the following equipment in the room:
  Stethoscope, manometer, thermometer (to measure vital signs)
  IV pole
  Emesis basin
  Tissues
  A clean gown, washcloth, and towel
  Extra pillows for positioning the patient

INTRAOPERATIVE CARE

The **intraoperative phase** begins when the patient enters the operating suite and ends when she is admitted to the postanesthesia care unit.

Theoretical Knowledge
knowing **why**

To provide intraoperative care, you will need theoretical knowledge of the roles of the various members of the

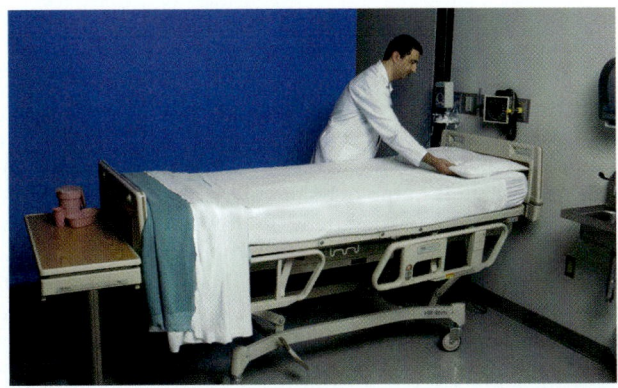

FIGURE 40-3 Open bed prepared for a patient's return from surgery.

intraoperative team and of the different types of anesthesia that are used.

Operative Personnel

The personnel who attend the client during the surgical procedure are called the *intraoperative team*. The team is divided into members who must use sterile technique and those who use clean technique (see Chapter 22 if you need to review medical and surgical asepsis). During the intraoperative phase, registered nurses (RNs) can function as the scrub nurse, circulating nurse, or registered nurse first assistant. Each of these roles contributes to the safe care of surgical clients.

Sterile Team. Members of the sterile intraoperative team include the surgeon, surgical assistant, and scrub person. Before beginning the surgery, they perform a surgical scrub of the hands and arms, dry with sterile towels, and don sterile gowns and gloves. (To review these procedures,

see Chapter 22.) Sterile team members are the only persons allowed to enter the sterile field (that is, the client and the area immediately surrounding the client). Creation of the operative field is explained in Clinical Insight 40-2.

The **scrub nurse** can be an RN, licensed vocational nurse (LVN), licensed practical nurse (LPN), or a surgical technician. The scrub nurse sets up the sterile field, prepares the surgical instruments, assists with the sterile draping of the patient, anticipates and responds to the surgeon's needs, and maintains the integrity of the sterile field. A **registered nurse first assistant (RNFA)** is an RN with additional education and training in surgical technique. The RNFA serves as an assistant to the surgeon to perform the surgical procedure, a role that has historically been filled by physicians.

Clean Team. Team members who abide by clean technique (medical asepsis) include the anesthesiologist or nurse anesthetist, the circulating RN, biomedical technicians, and radiology technicians. These personnel never enter the sterile field, but instead function around and beyond it.

An **anesthesiologist** or a **nurse anesthetist (CRNA)** induces amnesia, analgesia, and muscle relaxation or paralysis with anesthesia. His role is to continuously monitor and evaluate the patient's responses to the anesthetic agent and the surgical procedure. CRNAs administer more than half of all anesthetics in the United States.

The **circulating nurse** is an RN who applies the nursing process to coordinate all activities in the operating room. She is a client advocate who continuously monitors the client and the sterile field maintains a safe, comfortable environment; communicates with appropriate personnel outside the operating room; responds to emergencies; and, in some cases, administers sedation to the patient. An important aspect of the circulating nurse's role is to attend to the patient during the induction of anesthesia.

Clinical Insight 40-2 ► **Creating an Operative Field**

- A nonsterile team member (usually the circulating nurse) performs a surgical prep, using a scrub agent and "paint," to cleanse the operative site. Antiseptic agents must be approved by the U.S. Food and Drug Administration (FDA) and approved by the agency's infection control professional. Chlorhexidine and povidone-iodine solutions are most commonly used.
- The operative field encompasses the patient and the immediate surrounding area
  Creation of the sterile field proceeds as follows:
- Don head covering and shoe covers before entering the surgical suite.
- Perform a surgical scrub.
- Don sterile gown, gloves, and other surgical attire (e.g., mask).
- Cover the area surrounding the operative site with sterile drapes so that only the patient's operative area is exposed.
- Place sterile draping over the remainder of the patient's body.

- (In most cases) suspend a vertical drape at neck level so the client's head and airway are accessible to the anesthesiologist or nurse anesthetist (who is not sterile). For neurosurgery, even the head is draped, and the anesthesiologist or nurse anesthetist sits to the side of the head.

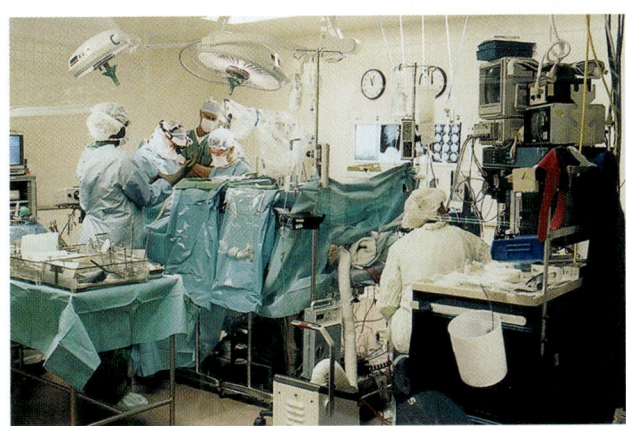

KnowledgeCheck 40-5

- Identify the intraoperative nursing roles that are part of the sterile intraoperative team and those that are part of the clean intraoperative team.
- Which nursing roles are always held by a registered nurse?

Types of Anesthesia

During surgery, anesthesia is used to obtain **analgesia** (control of pain), muscle relaxation or paralysis, and **amnesia** (memory loss). Anesthesia is classified as general, conscious sedation, or regional.

General Anesthesia

General anesthesia produces rapid unconsciousness and loss of sensation. The anesthesiologist or nurse anesthetist administers inhaled and intravenous medications that depress the patient's central nervous system (CNS) and relax the musculature. Muscle relaxants, paralyzing agents, narcotics, barbiturates, and inhaled gases are some of the agents used during general anesthesia.

Advantages of General Anesthesia

- The patient is unconscious, so she experiences no anxiety that might affect cardiac and respiratory functioning.
- The muscles are relaxed, so the patient remains completely motionless during the surgical procedure.
- Anesthesia can be adjusted to accommodate age, physical condition, and the length of the procedure. The anesthetist can increase or decrease the dosage without interrupting the procedure. Also, if surgical complications occur, the anesthesia can be continued for longer than originally planned.

Disadvantages of General Anesthesia

- The respiratory and circulatory muscles are depressed, so mechanical ventilation is needed while the patient is under the effects of the anesthetic.
- General anesthesia predisposes the patient to pneumonia and thrombophlebitis in the postoperative period.
- General anesthesia creates a risk for death, heart attack, stroke, and malignant hyperthermia. **Malignant hyperthermia** is a rare, often fatal, metabolic condition that can occur during the use of muscle relaxants and inhalation anesthesia. Metabolism increases in the skeletal muscles, they become rigid, and body temperature rises rapidly. Predisposition to this condition is inherited.
- Frequent minor complaints after general anesthesia include sore throat (from intubation), nausea and vomiting (from relaxation of gastrointestinal smooth muscle), headache, uncontrollable shivering, and confusion.

Conscious Sedation

Conscious sedation is an alternative form of anesthesia that provides intravenous sedation and analgesia without producing unconsciousness. During conscious sedation, the patient may feel sleepy but is aware of his surroundings, can be easily aroused by touch or speech, and can talk with the surgical team. Nevertheless, blood pressure, heart rate, respiratory rate, and oxygen saturation are monitored, and the patient usually receives oxygen via nasal cannula during the procedure. Because of the amnesic effect of many of the medications, the patient may not recall aspects of the procedure afterward. Advantages are that (1) pain and anxiety are adequately controlled without the risks of general anesthesia, and (2) recovery is rapid. Conscious sedation is used for procedures such as bronchoscopy and cosmetic surgery, but it is not practical for highly anxious patients.

Regional Anesthesia

Regional anesthesia prevents pain by interrupting nerve impulses to and from the area of the procedure. The patient remains alert but is numb in the involved area. Regional anesthesia may be administered by infiltration of the surgical site and surrounding tissue with local anesthetics, such as lidocaine (Xylocaine) or bupivacaine (Marcaine). These medications may also be injected into and around specific nerves to depress the sensory, motor, and/or sympathetic impulses of a limited area of the body.

Regional anesthesia is low in cost, simple to administer, and requires a minimal recovery period. It is especially suitable for minor, ambulatory procedures. However, many patients are apprehensive about being able to see and hear the procedure. Regional anesthesia may not be practical if the patient is highly anxious or if adequate pain control cannot be achieved. Techniques for achieving regional anesthesia include the following.

Peripheral Nerve Block. A **nerve block** is the injection of an anesthetic into and around a nerve or group of nerves (e.g., the facial nerve). A **Bier (intravenous) block** is a technique in which the anesthetist places a tourniquet on an arm or leg, and then injects a local anesthetic agent intravenously below the level of the tourniquet. The tourniquet is maintained at a pressure that limits venous return but continues to allow arterial circulation. The patient feels no pain in the extremity as long as the tourniquet is in place. Advantages of the Bier block are its rapid onset and recovery time. Also, the tourniquet decreases bleeding during the surgical procedure and prevents systemic absorption of the local anesthetic. However, when the procedure is finished, the tourniquet is deflated, and there is potential for systemic absorption of the anesthetic. To prevent tissue damage, the tourniquet must not be left in place for more than 2 hours.

Spinal Anesthesia. The injection of an anesthetic into the cerebrospinal fluid (CSF) in the subarachnoid space is known as **spinal anesthesia** (Fig. 40-4A). This injection blocks sensation and movement below the level of the injection. Spinal anesthesia is often used for surgical procedures in the lower abdomen, pelvis, and lower extremities. This technique allows the patient to remain conscious during the procedure and usually does not depress respirations. Occasionally a higher level of spinal anesthesia is achieved than intended—that is, the medication may migrate upward in the spinal fluid. This can depress respirations and cardiac rate. Placing the patient in Fowler's position may prevent respiratory paralysis.

Side effects of spinal anesthesia include hypotension, nausea, vomiting, urinary retention, and headache from leakage of CSF. A headache after spinal anesthesia must be closely monitored and may require additional treatment by the anesthesia staff.

The blood pressure may also decrease suddenly due to pervasive vasodilatation—the anesthesia blocks the sympathetic vasomotor nerves, which normally maintain muscle tone in peripheral blood vessels. Patients with these complications often require ventilation and support of blood pressure during surgery, so they must be carefully monitored during surgery and in the recovery period.

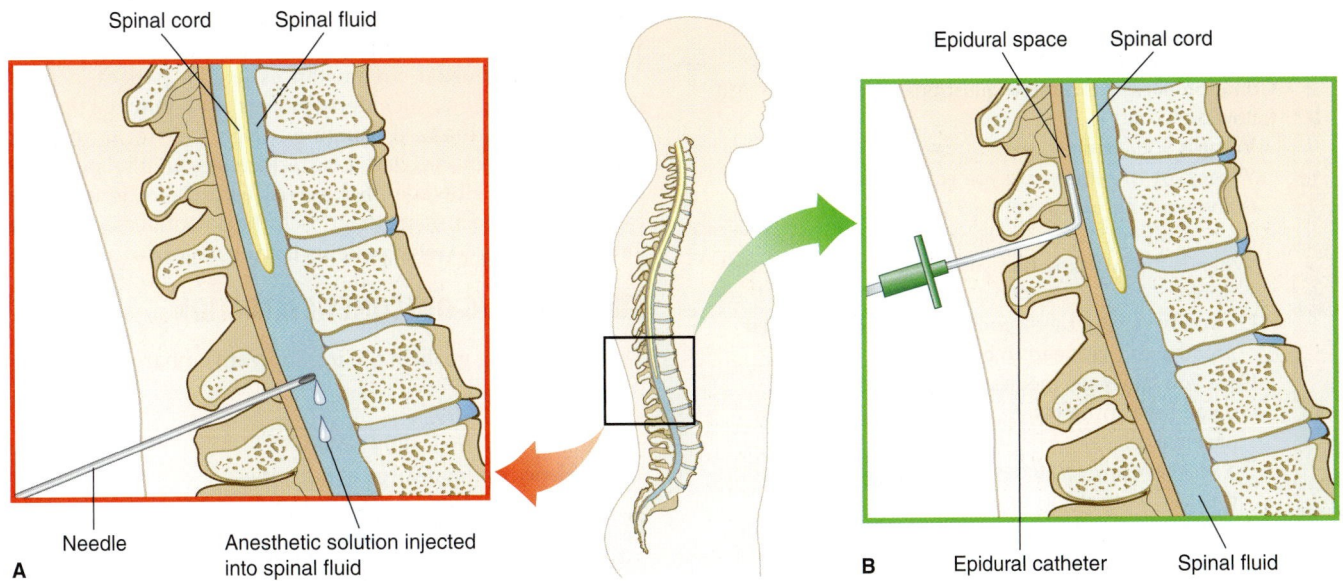

FIGURE 40-4 A. Spinal anesthesia is the injection of a local anesthetic into the subarachnoid space to block sensation and movement. B. Continuous epidural anesthesia can be used to provide postoperative analgesia.

Epidural Anesthesia. Epidural anesthesia requires insertion of a thin catheter into the epidural space (Fig. 40-4B). Anesthetic agents are infused through the catheter to produce loss of sensation. Epidural anesthesia can be used as a surgical anesthetic and to provide postoperative analgesia. Advantages and disadvantages of epidural anesthesia are similar to those of spinal anesthesia. Epidural anesthesia is safer than spinal anesthesia because the anesthetic does not enter the subarachnoid space and the depth of anesthesia is not as great. However, drugs intended for epidural administration are of a higher concentration than those for spinal administration; so if the medication is inadvertently injected too deeply (into the subarachnoid space), hypotension and respiratory paralysis occur, and temporary mechanical ventilation is necessary.

Local Anesthesia

Local anesthesia produces loss of pain sensation at the desired site (e.g., a wound to be sutured, a skin growth to be removed). It is typically used for minor procedures. However, after finishing a major surgery, the surgeon may infiltrate the operative area with local anesthetics to provide postoperative pain relief. Local anesthetics may be applied topically or injected. A **topical anesthetic** is applied directly to the skin and mucous membranes. Lidocaine (Xylocaine) and benzocaine (EMLA cream, T-caine) are commonly used because they are rapidly absorbed and rapid acting.

KnowledgeCheck 40-6

- What is the purpose of anesthesia?
- Under what type(s) of anesthesia does the client remain conscious?

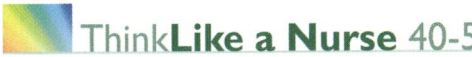 ThinkLike a Nurse 40-5

What form of anesthesia is Mr. Singh (Meet Your Patient) most likely to receive? Why?

PracticalKnowledge
knowing **how**

When a patient arrives in the surgical suite the nursing focus is on safe and successful completion of the surgery.

ASSESSMENT

The circulating nurse greets the client in the preoperative holding area and performs a brief assessment. The nurse first verifies that the surgical consent has been signed and witnessed and that the preoperative checklist is complete. The nurse then assesses the client's anxiety level and physical condition. The next steps are to measure the vital signs; examine the surgical site; and inspect IV lines, drainage tubes, and catheters. Often the circulating nurse or the anesthetist starts an IV line in the holding area if one is not already present. A preoperative medication may be given in the holding area. Vital signs are monitored often, or even continuously, during the intraoperative period.

For common interview questions to use in the intraoperative period, see the accompanying Assessment Box, Intraoperative Care Questionnaire. In addition to the checklist completed in the preoperative period, the surgery team will also probably complete a checklist, with one staff member functioning as the checklist coordinator. Figure 40-5 shows the World Health Organization's checklist. It covers three phases of a surgical procedure (WHO, 2008):

- Sign in (before anesthesia is given)
- Time out (before the skin incision)
- Sign out (before the patient leaves the surgical suite).

ANALYSIS/NURSING DIAGNOSIS

As in the preoperative phase, most intraoperative nursing care consists of standard activities to be used for all patients; and most intraoperative patients, regardless of the surgery, have

Intraoperative Care Questionnaire

Common nursing interview questions include the following:

What is your name?

What type of surgery are you going to have today?

Is someone here with you?

Are you allergic to any medications, latex, or tape?

When is the last time that you had anything to eat or drink?

Do you have false teeth, contact lenses, or any other prostheses that need to be removed?

Have you taken any medications today?

Do you have any implants, such as metal plates or a pacemaker?

Do you have any scratches, bruises, or other wounds on your body at this time?

Are there any parts of your body that are painful, such as a stiff shoulder or leg?

Also see the WHO Surgical Safety Checklist.

the potential complications (collaborative problems) or nursing diagnoses shown in Table 40-5, as well as the following Potential complications of anesthesia:

- Aspiration
- Vasomotor instability (and resultant hypotension and diminished peripheral perfusion)

- Respiratory depression
- Cardiovascular compromise

Except in unusual circumstances (e.g., a patient in poor nutritional status, a frail elderly patient), you may not need to identify individualized nursing diagnoses for a patient because the standardized care addresses all the potential complications. However, for nurses who prefer to organize care according to nursing diagnoses, the potential diagnoses in Table 40-5 apply to most patients having major surgery:

PLANNING OUTCOMES/EVALUATION

The overarching goals in the intraoperative phase are that the patient will:

- Be free from injury.
- Remain physiologically stable.
- Experience optimal surgical outcomes.

For *associated NOC standardized outcomes* for intraoperative patients, along with examples of goals created with NOC indicators and scales, refer to Table 40-5. Notice that the goals are appropriate for nearly all surgical patients.

Individualized goals/outcome statements are formulated from the patient's nursing diagnoses. The following are examples:

- Maintains body temperature within the normal range.
- Has clear lung sounds and patent airway.
- Has urine output of at least 30 mL/hr.
- Will have no skin, tissue, or neuromuscular injury as a result of positioning.
- Will not acquire healthcare-related infection.

| World Health Organization | **SURGICAL SAFETY CHECKLIST** (First Edition) |

Before induction of anaesthesia ▶▶▶▶▶▶▶ **Before skin incision** ▶▶▶▶▶▶▶▶▶▶ **Before patient leaves operating room**

SIGN IN	TIME OUT	SIGN OUT
☐ PATIENT HAS CONFIRMED • IDENTITY • SITE • PROCEDURE • CONSENT	☐ CONFIRM ALL TEAM MEMBERS HAVE INTRODUCED THEMSELVES BY NAME AND ROLE	NURSE VERBALLY CONFIRMS WITH THE TEAM:
☐ SITE MARKED/NOT APPLICABLE	☐ SURGEON, ANAESTHESIA PROFESSIONAL AND NURSE VERBALLY CONFIRM • PATIENT • SITE • PROCEDURE	☐ THE NAME OF THE PROCEDURE RECORDED
☐ ANAESTHESIA SAFETY CHECK COMPLETED		☐ THAT INSTRUMENT, SPONGE AND NEEDLE COUNTS ARE CORRECT (OR NOT APPLICABLE)
☐ PULSE OXIMETER ON PATIENT AND FUNCTIONING	ANTICIPATED CRITICAL EVENTS	☐ HOW THE SPECIMEN IS LABELLED (INCLUDING PATIENT NAME)
DOES PATIENT HAVE A:	☐ SURGEON REVIEWS: WHAT ARE THE CRITICAL OR UNEXPECTED STEPS, OPERATIVE DURATION, ANTICIPATED BLOOD LOSS?	☐ WHETHER THERE ARE ANY EQUIPMENT PROBLEMS TO BE ADDRESSED
KNOWN ALLERGY? ☐ NO ☐ YES	☐ ANAESTHESIA TEAM REVIEWS: ARE THERE ANY PATIENT-SPECIFIC CONCERNS?	☐ SURGEON, ANAESTHESIA PROFESSIONAL AND NURSE REVIEW THE KEY CONCERNS FOR RECOVERY AND MANAGEMENT OF THIS PATIENT
DIFFICULT AIRWAY/ASPIRATION RISK? ☐ NO ☐ YES, AND EQUIPMENT/ASSISTANCE AVAILABLE	☐ NURSING TEAM REVIEWS: HAS STERILITY (INCLUDING INDICATOR RESULTS) BEEN CONFIRMED? ARE THERE EQUIPMENT ISSUES OR ANY CONCERNS?	
RISK OF >500ML BLOOD LOSS (7ML/KG IN CHILDREN)? ☐ NO ☐ YES, AND ADEQUATE INTRAVENOUS ACCESS AND FLUIDS PLANNED	HAS ANTIBIOTIC PROPHYLAXIS BEEN GIVEN WITHIN THE LAST 60 MINUTES? ☐ YES ☐ NOT APPLICABLE	
	IS ESSENTIAL IMAGING DISPLAYED? ☐ YES ☐ NOT APPLICABLE	

THIS CHECKLIST IS NOT INTENDED TO BE COMPREHENSIVE. ADDITIONS AND MODIFICATIONS TO FIT LOCAL PRACTICE ARE ENCOURAGED.

FIGURE 40-5 World Health Organization's Surgical Safety Checklist. (*Source:* Reprinted with permission from the World Health Organization. Retrieved August 7, 2011, from http://www.who.int/patientsafety/safesurgery/tools_resources/SSSL_Checklist_finalJun08.pdf)

Table 40-5 ➤ Intraoperative Patients: Selected Standardized Nursing Diagnoses, Outcomes, and Interventions

NURSING DIAGNOSES (NANDA-I) AND COLLABORATIVE PROBLEMS	NOC OUTCOMES AND INDICATORS	NIC INTERVENTIONS AND ACTIVITIES (NOTE: HIGHLIGHTED INTERVENTIONS ARE ROUTINELY PERFORMED FOR ALL SURGERY PATIENTS.)
Nursing diagnosis: Risk for Aspiration related to depressed respirations and reflexes secondary to anesthesia **Collaborative problem:** Potential Complication of anesthesia: aspiration **Comments:** This is especially relevant for patients who have weak muscles for coughing or a poor gag reflex.	**NOC outcome:** Respiratory Status: Airway Patency **NOC goal:** (5) No choking or adventitious breath sounds	**Artificial Airway Management** ■ Institute endotracheal suctioning, as appropriate. **Aspiration Precautions** ■ Monitor pulmonary status. ■ Keep suction setup available. ■ Maintain an airway. **Sedation Management** ■ Ensure that emergency resuscitation equipment is readily available, specifically source to deliver 100% O_2, emergency medications, and a defibrillator. ■ Initiate an IV line. ■ Ensure availability of and administer antagonists as appropriate, per physician's order, or protocol. **Vomiting Management** ■ Position to prevent aspiration.
Nursing diagnosis: Risk for Imbalanced Body Temperature related to exposure in cool environment and administration of cool IV fluids **Collaborative problem:** Potential Complication of surgery and anesthesia: hyperthermia, hypothermia **Comments:** Applies especially to very young, very old, and very thin patients	**NOC outcome:** Thermoregulation **NOC goals:** ■ (5) No hyperthermia ■ (5) No hypothermia ■ (4) Mild increased (or decreased) skin temperature	**Temperature Regulation: Intraoperative** ■ Begin warming preoperatively and continue during intraoperative phase. ■ Adjust operating room temperature for therapeutic effect. ■ Apply head covering. ■ Cover exposed body parts. ■ Warm or cool all irrigating, IV, and skin preparation solutions, as appropriate. ■ Continuously monitor the patient's temperature. ■ Cover patient with heated blanket for transport to postanesthesia care unit. **Malignant Hyperthermia Precautions** ■ Maintain emergency equipment for malignant hyperthermia, per protocol, in operative areas. ■ Notify anesthesiologist and surgeon of patient history. ■ Provide a cooling blanket. **Vital Signs Monitoring** ■ Monitor blood pressure, pulse, temperature, and respiratory status, as appropriate. ■ Monitor skin color, temperature, and moistness.

(Continued)

Table 40-5 ➤ Intraoperative Patients: Selected Standardized Nursing Diagnoses, Outcomes, and Interventions—cont'd

NURSING DIAGNOSES (NANDA-I) AND COLLABORATIVE PROBLEMS	NOC OUTCOMES AND INDICATORS	NIC INTERVENTIONS AND ACTIVITIES (NOTE: HIGHLIGHTED INTERVENTIONS ARE ROUTINELY PERFORMED FOR ALL SURGERY PATIENTS.)
Nursing diagnosis: Risk for Imbalanced Fluid Volume related to NPO status and blood loss from surgery. **Collaborative problem:** Potential complication of surgery: fluid and electrolyte imbalance *Comments:* Clients undergoing surgery are at risk for vascular, cellular, and/or intracellular dehydration. Patients with renal or cardiac problems are at higher than normal risk for fluid and electrolyte imbalance.	*NOC outcomes:* Blood Loss Severity Fluid Balance Urinary Elimination Vital Signs *NOC goals:* ■ (4) Systolic and diastolic blood pressures, mild deviation from normal range ■ (5) Mean arterial pressure not compromised ■ (5) Central venous pressure not compromised ■ (5) Pulmonary wedge pressure not compromised ■ (4) Peripheral pulses mildly compromised ■ (4) 24-hr intake and output balance mildly compromised ■ (5) Adventitious breath sounds not present ■ (5) Neck vein distension not present ■ (5) Peripheral edema not present	**Fluid Management** ■ Maintain accurate intake and output record. ■ Insert urinary catheter, if appropriate. ■ Administer IV therapy, as prescribed. ■ Monitor hemodynamic status, including CVP, MAP, PAP, and PCWP, if available. ■ Prepare for administration of blood products (e.g., check blood with patient identification and prepare infusion setup), as appropriate. **Fluid Monitoring** ■ Determine possible risk factors for fluid imbalance (e.g., renal pathologies, liver dysfunction . . .). ■ Monitor color, quantity, and specific gravity of urine. ■ Monitor for distended neck veins, crackles in the lungs, peripheral edema, and weight gain. ■ Monitor blood pressure, heart rate, and respiratory status. ■ Monitor serum and urine electrolyte values. **Intravenous (IV) Therapy** ■ Monitor IV flow rate and IV site during infusion. ■ Monitor for IV patency before administration of IV medication.
Nursing diagnosis: Risk for Latex Allergy Response; or Latex Allergy Response related to multiple previous exposures to latex *Comments:* Use these diagnoses only if the patient has the necessary defining characteristics or risk factors. Do not use them routinely for all patients.	*NOC outcomes:* Immune Hypersensitivity Response Symptom Severity *NOC goals:* (5) No localized inflammatory responses (5) Respiratory, cardiac, renal, and neurological functions not compromised	**Latex Precautions (Intraoperative)** ■ Place allergy band on patient [if not already done preoperatively]. ■ Record allergy or risk in patient's medical record [or check to see that it was done]. ■ Post sign indicating latex precautions. ■ Survey environment and remove latex products. ■ Monitor latex-free environment. ■ Report information to physician, pharmacist, and other care providers, as indicated. **Preoperative Interventions** ■ Question patient or appropriate other about history of neural tube defect (e.g., myelomeningocele) or congenital urological condition (e.g., extrophy of the bladder). ■ Question patient or appropriate other about systemic reactions to natural rubber latex (e.g., facial or scleral edema, tearing eyes, urticaria, rhinitis, and wheezing). ■ Question patient or appropriate other about allergies to foods such as bananas, kiwi, avocado, mango, and chestnuts.

Table 40-5 ➤ Intraoperative Patients: Selected Standardized Nursing Diagnoses, Outcomes, and Interventions—cont'd

NURSING DIAGNOSES (NANDA-I) AND COLLABORATIVE PROBLEMS	NOC OUTCOMES AND INDICATORS	NIC INTERVENTIONS AND ACTIVITIES (NOTE: HIGHLIGHTED INTERVENTIONS ARE ROUTINELY PERFORMED FOR ALL SURGERY PATIENTS.)
Nursing diagnosis: Risk for Perioperative Positioning Injury related to patient factors such as edema, emaciation, obesity, and sensory perceptual disturbances secondary to anesthesia **Collaborative problem:** Potential complication of surgery: neuromuscular, skeletal, or skin injury	**NOC outcomes:** Circulation Status Mobility Neurological Status Physical Injury Severity Tissue Perfusion: Peripheral **NOC goals:** ■ (4) PaO_2 mild deviation from normal range ■ (4) $PaCO_2$ mild deviation from normal range ■ (4) Pallor and dependent rubor mild ■ (5) Joint movement not compromised ■ (5) Spinal sensory/motor function not compromised ■ (5) Central motor control not compromised ■ (5) No burns, bruises, extremity or back sprains, impaired mobility ■ (4) Capillary refill (fingers and toes) mild deviation from normal range ■ (5) No numbness ■ (5) All pulses no deviation from normal range ■ (5) Skin integrity not compromised	**Circulatory Precautions** ■ Perform a comprehensive appraisal of peripheral circulation (e.g., check peripheral pulses, edema, capillary refill, color, and temperature of extremity). **Positioning: Intraoperative** ■ Use assistive devices for immobilization. ■ Lock wheels of stretcher and operating room bed. ■ Use an adequate number of personnel to transfer patient. ■ Support the head and neck during transfer. ■ Immobilize or support any body part, as appropriate. ■ Maintain patient's proper body alignment. ■ Apply padding to bony prominences. ■ Apply safety strap and arm restraint, as needed. ■ Record position and devices used. **Surgical Precautions** ■ Verify surgical consent. ■ Verify surgical site. ■ Verify client's blood type. ■ Verify that there is blood on reserve. ■ Verify client's identity. ■ Verify patient's allergies. ■ Check ground isolation monitor. ■ Verify the correct functioning of equipment. ■ Check suction for adequate pressure and complete assembly of canisters, tubing, and catheters. ■ Count sponges, sharps, and instruments before, during, and after surgery, per agency policy; record results of counts. ■ Provide an electrosurgical unit, grounding pad, and active electrode, as appropriate. ■ Verify the integrity of electrical cords. ■ Verify the proper functioning of electrosurgical unit. ■ Verify that the client is not in contact with metal. ■ Check for the presence of implants, pacemakers, and metal prostheses pacemakers contraindicating use of electrosurgical cautery. ■ Verify the patient's skin integrity at site of [electrocautery] grounding pad. ■ Verify that skin prep solutions are non-flammable. ■ Adjust coagulation and cutting currents, as instructed by physician or per agency policy. ■ Inspect the patient's skin for injury [at conclusion of procedure]. ■ (non-NIC) Monitor sterile technique throughout procedure.

Sources: Bulechek, G. M., Butcher, H. K., & Dochterman, J. M. (Eds.). (2008). *Nursing interventions classification (NIC)* (5th ed.). St. Louis, MO: C.V. Mosby; Moorhead, S., Johnson, M., Maas, M., et al. (Eds.). (2008). *Nursing outcomes classification (NOC)* (4th ed.). St. Louis, MO: C.V. Mosby; and NANDA-I. (2012). *Nursing diagnoses: Definitions and classification 2012–2014.* Ames, IA: Wiley-Blackwell.

PLANNING INTERVENTIONS/IMPLEMENTATION

Intraoperative care focuses on maintaining a safe environment and assisting the surgery team to provide appropriate care for the client. The nurse anesthetist manages the interventions for most of the patient's potential problems, for example, fluid volume status, airway protection, and vital signs monitoring.

NIC standardized interventions for the intraoperative period come from the domain of Perioperative Care. They include interventions for all intraoperative patients, regardless of their individual nursing diagnoses. One intervention, Anesthesia Administration, must be performed by an anesthesiologist or nurse anesthetist. The nurse assists in implementing a number of interventions:

- Anesthesia Administration
- Autotransfusion
- Infection Control: Intraoperative
- Positioning: Intraoperative
- Surgical Assistance
- Surgical Precautions
- Surgical Preparation
- Temperature Regulation: Intraoperative

For *NIC standardized interventions* for specific intraoperative nursing diagnoses, refer to Table 40-5. Notice, however, that most of the interventions apply to all surgical patients and are subsumed by (or fall under) the preceding NIC Perioperative Care interventions. As in all of healthcare, you should be always mindful of using hand hygiene. Sterile asepsis is an important focus in the intraoperative period; you can review that in Chapter 22.

The following sections explain in more detail how to carry out "routine" interventions, such as providing skin preparation, positioning, and intraoperative safety measures. Note that "routine" in this context means that the activities are planned and performed for all patients. Nursing interventions are *never* routine in the general sense; they must always be performed with thought and skill.

Skin Preparation

Surgical skin preparation reduces the risk of postoperative wound infection by reducing the microbial count at the operative site. Skin preparation may begin in the preoperative phase, when the client cleanses the skin with an antimicrobial solution the evening before and the morning of surgery. The intraoperative nurse provides additional skin preparation as follows:

Assess the Skin. Assess skin for signs of infection, rash, or other forms of skin irritation. Document the condition of the skin on the intraoperative record.

Remove Hair From the Site Only If Necessary. Historically, the surgical site was always shaved. Now, however, you will remove hair only if there is a large amount of it in the area of the surgery or if the surgeon specifies a preference for hair removal. Hair removal increases the risk of abrasions or nicks in the skin, which provide a portal of entry for bacteria. If you do remove hair, you will likely do it in the preoperative holding area immediately before surgery to reduce the time for bacterial growth. Use clippers or depilatory cream to trim hair because they are less likely than a razor to cause skin irritation (Joanna Briggs Institute, 2007).

Cleanse the Surgical Site. In the operative suite, skin preparation precedes draping of the client. Cleanse the surgical site and a generous part of surrounding area with the recommended anti-infective solution. Povidone-iodine (Betadine) is commonly used for the scrub; then the skin is painted with Betadine solution. ✚ **If the client is allergic to iodine, use an alternative preparation solution.**

Positioning

Five variables determine the position of the patient in the OR: the surgical site, access to the patient's airway, the need to monitor vital signs, comfort, and safety. A position that is ideal for accessing the surgical site may not be used if any of the other factors are compromised. If the patient has preexisting injuries or discomfort, factor this information into the decision about how to position. For example, a patient with chronic cervical spine pain may be positioned using a neck roll.

The patient is usually positioned after anesthesia has begun. Use straps, wedges, pillows, and surgical table attachments to maintain the position during the surgery. To prevent shearing, lift—do not slide—the patient into position. In many cases, the surgical team assists with positioning.

The circulating nurse is responsible for preventing positioning injuries. Surgical patients often spend 3 to 4 hours, or even longer, in the same position. This places them at risk for pressure ulcer formation. Some anesthetic agents decrease tissue perfusion, further increasing the patient's risk for sustaining positioning injuries. For nursing interventions to address the NANDA-I diagnosis Risk for Perioperative Positioning Injury, see Table 40-5.

Intraoperative Safety Measures

Just before starting any surgical or invasive procedure, you should conduct a final verification process to confirm the correct patient, procedure, and site (The Joint Commission, 2011). The circulating nurse is responsible for a variety of other measures that protect the patient in the intraoperative phase. These measures are briefly explained here.

Assist the Scrub Nurse to Prepare and Maintain the Sterile Field. The circulating nurse gathers surgical supplies and equipment for use during surgery. She works with the scrub nurse to transfer the supplies to the sterile field.

Provide Supplies and Materials During Surgery. If additional supplies are needed during surgery, the circulating nurse obtains them and opens them onto the sterile field. Supplies may include dressings, surgical equipment, medications, irrigating solutions, or sutures.

Monitor Intake and Output of the Client. Together with the anesthetist, the circulating nurse monitors the fluid infused, urine output, drainage, and blood loss.

Handle Specimens. The circulating nurse handles specimens and sends them to the lab or pathology for evaluation after the surgery is complete. The surgeon may sometimes obtain a tissue sample that must be analyzed during the operative procedure. The circulator receives the specimen, coordinates with the pathologist to review the sample, and reports the pathology findings to the surgeon.

Perform Sponge, Sharps, and Instrument Counts. ✚ The circulating nurse and the scrub nurse count the supplies that are added to the sterile field. As the surgery comes to an end, a repeat count is performed to ensure that no instruments, sponges, or sharps are left inside the client. A retained sponge can lead to infection and additional surgeries.

A major surgery, such as a heart surgery, can use several hundred sponges. Once soaked in blood, sponges can blend in with the body cavity and be difficult to see. Some agencies are now using sponges with barcodes, which the nurse scans before and after use. The system alerts the surgical team if a sponge is left behind. In another system, the surgical team relies on

chip-embedded sponges with radiofrequency identification technology to count sponges and locate any that are left behind.

Document. Record the care provided and the client's response to care on the surgical record. This is usually a graphic or a checklist form, perhaps with some space for narrative notes about anything the form does not address.

KnowledgeCheck 40-7

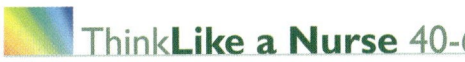

- What activities is the circulating nurse responsible for in the surgical suite prior to the skin incision?
- Describe six intraoperative safety measures performed by the circulating nurse.

ThinkLike a Nurse 40-6

What special concerns, if any, may affect Mr. Singh (Meet Your Patient) during the intraoperative phase of care?

POSTOPERATIVE CARE

The postoperative phase begins when the client enters the postanesthesia care unit and ends when he has healed from the surgical procedure.

TheoreticalKnowledge
knowing **why**

The postoperative phase consists of two parts: recovery from anesthesia and recovery from surgery.

Recovery From Anesthesia

The first postoperative phase is often known as the *postanesthesia phase* or the *immediate postoperative phase*. When the surgery is completed, the surgical team moves the client from the operating table to a bed (or gurney). They then transport him to the postanesthesia care unit (PACU), also called the *recovery room*. During this period, the client is at high risk for respiratory and cardiovascular compromise. As a precaution, the anesthetist and the circulating nurse accompany the client and attend to his needs during transport to the PACU.

The PACU, located near the OR, is typically an open unit that allows nurses to observe clients easily (Fig. 40-6). PACU nurses have specialized education and experience in caring for postoperative clients. The PACU nurse receives a comprehensive report from the anesthesia provider and circulating nurse, which should contain the following information:

- Procedure performed
- Type of anesthesia
- Medications administered in the surgical suite
- Duration of the procedure and anesthesia
- Postoperative vital signs
- Pulse oximetry values
- Allergies
- Lab values
- Estimated blood loss
- Fluid intake and output, including urine, stool, gastric losses
- Preoperative mobility status, skin integrity, and sensory perception abilities
- Surgical complications
- Presence of tubes, drains, catheters
- Existing IV lines
- Postoperative prescriptions

Recovery From Surgery

The second phase of postoperative care begins when the patient is discharged from the PACU and admitted to the surgical nursing unit. The patient is transported to the surgical unit only after he has recovered from anesthesia and his condition is stable. The goal of this phase is to facilitate healing and prevent postoperative complications (see Box 40-4).

PracticalKnowledge
knowing **how**

In the next sections we discuss nursing care associated with both phases of postoperative care.

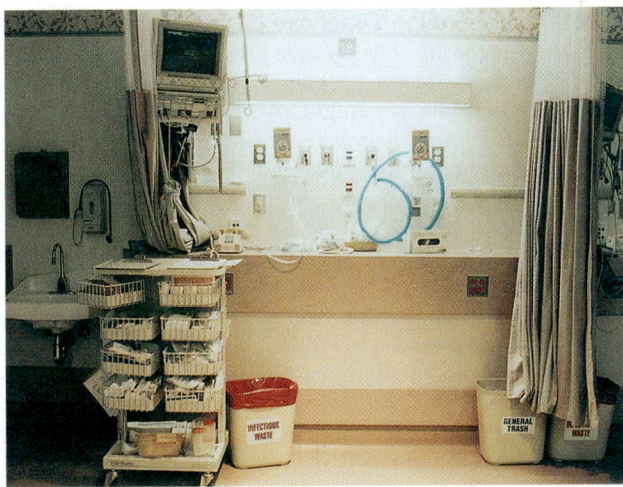

FIGURE 40-6 Postanesthesia care unit.

BOX 40-4 ■ Evidence of Recovery From Anesthesia

Airway—The patient is able to maintain a patent airway independently and to deep-breathe, cough, and expectorate secretions.

Level of consciousness—The patient is conscious and easily reoriented. Often patients will drift off to sleep between arousals; however, they easily reorient and are generally aware of circumstances and surroundings.

Vital signs—Vital signs are stable and within an acceptable range. The blood pressure may be markedly different from that taken during the immediate preoperative measures, because BP is often elevated preoperatively. This can also be due to anxiety, pain, and not administering routine BP medications because of NPO status. The patient may require medication to control pain or BP before he can be discharged from the PACU.

Mobility and sensation—The patient is able to move all extremities that he could move preoperatively. The patient regains movement and sensation once spinal or epidural anesthesia has worn off.

Fluid balance (I&O)—The patient is urinating at least 30 mL/hr and is in relative fluid balance. Consider blood loss, urine output, gastric drainage, and emesis when calculating fluid balance.

Dressings and drains—Dressings are dry and intact, or wound drainage is considered appropriate for the procedure. The patient should have no overt signs of excessive blood or fluid loss before he is transferred to the surgical unit.

Nursing Care in the Postanesthesia Care Unit

The PACU nurse performs a quick, focused initial assessment of the surgical patient in the presence of the anesthesia provider and circulating nurse. After that, she assesses the patient every 5 to 15 minutes. AORN (2009) has identified the essential elements of assessment in the PACU. For that information, refer to the Focused Assessment box, Postanesthesia Assessments: Essential Elements.

Focused Assessment

Postanesthesia Assessment: Essential Elements

The AORN (2009) has identified the essential elements of assessment in the PACU.

Vital signs
- ➤ Blood pressure, cuff or arterial
- ➤ Respiratory rate, respiratory competence, and breath sounds
- ➤ Respiratory adequacy, including skin color and condition
- ➤ Temperature (record type of measurement used, e.g., skin, tympanic, oral)
- ➤ Pulse (apical and peripheral)
- ➤ Oxygen saturation (e.g., pulse oximeter reading)

Peripheral circulation (postoperative tissue perfusion), for example, peripheral pulses and sensation at extremities

Neurological status, including pupil response and intracranial pressure (if indicated)

Mental status: Level of consciousness, alertness, lucidity, orientation

Intravenous therapy: Patency, location of sites, rates of solution(s), and/or blood products infusing

Allergies and sensitivities

Pain

Motor abilities, including return of sensory and motor control in areas affected by local or regional anesthetics

Skin integrity

Temperature regulation

Positioning

Surgical incision site, including condition of suture line(s) if visible

Nausea and vomiting

Fluid and electrolyte balance

Safety needs (e.g., siderails raised)

Central venous pressure (CVP), pulmonary wedge pressure

Airway: patency, presence of artificial airway, mechanical ventilator settings

Condition of dressing(s)

Drainage: Type, patency, and amount and type of drainage from dressings, tubes, and catheters

✚ An unconscious client is usually positioned on his side to help maintain an open airway. This decreases the likelihood of aspirating mucus or saliva by allowing it to drain out instead of back into the throat. Elevating the superior arm on a pillow allows for good chest expansion so the patient can breathe deeply and expand the lungs fully.

NIC: Postanesthesia Care. The only postoperative intervention from NIC's Perioperative Care category is Postanesthesia Care. Postanesthesia Care encompasses the preceding assessments and adds measures such as providing for safety and administering oxygen. Many patients arrive in the PACU with an artificial airway or endotracheal tube in place. For most, the patient remains in the PACU until he has recovered from the effects of anesthesia (Box 40-4). When the nurse determines that the patient is able to maintain his own airway, she removes the airway and transfers him to the surgical unit.

Postoperative Nursing Care on the Surgical Unit

The assigned nurse admits the patient to the surgical unit. If the patient is transported by gurney, assist him to the bed. As soon as the patient has arrived, perform an assessment, and listen to a summary report from the PACU nurse.

▇ ASSESSMENT

The initial postoperative assessment is identical to the assessment performed by the PACU nurse. However, the patient has undergone a period of stabilization since surgery, so the frequency of assessment can be less than in the PACU, where the patient was assessed every 5 to 15 minutes. You may increase the frequency if the patient's condition changes. Of course agency protocols vary, but a common pattern is to assess the patient:

On arrival to the nursing unit
Every 15 minutes for the first hour
Every 30 minutes for the next 2 hours
Every hour for the next 4 hours
Then every 4 hours

Knowledge Check 40-8
- What are the two phases of the postoperative phase of care?
- How often is a patient typically assessed after surgery?
- What assessments are made?

▇ ANALYSIS/NURSING DIAGNOSIS

If healing proceeds normally and no complications develop, most postoperative patients have a common set of collaborative problems (Table 40-6), regardless of the type of surgery they underwent. You will not need to write potential ("risk for") nursing diagnoses, except in special situations (e.g., patients with comorbid conditions, such as diabetes or asthma).

Potential Nursing Diagnoses. Write potential nursing diagnoses (instead of collaborative problems) only if a patient has a higher risk for the problem than the average surgical patient. For example, you might use:

- *Risk for Ineffective Peripheral Tissue Perfusion* for patients who have a history of peripheral arterial disease or cardiac insufficiency.
- *Risk for Deficient Fluid Volume* for patients who have lost a large amount of blood in surgery or who are dehydrated on admission.
- *Risk for Ineffective Breathing Pattern* for patients with weak accessory muscles for breathing, with a decreased level of consciousness, or with a respiratory condition such as emphysema.
- *Risk for Infection* for patients who have compromised immune status or who may not be capable of managing their own wound care at home.

Table 40-6 ➤ Potential Postoperative Complications (Collaborative Problems)

POTENTIAL COMPLICATION	DESCRIPTION	CLINICAL SIGNS	INTERVENTIONS FOR PREVENTION AND EARLY DETECTION
Respiratory System			
Aspiration Pneumonia	Airway inflammation caused by inhaling gastric secretions (especially hydrochloric acid from the stomach) because of absent gag reflex secondary to anesthesia	Cough, fever, elevated WBC, decreased or absent breath sounds, decreased oxygen saturation (SaO_2), tachypnea, dyspnea, blood-tinged sputum.	*Preoperative:* Institute NPO for at least 8 hours prior to surgery. *Postoperative:* Continue NPO until intestinal motility returns; carefully monitor sedated patient and place in side-lying position.
Atelectasis	Collapse of alveoli due to hypoventilation, airways blocked by mucus plugs, opioid analgesics, immobility	Decreased or absent breath sounds, noisy respirations, decreased O_2 saturation (SaO_2), chest asymmetry, sternal retractions, accessory muscle use, trachea deviated from midline, fever, tachypnea, dyspnea, tachycardia, diaphoresis, pleural pain, increased restlessness, anxiety	▪ Monitor for clinical signs (Column 3) ▪ Monitor rate, rhythm, depth, and effort of respirations. ▪ Monitor ability to cough effectively. ▪ Determine need for suctioning by listening for crackles and rhonchi over major airways. ▪ Suction, as needed. Auscultate lung sounds after suctioning and other respiratory treatments to determine effectiveness. ▪ Encourage deep breathing, coughing, moving in bed, ambulation, use of incentive spirometry. ▪ See interventions for NIC category Respiratory Monitoring.
Pneumonia	Inflammation of the alveoli due to infection with bacteria or viruses, toxins, or irritants. Caused by hypoventilation secondary to anesthesia and opioid analgesics, and by poor cough effort as a result of aging or weakness.	Productive cough with blood-tinged or purulent sputum, fever, elevated WBC, decreased or absent breath sounds, decreased SaO_2, chest pain, tachypnea, dyspnea	▪ Monitor for clinical signs. ▪ Encourage and assist with deep breathing, coughing, moving in bed, ambulation, use of incentive spirometry.
Pulmonary Embolus	A clot that occludes blood flow to a portion of the lungs; usually a result of clot formation in the lower extremities, which breaks loose and migrates to the lungs. May also be due to venous injuries, hypercoagulable state, use of high-dose estrogen, preexisting circulatory disorders.	Sudden onset of dyspnea, shortness of breath, chest pain, hypotension, tachycardia, decreased SaO_2, cyanosis	▪ Prevent thrombophlebitis: Encourage and assist with leg exercises, ambulation, antiembolism stockings, sequential compression devices, hydration. See Procedures 40-2 and 40-3. ▪ If thrombophlebitis occurs, position and immobilize the limb; do not massage calves.

(Continued)

Table 40-6 ➤ Potential Postoperative Complications (Collaborative Problems)—cont'd

POTENTIAL COMPLICATION	DESCRIPTION	CLINICAL SIGNS	INTERVENTIONS FOR PREVENTION AND EARLY DETECTION
Cardiovascular System			
Thrombophlebitis	Blood clot and inflammation of a vein or artery, usually in the legs. Results from increased coagulability and venous stasis due to immobility during and after surgery.	*Superficial:* Vein is red, hard, and hot to touch. *Deep:* Limb is pale and edematous; aching, cramping in limb; Homans' sign (pain in calf when foot is dorsiflexed).	Refer to Pulmonary Embolus actions, above.
Embolus	▪ Movement of a thrombus or foreign body from its original location. ▪ Movement in the arterial system results in symptoms in the area affected (e.g., cerebrovascular accident (CVA), myocardial infarction (MI), or loss of circulation to an area). ▪ In the venous system, often results in pulmonary embolus (see Pulmonary Embolus, above).	See Pulmonary Embolus, above. For arterial emboli, symptoms depend on the location.	▪ Monitor for clinical signs. ▪ Prevent thrombophlebitis. If thrombophlebitis occurs, position and immobilize the limb. ▪ Do not massage calves.
Hemorrhage	Bleeding may be internal or external. May be caused by slipped ligature, uncontrolled bleeder, or infection.	*If external:* Dressings saturated with bright red blood; increased output in drains or chest tubes *If internal:* Increased pain, increasing abdominal girth, ecchymosis or swelling around incision, tachycardia, hypotension	Frequently monitor vital signs, dressings, and wound drainage.
Hypovolemia	Decreased blood volume. May be due to blood loss during and after surgery; dehydration; or excess loss through vomiting, diarrhea, or drains	Hypotension, tachycardia, decreased urine output, fatigue, thirst, dehydration	▪ Monitor vital signs and I&O. ▪ Insert urinary catheter, if appropriate. ▪ Monitor skin color, temperature, and moistness; central and peripheral cyanosis. ▪ Identify possible causes of changes in vital signs. ▪ Administer IV therapy as prescribed. ▪ Promote oral intake when tolerated. ▪ Prepare to administer blood or blood products, as prescribed.
Gastrointestinal System			
Nausea and Vomiting	Stomach upset or vomiting related to pain, anxiety, anesthesia, medications, or oral intake before peristalsis returns	Vomiting, retching, stated nausea	▪ Have patient remain NPO until return of bowel sounds. ▪ Advance diet slowly. ▪ Treat pain.

Table 40-6 ▸ Potential Postoperative Complications (Collaborative Problems)—cont'd

POTENTIAL COMPLICATION	DESCRIPTION	CLINICAL SIGNS	INTERVENTIONS FOR PREVENTION AND EARLY DETECTION
Abdominal Distention (Tympanites)	Excess gas within the intestines; may be due to a slow return of peristalsis or from handling of the intestines during surgery	Abdominal discomfort, bloating, hypoactive or absent bowel sounds	▪ Encourage and assist to move in bed and ambulate. ▪ Maintain NPO until return of bowel sounds; avoid drinking with a straw. ▪ Provide fluids at room temperature.
Constipation	A decrease in the frequency of bowel movements, resulting in the passage of hard stool. Usually related to use of opioids, immobility, inadequate fluid intake, or low-fiber diet	Abdominal discomfort, bloating, hypoactive or absent bowel sounds	Encourage and assist the patient to move in bed, ambulate, and increase fluid and fiber intake after bowel sounds return.
Ileus	Loss of the forward flow of intestinal contents due to decreased peristalsis secondary to anesthesia, handling of the intestines during surgery, electrolyte imbalances, infection, or ischemic bowel	Abdominal pain, distention, absent bowel sounds, vomiting	There are few independent preventive measures. Observe for symptoms; notify the surgeon.
Genitourinary System			
Renal Failure	Decreased or absent urine output due to hypovolemia, shock, or toxic reaction to medications.	Urine output < 30 mL/hr; rising BUN and creatinine levels	Carefully monitor I&O and lab values.
Urinary Retention	Accumulation of urine in the bladder. May result from poor muscle tone as a result of anesthesia and anticholinergic medications, handling of tissues during surgery, or inflammation in the pelvic region.	Bladder distention, suprapubic pain, diminished urine output or output less than fluid intake, inability to void or small, frequent voidings, hypertension, restlessness	▪ Monitor for clinical signs. ▪ Provide privacy and adequate time to urinate. ▪ Catheterize if needed.
Urinary Tract Infection	Infection in the urinary tract related to catheterization, stagnant urine in the bladder secondary to immobility or anticholinergic medications, or instrumentation of the urinary tract	Urinary frequency, suprapubic discomfort, burning on urination, cloudy urine	▪ Monitor for clinical signs. ▪ Monitor I&O. ▪ Use aseptic technique with catheterization and perineal care. ▪ Provide adequate IV and oral fluids.
Surgical Incision			
Dehiscence	Separation of one or more layers of the wound due to poor nutritional status, obesity, or other strain on suture line, inadequate closure of the muscles, or wound infection	A pop or tearing sensation, especially with sudden straining from coughing, vomiting, or changing positions in bed. Usually an immediate increase in serosanguinous drainage occurs.	▪ Provide adequate nutrition. ▪ Use binders to support the incision. ▪ Have client avoid strain. ▪ Monitor for infection.

(Continued)

Table 40-6 ➤ Potential Postoperative Complications (Collaborative Problems)—cont'd

POTENTIAL COMPLICATION	DESCRIPTION	CLINICAL SIGNS	INTERVENTIONS FOR PREVENTION AND EARLY DETECTION
Evisceration	Protrusion of organs or tissues through the separated incision. For causes, see Dehiscence.	Visible protrusion of organs through incision	Same as for Dehiscence
Wound Infection	Inflammation or drainage from a wound due to growth of microorganisms secondary to poor aseptic technique or pathogens already present in surgical area	Localized swelling, redness, heat, pain, fever > 100.4°F or 38°C), foul-smelling drainage, or a change in the color of the drainage.	■ Effective skin prep in preoperative period ■ Surgical scrub according to guidelines in the intraoperative period ■ Monitor for systemic and localized signs and symptoms of infection. ■ Inspect incision and drain areas for redness and extreme warmth. ■ Inspect surgical dressings for drainage and odor. ■ Monitor vital signs, especially temperature. ■ Assess vulnerability to infection. ■ Maintain aseptic nontouch technique with surgical dressing changes. ■ Use and teach good hand hygiene. ■ Use sterile saline for wound cleansing up to 48 hours post-op (NICE, 2008). ■ See interventions for NIC category Infection Protection. ■ Limit the number of visitors, as appropriate. ■ Obtain cultures as needed. ■ Encourage sufficient nutritional and fluid intake. ■ Teach client about signs of infection.

Actual Nursing Diagnoses. Of course, you will use a nursing diagnosis whenever a problem becomes actual instead of merely potential. Nursing diagnoses will vary based on the surgical procedure and the client situation. There is usually no need for a Deficient Knowledge diagnosis because patient teaching is a routine intervention for all postoperative patients.

A common postoperative nursing diagnosis is Acute Pain. There are independent nursing interventions to relieve pain (e.g., teaching the patient to splint the incision). However, they do not usually provide adequate relief in the early post-op period. You will nearly always need to administer analgesics, which require a medical prescription. For other frequently used diagnoses, refer to Table 40-7.

■ PLANNING OUTCOMES/EVALUATION

A comprehensive plan of care for common postoperative nursing diagnoses includes NOC standardized outcomes as well as individualized goals. Because of shortened hospital stays, the postoperative period now extends well past the patient's discharge from the hospital. Often, especially for those who have had major or complex procedures, a home health nurse continues to follow the patient at home to facilitate a smoother transition through the postoperative process.

For postoperative *NOC standardized outcomes and individualized goals*, see Table 40-7.

■ PLANNING INTERVENTIONS/IMPLEMENTATION

Most postoperative interventions focus on prevention and early detection of potential complications (collaborative problems). Many such interventions are done as a part of the preoperative teaching. Others are described in Tables 40-6 and 40-7. These are routines that are followed for all postoperative patients, regardless of type of surgery. Also see Table 40-7 for *NIC interventions for postoperative nursing diagnoses.*

Specific nursing activities should be designed to relieve identified nursing diagnoses. In the next sections, we discuss pain management, routine postoperative teaching, and the use of sequential compression devices.

Table 40-7 ➤ Selected Standardized Nursing Diagnoses, Outcomes, and Interventions for Postoperative Patients

NURSING DIAGNOSES	OUTCOMES AND GOALS	NURSING INTERVENTIONS AND ACTIVITIES
Activity Intolerance r/t pain and the surgical procedure and stressors of surgery	***NOC outcomes:*** Activity Tolerance Endurance Energy Conservation Psychomotor Energy ***NOC goals:*** ■ O_2 saturation, heart rate, respiratory rate, systolic and diastolic blood pressure not compromised with activity ■ Ease of breathing with activity not compromised ■ Walking pace and distance not compromised ■ Ease of performing activities of daily living (ADLs) not compromised ■ Ability to speak with physical activity not compromised ■ Energy restored after rest, not compromised ■ Uses naps to restore energy, often demonstrated. ■ Exhibits concentration, consistently demonstrated.	***NIC interventions:*** Activity Therapy Energy Management Exercise Promotion: Strength Training ***Nursing activities:*** ■ Collaborate with other disciplines to plan and monitor activity program as appropriate. ■ Assist to choose appropriate activities. ■ Assist to focus on strengths rather than weaknesses. ■ Assist to identify activity preferences. ■ Instruct the client and family how to perform desired activities. ■ Refer to community centers, programs as appropriate. ■ Arrange physical activities to reduce competition for oxygen supply to vital body functions (e.g., avoid activity immediately after meals). ■ Avoid care activities during scheduled rest periods. ■ Assist to sit on side of bed ("dangle"), if unable to transfer or walk. ■ Monitor location and nature of pain during activity. ■ Teach activity organization and time management techniques to prevent fatigue.
Acute Pain r/t (1) inflammation or injury in the surgical area (2) abdominal distention secondary to decreased peristalsis (3) muscle pain secondary to positioning and tension	***NOC outcomes:*** Pain Level Pain Control ***NOC goals:*** ■ Consistently rates pain as controlled. ■ No moaning or crying ■ No facial expressions of pain ■ Describes causal factors. ■ Uses preventive measures. ■ Uses nonanalgesic relief measures. ■ Uses analgesics as recommended. ■ Reports changes in symptoms to a health professional. ***Other goals:*** No guarding of incision	***NIC interventions:*** Analgesic Administration Pain Management Patient-Controlled Analgesia (PCA) Assistance ***Nursing activities:*** ■ Assess location, characteristics, onset, duration, frequency, quality, and intensity of pain and predisposing factors. ■ Observe for nonverbal discomfort cues. ■ Assure the client of analgesic availability. ■ Consider cultural influences of responses to pain. ■ Utilize developmentally appropriate assessment method. ■ Determine necessary frequency of pain assessment and formulate pain assessment plan. ■ Provide information about the pain, such as causes, anticipated duration. ■ Control environmental factors that may contribute to the client's response.

(Continued)

Table 40-7 ➤ Selected Standardized Nursing Diagnoses, Outcomes, and Interventions for Postoperative Patients—cont'd		
NURSING DIAGNOSES	**OUTCOMES AND GOALS**	**NURSING INTERVENTIONS AND ACTIVITIES**
		■ Provide information about the pain, such as causes of the pain, how long it will last, and anticipated discomforts from procedures (e.g., teach the client to splint incision when ambulating). ■ Provide optimal pain relief with analgesics as appropriate. ■ Implement PCA as appropriate. ■ Intervene before pain becomes severe. ■ Medicate before activity to increase participation. ■ Teach nonpharmacological pain relief measures (e.g., visualization, progressive muscle relaxation). ■ Utilize multidisciplinary approach to pain management.
Anxiety r/t change in health status, hospital environment	**NOC outcomes:** Anxiety Level Anxiety Self-Control **NOC goals:** ■ Consistently uses effective coping strategies. ■ Often seeks information to reduce anxiety. ■ Consistently uses relaxation techniques to reduce anxiety. ■ Often maintains concentration. ■ Verbalizes that anxiety is mild. ■ Minimal restlessness, hand wringing, muscle tension, facial tension, difficulty concentrating. Minimal changes in vital signs; no dilated pupils, sweating or dizziness ■ Controls anxiety response consistently.	**NIC intervention:** Anxiety Reduction **Nursing activities:** ■ Use calm, reassuring approach. ■ Observe for verbal and nonverbal signs of anxiety. ■ Explain all procedures and activities. ■ Provide information concerning diagnosis, treatment, prognosis. ■ Administer back rub or neck rub as appropriate. ■ Listen attentively. ■ Create trusting atmosphere. ■ Assist the client to identify stressful situations. ■ Assist the client to recognize that she is anxious. ■ Assess the client's ability to make decisions. ■ Encourage verbalization of feelings, perceptions, and fears related to the surgical procedure. ■ Encourage family visits if these ease the client's stress. ■ Support use of appropriate defense mechanisms. ■ Instruct the client in use of relaxation techniques.
Nausea r/t manipulation of gastrointestinal tract, decreased peristalsis secondary to anesthesia	**NOC outcomes:** Nausea & Vomiting Control Nausea & Vomiting: Disruptive Effects Nausea & Vomiting Severity Nutritional Status: Food & Fluid Intake **NOC goals:** ■ No nausea, or intensity only mild ■ Reports nausea, retching, and vomiting controlled.	**NIC interventions:** Nausea Management Medication Management **Nursing activities:** ■ Provide information about the cause of nausea and vomiting and the expected duration. ■ Provide information about the goals, effects, and possible side effects of treatment with antiemetics. ■ Describe the limited role of administering parenteral fluids to prevent dehydration and

Table 40-7 ➤ Selected Standardized Nursing Diagnoses, Outcomes, and Interventions for Postoperative Patients—cont'd

NURSING DIAGNOSES	OUTCOMES AND GOALS	NURSING INTERVENTIONS AND ACTIVITIES
	■ Mild or no intolerance of odors ■ Mild or no intolerance of movement ■ Recognizes onset of nausea. ■ Recognizes precipitating stimuli. ■ Frequency, intensity, and distress of nausea are mild. ■ Uses preventive measures often. ■ Only mild decrease in food and fluid intake ■ No weight loss ■ Reports bothersome side effects from antiemetics. ■ Reports failure of antiemetic treatment.	to administer supplemental electrolytes (e.g., potassium). ■ Encourage the client to monitor own nausea experience, including use of a symptom diary. ■ Encourage the client to learn strategies for managing own nausea. ■ Perform complete assessment including frequency, duration, severity, and precipitating factors. ■ Observe for nonverbal cues of discomfort. ■ Evaluate past experiences with nausea. ■ Identify strategies that have been successful in relieving nausea. ■ Discuss relaxation and distraction techniques if anxiety is suspected of playing a role (e.g., guided imagery, self-hypnosis, biofeedback, music therapy). ■ Encourage frequent oral hygiene unless it stimulates nausea. Keep tissues and water to rinse the mouth nearby. ■ Give cold, clear, odorless foods, as appropriate. ■ Encourage the client to eat high-carbohydrate and low-fat foods and to eat small, frequent meals. ■ Drink cola, but not too cold; suck on an ice cube, sorbet, or a piece of frozen fruit. ■ Have the client sit in an upright position for 30 to 45 min after eating. ■ Control odors and unpleasant visual stimuli in the room. ■ Administer antiemetic medications. ■ Refer to a dietician as needed.
Constipation r/t decreased activity, decreased food or fluid intake, decreased peristalsis secondary to anesthesia, pain medication	***NOC outcome:*** Bowel Elimination ***NOC goals:*** ■ Elimination pattern not compromised ■ Reports ease of stool passage not compromised. ■ Bowel sounds not compromised ■ Muscle tone to evacuate stool not compromised ■ Passes soft, formed stool in amount appropriate for diet. ■ No pain with passage of stool ***Other:*** ■ Bloating not present	***NIC interventions:*** Bowel Management Constipation/Impaction Management ***Nursing activities:*** ■ for signs and symptoms of constipation. ■ Note date of last bowel movement. ■ Monitor bowel sounds. ■ Monitor frequency, consistency, shape, volume, and color of bowel movements. ■ Teach the client about specific foods that assist promotion of bowel regularity. ■ Insert a rectal suppository, enema, or irrigation, as needed. ■ Evaluate medication profile for GI side effects (e.g., narcotic analgesics). ■ Give warm liquids after meals. ■ Instruct the client in foods high in fiber.

(Continued)

Table 40-7 ➤ Selected Standardized Nursing Diagnoses, Outcomes, and Interventions for Postoperative Patients—cont'd

NURSING DIAGNOSES	OUTCOMES AND GOALS	NURSING INTERVENTIONS AND ACTIVITIES
Urinary Retention r/t anesthesia, preoperative medications (anticholinergics), pain, fear, unfamiliar surroundings, client's position	**NOC outcome:** Urinary Elimination **NOC goals:** ■ Empties bladder completely. ■ Fluid intake not compromised ■ No hesitancy with urination **Other:** ■ Bladder not palpable ■ Reports subjective feeling of empty bladder. ■ 24-hr intake and output balanced	**NIC interventions:** Urinary Retention Care Urinary Catheterization **Nursing activities:** ■ Perform comprehensive urinary assessment (fluid intake, urinary output, voiding pattern, cognitive function, preexisting urinary problems). ■ Provide privacy for elimination. ■ Use power of suggestion (run water, flush toilet). ■ Provide ample time (at least 10 minutes) for client to empty bladder. ■ Use spirits of wintergreen in bedpan or urinal. ■ Insert urinary catheter as appropriate. ■ Use percussion and palpation to estimate degree of bladder distention. ■ Catheterize for post-voiding residual as appropriate.
Delayed Surgical Recovery (etiologies will vary with pathology) (*Note:* This diagnosis is broad and encompasses some of the other diagnoses. If the client has Delayed Surgical Recovery, you will not, for example, need a diagnosis of Nausea on the plan of care. This diagnosis is appropriate when the patient requires more days to recover than the anticipated length of stay for the surgery.	**NOC outcomes:** Post-Procedure Recovery Wound Healing: Primary Intention Ambulation Blood Loss Severity Endurance Hydration Infection Severity Nausea & Vomiting Severity Pain Level **NOC goals:** ■ Systolic BP within 20 mm Hg of baseline ■ Ambulation tolerance in normal range ■ No nausea, vomiting, shivering ■ Only mild pain **Other:** ■ Ready for discharge within prescribed length of stay for surgery performed ■ No postoperative complications (e.g., bleeding, infection, delayed wound healing, pneumonia)	**NIC interventions:** Embolus Precautions Exercise Therapy: Ambulation Incision Site Care Nutrition Management Pain Management Self-Care Assistance **Nursing activities:** ■ Monitor for postoperative complications. ■ Monitor the healing process in the incision site. ■ Provide incision care as needed. ■ Teach the client and family how to care for the incision. ■ Facilitate early ambulation postoperatively. ■ Encourage increased intake of protein, iron, and vitamin C, as appropriate. ■ Determine, in collaboration with the dietician as appropriate, number of calories and type of nutrients needed to meet nutrition requirements. ■ Select and implement a variety of measures (e.g., pharmacological, nonpharmacological, interpersonal) to facilitate pain relief, as appropriate. ■ Teach principles of pain management. ■ Encourage independence, but intervene when the client is unable to perform.

Sources: Bulechek, G. M., Butcher, H. K., & Dochterman, J. M. (Eds.). (2008). *Nursing interventions classification (NIC)* (5th ed.). St. Louis, MO: C.V. Mosby; Moorhead, S., Johnson, M., Maas, M., et al. (Eds.). (2008). *Nursing outcomes classification (NOC)* (4th ed.). St. Louis, MO: C.V. Mosby; and NANDA-I. (2012). *Nursing diagnoses: Definitions and classification 2012–2014.* Ames, IA: Wiley-Blackwell. Used with permission.

Pain Management

Tissue damage in surgery is associated with inflammation and acute pain. Good pain management facilitates recovery.

One systematic evidence synthesis has found that there is no strong evidence to support that any particular nursing intervention is better than any other in relieving postoperative pain. Interventions included medication administration, preoperative education, regular assessment and documentation of pain intensity, use of protocols and flow sheets, and nonpharmacological interventions (e.g., massage) (Crowe, Chang, Fraser, et al., 2008). Therefore, when interventions seem to be equally effective, you will need to weigh the potential benefits, possible adverse events, and patient preferences to decide which to use.

Postoperatively, a patient usually receives analgesics by more than one route. For example, in the immediate postoperative period, the patient may receive intravenous or epidural medications, progress to oral opioids in a day or two, and then to nonopioid analgesics (e.g., acetaminophen). For a complete discussion of types of pain relief, refer to Chapter 32. Also refer to Procedure 32-1, Setting Up and Managing Patient-Controlled Analgesia by Pump; and Clinical Insight 32-2, Nursing Care of the Patient With an Epidural Catheter. Keep in mind that no one drug is likely to work for every person with pain.

CAM for Pain and Anxiety: Reflexotherapy for Acute Postoperative Pain and Anxiety

Tsay, Chen, Chen, and colleagues (2008) collected data from 61 patients in Taipei, Taiwan, who received surgery for gastric and liver cancer. Thirty of the patients received 20 minutes of foot reflexotherapy in addition to the usual pain management during postoperative days two, three, and four. They reported less pain and less anxiety than did the control group, who did not receive foot reflexotherapy.

One recent development is a single-use pain relief pump that administers a continuous, regulated flow of local anesthetic through a thin catheter directly into the patient's surgical site. A dressing holds the tubing in place, and the pump can be carried in a small bag and used after the patient returns home. It reduces the need for opioids, thus reducing complications such as nausea, vomiting, and respiratory depression. It is said to hasten ambulation and the return to normal activities. Depending on the type, the pump is filled with 65 to 750 mL of medication and can remain in place for up to 5 days, depending on the amount of anesthetic included (Fig. 40-7).

Postoperative Teaching

Teaching is especially important postoperatively because most patients must perform quite a bit of self-care. Postoperative teaching should reinforce content taught preoperatively. In addition, you should teach the patient about the applicable topics in Clinical Insight 40-1. To prepare the patient for self-care, your teaching should include the following topics:

- Postoperative treatment regimen (e.g., dressing changes, exercises), including rationale for the treatments
- Expected results and effects of the surgery
- The prescribed diet, and how to select foods on the diet
- Prescribed activity
- Signs and symptoms of complications that require the patient to notify the surgeon or primary care provider
- Return office or clinic visits
- Lifestyle changes that may be needed
- Community resources available (e.g., Reach for Recovery)

To use time efficiently, try to do some teaching each time you are at the bedside for other care. Be sure the patient is comfortable but alert. Do not attempt teaching when the patient is in pain, needs to void, or is drowsy from opioid analgesics.

Incentive Spirometry

Incentive spirometry may be prescribed for patients who are at high risk for atelectasis and pneumonia (e.g., the patient has a history of lung problems or smoking or will experience a prolonged period of inactivity). Incentive spirometry facilitates deep breathing, increases lung volume, and promotes coughing

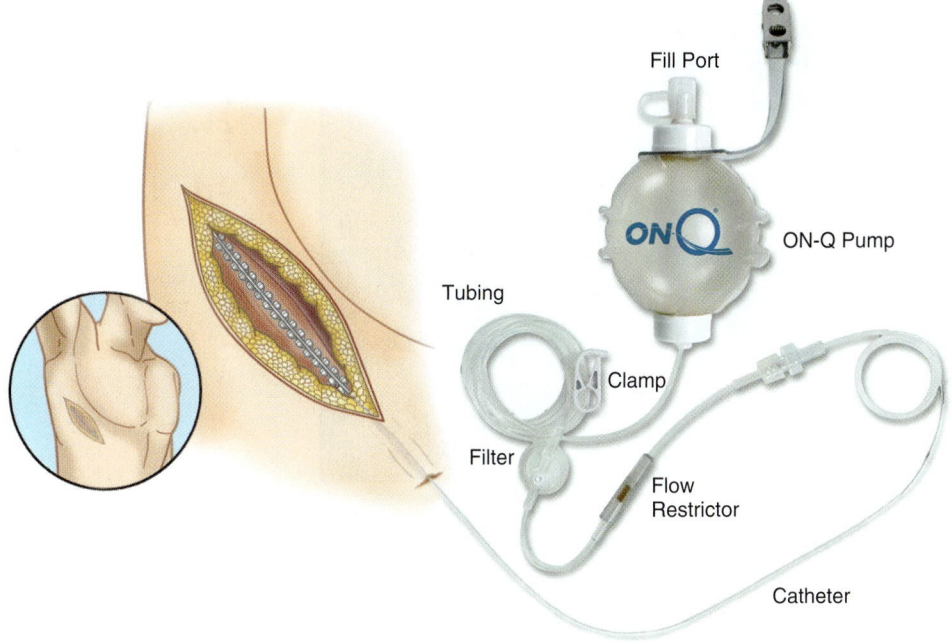

FIGURE 40-7 A single-use pain relief pump delivers a local anesthetic directly into the patient's surgical site.

Fill Port

ON-Q Pump

Tubing

Clamp

Filter

Flow Restrictor

Catheter

to clear mucus from the respiratory tree. The equipment varies in appearance, but all devices include a gauge to monitor the patient's progress visibly (Fig. 40-8). Also refer to the Self-Care box Teaching Your Patient About Incentive Spirometry.

Antiembolism Stockings and Sequential Compression Devices

More than half of hospitalized patients are at risk for venous thromboembolism, and surgical patients seem to be at higher risk than medical patients (Cohen, Tapson, Bergman, et al.,

2008). Preventive measures include anticoagulant medications (so-called "blood thinners"), postoperative exercises, and antiembolism stockings. You may also hear these called TED (thromboembolic disorder) hose. Antiembolism stockings have been discussed as a preoperative care intervention at the end of the section Prepare the Patient Physically for Surgery. Encourage postoperative patients to ambulate as soon and as much as possible to promote peripheral circulation and prevent thrombophlebitis. Antiembolism stockings are not a substitute for activity. To learn how to apply antiembolism stockings, see Procedure 40-2.

Sequential Compression Devices (SCDs). In addition to the preceding measures, a sequential compression device (SCD) may be prescribed for patients at high risk for thrombophlebitis. The SCD is a plastic sleeve with chambers. The sleeve is wrapped around the patient's legs, and provides sequential pressure to the chambers of the plastic sleeve. Starting at the ankle, the first chamber is inflated. When the second chamber inflates, the first chamber deflates, and so on. SCDs apply brief pressure to each segment of the leg. The pressure compresses the veins and promotes venous return to the heart. To learn to apply SCDs, refer to Procedure 40-3.

Gastrointestinal Suction

In addition to causing pain, abdominal distention can increase postoperative respiratory problems, place a strain on suture lines, and interfere with wound closure. Patients having certain surgeries, such as a procedure to relieve a bowel obstruction, are at high risk for abdominal distention. Such patients will return from surgery with a nasogastric (NG) or nasointestinal tube in place for gastric or intestinal decompression. If prolonged intestinal decompression is anticipated, a gastrostomy may be performed instead of using an NG tube.

Decompression tubes are typically connected to either intermittent or continuous suction (Figs. 40-9 and 40-10) to collect excess fluid and gas. Suction is continued until peristalsis resumes, bowel sounds are audible, and the patient is passing flatus. While suction is in place, the patient remains NPO. To review insertion and care of NG and nasoenteric tubes, see Chapter 29. To learn how to manage gastrointestinal suction, see Procedure 40-4.

<table>
<tr><td>

Self-Care

Teaching Your Patient About Incentive Spirometry

➤ Explain to the patient that the machine will enable him to monitor the depth of his breathing.
➤ Patients with abdominal or chest incisions may require pain medication to use the incentive spirometer.
➤ Assist the patient to an upright position in the bed or chair.
➤ Instruct the patient to do the following:
  1. Breathe out normally.
  2. Place the mouthpiece in the mouth and create a seal with the lips.
  3. Breathe in slowly and as deeply as possible through the mouthpiece. Monitor the depth of inspiration by viewing the gauge. (Establish goals for the patient so that progress can be monitored.)
  4. Hold your breath as long as possible, at least to a slow count of 3.
  5. Remove the mouthpiece from your mouth, and exhale.
  6. Rest for a few seconds
  7. Repeat this process 10 times every hour while awake, if possible.
  8. After each set of 10 deep breaths, cough to be sure lungs are clear. Support any incision when coughing by holding a pillow firmly against it.

</td></tr>
</table>

KnowledgeCheck 40-9

- Identify six potential postoperative complications.
- Why are sequential compression devices used?

CarePlanning & MappingPractice

For Care Planning & Mapping practice,

 Go to **Care Planning and Care Mapping Practice Exercises** on Davis*Plus*.

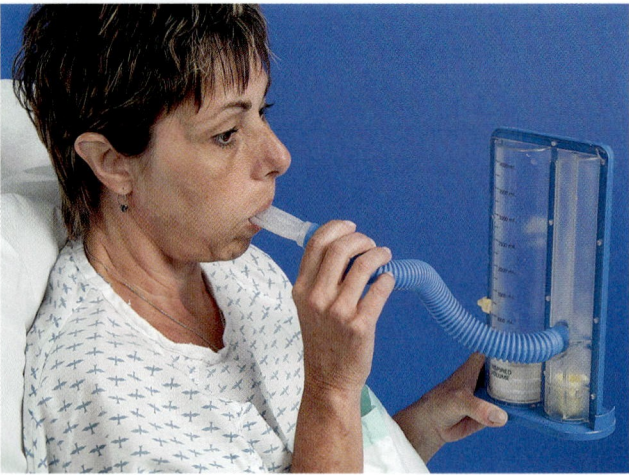

FIGURE 40-8 Incentive spirometry facilitates lung expansion and coughing to clear mucus from airways.

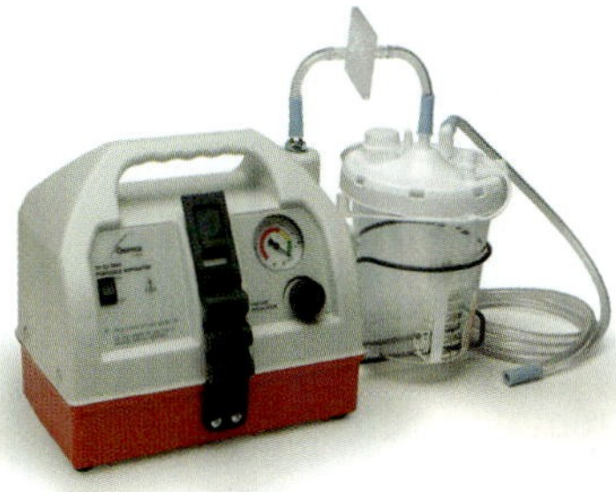

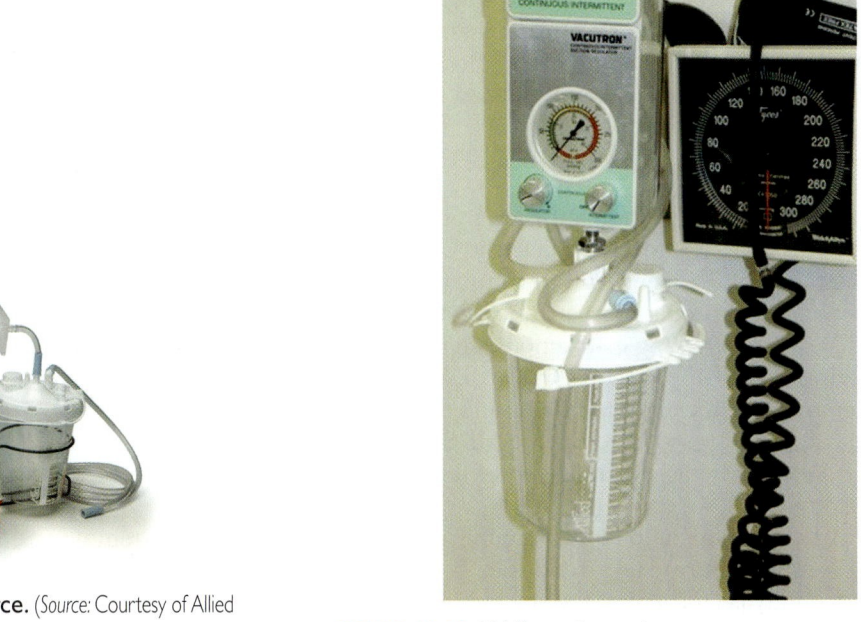

FIGURE 40-9 Portable suction source. (*Source:* Courtesy of Allied Healthcare Products, St. Louis, MO.)

FIGURE 40-10 Wall suction unit.

CLINICALREASONING
Applying the **Full-Spectrum Nursing Model**

Because the following critical thinking activities allow you to practice the kind of thinking you will use as a full-spectrum nurse, they usually have no single right answer. Discuss them with your peers—if you have difficulty with any of the questions, consult your instructor.

PATIENT SITUATION

Recall Nishad Singh (Meet Your Patient). He is a 68-year-old man who came to the emergency department (ED) with sudden onset of rectal bleeding. He had been "tired and dragging for several months." The ED nurse identified nursing diagnoses of Mild Anxiety, Pain, and Risk for Bleeding. Preoperatively, his vital signs were as follows:

BP: 138/88 mm Hg
Pulse: 104 beats/min and regular; 120 beats/min; 134 beats/min
Respiratory rate: 20 breaths/min
Temperature: 36.7°C (98.0°F)
Oxygen saturation: 98%

Mr. Singh was admitted to the hospital, where he received an IV of 1,000 mL of lactated Ringer's solution and a unit of packed red blood cells. He was to undergo emergency colon resection surgery; however, a left hemicolectomy including the sigmoid colon and the anus was required. He spent 4 hours in the PACU, until his vital signs stabilized. Mr. Singh now has a colostomy high in his descending colon, with a stoma on his left abdomen slightly superior to the level of his umbilicus. He also has an abdominal incision that was made for exploration. On the next day after the surgery, the surgeon informed Mr. Singh that he has widespread adenocarcinoma (cancer) of the colon with metastasis to the liver. The nurse has identified these four nursing diagnoses (among others):

Deficient Knowledge (colostomy care) r/t lack of prior experience and no preparation prior to surgery
Fear r/t diagnosis of colon cancer, liver metastasis, and possible terminal illness
Pain secondary to surgical incision and manipulation of abdominal organs during the surgical procedure
Risk for Impaired Skin Integrity r/t irritation from fecal drainage and ostomy pouch

THINKING

1. *Theoretical Knowledge:*
   a. What is a left hemicolectomy? If you do not know the answer, consult an appropriate reference.
   b. What does "metastasis to the liver" mean? If you do not know the answer, consult an appropriate reference.

(continued on next page)

2. *Critical Thinking (Inquiry):*
   a. Why might Mr. Singh have needed a colostomy instead of having his transverse colon reconnected to the remaining lower colon or rectum? State the reference you used to answer this question.
   b. Why do you think Mr. Singh has a colostomy above the level of the umbilicus and not lower down in his abdomen? State the reference you used to answer this question.

DOING

3. *Practical Knowledge:* Mr. Singh returned from surgery with knee-high antiembolism stockings.
   a. You notice that the stockings have slid down and become wrinkled between his knees and ankles. After you straighten them and pull them up, the tops reach to about 7.6 cm (3 in.) below Mr. Singh's knees. What does this probably mean, and what should you do?
   b. Which of the following instructions should you give when delegating care of Mr. Singh's antiembolism stockings to the nursing assistant? (Mr. Singh's stockings have closed toes.)
      - Remove the stockings and bathe and dry the legs every 8 to 12 hours.
      - Massage the legs after removing Mr. Singh's stockings.
      - Before reapplying stockings, report the presence of any lesions, sores, or redness of the lower extremities.
      - Instruct the patient to remain supine for at least 15 minutes after removing the stockings.
      - Make sure there are no wrinkles in the stockings once they have been applied.
      - Tug gently on the end of the stocking to create a small space between the end of the toes and the stocking.
4. *Nursing Process (Nursing Diagnosis):* List Mr. Singh's four nursing diagnoses in order of priority. List the highest priority first. Explain how you decided the priorities.

CARING

5. *Self-Knowledge:*
   a. If you were assigned to care for Mr. Singh today, what aspect of care would you feel best prepared to give? Explain your thinking.
   b. What aspect of Mr. Singh's care would you be most uncomfortable providing? Explain your thinking.
6. *Ethical Knowledge:* You want to provide culturally competent care. What is the first thing you will need to do in order to address Mr. Singh's cultural needs? Review Chapter 15 if you need to.

 Go To Chapter 40, **Clinical Reasoning: Applying the Full-Spectrum Nursing Model Response Sheet,** on Davis*Plus.*

PracticalKnowledge
procedures

Perioperative nursing care includes procedures and techniques designed for prevention and early detection of complications. Recall that full-spectrum nursing involves thinking, doing, and caring—all are equally important in perioperative care.

Procedure 40–1 ■ Teaching a Patient to Deep Breathe, Cough, Move in Bed, and Perform Leg Exercises

➤ For steps to follow in *all* procedures, refer to the Universal Steps for All Procedures found on the page facing the inside back cover.

Equipment

For teaching deep breathing and coughing:

- Folded blanket or a pillow (if teaching will include splinting of a surgical incision site)
- Tissues

For moving in bed:

- Small pillow or folded blanket
- Pillows

Delegation

A registered nurse (RN) should perform the initial teaching. You may delegate reinforcement of the teaching to a licensed vocational/practical nurse (LVN/LPN) or nursing assistive personnel (NAP).

Pre-Procedure Assessments

- Assess cognitive level and level of consciousness.
  Helps assess the patient's ability to understand and follow directions and select the appropriate teaching method.
- Assess pain level.
  Even preoperatively, pain must be well controlled to ensure full patient participation.

- Determine whether the surgical procedure and/or a physical disability will limit the patient's participation.
  For example, a fractured arm that has not yet been repaired will impair the patient's ability to hold a pillow for splinting.
- Determine whether the surgical procedure may entail special exercises or equipment. In addition, assess for any special equipment, such as braces, slings, or abductor wedges that may be needed when turning a patient in bed.
  Knee and hip surgeries often involve special exercises or equipment postoperatively. Consult the surgeon before teaching leg exercises. Spinal and neurological surgeries often limit movement in the postoperative period. For example, some spinal surgeries require the patient to logroll (move from head to toe as one unit). Some neurological procedures require limiting the amount of time the patient's head of bed is above 30°. Identify these restrictions preoperatively, and inform the patient and family about them during your teaching session.
- Assess the patient's belief about the ability of the surgical incision to remain intact.
  This is a common fear. If the patient believes that the incision will not stay together when he coughs or moves, he is less likely to comply.

Procedure 40-1A ■ Teaching a Patient to Deep Breathe and Cough

➤ When performing the procedure, always identify your patient according to agency policy and be attentive to standard precautions, hand hygiene, patient safety and privacy, body mechanics, and documentation.

Deep breathing and coughing expand the lungs, improve ventilation, promote gas exchange, and help prevent atelectasis and pneumonia. Coughing after deep breathing mobilizes secretions, which keeps airways and alveoli open and provides greater surface area for gas exchange.

Procedure Steps

1. **Assist the patient to a Fowler's** or semi-Fowler's position, with the shoulders relaxed.
   Allows for best chest and lung expansion.
2. **Assist the patient who will have** a chest or abdominal incision to practice splinting the site with a folded blanket or pillow.

Counterpressure supports the incision and decreases pain. ▼

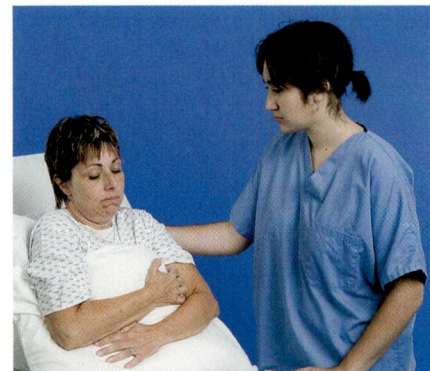

3. **Teach the patient diaphragmatic/** deep breathing. Tell the patient to:
   a. Place her hands anteriorly, along the lower end of the rib cage. The tips of the third fingers should touch at the midline.
   b. Slowly take a deep breath in through the nose. Tell the patient that she should feel her chest expanding as the diaphragm moves down.
   c. Hold her breath for 2 to 5 seconds.
      Stimulates surfactant production and helps prevent alveolar collapse.
   d. Slowly and completely exhale the breath through her mouth.

(continued on next page)

Procedure 40–1 ■ Teaching a Patient to Deep Breathe, Cough, Move in Bed, and Perform Leg Exercises (continued)

4. Teach the patient to cough in conjunction with diaphragmatic breathing. Instruct her to:
  a. Complete two or three cycles of diaphragmatic breathing.
  b. On the next breath in, have the patient lean forward and cough rapidly, through an open mouth, using the muscles of the abdomen,

thighs, and buttocks. Cough several times on that breath.
Helps the patient to distinguish coughing from merely clearing her throat.

Patient Experiencing Weakness
If the patient is too weak to perform this maneuver, have the patient inhale

deeply, bend forward slightly, and perform three or four "huffs" against an open glottis to move secretions forward.

Procedure 40-1B ■ Teaching a Patient to Move in Bed

➤ When performing the procedure, always identify your patient according to agency policy and be attentive to standard precautions, hand hygiene, patient safety and privacy, body mechanics, and documentation.

Moving in bed promotes blood circulation, stimulates respiratory function, and helps mobilize gas in the intestines.

Procedure Steps

1. **Start with the patient in the supine** position, bedrails up. Then instruct the patient as follows.
2. **To turn to the left side**: Bend the right leg, sliding the foot flat along the bed and flexing the knee.
   Enables the patient to push herself over to the opposite side.
3. **Reach the right arm across** the chest, and grasp the opposite bedrail.
   Helps the patient to turn, reduces the need to use the abdominal muscles for turning, and minimizes incision pain.

4. **Breathe deeply, and practice** splinting any potential abdominal or chest incisions. Assist the patient to practice as needed.
   Facilitates comfort during movement.
5. **Pull on the bedrail** while pushing off with the right foot.
   Assists patient to turn to the left. ▼

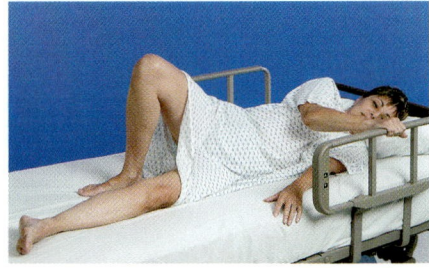

6. **If the patient cannot maintain** this position independently, place a folded pillow or blanket along her back for support.
7. **Change positions every 2 hours**, repeating the turning process with the opposite arm and leg. You will need to assist the patient who needs pillows placed for support.

Procedure 40-1C ■ Teaching Leg Exercises

➤ When performing the procedure, always identify your patient according to agency policy and be attentive to standard precautions, hand hygiene, patient safety and privacy, body mechanics, and documentation.

Leg exercises flex and extend the leg muscles to increase peripheral circulation and help prevent thrombus formation. Thrombus formation is a common postoperative complication.

Procedure Steps

1. **Instruct the patient to lie supine** in the bed.

   NOTE: These exercises can be done when the patient is up in a chair, but the effects of gravity will diminish the effect.

2. **Perform ankle circles.** Instruct the patient to:
   a. Start with one foot in the dorsi-flexed position.

b. Slowly rotate the ankle clockwise.
c. After three rotations, repeat the procedure in a counterclockwise direction.
d. Repeat this exercise at least three times in each direction, then switch and exercise the other ankle. ▼

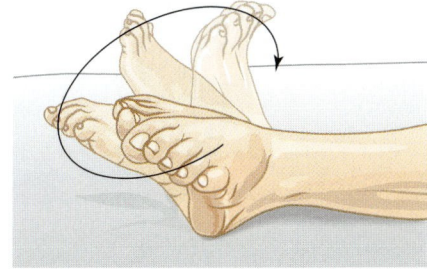

3. **Perform ankle pumps.** Instruct the patient to:
   a. Start with one foot, leg extended.
   b. Point the toe until her foot is plantar flexed.
   c. Pull the toes back toward her head until the foot is dorsiflexed; at the same time, press the back of the knee into the bed.
   d. Make sure she feels a pull, or a stretch, in the calf.
   e. Repeat the alternation between plantar and dorsiflexion several times.
   f. Repeat the cycle with the other foot.

4. Perform leg exercises. Instruct the patient to:
a. Lie supine in the bed.
b. Slowly begin bending the knee, sliding the sole of the foot along the bed until the knee is in a flexed position. ▼

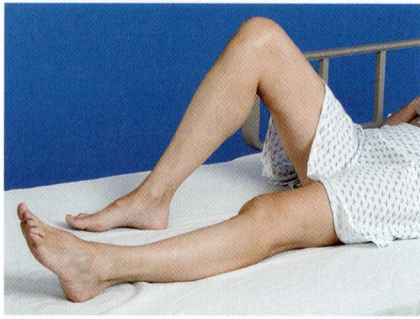

c. Reverse the motion, extending the knee until the leg is once again flat on the bed. ▼

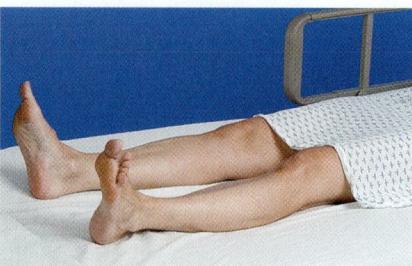

d. Repeat several times.
e. Repeat using the opposite leg.

? What if . . .

- **The patient has had knee, hip, or back surgery?**

  Leg exercises may be contraindicated in patients having knee, hip, or back surgery. Check the surgeon's prescriptions and/or collaborate with the physical therapist.

- **The patient has had nasal, ophthalmic, or neurological surgery?**

  Coughing and deep-breathing exercises are contraindicated.

  To avoid increasing intracranial pressure.

Evaluation

Make sure that the patient performs correctly a return demonstration of the procedures taught.

Documentation

In many healthcare facilities, checklists and charts have special areas in which to document patient teaching. Documentation should identify the person who completed the teaching, the person to whom the procedures were taught, what procedures were taught, and whether the patient understood the teaching. Also include the name and type of any printed materials given.

Practice Resources

Best practices, 2007.

Thinking About the Procedure

 Go to the *Fundamentals of Nursing Skills Videos,* **Perioperative Nursing: Teaching. Coughing and Deep Breathing With Splinting.**

1. What position did the nurse use to teach coughing and deep breathing?

 Go to the *Fundamentals of Nursing Skills Videos,* **Perioperative Nursing: Teaching. Leg Exercises.**

1. How was the patient positioned for the leg exercises?
2. Which exercise was taught first?

 Go to the *Fundamentals of Nursing Skills Videos,* **Perioperative Nursing: Teaching Moving in Bed.**

1. How did the nurse demonstrate the leg exercises to the patient?

 For suggested responses for all three exercises, go to Chapter 40, **Thinking About the Procedure Suggested Responses,** on Davis*Plus.*

Procedure 40–2 ■ Applying Antiembolism Stockings

➤ For steps to follow in *all* procedures, refer to the Universal Steps for All Procedures found on the page facing the inside back cover.

Equipment

- Measuring tape
- Antiembolism stockings
- Washcloth and towel (if needed to cleanse legs)
- Talcum powder (optional: check manufacturer's recommendations)

Delegation

You can delegate application of antiembolism stockings to nursing assistive personnel who have been trained in the task. Instruct the NAP as follows:

- Report the presence of any abnormalities on the lower extremities, such as lesions, sores, or redness, before applying the stockings.
- Instruct the patient to maintain a recumbent position for at least 15 minutes before applying the stockings.
- Do not massage the legs.
- Make sure there are no wrinkles in the stockings once they have been applied.

Pre-Procedure Assessment

- Assess the level of consciousness and cognitive ability.
  If the patient is unconscious or confused, you will need to call for assistance to hold and stabilize the lower extremities as you apply the stockings.
- Assess for signs and symptoms of severe peripheral arterial disease, such as weak or absent pulses, discoloration or cyanosis, or gangrene.
  Antiembolism stockings should not be used in patients with any of these findings because they compress the vessels and, therefore, further impede the already compromised arterial flow.
- Assess skin condition. Note of lesions, dermatitis, or major edema, as evidenced by shiny, taut skin.
  If skin is overstretched by edema, antiembolism stockings may irritate or worsen skin conditions and cause skin breakdown.
- Note the patient's position and length of time she has been in that position.
  Place the patient supine for at least 15 minutes before stocking application. This prevents trapping of pooled venous blood.

➤ When performing the procedure, always identify your patient according to agency policy and be attentive to standard precautions, hand hygiene, patient safety and privacy, body mechanics, and documentation.

➤ If possible, apply stockings in the morning, before the patient gets out of bed. This prevents venous distention and edema that occur when the patient is sitting or standing.

Procedure Steps

1. **Measure the patient's lower extremity.**
   Stockings must be sized correctly in order to apply the correct amounts of pressure at the ankle, mid-calf, and upper thigh. If they are not tight enough, they will not improve venous return effectively. If they are too tight, they may compress the veins and impair circulation to the skin. ▼

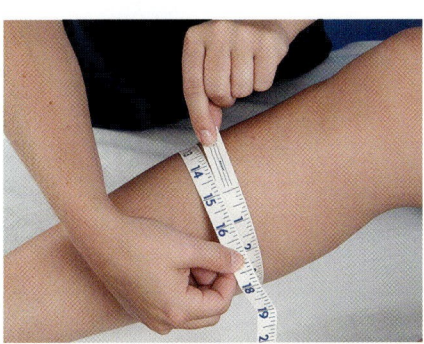

Thigh-High Stockings

a. Measure the circumference of the thigh at the widest section.
   The manufacturer of T.E.D.® brand stockings recommends that stockings not be applied if the thigh circumference exceeds 100 cm (25 in.).
b. Measure the calf circumference at the widest section.
c. Measure the distance from the gluteal fold to the base of the heel.

Knee-High Stockings

a. Measure the circumference of the calf at the widest section.
b. Measure the distance from the base of the heel to the middle of the knee joint.
   Evidence is not conclusive, but increasingly supports the use of knee-high instead of thigh-high hose.

2. **Assist the patient to a supine** position, and instruct him to maintain that position for at least 15 minutes before you apply the stockings.
   Prevents trapping of pooled venous blood by the antiembolism stockings.

3. **Cleanse the patient's legs and feet** if necessary. Dry well.
   Decreases the likelihood of infection and odor.

4. **Lightly dust the legs and feet** with talcum powder if desired and if recommended by the manufacturer. Do not use powder if the patient is or is likely to become diaphoretic.
   Powder eases the application of the stockings, but perspiration will cause the powder to clump.

5. **Holding one stocking at the top cuff in your dominant hand, slide your nondominant arm down and into the stocking until your hand reaches the heel of the stocking.**

6. **Grasp the center of the heel with your hand inside the stocking,**

and then slowly turn the stocking inside out to the level of the heel with your other hand.

The elastic in the stockings is very strong; this method is the easiest way to fit it over the foot and calf. ▼

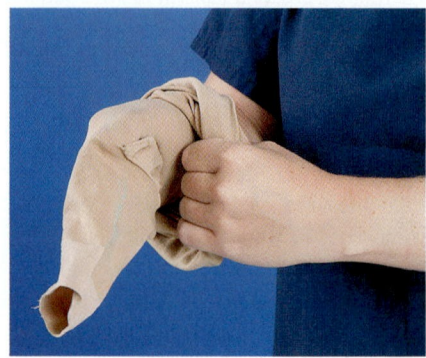

7. **Ask the patient to point his toes** as you grasp the turned foot of the stocking and ease it onto his foot and heel (like putting on a sock). Center the patient's heel in the heel of the stocking.

Ensures that the pressure of the stocking is over the correct anatomical areas.

8. **Gradually pull the remainder** of the stocking up and over the leg, turning it right side out as you

proceed. Be certain the stocking is straight. ▼

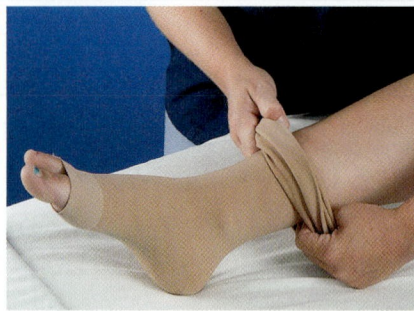

Knee-High Stockings
Pull up to 2.5 to 5 cm (1 to 2 in.) below the knee

Thigh-High Stockings
Pull up to the gluteal fold of the thigh, rotating inward so the gusset is centered over the femoral artery, slightly toward the inside of the leg.

Stockings apply varying amounts of compression between ankle, calf, and thigh areas. Keeping the stocking straight ensures that the pressure occurs over the correct areas.

9. **Smooth out any excess material**; keep stockings free of wrinkles and bunching.

Decreases the risk of skin breakdown and areas of potentially dangerous constriction.

10. **When using stockings with** closed toes, tug gently on the end of the stocking over the toes to create a small space between the end of the toes and the stocking.

Prevents compression of small vessels in the toes.

11. **Repeat the procedure** on the other leg.

12. **Remove the stockings** and bathe and dry the legs daily.

13. **Launder the stockings** at least every 3 days; dry them on a flat surface.

Soiled stockings can irritate the skin; dry flat to prevent stretching.

? What if . . .

- **Both legs do not measure the same?**

Order two different sizes of stockings and use one from each package to make two pairs.

Evaluation

- Evaluate patient comfort.
  Severe, continuous discomfort may indicate that the stockings are the wrong size.
- Check the stockings for wrinkles and/or rolling down at the top, especially when sitting.
  Wrinkles and rolling down can cause skin breakdown and areas of constriction.
- Evaluate and monitor skin condition.
  Elastic stockings should be removed for 20 to 30 minutes every 8 to 12 hours to allow you to inspect the patient's skin and evaluate the adequacy of his circulation.
- Evaluate the patient's ability to ambulate.
  It is important to reduce the time the patient is immobile due to pain, sedation, mechanical ventilation, and so on.
- Remeasure the legs regularly.
  To prevent complications related to swelling and weight gain.

Home Care

- Teach the client and/or caregiver to apply the stockings.
- Encourage the client to have two pairs of stockings on hand so that one pair can be used while the other is being laundered.
- Instruct the client to follow the manufacturer's directions for washing the stockings.
- Teach the client not to roll down the tops of the stockings.

Documentation

- Document leg measurements and size of the stockings used, to provide a baseline.
- Document the time and date applied.
- Note the condition of the skin, including any abnormalities.

Practice Resources
American Association of Critical-Care Nurses (AACN), 2010; Joanna Briggs Institute (2008b); Winslow & Brosz, 2008.

Thinking About the Procedure

Go to the *Fundamentals of Nursing Skills DVDs*, **Perioperative Nursing: Antiembolism Stockings.**

1. In what position did the nurse place the patient to measure leg length from the gluteal fold to the base of the heel?
2. How did the nurse position the patient to measure her leg length for knee-high stockings?
3. Did the nurse apply thigh-high or knee-high stockings?

For suggested responses, go to Chapter 40, **Thinking About the Procedure Suggested Responses,** on Davis*Plus*.

Procedure 40–3 ■ Applying Sequential Compression Devices

➤ For steps to follow in *all* procedures, refer to the Universal Steps for All Procedures found on the page facing the inside back cover.

Equipment

NOTE: Sequential compression devices may be referred to by several different brand names, including SCDS (sequential compression decompression stockings), Flowtrons, and PAS (pneumatic air stockings).

- Compression pump, motor, or machine
- Connecting tubing, if applicable (In some devices, the tubing is preconnected to the sleeves.)
- Compression sleeve (knee-high or thigh-high, depending on the order and the type of device)
- Elastic stockings (if also prescribed)
- Washcloth and towel
- Measuring tape

Delegation

You may delegate the application of the sequential compression device to a NAP who has had training in that task. Instruct the NAP to report any redness, irritation, or open areas on the lower extremities. SCDs should not be removed for long periods of time because they are needed to support the patient's peripheral circulation.

✚ Instruct the NAP to ensure that all cords and connecting tubing are in a place that will not create a fall risk for the patient or visitors.

Pre-Procedure Assessment

- Assess cognitive level and level of consciousness.
  Patients with altered cognition may be at higher risk for falls related to the presence of the connecting tubing and attachment to the compression pump. Patients who are unconscious will not be able to report a device that is creating too much pressure.
- Assess signs and symptoms of severe peripheral arterial disease, such as weak or absent pulses, discoloration or cyanosis, or gangrene.
  Increased compression of vessels by the sequential device may further impede arterial flow.
- Assess skin condition. Note of lesions, dermatitis, or major edema, as evidenced by shiny, taut skin.
  If skin is overstretched by edema, the sequential compression sleeve may irritate or worsen skin conditions and cause skin breakdown.

➤ When performing the procedure, always identify your patient according to agency policy and be attentive to standard precautions, hand hygiene, patient safety and privacy, body mechanics, and documentation.

Procedure Steps

1. **Cleanse the lower extremities**, if necessary.
   Remove surface dirt and/or bacteria, decreasing the likelihood of infection and odor.
2. **If elastic stockings have been ordered in conjunction with the sequential compression device,** apply them, following the steps in Procedure 40-2.
3. **For thigh-high SCD sleeves,** measure the thigh to ensure that the sleeves are of the proper size. Follow the manufacturer's instructions.
4. **Position the patient supine.**
   Prevents venous pooling. Allows for easier application of the compression sleeve.
5. ✚ **Place the compression device** pump in a location near an electrical outlet so that the cord will not pose a fall risk. Plug it in.

   NOTE: Many compression pumps come equipped with hangers so you can hang the device at the bottom of the patient's bed.

6. **Apply the compression sleeve.** ➤

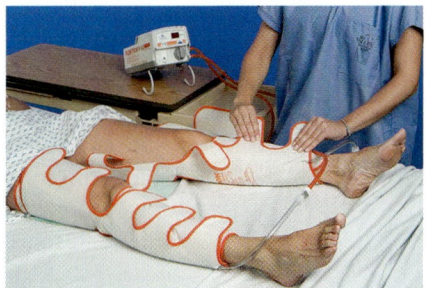

For Flowtron Brand (available in knee-length only):
   a. Open the Velcro fasteners on the sleeve.
   b. Place the sleeve under the lower leg below the knee, with the "air bladder" side down on the bed.
   c. Bring the ends of the sleeve up, and wrap them around the lower leg, leaving one to two fingerbreadths of space between the leg and the sleeve.
   Prevents excess pressure and overcompression.

For SCDS/PAS Brands
   a. Open the Velcro fasteners on the sleeve.

   b. Place the sleeve under the leg, ensuring that the fastener will close on the anterior surface. For thigh-high sleeves, place the opened sleeve under the leg, ensuring that the knee opening is at the level of the knee joint.
   Ensures that compression occurs over the correct structures. Prevents restricted range of motion (ROM) of the knee joint.
   c. Bring the ends of the sleeve up, and wrap them around the leg, leaving one to two fingerbreadths of space between the leg and the sleeve.
   Prevents excess pressure and overcompression.

7. **Connect the sleeve** to the compression pump.
8. **Turn the pump on** and, if applicable, set the compression pressure on the pump device to the manufacturer's recommended setting. *Note:* In some facilities, the compression pressure amount is preset and can be changed only by the central supply/equipment department.

Evaluation

After applying the device, make the following ongoing assessments:

- Inflation and deflation of the sleeve
  Ensures that the device is actually working.
- Kinking or pinching of the connecting tubing
  Interferes with inflation of sleeves and may cause overheating or malfunction of the unit.
- Circulation, sensation, and motion of the foot, including skin color, pulses, temperature, capillary refill, motion, and sensation
- Patient comfort
  Increasing discomfort may indicate excess or incorrect pressure.
- Skin condition. Remove the compression sleeves at intervals so that you can inspect skin and evaluate the adequacy of circulation. *Note:* If elastic stockings are being used in conjunction with the sequential compression device, follow the recommendations in Procedure 40-2.
- Signs and symptoms of deep vein thrombosis
  Even with sequential compression device therapy, a patient can still develop thrombi.

Patient Teaching

 Teach the patient to call for assistance when disconnecting the tubing from the compression pump in order to ambulate.
Prevents patient falls. The SCD tubing is a tripping hazard, and injuries from falls involving SCDs are likely to be more severe than injuries associated with general patient falls (Johnston & Davis, 2008).

Documentation

- Document the date and time you applied the device.
- Note the type and size (if applicable) of the compression sleeve used.
- Document the skin condition, including any abnormalities.

Sample documentation:

11/11/14   1100   Knee-high SCD applied per order. Skin warm, dry, and intact at time of application. Peripheral pulses palpable. Pt's wife instructed on use of SCD. Pt. unresponsive. No evidence of discomfort, no grimace or movement with application. ———————S. Bee, RN

Practice Resources

Berliner, Ozbilgin, & Zarin, 2003; Johnston & Davis, 2008; Larry, 2003; Markel & Morris, 2002. (*Note:* Some of these references are manufacturers and are not evidence based.)

Thinking About the Procedure

 Go to the *Fundamentals of Nursing Skills DVDs*, **Perioperative Nursing: Sequential Compression Device.**

1. Where did the nurse place the compression pump?
2. What kind of compression sleeve was used: knee-high or thigh-high?

For suggested responses, go to Chapter 40, **Thinking About the Procedure Suggested Responses,** on Davis*Plus.*

Procedure 40–4 ■ Managing Gastric Suction

➤ For steps to follow in *all* procedures, refer to the Universal Steps for All Procedures found on the page facing the inside back cover.

Equipment

Procedure 40-4A: Initial Equipment Setup

- Nonsterile procedure gloves
- Suction source (either a portable machine or piped-in wall source) (See Figures 40-9 and 40-10.)
- Suction container and tubing
- Stopcock (to connect the NG tube to suction tubing)

Procedure 40-4B: Emptying the Suction Container

- Clean nonsterile procedure gloves
- Graduated container
  To measure gastric output when emptying the suction container. Not needed if suction canister is marked for measuring.
- Alcohol wipes or chlorhexidine/alcohol antiseptic product

Procedure 40-4C: Irrigating the Nasogastric Tubing

- Nonsterile procedure gloves
- Irrigating set (basin and bulb syringe or catheter-tipped syringe)

- Normal saline irrigant (unless another irrigant is prescribed)
- Linen-saver pads

Procedure 40-4D: Providing Comfort Measures

- Nonsterile procedure gloves
- Emesis basin, cup, and water for mouth care
- Water-soluble lubricant
- Cotton-tip applicators
- Tissues or damp washcloth

NOTE: This procedure assumes an NG or other enteric tube is already in place and that its correct placement has already been verified. If you need to insert an NG tube or check placement, refer to Chapter 28. Tubes for gastric decompression are typically large-lumen tubes such as a Salem sump or Levin tube. See the table at the end of this procedure for more information about tubes.

Delegation

A registered nurse should do the initial setup and any subsequent irrigation. You may delegate a NAP to empty and measure

(continued on next page)

Procedure 40-4 ■ **Managing Gastric Suction** (continued)

drainage and perform comfort measures. You must monitor equipment functioning and the patient's responses to the decompression. Instruct the NAP about observations that should be reported to you.

Pre-Procedure Assessments

- Determine that the NG tube has been inserted and placement has been verified.

- Verify the prescriber's order for type of tube and whether it is to be placed to suction or a drainage bag; also verify the type of suction to be used (low, high, continuous, intermittent).
- Auscultate for bowel sounds.
- Assess the patient's ability to cooperate with the procedure and understand explanations.
- Refer to the Evaluation section of this procedure. This procedure assumes an NG tube is already in place, so assessments are ongoing.

Procedure 40-4A ■ **Initial Equipment Setup**

➤ When performing the procedure, always identify your patient according to agency policy and be attentive to standard precautions, hand hygiene, patient safety and privacy, body mechanics, and documentation.

Procedure Steps

1. **Place the collection container** in the holder (on the portable suction machine or on the wall). Plug the power cord into a grounded outlet if using a portable suction machine.
2. **Connect the short tubing** between the container and the suction source. In some systems, the port will be marked "vacuum."
3. **Connect the long suction tubing** to the container (it may be marked "patient"); if a stopcock is available, connect it to the open end nearest the patient.
4. **Don nonsterile procedure gloves.**
   Helps prevent transfer of microorganisms.
5. **After the nasogastric (NG) tube** has been inserted and placement verified, attach the end of the NG tube to the suction tubing.
   See Chapter 28 to review importance of tube placement. You must be certain the NG tube is in the stomach, not in the esophagus or airways.

6. **If using a double lumen** catheter (e.g., Salem sump), instill 10 to 20 mL of air into the vent lumen to make sure it is patent. This should create a soft hissing sound.
7. **Secure the NG tube** to the client's nose and gown (see Chapter 28 to review).
   Minimizes movement of the tube, helping to prevent irritation of the nares or other insertion site, as well as helping to keep the tube from migrating up out of the stomach.
8. **Turn on the suction source** to the prescribed amount. In an emergency when there is no order, always use low suction. Open the stopcock—note the direction of the arrows.
9. **Observe that drainage appears** in the collection container.
   It may take up to 5 minutes for air to be removed from the canister before the stomach contents will drain. ➤

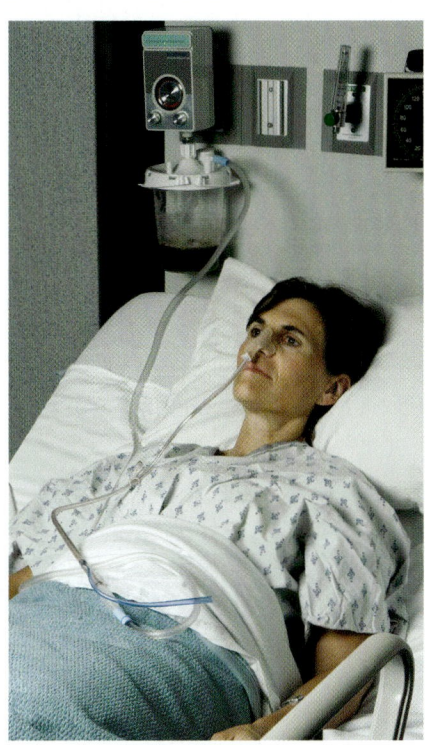

Procedure 40-4B ■ **Emptying the Suction Container**

➤ When performing the procedure, always identify your patient according to agency policy and be attentive to standard precautions, hand hygiene, patient safety and privacy, body mechanics, and documentation.

1. **Don clean nonsterile gloves.**
   Limits the transfer of microorganisms; protects your hands from contact with body secretions.
2. **Turn off the suction source** and close the stopcock on the tubing (or clamp the tubing, if there is no stopcock).
   Prevents suction flow during emptying of the container.

3. **Empty the suction canister.**

   Suction container is marked with measurements.
   Note the amount, color, and odor of the contents. Empty and rinse the container.

   Suction container is not marked incrementally.
   Remove the cap from the lid of the suction container and pour the drainage

into a graduated measuring container. Note color, odor, and amount.
A container with graduated markings enables you to monitor intake and output (I&O) accurately. Rinsing removes organic material that could be a reservoir for microorganisms.

4. **Wipe the port of the suction** container with an alcohol wipe. Place the

suction container back in its holder and close the stopper on the lid.

5. **Turn on the suction source** to the prescribed amount. Turn on the

stopcock (or unclamp the tubing), noting the direction of the arrows.

6. **Observe for proper functioning** of the suction and patency of the tubing.

7. **Remove and discard gloves**. Perform hand hygiene.

Procedure 40-4C ■ Irrigating the Nasogastric Tubing

➤ When performing the procedure, always identify your patient according to agency policy and be attentive to standard precautions, hand hygiene, patient safety and privacy, body mechanics, and documentation.

1. **Place a linen-saver pad** on the bed under the NG tube.
2. **Open the irrigation set** and pour saline into the basin.
   Water is not used because it may cause electrolyte imbalances.
3. **Don clean procedure gloves.**
   Limits the transfer of microorganisms; protects your hands from contact with body secretions.
4. **Check for correct placement** of the NG tube (see Chapter 28 as needed).
   Prevents accidental instillation of irrigant into the airways.
5. **Fill the syringe with 30 to 50 mL** of saline and lay it on the linen-saver pad.
6. **Clamp the NG tube** or turn off the stopcock connecting to the suction tubing. Disconnect the NG tube from the suction tubing.
   Prevents backflow of drainage and soiling of linens and clothing.
7. **Hold the drainage tubing up** until suction clears it. Then lay it on the

linen-saver pad or hook it over the suction machine.
   Keeps secretions from soiling the bed linens or clothing.
8. **Turn off the suction machine.**
9. **Unclamp the NG tube** or turn on the stopcock.
10. **Unpin the NG tube** (or remove tape) from the patient's clothing.
11. **With the syringe, instill** the irrigant slowly into the NG tube. Do not force the solution. Be careful not to instill fluid into the air vent.
    Clears the NG tube of gastric contents to keep it patent and helps keep the tube from adhering to the gastric mucosa. Partially digested food, clotted blood, or tissue debris may clog the tube and prevent effective drainage.
12. **Lower the end of the NG tube** and then release the syringe bulb (or pull back the plunger) to withdraw fluid. Instill and withdraw until fluid flows in and out freely.
    Uses the force of gravity with negative pressure to withdraw instilled fluid and gastric contents.

Double-Lumen NG Tube
Draw 30 mL of air into the syringe and inject it into the "pigtail" (the smaller-bore tube). Follow agency policy for this.
This clears the air-vent tube of any secretions. It must be patent in order to equalize pressure and prevent gastric tissue trauma at the drainage ports. The air also keeps the tube from draining fluid out of the stomach by capillary action.

13. **Reclamp the NG tube** or turn off the stopcock.
    Prevents backflow of drainage.
14. **Reconnect the NG tube** to the suction tube. Then release the clamp or turn on the stopcock.
15. **Reattach the NG tube** to the patient's clothing (with a pin or tape—see Chapter 28 as needed).
    Prevents irritating the patient's nostril.
16. **Provide comfort measures** (e.g., mouth care).
17. **Remove and discard gloves.** Perform hand hygiene.

Procedure 40-4D ■ Providing Comfort Measures

➤ When performing the procedure, always identify your patient according to agency policy and be attentive to standard precautions, hand hygiene, patient safety and privacy, body mechanics, and documentation.

1. **Don clean nonsterile procedure gloves.**
2. **Provide mouth care** (see Procedures 24-6, 24-7, and 24-8 if you need to review). Use mouthwash as desired. Avoid using lemon-glycerin swabs. Apply water-soluble lubricant to the lips if they become dry and crusty.
   The patient most likely has a dry mouth from not receiving oral intake and from mouth breathing. Lemon-glycerin swabs cause even more drying of tissues.
3. **Remove nasal secretions** with a tissue or a damp washcloth. Moisten

a cotton-tip applicator and wipe the inside of each nostril. If secretions are encrusted, moisten the applicator with hydrogen peroxide, then follow with an applicator moistened with water.
   To soften, dissolve, and remove secretions and prevent tissue irritation.
4. **Apply a small amount of** water-soluble lubricant to the inside of each nostril.
   Soothes and softens dried skin. Avoid petroleum-based lubricants, as complications may occur if they are inhaled.

5. **Check that the tape or tube** fixation device is secure. If it is not, replace it (see Procedure 28-2 as needed).
   Prevents irritation of the nasal skin and mucosa. Helps prevent migration of the NG tube from the stomach.

? What if . . .

■ **Resistance is met when you irrigate the NG tube?**

Check the tubing for kinks or evidence of obstruction. Have the patient to turn to the left side.
Turning to one side changes the position of the distal tip of the NG tube.

(continued on next page)

Procedure 40–4 ■ Managing Gastric Suction (continued)

■ **The patient complains that the NG tube is pulling against her nostril?**

The tube may not be properly anchored to her clothing. Reattach the safety pin (or tape) closer to the nose so that there is more slack in the tube.

■ **The NG tube causes excoriation of the nares?**

Remove the tape or fixation device from the nose. Remove the residual adhesive from the skin. Apply skin sealant and anchor the tube so that the adhesive touches in a different place on the skin. Keep the excoriated areas clean and dry.

■ **The NG tube does not drain?**

Check tubing for kinks or blockage. Check the suction apparatus. If the collection container is higher than the patient's abdomen, lower it. If these aspects are working properly, irrigate the tube (see Procedure 40-4C, preceding). If the tube still is not draining and the patient is uncomfortable, document and notify the primary care provider. Encourage the patient to relax and breathe slowly through her nose. If the patient has abdominal distention, pain, or vomiting, notify the provider immediately.

If the container is too high, the negative pressure of low suction may not be enough to overcome the force of gravity. Abdominal distention, pain, or vomiting may mean the system is not working. Continued distention creates undue strain on the suture line. You should notify the care provider of these symptoms even when the mechanical aspects of the suction seem in working order.

Gastric Decompression Tubes				
TYPE	**LUMEN(S)**	**USE**	**MANAGEMENT**	**DISCUSSION**
Levin	I, unvented	Decompression, feedings, or irrigation	Use low intermittent suction; may require irrigation.	If the tube opening(s) rest(s) against the gastric mucosa, the suction may irritate or injure the tissue.
Salem Sump		Decompression, suction, gastric lavage	Vented. May use high continuous suction.	The air vent helps keep the tube away from the gastric mucosa during suction.
Sengsten–Blakemore	2	Decompression; treatment of active bleeding from esophageal or gastric varices	Use low intermittent suction.	Gastric or esophageal balloons hold the tube in place.
Cantor	I, unvented	Decompression	Use intermittent suction.	Distal end is weighted with a balloon. Used in bowel obstruction. Rarely used because of the hazard posed by the mercury in the weighted balloon.
Miller–Abbott	2	Decompression	Use intermittent suction.	Distal end weighted with a balloon. Used in bowel obstruction. Rarely used because it contains mercury in the weighted balloon.
Ewald or Other Very Large-Bore Tube	May be passed orally for emergency evacuation of stomach contents to prevent absorption of ingested medications, poisons, or products. A piston tip syringe is placed on the end of the tube for manual suction. Typically, the stomach is washed repeatedly with saline and all contents are withdrawn. Because of its large diameter, this type of tube is not tolerated by patients who are alert, and is not left in place after lavage is completed.			
Weighted Small-Bore Tubes (e.g., Keofeed)	For feedings only. Suction collapses the tube.			

Evaluation and Maintenance

- Periodically assess placement of the tube by a combination of methods (i.e., checking pH of aspirate, by listening over the stomach with a stethoscope while injecting air into the tube, and by reviewing radiographic reports). See Chapter 28 for review, as needed.
- Monitor patency of the tube and the effectiveness of the suction. Check tube connections.
- Monitor patient comfort (e.g., sore throat).
  The continuing presence of a tube in the nose and throat is bothersome to patients. The major nuisance is the pressure of the tube against the internal mucous membranes, irritating the nostril, pharynx, and esophagus.
- Auscultate for bowel sounds; turn off suction while auscultating.
  Bowel sounds indicate the return of peristalsis and the success of gastric decompression. You may hear the sound of the suction apparatus and misinterpret it as bowel sounds.
- Monitor for gastric distention, vomiting, and abdominal pain.
  These symptoms probably indicate the suction is not working effectively. See the What if . . . ? section, preceding.
- Examine skin and mucous membranes around the insertion site (e.g., nares, abdomen).
- Follow agency policy or the primary care provider's prescription for irrigation of the gastric tube. It is common to irrigate with 30 to 60 mL of normal saline every 4 to 6 hours.
- Monitor the color of the drainage (should be green to gold). If there is blood in the drainage, notify the primary care provider.
- For clients undergoing prolonged GI suction, observe for signs and symptoms of hyponatremia and hypokalemia (i.e., fatigue, lethargy, confusion, seizures, muscle weakness, paresthesia, and cardiac dysrhythmias). Review lab results and report any symptoms to the primary care provider.
- Assess the patient's ability to move about in bed while attached to the suction source.

Patient Teaching

- Instruct the patient to notify you of any discomfort, and to not tug on or try to reposition the NG tube if it becomes uncomfortable.
- Instruct the patient to notify you if feeling nauseated.
  This could mean the tube is blocked and not draining effectively.

Home Care

Usually, gastric suction is performed in a hospital. If the client is to go home with gastric suction (e.g., a terminally ill person who has a bowel obstruction and wants to be in her own home), teach the family how to use the device before the person is discharged. Also arrange for home healthcare.

Documentation

- Record all drainage as output on the I&O record.
- Record the time, type, and volume of irrigations and the drainage returned.
- Be sure to include irrigation fluids as input on the I&O record.
- Note color, odor, and consistency of drainage.
- Document emotional and physical responses to NG intubation.
- Document any evidence of tube or equipment malfunction.
- Document epigastric pain, discomfort, distention, or vomiting.

Practice Resources

Best practices, 2007; Green, Harris, & Singer, 2008; Sarasota Memorial Hospital, reviewed 2010.

Thinking About the Procedure

 Go to the *Fundamentals of Nursing Skills Videos,* **Nutrition: Gastrointestinal Suction.**

1. What type of suction source was demonstrated in the Videos?
2. Why did the nurse not clamp the NG tube before disconnecting it from the suction tubing?

 For suggested responses, go to Chapter 40, **Thinking About the Procedure Suggested Responses,** on Davis*Plus.*

 To explore learning resources for this chapter,

 Go to Davis*Plus* at http://davisplus.fadavis.com/, keyword Treas.
Chapter Resources for Chapter 40:
  Knowledge Check and Think Like a Nurse Response Sheets
  Knowledge Check Answers
  Resources for Caregivers and Health Professionals
  Reading More About Perioperative Care (Suggested Readings)
  What Are the Main Points in This Chapter?
NCLEX-Style Review Questions
Care Planning and Care Mapping Exercise
Chapter Overview Podcasts

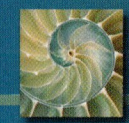

Concept Map

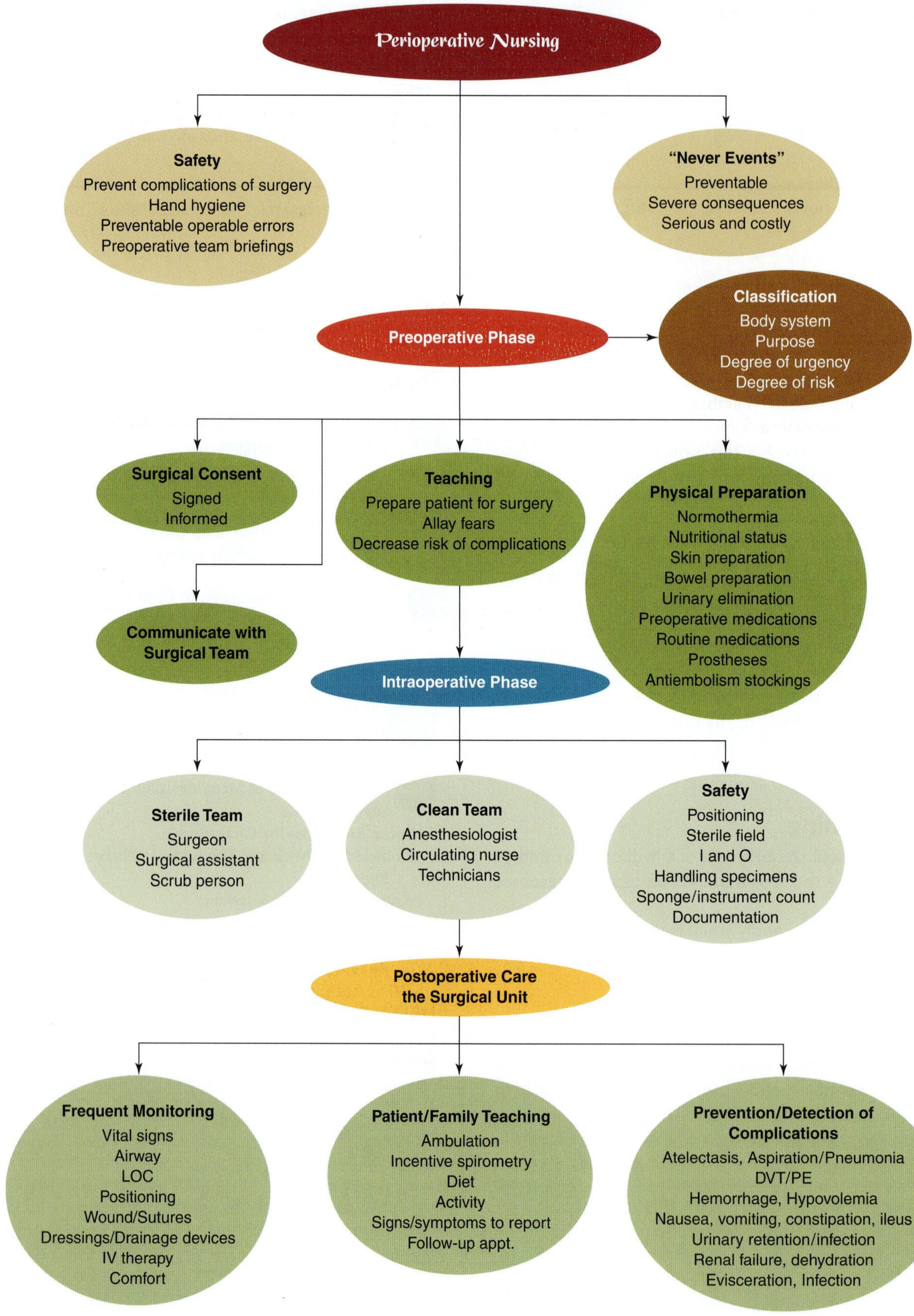

Perioperative Nursing

Safety
Prevent complications of surgery
Hand hygiene
Preventable operable errors
Preoperative team briefings

"Never Events"
Preventable
Severe consequences
Serious and costly

Preoperative Phase

Classification
Body system
Purpose
Degree of urgency
Degree of risk

Surgical Consent
Signed
Informed

Teaching
Prepare patient for surgery
Allay fears
Decrease risk of complications

Physical Preparation
Normothermia
Nutritional status
Skin preparation
Bowel preparation
Urinary elimination
Preoperative medications
Routine medications
Prostheses
Antiembolism stockings

Communicate with Surgical Team

Intraoperative Phase

Sterile Team
Surgeon
Surgical assistant
Scrub person

Clean Team
Anesthesiologist
Circulating nurse
Technicians

Safety
Positioning
Sterile field
I and O
Handling specimens
Sponge/instrument count
Documentation

Postoperative Care the Surgical Unit

Frequent Monitoring
Vital signs
Airway
LOC
Positioning
Wound/Sutures
Dressings/Drainage devices
IV therapy
Comfort

Patient/Family Teaching
Ambulation
Incentive spirometry
Diet
Activity
Signs/symptoms to report
Follow-up appt.

Prevention/Detection of Complications
Atelectasis, Aspiration/Pneumonia
DVT/PE
Hemorrhage, Hypovolemia
Nausea, vomiting, constipation, ileus
Urinary retention/infection
Renal failure, dehydration
Evisceration, Infection

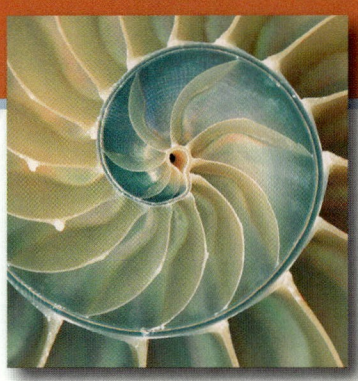

CHAPTER 41

Community & Home Nursing

Learning Outcomes

After completing this chapter, you should be able to:

➤ Define the meaning of *community*.

➤ Identify at least four factors by which you can recognize a healthy community.

➤ Discuss factors that create vulnerability for a population.

➤ Compare and contrast community-based care, community health nursing, public health nursing, and community-oriented nursing.

➤ Distinguish primary, secondary, and tertiary interventions in regard to a community health scenario.

➤ Discuss at least three strategies that nurses use to gather community data.

➤ Describe the roles of nurses in the community setting.

➤ Use standardized nursing language taxonomies (NANDA-I, NOC, NIC, Omaha, and CCC) to describe care planning in community and home care.

➤ Identify the primary goal of home care.

➤ Describe ways in which home healthcare differs from hospital nursing.

➤ Categorize the various agencies that deliver home healthcare according to purpose, client served, and funding source.

➤ Describe how the nurse's emphasis differs in hospice nursing as compared to home health nursing.

➤ List at least four criteria clients must meet in order for home care to be reimbursed by Medicare.

➤ Outline the steps required to prepare for a home visit, including considerations for the nurse's safety.

➤ Discuss ways in which the assessment process is unique in home care.

➤ Explain the role of the nurse in helping clients and families manage medications.

➤ Describe how infection control measures differ in the home and in the hospital.

➤ State two important safety concerns in home care that arise out of The Joint Commission 2012 home-care safety goals.

➤ Describe the nurse's role in treating caregiver strain.

Key Concepts

Community nursing

Home healthcare

Population

Related Concepts

See the Concept Map at the end of this chapter.

Caring for the Nguyens

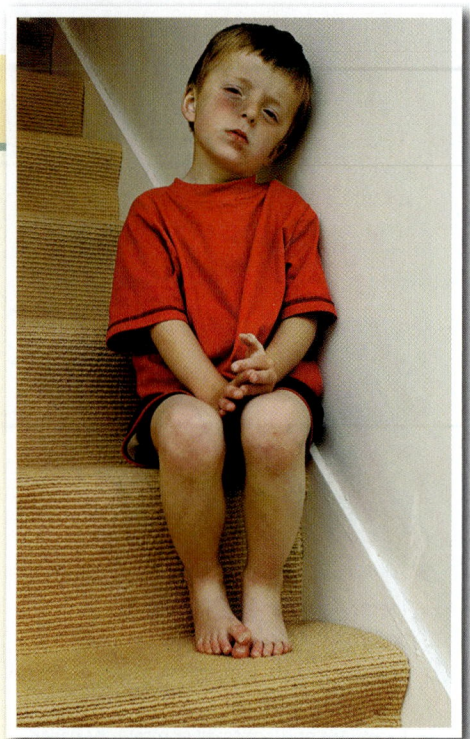

This feature allows you to practice the kind of thinking you will use as a full-spectrum nurse. There is usually more than one correct answer to a critical thinking question, so we do not provide answers for these features. It is more important to develop your nursing judgment than to "cover content." Discuss the questions with your peers. If you are still unsure, consult your instructor.

Yen Nguyen works as preschool teacher in her community. Andre is a 4-year-old boy in her class. Over the last few months, she has noticed that Andre has many bruises in various stages of healing. He seems withdrawn and does not interact much with the other children. She is concerned that Andre might be a victim of child abuse, but she is reluctant to make that accusation, especially because her assistant doesn't seem to have noticed anything amiss.

Mrs. Nguyen talks to her husband, Nam, about her concerns: "I'm worried about a child at school, but I'm afraid to say anything. What if I'm wrong? I'd probably lose my job. But if I'm right and I don't say anything, I could still lose my job, and this boy could be hurt even worse." Nam suggests that she contact the clinic nurse at the Family Medicine Center for confidential advice on how to proceed.

A. Imagine that you are the clinic nurse. Use the full-spectrum nursing model to identify at least 10 questions that you would need to answer to investigate Yen's concerns further.

B. *Self-knowledge:* What personal values do you have that would affect the manner in which you handle this situation? Explain.

C. *Ethical knowledge:* What is the most important ethical issue in this situation? That is, what is the most important goal? Note that there may be several moral and legal issues, but you are being asked to identify the *most*

important one. Note also that we are not asking you what the nurse *can* do, but rather what the nurse ideally *should* do.

D. You share the questions you have with Yen. She believes that there is a real need to investigate child abuse. You advise her to call the local child protective services (CPS) agency. Based on your knowledge of community and public health nursing, what aspects of the community health role will the nurse from CPS use as she investigates this situation?

 Go to **Caring for the Nguyens Response Sheet** on *DavisPlus.*

Meet Your Patients

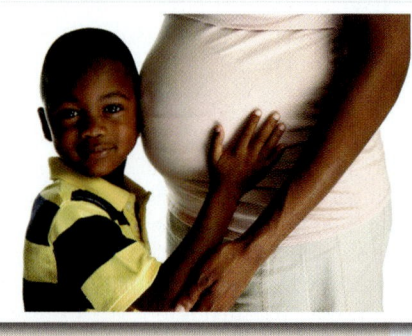

Your Neighbor, Tanya

You are nearing completion of your fundamentals course. One night while you are preparing for your next clinical, the telephone rings. It is your neighbor, Tanya. Her 5-year-old son, Jacob, attends kindergarten at the local public school. Jacob came home with a letter from the school nurse stating that another child in the class was ill with H1N1 influenza and that all the students in the class had been exposed to the disease.

Tanya is concerned about the risks to Jacob and the rest of the family. Tanya is 8 months pregnant, and the family has no health insurance. She states that because you are a nursing student, she thought you might know what she should do or where she might go for assistance.

Although you are flattered that your neighbor has consulted you, you need to consider whether you have the expertise to answer her questions. This complex situation requires knowledge from many aspects of nursing

Meet Your Patients (continued)

(e.g., immunizations, pregnancy, microbiology, pathophysiology). Though you may not have all of the information you need to answer her questions, you should be able to help your neighbor resolve her concerns. You will need to consider the following questions:

- What is going on in the situation that may influence the outcome?
- Who should be involved to improve the outcome?
- What theoretical knowledge do I need to answer my neighbor's questions? Where would I find this information?
- What additional data do I need to collect from my neighbor?
- What suggestions and/or referrals should I offer to my neighbor?

Your Patients, the Escobars

Flora Escobar is 78 years old. She lives at home with her husband, Roland, age 78. Both enjoyed good health until Roland suffered a cerebrovascular accident (CVA, or stroke) 3 weeks ago. He was hospitalized and then spent 2 weeks in a skilled nursing facility (SNF). He returned home yesterday and will be followed by the local home health agency for physical therapy and nursing care.

At your initial visit, Mrs. Escobar greets you at the door. She is a petite woman who appears exhausted. She is wearing an apron with the pockets stuffed with pill bottles. The hallway is partially blocked with a bedside commode, walker, and tray table. Mr. Escobar, wearing pajamas and a robe, is in a hospital bed in the living room. He is a tall, stocky man who is sitting up in bed but is slumped and leaning to the left.

After introducing yourself, you ask an open-ended question to build rapport: "How have things been going since you came home yesterday?" Mrs. Escobar nods, sighs, and says, "I'm worried that I'm doing things wrong. I have a hard time helping him move. He is so much bigger than me, and I don't want to hurt him. He is frustrated with me, but he has difficulty talking and can't tell me what he needs." Tears fill Mrs. Escobar's eyes. Her husband turns away to avoid eye contact with you. To refocus their attention, you suggest that you go over some information and then begin to look at what additional services might be helpful.

Imagine how stressed Mrs. Escobar must feel. How do you think you could best help this family? In this chapter, as you read the section on home health nursing, you should find it easier to answer those questions.

Theoretical Knowledge
knowing why

In this chapter, we begin with a discussion of community nursing, where you will frequently encounter problems such as Tanya presented in the Meet Your Patients scenario. An aging population and cost-cutting efforts to reduce hospital stays have resulted in the rapid growth of community-based healthcare, including home nursing care. We will explore the roles, interventions, and career opportunities for nurses who work within communities and in home healthcare. You might not have considered working outside the hospital, but perhaps your career path will lead you to caring for clients in one of the many community or home healthcare settings

ABOUT THE KEY CONCEPTS

In this chapter, you will learn about the concepts of *community nursing* and *home healthcare* and how different *populations* have unique healthcare needs. You will learn how these concepts are related to each other and to subconcepts such as public health nursing, vulnerable populations, and home visits. The concepts and their interrelationships will help you understand and recall chapter content.

UNDERSTANDING THE CONCEPT OF COMMUNITY

The word **community** comes from the Latin term *communis,* meaning "the gift or fellowship of common relations and feelings." Historically, it meant a body of like-minded people or the inhabitants of a town. Then and now, the term suggests a general sense of selflessness, sharing, relationship, and doing good that comes from working together. Most members of a community share a common language, certain rituals, and special customs.

In contrast to community, we tend to think of a **population** as a certain geographic region. But the term *population* has other meanings as well.

- It can mean the group of people of a particular race or class in a place (e.g., "There are 1,500 Latino people living in Edwards County").
- It can also mean *any* aggregation of people subject to statistical or other study (e.g., all the homeless people in Edwards County, or all the pregnant adolescents living in Edwards County).

The United States Bureau of the Census conducts a survey and count of the American people (the population of the United States) every 10 years. The most recent census is the one conducted in the year 2010. For results,

 Go to the **U.S. Census Bureau** Web site at http://www.census.gov/2010census/

When the census is completed, the U.S. Census Bureau groups the data into sections of 1,500 to 8,000 people, known as **census tracts.** The area of individual census tracts varies according to the density of the population. In urban centers, a census tract covers a small area. Rural census tracts are large. Census tracts are useful to public officials, market analysts, and anyone—including community nurses who study the characteristics and concerns of smaller sections of people.

Maps and census tracts show the *geopolitical* boundaries of a community. But as we noted earlier, a community can also be

a group of people with a common purpose. They may live in different geographical areas, but they have a "sense of belonging" to their group (community).

An **aggregate** is a group of individuals with at least one shared characteristic, either personal or environmental. For example, a community health nurse may work with a class of high school girls to reduce the incidence of adolescent pregnancy. The shared characteristics of this aggregate are that they are female, are of childbearing age, and attend a particular school. As another example, the nursing students in your school are an aggregate. What characteristics and goals do you share?

KnowledgeCheck 41-1
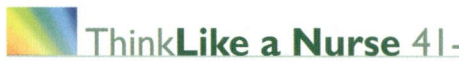

- Give several examples of a community.
- How is a population different from a community?

ThinkLike a Nurse 41-1

- Why might the boundaries of a census tract change every 10 years?
- How could you figure out what census tract you live or go to school in?

What Are the Components of a Community?

To understand a particular community and its needs, you will need information about its three components, the concepts of structure, status, and process.

- **Structure** refers to the general characteristics of a community. These include demographic data, such as gender, age, ethnicity, and educational and income levels, as well as data about healthcare services, such as the number of primary care providers or emergency care facilities in the area.
- **Status** describes the biological, emotional, and social outcome components of a community. *Biological* data include morbidity (illness) and mortality (death) rates, life expectancy ratios, and risk factor profiles for the respective age groups within a community. *Emotional* data include general indications of mental health and consumer satisfaction survey results about various aspects of the community as compared to other locales. *Social* data include crime rates, citizenship involvement in community-wide activities, and general functioning levels of the community members.
- **Process** describes the overall effectiveness level of the community. For example, do the members of the community perceive that they are part of a group with common purpose, values, or interests? What is the extent of interaction among community members? Does the community have an established forum for conflict resolution?

What Makes a Community Healthy?

As with individuals, the meaning and perception of health varies among aggregates. For nurses, it is important to understand what a particular community defines (and values) as health rather than relying on personal definitions. Health is whatever the client community defines it to be.

When determining what makes a community healthy from a traditional biomedical perspective, the national consensus paper *Healthy People 2020* provides useful guidelines. An earlier version of this document was produced in response to a 1979 report from the Surgeon General indicating that many of the health problems of Americans were preventable. *Healthy People 2020* identifies leading indicators for measuring the

health of our nation. Some examples affecting community health include the following:

- Physical activity
- Overweight and obesity
- Tobacco use
- Substance abuse
- Responsible sexual behavior
- Mental health
- Injury and violence
- Environmental quality
- Immunizations
- Access to healthcare

For the complete list of indicators, see Box 27-2, Focus Areas of *Healthy People 2020.*

The four overarching goals of the *Healthy People 2020* initiative are to (1) increase years of healthy life; (2) eliminate health disparities among different populations, including accessibility of healthcare; (3) create an environment conducive to social and physical health; and (4) promote healthy living for people across all life stages.

These aggregate goals are to be achieved through promoting healthy behaviors, increasing access to quality healthcare, and strengthening community health resources. For more information and for the complete set of *Healthy People 2020* objectives,

 Go to the **Healthy People 2020** Web site at http://www.healthypeople.gov/2020/

KnowledgeCheck 41-2

- What makes up the "structure" of a community?
- What is community "status"?
- What is community "process"?
- Use the guidelines from *Healthy People 2020* to compile a list of several characteristics that make a community healthy.

What Makes a Population Vulnerable?

A **vulnerable population** is defined as an aggregate that is at increased risk of adverse health outcomes. Members of vulnerable populations have a higher probability of developing illness than do members of the general population. Because of their increased risk of health problems, vulnerable populations are a major focus of community health efforts. Vulnerability involves multiple factors:

Limited Economic Resources. Income is a major predictor of health risk. People with higher incomes typically have greater access to health services and greater selection of providers, treatment options, and location of health services. In contrast, the more limited a person's income, the more limited her healthcare options. Consequently, many persons of low income forgo preventive or health maintenance care and seek healthcare services only when they are quite ill.

Limited Social Resources. Friends and family are valuable resources to help a person deal with day-to-day stress as well as the demands associated with illness. They often provide feedback, listen to concerns, and offer emotional and physical assistance. Unfortunately, not everyone has social resources. Older adults who live alone and people with mental illness are examples of groups at increased risk because of social isolation.

Age. The very young and the very old are less able to adapt to physiological stress and are at increased risk of disease. They are more prone to infections and may not be able to protect themselves environmental hazards, such as cold or heat. These age groups are also more often living in poverty.

Chronic Disease and Obesity. People who have chronic diseases are at greater risk for many health problems. For example, people with obesity are at increased risk for heart disease, diabetes, impaired mobility, joint pain, and other complications. People with diabetes are at risk for blindness, impaired wound healing, and other complications.

History of Abuse or Trauma. People who have experienced abuse or traumatic events often feel they have limited control over their health and circumstances. They may experience powerlessness and/or hopelessness and be unable to initiate activities that promote health or lead to early treatment of illness. These circumstances also tax their reserves and place them at risk for mental health problems.

Other vulnerable populations include people who are poor or homeless, migrant workers, people with disabilities, premature infants, women with high-risk pregnancy and pregnant adolescents, people with communicable disease, people who abuse substances, members of certain ethnic/racial groups, and the untreated mentally ill.

UNDERSTANDING THE CONCEPT OF COMMUNITY-BASED NURSING

A community can be either a *site* for healthcare delivery or a *recipient* of healthcare services. In fact, the first hospitals in the United States were established only in the late 1860s to protect society from contagious disease. Several decades passed before hospitals and other freestanding clinics became the predominant settings for providing healthcare. However, as the technological advances of the past 30 years have escalated the costs of delivering health services, efforts to lower costs have created a move back to more community-based care, including complementary and alternative care.

Community-based care refers to acute care or rehabilitative services performed in clinics, offices, mobile care units, and other facilities in the community—rather than in acute care settings, such as hospitals (although acute care settings also exist within the community). For example, many surgeries and diagnostic procedures are now performed in privately owned surgical centers, health clinics, and physicians' offices rather than in hospitals. People also receive mental, physical, cardiac, and pulmonary rehabilitation services in outpatient settings. Extended care facilities, or nursing homes, commonly provide rehabilitative care for patients after acute traumatic injuries, as well as continuous skilled care for older adults and people with chronic illness. The following sections describe three approaches to community-based nursing care: community health nursing, public health nursing, and community-oriented nursing.

Community Health Nursing

Although many people use the terms *community health nursing* and *public health nursing* interchangeably, the two are not identical. **Community health nursing** focuses on how the health of individuals, families, and groups affects the community as a whole. Community health nurses strive to promote, protect, preserve, and maintain the health of the population through the delivery of personal health services to individuals, families, and groups. For example, a community health nurse may work in a prenatal clinic providing free services for low-income women. The nurse provides a direct service to each pregnant woman, yet she is doing that to improve the general health of the entire community. By encouraging the mother to eat balanced meals, exercise, and avoid harmful substances, the nurse improves the health of both mother and baby—who

are members of the community—and, therefore, improves the overall health of the community.

Public Health Nursing

Public health nursing focuses on the community at large and the eventual effect of the community's health status on the health of individuals, families, and groups. The goal of public health is to prevent individual disease and disability, in addition to promoting and protecting the health of the community as a whole. For example, a public health nurse may be employed by a county health department to provide tuberculosis (TB) **surveillance services.** The nurse helps to protect the entire community by screening for TB at the local school, by testing high-risk individuals for TB, and by identifying and tracking clients with active disease to ensure that they complete the prescribed 6- to 9-month medication regimen.

Because public health focuses on large-scale programs that address the entire community, government-based agencies often provide these services. The United States Public Health Service (USPHS) is an example of a public health agency based within the federal government. Some examples of successful public health programs are HPV immunizations for adolescents, smoking cessation for healthcare workers, motor vehicle and infant car-seat safety, and obesity prevention programs for children.

For additional information on the USPHS,

 Go to Chapter 41, **Supplemental Materials: United States Public Health Service,** on Davis*Plus.*

Community-Oriented Nursing

Community-oriented nursing combines components of community and public health. It focuses on health promotion, illness prevention, early detection, and treatment provided within the community setting. The practice is evidence based and collaborative with other community health disciplines. The approach is a comprehensive look at the individual, family, group, and community at large. For example, a nurse with a community-oriented approach might work in a comprehensive adolescent prenatal program. The nurse provides individual care at the local clinic 2 days per week. While at the clinic, she gathers data from adolescent clients about the schools they attend; their knowledge of birth control, pregnancy, and childbirth; as well as the issues these girls face with pregnancy. On the remaining 3 days of the week, she meets with school officials to identify pregnant teens who need prenatal care; teaches a class about sexuality in the local high school; works with teachers to identify strategies to keep pregnant teens in school; provides parenting education to adolescents who have children; and advocates changing a bus route so that teens can easily get to the local clinic. Each aspect of care allows the nurse to gather more data about the needs of the individuals and the community as a whole. Figure 41-1 provides a schematic of the relationship of the various community-based nursing approaches identified in this section.

KnowledgeCheck 41-3

- What is the distinction between an aggregate population and a vulnerable population?
- Identify practice differences between a community-based nurse and an acute care nurse.
- How is public health nursing different from community health nursing? How is it the same?
- How is community-oriented nursing related to community health nursing and public health nursing?

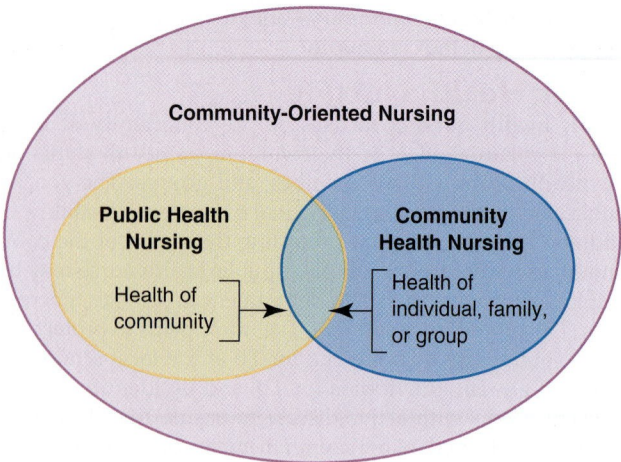

Community-Oriented Nursing

Public Health Nursing

Health of community

Community Health Nursing

Health of individual, family, or group

FIGURE 41-1 Schematic relationship of community nursing approaches.

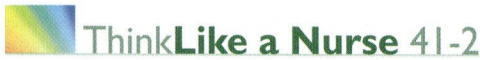

Think Like a Nurse 41-2

Review the scenario of Tanya and Jacob (Meet Your Patients). Which form of community-based nursing would be most appropriate to address Tanya's concerns?

Who Were Some Pioneers of Community Nursing?

The following are some of the most notable people who have contributed to the development of community-based nursing care.

Florence Nightingale—Established the importance of promoting health by manipulating the environment (e.g., light, warmth, sanitation, cleanliness) and nursing the whole person.

Lillian Wald—Known as the first community health nurse; founded the first visiting nurses association in New York.

Clara Barton—Founder of the American Red Cross.

Margaret Sanger—Founded the International Planned Parenthood Federation. Pioneered the use of family planning and birth control education.

If you would like to learn more about the achievements of these community health pioneers,

 Go to Chapter 41, **Supplemental Materials: Pioneers of Community-Based Nursing,** on *DavisPlus.*

WORKING WITHIN COMMUNITIES

In the community setting, nurses' roles vary depending on the community and its identified needs. Community nursing care is by nature holistic, and it serves a large client population. Therefore, one of the most effective nursing interventions is **empowerment.** This means assisting the client (individual or community) to recognize and use available resources to achieve or maintain the desired level of health, achieve autonomy, and maintain positive self-esteem.

What Are the Roles of Community Nurses?

Community health nurses function as client advocates, educators, collaborators, counselors, and case managers. All of these roles require excellent written and oral communication skills.

Although electronic health records and widespread use of e-mail, text messaging, and other forms of electronic communication have made it possible to communicate with large numbers of people, computer or Internet access might be a problem in some areas. In addition, there are still some people with limited or no computer skills.

Client Advocate. The effective community health nurse consistently supports the identified or expressed concerns of the client and/or community. Advocating for a community often requires political involvement at the local, state, or national levels. The challenge is in knowing whom to approach for political support and how to gain their support. As a community health nurse you can effect change by getting involved in your local student nurses association, professional nursing organizations, school board, citizen committees, or by attending council meetings.

Educator. Because community nursing focuses on wellness and disease prevention, much of what the nurse does involves client education—of individuals, aggregates at risk of disease, politicians, or a community at large. However, it is difficult to evaluate the effect of the education because people may not act on the knowledge for months or years after the teaching situation. When planning teaching, you must be aware of the stage of development, educational level, and learning style of the community group you intend to educate. The best learning programs are short; provide relevant, practical information; and can be easily incorporated into the learner's daily routine. For more information about teaching clients, see Chapter 26.

Collaborator. A primary task of a community health nurse is to serve as a collaborator. Partnerships and coalitions can effectively address common concerns among different communities. Consider the following example: A community health nurse is concerned about poor compliance with recommended immunization schedules for 2-year-olds in a particular community. He surveys some of the parents to determine their reasons for not obtaining vaccinations. The nurse discovers that the clinic's operating hours are limited and the automated call routing system is frustrating for people trying to schedule an appointment. The nurse also discovers that some offices are not reminding clients to return for missed appointments. The community nurse schedules a meeting of clinic staff, practice managers, and patients to resolve these issues. At the meeting, some larger issues are revealed, such as failure of state Medicaid agencies to reimburse the providers adequately and in a timely manner. In addition, there are not enough Medicaid providers to serve the community.

Counselor. Once you have established rapport with a group, members may consult you about a variety of health and non–health-related concerns. You must be careful to offer counsel only in areas within your scope of practice and make recommendations that are practical yet meet the needs of the community. Often, you may need only to serve as a witness to the group's concerns. Letting clients debate or work through issues empowers them and fosters self-reliance.

Case Manager. Community nurses commonly make referrals to or collaborate with other health and social agencies. Be cautious in referring clients to these resources, because agency policies and financing change frequently. Also, because community agencies often operate on grants and time-limited funding, a program that is available at one time may be dissolved at another. As a nurse, you will need to remain in contact with agencies to which clients are referred so that you

remain aware of the current restrictions and availability of services. For example, a local group has established a free healthcare program for resident children who are underinsured. Pediatricians and nurses volunteer their time to provide the care. Pharmaceutical representatives provide the medical supplies and routine medications. Local specialists (e.g., surgeons) provide services to those with complex or specialized needs. However, in such a clinic the appointment times fill up quickly, and often clients have to wait more than a month or two for an appointment. Before enrolling families in the program, you would need to be aware of these limitations and share this information with clients.

KnowledgeCheck 41-4

Give an example of a nursing activity involved in each of the following community health roles: educator, advocate, case manager, counselor, and collaborator.

How Are Community Nursing Interventions Classified?

There are three basic levels of care in which nursing interventions can be classified: primary, secondary, and tertiary. Most community-oriented nursing practices are aimed at the primary (prevention) level.

Primary Interventions

The goal of primary (first-level) interventions is to promote health and prevent disease. Educating susceptible individuals with no known disease process is an example of a routine, primary intervention that community health nurses practice. For example, a nurse may educate 9th grade students about the risk of hepatitis B and human papillomavirus (HPV), the benefits of vaccination, and strategies to reduce the likelihood of exposure to contaminated body fluids. Other examples include collaborating with local agencies to provide clean and secure temporary housing for migrant farm workers; or lobbying elected representatives for a ban on smoking in restaurants.

Secondary Interventions

Secondary (second-level) interventions aim to reduce the impact of the disease process by early detection and treatment. For example, a community health nurse may screen a sexually active adolescent girl for hepatitis B and/or HPV. She has known risk factors for sexually transmitted infection but no apparent disease symptoms. The nurse will also teach the client how to protect herself from sexually transmitted infections (STIs), hepatitis B, and HIV in the future. Other examples of secondary interventions include providing outreach screening programs offering mammography, scoliosis screening, lipid testing (Fig. 41-2), or prostate-specific antigen (PSA) testing for prostate cancer.

Promoting Patient-Centered Care in Community Health

Competency: Patient-Centered Care (Knowledge, Skills, Attitudes)*

Scenario: Nurses at a public clinic note an increased number of Hispanic clients seeking services. To best serve this growing community, one of the nurses researches healthcare issues affecting urban Hispanic populations. One statistic that surprises her is that Latino men are more likely to be diagnosed with late-stage prostate cancer and then to die from the disease than non-Latino men. Clinic staff therefore plans to develop a flyer about prostate cancer screening, directed at Hispanic men aged 50 and older. The nurse asks a male co-worker, Mr. Sanchez, what cultural norms might influence health behaviors. Mr. Sanchez explains that many Latino men view seeking healthcare as a sign of weakness. He explains "machismo" and "caballerismo," concepts of manliness in the Latino culture that value courage, honor and dignity. This means that for many Latino men, a digital rectal exam would be emasculating, embarrassing, and an affront to dignity.

The nurse searches the literature for more information and learns that many Hispanic men feel healthcare providers do not understand their culture and do not take time to develop a relationship with them. After synthesizing the literature, the nurses decided to adopt the following strategies:

➤ They will create educational materials, which will be available in Spanish.
➤ Educational materials will specifically address culture-based fears that the exam is a threat to manliness.
➤ To reach the men (who tend to avoid healthcare), nurses will educate the women in the family. They believe the women will then encourage their men to get screened.

➤ The nurses will use community leaders, public service announcements, and churches to spread information.

Think about it:

➤ In what ways did the nurses make the planned educational materials patient-centered?
➤ How could the nurses evaluate the patient-centeredness of the educational materials? What information would they need? Where might they obtain the information?
➤ Patient-centered care often correlates to improvements in care. How can the clinic staff evaluate improvements in the healthcare of Latino men in their community after the educational campaign?
  ➤ What goals are reasonable for this educational effort?
  ➤ What assessments would be used to determine effectiveness?

Sources: AHRQ 2010 National Healthcare Disparities Report. Table 1_3_1.2b. Accessed 3/3/12 at http://www.ahrq.gov/qual/qrdr10/index.html

Center for Research Strategies. (2004). Barriers to prostate screening for African-American and Latino men. Accessed 3/3/12 at http://www.cdphe.state.co.us/pp/ccpc/ProstateCancerFocusGroupReport2002.pdf

Rivera-Ramos ZA, Buki, LP. (2011). I will no longer be a man! Manliness and prostate cancer screenings among Latino men. *Psychology of Men & Masculinity, 12*(1), 13–25.
*For specific Knowledge, Skills, and Attitudes,

 Go to the QSEN web site at **http://www.qsen.org/**

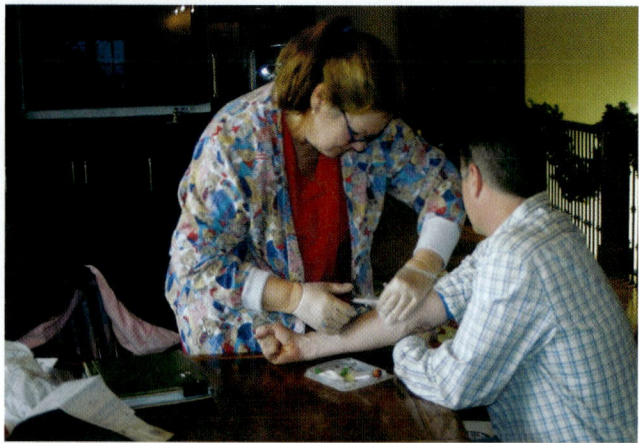

FIGURE 41-2 Secondary interventions. Early detection of heart disease with lipid screening.

Tertiary Interventions

The goal of tertiary (third-level) intervention is to halt disease progression and/or restore client functioning to the pre-disease state. The disease process is clinically apparent and client debilitation, including death, is likely without intervention. Tertiary-level interventions are usually the most invasive and require the nurse to collaborate with members of other disciplines to provide treatment. For example, a student may report to a school nurse that she has been involved in unprotected sexual activities. The school nurse may refer the student to the public health clinic for a pelvic exam and lab testing to detect STIs and for hepatitis B, HPV, and HIV screening. The student has an abnormal Pap smear, showing cells suggestive of HPV exposure. The nurse, in collaboration with the provider, provides medical treatment. There is no cure for HPV, so the teen also needs to learn how to prevent the spread of the disease to others and obtain regular Pap and pelvic exams to detect cervical cancer and other STIs.

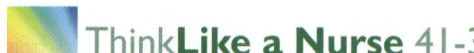

ThinkLike a Nurse 41-3

What level of intervention is required to address Tanya's concerns (Meet Your Patients)? Discuss your response.

KnowledgeCheck 41-5

For each of the nursing actions listed, identify the level of the nursing intervention as primary, secondary, or tertiary.

- Taking a client's blood pressure at a health fair
- Administering insulin to an elderly person at an extended care facility
- Teaching second-grade students to wash their hands correctly

What Career Opportunities Are Available for Community-Based Nurses?

The following are only a few of the many career opportunities for nurses who want to practice from a community-based perspective.

School Nursing

Nursing practice in the school setting began when educators realized that children with health problems had more difficulty learning. School nurses provide direct care for children with chronic health conditions, such as asthma, hyperactivity disorder, and diabetes. They also help children who need routine procedures, such as catheterization, during the school day. School nurses perform mandated vision and hearing screenings. They also administer prescribed medication and ensure that age-appropriate immunizations are documented. Some school nurses offer health education on topics such as sexual and reproductive health. The nurse may also serve as a role model for students who lack parental support or who are struggling with peer pressure. For the most part, a school nurse is autonomous and must be capable of prioritizing and making decisions (American Nurses Association [ANA] and the National Association of School Nurses [NASN], 2005).

Toward Evidence-Based Practice

Hicks, P., Tarr, G. M., & Hicks, X. P. (2007). Reminder cards and immunization rates among Latinos and the rural poor in northeast Colorado. *Journal of the American Board of Family Medicine, 20*(6), 581–586.

Reminder cards have been shown to increase immunization rates in urban settings. However, researchers wanted to investigate the effectiveness of reminder cards among impoverished Latino children living in rural areas. Language-appropriate reminder cards were mailed to patients with missing vaccines. These cards increased the rate of up-to-date immunization from 61.3% to 73.4%.

Moore, M. L., & Parker, A. L. (2006). Influenza vaccine compliance among pediatric asthma patients: What is the better method of notification? *Pediatric Asthma and Allergy Immunology, 19*(4), 200–204.

This study was conducted to find a better way to notify parents of changes in American Academy of Pediatrics

vaccine requirements in order to improve compliance. Researchers mailed a reminder card informing parents of asthmatic children at a military base about the need for influenza immunization. After the mailing the percentage of children ages 5 to 10 years receiving the vaccine increased significantly as compared to those receiving verbal reminders.

---

1. What would you anticipate to be patient-related obstacles to optimal vaccine coverage?

2. What would you anticipate to be some other factors in the medical clinic or office practice that could contribute to a less effective immunization program?

3. What are some ideas you have to improve the effectiveness of an immunization program in the setting where you might work?

 Go to Chapter 41, **Toward Evidence-Based Practice Suggested Responses,** on Davis*Plus.*

Occupational Health

Occupational health nurses work primarily in industrial or corporate settings. Traditionally, occupational health nurses provided health teaching for employees and their families in an effort to reduce absentee hours and increase productivity. Few industries still use the occupational nurse in this manner. Instead, most employ nurses to fulfill union contracts and to complete required medical documentation for disability claims or occupational hazardous events. Thus, the responsibilities of the occupational health nurse may be limited to performing new-hire and annual screenings, providing care to injured workers, completing random drug testing, and filing worker's compensation claims. To reduce costs, most large industries hire a staffing agency to provide trained occupational health nurses. Nursing autonomy and responsibility vary with the employer and the negotiated contract.

Parish Nursing

Parish nursing, also known as faith community nursing, is a community-oriented nursing specialty, defined by the American Nurses Association (ANA) and Health Ministries Association (HMA) (2005) as "the specialized practice of professional nursing that focuses on the intentional care of the spirit as part of the process of promoting holistic health and preventing or minimizing illness in a faith community." The major accountabilities and job activities of the parish nurse role revolve around integrating faith with health. The parish nurse acts as health educator, and personal health counselor (Fig. 41-3). She develops support groups, trains of volunteers, and provides community referrals as needed. The level of autonomy and responsibility of parish nurses varies, depending on the faith community setting.

Nursing in Correctional Facilities

Corrections nurses deliver patient care within the criminal justice system, for example, in juvenile detention, substance abuse treatment facilities, and prisons. In this environment, the nurse provides primary care services to patients of all ages in an unbiased and nonjudgmental manner (ANA, 2007). Correctional facilities have a medical team that provides routine examinations and acute and chronic healthcare on a scheduled or as-needed basis. The level of nursing autonomy is high in most correctional or substance rehabilitation facilities. The nurse also commonly performs occupational health duties for facility staff. For personal safety, nurses must meet certain physical requirements and complete special weapons training before working in most correctional facilities.

Public Health Clinics

Many community nurses practice within local and state departments of health, including public health clinics. Services offered by health departments can range from basic to comprehensive, based on financial constraints, such as the tax base of the community. Large cities tend to have many nurses who may specialize in an area, such as immunizations, prenatal health, school health, or epidemiological survey. Smaller communities may have only one nurse (or full-time equivalent) providing all services. The autonomy and scope of practice of public health nurses are often limited by the philosophy of the political administration and availability of funding.

Disaster Services Nursing

A **disaster** is any event inflicting widespread loss of life, health, and destruction of property. Features characterizing a disaster typically involve unpredictability, urgency, threat, speed, and uncertainty. They are typically classified as natural

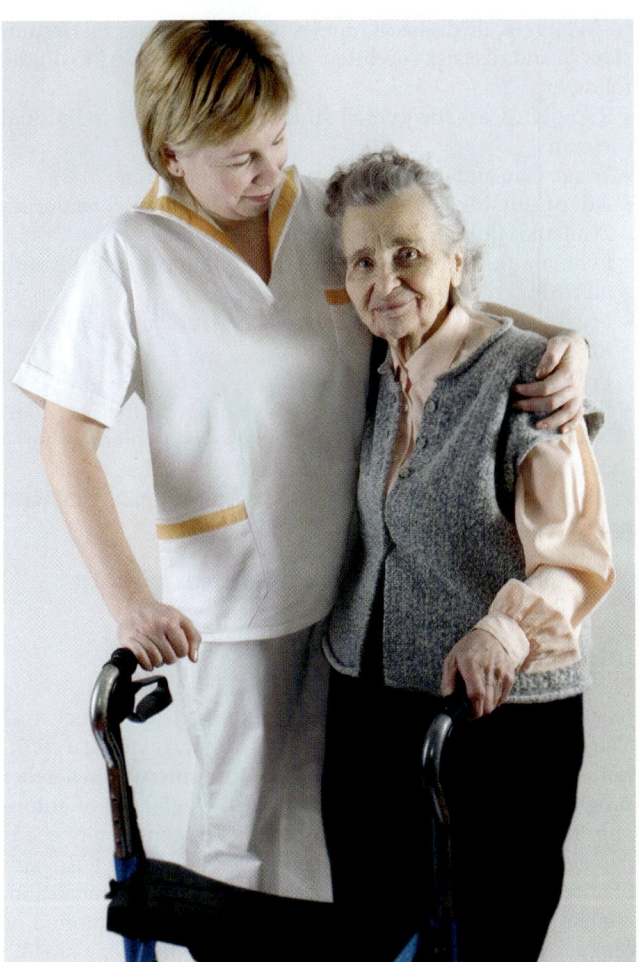

FIGURE 41-3 Parish nursing. Caring for an elderly woman in her home.

or human-made disasters, and may develop as sudden-onset or slow-onset. *Human-generated disasters* might be the result of activities such as a terrorist attack, war, or use of nuclear energy to cause harm or fear. *Technological disasters* cause damage or disruption on a large scale (e.g., computer systems failure, mass power outage, explosion, or hazardous substance exposure). Examples of *natural* or *ecological disasters* include hurricanes, earthquakes, tsunamis, and floods, or even environmental degradation, such as deforestation. Biological disaster may involve exposure to pathogenic microorganism, toxin, or other bioactive substance, for instance, an outbreak of endemic disease or plant contagion. Community-oriented nursing emphasizes community assessment and education to reduce the number of casualties when disasters occur and to achieve the best possible level of health for the people and community involved in a disaster.

Disasters affect the health status of a community in the following ways:

- Lead to premature death, illness or injury.
- Disrupt healthcare services offered within the community.
- Cause environmental issues, such as outbreaks of communicable disease or food/water-borne illness.
- Cause shortages of safe food and drinking water.
- Burden other healthcare systems when displaced populations shift to a host community for basic needs of living (Veenema, 2007).

In large-scale disasters, nurses practicing in special circumstances and disaster conditions are typically needed to do the following:

- Rapidly assess the overall situation and that of individual victims.
- Triage care and initiate life-saving measures first.
- Adapt nursing skills to the disaster situation, considering available equipment, supplies, and personnel.
- Evaluate the safety of the environment and remove health hazards.
- Provide leadership in coordinating care, assigning priorities for care, and transporting victims.
- Prevent further injury or illness.
- Provide compassionate support to victims and their families.

Good Samaritan laws protect nurses when volunteering—in any state—just as long as actions are reasonable.

For additional information on disaster preparedness and preparation for terrorist attacks,

 Go to Chapter 41, **Supplemental Materials: Disaster Preparedness,** on Davis*Plus.*

International Nursing

Nurses working in an international setting commonly provide relief services after a natural or human-made disaster. They may also offer health or human aid services through a medical clinic, faith-based mission, orphanage, or other international relief program. International nursing requires a high level of autonomy, flexibility, and ingenuity, depending on community needs and available resources. Common problems affecting the health of international communities are related to poor sanitation, contaminated food and water, waste management, limited or dangerous transportation, communicable disease, parasitic infections, cultural practices, and limited education. Nurses working globally commonly treat people with malnutrition, dehydration, mosquito and other insect-related illnesses, parasitic infestation, and HIV, to name a few (Fig. 41-4). Because of poor access to healthcare and limited or no resources to pay for medication, many people do not receive adequate healthcare.

 ThinkLike a Nurse 41-4

Increase your self-knowledge: Assume you are going to be a community-based nurse. Of the many career opportunities available, which work do you think you would rather do? Explain why.

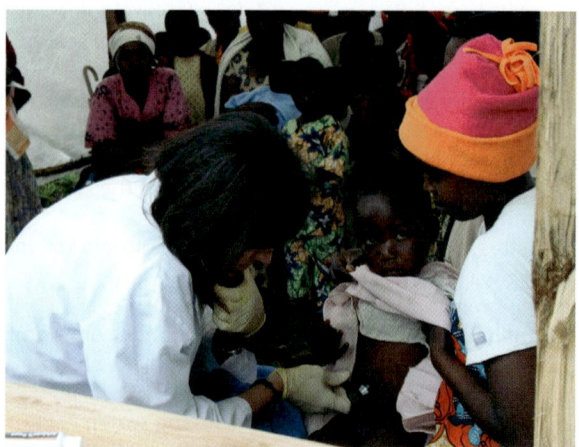

FIGURE 41-4 International nursing. Health and nutrition program for women and children at an African health clinic.

Practical Knowledge knowing **how**

Community nursing care should be delivered in a logical, culturally sensitive manner. The nursing process follows the same steps you have studied in the previous chapters but uses different forms and different language when your client is a community.

The ANA, in the *Standards for Community Health Nursing* (1986), defines the role of the community health nurse as it relates to theory, data collection, diagnosis, planning, intervention, evaluation, quality assurance and professional development, interdisciplinary collaboration, and research. If you need more information about community health nursing standards,

 Go to Chapter 41, **Resources for Caregivers and Health Professionals, Supplemental Materials,** on Davis*Plus.*

ASSESSMENT

Community assessment is usually ongoing and requires the nurse to collaborate with and compile information from a variety of sources. The assessment approach is based on the type of community, the purpose of the assessment, and personal preference. Most beginning students elect to assess a geopolitical community because the data are more readily available than data from aggregate groups. Therefore, we focus on the geopolitical community assessment procedure.

Windshield Survey. Community assessment usually begins with a **windshield survey,** which is performed by observing the community through your automobile window, on foot, or otherwise being physically present in the area. It is similar to general observation of the individual client in that it provides an overview and allows you to see the community in its natural state. As you observe, make note of the condition of buildings and public facilities, residences, religious facilities, streets and sewers, modes of transportation, lighting, outward signs of crime or violence, pollution, waste disposal, and other signs of the well-being of the community. Protective services, such as police and fire services, should be included. You may need to repeat the survey over a period of time at different times of the day, month, or year to get an accurate picture of the community. For more reliable survey results, observers should be trained.

- Begin by describing the neighborhood and the people you see in the community.
- Strive to remain objective in your observations; avoid using personal opinions and biases
- Route your course prior to conducting the visit.
- Record your findings as soon as possible after your survey.
- Document the observation with photographs and videography when possible.

Databases and Public Records. You can also obtain data from publicly available resources, such as birth records, marriage licenses, newspapers, and community Web sites. Internet search engines can help you obtain demographic information, morbidity and mortality data, vital statistics, educational levels, criminal activity, political leadership issues, and/or information about community resources.

Client Perceptions. You will also gather information about how individuals in the community perceive the community and its state of health. Through community gatherings and informal conversations, you can assess a cross section of the population. This is not only an important part of your

assessment, but also is an excellent way to establish rapport, convey your concerns, and develop a working relationship with key community members. All of this encourages more members of the community to participate in the resulting plan.

ANALYSIS/NURSING DIAGNOSIS

After a thorough assessment, you will analyze the complete set of data and compile a list of community strengths and limitations. Work with the community to develop a list of their priorities, considering needs identified by the client, and based on availability of funding and political feasibility.

The NANDA-I Taxonomy

In community practice, you need nursing diagnoses that describe the health status of individuals, families, groups, and entire communities. Recall from Chapter 4 that the NANDA-International (NANDA-I) taxonomy of nursing diagnoses can be used in any nursing setting or specialty. You would simply add the term *community* to other NANDA-I labels when creating a community-based diagnosis: for example, Decisional Conflict (Community) related to safety needs of the homeless population. In addition, the NANDA-I taxonomy includes three diagnoses that specifically describe the health status of a community:

- Deficient Community Health
- Ineffective Community Coping
- Readiness for Enhanced Community Coping

The Omaha Problem Classification System

The Omaha system was developed specifically for use in community settings (Martin & Norris, 1996). In addition to nursing diagnoses, it contains standardized terminology for outcomes and interventions. For a complete overview,

 Go to the **Omaha System** Web site at http://www.omahasystem.org/

The Omaha taxonomy consists of *diagnostic labels* organized into four *domains* (categories), along with two sets of *modifiers*. Within those domains, the system classifies 42 client problems or areas of concern. Refer to Box 41-1 for the four Omaha categories, examples of diagnosis (problem) labels, and problem modifiers.

As you can see, the problem labels in the environment domain are especially useful in community nursing.

To create a diagnostic statement, choose an appropriate label, and add a modifier to it from each of the two sets in Box 41-1. For example, a group Environment diagnosis for workers in a meatpacking plant with lax safety standards might read *Deficit in Group Workplace Safety*. If only one worker were at risk (perhaps because of her inattention to safety rules), you could write *Potential Deficit in Individual Workplace Safety*.

> *Domain:* Environment
> *Problems:* Income, Sanitation, Residence, and Workplace Safety
> *Modifiers:* (1) Health Promotion, Potential Deficit, or Deficit
> (2) Family, Individual, or Group
> *Diagnostic Statements:*
> Deficit in Group Workplace Safety
> Potential Deficit in Individual Workplace Safety

PLANNING OUTCOMES/EVALUATION

In the community you will need to write goals and outcomes for aggregates. The *Healthy People 2020* goals are aggregate goals, for example. The following are guidelines for using the Omaha and NOC taxonomies provide standardized terms for stating community goals.

Using NOC Outcomes

NOC standardized outcomes in the Community Health domain include the following (Moorhead, Johnson, Maas, et al., 2008):

- Community Competence
- Community Disaster Readiness
- Community Disaster Response
- Community Health Status
- Community Health Status: Immunity
- Community Risk Control: Chronic Disease
- Community Risk Control: Communicable Disease
- Community Risk Control: Lead Exposure
- Community Risk Control: Violence
- Community Violence Level

You can use these NOC labels to write goals by adding the appropriate NOC indicators and scales (see the Standardized Language section of Chapter 5).

BOX 41-1 ■ Omaha System: Domains and Examples of Problem Labels

Environmental Domain—The material resources, physical surroundings, and substances both internal and external to the client, home, neighborhood, and broader community
Problem (Diagnosis) Labels: Income, Sanitation, Residence, Neighborhood/Workplace Safety

Psychosocial Domain—Patterns of behavior, communication, relationships, and development.
Problem (Diagnosis) Labels: Social Contact, Role Change, Interpersonal Relationships, Spirituality, Grief, Mental Health, Sexuality, Caretaking/Parenting, Neglect, Abuse

Physiological Domain—Functional status of processes that maintain life.
Problem (Diagnosis) Labels: Hearing, Vision, Oral Health, Speech and Language, Pain, Respiration, Digestion-Hydration, Communicable/Infectious Condition

Health Related Behaviors Domain—Activities that maintain or promote wellness, promote recovery, or maximize rehabilitation potential.

Problem (Diagnosis) Labels: Nutrition, Personal Hygiene, Prescribed Medication Regimen, Sleep and Rest Patterns, Family Planning, Physical Activity

Problem Modifiers

Set 1—Health Promotion, Potential Deficit, Deficit

Set 2—Family, Individual, Group*

---

*Martin and Scheet (1992, p. 67) suggest that *Group* be added to these modifiers.

Source: Martin, K. S., & Scheet, N. J. (1992). *The Omaha system: Applications for community health nursing.* Philadelphia: W. B. Saunders, pp. 67–74. Used with permission.

Using Omaha System Outcomes

Using the Omaha system, you will develop goals/outcomes from the words in the nursing diagnosis. Recall that all nursing diagnoses are identified as *individual, family,* or *group,* so a group nursing diagnosis will automatically indicate a group goal. For example, for the diagnosis Deficit in Group Workplace Safety, you would build the outcomes around the words *Group Workplace Safety.* The Omaha system includes a five-point "Problem Rating Scale for Outcomes" (see Table 41-1) that describes what you expect to achieve in terms of the client's knowledge, behavior, and status. Using Table 41-1, you would create expected outcomes by applying this scale to Group Workplace Safety (shown in Table 41-2).

Table 41-2 indicates that after your interventions, because you have assigned (4) to the outcomes, you expect the group to demonstrate adequate knowledge of workplace safety, demonstrate usually appropriate behaviors (e.g., usually follow the safety rules), and demonstrate minimal accidents or injuries. To evaluate the client's progress, you would assign a scale number to the group's actual knowledge, behavior, and status *after interventions.*

As a community health nurse, you will need interventions to promote and preserve the health of individuals, aggregates, and communities. Both the NIC and the Omaha systems provide standardized vocabularies for aggregate interventions.

NIC Interventions

The NIC taxonomy includes 16 interventions specifically designed for community health. See the list of NIC Community Health Classes and Interventions in Box 41-2.

Omaha Interventions Labels

The Omaha taxonomy provides four intervention categories that you can use in community-oriented nursing practice:

Health Teaching, Guidance, and Counseling. These primary prevention activities include giving information; anticipating client problems; encouraging client action and responsibility for self-care; and assisting with coping, decision making, and problem-solving. As a community-oriented nurse, you should spend most of your time offering this level of intervention.

Table 41-1 ▸ Omaha Problem Rating Scale for Outcomes

CONCEPT	1	2	3	4	5
Knowledge The ability of the client to remember and interpret information	No knowledge	Minimal knowledge	Basic knowledge	Adequate knowledge	Superior knowledge
Behavior The client's observable responses, actions, or activities fitting the occasion or purpose	Never appropriate	Rarely appropriate	Inconsistently appropriate	Usually appropriate	Consistently appropriate
Status The condition of the client in relation to objective and subjective defining characteristics	Extreme signs/ symptoms	Severe signs/ symptoms	Moderate signs/ symptoms	Minimal signs/ symptoms	No signs/ symptoms

Source: The Omaha System. (2009, May 11; updated). *Solving clinical data-information puzzle: Problem rating scale for outcomes.* Retrieved from http://www.omahasystem.org/problemratingscaleforoutcomes.html. Used with permission.

Table 41-2 ▸ Creating Outcomes for Nursing Diagnosis: Deficit in Group Workplace Safety

RATING SCALE CONCEPT	PRESENT STATUS, BEFORE INTERVENTIONS	EXPECTED OUTCOME, AFTER INTERVENTIONS
Knowledge	(2) Minimal knowledge of workplace safety	(4) Adequate knowledge of workplace safety
Behavior	(2) Rarely appropriate safety behaviors	(4) Usually appropriate group safety behaviors
Status	(2) Severe signs/symptoms (e.g., frequent accidents or injuries)	(4) Minimal signs/symptoms (e.g., few accidents or injuries)

BOX 41-2 ■ NIC Community Health Classes and Interventions

Class: Community Health Promotion—Interventions that promote the health of the whole community

Interventions:

Case Management
Community Health Development
Fiscal Resource Management
Health Education
Health Policy Monitoring
Immunization/Vaccination Management
Program Development
Social Marketing

Class: Community Risk Management—Interventions that assist in detecting or preventing health risks to the whole community

Interventions:

Bioterrorism Preparedness
Community Disaster Preparedness
Communicable Disease Management
Environmental Management: Community
Environmental Management: Worker Safety
Environmental Risk Protection
Health Screening
Risk Identification
Surveillance: Community
Vehicle Safety Promotion

Source: Bulechek, G. M., Butcher, H. K., & Dochterman, J. M. (Eds.). (2008). *Nursing interventions classification (NIC)* (5th ed.). St. Louis, MO: C.V. Mosby. Used with permission from Elsevier Science.

Treatments and Procedures. These are secondary interventions directed toward preventing disease, identifying risk factors and early signs and symptoms, and decreasing or alleviating signs and symptoms.

Case Management. Case management is a tertiary intervention that includes coordination, advocacy, and referral. These activities involve facilitating service delivery on behalf of the client, communicating with health and human service providers, promoting assertive client communication, and guiding the client toward appropriate community resources.

Surveillance. These nursing activities include detection, measurement, critical analysis, and monitoring to indicate client status in relation to a given condition or phenomenon.

To write an intervention statement, you must combine one of those four "categories" of interventions with 75 "targets" (objects of the nursing interventions), such as bowel care and nutrition. Then you must add patient-specific information to individualize the nursing order. See Box 41-3 for intervention

categories, examples of targets, and intervention statements (nursing orders). To see the entire set of intervention targets,

 Go to the **Omaha System Web site** at http://www. omahasystem.org/shminter.htm

You will notice that the targets can be used for individuals as well as groups. It is the designation of the nursing diagnosis as *individual, family,* or *group* that determines this.

APPLYING THE NURSING PROCESS IN COMMUNITY-BASED CARE

Community assessment and care planning may at first seem different from what you have been doing for individual patients. But it does follow the same problem-solving process. This section illustrates how the process is applied in a situation you might easily encounter in the community.

BOX 41-3 ■ Omaha Intervention Categories and Examples of Targets

Categories

I. Health Teaching, Guidance, and Counseling
II. Treatments and Procedures
III. Case Management
IV. Surveillance

Examples of Targets

Anatomy/physiology
Behavior modification
Communication
Discipline
Feeding procedures
Homemaking/housekeeping
Substance use cessation
Wellness

Examples of Aggregate Targets

Caretaking/parenting skills
Day-care/respite

Durable medical equipment
Education
Employment
Environment
Finances
Housing
Legal system
Transportation
Other community resource

Examples of Nursing Intervention Statements

Treatments and Procedures (II): Feeding procedures (Demonstrate to Mrs. Adams how to feed Mr. Adams at the next visit.)
Surveillance (IV): Feeding procedures (After teaching, observe a feeding. Monitor for choking.)

Source: The Omaha System. (2009, May 11; updated). Solving the clinical data-information scheme: Intervention scheme. Retrieved from http://www.omahasystem.org/interventionscheme.html

Scenario: As a nurse employed by a local immunization clinic, you have been hired into a new position created by federal and state grant monies to investigate why immunization levels are low among 2-year-olds in Census Tract 15. The following is an example of how you might approach and work through the problem. You would begin with an assessment.

1. **Gather data about the community.**
   - *Define the community.* Determine the physical boundaries of Census Tract 15, a geopolitical community.
   - *Learn the community.* Start interacting with the community to build rapport. Begin the ongoing assessment by conducting windshield surveys, searching for information through reputable databases, and talking with community members.
   - *Focus the data collection.* Focus on the information that will help you determine possible causes of low immunization rates. In this case, the priority problem has already been defined by the financing agency.

ThinkLike a Nurse 41-5

What data would you want to look at? What are possible reasons for low immunization rates?

2. **Analyze the Data.** Next, examine the characteristics of the families failing to provide immediate immunization for children, including the following:
   - Family demographics
   - Age of children
   - Number of immunizations needed and the cost
   - Beliefs about negative effects of vaccines
   - Availability of transportation
   - Public sites providing vaccinations
   - Overall continuity of general healthcare for children

Assume that after working with the community for 6 months, you have spoken at parenting classes about the need to vaccinate children. Several community members have told you they thought their child had already received all necessary immunizations or that their doctor had said to wait until they have better insurance. You will need to arrange a meeting with the local providers to discuss low immunization status. They explain that many vaccinations are too expensive to provide based on the reimbursement they receive from government funding sources.

3. **Plan care.** Your next move is to do some planning. Using the Omaha system you could generate a care plan to address some of the issues raised by community members and physicians.

4. **Evaluate results and follow up.** Community assessment is never complete because the community is constantly changing. However, you need to define the identified needs and desired outcomes during a given period of time, based on best data available at the time of data collection. In this case, you would share with local healthcare providers, the health department, and local health policy committee your approach to addressing the factors suspected of contributing to poor immunization compliance. An important part of a community health nurse's role is to continue to monitor and evaluate the data and provide updates to the appropriate groups.

Now that you have some understanding of community healthcare, the rest of the chapter will focus on a specific type of community nursing: delivering healthcare in the patient's home.

TheoreticalKnowledge
knowing why

UNDERSTANDING THE CONCEPT OF HOME HEALTHCARE?

Recall that community-based healthcare refers to services performed outside of acute care settings. Home healthcare is one such service. **Home healthcare** is the delivery of health-related services in the client's home. Home healthcare is appropriate when a client needs ongoing care that exceeds the abilities of friends and family. It may supplement the skills a family member is providing or serve as a backup for safety or additional assessment. Older adults may use home healthcare services when they need ongoing care but want to avoid moving to a skilled nursing facility. People of any age may require home-care service when they are recovering from illness or surgery or when they are terminally ill. Chronically ill adults and children may receive home healthcare for ongoing care or to avoid hospitalization.

Goals of Home Healthcare

Nurses provide care to clients with complex, chronic, or terminal illness in the home. The primary goal in home healthcare is to promote self-care. Nursing activities are also directed at fostering client independence and teaching the caregivers to assist the client with ongoing health needs. This approach may be very different from what you have experienced in other clinical settings. For example, in the Meet Your Patients scenario, as the nurse you would help the couple to manage Mr. Escobar's care independently at home. Initially you might show Mrs. Escobar how to administer medications and explain their function; and demonstrate strategies for moving and turning Mr. Escobar. However, your goal would be for her to progress to handling these tasks independently.

Distinctive Features of Home Healthcare

Home health nursing differs from hospital nursing in several ways. The hospital environment is controlled. Surfaces are regularly disinfected; supplies are stocked; and foods, medications, and other therapies are readily available. Computers are conveniently located, containing information about the patient that is almost immediately accessible. In addition, the hospital-based nurse can consult almost immediately with a large team of healthcare providers (i.e., other nurses, the primary care provider, various therapists, social workers, a pastoral care provider, and even a business office staff to ensure that reimbursement will be forthcoming).

In contrast, when you are in a patient's home, surprisingly little is within your control. The home may be spotless or filthy, food plentiful or scarce, and supplies readily available or unreliable. The television may be on at full volume or loud music may be playing; a dog may bark continually; or several young children may be playing nearby and repeatedly interrupting your interactions with the client or caregiver. You will find nursing care in the home environment to be different from inpatient settings in the following ways:

- You are a guest in the client's home. The client and family determine whether they are willing to let you enter the home to deliver care.
- You are responsible for making the assessments and determining whether the primary care provider should be advised of client changes.

- You must bring all necessary supplies or arrange to have them delivered ahead of time.
- You must be able to distinguish between skilled services, which are eligible for reimbursement from Medicare, and homemaker services. **Skilled services** are services that must be performed or supervised by a licensed healthcare professional (Box 41-4). **Homemaker services** (e.g., cleaning, meal preparation) are available to clients only if the principal reason for home care is a skilled service. These services are provided by home health aides.
- You must be more self-sufficient and function more independently. Often there are no other team members immediately available for support, assistance, or consultation.
- You must be aware of and comfortable with the family observing you and the situation as you provide care.
- You will need to adapt to varying family relationships and some home environments that are difficult or even dysfunctional.
- You will need to encourage the family to help in providing care and in taking over care when you leave the home. Overburdened caregivers may need your help as much as does the client.
- You must preplan your visit by figuring out the directions to sites in advance and arranging appointments efficiently.
- Your personal safety is more of a concern when making home visits. You must always be aware of the environment around you and alert to possible dangers.
- As things do not always go as planned in a less controlled, home environment, you will need to be flexible, and learn to modify your plan.

One advantage of home healthcare is that it allows you to see the client differently. The home is a window into the client's life, through which you can see his personal environment—how he lives, eats, and negotiates his world (Fig. 41-5). The photos, mementos, personal belongings, and other things the client values and cherishes make cultural beliefs and practices more visible. These things provide clues to his lifestyle, strengths, resources, and motivation.

Home health nursing also differs from community healthcare. Community health nurses provide care for individuals, families, and groups with an emphasis on population-based care. In contrast, home health nursing focuses on the individual and his support system.

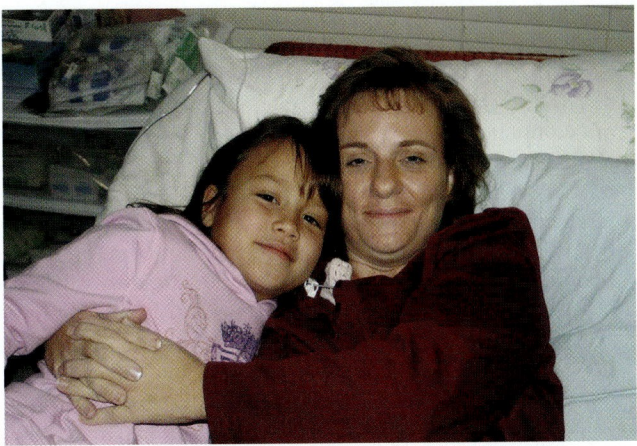

FIGURE 41-5 The home is a window into the client's life.

KnowledgeCheck 41-6

Identify at least four skilled services that may be provided in the home.

WHO PROVIDES HOME HEALTHCARE?

Home healthcare is provided by a variety of healthcare professionals employed by or working in cooperation with home healthcare agencies.

Home Health Agencies

Home health agencies coordinate the services of various professionals and paraprofessionals. The various types of agencies may be categorized by purpose, by type of client served, or by funding source.

Purpose. In this category, **direct care agencies** are the most common. They focus on direct client interaction by providing skilled care, associated therapies and health services, home health aides, chore workers, and delivery of **respite care** (relief for family caregivers). **Indirect service agencies** also play a vital role in home healthcare. Examples of indirect home services include pharmaceutical and infusion companies and suppliers of durable medical equipment. **Durable medical equipment (DME)** is reusable equipment (e.g., walkers, wheelchairs, apnea monitors). Medicare pays for some, but not all, such devices. It is expensive, so before ordering it, be sure the DME is covered or the client is able to pay for it.

Type of Client Served. An important specialty home service agency is hospice care. This may be a separate agency or a division of a home health agency. Still other agencies specialize in caring for patients with complex diseases, such as AIDS, or ventilator-dependent clients, or patients of a certain age group (services for older adults or chronically ill children).

Funding Source. Agencies may take on many forms based on funding source, profit or nonprofit status, and relationship with other healthcare organizations.

- **Public agencies** are official or governmental agencies organized at the city, county, state, or national level. They are usually funded by taxes, along with reimbursement from insurance companies. The local health department is a good example of a public agency. Health departments focus chiefly on community needs, although they often also offer some home health services, especially when tracking clients in some of their disease management programs.
- **Voluntary agencies** are prominent in the delivery of home healthcare. These agencies are normally governed by a

board of directors and funded by donations, endowments, and third-party (insurance) reimbursement. Many **hospice organizations** (groups that provide care for people who are frail, terminally ill, dying, or not expected to improve) are voluntary organizations.

- **Proprietary organizations** are corporate or privately owned businesses that aim to make a profit. These agencies receive payment from insurance companies but also accept private-pay clients. Proprietary organizations may provide traditional home health services as well as private-duty care and other services that assist individuals to remain independent.
- **Hospital-based agencies** are an extension of the services provided by a hospital. Clients who no longer meet the criteria for continued hospitalization may be transferred to home care for continued services. A benefit of this type of home health agency is in the ease of transition between hospital and home.

The Home Health Team

In home healthcare, the registered nurse serves as the coordinator of health services, but other members of the healthcare team may also provide care. The team varies according to the needs of the client but is usually multidisciplinary. It may include physicians; nurse practitioners; registered nurses; licensed practical or vocational nurses; home health aides; physical, speech, occupational, or respiratory therapists; nutritionists; social workers; pharmacists; podiatrists; dentists; chaplains; and family members.

Home Health Nurses

To succeed in home healthcare, you must have the ability to work independently and collaboratively, be flexible and resourceful, and adapt to different home environments and family interactions. The ANA asserts that because of the level of independence, knowledge, and expertise required to meet the demands of home care, baccalaureate nurses are better prepared for that role. However, they also say that the necessary knowledge and skills can be developed through formal orientation programs, structured preceptor programs, and guided clinical experiences (ANA, 2008, p. 8).

Home health nurses provide a broad range of services to clients of all ages. Your principal roles as a home health nurse (also called visiting nurse) are discussed in this section. Each role requires you to function as a skillful communicator. Communication is crucial in home care because of the need to establish good rapport with the client and family and to communicate frequently with other members of the healthcare team.

Direct Care Provider. As a direct care provider, you may administer medications, dress wounds, or perform other skilled, complex tasks.

Client and Family Educator. Recall that the goal of home healthcare is to promote self-care. Instead of focusing on

performing the procedures, you will be helping the client or family take over the care. You can easily see how you will need to communicate skillfully in this role. You must be able to clearly explain the care required, the rationale for the care, and how to safely perform the care. This requires patience, skill, and repetition.

Client Advocate. In home care, the client and family are directly in charge of the plan of care. As client advocate, you support the client's right to make healthcare decisions yet protect the client from harm if he is unable to make decisions. In the event family members disagree with the client's decisions, remember that as the client's advocate, you must try to see that his wishes are respected and his rights upheld. You must also advocate for services the client needs. This may mean trying to secure additional home health support to avoid hospitalization, or it may mean advocating for another level of service, such as referral to hospice or placement in the hospital, based on your assessment of the client and discussion with the client and family.

Care Coordinator. Patients at home may receive care from an array of healthcare providers. Therefore, home health nurses must manage and coordinate care. As the case manager, you will need to gather data at an initial visit and develop a plan of care that addresses the client's needs. Your plan may require you to make additional visits, as well as delivery of therapies and services by other professionals in the home.

KnowledgeCheck 41-7

What roles does the nurse assume in home care? List and describe them.

Hospice Nurses

As you learned in Chapter 17, **hospice nursing** focuses on care of patients who are dying or whose condition is not expected to improve. Hospice services are provided in the home, in the hospital, in nursing homes, and in homes specifically designed as hospices. The goal of hospice care is to promote comfort and quality of life. For these reasons, most hospice services are provided in the client's home. Because the client is not expected to regain health, the focus of home hospice care is quite different from traditional home care. More than promoting self-care and independence, hospice care focuses on providing comfort and managing symptoms (Table 41-3).

The roles of hospice nurse and home health nurse differ mainly in their emphasis. As a direct care provider, the hospice nurse assesses the client's condition and monitors responses to interventions aimed at relieving distress. As an educator, the hospice nurse teaches the client and family how to adjust medications and care to control pain and other symptoms. The roles of communicator and client advocate assume prime importance as the client's condition deteriorates. The nurse shares these roles

Table 41-3 ▶ Home Healthcare and Home Hospice Care		
	HOME HEALTHCARE	**HOME HOSPICE CARE**
Purpose	Promote self-care and independence.	Promote comfort and quality of life.
Focus of Nursing Interventions	Teach the family or other caregivers to assist the client with ongoing health needs and activities of daily living.	Provide comfort and manage symptoms.

with the family and other home caregivers. Generally, there is less coordination of multiple services in home hospice care. Instead, there may be greater emphasis on pain management. If you need more information on hospice care, see Chapter 17.

WHO PAYS FOR HOME HEALTHCARE?

Medicare, Medicaid, private insurance, and individual payments (private pay) help pay for home-care services. Medicare and Medicaid are the largest payers for home healthcare. Keep in mind the federal healthcare act passed in 2010 will likely change reimbursement in a variety of ways over the coming years (U.S. Congress, 2010).

Medicare is a federally funded healthcare system designed to provide health coverage for persons who are older than 65 years, disabled, or diagnosed with end-stage renal disease.

Medicare Reimbursement

Reimbursement by Medicare for home care depends on the following strictly applied criteria:

- *The client must need skilled care.* Other services may also be provided, but the primary purpose for establishing care must be based on a skilled care need. This means that Medicare will not pay for personal care such as bathing and dressing when this is the only care that the client needs.
- *The client must be homebound.* This means (1) the client must have a condition that restricts the ability to leave the home; and (2) leaving the home requires special assistance, transportation, supportive devices, or an escort.
- *The client must require nursing care that is part-time and intermittent.* This means Medicare will pay for a limited number of hours per day or days per week that the client can get skilled nursing care or home health aide services.
- *The plan of care must be authorized by the physician and recertified every 62 days.* For the client to continue to receive care, there must be evidence of continued need that remains acute.
- *The care must be medically necessary and reasonable.* The plan of care must address the client's health concerns and have clearly delineated outcomes. The expectations of the patient must be reasonable.
- *Medicare will pay only for interventions identified on the treatment plan.* The payer may periodically request patient records to verify that the care was given.
- *The home health agency must be approved by Medicare.* An agency must show that it meets the Medicare definitions and requirements in order to become Medicare certified.

Medicaid is a program sponsored jointly by the federal government and the states to provide services to people whose income is below a mandated level. In many states, the criteria for reimbursement are the same as those required by Medicare. However, at present each state determines what services will be part of its medical assistance plan.

Private Insurance and Self-Payment

Private insurance companies may also offer home health services. The type and extent of covered services are specified in each separate insurance group and plan.

Many people require assistance in the home but do not meet criteria for reimbursement from Medicare, Medicaid, or their private insurer. Others simply do not have health insurance. (This was true when this book was published; however, it may change over the next few years as new healthcare regulations are gradually put into effect.) Frequently, older clients require home health assistance but may not need skilled services. For

example, they may need assistance with grocery shopping, meal planning and preparation, or transportation. The client or family may contact an agency to provide chore worker assistance for these services. Services are billed directly to the client. Unfortunately, these services are usually available only to affluent clients and families. Those with limited income may be forced to do without needed services. This disparity may lead to inadequate care and illness, hospitalizations, and even death.

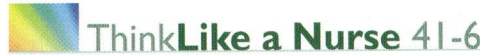

ThinkLike a Nurse 41-6

Review the scenario focused on Mr. Escobar (Meet Your Patients). What members of the home health team may be required to provide care? Why?

WHAT IS THE FUTURE OF HOME HEALTHCARE?

Healthcare analysts have predicted several changes in home care over the next few decades:

- **Increased need for home healthcare.** Over the next several decades, the demand for home care is expected to rise sharply. Considering the growing number of older adults in the United States, it is more cost effective to provide healthcare in the home than in an inpatient setting.
- **Increased use of the home for hospice care.** Public acceptance of the home as a place of comfort and care, as well as concerns about the cost of inpatient care, has increased the number of persons who choose this compassionate option for end-of-life and palliative care.
- **Increased technology.** Technological advances, such as online or telemedicine consultation, make it safer and more affordable to deliver complex care in the home and allow home health nurses to provide a growing array of services. Computerized monitoring and charting allow home health agencies to better coordinate care, receive needed supplies, and closely monitor costs.
- **Continued research.** Research is needed in the area of strategies to improve the effectiveness of care, identify predictors of need for rehospitalization, and integrate home care into overall community-based services.

The home healthcare industry has grown into big business, and it is expected to continue its growth through 2015 (Borger, Smith, Truffer, et al., 2006), and perhaps beyond. However, the future of home care may depend mostly on the state of the U.S. economy, recent federal legislation that will change how healthcare is structured, and the portion of the federal budget that is allocated to healthcare in general. There is some indication that the healthcare act of 2010 provides less support for some home health services, which will shift older adults to the more expensive inpatient services (U.S. Congress, 2010).

HOW ARE CLIENTS REFERRED TO HOME HEALTHCARE?

Referrals to home healthcare come from a variety of sources. However, for home care to begin, there must be a medical prescription and a physician-approved treatment plan.

Hospital-based agencies have a built-in referral base. If the primary provider or nursing staff determine the client would benefit from home health services, they refer the patient to the agency for evaluation while he is still hospitalized. Many agencies have *intake coordinators* who work in the hospital and review clients for suitability of services, gathering information

from the chart, the client, the family, and the hospital team. Home services are arranged before discharge from an inpatient facility.

Even if the hospital does not have its own home agency, the client may still be referred to home health services during a hospital stay. Ideally, a discharge planner gathers information, secures the prescription from the provider, and makes arrangements. In some smaller hospitals, this task falls to the staff nurse providing predischarge care.

Referrals may also come from doctors, nurses, primary care offices and clinics, mental health workers, and other healthcare providers in the community, as well as directly from families and clients. Most home health agencies evaluate clients to determine whether they are eligible for services that are reimbursable by insurance. They may also offer services that the client may pay for independently.

Practical Knowledge
knowing **how**

As a home healthcare nurse, your days will vary. Normally your caseload will be contained within a limited geographic boundary, so that you can schedule your visits efficiently, spending less time driving to visits, and have more time for delivering care. If you want to envision what it would be like to be a home health nurse, you need only to look at the list of services that Medicare recognizes as skilled; see Box 41-4.

HOW DO I MAKE A HOME VISIT?
The home visit has three phases: preparation before the visit, nursing care during the visit, and evaluation after the visit.

Before the Visit
You should first review the client's chart and referral form to determine why you are making the visit. You may also need to review material about the client's health problem, medications, or treatment plan. Then you can begin to plan for the visit. What supplies will you need? What teaching materials will you need? What are the goals of the visit? Does the agency require additional client information, such as insurance data, to provide care? The agency will probably have a set of forms (e.g., HIPAA privacy forms, billing information) for you to complete during the first visit. Be sure you have those with you.

Before the visit you will need to find the address, get directions to the home, and determine whether there are safety concerns. Contact the client to notify him of the planned date and time of the visit and to determine whether his health status has changed since the referral was made. This will allow you to bring additional equipment or personnel along if needed.

Prepare Supplies
Home health nurses usually carry a nursing bag (Fig. 41-6). The nursing bag is often customized to the needs of the clients in the nurse's case load, and normally contains the following:
- Handwashing supplies (e.g., soap or antibacterial hand rub, paper towels)
- Stethoscope
- Sphygmomanometers (with cuffs in a variety of sizes)
- Thermometers (oral and rectal)
- Small equipment (scissors, forceps, penlight, staple remover)

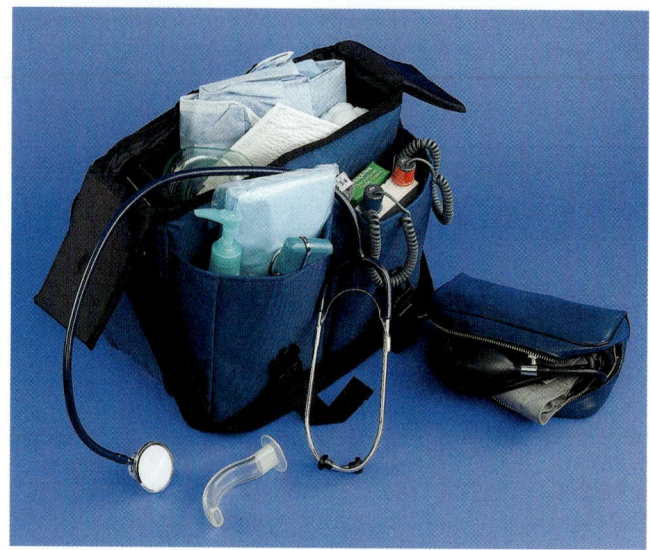

FIGURE 41-6 The home health nursing bag contains some standard items but is usually customized according to the requirements of the clients in the nurse's case load.

- Tape measure (with plastic coating that can be cleaned, or several disposable paper ones)
- Plastic apron
- Gloves, sterile and clean
- An assortment of gauze dressings, tape, and cotton balls
- Occupational Safety and Health Administration (OSHA) supplies: mask, protective eyewear, disinfectant spray, disposable gowns to protect clothing
- A variety of syringes and safety needles (this varies widely among agencies)
- Venipuncture supplies
- Airway and resuscitation mask
- Paper supplies (e.g., agency forms, business cards, local maps)

You may need other supplies, such as medications, a scale, and a transfer belt, depending on the requirements of the clients in your caseload. If the client needs frequent dressing changes or treatments that need supplies (e.g., tube feedings) it is best to have the supplies delivered directly to the client's house to reduce the number of materials you must carry. Note that in some states, nurses are not permitted to carry medications because of safety concerns. You will need to check on the rules that apply to your state.

Provide for Your Safety

As you drive to the home, begin to make your assessment. Locate the stores, hospital, and community resources. What is the overall character of the neighborhood? Does this appear to be a safe neighborhood? What are the conditions of the approach to the home?

Safety for yourself and the client is an essential consideration in home healthcare. Bring your impressions about neighborhood safety and home safety with you into the home. You should evaluate whether the environment contributes to the client's health problems. In addition, you must also assess the implications for your own safety. For suggestions about the safe delivery of home healthcare, see Clinical Insight 41-1.

Clinical Insight 41-1 ▶ **Safety Considerations in Home Care**

Before the Visit

- ✚ **Plan ahead.** Know where you are headed. Use a map or global positioning system (GPS). Contact the client or family for directions if it is unclear where you are headed. File a visit plan with your office each day.
- **Dress in appropriate clothing** as dictated by your agency. Wear a nametag clearly identifying you and the agency. Wear shoes that will allow you to run if necessary.
- **Carry a cell phone.**
- **Do not carry a purse,** multiple credit cards, or excess cash. Instead, use a waist or fanny pack and conceal it under clothing. Carry enough money for emergency transportation, telephone numbers for clients and home health agency, and emergency contact information.
- **Keep your car in good repair,** and always have enough gasoline in the tank. Be prepared for inclement weather, and always carry an emergency car safety pack.
- **Do not get out of your car for any reason if driving in an area that might not be safe.** Carjacking involves minor car impact ("fender bender") as a strategy to get a person to get out of the vehicle, leaving her vulnerable for attack, assault, or theft.
- **Observe your surroundings** as you drive to the visit. Notice the location of emergency services, local gas stations, and public places if help is required.
- **Program 911 into your cell phone** in case of an emergency. Carry mace or other items to aid in self-defense in case of situations in which you feel threatened.
- **Park as close to your destination as possible.** If possible, park your car facing the direction you wish to go when you leave. Never enter dead end streets or alleys.
- **Check your surroundings before you leave your car.** If you feel unsafe, leave the area immediately and call your office.
- **Lock the car. Leave no valuables in sight.**
- **Prepare your bag while you are still in the car.**
- **Carry your bag on one arm. In the opposite hand, carry your keys.** Always have them ready. You may need them if you decide to exit quickly. Also, you can use keys to defend yourself by placing the pointed ends of the keys between your fingers.
- **Walk directly to the client's house.** Walk in the middle of the sidewalk. Use common walkways. Avoid isolated and poorly lighted areas. Do not take shortcuts.
- **Knock or ring the doorbell before entering.** Never enter without being invited. If there is no answer at the door, call the patient using your cell phone, or return to a secure public pay phone and dial the client.
- **If for any reason you feel that the neighborhood is unsafe, do not get out of the car.** Instead, leave the neighborhood immediately and phone your agency.

At the Visit

- **Introduce yourself** and clearly identify your agency. Show your name badge.
- **Sit where you have access to an exit.** When you enter the home, observe all exits.
- **Notice who is present in the home. Request introductions.** This information is useful for planning care as well as for ensuring safety.
- **Leave immediately if you suspect substance use,** drug dealing, or drunken behavior.
- **Leave immediately if there is a violent domestic argument.** Do not attempt to intervene. When you return to your car, use your cell phone to dial 911, or drive to a phone booth in a safe location and place the call.
- **Request that animals be kept in another room** while you make your visit.
- **If weapons are visible, request that they be put away** immediately. Leave the home if this request is not met.
- **If household members interfere with the visit,** discuss the problem with the client. You may need to arrange a time to visit when they are not present.

After the Visit

- **Continue to observe the safety precautions** you used when getting to the visit. Do not let down your guard as you return to your car.
- **If you are in an unsafe neighborhood or poorly lighted area, leave immediately and do not consult the map** for directions to your next visit. Drive to a secure public location, and then consult the map.
- **Inform your agency** if you believe the home or neighborhood is potentially hazardous.
- **Request a security escort service** if future visits are required.
- **Document your assessments** and the care delivered.
- **Report abuse** if you suspect it in the home.

Other

The preceding tips focus on avoiding harm inflicted by others. However, you also need to protect yourself from infection and accidental injury, as you would in a hospital (see Clinical Insight 41-2). Use safe lifting techniques, and safe needle-handling techniques (see Chapters 25 and 33 if you need to review those). A small pilot study found that 13% of home healthcare nurses had experienced needlesticks in a 12-month period. Nurses attributed the sticks primarily to patient actions, followed by disposal-related activities (Gershon, Pogorzelska, Qureshi, et al., 2008).

KnowledgeCheck 41-8

What are the major tasks that must be completed before making a home visit?

At the Visit

When you arrive at the home, you must remember this is the client's domain. Knock or ring the doorbell, and wait to be invited in. Observe common courtesies. Introduce yourself to the client and family. Be respectful of their home, as well as their beliefs, values, practices, and cultural preferences.

The first few minutes of the initial visit set the tone for the relationship among client, family, nurse, and agency. This is your opportunity to develop rapport and trust. Introducing yourself, waiting for permission to enter, and treating the client and family members with respect are ways to help to establish rapport (Fig. 41-7).

You should also offer your card to identify yourself, and provide contact information for the home health agency. Generally, agencies have information packets that include the client's bill of rights, client responsibilities, billing information, information on the frequency and duration of services, how to reach the agency, and the date and time of the next visit.

As you do all this, you also gather data. Who answered your questions? What is the relationship between the caregiver and the client? How do they interact? What other people live there?

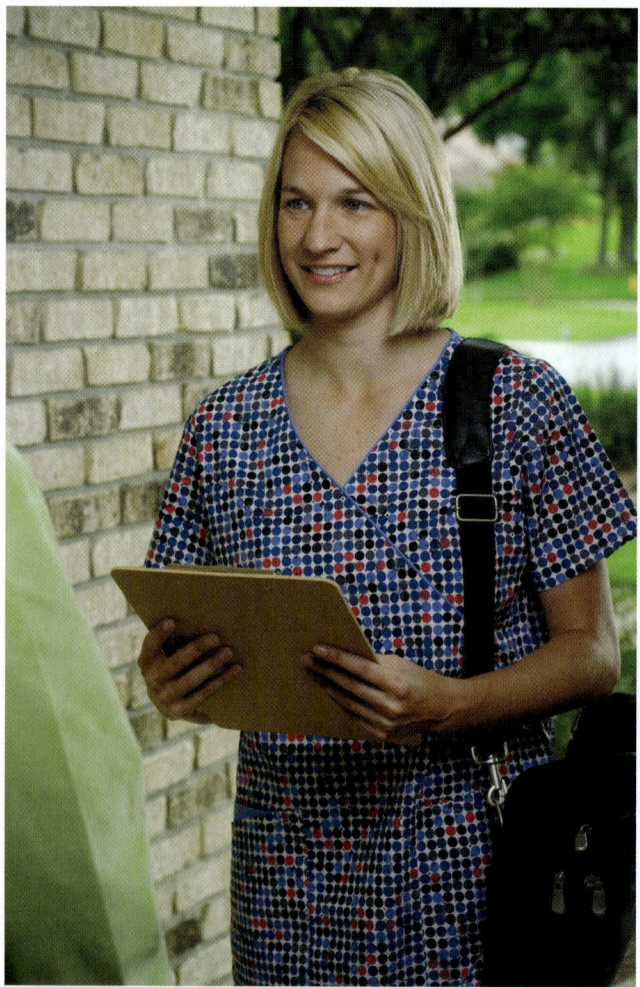

FIGURE 41-7 The first few minutes of the initial visit set the tone for the relationship among client, family, nurse, and agency.

What is the condition of the home? If this is an initial visit, you may need to verify or complete client data on the referral form. In the hospital, admissions personnel usually gather admitting data and obtain consent for treatment. In home care you need to collect and document this information.

At a home visit, you might do a variety of things, such as performing physical care; drawing blood sample for lab work; checking weight; administering medication, IV fluid, or tube feedings; providing wound or ostomy care; or whatever is needed.

ThinkLike a Nurse 41-7

Review the case of Mr. Escobar (Meet Your Patients). What information did you gain from the first few minutes of the visit?

- Both Mr. and Mrs. Escobar are in need of nursing interventions. However, this is your agency's first home visit to them, and you have other clients you must visit today, so you will need to prioritize. What must the home health nurse do on the initial visit to a client?
- In addition to completing your assessment and talking about a plan of care with the Escobars, what do you think is the single most important thing you can do for them today? Explain your thinking.
- When Mrs. Escobar meets you at the door and brings you into the living room, you notice a large German shepherd dog lying beside Mr. Escobar's bed. Mrs. Escobar says, "Stay, King"; and then to you, "Roland likes having him nearby." What should you do?

After the Visit

After you leave the home, there is still a lot of work for you to do. Often you will need to complete the documentation for the visit. In Chapter 18, you learned about documentation techniques, various forms of charting, and legal aspects of documentation. In home care all of these rules apply; however, some aspects of home-care documentation are unique.

Home health agencies often use Medicare's Outcome and Assessment Information Set (OASIS) to record initial assessment data. To continue to provide needed services to the client, you must include in your documentation (1) evidence of homebound status, and (2) evidence of continued need for skilled care.

Other post-visit activities include ordering supplies needed for the next visit, making referrals to additional services (e.g., occupational therapy), coordinating care among the various services, and scheduling the next visit.

NURSING PROCESS IN HOME CARE

The nursing process moves through the same phases in all patient care settings. The difference in home care is that you must use forms structured to satisfy Medicare and other insurance requirements. Nevertheless, you need to assess the client, the family, the home, and the community in order to **identify** nursing diagnoses and other health problems. You will work from a plan of care prescribed by a medical provider, but individualize it with suitable nursing diagnoses and interventions. Periodically, you must evaluate the client's continued homebound status and ongoing need for medical treatment and skilled nursing care.

ASSESSMENT

On the initial visit, you need to perform an assessment to establish a baseline and determine the type of care required. This assessment includes a health history, review of all

medications—prescribed, over-the-counter, and alternative—pertinent family and social history, mental status, functional ability, availability of family and informal support and caregivers, nutritional status, and assessment of the home environment. Often a full assessment requires multiple visits.

Medicare requires home health agencies to collect specific information for all Medicare clients they serve using OASIS. The OASIS data must be collected at the start of care, with each recertification (every 60 days), and at the termination of care. Medicare uses these data to determine the effectiveness of care and to monitor client outcomes. In addition to the required OASIS information, many agencies use other assessment tools created specifically for their needs. For an example of the OASIS form,

 Go to Chapter 18, **Tables, Boxes, Figures: ESG Figure 18-4, Outcome and Assessment Information Set (OASIS),** on Davis*Plus.*

It is also important to assess the needs of the caregivers—the family members, friends, and support system in the home. To be successful in home care, you must work *with* the caregivers. Take time at each visit to speak with them, making sure to include them in your assessment, plan of care, and teaching. Assessment of the caregivers often allows you to determine what services are needed in the home. Caregivers may have health problems of their own that affect their ability to provide care for another. This is common among older couples.

■ ANALYSIS/NURSING DIAGNOSIS

As in any setting, the nursing diagnoses are based on the client's responses to illness and care. As a home healthcare nurse, you will work with clients with numerous medical and nursing diagnoses. Two frequent nursing diagnoses, Caregiver Role Strain and Deficient Knowledge, are discussed below. Safety and Risk for Infection, also key concerns in the home, are thoroughly discussed in Chapters 22 and 23. Infection control measures in the home are also presented below, in the section Infection Control in the Home.

Caregiver Role Strain. Providing care to a loved one at home can be a challenge, especially when finances don't allow a family to hire home health aides. Around-the-clock caregiving duties can lead to physical exhaustion, social isolation, resentment, sadness, or depression. In addition, family members themselves may become seriously ill and no longer be able to function as caregiver. These role changes may be difficult for both the ill person and the caregiver. For example, imagine that your mother suddenly became very ill and you became her primary caregiver. This would be a reversal of the roles you both are used to, and it would be emotionally taxing, especially if you are already exhausted and isolated from your friends. In addition, a primary caregiver may worry that caring for the client interferes with other responsibilities (e.g., as a parent, spouse, friend, worker).

Given these factors, it is not surprising that the two nursing diagnoses most commonly applicable to loved ones providing care at home are Caregiver Role Strain and Risk for Caregiver Role Strain. These diagnoses identify those for whom the burden of delivering care has become—or is at risk for becoming—overwhelming. Common signs of caregiver role strain include difficulty adjusting to role changes, fatigue, isolation, depression, and difficulty in performing routine care for the client.

Deficient Knowledge. Client and family teaching is especially important in home care because most of the caregiving is performed by the client and significant others. You will spend much of your time teaching them the skills necessary for self-care (e.g., how to administer insulin, how to manage the oxygen equipment). Recall that to be eligible for home nursing care, clients must require skilled nursing care. Client education is a service that Medicare and other insurers will reimburse. You must be certain to include a Deficient Knowledge diagnosis on the care plan in order to ensure the client's continued eligibility and reimbursement for the service. In other chapters we caution against indiscriminate use of the Deficient Knowledge diagnosis. However, an exception must be made for home care.

Knowledge Check 41-9

- Why are the first few minutes of the initial visit so important?
- Identify five things that should be assessed at an initial home visit.

Think Like a Nurse 41-8

- Based on the information in the scenario, what nursing diagnoses might Mr. Escobar (Meet Your Patients) have? There may not be enough data to make definite diagnoses, but what probable diagnoses are there for which you would want to gather confirming data? Do not include potential diagnoses, such as Risk for Imbalanced Nutrition.
- Mr. Escobar has a potential problem, Risk for Falls. What are two interventions you would probably be able to do today to reduce his falls risk?
- What, if any, evidence of caregiver strain does Mrs. Escobar exhibit?

Standardized Terminology for Home Health Nursing Diagnoses

Recall from the nursing process chapters of this text that various disciplines, including nursing, have developed classifications of standardized terminology (also called *taxonomies, vocabularies,* and *languages*) for describing their work and for planning and documenting care. You are familiar with the NANDA-I taxonomy of nursing diagnoses; however, home-care nurses more commonly use the Clinical Care Classification (CCC) because it is closely related to the OASIS reporting forms required by Medicare. If you need to review the concept of standardized nursing language, see Chapters 4, 5, and 6.

The CCC also contains 182 diagnostic concepts—59 major categories and/or 123 subcategories—that describe nursing diagnoses and patient problems (Saba, 2007, p. 159). Approximately 50 labels are also NANDA-I diagnostic categories. About 50 of the 182 terms are especially applicable to home healthcare. Common CCC nursing diagnoses used in the home include the following:

Activities of Daily Living (ADLs) Alteration
Caregiver Role Strain
Family Processes Alteration
Home Maintenance Alteration
Knowledge Deficit
Physical Mobility Impairment
Self-Care Deficit

The CCC system consists of 21 care components to classify diagnoses and interventions. An accompanying coding structure and framework parallels the steps of the nursing process and links the CCC diagnoses to interventions and outcomes. To see the CCC Care Components, see Box 41-5. To see an example of a CCC nursing diagnosis and interventions, see

Box 41-6. For complete information on the CCC and complete lists of diagnoses, outcomes, and interventions,

 Go to the **Clinical Care Classification** Web site at http://www. sabacare.com

---

BOX 41-5 ■ Clinical Care Classification: 21 Care Components (Version 2.0) Coded by Alphabetic Classes*

A Activity Component
B Bowel Gastric Component
C Cardiac Component
D Cognitive Component
E Coping Component
F Fluid Volume Component
G Health Behavior Component
H Medication Component
I Metabolic Component
J Nutritional Component
K Physical Regulation Component
L Respiratory Component
M Role Relationship Component
N Safety Component
O Self-Care Component
P Self-Concept Component
Q Sensory Component
R Skin Integrity Component
S Tissue Perfusion Component
T Urinary Elimination Component
U Life Cycle Component

---

*The Clinical Care Classification system is copyrighted, placed in public domain, and cannot be sold, but is available with written permission (Saba, V., 2007. *Clinical Care Classification (CCC) system manual*. New York: Springer Publishing Co., p. 162).

BOX 41-6 ■ An Example of Clinical Care Classification Nursing Diagnoses and Interventions

A—ACTIVITY COMPONENT (*1 of 21 Care Components*)—
A cluster of elements that involve the use of energy in carrying out musculoskeletal and bodily actions.
01 Activity Alteration (*Major Nursing Diagnosis*)—
Change in or modification of energy used by the body.

Subcategories that provide greater definition of the problem (of "01 Activity Alteration")

01.1 Activity Intolerance
01.2 Activity Intolerance Risk
01.3 Diversional Activity Deficit
01.4 Fatigue
01.5 Physical Mobility Impairment
01.6 Sleep Pattern Disturbance
01.7 Sleep Deprivation

Actions performed to carry out physiological or psychological daily activities.
Example: Teach Passive Range of Motion

Source: Obtained from Saba, V. K. (n.d.). About. Clinical Care Classification System. Retrieved from http://sabacare.com/About/

PLANNING OUTCOMES/EVALUATION

The CCC defines an outcome as "a measurable outcome of the therapeutic nursing care that alters the health status of the patient" (Saba, 2007, p. 154). Others conceptualize a CCC outcome as being "What really happened to the recipient of services in terms of the particular problem for which care was provided" (Head, Maas, & Johnson, 1997, p. 51). To formulate a goal/outcome in the CCC system, attach one of the three CCC "modifiers" (*improve, stabilize, deteriorate*) to the diagnosis. The outcome describes the *desired* client health status. To evaluate client progress, you again use one of the three modifiers to describe the client's *actual* health status. The following is an example:

CCC nursing diagnosis:	Knowledge Deficit
Goal/expected outcome:	Knowledge Deficit, Improve
Actual status on evaluation:	Knowledge Deficit, Stabilized

Medicare requires that the client's status be evaluated and coded as improved, stabilized, or deteriorated, the same as the CCC system. In your nursing notes, you would include additional narrative to support your evaluation.

The Nursing Outcomes Classification (NOC) can also be used in home health nursing (Moorhead, Johnson, Maas, et al., 2008). A few of the outcomes that pertain to home and families are Caregiver Home Care Readiness, Caregiver Performance: Direct Care, Caregiver Stressors, Family Coping, and Family Functioning.

To prepare the client and family for self-care, inform them of the needs you have identified, and involve them in setting goals and planning care. They may be able to identify strategies to solve problems or to help you identify needs that are not readily apparent.

PLANNING INTERVENTIONS/IMPLEMENTATION

Medicare requires that the physician-prescribed plan of care include the following, as applicable:

- Parameters for notifying the primary provider of changes in vital signs and other clinical findings
- Diabetic foot care, including education
- Falls prevention interventions
- Depression interventions
- Interventions to monitor and treat pain
- Interventions to prevent pressure ulcers
- Pressure ulcer treatments

Once the plan of care has been agreed on, you will document it and forward it to the client's physician for certification. At the first visit, you will determine the specific skilled care required and make referrals to other required services such as physical, occupational, or speech therapy, social services, nutritional support, or home health aide services.

CCC Nursing Interventions

The CCC contains 198 nursing interventions organized according to the care components. For an example, see Box 41-6. An intervention consists of a label (e.g., Activity Care) and a definition (e.g., Actions performed to carry out physiological or psychological daily activities). In addition to the label, you must specify the type of intervention action from among four qualifiers:

Assess/Monitor/Evaluate/Observe
Care/Perform/Provide/Assist
Teach/Educate/Instruct/Supervise
Manage/Refer/Contact/Notify

The CCC nursing interventions include only skilled services because this type of service is the only type of care reimbursed by Medicare and most insurers in home health. In the case of the Escobars in the Meet Your Patients scenario, Mrs. Escobar is clearly experiencing Caregiver Strain. This is a nursing diagnosis under the Care Component of Coping. Several interventions are possible:

> **Coping Support:** Actions to sustain a person dealing with responsibilities, problems, or difficulties
>> Assess for Caregiver Strain.
>> Provide (perform) emotional support.
>> Refer to community services: caregiver support groups, Meals on Wheels, and respite care services.

NIC Interventions for Home Health

The Nursing Interventions Classification (NIC) may also be used in home health nursing (Bulechek, Butcher, & Dochterman, 2008). A few of the interventions that pertain to home and families are Caregiver Support, Family Integrity Promotion, Home Maintenance Assistance, and Respite Care.

Assisting With Medication Management

One of The Joint Commission 2012 safety goals for home care is to use medications safely. This involves preventing errors with look-alike and sound-alike medications, educating patients about anticoagulant therapy, and keeping a list and reconciling medications when a client transfers from one agency to another. Nurses taking care of patients in the home setting must be careful to avoid error when recording and communicating information about patients' medications. The Joint Commission also advises nurses to diligently compare those medications the patient is already taking to new ones to be given in the home. Nurses need to make sure patients know about medications they take at home; and that they should bring an updated list every time they visit a healthcare provider.

Some patients, particularly older adults, have visual and motor deficits that limit their ability to read labels and manipulate bottle caps, syringes, and so on. Other reasons for noncompliance include lack of outward symptoms, inability to tolerate side effects, pain, forgetfulness, low motivation, and impaired mental capacity. Always investigate the patient's reasons for nonadherence so that you can take appropriate actions. You may need to teach clients and caregivers skills such as measuring dosages, giving injections, and managing intravenous therapy. Or they may need tips on how to take oral medications if the client has difficulty swallowing. For example, for some clients, pills may be crushed and mixed in a small amount of applesauce. Involve family members in the care of the older adult, including giving medication, provided they are competent in doing so (Hall & Maslow, 2007).

Older adults and caregivers may have difficulty remembering when to take their pills, remembering which ones to take, and even remembering whether they have already taken them. Suggest they use a medication organizer with a compartment for each day of the week. You may need to prepare a week's worth of oral medications for them during your visits. To help them remember which drug is used for each of their illnesses or symptoms, you can write the medical condition, names of medication, and doses on a large card. Then use clear tape to attach a sample of each drug next to its name on the card.

Infection Control in the Home

The Joint Commission 2012 safety goals for home care include reducing the risk of healthcare-associated infections. In the hospital, you have ready access to supplies that facilitate infection control. The home presents unique challenges. Hand cleaning is one of the most important home interventions to prevent the transmission of infection. You will need to follow Standard Precautions but recognize how to modify infection control techniques for the home environment. For suggestions to help you maintain infection control during a home visit, see Clinical Insight 41-2.

Homes vary widely. Do not assume that a client lives in a clean residence or that running water and electricity are readily available. Some people with limited financial resources, especially in urban environments, live in single-room occupancy hotels (SROs). Residents of SROs live in a small room with shared bath and shower areas. Conditions can vary from clean and orderly to unclean and even detrimental to health. To provide optimal care, you need to bring infection control supplies and personal protective equipment to the visit or order them to be delivered to the home.

Barrier Precautions

Rationales for using barrier precautions differ from those in hospitals. As a rule, you will use gowns, gloves, and masks in home care to protect yourself, rather than the patient. You will need to use standard precautions, but will usually need a mask only when caring for clients who have pulmonary tuberculosis or multidrug-resistant infections. These organisms may be transmitted to other home-care patients through inanimate objects or hands, so use appropriate barrier precautions (Lescure, Locher, Eveillard, et al., 2009). See Chapter 22 if you need to review infection control.

Clean and Sterile Technique

Infection control in home care is different in many ways from that in acute care. In acute care, the patient is at risk from exposure to invasive interventions and environmental risks, including other patients and contaminated inanimate objects. Generally, patients have developed some resistance to the microorganisms in their own homes and are less likely to acquire infections there than in the hospital environment. You may find differences in how you handle home infusion therapy, urinary tract care, respiratory care, wound care, and enteral therapy. It is safe, in many instances, to replace sterile with clean technique, as in some of the following examples (Rhinehart, 2001):

- **Intravenous therapy.** Sterile practices should be the same at home as in the hospital because the associated risk of asepsis is so high.
- **Insulin injections.** Many people (e.g., those who have diabetes) must give themselves repeated injections, perhaps several each day. Supplies for home use are expensive. Insurance may or may not cover the cost, or the person may not have insurance. Therefore, although manufacturers recommend that disposable syringes and needles be used only once, and it is safest to do that, some people find it practical to reuse needles and syringes. For guidelines for patient teaching about this, see Clinical Insight 25-2, Reusing Needles and Syringes: Home Care.
- **Urinary catheters.** Clients and family typically use clean, rather than sterile, gloves to perform catheterization. In the home, clients frequently interrupt the drainage system to empty a leg bag, or to change or disinfect the

Clinical Insight 41-2 ▶ Infection Control in the Home

The following suggestions can help you maintain infection control during a home visit.

Hand Hygiene

- Keep antibacterial cleanser and OSHA-approved protective equipment in your nursing bag.
- Perform hand hygiene using soap and warm water or an antibacterial hand-rub at the beginning and end of each visit and before and after any treatment.
- If the home conditions are very dirty or your hands become grossly soiled, wash your hands with soap and warm water as soon as possible after (if not during) the visit.

Supplies

- In homes that you know are not very clean, limit the supplies you bring into the home. For example, leave your nursing bag in the car, and bring only the supplies you need for the visit.
- Some infection control experts believe the "bag technique" (i.e., placing a newspaper under the nursing bag before placing it on a surface) is not routinely needed, but should be used when home conditions warrant.
- If necessary, use a 1:10 dilution of chlorine bleach in water to disinfect surfaces or equipment in the home. Some equipment may need to be disinfected by boiling in a covered pan of water for 15 to 20 minutes. Do not boil plastic or rubber items.
- You can disinfect hard plastic items by wrapping them with a wet paper towel and placing them in a zippered plastic bag. Microwave the entire bag on high for 10 minutes.

Biohazard and Sharps Disposal

- Flush wound irrigation or potentially contaminated liquids down the toilet while wearing gloves and any other appropriate protective equipment.
- Double-bag dressings, equipment, or disposable supplies that have been contaminated with body secretions to prevent leakage. The bags should be labeled *Biohazard*.
- ✚ Carry small biohazard sharps containers. Place syringes and sharps in the container without recapping. If clients or family must use syringes or sharps, you may wish to leave a sharps container in the home. An alternative solution is to have them use a metal coffee can with lid or a thick plastic milk jug with lid.

Client Teaching

- Provide instruction on home cleanliness, hygiene, handwashing, food preparation, and instructions to avoid contact with persons who are ill, as needed.
- If the client is immunocompromised, teach the signs and symptoms of infection and the process for immediate notification of the primary care provider.

Special Situations

- If the patient has a multidrug-resistant infection or pulmonary tuberculosis, use appropriate barrier precautions. Leave reusable equipment (e.g., stethoscope, blood pressure cuff) in the home; and if possible, schedule these clients as the last appointment of the day.

---

drainage bag. They may also disinfect and reuse urinary catheters.

- **Respiratory care.** As an example, tracheostomy care in the home is nearly always performed using clean, not sterile, technique.
- **Wound care.** Procedures for wound care should be based on the potential for contamination and infection. Usually clean technique is adequate. For example, a surgical site that is primarily closed and has no drains should be low risk for home-care-acquired infection. However, if the incision has drains or is open, the risk for infection increases, and your wound care procedures must address the risk. Also, you do not need to arbitrarily "always" discard irrigation fluids at set intervals (e.g., every 24 hours). Recommend that caregivers to buy, small containers (e.g., no more than 500 mL) that can be used up in two or three visits. Teach them how to avoid contaminating the fluids (e.g., how to handle the cap, always recap the bottle, and store the bottle away from children and pets).
- **Enteral therapy.** Emphasize the need to refrigerate the feedings after opening and store solutions until expiration. Teach

caregivers to keep the kitchen appliances (e.g., blenders) and tools used in preparation meticulously clean. Sterilization of blender parts, measuring cups, and spoons is probably not necessary, but they should be washed in a dishwasher after use.

KnowledgeCheck 41-10

Identify three infection control supplies that you should bring in your nursing bag on a home health visit.

Safety in the Home

The two following Joint Commission 2012 home-care safety goals are also important to keep in mind:

- ✚ *Reduce the risk of client harm resulting from falls.* You will need to assess the client and the home for risk factors (e.g., dimly lit stairs, clutter on the floors) and teach caregivers falls reduction measures. You will find extensive discussion of falls prevention in Chapter 23 if you need more information about that.

■ ***Identify risks associated with oxygen therapy*** *(e.g., fire).* Be certain the home has working smoke detectors, fire extinguishers, and a fire safety plan. Assess the client and family's ability to understand and comply with fire prevention activities, and report any concerns to the physician.

If you need a checklist to use in assessing for safety hazards in the home,

 Go to Chapter 23, **Tables, Boxes, and Figures: ESG Figure 23-2, Home Safety Checklist,** on *DavisPlus.*

Supporting Caregivers

Even when the client is receiving in-home care from an agency, it is not around-the-clock care. If the client cannot perform self-care, most of the duties fall to family members. One study found that even with short-term formal services, family caregivers provided three-fourths of the care of homebound patients. Half of the caregivers said they were not adequately prepared when it was time for their home health services to

be discontinued. And at all stages, they expressed significant isolation, anxiety, and depression (Levine, Albert, Hokenstad, et al., 2006).

Recall that unrelieved caregiving duties are physically and emotionally taxing. Caregivers may become depressed, physically exhausted, isolated from friends, and neglectful of their own health. If the primary caregiver becomes unable to function, the client must be institutionalized. Clearly, it is important to provide caregiver support.

There is some evidence to indicate that caregiver support and training workshops can relieve depression, reduce the perceived burden of caregiving, and better prepare the caregivers for their role. However, those with more independent lives and social support showed the most improvement . Furthermore, not everyone can—or will want to—attend a workshop. Some cannot leave their caregiving duties; others haven't the time or energy; and still others may not have transportation (Huynh-Hohnbaum, Villa, Aranda, et al., 2008; Leutz, Capitman, Ruwe, et al., 2002). See Box 41-7 for suggestions to help caregivers.

BOX 41-7 ■ Ways to Help Caregivers

Provide a listening ear. Encourage caregivers to talk about what they do and how they feel, and listen actively to their concerns. Find time to focus on the caregiver's needs, rather than on those of the care recipient.

Give positive feedback and validate its importance to the client's health.

Help the caregiver identify people who may be able to help, for example, family members living outside the home, neighbors, church members, community support groups.

Talk with family and friends, if the caregiver wishes. Teach them how to support the caregiver, for example by telephoning regularly, visiting, sending cards, or staying with the client a few hours (or days) so the caregiver can rest or take a vacation. Encourage them to listen to the caregiver without giving advice, and to help her feel appreciated (e.g., "I really appreciate all you do for Dad.")

Arrange for a home health aide, if possible. This relieves the caregiver of housekeeping and grocery shopping.

Remind family members and significant others to take care of themselves. Explain that their health is important to both them and the patient. Even the most devoted and self-sacrificing person may understand when you explain, "You must take care of yourself in order to be able to take care of your loved one."

■ Stress the need for the person to eat nutritious meals. Arrange for meals to be delivered to the home, if needed.

■ Encourage the caregiver to rest as much as possible, perhaps while the home health aide is there; or ask family members

and acquaintances to take turns staying an hour or two with the patient while the caregiver rests or "gets away." Help contact these people and make a schedule, if needed.

■ Stress the need for the caregivers to take some time for themselves, even if it is just an hour alone, or coffee with a neighbor.

■ Encourage caregivers to take a vacation, if they can afford it. Reassure them that competent help can be obtained and that it is fine to delegate caregiving to others for a while.

■ Some agencies have a weekend respite program for caregivers. The client is admitted to a skilled care unit for 2 or 3 days so the caregiver can have a break.

Encourage the caregiver to maintain spiritual connections, for example, to take time to go to church or temple; or ask the spiritual adviser to visit the home.

Communicate medical updates about the client—lab results, new treatment plans, and so on.

Help the family understand the goals of care and solve problems when needed.

Teach the family what to expect with regard to medications, treatments, and signs of approaching death. If family members know what to expect, they will be less likely to panic or fear the inevitable.

Follow up with other healthcare team members promptly if the family has questions that are outside your scope of practice.

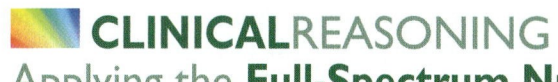

CLINICALREASONING
Applying the **Full-Spectrum Nursing Model**

Because the following critical thinking activities allow you to practice the kind of thinking you will use as a full-spectrum nurse, they usually have no single right answer. Discuss them with your peers—if you have difficulty with any of the questions, consult your instructor.

PATIENT SITUATION

Rachel, a freshman at State University, participated in a sorority rush activity during the second week of school. The event was attended by nearly 150 other freshman girls to socialize in the student union. About 2 or 3 days later, Rachel learned that six of the students at the party tested positive for the H1N1 virus and displayed signs of illness. Cite the resources you used to answer the following questions. Be sure they are of professional quality.

THINKING

1. *Theoretical Knowledge:*
   a. What is another name for the H1N1 virus?
   b. Name six common outward signs of an H1N1 infection that you might see in a college student.
2. *Critical Thinking (Contextual Awareness):*
   Why is it important to detect and treat H1N1 in a healthy population of young adults?

DOING

3. *Nursing Process (Assessment):*
   How might you assess the extent of the problem of H1N1 illness within the campus community?
4. *Practical Knowledge:*
   a. As the community health nurse, you design a *primary* intervention program to prevent an outbreak of H1N1 virus on campus. What might you do for this program?
   b. What interventions would you likely implement to deliver a *secondary* intervention program?
   c. Or a *tertiary* program?

CARING

5. *Self-Knowledge:*
   How would you feel if you were one of the first detected cases of H1N1 as the illness spread across the college campus?

To explore learning resources for this chapter,

Go to DavisPlus at http://davisplus.fadavis.com/, keyword Treas

Chapter Resources for Chapter 41:
    Knowledge Check and Think Like a Nurse Response
      Sheets
    Knowledge Check Answers
    Resources for Caregivers and Health Professionals
    Reading More About Community & Home Nursing
      (suggested readings)
    What Are the Main Points in This Chapter?
NCLEX-Style Review Questions

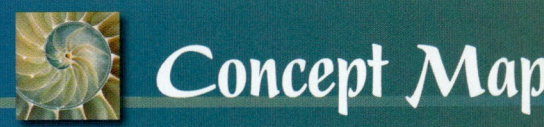

Concept Map

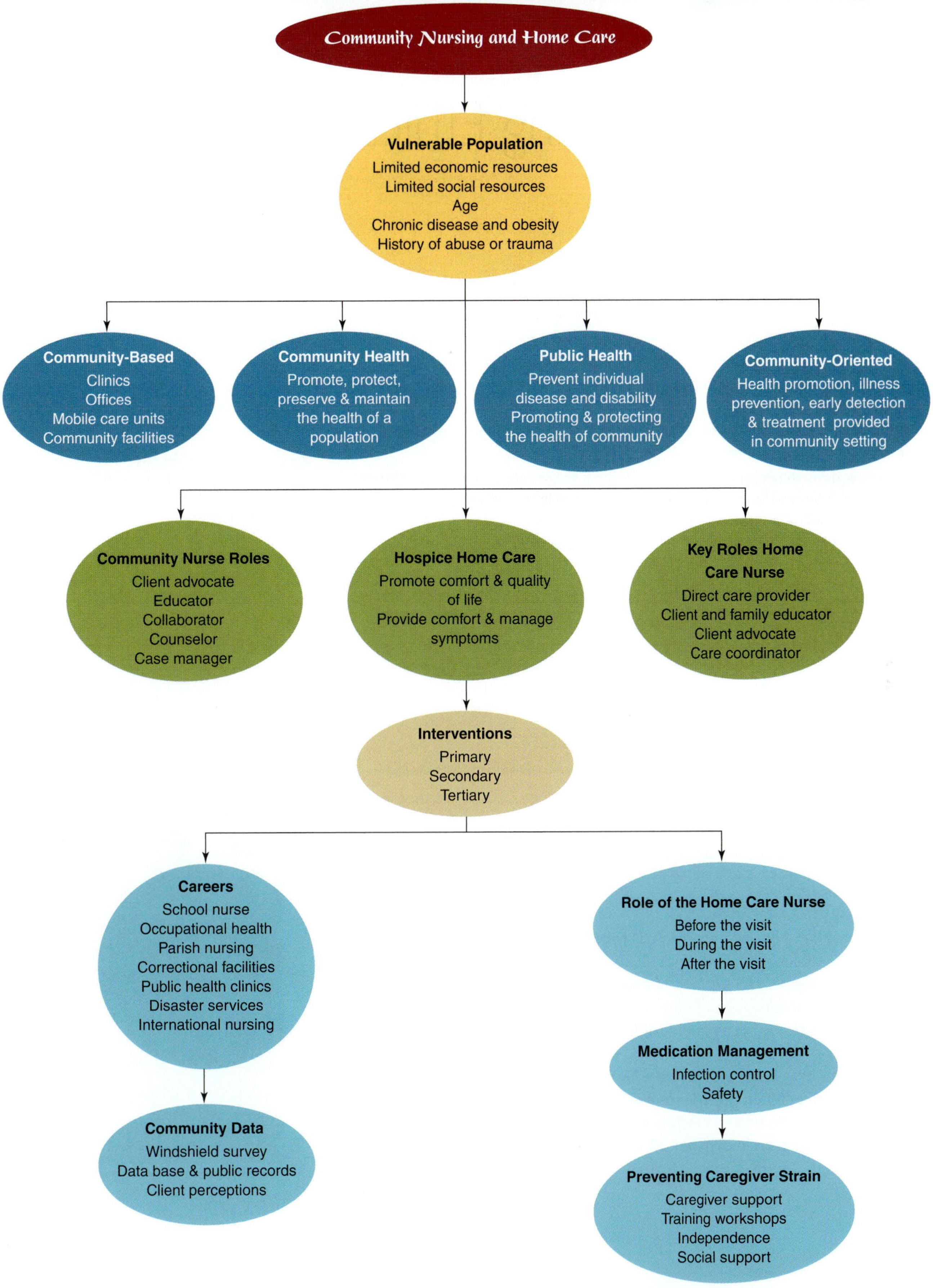

Community Nursing and Home Care

Vulnerable Population
Limited economic resources
Limited social resources
Age
Chronic disease and obesity
History of abuse or trauma

Community-Based
Clinics
Offices
Mobile care units
Community facilities

Community Health
Promote, protect,
preserve & maintain
the health of a
population

Public Health
Prevent individual
disease and disability
Promoting & protecting
the health of community

Community-Oriented
Health promotion, illness
prevention, early detection
& treatment provided
in community setting

Community Nurse Roles
Client advocate
Educator
Collaborator
Counselor
Case manager

Hospice Home Care
Promote comfort & quality
of life
Provide comfort & manage
symptoms

**Key Roles Home
Care Nurse**
Direct care provider
Client and family educator
Client advocate
Care coordinator

Interventions
Primary
Secondary
Tertiary

Careers
School nurse
Occupational health
Parish nursing
Correctional facilities
Public health clinics
Disaster services
International nursing

Role of the Home Care Nurse
Before the visit
During the visit
After the visit

Medication Management
Infection control
Safety

Community Data
Windshield survey
Data base & public records
Client perceptions

Preventing Caregiver Strain
Caregiver support
Training workshops
Independence
Social support

CHAPTER 42

Nugyens Ethics

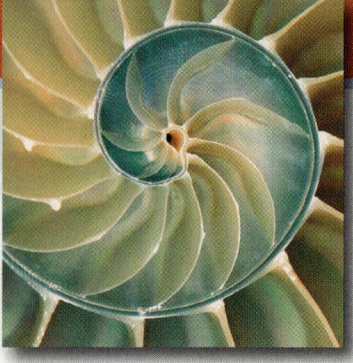

Learning Outcomes

After completing this chapter, you should be able to:

➤ Define *morals, ethics, bioethics,* and *nursing ethics.*

➤ Discuss what is meant by *ethical agency.*

➤ Identify at least four factors that contribute to the frequency of nurses' moral problems.

➤ Differentiate personal values and morality from professional values.

➤ Explain how developmental stages, values, moral frameworks, professional guidelines, and moral principles affect moral decisions.

➤ Describe five major ethical principles that are used in reasoning about healthcare.

➤ Compare and contrast four moral frameworks: consequentialism

(e.g., utilitarianism), deontology, an ethics of care, and feminist ethics.

➤ Identify the moral issues and principles involved in a given ethical situation.

➤ Describe what is meant by an integrity-producing compromise.

➤ Describe the nurse's obligations in ethical decisions.

➤ Discuss the role of the nurse as client advocate in the delivery of ethical nursing care.

➤ Apply the steps identified in the MORAL model for ethical decision making to issues nurses encounter in patient care.

Key Concepts

Morals
Nursing ethics
Values

Related Concepts

See the Concept Map at the end of this chapter.

Example Problems

Moral distress
Whistleblowing

Caring for the Nguyens

This feature allows you to practice the kind of thinking you will use as a full-spectrum nurse. There is usually more than one correct answer to a critical thinking question, so we do not provide answers for these features. It is more important to develop your nursing judgment than to "cover content." Discuss the questions with your peers. If you are still unsure, consult your instructor.

Mai Nguyen, Nam Nguyen's mother, has hypertension. She is forgetful about taking her medicines. Since her husband died, she has experienced periods of depression. When asked about her medicines she often replies, "It doesn't really matter since my husband died. If I die, what difference will it make?"

  Mai Nguyen was scheduled to have lunch with friends but did not arrive. When her friends called the house, they got no answer. At the end of lunch, one of Mai's friends decided to call Nam to inform him of her concerns about

his mother. Nam found his mother unresponsive on the kitchen floor. He called 911, and she was brought to the hospital by ambulance. At the hospital, the emergency department (ED) doctor tells Nam that his mother has had a massive stroke brought on by uncontrolled

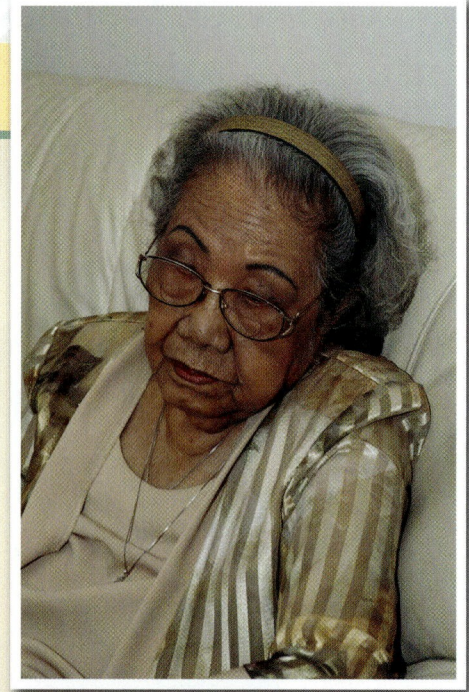

Caring for the Nguyens (continued)

hypertension. He asks Nam whether Mrs. Nguyen has an advance directive or living will. She has neither. The physician asks Nam to consider what level of care to offer his mother. He tells Nam that comprehensive treatment would include intubation, mechanical ventilation, and tube feeding support. The physician feels it is unlikely that she will experience significant recovery from this stroke.

Nam tells you, "I want everything done for my mother. I lost my father this year, and I'm not going to lose her, too."

Yen, Nam's wife, reminds you that Mai has been depressed since her husband died and has expressed a desire to die. Because Nam and Yen are not in agreement about the course of action, no decision is communicated. Mai Nguyen's condition continues to deteriorate, and the ED physician feels he must intubate her, place her on a ventilator, and admit her to the ICU according to hospital protocol.

A. You are aware of Mai Nguyen's statements and her poor compliance with treatment. What, if any, concerns do you have about this course of action?

B. Mai continues to decline. Nam Nguyen is informed that the "only thing keeping his mother alive is the ventilator and IV medicines." Do you consider this heroic treatment?

C. How would you approach Mr. Nguyen to speak with him about how he is feeling?

D. Nam and Yen have asked to meet with the team providing care to Mai. They announce that they would like all the "heroic measures to end." They request that Mai be allowed to die. Could you participate in this care? What actions would you be comfortable with? What actions would you be uncomfortable with?

Go to **Caring for the Nguyens Response Sheet** on *DavisPlus.*

Meet Your Patients

Angie and Edward Frese are a couple with two teenaged children. They are a close and loving family with a large network of family and friends. Alan, 15 years old, has just been severely injured in a high school soccer game. Angie and Edward are summoned to the hospital, where they are told that Alan has multiple bone fractures and active internal bleeding.

The surgeon informs the distressed parents that Alan will need a blood transfusion to survive. Although genuinely devastated, the parents adamantly refuse to consent to a lifesaving blood transfusion, stating they are Jehovah's Witnesses and that receiving blood is against their religious beliefs. The surgeon asks you, Alan's nurse, to get the parents to change their minds right away. You talk with the couple, but they continue to refuse a blood transfusion. You immediately contact your charge nurse. Try to answer the following critical-thinking questions about Alan and his parents. You may not have the experience or theoretical knowledge to answer them all—you will acquire that in this and the following chapter—but do your best based on the background you have.

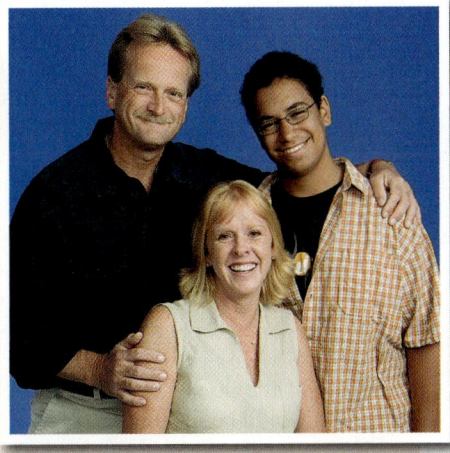

ThinkLike a Nurse 42-1

- Do Alan's parents have the right to refuse a blood transfusion based on their religious beliefs?
- Do you think the fact that Alan is a minor (under 18 years old) may make a difference in this situation?
- What actions do you think the charge nurse should take?
- Can an ethical conflict such as this be resolved to everyone's satisfaction?

Theoretical Knowledge
knowing **why**

The theoretical knowledge you will need to begin professional practice includes an understanding of the nature of morals and ethics (and especially nursing ethics) and basic information about factors that affect moral decisions (i.e., values, moral frameworks, professional guidelines, and ethical principles).

ABOUT THE KEY CONCEPTS

Nursing ethics, morals, and values are key concepts in this chapter because everything in the chapter is related to those concepts in some way—as you will discover. The subconcepts of advocacy and compromise, for example, are intimately integrated in the implementation of nursing ethics in clinical practice. Remember to use the key concepts to help you organize chapter content in your memory. As you read, try to understand how each subconcept you encounter relates to nursing ethics, morals, and values.

ETHICS AND MORALS

To understand nursing ethics, we must first understand the broader meaning of ethics. Although the terms *ethics* and *morals* have similar meanings, in modern theory **morals** refers to private, personal, or group standards of right and wrong. **Moral behavior** is behavior that is in accordance with custom or tradition and usually reflects personal or religious beliefs. An example of morality is the "Golden Rule," which says that you should treat others as you wish to be treated.

> Can you think of another example of moral behavior that you may have learned as a child?
>
> Can you identify any morals that are evident in the scenario about Alan at the beginning of the chapter?
>
> How do his parents' morals influence Alan's care?

Ethics, in contrast, is a systematic study of right and wrong conduct in situations that involve issues of values and morals. Ethics is a formal process for making logical and consistent moral decisions. In contrast, morals consider in a broad, general manner what is good or bad, right or wrong (e.g., "In general, it is wrong to steal"). Ethics answers the question, "What should I do in a given situation?" (e.g., "Is it wrong to steal if you have to do it to feed your children?"). Ethics uses specific rules, theories, principles, and perspectives to inquire into the justification of an individual's actions in a particular situation. It seeks to discover what we "ought" to do in certain circumstances.

In the case of Alan and his family (Meet Your Patients), the ethical decision making is quite different from the moral perspective of Alan's parents. The parents believe a blood transfusion is morally wrong; this fits with their religious beliefs. The surgeon and the nurse, however, believe withholding blood from Alan would be unethical.

Ethics and the Law. How are laws related to ethics and morals? Think about the following:

- *Law:* It is illegal to drive faster than the speed limit.
  Situation: A child is bleeding profusely and may have cut an artery. The driver drives very fast and even drives through a red light.
  Question: Was that illegal? Was it immoral?
- *Law:* In the United States, it is legal in certain situations to have an abortion.
  Fact: Although everyone would have to agree that the act is legal, people are about evenly divided as to whether they believe it is moral.

Ethics reflects the political and legal values of a society. However, you should be able to see that ethics is not the same as law, religion, institutional practices, or customs. An action that is legal or customary may not be morally right or ethically justifiable. The same holds true of religion. You cannot assume that an accepted practice of a certain religion is an ethical practice in every situation.

WHAT IS NURSING ETHICS?

Bioethics refers to the application of ethical principles to every aspect of healthcare, including direct care of patients, allocation of resources, utilization of staff, and medical and nursing research. **Nursing ethics** is a subset of bioethics. It refers to ethical questions that arise out of nursing practice. The first things to come to your mind may be dramatic questions such as, "Should we turn off the ventilator and allow this patient to die?" and "Is abortion moral?" In reality, you may have some input, but the patient, physician, and family will make the final decision in such situations. As a nurse, you are responsible for deciding the nature and extent of your own participation in each situation, and you must support patients who are making ethical decisions or perhaps coping with the results of decisions made by others. Consider the following true story paraphrased from Curtin and Flaherty (1982, pp. 3–4):

Example:

> *A woman took her 6-year-old son to the emergency department (ED) to have a scalp laceration sutured. On the way to the hospital, she tried to calm him by telling him that the doctors would "numb" him and no one would hurt him "on purpose." When they arrived in the ED, they were placed in a cubicle next to another little boy who was awaiting treatment for a similar laceration. His father was also trying to reassure his son, as the woman had done.*
>
> *A nurse entered the cubicle of the father and son. She roughly cleansed the cut with no explanation or words of comfort. The physician sutured the laceration without a word and without waiting for the local anesthetic to take effect. The boy screamed in pain and terror the whole time. The woman was horrified, and her son was scared. But when the very same nurse approached the woman and her son, she was kind and gentle. The same physician carefully injected a local anesthetic and waited for it to take effect before suturing.*

Why do you think there was such difference in the treatment? Was it because the man and boy appeared to be of lower socioeconomic status? Was it the presence of a father rather than a mother? Was it because the father and son were from a minority group and the woman and son were not? Regardless of why it happened, what makes this case important? After all, both boys received medical treatment; both incisions will heal; no one's life or health was threatened; no life-and-death decisions were made. But the first child's humanity and dignity were violated, and the actions were not fair. *This case is a perfect example of nursing ethics:* questions that have to do with *the nurse's* actions, not the actions of others. The nurse did not need a medical order or permission from hospital administration to act ethically.

In the Meet Your Patients scenario, you, as the nurse, are not responsible for deciding the broad questions: "Is blood transfusion right or wrong?" or "Do the parents have a right to refuse blood transfusion?" Your decision is "What should *I* do? Should I try to persuade the parents to change their minds, as the surgeon directs, or not?" That is the *nursing ethics* question. And in that scenario, you will need to deal with the effects of the final decision on Alan. He may be frightened; he may be angry; he may die. The nurse is there for patients' most human and vulnerable moments.

Why Should Nurses Study Ethics?

Nurses should study ethics for a variety of reasons.

- *You will encounter ethical problems frequently in your work.* A consciously made, informed decision must surely

be better than one made without awareness of the ethical issues involved. The most difficult question you will face as a nurse will not be "How do I do this?" but "Should I do this?"

- **Ethics is central to nursing.** Commitment to caring for other human beings supports the claim that nursing is a moral art (Curtin & Flaherty, 1982). Traditionally, people have expressed idealism by helping the sick; health and compassion are central values in nursing.

- **Multidisciplinary input is important.** As situations become more complex, multidisciplinary input becomes increasingly important. For example, surgeons are responsible for knowing what surgery to perform and obtaining consent, but the nurse has a part in being sure the patient is adequately informed so that true consent is obtained. No one profession is responsible for an ethical decision.

- **Ethical knowledge is necessary for professional competence.** Being a professional includes being accountable to others in the profession for the ethical conduct of your work. Using professional expertise for social good is one hallmark of a profession. Therefore, to conduct our work well and have it stand the test of public scrutiny, we need to be clear about the ethics of our work.

- **Ethical reasoning is necessary for nursing credibility among other disciplines.** For your opinion to be valued by others, you must be able to clearly express your moral position in a logical way. You must be able to (1) understand your own values as they relate to basic morality and (2) use ethical reasoning to articulate your moral position.

- **Ethical proficiency is essential for providing holistic care.** Nurses care for the whole person—that includes providing support for spiritual and moral concerns.

- **Nurses have a responsibility to be advocates for patients.** **Advocacy** is the communication and defense of the rights and interests of another. Since the 1960s, schools have socialized nurses to include patient advocacy in their role conceptions (Wilkinson, 1997). Currently, the American Nurses Association (ANA) Code of Ethics for Nurses (2001), provision 3, states: "The nurse promotes, advocates for and strives to protect the health, safety and rights of the patient." Advocacy includes taking appropriate action when the actions of a healthcare team member jeopardize the patient's rights or best interests. However, you can advocate for patients in everyday practice, for example by contacting a primary provider to request a new prescription when a pain medication is not effective. To advocate for patients in ethical situations, you must be able to identify the ethical issues and communicate the patient's wishes.

- **Studying ethics will help you to make better decisions.** The study of ethics prepares you to analyze moral problems from multiple perspectives rather than relying entirely on your personal values, intuition, and emotions. Practice in analyzing dilemmas will help you to become an informed decision maker, capable of understanding the perspectives of all the people in each situation—to understand, for example, why the Freses (Meet Your Patients) are refusing a blood transfusion.

Most nursing problems have more than one acceptable answer. This is especially true of ethical problems. Each situation is unique in its details—for example, the people differ in how they evaluate what is and is not beneficial for themselves. By thinking it through critically from several different angles, you will be assured that you have done all that you can to provide your client with the highest quality of ethical care.

KnowledgeCheck 42-1

- Define *morals*, and give an example that is not in the text.
- Define *ethics*, and give an example that is not in the text.
- How is bioethics different from ethics?
- Why do nurses need to study ethics?

What Is Ethical Agency?

Moral agency, or **ethical agency,** for nurses is the ability to base their practice on professional standards of ethical conduct and to participate in ethical decision making. Simply stated, it means that nurses have choices and are responsible for their actions. An ethical agent must be able to do the following:

- Perceive the difference between right and wrong.
- Understand abstract moral principles.
- Reason and apply moral principles to make decisions, weigh alternatives, and plan sound ways to achieve goals.
- Decide and choose freely.
- Act according to choice (this assumes both the power and the capability to act).

For more an expanded discussion of ethical agency,

 Go to Chapter 42, **Supplemental Materials: Elements of Ethical Agency,** on Davis*Plus.*

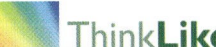 Think**Like a Nurse** 42-2

Consider the five components of ethical agency. To what extent do you believe nurses possess those abilities? Explain your thinking.

1. Perceive the difference between good and evil, right and wrong.
2. Understand abstract moral principles.
3. Reason and apply moral principles to make decisions, weigh alternatives, and plan sound ways to achieve goals.
4. Decide and choose freely.
5. Act according to choice (this assumes both the power and the capability to act).

Example Problem: Moral Distress

In practice, nurses often make but are unable to carry out their moral decisions. A seminal study by Wilkinson (1987/1988) identified this as **moral distress.** Situational pressures (constraints) influence nurses' moral decisions as well as their ability to carry out their decisions (e.g., Corley & Minick, 2002; Erlen, 2001; Georges & Grypdonck, 2002; Hamric, Davis, & Childress, 2006; Hart, 2009; Jameton, 1984; Zuzelo, 2007). Whether these constraints are real or merely perceived, nurses in various studies have named the following as obstacles to carrying out their moral decisions: physicians, nurse administrators, other nurses, institutional policies, the law, threat of lawsuits, being socialized to follow orders, and doubting their own knowledge (Catlin, Volat, Hadley, et al., 2008; Glasberg, Eriksson, & Norberg, 2008; Schluter, Winch, Holzhauser, et al., 2008; Wilkinson, 1987/1988).

This problem is not unique to nurses, and recent studies describe moral distress among other healthcare professionals (e.g., Schwenzer & Wang, 2006). No one is 100% "free" to

choose and act. Actions always have consequences: for you and for others. Nevertheless, if you are confident you have made a good decision and can express it rationally and clearly to others, you can at least enter into a conversation with nurse administrators, physicians, and families about what ought to be done. Then you will be comfortable knowing that you have done all you could do, even if it is not all you wished to do.

If you would like an optional, expanded discussion of moral distress,

 Go to Chapter 42, **Supplemental Materials: Moral Distress,** on Davis*Plus.*

Example Problem: Whistleblowing

Nurses experience **moral outrage** when they perceive that others are behaving immorally (Wilkinson, 1987/1988). Moral outrage is similar to moral distress, except that in cases of moral outrage, nurses do not participate in the act. Therefore, they do not believe that they are responsible for doing wrong, but that they are powerless to prevent the wrongdoing (Burkhardt & Nathaniel, 2008).

A nurse may respond to moral outrage by "blowing the whistle." A **whistleblower** is specifically defined as a person "who identifies an incompetent, unethical, or illegal situation, or actions of others, in the workplace and reports it to someone who may have the power to stop the wrong" (Ahern & McDonald, 2002, p. 314; Wilmot, 2000). The "others" in question may be an individual or an entire organization. When the wrongdoing involves an organization, the whistleblower must hold the situation up to public scrutiny, for example, by going to the news media or pursuing legal recourse.

At some point in your nursing career, you may become aware that a health team member or organization is doing something illegal, unethical, or incompetent. In deciding what to do, you will need to consider the consequence of the action, the competence of the person involved, and the completeness of your data about the incident. Before deciding to report the person, you will want to be sure that the information has been confirmed through another source and that reporting the problem will be likely to correct the wrongdoing or prevent future problems (Attree, 2007; Peternelj-Taylor, 2003). Weigh the risks against the benefits.

Impaired Nursing Practice. Whistleblowing is a difficult matter in the case of an impaired colleague. **Impaired nursing practice** occurs when the nurse's ability to perform the essential nursing functions is diminished by chemical dependence or by mental illness. Impairment is a threat to patients, and the impaired nurse may have difficulty being accountable to herself or assessing her self-competence. Therefore, the Code of Ethics for Nurses and an ANA resolution propose that as a compassionate colleague, you must ensure that an impaired nurse receives assistance in regaining optimal function by reporting the behaviors to the appropriate entity within the employment setting (ANA, 2001, 2002).

KnowledgeCheck 42-2

- Define *ethical agency.*
- What five abilities must be present for ethical agency to exist?
- List at least three constraints that can keep nurses from carrying out their moral decisions.

What Are Some Sources of Ethical Problems for Nurses?

Factors contributing to the frequency of nurses' ethical problems include societal factors, the nature of nursing work, and the nature of the nursing profession itself.

Societal Factors

This section discusses how some ethical problems for nurses are created by the ever-changing nature of our dynamic, multicultural society.

Increased Consumer Awareness. Historically, sick people sought the advice of a physician and then usually followed the physician's orders without question. Partly as a result of increased consumer awareness and availability of information online, professionals now are expected to share knowledge with patients and to obtain truly informed consent for treatments.

Technological Advances. With every new technology, new issues arise. Ethical questions surround organ transplants, amniocentesis capable of revealing fetal defects, in vitro fertilization and embryo transfer, genetic engineering, human embryonic stem cell research, cryogenics, and technical advances that allow loved ones to be maintained on life support beyond what anyone might have imagined 20 years ago (Brock, 2006).

Multicultural Population. We live in a multicultural, multifaith society; you cannot assume that your values and

---

Toward Evidence-Based Practice

Attree, M. (2007). Factors influencing nurses' decisions to raise concerns about care quality. *Journal of Nursing Management, 15*(4), 392–402.

Professional ethics require nurses to raise concerns about standards of practice; however, under-reporting is the norm. This qualitative study analyzed data from interviews with 142 nurses and found that nurses perceived reporting concerns to be a high-risk: low-benefit action. They lacked confidence in reporting systems. Nurses named fear of repercussions, retribution, labeling, and blame as reasons for

not raising concerns, as well as the belief that nothing would be done about the concerns.

1. What type of moral situation (for the nurse) is best illustrated by this study: moral distress or whistleblowing? Explain your reasoning.

 Go to Chapter 42, **Toward Evidence-Based Practice Suggested Responses,** on DavisPlus.

beliefs are similar to those of your patients and colleagues. You will need to respect a variety of belief systems, and serve as a patient advocate even when the patient's value system is strikingly different from your own. There are nursing theories that can help you recognize various cultural values, for example, Leininger's (2002) theory of cultural care diversity and universality (for a review, see Chapters 8 and 15).

Cost Containment. The emphasis on cutting healthcare costs creates many morally questionable situations. For example, patients are being sent home from the hospital while they are still very ill. On being discharged, they may learn that insurance payments are limited for services outside the hospital, including specialists, home care, and medical supplies (e.g., bandages, walkers). Cost containment efforts have led healthcare agencies to increase the number of patients each nurse is expected to care for. As a nurse, you will undoubtedly find yourself in situations where fewer nurses are available than patient acuity requires. You will have to make personal decisions about how far you will stretch your own resources.

The Nature of Nursing Work

Ethical problems exist in all kinds of work. However, the nature of nursing work can create unique ethical problems.

Nurses' Moral Problems

Nurses' moral problems are immediate, serious, and frequent. In the classroom, you have the luxury to leave questions unsettled. In the real world, you must always decide: either you take action, or you do not. For a nurse, deciding *not* to act is, in effect, an act. For example, suppose the family wishes a patient to have aggressive "code blue" (resuscitation) efforts; however, you know the patient does not want this. When the patient's heart stops, whether or not you know the "right" thing to do, you must decide immediately to carry out or not carry out the code blue. If you wait too long to ponder the ethical issues, the patient may die before you decide. If you do not decide, the effect is the same as though you had decided it was wrong to code.

Nurses' Unique Position in Healthcare Organizations

Nurses have multiple obligations and relationships, and sometimes conflicting loyalties. They are employees (with a relationship with the agency) as well as professionals (with a special relationship with patients). In addition, they have peer relationships and a unique relationship with physicians. Although most nurses are not employed by a physician, they are expected to follow physician prescriptions for patient care. In addition, in most organizations, physicians are higher on the power and status hierarchy than are nurses. Ethical questions arise when nurses experience conflicts among their loyalties to patients, families, physicians, employers, and other nurses. Consider the following example: a patient wants to know his test results; the physician is reluctant to tell him. What are the conflicting loyalties? Should the nurse give the patient the information or not? There are two options: tell or don't tell.

Tell. By telling the patient his test results, the nurse would honor the principle of personal autonomy and fulfill her obligation to the patient. But this might harm the patient's relationship with the physician, which is important to the patient's well-being. Furthermore, if the nurse tells the patient his test results, it may affect her relationship with the physician, and perhaps create problems between the physician and the employer (e.g., the hospital). In addition, if this action violates hospital policies, it would harm the nurse's relationship with the hospital.

Don't tell. The nurse could preserve the patient–physician relationship by withholding the test results from the patient. This choice does not honor her relationship with the patient. Also, if the nurse does not tell the patient his test results, the patient may find out anyway and be angry at the physician, the nurse, and the hospital.

According to professional ethics, your first allegiance is to the patient. However, the patient's needs often conflict with institutional policies, family desires, or even state laws. There may also be conflicts in your relationships with the patient and his family. You can see an example of this in the Meet Your Patients scenario, wherein the nurse finds it impossible to honor the parents' autonomy and at the same time advocate for Alan. You may also encounter this type of conflict when a patient does not want any heroic measures and wishes only to die peacefully, but the family has not yet been able to accept the imminent death and are insisting on full resuscitation.

The Nature of the Nursing Profession

Some ethical problems arise because of value conflicts and a lack of clarity within the nursing profession. We have unresolved questions about the nature, scope, and goals of our practice, as well as our professional values. In most of the following examples, we value both of the opposites. We would not wish to give up either one. But specific situations require us to choose between them, and that is one source of our discomfort.

- *Caring versus time spent with patients.* Nursing values caring, humanistic care, and nurse–patient relationships—but nurses now spend less time at the bedside (with patients) than ever before. One reason is understaffing and heavier patient loads, but there are other factors: the use of technology; the need for careful documentation; and the nursing emphasis on leading, managing, and delegation instead of hands-on care.
- *Caring versus professionalism.* On one hand, we claim the nurse is a professional, citing critical-thinking, knowledge, and management skills—on the other hand, we emphasize caring, with the nurse at the bedside offering comfort and doing hands-on tasks.
- *Autonomy versus escaping hard choices.* On one hand, we believe that nurses should have an equal status with other healthcare professionals—on the other hand, many nurses want to escape hard choices by "letting the doctor decide."
- *Higher pay versus cost effectiveness.* Most nurses believe we deserve higher pay—yet we claim nurses are cost effective because we work less expensively than do physicians.

WHAT FACTORS AFFECT MORAL DECISIONS?

By now, you should have an idea of the nature of morals and ethics and of the need to study nursing ethics. Focus now on some basic theoretical knowledge about factors that are involved in making moral decisions: developmental stages, values, moral frameworks, ethical principles, and professional guidelines. As you learn about each of these concepts, consider how it affects moral decision making.

Developmental Stage

A person's stage of moral development affects the way he reasons about moral issues. We learn and internalize our morals throughout the life span, beginning in childhood.

Kohlberg's (1968, 1981) studies led to his view that children go through a sequence of progressively higher levels of moral reasoning ability. They proceed gradually through several stages to a final level in adulthood, in which they base moral principles on universal and impartial principles of justice (Table 42-1). If you would like more information about moral development theory,

 Go to Chapter 42, **Tables, Boxes, Figures: ESG Table 42-1, Stages of Moral Development,** on Davis*Plus*.

The stages overlap. Kohlberg found that more than half of a person's thinking always reflects the stage he is in, with the remainder at the stage he is leaving or the stage into which he is moving. Although some people never achieve Kohlberg's highest levels, progression through the stages is always forward—except in extreme trauma, it is never backward—and people do not skip stages.

Gilligan (1993) challenged Kohlberg's perspective of moral development, citing it as being male biased. Gilligan's research found that girls develop morally by paying attention to community and to relationships, whereas boys tend to process dilemmas through more abstract ideals or principles. If you need a review of Gilligan's three stages: caring for oneself, caring for others, and caring for self and others, refer to Chapter 9.

Values, Attitudes, and Beliefs

Your values influence what you think and do. This is important to know because values are entangled in all ethical situations. If asked, could you say what your values are? Could you explain how they affect your decisions about right and wrong in a given situation? If so, that's a great beginning. If not, you will learn more as you move through this section.

Values and morals are learned in conscious and unconscious ways and become a part of your makeup. When we evaluate right and wrong, or good and bad, we are using moral judgment. Therefore, our individual preferences (values) of right or wrong become our moral values. Whether or not you are aware of it, your morals and values shape the manner in which you make ethical decisions in your nursing practice (Burkhardt & Nathaniel, 2008).

So, although ethics are based on a structured set of principles and theories, and ethical decisions are publicly stated in terms of possible alternative behaviors, such decisions are always influenced unconsciously by our own personal values and morals. It is important to clarify the influence of your values and morals each time you enter into a situation where you are called on to be objective in your decision making.

What Are Values?   A **value** is a belief you have about the worth of something; it serves as a principle or a standard that influences your decision making. Values are ideals, beliefs,

Table 42-1 ➤ Kohlberg's Stages of Moral Development	
LEVELS	**STAGES**
I. Preconventional Level	
The person conforms to cultural rules and labels of good and bad but interprets them in terms of (1) punishment and reward or (2) the physical power of those who enforce the rules. Children ages 4 to 10 yr are usually at this level; some adults never progress beyond it.	*Stage 1*—Punishment–obedience orientation. (It is a right action if it avoids punishment.) *Stage 2*—Personal interest orientation. (It is a right action if it satisfies your personal needs.)
II. Conventional Level	
Meeting family, group, or societal expectations is valuable in its own right, regardless of the consequences of the actions. The person goes beyond conforming to loyalty to the social order and identifying with those involved in it. Others set the standards, but the person is internally motivated to follow them.	*Stage 3*—Good boy–nice girl orientation. (It is a right action if it pleases others.) *Stage 4*—Law-and-order orientation. (It is a right action if it follows the rules.)
III. Postconventional, Autonomous, or Principled Level	
The person begins to define moral values and principles that have validity apart from society, groups, or persons in power. At this level, it becomes possible for the person to experience conflict between two socially accepted standards, and the person tries to decide rationally between them. Both the standards and the decision are internal. Moral principles have validity apart from the authority of groups and persons.	*Stage 5*—Legalistic, social contract orientation. (A right action is decided in terms of individual rights and standards agreed on by the whole society.) *Stage 6*—Universal ethical principles orientation. (A right action is determined by conscience and abstract principles such as the Golden Rule.)

Source: Adapted from: Gibbs, J. (2009). *Moral development & reality: Beyond the theories of Kohlberg and Hoffman.* Upper Saddle River, NJ: Pearson Education; Hoffman, M. (2000). *Empathy and moral development: Implications for caring and justice.* Cambridge: Cambridge University Press; Kohlberg, L. (1968). Moral development. In *International encyclopedia of social science.* New York: Macmillan; Kohlberg, L. (1981). *Essays on moral development.* Volumes 1–3. San Francisco: Harper & Row; Power, F., Higgins, A., & Kohlberg, L. (1989). *Lawrence Kohlberg's approach to moral education.* New York: Columbia University Press; and Waugh, D. (1978). Moral development: Theory and process. In *Teaching and evaluating the affective domain in nursing programs* (pp. 17–30). New York: Charles B. Slack.

customs, modes of conduct, qualities, or goals that are highly prized or preferred by individuals, groups, or society. You can value an idea, a person, a way of doing things, or even an object (e.g., money). People express their values through behaviors, feelings, knowledge, and decisions. For example, the nurse who values compassion will interact with patients in a sensitive, caring manner. Values can change over time through experience and thoughtful consideration.

Your **value set** is your "list" of values. It gives direction for your life and forms a basis for behavior. Your **value system** is your value set with the values ranked from most important to least important. The total number of values a person has is rather small. The number of significant ones is even smaller. It is easy enough to identify values—for example, love, freedom, courage, and responsibility—but how many of them have a consistent and predictable impact on your actions? Those are the significant values.

KnowledgeCheck 42-3

- What are values?
- What are three characteristics of values?

 Think**Like a Nurse** 42-3

- Think about what you value personally in your own life. What are the five ideals, principles, or things that are most important to you?
- Now refer back to Chapter 15, where you were asked to list five ideals, principles, or things that were most important to you. What did you list then? Is your list any different now that you have gained some clinical experience and theoretical knowledge?

What Are Attitudes?   Attitudes are mental dispositions or feelings toward a person, object, or idea. Attitudes can be cognitive (thinking), affective (feeling), and behavioral (doing). For example, you might have a positive attitude about cleanliness—that is, you may think it is a good thing (e.g., "The floor is clean. I like that.") But if you value cleanliness, you would be willing to scrub the floor. You would also wash your hands at appropriate times, bathe regularly, and teach others about hygiene.

What Are Beliefs?   A belief is something that one accepts as true (e.g., "I believe that germs cause disease and that by washing my hands I remove germs"). Beliefs are sometimes based on faith and sometimes on facts. A belief may or may not be true. Beliefs may or may not involve values. Consider the following statements of belief. The first does not involve a value; the second one does.

"I believe the Earth is round."

"Working hard to achieve goals is important to me; therefore, I believe that I must work during the summer to save money for college."

From those examples, can you see how values, beliefs, and behaviors are related?

 Think**Like a Nurse** 42-4

- Consider Alan and his family (Meet Your Patients). What do you think were the values of Alan's parents that influenced their behavior at the hospital? First, identify their behaviors specifically. Then speculate about the values underlying each behavior.
- How do you think values can influence health?

KnowledgeCheck 42-4

- Define *belief*; give a new example.
- Define *attitude*; give a new example.

Professional versus Personal Values

Your **personal value system** is a set of values that you have reflected on and chosen that will help you to lead a good life (Purtilo, 2005). You have internalized some *societal values* and have come to perceive them as your own (e.g., good manners). In addition, you probably have some *personal values* (e.g., friendship, fairness, creativity) that are important to you but may or may not be important to society at large.

As you move forward in your profession, you will integrate what you learn and experience and form **professional values.** Many of these will simply expand your personal values. The American Association of Colleges of Nursing (AACN) has identified five professional values (2008):

Altruism
Autonomy
Human dignity
Integrity
Social Justice

If you would like definitions and examples of professional behaviors for the AACN values,

 Go to Chapter 42, **Tables, Boxes, Figures: ESG Table 42-2, AACN and Other Professional Nursing Values and Behaviors,** on Davis*Plus.*

Additional professional values frequently cited for nursing include: caring, diversity, equality (or rights, privileges, or status), aesthetics, freedom (to choose), truth, service (commitment to useful work to others), basic and lifelong education, holism, competence, and loyalty.

Personal and professional values are not always congruent, though. Consider the following situation:

Alexandra Jensen is a 17-year-old pregnant woman who comes in to your hospital for a voluntary termination of an early pregnancy. You are assigned to admit her to your unit and get her ready for this procedure. Imagine that your personal value is that you do not believe in abortion but that your professional value is guided by the ANA standards of professional practice, which state that the nurse "delivers care in a manner that preserves and protects patient autonomy, dignity, rights, values and beliefs" (ANA, 2010, p. 47). It is difficult to hold a personal value in high regard while under pressure to assume a conflicting professional value.

How might you feel in the situation just described? Do you think that your personal and professional values need to be compatible in order for you to be a competent nurse? Do you think that you should have the absolute right to refuse to participate in a situation (such as the one above) that may violate your personal values?

 Think**Like a Nurse** 42-5

- Name some other examples of societal values.
- What groups and social experiences have helped to form your values?
- Examine your personal values to see whether they match the AACN professional values mentioned above. Which of those values, if any, do you *not* share? Explain your thinking.

KnowledgeCheck 42-5

- What is the difference between personal and professional values?
- What is an example of professional values?
- What are some other types of values?

How Are Values Transmitted?

As you have learned, we acquire values from social interaction. So how does that work? Table 42-2 outlines the methods of value transmission. A recent study adds the information that values transmission between parents and adolescents can be reciprocal and that the presence of a receptive and supportive parent makes value transmission more likely (Pinquart & Silbereisen, 2004).

What Is Value Neutrality?

You have probably been taught that nurses need to be non-judgmental in working with their clients. As a nurse, you do have a duty to provide the best care to clients. You should not assume that your personal values are right, and you should not judge the client's values as right or wrong on the basis of whether they agree with your value system. Think back to the discussion regarding Alexandra, who was seeking to terminate her pregnancy. A nurse who does not believe in abortion could still provide competent nursing care to Alexandra even though his personal values about abortion are different from Alexandra's. **Value neutrality** means that we attempt to understand our own values regarding an issue and to know when to put them aside, if necessary, to become nonjudgmental when providing care to clients. However, you should know that many ethicists believe value neutrality is not possible to achieve. Further, they say it is not even desirable because it obligates healthcare providers to suppress their own deepest moral and religious beliefs (Balch, 2006; Beckwith & Peppin, 2000; Clark, 2006; Goldenberg, 2005; Pellegrino, 2000).

KnowledgeCheck 42-6

- What are some ways that values can be transmitted?
- What is value neutrality?

Moral Frameworks

Moral (or **philosophical**) **frameworks** are systems of thought (theories) that are the basis for the differing perspectives that people have in ethical situations. Many such frameworks are rooted in ancient works, of, for example, the Greek philosophers Plato and Aristotle. No matter how well you know the theories, though, they will not provide answers for specific patient situations. They simply offer a lens through which you can examine an ethical problem. See Chapter 8 if you need to review the purposes and uses of theories.

There is no single "best" theory that will give you all the answers or provide the one "true" answer to an ethical problem. Each provides a different perspective. Using more than one framework to analyze a situation enables you to perform a more comprehensive analysis of the problem.

What Is Consequentialism?

In **consequentialist** theories, the rightness or wrongness of an action depends on the consequences of the act rather than on the act itself. Theories of this type are also called **teleology,** from the Greek word *telos,* meaning "end" or the study of ends (also called *final causes*) (Beauchamp & Childress, 2008). **Utilitarianism,** the most familiar consequentialist theory, takes the position that the value of an action is determined by its usefulness. The *principle of utility* states that an act must result in the greatest good (positive benefit) for the greatest number of people. Any act can become the ethical choice if it delivers "good" results. In healthcare, the principle of "first, do no harm," is consequentialist in nature. Because of this principle, we are always concerned about weighing the risks and benefits of our care (e.g., a medication may kill cancer cells, but side effects may harm the patient's quality of life).

Using utilitarianism to resolve an ethical problem, you would evaluate every alternative action for its potential outcomes, both positive and negative—similar to a technique you may already use when making other decisions, that is, making a list of pros and cons. You would then select the action that results in the most benefits for the greatest number of people involved in the situation. The following is an example of utilitarian reasoning: The practice of triage is used in a disaster when emergency

Table 42-2 ➤ Modes of Value Transmission	
MODE	**DESCRIPTION**
Modeling	Children learn values from a variety of role models (parents, peers, rock stars, significant others) by observation. This modeling may lead to socially acceptable or unacceptable behaviors.
Moralizing	"This way is the only way." Children are taught a complete set of values in an authoritarian approach. If the child does not conform, the parent may inflict guilt and fear on him. This approach by parents, teachers, church leaders, and other authorities may make it difficult for young people to make independent choices because they have no experience selecting values that are good for them.
Laissez-faire	"Doing your own thing." Children are allowed to explore differing sets of values on their own with little guidance or discipline. This may lead to conflict and confusion on the part of the child.
Reward and punishment	The child's behavior is controlled by offering rewards for certain valued behaviors and punishing the child who fails to comply. Rewards can strengthen behavior, whereas physical punishment may teach that violence is an acceptable behavior.
Responsible choice	A balance of freedom and restriction allows children to select the values, explore new behaviors, and experience the consequences. This can lead to personal satisfaction and parental support.

workers sort patients to determine who will be treated first or who will receive limited resources (e.g., oxygen or intravenous therapy). If a victim has little potential for survival, he may not be treated at all, or his treatment may be postponed to allow the healthcare team to treat those victims (i.e., "the greatest number") with the greatest potential to survive.

ThinkLike a Nurse 42-6

- Describe a time in your life when you used consequentialism to resolve a difficult situation.
- What types of clinical dilemmas might be best resolved using this model?

What Is Deontology?

Deontology, unlike the utilitarian model, considers an action to be right or wrong regardless of its consequences. Decisions are based on moral rules and unchanging principles. There are a variety of deontological theories, but you will commonly find they make use of the following, or similar, principles:

The Categorical Imperative. This principle, established by the philosopher Immanuel Kant (1724–1804), states that one should act only if the action is based on a principle that is universal—or in other words, if you believe that everyone should act in the same way in a similar situation.

Treat People as Ends and Never as Means. This means that the person is more important than the goal you may be trying to accomplish. Can you imagine the ethical concerns of research situations in which the research subjects were exposed to some amount of risk (e.g., a new surgical procedure) to find a drug or treatment that will benefit many other people?

Rules and Principles. When using a deontological model, you would critically examine a situation to determine which actions are right or wrong according to rules and principles such as justice, autonomy, doing good, and doing no harm. These principles are regarded as unchanging and absolute, and they come from the same universal values that underlie all major religions.

Rights and Duties. Deontological frameworks also emphasize rights (e.g., the right to freedom, the right of self-determination) and duties (obligations). For example, you must help someone in need because you have a duty to help others, not because helping will produce good consequences. In fact, you have a duty to help even if your helping may produce some bad consequences.

Difficulties When Using a Deontology Framework. The following are two common difficulties in applying this framework:

- **Conflict of universal principles.** Sometimes you must choose between conflicting universal principles. It is not always clear which principle to follow. Allowing Alan's parents (Meet Your Patients) to refuse him blood honors the principle of autonomy, but their decision may interfere with a right: Alan's right to life. Can you see that it might be difficult to choose the appropriate principle to honor?
- **Knowing another's motives.** In deontology, it is important to consider motives. It is one thing for Alan's parents to refuse a blood transfusion because they are honoring a religious principle; it would be quite another thing if they refused the transfusion because they stood to inherit a large trust fund left to Alan by his grandfather. Motives may place more weight on one of the conflicting universal principles over the other and make a decision clearer. Unfortunately, it

is sometimes hard to recognize your own motives, much less to be sure about the motives of others.

Key Point: *As a nurse, you will almost never be able to decide only on the basis of principles and rules; you will always need to consider the consequences of your actions.*

KnowledgeCheck 42-7

- Describe utilitarianism.
- Define *deontology.*

What Is Feminist Ethics?

Feminist ethics is based on the belief that traditional ethical models provide a mostly masculine perspective, and that they devalue the moral experience of women. Traditional deontological models focus on abstract principles such as fairness, justice, and rights, which are more typical of male reasoning. In contrast, virtues such as love, relationships, caring, nurturing, and sympathy are more relevant to women but are rarely seen in traditional theories (Bandman & Bandman, 2002). Feminists assert that focusing on deontological principles distracts one from dealing with larger social issues. Feminist ethical reasoning uses relationships and stories rather than universal principles. Feminists argue that it is impossible to avoid being influenced by one's relationships. They see that influence as positive and believe it should not be lessened by trying to be objective—and in any case, that objectivity is impossible to achieve.

Feminist theories do use principles and consequences, but they also ask you to look at social issues in the ethical situation to ensure that social facts are considered, particularly the issues of gender equality (Noddings, 2003)—to think when reasoning, "How is this decision affecting the woman?" Consider an example of deciding whether to allocate federally funded healthcare resources to younger people or to older adults. Feminist reasoning might say that, all other considerations being equal:

- In the United States there are more older women than older men.
- Older women tend to be poorer and are more likely to be alone than are men.
- Therefore, if healthcare for older adults were to be rationed, it would negatively affect women more than men.
- Therefore, more healthcare resources should be allocated to older people.

What Is an Ethics of Care?

The **ethics of care,** a nursing philosophy, directs attention to the specific situations of individual patients, viewed within the context of their life narrative. You would think, "What is the story of this person's life? What is going on right now in his life? And what does that have to do with the morality of the action I'm considering?" Care theories grew directly out of feminist ethics and especially promote nurturing of patients and caregivers (i.e., caring) (Volbrecht, 2002). An ethics of care emphasizes the role of feelings, but also includes some of the principles that are part of traditional ethics, such as *autonomy* (self-determination) or *beneficence* (doing good).

Using an ethics of care perspective, nurses include a responsibility to care as a part of their professional behavior. Some aspects of care include the ability and duty to appreciate, understand, and even share the patient's pain or condition. Using a caring framework, your ethical analysis would focus

on relationships and client stories. The following are specific ethics of care perspectives:

- Viewing caring as the central force in nursing (Leininger, 1988)
- Promoting dignity and respect for patients as people
- Attending to the particulars of each individual patient, especially the marginalized and disenfranchised members of society (Myhrvold, 2006).
- Cultivating responsiveness to others
- Redefining fundamental moral principles to include virtues such as kindness, attentiveness, empathy, compassion, and reliability

Reasoning using the caring perspective and patient stories tends to focus discussion at the level where the relationships are located, rather than in an intellectual plane. Critics of the ethics of care suggest that the term *caring* can be misinterpreted to become too sentimental and, therefore, ineffective, causing nursing to be seen as less strong than medicine. The following is a question that reflects this model of reasoning:

- Should we provide free medical care to the homeless? An ethics of care position would probably say yes, even though it might not, for example, provide the greatest good for the greatest number of people.

KnowledgeCheck 42-8

- How does feminist ethics affect ethical decision making?
- What does the ethics of care model emphasize?

Moral Concepts and Principles

Remember from Chapter 8 that theories are made up of concepts and principles. The same is true for moral theories. Moral concepts and principles are useful in ethical discussions because even if people disagree about which action is right in a situation, they may be able to agree about which principles apply. Agreement "in principle" may provide common ground for a compromise or other resolution of the problem. The various moral frameworks use some of the same principles in ethical reasoning, discussed following.

Autonomy

Autonomy refers to a person's right to choose and ability to act on that choice. Autonomy ties in with respect for human dignity. You demonstrate respect for autonomy when you treat patients with consideration, believe their stories about the course and symptoms of their illnesses, and protect those who are unable to decide for themselves.

In the Meet Your Patients scenario, if you believed autonomy to be the most important principle in the situation, and that respecting their autonomy gives Alan's parents the right to refuse blood products to their son on the basis of their religious beliefs, would you still try to persuade them to change their minds?

Informed Consent. The principle of autonomy underlies informed consent. You honor autonomy when you respect the patient's or surrogate decision maker's right to decide, even when you believe those choices are not in the patient's best interest. You can support autonomy by informing patients about advance directives and durable powers of attorney for healthcare.

Privacy and Confidentiality. The principles of privacy and confidentiality also derive in part from the principle of autonomy. An autonomous person has control over the collection, use, and access of her personal information. Many patients share sensitive information with nurses that

they would not share with others, and it is important to maintain their trust. This means that you should not discuss patients in the elevator, halls, lunchroom, or anywhere it can be overheard, even if the discussion is relevant to the patient's care. You should communicate to others only the information needed to provide healthcare. Share other information only with the patient's consent. If you would like more information about privacy and confidentiality, see Chapters 18 and 43; also,

 Go to Chapter 42, **Supplemental Materials: Confidentiality and Privacy,** on Davis*Plus*.

Nonmaleficence

The principle of **nonmaleficence** is the twofold duty to do no harm and to prevent harm. Both the physicians' Hippocratic oath and the nurses' Nightingale Pledge state that care providers have a duty to cause no harm to patients. When you are careful to prevent medication errors, use an ambulation belt for assisting patients to walk, you honor the nonmaleficence principle. Nonmaleficence refers to both actual harm and risk of harm, as well as to intentional and unintentional harm. In nursing it is rare to find intentional harm, but unintentional harm does occur due to lack of careful planning and consideration and lack of knowledge, skill, or ability. Nonmaleficence requires that you think critically and weigh potential risks against potential benefits. When considering treatment regimens, ask the question, "Does this treatment cause more harm or more good to the patient?"

- **Risk of harm is not always clear.** Suppose you are about to get a patient out of bed for the first time after surgery. The benefit clearly is that this will prevent postoperative complications such as pneumonia and thrombophlebitis, but the risks, in terms of excessive pain or unintentional damage to the operative site, may be less clear.
- **Weighing risks and benefits is a value-laden exercise.** Who is to say what amount of pain is excessive—you or the patient? To honor the principle of nonmaleficence in this situation, you would need to be sure to premedicate the patient and carefully assess his status as you are helping him to ambulate.

Respect for Dignity. The value of respect for human dignity derives in part from the duty to do no harm. **Respect for dignity** refers to the nurse's respect for the intrinsic worth of each person, without respect to age, race, religion, or any other factors. Respect for dignity recognizes that patients are vulnerable; and that nurses should not abuse their relationships for personal gain, or enter into romantic, sexual, or other relationships with their patients.

 ThinkLike a Nurse 42-7

Think about the Meet Your Patients scenario in terms of nonmaleficence. The parents refuse to allow a blood transfusion. You, the nurse, have tried to persuade them to change their minds. You do not need to decide what you ought to do; just analyze the situation in terms of the risks.

- What is it that creates the risk for harm to Alan?
- What is the risk for harm to Alan's parents because of the nurse's actions?

Beneficence

Beneficence is the duty to do or promote good. You can think of this principle as being on a continuum with nonmaleficence. At one end of the continuum is the duty to do

no harm; beneficence, at the other end, is the duty to bring about positive good. The following simple examples illustrate the duties in priority order:

- *Do no harm.* (Don't push the man into the river.)
- *Prevent harm* when you can. (If the man is getting dangerously close to the river's edge, warn him that he is about to fall into the river.)
- *Remove harm* when it is being inflicted. (If you see a struggle and someone is trying to push the man into the river, interfere and try to stop it if you can do so without undue harm to yourself.)
- *Bring about positive good.* (If the man has fallen in the river, jump in and try to save him, or toss him a lifeline and call 911 if you can't swim.)

When weighing the risks and benefits of an action, you are actually balancing nonmaleficence with beneficence. Keep in mind that patients, family members, and health professionals may identify benefits and harms differently. A benefit to one may represent a burden to another. For example, in Meet Your Patients, you may see a blood transfusion as a benefit to Alan, but to the parents it may represent harm. Doing good very much depends on the context and the rights of the person for whom the action is being taken.

Paternalism. Although beneficence seems like such a positive goal, it can have negative consequences. One such outcome is **paternalism** (treating others like children). This would occur, for example, if you think you know what is best for a competent client and then coerce the client to act as you wish rather than to act as she wishes. Saying to a patient, for example, "Trust us; we know what is best for you to do in this situation," may seem to be beneficent because you are trying to support the patient. But it is actually paternalistic behavior that lacks respect for the patient's autonomy.

Fidelity

Fidelity (faithfulness) is the duty to keep promises. It is a basic part of every patient care situation. Sometimes the promises are of major significance, such as promising not to share certain information with other members of the healthcare team. At other times it may be only a promise to come back to check the effectiveness of a pain medication or to bring a requested item back to the client's room. **Key Point:** *The duty to keep a promise is the same regardless of its level of importance.*

In practice, you will often find that competing tasks prevent you from being able to deliver something exactly as you have promised. Make promises in a thoughtful, careful manner to maximize the likelihood that you can keep them. Instead of "I'll be right back with your medication," you might be a bit more vague and say, "I must go help another patient for a few minutes, but I'll get there with your medication as quickly as I can."

Veracity

Veracity is the duty to tell the truth. This seems straightforward, but there are times when veracity presents a challenge. For example, should you tell the truth when you know that it might cause harm to the client? Would it be appropriate to tell a lie in order to relieve extreme patient anxiety? Most nurses would agree that it isn't hard to tell the truth, but at times it may be very hard to determine how *much* of the truth to tell. For example, healthcare professionals may feel uncomfortable giving families "bad news." So instead of saying, "Your father has a fatal illness and is unlikely to live for more than a month," they may say, "Your father is very ill, but we will do everything we possibly can for him." In this, as in most situations, the risk of losing patient trust outweighs any benefit of withholding some of the truth.

Although you always presume the value of telling the truth, there may be times when you are justified to withhold information. In the United States, we tend to place a higher value on autonomy than in some cultures. For example, in some cultures, families go to great lengths to protect a dying patient from the harsh truth of his prognosis, and the patient himself may not wish to know. In such a situation, you need to be culturally sensitive in order to act on the family's values, not the dominant cultural values. **Key Point:** *Always consider the context.*

ThinkLike a Nurse 42-8

Review the Meet Your Patients scenario. Alan will not survive without a blood transfusion; the parents refuse. He asks the nurse, "Am I going to die?" You do not need to decide which response is best; just write an example that illustrates each of the following. What might the nurse say if she wishes to:

- Tell Alan the truth?
- Withhold or partially disclose the truth?
- Answer with an untruth?

Justice

Justice is the obligation to be fair. It implies equal treatment of all patients. Questions of justice will become a part of your everyday experience in patient care, from deciding how to allocate your time among patients to larger decisions, such as how to allocate limited healthcare resources.

Distributive Justice

Distributive justice requires fair distribution of both benefits and burdens (Husted & Husted, 2008). It is especially relevant to healthcare, as in the following issues.

Allocating Resources. Distributive justice questions come up when more than one person or group competes for the same resources. For example, consider organ transplantation. Human organs are scarce resources. How do we decide which patient should receive an available organ? Is an 18-year-old more deserving of a kidney than a 75-year-old? Is a person with liver disease due to alcoholism less deserving of a liver than someone with liver disease not caused by alcoholism? The decision of who should live and who may die is never an easy decision. In the United States, a national committee sets criteria for how organs will be distributed so the standard of justice can be considered.

Fair Access to Care. Access to care is a specific kind of healthcare resource. The principle of distributive justice holds that we should provide equal access to healthcare for all. As the baby boomer generation ages, at the same time the baby boomer nurses are retiring. There are already fewer nurses to care for more aging patients at a time when national healthcare dollars are stretched thin. How will the nation decide where to spend the limited dollars? How will nurse managers decide how to provide adequate care when they do not have enough nurses on their staff? The ability to develop sound criteria on which to allocate resources is the challenge of distributive justice.

Compensatory Justice

Compensatory justice focuses on making amends for wrongs that have been done to individuals or groups. Malpractice suits consider this type of justice when they decide how much money to award a victim for being harmed. Groups of

citizens may also be harmed. For instance, if a company's unintentional pollution of water was proven to cause cancer in members of the community, a monetary settlement might be made.

Procedural Justice

Procedural justice is important in processes that require ranking or ordering (Volbrecht, 2002). For example, institutional policies are written to ensure that the same procedures apply to all clients or employees in the same way (e.g., visiting hours, working on holidays, sick leave). Can you think of an example of procedural justice that you have experienced during your nursing education? Often the unwritten rule of "first come, first served" is used as a basis for delivery of services.

ThinkLike a Nurse 42-9

Look again at the emergency department situation described in "What Is Nursing Ethics?" at the beginning of this chapter. In this scenario, two little boys were treated for lacerations. Which principle of justice was violated: distributive, compensatory, or procedural? Explain your thinking.

KnowledgeCheck 42-9

List each of the six ethical principles and its definition.

Professional Guidelines

You should consult professional guidelines when making ethical decisions. Healthcare professionals have an obligation to society to be competent in their field; to allow only qualified persons entry into the profession; to discipline members of the profession who do not practice at an acceptable level; to do no harm; and to use high moral and ethical standards to resolve dilemmas (Husted & Husted, 2008). You can find ethical standards for nurses in codes of ethics, standards of practice, statements of patients' rights, and various laws.

Nursing Codes of Ethics

Professional codes of ethics are formal statements of a group's expectations and standards for professional behavior generally accepted by members of the profession. Codes of ethics set forth ideal behaviors, but they are only as effective as the behaviors of the nurses who live up to the codes. The following are purposes of a nursing code of ethics:

- Inform the public about the profession's minimum standards.
- Demonstrate nursing's commitment to the public it serves.
- Outline major ethical considerations of nursing.
- Provide general guidelines for professional behavior.
- Guide the profession's self-regulating functions.
- Remind us of the special responsibility we assume in caring for the sick.

Nursing codes are not legally binding. However, they often exceed legal obligations. In most states, the state board of nursing uses the nursing code of ethics as the standard against which to evaluate a nurse's ethical behavior. The board has the legal authority to censure or reprimand the nurse who does not practice within the boundaries of ethical practice.

The two following nursing organizations have had long-standing codes to guide nurses' ethical decision making. The codes differ in specific details, but they are based on similar principles.

International Council of Nurses (ICN). The ICN first adopted its Code of Ethics for Nurses in 1953 as "a guide for action based on social values and needs" (ICN, 2006). The ICN Code has since served as the standard for nurses worldwide. It stresses respect for human rights, including cultural rights, the right to life and choice, the right to dignity, and right to be treated with respect. The code is designed to guide nurses in everyday choices, and it supports their refusal to participate in activities that conflict with caring and healing. To see the revised code,

 Go to Chapter 42, **Tables, Boxes, Figures: ESG Box 42-1, ICN Code of Ethics,** on Davis*Plus*.

The American Nurses Association. The ANA revised its Code of Ethics for Nurses in 2001 (Box 42-1). ANA used input from a wide range of nurses and groups to ensure that the revised code would be relevant in many practice settings and reflect current ethical situations. The code has nine provisions, followed by interpretive statements to explain what is meant by each provision. If you would like more information about the ANA Code for Nurses, which is now being revised,

 Go to the ANA Web site at http://nursingworld.org/MainMenuCategories/EthicsStandards/CodeofEthicsforNurses.aspx

---

BOX 42-1 ■ American Nurses Association Code of Ethics for Nurses

1. The nurse, in all professional relationships, practices with compassion and respect for the inherent dignity, worth, and uniqueness of every individual, unrestricted by considerations of social or economic status, personal attributes, or the nature of health problems.
2. The nurse's primary commitment is to the patient, whether an individual, family, group, or community.
3. The nurse promotes, advocates for, and strives to protect the health, safety, and rights of the patient.
4. The nurse is responsible and accountable for individual nursing practice and determines the appropriate delegation of tasks consistent with the nurse's obligation to provide optimum patient care.
5. The nurse owes the same duties to self as to others, including the responsibility to preserve integrity and safety, to maintain competence, and to continue personal and professional growth.
6. The nurse participates in establishing, maintaining, and improving health care environments and conditions of employment conducive to the provision of quality healthcare and consistent with the values of the profession through individual and collective action.
7. The nurse participates in the advancement of the profession through contributions to practice, education, administration, and knowledge development.
8. The nurse collaborates with other health professionals and the public in promoting community, national, and international efforts to meet health needs.
9. The profession of nursing, as represented by associations and their members, is responsible for articulating nursing values for maintaining the integrity of the profession and its practice, and for shaping social policy.

ANA Standards of Care

In addition to its Code of Ethics, the ANA sets standards for all aspects of clinical practice. In *Nursing: Scope and Standards of Practice* (2010), standard 7 focuses on ethical practice. This standard (see Box 42-2) directs nurses to practice within the parameters described in the Code of Ethics for Nurses.

The Patient Care Partnership

When patients are admitted to hospitals or to extended care facilities, they are entitled to specific rights in terms of their treatment: the right to make their own decisions, to be active partners in the treatment process, and to be treated with dignity and respect. Because rights are rooted in values, and because values are derived from culture, patient rights are different throughout the world. The American Hospital Association (AHA) published a document called *Patient Care Partnership* (2003). Instead of using "rights" language, this document is written in terms of patient expectations and responsibilities. The *Patient Care Partnership* encourages healthcare providers to be more aware of the need to treat patients in an ethical manner and to protect their rights. For a summary of the document, see Box 42-3.

The Joint Commission Standards for Accreditation

The Joint Commission standards contain sections on organizational ethics and individual rights. The section on organizational ethics requires ethical behavior in care, treatment, services, and business practices. It includes a statement about the need to provide for meeting patient needs in the event care must be denied in the institution. The standards state that an organization should (2008, p. 145):

- Manage relationships with patients and the public in an ethical manner.
- Consider patients' values and preferences, including decisions surrounding discontinuing care, treatment, and services.
- Help patients understand and exercise their rights.
- Inform patients of their responsibilities in care, treatment, and services.
- Recognize the organization's legal responsibilities.

BOX 42-2 ■ American Nurses Association Standards of Professional Performance Standard 7. Ethics

Definition: The registered nurse integrates ethical provisions in all areas of practice.

Measurement Criteria

The registered nurse:
- Uses the Code of Ethics for Nurses with Interpretive Statements (ANA, 2001) to guide practice.
- Delivers care in a manner that preserves and protects patient autonomy, dignity, and rights.
- Respects the centrality of the patient/family as core members of any health care team.
- Upholds and advocates for patient confidentiality within legal and regulatory parameters.
- Serves as a patient advocate assisting patients in developing skills for self-advocacy and informed decision making.
- Maintains a therapeutic and professional patient–nurse relationship with appropriate professional role boundaries.
- Demonstrates a commitment to practicing self-care, managing stress, and connecting with self and others.

- Contributes to resolving ethical issues of patients, colleagues, community groups, systems and other stakeholders.
- Takes appropriate action regarding instances of illegal, unethical, or inappropriate behavior that can endanger or jeopardize the best interests of the patient or situation.
- Cooperates in an interprofessional team to make ethical decisions regarding the application of technologies and the acquisition and sharing of data.
- Demonstrates professional comportment (openness, honesty, integrity, and authenticity). (Mass. Board of Higher Education Nursing Initiative, 2007)
- Speaks up when appropriate to question health care practice when necessary for safety and quality improvement.

―――――――――

Source: Excerpted from American Nurses Association. (2010). *Nursing: Scope and standards of practice* (2nd ed.). Silver Spring, MD: Nursebooks.org.

BOX 42-3 ■ American Hospital Association: The *Patient Care Partnership*

Patients, when hospitalized, should expect the following:
- High-quality care, including the right to know the identity of caregivers
- A clean, safe environment, including freedom from abuse and neglect, and discussion of any changes in care
- To be involved in making decisions about their care and treatment. This includes receiving information about:
  Health condition and treatments
  The benefits and risks of treatments, and whether a treatment is experimental or part of a research study
  What the patient and family will need to do regarding treatment follow-up after leaving the hospital
- Information about the right to make decisions and to refuse care, including advance directives and counselors or chaplains available to help with decision making

- Protection of privacy and confidentiality
- Help reviewing the bill and filing insurance claims
- Preparation and information when leaving the hospital, including:
  Identification of sources for follow-up care and whether the hospital has a financial interest in any of the referrals
  Coordination of hospital activities with caregivers outside the hospital
  Information and training about the self-care the person will need at home

―――――――――

Source: Excerpted and adapted from American Hospital Association. (2003). *The patient care partnership: Understanding expectations, rights and responsibilities.* Chicago: Author.

KnowledgeCheck 42-10

- How would the nurse use a professional guideline or code of ethics to assist in the ethical decision-making process?
- What are some examples of such resources?

ETHICAL ISSUES IN HEALTHCARE

As a nurse, you are likely to encounter a variety of ethical issues that occur in healthcare. For example, ethical questions arise in the following situations:

Abortion

Acquired immune deficiency syndrome (AIDS)

Advance directives

Allocation of healthcare goods and services

Assisted suicide and euthanasia

Compelling unwanted treatment

Confidentiality and privacy (e.g., reporting gunshot wounds and child abuse)

Do Not Attempt Resuscitation (DNAR) orders

Extraordinary (heroic) measures to prolong life

Informed consent

Organ transplantation

Reproductive technology (e.g., in vitro fertilization, surrogate mothering, sex preselection)

Withdrawing or withholding life-sustaining treatments (e.g., ventilators, artificial nutrition and hydration)

Extended discussion of those specific issues is best handled in an ethics text or an ethics course. However, if you wish to learn more about these situations and the specific ethical conflicts surrounding them,

 Go to Chapter 42, **Supplemental Materials: Ethical Issues in Healthcare,** on Davis*Plus*.

Practical Knowledge
knowing **how**

To fulfill your professional obligations for ethical practice, you will need practical knowledge of the concepts and processes of values clarification, moral decision making, patient advocacy, and integrity-producing compromise.

ASSESSMENT/ANALYSIS/DIAGNOSIS

A holistic, comprehensive patient assessment will help you establish the context in which ethical decisions are made. For patients struggling with moral issues, the following diagnoses may apply:

- *Decisional Conflict*—Use this label when the patient is uncertain about which course of action to take. The patient may verbalize distress and uncertainty; may delay decision making; may show physical signs of distress (e.g., increased heart rate); and may question moral rules, values, and personal beliefs.
- *Moral Distress*—Use this label when the patient has made a moral decision but is unable to carry out the chosen action. Cues include expressions of powerlessness, guilt, frustration, anxiety, self-doubt, and fear.

NANDA-I also lists other diagnoses in the Value/Belief/Action Congruence class, including Impaired Religiosity, Readiness for Enhanced Religiosity, Risk for Impaired Religiosity, Spiritual Distress and Risk for Spiritual Distress.

VALUES CLARIFICATION

Values clarification refers to the process of becoming conscious of and naming one's values (Burkhardt & Nathaniel, 2008). If you are clear about your values, you will be more able to make good decisions and to avoid imposing your values on others. Because each person has his own unique values set, it is also important that you appreciate how others' values influence their decisions. Clarifying values should be a positive process of growth that results in more awareness, empathy, and insight (Seroka, 1994; Steele & Harmon, 1983). A values clarification process does not tell you what your values ought to be; it merely helps you discover what they are and examine their relevance in your personal and professional life. There are no right or wrong answers to values clarification exercises. They are only to assist you in identifying your values. Values change over time, so you may need to repeat the process more than once in your lifetime.

How Can I Clarify My Values?

As a nurse, you will need to examine your values regarding life, death, wellness, and illness. A good place to start is to ask yourself questions about situations in which you think you may be uncomfortable, such as caring for a substance abuser seeking drugs in the emergency department, an unwed adolescent mother pregnant for the second time in 11 months, or parents such as the Freses (Meet Your Patients), who refuse treatment for a child because of religious beliefs. Ask yourself questions such as:

- Could I take care of this person?
- Does this bother me?
- What would I do if confronted with such a situation?
- Could I provide the same quality care as for my other patients?

If you would like to use some exercises that can help you begin to clarify your values related to healthcare,

 Go to Chapter 42, **Tables, Boxes, Figures: ESG Box 42-2, Rank-Ordering Values and ESG Box 42-3, Values Preference Exercise,** on Davis*Plus*.

How Can I Help Clients to Clarify Their Values?

Some clients may exhibit behaviors that indicate that their values are not clear. Consider this example:

Jon White is the chief executive officer of a large healthcare facility. Jon has had two myocardial infarctions (heart attacks) in the past 5 years. He also has hypercholesterolemia (high cholesterol) and hypertension (high blood pressure). Jon's physician has prescribed a cardiac medicine, low-dose aspirin, and medications to control his hypertension and cholesterol. Jon has repeatedly been taught about his diet, medications, and activity. He insists he is compliant. Jon's wife tells you that he has stopped exercising and is eating whatever he wants, including saturated fats. Jon tells her it is OK to eat what he wants because he is taking a "cholesterol-buster" pill.

The following patient behaviors may indicate that a patient needs values clarification:

- Ignoring the advice of a health professional
- Patient's words not consistent with his actions
- Numerous admissions to the agency for the same problem
- Uncertainty or confusion about which action to take

Which of those behaviors did Jon exhibit? To help Jon clarify his values, you might ask him to list the three things that

are most important to him in life. Or you could help him work through the steps in Table 42-3 (choosing, prizing, and acting).

KnowledgeCheck 42-11
- What is values clarification?
- What are the steps in values clarification?

ETHICAL DECISION MAKING

Decision models used in bioethics do not offer pat, easy decisions, but they do provide a guiding structure to follow to try to arrive at the best answer in specific situations. Decision models can help you decide on a course of action even if they do not tell you absolutely that the action is right or wrong.

How Can I Recognize Ethical Issues? We have said it is important to be aware of the ethical issues in patient care situations, but how will you recognize them? The key is that there is usually a conflict. Conflict may occur:
- About the right action to take
- Among the duties and obligations of healthcare professionals (or they are unclear)
- Between the needs and interests of an individual and a group of clients
- Between what the family wants and what the client wants or needs
- Between the family and health professionals
- Among ethical principles or values (e.g., autonomy versus nonmaleficence, as in the Meet Your Patients scenario)

Problem or Dilemma?

In the best of all possible worlds, you could easily apply moral principles and decide what to do. However, often in moral situations one ethical principle is at odds with another equally

Table 42-3 ➤ Values Clarification	
STEP AND DESCRIPTION	**QUESTIONS TO ASK YOUR PATIENT**
Choosing (cognitive)	
Beliefs are chosen:	Do (did) you have any choice about what you do?
Freely (allows you to cherish your choice)	Do you have any control over what happens?
From alternatives	What have you decided to do?
After considering all consequences (ensures that the alternative is right for you)	Can you list some alternative actions?
	What are your options?
	What could you do instead of ...?
	What do you think will happen if you do that?
	What will you gain by doing that?
	What is the disadvantage of doing that?
Prizing (affective)	
Beliefs and behaviors that are chosen are prized:	How do you feel about your decision?
With pride (feeling good about your choice)	People sometimes feel good after making such a decision. Others feel pressured. How is it for you?
With public affirmation	How do you intend to tell your family (friends) about this decision?
	What will you say to your wife (friends, family)?
	When will you announce your decision to ...?
Acting (behavioral)	
Beliefs are acted on:	Try to determine whether the client will act on the decision:
By incorporating the choice into one's own behavior	■ How do you think your wife (significant other) will react when you do that?
With consistency and repetition	■ When will you actually carry out this decision?
	Try to predict consistent behavior by asking:
	■ How many times in the past have you ...
	■ What kind of schedule have you worked out? How often and when will you ...?

Source: Adapted from Raths, L. E., Harmin M., & Simon, S. B. (1978). *Values and teaching: Working with values in the classroom.* Columbus, OH: Merrill.

important principle. It is also possible for a philosophical framework to produce more than one acceptable option. An **ethical dilemma** is a situation in which a choice must be made between two equally undesirable actions. There is no clearly right or wrong option. Such situations are emotionally painful for everyone in the situation, as you can see from the Meet Your Patients scenario at the beginning of this chapter. If you support Alan's parents' right to refuse a blood transfusion, you honor the principle of autonomy, but at the expense of the principle of nonmaleficence, which says we should prevent harm to Alan.

Fortunately, not all moral problems are dilemmas. In fact, you will confront a true dilemma only occasionally (Cahn, 1987; Curtin & Flaherty, 1982; Levine, 1989; White, 1983; Wilkinson, 1997). Not all moral problems are complex and difficult. Some questions are easily answered (e.g., "Should I take the patient's morphine to relieve my back pain?"). It is probably more accurate, then, to talk about *moral questions, moral problems,* or *moral situations* and not use the term *dilemma* loosely. Only problems that pose a question between competing and equally valuable interests are true dilemmas.

Ethical behavior and decision making do not deal only with dilemmas. They really involve choosing to be ethical in the everyday aspects of your practice: for example, treating colleagues and patients with respect, not passing up a room when you see a patient crying, or helping out a new graduate who is frustrated and anxious. The scenario about the two little boys in the emergency department (in the section What Is Nursing Ethics?) is more representative of everyday ethics than is the Meet Your Patients scenario.

How Do I Work Through an Ethical Problem?

Once you have identified an ethical problem, a decision model can help you think logically about the best action to take. Still, in the case of a true ethical dilemma, you will probably not be comfortable with any course of action, no matter how logically you think it through.

Ethical decision-making models will help you carefully consider several perspectives, guide your reasoning, and explain the reasons for your final action. As already mentioned, each approach may produce a different solution. One of the easiest to remember and use is the MORAL model. This model has been credited to two different authors: Thiroux (1977) and Crisham (in Scott, 1985). The letters MORAL will remind you of the steps in this model, which is described in the following section, which uses the Meet Your Patients scenario to illustrate ethical decision making.

First, Use Problem-Solving

As a first step in ethical decision making, use the nursing process approach to describe the problem and alternative approaches:

Assessment—What are the relevant facts? Alan needs a blood transfusion to survive. Both the surgeon and the nurse (you) have tried to persuade the parents to consent, but they still refuse. The parents' religion prohibits blood transfusions. Alan is 15 years old (a minor), so you cannot administer a transfusion without his parents' consent.

Analysis/Diagnosis—Identify the Problem; State the Conflict There is a values conflict: The healthcare professionals value preserving physical life; the parents place more value on preserving the soul. There is a moral dilemma, as well: If no transfusion is given, you violate

the principle of nonmaleficence (harm to Alan); if you somehow coerce the parents to consent, you have violated the principle of autonomy (respect for their values and their freedom to choose). So the decision to be made is whether to

- Follow the parents' wishes,
- Find a legal way to transfuse without their consent, or
- Find some compromise that will work.

Next, Use the MORAL Model

Now use the MORAL model to come up with alternative solutions for the Frese family (Meet Your Patients).

M—Massage the Dilemma

1. *First identify and define the issues in the dilemma, and consider the values and options of all the major players:* Mr. and Mrs. Frese, Alan, the surgeon, possibly a member of the clergy, and you, the nurse. You have already identified the values in the problem-solving approach: physical life versus spiritual life. You and the surgeon also value the principles of autonomy and nonmaleficence

2. *Then identify the information gaps.* In massaging the situation, you should ask yourself:
   - Do I fully understand the situation that is causing the need for blood?
   - How much time is available to make this decision—do the parents have to decide within a few minutes, or do they have enough time to discuss this with their clergy member?
   - Does the physician know that the family members are Jehovah's Witnesses?
   - Does the surgeon have any treatment that could be used to stabilize Alan while the parents discuss the situation?
   - Do Alan's parents fully understand the nature of Alan's physical emergency?
   - In the Freses' religious view, what is the consequence of receiving blood?
   - Do they understand what might happen if blood is not administered (i.e., do they understand the consequence of their action or inaction)?
   - Is this what Alan would want? Has Alan discussed in the past what he feels about blood transfusions? Have they ever had family discussions when other young Jehovah's Witnesses have been faced with such a decision? Where did Alan stand in those discussions?
   - How is this situation like other situations they have experienced in their lives?
   - Have they thought about their opposing duties: the duty to uphold their religious values and the duty to protect their son from harm?
   - Has everyone's voice been heard?
   - Have the parents contacted their clergy member and discussed the situation?
   - What emotions are coming into play in this situation?
   - How is this decision affecting the parents as individuals? Are they in agreement on the issue, or is there dissension? If there is dissension, are both sides being supported fairly?
   - Is there some common ground between what the surgeon wants and what the parents feel they need to do to uphold their religious convictions?

O—Outline the Options

At this step in the MORAL model, you (or the charge nurse or a member of the ethics committee) should outline all of the options to all parties, including those that are less realistic and

conflicting. You might ask a member of the ethics committee or the hospital chaplain to help the family and the doctor understand the opposing viewpoints.

The surgeon needs to outline the state of emergency that exists for Alan and to explain what the limited medical options are: to transfuse blood or, if no blood is given, what other treatments are available (e.g., volume enhancers). The surgeon will need to say how soon the decision must be made, based on Alan's condition. He should clearly describe the consequences of each action. Carefully, and with as little emotion as possible, explain the consequences of each action to the parents. The physician should state whether one administration of blood will likely fix the situation or whether continued administration may be required.

The family (or a member of the clergy) should explain for the doctor and nurse the basis for their refusal to consent and what they believe the consequence would be if blood were given.

R—Resolve the Dilemma

Now carefully review the issues and options. Apply basic moral principles. If you can, also look at the situation using alternate ethical frameworks.

- **Autonomy.** By their refusing to give consent, the Freses are exercising their autonomy. How far will we go to honor their autonomy?
- **Beneficence and Nonmaleficence.** How are we defining "good" (beneficence) and "harm" (nonmaleficence) in this situation? The physician defines "good" as Alan receiving the needed blood. He defines "harm" as the outcome for Alan without the blood, even if he uses a less effective alternative. Alan's parents would define "good" as following their religious mandates and making sure their son will remain pure in the eyes of God. They might explain that a Jehovah's Witness who willingly accepts a blood transfusion might forfeit his or her eternal life. They might believe the taking of blood to be more harmful than death, because they believe that would affect Alan's eternal life, not just his physical life.
- **Fidelity.** The surgeon is being loyal (exhibiting fidelity) to the principles of medicine and evidence-based practice, which mandate the administration of the blood. To the parents, their loyalty to their religious principles to ensure that Alan has eternal life may be more important than the loss of the physical life itself.
- **Veracity.** The principle of veracity holds that the surgeon should not exaggerate the need for the blood, and he should be honest with the parents in terms of the consequences of the alternative actions. Another question of veracity involves the parents: Are they being honest with each other regarding their feelings?

Your role as a nurse is to be an advocate for the patient and the family. Talk with the family and their religious representative, if available, about what they are thinking about their opposing duties: the duty to uphold their religious values and the duty to protect their son from physical harm. If you are in a position to do so, explain to the surgeon the reasoned position of Alan's parents.

Key Point: *Ensure that everyone's viewpoint has been respected and considered. This may be as important as the final decision that is reached. In this and other difficult situations, always look for the opportunity for a good compromise (to be discussed later in this chapter).*

A—Act by Applying the Chosen Option

This step is the first one that actually requires action. The hospital is bound to follow the parents' decision because Alan is a minor. However, if there is time, many agencies might refer this situation to the hospital ethics committee. The hospital might also ask a legal court authority to resolve the situation. If an emergency requires an immediate decision, the only *legal* action is to follow the parents' decision, whether or not you consider it the best moral action.

Whatever happens, Alan's parents will need emotional support. If they decide to refuse the blood transfusion, you must remain nonjudgmental in supporting them, even if you do not agree with their decision. If they, or the court, decide that the blood will be given, they may need even more support. They may feel overwhelming guilt, and they may fear that Alan will be forever burdened with guilt at the realization that they violated church doctrine with the medical care. If their extended family is not present, you could volunteer to call in extended family, friends, and church members if they wish. They will need a quiet, private place to await the outcome of the treatment.

L—Look Back and Evaluate

This phase calls for evaluation of the entire process, not just the consequence of the decided action.

- How well did the process work? Were processes in place for the dilemma to be discussed respectfully without undue delay in treatment?
- Were all parties' expectations realistic?
- How are all of the affected parties feeling now (doctor, parents, family, Alan, you)? Regardless of the outcome of the decision, do all involved feel they had a voice and their views were respected?
- How well did you do in the situation? Did you act as an effective advocate for the rights of Alan and his parents? Did the power and authority of the physician or hospital in the situation unduly influence you?
- Were policies and procedures in place to guide you in the process of working out this situation?
- Has anything changed since the dilemma came to light? Has a greater good been achieved for future situations? Have future situations been made easier as a result of the things learned in this situation? Has any aspect of this ethical decision now become a universal policy at the institution?
- Are further actions required in terms of this or like situations?

If you would like some guidelines to help you avoid common errors of moral reasoning,

 Go to Chapter 42, **Supplemental Materials: Common Errors in Decision Making,** on Davis*Plus.*

Look for a Good Compromise

Even if you believe you know the right thing to do, others may not agree with you, or there may be constraints that prevent you from doing it. For example, in the case of Alan, even if you decided the right thing to do is give him a blood transfusion, (1) his parents do not agree with you, and (2) the law says you cannot do so without his parents' consent. This will happen often—much more often than a true dilemma, in which you cannot *decide* the right thing to do. No matter how well we work together, there will always be ethical problems and disagreements. Many cases are full of complexity and uncertainty, and sometimes the price of acting on your beliefs is extremely high. For example, what might have happened if the surgeon had infused blood without the Freses' consent? What might have happened if you had refused to talk to the parents as the surgeon asked you?

Many times, it will be possible to reach a "good" compromise. A **good compromise** is one that preserves the integrity of all parties. This means that:

- **The discussions are carried out in a spirit of mutual respect**—all viewpoints are respected and considered.
- **The compromise solution itself is ethically sound;** that is, you should be able to provide a principles-based rationale for the compromise, as well as for each of the opposing positions. In the case of Alan and his parents, there probably is no compromise position between "give blood" and "don't give blood." Perhaps the parents would agree to one, but no more than one, transfusion; but that is hard to justify ethically. If one transfusion is acceptable (to honor nonmaleficence), why not two or three? If two transfusions are against their religious beliefs, why would one be acceptable? Nevertheless, in many other cases compromise is possible.

So how do you compromise without losing moral integrity? Begin by realizing there is more at stake than the issue itself ("Is a blood transfusion right or wrong?"). There are some things that are inherently good in compromising.

- First, it is never good to settle things by force (as you would if you got a court order to transfuse Alan without his parents' consent). You have probably heard the old saying "Might doesn't make right." A compromise can preserve the rights of the less powerful party in a disagreement.
- Keeping peace on a nursing unit is good for both the nurses and patients. When there is upheaval and moral suffering, care quality throughout the unit can suffer. A compromise can bring peace.
- There is intrinsic good in taking part in a process in which we must try to see things from others' points of view. It may make us more open-minded, more creative, and less judgmental.
- Keep in mind that most issues do contain room for reasonable differences of opinion. In the Meet Your Patients scenario, can you see that both sides are people of good will who have ethical reasons to justify their opinion? Also, there is often room for doubt, on your own part, about the morally best action to take.
- A compromise may achieve mutual respect. It is a significant thing to reach a settlement in which each party feels assured of the other's respect for its seriousness and sincerity.

Given all those ideas, a person of good will might want to reexamine and back away from a very strong opinion. Remember, sometimes your position isn't all that strong, and the other position isn't all that weak (as in the case of Alan). There is also always the chance that you may have made an error in your reasoning or have not completely understood some facts of the case. Ethical disputes can be settled only if you are willing to engage in discussion and admit the other people might have a point! There may be cases in which you cannot compromise (perhaps Alan's case is one), but don't listen to people who say, "You can never reach agreement on ethical issues. They are too complex." It is possible to achieve integrity-producing compromises, and in nursing, it is often necessary.

What Are My Obligations in Ethical Situations?

As you can see, in making ethical decisions nurses rarely act alone. Usually you will be one of several healthcare professionals and family members who will jointly arrive at the best decision. Your role when an ethical decision is needed includes the following:

- *Be aware of and sensitive to issues,* so you can identify them when they arise. Educate yourself—attend workshops, read, and talk to other nurses.
- *Assume responsibility for your own moral actions.* Even if you do not have the "last word" about what happens to a patient or about what others do, you are always responsible for your own actions in every situation.
- *Function as a team member* when ethical problems arise. Realize you should have input—no one profession has full moral expertise—and realize that your input can be valuable.
- *Support the patient and family members* while they are making the decision and afterward. Listen. Ask questions. Provide unbiased information. Be helpful without being too directive or judgmental.
- *Support patients who are not being allowed to decide.* For example, in the Meet Your Patients scenario, you would want to be sure Alan's wishes were considered, if possible. However, if the parents insist on deciding for him, against his wishes, he may need a great deal of emotional support.
- *Use and participate in institutional ethics committees* if you are given the opportunity.
- *Most important, advocate for your client.* You may need to balance your client's autonomy with the wishes of family members or the responsibilities of other healthcare professionals to the patient. As an advocate, you may find yourself in conflict with other team members or family members. Frequently you and the others involved will have different ethical perspectives.
- *Improve your ethical decision making.*

The following three sections discuss more fully the last three points above.

Use and Participate in Institutional Ethics Committees

There is no easy way to decide which principle should outrank another principle, or which person's values are best in a given situation. For this reason, many healthcare institutions have ethics committees. These typically interdisciplinary committees include nurses, doctors, clergy, ethicists, and lay representatives. Ethics committees develop guidelines and policies, provide education and counseling; and, in the case of ethical dilemmas, review the case and provide a forum for the expression of the diverse perspectives of those involved. Ethics committees usually follow one of three models when discussing a dilemma: the autonomy model, the patient benefit model, and the social justice model.

Autonomy Model. This model is useful when the patient is competent to decide. This model emphasizes patient autonomy and choice as the highest value. For example, if this committee knew Alan's (Meet Your Patients) wishes, they might be inclined to try to persuade his parents to do as Alan wants.

Patient Benefit Model. This model assists in decision making for the incompetent patient by using substituted judgment (i.e., what the patient would want for himself if he were capable of making these issues known). If Alan is unconscious and cannot say what he wants, this committee would probably ask Alan's parents, family, and friends, "What do you think Alan would want? Have you ever heard him talk about a situation such as this?"

Social Justice Model. This model focuses more on broad social issues involving the entire institution, rather than on a single patient issue (Yoder-Wise, 2007). Such a committee might consider whether, in general, an institution ought ever to seek a legal order to act against the wishes of the parents. Or they might discuss whether supporting parents' religious beliefs in this instance might have implications for supporting other types of religious beliefs in future cases.

KnowledgeCheck 42-12

- Define *ethical dilemma*.
- How can you recognize an ethical problem?
- What is an integrity-producing compromise?
- What are the functions of an ethics committee?
- What does the mnemonic *MORAL* stand for?

Be a Patient Advocate

The role of an advocate is to safeguard clients against abuse and violation of their rights. When you think of the rights and values described, for example, in the *Patient Care Partnership* and in nursing codes of ethics, you can see how important this role is. Be aware that advocacy in everyday clinical practice is less about the patient's legal rights and moral theory, and more about such seemingly "routine" measures as obtaining a new prescription when an analgesic is ineffective, even if it does mean telephoning the prescriber for the third time on your shift. The advocacy role requires you to be respectful, considerate, courageous, persistent, and concerned with justice.

Why do you think advocacy is so important? Why can't patients do these things for themselves? The following are some of the reasons.

You Have Special Knowledge That the Patient Does Not Have. Diseases, treatments, and the healthcare system are so complex that when patients become ill, they may not have the energy to deal with the complexity, even if they do have the necessary knowledge. You may need to help them to "jump through the necessary hoops" to get what they need. When patients' rights are denied or when they do not have the ability to exert their rights, nurses have a responsibility to step in. "Without the advocacy and protection of rights there really are no rights" (Bandman & Bandman, 2002, p. 23).

One Aspect of Your Professional Role Is to Defend Patients' Autonomous Decisions. Recall that the ANA Code of Ethics requires you to be a patient advocate (see Boxes 42-1 and 42-2). As a nurse, you will be called on to defend your patient's autonomous decisions even if you do not agree with them and even if they conflict with the opinions of others involved in the patient's care. You may find yourself the sole supporter of a patient's right to choose for himself the direction of his care.

Nurses Have a Special Relationship With Patients. You may find that you are able to obtain information about a patient that is not available to professionals of other disciplines. In general, nurses interact with patients over longer time intervals and are involved in very personal activities, especially in inpatient settings. They often become the most trusted caregivers. Details about family life, coping styles, personal preferences, fears, and insecurities are all more likely to come out over the time involved in nursing interventions than in the brief minutes of interaction when a physician makes rounds. In addition, patients may perceive less social distance between themselves and the nurse and, therefore, feel freer to confide in them. The nurses' point of view can be a valuable asset to resolving an ethical problem satisfactorily. Of course, many providers have long-standing relationships with their patients; however, this does not negate the importance of the nurse's input, which may provide a different perspective.

Your Role as an Advocate Is to Inform, Support, and Communicate. You should inform clients of their rights and provide the information they need to make informed decisions, if they are capable of doing so. Then you must remain objective and support them in the decisions they make. If others are not respecting client choices, you will need to intervene. This may simply be a matter of conveying information and clarifying the client's wishes to family or healthcare professionals (e.g., "I know how hard it is for you to let him go, but your dad says he has made peace and is ready to die. His treatments make him feel even more ill, and he simply does not want to fight anymore.") Advocacy may require you to arrange for the client to consult with a religious leader or an attorney for advice and support, or may require you to consult an institutional ethics committee.

Patients May Need Support With Regard to Advance Directives. In 2004, three of every 10 U.S. nursing home residents did not have advance directives (Resnick, Schuur, Heineman, et al., 2008), so there is work to be done in this area. Advocacy includes asking patients whether they have an advance directive and informing them about advance directives if they do not. Even people who have an advance directive do not always, or even often, understand the statements they have checked in the boxes on the form. Take the time to go over the form with them if they are able to do so. See Chapters 17 and 43 if you need further discussion of advance directives. For guidelines that will help you to function effectively as an advocate, see Box 42-4.

Improve Your Ethical Decision Making

By now, you should understand that you cannot avoid making moral decisions in nursing. A recent study pointed out the need to promote nurses' development from the conventional (rules-bound) to the post-conventional (reasoning) stage of moral development. The study found that when nurses were faced with ethical dilemmas they tended to use conventions (e.g., rules, procedures) as criteria for decision making rather than patients' personal needs and well-being (Dierckx de Casterlé, Izumi, Godfrey, et al., 2008). As a full-spectrum nurse, you should use the following suggestions so you will be prepared when ethical issues arise.

- **Use Theoretical Knowledge.** Review nursing and other literature for discussion of cases and experiences of other nurses. This will give you a broader view of the problems you may confront and the strategies for managing them. Become familiar with the various codes of ethics and the *Patient Care Partnership*, as well as the moral frameworks and principles.
- **Use Self-Knowledge.** Examine your personal value system. Explore the influences of your religion, cultural beliefs, and personal experiences. This will help you to recognize your comfort zone with specific ethical issues.
- **Use Practical Knowledge.** While still a student, you should ask to attend either ethical rounds or an ethics committee meeting. As a graduate nurse, you could volunteer

BOX 42-4 ■ Guidelines for Advocacy

The following principles will help you to function effectively as an advocate.

- **Keep the moral principle of patient autonomy always in mind.**
- **Know and document the facts** of the case.
- **Know the arguments** of those who oppose the patient.
- **Use role-playing** to develop a strategy for responding to the arguments.
- **Have a sound base of support for your actions.** Be familiar with any policies or laws that apply.
- **Form a coalition of allies,** if you can. Engage in consultation. Communicate, inform, and clarify their collaborative roles.
- **Intervene high enough in the hierarchy** to get the job done. If the difficulty is with a physician or an organizational policy, merely going to the charge nurse will

not be enough. You will need to communicate with nurse administrators or other agency administrators.

- **Demonstrate to the system** how it is defeating its own goals (e.g., for patient care).
- **Avoid getting into a power struggle** if possible (use the preceding steps first). If you must, decide how far you need to go and whether you are willing to go that far. You will need to enlist people with more power in the system than you have (e.g., family members, physicians, administrators).
- **Be aware of client vulnerability.** When possible, avoid confrontation. If there is risk for the client (as in a power contest), be sure the client is aware of his risks and possible gains; then let him choose how far to take the situation.
- **Have alternative actions.** Assess risks realistically. Weigh them against potential gains.

to be a member of your institution's ethics committee or plan to attend nursing ethics rounds to familiarize yourself with the types of ethical problems that occur at your institution.

- **Consult Reliable Sources.** Attend ethics education programs and talk about issues with other healthcare providers. Attorneys, ethicists, and members of the clergy can provide helpful perspectives.
- **Share.** Regularly engage in discussions with the staff on your unit to determine differences in value systems and to collaborate proactively to work out methods that can be used to resolve ethical dilemmas effectively. When you are faced with a difficult moral decision, consult

with peers, coworkers, and teachers. Seek guidance and support.

- **Evaluate.** After a situation is resolved, evaluate your decision and the effects of your actions. You should be able to learn from even the worst decision. And when everything goes well, you can file your strategies away to use in similar future situations.

KnowledgeCheck 42-13

- What are three reasons why patients may need a nurse advocate?
- Briefly describe the nurse's role as a patient advocate.

CLINICALREASONING:
Applying the **Full-Spectrum Nursing Model**

Because the following critical thinking activities allow you to practice the kind of thinking you will use as a full-spectrum nurse, they usually have no single right answer. Discuss them with your peers—if you have difficulty with any of the questions, consult your instructor.

PRACTICE SITUATION

Read the following summary of the Kothari and Kirschner article:

Kothari, S., & Kirschner, K. (2006). Abandoning the Golden Rule: The problem with "putting ourselves in the patient's place." *Topics in Stroke Rehabilitation, 13*(4), 68–73.

A large body of evidence documents the difficulties healthcare professionals have in predicting what their patient believes or wishes. These difficulties extend from the predictions of:

- Very specific patient wishes, such as for life-sustaining therapies
- More global assessments of patients' lives as a whole (for instance, their quality of life)

One explanation for this phenomenon is that healthcare professionals, either consciously or unconsciously, adopt "Golden Rule thinking." This refers to our attempts to understand another person's situation by imagining what we would believe or want under similar circumstances, in other words, "putting ourselves in the patient's place."

Although Golden Rule thinking would seem to be a promising strategy, studies show that it actually results in inaccurate presumptions of patients' wishes or beliefs. These presumptions, in turn, have significant clinical and ethical implications. That is, they cause healthcare professionals and families to make decisions for the patient that are, in reality, *not* what the patient would want. The thinking goes:

I should put myself in the patient's place.

If I were the patient, I would want X.

Therefore, the patient probably wants X.

Because the patient probably wants X, we will do X.

This thinking process can have different results: (1) The patient really does want X, so you have met his needs. (2) The patient really wanted Y, so you did not meet his needs.

THINKING

1. *Theoretical Knowledge:* What is the Golden Rule, or what does it say?
2. *Critical Thinking (Inquiry):* What is one thing that could be done ahead of time to prevent the need for Golden Rule thinking? Explain why that would work.

DOING

3. *Nursing Process (Assessment):* If you do not know what the patient would want, instead of thinking what *you* would want, how might you get an idea of what the patient might want?

CARING

4. *Self-Knowledge:* What is your earliest memory of being taught the Golden Rule?
5. *Ethical Knowledge:* Which moral principle does the Golden Rule seem to try to follow: autonomy, nonmaleficence/beneficence, fidelity, veracity, or justice?

 Go To Chapter 42, **Clinical Reasoning: Applying the Full-Spectrum Nursing**

 To explore learning resources for this chapter,

 Go to Davis*Plus* at http://www.Davisplus.fadavis.com, keyword Treas.

Chapter Resources for Chapter 42:
   Knowledge Check and Think Like a Nurse Response Sheets
   Knowledge Check Answers
   Resources for Caregivers and Health Professionals
   Reading More About Nursing Ethics (Suggested Readings)
   What Are the Main Points in This Chapter?
NCLEX-Style Review Questions
Chapter Overview Podcasts

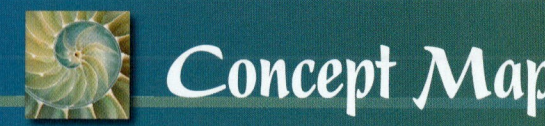

Concept Map

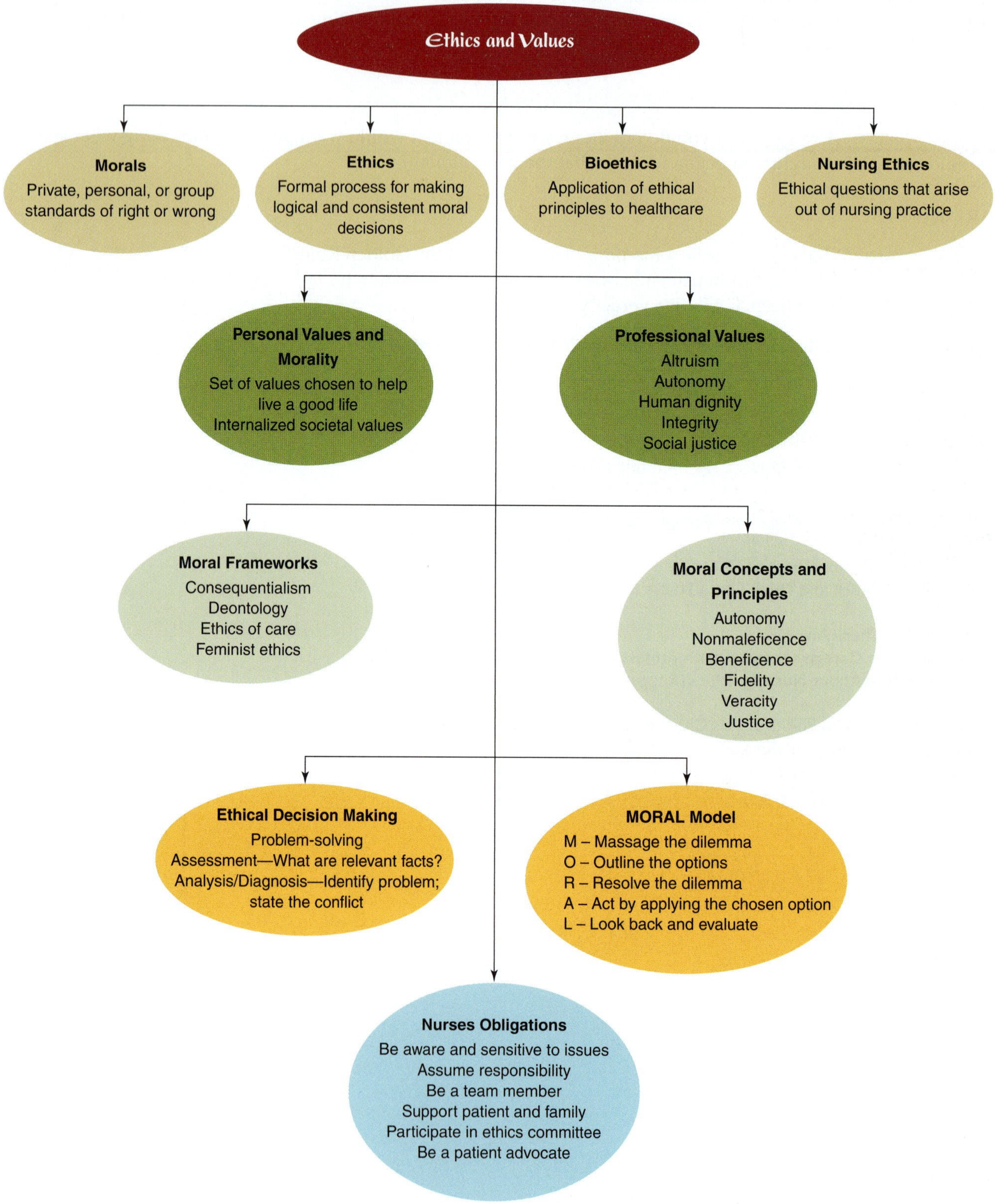

Ethics and Values

Morals
Private, personal, or group standards of right or wrong

Ethics
Formal process for making logical and consistent moral decisions

Bioethics
Application of ethical principles to healthcare

Nursing Ethics
Ethical questions that arise out of nursing practice

Personal Values and Morality
Set of values chosen to help live a good life
Internalized societal values

Professional Values
Altruism
Autonomy
Human dignity
Integrity
Social justice

Moral Frameworks
Consequentialism
Deontology
Ethics of care
Feminist ethics

Moral Concepts and Principles
Autonomy
Nonmaleficence
Beneficence
Fidelity
Veracity
Justice

Ethical Decision Making
Problem-solving
Assessment—What are relevant facts?
Analysis/Diagnosis—Identify problem; state the conflict

MORAL Model
M – Massage the dilemma
O – Outline the options
R – Resolve the dilemma
A – Act by applying the chosen option
L – Look back and evaluate

Nurses Obligations
Be aware and sensitive to issues
Assume responsibility
Be a team member
Support patient and family
Participate in ethics committee
Be a patient advocate

society by establishing acceptable patterns of behaviors, and are enforceable by a controlling authority. Nurses are legally responsible for their own actions and this legal responsibility cannot be delegated—this is the basis for liability in nursing practice. **Liability** means that the person is financially or legally responsible for something. **Malpractice** is one source of legal liability. It means that a professional person has failed to act in a reasonable and prudent manner. If someone is harmed, the professional may be held liable.

WHAT ARE THE SOURCES AND TYPES OF LAW?

The United States Constitution establishes three branches of government: executive, legislative, and judicial. Each branch has specified authority, designed to equalize power among the three and to provide a system of checks and balances (Table 43-1).

Laws are derived primarily from four sources: (1) the Constitution, (2) statutes, (3) administrative bodies, and (4) the courts (Table 43-1).

Constitutional Law. A **constitution** is a system of fundamental laws and principles that prescribes the nature, functions, and limits of a government. The U.S. Constitution is the superior law of the land and applies to all states and territories throughout the United States. Thus, all state and federal laws must comply with the U.S. Constitution. The U.S. Constitution limits the powers of the federal government and gives each state the power to govern itself and to pass laws to promote the health, welfare, order, and security of its citizens.

Statutory Law. A **statute** is a law passed by the federal Congress or by a state legislative body. Congress (Senate and House of Representatives) passes laws for the benefit of society

as a whole, whereas states use their police power to enforce laws to ensure the general health, safety, and welfare of their specific citizens. The Nurse Practice Act (NPA) is an example of statutory law. The legislative body of each state passes regulations (laws) that govern the profession of nursing, known as Nurse Practice Acts. These NPAs can be found in each state's Revised Statutes.

Administrative Law. Formally defined, **administrative law** refers to the laws that govern administrative agencies. Administrative agencies are created at the federal level by Congress and at the state level by a state's legislative bodies. As applied to nursing, administrative law comprises the rules and regulations passed by administrative bodies or agencies to fulfill their statutory missions. Within each state's Nurse Practice Act, the state legislative body has created a state board of nursing to enforce the NPA by passing the rules and regulations that are necessary to ensure compliance. These rules and regulations can be found in each state's administrative code.

Common (Judicial) Law. A compilation of laws made by judges or courts is known as **common law.** Also referred to as *case law*, common law is based on common customs and traditions. It comes from legal principles and guidelines that judges use to determine the outcome of legal cases.

WHAT LAWS AND REGULATIONS GUIDE NURSING PRACTICE?

As a professional nurse, you will need to understand the various laws and regulations that guide nursing practice. Laws and regulations at the federal and state levels have a direct impact on the nurse's actions and decisions.

Table 43-1 ▶ Structure for Law and Common Questions That Apply to Nursing

BRANCHES OF GOVERNMENT		
	EXAMPLE	**DESCRIPTION**
Executive	The president of the United States, attorney general, secretary of state, state governors	Authority to execute and/or enforce laws.
Legislative	Congress (House of Representatives + Senate)	Make or formulate laws.
Judicial	U.S. Supreme Court; state and local courts	Interpret statutory law and decide cases and controversies.

TYPE/SOURCE OF LAW		
	EXAMPLE	**QUESTION POSED**
Constitutional Law	Freedom of speech	Can an employer prevent internationally educated nurses from speaking in their native language in the work environment?
Statutory Law	Definition of *nursing*	What is the nurse's scope of practice (duties and responsibilities)?
Administrative Law	Delegation and supervision	Is the registered nurse legally responsible for tasks or assignments delegated to other nurses?
Common Law	Affirmative duty	Does a registered nurse have a responsibility to exercise an independent judgment to prevent harm to patients?

Federal Law

State NPAs typically require you to have knowledge of federal laws affecting nursing practice.

Bill of Rights

The first ten amendments to the U.S. Constitution are known as the **Bill of Rights**. The Bill of Rights clearly identifies, and in many ways limits, the role of government in individuals' lives. Many of these rights have direct implications for patients receiving healthcare, such as patients' right to be informed, make decisions affecting health and welfare, and protect personal property. Protecting patients' privacy rights is a fundamental role of the professional nurse and is derived from the Bill of Rights. If you would like to review a few of the amendment under the Bill of Rights that pertain to patients and nurses,

 Go to Chapter 43, **Tables, Boxes, Figures: ESG Box 43-1, Select Amendments Under the Bill of Rights,** on Davis*Plus.*

 Think**Like a Nurse** 43-1

- Develop a scenario illustrating how a nurse might protect a patient's right to privacy.
- What is one thing a nurse can do to respect a patient's property rights?

Health Insurance Portability and Accountability Act (HIPAA)

The Health Insurance Portability and Accountability Act (HIPAA) was passed by Congress in 1996 to protect patients:
- Protect health insurance benefits for workers who lose or change their jobs.
- Protect coverage to persons with preexisting medical conditions.
- Establish standards to protect the privacy of personal health information.

Nurses and other healthcare providers must protect the patient's right to privacy by not sharing patient information with unauthorized individuals. Under HIPAA rules, healthcare agencies and their employees must take steps to ensure the confidentiality of the patient information and medical records. In addition, HIPAA allows for patients to see, make corrections to, and obtain copies of their medical records.

Case: Violation of a Patient's Privacy

Patients at a state-operated psychiatric facility filed a lawsuit in the U.S. District Court for the Eastern District of New York, challenging the facility's practice of supervising some of the patients' visitations by video (not audio) when ordered by the provider. The guard in this particular case was not close enough to hear conversations, nor did he make an attempt to listen. The court ruled that the patients' privacy rights were not being violated by the practice for prescribed supervised visits in effect at this facility
Sparks v. Seltzer, F. Supp. 2d, 2009 WL 1039886 (E.D. N.Y., April 20, 2009)

Emergency Medical Treatment and Active Labor Act (EMTALA)

The Emergency Medical Treatment and Active Labor Act (EMTALA) requires healthcare facilities to provide emergency medical treatment to patients who seek healthcare in the emergency department, regardless of their ability to pay, legal status, or citizenship status. The obligation is for the medical facility to provide medical screening to determine if an emergency exists and to stabilize the patient before transferring him or her to another healthcare facility.

 Think**Like a Nurse** 43-2

A 54-year-old uninsured and unemployed woman arrives at the emergency department of a small private hospital complaining of chest pain and nausea. The triage nurse calls the on-call physician, who instructs the nurse to send the patient to the county hospital several blocks away. The nurse assesses the patient and contacts her supervisor, who tells her to contact the medical chief of staff to inform him that the patient is in need of emergency treatment.

- Discuss whether the nurse's action was appropriate or inappropriate.

Patient Self-Determination Act (PSDA)

The Patient Self-Determination Act (PSDA) of 1991 recognizes the patient's right to make decisions regarding his own healthcare, based on the information provided to him by the healthcare provider, regarding the medical or surgical treatment options available, the benefits, risks, and alternatives. Box 43-1 describes agency and healthcare workers' responsibilities under the PSDA.

There are two types of legal written advance directives, the living will and the durable power of attorney for healthcare.

A **living will** is prepared by an alert and oriented (competent) individual to give directions to others about that person's wishes regarding life-prolonging treatments if the person becomes unable to make those decisions. The requirements that make a living will a legal document may vary from state to state. However, language common in the living will gives the person the opportunity to specify treatment in numerous areas (Box 43-2).

A **durable power of attorney for healthcare (DPOA)** identifies a person who will make healthcare decisions in the event

BOX 43-1 ■ The Patient Self-Determination Act

The Patient Self-Determination Act requires healthcare facilities to do the following:
- Provide written information to each patient regarding the right to make decisions, including the right to accept or to refuse medical treatment, and the right to make advance directives.
- Document in the patient's medical record the presence or absence of advance directives.
- Provide education to the staff, healthcare providers, and community on advance directives.
- Follow state law as it relates to advance directives.
- Treat everyone the same regardless of the presence or absence of advance directives (Do not discriminate)

BOX 43-2 ■ Sample Living Will Language

If I am in a terminal condition, irreversible coma, or in a persistent vegetative state, my wishes are as follows:

I □ **do** □ **do not** want to be in or taken to a hospital.

I □ **do** □ **do not** want pain medications to keep me comfortable.

I □ **do** □ **do not** want cardiac resuscitation, including drugs and electrical shock.

I □ **do** □ **do not** want mechanical respiration/artificial respiration.

I □ **do** □ **do not** want tube feeding or any other artificial or invasive form of nutrition (food).

I □ **do** □ **do not** want hydration (water), via tube or intravenous.

I □ **do** □ **do not** want blood or blood products.

I □ **do** □ **do not** want any form of surgery or invasive diagnostic tests.

I □ **do** □ **do not** want kidney dialysis.

I □ **do** □ **do not** want antibiotics.

Case: Durable Power of Attorney

Mrs. Terry Schiavo collapsed in her Florida home in 1990 after she was without oxygen for about 5 minutes because of a suspected potassium imbalance secondary to bulimia. She suffered severe brain damage. Terry Schiavo did not have a living will. According to Florida law, her husband became her legal guardian, and thus the decision maker regarding her medical treatments. In November 1992, Mr. Schiavo won a medical malpractice lawsuit for $1 million from her physician on the theory that he failed to diagnose Mrs. Schiavo's bulimia.

In 2000, Mr. Schiavo petitioned the court to have Terri's feeding tube removed. Her parents opposed the action. Over the next 5 years, extensive legal battles ensued. Finally, the court ruled in favor of removing the feeding tube. Mrs. Schiavo died on March 31, 2005. It was lack of a living will that (1) permitted the prolonged legal battle between Mrs. Schiavo's husband and her parents and (2) made it impossible to know for sure what Terry Schiavo would have wanted. It's all guesswork without a living will (Quill, 2005).

that the patient is unable to do so. The person given the right to make decisions is called the *surrogate decision maker*. The surrogate has the right to make the medical decisions for as long as the person is not able to do so for himself (is considered incompetent).

Case: Durable Power of Attorney (DPOA)

Mr. Green was in a coma as a result of suffering head trauma during a motor vehicle accident. In his DPOA, he had designated his brother, Joey, as his surrogate. Although Mr. Green was married with two adult children, Joey was the person legally recognized to make decisions regarding Mr. Green's healthcare. Two weeks later, Mr. Green became conscious and regained the ability to make decisions. At that point, Mr. Green no longer required Joey as a surrogate.

The American Nurses Association (ANA) highlighted the nurse's role in implementing the PSDA in a 1991 position statement. As a nurse, you have the following responsibilities:

- Facilitate informed decision making for patients making choices about end-of-life care.
- Know the laws pertaining to advance directives in the state in which you are practicing.
- Make sure the patient's advance directives are current and reflect the patient's desires.
- Ask the following questions about advance directives as a part of the nursing admission assessment:

  Do you have basic information about advance care directives, including living wills and durable power of attorney?

  Do you wish to initiate an advance care directive? If you have already prepared an advance care directive, can you provide it now?

  Have you discussed your end of life choices with your family and/or designated surrogate and healthcare team worker?" (ANA, 1991)

Americans With Disabilities Act (ADA)

The Americans With Disabilities Act (ADA) of 1990 provides protection against discrimination of individuals with disabilities. A person has a **disability** if he has a physical or mental impairment that substantially limits one or more major life activities (Equal Employment Opportunity Commission [EEOC], 1992). In general, the ADA provides that employers must provide reasonable accommodations within the work setting to allow employees with disabilities to perform their jobs.

Case: ADA Accommodations

- A nurse with a substance abuse addiction after rehabilitation was restricted from dispensing medication after she was caught using illegal drugs. Her employer had a policy allowing employees to participate in drug rehabilitation and return to work with a last-chance agreement. When the nurse returned to work after rehabilitation, she was reassigned to a job that did not require her to dispense medication. She was given periodic drug tests.
- An intensive care unit (ICU) nurse with leukemia had difficulty tolerating rotating schedules. The nurse manager accommodated her by assigning a permanent day schedule.
- A nurse with cerebral palsy worked for an insurance company investigating medical claims. Her employer adapted the workstation by installing an adjustable keyboard tray, ergonomic chair, and room for mobility braces nearby. The employer also allowed regular rest periods. She was repositioned closer to the restroom to help reduce fatigue.
- A nurse with insulin-dependent diabetes had difficulty maintaining glucose control. Her employer provided consistent times for breaks and lunch and privacy to check blood sugar levels and administer insulin as needed (Job Accommodation Network, 2006).

For a list of additional strategies to accommodate nurses with various disabilities,

 Go to the Job Accommodation Network at http://www.jan. wvu.edu/media/nurses.html

KnowledgeCheck 43-1

- Which federal law requires healthcare agencies to provide patients with information about advance directives?
- Which federal law ensures that patients can receive emergency treatment regardless of their ability to pay?
- What protections are provided to patients by the Department of Health and Human Services "privacy rule" of the HIPAA?

State Laws

In addition to federal law, many states have laws that directly impact nurses' actions and behaviors. These include mandatory reporting laws, Good Samaritan laws, NPAs, and medical malpractice statutes.

Mandatory Reporting Laws

The law in various states requires healthcare workers to report communicable diseases. You also have a duty to report physical, sexual, or emotional abuse or neglect of children, older adults, or the mentally ill, whether you suspect it or have actual evidence of it. The intent is to protect people who cannot protect themselves and to protect society against the spread of communicable diseases. Mandatory reporting laws also protect you when reporting abuse. In most instances, the identity of the reporter is kept confidential. If you fail to report certain communicable diseases in a patient whom you are caring for in the clinic, or if you fail to report abuse when you have reason to believe a child was abused, you are actually liable in a court of law and could be charged for criminal misdemeanor.

The duty to report is an act of protection that takes priority over the patient's right to privacy. Therefore, if you report abuse or neglect, you cannot be charged with violating a patient's right to privacy (e.g., under HIPAA). Since the mandatory reporting laws vary from state to state, you should be familiar with the law in your state.

Case: Mandatory Reporting

In Texas, two school administrators were charged with a misdemeanor for failing to report to police or to Child Protective Services that the mother of a student had twice reported seeing a teacher molest another student (Vaughn, 1998).

Good Samaritan Laws

Good Samaritan laws are designed to protect from liability those who provide emergency care to someone who has been injured. To successfully use the Good Samaritan defense, the following elements must be present:
- Care was provided in an emergency situation.
- Person(s) providing the care did not cause the emergency or injury.
- Care was provided in a reasonably competent manner.
- Care provided must be voluntary (not paid).
- Person receiving care did not object to receiving care.

Nurses should follow these guidelines to ensure their protection by Good Samaritan laws:
- Call 911, or have someone else call, as soon as you can.
- Do not leave the person unless you transfer care to an equally competent professional.
- Place the person under the care of emergency personnel, physicians, or advanced practice nurses as soon as possible and follow their instructions.
- Do not accept money or any other form of compensation for the services provided.

Good Samaritan laws vary from state to state. You should be familiar with the law in your state.

Case: Good Samaritan

A registered nurse was leaving the hospital after working a 12-hour shift, when she witnessed a single-person motor vehicle accident. She called 911, stopped, and approached the accident scene, where she smelled gasoline. Fearing that the car would explode, she pulled the accident victim from the car, put him flat on the ground, and assessed his injuries. She put pressures on his bleeding femoral artery and stayed with him until the ambulance arrived. The victim had spinal cord injuries and sued the nurse for removing him from the car. However, the nurse was protected from liability by the Good Samaritan law.

Key Point: *Nurses working in healthcare environments may not be protected by Good Samaritan laws if they already have a responsibility to provide care to those in need.*

Case: Good Samaritan

June, an RN, was working in the emergency department (ED) when a patient walked in and collapsed. She performed CPR on the patient until the medical treatment team arrived in the ED. June had a legal duty or obligation to provide care to the patient and could not rely on the Good Samaritan law as a defense in any lawsuit.

Nurse Practice Acts

Nurse Practice Acts are statutory laws passed by each state's legislative body that define the practice of nursing. Nurse Practice Acts are designed to do the following:
- Protect patients or society.
- Define the scope of nursing practice.
- Identify the minimum level of nursing care that must be provided to clients.

The components of NPAs are discussed in more detail later in the chapter.

Medical Malpractice Statutes

Medical malpractice refers to a lawsuit brought against a healthcare provider for damages due to the death, injury, or other loss of the person being treated. Laws governing medical malpractice vary from state to state, primarily regarding the time frame for bringing a lawsuit (statute of limitations) and the amount of monetary compensation allowed. To protect themselves from personal losses, many healthcare providers purchase malpractice insurance, which provides them with an

attorney to defend against the claim and pay the damages (money) awarded to the claimant by a judge or jury. Malpractice is discussed in more detail later in this chapter.

Other Guidelines for Practice

In addition to federal and state laws, other practice guidelines may also factor into what constitutes reasonable and prudent nursing care.

Institutional Policies and Procedures

Institutional policies and procedures usually are more specific and detailed than standards set by professional organizations. They describe care that is reasonable, appropriate, and expected in the context of that facility. You must be familiar with these policies and procedures because they can be used as evidence of a violation of a standard of care if you failed to follow them. Healthcare facilities should not have policies and procedures that conflict with the Nurse Practice Act, professional standards of practice, the ANA Code of Ethics for Nurses, and other documents that guide nursing practice. If you encounter any conflicts, or if a policy is not working well, you should bring the matter to your supervisor's attention and/or contact the board of nursing in your state for an advisory opinion.

American Nurses Association Code of Ethics

The ANA Code of Ethics (2001) describes the standards of professional responsibility for nurses and provides insight into ethical and acceptable behavior. It describes nurses' obligations for safe, compassionate, nondiscriminatory, and quality care, while defining commitments to self, the patient, the employer, and the profession.

The Code of Ethics is not a law, so you would not be charged with criminal offenses for violating the code's provisions. In many situations, there is a fine line between what is legal and what is ethical. When confronted with a situation, you should ask yourself, "Is there a law that relates to this situation?" and "What guidance is provided under the Code of Ethics?" Your action should then be consistent with the code. The ANA code guarantees the patient the right to dignity, privacy, and safety. The ANA code also guarantees the nurse will do the following:

- Be accountable and competent.
- Use informed judgment.
- Maintain employment conditions conducive to quality patient care.
- Protect the client from misinformation and misrepresentation.
- Collaborate with other healthcare professions to meet the patient's healthcare needs.

Key Point: *A nurse who violates a provision of the code of ethics may have to defend her action to her state board of nursing.* Likewise, in a malpractice suit, courts may look to these codes to judge whether the nurse's action was at the level expected by the profession. However, the code will not likely protect you if you break a law or fail to follow agency policies, even if you believe the law to be immoral. If you need more information on nursing codes of ethics, see Chapter 42.

Patient Care Partnership

The Patient Care Partnership (PCP) replaced the American Hospital Association's Patient Bill of Rights. This updated brochure is available in eight languages. It explains to patients in plain language that during hospitalization, they should expect the following:

- High-quality care
- A clean and safe environment
- Involvement in care
- Protection of privacy

- Help when leaving the hospital
- Help with billing claims

Like the ANA Code of Ethics, these rights are not necessarily legally binding, but they can provide evidence by which to judge whether the patient's care and environment met reasonable and appropriate standards. For more information on the Patient Care Partnership, see Box 42-3.

American Nurses Association Bill of Rights for Registered Nurses

The Nurse's Bill of Rights is a policy statement adopted by the ANA to identify the seven conditions nurses should expect from their workplace that are necessary for sound professional practice. It provides a framework for employers to understand what nurses need for a safe work environment and to support nurses as they address such issues as unsafe staffing, workplace violence, and mandatory overtime (ANA, 2009). The Bill of Rights highlights that nurses have the right to:

- Practice in a manner that fulfills their obligations to society and to those who receive nursing care
- Practice in environments that allow them to act in accordance with professional standards and legally authorized scopes of practice
- A work environment that supports and facilitates ethical practice in the Code of Ethics for Nurses
- Freely and openly advocate for themselves and their patients, without fear of retribution
- Fair compensation for their work, consistent with their knowledge, experience, and professional responsibilities
- A work environment that is safe for themselves and for their patients
- Negotiate the conditions of their employment, either as individuals or collectively, in all practice settings

American Nurses Association Standards of Practice

The ANA (2010) Standards of Practice have three components:

1. *Professional standards of care* that incorporate the nursing process in the diagnostic, intervention, and evaluation aspect of patient care
2. *Professional performance standards* that identify the various role functions of the nurse in direct patient care, quality of practice, ethics, education, communication, research, leadership, collaboration, resource management, collegiality, and environmental health
3. *Practice guidelines* for the various specialty areas that are developed by professional organizations (e.g., American Association of Critical Care Nurses).

If you need to review the ANA Standards of Clinical Nursing Practice, refer to Chapter 1, Table 1-5. Standards establish the minimum level of competency for nurses. Nurses are expected to follow the standards that apply to their specialty areas. For example, ANA has standards for gerontological nursing, home health nursing, and nursing informatics.

Think**Like a Nurse** 43-3

Recall the opening scenario (Meet Your Nurse Role Model). Would the nurse have done the right thing if she had decided not to accept the assignment and leave the facility immediately?

- What standards, guidelines, and laws would apply to determine whether the nurse's behavior was in accordance with standards of practice?
- Which statements in the ANA Bill of Rights for Registered Nurses might the nurse use to justify her actions?

Nurse Practice Acts

As you have learned, Nurse Practice Acts contain a provision that creates and empowers a state board of nursing to regulate the practice of nursing in that state. All 50 states, the District of Columbia, and the five U.S. territories have established boards of nursing. Although NPAs can vary from state to state, they all have common components, because states used American Nurses Association guidelines in developing their regulations. A state's Nurse Practice Act usually includes the following:

- The authority of the board of nursing, its composition and powers
- A definition of *nursing* and the boundaries of nursing practice
- Standards for the approval of nursing education programs
- The requirements for licensure of nurses
- Grounds for disciplinary action against a nurse's license

Case: Nurse Practice Act

Mejonus X Institute advertised an associate degree nursing program that could be completed in 12 months at a cost of $45,000. You are interested in the program, but are not sure if the program is legitimate. Your initial investigation of the program should start with the state board of nursing, which approves nursing education programs. A list of approved nursing programs can usually be found on the state board of nursing Web site in many states.

Requirements for Licensure

Perhaps the most important function of state boards of nursing is establishing and enforcing the requirements for licensure. Unlicensed health providers pose a danger to the health, safety, and welfare of the general public because they have not met the specified standards to ensure a minimum level of competency to enter the nursing profession. In most states, the applicant for licensure must do the following:

- Graduate from an approved or accredited nursing program.
- Meet the established character criteria.
- Undergo a criminal background check and fingerprinting.
- Pass the NCLEX-RN® or -PN exam.
- Pay an application fee.
- Some states, such as Texas, may require applicants to pass a jurisprudence examination before receiving a permanent license.

Some states give a temporary license pending the results of the first attempt at the licensure exam.

Special Cases of Licensure

To protect the public, licensing is meant to ensure to practicing nurses have met the minimum competencies set by the state.

Mutual Recognition Model (MRM)/Multi-State Licensure Compact. Certain states, through a multistate agreement, allow nurses who are licensed to practice in one state to practice in all other states participating in the agreement. The nurse does not have to retake the NCLEX-RN® or -PN examination, but must apply to the new state and fulfill any of that state's application requirements such as fingerprinting, background check, transcripts, and fees. When two states enter into the multistate licensure compact, you do not have to obtain a separate license to practice in either state.

Case: Multi-State Compact

Roberto was a clinical nurse residing in Overland Park, Kansas, and originally licensed in the state of Kansas after passing the NCLEX-RN®. He subsequently became employed at the Children's Hospital on the other side of the state line in Missouri. Roberto was required to maintain active licensure in the state where he was employed. He received an RN licensure in the state of Missouri by meeting the requirements of the Missouri State Board of Nursing, but did not have to retake the NCLEX-RN®.

Government/Military Personnel. Another special case of licensure involves nurses employed by the military, Veterans Administration, U.S. Public Health Service, or other entities of the federal government. These nurses may practice in other states without obtaining a new license as long as they are practicing within the parameters or scope of their employment.

Case: Special Case of Licensure

Jane was a clinical nurse in the United States Air Force Reserve. She was licensed in the state of Texas, but was assigned to a military hospital in Nevada for her 2-week annual military tour. Jane would not need to obtain a license in the state of Nevada to practice at the military hospital.

Scope of Practice

The scope of nursing practice is found in the definition of nursing at the various levels. Nurses must be familiar with the definition of nursing at their level to appropriately plan and implement care that is consistent with their scope of practice. Any nurse who practices outside the scope of practice can be charged with violation of the Nurse Practice Act. Nurse Practice Acts vary slightly state by state. However, in most states, licensed practical nurse/licensed vocational nurse (LPN/LVN) scope of practice is limited in assessment privileges and interpretation of clinical data. Typically, LPN/LVNs do not have authority to alter nursing care plans.

Understanding the definition of nursing practice in your state is important, because it determines the legal limits of your practice, as illustrated in this landmark case.

Case: Scope of Practice

A physician delegated to an LPN the task of administering a polio booster to a 2-year-old boy. The nurse put the boy over her knee and proceeded to give the injection. The boy moved and the needle broke off in his buttocks, where it remained for 9 months despite attempts to surgically remove it. Because the Washington State Nurse Practice Act at that time did not allow LPNs to give injections, the nurse was in violation of the Nurse Practice Act by performing a task that was outside of her legal limits (Barber v. Reinking, 68 Wash. 2d 122, 411. P. 2d 861 (1966)).

This case should make clear that no one, including an employer or physician, can increase a nurse's legal scope of practice.

Disciplinary Actions

The state board of nursing can take disciplinary actions against your license for violation of the Nurse Practice Act. A disciplinary action usually involves some or all of the following:

- The process begins with a complaint from an individual, employer, or professional organization that the nurse has engaged in unprofessional conduct.
- The complaint is then assigned to an investigator to determine its legitimacy or validity.

  If the investigator decides the complaint is invalid or does not constitute a violation of the NPA, it will be dismissed.

  If the complaint may violate the NPA, the investigator gathers additional information by contacting the nurse, interviewing witnesses, and reviewing documents and records.

- The case may be heard by the board of nursing, who will decide if the nurse violated the NPA and the appropriate punishment. The board of nursing must provide you with the following to fulfill the due process requirements of the Fourteenth Amendment:

  Notice of the charges against you

  The evidence that supports the charges

  A hearing in which you have the opportunity to cross-examine the witnesses and to present your own evidence and witnesses

- If you are not satisfied with the board's actions and punishment, you can appeal your case to the appropriate state court.
- At every stage during the disciplinary process, you have the right to have an attorney present. You should ask a potential attorney two questions: (1) How many of your cases were in the area of administrative law and procedures? (2) How many times have you represented clients in front of professional boards, such as the board of nursing?

For examples of nursing actions that constitute unprofessional conduct,

 Go to Chapter 43, **Tables, Boxes, Figures: ESG Box 43-2, Actions, Behaviors, or Omissions that Constitute Unprofessional Conduct,** on Davis*Plus.*

 Think**Like a Nurse** 43-4

A registered nurse was assigned to care for a 76-year-old patient who had a stroke. On entering the room, the nurse found the patient surrounded by 10 family members. The nurse requested the family members leave the room so she could conduct her initial assessment and perform any related treatments. They did so. The nurse provided care in a professional, unhurried, and gentle manner. As she was leaving, the patient said, "Thank you. You are a wonderful nurse." Later, the nursing supervisor told her the patient told his family members that the nurse had spoken harshly to him and had yanked his arms. The family stated they would file a complaint with the hospital administrator and the board of nursing.

- Are there grounds for disciplinary actions? What should the nurse do?

Knowledge**Check** 43-2

How does each of the following protect patients?
- The Patient Care Partnership
- Nursing codes of ethics
- Mandatory reporting laws

Credentialing

Many healthcare disciplines, including nursing, use a voluntary form of self-regulation called **credentialing.** In the legal sense, credentialing includes accreditation and certification. Having credentials implies that the person or agency has met higher standards than the minimum required (e.g., licensure).

Accreditation. Most nursing boards establish educational requirements for nursing programs and continuing education courses within a given state. The board usually requires that for a nursing program to be **accredited,** it must meet the requirements for accreditation established by the National League for Nursing (NLN) or the American Association of Colleges of Nursing (ACCN) and by the state NPA. This helps ensure students receive education that meets the minimum standard for quality and that patients are cared for by safe practitioners.

Accreditation also applies to other than educational facilities; for example, hospitals seek accreditation by The Joint Commission. This is intended to ensure a minimum standard quality of care is provided.

Certification. Another form of credentialing is **certification**. Through certification and licensing, the board identifies nurses who are qualified for advanced practice (e.g., clinical nurse specialists, midwives, and nurse practitioners) or for certification in a subspecialty, such as emergency nursing or pediatric nursing. In some states, the board establishes the criteria for certification, including (1) educational preparation, (2) clinical experience, and (3) certification by other professional organizations. In other states, the nurse may obtain an advanced practice license only if she is first certified by a national organization, such as the American Nurses Credentialing Corporation (ANCC) or a specialty organization. Not all states require certification for advanced practice nurses.

WHAT IS CRIMINAL LAW?

Criminal law deals with wrongs or offenses against society. It may result in prosecution (legal action) by the state or federal government for engaging in behavior that constitutes a crime. A **crime** is a violation of a law as defined by a legislative body. The legislature also specifies the punishments for the crime. State-level criminal laws vary from state to state.

There are two "levels" of crimes: misdemeanors and felonies. The primary difference is the possible punishment.

- **Felonies** involve crimes punishable by more than one year in jail (e.g., murder, assisted suicide, rape/sexual assault, stealing drugs and equipment, felony abuse). A person convicted of a felony loses the right to vote, hold public office, serve on a jury, and to possess firearms. The person may also lose any professional license.
- Compared to a felony, a **misdemeanor** is a minor charge. Misdemeanors involve less than a year in jail. They include crimes such as assault, battery, and petty theft. You may also lose your nursing license if you are convicted of a misdemeanor that involves crimes against persons or that can cause harm to others.

An emerging issue in the nursing profession is whether nurses who accidentally cause harm to patients should be charged with criminal offenses (e.g., a nurse accidentally administers the wrong drug to a patient and the patient dies). In the past, these cases have been dealt with under civil law and by the board of nursing. Now state prosecutors are beginning to bring felony and misdemeanor charges against these nurses.

Case: Criminal Law, Impaired Nurse

Several patients complained that their pain medication was not working. A review of the medical records of the patients assigned to the nurse revealed that all but one of her patients who received pain medication had similar complaints. When confronted, the nurse admitted to stealing the patients' pain medication and giving them saline. She also admitted to using other nurses' passwords for stealing narcotics. The nurse was terminated and reported to the board of nursing. She refused to enter the impaired nurse's program. Her license was revoked after a hearing. She also faced criminal charges for theft of controlled substances.

Case: Criminal Law, Theft

Joan, an RN, was arrested for stealing computer equipment and wound supplies, valued at $55,000, from the hospital. She was charged with grand larceny, a felony. Two weeks before her trial, she entered into a plea deal that reduced the charge to a misdemeanor with probation for 6 months.

For an expanded discussion of criminal law,

 Go to Chapter 43, **Supplemental Materials,** on Davis*Plus*.

WHAT IS CIVIL LAW?

In contrast to criminal law, in which the state or federal government brings charges against a person, civil law involves a dispute between individuals or entities. A settlement in civil law often results in the guilty party paying monetary damages. The two types of civil law are contract law and tort law.

- **Contract law** involves a written or oral agreement between two parties in which one party accepts an offer made by the other party to perform (or not perform) certain acts in exchange for something of value. A breach of contract occurs if either party does not comply with the terms of the agreement. An example would be an employment contract.
- **Tort law,** on the other hand, deals with wrongs done to one person by another person that does not involve contracts. A tort is a civil wrong and there are three types of tort: quasi-intentional torts, intentional torts, and non-intentional torts.

What are Quasi-Intentional Torts?

Quasi-intentional torts involve actions that injure a person's reputation. The overall concept for these torts is defamation of character. All four of the following essential elements of **defamation of character** must be present. The communication (written or oral) about the person:

- Was false
- Was made to another person or persons
- Caused the defamed person to experience shame and ridicule and had a negative impact on the person's reputation
- Was made as a statement of fact rather than as an opinion

Libel is the written or published form of defamation of character. **Slander** is the spoken or verbal form of defamation of character. A person is not guilty of defamation of character if the statement made about the other person is true or if the person has the protection of a "privilege," such as reporting possible child abuse.

Case: Quasi-intentional torts

The nursing supervisor called you into an empty conference room and stated, "I know that you have been stealing (diverting) narcotics from the unit and injecting yourself with it while at work. It shows, because your work is sloppy and you are falsifying your documentation. You are a poor excuse for a nurse." Before you were able to defend yourself, the supervisor left the room. The statements were not true. The supervisor committed slander.

What Are Intentional Torts?

An **intentional tort** is an action taken by one person with the intent to harm another person. The harm does not have to be violent, hostile, or cause a significant amount of pain or distress to the other person. The person must have merely intended to cause harm or known the action would bring about the harm. Intentional torts may be prosecuted under civil and criminal law. For example, a nurse who is sued for malpractice in civil court may also be charged with a homicide if a patient died because of the nurse's actions. Intentional torts most commonly encountered in nursing are assault, battery, false imprisonment, and invasion of privacy.

Assault

An assault occurs when a nurse intentionally places a patient in immediate fear of personal violence or offensive contact. An assault must include words expressing an intention to cause harm and some type of action. For example, a nurse has committed an assault if she says to the patient, "I will slap you" and raises her hand as if to slap the patient. The combination of the words and action causes the patient to believe the threat will be carried out.

Battery

A **battery** is committed when (1) an offensive or harmful physical contact is made with the patient without his consent, or (2) there is unauthorized touching of a person's body by another person. To avoid charges of battery, always obtain informed consent before providing certain treatments. On admission to healthcare facilities, patients sign a general consent form, which usually covers routine aspects of nursing care, such as vital signs and patient assessments. However, when performing any invasive procedure, such as insertion of catheters or intravenous lines, you should always explain the procedure to the patient and obtain his consent before starting.

Assault and Battery

An **assault and battery** occurs when there is the intent to cause a person fear combined with an offensive or harmful contact.

Case: Assault and Battery

A patient admitted for an elective surgical procedure complained that the automatic blood pressure cuff was causing her extreme pain and demanded it be removed. The nurse did not immediately remove the cuff as requested by the patient. The nurse was guilty of a battery, but not assault, because there was no evidence that the nurse intended to create or cause fear or pain

Coulter v. Thomas, 33 S.W.3d 522 (Ky. 2000)

False Imprisonment

False imprisonment is the restraint of a person without proper legal authorization. It includes any type of unjustified restriction on a person's freedom of movement—for example, when nurses restrain patients without their permission or when patients are involuntarily committed to mental health units. False imprisonment can involve the use of physical restraints (e.g., wrist restraints) or chemical restraints (e.g., sedatives or opioids). You may restrain patients who pose a threat to themselves or others. However, you must immediately obtain the proper authorization to continue the restraint.

Against Medical Advise (AMA). If a competent patient wishes to leave the healthcare facility, you should contact the nursing supervisor and the primary care provider. Inform the patient of the risks associated with leaving, and give her the choice to stay and receive treatment or to sign out against medical advice (AMA). You need to be aware of the hospital policy and procedures on AMA discharges.

Invasion of Privacy

Invasion of privacy violates a person's right to be left alone. The law recognizes that a person's personal life should not be opened up for public scrutiny and the person has the right to freedom from unwanted interference in her private affairs. A person has the right to:

- Have her private information protected
- Not be falsely portrayed or intentionally misrepresented in character, beliefs, or actions
- Be free from unwanted intrusion (spying, eavesdropping).

Examples of violating right to privacy include discussing patients in public places (e.g., elevators, cafeterias), photographing patients without their permission, providing information to news media without consent, searching a patient's personal belongings without permission, and releasing medical information without the patient's consent.

Fraud

Fraud is the false representation of significant facts by words or by conduct. It can occur through making false statements, falsifying documentation, or concealing information that should have been disclosed. It is intentionally misleading or deceiving another person to act (or not act) for the personal gain of the one committing the fraud.

Case: Fraud

A nurse admitted receiving more than $70,000 in Medicaid funds for private nursing services that she never provided. She submitted Medicaid reimbursement claims that falsely indicated that she provided nursing services to seven children and three young adults. The nurse entered a guilty plea to a felony (fraud) ("Rochester Nurse Guilty of Medicaid Fraud," 2007).

What are Non-Intentional Torts?

The most common type of non-intentional torts involving healthcare professionals are negligence or malpractice. **Negligence** is the failure to use ordinary or reasonable care or the failure to act in a reasonable and prudent (careful) manner. **Malpractice** has a similar definition, but applies only to professionals, such as nurses and physicians. It is defined as the failure of a professional person to act in a reasonable and prudent

manner. A malpractice lawsuit may occur when such actions cause injury or death to the patient. The person bringing the lawsuit is the **plaintiff** and the person who must defend against the lawsuit is the **defendant**.

Malpractice/Negligence Liability

To win and recover damages (money) in a malpractice lawsuit, the plaintiff must prove four elements (duty, breach of duty, causation, and damages) by a "preponderance of the evidence," in other words, with enough evidence to tip the scale in his favor.

Duty. A duty forms when the patient is assigned to the nurse or seeks treatment from the nurse, or when the nurse observes another person doing something that could harm the patient.

Breach of Duty. A breach of duty occurs when the nurse fails to meet standards of care. Attorneys look to several sources of information to identify the standards of care and to determine what a reasonable and prudent (careful) nurse would have done in the situation. These sources include the Nurse Practice Act, job descriptions, hospital policies and procedures, textbooks, professional standards and guidelines developed by professional organizations, and nursing codes of ethics.

Causation. The breach of duty or deviation from acceptable standards of care by the nurse must be the direct and proximate cause of the injury suffered by the patient. Causation is usually established based on the testimony of experts, such as advanced practice nurses, or other healthcare professionals, who can clearly show the connection between the nurse's action or omission and the resulting injury to the patient.

Case: Causation

A nurse forgot to change a patient's dressing at the scheduled time, but did change it 3 hours later. The hospital policy read that nurses must administer medications or perform prescribed treatments within 30 minutes before or 30 minutes after the scheduled time. The patient did not experience any harm or infection. In this case, there was the existence of a duty and a breach of duty, but the breach of duty did not cause any harm or injury to the patient. Therefore, if a malpractice action had been brought, the plaintiff would not receive an award. Nurses are encouraged to report medication and treatment errors as promptly as possible so that actions can be taken to prevent and/or minimize injury to the patient.

Damages. In civil cases, the remedy for the harm the patient suffered is money. The judge or jury will award the plaintiff money to compensate him for pain and suffering, lost wages, additional medical bills, and other losses. In some cases, the plaintiff may be awarded punitive damages (additional money) for grossly negligent or wrongful behavior by the healthcare provider.

Case: Damages

A 16-year-old pregnant female went into labor and was admitted to the hospital. She was diagnosed with a strep infection and an intravenous (IV) antibiotic was prescribed. The nurse mistakenly administered an epidural pain medication into the IV line. The patient began having seizures and

(Continued)

Case: Damages—cont'd

subsequently died; however, the baby was safely delivered by an emergency cesarean section. Several safeguards were in place to prevent medication errors, such as a computerized system that scans medications to ensure accuracy, and a bright pink label on the epidural pain medication warning against IV administration. A lawsuit was brought by the family (plaintiff) against the hospital and nurse (defendants).

Analysis of the case:

Duty: Based on the nurse–patient relationship

Breach of Duty: Administering an incorrect medication via the wrong route

Causation: Medication caused the female to have seizures and die.

Damages: In the above case, a settlement was reached with a present value of about $1.9 million.

(Frew, 2006; Nurses Service Organization [NSO], 2008b).

KnowledgeCheck 43-3

- Distinguish negligence from malpractice.
- Distinguish civil law from criminal law.
- Under which type of law (constitutional, statutory, administrative, or common law) does each of the following fall?
  A defendant claiming the right not to incriminate himself under the Fifth Amendment
  A nurse having her license revoked by the state board of nursing
  The wording of a state nurse practice act
- Define *plaintiff* and *defendant* in the context of civil law.

ThinkLike a Nurse 43-5

- Give one nursing example of each: negligence, malpractice, damages.
- Can you think of one nonfraudulent example of a nurse being untruthful with a patient? Do you think that the circumstances described in your example make the untruthfulness justifiable?
- Can you think of an example of a nurse committing assault, other than the one given in the text?

Vicarious Liability

You are legally accountable for your actions or inactions. This is a common legal principle that should guide your behavior. It means that you can be sued for behavior or omissions that deviate from acceptable standards. In certain circumstances, though, the law will assign liability to a person or entity that did not directly cause the injury, but with whom you have a specific kind of relationship (e.g., a physician or a hospital). This type of liability is known as **vicarious** or **substituted liability.** The various types of vicarious liability existing under common law are discussed below.

Captain of the Ship. This principle applies to situations where a physician (e.g., surgeon or obstetrician) is held liable for the negligence of another healthcare provider. *Captain of the Ship* usually applies to surgical suite situations. Many states no longer recognize it as protection for the nurse because the nurse is still liable for her own actions.

Borrowed Servant Doctrine. For situations involving liability for acts of a nonemployed worker, the *borrowed servant doctrine* relieves the primary employer of liability for the actions or omission of its employee when the employee was borrowed by another person. This would apply, for example, to agency nurses.

Respondeat Superior. The Latin term *respondeat superior* means "let the master answer." The employer must answer for the negligent acts or omissions of its employees who are functioning within the scope of their employment. For example, a nurse is working within the scope of her practice as a labor and delivery nurse but she makes a medication error; the hospital can be sued for the nurse's error.

KnowledgeCheck 43-4

- Define these terms: *assault, battery, fraud, slander, libel, negligence, malpractice.*
- State the four elements of malpractice.

LITIGATION IN CIVIL CLAIMS

Litigation is the formal process wherein the legal issues, rights, and duties between the parties are heard and decided (adjudicated). The litigation process follows several stages: (1) pleading and pretrial motions, (2) discovery, (3) alternative dispute resolution, (4) trial, and (5) appeal.

Pleading and Pretrial Motions

The litigation process starts when the plaintiff files a complaint. A **complaint** is a legal document outlining how the plaintiff has been harmed by another person. Once the case is filed with the court, the complaint is served on (delivered to) the defendant.

If you are served with a complaint, you must immediately notify your employer. In addition, if you have malpractice insurance, you must notify your insurance company. You will need an attorney to defend you. Your attorney has a specified time within which to file an "answer" to the complaint and address each of the *allegations* (unproven accusations). As a defendant, you should not contact the plaintiff or the plaintiff's attorney or discuss the case with coworkers or friends. Cooperate fully and be honest in all your answers. The facility's risk manager and your attorney will advise you.

Discovery Phase

The discovery process allows for both parties to gather facts and evidence about the case that can be used at trial. Discovery is designed to make sure there are no "surprises" during the trial. Attorneys may obtain discovery through written questions *(interrogatories),* requests for documents and other evidence, and by *depositions* (attorneys orally question parties to the lawsuit under oath, as though they were testifying in court). You may be deposed (questioned) as either a fact witness, a party to the lawsuit (defendant), or an expert witness. A *fact witness* is someone who was present when the incident occurred, whereas the defendant will testify as to the care provided and the actions taken.

Deposition may occur several years after the incident, so you may not remember specific information. You should prepare for the deposition by reviewing the medical records and any other evidence that may exist regarding the lawsuit. During the deposition, listen to your attorney, do not volunteer information, take your time before answering each question, and provide only objective information. Always tell the truth, but base your answers on facts; do not speculate. If your attorney objects to any question, immediately stop and do not provide an answer unless directed to do so by your attorney.

Alternative Dispute Resolution

Lawyers and involved parties usually try to resolve disputes before going to trial. The three most common methods of alternative dispute resolution are as follows:

- **Negotiation** takes place informally between the lawyers for the plaintiff and the defendant in an attempt to settle the case prior to trial.
- **Mediation** is the attempt to resolve the dispute using a neutral third party. The primary role of the mediator is to help the parties focus on the issues and to facilitate communication to identify what is needed to reach a resolution.
- **Arbitration** involves a third party making a decision after hearing the evidence and information from both parties.

Trial Process

If the dispute cannot be resolved and is not dismissed by the court during pretrial motions, the case goes to trial. Malpractice cases are usually heard by a jury. After hearing all the evidence and reviewing submitted documents, the judge or jury makes a decision, which is either dismissal or the award of damages.

Appeal

After the judge or jury has made a decision, either party has the opportunity to present post-trial motions, move for a new trial, or appeal the verdict and/or damages to an appeals court. The appeals court will review the transcript and documents from the trial and determine if a correct verdict (decision) was made.

KnowledgeCheck 43-5

- Identify the phases of the trial process.
- How is arbitration different from mediation?

PracticalKnowledge
knowing **how**

To decrease your chances of being involved in a malpractice suit, you should know the most common causes of malpractice claims and some practical preventive actions you can take. Keep in mind that causes are often difficult to categorize because they overlap; an error usually results from interlocking causes.

WHAT ARE THE MOST COMMON MALPRACTICE CLAIMS?

Nurses must use the nursing process to provide safe and efficient care to patients. The most common causes of nursing malpractice claims can be categorized according to where they fall in the nursing process; failure to assess and diagnose, failure to plan, failure to implement, and failure to evaluate (O'Keefe, 2001) (Box 43-3).

Failure to Assess and Diagnose

Failure to conduct an adequate assessment can lead to numerous breaches of duty. Failure to analyze the data and make correct nursing diagnoses can lead to incorrect or no actions.

> ### Case: Failure to Assess and Diagnose
>
> In an actual case, the healthcare provider's failure to properly diagnose and treat status asthmaticus, intubate the patient, properly sedate the patient, administer oxygen, administer the correct amounts of medication, and follow the hospital's protocols and standards of care resulted in the death of a 10-year-old child. A $3.5 million award of damages was made to the family (Nursing Service Organization [NSO], 2008a).

Safe and competent assessment and diagnosis practices require the nurse to do the following:

- Perform an admission assessment. This duty cannot be delegated to a nursing assistant.
- Analyze the assessment data to clearly identify problems.

BOX 43-3 ■ Common Causes of Malpractice Litigation

Failure to respond, such as not intervening to care for the patient's specific symptoms or expressed request for care.

Failure to educate, such as not answering questions, not teaching self-care measures, or not explaining procedures or equipment adequately on the patient's discharge.

Failure to follow standards of care and institutional policies and procedures. This most commonly occurs in the form of medication errors and failure to follow a provider's orders. It also frequently occurs from failure to use equipment responsibly. Among other reasons, a nurse may fail to follow standards of care when the unit is understaffed or the nurse is inexperienced.

Failure to communicate often comes up when a nurse fails to seek medical authorization for a treatment or fails to notify a physician in a timely manner when a patient's condition warrants action.

Failure to document the following in the patient's record: assessment data (e.g., drug allergies), patient injuries, medication administration details, patient progress and response to treatment, physicians' orders, and telephone conversations with physicians.

Failure to act as an advocate. Nurses must frequently intervene to prevent harm to the patient by other healthcare providers and by relatives and significant others. The following are examples of advocacy errors:

a. *Medical and discharge orders.* As an example of failure to advocate, suppose two physicians order the same drug for a patient, but under different brand names. The nurse does not recognize that two drugs are the same, so the patient receives twice the normal amount and has a toxic reaction. Other errors occur when the nurse does not question incomplete or illegible orders or does not question discharge orders when she believes the patient is not well enough to be discharged.

b. *Impaired nurses.* You have a duty under most state nursing practice acts to report impaired nursing practice (e.g., as a result of alcoholism or mental illness) to the appropriate licensing agency. Failure to do so is a failure to advocate for patients.

c. *Family and significant others.* Advocacy includes reporting neglect and intentional injuries to children, the elderly, and the disabled. Failure to do so may constitute negligence and/or violation of state statutes.

Clinical Insight 43-1 ➤ Tips for Avoiding Malpractice

- **Develop open, honest, respectful, caring relationships** with patients and families. Patients are less likely to sue if they feel that you were caring and professional. Angry patients who feel mistreated are more likely to bring suit.
- **Careful, thorough documentation** is the best defense if a lawsuit does occur:
  - Use and document all steps of the nursing process.
  - Be especially thorough when documenting care for patients who will not comply with treatments or who complain a lot.
  - Courts assume that if care is not documented, it was not given.
- **Know and follow applicable laws:** (1) federal and state laws, (2) your state's nurse practice act (perform only the activities within your scope of practice and competence).
- **Know and follow agency policies and procedures.**
- **Know and follow standards of care** set forth in the state nurse practice act, professional organizations, professional literature, agency policy, and so on.
- **Follow the "rights" of medication administration** (see Chapter 25).
- **Perform falls risk assessments,** document, and take measures to ensure patient safety.
- **Recognize "problem" patients.** Try to identify the basic problem or complaint and intervene to resolve it.
- **Follow medical orders,** but clarify them as needed. Do not implement a questionable order or one you do not understand.

- **Don't blame or criticize other healthcare providers** in the presence of patients (e.g., "Sorry you didn't get your pain medication. The night shift was a little short-staffed last night.")
- **Maintain patient privacy and confidentiality.**
- **Don't make statements that may appear to be an admission of guilt** (e.g., "Omigosh, I forgot to shut off that IV!"). Errors should not be included on the patient's health record, but instead recorded in an incident report.
- **Stay competent in your area of practice;** for example, attend continuing education and inservice programs to improve your knowledge and skills.
- **Don't accept a clinical assignment that you think you are not competent to perform.** Evaluate your assignment with your supervisor if there is a question.
- **Recognize significant assessment cues,** and notify primary care providers of changes in the patient's condition or patient complaints.
- **Document the time and content of telephone conversations with other healthcare providers.**
- **Send copies only,** never originals, of records and reports requested by other professionals.

Practice Resources

Aiken, 2004; Austin, 2008.

- Apply theoretical knowledge to ensure a correct diagnosis. The presenting signs and symptoms should be consistent with the disease process or medical problem. Remember that the nursing diagnosis consists of Patient Response related to Etiology. When the assessment reveals adverse symptoms, the nurse must report the symptoms to the appropriate provider and carry out the standard nursing care and prescribed interventions.
- Conduct frequent, focused assessments until the end of your shift or until the problem is resolved.

Failure to Plan

The American Nurses Association standards specifically require nurses to formulate a plan of care. The plan may be written or unwritten, depending on state regulations. Many agencies require nurses to complete nursing care plans or patient care tools as a means of measuring patient outcomes and progress. The plan of care should be consistent with standards of treatments acceptable for the given diagnosis or problem. Safe and competent practices in this category require the nurse to do the following:

- Know the correct approach to treat patient actual or potential problems.

- Have the theoretical knowledge base to successfully plan nursing care for patients.
- Develop a plan of care that is individualized to the patient.

Failure to Implement a Plan of Care

Implementation is the nursing process step in which the nurse performs the care or nursing interventions. Failure to implement encompasses a variety of actions, shown in Box 43-3, Common Causes of Malpractice Litigation.

Failure to Evaluate

Evaluation is the last step in the nursing process. It requires you to make a decision or judgment about the success of your interventions in addressing the client's problems. The duty to evaluate requires an ongoing cycle of the following:

- *Observing for changes* after interventions and treatments. You must know the expected outcomes and side effects of medications and treatments, so you can accurately interpret and document anticipated and adverse responses.
- *Recognizing significance of the change.* For example, if Mr. Adkins's blood pressure (BP) is usually 140/88 mm Hg, a change to 150/90 mm Hg after exercise would not be significant for him. But for Mrs. Jonas, whose BP is usually

100/64 mm Hg, a change to 150/90 mm Hg would be cause for concern.

- *Documenting or reporting symptoms* to the appropriate person. If a change is significant, you have a legal duty to report the change to the appropriate provider and to document this change in the appropriate medical record.
- *Following up on patient responses* to nursing interventions requires you to know the expected outcomes and side effects of medications and treatments.

KnowledgeCheck 43-6

- State the four requirements of the nurse's duty to assess.
- State four ways in which the nurse may fail to implement a plan of care.
- Give one example of the duty to advocate for a patient.
- List the four components of the nurse's legal duty to evaluate.

HOW CAN YOU MINIMIZE YOUR MALPRACTICE RISKS?

The best way to minimize your risk of malpractice is to practice in a safe and competent manner. You must have the appropriate body of theoretical knowledge for clinical practice, which you are already beginning to acquire. You should also be familiar with (1) your state's nurse practice act, (2) professional standards of practice, and (3) institutional policies and procedures. These provide the legal framework for your practice and help you to evaluate the quality of the care you deliver. Ignorance of the law and of practice standards is no excuse for failing to comply with the law, and it is no defense in a malpractice suit.

You may significantly reduce your risk exposures when you follow these three guidelines:

- Perform timely patient assessments and document your findings for every patient interaction.
- Communicate all changes in your patient's status to the primary healthcare provider and document those changes.
- Use the proper chain of command to ensure appropriate and timely care when the primary healthcare provider is not available ("Legal Liability: New Study," 2009; p. 21).

You will find discussion of other helpful suggestions in the remainder of this chapter. For more tips, see Clinical Insight 43-1.

If you would like to see the typical standards of care found in a nurse practice act,

Go to Chapter 43, **Tables, Boxes, Figures: ESG Box 43-3, Minimum Acceptable Standards of Care Required by a Typical State Nurse Practice Act,** on *DavisPlus*.

Use the Nursing Process and Follow Professional Standards of Care

The nursing process provides you with a systematic approach to patient care and is the legally acceptable model of decision making in nursing practice. Your documentation should reveal that you have assessed, diagnosed, planned, implemented, and evaluated care based on current and acceptable standards.

Avoid Medication and Treatment Errors

Medication errors are among the most common healthcare errors. To accurately administer medications, you must know the rationale for administering the drug, safe dosage ranges, side effects of the medications, and relevant information to teach the patient about the medication. To prevent medication errors, you should do the following:

- Follow the "rights of medication administration" (see Chapter 25).
- Investigate any patient concerns before giving the medication (e.g., the patient might say, "Is this a new medication? I have not taken this one before.")
- Question prescriptions that are incomplete or that seem inappropriate.
- Make sure the equipment used to administer drugs is working properly.
- Use the correct technique to provide patient treatment (e.g., failure to maintain a sterile field during wound care could lead to an infection).

For tips to help you use equipment properly and safely, refer to Clinical Insight 43-2.

Report and Document

For every suggestion for minimizing malpractice risk, add the reminder: "Document what happened." Remember the old adage: "If it isn't documented, it wasn't done." If you are ever required to appear in court the patient record may be the only proof you have of the care you gave. It is unlawful to make false entries or destroy entries in medical records, but do carefully record in detail all care you provide.

Charting

A basic principle of charting is that a third person should be able to read your documentation and form a mental picture of your patient and the care provided during your shift. Record all interactions with clients, as well as patients' refusal of or noncompliance with treatment. Document telephone conversations with primary care providers, including time, content of the conversation and the action you took. Document the facts;

Clinical Insight 43-2 ➤ Using Equipment Safely

The following will help you to ensure proper and safe use of equipment:

1. Obtain appropriate training on equipment use.
2. Follow the healthcare agency's protocols, policies, and procedures on the use of the equipment.
3. Follow the manufacturer's operating instructions.
4. Be sure medical equipment has been properly inspected.
5. Perform safety checks regularly and before use.

6. Position and use equipment properly during treatment.
7. Know how the equipment functions; be alert to signs that it is not working properly.
8. Make sure rooms are not cluttered with equipment.
9. Follow agency policies regarding equipment brought from the patient's home (e.g., hair dryers, electric shavers, radios); usually these should be inspected for proper grounding and safe cords.

Toward Evidence-Based Practice

Snyder, E. K. (2008, October). Psych: No fall-risk assessment done, negligence found. *Legal Eagle Eye Newsletter for the Nursing Profession, 16(10), 8.*

A 57-year-old woman was admitted for inpatient psychiatric care for suicidal ideation. The day before hospitalization she had fallen and fractured her right tibia and fibula. The nurses admitting the patient marked through the risk assessment and fall precautions section of the admission nursing assessment form with letters "N.A.," signifying the risk assessment and fall precautions were not relevant to the care of this patient. Yet her other nursing documentation noted the patient's unsteady gait, muscle weakness, confused mental state, and poor judgment. While hospitalized, the patient reportedly awoke during the night and alerted the nurse for help to the restroom. When she got no response, she attempted to get up on her own and fell. The jury in the Supreme Court, Richmond County, New York awarded her $598,000 for negligence of the nurse.

Cifelli v. St. Vincent's, 2008 WL 4093163 (Sup. Ct. Richmond Co., N.Y., July 17, 2008).

1. The nurse noted the client to be unsteady on her feet, weak, confused, and making poor judgments. What do you think was the basis for the court decision that the patient's injury was due to negligence of the nurse?

Snyder, E. K. (2006, April). Falls: Court finds substandard precautions. Negligence found. *Legal Eagle Eye Newsletter for the Nursing Profession, 14(4), 8.*

The New York Supreme Court, Appellate Division, made note that the elderly patient had right-sided weakness, dementia, psychosis, and aphasia and was on multiple medications. After this patient had fallen numerous times during unassisted ambulation, the nurse reminded him repeatedly to ring the call bell and wait for assistance. The court ruled the nurse did not properly evaluate the patient's risk of falling in light of his medical history, medications, prior falls, and the fact that additional safeguards other than simple verbal reminders are necessary to ensure the patient's safety. Negligence was found.

Hranek v. United Methodist Homes, __ N.Y.S.2d __, 2006 WL 560208 (N.Y. App., March 9, 2006).

2. In this case, what was the basis for the court decision that the patient's injury was due to negligence of the nurse?

Snyder, E. K. (2006, June). Patient falls while nurses were busy with another patient: Court finds negligence. *Legal Eagle Eye Newsletter for the Nursing Profession, 14(6), 6.*

The patient, Mrs. McLaughlin, was admitted to an inpatient psychiatric facility for electroconvulsive therapy (ECT) as treatment of depression. Side effects of ECT can include headaches, memory difficulties, confusion, and hallucinations. In addition, the patient had a history of osteoarthritis, scoliosis, and Parkinson's disease that also make a falls-risk assessment appropriate while receiving hospital care. The psychiatrist ordered a vest restraint because the patient was combative with staff and hallucinating. The patient's antidepressant was increased and an anti-hallucinogen was added.

Meanwhile, another patient was admitted to the psychiatric unit who was in a highly agitated state. Nursing staff on the unit provided care to the newly admitted man with paranoid schizophrenia, leaving Mrs. McLaughlin unattended in her room. During this time she suffered a fall. No one had checked on Mrs. McLaughlin since the man was brought into the unit, although they were required to do so every 15 minutes.

The nurses were clearly aware of their duty toward the patient, who was in a highly confused state and had hallucinated for the past several days. She was at high risk for falling. The Court of Appeals of Ohio ruled that the hospital's psychiatric specialty nurses were negligent and that their negligence was the legal cause behind the patient's injuries resulting from a fall.

McLaughlin v. Firelands Community Hosp, 2006 WL 1047499 (Ohio App., April 21, 2006)

3. In the case in which the nurse was caring for a patient at high risk for falls but got busy taking care of another patient at the time of the fall, what was the basis for the court decision that the patient's death was due to negligence of the nurse?

4. In retrospect, what could the nurse have done differently to protect the patient from injury?

 Go to Chapter 43, **Toward Evidence-Based Practice Suggested Responses,** on Davis*Plus*.

---

do not editorialize (e.g., do not write, "I could not check on the patient as often as ordered because we were understaffed"). Refer to Chapter 18 for a review of your documentation responsibilities. When charting, use the letters F-A-C-T as a reminder that information must be factual, accurate, complete, and timely. Also refer to Clinical Insight 43-3 for guidelines to help you document patient care.

Incident Reports

If a standard of care is breached or an unusual incident occurs (e.g., a visitor or patient falls or is injured), you should complete an **incident report** (also called *variance report* or *occurrence report*). These reports are used, in part, for quality improvement in the agency and should not be used to discipline staff members or be placed in employees' files. The goal is to prevent the incident

Clinical Insight 43-3 ➤ Guidelines for Documenting Care

To be accurate and complete, your reporting and documentation of patient care must address the following:
1. Patient status (e.g., symptoms and responses to treatments)
2. The nursing care given
3. Physician, advance practice nurse, dentist, and podiatrist prescriptions
4. Medications and treatments
5. Patient responses
6. Consultations with other members of the healthcare team regarding patient status

You might find helpful the FACT mnemonic for documenting care. When documenting care, you must be:

F— Factual: Don't chart your opinions; chart facts.

A—Accurate: For example, record the vital signs accurately.

C—Complete: Don't omit any important information.

T—Timely: Chart care as soon as possible after doing it; don't wait until the end of your shift and then try to remember everything that happened.

Another way to remember how to document is to use the 5 Cs.

Charting should be:

Complete
Clear
Correct
Comprehensive
Chronological

Reference

Helm, A. (2003). *Nursing malpractice: Sidestepping legal minefields.* Philadelphia: Lippincott, Williams & Wilkins, pp. 1–33.

---

from occurring again. In some states, an incident report must be made available as a part of discovery in litigation. In other states, only the chart may be subpoenaed. However, in those states if the incident report is mentioned in the chart, the otherwise confidential report may be used as evidence. Therefore, do not write "Incident report completed" in the patient record.

When reporting an incident, be sure to clearly identify the patient, date, time, and location. Briefly describe the incident in factual terms. Use the exact words of the patient or persons involved and put the information in quotes. Do not speculate, draw conclusions, or place blame. Identify any witnesses to the event or equipment involved.

For example:

1900 Demerol 50 mg given intramuscularly. Physician order: Demerol 15 mg.

1930 Patient's respirations: 8 breaths/min; BP 100/60 mm Hg; skin pale.

2000 Called Dr. Smith. Orders for naloxone (Narcan) 1 mg IV STAT

2005 Narcan given as ordered. Resp 12 breaths/min, BP 118/70 mm Hg

You should be prepared to discuss the 30-minute delay between the patient's findings and contacting the physician. The standard of care would require that the physician be notified immediately. Chapter 18 presents additional information on occurrence reports.

Obtain Informed Consent

Informed consent is the permission for any and all types of care, given by the patient with full knowledge of the risks, benefits, costs, and alternatives. For hospital admission and for invasive or specialized treatments or diagnostic procedures, the consent must be written and signed by the patient or the person legally responsible for the patient. The law provides for implied or assumed consent in emergency situations; therefore, written consent is not necessary in an emergency if experts would agree that there was an immediate threat to life or health.

Elements of Consent

To be legally valid, the informed consent should fulfill the following requirements:

- **Completeness.** Healthcare consumers need a great deal of information to make educated decisions. Be sure they get all the information needed to make decisions regarding the treatment. This includes the nature of the procedure, risks, benefits, post-procedure care and considerations, and alternatives.

- **Clarity and Comprehension.** Language should be appropriate to the patient's educational level, so the patient (or his surrogate decision maker) can understand the explanation. Always ask the patient to describe in his own words the procedure to which he is consenting. If the patient asks, "What will the doctor do during surgery?" the nurse is aware that the patient does not understand the nature of the surgery. She could contact the surgeon.

- **Voluntariness.** The patient must be free to accept or reject the treatment. He must not be pressured or coerced to give consent. There must be no actual or implied threat by anyone to force the patient into having the surgery (e.g., "Mom, if you don't let them do this, I'm never coming back to see you."). Otherwise, the consent is not valid.

- **Competence.** The person must have the ability to understand the information and make a choice about the particular situation (e.g., the ability to decide what clothing to wear does not necessarily mean that the person is competent to decide whether to have surgery). If the person is confused and disoriented, you should contact the case manager or your supervisor for guidance. State law identifies the order of individuals who can make decisions for individuals who are judged incompetent. It is usually the spouse, then parents, then sisters and brothers, and so on. If the person does not have relatives, the court will appoint a legal guardian to make healthcare decisions.

Generally speaking, a competent adult has the legal right to consent to or refuse any treatment. However, this right does

not always extend to situations where an adult is making the decision for a minor. A court sometimes will authorize treatment of a child against his parents' wishes. In some states, a minor who is married or living independently is considered emancipated and can make his/her own healthcare decisions.

The Nurse's Role

As a nurse, your legal role regarding written consent is to collaborate with the primary provider, usually a physician or advanced practice nurse. You may witness a patient's signature on a consent form, but you are not legally responsible for explaining the treatments and options, or for evaluating whether the provider has adequately explained them. You must, however, determine that the elements of a valid informed consent are in place, communicate the patient's needs for more information to the care provider, and provide feedback if the patient wishes to change her consent.

Be sure you have the patient's informal, verbal consent for nursing interventions that you perform (e.g., urinary catheterization). Coming to the agency for healthcare implies that the patient consents to usual treatment, such as injections and vital signs. However, you should explain all procedures to the patient before their implementation. If the patient objects, identify the reasons for the refusal, correct any misinformation, and explain the benefits of the treatment. If the patient still objects or refuses, do not proceed and contact the primary care provider.

In addition to state statutes, case law, and agency policy, The Joint Commission standards provide valuable guidance regarding informed participation in decision making. See Chapter 42 for discussion of informed consent from an ethical perspective.

Maintain Patient Safety

Falls are by far the most common incident reported in hospitals and long-term care facilities. On admissions to the facility, all patients should be assessed for risks of falls and "fall precautions" instituted when needed. Simply raising the siderails on the bed is not enough to prevent falls. You may still be found negligent if the patient falls because he called for help and no one came to assist him out of bed, or if the call bell was not placed within the patient's reach and he was unable to call for assistance. Several useful tools have been developed for assessing falls, including the Morse Fall Scale. See Chapter 23 for information about meeting patients' safety needs, including falls and use of restraints. For a falls risk assessment tool,

 Go to Chapter 23, **Tables, Boxes, Figures: ESG Figure 23-1,** on Davis*Plus*.

Maintain Confidentiality and Privacy

Always maintain patient confidentiality unless directed by law to do otherwise (e.g., when a patient is threatening to harm someone). Family members and significant others do not have an automatic right to information about the patient. For example, parents do not have an automatic right to see the medical records of their child if that child is married and/or declared legally competent to make independent decisions. Of course, you need to discuss clients' medical conditions with other health team members, but this does not include chatting about the client's personal life or talking about the patient in the lunchroom. The general nursing principle is that you should discuss the patient's health status with those who have a need to know (those involved in the patient's care).

Another aspect of privacy is to maintain the confidentiality of patient records (e.g., do not leave a patient's health record in locations that are accessible to visitors or nonauthorized staff). Do not give information about patients over the phone unless the agency has a system that enables you to know you are speaking to a person authorized by the patient. Refer to Chapter 44 if you require advice about maintaining confidentiality of electronic records. Also, refer to Clinical Insight 18-3, Guidelines for Documenting in the Electronic Health Record, in Chapter 18.

Provide Education and Counseling

Part of your role as a nurse is to provide information to patients and caregivers about their illness, medications, and other treatments. This helps to fulfill informed consent requirements and to involve patients in their own healthcare. Use teaching-learning principles to make sure the patient understands, retains the knowledge, and can demonstrate any skills. Ask the patient to repeat instructions to you or to provide a return demonstration of a skill, such as self-injection of insulin. To reinforce understanding, always review written information with the patient.

Assign, Delegate, and Supervise According to Guidelines

As a nurse, you are expected to make assignments and delegate tasks to ensure patients receive timely and quality care. To do this safely, you must know the education background, knowledge, experience, and physical and emotional capability of those to whom you delegate. In addition, you must consider the condition and requirements of the patient. For example, it would be negligent to assign a practical nurse to care for a patient on a ventilator without checking to ensure that the nurse has had training and experience with such patients.

The duty to delegate has a corresponding duty to supervise the care. For example, if you assign an aide to take vital signs, you must check periodically to see that the vital signs are taken, accurately reported, and recorded. If you need to review specific guidelines for delegating, see Chapter 7. For the ANA and other relevant Web sites,

 Go to Chapter 43, **Resources for Caregivers and Health Professionals,** on Davis*Plus*.

Accept Assignments for Which You Are Qualified

As a nurse, when you accept an assignment, you must consider whether the assignment is within your level of education, experience, and physical and emotional capability. The refusal to accept an assignment does not mean that you have abandoned the patient. Your duty to the patient begins once you accept the assignment. Remember the general principle that you are legally responsible for the assignment that you accept. If your assignment becomes overwhelming and unmanageable, immediately contact the charge nurse or nursing supervisor for assistance.

Nursing supervisors have a duty to ensure adequate staffing and patient coverage. This means that you must report to the nurse in charge when leaving the patient care unit. Failure to do this may result in charges of patient abandonment. A nurse should never leave the patient care unit without making certain there is another nurse available to provide care to the patient. This does not mean that you must work overtime (e.g., a double shift), as long as you follow established policies and procedures, which will include giving notice and explaining your reasoning (e.g., that you are too fatigued to provide safe care).

If you work a double shift or if a unit is understaffed, you are still liable for any malpractice that you commit. Unfortunately, being "busy" and overwhelmed is not a defense for error. In addition, you have the duty to tell supervisors that staffing is inadequate; be sure to do it in writing. You should know and follow agency policy on how to address short-staff issues.

Participate in Continuing Education

As a nurse, you have a duty to participate in ongoing education in your area of practice and to keep up with new laws, equipment, treatments, and procedures. Be sure to obtain documentation of your attendance. In some states, continuing education is mandatory for relicensure. In states where it is not mandatory, other standards of care still require that you obtain the education and training necessary to implement current nursing procedures and practices. In malpractice cases, the nurse's competency in providing nursing care is frequently an issue. Continuing education is available "for credit" through colleges and universities, other healthcare agencies, conferences, in some nursing journals (e.g., *The American Journal of Nursing*), and online.

Observe Professional Boundaries

Nurses must be careful to maintain professional boundaries, not only with the patient but also with other healthcare providers. Do not accept gifts from vulnerable patients or encourage attempts to have close personal relationships outside the healthcare setting. Violations of professional boundaries may be physical, sexual, emotional, or financial in nature. Cues to possible overstepped boundaries are listed in Box 43-4.

If you would like more specific information on professional boundaries,

 Go to the National Council on State Boards of Nursing Web site at https://www.ncsbn.org/ ProfessionalBoundariesbrochure.pdf.

BOX 43-4 ■ Potential Boundary Violations Between Nurse and Client

Excessive Self-Disclosure—Discussing personal problems or intimate details with the client

Flirtation—Communication that is sexual in nature or reveals personal attraction between client and nurse

Secretive Behavior—When the nurse is defensive or guarded about the interaction between client and nurse

"Super Nurse" Attitude—The nurse that acts as though she is the only one who understands and can meet the client's needs

Excessive Attention to Client—When the nurse spends an unusually greater amount of time with a particular client than is required by his needs; personal gifts, off-duty visits, or trading assignments are signs of boundary violation

Unclear Communication—When only part of the story is told with client care. The client might repeatedly seek out the nurse, even when not assigned to his care.

Source: Used with permission from: National Council of State Boards of Nursing (NCSBN). (n.d.). Professional boundaries: A nurse's guide to the importance of appropriate professional boundaries. Retrieved January 19, 2012, from https://www.ncsbn.org/ ProfessionalBoundariesbrochure.pdf

Sexual Harassment. Be aware of and report the behaviors of staff members who commit sexual harassment. **Sexual harassment** involves the use of power over people lower in the power structure of the organization. It is defined as "unwelcome sexual advances, requests for sexual favors, and other verbal or physical conduct of a sexual nature" if submission (1) is a condition of employment, (2) interferes with job performance, (3) is the basis for employment decisions, or (4) creates a hostile and intimidating work environment (EEOC, 2002, modified 2009).

If you witness or experience sexual harassment, your first step is to consult the agency's sexual harassment policy. Every agency receiving federal funding must have such a policy in place. It will tell you how to file a grievance, what forms you need to use, to whom the incident is reported, and what the procedure is for hearing and resolution.

Observe Mandatory Reporting Regulations

As noted earlier in the chapter, most states have laws requiring the nurse to report communicable diseases, known or suspected abuse of patients, and impaired or unsafe professional practice. When you observe violations of the state's licensing regulations, you have a professional and legal responsibility to report them to the appropriate authority. The "authority" varies among states; it may be your immediate supervisor, the board of nursing, or a peer assistance program, often sponsored by the state nurses association. See the section Mandatory Reporting Laws, earlier in the chapter. Also see the following discussion regarding impaired nurses.

Impaired Nurses

Nurses who come to work under the influence of alcohol or mind-altering substances pose a danger to the health, safety, and welfare of the patients. You have a legal obligation to protect patients from impaired nurses. Always pay attention to the possibility of a coworker using or stealing narcotics. Impaired nurses account for a major percentage of disciplinary actions against nurses. For example, the Kansas Board of Nursing reported that in a 2-year period, 325 cases were investigated that involved substance abuse by nurses. Of these cases, 72% involved drug use, 22% alcohol abuse, and 6% involved a combination of both alcohol and drugs (Sidlinger & Hornberger, 2008). See Box 43-5 for signs of chemical dependence in the workplace. To determine the magnitude of the problem in your state, go to the state board of nursing's Web site and click on *disciplinary actions*.

Unauthorized Practice

Your employer will require you to submit verification of current licensure in the state where you are working. If your license expires and you continue to practice nursing, you can be charged with unauthorized practice of nursing. You must report the unauthorized practice of nursing, which means reporting persons practicing nursing without a proper license. In addition, you must know the scope of practice for LPNs/LVNs and nursing assistive personnel to ensure that they practice within their professional boundaries. For example, unlicensed personnel cannot perform the initial patient assessment on a newly admitted patient.

Abuse and Communicable Diseases

State laws also require you to report known or suspected child, elder, and spousal abuse, and communicable disease. Because state laws may vary, you need to be familiar with them in order to know what and to whom to report in your area. If you are

BOX 43-5 ■ Signs of Potential Chemical Dependence in the Workplace

Absenteeism
- Frequent unscheduled absences with improbable excuses
- Frequent late arrivals or early departures
- Absences after payday or days off
- Higher than average absences for cold, flu, and minor illnesses

Absent "On the Job"
- Long shift breaks
- "Locked door syndrome" (excessively long use of restroom)
- Frequent visits to Occupational Health Services for illness on the job

Difficulty Concentrating
- Errors, particularly involving medication or with taking and transcribing verbal orders
- Omitted, illogical, incomplete, or illegible charting
- Taking more time to carry out assignments than is expected given the nurse's skill and experience
- Deterioration of handwriting during the shift
- Overlooking the signs of patient's deteriorating condition

Inconsistent Work Patterns
- Alternating periods of high and low efficiency
- Minimal or substandard work compared to that of peers
- Frequent requests for help with patient assignments

Physical or Emotional Problems
- Nervousness, excessive sweating, tremors of the hands
- Physical or emotional condition changes during shift
- Deteriorating personal appearance, grooming, and hygiene

Decreasing Efficiency
- Omitting treatments; making bad decisions; showing poor judgment related to patient care
- Requests to be changed to a less supervised shift

Poor Relationships on the Job
- Mood swings, from isolation to angry outbursts
- Uncooperativeness
- Avoidance of contact with supervisors
- Patient complaints of irritability, roughness, or verbal abuse
- Lethargy and hyperactivity
- Emotional hypersensitivity

Medication-Centered Problems
- Excessive use of PRN psychoactive medications or narcotics recorded for patients
- Increased waste or breakage of controlled substances
- Missing drugs, unaccounted-for doses
- Omission of dates or times from narcotic sign-out sheets
- Patient complaints about lack of pain relief

Personal Life Interferes with Job
- Frequent or excessively long phone calls
- Visitors or unexplained errands during work shift
- Legal problems
- Increased number of accidents

Source: Georgia Nurses Association. (n.d.). Nurse Advocate Program. Checklist for detecting potential chemical dependence in an employee. Retrieved January 19, 2012, from http://www.georgianurses.org/impaired_nurse.htm#pabi

---

working for a healthcare agency when you suspect abuse, always report it to your supervisor. If you need to review signs of abuse, refer to Procedure 9-1, Assessing for Abuse, in Chapter 9.

Other Safeguards for Nurses

In addition to the Good Samaritan laws and the ANA Bill of Rights for Registered Nurses (previously discussed), safe harbor laws and professional liability insurance offer some legal protection for nurses.

Safe Harbor Laws

Safe harbor laws, found in the Nurse Practice Act or other state laws, provide for exceptions to certain laws. They protect you from being suspended, terminated, disciplined, or discriminated against for refusing to do (or not do) something you believe would be harmful to a patient. Under these laws, you also have a right to ask for peer review of either the situation or directives that you believe would violate the nursing practice act. You must follow the guidelines required under the safe harbor provisions.

Case: Prepping a Patient for a Surgical Procedure

The nurse could not find documentation of informed consent in the patient's medical record. Knowing her legal role in informed consent, she refused to assist with treatment of the patient, who had not given informed consent. Safe harbor laws protected her from dismissal for denying the surgeon's request for her to obtain it.

Professional Liability Insurance

If you are sued for malpractice, the insurance company pays for the attorney's fees and for any judgment or settlement, up to the limits. You should carefully review your insurance policy because most insurance policies have **exclusions** (items not covered by the policy). If the patient's claim arises out of excluded activities, the insurance company will not pay for the costs of litigation and damages. The following are examples of exclusions:
- Sexual abuse of a patient, assault and battery, and other intentional torts
- Injury caused while the nurse is under the influence of drugs or alcohol
- Criminal activity
- Transmission of acquired immunodeficiency syndrome (AIDS) from the nurse to a patient
- Actions that can lead to an award of punitive damages (damages awarded to punish the defendant for egregious acts or omissions)

Types of Coverage

There are two types of malpractice coverage. **Occurrence-type insurance** is most often recommended for nurses, because this policy covers malpractice claims for any injury or damage that occurred during the time the policy was in force, regardless of when the claim was reported and the lawsuit occurred. In contrast, **claims-made insurance** covers only those claims in which the negligent action or omission occurred and the claim was filed or reported during the policy period. To maintain coverage under a claims-made policy after it has lapsed or

been canceled, some insurers will offer "tail" insurance. You should consult an attorney to decide which type of policy is best for you.

As a rule, if you work for a hospital or other institution, you will be covered by the institution's insurance. However, it covers you only while you are working within the scope of your employment. For example, you would not be covered during the one day a week that you volunteer at a free clinic. Some legal experts recommend that you purchase individual liability insurance in addition to the coverage provided by your employer. Again, consult a lawyer before making a decision.

ThinkLike a Nurse 43-6

Susan, an RN, was employed by Landold Nursing Service and assigned to Alvalup Hospital from June 1, 2012 to May 30, 2013. Susan carried her own professional liability claims-made policy during this time. She decided to attend real estate school and not renew her policy. On August 10, 2008, a medical malpractice claim was filed against Susan.

■ Based on this scenario, would Susan have coverage under her policy? What kind of policy would she have to obtain in order to be protected from a claim made against her?

Student Responsibilities

As a student, you are held to the same standards of care as are licensed nurses. You must be familiar not only with your state's standards of practice, but also with the policies and procedures in the agency in which you have your clinical experiences. Your instructor is responsible for making assignments that are within your competence and for providing clinical supervision. However, this does not release you from your own legal responsibilities. To help protect yourself and your patients:

■ Prepare carefully for each clinical experience.
■ Never attempt a procedure or make a judgment about which you feel unsure. If you lack the theoretical or practical

knowledge for an assignment, notify your clinical instructor immediately.
■ Notify your instructor or a staff nurse if your patient's condition changes significantly.
■ Unless otherwise arranged, take instructions only from your clinical instructor.

Your nursing school may require you to carry personal professional liability insurance. The school's policy will cover you only for the nursing care you give in your educational experiences. If you work, for example, as an aide, the school's policy will not provide coverage for you at work. Furthermore, you are legally permitted to perform only the procedures contained in your job description. For example, even though you administer injections in your student role, you are not licensed to do so in your role as an aide.

SUMMARY

Ethical and legal issues are a major source of conflict for nursing practice. This chapter discusses only the legal aspects of the major issues. See Chapter 42 for ethical considerations. It is important to be clear in your mind that what is legal and what is ethical are not always the same thing. On the one hand, an act may be legal (e.g., abortion) even though you may consider it unethical. On the other hand, you may believe an action (e.g., assisted suicide) is ethically necessary, but the law may forbid it. You should be aware of the legal consequences that your ethical decisions may bring about.

For a more detailed discussion of some major legal issues in nursing (e.g., stem cell research, cloning, reproductive issues, life-sustaining medical treatment),

 Go to Chapter 43, **Supplemental Materials: What are the Major Legal Issues in Nursing Practice?** on Davis*Plus.*

CLINICALREASONING
Applying the **Full-Spectrum Nursing Model**

Because the following critical thinking activities allow you to practice the kind of thinking you will use as a full-spectrum nurse, they usually have no single right answer. Discuss them with your peers—if you have difficulty with any of the questions, consult your instructor.

PATIENT SITUATION

A nurse employed by a temporary agency is assigned to a neurology unit for a 12-hour shift. On arrival, she discovers that the registered nurse assigned for the shift called in sick, leaving her with two nursing assistive personnel (NAPs) to provide patient care and administer medication, including controlled substances. The nursing supervisor informs her that she will be responsible for the unit with 22 patients, 12 of whom are acutely ill and require close observation and frequent care. The nursing supervisor is not available to work on the unit and has no additional RNs to provide patient care. The nurse decides not to accept the assignment, to report the decision and reasons to her agency supervisor, and to leave the neurology unit immediately before starting the shift.

THINKING

1. *Theoretical Knowledge:*
   a. In addition to protecting her nursing license, what other factors should the nurse have considered in deciding whether to stay or leave the unit?
   b. Because the nurse decided not to accept the assignment, would this have been considered as abandonment?
   c. What standards, guidelines, and laws would apply to determine whether the nurse's behavior was in accordance with standards of practice?

(continued on next page)

2. *Critical Thinking (Contextual Awareness):*
   a. Which statements in the ANA Bill of Rights for Nurses should the nurse have considered before deciding whether to accept the assignment?
   b. What factors in this situation could create legal problems for the nurse?

DOING

3. *Nursing Process (Planning/Intervention):* The nurse's action (leaving the unit) might be viewed, under some laws in some situations, as abandonment of patients. What are some alternative actions the nurse might have taken to avoid that risk?

CARING

4. *Self-Knowledge:* Have you ever been in a situation where you felt a moral obligation to help out but yet knew you would be in over your head? Describe your experience.

5. *Ethical Knowledge:* In your opinion, did the nurse do the right thing when she decided not to accept the assignment and to leave the nursing unit immediately? Explain your thinking.

 Go To Chapter 43, **Clinical Reasoning: Applying the Full-Spectrum Nursing Model Response Sheet,** on Davis*Plus*.

 To explore learning resources for this chapter,

 Go to DavisPlus at http://davisplus.fadavis.com/ keyword Treas

Chapter Resources for Chapter 43:
   Knowledge Check and Think Like a Nurse Response Sheets
   Knowledge Check Answers
   Resources for Caregivers and Health Professionals
   Reading More About Legal Issues (Suggested Readings)
   What Are the Main Points in This Chapter?
NCLEX-Style Review Questions
Chapter Overview Podcasts

Concept Map

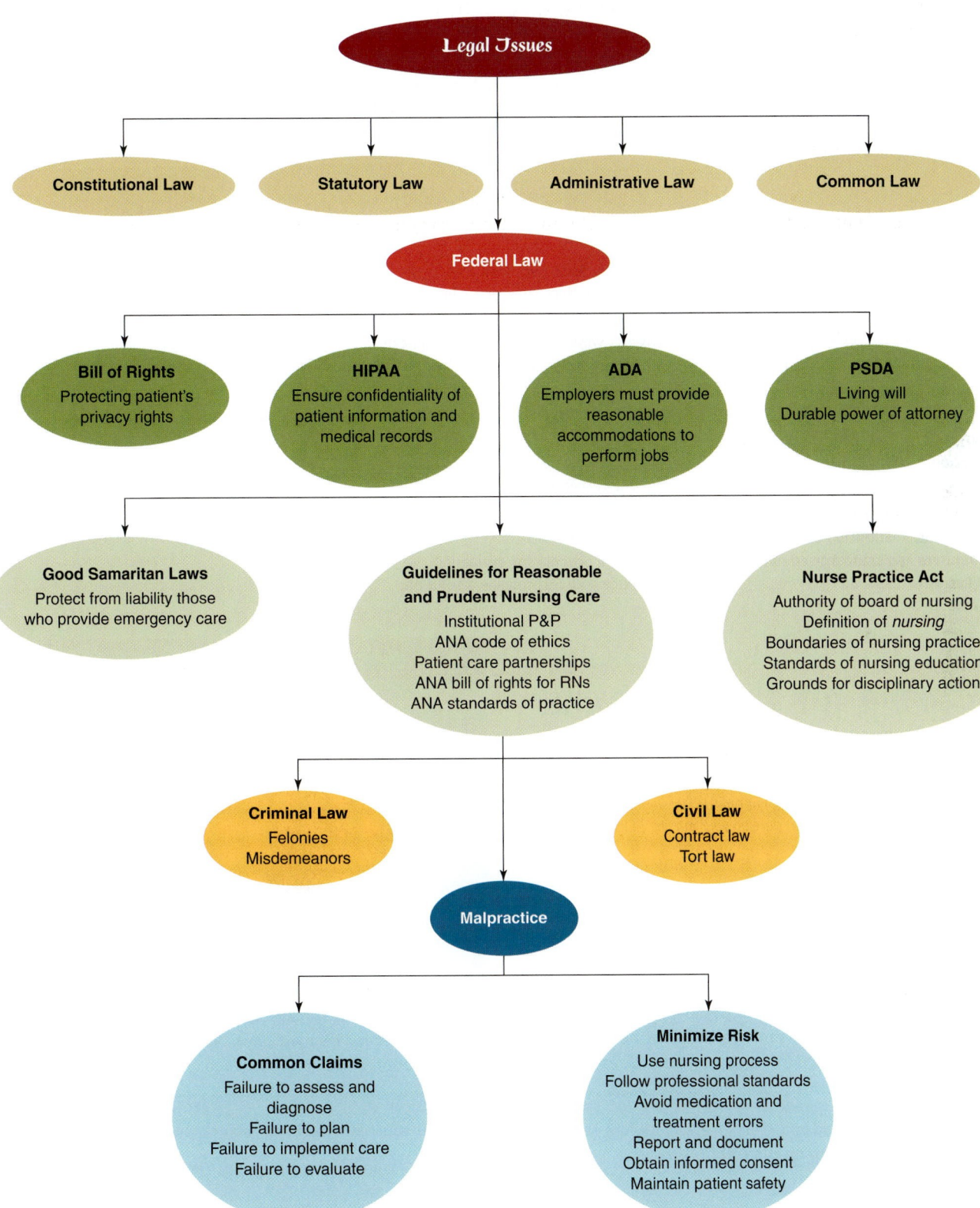

Legal Issues

- Constitutional Law
- Statutory Law
- Administrative Law
- Common Law

Federal Law

Bill of Rights
Protecting patient's privacy rights

HIPAA
Ensure confidentiality of patient information and medical records

ADA
Employers must provide reasonable accommodations to perform jobs

PSDA
Living will
Durable power of attorney

Good Samaritan Laws
Protect from liability those who provide emergency care

Guidelines for Reasonable and Prudent Nursing Care
Institutional P&P
ANA code of ethics
Patient care partnerships
ANA bill of rights for RNs
ANA standards of practice

Nurse Practice Act
Authority of board of nursing
Definition of *nursing*
Boundaries of nursing practice
Standards of nursing education
Grounds for disciplinary action

Criminal Law
Felonies
Misdemeanors

Civil Law
Contract law
Tort law

Malpractice

Common Claims
Failure to assess and diagnose
Failure to plan
Failure to implement care
Failure to evaluate

Minimize Risk
Use nursing process
Follow professional standards
Avoid medication and treatment errors
Report and document
Obtain informed consent
Maintain patient safety

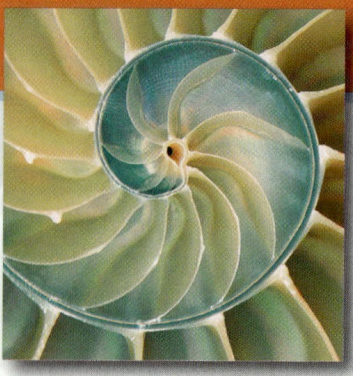
Nursing Informatics

Learning Outcomes

After completing this chapter, you should be able to:

- ➤ Define *informatics* and its four components.
- ➤ Describe the importance of computers in evidence-based nursing practice.
- ➤ Discuss the benefits of the electronic health record.
- ➤ Discuss the impact of legislative efforts to encourage electronic health record adoption.
- ➤ Describe the importance of protecting personal health information.
- ➤ Explain the relationship between computers and standardized nursing languages.

- ➤ Identify at least two ways that automation decreases error in healthcare.
- ➤ Discuss ways that computerization can increase the risk for error in healthcare.
- ➤ Explain how computers can reduce some of the barriers to evidence-based practice.
- ➤ Identify at least four online sources of nursing research.
- ➤ Describe the process of literature database searching.
- ➤ Outline a process for evaluating evidence and determining a solution.

Key Concepts

Electronic Communication

Informatics

Healthcare Technology

Related Concepts

See the Concept Map at the end of this chapter.

Caring for the Nguyens

This feature allows you to practice the kind of thinking you will use as a full-spectrum nurse. There is usually more than one correct answer to a critical thinking question, so we do not provide answers for these features. It is more important to develop your nursing judgment than to "cover content." Discuss the questions with your peers. If you are still unsure, consult your instructor.

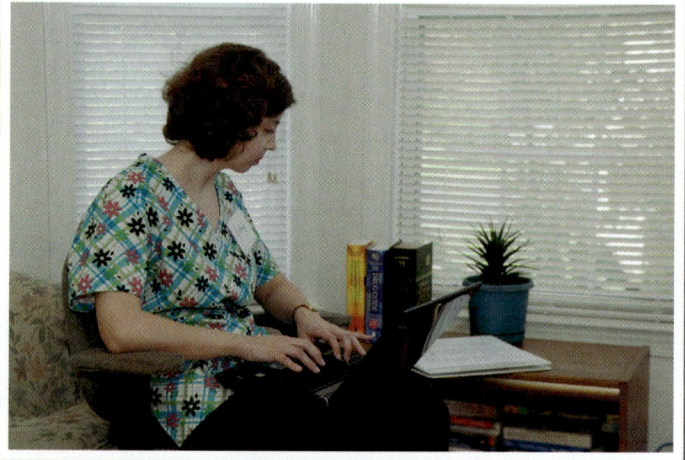

Nam Nguyen, a patient you have been caring for at the Family Medicine Center, has been devastated by his recent diagnoses of type 2 diabetes mellitus and hypertension. "Oh my, this is bad. This stuff kills you. I don't understand what I did to cause this," he sighs. He is having difficulty following his medication regimen and says he doesn't understand what he is supposed to do. You have supplied him with information at each of his clinic visits as well as handouts, medication information, and a reminder sheet for his medicines. Nam asks you if there is any information available on the Web.

A. What advice would you give him about looking up medical information on the Web?

B. What sources would you recommend to Nam?

 Go to **Caring for the Nguyens Response Sheet** on *DavisPlus.*

Meet Your Nurse Role Model

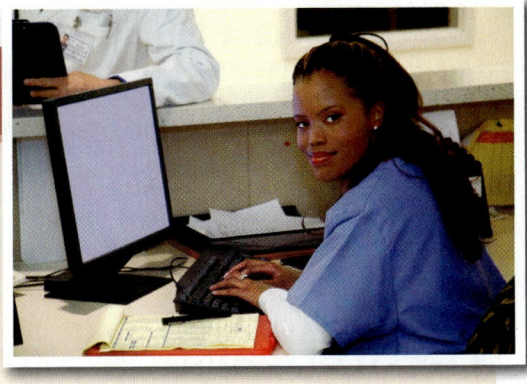

Six week ago, Ted Samuels, 67 years old and a business executive, began experiencing headaches, occasional palpitations, blurred vision, and increased thirst. Mr. Samuels accesses the **patient Web portal** of his **personal health record** (PHR) and sends an e-mail to his physician's scheduling service requesting an appointment. Within an hour, an appointment is confirmed with the family nurse practitioner (FNP) for the next day.

The physician's office has just installed an electronic health record (EHR) system that is **integrated** with the hospital record for seamless communication among Mr. Samuels's caregivers. At his appointment, the registrar enters his insurance and contact information into the system, and explains that the system is **encrypted** (special security coding) to protect his privacy. In the exam room, the medical assistant weighs Mr. Samuels, takes his vital signs, and enters the information in the EHR. Next, Karen Shock, FNP, arrives. As she takes Mr. Samuels's history and completes a physical examination, she updates the information in the computer. Noting his family history of diabetes, the increased thirst, and slight weight gain, she checks a random glucose via the office glucometer and finds a blood sugar level of 300 mg/dL. The **decision support algorithms** built into the software alert her that Mr. Samuels's blood pressure was also elevated at 170/98 mm/Hg. The software suggests possible medical diagnoses of hyperglycemia and hypertension. Following the evidence-based care guidelines in the computer, Ms. Shock uses computerized provider order entry (**CPOE**) to enter requests for a basic metabolic profile, lipid profile, electrocardiogram (ECG), blood urea nitrogen (BUN), creatinine, and hemoglobin (Hgb) A1c. She asks that Mr. Samuels fast for the blood work, and prints patient education instructions. Ms. Shock instructs Mr. Samuels to check his blood pressure two to three times daily for one week and to enter the results in the online log in his PHR. She asks Mr. Samuels to grant viewing rights to the log for her and Dr. Gregg.

The next morning Mr. Samuels arrives at the hospital for his lab work and ECG. His registration information is automatically updated from the information provided with a previous health visit. The **online order requisitions** that Ms. Shock entered yesterday provide the technicians with the information needed, the tests are completed, and Mr. Samuels is quickly on the way back to his office. At the end of the day, he receives an e-mail notification that his lab results are available for review. He logs into the PHR portal to view the results. He also finds a message from Ms. Shock confirming the preliminary diagnosis of type 2 diabetes. The office is scheduling diabetic instruction, and they have e-mailed a prescription to Mr. Samuels's pharmacy for metformin, an antidiabetes drug. An education leaflet explaining the medication and potential side effects is attached to the message. Mr. Samuels notices that metformin is now showing on his **medication list** in his PHR.

Over the course of the week, Ms. Shock monitors Mr. Samuels's blood pressure log entries. A **trending graph** shows consistently high blood pressure readings. She orders Lisinopril, an antihypertensive, 5 mg daily, and requests that he continue to check his blood pressure frequently. A follow-up appointment is scheduled for 6 weeks.

A few weeks later, Mr. Samuels wakes up with severe chest pain and calls 911. En route to the emergency department (ED), the paramedic transmits an ECG tracing via satellite to the ED physician. Using telehealth technology, the physician interprets the ECG, determines that Mr. Samuels is having a myocardial infarction, and has notifies the cardiac catheterization team to be on standby. The ED physician sees that Mr. Samuels has recently completed tests at the hospital, and reviews his medication list, allergies, and medical history online. Within 30 minutes Mr. Samuels is sent to the cath lab for percutaneous transluminal coronary angioplasty.

Four hours later, Mr. Samuels is resting in the progressive care unit. Throughout the next 48 hours, the bedside nurse monitors his vital signs and cardiac rhythm. An **interface** allows the nurse to directly import vital signs data from the cardiac monitor directly into his electronic health record. Caregivers document electronically at the bedside, and the physician uses CPOE to manage Mr. Samuels's prescriptions. At discharge, the nurse gives Mr. Samuels a printed copy from the EHR of his medication list, discharge instructions, and follow-up appointments are made with Dr. Gregg and the cardiologist.

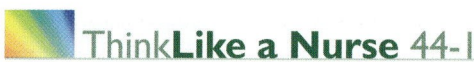

ThinkLike a Nurse 44-1

Reflect on this Meet Your Nurse Role Model scenario. Identify how information was managed and processed.

■ What mechanisms for gathering and disseminating information were used?

■ How did automation assist decision making?

■ How was evidence used in decision making?

■ What characteristics make it more likely for patients to use personal health records?

TheoreticalKnowledge
knowing why

Computers are becoming as much of a diagnostic tool as stethoscopes. The Meet Your Nurse Role Model scenario is an example of how healthcare professionals use these tools to make decisions in practice. This chapter gives you an overview of how this works.

ABOUT THE KEY CONCEPTS

Healthcare is increasingly complex, expanding, and ever changing. Patients and payors alike demand more efficient and effective healthcare. You may already feel the push and pull on your time and knowledge. And why work harder, when you can work smarter using technology-based tools? **Nursing informatics** and **healthcare technology** (e.g., mechanical ventilators, implantable insulin pumps) support your passion for nursing and innovation, leading to improved patient outcomes and higher quality care. **Electronic communication** (e.g., electronic health records and telehealth) is also an important part of this equation.

WHAT IS NURSING INFORMATICS?

Whether you become a staff nurse, an administrator, a researcher, primary healthcare provider, or an educator, you will need current, accurate, and "best available" information to do your job well. The good news is that plenty of information is available. PubMed, a vast medical literature database supported through the National Institutes of Health, currently contains more than 21 million citations for biomedical literature from MEDLINE, life science journals, and online books (National Institutes of Health [NIH], 2012). If you read two new nursing articles every day, by the end of the year you would be 918 years behind in keeping up with the literature. The bad news (if you want to call it that) is that we are drowning in information while still lacking in knowledge. Do you ever feel that way as a student?

It is not possible to keep all the necessary information in your head. No one can. We need critical thinking and electronic tools to make it useful to us. No one can learn and retain all the information, so you must know how to find, process, and manage it to arrive at the best decisions for your practice. In essence, this is the definition of **informatics:** the managing and processing of information necessary to make decisions.

The American Nurses Association (ANA) describes **nursing informatics** as the specialty where nurses use *data, information, knowledge,* and *wisdom* to support patients, nurses, and other healthcare providers in decision making in all roles and settings (ANA, 2008, p. 65). Communication and transmitting information is a big part of nursing informatics.

Nursing informatics specialists (NIS) work with informatics technicians and others to provide clinical information and data analysis for effective patient care. In addition, they work with computers, data analysis systems, and nursing knowledge and experience to be sure the best possible care is provided. This role involves good understanding of basic nursing techniques and standards. Functions of the NIS include data collection, analysis of different types of data, information sharing, and research dissemination. The nursing informatics specialist also acts as a manager or team leader to bring together all aspects of treatment options and best practice research. In sum, the NIS uses nursing science, computer science, and information science to manage and communicate data, information, knowledge, and wisdom in nursing practice. The sections that follow describe these four elements of informatics.

Data

Data are "discrete entities that are described objectively without interpretation" (ANA, 2008). In other words, data are raw, unprocessed numbers, symbols, or words that have no meaning by themselves. For example, what does 101 mean? It could indicate the movie title *101 Dalmatians;* a piece of programming language; or someone's body temperature, pulse rate, weight, or age. Without a context, data are meaningless.

In nursing, we speak of data as the primary facts and observations acquired when providing services, such as the numerical value of a blood pressure measurement, or facts such as "Father died of prostate cancer." Notice that even this information has no meaning until the nurse interprets it: The meaning of "Father died of prostate cancer" changes if the client is a healthy 24-year-old female sharing this information versus a 74-year-old male experiencing blood in his urine.

Information

Information consists of groupings of data processed into a meaningful, structured form (ANA, 2001). If you combine 300 with a unit of measure, you know that the number represents a blood sugar result. If other data—gender (male), age (67), and family history—are grouped together, information is formed. You now know that this man has most likely developed type 2 diabetes.

Data:	300 mg/dL glucose, male, 67, thirst
Grouped data:	Male gender, age 67, family history of diabetes
Information:	Man with probable new onset of diabetes

Knowledge

In the opening Meet Your Nurse Role Model scenario, what *information* did the FNP receive that triggered an alert? What information did the FNP use to create *knowledge* of Mr. Samuels's condition? Take a minute to write your answer.

You should have written that the FNP received information on the blood sugar (300 mg/dL) and blood pressure (170/98). Grouping this with other information (e.g., the history of headaches, blurred vision, palpitations, family history of diabetes), the FNP created *knowledge* of the potential for a diagnosis of type 2 diabetes and hypertension.

Knowledge is formed when data are grouped, creating meaningful information and relationships, which are then added to other structured information (ANA, 2008). The knowledge can either be previously known or new. In the preceding scenario of the 67-year-old man with blood sugar of 300 mg/dL, we can add information about pathophysiology,

pharmacokinetics (how medications work), patient history, and physical assessment, providing the knowledge to make an informed decision about the patient's current condition and further treatment.

Figure 44-1 depicts the transformation of data into knowledge. As we have come to realize that the gathering of data and information to make decisions is never ending, the model has evolved to depict overlapping circles and both forward and backward movement.

Wisdom

Nelson and Joos (1989) added *wisdom* to the Graves and Corcoran model. **Wisdom** is defined as the *appropriate use* of knowledge in managing or solving human problems. As we discussed in Chapter 1, wisdom develops as an outcome of your clinical experience, theoretical knowledge, critical thinking, and intuition—as you progress from novice to expert in the practice of full-spectrum nursing.

KnowledgeCheck 44-1

- What is the difference between knowledge and wisdom?
- Define the following: *data, information, knowledge.*
- Give an example of each: data, information, knowledge.

UNDERSTANDING COMPUTERS

Computers are vital to the functioning in our daily lives. We rely on them for communication (e.g., e-mail, texting, blogs, social networking), access to information (e.g., personal and business contacts, education, general information), business operations (e.g., scheduling, purchasing), to name but a few. By definition, a **computer** is an electronic device with four main functions: input, process, output, and storage. Collectively, these operations are known as **information processing** (or *data processing*). The power of a computer is based on:

- The speed, accuracy, and reliability with which it operates
- The enormous amounts of data it is capable of storing and keeping readily available for processing

Computers consist of hardware (machines and monitors), memory (data storage), processors (translators), and software (coded programs or applications that support specific functions). They can exist as a stand-alone device, or as part of a network of computers that share a common purpose. Power in computing is enhanced by the ability to connect to other computers. Devices can either be *wired* (connected with physical wires) or *wireless* (connected through electromagnetic waves).

Data are stored either internally (in the memory) or externally on some form of storage media (discs, flash drives, portable hard drives, network drives). If you are a savvy computer user, you probably already know how a computer functions. See if you can answer questions about computer basics.

 Go to Chapter 44, **Supplemental Materials: Pretest: Computer Basics and Pretest Answer Key,** on Davis*Plus*.

If you had difficulty answering the questions,

 Go to Chapter 44, **Supplemental Materials: How Does a Computer Work?** on Davis*Plus*.

COMPUTERS IN THE WORKPLACE

Because computers are so important and so widely used in healthcare, it is essential that nurses develop a set of core computer competencies or skills (Hart, 2008). These include a basic understanding of computer logic, data entry, data retrieval, information literacy, and troubleshooting hardware and software issues. In your work as a nurse, you will use computers to provide and manage patient care, for continuing education, and for communication. Consider the following examples.

Tools for Providing and Managing Care

As a nurse, you will be called on to use a wide variety of computerized devices in the workplace. Digital thermometers, cardiorespiratory monitors, glucometers, cell phones, smart IV pumps, bar code scanners, and electronic bed scales are all types of computers.

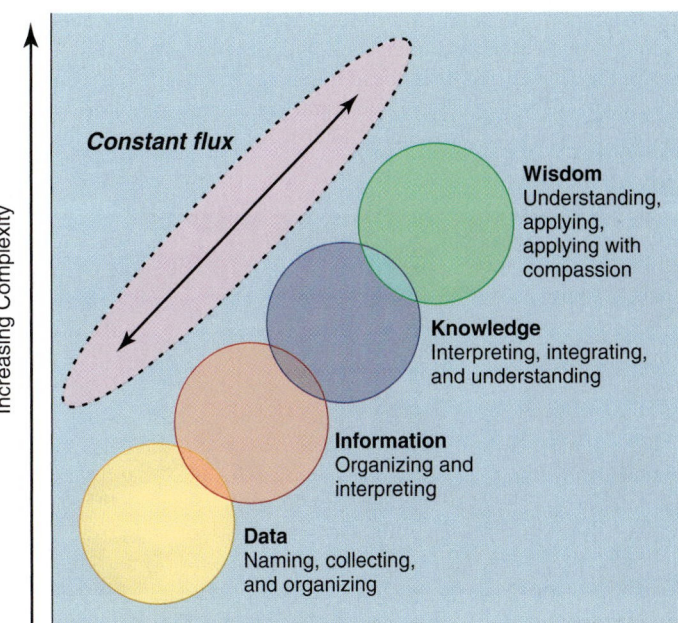

FIGURE 44-1 The relationship of data, information, knowledge, and wisdom. Each level increases in complexity. (Reprinted from Englebardt, S., & Nelson, R. *Health care informatics: An interdisciplinary approach.* Copyright 2002. With permission from Elsevier.)

Some agencies are using **real time location systems** (RTLS) or radio frequency identification detectors (RFID) to assist in locating patient care equipment throughout the building. These systems save nurse time, discourage staff from storing equipment on a particular unit rather than a centrally accessible location, and decrease costs of lost items (Turisco & Rhoads, 2008). Other efficiency-enhancing devices include hands-free communication badges and wireless phones, which may be interfaced with alerts from bedside equipment. These devices can save nurses several minutes on a busy day.

Internet-based tools for staff scheduling, patient flow, access to evidence-based references, policy and procedures, and staff education are fast becoming the norm. Many hospitals have developed internal resources, special intranet pages of references specific to nursing.

Computers in Nursing Education

New trends in nursing education include the use of clinical simulation mannequins and Web programs (Cannon-Diehl, 2009) (Fig. 44-2). Research indicates that these methods are effective in teaching critical thinking, problem-solving, physical assessment, and some clinical skills. You may have already been using clinical simulation mannequins in your nursing program. Would it surprise you to know that practicing nurses also use them in continuing education provided in their workplaces? What kind of computer programs and devices are available in your clinical setting?

Electronic Communication

Electronic communication can be very simple (e.g., text messaging), or very complex (e.g., long-distance telehealth) and can sometimes replace face-to-face interaction between people.

Electronic Mail and Text Messaging

In many facilities electronic mail (e-mail) allows for rapid, simultaneous distribution of information and messaging to a large number of recipients. Nurses and other healthcare providers can use e-mail to interact with patients; consult with colleagues; and communicate with insurance industry representatives, pharmacies, and hospitals. E-mail and mobile text messaging offer convenient, up-to-the-minute patient updates among nurses, other providers, and patients and their families. However, it is critical that these transmissions occur only on secure or encrypted sites if personal patient information is involved. A patient's **protected health information** includes any individually identifiable health information; current, past, or potential physical or mental conditions; and any payment information, such as Social Security numbers or insurance.

Be aware that privacy is not ensured with electronic mail. For example, it is entirely legal and not uncommon for employers to read incoming and outgoing employee messages sent on company equipment. In addition, once a message has been sent, you have no control over who may actually read it or to whom it might be forwarded. You also don't know if other people receive a blind copy of the message without your knowledge. Most facilities have policies governing use of company e-mail for personal use. You always check facility policies before sharing e-mail addresses with persons outside of the organization. For more information about e-mail security,

 Go to Chapter 44, **Supplemental Materials: E-mail Security,** on Davis*Plus.*

How was e-mail used to facilitate communication between the patient and providers in the Meet Your Nurse Role Model situation?

Web Conferencing and Webinars

Web conferencing is used to conduct or participate in live or synchronous meetings or presentations via the Internet. Attendees download a Web-based application onto their local computers. These interactions are most often two-way communication. To access the meeting, an e-mail is distributed to the attendee(s) that contains a link to enter the conference at the arranged time. A **Webinar,** or **Webcast,** is a specific type of Web conference that is one way from the speaker to the audience. These tools can be useful in helping staff obtain updated clinical information (e.g., continuing education, inservice) for patient care.

Listserv

Electronic mailing lists are an extension of e-mail use. The most common mailing list application is called a **listserv** (short for *list server*). The names and addresses of the people on the mailing list, called **subscribers,** are stored by the listserv on a single server. A single address is then designated for the group to use. When a message is sent to that address, it is delivered to the listserv server, which then distributes the message via e-mail to all subscribers.

Nearly all subspecialties and special interest groups in healthcare have a listserv. Interested professionals subscribe to the list and receive mailings from others on the list. Be aware that any message you send through the mailing list goes to *everyone* on the mailing list. Like sending any e-mail, be careful when you hit the Reply All command!

Listservs are a powerful communication tool. Communication is global and almost instantaneous. Ideas and protocols can be shared, questions asked and answered, and surveys taken. Everyone on the list can share in the discussion. Numerous nursing listservs are available, representing a wide variety of topics and health specialty areas. Use a Web search engine and search using the keywords "nursing listservs." Look for a site that interests you. What kind of information do you see? Visit one of the sites.

Social Networking

Social networking tools allow people to connect interactively with others who have similar interests. This can be done through **blogging** (posting open messages that can

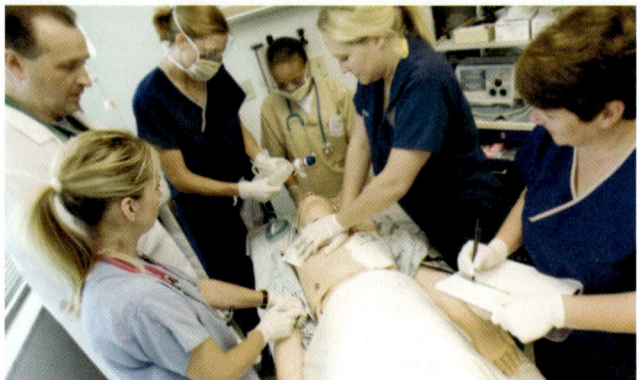

FIGURE 44-2 Human patient simulator offers practical experience before caring for patients or training special skills.

be read by anyone with permissions to access the site), sharing pictures or videos, or **instant messaging** (real-time conversations with another person who is online). Sites generally require you to register, create a profile, and be granted access privileges by the Web page administrator. MySpace, Twitter, Facebook, YouTube, and LinkedIn are examples of popular social networking sites. You can go to YouTube to view video demonstrations of nursing skills. Be cautious about whether the source of information is expert and reliable; for example, some of the YouTube skills videos have errors in the demonstrations. To find reliable nursing videos, often it's easiest to search the specific topic, not simply nursing videos in general.

As with many Web-based tools, social networking sites are searchable by anyone with access. Many employers now regularly include searches of these sites as part of their applicant verification process. A wise rule of thumb is not to post anything on these sites that you would not want an employer to see. ✚ In addition, posting pictures or descriptions of patient information represents significant risk of violating federal privacy laws.

Another tool gaining popularity is a wiki. **Wikis** are Web pages, such as Wikipedia, that can either be public or limited to specific groups through user name and passwords. Many schools have created Wikis to support communication among student groups. Support group Wikis are becoming common for use by patients with chronic health conditions, such as diabetes or congestive heart failure. It is important to note that anyone with access can add information to these sites, creating the potential for including inaccurate information. It is useful to know if support groups are being facilitated or at least monitored by a professional before recommending them to patients.

As we are shifting from the Information Age to the Interaction Age, educators are resorting to new, more engaging and collaborative methods for teaching and learning. One example is a Web-based, three-dimensional, virtual world called *Second Life,* which digitally simulates the human experience. Residents, or participants in Second-Life, also called **avatars,** can interact with one another in a social networking–type community that the residents refer to as the Grid. Educators use this game-like environment to simulate a nurse–patient experience and clinical care as well as to evaluate a variety of nursing skills.

Telehealth

Telehealth is the use of telecommunication to send healthcare information between patients and professionals at different locations (Fig. 44-3). It improves access to healthcare by providing long-distance clinical healthcare, patient and professional education, and health administration. For instance, the U.S. Department of Defense pioneered telehealth technology and now uses it to provide healthcare services to soldiers in combat and dependent families in outlying posts. The following are other examples of the use of telehealth.

- **Rural Healthcare.** In rural healthcare sites there may not be a specialist located in the area. Telecommunications equipment at the rural site and the specialist's site allow the specialist and patient to see and talk to each other. The specialist can also view the health records, x-ray films, lab results, and so on. This reduces the cost of traveling to a distant site, and the stress on a patient who may not feel well enough to travel.

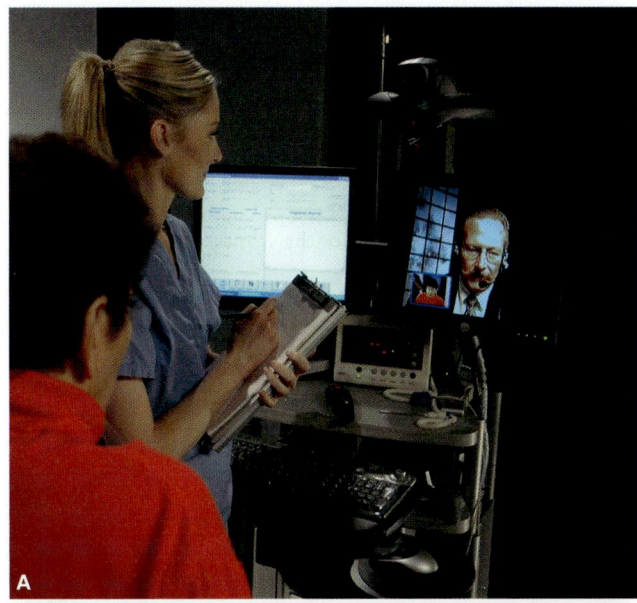

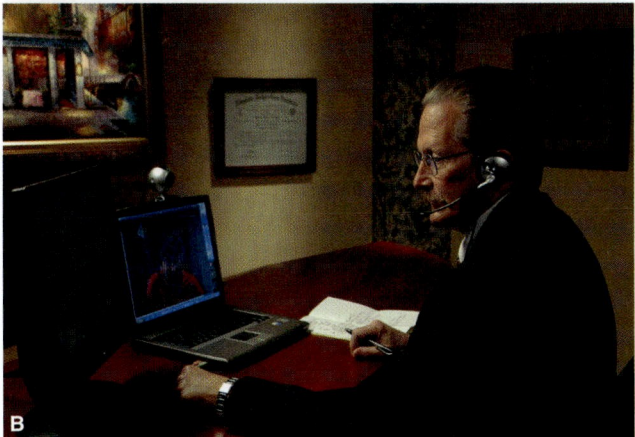

FIGURE 44-3 A. B. Telehealth improves access among healthcare providers at remote and central sites.

- **Home Health Monitoring.** A more common use of telehealth is the use of home health monitoring devices. These devices allow the healthcare professional to monitor vital signs and other indicators without physically entering a home or requiring a patient to make a clinic trip. Therefore, patients can be monitored more frequently, providing better follow-up care and allowing for earlier discharge from the hospital. See the Home Care box, Use of Informatics in Home Care.

- **Shortage of Healthcare Providers.** In the hospital, critically ill patients can be remotely monitored by a hospital **intensivist** (physician employed by the hospital to provide healthcare to patients in intensive care) and critical care nurses from a central location. These systems enhance patient safety and provide an extra set of eyes for a busy nurse who cannot remain constantly at a patient's bedside.

- **Emergency Care Triage.** Some cities have incorporated telehealth nurse triage into their emergency 911 call system. Telenurses use a set of protocols to manage patient calls. These cities report a significant decrease in need for ambulance services and emergency room visits (Enrado, 2009).

Despite barriers, such as cost and issues surrounding cost, privacy, licensing, and reimbursement, telehealth applications

Home Care

Use of Informatics in Home Care

A computer or mobile phone application for documentation has been developed for home health aides. On arriving at a patient's home, the aide uses a phone to dial in to a central number and keys in her identification. The time of the call, number from which it came, and identification of the worker are automatically recorded.

At the end of the visit, the aide again calls from the phone. Again, the location, time, and identification of the caller are recorded. Using the keypad, the aide then enters codes indicating the tasks accomplished. This reduces the time spent documenting care, improves accuracy, allows access by the healthcare team, and prevents lost records.

will continue to expand in the future. For information about barriers that slow the growth of telehealth,

 Go to Chapter 44, **Supplemental Materials: Barriers to Telehealth,** on Davis*Plus*.

 Think**Like a Nurse** 44-2

- As a patient, would you prefer a telehealth or a face-to-face consultation? Why?
- Now imagine that you are an accident victim brought to a rural clinic staffed only with paraprofessionals. Does your answer change? If so, why?

COMPUTERS AND HEALTHCARE REFORM

The rising cost of healthcare affects nearly every sector of the population and the economy of the nation. As costs have steadily increased, consumers and third-party payers have expressed concerns about the quality of care and the outcomes associated with chronic health conditions. Government agencies and private organizations emerged to seek information technology solutions to assist in decreasing costs, improving efficiency, and improving patient outcomes.

Electronic Health Record Adoption

The United States healthcare community has been slow to embrace EHR, due in large part to fears of loss of physician autonomy, purchase and installation costs, user adoption and systems training, and uncertainty about the ability of the EHR vendors to remain in business and support their software (Ford, Menachemi, Peterson, et al., 2009). Some people adopt early, some more slowly. If you would like to know the categories of how people tend to respond to innovation.

 Go to Chapter 44, **Tables, Boxes, Figures: ESG Box 44-1, Adopters of Innovation** on Davis*Plus*.

In 2004, a national plan was set in motion to establish a nationwide system for exchange of medical information through electronic health records. **Interoperability** refers to the ability of computers to talk with each other through standard languages or formats without losing the meaning of the information. If information about heart rate is to be exchanged, for example,

consistent languages are needed. For example the EHR system in Hospital A might refer to "heart rate," while the EHR system in a physician's office might refer to "pulse rate," which could interfere with clear communication. The computers need a language that allows each to recognize the other's terminology. The rationale for government support of a nationwide interoperable system of health records is to do the following:

- *Provide patient-focused healthcare.* Patient-focused healthcare is assumed to be higher quality and more cost efficient than a paper documentation system. It is to be accomplished through wider use (access) of electronic health information by care providers and patients.
- *Improve population health.* The nationwide interoperable system of EHR is expected to allow more timely access and use of patient information—information that would be used in research, quality improvement, and emergency preparedness.

In early 2009, legislation intended to stimulate the U.S. economy designated a multibillion-dollar program for healthcare reform. By providing financial incentives and, in later phases, penalties, the federal government's goal is an EHR for all Americans by 2015. Hospitals and physician offices will need to devote considerable time and resources to meet this aggressive time line.

Patients Are Using Computers Too

Roughly two-thirds of American adults have gone online to find healthcare-related information (Taylor, 2008). Patients who look for this information may be seeking information about conventional, alternative, or complementary therapies and treatments, or looking for shared experiences of others with similar conditions. Patients may not always share their findings from online searches with their healthcare providers, which can lead to confusion or adverse reactions to prescribed treatment.

You can help guide your patients in their searches by educating them about how to use online sources and choose reputable, trustworthy sites. You may also need to help interpret information that patients find. Many hospitals have patient education materials on their Web sites that provide links to reputable sources.

T.I.G.E.R.

The Technology Informatics Guiding Education Reform (TIGER) initiative was launched in 2006, when a group of nursing educators, government and industry leaders, and representatives met. They formed a think tank to develop a shared vision, strategies, and specific actions to improve nursing education, nursing practice guidelines, and clinical care of patients through the use of health information technology (DuLong, 2009), primarily by developing a stronger health information technology (IT) infrastructure. More than 70 professional nursing organizations formed this organization to make healthcare safer, more effective and efficient, and more patient-centered and equitable.

INFORMATICS IN NURSING PRACTICE

You have been introduced to several ways in which computer information systems are used in nursing care. In this section, we describe the role of informatics and standardized nursing languages in communicating health information, promoting evidence-based practice, using health records, decreasing medical error, and protecting patient privacy and confidentiality. Table 44-1 summarizes the use

Table 44-1 ➤ Use of Computer Information Systems in Nursing

NURSING PRACTICE	NURSING EDUCATION	NURSING ADMINISTRATION	NURSING RESEARCH
Literature access and retrieval (e.g., for evidence-based practice)	Literature access and retrieval	Quality assurance and utilization review	Literature review
Care planning	Computer-assisted instruction (CAI) programs	Employee records (e.g., to track licenses, immunizations)	Data collection
Client records (e.g., documenting, order entry, retrieving lab results)	Classroom technology	Staffing patterns, hiring	Data analysis (both qualitative and quantitative)
Telenursing (e.g., in home health)	Distance learning	Buildings and facilities management	Research dissemination
Case management	Testing and grading	Finance and budgets	Applying for grants
Documenting medications	Student records	Accreditation reviews (e.g., monitoring quality indicators for The Joint Commission)	
Transcribing orders	Development of electronic and learning communities using the World Wide Web		
Reordering medications			
Identifying drug interactions			
Warning practitioners about drug incompatibilities			

of computers in practice, education, administration, and research.

Why Are Computers Important for Evidence-Based Practice?

Rapid access to the ever-increasing volume of knowledge changes the way decisions are made in healthcare. The **traditional model of healthcare decision making** relies on each practitioner's personal experience and judgment. But healthcare is now so complex that problems routinely exceed the clinical decision-making capacity and reliability of individual practitioners. A better model of decision making is **evidence-based practice.** As we discussed in Chapters 6 and 8, evidence-based practice uses a knowledge base of

---

QSEN

Are Information Technologies Living Up to Their Promise?

Competency: Informatics (Knowledge, Skills, Attitudes); Safety (Knowledge, Skills, Attitudes)*

Background: Billions of dollars have been allocated for the development of electronic information systems (which are made up of electronic health records, digitized images, decision-support systems, computerized provider order entry, communication systems, and more). The totally electronic health information system has been promised to enhance the quality and safety of health care and provide information for clinical research. But is it really possible to develop a reliable, error-proof system that everyone understands and uses correctly?

Research: A recent article (Black, Car, Pagliari, et al., 2011) questions whether we should automatically assume the usefulness of an all-electronic information system. Using 53 high-quality studies, researchers evaluated the evidence to support the use of information technologies to improve the quality and safety of health care. They concluded that existing evidence was weak and inconsistent. Not only did very few of the promised benefits materialize, but new sources of errors were created. They found one particularly troubling effect: the tendency for prescribing errors, which resulted when prescribers overestimated the capabilities of clinical decision-support systems.

Think about it:

The informatics competency stresses the need for nurses to understand the time, effort, and skill required for information

technologies to become reliable, effective tools for patient care system. What do you see as the nurse's role in developing and evaluating the electronic health record?

Consider the following questions to help develop your knowledge, skills and attitudes about informatics and safety:

➤ What thinking skills will be necessary for nurses and other providers to respond appropriately to decision supports and alerts?

➤ How will nurses, in particular, use an electronic health record?

➤ How might electronic health records be used to improve care?

➤ How might the electronic health record improve the safety of an individual patient's care?

➤ What information should be included in an electronic database to make it useful for clinical research?

Source: Black AD, Car J, Pagliari C, Anandan C, Cresswell K, et al. (2011). The impact of eHealth on the quality and safety of health care: a systematic overview. PLoS Medicine 8(1). Accessed 1/22/12 from http://www.plosmedicine.org/article/info%3Adoi%2F10.1371%2Fjournal. pmed.1000387;jsessionid=9E4ABB296687D9F6E327E841FD3622B3

*For specific Knowledge, Skills, and Attitudes,

 Go to the QSEN web site **at http:www.qsen.org.ksas_ prelicensure.php**

accumulated "best evidence" that can change quickly and continuously. To find the current *best* evidence, you must be able to locate the evidence, evaluate its quality and relevance to the problem, and apply the solution.

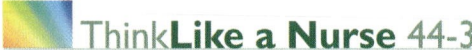

ThinkLike a Nurse 44-3

Analyze the Meet Your Nurse Role Model scenario. What example of evidence-based practice do you find in it?

WHAT ARE THE BENEFITS OF AN ELECTRONIC HEALTH RECORD?

Electronic health records (EHRs) as part of networked information systems software allows clinicians to create, store, edit, and retrieve patient charts on a computer. Figure 44-4 is an example of a computer screen using EHR software. Notice the electronic view uses combinations of tabs and icons to support logical navigation through the patient chart. These tabs are often named and arranged to match tabs from a traditional paper chart, including patients' clinical and personal data.

A successful EHR project allows an organization to replace paper charts and care plans with electronic health records. Other benefits of the EHR are discussed in following section and also in Chapter 18.

Improved Efficiency. Improved data access can increase efficiency, productivity, and continuity of care. A paperless health record conveniently stores all patient information in one location, rather than in bits and pieces in many different files and locations.

Privacy. Access to sensitive patient information can be limited only to individuals with proper authorization, and each retrieval of data can be logged electronically—a vast improvement over the folders and charts that can pass through many hands without a record of who examines them.

Accessibility. Have you ever needed to write your nursing notes before leaving the clinical setting, only to discover that the chart was in the x-ray department with the patient? Or that the physician was making rounds with it in her hands? In contrast to a paper record, any number of people in different locations can access a computerized record—and all at the same time. A physician can view lab results from the office while a nurse views them in the hospital and a lab technician adds more data. A variety of hardware supports the need to access patient health information, from stationary bedside terminals, wireless laptops mounted on mobile carts, and handheld devices such as smart phones (Fig. 44-5).

Reduced Errors. Computer physician order entry (CPOE) allows healthcare providers to enter orders into a computerized system instead of handwriting them, thus reducing errors resulting from illegible handwriting.

Research and Public Health Benefits. Computerized records place data in repositories (storage areas) so that the information can be sorted and collated to create the information and knowledge necessary to aid decision-making research. For example, state health departments can access population-based medical information to track communicable diseases, possibly preventing epidemics. Health researchers and analysts can also use aggregate health information to judge, for example, which treatment is most effective for a disease, thus improving patient outcomes over time. To protect patient privacy and ethical practice of research, review boards govern access to population data.

Planning Care. Some EHR systems are designed for planning as well as for documenting care. Standardized care plans are typically incorporated in EHR systems. Other applications are designed to support efficient patient care workflow. Studies demonstrate that nurses who understand the nursing process and are familiar with computers are more accepting of automated

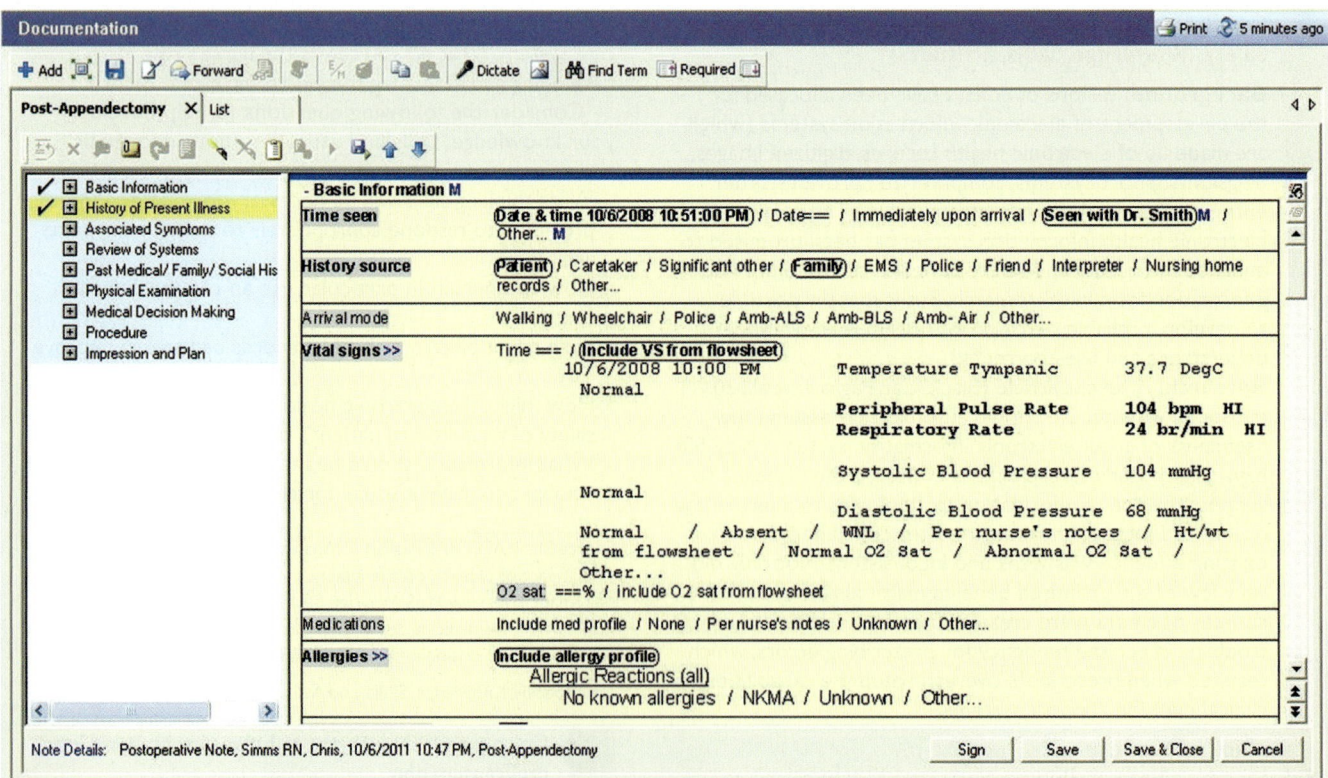

FIGURE 44-4 Computer screen from an electronic health record. (Courtesy of Cerner Corporation, Kansas City, MO.)

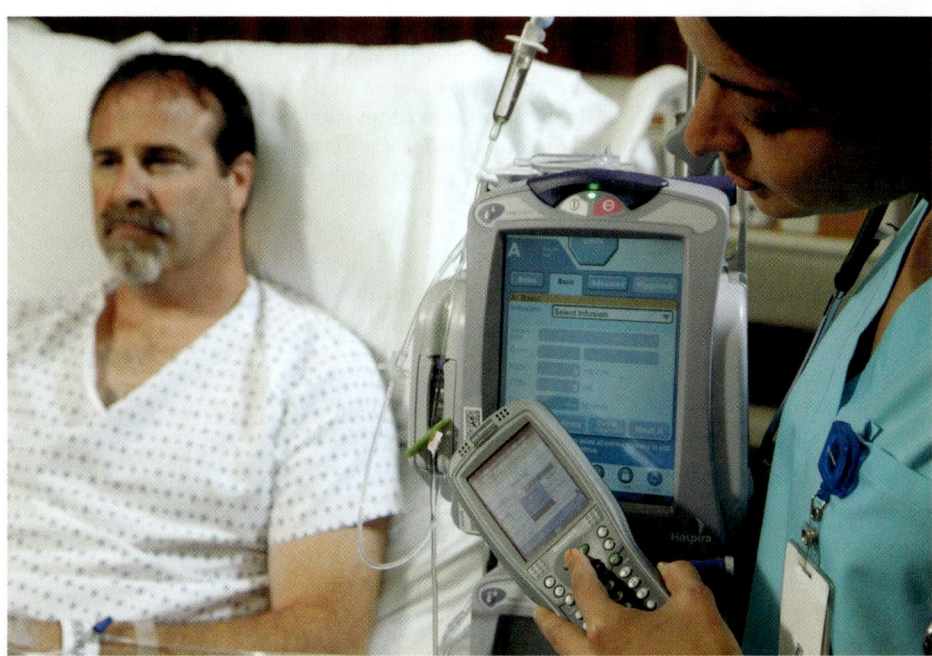

FIGURE 44-5 Point-of-access computing. A. Handheld device. B. Terminal unit for accessing patient data.

documentation (Kossman & Scheidenhelm, 2008). As more people are comfortable with computers and use them daily, nurses' acceptance of computers in the workplace also is increasing.

Unintended Consequences. Little research has been done on the unintended consequences of EHR implementations. Consider the following examples:

- Although the intent of computerization is to decrease cost through improved efficiency and communication, instituting an EHR system without addressing *changes in nursing workflow* and *communication patterns* can actually make unit operations less effective (Kossman & Scheidenhelm, 2008).
- *Software upgrade* and *periodic new releases* are inevitable, some of which may require more robust hardware than previous editions. New, expensive equipment to replace perfectly serviceable hardware, which has been rendered obsolete by your EHR, is a factor when considering the cost of an EHR.
- The *portability* of EHR can lead to *decreased face-to-face communication* among the healthcare team.

The nurse informatics specialist, a nurse who has gained additional education and experience in informatics, often provides guidance for clinicians in identifying gaps between how the EHR system functions and how clinical processes work. Successful changes from paper to electronic systems are those that provide opportunities for nurses to have a voice in choosing systems and planning the change.

KnowledgeCheck 44-2

- What are some of the benefits of EHR implementation?
- What is personal health information, and why is it important to protect it?
- How is a listserv different from regular e-mail?

Why Are Standardized Nursing Languages Needed for Electronic Health Records?

Suppose you wanted to find out how many patients on your hospital unit had a nursing diagnosis of Impaired Skin Integrity during the past year. If the hospital uses paper

medical records, how could you find out? If the records are computerized, would that make a difference?

You probably said something such as "Pull all the charts, and look at the nursing notes." Or maybe, search for the words *Impaired Skin Integrity* in the electronic health records. That's a beginning. But think about this: Nurses use a variety of terms to describe the same data. For example, in some charts you would find the term *skin breakdown;* in others, *a reddened area, bedsore,* or a *stage III pressure ulcer.* Would you count all of these as Impaired Skin Integrity? What if the nurses used some terms you didn't think to search for? Do you see how the lack of a uniform way to describe patient problems can hamper efforts to create and retrieve nursing data from automated documentation systems? Recall the goal for interoperability among EHR systems discussed previously in the chapter. Standardized language—using the same terms to describe a phenomenon in all EHRs—helps to achieve that goal.

Nurses do not describe clinical interventions any more uniformly than they describe nursing diagnoses. Inconsistent language and meaning make it difficult to compare and research nursing contributions to patient care (Beyea, 2000). Use of standardized nursing languages helps to ensure that nursing activities are an integral component of any electronic health record. As research and teaching of standardized interventions promotes wider understanding of them, they will help to further define the scope of nursing practice. When nursing terminology is visible in the EHR, it becomes possible to recognize the contribution that nurses make to achieving patient outcomes and organizational goals.

The first use of standardized nursing language began in the 1970s, with the NANDA International (NANDA-I) classification of nursing diagnoses. Since then, several initiatives to develop standardized languages for nursing practice have arisen (Wilkinson, 2011). By 2003, the American Nurses Association Committee for Nursing Practice Information Infrastructure had recognized 13 standardized languages.

 Go to Chapter 44, *Standardized Language: American Nurses Association Recognized Languages for Nursing,* on Davis*Plus*.

Each of these languages makes a unique contribution to knowledge development in nursing. At this time, it appears that no single language has captured nursing practice in its entirety. Each language is currently in the process of revision and further development. This is, of course, true of *all* languages, including English and Spanish and other spoken languages.

This text primarily uses the NANDA-I, NIC, and NOC classifications for describing patient problems, outcomes, and interventions (see Chapters 4, 5, and 6 if you need a review). Other classifications, such as the Omaha system and Community Care Classification, were created for specific settings (i.e., community health and home health, respectively), but can actually be used in all settings. Adoption of a single standardized language system would enhance communication among nurses, with other healthcare professionals, and with the public. Because this does not appear likely, however, nurses are working to "map" terms from each system to their equivalents in other systems (e.g., Impaired Skin Integrity in NANDA-I might map to Integument in the Omaha system). This contributes to the interoperability mentioned earlier in the chapter.

How Does Computerization Reduce Error in Healthcare?

As healthcare becomes more complex, the opportunities for error significantly increase. A hospital stay can be prolonged or injury and even death can result from a seemingly simple mistake. Administering incompatible medications, or erroneously transcribing a medication order can carry serious consequences. These are *errors of commission,* meaning that the wrong action occurs. There are also *errors of omission*—errors in which the correct action does not occur, such as overlooking a serious medication allergy, or failing to put up the bed rails for a confused patient.

Another way to look at errors is by asking, "Is it an *error in planning,* say, when the original intended action or plan is not correct?" Or, "Is it an *error of execution*—that is, when the correct action does not proceed as intended?"

 Illegible or confusing handwriting by clinicians can lead to medication errors and other sentinel events. Mistaken abbreviations or acronyms, look-alike, and sound-alike medication mix-ups are errors that can be prevented with computer-entry prescriptions. Other times errors result from faulty communication among healthcare providers, which, in some cases, can also be prevented by electronic prescribing.

Automation (e. g., EHR) provides a secure way to integrate all patient information, including allergy history, laboratory workups, and other prescriptions. It improves communication among those who prescribe, dispense, and administer medication to patients. For example, new prescriptions are automatically checked for potential errors or problems. The system can detect dosing errors by flagging medication dilution or dosages that fall outside normal standards and alert providers of the possibility of a drug interaction, allergy, or incorrect dose. In addition, some drug names sound like other drugs; the EHR can notify prescribers and help avoid a serious drug error.

Three examples of error-prevention technologies:
Computerized physician order entry (CPOE) helps prevent errors in reading and transcribing orders.

Bar coding medications at the unit-dose level helps to prevent nurses from selecting an incorrect medication (Bell, 2009).
Use of smart technologies (e.g., infusion devices) at the point of care helps to ensure that the correct dose is delivered to the patient.

To read more about ways to decrease medication error,

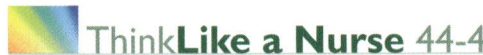
Go to Chapter 44, **Supplemental Materials: How Does Automation Decrease Medication Error?** on *DavisPlus.*

How Can Computerization Increase the Risk of Error in Healthcare?

Although convenient and time saving, some risks for error are inherent in EHRs.

- EHR documentation tools can contribute to loss of detail in nurses' notes, which in turn can lead to failure to meet unique patient needs.
- When documentation is copied numerous times, there also may be questions about the accuracy or specificity of the assessments over time. Copy and paste errors can lead to safety hazards, such as obtaining the wrong tests, interpreting the wrong results, performing the wrong treatments, and even administering the wrong medication to patients.

Remember, good documentation does more than provide a record of patient data; but it also serves as a communication tool for the multidisciplinary team for devising the patient's plan of care.

Because of the way data is entered into the patient's record using fields, pull-down lists, check boxes, and standardized language, EHRs can contribute to premature labeling of patient problems without critical reflection of the patient's individual needs. Once a patient's condition is pigeon-holed, the plan for care tends to "stick" without consideration of new information as it occurs, or without adequately representing the patient's progress. For instance, without a field to document in the patient's own words, the nurses' notes may fail to reveal insight in the patient's response to care.

When relying on the EHR for documentation of all patient data, inadequate verbal communication may occur. Handoff reports then might be abbreviated without adequate discussion of relevant patient information.

ThinkLike a Nurse 44-4

How does automation contribute to or decrease errors in healthcare?

How Can I Use Electronic Health Records Ethically?

Medical records contain highly sensitive information. Patients confide in nurses and physicians, trusting that their information will remain private. Most facilities have policies in place to manage security breaches and assign fines or prosecution when patient privacy is violated. Strong personal integrity and adherence to nursing and other codes of ethics are necessary to protect patient privacy within healthcare organizations.

Only one person at a time can view a paper record, and that person and the record must be in the same geographical

Toward Evidence-Based Practice

Fowler, S. B., Sohler, P., & Zarillo, D. F. (2009). Bar code technology for medication administration: Medication errors and nurse satisfaction. *MEDSURG Nursing, 18*(2), 103–109.

A bar code administration system provides a safe mechanism for delivering medications to the unit for the nurse to administer. This study compared nurse satisfaction with this system pre-implementation, 3 months post-implementation, and 6 months post-implementation. The new bar code medication administration system was piloted in a 53-bed medical surgical unit. The sample studied was small and did not show significant differences in satisfaction between nurses trained without technology versus those recently trained with the use of other computer-based programs.

1. What is a bar code medication system? And how does it work?

2. What are a few of the major benefits of using a bar code medication system?

3. What drawbacks or risks can you think of when using this type of system?

4. At first glance, what conclusion might you draw about the study of nurses' satisfaction with the bar code system?

5. How might you explain why some of the nurses in the study did not express overwhelming satisfaction when using the bar code technology?

6. Before drawing conclusions about whether the bar code technology has merit or not, though, what questions do you need to ask about the group of nurses sampled in this study? Should further research be recommended?

 Go to Chapter 44, **Toward Evidence-Based Practice Suggested Responses,** on Davis*Plus*.

---

location. With an automated record, many people can view the information at the same time, and they can be in many different locations. Still, in some ways the automated record is more secure than the paper record. Almost anyone in the clinical unit can view the paper record. There is no documentation to show who has seen the information. In contrast, several measures protect the confidentiality of the EHR.

Passwords

Passwords for all users are probably the most obvious protection. Most institutions tie passwords to the responsibilities of the job description. For example, the business office does not have access to clinical information, and nurses do not have access to data about the patient's bill paying. The following are some simple rules for password management:
- Never share passwords with others.
- The more complex the password is, the harder it is for hackers to break it or onlookers to remember it. Use combinations of letters, numbers, and symbols for maximum protection.
- Don't use words that are easy to guess (e.g., pet names, birthdays).
- Change passwords frequently.
- Do not record passwords in places that are easily accessible to others.

It is important to protect the privacy of healthcare records not only from outside observers, but also from professionals who are not assigned to care for the patient. In fact, those are the people who are most likely to breach confidentiality.

Audit Trails

Organizations are required to have software that tracks each person who accesses information. This is called an **audit trail.** Anything a person adds to or changes in the record is recorded automatically on the audit trail and can be investigated.

HIPAA Regulations

The Health Insurance Portability and Accountability Act (HIPAA) of 1996 was the first comprehensive federal protection for the privacy of individually identifiable health information. Most health insurance plans and care providers must now comply with the U.S. Department of Health and Human Services (USHHS) Privacy Rule ("the HIPAA regulations"). The two important requirements are that health plans and providers must:
- Obtain consent before disclosing health information used for treatment or payment options.
- Limit disclosure of information to the minimum necessary to accomplish intended purposes.

Subsequent rules increased fines to organizations for each reported breach of personal health information, and gave authority to individual states to monitor compliance with the rules. These rules apply to all forms of communication: electronic, written, and verbal. For full information,

 Go to the **U.S. Department of Health and Human Services** Web site at http://www.hhs.gov/ocr/privacy/

If you would like further discussion of EHR privacy issues, review How Do I Maintain Confidentiality and Data Security? in Clinical Insight 18-3.

KnowledgeCheck 44-3
- List at least three ways in which computers can help reduce healthcare errors.
- Discuss at least three measures the nurse can take to protect the confidentiality of patients' electronic health records.

PracticalKnowledge
knowing how

Professional standards require accountable practitioners to keep up to date with research and new knowledge. For example, criteria in ANA Professional Performance standard 8 state that the nurse should demonstrate a commitment to lifelong learning and seek experiences that reflect current practice

to maintain skills and competence (ANA, 2010). You can accomplish this by knowing how to search literature databases efficiently and use Web resources discriminatingly to complement your use of the EHR in providing quality patient care.

USING INFORMATICS TO SUPPORT EVIDENCE-BASED PRACTICE

As you have learned in previous chapters, evidence-based practice involves (1) identifying a clinical question or need for change, (2) searching the literature, (3) evaluating evidence, and (4) translating the results into practice (Pipe, Cisar, Caruso, et al., 2008). It is not enough to find one journal article in support of an intervention. Instead, you need to search broadly for high-quality, scientific evidence. Managing and processing information are essential for these tasks. Nurses require the most current, best-quality information for making decisions in their practice. In hospital settings, nurses need information on a wide variety of topics including clinical nursing issues, drug therapy, improving patient outcomes, innovative practice changes, and leadership skills. But how do nurses use automated systems to access that information? See Box 44-1 for a profile of an information-literate person.

How Do Computers Reduce Barriers to Evidence-Based Practice?

Most nurses are action oriented, preferring to learn by looking, listening, and talking. It may seem easier to seek information from colleagues, rely on past experience, draw on knowledge of pathophysiology, and read whatever references are closest at hand. However, in the clinical setting, the closest reference book may not contain the most current information or the best possible evidence. Computers at the workplace help overcome this barrier to evidence-based practice by providing fast, easy access to current practice information from around the world. For example, you could quickly use a computer to look up the latest, tested interventions for a patient who is incontinent of urine.

How Do I Use Computers to Search the Literature?

Lack of literature-searching skills is another reason many nurses fail to take advantage of automated information available to them to enrich their practice. There are several steps to conducting an automated search of the literature.

- **Identify the information.** When you clearly know what information you want to gather and how it will be used, it is easier and more efficient to search, locate, evaluate, retrieve, organize, and manage the resources required to answer your question.
- **Formulate a precise definition of the problem.** This is usually in the form of a question, for example, "What are the leading causes of falls in older adults?" This question guides your search for information.
- **Conduct a search** of the most recent literature and most relevant studies using a key word or question. To learn about or review the PICO method of defining and stating questions, go to Chapter 8, Formulate a Searchable Question, and Box 8-4, PICO Questions.

ThinkLike a Nurse 44-5

Before reading the next section, see whether you can puzzle out the answers to the following two questions. Consult with your classmates and instructors, if necessary, after finishing the chapter.

- Why must a question be formed before initiating the search?
- The suggested question in the preceding section was "What are the leading causes of falls in older adults?" Why can't you use a general topic such as "falls" for your search topic?

BOX 44-1 ■ Profile of an Information-Literate Person

An information literate person accesses information:

- Recognizes the need for information
- Understands accurate and complete information is the basis for intelligent decision making
- Formulates questions based on information needs
- Identifies potential sources of information and selects those with credibility
- Accesses print and technology-based sources of information

An information literate person evaluates information:

- Accepts authoritative, current reliable information
- Sorts information based on accuracy and relevance
- Distinguishes opinion from factual knowledge
- Rejects inaccurate and misleading information
- Rejects biased information
- Creates new information to replace inaccurate or missing information as needed

An information-literate person manages information:

- Develops successful search strategies.
- Organizes information so the most important points are clear.

- Breaks complex information into understandable chunks.
- Sorts out language and technical points into meaningful terms.
- Tracks sources of information responsibly and credits appropriately.

An information literate person uses information:

- Organizes information for practical application.
- Integrates new information into an existing body of knowledge.
- Applies information in critical thinking and problem-solving.

Other characteristics:

- A resourceful and independent learner
- Competent reader
- Confident in his or her ability to solve problems
- Able to function independently and work well in groups
- Creative and able to adapt to change

Source: Adapted from: Doyle, C. S. (1992). *Final report to National Forum on Information Literacy.* University of Calgary. Information Literacy Group, 1998. Retrieved February 6, 2012; and Krumsieg, K., & Baehr, M. (2002). *Foundations of learning* (3rd ed.). Corvallis, OR: Pacific Crest.

Sources of Nursing Research

You must evaluate the type of literature you need to answer your clinical or research question. For instance, a research report provides better support for an intervention than does an opinion article. Although some information is classic and timeless, it is usually best to find the most current studies from reliable sources, such as government agencies, clinical organizations, or professional, refereed, peer-reviewed sources.

Textbooks. Textbooks are excellent when looking for a compilation of information, but are not a dynamic source of information because of the time it takes for publication.

Printed Journal Articles. Printed journal articles are more current, but the information may still be 6 months to 2 years old by the time the article is published. Journals may vary in their degree of academic rigor. You must discriminate among scholarly, general interest, and popular periodical literature, depending on the purpose of your literature search.

- *Scholarly Journals.* A scholar, clinical expert, or scientific researcher in the field submits topical articles that adhere to professional standards, carefully footnoting and citing references. Articles submitted to scholarly journals are reviewed by a group of experts to determine if they are suitable for publication. This process is known as *peer review.* The main purpose of a scholarly journal is to report on original research to make the information available to others. Examples of scholarly journals include *Journal of Nursing Scholarship, Journal of Clinical Nursing, Nursing Research, Nurse Educator,* and *International Journal of Nursing Terminologies and Classifications.*
- *General interest periodicals.* General interest periodicals are usually attractive. Articles tend to be heavily illustrated, often with photographs. News and general interest periodicals sometimes cite sources, but not always. Articles may be written by a member of the editorial staff, a scholar, or a freelance writer and are often peer reviewed. The language is geared to any educated audience. A specialty is not assumed. Some examples of general interest nursing periodicals include the *American Journal of Nursing, RN,* and *Nursing* [current year].
- *Popular periodicals.* Popular periodicals are usually slick and attractive in appearance and informal in style. They include many colorful graphics and photographs. These publications rarely, if ever, cite sources. Information in such journals is often second- or third-hand, and the original source is sometimes obscure. Articles are usually short, lack depth, and are written in common language at a 5th-grade reading level. The main purpose is to promote a product or viewpoint. Examples include *Parents, Women's Health,* and *Modern Healthcare.*

The World Wide Web. By accessing the Internet, you can find current information on about any topic from a variety of sources from a variety of sources, ranging from government sources, such as the Centers for Disease Control and Prevention (CDC), all the way to informal sources, such as blogs. Because the quality of content is not monitored for accuracy on many sites, be sure to select credible sources.

Literature Databases

Literature databases are powerful tools for finding information. Literature databases are catalogues of articles, usually sorted by discipline. Databases exist for engineering, education, law, medicine, nursing, and other disciplines. These databases often overlap—what is found in one database might also be found in another. For example, MEDLINE is the largest medical database and lists internationally published articles from journals in all areas of biomedicine. The Cumulative Index for Nursing and Allied Health Literature (CINAHL) is a smaller database covering nursing, allied health, biomedical, and consumer health journal articles. Most of the articles in CINAHL are also listed in MEDLINE. If, however, you are looking for a nursing-focused article, it is more efficient to use CINAHL because the search is already narrowed to nursing and allied health.

Each entry in a database contains an article citation, subject headings describing the article, and a text summary of the article called an **abstract.** Other information about the article may also be included, such as the name of the author(s), the name of the institution at which the research was done, and the language in which the article was published (Box 44-2). Many full-text journal articles are available online, some for free and some for a fee. Some are available in the school or hospital's library for nurses to access. Table 44-2 includes descriptions of some commonly used databases in healthcare. Do not limit your search to a single database. You will find valuable information in the databases of other disciplines (e.g., psychology, education, business, law, and general science).

How Do I Evaluate Evidence and Determine a Solution?

Evaluating the evidence is sometimes as simple as reading a descriptive research study and applying the results to your current situation. For example, in the search for information about falls in older adults, you may find research to indicate a number of safety measures that can be easily implemented to create a safer environment for your patients. However, at other times evaluating evidence can be complicated, requiring an understanding of statistics and research methods. Just because one study indicates that sugar causes cancer does not mean that the study was valid or reliable; therefore, you must not base conclusions on the results of only one study. Experience and further study of research will increase your ability to evaluate what you find in the literature.

BOX 44-2 ■ Example of a Database Entry

Author(s):	Ward, Kathleen R. Koerner, Dianna K.
Title:	Sink or swim: the Titanic medication administration fair.
Source:	Journal of Continuing Education in Nursing. 39(4):179-84, 2008 Apr.
Standard No:	ISSN: 0190-535X Serial Identifier: 006740000
	NLM Unique Identifier: 7809033
Language:	English
Descriptor:	Medication safety
	Decision Making, Patient
Document Type:	Journal article; research; tables/charts
Database:	CINAHL

The search results may also contain an abstract of the article, and in some instances, the full-text article is available either for a fee or at no charge.

Table 44-2 ▶ Selected Databases for Health Literature

DATABASE	DESCRIPTION
CINAHL (Cumulative Index for Nursing and Allied Health Literature)	Covers nursing, allied health, biomedical, and consumer health journals; publications of the American Nursing Association; and the National League for Nursing. Coverage with abstracts is from January 1986 to the present. Coverage with indexing from 1982 to the present. Updated monthly.
Cochrane Library	A regularly updated collection of evidence-based medicine databases, including systematic reviews, reviews of effectiveness, and a controlled-trials register. This is a source of reliable evidence about the effects of healthcare.
Health and Wellness Resource Center	Provides integrated access to medical, health, and wellness information from reference sources, magazine and journal articles, pamphlets, and some Web resources. Quick Start links include a medical encyclopedia, dictionary, drug and herb finder, health organization directory, health assessment links, health news, and a few select medical Web sites.
MEDLINE	Produced by the U.S. National Library of Medicine, MEDLINE is world's largest medical library in all areas of biomedicine and healthcare.
PsycINFO 1887	Covers worldwide literature in psychology and related disciplines, such as psychiatry, sociology, anthropology, education, linguistics, and pharmacology. Journal articles, technical reports, and dissertations are included. Coverage is from 1887 to the present. Updated weekly.

Key point: *Although an article you find on the Web may be current, it is not necessarily complete, accurate, valid, or reliable.* Many sites are created by people with questionable credentials or by companies attempting to sell their product or service. Such sites may not provide the best information to support your research. See Box 44-3 for suggestions on evaluating materials you obtain from a Web site. For ethical principles to guide health information Web sites,

 Go to Chapter 44, **Tables, Boxes, Figures: ESG Box 44-2, Guiding Ethical Principles for Health Information Web Sites,** on Davis*Plus*.

If you would like to review the process for evaluating the quality of research articles you find in your searches, or for a process to find the best evidence for a nursing intervention, refer to Chapter 8, How Can I Base My Practice on the Best Evidence?

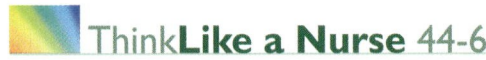 Think**Like a Nurse** 44-6

What factors can make the Web an unreliable source of information? What factors can help you find reliable information?

BOX 44-3 ■ How to Evaluate a Health Information Web Site

Remember, anyone can publish anything on the Web. The information you obtain may have been created by an expert, but most World Wide Web sites are authored by nonexperts. They may contain fact or opinion. Do not believe everything you read on the Web! Use the following questions to guide your evaluation.

Evaluate For

Questions to Ask

Authority
- *Who is the author?* What are his credentials and qualifications to speak on this topic? Are the sources of information stated? Don't confuse the author with the Webmaster.
- *Check the URL domain* (e.g., *www.nih.gov*). What institution published the document? The Web address provides clues to this:

  .com—a company.   .mil—the U.S. military
  .edu—a school or university .net—a network of computers
  .gov—the U.S. government   .org—a nonprofit organization
  The domain symbols ~ or % or a name (e.g., jsmith), "users," or "members" indicate a personal Web page.

- *Who is the sponsor?* The name right after "www" will provide a clue (e.g., see "nih"), but the full name (e.g., National Institutes of Health) should be on the page.
- *Can you contact the author* for clarification or more information?

Currency
- *When was it produced?* For some topics, you need current information.
- *When was it updated?* Note that the fact that the Web page was "updated" may not mean that the information was updated at the same time. It may simply mean that the physical file was changed in some way (e.g., a misspelled word corrected)
- *Are the links up to date?* Check the links to see whether they work.

BOX 44-3 ■ How to Evaluate a Health Information Web Site—cont'd

Evaluate For	Questions to Ask
Purpose	■ Why was the page put on the Web? Remember that many sites are designed to a product or an idea. Other purposes may be to entertain, to give facts, to share humor, or to provide a forum for ideas and opinions. ■ Look for words such as "about our company," "mission," "philosophy," "who am I," and so on. ■ Who are the intended users of the page? Students, experts, patients? ■ Are there advertisements on the page? This may be a clue.
Availability	■ Can you view or download the information without a special browser or special software? ■ Are there fees for viewing the full content?
Content quality (accuracy, objectivity, coverage)	■ Are the sources documented with footnotes or links? Are they scholarly links or information sources? ■ Is the information provided by the site, or is it reproduced from another source? ■ Are there links to the original sources (if they are online)? Or a reason for not providing a link? Do they work? ■ Look for bias (e.g., political or ideological), especially when you agree with it! Are there links to opposing views if it is an opinion page? ■ Is the information reliable and error free? Is there someone who verifies or checks the information? ■ How comprehensive is the material? ■ What does the page offer that you can't find elsewhere? ■ Look up the page in a directory that evaluates the Web site contents. For example: http://www.lib.umd.edu/ues/guides/evaluating-web http://olinuris.library.cornell.edu/ref/research/webcrit.html
Usability	■ Is it easy to read and navigate? ■ Are Help screens available? ■ Is there a search engine on the site? ■ Is it frequently offline or slow to load?

CLINICALREASONING
Applying the **Full-Spectrum Nursing Model**

Because the following critical thinking activities allow you to practice the kind of thinking you will use as a full-spectrum nurse, they usually have no single right answer. Discuss them with your peers—if you have difficulty with any of the questions, consult your instructor.

PATIENT SITUATION

Sarita, a nurse working in the surgical ICU, is ordering patient lab and recording patient information in the electronic health record (EHR). While at the computer terminal, a physician walks over to her and requests an update on a postsurgery patient's condition. They go to the bedside to assess the patient's color and perfusion after surgery. Another nurse, Janelle, needs to order a STAT x-ray using the central computer in the unit. When Sarita goes back to the computer screen to order lab work and finish her documentation, Janelle has stepped in and is now accessing another patient's record.

THINKING

1. *Theoretical Knowledge:*
   a. Name five benefits of using an electronic health record for storing and retrieving patient data in a busy critical care unit.
   b. List five potential areas of difficulty in using this same electronic health record.
2. *Critical Thinking (Considering Alternatives):*
   a. Brainstorm about possible solutions for dealing with bottlenecks among staff using a centralized computer.

DOING

3. *Practical Knowledge:*
   a. Where would you look to find out who has accessed the patient record?

(continued on next page)

CARING

4. *Ethical Knowledge:*
   a. What violation has Sarita committed in this situation? What should she have done instead?
   b. What is the nurse's responsibility in protecting patient information in the electronic record? What kinds of things should the nurse do?
5. *Self-Knowledge:*
   a. Have you ever been so busy that you feel like you just needed to take a "necessary" shortcut to save time? Describe your experience.

 Go To Chapter 44, **Clinical Reasoning: Applying the Full-Spectrum Nursing Model Response Sheet** on Davis*Plus*.

 To explore learning resources for this chapter,

 Go to Davis*Plus* at http://davisplus.fadavis.com/ keyword Treas
Chapter Resources for Chapter 44:
   Knowledge Check and Think Like a Nurse Response Sheets
   Knowledge Check Answers
   Resources for Caregivers and Health Professionals
   Reading More About Informatics (Suggested Readings)
   What Are the Main Points in This Chapter?
NCLEX-Style Review Questions
Chapter Overview Podcasts

Concept Map

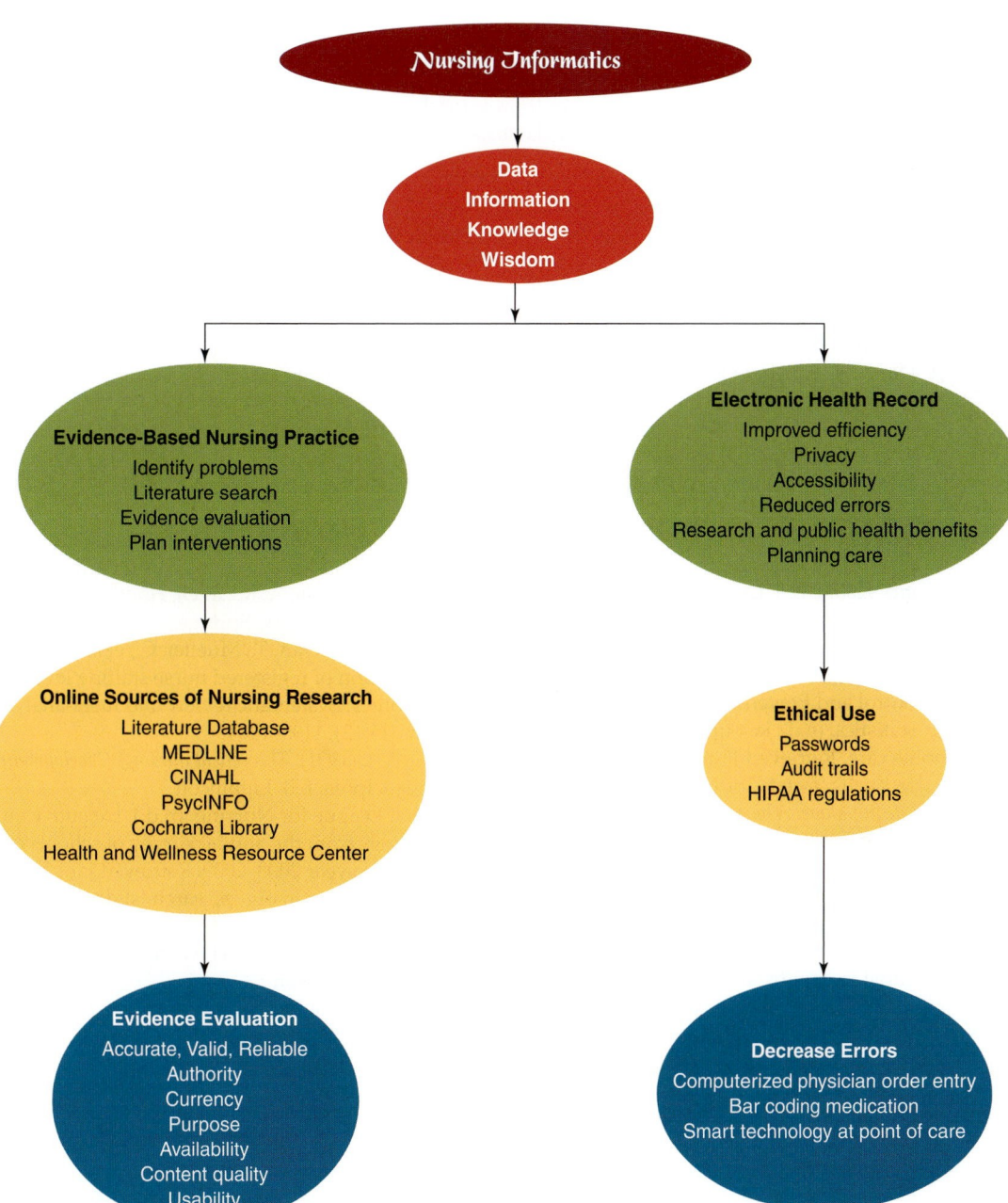

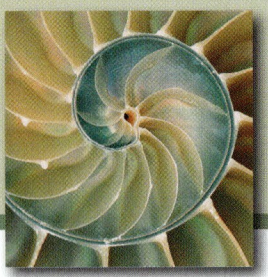

Cited Bibliography

NOTE: For a complete bibliography,

 Go to **Student Resources, Bibliography,** on Davis*Plus*.

Caveat: The URLs in this Bibliography were checked prior to publication; however, some links will be broken over time. When you find a non-working URL, try going back to the main page, or browse for the article on your preferred search engine. You might also lookup the citation in your school's library or online library database.

CHAPTER I

American Nurses Association (ANA). (1980). *Nursing's social policy statement.* Washington, DC: Author.

American Nurses Association (ANA). (2010). *Nursing: Scope and standards of practice* (2nd ed.). Silver Spring, MD: Nursebooks.org.

Benner, P. (1984). *From novice to expert: Excellence and power in clinical nursing practice.* Menlo Park, CA: Addison-Wesley.

Benner, P., & Wrubel, J. (1989). *The primacy of caring.* Menlo Park, CA: Addison-Wesley.

Bright, M. A. (2002). *Holistic health and healing.* Philadelphia: F. A. Davis.

Bureau of Labor Statistics (2009). U.S. Department of Labor. *Occupational outlook handbook,* 2010-2011 Edition. Registered Nurses. Retrieved January 9, 2011, from http://www.bls.gov/oco/ocos083.htm

Centers for Disease Control and Prevention (CDC), National Center for Health Statistics. (n.d., last updated April 15, 2010). Nursing home care. Retrieved January 9, 2011, from http://www.cdc.gov/nchs/fastats/nursingh.htm

Chambers, P. (1958). *A doctor alone: A biography of Elizabeth Blackwell, the first woman doctor.* London: Abelard-Schuman.

Cronenwett, L., Sherwood, G., Barnsteiner, J., et al. (2007). Quality and safety education for nurses. *Nursing Outlook, 55*(3), 122–131.

Darcé, K. (2007, November 7). Are retail clinics a healthy choice? Outlets opening in county could fill niche; physicians warn of drawbacks. *The San Diego Union-Tribune.* Retrieved January 9, 2011, from http://www.signonsandiego.com/news/business/20071107-9999-1n7clinics.html

Disch, J., Bellman, G., & Ingbar, D. (2001). Medical directors as partners in creating healthy work environments. *AACN Clinical Issues, 12*(3), 366–377.

Dock, L. L., & Stewart, I. M. (1938). *A short history of nursing* (4th ed.). New York: Putnam.

Donahue, M. P. (1985). *Nursing: The finest art. An illustrated history.* St. Louis, MO: C. V. Mosby.

Health Resources and Services Administration. (2004). The registered nurse population: Findings from the March 2004 national sample survey of registered nurses. Washington, DC: U.S. Department of Health and Human Services, Bureau of Health Professions. Retrieved December 1, 2010, from http://bhpr.hrsa.gov/healthworkforce/rnsurvey04/

Health Resources and Services Administration (HRSA). (2010, September). *The registered nurse population. findings from the 2008 National Sample Survey of Registered Nurses.* Retrieved January 6, 2011, from http://bhpr.hrsa.gov/healthworkforce/rnsurvey/2008/nssrn2008.pdf

Henderson, V. (1966). *The nature of nursing.* New York: Macmillan.

Hobbs, F. (2001). The elderly population. U.S. Census Bureau. Retrieved January 7, 2011, from http://www.census.gov/population/www/pop-profile/elderpop.html

International Council of Nurses. (2007, last updated 2010, April 12). ICN definition of nursing. Retrieved December 1, 2007, from http://www.icn.ch/definition.htm

Jonas, S., & Kovner, A. R. (2005). *Health care delivery in the U.S.* (8th ed.). New York: Springer.

Kane, R., Shamliyan, T., Mueller, C., et al. (2007). The association of registered nurse staffing levels and patient outcomes: Systematic review and meta-analysis. *Medical Care, 45*(12), 1195–1204.

Meleis, A. I. (1991). *Theoretical nursing: Development and progress.* Philadelphia: J. B. Lippincott.

National League for Nursing. (n.d.). Executive summary. Findings from the annual survey of schools of nursing, academic year 2008–2009. Retrieved January 7, 2011, from http://www.nln.org/research/slides/exec_summary_0809.pdf

Nightingale, F. (1876). *Notes on nursing for the labouring classes.* London: Harrison.

Potera, C. (2007). In the news. Infections and deaths down, quality up. *American Journal of Nursing, 107*(4), 19.

Pullen, R. L., Jr. (2006). Why choose nursing education? *Men in Nursing, 1*(5), 36–39.

Quadagno, J. S. (2004). Physician sovereignty and the purchasers' revolt. *Journal of Health Politics, Policy and Law, 29*(4), 815–834.

Rockwell, L. H., Jr. (1994). The American Medical Association: A sordid history. Retrieved December 5, 2010, from http://www.healthe-livingnews.com/articles/american_medical_association_sorbid_history.html

Safriet, B. J. (1994). Impediments to progress in healthcare work-force policy: License and practice laws. *Inquiry, 31*(3), 310–317.

Starr, P. (1982). *The social transformation of American medicine.* New York: Basic Books.

Sterchi, S. (2007). Perceptions that affect physician-nurse collaboration in the perioperative setting. *AORN Journal* (July). Retrieved January 8, 2011, from http://findarticles.com/p/articles/mi_m0FSL/is_1_86/ai_n19448209/pg_1

Sultz, H., & Young, K. (2008). *Health care USA: Understanding its organization and delivery* (6th ed.). Burlington, MA: Jones & Bartlett Learning.

Tourangeau, A., Doran, D., Hall, L., et al. (2007). Impact of hospital nursing care on 30-day mortality for acute medical patients. *Journal of Advanced Nursing, 57*(1), 32–44.

U.S. Census Bureau. (last modified 2007, May 31). U.S. interim projections by age, sex, race, and Hispanic origin Summary tables. Retrieved January 8, 2011, from http://www.census.gov/ipc/www/usinterimproj/

U.S. Department of Labor. Bureau of Labor Statistics. (2009). Registered nurses. *Occupational outlook handbook* (2010–2011 ed.). Retrieved January 9, 2011, from http://www.bls.gov/oco/ocos083.htm

Venes, D. (2009). *Taber's cyclopedic medical dictionary* (21st ed.). Philadelphia: F. A. Davis.

Wilkinson, J. M. (1996). The C word: A curriculum for the future. *N&HC: Perspectives on Community, 17*(2), 72–77.

World Health Organization (WHO). (2007). Frequently Asked Questions. Preamble to the Constitution of the World Health Organization as adopted by the International Health Conference, New York, June 19–July 22, 1946; signed on July 22 by the representatives of 62 States (*Official Records of the World Health Organization,* no. 2, p. 100) and entered into force on April 7, 1948. Retrieved January 8, 2011, from http://www.who.int/suggestions/faq/en/

CHAPTER 2

American Nurses Association (ANA). (2010). *Nursing: Scope and standards of practice* (2nd ed.). Silver Spring, MD: Nursebooks.org

American Philosophical Association. (1990). *Executive summary of: Critical thinking: A statement of expert consensus for purposes of educational assessment.* Millbrae, CA: California Academic Press.

Brookfield, S. D. (1991). *Developing critical thinkers.* San Francisco: Jossey-Bass.

Ennis, R. H. (2004). A super-streamlined conception of critical thinking. Retrieved January 9, 2011, from http://www.criticalthinking.net/SSConcCTApr3.html

Heaslip, P. (1992). Creating the thinking practitioner: Critical thinking in clinical practice. Unpublished manuscript. (ERIC Document Reproduction Service No. ED354822).

McDonald, M. E. (2002). *Systematic assessment of learning outcomes: Developing multiple-choice exams.* Boston: Jones & Bartlett.

Moore, B. N., & Parker, R. (2009). *Critical thinking* (9th ed.). Columbus, OH: McGraw-Hill.

Paul, R. W. (1990). *Critical thinking.* Rohnert Park, CA: Center for Critical Thinking and Moral Critique, Sonoma State University.

Paul, R. W. (1993). *Critical thinking: What every person needs to survive in a rapidly changing world* (3rd ed.). Santa Rosa, CA: Foundation for Critical Thinking.

Paul, R. W., Ennis, R. H., & Norris, S. (1996). In: B. Fowler (Ed.), *Critical thinking definitions* (Critical Thinking Across the Curriculum Project). Lee's Summit, MO: Longview Community College.

Raingruber, B., & Haffer, A. (2001). *Using your head to land on your feet.* Philadelphia: F. A. Davis.

Swanson, K. M. (1990). Providing care in the NICU: Sometimes an act of love. *Advances in Nursing, 13,* 60–73.

Wilkinson, J. M. (2011). *Nursing process & critical thinking* (5th ed.). Upper Saddle River, NJ, Prentice-Hall.

CHAPTER 3

American Nurses Association (ANA). (2008) *Guide to the Code of Ethics for Nurses—interpretation and application.* Silver Spring, MD: Author.

American Nurses Association (ANA). (2010). *Nursing: Scope and standards of practice* (2nd ed.). Silver Spring, MD: Nursebooks.org.

Cronenwett, L., Sherwood, G., Barnsteiner, J., et al. (2007). Quality and safety education for nurses. *Nursing Outlook, 55*(3), 122–131.

Dochterman, J. M., & Jones, D. A. (Eds.). (2003). *Unifying nursing languages: The harmonization of NANDA, NIC, and NOC.* Washington, DC: American Nurses Association, Nursesbooks.org

Gordon, M. (1994). *Nursing diagnosis: Process and application* (3rd ed., p. 70). St. Louis, MO: C. V. Mosby.

Graf, C. (2008). How to try this: The Lawton Instrumental Activities of Daily Living Scale. *American Journal of Nursing, 108*(4), 52–62.

The Joint Commission (TJC). (2008). *Hospital accreditation standards.* Oakbrook Terrace, IL: Author.

Karnofsky, D. A., & Burchenal, J. H. (1949). The clinical evaluation of chemotherapeutic agents in cancer. In: C. M. MacLeod (Ed.), *Evaluation of chemotherapeutic agents.* New York: Columbia University Press.

Lawton, M. P., & Brody, E. M. (1969). Assessment of older people: Self-maintaining and instrumental activities of daily living. *The Gerontologist, 9*(3), 179–186.

Maslow, A. (1970). *Motivation and personality* (2nd ed.). New York: Harper & Row.

Maslow, A., & Lowery, R. (Eds.). (1998). *Toward a psychology of being* (3rd ed.). New York: John Wiley & Sons.

NANDA International (NANDA-I). (2009). *Nursing diagnoses: Definitions and classification 2009–2011.* Philadelphia: Author.

National Council of State Boards of Nursing (NCSBN). (2011). *Model nursing practice act.* Retrieved March 31, 2011, from https://www.ncsbn.org/Model_Nursing_Practice_Act_March2011.pdf

Orem, D. (1991). *Nursing: Concepts of practice* (4th ed., p. 126). St. Louis, MO: Mosby Year Book.

Orem, D.E. (1995). *Nursing: Concepts of practice* (5th ed.). St. Louis, MO: Mosby.

Purnell, L. D., & Paulanka, B. J. (2008). *Transcultural health care: A culturally competent approach* (3rd ed.). Philadelphia: F. A. Davis.

Roy, C., & Andrews, H. (1991). *The Roy adaptation model: The definitive statement* (pp. 15–17). Norwalk, CT: Appleton & Lange.

Roy, C., & Andrews, A. A. (1999). *The Roy adaptation model* (2nd ed.). Norwalk, CT: Appleton & Lange.

Shelkey, M., & Wallace, M. (2007). Katz index of independence in activities of daily living (ADL). *Try this: Best practices in nursing care to older adults,* 2. Hartford Institute for Geriatric Nursing, New York University College of Nursing. Retrieved March 31, 2011, from http://consultgerirn.org/uploads/File/trythis/try_this_2.pdf

CHAPTER 4

American Medical Association (AMA). (2010). *Current procedural terminology: CPT 2010* (professional ed.). Chicago: Author.

American Nurses Association (ANA). (1980). *ANA social policy statement.* Washington, DC: Author.

American Nurses Association (ANA). (2010). *Nursing: Scope and standards of practice* (2nd ed.). Silver Spring, MD: Nursebooks.org.

American Psychiatric Association. (2000). *Diagnostic and statistical manual of mental disorders.* Arlington, VA: Author.

Bates, D. W., Ebell, M., Gotlieb, E., et al. (2003). A proposal for electronic medical records in U.S. primary care. *Journal of the American Medical Informatics Association, 10*(1), 1–10.

Beyea, S. (2000, May). Standardized nursing vocabularies and the perioperative nursing data set: Making clinical practice count. *CIN plus, 3*(2), 1, 5, 6.

Carpenito, L. J. (2006). *Nursing diagnosis: Application to clinical practice* (11th ed.). Philadelphia: J. B. Lippincott.

Gordon, M. (1994). *Nursing diagnosis: Process and application* (3rd ed.). St. Louis, MO: C. V. Mosby.

International Council of Nurses (ICN). (2005). *International classification for nursing practice.* Geneva, Switzerland: Author.

Lunney, M. (2008). Critical need to address accuracy of nurses' diagnoses. *Online Journal of Issues in Nursing, 13.*

Maslow, A. (1971). *The farther reaches of human nature.* New York: Viking Press.

Maslow, A., & Lowery, R. (Eds.). (1998). *Toward a psychology of being* (3rd ed.). New York: John Wiley & Sons.

Müller-Stauber, M., Lavin, M. A., Needham, I., et al. (2006). Nursing diagnoses, interventions and outcomes—application and impact on nursing practice: Systematic review. *Journal of Advanced Nursing, 56*(5j), 514–531.

NANDA International (NANDA-I). (2009). *NANDA nursing diagnoses: Definitions & classification 2009–2011.* Philadelphia: Author.

Wilkinson, J. M. (2011). *Nursing process and critical thinking* (5th ed.). Upper Saddle River, NJ: Prentice-Hall.

World Health Organization (WHO). (1992). *Manual of the international classification of diseases and related health problems* (10th rev. ed.). Geneva, Switzerland: Author.

CHAPTER 5

American Nurses Association (ANA). (2010). *Nursing: Scope and standards of practice* (2nd ed.). Silver Spring, MD: Author.

Green, C., & Wilkinson, J. (2004). *Maternal newborn nursing care plans.* St. Louis: Mosby.

Harris, B. L. (1990). Becoming deprofessionalized: One aspect of the staff nurse's perspective on computer-mediated nursing care plans. *Advances in Nursing Science, 13*(2), 63–74.

Healthy People 2020. (2010). Washington, DC: U.S. Department of Health and Human Services. Retrieved April 8, 2011, from http://healthypeople.gov/2020/about/default.aspx

Johnson, M., Moorhead, S., Bulechek, C., et al. (2012). *NOC and NIC linkages to NANDA-I and clinical conditions* (3rd ed.). St. Louis, MO: C. V. Mosby.

Moorhead, S., Johnson, M., Maas, M., et al. (2008). *Nursing outcomes classification* (4th ed.). St. Louis, MO: C. V. Mosby/Elsevier.

Mueller, A., Johnston, M., & Bligh, D. (2002). Viewpoint: Joining mind mapping and care planning to enhance student critical thinking and achieve holistic nursing care. *Nursing Diagnosis: The International Journal of Nursing Language and Classification, 13*(1), 24–27.

NANDA International (NANDA-I). (2009). *Nursing diagnoses: Definitions and classification 2009–2011.* Ames, IA: Wiley-Blackwell.

NSW Department of Health. (2011). Policy directive. Care coordination: Planning from admission to transfer of care in NSW public hospitals. Retrieved April 6, 2011, from http://www.health.nsw.gov.au/policies/pd/2011/pdf/PD2011_015.pdf

Walker, C., Hogstel, M., & Curry, L. (2007). Hospital discharge of older adults. *American Journal of Nursing, 107*(6), 60–71.

Wilkinson, J. M. (2011). *Nursing process & critical thinking* (5th ed.). Upper Saddle River, NJ: Prentice-Hall.

CHAPTER 6

Agency for Healthcare Research and Quality (AHRQ). (2003, updated 2008). Guideline summary. Preventing pressure ulcers and skin tears. In: *Evidence-based geriatric nursing protocols for best practice.* Retrieved April 10, 2011, from http://www.guideline.gov/content.aspx?id=12262&search=pressure+ulcer#Section442.

American Nurses Association (ANA). (2006). ANA-recognized terminologies and data element sets. Retrieved April 10, 2011, from http://nursingworld.org/npii/terminologies.htm

American Nurses Association (ANA). (2010). *Nursing: Scope and standards of practice* (2nd ed.). Silver Spring, MD: Author.

Barton, M. B., Miller, T., Wolff, T., et al. (2007). How to read the new recommendation statement: methods update from the U.S. Preventive Services Task Force. Originally published in *Annals of Internal Medicine, 147,* 123–127. Retrieved April 10, 2011, from http://www.uspreventiveservicestaskforce.org/uspstf07/methods/methupd.htm

Bulechek, G. M., Butcher, H. K., & Dochterman, J. C. (Eds.) (2012). *Nursing interventions classification (NIC)* (6th ed.). St. Louis, MO: C. V. Mosby.

Cronenwett, L. R. (2002). Research, practice and policy: Issues in evidence-based care. *Online Journal of Issues in Nursing, 7*(2). Retrieved April 23, 2011, from http://www.nursingworld.org/MainMenuCategories/ANAMarketplace/ANAPeriodicals/OJIN/Columns/KeynotesofNote/EvidenceBasedCare.aspx

Cronenwett, L., Sherwood, G., Barnsteiner, J., et al. (2007). Quality and safety education for nurses. *Nursing Outlook, 55*(3), 122–131.

Fain, J. A. (2008). *Reading, understanding, and applying nursing research: A text and workbook* (3rd ed.). Philadelphia: F. A. Davis.

Frisch, N. C. (2001, May 31). Nursing as a context for alternative/complementary modalities. *Online Journal of Issues in Nursing, 6*(2), Manuscript 2, p. 2. Retrieved April 10, 2011, from http://www.nursingworld.org/MainMenuCategories/ANAMarketplace/ANAPeriodicals/OJIN/TableofContents/Volume62001/No2May01/AlternativeComplementaryModalities.aspx

Institute of Medicine. (1992). Guidelines for clinical practice: From development to use. In: M. J. Field & K. N. Lohr (Eds.). Washington, DC: National Academies Press.

Joanna Briggs Institute. (2007). Topical skin care in aged care facilities. *Best Practice Information Sheet, 11*(3). Retrieved April 10, 2011, from http://connect.jbiconnectplus.org/ViewSourceFile.aspx?0=4346

Johnson, M., Moorhead, S., Bulechek, G., Butcher, H., et al. (2012). *NOC and NIC linkages to NANDA-I and clinical conditions* (3rd ed.). St. Louis, MO: C. V. Mosby.

Martin, K. (2005). *The Omaha System: A key to practice, documentation, and information management* (2nd ed.). Philadelphia: W. B. Saunders.

McCloskey, J. C., & Bulechek, G. M. (Eds.). (1992). *Nursing interventions classification (NIC)*. St. Louis, MO: C. V. Mosby.

Quality and Safety Education for Nurses. (2011). Quality and safety competencies. Retrieved April 9, 2011, from http://www.qsen.org/ksas_prelicensure.php

Saba, V. K. (1995). Home Health Care Classifications (HHCCs): Nursing diagnoses and nursing interventions. In: *An emerging framework: Data system advances for clinical nursing practice*. ANA Publication No. NP-94. Washington, DC: American Nurses Association (ANA). Also available at http://www.sabacare.com/

Saba, V. K. (2006). *Clinical care classification system manual: A guide to nursing documentation*. New York: Springer.

Titler, M. G., Mentes, J. C., Rakel, B. A., et al. (1999). From book to bedside: Putting evidence to use in the care of the elderly. *Joint Commission Journal of Quality Improvement, 25*, 545–556.

Wilkinson, J. M. (2011). *Nursing process & critical thinking* (5th ed.). Upper Saddle River, NJ: Prentice-Hall.

CHAPTER 7

American Nurses Association (ANA). (1996). *Registered professional nurses and unlicensed assistive personnel* (2nd ed.). Washington, DC: Author.

American Nurses Association (ANA). (2001). *Code of ethics for nurses with interpretive statements*. Washington, DC: Author.

American Nurses Association (ANA). (2007). Revised position statement: Registered nurses utilization of nursing assistive personnel in all settings. Retrieved March 1, 2008, from http://www.nursingworld.org/MainMenu Categories/HealthcareandPolicyIssues/ANAPosition Statements/uap/UnlicensedAssistivePersonnel.aspx

American Nurses Association (ANA). (2010). *Nursing: Scope and standards of practice* (2nd ed.). Silver Spring, MD: Author.

American Nurses Association (ANA) and the National Council of State Boards of Nursing (NCSBN). (2006). Joint statement on delegation. American Nurses Association (ANA) and the National Council of State Boards of Nursing (NCSBN). Retrieved February 1, 2008, from https://www.ncsbn.org/1056.htm

Ayers, D. M. M., & Montgomery, M. (2008). Delegating the "right" way. *Nursing2008, 38*(4), 57–58.

Bulechek, G. M., Butcher, H. K., & Dochterman, J. M. (Eds.) (2012). *Nursing interventions classification (NIC)* (6th ed.). St. Louis, MO: C. V. Mosby.

Cronenwett, L., Sherwood, G., Barnsteiner, J., et al. (2007). Quality and safety education for nurses. *Nursing Outlook, 55*(3), 122–131.

Dickens, G., Stubbs, J., & Haw, C. (2008). Delegation of medication administration: An exploratory study. *Nursing Standard, 22*(22), 35–40.

Draper D. A, et al. (2008) The role of nurses in hospital quality improvement. HSC Research Brief No. 3. Accessed September 18, 2011, from http://hschange.org/CONTENT/972/

Johnson, K., Hallsey, D., Meredith, R. L., et al. (2006). A nurse-driven system for improving patient quality outcomes. *Journal of Nursing Care Quality, 21*(2), 168–175.

London, F. (1998). Improving compliance. What you can do. *RN, 61*(1), 43–46.

National Council of State Boards of Nursing. (1995). *Delegation: Concepts and decision-making process*. National Council position paper. Chicago: Author.

Wilkinson, J. (2011). *Nursing process & critical thinking* (5th ed.). Upper Saddle River, NJ: Prentice-Hall.

CHAPTER 8

American Nurses Association (ANA). (1981). *Guidelines for the investigative functions of nurses*. Washington, DC: Author.

American Nurses Association (ANA). (1994). Position statement: Education for participation in nursing research—4/94. Retrieved March 2, 2008, from http://nursingworld.org/MainMenuCategories/HealthcareandPolicyIssues/ANAPositionStatements/Archives/rseducat14484.aspx

American Nurses Association (ANA). (2010). *Nursing: Scope and standards of practice* (2nd ed.). Silver Spring, MD: Nursebooks.org.

Benner, P. (1984). *From novice to expert. Excellence and power in clinical nursing practice*. Menlo Park, CA: Addison-Wesley.

Benner, P., & Wrubel, J. (1989). *The primacy of caring: Stress and coping in health and illness*. Menlo Park, CA: Addison-Wesley.

Brockopp, D. Y., & Hastongs-Tolsma, M. T. (2003). *Fundamentals of nursing research* (3rd ed.). Sudbury, MA: Jones & Bartlett.

Bulechek, G. M., Butcher, H. K., & Dochterman, J. M. (Eds.) (2012). *Nursing interventions classification (NIC)* (6th ed.). St. Louis, MO: C. V. Mosby.

Center for Evidence Based Medicine. Asking focused clinical questions. Page last edited April 7, 2009. Retrieved January 12, 2011, from http://www.cebm.net/index.aspx?o=1036

Chinn, P., & Kramer, M. (1991). *Theory and nursing: A systematic approach*. St. Louis, MO: Mosby Year Book.

Chinn, P. L., & Kramer, M. K. (2007). *Theory and nursing: Integrated knowledge development* (7th ed.). St. Louis, MO: C. V. Mosby.

Cronenwett, L., Sherwood, G., Barnsteiner, J., et al. (2007). Quality and safety education for nurses. *Nursing Outlook, 55*(3), 122–131.

Dossey, B. M. (1999). *Florence Nightingale: Mystic, visionary, healer*. Springhouse, PA: Springhouse.

Fain, J. A. (2009). *Reading, understanding, and applying nursing research: A text and workbook* (3rd ed.). Philadelphia: F. A. Davis.

Feil, N. (2003). *V/F validation* (rev. ed.). Cincinnati, OH: Feil Productions. Also available from http://www.edwardfeilproductions.com/catalogue.html#books

Flaskerud, J. H., & Halloran, E. J. (1980). Areas of agreement in nursing theory development. *Advances in Nursing Science, 3*(1), 1–7.

Goode, C., Butcher, L., Cipperley, J., et al. (1996). *Research utilization: A study guide* (2nd ed.). Ida Grove, IA: Horn Video Productions.

Hall, L.E. (1966). Another view of nursing care and quality. In: M.K. Straub, *Continuity of patient care. The role of nursing*. Washington, D.C.: Catholic University of America Press.

Henderson, V. (1966). *The nature of nursing*. New York: Macmillan.

Horsley, J.A. (1983). *Using research to improve nursing practice.* NY: Grune & Stratton.

Johnson, D. E. (1968). Theory in nursing: Borrowed and unique. *Nursing Research, 11,* 206.

Johnson, D. E. (1980). The behavioral system for nursing. In: J. P. Riehl & C. Roy (Eds.), *Conceptual models for nursing practice* (2nd ed., pp. 207–216). New York: Appleton-Century-Crofts.

King, I. M. (1971). *Toward a theory for nursing: General concepts of human behavior.* New York: John Wiley & Sons.

Kolcaba, K. Y. (1994). A theory of holistic comfort for nursing. *Journal of Advanced Nursing, 19,* 1178–1184.

Leininger, M. M. (1978). *Transcultural nursing: Concepts, theories and practices.* New York: John Wiley & Sons.

Leininger, M. M. (1981). The phenomenon of caring: Importance, research questions, and theoretical considerations. In *Caring: An essential human need* (Proceedings of the three national caring conferences; pp. 3–15). Thorofare, NJ: Charles B. Slack.

Levine, M. E. (1967). The four conservation principles of nursing. *Nursing Forum, 6,* 45–59.

Levine, M. E. (1969). *Introduction to clinical nursing.* Philadelphia: F. A. Davis.

Marriner-Tomey, A., & Raile-Alligood, M. (2006) *Nursing theorists and their work* (6th ed.). St. Louis, MO: C. V. Mosby.

Maslow, A. (1970). *Motivation and personality* (2nd ed.). New York: Harper & Row.

Maslow, A. (1971). *The farther reaches of human nature.* New York: Viking Press.

Maslow, A., & Lowery, R. (Eds.). (1998). *Toward a psychology of being* (3rd ed.). New York: John Wiley & Sons.

National Heart, Lung, and Blood Institute & Boston University. (n.d., last updated 2012). *Framingham Heart Study.* Available at http://www.framinghamheartstudy.org/index.html. Updated September 20, 2007. Retrieved February 8, 2012.

National Institute of Nursing Research (NINR). (n.d., page last updated 2007, April 18). 2004 areas of research opportunity. Retrieved February 15, 2011, from http://www.nih.gov/ninr/research/dea/2004AoRO.html

National Institute of Nursing Research (NINR). (2005). *Mission statement.* Retrieved January 28, 2011, from http://www.ninr.nih.gov/NR/rdonlyres/9021E5EB-B2BA-47EA-B5DB-1E4DB11B1289/4894/NINR_StrategicPlanWebsite.pdf

National Institute of Nursing Research (NINR). (2010, December 24). Weekly funding opportunities and notices, table of contents (TOC). Retrieved February 15, 2011, from http://grants1.nih.gov/grants/guide/WeeklyIndex.cfm/12-24-2010/

National Institutes of Health (NIH). (n.d.a, last reviewed 2010, February 9). The NIH almanac—organization. National Institute of Nursing Research. Retrieved February 10, 2008, from http://nih.gov/about/almanac/organization/NINR.htm

National Institutes of Health (NIH). (n.d.b). Nuremberg Code: Directives for human experimentation. *Regulations and ethical guidelines.* Office of Human Subjects Research. Retrieved January 13, 2011, from http://ohsr.od.nih.gov/guidelines/nuremberg.html

Neuman, B. M., & Young, R. J. (1972). A model for teaching total person approach to patient problems. *Nursing Research, 21,* 264–269.

Nieswiadomy, R. M. (2008). *Foundations of nursing research* (5th ed.). Upper Saddle River, NJ: Prentice-Hall.

Nightingale, F. (1859/1992). *Notes on nursing: What it is and what it is not.* Philadelphia: J. B. Lippincott.

NurseScribe©. (2000–2007, updated 2007, July 20). Nursing theory page. Retrieved January 13, 2011, from http://www.enursescribe.com/ (Page under construction at time of publication).

Orlando, I. J. (1972). *The dynamic nurse-patient relationship: Function, process, and principles.* New York: G. P. Putnam's Sons.

Parse, R. R. (1981). *Man-living-health: A theory of nursing.* New York: John Wiley & Sons.

Pender, N. J., Murdaugh, C. L., & Parsons, M. A. (2006). *Health promotion in nursing practice* (5th ed.). Upper Saddle River, NJ: Prentice-Hall.

Peplau, H. E. (1952). *Interpersonal relations in nursing.* New York: G. P. Putnam's Sons.

Polit, D. F., & Beck, C. T. (2007). *Nursing research: Generating and assessing evidence* (8th ed.). Philadelphia: Lippincott Williams & Wilkins.

Rigdon, I. S., Clayton, B. D., & Dimond, M. (1987). Toward a theory of helpfulness for the elderly bereaved: An invitation to a new life. *Advances in Nursing Science, 9*(2), 32–43.

Rogers, M. (1970). *An introduction to the theoretical basis of nursing.* Philadelphia: F. A. Davis.

Sacket, D., Richardson, W., Rosenberg, W., et al. (1997). *Evidence-based medicine: How to practice and teach EBM.* New York: Churchill Livingstone.

Selye, H. (1993). *Neuroendocrinology and stress.* New York: New York Academy of Science.

Stilwell, S., Fineout-Overholt, E., Melnyk, G., et al., (2010). Evidence-based practice, step by step: Asking the clinical Question: A key step in evidence-based practice. *American Journal of Nursing, 110*(3): 58-61.

Sullivan, D. T., & Warren, J. (2007). Quality and safety education for nurses. *Nursing Outlook, 55*(3), 122–131. Retrieved February 1, 2011, from http://www.nursingoutlook.org/article/S0029-6554(07)00062-0/abstract

University of Southern California, Health Sciences, Los Angeles. (n.d.) Evidence based decision making, asking a good question (PICO). Retrieved January 12, 2011, from http://www.usc.edu/hsc/ebnet/ebframe/PICO.htm

Von Bertalanffy, L. (1976). *General system theory: Foundations, development and applications* (rev. ed.). New York: George Braziller.

Watson, J. (1988). *Nursing: Human science and human care. A theory of nursing* (Publication No. 15–2236). New York: National League for Nursing Press.

Watson, J. (2007). Theory evolution. Dr. Jean Watson's Theory of Human Caring. Denver: University of Colorado Health Sciences Center School of Nursing. Retrieved February 3, 2011, from http://www.nursing.ucdenver.edu/faculty/jw_evolution.htm

Wiedenbach, E. (1964). *Clinical nursing: A helping art.* New York: Springer.

Wilson, H. S. (1993). *Introducing research in nursing* (2nd ed.). Redwood City, CA: Addison-Wesley Nursing.

Yura, H., & Torres, G. (1975). *Today's conceptual frameworks with the baccalaureate nursing programs* (NLN Publication No. 15-1558). New York: National League for Nursing.

CHAPTER 9

About Teen Depression [Fact sheet]. (n.d.). Educational Web site sponsored by CRC Health Group. Retrieved March 29, 2011, from http://www.about-teen-depression.com/teen-depression.html

Advisory Committee on Immunization Practices (ACIP). (2008). Prevention and control of influenza. Recommendations of the Advisory Committee on Immunization Practices (ACPI), 2007. *MMWR Recommendations and Reports, 57*(RR-07), 1–60. Retrieved March 18, 2011, from http://www.cdc.gov/mmwr/preview/mmwrhtml/rr5707a1.htm

American Academy of Family Physicians (AAFP). (2006, updated 2010). Toilet training your child. (Written by familydoctor.org editorial staff.) Retrieved March 26, 2011, from http://familydoctor.org/online/famdocen/home/children/parents/toilet/179.html

American Academy of Pediatrics (AAP). (2005). Policy statement: AAP Publications reaffirmed, October 2004: Condom use by adolescents. *Pediatrics, 107,* 1451–1455. Retrieved March 3, 2011, from http://aappolicy.aappublications.org/cgi/reprint/pediatrics;115/5/1438.pdf

American Academy of Pediatrics (AAP). (2006). Policy statement. Active healthy living: Prevention of childhood obesity through increased physical activity. *Pediatrics, 117*(5), 1834–1842.

American Academy of Pediatrics (AAP). (2011). Children's health topics. Car safety seats: A guide for families 2010. Retrieved March 26, 2011, from http://www.aap.org/healthtopics/carseatsafety.cfm

American Cancer Society. (n.d.a, last reviewed, 2010). How to examine your breasts. Retrieved March 10, 2011, from http://www.cancer.org/docroot/CRI/content/CRI_2_6x_How_to_perform_a_breast_self_exam_5.aspAmerican Cancer Society (2010, last revised).

American Cancer Society. (n.d.b, last revised July 2010). Guidelines for the early detection of cancer. Retrieved February 20, 2011, from http://www.cancer.org/docroot/PED/content/PED_2_3X_ACS_Cancer_Detection_Guidelines_36.asp?sitearea+PED

American Cancer Society (ACS). (2010). Detailed guide: Breast cancer. American Cancer Society recommendations for early breast cancer detection. Retrieved March 28, 2011, from http://www.cancer.org/acs/groups/cid/documents/webcontent/003090-pdf.pdf

American Heart Association (AHA). (2011a). Overweight in children. Retrieved March 7, 2011, from http://www.americanheart.org/presenter.jhtml?identifier=4670

American Heart Association (AHA). (2011b). Physical activity. Retrieved March 4, 2011, from http://www.americanheart.org/presenter.jhtml?identifier=4563

American Lung Association (ALA). (2010). Trends in tobacco use. Retrieved March 29, 2011, from http://www.lungusa.org/finding-cures/our-research/trend-reports/Tobacco-Trend-Report.pdf

APGAR. (n.d., last updated 2009, November 30). MedlinePlus: Medical encyclopedia. U.S. National Library of Medicine, National Institutes of Health. Retrieved March 27, 2011, from http://www.gov/medlineplus/ency/article/003402.htm#top

Balkaya, N., Memis, S., & Demirkiran, F. (2007). The effects of breast self-exam education on the performance of nursing and midwifery students: A 6-month follow-up study. *Journal of Cancer Education, 22*(2), 77–79.

Broderick, P. (1998). Pediatric vision screening for the family physician. (Includes American Academy of Pediatrics vision screening guidelines). *American Family Physician, 58*(3). Retrieved March 27, 2008, from http://www.aafp.org/afp/980901ap/broderic.html

Brodowski, M. L., Nolan, C. M., Gaudiosi, J. A., et al. (2008, April 4). Nonfatal maltreatment of infants—United States, October 2005–September 2006. *Morbidity and Mortality Weekly Report, 57*(13), 336–339.

Bureau of Justice Statistics. (n.d., last reviewed 2011). Homicide trends in the U.S., intimate homicide. U.S. Department of Justice, Office of Justice Programs. Retrieved March 15, 2011, from http://bjs.ojp.usdoj.gov/content/homicide/intimates.cfm

Centers for Disease Control and Prevention (CDC). (n.d., last updated 2011, February 15). About BMI for children and teens. Retrieved March 3, 2011, from http://www.cdc.gov/healthyweight/assessing/bmi/childrens_bmi/about_childrens_bmi.html#My%20two%20children

Centers for Disease Control and Prevention (CDC). (2002). Infant mortality statistics from the 1999 period linked birth/infant death data set. *National Vital Statistics Reports, 50*(4). Retrieved March 2, 2011, from http://www.cdc.gov/nchs/fastats/infant_health.htm

Centers for Disease Control and Prevention (CDC). (2005a). 10 Leading causes of unintentional injury deaths, United States, 2005; and WISQARS injury mortality reports, 1999–2005. (Last reviewed 2008, January 23). *National Center for Injury Prevention and Control.* Retrieved March 28, 2011, from http://webappa.cdc.gov/sasweb/ncipc/mortrate10_sy.html

Centers for Disease Control and Prevention (CDC). (2005b). Sexual behavior and selected health measures: Men and women 15–44 years of age, United States, 2002. Advance data from *Vital and Health Statistics, 362.* Retrieved March 28, 2011, from http://www.cdc.gov/nchs/data/ad/ad362.pdf

Centers for Disease Control and Prevention (CDC). (2006). The state of childhood asthma, United States, 1980–2005. Advance data from *Vital and Health Statistics, 381.* Retrieved March 28, 2011, from http://www.cdc.gov/nchs/data/ad/ad381.pdf

Centers for Disease Control and Prevention (CDC). (2007a). Summary health statistics for U.S. children: National health interview survey, 2006. *Vital and Health Statistics, 10*(234). Retrieved March 28, 2011, from http://www.cdc.gov/nchs/data/series/sr_10/sr10_234.pdf

Centers for Disease Control and Prevention (CDC). (2007b). Adolescent reproductive health home. Teen pregnancy. Retrieved March 29, 2011, from http://www.cdc.gov/reproductivehealth/AdolescentReproHealth/

Centers for Disease Control and Prevention (2008). HIV/AIDS among persons aged 50 and older. Retrieved March 3, 2011, from http://www.cdc.gov/hiv/topics/over50/resources/factsheets/over50.htm

Centers for Disease Control and Prevention (CDC). (2010a). State disparities in teenage birth rates in the United States. NCHS Data Brief No. 46. Retrieved March 17, 2012, from http://www.cdc.gov/nchs/data/databriefs/db46.pdf

Centers for Disease Control and Prevention (CDC). (2010b). HIV in the United States. Retrieved March 3, 2011, from http://www.cdc.gov/hiv/resources/factsheets/us.htm

Centers for Disease Control and Prevention (CDC). (2011b). Vital signs: Teen pregnancy—United States, 1991–2009. *Morbidity and Mortality Weekly Report, 60*(13), 414–420.

Centers for Disease Control and Prevention (CDC). (2011a). 2011 Child & adolescent immunization schedules. Department of Health and Human Services. Retrieved January 7, 2011, from http://www.cdc.gov/vaccines/recs/schedules/child-schedule.htm#printable

Centers for Disease Control and Prevention (CDC). (2012, updated). About Teen Pregnancy. Retrieved March 17, 2012, from http://www.cdc.gov/TeenPregnancy/AboutTeenPreg.htm

Dembrow, M., Golden, A., Paulk, D., et al. (2007, November 12). How to recognize and diagnose child abuse. *The Clinical Advisor.* Retrieved March 4, 2011, from http://www.clinicaladvisor.com/how-to-recognize-and-diagnose-child-abuse/article/117515/

Eaton, D. K., Kann, L., Kinchen, S., et al. (2008). Youth risk behavior surveillance—United States, 2007. *Morbidity and Mortality Weekly Report, 57*(SS-04), 1–131.

Fingerhut, L., & Anderson, R. (n.d., last reviewed 2009). National Center for Health Statistics (NCHS), Division of Vital Statistics. NCHS health e-stat. The three leading causes of injury mortality in the United States, 1999–2005. Retrieved March 3, 2011, from http://www.cdc.gov/nchs/data/hestat/injury99-05/injury99-05.htm

Fowler, J. W. (1981). *Stages of faith: The psychology of human development and the quest for meaning.* New York: Harper & Row.

Garofalo, R., Herrick, A., Mustanski, B. S., et al. (2007). Tip of the iceberg: Young men who have sex with men, the Internet, and HIV risk. *American Journal of Public Health, 97*(6), 1113–1117.

Gavin, L., MacKay, A., Brown, K., et al. (2009). Sexual and reproductive health of persons aged 10–24 years—United States, 2002–2007. *MMWR Surveillance Summaries, 58* (SS-06), 1–58.

Gilligan, C. (1982). *In a different voice: Psychological theory and women's development.* Cambridge, MA: Harvard University Press.

Gilligan, C. (1993). *In a different voice: Psychological theory and women's development.* Cambridge, MA: Harvard University Press.

Green, B. B., & Taplin, S. H. (2003). Breast cancer screening controversies. *Journal of the American Board of Family Practice, 16,* 233–241.

The guide to clinical preventive services 2010–2011 (AHRQ Publication No. 10–05145). (2010, August). Rockville, MD: Agency for Healthcare Research and Quality. Retrieved March 30, 2011, from http://www.ahrq.gov/clinic/pocketgd1011/pocketgd1011.pdf

Hackshaw, A. K., & Paul, E. A. (2003). Breast self-examination and death from breast cancer: A meta-analysis. *British Journal of Cancer, 88,* 1047–1053.

Havighurst, R. J. (1971). *Developmental tasks and education* (3rd ed.). New York: Longman.

Heron, M., Hoyert, D., Murphy, S., et al. (2009). Deaths: Final data for 2006. *National Vital Statistics Reports, 57*(14). April 17, 2009. DHHS Publication No. (PHS) 2009-1120. U. S. Department of Health & Human Services, Centers for Disease Control and Prevention, National Center for Health Statistics. Retrieved March 19, 2012, from http://www.cdc.gov/nchs/data/nvsr/nvsr57/nvsr57_14.pdf

Hussey, J. M., Chang, J. J., & Kotch, J. B. (2006). Child maltreatment in the United States: Prevalence, risk factors, and adolescent health consequences. *Pediatrics, 118*(3), 933–942.

Institute of Medicine, Food and Nutrition Board. (2010). Dietary reference intakes for calcium and vitamin D. Washington, DC: The National Academies of Sciences. Also available at http://www.iom.edu/Reports/2010/Dietary-Reference-Intakes-for-Calcium-and-Vitamin-D.aspx

The Joint Commission (TJC). (2008). *Hospital accreditation standards.* Oakbrook Terrace, IL: Author.

Knutson, D., & Steiner, E. (2007). Screening for breast cancer: Current recommendations and future directions. *American Family Physician, 75*(11), 1660–1666.

Kohlberg, L. (1968). Moral development. In: *International encyclopedia of social science.* New York: Macmillan.

Kohlberg, L. (1981). *Essays on moral development* (Vols. 1–3). San Francisco: Harper & Row.

Lippert, J., Shea, J., & Seagrave, M. (2008). Anorexia nervosa: Dying to be thin. *The Clinical Advisor, 11*(1), 67–70.

McFarlane, J. H., & Miller, A. (2005). Promoting community protection of adolescents. Juvenile Rights Project, Inc. Retrieved March 29, 2011, from http://www.jrplaw.org/Documents/CJA%20final%20part%201.pdf

Miller, J. L., & Silverstein, J. H. (2007). Management approaches for pediatric obesity. *Nature Clinical Practice Endocrinology & Metabolism, 312,* 810–818.

Moracco, K., Runyan, C., Bowling, J., et al. (2007). Women's experiences with violence: A national study. *Womens Health Issues, 17*(1), 3–12.

Mosher, W., Chandra, A., & Jones, J. (2005). Sexual behavior and selected health measures: Men and women 15–44 years of age, United States 2002. Advance data from *Vital and Health Statistics, 362.* Centers for Disease Control and Prevention (CDC). Division of Vital Statistics. Retrieved March 12, 2011, from http://www.cdc.gov/nchs/data/ad/ad362.pdf

National Cancer Institute (NCI). (2008). Breast cancer screening (PDQ®). Retrieved March 28, 2011, from http://www.cancer.gov/cancertopics/pdq/screening/breast/HealthProfessional/page10

National Cancer Institute (NCI). (2009). What you need to know about breast cancer: Risk factors. Retrieved April 18, 2011, from http://www.cancer.gov/cancertopics/wyntk/breast/page4

National Center for Health Statistics (NCHS). (n.d., updated 2010). Prevalence of overweight among children and adolescents: United States, trends 1963–1965 through 2007–2008. Retrieved March 27, 2011, from http://www.cdc.gov/nchs/products/hestats.htm

National Center for Health Statistics (NCHS). (2007a). *National Vital Statistics Reports, 56*(7). Retrieved March 15, 2011, from http://www.cdc.gov/nchs/pressroom/07newsreleases/teenbirth.htm

National Guideline Clearinghouse (NGC). (1998; revised 2012). Guideline synthesis: Screening for breast cancer in women at average risk. In: National Guideline Clearinghouse (NGC) [Web site]. Agency for Healthcare Research and Quality (AHRQ). Retrieved March 17, 2012, from http://guideline.gov/syntheses/synthesis.aspx?id=35115

National Guideline Clearinghouse (NGC). (2007b). Guideline summary: Evaluation of suspected child physical abuse. National Guideline Clearinghouse (NGC). Retrieved March 4, 2011, from http://www.guideline.gov/content.aspx?id=11057.

National Institutes of Health (NIH). (2008). NIH news. WHI follow-up study confirms health risks of long-term combination hormone therapy outweigh benefits for postmenopausal women. U.S. Department of Health and Human Services. Retrieved April 18, 2011, from http://www.nih.gov/news/health/mar2008/nhlbi-04.htm

National Center for Health Statistics (NCHS). (2009). Health, United States, 2008: With special feature on the health of

young adults. With chartbook. Hyattsville, MD: Author. Retrieved February 20, 2011, from http://www.cdc.gov/nchs/data/hus/hus08.pdf

Nelson, H., Nygren, P., & McInerney, Y. (2004). Screening for family and intimate partner violence (Systematic Evidence Reviews, No. 28). Rockville, MD: Agency for Healthcare Research and Quality. Retrieved March 4, 2011, from http://www.ncbi.nlm.nih.gov/books/NBK42851/

Office on Child Abuse and Neglect, U.S. Deparment of Health and Human Services; Goldman, J., Salus, M., Wolcott, D., et al. (2003). What factors contribute to child abuse and neglect? In: *A coordinated response to child abuse and neglect: The foundation for practice.* Retrieved March 2, 2011, from http://www.childwelfare.gov/pubs/usermanuals/foundation/foundatione.cfm

Office of Dietary Supplements, National Institutes of Health. (2011). Dietary supplement fact sheet: Vitamin D. Retrieved March 4, 2011, from http://ods.od.nih.gov/factsheets/vitamind

Polan, E., & Taylor, D. (2007). *Journey across the life span: Human development and health promotion* (3rd ed.). Philadelphia: F. A. Davis.

Recommended immunization schedules for persons aged 0–18 years—United States, 2008. (2008). *Morbidity and Mortality Weekly Report, 57,* Q1. Retrieved April 21, 2008, from http://www.cdc.gov/mmwr/preview/mmwrhtml/mm5701a8.htm

Remez, L. (2000). Oral sex among adolescents: Is it sex or is it abstinence? *Family Planning Perspectives, 32,* 298–304.

Rosolowich, V. (2006). Breast self-examination. *Journal of Obstetrics and Gynaecology Canada, 28,* 728–730.

Sadock, B., & Sadock, V. (2007). *Kaplan & Sadock's synopsis of psychiatry* (10th ed.). Philadelphia: Lippincott Williams & Wilkins.

Schnitzer, P. G., & Ewigman, B. G. (2005). Child deaths resulting from inflicted injuries: Household risk factors and perpetrator characteristics. *Pediatrics, 116*(5), e687–e693.

Smith, C. A., Ireland, T. O., & Thornberry, T. P. (2005). Adolescent maltreatment and its impact on young adult antisocial behavior. *Child Abuse & Neglect, 29*(10), 1099–1119.

Substance Abuse and Mental Health Services Administration (SAMHSA), Office of Applied Studies, Department of Health and Human Services. (2009). *Results from the 2009 national survey on drug use and health: Vol. 1. Summary of national findings.* Retrieved March 28, 2011, from http://www.oas.samhsa.gov/NSDUH/2k9NSDUH/2k9ResultsP.pdf

Tanner, J. (1962). *Growth at adolescence* (2nd ed.). Oxford: Blackwell.

Task force says men age 75 and older should not be screened for prostate cancer [Press release]. (2008, August 4). Rockville, MD: Agency for Healthcare Research and Quality. Retrieved March 4, 2011, from http://www.ahrq.gov/news/press/pr2008/tfproscanpr.htm

Thompson, R., Bonomi, A., Anderson, M., et al. (2006). Intimate partner violence. *American Journal of Preventive Medicine, 30*(6), 447–456.

Uphold, C. R., & Grahan, M. V. (2004). *Clinical guidelines in family practice.* Gainsville, FL: Barmarrae Books.

U.S. Department of Health and Human Services (USDHHS). (2008). 2008 Physical activity guidelines for Americans. Retrieved March 3, 2011, from http://www.health.gov/paguidelines/pdf/paguide.pdf

U.S. Department of Health and Human Services (USDHHS). (2010). Maternal, infant and child health. *Healthy People 2020.* Retrieved March 2, 2011, from http://www.healthypeople.gov/2020/topicsobjectives2020/objectiveslist.aspx?topicid=26

U S. Department of Justice (2000). Extent, nature, and consequences of intimate partner violence. Retrieved March 4, 2011, from http://www.ncjrs.gov/pdffiles1/nij/181867.pdf

U.S. Environmental Protection Agency (EPA). (last updated 2010, October). Asthma. Indoor environmental asthma triggers. Retrieved March 28, 2011, from http://www.epa.gov/asthma/triggers.html

U.S. Preventive Services Task Force (USPSTF). (2004). *Screening for testicular cancer: Recommendation statement.* Rockville, MD: Agency for Healthcare Research and Quality. Retrieved February 12, 2011, from http://www.uspreventiveservicestaskforce.org/3rduspstf/testicular/testiculrs.htm

U.S. Preventive Services Task Force (USPSTF). (2009). *Screening for breast cancer: Clinical summary.* Rockville, MD: Agency for Healthcare Research and Quality. Retrieved March 11, 2011, from http://www.ahrq.gov/clinic/uspstf09/breastcancer/brcansum.htm

Waldrop, J. (2008). Stopping childhood obesity before it begins. *The Clinical Advisor, 11*(1), 35–36, 39–41.

Waugh, D. (1978). Moral development: Theory and process. In: *Teaching and evaluating the affective domain in nursing programs* (pp. 17–30). Thorofare, NJ: Charles B. Slack.

Whitaker, R. C., Phillips, S. M., Orzol, S. M., et al. (2007). The association between maltreatment and obesity among preschool children. *Child Abuse & Neglect, 31*(11–12), 1187–1199.

Wilkinson, J. (2009). *Nursing diagnosis handbook* (9th ed.). Upper Saddle River, NJ: Prentice-Hall.

CHAPTER 10

Alley, D., Liebig, P., Pynoos, J., et al. (2007). Creating elder-friendly communities: Preparations for an aging society. *Journal of Gerontological Social Work, 49*(1/2), 1–18.

Al Omari, H., Kramer, K., Hronek, C., et al. (2005) The Wheat Valley assisted living culture: Rituals and rules. *Journal of Gerontological Nursing, 31*(1), 9–16.

Alzheimer's Association. (2008). Risk factors. Retrieved November 2, 2008, from http://www.alz.org/alzheimers_disease_causes_risk_factors.asp

American Cancer Society guidelines for the early detection of cancer. (n.d., last revised 2010, July) Retrieved February 20, 2011, from http://www.cancer.org/docroot/PED/content/PED_2_3X_ACS_Cancer_Detection_Guidelines_36.asp?sitearea+PED

American College of Obstetricians and Gynecologists (ACOG). (2003, reaffirmed 2006). *Breast cancer screening* (ACOG Practice Bulletin No 42). Washington, DC: Author. Retrieved March 14, 2011, from http://www.guideline.gov/content.aspx?id=3990&search=breast+cancer+screening

American College of Obstetricians and Gynecologists (ACOG) (2011). Breast cancer screening. Washington (DC): American College of Obstetricians and Gynecologists (ACOG); (ACOG practice bulletin; no. 122). Retrieved March 19, 2012, from http://guideline.gov/content.aspx?f=rss&id=34275#Section420

American Diabetes Association. (2011). Diabetes statistics. Data from the 2011 national diabetes fact sheet. Retrieved March 25, 2011, from http://www.diabetes.org/diabetes-basics/diabetes-statistics/

Assisted Living Quality Coalition. (1998). *Assisted living quality initiative: Building a structure that promotes quality.* Washington, DC: Author.

Badgwell, B., Giordano, S., Duan, Z., et al. (2008). Mammography before diagnosis among women age 80 years and older with breast cancer. *Journal of Clinical Oncology, 26*(15), 2482–2488.

Bartali, B., Semba, R., Frongillo, E., et al. (2006). Low micronutrient levels as a predictor of incident disability in older women. *Archives of Internal Medicine, 166*(21), 2335–2340.

Centers for Disease Control and Prevention (CDC). (2011). Recommended adult immunization schedule, United States 2011. U.S. Department of Health and Human Services. Retrieved March 8, 2011, from http://www.cdc.gov/vaccines/recs/schedules/downloads/adult/adult-schedule.pdf

Cherkas, L., Hunkin, J., Kato, B., et al. (2008). The association between physical activity in leisure time and leukocyte telomere length. *Archives of Internal Medicine, 168*(2), 154–158.

Cumming, E., & Henry, W. (1961). *Growing old, the process of disengagement.* New York: Basic Books.

Erikson, E. H. (1963). *Childhood and society* (2nd ed.). New York: W. W. Norton.

Ertel, K., Glymour, M., & Berkman, L. F. (2008). Effects of social integration on preserving memory function in a nationally representative US elderly population. *American Journal of Public Health, 98*(7), 1215–1220.

Faber, M., Bosscher, R., Paw, M., et al. (2006). Effects of exercise programs on falls and mobility in frail and pre-frail older adults: A multicenter randomized controlled trial. *Archives of Physical Medicine and Rehabilitation, 87*(7), 885–896.

Federal Interagency Forum on Aging Related Statistics. (2008). Older Americans 2008: Key indicators of well-being. Retrieved March 7, 2011, from http://www.agingstats.gov/agingstatsdotnet/Main_Site/Data/Data_2008.aspx

Flaherty, J., Morley, J., Murphy, D., et al. (2002). The development of outpatient clinical glidepaths. *Journal of the American Geriatrics Society, 50*, 1886–1901.

Folstein, M. F., Folstein, S., & McHugh P. R. (1975). Mini mental state: A practical method for grading the cognitive state of patients for the clinician. *Journal of Psychiatric Research, 12*, 189–198.

Fong, T., Jones, R., Rudolph, J., et al. (2010) Development and validation of a brief cognitive assessment tool. *Archives of Internal Medicine.* doi:10.1001/archinternmed.2010.423 Frailty in older adults. (2006). JAMA patient page. *JAMA, 296*(18). Retrieved March 13, 2011, from http://jama.ama-assn.org/cgi/content/full/296/18/2280?maxtoshow5&_HITS510&hits510&RESULTFORMAT5&fulltext5patient1page1frail&searchid51&FIRSTINDEX50&resourcetype5HWCIT

Futterman, M. (2008, October 30). Over 80, it's anyone's race. *The Wall Street Journal,* pp. W1, W4.

Guide to clinical preventive services, 2010–2011 (AHRQ Publication No. 08–05122). (2010). Rockville, MD: Agency for Healthcare Research and Quality. Retrieved March 30, 2011, from http://www.ahrq.gov/clinic/pocketgd1011/gcp10s2.htm

Houser, A., Fox-Grage, W., & Gibson, M. J. (2009). *Across the states: Profiles of long-term care and independent living* (8th ed.). Washington, DC: AARP Public Policy Institute.

Kung, H-C., Hoyert, D. L., Xu J., et al. (2008, April 24). [US Department of Health and Human Services, Centers for Disease Control and Prevention] Deaths: Final data for 2005. *National Vital Statistics Reports, 56*(10), 1–121. Retrieved March 7, 2011, from http://www.cdc.gov/nchs/data/nvsr/nvsr56/nvsr56_10.pdf

Laumann, E. O., Leitsch, S. A., & Waite, L. J. (2008). Elder mistreatment in the United States: Prevalence estimates from a nationally representative study. *Journal of Gerontology: Social Sciences, 63B*(4), S248–S254.

Macko, R., Benvenuti, F., Stanhope, S., et al. (2008). Adaptive physical activity improves mobility function and quality of life in chronic hemiparesis. *Journal of Rehabilitation Research and Development, 45*(2), 323–328.

Martin, F. C., & Brighton, P. (2008). Frailty: Different tools for different purposes? *Age and Ageing, 37*, 129–131.

National Cancer Institute (NCI). (2007). The prostate-specific antigen (PSA) test: Questions and answers. U.S. National Institutes of Health. Retrieved April 18, 2011, from http://www.cancer.gov/cancertopics/factsheet/Detection/PSA

National Cancer Institute (NCI). (2008). Breast cancer screening (PDQ®). Retrieved March 28, 2011, from http://www.cancer.gov/cancertopics/pdq/screening/breast/HealthProfessional/page10

Perls, T. (2006). The different paths to 100. *American Journal of Clinical Nutrition, 83*(Suppl.), 484S–487S.

Perls, T., Silver, M. H., & Lauerman, J. F. (1999). *Living to 100: Lessons in living to your maximum potential at any age.* New York: Basic Books.

Rockwood, K. (2005). What would make a definition of frailty successful? *Age and Ageing, 34*, 432–434.

Shelkey, M., & Wallace, M. (2007). Katz index of independence in activities of daily living (ADL). (2007). *Try this: Best practices in nursing care to older adults, 2.* Hartford Institute for Geriatric Nursing, New York University College of Nursing. Retrieved March 7, 2011, from http://consultgerirn.org/uploads/File/trythis/try_this_2.pdf

Shephard, R. J. (2008, April). Maximal oxygen intake and independence in old age. *British Journal of Sports Medicine, 10.* Retrieved December 12, 2008, from http://bjsm.bmj.com/cgi/content/abstract/bjsm.2007.044800v1

Smith, R., Cokkinides, V., & Eyre, H.; American Cancer Society. (2003). American Cancer Society guidelines for the early detection of cancer. *CA–A Cancer Journal for Clinicians, 53*, 27–43.

Snowdon, D. A. (2003). Healthy aging and dementia: Findings from the Nun study. *Annals of Internal Medicine, 139*(5, Pt. 2), 450–454.

Task force says men age 75 and older should not be screened for prostate cancer [Press release]. (2008, August 4). Rockville, MD: Agency for Healthcare Research and Quality. Retrieved March 7, 2011, from http://www.ahrq.gov/news/press/pr2008/tfproscanpr.htm

Tomita, M., Mann, W., Stanton, K., et al. (2007). Use of currently available smart home technology by frail elders. Process and outcomes. *Topics in Geriatric Rehabilitation, 23*(1), 24–34.

U.S. Census Bureau. (2006). National populations estimates for the 2000s. Washington, DC: Author. Retrieved March 7, 2011, from http://www.census.gov/population/www/projections/usinterimproj/

U.S. Census Bureau. (2007). Census Bureau releases new data on residents of adult correctional facilities, nursing homes, and other group quarters. Retrieved March 7, 2011, from

http://www.census.gov/newsroom/releases/archives/american_community_survey_acs/cb07-cn11.html

U.S. Census Bureau. (2008). 2008 national population projections. Washington, DC: Author. Retrieved March 7, 2011, from http://www.census.gov/population/www/projections/2008projections.html

U.S. Department of Health and Human Services (USDHHS). (2008). Physical activity guidelines for Americans. At-a-glance: A fact sheet for professionals. Retrieved November 3, 2008, from http://www.health.gov/paguidelines/factsheet prof.aspx

U.S. Department of Health and Human Services, Public Health Service, National Institutes of Health. (2003). *What's your aging IQ*. Retrieved March 26, 2011, from http://www.niapublications.org/tipsheets/pdf/Whats_Your_Aging_IQ.pdf

U.S. Preventive Services Task Force (USPSTF). (2002). *Screening for breast cancer: Systematic evidence review*. Rockville, MD: Agency for Healthcare Research and Quality. Retrieved April 15, 2011, from http://www.cdc.gov/cancer/breast/basic_info/screening.htm. http://www.uspreventive servicestaskforce.org/uspstf/uspscerv.htm

U.S. Preventive Services Task Force (USPSTF). (2009, March). Screening for colorectal cancer. Topic page. Retrieved July 7, 2011, from http://www.uspreventiveservicestaskforce.org/uspstf/uspscolo.htm

Villareal, D., Banks, M., Sinacore, D., et al. (2006). Effect of weight loss and exercise on frailty in obese older adults. *Archives of Internal Medicine, 166*(8), 860–866.

Wilson, D. M., & Palha, P. (2007, Fourth Quarter). A systematic review of published research articles on health promotion at retirement. *Journal of Nursing Scholarship*, 330–337.

Woodhouse, K. W., & O'Mahony, M. S. (1997). Frailty and ageing. *Age and Ageing, 26*, 245–246.

Zimmerman, S., & Sloane, P. D. (2007). Improving practice through research in and about assisted living: Definition and classification of assisted living. *The Gerontologist, 47*(Special issue III), 33–39.

CHAPTER 11

Agency for Healthcare Research and Quality (AHRQ). (2009). Educating patients before they leave the hospital reduces readmissions, emergency department visits and saves money [Press release]. Retrieved Feburary 4, 2011, from http://www.ahrq.gov/news/press/pr2009/redpr.htm

Albom, M. (1997). *Tuesdays with Morrie*. New York: Doubleday.

American Geriatrics Society. (n.d.). *AGS/BGS clinical practice guideline: Prevention of falls in older persons*. American Geriatrics Society, British Geriatrics Society, and American Academy of Orthopaedic Surgeons Panel on Falls Prevention. Retrieved February 2, 2011, from http://www.americangeriatrics.org/health_care_professionals/clinical_practice/clinical_guidelines_recommendations/prevention_of_falls_summary_of_recommendations/

Benner, P., & Wrubel, J. (1989). *The primacy of caring*. Menlo Park, CA: Addison-Wesley.

Bettelheim, B. (1979). *Surviving and other essays*. New York: Knopf.

Centers for Disease Control and Prevention (CDC). (n.d.). Chronic disease prevention and health promotion. Last updated January 5, 2011. Retrieved January 15, 2011, from http://www.cdc.gov/chronicdisease/resources/publications/index.htm

Centers for Disease Control and Prevention (CDC). (2002, October). Prevalence of self-reported arthritis or chronic joint symptoms among adults—United States, 2001. *Morbidity and Mortality Weekly Report, 51*(42), 948. Retrieved January 13, 2011, from http://www.cdc.gov/mmwr/preview/mmwrhtml/mm5142a2.htm

Centers for Disease Control and Prevention (CDC). (2009). Chronic disease prevention and health promotion. Retrieved January 13, 2011, from http://www.cdc.gov/chronicdisease/overview/index.htm

Centers for Disease Control and Prevention (CDC). (2010). Health effects of secondhand smoke. Retrieved February 1, 2011, from http://www.cdc.gov/tobacco/data_statistics/fact_sheets/secondhand_smoke/health_effects/index.htm

Centers for Disease Control and Prevention (CDC). (2010, updated). NCHS health e-stat. Prevalence of obesity among children and adolescents: United States, trends 1963–1965 through 2007–2008.

Centers for Medicare & Medicaid Services (CMS). (2007, May 8). Medicare program: Inpatient rehabilitation facility prospective payment system for FY 2008. *Federal Register, 72*(88), 26230.

Chan, I. W. S., Lai, J. C. L., & Wong, K. W. N. (2006). Resilience is associated with better recovery in Chinese people diagnosed with coronary heart disease. *Psychology and Health, 21*(3), 335–349.

Cockerham, W. (2000). *Medical sociology*. Upper Saddle River, NJ: Prentice-Hall.

Drummond-Dye, R. (2007, December). Medicare focuses on home health policies. *PT: Magazine of Physical Therapy*. Retrieved January 13, 2011, from the American Physical Therapy Association, http://www.apta.org/AM/Template.cfm?Section=Home&TEMPLATE=/CM/HTMLDisplay.cfm&CONTENTID=45281

Dudas, V. (2001). The impact of follow-up telephone calls to patients after hospitalization. *The American Journal of Medicine, 111*(9), 26–30.

Dunn, H. L. (1959). High-level wellness for man and society. *American Journal of Public Health, 49*(6), 786–788.

Ellis, B. H., Shannon, E. D., Cox, J. K., et al. (2004). Chronic conditions: Results of the Medicare health outcomes survey, 1998–2000. *Health Care Financing Review* (Summer). Retrieved March 1, 2011, from http://findarticles.com/p/articles/mi_m0795/is_4_25/ai_n6332418

Frankl, V. (1959/1962/1984). *Man's search for meaning*. New York: Washington Square Press.

Frankl, V. (2004). *Man's search for meaning*. London: Rider.

Glod, C. A. (1998). *Contemporary psychiatric-mental health nursing: The brain-behavior connection*. Philadelphia: F. A. Davis.

Godress, J., Ozgul, S., Owen, C., et al. (2005). Grief experiences of parents whose children suffer from mental illness. *Australian and New Zealand Journal of Psychiatry, 39*, 88–94.

Greenwald, J. L., Denham, C. R., & Jack, B. W. (2007). The hospital discharge: A review of a high risk care transition with highlights of a reengineered discharge process. *Journal of Patient Safety, 3*(2), 97–106.

The Joint Commission (TJC). (2008a). *2008 Hospital accreditation standards* (pp. 216–218, 366–367). Oakbrook Terrace, IL: Author.

The Joint Commission (TJC). (2008b). 2008 National patient safety goals. Retrieved February 22, 2008, from http://www.jcaho.org/PatientSafety/

Kokanovic, R., Petersen, A., & Klimidis, S. (2006). "Nobody can help me . . . I am living through it alone": Experiences of caring for people diagnosed with mental illness in ethno-cultural and linguistic minority communities. *Journal of Immigrant and Minority Health, 8*(2), 125–135.

Lewis, C. S. (1961). *A grief observed*. London: Faber and Faber.

Lifton, R., & Olson, E. (1974). *Living and dying*. New York: Praeger.

McFetridge, B., Gillespie, M., Goode, D., et al. (2007). An exploration of the handover process of critically ill patients between nursing staff from the emergency department and the intensive care unit. *Nursing in Critical Care, 12*(6), 261–269.

Moltmann, J. (1983). *The power of the powerless*. San Francisco: Harper & Row.

Myers, J., Sweeney, T., & Witmer, J. (2000). The wheel of wellness counseling for wellness: A holistic model for treatment planning. *Journal of Counseling & Development, 78*(3), 251–267.

National Institute of Mental Health. (2003). Older adults: Depression and suicide facts, 2003. Retrieved March 1, 2011, from http://www.nimh.nih.gov/publicat/elderly depsuicide.cfm

Naylor, M., Brooten, D., Jones, R., et al. (1994). Comprehensive discharge planning for the hospitalized elderly. A randomized clinical trial. *Annals of Internal Medicine, 120,* 999–1006.

Neuman, B. (2002). The Neuman systems model. In: B. Neuman, *The Neuman systems model* (4th ed.). Norwalk, CT: Appleton & Lange.

Ottawa Charter for Health Promotion. (1986). First International Conference on Health Promotion, Ottawa, Canada, November 21, 1986. World Health Organization (WHO). Retrieved February 1, 2011, from http://www.who.int/healthpromotion/conferences/previous/ottawa/en/

Parsons, T. (1975). The sick role and role of the physician reconsidered. *Milbank Memorial Fund Quarterly, 53,* 257–278.

Phillips, C. O., Wright, W. M., Kern, D. E., et al. (2004). Comprehensive discharge planning with postdischarge support for older patients with congestive heart failure—a meta-analysis. *JAMA, 291,* 1358–1367.

Reeve, C. (1998). *Still me*. New York: Random House.

Seigel, B. (1986). *Love, medicine and miracles*. New York: Harper & Row.

Sheinfeld-Gorin, S., & Arnold, J. (2006). *Health promotion in practice*. San Francisco: Jossey-Bass.

Smith, P. (1992). *Living the disrupted life: A symphony of survival*. Unpublished doctoral dissertation, University of Kansas.

Stuck, A. E., Walthert, J. M., Nikolaus, T., et al. (1999). Risk factors for functional status decline in community living elderly people: A systematic literature review. *Social Science and Medicine, 48*(4), 445–469.

Suchman, E. A. (1972). Stages of illness and medical care. In: E. G. Jaco (Ed.), *Patients, physicians, and illness* (2nd ed.). New York: Free Press.

Thompson, C. W., Durrant, L., Barusch, A., & Olson, L. (2006). Fostering coping skills and resilience in home enteral nutrition (HEN) consumers. *Nutrition in Clinical Practice, 21*(6), 557–565.

Thompson, J., & Manore, M. (2009). *Nutrition: An applied approach* (2nd ed.). San Francisco: Benajmin Cummings.

Valladares, A. (2001). *Against all hope: A memoir of life in Castro's gulag*. San Francisco: Encounter Books.

Vanauken, S. (1977). *A severe mercy*. New York: Bantam Books.

Watson, J. (1979). *Nursing: The philosophy and science of caring*. Boston: Little, Brown; 2nd printing 1985, Boulder, CO: University Press of Colorado.

Wilber, T. (2000). *Grace and grit: Spirituality and healing in the life and death of Treya Killam Wilber* (rev. ed.). Boston: Shambhala Publications.

World Health Organization (WHO). (1948). Preamble to the Constitution of the World Health Organization as adopted by the International Health Conference, New York, June 19–22, 1946, and entered into force on April 7, 1948. Retrieved January 8, 2011, from http://www.who.int/suggestions/faq/en/

Zwicker, D., & Picariello, G. (2003). Discharge planning for the older adult. In: M. Mezey, T. Fulmer, I. Abraham, & D. A. Zwicker (Eds.), *Geriatric nursing protocols for best practice* (2nd ed., pp. 292–316). New York: Springer.

CHAPTER 12

Alford, L. (2007). Findings of interest from immunology and psychoneuroimmunology. *Manual Therapy, 12*(2), 176–180.

Badger, J. (2008). Critical care nurse intern program: Addressing psychological reactions related to critical care nursing. *Critical Care Nursing Quarterly, 31*(2), 184–187.

Bennett, M., & Lengacher, C. (2007). Humor and laughter may influence health: IV. Humor and immune function. *Evidence-Based Complementary and Alternative Medicine, 6*(2), 159–164. Retrieved February 19, 2011, from http://www.hindawi.com/journals/ecam/2009/143853.abs.html

Bost, N., & Wallis, M. (2006). The effectiveness of a 15-minute weekly massage in reducing physical and psychological stress in nurses. *Australian Journal of Advanced Nursing, 23*(4), 28–33.

Brammer, L. M., & MacDonald, G. (2003). *The helping relationship: Process and skills* (8th ed.). Old Tappan, NJ: Pearson.

Bulechek, F., Butcher, H., & Dochterman, J. (2012). *Nursing interventions classification (NIC)* (6th ed.). St. Louis, MO: C. V. Mosby.

Cousins, N. (1979). *Anatomy of an illness*. New York: Bantam Books.

Davidson, R., Kabat-Zinn, J., Schumacher, J., et al. (2003). Alterations in brain and immune function produced by mindfulness meditation. *Psychosomatic Medicine, 65,* 564–570.

Hall, L., Doran, D., & Pink, L. (2008). Outcomes of interventions to improve hospital nursing work environments. *Journal of Nursing Administration, 38*(1), 40–46.

Hegge, M., & Larson, V. (2008). Stressors and coping strategies of students in accelerated baccalaureate nursing programs. *Nurse Educator, 33*(1), 26–30.

Holmes, T., & Rahe, R. (1967). The social readjustment and rating scale. *Journal of Psychosomatic Research, 11,* 213–218.

Johnson, M., Moorhead, S., Bulechek, C., et al. (2012). *NOC and NIC linkages to NANDA-I and clinical conditions* (3rd ed.). St. Louis, MO: C. V. Mosby.

Johnson, P. (2002). The use of humor and its influences on spirituality and coping in breast cancer survivors. *Oncology Nursing Forum, 29*(4), 691–695.

Keegan, L. (2003). Therapies to reduce stress and anxiety. *Critical Care Nursing Clinics of North America, 15*(3), 321–327.

Maddi, S. (1987). Hardiness training at Illinois Bell Telephone. In: J. P. Opatz (Ed.), *Health promotion evaluation* (pp. 1101–1115). Stevens Point, WI: National Wellness Institute.

Maddi, S. (2002). The story of hardiness: Twenty years of theorizing, research and practice. *Consulting Psychology Journal, 54,* 173–185.

Maville, J., Bowen, J., & Genham, G. (2008). Effect of healing touch on stress perception and biological correlates. *Holistic Nursing Practice, 22*(2), 103–110.

Moorhead, S., Johnson, M., & Maas, M., et al. (Eds.). (2012). *Nursing outcomes classification (NOC)* (5th ed.). St. Louis, MO: C. V. Mosby.

Morgan, P., Fogel, J., Rose, L., et al. (2005). African American couples merging strengths to successfully cope with breast cancer. *Oncology Nursing Forum, 32*(5), 979–987.

NANDA International (NANDA-I). (2009). *Nursing diagnoses: Definitions and classification 2009–2011.* Oxford: Wiley-Blackwell.

Neeb, K. (2006). *Fundamentals of mental health nursing* (3rd ed.). Philadelphia: F. A. Davis.

Olson, R. (2003). Definitions of biofeedback. In: M. S. Schwartz & F. Andrasik (Eds.), *Biofeedback: A practitioner's guide* (3rd ed.). New York: Guilford Press.

Robinson, F. P., Mathews, H. L., & Witek-Janusek, L. (2000). Stress reduction and HIV disease: A review of intervention studies using a psychoneuroimmunology framework. *Journal of the Association of Nurses in AIDS Care, 11*(2), 87–96.

Scanlon, V., & Sanders, T. (2007). *Essentials of anatomy and physiology* (5th ed., pp. 239, 241). Philadelphia: F. A. Davis.

Selye, H. (1974). *Stress without distress.* Philadelphia: J. B. Lippincott.

Selye, H. (1976). *The stress of life* (rev. ed.). New York: McGraw-Hill.

Stuart, B., & Sundeen, S. (2009). *Nurse-client interaction: Implementing the nursing process* (6th ed.). St. Louis, MO: C. V. Mosby.

Sullivan, M., Hawes, K., Winchester, S., et al. (2008). Developmental origins theory from prematurity to adult disease. *JOGNN: Journal of Obstetric, Gynecologic, & Neonatal Nursing, 37*(2), 158–164.

Townsend, M. C. (2009). *Psychiatric mental health nursing* (6th ed.). Philadelphia: F. A. Davis.

CHAPTER 13

Albom, M. (1997). *Tuesdays With Morrie.* New York: Doubleday.

American Psychiatric Association (APA). (2000). *Diagnostic and statistical manual of mental disorders* (4th ed., text rev.). Washington, DC: Author. Also available from http://www.psychiatryonline.com/

Association of Saskatchewan Home Economists. (n.d.). Help your child develop a positive body image. Retrieved March 26, 2011, from http://www.homefamily.net/index.php?/categories/results/help_your_child_develop_a_positive_body_image1

Blanchflower, D. B., & Oswald, A. J. (2008), Is well-being U-shaped over the life cycle? *Social Science & Medicine, 66,* 1733–1749.

Bourne, E. J. (2005). *The anxiety and phobia workbook* (4th ed.). Oakland, CA: New Harbinger.

Bracken, B. A. (Ed.). (1996). *Handbook of self-concept.* New York: John Wiley & Sons.

Brigham and Women's Hospital. (2001). *Psychosocial approaches to deeply disturbed persons.* Boston: Author.

Bulechek, G. M., Butcher, H. K., & Dochterman, J. M. (Eds.). (2012). *Nursing interventions classification (NIC)* (6th ed.). St. Louis, MO: C. V. Mosby.

Center for Food Safety and Applied Nutrition, U.S. Food and Drug Administration. (2002, March 25). Consumer advisory. Kava-containing dietary supplements may be associated with severe liver injury. Retrieved March 20, 2011, from http://www.fda.gov/Food/ResourcesForYou/Consumers/ucm085482.htm

Centers for Disease Control and Prevention (CDC). (2002). Hepatic toxicity possibly associated with kava-containing products—United States, Germany, and Switzerland, 1999–2002, *Morbidity and Mortality Weekly Report, 51*(47), 1065–1067. Retrieved March 20, 2011, from http://www.cdc.gov/mmwr/PDF/wk/mm5147.pdf

Centers for Disease Control and Prevention (CDC). (2007). Suicide. Facts at a glance. Retrieved January 20, 2008, from http://www.cdc.gov/ncipc/dvp/Suicide/SuicideDataSheet.pdf

Chen, T. M., Huang, F. Y., Chang, C., et al. (2006). Using the PHQ-9 for depression screening and treatment monitoring for Chinese Americans in primary care. *Psychiatric Services, 57,* 976–981.

Cheung, Y. B., Law, C. K., Chan, B., et al. (2006). Suicidal ideation and suicidal attempts in a population-based study of Chinese people: Risk attributable to hopelessness, depression, and social factors. *Journal of Affective Disorders, 90*(2–3), 193–199.

Clark, M. M., Croghan, I. T., Reading, S., et al. (2005). The relationship of body image dissatisfaction to cigarette smoking in college students. *Body Image, 2*(3), 263–270.

Dickstein, E. (1977). Self and self-esteem: Theoretical foundations and their implications for research. *Human Development, 20,* 129–140.

Edwards, N. (2003). Differentiating the three D's: Delirium, dementia, and depression. *MedSurg Nursing.* Retrieved February 18, 2011, from http://findarticles.com/p/articles/mi_m0FSS/is_6_12/ai_n18616788

Erikson, E. (1963). *Childhood and society* (2nd ed.). New York: W. W. Norton.

Goldston, D. B., Reboussin, B. A., & Daniel, S. S. (2006). Predictors of suicide attempts: State and trait components. *Journal of Abnormal Psychology, 115*(4), 842–849.

Gorman, L. M., & Sultan, D. E. (2008). *Psychosocial nursing for general patient care* (3rd ed.). Philadelphia: F. A. Davis.

Howarth, D., Heath, J., & Snope, F. (1999). Beyond the Folstein: Dementia in primary care. *Primary Care: Clinics in Office Practice, 26,* 299–314.

Hulisz, D. T. (2008). Top herbal products: Efficacy and safety concerns. Medscape Nurses. ©2007. Retrieved March 20, 2008, from http://www.medscape.org/viewprogram/8494

International Society for Mental Health Online (ISMHO). (last updated September 2004). All about depression. Retrieved March 20, 2008, from http://www.allaboutdepression.com/gen_01.html#3

Jamison, K. R. (1997). *An unquiet mind: A memoir of moods and madness.* London: Picador.

Johnson, M., Bulechek, G., Dochterman, J., et al. (2006). *NANDA, NOC, & NIC linkages: Nursing diagnoses, outcomes, and interventions* (2nd ed.). St. Louis, MO: C. V. Mosby.

Kroenke, K., Spitzer, R. L., & Williams, J. B. W. (2001). The PHQ-9. Validity of a brief depression severity measure. *Journal of General Internal Medicine, 16*(9), 606–613.

Kurlowicz, L. H. (2008). Depression. In: E. Capezuti, D. Zwicker, M. Mezey, & T. Fulmer (Eds.), *Evidence-based*

geriatric nursing protocols for best practice (3rd ed., pp. 57–82). New York: Springer.

Maslow, A. (1968). *Toward a psychology of being* (2nd ed.). New York: Van Nostrand-Reinhold.

Maybury, B. C. (2008, March 10). Suicide prevention: Every nurse's responsibility. Nurse.com. Retrieved January 22, 2011, from http://news.nurse.com/apps/pbcs.dll/article?AID=200880305017

McCabe, M. P., Ricciardelli, L. A., Sitaram, G., et al. (2006). Accuracy of body size estimation: Role of biopsychosocial variables. *Body Image, 3*(2), 163–171.

Moorhead, S., Johnson, M., Maas, M. L., et al. (Eds.). (2008). *Nursing outcomes classification (NOC)* (4th ed.). St. Louis, MO: C. V. Mosby.

Moser, D. K. (2007). "The rust of life": Impact of anxiety on cardiac patients. *American Journal of Critical Care, 16,* 361–369.

NANDA International (NANDA-I). (2009). *Nursing diagnoses: Definitions and classification 2009–2011.* Philadelphia: Author.

National Guideline Clearinghouse (NGC). (2010). Major depression in adults in primary care. Retrieved March 22, 2011, from http://www.guideline.gov/content.aspx?id=23857&search=major+depression+in+adults+in+primary+care

National Institute of Mental Health (NIMH). (n.d.a) Older adults: Depression and suicide (NIH Publication No. 4593) [Fact sheet]. Revised 2007, April. Retrieved February 26, 2011, from http://www.nimh.nih.gov/publicat/elderly depsuicide.cfm

National Institute of Mental Health (NIMH). (n.d.b) Suicide in the U.S.: Statistics and prevention (Page last reviewed 2008, March 20). Retrieved January 22, 2008, from http://www.nimh.nih.gov/health/publications/suicide-in-the-us-statistics-and-prevention.shtml

Neeb, K. (2001). *Fundamentals of mental health nursing* (2nd ed., pp. 365–378). Philadelphia: F. A. Davis.

Peplau, H. (1963). A working definition of anxiety. In: S. Burd & M. Marshall (Eds.), *Some clinical approaches to psychiatric nursing.* New York: Macmillan.

Plassman, B., Langa, K., Fisher, G., et al. (2007). Prevalence of dementia in the United States: The aging, demographics, and memory study. *Neuro-epidemiology, 29* 125–132. Retrieved January 25, 2011, from http://content.karger.com/ProdukteDB/produkte.asp?doi=109998

Pleis, J. R., & Lethbridge-Cejku, M. (2006, December). Summary health statistics for U.S. Adults: National health interview survey, 2005. *Vital and Health Statistics, 10*(232), Centers for Disease Control. Retrieved March 17, 2008, from http://www.cdc.gov/nchs/data/series/sr_10/sr10_232.pdf

Richardson, S. (2003). Delirium: Assessment and treatment of the elderly patient. *The American Journal for Nurse Practitioners, 7*(1), 9–15.

Shen, B. J., Avivi, Y. E., Todaro, J. F., et al. (2008). Anxiety characteristics independently and prospectively predict myocardial infarction in men. The unique contribution of anxiety among psychologic factors. *Journal of the American College of Cardiology, 51,* 113–119.

Stanley, M., Blair, K. A., & Beare, P. G. (2005). *Gerontological nursing* (3rd ed.). Philadelphia: F. A. Davis.

Steptoe, A. (Ed.). (2007). *Depression and physical illness.* New York: Cambridge University Press.

Stice, E., & Shaw, H. (2003). Prospective relations of body image, eating, and affective disturbances to smoking onset in adolescent girls: How Virginia slims. *Journal of Consulting and Clinical Psychology, 71*(1), 129–135.

Stokes, R., & Frederick-Recascino, C. (2003). Women's perceived body image: Relations with personal happiness. *Journal of Women & Aging, 15*(1), 17–29.

Stuart, G. W., & Laraia, M. T. (2001). *Principles and practice of psychiatric nursing* (7th ed.). St. Louis, MO: C. V. Mosby.

Townsend, M. C. (2008). *Essentials of psychiatric mental health nursing* (4th ed.). Philadelphia: F. A. Davis.

U.S. Preventive Services Task Force (USPSTF). (2004). Screening for suicide risk. Retrieved March 18, 2008, from http://www.uspreventiveservicestaskforce.org/uspstf/uspssuic.htm

Wingood, G. M., DiClemente, R. J., Harrington, K., et al. (2002). Body image and African American females' sexual health. *Journal of Women's Health and Gender Based Medicine, 11*(5), 433–439.

CHAPTER 14

Bulechek, F., Butcher, H., & Dochterman, J. (2012). *Nursing interventions classification (NIC)* (6th ed.). St. Louis, MO: C. V. Mosby.

Centers for Disease Control and Prevention (CDC). (2005, updated 2010, July 12). Burden of chronic disease on minority racial populations and women. Retrieved January 10, 2011, from http://www.cdc.gov/nccdphp/overview.htm#4

Centers for Disease Control and Prevention (CDC). (2010, August 27). Births, marriages, divorces, and deaths: Provisional data for 2009. *National Vital Statistics Report, 58*(25), 1–6. Retrieved January 14, 2011, from http://www.cdc.gov/nchs/nvss.htm

Friedman, M. M., Bowden, V. R., & Jones, E. G. (2003). *Family nursing: Research, theory, and practice* (5th ed.). Upper Saddle River, NJ: Prentice-Hall.

Hanson, S. M. (2005). *Family health care nursing: Theory, practice, and research* (3rd ed.). Philadelphia: F. A. Davis

Huges, M. E., Waite, L. J., LaPierre, T. A., et al. (2007). All in the family: The impact of caring for grandchildren on grandparents' health. *Journals of Gerontology Series B: Psychological Sciences and Social Sciences, 62,* S108–119.

McGoldrick, M., & Carter, E. (1985). The stages of the family life cycle. In: J. Henslin (Ed.), *Marriage and family in a changing society.* New York: Free Press.

Moorhead, S., Johnson, M., & Maas, M. (Eds.). (2008). *Nursing outcomes classification (NOC)* (4th ed.). St. Louis, MO: C. V. Mosby.

Rehabilitation and Training Research Center on Disability Demographics Statistics. (2007). *The 2006 annual disability status report.* Ithaca, NY: Cornell University.

U.S. Census Bureau. (2006). Households by size: 1960 to present and households by type: 1940 to present. Table HH1. Retrieved December 5, 2009, from http:// http://www.census.gov/population/socdemo/hh-fam/hh1.pdf

U.S. Census Bureau. (2007; updated August 27, 2008). America's families and living arrangements: 2006 (Current Population Reports P20-553). Table HH-1. Retrieved January 5, 2011, from http://www.census.gov/population/www/socdemo/hh-fam/cps2006.html

U.S. Census Bureau. (2009, September). America's families and living arrangements: 2007 (Current Population Reports P20-561). Retrieved February 19, 2013, from http://www.census.gov/hhes/families/files/p20-561.pdf

CHAPTER 15

Agency for Healthcare Research and Quality (AHRQ). (2007). *National healthcare disparities report* (AHRQ Publication No. 08-0041). Rockville, MD: U.S. Department of Health and Human Services, Agency for Healthcare Research and Quality. Retrieved January 26, 2011, from http://www.ahrq.gov/qual/nhdr07/nhdr07.pdf

American Nurses Association (ANA). (1991). *Position statements: Cultural diversity in nursing practice.* Retrieved January 25, 2011, from http://www.nursingworld.org/MainMenuCategories/HealthcareandPolicyIssues/ANAPositionStatements/EthicsandHumanRights/prtetcldv14444.aspx

American Nurses Association (ANA). (2010). *Nursing: Scope and standards of practice* (2nd ed.). Silver Spring, MD: Author.

Andrews, M. M., & Boyle, J. S. (2007). *Transcultural concepts in nursing care* (5th ed.). Philadelphia: Lippincott Williams & Wilkins.

Bulechek, G. M., Butcher, H. K., & Dochterman, J. M. (Eds.). (2012). *Nursing interventions classification (NIC)* (6th ed.). St. Louis, MO: C. V. Mosby.

Burns, T., Catty, J., Becker, T., et al. (2007). The effectiveness of supported employment for people with severe mental illness: A randomized controlled trial. *The Lancet, 370*(9593), 1146–1152.

Campinha-Bacote, J. (2007, November 9). *Cultural competence in nursing curricula: How are we doing 20 years later?* Paper presented at the annual convention of the National Organization for Associate Degree Nursing, Las Vegas, NV.

Canadian Census. (2007a). Ethnic diversity and immigration. Statistics Canada. Last modified September 7, 2007. Retrieved February 22, 2011, from http://www41.statcan.ca/2007/30000/ceb30000_000_e.htm

Canadian Census. (2007b). Population. Statistics Canada. Retrieved February 22, 2011, from http://www41.statcan.ca/2007/3867/ceb3867_000_e.htm

Carballeira, N. (1997). The LIVE and LEARN model for cultural competent family services. *Continuum, 17*(1), 7–12.

Cloyes, K. (2007). Prisoners signify: A political discourse analysis of mental illness in a prison control unit. *Nursing Inquiry, 14*(3), 202–211.

Cronenwett, L., Sherwood, G., Barnsteiner, J., et al. (2007). Quality and safety education for nurses. *Nursing Outlook, 55*(3), 122–131.

Geissler, E. M. (1991). Transcultural nursing and nursing diagnosis. *Nursing and Health Care, 12*(4), 190–203.

Giger, J. N., & Davidhizar, R. (2008). *Transcultural nursing: Assessment and intervention* (5th ed.). St. Louis, MO: C. V. Mosby.

Hanson, S. (2001). *Family health care nursing: Theory, practice, and research* (2nd ed., p. 39). Philadelphia: F. A. Davis.

Healthy People 2020. (n.d.). Disparities. Retrieved January 26, 2011, from http://healthypeople.gov/2020/about/DisparitiesAbout.aspx

Leininger, M. (1978). *Transcultural nursing: Concepts, theories, and practices.* New York: John Wiley & Sons.

Leininger, M. (2007). Theoretical questions and concerns: Response from the Theory of Culture Care Diversity and Universality perspective. *Nursing Science Quarterly, 20*(1), 9–13.

Leininger, M. M., & McFarland, M. R. (2002). *Transcultural nursing: Concepts, theories, research and practices* (3rd ed.). New York: McGraw-Hill.

Leininger, M. M., & McFarland, M. R. (2006). *Culture care diversity and universality: A worldwide nursing theory.* Sudbury, MA: Jones & Bartlett.

Leppa, C. (2000). Transcultural communication within the health care subculture. In: J. Luckmann (Ed.), *Transcultural communication in health care* (pp. 74–83). Clifton Park, NY: Thomson Delmar Learning.

Lipson, J., & Meleis, A. (1985). Culturally appropriate care: The case of immigrants. *Topics in Clinical Nursing, 7*(3), 48–56.

Munoz, C., & Luckmann, J. (2004). *Transcultural communication in health care* (2nd ed.). Clifton Park, NY: Thomson Delmar Learning.

Purnell, L. (2000). A description of the Purnell model for cultural competence. *Journal of Transcultural Nursing, 11,* 40–46.

Purnell, L. (2002). The Purnell model for cultural competence. *Journal of Transcultural Nursing, 13*(3), 193–196.

Purnell, L. D., & Paulanka, B. J. (2008). *Transcultural health care: A culturally competent approach* (3rd ed.). Philadelphia: F. A. Davis.

Spector, R. E. (2004). *Cultural diversity in health and illness* (6th ed.). Upper Saddle River, NJ: Prentice-Hall.

Strickland, O. L., Giger, J. N., Nelson, M. A., et al. (2007). The relationships among stress, coping, social support, and weight class in premenopausal African American women at risk for coronary heart disease. *Journal of Cardiovascular Nursing, 22*(4), 272–278.

Suzuki, L. A., & Ponterotto, J. G. (2007). *Handbook of multicultural assessment: Clinical, psychological, and educational applications* (3rd ed.). San Francisco: Jossey-Bass.

Urban Indian Health Commission. (2007). Invisible tribes: Urban Indians and their health in a changing world (Robert Wood Johnson Foundation report). Retrieved January 26, 2011, from http://www.uihi.net/Public/UIHC%20Publications/UIHC_Report_FINAL.pdf

U.S. Census Bureau (n.d.). Minority census population. Retrieved January 26, 2011, from http://2010.census.gov/mediacenter/awareness/minority-census.php

U.S. Census Bureau. (2010). *United States Census 2010. 2010 census questionnaire reference book.* Retrieved February 22, 2010, from http://2010.census.gov/partners/pdf/langfiles/qrb_English.pdf

U.S. Department of Health and Human Services, OPHS, Office of Minority Health. (2001). National standards for culturally and linguistically appropriate services in health care: Final report. Washington, DC: Author. Retrieved February 1, 2011, from http://minorityhealth.hhs.gov/assets/pdf/checked/finalreport.pdf

Zborowski, M. (1969). *People in pain.* San Francisco: Jossey-Bass.

CHAPTER 16

American Nurses Association (ANA). (2010). *Nursing: Scope and standards of practice* (2nd ed.). Silver Spring, MD. Nursebooks.org.

Aspen Reference Group. (2002). *Palliative care: Patient and family counseling manual* (2nd ed.). Clifton Park, NY: Thomson Delmar Learning.

Beckman, S., Boxley-Harges, S., Bruick-Sorge, C., et al. (2007). Five strategies that heighten nurses' awareness of spirituality to impact client care. *Holistic Nursing Practice, 21*(3), 135–139.

Benson, H., Dusek, J. A., Sherwood, J. B., et al. (2006). Study of the therapeutic effects of intercessory prayer (STEP) in cardiac bypass patients: A multicenter randomized trial of

uncertainty and certainty of receiving intercessory prayer. *American Heart Journal, 151*(4), 934–942.

Bodhi, B. (2007). The Buddhist way of life on the eightfold path. Retrieved March 26, 2011, from http://www.hinduwebsite.com/buddhism/eightfoldpath.asp

Boyd, D. (1974). *Rolling thunder.* New York: Random House.

Brussat, F., & Brussat, M. A. (1996). *Spiritual literacy: Reading the sacred in everyday life.* New York: Simon & Schuster.

Bulechek, G. M., Butcher, H. K., & Dochterman, J. M. (Eds.). (2012). *Nursing interventions classification (NIC)* (6th ed.). St. Louis, MO: C. V. Mosby.

Cavendish, R., Konecny, L., Mitzeliotis, C., et al. (2003). Spiritual care interventions of nurses using Nursing Interventions Classification (NIC) labels. *International Journal of Nursing Terminologies and Classifications, 14*(4), 113–124.

Cenkner, W. (1990). Hinduism. In: J. A. Komonchak, M. Collins, & D. A. Lane (Eds.), *The new dictionary of theology* (pp. 466–469). Collegeville, MN: Liturgical Press.

The Collected Works of Florence Nightingale. (2007). University of Guelph, Ontario, Canada. Retrieved February 22, 2011, from http://www.sociology.uoguelph.ca/fnightingale

Donahue, M. P. (1985). *Nursing: The finest art. An illustrated history.* St. Louis, MO: C. V. Mosby.

Dunn, K., & Horgas, A. (2000). The prevalence of prayer as a spiritual self-care modality in elders. *Journal of Holistic Nursing, 18*(4), 337–351.

Esposito, J. L. (1990). Islam. In: J. A. Komonchak, M. Collins, & D. A. Lane (Eds.), *The new dictionary of theology* (pp. 527–529). Collegeville, MN: Liturgical Press.

Gaskamp, C., Sutter, R., Meraviglia, M., et al. (2006). Evidence-based guideline: Promoting spirituality in the older adult. *Journal of Gerontological Nursing, 32*(11), 8–13. Retrieved February 1, 2011, from http://www.ncbi.nlm.nih.gov/pubmed/17112133.

Gowri, A., & Hight, E. (2001). Spirituality and medical practice: Using the HOPE questions as a practical tool for spiritual assessment. *American Family Physician, 63,* 81–88.

Harris, W., Gowda, M., Kilb, J., et al. (1999). A randomized, controlled trial of the effects of remote, intercessory prayer on outcomes in patients admitted to the coronary care unit. *Archives of Internal Medicine, 159*(19), 2273–2278.

Harrison, M. O., Edwards, C. L., Koenig, H. G., et al. (2005). Religiosity, spirituality, and pain in patients with sickle cell disease. *Journal of Nervous and Mental Disorders, 193,* 250–257.

Highfield, M. E. F. (1992). Spiritual healing of oncology patients: Nurse and patient perspectives. *Cancer Nursing, 15*(1), 1–8.

Highfield, M. E. F. (2000). Providing spiritual care to patients with cancer. *Clinical Journal of Oncology Nursing, 4*(3), 115–120.

Highfield, M. E. F., & Cason, C. (1983). Spiritual needs of patients: Are they recognized? *Cancer Nursing, 6*(3), 187–192.

Hungelmann, J., Kenkel-Rossi, E., Klassen, L., et al. (1996). Focus on spiritual well-being: Harmonious interconnectedness of mind-body-spirit—use of the JAREL spiritual well-being scale. *Geriatric Nursing, 17*(6), 262.

The Joint Commission (TJC). (2008). *2008 hospital accreditation standards.* Oakbrook Terrace, IL: Author.

Keddington, R. K. (2007). Caring for members of the Church of Jesus Christ of Latter-Day Saints (Mormons) in the emergency department. *Journal of Emergency Nursing, 33*(3), 252–256.

Keegan, L. (2000). A comparison of the use of alternative therapies among Mexican Americans and Anglo-Americans in the Texas Rio Grande Valley. *Journal of Holistic Nursing, 18*(3), 280–295.

Kirkwood, N. A. (2005). *A hospital handbook on multiculturalism* (rev. ed.). Harrisburg, PA: Morehouse.

Kluckhohn, C., & Leighton, D. (1962). *The Navajo.* Garden City, NY: Doubleday.

Knierim, T. (last updated 2011, January). The noble eightfold path. Retrieved April 26, 2008, from http://www.thebigview.com/buddhism/eightfoldpath.html

Koenig, H. G., McCollough, M. E., & Larson, D. B. (2001). *Handbook of religions and health.* New York: Oxford University Press.

Krishnamurti, J. (1989). *Think on these things.* New York: Harper Perennial.

le Gallez, P., Dimmock, S., & Bird, H. (2000). Spiritual healing as adjunct therapy for rheumatoid arthritis. *British Journal of Nursing, 9*(11), 695–700.

Macquarrie, J. (1977). *Principles of Christian theology* (2nd ed.). New York: Scribner.

Macrae, J. (1995). Nightingale's spiritual philosophy and its significance for modern nursing. *Image: Journal of Nursing Scholarship, 27*(1), 8–10.

Matthews, D., Marlowe, S., & MacNutt, F. (2000). Effects of intercessory prayer on patients with rheumatoid arthritis. *Southern Medical Journal, 93*(12), 1177–1186.

Matthews, W., Conti, J., & Sireci, S. (2001). The effects of intercessory prayer, positive visualization, and expectancy on the well-being of kidney dialysis patients. *Alternative Therapies in Health and Medicine, 7*(5), 42–52.

McCaffrey, A. M., Eisenberg, D. M., Legedza, A. T. R., et al. (2004). Prayer for health concerns: Results of a national survey on prevalence and patterns of use. *Archives of Internal Medicine, 164*(8), 858–862.

Millspaugh, C. D. (2005). Assessment and response to spiritual pain: Part II. *Journal of Palliative Medicine, 8*(6), 1110–1117.

Moorhead, S., Johnson, M., & Maas, M. L., et al. (Eds.). (2008). *Nursing outcomes classification (NOC)* (4th ed.). St. Louis, MO: C. V. Mosby.

NANDA International (NANDA-I). (2009). *Nursing diagnoses: Definitions and classification 2009–2011.* Philadelphia: Author.

Oxtoby, W. G., & Segal, A. G. (2007). *A concise introduction to world religions.* Cary, NC: Oxford University Press.

Palmer, R. F., Katerndahl, D., & Morgan-Kidd, J. (2004). A randomized trial of the effects of remote intercessory prayer: Interactions with personal beliefs on problem-specific outcomes and functional status. *Journal of Alternative and Complementary Medicine, 10*(3), 438–448.

Pawlikowski, J. (1990). Judaism. In: J. Komonchak, M. Collins, & D. A. Lane (Eds.), *The new dictionary of theology* (pp. 543–548). Collegeville, MN: Liturgical Press.

Reeve, C. (2002). *Nothing is impossible: Reflections on a new life.* New York: Random House.

Roberts, L., Ahmed, I., & Hall, S. (2000). Intercessory prayer for the alleviation of ill health. *Cochrane Database of Systematic Reviews,* Issue 2. Art. No.: CD000368.

Ryan, P. (1992). Perception of the most helpful nursing behaviors in a home-care hospice setting: Care-givers and nurses. *American Journal of Hospice and Palliative Care, 9*(5), 22–31.

Sodestrom, K., & Martin, I. M. (1987). Patients' spiritual coping strategies: A study of nurse and patient perspectives. *Oncology Nursing Forum, 14*(2), 41–46.

Sparber, A., Bauer, L., Curt, G., et al. (2000). Use of complementary medicine by adult patients participating in cancer clinical trials. *Oncology Nursing Forum, 27*(6), 887–888.

CHAPTER 17

Ahrens, T., Yancey, V., & Kollef, M. (2003). Improving family communications at the end of life: Implications for length of stay in the intensive care unit and resource use. *American Journal of Critical Care, 12*(4), 317–324.

American Nurses Association (ANA). (1994a). Position statement: Active euthanasia. Washington, DC: Author. Retrieved February 5, 2011, from http://www.nursing world.org/MainMenuCategories/HealthcareandPolicy Issues/ANAPositionStatements/EthicsandHumanRights/ prteteuth14450.aspx

American Nurses Association (ANA). (1994b). Position statement: Assisted suicide. Washington, DC: Author. Retrieved February 5, 2011, from http://www.nursingworld.org/ MainMenuCategories/HealthcareandPolicyIssues/ANA PositionStatements/EthicsandHumanRights/prtetsuic 14456.aspx

American Nurses Association (ANA). (2003). Position statement: Pain management and control of distressing symptoms in dying patients. Retrieved February 3, 2011, http://www.nursingworld.org/MainMenuCategories/ HealthcareandPolicyIssues/ANAPositionStatements/ EthicsandHumanRights/etpain14426.aspx

American Nurses Association (ANA). (2004). Position statement: Nursing care and do-not-resuscitate decisions. Washington, DC: Author. Retrieved February 2, 2011, from http://www.nursingworld.org/MainMenuCategories/ EthicsStandards/Ethics-Position-Statements/Copy%20 of%20dnr0414405.aspx

Bednash, G., & Ferrell, B. (2000). *The end-of life nursing education consortium (2000). The ELNEC curriculum.* Washington, DC: American Association of Colleges of Nursing and City of Hope National Medical Center.

Bowlby, J. (1982). *Attachment and loss* (Vols. 1–3). New York: Basic Books.

Boyle, D. K., Miller, P. A., & Forbes-Thompson, S. A. (2005). Communication and end-of-life care in the intensive care unit. Patient, family, and clinician outcomes. *Critical Care Nursing Quarterly, 28*(4), 302–316.

Boyle, J. S., Bunting, S. M., Hodnicki, D. R., et al. (2001). Critical thinking in African American mothers who care for adult children with HIV: A cultural analysis. *Journal of Transcultural Nursing, 12*(3), 193–202.

Briggs, D. A., & Pehrsson, D-E. (2008). Use of bibliotherapy in the treatment of grief and loss: A guide to current counseling practices. *Theory, Research & Practice, 71,* 32–42.

Bulechek, G., Butcher, H., & Dochterman, J. M. (2008). *Nursing interventions classification (NIC)* (5th ed.). St. Louis, MO: C. V. Mosby.

College of American Pathologists. (last updated 2007). Autopsy. Postmortem flow chart. College of American Pathologists, Autopsy Committee. Retrieved August 21, 2009, from http://capstaging.cap.org/apps/docs/committees/ autopsy/POSTMORTEM_FLOW_CHART.pdf

DeSpelder, L., & Strickland, A. (1996). *The last dance.* Mountain View, CA: Mayfield.

Duffy, S., Jackson, F., Schim, S., et al. (2006). Cultural concepts at the end of life. *Nursing Older People, 18*(8), 10–14.

Eisenhandler, S. A. (2004). The arts of consolation: Commemoration and folkways of faith. *Generations, 28*(2), 37.

Emanuel, L., Ferris, F., von Gunten, C., et al. (2008). The last hours of living: Practical advice for clinicians CME/CE. From: L. Emanuel, F. Ferris, C. von Gunten, et al. (2005), EPEC™-O: Education in Palliative and End-of-life Care for Oncology. (Module 6: Last Hours of Living © The EPEC Project™, Chicago, IL). Major funding provided by the National Cancer Institute; Supplemental funding provided by the Lance Armstrong Foundation. Retrieved August 30, 2008, from http://www.medscape.com/ viewarticle/542262

Engel, G. L. (1961). Is grief a disease? A challenge for medical research. *Psychosomatic Medicine, 23*(1), 18–22.

Ferrell, B., Grant, M., & Virani, R. (1999). Strengthening nursing education to improve end-of-life care. *Nursing Outlook, 47*(6), 252.

Ferszt, G. G., & Leveillee, M. (2006). How do you distinguish between grief and depression? *Nursing2006, 36*(9), 60–61.

Florczak, K. L. (2008). The persistent yet ever changing nature of grieving a loss. *Nursing Science Quarterly, 21*(1), 7–11.

Gambles, M., Crooke, M., & Wilkinson, S. (2002). Evaluation of a hospice based reflexology service: A qualitative audit of patient perceptions. *European Journal of Oncology Nursing, 6*(1), 37–44.

Goldsmith, B., Morrison, R. S., Vanderwerker, L. C., et al. (2008). Elevated rates of prolonged grief disorder in African Americans. *Death Studies, 32,* 352–365.

Hancock, K., Clayton, J., Parker, S., et al. (2007). Truth-telling in discussing prognosis in advanced life-limiting illnesses: A systematic review. *Palliative Medicine, 21,* 507–517.

Hudson, P. L. (2006). How well do family caregivers cope after caring for a relative with advanced disease and how can health professionals enhance their support? *Journal of Palliative Medicine, 9*(3), 694–703.

Johnson, M., Moorhead, S., Bulechek, C., et al. (2012). *NOC and NIC linkages to NANDA-I and clinical conditions* (3rd ed.). St. Louis, MO: C. V. Mosby.

Johnstone, P., Polston, G., Niemtzow, R., et al. (2002). Integration of acupuncture into the oncology clinic. *Palliative Medicine, 16*(3), 235–239.

The Joint Commission (TJC). (2008). *Hospital accreditation standards.* Oakbrook Terrace, IL: Author.

Karnes, B. (1995). *Gone from my sight: The dying experience.* Stillwell, KS: Barbara Karnes Books.

Kruse, B. (2004). The meaning of letting go: The lived experience for caregivers of persons at the end of life. *Journal of Hospice and Palliative Nursing, 6*(4), 215–222.

Kurtz, S. F., Strong, C. W., & Gerasimow, D. (2007, February). The 2006 Revised Uniform Anatomical Gift Act—a law to save lives. *Health Law Analysis.* Retrieved April 1, 2011, from http://www.law.upenn.edu/bll/archives/ulc/uaga/ kurz032106.pdf

Matzo, M., & Sherman, D. (2006). *Palliative care nursing* (2nd ed.). New York: Springer.

Moorhead, S., Johnson, M., Maas, M., et al. (2007). *Nursing outcomes classification (NOC)* (4th ed.). St. Louis, MO: C. V. Mosby.

National Guideline Clearinghouse (NGC). (2006). Providing spiritual care to the terminally ill older adult. Retrieved February 26, 2011, from http://www.guideline.gov/ content.aspx?id=10552&search=promoting+spirituality+ in+the+older+adult

National Hospice and Palliative Care Organization (NHPCO). (2009). NHPCO facts and figures: Hospice care in America. Retrieved February 2, 2011, from http://www.nhpco.org/files/public/Statistics_Research/NHPCO_facts_and_figures.pdf

National Office, Partnership for Caring, 1620 Eye St. NW, Suite 202; Washington, DC 20006. 202-296-8071. Not for reproduction. Note that forms are updated annually, so the current version must be found online at http://caringinfo.org/i4a/pages/index.cfm?pageid=3289

O'Connor, L., & Lunney, M. (1998). Care of the caregiver—family member with a chronic illness. *Nursing Diagnosis, 9*(4), 152.

Pitorak, E. (2003). Care at the time of death. *American Journal of Nursing, 103*(7), 42–52.

President's Commission for the Study of Ethical Problems in Medicine and Biomedical and Behavioral Research. (1981). *Defining death: A report on the medical, legal, and ethical issues in the determination of death.* Washington, DC: U.S. Government Printing Office.

Qaseem, A., Snow, V., Shekelle, P., et al. (2008). Evidence-based interventions to improve the palliative care of pain, dyspnea, and depression at the end of life: A clinical practice guideline from the American College of Physicians. *Annals of Internal Medicine, 148*(2), 141–146.

Rando, T. (1984). *Grief, dying and death: Clinical interventions for caregivers.* Champaign, IL: Research Press.

Rando, T. (1986). *Loss and anticipatory grief.* Lexington, MA: Lexington Books.

Rando, T. (1993). *Treatment of complicated mourning.* Champaign, IL: Research Press.

Rando, T. (2000). *Clinical dimensions of anticipatory mourning: Theory and practice in working with the dying, their loved ones, and their caregivers.* Champaign, IL: Research Press.

Teno, J. M., Casey, V. A., Welch, L. C., et al. (2001). Patient-focused, family-centered end-of-life medical care: Views of the guidelines and bereaved family members. *Journal of Pain and Symptom Management, 22*, 738–751.

Thompson, E., & Reilly, D. (2002). The homeopathic approach to symptom control in the cancer patient: A prospective observational study. *Palliative Medicine, 16*(3), 227–233.

Traylor, E., Hayslip, B., Kaminski, P. L., et al. (2003). Relationships between grief and family system characteristics: A cross lagged longitudinal analysis. *Death Studies, 27*(7), 575–601.

U.S. Department of Health and Human Services. (n.d.) Organ and Tissue Donation. Retrieved April 2, 2011, from http://dying.about.com/od/livingafteradeath/ss/organdonate_3.htm

Verheijde, J. L., Rady, M. Y., & McGregor, J. L. (2007). The United States Revised Uniform Anatomical Gift Act (2006): New challenges to balancing patient rights and physician responsibilities. *Philosophy, Ethics, and Humanities in Medicine.* Retrieved May 5, 2008, from http://www.pubmedcentral.nih.gov/articlerender.fcgi?artid=2001294

Von Gunten, C. F., Ferris, F. D., & Emanuel, L. L. (2000). Ensuring competency in end-of-life care: Communication and relational skills. *JAMA, 284*(23), 3051–3057.

Worden, J. W. (2002). *Grief counseling and grief therapy: A handbook for the mental health practitioner* (3rd ed.). New York: Springer.

CHAPTER 18

American Nurses Association (ANA). (2010). *Nursing: Scope and standards of practice* (2nd ed.). Silver Spring, MD: Author.

AMNews. (2007, March 19). Hospital EMR not widespread yet. Retrieved February 10, 2011, from http://www.ama-assn.org/amednews/2007/03/19/bicb0319.htm

Collins, S. A., Stein, D. M., Vawdrey, D. K., et al. (2011) Content overlap in nurse and physician handoff artifacts and the potential role of electronic health records: A systematic review. *Journal of Biomedical Informatics, 44*(4), 704–712.

Currie, J. (2002). Improving the efficiency of patient handover. *Emergency Nurse, 10*(3), 24–28.

Haig, K., Sutton, S., & Whittington, J. (2006). SBAR: A shared mental model for improving communication between clinicians. *Joint Commission Journal of Quality and Patient Safety, 32*(3), 167–175.

Hing, E., Burt, C. & Woodwell, D. (2006, October 26). Electronic medical record use by office-based physicians and their practices: United States, 2006. *Vital Health Statistics, 393.* Washington, DC: Centers for Disease Control Advance Data.

Jamoom, E., Beatty, P., & Bercovitz, A., et al. (2012). Physician adoption of electronic health record systems: United States, 2011. National Center for Health Statistics, Centers for Disease Control and Prevention. Retrieved December 20, 2012, from http://www.cdc.gov/nchs/data/databriefs/db98.pdf

The Joint Commission (TJC). (2008a). The official "do not use" list. Retrieved August 27, 2008, from http://www.jointcommission.org/Do_Not_Use_List_of_Abbreviations/

The Joint Commission (TJC). (2008b). *2008 hospital accreditation standards* (pp. 116–117). Oakbrook Terrace, IL: Author.

The Joint Commission (TJC). (2010). Accreditation Program: Hospital; national patient safety goals, effective January 1, 2011. Retrieved February 4, 2011, from http://www.jointcommission.org/assets/1/6/2011_NPSGs_HAP.pdf

The Joint Commission (TJC). (2011). 2011 Joint Commission Standards for acute care hospitals, revised December 2010. Retrieved February 27, 2011, from http://www.cihq-hacp.org/images/pdf/2011_TJC_Acute_Care_Standards_-_Rev12.10.pdf

Kaiser Permanente of Colorado. (n.d.). SBAR technique for communication. Institute for Healthcare Improvement. Retrieved August 16, 2008, from http://www.ihi.org/IHI/Topics/PatientSafety/SafetyGeneral/Tools/SBARTechniqueforCommunicationASituationalBriefingModel.htm

Kitch, B., Cooper, J., Zapol, W., et al. (2008). Handoffs causing patient harm: A survey of medical and surgical house staff. *The Joint Commision Journal on Quality and Patient Safety, 34*(10), 563–570.

Moody, L., Slocomb, E., Berg, B., et al. (2004). Electronic health records documentation in nursing: Nurses' perceptions, attitudes, and preferences. *Computers, Informatics, Nursing, 22*(6), 337–344.

Riesenberg L., Leisch J., Cunningham J., et al. (2010). Nursing handoffs: A systematic review of the literature. *American Journal of Nursing, 110*(4), 24-34.

Schroeder, S. (2006). Picking up the PACE: A new template for shift report. *Nursing2006, 36*(10), 22–23.

CHAPTER 19

American Association of Critical-Care Nurses (AACCN). (2010). *AACN practice alert. Noninvasive blood pressure monitoring.* Retrieved February 10, 2011, from http://www.aacn.org/WD/Practice/Docs/PracticeAlerts/NIBP%20Monitoring%2004-2010%20final.pdf

American Heart Association (AHA). (n.d.). *Blood pressure—buying and caring for home equipment.* Retrieved February 8, 2011, from http://www.americanheart.org/presenter.jhtml?identifier=4495

Best practices: Evidence-based nursing procedures (2nd ed., pp. 59–62). (2007). Philadelphia: Lippincott Williams & Wilkins.

British Hypertension Society, Hypertension Influence Team. (2006). *"Let's do it well" nurse learning pack.* Retrieved February 10, 2011, from http://www.bhsoc.org/pdfs/hit.pdf

Centers for Disease Control and Prevention (CDC). (2008). Guideline for disinfection and sterilization in healthcare facilities, 2008. Retrieved February 7, 2011, from http://www.cdc.gov/hicpac/pdf/guidelines/Disinfection_Nov_2008.pdf

Centers for Disease Control and Prevention (CDC). (2011). Vital signs: Prevalence, treatment, and control of hypertension—United States, 1999–2002 and 2005–2008. *Morbidity and Mortality Weekly Report, 60*(4), 103–108. Retrieved February 16, 2001, from http://www.cdc.gov/mmwr/preview/mmwrhtml/mm6004a4.htm?s_cid=mm6004a4_w

De Curtis, M., Calzolari, F., Marciano, A., et al. (2008). Comparison between rectal and infrared skin temperature in the newborn. *Archives of Disease in Childhood—Fetal and Neonatal Edition, 93*, F55–F57.

Gomolin, I. H., Aung, M. M., Wolf-Klein, G., et al. (2005). Older is colder: Temperature range and variation in older people. *Journal of the American Geriatrics Society, 53*(12), 2170–2172.

Gyi, A. A. (2007). Vital signs (JBI Evidence Summary No. ES6699). Retrieved February 9, 2011, from http://www.jbiconnect.org/connect/docs/cis/es_html_viewer.php?SID=6699&lang=en&region=AU

Heusch, A. I., & McCarthy, P. W. (2005). The patient: A novel source of error in clinical temperature measurement using infrared aural thermometry. *Journal of Alternative & Complementary Medicine, 11*(3), 473–476.

Hwu, Y. J., Coates, V. E., & Lin, F. Y. (2000). A study of the effectiveness of different measuring times and counting methods of human radial pulse rates. *Journal of Clinical Nursing, 9*(1), 146–152.

Jevon, P., Ewens, B., & Lowe, R. (2000). Practical procedures for nurses. Measuring apex and radial pulse. *Nursing Times, 96*(50), 43–44.

Johnson, M., Moorhead, S., Bulechek, C., et al. (2012). *NOC and NIC linkages to NANDA-I and clinical conditions* (3rd ed.). St. Louis, MO: C. V. Mosby.

Joint National Committee on Prevention, Detection, Evaluation, and Treatment of High Blood Pressure. (2004). *JNC 7 Complete Report. The seventh report of the Joint National Committee on Prevention, Detection, Evaluation, and Treatment of High Blood Pressure.* Bethesda, MD: National Institutes of Health. Retrieved February 22, 2011, from http://www.nhlbi.nih.gov/guidelines/hypertension/index.htm

Kennedy, K. J., Dreimanis, D. E., Beckingham, W. D., et al. (2003). *Staphylococcus aureus* and stethoscopes [Letter to the editor]. *Medical Journal of Australia, 178*(9), 468.

Lockwood, C., Conroy-Hiller, T., & Page, T. (2004). Vital signs. *JBI Database of Systematic Reviews,* ID No. SR0115. Retrieved February 8, 2011, from http://onlinelibrary.wiley.com/doi/10.1111/j.1479-6988.2004.00012.x/abstract

Ma, G., Sabin, N., & Dawes, M. A. (2008). A comparison of blood pressure measurement over a sleeved arm versus a bare arm. *Canadian Medical Association Journal, 178*(5), 585–589.

Mackowiak, P. A. (1998). Concepts of fever. *Archives of Internal Medicine, 158*(17), 1870–1881.

McCance, K. L., & Huether, S. E. (2006). *Pathophysiology: The biologic basis for disease in adults and children* (5th ed.). St. Louis, MO: C. V. Mosby.

McKay, D. W. (2008). Measuring blood pressure: A call to bare arms? *Canadian Medical Association Journal, 178*(5), 591–592.

NANDA International (NANDA-I). (2009). *Nursing diagnoses: Definitions and classification 2009–2011.* Philadelphia: Author.

National Guideline Clearinghouse (NGC). (2007). Guideline summary: 2007 guidelines for the management of arterial hypertension. Rockville, MD: Author. Retrieved February 8, 2011, from http://www.guideline.gov/content.aspx?id=10952&search=arterial+hypertension+management

National Heart, Lung, and Blood Institute (NHLBI). (1996, revised 2005). *The fourth report on the diagnosis, evaluation, and treatment of high blood pressure in children and adolescents* (NIH Publication No. 05-5267). U.S. Department of Health and Human Services. Retrieved February 8, 2011, from http://www.nhlbi.nih.gov/health/prof/heart/hbp/hbp_ped.pdf

National Heart Lung and Blood Institute (NHLBI). (2007). *A pocket guide to blood pressure measurement in children.* From the National High Blood Pressure Education Program Working Group on High Blood Pressure in Children and Adolescents. National Institutes of Health. Retrieved February 24, 2011, from http://www.nhlbi.nih.gov/health/public/heart/hbp/bp_child_pocket/bp_child_pocket.pdf

Perk, G., Stessman, J., Ginsberg, G., et al. (2003). Sex differences in the effect of heart rate on mortality in the elderly. *Journal of the American Geriatrics Society, 51*(9), 1260–1264.

Perloff, D., Grim, C., Flack, J., et al. (1993). Human blood pressure determination by sphygmomanometry. AHA Medical/Scientific Statement, Product Code: 88:2460–2467. Dallas, TX: American Heart Association.

Pickering, T., Hall, J., Appel, L., et al. (2005). Recommendations for blood pressure measurement in humans and experimental animals: Part 1: Blood pressure measurement in humans: A statement for professionals from the subcommittee of Professional and Public Education of the American Heart Association Council on High Blood Pressure Research. *Hypertension, 45*(1), 142–161.

Quatrara, B., Coffman, Z., Jenkins, T., et al. (2007). The effect of respiratory rate and ingestion of hot and cold beverages on the accuracy of oral temperatures measured by electronic thermometers. *MedSurg Nursing, 16*(2), 105–108.

Robinson, J. L., Jou, H., & Spady, D. W. (2005). Accuracy of parents in measuring body temperature with a tympanic thermometer. *Family Practice, 6*(1), 3.

Rutala, W. A., & Weber, D. J. (2004). Disinfection and sterilization in health care facilities: What clinicians need to know. *Clinical Infectious Diseases, 39*, 702–709.

Siegel, J. D., Rhinehart, E., Jackson, M., et al. (2006). Healthcare Infection Control Practices Advisory Committee (HICPAC). Management of multidrug-resistant organisms in healthcare settings, 2006. Atlanta, GA: Centers for Disease Control & Prevention. Retrieved February 10, 2011, from http://www.cdc.gov/ncidod/dhqp/pdf/ar/mdroguideline2006.pdf

Stomski, N. (2009). Vital signs. Evidence summaries—Joanna Briggs Institute. Retrieved February 9, 2011, from http://connect.jbiconnectplus.org/ViewDocument.aspx?0=1335

Sund-Levander, M., Forsberg, C., & Wahren, L. K. (2002). Normal oral, rectal, tympanic and axillary body temperature in adult men and women: A systematic literature review. *Scandinavian Journal of Caring Sciences, 16*(2), 122–128.

Therapeutic Research Center. (2007). Thermometer comparison. *Healthcare Professional Information, 23*(231006). Stockton, CA: Author. Retrieved June 1, 2008, from http://www.pharmacistsletter.com

Trim, J. (2005). Monitoring pulse. *Nursing Times, 101*(21), 30–31.

U.S. Environmental Protection Agency (EPA). (2001). Memorandum of understanding between the American Hospital Association & the U.S. Environmental Protection Agency. Retrieved February 16, 2011, from http://www.h2e-online.org/docs/h2emou101501.pdf

Vital signs. (1999). *Best Practice, 3*(3), 1–6. Retrieved February 18, 2011, from http://www.joannabriggs.edu.au/pdf/BPISEng_3_3.pdf

Wunderlich, C. A. (1871). *On the temperature in diseases* (2nd ed., W. Bathurst Woodman, Trans.). London: New Sydenham Society. Retrieved May 30, 2012, from http://books.google.com/books?hl=en&lr=&id=3-wHAAAAIAAJ&oi=fnd&pg=PA1&dq=wunderlich_temperature&ots=97uPlXqxky&sig=NmJTwucR4Q0Bep7MfFxfvGAoDUE#PPR10,M1

CHAPTER 20

Adams-Wendling, L., & Pimple, C. (2007, June). *Nursing management of hearing impairment in nursing facility residents* (p. 56). Iowa City: University of Iowa Gerontological Nursing Interventions Research Center. Research Dissemination Core. Brief summary of guideline, National Guideline Clearinghouse. Retrieved March 20, 2011, from http://www.guideline.gov/summary/summary.aspx?doc_id=11053&nbr=005832&string=hearing

American Association of Critical-Care Nurses (AACN). (2005). *AACN standards for establishing and sustaining healthy work environment: A journey to excellence.* Aliso Viejo, CA: Author.

American Nurses Association (ANA). (2010). *Nursing: Scope and standards of practice* (2nd ed.). Silver Spring, MD: Nursebooks.org.

Ammentorp, J., Sabroe, S., Kofoed, P. E., et al. (2007). The effect of training in communication skills on medical doctors' and nurses' self-efficacy: A randomized controlled trial. *Patient Education and Counseling, 66*(3), 270–277.

Apker, J., Propp, K. M., Ford, W. S. Z., et al. (2006). Collaboration, credibility, compassion, and coordination: Professional nurse communication skill sets in health care team interactions. *Journal of Professional Nursing, 22*(3), 180–189.

Beyea, S. (2004). Improving verbal communication in clinical care. *AORN Journal 79*(5), 1053–1057.

Cronenwett, L., Sherwood, G., Barnsteiner, J., et al. (2007). Quality and safety education for nurses. *Nursing Outlook, 55*(3), 122–131.

Edwards, N., Peterson, W. E., & Davies, B. L. (2006). Evaluation of a multiple component intervention to support the implementation of a "Therapeutic Relationships" best practice guideline on nurses' communication skills. *Patient Education and Counseling, 63*(1–2), 3–11.

Haig, K. M., Sutton, S., & Whittington, J. (2006). National Patient Safety Goals. SBAR: A shared mental model for improving communication between clinicians. *The Joint Commission Journal on Quality and Patient Safety, 32*(3), 167–175.

Hall, E. T. (1992). *The hidden dimension.* Gloucester, MA: Peter Smith.

Hall, K. (2011) Professional boundaries: building a trusting relationship with patients. *Home Healthcare Nurse, 29*(4), 210–217.

Holder, K., & Schenthal, S. (2007). Watch your step: Nursing and professional boundaries. *Nursing Management, 38*(2), 24–29.

Jayasekara, R. (2009, August). Dementia: Communication skills for staff. Evidence summaries—Joanna Briggs Institute. Retrieved February 20, 2013, from http://www.jbiconnect.org/connect/docs/cis/es_html_viewer.php?SID=6786&lang=en&region=AU

The Joint Commission (TJC). (2009). *Hospital accreditation standards 2010: Accreditation policies, standards, elements of performance, scoring.* Oakbrook Terrace, IL: Author.

The Joint Commission (TJC). (2012). *2013 National patient safety goals.* Retrieved February 20, 2013, from http://www.jointcommission.org/hap_2013_npsg/

Miller, C. A. (2008). How to try this. Communication difficulties in hospitalized older adults with dementia. *American Journal of Nursing, 108*(3), 58–62.

Miller, L. (2010, September 21). *Overheard: What we say, what we mean, what families hear.* Poster session presented at the 26th annual educational conference of the National Association of Neonatal Nurses (NANN).

National Council of State Boards of Nursing. (2007). Professional Boundaries—a nurse's guide to the importance of appropriate professional boundaries. Retrieved September 22, 2011, from https://www.ncsbn.org/Professional_Boundaries_2007_Web.pdf

Pope, B. B., Rodzen, L., & Spross, G. (2008). Raising the SBAR: How better communication improves patient outcomes. *Nursing2008, 38*(3), 41–43.

Stein, L., Watts, D., & Howell, T. (1990). Sounding board: The doctor-nurse game revisited. *New England Journal of Medicine, 322*(8), 546–549.

Tannen, D. (2001). *You just don't understand: Women and men in conversation.* New York: HarperCollins.

Venes, D. (2009). *Taber's cyclopedic medical dictionary* (21st ed.). Philadelphia, F. A. Davis.

Williams, K., Herman, R., Gajewski, B., et al. (2009). Elderspeak communication: Impact on dementia care. *American Journal of Alzheimer's Disease and Other Dementias, 24*, 11–20.

CHAPTER 21

Agency for Healthcare Research and Quality (AHRQ). (n.d.). Recommendation: Cervical cancer. Retrieved February 21, 2011, from http://epss.ahrq.gov/ePSS/RecomDetail.do?tab=1&sid=32&age=70&sex=Female&sexuallyActive=yes&tobacco=no

American Cancer Society. (2010, last revised). American Cancer Society guidelines for the early detection of cancer.

Retrieved February 20, 2011, from http://www.cancer.org/docroot/PED/content/PED_2_3X_ACS_Cancer_Detection_Guidelines_36.asp?sitearea+PED

American Cancer Society. (2011, last revised). Detailed guide. Breast cancer: American Cancer Society recommendations for early breast cancer detection. Retrieved February 20, 2011, from http://www.cancer.org/docroot/CRI/content/CRI_2_4_3X_Can_breast_cancer_be_found_early_5.asp

American College of Obstetricians and Gynecologists (ACOG). (2003, reaffirmed 2006). *Breast cancer screening* (ACOG Practice Bulletin No. 122). Washington, DC: Author.

American College of Obstetricians and Gynecologists (ACOG). (2009a). Interpreting the U.S. Preventive Services Task Force breast cancer screening recommendations for the general population. Retrieved February 20, 2011, from http://www.acog.org/from_home/Misc/uspstfinterpretation.cfm

American College of Obstetricians and Gynecologists (ACOG). (2009b). First cervical cancer screening delayed until age 21; less frequent Pap tests recommended [Press release]. Retrieved February 21, 2011, from http://www.acog.org/from_home/publications/press_releases/nr11-20-09.cfm

Anderson, B., Kelly, A. M., Kerr, D., et al. (2008). Impact of patient and environmental factors on capillary refill time in adults. *American Journal of Emergency Medicine, 26*(1), 62–65.

Balkaya, N. A., Memis, S., & Demirkiran, F. (2007). The effects of breast self-exam education on the performance of nursing and midwifery students: A 6-month follow-up study. *Journal of Cancer Education, 22*(2), 77–79.

Centers for Disease Control and Prevention (CDC). (n.d.). Glasgow Coma Scale. Last reviewed June 23, 2006. Retrieved February 26, 2011, from http://www.bt.cdc.gov/masscasualties/gscale.asp

Centers for Disease Control and Prevention (CDC). (2008). Guideline for disinfection and sterilization in healthcare facilities, 2008. Retrieved February 20, 2011, from http://www.cdc.gov/hicpac/Disinfection_Sterilization/2_approach.html

Doerflinger, M. (2007). How to try this: The Mini-Cog. *American Journal of Nursing, 107*(12), 62–71. Retrieved February 26, 2011, from http://www.nursingcenter.com/prodev/ce_article.asp?tid=756614

Fulmer, T. (1991). The geriatric nurse specialist role: A new model. *Nursing Management, 22*(3), 91–93.

Fulmer, T. (2007). How to try this: Fulmer SPICES. *American Journal of Nursing, 107*(10), 40–49.

Green, B., & Taplin, S. (2003). Breast cancer screening controversies. *Journal of the American Board of Family Practice, 16*(3), 233–241.

Hackshaw, A., & Paul, E. (2003). Breast self-examination and death from breast cancer: A meta-analysis. *British Journal of Cancer, 88*(7), 1047–1053.

Kennedy, K. J., Dreimanis, D. E., Beckingham, W. D., et al. (2003). *Staphylococcus aureus* and stethoscopes [Letter to the editor]. *Medical Journal of Australia, 178*(9), 468.

Knutson, D., & Steiner, E. (2007). Screening for breast cancer: Current recommendations and future directions. *American Family Physician, 75*(11), 1660–1666.

Kösters, J., & Gøtzsche, P. (2003). Regular self-examination or clinical examination for early detection of breast cancer. *Cochrane Database of Systematic Reviews*, Issue 2. Art. No.: CD003373.

Management of Overweight and Obesity Working Group. (2006). VA/DoD clinical practice guideline for screening and management of overweight and obesity. Washington, DC: Department of Veterans Affairs, Department of Defense. Retrieved February 21, 2011, from http://www.guideline.gov/content.aspx?id=10714

National Guideline Clearinghouse (NGC). (2005, revised 2011). Guideline synthesis: Screening for cervical cancer. Rockville, MD: Author. Retrieved February 21, 2011, from http://guideline.gov/syntheses/synthesis.aspx?f=rss&id=25623.

National Heart Lung and Blood Institute (NHLBI), Obesity Education Initiative. (n.d.). Body mass index table. Retrieved February 21, 2011, from http://www.nhlbi.nih.gov/guidelines/obesity/bmi_tbl.htm

Rauen, C., Chulay, M., Bridges, E., et al. (2008). Seven evidence-based practice habits: Putting some sacred cows out to pasture. *Critical Care Nurse, 28*(2), 98–124.

Rosolowich, V. (2006). Breast self-examination. *Journal of Obstetrics & Gynaecolocy Canada: JOGC, 28*(8), 728–730.

Rowley, G., & Fielding, K. (1991). Reliability and accuracy of the Glasgow Coma Scale with experienced and inexperienced users. *The Lancet, 337*, 55–538.

Rutala, W. A., & Weber, D. J. (2004). Disinfection and sterilization in health care facilities: What clinicians need to know. *Clinical Infectious Diseases, 39*, 702–709.

Tanner, J. (1962). *Growth at adolescence* (2nd ed.). Oxford: Blackwell Scientific.

Tarrant, M. (2006). Why are we still promoting breast self-examination? *International Journal of Nursing Studies, 43*(4), 519–520.

Teasdale, G., & Jennett, B. (1974). Assessment of coma and impaired consciousness. *The Lancet, 2*(7872), 81–84.

Teasdale, G., Kril-Jones, R., & van der Sande, J. (1978). Observer variability in assessing impaired consciousness and coma. *Journal of Neurology, Neurosurgery, and Psychiatry, 41*, 603–610.

U.S. Preventive Services Task Force (USPSTF). (2009). *Screening for breast cancer: Clinical summary*. Rockville, MD: Agency for Healthcare Research and Quality. Retrieved December 13, 2009, from http://www.ahrq.gov/clinic/uspstf09/breastcancer/brcansum.htm

Van Leeuwen, A. M., Kranpitz, T. R., & Smith, L. S. (2011). *Davis's comprehensive handbook of laboratory and diagnostic tests: With nursing implications* (4th ed.). Philadelphia: F. A. Davis.

Weiss, N. S. (2003). Breast cancer mortality in relation to clinical breast examination and breast self-examination. *Breast Journal, 9*(Suppl. 2), S86–S89.

Wijdicks, E. F. M., Bamlet, W. R., Maramattom, B. V., et al. (2005). Further validation of the FOUR score coma scale by intensive care nurses. *Annals of Neurology, 58*(4), 585–593.

Wolf, C., Wijdicks, E., Bamlet, W., et al. (2007). Further validation of the FOUR score coma scale by intensive care nurses. Mayo Clinic proceedings. Retrieved February 26, 2011, from http://www.mayoclinicproceedings.com/content/82/4/435.full

Yifan, Xue. (2007). Dehydration: Assessment. Evidence summaries—Joanna Briggs Institute. Retrieved February 22, 2011, from http://www.jbiconnect.org/connect/docs/cis/es_html_viewer.php?SID=5104&lang=en&region=AU

CHAPTER 22

Agency for Healthcare Research and Quality (AHRQ). (2009). Health care–associated infections. Retrieved March 21, 2011, from http://www.ahrq.gov/qual/hais.htm

American Heart Association (AHA). (2008). Hypertension: Ambulatory blood pressure monitoring in children and adolescents: Recommendations for standard assessment. *Hypertension, 5*(3), 433–451. Retrieved March 26, 2011, from http://hyper.ahajournals.org/cgi/content/full/52/3/433

American Institute of Architects. (2006). *Guidelines for design and construction of hospital and health care facilities.* Washington, DC: American Institute of Architects Press.

American Nurses Association (ANA). (2010). *Nursing: Scope and standards of practice* (2nd ed.). Silver Spring, MD: Author.

Association of periOperative Registered Nurses (AORN). (2004). Recommended practices for surgical hand antisepsis/hand scrubs. *AORN Journal, 79*(2), 416–431.

Association of periOperative Registered Nurses (AORN). (2005a). Recommended practices for surgical attire. In: *Standards, recommended practices, and guidelines* (pp. 377–385). Denver: Author.

Association of periOperative Registered Nurses (AORN). (2005b). Recommended practices for surgical hand antisepsis/hand scrubs. In: *Standards, recommended practices, and guidelines* (pp. 299–305). Denver: Author.

Association of periOperative Registered Nurses (AORN). (2006). Recommended practices for maintaining a sterile field. In: *Standards, recommended practices, and guidelines* (pp. 402–416). Denver: Author.

Association for Professionals in Infection Control and Epidemiology (APIC). (2010). *Guide to the elimination of methicillin-resistant* Staphylococcus aureus *(MRSA) transmission in hospital settings* (2nd ed.). Washington, DC: Author. Retrieved March 22, 2011, from http://www.apic.org/downloads/MRSA_elimination_guide_27030.pdf

Bauman, R. W., Machunis-Masuoka, E., & Tizard, I. R. (2006). *Microbiology: Alternate edition with disease by body system.* San Francisco: Benjamin Cummings.

Best practices: Evidence-based nursing procedures (2nd ed.). (2007). Philadelphia: Lippincott Williams & Wilkins.

Boyce, J. M., & Pittet, D. (2002, October 25). Guideline for hand hygiene in health-care settings. Recommendations of the Healthcare Infection Control Practices Advisory Committee, & the HICPAC/SHEA/APIC/IDSA Hand Hygiene Task Force. *Morbidity and Mortality Weekly Report, 51*(RR16), 1–44.

Bulechek, G. M., Butcher, H. K., & Dochterman, J. M. (Eds.) (2012). *Nursing interventions classification (NIC)* (6th ed.). St. Louis, MO: Mosby.

Burke, J. P., Garibaldi, R. A., Britt, M. R., et al. (1981). Prevention of catheter-associated urinary tract infections: Efficacy of daily mental care regimens. *American Journal of Medicine, 70,* 655–658.

Calfee, D., Salgado, C., Classen, D., et al. (2008). Guideline summary. Strategies to prevent transmission of methicillin-resistant *Staphylococcus aureus* in acute care hospitals. *Infection Control and Hospital Epidemiology, 29*(Suppl. 1), S62–S80. Rockville, MD: National Guideline Clearinghouse. Retrieved May 18, 2009, from http://www.guideline.gov/summary/summary.aspx?view_id=1&doc_id=13397

Carling, P. C., Parry, M. F., & Von Beheren, S. M.; for the Healthcare Environmental Hygiene Study Group (2008). Identifying opportunities to enhance environmental cleaning in 23 acute care hospitals. *Infection Control & Hospital Epidemiology, 29*(1), 1–7.

Centers for Disease Control and Prevention (CDC). (n.d.a, last modified 2010, March). Multidrug-resistant organisms in non-hospital healthcare settings. Retrieved March 21, 2011, from http://www.cdc.gov/ncidod/dhqp/ar_multidrugFAQ.html

Centers for Disease Control and Prevention (CDC). (n.d.b, last updated 2010, November). Vancomycin-resistant enterococci (VRE) in healthcare settings. Retrieved March 22, 2011, from http://www.cdc.gov/HAI/organisms/vre/vre.html#a3

Centers for Disease Control and Prevention (CDC). (n.d.c, last updated 2011, February). *Clostridium difficile (C. diff)* in healthcare settings. Retrieved March 22, 2011, from http://www.cdc.gov/HAI/organisms/cdiff/Cdiff.html

Centers for Disease Control and Prevention (CDC). (n.d.d, last updated 2009, June). Antibiotic resistance questions & answers. Retrieved March 24, 2011, from http://www.cdc.gov/getsmart/antibiotic-use/anitbiotic-resistance-faqs.html#h

Centers for Disease Control and Prevention (CDC). (n.d.e). Emergency preparedness & response: Emergency preparedness and you. Retrieved March 27, 2011, from http://emergency.cdc.gov/preparedness/

Centers for Disease Control and Prevention (CDC). (2002). Guidelines for hand hygiene in health-care settings, Recommendations and reports, *Morbidity and Mortality Weekly Report, 51*(RR-16). Retrieved March 28, 2011, from http://www.cdc.gov/mmwr/preview/mmwrhtml/rr5116a1.htm

Centers for Disease Control and Prevention (CDC). (2008). Guideline for disinfection and sterilization in healthcare facilities, 2008. Infection Control Practices Advisory Committee (HICPAC). Retrieved March 24, 2011, from http://www.cdc.gov/ncidod/dhqp/pdf/guidelines/Disinfection_Nov_2008.pdf

Centers for Disease Control and Prevention (CDC). (2009a). CDC estimates of 2009 H1N1 influenza cases, hospitalizations and deaths in the United States, April–November 14, 2009. Retrieved March 29, 2011, from http://www.cdc.gov/h1n1flu/estimates_2009_h1n1.htm

Centers for Disease Control and Prevention (CDC). (2009b). 2009 H1N1 and seasonal flu: What you should know about flu antiviral drugs. Retrieved March 29, 2011, from http://www.cdc.gov/H1N1flu/antivirals/geninfo.htm#box

Centers for Disease Control and Prevention. (2009c). *Guideline for prevention of catheter-associated urinary tract infections, 2009.* Retrieved March 29, 2011, from http://www.cdc.gov/hicpac/cauti/001_cauti.html

Cousins, N. (1979). *Anatomy of an illness.* New York: Bantam.

Davey, V. (2007). Disaster care. Questions and answers on pandemic influenza. *American Journal of Nursing, 107*(7), 50–57.

Davidson, S. J., & Malkary, G. (2008, January 9). Dangerous devices. *Most Wired Magazine.* Retrieved March 24, 2011, from http://www.hhnmostwired.com/hhnmostwired_app/jsp/articledisplay.jsp?dcrpath=HHNMOSTWIRED/Article/data/Fall2007/080109MW_Online_Davidson&domain=HHNMOSTWIRED

Elixhauser, A., & Steiner, C. (2007). Infections with methicillin-resistant *Staphylococcus aureus* (MRSA) in U.S. hospitals, 1993–2005 (Statistical Brief No. 35). Healthcare

Cost and Utilization Project. Retrieved March 22, 2011, from http://www.hcup-us.ahrq.gov/reports/statbriefs/sb35.jsp

Foxwell, A., Roberts, L., Lokuge, K., & Kelly, P. (2011). Transmission of influenza on international flights, May 2009. *Emerging Infectious Diseases, 17*(7). Retrieved November 16, 2011, from http://wwwnc.cdc.gov/eid/article/17/7/10-1135_article.htm.

Franco, G. P., de Barros, A. L., Nogueira-Martins, L. A., et al. (2003). Stress influence on genesis, onset and maintenance of cardiovascular diseases: Literature review. *Journal of Advanced Nursing, 43*(6), 548–554.

Halcomb, E. J., Griffiths, R., & Fernandez, R. (2008a). Evidence synthesis. Role of MRSA reservoirs in the acute care setting. *International Journal of Evidence Based Healthcare, 6*(2), 50–62.

Halm, M., Hickson, T., Stein, D., et al. (2011). Blood cultures and central catheters: Is the "easiest way" best practice? *American Journal of Critical Care, 20*(4), 335–338.

Hutchins K., Karras, G., Erwin, J., et al. (2009) Ventilator-associated pneumonia and oral care: A successful quality improvement project. *American Journal of Infection Control, 37*(7), 590–597.

Institute for Healthcare Improvement. (2006). Protecting 5 million lives from harm. Retrieved March 26, 2011, from http://www.ihi.org/IHI/Programs/Campaign/

Johnson, M., Bulechek, G., Butcher, H., et al. (2006). *NANDA, NOC, and NIC linkages* (2nd ed.). St. Louis, MO: C. V. Mosby.

The Joint Commission (TJC). (2008a). *2008 hospital accreditation standards.* Oakbrook Terrace, IL: Author.

The Joint Commission (TJC). (2008b). *Hospital accreditation program. 2011 chapter: National patient safety goals.* Retrieved March 11, 2011, from http://www.jointcommission.org/assets/1/6/2011_NPSGs_HAP.pdf

The Joint Commission. (2010). Accreditation program: Hospital. National Patient Safety Goals. Effective January 1, 2011. Retrieved April 10, 2012, from http://www.jointcommission.org/assets/1/6/2011_NPSGs_HAP.pdf

Klevens, R. M., Morrison, M. A., & Nadle, J., et al. (2007). Invasive methicillin-resistant *Staphylococcus aureus* infections in the United States. *JAMA, 298*(15), 1763–1771.

Larson, E., Girard, R., & Pessoa-Silva, C. L., et al. (2006). Skin reactions related to hand hygiene and selection of hand hygiene products. *Association for Professionals in Infection Control and Epidemiology, 34,* 627–635.

Maki, D. G. (2001). Engineering out the risk of infection with urinary catheters. *Emerging Infectious Diseases, 7*(2), 342–347.

Maki, D. G., Knasinski, V., & Tambyah, P. A. (2000). Risk factors for catheter-associated urinary tract infection: A prospective study showing minimal effects of catheter care violations on the risk of CAUTI [Abstract]. *Infection Control Hospital Epidemiology, 21,* 165.

Manges, A. R., Perdreau-Remington, F., Solberg, O., et al. (2005). Multidrug-resistant *Escherichia coli* clonal groups causing community-acquired bloodstream infections. *Journal of Infection, 53*(1), 25–29.

McKibben, L., Horan, T., & Tokars, M. D. (2005). Guidance on public reporting of healthcare-associated infections: Recommendations of the Healthcare Infection Control Practices Advisory Committee. *American Journal of Medical Quality, 33*(4), 217–226. Retrieved March 9, 2011, from http://www.cdc.gov/ncidod/hlp/PublicReportingGuide.pdf

Minnesota Department of Health. (n.d.). Components of personal protective equipment. Retrieved March 28, 2011, from http://www.health.state.mn.us/divs/idepc/dtopics/infectioncontrol/ppe/comp/index.html

Moorhead, S., Johnson, M., Maas, M. L., et al (2008). *Nursing outcomes classification (NOC)* (4th ed.). St. Louis, MO: C. V. Mosby.

New York State Department of Health. (2011). Emergency preparedness. Retrieved March 27, 2011, from http://www.health.state.ny.us/environmental/emergency/

Occupational Safety & Health Administration, U.S. Department of Labor. (n.d., last reviewed 2009, January). Bloodborne pathogens and needlestick prevention. Post-exposure evaluation. Retrieved March 26, 2011, from http://www.osha.gov/SLTC/bloodbornepathogens/index.html

Orrett, F. A., Brooks, P. J., & Richardson, E. G. (1998). Nosocomial infections in a rural regional hospital in a developing country: Infection rates by site, service, cost, and infection control practices. *Infection Control Hospital Epidemiology, 19*(2), 136–140.

Perry, C., Marshall, R., & Jones, E. (2001). Bacterial contamination of uniforms. *Journal of Hospital Infection, 48*(3), 238–241.

Pitout, J. D. D., & Laupland, K. B. (2008). Extended-spectrum B-lactamase-producing Enterobacteriaceae: An emerging public-health concern. *The Lancet Infectious Diseases, 8,* 159–166.

Pratt, R. J., Pellowe, C. M., Wilson, J. A., et al. (2007). Epic2: National evidence-based guidelines for preventing healthcare-associated infections in NHS hospitals in England. *Journal of Hospital Infection, 65*(Suppl. 1), S1–S64.

Rice, L. B. (2001). Emergence of vancomycin-resistant enterococci. *Emerging Infectious Diseases, 7*(2), 183–187.

Rupp, M. E., Fitzgerald, T., Puumala, S., et al. (2008). Prospective, controlled, cross-over trial of alcohol-based hand gel in critical care units. *Infection Control and Hospital Epidemiology, 29*(1), 8–15.

Saint, S., & Lipsky, B. A. (1999, April 26). Preventing catheter-related bacteremia. *Archives of Internal Medicine, 159,* 800–808.

Schneider, R., Alexander, C., Staggers, F., et al. (2005). Long-term effects of stress reduction on mortality in persons 55 years of age with systemic hypertension. *American Journal of Cardiology, 95*(9), 1060–1064.

Siegel, J. D., Rhinehart, E., Jackson, M., et al. (2006). *Management of multidrug-resistant organisms in healthcare settings, 2006.* Retrieved March 26, 2011, from http://www.cdc.gov/ncidod/dhqp/pdf/ar/mdroGuideline2006.pdf

Siegel, J. D., Rhinehart, E., Jackson, M., et al. (2007). *2007 Guideline for isolation precautions: Preventing transmission of infectious agents in the healthcare setting.* Retrieved March 11, 2011, from http://www.cdc.gov/ncidod/dhqp/pdf/guidelines/Isolation2007.pdf

Smith, G., Vijaykrishna, D., Bahl, J., et al. (2009). Origins and evolutionary genomics of the 2009 swine-origin H1N1 influenza A epidemic. *Nature, 459,* 1122–1125.

Spahr, A., Klein, E., Khuseyinova, N., et al. (2006). Periodontal infections and coronary heart disease. *Archives of Internal Medicine, 166*(5), 554–559.

U.S. Department of Health & Human Services. (n.d.). Flu pandemics. Retrieved March 27, 2011, from http://www.flu.gov/individualfamily/about/pandemic/index.html

U.S. Department of Homeland Security. (2010). Make a plan. Retrieved August 8, 2008, from http://www.ready.gov/america/makeaplan/index.html

U.S. Department of Labor. (n.d.a). *Occupational safety and health standards: General description and discussion of the levels of protection and protective gear.* 1910.120 App B. Retrieved March 26, 2011, from http://www.osha.gov/pls/oshaweb/owadisp.show_document?p_table=STANDARDS&p_id=9767

U.S. Department of Labor. (n.d.b). (Lack of) personal protective equipment. *Occupational Safety and Health Standards.* 1910.1030(d)(3)(xii). Retrieved March 28, 2011, from http://www.osha.gov/SLTC/etools/hospital/hazards/ppe/ppe.html

Veneema, T. G., & Tõke, J. (2006). Early detection and surveillance for biopreparedness and emerging infectious diseases. *Online Journal of Issues in Nursing, 11*(1).

Warren, J. W. (1997). Catheter-associated urinary tract infections. *Infectious Disease Clinics of North America, 11*(3), 609–622.

Whyte, J. (2008). MRSA: Not a new crisis. *The Clinical Advisor, 11*(1), 100.

World Health Organization (WHO). (2007). *Epidemic and pandemic alert and response (EPR): avian influenza.* Retrieved March 29, 2011, from http://www.who.int/csr/disease/avian_influenza/en/index.html

World Health Organization (WHO). (2008). *The world health report 2007—a safer future: Global public health security in the 21st century.* Retrieved April 1, 2011, from http://www.who.int/whr/2007/en/index.html

CHAPTER 23

Ackley, B., & Ladwig, G. (2008). *Nursing diagnosis handbook* (8th ed.). St. Louis, MO: C. V. Mosby.

Adams, P., Barnes, P., & Vickerie, J. (2008). Summary health statistics for the U.S. population: National Health interview survey, 2007. *Vital Health Statistics 2008, 10*(238). Retrieved May 10, 2011, from http://www.cdc.gov/nchs/data/series/sr_10/sr10_238.pdf

AHI of Indiana. (n.d.). Upright® program overview. Retrieved May 11, 2011, from http://www.ahiofindiana.com/index.php

Akyol, A. D. (2007). Falls in the elderly: What can be done? *International Nursing Review, 54*(2), 191–196.

American Academy of Neurology (AAN). (2008a, February). Get Up and Go Test. Retrieved May 11, 2011, from http://www.aan.com/practice/guideline/uploads/273.pdf

American Academy of Neurology (AAN). (2008b, February). Get Up and Go Test. Retrieved May 11, 2011, from http://www.aan.com/practice/guideline/uploads/274.pdf

American Academy of Pediatrics (AAP). (2011). *Car safety seats: A guide for families for 2011.* Retrieved May 12, 2011, from http://www.aap.org/healthtopics/carseatsafety.cfm

American Association of Poison Control Centers. (n.d.a). *Out-of-hospital patient management guidelines: Ipecac syrup.* Retrieved May 10, 2011, from http://www.aapcc.org/archive/FinalizedPMGdlns/Ipecac%20Guideline%20-%20final%20for%20JTCT.pdf

American Association of Poison Control Centers. (n.d.b). *First aid tips.* Retrieved May 11, 2011, from http://www.aapcc.org/dnn/FirstAid/tabid/115/Default.aspx

American Heart Association (AHA). (2006). 2005 American Heart Association (AHA) guidelines for cardiopulmonary resuscitation (CPR) and emergency cardiovascular care (ECC) of pediatric and neonatal patients: Pediatric basic life support. *Pediatrics, 1176,* e989, doi:10.1542/peds.2006-0219

American Heart Association (AHA). (2005). Part 2: Adult basic life support. *Circulation, 112,* III-5–III-16. Retrieved May 15, 2011, from http://circ.ahajournals.org/cgi/content/full/112/22_suppl/III-5?maxtoshow=&HITS=10&hits=10&RESULTFORMAT=1&title=Part+2%3A+adult+basic+life+support&andorexacttitle=and&andorexacttitleabs=and&andorexactfulltext=and&searchid=1&FIRSTINDEX=0&sortspec=relevance&resourcetype=HWCIT

American Nurses Association (ANA). (2001). Position statement: Reduction of patient restraint and seclusion in health care settings—10/17/01. Retrieved May 15, 2011, from http://www.nursingworld.org/MainMenuCategories/HealthcareandPolicyIssues/ANAPositionStatements/EthicsandHumanRights/prtetrestrnt14452.aspx

American Nurses Association (ANA). (2002). Needlestick prevention guide. Retrieved May 11, 2011, from http://www.nursingworld.org/MainMenuCategories/OccupationalandEnvironmental/occupationalhealth/SafeNeedles/NeedlestickPrevention.aspx

American Nurses Association (ANA). (2003, September 17). ANA launches "handle with care" ergonomics campaign [Press release]. Retrieved July 28, 2011, from http://www.nursingworld.org/MainMenuCategories/OccupationalandEnvironmental/occupationalhealth/handlewithcare/HandleWCarePressRelease.aspx

American Nurses Association (ANA). (2008a). *ANA's health system reform agenda.* Retrieved May 9, 2011, from http://www.nursingworld.org/MainMenuCategories/HealthcareandPolicyIssues/HealthSystemReform/Agenda/Principles/ANAsHealthSystemReformAgenda.aspx

American Nurses Association (ANA). (2008b). Position statement (revised). Elimination of manual patient handling to prevent work-related musculoskeletal disorders. Retrieved May 11, 2011, from http://nursingworld.org/MainMenuCategories/OccupationalandEnvironmental/occupationalhealth/handlewithcare/Work-Related-Musculoskeletal-Disorders-PDF.aspx [Note: This URL requires log-in]

American Red Cross. (2007). Be Red Cross ready. Conscious choking. Retrieved May 15, 2011, from http://www.redcross.org/flash/brr/English-html/conscious-choking.asp

Berg, J., McConnell, R., Milam, J., et al. (2008). Rodent allergen in Los Angeles inner city homes of children with asthma. *Journal of Urban Health, 85*(1), 52–61.

Bruce, D. G., Devine, A., & Prince, R. L. (2002). Recreational physical activity levels in healthy older women: The importance of fear of falling. *Journal of the American Geriatrics Society, 50*(1), 84–89.

Brush, B., & Capezuti, E. (2001). Historical analysis of siderail use in American hospitals. *Journal of Gerontological Nursing, 25,* 26–34.

Bulechek, G., Butcher, H., & Dochterman, J. (Eds.). (2008). *Nursing interventions classification (NIC)* (5th ed.). St. Louis, MO: C. V. Mosby.

Bureau of Labor Statistics. (2006). Economic news release. Nonfatal occupational injuries and illnesses requiring days away from work, 2006. Retrieved July 28, 2011, from http://www.bls.gov/news.release/osh2.nr0.htm

Campbell, A. J., Robertson, M. C., Gardner, M. M., et al. (1999). Falls prevention over 2 years: A randomized controlled

trial in women 80 years and older. *Age and Ageing, 28,* 513–518.

Capezuti, E., Wagner, L., Brush, B., et al. (2007). Consequences of an intervention to reduce restrictive side rail use in nursing homes. *Journal of the American Geriatrics Society, 55*(3), 334–342.

Centers for Disease Control and Prevention (CDC). (n.d., last updated December 8, 2010). Falls among older adults: An overview. Retrieved May 10, 2011, from http://www.cdc.gov/HomeandRecreationalSafety/Falls/adultfalls.html

Centers for Disease Control and Prevention (CDC). (2005). Foodborne illness. Frequently asked questions. Retrieved May 12, 2011, from http://www.cdc.gov/ncidod/dbmd/diseaseinfo/files/foodborne_illness_FAQ.pdf

Centers for Disease Control and Prevention (CDC). (2011). Measures to prevent bites from mosquitoes, ticks, fleas and other insects and arthropods . Retrieved May 12, 2011, from http://www.cdc.gov/ticks/index.html

Centers for Disease Control and Prevention (CDC), National Center for Injury Prevention and Control .(n.d.a). Falls among older adults: An overview. Web-based injury statistics query and reporting system (WISQARS). Retrieved May 9, 2011, from http://www.cdc.gov/HomeandRecreationalSafety/Falls/adultfalls.html

Centers for Disease Control and Prevention (CDC), National Center for Injury Prevention and Control (n.d.b). 2007, United States: Unintentional injuries, all ages, all races, both sexes. Web-based injury statistics query and reporting system (WISQARS). Retrieved May 10, 2011, from http://webappa.cdc.gov/cgi-bin/broker.exe?_service=v8prod&_server=app-v-ehip-wisq.cdc.gov&_port=5081&_sessionid=tZiXtTZ7M52&_program=wisqars.details10.sas&_service=&type=U&prtfmt=STANDARD&age1=.&age2=.&agegp=AllAges&deaths=123706&_debug=0&lcdfmt=lcd1age&ethnicty=0&ranking=10&deathtle=Death

Centers for Disease Control and Prevention (CDC), National Center for Injury Prevention and Control. (2006). Child passenger safety [Fact sheet]. Retrieved May 12, 2011,from http://www.cdc.gov/ncipc/factsheets/childpas.htm

Centers for Disease Control and Prevention (CDC), National Center for Injury Prevention and Control. (2007). National child passenger safety week, September 16–22, 2007. Last updated May, 2008. Retrieved August 26, 2008, from http://www.cdc.gov/ncipc/duip/spotlite/chldseat.htm

Centers for Disease Control and Prevention (CDC), National Center for Injury Prevention and Control. (2008). Preventing falls: How to develop community-based fall prevention programs for older adults. Retrieved May 13, 2011, from http://www.cdc.gov/ncipc/preventingfalls/CDC_Guide.pdf

Centers for Disease Control and Prevention (CDC), National Center for Injury Prevention and Control. (2010a). Injury prevention & control: Home and recreational safety: Unintentional poisoning. Web-based injury statistics query and reporting system (WISQARS). Retrieved May 9, 2011, from http://www.cdc.gov/HomeandRecreationalSafety/Poisoning/index.html

Centers for Disease Control and Prevention (CDC), National Center for Injury Prevention and Control. (2010b). Poisoning in the United States [Fact sheet]. Web-based injury statistics query and reporting system (WISQARS). Retrieved May 9, 2011, from http://www.cdc.gov/HomeandRecreationalSafety/Poisoning/poisoning-factsheet.htm

Centers for Disease Control and Prevention (CDC), National Center for Injury Prevention and Control. (2010c). Teen drivers [Fact sheet]. Web-based injury statistics query and reporting system (WISQARS). Retrieved May 10, 2011, from http://www.cdc.gov/MotorVehicleSafety/Teen_Drivers/teendrivers_factsheet.html

Centers for Disease Control and Prevention (CDC), National Center for Injury Prevention and Control. (2010d). Child passenger safety. Retrieved May 12, 2011,from http://www.cdc.gov/features/passengersafety/

Centers for Medicare & Medicaid Services. (2006a). Eliminating serious, preventable, and costly medical errors—never events [Press release]. Department of Health & Human Services. Retrieved August 20, 2011, from http://www.cms.hhs.gov/apps/media/press/release.asp?Counter=1863

Centers for Medicare & Medicaid Services. (2006b, December 8). Rules and Regulations. Part IV. Department of Health and Human Services, CMMS, 42 CFR Part 482. Medicare and Medicaid programs; Hospital conditions of participation: Patients' rights; Final rule. *Federal Register, 71*(236), 71428.

Centers for Medicare & Medicaid Services. (2008, July 31). Medicare and Medicaid move aggressively to encourage greater patient safety in hospitals and reduce never events [Press release]. CMS Office of Public Affairs. Retrieved May 9, 2011, from http://www.cms.hhs.gov/apps/media/press/release.asp?Counter=3219&intNumPerPage=10&checkDate=&checkKey=&srchType=1&numDays=3500&srchOpt=0&srchData=&keywordType=All&chkNewsType=1%2C_2%2C_3%2C_4%2C_5&intPage=&showAll=&pYear=&year=&desc=&cboOrder=date

Centers for Medicare & Medicaid Services. (2011). HAC posting on Hospital Compare. Retrieved May 15, 2011, from http://www.cms.gov/HospitalQualityInits/06_HACPost.asp

Choking—adult or child over 1 year. (n.d.). MedlinePlus: Medical encyclopedia. U.S. National Library of Medicine, National Instutes of Health. Retrieved May 15, 2011, from http://www.nlm.nih.gov/MEDLINEPLUS/ency/article/000049.htm

Choking—infant under 1 year. (n.d.). MedlinePlus: Medical encyclopedia. U.S. National Library of Medicine, National Instutes of Health. Retrieved May 15, 2011, from http://www.nlm.nih.gov/MEDLINEPLUS/ency/article/000048.htm

Choking—unconscious adult or child over 1 year. (n.d.). MedlinePlus: Medical encyclopedia. U.S. National Library of Medicine, National Instutes of Health. Retrieved May 15, 2011, from http://www.nlm.nih.gov/MEDLINEPLUS/ency/article/000051.htm

Ciencewicki, J., & Jaspers, I. (2007). Air pollution and respiratory viral infection. *Inhalation Toxicology, 19*(14), 1135-1146.

Committee on Quality of Health Care in America. (1999). In: L.T. Kohn, J. M. Corrigon, & M. S. Donaldson (Eds.), *To err is human: Building a safer health system.* Washington, DC: The National Academies Press, National Academy of Sciences.

Cooper, M., & Kulkarni, R. (2011, updated). Lightning injuries in emergency medicine. *Nedscape Reference.* Retrieved July 30, 2011, from http://emedicine.medscape.com/article/770642-overview

Cronenwett, L., Sherwood, G., Barnsteiner, J., et al. (2007). Quality and safety education for nurses. *Nursing Outlook, 55*(3), 122–131.

Delahanty, K., & Myers, F., III (2007). Infection control survey report. *Nursing 2007, 37*(6), 28–38.

Deshpande, N., Metter, E., Bandinelli, S., et al. (2008). Psychological, physical, and sensory correlates of fear of falling and consequent activity restriction in the elderly: The InCHIANTI study. *American Journal of Physical Medicine & Rehabilitation, 87*(5), 354–362.

Deshpande, N., Metter, E., Lauretani, F., et al. (2008). Activity restriction induced by fear of falling and objective and subjective measures of physical function: A prospective cohort study. *Journal of the American Geriatrics Society, 56*(4), 615–620.

Doenges, M., Moorhouse, M., & Geissler-Murr, A. (2005). *Nursing diagnosis manual*. Philadelphia: F. A. Davis.

Evans, L., & Cotter, V. (2008). Avoiding restraints in patients with dementia. *American Journal of Nursing, 108*(3), 40–50.

Evergreen Industries & Obviously Enterprises. (2006). The Internet consumer recycling guide. The world's shortest comprehensive recycling guide. Retrieved May 16, 2011, from http://www.obviously.COM/recycle/guides/shortest.html

First aid tips. (n.d.). American Association of Poison Control Centers. Retrieved July 28, 2011, from http://www.aapcc.org/dnn/FirstAid/tabid/115/Default.aspx

Flores, N. (2008). Dealing with an angry patient. *Nursing2008, 38*(5), 30–31.

Fonad, E., Wahlin, T., Winblad, B., et al. (2008). Falls and fall risk among nursing home residents. *Journal of Clinical Nursing, 17*(1), 126–134.

FoodSafety.gov, U.S. Department of Health and Human Services. (n.d.). Keep food safe. Retrieved May 12, 2011, from http://www.foodsafety.gov/keep/index.html

Friedman, S. M., Munoz, B., West, S. K., et al. (2002). Falls and fear of falling: Which comes first? A longitudinal prediction model suggests strategies for primary and secondary prevention. *Journal of the American Geriatrics Society, 50*(8), 1329–1335.

Gardner, M. M., Robertson, M. C., & Campbell, A. J. (2000). Exercise in preventing falls and fall-related injuries in older people: A review of randomized controlled trials. *British Journal of Sports Medicine, 34*(1), 7–17.

Gates, S., Fisher, J., Cooke, M., et al (2008). Multifactorial assessment and targeted intervention for preventing falls and injuries among older people in community and emergency care settings: Systematic review and meta-analysis. *BMJ, 336*, 130–133

Gray-Micelli, D. (2008). Preventing falls in acute care. In: E. Capezuti, D. Zwicker, M. Mezey, et al. (Eds.), *Evidence-based geriatric nursing protocols for best practices* (3rd ed., pp. 161–198). New York: Springer.

Grossman, V. (2003). Gang members in the ED. *American Journal of Nursing, 103*(2), 52–53.

Haumschild, M. J., Karfonta, T., Haumschild, M. S., et al. (2003). Clinical and economic outcomes of a fall-focused pharmaceutical intervention program. *American Journal of Health-System Pharmacy, 60*(10), 1029–1032.

Hendrich, A. (2007). How to try this: Predicting patient falls. *American Journal of Nursing, 107*(11), 50–59.

Hizel, S., Ozcebe, H., Sanli, C., et al. (2008). Children and firearms in Turkish homes. *Child: Care, Health & Development, 34*(1), 32–34.

Hughes, K., van Beurden, E., Eakin, E., et al (2008). Older persons' perception of risk of falling: Implications for fall-prevention campaigns. *American Journal of Public Health, 98*(2), 351–357.

Injury Center, Centers for Disease Control and Prevention (CDC). (n.d., last updated 2008, March). *Tips to prevent poisonings.* Retrieved May 15, 2011, from http://www.cdc.gov/ncipc/factsheets/poisonprevention.htm

Institute for Clinical Systems Improvement (ICSI). (2008). Prevention of falls (acute care). Health care protocol. Bloomington, MN: Author. Retrieved May 13, 2011, from http://www.guideline.gov/content.aspx?id=16005&search=prevention+of+falls+(acute+care)

Institute for Healthcare Improvement. (n.d.). Overview of the 100,000 lives campaign. Retrieved May 15, 2011, from http://www.ihi.org/IHI/Programs/Campaign/100k CampaignOverviewArchive.htm. Used by permission.

Institute of Medicine (IOM). (2001). *Crossing the quality chasm: A new health system for the 21st century*. Washington, DC: The National Academies Press. Retrieved November 17, 2011, from http://www.nap.edu/openbook.php?record_id=10027&page=R1

Institute of Medicine (IOM). (2011). *The future of nursing: Leading change, advancing health*. Washington, DC: The National Academies Press. Retrieved November 17, 2011, from http://books.nap.edu/openbook.php?record_id=12956

Joanna Briggs Institute. (2010). Interventions to reduce the incidence of falls in older adult patients in acute care hospitals. *Best Practice, 14*(1).

Johnson, M., Moorhead, S., Bulechek, C., et al. (2012). *NOC and NIC linkages to NANDA-I and clinical conditions* (3rd ed.). St. Louis, MO: C. V. Mosby.

The Joint Commission (TJC). (2008). *2008 Hospital accreditation standards.* Oakbrook Terrace, IL: Author.

The Joint Commission (TJC). (2011). The Joint Commission, accreditation program: Hospital. National patient safety goals (effective January 1, 2011). Retrieved May 9, 2011, from http://www.jointcommission.org/assets/1/6/2011_NPSGs_HAP.pdf

Kenny, R., Rubenstein, L., Martin, F., et al. (2001). American Geriatrics Society (AGS) Panel on Falls in Older Persons. Special series: Clinical practice. Guideline for the prevention of falls in older persons. *Journal of the American Geriatrics Society, 49*(5), 644–672.

King, M., & Bailey, C. (2007, December 21) Carbon-monoxide-related deaths: United States, 1999–2004. *Morbidity and Mortality Weekly Report, 56*(50), 1309–1312. Retrieved May 10, 2011, from http://www.cdc.gov/mmwr/preview/mmwrhtml/mm5650a1.htm

Krieger, J., & Higgins, D. (2002). Housing and health: Time again for public health action. *American Journal of Public Health, 92*(5), 758–768.

leBel, J., & Goldstein, R. (2005). Special section on seclusion and restraint: The economic cost of using restraint and the value added by restraint reduction or elimination. *Psychiatric Services, 56*, 1109–1114.

Lee, M., & Ernst, E. (2010). Systematic reviews of t'ai chi: An overview. *British Journal of Sports Medicine*. doi:10.1136/bjsm.2020.080622

Lopes, M. I. L., Miranda, P. J., & Sarinho, E. (2006). Use of the skin prick test and specific immunoglobulin E for the diagnosis of cockroach allergy. *Journal of Pediatrics, 82*(3), 204–209.

Miniño, A. M., Heron, M. P., Murphy, S. L., et al. (2007). Deaths: Final data for 2004. *National Vital Statistics Reports, 55*(19). Hyattsville, MD: National Center for Health Statistics.

Moorhead, S., Johnson, M., Maas, M., et al. (Eds.). (2008). *Nursing outcomes classification (NOC)* (4th ed.). St. Louis, MO: C. V. Mosby.

Morse, J. (1997). *Preventing patient falls.* Thousand Oaks, CA: Sage.

Morse, J. (2001, First Quarter). Preventing falls in the elderly. *Reflections on Nursing Leadership, 26–27.*

Morse, J. (2009). *Preventing patient falls: Establishing a fall intervention program* (2nd ed.). New York: Springer

Murphy, S., Williams, C., & Gill, T. (2002). Characteristics associated with fear of falling and activity restriction in community-living older persons. *Journal of the American Geriatrics Society, 50*(3), 516–520.

NANDA International (NANDA-I). (2009). *NANDA nursing diagnoses: Definitions and classification 2009–2011.* Ames, IA: Wiley-Blackwell.

National Ag Safety Database (NASD). (1998). How does safety rate on your farm or ranch? Check lists: Home safety 1, 2, and 3. Retrieved May 15, 2011, from http://nasdonline.org/document/1634/d001509/how-does-safety-rate-on-your-farm-or.html

National Cancer Institute. (n.d.). Secondhand smoke: Questions and answers [Fact sheet]. Retrieved July 29, 2011 , from http://www.cancer.gov/cancertopics/factsheet/Tobacco/ETS

National Center for Injury Prevention and Control, Centers for Disease Control and Prevention (CDC). (2006). Injury—A risk at any stage of life. In *CDC injury fact book.* Retrieved July 29, 2011, from http://www.cdc.gov/Injury/publications/FactBook/Injury—A_Risk_at_Any_Stage_of_Life2006-a.pdf

National Institute for Occupational Safety and Health (NIOSH). (n.d.). Safer medical device implementation in health care facilities. Centers for Disease Control and Prevention, Department of Health and Human Services. Retrieved May 11, 2011, from http://www.cdc.gov/niosh/topics/bbp/safer/

National Institute for Occupational Safety and Health (NIOSH). (2003). *Protect your family: Reduce contamination at home* (DHHS [NIOSH] Publication No. 97-125). Retrieved May 10, 2011, from http://www.cdc.gov/niosh/thttext.html

National Institute for Occupational Safety and Health (NIOSH). (2004). *Worker health chartbook 2004* (NIOSH Publication No. 2004-146). Centers for Disease Control and Prevention, Department of Health and Human Services. Retrieved May 10, 2011from http://www.cdc.gov/niosh/docs/2004-146/

The National Rifle Association Headquarters. (n.d.). What is the Eddie Eagle GunSafe® Program? Retrieved May 12, 2011, from http://www.nrahq.org/safety/eddie/

The National Rifle Association Headquarters. (2011). Education & training programs. NRA gun safety rules. Retrieved May 12, 2011, from http://www.nrahq.org/education/guide.asp

National Safety Council (2010). Summary from *Injury facts,* 2020 edition. Retrieved May 9, 2011, from http://www.nsc.org/news_resources/injury_and_ death_statistics/Documents/Summary_2010_Ed.pdf

National Safety Council. (2011). NSC injury facts®. Itasca, IL: National Safety Council. Also available for purchase at http://shop.nsc.org/Product.aspx?ProductId=2310&CategoryId=62

O'Keefe, L. (2009). What to consider when positioning carseats for toddlers. *AAP News, 30*(4), 12. American Academy of Pediatrics. Retrieved July 15, 2011, from http://aapnews.aappublications.org/cgi/content/full/30/4/12-a

Overview of the 100,000 lives campaign. (n.d.). Institute for Healthcare Improvement. Retrieved May 10, 2011, from http://www.ihi.org/IHI/Programs/Campaign/100kCampaignOverviewArchive.htm

Park, M., & Tang, J. (2007). Changing the practice of physical restraint use in acute care. *Journal of Gerontological Nursing, 33*(2), 9–16.

Rhodes, K. V., & Iwashyna, T. J. (2007). Child injury risks are close to home: Parent psychosocial factors associated with child safety. *Maternal & Child Health Journal, 11*(3), 269–275.

Shever, L., Titler, M., Kerr, P., et al. (2008). The effect of high nursing surveillance on hospital cost. *Journal of Nursing Scholarship, 40*(2), 161–169.

Stevens, J., & Sogolow, E. (2008). *Preventing falls: What works.* Atlanta, GA: Centers for Disease Control and Prevention (CDC), National Center for Injury Prevention and Control. Retrieved May 13, 2011, from http://www.cdc.gov/ncipc/preventingfalls/CDCCompendium_030508.pdf

Talerico, K., & Capezuti, E. (2001). Myths and facts about side rails. *American Journal of Nursing, 101*(7), 43–48.

Tilly, J., & Reed, P. (2008). Falls, wandering, and physical restraints: A review of interventions for individuals with dementia in assisted living and nursing homes. *Alzheimer's Care Today, 9*(1), 45–50.

U.S. Department of Health and Human Services (USDHHS). (2006). *The health consequences of involuntary exposure to tobacco smoke: A report of the Surgeon General.* Rockville, MD: Centers for Disease Control and Prevention (CDC), Coordinating Center for Health Promotion, National Center for Chronic Disease Prevention and Health Promotion, Office of Smoking and Health.

U.S. Department of Labor, Occupational Safety and Health Administration (OSHA). (2001). Enforcement procedures for the occupational exposure to bloodborne pathogens (CPL 02-02-069). Retrieved May 11, 2011, from http://www.osha.gov/pls/oshaweb/owadisp.show_document?p_table=DIRECTIVES&p_id=2570

U.S. Environmental Protection Agency (EPA). (2007). *Methods of mosquito control.* Retrieved May 12, 2011, from http://www.epa.gov/pesticides/health/mosquitoes/mosquito.htm

U.S. Environmental Protection Agency (EPA). (2008). Wastes. Retrieved May 12, 2011, from http://www.epa.gov/epawaste/

U.S. Food and Drug Administration (FDA). (n.d.). Food. Retrieved May 12, 2011, from http://www.fda.gov

Walker, B., Jr., & Mouton, C. P. (2008). Environmental influences on cardiovascular health. *Journal of the National Medical Association, 100*(1), 98–102.

Weber, V., White, A., & McIlvried, R. (2008). An electronic medical record (EMR)-based intervention to reduce polypharmacy and falls in an ambulatory rural elderly population. *Journal of General Internal Medicine, 23*(4), 399–404.

Wijlhuizen, G., de Jong, R., & Hopman-Rock, M. (2007). Older persons afraid of falling reduce physical activity to prevent outdoor falls. *Preventive Medicine, 44*(3), 260–264.

Wilburn, S. (2004). Needlestick and sharps injury prevention. *Online Journal of Issues in Nursing, 9*(3), 104.

Wilkinson, J., & Ahern, N. (2009). *Prentice-Hall nursing diagnosis handbook* (9th ed.). Upper Saddle River, NJ: Prentice-Hall.

CHAPTER 24

American Academy of Orthopedic Surgeons (AAOS). (2001, 18 September). 85% of women changed shoe-wear habits due to foot problems. *Newswise.* Retrieved June 11, 2011, from http:www.newswise.com/articles/view/26033/

American Association of Critical-Care Nurses (AACN). (2013). AACN practice alert. Bathing the adult patient. Retrieved April 29, 2013, from http://www.aacn.org/wd/practice/docs/practicealerts/bathing-the-adult-patient-practice-alert.pdf.

American Association of Critical-Care Nurses (AACN). (2007). AACN practice alert. Oral care in the critically ill. Retrieved June 12, 2011, from http://classic.aacn.org/AACN/practiceAlert.nsf/Files/OC/$file/Oral%20Care%20in%20the%20Critically%20Ill%20.pdf

American Dental Association (ADA). (n.d.). Cleaning your teeth and gums (oral hygiene). Retrieved June 15, 2011, from http://www.ada.org/2624.aspx

Bausch & Lomb. (2008). Official home page. Retrieved June 15, 2011, from http://www.bausch.com

Bausch & Lomb. (2009). Inserting and removing your GP contact lenses. Retrieved June 15, 2011, from http://www.bausch.ca/en_CA/consumer/visioncare/product/rgpinsert.aspx

Berry, A., & Davidson, P. (2007). Consensus-based clinical guideline for the provision of oral care for the critically ill adult. Intensive Care Coordination & Monitoring Unit. Retrieved June 18, 2011, from http://intensivecare.hsnet.nsw.gov.au/five/doc/intensive%20care%20collaborative%20guidelines/8%20%20Final%20oral%20guideline%20December%205_1.pdf

Birch, S., & Coggins, T. (2003). No-rinse, one-step bed bath: The effects on the occurrence of skin tears in a long-term care setting. *Ostomy Wound Management, 49*(1), 64–67.

Bliss, D., Zehrer, C., Savik, K., et al. (2006). Incontinence-associated skin damage in nursing home residents: A secondary analysis of a prospective multicenter study. *Ostomy and Wound Management, 52*(12), 46–55.

Bloomfield, J., Pegram, A., & Jones, A. (2008). Recommended procedure for bedmaking in hospital. *Nursing Standard, 22*(23), 41–44.

Bulechek, G., Butcher, H., & Dochterman, J. (Eds.). (2008). *Nursing interventions classification (NIC)* (5th ed.). St. Louis, MO: C. V. Mosby.

Cason, C., Tyner, T., Saunders, S., et al. (2007). Nurses' implementation of guidelines for ventilator-associated pneumonia from the Centers for Disease Control and Prevention (CDC). *American Journal of Critical Care, 16*(1), 28–38.

Chalmers, J. (2005). Oral hygiene care for residents with dementia: A literature review. *Journal of Advanced Nursing, 52*(4), 410–419.

Chu, J. (2004). Customary vs disposable baths. *American Journal of Nursing, 104*(9), 72.

Collins, J., Nelson, A., & Sublet, V. (2006). *Safe lifting and movement of nursing home residents* (DHHS [NIOSH] Publication No. 2006-117). National Institute for Occupational Safety and Health. Retrieved June 15, 2011, from http://www.cdc.gov/niosh/docs/2006-117/pdfs/2006-117.pdf

Coughlan, M., & Healy, C. (2008). Nursing care, education and support for patients with neutropenia. *Nursing Standard, 22*(46), 35–41.

De Castro, A. (2004). Handle With Care®. The American Nurses Association's campaign to address work-related musculoskeletal disorders. *Online Journal of Issues in Nursing, 9*(3), Manuscript 2. Retrieved June 11, 2011, from http://nursingworld.org/MainMenuCategories/ANA Marketplace/ANAPeriodicals/OJIN/TableofContents/Volume92004/No3Sept04/HandleWithCare.aspx

Department of Veteran Affairs. (n.d.). Your VA hearing aid. Retrieved June 15, 2011, from http://www.ncrar.research.va.gov/ForVets/documents/HearingAidbook.pdf

Downey, L., & Lloyd, H. (2008). Bed bathing patients in hospital. *Nursing Standard, 22*(34), 35–40.

Dunn, J., Thiru-Chelvam, B., & Beck, C. (2002). Bathing. Pleasure or pain? *Journal of Gerontological Nursing, 28*(11), 6–13.

Erikson Labs Northwest. (n.d.). Handling your ocular prosthesis. Retrieved June 15, 2011, from http://www.ericksonlabs.com/v/Artificial_Eyes/care_handling.asp

EZ-Shampoo instructions for use [Package insert]. (2005). EZ-Access, a division of Homecare Products. Retrieved June 15, 2011, from http://www.ezaccess.com/dealers/Instr_Sheets/EZ-SHAMPOO_IS.pdf

Fitch, J. A., Munro, C. L., Glass, C. A., et al. (1999). Oral care in the adult intensive care unit. *American Journal of Critical Care, 8*(5), 314–318.

Flori, L. (2007). Don't throw in the towel: Tips for bathing a patient who has dementia. *Nursing2007, 37*(7), 22–23.

George, M., & Naik, A. (2006). Clinician's role in the treatment of bathing disability. *Geriatrics Aging, 9*(9), 642–645.

Gordon, M. (2006). *Manual of nursing diagnosis* (11th ed., p. 175). Sudbury, MA: Jones & Bartlett.

Gray, M., Bliss, D., Doughty, D., et al. (2007). Incontinence-associated dermatitis: A consensus. *Journal of Wound, Ostomy and Continence Nursing, 34*(1), 45–54.

Haas, J., & Larson, E. (2008). Compliance with hand hygiene guidelines. *American Journal of Nursing, 108*(8), 40–44.

Harris D., Eilers J., Harriman, A., et al. (2008). Putting evidence into practice: Evidence-based interventions for the management of oral mucositis. *Clinical Journal of Oncology Nursing, 12*(1), 141–152.

Holman, C., Roberts, S., & Nicol, M. (2005). Promoting healthy sight and eye care. *Nursing Older People, 17*(1), 37–38.

Hospital Info. (2010). Artificial eye service (ocular prosthetics). Norfolk and Norwich University Hospitals, NHS Foundation Trust. Retrieved June 15, 2011, from http://www.nnuh.nhs.uk/Dept.asp?ID=517&q=prosthetic,eye

Human, L., & Bell, J. (2007). Oral hygiene in critically ill patients. *Southern African Journal of Critical Care, 23*(2), 61–65. Retrieved June 15, 2011, from http://findarticles.com/p/articles/mi_6870/is_2_23/ai_n32398569/

Joanna Briggs Institute. (2004). Oral hygiene care for adults with dementia in residential aged care facilities. *Best Practice, 8*(4), 1–6. ISSN 1329-1874. Retrieved June 12, 2011, from http://www.joannabriggs.edu.au/

Joanna Briggs Institute. (2007). Topical skin care in aged care facilities. *Best Practice, 11*(3), 1–3.

Johnson, D., Lineweaver, L., & Maze, L. (2009). Patients' bath basins as potoential sources of infection: A multicenter sampling study. *American Journal of Critical Care, 18*, 31–40.

Johnson, M., Bulechek, G., Dochterman, J., et al. (2001). *Nursing diagnoses, outcomes, and interventions: NANDA, NOC, & NIC linkages.* St. Louis, MO: C. V. Mosby

Katz, S., Down, T., Cash, H., et al. (1970). Progress in the development of the Index of ADL. *The Gerontologist, 10*(1), 20–30. Retrieved June 18, 2011, from http://consultgerirn.org/uploads/File/trythis/try_this_2.pdf

Kovach, C., & Meyer-Arnold, E. (1997). Preventing agitated behaviors during bath time. *Geriatric Nursing, 18*(3), 112–114.

Larson, E., Ciliberti T., Chantler, C., et al. (2004). Comparison of traditional and disposable bed baths in critically ill patients. *American Journal of Critical Care, 13*(3), 235–241.

Lentz, J. (2003). Daily baths: Torment or comfort at end of life? *Journal of Hospice and Palliative Nursing, 5*(1), 34–40.

Massachusetts Eye and Ear Infirmary. (n.d.). Contact lens options. Retrieved June 15, 2011, from http://www.masseyeandear.org/specialties/ophthalmology/contact-lens/about/

Meade, C., Bursell, A., & Ketelsen, L. (2007). Effects of nursing rounds: On patients' call light use, satisfaction, and safety. *American Journal of Nursing, 107*(2), 58–70; quiz, 70–71.

Moorhead, S., Johnson, M., & Maas, M., et al. (Eds.). (2012). *Nursing outcomes classification (NOC)* (5th ed.). St. Louis, MO: C. V. Mosby.

Munro, C. L., & Grap, M. J. (2004). Oral health and care in the intensive care unit: State of the science. *American Journal of Critical Care, 13*(1), 25–34.

NANDA International (NANDA-I). (2009). *NANDA nursing diagnoses: Definitions and classification, 2009–2011.* Oxford: Wiley-Blackwell.

NANDA International (NANDA-I). (2012). *NANDA nursing diagnoses: Definitions and classification, 2012–2014.* Oxford: Wiley-Blackwell.

National Collaborating Centre for Primary Care. (2004, June). Clinical guidelines for type 2 diabetes. Prevention and management of foot problems. London: National Institute for Clinical Excellence (NICE). Retrieved June 13, 2011, from http://www.nice.org.uk/nicemedia/live/10934/29241/29241.pdf

National Collaborating Centre for Primary Care. (2006). Postnatal care. Routine postnatal care of women and their babies. London: Royal College of General Practitioners. Retrieved June 13, 2011, from http://www.guideline.gov/content.aspx?id=9630&search=postnatal+care

National Institute on Deafness and Other Communication Disorders (NIDCD). (2007). Hearing aids [Fact sheet]. Retrieved June 15, 2011, from http://www.nidcd.nih.gov/staticresources/health/hearing/HearingAids07.pdf

Nelson, A., Lloyd, J., Menzel, N., et al. (2003). Preventing nursing back injuries: Redesigning patient handling tasks. *Journal of the American Association of Occupational Health Nurses, 51*(3), 126–134.

Nelson, A., Pragala, G., & Menzel, N. (2003). Myths and facts about back injuries in nursing. *American Journal of Nursing, 103*(2), 32–40.

Neppelenbroek, K., Pavarina, A., Spolidorio, D., et al. (2008). Effectiveness of microwave disinfection of complete dentures on the treatment of *Candida*-related denture stomatitis. *Journal of Oral Rehabilitation, 35*(11), 836–846.

O'Flynn, J. (2007). Prospective sampling of patient bath basins in acute care setting: Qualitative evaluation of bacterial colonization. *American Journal of Infection Control, 35*(5), E50–E51.

Pappas, P., Rex, J., Sobel, J., et al. (2009). Clinical practice guidelines for treatment of candidiasis: 2009 update by the Infectious Diseases Society of America. *Clinical Infectious Disease, 38*(2), 161–189. Retrieved June 14, 2011, from http://www.guidelines.gov/content.aspx?id=14174&search=treatment+of+candidiasis

Peters, R. (2010). Artificial eyes of glass and plastic and suggestions regarding their care. Center for Ocular Prosthetics. Retrieved June 15, 2011, from http://www.artificialeyesplastic.com/new-eye-care.htm

Plummer, E., & Albert, S. (2008). Diabetic foot care management in the elderly. *Clinics in Geriatric Medicine, 24*(3), viii, 551–567.

Procter & Gamble. (2008). How to shave. Trim and shape. Retrieved June 15, 2011, from http://www.gillette.com/en/us/mens-style/how-to-shave.aspx?utm_source=Bing&utm_medium=cpc&utm_term=for%2Bshaving%2B&utm_campaign=Gillette.BR_Search_Category%2BInterest_06.2010

Rasin, J., & Barrick, A. L. (2004). Bathing patients with dementia. *American Journal of Nursing, 104*(3), 30–33.

Robles, R., Corcoles, G., Torres, L., et al. (2002). Frequency of the adverse events during the hygiene of the critical patients. *Enfermia Intensiva, 13*(2), 47–56.

Rose, M., & Drake, D. (2008). Best practices for skin care of the morbidly obese. *Bariatric Nursing and Surgical Patient Care, 3*(2), 129–134.

Sehulster, L., Chinn, R., Arduino, et al. (2003). Guidelines for environmental infection control in health-care facilities. Recommendations of CDC and the Healthcare Infection Control Practices Advisory Committee (HICPAC). *Morbidity and Mortality Weekly Report, 52*(RR-10), 1–42.

Shiomori, T., Miyamoto, H., Makishima, K., et al. (2002). Evaluation of bedmaking-related airborne and surface methicillin-resistant *Staphylococcus aureus* contamination. *Journal of Hospital Infection, 50*(1), 30–35.

Siegel, J., Rhinehart, E., Jackson, M., Chiarello, L.; & the Healthcare Infection Control Practices Advisory Committee (2007). *2007 guideline for isolation precautions: Preventing transmission of infectious agents in the healthcare setting.* Retrieved June 12, 2011, from http://www.cdc.gov/hicpac/pdf/isolation/Isolation2007.pdf

Singapore Ministry of Health. (2004). *Nursing management of oral hygiene.* Singapore: Singapore Ministry of Health. Retrieved June 18, 2011, from http://guidelinecentral.com/_webapp_1825298/Nursing_management_of_oral_hygiene

Slot, D., Dörfer, C., & Van der Weijden, G. (2008). The efficacy of interdental brushes on plaque and parameters of periodontal inflammation: A systematic review. *International Journal of Dental Hygiene, 26*(4), 253–264.

Sona, C., Zack, J., Schallom, M., et al. (2008, November 17). The impact of a simple, low-cost oral care protocol on ventilator-associated pneumonia rates in a surgical intensive care unit [Abstract]. *Journal of Intensive Care Medicine.* Retrieved June 12, 2011, from http://www.ncbi.nlm.nih.gov/pubmed/19017665

Stern, C. (2007). Older adults: Bathing & skin care. Evidence summaries—Joanna Briggs Institute. Retrieved June 12, 2011, from http://www.jbiconnect.org/connect/docs/cis/es_html_viewer.php?SID=6298&lang=en&region=AU

Stiefel, K. A., Damron, S., Sowers, N. J., & Velez, L. (2000). Improving oral hygiene for the seriously ill patient: Implementing research-based practice. *Medical-Surgical Nursing Journal, 9*(1), 40–43, 46.

Thompson Healthcare. (2008). How to shampoo the hair of a person in bed. Retrieved June 18, 2011, from http://www.drugs.com/cg/how-to-shampoo-the-hair-of-a-person-in-bed.html

Trieger, N. (2004). Oral care in the intensive care unit. *American Journal of Critical Care, 13*(1), 24.

Trinkoff, A., Brady, B., & Nielsen, K. (2003). Workplace Prevention and Musculoskeletal Injuries in Nurses. *Journal of the Association of Occupational Health Professionals in Healthcare, 23*(4), 26–30.

U.S. Food and Drug Administration (FDA). (2009, October). A new online guide to hearing aids. Retrieved June 15, 2011, from http://www.fda.gov/downloads/ForConsumers/ConsumerUpdates/UCM187245.pdf

Vernon, M., Hayden, M., Trick, W., et al. (2006). Chlorhexidine gluconate to cleanse patients in a medical intensive care unit: The effectiveness of source control to redice the bioburden of vancomycin-resistant enterococci. *Archives of Internal Medicine, 166,* 306–312.

Warshaw, E., Nix, D., Kula, J., et al. (2002). Clinical and cost effectiveness of a cleanser protectant lotion for treatment of perineal skin breakdown in low-risk patients with incontinence. *Ostomy and Wound Management, 48*(6), 44–51.

Watando, A., Ebihara, S., Ebihara, T., et al. (2004). Daily oral care and cough reflex sensitivity in elderly nursing home patients. *Chest, 126*(4), 1066–1070.

CHAPTER 25

Ahlin, C., Klane-Soderlvist, B., Brundin, S., et al. (2006). Implementation of a written protocol for management of central venous access devices: A theoretical and practical education, including bedside examination. *Journal of Infusion Nursing, 29*(5), 253–259.

Amarasingham, R., Plantinga, L., Diener-West, M., et al. (2009). Clinical information technologies and inpatient outcomes: A multiple hospital study. *Archives of Internal Medicine, 169,* 108–114.

American Academy of Family Physicians (AAFP). (2004, updated 2011, February). Nasal sprays: How to use them correctly. *Family Doctor.* Retrieved August 5, 2011, from http://familydoctor.org/online/famdocen/home/common/allergies/treatment/104.html

American Academy of Family Physicians (AAFP). (2006). Metered-dose inhaler: How to use it correctly. *Family Doctor.* Retrieved August 5, 2011, from http://familydoctor.org/online/famdocen/home/common/asthma/medications/040.html

American Society of Health-System Pharmacists. (n.d.). How to use rectal suppositories properly. Retrieved August 6, 2011, from http://www.safemedication.com/safemed/MedicationTipsTools/HowtoAdminister/HowtoUseRectalSuppositoriesProperly.aspx

Best practices: Evidence-based nursing procedures (2nd ed., pp. 117–124). (2007). Philadelphia: Lippincott Williams & Wilkins.

Bollinger, M. B. (2005). How do patients determine that their metered-dose inhaler is empty? *Pediatrics, 116,* 563–564. Retrieved August 4, 2011, from http://pediatrics.aappublications.org/content/116/Supplement_2/563.1.full?ck=nck

Bradshaw, A. Dip, N., & Price, L. (2006). Rectal suppository insertion: The reliability of the evidence as a basis for nursing practice. *Journal of Clinical Nursing, 16*(1), 98–103.

Brock, T. P., Wessell, A. M., Williams, D. M., et al. (2004). Accuracy of float testing for metered-dose inhaler canisters. *Journal of the American Pharmaceutical Association, 42*(4), 582–586.

Bulecheck, G., Butcher G., & Dochterman, J. (Eds.). (2007). *Nursing interventions classification (NIC)* (5th ed.). St Louis, MO: C. V. Mosby.

Chan, H. (2001). Effects of injection duration on site-pain intensity and bruising associated with subcutaneous heparin. *Journal of Clinical Nursing, 25*(6), 882–892.

Cocoman, A., & Barron, C. (2008). Administering subcutaneous injections to children: What does the evidence say? *Journal of Children's and Young People's Nursing, 2*(2), 84–89.

Davanport, D. E., & Utterback, V. A. (2011). Physics and flushes: The science supporting why we do what we do. *Nursing2011, 41*(8), 65–66.

Elias, B. L., & Moss, J. A. (2011, April). Smart pump technology: What we have learned. *Computers in Informatics Nursing, 29*(3), 184–190.

Floyd, S., & Meyer, A. (2007). Intramuscular injections—what's best practice? *Nursing, 13*(6), 20–2.

Goedert, J. (2010). CPOE tester shows high error rates. HDM Breaking News, June 30, 2010.

Greenway, K. (2004). Using the ventral gluteal site for intramuscular injection. *Nursing Standard, 18*(29), 39–42.

Hadaway, L. (2008). Targeting therapy with central venous access devices. *Nursing2008, 38*(6), 34–41.

Han, Y. Y., Carcillo, J. A., Venkataraman, S. T., et al. (2005). Unexpected increased mortality after implementation of a commercially sold computerized order entry system. *Pediatrics, 116,* 1506–1512.

Heller, J. L. (2011, updated). Eye emergencies. MedlinePlus: Medical encyclopedia. National Library of Medicine, National Institutes of Health. Retrieved August, 5, 2011, from http://www.nlm.nih.gov/medlineplus/ency/article/000054.htm

Hitchen L. (2008). Frequent interruptions linked to drug errors. *BMJ, 336*(7654), 1155.

Hockenberry-Eaton, M. J., & Tashiro, J. (2012). *Wong's essentials of pediatric nursing* (9th ed.). St. Louis, MO: C. V. Mosby.

Howard, A., Mercer, P., Nataraj, H. C., et al. (1997). Bevel-down superior to bevel-up in intradermal skin testing. *Annals of Allergy, Asthma, & Immunology, 78,* 594–596.

Infusion Nurses Society (INS). (2006a). *Infusion nursing standards of practice.* Norwood, MA: Gardner Foundation.

Infusion Nurses Society (INS). (2006b). Infusion nursing standards of practice. *Journal of Infusion in Nursing, 29*(Suppl. 1), S1–S9.

Institute for Safe Medication Practices. (2004). *IMSP list of error-prone abbreviations, symbols, and dose designations.* Retrieved December 22, 2011, from www.ismp.org/PDF/ErrorProne.pdf

Joanna Briggs Institute. (2005). Strategies to reduce medication errors with reference to older adults. *Best Practice, 9*(4), 1–6.

The Joint Commission (TJC). (2006). Using medication reconciliation to prevent errors. *Sentinel Event Alert, 35.*

The Joint Commission (TJC). (2008). Preventing pediatric medication errors. *Sentinel Event Alert, 39.* Retrieved August 6, 2011, from http://www.jointcommission.org/sentinel_event_alert_issue_39_preventing_pediatric_medication_errors/

The Joint Commission (TJC). (2011). *2011–2012 National patient safety goals.* Retrieved December 16, 2011, from http://www.jointcommission.org/assets/1/6/NPSG_EPs_Scoring_CAH_20110707.pdf

Kroger A. T., Sumaya, C. V., Pickering, L. K., et al.; & Advisory Committee on Immunization Practices (ACIP), Centers for Disease Control and Prevention (CDC). (2012). General recommendations on immunization: Recommendations of the Advisory Committee on Immunization Practices (ACIP). *Morbidity and Mortality Weekly Report, 60*(RR02), 1–60. Retrieved February 20, 2013, from www.cdc.gov/mmwr/preview/mmwrhtml/rr6002a1.htm

Moorhead, S., Johnson, M., & Maas, M. (2007). *Nursing outcomes classification (NOC)* (4th ed.). St. Louis, MO: C. V. Mosby.

National Center for HIV, STD, and TB Prevention, Division of Tuberculosis Elimination. (2008). Mantoux tuberculosis skin test facilitator guide. Part one: Administering the Mantoux tuberculin skin test. Retrieved December 15, 2011, from http://www.cdc.gov/tb/education/Mantoux/part1.htm

Nicholl, L. H., & Hesby, A. (2002). Intramuscular injection: An integrative research review and guideline for evidence-based practice. *Applied Nursing Research, 15*(3), 149–162.

Nisbet, A. C. (2006). Intramuscular injections in the increasingly obese population: Retrospective study. *BMJ, 332,* 637–638. Retrieved December 21, 2011, from http://www.bmj.com/cgi/reprint/332/7542/637

Phillips, D. (2010). *Manual of IV therapeutics* (5th ed.). Philadelphia: F. A. Davis.

Phillips, N., & Nay, R. N. (2007). Nursing administration of medication via enteral tubes in adults: A systematic review. *International Journal of Evidence-Based Healthcare, 5*(3), 324–353.

Phillips, N., & Nay, R. N. (2008). A systematic review of nursing administration of medication via enteral tubes in adults. *Journal of Clinical Nursing, 17*(17), 2257–2265.

Poon, E. G., Keohane, C. A., Yoon, C. S., et al. (2010, May 6). Effect of bar-code technology on the safety of medication administration. *New England Journal of Medicine, 362*(18), 1698–707.

Ram, F. S. F., Brocklebank, D. M., White, J., et al. (2002). Pressurized metered dose inhalers versus all other hand-held inhaler devices to deliver beta-2 agonist bronchodilators for non-acute asthma. *Cochrane Database of Systematic Reviews,* Issue 2. Art. No.: CD002158. doi:10.1002/14651858

Rowan, N. (2006, September). Insulin (subcutaneous). Evidence summaries—Joanna Briggs Institute (p. 1). Retrieved December 21, 2011, from ProQuest Nursing & Allied Health Source database (Document ID: 1446922971).

Roy, V., Gupta, P., & Srivastava, S. (2005). Medication errors: Causes & prevention. *Health Administrator, 19*(1), 60–64.

Sittig, D. F., & Singh, H. (2011). Defining health information technology–related errors: New developments since To Err Is Human. *Archives of Internal Medicine, 171,* 1281–1284.

Stevens, S. (2005). Ophthalmic practice: Irrigating eyes. *Community Eye Health, 8*(55), 109–110.

Trbovich, P. L., Pinkney, S., Cafazzo, J. A., et al. (2010, October 19). The impact of traditional and smart pump infusion technology on nurse medication administration performance in a simulated inpatient unit. *Quality and Safety in Health Care, 19*(5), 430–434.

U.S. Department of Health and Human Services (USDHHS), Division of Healthcare Quality Promotion (DHQP). (1991, last updated 2008, November). Regulations (Standards—29 CFR) Bloodborne pathogens—1910.1030. Retrieved August 14, 2011, from http://www.osha.gov/Publications/osha3187.pdf

U.S. Department of Health and Human Services (USDHHS), National Institute for Occupational Safety and Health (NIOSH). (n.d.). *What every worker should know—how to protect yourself from needlestick injuries* (Publication No. 2000–135). Retrieved August 5, 2011, from http://www.cdc.gov/niosh/docs/2000-135/

U.S. Department of Labor, Occupational Safety & Health Administration (OSHA). (n.d.). Hospital eTool—healthcare wide hazards module: Needlesticks/sharps injuries. Retrieved February 20, 2013, from http://www.osha.gov/SLTC/etools/hospital/hazards/sharps/sharps.html

U.S. Food and Drug Administration, Center for Evaluation and Research. (2008). Metered-dose inhalers (MDI). Retrieved August 5, 2011, from http://www.fda.gov/Drugs/DrugSafety/InformationbyDrugClass/ucm063054.htm

Wynaden, D., Landsborough, I., McGowan, S., et al. (2006). Best practice guidelines for the administration of intramuscular injections in the mental health setting. *International Journal of Mental Health Nursing, 15*(3), 195–200.

Zaybak, A., & Khorshid, L. (2008). A study on the effect of the duration of subcutaneous heparin injection on bruising and pain. *Journal of Clinical Nursing, 17*(3), 378–385.

Zwicker, D., & Fulmer, T. (2008). Reducing adverse drug events. In: E. Capezuti, D. Zwicker, M. Mezey, & T. Fulmer (Eds.), *Evidence-based geriatric nursing protocols for best practice* (3rd ed.). New York: Springer.

CHAPTER 26

American Hospital Association. (2003). *The patient care partnership: Understanding expectations, rights, and responsibilities.* Chicago, IL: Author. Retrieved February 10, 2011 from http://www.aha.org/aha/issues/Communicating-With-Patients/pt-care-partnership.html

American Nurses Association (ANA). (2001). *Code of ethics for nurses with interpretive statements.* Washington, DC: American Nurses Publishing. Retrieved February, 8, 2011 from http://www.nursingworld.org/MainMenu Categories/ThePracticeofProfessionalNursing/Ethics Standards/CodeofEthics.aspx.

American Nurses Association (ANA). (2010). *Nursing: Scope and standards of practice* (2nd ed.). Public comment draft, January 2010. Silver Spring, MD: Nursebooks.org.

Bader, J. L., & Strickman-Stein, N. (2003). Evaluation of new multimedia formats for cancer communication. *Journal of Medical Internet Research, 5*(3), e19. Retrieved February 15, 2010, from http://www.jmir.org/2003/3/e16/

Bastable, S. B. (2008). Nurse as educator: *Principles of teaching and learning for nursing practice.* (3rd ed.) Boston: Jones & Bartlett.

Berkman, N. D., Sheridan, S. L., Donahue, K. E., et al. (2011). *Health literacy interventions and outcomes: An updated systematic review* (Evidence Report/Technology Assessment No. 199). (Prepared by RTI International—University of North Carolina Evidence-based Practice Center under Contract No. 290-2007-10056-I.) AHRQ Publication No. 11-E006. Rockville, MD: Agency for Healthcare Research and Quality. Retrieved April 1, 2011, from http://www.ahrq.gov/clinic/tp/lituptp.htm

Bloom, B. S., & Krathwohl, D. R. (1956). Taxonomy of educational objectives: The classification of educational goals. *Handbook I: Cognitive domain.* New York: Longmans, Green.

Bloom, B. S., Mesia, B. B., & Krathwohl, D. R. (1964). Taxonomy of educational objectives (*Vol. 1, The Affective Domain* and *Vol. 2, The Cognitive Domain*). New York: David McKay.

Bulechek, G., Butcher, H., & Dochterman, J. M. (2008). *Nursing Interventions Classification (NIC)* (5th ed.). St. Louis, MO: Mosby.

Clarke-Tasker, V. A., & Wade, R. (2002, May–June). What we thought we knew: African American males' perception of prostate cancer and screening methods. *Association of Black Nursing Faculty Journal, 13*(3), 56-60.

The Communication Initiative (TCI). (2003, July 29). Health belief model. Retrieved April 20, 2004, from http://www.comminit.com/ctheories/sid-8180.html

Janda, M., Stanek, C., Newman, B., et al. (2002). Impact of videotaped information on frequency and confidence of breast self-examination. *Breast Cancer Research and Treatment, 73*(1), 37–43.

Jarrell, K., Alpers, R., & Wotring, R. (2011). Is knowledge deficit helpful or hindering nursing diagnosis? *Teaching and Learning in Nursing, 6*(2), 89–91.

The Joint Commission (TJC). (2006). *Patient-centered communication standards for hospitals.* Retrieved February 10, 2011 from http://www.jointcommission.org/Advancing_Effective_Communication/

The Joint Commission (TJC). (2007). What did the doctor say? Improving health literacy to protect patient safety. Retrieved April 6, 2011, from http://www.jointcommission.org/What_Did_the_Doctor_Say/

Krathwohl, D. R. (2002, Autumn). A revision of Bloom's taxonomy: An overview. *Theory Into Practice, 41*(4), 212–224.

Lee, J. C., Boyd, R., & Stuart, P. (2007). Randomized controlled trial of an instructional DVD for clinical skills teaching, *Emergency Medicine Australasia, 19*(3), 241–245.

London, F. (1999). *No time to teach.* Philadelphia: J. B. Lippincott.

Moorhead, S., Johnson, M., Maas, M., & Swanson, E. (Eds.). (2008). *Nursing outcomes classification (NOC)* (4th ed.). St Louis: Mosby.

Muilenburg, L. Y., & Bergeb, Z. L. (2005). Student barriers to online learning: A factor analytic study. *Distance Education, 26*(1), 1475–1498.

NANDA International (NANDA-I). (2009). *NANDA nursing diagnoses: Definitions and classification 2009–2010.* Philadelphia: Author.

National Network of Libraries of Medicine. (2008). Health literacy. Retrieved September 19, 2008 from http://nnlm.gov/outreach/consumer/hlthlit.html

Nightingale, F. (1860/1992). *Notes on nursing: What it is and what it is not.* Philadelphia: J. B. Lippincott.

Piaget, J. (1966). *Origins of intelligence in children.* New York: W. W. Norton.

Rankin, S.H., Stallings, K.D., & London, F. (2005). *Patient education in health and illness* (5th ed.). Philadelphia: Lipppincott Williams & Wilkins.

U.S. Department of Health and Human Services, the Secretary's Advisory Committee on National Health Promotion and Disease Prevention Objectives for 2020. (2009). Topics and objectives - *Healthy People 2020* (p. 130). Washington, DC: U.S. Government Printing Office. Retrieved on February 19, 2013, from http://healthypeople.gov/2020/topicsobjectives2020/objectiveslist.aspx?topicId=18

Wiljer, D., & Catton, P. (2003). Multimedia Formats for patient education and health communication: Does user preference matter? *Journal of Medical Internet Research, 5*(3), e19.

Yekta, Z. P., & Nasrabadi, A. N. (2004). Concept mapping as an educational strategy to promote meaningful learning. *Journal of Medical Education, 5*(2), 47–45.

CHAPTER 27

Agency for Healthcare Research and Quality (AHRQ). (2012, November). *The guide to clinical preventive services, 2012: Recommendations of the U.S. Preventive Services Task Force* (AHRQ Publication No. 12-05145). Rockville, MD: Author. Retrieved February 5, 2011, from http://www.ahrq.gov/clinic/pocketgd.htm

American Academy of Family Physicians (AAFP). (2012, October). *Summary of recommendations for clinical preventive services.* Revision 6.8. Leawood, KS: American Academy of Family Physicians (AAFP). Retrieved February 5, 2011, from http://www.aafp.org/online/etc/medialib/aafp_org/documents/clinical/CPS/rcps08-2005.Par.0001.File.tmp/June2010.pdf

American Cancer Society. (2009a, last revised 2013, January 25). *Skin cancer prevention and early detection.* Atlanta, GA: American Cancer Society. Retrieved February 15, 2013, from http://www.cancer.org/acs/groups/cid/documents/webcontent/003184-pdf.pdf

American Cancer Society. (2009b, last revised 2013, February 6). *Breast cancer: Early detection.* Atlanta, GA: American Cancer Society. Retrieved February 20, 2013, from http://www.cancer.org/acs/groups/cid/documents/webcontent/003165-pdf.pdf

American Cancer Society. (2009c, last revised 2013, January 11). *American Cancer Society guidelines for the early detection of cancer.* Atlanta, GA: American Cancer Society. Retrieved February 20, 2013, from http://www.cancer.org/Healthy/FindCancerEarly/CancerScreeningGuidelines/american-cancer-society-guidelines-for-the-early-detection-of-cancer

American Cancer Society. (2010a). *Cancer facts and figures 2010.* Atlanta, GA: American Cancer Society. Retrieved February 8, 1109, from http://www.cancer.org/acs/groups/content/@epidemiologysurveilance/documents/document/acspc-026238.pdf

American Cancer Society. (2010b, last revised). *Detailed guide: Can testicular cancer be found early?* Atlanta, GA: American Cancer Society. Retrieved February 12, 2011, from http://www.cancer.org/Cancer/TesticularCancer/DetailedGuide/testicular-cancer

American College of Sports Medicine (ACSM). (2009). *ACSM'S guidelines for exercise testing and prescription* (8th ed.). New York: Lippincott Williams & Wilkins.

Bulechek, G., Butcher, H., & Dochterman, J. (2012). *Nursing interventions classification (NIC)* (6th ed.). St. Louis, MO: C. V. Mosby.

Centers for Disease Control and Prevention (CDC). (2009a). Smoking-attributable mortality, years of potential life lost, and productivity losses—United States, 2000–2004. *JAMA, 301*(6), 593–594.

Centers for Disease Control and Prevention (CDC). (2009b). Deaths. *National Vital Statistics Reports, 58*(1). Retrieved January 30, 2011, from http://www.cdc.gov/nchs/products/nvsr.htm#vol58

Daniels, S. R., Greer, F. R., and the Committee on Nutrition (2008, July). Lipid screening and cardiovascular health in childhood. *Pediatrics, 122*(1), 198–208. Retrieved February 9, 2011, from http://pediatrics.aappublications.org/cgi/content/full/122/1/198

Division of Nutrition, Physical Activity and Obesity, National Center for Chronic Disease Prevention and Health Promotion. (2010, February 9). *U.S. physical activity statistics,*

behavioral risk factor surveillance system (BRFSS). Centers for Disease Control and Prevention, Department of Health and Human Services. Retrieved on April 29, 2012, from http://apps.nccd.cdc.gov/PASurveillance/StateSum ResultV.asp?CI=&Year=2008&State=0#data

Ford, E. S., van Dam, R. M., & Fonarow, G. C. (2009). Trends in the prevalence of low risk factor burden for cardiovascular disease among United States adults. *Circulation, 120,* 1181–1188 Retrieved February 19, 2011, from http://circ. ahajournals.org/cgi/content/abstract/CIRCULATION AHA.108.835728v1

Gepner, A. D., Piper, M. E., & Johnson, H. M. , et al. (2011). Effects of smoking and smoking cessation on lipids and lipoproteins: Outcomes from a randomized clinical trial. *American Heart Journal, 161*(1), 145–151. doi: 10.1016/j.ahj. 2010.09.023.

Hall, D. R. (2004). *Lifestyle check assessment.* Vanderbilt University Health and Wellness. Retrieved on April 30, 2012, from http://healthandwellness.vanderbilt.edu/ news/2011/09/the-health-risk-assessment-tool/

Halls, C., & Rhodes, J. (2002, September). Employee wellness and beyond at Appleton Papers Inc. *Athletic Therapy Today,* 46–47.

Hettler, W. (1984). Wellness: Encouraging a lifetime pursuit of excellence. *Health Values: Achieving High Level Wellness, 8,* 13–17.

Janssen, I., Katzmarzyk, P. T., & Ross R. (2004, March). Waist circumference and not body mass index explains obesity related health risk. *American Journal of Clinical Nutrition, 79*(3), 379–384.

Kobasa, S. (1979). Stressful life events, personality, and health: An inquiry into hardiness. *Journal of Personality and Social Psychology, 37*(1), 1–11.

Lazarus, R. S. (1966). *Psychological stress and the coping process.* New York: McGraw-Hill.

Leavell, H., & Clark, E. (1965). *Preventive medicine for doctors in the community.* New York: McGraw-Hill.

Linn, H. H., Ezzati, M., Chang, H. Y., et al. (2009). Association between tobacco smoking and active tuberculosis in Taiwan: Prospective cohort study. *Journal of Respiratory Critical Care Medicine, 180*(5), 475–480.

Maddi, S. R., Koshaba, D. M., Fazel, M., et al. (2009, July 1). The personality construct of hardiness, IV. *Journal of Humanistic Psychology, 49*(3), 292–305.

Moorhead, S., Johnson, M., Maas, M., et al. (2008). *Nursing outcomes classification (NOC)* (4th ed.). St. Louis, MO: C. V. Mosby.

Myers, J., Sweeney, T., & Witmer, J. (2000). The wheel of wellness counseling for wellness: A holistic model for treatment planning. *Journal of Counseling & Development, 78*(3), 251–267.

NANDA International (NANDA-I). (2009). *Nursing diagnoses: Definitions and classification 2009–2011.* Philadelphia: Author.

National Cancer Institute. (2009). Prostate-specific antigen (PSA) test. Retrieved February 13, 2011, from http:// cancertrials.nci.nih.gov/cancertopics/factsheet/ Detection/PSA

National Institutes of Health (NIH). (2004). *Third report of the National Cholesterol Education Program (NCEP) expert panel on detection, evaluation, and treatment of high blood cholesterol in adults (adult treatment panel III)* (NIH Publication No. 01– 3670). Washington, DC: Author. Retrieved February 19,

2011, from http://www.nhlbi.nih.gov/guidelines/ cholesterol/index.htm

Neuman, B. (1995). *The Neuman systems model* (3rd ed.). Stamford, CT: Appleton & Lange.

Olson, M. B., Krantz, D. S., Kelsey, S. F., et al. (2005, July– August). Hostility scores are associated with increased risk of cardiovascular events in women undergoing coronary angiography: A report from the NHLBI-Sponsored WISE Study. *Psychosomatic Medicine, 67*(4), 546–552.

Pender, N. J., Murdaugh, C. L., & Parsons, M. A. (2010). *Health promotion in nursing practice* (6th ed.). Upper Saddle River, NJ: Prentice-Hall.

Pope, M. A., Burnett, R. T., Krewski, D., et al. (2009). Cardiovascular mortality and exposure to airborne fine particulate matter and cigarette smoke. Shape of the exposure-response relationship. *Circulation, 120*(6), 941– 948. Retrieved February 17, 2011, from http://circ. ahajournals.org/cgi/content/abstract/120/11/941

Prochaska, J., & DiClemente, C. (1982). Transtheoretical therapy: Toward a more integrative model of change. *Psychotherapy: Theory, research and practice, 19*(3), 276–288.

Qureshi, N., Wilson, B., Santaguida, P., et al. (2009, August). *NIH State-of-the-Science Conference: Family history and improving health* (Evidence Report/Technology Assessment No. 186). (Prepared by the McMaster University Evidence-based Practice Center, under Contract No. 290-2007-10060-I.) AHRQ Publication No. 09-E016. Rockville, MD: Agency for Healthcare Research and Quality. Retrieved February 17, 2011, from http://www.ahrq.gov/clinic/tp/famhimptp.htm

Rahe, R. (1974). Life change and subsequent illness reports. In: E. K. Gunderson & R. H. Rahe (Eds.), *Life stress and illness.* Springfield, IL: Charles C Thomas.

Selye, H. (1976). *The stress of life.* New York: McGraw-Hill.

Singh, M., & Das, R. R. (2011). Zinc for the common cold. *Cochrane Database of Systematic Reviews,* Issue 2. Art. No.: CD001364. doi:10.1002/14651858.CD001364.pub3

Sinha, V. (2009). Immunological role of hardiness on depression. *Indian Journal of Psychological Medicine, 31*(1), 39–44. Retrieved May 8, 2011, from http://www.ijpm.info/ article.asp?issn=0253-7176;year=2009;volume=31;issue=1; spage=39;epage=44;aulast=Sinha

Tindle, H. A., Chang, Y. F., Kuller, L. H., et al. (2009, August 10). Optimism, cynical hostility, and incident coronary heart disease and mortality in the Women's Health Initiative. *Circulation, 120*(8), 656. Retrieved February 5, 2011, from http://circ.ahajournals.org/cgi/content/abstract/ CIRCULATIONAHA.108.827642v1

U.S. Department of Agriculture (USDA). (2009, last updated.). MyPyramid: Steps to a healthier you. Retrieved February 19, 2011, from http://www.mypyramid.gov/

U.S. Department of Health and Human Services (USDHHS), The Secretary's Advisory Committee on National Health Promotion and Disease Prevention Objectives for 2020. (2008a). Phase I report: Recommendations for the framework and format of *Healthy People 2020.* Retrieved February 20, 2013, from http://healthypeople.gov/2020/ about/advisory/PhaseI.pdf

U.S. Department of Health and Human Services (USDHHS). (2008). 2008 physical activity guidelines for Americans. Retrieved February 5, 2011, from http://www.health.gov/ paguidelines/

U.S. Department of Health and Human Services (USDHHS), Office of Disease Prevention & Health Promotion and

Human Services. (2009, October 30, revised). Proposed *Healthy People 2020* objectives. Retrieved February 12, 2011, from http://www.healthypeople.gov/hp2020/Objectives/TopicAreas.aspx

U.S. Department of Health and Human Services (USDHHS), Office of Disease Prevention & Health Promotion and Human Services. (2010). *Healthy People 2020* objectives. Retrieved May 1, 2012, from http://healthypeople.gov/2020/topicsobjectives2020/pdfs/HP2020objectives.pdf

U.S. Department of Health and Human Services (USDHHS), U.S. Department of Agriculture. (2011). Dietary guidelines for Americans 2010. Retrieved May 1, 2012, from http://www.health.gov/dietaryguidelines/dga2010/DietaryGuidelines2010.pdf

Wallston, K. A., Wallston, B. S., & DeVellis, R. (1978, last modified 2007, June 15). Development of the multidimensional health locus of control (MHLC) scales. *Health Education Monographs, 6,* 160–170. (MHLC scales available at Vanderbilt University, Multidimensional Health Locus of Control Scales.) Retrieved February 17, 2011, from http://www.vanderbilt.edu/nursing/kwallston/mhlcscales.htm

Watson, J. (1979). *Nursing: The philosophy and science of caring.* Boston: Little, Brown.

Witmer, J., & Sweeney, T. (1992). A holistic model for wellness and prevention over the life span. *Journal of Counseling & Development, 71,* 140–148.

World Health Organization (WHO). (1948). Preamble to the constitution of the World Health Organization as adopted by the International Health Conference, New York, June 19–22, 1946; signed on July 22, 1946 by the representatives of 61 states (*Official Records of the World Health Organization,* no. 2, 100) and entered into force on 7 April 1948.

World Health Organization (WHO). (1986). Ottawa charter for health promotion. First International Conference on Health Promotion, Ottawa, November 21, 1986. Retrieved April 19, 2012, from http://www.who.int/hpr/NPH/docs/ottawa_charter_hp.pdf

CHAPTER 28

A Report of the Panel on Macronutrients, Subcommittees on Upper Reference Levels of Nutrients and Interpretation and Uses of Dietary Reference Intakes, and the Standing Committee on the Scientific Evaluation of Dietary Reference Intakes. (2005). Dietary Reference Intakes for energy, carbohydrate, fiber, fat, fatty acids, cholesterol, protein, and amino acids (macronutrients). National Academy of Science, Institute of Medicine, Retrieved January 1, 2012, from http://books.nap.edu/openbook.php?record_id=10490&page=R1

Agency for Healthcare Research and Quality (AHRQ). (2003, June). *Routine vitamin supplementation to prevent cancer and cardiovascular disease. What's new from the USPSTF* (AHRQ Publication No. APPIP03–0012). Rockville, MD: Author. Retrieved June 8, 2011, from http://www.ahrq.gov/clinic/3rduspstf/vitamins/vitaminswh.htm

Aghdassi, E., Royall, D., & Allard, J. (1999). Oxidative stress in smokers supplemented with vitamin C. *International Journal of Vitamin and Nutrition Research, 69,* 45.

Amella, E. (2007). Eating and feeding issues in older adults with dementia: Part II: Interventions. *Try this: Best practices in nursing care for hospitalized older adults with dementia. D11.2.* The Hartford Institute for Geriatric Nursing and the Alzheimer's Association. Retrieved June 18, 2011, from http://consultgerirn.org/uploads/File/trythis/try_this_d11_1.pdf

American Academy of Pediatrics (AAP). (2006). Policy statement. Dietary recommendations for children and adolescents: A guide for practitioners. *Pediatrics, 117*(2), 544–559. Retrieved June 8, 2011, from http://aappolicy.aappublications.org/cgi/content/full/pediatrics;117/2/544

American Academy of Pediatrics (AAP). (2010). AAP publishes new recommendations for iron intake among infants, toddlers. Retrieved June 8, 2011, from http://www.aafp.org/online/en/home/publications/news/news-now/clinical-care-research/20101020aapironrpt.html

American Association of Critical-Care Nurses (AACCN). (2005a). Practice alert. Verification of feeding tube placement. Retrieved June 16, 2011, from http://www.aacn.org/wd/practice/content/practicealerts.pcms?menu=practice

American Association of Critical-Care Nurses (AACCN). (2005b). Practice alert. Dye in enteral feeding. Retrieved June 16, 2011, from http://www.aacn.org/wd/practice/content/practicealerts.pcms?menu=practice

American Diabetes Association. (n.d.). Managing diabetes. Checking blood glucose. Retrieved June 9, 2011, from http://www.diabetes.org/living-with-diabetes/treatment-and-care/blood-glucose-control/checking-your-blood-glucose.html

American Diabetes Association. (2011). Summary of revisions to the 2011 clinical practice recommendations. *Diabetes Care, 34*(Suppl. 1), S3.

American Gastroenterological Association. (1995). American Gastroenterological Association medical position statement: Guidelines for the use of enteral nutrition. Retrieved June 17, 2011, from http://www3.us.elsevierhealth.com/gastro/policy/v108n4p1280.html

American Heart Association (AHA). (n.d.a, updated 2011, June 29). Fats and oils: AHA recommendation. Retrieved February 20, 2013, from http://www.heart.org/HEARTORG/GettingHealthy/FatsAndOils/Fats101/Fats-and-Oils-AHA-Recommendation_UCM_316375_Article.jsp

American Heart Association (AHA). (n.d.b). Fat substitutes. Retrieved February 15, 2013, from http://www.heart.org/HEARTORG/GettingHealthy/NutritionCenter/Fat-Substitutes_UCM_305978_Article.jsp

American Heart Association (AHA). (n.d., updated 2010, May 21). Consumer FAQ: "Better" fats (monounsaturated and polyunsaturated fats). Retrieved June 16, 2011, from http://www.heart.org/HEARTORG/GettingHealthy/NutritionCenter/Frequently-Asked-Questions-About-Better-Fats_UCM_305985_Article.jsp

American Society for Parenteral and Enteral Nutrition (A.S.P.E.N.) Board of Directors. (2009a). Clinical guidelines for the use of parenteral and enteral nutrition in adult and pediatric patients, 2009. *Journal of Parenteral and Enteral Nutrition, 33*(3), 255–259. Retrieved June 8, 2011, from http://online.sagepub.com/search/results?src_selected=selectComplete&submit=yes&src=selected&andorexactfulltext=and&journal_set=sppen&fulltext=guidelines+for+the+use+of+parenteral

A.S.P.E.N. Board of Directors and Task Force on Parenteral Nutrition Standardization. (2007). A.S.P.E.N. statement on parenteral nutrition standardization. *Journal of Parenteral and Enteral Nutrition, 31*(5), 441–448. Retrieved June 8,

2011, from http://www.nutritioncare.org/Index.aspx?id=5706

Bankhead, R. Boullata, J., Brantley, S., et al., and American Society for Parenteral and Enteral Nutrition (A.S.P.E.N.), Board of Directors. (2009b). Special report: Enteral nutrition practice recommendations. *Journal of Parenteral and Enteral Nutrition, 20*(10). Retrieved February 20, 2013, from http://pen.sagepub.com/content/early/2009/01/27/0148607108330314.full.pdf+html

Barberger-Gateau, P., Raffaitin, C., Letenneur, L., et al. (2007). Dietary patterns and risk of dementia. The three-city cohort study. *Neurology, 69*, 1921–1930.

Barclay, L., & Lie, D. (2008). Calcium may improve bone mineral density in men. *Medscape Medical News.* Retrieved June 14, 2011, from http://www.medscape.com/viewarticle/583343 . Also published in 2008 in *Archives of Internal Medicine, 168*, 2276–2282.

Barone, L., Milosavljevic, M., & Gazibarich, B. (2003). Assessing the older person: Is the MNA a more appropriate nutritional assessment tool than the SGA? *Journal of Nutritional Health Aging, 7*(1), 13–17.

Berkowitz, B., & Borchard, M. (2009). Advocating for the prevention of childhood obesity: A call to action for nursing. *Online Journal of Issues in Nursing, 14*(1), Manuscript 2. Retrieved June 13, 2011, from http://www.nursingworld.org/MainMenuCategories/ANAMarketplace/ANAPeriodicals/OJIN/TableofContents/Vol142009/No1Jan09/Prevention-of-Childhood-Obesity.aspx

Best practices: Evidence-based nursing procedures (2nd ed.). (2007). Philadelphia: Lippincott Williams & Wilkins.

Boitano, M., Bojak, S., McCloskey, S., et al. (2010). Improving the safety and effectiveness of parenteral nutrition. *Nutrition in Clinical Practice, 25*(6), 663–671.

Brody, J. (2008, August 5). Health. Sorting out coffee's contradictions. *The New York Times.* Retrieved June 15, 2011, from http://www.nytimes.com/2008/08/05/health/05brod.html?_r=science&oref=slogin

Bulechek, G., Butcher, H., & Dochterman, J. (2007). *Nursing interventions classification (NIC)* (5th ed.). St. Louis, MO: C. V. Mosby.

Centers for Disease Control and Prevention (CDC). (2005). Recommended infection-control and safe injection practices to prevent patient-to-patient transmission of blood-borne pathogens. Diabetes care procedures & techniques. *Morbidity and Mortality Weekly Report, 54*(09), 220–223. Retrieved June 16, 2011, from http://www.cdc.gov/hepatitis/Populations/PDFs/diabetes_handout.pdf

Centers for Disease Control and Prevention (CDC). (2008, reviewed and updated 2013, January 11). Overweight and obesity. Obesity prevalence. Retrieved February 20, 2013, from http://www.cdc.gov/nccdphp/dnpa/obesity/childhood/prevalence.htm

Centers for Disease Control and Prevention (CDC). (2009). Application of lower sodium intake recommendations to adults—United States, 1999–2006. *Morbidity and Mortality Weekly Report, 58*(11), 281–283. Retrieved June 8, 2011, from http://www.cdc.gov/mmwr/preview/mmwrhtml/mm5811a2.htm

Cincinnati Children's Hospital Medical Center. (2011). Best evidence statement (BESt). Confirmation of nasogastric/orogastric tube placement. Cincinnati, OH: Author. Retrieved February 20, 2013, from http://www.guideline.gov/content.aspx?id=35117

Clark, R., Birks, J., Nexo, E., et al. (2007). Low vitamin B_{12} status and risk of cognitive decline in older adults. *American Journal of Clinical Nutrition, 86*(5), 1384–1391.

Clarke, S. (2008). Drug administration via nasogastric tube. *Paediatric Nursing, 20*(7), 32.

Cullen, L., Taylor, D., Taylor, S., et al. (2004). Nebulized lidocaine decreases the discomfort of nasogastric tube insertion: A randomized, double-blind trial. *Annals of Emergency Medicine, 44*(2), 131–137.

Detsky, A., McLaughlin, J., Baker, J., et al. (1987). What is subjective global assessment? *Journal of Parenteral and Enteral Nutrition, 11*(1), 813–817.

DiMaria-Ghalili, R. (2008). Nutrition. In: E. Capezuti, D. Zwicker, M. Mezey, et al. (Eds.), *Evidence-based geriatric nursing protocols for best practice* (3rd ed., pp. 353–367). York: Springer.

DiMaria-Ghalili, R., & Guenter, P. (2008). The mini nutritional assessment. *American Journal of Nursing, 108*(2), 50–59; quiz, 60.

Donnelly, J. E., Blair, S. N., Jakicic, J. M., et al. (2009, June). Appropriate physical activity intervention strategies for weight loss and prevention of weight regain for adults. American College of Sports Medicine position stand. *Medicine & Science in Sports & Exercise, 41*(2), 459–447, Retrieved June 13, 2011, from http://journals.lww.com/acsm-msse/Fulltext/2009/02000/Appropriate_Physical_Activity_Intervention.26.aspx

Ebersole, P., Hess, P., Touhy, T., et al. (2009). *Ebersole and Hess' gerontological nursing & healthy aging* (3rd ed.). Philadelphia: Elsevier.

Editorial Board Palliative Care, Association of Comprehensive Cancer Centres (ACCC). (2006, January 12). Practice guidelines: Nausea and vomiting. Utrecht, The Netherlands: Author.

Elpern, E., Killeen, K., Talla, E., et al. (2007). Capnometry and air insufflations for assessing initial placement of gastric tubes. *American Journal of Critical Care, 16*(6), 544–550.

Flicker, L. L., McCaul, K. A., Hankey, G. J., et al. (2010). Body mass index and survival in men and women aged 70 to 75. *Journal of the American Geriatrics Society, 58*(2), 234–241.

Food and Nutrition Board, Institute of Medicine, National Academies. (2011). Dietary Reference Intakes (DRIs): Recommended Dietary Allowances and Adequate Intakes, vitamins. Retrieved June 7, 2011, from http://www.iom.edu/Reports/2010/Dietary-Reference-Intakes-for-Calcium-and-Vitamin-D.aspx

Friedman, N., & Zeiger, R. (2005). The role of breast-feeding in the development of allergies and asthma. *Journal of Allergy and Clinical Immunology, 115*(8), 1238–1248.

Garibalia, S. E., & Forster, S. J. (2008). Dietary intake of older patients in hospital and at home: The validity of patient kept food diaries. *Journal of Nutrition, Health & Aging, 12*(2), 102–106.

GlaxoSmithKline. (last updated 2008). Diabetes.com. How to test your blood sugar. Retrieved June 8, 2011, from http://www.diabetes.com/blood-sugar-control-matters/low-blood-sugar.html

Glucose monitoring. A guide to checking your blood sugar. (2008). *Advance for Nurse Practitioners, 16*(12), 28.

Griffiths, R., Thompson, D., Chau, J., et al. (2006). Systematic reviews. Insertion and management of nasogastric tubes for adults. Joanna Briggs Institute. Retrieved June 15, 2011,

from http://www.joannabriggs.edu.au/protocols/protnasotube.php

Guedon, C. (2000). Enteral nutrition: Techniques and indications. *Annales de Médecine Interne, 151*(8), 658–663.

Guyton, A. C., & Hall, J. E. (2011). *Textbook of medical physiology* (12th ed.). Philadelphia: W. B. Saunders.

Hollis, J., Gullion, C., Stevens, V., et al.; and Weight Loss Maintenance Trial Research Group. (2008). Weight loss during the intensive intervention phase of the weight-loss maintenance trial. *American Journal of Preventive Medicine, 35*(2), 118–126.

Honenyard, D. (2008). Dietary strategies for preventing cancer. *The Clinical Advisor, 11*(3), 23–25, 29–30.

Infusion Nurses Society (INS). (2006a). *Policies and procedures for infusion nurses* (3rd ed.). Norwood, MA: Author.

Infusion Nurses Society (INS). (2011,). Infusion nursing standards of practice. *Journal of Infusion Nursing, 34*(Suppl. 1).

Institute of Medicine. (2000). Dietary intakes of vitamin C, vitamin E, selenium, and carotenoids. *Pharmacist's Letter, 16*(5), 26–27.

Joanna Briggs Institute. (2007a). Effective dietary interventions for overweight and obese children. *Best Practice, 11*(1), 69–72.

Joanna Briggs Institute. (2007b). Effectiveness of interventions for undernourished older inpatients in the hospital setting. *Best Practice, 11*(2), 1–4.

Jockers, B. (2007). Vitamin D sufficiency: An approach to disease prevention. *American Journal for Nurse Practitioners, 11*(10), 43–50.

The Joint Commission (TJC). (2006). Sentinel event alert: Tubing misconnections—a persistent and potentially deadly occurrence. Retrieved January 2, 2012 , from http://www.jointcommission.org/sentinel_event_alert_issue_36_tubing_misconnections—a_persistent_and_potentially_deadly_occurrence/

The Joint Commission (TJC). (2007). Avoiding catheter and tubing misconnections. *Patient Safety Solutions, 1*(7). Retrieved June 12, 2011, from http://www.ccforpatientsafety.org/common/pdfs/fpdf/presskit/PS-Solution7.pdf

Kaushik, N., Pietraszewski, M., Holst, J., et al. (2005). Enteral feeding without pancreatic stimulation. *Pancreas, 31*(4), 353–359.

Leydon, N., & Dahl, W. (2008). Improving the nutritional status of elderly residents of long-term care homes. *Journal of Health Services & Research Policy, 13*(Suppl. 1), 25–29.

Lim, L. S., Hoeksema, L. J., Sherin, K.; and the ACPM Prevention Practice Committee. (2009, April). Screening for osteoporosis in the adult U.S. population: ACPM position statement on preventive practice. *American Journal of Preventative Medicine, 36*(4), 366–375.

Lutz, C., & Przytulski, K. (2011). *Nutrition and diet therapy* (5th ed.). Philadelphia: F. A. Davis.

Marion County Children's Alliance. (n.d.). 5-2-1-0 brochure. Retrieved May 5, 2012, from http://www.mcchildrensalliance.org/5210/assets/5210%20brochure.pdf

May, S. (2007). Testing nasogastric tube positioning in the critically ill: Exploring the evidence. *British Journal of Nursing, 16*(7), 414–418.

Metheney, N. (2006). Preventing respiratory complications of tube feedings: Evidence based-practice. *American Journal of Critical Care, 16,* 360–369. Retrieved June 15, 2011, from http://ajcc.aacnjournals.org/cgi/content/full/15/4/360

Mitrou, P., Kipnis, V., Thiébaut, A., et al. (2007). Mediterranean dietary pattern and prediction of all-cause mortality in a US population. *Archives of Internal Medicine, 167*(22), 2461–2468.

Moorhead, S., Johnson, M., Maas, M., et al. (2012). *Nursing outcomes classification (NOC)* (5th ed.). St. Louis, MO: C. V. Mosby.

MyPlate for older adults. (2011). Tufts University, Gerald J. and Dorothy R. Friedman School of Nutrition Science and Policy. Retrieved January 1, 2012, from http://hnrc.tufts.edu/images/MYplate_OlderAdults.pdf

NANDA International (NANDA-I). (2012). *Nursing diagnoses: Definitions and classification 2012–2014*. Ames, IA: Wiley-Blackwell.

National Association of Anorexia Nervosa and Associated Disorders. (n.d.). Eating disorders and the Internet. Retrieved June 8, 2011, from http://bespin.stwing.upenn.edu/~upsych/Perspectives/2002/Laksmana.pdf

National Center for Health Statistics. (2008a [reviewed]). Faststats A to Z. Overweight. Centers for Disease Control and Prevention. Retrieved June 23, 2011, from http://www.cdc.gov/nchs/fastats/overwt.htm

National Center for Health Statistics. (2008b). Prevalence of overweight, obesity and extreme obesity among adults: United States, trends 1976–80 through 2005–2006. Centers for Disease Control and Prevention. Retrieved June 22, 2011, from http://www.cdc.gov/nchs/data/hestat/overweight/overweight_adult.pdf

National Digestive Diseases Information Clearinghouse (NDDIC). (2006). Lactose intolerance. National Institute of Diabetes and Digestive and Kidney Diseases, National Institutes of Health. Retrieved June 8, 2011, from http://digestive.niddk.nih.gov/ddiseases/pubs/lactoseintolerance/#cause

National Guideline Clearinghouse (NGC). (2003, updated June 2008). Brief summary: Mealtime difficulties. In: Evidence-based geriatric nursing protocols for best practice. Rockville, MD: Author. Retrieved June 16, 2011, from http://www.guideline.gov/content.aspx?id=12267

National Guideline Clearinghouse (NGC). (2006a). Assessment and management of obesity and overweight in adults Rockville, MD: Author. Retrieved June 2, 2011, from http://www.guideline.gov/syntheses/synthesis.aspx?id=25323

National Guideline Clearinghouse (NGC). (2006b). Critical illness evidence-based nutrition practice guideline. Rockville, MD: Author. Retrieved June 17, 2011, from http://www.guideline.gov/content.aspx?id=12818

National Guideline Clearinghouse (NGC). (2006c). Brief guideline summary: Nutrition support in adults: Oral nutrition support, enteral tube feeding and parenteral nutrition. Rockville, MD: Author. Retrieved January 1, 2012, from http://www.guideline.gov/summary/summary.aspx?doc_id=8739&nbr=004851&string=parenteral_AND_nutrition_AND_guide

National Guideline Clearinghouse (NGC). (2008a). Brief guideline summary: Parenteral nutrition administration. In: Safe practices for parenteral nutrition. Rockville, MD: Author. Retrieved June 8, 2011, from http://www.guideline.gov/summary/summary.aspx?view_id=1&doc_id=12513

National Guideline Clearinghouse (NGC). (2008b). Brief guideline summary: Prevention of bloodstream infections. In: Prevention and control of healthcare-associated infections in Massachusetts. Rockville, MD: Author. Retrieved June 12, 2011, from http://www.guideline.gov/content.aspx?id=12922

National Guideline Clearinghouse (NGC). (2009, April). Guideline summary: Screening for osteoporosis in the adult U.S. population: ACPM position statement on preventive practice. Rockville, MD: Author. Retrieved June 18, 2011, from http://www.guideline.gov/summary/summary.aspx?view_id=1&doc_id=15270

National Heart, Lung and Blood Institute (NHLBI). (n.d.). Body mass index table. Retrieved June 8, 2011, from http://www.nhlbi.nih.gov/guidelines/obesity/bmi_tbl.htm

National Heart, Lung and Blood Institute (NHLBI). (n.d.). Classification of overweight and obesity by BMI, waist circumference, and associated risks. Retrieved June 8, 2011, from http://www.nhlbi.nih.gov/health/public/heart/obesity/lose_wt/bmi_dis.htm

National Heart, Lung and Blood Institute (NHLBI). (1998). Clinical guidelines on the identification, evaluation, and treatment of overweight and obesity in adults: The evidence report. Washington, DC: U.S. Department of Health & Human Services. Retrieved June 18, 2011, from http://www.nhlbi.nih.gov/guidelines/obesity/ob_gdlns.htm

National Institutes of Health (NIH), Office of Dietary Supplements. (2002/2005). Nutrient recommendation: Dietary Reference Intakes (DRI) and Recommended Dietary Allowances (RDA). Food and Nutrition Board of the Institute of Medicine, National Academy of the Sciences. Retrieved March 1, 2013, from http://ods.od.nih.gov/Health_information/Dietary_Reference_Intakes.aspx

National Institutes of Health, Office of Dietary Supplements. (2005). Nutrient recommendation: Dietary Reference Intakes (DRI) Tolerable upper level intake levels: Vitamins. Food and Nutrition Board of the Institute of Medicine, National Academy of Sciences. Retrieved January 1, 2012, from http://ods.od.nih.gov/Health_information/Dietary_Reference_Intakes.aspx

National Institutes of Health, Office of Dietary Supplements. (2011). Dietary Reference Intakes for calcium and vitamin D. Food and Nutrition Board of the Institute of Medicine, National Academy of Sciences. Retrieved January 1, 2012, from http://ods.od.nih.gov/Health_Information/Dietary_Reference_Intakes.aspx

Newman, A. (2009, January 31). Obesity in older adults. *OJIN*, *14*(1), Manuscript 3. Retrieved January 2, 2012, from http://www.nursingworld.org/MainMenuCategories/ANAMarketplace/ANAPeriodicals/OJIN/TableofContents/Vol142009/No1Jan09/Obesity-in-Older-Adults.aspx

Nutrition Screening Initiative. (2003). *Determine your nutritional health*. Washington, DC: National Council on Aging.

Owen, C., Martin, R., Whincup, P., et al. (2007). Does breastfeeding influence risk of type 2 diabetes in later life? A quantitative analysis of published evidence. *American Journal of Clinical Nutrition, 84*(5), 1045–1054.

Peter, S., & Gill, F. (2009). Development of a clinical practice guideline for testing nasogastric tube placement. *Journal for Specialists in Pediatric Nursing, 14*(1), 3–11.

Preston, A., Rodriguez, C., Rivera, C., et al. (2003). Influence of environmental tobacco smoke on vitamin C status in children. *American Journal of Clinical Nutrition, 77*(1), 167–172.

Rauen, C., Chulay, M., Bridges, E., et al. (2008). Seven evidence-based practice habits: Putting some sacred cows out to pasture. *Critical Care Nurse, 28*(3), 98–124.

Rosenbauer, J., Herzig, P., Kaiser, P., et al. (2007). Early nutrition and risk of type 1 diabetes mellitus—a nationwide case-control study in preschool children. *Experimental & Clinical Endocrinology & Diabetes, 115*(8), 502–508.

Russell, R., Rasmussen, H., & Lichtenstein, A. (1999). Modified food guide pyramid for people over seventy years of age. *Journal of Nutrition, 129*(3), 751–753.

Scarmeas, N., Luchsinger, J., Mayeux, R., et al. (2007). Mediterranean diet and Alzheimer disease mortality. *Neurology, 69*, 1084–1093.

Schardt, D. (2008, March). Caffeine. The good, the bad, and the maybe. *Nutrition Action Health Letter*. Center for Science in the Public Interest. Retrieved June 15, 2011, from http://www.cspinet.org/nah/02_08/caffeine.pdf

Schlenker, E., & Roth, S. (2006). *Williams' essentials of nutrition & diet therapy* (9th ed.). St. Louis, MO: C. V. Mosby.

Schmiedling, N., Waldman, R., & Desaulles, C. (1997). Nasogastric tubes: Insertion, placement, and removal in adult patients. *Gastroenterological Nursing, 20*(1), 15–19.

Shaw, A., Fulton, L., Davis, C., et al. (n.d.). *Using the Food Guide Pyramid: A resource for nutrition educators.* U.S. Department of Agriculture Food, Nutrition, and Consumer Services. Retrieved June 7, 2011, from http://www.cnpp.usda.gov/Publications/MyPyramid/OriginalFoodGuidePyramids/FGP/FGPResourceForEducators.pdf#xml=http://65.216.150.153/texis/search/pdfhi.txt?query=SERVING+SIZE&pr=MyPyramid&sufs=2&order=r&cq=&id=4592b7130

Shlamovitz, G. Z., & Shah, N. R. (2008). Nasogastric tube. *Emedicine*. Retrieved June 16, 2011, from http://emedicine.medscape.com/article/80925-overview

Simons, S. R., & Abdallah, L. M. (2012). Bedside assessment of enteral tube placement: Aligning practice with evidence. *American Journal of Nursing, 112*(2), 40–48.

Speroni, K., Earley, C., & Atherton, M. (2007). Evaluating the effectiveness of the Kids Living FitTM program: A comparative study. *Journal of School Nursing, 23*(6), 329–336.

Swinburn, B., Sacks, G., Lo, S., et al. (2009). Estimating the changes in energy flux that characterize the rise in obesity prevalence. *American Journal of Clinical Nutrition, 89*(6), 1723–1728.

Task Force for the Revision of Safe Practices for Parenteral Nutrition. (2004). Safe practices for parenteral nutrition. *Journal of Parenteral and Enteral Nutrition, 28*(6), S39–S70.

Thompson, J., & Manore, M. (2011). *Nutrition: An applied approach* (3rd ed.). San Francisco: Benjamin Cummings.

U.S. Department of Agriculture (USDA). (n. d.). SuperTracker, MyPlan. Retrieved January 2, 2012, from https://www.choosemyplate.gov/SuperTracker/myplan.aspx

U.S. Department of Agriculture, Food and Nutrition Center. (2002–2005). *Dietary guidance. DRI tables. Dietary Reference Intakes: Macronutrients.* National Academy of Sciences. Institute of Medicine. Food and Nutrition Board. Retrieved April 17, 2013 from http://www.iom.edu/Global/News%20Announcements/~/media/C5CD2DD7840544979A549EC47E56A02B.ashx

U.S. Department of Agriculture (USDA). (2011a, June). Be a healthy role model for children: Ten tips for setting good examples. 10 Tips Education series. DG Tipsheet 12. Retrieved March 10, 2013, from http://www.choosemyplate.gov/food-groups/downloads/TenTips/DGTipsheet12BeAHealthyRoleModel.pdf

U.S. Department of Agriculture (USDA). (2011b, June). Build a healthy meal: Ten tips for healthy meals. 10 Tips Education Series. Retrieved March 3, 2013, from http://www.choosemyplate.gov/downloads/TenTips/DGTipsheet7BuildAHealthyMeal.pdf

U.S. Department of Agriculture (USDA). (2011c, June). ChooseMyPlate.gov. Retrieved January 2, 2012, from http://www.choosemyplate.gov/

U.S. Department of Agriculture (USDA). (2011d, June). Healthy eating for vegetarians: Ten tips for vegetarians. 10 Tips Education series. Tip sheet 8. Retrieved March 3, 2013, from http://www.choosemyplate.gov/food-groups/downloads/TenTips/DGTipsheet7BuildAHealthy Meal.pdf

U.S. Department of Agriculture (USDA). (2011e, June). Steps to a healthier weight. Retrieved June 10, 2011, from http://www.choosemyplate.gov/STEPS/stepstoahealthier weight.html

U.S. Department of Agriculture (USDA) and U.S. Department of Health and Human Services (USDHHS). (2010, December). *Dietary Guidelines for Americans, 2010* (7th ed.). Washington, DC: U.S. Government Printing Office. Retrieved January 1, 2012, from http://health.gov/dietaryguidelines/dga2010/dietaryguidelines2010.pdf

U.S. Department of Health and Human Services (USDHHS). (2008). *2008 Physical activity guidelines for Americans* (ODPHP Publication No. U0036). USDHHS, Office of Disease Prevention and Health Promotion. Retrieved January 1, 2012, from http://www.health.gov/paguidelines/guidelines/default.aspx

U.S. Department of Health and Human Services (USDHHS). (2010a). *Healthy People 2020,* Topics and objectives. Nutrition and weight status. Washington, DC: U.S. Government Printing Office. Retrieved May 1, 2012 , from http://healthypeople.gov/2020/topicsobjectives2020/overview.aspx?topicid=29

U.S. Department of Health and Human Services (USDHHS). (2010b, updated November 23, 2011). *Healthy People 2020,* Topics and objectives: Food safety. Retrieved January 2, 2012, from http://healthypeople.gov/2020/topics objectives2020/overview.aspx?topicid=14

U.S. Food and Drug Administration (FDA). (2005). Luer lock misconnections can be deadly. Retrieved March 2, 2013, from http://www.premierinc.com/quality-safety/tools-services/safety/topics/tubing-misconnections/downloads/fda-luer-lock-misconnections.pdf

U.S. Preventive Services Task Force (USPSTF). (2009). Folic acid for the prevention of neural tube defects. Clinical summary of U.S. Preventive Services Task Force recommendation. Agency for Healthcare Research and Quality. Retrieved June 13, 2011, from http://www.ahrq.gov/zclinic/uspstf09/folicacid/folicsum.htm

Vegetarian Diet Information. (n. d.). U.S. Vegetarian dietary guideline. Retrieved March 1, 2013, from http://www.vegetarian-diet.info/vegetarian-dietary-guidelines.htm

Vegetarian Diet Pyramid©. (n. d.). Mayo Foundation for Medical Education and Research (MFMER), with permission. Retrieved January 1, 2012, from http://www.mayoclinic.com/health/medical/IM02769

Vogiatzoglou, A., Refsum, H., Johnston, C., et al. (2008). Vitamin B_{12} status and rate of brain volume loss in community-dwelling elderly. *Neurology, 71*(11), 826–832.

Wagner, C., and Greer, F.; and the Section on Breastfeeding and Committee on Nutrition. (2008). Prevention of rickets and vitamin D deficiency in infants, children, and adolescents. *Pediatrics, 122*(5), 1142–1152. Retrieved June 6, 2011, from http://aappolicy.aappublications.org/cgi/content/full/pediatrics;122/5/1142

Wiegand, D., & Carlson, K. (Eds.) (2005). *AACN procedure manual for critical care* (5th ed.). St. Louis, MO: Elsevier Saunders.

Wilkinson, J. M., & Ahern, N. (2013). *Prentice-Hall nursing diagnosis handbook with NIC interventions and NOC outcomes* (10th ed.). Upper Saddle River, NJ: Prentice-Hall Health.

Wolfe, T., Fosnocht, D., & Linscott, M. (2000). Atomized lidocaine as topical anesthesia for nasogastric tube placement: A randomized, double-blind, placebo-controlled trial. *Annals of Emergency Medicine, 35*(5), 421–425.

World Health Organization (WHO). (2006a). BMI classification. Global database on body mass index. Retrieved June 8, 2011, from http://apps.who.int/bmi/index.jsp?introPage=intro_3.html

World Health Organization (WHO). (2006b). WHO child growth standards length/height-for-age, weight-for-age, weight-for-length, weight-for-height and body mass index-for-age. Retrieved March 1, 2011, from http://www.who.int/childgrowth/standards/Technical_report.pdf

CHAPTER 29

Allison, J. (2005). Colon cancer screening guideline: The fecal occult blood test has become a better fit. *Gastroenterology, 129*(2), 745–748.

American Cancer Society. (2010). Cancer facts and figures 2010. Retrieved June 13, 2011, from http://www.cancer.org/Research/CancerFactsFigures/CancerFactsFigures/cancer-facts-and-figures-2010

American Cancer Society. (2011). Detailed guide: Colon and rectum cancer: Revised March 2, 2011. Retrieved May 3, 2011, from http://www.cancer.org/acs/groups/cid/documents/webcontent/003096-pdf.pdf

American Gastroenterological Association. (2007). Understanding constipation [Brochure]. Retrieved June 22, 2011, from http://www.gastro.org/patient-center/digestive-conditions/AGAPatientBrochure_Constipation.pdf

Atkins, D. (2008). The periodic health examination. In: L. Goldman & D. Ausiello (Eds.), *Cecil medicine* (23rd ed.). Philadelphia: Saunders Elsevier.

Ayello, E., & Sibbald, R. (2008). Preventing pressure ulcers and skin tears. In: E. Capezuti, D. Zwicker, M. Mezey, et al. (Eds.), *Evidence-based geriatric nursing protocols for best practice* (3rd ed., pp. 403–429). New York: Springer. Retrieved June 21, 2011, from http://www.guideline.gov/summary/summary.aspx?doc_id=12262&nbr=006346&string=Bedpan

Balas, M., Casey, C., & Happ, M. (2008). Comprehensive assessment and management of the critically ill. In: E. Capezuti, D. Zwicker, M. Mezey, et al. (Eds.), *Evidence-based geriatric nursing protocols for best practice* (3rd ed., pp. 565–593). New York: Springer. Retrieved June 15, 2011, from http://www.guideline.gov/summary/summary.aspx?doc_id=12253&nbr=006337&string=Bedpan

Baldwin, C., Grant, M., Wendel, C., et al. (2008). Influence of intestinal stoma on spiritual quality of life of U.S. veterans. *Journal of Holistic Nursing, 26*(3), 185–194. Retrieved June 22, 2011, from http://jhn.sagepub.com/cgi/content/abstract/26/3/185

Beltz, J. (2006). Fecal incontinence in acutely and critically ill patients: Options in management. *Ostomy Wound Management, 52*(12), 56–58, 60, 62–66.

Benoit R., & Watts, C. (2007). The effect of a pressure ulcer prevention program and the bowel management system in reducing pressure ulcer prevalence in an ICU setting.

Journal of Wound, Ostomy, & Continence Nursing, 34(2), 163–175.

Black, P. (2008). Peristomal skin care: An overview of available products. *British Journal of Nursing, 16,* 1048–1056.

Brink, D., Barlow, J., Bush, K., et al. (2012). *Colorectal cancer screening.* Bloomington, MN: Institute for Clinical Systems Improvement (ICSI).

Bulechek, F., Butcher, H., & Dochterman, J. (2012). *Nursing interventions classification (NIC)* (6th ed.). St. Louis, MO: C. V. Mosby.

Burch, J., & Sica, J. (2008). Common peristomal skin problems and potential treatment options. *British Journal of Nursing, 17,* S4–11.

Chapman, J., Bernstein, L., Lee, R., et al. (Eds.). (2006). Food allergy: A practice parameter. *Annals of Allergy, Asthma & Immunology, 96,* S1–S68.

Creason, N., & Sparks, D. (2000). Fecal impaction: A review. *Nursing Diagnosis, 11*(15), 15–23.

Cronin, E. (2008). Colostomies and the use of colostomy appliances. *British Journal of Nursing, 17,* S12–16.

Foran, M., Petersen, J., & Llewandrowski, K. (2006). Occult blood. In: *Laboratory medicine practice guidelines: Evidence-based practice for point-of-care testing* (pp. 95–104). Washington, DC: National Academy of Clinical Biochemistry (NACB). Retrieved June 20, 2011, from http://www.guideline.gov/summary/summary.aspx?doc_id=10819&nbr=005644&string=fecal_AND_occult_AND_blood

Gallagher, P., O'Mahony, D., & Quigley, E. (2008). Management of chronic constipation in the elderly. *Drugs & Aging, 25*(10), 807–822.

Ginsberg, D., Phillips, S., Wallace, J., et al. (2007). Evaluating and managing constipation in the elderly. *Urologic Nursing, 27*(3), 191–200.

Gomella L., & Haist, S. (n.d.). Laboratory diagnosis: Chemistry, immunology, serology. In: *Clinician's pocket reference: The scut monkey* (11th ed.). New York: McGraw-Hill Professional.

Gray-Micelli, D. (2008). Preventing falls in acute care. In: E. Capezuti, D. Zwicker, M. Mezey, et al. (Eds.), *Evidence-based geriatric nursing protocols for best practice* (3rd ed., pp. 161–198). New York: Springer. Retrieved June 15, 2011, from http://www.guideline.gov/summary/summary.aspx?doc_id=12265&nbr=006349&string=Bedpan

Joanna Briggs Institute. (2008). Management of constipation in older adults. *Best Practice, 12*(7), 33–36. Retrieved March 3, 2013, from http://connect.jbiconnectplus.org/ViewSourceFile.aspx?0=453

The Joint Commission Accreditation Program. (2011). Critical Access Hospital National Patient Safety Goals 2011. Retrieved June 23, 2011, from http://www.jointcommission.org/cah_2011_npsgs/

Kaiser Permanente Care Management Institute. (2008). Colorectal screening clinical practice guideline. Oakland, CA: Author. In: Brief Summary. National Guidelines Clearinghouse (NGC). Retrieved March 3, 2013, from http://guideline.gov/content.aspx?id=14345

Karadag, A., Mentex, B., & Ayaz, S. (2005). Colostomy irrigation: Results of 25 cases with particular reference to quality of life. *Journal of Clinical Nursing, 14*(4), 479–485.

Kent, M. (2008). Changing an ostomy pouching system. *Nursing2008, 38*(12), 50–54.

Keshava, A., Renwick, A., Stewart, P., et al. (2007). A nonsurgical means of fecal diversion: The Zassi bowel management system. *Diseases of the Colon & Rectum, 50,* 1017–1022.

Korzenik, J. (2008). Diverticulitis: New frontiers for an old country: Risk factors and pathogenesis. *Journal of Clinical Gastroenterology, 42*(10), 1128–1129.

Lutz, C., & Przytulski, K. (2010). *Nutrition and diet therapy: Evidence-based applications* (5th ed.). Philadelphia: F. A. Davis.

Moorhead, S., Johnson, M., & Maas, M., et al. (Eds.). (2012). *Nursing outcomes classification (NOC)* (5th ed.). St. Louis, MO: C. V. Mosby.

Müeller-Lissner, S., Kamm, M., Scarpignato, C., et al. (2005). Myths and misconceptions about chronic constipation. *American Journal of Gastroenterology, 100,* 232–242.

NANDA International (NANDA-I). (2009). *NANDA nursing diagnoses: Definitions and classification 2009–2011.* Ames, IA: Wiley-Blackwell.

National Guideline Clearinghouse (NGC). (n.d.). Brief guideline summary: Evaluation and treatment of constipation in infants and children: Recommendations of the North American Society for Pediatric Gastroenterology, Hepatology and Nutrition (2006). Rockville, MD: Author. Retrieved February 8, 2009, from http://www.guideline.gov/summary/summary.aspx?doc_id=9792&nbr=005245&string=fecal_AND_impaction

National Guideline Clearinghouse (NGC). (2008). Brief guideline summary: Screening for colorectal cancer: U.S. Preventive Services Task Force recommendation statement. Rockville, MD: Author. Retrieved June 23, 2011, from http://www.guideline.gov/summary/summary.aspx?view_id=1&doc_id=13133

National Institute of Allergy and Infectious Diseases (NIAID). (2001, June). Food allergy and intolerances [Fact sheet]. Retrieved June 29, 2011, from http://www.wrongdiagnosis.com/artic/food_allergy_and_intolerances_niaid_fact_sheet_niaid.htm

Norton, C., & Chelvanayagam, S. (2000). A nursing assessment tool for adults with fecal incontinence. *Journal of Wound, Ostomy and Continence Nursing, 27,* 279–291.

Norton, W. (2008). An overview of bowel incontinence: What can go wrong? *The Exceptional Parent, 38*(9), 67–70.

Pullen, R. (2006). Teaching your patient to irrigate a colostomy. *Nursing2006, 36*(4), 22.

Richbourg, L., Fellows, J., & Arroyave, W. (2008). Ostomy pouch wear time in the United States. *Journal of Wound, Ostomy and Continence Nursing, 35*(5), 504–508.

Scarlett, Y. (2004). Medical management of fecal incontinence. *Gastroenterology, 126,* S55–S63.

Schnelle, J. F., & Leung, F. W. (2004). Urinary and fecal incontinence in nursing homes. *Gastroenterology, 126*(1 Suppl. 2), S41–S47.

Shakil, A., Church, R., & Rao, S. (2008). Gastrointestinal complications of diabetes. *American Family Physician, 77*(12), 1697–1703.

Siegel, J., Rhinehart, E., Jackson, M., et al.; and the Healthcare Infection Control Practices Advisory Committee. (2007). Guideline for isolation precautions: Preventing transmission of infectious agents in healthcare settings, 2007. Centers for Disease Control and Prevention (CDC). Retrieved June 24, 2011, from http://www.cdc.gov/ncidod/dhqp/pdf/guidelines/Isolation2007.pdf

Simmons, K., Smith, J., Bobb, K-A, et al. (2007). Adjustment to colostomy: Stoma acceptance, stoma care self-efficacy and interpersonal relationships. *Journal of Advanced Nursing, 60*(6), 627–635.

United Ostomy Associations of America. (2005). *Ostomates food reference chart.* Retrieved from http://www.uoaa.org/ostomy_info/pubs/uoa_diet_nutrition_en.pdf

Van Leeuwen, A., Kranpitz, T., & Smith, L. (2009). *Davis's comprehensive handbook of laboratory and diagnostic tests with nursing implications* (3rd ed.). Philadelphia: F. A. Davis.

Van Leeuwen, A., Poelhuis-Leth, D., & Bladh, M. (2011). *Davis's comprehensive handbook of laboratory and diagnostic tests with nursing implications* (4th ed.). Philadelphia: F. A. Davis.

Wilkinson, J. (2009). *Nursing diagnosis handbook with NIC interventions and NOC outcomes* (9th ed.). Upper Saddle River, NJ: Prentice-Hall.

Wilson, L. (2005). Understanding bowel problems in older people. Part I. *Nursing Older People, 17*(8), 25–29.

Wishin, J., Gallagher, T., & McCann, E. (2008). Emerging options for the management of fecal incontinence in hospitalized patients. *Journal of Wound, Ostomy and Continence Nursing, 35*(1), 104–110.

Wound, Ostomy and Continence Nurses Society. (2003). *Guideline for prevention and management of pressure ulcers.* Glenview, IL: Author.

Yuan, C. (Ed.). (2005). *Handbook of opioid bowel dysfunction.* New York: Haworth Reference Press.

CHAPTER 30

Agency for Healthcare Research and Quality. (2007, November). *Patient self-management support programs: An evaluation.* Retrieved January 7, 2012 from http://www.ahrq.gov/qual/ptmgmt/

Agency for Healthcare Research and Quality, National Guideline Clearinghouse. (2006, revised 2010 March). Guideline synthesis: Evaluation and management of urinary incontinence. Retrieved June 3, 2011, from http://www.guideline.gov/syntheses/synthesis.aspx?id=16411

Barbosa-Cesnik, C., Brown, M. B., Buxton, M., et al. (2011). Cranberry juice fails to prevent recurrent urinary tract infection: Results from a randomized placebo-controlled trial. *Clinical Infectious Disease, 52*(1), 23-30.

Beers, M. H., Jones, T.V., Berkwits, M. & Kaplan, J. L., et al. (2000, updated 2009). Table 307-1. Selected physiologic age-related changes. In: *The Merck manual of geriatrics* (3rd ed.). Philadelphia: F.A. Davis. Retreived May 28, 2011, from http://www.merckmanuals.com/media/professional/pdf/Table_337-1.pdf

Best practices: Evidence-based nursing procedures (pp. 117–124). (2008). Philadelphia: Lipppincott Williams & Wilkins.

Bulechek, G., Butcher, H., & Dochterman, J. (2008). *Nursing interventions classification (NIC)* (5th ed.). St. Louis: Mosby.

Burgio, K. L., Goode, P., Urban, et al. (2007). Postoperative biofeedback assisted behavioral training to decrease prostatectomy incontinence: A randomized, controlled trial. *Journal of Urology, 175*(1), 196—210.

Corna, L. M., & Cairney, J. (2005). The role of social support in the relationship between urinary incontinence and psychological distress in older adults. *Canadian Journal of Aging, 24*(3), 285–294.

Doughty, D. B. (2006). *Urinary & fecal incontinence: Current management concepts.* St. Louis, MO: Mosby.

Dowling-Castronovo, A. (2007). Urinary incontinence assessment in older adults: Part I. Transient urinary incontinence. *Try this: Best practices in nursing care to older adults, 11.2.* Retrieved June 3, 2011, from http://consultgerirn.org/uploads/File/trythis/try_this_11_1.pdf

Dowling-Castronova, A. (2008). Urinary incontinence assessment in older adults: Part II. Established urinary incontinence. *Try this: Best practices in nursing care to older adults, 11.2* Retrieved June 3, 2011, from http://consultgerirn.org/uploads/File/trythis/issue11-2.pdf

Dowling-Castronovo, A., & Bradway, C. (2003; updated 2008, November). Urinary incontinence. In: M. Mezey, T. Fulmer, I. Abraham, & D. A. Zwicker (Eds.), *Geriatric nursing protocols for best practice* (pp. 83–98). New York: Springer. Retrieved June 3, 2011, from http://consultgerirn.org/topics/urinary_incontinence/want_to_know_more

Dowling-Castronovo, A, ,& Bradway, C. (2008). Urinary incontinence (UI) in older adults admitted to acute care. In: Capezuti, E., Zwicker, D., Mezey, M., et al. (Eds.), *Evidence-based geriatric nursing protocols for best practice* (3rd ed., pp. 309–336). New York: Springer. Retrieved August 29, 2011, from http://www.guideline.gov/summary/summary.aspx?doc_id=13163.

Finnish Medical Society. (2008, August). Urinary incontinence in women. In: *EBM guidelines. Evidence-based medicine.* Helsinki, Finland: Wiley Interscience. John Wiley & Sons. In: Guideline Summary (2009, May). Rockville, MD: National Guideline Clearinghouse (NCG). Retrieved March 3, 2013, from http://www.guideline.gov/content.aspx?id=13195&search=urinary+incontinence+women

Gamiero, M. O., Gamiero, E. H., Gamiero, F. O., et al. (2010, January). Vaginal weight cone versus assisted pelvic floor muscle training in the treatment of female urinary incontinence. A prospective, single-blind, randomized trial. *International Urogynecology Journal.* Retrieved June 2, 2011, from http://www.springerlink.com/content/f30811hl28g8733t/

Gould, C. V., Umshied, C. A., Agarwal, R. K., et al.; and the Healthcare Infection Control Practices Advisory Committee (HICPAC). (1981, updated 2010). Guideline for prevention of catheter-associated urinary tract infections 2009. Centers for Disease Control and Prevention, Healthcare Infection Control Practices Advisory Committee. Retrieved June 4. 2011, from http://www.cdc.gov/hicpac/pdf/CAUTI/CAUTIguideline2009final.pdf

Grabe, M., Bishop, M.C., Bjerklund-Johansen, T.E., et al. (2008, March). Catheter-associated urinary tract infections. In: *Guidelines on the management of urinary and male genital tract infections.* ARNHEM, Netherlands: European Association of Urology. In: Guideline Summary. Rockville, MD: National Guideline Clearinghouse (NGC). Retrieved June 5, 2011, from http://www.uroweb.org/fileadmin/user_upload/Guidelines/The%20Management%20of%20Male%20Urinary%20and%20Genital%20Tract%20Infections.pdf

Griffith, R. & Fernandez, R. (2007, republished 2009, January). Strategies for the removal of short-term indwelling urethral catheters in adults. *Cochrane Database of Systematic Reviews,* Issue 2. Art. No.: CD004011. doi:10.1002/14651858.CD004011.pub3

Hartmann, K. E., McPheeters, M. L., Biller, D. H., et al. (2009, August). Treatment of overactive bladder in women (Evidence Report/Technology Assessment No. 187.) (Prepared by the Vanderbilt Evidence-based Practice Center under Contract No. 290-2007-10065-I.) AHRQ Publication No. 09-E017. Rockville, MD: Agency for Healthcare Research and Quality.

Hayder, D., & Schnepp, W. (2010). Experiencing and managing urinary incontinence: A qualitative study. *Western Journal of Nursing Research, 32*(4), 480–496.

Hay-Smith, J. (2000, November/December). Pelvic floor re-education. *Evidence Based Medicine, 5,* 183.

Hunter, K. F., Moore, K. N., Cody, D. J., et al. (2007, February 21). Conservative management for postprostatectomy urinary incontinence. *Cochrane Database of Systematic Reviews.* In the Cochrane Library. Chichester, UK: John Wiley & Sons, Ltd. Retrieved June 3, 2011, from http://www.cochrane.org/reviews/en/ab001843.html

Institute of Medicine (IOM). (2004). *Dietary reference intakes for electrolytes and water.* Washington, DC: National Academies Press.

Jahn, P., Preuss, M., Kernig, A., et al. (2007). Types of indwelling urinary catheters for long-term bladder drainage in adults. *Cochrane Database of Systematic Reviews,* Issue 3. Art. No.: CD004997. doi:10.1002/14651858.CD004997.pub2

Joanna Briggs Institute. (2010). Management of short-term indwelling urethral catheters to prevent urinary tract infections. *Best Practice, 14*(12), 51–54.

Kessler, T. M., Ryu, G. R., & Burkhard, F. C. (2008). Clean intermittent self-catheterization: A burden for the patient? *Neurourology and Urodynamics, 27*(8). Retrieved June 4, 2011, from http://www3.interscience.wiley.com/journal/121385630/abstract. DOI 10.1002/nau.20610

Kiel, R. J., & Nashelsky, J. (2003, February). Does cranberry juice prevent or treat urinary tract infection? *Journal of Family Practice,* Retrieved June 2, 2011, from http://www.jfponline.com/pages.asp?aid=1391&UID=

Lewis, L. (2003). Managing incontinence at home. *American Journal of Nursing, 3*(Suppl.), S41.

Lo, E., Nicolle, L., Classen, D., et al. (2008). Strategies to prevent catheter-associated urinary tract infections in acute care hospitals. *Infection Control Hospital Epidemiology* (Suppl. 1), 41–50. In the Cochrane Library. Chichester, UK: John Wiley & Sons, Ltd.

Madigan, E., & Neff, D. (2003). Care of patients with long-term indwelling urinary catheters. *Online Journal of Issues in Nursing, 8*(3). Retrieved June 1, 2011, from http://www.nursingworld.org/MainMenuCategories/ANAMarketplace/ANAPeriodicals/OJIN/TableofContents/Volume82003/No3Sept2003/HirshArticle/CareofPatientswithLongTermIndwellingUrinaryCatheters.aspx

McConnell, E. A. (2001). Clinical do's and don'ts: Applying a condom catheter. *Nursing, 31*(1), 70.

Moore, K. N., Fader, M. & Getliffe, K. (2007). Long-term bladder management by intermittent catheterisation in adults and children. *Cochrane Database Systems Review,* Issue 4. Art. No.: CD006008.

NANDA International (NANDA-I). (2009). *Nursing diagnoses: Definitions and classification 2009–2011.* Philadelphia: Author.

NANDA International (NANDA-I). (2012). *Nursing diagnoses: Definitions and classification.* Ames, IA: Wiley-Blackwell.

National Collaborating Centre for Women's and Children's Health. (2006, October). Urinary incontinence: The management of urinary incontinence in women. London: *Royal College of Obstetricians and Gynaecologists* (RCOG), 221. In National Guideline Clearinghouse Summary. Retrieved June 3, 2011, from http://www.guideline.gov/summary/summary.aspx?view_id=1&doc_id=9926

National Institute for Health and Clinical Excellence (NICE). (2006). Urinary incontinence. The management of urinary incontinence in women. Quick reference guide. National Collaborating Centre for Women's and Children's Health, Retrieved June 12, 2011, from http://www.nice.org.uk/nicemedia/pdf/word/CG40quickrefguide1006.pdf

National Institutes of Health, Clinical Center. (2010, updated). Clean intermittent self-catheterization. Patient Information Publications. Retrieved June 1, 2011, from http://www.cc.nih.gov/ccc/patient_education/pepubs/bladder/ciscmen5_22.pdf

National Institutes of Health, Warren Grant Magnuson Clinical Center. (1999, last updated 2009, March 31). 24-hour urine collection. *Procedures/Diagnostic Tests.* Retrieved May 29, 2011, from http://clinicalcenter.nih.gov/ccc/patient_education/procdiag/24hr.pdf

National Kidney and Urologic Diseases Information Clearinghouse (NKUDIC). (2005). Urinary tract infection in adults. Retrieved May 22, 2011, from http://kidney.niddk.nih.gov/Kudiseases/pubs/utiadult/.

Nazarko, L. (2008). Reducing the risk of catheter-related urinary tract infection. *British Journal of Nursing, 17*(16), 1002–1010.

Newman, D. K., & Palmer, M. H. (Eds.). (2003, March). State of the science on urinary incontinence. *American Journal of Nursing* (Suppl.), 1–56.

Ord, J., Lunn, D., & Reynard, J. (2003). Bladder management and risk of bladder stone formation in spinal cord injured patients. *Journal of Urology, 170*(5), 1734–1737.

Pilloni, S., Krhut, J., Mair, D., et al. (2005). Intermittent catheterisation in older people: A valuable alternative to indwelling catheterization. *Age and Ageing, 34,* 57–60.

Prevention of catheter-associated urinary tract infections. (2008, January 31). In: *Betsy Lehman Center for Patient Safety and Medical Error Reduction, JSI Research and Training Institute, Inc. Prevention and control of healthcare-associated infections in Massachusetts. Part 1: Final recommendations of the Expert Panel* (pp. 83–89). Boston: Massachusetts Department of Public Health;. Retrieved on May 11, 2012, from http://www.guideline.gov/content.aspx?id=12923

Ramakrishnan, K., & Mold, J. W. (2005). Urinary catheters: A review. *Internet Journal of Family Practice, 3*(2). Retrieved May 9, 2012, from http://www.ispub.com/journal/the-internet-journal-of-family-practice/volume-3-number-2/urinary-catheters-a-review.html

Saint Jude's Children's Research Hospital. (2004). Collecting urine cultures from infant girls. Do you know. . . An educational series for patients and their families. Retrieved March 3, 2013, from http://www.stjude.org/SJFile/sedation_collecting_urine_cultures_infant_girls.pdf.

Sampselle, C.M., Wyman, J.G., Thomas, K.K., et al. (2006). Evidence-based clinical practice guideline: Continence for women. *Journal of Obstetric and Neonatal Nurses, 29*(1), 18–26.

Scanlon, V. C., & Sanders, T. (2011). *Essentials of anatomy and physiology,* (6th ed.). Philadelphia: F. A. Davis.

Schröder, A., Abrams, P., Andersson, K. E., et al. (2009, March). Incontinence in women. In: *Guidelines on urinary incontinence* (pp. 28–43). Arnhem, The Netherlands: European Association of Urology (EAU).

Schumm, K., & Lam, T. B. (2008). Types of urethral catheters for management of short-term voiding problems in hospitalised adults. *Cochrane Database of Systematic Reviews, 16*(2), Art. No.: CD004013.

Siegel, J. D., Rhinehart, E., Jackson, M., et al. (2007). *Healthcare Infection Control Practices Advisory Committee. Guideline for*

isolation precautions: Preventing transmission of infectious agents in healthcare settings, 2007. Standard precautions. Atlanta, GA: Centers for Disease Control and Prevention. Retrieved May 10, 2012, from http://www.cdc.gov/hicpac/2007ip/2007 isolationprecautions.html

Stuempfle, K. J. & Drury, D. G. (2003). Comparison of 3 methods to compare urine specific gravity in college athletes. *Journal of Athletic Training, 38*(4), 315–319.

Sublett, C. M. (2008). Adding to the evidence base: A review of two qualitative studies. *Urologic Nursing, 28*(2), 130–131.

Thiedke, C. C. (2003). Nocturnal enuresis. *American Family Physician, 67*(7), 1499–1506. Retrieved March 2, 2013, from http://www.aafp.org/afp/20030401/1499.html

Thompson, J. & Manore, M. (2012). *Nutrition and health: An applied approach* (3rd ed.). San Francisco: Benjamin Cummings.

Urinary Continence Guideline Panel (UCGP). (1992). *Urinary incontinence in adults.* Rockville, MD: Agency for Healthcare Policy and Research, Public Health Service, U.S. Department of Health and Human Services.

VanKampen, M., DeWeerdt, W., VanPoppel, H., et al. (2000, January 8). Effect of pelvic-floor re-education on duration and degree of incontinence after radical prostatectomy: A randomised controlled trial. *The Lancet, 355,* 98–102.

Van Leeuwen, A., Kranpitz, T., & Smith, L. (2010). *Davis's comprehensive handbook of laboratory and diagnostic tests with nursing implications.* Philadelphia: F. A. Davis.

Van Leeuwen, A., Poelhuis-Leth, D., & Bladh, M. (2011). *Davis's comprehensive handbook of laboratory and diagnostic tests with nursing implications* (4th ed.). Philadelphia: F. A. Davis.

Wilde, M. H., & Getliffe, K. (2006). Urinary catheter care for older adults. *Annals of Long-term Care: Clinical Care and Aging, 8*(14), Retrieved June 1, 2011, from http://www.annalsoflongtermcare.com/article/6051

Wilson, M. (2004). Urinary incontinence: A treatise on gender, sexuality, and culture. *Clinical Geriatric Medicine, 20*(3), 565–570.

Wong, E. S., & Hooten, T. M. (1981, updated 2005). Guideline for prevention of catheter-associated urinary tract infections. Centers for Disease Control and Prevention (CDC). Retrieved December 10. 2009, from http://hica.jp/cdcguideline/UTI.htm

Wooten, T. M., Bradley, S. F., Cardenas, D. D., et al. (2010, March 1). Diagnosis, prevention, and treatment of catheter-associated infection in adults: 2009 international clinical practice guidelines from the Infectious Diseases Society of America. *Clinical Infectious Diseases, 50*(5), 625–663.

Wound, Ostomy, and Continence Nurses Society. (2008). Catheter associated urinary tract infections (CAUTI) [Fact sheet]. Retrieved June 3, 2011, from http://www.wocn.org/pdfs/WOCN_Library/Fact_Sheets/cauti_fact_sheet.pdf

Wyman, J. F. (2003). Treatment of urinary incontinence in men and older women. *American Journal of Nursing, 103*(Suppl. 3), 26–35.

CHAPTER 31

American Association of Neuroscience Nurses. (2007). *Care of the patient with seizures.* Glenview, IL: Author. Retrieved August 29, 2011, from http://www.aann.org/pubs/cpg/seizures.pdf

Borson, S., Scanlan, J., Brush, M., et al. (2000). The Mini-Cog: A cognitive "vital signs" measure for dementia screening in multi-lingual elderly. *International Journal of Geriatric Psychiatry, 15*(11), 1021–1027.

Braun, C., Stangler, T., Narveson, J., et al. (2009). Animal-assisted therapy as a pain relief intervention for children. *Complementary Therapies in Clinical Practice, 15*(2), 105–109.

Bulechek, G., Butcher, H., & Dochterman, J. (2012). *Nursing interventions classification (NIC)* (6th ed.). St. Louis, MO: C. V. Mosby.

Burtin, M., & Doree, C. (2009). Ear drops for the removal of ear wax. *Cochrane Database of Systematic Reviews,* Issue 1. Art. No.: CD0043326. doi:10.1002/14651858.CD004326.pub2 Retrieved September 2, 2011, from http://www.mrw.inter science.wiley.com/cochrane/clsysrev/articles/CD004326/frame.html

Epilepsy Foundation of America. (n.d). About epilepsy. Retrieved September 6, 2011, from http://www.epilepsyfoundation.org/about/

Foundation of the American Academy of Ophthalmology. (2007). Eye exams: What to expect. Retrieved August 26, 2011, from Eyecare America, http://www.eyecareamerica.org/

Gleeson, M., & Higgins, A. (2009). Touch in mental health nursing: An exploratory study of nurses' views and perceptions. *Journal of Psychiatric & Mental Health Nursing, 16*(4), 382–389.

Gleeson, M., & Timmins, F. (2005). A review of the use and clinical effectiveness of touch as a nursing intervention. *Clinical Effectiveness in Nursing, 9*(1–2), 69–77.

Harkin, H. (n.d.). Ear care guidance from the NHS Modernisation Agency. Retrieved March 3, 2013, from http://www.wales.nhs.uk/sitesplus/documents/863/Package-for-GPs-no-PIL.PDF

Hooker, S. D., Freeman, L. H., & Stewart, P. (2002). Pet therapy research: A historical review. *Holistic Nursing Practice, 17*(1), 17–23.

Huntley, A. (2008). Documenting level of consciousness. *Nursing 2008, 38*(8), 63–64.

Jayasekara, R. (2008). Dementia: Wandering. Evidence summaries—Joanna Briggs Institute. Retrieved September 2, 2011, from http://www.guideline.gov/summary/summary.aspx?ss=15&doc_id=13192&nbr=6688

Jirovetz, L., Buchbauer, G., Stoilova, I., et al. (2006). Chemical composition and antioxidant properties of clove leaf essential oil. *Journal of Agricultural and Food Chemistry, 54*(17), 6303–6307.

Johnson, M., Bulechek, G., Dochterman, J. M., et al. (2012). *NOC and NIC Linkages to NANDA-I and Clinical Conditions* (3rd ed.). St. Louis, MO: C. V. Mosby.

The Joint Commission (TJC). (2008). *2008 hospital accreditation standards.* Oakbrook Terrace, IL: Author.

Kyle, G. (2005). Evaluating the effectiveness of aromatherapy in reducing levels of anxiety in palliative care patients: Results of a pilot study. *Complementary Therapies in Clinical Practice, 12*(2), 148–155.

McCaffrey, R., Thomas, D., & Kinzelman, A. (2009). The effects of lavender and rosemary essential oils on test-taking anxiety among graduate nursing students. *Holistic Nursing Practice, 23*(2), 88.

Moorhead, S., Johnson, M., Maas, M., et al. (2012). *Nursing outcomes classification (NOC)* (5th ed.). St. Louis, MO: C. V. Mosby.

NANDA International (NANDA-I). (2012). *Nursing diagnoses: Definitions and classification 2012–2014.* Ames, IA: Wiley-Blackwell.

Polan, E., & Taylor, D. (2007). *Journey across the life span: Human development and health promotion* (3rd ed.). Philadelphia: F. A. Davis.

Roland, P. S., Smith, T. L., Schwartz, S. R., et al. (2008). Clinical practice guideline: Cerumen impaction. *Otolaryngology—Head and Neck Surgery, 139,* S1–S21.

Scanlon, V., & Sanders, T. (2007). *Essentials of anatomy and physiology* (6th ed.). Philadelphia: F. A. Davis.

Sonboli, A., Babakhani, B., & Mehrabian, A. (2006). Antimicrobial activity of six constituents of essential oil from *Salvia. Zeitschrift für Naturforschung, 61*(3–4), 160–164.

Wiegand, L. (2005). *AACN procedure manual for critical care.* Philadelphia: W. B. Saunders.

Zervakis, J., & Schiffman, S. (2004). Adverse taste side effects of cardiovascular medications. *Geriatric Times, 5*(1), 405–413.

CHAPTER 32

Agency for Healthcare Policy and Research (AHCPR), Public Health Service, U.S. Department of Health and Human Services. (1994). *The clinical practice guideline for the management of cancer pain.* AHCPR Publication No. 94-0592. Rockville, MD: Author.

American Academy of Pain Management. (2008, September 8–11). Annual meeting of the American Academy of Pain Management (AAPM), Nashville, TN.

American Academy of Pediatrics (AAP), Committee on Psychological Aspects of Child and Family Health and American Task Force on Pain in Infants, Children, and Adolescents. (2001). The assessment and management of acute pain in infants, children and adolescents. *Pediatrics, 108*(3), 793–797.

American Geriatrics Society, Panel on Persistent Pain in Older Persons. (2002). The management of persistent pain in older persons. *Journal of the American Geriatric Society, 50*(Suppl. 6), S205–S224.

American Geriatrics Society, Panel on Persistent Pain in Older Persons. (2009). Pharmacological management of persistent pain in older persons. *Journal of the American Geriatrics Society, 57*(8), 1331–1346.

American Pain Society. (1994). Part III: Pain terms, a current list with definitions and notes on usage. In: H. Merskey & N. Bogduk; and IASP Task Force on Taxonomy (Eds.), *Classification of chronic pain* (2nd ed.). Seattle: IASP Press.

American Pain Society. (2009). *Principles of analgesic use in the treatment of acute pain and cancer pain* (6th ed.). Glenview, IL: Author.

American Pain Society. (2008). *Principles of analgesic use in the treatment of acute pain and cancer pain* (6th ed.). Shobie, IL: Author.

American Society for Pain Management Nursing. (n.d.) Position papers. Retrieved September 6, 2011, from http://www.aspmn.org/Organization/position_papers.htm

Baldridge, K., & Andrasik, F. (2010). Pain assessment in people with intellectual or developmental disabilities. *American Journal of Nursing, 110*(12), 28–37.

Barnes, P. M., Bloom, B., & Nahin, R. L. (2008). Complementary and alternative medicine use among adults and children: United States, 2007. *National Health Statistics Reports,* no. 12. Hyattsville, MD: National Center for Health Statistics.

Berdine, H. J. (2002). The fifth vital sign: Cornerstone of a new pain management strategy. *Disease and Management Outcomes, 10*(3), 155–156.

Best practices: Evidence-based nursing procedures (pp. 117–124). (2008). Philadelphia: Lippincott Williams & Wilkins.

Bishop, F. L., Yardley. L., & Lewith, G. T. (2008). Treat or treatment: A qualitative study analyzing patients' use of complementary and alternative medicine. *American Journal of Public Health, 98*(9), 1700–1705.

Bjoro, K., Bergen, K., & Herr, K. (2008). Tools for pain assessment in older adults with end-stage dementia. *American Academy of Hospice and Palliative Medicine Bulletin, 9*(3), 1–4.

Bulechek, G., Butcher, G., & Dochterman, J. (Eds.). (2012). *Nursing interventions classification (NIC)* (6th ed.). St. Louis, MO: C. V. Mosby.

Cassileth, B., Trevisan, C., & Jyothirmai, G. (2007). Complementary therapies for cancer pain. *Current Pain & Headache Reports, 11*(4), 265–269.

Christo, P. J. (2009, January 31). *Clinical concepts in pain and aging.* Paper presented at the annual meeting of the American Academy of Pain Management (AAPM), Honolulu, HI.

Cohen, M., Weber, R., & Moss, J. (2006, April 1). Patient-controlled analgesia: Making it safer for patients. Institute of Safe Medicine Practice (ISMP). Retrieved May 14, 2012, from http://www.ismp.org/profdevelopment/PCA Monograph.pdf

D'Arcy, Y. (2008a, January). Keep your patient safe during PCA. *Nursing, 38*(1), 50–55.

D'Arcy, Y. (2008b, February). What you need to know about opioids. *Nursing, 38*(2), 26–28.

Ernst, E. (2008). *Complementary therapies for pain management: An evidence-based approach.* St. Louis, MO: Elsevier.

Evans, D. (2002). The effectiveness of music as an intervention for hospital patients: A systematic review. *Journal of Advanced Nursing, 37*(1), 8–18.

Evans, F. J. (1974). The placebo response in pain reduction. *Advances in Neurology, 4,* 289–296.

Flaherty, E. (2007). Pain assessment in older adults. *Try this: Best practices in nursing care to older adults, 7,* 1–2. The Hartford Institute for Geriatric Nursing, New York University College of Nursing. Retrieved March 7, 2011, from http://consultgerirn.org/uploads/File/trythis/try_this_2.pdf

Hagle, M., Lehr, V., Brubakken, K., et al. (2004). Respiratory depression in adult patients with intravenous patient-controlled analgesia. *Orthopedic Nursing, 28*(1), 18–25.

Hart, J. (2008, April 1). Complementary therapies for chronic pain management. *Alternative and Complementary Therapies, 14*(2), 64–68.

Herr, K. (2004). Evidence-based assessment of acute pain in older adults: Current nursing practices and perceived barriers. *Clinical Journal of Pain, 20,* 331–340.

Herr, K., Bjoro, K., & Decker S. (2006). Tools for assessment of pain in nonverbal older adults with dementia: A state-of-the-science review. *Journal of Pain Symptom Management, 31*(2), 170–192.

Herr, K., Coyne, P. J., Key, T., et al. (2006). Pain assessment in the nonverbal patient: Position statement with clinical practice recommendations. *Pain Management Nursing, 7*(2), 44–52.

Hockenberry, M. J., & Wilson, D. (2009). *Wong's essentials of pediatric nursing* (8th ed.). St. Louis, MO: C. V. Mosby.

Horgas, A. L. (2007). Assessing pain in older adults with dementia. *Try this: Best practices for nursing care for hospitalized older adults, D2,* 1–2. The Hartford Institute for Geriatric Nursing and the Alzheimer's Association. Retrieved March 7, 2011, from http://consultgerirn.org/uploads/File/trythis/try_this_d2.pdf

Institute for Clinical Systems Improvement (ICSI). (2011, November). *Health care guideline: Assessment and management of acute pain* (5th ed.). Retrieved September 10, 2011, from https://www.icsi.org/_asset/bw798b/ChronicPain-Interactive1111.pdf

Jacox, A. (1994). Management of cancer pain (AHCPR Publication No. 94-0592). Rockville, MD: Agency for Healthcare Policy and Research, Public Health Service, U.S. Department of Health and Human Services.

Jarqyna, D., Jungquist, C., Pasero, C., et al. (2011). American Society for Pain Management nursing guidelines on monitoring for opioid-induced sedation and respiratory depression. *Pain Management Nursing, 12*(3), 118–145.e10.

Johnson, M., Moorhead, S., Bulechek, G., et al. (2012). *NOC and NIC linkages to NANDA-I and clinical conditions* (3rd ed.). St. Louis, MO.

Lewandowski, C. S., Good, M., & Draucker, C. B. (2005). Changes in the meaning of pain with the use of guided imagery. *Pain Management Nursing, 6*(2), 58–67.

Mailis-Gagnon, A. F., Sandoval, J. A., & Taylor, R. S. (2009, January 21). Spinal cord stimulation for chronic pain. *Cochrane Database of Systematic Reviews*, Issue 3. Art. No.: CD003783. DOI: 10.1002/14651858.CD003783.pub2. Retrieved March 3, 2013, from http://www.cochrane.org/reviews/en/ab003783.html

McCaffery, M. (1968). *Nursing practice theories related to cognition, bodily pain, and man-environment interactions.* Los Angeles: UCLA Students Store.

McCaffery, M., & Pasero, C. (1999). *Pain clinical manual* (2nd ed.). St. Louis, MO: C. V. Mosby.

Melzack, R., & Wall, P. (1965). Pain mechanisms: A new theory. *Science, 150,* 971–979.

Merskey, H. (1979). Pain terms: A list with definitions and notes on usage recommended by the IASP Subcommittee on Taxonomy. *Pain, 6*(3), 249–252.

Merskey, H., & Bogduk, N. (Eds.). (1994). *Classification of chronic pain* (2nd ed.). Seattle, WA: International Association for the Study of Pain.

Molony, S. L., Kobayashi, M., Holleran, E. A., et al. (2005, March). Assessing pain as a fifth vital sign in long-term care facilities: Recommendations from the field. *Journal of Gerontological Nursing, 31*(3), 16–24.

NANDA International (NANDA-I). (2011). *Nursing diagnoses: Definitions and classification 2012-2014*, Oxford: Wiley-Blackwell.

National Guideline Clearinghouse (NGC). (2003; updated 2009, May 1). Assessment and management of pain. Rockville, MD: Author. Retrieved September 5, 2011, from http://www.guideline.gov/summary/summary.aspx?doc_id=11507&nbr=005960&string=assessment+and+%22Management+of+pain%22

National Institutes of Health (NIH), National Institute on Drug Abuse. (2005, revised.). Research report series: Prescription drugs abuse and addiction. Retrieved August 28, 2011, from http://www.nida.nih.gov/ResearchReports/Prescription/prescription.html

O'Rourke, D. (2004). The measurement of pain in infants, children, and adolescents: From policy to practice. *Physical Therapy, 84*(6), 560–570.

Pasero, C. (1997). Pain ratings: The fifth vital sign. *American Journal of Nursing, 97*(2), 15–16.

Pasero, C., Manworren, R. C. B., & McCaffery, M. (2008). IV opioid range orders for acute pain management. *American Journal of Nursing, 107*(2), 52–60.

Pasero, C., & McCaffery, M. (2010). *Pain assessment and pharmacological management.* Philadelphia: Elsevier Mosby.

Patterson, C. (2008). Six myths about opioid use. *Nursing2008, 38*(11), 60–61.

Schneider, J. P. (2006–2007, Winter). Opioids, pain management, and addiction. *Pain Practitioner, 16,* 17–24.

Shin, S. Y., & Kolanowski. A. M. (2010). Best evidence of psychosocially focused nonpharmacologic therapies for symptom management in older adults with osteoarthritis. *Pain Management Nursing, 11*(4), 234–244.

Slater, R., Cantarella, A., Fanck, L., et al. (2008, June 24th). How well do clinical pain assessment tools reflect pain in infants? *PLoS Medicine, 5*(6), e129. Retrieved September 5, 2011, from http://www.asianhhm.com/Knowledge_bank/research_insights/clinical_pain_assessment_tools_reflect_pain.htm

Smith, C. A., Collins, C. T., Cyna, A. M., et al. (2006). Complementary and alternative therapies for pain management in labour. *Cochrane Database of Systematic Reviews*, Issue 4. Retrieved September 5, 2011, from http://www.cochrane.org/reviews/en/ab003521.html

Spies, C., Rehberg, B., Schug, S. A., et al. (2009). *Pocket guide to pain management.* New York: Springer.

Spragud, L. J., Piira, T., & Baeyer, C. L. (2003). Children's self-report of pain intensity. *American Journal of Nursing, 103*(12), 62–64.

Taddio, A., Katz, J., Hersich, A., et al. (1997). Effects of neonatal circumcision on pain response during subsequent routine vaccination. *The Lancet, 349,* 599–603.

Takai, Y., Yamamoto-Mitani, N. Okamoto, Y., et al. (2010). Literature review of pain prevalence among older residents of nursing homes. *Pain Management Nursing, 11*(4), 209–223.

Warden, V., Hurley, A. C., & Volicer, L. Development and psychometric evaluation of the Pain Assessment in Advanced Dementia (PAINAD) scale. *Journal of the American Medical Directors Association, 4*(1), 9–15.

Webster, L. R., & Webster, R. M. (2005). Predicting aberrant behaviors in opioid-treated patients: Preliminary validation of the Opioid Risk Tool. *Pain Medicine, 6*(6), 432–442.

World Health Organization (WHO). (1990). *Cancer pain relief and palliative care: Report of a WHO expert committee.* WHO Technical Report series, No. 804. Geneva, Switzerland: Author.

CHAPTER 33

American College of Sports Medicine (ACSM). (2009, February). Appropriate physical activity intervention strategies for weight loss and prevention of weight regain for adults. Position stand. *Medicine & Science in Sports & Exercise, 41*(12). Retrieved September 29, 2011, from http://www.acsm-msse.org/pt/pt-core/template-journal/msse/media/0209.pdf

American Nurses Association (ANA). (2006). Preventing back injuries: Safe patient handling and movement. Retrieved October 1, 2011, from http://www.nursingworld.org/MainMenuCategories/OccupationalandEnvironmental/occupationalhealth/OccupationalResources/PreventingBackInjuries.aspx

Borg, G. (1998). *Borg's perceived exertion and pain scales.* Stockholm, Sweden: Human Kinetics.

Bulechek, G., Butcher, H., & Dochterman, J. (2012). *Nursing interventions classification (NIC)* (6th ed.). St. Louis, MO: C. V. Mosby.

Bunting-Perry, L. K. (2006, April). Palliative care in Parkinson's disease: Implications for neuroscience nursing. *Journal of Neuroscience Nursing, 38*(2), 106–113.

Caap-Ahlgren, M., Lannerheim, L., & Dehlin, O. (2002). Older Swedish women's experiences of living with symptoms related to Parkinson's disease. *Journal of Advanced Nursing, 39*(1), 87–95.

Caspersen, C. J., Powell, K. E., & Christenson, G. M. (1985). Physical activity, exercise, and physical fitness: Definitions and distinctions for health-related research. *Public Health Report, 100*(2), 126–131.

Centers for Disease Control and Prevention (CDC). (2008, updated 2011). Physical activity for everyone. Retrieved October 2, 2011, from http://www.cdc.gov/physical activity/everyone/guidelines/olderadults.html

Collins, J. W., Nelson, A., Sublet, V. (2006). Safe lifting and movement of nursing home residents (DHHS [NIOSH] Publication No. 2006-117). Department of Health and Human Services

Foster, C. (2004). "Talk test" measures exercise intensity. *Medicine & Science in Sports & Exercise, 36*(9), 1632–1636.

Frimel, T. N., Sinacore, D. R., & Villareal, D. T. (2008, July). Exercise attenuates the weight-loss induced reduction in muscle mass in frail obese older adults. *Medicine & Science in Sport & Exercise, 40*(7), 1213–1219.

Herlofson, K., & Larsen, J. P. (2003). The influence of fatigue on health-related quality of life in patients with Parkinson's disease. *Acta Neurologica Scandinavica, 107*, 1–6.

Jitramontree, N. (2002, updated 2007, August). *Evidence-based practice guideline. Exercise promotion: Walking in elders* (p. 57). Iowa City: University of Iowa Gerontological Nursing Interventions Research Center, Research Dissemination Core. Retrieved October 1, 2011, from http://www.guideline. gov/summary/summary.aspx?ss=15&doc_id=10948& nbr=5728

Koukouli, S., Vlachonikolis, I. G., & Philalithis, A. (2002). Socio-demographic factors and self-reported functional status: The significance of social support. *BMC Health Services Research, 2*, 20. [Note: available open source at http://www.biomedcentral.com/1472-6963/2/20]

Maddalozzo, G. F., & Snow, C. M. (2000). High intensity resistance training: Effects on bone in older men and women. *Calcified Tissue International, 66*, 399–404.

Management of osteoporosis in postmenopausal women: 2010 position statement of the North American Menopause Society. (2010). *Menopause, 17*(1), 25–54.

Moorhead, S., Johnson, M., Maas, M., et al. (2008). *Nursing outcomes classification (NOC)* (4th ed.). St. Louis, MO: C. V. Mosby.

National Institutes of Health, National Institute on Aging. (2006, October, updated 2011, June). Exercise and physical activity: Getting fit for life. Retrieved March 1, 2013, from http://www.nia.nih.gov/HealthInformation/Publications/ exercise.htm

National Osteoporosis Foundation. (2010). Calcium: What you should know. Retrieved March 4, 2013, from http:// www.nof.org/aboutosteoporosis/prevention/calcium

Nelson, A., & Baptiste, A. (2004, September 30). Evidence-based practices for safe patient handling and movement. *Online Journal of Issues in Nursing, 9*(3). Retrieved March 1, 2013, from http://www.nursingworld.org/MainMenu Categories/ANAMarketplace/ANAPeriodicals/OJIN/ TableofContents/Volume92004/No3Sept04/Evidence BasedPractices.aspx

Nelson, A., Fragala, G., & Menzel, N. (2003). Myths and facts about back injuries in nursing. *American Journal of Nursing, 103*(2), 32–40.

Occupational Safety and Health Administration, U. S. Department of Labor. (2009). Ergonomics for the prevention of musculoskeletal disorders: Guidelines for nursing homes. OSHA 3182-2009. Retrieved on October 2, 2011, from http:// www.osha.gov/ergonomics/guidelines/nursinghome/ final_nh_guidelines.pdf

Simoes, E. J., Kobau, R., Waterman, B., et al. (2006, December). Associations of physical activity and body mass index with activities of daily living in older adults. *Journal of Community Health, 31*(6), 453–467.

Sunvisson, H., & Ekman, S. (2001). Environmental influences on the experiences of people with Parkinson's disease. *Nursing Inquiry, 8*, 41–50.

Sunvisson, H., Ekman, S., Hagberg, H., et al. (2001). An educational program for individuals with Parkinson's disease. *Scandinavian Journal of Caring Sciences, 15*, 311–317.

Swann, J. (2007). Rheumatoid arthritis: When the body rebels against itself. *Nursing & Residential Care, 9*(5), 222–224.

Taber's cyclopedic medical dictionary (last updated 2009). Taber'sOnline. Retrieved October 17, 2011, from http:// www.tabers.com/tabersonline/ub/view/Tabers/143638/ 8/mobility

U.S. Department of Health and Human Services (USDHHS). (2008, updated 2011). 2008 physical activity guidelines for Americans. Retrieved March 4, 2013, from http://www. health.gov/paguidelines

U.S. Department of Health and Human Services (USDHHS). (2011). *Implementing Healthy People 2020.* Retrieved March 1, 2013, from http://www.healthypeople.gov/2020/ Implement/default.aspx

Wade, D. T., Gage, H., Owen, C., et al. (2003). Multidisciplinary rehabilitation for people with Parkinson's disease: A randomized controlled study. *Journal of Neurology Neurosurgery and Psychiatry, 74*, 158–162.

CHAPTER 34

Alan Guttmacher Institute. (2002, updated 2006, December). Sexual and reproductive health: Women and men. In: *Facts in brief.* Washington, DC: Author.

American Academy of Pediatrics (AAP), Committee on Adolescents. (2001). Care of the adolescent sexual assault victim. *Pediatrics, 107*(6), 1476–1479. Retrieved September 15, 2011, from http://pediatrics.aappublications.org/cgi/ content/full/107/6/1476

American Cancer Society. (2010). Breast awareness and self-exam. Retrieved March 4, 2013, from http://www.cancer. org/Cancer/BreastCancer/MoreInformation/BreastCancer EarlyDetection/breast-cancer-early-detection-acs-recs-bse

American Cancer Society. (2011, January). Testicular self exam. Retrieved March 4, 2013, from http://www. cancer.org/Cancer/TesticularCancer/MoreInformation/ DoIHaveTesticularCancer/do-i-have-testicular-cancer-self-exam

American Geriatrics Society Foundation for Health in Aging. (n.d.). Aging in the know. Sexual problems. Retrieved September 12, 2011, from http://consultgerirn.org/topics/ advance_directives/topic_resources/patient_and_family_ resources/

American Psychiatric Association (APA). (2000). *Diagnostic and statistical manual of mental disorders* (4th ed., text rev.). Washington, DC: Author.

Annon, J. (1974). *The behavioral treatment of sexual problems.* Honolulu, HI: Enabling Systems.

Arena, J. M., & Wallace, M. (2008, updated 2012, July). Sexuality issues in aging: Nursing standard of practice protocol sexuality in older adults. Hartford Institute for Geriatric Nursing. Retrieved March 4, 2013, from http://www.consultgerirn.org/topics/sexuality_issues_in_aging/want_to_know_more

Basson, R. (2001). Using a different model for female sexual response to address women's problematic low sexual desire. *Journal of Sex and Marital Therapy, 27,* 395–403.

Beach, E. K., Maloney, B. H., Plocica, A. R., et al. (1992). The spouse: A factor in recovery after acute myocardial infarction. *Heart & Lung, 21*(1), 30–38.

Beckman, N., Waern, M., & Gustafson, D. (2008). Secular trends in self reported sexual activity and satisfaction in Swedish 70 year olds: Cross sectional survey of four populations, 1971–2001. *BMJ, 337,* A279.

Bulechek, G., Butcher, H., & Dochterman, J. (2012). *Nursing interventions classification (NIC)* (6th ed.). St. Louis, MO: C. V. Mosby.

Centers for Disease Control and Prevention (CDC). (2007a). National Center for Health Statistics Health, 2007 with chartbook trends on the health of Americans. Hyattsville, MD: U.S. Department of Health and Human Services. Retrieved September 15, 2011, from http://www.cdc.gov/nchs/data/hus/hus07.pdf#051

Centers for Disease Control and Prevention (CDC). (2007b). National Center for Health Statistics Sexually Transmitted Diseases Surveillance, 2007. Hyattsville, MD: U.S. Department of Health and Human Services. Retrieved March 4, 2013, from http://www.cdc.gov/std/stats07/natoverview.htm

Centers for Disease Control and Prevention (CDC). (2009). *National Vital Statistics Reports, 58*(1). Retrieved March 4, 2013, from http://www.cdc.gov/nchs/products/nvsr.htm#vol58

Centers for Disease Control and Prevention (CDC). (2010, December 17). Sexually transmitted treatment guidelines, 2010. *Morbidity and Mortality Weekly Report, 59*(RR-12), 1–110. Retrieved March 4, 2013, from http://www.cdc.gov/mmwr/pdf/rr/rr5912.pdf

Cooper, A., Skinner, J., Nherera, L., et al. (2007). *Clinical guidelines and evidence review for post myocardial infarction: Secondary prevention in primary and secondary care for patients following a myocardial infarction.* London: National Collaborating Centre for Primary Care and Royal College of General Practitioners.

Davidson, M. R. (2004). Sexually transmitted infections: Screening and counseling. *Clinician Reviews, 14*(6), 56–62.

DeBusk, R., Drory, Y., Goldstein, I., et al. (2000). Management of sexual dysfunction in patients with cardiovascular disease: Recommendations of the Princeton Consensus Panel. *American Journal of Cardiology, 86*(2), 175–181.

EngenderHealth. (2007). Sexual response and sexual practices: Normal changes in response with aging. *Sexuality and Sexual Health: An Online MiniCourse.* Retrieved March 4, 2013, from http://www.engenderhealth.org/res/onc/sexuality/response/miw/pg5.html

Friedman, S. (2000). Cardiac disease, anxiety and sexual functioning. *American Journal of Cardiology, 86* (Suppl. 2A), 46F–50F.

Homor, G. (2010). Child sexual abuse: Consequences and implications. *Journal of Pediatric Health Care, 24*(6), 358–364.

Hyde, J. S., & DeLamater, J. D. (2008). *Understanding human sexuality* (10th ed.). Columbus, OH: McGraw-Hill.

Iannacchione, M. A. (2004). The vagina dialogues: Do you douche? *American Journal of Nursing, 104*(1), 40–46.

Jackson, G. (2000). Sexual intercourse and stable angina pectoris. *American Journal of Cardiology, 86*(Suppl. 2A), 35F–37F.

Kaufman, J., & American Academy of Pediatrics, Committee on Adolescence. (2008). Care of the adolescent sexual assault victim. *Pediatrics, 122*(2), 462–470.

Kennedy-Malone, L., Fletcher, K., & Plank, L. (2004). *Management guidelines for nurse practitioners working with older adults.* Philadelphia: F. A. Davis.

Klein, F., Sepekoff, B., & Wolf, T. J. (1985, Spring). Sexual orientation: A multi-variable dynamic process. *Journal of Homosexuality, 11*(1–2), 35–49.

Kleinplatz, P. J. (2008). Sexuality and older people. *BMJ, 337,* a239.

Laumann, E. O., Paik, A., Glasser, D. B., et al. (2006). A cross-national study of subjective sexual well-being among older women and men: Findings from the Global Study of Sexual Attitudes and Behaviors. *Archives of Sexual Behavior, 35,* 145–161.

Lindau, S. T., Schumm, P., Laumann, E. O., et al. (2007). A study of sexuality and health among older adults in the United States. *New England Journal of Medicine, 357*(8), 762–774. Retrieved March 4, 2013, from http://www.nejm.org/doi/full/10.1056/NEJMoa067423

Masters, W. H., & Johnson, V. E. (1966). *Human sexual response.* Philadelphia. Lippincott Williams & Wilkins.

Miner, M. M. (2006). Sexual activity after myocardial infarction: When to resume the use of erectogenic drugs. *Current Sexual Health Reports, 3*(1), 30–34.

Moorhead, S., Johnson, M., Maas, M., et al. (Eds.). (2008). *Nursing outcomes classification (NOC)* (4th ed.). St. Louis, MO: C. V. Mosby.

Moser, D. K. (2007). The rust of life: Impact of anxiety on cardiac patients. *American Journal of Critical Care, 16*(4), 361–369. Retrieved May 16, 2012, from http://ajcc.aacnjournals.org/content/16/4/361.abstract

Muller, J. E. (2000). Triggering of cardiac events by sexual activity: Findings from a case-crossover analysis. *American Journal of Cardiology, 86* (Suppl. 2A), 14F–18F.

Parashar, S., Rumsfeld, J. S., Reid, K. J., et al. (2008). Impact of depression on sex differences in outcome after myocardial infarction. *Circulation: Cardiovascular Quality and Outcomes, 2,* 33–40.

Penhollow, T. M., Young, M., & Denny, G. (2009, January/February). Predictors of quality of life, sexual intercourse, and sexual satisfaction in older adults. *American Journal of Health Education, 40*(1), 13–22.

Rennison, C. M., & Rand, M. R. (2008). *Crime victimization, 2007: Findings from the National Crime Victimization Survey.* Washington, DC: Bureau of Justice Statistics, U.S. Department of Justice. Retrieved March 4, 2013, from http://bjs.ojp.usdoj.gov/index.cfm?ty=dcdetail&iid=245

Rodgers, J. E. (2003). *Sex: A natural history.* New York: Times Books.

Running, A., & Berndt, A. (2003). *Management guidelines for nurse practitioners working in family practice.* Philadelphia: F. A. Davis.

Salaman, M. (2008). Sex after a heart attack—for men: Be careful with performance enhancing drugs. About.com: Heart Disease. Retrieved March 4, 2013, from http://heartdisease. about.com/lw/Health-Medicine/Conditions-and-diseases/ Sex-after-a-Heart-Attack-for-Men.htm

Stanley, M., Blaire, K. A., & Beare, P. G. (2005). *Gerontological nursing: Promoting successful aging with older adults* (3rd ed.). Philadelphia: F. A. Davis.

Stehle, B. F. (1985). *Incurably romantic*. Philadelphia: Temple University Press.

Steinke, E. E. (2000). Sexual counseling after myocardial infarction. *American Journal of Nursing, 100*(12), 38–43.

Steinke, E. E. (2002). A videotape intervention for sexual counseling after myocardial infarction. *Heart & Lung, 31*(5), 348–354.

Steinke, E. E., & Patterson-Midgley, P. (1996). Sexual counseling of MI patients: Nurses' comfort, responsibility, and practice. *Dimensions of Critical Care Nursing, 15*(4), 216–223.

Taverner, W. (2007). *Taking sides: Clashing views in human sexuality*. New York: McGraw-Hill.

U.S. Department of Health and Human Services, Centers for Disease Control and Prevention, National Center for Health Statistics. (2006, updated 2010). Recent trends in teenage pregnancy in the United States, 1990–2002. Retrieved March 4, 2013, from http://www.cdc.gov/nchs/data/ hestat/teenpreg1990-2002/teenpreg1990-2002.htm

Wallace, M. A. (2008). Assessment of sexual health in older adults. *American Journal of Nursing, 108*(7), 52–60.

World Health Organization (WHO). (2002). Gender and reproductive rights. WHO draft working definition, October 2002. Retrieved March 4, 2013, from http://www. who.int/reproductive-health/gender/glossary.html

World Health Organization (WHO). (2010). Female genital mutilation [Fact sheet #241]. Retrieved September 12, 2011, from http://www.who.int/mediacentre/factsheets/ fs241/en/

Zucker, K. J. (2000). Gender identity disorder. In: A. J. Sameroff, M. Lewis, & S. M. Miller (Eds.), *Handbook of developmental psychopathology* (2nd ed., pp. 671–686). New York: Plenum.

CHAPTER 35

American Sleep Apnea Association. (n.d.). Sleep apnea. Retrieved March 4, 2013, from http://www.sleepapnea. org/learn/sleep-apnea.html

Ball, E., & Caivano, C. K. (2008). Internal medicine: Guidance to the diagnosis and management of restless legs syndrome. *Southern Medical Journal, 101*(6), 631–634.

Birath, J. B., & Martin, J. L. (2008). Common sleep problems affecting older adults. *Annals of Long-Term Care, 12*. Retrieved March 4, 2013, from http://www.annalsoflongtermcare. com/article/8100

Bulechek, G., Butcher, H., & Dochterman, J. (2012). *Nursing interventions classification (NIC)* (6th ed.). St. Louis, MO: C. V. Mosby.

Chee, M. W., & Chuah, L. Y. (2008). Functional neuroimaging insights into how sleep and sleep deprivation affect memory and cognition. *Current Opinion in Neurology, 21*(4), 417–423.

Cohen, G. (2004). *American Academy of Pediatrics guide to your child's sleep*. New York: Villard Books.

Cohen, S., Doyle, W. J., Alper, C. M., et al. (2009). Sleep habits and susceptibility to the common cold. *Annals of Family Medicine, 169*(1), 62–67.

Germann, W. J., & Stanfield, C. L. (2008). *Principles of human physiology* (3rd ed.). San Francisco: Benjamin Cummings.

Haesler, E. J. (2004). Effectiveness of strategies to manage sleep in residents of aged care facilities. *Joanna Briggs Institute Reports, 2*(4), 115–183. Retrieved September 28, 2011, from http://www.joannabriggslibrary.org/index. php/jbisrir/article/view/377

Hening, W. A. (2007). Current guidelines and standards of practice for restless legs syndrome. *American Journal of Medicine, 230*(Suppl. 1), S22–27.

Holcomb, S. S. (2006). Recommendations for assessing insomnia. *Nurse Practitioner, 31*(2), 55–60.

Holcomb, S. S. (2007). Putting insomnia to rest. *Nurse Practitioner, 32*(4), 28–34.

Hui, L., Hua, F., Diandong, H., et al. (2007). Effects of sleep and sleep deprivation on immunoglobulins and complement in humans. *Brain, Behavior, & Immunity, 21*(3), 308–310.

Johnson, M., Moorhead, S., Bulechek, C., et al. (2012). *NOC and NIC linkages to NANDA-I and clinical conditions* (3rd ed.). St. Louis, MO: C. V. Mosby.

Kazuo, E., Pickering, T. J., Phil, D., et al. (2008). Short sleep duration as an independent predictor of cardiovascular events in Japanese patients with hypertension. *Archives of Internal Medicine, 168*, 2225–2231.

Lockley, S. W., Barger, L. K., Ayas, N. T., et al. (2007). Effects of health care provider work hours and sleep deprivation on safety and performance. *Joint Commission Journal on Quality & Patient Safety, 33*(Suppl. 11), 7–18.

Marshall, N. S., Glazier, N., & Grunstein, R. R. (2008). Is sleep duration related to obesity? A critical review of the epidemiological evidence. *Sleep Medicine Review, 12*(4), 299–302.

McCance, K. L., & Huether, S. E. (2005). *Pathophysiology: The biologic basis for disease in adults and children* (5th ed.). St. Louis, MO: C. V. Mosby.

Moorhead, S., Johnson, M., & Maas, M., et al. (Eds.). (2012). *Nursing outcomes classification (NOC)* (5th ed.). St. Louis, MO: C. V. Mosby.

National Institute of Neurological Disorders and Stroke (NINDS). (2009, updated 2011, December 28). Narcolepsy [Fact sheet]. National Institutes of Health. Retrieved March 4, 2013, from http://www.ninds.nih.gov/disorders/ narcolepsy/detail_narcolepsy.htm

National Sleep Foundation (NSF). (n.d.). Restless leg syndrome (RLS) and sleep. Retrieved March 4, 2013, from http:// www.sleepfoundation.org/article/sleep-related-problems/ restless-legs-syndrome-rls-and-sleep

National Sleep Foundation (NSF). (2008). 2008 Sleep in America poll: Summary of findings. Retrieved March 4, 2013, from http://www.sleepfoundation.org/article/ press-release/sleep-america-poll-summary-findings

Ong, J. C., Stepanski, E. J., & Gramling, S. E. (2009, February 15). Pain coping strategies for tension-type headache: Possible implications for insomnia. *Journal of Clinical Sleep Medicine, 5*(1), 52–56.

Polan, E., & Taylor, D. (2007). *Journey across the life span* (2nd ed.). Philadelphia: F. A. Davis.

Ranjbaran, Z., Keefer, L., Stepanski, E., et al. (2007). The relevance of sleep abnormalities to chronic inflammatory conditions. *Inflammatory Resource, 56*, 51–57.

Roth, T., Roehrs, T., & Pies, R. (2007). Insomnia: Pathophysiology and implications for treatment. *Sleep Medicine Reviews, 11*(1), 71–79.

Smyth, C. A. (2008). Evaluating sleep quality in older adults. *American Journal of Nursing, 108*(5), 42–50.

Tuller, D. (2004, March 30). Poll finds even babies don't get enough rest. *The New York Times.*

U.S. Department of Health and Human Services (USDHHS), National Institutes of Health (NIH). (2010, November). Explore restless legs syndrome. National Heart Lung and Blood Institute. Retrieved March 4, 2013, from http://www.nhlbi.nih.gov/health/health-topics/topics/rls/

CHAPTER 36

Agency for Healthcare Research and Quality (AHRQ). (1994). *Clinical practice guidelines: Pressure ulcer treatment.* Rockville, MD: Author.

Armstrong, D. G., Attinger, C. E., Boulton, A. J., et al. (2004). Guidelines regarding negative pressure wound therapy (NPWT) in the diabetic foot: Results of the Tucson expert consensus Conference (TECC) on V.A.C. therapy. *Ostomy Wound Management, 50*(4, Suppl. B), 3S–27S.

Armstrong, D. G., Ayello, E. A., Capitulo, K. L., et al. (2008). New opportunities to improve pressure ulcer prevention and treatment: Implications of the CMS inpatient hospital care present on admission indicators/hospital-acquired conditions policy—a consensus paper from the International Expert Wound Care Advisory Panel. *Advances in Skin Wound Care, 21*, 469–70, 472–478.

Association of periOperative Registered Nurses (AORN). (2008). Perioperative standards and recommended practices. Denver: Author.

Atiyeh, B. S., & Hayek, S. N. (2004). An update on management of acute and chronic open wounds: The importance of moist environment on optimal wound healing. *Medicinal Chemistry Reviews, 1*, 111–121.

Autio, L., & Olsen, K. K. (2002). The four S's of wound management: Staples, sutures, steri-strips, and sticky stuff. *Holistic Nursing Practice, 16*(2), 80–88.

Ayello, E. A., & Lyder, C. H. (2008). A new era of pressure ulcer accountability in acute care. *Advances in Skin & Wound Care, 21*(3), 134–140.

Baranoski, S. (2008). Choosing a wound dressing, part 2. *Nursing2008, 38*(2), 14–15.

Bates-Jensen, B. M. (2007). Quality indicators for the care of pressure ulcers in vulnerable elders. *Journal of the American Geriatrics Society* (Suppl. 2), S409–S416.

Bergeron, J. D., Bizjak, G., Le Badour, G., et al. (2009). *First responder* (8th ed.). Upper Saddle River, NJ: Prentice-Hall.

Bergstrom, N., Bennett, M. A., Carlson, C., et al. (1994). *Treatment of pressure ulcers. Clinical practice guideline 15* (AHCPR Publication No. 95–0622.). Rockville, MD: U.S. Department of Health and Human Services, Public Health Service, Agency for Health Care Policy and Research.

Bill, T. J., Ratliff, C. R., Donovan, A. M., et al. (2001). Quantitative swab culture versus tissue biopsy: A comparison in chronic wounds. *Ostomy Wound Management, 47*(1), 34–37.

Black, J., Baharestani, M., Cuddigan, J., et al. (2007a). National Pressure Ulcer Advisory Panel's Updated Pressure Ulcer Staging System. *Dermatology Nursing, 19*(4), 343–349.

Black, J., Baharestani, M., Cuddigan, J., et al. (2007b). National Pressure Ulcer Advisory Panel's Updated Pressure Ulcer Staging System. *Advances in Skin and Wound Care, 20*(5), 269–274.

Branom, R. (2002). Is this wound infected? *Critical Care Nursing Quarterly, 25*(1), 55–62.

Brown, G. (2003). Long-term outcomes of full-thickness pressure ulcers: Healing and mortality. *Ostomy Wound Management, 49*(10), 42–50.

Bryant, R. A., & Nix, D. P. (2006). *Acute and chronic wounds: Current management concepts,* (3rd ed., pp. 100–129). St. Louis, MO: C. V. Mosby Year Book.

Bulechek, F., Butcher, H., & Dochterman, J. (2012). *Nursing interventions classification (NIC)* (6th ed.). St. Louis, MO: C. V. Mosby.

Buss, I. C., Halfens, R. J. G., & Abu-Saad, H. H. (2002). The most effective time interval for repositioning subjects at risk of pressure sore development: A literature review. *Rehabilitation Nursing, 27*(2), 59–63.

Campton-Johnston, S. M., & Wilson, J. A. (2001). Infected wound management: Advanced technologies, moisture-retentive dressings, and die-hard methods. *Critical Care Nursing Quarterly, 24*(2), 64–77.

Chariker, M. (2009). Moisture balance: Exploring options in negative pressure wound therapy. *Skin and Wound Care, 22*(Suppl. 1), 10–12.

Cutting, K. F., & White, R. J. (2005, January). Criteria for identifying wound infection—revised. *Ostomy Wound Management, 51*(1), 28–34.

Dunaway, E., & Goldrick, B. A. (2007, July/August). Sternal wound infections: What every nurse should know. *OR Nurse Online*, 28–34.

European Pressure Ulcer Advisory Panel (EPUAP) and National Pressure Ulcer Advisory Panel (NPUAP). (2009a). Treatment of pressure ulcers: Quick reference guide. Washington, DC: National Pressure Ulcer Advisory Panel.

European Pressure Ulcer Advisory Panel (EPUAP) and National Pressure Ulcer Advisory Panel (NPUAP) (2009b). Prevention and treatment of pressure ulcers: Quick reference guide. Washington DC: National Pressure Ulcer Advisory Panel. Retrieved March 4, 2013, from http://www.npuap.org/Final_Quick_Prevention_for_web_2010.pdf

Fernandez, R., & Griffiths, R. (2010, March 14). Water for wound cleansing. *Cochrane Database of Systematic Reviews,* Issue 1. Art. No.: CD003861. doi:10.1002/14651858. CD003861.pub2

Fletcher, R. K. (1999). Physical and laboratory assessment. In: J. T. Stone, J. F. Wyman, & S. A. Salisbury (Eds.), *Clinical gerontological nursing: A guide to advanced practice* (2nd ed., pp. 85–128). Philadelphia: W. B. Saunders.

Franz, R. A. (2008). Identifying infection in chronic wounds. *Nursing 2008, 37*(7), 73.

Gardner, S. E., Frantz, R. A., Saltzman, C. L., et al. (2006). Diagnostic validity of three swab techniques for identifying chronic wound infection. *Wound Repair Regeneration, 14*(5), 548–557.

Health Leaders Media. (2007, January). New-age wound care solutions drive improved efficiency, outcomes, and patient satisfaction. Retrieved March 4, 2013, from http://www.healthleadersmedia.com/HOM-67349-4625/Newage-wound-care-solutions-drive-improved-efficiency-outcomes

Hess, C. T. (2007). *Clinical guide: Skin and wound care.* Philadelphia: Lippincott Williams & Wilkins.

Immunization Action Coalition. (2007, reviewed 2009, February). Tetanus vaccine questions and answers. Reviewed by Centers for Disease Control and Prevention (CDC). Retrieved October 23, 2011, from http://www.vaccineinformation.org/tetanus/qandavax.asp

Institute for Clinical Systems Improvement (ICSI). (2012, January). Health care protocol: *Pressure ulcer prevention and treatment* (3rd ed.). Bloomington, MN: Author. Retrieved March 4, 2013, from https://www.icsi.org/_asset/6t7kxy/PresUlcerTrmt-Interactive0112.pdf

Joanna Briggs Institute. (2007). Topical skin care in aged care facilities. *Best Practice, 3*(3), 1–4. Retrieved March 4, 2013, from http://connect.jbiconnectplus.org/ViewSourceFile.aspx?0=4346

Joanna Briggs Institute. (2008a). Pressure ulcers: Management of pressure-related tissue damage. *Best Practice*, *12*(3), 1–4. Retrieved March 4, 2013, from http://connect.jbiconnectplus.org/ViewSourceFile.aspx?0=431

Joanna Briggs Institute. (2008b). Pressure ulcers: Prevention of pressure-related damage. *Best Practice, 12*(2), 1–4. Retrieved March 4, 2013, from http://www.westicu.cn/wxd_hxa/exam/exam_pic/2009114162230650.pdf

Kayser-Jones, J. S., Beard, R. L., & Sharpp, T. J. (2009). Dying with a stage IV pressure ulcer. *American Journal of Nursing, 109*(1), 40–49.

Kinetic Concepts Incorporated (KCI). (2007). *V.A.C. therapy clinical guidelines: A reference source for clinicians.* San Antonio, TX: Author.

Kinetic Concepts Incorporated (KCI). (2008). *Basic V.A.C. dressing application pocket guide.* Retrieved October 25, 2011, from http://www.kci1.com/Pocket_Guide.pdf

Krasner, D. L., Shapshak, D., & Hopf, H. W. (2007). Managing wound pain. In: R. A. Bryant & D. P. Nix (Eds.), *Acute and chronic wounds: Current management concepts* (3rd ed., pp. 539–565). St. Louis, MO: C. V. Mosby/Elsevier.

Medica-Rents Co. (2008). *Prospera PRO-I: Negative pressure wound therapy.* Fort Worth, TX: Medica-Rents.

Moore, Z., & Cowman, S. (2007). Effective wound management: Identifying criteria for infection. *Nursing Standard, 21,* 24, 68–76.

Moorhead, S., Johnson, M., & Maas, M., et al. (Eds.). (2012). *Nursing outcomes classification (NOC)* (5th ed.). St. Louis, MO: C. V. Mosby.

Myers, B. A. (2008). *Wound management: principles and practice* (2nd ed.). Upper Saddle River, NJ: Pearson Education.

NANDA International (NANDA-I). (2012). *Nursing diagnoses: Definitions and classification 2012–2014.* Ames, IA: Wiley-Blackwell.

National Guideline Clearinghouse (NGC). (2006; revised 2008, December). Guideline synthesis: Management and treatment of pressure ulcers. Rockville, MD: Author. Retrieved October 25, 2011, from http://www.guideline.gov/summary/summary.aspx?doc_id=11013&nbr=005793&string+Management+and+%22treatment+of+pressure+ulcers%22

National Pressure Ulcer Advisory Panel (NPUAP). (2003). Updated staging system. Retrieved April 18, 2013 from http://www.npuap.org/push3-0.htm

National Pressure Ulcer Advisory Panel (NPUAP). (2007a). NPUAP recommendation on measurement of wound area. *Inside the NPUAP,* Volume 21. Retrieved October 29, 2011, from http://www.npuap.org/Fall07.pdf

National Pressure Ulcer Advisory Panel (NPUAP). (2007b). Pressure ulcer stages revised by NPUAP. Retrieved October 26, 2011, from http://www.npuap.org/pr2.htm

National Pressure Ulcer Advisory Panel (NPUAP). (2007c). Terms and definitions related to support surfaces. Retrieved October 29, 2011, from http://www.npuap.org/NPUAP_S3I_TD.pdf

National Pressure Ulcer Advisory Panel (NPUAP). (2007d). Frequently asked questions. Retrieved October 29, 2011, from http://www.npuap.org/woundinfection.htm

National Pressure Ulcer Advisory Panel (NPUAP). (2007e). Updated staging systems. Retrieved March 4, 2013, from http://www.npuap.org/pr2.htm

National Pressure Ulcer Advisory Panel (NPUAP). (2010). Registered nurse competency-based curriculum: Pressure ulcer prevention. Revision of the 2001 Registered nurse competency-based curriculum: Pressure ulcer prevention. Based on National Pressure Ulcer Advisory Panel and European Pressure Ulcer Advisory Panel. (2009). *Prevention and treatment of pressure ulcers: Clinical practice guideline.* Washington DC: National Pressure Ulcer Advisory Panel.

National Pressure Ulcer Advisory Panel, European Pressure Ulcer Advisory Panel. (2009). Pressure ulcer treatment recommendations. In: *Prevention and treatment of pressure ulcers: Clinical practice guideline* (pp. 51–120). Washington, DC: Author. Retrieved March 4, 2013, from http://www.guideline.gov/content.aspx?id=25139&search=pressure+ulcer+treatment

Pieper, B., Langemo, D., & Cuddigan, J. (2009). Pressure ulcer pain: A systematic literature review and National Pressure Ulcer Advisory Panel white paper. *Ostomy Wound Management, 55*(2). Retrieved March 4, 2013, from http://www.o-wm.com/content/pressure-ulcer-pain-a-systematic-literature-review-and-national-pressure-ulcer-advisory-pane

Rolstad, B. S., & Ovington, L. G. (2007). Principles of wound management. In: R. A. Bryant & D. P. Nix (Eds.), *Acute and chronic wounds: Current management concepts* (3rd ed., pp. 391–426). St. Louis, MO: C. V. Mosby Elsevier.

Russo, C. A., Steiner, C., & Spector, W. (2008, December). Hospitalizations related to pressure ulcers among adults 18 and older, 2006. *HCUP Statistical Brief #64.* Rockville, MD: Agency for Healthcare Research and Quality. Retrieved March 4, 2013, from http://www.hcup-us.ahrq.gov/reports/statbriefs/sb64.pdf

Samson, D., Lefevre, F., & Aronson, N. (2004, December). *Wound-healing technologies: Low-level laser and vacuum-assisted closure. summary* (Evidence Report/Technology Assessment No. 111). AHRQ Publication No. 05-E005-1. December 2004. Rockville, MD: Agency for Healthcare Research and Quality. Retrieved March 4, 2013, from http://archive.ahrq.gov/clinic/epcsums/woundsum.pdf

Siegel, J. D., Rhinehart, E., Jackson, M., et al.; and the Healthcare Infection Control Practices Advisory Committee. (2007, June, updated 2010, September 29). 2007 guideline for isolation precautions: Preventing transmission of infectious agents in healthcare settings. Retrieved March 4, 2013, from http://www.cdc.gov/hicpac/2007IP/2007isolationPrecautions.html

Stotts, N. A., & Gunningberg, L. (2007). Predicting pressure ulcer risk, using the Braden scale with hospitalized older adults; the evidence supports it. *American Journal of Nursing, 107*(11), 40–49.

Sullivan, N., Snyder, D. L., Tipton, K., et al. (2009, May 26; correction 2009, November 12). *Negative pressure wound therapy devices: Technology assessment report.* Rockville, MD: Agency for Healthcare Research and Quality, U.S. Department of Health and Human Services. Retrieved March 4,

2013, from http://www.ahrq.gov/research/findings/ta/negative-pressure-wound-therapy/index.html

Sussman, C., & Bates-Jensen, B. M. (2007). *Wound care: A collaborative practice manual for health care professionals* (3rd ed.). Gaithersburg, MD: Aspen.

3M. (2004, December). 3M surgical tapes and adhesive skin closures. Retrieved October 25, 2011, from http://solutions.3m.com/wps/portal/3M/en_US/wound-care/skin/

U.S. Department of Health and Human Services (UDSHHS). (1992). *Clinical practice guideline. Pressure ulcers in adults: Prediction and prevention* (pp. 16–17) (PPPPUA Publication No. 92-0047). Rockville, MD: U.S. Public Health Service.

U.S. Department of Health and Human Services (UDSHHS). (2010). *Healthy People 2020* objectives. Retrieved March 4, 2013, from hypeople.gov/2020/topicsobjectives2020/default.aspx

Wound, Ostomy and Continence Nurses Society (WOCN) , Wound Committee 2011. (2001, updated 2005, revised 2011). Clean versus sterile dressing techniques for management of chronic wounds [Fact sheet]. Wound, Ostomy and Continence Nurses Society and the Association for Professionals in Infection Control and Epidemiology. Retrieved on March 4, 2013, from http://www.wocn.org/news/76597/

Wound, Ostomy and Continence Nurses Society (WOCNS). (2007). *Position statement: Pressure ulcer staging* (p. 52). Mount Laurel, NJ: Author.

CHAPTER 37

American Academy of Pediatrics.(2011). Pulse oximetery: A viable, readily available screening tool for infants with suspected critical congenital heart disease. Healthy Children. Retrieved January 23, 2012, from http://www.aap.org/en-us/about-the-aap/aap-press-room/Pages/Pulse-Oximetry-a-Viable,-Readily-Available-Screening-Tool-for-Infants-with-Suspected—Critical-Congenital-Heart-Disease.aspx

American Association of Critical-Care Nurses (AACN). (2005). *AACN procedure manual for critical care* (5th ed.). Philadelphia: W. B. Saunders.

American Association of Critical-Care Nurses (AACN). (2007). AACN practice alert. Oral care in the critically ill. Retrieved July 2, 2011, from http://classic.aacn.org/AACN/practiceAlert.nsf/Files/OC/$file/Oral%20Care%20in%20the%20Critically%20Ill%20.pdf

American Association of Critical-Care Nurses (AACN). (2008). AACN practice alert. Ventilator associated pneumonia. Retrieved July 2, 2011, from http://www.aacn.org/WD/Practice/Docs/Ventilator_Associated_Pneumonia_1-2008.pdf

American Association for Respiratory Care (AARC). (2004a). AARC clinical practice guideline. Nasotracheal suctioning—2004 revision and update, 2004. Retrieved July 3, 2011, from http://www.rcjournal.com/cpgs/pdf/09.04.1080.pdf

American Association for Respiratory Care (AARC). (2004b). AARC clinical practice guideline: Resuscitation and defibrillation in the health care setting. *Respiratory Care, 49*(9), 1085–1099.

American Heart Association (AHA). (2005). 2005 American Heart Association guidelines for cardiopulmonary resuscitation and emergency cardiovascular care. Part 3: Overview of CPR; Part 4: Adult basic life support; Part 5: Electrical therapies: automated external defibrillators, defibrillation, cardioversion, and pacing; Part 7.1: *Circulation*

112: IV-12–57. Retrieved July 3, 2011, from http://circ.ahajournals.org/cgi/content/full/112/24_suppl/IV-51?maxtoshow=&hits=10&resultformat=&fulltext=oropharyngeal+airway&searchid=1&firstindex=0&resourcetype=HWCIT#Sec2

American Lung Association (ALA). (2008a). Asthma action plan. Retrieved June 23, 2011, from http://www.lungusa.org/lung-disease/asthma/living-with-asthma/take-control-of-your-asthma/AsthmaActionPlan-JUL2008-high-res.pdf

American Lung Association (ALA). (2008b). Asthma & allergy: Peak flow meters. Retrieved from http://www.lungusa.org/lung-disease/asthma/living-with-asthma/take-control-of-your-asthma/AsthmaActionPlan-JUL2008-high-res.pdf

American Lung Association (ALA). (2010). Trends in lung cancer morbidity and mortality. Retrieved June 19, 2011, from http://www.lungusa.org/finding-cures/our-research/trend-reports/lc-trend-report.pdf

American Lung Association (ALA). (2011). Children and teens. Retrieved June 19, 2011, from http://www.lungusa.org/stop-smoking/about-smoking/facts-figures/children-teens-and-tobacco.html

American Thoracic Society and the Infectious Diseases Society of America. (2005). Guidelines for the management of adults with hospital-acquired, ventilator-associated, and healthcare-associated pneumonia. *American Journal of Respiratory and Critical Care Medicine, 171,* 388–416.

Attin, M., Cardin, S., Dee, V., et al. (2002). An educational project to improve knowledge related to pulse oximetry. *American Journal of Critical Care, 11,* 529–534.

Bailey, P. L., Lu, K. J., Pace, N. L., et al. (2000). Effects of intrathecal morphine on the ventilatory response to hypoxia.*New England Journal of Medicine, 343,* 1228–1234.

Barnett, M. (2005). Tracheostomy management and care. *Journal of Community Nursing, 19*(1), 4–8.

Best practices: Evidence-based nursing procedures (2nd ed., pp. 59–62). (2007). Philadelphia: Lippincott Williams & Wilkins.

Birmingham East and North Primary Care Trust. (2009). Oral and tracheostomy suctioning policy. Retrieved July 1, 2011, from http://www.bpcssa.nhs.uk/policies/_ben%5Cpolicies%5C607.pdf

Bozyk, P., & Hyzy, R. (2008). Modes of mechanical ventilation. *UpToDate for Patients.* Retrieved July 2, 2011, from http://www.uptodate.com/contents/modes-of-mechanical-ventilation

Bulechek, G., Butcher, H., & Dochterman, J. (2012). *Nursing interventions classification (NIC)* (6th ed.). St. Louis, MO: C. V. Mosby.

California Department of Public Health. (2007). Guidelines for collecting and shipping specimens for influenza A (H5N1) diagnostics. Retrieved June 25, 2011, from http://www.co.fresno.ca.us/uploadedFiles/Departments/Public_Health/Divisions/CH/content/CD/content/Diseases/Avian_Flu/H5N1specimencollectionguidelines08.13.07%5B1%5D.pdf

Centers for Disease Control and Prevention (CDC). (n.d., revised 2011, April). Pneumococcal disease in-short. Retrieved June 23, 2011, from http://www.cdc.gov/vaccines/vpd-vac/pneumo/in-short-both.htm#who

Centers for Disease Control and Prevention (CDC). (2004). Guidelines for preventing health-care-associated pneumonia, 2003. *Morbidity and Mortality Weekly Report, 53,* 1–36.

Centers for Disease Control and Prevention (CDC). (2010). Prevention and control of influenza with vaccines. Recommendations of the Advisory Committee on Immunization Practices (ACIP), 2010. Retrieved June 23, 2011, from http://www.cdc.gov/mmwr/preview/mmwrhtml/rr5908a1.htm?s_cid=rr5908a1_e

Centers for Disease Control and Prevention (CDC). (2008). Using over-the-counter cough and cold products in children. Atlanta, GA. Retrieved June 23, 2011, from http://www.fda.gov/ForConsumers/ConsumerUpdates/ucm048515.htm#TipsforParentsandCaregivers

Centers for Disease Control and Prevention (CDC). (2012). Work-related asthma—38 states and District of Columbia, 2006–2009. *Morbidity and Mortality Weekly Report (MMWR)*, *61*(20), 375–378. Retrieved May 27, 2012, from http://www.cdc.gov/mmwr/preview/mmwrhtml/mm6120a4.htm

Centers for Disease Control and Prevention (CDC)/National Center for Health Statistics (NCHS). (2008, last updated February, 2011). In: FastStats, Centers for Disease Control and Prevention (CDC), U.S. Department of Health and Human Services. Retrieved June 19, 2011, from http://www.cdc.gov/nchs/fastats/smoking.htm

Chronic obstructive pulmonary disease. (n.d., last updated 2009, October 9). MedlinePlus: Medical encyclopedia. U.S. National Library of Medicine, National Institutes of Health. Retrieved June 19, 2011, from http://www.nlm.nih.gov/medlineplus/ency/article/000091.htm

Cleveland Clinic. (2009). Tracheal suction guidelines. Retrieved July 13, 2011, from http://my.clevelandclinic.org/services/tracheostomy/hic_tracheal_suction_guidelines.aspx

Coffin, W., Klompas, M., Classen, D., et al.; and the Healthcare-Associated Infections Task Force. (2008). Guideline summary: Strategies to prevent ventilator-associated pneumonia in acute care hospitals. *Infection Control and Hospital Epidemiology*, *29*(Suppl. 1), S31–S40. Rockville, MD: National Guideline Clearinghouse (NGC). Retrieved July 2, 2011, from http://www.guideline.gov/content.aspx?id=13396

Dennis-Rouse, M. D., & Davidson, J. E. (2008). An evidence-based evaluation of tracheostomy care practices. *Critical Care Nursing Quarterly*, *31*(2), 150–160.

Fields, L. (2008). Oral care intervention to reduce incidence of ventilator-associated pneumonia in the neurologic intensive care unit. *Journal of Neuroscience Nursing*, *40*(5), 291–298.

Fiore, A., Shay, D., Broder, K., et al. (2008). Prevention and control of influenza. Recommendations of the Advisory Committee on Immunization Practices (ACIP), 2008. *Morbidity and Mortality Weekly Report*, *57*(RR-07), 1–60. Retrieved June 23, 2011, from http://www.cdc.gov/mmwr/preview/mmwrhtml/rr57e717a1.htm

Fiore, M., Jaén, C., Baker, T., et al. (2008). *Treating tobacco use and dependence: 2008 update*. Clinical Practice Guideline. Rockville, MD: U.S. Department of Health and Human Services. Public Health Service. Retrieved June 23, 2011, from http://www.surgeongeneral.gov/tobacco/treating_tobacco_use08.pdf

Foxwell, A., Roberts, L., Lokuge, K., & Kelly, P. (2011). Transmission of influenza on international flights, May 2009. *Emerging Infectious Diseases*, *17*(7) [serial on the Internet]. Retrieved February 19, 2013, from http://dx.doi.org/10.3201/eid1707.101135.

Green, C. (2000). *Critical thinking in nursing: Case studies across the curriculum*. Upper Saddle River, NJ: Prentice-Hall Health.

Hall, J. E. (2006). *Guyton and Hall textbook of medical physiology* (12th ed.). New York: Saunders.

Hemilä, H., Chalker, E., Treacy, B., et al. (2007). Vitamin C for preventing and treating the common cold. *Cochrane Database of Systematic Reviews*, Issue 3. Art. No.: CD000980. doi:10.1002/14651858CD000980.pub3

Herbal solution hastens resolution of common cold. (2008). Evidence-based medicine. *The Clinical Advisor*, *11*(5), 110.

Hill, E., & Stoneham, M. (2000). Practical applications of pulse oximetry. *Update in Anaesthesia*, *11*(4). Retrieved June 15, 2011, from http://www.nda.ox.ac.uk/wfsa/html/u11/u1104_01.htm

Hugonnet, S., Uckay, I., & Pittet, D. (2007). Staffing level: A determinant of late-onset ventilator-associated pneumonia. *Critical Care*, *11*(4), R80.

Johnson, M., Moorhead, S., Bulechek, C., et al. (2012). *NOC and NIC linkages to NANDA-I and clinical conditions* (3rd ed.). St. Louis, MO: C. V. Mosby.

Johnston, J., Davis, S., & Sherman, J. (n.d.). Care of the child with a chronic tracheostomy. Retrieved November 12, 2011, from http://www.thoracic.org/education/care-of-the-child-with-chronic-tracheostomy/index.php

Kuriakose, A. (2008). Using the synergy model as best practice in endotracheal tube suctioning of critically ill patients. *Dimensions of Critical Care Nursing*, *27*(1), 10–15.

Larsson, I., Sahlsten, M., Segesten, K., et al. (2011). Patients' perceptions of barriers for participation in nursing care. *Scandinavian Journal of Caring Sciences*, *25*(3), 575–582.

Lazzara, D. (2002). Eliminate the air of mystery from chest tubes. *Nursing2002*, *32*(6), 36–45.

Lewarski, J. (2005). Long-term care of the patient with a tracheostomy. *Respiratory Care*, *50*(4), 534–537.

Linde, K., Barrett, B., Bauer, R., et al. (2006). Echinacea for preventing and treating the common cold. *Cochrane Database of Systematic Reviews*, Issue 1. Art. No.: CD000530. doi:10.1002/14651858.CD000530.pub2

Maselli, D., & Restrepo, M. (2011). Strategies in the prevention of ventilator-associated pneumonia. *Therapeutic Advances in Respiratory Disease*, *5*(2), 131–141.

Mateoso, J., Gonzalez, N., Sadaba, M., et al. (2011). Nursing care in the prevention of ventilator-associated pneumonia. *Enferm Intensive*, *22*(1), 22-30.

Moorhead, S., Johnson, M., Maas, M., et al. (2012). *Nursing outcomes classification (NOC)* (5th ed.). St. Louis, MO: C. V. Mosby.

Morrow, B., & Argent, A. (2008). A comprehensive review of pediatric endotracheal suctioning: Effects, indications, and clinical practice. *Pediatric Critical Care Medicine*, *9*(5), 465–477.

Munro, C., Grap, M., Jones, D., et al. (2009). Chlorhexidine, toothbrushing, and preventing ventilator-associated pneumonia in critically ill adults. *American Journal of Critical Care*, *18*, 425–437.

NANDA International (NANDA-I). (2012). Nursing diagnoses: Definitions and classification 2012–2014. Ames, IA: Wiley-Blackwell.

National Guideline Clearinghouse (NGC). (2001, July 29; revised 2008, October). Guideline synthesis: Tobacco use cessation and prevention. Rockville, MD: Author. Retrieved June 23, 2011, from http://www.guideline.gov/syntheses/synthesis.aspx?id=16422

National Institutes of Health (NIH). (2000). *Critical care therapy and respiratory care section: Airway suctioning and the*

use of the Ballard closed tracheal suctioning system. Bethesda, MD: National Institutes of Health, Critical Care Medicine Department. Retrieved July 1, 2011, from http://www.cc.nih.gov/ccmd/cctrcs/pdf_docs/Airway%20Management/01-aiarwaysuctioning-bal.pdf

Paul, I., Beiler, J., McMonagle, A., et al. (2007). Effect of honey, dextromethorphan, and no treatment on nocturnal cough and sleep quality for coughing children and their parents. *Archives of Pediatrics & Adolescent Medicine, 161*(12), 1140–1146.

Pierson, D., Epstein, S., Durbin, C., Jr., et al. (2005). Symposium: Tracheostomy from A to Z. *Respiratory Care, 50*(4), 473–559.

Porth, C. M., & Matfin, G. (2010). *Pathophysiology: Concepts of altered states* (8th ed.). New York: Lippincott Williams & Wilkins.

Rajkumar, A., Karmarkar, A., & Knott, J. (2006). Pulse oximetry: An overview. *Journal of Perioperative Practice, 16*(10), 502–504.

Rauen, C., Chulay, M., Bridges, E., et al. (2008). Seven evidence-based practice habits: Putting some sacred cows out to pasture. *Critical Care Nurse, 28*(2), 98–124.

Rice, V., & Stead, L. (2008). Nursing interventions for smoking cessation. *Cochrane Database of Systematic Reviews,* Issue 1. Art. No.: CD001188. doi:10.1002/14651858.CD001188.pub3

Roberts, K., Whalley, H., & Bleetman, A. (2005). The nasopharyngeal airway: Dispelling myths and establishing the facts. *Emergency Medicine Journal, 22,* 394–396.

Rodden, A., Spicer, L., Diaz, V., et al. (2007). Does fingernail polish affect pulse oximeter readings? *Intensive & Critical Care Nursing, 23*(1), 51–55.

Roman, M., & Mercado, D. (2006). Review of chest tube use. *MedSurg Nursing, 15*(1), 41–43.

Schick, S., & Glantz, S. (2005). Philip Morris toxicological experiments with fresh sidestream smoke: More toxic than mainstream smoke. *Tobacco Control, 14*(6), 396–404. Retrieved June 19, 2011, from http://www.ncbi.nlm.nih.gov/pmc/articles/PMC1748121/

Siegel, J., Rhinehart, E., Jackson, M., et al.; and the Healthcare Infection Control Practices Advisory Committee. (2007). 2007 Guideline for isolation precautions: Preventing transmission of infectious agents in healthcare settings. Retrieved June 30, 2011, from http://www.cdc.gov/ncidod/dhqp/pdf/guidelines/Isolation2007.pdf

Stich, J., & Cassella, D. (2009). Getting inspired about oxygen delivery devices. *Nursing2009, 39*(9), 51–54.

Tablan, O., Anderson, L., Besser, R., et al. (2004). Guidelines for preventing healthcare-associated pneumonia, 2003. Recommendations of CDC and the Healthcare Infection Control Practices Advisory Committee. *Morbidity and Mortality Weekly Report, 53*(RR-03), 1–36. Retrieved June 23, 2011, from http://www.cdc.gov/mmwr/preview/mmwrhtml/rr5303a1.htm

Texas Department of State Health Services. Laboratory Services Section Home. (2009). Guidelines for specimen collection and submission: Mycobacteriology (AFB) collection, transport, and storage. Retrieved June 25, 2011, from http://www.dshs.state.tx.us/LAB/myco_guidelines.shtm

Thille, A., Rodriguez, P., Cabello, B., et al. (2006). Patient-ventilatory asynchrony during assisted mechanical ventilation. *Intensive Care Medicine, 32*(10), 1515–1522.

Thompson, L. (2000). Suctioning adults with an artificial airway. The Joanna Briggs Institute for Evidence Based Nursing and Midwifery. Systematic Review No. 9, 4(4), 1–6.

U.S. Environmental Protection Agency. (2004). Revisions to the air quality index [Fact sheet]. Retrieved July 4, 2011, from http://www.epa.gov/ttn/caaa/t1/fact_sheets/factsht.pdf

U.S. Food and Drug Administration/Consumer Health Information. (2008). Using over-the-counter cough and cold products in children. Retrieved June 23, 2011, from http://www.fda.gov/ForConsumers/ConsumerUpdates/ucm048515.htm#TipsforParentsandCaregivers

Vandenberg, J., Lutz, R., & Vinson, D. (1999). Large-diameter suction system reduces oropharyngeal evacuation time. *Journal of Emergency Medicine, 17*(6), 941–944.

Vandenberg, J., & Vinson, D. (1999). The inadequacies of contemporary oropharyngeal suction. *American Journal of Emergency Medicine, 17*(6), 611–613.

Vargo, J. J., Zuccaro, G., Dumot, J. A., et a;. (2002). Automated graphic assessment of respiratory activity is superior to pulse oximetry and visual assessment for the detection of early respiratory depression during therapeutic upper endoscopy. *Gastrointestinal Endoscopy, 55,* 826–831.

Vital signs: Current cigarette smoking among adults aged ≥ 18 years—United States, 2005–2010. (2011). *Morbidity and Mortality Weekly Report, 60.* Early release. Retrieved September 7, 2011, from http://www.cdc.gov/mmwr/preview/mmwrhtml/mm60e0906a1.htm?s_cid=mm60e0906a1_w

CHAPTER 38

American Heart Association (AHA). (2005). 2005 American Heart Association guidelines for cardiopulmonary resuscitation and emergency cardiovascular care: International consensus on science. Part 3: Overview of CPR; Part 4: Adult basic life support; Part 5: Electrical therapies: automated external defibrillators, defibrillation, cardioversion, and pacing; Part 7.1: Circulation *112*(Suppl. 24), IV-12–57. Retrieved March 4, 2013, from http://circ.ahajournals.org/content/112/24_suppl/IV-12.full?sid=37e55c1f-b260-40b9-baae-79d762c38be1

American Heart Association (AHA). (2011a, November 14). Cigarette smoking and cardiovascular diseases. Retrieved November 20, 2011, from http://newsroom.heart.org/pr/aha/smoking-tip-sheet-nov-14-2011-217833.aspx

American Heart Association (AHA). (2011b, February 24). Hands Only™ CPR. Retrieved March 4, 2013, from http://handsonlycpr.eisenberginc.com/

American Heart Association (AHA). (2011c, updated 2012, October 12). Heart failure medications. Retrieved March 4, 2013, from http://www.heart.org/HEARTORG/Conditions/HeartFailure/PreventionTreatmentofHeartFailure/Heart-Failure-Medications_UCM_306342_Article.jsp#.TsLKAmAqnL4

American Lung Association (ALA). (2010, February). Children and teens. Retrieved March 4, 2013, from http://www.lungusa.org/stop-smoking/about-smoking/facts-figures/children-teens-and-tobacco.html

Bulechek, G., Butcher, H., & Dochterman, J. (2012). *Nursing interventions classification (NIC)* (6th ed.). St. Louis, MO: C. V. Mosby.

Centers for Disease Control and Prevention (CDC). (2008). Health, United States, 2008. In: FastStats, Centers for Disease Control and Prevention (CDC), U.S. Department

of Health and Human Services. Retrieved November 15, 2011, from http://www.cdc.gov/nchs/fastats/smoking.htm

Jenkins, D., Kendall, C., Faulkner, D., et al. (2008). Long-term effects of a plant-based dietary portfolio of cholesterol-lowering foods on blood pressure. *European Journal of Clinical Nutrition, 62,* 781–788.

Johnson, M., Moorhead, S., Bulechek, G., et al. (2012). *NOC and NIC linkages to NANDA-I and clinical conditions.* St. Louis, MO: C. V. Mosby:

Kuriyama, S., Shimazu, T., Ohmori, K., et al. (2007). Green tea consumption and mortality due to cardiovascular disease, cancer, and all causes in Japan: The Ohsaki study. *JAMA, 296*(10), 1255–1265.

Moorhead, S., Johnson, M., Maas, M., et al. (2012). *Nursing outcomes classification (NOC)* (5th ed.). St. Louis, MO: C. V. Mosby.

Moser, D. (2007). "The rust of life": Impact of anxiety on cardiac patients. *American Journal of Critical Care, 16,* 361–369.

NANDA International (NANDA-I). (2012). *Nursing diagnoses: Definitions and classification 2012–2014.* Ames, IA: Wiley-Blackwell.

National Heart, Lung, and Blood Institute (NHLBI). (2002, update in development). Third report of the expert panel on detection, evaluation, and treatment of high blood cholesterol in adults (Adult Treatment Panel III). Retrieved November 18, 2011, from http://www.nhlbi.nih.gov/guidelines/cholesterol/

National Heart, Lung, and Blood Institute (NHLBI). (2011). Integrated guidelines for cardiovascular health and risk reduction in children and adolescents. Retrieved March 4, 2013, from http://www.nhlbi.nih.gov/guidelines/cvd_ped/

Porth, C. M. (2008). *Pathophysiology: Concepts of altered states* (8th ed.). New York: Lippincott Williams & Wilkins.

Rasavong, C. (2009). Reliability and validity for Homan's sign for the detection of deep vein thrombosis. *CyberPT.* Retrieved January 15, 2012, from http://www.cyberpt.com/homansign.asp

Sayre, M., Berg, R., Cave, D., et al. (2008). Hands-only (compression-only) cardiopulmonary resuscitation: A call to action for bystander response to adults who experience out-of-hospital sudden cardiac arrest: A science advisory for the public from the American Heart Association Emergency Cardiovascular Care Committee. *Circulation, 117,* 2162–2167. Retrieved March 4, 2013, from http://circ.ahajournals.org/cgi/reprint/CIRCULATIONAHA.107.189380

Sesso, H., Buring, J., Christen, W., et al. (2008, Novmeber 12). Vitamins E and C in the prevention of cardiovascular disease in men. *JAMA, 300*(18). Retrieved March 4, 2013, from http://jama.ama-assn.org/cgi/content/full/300/18/2123

Spangler, L., Newton, K., Grothaus, L., et al. (2007). The effects of black cohosh therapies on lipids, fibrinogen, glucose and insulin. *Maturitas, 57*(2), 195–204.

Wood, S., & Nghiem, H. (2007). Raw garlic and garlic supplements offer no effect on lipids. *Archives of Internal Medicine, 167,* 125–126, 346–353.

CHAPTER 39

AABB. (n.d.). FAQ. Retrieved November 28, 2011, from http://www.aabb.org/resources/bct/Pages/bloodfaq.aspx

AABB. (2008). Blood management: Options for better patient care. MD: AABB.

The Association of periOperative Registered Nurses (AORN). (2009). *Safe environment of care, Recommendation XVI, Perioperative standards and recommended practices* (pp. 431–432). Denver, CO: Author.

Betsy Lehman Center for Patient Safety and Medical Error Reduction, JSI Research and Training Institute, Inc. (2008, January 31). *Prevention and control of healthcare-associated infections in Massachusetts. Part 1: Final recommendations of the Expert Panel* (pp. 69–82). Boston, MA: Massachusetts Department of Public Health. National Guideline Clearinghouse Brief Summary. Prevention of bloodstream infections. Retrieved November 29, 2011, from http://www.guideline.gov/summary/summary.aspx?doc_id=12922&nbr=006636&string=intravenous_AND_administration

Blest, A., Roberts, M., Murdock, J., et al. (2007). How often should a red blood cell administration set be changed while a patient is being transfused? A commentary and review of the literature. *Transfusion Medicine, 18,* 121–133.

Bulechek, G., Butcher, H., & Dochterman, J. (Eds.). (2012). *Nursing interventions classification (NIC)* (6th ed.). St. Louis, MO: C. V. Mosby.

Camp-Sorrell, D. (Ed.). (2011). *Access device guidelines: Recommendations for nursing practice and education* (3rd ed.). Pittsburgh, PA: Oncology Nursing Society.

Centers for Disease Control and Prevention (CDC). (2002). Guidelines for the prevention of intravascular catheter-related infections. *Morbidity and Mortality Weekly Report, 51*(RR-10), 1–26. Retrieved November 28, 2011, from http://www.cdc.gov/mmwr/preview/mmwrhtml/rr5110a1.htm

Finnish Medical Society Duodecim. (2000, updated 2008; update pending). Guidelines: Blood transfusion: Indications and administration. Retrieved November 22, 2011, from http://www.guidelines.gov/content.aspx?id=12787&search=blood+transfusions+indications+administration

Foster, J. P., Richards, R., & Showell, M. G. (2006, updated 2009). Intravenous in-line filters for preventing morbidity and mortality in neonates. *Cochrane Database of Systematic Reviews,* Issue 2. Art. No.: CD005248. doi:10.1002/14651858.CD005248.pub2

Gillies, D., Wallen, M., Morrison, A., et al. (2005). Optimal timing for intravenous administration set replacement. *Cochrane Database of Systematic Reviews,* Issue 4. Art. No: CD003588.

Gorski, L. (2007). Infusion nursing standards of practice: Standard 43: catheter stabilization. *Journal of Infusion Nursing, 30*(1), 20–21.

Hadaway, L. (2006). Technology of flushing vascular access devices. *Journal of Infusion Nursing, 29*(3), 137–145.

Hadaway, L. (2007). Infiltration and extravasation. *American Journal of Nursing, 107*(8), 64–72.

Hadaway, L. (2010). Don't disconnect IV administration sets. Lynn Hadaway Associates, Inc. [Web log]. Retrieved December 22, 2011, from http://hadawayassociates.blogspot.com/2010/03/dont-disconnect-iv-administration-sets.html

Houck, D., & Whiteford, J. (2007). Transfusion with infusion pump for peripherally inserted central catheters and other vascular access devices. *Journal of Infusion Nursing, 30*(6), 341–344.

Infusion Nurses Society (INS). (2006a). Infusion nursing standards of practice. *Journal of Infusion Nursing, 29*(1S), S1–S92. Norwood, MA: Author.

Infusion Nurses Society (INS). (2006b). *Policies and procedures for infusion nurses* (3rd ed.). Infusion Nurses Society Clinical Practice Committee. Norwood, MA: Author.

Institute for Healthcare Improvement (IHI). (n.d.). Implement the central line bundle. Retrieved November 26, 2011, from http://www.ihi.org/IHI/Topics/CriticalCare/Intensive Care/Changes/ImplementtheCentralLineBundle.htm

Institute of Medicine (IOM). (2004). *Dietary reference intakes for electrolytes and water.* Washington, DC: National Academies Press.

Joanna Briggs Institute. (2008). Management of peripheral intravascular devices. *Best Practice, 12*(5). Retrieved November 30, 2011, from http://connect.jbiconnectplus. org/ViewSourceFile.aspx?0=439

The Joint Commission (TJC). (2011). Hospital: 2011 national patient safety goals. Retrieved November 28, 2011, from http://www.jointcommission.org/assets/1/6/HAP_NPSG_6-10-11.pdf

LeDuc, K. (1997). Efficacy of normal saline solution versus heparin solution for maintaining patency of peripheral intravenous catheters in children. *Journal of Emergency Nursing, 23*(4), 306–309.

Lim, L. S., Hoeksema, L. J., Sherin, K.; and ACPM Prevention Practice Committee. (2009, April). Guideline summary: Screening for osteoporosis in the adult U.S. population: ACPM Position statement on preventive practice. Rockville, MD: National Guideline Clearinghouse. Retrieved November 28, 2011, from http://www.guideline.gov/summary/summary.aspx?view_id=1&doc_id=15270

Macklin, D. (2003). Phlebitis. *American Journal of Nursing, 103*(2), 55–60.

Marschall, J., Mermel, L., Classen, D., et al. (2008, October. Guideline Summary. Strategies to prevent central line-associated bloodstream infections in acute care hospitals. *Infection Control and Hospital Epidemiology, 29*(Suppl. 1), S22–S30. Retrieved November 29, 2011, from http://www.guideline.gov/summary/summary.aspx?view_id=1&doc_id=13395

Mentes, J. (2008). Managing oral hydration. In: E. Capezuti, D. Zwicker, M. Mezey, et al. (Eds.). *Evidence-based geriatric nursing protocols for best practice* (3rd ed., pp. 369–390). New York: Springer. Retrieved November 27, 2011, from http://www.guideline.gov/content.aspx?id=12256&search=dehydration

Moorhead, S., Johnson, M., Maas, M., et al. (Eds.). (2008). *Nursing outcomes classification (NOC)* (4th ed.). St. Louis, MO: C. V. Mosby.

MyFoodDiary.com. (2003–2011). Recommended daily water intake. Retrieved December 20, 2011, from http://www.myfooddiary.com/resources/ask_the_expert/recommended_daily_water_intake.asp

NANDA International (NANDA-I). (2012). *Nursing diagnoses: Definitions and classification 2012–2014.* Ames, IA: Wiley-Blackwell.

National Guideline Clearinghouse (NGC). (2008). Guideline summary: Prevention of bloodstream infections. In: *Prevention and control of healthcare-associated infections in Massachusetts.* Rockville, MD: Author. Retrieved November 27, 2011, from http://www.guideline.gov/summary/summary.aspx?doc_id=12922

National Institutes of Health, Office of Dietary Supplements. (2011). Dietary reference intakes for calcium and vitamin D. Food and Nutrition Board of the Institute of Medicine, National Academy of Sciences. Retrieved January 1, 2012, from http://ods.od.nih.gov/Health_Information/Dietary_Reference_Intakes.aspx

National Osteoporosis Foundation. (2008, revised 2010, January). *Clinician's guide to the prevention and treatment of osteoporosis.* Washington, DC: National Osteoporosis Foundation. Retrieved November 25, 2011, from http://www.nof.org/sites/default/files/pdfs/NOF_Clinician Guide2009_v7.pdf

Niesen, K. M., Harris, D. Y., Parkin, L. S., et al. (2003). The effects of heparin versus normal saline for maintenance of peripheral intravenous locks in pregnant women. *Journal of Obstetrics, Gynecology, & Neonatal Nursing, 32*(4), 503–508.

O'Grady, N. P., Alexander, M., Burns, L. A., et al.; and Healthcare Infection Control Practices Advisory Committee (HICPAC). (2011). *Guidelines for the prevention of intravascular catheter-related infections,* 2011. Atlanta, GA: Centers for Disease Control and Prevention (CDC).

Oncology Nursing Society (ONS). (2004). *Access device guidelines: Recommendations for nursing practice and education* (2nd ed.). Pittsburgh, PA: Author.

Pflaum, S. (1979). Investigation of intake-output as a means of assessing body fluid balance. *Heart & Lung: Journal of Acute & Critical Care, 8*(3), 495–498.

Pflaum, S. (2000). Evaluating the reliability and utility of cumulative intake and output. *Journal of Nursing Care Quality, 14*(3), 37–42.

Pflaum, S. (2006). Evaluating the reliability of recorded fluid balance to approximate body weight change in patients undergoing cardiac surgery. *Heart & Lung: Journal of Acute & Critical Care, 35*(1), 27–33.

Phillips, L. (2010). *Manual of IV therapeutics* (5th ed.). Philadelphia: F. A. Davis.

Polovich, M., White, J., & Kelleher, L. (Eds.) (2006). Chemotherapy and biotherapy guidelines and recommendations for practice, *Journal of Infusion Nursing, 29*(Suppl. 1), S1–S92.

Pronovost, P., Needham, D., Berenholtz, S., et al. (2006). An intervention to decrease catheter-related bloodstream infections in the ICU. *New England Journal of Medicine, 355,* 2725–2732.

Pronovost, P., Goeschel, C., Colantuoni, E., et al. (2010). Sustaining reductions in catheter-related bloodstream infections in Michigan intensive care units: Observational study. *BMJ, 340,* c309. Retrieved November 22, 2011, from http://www.bmj.com/cgi/content/full/340/feb04_1/c309

Rhoads, J., & Meeker, B. (2008). *Davis's guide to clinical nursing skills.* Philadelphia: F. A. Davis

Smith, B., & Royer, T. (2007). New standards for improving peripheral IV catheter securement. *Nursing2007, 37*(3), 72–74.

Society for Healthcare Epidemiology of America. (2008). SHEA/IDSA practice recommendation. Strategies to prevent central line–associated bloodstream infections in acute care hospitals. *Infection Control & Hospital Epidemiology, 29*(Suppl.), S22–S30. Retrieved November 26, 2011, from http://www.journals.uchicago.edu/doi/pdf/10.1086/591059

Timsit, J-F, Schwebel, C., Boudma, L., et al. (2009). Chlorhexidine-impregnated sponges and less frequent dressing changes for prevention of catheter-related infections in critically ill adults: A randomized controlled trial. *JAMA, 301*(12), 1231–1241, 1285–1287.

U.S. Department of Agriculture (USDA), Center for Nutrition Policy and Promotion. (2011, January, 31). *2010 Dietary*

guidelines for Americans. Retrieved December 20, 2011, from http://www.cnpp.usda.gov/DGAs2010-Policy Document.htm

U.S. Department of Agriculture (USDA). (2004, updated 2010). Dietary Reference Intakes: Recommended intakes for individuals. National Academy of Sciences. Retrieved November 29, 2011, from http://www.iom.edu/Activities/Nutrition/SummaryDRIs/~/media/Files/Activity%20Files/Nutrition/DRIs/5_Summary%20Table%20Tables%201-4.pdf

U.S. Department of Health and Human Services (USDHHS). (updated, 2009). *Osteoporosis* (NIH Publication No. 07–5158). Bethesda, MD: National Institute of Arthritis and Musculoskeletal and Skin Diseases, NIAMS/National Institutes of Health. Retrieved November 20, 2011, from http://www.niams.nih.gov/Health_Info/Bone/Osteoporosis/default.asp

Uslusoy, E., & Mete, S. (2008). Predisposing factors to phlebitis in patients with peripheral intravenous catheters: A descriptive study. *Journal of the American Academy of Nurse Practitioners, 20*(4), 172–180.

Wenzel, R., & Edmond, M. (2006). Team-based prevention of catheter-related infections. *New England Journal of Medicine, 355,* 2781–2783.

CHAPTER 40

Agency for Healthcare Research and Quality (AHRQ). (2003, December). AHRQ's patient safety initiative: Building foundations, reducing risk. Interim Report to the Senate Committee on Appropriations. AHRQ Publication No. 04-RG005. Rockville, MD: Author. http://www.ahrq.gov/qual/pscongrpt/

Agency for Healthcare Research and Quality (AHRQ). (2008). New AHRQ study finds surgical errors cost nearly $1.5 billion annually [Press release]. Retrieved August 3, 2011, from http://www.ahrq.gov/news/press/pr2008/surgerrpr.htm

American Association of Critical-Care Nurses (AACN). (2010). AACN practice alert. Venous thrombosis prevention. Retrieved August 8, 2011, from http://www.aacn.org/WD/Practice/Docs/PracticeAlerts/VTE%20Prevention%2004-2010%20final.pdf

Association of periOperative Registered Nurses (AORN). (2009). *Perioperative standards and recommended practices.* Denver, CO: Author.

Bartley, M. (2006). Keep venous thromboembolism at bay. *Nursing2006, 36*(10), 36–43.

Berliner, E., Ozbilgin, B., & Zarin, D. (2003). A systematic review of pneumatic compression for treatment of chronic venous insufficiency and venous ulcers. *Journal of Vascular Surgery, 37*(3), 539–544.

Best practices: Evidence-based nursing procedures (2nd ed.). (2007). Philadelphia: Lippincott Williams and Wilkins.

Boyce, J., & Pittet, D. (2002). Guideline for hand hygiene in health-care settings. Recommendations of the Healthcare Infection Control Practices Advisory Committee and the HICPAC/SHEA/APIC/IDSA Hand Hygiene Task Force. *Morbidity and Mortality Weekly Report, 51*(RR-16), 1–44. Retrieved August 3, 2011, from http://www.cdc.gov/mmwr/preview/mmwrhtml/rr5116a1.htm

Bulechek, G. M., Butcher, H. K., & Dochterman, J. M. (Eds.). (2012). *Nursing interventions classification (NIC)* (6th ed.). St. Louis, MO: C. V. Mosby

Centers for Disease Control and Prevention (CDC). (n.d., updated 2010). Having surgery? What you should know before you go. Retrieved August 6, 2011, from http://www.cdc.gov/features/SafeSurgery/

Centers for Disease Control and Prevention (CDC) National Center for Health Statistics. (2009). U.S. outpatient surgeries on the rise [Press release]. Retrieved August 3, 2011, from http://www.cdc.gov/nchs/pressroom/09newsreleases/outpatientsurgeries.htm

Centers for Medicare & Medicaid Services. (2006). Eliminating serious, preventable, and costly medical errors—never events [Press release]. Department of Health & Human Services. Retrieved August 3, 2011, from http://www.cms.hhs.gov/apps/media/press/release.asp?Counter=1863

Centers for Medicare & Medicaid Services. (2008, July 31). Medicare and Medicaid move aggressively to encourage greater patient safety in hospitals and reduce never events [Press release]. CMS Office of Public Affairs. Retrieved August 3, 2011, from http://www.cms.hhs.gov/apps/media/press/release.asp?Counter=3219&intNumPerPage=10&checkDate=&checkKey=&srchType=1&numDays=3500&srchOpt=0&srchData=&keywordType=All&chkNewsType=1%2C_2%2C_3%2C_4%2C_5&intPage=&showAll=&pYear=&year=&desc=&cboOrder=date

Cohen, A., Tapson, V., Bergman, J-F., et al. (2008). Venous thromboembolism risk and prophylaxis in the acute hospital care setting (ENDORSE study): A multinational cross-sectional study. *The Lancet, 371*(9610), 387–394.

Crenshaw, J. T. (2011). Preoperative fasting: Will the evidence ever be put into practice? *American Journal of Nursing, 111*(10), 38–45.

Crowe, L., Chang, A., Fraser, J., et al. (2008). Systematic review of the effectiveness of nursing interventions in reducing or relieving post-operative pain. *International Journal of Evidence-Based Healthcare, 6*(4), 396–430.

Dale, A., Rothrock, J., & McEwen, D. (Eds.). (2003). *Alexander's care of the patient in surgery* (12th ed.). St. Louis, MO: C. V. Mosby.

Green, S., Harris, C., & Singer, J. (2008). Gastrointestinal decontamination of the poisoned patient. *Pediatric Emergency Care, 24,* 176–178.

Haynes, A., Weiser, T., Berry, W., et al. (2009). A surgical safety checklist to reduce morbidity and mortality in a global population. *New England Journal of Medicine, 360*(5), 491–499.

Hendrickson, S., Wadhera, R., & El Bardissi, A. (2008). Development and pilot evaluation of a preoperative briefing protocol for cardiovascular surgery. *Journal of the American College of Surgeons, 208*(6), 1115–1123.

Hooper, V., Chard, R., Clifford, T., et al. (2009). ASPAN's evidence-based clinical practice guideline for the promotion of perioperative Normothermia. *Journal of PeriAnesthesia Nursing, 24*(5), 271–287. Retrieved August 6, 2011, from https://www.aspan.org/Portals/6/docs/ClinicalPractice/Guidelines/Normothermia_Guideline_10-09_JoPAN.pdf

Institute for Healthcare Improvement (IHI). (2011). Protecting 5 million lives. Retrieved August 3, 2011, from http://www.ihi.org/offerings/Initiatives/PastStrategicInitiatives/5MillionLivesCampaign/Pages/default.aspx

Joanna Briggs Institute. (2007). Pre-operative hair removal to reduce surgical site infection. *Best practice, 11*(4).

Joanna Briggs Institute. (2008a). Graduated compression stockings for the prevention of post-operative venous thromboembolism. *Best Practice, 12*(4).

Joanna Briggs Institute. (2008b). Preoperative fasting for preventing perioperative complications in children. *Best Practice, 12*(1), 29–32.

Johnston, J., & Davis, M. (2008). When sequential-compression devices cause falls. *American Journal of Nursing, 108*(4), 37-38.

The Joint Commission (TJC). (2011). *National patient safety goals for 2009.* Retrieved August 3, 2011, from http://www.jointcommission.org/assets/1/6/HAP_NPSG_6-10-11.pdf

Larry, C. (Ed.). (2003). Applying anti-embolism stockings. Retrieved August 9, 2011, from http://www.newlook.com.sg/info.asp?key=TED%20ApplyTh

Makary, M., Mukherjee, A., Sexton, J., et al. (2007). Operating room briefings and wrong-site surgery. *Journal of the American College of Surgeons, 204*(2), 236–243.

Mangram, A., Horan, T., Pearson, M., et al. (1999). The Hospital Infection Control Practices Advisory Committee. Guideline for prevention of surgical site infection, 1999. *Infection Control and Hospital Epidemiology, 20*(4), 247–278. Retrieved August 6, 2011, from http://www.cdc.gov/ncidod/dhqp/pdf/guidelines/SSI.pdf

Markel, D., & Morris, G. (2002). Effect of external sequential compression devices on femoral venous blood flow. *Journal of the Southern Orthopaedic Association, 11*(1), 2–9.

Moorhead, S., Johnson, M., Maas, M., et al. (Eds.). (2008). *Nursing outcomes classification (NOC)* (4th ed.). St. Louis, MO: C. V. Mosby.

NANDA International (NANDA-I). (2009). *Nursing diagnoses: Definitions and classification 2009–2011.* Oxford: Wiley-Blackwell.

NANDA International (NANDA-I). (2012). *Nursing diagnoses: Definitions and classification 2012–2014.* Philadelphia: Author. Used with permission.

National Guideline Clearinghouse (NGC). (2009). *Guideline summary: Strategies to prevent surgical site infections in acute care hospitals.* Rockville, MD. Author. Retrieved August 6, 2011, from http://www.guideline.gov/content.aspx?id=13399

National Institute for Health and Clinical Excellence (NICE). (2008, updated 2011). Surgical site infection: Prevention and treatment of surgical site infection (NICE Clinical Guideline 74). Retrieved August 6, 2011, from http://www.nice.org.uk/CG74

Practice guidelines for preoperative fasting and the use of pharmacologic agents to reduce the risk of pulmonary aspiration: Application to healthy patients undergoing elective procedures: An updated report by the American Society of Anesthesiologists Committee on Standards and Practice Parameters. (2011). *Anesthesiology, 114*(3), 495–511.

Ridge, R. (2008). Doing right to prevent wrong-site surgery. *Nursing2008, 38*(3), 24–25.

Sarasota Memorial Hospital. (reviewed 2010). Nursing procedure: Gastric suction—GOMCO. SMH Nursing Procedures. Retrieved August 9, 2011, from http://home.smh.com/sections/services-procedures/medlib/nursing/NursPandP/ped15_GastricSuction_052410.pdf

Siegel, J., Rhinehart, E., Jackson, M., et al.; and the Healthcare Infection Control Practices Advisory Committee. (2007). *2007 Guideline for isolation precautions: Preventing transmission of infectious agents in healthcare settings.* Retrieved August 3, 2011, from http://www.cdc.gov/hicpac/2007IP/2007isolationPrecautions.html

Tsay, S.-L., Chen, H.-L., Chen, S.-C., et al. (2008). Effects of reflexotherapy on acute postoperative pain and anxiety among patients with digestive cancer. *Cancer Nursing, 31*(2), 109–115.

Winslow, E., & Brosz, D. (2008). Graduated compression stockings in hospitalized postoperative patients: Correctness of usage and size. *American Journal of Nursing, 108*(9), 40–51.

World Health Organization (WHO). (2008). *Surgical safety checklist.* Retrieved August 7, 2011, from http://www.who.int/patientsafety/safesurgery/tools_resources/SSSL_Checklist_finalJun08.pdf

CHAPTER 41

American Nurses Association (ANA). (1986). *Standards of community health nursing practice.* Washington, DC: Author.

American Nurses Association (ANA). (2007). *Corrections nursing: Scope and standards of practice.* Silver Spring, MD: Author.

American Nurses Association (ANA). (2008). *Home health nursing: Scope and standards of practice.* Silver Spring, MD: Author.

American Nurses Association (ANA) and the Health Ministries Association (HMA). (2005). *Faith community nursing: Scope and standards of practice.* Silver Spring, MD: Author.

American Nurses Association (ANA) and the National Association of School Nurses (NASN). (2005). *School nursing: Scope and standards of practice.* Silver Spring, MD: Author.

Borger, C., Smith, S., Truffer, C., et al. (2006). Health spending projections through 2015: Changes on the horizon. *Health Affairs, 25,* w61–w72. Retrieved March 4, 2013, from http://www.commed.vcu.edu/IntroPH/Introduction/percentgdp2015hamar06.pdf

Broadway, R. L. (2002, July). Anthrax threat intensifies focus on disaster preparedness. *Healthcare Financial Management,* 28–31.

Bulechek, G., Butcher, H., & Dochterman, J. (Eds). (2012). *Nursing interventions classification (NIC)* (6th ed.). St. Louis, MO: C. V. Mosby.

Centers for Disease Control and Prevention (CDC). (modified 2008). *Guidelines for infection control in home care settings.* Atlanta, GA: Author. Retrieved January 15, 2012, from http://www.cdc.gov/ncidod/dhqp/gl_home_care.html

Gershon, R., Pogorzelska, M., Qureshi, K., et al. (2008). Home health care registered nurses and the risk of percutaneous injuries: A pilot study. *AJIC: American Journal of Infection Control, 36*(3), 165–172.

Hall, G. H., & Maslow, K. (2007). Working with families of hospitalized older adults with dementia. *Try this: Best practices for older adults with dementia, D10.* New York: The Hartford Institute for Geriatric Nursing, College of Nursing, New York University. Retrieved March 7, 2013, from http://consultgerirn.org/uploads/File/trythis/try_this_d10.pdf

Head, B., Maas, M., & Johnson, M. (1997). Outcomes for home and community nursing in integrated delivery systems. *Caring, 16*(1), 50–56.

Hicks, P., Tarr, G. M., & Hicks, X. P. (2007). Reminder cards and immunization rates among Latinos and the rural poor in northeast Colorado. *Journal of the American Board of Family Medicine, 20*(6), 581–586.

Huynh-Hohnbaum, A-L., Villa, V., Aranda, M., et al. (2008). Evaluating a multicomponent caregiver intervention. *Home Health Care Services Quarterly, 27*(4), 299–325.

The Joint Commission (TJC). (2012). 2013 Home care national patient safety goals. Retrieved March 4, 2013, from http://www.jointcommission.org/assets/1/18/NPSG_Chapter_Jan2013_OME.pdf

Larsson, L. S., & Butterfield, P. (2002). Mapping the future of environmental health and nursing: Strategies for integrating national competencies into nursing practice. *Public Health Nursing, 19*(9), 301–308.

Lescure, F-X., Locher, G., Eveillard, M., et al. (2009). Community-acquired infection with healthcare-associated methicillin-resistant *Staphylococcus aureus*: The role of home nursing care. *Infection Control & Hospital Epidemiology, 27,* 1213–1218. Retrieved March 4, 2013, from http://www.journals.uchicago.edu/doi/pdf/10.1086/507920

Leutz, W., Capitman, J., & Ruwe, M. et al. (2002). Caregiver education and support: Results of a multi-site pilot in an HMO. *Home Health Care Services Quarterly, 21*(2), 49–72.

Levine, C., Albert, S., Hokenstad, A., et al. (2006). "This case is closed": Family caregivers and the termination of home health care services for stroke patients. *Milbank Quarterly, 84*(2), 305–331.

Martin, K. S., & Norris, J. (1996). The Omaha system: A model for describing practice. *Holistic Nursing Practice, 11*(1), 75–83.

Martin, K. S., & Scheet, N. J. (1992). *The Omaha system: Applications for community health nursing.* Philadelphia: W. B. Saunders. Retrieved March 4, 2013, from http://www.omahasystem.org/interventionscheme.html

Moore, M. L., & Parker, A. L. (2006). Influenza vaccine compliance among pediatric asthma patients: What is the better method of notification? *Pediatric Asthma and Allergy Immunology, 19*(4), 200–204.

Moorhead, S., Johnson, M., Maas, M., et al. (Eds.). (2012). *Nursing outcomes classification (NOC)* (5th ed.). St. Louis, MO: C. V. Mosby.

Nightingale, F. (1860/1969). *Notes on nursing: What it is, and what it is not.* New York: Dover.

The Omaha System. (2009, May 11; updated). *Solving clinical data-information: Problem rating scale for outcomes.* Retrieved March 4, 2013, from http://www.omahasystem.org/problemratingscaleforoutcomes.html

Pryor, E. (1987). *Clara Barton: Professional angel.* Philadelphia: University of Pennsylvania Press.

Rhinehart, E. (2001, March–April). Infection control in the home. *Emerging Infectious Diseases, 7*(2), 1–12. Retrieved March 4, 2013, from http://wwwnc.cdc.gov/eid/article/7/2/70-0208.htm

Saba, V. K. (n.d.). Clinical Care Classification System. About. Retrieved March 4, 2013, from http://sabacare.com/About/

Saba, V. (2007). *Clinical care classification (CCC) system manual: A guide to nursing documentation.* New York: Springer.

Sabas, V. K. (2012). Clinical Care Classification System (version 2.5). Retrieved March 4, 2013, from http://sabacare.com/Tables/Diagnoses.html

Siegel, B. (1983). *Lillian Wald of Henry Street.* New York: Macmillan.

U.S. Congress. (2010). *H.R.3962, the Affordable Health Care for America Act.* 111th Cong., 1st sess. Retrieved March 4, 2013, from http://housedocs.house.gov/rules/health/111_ahcaa.pdf

U.S. Department of Health and Human Services. Office of Disease Prevention and Health Promotion. *Healthy People 2020.* Washington, DC. Retrieved January 13, 2012, from http://healthypeople.gov/2020/topicsobjectives2020/pdfs/HP2020objectives.pdf

Veenema, T. G. (Ed.) (2007). *Disaster nursing and emergency preparedness for chemical, biological, and radiological terrorism and other hazards* (2nd ed.). New York: Springer.

West Virginia Department of Military Affairs and Public Safety. (n.d.). *Ready WV: A family emergency guide.* West Virginia Office of Emergency Services. Retrieved March 4, 2013, from http://www.volunteerwv.org/nd/assets/downloads/CC/Ready_WV_Family_Emergency_Guide_March2011.pdf

CHAPTER 42

Ahern, K., & McDonald, S. (2002). The beliefs of nurses who were involved in a whistleblowing event. *Journal of Advanced Nursing, 38*(3), 303–309.

American Association of Colleges of Nursing Association (AACN). (2008). *The essentials of baccalaureate education for professional nursing practice.* Washington, DC: Author. Retrieved August 12, 2011, from http://www.aacn.nche.edu/Education/pdf/BaccEssentials08.pdf

American Hospital Association (AHA). (2003). *Patient care partnership: Understanding expectations, rights and responsibilities.* Retrieved August 14, 2011, from http://www.aha.org/aha/issues/Communicating-With-Patients/pt-care-partnership.html

American Nurses Association (ANA). (1988). *Nursing and the human immunodeficiency virus: A guide for nursing's response to AIDS.* Kansas City, MO: Author.

American Nurses Association (ANA). (1991). American Nurses Association: Position statement on HIV testing. Retrieved August 14, 2011, from http://www.nursingworld.org/BloodborneandAirborneDiseases

American Nurses Association (ANA). (1992). Ethics and human rights position statements: Forgoing nutrition and hydration. Retrieved August 14, 2011, from http://www.nursingworld.org/EthicsHumanRights

American Nurses Association (ANA). (1994a). Ethics and human rights position statements: Active euthanasia. Retrieved August 14, 2011, from http://www.nursingworld.org/EthicsHumanRights

American Nurses Association (ANA). (1994b). Ethics and human rights position statements: Assisted suicide. Retrieved August 14, 2011, from http://www.nursingworld.org/EthicsHumanRights

American Nurses Association (ANA). (2001). *Code of ethics for nurses with interpretive statements.* Washington, DC: American Nurses Publishing. Retrieved August 12, 2011, from http://nursingworld.org/MainMenuCategories/EthicsStandards/CodeofEthicsforNurses/2110Provisions.aspx

American Nurses Association (ANA). (2002). The profession's response to the problems of addictions and psychiatric disorders in nursing. Resolution by the House of Delegates. Retrieved August 12, 2011, from http://www.nursingworld.org/MemberCenterCategories/ANAGovernance/HODArchives/2002-HOD/2002-Actions/The-Professions-Response-to-the-Problem-of-Addictions-and-Psychiatric-Disorders-in-Nursing.aspx

American Nurses Association (ANA). (2003). Position statement on nursing care and do-not-resuscitate (DNR) decisions. Retrieved August 14, 2011, from http://www.nursingworld.org/EthicsHumanRights

American Nurses Association (ANA). (2010). *Nursing: Scope and standards of practice* (2nd ed.). Silver Spring, MD: Author.

Attree, M. (2007). Factors influencing nurses' decisions to raise concerns about care quality. *Journal of Nursing Management, 15*(4), 392–402.

Balch, S. (2006). The dubious value of value neutrality. *Academic Questions, 19*(4), 44–48.

Bandman, E., & Bandman, B. (2002). *Nursing ethics through the life span* (4th ed.). Upper Saddle River, NJ: Prentice-Hall.

Bayles, M. (1984). *Reproductive ethics.* Englewood Cliffs, NJ: Prentice-Hall.

Beauchamp, T. L., & Childress, J. F. (2008). *Principles of biomedical ethics* (6th ed.). New York: Oxford University Press.

Beckwith, F. J., & Peppin, J. F. (2000). Physician value neutrality: A critique. *Journal of Law, Medicine, and Ethics, 28*(1), 67–75.

Brock, D. W. (2006). Is a consensus possible on stem cell research? Moral and political obstacles. *Journal of Medical Ethics, 32*, 36–42.

Burkhardt, M., & Nathaniel, A. (2008). *Ethics and issues in contemporary nursing* (3rd ed.). Clifton Park, NY: Thomson Delmar Learning.

Cahn, M. T. (1987). The nurse as moral hero: A case for required dissent. *Dissertation Abstracts International, 50*(3). (University Microfilms International No. 88–22134).

Cameron, B. (2004). Ethical moments in practice: The nursing "how are you" revisited. *Nursing Ethics, 11*(1), 53–62.

Canadian Nurses Association (CNA). (2008). *Code of ethics for registered nurses.* Retrieved August 12, 2011, from http://www.cna-nurses.ca/CNA/practice/ethics/code/default_e.asp

Catalano, J. T. (2008). *Nursing now!* (5th ed.). Philadelphia: F. A. Davis.

Catlin, A., Volat, D., Hadley, M., et al. (2008). Conscientious objection: A potential neonatal nursing response to care orders that cause suffering at the end of life? Study of a concept. *Neonatal Network®: Journal of Neonatal Nursing, 27*(2), 101–108.

Clark, C. (2006). Moral character in social work. *British Journal of Social Work, 36*(1), 75–89.

Corley, M. C., & Minick, P. (2002). Moral distress or moral comfort. *Bioethics Forum, 18*(1–2), 7–14.

Curtin, L., & Flaherty, J. (1982). *Nursing ethics: Theories and pragmatics.* Bowie, MD: Robert J. Brady.

Dierckx de Casterlé, B., Izumi, S., Godfrey, N., et al. (2008). Nurses' responses to ethical dilemmas in nursing practice: Meta-analysis. *Journal of Advanced Nursing, 63*(6), 540–549.

Epstein, E., & Delgado, S. (2010). Understanding and addressing moral distress. *The Online Journal of Issues in Nursing.* doi:10.3912/OJIN.Vol15No03Man01

Erlen, J. (2001). Moral distress: A pervasive problem. *Orthopaedic Nursing, 20*(2), 76–82.

Georges, J. J., & Grypdonck, M. (2002). Moral problems experienced by nurses when caring for terminally ill people: A literature review. *Nursing Ethics, 9*(2), 155–178.

Gibbs, J. (2009). *Moral development & reality: Beyond the theories of Kohlberg and Hoffman.* Upper Saddle River, NJ: Pearson Education.

Glasberg, A-L, Eriksson, S., & Norberg, A. (2008). Factors associated with "stress of conscience" in healthcare. *Scandinavian Journal of Caring Sciences, 22*(2), 249–258.

Goldenberg, M. (2005). On evidence and evidence-based medicine: Lessons from the philosophy of science. *Social Science & Medicine, 62*(11), 2621–2632.

Gutierrez, K. M. (2005). Critical care nurses' perceptions of and responses to moral distress. *Dimensions of Critical Care Nursing, 24*, 229–241.

Hamric, A., Davis, W. S., & Childress, M. D. (2006). Moral distress in health care professionals. *Pharos of Alpha Omega Alpha Honor Medical Society, 69*(1), 16–23.

Hart, T. J. (2009, September 2). Moral distress in a non-acute continuing care setting: The experience of registered nurses. Master's thesis, Queen's University, Kingston, Ont., Canada. Retrieved August 12, 2011, from https://qspace.library.queensu.ca/jspui/handle/1974/5115

Hoffman, M. (2000). *Empathy and moral development: Implications for caring and justice.* Cambridge: Cambridge University Press.

Husted, J., & Husted, G. (2008). *Ethical decision making in nursing and healthcare* (4th ed.). New York: Springer.

International Council of Nurses (ICN). (2006). *The ICN code of ethics for nurses.* Geneva, Switzerland: Author. Retrieved August 13, 2011, from http://www.icn.ch/about-icn/code-of-ethics-for-nurses/

Jameton, A. (1984). *Nursing practice: The ethical issues.* Englewood Cliffs, NJ: Prentice-Hall.

The Joint Commission (TJC). (2008). *2008 Hospital accreditation standards.* Oakbrook Terrace, IL: The Joint Commission on Accreditation of Healthcare Organizations.

Kohlberg, L. (1968). Moral development. In: *International encyclopedia of social science.* New York: Macmillan.

Kohlberg, L. (1981). *Essays on moral development* (Vols. 1–3). San Francisco: Harper & Row.

Kothari, S., & Kirschner, K. (2006). Abandoning the Golden Rule: The problem with "putting ourselves in the patient's place." *Topics in Stroke Rehabilitation, 13*(4), 68–73.

Leininger, M. (1988). Leininger's theory of nursing: Cultural care diversity and universality, *Nursing Science Quarterly, 1*(4), 150–152.

Leininger, M. (2002). Culture care theory: A major contribution to advance transcultural nursing knowledge and practice. *Journal of Transcultural Nursing, 13*(3), 189–192.

Levine, M. E. (1989). Beyond dilemma. *Seminars in Oncology Nursing, 5*(2), 124–128.

McCue, C. (2010). Using the AACN framework to alleviate moral distress. *Online Journal of Issues in Nursing, 16*(1). doi:10.3912/OJIN. Vo. 16No01PPT02

Myhrvold, T. (2006). The different other—towards an including ethics of care. *Nursing Philosophy, 7*(3), 125–136.

National Conference of Commissioners on Uniform State Laws. (2006). Revised Uniform Anatomical Gift Act. Retrieved August 14, 2011, from http://www.law.upenn.edu/bll/archives/ulc/fnact99/uaga87.htm

National League for Nursing. (2007). *Core values.* Retrieved August 12, 2011, from http://www.nln.org/aboutnln/corevalues.htm

Noddings, N. (2003). *Caring: A feminine approach to ethics and moral education* (2nd ed.). Berkeley: University of California Press.

O'Keefe, M. E. (Ed.). (2000). *Nursing practice and the law: Avoiding malpractice and other legal risks.* Philadelphia: F. A. Davis.

Olsen, D. (2007). Ethical issues. Unwanted treatment: What are the ethical implications? *American Journal of Nursing, 107*(9), 51–53.

Pellegrino, E. D. (2000). Commentary: Value neutrality, moral integrity, and the physician. *Journal of Law, Medicine, and Ethics, 28*(1), 78–81.

Peternelj-Taylor, C. (2003). Whistleblowing and boundary violations: Exposing a colleague in the forensic milieu. *Nursing Ethics, 10*(5), 526–540.

Pinquart, M., & Silbereisen, R. K. (2004). Transmission of values from adolescents to their parents: The role of value content and authoritative parenting. *Adolescence, 39*(153), 83–100.

Power, F., Higgins, A., & Kohlberg, L. (1989). *Lawrence Kohlberg's approach to moral education.* New York: Columbia University Press.

Purtilo, R. (2005). *Ethical dimensions in the health professions* (4th ed.). Philadelphia: W. B. Saunders.

Raths, L., Harmin, M., & Simon, S. (1978). *Values and teaching.* Columbus, OH: Merrill.

Resnick, H., Schuur, J., Heineman, J., et al. (2008). Advance directives in nursing home residents aged > or=65 years: United States 2004. *American Journal of Hospice and Palliative Care, 25*(6), 476–482.

Roe v. Wade, No. 70-18, 410 U.S. 113. (1973). Roe et al., v. Wade, District Attorney of Dallas County *Appeal from the United States District Court for the Northern District of Texas.* Retrieved August 14, 2011, from http://caselaw.lp.findlaw.com/scripts/getcase.pl?court=us&vol=410&invol=113

Schluter, J., Winch, S., Holzhauser, K., et al. (2008). Nurses' moral sensitivity and hospital ethical climate: A literature review. *Nursing Ethics, 15*(3), 304–321.

Schwenzer, K., & Wang, L. (2006). Assessing moral distress in respiratory care practitioners. *Critical Care Medicine, 34*(12), 2967–2973.

Seroka, A. M. (1994). Values clarification and ethical decision making. *Seminars for Nurse Managers, 2*(1), 8–15.

Steele, S. M., & Harmon, V. M. (1983). *Values clarification in nursing* (2nd ed.). New York: Appleton & Lange.

Thiroux, J. (1977). *Ethics, theory and practice.* Philadelphia: MacMillan.

Volbrecht, R. M. (2002). *Nursing ethics: Communities in dialogues* (3rd ed.). Upper Saddle River, NJ: Prentice-Hall.

Watson, J. (1981, Summer). Socialization of the nursing student in a professional nursing education programme. *Nursing Papers, 13,* 19–24.

Waugh, D. (1978). Moral development: Theory and process. In: *Teaching and evaluating the affective domain in nursing programs* (pp. 17–30). New York: Charles B. Slack.

Webster, G. C., & Baylis, F. E. (2000). Moral residue. In: S. B. Rubin & L. Zoloth (Eds.), *Margin of error: The ethics of mistakes in the practice of medicine* (pp. 217–230). Hagerstown, MD: University Publishing Group.

White, G. B. (1983). Philosophical ethics and nursing: A word of caution. In: P. L. Chinn (Ed.), *Advances in nursing theory development.* Rockville, MD: Aspen Systems.

Wilkinson, J. M. (1987/1988). Moral distress in nursing practice: Experience and effect. *Nursing Forum, 23,* 16–29.

Wilkinson, J. M. (1997). Toward a context-sensitive theory of nursing ethics: Classification and comparison of nurses' narratives from four time periods (1934, 1979, 1989 & 1995). Unpublished doctoral dissertation, University of Kansas, Kansas City.

Wilmot, S. (2000). Nurses and whistleblowing: The ethical issues. *Journal of Advanced Nursing, 32*(5), 1051–1057.

Yoder-Wise, P. (2007). *Leading and managing in nursing* (4th ed.). St. Louis, MO: C. V. Mosby.

Zuzelo, P. R. (2007). Exploring the moral distress of registered nurses. *Nursing Ethics, 14,* 344–359.

CHAPTER 43

Aiken, T. D. (2004). *Legal, ethical, and political issues in nursing* (2nd ed.). Philadelphia: F. A. Davis.

American Nurses Association (ANA). (2001; updated in development). *Code of ethics for nurses with interpretive statements.* Washington, DC: Author. Retrieved January 19, 2012, from http://ana.nursingworld.org/MainMenu Categories/EthicsStandards/CodeofEthicsforNurses/Code-of-Ethics.aspx

American Nurses Association (ANA). (2009). Nurses' bill of rights FAQs. Retrieved March 4, 2013, from http://nursingworld.org/DocumentVault/NursingPractice/FAQs.aspx

American Nurses Association (ANA). (2010). *Nursing: Scope and standards of practice* (2nd ed.). Silver Spring, MD: Nursebooks.org.

American Nurses Association (ANA), Task Force on End of Life Decisions (1991). Position statement: Nursing and the patient self-determination acts. Retrieved on March 4, 2013, from http://ana.nursingworld.org/MainMenu Categories/EthicsStandards/Ethics-Position-Statements/prtetsdet14455.aspx

Americans With Disabilities Act (ADA) of 1990, Pub. L. No. 101-336, 104 Stat. 327, codified at 42 U.S.C. § 12101 *et seq.* (1990). Retrieved March 4, 2013, from http://www.ada.gov/statute.html

Austin, S. (2008). 7 tips for safe nursing practice. *Nursing2008, 28*(3), 34–39.

Barber v. Reinking. No. 37921. (1966). *The Supreme Court of Washington, Department Two. Legal Eye.* 411 P.2d 861. Retrieved March 4, 2013, from http://www.leagle.com/xmlResult.aspx?xmldoc=196620768Wn2d139_1187.xml&docbase=CSLWAR1-1950-1985

Coulter v. Thomas. No. 1998-SC-000795-DG. (2000). *Supreme Court of Kentucky. Legal Eye.* Retrieved March 4, 2013, from http://www.leagle.com/xmlResult.aspx?xmldoc=2000555 33SW3d522_1553.xml&docbase=CSLWAR2-1986-2006

Doe v. Bolton. No. 70-40. (1973). *Appeal from the United States District Court for the Northern District of Georgia. Legal Information Institute.* Retrieved March 4, 2013, from http://www.law.cornell.edu/supct/search/display.html?terms=Doe%20v.%20Bolton&url=/supct/html/historics/USSC_CR_0410_0179_ZS.html

Equal Employment Opportunity Commission (EEOC). (1992). *A technical assistance manual on the employment provisions (title I) of the Americans With Disabilities Act.* Retrieved March 4, 2013, from http://www.jan.wvu.edu/links/ADAtam1.html

Equal Employment Opportunity Commission (EEOC). (2002, modified 2009, March 11). *Guidelines on discrimination because of sex.* (Section 1604.11, Sexual harassment. Code of Federal Regulations, Title 29, Vol. 4). Retrieved March 4, 2013, from http://www.access.gpo.gov/nara/cfr/waisidx_06/29cfr1604_06.html

Fedorka, P., & Resnick, L. K. (2001). Defining nursing practice. In: M. O'Keefe (Ed.), *Nursing practice and the law: Avoiding malpractice and other legal risks* (pp. 97–117). Philadelphia: F. A. Davis.

Ferrell, K. G. (2007). Documentation, part 2: The best evidence of care. Complete and accurate charting can be crucial to exonerating nurses in civil lawsuits. *American Journal of Nursing, 107*(7), 61–64.

Frew, S. A. (2006, November). Nurse charged with felony in medication error death. Retrieved March 4, 2013, from http://www.medlaw.com/healthlaw/MEDMAL/nurse-charged-with-felony.shtml

Georgia Nurses Association. (n.d.). Nurse Advocate Program. The impaired nurse: Checklist for detecting potential chemical dependence in an employee. Retrieved March 4, 2013, from http://www.georgianurses.org/impaired_nurse.htm#pabi

Job Accommodation Network. (2006, updated 2011, May 31). *Office of Disability Employment Policy, Accommodation and Compliance Series: Nurses with disabilities*. Morgantown, WV: Job Accommodation Network. Retrieved March 4, 2013, from http://www.jan.wvu.edu/media/nurses.html

Kansas State Board of Nursing, (1993, last amended 2007, April 20). Unprofessional conduct. Retrieved March 4, 2013, from http://www.ksbn.org/npa/pages/60-7-106.pdf

Legal liability: New study alerts RNs to daily practice risks. (2009). *Nursing 2009, 39*(9), 21–23.

Marchand, D. V. (2001). American jurisprudence. In: M. O'Keefe (Ed.), *Nursing practice and the law: Avoiding malpractice and other legal risks* (pp. 3–22). Philadelphia: F. A. Davis.

Missouri Revised Statutes, 335 Mo. Rev. Stat. § 335.016 (2012, August 28). Retrieved March 4, 2013, from http://www.moga.mo.gov/statutes/C300-399/3350000016.HTM

National Council of State Boards of Nursing (NCSBN). (n.d.). Professional boundaries: A nurse's guide to the importance of appropriate professional boundaries. Retrieved March 4, 2013, from https://www.ncsbn.org/ProfessionalBoundaries brochure.pdf

National Council of State Boards of Nursing (NCSBN). (2005). Working with others: A position paper. Retrieved March 4, 2013, from https://www.ncsbn.org/Working_with_Others.pdf

Nurses Service Organization (NSO). (2008a). Legal case study: Case Study: Failure to properly assess patient; failure to properly monitor patient's vital signs and intake/output; failure to recognize and respond to signs and symptoms of sepsis; failure to communicate with the patient's physician; and failure to direct the patient to emergency care. Retrieved March 4, 2013, from http://www.nso.com/case-studies/casestudy-article/240.jsp

Nurses Service Organization (NSO). (2008b). Legal case study: Case study: Failure to report patient's deteriorating condition to the attending physician and administration of anxiolytic medication in the presence of respiratory distress. Retrieved March 4, 2013, http://www.nso.com/case-studies/article/237.jsp

O'Keefe, M. E. (Ed.). (2001). *Nursing practice and the law: Avoiding malpractice and other legal risks*. Philadelphia: F. A. Davis.

Quill, T. E. (2005). Terry Schiavo—a tragedy compounded. *New England Journal of Medicine, 352*(16), 1630–1633.

Reising, D. L., & Allen, P. N. (2007). Protecting yourself from malpractice claims. *American Nurse Today, 2*(2). Retrieved March 4, 2013, from http://www.americannursetoday.com/article.aspx?id=4186&fid=4172#

Rochester nurse guilty of Medicaid fraud. (2007, March 16). The Water Buffalo Press [Web log]. Retrieved January 19, 2012, from http://waterbuffalopress.blogspot.com/2007/03/rochester-nurse-guilty-of-medicaid.html

Roe v. Wade, No. 7-18. (1973). *Appeal from the United States District Court for the Northern District of Texas. Legal Information Institute*. Retrieved March 4, 2013, from http://www.law.cornell.edu/supct/search/display.html?terms=roe%20v%20wade&url=/supct/html/historics/USSC_CR_0410_0113_ZS.html

Sidlinger, L., & Hornberger, C. (2008). Current characteristics of the investigated impaired nurse in Kansas. *The Kansas Nurse, 83*(1), 3–5.

Snyder, E. K. (n.d.). Emergency Medical Treatment and Active Labor Act: What every healthcare negligence lawyer should know. *Legal Eagle Eye Newsletter for the Nursing Profession*. Retrieved March 4, 2013, from http://www.nursinglaw.com/EMTALA022306.htm#_ednref13

Snyder, E. K. (2006, April). Falls: Court finds substandard precautions. Negligence found. *Legal Eagle Eye Newsletter for the Nursing Profession, 14*(4), 8.

Snyder, E. K. (2007). December). Fall: Patient not restrained, court does not fault nurses. *Legal Eagle Eye Newsletter for the Nursing Profession, 15*(12), 8.

Snyder, E. K. (2008, October). Psych: No fall-risk assessment done, negligence found. *Legal Eagle Eye Newsletter for the Nursing Profession, 16*(10), 8.

Supervised visits: Patients' privacy rights. (2009, June). *Legal Eagle Eye Newsletter*, p. 3. Retrieved March 4, 2013, from http://www.nursinglaw.com/supervisedvisits.pdf

Vaughn, C. (1998, May 1). Accused of failure to report suspected abuse by colleague—Charges filed against 2 Fort Worth educators. *Star-Telegram*. Retrieved March 4, 2013, from http://www.nospank.net/n-c38.htm

Webster v. Reproductive Health Services. No. 88-605. (1989). *Appeal from the United States Court of Appeals for the Eight Circuit. Legal Information Institute*. Retrieved March 4, 2013, from http://www.law.cornell.edu/supct/html/historics/USSC_CR_0492_0490_ZS.html

CHAPTER 44

American Nurses Association (ANA). (2008). *Scope and standards of nursing informatics practice* (ANA Publication No. NIP21). Washington, DC: American Nurses Publishing/American Nurses Foundation.

American Nurses Association (ANA). (2010). *Nursing: Scope and standards of practice* (2nd ed.). Silver Spring, MD: Author.

American Nurses Association (ANA) Expert Panel. (2007). *Nursing informatics: Scope of practice*. Silver Springs, MD: Author.

Bell, M. M. (2009, May). Bar code point of care systems: Benefits and pitfalls. *Pennsylvania Nurse*, 9–10.

Beyea, S. (2000, May). Standardized nursing vocabularies and the perioperative nursing data set: Making clinical practice count. *CIN Plus, 3*(2), 1, 5, 6.

Cannon-Diehl, M. R. (2009). Simulation in healthcare and nursing. *Critical Care Nursing Quarterly, 32*(2), 128–136.

Doyle, C. S. (1992). Final report to National Forum on Information Literacy. University of Calgary. Information Literacy Group, 1998. Retrieved February 6, 2012, from http://www.asla.org.au/pubs/ws/accommat5.htm

DuLong, D. (2009). *The TIGER Initiative: Collaborating to integrate evidence and informatics into nursing practice and education: An executive summary* (pp. 1–30). Retrieved

March 4, 2013, from http://www.tigersummit.com/uploads/TIGER_Collaborative_Exec_Summary_040509.pdf

Enrado, P. (2009, May 1). Tele-nurses help with 911 calls as cities cope with tight budgets. Retrieved March 4, 2013, from http://www.healthcareitnews.com/news/tele-nurses-help-911-calls-cities-cope-tight-budgets

Ford, E. W., Menachemi, N., Peterson, L. T., et al. (2009). Resistance is futile: But it is slowing the pace of EHR adoption nonetheless. *Journal of the American Medical Informatics Association, 16*(3), 274–281.

Fowler, S. B., Sohler, P., & Zarillo, D. F. (2009). Bar code technology for dedication administration: Medication errors and nurse satisfaction. *MedSurg Nursing, 18*(2), 103–109.

Hart, M. D. (2008). Informatics competency and development within the US nursing population workforce. *Computers, Informatics, Nursing, 26*(6), 320–329.

Kossman, S. P., & Scheidenhelm, S. L. (2008). Nurses' perceptions of the impact of electronic health records on work and patient outcomes. *Computers, Informatics, Nursing, 26*(2), 69–77.

Krumsieg, K., & Baehr, M. (2002). *Foundations of learning* (3rd ed.). Corvallis, OR: Pacific Crest.

National Institutes of Health (NIH). (2012). The National Library of Medicine PubMed. Retrieved March 4, 2013, from http://www.ncbi.nlm.nih.gov/pubmed/

Nelson, R., & Joos, I. (1989, Fall). On language in nursing: From data to wisdom. *PLN Visions, 6*, 7.

Pipe, T. B., Cisar, N. S., Caruso, E., et al. (2008). Leadership strategies: Inspiring evidence-based practice at the individual, unit, and organizational levels. *Journal of Nursing Care Quality, 23*(5), 265–271.

Rippen, H., & Risk, A. (2000). e-Health code of ethics. *Journal of Medical Internet Research, 2*(1), e2. Retrieved March 4, 2013, from http://www.jmir.org/2000/2/e9/

Rogers, E. M. (2005). *Diffusion of innovations* (pp. 282–285). New York: Free Press.

Taylor, H. (2008). Number of "cyberchondriacs" adults going online for health information has plateaued or declined. *Healthcare News, 8*(8), 1–6.

Turisco, F., & Rhoads, J. (2008). Equipped for efficiency: Improving nursing care through technology. Retrieved March 4, 2013, from http://www.chcf.org/publications/2008/12/equipped-for-efficiency-improving-nursing-care-through-technology

Wilkinson, J. (2012). *Nursing process and critical thinking* (5th ed.). Upper Saddle River, NJ: Pearson.

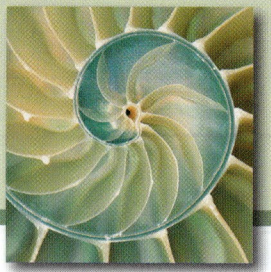

Credits

*Note: Unless cited below, text credits appear within the text

CHAPTER 1

Nurses Make a Difference 1-1: The National Library of Medicine

Nurses Make a Difference 1-2: © BananaStock

Figures 1-1 through 1-3: National Library of Medicine

Figure 1-4: © Kseniya Abramova, www.istockphoto.com

Figure 1-5: From Wilkinson, J.W., & Treas, L. (2011). *Fundamentals of nursing* (2nd ed.). Philadelphia: F.A. Davis.

CHAPTER 2

Meet Your Patient: Royalty-Free/Corbis

CHAPTER 3

Meet Your Patient: Everyday Faces, Photo Copyright Photodisc.

Figure 3-1: From Wilkinson, J.W., & Treas, L. (2011). *Fundamentals of nursing* (2nd ed.). Philadelphia: F.A. Davis.

Figure 3-2: From Wilkinson, J.M. (2011). *Nursing process and critical thinking* (5th ed., p. 78, Fig. 3.3), Philadelphia: F.A. Davis.

Figure 3-3: Courtesy Smith Northview Hospital, Valdosta, GA.

Figure 3-4: Courtesy Shore Memorial Hospital, Somers Point, NJ.

CHAPTER 4

Meet Your Patient: Photo © BananaStock

Figures 4-1 through 4-5: From Wilkinson, J.W., & Treas, L. (2011). *Fundamentals of nursing* (2nd ed.). Philadelphia: F.A. Davis.

Figure 4-6: Adapted from Maslow, A. (1971). *The farther reaches of human nature*. New York: Viking Press; and Maslow, A., & Lowery, R. (Eds.). (1998). *Toward a psychology of being* (3rd ed.). New York: Wiley & Sons.

CHAPTER 5

Meet Your Patient: Ryan McVay/Photodisc/PunchStock

Figure 5.1: From Wilkinson, J.W., & Treas, L. (2011). *Fundamentals of nursing* (2nd ed.). Philadelphia: F.A. Davis.

Figure 5-2: Courtesy Shawnee Mission Health System, Shawnee Mission, KS.

Figure 5-3: From Wilkinson, J.W., & Treas, L. (2011). *Fundamentals of nursing* (2nd ed.). Philadelphia: F.A. Davis.

Figure 5-4: Courtesy Shawnee Mission Health System, Shawnee Mission, KS.

Figure 5-5: Adapted from Genesis Medical Center, Davenport, IA 52804. Used with permission.

CHAPTER 6

Meet Your Patient: Ryan McVay/Photodisc/PunchStock

Figure 6-2: Courtesy Fain, J.A. (2003). *Reading, understanding, and applying nursing research: A text and workbook* (2nd. ed., p. 82). Philadelphia: F.A. Davis.

Figure 6-3: From Wilkinson, J.W., & Treas, L. (2011). *Fundamentals of nursing* (2nd ed.). Philadelphia: F.A. Davis.

Figure 6-4: Copyright © Ergo Partners, L.C. All rights reserved. Use with permission.

CHAPTER 7

Meet Your Patients: Thinkstock/Getty Images

Figure 7-1: From Wilkinson, J.W., & Treas, L. (2011). *Fundamentals of nursing* (2nd ed.). Philadelphia: F.A. Davis.

Figure 7-2: Courtesy Ergo Partners, L.C., Boulder, CO. Used with permission.

CHAPTER 8

Meet Your Patient: From Wilkinson, J.W., & Treas, L. (2011). *Fundamentals of nursing* (2nd ed.). Philadelphia: F.A. Davis.

Figure 8-2: Courtesy Jean Watson.

Figures 8-3 and 8-4: From Wilkinson, J.W., & Treas, L. (2011). *Fundamentals of nursing* (2nd ed.). Philadelphia: F.A. Davis.

Figure 8-5: Adapted from Maslow, A. (1970). *The farther reaches of human nature*. New York: Viking Press; and Maslow, A., & Lowery, R. (Eds.). (1998). *Toward a psychology of being* (3rd ed.). New York: Wiley & Sons.

CHAPTER 9

Meet Your Patient: Photodisc Blue/Getty Images

Figures 9-1, 9-2, and 9-4: From Dillon, P.M. (2007). *Nursing health assessment: A critical thinking case studies approach* (2nd ed.). Philadelphia, F.A. Davis.

Figure 9-3: Polan, E., & Taylor, D. (2007). *Journey across the lifespan* (3rd ed.). Philadelphia: F.A. Davis.

Figure 9-5: Getty Images, Royalty Free

Figure 9-6: Centers for Disease Control and Prevention, www.cdc.gov/vaccines

Figure 9-7: © Robert Dant, www.istockphoto.com

Figure 9-8: © PunchStock

Figure 9-9: Photodisc Red/Getty Images, Scott T. Baxter

Figure 9-10: Centers for Disease Control and Prevention, www.cdc.gov

Figure 9-11: Everyday Faces, Photodisc

Figure 9-12: Photodisc Green/Getty Images

Figure 9-13: Photodisc Green/Getty Images, Anderson Ross

Figure 9-14; Procedure 9-1 (girl): From Wilkinson, J.W., & Treas, L. (2011). *Fundamentals of nursing* (2nd ed.). Philadelphia: F.A. Davis.

CHAPTER 10

Meet Your Patient: © Silvia Jansen, www.istockphoto.com
Figure 10-3: Photodisc/Getty Images

CHAPTER 11

Figure 11-4: Senior Lifestyles, Photodisc
Figure 11-6: Fishermen's Hospital, Marathon, FL. Used with permission.
Clinical Insight 11-1: From Wilkinson, J.W., & Treas, L. (2011). *Fundamentals of nursing* (2nd ed.). Philadelphia: F.A. Davis.

CHAPTER 12

Meet Your Patient: © Digital Vision
Figures 12-1, 12-2, 12-4, and 12-6: From Wilkinson, J.W., & Treas, L. (2011). *Fundamentals of nursing* (2nd ed.). Philadelphia: F.A. Davis.
Figure 12-7: Getty Images Photodisc

CHAPTER 13

Figure 13-5: Townsend, M.C. (2009). *Psychiatric mental health nursing. Concepts of care* (5th ed., p. 248). Philadelphia: F.A. Davis.

CHAPTER 14

Figures 14-1 through 14-5: From Wilkinson, J.W., & Treas, L. (2011). *Fundamentals of nursing* (2nd ed.). Philadelphia: F.A. Davis.
Figure 14-6: From Dillon, P.M. (2007). *Nursing health assessment: A critical thinking case studies approach* (2nd ed.). Philadelphia: F.A. Davis.

CHAPTER 15

Figures 15-2 through 15-5: © www.istockphoto.com

CHAPTER 16

Meet Your Patient: © Photodisc, Senior Lifestyles
Figures 16.1 and 16.2: From Wilkinson, J.W., & Treas, L. (2011). *Fundamentals of nursing* (2nd ed.). Philadelphia: F.A. Davis.

CHAPTER 17

Figure 17-1: © Gina Guarnieri, www.istockphoto.com
Clinical Insight 17-3: From Wilkinson, J.W., & Treas, L. (2011). *Fundamentals of nursing* (2nd ed.). Philadelphia: F.A. Davis.

CHAPTER 18

Meet Your Patient; Figures 18-1, 18-6, 18-7, and 18-10: From Wilkinson, J.W., & Treas, L. (2011). *Fundamentals of nursing* (2nd ed.). Philadelphia: F.A. Davis.

CHAPTER 19

Meet Your Patient: Photo © BananaStock
Figures 19-1 through 19-12: From Wilkinson, J.W., & Treas, L. (2011). *Fundamentals of nursing* (2nd ed.). Philadelphia: F.A. Davis.
Procedures 19-1 (A–F), 19-2 (A–H) through 19-6: From Wilkinson, J.W., & Treas, L. (2011). *Fundamentals of nursing* (2nd ed.). Philadelphia: F.A. Davis.

CHAPTER 20

Meet Your Patient; Figures 20-1 through 20-3: From Wilkinson, J.W., & Treas, L. (2011). *Fundamentals of nursing* (2nd ed.). Philadelphia: F.A. Davis.

CHAPTER 21

Figures 21-1 through 21-10; Box 21-1: From Dillon, P.M. (2007). *Nursing health assessment: A critical thinking case studies approach* (2nd ed.). Philadelphia, F.A. Davis.
Figure 21-11; Procedure 21-12 (Step 5): From Scanlon, V.C., & Sanders, T. (2003). *Essentials of anatomy & physiology* (4th ed.). Philadelphia, F.A. Davis.
Clinical Insight 21-1a and b; Clinical Insight 21-3 (all figures); Procedure 21-2b (Step 7 [Malignant Melanoma]); Documentation; Procedure 21-5 (all figures); Procedure 21-6 (Steps 3–8 [all figures]); Procedure 21-7 (Steps 1 through 3e, 5 [Weber Test], and 6); Procedure 21-10 (all figures); Procedure 21-13 (Steps 1b, c, and 2 [adapted]); Procedure 21-14 (Step 7c, Deep Palpation Techniques [1, 2]); Procedure 21-15 (Steps 1c [1] [2], 1d, 2 [all], 6c [1], and 6c [2]): From Dillon, P.M. (2007). *Nursing health assessment: A critical thinking case studies approach* (2nd ed.). Philadelphia: F.A. Davis.
Meet Your Patient; Table 21-1; Procedure 21-1 (all figures); Procedure 21-2 (Step 3); Procedure 21-4 (Steps 1 and 3); Procedure 21-6 (Preliterate, Snellen standard, Snellen E); Procedure 21-7 (Structures); Procedure 21-12 (Step 2a, b); Normal Lung Sounds (all figures); Abnormal Lung Sounds (all figures); Procedure 21-14 (Step 3d [1] [2], Step4b [1], Step4c [3] (Four Abdominal Quadrants); Procedure 21-19 (drawing): From Wilkinson, J.W., & Treas, L. (2011). *Fundamentals of nursing* (2nd ed.). Philadelphia: F.A. Davis.
Describing Skin Lesions; Procedure 21-8 (Steps 4d, and 5a, b); Procedure 21-9 (Step 2b[1] and [3]); Procedure 21-11 (Steps 4 a, b, c, and 6); Procedure 21-14 (Steps 5, 6, and 7d); Procedure 21-15 (Steps 3a, b [1], 3b [2], 4a, 8 [all], and 9); Procedure 21-16 (Steps 11c, 13a, 18a, 20, 21a, b, c, 22c, 23 [all], and 24); Procedure 21-17 (Steps 5a, c, and 6); Procedure 21-18 (Steps 2, and 3b, c); Procedure 21-19 (Step 2b [photo]: From Dillon, P. (2007). *Nursing health assessment* (2nd ed.). Philadelphia: F.A. Davis.
Procedure 21-7 (Step 3f [1, 2, and 3]): Courtesy Ann Marie Ramsay, RN, MSN, CPNO, Section of Pediatric Otolaryngology, University of Michigan, Ann Arbor.
Procedure 21-17 (Tanner Staging and Maturation Status in Females, Stages 1 through 5): From Tanner, J.M. (1962). *Growth at adolescence* (2nd ed.). Oxford: Blackwell Scientific.
Abnormal Atlas:
Alopecia Areata, Cyanosis, Fungal Infection, Half-and-Half Nails, Herpes Simplex, Kyphosis, Lordosis, Locations of Direct and Indirect Hernias, Propulsive Gait, Ringworm, Scissors Gait, Scoliosis, Spastic Gait, Steppage Gait, Vitiligo, Waddling Gait, Locations of Direct and Indirect Hernias, Petechiae, Venous Star: From Dillon, P. (2007). *Nursing health assessment* (2nd ed.). Philadelphia: F.A. Davis.
Capillary Hemangioma, Port-Wine Stain, Syphilitic Chancre, Vesicles (blisters): From Goldsmith, L.A., Tharp, M.D., & Lazarus, G. (1997). *Adult and pediatric dermatology: A color guide to diagnosis and treatment*. Philadelphia: F.A. Davis.

Degenerative Joint Disease: Courtesy MCP Hahneman University, Department of Dermatology, Philadelphia, 2007.

Gingival Recession: Courtesy Robert A. Levine, DDS, and Sheryl Radn, DDS.

Jaundice: From Linda Chapman and Roberta F. Durham (2010), *Maternal-Newborn Nursing: Critical Components of Nursing Care*. Philadelphia: F.A. Davis.

Leukoplakia and Cancer of the Tongue: Tina S. Liang, DMD.

Pediculosis, Pterygium, Subconjuntival Hemorrhage: Courtesy Will's Eye Institute, Philadelphia.

Gingival Recession: Courtesy Robert A. Levine, DDS, and Sheryl Radin, DDS, Pediatric Dentistry.

Enlarged Tonsil with Exudates: Courtesy SIU BIOMED, CMSP Clearing House 071-2786.

Black Hairy Tongue, Genital Warts, Heberden's Nodes, Rheumatoid Arthritis, Syphilitic Chancre, and Herpes Vulvovaginitis: Courtesy MCP Hahneman University, Department of Dermatology.

CHAPTER 22

Meet Your Patient: www.istockphoto.com

Figure 22-1: From Wilkinson, J.W., & Treas, L. (2011). *Fundamentals of nursing* (2nd ed.). Philadelphia: F.A. Davis.

Figures 22-2 and 21-3: From Scanlon, V.C., & Sanders, T. (2003). *Essentials of anatomy and physiology* (4th ed.). Philadelphia: F.A. Davis.

Clinical Insight 22-6; Procedure 22-1A (Steps 3, 5, and 9); Procedure 22-1B (Step 4); Procedure 22-3 (Steps 1A and B, 2B, and 3); Procedure 22-4 (Steps 7, 10, 12, and 15); Procedure 22-5 (Step 8); Procedure 22-6 (Steps 1, 2, 5a [2] and [3], and 5c [2]); Sterile Glove Sizes; Procedure 22-7 (Steps 5, 7 through 9); Procedure 22-8a (Steps 3 through 6, and 10); Procedure 22-8B (Step 2); Procedure 22-8c (Step 4): From Wilkinson, J.W., & Treas, L. (2011). *Fundamentals of nursing* (2nd ed.). Philadelphia: F.A. Davis.

CHAPTER 23

Meet Your Patient: © Jay Freis/Digital Vision/ Getty Images

Figures 23-1, 23-4, and 23-5 (all figures); Procedure 23-1 (Step 1, Leg Sensors); Procedure 23-4 (Step 4 [all figures]): From Wilkinson, J.W., & Treas, L. (2011). *Fundamentals of nursing* (2nd ed.). Philadelphia: F.A. Davis.

Figure 23-3: © Scott Rothstein, www.istockphoto.com

CHAPTER 24

Meet Your Patient: Getty Images

Figures 24-1, 24-4, 24-5a, b, and c, and 24-6; Self-Care 24-3; Clinical Insight 24-1 (all); Procedure 24-1 (Steps 4, 5b, 7c, 9f, 10b, and 10d); Procedure 24-2 (Step 5b); Procedure 24-3 (Equipment); Procedure 24-4 (Steps 3c [3][4], 3f); Procedure 24-5 (Pre-assessment, Steps 6 and 12); Procedure 24-6 (Steps 10 and 11a, b, and c); Procedure 24-7 (Steps 1a, b, and 7); Procedure 24-8 (Equipment, Step 5a); Procedure 24-9 (Step 10); Procedure 24-9c (What If); Procedure 24-10 (Step 4); Procedure 24-11 (Step 4c); Procedure 24-12 (all figures); Procedure 24-13 (all figures); Procedure 24-14 (all figures): From Wilkinson, J.W., & Treas, L. (2011). *Fundamentals of nursing* (2nd ed.). Philadelphia: F.A. Davis.

Figure 24-3: From Dillon, P.M. (2007). *Nursing health assessment: A critical thinking case studies approach* (2nd ed.). Philadelphia: F.A. Davis.

CHAPTER 25

Meet Your Patient; Figures 25-1 through 25-11, 25-14 through 25-21, 25-24 through 25-26; Medication Guidelines (Step 12b); Procedure 25-1 (Steps 1h, 2e, 2f, and 7); Procedure 25-2 (Steps 6, 8, and 11); Procedure 25-2A (Step 6c); Procedure 25-3 (Step 6a and b); Procedure 25-4 (Step 4b and c); Procedure 25-5 (Steps 3, 6c and j); Procedure 25-6 (Step 9a, c); Procedure 25-7A (Step 4); Procedure 27-7D (Step 5); Procedure 25-8 (Steps 7 and 11); Procedure 25-9 (Equipment); Procedure 25-9A (Steps 2, 4a and b); Procedure 25-9B (Steps 6a through 9); Procedure 25-9C (Steps 2, 4, and 5); Procedure 25-9E (Step 5); Procedure 25-10 (Equipment 2 and 3, Step 3, and 3a, b, c); Procedure 25-10B (Steps 2 through 5); Procedure 25-11 (Equipment, Step 11); Procedure 25-12 (Step 1b); Procedure 25-13A (Steps 3 and 4); Procedure 25-13B (Step 2); Procedure 25-13C (Step 4); Procedure 25-14B (Steps 8 and 11); Procedure 25-15A (Steps 6 and 8); Procedure 25-15B (Step 5); Procedure 25-16 (Step 5); Procedure 25-16B (Steps 9 and 12); Procedure 25-16C (Step 7); Procedure 25-17 (Step 8); Procedure 25-17B (Step 7); Procedure 25-17C (Step 6); Clinical Insight 25-3 (all); Clinical Insight 25-4 (Step 6); Clinical Insight 25-5 (Steps 6 and 7); Clinical Insight 25-6: From Wilkinson, J.W., & Treas, L. (2011). *Fundamentals of nursing* (2nd ed.). Philadelphia: F.A. Davis.

Figure 25-12: Courtesy Hospira, Lake Forest, IL.

Figures 25-13 and 25-23: Courtesy Medi-Dose®, Inc., EPS®, Inc.

Procedure 25-10 (Equipment 1): Courtesy Edward Lin, MD, Ingenious Technologies Corporation. Training video link: http://ingenious.com/NS/ns.htm

CHAPTER 26

Meet Your Patient: Photo © BananaStock

Figures 26-1 and 26-2: From Wilkinson, J.W., & Treas, L. (2011). *Fundamentals of nursing* (2nd ed.). Philadelphia: F.A. Davis.

Figure 26-3: Photo courtesy Laerdal Medical Corporation.

Figure 26-5: Courtesy Merck & Co., Inc. #994795(1)-05-COZ

CHAPTER 27

Meet Your Peer: © Thomas Eyedesign, www.istockphoto.com

Figures 27-1, 27-2, and 27-3: From Wilkinson, J.W., & Treas, L. (2011). *Fundamentals of nursing* (2nd ed.). Philadelphia: F.A. Davis.

CHAPTER 28

Figures 28-3 and 28-4A and B: Courtesy Covidine, Mansfield, MA.

Figures 28-5 through 28-7; Clinical Insight 28-3; Clinical Insight 28-5; Procedure 28-1 (Steps 10g, 13, and 16); Procedure 28-2 (Steps 3, 13, and 20e); Procedure 28-3 (Steps 11 and 18): From Wilkinson, J.W., & Treas, L. (2011). *Fundamentals of nursing* (2nd ed.). Philadelphia: F.A. Davis.

Clinical Insight 28-2a and b: From Lutz, C., & Przytulski, K. (2006). *Nutrition and diet therapy* (4th ed.). Philadelphia: F.A. Davis.

Procedure 28-2 (Step 11): From Scanlon, V.C., & Sanders, T. (2003). *Essentials of anatomy and physiology* (4th ed.). Philadelphia: F.A. Davis.

Procedure 28-2 (Step 20g): Courtesy Dale Medical Products, Inc. Plainville, MA.

Procedure 28-5 (Equipment): Permission for use granted by Cook Medical Incorporated, Bloomington, IN.

CHAPTER 29

Meet Your Patient: © The Linke, www.istockphoto.com

Figures 29-5 and 29-6; Procedure 29-1 (Step 9); Procedure 29-2A (Regular and Fracture Bedpan); Procedure 29-3A (Step 12); Procedure 29-3B (Step 3); Procedure 29-4 (Steps 7 and 9); Procedure 29-7 (Steps 5 and 9); Procedure 29-8 (Step 10): From Wilkinson, J.W., & Treas, L. (2011). *Fundamentals of nursing* (2nd ed.). Philadelphia: F.A. Davis.

Figure 29-7; Procedure 29-7 (Equipment): From Williams, L., & Hopper, P. (2007). *Understanding medical surgical nursing* (2nd ed.). Philadelphia: F.A. Davis.

Procedure 29-6 (Equipment and Indwelling Fecal Device); Procedure 29-8B (Step 11): Courtesy Hollister, Inc., Libertyville, IL.

CHAPTER 30

Meet Your Patient: © BananaStock

Figures 30-1 through 30-4: From Scanlon, V.C., & Sanders, T. (2003). *Essentials of anatomy and physiology* (4th ed.). Philadelphia: F.A. Davis.

Figures 30-5 through 30-12; Procedure 30-1B (Steps 2 and 5); Procedure 30-2A (Step 3c and What If [Step 4]); Procedure 30-4 (Equipment); Procedure 30-4A (Steps 3, 9b, and 11); Procedure 30-4B (Steps 10 and 12 and What If); Procedure 30-5 (Steps 9 [1] and [2], and 13); Procedure 7A (Step 19); Procedure 7B (Step 9 [1] and [2]): From Wilkinson, J.W., & Treas, L. (2011). *Fundamentals of nursing* (2nd ed.). Philadelphia: F.A. Davis.

Focused Assessment (Guidelines Urinary Elimination): From Williams, L., & Hopper, P. (2007). *Understanding medical surgical nursing* (2nd ed.). Philadelphia: F.A. Davis.

CHAPTER 31

Meet Your Patient: © Aguru, www.istockphoto.com

Procedure 31-1 (Step 9d): From Wilkinson, J.W., & Treas, L. (2011). *Fundamentals of nursing* (2nd ed.). Philadelphia: F.A. Davis.

CHAPTER 32

Meet Your Patient: © Jason Doiy, www.istockphoto.com

Figures 32-1 through 32-3, 32-5: From Wilkinson, J.W., & Treas, L. (2011). *Fundamentals of nursing* (2nd ed.). Philadelphia: F.A. Davis.

Wong Baker FACES Scale: From Hockenberry, M.J., & Wilson, D. (2009). *Wong's essentials of pediatric nursing* (8th ed.). St. Louis, MO: C.V. Mosby. Used with permission. Copyright Mosby. http://www1.us.elsevierhealth/FACES

CHAPTER 33

Meet Your Patient: © Christopher Futcher, www.istockphoto.com

Figures 33-1 and 33-2: From Scanlon, V.C., & Sanders, T. (2003). *Essentials of anatomy and physiology* (4th ed.). Philadelphia: F.A. Davis.

Figures 33-3 through 33-7, 33-14 through 33-18A and B; Tables 33-2 and 33-3 (all figures); Clinical Insight 33-6 (all); Clinical Insight 33-2 (unnumbered figure 1 and parts 1 through 3, Hand Roll, and Cradle Boot); Procedure 33-1A (Steps 8, 16, and 19); Procedure 33-1B (Steps 2c and 7); Procedure 33-1C (Steps 3 and 9); Procedure 33-2A (Steps 4b, 6, and 16); Procedure 33-2B (Steps 4 and 6); Procedure 33-2C (Steps 5 and 11); Procedure 33-3A (Steps 8 and 10); Procedure 3C (Step 8): From Wilkinson, J.W., & Treas, L. (2011). *Fundamentals of nursing* (2nd ed.). Philadelphia: F.A. Davis.

Figures 33-8 and 33-9, 33-11 through 33-13: Courtesy EZ Way, Inc., Clarinda, IA.

Clinical Insight (Hip Abduction): From Williams, L., & Hopper, P. (2007). *Understanding medical surgical nursing* (2nd ed.). Philadelphia: F.A. Davis.

CHAPTER 34

Meet Your Patients: © Cheryl Casey, © Steve Luker, © C. Glade, www.istockphoto.com

Figures 34-1 and 34-2: From Scanlon, V.C., & Sanders, T. (2003). *Essentials of anatomy and physiology* (4th ed.). Philadelphia: F.A. Davis.

Figure 34-5: © Photos.com/Getty Images

Figures 34-3, 34-4, 34-6 through 34-8: From Wilkinson, J.W., & Treas, L. (2011). *Fundamentals of nursing* (2nd ed.). Philadelphia: F.A. Davis.

CHAPTER 35

Meet Your Patient: © Diane Diederich, www.istockphoto.com

Figures 35-1 through 35-4; Procedure 35-1 (Steps 5 through 9, 11): From Wilkinson, J.W., & Treas, L. (2011). *Fundamentals of nursing* (2nd ed.). Philadelphia: F.A. Davis.

Figure 35-5: From Guyton, A.C., & Hall, J.E. (2006). *Medical physiology* (10th ed.). Philadelphia: W.B. Saunders.

CHAPTER 36

Meet Your Patient: From Photodisc, Everyday Faces.

Figure 36-1: From Scanlon, V.C., & Sanders, T. (2003). *Essentials of anatomy and physiology* (4th ed.). Philadelphia: F.A. Davis.

Figures 36-2 through 36-7, 36-9 through 36-16; unnumbered figures 36-B through 36F (Table 36-3); Procedure 36-1 (Steps 7 and 11); Procedure 36-2 (Steps 7, 8, and 10); Procedure 36-3 (Steps 5 and 11); Procedure 36-5 (Steps 14 and 17); Procedure 36-6 (Steps 4, 16, 18, and 19); Procedure 36-7A (Steps 2, 8, 9, and 15); Procedure 36-8 (Step 7); Procedure 36-9 (Steps 8 and 9); Procedure 36-10 (Step 8e); Procedure 36-11 (Steps 8b, 12, 19, 20, and 22); Procedure 36-12 (Steps 15, 18, 21–23, 26, and 29); Procedure 36-13A (Steps 2 and 4); Procedure 36-13B (Step 3); Procedure 36-14 (Steps 7, 8, and 10); Procedure 36-15 (Steps 4 and 7): From Wilkinson, J.W., & Treas, L. (2011). *Fundamentals of nursing* (2nd ed.). Philadelphia: F.A. Davis.

Figure 36-8: Adapted from AHRQ Clinical Practice Guidelines.

Unnumbered figure 36-A (Table 36-3): Courtesy WoundEducators.com, LLC, Great River, NY.

Procedure 36-7B (Step 10): Courtesy Talley Group Limited, Hampshire, England.

CHAPTER 37

Meet Your Patient: © BananaStock

Figures 37-1, 37-2, and 37-3: From Scanlon, V.C., & Sanders, T. (2003). *Essentials of anatomy and physiology* (4th ed.). Philadelphia: F.A. Davis.

Figures 37-4, 37-5, 37-7, and 37-9: From Williams, L., & Hopper, P. (2007). *Understanding medical surgical nursing* (2nd ed.). Philadelphia: F.A. Davis.

Figures 37-6, 37-8, 37-10, and 37-11; Procedure 37-1 (Steps 8, 10, and 17); Procedure 37-2 (Step 6); Procedure 37-3 (Steps 1a–f and 4); Procedure 37-4 (Steps 1, 1 [Variation], 6, 8, and 10, Oxygen Delivery Systems [all]); Procedure 37-5 (Equipment [all], 9, 14c, 15, and 15 [Rationale]); Procedure 37-6 (Step 12b); Procedure 37-7 (Step 5); Procedure 37-8 (Steps 13a, 15, and 16); Procedure 37-9 (Step 13b and e); Procedure 37-10 (Steps 1, 4, and 13); Procedure 37-11 (Steps 1a, b, 20, 25, and 27); Clinical Insight 37-3a and b; Clinical Insight 37-4: From Wilkinson, J.W., & Treas, L. (2011). *Fundamentals of nursing* (2nd ed.). Philadelphia: F.A. Davis.

Procedure 37-7 (Equipment): © Unomedical A/S, used with permission.

CHAPTER 38

Meet Your Patient: www.istockphoto.com

Figures 38-1 and 38-2: From Scanlon, V.C., & Sanders, T. (2003). *Essentials of anatomy and physiology* (4th ed.). Philadelphia: F.A. Davis.

Figures 38-3 and 38-4; Procedure 38-1 (Steps 2 and 11): From Wilkinson, J.W., & Treas, L. (2011). *Fundamentals of nursing* (2nd ed.). Philadelphia: F.A. Davis.

CHAPTER 39

Meet Your Patient: Getty Images, Photodisc

Figure 39-1: From Scanlon, V.C., & Sanders, T. (2003). *Essentials of anatomy and physiology* (4th ed.). Philadelphia: F.A. Davis.

Figures 39-2 through 39-14; Procedure 39-1 (Equipment, Steps 2d, g, and h, 12, 14 [Variations], 20, and 25b and c); Procedure 39-2 (Step 7); Procedure 39-3 (Steps 10 and 11); Procedure 39-4B (Step 6); Procedure 39-6 (Steps 3, 9, and 11); Procedure 39-7 (Step 6); Procedure 39-8A (Steps 5c and 13); Clinical Insight 39-2 (all figures); Clinical Insight 39-4 (Veins): From Wilkinson, J.W., & Treas, L. (2011). *Fundamentals of nursing* (2nd ed.). Philadelphia: F.A. Davis.

Procedure 39-1 (Steps 14 and 18 [Variation]): From Rhoads, J., & Meeker, B.J. (2008). *Davis's guide to clinical nursing skills*. Philadelphia: F.A. Davis.

CHAPTER 40

Meet Your Patient: © Vikram Raghuvanshi, www.istockphoto.com

Figures 40-1, 40-3, 40-4a and b, 40-8, and 40-10; Procedure 40-1A (Step 2); Procedure 40-1B (Step 5); Procedure 40-1C (Steps 2d, and 4b and c); Procedure 40-2 (Steps 1, 6, and 8); Procedure 40-3 (Step 6); Procedure 40-4 (Step 9 and unnumbered table). From Wilkinson, J.W., & Treas, L. (2011). *Fundamentals of nursing* (2nd ed.). Philadelphia: F.A. Davis.

Figures 40-2 and 40-6; Clinical Insight 40-3 (Operating Room): From Williams, L., & Hopper, P. (2007). *Understanding medical surgical nursing* (2nd ed.). Philadelphia: F.A. Davis.

Figure 40-7: Courtesy I-Flow Corporation, Lake Forest, CA.

CHAPTER 41

Caring for the Nguyens: © Agostinos Angel, www.istockphoto.com

Meet Your Patient: © Photo Euphoria, www.istockphoto.com

Figures 41-1, 41-4 through 41-6: From Wilkinson, J.W., & Treas, L. (2011). *Fundamentals of nursing* (2nd ed.). Philadelphia: F.A. Davis.

Figure 41-3: © Alexander Raths, www.istockphoto.com

Figure 41-7: © Photos.com/Getty Images

CHAPTER 42

Meet Your Patient: From Wilkinson, J.W., & Treas, L. (2011). *Fundamentals of nursing* (2nd ed.). Philadelphia: F.A. Davis.

CHAPTER 43

Meet Your Patient: © Nathan Watkins, www.istockphoto.com

CHAPTER 44

Meet Your Patient: © S.J. Locke, www.istockphoto.com

Figure 44-1: Adapted from Englebardt, S., & Nelson, R. *Health care informatics: An interdisciplinary approach.* Copyright (2002). With permission from Elsevier.

Figure 44-2: Courtesy Laerdal Medical Corp., Wappingers Falls, NY.

Figure 44-3: Courtesy Doctors Telehealth Network, Newport Beach, CA.

Figures 44-4 and 44-5A: Courtesy Cerner Corporations.

Figure 44-5b: © Adivin, www.istockphoto.com

INDEX

Universal Steps for All Procedures

> ➤ You should consider the following nursing activities to be a part of every procedure in this text.

Before Approaching a Patient

- Check the medical order or obtain an order, if necessary.
- Refer to agency protocols unless you already know them.
- Get a signed, informed consent, if needed.
- Wash your hands. Follow agency policy and CDC (2002) guidelines* for hand hygiene.
- Gather the necessary supplies and equipment.
- Obtain assistance from another healthcare worker, if it will be needed (e.g., to lift a patient).

Preparing the Patient

- Identify the patient: Read the wrist band, and ask the patient to state his or her name.
- Explain the procedure to the patient: What you will do, what the patient will feel, and what he or she is expected to do (e.g., "You will need to lie very still.")
- Provide privacy. For example, ask visitors to step out of the room, draw bed curtains, and close the door.
- Position the bed or treatment table to a working level; lower the near siderail.
- Make any relevant assessments (e.g., take vital signs) to ensure that the patient (1) still requires the procedure and (2) is able to tolerate it.

During the Procedure

- Wash your hands before touching the patient, before gloving, and after removing gloves. Wash them again before leaving the room.*
- Maintain correct body mechanics.
- Continue to observe the patient while performing the procedure steps.

After the Procedure

- Evaluate the patient's response to the procedure.
- Leave the patient in a comfortable, safe position, with the call light within reach.
- If the patient is in bed, return the bed to its original position and raise the siderail (if the patient requires this precaution).
- Document that the procedure was done; document the patient's responses.
- Dispose of supplies and materials according to agency policy.

Remember:

All procedures are "rules of thumb." Everything you learn can be altered by medical orders, agency policies, and individual patient needs.

Everything you do requires nursing judgment!

---

*Boyce, J. M., & Pittet, D. (2002, October 25). Guidelines for hand hygiene in health-care settings. Recommendations of the Healthcare Infection Control Practices Advisory Committee and the HICPAC/SHEA/APIC/IDSA Hand Hygiene Task Force. *Morbidity and Mortality Weekly Reports, Recommendations and Reports, 51*(RR16), 1–44. Retrieved from www.cdc.gov/mmwr/preview/mmwrhtml/rr5116a1.htm